AAOS
AMERICAN ACADEMY OF ORTHOPAEDIC SURGEONS

NINTH EDITION

Nancy Caroline's Emergency Care in the Streets

Volume 1

Preparatory
The Human Body and Human Systems
Patient Assessment
Pharmacology
Airway Management
Medical

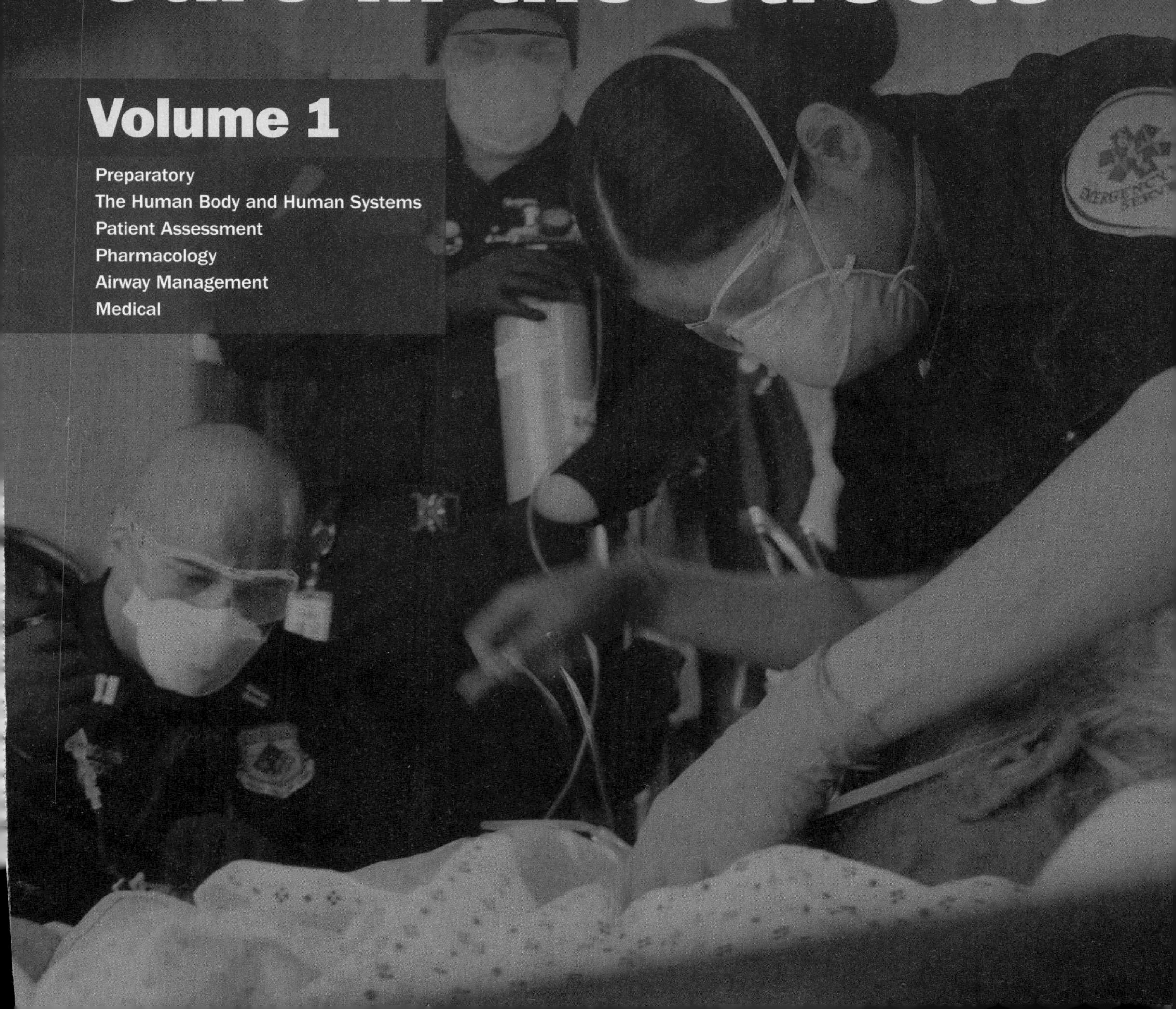

AAOS

American Academy of Orthopaedic Surgeons

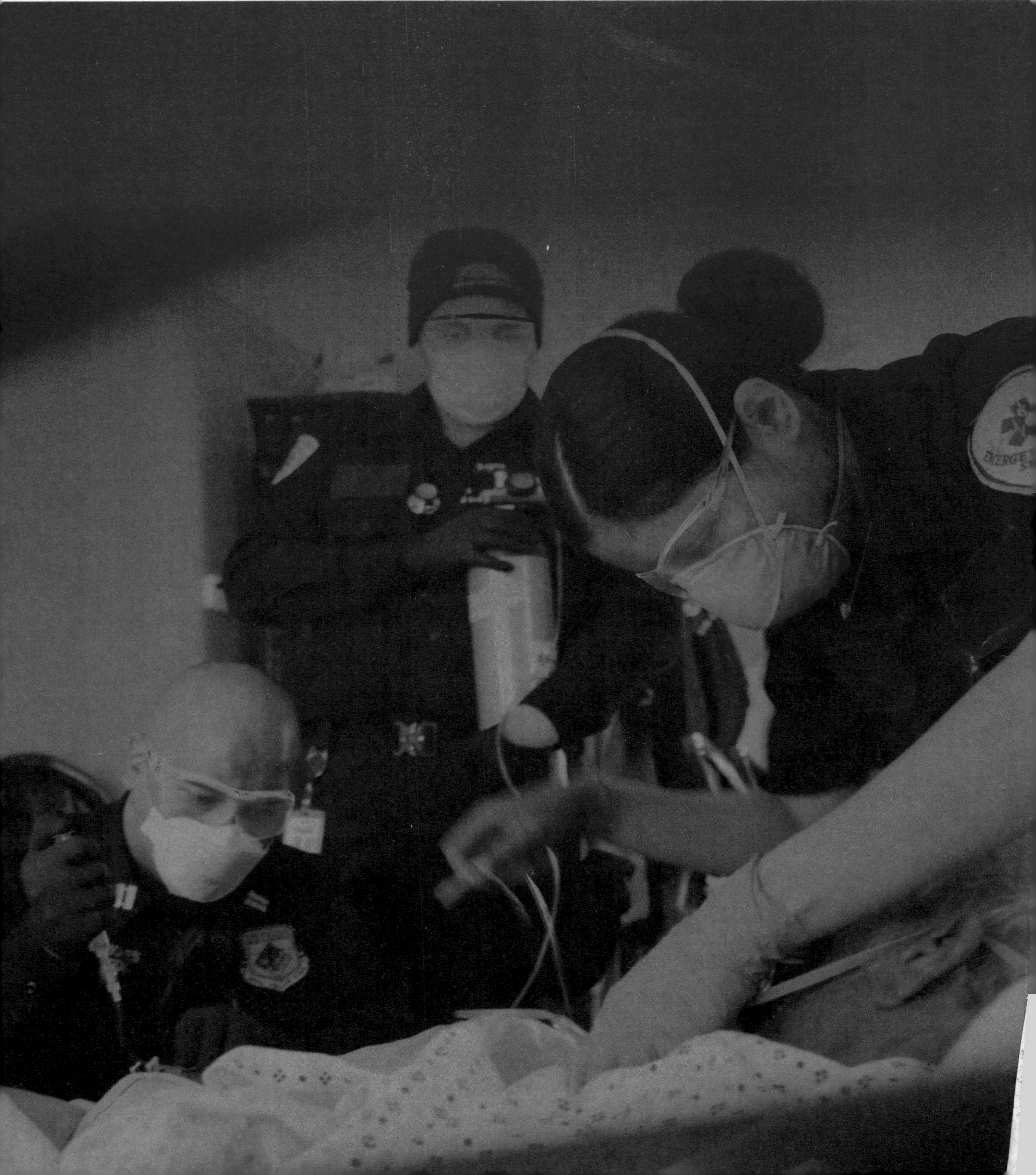

NINTH EDITION

Nancy Caroline's Emergency Care in the Streets

AAOS

American Academy of Orthopaedic Surgeons

Series Editor:

Alfonso Mejia, MD, MPH, FAAOS

Lead Editors:

Barbara Aehlert, MSEd, BSPA, RN

Bob Elling, MPA, EMT-P

JONES & BARTLETT LEARNING

World Headquarters
Jones & Bartlett Learning
25 Mall Road
Burlington, MA 01803
978-443-5000
info@jblearning.com
www.jblearning.com
www.psglearning.com

Editorial Credits
Chief Commercial Officer: Anna Salt Troise, MBA
Director, Publishing: Hans J. Koelsch, PhD
Senior Manager, Editorial: Lisa Claxton Moore
Senior Editor: Steven Kellert

Jones & Bartlett Learning books and products are available through most bookstores and online booksellers. To contact the Jones & Bartlett Learning Public Safety Group directly, call 800-832-0034, fax 978-443-8000, or visit our website, www.psglearning.com.

Substantial discounts on bulk quantities of Jones & Bartlett Learning publications are available to corporations, professional associations, and other qualified organizations. For details and specific discount information, contact the special sales department at Jones & Bartlett Learning via the above contact information or send an email to specialsales@jblearning.com.

23747-4

Production Credits
Vice President, Product Management: Marisa R. Urbano
Vice President, Content Strategy and Implementation: Christine Emerton
Director, Product Management: Cathy Esperti
Director, Product Management: Laura Carney
Director, Content Management: Donna Gridley
Manager, Content Strategy: Tiffany Sliter
Developmental Editor: Mike Boblitt
Content Coordinator: Mark Restuccia
Director, Project Management and Content Services: Karen Scott
Manager, Program Management: Kristen Rogers
Project Manager: John Fuller
Senior Digital Project Specialist: Angela Dooley
Director of Marketing: Brian Rooney
Vice President, International Sales, Public Safety Group: Matthew Maniscalco
Director of Sales, Public Safety Group: Brian Hendrickson
Content Services Manager: Colleen Lamy
Vice President, Manufacturing and Inventory Control: Therese Connell
Composition: S4Carlisle Publishing Services
Cover and Text Design: Scott Moden
Senior Media Development Editor: Troy Liston
Rights & Permissions Manager: John Rusk
Rights Specialist: Benjamin Roy
Cover Image and Title Pages: © John Moore/Getty Images News/Getty Images
Printing and Binding: LSC Communications

Library of Congress Cataloging-in-Publication Data
Names: American Academy of Orthopaedic Surgeons, author, issuing body. | Aehlert, Barbara, editor. | Elling, Bob, editor. | Caroline, Nancy L.
Title: Nancy Caroline's emergency care in the streets / AAOS ; Nancy Caroline ; series editor, Alfonso Mejia ; lead editors, Barbara Aehlert, Bob Elling.
Other titles: Emergency care in the streets
Description: Ninth edition. | Burlington, MA : Jones & Bartlett Learning, [2023] | Includes index.
Identifiers: LCCN 2021039667 | ISBN 9781284256789 (hardcover)
Subjects: MESH: Emergency Treatment | Emergency Medical Services | Emergency Medical Technicians
Classification: LCC RC86.7 | NLM WB 105 | DDC 616.02/5--dc23
LC record available at https://lccn.loc.gov/2021039667

6048

Printed in the United States of America
26 25 24 23 22 10 9 8 7 6 5 4 3 2 1

Brief Contents

VOLUME 1

Brief Contents

VOLUME 2

Contents

VOLUME 1

Skill Drills

VOLUME 1

Acknowledgments

AAOS
American Academy of Orthopaedic Surgeons

The American Academy of Orthopaedic Surgeons and the Public Safety Group would like to acknowledge the editors, authors, and reviewers of previous editions of *Nancy Caroline's Emergency Care in the Streets* who were involved in the development of this textbook.

Series Editor

Alfonso Mejia, MD, MPH, FAAOS
Program Director, Orthopedic Surgery Residency Program
Vice Head, Department of Orthopedic Surgery
University of Illinois College of Medicine
Medical Director
Tactical Emergency Medical Support Physician
South Suburban Emergency Response Team
Chicago, Illinois

Lead Editors

Barbara Aehlert, MSEd, BSPA, RN
President
Southwest EMS Education, Inc.
Dallas, Texas

Bob Elling, MPA, EMT-P (ret.)
Author, Educator, Advocate, and Paramedic
Hernando, Florida

Authors

Barbara Aehlert, MSEd, BSPA, RN
Chapters 7, 13, 14, 15, 18
President
Southwest EMS Education, Inc.
Dallas, Texas

Chuck Allias, MS, NRP
Chapters 9, 45
Director of Emergency Services
Program Director
Indiana University of Pennsylvania
Indiana, Pennsylvania

Andrew Bartkus, JD, MSN, RN, NRP, CEN, CCRN, CFRN, Esq.
Chapter 28
Emergency Department Director
Sandoval Regional Medical Center
Rio Rancho, New Mexico

Dave Bledsoe, NREMT-P, RN, LNC (ret.)
Chapters 4, 6
Lieutenant/Paramedic
Orlando Fire Department
Orlando, Florida

Andrew G. Dubina, MD
Chapter 38
Resident Physician
University of Maryland School of Medicine
Department of Orthopaedics
Baltimore, Maryland

Rommie L. Duckworth, MS, LP
Chapters 49, 50, 51, 53
Captain/EMS Coordinator
Ridgefield Fire Department
Ridgefield, Connecticut

Bob Elling, MPA, EMT-P (ret.)
Chapters 2, 8, 11, 12, 40, 41
Author, Educator, Advocate, and Paramedic
Hernando, Florida

Wm. Travis Engel, DO, MSc, NRP, FP-C, CCP-C
Chapters 37, 42, 43, 44
Pediatric Critical Care Medicine Fellow
Children's Mercy Hospital
Kansas City, Missouri

Jason Ferguson, EdD, NRP
Chapters 17, 31
Associate Vice President
Central Virginia Community College
Lynchburg, Virginia

Seth Hawkins, MD, FACEP, FAEMS, MFAWM
Chapter 39
Assistant Professor of Emergency Medicine, Wake Forest University
Medical Director, Burke County EMS and Burke County Communications
Medical Director, Western Piedmont Community College Emergency Services Programs
Medical Director, North Carolina State Parks
Chief, Appalachian Mountain Rescue Team
Winston-Salem, North Carolina

Matt Hunt, BSEd, EMT-P
Chapters 1, 5
Paramedic Instructor
Albany State University
Albany, Georgia

Rhonda J. Hunt, MEd, NRP
Chapters 3, 25, 29, 32, 34, 35
EMS Program Director
Assistant Professor
Albany State University
Albany, Georgia

Michael Kaduce, MPS, NRP
Chapters 20, 36, 46
EMT Program Director
UCLA Center for Prehospital Care
David Geffen School of Medicine
Los Angeles, California

William J. Leggio, EdD, NRP
Appendix
Office of the Chief Medical Officer
Austin, Texas

Stephen J. Rahm, NRP
Chapter 16
Chief, Office of Clinical Direction
Co-Chair, Centre for Emergency Health Sciences
Spring Branch, Texas

Charles Sowerbrower, MEd, NRP, NCEE, CCP-C
Chapter 21
Chairperson
Sinclair Community College
Dayton, Ohio

Bryan Ware, BS, EMT-P
Chapters 10, 19, 30, 33, 47, 48, 52
Fire Chief
Beulah Fire Protection and Ambulance District
Beulah, Colorado

Katherine H. West, MSEd, RN, DICO-C
Chapter 27
Infection Control Consultant
Infection Control Emerging Concepts
Palm Harbor, Florida

Brittany Williams, DHSc, RRT-ACCS, NPS, AE-C, REMT-P
Chapters 13, 14, 22, 23, 24, 26, Appendix
Professor, Respiratory Care
Director, Clinical Education
Santa Fe College
Gainesville, Florida

Contributors

Andrew N. Pollak, MD, FAAOS
The James Lawrence Kernan Professor and Chairman
Department of Orthopaedics
University of Maryland School of Medicine
Senior Vice President for Clinical Transformation and Chief of Orthopaedics
University of Maryland Medical System
Medical Director
Baltimore County Fire Department
Director, Shock Trauma Go Team
Special Deputy US Marshal
Baltimore, Maryland

Rebecca Ridenhour, PharmD
BJC-Progress West Hospital
O'Fallon, Missouri

Reviewers

Jonathan A. Alford, NRP
Center for Trauma and Critical Care Education, School of Medicine
Virginia Commonwealth University
Richmond, Virginia

Nick Baker, AASN, RN, EMT-P
Austin/Travis County EMS
Austin, Texas

Jeannett Banks, EdS, MEd, NRP
Children's Hospital of the King's Daughters
Norfolk, Virginia

Ryan Batenhorst, MEd, NRP
Creighton University
Omaha, Nebraska

Alan M. Batt, PhD(c), MSc, CCP, PGCME, FHEA
Fanshawe College
Ontario, Canada

Edward L. Bays, BS, NRP
Mountwest Community & Technical College
Huntington, West Virginia

Mark A. Boisclair, MPA, NRP
Chattahoochee Valley Community College
Phenix City, Alabama

Jason Brooks, EdD, NRP
University of South Alabama, Department of EMS Education
Mobile, Alabama

Chad Burkhart, AS, Paramedic
School of EMS
New Windsor, New York

Ted Chialtas, BA, Fire Captain/Paramedic
San Diego Fire-Rescue Department, Paramedic Program
San Diego, California

Sharon F. Chiumento, BSN, BS, EMT-P
Monroe Community College
Rochester, New York

Kevin T. Collopy, MHL, FP-C, NRP, CMTE
AirLink/VitaLink Critical Care Transport
Novant Health New Hanover Regional Medical Center
Wilmington, North Carolina

Kent Courtney, Paramedic/Firefighter
Essential Safety Training and Consulting
Rimrock, Arizona

Anthony Cuda, NRP
Community College of Allegheny County
Pittsburg, Pennsylvania

Kevin Curry, AS, NRP, CCEMTP
United Training Center
Lewiston, Maine

Reuben Farnsworth, BS, NRP, CCP/CP-C
RockStar Education and Consulting
Delta, Colorado

David Fifer, MS, NRP, FAWM
Eastern Kentucky University Paramedic Program
Richmond, Kentucky

Charles Foat, PhD, NRP
Johnson County Community College
Overland Park, Kansas

Lori Gallian, BS, EMT-P
Summit Science
Sacramento, California

Fidel O. Garcia, Paramedic
Professional EMS Education, LLC
Grand Junction, Colorado

Rodney L. Geilenfeldt II, BS, EMT-P
Division Chief of Clinical Services
Kootenai County EMS System
Coeur d'Alene, Idaho

Craig Gesterling, BS, NRP
School of EMS
St. Petersburg, Florida

Jeffery D. Gilliard, MEd, NRP, CCEMTP, FPC
EMETSEEI Institute
Rockledge, Florida

Jamie O. Gray, BS, AAS, NRP, FF
Alabama Office of Emergency Medical Services
Prattville, Alabama

James E. Gretz, MBA, NRP, CCP-C
JeffSTAT–Thomas Jefferson University Hospital
Philadelphia, Pennsylvania

Kevin M. Gurney, MS, CCEMTP, I/C
Delta Ambulance
Waterville, Maine

Katie E. Hall, BA, NRP, CCP, IC
Roane State Community College
Knoxville, Tennessee

Kirk Hallett, EMT-P
Richmond Ambulance Authority
Richmond, Virginia

Jennifer Hannigan, MEd, Paramedic, CIC
Fire Department of the City of New York
Emergency Medical Services Bureau of Training
Bayside, New York

Anthony S. Harbour, MEd, BSN, RN, NRP
Southern Virginia EMS
Roanoke, Virginia

Greg Helmuth, MA, NRP
Hawkeye Community College
Waterloo, Iowa

Thomas Herron, AAS, NRP
Roane State Community College
Knoxville, Tennessee

Paul Hitchcock, NRP
Department of Homeland Security
Herndon, Virginia

Michele M. Hoffman, MSEd, RN, EMT
James City County Fire Department
James City County, Virginia

Suh Hughart, EMT-P
San Marcos Hays County EMS
San Marcos, Texas

Sandra Hultz, BS, NRP
Holmes Community College
Ridgeland, Mississippi

Joseph L. Hurlburt, BS, NREMT-P
Manton, Michigan

Darin (DJ) Jackson, MDiv, Paramedic
Asheville–Buncombe Technical Community College
Asheville, North Carolina

Adam Johnson, NRP
Rhinelander Fire Department
Oneida County Special Response Team
Nicolet Area Technical College
Northcentral Area Technical College
Rhinelander, Wisconsin

William Johnston, BA, AEMCA
Ottawa Paramedic Service
Ottawa, Ontario, Canada

Brian D. Katcher, NRP, FP-C
PHI Air Medical
Lord Fairfax Community College
Front Royal, Virginia

Jared Kimball, MPS, NRP
Tulane Trauma Education
New Orleans, Louisiana

Timothy M. Kimble, BA, AAS, NRP, CEM
Washington Township Fire and Rescue
Waynesboro, Pennsylvania
LifeCare Medical Transports
Fredericksburg, Virginia

Don Kimlicka, NRP, CCEMTP
Regional EMS Coordinator, State of Wisconsin DPH/DHS, Madison, Wisconsin
Adjunct Faculty, Mid-State Technical College
Wisconsin Rapids, Wisconsin

Mark A. King, MEMS, Paramedic/IC (ret.)
Kennebec Valley Community College
Fairfield, Maine

Blake E. Klingle, MS, RN, CEN, CCEMTP
Waukesha County Technical College
Pewaukee, Wisconsin

Karen (Keri) Wydner Krause, RN, EMT-P, CCRN
Lakeshore Technical College
Cleveland, Wisconsin

Jim Ladle, BS, FP-C, CCP-C (ret.)
South Jordan Fire Department
University of Utah AirMed
Salt Lake City, Utah

Tony Lipari, EMT-P
Bolton Emergency Medical Services
Bolton Landing, New York

Ricky Lyles, NRP
Southside Virginia Community College
Keysville, Virginia

Monica Malec, MD
University of Chicago
Chicago, Illinois

Paul Mallon, BSN, RN, LP, CFRN
Austin/Travis County EMS
Austin, Texas

John Morrissey, BS, NREMT-P (ret.)
Clay, New York

Patrick Murphy, BA, EMT-P, FP
Austin Travis County EMS
Austin, Texas

Jim O'Connor
Columbus Division of Fire
Columbus, Ohio
Ohio Fire Academy
Reynoldsburg, Ohio

Keito Ortiz, Paramedic, NYS CIC
Jamaica Hospital Medical Center, Level 1 Trauma Center
Jamaica, New York

Jose A. Perez, Paramedic, Certified Instructor Coordinator (CIC)
Fire Department of New York EMS Academy
Bureau of Training
Queens, New York

Joyce M. Pettengill, AAS, NRP
Fayetteville Technical Community College
Fayetteville, North Carolina

Ian Pleet
MedStar Simulation and Training Education Lab (SiTEL)
Washington, DC

Alexander Price, BSN, RN, CEN
Sandoval Regional Medical Center
Rio Rancho, New Mexico

Ernest K. Ralston, PG, EMTP-T, CMAS, NAEMSP
Center for Asymmetric Emergency Medicine
Centreville, Virginia

Kevin Ramdayal, Paramedic
New York City Fire Department
Borough of Manhattan Community College
New York City, New York

Curtis A. Rhodes, NRP, CCEMTP
Gordon Cooper Technology Center
Shawnee, Oklahoma

Chris Rock, MSN, RN
City of Tacoma Fire Department
Tacoma, Washington

Keith A. Sharisky, NRP
Aberdeen Fire Rescue, Advanced Care Ambulance
Aberdeen, South Dakota

Douglas Skinner, MPA, NRP, NCEE
SCS Safety Health and Security Associates LLC
Leesburg, Virginia

Jeremy H. Smith, NRP
Joint Special Operations Medical Training Center
Fort Bragg, North Carolina

Scott A. Smith, MSN, APRN-CNP, ACNP-BC, NRP, I/C
Medical Education Solutions, LLC
Portland, Maine

Sara Sproule, CCEMTP
Prince William County Department of Fire and Rescue
Woodbridge, Virginia

Robert Stanley, MPH, NRP
School of EMS
St. Petersburg, Florida

Andrew W. Stern, MPA, MA, NRP, CCEMTP
Town of Colonie Emergency Medical Services
Colonie, New York
Hudson Valley Community College
Troy, New York

Stephanie Stewart, DNP, APRN, CRNA
Central Connecticut State University
New Britain, Connecticut

Jonathan C. Stone, MPA, NRP, FP-C
Utah Valley University
Orem, Utah

Frank Strange Jr, MS
Oklahoma State University
Oklahoma City, Oklahoma

Justin G. Tilghman, PhD, Paramedic, CEM
Lenoir Community College
Kinston, North Carolina

Laura Tipping-Wilhelm, MSN, BSN, APRN-C, CEN, CCRN, CAPA, CPAN
New Haven, Connecticut

Scott Tomek, EdS, MA, FP-C, CCP-C
Allina Health EMS
St. Paul, Minnesota

Amy E. V. Trujillo, MA, NRP
Fielding Fire Department
Fielding, Utah

Brian Turner, RN, CCEMTP
UnityPoint Health
Princeton, Iowa

Jerad Warlick, BS, NRP, FP-C
Oklahoma State University
Oklahoma City, Oklahoma

Thomas F. (Tom) Watson, AS, AAS, Paramedic
Thomas Nelson Community College
Hampton, Virginia

Gregory West, EdD, JD, NRP
Waukesha County Technical College
Pewaukee, Wisconsin

Michael H. Wilhelm, DNP, APRN, CRNA
UCONN Health–John Dempsey Hospital
Farmington, Connecticut

David Yarmesch, BSOL, AAS-EMS, CSSGB, EMSI, Paramedic
MetroHealth Medical Center
Cleveland, Ohio

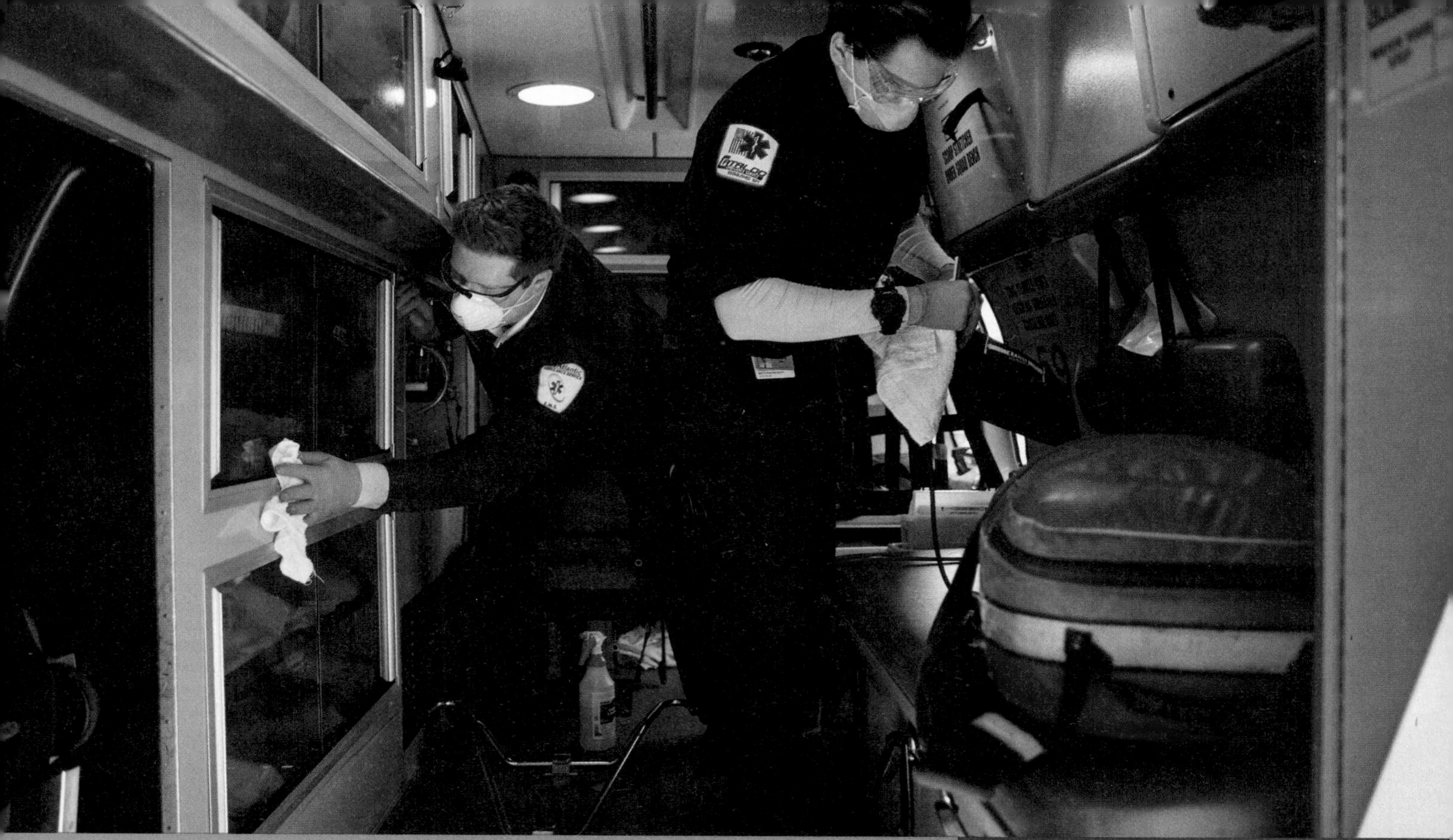

Preparatory

VOLUME 1

SECTION

1

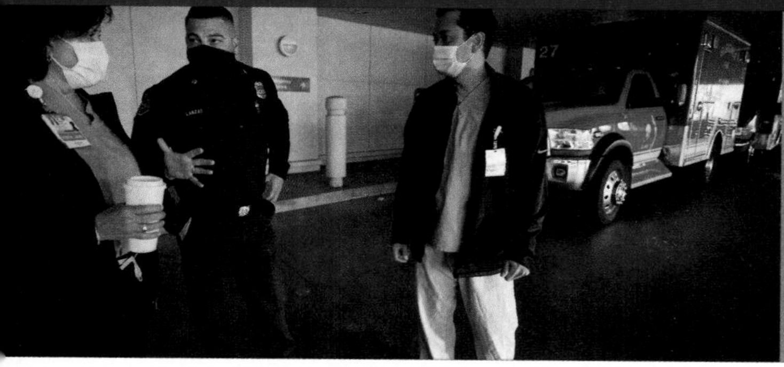

Chapter 1

EMS Systems

NATIONAL EMS EDUCATION STANDARD COMPETENCIES

Preparatory

Integrates comprehensive knowledge of the EMS system, safety/well-being of the paramedic, and medical/legal and ethical issues, which is intended to improve the health of EMS personnel, patients, and the community.

Emergency Medical Services (EMS) Systems

- EMS systems (p 4)
- History of EMS (pp 5, 14–15)
- Roles/responsibilities/professionalism of EMS personnel (pp 23–26)
- Quality improvement (pp 27–30)
- Patient safety (pp 4, 10, 19)

Research

- Impact of research on emergency medical responder (EMR) care (p 16)
- Data collection (p 33)
- Evidence-based decision making (pp 36–37)
- Research principles to interpret literature and advocate evidence-based practice (p 30)

KNOWLEDGE OBJECTIVES

1. List key developments in the history of emergency medical services (EMS). (p 5)
2. Discuss the processes of licensure and certification. (pp 10–12)
3. Define reciprocity, including its relevance to the practice of emergency medical care. (p 12)
4. List the five main types of services that provide emergency medical care. (pp 12–14)
5. Discuss the critical points, required components, and system elements of EMS. (pp 14–15)
6. Describe the EMS education levels in terms of skill sets needed for each of the following: emergency medical responder, emergency medical technician, advanced emergency medical technician, and paramedic. (pp 15–17)
7. Discuss the role of the *National EMS Scope of Practice Model* and the *National EMS Education Standards* as they relate to EMS education levels. (p 17)
8. Discuss initial paramedic education and the importance of continuing education. (pp 17–18)
9. Describe various types of transports the paramedic may perform, including transports to specialty centers and interfacility transports. (pp 18–19)
10. Discuss the paramedic's role in working with other health care providers and public safety agencies. (pp 19–20)
11. Characterize the EMS system's role in prevention and public education in the community. (p 20)
12. Describe the attributes that a paramedic is expected to possess. (pp 22–23)
13. Describe the roles and responsibilities of the paramedic. (pp 23–26)

14. Discuss issues relating to the appropriate method of transport, as well as nontransport situations. (pp 18–19, 28)
15. Describe how medical direction of an EMS system works and the paramedic's role in the process. (pp 26–27)
16. Discuss the purpose of the EMS continuous quality improvement (CQI) process. (pp 27–28)
17. Discuss examples of how errors can be prevented when providing EMS care. (pp 28–30)
18. Discuss the importance of medical research and its role in refining EMS practices. (pp 30–32)
19. List the types of research and subtypes within each category. (pp 32–34)
20. Discuss ethical considerations related to conducting medical research. (pp 34–35)
21. Define peer-reviewed literature and describe how this relates to a practicing paramedic. (pp 35–36)
22. Discuss evidence-based medicine and how to incorporate this concept into everyday paramedic practice. (pp 36–37)

SKILLS OBJECTIVES

There are no skills objectives for this chapter.

Introduction

The **emergency medical services (EMS)** system is no longer considered to be in its infancy; nonetheless, it continues to evolve. When it was initially established, a responder was called to a location for people who were ill or injured and simply transported them rapidly to a medical facility; this practice was often called "load and go." As awareness of EMS capabilities grew, the need for improved systems in various, primarily rural, locations became evident. This awareness, along with research and guidelines from national organizations, has led to the advancement of EMS.

As a paramedic, you will encounter many different types of patients and many different types of situations. The most important thing to remember is that your call is a true emergency in the eyes of the callers or patients, so do not judge them negatively if you feel the situation is not really an emergency. In reality, most of your calls will not entail actual life threats, but they are still important events to your patients **FIGURE 1-1**. The public's perception of you will often be compared with what is seen on television, read in published articles, and encountered in patients' previous experiences; it will also be based on your treatment of their loved ones. Whenever you are in uniform or representing your profession, whether on duty or off, treat all people you encounter with respect and dignity.

As you move forward in your education and career, always be ready for change: EMS is a continually evolving field. Regardless of whether you will be

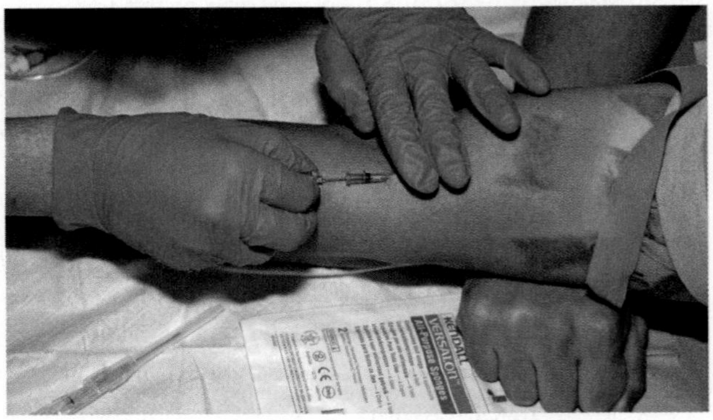

FIGURE 1-1 Today's prehospital providers are highly trained to provide a wide variety of emergency medical services to the public.

SAFETY

Rescuer safety is paramount, but so is the patient's safety! Why all this emphasis on patient safety? A patient's care process is complex, comprising many separate components (eg, prehospital care, emergency department (ED) providers, radiology, laboratory, transport). All of these provider groups must coordinate their actions as part of the joint effort that makes up the patient's overall health care experience. In an ideal world, a patient would move seamlessly from the field through the various departments and from initial presentation to disposition. Of course, we do not live in such an ideal world, and the complexity of the many steps involved opens up many opportunities for process failures, errors, and adverse outcomes.

a volunteer or serve with a paid career department, continuing education is a must; some of what you learn today may not be applicable tomorrow.

EMS System Development

The History of EMS

Much of the prehospital emergency medical care you will deliver as a paramedic can be attributed directly or indirectly to pioneers' visionary advances in the field, including the work of Drs. Peter Safar and Nancy Caroline. You will read more about them later in this chapter. If you research the history of EMS, you may be surprised to learn how long organized systems have been in place. For example, the first recorded use of an ambulance was by the military during the Siege of Málaga in 1487. It was used strictly for transport, and there was no documentation that any actual medical care was provided. During the 1800s, EMS started to make some headway with the following key developments:

- 1800—Baron Dominique-Jean Larrey, chief physician in Napoleon's army, is credited with establishing the first prehospital system for triaging and transporting patients.
- 1860 to 1870—Civilian ambulance services began in Cincinnati, Ohio, in 1865 and in New York City in 1869. In New York City, ambulances (horse-drawn carriages) were dispatched by telegraph from Bellevue Hospital's Centre Street branch. In the first year alone, these ambulances responded to more than 1,800 calls for help throughout the city.
- 1899—The first operated automobile-type ambulance came out of Michael Reese Hospital in Chicago, Illinois.

The 1900s continued to see the evolution of EMS, with significant changes occurring between World Wars I and II. During this time, a major shift occurred; many hospital-based ambulance services did not survive due to the lack of workforce resulting from the wars. Some key developments in EMS before 1950 included the following:

- 1926—The Phoenix Fire Department added service similar to present-day EMS.
- 1928—Julian Stanley Wise launched the first rescue squad out of Roanoke, Virginia, called Roanoke Life Saving and First Aid Crew. Numerous other rescue squad organizations were soon developed along the East Coast, primarily in New Jersey.
- 1940s—Because of a shortage of medical personnel, the role of EMS was turned over to fire and police departments. Unfortunately, no minimum training standards were set for this role. Also, the role of providing emergency medical care was not always immediately accepted or welcomed by these departments.

YOU are the Paramedic

PART 1

At 1618 hours you are dispatched to the 300 block of Hunt Road for a report of a collision between a car and a motorcycle; you notify dispatch that you are en route. Three minutes later as you are nearing the crash scene, you notice a car parked diagonally across the road and a motorcycle lying on its side about 20 feet (6 m) farther up from the car. You note fluid leaking from underneath the car, but it appears no one is inside the car. A crowd of bystanders is gathered at a driveway and you notice a man holding a motorcycle helmet. You think this may be the rider until the man steps to the side of the crowd and you see someone lying supine on the ground. You also note two women trying to talk to a young woman who is screaming hysterically. No other public safety agencies have arrived on scene. You do not notice any hazards at this time.

As you exit the ambulance and approach the scene, you see damage to the right front fender and the car's passenger door. The man holding the helmet turns and calls to you to hurry. He tells you he was driving the car and that he is fine, but the motorcycle rider is "hurt bad."

1. What is your first action as you are approaching the scene and conducting a scene size-up?
2. What role does the emergency medical services system play in this call?

Words of Wisdom

Nancy Lee Caroline was born in a Boston suburb to Leo and Zelda Caroline in 1944. Nancy had a strong social conscience and devoted her life to medicine, teaching, and her patients—and she had a superb sense of humor. She has often been rightly called the "Mother of Paramedics" because of her dedication to paramedic education **FIGURE 1-2**. Nancy died of multiple myeloma at age 58 in 2002.

Nancy's medical career began at the young age of 15 in the pathology laboratory of the famous Benjamin Castleman, MD, at Massachusetts General Hospital, where she conducted medical research long before she entered college. Nancy majored in linguistics at Radcliffe College and received her MD degree from Case Western Reserve University in 1977. She eventually took a fellowship in critical care medicine at the University of Pittsburgh, where she began her groundbreaking work in paramedicine.

Around that time, the late Peter Safar, MD, was overseeing a US Department of Transportation grant to create a curriculum for paramedics. Dr. Safar offered Nancy an opportunity, as medical director of Freedom House Enterprises Ambulance Service, to train paramedics chosen from a group of African American men who did not have a chance to complete their high school educations. Nancy was extremely successful—so successful that she was asked to write a curriculum for paramedic training. That curriculum was published as the first edition of the textbook you are reading: *Emergency Care in the Streets*.

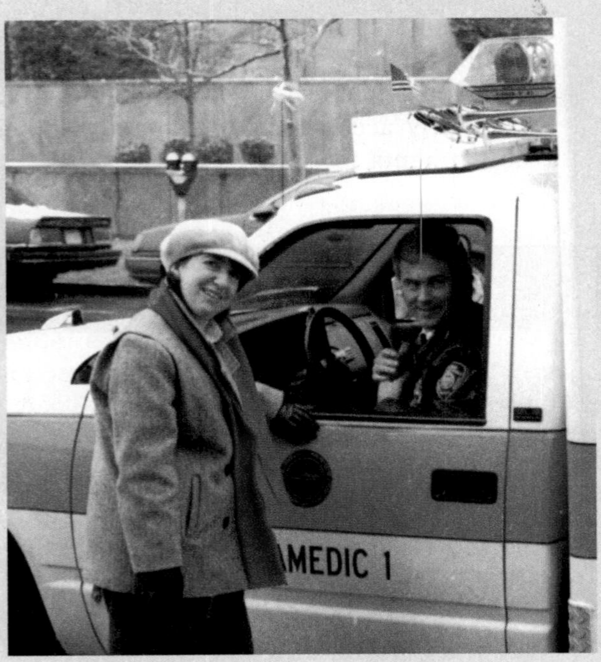

FIGURE 1-2 Nancy L. Caroline with an ambulance from the Boston Department of Health and Hospitals.

The list of Nancy's other accomplishments is long. She served as the first medical director of Israel's Red Cross Society (Magen David Adom), where, in addition to training the first Israeli paramedics, she took extensive Hebrew lessons (it was a point of pride for her to develop a knowledge of the languages in whatever country she was working). After her tenure there ended in 1981, Nancy relocated to Nairobi, Kenya, to become Senior Medical Officer of the African Medical and Research Foundation (AMREF), the foundation that oversees the famous Flying Doctors service. When she became aware of the devastating famine that overtook Ethiopia in the early 1980s, Nancy became a consultant for the League of Red Cross Societies, writing a handbook on basic life support and running classes on first aid for African nations. She worked with the Ethiopian Orthodox Church to provide better nourishment and health care to children in more than 600 orphanages. In addition, Nancy served as director of medical programs for the American Jewish Joint Distribution Committee in Addis Ababa.

In 1987, Nancy returned to Israel to serve as medical consultant for the Center for Educational Technology and for AMREF, developing training materials in emergency medicine and writing correspondence courses for rural health workers in Africa. She also served as an adjunct professor at the University of Pittsburgh's medical school. While volunteering in the Department of Oncology in Tel Hashomer, Nancy collaborated with Alexander Waller, MD, to create the *Handbook of Palliative Care in Cancer*.

Nancy settled in Metula, Israel. She realized there was a need for special care in northern Israel for people with advanced cancer. In 1995, Nancy founded the Hospice of the Upper Galilee (HUG). In 2002, she married geneticist and molecular biologist Lazarus Astrachan.

Nancy left the world too soon, but unquestionably left the world a better place. Despite all her accomplishments, the compliment that meant the most to her was to be called the Mother of Paramedics. Nancy was, no doubt, the best mother paramedics could have.

The 20th Century and Modern Technology

During World Wars I and II, battlefield corps (systems for field treatment and transport) continuously evolved as new techniques were learned that improved field care. In the 1950s and 1960s, EMS began to make significant strides forward. During the 1950s and the Korean War, military medical researchers recognized that bringing hospital-type services closer to the field might give patients a better chance of survival. Helicopters were first used in 1951 during the Korean War. They brought patients to Mobile Army Surgical Hospitals (MASH units), which helped thousands of soldiers and civilians survive their injuries in that war **FIGURE 1-3**.

In 1956, Drs. James Elan and Peter Safar developed mouth-to-mouth resuscitation. Three year later, Frank Pantridge developed the first portable defibrillator in 1959. Both of these advances proved instrumental in saving lives in the field.

In the late 1950s and early 1960s, the focus moved back to bringing the hospital to the patient in some European countries. In these countries, **mobile intensive care units (MICUs)** were developed and staffed by specifically trained physicians. This concept quickly spread to the United States. At that time, however, US physicians were in short supply, and physicians who were interested in participating in such units had minimal expertise outside of the hospital. Physicians were then asked, "Can a person who is not a physician be trained to perform advanced medical skills?" Many answered "Yes."

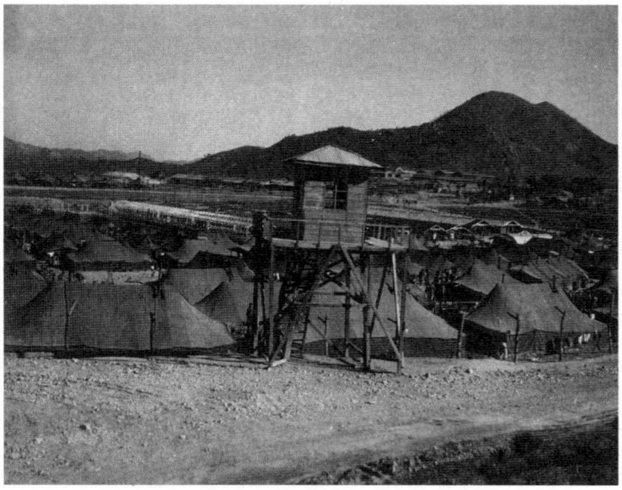

FIGURE 1-3 Temporary hospitals, such as this one in use during the Korean War, were set up to provide more rapid care for the injured.

In 1965, the National Academy of Sciences and the National Research Council released "The White Paper," formally titled *Accidental Death and Disability: The Neglected Disease of Modern Society*; the paper was subsequently published in 1966. Some of the findings related to medical care highlighted in this paper include the following:

- A lack of uniform laws and standards
- Ambulances and equipment were of poor quality or nonexistent
- Lack of communication between EMS and hospitals
- Lack of personnel training
- Hospitals only had part-time staff
- More people died in motor vehicle crashes in the United States each year than in the Vietnam War

Based on these findings, the White Paper outlined 10 critical points to establish a functioning system.

As a response to the unmet needs related to field-based medical care identified in the White Paper, the US Congress passed the National Highway Safety Act of 1966. As part of this act, the US Department of Transportation (US DOT) was created to provide authority and financial support to develop basic and advanced life support programs. In 1968, the Task Force of the Committee of EMS drafted basic training standards, and the principles of a 9-1-1 system to provide universal access to emergency services were created. **TABLE 1-1** lists the critical points, required components, and system elements of EMS that were ultimately developed as a result of the White Paper's publication.

In 1969, a year after basic training standards were developed, Dr. Eugene Nagel, then of Miami, Florida, began training firefighters from the Miami Fire Department with advanced emergency medical skills, thus creating the first true paramedic program **FIGURE 1-4**. Dr. Nagel then took the use of advanced emergency medical treatment one step further: He developed a telemetry system that enabled firefighters to transmit a patient's electrocardiogram (ECG) to physicians at Jackson Memorial

Hospital and to receive radio instructions from the physicians regarding what measures to take. Dr. Nagel is often called the "Father of Paramedicine." Standards for ambulance design and equipment were also published in 1969.

During the 1970s, advancements in EMS continued, helicopters for medical transport became more widely available, and the National Registry of Emergency Medical Technicians (NREMT) was established. The first emergency medical technician

TABLE 1-1 Critical Points, Required Components, and System Elements of EMS

Year	Source	Item
1966	*Accidental Death and Disability: The Neglected Disease of Modern Society* (The White Paper)	Critical points for establishing a functioning EMS system: 1. Develop collaborative strategies to identify and address community health and safety issues. 2. Align the financial incentives of EMS and other health care providers and payers. 3. Participate in community-based prevention efforts. 4. Develop and pursue a national EMS research agenda. 5. Pass EMS legislation in each state to support innovation and integration. 6. Allocate adequate resources for medical direction. 7. Develop information systems that link EMS across its continuum. 8. Determine the costs and benefits of EMS to the community. 9. Designate a single nationwide emergency telephone number. 10. Ensure all calls for emergency help are automatically accompanied by location-identifying information.
1973	Emergency Medical Services Systems Act	Required components of an EMS system: 1. Integration of health services 2. EMS research 3. Legislation and regulation 4. System finance 5. Human resources 6. Medical direction 7. Education and training systems 8. Public access and education 9. Prevention 10. Transportation 11. Communication systems 12. Clinical care facilities 13. Patient information and education systems 14. Mutual aid agreements 15. Evaluation
1988	National Highway Traffic Safety Administration (NHTSA)	NHTSA's essential EMS elements: 1. Regulation and policy 2. Resource management 3. Human resources and training 4. Transportation 5. Facilities 6. Communication 7. Public information and education 8. Medical direction 9. Trauma systems 10. Evaluation

Year	Source	Item
1996	National Highway Traffic Safety Administration	System attributes from the EMS Agenda for the Future: 1. Integration of health services 2. EMS research 3. Legislation and regulation 4. System finance 5. Human resources 6. Medical direction 7. Education systems 8. Public education 9. Prevention 10. Public access 11. Communication systems 12. Clinical care 13. Information systems 14. Evaluation
2019	National Highway Traffic Safety Administration	NHTSA's EMS Agenda 2050: EMS should be: 1. Inherently safe and effective 2. Integrated and seamless 3. Socially equitable 4. Reliable and prepared 5. Sustainable and efficient 6. Adaptive and innovative

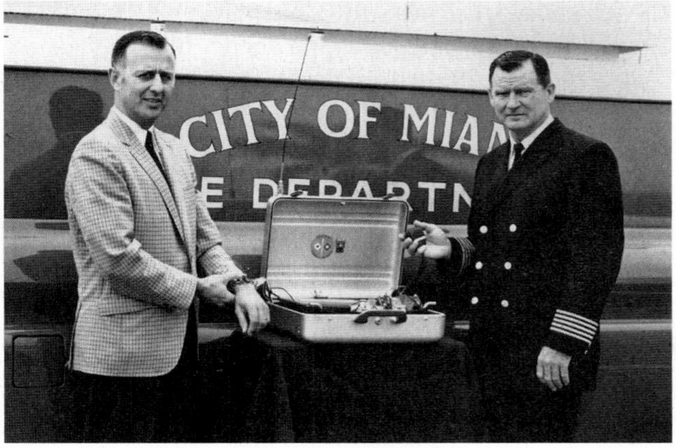

FIGURE 1-4 Dr. Eugene Nagel, widely considered the Father of Paramedicine, provided much-needed leadership to the developing field of EMS training. Here he is shown (at left) in 1967 with Chief Larry Kenney of the Miami Fire Department, with the first telemetry package used by paramedics.

Courtesy of Eugene L. Nagel and the Miami Fire Department.

(EMT) textbook, *Emergency Care and Transportation of the Sick and Injured*, was published by the American Academy of Orthopaedic Surgeons (AAOS) in 1971. In that same year, the AAOS began training EMTs nationwide through a national workshop. The following year, the first television series focused on EMS, *Emergency!*, started a very successful 8-year run. The lead characters, John Gage and Roy DeSoto, became household names. Many EMS providers still reflect on this series because of its realistic depiction of modern-day EMS.

In 1973, the Emergency Medical Services Systems Act defined 15 required components of an EMS system, listed in Table 1-1, emphasizing regional development and trauma care. This act provided a structure and uniformity to the EMS system that came out of pioneering programs in Miami, Seattle, Pittsburgh, and the Illinois Trauma System (Dr. David Boyd). In 1974, after a federal report disclosed that fewer than one-half of ambulance personnel had completed sufficient training, guidelines were published to develop and implement EMS systems. In 1975, the American Medical Association recognized emergency medicine as its own specialty branch within medicine. Many cities set up individual advanced EMS training, and regions added their own spin to what they thought was the essential standard of care. However, it was not until

1977 that the US DOT developed the first National Standard Curriculum for paramedics—a curriculum based on the work of Dr. Nancy Caroline.

Through the 1980s and 1990s, changes continued in EMS and the number of trained personnel grew significantly. The National Highway Traffic Safety Administration (NHTSA) developed 10 system elements, listed in Table 1-1, to sustain EMS systems. Unfortunately, federal funding and staff to support these efforts were reduced, and the responsibility for EMS was transferred to the states. Although it was made clear that the federal funding provided was just "seed money" and that long-term local funding strategies needed to be developed, many states apparently believed the federal dollars would not go away. Unfortunately, the money stopped, and to this day, funding of EMS systems remains a significant challenge for local governments and states.

Several other major legislative initiatives also came about during this time, such as the Emergency Medical Services for Children (EMSC) program grant funding that was implemented in 1985.[1] In 1986, an amendment was made to the Public Safety Officers' Benefits Program so that families of firefighters, members of a rescue squad, and members of an ambulance crew would be compensated if the provider was killed in the line of duty. As progress continued into the 1990s, **trauma systems** started making headway as part of EMS. Some of these secondary programs received federal funding, but they continue to struggle to prove their necessity and maintain this funding. Their expertise is vital to the further advancement of EMS, but a lack of funding has often curtailed their practical impact.

EMS continues to evolve and change in the 21st century. Numerous initiatives are appearing, such as the National EMS Quality Alliance (NEMSQA), formerly called EMS Compass. This organization develops and endorses evidence-based quality measures for EMS and health care partners that improve the experience and outcomes of patients and care providers.[2] The idea that EMS training can be used in many other health care areas, instead of strictly in an ambulance, is also being recognized. Paramedics are being used to provide care in hospital EDs, health care clinics, vaccination sites, and physicians' offices. Community paramedicine, a health care model in which experienced paramedics receive advanced training to provide additional services in the prehospital environment, is becoming a reality, and advances are continually being made in this area. It is important to note that these additional capabilities are not being developed to replace current health care modalities, but rather to apply the capabilities of paramedics in areas not served previously—for example, assisting a home health nurse.

SAFETY

Each hospital and EMS system manages its safety culture locally; both choose which programs they will to implement to manage safety concerns. A **safety culture** has several key features:

- Acknowledges organizations that engage in high-risk activities and determines the importance of consistent, safe operations to counteract these risks
- Supports a blame-free environment where errors can be reported without fear of punishment
- Maintains organizational commitment to address reported errors and safety concerns

An organization's safety culture can be measured using validated surveys given to providers, such as the Patient Safety Culture Survey and the Safety Attitudes Questionnaire developed by the Agency for Healthcare Research and Quality (AHRQ). These surveys ask providers to rate the safety culture of their workplace and the organization in its entirety. The AHRQ provides yearly updates of benchmark data from its hospital survey. Specific activities, such as teamwork training, executive walk-rounds, and established safety teams, have been associated with some improvements in safety culture measurements but are not yet linked to lower error rates.

Licensure, Certification, Registration, and Credentialing

Throughout this section, we will use the terms *licensure* and *registration* interchangeably, though they mean entirely different things. Depending on your state or location, you may be licensed or you may be registered. **Registration** means that a recognized board of registration holds records of your education, state, or local licensure, and recertification.

Licensure is how states control who is allowed to practice as a health care provider. Once you complete your initial paramedic education, you will be eligible to take your state's certification examination, depending on your state.

Credentialing occurs at a local level, where your medical director determines which skills health care providers in the EMS system are allowed to perform. Those skills cannot supersede those determined by the state. In general, those skills do not transfer from service to service. The medical director can approve the skills of only those medics who are under the director's span of control. In particular, some providers can be trained to perform further invasive procedures or monitoring and receive special credentialing.

Words of Wisdom

The terms medical *director* and medical *direction* can be easily confused. The medical *director* oversees guidelines and protocols for an agency—that is, medical *direction*. While in the field, a paramedic will operate under medical direction but is unlikely to communicate directly with the medical director.

Some states require EMS providers to take a test and establish licensure through a registry system such as the NREMT. A **certification** examination is used to ensure health care providers have at least the same basic level of knowledge and skill. Once you have passed the required examinations, your state and/or NREMT will give you a certificate or license.

Different states refer to the authority granted to EMS providers to function as a paramedic as licensure, certification, or credentialing. For the purposes of this text, the term *licensure* will be used. It is unlawful to perform a paramedic's functions before licensure; to be more specific, doing so is considered practicing medicine without a license unless a paramedic program internship preceptor directly supervises you as a part of your training program. Although holding a license shows you have successfully completed the education and testing requirements to achieve such a license, it does not mean that you can perform as a paramedic without or outside the supervision of your service's physician medical director. Agencies (state, local, and national) still require that paramedics receive **medical direction** (both online and off-line). The concept and principles of medical control are discussed later in the chapter.

YOU are the Paramedic

PART 2

Your initial impression of the patient is that he is a young man and appears to be unresponsive. He is not wearing any protective clothing, and some of the bystanders tell you they took off his helmet "so he could breathe." You note that the patient is breathing, but his breaths are very shallow and he has some minor bleeding from an obvious fracture of his left lower leg. Before you reach the patient, the hysterical woman runs to you and begs you to hurry up and do something because "My boyfriend is dying!" She does not think you are moving fast enough. The two women try again to console her, but she is frantic. You have been told she was not involved in the crash.

Recording Time: 1 Minute	
Appearance	Pale, not moving, obvious deformity of left lower leg
Level of consciousness	Unresponsive to all stimuli
Airway	Patent
Breathing	Rapid and shallow, with what appears an asymmetric pattern
Circulation	Rapid and weak radial pulses

3. What aspects of professionalism must be employed in this situation?
4. Aside from those noted in the previous question, what roles and responsibilities are vital as a prehospital health care provider?

If your state requires you to pass the NREMT cognitive and psychomotor examinations to become licensed, you will have to pass a written exam and demonstrate several practical skills. To be eligible, you must first successfully complete initial paramedic education through an accredited program. Your school is required to verify your course completion before you can sit for the exam. The NREMT exam tests the candidate on the Paramedic Psychomotor Competency Portfolio, a comprehensive collection of skills and scenarios crucial to paramedic practice. Detailed information on the examination requirements can be found at the NREMT website, nremt.org.

The Committee on Accreditation of Educational Programs for the EMS Professions (CoAEMSP) is currently the only accrediting body for paramedic programs. Its mission is to continuously improve EMS education quality through accreditation and recognition services for the full range of EMS professions. Because of changes to the *National EMS Scope of Practice Model*, the need to expand the professional image of EMS, and the desire to establish consistent guidelines for paramedicine, the number of accredited paramedic training facilities is expected to grow significantly in the coming years.

Reciprocity

Each state has different licensing or certification requirements and procedures regardless of whether it follows the *National EMS Scope of Practice Model*. Granting certification to a provider from another state or agency is known as **reciprocity**. If you are planning to relocate to another state or country, investigate the licensure process beforehand. Keep in mind that many other countries will not accept the training provided in the United States and reciprocity will not be automatic. Common reciprocity requirements include holding current state licensure or NREMT certification, being in good standing, and meeting all training requirements for the state in which you are applying. You may be asked to provide your education transcript, continuing education hours, and/or evidence of refresher course completion. Some states may require practical skills testing, but others may waive this requirement if you hold NREMT certification. Training regarding state-specific protocols and procedures may be required. You will also likely be required to provide information for a criminal background check. Because you will be an integral part of the health care system, most states want to ensure you do not have previous issues that could call into question your integrity or professionalism. Finally, some states will require a fee to process your reciprocity application and provide a license.

Words of Wisdom

In 2020, the NREMT launched the National EMS-ID number system. An EMS-ID is a 12-digit identification number issued at no charge to all EMS providers, from emergency medical responders to paramedics, and to students entering the profession. The number is automatically generated by the NREMT when a person creates an account. For EMS providers with an existing account, an EMS-ID is retroactively created. Unlike the number issued by the NREMT (NR number) when an individual becomes certified, EMS-IDs do not change as the person's certification level changes. Thus, the various certification numbers that providers may obtain over the course of their careers are all tied back to the single EMS-ID.

Words of Wisdom

NREMT certification often facilitates licensure in other states. The Interstate Commission for EMS Personnel Practice aims to increase the ability of EMS providers to practice in other states through the Recognition of EMS Personnel Licensure Interstate CompAct (REPLICA). REPLICA is not a form of EMS licensure reciprocity, but simply extends a privilege to EMS personnel from member states to practice on a short-term or intermittent basis under approved circumstances in other member states. Examples include EMS providers responding as part of an agency with a multistate footprint, staffing for large unplanned events that do not reach the level of a governor-declared disaster, and staffing for large planned events such as concerts and races.

Traditional EMS Employment

Once you become a licensed paramedic, you will have a variety of career options available to you. Although, in general, your scope of practice will remain the same, there may be slight modifications of what will be expected of you. Working hours can vary greatly, from 24-hour to 12-hour to 8-hour shifts, or any number of scheduled shifts. Some career possibilities include the following:

- **Fire-based EMS.** In general, most EMS providers who are integrated into a fire department are paid by and operate under the municipal government. Depending on your state, however, this may not always be the case. Some locations operate entirely with nonpaid volunteers, while others use providers who are paid per call; they do not receive compensation until a call comes in. EMS may have a separate management system within these organizations and operate independently from the organization's fire side. Depending on the specific situation in any one agency, maintaining separate operations management systems may or may not be valuable due to both areas' numerous expectations. If there is separate management, the managers often report to a main chief or director to ensure consistency of department operations. Fire and EMS personnel may respond together to major incidents when additional staffing is required; you may have a dual role of working with both fire and EMS providers. Recently, the trend toward fire-based EMS roles has increased: The incidence of fires is declining thanks to prevention efforts, so fire departments can better justify keeping a staffed in-house department if they add EMS to their array of services.
- **Third-service EMS (municipalities): single or shared.** Depending on their financial capabilities, some municipalities may establish and operate their own ambulance services independent of fire, police, and other public safety entities. In some cases, independent ambulance agencies offer their services under contract to municipalities that cannot afford to provide their own services. Some states allow multiple municipalities to share services under agreements, with each being an equal owner of the resulting system. These shared services reduce the cost to all, which allows them to cover the cost of providing paramedic service. Third-service systems typically function independently of the fire service. Consequently, you may need to explicitly request a response if you need fire or rescue assistance; they may not be sent automatically. This works both ways: The fire department may need to request EMS response for medical support, unless the agencies have established a prearranged response process.
- **Private EMS agency: for-profit or nonprofit.** In general, private services operate similarly to third-service EMS agencies. The primary difference is that they contract their services to municipalities. This kind of contract can include anything from managing an existing service to providing full service to the communities. Operations of private service vary greatly. Some follow standard 24-hour shift practices, while others follow a "status systems management" structure. With the latter structure, providers report to a central location at the beginning of the shift, pick up an ambulance, and are sent to a staging area within the service area. The location of the staging area is often established depending on past requests for service. Although this approach functions well in most cases, emergencies cannot be predicted, so there is the potential that a serious call may have to wait a significant length of time for a unit to arrive.
- **Hospital-based EMS.** These services can vary greatly, but, in most cases, hospital-based services tend to offer interfacility-type transports, as well as aeromedical services, which are typically available in larger and remote organizations. Some hospitals also offer 9-1-1 response and paramedic intercept service in some locations. As a paramedic working in a hospital-based system, you will often be required to assist with patient care in other areas of the hospital during your down time. Typically, you will work from an ED, but you may also be part of an internal emergency response team. One benefit of being part of a hospital-based team is the access to information that is available from various medical providers, especially in complex cases.
- **Hybrid or other.** As paramedicine continues to grow, so will the various expectations and jobs you may encounter. Many large companies, such as those operating oil drilling platforms and factories with hundreds or thousands of employees, have their own medical response and care facilities. In some

areas, paramedics work in conjunction with primary care providers, physician assistants, and nurse practitioners. Numerous companies have been established to hire personnel to fill medical positions at specific locations, such as national parks, amusement parks, and other venues.

Regardless of where you work as a paramedic, you need to keep your training and skills current to ensure you are ready to respond at all times.

The EMS System

Today's EMS system is a complex network of coordinated services providing various care levels to a community. These services work in unison to meet both the new and standing needs of the citizens in the community in which they reside. As a paramedic, you are part of this network; in turn, you must stay active in your community to meet its ever-changing needs.

The EMS network begins with citizen involvement in the complex EMS system. In most cases, the public does not understand EMS and knows only what is seen in newspapers, television, and movies. Be prepared: They may assume the inappropriate behaviors of actors on EMS TV series reflect reality, so you will also have the task of educating them on the truth. Members of the community may need to be taught what is an emergency and what is not, how to activate the EMS system, and how basic care can be provided before EMS arrives. Remember, the public usually does not have medical training or knowledge, so in their eyes a superficial cut may be an emergency.

Street Smarts

Many members of the public possess smartphones equipped with cameras, so your actions at the scene may be broadcast to a much larger audience, sometimes in real time. Always be professional and keep your cool.

When you are called to a "sick person" at 0200 hours who has only a common cold and cannot sleep, you must avoid becoming angry with the patient, your career, or your EMS system. You will encounter many general symptoms in your career and education that could cause you to overlook a serious problem. Be compassionate and caring with your patient; this will build the patient's trust in both you and the EMS system.

Street Smarts

A patient may experience only once what you as a paramedic may experience hundreds of times. Recognize the patient's fear and anxiety and demonstrate empathy and understanding while providing care.

Factors that play a role in determining the outcome or likelihood of your patient's survival include the following:

- Bystander care
- Dispatch (including prearrival directions)
- Response (both mode and distance)
- Prehospital assessment and care provided (level of EMS-trained personnel)
- Transportation (ground ambulances, critical care units, air transport)
- ED care (on-duty trained emergency physicians and staff)
- Definitive care (including trauma, pediatric, and neurologic specialists)
- Rehabilitation

When members of the public activate the EMS system, their first contact is usually a dispatcher. Requirements for dispatcher training vary from state to state, and dispatchers must often cover police and fire communications as well as all general department phone calls. Dispatchers must interpret the caller's needs to determine if it is an emergency by extracting appropriate information, and then decide what resources need to be sent. Scene findings do not always accurately reflect the information received by dispatch and relayed to you. You must remember that dispatch can provide you with only the information that the caller provides to them; never underestimate or overestimate that information or get angry with dispatch if their information is completely different from what you encounter on scene.

Being active in your community increases your awareness of local resources and their capabilities.

For example, consider a patient who may be suffering from an acute stroke. This patient should be transported to a facility capable of performing computed tomography (CT). If your local facility does not have this capability, you should transport the patient to a facility with those capabilities within a reasonable time and distance. Of course, in some regions, competent adult patients may request the facility to which they wish to be transported. However, if it is different from the facility you feel would be most appropriate, this is the time for you to educate your patient, but not to argue. If you cannot talk the patient into going to the facility you feel is best, consider seeking assistance from online (direct) medical control. If that fails, document the patient's choice and your efforts to educate the patient and/or family on your prehospital care report.

Special Populations

EMS systems must be capable of handling many different situations, including obstetric, pediatric, and geriatric emergencies. Proper procedures, drug dosages, and even assessment techniques may vary depending on patient characteristics such as age and gender.

Levels of Education

Licensure of EMS personnel is usually a state function, subject to the laws and regulations of the state in which the EMS provider practices. For this reason, there are variations from state to state in the scope of practice and in education and relicensure requirements. The following information explains how the system is supposed to work from the federal level to the local level.

At the federal level, NHTSA brought in experts from around the country to create the *National EMS Scope of Practice Model.*[3] This document provides overarching guidelines as to what skills each level of EMS provider should be able to accomplish. The next step is the state level. Because licensure is usually a state function, laws and regulations are enacted to specify how EMS providers will operate. These laws are then executed by the state EMS administrative offices, which control licensure. Many states have a set of statutes or rules to be followed and a scope of practice for every EMS level. Finally, the service's medical director normally develops a set of patient care guidelines that outline each level's approved skills and treatments. For example, the medications that will be carried on your emergency vehicle or where patients are transported are day-to-day operational concerns in which the medical director may have direct input. States may define the role of the medical director differently, so ensure you understand and follow your state's processes.

The national guidelines are intended to ensure a more consistent delivery of EMS across the country. The medical director can limit the scope of practice but cannot expand it beyond state law. Expanding the scope of practice requires state approval.

In 2009, the National Standard Curricula for all levels of EMS providers were revised to a new format and renamed the *National EMS Education Standards.*[4] In the United States, NHTSA is the federal administrative source for these standards and related documents. The *National EMS Education Standards* for the four levels of EMS providers can be downloaded from the NHTSA website at ems.gov.

The Dispatcher

The dispatcher plays a vital role in an EMS call. This staff member receives and enters all information on the call, interprets the information, and then relays it to the appropriate resources **FIGURE 1-5**. In some locations, the dispatcher may be trained as an emergency medical dispatcher. This person will

FIGURE 1-5 The dispatcher coordinates the entire rescue effort. This staff member interprets a caller's information and then sends appropriate personnel and resources to the scene.

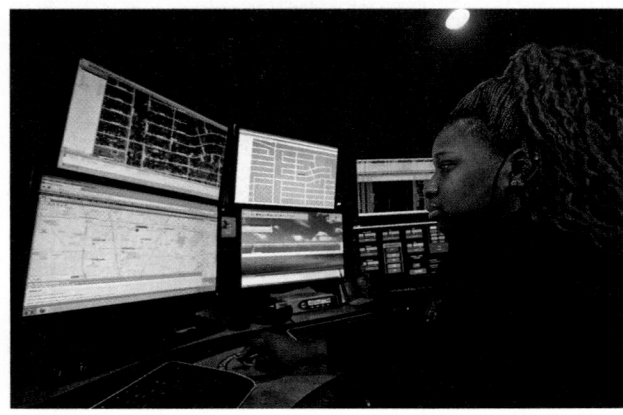

have the added task of giving prearrival instructions (eg, cardiopulmonary resuscitation [CPR], bleeding control) after asking a series of questions of the caller in hopes that the instructions provided may benefit the patient until you arrive on scene.

Emergency Medical Responder

Until recently, the emergency medical responder (EMR) level was known as the "first responder." Not all states incorporate this certification and/or licensing level, and for those states that do, there can be considerable variability in requirements and allowed skills. In the generic use of the term, an EMR is usually a person trained in CPR and/or first aid. In some states, EMRs can function only as part of an organized group, and that group must be affiliated with a transporting ambulance service. As a paramedic, you will need to familiarize yourself with the level of training of the EMRs in your system.

An EMR has completed a course covering the *National EMS Education Standards* for the EMR level. This training will help the EMR recognize the seriousness of a patient's condition, administer appropriate basic care, and relay information to the paramedic. EMRs are an essential level of provider to the EMS system, especially in rural areas **FIGURE 1-6**.

EMT

Historically called the EMT-Basic (EMT-B), the EMT is the backbone and primary provider level in many EMS systems **FIGURE 1-7**. This is also the level of certification required for an individual to enter a paramedic education program. Much life-saving care is provided at this level.

The skills and treatments that EMTs are permitted to perform vary from state to state. EMTs may be trained in advanced airway intervention, limited medication administration, and intravenous (IV) fluid therapy; however, EMTs with this expanded scope of practice are not recognized at a different certification level per the *National EMS Education Standards*. There are more providers trained and certified as an EMT than at any other EMS level.

Advanced EMT

The level formerly called EMT-Intermediate (EMT-I) has gone through numerous changes over the years. It was initially developed in 1985, when it was known as the EMT-I 85 level. The EMT-I skill level saw a significant change in 1999, when the 1985 curriculum underwent substantial revision. More recently, changes made within the *National EMS Scope of*

Controversies

Some argue that all that is needed in an urban setting are AEMTs rather than paramedics. In contrast, others argue that AEMTs perform ALS skills without having adequate academic preparation and should be phased out. The jury is still out on whether this level of training will become an attractive option for jurisdictions and EMS providers.

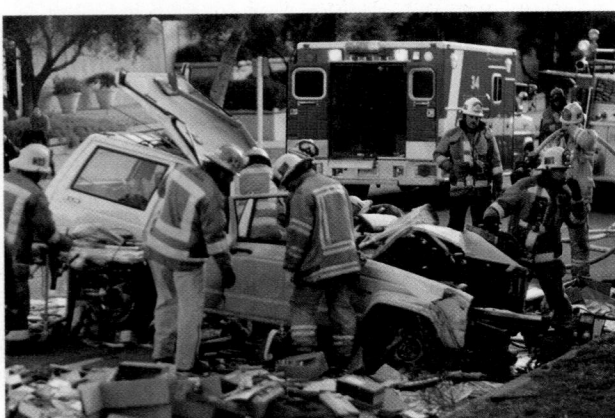

FIGURE 1-6 The emergency medical responder is critical for providing the initial emergency patient care, particularly when medical personnel must travel long distances to a scene.

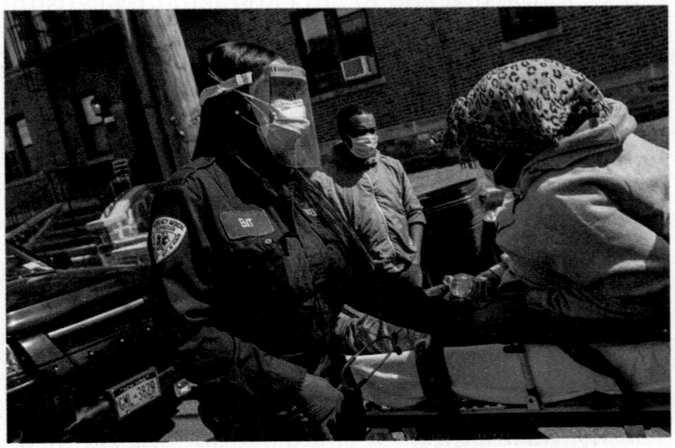

FIGURE 1-7 Emergency medical technicians comprise the largest number of EMS providers.

Practice Model have eliminated the intermediate level, and it has been replaced with the Advanced EMT (AEMT) level in most states. AEMTs are trained in more advanced pathophysiology and some advanced procedures such as establishing IV access, administering IV fluids, performing blood glucose monitoring, administering several medications, and performing some advanced airway management.

Paramedic

Currently, paramedic is the highest EMS skill level at which you can be certified or licensed at the national level. In 1998, the US DOT paramedic curriculum underwent major revisions and the level of training and skills increased greatly. In 2009, when the *National EMS Education Standards* were completed, the skills allowed at the paramedic level changed to some extent. Starting in 2013, a paramedic student must have attended and successfully completed training at an accredited institution to test through NREMT. States that do not employ NREMT as their testing mechanism may not require EMS training institutions to be accredited. Although a paramedic may hold a license or certification independently, states require paramedics to function directly under a licensed physician's guidance and to be affiliated with a paramedic-level service. Paramedics are allowed to complete further education and earn the title of critical care paramedic in some states. Research your state's laws to see if this is allowed.

Paramedic Education

Initial Education

Education may vary from state to state, but for the most part, all states base their paramedic education programs on the *National EMS Education Standards* for the paramedic. As mentioned, significant changes were made to these standards (formerly called curricula) in 2009. A major recommendation was the inclusion of a college-level anatomy and physiology course. Some training institutions offer this as part of a paramedic training program; for others, it is a prerequisite. The *National EMS Education Standards* outline the minimum of what a paramedic must know to practice. States require varying hours of education, but the national average falls between 1,000 and 1,500 hours of combined classroom, clinical, and field education. Some leaders want to structure education so the paramedic designation is achieved through an associate or bachelor's degree accredited program. This approach's distinct benefit is that it can give paramedics credits to earn higher-level college degrees.

> **Words of Wisdom**
>
> The number of calls you go on is not the deciding factor on how much more education you need.

Continuing Education

Most states require paramedics to complete a certain number of continuing education hours and/or a refresher program. Such programs keep you up-to-date on new research findings, new techniques and skills, and help prevent degradation of the skills you use less frequently **FIGURE 1-8**. Continuing education can also showcase current issues in your state that impact you and your system's ability to provide quality emergency medical care. Continuing education can be enjoyable, and it should be.

Whenever possible, you should attend conferences and seminars, ideally with some of them being out of your region and/or state, which helps broaden your knowledge base and EMS network. Consider attending conferences that may not be designed for paramedics, such as those targeted at nurses or physicians. Read EMS journals and research publications to stay current. Due to advances

FIGURE 1-8 Continuing education can keep you up-to-date on the technologic improvements that are continually made available to paramedics.

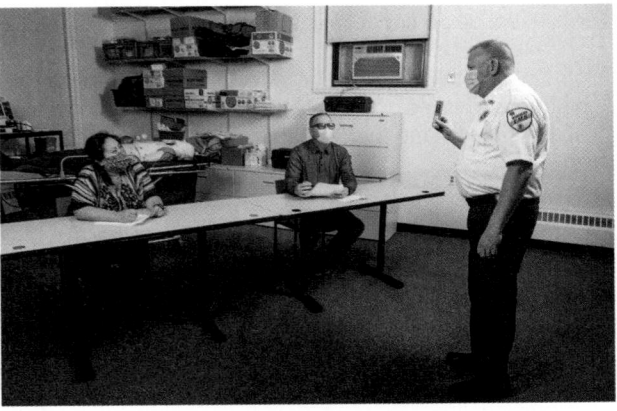

in technology, Internet-based continuing education resources have expanded greatly, but you must ensure these programs meet your state or national requirements. When you are investigating continuing education options, consider seeking out courses from those organizations that have made the effort to become accredited through the Commission on Accreditation for Pre-Hospital Continuing Education (CAPCE), formerly called the Continuing Education Coordinating Board for EMS (CECBEMS). This organization develops continuing education standards and is involved in setting accreditation standards for prehospital providers.[5]

Get everyone in your service involved in postrun critiques, which can help identify problem areas in your practice. Postrun critiques are considered to be a form of continuing education in some states.

No matter what requirements are mandated by your state licensing agency, responsibility for continuing medical education ultimately rests with you. You know which areas of your knowledge have diminished and which skills require additional refresher efforts. You are the person who will have to live with the questions and doubts that inevitably arise after something goes wrong in the field. If something does go wrong, after the call is not the time to realize you should have done something differently or attended extra training. Continuing medical education is a way to help ensure you are following the latest best practices and will build confidence in your skills.

Additional Types of Transports

Transport to Specialty Centers

In addition to hospital EDs, many EMS systems include specialty centers that focus on specific types of care (eg, trauma, burns, poisoning, and

YOU are the Paramedic

PART 3

An initial assessment reveals that the patient is unresponsive and the only visible injury is to the patient's leg. You also note damage to the left side of the helmet. While your partner is gathering the immobilization equipment, fire department rescue personnel arrive and you ask one of them to talk with the girlfriend and find out as much information about the patient as possible.

Further assessment reveals diminished breath sounds on the patient's left side, distended neck veins, and asymmetric movement of the left chest. His radial pulses are weakening and increasing in rate. Recognizing signs of a tension pneumothorax and following your local protocols, you quickly perform a needle thoracostomy on the affected side. You hear a rush of air, and the patient's color and pulse rate improve.

Your partner inserts an oral airway and begins ventilating the patient with a bag-mask device and 100% oxygen while rescue personnel assist you in packaging the patient on the long backboard. His left leg is secured to his right leg, and bleeding is controlled with direct pressure and a dressing. The patient is loaded into the ambulance and you quickly obtain his vital signs. The rescuer who was talking to the girlfriend tells you the patient is 22 years old, has no medical history, and takes no medications. The girlfriend does not think he is allergic to anything. He has a blood glucose level of 102 mg/dL, and the cardiac monitor shows sinus tachycardia without ectopy.

Recording Time: 6 Minutes	
Respirations	12 breaths/min assisted with ventilations
Pulse	138 beats/min, weak radial pulses
Skin	Pale, cool, diaphoretic
Blood pressure	96/54 mm Hg
Oxygen saturation (Spo_2)	92% with ventilations by a bag-mask device and 100% oxygen
Pupils	Equal but sluggish to react

5. How will you determine how and where to transport this patient?

cardiac or psychiatric conditions) or specific types of patients (eg, children). Specialty centers normally have in-house specialists, while other facilities must page operating teams, surgeons, or other specialists from outside the hospital. Typically, only a few hospitals in a region are designated as specialty centers. Transport time to a specialty center may be slightly longer than the time to an ED, but patients will receive definitive care more quickly at a specialty center.

Know the location of the centers in your area and when you should transport the patient directly to one. Sometimes, air medical transport will be necessary. Local, regional, and state protocols may guide your decision in these instances.

SAFETY

Some recent adverse events associated with interfacility transfers have brought closer scrutiny of these transports. A recent Canadian study suggests that the rate of such events is lower when transports are staffed with specifically trained critical care transport providers.[6] Overall, data indicate that 1 in 15 patients experienced serious adverse events during transport, including hypotension, initiation of vasopressor therapy, and respiratory events. An analysis showed that hemodynamic instability requiring intervention such as fluids or vasopressors was by far the most common adverse event, followed by respiratory instability or hypoxia. Additionally, in-transit critical care events were independently associated with mechanical ventilation and baseline hemodynamic instability.

Some problematic events have been identified concerning specific types of transports. The most common adverse events noted for pediatric transports were hypothermia, medication errors, tachycardia, procedure error, loss of IV access, and cyanosis. Interestingly, the adverse event rate was lower in this population when specialized teams performed the transport.

The value of employing specialty-trained teams in interfacility transport of complex cases is increasing as newer and more advanced therapies become more widely employed during transport, such as inhaled nitric oxide and extracorporeal membrane oxygenation. In a review of adult transports, one group of authors found that 70% of adverse events could have been avoided by better preparation before transport, communication between the sending and receiving facilities, and the use of checklists and protocols.[7]

Interfacility Transports

Many EMS agencies provide interfacility transportation for patients. Examples include transfer from a clinic to a hospital, from a hospital to a rehabilitation center, from a hospital to a long-term care facility, or from one hospital to another hospital. During such a transport, the health and well-being of the patient is your responsibility. If medical control is required during transport, it comes from the transporting facility until you arrive at the receiving facility and hand off care with a report. Obtain the patient's medical history, chief complaint, and latest vital signs before the transport and provide ongoing patient care during transport. When a patient is critically ill or injured and requires transport with supplies and services beyond a paramedic's scope of practice, a specialty care transport team may be necessary. Depending on the patient's needs, the team may consist of one or more nurses or critical care paramedics, a respiratory therapist, or a physician.

Working With Other Professionals

Working With Hospital Staff

Become familiar with the receiving hospitals to which you will transport patients, staff members' functions, and their routine operating procedures in all hospital areas, especially the ED. Also, learn about advances in emergency medical care and how to interact with hospital personnel. This experience will help you understand how your care influences a patient's recovery and will emphasize the importance and benefits of proper prehospital care. It will also show you the consequences of delay, inadequate care, or poor judgment. You are an integral part of a patient's care plan; therefore, you must interact professionally with all hospital personnel who will be part of your patient's care. Never ridicule or undermine any member of the hospital staff. Sometimes, the hospital staff may not realize the EMS provider's capabilities or the situation in which the care was provided; a little explanation can go a long way toward educating them. You should also recognize that the care a patient receives in the hospital may differ from what you do in the field.

Physicians are not likely to be in the field with you to provide personal, on-the-spot instructions. However, you may consult with appropriate medical staff by using the radio through established (online) medical control procedures. In addition, a physician or nurse may serve as an instructor for medical subjects in your education program. Through these experiences, you will become more comfortable using medical terms, interpreting patient signs and symptoms, and developing patient management skills.

Working With Public Safety Agencies

Some public safety personnel have EMS training, and you should become familiar with the roles and responsibilities of these workers. Personnel from certain agencies are often better prepared than you are to perform particular functions. For example, employees of a utility company are better equipped to control downed power lines than are you or your partner. Law enforcement personnel can better handle violent scenes and traffic control, while you and your partner provide emergency medical care **FIGURE 1-9**. If you work together, recognizing that each person has special training and a job to do at the scene, effective scene and patient management will prevail. Remember, the best, most efficient patient care is achieved through cooperation among agencies.

Community Expectations

In addition to responding to EMS calls, taking care of the patient, transporting, and returning to service, EMS providers have responsibilities to the community. The community has expectations of EMS providers and, as a health care provider and public servant, you must project confidence to the community you serve. As previously mentioned, the general public usually has no idea what EMS does, so your encounters with community members are opportunities to educate them.

FIGURE 1-9 You will work with law enforcement personnel when dealing with violent patients.

Whether you are working in the public or private sector, encourage people in the community to become involved in your service to some level. Present-day medicine focuses on prevention; getting involved in community efforts gives you an opportunity to use your medical expertise to help the people you serve. For example, you might review the types of calls you respond to most commonly, and then use this information to develop prevention strategies or activities within your community to reduce those types of calls. Perhaps your community has many calls relating to accidental falls. A variety of training programs are available to help identify possible causes of falls, known as "fall prevention programs." As part of such a program, you can visit homes in your community, especially housing developments and facilities catering to older adults, to offer prevention suggestions.

As a new paramedic, you will be considered part of the health care and emergency services community. You will work side by side with other professionals and groups. For example, you will integrate your work with that of other medical professionals; law enforcement; public health services; emergency management and disaster services; home health groups, such as hospice; and, of course, emergency responders. You must understand your role and the roles of those with whom you interact to ensure calls run as smoothly as possible. You must also be prepared for any number of situations, and establish expectations for each role at each scene.

> **Words of Wisdom**
>
> The best paramedics continually seek out education and refresh their basic life support skills as well as advanced life support skills.

National EMS Group Involvement

Many national and state EMS organizations exist, and many invite paramedic membership. These organizations impact the future direction of EMS, so it

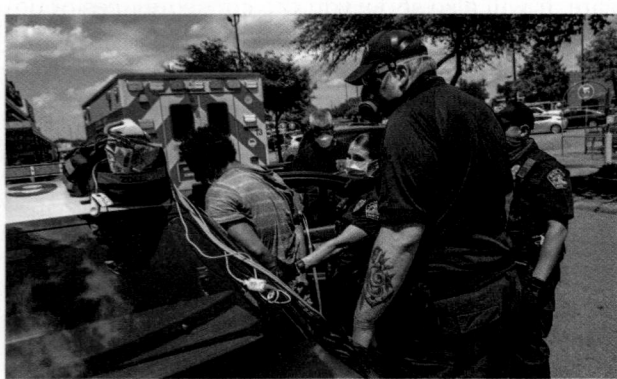

TABLE 1-2 National EMS Organizations

- National Highway Traffic Safety Administration (NHTSA)
- National Association of Emergency Medical Service Physicians (NAEMSP)
- National Association of State EMS Officials (NASEMSO)
- National Association of EMS Educators (NAEMSE)
- National Registry of EMTs (NREMT)
- National Association of EMTs (NAEMT)
- Emergency Medical Services for Children (EMSC)
- American College of Emergency Physicians (ACEP)
- American Ambulance Association (AAA)
- Committee on Accreditation of Educational Programs for the Emergency Medical Services Professions (CoAEMSP)
- International Association of Flight and Critical Care Paramedics (IAFCCP)

is essential for you to identify and become involved in them. Through these groups, you can also gain access to valuable resources to help you develop yourself and your service area and to improve your problem-solving skills. One common goal advocated by many national and state organizations is to promote uniformity of EMS standards and practices. Some of these organizations are listed in **TABLE 1-2**.

Professionalism

During your paramedic education, you will learn a vast amount of information designed to make you a **health care professional**, practicing at the paramedic level. A **profession** is a field of endeavor that requires a specialized set of knowledge, skills, and expertise, often gained after lengthy education.

A health care professional has the following attributes:

- Conforms to the same standards of other health care professions
- Provides quality patient care
- Instills pride in the profession
- Strives continuously for high standards
- Earns respect from others in the profession
- Meets high societal expectations of the profession whether on or off duty

As an EMS provider, you must meet numerous standards, competencies, and continuing education

FIGURE 1-10 Adopting a professional attitude and appearance is a critical part of working with the public and earning their trust.

requirements. The paramedic profession also has expected standards and performance parameters as well as a code of ethics. Collectively, these are the criteria by which you will be measured.

You must remember that you are in a highly visible role in the community **FIGURE 1-10**. Consequently, professional image and behavior must be a priority whether you are in uniform on duty or are off duty in street clothes. You represent the agency, city, county, district, or state in which you work. It has been said that people will make an initial judgment of you within the first 10 seconds of meeting you, even if you say nothing. A positive impression will usually win complete trust from your patients and their family. Conversely, a negative impression will reflect poorly not only on you, but also on your service—and a negative image can be very hard to change. As a paramedic, you will meet new people every day as part of your career. To provide the best possible care, you must instill confidence in them, as well as establish and maintain credibility. Whenever you walk into a situation, remember that a significant part of your job is to continually show your concern for your patients and their families' well-being. Your appearance is also of utmost importance and has more effect than you may think. It is not appropriate to arrive at a call in dirty clothes, with dirty hands, and smelling offensively. Appear and act like a professional at all times. Professionalism has no boundaries; saying you are "only a volunteer" or "only a part-time worker" is no excuse for unprofessional behavior.

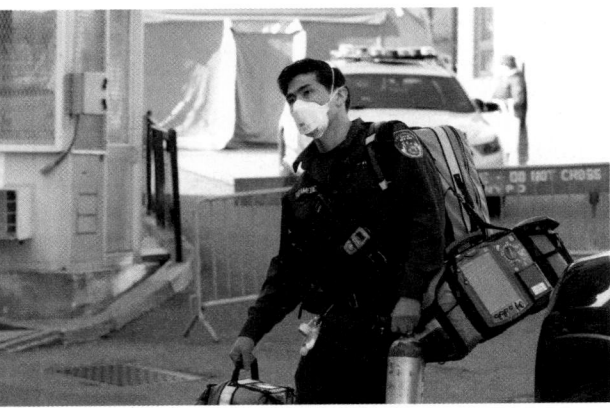

Words of Wisdom

Earning paramedic licensure brings new prestige, but it also imposes new responsibilities. Paramedics are entrusted with the lives of other people and, although some calls will be terrifying and challenging to you, there is no more awesome or sacred responsibility than that. Your education as a paramedic must not stop with this textbook. Continue to read and study and ask questions. Refine your knowledge and skills, so you can give to each patient the best of which you are capable. Realize that having a wealth of knowledge and skills does not mean you can and must use them on every call. Like a physician, you have a vast array of capabilities, so learn when and when not to use them and how to do so appropriately. Learn to conduct yourself with humility, to accept criticism, to learn from mistakes as well as from triumphs, and to demand of yourself and your colleagues nothing less than the best. Only then will the title of paramedic signify what it is meant to signify: a commitment to other people.

As a paramedic, you are an integral part of the entire health care system; in this role, you must present a professional image and treat others in the profession with the respect you would want to be treated with. Although it is inappropriate to argue with other health care providers or hospital staff, you can certainly have professional discussions regarding patient care. Remember, you are a patient advocate, and it is appropriate for you to raise concerns about patient care professionally at appropriate times and locations. On some occasions, differences of opinion may arise; these are best addressed by contacting a supervisor. Such conversations may identify instances when other branches of health care do not follow the same practices as EMS, due to different expectations or requirements.

Other attributes of professionalism as a paramedic include the following:

- **Integrity.** This is the single most important attribute for all paramedics. Be open, honest, and truthful with your patients and coworkers.
- **Empathy.** Show your patients, their families, and other health care professionals that you identify and understand their feelings. It is okay to show emotions to some extent.
- **Self-motivation.** Have an internal drive for excellence, which is often a driving force to ensure you always behave professionally. Continuously educate yourself, accept negative or constructive feedback, and perform with minimal supervision.
- **Confidence.** Show you are confident in your abilities and skills, so that you instill confidence in your patients and colleagues. Continually strive to be the best paramedic you can; attend educational sessions and perform self-critiques. These measures are only a few of the ways to build confidence and, in turn, help you run your calls smoothly and effectively.
- **Communications.** Express and exchange your ideas, thoughts, and findings with other professional colleagues effectively. Consciously remind yourself to listen well and speak directly, without using confusing medical terms, when you interact with patients and their families. Completing clear, professional written or electronic documentation is also essential. Record keeping and reporting is a responsibility of all EMS providers.
- **Teamwork and respect.** Teamwork is required in EMS. On every call, everyone must work together to achieve a common goal: to provide the best possible prehospital care to ensure the patient's overall well-being. Most often in the field, you as the paramedic are considered the team leader. Being the team leader does not entitle you to undermine other team members, regardless of their level; instead, you must help guide and support the team. Remain flexible and open to change at any moment, and communicate at an appropriate place and time with other team members to resolve problems. Always be as respectful of others as you would expect them to be with you.
- **Patient advocacy.** Advocacy includes advocating for the patients you treat, and advocating for changes in the EMS system that will improve care or save lives. Always act in your patients' best interest while respecting their wishes and beliefs, regardless of your own. This includes patients with special needs and those with different lifestyles, values, and cultures from your own. Never allow your personal feelings about a patient to impact the care you provide. Respect the people you serve. While you need to communicate to do

your job, make sure you maintain a high level of confidentiality. Whatever details you have to communicate about your patient, ensure your communication about the patient does not occur in front of anyone who is not part of your team. When you talk to your team members, do so in private and away from the public's ear, quietly and with appropriate respect. Your role as a patient advocate also means you should always be on the lookout for spousal abuse, child abuse or neglect, and elder abuse or neglect. If you suspect abuse, report and communicate your findings to the appropriate authorities or as outlined in your state's law.

- **Injury prevention.** As a paramedic, you are in the unique position of seeing the patient's surroundings before transport. If you spot a potential hazard (such as a loose rug at the top of the stairs), use your diplomatic skills and talk about your findings with the patient or a family member. Get involved with training programs such as focusing on fall prevention or child passenger safety. By educating the public on these issues, you may prevent a potential injury. Discuss the importance of using bike helmets, safety belts, and child car seats whenever you can: Sharing such information is another way of preventing injuries.
- **Careful delivery of service.** Paramedics must deliver the highest-quality patient care possible. Pay careful attention to details, and continuously evaluate and reevaluate your performance. Use other medical professionals as resources rather than seeing them as adversaries. Follow policies, protocols, and procedures as well as the orders of your superiors.
- **Time management.** Time management is an essential skill in any profession. Use your time wisely. For example, prioritize your patient's needs, always keep your emergency vehicle ready to go, and ensure you document each emergency call as soon as it has concluded. Each of these elements is a component of professional delivery of service. Use down time to research and retrain yourself on rarely used skills or topic areas.
- **Administration.** Part of your role as a paramedic will be administrative. In addition to documenting each call thoroughly and professionally, you may be asked to take on special projects or station duties. As you advance in your career, you may play a role in working with other agencies and forging partnerships with other public safety resources. You may be appointed to a leadership position within your organization; this is your opportunity to shine and to help others achieve their goals within your service.

Street Smarts

One of your responsibilities as an EMS provider is to provide emotional support. Remember, calming and reassuring the patient, the family, and other responders can go a long way toward making you an effective paramedic.

As the health care industry gains a better understanding of paramedics' skills and abilities, more health care locations are using paramedic services within their organizations. For example, many hospitals now incorporate paramedics in their EDs and clinics. Physician offices also are identifying the benefits of using paramedic services within their organizations. As new forms of influenza and coronavirus have emerged in recent years, some clinics and local public health departments have engaged paramedics to administer vaccines against these infections. In other locations, paramedics may help home health organizations deliver care to patients in their own homes. You may also perform special types of transports beyond the standard 9-1-1 emergency calls. For example, your service may provide transfers between health care locations, including specialty services such as critical care, neonatal, or high-risk obstetric transfers. The expertise that a paramedic acquires is a vital part of the entire emergency medical environment; offer your abilities in all ways possible.

Roles and Responsibilities

So what does it mean to be a paramedic? What are your roles? What are your responsibilities? These are the questions you should ask yourself throughout your career. The EMS system continues to grow and mature, and with those changes will come new roles and additional responsibilities. Some of

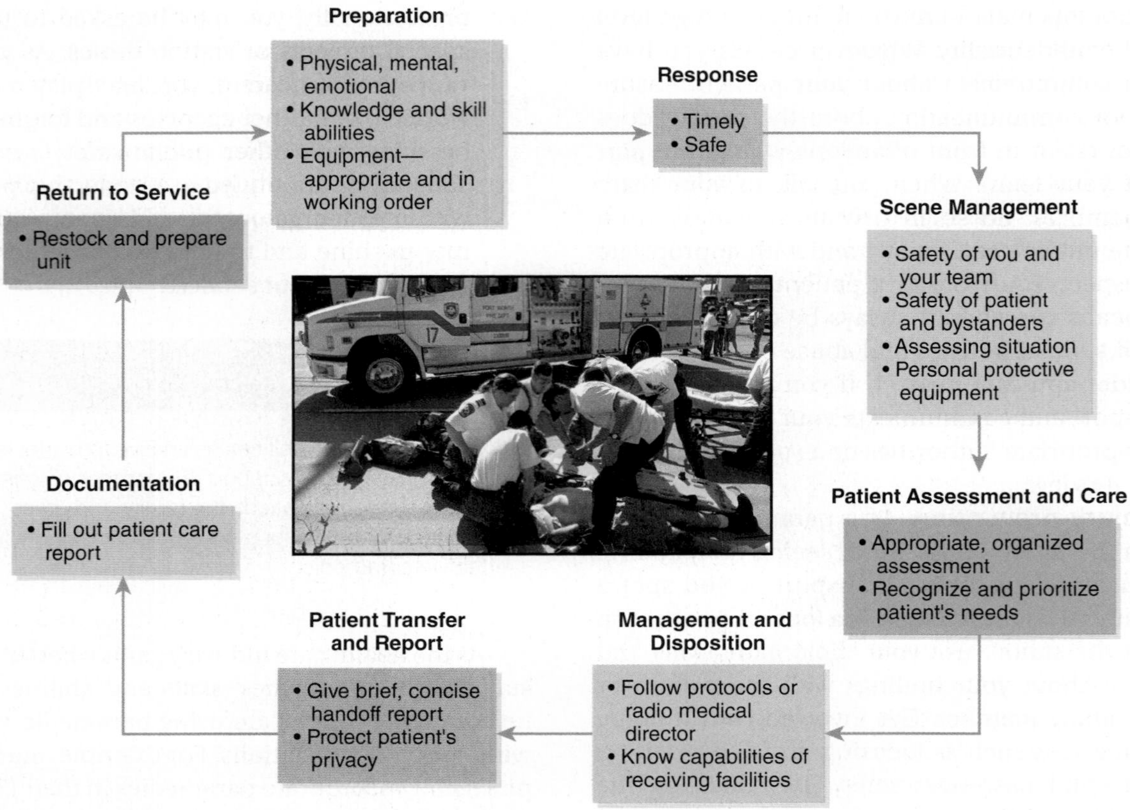
Preparation
• Physical, mental, emotional
• Knowledge and skill abilities
• Equipment—appropriate and in working order
Response
• Timely
• Safe
Scene Management
• Safety of you and your team
• Safety of patient and bystanders
• Assessing situation
• Personal protective equipment
Patient Assessment and Care
• Appropriate, organized assessment
• Recognize and prioritize patient's needs
Management and Disposition
• Follow protocols or radio medical director
• Know capabilities of receiving facilities
Patient Transfer and Report
• Give brief, concise handoff report
• Protect patient's privacy
Documentation
• Fill out patient care report
Return to Service
• Restock and prepare unit

FIGURE 1-11 Paramedics follow a sequence of procedures for each emergency call.

the primary responsibilities include the following **FIGURE 1-11**:

- **Preparation.** Be prepared physically, mentally, and emotionally. Keep up your knowledge and skill abilities. Ensure that you have the appropriate equipment for your call and that it is in good working order. When the call comes in, your chance to prepare has ended.
- **Response.** Responding to the event in a timely, safe manner is very important. High vehicle speed—running "hot" without due regard for your safety and the safety of your partner, your patient, and other people on the highway (even if they should get out of your way but do not)—is not acceptable. In most cases, running "hot" offers no measurable benefit for the patient's outcome.
- **Scene management.** Your priority is to ensure your safety and the safety of your team. Then you must ensure the patient is safe, as well as any bystanders. Part of your preparation before reaching the scene should include considering all possibilities from dispatch information; however, never unwaveringly set your mind on a single possibility based on that initial information. Once you are at the scene, assess the situation thoroughly, as the nature of the call may give valuable information about its safety. Scene safety measures include but are not limited to wearing personal protective equipment (PPE) such as gloves, masks, and goggles. The paramedic often sets the example for safety to the members of the EMS team.
- **Patient assessment and care.** Perform an organized assessment of all patients. Although a patient assessment is similar at all EMS levels, you will learn additional assessment concepts in this textbook. Recognize and prioritize the patient's needs based on the injuries or the illness most in need of urgent treatment.
- **Management and disposition.** Follow the medical guidelines or protocols approved by your medical director and possibly your state.

When you are in the field, you will sometimes discover that these protocols or guidelines do not cover your particular situation. In such a case, make online contact with your medical control physician and use your critical thinking skills. Having a good working relationship with your medical director is critical. You are the eyes, ears, and touch for the medical director. Situations that require a protocol or guideline variance or a decision that may be outside of your scope of practice need to be communicated with your medical director. If you cannot make contact, you must carefully weigh your choices before you perform any intervention, and communicate with your medical director as soon as possible. Although most calls will require transport to an ED, you must also be aware of other transport and destination decisions. For example, a patient with carbon monoxide poisoning may need to be transported to a hospital with a hyperbaric chamber: do you know where it is and how to access it? Your local receiving facilities may not keep you apprised of changes in their capabilities; therefore, it is your responsibility to keep up-to-date with your area's health care abilities. Know which facilities have specialty cardiac programs and which are capable of handling trauma or pediatric emergencies. Know the capabilities of all receiving facilities you may interact with before a call; this will help you make the right decision or provide information to the patient and any family members. You may also respond to calls where the patient refuses your care. Patient refusal of care is covered further in Chapter 4, *Medical, Legal, and Ethical Issues*.

- **Patient transfer and report.** Once you arrive at the receiving facility, continue to act as a patient advocate and give the appropriate facility staff a brief, concise handoff report. Once again, use discretion so you protect your patient's privacy. If the receiving facility is extremely busy, the staff there may not always offer you as much time as you prefer to do a handoff report. Do not become frustrated or angry; instead, do your best to get as much pertinent information to them as possible and ensure the facility is aware and ready to take over patient care.
- **Documentation.** After you transfer the patient, it is imperative to fill out a patient care report, preferably immediately. Many states require some sort of written report to be left at the facility. If this is not possible or required, inform the facility how to reach you if providers there have a question. Recognize that your patient care report serves as a legal record of all aspects of the call. Just as physicians must document their care of patients, so must you. Guidelines for documentation are covered in Chapter 6, *Documentation*.
- **Return to service.** Every person on the EMS team is responsible for restocking and preparing the unit for the next call as quickly as possible. Preparing for the next call should be the first item you complete when you return from a call. Failure to do so can bring about serious legal consequences if another call comes in and the unit is not fully restocked and ready to respond.

Documentation and Communication

Documentation of equipment repairs and checks is nearly as important as documenting patient care.

As a paramedic, you are looked on as a health care professional, so take advantage of this role. Educate the public about what you do and its importance. Get involved with prevention, community, and leadership activities whenever possible **FIGURE 1-12**. Never miss an opportunity to teach the community about injury and illness prevention. Explain to people how to appropriately use your services. In the areas where trained EMS staff are limited, use your abilities to promote programs that get the public involved, such as CPR and automated external defibrillator (AED) training, which is one of the proven determinants of whether a person in cardiac arrest will live or die.

Some paramedics may have other health care responsibilities, such as working in clinics, freestanding emergency facilities, and hospitals. Home visits by paramedics under direct medical control (mobile integrated health care) also exist. In recent years, with the increased concerns about influenza

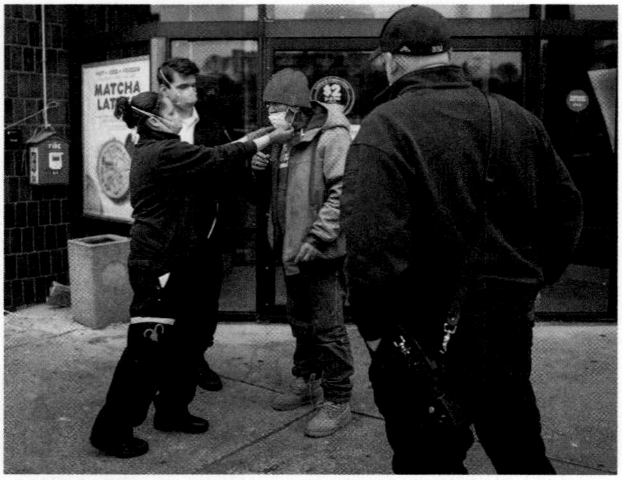

FIGURE 1-12 Part of your role as a public servant is to interact with and educate the public.

and pandemic issues, paramedics and home health nurses have been asked to evaluate people at home and provide some immunization and medication administration.

Providers at all EMS levels need to be advocates for prehospital health care, which often means setting well-thought-out campaigns for EMS. Research your community, look at the system's strengths and weaknesses, and develop plans for initiatives to improve it. Many people do not truly understand the role of EMS and do not recognize how vital EMS is until a loved one becomes ill unexpectedly. By involving yourself in your community, you can both educate and advocate. It is up to all EMS personnel to educate the media and public. Strive to stay at the top of your profession. Continue your education and become a mentor for new EMS providers.

Medical Direction

One important difference between providers with different EMS education levels is that paramedics possess advanced cardiologic, pharmacologic, and trauma care skills. However, paramedics do not have independent authority to act. Instead, they are subject to the authority of physicians who are educated about the levels and the extent of the education of EMS personnel; these physicians play a vital role in the medical direction of an EMS system. The best medical directors are active in all aspects of the service they oversee, a role that goes far beyond merely signing forms. The role of an EMS medical director may include the following responsibilities:

- Educate and train personnel.
- Participate in the recommendation or selection of new personnel.
- Participate in the recommendation or selection of equipment.
- Develop clinical protocols or guidelines in collaboration with other EMS personnel who are considered experts in the field.
- Develop and assist in a quality improvement program.
- Provide input into patient care.
- Act as a liaison between EMS systems and other health care agencies.
- Serve as an EMS advocate to the community.
- Serve as the "medical conscience" of the EMS system.

The medical director provides online and off-line medical control for the EMS system. **Online (direct) medical control** is medical direction given in real time to an EMS service or provider, either by radio or other electronic communication. It is typically provided by an emergency physician working in a hospital ED that serves as a base station for EMS units in the area, rather than directly by your medical director. Online medical control has multiple benefits: It provides immediate and specific patient care resources, allows telemetry transmission, allows for continuous quality improvement, and can offer on-scene assistance. In some locations, video telemetry is available, allowing the medical control physician to see what the EMS team sees.

Off-line (indirect) medical control is medical direction given through a set of protocols, policies, and/or standards developed by or with the approval of your medical director. Off-line medical control allows for the development of protocols or guidelines, standing orders, procedures, and training. A **protocol** or guideline is a treatment plan for a specific illness or injury. A **standing order** is a type of protocol or guideline that is a written document signed by the EMS system's medical director; it outlines specific directions, permissions, and sometimes prohibitions regarding patient care that is rendered before contacting medical control (eg, chest decompression). Protocols or guidelines are usually developed in conjunction with national standards. For example, EMS personnel often use the American Heart Association's advanced cardiac life support algorithms as a guide for developing a treatment protocol for cardiac patients. Protocols dictate which types of equipment and supplies are approved and needed as well as minimum expectations of personnel.

The medical director also plays a role after an emergency call ends. This physician can help with patient care report reviews or even personally perform such reviews to ensure continuous quality improvement.

> **Words of Wisdom**
>
> On some calls, you may encounter a physician on scene. If the physician is familiar with EMS protocols or happens to be your medical director, it can be a great help. In other cases, you may be caught between what the physician on the scene wants to do and the protocols that your medical director has given your service. Remember, you work with your physician medical director and you must adhere to local protocols and standing orders.
>
> Remain calm and composed should the physician on the scene demand medical control of the situation. Politely explain all your actions must be in accordance with your EMS medical director's protocols. Point out that you can transfer care of the patient to an on-site physician only if that physician takes full responsibility for the patient and will be present during transport, riding with the patient in the ambulance to the ED, as well as signing for any orders given.
>
> Most states and services have rules that EMS must follow in these cases. They also require the on-site physician to sign release forms. The only exception occurs when the on-site physician is also the service's medical director.

Improving System Quality

Continuous Quality Improvement and Quality Control

Making a good thing better should always be part of your paramedic career. One tool often used to continually evaluate EMS care is **continuous quality improvement (CQI)**. CQI focuses on assessing current practices and looking for ways to create ongoing improvement, thereby reducing the chance of a problem arising in the first place. A CQI program can help both you as a paramedic and your service when properly developed and followed.

The CQI process is dynamic, and your EMS system should develop a structure for it before launching its CQI assessment program. Also, check with your state or region to identify any requirements it may have for CQI. A good CQI process should include the following steps:

- Identify any departmental or system-wide issues.
- Identify specific items that need to be measured.
- Conduct an in-depth review of the issue(s).
- Evaluate the issue(s) and develop a list of remedies.
- Develop an action plan for correction of issue(s).
- Enforce a plan of action, including time frames.
- Reexamine the issue.
- Identify and promote excellence found in patient care during the evaluation.
- Identify modifications that may be needed to protocols and standing orders.
- Identify situations that are currently not addressed by protocols and standing orders.

A comprehensive CQI program can help prevent problems from arising by evaluating day-to-day operations and identifying possible stress points in these operations. These may include the following elements:

- Medical direction issues
- Education
- Communications
- Prehospital treatment
- Transportation issues
- Financial issues
- Receiving facility review
- Dispatch
- Public information and education
- Disaster planning
- Mutual aid

Although it may not always be feasible, all emergency calls should be reviewed. Ultimately, the focus of CQI needs to be on improving patient care. Often providers show hesitation when faced with a CQI process because of fear of being ridiculed or reprimanded. To avoid this reluctance to participate, it is essential to use your CQI process not as a punitive tool, but rather as a constructive tool for continuous improvement.

FIGURE 1-13 Peer reviews should be seen as a constructive part of paramedic practice.

Quality control is another process that evaluates problems and finds solutions to them. Some services choose to perform quality control through peer reviews **FIGURE 1-13**. A peer review can be a good learning experience if the people performing the reviews have proper and consistent guidelines to follow and keep an open mind. No matter how good your education, you will inevitably make mistakes and miss things from time to time. When a peer reviewer finds things you can improve, you should look at that feedback as an educational tool. In an ideal system, the peer review team members will rotate on and off, meaning at some point, you will also serve as a reviewer.

Street Smarts

Never use the peer review process as a tool to demean or belittle a fellow EMS provider, and do not discuss your findings with anyone who is not identified as part of the review process. Be professional.

Minimizing Errors

A function of the evaluation process for ensuring quality control is to determine ways to eliminate human error. To cut down on the potential for errors, ensure adequate lighting when handling medications and keep interruptions to a minimum. In addition, keep medications in a specific location and in their original packaging.

High-risk activities include handing off patients. You must deal with issues related to the physical transfer of the patient from your stretcher and communication with the next caregiver in line. Provide a written copy of your assessment and treatment along with the verbal report to help ensure continuity of care. You must report your care of the patient and any changes that may have occurred since you took over the patient's care. Other safety issues revolve around advanced airway management, medication administration, and safe transport (such as avoiding ambulance crashes and providing proper immobilization) of patients who may potentially have traumatic injuries.

You must strive to identify potential errors and eliminate them as much as possible. Understanding the circumstances that cause errors can help you identify those that can be prevented. There are three primary sources of errors, which may occur singly or in combination: rules-based failure, knowledge-based failure, and skills-based failure. For example, does the paramedic have the legal right to administer the particular medication needed by the patient? If not, a rules-based failure has occurred if a paramedic assists with the administration. Does the paramedic know all of the pertinent information about the medication being delivered? If not, a breakdown at this point, such as the administration of the wrong medication, would be referred to as a knowledge-based failure. Finally, is the equipment operating and being used properly? If not, a skills-based error has occurred. Any error can come from multiple sources.

As noted earlier, agencies need to have clear protocols—that is, detailed plans that describe how specific patient issues, such as chest pain or shortness of breath, are to be managed. In some states, guidelines are used instead of protocols. Each has a different meaning. Services with active medical directors will offer guidelines that describe allowable treatment plans that you as a paramedic can use to determine what you need to do and when, without contacting medical control first. Protocols typically outline a care plan in a specific order and do not allow you to flex outside of the medical director's treatment plan without contacting them first. Protocols and guidelines need to be understood by all paramedics within the service. You may fail to help the patient if you follow a protocol or guideline to exactness, but you may also fail if you do not. Be

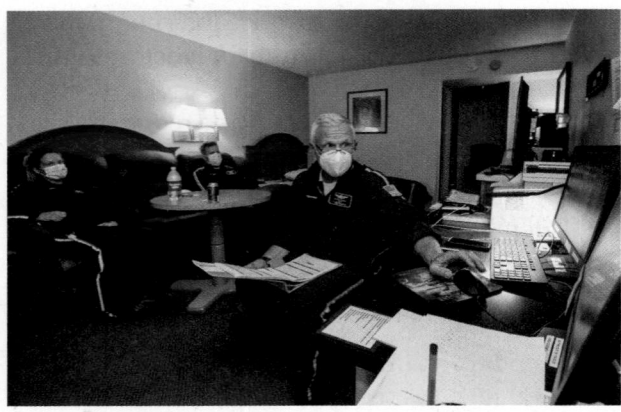

prepared to make modifications and use the best resource you have available: online (direct) medical control.

The environment can be part of the reason for errors. Are there ways to limit distractions? Can paramedics find what they need promptly? Sometimes the solution is as easy as ensuring flashlights are available on all emergency vehicles. Make sure all medications and equipment are properly labeled and organized.

Words of Wisdom

Whenever the environment is in CHAOS:

- Control
- Has
- Advantage
- Over
- Stress

When you are about to perform a skill, ask yourself, "Why am I doing this?" Consider the reason for your actions to allow you time to reflect and make a more informed decision. Just because you *can* perform a large variety of procedures, that does not mean you *should*. It should be clear in your mind why you are using a skill or administering a medication. If you cannot come up with a solution to the patient's problem, ask for help. Talk with your partner, contact medical control, or call your EMS supervisor.

Another way for you to help limit medical errors is to use "cheat sheets." Have a copy of your protocol book with you or have the protocols for your system available on your smartphone. Although some may suggest that reviewing a protocol during a call is equivalent to admitting you do not know what you are doing, in actuality, you cannot memorize all aspects of your protocols. Choosing to review and confirm that your decision is correct shows professionalism and concern for your patient. Emergency physicians have many reference materials available to them. Physicians recognize that they cannot memorize everything, so referencing a book or other reliable resources helps ensure the use of accurate information.

YOU are the Paramedic

PART 4

Due to the urgency of the situation, you ask one of the rescue personnel who has been cleared to drive your unit to drive the ambulance and to start transport to the Mayfield Medical Center, a trauma center that is 9 miles (14 km) away. It is 1628 hours. You call medical control and give a thorough description of the patient's mechanism of injury, signs and symptoms, presentation, and vital signs. You report that you successfully decompressed the patient's left chest, which improved the patient's BP and pulses, although he is still unresponsive.

You arrive at the trauma center at 1638 hours. You give a verbal and a written report to the receiving facility. You and your partner clean and ready the ambulance in case you receive another call before you get back to your station. You save a copy of the report for your supervisor to add to a study being done on the benefits of prehospital needle decompression. Ten minutes later, you are in service and dispatched immediately to another call.

Recording Time: 13 Minutes	
Respirations	12 breaths/min assisted with bag-mask ventilation
Pulse	118 beats/min
Skin	Pale, slightly diaphoretic
Blood pressure	104/62 mm Hg
Oxygen saturation (Spo_2)	98% on oxygen via bag-mask
Pupils	Equal but sluggish to react

6. Explain why this situation is a good example of how EMS research may help future patients through evidence-based practice.

7. How is retrospective research beneficial for educating EMS personnel?

Preventing errors requires being conscientious about protocols and not allowing interruptions while providing patient care. Use decision-making aids, such as algorithms, and reflect on what has been done as an informal critique for future improvement of your performance. Finally, after a troublesome call, sit down and talk. Talk with your partner and/or your supervisor. Discussing events that recently happened provides an excellent avenue for learning. Your discussions can help lead to changes in protocols, changes in how equipment is stocked, or even the purchase of new equipment.

EMS Research

As medicine has increasingly been drawn toward **evidence-based practice**, so has the EMS system. Although EMS systems have been used for more than 40 years, minimal research has been conducted to prove that what you will do as a paramedic will truly improve patient outcomes. Due to the emphasis by numerous organizations and the public's eye on this care process, patient care protocols must be based on scientific findings as often as possible.

An essential step in the effort to link scientific findings to patient care was taken in 2001 with the publication of the *National EMS Research Agenda*,[8] a document commissioned by the Department of Transportation and the Department of Health and Human Services, which described processes and set goals for the optimization of prehospital emergency medical care. A publication at the ems.gov website titled *Progress of Evidence-Based Guidelines for Prehospital Emergency Care*[9] outlines some of the progress in relation to research findings.

Research can force a dramatic departure from the standardized, non-evidence-based method of operation historically used in EMS. For example, studies have continued to show that a "hands only" CPR technique by bystanders, along with early use of an AED, greatly improves the chances that a victim of sudden cardiac arrest will survive to release from the hospital. Previously, the treatment protocol dictated care for airway and breathing problems first for all patients, followed by care for circulation issues (the ABCs). However, research has shown that to achieve the best outcome for patients in cardiac arrest, circulation should be addressed first, which means changing the ABCDE acronym in the context of cardiac arrest to CABDE. Similar studies are planned or in progress to either change or reaffirm the standards of care provided in prehospital medicine.

It is essential to ensure that properly educated researchers perform research. Although the majority of researchers have a PhD or MD degree and a vested interest in EMS research, in reality, anyone can be part of research if properly trained. The NREMT and the Robert Wood Johnson Foundation continue to research various topics that relate to emergency medical care and emergency services in general.

An increase in the number of accredited colleges and universities that provide an EMS track for paramedics is a tremendous benefit to both the EMS system and EMS research. You can now enter the EMS field trained as a paramedic and hold a bachelor's degree. Although the EMS field is currently primarily composed of providers who hold a license or certification, paramedic students who have bachelor's degrees will further enhance the professional image within the medical community. Many higher learning institutions also produce high-quality research, which then feeds back into the educational system and practice. As a paramedic student, you may have the opportunity to assist in a research project related to your career in the EMS field; this is an opportunity you should not pass up. You may be part of something that will eventually change the future of EMS.

Evidence-Based Medicine

Evidence-based research can be found in the following publications: *Journal of Trauma and Acute Care Surgery, New England Journal of Medicine, Journal of the American Medical Association, Prehospital Emergency Care, Circulation,* and *Annals of Emergency Medicine.*

The Research Process

The first step in conducting research is to identify the specific problem, procedure, or question to be investigated. In general, a research topic usually arises when a specific practice is questioned. You may identify items during your paramedic calls that could initiate valid research projects. For example, the efficacy of endotracheal intubation and rapid sequence intubation in the field has been a popular research topic, as have "lights and siren" responses. Even if the topic has been investigated before, it can often be revisited from a new angle. Research findings are sometimes flawed, and a new study may identify those flaws or enhance previous research findings. Some research topics are driven by a product manufacturer or an entity that is strictly out to prove something right or wrong regardless of its importance in EMS. Therefore, carefully reviewing the research—in its entirety and not just the summary—is very important.

Once the question has been determined, a **research agenda** is developed. This agenda specifies the questions to be answered, the specific aims to be addressed, and the precise methods by which the study will be carried out and the data will be gathered. Although numerous additional questions may arise from results found during the study, the researcher must adhere to the research agenda and answer the specific questions at hand. Other items of interest encountered during the course of the research may themselves become research topics in a separate study.

After the qualified researcher has decided on a specific question to be answered and developed the research agenda, the next step is to determine the **research domain** in which the study should be conducted. A research domain is the research area to be addressed—clinical, basic science, systems, or education. The clinical domain, for example, would include stroke research involving clinical trials that seek to improve patient care. An example of basic science research is a study of the effectiveness of a new drug in limiting carbon monoxide poisoning in an animal model. The systems domain in EMS research would focus on operations, such as the effects of sleep-deprived EMS providers on patient care. The education domain would focus on how programs are taught, such as in a study of the components that make up high-performing paramedic programs. This domain may also include research on education competency standards.

EMS providers may perform EMS research, but it is more commonly performed by people who are studying a particular branch of medicine or science. In many cases, research will be performed within a **research consortium**, a group of agencies working together to study a particular topic. Paramedics may become involved in this kind of collaborative research by gathering data. For example, you may be part of a study to determine the outcomes for patients with STEMI (ST-segment elevation myocardial infarction) who are transported to a facility that does not offer cardiac specialty services such as a cardiac catheterization lab, or to establish whether the time saved via helicopter transport improves outcomes.

You may be asked to identify certain populations for research or even gather volunteers from your calls in some cases. If you are asked to identify patients who might be candidates for inclusion in a study, carry some information with you regarding the research. If a patient agrees to become part of the research, obtain informed consent from the patient specifically for the research; the informed consent that patients give you to treat them during an emergency is not the same as authorization to use their data in research. *It is crucial that initiatives associated with research never take priority over the care the patient may need.* If the patient agrees to participate, note this in your patient care report. Your job is to ensure you accurately gather and report data about the patients you encounter who fit within the study's parameters. The information gathered will then be analyzed by the researchers to answer the question at hand. The results could then be shared with the rest of the EMS and scientific community, and thereby improve patient care practices. Evidence-based medical practice is based on such research.

Funding

Before a research project involving any human research subjects can begin, approval from an **institutional review board (IRB)** is required to ensure that the rights of study subjects are protected throughout the study. An IRB comprises a group or institution that reviews the research. The requirements for IRB review, which makes research legal, ethical, and potentially eligible for federal funding, were devised in 1966 by the US Public Health Service.

Major research requires specific funding. In particular, large clinical trials or systems research can carry a significant financial cost. This cost is funded through various sources, such as local or federal government, nonprofit foundation grants, and industry or corporate funding. To qualify for a federal or public grant, the study must first go through a rigorous evaluation process to ensure it will answer a question within the domain covered by the grant. The methods and results are then subject to stipulations placed on them by the grantor. Similarly, nonprofit organizations or foundations will fund research in their specific areas of interest, and typically will have some control over the methods used. Corporate support can take the form of a grant to a nonprofit research organization but more commonly will be a chartered research project to validate a product manufactured by the corporation, such as a new medication or piece of medical equipment. When you are seeking funding, keep in mind that some grants have stipulations that may be perceived as trying to alter outcomes in favor of the grantor. Before applying for a grant, ensure you meet all the criteria and adhere to the entire project's expectations.

Any type of support given to a researcher is considered funding, including free lab space, travel, or assistants to help with the research. To prevent the appearance of bias or potential conflicts of interest, researchers should disclose all sources of funding and support and maintain total transparency with regard to their research methods.

Types of Research

Several different types of research are possible, including quantitative and qualitative research. The type of research that will yield the best results may depend on the research topic and what the researcher wishes to learn.

Qualitative research focuses on questions within a context of surrounding events and concurrent processes and attempts to build a more complete, holistic picture. In other words, qualitative research considers the real-world factors that may have influenced the results of a study and may attempt to interpret the results to account for these factors. Such research is often undertaken when specific answers cannot be identified in quantitative research. Qualitative research often relies on the researcher's interpretation of previously published data and yields a statement of the findings. Qualitative methods investigate the why and how of decision making, not just the what, where, and when. It is challenging to evaluate qualitative studies by using set guidelines. Rather, each study must have a set of parameters specific to the question. Some medical research falls into the qualitative category.

Quantitative research is based on numeric data. Types of quantitative research include the following:

- **Experimental research.** A scientific approach to research in which a researcher controls, manipulates, and then measures one or more variables to ascertain how manipulating the variables affects the subjects. Experimental research is concerned with cause-and-effect relationships.
- **Nonexperimental research.** Descriptive research that does not involve experimentation using patients and manipulating variables to reach a conclusion. For example, a study on the effectiveness of different levels of pain management would be unethical or even difficult to conduct on humans; instead, data would be gathered through interviewing patients and watching vital signs parameters.
- **Survey research.** In this type of research, conclusions are based on survey results. To be valid, researchers must identify what is being measured and determine the appropriate sample size. Additionally, the sample population must reflect the composition of the population being researched. For example, if a study of the incidence of cancer were conducted in an area that had a particularly high incidence of cancer, the results of that study would not be indicative of the whole country. Therefore, it is imperative that when you review a research report, you identify whether the outcome would be similar in your location—that is, whether the findings can be generalized to your patient population.

Retrospective research uses available data, such as from medical records or patient care reports. This research may involve examining those records to determine the types of calls that occur at night versus daytime, or the number of calls where substance abuse was the cause of the patient's complaint. This information may then be used to develop educational sessions for EMS personnel or to plan public education and public prevention strategies. Sometimes the researcher may need to collaborate with a hospital or group of hospitals in gathering the necessary patient outcome information. To comply with federal laws such as the Health Insurance Portability and Accountability Act (HIPAA), patient identification information may have to be deleted from records before the data are shared between agencies. However, in some states, governmental or municipal agencies have rules that supersede HIPAA requirements and establish that all information held by these agencies is part of the public record.

Many large retrospective studies collect and analyze data from widespread, sometimes nationwide, databases. Such databases may link EMS, hospitals, and even post-hospitalization providers into the system and allow for constructing a broad, total picture of the patient population in question. National databases for patients who have experienced cardiac arrest, patients requiring extracorporeal membrane oxygenation, children, and trauma registries exist within the United States. Such databases are typically overseen by a centralized agency, typically within the federal government; state or local governments usually collect data to populate the databases. The same techniques of data collection and analysis can be used at the local level for smaller research projects: Data from various hospitals and EMS agencies can be entered into a centralized database, which can then be used to study specific patient populations. To ensure accurate research results, clear-cut guidelines for data entry must be established and enforced to allow data comparisons.

In addition to retrospective research, other types of research include prospective research, cohort research, and case studies. **Prospective research** studies gather information as events occur in real time. **Cohort research** examines patterns of change, a sequence of events, or trends over time within a specific population or "cohort" of study subjects. Inversely, a **case study** method is the investigation and documentation of a single case over a specific period. A case-control study is typically a retrospective study that compares groups of people known to have the disease or condition being studied (cases) to a similar group of people who do not have the disease or condition (controls) to help identify the likely cause and risk factors for the condition.

Additionally, these categories of research can be subgrouped as cross-sectional or longitudinal. A **cross-sectional design** collects all data at one point in time, essentially serving as a "snapshot" of events and information. A **longitudinal design** collects information at various set time intervals. Therefore, a prospective study must have, by design, a longitudinal data-gathering method. In contrast, retrospective, cohort, or case study research can utilize either a cross-sectional or longitudinal data collection technique.

Finally, a **literature review** is a form of research in which the existing literature is reviewed, and the researcher analyzes this collection of research to draw a conclusion. More formal methods of reviewing the literature include systematic case reviews and meta-analyses. In systematic case reviews, researchers evaluate and synthesize relevant literature on a topic through a structured, comprehensive approach. In meta-analyses, researchers combine and statistically analyze the results of multiple studies.

Research Methods

A beginning step in conducting research is identifying the group or groups of people necessary for the research. Once a group is identified, it may be refined further, such as by limiting the research to people in a specific age bracket, with a particular medical condition, or of a specific gender. For example, a researcher may wish to study men older than age 50 years who have high blood pressure.

Once a list of eligible subjects has been identified, researchers randomly choose who will be part of the research, using one of many different techniques. A list of subjects or groups can be computer-generated (**systematic sampling**) or time frame parameters can be set (**alternative time sampling**). The least preferred method is when subjects are manually assigned to a specific researcher (**convenience sampling**), rather than being randomly assigned. Even in the best cases, **sampling errors** can occur. For example, a study may fail to include all of the needed subjects, or some people in the study may meet the criteria yet not be the best representation of the population of interest. The researchers must also consider the number of people who are asked to participate. It is recommended that researchers select a much higher sample size than is actually needed, which allows for a margin in case not all participants complete the study or some fall out of the research parameters. For example, if the researchers need 500 participants, they might want to consider searching for 600 candidates.

For sampling to yield meaningful, reliable results, the population size must be appropriate. So how do researchers know how many people they need? To avoid a type II error (not finding a difference between two or more groups when one actually exists), the study must be adequately powered, which requires a power analysis. To formulate the power analysis, researchers must know the variance, which is the variability of findings in your target population. To estimate the variance, researchers conduct a pilot study. Without these initial steps, the randomized prospective study will not yield the accurate data that people associate with this research method.

> **Words of Wisdom**
>
> Lower-level research lays the foundation for higher-level research.

The researchers must also identify the **parameters** for their study—that is, the type of people who are appropriate for the study. Another tool to consider is **blinding**, in which the patient and providers do not know if the subject (patient) is receiving the intervention being evaluated or a placebo. In single-, double-, and triple-blinded studies, one, two, or all parties involved in the research are blinded, respectively. When participants in the research project are advised of all aspects of the project, it is known as an **unblinded study**.

As research continues, data will be acquired. The gathered statistics can be presented in either a **descriptive** or **inferential** format. In a descriptive format, observations are made, but no attempts are made to alter or change an event. In an inferential format, a hypothesis is used to prove one finding versus another. Descriptive statistics can also be presented in either a qualitative or quantitative style. The quantitative approach covers additional variables, such as the mean, median, and mode. For example, in a study on diabetes in women who are between 30 and 40 years old, the mean age of study participants equals the average age of the subjects, the median age is the midpoint age of the subjects, and the mode is the most frequent age of the subjects. Finally, the **standard deviation** indicates how much the values in a data set differ from the mean.

Ethical Considerations

As in many aspects of a profession, **ethical** issues must be considered when conducting research. One entity that monitors whether a study is conducted ethically is the organization's IRB; its primary purpose is to ensure that study participants are protected and that the researchers engage in proper conduct.

Researchers must ensure that any risks to study subjects will not outweigh the potential benefits in any study. They must acquire informed consent from all subjects and be sure their rights and welfare are adequately protected. Any potential conflicts of interest related to the study should be identified. For example, if a person is involved in a similar study, or is employed by the person or company sponsoring the study, this would be considered a conflict of interest and that person should be removed from the study.

Subjects must participate voluntarily in any research, without being coerced to do so. They must also be informed of all potential risks that may occur and be allowed to withdraw from the research at any time **FIGURE 1-14**. At a minimum, subjects should be advised they are protected by the Office of Human Research Protections, and offered this agency's educational materials for those persons involved in research. (The Food and Drug Administration also offers guidance for researchers on a variety of topic areas.) The potential for subject withdrawal or any other possible variable that may

FIGURE 1-14 Any person who participates in a research study should be well informed of the study's goals as well as the potential risks and any potential benefits associated with participation.

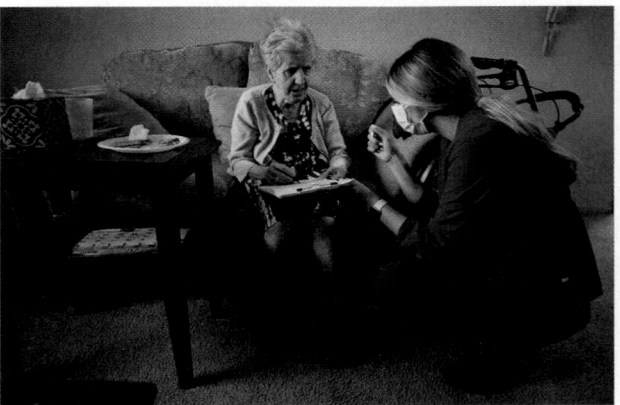

affect the outcome should be identified before the study begins to ensure the research is not flawed.

Patients who are potential participants in a clinical domain research trial must be informed about the study protocols before enrolling in the study. For example, a pharmaceutical corporation may have introduced a new respiratory medication. Patients may be recruited to join a trial in which they will receive either the new medication, a more well-studied medication, or a placebo to validate the medication's effectiveness. Each patient would have to be informed of the potential effects (positive or adverse) of participating in the study and sign a waiver to be entered into the program. In some cases, a treatment that is being studied may be administered in emergency situations under a waiver of informed consent; it is assumed the patient would want the treatment to be given because of its life-saving potential.

Evaluating Medical Research

Paramedics must know how to evaluate what is true medical research and what is a printed personal preference. When you are evaluating a research article, look for specific criteria to determine the quality of the research. **TABLE 1-3** provides 15 questions to answer when evaluating and interpreting research. Once you have identified the type of study, its methods, and its strengths, it is time to look at the body of the study itself. Most important, you must avoid the temptation to skim through the study and look at only a couple of findings. If you do not read the entire study, you may miss key points that will alter your understanding of the information presented.

TABLE 1-3 Fifteen Questions to Answer When Evaluating and Interpreting Research

1. Was the research peer reviewed?
2. What was the research hypothesis?
3. Was the study approved by an institutional review board and conducted ethically?
4. What was the population being studied?
5. What were the inclusion and exclusion criteria?
6. What method was used to acquire a sample of patients?
7. How many groups were the patients divided into?
8. How were the study subjects assigned to the groups?
9. What type of data was gathered?
10. Did the study have enough subjects involved?
11. Are there any confounding variables unaccounted for?
12. Were the data analyzed correctly?
13. Is your conclusion logically supported by the data?
14. Will it apply in your local EMS systems?
15. Were the subjects similar to the patients in your local EMS systems?

To start, determine the study's hypothesis and whether the population base matches your region. For example, if you work in an area where environmental temperatures are high, such as Arizona, how relevant would a study on hyperthermia be if performed in an ordinarily cold environment such as Alaska? Valid studies have a clearly stated hypothesis and clearly defined outcome measurements. Avoid studies with vague hypotheses or outcome measurements, as those are frequently subject to manipulation. The larger the number of subjects who are involved in a study, the more relevant the data are likely to be. For example, if you were reading two studies on aspirin's validity for active chest pain, and one study includes a patient base of 1,000 while the other has a patient base of 15,000, the information gathered from the latter study will likely be more relevant.

Next, look at the patient profiles and selection criteria. How were they decided on, and were the patients selected at random? What inclusion criteria existed for entry into the study? For a study to be valid, all subjects need to be accounted for, even if they did not make it into the final outcome. If subjects were dropped from the study, clear reasons should be offered as to why they were removed. Then, consider the number of subjects. Is the number the same at the beginning and at the end, including any patients who dropped out? If the numbers do not match, the data are essentially invalid and should not be considered. Basically, any discrepancies during a study should be reported and explained.

Determine how the data were analyzed. Ensure the methods of analysis are appropriate for what the study is designed to measure.

Identify the authors of the study and their conclusions. Make certain their conclusions are not biased in any way based on financial or other conflicts of interest that might sway the final analysis.

Finally, determine whether the outcomes and results are significant, both statistically and clinically. Statistical significance describes how often the results of a study might happen by chance. For example, if the likelihood that different outcomes between different groups of subjects are due to chance alone is less than 5%, the difference is said to be statistically significant. Of equal importance is the clinical significance. Is the finding effective in enough patients to make it a useful treatment for the majority? For example, if a new medication resulted in a benefit for only 1 of every 1,000 patients and costs $5,000 per dose, would this be considered statistically significant? Would that medication be worth it? If that same medication resulted in an 80% likelihood of a positive outcome, therefore showing clinically significant results, would that cost now be worth it?

The type of journal in which the research is published is another vital part of determining quality and validity. One method of ensuring quality and validity is through the **peer review** process. Many medical journals accept research studies from a wide variety of sources. Before publication, these studies are sent to other subject-matter experts (the author's "peers") to review the content and research methods. The research and its conclusions are then accepted, revised, or rejected based on the peer review findings. This method allows for greater checks and balances in ensuring the quality of the research methods and the validity of the research conclusions. Many EMS and medical peer-reviewed journals are available in print as well as online.

More broadly, the proliferation of medical information on the Internet has resulted in specific Internet sites becoming useful tools for accessing research. Sources range from comprehensive sources, such as Google Scholar, to more medically specific sources, such as Medscape and PubMed, which contain a substantial number of published articles from various journals and publications. When reviewing the research available on a particular topic, such sites can be useful for finding peer-reviewed research.

As discussed, a research study must follow a structured process. A good study will define precisely what it is intended to be measured, the population affected, and the goal of the research. A good research article will have adequate data; for example, 5,000 people were identified and followed over a 5-year period, with data available from all people involved. With any research topic, there are limitations as to what can be measured and how accurately. If in reviewing a research article, you find that some people backed out, died, or were omitted for any reason not originally anticipated or outlined, then the results may be flawed.

As a new paramedic, you must review research carefully and use only credible sources. You owe it to yourself as well as your patients to thoroughly read and understand relevant studies.

Evidence-Based Medicine

It is important to ensure that the research you are using for decisions is credible and follows proper research processes.

For example, a supposedly well-designed and well-conducted study submitted in 1998 on the topic of a potential link between vaccines and autism did not outline a control group or actual studies.[10] It was devised through personal recollection of people and vague conclusions that offered no statistical proof. The *Lancet*, the journal that published the study's findings, retracted the article in 2010, and the study creator's (Dr. Andrew Wakefield) medical license was revoked soon after.[11]

Extensive research ensued over the following years. Although the original 1998 "study" claimed there was a direct link, more than 48 validated studies had been performed as of 2018, including studies involving millions of children, clearly demonstrating no link between vaccination and autism.[11]

Similarly, many research papers on the efficacy of vaccines have been published. Valid research shows that vaccines greatly reduce the risk of death and disability, with no link to autism.

This example shows the importance of reviewing research papers referenced in a current study.

Evidence-Based Practice

Evidence-based practice is becoming an integral part of functioning as a paramedic. Your patient care should focus on the procedures that have proved useful in improving patient outcomes. Only a limited amount of prehospital EMS research exists concerning other medical research areas;

however, as EMS research continues to expand, evidence-based practice will have a correspondingly greater role in EMS.

High-quality patient care should focus on procedures useful in improving patient outcomes through sound research. EMS providers need to stay up-to-date on the latest advances in health care. The International Liaison Committee on Resuscitation (ILCOR) revises CPR and other resuscitation guidelines based on a review of new evidence published throughout the world. Although once revised every 5 years, ILCOR has moved to a more frequent review schedule since 2015, updating guidelines every other year. These revised guidelines are then published by the American Heart Association (AHA). These guidelines are an excellent example of using medical evidence to develop specific treatment guidelines for application in the prehospital care environment. To learn more about the science of developing consensus guidelines for resuscitation, refer to the ILCOR website (ilcor.org).

Evidence-Based Medicine

In 2020, ILCOR, along with the AHA, a member of ILCOR, released an updated consensus document on the science of resuscitation that supports the 2020 Guidelines for Cardiopulmonary Resuscitation and Emergency Cardiovascular Care. Those Guidelines are referenced throughout this book, especially in the sections related to cardiology, neurology, pediatrics, and resuscitation.

One word of caution: When reading new research results, make sure you understand what the results mean. Ask questions and critically evaluate published studies. Conclusions that seem too good to be true may very well be.

To link medical research and evidence to patient care, you must ensure that the quality of the evidence is sufficient to justify changing patient care protocols. To ensure quality evidence, researchers often rate the quality of a study. Many different rating systems may be used. For example, the American Heart Association assigns classes (strength) of recommendation and levels (quality) of evidence **TABLE 1-4**.

TABLE 1-4 American Heart Association Classes of Recommendations and Levels of Evidence

Class (Strength) of Recommendation	Level (Quality) of Evidence
Class I (Strong)	Level A (Highest-quality evidence)
Class IIa (Moderate)	Level B-R (Randomized)
Class IIb (Weak)	Level B-NR (Nonrandomized)
Class III (No Benefit—Moderate)	Level C-LD (Limited Data)
Class III (Harm—Strong)	Level C-EO (Expert Opinion)

Data from: American Heart Association. Highlights of the 2020 American Hospital Association guidelines for CPR and ECC. https://cpr.heart.org/-/media/cpr-files/cpr-guidelines-files/highlights/hghlghts_2020_ecc_guidelines_english.pdf. Accessed January 28, 2021.

Quality EMS research has many benefits for the future. Research determines the effectiveness of treatment in all health care fields: what works and what does not work. Because funding for EMS continues to be a challenge and many aspects of what you will do are coming under increasing scrutiny, it will be vital that you and EMS in general can prove that your actions make a difference. Proper research achieves this when it is outcome-based, which means the topic generates conclusions on improving patient outcomes. Research can help identify which procedures, medications, and treatments work and which do not. Once a study is released and your medical director has decided to follow its recommendations, your service should measure the results of these new practices as part of your CQI program. These practice changes can be as simple as changing the jump kit design to provide a faster door-to-drug administration time for cardiac patients or adding equipment such as transport ventilators. In combination, these efforts eventually will lead to a higher professional image to the community of the services you provide, regardless of whether you are a volunteer or a paid career paramedic.

YOU are the Paramedic SUMMARY

1. What is your first action as you are approaching the scene and conducting a scene size-up?

As you are approaching the scene, look for hazards and consider the need for any additional resources. Have the fire department dispatched for scene hazards, extrication (eg, from a vehicle), and additional help. Request law enforcement personnel for traffic control and/or crowd control. Are there any other hazards requiring specialized care, such as downed power lines or spilled hazardous materials such as oil or gasoline? Do a quick visual inspection to determine the mechanism of injury. How many patients do you see? Call for additional units as soon as possible to minimize scene time and the length of time it will take for all patients to reach definitive care.

2. What role does the EMS system play in this call?

The EMS system's role at this call will be the same as for all calls: to provide high-quality patient care and transport within the scope of practice for the level of licensure. The EMS network begins with citizen involvement. The public must recognize a need and be aware of how to access the EMS system in their community. The public must also be educated on what to do, and what not to do, to patients before your arrival. Once the EMS system has been activated, a dispatcher receives the information, processes or interprets the information, identifies whether this is an actual emergency, and then dispatches appropriate units.

The role of the EMS system continues when providers, such as paramedics, arrive on scene. Roles at the scene will include determining what is happening at the scene and developing a care plan for the patients, including deciding on the appropriate transport method and receiving facility.

3. What aspects of professionalism must be employed in this situation?

As a health care provider, you must provide care appropriate for your level of licensure and do so in a manner that builds confidence in your patient and others on scene. You are in a highly visible role and will be judged on your level of professionalism and your overall appearance. You are a representative of your profession and your agency. You must continually show that you are genuinely concerned for the patient's well-being and their family.

In this situation, you must employ integrity and empathy when dealing with the patient's girlfriend. She is scared and upset, as most people are when faced with an unfamiliar traumatic situation. Communicating with her should not take precedence over patient care, but a kind word can make all the difference. Be aware the girlfriend may be a valuable source of information regarding the patient's history. If you deem the situation serious enough that the patient needs your immediate care, ask another responder to gather this information from her. Work as a team with your partner and, in this case, rescue personnel to help assess, treat, and transport this patient. Ask one of the rescue personnel to talk with the girlfriend and let her know you are doing everything possible to help the patient. Also, let her know which hospital you are transporting him to. You should act as an advocate for this patient because he cannot speak for himself and advise the hospital of any information received from the girlfriend on scene.

4. Aside from those noted in the previous question, what roles and responsibilities are vital as a prehospital health care provider?

Educating the public is a large part of your responsibility as a paramedic. You should involve yourself in prevention, community, and leadership activities whenever possible. The public should know how to appropriately use your services, and promotion of public involvement in activities such as CPR training is vital in areas where EMS resources are limited.

5. How will you determine how and where to transport this patient?

Appropriate transport and destination decisions are often made through cooperation with other medical professionals. The patient's injuries and presentation should dictate whether he is taken to the closest facility (ie, cardiac arrest) or to a more appropriate location that may be farther away (ie, a trauma center in this patient's case).

The patient in this scenario has an altered mental status and respiratory compromise, making this an emergency transport. If definitive care is a great distance away, air transport may be a better option. Know your local hospitals' capabilities; many can provide life-saving and stabilizing care in the ED and then arrange to transfer the patient to a more definitive location. However, if the patient potentially needs surgical intervention for stabilization, then transporting him to a facility other than a trauma center may only delay definitive care and increase the risk of morbidity or mortality.

YOU are the Paramedic SUMMARY continued

6. Explain why this situation is a good example of how EMS research may help future patients through evidence-based practice.

With evidence-based practice, patient care focuses on the procedures that have proved useful in improving patient outcomes—needle decompression in this instance. Documenting procedures that have benefited patients in the past helps provide information so research may lead to establishing protocols or standing orders for similar patients in the future.

7. How is retrospective research beneficial for educating EMS personnel?

Retrospective research uses currently available information. Continuous quality improvement (CQI) is a form of retrospective research; examining patient care records helps determine opportunities for improvement and provides information to guide the educational needs for EMS personnel. It can also be used to plan public education and prevention strategies.

EMS Patient Care Report (PCR)

Date: 04-20-22		**Nature of Call:** MVC		**Location:** 300 block of Hunt Road	
Dispatched: 1618	**En Route:** 1618	**At Scene:** 1621	**Transport:** 1628	**At Hospital:** 1638	**In Service:** 1648

Patient Information

Age: 22 **Sex:** M **Weight (in kg [lb]):** 78 kg (172 lb)	**Allergies:** NKDA **Medications:** None **Past Medical History:** None **Chief Complaint:** AMS, possible pneumothorax, possible open fx of L lower leg

Vital Signs

Time: 1627	**BP:** 96/54	**Pulse:** 138	**Respirations:** 12	**Spo_2:** 92% on O_2 via bag-mask
Time: 1634	**BP:** 104/62	**Pulse:** 118	**Respirations:** 12	**Spo_2:** 98% on O_2 via bag-mask
Time:	**BP:**	**Pulse:**	**Respirations:**	**Spo_2:**

EMS Treatment (circle all that apply)

Oxygen @ 15 L/min via (circle one): NC NRM (**Bag-mask device** — circled)		(**Assisted Ventilation** — circled)	(**Airway Adjunct:** Oral — circled)	**CPR**
Defibrillation	(**Bleeding Control** — circled)	(**Bandaging** — circled)	(**Splinting** — circled)	(**Other:** Cardiac monitor — circled)

Narrative

22-year-old man involved in an MVC—motorcycle rider who hit car, unresponsive, possible tension pneumothorax, and open fx of L lower leg with minor bleeding. Helmet removed by bystanders before EMS arrival. On arrival, pt supine on ground unresponsive, pupils equal but sluggish to react, presents with very diminished breath sounds on the left, hyperresonance to percussion, JVD. Radial pulses weakened, increased in rate, and asymmetric movement of L chest noted. Needle thoracostomy performed per local protocol. Ventilations improved, neck veins now flat, Spo_2 increased to 98%, radial pulses stronger, BP increased but no change in mental status, cardiac monitor showing sinus tach without ectopy, glucose 102 mg/dL. Skin pale, cool, diaphoretic. Inserted oropharyngeal airway, assisted ventilations with bag-mask, splinted L leg to R leg—bleeding controlled with direct pressure and bandaging, full spine immobilized on scoop stretcher with c-collar and blocks, circulation grossly intact in all extremities before and after immobilization. Transported to Mayfield Medical Center without incident.

End of report

Prep Kit

Ready for Review

- World Wars I and II saw the development of ambulance corps to rapidly care for and remove injured soldiers from the battlefields.
- During the Korean and Vietnam Wars, wounded soldiers could be saved by using helicopters to rapidly move them from the battlefield to a medical unit.
- In 1966, the National Academy of Sciences and the National Research Council published "The White Paper" outlining 10 critical points related to medical care. Based on these points:
  - The National Highway Safety Act was passed in 1966.
  - The US Department of Transportation was created.
- Paramedics are required to be licensed, which may also be called certification or credentialing. Performing functions as a paramedic before obtaining licensure is unlawful.
- The standards for prehospital emergency medical care and the people who provide it are governed by the laws in each state and are typically regulated by a state office of EMS.
- A paramedic has a variety of career options. Traditional employment options include fire-based EMS, third-service EMS, private EMS agencies, hospital-based EMS, and hybrid models in which paramedics work alongside other providers or for specific venues.
- There are generally four EMS training levels: emergency medical responder, emergency medical technician, advanced emergency medical technician (AEMT), and paramedic. Variations exist from state to state. At the advanced life support levels (paramedic and AEMT), personnel may perform invasive procedures under standing orders or guidance from online (direct) medical control.
- Paramedics may be involved in various types of transports, including transports to specialty centers that focus on specific types of care of certain populations. They may also perform interfacility transports.
- Paramedics work with other health care providers and other public safety agencies. Becoming familiar with their roles and responsibilities is beneficial when on EMS calls.
- Continuing education programs expose paramedics to new research findings and refresh their skills and knowledge; consider those accredited through the Commission on Accreditation for Pre-Hospital Continuing Education (CAPCE).
- Each EMS system has a physician medical director who authorizes the providers in the service to provide medical care in the field. Medical control is typically both online (direct) and off-line (indirect).
- Members of the paramedic profession are expected to adhere to standards and performance parameters as well as a code of ethics.
- Professional attributes that a paramedic is expected to have include integrity, empathy, self-motivation, confidence, communication skills, teamwork, respect, patient advocacy, injury prevention efforts, careful delivery of service, time management skills, and administrative skills.
- Some of the primary paramedic responsibilities include preparation, response, scene management, patient assessment and care, management and disposition, patient transfer and report, documentation, and return to service.
- Quality control and continuous quality improvement are tools paramedics use to evaluate and improve the care they provide to patients.
- Research helps bring together the findings of many professionals involved in EMS and reach

Prep Kit continued

a consensus on what EMS personnel should or should not do. Types of research include quantitative and qualitative research.

- There are many ethical considerations in conducting medical research. Researchers must obtain consent from study subjects, fully inform them of the research parameters, and ensure that subjects' rights and welfare are protected.
- Paramedics must know how to evaluate medical research. Become familiar with criteria for determining the quality of the research, including how to recognize peer-reviewed literature and how to use the Internet for finding quality research articles.
- Evidence-based practice is becoming an integral part of functioning as an EMS provider. Engage in reviewing medical literature as it becomes available, and make efforts to stay on top of changing guidelines related to your practice of paramedicine.

Vital Vocabulary

alternative time sampling Time parameters that are set during a research project.

blinding A research design in which the patient and providers do not know if the subject (patient) is receiving the intervention being evaluated or a placebo. All other aspects of the study (ie, consent) must follow the requirements of the approving IRB.

case study A type of research in which a single case is investigated and documented over a specified period.

certification A process in which a person, an institution, or a program is evaluated and recognized as meeting certain predetermined standards to provide safe and ethical care.

cohort research A type of research that examines patterns of change, a sequence of events, or trends over time within a certain population of study subjects.

continuous quality improvement (CQI) A system of internal and external reviews and audits of all aspects of an EMS system.

convenience sampling A type of research in which subjects are manually assigned to a specific person or crew, rather than being randomly assigned; the least-preferred component of research.

credentialing The process of obtaining, verifying, and assessing a practitioner's qualifications to provide care for a specific health care agency.

cross-sectional design A data collection method in which all data at one point in time are collected, essentially serving as a "snapshot" of events and information.

descriptive A research format in which an observation of an event is made, but without attempts to alter or change it.

emergency medical services (EMS) A health care system designed to bring immediate on-scene care to those in need, along with transport to a definitive medical care facility.

ethical A behavior expected by a person or group following a set of rules.

evidence-based practice The use of practices that have been proven to be effective in improving patient outcomes; strongly relies on the reviewed literature but incorporates the provider's experience and training, and characteristics of the population.

health care professional A person who follows specific professional attributes that are outlined in this profession.

inferential A research format that uses a hypothesis to prove one finding from another.

Prep Kit continued

institutional review board (IRB) A group or institution that follows a set of requirements for reviewing proposed research that the US Public Health Service devised.

licensure The process whereby a state allows qualified people to perform a regulated act.

literature review A form of research in which the existing literature is reviewed, and the researcher analyzes the collection of research to draw a conclusion.

longitudinal design A data collection method in which information is collected at various set time intervals, and not just at one time.

medical direction Direction given to an EMS system or provider by a physician.

mobile intensive care units (MICUs) An early title given to an ambulance-style unit.

off-line (indirect) medical control Medical direction given through a set of protocols, policies, and/or standards.

online (direct) medical control Medical direction given in real time to an EMS service or provider.

parameters Outlined measures that may be difficult to obtain in a research project.

peer review The process used by medical magazines, journals, and other publications to ensure the quality and validity of an article before it is published, and which involves sending the article to subject-matter experts for review of the content and research methods.

profession A specialized set of knowledge, skills, and/or expertise.

prospective research A type of research that gathers information as events occur in real time.

protocol A treatment plan developed for a specific illness or injury.

qualitative A type of descriptive statistic in research that does not use numeric information.

quality control The medical director's responsibility to ensure the appropriate medical care standards are met by EMS personnel on each call.

quantitative A type of measurement in research that uses numerical data and statistics, including the mean, median, mode, and standard deviation.

reciprocity The process of granting licensure or certification to a provider from another state or agency.

registration Providing information to an entity that stores it in some form of record book. In the context of EMS, records of your education, state or local licensure, and recertification are held by a recognized board.

research agenda The specific questions that a study aims to answer, and the precise methods through which the data will be gathered.

research consortium A group of agencies working together to study a particular topic.

research domain The area (clinical, basic science, systems, or education) that a study will impact.

retrospective research Research performed from currently available information.

safety culture In an EMS organization, a system of beliefs and practices that (1) acknowledges that organizations engage in high-risk activities, (2) determines the importance of consistent, safe operations to counteract these activities, (3) supports a blame-free environment where errors can be reported without fear of punishment, and (4) maintains organizational commitment to address reported errors and safety concerns.

sampling errors Expected errors that occur in the sampling phase of research.

standard deviation A measure of the range of scores in a set of data relative to the mean score.

standing order A type of written protocol signed by the EMS system's medical director that outlines specific directions, permissions, and sometimes prohibitions regarding patient care that is rendered before contacting medical control.

Prep Kit continued

systematic sampling A computer-generated list of subjects or groups for research.

trauma systems The collaboration of prehospital and in-hospital medicine that focuses on optimizing the use of resources and assets of each, with a primary goal of reducing the mortality and morbidity of trauma patients.

unblinded study A type of study in which the subjects are advised of all aspects of the study.

References

1. EIIC. Emergency Medical Services for Children Innovation & Improvement Center website. https://emscimprovement.center. Accessed March 3, 2021.
2. About NEMSQA. NEMSQA website. https://www.nemsqa.org/about/. Accessed March 2, 2021.
3. National Highway Traffic Safety Administration. National EMS Scope of Practice Model. https://www.ems.gov/education/EMSScope.pdf. Published February 2007. Accessed January 29, 2021.
4. National Highway Traffic Safety Administration, Office of EMS. National Emergency Medical Services Education Standards. https://www.ems.gov/pdf/National-EMS-Education-Standards-FINAL-Jan-2009.pdf. Published January 2009. Accessed January 29, 2021.
5. CAPCE. Commission on Accreditation for Pre-Hospital Continuing Education website. https://www.capce.org. Accessed March 3, 2021.
6. Singh JM, MacDonald RD, Ahghari M. Critical events during land-based interfacility transport. *Ann Emerg Med.* 2014:64(1):9-15.
7. Ligtenberg JM, Arnold LG, Stienstra Y, et al. Quality of interhospital transport of critically ill patients: a prospective audit. *Crit Care.* 2005;9(4):R446-R451.
8. National Highway Traffic Safety Administration, Department of Transportation, and Maternal and Child Health Bureau, Health Resources Services Administration, Department of Health and Human Services. National EMS Research Agenda. https://one.nhtsa.gov/people/injury/ems/Archive/EMS03-ResearchAgenda/home.htm. Published December 31, 2001. Accessed January 29, 2021.
9. Office of Emergency Medical Services, National Highway Traffic Safety Administration. Progress of Evidence-Based Guidelines for Prehospital Emergency Care. https://www.ems.gov/pdf/2012/EBG_Project_Overview_Dec2011.pdf. Published December 2011. Accessed January 29, 2021.
10. Federman RS. Understanding vaccines: a public imperative. *Yale J Biol Med.* 2014;87(4):417-422.
11. American Academy of Pediatrics. Vacine safety: examine the evidence. Healthy Children website. https://www.healthychildren.org/English/safety-prevention/immunizations/Pages/Vaccine-Studies-Examine-the-Evidence.aspx. Updated July 24, 2018. Accessed May 10, 2021.

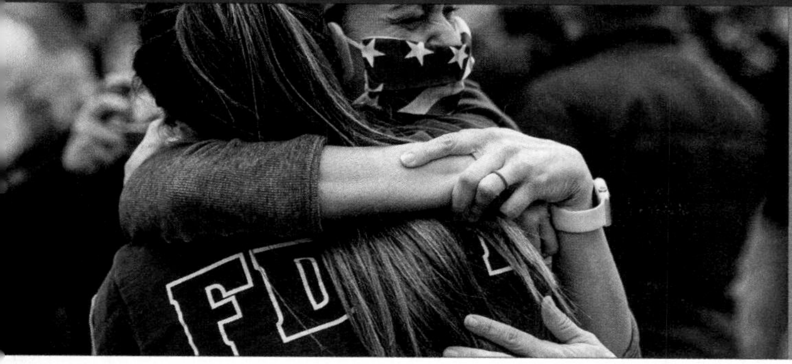

Chapter 2

Workforce Safety and Wellness

NATIONAL EMS EDUCATION STANDARD COMPETENCIES

Preparatory

Integrates comprehensive knowledge of the EMS system, safety/well-being of the paramedic, and medical/legal and ethical issues which is intended to improve the health of EMS personnel, patients, and the community.

Workforce Safety and Wellness

- Provider safety and well-being (pp 47–48)
- Standard safety precautions (pp 47, 48)
- Personal protective equipment (pp 60–66)
- Stress management (pp 70–79)
  - Understanding and dealing with death and dying (pp 79–82)
- Prevention of response-related injuries (pp 75–76)
- Prevention of work-related injuries (p 83)
- Lifting and moving patients (pp 53–54)
- Disease transmission (pp 56–57)
- Wellness principles (pp 47–56)

Medicine

Integrates assessment findings with principles of epidemiology and pathophysiology to formulate a field impression and implement a comprehensive treatment/disposition plan for a patient with a medical complaint.

Infectious Diseases

Awareness of

- A patient who may have an infectious disease (p 57)
- How to decontaminate equipment after treating a patient (Chapter 47, *Transport Operations*)

Assessment and management of:

- A patient who may have an infectious disease (Chapter 27, *Infectious Diseases*)
- How to decontaminate the ambulance and equipment after treating a patient (Chapter 47, *Transport Operations*)
- A patient who may be infected with a bloodborne pathogen (Chapter 27, *Infectious Diseases*)
  - Human immunodeficiency virus (HIV) (Chapter 27, *Infectious Diseases*)
  - Hepatitis B (Chapter 27, *Infectious Diseases*)
- Antibiotic-resistant infections (Chapter 27, *Infectious Diseases*)
- Current infectious diseases prevalent in the community (Chapter 27, *Infectious Diseases*)

Anatomy, physiology, epidemiology, pathophysiology, psychosocial impact, presentations, prognosis, and management of:

- HIV-related disease (Chapter 27, *Infectious Diseases*)
- Hepatitis (Chapter 27, *Infectious Diseases*)
- Pneumonia (Chapter 17, *Respiratory Emergencies*)
- Meningococcal meningitis (Chapter 27, *Infectious Diseases*)
- Tuberculosis (Chapter 27, *Infectious Diseases*)
- Tetanus (Chapter 27, *Infectious Diseases*)

- Viral diseases (see Chapter 17, *Respiratory Emergencies*; Chapter 27, *Infectious Diseases*; and Chapter 44, *Pediatric Emergencies*)
- Sexually transmitted diseases (Chapter 27, *Infectious Diseases*)
- Gastroenteritis (Chapter 21, *Abdominal and Gastrointestinal Emergencies*, and Chapter 27, *Infectious Diseases*)
- Fungal infections (Chapter 27, *Infectious Diseases*)
- Rabies (Chapter 27, *Infectious Diseases*)
- Scabies and lice (Chapter 27, *Infectious Diseases*)
- Lyme disease (Chapter 27, *Infectious Diseases*)
- Rocky Mountain spotted fever (Chapter 27, *Infectious Diseases*)
- Antibiotic-resistant infections (Chapter 27, *Infectious Diseases*)

KNOWLEDGE OBJECTIVES

1. Describe components of personal well-being and their importance in managing stress. (pp 48–56)
2. List seven factors that have been found to improve heart health, according to the American Heart Association. (p 48)
3. Explain how mental, emotional, and spiritual well-being pertains to your paramedic career. (pp 55–56)
4. Define infectious disease and communicable disease. (p 57)
5. Discuss the various routes of disease transmission. (p 57)
6. Describe standard precautions that are used to prevent infection when treating patients. (pp 58–59)
7. Explain the importance of immunizations. (p 58)
8. Describe the various types of personal protective equipment used to protect against airborne and bloodborne pathogens. (pp 60–63)
9. Discuss the importance of ambulance cleaning and disinfection. (p 64)
10. Explain postexposure management when exposed to patient blood or body fluids, including completing a postexposure report. (p 58)
11. Recognize the possibility of hostile situations and steps to deal with them. (pp 67–68)
12. Discuss how to determine scene safety and prevent work-related injuries at the scene of a traffic incident. (pp 68–69)
13. Describe physiologic, physical, and psychological responses to stress. (p 70)
14. Describe reactions to expect from ill and injured patients, including how you can effectively work with people exhibiting a range of stress-related behaviors. (pp 73–76)
15. Discuss techniques for working at particularly stressful situations, including multiple-casualty incidents and the death of a child. (pp 81, 82)
16. Describe issues concerning care of a dying patient, death, and the grieving process of family members. (pp 79–81)
17. Describe posttraumatic stress disorder (PTSD) and steps that can be taken, including critical incident stress management (CISM), to decrease the likelihood that PTSD will develop. (p 82)

SKILLS OBJECTIVES

1. Demonstrate how to properly remove gloves. (p 61, Skill Drill 2-1)
2. Demonstrate proper handwashing techniques. (p 62, Skill Drill 2-2)
3. Demonstrate the necessary steps to manage a potential exposure situation. (pp 58–66)

Introduction

As a paramedic, you have taken steps to ensure that you can provide a higher level of care to the community. You are dedicated to providing prehospital emergency care and transport for those in need, which makes your job gratifying, but also very demanding. Although you will learn many skills to assist with delivery of emergency medical care, you should never lose sight of the most important factor—your own personal wellness and safety, both on scene and off. Scene safety is crucial because of the risks posed by scene hazards, environmental conditions, human-made threats, violence aimed at first responders, and infectious diseases. The demands placed on you as a paramedic can be either minimal or extreme. For example, you may find yourself working a double shift or holding more than one job, which can compromise your safety because of a lack of rest. Even a single shift may be so busy that you never get time to sit down. Add to that the challenge of making sure you eat proper meals, and you can easily find yourself overworked, undernourished, and at risk for numerous health issues.

Given the increasing demands placed on paramedics, your preparation is of the utmost importance. As you begin your career, you may be assigned to a veteran paramedic who will serve as your mentor. Many veterans may have been trained before wellness and safety training were given such high importance in EMS. Regardless of whom you will work with, this chapter is designed to highlight current wellness recommendations and ways to keep yourself ready for any emergency. Maintaining your health from the beginning will help ensure that you have had a long, healthy, and satisfying career when you become that veteran in 20 or more years.

> **Words of Wisdom**
>
> Some diseases may result in a patient being tracked or traced, isolated, or quarantined. These practices are not the same. According to the Centers for Disease Control and Prevention (CDC), isolation separates a sick person with a contagious disease from people who are not sick. In contrast, quarantine refers to the restriction of the movements of a person who may have been exposed to a contagious disease to monitor them for signs of illness.[1]

Several studies have assessed injury, illness, and death among EMS workers. A 2013 study found that EMS has one of the lowest overall fatality rates compared with other emergency services, such as law enforcement and fire service.[2] In these data, fatalities tended to be linked to transportation crashes, with ambulance crashes resulting in the highest number of deaths. These ambulance crashes primarily occurred during emergent responses. The same study reported that EMS also exceeds all other emergency professions in the number of nonfatal injuries experienced. The common injuries were strains and sprains, usually sustained during the initial scene response and while moving a patient. The most common injury site was the back. The authors concluded that injuries are costly and place a burden on the EMS system, decreasing the number of providers available to assist patients. Finally, the authors found fatigue and sleep deprivation were the major contributing factors to injuries and fatalities. According to this study, being awake for 21 hours results in a state equal to being legally intoxicated.

> **Words of Wisdom**
>
> According to the Bureau of Labor Statistics, approximately 4.1 million serious injuries and 4,500 deaths occur in US workplaces each year, which have a direct cost of more than $50 billion annually.[3] EMS providers visit EDs for work-related injuries and exposures more than 20,000 times each year.[3] As a paramedic, you are most at risk for sprains and strains, exposures to blood and body fluids, and falls. Simple measures such as practicing safe lifting, using appropriate personal protective equipment (PPE), and wearing slip-resistant footwear can greatly reduce the risks of these injuries.

Data from the National Highway Traffic Safety Administration suggest that 1,500 ambulance crashes occur in the United States each year. Of these crashes, 59% occur during an emergent response, while 34% happen during a nonemergent transport. From 2007 to 2011, there were more than 3,000 crashes involving ambulances in the United States, causing 1,400 injuries. Of this number, 29 crashes were fatal, with a total of 33 deaths reported from these events.[4] Additional information about the safe operation of EMS vehicles can be found in the EMS Vehicle Operator Safety course, sponsored by the National Association of Emergency Medical Technicians.

These findings emphasize that, as a new paramedic, you must be aware of your health and well-being while also being aware of your limitations. Never push yourself beyond your normal limits, and seek assistance whenever possible. Finally, always be aware of hazards and other traffic. One point that needs to be emphasized with every response is that *the scene is never safe, and EMS providers should never let their guard down!*

Components of Well-Being

Wellness was first defined in 1654, by Sir Archibald Johnston, a Scottish judge, as the quality or state of being in good health, especially as an actively sought goal. A focus on wellness is indeed an essential component of any EMS training program because it will enable providers to have a long, rewarding career in patient care.

Wellness is often considered to have three components: physical, mental, and emotional. Some believe that a fourth component, spiritual, is also essential.

Physical Well-Being

If you are in top physical condition and become injured, then you will tend to heal more quickly and with fewer complications than if you were in poor physical condition. Muscle strength, flexibility, cardiac endurance, emotional equilibrium, posture (both sitting and standing), state of hydration, the foods you eat, and the amount of sleep you get will all affect your quality of life. Each of these factors may also directly affect your chances of avoiding injury or illness on the job. For example, the Life's Simple 7 list from the American Heart Association (AHA) includes seven factors that have been found to improve heart health: get active, control cholesterol, eat better, manage blood pressure (BP), lose weight, reduce blood sugar, and stop smoking **FIGURE 2-1**. Taking these steps can improve your overall physical and mental well-being.

Nutrition

As a paramedic, you will encounter many patients in poor health due to poor nutrition; however, some EMS providers practice extremely poor nutritional habits themselves. Even though nutritional information changes regularly, current nutritional guidelines are readily available. Research often points out the consequences of poor nutrition, including heart disease, type 2 diabetes, obesity, and various medical conditions. Although EMS providers are strongly encouraged to maintain good health, many services still require providers to work 24-hour shifts, during which they often must go without meals or rest breaks. Situations like this will challenge you as you try to live a healthy lifestyle.

The US Department of Agriculture's (USDA) *Dietary Guidelines for Americans, 2020–2025* suggests eating foods from six categories—vegetables,

YOU are the Paramedic

PART 1

You are performing your morning ambulance check when a call comes in at 0712 hours for a possible cardiac arrest at 984 Solomon Street. You are en route 1 minute later. The traffic is very heavy at this time, and you become agitated as you try to navigate through it. The frustration builds as you think about the dispatch information and the potential of running a field code. You have not had much rest because you just came from another EMS job where you were busy all night. Besides your lack of rest, you have not been eating well lately, frequently relying on drive-through meals. You also have been slacking on your workout routine; you have gained a few pounds and notice that you get winded more easily than in the past. Your coworkers have noted this change and have brought it to your attention, but you tell them you are young and can handle it.

1. The decline of your physical well-being will eventually affect your attitude and, in turn, put your job at risk. What steps can you take to avoid this outcome?
2. Why is it so important to also find ways to enhance your mental, emotional, and spiritual well-being?

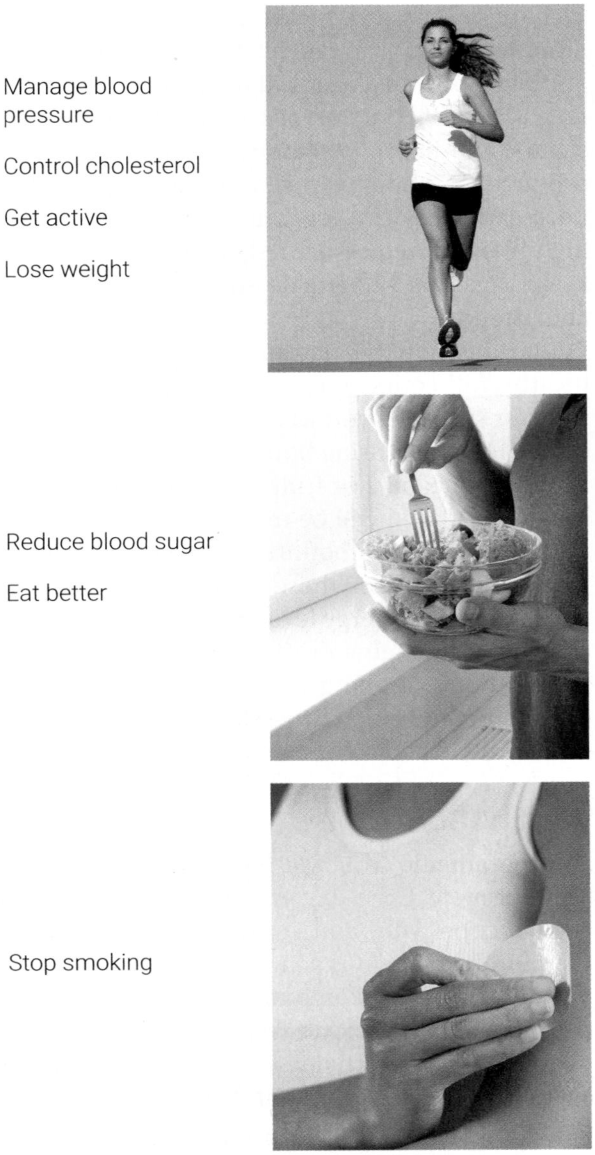

FIGURE 2-1 The American Heart Association's Life's Simple 7 includes key factors that have been found to improve your heart health.

fruits, grains, dairy, protein foods, and oils—in suggested portions.[5] Research has shown that each person's nutritional requirements are different; therefore, you should tailor your eating style to your individual needs. For example, a moderately active woman age 19 to 30 years requires around 2,000 calories per day. By comparison, eating 2,200 calories per day is the limit suggested for sedentary men older than 50 years. On the MyPlate website produced by USDA (MyPlate.gov), the MyPlate icon

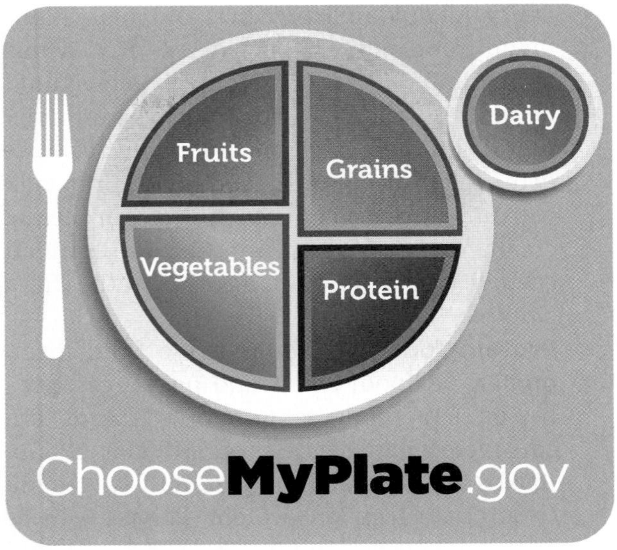

FIGURE 2-2 The USDA's MyPlate icon emphasizes healthy portions of vegetables, fruits, grains, proteins, and dairy.

provides a quick look at the recommended relative portion sizes of five food groups **FIGURE 2-2**.[6] The amount you need from each of these groups is directly dependent on your age, sex, and level of physical activity.[5] Follow these guidelines to get the nutrients you need:

- **Vegetables.** Any vegetable or 100% vegetable juice counts as a member of the Vegetable Group. Vegetables may be raw or cooked; fresh, frozen, canned, or dried/dehydrated; and whole, cut-up, or mashed. Vary the vegetables you eat; eat more dark green vegetables and orange vegetables, as well as beans and peas. It is suggested that one-half of your plate should be fruits and vegetables.
- **Fruits.** Any fruit or 100% fruit juice counts as part of the Fruit Group. Fruits may be fresh, canned, frozen, or dried, and may be whole, cut-up, or pureed.
- **Grains.** Any food made from wheat, rice, oats, cornmeal, barley, or another cereal grain is a grain product. Bread, pasta, oatmeal, breakfast cereals, tortillas, and grits are examples of grain products. Make one-half your grains whole. Whole grains are healthier because they contain important nutrients that reduce the risk of disease, as well as more protein and more fiber.

- **Dairy.** All fluid milk products and many foods made from milk are considered part of this food group. Most Dairy Group choices should be fat-free or low-fat. Foods made from milk that retain their calcium content are also part of the group. In contrast, foods made from milk with little to no calcium, such as cream cheese, cream, and butter, are not. Calcium-fortified soymilk (soy beverage) is also part of the Dairy Group.
- **Protein foods.** All foods made from meat, poultry, seafood, beans and peas, eggs, processed soy products, nuts, and seeds are considered part of the Protein Foods Group. (Beans and peas are also part of the Vegetable Group.) Go lean on protein; choose low-fat or lean meats and poultry. Bake, broil, or grill these items. Vary your choices by consuming more fish, beans, peas, nuts, and seeds.
- **Oils.** Oils are fats that are liquid at room temperature, like the vegetable oils used in cooking. Oils come from many different plants and from fish. Oils are *not* a food group, but they provide essential nutrients. For this reason, oils are included in USDA dietary patterns. Know your fats; make most fat sources from fish, nuts, and vegetable oils. Limit solid fats, like butter, stick margarine, shortening, and lard; avoid trans fats such as partially hydrogenated oils **FIGURE 2-3**.

Finally, it is essential to read the nutrition label of prepared or processed foods. Many such foods include sodium as a preservative and will have sodium levels that can reach 50% of your daily allowance with one meal. Look at the amount and type of fat and the make-up of the carbohydrates (starches, sugars, and fiber). Remember, even though a food product may be advertised as "fat free," it is not necessarily healthy for you. Look for foods with high fiber content; fiber helps you feel full longer, keeps digestive bacteria healthy, and lowers BP and cholesterol.

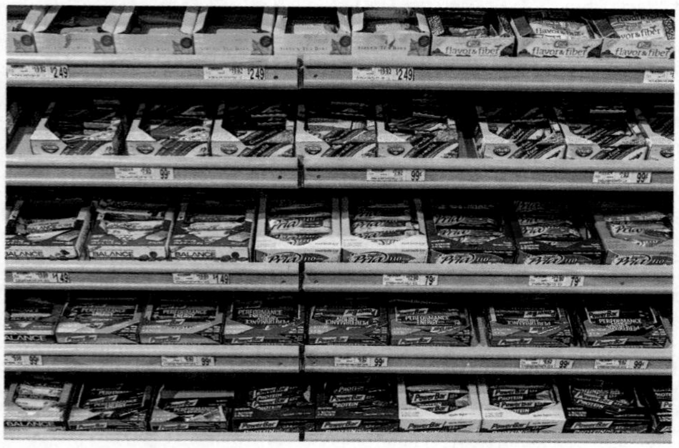

FIGURE 2-3 Health bars are a quick, healthy alternative to fast food. When selecting a health bar, read the ingredients to make sure it truly is healthy.

Because of the nature of your job, planning healthy, full-course meals will be challenging. Plan for your shift as if you will get minimal time to rest or to eat a meal. Bring bottles of water and various healthy snack bars or fruit with you. When you are hungry, fast food will be tempting, but try to avoid it. Due to the high amounts of fat found in most fast food, the nutrition in these items will not be enough to sustain your energy level. Also avoid candy bars, caffeine, and energy drinks; they may give you an instant burst of energy, but after that initial rush of caffeine and sugars runs out, you will feel even more exhausted.[7]

Weight Control

As a paramedic, you will have to act quickly and appropriately. Each day you must observe, assess, access, cope with, and control chaotic situations; therefore, staying fit is an important component for all people who work in public service. Many habits you practice as an adult were formed during your youth. Often, the activities that made you happiest as a child are the ones that drive you later in life, including eating well and staying active. Although it may be challenging, you can change habits developed in childhood.

The USDA's dietary guidelines include the following key principles:

- Follow a healthy eating pattern across the lifespan.
- Focus on variety, nutrient density, and amount.
- Limit calories from added sugars and saturated fats, and reduce sodium intake.
- Shift to healthier food and beverage choices.
- Support healthy eating patterns for all.[5]

The dietary guidelines further define a healthy eating pattern and deemphasize dieting.[5] Diets are generally not as effective as making healthy food choices. The typical American consumes far too many calories, which are ultimately stored as fat. As you age, this fat storage occurs more readily and becomes much harder to eliminate. The goal should be gradual weight reduction, which is much safer than crash dieting. Gradual weight loss requires you to make a plan for nutrition and fitness and stick to it. Rather than taking coffee breaks, take a walk or perform other forms of activity. For example, if you work in a multilevel building, take the stairs rather than an elevator. Stand up and move around as much as you can; avoid sitting for hours while watching TV, browsing the Internet, or using social media. If you must eat out, consider choosing smaller meals or even sharing a meal with your partner. Eat oatmeal or cold cereal for breakfast, a salad with minimal or no dressing and one-half sandwich for lunch, and a sensible dinner that consists of baked or broiled foods.

Words of Wisdom

Tips for healthy eating include:

- Avoid oversized portions, eat slowly, and allow your body time to identify fullness.
- Focus on fruits and vegetables.
- Vary the types of foods you eat. For example, alternate between seafood, meat, and beans as your protein sources.
- Drink water instead of soda (including diet soda) or other sugary drinks (which are associated with weight gain/obesity, type 2 diabetes, heart disease, kidney disease, nonalcoholic liver disease, tooth decay and cavities, and gout).
- Read food labels closely. Choose foods with fewer calories; low amounts of fat, sugar, and sodium; and high amounts of fiber.

Exercise

Regular exercise is associated with overall body weight, nutritional status, and hydration. It has been shown to improve sleep, mental capacity, ability to cope with stress, sex life, and overall long-term health. The exercise program you choose depends on your personal preferences and fitness goals. You are more likely to stick with an exercise program if it is something you enjoy. Aim to maintain, or improve, three areas: your cardiovascular endurance, your flexibility, and your overall physical strength. If you are just beginning an exercise program, then it is recommended that you consult with your primary care physician (PCP). Although you may be eager to achieve weight loss and get in shape, you must take it slowly to avoid injury. Remember, you did not gain all that weight overnight; nor you will not lose it overnight.

In general, it is recommended that adults engage in at least 30 minutes of moderate to vigorous physical activity *every day* to help build optimal cardiovascular endurance. However, any planned physical activity is helpful. Although you may feel you get enough of a workout during your shift at a busy department, the activity on an EMS call is not sufficient to meet the suggested activity requirements for wellness. To stay in good physical condition, you need to find a healthy balance between full-out physical activity (when you are "running hot") and no activity at all **FIGURE 2-4**. Many departments, realizing peak physical condition of their staff is essential, may provide their employees with workout equipment to use both on and off duty.

Depending on your level of health, you should attempt to reach your target heart rate every time you exercise; however, this should not be the goal if you are just beginning an exercise program. The goal is to gradually increase your activity to meet your target heart rate. The AHA suggests that your

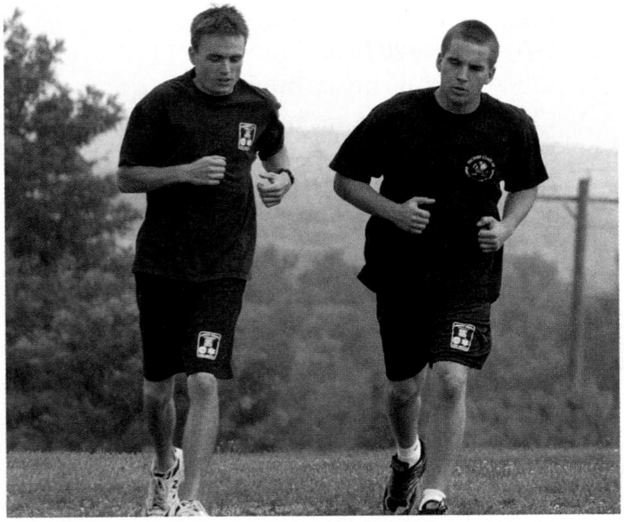

FIGURE 2-4 Regular exercise—apart from the work you do on EMS calls—should be part of your daily or weekly routine.

target be between 50% and 69% of your maximum heart rate.[7] The method to find your target heart rate is as follows:

1. Take 220 and subtract your age in years to find your estimated maximum heart rate (not target range). For example, if you are 40 years old, then your maximum heart rate would be 180 beats/min.
2. Multiply your maximum heart rate by 0.5 and 0.69 to find your target range. In this case, it would be 90 to 124 beats/min.

If you know your resting heart rate, which would be your pulse on first waking up in the morning and before getting out of bed, then calculate your target heart rate as follows:

1. Subtract your age in years from 220. Next, subtract your resting heart rate.
2. Multiply this number by 0.5 to 0.8, and then add your resting heart rate to find your target range.

For example, suppose a 40-year-old has a resting heart rate of 60 beats/min. Calculations would be as follows:

1. **Resting heart rate**
   60 beats/min
2. **Maximum heart rate** (for a healthy patient without coronary artery disease)
   220 − 40 = 180 beats/min
3. **Maximum heart rate minus resting heart rate**
   180 − 60 = 120 beats/min
   120 × 0.5 = 60 beats/min
   120 × 0.8 = 96 beats/min
4. **Target heart rate**
   60 + 60 = 120 beats/min
   96 + 60 = 156 beats/min
   Range: 120 to 156 beats/min

Street Smarts

Being a paramedic in the field is physically and mentally demanding. Following simple guidelines for nutrition, exercise, and mental health will greatly enhance and prolong your career. Consider establishing a group of coworkers who share wellness ideas or start a friendly weight-loss or activity-level competition. Remember, the only way to benefit from these wellness goals is to commit to them for the long haul.

Smoking and Tobacco

Knowledge about the harmful effects of smoking in relation to health continues to grow. As mentioned earlier, our behavior as adults is often linked to our youth. Some studies suggest that the presence of smokers in the family increases your likelihood of smoking. If you don't smoke now, then don't start! With the numerous regulations that have been placed on smoking and advertising cigarettes over the years, the number of smokers has dropped. Unfortunately, with the introduction of vapor-type smoking devices, this habit has seen a resurgence, especially among the Millennial generation. The use of e-cigarettes (vaping) is banned on airplanes and in many public spaces. Research is under way on the effects of these new devices, but they have already been linked to serious lung diseases.[8] You must also understand that everyone responds differently to smoke, and some of your patients may be highly sensitive to its odor. If you smoke right before a call, then the odor on your uniform may be enough to cause serious effects in an already sick patient.

If you do smoke and are trying to quit, then first understand that smoking is an addiction and quitting may not be easy. Seek help. Many EMS agencies now offer smoking cessation classes for their employees. Talk to your PCP. A variety of programs exist that can help to reduce a smoker's psychological dependency. These programs may include instructions, electronic media (eg, DVDs), medications, and counseling to provide ongoing support. Other options include psychotherapy, hypnotism, and acupuncture. The effectiveness of these options appears to be dependent on the individual.

As noted earlier, in recent years, electronic cigarettes (e-cigarettes) have become a popular alternative to tobacco cigarettes. Also called electronic nicotine delivery systems or personal vaporizers, these devices simulate smoking tobacco by producing an aerosol made by vaporizing a flavored liquid solution. Although the full extent of their danger has not been determined,[9] these devices are certainly not healthful and should be avoided.

Alcohol Use

As a paramedic, you may notice some people express the common idea that drinking alcohol can alleviate stress, particularly after a "bad call." Alcohol is a drug that can modify how the brain perceives stress. Unfortunately, alcohol cannot alleviate stress, and the uncomfortable nature of stress persists beyond the duration of the effects of alcohol. Be aware that using alcohol to cope with stress can lead to dependence and magnify the effect of stressful situations on your life. The CDC website provides resources to help people assess their drinking habits. Recognizing unhealthy drinking habits early is vital to the EMS provider's career and long-term health.

Circadian Rhythms and Shift Work

Your job as a paramedic will often conflict with your body's circadian rhythm, or natural timing system. Suprachiasmatic nuclei are areas of your brain that control your circadian rhythm, which governs your so-called internal clock. Ignoring your circadian rhythm can cause you to experience consistent difficulties with sleep, higher thought functions, physical coordination, and even social functions. Ideally, you should determine what your natural rhythms are and design your schedule to match them. Research on circadian rhythms is only beginning to appear in medical journals, suggesting that someday a person might be able to alter their internal clock.

Some tips for dealing with shift work are as follows:

- Avoid caffeine.
- Eat healthy meals and try to eat at the same times every day.
- Keep a regular sleep schedule.

Most important, do not overlook the need for rest, whatever your individual rhythm may be. Current research and literature have shown that inadequate sleep has the same effect on your body and mind as intoxication. Many employers are finally realizing that inadequate sleep can result in serious consequences while you are operating an emergency vehicle or selecting and administering medications. In turn, many EMS agencies have adopted policies to ensure work schedules allow sufficient time for rest and sleep, with the goal of reducing work-related errors such as ambulance crashes.

Periodic Health Risk Assessments

Besides sleep, diet, exercise, hydration, and all the other things that make up a healthy lifestyle, hereditary factors may affect your overall health. Research your family's health history. Alzheimer disease, chemical addiction, cancer, cardiac illness, hypertension, migraine, mental illness, and stroke all feature prominent hereditary factors. The most common of all heredity health risk factors are heart disease and cancer. Although family history cannot be changed, you can modify your lifestyle to help you deal with any hereditary issues that arise.

Share this information with your personal physician. Work to set up a schedule for your health assessments, building them into your routine physical checkups. Your physician should be your ally in screening for these diseases and in assessing your lifestyle as well as your hereditary factors.

Body Mechanics

As a paramedic, you will be required to lift and move a variety of patients. Some patients are small and lightweight, whereas others may have morbid obesity. You can develop several habits to prepare yourself to safely lift most patients, no matter their weight, including the following actions:

- **Minimize the number of total body lifts you have to perform.** When patients need to be lifted, be prepared and plan the lift. In many cases, patients do not need to be lifted to a cot or any other location. For example, a patient with an isolated arm laceration and no other issues can walk to the ambulance. Evaluate every situation to identify the easiest and safest way to lift or move a patient.
- **Coordinate every lift before performing the lift.** Advise your patients regarding what they may experience during the lift so they do not panic. Once the lift is planned, use clear communication to execute it, such as "On the count of three, lift." Be sure to plan and clarify with your team members, in advance, whether the lift will occur *on* "three," or *after* you say "three."
- **Minimize the total amount of weight you have to lift.** If you have extra people available, then ask for assistance. In some cases, the patient might be able to offer some assistance with moving. If possible, remove any unneeded equipment from the cot.
- **Never lift with your back.** A back injury can be a career-ending event, but you can prevent

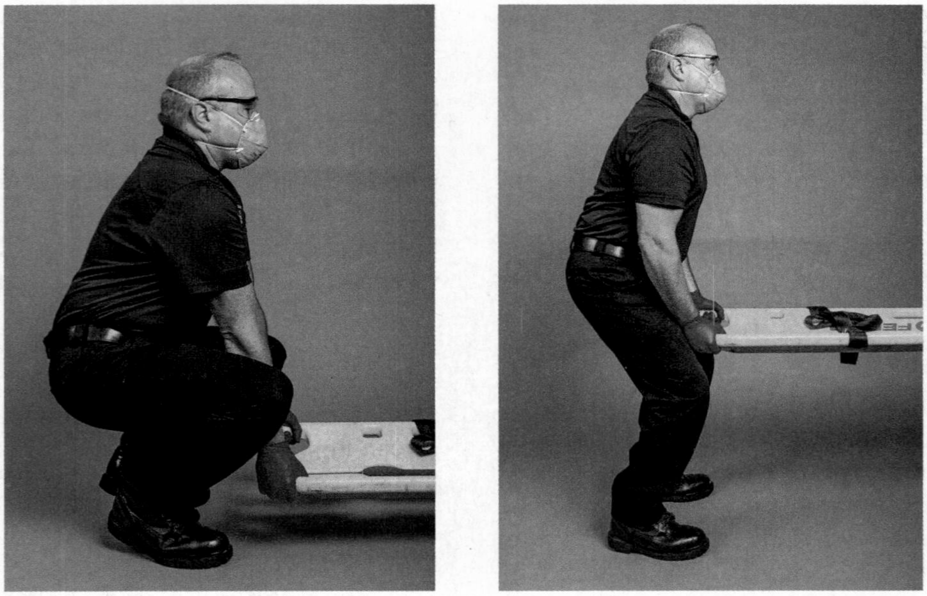

FIGURE 2-5 If your body is properly aligned when you lift, then the line of force exerted against the spine occurs in an essentially straight line down the vertebrae. In this way, the vertebrae support the lift.

issues if you do not lift with your back. To help protect your back, follow these precautions **FIGURE 2-5**:

- Always keep your back in a straight, upright position and lift without twisting.
- When lifting, spread your legs about 15 inches (38 cm) apart (shoulder width), and place your feet so your center of gravity is properly balanced. Keep your head upright and facing forward.
- Hold your back upright as you bring your upper body down by bending your knees.
- Lift by raising your upper body and arms and by straightening your legs until you are standing.
- Always lift with your legs, not with your back!
- Remember to breathe while lifting; do not hold your breath.
- If you are working with a partner while lifting, then plan both your counting style and exactly how the lift will be performed.

- **Do not carry what you can put on wheels.** Position the ambulance, and the cot, as close to the patient as you can. Many services have switched to stretchers with air- or battery-powered lifting mechanisms to reduce the physical exertion required of providers to lift the stretcher into the ambulance. Most stair chairs now have tracks to make going down stairs easier and safer.
- **Ask for help.** Anytime you need to move a patient who cannot or should not walk, consider the possibility of asking an extra person to help you **FIGURE 2-6**. Many services have specialty units to help transport patients who are obese. These units carry special equipment (eg, lifts, air-mattress, bariatric stretcher) designed to facilitate movement of these patients.

SAFETY

Back injuries can be career ending. These injuries tend to happen early in providers' careers, with one-quarter of EMS providers experiencing a career-ending back injury within their first 4 years on the job. The fact that these injuries occur less frequently later in providers' careers suggests proper lifting technique, which is learned and reinforced with practice, is the key to safety.[10]

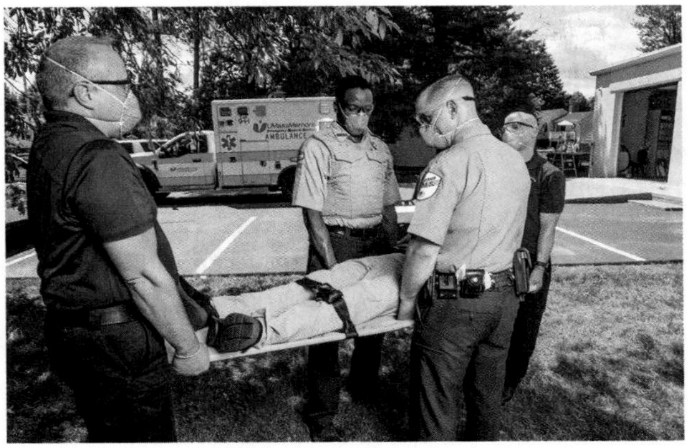

FIGURE 2-6 Never hesitate to ask for help from your coworkers, or to provide it when you are asked.

Mental Well-Being

As a paramedic, you will be exposed not only to diseases and injuries, but also to stress. When you are subjected to stress, your **fight-or-flight response** is activated. This is the same system that comes into play when you exercise or do something fun to promote the feeling of well-being (known as positive stress). It is crucial that you prepare yourself for how you will react when the fight-or-flight response kicks in. If you are unconditioned or unprepared for stress, then you will not adapt effectively to the physiologic responses triggered by your stressor. Those responses may include increased sympathetic tone, which results in dilation of the pupils, increased heart rate, dilation of the bronchi, mobilization of glucose, shunting of blood away from the gastrointestinal (GI) tract and cerebrum, and increased blood flow to the skeletal muscles. Collectively, these physiologic responses help you deal with stressful situations as they are happening—a period in which you should rely on preplanning and gut instinct as your primary resources. However, to maintain your mental well-being for the long term, you need to handle stressful situations using appropriate coping skills.

As a paramedic, you will need to control your emotions at all times, regardless of the situation. Remember, a professional is someone who can remain calm and think clearly when everything else is in disarray. The most important step you can take to control your fight-or-flight response is to plan for it. Many resources are available to help you prepare for stressful situations, such as physical exercise programs and counseling. Stress management is discussed in more detail later in this chapter.

Emotional Well-Being

Paramedics have a genuine interest in helping people. To remain healthy throughout your EMS career, you need to make a deliberate effort to create a healthy balance between your work and home life. Although you may be very dedicated to your work, you must separate yourself from your career from time to time—regardless of how much you enjoy it—and focus on your personal life and family. Family members may not understand your EMS life and may feel neglected, or may be otherwise impacted by the effects of your stress. Even if you share the same career as family members and friends, it is unhealthy to live this lifestyle “24/7/365” without taking time to step back and reassess your relationship to your work.

As an EMS practitioner, you will pour a large amount of energy into your work. Although this dedication is admirable, you still need to effectively deal with the stress that comes with the job. A common stressor in EMS is the ever-present need to deal with patient disability and death. Another common stressor is “frequent flyer” and “combative and/or belligerent” patients. Although many of these patients have medical conditions or traumatic injuries that cause their behaviors, such situations will nonetheless be stressful for you. As a new paramedic, you may feel that you can or must save every life or have a positive effect on every patient, but outcomes for some patients will undoubtedly be negative, even with your best efforts. It is important to learn not to take such situations personally.

Good paramedics are strong, sensitive people **FIGURE 2-7**. However, these traits are also intertwined with normal emotional reactions to job stressors, so you need to develop coping strategies to handle the pressures of the EMS life. If you are approached by a coworker or leader who has noticed changes in your behavior, then take their concerns seriously; these could be warning signs that indicate you need to seek assistance. Likewise, if you note changes in your coworkers, then do not ignore them; pick an appropriate time and, in a calm manner, express to them what you are noticing.

Put aside any discomfort you may have about voicing your observations or fear of their reaction, because the action you are taking may be a first step toward moving someone back to emotional and physical well-being.

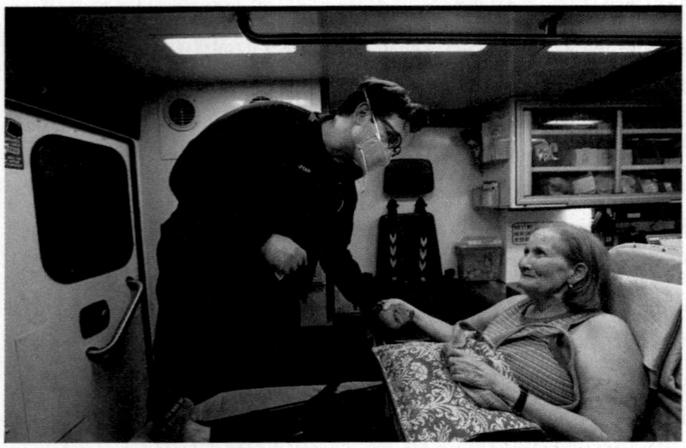

FIGURE 2-7 One thing that draws people to work as a paramedic is the pleasure of interacting closely with people.

Spiritual Well-Being

Spirituality is an unseen dimension of human experience that influences a person's beliefs, attitudes, emotions, and behavior. Some people address their spirituality with formal religion, while others embrace reflective moments by taking a walk, practicing meditation, or engaging in yoga. Medical care supports the dignity and value of life and the sacredness of all people. As a paramedic, respecting patients' spiritual (and cultural) practices is essential to providing effective patient care.

Disease Transmission

As a paramedic, you will be called on to treat and transport patients with various infectious or communicable diseases. At times, you may have to transport a chronically ill patient without knowing that they have an infectious or contagious disease until well after the call. Given these possibilities, you must make every attempt to identify a disease if you have an indication that one may be present.

YOU are the Paramedic

PART 2

You arrive on scene 7 minutes later, only to realize that you have been to this residence before, and that a 23-year-old man with a history of leukemia lives here. When you arrive, family members inform you that the patient is the same young man, whose condition has deteriorated rapidly over the past few weeks. Your heart drops as you remember the times you transported him and the conversations you had. You remember thinking to yourself how lucky you are to be healthy and have a good job. This courageous young man has always remained optimistic about his condition, making you and everyone around him feel better. You start to feel a little guilty for how you reacted while responding; obviously, your frustrations are nothing compared with the magnitude of this family's emotions.

His mother allows you into the patient's home and tells you he began feeling ill yesterday and would not eat last night. She just came in to check on him and found him not breathing.

Recording Time: 0 Minutes	
Appearance	Pale, cyanotic, appears lifeless
Level of consciousness	Unresponsive
Airway	Open and clear
Breathing	Apneic
Circulation	Pulseless
Skin	Cold to touch

3. According to his mother's report, the patient has been apneic for an unknown amount of time. What should be your next action?

4. On the basis of your previous interactions with the patient, which stage of grieving do you feel he reached?

An **infectious disease** is a medical condition caused by the growth and spread of small, harmful organisms within the body. A **communicable disease** is a disease that can be spread from one person or species to another. Chapter 27, *Infectious Diseases,* covers emergency medical care of patients with infectious diseases and protection from specific diseases in greater depth, whereas this chapter covers general protection of paramedics against such diseases.

Words of Wisdom

Many people confuse the terms *infectious* and *contagious*. In fact, all contagious diseases are infectious, but only some infectious diseases are contagious. For example, pneumonia caused by pneumococcal bacteria is an infectious process, but it is not contagious. In other words, it will not be transmitted from one person to another. Some infectious agents, such as the hepatitis B virus (HBV) and COVID-19, are contagious because they can be transmitted from one person to another.

Immunizations, personal protective equipment (PPE), and simple handwashing can dramatically minimize your risk of **infection**. When you use these protective measures, your risk of contracting a serious infectious or communicable disease is significantly reduced. Proper cleaning and disinfecting of the ambulance and equipment after each call will also help to prevent transfer of diseases to other patients.

When you come in contact with a patient who poses a potential risk of infection to you, discretion is imperative while communicating with other health care providers and your coworkers. Do not give out sensitive patient history over the radio during your patient care report or to anyone who is not directly involved with the patient's care. However, during your transfer of care, provide a complete patient history for the receiving facility and include appropriate patient history in your written or electronic PCR.

Whereas all infections result from an invasion of body spaces and tissues by germs, different germs use different means of attack. These means are known as mechanisms of transmission. **Transmission** is the spread of an infectious agent from one organism to another. Infectious diseases can be transmitted in several ways, specifically, through contact (direct or indirect), airborne, foodborne, and vector-borne (transmitted through insects or parasitic worms) transmission.

Contact transmission is movement of an organism from one person to another through physical touch. The two types of contact transmission are direct and indirect. **Direct contact** occurs when an organism is moved from one person to another through touching without any intermediary. For example, **bloodborne pathogens** are microorganisms that are present in human blood; they can cause disease if blood of one person containing the pathogen contacts and enters the bloodstream of another person. Another example of direct contact is sexual transmission. Patients who are infected with the human immunodeficiency virus can transfer the virus to their partners during sex.

Indirect contact involves spreading infection between the patient with an infection to another person through a contaminated, inanimate object. The object that transmits the infection is called a fomite. A needlestick is an example of the spread of infection through indirect contact. In this case, the virus moves from the patient to the needle to the health care provider. Many years ago, this transmission route was common before the advent of safety equipment such as needleless IV systems.

Airborne transmission involves the spread of an infectious agent through mechanisms such as droplets or dust. Both the common cold and COVID-19 are moved from person to person by coughing and sneezing. Because of the risk of airborne transmission, it is unsanitary to use your hands to cover a cough or sneeze: the organism travels onto your hands and can spread from there. Using a tissue when coughing or sneezing is better for controlling the spread of organisms; of course, because you then have a piece of tissue full of organisms in your hand, you must wash your hands after disposing of the tissue. If you are wearing long sleeves, an effective technique to avoid contaminating your hands is coughing or sneezing into the fabric of your inner sleeve. Because you do not touch objects with your inner arms, the risk of moving the organism to an object or person is reduced. The organisms are trapped in the fabric and will eventually die.

Street Smarts

The COVID-19 pandemic has had a profound effect on EMS agencies and EMS providers across the globe. About 6 months into the pandemic, a small study found the fatality rate for COVID-19 to be almost 50% higher for EMS providers than for the general population.[11] Each EMS agency needs to have a plan in place for the safety of its personnel in all aspects of the job, including while in the station, on calls, and providing care, as well as follow-up and testing.

Management of an Exposure

If you have been exposed to a patient's blood or body fluids, follow your department's infection control plan. Generally, any EMS provider who has had significant exposure should do the following:

- Turn patient care over to another EMS provider.
- Wash the affected area immediately with soap and water.
- If your eyes were exposed, rinse them with water for at least 20 minutes as soon as possible.
- Comply with all reporting requirements.
- Get a medical evaluation.
- Obtain the proper immunization boosters.
- Document the incident, including the actions taken to reduce chances of infection.

The topic of postexposure protocols is covered in more detail in Chapter 27, *Infectious Diseases*.

Protecting Yourself

Much has changed in EMS since its inception. The use of PPE was uncommon in the early years. In fact, being coated with blood and dirt was considered a status symbol. Surgeons in the 1800s took similar pride in their messy operating aprons but were actually transmitting infectious diseases. Present-day EMS practices are changing rapidly, especially in light of the worldwide COVID-19 pandemic. In particular, recommendations for protection are being updated as research and best practices are shared among health professionals.

Thanks to the CDC's research and reporting, EMS providers are now more keenly aware that biohazards are an integral part of their profession and can have long-term effects on health care workers if they do not adhere to the recommended precautions.[12,13] EMS follows **standard precautions**. Standard precautions approach all body fluids as being potentially infectious. **TABLE 2-1** summarizes the CDC's recommendations in regard to standard precautions.

Immunizations

As a paramedic, you are at increased risk for acquiring an infectious or communicable disease. Using basic protective measures can minimize the risk.

Prevention begins by maintaining your personal health. You should receive annual health exams. A history of all your childhood infectious diseases—for example, chickenpox, mumps, measles, rubella, and whooping cough—should be recorded and kept on file. If you have not had one of these diseases, then you must be immunized against it.

The CDC and the Occupational Safety and Health Administration (OSHA) have developed requirements for protection from bloodborne pathogens such as HBV.[14] Your EMS system should have its own immunization program in place. Immunizations should be kept up-to-date and recorded in your file. Recommended immunizations include the following:

- Tetanus and diphtheria boosters (every 10 years)
- Measles, mumps, rubella (MMR) vaccine
- Influenza vaccine (yearly)
- HBV vaccine and, if applicable, hepatitis C screening
- Varicella (chickenpox) vaccine or having had chickenpox
- COVID-19 vaccine[15]

You should also have a skin test for tuberculosis (TB) before you begin working as a paramedic. The purpose of this test is to identify anyone who has been exposed to the TB pathogen in the past. Testing should be repeated every year if you have been exposed to TB disease. Be aware that routine testing may cause an individual to build up a reactive tolerant level, resulting in a positive skin test even

TABLE 2-1 Standard Precautions for Care of All Patients in All Health Care Settings

Component	Recommendation
Hand hygiene	• After touching blood, body fluids, secretions, excretions, or contaminated items • Immediately after removing gloves or other PPE • Before, after, and between patient contacts
Personal Protective Equipment (PPE)	
Gloves	• For touching blood, body fluids, secretions, excretions, or contaminated items • For touching mucous membranes and nonintact skin
Gown	• During procedures and patient care activities when contact of the paramedic's clothing/exposed skin with blood, body fluids, secretions, excretions, or contaminated items is anticipated
Mask, eye protection, face shield	• During procedures and patient care activities likely to generate splashes or sprays of blood, body fluids, secretions, or excretions (eg, suctioning, ET intubation, and aerosolized medication administration); during aerosol-generating procedures, including care for COVID-19 patients
HEPA respirator or N95 mask	• When working with a patient with TB or any other respiratory illness (eg, COVID-19)
Patient Care Environment	
Soiled patient care equipment	• Handle in a manner that prevents transfer of microorganisms to others and to the environment • Wear gloves if visibly contaminated • Hand hygiene
Environmental controls	• Have procedures for routine care, cleaning, and disinfection of environmental surfaces • Special attention to frequently touched surfaces within the ambulance (eg, handrails, seats, cabinets, doors) • Have patients with TB or COVID-19 wear a surgical mask • Have ventilation/exhaust fans working in the patient compartment
Textiles and laundry	• Handle in a manner that prevents transfer of microorganisms to others and to the environment
Needles and other sharp objects	• Do not recap, bend, break, or hand-manipulate used needles • Use safety features when available (eg, needleless IV systems) • Place sharps in puncture-resistant containers
Special Circumstances	
Patient resuscitation	• Use a resuscitation bag or other ventilation device to prevent contact with mouth and oral secretions
Respiratory hygiene/cough etiquette	• Instruct symptomatic patients to cover the mouth/nose when sneezing or coughing • Use tissues and dispose of them in a no-touch receptacle • Perform hand hygiene after touching tissues • Place surgical masks on the patient and provider • If a mask cannot be used, maintain special separation distance (more than 3 ft [about 1 m]) if possible

Abbreviations: ET, endotracheal; HEPA, high-efficiency particulate air; IV, intravenous; TB, tuberculosis.

Data from Centers for Disease Control and Prevention. Guideline for Hand Hygiene in Health-Care Settings: Recommendations of the Healthcare Infection Control Practices Advisory Committee and the HICPAC/SHEA/APIC/IDSA Hand Hygiene Task Force. *MMWR.* 2002;51(No. RR-16). Siegel JD, Rhinehart E, Jackson M, Chiarello L, Healthcare Infection Control Practices Advisory Committee. 2007 Guideline for Isolation Precautions: Preventing Transmission of Infectious Agents in Healthcare Settings. http://www.cdc gov/hicpac/pdf/Isolation/Isolation2007.pdf. Accessed February 26, 2021.

if the person is not actually infected. Thus, a positive skin test does not necessarily mean you have TB; it simply indicates that you may have been exposed to this pathogen. Additional follow-up will be needed to determine whether the disease is active, such as radiologic or even blood tests to confirm or clear the results. Other vaccines now suggested for paramedics may also include pertussis (whooping cough).[16]

If you know you will be transporting a patient with a communicable disease, you have a definite advantage. In this situation, your health record will be valuable. If you have already had the disease or been vaccinated, then your risk is significantly reduced or eliminated. However, you will not always know whether a patient has a communicable disease. Given this reality, you should always adhere to standard precautions if the possibility of exposure to blood or other body fluids exists.

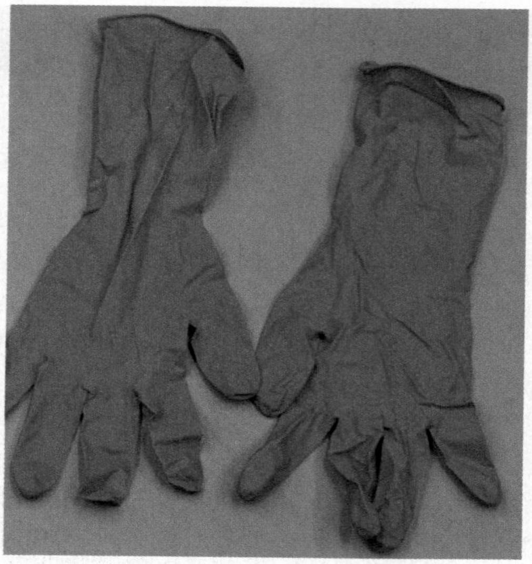

FIGURE 2-8 Use medical gloves on every EMS call.

Personal Protective Equipment and Practices

At a minimum, each ambulance should be equipped with specific PPE—not just because it is the law under OSHA, but also because it is an essential part of ensuring your safety. At a minimum, you should have access to gloves, facial protection (masks and eyewear), gowns, and N95 or N100 respirators. This section focuses on the importance of using **infection control** practices.

> **Words of Wisdom**
>
> If you do not have access to soap and water, then carry waterless hand wipes in your ambulance and use them instead. Isopropyl alcohol, the active ingredient they contain, is a very effective bactericide. Whatever else you do, always wash your hands.

Wear Gloves

Gloves are absolutely essential on any EMS call, and some patient encounters may warrant more than one set of gloves for a provider, depending on the procedure, patient's history, and environment **FIGURE 2-8**. Anytime you could be exposed to a patient's body fluids, consider donning a new set of gloves before loading the patient in the ambulance. Be sure to take off your gloves before you drive or leave the ambulance. Use nitrile (nonlatex) gloves if possible to avoid developing a sensitivity to latex or exposing a patient who may have a latex allergy.

Change medical gloves if they have been exposed to motor oil, gasoline, or any petroleum-based product. Do not perform tasks such as using a radio, driving, writing a PCR, or using any monitoring device such as a cardiac monitor or pulse oximeter when wearing contaminated gloves.

Removing used medical gloves requires a methodical technique to avoid contaminating yourself with the materials from which gloves have protected you **SKILL DRILL 2-1**.

Wash Your Hands

Proper handwashing is one of the simplest, yet most effective, ways of controlling disease transmission. Get used to washing your hands before and after using the bathroom, before ingesting anything by mouth, before getting into your personal vehicle after a call or shift, and before and after any physical contact between you and a patient or an instrument. Also wash your hands after you remove your gloves.

Skill Drill 2-1 Proper Glove Removal Technique

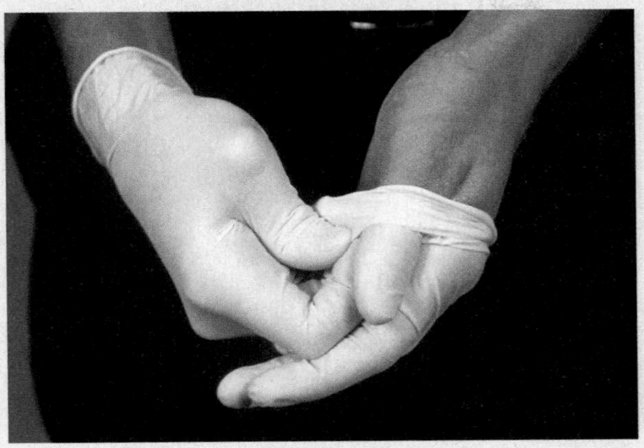

Step 1

Begin by partially removing one glove. With the other gloved hand, pinch the first glove at the wrist—being certain to touch only the outside of the first glove—and start to roll it back off the hand, inside out. Leave the exterior of the fingers on the first glove exposed.

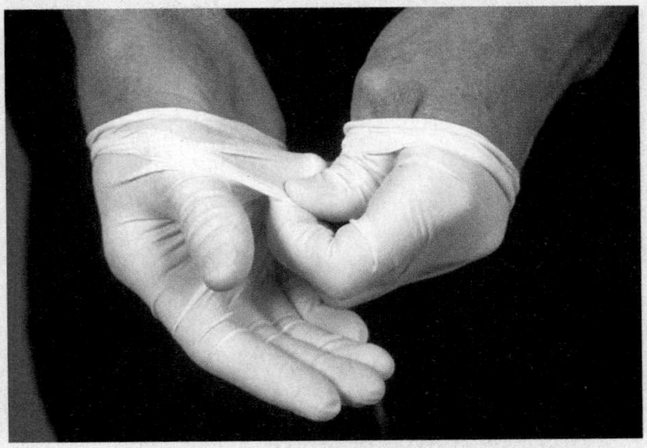

Step 2

Use the partially gloved fingers to pinch the wrist of the second glove and begin to pull it off, rolling it inside out toward the fingertips as you did with the first glove.

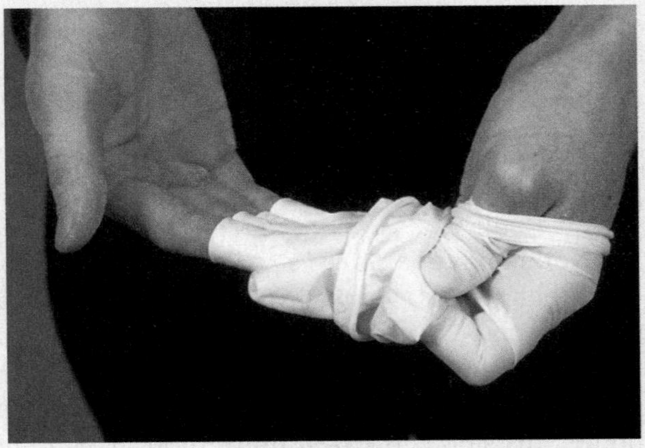

Step 3

Continue pulling the second glove off until you can pull the second hand free.

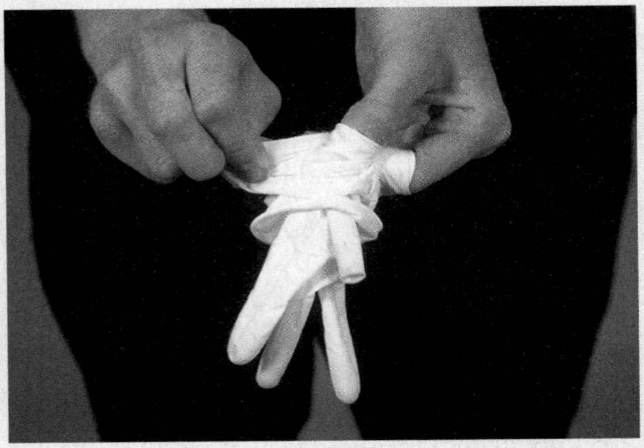

Step 4

With your now-ungloved second hand, grasp the exposed inside of the first glove and pull it free of your first hand and over the now-loose second glove. Be sure that you touch only clean, interior surfaces with your ungloved hand.

Skill Drill 2-2 Handwashing

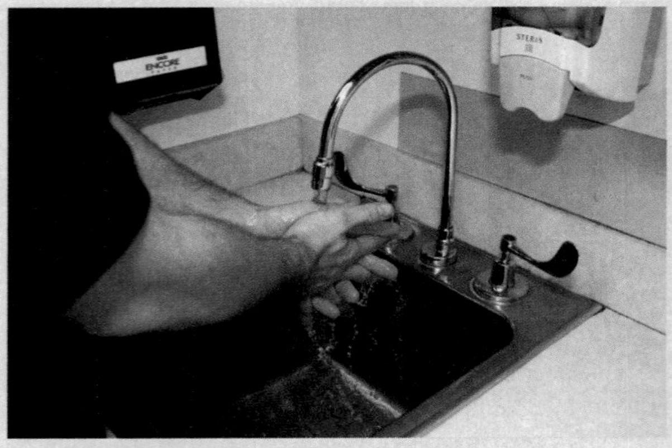

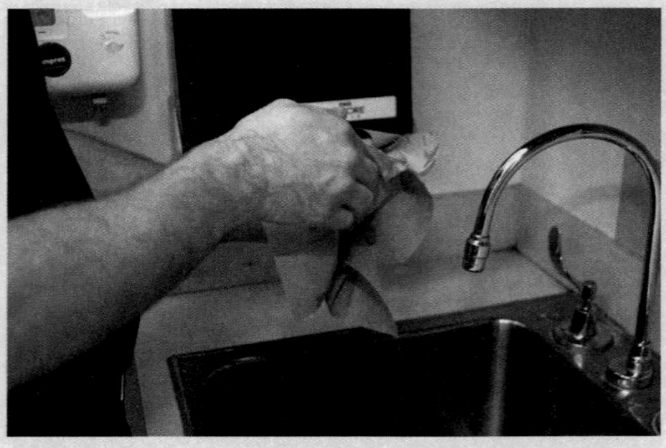

Step 1

Apply soap to hands. Rub hands together for at least 15 seconds to work up a lather. Pay particular attention to your fingernails. Rinse both hands using warm water.

Step 2

Dry your hands with a paper towel and use the paper towel to turn off the faucet.

When you wash your hands, wash them vigorously with antimicrobial foam or gel for at least 20 seconds before rinsing with clean water.[17,18] Wash your hands routinely and often. Turn handwashing into a habit. Habits are reliable, even when you are stressed.

Follow the steps shown in **SKILL DRILL 2-2** for proper handwashing.[17,18]

Use Hand Lotion

When you engage in frequent handwashing, your hands may begin cracking because natural oils are also washed off your skin during this process. Use hand lotion several times per day, both on and off duty. Your skin is a very effective barrier to pathogens, as long as it has not been breached by the drying effects of frequent washing.

Use Eye Protection

Many seasoned paramedics make it their standard practice to wear anti-splash eyewear throughout any patient contact. That is a good idea. Eye protection is an absolute necessity during suctioning or intubation procedures. In fact, during intubation, a face shield may offer better protection. Prescription eyeglasses do not offer the same level of protection; use goggles or shields to cover them.

Wear a Mask

If anyone on scene shows signs of an airborne disease, then protect yourself with a surgical mask at a minimum. A surgical mask protects against additional infections during a weakened state. If you are sick (eg, fever, GI symptoms, cough), then stay at home; this step is the best prevention to avoid illness. In particular, you should not respond to calls involving patients with compromised immune systems when you are sick.

Protect Your Body

Masks and gowns are appropriate whenever you care for an extremely messy or bloody patient **FIGURE 2-9**. A 30-gallon (114-L) trash bag can be used as a two-armed glove to slide a patient from a couch or bed onto an ambulance cot if the patient is covered with feces, urine, or blood. After the

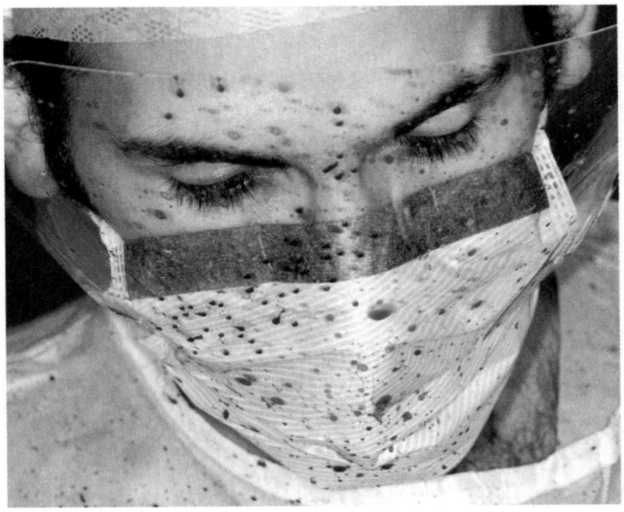

FIGURE 2-9 You must always protect yourself from contact with any type of body fluids.

© Dr. P. Marazzi/Photo Researchers, Inc..

Words of Wisdom

Aerosol-generating procedures (AGPs) are treatments that increase the risk for transmission of infections that are spread through the air or by droplets. During an AGP, small particles and droplets from the patient's respiratory tract become airborne. Nearby EMS providers who are not wearing appropriate PPE can inhale those particles or droplets or get them into their eyes or mouth, thereby exposing them to viruses or bacteria. When a patient has an infectious respiratory disease or in situations of community spread of communicable diseases, AGPs pose a high risk for caregivers. Examples of AGPs include CPR and some basic and advanced airway procedures.

patient has been moved, you can simply turn the bag inside-out, squeeze the air out of it, tie a knot in its open end, and place it in a hazardous materials (hazmat) bag.

Incontinence barriers should be laid out on a surface if the patient is leaking any type of fluid or has skin lesions.

N95 or N100 Respirators

Read some of the recent statistics on TB and you will quickly realize this is one of the most common diseases contracted around the world. According

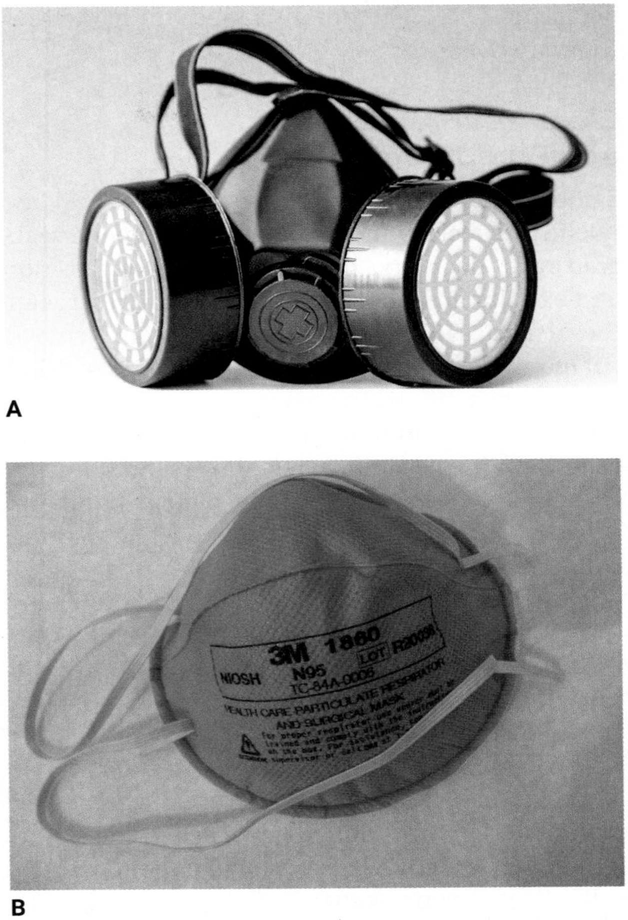

FIGURE 2-10 Specially designed respirator masks, such as an N95 or N100 respirator, protect against infection from tuberculosis bacteria and coronavirus. **A.** High-efficiency particulate air (HEPA) mask with filter canisters. **B.** N95 masks.

A: © science photo/Shutterstock; B: © The Venusian One/Shutterstock.

to World Health Organization estimates, there were 10 million new cases of this disease in 2019, and 1.4 million deaths from TB.[19] The risk posed by contact with the TB bacillus makes it that much more important to wear an N95 or N100 respirator **FIGURE 2-10** and not just a simple surgical mask. These respirators often require fit testing, which may be offered at your service.

When the COVID-19 pandemic hit the world in 2020, the need to use N95 and N100 respirators became even more urgent. The lessons from this pandemic for the entire health care community are only now being fully digested, but they will have a lasting effect on how we interact with patients and the community for years to come. More specific details on COVID-19 are discussed in Chapter 27, *Infectious Diseases.*

Clean Your Ambulance and Equipment

Sanitize your patient compartment surfaces frequently, especially the ambulance cot, bench seat, grab rails, deck and deck hardware, and interior and exterior areas around the door handles. Clean these surfaces daily and after every call. Remove cot mounts at least once per week to get rid of dried blood and vomit, which tend to accumulate there. Clean this area more often if you have had messy calls. Routinely sanitize telephones and microphones, especially ones in the patient compartment, which you may have handled while wearing contaminated gloves.

Sanitize or replace your pen often. You typically handle it several times during every call, with your gloves on. Then, you handle it after the call, after you have washed your hands. Do not put your pen in your mouth! Likewise, sanitize your stethoscope with alcohol or disinfectant wipes after *every* call. Many agencies have started using ultraviolet light to sanitize pens, cell phones, and other items potentially exposed to patients during calls. Follow your agency policies with any specialty procedures.

Discard any piece of equipment that is intended for single use in an appropriate hazmat bag (per your service exposure control plan). For any reusable piece of equipment that has had direct contact with the patient or the patient's body fluids, use a commercial disinfecting agent for decontamination. You can also use bleach diluted in water (1:10) as a disinfecting agent. Disinfection will kill many microorganisms on the surface of your equipment. But be aware of the type of disinfecting agent you use: Not all disinfectants can be used on every surface, and some are harmful if they come in contact with your skin. Depending on the agent, you may need to keep the surface wet with the disinfectant for 5 minutes or more to ensure adequate decontamination.

Properly Dispose of Sharps

Disposal containers (large for the ambulance and small for carry-in gear) for sharps, such as needles and blades, are essential to protect crews against needlesticks or cuts **FIGURE 2-11**.

FIGURE 2-11 Any needles or blades must be disposed of in a sharps container.

Wear Appropriate Turnout Gear for the Situation

Turnout (or bunker) gear is a fire service term for protective clothing designed for structural firefighting environments. Turnout gear provides some protection by using different layers of fabric or other material to protect from the heat of a fire, to reduce trauma from impact or cuts, and to keep water away from the body. Like most protective clothing, however, turnout gear adds weight and reduces the wearer's range of motion to some degree. Also, turnout gear is hard to clean, so you should avoid using it in situations that will likely expose you to a patient's blood or body fluids.

The exterior fabrics of turnout gear provide increased protection from cuts and abrasions. They also act as a barrier against high external temperatures. In cold weather, an insulated thermal inner layer of material that helps retain body heat is recommended.

Turnout gear or a bunker jacket provides minimal protection from electrical shock, but it does protect you from heat, fire, possible flashover, and flying sparks. The jacket's front opening should be fastened, and the jacket should be worn with the collar up and closed in front to protect your neck

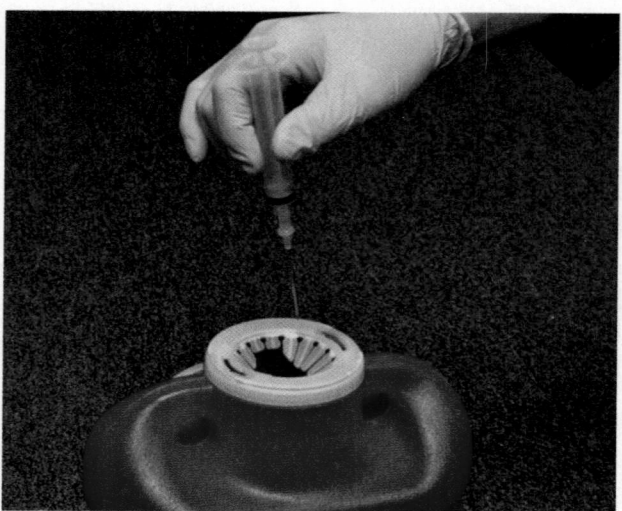

SAFETY

The American National Standards Institute (ANSI) requires that all EMS providers use an approved high-visibility public safety vest while on or near the roadway.

and the upper part of your chest. Proper fit is essential so that you can move freely.

Gloves, Helmets, and Boots

Firefighting gloves provide the best protection from heat, cold, and cuts, but they also reduce manual dexterity. In addition, firefighting gloves will not protect you from electrical hazards. In rescue situations, you must be able to use your hands freely to operate rescue tools, provide patient care, and perform other duties. Puncture-proof leather gloves, with latex gloves underneath, will permit free use of your hands while also offering added protection from injury and body fluids.

You should wear a helmet anytime you are working in a fall zone. A fall zone is an area where you are likely to encounter falling objects. The helmet should provide top and side impact protection. It should also have a secure chin strap. Objects will often fall one after another: If the strap is not secure, the first falling object may knock off your helmet, leaving your head unprotected as the remaining objects fall.

Construction-type helmets are not well suited for rescue situations. They offer minimal impact protection and have inadequate chin straps. Modern fire helmets afford the best thermal and impact protection.

You can lose a significant amount of body heat in cold weather if you are not wearing a hat or helmet. An insulated hat made from wool or synthetic material can be pulled down over the face and the base of the skull to reduce heat loss in extremely cold weather.

In situations that may involve an electrical hazard, you should always wear a helmet with a chin strap and face shield. The shell of the helmet should be made of a certified electrical nonconductor. The chin strap should not stretch, but rather should fasten securely so that the helmet will stay in place if you are knocked down or a power line hits your head. You should also be able to lock the face shield on the helmet; this will protect your face and eyes from power lines and flying sparks. A standard fire turnout helmet should meet all of these needs.

Boots should be water resistant, well fitting, and flexible so that you can walk long distances comfortably. If you will be working outdoors, you should choose boots that cover and protect your ankles, while keeping out stones, debris, and snow. Steel-toed boots are preferred. In cold weather, your boots must also protect you from the cold. Leather is one of the best materials for boots. However, boots made of other materials, such as waterproof, windproof, and breathable fabrics, are also very good choices. The soles of your boots must provide traction. Lug-type soles may grip well in snow, but they become very slippery when caked with mud.

Properly fitted boots and shoes are extremely important because a minor annoyance can become a disabling injury if it continues over time. You may develop painful blisters if your feet slip around inside your boots. However, make sure you have enough room to wiggle your toes.

Boots should be puncture-resistant, protect the toes, and provide foot and ankle support. It may be challenging to obtain a good fit with firefighting boots; shoe inserts or sock layering may be needed to ensure a comfortable fit. Make sure the tops of your boots are sealed off to prevent the entry of rain, snow, glass, or other materials. Moisture increases blistering—wool or wicking socks help prevent feet from becoming wet.

Socks will keep your feet warm and provide some cushioning for you as you walk. In cold weather, two pairs of socks are generally preferable to one thick pair. A thin sock next to the foot helps to wick perspiration away to a thicker, outer sock. This tends to keep your feet warmer, drier, and generally more comfortable. Keep these points in mind when purchasing new shoes or boots.

Eye, Ear, and Skin Protection

The human eye is fragile, and permanent loss of sight can occur from even very minor injuries. As a paramedic, you will need to protect your eyes from blood and other body fluids, foreign objects, plants, insects, and debris from extrication. You may wear eyeglasses with side shields during routine patient care. In contrast, when tools are being used during extrication, you should wear a face shield or goggles. In these instances, prescription eyeglasses do not provide adequate protection.

In snow or white sand, particularly at higher altitudes, you must also protect your eyes from ultraviolet exposure. Specially designed eyeglasses or goggles can provide this protection. In addition, your eye protection must be adaptable to the weather and the physical demands of the task. It is crucial that you have clear vision at all times.

Exposure to loud noises for long periods can cause permanent hearing loss. Specific equipment, such as helicopters, some extrication tools, and sirens, produce high noise levels. Wearing soft foam industrial-type earplugs usually provides adequate protection.

Your skin needs protection against sunburn while you are working outdoors. Long-term exposure to the sun increases the possibility of skin cancer. It might be considered an annoyance, but sunburn is a type of thermal burn. In reflective areas such as sand, water, and snow, your risk of sunburn increases. Protect your skin by applying sunscreen with a minimum sun protection factor (SPF) of 15.

Body Armor

Although you are trained to avoid any situation that may involve violence, scenes are dynamic, and a situation that appears safe initially may quickly deteriorate and become dangerous. For this reason, EMS responders sometimes wear ballistic-resistant or stab-resistant armor for personal protection.

SAFETY

Remember, ballistic protection is not fail-proof and has the potential to provide a sense of false security.

The National Institute of Justice (NIJ) has developed a scale that identifies the global minimum for performance requirements and testing methods for personal body armor.[20] The resulting score, known as the NIJ threat level, can be found on the product's label, along with an expiration date. There are five general classifications of protection, ranging from extremely lightweight and flexible to heavy and bulky **TABLE 2-2**.[20] The lighter vests do not stop large-caliber bullets, but they offer more flexibility and are preferred by most EMS and law enforcement personnel. Such vests are commonly worn under a uniform shirt or jacket. The larger, heavier vests are worn outside of your uniform and may be bulky and difficult to wear in hot temperatures and high humidity. They are also costly and require replacement at various intervals.

TABLE 2-2 National Institute of Justice Threat Levels

Threat Level	Protection Offered
Type IIA	Higher-velocity and mass ammunition. Examples: 9 mm and .40 Smith & Wesson.
Type II	High-velocity ammunition and rounds that travel up to 1,400 feet/second. Examples: 9 mm and .357 Magnum.
Type IIIA	Better protection from jacketed hollow-point rounds. Examples: .44 Magnum and high-velocity 9 mm.
Type III	Often used in tactical situations. Examples: Protection from rifles and other high-velocity rounds.
Type IV	Highest protection level made with heavy ceramic plates. Example: Armor-piercing bullets.

Data from: National Institute of Justice. Ballistic Resistance of Body Armor, NIJ Standard 0101.06. https://www.ncjrs.gov/pdffiles1/nij/223054.pdf#page=17. Published July 2008. Accessed December 30, 2020.

While body armor may protect the wearer's underlying organs from penetrating injury, the blunt force trauma may still be significant, especially from high-powered gunfire rounds. Vests also offer little or no protection from fragments that are generated during an explosion or against stabbing attacks. While body armor may not be practical in all circumstances, it still offers a measure of protection that is better than nothing at all.

Familiarize yourself with the type of body armor used by your department, and remember that scene safety is always your first concern. Body armor is used for additional protection; it does not take the place of surveying the scene and avoiding dangerous conditions. Like all EMS equipment, training should be done while wearing your vest to ensure ease of use in real-life situations.

Hostile Situations

As a paramedic, you may be involved with or asked to assist during hostile situations. Potential hostile situations can often be identified using dispatch information, such as a report that "The patient is uncooperative" or "The patient is making verbal threats." In 2003, the National Association of EMS Physicians released a position statement that, for the first time, offered an official endorsement of *rights to safety* not only of patients but also of EMS providers.

Street Smarts

Some of the most dangerous calls are those with limited or vague information. If a 9-1-1 caller refuses to give a dispatcher adequate information, then the dispatcher should communicate that fact to you. Ensure law enforcement has been dispatched or request law enforcement to respond to the scene first or with you to ascertain safety.

If you must respond to a hostile situation, then it is best to stage a safe distance away and wait for law enforcement to secure the scene. Specifically, be wary of any call dispatched as a fight, stabbing, shooting, possible rioting, domestic disturbance, "person down," or "unknown medical aid." Every one of these calls is suspicious and warrants an initial response by police. In addition, you should request law enforcement to any call that your gut instincts suggest could be violent.

You must seek any necessary training to help you understand how to handle hostile situations safely. Numerous resources are available, including Tactical Emergency Medical Services or Rescue Task Force programs. Many law enforcement agencies have used these courses to develop their own systems tailored to their regions. If you will be routinely involved in hostile situations, then your EMS agency should first work with your local law enforcement agencies to identify needs, and then fill those needs, preferably based on their recommendations.

Never enter the scene first if the element of hostility is known or can be anticipated in advance. Discipline yourself to scrutinize all information that comes to you from others, and keep yourself on "yellow alert" whenever you are on duty.

Words of Wisdom

In some cases, emergency responders might be the direct target of violence. The rate of violence-related injuries with work loss for emergency responders is 22 times higher than the overall rate for other employees in the United States.[21] Ensuring health and wellness in the face of violence against EMS providers demands prevention strategies and protection strategies.

Recommendations for prevention of violence include the following:

- Training and practice in identifying scenes of potential violence
- Training and practice in de-escalation strategies and techniques
- Training and practice to improve interpersonal communications
- Practice in ongoing scene assessment
- Dispatch identification and alerting of past or potential threats of violence

Recommendations for protection against violence include the following:

- Training and practice in self-defense and escape techniques
- Training and practice in physical and chemical restraint techniques
- Fitting and use of body armor
- Training and practice in operations with law enforcement personnel

If you experience physical or verbal violence, report it on the appropriate incident form. Follow your state laws and department policies to report instances of physical assault.

Remember, waiting for law enforcement to arrive does not make you an uncaring provider. If you get hurt, then you will be unable to help other patients.

Before you come in contact with a hostile patient, carefully review your surroundings. First identify the fastest way to exit the area (egress plan), then look for potential weapons in the general area and within reach of the patient. After you make contact with a hostile patient, listen more than you talk, and do not argue with or ridicule the patient. Concentrate on de-escalating the patient's emotions. Many hostile patients who start out unwilling to go to the hospital will agree to transport as a result of your patience, tactful reasoning, and reassurance. Show empathy and understanding on the scene and you will earn the trust of your patients.

Remember that whenever you are on someone else's turf, that individual has a clear advantage. You can expect the person to know everything about the environment while you know nothing (including the location of any weapons). Hostile patients in their home environments are much more dangerous there than anywhere else, especially in poor lighting.

Words of Wisdom

If you are the first unit to arrive on the scene, then perform a scene size-up and notify other responding units of any actual or potential hazards that may be present. Your first job is to ensure your safety as well as the safety of your crew and any bystanders.

Street Smarts

Knowledge of diverse cultures plays a significant role in effective communication. The more you know about the people you serve, the more likely you will know their customs and expectations. Be diligent in your pursuit of treating all patients with respect and dignity, putting your personal prejudices aside. By doing so, you can potentially lessen the stress of the emergency situation.

Traffic Incidents

Regardless of where you live or work, motor vehicles may move at high speeds, may carry hazardous substances, and may collide with one another in locations that are dangerous for you and all involved. It is essential to stay aware of your surroundings, including the familiar ones you see day in and day out. With the widespread use of various technologies in motor vehicles (eg, smartphones and global positioning systems), distracted driving is becoming as problematic as driving under the influence of drugs or alcohol. At many scenes, bystanders or other motorists want to see, or use their phone to record, what the action is all about. While focusing intently on a traffic incident, they may not pay attention to you; therefore, you always need to be aware of other vehicles and onlookers.

Begin making physical observations a mile or so before you approach the scene of a traffic incident. Watch the traffic, pay attention to the wind direction, look for smoke, and begin planning for lighting and weather-related issues. As you get closer, note the kinds of vehicles and obstacles involved. If traffic is not yet handled, then determine how traffic flow is moving and how to control it initially. Important considerations include the following: How big an incident do you have, both in size and scope? Are you dealing with commercial carriers of industrial products? What resources will you need immediately? What is the topography? Where will leaking fluids drain naturally (if evident)? Where do you eventually want to park the ambulance? What will your working space be?

As at any scene, your approach at a traffic incident should include a visual assessment of your entire surroundings. Look for hazards before you enter the scene. These hazards may include downed power lines or poles, leaking fuel, and potential for fire. Becoming familiar with your response area to determine your best and safest route is critical because it also alerts those who might be available to help you with traffic control, air support, hazmat response, terrain issues, and potential destinations. Some states have programs in place that are designed to help with traffic incident management. For example, the state of Wisconsin initiated the Traffic Incident Management Enhancement (TIME) Program, which teaches all emergency responders the safest way to set up a scene and how to identify hazards. As a new paramedic, seek out any programs and resources your state or region may offer—your life could depend on it.

Traffic may be only one of the many hazards at the scene of a motor vehicle crash **FIGURE 2-12**. For example, parking a hot, running ambulance over dry grass may initiate a grass or vehicle fire. Remember, your primary concern at any scene is safety for yourself as well as for those around you. Identify as many hazards as possible while you drive up and before leaving your unit.

Words of Wisdom

Scene safety begins with preparation. As you and your partner or crew prepare to respond to the scene, make sure you fasten your seat belts and shoulder harnesses before you move the ambulance.

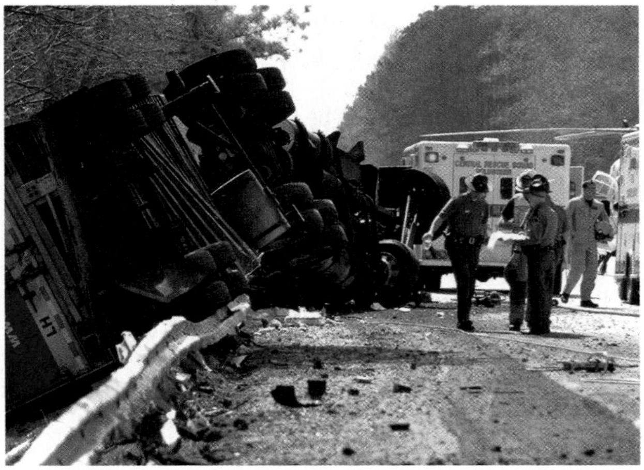

FIGURE 2-12 It is crucial to place your vehicle in a safe, visible location from which you can easily exit and one that is not too close to potential hazards to minimize the risk of any additional incidents at a busy crash scene.

Words of Wisdom

The safe operation of emergency vehicles is an integral part of any EMS provider's job. Principles of properly and safely operating an emergency vehicle include judicious use of lights and siren, proceeding cautiously through intersections, always remaining calm, and never assuming that other drivers will yield. These and other principles are covered in greater detail in Chapter 47, *Transport Operations*.

Driving with lights and siren *does not* authorize you to ignore due regard for other motorists on the roadway or to drive at excessive speeds. Remember that ambulances do not handle like smaller, lighter motor vehicles. They require significantly more time and distance to stop, and you can more easily lose control of an ambulance. Most states have specific rules or statutes about using lights and siren, which are your responsibility to know.

Power Lines and Lightning Hazards

You should never touch downed power lines. Dealing with power lines is beyond the scope of paramedic training. However, you should mark off a danger zone around such lines. Energized ("live") power lines, especially high-voltage lines, behave in unpredictable ways. You need in-depth training to be able to handle the equipment used in an electrical emergency. This equipment also has specific storage needs and requires careful cleaning. Dirt or other contaminants can make this equipment useless or dangerous.

At the scene of a motor vehicle collision (MVC), above-ground and below-ground power lines may become hazards. Disrupted overhead wires may or may not be a visible hazard. You must be careful even if you do not see sparks coming from lines. Visible sparks are not always present in charged wires. The area around downed power lines is always a danger zone, and this danger zone extends well beyond the immediate accident scene.

Use utility poles as landmarks for establishing the perimeter of the danger zone. The danger zone must be a restricted area. Remember, the safety zone is generally one span of the power pole's distance. Only emergency personnel, equipment, and vehicles are allowed inside this area.

Do not approach downed wires or touch anything that downed wires have come in contact with until qualified personnel have concluded that no risk of electrical injury exists. This may mean that you cannot access a severely injured victim of an MVC even though you can see and talk to the patient.

Lightning is a complex natural phenomenon. It is not true that "lightning never strikes in the same place twice." If the right conditions remain present, a repeated strike in the same area can occur.

Lightning is a threat in two ways: through a direct hit and through ground current. After a lightning bolt strikes, current moves along the earth, following the most conductive pathway. To avoid being injured by a ground current, stay away from drainage ditches, moist areas, small depressions, and wet ropes. If you are involved in a rescue operation, you may need to delay it until the storm has passed. Recognize the warning signs just before a lightning strike. As your surroundings become charged, you may feel a slight tingling sensation on your skin, or your hair may even stand on end. In this situation, a strike may be imminent. Move immediately to the lowest possible area.

If you are caught in an open area, try to make yourself the smallest possible target for a direct hit or for ground current. To keep from being hit by the initial strike, stay away from ground projections, such as a single tree. Drop all equipment, particularly metal objects that project above your body. Avoid fences and other metal objects, as they can transmit current from the initial strike over a long distance. Distance yourself from other people, and position yourself in a low crouch, which exposes only your feet to the ground current. By comparison, if you sit, both your feet and your buttocks are exposed. Place an object made of nonconductive material, such as a blanket, under your feet. Get inside a vehicle or your unit, if possible, as vehicles will protect you from lightning.

SAFETY

Recognize the warning signs before a lightning strike. If you feel a tingling sensation on your skin or your hair stands on end, move immediately to a low-lying area. If you are caught in an open area, make yourself as small a target as possible.

Stress

As discussed previously, EMS is a high-stress job. Understanding the causes of stress and knowing how to deal with stress is crucial to your job performance, health, and interpersonal relationships. To prevent stress from negatively affecting your life, you need to understand what stress is, how its physiologic effects unfold, what you can do to minimize these effects, and how to deal with stress on an emotional level.

Any event that causes you to react physically, emotionally, or mentally is considered **stress**. Stress events may be pleasant, unpleasant, mild, or intense. Hans Selye, MD, PhD, considered the "father of stress theory," defined biologic stress as the "nonspecific response of the body to any demand made upon it."[22]

Words of Wisdom

As a paramedic, you may be led to believe that showing emotion is a sign of weakness. In reality, showing appropriate emotions in certain situations can help a grieving family or patient. Everyone reacts differently to stressful events. Some people may get angry, whereas others may laugh or be silent. Do not assume that people are not affected by stress because they do not react in a way you feel they should.

Stress is a bodily reaction to any agent or situation (**stressor**) that requires a person to adapt. Adaptation is necessary for meeting the demands of everyday life. By itself, stress is neither a good thing nor a bad thing, nor should stress be avoided at all costs. Selye classified stress into two categories: eustress (positive stress), the kind of stress that motivates a person to achieve; and distress (negative stress), the stress that a person finds overwhelming and debilitating **FIGURE 2-13**.

What Triggers Stress

A stress response often begins with events that are perceived as threatening or demanding, but the specific events that trigger this reaction vary enormously from person to person. The following factors are the most common stress triggers in most people:

- Loss of a loved one (eg, death of a spouse, family member, close friend, or colleague) or of a valued possession
- Personal injury or illness

YOU are the Paramedic

PART 3

Your partner attaches the cardiac monitor to the patient, and you note asystole in two leads. As you were lifting the patient's shirt for your partner to attach the electrodes, you also noticed some lividity. Family members are starting to arrive. The patient's mother is becoming hysterical and asks you to do something. She tells you her son cannot be dead because she asked God to give him just a few more months. Your partner steps outside to call the dispatcher, law enforcement, and the coroner, and leaves you to talk with the family.

5. How will you explain the situation to the family, and what is your responsibility to them?
6. Which stage of the grieving process is the patient's mother exhibiting?

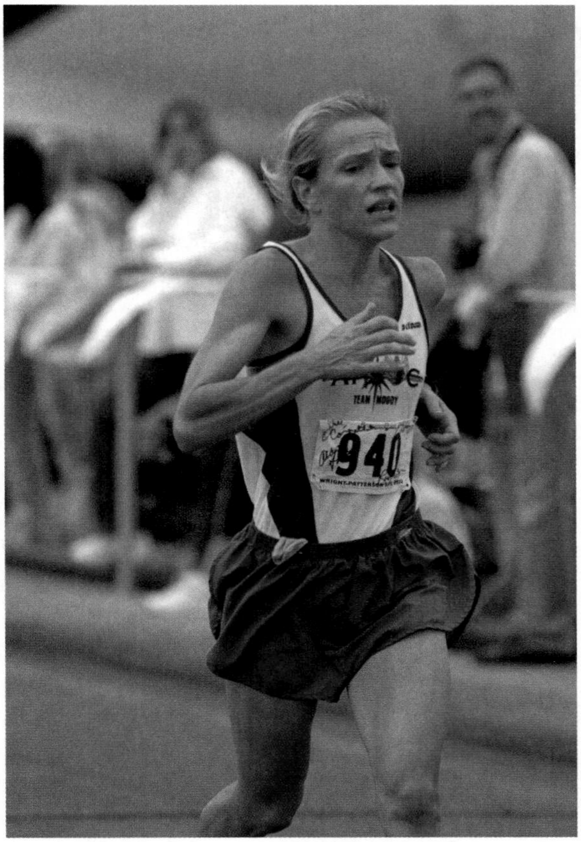

FIGURE 2-13 Positive stress (eustress) can push you to greater achievements.

Courtesy of Island Photography/US Air Force.

- A major life event (eg, starting or finishing school, marriage, divorce, pregnancy, or having children leave home)
- Job-related stress (eg, conflicts with others, excessive responsibility, the possibility of losing a job, or changing a job)

During the past 4 decades, several studies have assessed psychological stress levels in paramedics. The studies that seek to evaluate stress levels and compare them usually examine life-change units (LCUs). These LCUs were originally described by Adolf Meyer and further explored by researchers Thomas Holmes and Richard Rahe.[23] These researchers used the "Social Readjustment Rating Scale," which ranks 43 stress-producing events in a person's life and provides a weighted score for each event **TABLE 2-3**.[23] They predicted that a score greater than 150 LCU could cause or be associated with the development of disease and illness (eg, heart attack, stroke).[23]

To deal effectively with stress, as a paramedic, you need to make a personal appraisal of stress triggers in your life and take or plan appropriate actions to minimize their effects.

SAFETY

Human errors often occur in the context of a poorly designed system. For example, lapses in human tasks may occur secondary to long work hours, and predictable mistakes occur when inexperienced staff members face complex cognitive decisions. Instead of punishing a paramedic, the systems approach to EMS seeks to identify the situations that give rise to human error and change the underlying problem.

Physiology of Acute Stress

One fundamental model for stress evolved from studies of how humans respond to threats. It was observed that when a person perceived an event as threatening, the same set of physiologic reactions was triggered, whatever the threat (this is why Selye referred to stress as a "nonspecific" response).

Typically, these physiologic reactions prepare the body for the fight-or-flight response by activating the sympathetic nervous system. The fight-or-flight response was a beneficial survival mechanism for early humans, mobilizing a person to either defend (fight) or to run away (flight) in the face of possible danger. In today's world, however, an automatic fight-or-flight response to stressful circumstances is not as helpful as it was once thought to be. Most stressors that you face today should not be solved by fighting or running away. In fact, most negative stress responses result from an accumulation of smaller stress events, thereby placing the body in a continuous, unrelieved state of alert. Chronic exhaustion and ill health can result. To avoid these unwanted outcomes, you should evaluate and handle every stress event immediately, especially if it is negative in nature. Running away or ignoring the problem will not make it go away. These physiologic reactions are discussed further in Chapter 8, *Anatomy and Physiology*.

Reactions to stress can be categorized as acute, delayed, or cumulative. An **acute stress reaction** occurs during a stressful situation. As a paramedic, you may feel nervous and excited, and your ability

TABLE 2-3 Social Readjustment Rating Scale

Rank	Life Event	LCU	Rank	Life Event	LCU
1	Death of a spouse	100	23	Son or daughter leaving home	29
2	Divorce	73	24	Trouble with in-laws	29
3	Marital separation	65	25	Outstanding personal achievement	28
4	Jail term	63	26	Spouse begins or stops work	26
5	Death of close family member	63	27	Begin or end school	26
6	Personal injury or illness	53	28	Change in living conditions	25
7	Marriage	50	29	Revision of personal habits	24
8	Fired at work	47	30	Trouble with boss	23
9	Marital reconciliation	45	31	Change in work hours or conditions	20
10	Retirement	45	32	Change in residence	20
11	Change in health of family member	44	33	Change in schools	20
12	Pregnancy	40	34	Change in recreation	19
13	Sexual dysfunction	39	35	Change in church activities	19
14	Gain of new family member	39	36	Change in social activities	19
15	Business readjustment	39	37	Small loan, such as for a household appliance or vehicle	17
16	Change in financial status	38	38	Change in sleeping habits	16
17	Death of close friend	37	39	Change in number of family get-togethers	15
18	Change to different line of work	36	40	Change in eating habits	13
19	Change in number of arguments with spouse	35	41	Vacation	13
20	Large loan, such as a home mortgage	31	42	Christmas	12
21	Foreclosure of mortgage or loan	30	43	Minor violation of the law	11
22	Change in responsibilities at work	29			

Check off those events that currently apply to your life and add up the corresponding points. A score less than 150 is thought to be within the range of normal stress. A score between 150 and 199 suggests a mild stress; between 200 and 299 points suggests a moderate stress; and greater than 300 points is indicative of a major stress.

Abbreviation: LCU, life-change unit.

Reprinted from *Journal of Psychosomatic Research*, vol. II, T. H. Holmes and R. Rahe, "The Social Readjustment Rating Scale," pp. 213–218. Copyright 1967, with permission from Elsevier.

to focus may increase. If the stress of the situation becomes too great, however, then you may experience negative emotional and physical reactions.

A **delayed stress reaction** manifests after the stressful event. During a crisis, you will be able to focus and function, but afterward, you may be left with nervous, excited energy that continues to build. As a new paramedic, you must identify events that may cause a delayed stress reaction in you and learn stress management techniques to improve your ability to effectively manage stress when it occurs.

Cumulative stress reactions can occur when you are exposed to prolonged or excessive stress. After the stressful event is over, you may be unable to shake off its effects, even with the aid of stress management techniques. Inevitably, another stressful situation occurs, and then another. Each time, you may find it harder to recover from an event, and you may become exhausted and overwhelmed. Cumulative stress can result in physical symptoms, which are your body's way of saying there is a problem. These symptoms often include fatigue, changes in appetite, GI problems, or headaches. Stress may also cause insomnia or hypersomnia, irritability, inability to concentrate, and hyperactivity or underactivity. In addition, stress may manifest itself through psychological reactions such as fear, dull or nonresponsive behavior, depression, oversensitivity, anger, irritability, frustration, isolation, inability to concentrate, alcohol or drug abuse, and loss of interest in work or sexual activity. Your fast-paced lifestyle as a paramedic may compound these effects by not allowing you to rest and recover fully after periods of stress. Prolonged or excessive stress has been shown to be a strong contributor to heart disease, hypertension, cancer, and depression.[24] Moreover, cumulative stress can eventually lead to job burnout, a topic discussed later in this chapter.

Words of Wisdom

Learn to look for or recognize signs of stress in yourself, your coworkers, and your patients. Early discovery can often allow you to practice techniques to prevent stress from worsening.

How People React to Stressful Situations

Anyone—the patient, the family, bystanders, or health care professionals—who confronts critical illness or injury responds in some way to the stresses of each emergency.

Responses of Patients to Illness and Injury

Patients' responses to emergencies are determined by their personal methods of adapting to stress. As a paramedic, it will help you to recognize certain common patterns of coping. A response shown by many patients is anxiety. Some people will exhibit their anxiety by denying it; others may become irritable or angry and perhaps direct this hostility toward you. Do not take such behavior personally. Remaining calm and reassuring is one of the best de-escalation techniques. Be aware that common reactions to illness and injury include the following:

- **Fear.** Patients may have realistic fears, such as fear of pain, disability, or death (or fear of their economic effects). Patients may also fear the actions you need to take to care for them, such as using needles to start an IV line or give medications.
- **Depression.** Depression is a natural response to loss. A patient who has experienced a stroke, for example, may have lost the ability to move an arm or leg on one side of the body and even the ability to speak, but can understand everything you say and do. Depression may also be evident when you are on a scene where you have just ceased efforts to resuscitate a loved one.
- **Anxiety.** Patients may exhibit diffuse anxiety, a feeling of helplessness or a loss of control. People whose self-esteem depends on being active, independent, and aggressive are particularly vulnerable to anxiety when they become ill or injured. At times, anxiety may appear similar to anger; you must recognize the difference. Incorrectly identifying someone as angry may put you in a defensive position and prevent you from addressing the patient's anxiety and individual care needs.
- **Anger.** Anger is a challenging problem for many EMS providers to deal with **FIGURE 2-14**. You may have a natural tendency to think, "I am trying to help this person, so why is he taking it out on me?" It is crucial to remember that some patients respond to fear, discomfort, or limitation of function by becoming angry, and their extreme reactions are not your fault or that of your team.
- **Confusion.** Confusion can occur with anyone but is more common among older patients, in whom illness or injury frequently causes disorientation. Confusion may be exacerbated by the presence of unfamiliar people and equipment, which may seem overwhelming to the

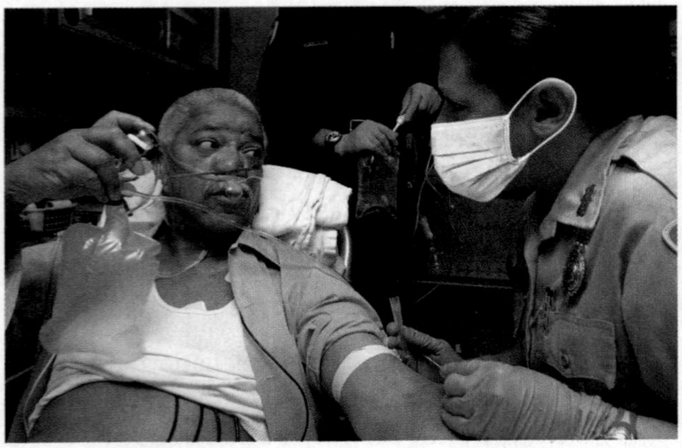

FIGURE 2-14 The sudden loss of control a patient feels when being treated during an emergency can lead to unexpected and sometimes extreme reactions.

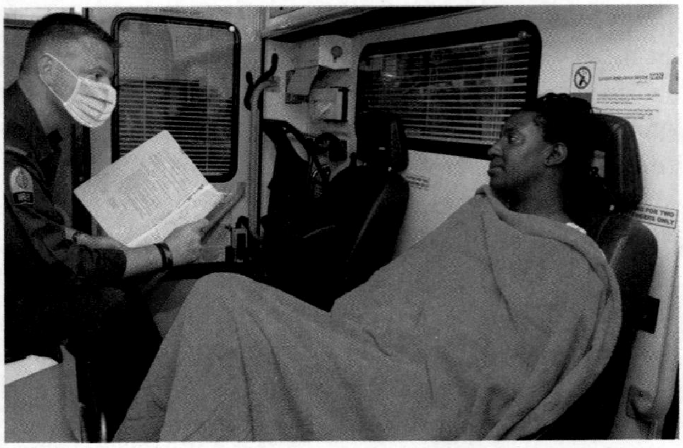

FIGURE 2-15 Particularly when serving people whose backgrounds are different from your own, you must always maintain an open, nonjudgmental attitude.

patient. If a patient appears confused, it is essential to explain carefully at the outset who you are and what you plan to do. Allow the patient enough time (within reason) to gather their thoughts and become comfortable with the situation.

In addition to experiencing the reactions just described, some patients may show one or more of the following psychological **defense mechanisms**:

- **Denial**. Patients often ignore or diminish the seriousness of an emergency situation. Some patients may downplay their symptoms with words such as "only" or "a little," whereas others may dismiss their symptoms altogether, only to describe them to hospital staff after arrival at the ED. You may have to seek out other sources to obtain reliable information in these cases.
- **Regression**. Regression is a return to an earlier age level of behavior or emotional adjustment. Children often exhibit this defense mechanism when under stress because of fear of "getting in trouble." Adults may also revert to childlike behaviors when under stress. Patients with other psychological disorders may exhibit regression as part of their normal responses.
- **Projection**. Projection is attributing personal (sometimes unacceptable) feelings, motives, desires, or behavior to others. Patients who express vehement indignation or anger may unconsciously be denying their own "bad" behavior by attributing it to other people.
- **Displacement**. Displacement occurs when someone redirects an emotion from the original cause of emotion (eg, a cardiac condition) to a more immediate substitute (eg, a paramedic). Displacement is often the operative mechanism when patients express anger toward you, but in reality are angry at someone else—themselves, a family member, fate, or just the situation.

As noted, most psychological stress responses are not under your patients' conscious control. It is common for ill or injured patients to respond angrily toward EMS providers, only to forget about it after the situation has passed.

Often, reactions to illness or injury are rooted in the patient's culture. Modern society is becoming more multicultural, and people of some cultures may openly exhibit behaviors that might be considered inappropriate in another culture. You need to respect every patient's cultural background. Never attempt to change someone's behavior just because it is different from your own.

Many Americans place great emphasis on making eye contact, having a firm handshake, and respecting personal space. Some patients may not make eye contact because their culture believes that lowered eyes show deference to your authority and uniform. When making physical contact, obtain permission to do so, if possible, beforehand. Identify and understand the cultural characteristics of the populations you serve **FIGURE 2-15**.

Special Populations

When children are seriously ill or injured, family members and other people at the scene may become frantic. You need to remain calm and confident in your skills; that may be all that is needed to provide reassurance to everyone at the scene. Children will often respond better to people who are calm, even if their illnesses or injuries are significant.

Responses of Family, Friends, and Bystanders

Bystanders and family members may exhibit responses that are similar to those shown by patients. Family members may be anxious, panicky, or angry, especially if they are struggling with guilt. Consciously or unconsciously, family members may feel responsible for what has happened. For instance, they may believe that if they had kept a closer eye on a child, they would not have run out into the street and become injured. Some family members may insist that you do something differently or act more quickly during an emergency.

As a paramedic, you must recognize that the patient's family and friends have concerns, too, and that their behavior, however unpleasant, results from distress. Do not take it personally, and remain calm. Reassure family members that you are doing everything you can and that you have physician guidance available at all times. You will often enter situations where everyone is under stress, and you have no guarantee that people will behave appropriately.

In a situation involving mass casualties, such as a multiple-vehicle collision, building collapse, or natural disaster (eg, a tornado, flood, or earthquake), both patients and bystanders may react by becoming dazed, disorganized, or overwhelmed. Reactions to stress are defined differently depending on the organization or resource; following are five of the most common reactions. In general, people with these reactions (including your coworkers) should be removed from the scene, but not left alone—find someone who is capable of handling them.

- **Anxiety.** Signs of anxiety include sweating, trembling, weakness, nausea, and sometimes vomiting. People experiencing this response can recover fully within a few minutes and provide helpful assistance if properly directed. You are also not immune to anxiety, so you must be able to identify this response and accept assistance as needed.
- **Blind panic.** A more worrisome reaction is **blind panic**, in which a person's judgment seems to disappear entirely. They may not fully understand the situation at hand or its dangers. Blind panic is particularly dangerous because it may cause mass panic among others present.
- **Depression.** Depression is seen in people who sit or stand in a numbed, dazed state. Depressed bystanders need to be brought back to reality as soon as possible; do not leave them to sit and dwell on the situation.
- **Overreaction.** People who overreact to stress tend to talk compulsively, joke inappropriately, become overly active, and race from one task to another without accomplishing anything useful.
- **Conversion hysteria.** In **conversion hysteria**, the patient subconsciously converts anxiety into a bodily dysfunction; they may be unable to see or hear or may become paralyzed in an extremity.

More details on how to cope with bystanders are found in Chapter 48, *Incident Management and Mass-Casualty Incidents.*

Words of Wisdom

Do not assume that seemingly nonemergency complaints are not a sign of something wrong. Tunnel vision can cause many mistakes in patient assessments and ultimately in patient outcomes.

Paramedic Responses

As a paramedic, you are not immune to the stresses of emergency situations. Expect that you will sometimes experience a multitude of feelings, not all of them pleasant. Even unpleasant feelings are natural, and although it may be difficult, you must keep control of them during an emergency or when dealing with patients and their loved ones. An attitude of outward calm and confidence on your part will do much to relieve others' anxiety at the scene, which is also part of a paramedic's therapeutic role.

One common reaction among health care professionals is a feeling of irritation at the patient who does not appear to be particularly ill or injured. Consider the possibility that people who call 9-1-1 with seemingly minor complaints are calling because the situation is an emergency in their eyes. For example, imagine a woman calls 9-1-1 because she cannot get to sleep. Her problem is that it is her first night back home after her husband's funeral. She is afraid of her first night alone in the house and did not know who else to call. Recognize that situations like these are teachable moments and take the time to educate and politely remind people that their nonemergent issue can prevent you from being available for someone who may genuinely need you.

Sometimes described as "the cost of caring," **compassion fatigue** is common among those who work in health care and disaster and emergency services. Compassion fatigue, also known as secondary stress disorder, is characterized by a gradual lessening of compassion over time. It differs from posttraumatic stress disorder, which is caused by direct exposure to a traumatic incident or series of traumatic incidents. Compassion fatigue is a reaction to caring for others who have experienced trauma. It may be characterized by the following symptoms:

- High absenteeism
- Difficult relationships with colleagues and coworkers
- Inability to work in teams
- Aggressive behavior toward patients
- Strong negative attitudes toward work
- Lack of empathy for patients
- Judgmental attitude toward patients
- Preoccupation with nonwork issues while on duty
- Other symptoms of increased stress

Supporting patients in emergency situations can be difficult. It is stressful both for them and for you. As a caring paramedic, you are vulnerable to all the stresses that go with your profession. You must recognize the signs of compassion fatigue so that it does not interfere with your work or your life away from work, including your family life. The signs and symptoms are similar to those of cumulative stress. They may not be obvious at first, but rather may be subtle and not be present all of the time.

Coping With Your Own Stress

Early warning signs of your own stress may include heart palpitations, rapid breathing, chest tightness, and sweating. You may find that you no longer enjoy your career or that you lack the energy or the desires you once had. It is important that you recognize your body's reaction to the fight-or-flight response. You may notice rapid breathing and breathlessness, unnecessary shouting, and perhaps the use of inappropriate language that you would not usually use. As discussed previously, others may notice these signs of stress and alert you to them; do not become offended because this observation can help you take appropriate and immediate action.

You can prepare for or handle stress in many different ways. Remember that once you are in fight-or-flight mode, you are primarily functioning by instinct. Consider the following stress management techniques to head off this reaction:

- **Controlled deep breathing.** Take deep breaths in through the nose and out through the mouth. Controlled deep breathing may flood the body and brain with oxygen just before activation of the fight-or-flight response and may help prevent it from engaging.
- **Progressive relaxation.** Progressive relaxation is a strategy in which you tighten and then relax specific muscle groups to initiate muscle relaxation throughout the body. This technique may be performed before, during, or after a call.
- **Professional assistance.** Even the best paramedic may not be able to handle the continuous onslaught of stressful events associated with the EMS environment. Seek out professional services such as employee assistance programs or critical incident stress management services, described later in this chapter **FIGURE 2-16**.

Other coping strategies include focusing on the immediate situation while on duty. Remind yourself, "I will do my very best, even if a situation does not turn out well."

As discussed previously, avoid excessive amounts of stimulants such as caffeine or the urge to use alcohol, cigarettes, or sleeping aids after a stressful event. Attempt to get enough natural rest. Exercise vigorously and regularly (although not

FIGURE 2-16 Consulting with a professional counselor or therapist can be a vital part of dealing with stress and maintaining your emotional well-being. Consulting a professional does not mean you are weak and unable to handle stress; every professional, including you, has a breaking point.

right before bedtime). Identify people and activities that make you laugh or feel good, or befriend a coworker who can relate to you and offer support when needed.

Burnout

Another sign of stress is job burnout. Why should you start worrying now about something that may not ever happen? You must understand that the beginning of your EMS career is the right time for you to start developing attitudes and habits to help prevent burnout.

Burnout is exhaustion of physical or emotional strength. You may find that you no longer enjoy your career or that you lack the energy or desires you once had. Burnout may be a consequence of chronic, unrelieved stress. Your job as a paramedic is full of potential stressors. Of course, EMS professionals are not the only people susceptible to burnout; it can happen to anyone, in any field. Burnout develops because of how a person reacts to stress, but it does not occur solely because of stress. EMS-related stress is often associated with interpersonal relationships, pay, prestige, fringe benefits, and other legitimate issues. The timeline for burnout varies among people; a situation that burns out one paramedic in 1 year may take 10 years to affect another paramedic, or not cause burnout at all. A paramedic who never takes a vacation may experience burnout more quickly than colleagues who do. One technique to prevent burnout is to turn off your phone or other alerting devices when off duty and make yourself unavailable from time to time.

YOU are the Paramedic

PART 4

You hold the patient's mother and tell her and the family that the patient has been down too long, that there is nothing that can be done, and that he has died. You explain that he has no cardiac activity and blood has started to pool in his body's dependent areas. The mother is hysterical and begs you to do something. You calmly repeat that there is nothing you can do and ask her if there is someone you can call to help with her grieving. You also ask if her son was a hospice patient. She tells you that they did not think it was time for that. Her 19-year-old nephew steps in and accuses you of not knowing your job. He is becoming increasingly hostile. You know that law enforcement personnel are en route, but it may be a few minutes before they arrive.

7. How should you deal with the nephew's hostility?

8. How will you deal with your own feelings and stress related to this call?

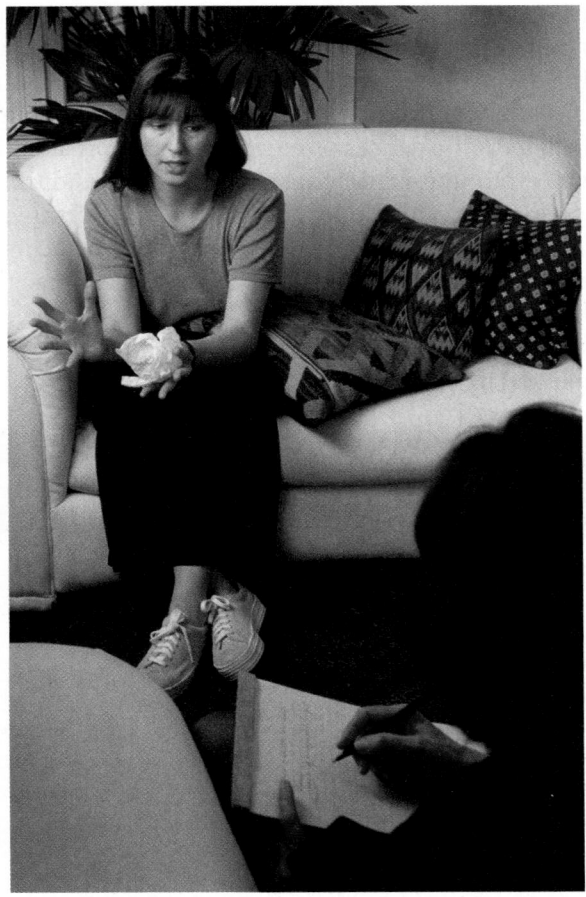

One person's eustress may be another's distress. The reason is that distress is a learned reaction based on how a person perceives and interprets the world around them. In other words, distress is nearly always the result of what a person believes. Here are some beliefs that are common among EMS personnel:

- I have to be *perfect* all the time.
- My safety depends on being able to anticipate every possible danger.
- I am totally responsible for what happens to patients; if they die, then it is my fault.
- If there is something I do not know, then people will think less of me.
- If I show emotions, then I am weak and unable to handle stress.
- A good paramedic never makes mistakes.

These are all false beliefs and can lead to burnout. Prevention and relief of stress among EMS personnel begin with recognizing that such beliefs are unrealistic and invalid.

Like many of the medical conditions you will study in this text, burnout is a type of illness and has its own signs and symptoms. These signs and symptoms may seem trivial at first, but if they are ignored, the illness grows in nature until it becomes debilitating. Symptoms of impending burnout include the following:

- Chronic fatigue and irritability
- Cynical, negative attitude
- Lack of desire to report to work
- Emotional instability (crying easily, losing your temper without provocation, laughing inappropriately)
- Changes in sleep patterns (insomnia or sleeping more than usual) and waking without feeling refreshed
- Feelings of being overwhelmed or being helpless or hopeless
- Loss of interest in hobbies
- Decreased ability to concentrate
- Declining health (having frequent colds, stomach upsets, and muscle aches and pains, especially headaches or backaches)
- Constant tightness in your muscles
- Overeating, smoking, or abusing drugs or alcohol

Some paramedics have been in the field for 20 years and show no signs of burnout, reporting to work every day with the same enthusiasm they had as a rookie. What is their secret? In general, the paramedics who do not experience burnout are those who have learned to respect and value themselves. These paramedics have also identified and dealt with the causes of burnout and taken actions to prevent it. It is truly not as easy as it sounds, but as a new paramedic, you should learn from these veterans. Practically speaking, what does it mean to respect and value yourself? How can you translate that attitude into concrete action? Some steps you can take to protect yourself from burnout are summarized in **TABLE 2-4**.

TABLE 2-4 Dr. Caroline's Guidelines for Preventing Burnout

1. Paramedic heal thyself! Take care of your own health.
   - Get enough rest.
   - Eat a balanced diet.
   - Get regular physical exercise—at least 30 minutes of aerobic activity (walking, running, or swimming) three to four times per week.
   - Do not abuse your body. Smoking, overindulgence in alcohol, taking recreational drugs, and self-prescribing any other drugs are all forms of self-abuse.
2. Give yourself some "me" time every day. Some of the most stress-resistant paramedics are those who have learned techniques of meditation and can use them to escape now and then to a quiet place within themselves. Try different methods of meditation or relaxation and see which one works best for you.
3. Learn how to relax **FIGURE 2-17**.
   - Take time for hobbies.
   - Engage in social activities with people not involved in EMS.
   - Leave your job behind when your shift is over.
4. Do not make unreasonable demands on yourself.
   - Forget the idea that you have to be perfect. No one is perfect. If you do the best job you can, then that is good enough.
   - You do not have to be right all the time. Accept the fact that now and then you will make a mistake—and that the world will not come to an end on account of it.
5. Do not make unreasonable demands on others.
6. Stay in touch with your feelings.
   - Find someone you can talk to. Share stress.
   - Cry when you need to. There is no shame in being sad sometimes.
7. Learn techniques for managing stress while on duty. Do not let stress accumulate.
8. Debrief after tough calls.

FIGURE 2-17 One of the best ways of dealing with the stress of working as a paramedic is to invest in relationships and activities outside of work that are meaningful to you. Make the most of your time off; it is an opportunity to refresh yourself.

Words of Wisdom

Dealing with stress as a paramedic requires the ability to emotionally distance yourself from the situation and accept the limits of what you can personally do.

Coping With Death and Dying

As a paramedic, you will deal with death sometime in your career. What do you say to people who know they are dying? What do you say to a bereaved parent, spouse, or other family member? How do you deal with your own feelings when a patient has died while under your care? These are all questions you need to answer for yourself eventually, and it may take a lifetime to sort them out.

Death in the Western world is generally regarded as a traumatic experience, something to be feared and postponed as long as possible. Think about it: an average person's only experience with death is through the death of another. As a paramedic, you will be there when people are born and you will be there when many of them die. Every one of these encounters is an honor—a most private moment in someone's life, to which you and a small number of your coworkers are invited. In some cultures, these moments are a holy time; regardless of culture, death is likely one of the most important passages in a person's life. Many patients will exhibit great dignity while dying, which may show you how to die with dignity someday.

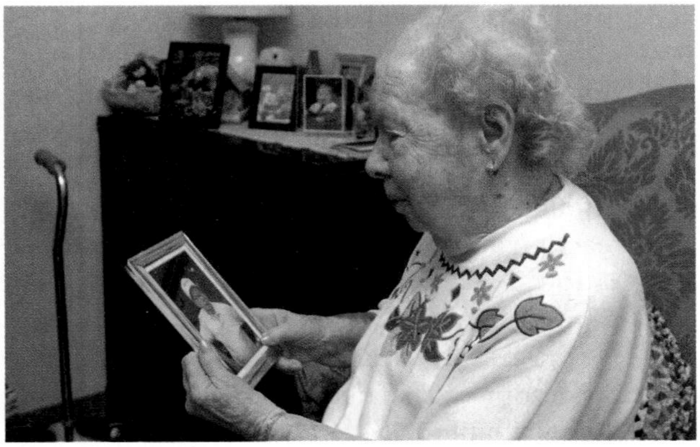

FIGURE 2-18 People usually go through a lengthy process of grieving before fully accepting the death of a loved one.

As a paramedic, you will have the opportunity to help a great many people—but few resuscitations will be successful, no matter how long your career. Yours may be the last face a dying person sees, so make it count. Show compassion and concern for the individual as well as for their family and friends. What follows are some general guidelines and techniques for dealing with the dying, their families, and your own stress.

Stages of the Grieving Process

In her classic study, *On Death and Dying*, Elisabeth Kübler-Ross, MD, defined five stages through which grieving people—usually dying individuals, but sometimes their survivors—often proceed **FIGURE 2-18**.[25] Each of these stages in some way helps the dying or their family members adapt to their own reality. It helps to be aware of these stages and to consider the behavior of dying patients or their families in the context of the grieving process. Be aware that all people do not follow the stages in order or experience every stage and that you may arrive after a stage has already passed.

- **Stage 1: Denial.** As discussed earlier, denial is a mechanism by which people attempt to ignore a problem or pretend it does not exist. Denial is a way of buffering bad news until the person can mobilize resources to deal with that news more effectively. Allow people enough time to work through this stage and offer assistance only if they ask for it.
- **Stage 2: Anger.** When people can no longer deny the reality of a situation, anger over the

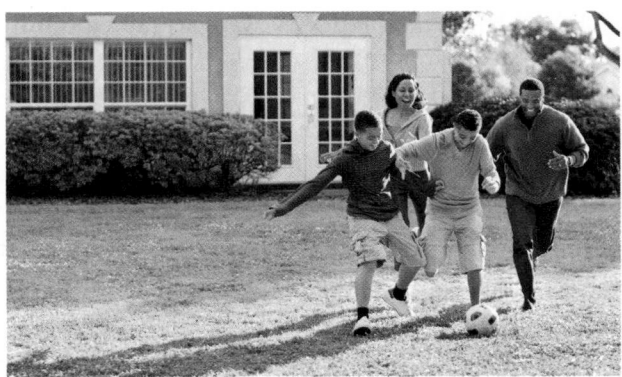

loss may replace denial. They may ask, "Why me?" and displace their anger randomly to those around them. As mentioned earlier, such anger may be challenging for you to deal with. Some people may manifest their anger through physical actions; be prepared for that reaction and keep yourself and others safe.

- **Stage 3: Bargaining.** When anger does not change the painful reality of a situation, people may resort to bargaining—that is, trying to make some sort of deal in hopes of postponing the inevitable ("If I can just live long enough to see my daughter's wedding, then I'll die in peace.").
- **Stage 4: Depression.** When bargaining fails to change the reality of a loss and people must come to terms with dying, a sudden and enormous sense of loss occurs. They may become very quiet. Depression in the face of dying is common among couples who have been married or together for most of their lives and have rarely spent time apart. People may want permission to express their sorrow—in words, in tears, or in what Kübler-Ross calls "the silence that goes beyond words." Acknowledge their loss and sadness, and if they act like they want to cry, offer some tissues, a towel, or a shoulder to cry on. If they seem to want a hug, then offer it. If they seem to just want to be quiet by themselves, then do what you can to accommodate that as well. It is not wrong for you to appropriately exhibit emotions to a grieving person.
- **Stage 5: Acceptance.** In the final stage of grief, people who are dying prepare to disengage from the world around them. They shed their fears and most of their other feelings and begin to loosen the ties that bind them to the living. When a dying person enters the acceptance stage, the family is often in need of the most help. Although families may know of an impending death, their emotions and reactions may change completely when that time comes. The process of dying is not pleasant and it may be shocking when death occurs.[25]

Dealing With a Dying Patient

People who are dying generally know, at least, that their situation is serious; they may be well aware that they are dying and may want to talk about it. Some health care professionals are reluctant to discuss death with patients, so they try to maintain an attitude of reassurance by saying, "Everything will be okay." That is making a promise you are not able to keep. Do not give a false sense of hope to a situation; do not say a patient will recover when they may not. Perhaps the most important thing you can do for dying patients is to let them know that you understand and will talk about death if they wish. You do not need to come right out and ask, "Do you want to talk about dying?" You can simply say, "If there is anything you would like to talk about, then I will listen."

Let patients talk as much as they wish **FIGURE 2-19**. Make some appropriate physical contact. Hold their hand, put a hand on their shoulder, or make some other unmistakable gesture of empathy.

What if patients come straight out and ask you, "Am I going to die?" Your answer should acknowledge the seriousness of their condition without taking away all hope. For example, you might say, "Your illness is serious, but we will give you the best care available."

Dying patients also need to feel that they still have some control over their lives. When people lose all control over their lives, they may lose a measure of their dignity and self-respect. Explain to them what you are doing and allow them to participate in their treatment as much as possible. Ask them if

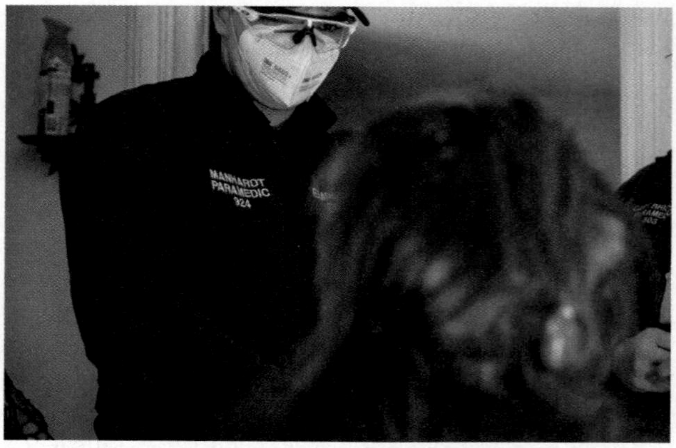

FIGURE 2-19 Patients will have different ways of dealing with their immediate situation. Some patients may be relieved to talk openly about how they feel, whereas others may have a greater sense of privacy or stoicism.

there is anyone they would like you to contact or if they have any special instructions they want conveyed to someone. If they ask you to convey a message, then write it down word-for-word as they state it to you. You will find that people who know they are going to die will often look you in the eye and say, "I think I am going to die." Regardless of the situation, always provide the best emergency medical care you can.

Dealing With a Grieving Family

Suppose you are called to a scene where a child has been run over by a truck. You can see at a glance that the child is dead. Two police officers are with the child's mother, who is crying hysterically. The fact that there is nothing you can do for the child does not mean that the call is over. There is another patient at the scene—the child's mother—and the call is not over until you have done all you can for her **FIGURE 2-20**.

Your local protocol may state that you have to verify a death by obtaining a cardiac monitor strip. Be aware that in a case like this, such an action may give the mother false hope that you can or will resuscitate her child.

What kinds of things can you do for a grieving family? How can you help them begin the process of dealing with their loss? Here are a few guidelines:

- Do not try to hide the deceased patient's body from the family, even if the body has been badly mutilated. In situations where the deceased patient's appearance may be disfigured, attempt to warn or educate the family beforehand about what they may see. People who are prevented from seeing a loved one's body may later have enormous difficulty working through their grief because they may be unable to get beyond their denial. Seeing the body helps the person achieve closure of the situation.
- For similar reasons, do not use euphemisms for death, such as "expired" or "passed away." The family needs to hear the word "dead."
- Do not hurry to clear away all your resuscitation equipment. Let the family see the equipment before you start tidying up and packing away your gear so that they will know that everything possible was done.
- Give the family some time with their loved one, especially when the deceased patient is a child. If the death occurred in a public place, then move the deceased into the ambulance or protect the scene from onlookers, and let the family say goodbye in their own way.
- Try to arrange for further emotional support. Offer to contact a neighbor, friend, or the family's clergy.
- Accept the family's right to experience a variety of feelings—guilt, shock, denial, or anger.

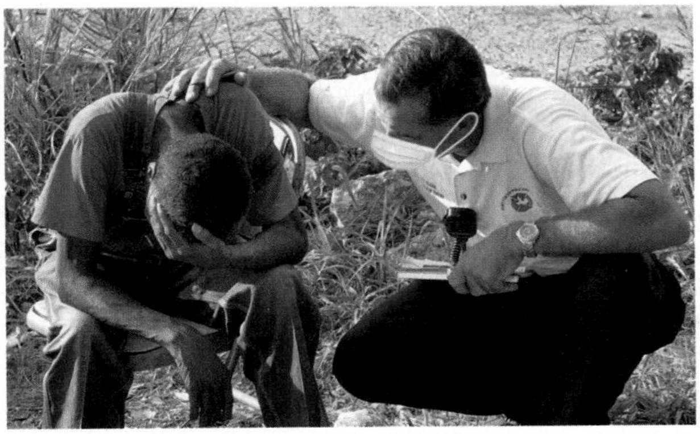

FIGURE 2-20 While on scene, one of your responsibilities is to help family members through the initial period after the death of a loved one.

Dealing With a Grieving Child

You need to be particularly sensitive to children's emotional needs and how they differ depending on their age group. When they are exposed to the death of a family member, children up to age 3 years will be aware that something has happened and that people are sad. Children age 3 to 6 years of age believe that death is temporary and may continually ask when the person will return. The family should emphasize to the child that they are not responsible for the death, that the family member will not be coming home, and that it is okay to cry when you are sad.

Children age 6 to 9 years may mask their feelings to not look babylike. Family members should discuss the usual feelings of grieving with the child. Also, they should not hesitate to cry in front of a child.

Children age 9 to 12 years may want to know the details surrounding the incident. Family members should encourage sharing of feelings and memories to facilitate the grieving process.

After the Call Is Over

Many calls can be shocking. In those cases, everyone involved in the call is likely to experience some intense feelings. If these feelings stay bottled up, then many different kinds of problems may result later. For this reason, every ambulance service needs to develop routine procedures for debriefing after any call, especially those that involve the death of a patient. All those who participated in the call need a chance to sit down together, in an atmosphere of confidentiality, and air their feelings about what happened.

Most calls should not disrupt your everyday life functions. But some especially traumatic calls can preoccupy even well-adjusted providers for weeks or even months afterward. This type of delayed stress reaction is called **posttraumatic stress disorder (PTSD)**. A **critical incident** is one that overwhelms the ability of an EMS worker or an EMS system to cope with the experience, either at the scene or later.

Most paramedics never experience PTSD, but it can occur. Let your superiors know if you or a coworker is experiencing one or more of the following signs of PTSD:

- You have trouble getting an incident out of your thoughts.
- You keep having flashbacks of an incident.
- You have nightmares or other sleep disturbances after an incident.
- Your appetite is not the same after an incident.
- After an incident, you laugh or cry for no good reason.
- You find yourself withdrawing from coworkers and family members after an incident.
- You rely on alcohol or cigarettes, or make other unhealthy choices to calm yourself down.

Critical incident stress management (CISM) is a resource available for emergency personnel who have been involved in particularly traumatic calls or incidents. The CISM process was developed to address acute stress situations and potentially decrease the likelihood that PTSD will develop after such an incident. Although public safety organizations have used CISM for more than 30 years, no concrete evidence exists on its efficacy in preventing PTSD or burnout. The following are suggested events where some sort of debriefing or management may be considered:

- Serious injury or death of a fellow worker in the line of duty
- Suicide of a fellow worker
- Mass-casualty incidents, such as an airliner crash or train wreck
- Serious injury or death of a child
- Intense media attention to an incident

Controversies

Psychology professionals and EMS professionals alike have debated the effectiveness of CISM for some time. Be open-minded about the experience and then draw your own conclusion.

It is impossible to predict how any given person will react. People should be offered opportunities to debrief, but it should never be forced on them or made mandatory.

Some EMS systems still have CISM teams or a form thereof to provide support after a traumatic call—and sometimes even during the incident. The intervention may take the form of a brief (usually about 30 minutes) defusing session right after the call, in which all who were involved in the incident are offered an opportunity to express their feelings about what happened. A formal debriefing is usually coordinated and should be handled by one or more professional counselors 24 to 72 hours after an incident, when it becomes clear that the incident has had a serious effect and is causing persistent symptoms among the crew. Again, this process should be optional and not open to the media.

Some services may offer an **employee assistance program (EAP)**. This resource is usually provided by a trained, professional counselor who works outside of the service and is available off duty. Successful EAPs do not focus only on "work-related" behaviors, as some personal issues (eg, childcare, finances, dependency, relationship stress) may lead to poor work choices and unacceptable behaviors. The EAP is successful only if those who attend do so by their own choice and are willing to share every issue that may bother them. If you or your coworkers note changes in your behavior at work and an EAP is available, then it is a worthwhile venture to pursue for the betterment of your health and career.

SAFETY

A debriefing may occur shortly after a serious adverse event or sentinel event (an unanticipated patient safety incident that results in patient harm or death). The debriefing is a powerful inquiry tool in which a brief exchange occurs to identify what happened, what was learned, and what can be done better in the future. A member of senior leadership usually leads a debriefing. The senior leadership should also use a debriefing to provide emotional support to staff and/or family, determine reporting obligations, and perhaps visit the event site. The debriefing does not focus on system changes and it should not be used for disciplinary purposes.

Peer Support and Suicide Prevention

Like all populations, EMS providers are not immune to thoughts of suicide or suicide attempts. Because prolonged stress is a risk factor for suicide, prevention starts with recognizing that you or your colleagues are becoming overwhelmed. Even if you do not identify suicidal tendencies in yourself, you may receive input from colleagues. Do not disregard what you recognize or what others note to you. A survey of more than 4,000 respondents showed that 37% of EMS respondents contemplated suicide and 6.6% attempted it.[26] Although that attempt number may seem relatively low, in comparison, CDC showed suicide contemplation and attempt levels for the general population to be 3.7% and 0.5%, respectively.[26] Its study suggests that emergency workers are at higher risk for suicidal thoughts and attempts than nonemergency workers.[26]

A combination of cumulative stress and acute, intense stress can weigh heavily on EMS providers. While awareness of EMS provider suicide has grown over the years, you should understand and select strategies to deal with stress constructively. It is essential to be aware of the signs of stress and burnout in yourself and your coworkers. Any suicidal thoughts or attempts must be taken seriously. If you experience any suicidal ideations or if a colleague expresses such ideations, you should seek help, including professional counseling.

Peer support is the process by which a properly trained member of your department provides confidential support to another member who is experiencing personal, emotional, or work-related problems and acts as a bridge to outside professional services. Many departments provide both critical incident stress debriefing (CISD) programs and peer support programs. Whereas CISD is especially valuable following stressful incidents that involve multiple members of a department, peer support is more appropriate for assisting individuals and for situations where ongoing follow-through is needed. Both types of programs provide valuable assistance for dealing with stressful situations.

One advantage of peer support is that it can build on the existing mutual trust and understanding between two members of the same department. Peer support provides a safe and nurturing environment for all affected members. Trained peer counselors understand the unique needs of public safety providers. They understand the importance of confidentiality and the physical requirements and mental stressors of being a first responder. In addition, they are prepared to adjust to the irregular schedules and other logistical challenges of first responders. Peer counselors can respond in a moment of crisis. They can help to direct a member to self-care, or they can help to provide a bridge to outside professional help when needed.

Peer support is voluntary. It can be initiated at the request of the member, a concerned coworker, or a supervisor, and may follow a potentially traumatic call. People with whom you work may be able to identify warning signs of stress early and reach out to other team members before these signs become significant problems. Peer counselors can follow up with members weeks or months after a troubling event occurs.

Peer support is not limited to work-related problems. Family issues, financial difficulties, stress or anxiety, and substance abuse are all issues that may be addressed through a peer support

Words of Wisdom

Some peer support programs use the acronym LOVE to describe the role of the peer counselor:

L Listen carefully.
O Offer assistance.
V Validate through understanding.
E Encourage the person never to give up and to seek assistance.

program. Properly trained peer support personnel can be available to the first responder's family members, too.

The effectiveness of peer support relies on confidentiality. This confidentiality is carefully maintained except in cases where there is a risk of harm to the member or to others, or where there is criminal activity. Check with your supervisor to see if a peer support program is available for members of your department.

YOU are the Paramedic SUMMARY

1. The decline of your physical well-being will eventually affect your attitude and, in turn, put your job at risk. What steps can you take to avoid this outcome?

Physical well-being components include proper nutrition, exercise, adequate sleep, and the avoidance of unhealthy habits or substances. Eat healthy meals, preferably at the same time each day. Plan meals in advance and account for the possibility that you may not be near a microwave or refrigerator. Follow the USDA's MyPlate dietary guidelines. Carry bottled water and snacks such as raisins, nuts, and fruits.

Exercise is essential for weight management and stress management. If you choose an activity you enjoy, you will be more likely to stick with it. Your exercise regimen should focus on three areas: cardiovascular endurance, flexibility, and physical strength. Try to engage in at least 30 minutes of moderate to vigorous physical activity most days of the week. Avoid caffeine, tobacco use, and excessive alcohol consumption.

It is also important to keep a regular sleep schedule, even though this is virtually impossible when performing shift work. Get as much sleep as possible as time permits.

2. Why is it so important to also find ways to enhance your mental, emotional, and spiritual well-being?

The ability to think clearly and react properly is strongest when your mental well-being is in balance. Practice techniques for coping with the fight-or-flight response before they are needed to help guide you when an emergency situation arises. To maintain your emotional health, you need a balance between your life at work and life away from work. When you are off duty, try to stay off duty.

Maintain your skills and education, but accept the fact that patients may not do well or die. This reality is not something that you can control (unless you are directly responsible for that death through negligence). Strive to do your best and remember that you are valuable and what you do makes a difference.

You may not be a member of an organized religious group, but if you are, then you may find comfort in these beliefs. Medical care supports the dignity and value of life, and the sacredness of individuals. Having a rich sense of your own spirituality will help to keep your life in good perspective.

3. According to his mother's report, the patient has been apneic for an unknown amount of time. What should be your next action?

The first step is to ensure that patient cannot be resuscitated. Attach a cardiac monitor and check for asystole in two leads. If you find electrical activity, then consider proceeding with CPR and follow your local protocols for the presenting rhythm. If the patient presents with asystole, or if other signs of obvious death are present, then refrain from disturbing the body and tell the family that your findings clearly show the person has died and it is not possible to change the situation.

Also, notify the dispatcher, who should send law enforcement personnel (if not already done) and contact the coroner. In most states, the coroner or medical examiner will make decisions on death scenes (ie, whether an autopsy is needed, where to transport the deceased person, and who will sign the death certificate). If you note anything of a suspicious nature, then do not attempt to address your concerns with anyone related to the deceased. Document your findings and address your concerns with law enforcement or the coroner. In most areas it is also standard practice for law enforcement personnel to

YOU are the Paramedic SUMMARY continued

write a report, even for instances of death from obvious natural causes—such as an older person with a history of cancer.

4. On the basis of your previous interactions with the patient, which stage of the grieving process do you feel he reached?

This patient had reached the acceptance stage of grief. During your previous interactions with him, you observed that he appeared to be prepared for his inevitable death, yet maintained a positive outlook despite this.

5. How will you explain the situation to the family, and what is your responsibility to them?

Telling the family that a loved one has died is never easy. Be direct. Do not "sugarcoat" the situation and do not use euphemisms for death. It is important to use the word "dead" or "died" to help the family move past their denial. Allow the family to see the body if they choose, unless it is a potential crime scene. Give the family some time with the patient to allow them the chance to say goodbye. Try to arrange for further support as needed. If they request it, then call a neighbor, religious person, or other family members to come over. Never contact people on behalf of the family without their request.

Probably the most challenging part is to remind yourself not to take things personally if the family becomes upset with you. They may experience guilt, shock, denial, or anger, and you have to recognize that these are coping mechanisms that are not directed at you. Treat them with respect and empathy and allow them to work through their grief while offering to assist with whatever they may need. Often, after family members become accustomed to the situation, they will realize how they treated you and offer apologies. If that occurs, then accept the apology without recourse.

6. Which stage of the grieving process is the patient's mother exhibiting?

She appears to be in two stages. She is still in denial, but is also trying to bargain. She understands that her son is terminally ill, but is still hopeful that the problem can be fixed. Her son's death is reality, however, and she may move rapidly into the depression stage.

The loss of a child is a traumatic experience, no matter what the child's age. The patient you can help in this situation is the mother. Ask her what you can do to help. If she asks you for help, then suggest support groups that may be offered through the local hospital or other agencies. Each situation is different and should be handled based on the needs of the bereaved.

7. How should you deal with the nephew's hostility?

The first step is to make sure that you remove yourself from a dangerous situation and request law enforcement personnel if they are not already en route or on scene. Removing yourself from a dangerous situation does not mean that you are abandoning your patient.

A person's behavior can change in the blink of an eye during critical situations or when faced with death. Use your intuition or gut instincts to help predict when a hostile situation is developing. If you are in contact with an aggressive person, then listen without arguing. Concentrate on de-escalating their emotions. An upset person does not listen or reason well; often their fight-or-flight-response has been activated. It is vital to build a rapport with the person. Rapport is based on empathy and understanding. Although you do not want to say, "I know how you feel," it is important to stress, "I will help you if you would like. Let me know how I can help you." Remember to put aside any personal prejudices and do your best to be understanding and accepting.

8. How will you deal with your own feelings and stress related to this call?

As a new paramedic, understand that you cannot save every patient. You need to frequently remind yourself, "I will always provide the best care possible in all situations, but not all patients will have a positive outcome in spite of that." Dealing with stress is part of being a paramedic. When the situation involves a child, coworker, or family member, it can be much more difficult to handle.

This call could be particularly stressful because of your frustrated frame of mind en route to the call, followed by your sudden change of emotions when you arrived on scene. Although death can be stressful, this situation could very easily be a trigger for acute stress. Talking with your partner should be the first step and possibly all that will be needed. However, if you find yourself becoming more irritable, losing sleep, or drinking more, or if you recognize any other signs that indicate you are not coping well, then you must seek professional assistance. Most calls should not disrupt your normal daily functions, but if you find yourself preoccupied for weeks or months afterward, then you may be experiencing PTSD. Report any concerns to your supervisor immediately and follow departmental policies for seeking help.

YOU are the Paramedic SUMMARY continued

EMS Patient Care Report (PCR)					
Date: 01-12-22	**Incident No.:** 1101034	**Nature of Call:** Possible cardiac arrest		**Location:** 984 Solomon Street	
Dispatched: 0712	**En Route:** 0713	**At Scene:** 0720	**Transport:**	**At Hospital:**	**In Service:** 0735
Patient Information					
Age: 23 **Sex:** M **Weight (in kg [lb]):** 70 kg (154 lb)			**Allergies:** NKDA **Medications:** See list (attached to report) **Past Medical History:** Leukemia **Chief Complaint:** Cardiac arrest		

Vital Signs				
Time: 0721	**BP:** 0	**Pulse:** 0	**Respirations:** 0	**Spo_2:**
Time:	**BP:**	**Pulse:**	**Respirations:**	**Spo_2:**
Time:	**BP:**	**Pulse:**	**Respirations:**	**Spo_2:**

EMS Treatment (circle all that apply)				
Oxygen @ ____ L/min via (circle one): **NC NRM Bag-mask device**		**Assisted Ventilation**	**Airway Adjunct**	**CPR**
Defibrillation	**Bleeding Control**	**Bandaging**	**Splinting**	**Other:** Cardiac monitor

Narrative

Dispatched to a possible cardiac arrest. Arrived on scene to find a 23 y/o man supine in bed apneic and pulseless. Pt has been down for an unknown amount of time. Mother states that pt refused to eat last night and she found him "not breathing" just before calling EMS. Pt cold to touch, no obvious signs of injury, presents with dependent lividity. Cardiac monitor shows asystole in two leads. Pt has history of leukemia and mother states "he has been getting worse over the past month." He was not a hospice pt. Mother also stated that he was not "feeling well" last night. Contacted Medical Control with information and was approved to withhold resuscitation @ 0722. Advised dispatch to notify law enforcement and coroner of death. Stayed on scene with pt and family until turned over to coroner.

End of report

Prep Kit

Ready for Review

- As a paramedic, you need to know how to ensure your own well-being.
- Wellness has at least four dimensions: physical, mental, emotional, and spiritual. It is essential to keep all four dimensions healthy and balanced.
- The Life's Simple 7 list from the American Heart Association identifies seven factors found to improve heart health: get active, control cholesterol, eat better, manage BP, lose weight, reduce blood sugar, and stop smoking.

Prep Kit continued

- Nutrition plays a key role in maintaining day-to-day energy and maintaining a healthy body for life. The *Dietary Guidelines for Americans, 2020–2025* from the US Department of Agriculture outline guidelines for nutrition.
- Practice proper lifting and moving techniques to protect your body and lengthen your career.
  - Minimize the number of total body lifts you have to perform.
  - Coordinate every lift before performing the lift.
  - Minimize the total amount of weight you have to lift.
  - Never lift with your back.
  - Do not carry what you can put on wheels.
  - Ask for help anytime you need it.
- A communicable disease is any disease that can be spread from person to person or animal to person. Infectious diseases can be transmitted by contact (direct or indirect), or can be spread through airborne, foodborne, or vector-borne transmission.
- Even if you are exposed to an infectious disease, your risk of becoming ill is low. Whether an acute infection occurs after exposure depends on several factors, including the amount and type of infectious organism and your resistance to that infection.
- You can take several steps to protect yourself against exposure to infectious diseases, including keeping up-to-date with recommended vaccinations, taking standard precautions at all times, and handling all needles and other sharp objects with great care.
- Because it is often impossible to tell which patients have infectious diseases, avoid direct contact with all patients' blood and body fluids.
- Standard precautions are protective measures designed to prevent health care workers from coming in contact with infectious organisms carried by patients. Proper handwashing is one of the simplest, yet most effective, ways of controlling disease transmission. Also use the proper PPE for the situation, including gloves, gowns, eye protection, masks, and possibly other specialized equipment.
- Infection control should be an essential part of your daily routine. Be sure to follow proper steps when dealing with potential exposure situations. Know what to do if you are exposed to an airborne or bloodborne disease.
- Cleaning your ambulance and equipment is part of protecting yourself and your patients. Decontamination of equipment and supplies that have been potentially exposed to body substances requires a different cleansing routine than just soap and water; disinfectant may be required.
- Some situations may require that EMS providers wear turnout gear; firefighting gloves, helmets, and boots; eye, ear, and skin protection; or body armor.
- Keep yourself on alert while you are on duty. Do not be afraid to ask for police to respond to or enter a scene first.
- During your career, you will be exposed to many hazards. Some situations will be dangerous to you or your crew. In these cases, you should be properly protected, or you must avoid the situation altogether.
- Scene hazards may include traffic hazards, unstable vehicles, other traffic, bystanders, potential exposure to hazardous materials, electricity, fire, and lightning. Your safety is the most critical consideration. Never approach a scene without first observing it from a safe distance.
- The most dangerous calls are your everyday ones because you become comfortable with them and may let down your guard.
- Your primary concern at any scene is safety for yourself as well as those around you.
- Safe emergency vehicle operation is crucial to the paramedic, crew, patient, and other motorists' safety.
- Stress reactions can be acute, delayed, or cumulative. Posttraumatic stress disorder is a syndrome with onset following a traumatic, usually life-threatening event. Critical incident stress

Prep Kit continued

management is a process developed to address acute stress situations. You may also seek help through an employee assistance program.

- Compassion fatigue, also known as secondary stress disorder, is characterized by a gradual lessening of compassion over time. Its signs and symptoms are similar to those of cumulative stress.
- Learn how to effectively control stress so that it does not affect your wellness. Take appropriate action. Initial stress management techniques include the following:
  - Controlled deep breathing
  - Progressive relaxation
  - Professional assistance
- Patients' reactions to stress may include fear, anxiety, depression, anger, confusion, denial, regression, projection, and displacement.
- You are not immune to the stresses of emergency situations and may experience many feelings; not all of them will be pleasant.
- Burnout is a consequence of chronic, unrelieved stress.
- As a paramedic, you will be present when people are born and you will be there when people die. The patient who is dying may be aware of that fact and may want to talk about it. Be prepared to listen and provide empathy; you may be the last person the patient sees or talks to.
- Be aware of behavioral changes in yourself and your coworkers, which may indicate a risk for suicide. Reach out to professionals who are specifically trained to assist, and take advantage of resources such as EAPs and the CISM process.

Vital Vocabulary

acute stress reaction Reaction to stress that occurs during a stressful situation.

airborne transmission The spread of an organism in aerosol form, such as droplets or dust.

blind panic A fear reaction in which a person's judgment seems to disappear entirely; it is particularly dangerous because it may cause mass panic among others.

bloodborne pathogens Pathogenic microorganisms that are present in human blood and can cause disease in humans; they include, but are not limited to, hepatitis B virus and human immunodeficiency virus.

burnout The exhaustion of physical or emotional strength.

communicable disease Any disease that can be spread from person to person or from animal to person.

compassion fatigue Also known as secondary stress disorder; a disorder characterized by gradual lessening of compassion over time.

conversion hysteria A reaction in which a person subconsciously transforms their anxiety into a bodily dysfunction; the person may be unable to see or hear or may become partially paralyzed.

critical incident An event that overwhelms the ability to cope with the experience, either at the scene or later.

critical incident stress management (CISM) A process that utilizes trained counselors who confront responses to critical incidents and help to defuse them, directing emergency services personnel toward physical and emotional equilibrium.

cumulative stress reaction Prolonged or excessive stress.

defense mechanisms Psychological ways to relieve stress, which are usually automatic or subconscious; they include denial, regression, projection, and displacement.

delayed stress reaction Reaction to stress that occurs after a stressful situation.

denial An early response to a serious medical emergency, in which the severity of the emergency is diminished or minimized. Denial is the first coping mechanism for people who believe they are going to die.

Prep Kit continued

direct contact Exposure to or transmission of a communicable disease from one person to another by physical contact.

displacement A defense mechanism characterized by redirection of an emotion from one person to another.

employee assistance program (EAP) A counseling program to help with situations that may affect the health and well-being of EMS professionals.

fight-or-flight response A physiologic response to a profound stressor that helps a person deal with the situation at hand; features increased sympathetic tone and results in dilation of the pupils, increased heart rate, dilation of the bronchi, mobilization of glucose, shunting of blood away from the GI tract and cerebrum, and increased blood flow to the skeletal muscles.

indirect contact Exposure or transmission of disease from one person to another by contact with a contaminated, inanimate object.

infection The invasion of a host or host tissues by organisms such as bacteria, viruses, or parasites, with or without signs or symptoms of disease.

infection control Procedures to reduce transmission of infection among patients and health care personnel.

infectious disease A disease that is caused by growth and spread of small, harmful organisms within the body, or that is capable of being transmitted with or without direct contact.

posttraumatic stress disorder (PTSD) A delayed stress reaction to a previous incident, often the result of one or more unresolved issues concerning the incident.

projection A defense mechanism characterized by blaming unacceptable feelings, motives, or desires on others.

regression A defense mechanism characterized by a return to more childlike behavior while under stress.

standard precautions Protective measures that have traditionally been developed by the Centers for Disease Control and Prevention for use in dealing with objects, blood, body fluids, or other potential exposure risks of communicable disease.

stress A reaction of the body to any agent or situation that requires the person to adapt.

stressor Any agent or situation that causes stress, whether good or bad.

transmission The spread of an infectious agent from one organism to another; mechanisms of transmission may be classified as contact (direct or indirect), airborne, foodborne, or vector-borne.

References

1. Centers for Disease Control and Prevention. Quarantine and isolation. https://www.cdc.gov/quarantine/. Updated September 29. 2017. Accessed February 25, 2021.
2. Maguire BJ, Smith S. Injuries and fatalities among emergency medical technicians and paramedics in the United States. *Prehosp Disaster Med.* 2013;28(4):376-382.
3. Bureau of Labor Statistics. Occupational employment statistics. https://www.bls.gov/oes/current/oes_nat.htm. Modified March 31, 2020. Accessed December 30, 2020.
4. National Highway Traffic Safety Administration. The National Highway Traffic Safety Administration and ground ambulance crashes. April 2014. https://www.naemt.org/Files/HealthSafety/2014%20NHTSA%20Ground%20Amublance%20Crash%20Data.pdf. Accessed February 25, 2021.
5. US Department of Agriculture. Dietary guidelines for Americans, 2020–2015. 9th ed. https://www.dietaryguidelines.gov/sites/default/files/2020-12/Dietary_Guidelines_for_Americans_2020-2025.pdf. Published December 2020. Accessed February 25, 2021.
6. US Department of Agriculture. Choose MyPlate. https://www.myplate.gov/. Accessed February 25, 2021.
7. American Heart Association. Target heart rates chart. https://www.heart.org/en/healthy-living/fitness/fitness-basics/target-heart-rates#.V9q9TpgrKhc. Updated January 4, 2015. Accessed February 25, 2021.
8. Centers for Disease Control and Prevention. Outbreak of lung injury associated with the use of e-cigarette, or vaping, products. https://www.cdc.gov/tobacco/basic_information/e-cigarettes/severe-lung-disease.html.

Prep Kit continued

Updated February 25, 2020. Accessed February 25, 2021.

9. Shmerling RH. Can vaping damage your lungs? What we do (and don't) know. Harvard Health Publishing blog. https://www.health.harvard.edu/blog/can-vaping-damage-your-lungs-what-we-do-and-dont-know-2019090417734. Updated December 10, 2019. Accessed February 25, 2021.
10. National Institute for Occupational Safety and Health. Emergency medical services workers: injury data. Centers for Disease Control and Prevention website. https://www.cdc.gov/niosh/topics/ems/data.html. Accessed May 10, 2021.
11. Maguire BJ, O'Neill BJ, Phelps S, Maniscalco PM, Gerard DH, Handal KA. COVID-10 fatalities among EMS clinicians. EMS1. https://www.ems1.com/ems-products/personal-protective-equipment-ppe/articles/covid-19-fatalities-among-ems-clinicians-BMzHbuegIn1xNLrP/. Published September 25, 2020. Accessed October 13, 2020.
12. Centers for Disease Control and Prevention. Guideline for hand hygiene in health-care settings: Recommendations of the Healthcare Infection Control Practices Advisory Committee and the HICPAC/SHEA/APIC/IDSA Hand Hygiene Task Force. *MMWR.* 2002;51(RR-16):1-45, quiz CE1-4.
13. Siegel JD, Rhinehart E, Jackson M, Chiarello L, Healthcare Infection Control Practices Advisory Committee. 2007 guideline for isolation precautions: preventing transmission of infectious agents in healthcare settings. https://www.cdc.gov/infectioncontrol/pdf/guidelines/isolation-guidelines-H.pdf. Updated July 2019. Accessed February 26, 2021.
14. Centers for Disease Control and Prevention, National Institute for Occupational Safety and Health. Bloodborne infectious diseases: HIV/AIDS, hepatitis B, hepatitis C. http://www.cdc.gov/niosh/topics/bbp/default.html. Updated September 7, 2016. Accessed February 26, 2021.
15. Centers for Disease Control and Prevention. COVID-19 vaccination. https://www.cdc.gov/vaccines/covid-19/index.html. Updated December 20, 2020. Accessed February 26, 2021.
16. Centers for Disease Control and Prevention. Vaccines & immunizations. http://www.cdc.gov/vaccines/index.html. Updated February 16, 2021. Accessed February 26, 2021.
17. Centers for Disease Control and Prevention. When and how to wash your hands. http://www.cdc.gov/handwashing/when-how-handwashing.html. Updated November 24, 2020. Accessed February 26, 2021.
18. Centers for Disease Control and Prevention. Clean hands count for healthcare providers. https://www.cdc.gov/handhygiene/providers/index.html. Reviewed January 31, 2020. Accessed December 30, 2020.
19. World Health Organization. Global tuberculosis report 2020. https://apps.who.int/iris/bitstream/handle/10665/336069/9789240013131-eng.pdf. Accessed February 26, 2021.
20. National Institute of Justice. Ballistic Resistance of Body Armor, NIJ Standard 0101.06. https://www.ncjrs.gov/pdffiles1/nij/223054.pdf#page=17. Published July 2008. Accessed December 30, 2020.
21. Maguire BJ, O'Neill BJ. Emergency medical service personnel's risk from violence while serving the community. *Am J Public Health.* 2017;107(11):1770-1775.
22. Selye H. Stress without distress. In: Serban G, ed. *Psychopathology of Human Adaptation.* Boston, MA: Springer; 1976. https://doi.org/10.1007/978-1-4684-2238-2_9.
23. Holmes TH, Rahe RH. The Social Readjustment Rating Scale. *J Psychosom Res.* 1967;11(2):213-218.
24. American Psychological Association. Stress effects on the body. https://www.apa.org/topics/stress/body. Published November 1, 2018. Accessed February 26, 2021.
25. Kübler-Ross E. *On Death and Dying.* New York, NY: Macmillan; 1969.
26. Newland C, Barber E, Rose M, Young A. Survey reveals alarming rates of EMS provider stress and thoughts of suicide. *JEMS.* 2015;40(10):30-34. https://www.jems.com/special-topics/survey-reveals-alarming-rates-of-ems-provider-stress-and-thoughts-of-suicide/. Accessed February 26, 2021.

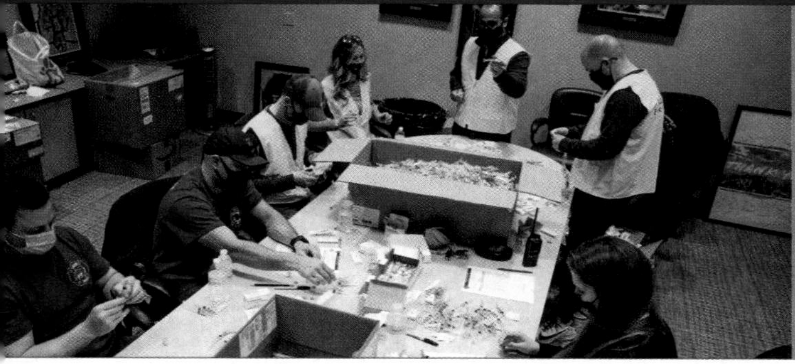

Chapter 3

Public Health

NATIONAL EMS EDUCATION STANDARD COMPETENCIES

Public Health

Applies fundamental knowledge of principles of public health and epidemiology including public health emergencies, health promotion, and illness and injury prevention.

KNOWLEDGE OBJECTIVES

1. Define public health and its role in the health care system. (p 92)
2. Define intentional injuries and unintentional injuries. (p 92–93)
3. Discuss the detrimental effects of injuries as related to public health. (pp 92–93)
4. Discuss pediatric injuries and risk factors for them. (pp 93–94)
5. Discuss the detrimental effects of chronic and acute illness as related to public health. (pp 94–95)
6. Explain the concept of years of potential life lost. (pp 95–96)
7. Explain the relevance of a teachable moment in EMS. (pp 96–97)
8. Discuss the principles of injury prevention, including education, enforcement, engineering/environment, and economic incentives. (pp 97–100)
9. List the major public health laws, regulations, and guidelines in place in the United States, including the purpose of each. (pp 98–99)
10. Explain the paramedic's unique role in promoting public health, in terms of both illness and injury. (pp 92–95)
11. Define primary prevention and secondary prevention; include examples of each. (pp 101–102)
12. Define morbidity and mortality. (p 103)
13. Discuss the concept of injury surveillance and how it relates to EMS. (p 104)
14. Explain the Haddon matrix and how it can be used in the understanding and prevention of injury. (pp 105–106)
15. List ways a paramedic can promote injury prevention in the community. (pp 107–108)
16. Describe the steps involved in organizing a community prevention program. (pp 109–110)

SKILLS OBJECTIVES

There are no skills objectives for this chapter.

Introduction

In 1996, San Diego paramedic Paul Maxwell responded to a call for a possible drowning.[1] A 2-year-old boy had wandered away from a daycare facility and fallen into a neighbor's backyard pool. Despite everyone's best efforts, he could not be resuscitated. The mother was inconsolable and her cries haunted the paramedic.

Maxwell wondered how such tragedies could be prevented. If he could help it, he never wanted to go on another call like that again. Doing a little investigation, and looking up incidents on his emergency medical services (EMS) system's database, he discovered a pattern of increased drownings in his region. Maxwell decided to get involved. In cooperation with his EMS agency, he and fellow paramedics created Medics Eliminating Preventable Injury in Children, EPIC Medics. Their organization then collaborated with other groups in his community with an interest in child safety. Using his system's data and motivated by his firsthand knowledge of the suffering that such deaths inflict, Maxwell began a coordinated effort to reduce backyard pool drownings in his community. In time, through the development of legislation and education, Maxwell's program successfully contributed to a significant reduction in drownings.

This story illustrates the influential and powerful role that an EMS provider can have in injury or illness prevention. This chapter discusses injury and illness prevention as they relate to public health, and defines the EMS provider's role in promoting public health in the community.

Role of Public Health

For decades, the health care system in the United States concentrated on treating illnesses and injuries as opposed to preventing them. However, due in part to skyrocketing health care costs, the incidence of chronic disease, and health care reform, there has been a recent shift toward greater emphasis on prevention.

According to the American Public Health Association, **public health** is defined as "the practice of preventing disease and promoting good health within groups of people."[2] A common misconception regarding public health agencies is the notion that their primary mission is to provide clinical services for individuals who are otherwise unable to access health care services elsewhere. In reality, public health professionals examine the overall needs of the population at large to determine the best use of health resources to enhance the quality of life for the public in general. Traditionally, this has included efforts to prevent and control communicable disease and promote health within a community. Examples include immunization and nutrition programs for children; environmental health monitoring, regulation, and remediation; community planning; and exploration of the social determinants of health.

Public Health Threats

TABLE 3-1 shows the top 10 causes of death in the United States in 2019. In that year, almost 74% of all deaths were caused by one of the conditions in this list.[3] This information is crucial in understanding the impact of injuries and illnesses on different age groups.

Injuries

Injuries can be classified as intentional or unintentional. **Intentional injuries** include any injury or death that is self-inflicted or perpetrated by another person, usually in the context of violence. Examples

YOU are the Paramedic

PART 1

You are dispatched to a motor vehicle crash scene involving two patients and a possible ejection. You are very familiar with this stretch of roadway, as you have responded to many other crashes there. A sharp curve in the road has a reputation for leaving drivers in a ditch or worse; thus, you suspect the injuries may be serious, and you request an additional unit be dispatched.

1. What is the most appropriate way to respond to this scene?
2. Based on the information provided, what potential injuries and complications should you anticipate?

TABLE 3-1 Top 10 Causes of Death in 2019

1. Heart disease
2. Cancer
3. Unintentional injuries
4. Chronic lower respiratory disease
5. Stroke (cerebrovascular diseases)
6. Alzheimer disease
7. Diabetes
8. Kidney disease (ie, nephritis, nephrotic syndrome, and nephrosis)
9. Influenza and pneumonia
10. Intentional self-harm (eg, suicide)[a]

[a]Provisional mortality data for 2020 indicate that COVID-19 was the third leading cause of death in the United States in that year, bumping suicide from the top 10 list.

Data from: Ahmed FB, Cisewski JA, Minino A, et al. Provisional mortality data—United States, 2020. *MMWR.* 2021;70(14):519-522; and Kochanek KD, Xu J, Arias E. *Mortality in the United States, 2019.* National Center for Health Statistics Data Brief, December 2020. https://www.cdc.gov/nchs/data/databriefs/db395-H.pdf. Accessed April 28, 2021.

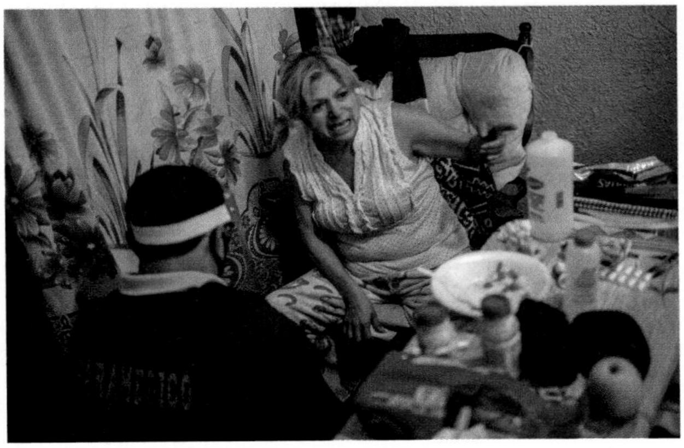

FIGURE 3-1 Intentional injuries include all cases of abuse of a spouse, child, or older adult. As a medical professional, you have an ethical, professional, and—in most states—a legal obligation to report these cases.

© PEDRO PARDO/AFP/Getty Images.

of intentional injuries include assault, self-harm behavior, intentional overdose, and suicide **FIGURE 3-1**. By contrast, **unintentional injuries** occur without intent to cause harm; these events might also be called accidents. Unintentional injuries account for the vast majority of all injuries **FIGURE 3-2**.

An injury or illness **risk** is a potentially hazardous situation in which the well-being of people can be harmed. **Risk factors** are characteristics that increase the likelihood that a person will experience a particular disease or injury. Research into risk factors can reveal crucial information that can aid in recognizing and perhaps even preventing certain kinds of injuries.

8% (2,087,176)

92% (24,823,156)

- Unintentional
- Intentional

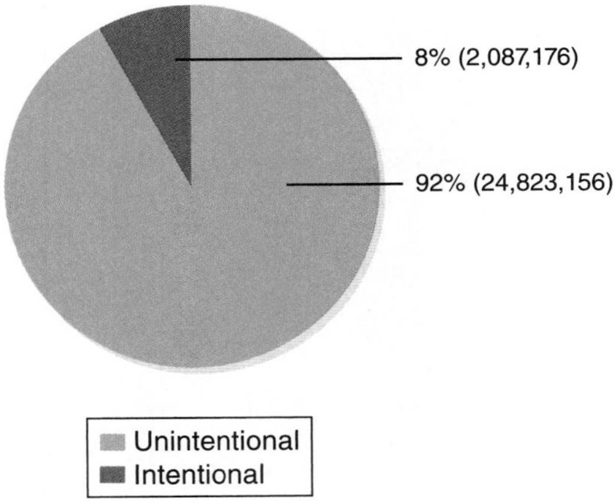

FIGURE 3-2 Most injuries are unintentional.

Data from: WISQARS: nonfatal injury reports, 2000–2019. Centers for Disease Control and Prevention website. https://webappa.cdc.gov/sasweb/ncipc/nfirates.html. Updated November 20, 2020. Accessed May 28, 2021.

TABLE 3-2 Top 10 Causes of Death by Unintentional Injury, 2019

1. Drug poisoning
2. Falls
3. Motor vehicle/traffic
4. Suffocation
5. Unspecified
6. Drowning
7. Nondrug poisoning
8. Fire/flames
9. Natural/environmental
10. Other specified and classifiable

Data from: Causes of injury-related death. WISQARS. Centers for Disease Control and Prevention website. https://wisqars-viz.cdc.gov:8006/explore-data/home. Accessed May 28, 2021.

As the third leading cause of death for all age groups,[3] injury is one of the greatest threats to public health in the United States. **TABLE 3-2** shows the top 10 causes of death from unintentional injury in 2019. Does anything about the list surprise you?

Unintentional Injuries in Children

In the United States, injury is the leading cause of death in children ages 19 and younger.[4] In 2015, children and teens accounted for an estimated 30 million emergency department (ED) visits, with almost 8 million of these visits involving injuries.[5] Compared to adults, children have thinner skin, a smaller airway, a larger head in proportion to their bodies, and a lesser ability to protect themselves from harm **FIGURE 3-3**. Such differing characteristics put them at greater risk for sustaining injuries or being more seriously affected by them.

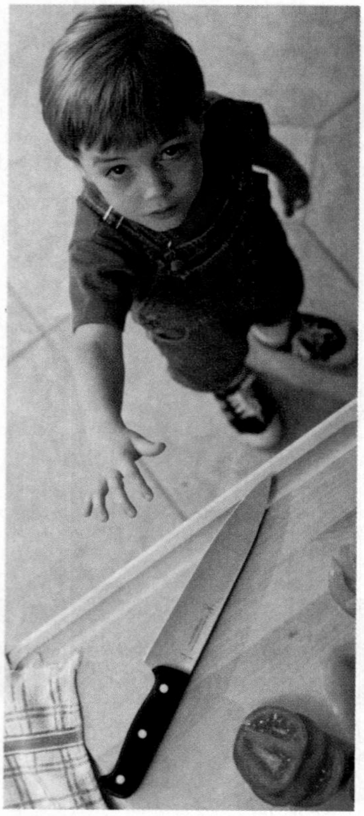

FIGURE 3-3 Children are at higher risk of sustaining serious injuries from an accident. Parents should always be on the alert for potential dangers within reach of a child.

Risk Factors for Children

Injury patterns vary widely depending on a child's age, sex, socioeconomic status, developmental stage, family environment, and a whole host of other factors.[6] Thus, it is imperative for parents, teachers, and health care providers to be aware of the threats to children's health and remain vigilant in taking preventive measures.

Many people believe that schools are becoming increasingly violent, making the risk of *intentional* injuries an ever-present and growing threat to students' safety. Certainly, the very real tragedies that have occurred, from school shootings to bullying and suicide, have captured our attention on multiple occasions. However, despite these distressing stories, *unintentional* injuries—accidents—are much more common and therefore represent a much greater threat to children.

Most frequently, injuries received at school occur during sports activities, industrial arts classes, and playground activities. Each year approximately 200,000 children 14 years of age and younger sustain injuries while playing on playgrounds, with more than 20,000 of these children suffering traumatic brain injuries.[7] The Centers for Disease Control and Prevention (CDC) also reports that more than 2.6 million children and teenagers are evaluated in the ED each year for sports-related injuries.[8]

Chronic Illness

Experts define a chronic condition as "a physical or mental health condition that lasts more than one year and causes functional restrictions or requires ongoing monitoring or treatment."[9] Chronic illnesses and diseases (eg, cancer, heart disease, stroke, chronic obstructive pulmonary disease, arthritis, hypertension, obesity, diabetes) represent a significant threat to public health. In 2018, more than one-half of all Americans had at least one chronic illness.[9,10] Individuals with multiple chronic conditions have a worse health-related quality of life, higher health care costs, and increased risk of death compared to those without chronic conditions.[10] **TABLE 3-3** summarizes US chronic illness statistics.

Acute Illness

On December 31, 2019, the first report of an emerging new respiratory illness in Wuhan, China, was made.[11] This viral illness caused severe respiratory symptoms, resulting in respiratory failure and, in some cases, death. The disease spread rapidly, infecting family members of ill people and the health care workers caring for them. Cases began occurring in people with no known contact with other ill people, indicating that the virus was spreading in the general population. The virus was soon identified as a novel (new) coronavirus and named severe acute respiratory syndrome coronavirus 2 (SARS-CoV-2) because it is a close cousin to the Middle East respiratory syndrome–related coronavirus (MERS-CoV) and the SARS virus. The disease it causes was called coronavirus disease 2019 (COVID-19).

Within 3 weeks of the initial report, cases of the new disease had been reported in Japan, Korea, Thailand, and the United States. On March 11, 2020, the World Health Organization (WHO) characterized COVID-19 as a pandemic.[12] Despite applying lessons learned from previous pandemics and

TABLE 3-3 Chronic Illnesses in the United States

- Seven of every 10 US deaths each year result from chronic diseases.
- An estimated 25% of US adults have two or more chronic conditions; more than half of older adults have three or more chronic diseases.
- Women are more likely to have multiple chronic conditions compared to men.
- Adults living in rural areas have a higher prevalence of multiple chronic conditions compared to those living in urban areas.
- Diabetes is the leading cause of kidney failure, blindness, and amputations of the lower extremities in the United States for people 20 years of age and older. Experts predict that the population with diabetes will increase by 100% by 2034.
- Arthritis is the most common cause of disability, significantly impairing the lives of more than 8.6 million people in the United States.
- In 2017–2018, the prevalence of obesity among US adults was 40.0% among younger adults between the ages of 20 and 39 years, 44.8% among middle-aged adults between the ages of 40 and 59 years, and 42.8% among adults age 60 years and older.
- In 2017–2018, women had a higher prevalence of severe obesity than men did; the prevalence was highest among adults between the ages of 40 and 59 years.
- One-third of people with a chronic illness encounter basic or social problems that impair daily life.

Data from: Raghupathi W, Raghupathi V. An empirical study of chronic disease in the United States: a visual analytics approach to public health. *Int J Environ Res Public Health*. 2018;15(3):431; Boersma P, Black LI, Ward BW. Prevalence of multiple chronic conditions among US adults, 2018. *Prev Chronic Dis*. 2020;17:200130; *National Diabetes Statistics Report 2020: Estimates of Diabetes and Its Burden in the United States*. Centers for Disease Control and Prevention; 2020. https://www.cdc.gov/diabetes/pdfs/data/statistics/national-diabetes-statistics-report.pdf. Accessed April 28, 2021; Chronic diseases: the leading causes of death and disability in the United States. Centers for Disease Control and Prevention website. http://www.cdc.gov/chronicdisease/overview/. Updated January 12, 2021. Accessed April 28, 2021; Hootman J, Brault M, Helmick C, Theis K, Armour B. Prevalence and most common causes of disability among adults—United States, 2005. *MMWR*. 2009;58(16):421-426; Hales CM, Carroll MD, Frayar CD, Ogden CL. Prevalence of obesity and severe obesity among adults: United States, 2017–2018. *NCHS Data Brief*. 360: February 2020. https://www.cdc.gov/nchs/products/databriefs/db360.htm. Accessed June 1, 2021; and Houtum L, Rijken M, Groenewegen P. Do everyday problems of people with chronic illness interfere with their disease management? Biomed Central website. http://bmcpublichealth.biomedcentral.com/articles/10.1186/s12889-015-2303-3. Accessed April 28, 2021.

natural disasters, governments, public health systems, and health care delivery systems across the world were initially unprepared for the COVID-19 pandemic. Efforts to respond to and control the pandemic have required cooperation at all levels of the US government and among international governments and health organizations. Through these joint efforts, vaccines were developed at a record pace (Operation Warp Speed) to help protect against COVID-19 infection, with the first of these vaccines being approved for use in the United States in December 2020.

The COVID-19 pandemic illustrates the devastating effects when a public health threat turns into reality. Similarly widespread illnesses may result from a contaminated water supply, contaminated seafood (eg, from oil leaks), radiation leak, unsanitary conditions after a natural disaster, or increased cancer incidence after major public disasters, to name just a few causes. All public health stakeholders must be vigilant for such threats, participate in prevention efforts, and join in the prompt, concerted response when they do occur.

The Cost of Public Health Threats

Beyond the unquestionable physical and emotional pain and suffering that they cause among patients and their families, injury and illness have far-reaching consequences. The financial effect on families and communities cannot be understated, as the costs of health care, insurance, and additional governmental assistance programs rise in response.

Societal costs of injuries can be measured using the concept of **years of potential life lost (YPLL)**. YPLL is based on an average of life expectancies, where 75 years is typically the reference life expectancy. To calculate YPLL, researchers sum the total deaths in a population occurring at each age; they then multiply this total by the number of years remaining up to age 75 years. Thus, if 10 people in the population died at 65 years, the YPLL would be 100:

$$10 \times (75 - 65) = 100$$

YPLL can be calculated for a specific cause of death as a proportion of the total YPLL lost in the population. This total lends insight into the relative importance of different causes of premature deaths within a population that can guide public health planning, including prevention efforts.[13]

The YPLL associated with injuries is far greater than the YPLL linked with cancer or heart disease. Several reasons exist for this discrepancy. First, younger people typically participate in more risk-taking activities than older people do, and are more susceptible to fatal injuries. Further, when older people die from injuries, fewer YPLL are lost than is the case with a younger person.

Because medical conditions such as heart disease and cancer often cause death at a later age, they typically result in a lower YPLL than occurs with trauma. However, in some instances, such as congenital heart disease, a medical condition can cause significant YPLL.

Finally, years of life lost are associated with death secondary to injury or illness as well as disability. Consider the scenario of a 22-year-old in a bicycle crash. If the patient did not die but instead remained in a comatose state for the rest of his life, the term *YPLL* could still be applied. Although the patient did not lose potential life, he did lose years in which he would be productive, such as earning income, paying taxes, and making other contributions to society.

Who pays for these costs? Unfortunately, *everyone* does. Through higher taxes and higher insurance premiums, we *all* pay the price.

The Teachable Moment

Imagine you are on the scene of a motor vehicle collision (MVC). No one is seriously injured, but the driver admits he was not wearing his seat belt. As you prepare for transport, you look this patient in the eye and say, "You were very lucky this time. I've seen a lot of very severe injuries and even deaths caused by crashes much less serious than this one. You really need to wear your seat belt *every* time you get into a vehicle. It could save your life."

Near misses like these cause people to realize just how vulnerable they truly are and how perilous their actions could have been; thus, the lesson is more likely to stick. This scenario is an example of a *teachable moment*: the time immediately following an event, when the sense of distress and danger is still very real and everyone concerned is perhaps more receptive to instruction on how the event or illness could have been prevented. In that moment, the role of the EMS provider as a caregiver and protector is perhaps at its strongest, putting you in an optimal position to convey and reinforce the message. However, the concept of the teachable moment also extends well beyond the realm of trauma, to include frightening and potentially devastating medical incidents such as a person with diabetes who develops a coma after missing breakfast. The coma is easily reversed with medication, but it could have resulted in the patient's death if not discovered in time, and could have been prevented altogether with more diligent attention to meal timing.

During a teachable moment, you can penetrate the usual facade and reach a person's core values. However, when you do so, tread carefully. Lecturing a mother immediately after her child has been seriously injured is unlikely to be effective; in fact, it might cause her to become defensive or even hostile toward you. Therefore, you must choose your moment wisely. Use good judgment, be nonjudgmental, and be sensitive to the situation's emotionally charged nature **FIGURE 3-4**. The following factors all contribute to creating a teachable moment:

- The injuries or illnesses are such that the parents, companions, or the patients themselves will be receptive to the message; you are aware that you must temper your message based on their ethnic and religious differences.
- The scene is conducive to delivering such a message in a nonthreatening, nonjudgmental way. You are not intruding inappropriately or causing embarrassment that could lead to the opposite reaction.
- A definitive prevention measure could have helped, such as using a seat belt, getting a flu shot, installing a car seat correctly, stopping smoking, wearing a helmet, or keeping firearms locked and safe. Vague advice is less likely to have a lasting effect.

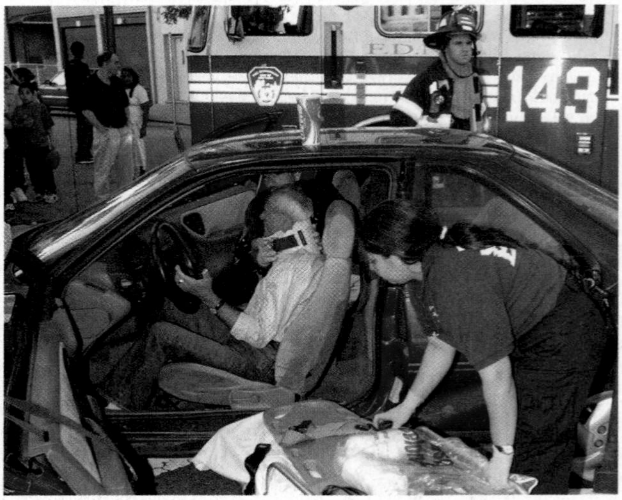

FIGURE 3-4 When injuries are not apparently serious, consider reinforcing the need for safety to prevent future injuries. Remind vehicle drivers and occupants of the importance of compliance with seat belt laws.

Sometimes, a teachable moment can be preemptive, taking place well before a tragic event occurs. For example, imagine you are providing a wellness check in the home of an older patient when you notice a potential tripping hazard in the living room. Taking the time to inform the patient of the danger and then advising them how this threat can be averted may save the patient from a fall and injury in the future. The informal nature of this education makes it perhaps the most effective kind you can provide.

Prevention

Public health efforts aim to impact people within an entire city, community, state, or country. For example, a vaccination program conducted by a local health department may provide flu vaccines to

Street Smarts

Capitalizing on a teachable moment requires tact and empathy. It is essential to avoid communication that could be perceived as belittling, condescending, or otherwise disrespectful. For example, in a situation where the paramedic is relatively young and the patient is perhaps older, if the patient perceives the paramedic to be lecturing or scolding, the paramedic's efforts will be counterproductive. Use good communications skills, be culturally sensitive, and remain nonjudgmental at all times.

The best teachable moments are actually those that convey positive reinforcement. If people wear seat belts properly and survive a crash with little or no injury, tell them, "It's a good thing you had your seat belts on." You will notice smiles on their faces and they will likely remember your statement forever.

YOU are the Paramedic

PART 2

On arrival, you find a single vehicle angled downward in a ditch, with severe front-end damage that resulted from a high-speed impact with a tree. You can see a woman sitting in the driver's seat with a volunteer firefighter holding her cervical spine in a neutral, in-line position. Another woman stands several feet away from the vehicle, holding a crying infant with several evident abrasions and blood on his face. The woman who is holding the infant states that she was not involved in the crash, but she and her husband saw it happen. She says that the infant, still in his car seat, was thrown from the vehicle on impact with the tree, landing in the ditch. The bystander raced across the street and removed the child from the car seat. At the same time, her husband hurried over to check on the driver and then called 9-1-1.

Your partner is speaking with the driver, who is crying uncontrollably and shouting, "I'm fine. Please just take care of my baby!" She had been wearing her seat belt, and her only complaint is mild ankle pain. The second unit arrives and assumes care for the mother, at which time you and your partner focus on the infant, an 8-month-old boy. Immediately, you see he has a 1-inch-long laceration surrounded by a 2-inch-diameter hematoma on the right side of his forehead (the bleeding was controlled before your arrival). Additionally, you observe a slight degree of angulation in the infant's left forearm.

Recording Time: 0 Minutes	
Appearance	Agitated and crying
Level of consciousness	Awake and age appropriate
Airway	Open, clear, and patent
Breathing	Rapid rate, frequent gasping while crying
Circulation	Brachial pulse is strong, rapid, and regular. Skin is warm, dry, and normal color. Bleeding from head laceration has been controlled.

3. What are the risk factors associated with the infant's injuries?
4. Is this a teachable moment?

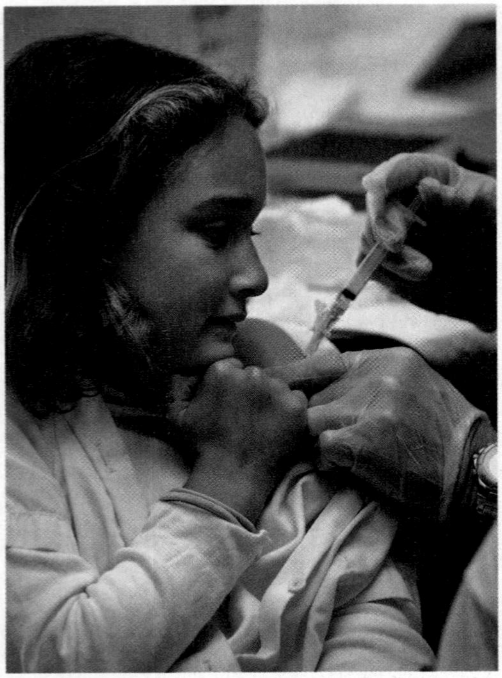

FIGURE 3-5 Vaccination programs allow the general public to receive flu vaccinations, helping to reduce the overall incidence of the flu.

children and adults in its community **FIGURE 3-5**. As a result of these efforts, people are more likely to stay well during flu season, use fewer health care resources, continue going to school, and remain productive in their jobs. The quality of life improves for the whole community, the economy is more stable because its workforce remains intact, and health care costs are lowered.

The 4 Es of Prevention: Education, Enforcement, Engineering/ Environment, and Economic Incentives

Interventions—specific actions intended to improve health and safety outcomes—need to combine *education* with three other types of interventions: *enforcement*, *engineering/environment*, and *economic incentives*. These are commonly referred to as the "4 Es of prevention" **FIGURE 3-6**. The most effective prevention efforts reflect a combination of these interventions.

Education

Most paramedics know that people can behave in ways that cause them to become injured or ill or that put others at risk. Many people do not recognize this relationship between behavior and consequence, however, and therefore cannot assess the risk of doing something: "I didn't know it was unsafe to put my baby's seat in the front passenger seat" or "I didn't think I needed a flu shot." Other people know the risk and disregard it anyway: "I don't wear seat belts because they are uncomfortable" or "I don't believe in giving my baby all of those shots." Through education, you can often inform people about potential dangers and then persuade them to change risky behavior. For example, you can show parents how to use an infant car seat. You can also tell people about the horrors of being thrown from a vehicle, or relate general information about people you have treated who were at risk of death from the flu. Similarly, you might explain how pertussis, once nonexistent in the United States due to adequate vaccinations, is once again being seen in this country and why childhood immunizations are necessary. **TABLE 3-4** lists several additional health and safety tips that you can share with your patients, their families, and the broader community.

Messages need to be tailored to particular groups and reinforced with meaningful rewards to be effective. Educational techniques that seem to be particularly promising include the use of contracts or participant commitment, incentives, behavioral feedback, and modeling.

Enforcement

Sometimes despite your best efforts, even though some members of your community may understand the risks, their behavior will not necessarily change. However, one advantage of any educational effort is that it can occasionally pave the way for legislative and environmental/technological changes.

For example, behavior change may be facilitated by changes in the law. Legislation/regulation can lead to the formulation of rules that require people, manufacturers, and governments to comply with certain safety practices. Elected government bodies routinely legislate, or enact laws, that require safe practices. Bureaucracies or agencies

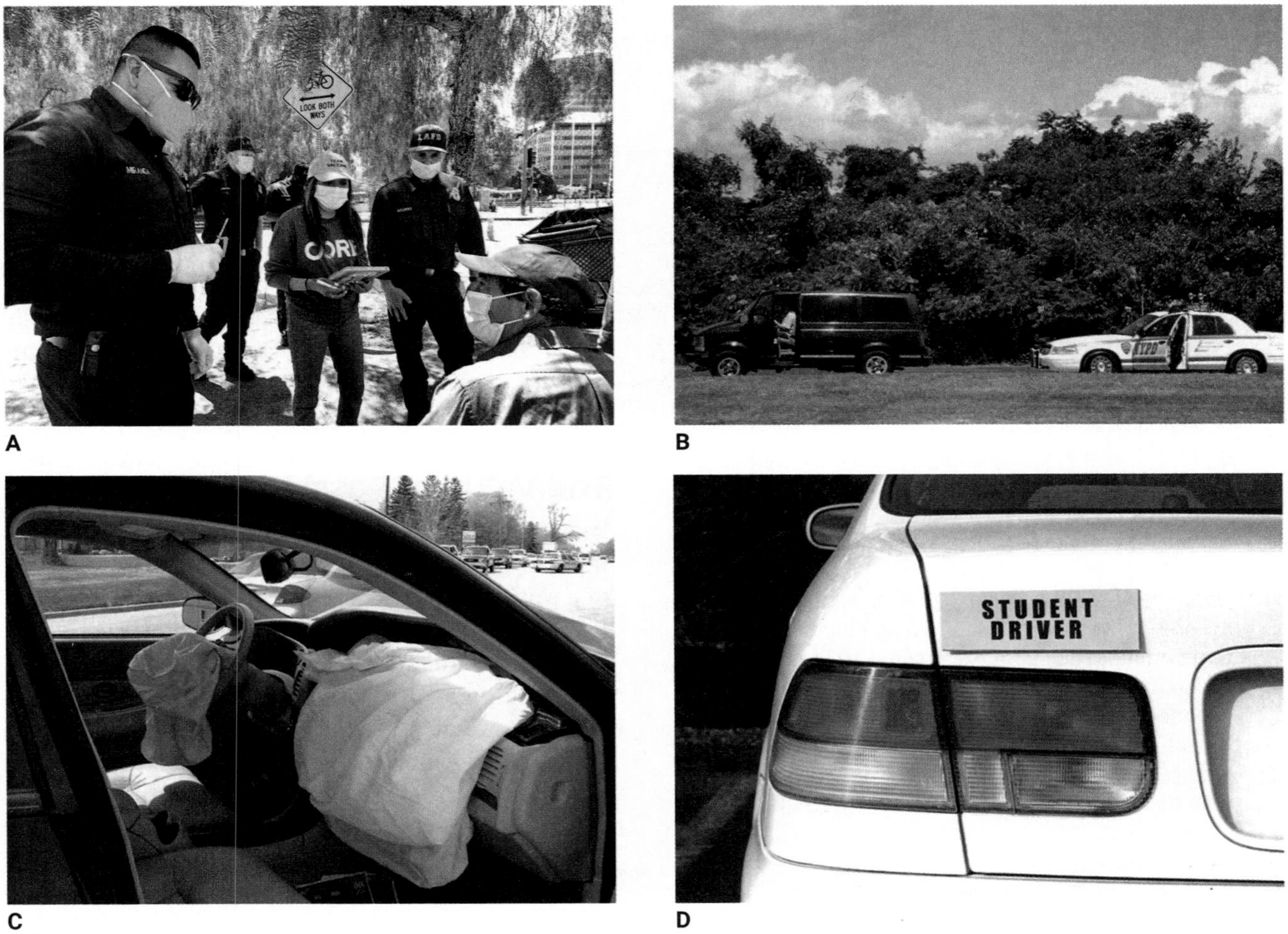

FIGURE 3-6 The 4 Es of prevention include education **(A)**, enforcement **(B)**, engineering/environment **(C)**, and economic incentives **(D)**. Examples of economic incentives include lower insurance rates for young drivers who have taken approved driver education programs or for adults who do not smoke.

that set policies and establish procedures also create regulations that control the manufacture, sale, and/or use of products. All these measures are helpful in the enforcement of safety regulations.

Many rules, regulations, guidelines, and laws govern public health. Some are generated by the federal government, whereas individual states or municipalities promulgate others. For example, there is currently no federal law requiring riders to use motorcycle helmets, and state laws on this issue vary widely. Similarly, there is no federal law requiring riders to wear a bicycle helmet; however, several states, municipalities, and counties have established child helmet laws. Most of these laws cover only bicyclists younger than 18 years.

Economic Incentives

Saving money by receiving a reduction in your insurance rates for being a careful driver or a nonsmoker is one example of how monetary incentives can reinforce safe behavior. Also, organizations often recognize the value of offering free or subsidized safety products (eg, bike helmets, fire extinguishers, carbon monoxide monitors, safety locks, smoking cessation kits, contraceptives), which may lead to a reduction in specific threats to public health.

Engineering/Environment

Most EMS providers can think of spots on the road where environmental changes such as

TABLE 3-4 Tips for Promoting Safety and Health

- Teach children about safety measures, such as never inserting their fingers into a wall socket, avoiding the oven and stove, and avoiding the pool when adults are not directly supervising them.
- Store drugs and chemicals out of children's reach.
- Store any firearms in the household in a locked location. Keep guns unloaded, and store the ammunition in a separate location.
- Install safety gates around stairs and swimming pools.
- Use window locks or guards for windows above ground level, and use stair gates to help prevent childhood fall injuries.
- To reduce the risk of childhood strangulation, ensure that drapery and window blind cords are out of reach.
- Once they are old enough to understand, teach children how to dial 9-1-1, and teach them when it is appropriate to do so.
- Program emergency phone numbers into your telephone. Include numbers for the local police department, fire department, EMS, and poison control center. If your phone is not programmable, post these phone numbers in a nearby visible location such as on the refrigerator.
- Ensure that your home and its exterior are well lit and that surfaces are even.
- Consider trip-and-fall hazards for older adults. Ensure all electrical cords are placed out of the flow of traffic, and avoid small rugs or runners that are not slip-resistant.
- Reduce bathroom hazards by installing grab bars in the shower and near the toilet. Minimize the likelihood of slipping by using rubber mats in showers and tubs.
- Install and maintain smoke alarms.
- If your home uses gas heat, install and maintain carbon monoxide detectors.
- Keep your water heater adjusted to less than 120°F (48.9°C) to prevent burns.
- Teach hands-only CPR to your family and friends.

Modified from: Home safety checklist. American College of Emergency Physicians website. https://www.emergencyphysicians.org/article/health--safety-tips/home-safety-checklist. Accessed May 28, 2021.

adding guardrails or smoothing out dangerous curves could prevent crashes. Indeed, making environmental changes or changing the way certain products are designed (eg, adding a new safety feature to vehicles) can offer automatic protection from injury, often without any conscious change in a person's behavior. These changes are called **passive interventions**. For example, the development of child-resistant medication bottles was a passive intervention intended to reduce poisonings; this blanket approach can be more effective and reliable than simply trying to keep the bottle out of a child's reach.

Strategies to modify environmental factors are often expensive and can include social, legal, political, and cultural approaches. Thus, they typically occur only after public awareness has been increased, thereby motivating the community to take responsibility for seeing positive changes made.

The Value of Passive Interventions

Passive interventions, or those preventive measures that do not require a conscious effort on the part of a potential victim, are often the most successful. Also referred to as automatic protection, passive interventions include sprinkler systems in commercial buildings, airbags in automobiles, and softer, yielding materials as playground surfaces. These measures can provide 24-hour protection without requiring any real effort on the part of the user.

Comparing education to automatic protection strategies, consider how each might aid in the prevention of head and chest injuries in MVCs:

- **Option 1.** Educate people on the importance of wearing their seat belts.
- **Option 2.** Mandate that all new vehicles be equipped with automatic seat belts and airbags.

The automatic protection offered by Option 2 is more likely to reduce injuries, because people do not have to do anything to make it work. However, the most effective strategies include a combination of education, enforcement, engineering/environmental modifications, and/or economic incentive programs. Education, in particular, is always a factor. Motor vehicle passengers need to know that airbags do not replace the need for seat belts.

Why EMS Should Be Involved

In the National Academy of Sciences/National Research Council's historic 1966 study, *Accidental Death and Disability: The Neglected Disease of Modern Society*, the commission noted that just as EMS could help with trauma *after* an event, injury prevention initiatives could help *before* an accident happened.[14] In 1996, representing every imaginable EMS constituency, the *Consensus Statement on the EMS Role in Primary Injury Prevention* contended that working toward this level of prevention should be seen as an "essential" activity "that must be undertaken by the leaders, decision-makers, and providers of every EMS system."[15]

Primary prevention is the name given to actions that stop injuries or illnesses before they occur. **Secondary prevention** measures take place after a patient has sustained an injury or developed an illness, in which case the goal is to "prevent" the problem from getting worse (eg, stabilizing a fractured extremity to prevent further tissue, nerve, or vascular damage; or administering epinephrine to a patient having an allergic reaction to a bee sting).

Historically, EMS has focused almost exclusively on *secondary* prevention. However, EMS culture has changed in recent years, and providers are now more involved in *primary* prevention efforts within their communities **FIGURE 3-7**.

Unlike other medical professionals, EMS providers see citizens in their homes and environments and during activities of daily life. As a result, EMS providers have more opportunities for prevention education than do other health care professionals. As previously stated, both the community and the health care system benefit more from efforts to prevent injuries and illness than from trying to treat them after they occur. EMS involvement in prevention education also has the following advantages:

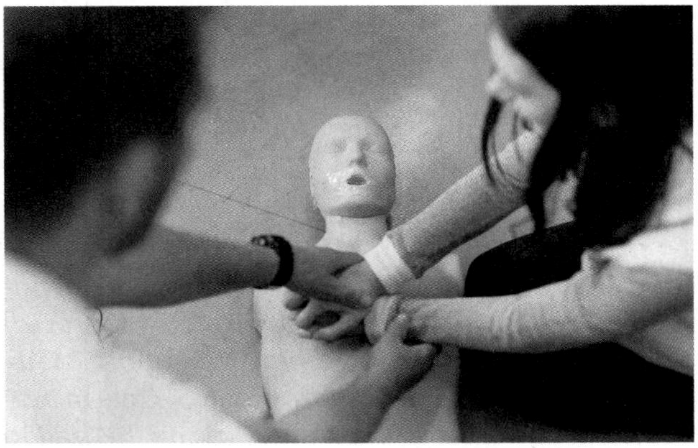

FIGURE 3-7 Embracing the full role of a paramedic means being involved in the concerns of your community.

- EMS providers are widely distributed among the population.
- In a remote setting, EMS providers may be the most medically educated people available. They may be the only source of help, whether they are a 1-hour drive down the mountain to the nearest ED or 200 miles offshore on an oil platform.
- EMS providers are considered advocates of the health care consumer. They work in concert with their patients and their patients' families.

YOU are the Paramedic

PART 3

Following your local protocol, you take measures to protect the infant's spine. Your partner informs you that, according to his mother, the child has no significant medical history, has no known allergies, and does not take any medications. The woman holding the infant tells you that she found him facedown, still strapped into his car seat, and crying when she got to him. However, no one on the scene can say with certainty whether the child lost consciousness.

Recording Time: 3 Minutes	
Respirations	42 breaths/min
Pulse	138 beats/min
Skin	Warm, dry, and normal color
Oxygen saturation (Spo_2)	99% on room air
Pupils	Pupals Equal, Round, and Reactive to Light and Accomodation (PERRLA)

5. What primary prevention measures might have helped to circumvent this traumatic incident? List any passive interventions that could have made a positive impact.

- EMS providers are welcome in schools and other environments.
- EMS providers are considered authorities on injury and prevention.

How EMS Can Get Involved

Motivated by their field experiences, EMS providers have emerged as strong advocates—and practitioners—of injury and illness prevention. Many paramedics have taken a more proactive role in new prevention programs, sometimes taking the lead in developing these programs.

For example, in 2016, paramedic Lisa Cassidy of the St. Charles County Ambulance District in Missouri led the charge in an awareness campaign called "Stop Heroin." Emboldened by a rising problem of heroin abuse in the community and the tragic deaths of many young users, Cassidy and more than 200 of her colleagues began every shift by donning "Stop Heroin" uniforms **FIGURE 3-8**. Every day across the county, the public saw paramedics on calls, at schools, and at other community events, wearing shirts that boldly proclaimed "Stop Heroin." This sparked a public awareness campaign that was ultimately featured in local and national publications. When asked why she became involved in the initiative, Cassidy stated her viewpoint quite eloquently:

> When it comes to drug use and overdoses, EMS has always been "reactive." Someone overdoses, we give Narcan, transport . . . the end. Since Narcan does not always work, I and the rest of my colleagues are all too often forced to deliver the worst news that a mother or father will ever receive: that we did everything we could, but their child is dead. This conversation was happening over and over, and with increasing frequency in our community. I decided that, as the organization that sees these situations firsthand, we should be part of the conversation, and hopefully, have a hand in developing a meaningful solution to the problem that is plaguing our county.

Strategies that promote interventions might include fundraisers to purchase and distribute free bicycle helmets to children, car seat checks and installations, appearing at health fairs, giving speeches to community groups and schoolchildren, BP checks, fall prevention services for older adults, or swimming safety education **FIGURE 3-9**.

One of the most visible ways in which EMS professionals have interacted with public health agencies is through the provision of immunizations. Consider how EMS professionals are ideally suited to reach at-risk populations. Their inherent mobility allows them to reach widely dispersed populations, something that might be especially helpful in rural areas where vaccination sites are either scarce, too far away, or impractical for people without a reliable means of transportation. Another benefit of EMS's involvement in immunizations may be

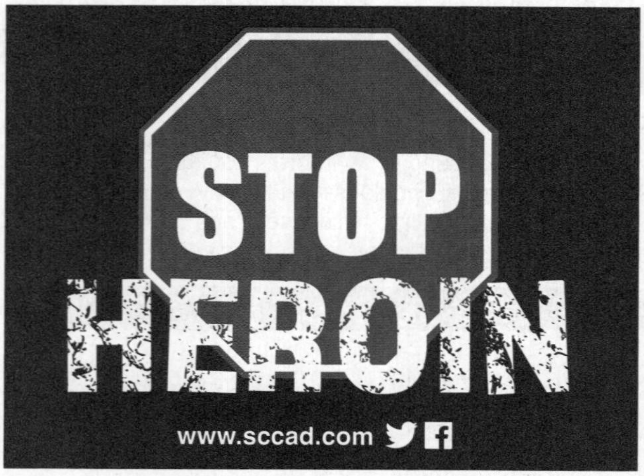

FIGURE 3-8 Inspired by the passionate convictions of paramedic Lisa Cassidy, the St. Charles County Ambulance District began an aggressive awareness and prevention campaign targeting heroin abuse in their community.

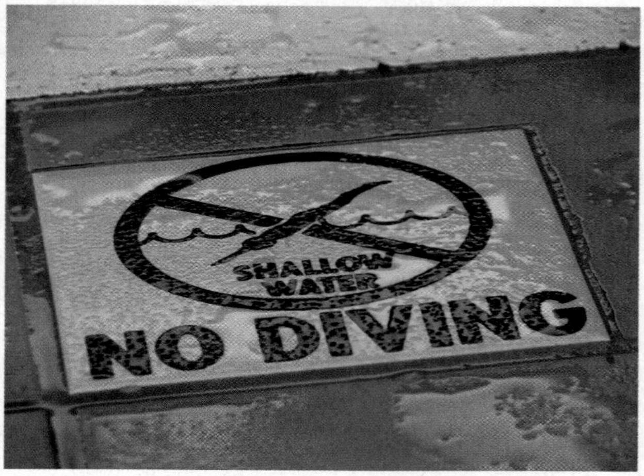

FIGURE 3-9 Many public safety rules exist because of the persistent efforts of medical professionals and other involved citizens.

the typically positive perception of EMS in small communities; this puts providers in an ideal position to bring aid to patients and families who are unable or unwilling to use private or governmental health care services. Many EMS providers have the requisite clinical training in medication security, aseptic technique, medication administration, post-injection care, documentation of informed consent for treatment, and ways to discuss risks, benefits, and possible side effects with the patient. Combined with the routine tasks performed by paramedics on the ambulance, this training makes them excellent candidates for the administration of vaccines to adults and children.

Of course, for such a program to work, EMS must work closely with the local public health agency to develop a plan that addresses all logistical matters, clearly defines each person's role and responsibilities, identifies and resolves any issues pertaining to the need for additional training, clearly explains the procedures for procuring the vaccine, and forestalls potential liability issues. Most of the time, these challenges are nowhere near as complicated as they may sound.

As the health care landscape continues to change in response to legislation like the Patient Protection and Affordable Care Act, paramedics across the United States have begun to witness the next evolution in the field of EMS. In particular, the terms *community paramedic* and *mobile integrated health care* have earned nationwide attention over the past several years. Several states have already implemented education requirements and legislation that recognizes the legitimacy of community paramedicine.

Words of Wisdom

In addition to being a health care provider, you—like any other health professional—must also be a health educator and advocate. Teaching helps keep your skills sharp; at the same time, it identifies you as a resource person in the community.

The concept of community paramedicine gives providers many new and expanded avenues for preventing illnesses and injuries as part of their regular daily duties. Conducting home health visits and well-being checks, providing wound care and other in-home therapies, ensuring medication compliance—the possibilities seem endless. EMS agencies that offer community paramedic services may eventually be recognized as a cost-effective supplement or alternative to ED visits and hospital admissions.

By offering these expanded services, EMS agencies could take a more proactive approach toward decreasing the **morbidity** (number of nonfatal injuries and subsequent disability) and **mortality** (death rate) among their patients. Providers could also play a significant role in reducing unnecessary hospital readmissions, wherein patients who were recently discharged from the hospital return only days later for conditions that could have been managed or prevented at home. These readmissions are expensive both for the patient and for hospitals (which may be at risk for the additional financial exposure under certain circumstances) and society at large, which will ultimately bear the financial burden through increases in insurance premiums and health care costs. As for the financial benefits for EMS systems that community paramedicine might bring, opportunities for reimbursement could exist through creative contracting with hospitals, managed care

Documentation and Communication

Do not forget special population groups in your safety and prevention programs. For instance, you may find different illness and injury patterns related to ethnicity, and can highlight these topics through the programs you offer to the public. Have printed materials available in the most common languages spoken in your community. Do not neglect people with physical or developmental challenges. Do your best to get the word out in every way possible.

Special Populations

With a growing geriatric population, a good flu prevention program may be one of the keys to preventing an overload of the health care system. Evaluate all community options available to the older population in your area, and bridge any gaps with programs to meet their needs and prevent illnesses related to the flu.

agencies, or other third-party payers that recognize the significant financial savings they could realize through a partnership with the EMS agency.

During the COVID-19 pandemic, the public health–related roles of EMS providers evolved quite rapidly. For instance, several state governors used their emergency powers to allow EMTs with additional training and paramedics to assist in vaccination programs across their jurisdictions. Paramedics also became involved in COVID-19 testing and contact tracing. Contact tracing includes monitoring those persons who have tested positive, alerting others who have been in close contact with the infected individual, and providing instructions for quarantining and/or seeking medical attention.[16,17]

Words of Wisdom

One manner in which EMS can assist public health efforts is by using dispatch data to perform **syndromic surveillance**. In a syndromic surveillance system, information regarding the number and nature of medical cases is compared with the expected volume of calls for the community at a given time and place. If cases exceed the expected numbers, epidemiologists are alerted to the possibility of an outbreak of disease.

Injury and Illness Surveillance

In the prevention setting, **surveillance** involves watching over society, and collecting and analyzing data. This kind of ongoing, systematic collection, analysis, and interpretation of data is essential to planning, implementing, and evaluating public health practice **FIGURE 3-10**.

The data are carefully analyzed and interpreted by **epidemiologists**, scientists who attempt to address health problems after studying the distribution and determinants of health-related events and conditions in a population—a field of study referred to as **epidemiology**. The epidemiologists' insights are used in developing interventions intended to prevent further injury or illness. For example, epidemiologists played a key role in recognizing and promoting the safety benefits of wearing seat belts.

A strong surveillance system is fundamental to creating an effective prevention program. In the case of injury surveillance, you need to know *who* is being injured, *where*, *by what* mechanism, and—if readily discernable—*why*. Thus, to create the most effective injury and disease surveillance program, you should begin by becoming familiar with the injuries and diseases common within your community.

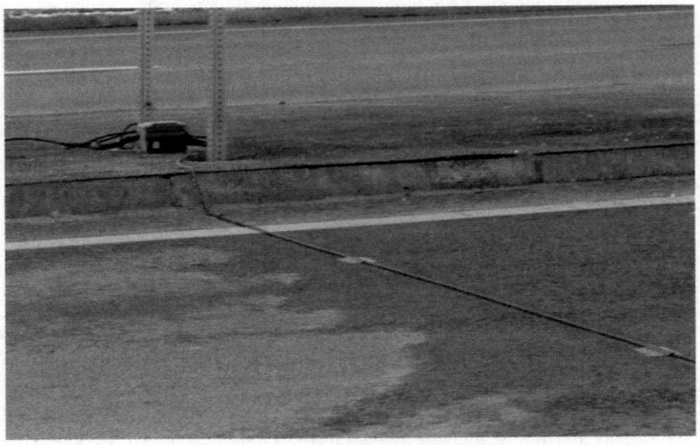

FIGURE 3-10 One type of surveillance that is familiar to anyone who drives is the use of technology that can tally the number of cars using a particular roadway.

Documentation and Communication

In the setting of a possible public health threat, the patient care reports that paramedics write following every call may be read and analyzed by epidemiologists to identify leading causes of injury or illness and then figure out ways to correct them. To guarantee "clean" data, you must fill out all the required fields in an EMS report, no matter how minute the details may seem. Including information such as a patient's sex or whether the patient was restrained during an MVC is imperative to facilitate accurate analysis.

Your narrative section is equally important, if not more so. Be as accurate and detailed as possible when reporting the circumstances behind an injury or illness. Although you may have checked the appropriate box in your care report, do not forget to describe the details. Narratives tell the story of what happened, helping the reader see how the incident unfolded. This firsthand information is often lost in hospital and police reports that rely on third- and fourthhand information hours or days later; thus, your reports must be clear and concise, yet thorough and detailed.

The Haddon Matrix

William Haddon, Jr, MD, the National Highway Traffic Safety Administration's first director, was given a clear, yet herculean mandate: to find ways to prevent people from being killed and injured on the nation's highways. In response, Haddon created a matrix that identified several principles of injury prevention.[18,19] This model proved so successful in helping researchers think about injuries that it was named after Haddon: the **Haddon matrix**. Haddon added the factor of *time* to the previous models used to address the causes of injury. The host, agent, and environment are seen as factors that interact over time to cause injury. These factors correspond to three phases of the event: pre-event, event, and post-event. Thus, the Haddon matrix uses nine separate components to analyze the injury, and encourages creative thinking to understand the causes of and potential interventions for injury. **TABLE 3-5** shows a Haddon matrix for the example of children who are occupants in vehicles that become involved in MVCs.

Most EMS providers are trained to respond in the *post-event* phase, after an injury or illness has taken place. This kind of response is *reactive*, not preventive. However, the post-event phase may be the optimal time to reflect on the event and apply your firsthand knowledge, asking, "*Why* did this happen?" and "*How* might this be prevented in the future?"

If you are willing to expend the extra effort needed to truly fulfill your role as your patients' advocate, you might be surprised at the difference you can make in motivating other medical professionals and organizations, your local government, and other members of your community to get involved.

TABLE 3-5 Childhood Motor Vehicle Occupant Injuries Using the Haddon Matrix

	Host (Human)	Agent (Car Seat/Vehicle)	Environment
Pre-event	• Wear seat belts and use car seats at all times. • Ensure the babysitter, daycare, and extended family members use car seat. • Drive defensively. • Reduce driving during high-risk times, such as rush hour, holiday weekends, or high-speed long-distance travel.	• Maintain up-to-date recall information on car seats. • Manufacture easy-to-use car seats. • Provide three-point seat belts in rear seating positions. • Regulate good maintenance and safety features of vehicle.	• Enforce seat belt and car seat laws. • Encourage safer roads with lower speeds, breakaway poles, and medians. • Encourage low-cost car seat programs. • Conduct media and education campaigns about seat belts, car seats, drunk driving, and enforcement.
Event	• Driver maintains control of vehicle. • Driver is belted. • Child is restrained.	• Seat belts and correctly used car seats restrain and protect. • Vehicle design provides crash protection.	• Breakaway signs and light poles are in place. • Guardrails and medians are in place.
Post-event	• Bystanders are trained in first response. • EMS personnel are expertly trained in treating pediatric injuries as well as car seat and seat belt extrications.	• Ambulances are outfitted with up-to-date supplies and equipment designed for children.	• Roadside call boxes are in place. • 9-1-1 and emergency medical dispatch systems are in place. • Adequate road shoulders for emergency use are in place. • There is quality EMS response and transport. • The patient is transported to a trauma center per protocol.

Abbreviation: EMS, emergency medical services

Through your eyes—the eyes of someone uniquely qualified to speak to the problem—perhaps they will be compelled to examine the problem more closely and ultimately to pursue and implement strategic solutions in the *pre-event* phase, sparing someone's son or daughter, or mother or father, from experiencing an event in the first place. Prevention is always better than crisis management.[20]

Words of Wisdom

Start your project with small, realistic goals. Contact other communities that have addressed similar problems. Learn from them, and perhaps you will avoid wasting time and energy creating something that already exists.

Getting Started in Your Community

Every community has its unique problems, many of which have a negative impact on the well-being of its residents. Trying to address all of these issues would be an overwhelming task. It would divide attention in so many different directions that it would be nearly impossible to research, develop, and implement any meaningful and effective interventions for every problem. Therefore, the most effective prevention programs elect to focus on problems that impair the health and well-being of the greatest number of people, thereby potentially *helping* the greatest number of people.

In time, perhaps you will get the opportunity to target other problems you want to address, even though they may affect only a minority of the population. However, by first tackling those issues that affect the greatest number of citizens, you and your community will feel a sense of pride at accomplishing a task that has had maximum impact on the community's well-being.

Recognizing Injury and Illness Patterns in Your Community

To be effective in prevention, you need to understand the specific and perhaps unique patterns of injuries and illnesses that occur in your community. Examine the characteristics of your community's population, environment, and the types of risks present. Your regional or state EMS office or public health department would be an excellent place to start, because it will likely have the most data, statistics, and other resources with relevant

YOU are the Paramedic

PART 4

Once the infant is immobilized and loaded into the ambulance, you decide the mechanism of injury alone is reason to commence rapid transport to the closest trauma center. En route, you start an intravenous (IV) line, clean and dress the wound on the patient's head, and splint his left arm. On arrival at the trauma center, you find the pediatric trauma team awaiting your report.

Recording Time: 10 Minutes	
Respirations	42 breaths/min
Pulse	126 beats/min
Skin	Warm, dry, and normal color
Cardiac monitor	Sinus tachycardia without ectopy
Oxygen saturation (Spo_2)	99% on room air
Pupils	PERRLA

6. Apply the Haddon matrix to this scenario.
7. What steps have you taken that would be considered secondary injury prevention?
8. What steps could you take to develop a prevention program to reduce similar incidents in the future?

information. Many state organizations even make this information available on the Internet.

Documentation and Communication

The importance of collecting data for measuring trends, validating interventions, assessing resources, and ultimately, persuading others to act, cannot be overstated. For the EMS provider, this process begins with the prehospital care report. By accurately describing the details of the scene, the mechanism of injury, the nature of the injury or illness, the status of the patient's immunizations, and the use or absence of protective devices, you are providing important evidence demonstrating the scope of the problem.

As an EMS provider, you can make a difference by being diligent in your documentation. Your first-hand observations may be relevant to other agencies such as law enforcement, the legal system, and social services seeking to intercede in settings of intentional violence. Paramedic training prepares you to recognize and report the signs and risk factors associated with, for example, intentional violence and empowers you to be proactive in the fight against suicide, domestic violence, and child abuse. This medical training and your unique perspective from being present at the scene put you among the few professionals who are able to provide this invaluable service.

SAFETY

As an EMS provider, you are continually taught to use personal protective equipment such as a helmet, reflective vest, and gloves and to observe traffic and other safety laws while on the job. The need for personal safety doesn't stop when your shift is over. Wear a seat belt and observe safety laws in everything you do. Practice a safe lifestyle both on and off the job.

As you make the journey from rookie paramedic to seasoned EMS veteran, never forget that your actions or inactions will influence other members of your crew, as well as the next generation of paramedics. The example you set will have an impact long after you retire.

Prevention Programs for Children

Many prevention programs focus on children. Numerous government and private grants, commercial sponsors, and nonprofit groups will support car seat inspections, helmet donations, fundraising events, and more, because they recognize the serious threat that injury poses to children. One such resource is Safe Kids Worldwide, a nonprofit organization made up of more than 400 coalitions in the United States and partners in over 30 countries. This organization's goal is to reduce the prevalence of preventable childhood injuries.[21] Its website is filled with helpful information, including examples of how other groups have addressed challenges similar to yours and resources that can assist you as you formulate new ideas.

SAFETY

Many EMS agencies have obtained certification for a few providers to offer no-cost child safety seat checks in their community.[22]

Sometimes, EMS providers' focus on children's issues can have other unintended benefits. One of these is the "pass-along effect," wherein other members of a child's family benefit from the message originally intended solely for the child's welfare. An example of this phenomenon occurs when a third-grader is educated on the importance of wearing a seat belt and later insists that Daddy buckle up, too.

Given the wide array of injuries that may affect children, how should you prioritize your prevention efforts? Experts in public health suggest focusing on injuries associated with a high rate of mortality, those that lead to hospitalizations and are frequently accompanied by long-term disability, or those known to have highly effective countermeasures. In other words, give priority to injuries that are common, severe, and readily preventable.

The Steps to Developing a Prevention Program

One step-by-step approach to establishing an injury prevention program, originally advocated by the Emergency Medical Services for Children

(EMSC) program, emphasizes the need to carefully establish goals and objectives with measurable outcomes. This initiative has since been adopted by various state offices and organizations such as the National Highway Traffic Safety Administration and the American Association for the Surgery of Trauma.[23] The following framework is described in terms of childhood prevention programs, but these methods can be applied to other age groups as well.

1. **Conduct a community assessment.** Bring people and groups together to assess what is already being accomplished in your region and to establish what resources (expertise, time, money) are potentially available. Ensure you invite people who represent the community at large, in all its diversity, including survivors of injuries or major illnesses and their families **FIGURE 3-11**. Recognize that some members of the community may have had a loved one die as a result of a preventable injury or illness; these people can be powerful advocates. Potential partners include:
   - EMS groups (private and public ground and air ambulance services, fire departments and firefighter unions, volunteer services, rescue squads, lifeguards)
   - Law enforcement (police departments and police officers, unions, sheriff's office, highway patrol, training academies)
   - School groups (parent-teacher associations, student clubs, school boards, faculty)
   - The media (management, editorial board members, staff reporters)
   - Public health officials and health care providers (groups representing emergency physicians and nurses, pediatricians, managed care organizations, hospitals, clinics) **FIGURE 3-12**
   - Members of the business community (including those related to insurance, cars, sports, home improvements, safety equipment, and local chambers of commerce)
   - Religious organizations, civic groups, and service clubs (such as the Kiwanis and the Boy Scouts and Girl Scouts)
   - Sports-related organizations (eg, Little Leagues or YMCAs)
   - Local chapters of nonprofit groups (eg, Safe Kids coalitions, Mothers Against Drunk Driving, the American Red Cross, the Alzheimer's Association)
   - Local and national celebrities, community leaders, and elected officials
   - Research groups (such as those at state universities, private colleges, community colleges)
2. **Define the problem.** On the basis of the community assessment and the data you have been able to gather, define the problem in specific, quantifiable terms. For example, you should be able to answer the following questions for your community:
   - What are the most frequent causes of fatal and nonfatal childhood injuries?
   - What are the most frequent diseases and chronic illnesses in the community?
   - Which populations (by age, location, and other characteristics) are at highest risk of

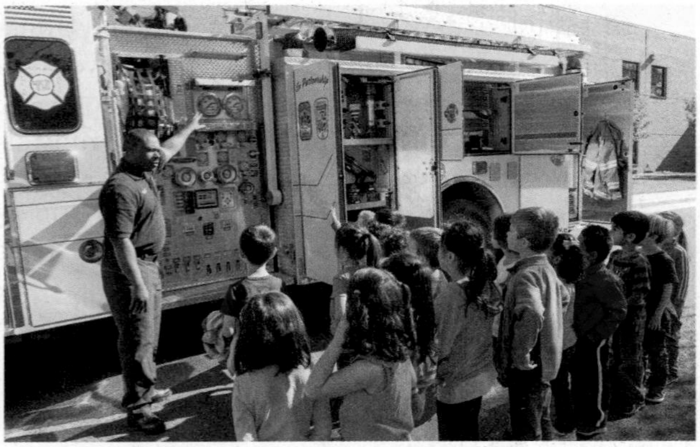

FIGURE 3-11 Fire safety training is one example of how public safety agencies engage in injury prevention activities.

FIGURE 3-12 Many organizations can serve as potential partners in an injury prevention campaign.

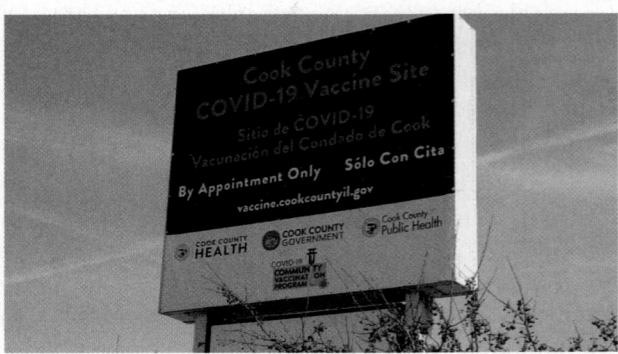

experiencing these injuries or illnesses? When and where are they occurring?
- What, if anything, is already being done to prevent these injuries or illnesses?
- Is an effective intervention available? What resources do you have to develop, implement, and evaluate different interventions?

3. **Set goals and objectives.**
   - **Goals.** Create a broad, general statement about the long-term changes the prevention initiatives are designed to make. For example, your goal might be to decrease preventable injuries to children on the community's roadways.
   - **Objectives.** These statements should be specific, time-limited, and quantifiable. There are two types of objectives: process and impact. A **process objective** might be to distribute 1,000 child safety seats to low-income families within the next 18 months, or to ensure that 500 older adult community members receive the flu vaccine. An **outcome (impact) objective** might be that the bicycle safety program will increase the rate of helmet use by children younger than 18 years from 30% to 50% within the next 18 months, or that the flu clinic will increase the number of flu vaccinations by 25% during the next year.
4. **Plan and test interventions.** Interventions are the actions you take to accomplish your goals and objectives. Using the 4 Es of prevention, brainstorm about options. Consider the resources you have available, and consider what other communities have done in similar situations. You may discover an intervention that proved successful for them, in which case you might be able to duplicate their actions. Experienced prevention specialists also suggest that you consider timing and cultural elements as you plan your intervention. Finally, getting a sample group together and testing the intervention before actually initiating the full program often helps to improve your chances of success.
5. **Implement and evaluate interventions.** There is a science to planning, implementing, and evaluating an intervention. To be credible, the results of your intervention must be measurable. A formal **evaluation** will definitively tell you whether you have met your goals and objectives. You want to spend your time and resources on efforts that you can *show* make a difference. For example, if your goal is to increase the use of seat belts, you could establish a measurable objective such as "Seat belt usage in the community will increase by 50%." To measure the effectiveness of your interventions, you could place volunteers at intersections throughout the city. These volunteers would then count every belted and non-belted motorist who stops in front of them, allowing you to measure the results of your interventions.

Finally, be aware that many—if not most—interventions demand ongoing attention to remain effective. The EMS service that had initial success in reducing backyard drownings saw the numbers go back up a few years after rolling out the program, as public interest and enthusiasm began to wane. Legislation to fence pools had a positive effect, but by itself, without continuing other interventions such as education, it was insufficient. The service had to redouble its efforts to reestablish the educational pieces of the program that had worked so well initially. This case illustrates why you should consider building a long-term maintenance plan into any intervention program, if you want to keep its momentum going.

Community Organizing

Members of the EMS community who have created successful prevention programs give the following advice, which can help you as you build your team and create an implementation plan:

- Identify a lead person to coordinate the effort.
- Build as broad a base of support as possible.
- Create a realistic timeline for any project, keeping in mind that most programs must be ongoing to be effective.
- Gather data and facts that pinpoint who is being injured where, with what, and how frequently, or data on which types of diseases are most common in your community.
- Choose goals and objectives that are SMART: Simple, Measurable, Accurate, Reportable, and Trackable; build consensus in the community on the need for action.

- Ensure you understand the religious, ethnic, cultural, and language challenges that you may face in implementing an intervention.
- Do not reinvent the wheel: seek out others who have had success with similar interventions or who have expertise in public health.
- Anticipate opposition and expect some losses; turf battles are common but not inevitable.
- When you lobby legislators, be brief during your phone calls, visits, and testimony.
- Set up your program so that you can measure results and make changes as needed.
- Establish self-sustaining funding sources.
- Keep a sense of humor and persist—change does not happen overnight.

Funding a Prevention Program

Ideally, EMS agencies should have the resources to incorporate primary prevention activities included within their normal operating budget. However, because this role represents a relatively new expansion of the EMS mission, this will take time. Even so, highly motivated and creative people have found a number of innovative ways to secure the resources they need:

- Partnering with the local media to create prevention messages, especially related to seasonal injuries or hazards.
- Seeking grants from regional, state, or national sources, such as the EMSC program. (Contacting your state EMS office about grant programs is a good place to start.)
- Seeking sponsorships from local nonprofit service organizations or commercial firms.

Networking with other organizations that are interested in prevention often provides greater leverage in seeking grants or sponsorships. Perhaps the EMS provider donates the time of volunteers and is a credible voice in the community, whereas the partner provides organizational resources and knowledge about establishing a scientifically credible injury intervention.

Summary

Today, the field of medicine continues to dedicate increasing attention and resources to the mission of public health—that is, promoting health and wellness and *preventing* injury and illness, rather than merely treating them after the fact. Efforts such as vaccination programs, helmet safety education, and disease screening can keep people well and decrease health care costs.

However, prevention is not a goal reserved solely for public health specialists. We can all play a part. Many EMS providers have embraced leadership roles in primary prevention after witnessing too many horrific examples of needless suffering. These leaders have recognized the unique opportunities afforded to them as first responders. How can *you* make a difference in your community?

YOU are the Paramedic SUMMARY

1. What is the most appropriate way to respond to this scene?

As with any call, you should wear your seat belt, stop at all red lights and stop signs, and operate with due regard for others. Keep in mind that despite the use of lights and siren, other drivers may not be able to hear or see your ambulance coming. A good rule of thumb is to perceive your lights and siren as a request for—not a guarantee of—the right-of-way. Other considerations include weather, road construction, traffic control, the presence of bystanders or children, and the need for additional specialty resources.

2. Based on the information provided, what potential injuries and complications should you anticipate?

Because there have been multiple crashes in this location, the environment may be a part of the problem. The negative bank of the curve, combined with the potential for excessive speed, increases the likelihood of an accident and serious injury. Anytime an ejection occurs, the assumption is that restraints were not used properly, which in turn greatly increases the threat of life-threatening trauma (eg, head and spine, severe external or internal blood loss). One other consideration is the possibility that

YOU are the Paramedic SUMMARY continued

drugs and/or alcohol contributed to the crash, in which case further scene safety issues arise.

3. What are the risk factors associated with the infant's injuries?

Having been ejected from the vehicle, the infant is at risk for significant injuries that could result in permanent disability or death. Beyond the visible injuries of a head hematoma/laceration and a forearm fracture, you should maintain a high index of suspicion for occult injuries—those not readily seen. Consider the mechanism of injury. Because the car seat was thrown from the vehicle, the patient may have come into contact with surfaces within the vehicle (eg, a window or windshield), and any object outside the vehicle, including the ground, trees, or something else.

4. Is this a teachable moment?

No. Because of the potentially critical status of the infant and the mother's level of distress over her baby's welfare, this is not the appropriate time to provide education on prevention. Under less severe circumstances, the improperly secured car seat would meet the criteria for a teachable moment.

5. What primary prevention measures might have helped to circumvent this traumatic incident? List any passive interventions that could have made a positive impact.

Some primary prevention measures in this scenario might include environmental changes such as improved warning systems (eg, reflective signs with flashing lights to alert drivers to the sharp curve ahead); installation of safety equipment such as reflective guardrails or other engineering projects such as reconstructing the roadway to eliminate the sharp degree of the problematic curve; greater enforcement of traffic laws, with higher fines for exceeding the speed limit (economic incentives) along with stronger law enforcement presence in the area; and/or educating parents on the proper installation of infant car seats, perhaps even offering free car seat inspections at fire and ambulance bases.

6. Apply the Haddon matrix to this scenario.

In this call you may view the event in the following manner:

- Pre-event:
  - Ensure a car seat is used and properly secured.
  - Drive defensively.
  - Car seat manufacturers must ensure that their products meet standards.
  - Vehicles should provide for easy installation of car seats.
  - Maintain the vehicle in proper working order.
  - Enforce car seat laws.
  - Install guardrails, traffic lights, and stop signs.
  - Provide law enforcement patrol in the area to enforce speed laws.
  - Offer education on the proper use of car seats.
- Event:
  - The child is properly restrained.
  - The driver maintains control of the vehicle.
  - The car seat is used correctly.
  - The vehicle design provides crash protection.
  - Guardrails, stop signs, and traffic lights are in place.
- Post-event:
  - First responders are trained and available.
  - Paramedics are up-to-date with pediatric certifications.
  - The ambulance is stocked with pediatric supplies.
  - Enhanced 9-1-1 is available.
  - The road shoulder is sufficient for emergency use.
  - A trauma center is nearby.

7. What steps have you taken that would be considered secondary injury prevention?

The mechanism of injury indicates the need for spinal precautions. Following your local protocol to ensure the patient's spine is protected and gaining IV access are secondary preventive measures you have taken to be prepared in the event that the infant's status deteriorates en route. Monitoring the infant's vital signs and electrocardiogram, and providing rapid transport to the closest, most appropriate facility are all crucial elements for secondary prevention in this case.

8. What steps could you take to develop a prevention program to reduce similar incidents in the future?

As part of your community assessment (your first step), researching call volume from this area would be a good place to start, as would retrieving information from local law enforcement and fire departments. Use these data to seek out identifiable patterns, then formulate a definition for the problem. Next, set a measurable and reasonable goal for reducing crashes and serious injuries in the designated area, and then define your objectives. These

YOU are the Paramedic SUMMARY continued

objectives might involve such interventions as offering free workshops for car seat installation and lobbying to have the roadway reconstructed and guardrails installed. Look for similar locales that have experienced similar problems under similar circumstances and learn how those communities addressed the matter. Was it effective? What did they learn along the way? Can they offer any helpful suggestions? Finally, put your plan into action, and after a predetermined period of time, evaluate the effectiveness of the interventions. Compare the new data you collect to the old data to see whether any positive changes have occurred. Regardless of the outcome, use your findings to adjust your goals and objectives as needed to become even more effective.

EMS Patient Care Report (PCR)

Date: 01-02-22	**Incident No.:** 1101234	**Nature of Call:** MVC		**Location:** Hwy 232 @ Needle Road	
Dispatched: 1420	**En Route:** 1422	**At Scene:** 1437	**Transport:** 1449	**At Hospital:** 1504	**In Service:** 1511

Patient Information

Age: 8 months **Sex:** M **Weight (in kg [lb]):** 10 kg (22 lb)	**Allergies:** NKDA **Medications:** None **Past Medical History:** None **Chief Complaint:** Lac/hematoma to R forehead, possible fx to L forearm

Vital Signs

Time: 1440	**BP:**	**Pulse:** 138	**Respirations:** 42	**Spo$_2$:** 99% on room air
Time: 1447	**BP:**	**Pulse:** 126	**Respirations:** 42	**Spo$_2$:** 99% on room air
Time:	**BP:**	**Pulse:**	**Respirations:**	**Spo$_2$:**

EMS Treatment (circle all that apply)

Oxygen @ _____ L/min via (circle one): **NC NRM Bag-mask device**		**Assisted Ventilation**	**Airway Adjunct**	**CPR**
Defibrillation	**Bleeding Control**	**Bandaging**	**Splinting**	**Other: Cardiac monitor**

Narrative

Unit 1 responded to a single-vehicle MVC with ejection. En route, EMS contacted dispatch to request an additional unit. Upon arrival, EMS found the vehicle in a ditch with moderate to severe damage, including a shattered window. A bystander stood several feet away from vehicle, holding a crying 8-month-old infant. Bystander said infant was thrown from vehicle, along with his car seat, landing face down in the ditch, still secured in car seat. Bystander removed patient from car seat before EMS arrival. Patient's mother was still in vehicle's driver seat. Mother is AAO×4 and denying injury. The second unit arrived soon after Unit 1 made patient contact, at which time they assumed care of the mother.

The infant patient had blood on his face from an approximately 3-cm lac superior to the right orbit with a hematoma surrounding the lac. Bleeding was controlled before arrival. Patient also presented with angulation to L forearm. Skin warm, dry, and normal color. Eyes PERRLA; it is unknown if patient experienced any loss of consciousness. Patient's spine secured according to local protocol. Vital signs normal for age (see vitals section). IV started, monitored ECG, dressed and bandaged wound, and splinted L forearm. Rapid transport to Midland Trauma Center due to MOI. No changes en route. Report given to Kathy RN on arrival.

End of report

Prep Kit

Ready for Review

- Public health is a field that encompasses health promotion and disease prevention for *groups* of people. Public health professionals examine the overall needs of the population to determine the best use of health resources and enhance quality of life for the public in general.
- Public health threats include both injuries and illnesses. The concept of years of potential life lost (YPLL) provides insight into the relative importance of different causes of premature deaths within a population that can guide public health planning, including prevention efforts.
- A teachable moment is an opportunity to convey and reinforce a message. Certain factors must be present for a teachable moment to exist. The best teachable moments are those that utilize positive reinforcement.
- The 4 Es of prevention are education, enforcement, engineering/environment, and economic incentives.
- Passive interventions are measures that do not require a conscious decision to act. An example is airbags in automobiles.
- The 1966 National Academy of Sciences/National Research Council study, *Accidental Death and Disability: The Neglected Disease of Modern Society*, noted that EMS could be a great asset in the post-event phase (secondary prevention) and that pre-event prevention (primary prevention) could significantly reduce the prevalence of injury or illness before it develops.
- The 1996 *Consensus Statement on the EMS Role in Primary Injury Prevention* emphasized that primary injury prevention is an essential activity of EMS.
- EMS providers can work with public health agencies on prevention efforts, such as providing immunizations. In the subfields of community paramedicine and mobile integrated health care, paramedics work in the community to prevent illness and injury as part of their regular daily duties.
- Surveillance is the ongoing systematic collection, analysis, and interpretation of data essential to the planning, implementation, and evaluation of public health practice. The data collected through such efforts are analyzed and interpreted by epidemiologists. Surveillance is crucial to an effective prevention program.
- The Haddon matrix uses nine separate components to analyze injury. The host, agent, and environment are factors that interact over time to cause injury during the pre-event, event, and post-event phases. The Haddon matrix encourages creative thinking to understand the causes and potential interventions for injury.
- The most effective prevention programs focus on problems that impair the health and well-being of the greatest number of people. To get started in your community, examine the population, environment, and types of risks present.
- Diligence in documentation is one way you can make a difference, especially in relation to cases involving intentional violence. Learn to recognize signs and risk factors associated with intentional violence, and include these factors as you create accurate, thorough documentation.
- Prevention programs often focus on children. Injury patterns in children vary widely depending on a range of factors, including the child's age, sex, socioeconomic status, development stage, and family environment.
- Steps in developing a prevention program include the following:
  - Conduct a community assessment.
  - Define the problem.
  - Set goals and objectives.
  - Plan and test interventions.
  - Implement and evaluate interventions.
- Creating a successful prevention program includes drafting an implementation plan that

Prep Kit continued

covers aspects such as data, goals, timelines, and funding sources. To fund a prevention program, consider partnering with local media, obtaining grants, or seeking sponsorship from local organizations or firms.

Vital Vocabulary

epidemiologists Public health professionals who investigate patterns and causes of disease and injury in a given population, and seek to reduce the risk, occurrence, and negative effects of these threats through research, public education, and legislative change.

epidemiology A scientific field devoted to studying the distribution and determinants of health-related events and conditions in a population in an attempt to address health problems.

evaluation Application of the appropriate methods, skills, and activities to determine whether a service or program is needed, likely to be used, conducted as planned, and actually helps people.

Haddon matrix A framework developed by William Haddon, Jr, MD, as a method to generate ideas about injury prevention that address the host, agent, and environment and their impact in the pre-event, event, and post-event phases of the injury process.

intentional injuries Injuries that are purposefully inflicted by a person on themselves or on another person; examples include suicide or attempted suicide, homicide, rape, assault, domestic abuse, elder abuse, and child abuse.

interventions In the context of prevention, specific measures or activities designed to meet a program objective; categories include education/behavior change, enforcement/legislation, engineering/technology, and economic incentives.

morbidity Number of nonfatally injured or disabled people; usually expressed as a rate, calculated as the number of nonfatal injuries in a certain population in a given time period divided by the size of the population.

mortality Deaths caused by injury and disease; usually expressed as a rate, calculated as the number of deaths in a certain population in a given time period divided by the size of the population.

outcome (impact) objective A statement of the intended effect of the program on participants or on the community in such terms as the participants' increased knowledge, changed behaviors or attitudes, or decreased injury rates.

passive interventions Something that offers automatic protection from injury or illness, often without requiring any conscious change of behavior by the person; child-resistant bottles and airbags are examples.

primary prevention Keeping an injury or illness from occurring.

process objective A statement of how a program will be implemented, describing the service to be provided, the nature of the service, and to whom it will be directed.

public health An industry whose mission is to prevent disease and promote good health within groups of people.

risk A potentially hazardous situation that puts people in a position in which they could be harmed.

risk factors Characteristics of people, behaviors, or environments that increase the chances of disease or injury; examples include alcohol use, poverty, smoking, and sex.

secondary prevention Reducing the effects of an injury or illness that has already happened.

surveillance The ongoing systematic collection, analysis, and interpretation of injury data essential to the planning, implementation, and evaluation of public health practice.

syndromic surveillance Monitoring and comparing the current number and nature of

Prep Kit continued

medical cases against the expected volume of these cases at a given time and place in the community.

unintentional injuries Injuries that occur without intent to harm (commonly called accidents); examples include motor vehicle collisions, poisonings, drownings, falls, and most burns.

years of potential life lost (YPLL) A way of measuring and comparing the overall impact of deaths resulting from different causes.

References

1. EPIC medics. California Paramedic Foundation website. https://caparamedic.org/epic-medics/. Accessed April 28, 2021.
2. American Public Health Association. Get the facts. What is public health? Our commitment to safe, healthy communities. https://www.apha.org/~/media/files/pdf/factsheets/whatisph.ashx. Accessed April 28, 2021.
3. Kochanek KD, Xu J, Arias E. *Mortality in the United States, 2019.* National Center for Health Statistics Data Brief: December 2020. https://www.cdc.gov/nchs/data/databriefs/db395-H.pdf. Accessed April 28, 2021.
4. Injury prevention and control: protect the ones you love—child injuries are preventable. Centers for Disease Control and Prevention website. https://www.cdc.gov/safechild/. Updated May 2, 2016. Accessed February 4, 2017.
5. McDermott KW, Stocks C, Freeman WJ. *Overview of Pediatric Emergency Department Visits, 2015.* HCUP Statistical Brief #242: August 2018. Agency for Healthcare Research and Quality website. https://hcup-us.ahrq.gov/reports/statbriefs/sb242-Pediatric-ED-Visits-2015.pdf. Accessed April 28, 2021.
6. Liller K. Unintentional injuries in children. *Pediatr Rev.* 2011;32(10):431-438; quiz 439.
7. Playground safety. Injury prevention and control: protect the ones you love—child injuries are preventable. Centers for Disease Control and Prevention website. https://www.cdc.gov/safechild/playground/index.html. Updated February 6, 2019. Accessed April 28, 2021.
8. Sports safety. Injury prevention and control: protect the ones you love—child injuries are preventable. Centers for Disease Control and Prevention website. https://www.cdc.gov/safechild/sports_injuries/index.html. Updated February 6, 2019. Accessed April 28, 2021.
9. Raghupathi W, Raghupathi V. An empirical study of chronic disease in the United States: a visual analytics approach to public health. *Int J Environ Res Public Health.* 2018;15(3):431.
10. Boersma P, Black LI, Ward BW. Prevalence of multiple chronic conditions among US adults, 2018. *Prev Chronic Dis.* 2020;17:200130.
11. A timeline of the coronavirus pandemic. *New York Times* website. https://www.nytimes.com/article/coronavirus-timeline.html. Published August 6, 2020. Accessed April 28, 2021.
12. COVID-19 dashboard. Johns Hopkins University, Center for Systems Science and Engineering, website. https://www.arcgis.com/apps/opsdashboard/index.html. Accessed April 28, 2021.
13. Years of life lost. Health Knowledge website. https://www.healthknowledge.org.uk/public-health-textbook/research-methods/1a-epidemiology/years-lost-life. Accessed August 18, 2021.
14. Committee on Trauma and Committee on Shock. *Accidental Death and Disability: The Neglected Disease of Modern Society*. Washington, DC: National Academy of Sciences; 1966:10.
15. National Highway Traffic Safety Administration (NHTSA), US Department of Transportation. *Consensus Statement on the EMS Role in Primary Injury Prevention*. Washington, DC: NHTSA; 1996.
16. Contract tracing for COVID-19. Centers for Disease Control and Prevention website. https://www.cdc.gov/coronavirus/2019-ncov/php/contact-tracing/contact-tracing-plan/contact-tracing.html. Updated February 25, 2021. Accessed April 28, 2021.
17. Lawrence E. Tracing a new pathway for EMS workers. EMS1 website. https://www.ems1.com/ems-products/financial-services/articles/tracing-a-new-pathway-for-ems-workers-2NckxMdO7A0udnXK/. Published May 28, 2020. Accessed April 28, 2021.
18. The facts. National Highway Traffic Safety Administration website. https://one.nhtsa.gov/nhtsa/Safety1nNum3ers/june2015/S1N_June15_ChangeTrafficSafety_3.html. Accessed April 28, 2021.
19. Runyan C. Using the Haddon matrix: introducing the third dimension. *Inj Prev.* 1998;4(4):302-307.
20. Dalton D. *Enough Is Enough: Finding Balance in an Imbalanced World.* Bloomington, IN: Xlibris Publishing; 2003.
21. Who we are. Safe Kids Worldwide website. https://www.safekids.org/who-we-are. Accessed April 28, 2021.
22. Become a tech. National Child Passenger Safety Certification website. https://cert.safekids.org/become-tech. Accessed June 1, 2021.
23. Ten steps for developing an injury prevention program: a community guide to injury prevention. American Association for the Surgery of Trauma website. https://www.aast.org/resources-detail/ten-steps-developing-injury-prevention-program. Accessed June 1, 2021.

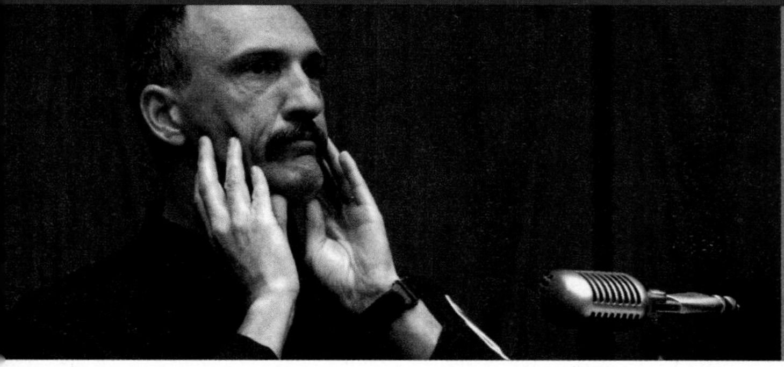

Chapter 4

Medical, Legal, and Ethical Issues

NATIONAL EMS EDUCATION STANDARD COMPETENCIES

Preparatory

Integrates comprehensive knowledge of the EMS system, safety/well-being of the paramedic, and medical/legal and ethical issues, which is intended to improve the health of EMS personnel, patients, and the community.

Medical/Legal and Ethics

- Consent/refusal of care (pp 135–136)
- Confidentiality (pp 129–130)
- Advance directives (pp 144–145)
- Tort and criminal actions (pp 124–125)
- Evidence preservation (pp 133–134)
- Statutory responsibilities (p 150)
- Mandatory reporting (p 134)
- Health care regulation (pp 129–131)
- Patient rights/advocacy (pp 136–138)
- End-of-life issues (pp 149–150)
- Ethical principles/moral obligations (pp 121–123)
- Ethical tests and decision making (pp 136–137)

KNOWLEDGE OBJECTIVES

1. Differentiate between laws and ethics. (pp 118–119)
2. Describe medical ethics, including the implications for paramedics. (pp 119–123)
3. Discuss the legal system in the United States and how it affects paramedics. (pp 123–124)
4. Differentiate between civil and criminal law relevant to paramedics. (pp 124–126)
5. Describe the process of a typical lawsuit against emergency medical services. (pp 126–127)
6. Discuss the legal and ethical accountability of paramedics. (pp 127–128)
7. Discuss legislation that affects paramedic practice. (p 128)
8. Differentiate between licensure and certification as they apply to paramedic practice. (pp 128–129)
9. Explain the importance and necessity of patient confidentiality and the standards for maintaining patient confidentiality applicable to paramedic practice. (pp 129–130)
10. Discuss the legal and ethical issues surrounding patient transport. (p 133)
11. Describe the actions that you should take to preserve evidence at a crime or motor vehicle crash scene. (pp 133–134)
12. Explain the mandatory reporting requirements for special situations, including abuse or neglect, drug-related injuries, childbirth, suicide, and crime scenes. (p 134)

13. Differentiate between expressed, informed, implied, and involuntary consent. (pp 135–136)
14. Describe the processes you should use to determine consent or valid refusal, especially relative to the patient's decision-making capacity. (pp 136–137)
15. Identify the steps to take if a patient refuses care, and when to transport a patient against the patient's will. (pp 137–138)
16. Identify methods for obtaining consent for minors, including exceptions for emancipated minors. (pp 138–139)
17. Discuss the legal ramifications of patient restraint, both physical and chemical, for patient and practitioner safety. (pp 139–140)
18. Define the four elements that must be present to prove negligence: duty, breach of duty, proximate cause, and damage (harm). (pp 140–143)
19. Discuss abandonment as it relates to paramedic practice. (pp 143–144)
20. Discuss patient rights, including autonomy, end-of-life decisions, and the moral and ethical implications of do not resuscitate orders and other advance directives. (pp 144–149)
21. Identify situations in which it would be appropriate for you to cease resuscitation efforts or not to initiate resuscitation efforts in the field. (pp 148–149)
22. Discuss your responsibilities relative to resuscitation efforts for patients who are potential organ donors. (pp 149–150)
23. Discuss common defenses to litigation, including contributory negligence. (p 150)
24. Describe forms of legal immunity that can apply to you as a paramedic. (pp 150–151)
25. Discuss employment legislation regarding sexual harassment, discrimination, disabilities, the Family and Medical Leave Act (FMLA), Occupational Safety and Health Administration law, and other legislation that applies to paramedic practice. (pp 152–155)

SKILLS OBJECTIVES

There are no skills objectives for this chapter.

Introduction

All medical professionals provide care under laws, which govern many human activities in a democracy. As a paramedic, you, too, will be governed by a set of laws that affect how you treat patients. Laws define our obligations and protect our rights and the rights of others. **Ethics** are principles, either personal or societal, that determine what is right and wrong. One of the major differences between laws and ethics is that laws include enforceable sanctions for violations **FIGURE 4-1**. As a paramedic responding to an emergency, you work within a framework of several types of laws that are set down by the federal government and/or the state government, including:

- Motor vehicle laws for the operation of an emergency vehicle
- Emergency medical services (EMS) legislation
- Medical licensing statutes and regulations

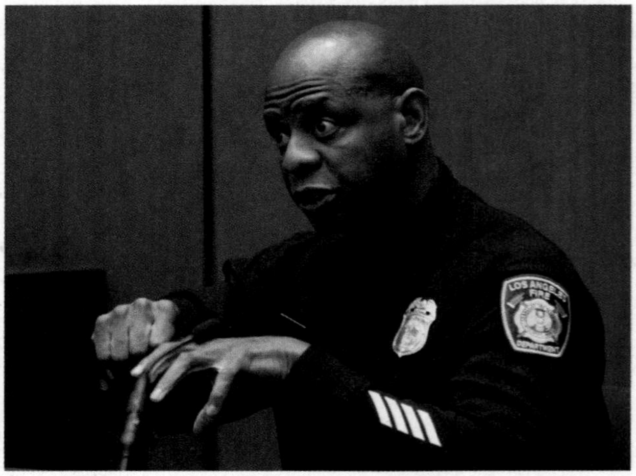

FIGURE 4-1 Unlike ethics, laws are enforceable rules that all citizens are obliged to follow. Paramedics are sometimes called into court to testify and provide evidence regarding cases that are under investigation or being litigated.

- Civil and criminal statutes about touching, treating, transporting, and possibly injuring another person
- Confidentiality laws such as the Health Insurance Portability and Accountability Act (HIPAA)

It is essential that you have a basic understanding of the laws and ethics applicable to prehospital emergency care. Failure to perform your job within the law can result in civil liability or even criminal liability. Indeed, malpractice lawsuits against EMS providers are increasing.[1] Practicing outside the law may also result in regulatory action within your state (a disciplinary hearing, for example) or action by your agency and medical director. An EMS provider can be prosecuted in any or all of these jurisdictions for the same case.

Ethics is the branch of philosophy that deals with the study and understanding of the distinction between right and wrong and how people apply concepts of right and wrong to their personal and professional lives. *Applied ethics* refers to the use of ethical values. In the past, the terms *ethics* and **morality** (pertaining to conscience, conduct, or character) were sometimes distinguished from one another, but today the two words are more commonly used interchangeably and little, if any, meaningful difference exists between the two. A moral paramedic is an ethical paramedic.

This chapter reviews important legal and ethical concepts affecting paramedic practice. However, this text is only a framework to help you understand these issues. It cannot substitute for competent legal advice because many laws and legal obligations differ from state to state. Contact an attorney specializing in the representation of medical professionals if you need legal advice related to your practice.

Words of Wisdom

Without question, your best legal protection is to provide appropriate patient assessment and emergency medical care, based on the patient's condition, followed by complete and accurate documentation. Be a strong advocate for your patient. Perform within your scope of practice and be respectful of patients, their property, and their privacy.

Words of Wisdom

Many state EMS offices have websites with information on laws that affect emergency medical responders, emergency medical technicians, and paramedics. It is a good idea for you to review the laws of the state in which you work.

Medical Ethics

It is essential to understand the difference between your personal ethics and the ethics of your profession. On the one hand, personal ethics are the product of your upbringing, family and community influences, your religious background, and

YOU are the Paramedic

PART 1

You are eating breakfast at 0737 hours when you are dispatched to 487 Lenore Street for an unresponsive person. While you are en route, you and your partner discuss what could possibly be wrong with this patient, such as cardiac arrest, hypoglycemia, or stroke.

You arrive on scene at 0742 hours and are met at the ambulance by a woman who tells you that her 64-year-old mother is "acting strangely" this morning. She says that her mother initially would not respond to her at all, but then started "talking out of her head." She also says her mother does not want to go to the hospital.

1. What type of consent is required to treat a patient with altered mental status?
2. What information must you determine prior to allowing a patient to refuse care?

your conscience. On the other hand, professional ethics arise out of your profession's standards and practices, the Code of Professional Conduct, and in some instances, various state and federal laws such as HIPAA (discussed later in this chapter). Situations may arise in which your personal ethical beliefs may come into conflict with your professional ethical standards. In almost every such case, you will be bound by professional ethics and must understand that your personal ethics must be temporarily set aside.

As a paramedic, you must always be ethical in your practice and be aware of your own moral standards in your daily work. The interests of your patient should take precedence over your personal beliefs and standards **FIGURE 4-2**.

Ethics related to the practice and delivery of health care are known as medical ethics (sometimes called bioethics). Your understanding of medical ethics must be formed as a part of, and consistent with, general codes established for health care professionals **FIGURE 4-3**. Throughout history, many codes of ethics for health professionals have been published. The Declaration of Geneva, first drafted by the World Medical Association in 1948, provides a good example; it is the oath taken by many medical students on completion of their studies, at the time of being admitted to the medical profession:

> I solemnly pledge myself to consecrate my life to the service of humanity; I will give to my teachers the respect and gratitude that is their due; I will practice my profession with conscience and dignity; the health of my patient will be my first consideration; I will respect the secrets which are confided in me, even after the patient has died; I will maintain by all the means in my power the honor and noble traditions of the medical profession; my colleagues will be my sisters and brothers; I will not permit considerations of age, disease or disability, creed, ethnic origin, gender, nationality, political affiliation, race, sexual orientation, social standing, or any other factor to intervene between my duty and my patient; I will maintain the utmost respect for human life; I will not use my medical knowledge to violate human rights and civil liberties, even under threat; I make these promises solemnly, freely, and upon my honor.[2]

Similar principles underlie the more detailed *Code of Ethics for EMS Practitioners*, which was

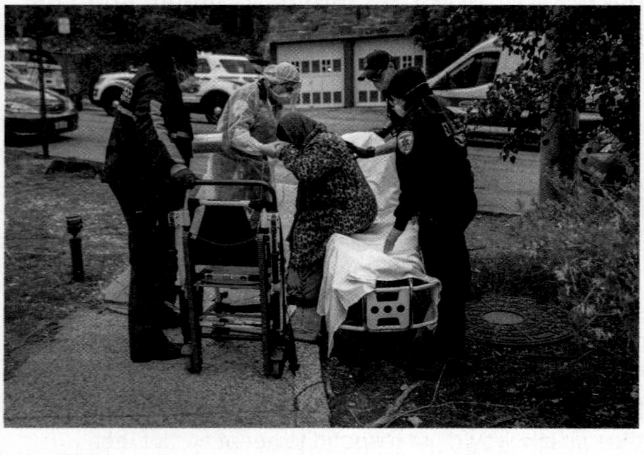

FIGURE 4-2 As a paramedic serving a diverse public, you will frequently work with people who have cultural backgrounds that differ from your own. Work to set aside your personal beliefs when making decisions on the patient's behalf.

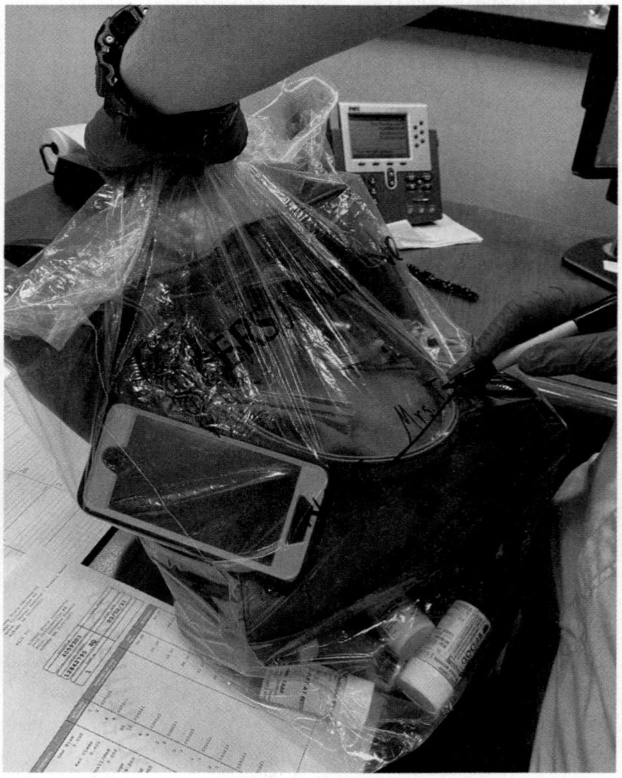

FIGURE 4-3 When people call 9-1-1, they trust you not only to provide proper emergency medical care, but also to use sound ethical judgment, which includes safeguarding their possessions.

issued by the National Association of Emergency Medical Technicians (NAEMT) in 1978 and is still in effect today:

> Professional status as an Emergency Medical Services (EMS) Practitioner is maintained and enriched by the willingness of the individual practitioner to accept and fulfill obligations to society, other medical professionals, and the EMS profession. As an EMS practitioner, I solemnly pledge myself to the following code of professional ethics:
>
> - To conserve life, alleviate suffering, promote health, do no harm, and encourage the quality and equal availability of emergency medical care.
> - To provide services based on human need, with compassion and respect for human dignity, unrestricted by considerations of nationality, race, creed, color, or status; to not judge the merits of the patient's request for service, nor allow the patient's socioeconomic status to influence our demeanor or the care that we provide.
> - To not use professional knowledge and skills in any enterprise detrimental to the public well-being.
> - To respect and hold in confidence all information of a confidential nature obtained in the course of professional service unless required by law to divulge such information.
> - To use social media in a responsible and professional manner that does not discredit, dishonor, or embarrass an EMS organization, coworkers, other health care practitioners, patients, individuals, or the community at large.
> - To maintain professional competence, striving always for clinical excellence in the delivery of patient care.
> - To assume responsibility in upholding standards of professional practice and education.
> - To assume responsibility for individual professional actions and judgment, both in dependent and independent emergency functions, and to know and uphold the laws which affect the practice of EMS.
> - To be aware of and participate in matters of legislation and regulation affecting EMS.
> - To work cooperatively with EMS associates and other allied health care professionals in the best interest of our patients.
> - To refuse participation in unethical procedures, and assume the responsibility to expose incompetence or unethical conduct in others to the appropriate authority in a proper and professional manner.[3]

Your state may also have its own code of ethics for EMS professionals. Likewise, the service or company you work for may have its own set of policies, rules, or regulations that will guide its employees' ethical expectations. The ICARE program, developed by a group of EMS students and educators, incorporates many of the finest qualities of EMS professionals.[4] ICARE (which stands for Integrity, Compassion, Accountability, Respect, and Empathy) is an excellent concept for you to remember and incorporate into the emergency medical care that you provide to your patients.[4] All of the various codes and rules of right and wrong ultimately stem from a concern for the patient's welfare. It is a safe generalization to say that if you place the patient's welfare ahead of all other considerations, you will rarely (if ever) commit an unethical act in the practice of emergency medical care.

It would be impossible to list all ethical dilemmas that you could encounter in your work as a paramedic. Regardless of the ethical circumstances that arise, you should always apply three basic ethical concepts when making a decision. These ethical principles, which have been considered an inherent part of health care for centuries, are (1) to do no harm, (2) to act in good faith, and (3) to always act in the patient's best interest.

The principle of "First, do no harm" (Latin: *primum non nocere*) essentially means that you should take due care to ensure that the patient receives the best possible care and that your actions do nothing to harm the patient. It requires you to take care of how you assess, treat, and transport patients so that you do nothing to exacerbate their medical condition or cause an additional injury or medical condition.

The two principles of acting in good faith and acting in the patient's best interest go hand in hand. These principles are simply a reinforcement of your commitment to always place the patient's interests above all else and to make decisions that are motivated by a clear desire to benefit the patient. Sometimes you may make decisions on behalf of an unconscious or otherwise incompetent patient that the patient or a family member will later question.

In such circumstances, you should be able to state confidently that the decision you made was motivated by your desire to benefit the patient.

As a paramedic, you must be accountable for your actions at all times. How you handle teamwork, your personal attitude on the job, justice and respect for patient autonomy, and cultural or lifestyle diversity will ultimately shape your career. Consider what type of paramedic you want to become **FIGURE 4-4**. It is helpful for you, as a new paramedic, to choose a mentor whose style and professionalism you wish to emulate.

Street Smarts

Some religious beliefs influence a patient's decision about treatment and may differ from what you think is best for a patient. For example, patients sometimes refuse standard life-saving therapies and treatments based on their religious convictions. Take the time to learn about the different religious communities in your service area and their beliefs.

Professional ethics are essential as the EMS profession continues its pursuit of being recognized and funded in the same manner as other medical professions. Immature, unprofessional behavior is unethical and has no place in this profession. Criminal acts, such as sexual misconduct, substance abuse, patient abuse, and harassment or stalking of coworkers, are both unethical and illegal. Likewise, inappropriate use of emergency vehicles, inappropriate visitors entertained at the station, and use of alcohol on duty are strictly forbidden. Off-duty misconduct can, and does, affect your reputation and may affect your employment status as well. News stories that depict EMS personnel engaged in any immature or illegal activities will only lessen the public's confidence in the services you provide.

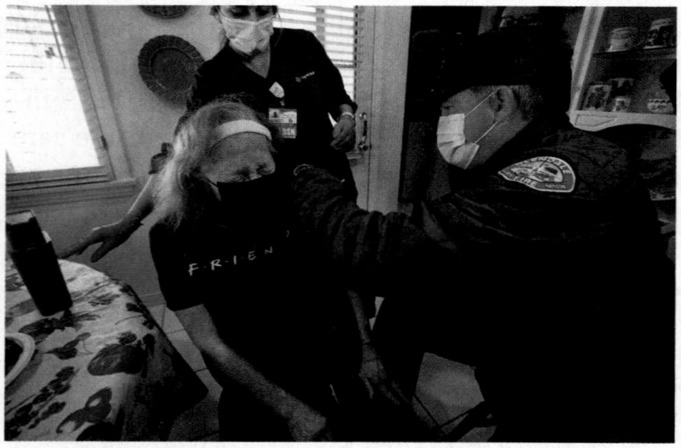

FIGURE 4-4 One of the best ways to hone your skills as a paramedic is to find a good mentor whose work ethic and attitude you admire.

Unfortunately, another significant ethical and legal problem in EMS is the falsification of training and certification; for example, falsely representing your level of certification or falsifying training records.[5,6] Practitioners who falsely represent themselves will face charges; any EMS instructor who signs off on such a falsification will face similar charges as well. These charges can result in punishments ranging from suspension and revocation of licensure to criminal and civil charges based on the patient's outcome.

Always be respectful of patients and never do anything to violate the trust that patients have placed in you. As a paramedic, you are expected to honor the trust that has been bestowed on you as a member of the health care profession, to act ethically and professionally in every circumstance, and to avoid any misconduct that could call into question your ethics or integrity. Regrettably, some paramedics have violated their profession's ethical standards and have mistreated patients in various ways. Such misconduct has included discriminatory and abusive treatment, embellishing patient assessment findings over the radio to obtain drug orders from a physician, and even sexual abuse. These violations of ethical standards harm the profession as a whole, not just those parties directly involved. Fortunately, these cases of misconduct are rare. Your profession's ethics require total commitment to acting in the best interest of patients and to otherwise conducting yourself professionally and ethically at all times—that is, caring about your patients, coworkers, and the EMS system as a whole. To meet this standard, you cannot overlook other EMS providers engaging in misbehavior. Instead, you must promptly report any misconduct using the appropriate chain of command. Similarly, you are obligated to report medical errors you either make or witness to the medical director as soon as possible.

Paramedics who choose to become patient advocates, who participate in and actively seek out the best in training and professional development, and who put the good of the team above their own aspirations will ultimately succeed and be rewarded with a fulfilling career in EMS. Good mentors can instill good ethics. People seem to perform best when they share themselves and work toward an end much more significant than themselves. EMS is an evolving specialty, and its future lies in your hands.

Ethics and EMS Research

EMS practices have largely evolved like the rest of EMS: with grassroots effort and precious little research to confirm the effectiveness of procedures used in the prehospital setting. Properly randomized controlled studies in EMS are uncommon, but they are emerging. Remember that the first principle of medical practice is to do no harm, which means you must continue to seek further education about the effectiveness of EMS practice. Some EMS care still relies on anecdotal experience and is unsupported by research. Some EMS procedures, however well intentioned, may prove not to be helpful to patients. As a health care provider, you must be aware of procedures that are not recommended, even if anecdotal evidence suggests those procedures worked for you or your colleagues in the past.

Conducting EMS studies on critically ill or injured patients without their **consent** (agreement to accept a medical intervention) poses a real ethical dilemma. These patients are usually unable to give consent, and their physical state is so compromised that even if they are conscious, they may be unable to absorb information to give informed consent (discussed later in this chapter). Research projects involving human subjects must be overseen by an institutional review board (IRB) that reviews and monitors the project and ensures adherence to ethical standards. In addition, the Food and Drug Administration has specific guidelines regarding exceptions to informed consent, such as research conducted in emergency settings. As part of your continuing education, monitor how researchers are handling this issue and other ethical debates concerning patients in research.

The Legal System in the United States

Both federal and state governments make, administer, and interpret laws that affect paramedics. Each level of government has three branches **FIGURE 4-5**. The legislative branch, made up of elected officials (Congress at the federal level; state legislatures at the state level), makes laws. The judicial branch (consisting of the court system) enforces and interprets those laws and resolves disputes based on the interpretation of laws. Common law can also affect EMS. **Common law** (case law) is defined as a decision that a judge has made through a court case based on interpretation of statutes and constitutions. A common law can be overturned either by another court with higher authority or by the issuing court at a later time.

Courts have several levels, including trial courts and appellate courts. Although many people believe that all law comes from statutes passed by the legislative branch, this notion is not entirely accurate. Court decisions, especially those issued by appellate courts, establish precedent and become the law of the state in which you live and practice as a paramedic. In most cases, these court decisions establish negligence standards (discussed later in this chapter) that will apply if a patient sues you.

The third branch—the executive or administrative branch—reports to the president (in Washington, DC) or the governor (in your state capital); it is made up of various cabinets and agencies (bureaucrats) that carry out and administer laws. The agencies often use regulations to establish how things should be done. Agencies such as the Occupational

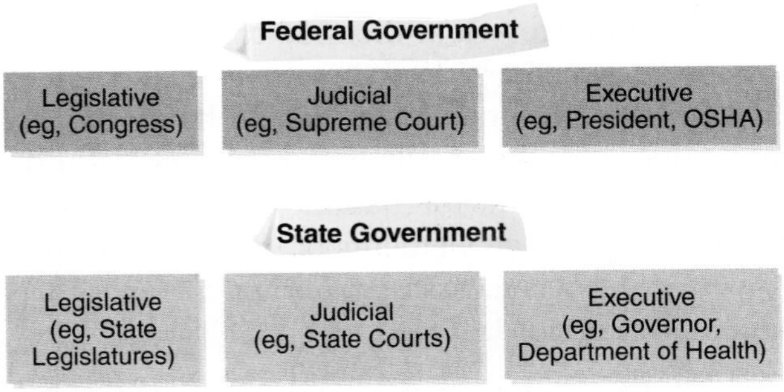

FIGURE 4-5 Both federal and state governments enact and review legislation specific to paramedics.

Safety and Health Administration (OSHA) and the US Department of Transportation at the federal level, as well as the Department of Health at the state level, are examples of parts of the administrative branch.

All states now have some type of legislation that sets out the framework for their EMS system. In addition, state agencies or county governments may establish administrative regulations that govern the practice of paramedics. You need to know and understand the laws and administrative regulations that affect your practice in your home state.

Types of Law

Two kinds of law apply to paramedics in the court setting: civil law, under which a patient can sue you for a perceived injury, and criminal law, under which the state can prosecute you for breaking a legal statute. Although some lawsuits may be based on state statutes, most claims will arise out of negligence principles established by prior court decisions. Malpractice lawsuits are tried under civil law, whereas many cases of medication misuse will be tried under criminal law.

A substantial part of civil law is concerned with establishing **liability**, or responsibility. When a person experiences an injury and seeks redress for that injury, the judicial process must determine who was responsible. For example, a patient or (if the patient died) a surviving relative may be dissatisfied with the medical care the patient received. The patient or surviving relative may believe that inadequate medical care led to a bad outcome. People have a constitutional right to take legal action against the physician, nurse, paramedic, or other parties involved in a patient's care. However, the person who is suing must prove that the medical providers being sued caused harm by failing to provide medical care that met accepted standards. A bad outcome alone does not necessarily mean the medical provider was negligent; the patient or surviving relative has to prove all elements of negligence before a lawsuit will be successful. A finding of negligence requires four criteria:

1. That a health care provider had a *duty to act*
2. That the provider committed a *breach of duty to act*
3. That the patient suffered *damages* as a result of the breach of duty
4. That the damages were *proximally caused* (foreseeable) from that breach of duty

A claim that contains all of these elements is sometimes referred to as an actionable cause.

A legal action based on such a claim is called a **civil lawsuit**—that is, an action instituted by a private person or entity (the **plaintiff**) against another private person or entity (the **defendant**)—and the wrongful act that gives rise to a civil lawsuit is called a **tort**. The law recognizes two classifications of torts: unintentional torts (commonly referred to as negligence) and intentional torts (which are wrongful acts that are performed on purpose). Examples of intentional torts include assault, battery, and false imprisonment, which are discussed later. The objective of a civil lawsuit is usually some sort of compensation (**damages**) for the injury the plaintiff sustained.

In medical liability cases, the plaintiff usually seeks monetary compensation for physical suffering, mental anguish, hospital and other medical bills, and sometimes loss of earnings or earning capacity. In some instances, the court may also award **punitive damages** (usually monetary compensation) if the EMS provider's misconduct was intentional or constituted a reckless disregard for the safety of the public. To succeed in a civil lawsuit, the plaintiff needs to show that a majority of the credible evidence favors their position, and then convince the jury of this position.

Lawsuits against EMS providers most often result from emergency vehicle crashes. Safe driving is a key to preventing lawsuits. Vehicle crashes are all too common and cause expensive property damage as well as serious harm to patients, bystanders, and EMS providers **FIGURE 4-6**.

Other kinds of lawsuits against EMS providers are also on the rise.[1] Many of these lawsuits involve dispatch and transport issues, such as a delayed transport response or deterioration of the patient's condition after not being transported. Other lawsuits address the quality of emergency medical care provided by EMS providers, especially paramedics.

Sometimes the same allegedly wrongful or harmful act that gave rise to a civil lawsuit may also result in criminal prosecution. A **criminal prosecution** is an action taken by the government against a person the prosecutors believe has violated criminal laws. In a criminal case, the government must prove guilt beyond all reasonable doubt

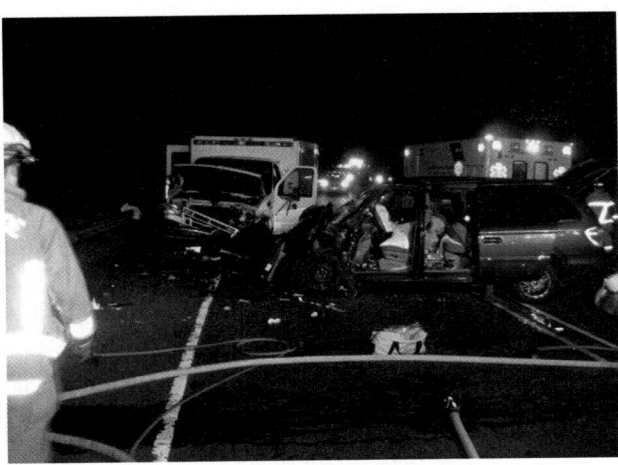

FIGURE 4-6 Civil lawsuits against paramedics often arise from emergency vehicle crashes.

Courtesy of Oregon State Police.

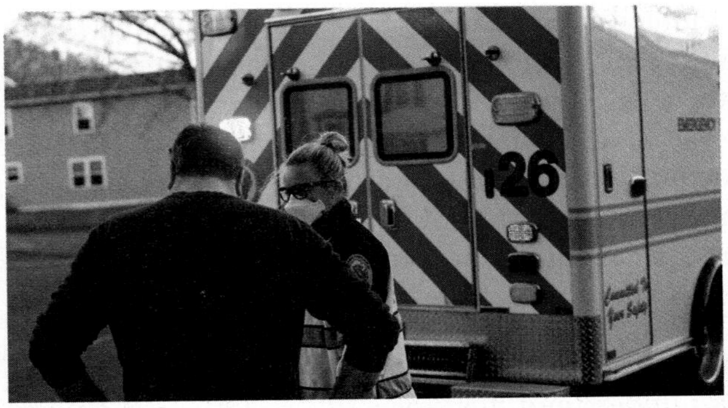

FIGURE 4-7 Your best prevention against any legal action is to obtain informed consent whenever possible, and to keep the needs of the patient as your priority.

© ALEX EDELMAN/AFP/Getty Images.

to a jury. If the government succeeds, then the defendant can be fined or imprisoned, or both.

The criminal laws most likely to apply to prehospital care include assault, battery, and false imprisonment.

- **Assault** occurs when a person (the EMS provider) instills a fear of immediate bodily harm or breach of bodily security (including loss of freedom) in another (the patient), regardless of whether the threat of harm is actually carried out. Threatening to restrain a patient who does not want to be transported could be considered assault.
- **Battery** occurs when the defendant (the EMS provider) touches another person (the patient) in a harmful or offensive way without the person's consent. Charges of battery may arise if you make physical contact before asking if you may touch the patient.
- **False imprisonment** occurs when a person (the patient) is intentionally and *unjustifiably* detained by another (the EMS provider). Charges of false imprisonment may arise if you transport a patient without their consent or wrongfully use restraints.

The difference between assault and battery can be summarized with the following example. Saying, "I'm going to kick your teeth in!" is assault; actually kicking the person's teeth in is battery. Just about any act of medical treatment performed without consent may be considered assault or battery, or both, because such acts constitute a threat to the patient's bodily security ("Now I'm going to stick you with this needle . . .") and unauthorized contact with the patient's body.

The prosecution generally needs to prove the defendant intended to cause harm to prosecute a criminal charge of assault or battery. In a civil case, the plaintiff need only establish that the conduct took place without consent.

The charge of false imprisonment is infrequently prosecuted in EMS. Courts tend to be lenient toward EMS personnel when they show that they were acting in the patient's best interest and believed that the patient did not have the capacity to provide informed consent. Occasionally, EMS providers may be charged with battery when they physically force someone to be transported, especially when they apply restraints, in the absence of just cause. In essence, the best way for EMS providers to protect themselves against these charges is to obtain informed consent for almost everything they do, or to clearly document the need to use restraints for the patient's protection **FIGURE 4-7**. All medical care providers must obtain informed consent. EMS providers, however, will need to consider specific guidelines and tips (presented later in this chapter) that may not apply to most hospital-based personnel. A rule of thumb is to use the least amount of restraint necessary when restraining or transporting patients against their will. The EMS provider's goal is always to prevent any further injury and to protect the patient's dignity.

In the past, EMS providers were taught that they should be aware of kidnapping and possible criminal or civil charges being brought against them in cases in which patients were transported against their will; however, no successful prosecution has ever been achieved against a paramedic for this action. As with kidnapping, no successful criminal prosecution has ever been achieved against a paramedic for false imprisonment. Successful civil prosecutions for false imprisonment are extremely rare.

Paramedics may also be sued for **defamation**, which is intentionally making a false statement through written or verbal communication that injures a person's good name or reputation. It must be emphasized that this must be a *false statement*. Truth is an absolute defense against any type of defamation claim. As a paramedic, you are encouraged to always make absolutely truthful statements. **Libel** is making a false statement in written form that injures a person's good name. Thus, when you complete your patient care report (PCR), you must avoid using terms that may be considered judgmental or offensive, such as "The patient appears to be drunk." Instead, you may write, "The patient smelled of ETOH." Whatever your personal views, think about how your PCR would sound if read aloud in court. Do not let thoughtless comments become evidence against you.

Slander is making a false oral statement that injures a person's good name. Once again, you must avoid using terms that could be considered judgmental or offensive to the patient when you are passing along prehospital care information to emergency department (ED) personnel. Always keep in mind that the patient is someone's son or daughter, husband or wife, brother or sister, or father or mother. How would you like information about your family members to be treated when information is relayed to the hospital? Slander can also occur when you make false or derogatory statements about other health professionals or entities, such as hospitals. Never make a derogatory statement to a patient or family member about a medical facility or provider when a decision is being made regarding where the patient will be transported.

Street Smarts

Being courteous, honest, and professional will prevent most patients from complaining or filing lawsuits.

The Legal Process

A civil lawsuit begins when a dissatisfied patient contacts an attorney, who then files a document for a lawsuit (called a complaint) on behalf of the patient with a local court. The court where the action is first filed is generally referred to as the court of original jurisdiction. In the context of EMS, the complaint will contain the general allegations against you and the EMS system, but may not contain much specific information about what the patient thinks went wrong. The patient's attorney (or the attorney's staff) must hand-deliver a copy of the complaint and a notice called a summons to all people or agencies named in the lawsuit, notifying them of the complaint and the need to respond. From start to finish, a lawsuit may take several years to unfold. Because the lawsuit may not begin until several years after you see the patient, good documentation is essential to defending a lawsuit.

Your attorney will usually be assigned to you by the insurance company that handles your employer's claims, whether the employer is a government or private agency. The response, or answer to the complaint, will be filed by your attorney. After the complaint is filed and you (through your attorney) have answered, an interval known as the discovery period begins. The discovery period can last anywhere from a few months to more than 2 years **FIGURE 4-8**. During the discovery period, attorneys on both sides seek to find out as much about the case as possible. They will exchange written

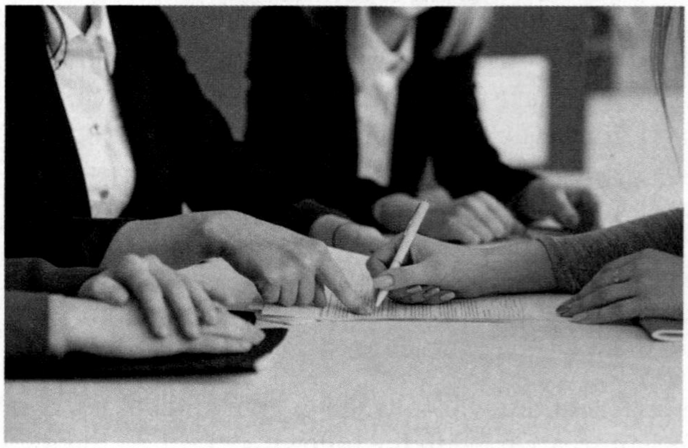

FIGURE 4-8 The process of a lawsuit can take years, and because of expenses associated with a trial, can result in out-of-court settlements.

questions that the parties must answer under oath, exchange documents such as the patient's medical record, and take depositions (statements recorded under oath). Stay in touch with your attorney during this time and ask for a full explanation of everything that is happening. Your attorney will also prepare you for a deposition, instructing you where to go, what to wear, and how to respond to certain types of questions.

Attorneys may also file motions (requests for the court to take an action) and argue them before the judge. Your attorney will seek to have the lawsuit dismissed by filing motions to that effect. The plaintiff's attorney may ask the court to rule on certain portions of the claim by filing other motions. Either side may file motions asking the court to compel the other side to produce documents or information that is being withheld.

Most civil cases are resolved during a settlement process because it is expensive and time-consuming to take a case through trial. Settlement processes bring the parties and their attorneys together for mediation, which is a conference set up to see if the parties can agree on a dollar amount that will resolve the case, or arbitration, which is a mini-trial in which a single arbitrator or a panel of arbitrators makes a decision based on the evidence presented by both sides.

If the case is not resolved during the settlement process, then it will proceed to trial. During a trial, the judge rules on what the law is and the jury decides what the facts are. Trial juries can be unpredictable; if they perceive that the EMS system has failed to meet community standards, then large monetary damages can be rewarded. In most cases, the trial will be the final step in the judicial process, but the party that loses at trial always has the right to have the decision reviewed by an appellate court. Appeals are costly and time-consuming, however, and only a small percentage of cases are ever appealed.

Legal Accountability of the Paramedic

The Paramedic and the Medical Director

The relationship between a paramedic and a medical director is complex and often not well understood. Ultimately, you have three lines of authority to answer to within the EMS system: your medical director, the licensing agency, and your employer. Although some overlap exists, it is essential to keep these distinctions in mind. State EMS legislation usually requires that you perform advanced procedures and skills only under a physician's supervision. Legislation may also require the EMS system to have a medical director. Although the medical director has a supervisory relationship with the paramedic, legally speaking, a paramedic is not an agent of the physician.

Your actions as a paramedic, therefore, are not the physician's actions, and you will be held accountable for your own actions. However, the medical director can be held legally accountable for failing to supervise you closely enough, or for failing to take action if your performance is not up to standard. The medical director may restrict your practice, or even withdraw supervision entirely, if the medical director does not believe you are performing as you should be. The medical director may also require specific remedial training if you are weak in some areas of practice. Although these remedial requirements may ultimately result in employment actions, medical directors are generally not held legally responsible for employers' disciplinary actions.

Many of your activities as a paramedic require an order from a licensed physician. Orders may be given by radio or mobile phone (online medical control), or they may be defined by protocols or standing orders (off-line medical control). In any case, you are not at liberty to disregard or reverse a physician's order unless you truly believe that carrying out the order will harm the patient. That fact may give rise to difficult situations, such as instances in which you find yourself at the scene of an emergency together with a physician who may not be knowledgeable in prehospital emergency care. Under those circumstances, you may feel that the orders of the on-scene physician are inappropriate. However, if you choose to disregard a physician's orders, you are on questionable legal ground, assuming the physician is licensed in that state and the order is appropriate. It is best to ask the service medical director to develop protocols ahead of time defining the paramedic's relationship with the medical director of the service and with other physicians in the community, including bystander physicians.

A physician is not required to ride to the ED with EMS personnel unless that physician has performed procedures above the EMS providers' level or has otherwise assumed responsibility for patient care. Always be sure that the physician is licensed in your state, and document the physician's name and contact information before allowing a physician to provide patient care. Also, beware of those who call themselves "doctor" but are not medical doctors, such as people with a PhD or PharmD. If conflicts do arise between you and physician bystanders in the field, then online medical control should resolve them. Do not follow a physician's order that falls outside of your scope of practice. Such action would fall under the **borrowed servant doctrine**, a principle that absolves your institution from liability when you act beyond your scope of certification or training by following someone else's orders.

Documentation and Communication

If you must deviate from your protocols because of unusual circumstances, then consult with online medical control and make sure you document it well on your PCR.

EMS-Enabling Legislation

Most states have EMS-enabling legislation, which defines how EMS is structured and designates responsibilities to government agencies. These laws also provide the state-based framework for the paramedic's actual practice—what you are permitted to do in the field. For example, EMS legislation may define the need for a medical director and define the scope of practice for different EMS personnel levels. Familiarize yourself with the EMS legislation in your state and any regulations that flow from those statutes.

Administrative Regulations

Administrative regulations set forth by bureaucracies at state and federal levels affect and define the specific rules under which paramedics practice. For example, regulations may set out the specific skills and medications to be used by each EMS provider level. Regulations, usually developed by either the state's Department of Health or the county agency responsible for regulating EMS practice, may further define your role in the emergency medical care of patients. Regulations may also define licensure or certification requirements, renewal requirements, continuing education requirements, and a list of behaviors that may subject you to suspension or revocation of your license or certification.

If you provide less than adequate care or fail to meet recertification requirements, then the administrative agency may also take action against your paramedic license. A license is not a right, but rather a privilege, granted by a government agency, allowing you to provide care to its citizens. Failure to abide by the regulations can have serious consequences.

Licensure and Certification

The terms *licensure* and *certification* are often confused because, in some states, paramedics are considered licensed, but in others, they are considered certified. Certification generally refers to a certain level of credentials based on hours of training and assessment exams, and addresses criteria that must be met for minimum competency. Certification may be granted by a governmental agency or a private organization (eg, American Heart Association, American Red Cross, Emergency Care and Safety Institute, Health and Safety Institute, National Safety Council). The fact that you have received certification from a private organization does not necessarily mean that you have the authority to practice the skills included in that certification.

Licensure refers to a carefully defined level of practice, usually granted by a government agency or local authority such as a state health department or county EMS authority. Often, these agencies themselves create and administer the licensing exams. A license is a privilege granted by a government authority on certain conditions. You must comply with the government's requirements for professional behavior, continuing education, and licensure renewal, or risk losing that privilege. The rights and privileges conferred by licensing in one state may not be conferred in other states that certify, rather than license, paramedics.

Another concept that you may encounter is credentialing. A specific EMS agency may adopt credentialing as part of its employment requirements. For example, although you may be licensed as a paramedic by your state, the service for which you are seeking to work may impose additional requirements as part of its eligibility standards. Typically, this may include certification in cardiopulmonary resuscitation (CPR), trauma, or advanced cardiac life support, or passing a regional protocol examination.

Discipline and Due Process

If you commit an infraction of the rules pertaining to licensure, then the agency that granted the license may seek to restrict, suspend, or even revoke your privilege to practice.

When an administrative agency proposes a licensing action, you have a right to **due process**. Due process is a right to a fair procedure for the action the agency proposes to take. Due process has two components: notice and opportunity to be heard. Notice means that the agency must notify you of the actions that allegedly constitute the infraction, usually by receipt of a certified letter containing a notice of contemplated action. The letter informs you of the proposed action to be taken and the sections of the regulations the agency is alleging were violated. The letter also informs you of your right to a hearing and the procedure for requesting a hearing. The hearing provides you with an opportunity to tell your side of the story. If the licensing agency still believes licensure action is warranted after the hearing, it will send a notice of final action. You may have appeal rights if a final licensure action is taken.

Medical Practice Act

In most states, physicians and other health care practitioners are allowed to function through the provisions of a **Medical Practice Act**. This act usually defines the minimum qualifications of those who may perform various health services, defines the skills that each type of practitioner is legally permitted to use, and establishes a means of licensure or certification for different categories of health care professionals. It may also include requirements for relicensure or recertification based on continuing education and other factors. In some cases, the Medical Practice Act may require that a physician assume responsibility for a paramedic's competency through mandatory training, skill competency testing, and run review. Become familiar with the terms of the Medical Practice Act in your state.

Scope of Practice

The **scope of practice** for paramedics may be spelled out in your state's EMS legislation or regulations. The scope of practice encompasses the emergency medical care that you are permitted to perform according to the state under its license or certification; however, a local medical director may limit the skills you may perform (eg, rapid sequence intubation).

Suppose you carry out a procedure that you are not authorized to perform under the enabling legislation. In that case, you are practicing outside your scope of practice, which may be considered negligence or, in some states, a criminal offense (considered practicing medicine without a license). The scope of practice is not the same as the standard of care, which is what a reasonable paramedic in a similar situation would do. This topic is discussed later in this chapter.

Health Insurance Portability and Accountability Act

The **Health Insurance Portability and Accountability Act (HIPAA)** outlines stringent privacy requirements for patient information. The act, enacted in 1996, provides for criminal sanctions and civil penalties for releasing a patient's private medical information in an unauthorized manner. The HIPAA Privacy Rule, which is the most relevant part of HIPAA for health care providers, is enforced by the Office for Civil Rights in the US Department of Health and Human Services. It protects a person's **protected health information (PHI)**, which is any identifiable health information created, disclosed, used, maintained, stored, or transmitted that is related to providing a health care service. By comparison, the HIPAA Security Rule is the portion of HIPAA that pertains to protecting electronic health information.

Medical information can be disclosed only if it is necessary for a patient's treatment, for payment or medical billing purposes, or when the release has been authorized in writing by the patient or a lawful patient representative. HIPAA was created not to stop the flow and continuity of a patient's health care information, but rather to control the distribution of information to ensure the patient's privacy. In essence, this act mandates that patient information should not be shared with entities or people not involved in the patient's care, although several special situations may require the release of patient information without the patient's authorization (discussed next). HIPAA requires each EMS agency to have a privacy officer responsible for ensuring that all PHI that the service deals with is not released in an unauthorized manner in either written, electronic, or oral/verbal form.

As a paramedic, you must be aware of where written patient information is at all times. You cannot casually discuss a patient in places where you might be overheard, such as in an elevator or hospital cafeteria **FIGURE 4-9**. Use caution when giving reports or discussing patient information in other public places such as crash scenes or common areas in the ED. Sharing patient stories with other paramedics may subject you to liability. Similarly, use caution when members of the media or the public are riding with your service to ensure PHI is not disclosed without the patient's consent.

HIPAA requires you to provide patients with a copy of your service's privacy policies. Although this step can often be challenging to perform in an emergency setting, you must do the best that you can to comply with the law. Most services create multipage leaflets that can be handed out to patients for this purpose.

Some states also have laws dealing with patient confidentiality; a breach of that confidentiality may allow patients to sue for unauthorized release of their medical information **FIGURE 4-10**. Confidentiality is also a part of the Code of Ethics for Emergency Medical Technicians issued by NAEMT. If your service receives a subpoena for a patient's PHI, then be sure to notify legal counsel before releasing the patient's medical record to anyone.

Special HIPAA Circumstances

Many EMS providers are confused about the legal issues surrounding HIPAA and mistakenly believe that any release of a patient's private medical information may result in penalties. In fact, the HIPAA Privacy Rule acknowledges that patient information must sometimes be shared to better society as a whole. Specifically, the Privacy Rule permits covered entities to disclose PHI to public health authorities who are legally authorized to receive such reports to prevent or control disease, injury, or disability. These exceptions include legally mandated reporting (eg, dog bites, gunshot wounds, alleged child abuse or neglect), authorized data collection and research by public health agencies (eg, births, deaths, diseases that are being investigated or are at risk of causing a public epidemic), authorized requests by law enforcement agencies, and information required to be disclosed pursuant to a valid subpoena.

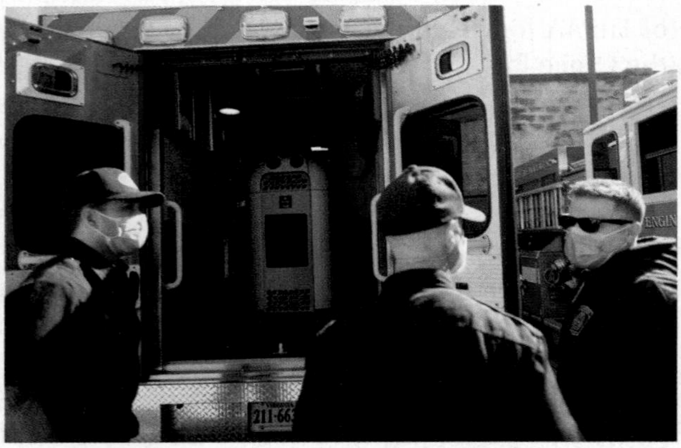

FIGURE 4-9 The Health Insurance Portability and Accountability Act guarantees a patient's confidentiality at all times. Be careful never to discuss a patient's condition in public.

FIGURE 4-10 When you communicate with a patient, be sensitive to the patient's point of view and the environment in which you choose to communicate.

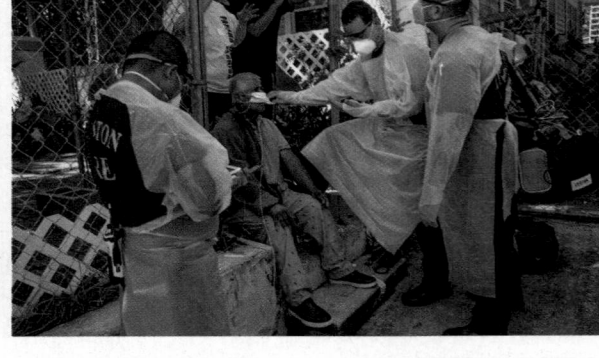

Exchange of health information for a medical need is allowed under HIPAA and is, in fact, ethical and necessary. For example, the electronic transfer of health information from your electronic PCR to the receiving hospital is entirely appropriate. It is also appropriate for a physician to dictate patient information into a dictation machine, which is then transcribed into the patient's medical record. Furthermore, it is permissible under HIPAA for hospitals to share information with EMS providers about patient outcome for the purposes of quality assurance, quality improvement, and education. For example, when you treat and transport a patient to the receiving facility, you may follow up to inquire about what further care your patient required after you transferred care. It is important and necessary for you to understand the outcome of your interventions so that you can learn and improve your own decision making. Finally, the exchange of health information for insurance and billing is appropriate. In most cases, the billing agency must sign an agreement indicating that health information will be used only for billing purposes and will not be shared with outside parties.

HIPAA Implications for Electronic Communications

Because of the popularity of social media networks, many EMS agencies have created policies to address issues associated with sharing patient care information over the Internet. Some agencies have gone as far as prohibiting EMS providers from carrying camera-enabled mobile phones while on duty. You must ensure that everyone on your call understands that patient information should never be posted (eg, in the form of photos, videos, comments, or other data) on any social media network due to HIPAA regulations.

As a paramedic, you have a unique perspective from which you treat patients. Many times, recordings of emergency scenes are captured by camera. For example, an EMS vehicle is equipped with a camera that records patient care, or EMS responders make take a photograph with their smartphone to illustrate the mechanism of injury at a crash scene. Make certain that if a camera is used on scene or during patient treatment, then no patient identifiers are present that could allow someone who was not involved in patient care to identify the patient.

HIPAA also regulates how you and your service transmit PHI electronically. In recent years, the widespread use of Bluetooth and other wireless technologies has increased the potential for patient information to be stolen by hackers. The Safeguards Principle of HIPAA requires that reasonable administrative, technical, and physical safeguards be put in place to protect patient information. If you are unsure whether the equipment you may be using is safeguarded, then seek the advice of your organization's administrators.

HIPAA Training

HIPAA rules and regulations should be taught to all entities involved in health care. Each agency in the United States that is a covered entity, as defined by the US Department of Health and Human Services, should follow HIPAA guidelines to protect both the patient and the provider. As mentioned previously, each agency must have a designated privacy officer who can help you better understand all of the rules and regulations of HIPAA and your role in EMS. Your employer is required to provide you with HIPAA training when you are hired and then again on an annual basis.

Emergency Medical Treatment and Active Labor Act

The **Emergency Medical Treatment and Active Labor Act (EMTALA)** was enacted in 1986 to combat the practice of so-called *patient dumping*. Patient dumping occurs when hospital ED staff deny medical screening or stabilizing treatment, or when staff inappropriately transfer a person whose condition is unstable. Historically, most patient dumping occurred when hospital staff discovered that the patient did not have health insurance or was otherwise unable to pay. EMTALA pays particular attention to the practice of sending women in labor to distant hospitals.

In recent years, *economic triage* has been introduced. This term refers to the practice of making health care decisions based on the ability of the patient or the insurance carrier to provide payment for services. Although such considerations may have a place in certain aspects of the health care field, an EMS provider should never decide to treat or transport based on financial considerations, regardless of the EMS employer's current financial state. As a paramedic, your only consideration should be the patient's needs; billing personnel should address reimbursement issues. Paramedics have occasionally been accused of providing a lower standard of care for indigent people or those on public assistance, but financial status should never become a deciding factor in your practice. Always provide the highest possible quality of emergency medical care to all patients, regardless of their financial status.

As a paramedic, it is also vital that you clearly understand local protocols regarding the choice of hospitals to which you may transfer patients. Only one hospital may be available in some rural areas, but several options may be available in other places. Some EMS systems require you to transfer the patient to the nearest hospital. In other systems, protocols dictate that hospital selection be based on the patient's specific needs. For example, some patients may require the services of a trauma center, a children's hospital, or a hospital with cardiac catheterization capabilities. Depending on your local protocols, you alone might choose the destination; in other EMS systems, you may be required to consult with medical control when making such decisions. You must become familiar with the protocols in your area of practice.

EMTALA issues are regulated by the Centers for Medicare and Medicaid Services (CMS) and carry severe monetary penalties—up to and including loss of Medicare funding—for hospitals that fail to comply with the regulations. The CMS also issues severe fines for hospitals and physicians who violate EMTALA provisions. In addition, EMTALA allows private citizens to sue for violations of the act. Under most circumstances, neither an ambulance service nor a paramedic can be sued or charged with a violation under EMTALA. However, an ambulance service that a hospital owns may be subject to a claim under EMTALA in some instances.

EMTALA includes complex language that appears to be medical language but is actually legal language. For example, an *emergency medical condition* under EMTALA refers to what most paramedics would call an *acute situation.* EMTALA guarantees a medical screening exam and treatment to stabilize any emergency medical conditions found, to any patient presenting to a hospital with an ED **FIGURE 4-11**. It prohibits discrimination for any reason, including the ability to pay. EMTALA may also cover some urgent care centers. Although this act does not directly regulate paramedics, EMS is often the vehicle, both figuratively and literally, by which patient dumping takes place.

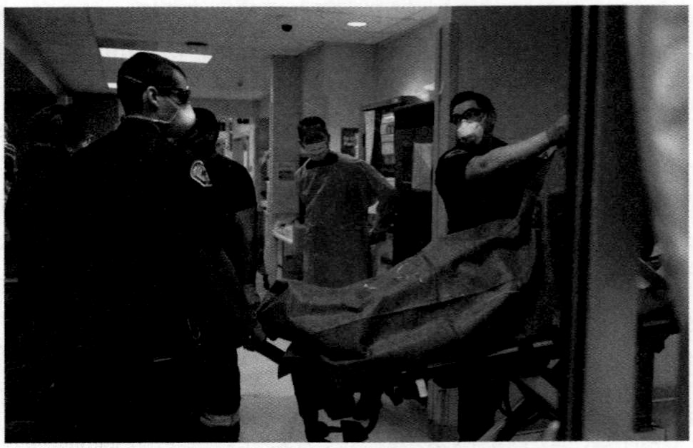

FIGURE 4-11 The Emergency Medical Treatment and Active Labor Act requires that every patient who presents to a hospital receive emergency medical treatment, regardless of ability to pay for medical treatment when it is received.

EMTALA also regulates patient transfers and applies to both the sending and receiving facilities. As a paramedic, you should never transfer a patient between facilities who needs emergency medical care that falls outside your scope of practice, and you must feel comfortable that the patient is stable enough to transfer. Transferring hospital staff must ensure that the transferring ambulance and crew can meet the patient's needs during transfer and request an appropriately staffed and equipped ambulance. It would be a potential EMTALA violation if hospital staff requested a basic life support (BLS) ambulance and crew to transport a patient with a serious cardiac condition requiring cardiac monitoring and medication administration during transport. Should a patient need a higher level of care, the sending hospital's responsibility is to ensure that the receiving facility agrees to accept the patient. It is also the transferring hospital staff's responsibility to provide someone to ride along if necessary to meet the patient's needs (eg, a nurse, a respiratory therapist, or even a physician).

Make sure you have received all appropriate paperwork before leaving on a patient transfer, including all pertinent medical records, laboratory results, radiographs, and other documents. The staff should have a bed ready for the patient when you arrive at the receiving hospital.

Emergency Vehicle Laws

Most states have specific statutes that define an emergency vehicle and indicate what traffic should do when an emergency vehicle approaches. Although the laws vary somewhat from state to state, all of these statutes still require emergency vehicles to operate safely and prudently. Laws governing emergency vehicle operations do not authorize speeding, running red lights, or driving the vehicle in an unsafe manner if any of those activities puts the public at unreasonable risk. Most state laws establish a higher standard for the emergency vehicle operator by making the operator responsible for operating the vehicle with *due regard* (proper consideration and attention) for all others' safety.[7] If a crash occurs, EMS providers will often be found at fault in civil cases brought against the drivers. Even worse, if you are the driver, then you might also be charged criminally in such situations. Although it is important to know your state's laws about emergency vehicle operation, recognize that the blue Star of Life and the flashing red lights on your vehicle do not exempt you from defensive driving and common courtesy; you will be held responsible for your actions while behind the wheel.

Emergency vehicle operators are professionals trained to operate their vehicle safely at all times, and to anticipate reactions from other drivers in stressful situations. A collision could result in injuries to innocent people, and it could injure or delay treatment of the original patient who needs your help. Collisions involving emergency vehicles are the most common cause of paramedics facing legal action, be it criminal, civil, or administrative.

Transportation

You should transport patients to the hospital of their choice when possible and reasonable; however, most EMS systems have protocols that direct paramedics to transport certain types of patients to particular hospitals. Examples of these patients include those who have experienced trauma, stroke, and cardiac events; homeless patients; mentally ill patients; and patients with obesity. Each hospital's capability to care for particular kinds of patients should guide the EMS system in developing transport protocols. Transport of patients to a facility that cannot care for their particular illness or injury can result in liability for the paramedic.

Decisions made by paramedics not to transport patients at all have been the subject of litigation. Several studies have demonstrated that paramedics should not be compelled to decide which patients need to be transported to the hospital for any health conditions. The EMS system, including paramedics, does not have access to sophisticated diagnostic tools or radiography in the prehospital setting. Failure to transport a patient whose condition later deteriorates can bring about a lawsuit that is difficult to defend. Again, most EMS systems have protocols outlining when it is acceptable not to transport a patient, and many require consultation with online medical control.

Crime Scene and Emergency Scene Responsibilities

In a situation involving a death, or at any potential crime scene, it may take law enforcement officials some time to figure out whether the scene involved a suicide, homicide, or some other form of criminal activity. It is vital for you to use extreme caution and not disturb or destroy potential evidence.

If the scene is a vehicle crash, then do not move anything unless doing so is absolutely necessary to provide care—including broken glass, pieces of metal, or even a beer can. Leave deceased people where they are until a coroner or medical examiner arrives to investigate.

If the incident scene is indoors, then do not touch anything you do not have to touch, such as telephones or doorknobs, because of the risk of eliminating fingerprints. Carefully document any statements made by witnesses and get their contact information. Limit the number of EMS personnel who enter the scene, because each person who enters the scene further contaminates what may later turn out to be a crime scene. If it is necessary to move furniture or other objects, then notify law enforcement personnel that you have done so. Preserve any clothing that you remove from the patient, and make every attempt not to alter evidence on the clothing (eg, do not cut through bullet or knife holes).

In cases of sexual assault, the patient may carry vital pieces of evidence such as fiber, hair, semen, or blood on the body. Take care to protect this evidence.

If the scene involves a death, then stay with the body until the police arrive. Protect the scene from contamination by bystanders, family members, media, or additional EMS personnel.

If you have any doubt about the possibility of saving the patient, then initiate resuscitation and transport to the hospital.

SAFETY

Be aware that the perpetrator may still be at or near the crime scene and could be a factor in when and how you care for the patient.

Mandatory Reporting

Each state has its own requirements regarding categories of cases that must be reported to the appropriate authorities. These cases include some of the most difficult ones you will see as a paramedic.

Virtually every state has laws requiring EMS providers to report suspected child and elder abuse. You need to be familiar with the reporting requirements established by your state. In most states, reporting laws also contain **immunity** provisions that protect health care providers who file reports from legal liability, provided those reports were not made with malicious intent. Failure to report is a crime and in many states carries severe implications. If your state requires you to report, then complete the reporting yourself; do not pass along the information and expect that someone else will make the report.

The obligation to report is most frequently applied to the following categories of cases:

- Neglect or abuse of children
- Neglect or abuse of older people
- Domestic violence
- Injury sustained during the commission of a felony, or specific injuries considered to be of suspicious origin (eg, gunshot wounds or stab wounds)
- Drug-related injuries
- Childbirth occurring outside a licensed medical facility
- Rape
- Animal bites
- Certain communicable diseases

Because reporting requirements vary widely from state to state, learn the laws of your state and observe reporting obligations that apply to you.

Documentation and Communication

Be observant and report any suspicious signs or symptoms to proper authorities.

Coroner and Medical Examiner Cases

Every EMS system should have a list of procedures for cases that involve the coroner and medical examiner **FIGURE 4-12**. Although coroner laws vary somewhat from state to state, generally you should notify the police of all coroner cases, including the following situations:

- Obvious or suspected homicide
- Obvious or suspected suicide
- Any other violent or sudden, unexpected death
- Death of a prison inmate

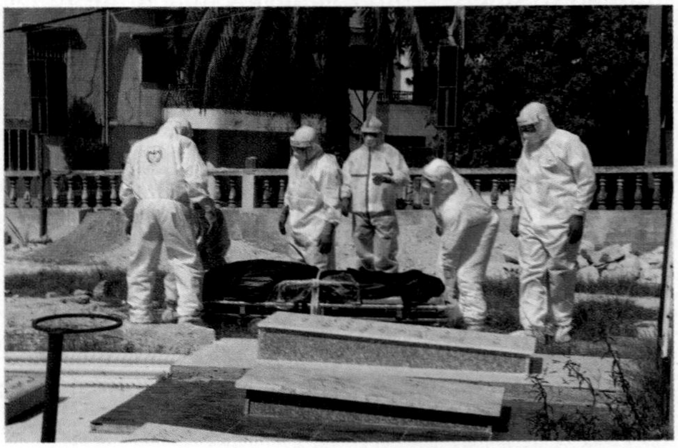

FIGURE 4-12 EMS providers assisting the coronor's office in moving a deceased patient with a highly infectious disease. In any situation involving the death of a person, contact the police or coroner with pertinent details, according to local protocols.

Paramedic–Patient Relationships

The most important premise affecting paramedics does not appear in any of the statute books; it is the rule of doing what is best for the patient. You are trained in emergency medical care, not law. Therefore, every decision regarding patient care that you make should be based on standards of good medical care, not on possible legal consequences. When you do what is best for the patient within your scope of practice, it is unlikely you will run afoul of the law. Even if a lawsuit is initiated, your defense will be significantly enhanced if you have always kept the patient's best interest in mind.

Consent and Refusal

Before providing emergency medical care, you must obtain the patient's consent. Any touching of a patient's body without consent may give rise to charges of assault and battery. The concept of consent refers to patients who are of legal age and who possess **decision-making capacity** (the capacity to make appropriate medical care decisions for themselves). Patients with decision-making capacity have the right to refuse all or part of the emergency medical care offered to them. Be familiar with the two types of consent: informed consent and implied consent.

Informed consent is a patient's voluntary agreement to be treated after being told about the nature of the disease, risks and benefits of the proposed treatment, alternative treatments, or the choice of no treatment at all. You must obtain informed consent from every adult patient who has decision-making capacity. To obtain informed consent, follow these four steps:

1. Describe the suspected injury or illness to the patient.
2. Describe the treatment you would like to administer, and list potential risks associated with the proposed treatment.
3. Discuss any alternative types of treatment available.
4. Advise the patient regarding the potential consequences of refusing treatment.

Patients' language barriers, emotional states, and mental abilities may impede your ability to give patients the information they need to make informed decisions. The key is to ensure each patient understands what you are trying to do and permits you to administer treatment. Although the informed consent process under emergency conditions may not include the same level of formality seen in a hospital, you must document the patient's consent in your PCR to protect yourself against potential legal action.

Informed patient consent is routinely obtained verbally but may also be communicated through patient conduct, such as patients rolling up their sleeves to allow you to take their blood pressure. **Expressed consent** is a type of informed consent that occurs when the patient does something, either by telling you or by taking some sort of action, that demonstrates you have permission to provide emergency medical care.

Implied consent is a form of consent assumed to be given by unconscious adults or by adults who are too ill or injured to consent verbally to emergency life-saving treatment. It also applies to minors if no parent or guardian is present. When operating under informed consent, you assume that the patients would want care because of the severity of their condition, but the patients do not have decision-making capacity when treatment is necessary. Suppose a patient shows convincing evidence that decision-making capacity is altered (eg, signs of mental illness, shock, stress, confusion, head injury). In that case, you may treat the patient under implied consent because treatment is in the patient's best interest.

Some EMS personnel incorrectly use the term **involuntary consent** to refer to situations in which a law enforcement officer or a legal guardian grants permission to treat someone who is under arrest (or otherwise in custody), incapacitated, a minor, or for other reasons. Involuntary consent is an oxymoron because consent can never be involuntary. People under arrest or in prison do not necessarily lose their right to be involved in medical treatment decisions. It is not uncommon for a law enforcement officer to direct EMS personnel to treat a person under arrest, but you should continue to follow informed consent guidelines. If a prisoner refuses treatment, then consult with medical control. Likewise, do not assume that a law enforcement officer has the right to refuse treatment for a patient. Always remember that no one, including law enforcement, relatives (unless they have power of attorney and you can verify it), businesses, and churches, has the right to refuse treatment for a patient. Your legal obligation is to your patients and to treating them as needed. If the patient desires treatment, then do everything in your power to treat the patient and document that care accordingly.

Decision-Making Capacity

Refusals, like consent, must be informed refusals, and all the same prerequisites apply. Patients must have decision-making capacity to be able to refuse care. Decision-making capacity is the ability of patients to understand the information you provide to them, coupled with the ability to process that information and choose medical care that is appropriate for them. You have several tools you can use to evaluate a patient's decision-making capacity, but the best one is your ability to talk to the patient to find out whether the patient understands what is happening. If pulse oximetry and blood glucose measurements are outside normal ranges, then these readings constitute measurable information regarding the patient's ability to understand and communicate. Detailed documentation of decision-making capacity is essential to include in your PCR to show that the patient understood your proposed treatment plan.

If a conscious patient with decision-making capacity refuses to consent to treatment, that person may not be treated without a court order **FIGURE 4-13**. In such instances, consult with medical control for instructions. The most prudent approach is to inform the person calmly and sympathetically of the possible consequences of refusing treatment. Many people who refuse medical treatment do so out of fear and emotional distress. You need to recognize and manage the patient's distress in an understanding way. Often patients refuse treatment and transportation to the hospital because of concerns about the costs associated with ambulance and hospital treatment. Addressing these concerns can be challenging for you and may require all of your "people skills."

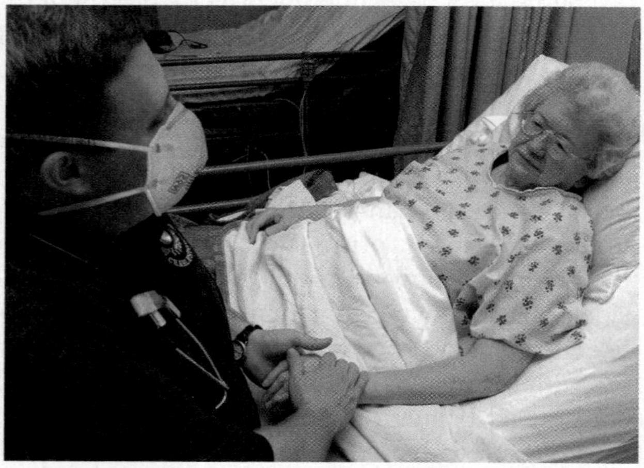

FIGURE 4-13 When a conscious patient with decision-making capacity makes a decision, you must respect that choice.

Be wary of situations when a patient refuses treatment and/or transport, but you believe that treatment and/or transport is in the patient's best interest. The patient may be alert and oriented but incapable of making an informed decision even after you communicate the need for care to the best of your ability. Examples of factors that may prevent a patient from making an informed refusal include the following:

- Head injury
- Altered mental status
- Unstable vital signs
- Abnormal blood glucose levels
- Abnormal oxygen saturation levels
- Cerebral ischemia
- Mental illness
- Drug or alcohol intoxication
- Urinary tract infection
- Suicidal or homicidal ideation
- Inability to cope with emotional distress
- Developmental disability

If you reasonably suspect that a patient has an issue that impedes the ability to give either informed consent or an informed refusal, then take aggressive steps in the patient's best interest. If you can contact medical control for direction, then immediately inform medical control of your concerns, and the basis for those concerns. Ask for guidance in transporting the patient without consent, and the best way to accomplish this. If you do not have access to medical control, then it is usually best to follow your instincts and transport the patient if forcible transport can be accomplished reasonably and safely. Consider calling for assistance from your EMS agency or law enforcement, and be keenly aware of your local protocols and resources in this regard. Use whatever resources you have available.

In particular, psychiatric emergencies present challenges with respect to consent. When a person's life is not in danger, a police officer is generally the only person given the authority to restrain and transport that person without consent. EMS providers should not do so except at the express request of the police. Notably, neither a physician nor the patient's family may authorize such transport in most regions; they may authorize involuntary commitment, but their authority does not extend to forcible transport. Therefore, every EMS system needs to establish protocols, based on local laws, for dealing with mentally impaired patients who refuse transport. Police participation will be required in many instances, and each agency's role should be clearly defined beforehand.

Courts have given EMS personnel substantial leeway in their decisions to transport patients against their will whenever the on-scene paramedics have acted in the patient's best interest and have proper documentation. The vast majority of court rulings reflect the courts' belief that the paramedic has a duty to act in the patient's best interest and suspect the worst. As a paramedic, you are not expected to establish a definitive diagnosis of the patient's condition in the field, and you are not held to the same standard as a medical professional with a higher degree. It is generally assumed that no harm is done if the patient is treated and transported without consenting to transport when paramedics have used their best judgment on the patient's behalf. If the patient is taken to the hospital and the physician determines that the patient has adequate mental capacity to refuse further treatment, then the patient has only lost time.

It is very challenging to decide when to transport patients against their will. If you believe that the patient is not competent to make a reasonable decision, and that treatment is necessary, then it is better to treat the patient. You are less likely to face legal consequences for treating a patient who should be treated—even without consent—than for abandoning that patient. (Abandonment is discussed later in this chapter.) Individual state statutes provide more guidance in this situation. Become familiar with the state statutes where you practice.

Sometimes patients refuse treatment as a way of denying that they have a problem; for example, a middle-aged man with chest pain may refuse treatment to deny the possibility that he may be experiencing a heart attack. A sympathetic ear and a little reassurance on your part will often convert an unconvinced patient into someone you can help. Remember this phrase: "It never hurts to have these things checked out."

Having a patient speak with medical control by radio or telephone may be helpful at times. Suppose the patient is still declining emergency medical care after you have explained the medical situation and the possible consequences of refusing treatment, and no evidence exists that the patient is impaired in any way that would prohibit an informed refusal. In that case, there is not much else that you can do. However, even at that point, you must maintain a courteous, sympathetic attitude. It is inappropriate for you to label the person who refuses treatment a "bad patient" or to behave in a hostile or aggressive manner. You are at the scene to help the patient, so try to find out what is bothering the patient and why the patient is rejecting help. Always respect the patient's rights.

Let patients know that your chief concern is their well-being and that it is perfectly fine to change their minds. Urge patients to seek further medical evaluation from the physician of their choice. Help them make concrete plans for follow-up. Some patients will agree to transport but will not consent to treatment (or some component of your treatment, such as pain medication or a cervical collar); others may consent to treatment but refuse transport. If patients refuse transport, then try to make sure that someone will remain with them after you leave and always advise them to call 9-1-1 again for help if needed.

Never threaten a patient in any way. Some examples include telling patients that they will be taken forcefully to the hospital if they call 9-1-1 again; threatening to cause pain to an uncooperative patient (ie, intravenous [IV] injection, nasogastric tube insertion); or threatening to restrain the patient. All of these actions not only would be highly unprofessional and inappropriate, but would also constitute assault. Following through—that is, acting on these threats—would constitute battery.

Documenting Informed Refusal

Your documentation of patient refusals is critical in case of subsequent litigation in which the patient claims you committed abandonment. Document all your assessment and mental status exam findings carefully, including the patient's history, the patient's stated reasons for refusing care, and all instructions and explanations given to the patient. Note how much time you spent attempting to provide emergency medical care. The report should be signed by the patient and by an impartial observer (eg, a police officer, if available). A witness or observer is expected to actually hear the exchange of information, not just sign a piece of paper. Soliciting signatures from others at the scene who may not have been paying attention to your conversation or the information exchanged with the patient may pose legal issues. The documentation of refusals is covered in detail in Chapter 6, *Documentation*.

It can be frustrating and difficult to accept that a patient may refuse all or part of emergency medical care. However, it is important to respect a patient's rights, regardless of whether it is contrary to your beliefs or what you think you should be doing. Courts have upheld patient refusals when paramedics carefully documented a patient's decision-making capacity and their explanation of the possible consequences of refusing care.

Documentation and Communication

Prehospital refusal of treatment forms must be supported with action. Legally, you must have undertaken the process of attempting to obtain informed consent to treat the patient. Just because a patient has signed a refusal form, that does not mean the patient has given you an informed refusal. You must have informed the patient of your proposed plan of care, as well as potential risks of refusing that care, and provided that information in a manner the patient is capable of understanding.

Minors

Caring for a **minor** presents unique issues for the paramedic. Because minors have no legal status, they can neither refuse nor consent to emergency medical care. In the case of children and adults who have legal guardians, consent must be obtained, if possible, from a parent or legal guardian of the patient. If a parent or guardian is unavailable, then emergency treatment to sustain life may be undertaken without direct consent under the implied

YOU are the Paramedic

PART 2

You are led into the kitchen and see an older woman sitting at the kitchen table drinking coffee. She looks up as you walk in and starts to yell at her daughter: "I told you not to call them! I'm not going!" She is pale, frail-looking, and very agitated. Her daughter tells you that her mother has had small strokes in the past due to a small brain tumor. She also tells you her mother does not have a do not resuscitate order, but she does have an advance directive. She also takes medication for high blood pressure, hypothyroidism, and elevated cholesterol levels.

Recording Time: 0 Minutes	
Appearance	Pale, agitated
Level of consciousness	Appears alert
Airway	Open and clear
Breathing	Appears normal
Circulation	Pale, but her nail beds are pink

3. What are the possible consequences of treating this patient without her consent?
4. On the basis of her history, what might be her problem?

consent doctrine. Also be aware of the legal principle known as in loco parentis, a term that means "in the place of the parent." This principle may also apply in school, day care, or summer camp if a parent is unavailable. For example, based on this principle, the school administrator or day care director may make treatment and transportation decisions on behalf of the minor.

A particularly difficult circumstance can arise if a parent or legal guardian refuses to grant consent to treat a minor who clearly requires life-saving or limb-saving treatment. Although adults have the right to refuse treatment for themselves, state laws generally do not permit a parent or guardian to deny treatment to a minor. The failure of a parent or guardian to allow such treatment may constitute neglect. If confronted with such a circumstance, then notify law enforcement and medical control. State law may permit the state to assume custody of the minor to ensure that necessary emergency treatment is provided.

An emancipated minor is younger than the legal age (generally 18 years) in a given state but can be treated as a legal adult because of qualifying circumstances. Individual state law determines which circumstances qualify a minor as emancipated, although most states recognize any minor who has been emancipated by court order. Other states add criteria such as marriage, pregnancy, or active military service. Emancipated minors may be treated as adults when obtaining consent or refusal.

As with adult patients who refuse transport, if you reasonably suspect the patient is a minor and the patient has no proof to the contrary, then be prepared to transport. Legally speaking, you are better off erring on the side of caution—that is, in favor of transport and acting in the best interest of the patient— rather than abandoning the patient.

Obtaining consent for medical treatment may be one of the more difficult skills to develop as a new paramedic, but you will find that your expertise increases over time. A patient or even a child's guardian may not want you to assess and treat for various reasons **FIGURE 4-14**. As a patient advocate, you must anticipate the potential challenges to obtaining permission and be prepared to discuss the need for emergency medical care.

Street Smarts

Generally, when treating mentally competent adult patients, do not *tell* the person that you are going to do a procedure. Instead, *ask* them if you can perform the procedure and *explain* why they need it.

Violent Patients and Restraints

The use of force by paramedics against patients has triggered numerous lawsuits in recent years. However, the reality of today's EMS practice is that

Special Populations

Although legislation varies in different areas, in most states, a pregnant teenager is considered emancipated during her pregnancy and can make all legal and medical decisions for herself and her unborn baby. However, if her own parents have not granted emancipation, she assumes the status of a minor again once she delivers her baby, and her parents or legal guardians can make all of her medical and legal decisions. The teenager does, however, remain the legal guardian for her baby and can make all medical and legal decisions for her baby. The rationale for this complicated scenario is that although the teenage mother is responsible for her child, her own parents maintain responsibility for her, which helps to ensure she has the stability the baby needs.[8] Because laws for emancipated minors vary among states, research the laws in your state.

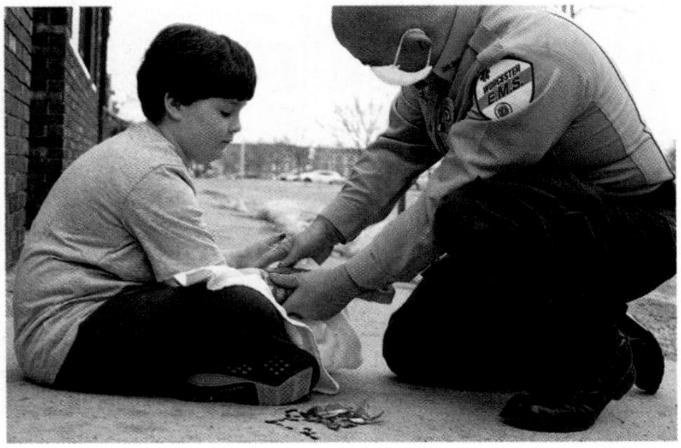

FIGURE 4-14 When you interact with a young child, explain the need for treatment, and consult a parent or guardian.

© Jones & Bartlett Learning. Courtesy of MIEMSS.

you will encounter violent patients who must be restrained to protect the patients themselves and to protect those who are trying to care for them.

Under the law, you can use force only in response to a patient's use of force against you. If you are attacked, then you may defend yourself against the attack. However, the use of temporary disabling sprays, knives, or firearms is generally outside the scope of paramedic practice and is usually prohibited by the EMS agency. The amount of force that you are allowed to use under the law is either equal to or slightly greater than the force offered by the patient, and must be in response to the patient's actions. The use of extreme force in patient restraint is a common source of legal actions against EMS, in both criminal and civil courts. Unfortunately, violence against EMS providers is on the rise. For your safety, do not enter an unsafe scene until law enforcement personnel can secure the scene and make it safe for you to enter.

In situations requiring patient restraint for medical reasons, it is important to understand that you may restrain patients only when they are a danger to themselves or others **FIGURE 4-15**. Violence can result from hypoxia, hypoglycemia, mental illness, brain injury, drug abuse or overdose, alcohol, or a variety of other underlying medical and psychiatric causes. Specific medical protocols should cover what is considered appropriate in your EMS system for restraining patients. They should spell out what medications or devices can be used in restraining patients. Many EMS systems administer medications (ie, chemical restraints), such as benzodiazepines or antipsychotics, to calm patients who are violent and need transportation to a hospital to discover the underlying medical or psychiatric cause of their outbursts.

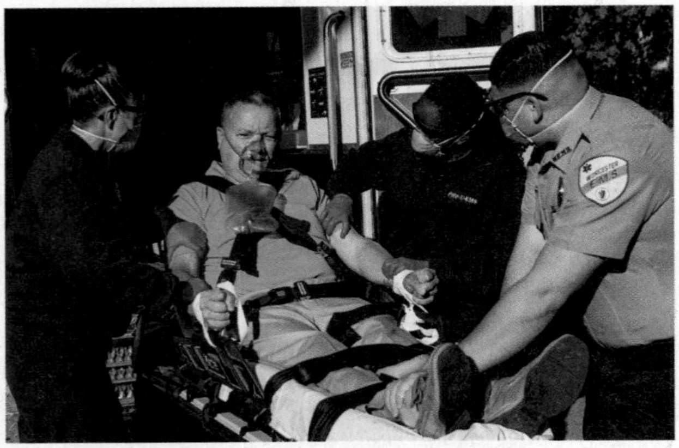

FIGURE 4-15 Use restraint only when absolutely necessary to ensure your safety and that of the patient. It will most likely take several strong people to fully restrain a patient. Never use restraint as a form of punishment.

Negligence and Protection Against Negligence Claims

Unless some type of immunity is present, nothing can protect the paramedic from liability for **negligence**, a serious charge. Negligence occurs when a series of events happens:

1. The paramedic—or, in some cases, the EMS system—had a legal duty to the patient (duty to act). For example, a paramedic hired to serve a community has a legal duty to the citizens of that community.
2. A breach of duty occurred; that is, the person accused of negligence failed to act as another person with similar training would have acted under the same or similar circumstances. Breach of duty may involve doing less than the person was trained to do (an error of omission; ie, a paramedic who fails to splint an injured extremity) or doing more than the person was trained to do (an error of commission; ie, a paramedic who sutures a laceration when that skill is not within the scope of practice).
3. The failure to act appropriately was the proximate cause (the first event in a chain of events) of the plaintiff's injury.
4. Harm resulted.

As a paramedic, you and the EMS system in which you work are protected from liability as long as you perform according to the standards for paramedics and EMS systems. Your best protection is to behave in all circumstances according to established procedures and standards set by national agencies, such as the guidelines for ambulance design and equipment from the National Highway Traffic Safety Administration. Although those standards are not law, they can be introduced as evidence in litigation and may affect a lawsuit's outcome. Therefore, it is in your best interest to ensure that your emergency vehicle is maintained in optimal condition and equipped according to prevailing standards.

Paramedics frequently ask if they should obtain their own insurance coverage even though they generally will be covered by the insurance provided by their employers. Although the insurance carried by your employer will generally cover you in any situation related to your employment, having additional insurance can be a good idea. Having your own liability policy will provide you with protection in several possible circumstances:

- If your employer's insurance carrier is required to pay out on a claim based on wrongdoing for which you are responsible, then it is possible (though rare) that the carrier will try to recover against you personally.
- If you are sued as a result of having provided off-duty emergency assistance.
- If you are an instructor teaching EMS-related classes outside the scope of your employment and are sued by a student or other party.

Insurance of this type is generally reasonably priced and may be a wise investment.

One aspect of negligence is the presence of *foreseeability*. This concept implies that the injury, or harm, could have been predicted and avoided if the proper precautions had been taken. For example, giving an incorrect dosage of a drug will foreseeably harm a patient, just as running a red light while en route to a call may foreseeably result in a motor vehicle crash.

Negligence is commonly divided into three categories: (1) malfeasance, (2) misfeasance, and (3) nonfeasance. **Malfeasance** occurs if you perform an act that you were never authorized to do, such as a medical intervention that is outside your scope of practice. **Misfeasance** occurs if you perform an act that you are legally permitted to do, but you do so improperly. For example, misfeasance occurs when you administer a medication that is clearly within the scope of practice but accidentally calculate an incorrect dose. **Nonfeasance** occurs if you fail to perform an act that you are required or expected to perform. Failure to perform CPR when a patient goes into cardiac arrest would be an example of nonfeasance.

Elements of Negligence

Duty

Duty is prescribed by the law: It is what you, as a paramedic, must do and how you must do it. Without question, your first duty as a paramedic is to do no further harm to a patient.

The first element of negligence a patient must prove for a lawsuit to be successful is **duty**. In relation to medical negligence, duty is defined as "an obligation, to which law will give recognition and effect; to conform to a particular standard of conduct toward another."[9] If a person fails to perform according to that standard, and this failure caused the injury, then that person may be considered legally liable.

Much confusion surrounds the concept of legal duty in EMS. For example, many paramedics think that they have a legal obligation to stop at roadside crashes simply because they are paramedics. However, in all but a few states, this is not the case. Although you may feel an ethical obligation to stop and assist, the law in most states does not require it. You are obligated to respond to calls when working a shift or while volunteering for a squad. Most services have a policy addressing the discovery of another incident while en route to a call or en route to the hospital with a patient. The key to legal duty is to make sure the appropriate personnel are dispatched if you cannot stop to render assistance due to the severity of the patient you are currently treating.

Another misconception is the idea that if you put a sticker that says "paramedic" on your personal vehicle, this identification somehow invokes a **legal obligation** (a duty enforceable in a court of law) to stop at all emergencies.[10] This is not true. However, you do have a legal obligation to perform within the standard of care if you decide to stop and provide assistance. In addition, you have a legal duty not to abandon the patient after you have begun treatment. It is essential to understand your legal obligations when you are off duty. Learn your state laws, and educate your peers regarding these off-duty obligations.

The concept of duty extends to maintaining licensure or certification, attending continuing education courses, and maintaining your skills. Maintaining your health and psychological well-being so that you are adequately prepared for the rigors of prehospital patient care is essential. Also, you have a duty to check your equipment at the beginning of each shift and ensure all equipment is functioning correctly. Finally, you have a duty to honor your patients' rights to privacy and their rights to refuse or limit the care you provide.

EMS agencies—and even entire EMS systems—can be held to a legal duty. EMS agencies have a duty to respond to calls for aid and to use mutual aid resources appropriately if call volume is too heavy to allow for making a response within an appropriate time frame. Some EMS agencies may operate with formal contracts that specify legal duties, such as minimum response times.

Legal duty is a concept in the law that tells you what your standards of practice are. It is an unpredictable legal concept, often defined in the context of a case tried in a court of law. Even so, the concept of legal duty is used by attorneys defending EMS providers. For example, in a lawsuit against an off-duty paramedic who stopped at a crash to render aid, the paramedic's attorney may attempt to show that the paramedic had no duty to the patient, but instead provided assistance that was not required by law.

Attorneys are often trained to work from the most general defense to the case's most specific elements. Lack of legal duty is a general defense; however general it is, it may still be true.

Breach of Duty

The second element a patient must prove for a lawsuit to be successful is that the paramedic failed to perform within the **standard of care**. The standard of care is what a reasonable paramedic would have done in the same or similar situation. In a lawsuit, a jury will listen to the testimony of expert witnesses on both sides and ultimately decide whether your care was reasonable. These expert witnesses will identify several bases for their testimony about whether your care was reasonable. Those sources will include their own training and experience; your training, experience, and continuing education; textbooks; protocols; national standards; standard operating procedures; and the PCR. Good documentation will go a long way toward proving you maintained a high standard of care **FIGURE 4-16**.

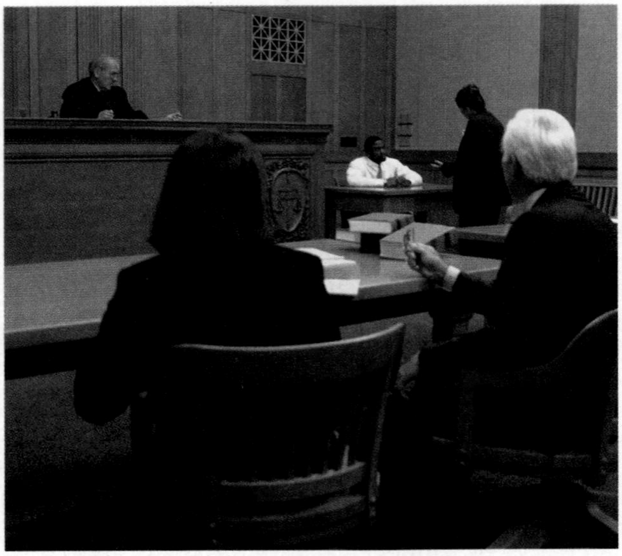

FIGURE 4-16 Court discussions will be based on your documentation and testimony. Make sure your documentation is neat, thorough, and accurate.

Some states differentiate between **ordinary negligence** and **gross negligence**. How high a standard of care you will be held to varies from one state to another. Some states provide immunity for all but the poorest emergency medical care given by the paramedic. This immunity often comes in the form of a **Good Samaritan law** (discussed later in this chapter) in those cases in which the paramedic was off duty and no compensation was paid for the assistance provided.

In states that follow a gross negligence standard, a lawsuit against a paramedic will not be successful unless that paramedic has seriously departed from the accepted standards. Actions are considered grossly negligent if they are willful or wanton (malicious) under the law. This standard is difficult for a plaintiff to meet. Usually, either intentional conduct or recklessness is essential to a finding of willful or wanton conduct. For example, *Black's Law Dictionary* defines willful misconduct as "intentional disregard to the safety of others,"[11] and wanton misconduct as "the reckless disregard for the safety and rights of others while knowing harm or injury may result."[12] Some states have defined wanton misconduct as "reckless disregard," "utter indifference," or "conscious disregard" for the safety of others. If you can convince the jury that you acted in good faith, then you will usually not be found negligent.

In other states, to succeed in a lawsuit, a plaintiff has to show only ordinary negligence, which can be a failure to act or a simple mistake that causes harm to a patient. It is much easier for a plaintiff to prove negligence under the ordinary negligence standard.

In certain circumstances, a unique theory of negligence known as **res ipsa loquitur** may apply even though the plaintiff cannot clearly demonstrate the exact manner by which an injury occurred. *Res ipsa loquitur* means "the thing speaks for itself." Under this theory, you could be held liable if it is shown that the plaintiff was injured, that the cause of the injury was in your control, and that such injuries do not ordinarily occur unless negligence is present. For example, you and your partner are called to the home of a patient who lost consciousness due to an apparent drug overdose. While loading the patient into the ambulance, your partner slips, causing the stretcher to tip over; the patient strikes the ground and sustains a large laceration to his head. The patient later sues for negligence. Because the patient was unconscious at the time of the incident, he cannot describe how the fall occurred. Under the doctrine of *res ipsa loquitur*, the patient can prevail in his lawsuit by showing that he was under your care, that he sustained an injury, and that his injury would not have occurred unless negligence was present.

Another type of negligence is known as **negligence per se**. The principle of negligence per se is generally applied in those circumstances in which a paramedic inexcusably violates a statute. An example might be treating a patient even though your license is expired. A finding that a statute has been violated can sometimes lead to an automatic finding of negligence.

Proximate Cause

Even in cases in which the paramedic had a legal duty to the patient, and the paramedic breached the standard of care, a plaintiff must still link the act that fell below the standard of care directly to the injury by showing that the act (or failure to act) proximately caused the harm. *Black's Law Dictionary* defines **proximate cause** as "that which, in a natural and continuous sequence, unbroken by any intervening cause, produces injury, and without which the result would not have occurred."[13] Simply stated, a plaintiff will have to prove that your improper action, or failure to act, was the cause of the injury. For example, failure to secure a patient on a backboard can be the proximate cause of severing the spinal cord.

Proving that an act or a failure to act caused an injury is the most challenging part of a lawsuit. For example, imagine treating a patient from a motor vehicle crash who has a spinal cord injury, and you drop the stretcher during patient care. The patient may try to show that the injury resulted from the dropped stretcher and not from the crash itself. In such a case, careful documentation of the patient's neurologic status when you first encountered the patient would be essential to your defense.

Words of Wisdom

As a paramedic, you may sometimes face ethical conflicts regarding allocating limited resources during triage situations. For example, would you give special consideration to an injured person whom you knew personally? Would you be more likely to provide prompt emergency medical care to an innocent victim of a crime while delaying care to a more seriously injured perpetrator? Would you be able to apply triage protocols objectively to a person who is abusive toward you? Triage requires you to be professional and ethical in every respect because decisions made during triage can affect life and death. Triage procedures are discussed in Chapter 48, *Incident Management and Mass-Casualty Incidents*.

Harm

The final element plaintiffs must prove in a negligence lawsuit is that they were harmed. Although physical injury is usually part of any lawsuit for medical negligence, patients may also claim damages for emotional distress, loss of income, loss of enjoyment of life, loss of spousal consortium, loss of household services, and loss of future earning capacity. They will have to show that your actions as a paramedic were proximate causes of each of these losses.

Abandonment

Abandonment is a form of negligence that involves the termination of medical care without the patient's consent. This term also implies that the patient had a continuing need for medical treatment and that the abrupt termination of treatment was the cause of subsequent injury or death. After you have responded to an emergency, you may not leave a patient in need of medical treatment until another competent health care professional with an equal or higher level of training has taken responsibility for that patient's care. Notify an appropriate health care professional of the patient's presence in the ED and that you are transferring responsibility for patient care to that person. Transfer of care should be properly documented.

It is also vital to complete a written report, which is often submitted electronically and frequently arrives after the call. The ED physician or nurse who is taking over the care of your patient must receive this report. The written report will permit the ED physician and staff to review your findings in the field, the medications you gave the patient, and the procedures you performed.

Some situations may not require transport and are not considered abandonment. EMS systems frequently receive calls for service for patients who may not need treatment or transportation. A patient may have fallen and needs help getting up from the floor or may want your help administering his medication. Or, a patient who has a legitimate medical emergency, such as hypoglycemia, may feel fine after treatment and may not require transport to a hospital. Your local medical director should provide protocols for these situations. However, in general, it is a good idea to encourage transport.

Some ambulance services, particularly in rural areas, may employ providers of various training levels and may not have a full staff of paramedics available at all times. In those areas, even if you make the initial response, you may not need to be part of the transport crew if the patient does not need advanced care. If in doubt, contact your medical control.

Many EMS systems provide a tiered response, with BLS providers reaching the patient quickly, followed by advanced life support (ALS) providers. If a BLS crew responds and makes an improper determination that a patient does not need ALS care, then the system may be exposed to liability. Your service needs to work with every provider involved to set up protocols that guide the situations in which a BLS crew may cancel an incoming ALS crew's response.

Patient Autonomy

It is well established that patients have the right to direct their care and decide how they want their end-of-life medical care provided to them. This right, known as **patient autonomy**, has come to the forefront of medical ethics. In almost every case, except where the patient is a minor or lacks decision-making capacity, you must respect and honor the patient's right to make medical decisions, however irrational or unsound those decisions may appear.

Patients' decisions may not be accepted by other members of the public or even by other members of their families. Nevertheless, the courts, including the US Supreme Court, have clearly recognized the right of patients to make decisions about their own medical care, even if that decision will bring about the patient's death. Ethics surrounding patient autonomy has become the subject of many discussions among paramedics, who find themselves in the unique position of being accountable to more systems than the average health care provider in trying to respect the patient's wishes. The EMS system, your medical director, the EMS agency for which you work, and your community's standard of care may all compete with the patient's wishes. These competing interests can create an ethical conflict that you will need to resolve through communication with all parties involved.

Occasionally, a physician will give an order that you feel is detrimental to the patient's best interests. You need to immediately discuss with the physician why you feel that way. As a paramedic, you are often in a better position to see what is really going on with the patient, and a big part of your job is to communicate fully with the physician. Never perform a procedure or administer a medication that you believe will be detrimental to the patient. For example, suppose a physician asks you to perform a procedure in which you are not trained or asks you to administer medication in a dose that is well outside the range of your protocols. In that case, it is essential to obtain clarification from the physician and communicate your objections. You could discuss your current standing orders and offer a feasible alternative within your scope of practice, or you could request that the physician speak with your medical director. In all circumstances, act in the patient's best interest as an advocate.

Advance Directives

An **advance directive** is usually a written document (but can also be an oral statement) that expresses the wants, needs, and desires of a patient about future medical care. Advance directives state what medical care the patient wants or does not want when the patient is unable to express these wishes. Living wills, do not resuscitate (DNR) orders, and organ donation orders are all types of advance directives.

Advance directives differ from state to state. In some states, a DNR order (also known as a resuscitation directive) may restrict any ALS care, whereas others provide for comfort care, including pain medications and oxygen therapy. In Colorado, a person designated as the medical durable power of attorney (discussed next) can revoke a resuscitation directive. In contrast, in Montana, the patient or physician is the only one who can revoke a resuscitation directive.

Whether advance directives bind EMS personnel is a function of state law. These laws, like those that cover DNR orders, are usually quite narrow, often limited to terminal patients in nursing homes or hospice care. Learning and following the laws of your state will provide a framework for decisions regarding advance directives.

Living Will and Health Care Power of Attorney

The **living will** and the **health care power of attorney** are types of advance directives through which patients can express their wishes regarding end-of-life medical care. These directives are sometimes called health care "durable" powers of attorney because they remain in effect after a patient loses decision-making capacity. Dealing with powers of attorney can sometimes be confusing for providers. First of all, various types of powers of attorney exist, and not all of them authorize the designated agent to make decisions regarding health care. Older patients commonly execute powers of attorney that enable others to conduct financial affairs on their behalf, which do not affect health care. It is also possible that a power of attorney may have been executed outside the state in which the patient now resides and its effect within your state may be questionable. As a paramedic, you should ask to see the power of attorney and then carefully review it to determine whether it authorizes the agent to make health care decisions. Most states recognize that advance directives, except for DNR orders, probably will not apply in emergency situations because the paramedic is unable to take the time to read and interpret a legal document on scene. When you are in doubt, contact medical control for assistance.

Living wills generally require some kind of precondition to activate their terms, such as a terminal illness or an irreversible coma. The living will should spell out precisely what kind of treatment a patient wishes to be given should that individual become incapacitated. A living will often contains a health care power of attorney, which designates another person (eg, a spouse, partner, adult sibling, or parent) to make health care decisions for the patient when the patient is unable to make those decisions. The person designated to make decisions does not have to be a relative, but may be someone close to the patient who understands the patient's wishes. In those cases where the living will does not contain a health care power of attorney, its use in the field will be limited and you should consult medical control.

The person who carries the health care power of attorney is often called the **surrogate decision maker** **FIGURE 4-17**. The surrogate decision maker is legally obligated to make decisions as the patient would want, and has presumably discussed these decisions with the patient. Bear in mind that the surrogate decision maker has no authority until the patient becomes incapable of making decisions. If you arrive on scene and find that a surrogate decision maker is attempting to make decisions that conflict with a competent patient's decisions, then always follow the patient's decisions. Do not refuse emergency medical care to a patient who desires it.

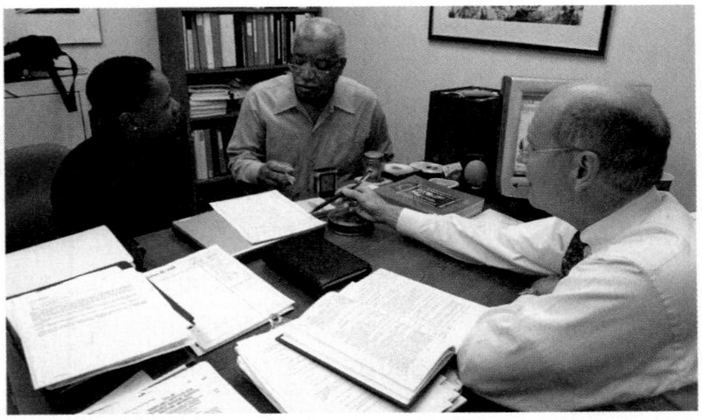

FIGURE 4-17 A surrogate decision maker (often a child or other close relative) is frequently designated when a person draws up a living will.

DNR Orders

As mentioned previously, a **do not resuscitate (DNR) order** (also referred to as *do not attempt resuscitation [DNAR]*) is an advance directive that describes which life-sustaining procedures, if any, should be performed if a patient's medical condition suddenly deteriorates. During the last 20 years, DNR orders have finally been recognized as valid in the prehospital setting **FIGURE 4-18**. EMS has now joined the medical community in recognizing that patients have the same rights to direct and refuse care outside the hospital that they do inside the hospital.

Words of Wisdom

Do not be confused: A living will is not the same as a DNR order. The living will allows for decisions to be made regarding DNR orders if patients become incapacitated or unable to make their own decisions.

Many states now have DNR forms specific to EMS, and most states have laws that govern the natural process of dying and what rights patients have to direct that process.

States have their own procedures for how to recognize a valid DNR order. Some states rely on a written physician order (which might not be available to the EMS provider), while others may require the patient to wear an identification bracelet or necklace. In some cases, such jewelry indicates that the patient has consented to the release of stored information, such as the patient's DNR status, to medical personnel **FIGURE 4-19**. In some states, DNR orders expire within a specified time frame and must be renewed to remain valid, whereas others may have no expiration date. It may also be a requirement that the DNR order be executed within your state by a physician licensed to practice medicine within the state. Be familiar with the documents used in your state and what you are expected to do if those documents are unavailable.

YOU are the Paramedic

PART 3

The patient's daughter brings you a list of her mother's medications and you quickly review it—carvedilol (Coreg), lisinopril (Prinivil), levothyroxine (Synthroid), and simvastatin (Zocor). She also hands you a copy of the advance directive, which states the patient wishes no heroic measures be taken if she is not breathing and does not have a pulse.

The patient tells you her name is Mary, but cannot tell you the day of the week or how old she is. She agrees to let you take her vital signs, but still says she will not go to the hospital. Measurement of her blood glucose level shows a reading of 138 mg/dL.

Her daughter tells you that her mother's symptoms have been present for several days, but today she is worse. She keeps forgetting basic things and is now refusing to eat. She thinks her mother might be having "ministrokes" and her confusion is getting worse.

Recording Time: 4 Minutes	
Respirations	20 breaths/min, regular
Pulse	108 beats/min, strong radial pulses
Skin	Cool and dry
Blood pressure	152/98 mm Hg
Oxygen saturation (Spo_2)	97% on room air
Pupils	Pupils Equal, Round, and Reactive to Light and Accommodation (PERRLA)

5. Would it be considered abandonment if you left the scene at this point?

6. Does the patient's advance directive take precedence over her current wishes?

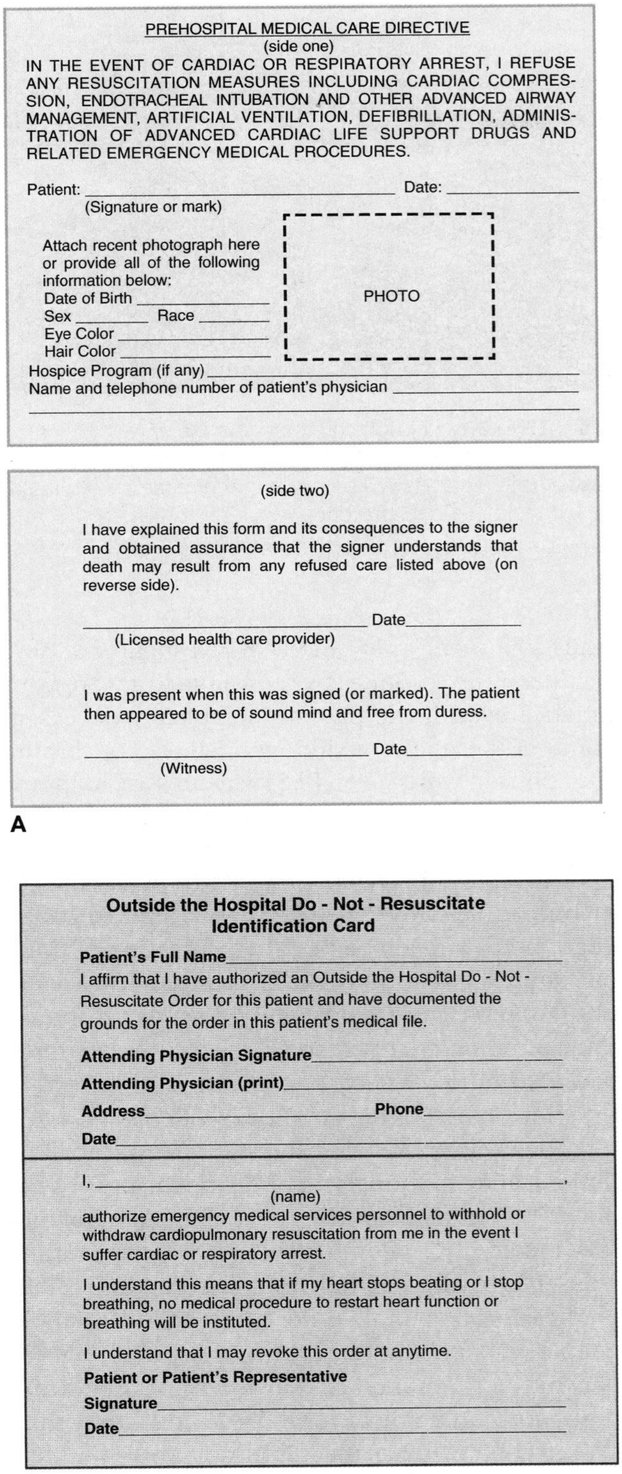

PREHOSPITAL MEDICAL CARE DIRECTIVE
(side one)
IN THE EVENT OF CARDIAC OR RESPIRATORY ARREST, I REFUSE ANY RESUSCITATION MEASURES INCLUDING CARDIAC COMPRESSION, ENDOTRACHEAL INTUBATION AND OTHER ADVANCED AIRWAY MANAGEMENT, ARTIFICIAL VENTILATION, DEFIBRILLATION, ADMINISTRATION OF ADVANCED CARDIAC LIFE SUPPORT DRUGS AND RELATED EMERGENCY MEDICAL PROCEDURES.

Patient: ______________________ Date: __________
(Signature or mark)

Attach recent photograph here or provide all of the following information below:
Date of Birth __________
Sex ______ Race ______
Eye Color __________
Hair Color __________

PHOTO

Hospice Program (if any) __________
Name and telephone number of patient's physician __________

(side two)

I have explained this form and its consequences to the signer and obtained assurance that the signer understands that death may result from any refused care listed above (on reverse side).

______________________ Date __________
(Licensed health care provider)

I was present when this was signed (or marked). The patient then appeared to be of sound mind and free from duress.

______________________ Date __________
(Witness)

A

Outside the Hospital Do - Not - Resuscitate Identification Card

Patient's Full Name __________
I affirm that I have authorized an Outside the Hospital Do - Not - Resuscitate Order for this patient and have documented the grounds for the order in this patient's medical file.

Attending Physician Signature __________
Attending Physician (print) __________
Address __________ **Phone** __________
Date __________

I, ______________________,
(name)
authorize emergency medical services personnel to withhold or withdraw cardiopulmonary resuscitation from me in the event I suffer cardiac or respiratory arrest.

I understand this means that if my heart stops beating or I stop breathing, no medical procedure to restart heart function or breathing will be instituted.

I understand that I may revoke this order at anytime.

Patient or Patient's Representative
Signature __________
Date __________

B

FIGURE 4-18 A. An example of a wallet-size do not resuscitate (DNR) order. **B.** An example of a pocket-size DNR order.

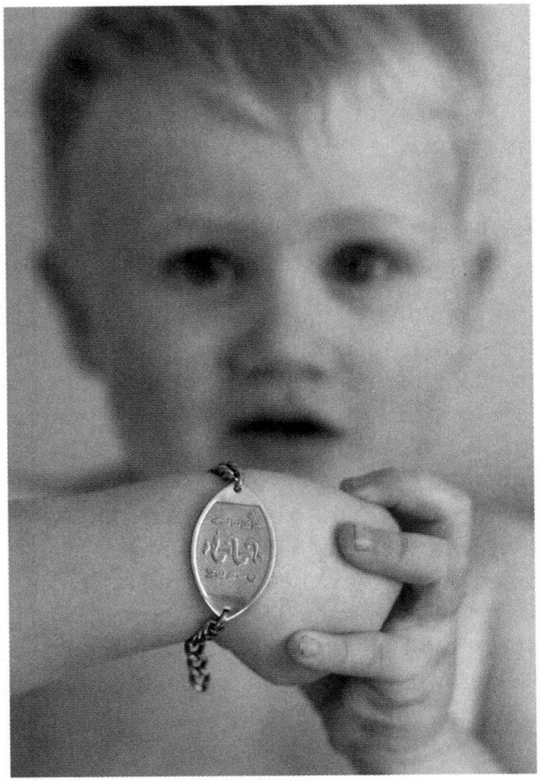

FIGURE 4-19 Medical identification bracelets can provide access to vital information about a patient, including important medical conditions and possible do not resuscitate orders. If the patient has a Medic Alert bracelet, the EMS provider can obtain stored patient information from the Medic Alert Foundation.

Although laws might differ from state to state, generally speaking, DNR orders must meet the following requirements to be valid:

- Clearly state the patient's medical condition(s).
- Include the signature of the patient or legal guardian.
- Include the signature of one or more physicians.
- DNR orders contain expiration dates in some states, whereas in others, no expiration date is included. DNR orders with expiration dates must be dated in the preceding 12 months to be valid.

Even if the patient has a valid DNR order, you are still obligated to provide supportive measures if indicated (eg, oxygen, pain relief, and comfort) to a patient who is not in cardiac arrest, whenever possible. In consultation with its medical director and legal counsel, each ambulance service must develop a protocol to follow in these circumstances.

Withholding or Withdrawing Resuscitation

Current bioethical guidelines rely on common sense and reasonable judgment in deciding when to stop CPR and resuscitation efforts, and when to decline to initiate them at all. The National Association of EMS Physicians has published data that demonstrate the benefits of on-scene resuscitation, along with guidelines for the termination of resuscitation of nontraumatic cardiopulmonary arrest.[14] These guidelines have been adopted by many EMS organizations across the United States, allowing for field personnel to make a clinical decision regarding resuscitation based on down time, poor outcome analysis, and family input. These guidelines represent a paradigm shift from previous resuscitation modalities, and some organizations have hesitated to implement such practices. Nevertheless, numerous studies document the benefit of adopting such practices.[14]

Each resuscitation should be based on the futility of such efforts. Futile resuscitation efforts—interventions that studies have shown do not benefit patients—are not medically or ethically indicated **FIGURE 4-20**. If you are unsure of the time of a cardiac arrest, begin care and immediately contact medical control to discuss termination of resuscitative efforts.

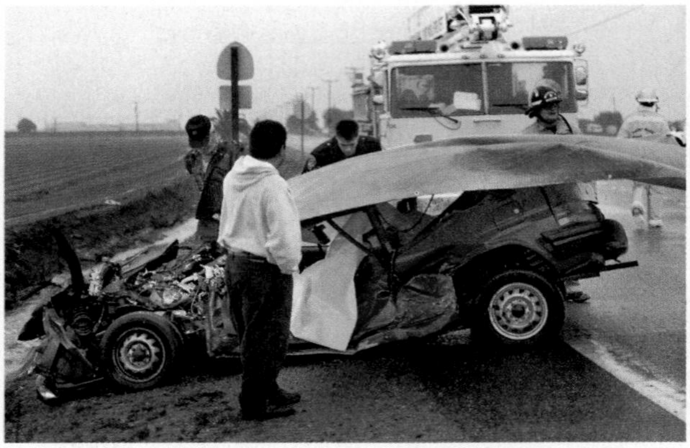

FIGURE 4-20 Although your instincts are always to try to sustain life at whatever cost, sometimes it is clear that resuscitation efforts will be futile. In that case, they should be withheld per local protocols.

You will need to consider the time it will take for a patient to reach definitive care at the hospital and the likelihood of survival, especially if you work in rural and wilderness areas. Occasionally, you will hear a story about a patient who recovered from what appeared to be a hopeless situation, providing motivation for you to attempt to save a patient under impossible circumstances. Such rare survival cases should not guide your decisions about resuscitation efforts, even though terminating life-saving efforts in the field may seem contrary to your instincts as a health care provider.

Each state has different laws that may define the role of the paramedic in regard to resuscitation. In some jurisdictions, you may be able to pronounce death; in others, only a medical investigator or physician may do so. State laws continue to govern your practice even if the patient is clinically deceased. Some of these laws include guidelines concerning situations in which even BLS measures are inappropriate. For example, do not attempt resuscitation for patients who are obviously dead (eg, livor or rigor mortis or putrefaction), or who have injuries incompatible with life (eg, decapitation). If resuscitation has already begun, then cessation of these efforts in the field may be appropriate in cases of blunt trauma arrest, a prolonged rescue or response time, or other lengthy medical resuscitation efforts. Termination of resuscitative efforts is discussed in Chapter 40, *Responding to the Field Code*.

The decision to halt resuscitation is particularly difficult and emotional when you are caring for a pediatric patient. Studies have shown that paramedics feel incredibly uncomfortable about terminating resuscitation in children. Paramedics and other medical professionals tend to be action-oriented people who feel that they must "do something" (as part of their moral code). However, in some situations, you can do more for the grieving family than for the child who has died. Ethically, you should be prepared to support the family, which can be the hardest part of the job.

Training, literature reviews, and open discussions about what actions are medically appropriate within EMS protocols should provide you with guidance and ease your concerns about difficult resuscitation situations. Continuing education regarding resuscitation issues may provide alternative viewpoints and a broader picture that allow you to make appropriate decisions in the field.

As a paramedic, you must thoroughly understand the consequences of typical EMS interventions. Ultimately, medical interventions and life-saving attempts may prolong suffering or fail to return a patient to a meaningful life. When in doubt, do not hesitate to consult medical control. If communication is hindered because of terrain or wilderness conditions, then your judgment will benefit from knowing about interventions and the consequences of those interventions ahead of time.

End-of-Life Decisions

Paramedics often deal with patients at the very end of their lives. These patients and their families should be treated with the utmost respect and empathy. You should never think: "Why did they bother to call 9-1-1 if they don't want us to do anything?" (This example represents the paramedic's moral code getting in the way of the paramedic's medical ethics.) Instead, understand that the family of a dying patient, even one under hospice care, may not know how to check a pulse, and may not understand that agonal gasps may continue for hours before a patient dies. Furthermore, despite knowing that death is near, a loved one may call for an ambulance, not knowing what else to do at the moment of death. Many people have never been with someone at the moment of death. If information and emotional support are what they need, then provide them; doing so is part of your job.

Avoid imposing your moral code on a patient whose value system may differ from your own. You will encounter dying patients with varied cultural beliefs, and must be prepared to respect their wishes even if their lifestyle or religious beliefs do not match your own.

You are also likely to encounter confusing scenarios when the DNR paperwork may not be immediately available. It is permissible, if not obligatory, that you begin resuscitation efforts and then discontinue them (with agreement from online medical control) if and when the paperwork is confirmed. In other situations, the paperwork may be readily available, but family members may disagree with the DNR order and insist that you begin resuscitation. In such cases, avoid any hostile encounters while carrying out the patient's wishes to the best of your ability. Contact medical control in confusing situations involving resuscitation questions. The medical control physician can be a valuable resource in such circumstances.

Medical Orders for Life-Sustaining Treatment

In recent years, a type of end-of-life document has emerged that is known as medical orders for life-sustaining treatment (MOLST) or physician orders for life-sustaining treatment (POLST). Although similar to a DNR order in many respects, the MOLST is more expansive. It is intended to be followed by all health care providers, not just EMS personnel. The DNR generally applies to patients who are in cardiac arrest, whereas MOLST may apply to patients with impending pulmonary failure who are not in cardiac arrest. MOLST documents typically contain provisions that address the initiation of CPR, intubation, feeding tubes, the use of antibiotics, and **palliative care** (intended to provide comfort and relief from pain). They apply only when the patient has lost decision-making capacity. *MOLST orders are not used in all states, and you must check whether your state has adopted such provisions.*

Organ Donation

A significant issue in medical ethics involves the potential for patients with mortal injuries to donate organs. Donor organs are badly needed within the medical system, with some patients waiting years for a match.

In specific circumstances, a patient who is not successfully resuscitated may be a potential organ donor. Some medical centers can procure organs, including the kidneys and liver, in certain situations from such patients. These situations typically occur after in-hospital cardiac arrest but may also be associated with certain specific out-of-hospital cardiac arrest situations that occur near specialized centers. Be aware of your local centers and their respective protocols and capabilities.

Organ donation and the parameters for viable organs should be spelled out within the individual EMS system. Also understand the state law

FIGURE 4-21 Most states have an organ donation designation on the driver's license, either on the front or reverse side (here, it is shown at lower right).

concerning organ donation: In many cases, a patient must have witnessed, informed consent (usually in writing) to donate organs.

In general, major organs such as the kidneys and liver are not appropriate for organ donation after prolonged hypotension or CPR. However, other tissues such as the corneas and skin may be valuable. Many states have programs that allow patients to agree to organ donation by making a notation on their driver's licenses **FIGURE 4-21**. If the patient's wishes regarding organ donation are unknown, then relay this information when transferring patient care and discuss with medical direction, if appropriate.

Continuing education workshops offered by organ transplant teams and EMS leaders to increase awareness of the vital role of EMS in securing transplants may be another resource available to your EMS system.

Defenses to Litigation

Over the last 10 years, the media and public education have made the public more aware of what to expect from the local EMS system. If citizens perceive your response as delayed or your efforts as incompetent, then they will often file lawsuits seeking compensation for injuries they believe were caused by inadequate EMS care. If you do not explain to your patients why you were delayed, or why a procedure is difficult, then you leave yourself open to the consequences of unanswered questions that can lead a patient to seek legal action. In essence, your first defense to litigation is an open, informative, trust-based relationship with your patients. When this relationship is not possible or fails in its intent, and litigation occurs, several legal defenses may be used in the courtroom.

If a lawsuit is filed against you, then you and the agency with which you are employed may implement one of two commonly used defenses: statute of limitations and contributory negligence. Every state has laws that limit the time within which a lawsuit may be filed. Such laws are called **statutes of limitations**. The time to file may be as short as 1 year in some states, or as long as 5 or 6 years in other states. A lawsuit that is filed beyond these statutory periods can be dismissed as untimely. However, these statutory periods are typically extended for minors until the minor reaches the age of majority.

Another potential defense is known as **contributory negligence**. This defense will apply when the plaintiff has done something that contributes to injuries. For example, you encounter a patient with chest pain that appears to be cardiac in nature. Before administering nitroglycerin, you inquire about any recent use of erectile dysfunction medications. The patient denies using any such medication, even though he actually used one of the medications several hours earlier. Shortly after you administer the nitroglycerin, the patient experiences a severe drop in blood pressure and almost dies due to the interaction between the nitroglycerin and erectile dysfunction medication. In the lawsuit that follows, you are able to assert the defense of contributory negligence because the patient failed to state that he had used the medication several hours earlier, and that usage clearly contributed to his adverse reaction to the nitroglycerin.

Good Samaritan Legislation

Although every state has some form of a Good Samaritan law, not every state extends such protection to all citizens and off-duty EMS personnel. As an EMS provider, you should contact your state legislators to determine which level of Good Samaritan protection is offered.[15] Although these statutes were initially passed to encourage the public to help at emergency scenes, many of them also provide some protection for EMS personnel who are off duty and assist at an emergency. Most states' laws limit the legal protection provided: Emergency care must be

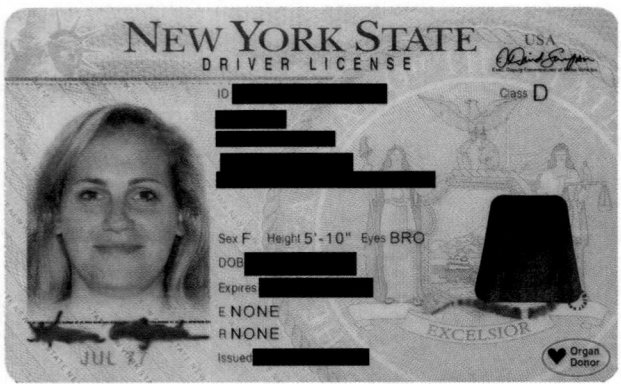

given free of charge (gratuitously). As a general rule, if you are on duty and have a legal duty to a patient, then the Good Samaritan law *will not* protect you. Good Samaritan laws may help cover you if you render assistance in another state, but they do not supersede the licensing agency's laws in your state.

Most Good Samaritan laws also require that people responding to an emergency do all that they can, within their knowledge, to support and sustain life and to prevent further injury. As a paramedic, you are not expected to function as a physician; however, you are expected to deploy those skills that any other paramedic with similar training would use under the same or similar circumstances.

Courts have not been generous in applying the Good Samaritan law during routine EMS work. Instead, they have applied the concept of immunity only during emergencies.

Governmental Immunity

An abiding principle of English law is that you cannot sue the queen (or king) because "the queen can do no wrong." In the United States, this concept, called sovereign immunity, has taken the form of legislation that identifies only limited types of lawsuits that can be filed against government agencies. Paramedics working for government agencies, such as a fire department, also have some governmental immunity for their actions. The immunity statutes may also set limited time frames in which lawsuits can be filed, and may limit the amount of money a plaintiff can recover.

Qualified Immunity

Governmental immunity does not cover civil rights violations, and attorneys can file lawsuits against paramedics in the public sector for violating a patient's civil rights. The most common type of complaint occurs when EMS personnel either improperly restrain a violent patient or use excessive force to restrain a patient. Civil rights lawsuits may also be filed if your conduct as a paramedic deviates so far from the standard of care that a civil rights violation is said to occur.

YOU are the Paramedic

PART 4

You talk to Mary and explain to her that she needs to be evaluated. She starts to cry and tells you, "They are just sending me to that hospital to die." You convince her that this is not true and that she needs to see a physician so that she will feel better. She reluctantly agrees to go with you and says that she has a slight headache but otherwise feels fine. You perform a stroke assessment and see no signs of deficits.

At 0752 hours, the patient is on a stretcher in the ambulance and you are en route to the hospital. You start a 20-gauge IV line in her left antecubital fossa and draw blood. You administer normal saline at a TKO (to keep open) flow rate. She will not tolerate a nasal cannula, so you monitor her oxygen saturation level. The cardiac monitor shows sinus tachycardia without ectopy.

You reassess her vital signs en route and transport her to Cedar's Medical Center, arriving at the hospital at 0804 hours. You give a report to the receiving nurse and are back in service at 0815 hours.

Recording Time: 14 Minutes	
Respirations	18 breaths/min, regular
Pulse	102 beats/min, strong radial pulses
Skin	Cool and dry
Blood pressure	162/94 mm Hg
Oxygen saturation (Spo_2)	98% on room air
Pupils	PERRLA

7. If the patient had continued to refuse treatment and transport, then what options might you have exercised?

8. Under which type of consent was this patient treated?

If paramedics work or volunteer for public agencies (eg, fire departments) and are sued by patients alleging civil rights violations, they may have another type of immunity called **qualified immunity**. Under this doctrine, you are held liable only when the plaintiff can show that you violated a clearly established law of which you should have known. This kind of immunity does not apply to tort cases.

Employment Law and the Paramedic

In addition to the legal issues that arise out of your role as a paramedic providing patient care, several laws affect your relationship with your employer. In fact, throughout your career as a paramedic, the chances of becoming involved in a legal issue regarding your employment are probably as great, if not greater, than your chances of being sued by a patient. The relationship between employer and employee involves an ever-growing web of state and federal laws and regulations of which you should have a basic understanding.

Americans With Disabilities Act

The Americans With Disabilities Act (ADA) is a federal law adopted in 1990 to protect qualified people with disabilities from being discriminated against in employment. This law generally applies to all employers with a minimum of 15 employees, but state laws providing similar protection may include those with even fewer employees. The ADA applies to all aspects of employment, including hiring, promotions, training, salary, benefits, and termination. A common misconception about the ADA is that it requires employers to hire employees with disabilities who may not be qualified for the job. This notion, of course, is not true.

To be protected by the ADA, a person must meet two basic qualifications:

1. Have a physical or mental disability that limits one or more major life activities such as hearing, seeing, walking, or speaking; and
2. Possess the basic qualifications for the job and be able to perform the essential functions of the job adequately, with or without reasonable accommodations.

An employer may not inquire about an applicant's disability or require a medical exam until after a job offer has been made. If a person with a disability would be able to perform the essential functions of the job using reasonable accommodations, then the employer may be required to provide and pay for the cost of these accommodations. The law does not require an employer to provide accommodations that would result in an undue hardship to the employer or to other employees.

The ADA does not require an employer to give preference to a person with a disability. It merely requires that an employer make employment decisions based on reasons unrelated to the disability (ie, the applicant's ability to perform the essential job functions).

Title VII of the Civil Rights Act

Title VII is the section of the Civil Rights Act of 1964 that prohibits discrimination in employment based on race, color, religion, sex, or national origin. In addition, this section of the law provides protection against sexual harassment in the workplace. The antidiscrimination provisions of Title VII apply to all aspects of employment, including recruiting, hiring, promotions, benefits, and termination. Like the ADA, Title VII applies only to businesses with more than 15 employees.

Today it is unusual for an employer to blatantly refuse to hire or promote someone based on race, sex, religion, color, or national origin. Successful discrimination claims often involve identifying a discriminatory hiring pattern that develops over time and demonstrating that a particular class of people, such as women or African Americans, are rarely hired or promoted and are vastly under-represented in the overall workforce.

Certain hiring practices violate Title VII even when these practices appear neutral. For example, imagine that an employer places a classified ad seeking to hire paramedics and states that one of the job qualifications is a minimum height of 5 feet 9 inches (175 cm). Although this qualification might seem neutral with respect to sex, it would have a negative effect on the ability of women to be considered for the job because only a small percentage of women would meet the minimum height requirement. The burden would be on the employer to prove that it was necessary for a paramedic to be at least 5 feet 9 inches (175 cm) tall to perform the job's functions effectively. Clearly, the employer could not meet this burden.

Sexual Harassment

Sexual harassment litigation is one of the most common claims filed under Title VII, and many such claims have been made against EMS agencies. Sexual harassment can occur between any combination of sexes, sexual orientations, or gender identities.[16] Two types of sexual harassment claims exist: (1) **quid pro quo** ("this for that") claims, in which a person in authority attempts to exchange some work-related benefit such as a raise or promotion for inappropriate employee actions (eg, sexual favors), and (2) **hostile environment** claims. In the latter claims, the plaintiff asserts that the employer or an agent of the employer either created an offensive practice or allowed it to continue, making it uncomfortable or impossible for the employee to continue working. Most sexual harassment claims fall into the hostile environment category.

No precise definition exists in the law of the types of conduct that would constitute sexual harassment. Nevertheless, court decisions over the years have identified several circumstances that can be considered harassment:

- Sexual jokes or comments
- Display of sexually offensive photographs or other material
- Unwelcome sexual advances
- Inappropriate and unwelcome touching or kissing
- Inappropriate inquiry into an employee's sex life

All employers must prevent sexual harassment from occurring and investigate all claims of sexual harassment promptly. As part of their obligation under the law, employers should provide training in sexual harassment for all newly hired employees and for all employees annually. As an employee, it is important to promptly report any conduct that you feel constitutes sexual harassment to your supervisor or to your organization's human resources department.

Additional Federal Laws Dealing With Discrimination

Several other federal laws prohibit various types of discrimination in the workplace. These include the following:

1. The *Pregnancy Discrimination Act* makes it illegal to discriminate in all employment areas based on pregnancy, childbirth, or any medical condition related to pregnancy. This law was adopted in 1978 as an amendment to Title VII. Before enacting this law, it was common for employers to refuse to hire women who were pregnant or to terminate women after they became pregnant. The law also requires employers to provide health benefits and medical leave for pregnancy and childbirth equal to those provided for other medical conditions.
2. The *Equal Pay Act of 1963* makes it illegal to pay different compensation rates to men and women if they perform equal work in the same workplace. Executives and managers are generally exempt from the provisions of the law.
3. The *Age Discrimination in Employment Act of 1967* protects people who are age 40 years or older from discrimination in all aspects of employment based on age. The law applies to businesses with 15 or more employees.

State Laws

Many states have also passed laws that deal with discrimination in the workplace. For the most part, these laws address the same issues covered under federal law. In some cases, these laws provide more rights than federal laws. For example, some state laws prohibit discrimination based on sexual orientation, marital status, or gender identity, which may not all be covered under federal law.[17] Also, many discrimination protections under federal law do not apply to employers with fewer than 15 employees, whereas many state laws do apply. It is essential to become familiar with the laws of your state.

Family and Medical Leave Act

The Family and Medical Leave Act (FMLA) of 1993 is a federal law that grants eligible employees the right to take up to 12 weeks of unpaid leave per year under certain circumstances. To be eligible for such leave, an employee must work for an employer with at least 50 employees and must have worked for that employer for at least 12 months. Leave may be taken to deal with a medical condition of the employee or a family member or a child's birth or adoption.

Some states have passed their own Family Leave Acts that may provide the employee with more rights than the federal law or that apply to employers with fewer than 50 employees.

Occupational Safety and Health Administration

The Occupational Safety and Health Administration (OSHA) is the federal agency regulating safety in the workplace. States may enforce tighter regulations than those set by OSHA but may not make regulations more lenient. All employers are covered either by OSHA or an OSHA-approved safety plan. Under the OSHA Act of 1970, all employers have several basic responsibilities, including the following:

- To comply with all OSHA standards, rules, and regulations that apply to the business
- To provide all employees with a workplace that is free from hazards
- To warn employees of potential hazards
- To ensure all employees are provided with appropriate safety equipment
- To establish and maintain a reporting system for all workplace injuries or illnesses
- To provide training for all employees

Health care employers have some additional responsibilities that are unique to the industry, including the following:

- Development of an exposure control plan to assist employees who may have been exposed to certain bloodborne pathogens
- Development of training programs for all newly hired employees as well as annual refresher training for all employees that address issues related to bloodborne pathogens
- Making the hepatitis B vaccine available at no charge to all employees
- Development of guidelines regarding the use of standard precautions

OSHA regulations and standards change quite frequently, and as a paramedic, you should do your best to keep up-to-date with these changes. In the EMS environment, thousands of EMS employees sustain injuries and illnesses each year. You share an obligation, along with your employer, to do all that you can to avoid injuries.

Ryan White Act

The Ryan White Act is a federal law that provides certain safeguards and protections for health care workers who are exposed or potentially exposed to certain designated diseases. The Centers for Disease Control and Prevention has specified the conditions covered by this act; they include human immunodeficiency virus infection, acquired immunodeficiency syndrome, tuberculosis, hepatitis B, meningitis, diphtheria, hemorrhagic fevers, plague, and rabies.

The Ryan White Act contains several important provisions, which include the following:

- Hospitals and emergency response employers are required to establish a notification system to be used when an exposure occurs.
- Employers must appoint a designated infection control officer to handle exposures and to assist all employees who may have been exposed.
- Access to the medical records of the patient who is the source of the exposure may be obtained to determine whether the patient has tested positively for, or is exhibiting signs and symptoms of, a covered infectious disease.

If you believe that you have been exposed to an infectious disease, promptly notify the infection control officer within your service. The infection control officer will be aware of any state-specific laws related to infectious disease exposure.

National Labor Relations Act

Many paramedics are employed by EMS agencies that are unionized. Unionization means that at some point, the employees have elected to have a union represent them as their collective bargaining agent for purposes of negotiating issues such as compensation, benefits, and work conditions. The National Labor Relations Act, also known as the Wagner Act, is the primary law that establishes unions and union workers' rights and specifies what are considered unfair labor practices by employers.

Under this law, employees have a wide variety of rights, with which they should become familiar.

In addition to the provisions of the National Labor Relations Act, each state has its own set of laws that affect union members' rights. In some states, so-called right to work laws do not allow an employer or a union to require you to join a union as a condition to being hired or retained on the job. You may be required to join the union within a specific period after being hired in other states.

YOU are the Paramedic SUMMARY

1. What type of consent is required to treat a patient with altered mental status?

Any patient who is incapacitated and cannot make decisions is treated under implied consent. This principle applies to any patient who is too ill or injured to consent to emergency life-saving treatment. It is assumed that the patient would want emergency medical care because of the severity of the condition. Implied consent is also applied to minors or those adults who have guardians when a serious illness or injury has occurred and a parent or guardian is not present.

2. What information must you determine prior to allowing a patient to refuse care?

First determine the patient's decision-making capacity by talking with her. Factors that will help you include the patient's orientation to person, place, and time; use of drugs or alcohol; potential head trauma; the patient's medical history; and the patient's vital signs, blood glucose level, and oxygen saturation level. To refuse treatment and/or transport, patients must be able to understand the information given regarding their condition and care and make a decision based on that information. As a general rule, patients with an altered mental status or unstable vital signs probably cannot be considered able to refuse transport. To avoid potential legal action, follow the protocols established by your service.

3. What are the possible consequences of treating this patient without her consent?

Touching and/or treating a patient without consent may be grounds for charges of assault, battery, and possibly false imprisonment. These charges may result from improper restraint methods, failing to ask for permission before touching or making physical contact, or transporting a patient without consent. However, the patient must be of legal age and demonstrate the ability to make informed decisions and refuse emergency medical care.

4. On the basis of her history, what might be her problem?

This patient has a history of transient ischemic attacks (TIAs), a brain tumor, hypothyroidism, hypertension, and hyperlipidemia. Any or all of these conditions could be the problem or could be contributing factors. She is exhibiting symptoms similar to TIAs with periods of unresponsiveness. However, because her confusion has lasted for more than 24 hours, another cause or an additional cause is likely. The brain tumor could also be a major factor. It may be growing or pressing on specific brain areas, leading to her signs and symptoms. Hypertension may be a contributing factor for TIAs, or could exacerbate the brain tumor. Hypothyroidism causes many signs and symptoms, and taking too much or too little of her medication may result in mental status changes. Hyperlipidemia indicates that the patient already has an excess of cholesterol. If any blockages in major vessels supplying the brain are present, then hypoxia and an altered mental status may result.

5. Would it be considered abandonment if you left the scene at this point?

Yes. The patient clearly has an altered mental status, and abiding by her wishes not to be transported would be considered abandonment. A patient with an altered mental status does not have decision-making capacity and cannot refuse care. After you respond to a call and make contact with a patient, you cannot legally release that patient's care unless the patient is competent to refuse care or you have turned care over to someone of an equal or higher level of training.

6. Does the patient's advance directive take precedence over her current wishes?

If she is capable of making informed decisions, then she can override the advance directive. In this situation, the patient is not in cardiac arrest so this is not an issue, because her advance directive is specific to a cardiac arrest.

YOU are the Paramedic SUMMARY continued

7. If the patient had continued to refuse treatment and transport, then what options might you have exercised?

Having her daughter talk to her may have helped, but if all else failed, then it would have become necessary to contact medical control for direction. She has an altered mental status and cannot refuse care because of her impaired decision-making capacity. In such a situation, follow local protocols, and before contacting medical control, ensure you have all of the information concerning the patient—vital signs, blood glucose level, medical history, medications, and any findings—readily available.

Not only can medical control direct you in the proper handling of the patient, but having the patient speak directly to the physician on the phone may be enough to convince her that transport is necessary. Continue to be patient but firm in expressing to her why she needs to be transported for emergency medical care.

8. Under which type of consent was this patient treated?

The patient was treated under informed consent as well as implied consent. She has an altered mental status, which technically means that she can be treated under implied consent.

She was also treated under informed consent. She is not completely disoriented and understands most of what you are telling her. She agrees initially to allow you to take vital signs. She understands what you are about to do and gives you permission to do it. These actions constitute informed consent.

EMS Patient Care Report (PCR)

Date: 02-02-22	**Incident No.:** 02110985	**Nature of Call:** Unresponsive person		**Location:** 487 Lenore Street	
Dispatched: 0737	**En Route:** 0738	**At Scene:** 0742	**Transport:** 0752	**At Hospital:** 0804	**In Service:** 0815

Patient Information

Age: 64 **Sex:** F **Weight (in kg [lb]):** 69 kg (152 lb)	**Allergies:** Penicillin **Medications:** Coreg, Synthroid, Zocor, Prinivil **Past Medical History:** HTN, brain tumor, TIAs, hyperlipidemia, hypothyroidism **Chief Complaint:** Slight headache, acting strangely, altered mental status

Vital Signs

Time: 0746	**BP:** 152/98	**Pulse:** 108	**Respirations:** 20	**Spo_2:** 97% on room air
Time: 0756	**BP:** 162/94	**Pulse:** 102	**Respirations:** 18	**Spo_2:** 98% on room air
Time:	**BP:**	**Pulse:**	**Respirations:**	**Spo_2:**

EMS Treatment (circle all that apply)

Oxygen @ ____ L/min via (circle one): **NC NRM Bag-mask device**		**Assisted Ventilation**	**Airway Adjunct**	**CPR**
Defibrillation	**Bleeding Control**	**Bandaging**	**Splinting**	**Other:** Cardiac monitor (circled)

Narrative

EMS responded to a possible unresponsive person to find a 64 y/o woman reporting "slight" headache and altered mental status. Pt awake, but confused, oriented to person, place, and event, but not time (verbal per AVPU scale). Daughter states that she has been this way for several days and has periods of not responding at all. Pt is ambulatory, no apparent distress noted, and no neuro deficits. PERRLA, glucose level is 138 mg/dL, heart monitor showing sinus tach without ectopy. Nothing else significant noted. Pt refused oxygen, but Spo_2 level on room air remains within normal limits. 20-gauge IV L antecubital fossa with blood drawn for labs and NS at TKO. Transported to Cedar's Medical Center, no changes en route.

End of report

Prep Kit

Ready for Review

- As a paramedic, you operate in a community that exposes you to professional liability, and that requires you to have a solid understanding of law and ethics. Failing to perform your job as expected within the medical community, the legal community, and the regulations of the jurisdiction in which you function will expose you to civil and/or criminal liability.
- When personal ethics conflict with professional ethics, you usually will be bound by professional ethics and must temporarily set aside your personal ethics.
- Three primary ethical principles apply to your practice: (1) to do no harm, (2) to act in good faith, and (3) to always act in the patient's best interest.
- EMS providers should stay aware of the latest EMS research to promote evidence-based practice.
- The foundation of the legal system in the United States is the federal government. The three branches of government are the executive, judicial, and legislative branches.
- The two types of law are civil and criminal.
  - Civil cases can result in professional and criminal consequences, fines, and monetary awards to the victim, or drug and alcohol rehabilitation for minor crimes.
  - Criminal cases result in the incarceration of a person.
- As a paramedic, you are particularly susceptible to charges of assault and battery. Assault occurs when you instill the fear of bodily harm in a person. Battery takes place when you unlawfully touch another person without consent.
- Charges of false imprisonment, although extremely rare, can occur if you unjustifiably restrain a patient or if you use excessive force. To protect against this charge, ensure that appropriate documentation and policy exist regarding the specific call.
- Defamation, slander, and libel present risks to you if you make statements, either verbal or written, that injure a person's good name; these same risks apply to statements about entities such as hospitals.
- Lawsuits follow a general process that starts with a complaint or notice of complaint, a response or answer by the defendant, discovery, settlement discussions, and trial process.
- As a paramedic, you are subject to multiple legal jurisdictions, including state law, state regulations, local medical protocol, and departmental policy.
- Medical directors have a supervisory relationship over paramedics, but you are held personally responsible for your actions.
- Your actions function as an extension of a series of medical directions from the medical director, provided on either an online or off-line basis. These directives are binding unless you believe that your actions will cause harm to the patient.
- State legislation enables paramedics to practice in every state. It is your responsibility to understand the statutes of the state in which you practice.
- State jurisdictions issue paramedics either licenses or certificates. The licensure or certification is a privilege—not a right—extended by the governing authority that allows you to practice within the enacting legislation.
- You have a right to due process, a fair procedure that includes appropriate legal notice of the action to be taken against you, and the opportunity to be heard before the licensing or certifying agency.
- State laws define paramedics' scope of practice, which specifies your limits of practice allowed under the Medical Practice Act.
- HIPAA was first enacted in 1996 to protect a person's private health information, but permits disclosure when necessary to better society as a whole, such as when data are used to protect or improve public health.

Prep Kit continued

- EMTALA, another federal law, is designed to prevent hospital emergency departments from turning patients away for any reason, including inability to pay for care.
- Emergency vehicle operations must be performed in a manner that protects the public from further injury. No call can justify driving in a manner that endangers the public.
- The decision to transport a patient to a specific medical facility should be based on the patient's preferences and medical needs.
- Crime scenes present the intersection between EMS and law enforcement. You have an obligation to assist the law enforcement community in preserving evidence and documentation of scenes or actions that may later be introduced on behalf of a criminal prosecution.
- You can be held legally responsible if you fail to report suspected abuse or neglect, domestic violence, gunshot or stab wounds, childbirth outside a medical facility, rape, infectious diseases, or animal bites.
- Immediately report suspected homicides, suicides, prison inmate deaths, and other violent or unexpected deaths to local law enforcement personnel to allow a coroner or medical examiner to examine the body.
- All patients of sound mind have the legal right under the US Constitution to privacy, consent, and refusal. You cannot infringe on these inalienable rights unless you believe that patients are not of sound mind and pose a harm to themselves or others.
- Patient refusals create an enormous potential legal liability for paramedics. Your only protection against a civil lawsuit over a refusal will be the documentation at the time of the incident.
  - A refusal signature without narrative and evidence of a physical assessment is worthless.
- No one, including law enforcement, family members (unless they have power of attorney and you can verify it), businesses, and churches, has the right to refuse treatment for a patient.
- Obtain informed consent from patients before beginning any medical process, including the physical exam.
- Obtain expressed consent—action demonstrating permission to provide care—from patients before initiating treatment.
- Implied consent is a form of consent assumed to be given by unconscious adults or by adults who are too ill or injured to consent verbally to emergency life-saving treatment. In those cases, you assume that the patients would want care because of their condition's severity.
- Determining the decision-making capacity of a patient can be tricky. Tools such as pulse oximetry and blood glucose measurements can provide factual documentation of patient awareness and the ability to make clear decisions regarding medical care. If you reasonably suspect that a patient has an issue that impedes the ability to give either informed consent or informed refusal, then take aggressive steps in the patient's best interest. In any questionable circumstance, thorough documentation and consultation with medical control will provide the best protection against lawsuits.
- Treatment of minors poses challenges that local jurisdictions must address before a call occurs. In general, if the patient is a minor, then the minor has neither the right to consent to care nor the right to refuse it, although exceptions for emancipated minors exist.
- Violent patients may be restrained using physical or chemical means if they are a danger to themselves or others. Always follow local medical and law enforcement protocols when addressing the needs of violent or potentially violent patients.
- Negligence occurs only when the following four processes have occurred:
  - Duty to act. The paramedic must have had a legal duty to the patient.

Prep Kit continued

- Breach of duty. The paramedic did not fulfill that duty.
- Proximate cause. The paramedic's breach of duty caused the plaintiff's injury.
- Injury resulted. An injury occurred as a result of the other processes.

- Negligence can be categorized as acts of commission (malfeasance and misfeasance) or acts of omission (nonfeasance).
- As the highest level of prehospital emergency care provider, you must ensure you do not abandon your patients. Abandonment can occur anytime you turn over patient care inappropriately or to a person with a level of training less than your own.
- Documentation is the only means to prevent the appearance of abandonment.
- Patients have the right to determine their care. You must understand your legal limitations based on any advance directives issued by the patient.
- DNR orders are a specific form of advance directive that generally define the care a patient wants when life-saving procedures are required. A DNR order is *not* a "do not care for the patient" order.
- Patients often make decisions about medical care and treatment issues before an emergency occurs. Be familiar with DNR orders, living wills, health care powers of attorney, surrogate decisions, and organ donation orders.
- Futile resuscitation efforts, which you may encounter, need to be addressed and considered before an emergency event. Weighing various ethical issues prior to their occurrence can help prevent and reduce suffering in patients.
- You may provide care when off duty and, in most jurisdictions, will be protected under the Good Samaritan laws in such circumstances. However, you are protected only if you perform within your training and education and if you do not receive any compensation.
- As a paramedic, you may be protected under specific governmental immunity clauses. These protections may be invalid if you commit negligence or if you are deemed to be personally liable for harm to a patient.
- Two common legal defenses are the statute of limitations (time in which to file a lawsuit) and contributory negligence (when a plaintiff contributes to the negative outcome by committing an act or failing to disclose relevant information to medical practitioners).
- Several federal and state laws affect the relationship between you and your employer. These laws promote a healthier, safer workplace by addressing discrimination, sexual harassment, family leave, and occupational safety regulations.

Vital Vocabulary

abandonment Termination of medical care for the patient without giving the patient sufficient opportunity to find another qualified health care professional to take over medical treatment.

advance directive A written document or oral statement that expresses the wants, needs, and desires of a patient in reference to future medical care; examples include living wills, do not resuscitate orders, and organ donation orders.

assault To create in another person a fear of immediate bodily harm or invasion of bodily security (including loss of freedom).

battery The act of carrying out a physical threat; the use of force against another person, resulting in harmful, offensive, or sexual contact.

borrowed servant doctrine A principle that absolves an institution of liability when one of its members acts beyond the scope of certification or training by following someone else's orders.

Prep Kit continued

civil lawsuit An action instituted by a person or entity against another person or entity.

common law A decision that a judge has made through a court case based on interpretation of statutes and constitutions; it can be overturned either by another court with a higher authority or the issuing court at a later time. Also called case law.

consent Agreement by the patient to accept a medical intervention.

contributory negligence Act(s) committed by a plaintiff that contribute to adverse outcomes.

criminal prosecution An action instituted by the government against a person for violation of criminal law.

damages Compensation for injury awarded by a court.

decision-making capacity The patient's ability to understand and process the information given and the proposed treatment plan.

defamation Intentionally making a false statement, through written or verbal communication, that injures a person's good name or reputation.

defendant In a civil lawsuit, the person against whom a legal action is brought.

do not resuscitate (DNR) order A type of advance directive that describes which life-sustaining procedures should be performed in the event of a sudden deterioration in the patient's medical condition.

due process The right to a fair procedure for a legal action against a person or agency. It has two components: notice and opportunity to be heard.

duty Legal obligation of public and certain other ambulance services to respond to a call for help in their jurisdiction.

emancipated minor A person who is younger than the legal age (generally 18 years) in a given state, but is legally considered an adult because of other circumstances.

Emergency Medical Treatment and Active Labor Act (EMTALA) A federal law enacted in 1986 to combat the practice of patient dumping—that is, hospitals refusing to admit seriously ill patients or women in labor who could not pay, forcing EMS providers to dump the patients at another hospital. Issues are regulated by the Centers for Medicare and Medicaid Services, and the law carries severe monetary penalties—up to and including loss of Medicare funding—for hospitals and physicians that fail to comply.

ethics A set of values in society that differentiates right from wrong.

expressed consent A type of informed consent that occurs when the patient does something, either through words (verbal or written) or by taking some sort of action, that demonstrates permission to provide emergency medical care.

false imprisonment Intentionally or unjustifiably detaining a person. Examples include transporting a patient without consent, or wrongfully using restraints.

Good Samaritan law A statute providing limited immunity from liability to people responding voluntarily and in good faith to the aid of an injured person outside the hospital.

gross negligence Negligence that is willful, wanton, intentional, or reckless; a serious departure from the accepted standards.

health care power of attorney A legal document that allows another person to make health care decisions for the patient, including withdrawal or withholding of care, when the patient is incapacitated.

Health Insurance Portability and Accountability Act (HIPAA) A federal law enacted in 1996 that provides for criminal sanctions and civil penalties for releasing a patient's protected health information in a way not authorized by the patient.

hostile environment Situation in which an employer or an employer's agent either creates an offensive practice related to sex or allows it to continue, making it uncomfortable or impossible for an employee to continue working.

Prep Kit continued

immunity Legal protection from penalties that could normally be incurred under the law.

implied consent Assumption on behalf of a person unable to give consent that the person would have done so.

informed consent A patient's voluntary agreement to be treated after being told about the nature of the disease, the risks and benefits of the proposed treatment, alternative treatments, or the choice of no treatment at all.

in loco parentis Phrase meaning "in the place of the parent"; used to describe situations in which a designated authority figure makes medical treatment and transport decisions for a minor child when a parent or guardian is unavailable.

involuntary consent An oxymoron, because consent is never involuntary; often used to describe a figure of authority dictating medical care be given to someone in custody, incapacitated, or a minor.

legal obligation A duty that is enforceable in a court of law.

liability A finding in civil cases that most of the evidence shows the defendant was responsible for the plaintiff's injuries.

libel Making a false statement in written form that injures a person's good name.

living will A type of advance directive, generally requiring a precondition for withholding resuscitation when the patient is incapacitated.

malfeasance Unauthorized act committed outside the scope of medical practice defined by law.

Medical Practice Act An act that usually defines the minimum qualifications of those who may perform various health services, defines the skills that each type of practitioner is legally permitted to use, and establishes a means of licensure or certification for different categories of health care professionals.

minor A person younger than 18 years of age who does not have the legal authority to refuse or consent to emergency care.

misfeasance An appropriate act performed in an improper manner, such as a medication administered at the wrong dose.

morality Pertaining to conscience, conduct, and character.

negligence Professional action or inaction on the part of the health care practitioner that does not meet the standard of ordinary care expected of similarly trained and prudent health care practitioners, resulting in injury to the patient.

negligence per se Inexcusable violation of a statute, such as practicing paramedicine without a valid license or certification.

nonfeasance Failing to perform a required or expected act.

ordinary negligence Negligence that involves a failure to act, or a simple mistake that causes harm to a patient.

palliative care A type of medical care intended to provide comfort and relief from pain, nausea, and shortness of breath.

patient autonomy The right to direct one's own medical care, and to decide how end-of-life medical care should be provided.

plaintiff In a civil lawsuit, the person who brings a legal action against another person.

protected health information (PHI) Any identifiable health information created, disclosed, used, maintained, stored, or transmitted related to providing a health care service.

proximate cause The specific reason that an injury occurred; one of the items that must be proven for a paramedic to be held liable for negligence.

punitive damages Compensation, usually monetary, awarded to a plaintiff for intentional or reckless acts committed by the defendant.

qualified immunity Protection in which the paramedic is only held liable when the plaintiff can show that a clearly established law, of which the paramedic should have known, has been violated.

Prep Kit continued

quid pro quo Circumstance in which a person in authority attempts to exchange some work-related benefit, such as a raise or promotion, for an inappropriate employee action (eg, sexual favors); literal translation from Latin is "this for that."

res ipsa loquitur Theory of negligence that assumes an injury can only occur when a negligent act occurs.

scope of practice Describes what a state permits a paramedic practicing under a license or certification to do.

slander Making a false oral statement that injures a person's good name.

standard of care Describes what a reasonable paramedic with training would do in the same or a similar situation.

statutes of limitations Laws that limit the period within which a lawsuit may be filed.

surrogate decision maker A person designated by a patient to make health care decisions as the patient would want when the patient becomes incapable of making decisions.

tort A wrongful act that gives rise to a civil lawsuit.

References

1. National Practitioner Data Bank. Statistics for National Practitioner Data Bank medical malpractice payment reports and adverse action reports. https://www.npdb.hrsa.gov/analysistool/. Accessed February 1, 2021.
2. WMA declaration of Geneva. World Medical Association website. https://www.wma.net/policies-post/wma-declaration-of-geneva/. Published October 14, 2017. Accessed February 1, 2021.
3. Code of ethics and EMT oath. National Association of Emergency Medical Technicians website. https://www.naemt.org/about-ems/emt-oath. Accessed February 1, 2021.
4. Smith M. Do you care enough to ICARE? *EMS Mag.* 2008;37(7):26-27. http://www.icarevalues.org/EMS_Mag.pdf. Accessed February 1, 2021.
5. Maggiore WA. Problem of fraudulent EMT certification growing. *J Emerg Med Serv*. 2010;35(8).
6. A matter of integrity. *J Emerg Med Serv*. 2010;35(9). https://www.jems.com/training/matter-integrity/. Accessed February 1, 2021.
7. Due regard. *Black's Law Dictionary.* 2nd ed. http://thelawdictionary.org/due-regard/. Accessed February 1, 2021.
8. English A, Bass L, Boly AD, Shragh F. *State Minor Consent Laws: A Summary*. 3rd ed. Center for Adolescent Health and the Law. FreeLists website. https://www.freelists.org/archives/hilac/02-2014/pdftRo8tw89mb.pdf. Published January 2010. Accessed May 11, 2021.
9. Keeton WP, Dobbs D, Keeton RE, Owen DG. *Prosser and Keeton on Torts*. 5th ed. St. Paul, MN: West Group; 1984.
10. Legal obligation. *Black's Law Dictionary.* 2nd ed. http://thelawdictionary.org/legal-obligation/. Accessed February 1, 2021.
11. Willful misconduct. *Black's Law Dictionary.* 2nd ed. http://thelawdictionary.org/willful-misconduct/. Accessed February 1, 2021.
12. Wanton misconduct. *Black's Law Dictionary.* 2nd ed. http://thelawdictionary.org/wanton-misconduct/. Accessed February 1, 2021.
13. Proximate cause. *Black's Law Dictionary*. 2nd ed. http://thelawdictionary.org/proximate-cause/. Accessed February 1, 2021.
14. Millin MG, Khandker SR, Malki A. Termination of resuscitation of nontraumatic cardiopulmonary arrest: resource document for the National Association of EMS Physicians position statement. *Prehosp Emerg Care.* 2011;15(4):547-554.
15. Emergency volunteer toolkit: volunteer protection acts and Good Samaritan laws fact sheet. Association of State and Territorial Health Officials website. https://www.astho.org/Programs/Preparedness/Public-Health-Emergency-Law/Emergency-Volunteer-Toolkit/Volunteer-Protection-Acts-and-Good-Samaritan-Laws-Fact-Sheet/. Accessed February 1, 2021.
16. Sex-based discrimination. US Equal Employment Opportunity Commission website. https://www.eeoc.gov/laws/types/sex.cfm. Accessed February 1, 2021.
17. What you should know about EEOC and the enforcement protections for LGBT workers. US Equal Employment Opportunity Commission website. https://www.eeoc.gov/eeoc/newsroom/wysk/enforcement_protections_lgbt_workers.cfm. Accessed February 1, 2021.

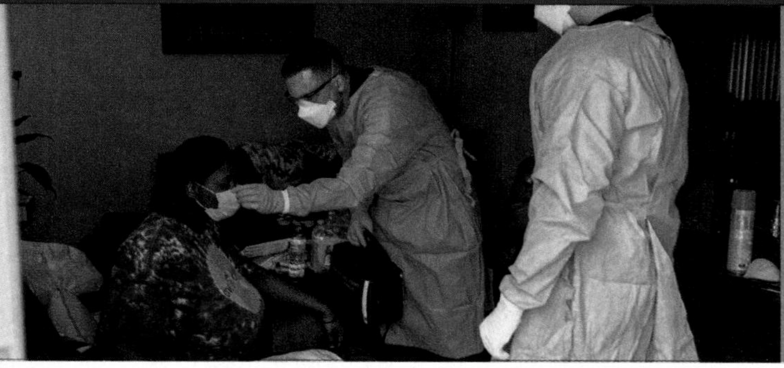

Chapter 5

Communications

NATIONAL EMS EDUCATION STANDARD COMPETENCIES

Preparatory

Integrates comprehensive knowledge of the EMS system, safety/well-being of the paramedic, and medical/legal and ethical issues, which is intended to improve the health of EMS personnel, patients, and the community.

EMS System Communication

Communication needed to

- Call for resources (pp 166–169)
- Transfer care of the patient (pp 183–185)
- Interact within the team structure (pp 166–167)
- EMS communication system (pp 170–171)
- Communication with other health care professionals (p 185)
- Team communication and dynamics (pp 165–167)

Therapeutic Communication

Principles of communicating with patients in a manner that achieves a positive relationship

- Interviewing techniques (pp 186–187)
- Adjusting communication strategies for age, stage of development, patients with special needs, and differing cultures (pp 187–188)
- Verbal defusing strategies (p 189)
- Family presence issues (pp 185–186, 193–194)
- Dealing with difficult patients (pp 189–190)
- Factors that affect communication (p 196)

Medical Terminology

Integrates comprehensive anatomic and medical terminology and abbreviations into written and oral communication with colleagues and other health care professionals.

KNOWLEDGE OBJECTIVES

1. Discuss the importance of effective communication while providing emergency medical care. (pp 164–165)
2. Describe the communication loop and how it is used to communicate effectively. (pp 165–166)
3. List barriers to effective verbal communication. (pp 165–166)
4. Explain the importance of emergency medical dispatch (EMD) and prearrival instructions in a typical emergency medical services (EMS) response. (pp 167–168)
5. Explain the role of the emergency medical dispatcher in a typical EMS response. (pp 167–170)
6. Describe the components, function, and use of the local dispatch communications system. (pp 171–173)
7. List the phases of EMD. (p 169)
8. Explain basic concepts of radio communications. (pp 170–171)
9. List the components of communications systems. (pp 171–173)

10. Differentiate between the following types of communications technologies:
    - Simplex radio systems (p 171)
    - Duplex radio systems (p 171)
    - Multiplex radio systems (p 172)
    - Digital radio systems (p 172)
    - Repeaters (p 172)
    - Digital trunked radio systems (p 173)
    - Cellular technology (p 174)
    - Biotelemetry (p 176)
    - Computer networks (pp 176–177)
11. Define interoperability, including its importance during large-scale events. (p 173)
12. Recognize the protected legal status of patient health information. (pp 175, 179, 186)
13. Describe the functions and responsibilities of the Federal Communications Commission. (p 170)
14. Describe the phases of communication necessary to complete a typical EMS response. (pp 180–181)
15. Describe the format for reporting essential patient assessment information to medical control. (pp 182–183)
16. Describe the importance of effective verbal communication of patient information to the hospital. (p 182)
17. List factors that may enhance verbal communication. (p 165)
18. Identify internal and external factors that affect patient/bystander interviews. (p 200)
19. Discuss the strategies for developing patient rapport. (pp 185–186)
20. Provide examples of open-ended and closed-ended questions. (pp 186–187)
21. Discuss interviewing strategies to obtain useful information from a patient. (pp 187–188)
22. Discuss common errors to avoid when interviewing a patient. (pp 188–189)
23. Identify the nonverbal skills that are used when interviewing a patient. (p 189)
24. Describe the strategies that are used when interviewing a patient who is hostile or potentially violent. (pp 189–190)
25. Summarize developmental considerations of various age groups that influence patient interviewing. (pp 190–191)
26. Discuss the techniques that are used when interviewing patients with special challenges. (pp 192–193)
27. Define cultural competence. (p 193)
28. Discuss interviewing considerations used in cross-cultural communications. (p 194)
29. Provide examples of traditional folk medicine, including why it is important to understand those practices. (pp 194–196)

SKILLS OBJECTIVES

There are no skills objectives for this chapter.

Introduction

This chapter discusses communication, including how to effectively communicate and how to use various communications technologies. The ability to communicate clearly is a core emergency medical services (EMS) skill and one of the most important factors in EMS operations. You must be able to communicate with the dispatch center to receive the information needed to respond to an emergency call. You will also need to communicate with other EMS system members, including your partner, other responders, and hospital personnel. In addition, you must communicate effectively with patients, family

Documentation and Communication

Communicate: To transmit information, thought, or feeling so that it is satisfactorily received or understood

Communication: A process by which information is exchanged between individuals through a common system of symbols, signs, or behavior

Communications: The technology of the transmission of information (as by print or telecommunication)[1]

members, and bystanders, often when they are under considerable stress.

Many factors can influence how effectively you can communicate, including your communication style, knowledge level, ability to listen and comprehend, ability to accurately convey information, and life experience. Communication can also be affected by your tone of voice (especially important on the radio or over a telephone), your body language (important in face-to-face interactions), and your ability to use technology.

Communication Theory

Communication is both an interactive and a circular process or loop **FIGURE 5-1**. It begins with the sender, who formulates and encodes the message to be sent. *Encoding* involves determining the words or ideas to be sent and formatting the information for transmission. The message is then transmitted to the receiver. The receiver receives and decodes the message to discover the information being relayed. Although many methods of transmitting information are available, the following are most commonly used in EMS:

- Verbal
- Nonverbal (body language, facial expressions, etc)
- Written
- Visual (photographs, images, charts, electrocardiogram [ECG] tracings, etc)
- Electronic (voice, data, text, images, and video)

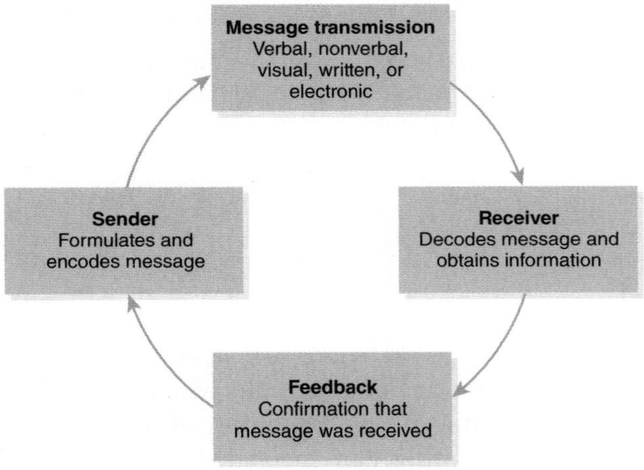

FIGURE 5-1 The communication loop.

The final step in effective communication is feedback, which is the receiver's confirmation that the message was accurately received. Feedback also permits clarification of the message if it was unclear. This step completes the communication loop. A simple example of the communication loop in action might take the following form:

- **Dispatcher:** *Medic 1, Central Dispatch, traffic collision, respond Priority 1 to the intersection of West Main and Third Street.* (Information is encoded and transmitted.)
- **Paramedic:** *Central Dispatch, Medic 1 copies, responding Priority 1 to West Main and Third.* (Information is received, decoded, understood, and confirmed.)

Barriers to Effective Communication

As an EMS provider, you will encounter a wide range of potential barriers to communication in your interactions with patients, family members, and bystanders. These challenges can include language barriers, vision or hearing impairments, impaired cognition or confusion, psychiatric

YOU are the Paramedic

PART 1

An older man is not feeling well. His family becomes concerned and activates the EMS system by calling 9-1-1.

1. As a paramedic in the EMS system, how will you be notified about the incident's location and nature?
2. What will the dispatcher be doing while you are en route to the call?
3. How will you communicate with the other responders and agencies involved in the emergency response?

conditions, substance abuse, preexisting medical conditions, lack of ability to comprehend, stress, and preconceptions.

To minimize these barriers, you must adjust how you communicate. If you are working with a patient who speaks another language and you have only a limited vocabulary in that language, then use a qualified interpreter whenever possible. This practice helps reduce the risk of missing crucial information or using the wrong word, which could cause confusion or be insulting to the patient.

You may also experience communication barriers when interacting with coworkers or other EMS system members, such as the use of different terminology or definitions by other agencies or jurisdictions, interoperability (technology compatibility) issues, and communications system failures. This chapter addresses how to deal with each of these challenges.

Finally, your attitude and demeanor can affect communication. For example, the message you send (either intentionally or unintentionally) when caring for a homeless patient may be different from the message you send to a well-dressed resident of an upscale neighborhood. Treat every patient you encounter professionally and to the best of your ability, regardless of their circumstances.

Response to the Call for Emergency Medical Services

Crew Resource Management

During the 1980s, several catastrophic airline crashes led the airline industry to examine what went wrong. One of the most significant issues identified was a lack of communication between the pilots and other crew members. Copilots and others often recognized the developing problems, but were unwilling to speak up or question the pilot's judgment due to the prevailing cockpit culture, or were ignored when they reported a hazardous situation. This lack of communication led to bad decisions by the pilots in command, which resulted in crashes that cost many lives.

Crew resource management (CRM) is an operational practice developed by the US Air Force and the airline industry that is designed to enhance communication and teamwork and reduce preventable errors. It involves all flight crew members in flight safety, encouraging all flight crew members to pay attention, voice concerns, and participate in the decision-making process. They are expected to question any decisions they think are unsafe or unwise. Flight services use a sterile cockpit concept, which means that all attention is placed on the safety of the crew and surroundings during takeoff and landings. EMS should also use this concept while responding to calls and during patient transport. Any unnecessary external stimuli should be eliminated, and extraneous conversation that does not have a bearing on the call should be avoided. The essence of CRM is teamwork, based on effective communication. It uses all available resources to maximize safety. CRM principles have been adapted by the military and many health care settings, including the air medical transport (helicopter and fixed-wing) industry.

SAFETY

The use of CRM in EMS involves teamwork and effective communication among all members of the response team. It keeps everyone on the same page and reduces the risk of errors resulting from a lack of awareness of real or possible risks to the patient or responders.[2]

In practice, CRM begins with a prebriefing while en route to the call. For example, when responding to a traffic collision with a report of multiple patients, preplanning can involve designating who will be in charge, who will perform triage, and who will begin treatment. After EMS providers arrive on scene, CRM involves frequent check-ins and updates, reassessments of the situation, and fine-tuning of the plan as necessary. Crew members should cross-check each other when a high risk of errors exists; for example, they should double-check medication doses when treating a pediatric patient. Every team member is responsible for maintaining situational awareness and letting others know about a potential problem or risky situation. Likewise, concerns voiced by any team member need to be taken seriously by the rest of the team.

CRM training and practice should be a part of EMS education. In fact, it is now incorporated into the National Registry of Emergency Medical Technicians' Paramedic Psychomotor Competency Portfolio.[3]

Phases of EMS Dispatch

Calls to 9-1-1 for emergency medical assistance are answered in most EMS systems by an **emergency medical dispatch (EMD)** system. This system is specifically designed to meet the unique needs of EMS response and of callers reporting a medical emergency. The term **dispatch** means to send to a specific destination or to send on a task; however, the emergency medical dispatcher does much more than simply order ambulances to emergencies. The dispatcher functions as a vital part of the EMS team. The dispatcher obtains as much information as possible about the emergency, determines which resources are needed, and dispatches the appropriate vehicles and personnel to the scene. In some systems, the EMD process also includes emergency medical care instructions to the 9-1-1 caller. The dispatcher monitors and coordinates communication with responders in the field during all phases of the response, locates and sends additional resources as needed, and maintains written and electronic records of the call.[4]

Emergency dispatch of EMS calls is a key component of the overall public safety system. An EMS response will almost always include an ambulance, but it may also include fire service, rescue, or law enforcement units. As a paramedic, you need to understand how the ambulance and overall dispatch systems in your area operate.

All EMS calls originate when someone—generally a member of the public—recognizes that a potential medical emergency exists and reports it to the local emergency response system. In most parts of the United States, this step is accomplished by calling 9-1-1. This telephone call is automatically routed to a **public safety answering point (PSAP)**. A primary PSAP may either dispatch resources directly or route the call to a secondary PSAP, such as a specialized EMS dispatch center.

Information Gathering

When someone calls for an ambulance, that person is often in distress. This emotional state can interfere with their ability to convey information. The most effective method of gathering information from a caller who is under stress is to use a series of short questions. When a 9-1-1 call comes in, the dispatcher will try to elicit the following information:

- **The exact location of the patient or patients.** This information includes the street name and number, the proper geographic designation (such as whether the street is East Maple or West Maple), and the community's name (because adjacent towns may have streets with the same name). If the call comes from a rural area, the dispatcher will try to establish landmarks (such as the nearest cross street or business establishment, water tower, or antenna).
- **The telephone number of the caller.** This information is essential if the call is disconnected or the dispatcher needs to call back for more information. It is common for responders to be unable to find the address and to need to ask for help from the original caller. Asking for the caller's telephone number also helps discourage nuisance calls, because prank callers are reluctant to supply their phone numbers.
  - Many areas have **enhanced 9-1-1 systems** in which much of this information, such as the phone number and location of the caller, is determined and displayed automatically by the computer dispatch terminal. Not all systems have this capability, however. Even if it is an enhanced system, the cell phone number generated may be generic, not the actual phone number of the caller. Dispatchers will double-check the information provided by the caller.
  - In areas with enhanced wireless (cellular) 9-1-1 systems, dispatchers can see the number of the wireless (mobile) phone from which the call was placed, and in many cases, the latitude and longitude of the caller's location from the global positioning system (GPS) receiver of the phone. This technology can be beneficial for pinpointing the source of wireless calls from remote locations.
- **Why EMS was called.** This information is the caller's perception of the nature of the emergency.
- **Information about the patient's condition.** Obtaining more specific information will help the dispatcher evaluate the urgency of the situation and decide whether the caller needs

to be provided with prearrival instructions by phone. The dispatcher should ask:
  - Is the patient conscious?
  - If not, then is the patient breathing?
  - Is the patient bleeding badly?
- **Details about the location.** The dispatcher will seek to obtain additional information that will help responders access the scene as quickly and safely as possible, such as whether the residence door is locked or whether any pets are present.
- **Information about the situation.** This information enables the dispatcher to estimate the emergency's magnitude and identify which resources are required. For example, if the emergency is a motor vehicle crash, then the dispatcher should ask about:
  - The types of vehicles involved (sedans, trucks, motorcycles, buses, etc).
  - If a commercial truck is involved, does the caller know what type of cargo it is carrying? A truck carrying hazardous materials (hazmat) requires a different approach from one carrying bananas.
  - The number of people injured and an estimate of the extent of injuries.
  - Apparent hazards at the scene, such as heavy traffic, downed power lines, fire, spilled chemicals, and peculiar odors. Information about such hazards enables the dispatcher to contact other agencies that may need to be involved, such as utility workers to manage downed wires or hazmat teams to deal with spilled fuel or chemicals.

Words of Wisdom

During the COVID-19 pandemic, dispatchers also sought out information about infectious diseases that the patient might have. If a possibility of exposure exists, the EMS team may decide to send only one provider on scene who has been fully encapsulated with the proper PPE to evaluate the patient. If additional resources are needed, they can be requested by the provider who has made contact with the patient. This approach lessens the possibility of exposure of the entire team on every call. Dispatchers may also ask the patient to meet EMS providers outside instead of having those responders enter the residence.

Dispatch

As soon as the dispatcher has obtained the address of the emergency, the telephone number of the caller, and the nature of the emergency, the dispatcher will ask the caller to wait on the line. The dispatcher determines which resources need to be dispatched based on the call's nature, location, and available resources. Next, the dispatcher notifies these resources and informs them about the call's nature and its exact location. Dispatch may be performed using a radio, telephone, push-to-talk (PTT) cellular device, pager, or computer terminal. Although this process generally occurs in a dispatch center, technology has allowed dispatchers for services that respond in remote or rural areas to perform this task from home with the use of a laptop and a dedicated phone line.

After the ambulance is dispatched, the dispatcher will return to the caller to obtain the rest of the information described earlier. Further questioning may reveal special circumstances that might affect the response. The dispatcher will relay this information while the responding unit is en route. This process permits the EMS crew to determine whether to respond using the lights and siren (based on local protocols), and to anticipate and prepare for any tasks that may need to be performed at the scene.

Computer-Assisted Dispatch

Most EMS systems utilize **computer-assisted dispatch (CAD)** systems, which make use of linked dispatch center computer consoles and vehicle-mounted mobile data terminals (MDTs). The CAD system enables the dispatcher to view all information about the call, including information received from the caller, times of events, and visual prompts that list key questions to ask the caller. It may also display additional information provided by the enhanced 9-1-1 system, such as maps, the fastest route to the location of the call, prior calls to the same address, and known hazards at the call location (eg, toxic chemicals stored at a business, potentially dangerous pets). The CAD system may make recommendations about which EMS units to dispatch based on location and response times. Using the CAD system, the dispatcher can send all of this information to the responding EMS crew via the MDT, with the crew then being able to see the information displayed on the CAD terminal.

Advice to the Caller

After directing the necessary resources (ambulance, fire, rescue, law enforcement, etc) to the scene and alerting responders to any special circumstances, the dispatcher will return to the telephone and inform the caller what is being done (eg, "An ambulance is on the way and should be there in about 5 minutes"). If the patient has a life-threatening emergency, the dispatcher may be able to provide prearrival medical instructions to the caller through the EMD program. These instructions can include a range of emergency medical care techniques, such as airway maintenance, abdominal thrusts, hands-only CPR, or hemorrhage control. The caller is likely to be agitated, so the dispatcher's instructions must be clear and straightforward.

Ongoing Communications With Responding Units in the Field

The dispatcher must always remain aware of what is occurring in the field and stay in contact with the ambulance and other responders. As mentioned previously, the dispatcher is the responding EMS providers' resource for contacting other agencies, such as fire, rescue, and law enforcement, whose presence may be required at the scene. The dispatcher can also request any specialized resources that may be needed, such as heavy extrication or air medical transport. The dispatcher can coordinate communications between the ambulance and medical control (discussed later in this chapter) or help determine the appropriate destination facility.

The phases of the emergency medical dispatch process and the dispatcher's roles are summarized in **TABLE 5-1**. It is routine practice to use 24-hour

TABLE 5-1 Phases of Emergency Medical Dispatch

Phases of Dispatch/Information Gathered	Dispatcher Action
• Initial receipt of 9-1-1 call	• Answers telephone promptly • Identifies agency
• Information gathering • Address/location of incident • Call-back number • Perceived emergency • Patient's name and condition • For traffic incidents: • Number of vehicles • Types of vehicles • Number of patients • Hazards at scene	• Obtains as much information as possible about the emergency
• Dispatch	• Dispatches ambulances and other resources (fire, law enforcement, etc) as needed • Notifies responding units of special situations • Contacts hazmat teams and other agencies as needed • Monitors communications from the field
• Advice to caller	• Informs caller what is being done • Gives patient care instructions by phone, if required
• Ongoing communications with responding units in the field	• Logs response and arrival times • Coordinates requests for additional resources • Facilitates communications with other agencies or medical facilities • Remains aware of location and status of all units in the field

Data from: Association of Public-Safety Communications Officials. Minimum training standards for public safety telecommunicators. APCO ANS 3.103.2.2015. https://www.apcointl.org/training-and-certification/comm-center-training-programs/training-standards-guidelines/. Accessed July 6, 2021.

(standard military) time in EMS dispatch and documentation (24-hour time is discussed in Chapter 6, *Documentation*).

EMS Communications Systems

During an emergency response, you will use a variety of communications equipment. Some EMS systems use basic two-way radio systems, whereas others use sophisticated, computerized radio systems. The use of cellular technology is common. All of these communications systems and devices rely on radio signals to send and receive information. As an EMT, you need to understand basic radio communications theory and how radio equipment operates.

EMS and public safety communications systems are generally dependable, but anything based on technology can (and at some point will) fail. Having backup communications systems is essential. Such backup systems may include independent radio frequencies and systems, cell phones, satellite telephones, or MDTs. Backup systems are discussed in more detail later in this chapter.

Basic Radio Communications Theory

Radio Waves

Radio waves are a type of electromagnetic radiation that may be encoded to transmit a wide variety of information. The basic radio wave in which a signal is encoded is called a carrier wave.[5,6]

Radio Frequencies

The radio **frequency** is the number of oscillations (or cycles) per second of the carrier wave, typically measured in **hertz (Hz)**. One hertz equals one cycle per second, one megahertz (MHz) equals 1 million cycles per second, and one gigahertz (GHz) equals 1,000 MHz, or 1 billion cycles per second. Thus, a radio wave with a frequency of 156.075 MHz is oscillating 156,075,000 times per second.[5,6]

Frequencies are grouped into bands by the **Federal Communications Commission (FCC)**. The FCC assigns each band for a specific purpose. EMS and public safety communications systems typically operate in the **very high frequency (VHF) band**, from 30 MHz to 300 MHz, and in the **ultra high frequency (UHF) band**, from 300 MHz to 3.0 GHz. The higher frequency bands generally have less interference, but also have a shorter transmission range.[5,6]

FCC Narrow-Band Standards

The number of agencies using radio systems has expanded over the years, and new technologies have been developed alongside this expansion. In turn, the FCC recognized the need to allocate more frequencies for public safety and EMS use. Under previous standards, individual frequency assignments were spaced 25 KHz (0.025 MHz) apart. Since January 1, 2013, however, frequencies in the public safety radio spectrum between 150 and 174 MHz and between 421 and 470 MHz have been reassigned with a spacing of 12.5 KHz, referred to as **narrow-band** technology. In consequence, radios that use the older 25 kHz technology are now obsolete.

Adoption of the narrow-band system effectively doubled the number of frequencies available for public safety and EMS use. It also supports newer, more sophisticated digital radio systems.[7] Narrow-band radio standards are discussed further in the *Interoperability* section of this chapter.

YOU are the Paramedic

PART 2

Your unit arrives at the residence. An older woman meets your crew at the door. She tells you that her husband has cancer and that he is not feeling well. After ensuring that the scene is safe, you enter the residence. You see a frail-looking older man sitting in a recliner in a tidy room with a television playing loudly in the corner. The wife tells you her husband does not hear well.

4. How will you initiate communication with this patient?
5. Is the television noise a consideration in your assessment?

Radio Signals

Radio communications require two types of devices. First, the transmitter takes data or sound, converts it into a radio signal, and transmits it on the designated frequency. Then, the receiver collects the radio signal and translates it back into data or sound. Most radios used in EMS communications contain both a transmitter and a receiver, and are referred to as **transceivers** (two-way radios).[5,6]

A limiting factor affecting all radio signals is range. The range of a transmitter depends on its output power, the frequency being used, its antenna's location and size, and whether an uninterrupted "line of sight" (path) to the receiver exists. The farther the receiver is from the antenna of the transmitter, the weaker the signal becomes. Anything that interrupts the radio signal, such as buildings, mountains, or other large objects, can reduce the radio's effective range.[5,6]

A constant level of static or background **noise** is present on all radio frequencies. Radio receivers are equipped with a filtering system known as **squelch**, which ensures that users do not have to listen to static when a radio signal is not being transmitted. The squelch setting can be adjusted to block out the background noise, but still allow radio signals to be heard.[5,6]

Communications Systems Components

Base Stations

Base station radios are the most powerful radios in the communications system, with a transmitter output power of up to 275 watts. They have a fixed location, such as a dispatch center or hospital. Base stations feature large antennas, which are usually placed on top of buildings or tall masts, giving them a longer range than mobile or portable radios. They are often capable of operating on multiple frequencies and bands. Some hospitals and dispatch centers have access to multiple radio systems.

Mobile Transceivers

Mobile transceivers are mounted in vehicles and aircraft, and their operation relies on the vehicle's power system. They use an antenna that is externally mounted on the vehicle. The transmitter output power can vary from 5 to 50 watts, and the line-of-sight range can extend up to 15 miles (24 km).

Portable Transceivers

Portable transceivers are small, battery-powered units (sometimes called "handhelds" or "walkie-talkies"). The transmitter output power is low, typically between 1 and 5 watts, and small, radio-mounted antennas typically limit the range to 3 to 5 miles (5 to 8 km). Most portable radios operate on one band and have either single- or multiple-channel capabilities. Portable, handheld radios are useful when you must work at a distance from your vehicle but need to stay in communication with the dispatch center, medical control, or other EMS providers **FIGURE 5-2**.

Radio Systems

Simplex is the most basic type of radio system, in which all radio transmissions occur on the same frequency. Simplex radios allow multiple users to communicate with each other using one common frequency. These systems are normally restricted to line of sight. In public safety and EMS communications, simplex radios are usually used only for short-range communications, such as for tactical use at an incident scene.

Duplex radio systems utilize a pair of frequencies. Radio signals are transmitted on one frequency and received on a second frequency. Semi-duplex

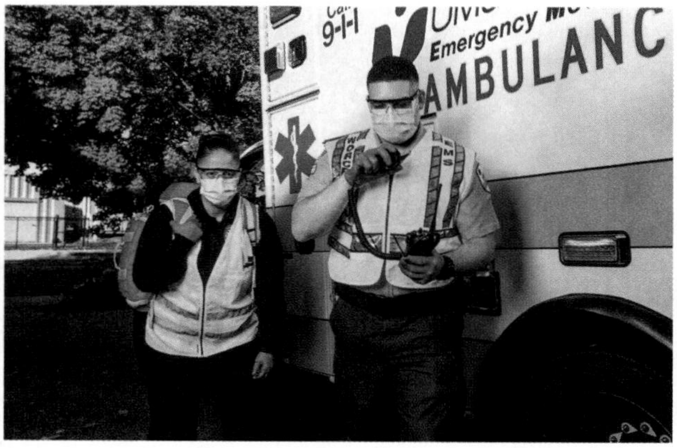

FIGURE 5-2 A portable radio is essential if you need to communicate with the dispatcher, other units on scene or responding to the scene, or medical control when you are away from the ambulance.

systems allow communication in only one direction at a time and the use of repeaters (discussed in the next section). In contrast, full-duplex systems allow continuous communication in both directions simultaneously (similar to a telephone).

Multiplex radio systems use radio signals to carry multiple audio and/or data streams at the same time. Commercial frequency modulation (FM) radio uses a multiplex signal to carry stereo sound. The most common use of multiplex technology in EMS communications systems is to transmit both voice and ECG tracings (biotelemetry). This topic is discussed later in this chapter.

Digital radio systems allow the transmission of digital signals (computer, etc) or analog (voice) signals that have been digitized and compressed by a computer. Digital signals are clearer than analog signals and allow the transmission of a greater volume of data in the same bandwidth. Digital radios can communicate with other digital radios and with analog radios.[6]

Repeaters

Repeaters are used in most semi-duplex radio systems. A **repeater** is a specialized base station transceiver with a powerful transmitter and a large antenna, typically located on a high spot such as a tower, mountaintop, or tall building **FIGURE 5-3**. It receives the radio signal on the transmit (input) frequency and rebroadcasts it at a higher power level on the receive (output) frequency. The use of repeaters allows the radio system to cover a much larger geographic area and to bypass obstructions such as hills, canyons, or buildings. It also enables lower-powered transceivers, such as portable units, to communicate over greater distances. Vehicles may also have repeaters to retransmit signals from a portable unit using the vehicle radio. Most radio systems have multiple repeaters placed in different locations throughout the service area.[6]

Encoded radio signals allow multiple users to share frequencies and repeaters. The most common type of encoding used in public safety and EMS radio systems is the Continuous Tone-Coded Squelch System (CTCSS), also known as the "PL" (short for private line) system. The CTCSS transmits a continuous, inaudible tone along with the regular radio signal. Receivers that have a CTCSS decoder set to that tone will be able to receive the transmission, whereas receivers without it will not. Encoding allows the use of multiple repeaters on the same frequencies. The CTCSS encoding specifies which repeater will "open" to receive and retransmit the signal.

Another encoding system used in some regions is the Dual-Tone Multi-Frequency (DTMF) system. DTMF tones are encoded using a keypad on the transmitter. These tones then "dial in" and activate the designated remote receiver, permitting it to receive the transmission. Systems using UHF-band Med channels frequently make use of this type of encoding.[8]

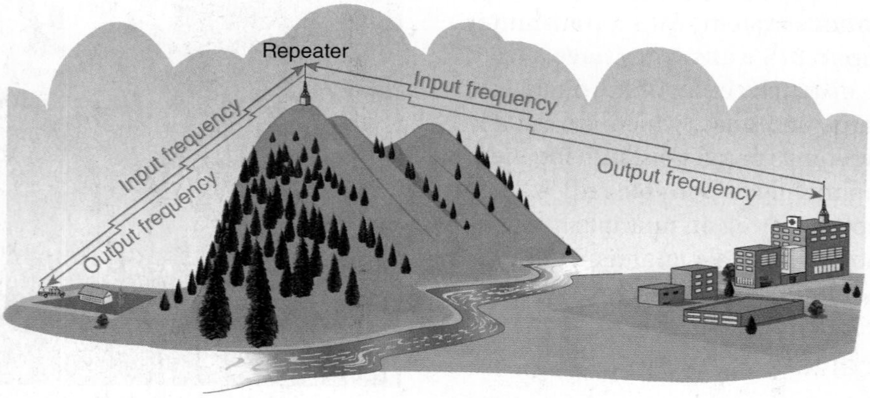

FIGURE 5-3 Repeaters utilize paired radio frequencies to bypass obstacles such as hills, and extend the range of portable transceivers.

Digital Trunked Radio Systems

Trunked radio systems are sophisticated digital communications networks, usually operating in the 800 and 900 MHz UHF bands. They use multiple repeaters and computers to route radio traffic within the system. Trunked radio systems can carry voice or data, such as CAD system information. In a trunked system, the transceiver is set to a channel or mode, rather than to a specific frequency. Each mode is designated for a particular purpose, such as dispatch, tactical operations, or hospital communications. The network frequencies are "pooled" by the computer. When a transceiver in the system needs to transmit on a selected mode, the network assigns that transmission to the next available frequency. When the transmission is completed, the frequency goes back into the pool.[6]

Radio Dead Spots

Radio dead spots are areas where mobile or portable radios cannot communicate with a repeater or with each other. These radio dead spots may be caused by distance, such as in rural areas, or by obstructions such as mountains, buildings, or other tall objects. You must learn the locations of radio dead spots in your service area.

There are many ways to establish or maintain communications in radio dead spots. One method is to use alternative communications systems, such as cell or **landline** (wired) phones. Additional repeaters can be installed in rural areas, or agreements can be established with federal or state agencies to use their radio systems as a backup. Use of another agency's radio frequencies and/or repeaters should occur only with prior permission, or in the event of an emergency during which no other option exists.

In urban settings, radio dead spots often occur in areas with tall buildings, inside large buildings, and in underground locations such as subways or basements. In locations where radio communications are used frequently, small local repeaters can be installed in building lobbies or subway stations. If a local repeater is unavailable, then a temporary relay station may be created by positioning an emergency responder with a portable radio at the top of the subway stairs or near a building exit, so that direct communications can be established with both responders on the inside and the incident commander or a local repeater on the outside.

Interoperability

During your career as a paramedic, you will likely be involved in one or more large-scale events, such as a natural disaster or mass-casualty incident (MCI). Such incidents may overwhelm the locally available resources and require help from outside agencies, referred to as **mutual aid**. Local agencies enter into mutual aid agreements with neighboring or regional jurisdictions to back up each other in the event of a large-scale incident.

Mutual aid requests can range from a call for additional ambulances from nearby communities, to a state- or national-level response, to a large-scale disaster. These events will require members of multiple agencies to work together under high-stress, high-stakes conditions. To achieve cooperation, each agency's communications system must be compatible with those of the other agencies participating in the response. This principle is referred to as **interoperability**.

The current drive for interoperability stems from several large-scale incidents in which mutual aid responders with incompatible radio systems could not communicate with local agencies or with one another. To address this situation, the US Department of Homeland Security developed the SAFECOM communications program. Its national interoperability standards were released in 2006 and are intended to develop "a system of interoperable public safety communications across all: local, tribal, state, and federal 'first responder' communications systems."[9]

An important component of these interoperability standards is the use of nationally standardized frequencies for disaster responses and other communications. These frequencies have been established as a part of the FCC's narrow-band system. Each state has also established its own internal standards for interoperability between local jurisdictions. The state standards are used for MCIs and other local mutual aid responses, whereas national standards are used for interstate and national events. State standards often also include designated statewide frequencies for specific purposes, such as air-to-ground communications.

The Association of Public-Safety Communications Officials has also established digital radio hardware standards, known as the Project 25 (P25) standards. These standards ensure the digital radio equipment supplied by different manufacturers to the public safety communications community are compatible with one another.[10] Radios that are P25 compliant meet the national standards for hardware design, narrow-band compliance, and interoperability. They are capable of communicating with both analog (legacy) radio systems and newer digital radio systems—a characteristic referred to as "backward compatibility."

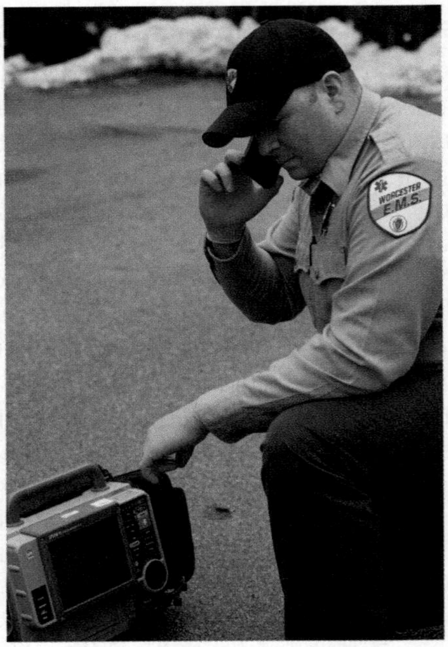

FIGURE 5-4 Cell phones are a common adjunct to the communications infrastructure of many EMS systems.

Words of Wisdom

During interoperable communications, there are a few things to keep in mind. Technology allows different agencies to communicate over one frequency while using their home frequency. However, this broadcast is subject to a delay because of the two-step process—the merger of two frequencies, followed by retransmission. You need to give the system a second or two to merge the two frequencies before you start speaking. Otherwise, the first part of your conversation will not be heard.

Cellular Technology

Cell phones have been used in EMS communications for many years. As the technology related to smartphones and tablet computers has advanced, cellular technology has become a more important component of EMS and public safety communications systems **FIGURE 5-4**. A cell phone is a low-power, portable radio that communicates through a series of interconnected repeaters called cells. These cells are linked by a sophisticated computer system and connected to the telephone network.

Cell phones should be programmed with important and commonly used telephone numbers such as medical control, local hospital EDs, and dispatch centers. Cell phones can directly access hospitals, poison control centers, and other services that may not have direct radio communications capabilities. Telephone calls may be patched into radio networks through dispatch centers or base stations, enabling direct communication between a paramedic using a radio in the field and another party using a telephone, such as a medical control physician. The phone patch is important when requesting orders or permission to perform a procedure. Simply contacting medical control with your cell phone does not allow for recording of the conversation, as would typically occur with standard radio communication. To reduce your liability while using your cell phone, make sure you have the ability to record the conversation.

Smartphones have brought previously unheard-of capabilities to the EMS provider. Smartphones allow users to communicate wirelessly using voice, text, and video, and to take and send photographs or videos to other devices. They frequently have built-in GPS receivers with mapping software and can access a vast range of medical applications (software), including local EMS protocols, pharmaceutical references, and medical reference books. Other types of cellular devices that may be used in EMS and public safety communications systems include PTT devices and tablet computers, which may be used for patient care reports (PCRs) and billing.

As a paramedic, you must be aware of the privacy implications of taking photographs or videos using smartphones or tablets. Although the ability to document the appearance of a wrecked vehicle to show to the receiving trauma surgeon might seem harmless, you still need to protect the patient's right to privacy as outlined in the Health Insurance Portability and Accountability Act (HIPAA). Sharing of these types of images must be done only in a secure fashion, following local EMS guidelines or protocols. Some EMS systems use mobile applications that capture the image and send it directly to secure medical charting software, so that the image is not stored on the individual phone or tablet. It is *always* inappropriate to post images, videos, or other individually identifiable patient information on social media. Paramedics and other health care providers have lost their jobs and faced other significant penalties for doing so.[11]

Another evolving use of cellular technology that is important for EMS is **automatic crash notification (ACN)**, also known as advanced automatic crash notification. ACN systems use specialized onboard computers in motor vehicles to send data to a monitoring station in the event of a crash. That information can include the following items:

- Geographic location of the crash
- Vehicle type
- Severity of the crash
- Principal direction of force at the point of impact
- Whether seat belts were in use
- Whether airbags were deployed

ACN systems may also allow direct two-way voice communication with the vehicle occupants. The data provided by these systems have been shown to accurately predict the severity of potential injuries to the vehicle's occupants and can help EMS providers make transport decisions (eg, whether a patient should be transported to a trauma center, or whether a helicopter should be dispatched to a remote motor vehicle crash scene).[12]

Satellite Communications

Satellite telephones can be valuable in rural and remote areas that lack reliable—or sometimes any—radio and cell phone coverage. They are also an invaluable resource in disaster situations. This technology is expensive, which can limit its use when other alternatives exist.

GPS is a satellite network that utilizes handheld or vehicle-mounted receivers to locate the user's position and provide directions to other locations, such as an emergency scene. GPS data may be used to track the locations of ambulances, other emergency vehicles, and aircraft. **Geographic information system (GIS)** technology utilizes computerized GPS mapping systems to perform the following functions:

- Track and predict ambulance response times
- Determine distance to the closest trauma center or other hospitals from specific locations
- Track frequency of motor vehicle crashes and the severity of injuries from different geographic locations
- Determine the location of emergency helipads
- Provide other information useful in EMS system operations and planning.

GIS data can be used to improve ambulance response and transport times by positioning resources where and when they are most likely to be needed, and to determine the types of resources that are sent to a given location, based on past responses.

Satellite distress beacons and messengers can be a worthwhile safety technology for ambulances and emergency medical personnel who operate in rural or remote locations, or during search and rescue or disaster operations. Most beacons and messengers have built-in GPS receivers that will transmit their location to the satellite. All such beacons can send emergency distress messages, and some are also able to send tracking data and text messages via the satellite system.

Backup Communications Systems

Any system that relies on technology has the potential to fail. The higher the consequences of such a failure, the more critical it is to have an effective backup system. As mentioned previously, all EMS and public safety communications systems need to have some type of backup plan. The most commonly used backup system is an alternative radio system, typically one that relies on basic technology such as VHF or UHF simplex and duplex radios and redundant repeaters, and which can be easily accessed by base, portable, and mobile radios. Almost every EMS system uses landline and cell phone networks as a backup to other communications technologies. Backup systems should also include generators at dispatch centers and hospitals to maintain radio communications in the event of power outages. Backup systems may be shared between several local agencies (EMS, fire, law enforcement, etc).

In disaster situations, the primary methods of communication may be out of service. Towers and repeaters may be damaged, cell sites may be disabled, and computer networks may be down. In these circumstances, having redundant or backup systems is essential. Local and regional disaster plans often use amateur radio groups such as the Amateur Radio Emergency Service (ARES) and the Radio Amateur Civil Emergency Service (RACES) as additional backup systems.[13] You must know how to access and use ARES, RACES, and all other backup communications systems utilized in your service area.

Biotelemetry

Biotelemetry is the measurement and transmission of vital signs and other physiologic data to a **remote terminal**. Biotelemetry, often referred to simply as telemetry, is used to monitor the health of astronauts in space and NASCAR drivers during a race.[14,15] In EMS, it is mostly used to send ECG data to the medical control physician or a hospital ED. ECG telemetry originated in Miami, Florida, during the early 1970s, and had an essential role in establishing the paramedic profession. Telemetry made it possible for physicians to supervise paramedics caring for patients in the field. The technical feasibility of such supervision convinced the medical community and the public to accept the idea of paramedics performing advanced procedures such as defibrillation. As EMS systems have matured and paramedics have become more skilled, the use of ECG telemetry to confirm cardiac rhythms before treatment has become much less common. Most EMS systems now rely on the paramedic to assess the patient's cardiac rhythm and make independent treatment decisions.

In recent years, advances in medicine and communications technology have again made ECG telemetry a valuable EMS tool. The current national standard of care for patients with an acute ST-segment elevation myocardial infarction (STEMI) is percutaneous coronary intervention (PCI). Rapid transport of patients directly to the closest primary PCI hospital/STEMI receiving center and short "door-to-balloon" times have resulted in much better patient outcomes.[16] Many EMS systems now have policies to bypass non-PCI hospitals and transport patients directly to a primary PCI center, if such a facility is readily available.[17] (See Chapter 18, *Cardiovascular Emergencies*, for more information on the care of patients with STEMI.)

YOU are the Paramedic

PART 3

You bend down to the patient's eye level and introduce yourself and your partner. The patient looks at you and smiles. You ask the patient for his name. The patient continues to smile and looks to his wife. The wife states her husband's name is John Smith. She leans over to her husband's left ear and yells, "They wanted to know your name, John!" Mr. Smith nods in acknowledgment. You continue with your assessment and ask, "May we call you John?" Mrs. Smith answers the question for her husband, "Yes, he goes by John."

Recording Time: 2 Minutes	
Appearance	Frail
Level of consciousness	Responds to voice
Airway	Open
Breathing	Adequate
Circulation	Adequate

6. What does it mean to "get on the same level as the patient"? What is the importance of this action?

7. How can you address the problem of a family member answering questions for the patient?

Cell phone networks, broadband networks, and digital radio systems can directly transmit 12-lead ECG tracings and other data from the field to the hospital.[16] New, highly secure systems can send the ECG tracing to anyone with access to an Internet connection. This practice permits the medical control physician to diagnose STEMI before the patient reaches the hospital and make appropriate destination and treatment decisions, such as transporting the patient directly to the cardiac catheterization lab. In some EMS systems, paramedics are responsible for interpreting ECG tracings and making the destination decision.

Another exciting area of advancement in EMS and other areas of health care is **telemedicine**. Telemedicine technology uses specialized computer terminals and networks that permit secure two-way transmission of sound, video, vital signs, ECG tracings, and other diagnostic data. This technology allows for an interactive exchange of information between the paramedic and the medical control physician.[18] Telemedicine technology can facilitate rapid assessment and treatment of a wide range of conditions and patients in the prehospital setting, including patients with stroke and STEMI, as well as pediatric and trauma patients.

New technology is constantly being introduced, and what was once considered new and cutting edge may quickly become the standard. Ambulances are now being outfitted with internal wireless networks that can communicate with onboard devices and multiple outside computer networks using broadband, cellular, wireless (Wi-Fi), and other communications networks.[19] It is crucial to familiarize yourself with the telemetry, telemedicine, and other communications technologies used in your area. EMS systems must keep up with advances in technology that can improve the communication of vital information and the quality of emergency medical care.

Communicating by Radio

The effectiveness of an EMS communications system depends on both the hardware/software in use and the people who use it. Communicating by radio under emergency conditions requires a knowledge of the process of communication and an understanding of the technical operations of radios and other devices described earlier. It also requires an appreciation of the conventions and etiquette of radio communications. Keep your communications simple, brief, and direct.

FCC Regulations

The FCC regulates all radio and television communications in the United States.[20] It issues radio station licenses, allocates frequencies, develops technical standards, and establishes and enforces rules and regulations for radio equipment operation. FCC officials monitor transmissions on various frequencies and conduct spot checks of base stations to ensure they are properly licensed. Fines and other penalties can be imposed on agencies and individual providers for failing to follow the rules and regulations of the FCC.

The FCC requires that frequencies allocated for public safety and EMS communications be used only for that purpose. The transmission of messages unrelated to the provision of EMS and the use of obscene language is forbidden. If it is necessary for a dispatcher to communicate a personal message to you (ie, call your home right away), then the dispatcher should call your personal cell phone, or notify you by radio to contact the base or dispatch center by phone.

Clarity of Transmission

Following are some basic guidelines that can help you improve the clarity of your radio communications:

- Know what you want to say before beginning your transmission.
  - Make notes (or use the PCR).
  - Anticipate what questions you may be asked.
- Before you begin to transmit, make sure the radio is turned on. Check the volume setting and listen to make sure the channel is clear.
  - If another transmission is in progress, wait until both parties have finished transmitting before you start to transmit.
- Keep your mouth close to the microphone, but not too close. About 2 to 3 inches (5 to 7 cm) is usually ideal.
- After the channel is clear, press the PTT key on the microphone or the side of the handheld radio for at least 1 second before you start

speaking, which ensures the beginning of your message is not cut off.

- Start your transmission with the identifier (number or name) of the unit being called, then your own identifier (*"Mercy Hospital, this is Medic 3."*).
  - This practice ensures the unit being called is alerted and will be listening when you give your own identification, thereby avoiding unnecessary delays.
  - If you initially say, *"Medic 3 calling Mercy Hospital,"* the recipients may not pay attention until you have mentioned their identifier and will miss who is calling. They would then respond, *"This is Mercy Hospital. What unit is calling?"*
  - This practice is a general radio convention. Some EMS systems may use a different format. Learn and use the accepted radio format for your area.
- Wait for a response to ensure the other station is listening.
- Speak slowly, clearly, and distinctly, pronouncing each word carefully.
- Do not shout; speaking at too high a volume distorts the signal. Speak in a normal pitch.
- Remain calm and speak in a normal and conversational tone. Keep your voice free of emotion.
- Use **clear text** (plain language), and use only radio codes that are specifically approved by your system and that everyone will understand. When in doubt, avoid using radio codes in your transmissions. Clear text communications and codes are discussed in more detail later.
- If you have a lot of information to convey, then break your transmission into short (30-second) chunks.
  - Pause periodically for questions, etc.
  - Say "break" to signify a pause.
- When speaking a word or name that might be misunderstood, spell it using the International Radiotelephony Phonetic Alphabet **TABLE 5-2** or a similar system.
- When speaking numbers that might be misunderstood, first transmit the number as a whole, then digit by digit. For example, if the patient's respirations are 16 breaths per minute, then you would say, "Respirations are sixteen, that is, one-six."
- Confirm receipt of all replies.
  - Repeat information back to ensure accuracy ("parroting").
- Indicate when your transmission is completed.

Content of Transmissions

The content of your radio communications needs to be accurate and concise **FIGURE 5-5**. Here are

TABLE 5-2 International Radiotelephony Phonetic Alphabet

A Alfa (or Alpha)	**J** Juliett (or Juliet)	**R** Romeo
B Bravo		**S** Sierra
C Charlie	**K** Kilo	**T** Tango
D Delta	**L** Lima	**U** Uniform
E Echo	**M** Mike	**V** Victor
F Foxtrot	**N** November	**W** Whiskey
G Golf	**O** Oscar	**X** X-ray
H Hotel	**P** Papa	**Y** Yankee
I India	**Q** Quebec	**Z** Zulu

Data from: International Civilian Aviation Organization. Alphabet—radiotelephony. https://www.icao.int/pages/alphabetradiotelephony.aspx. Accessed January 30, 2021.

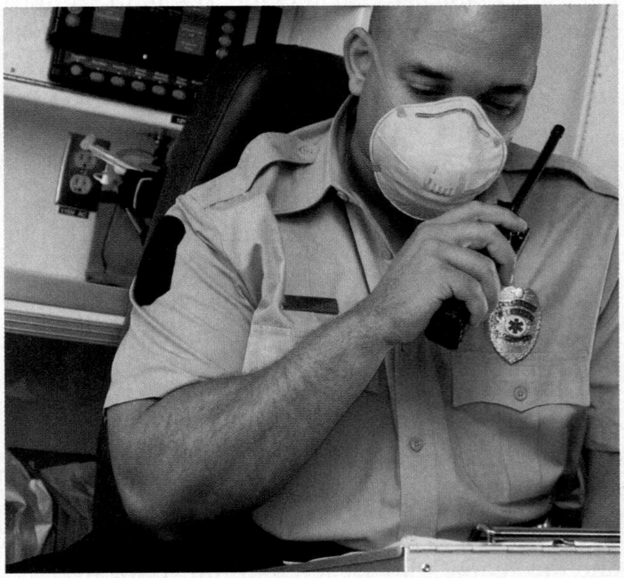

FIGURE 5-5 Give the radio report in an objective, accurate, and professional manner.

some other guidelines related to the content of EMS radio communications:

- Be aware that everything you say over the radio is being said in public. A patient or visitor in the ED hallway, a 12-year-old radio enthusiast playing with a scanner app on a smartphone, or a local reporter may be listening to your transmission. This consideration also applies to communications over cell phones or digital trunked systems. Do not say anything on the radio you do not want others to hear.
- It is essential to protect the patient's privacy at all times. As mentioned previously, this confidentiality is required by HIPAA regulations. Do not use the patient's name on air, and do not unnecessarily transmit personal information about the patient. Sensitive information is usually best given face to face to the receiving facility staff.
- Be impersonal. Use "we," not "I," to refer to yourself, and use proper names and titles ("Paramedic Smith") to refer to others.
- Use proper and correct medical terminology.
- Avoid using words that are difficult to hear. The words "yes" and "no" may be easily missed in transmission; use "affirmative" and "negative" instead.
- Act professionally. Do not try to be a comedian or a critic. The radio is not the place for sarcasm or other poor conduct. Use standard formats agreed on by your EMS agency for transmission of information. When the listeners know what they are listening for, they are less likely to miss parts of the transmission.
- When you receive instructions by radio from dispatch or medical control, "parrot" the order back to make certain you have understood it correctly. If the physician instructs you to "Administer lidocaine 75 milligrams slowly IV," then you would respond, "Copy lidocaine, 75 milligrams slowly IV."
- Question any orders you did not hear clearly or did not understand.
- If you have a long message to transmit, then break the message into 30-second segments, checking at the end of each segment to determine whether it was received and understood. The accepted way to signify a pause is to say "break," which lets the receiver know you are pausing and permits them to ask questions, if necessary.
- When you finish transmitting, notify the receiver that the transmission is finished by saying "over," "end of transmission," or "clear."

Codes

The **ten-code** system and other radio codes were once in everyday use, but have been phased out in most EMS systems. One of the biggest drawbacks of using radio codes is that the same code often has different meanings in different jurisdictions. For example, the code "10-55" can mean an intoxicated driver, a coroner's case (deceased person), or a bomb threat, depending on the jurisdiction.

A code system used by dispatchers in many EMS systems is the **medical priority dispatch system (MPDS)**. The MPDS uses a specific format to indicate the nature of the emergency (EMD protocol) and the priority (determinant level/number). The dispatcher uses this information to decide the priority and response mode when assigning the responding units. These codes may or may not be relayed to the responding units, based on the local system protocol. Although the general format is standardized, the specific priority codes may vary between jurisdictions.

The National Incident Management System (NIMS) discourages the use of all radio codes. The preferred format is clear text, which is discussed next. For radio codes to be of any use, everyone using the radio system must know the meaning of the code words. If codes or other specific terminology are used in your agency, then learn and use them correctly. The NIMS is discussed further in Chapter 48, *Incident Management and Mass-Casualty Incidents.*

Clear Text Communications

There is no room for misunderstandings and miscommunication during the response to an emergency incident. The larger the incident, the more important it is that responders, dispatchers, and incident commanders all use common terminology. For these reasons, the preferred communications format in many systems is clear text (also called plain language). This practice simply means using everyday language and accepted terms to communicate. For example, to request additional resources, you would say: "Dispatch, this is Medic 17. We will require two additional advanced life support ambulances. Request that they approach from the south."

Clear text is the format recommended by the NIMS interoperability standards.[21] Having interoperable radio equipment is of limited value if those using the equipment are essentially speaking different languages.

Communications Formats Used During the Different Phases of the Response

Each agency or region will have its own format for radio and other communications. The details may vary between different regions and agencies, but the basics are common to all systems. This section reviews the basic format for each phase of an EMS response, but you need to familiarize yourself with your area's expected format or formats.

Dispatch Communications

When you are alerted by dispatch about an EMS call, record the location and call information as it is provided. This step is essential to ensure you fully understand the dispatch. After the call is dispatched and you have recorded the details, respond to the dispatcher that you have received the information. A basic sequence is as follows:

- **Dispatch:** *Medic 2, Regional Dispatch. Priority 1: Motor vehicle collision, Second Street at Main Street. Possibly two patients. Time 2104.*
- **Medic 2:** *Regional Dispatch, Medic 2 copies, Priority 1: Motor vehicle collision, Second Street at Main Street, two patients.*

Your response to dispatch confirms that you have received the message and are preparing to respond to the appropriate location, ensures that an effective and accurate transfer of information has occurred, and establishes your dispatch time.

Response to the Scene Communications

After receiving the information and acknowledging the call, you need to determine how to get to the call location. This process may involve using the crew's knowledge of the area, a GPS-based electronic navigation system, or paper maps (which should still be carried in the event of Internet or GPS failure). As you begin to travel toward the scene, you need to notify dispatch. This step lets them know you are on the way and establishes your en-route time. This exchange could proceed as follows:

- **Medic 2:** *Regional Dispatch, Medic 2 en route to Second Street at Main Street.*
- **Dispatch:** *Medic 2, en route at 2105.*

Your next transmission should be your arrival on scene. This step allows you to update dispatch and establishes your arrival time. Your notification can be as follows:

- **Medic 2:** *Medic 2, on scene. Confirm two vehicles, moderate damage; both occupants are still in vehicles. Notify any other responders that access to Second Street is blocked and they need to approach from the north side of the street.*
- **Dispatch:** *Medic 2, arrived. Two vehicles, occupants inside, approach to Second Street is blocked. On-scene time is 2110.*

With this exchange, you have confirmed your unit's arrival, the number of vehicles and patients, and the patients' location. You have also provided critical prearrival instructions for the other responding units. Now is an appropriate time to request additional resources, if any are needed.

You may find that you need additional resources (eg, more ambulances, a heavy rescue unit, a hazmat team, a helicopter) at any point during a response. Any time that you determine that additional resources are needed is an appropriate time to request them. Other times to consider making such a request include while you are en route to the scene (based on either what you know or what you can anticipate about the scene), and after you have had the opportunity to determine the number of patients, the nature of their injuries, and the presence or absence of any physical entrapment.

On-Scene and Tactical Communications

While you are operating at the scene of an emergency medical call, you need to stay in contact with other responders at the scene. This contact is typically accomplished using a portable radio on an assigned tactical channel. Use of a tactical channel or frequency takes on-scene communications off of the main dispatch channel, leaving it open for other radio traffic. In the event of a large-scale incident, a more elaborate communications plan may be implemented, using different frequencies or channels for different purposes (triage, rescue operations, air medical, etc).

SAFETY

The **universal timeout** is a planned pause before the beginning of a procedure that improves safety and communication among all personnel and helps prevent human errors. It allows time for everyone to silently review important aspects of the procedure with minimal distraction, ensure all preparations and equipment are in place, and confirm the correct procedure is being performed on the correct site. As mentioned earlier, this concept is used in aviation (where it is known as a silent, or "sterile," cockpit during takeoff and landing) and is required in hospitals before surgical or other procedures. The timeout has been shown to reduce preventable errors, even under high-stress conditions.[22]

Use of the universal timeout has value in the EMS environment as well. Examples include performing a timeout before crucial decisions or procedures in the field, and on EMS arrival to the receiving facility for trauma and other critical patients so that no key information is lost during transfer of patient care. Many procedures that need to be performed during a 9-1-1 call are emergent and time critical, so a group pause may not always be possible. In these situations, you can perform a quick internal timeout to ensure you are ready. A version of this approach has been taught in EMS training programs for years, with the advice to "Stop, take a deep breath, think, and then act." More time may be available in a situation such as an interfacility transport, making a general timeout more feasible.

Patient Transport Communications

After you have assessed your patient and begun treatment, you need to prepare for transport. This process involves two further phases of communication. The first is advising dispatch of the transport, and the second is contacting medical control and/or the receiving facility.

You must inform dispatch that you are transporting the patient(s). This information lets dispatch know your status and establishes a time-stamp for departing the scene. When contacting dispatch, your radio report may be as follows:

- **Medic 2:** *Medic 2, leaving Second and Main, en route to Municipal Hospital, two patients on board, nonemergency traffic.*
- **Dispatch:** *Medic 2, received. I show you en route to Municipal Hospital, nonemergency traffic with two patients. Time 2134.*

This transmission documents the fact that you have completed operations at the scene and are on your way to the hospital, and that the response is nonemergent.

The next radio transmission to dispatch is to notify them of your arrival at the medical facility. This radio report can be as follows:

- **Medic 2:** *Medic 2, arrived at Municipal Hospital, out of service.*
- **Dispatch:** *Medic 2 received. I have you out at Municipal Hospital and unavailable for service. Time 2145.*

In this exchange, the EMS unit confirms arrival at the hospital and establishes its status. This step is important because it documents that your unit is unavailable for further responses at this time. You may not be available for service while you turn over patient care, give your report, and restock your ambulance.

After you have completed these tasks and are ready for another call, you need to update dispatch that you are back in service. Never assume that dispatch knows your status. For example, the update might take the following form:

- **Medic 2:** *Medic 2, we are clear of Municipal Hospital and available.*
- **Dispatch:** *Medic 2 received. I show you back in service and available. Time 2159.*

Relaying Information to Medical Control

The legal basis for paramedic practice is supervision by a physician. This supervision may take the form of **off-line medical control**, under which you may perform specific procedures or treatments based on protocols or standing orders without physician contact, and **online medical control**, in which the physician gives patient-specific orders and instructions directly to you by radio or telephone.

Many EMS systems rely on a hybrid of these two models—that is, protocols cover routine emergency medical care, but more complex situations require physician contact and guidance.

When you are in the field, your radio communications with the medical control physician need to be clear, concise, and accurate. Using a standard format for communicating patient information over the radio will ensure that essential information is relayed in a consistent manner and that nothing is omitted **FIGURE 5-6**.

The next section discusses essential patient assessment information to be included in your radio report to medical control. In larger EMS systems, paramedics commonly transport patients to hospitals other than the assigned medical control facility. In these cases, always follow your local protocol and notify both facilities of your destination. When the patient is being transported to a different facility, advise medical control of the reason for this destination choice and the receiving facility's name.

Format for Reporting Medical Information

The two keys to a good radio report are being organized and knowing what you want to say before beginning your transmission. You must include all required information. It is a good idea to write your reporting format on a notecard and affix the notecard to your handheld transmitter or in the ambulance near the radio so you can easily refer to it while making your report. The exact format will vary between EMS systems, but the following information needs to be included in all medical radio reports:

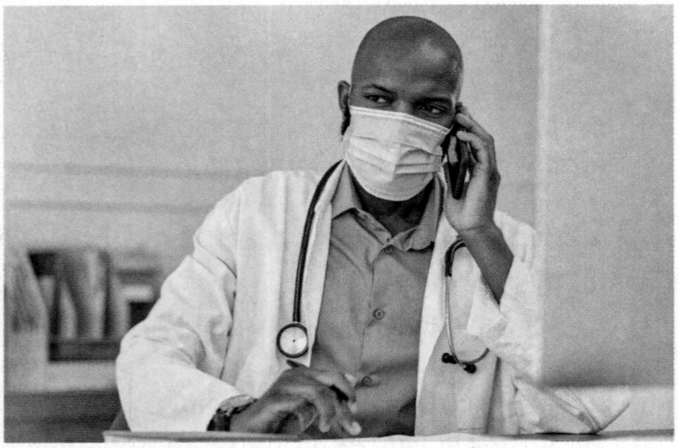

FIGURE 5-6 Use a standard format for communicating patient information to medical control.

- The destination facility and estimated time of arrival (ETA)
- The patient's age and sex
- The patient's chief complaint
- A brief, pertinent history of the present illness or injury
- Medications and important allergies
- Anything the physician needs to know about the patient's past medical history relative to the current situation, including major underlying medical conditions
- The patient's level of consciousness and degree of distress
- The patient's mental status
- The patient's vital signs
- The pertinent physical findings in head-to-toe order
- ECG findings
- Treatment given so far and response to treatment

Here is a clear, concise, and accurate medical control transmission regarding a patient experiencing heart failure:

- **Paramedic:** *Memorial Hospital, this is Medic 8.*
- **Hospital:** *Medic 8 go ahead, this is Dr. McCalla, time is 1643.*
- **Paramedic:** *Memorial Hospital, this is Paramedic Garcia on Medic 8. We are en route to your facility with an ETA of 11 minutes. Onboard we have a 53-year-old male patient reporting severe shortness of breath, which awakened him from sleep and is worse when he is lying down. He has a history of hypertension and takes hydrochlorothiazide. He is alert, denies chest pain, and is in significant respiratory distress. Cardiac monitor shows sinus tachycardia at 130 with a corresponding pulse, respirations of 36 and labored, BP of 190/120, and pulse oximetry is up from 88% to 96% after placing him on low-concentration oxygen. He has crackles and wheezes in both lung fields. There is no JVD. He has 2+ pitting ankle edema. We have established*

a saline lock. Do you have any questions or orders?

The preceding transmission was organized and to the point. The physician hearing it would readily recognize that this is a hypertensive patient with left-side heart failure, and would be able to make a sound decision about treatment orders.

When paramedics call in without using a standard reporting format, the physician may have to gather the information to know what is going on. Consider the following (*not recommended*) dialogue:

- **Paramedic:** *Memorial Hospital, we have a patient with a pulse of 130, a BP of 190/120, and respirations of 36. We're sending you a strip.*
- **Physician:** *Who is this calling?*
- **Paramedic:** *This is Medic 8.*
- **Physician:** *Medic 8, what's the patient's problem?*
- **Paramedic:** *He's short of breath.*
- **Physician:** *How long has this been going on?*
- **Paramedic:** *Just a minute* (pause). *He says it woke him up from sleep about an hour ago.*
- **Physician:** *Does he have any underlying medical conditions?*
- **Paramedic:** *He takes medicine for hypertension.*
- **Physician:** *Is he in any distress?*
- **Paramedic:** *Yes, he's having a hard time breathing.*
- **Physician:** *What do his lungs sound like?*
- **Paramedic:** *He has crackles and wheezes all over.*
- **Physician:** *Where are you taking him?*
- **Paramedic:** *To your hospital.*
- **Physician:** *What is your ETA?*
- **Paramedic:** *11 minutes.*

This exchange was disorganized, incomplete, and inefficient. Such an exchange wastes time, causes frustration, and creates a high risk of important information being missed or not clearly communicated. To avoid ineffective conversations, first gather your information at the scene, organize it clearly in your mind, and only then pick up the microphone. Listening to recorded medical control calls can be an effective way to learn the format preferred by your system.

It is essential to continue your assessment of the patient. After your radio report is completed, reassess the patient and be alert for any changes. All patients have the potential to worsen rapidly. Report any changes in an update to the receiving facility.

In-Person Report and Transfer of Care Communications

The final phase of your patient care communication is your bedside report. During this report, you must relay all pertinent patient information and then transfer (hand off) patient care to the receiving facility's medical and nursing staff. Use the same format as your radio report, but with additional detail as required, and include any updates to the information provided in your radio report.

Keep in mind that the patient, and possibly the family, will also be listening **FIGURE 5-7**. If you need to communicate sensitive information, it may be more appropriate to step outside the patient care room or to speak in a softer tone to the receiving staff. Always respect the patient's right to privacy. See Chapter 4, *Medical, Legal, and Ethical Issues,* for more on patient confidentiality and HIPAA.

The final step is to ensure that you have answered all questions from the medical and nursing staff. Patient handoff also involves written documentation. Your charting needs to reflect the emergency medical care you provided and be consistent with your verbal report. See Chapter 6, *Documentation,* for more information on documentation.

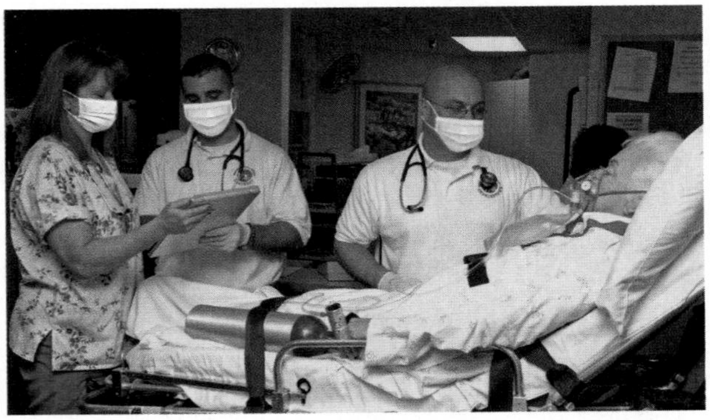

FIGURE 5-7 Be mindful of how you provide your report when the patient or family members are present.

SAFETY

Transfer of patient care, or handoff, is one of the highest-risk aspects of emergency (or any) medical care. Multiple handoffs may occur between various providers, including physicians, nurses, paramedics, EMTs, and other responders. It is easy for errors or omissions to occur during handoffs. Numerous studies of prehospital communications have examined the handoff between EMS and ED or hospital staff.[23] These studies have demonstrated a loss of key clinical information during handoff, such as changes in vital signs (eg, transient hypotension), medications administered, and changes in ventilator settings—all of which may directly result in patient harm. To help prevent such errors, you are strongly encouraged to use a standardized approach when transferring patient care.

One method used by many health systems is the **situation, background, assessment, and recommendation (SBAR)** technique. This technique has become a best practice in health care to relay crucial information accurately. The SBAR technique allows for a brief, yet complete and expected, handoff of information. Everyone involved in the handoff has a shared mental model, improving the safety of the transition of care. The elements of the SBAR technique are as follows[24]:

- **Situation.** Briefly describe the current situation. Give a clear, concise overview of the pertinent issues.
- **Background.** Briefly state the pertinent history. What got us to this point?
- **Assessment.** Summarize facts and give your best assessment. What is going on? Use your best judgment.
- **Recommendation.** Which actions are you asking for? What do you want to happen next?

Medical Terminology

Using medical terminology correctly is essential for effective EMS communication, and it improves the accuracy of your communication. Familiarize yourself with the accepted or approved medical terminology and abbreviations used in your EMS system. Medical terminology may seem to be a foreign language, and in fact, it is. Most medical terminology comes from Greek and Latin. A review of Chapter 7, *Medical Terminology,* can help you become proficient in using medical terminology.

YOU are the Paramedic

PART 4

Your partner asks Mrs. Smith to please take her to John's medications so she can make note of them. Mrs. Smith willingly complies. You are still on the same level as John and you slowly ask in a slightly louder voice, "Can you understand me, John?" After a pause, John answers, "Yes."

Recording Time: 5 Minutes	
Respirations	14 breaths/min
Pulse	76 beats/min, strong and regular
Skin	Pale, cool, dry
Blood pressure	110/66 mm Hg
Oxygen saturation (Spo_2)	93% room air
Pupils	Pupils Equal, Round, and Reactive to Light and Accommodation (PERRLA)

8. Give some examples of effective communication techniques for people with hearing impairment.

9. How can your body language affect your assessment of this patient?

Words of Wisdom

As a paramedic, you can be your own worst enemy when communicating with others on the health care team. Paramedics sometimes use big words to try to impress the person listening to or reading their reports. Some medical terminology can be misunderstood, especially over a radio or telephone. Words that contain the prefixes hyper-, hypo-, inter-, or intra- tend to sound the same when a person is excited or in a hurry. If they are misunderstood, orders for medications or procedures can be incorrect. In some cases, the orders may not be received at all. To avoid errors, remember to keep your communication simple and to the point. Moreover, make sure you use proper terminology, grammar, and spelling.

Therapeutic Communication

As a paramedic, your job will involve daily interactions with people, often when they are at their worst or most vulnerable. At least one-half of the calls you will run as a paramedic will take you into people's homes, day and night, and in the most private moments of their lives. Try to see every invitation into another's home as a personal honor in a time and place where few would be welcome **FIGURE 5-8**.

You will often work in noisy, chaotic, bizarre, and sometimes dangerous environments. Under these circumstances, communicating with patients (and their family members) can be particularly challenging. In these types of situations, other responders will look to you for leadership. If the scene is noisy, then do not shout. When you shout, so does everyone else. When people are shouting, they tend to get excited. If you remain calm and in control, then so will others.

If you answer a call in a dark, noisy place such as a bar, ask the bartender to turn off the music, turn up the lights, and keep an eye on the other patrons. If you must use a noisy compressor or run a diesel engine on the scene, then shut it off as soon as you can. Talk close to the patient's ears in a calm voice. This technique lets the patient know that you have your emotions under control, and it will help the patient stay calm as well.

Therapeutic communication involves using specific strategies to encourage the patient to express ideas and feelings. It is also a way to convey your respect, acceptance, and genuine concern for someone you have never met before. If you want people to tell you about their problems, then you need first to convince them you want to hear what they have to say. Give patients your undivided attention, listen and pay attention to what they say, and always carry a notepad and write things down. It is inefficient and erodes patient confidence to repeat questions because you did not record the answer the first time you asked.

An excellent way to demonstrate that you are genuinely listening is a technique called active listening. Active listening involves repeating back the key parts of a patient's responses to questions. Repeating this information back helps to assure the patient that you are indeed listening and confirms receipt of the information the patient is sharing.

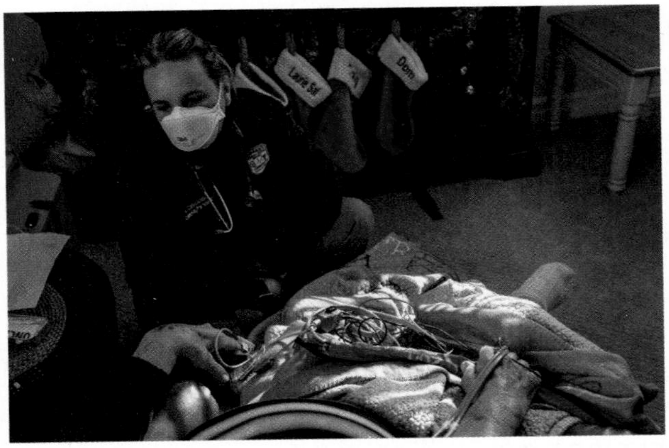

FIGURE 5-8 Think of it as an honor to be asked into a patient's home. Always be respectful and kind.

Developing Rapport

An essential first step in every patient encounter is to develop a good rapport. To treat a patient effectively, you need to obtain accurate information about the patient's condition and medical history. This process is much easier if the patient is calm and trusts you. Start by trying to put the patient in crisis at ease.

Information gathering is a learned skill. Even under the best circumstances, obtaining the necessary information can be a challenging task. Some patients may resist giving details about themselves. Others may have trouble focusing on you because of the chaos of the emergency scene, or they may be distracted by their physical or emotional conditions, or they may feel threatened by you or others at the scene.

For a patient who is reluctant to share personal information, start by explaining why you need their name and date of birth. Reassure the patient that all the information is confidential and will be protected as mandated by federal law. Moving the patient to the ambulance can help create a calmer atmosphere for the patient and make talking and listening easier. Ask personal questions quietly and in private whenever possible. Even if you have earned a patient's trust, many people just do not want to talk about certain things in front of others.

If the patient feels threatened and is reluctant to communicate, cautiously approach the patient and use open posturing (eg, stand with your palms facing out). Smile and be calm. Reassure the patient, and if possible, move and talk a little more slowly than usual. All of these actions can promote a less threatening environment.

Street Smarts

Patients will notice how you treat or are treated by other EMS personnel at the scene. If you are treated with respect and treat others with respect, then the patient will have more confidence in you.

Introductions

The first step in promoting open communication is the introduction. As soon as is reasonably possible, introduce yourself. A simple greeting will usually suffice; for example: "Good afternoon, sir. My name is Erica. I am a paramedic with the fire department. What is your name?"

Establishing eye contact can reassure the patient and help you begin your neurologic exam. Lack of a response may indicate altered mental status. A far-off stare may suggest substance abuse or a psychiatric condition. The eyes may also signal that someone is becoming hostile or potentially violent.

If no threat is evident, then get on the same level as the patient. Sit on a chair or squat next to the patient. This technique promotes trust and helps alleviate anxiety. Getting on the same level is especially helpful when dealing with children. Position yourself where the patient can easily see you, and so that a patient with hearing impairment may better observe your lips and facial expressions. Be aware of your body language, which can either put the patient at ease or make the patient uncomfortable. Use open-handed gestures, do not cross your arms, and do not react to the patient's responses with skepticism. Body language is discussed in more detail later in this chapter.

Use the patient's name in all interactions. A good rule of thumb is if the patient is your age or younger, then call the patient by their first name. If the patient is older than you, then address them as "sir," "ma'am," "mister," "missus," or "miss." Speak slowly and calmly, and always be honest, because a falsehood can permanently damage the patient's trust in you.

Respect and Protect People's Modesty

Modesty matters, no matter how acute the medical condition or injury may be. It is especially important to older adults, adolescents, and young children. If the patient is not personally sensitive to modesty, then the patient's family members most certainly will be **FIGURE 5-9**.

Conducting the Interview

Two types of questions are used in effective interviewing: open-ended and closed-ended. An **open-ended question** is one that does not allow for a simple yes or no answer. Always start with open-ended questions when interviewing patients. This technique allows the patient to freely give you information, and enables you to begin assessing the patient's mentation. Examples of open-ended questions are "How are you feeling right now?" and "Can you tell me what happened?" Ask one question at

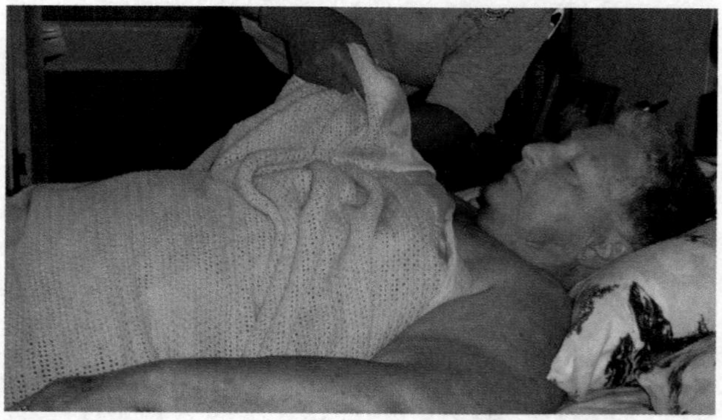

FIGURE 5-9 Show your patient the same respect you would want others to show your grandparents, parents, or siblings. Protect the patient's modesty with a blanket or towel.

Courtesy of Rhonda Hunt.

a time and do not rush patients; let them answer at their own pace. Many patients will answer all of your questions by describing what has happened over the past few days. You should be ready to document this response so that you do not have to ask questions that have already been answered.

A **closed-ended question**, also known as a direct question, is meant to elicit a specific answer. Examples of closed-ended questions are "What year were you born?" and "Does your arm hurt here?" (while you palpate the injured area). Closed-ended questions are very helpful for patients experiencing shortness of breath. By being specific with your questions and expecting yes or no responses, you can get the information you need without worsening the patient's shortness of breath.

It is a good idea to develop a standard set of medical history questions that you ask almost all patients. Use simple language that people without medical training can understand, but avoid talking down to them.

Strategies to Elicit Useful Responses to Questions

When people are in crisis, they may experience a breakdown in their ability to communicate. It can be almost impossible to think and organize your thoughts when you are terrified or in pain. In such a situation, asking simple open- and closed-ended questions may not yield the information you need to get a clear picture of what is going on. You can use various interviewing tools to get the answers you need from these patients.

Reflection

Reflection is the repetition of a word or phrase that a patient has used in previous statements to encourage more detail. For example, the patient may have said, "I could not catch my breath."

- **Paramedic:** *You say you could not catch your breath, ma'am?*
- **Ms. Williams:** *Well, my chest felt tight, and I could not breathe fully.*
- **Paramedic:** *What were you doing when this episode occurred?*
- **Ms. Williams:** *I was in my chair, and it started all of a sudden.*

This technique has given you vital information. Now you are aware that the onset was sudden and did not result from exertion, which is more information than was originally communicated by the patient.

Empathy

Empathy can be described as putting yourself in the patient's position and attempting to understand their feelings and perspective.

- **Paramedic:** *Why did you call us tonight, Mr. Smith?*
- **Mr. Smith:** *I feel so sad and depressed. I cannot seem to function.*
- **Paramedic:** *What do you think is making you feel this way, sir?*
- **Mr. Smith:** *I have not felt normal since my wife died of cancer last week. I just do not have the spirit to continue.*
- **Paramedic:** *I am sorry to hear about your wife, Mr. Smith. I understand how difficult this time must be. I am here to help you.*

This patient may or may not have other issues affecting his health, but he requires help.

Confrontation

Confrontation is the technique of making the patient aware that something is not consistent with the patient's story. Always consider whether using this technique could provoke the patient. The key is to remain professional and nonjudgmental. Consider a patient who has been involved in a traffic incident who is in your ambulance:

- **Paramedic:** *What caused you to lose control of your vehicle?*
- **Mr. Jones:** *I was just driving along when I skidded on something.*
- **Paramedic:** *Have you been drinking alcohol tonight?*
- **Mr. Jones:** *No, nothing tonight.*
- **Paramedic:** *Anything you tell me is confidential, and I detect the smell of alcohol on your breath. There were also some empty bottles in your vehicle. It is important you tell me the truth so I can make sure that we and the hospital staff can take proper care of you.*
- **Mr. Jones:** *Yes, I had four beers tonight.*

Interpretation

If you are not sure what a patient is trying to tell you, it can sometimes help to restate what you think the patient said. Then invite the patient to correct you. Interpretation can also be used when a patient refuses to give information that you need to determine a treatment plan.

With this method, you begin by diplomatically telling the patient what you think you heard and believe is going on, and then asking if you are right. For example, you are with a patient who is 16 years old. Her parents have called you because she was "acting depressed and we think she is on drugs." You remove her to the ambulance for transport, and she says, "I don't know how I got in this mess."

- **Paramedic:** *"What mess?"*
- **Patient:** *"I can't say. I don't want to hurt my parents."*
- **Paramedic:** *"Why do you think you are hurting your parents?"*
- **Patient:** *"They never liked my boyfriend, and now I'm in trouble."*
- **Paramedic:** *"Did your boyfriend hurt you?"*
- **Patient:** *"No, but I can't tell my parents what is wrong."*
- **Paramedic:** *"This may be totally wrong, but I must ask this question so I can inform the physician for your well-being. Do you think you are pregnant?"*
- **Patient:** *(starting to cry) "I don't know, but I think I may be."*

The skill of interpretation requires you to use your best intuition and diplomatic skills. One of the best phrases to begin with is, "So, if I understand correctly, what you are saying is . . ."

Facilitation

If patients hesitate to answer questions thoroughly, then encourage them to provide more information. One useful expression is simply "Please tell me more about that." Others include "Tell me what concerns you the most" and "What more do we need to know about you to be most helpful?" Allow the patient to speak without interruption, and nod as information is shared to acknowledge that you are following what is said.

Silence

If you sense that patients are trying to put something into words but are having trouble expressing themselves, then remember this famous advice: "Never miss a good opportunity to shut up." Be patient. Do not say anything at all for a few seconds. Let the patient talk.

Clarification

If you do not understand what patients have told you, ask them to explain what they mean. This method communicates that you are listening and taking their comments seriously. It may also help you understand what they are trying to tell you.

Redirection

Sometimes patients will mention something in passing or will avoid answering a specific question. You can politely redirect their attention to that question (several times, if necessary) until you get them to answer it.

Simplification and Summarization

Some patients have a difficult time speaking plainly, no matter how hard they try. It can be challenging to communicate with people who have psychiatric conditions, who fabricate their diseases, or who are afraid or upset. If patients give you a confusing or disorganized response, try putting their comments into simpler terms and see if they agree with your summary. This method can help them focus their thoughts and assist you as an interviewer.

Common Interviewing Errors

In addition to good interviewing techniques, the following are some common errors that should be avoided:

- **Never provide false assurance or make unlikely claims.** Your job is to be neutral and objective. Assuring someone that they will be fine seems like a caring and straightforward statement, but never make promises you cannot keep.
- **Do not offer a diagnosis or medical advice that is beyond your scope of practice.** It is appropriate to give your medical opinion and offer advice based on your individual scope of practice and your best judgment, such as the following: "I do not know if the pain in your chest is from your heart or from indigestion, but I am concerned that it may be your heart. I think we should take you to the hospital so that you can be fully evaluated."

- **Do not ask leading questions.** You may not get a reliable answer from a question such as "You have not been having any blurry vision, have you?"
- **Avoid interrupting the patient or talking too much.** You need to hear what the patient has to say.

Nonverbal Skills

As an EMS provider, you will also need to master some nonverbal communication skills. Always keep in mind the adage, "You only get one chance to make a first impression." People often form opinions of others at the first observation. If you look sloppy and unkempt, then the patient may assume that your knowledge and skills are also inferior. In contrast, a professional appearance and demeanor is likely to instill confidence in patients.

Be patient and calm, because acting impatient will make the patient feel uncomfortable and stressed. It is understood that most emergencies require quick action; however, you can still be efficient and fast while displaying an air of patience and calm.

Avoid a closed posture (eg, crossing your arms), because this type of body language sends negative signals. Be aware of your facial expressions and gestures. Avoid physical gestures that may convey disrespect, such as smirking at the patient's answers or rolling your eyes at your partner. Making the patient feel disrespected or uncomfortable could limit your ability to gain information. Maintain constant, nonjudgmental eye contact. Keep your tone of voice neutral, and encourage answers; do not demand them.

Some people do not like to be touched, whereas other people feel it is a valuable demonstration that someone cares about them. Try gently touching the patient on a neutral part of the body, such as a shoulder or arm. This technique can reassure the patient and reduce anxiety **FIGURE 5-10**. If the patient pulls away from you, it is likely that touch may not be a helpful strategy in this instance. If the patient reacts positively by leaning toward you or seeming to relax, then a therapeutic touch will work.

Special Interview Situations

Certain situations in your paramedic practice may require special communication techniques. Some of these situations include uncommunicative patients, hostile or violent patients, older patients, young children, and patients with special challenges. Avoid stereotyping any of these groups of patients, as doing so will hinder effective communication.

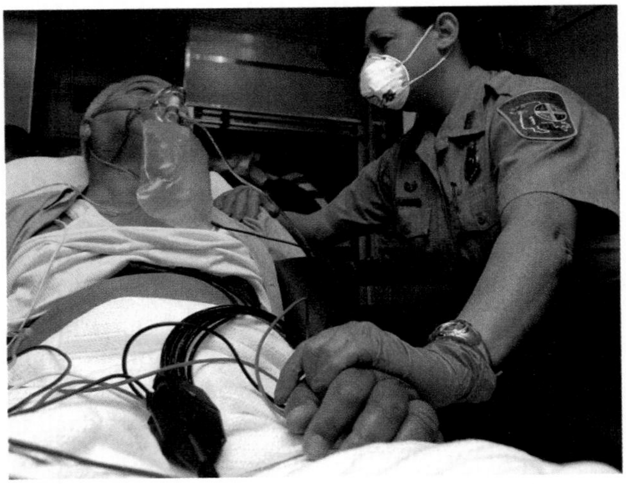

FIGURE 5-10 A gentle touch on the hand, arm, or shoulder can comfort someone who is sick or hurt and scared.

SAFETY

Patients who have been involved in a physically or psychologically traumatic event are affected by the actions and perceived attitude of those caring for them, including EMS personnel. Studies have demonstrated that showing empathy; explaining what is going on, what you need to do, and why you need to do it (eg, start an intravenous [IV] line); involving patients in their care; and giving patients choices when possible are actions that can reduce the potential severity of posttraumatic stress experienced by these patients. Do not underestimate the positive effect you can have by being emotionally supportive and caring for your patients.[25]

People Who Are Hostile or Violent

Emergency situations can be emotional for the people involved, particularly patients and their loved ones. This heightened emotion may cause some people to become hostile, even toward providers trying to help them, like you. Pay attention and always act in a manner to ensure your safety and the safety of others.

It is vital to acknowledge the hostile person's concerns and to empathize with that individual. Remain calm and try to understand the person's concerns. Use interpretation, clarification, and summarization to help the person feel heard and understood. Consider the possibility that you may be unable to defuse a situation involving a hostile person, in which case you may have to defer to law enforcement personnel.

During your career as a paramedic, you are guaranteed to receive some insults from people in crisis, probably on a near-daily basis. Such a reaction is especially predictable when you are dealing with people who are chemically impaired. Discipline yourself to never respond in kind. Nothing escalates a situation faster than trading insults with people, especially when witnesses are present. Not only does this type of behavior make no sense, but it is also unprofessional and can be dangerous. In this day of omnipresent smartphone cameras and social media, you do not want to lose your temper and have it show up minutes later on the Internet.

Hostile or angry patients may present a threat to you and others. Some may be under the influence of drugs or alcohol, or may have behavioral or mental health issues. These factors can make the patient's behavior unpredictable. Always approach a hostile or angry patient with caution and maintain eye contact. Also, avoid interviewing this person by yourself. It is a good idea for your partner to be present, but have them stay a little farther back to prevent the patient from feeling crowded. Have additional backup units, either law enforcement personnel or other EMS responders, close by when dealing with a potentially violent individual. If the patient becomes increasingly agitated or violent and backup is not available, consider leaving the scene to ensure your safety (follow local protocol).

The following are some additional tips for dealing with potentially violent patients:

- As you enter the scene, identify escape routes. Do not permit the patient to get between you and the only way out of the room.
- Approach the patient from the front, with your hands visible and palms open.
- Begin by introducing yourself, explaining your role, and asking for the patient's name.
- If safe to do so, get on the same level as the patient.
- Ask permission to ask questions and touch the patient.
- Always be honest.
- Be wary for signs of impending attack, such as clenched fists, hostile language, tensed neck and face muscles, and threatening gestures.

Street Smarts

Make it part of your routine to look for aggressive body language that signals increased anger and a possible attack. These signs include clenched fists, intense staring directed at you, and breathing heavily through clenched teeth.

Sexually Aggressive Patients

Occasionally, you will encounter a patient who is sexually aggressive toward you or other responders. This situation can occur with both male and female patients and male and female responders. Begin by making sure you have someone else present at all times when you are with the patient. Communicate professionally and politely. Make sure your words are not sexually ambiguous. Most of all, maintain professionalism at all times. Follow your agency's policies, document your encounter meticulously, and get witness names and signatures on the patient notes or run report. This topic is covered in further detail in Chapter 11, *Patient Assessment*.

Special Considerations of Age

Do not presume that older people are more challenging to communicate with than young people just because of their age. When sick, their illnesses do tend to be more complex than those of younger people. They may have more than one disease process, and they may be taking several kinds of medications. Members of the older adult population have a wide range of individual differences in hearing, eyesight, mentation, and mobility, to which you may need to adapt. At the same time, recognize that each patient is an individual, and that you need to base your assessment and treatment on the patient's individual needs, rather than a blanket set of assumptions. When communicating with an older adult patient, ask only one question at a time.

Remember that these patients may have depressed cognitive ability, and it may take a few moments for the patient to formulate an answer to your questions. If you ask rapid-fire questions to members of this patient group, it may lead to confusion and possibly aggravation on the part of the patient.

Children can pose communication challenges even to the best paramedics. They tend to protest pain vigorously, they may be afraid of strangers, they may panic when separated from their parents or caregivers, and their bodies may seem unfamiliar to you. Many paramedics are not as experienced or as comfortable with taking children's vital signs, starting IV lines, or intubating children as they are with adults. This hesitance is common, but with a little practice, you can become comfortable with these skills.

The most crucial aspects of your initial contact with children are friendly eye contact, a reassuring smile, and calm-voiced explanations geared to match the child's age and level of understanding. Minimize your movements, lower your voice, and touch as gently as you can. Start by talking with the patient's parent or caregiver. This step will show the child that the parent or caregiver trusts you, which can improve the child's trust in you as well.

Try keeping your eye level at or below the child's level. You might try sitting on the floor and placing the child on the cot or on a parent or caregiver's lap **FIGURE 5-11**. When you examine a toddler (age 1 to 3 years) or young child, follow the reverse order of your normal exam by starting at the feet and moving toward the head, as this process is often less intimidating for the child. Whenever possible, involve a parent or caregiver in the hands-on care of a conscious young child. This technique is more critical with infants and toddlers and less helpful with older children.

When parents or caregivers are unavailable or in other stressful situations, toys may be useful for bridging the gap between paramedics and some children **FIGURE 5-12**. Many EMS programs stock their ambulances with teddy bears for toddlers. Local public service groups or clubs often donate stuffed toys to hospitals and EMS agencies.

Generally, it is a good idea to treat adolescents as adults. You may gain more cooperation by offering adolescents options and honoring their choices, but never offer an option you know you cannot honor. Adolescents (beginning at around age 13 years) may not want their parents or caregivers present during questioning or the physical exam.

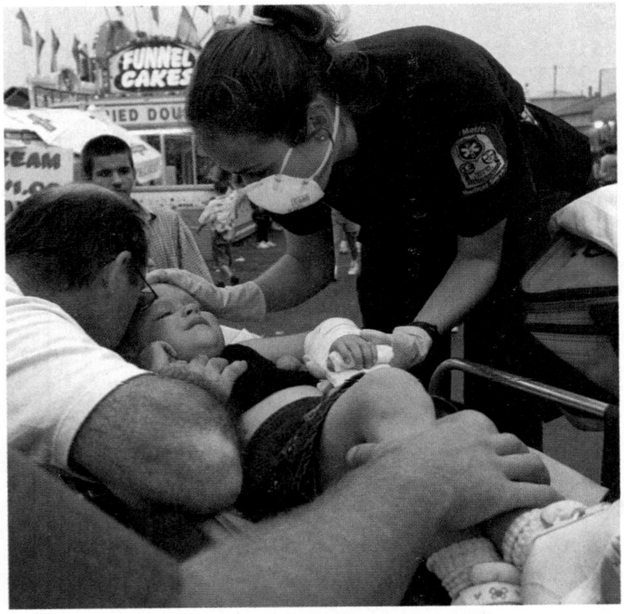

FIGURE 5-11 When you examine a young child, involve the parents or caregivers. Have a parent hold the child on their lap, or ask the parent to keep the child occupied while you work.

Photo illustration by Craig Jackson inthedarkphotography.com.

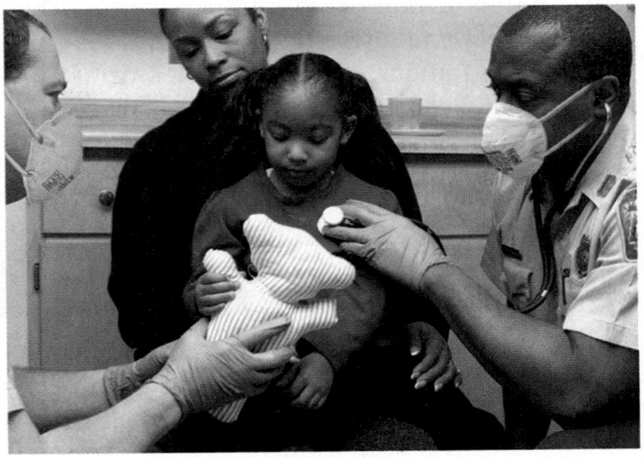

FIGURE 5-12 A stuffed animal or toy can put a young child at ease.

Make special efforts to protect the modesty of patients older than age 2 years, and of adolescents in particular. Patients in this age group are becoming more aware of their bodies and may be especially embarrassed during a physical exam. Avoid disrobing the patient unless necessary.

Street Smarts

A parent who presents as overly vigilant or controlling regarding their child's care may simply be stressed by the circumstances. It is expected for parents to want to be involved in their children's care. If, however, the parent insists on monitoring the conversation even when doing so is clearly not in the adolescent patient's best interest, and especially if the parent shows physical signs of aggression, you should document and communicate the parent's behavior to the appropriate person.

People With Special Challenges

Do not overlook the needs of people with difficulties with speech, hearing, sight, and/or other types of communication disorders. When you encounter a patient who has trouble communicating, remember that family members or primary caregivers who know these patients well can facilitate your efforts. For example, many caregivers enroll in sign language and lip-reading classes to facilitate communication with these patients. They can also help you alleviate the patient's fear and anxiety. If a patient wears eyeglasses or a hearing aid, then ensure those items are available and functional.

Many caregivers find that therapeutic touch and eye contact are helpful bridging mechanisms when caring for patients with special challenges. For example, a light touch on a patient's shoulder can convey kindness, whereas a firm grasp can express reassurance. Some patients respond well to brief, one-armed hugging.

A particularly challenging group of patients are those with autism. Autism can vary in severity and falls under a broader category known as **pervasive developmental disorders (PDDs)**. PDDs cause delays in many areas of childhood development, such as developing skills to communicate and interact socially, and the effects can be lifelong.

Children with autism may have difficulty developing language skills and understanding what others say to them. They also may have difficulty communicating nonverbally, such as through hand gestures, eye contact, and facial expressions. Not every person with autism will have difficulty with language. Some people with autism may be unable to speak, whereas others may have rich vocabularies and be able to talk about specific subjects in great detail. Most children with autism have little or no problem pronouncing words; however, they may have difficulty using language effectively, especially when they talk to other people. They also may be unable to understand body language and the nuances of vocal tones.

YOU are the Paramedic

PART 5

You find that John can hear you with some minor adjustments on your part. He tells you he feels weak and states his physician put him on a new "heart pill" within the last week. He thinks it is making him sick, and he cannot remember the name of it. You assemble oxygen via nasal cannula for the patient. When you go to put the cannula on the patient, he pushes your hand away and turns his head. You state, "John, it is just a cannula." He reluctantly lets you apply it.

Recording Time: 10 Minutes	
Respirations	14 breaths/min
Pulse	78 beats/min
Skin	Pale, cool, dry
Blood pressure	110/64 mm Hg
Oxygen saturation (Spo_2)	98% on 4 L/min via nasal cannula
Pupils	PERRLA

10. How could you have prevented the patient's reaction to the nasal cannula?

Children with autism who can speak will often say things that have no meaning or that seem out of context in conversations with others. One example is the use of continuous repetition of words or phrases. When you communicate with a patient with autism, it may be best to address questions to the parent or caregiver. They are often your best resource for communicating with the patient.

For additional information about communicating with and caring for these patients, refer to Chapter 46, *Patients With Special Challenges.*

Cross-Cultural Communication

Cultural Competence

When faced with a stressful situation, people will react differently. Often this response is driven by the individual's cultural background and upbringing. The reactions of members of some cultures to injury, illness, or death may seem strange (and sometimes even unsettling) to members of other cultures. As a health care provider, you must avoid viewing others from an ethnocentric perspective. **Ethnocentrism** is the belief that one's own culture or ethnic group is inherently superior to others, or that one's own cultural viewpoint is always "right" and the viewpoints of others are "wrong." An ethnocentric viewpoint interprets the actions and beliefs of persons from different cultural or ethnic groups based solely on the standards and values of one's own culture.

An ethnocentric viewpoint can lead to incorrect assumptions and may interfere with your ability to provide appropriate emergency medical care because you have misinterpreted key information. An example may be an Ethiopian patient with shortness of breath. If you apply oxygen, then the patient and family may become agitated and fearful. The dominant American cultural belief is that oxygen use is routine and comforting, but the Ethiopian cultural belief is that the use of oxygen signifies grave or near-fatal disease.[26] The ethnocentric response to this situation would be to assume that the patient and family are behaving irrationally. The culturally competent response is to understand why the patient is reacting in a manner you did not anticipate. The reactions of persons from different backgrounds may be unfamiliar to you, but they are not wrong. They are merely different and are dictated by expectations of the individual's culture. To be an effective EMS provider, you need to understand these differences.

Culture can be defined as the system of beliefs, attitudes, and behaviors that are learned and shared by members of a group. That group may be defined by a shared ethnic background, language, or religion; or it may be based on another shared identity, such as the military or the gay community. Health care and EMS have their own distinctive cultures, with their own languages, traditions, rituals, and rites of initiation.

Human beings are not born with a sense of culture; instead, it is learned from others. Your parents and family provided your first introduction to your culture. As time goes by, people learn other aspects of culture from friends, social and religious groups, the media, and many other sources. As an individual, you are a blend of many cultural influences. You may be a member of a cultural group based on ethnicity, language, or religion. You are also a member of your city's or region's cultures, your circle of friends, and your profession. People switch their cultural identities and practices depending on the circumstances. How you interact with your aging relatives, for example, will differ from how you relate to your friends, coworkers, or patients.

Every person you encounter has a similar mixture of cultural influences that influence how they behave and how they react when stressful situations arise. As a paramedic, it is your responsibility to recognize these differences and to understand how they may affect your interactions with the diverse population you serve. This understanding is referred to as **cultural competence**. In EMS, cultural competence may be defined as an understanding of the predominant cultures that exist in the geographic area in which you provide patient care.

The rest of this section focuses on developing your awareness of how cultural beliefs and practices affect people's views of health, illness, and health care. It also explores how you can effectively interact and communicate with patients and families from different cultures. The discussion here primarily examines ethnic and traditional cultural groups and their health beliefs and practices. In this limited space, it is impossible to provide detailed descriptions of all cultural health practices that you may encounter. Although this section highlights some examples that illustrate the wide range of cultural beliefs and practices, you will need to identify the primary cultural groups in your area and learn about their specific cultural and health care practices.

Cultural Awareness

Body Language

Body language and gestures are widely used by individuals from various groups, but they may be interpreted differently by members of different cultures. The intended meaning may not be recognized and lead to confusion, or an innocent gesture in one culture may be considered rude in another. Perhaps the most universal cross-cultural gesture is the smile: A smile is readily understood by most every culture and conveys goodwill.

Every culture has its own social norms, religious practices, and interpretation of body language. What may be perceived as rude or odd may simply be a difference of cultural standards. It is not possible in this chapter to cover all cultural norms you might potentially encounter, but the following list describes a few cultural practices that you should recognize:

- **Eye contact.** Members of some cultures may avoid making direct eye contact. Avoiding eye contact is a sign of respect in many Native American cultural groups, and in some Asian, African, Latin American, and Caribbean cultures. Prolonged eye contact is acceptable in the Arab world, Somalia, Brazil, and most European cultures.
- **Touching with the left hand.** Islamic and Hindu cultures avoid touching with the left hand because traditionally, this hand was used for unclean functions. It is considered rude to use the left hand in greeting.
- **Touching the head.** Members of many Asian cultures do not touch the head. The head is considered the most sacred part of the body and is the soul's residence. Touching the head may put the soul in jeopardy.
- **Feet.** Showing the bottom of the feet is considered offensive in many Muslim nations and most of Thailand.
- **Hands on hips.** This posture can be a sign of hostility in Mexico and Argentina.
- **Nodding.** Members of Indian and Arabic cultures may signal agreement by moving the head from side to side (the Western "no"). Some members of Asian cultures will nod to indicate "I acknowledge you are speaking to me," but that gesture does not necessarily indicate agreement.
- **Hand gestures.** Hand gestures can have very different meanings in different cultures. Some gestures may be innocent to one cultural group, but insulting to another. Learn about and be cautious with your use of hand gestures with members of different cultures in your community.

> **Words of Wisdom**
>
> It is essential to become familiar with the cultural groups that live in your service area. Some areas have organized cultural awareness training programs. If no such programs are available in your community, then consider organizing one. Invite representatives from local religious or cultural organizations to meet with your EMS agency and develop training classes. Other resources may include local hospitals, colleges, and community groups.

Traditional Folk Medicine and Understanding of Illness

Not every culture views health and illness in the same way. Most of the patients you will encounter will subscribe to the Western biomedical model, which emphasizes a biologic understanding of disease and injury, along with the use of scientifically proven diagnostic tests and treatments. It views illness as a battle to be won using laboratory tests, radiographs, medications, and surgical procedures.

Many immigrants to the United States follow the traditional folk medicine practices of their culture or homeland. Traditional models of illness typically involve a belief that health is the result of a balance of forces. If an imbalance occurs, then the individual becomes ill. Thus, treatments and remedies are aimed at restoring the balance. Other beliefs may view illness as a result of the loss of one's spirit or of magical influences **TABLE 5-3**. Humoral medicine practices were followed by Western medicine well

TABLE 5-3 Traditional Beliefs About Health, Illnesses, and Folk Treatments

Beliefs	Examples	Folk Treatments

Humoral balance	• Balance between humors: blood, yellow bile, black bile, phlegm
	• Each humor is associated with a season, element, organ, and/or specific qualities of heating/cooling and moisture/dryness
		• "Feed a cold, starve a fever."
		  • Foods thought to be heating or cooling
		• Imitative magic (drawing the sickness [poison] from the body):
		  • Coining: heated oil is applied to the skin, then coins are rubbed on the skin, creating red welts
		  • Cupping: heated glass jars or cups are placed on the skin; as the cups cool, they create suction, red marks, and sometimes bruises
		  • Ear candles: waxed paper cones are inserted into the ear canal and burned to remove earwax
		• Bleeding and blistering as treatments to restore balance

Illness as a loss of spirit	• The individual's spirit may flee the body because of:
	  • Sudden noises
	  • Physical trauma or injury
	  • Spiritual or emotional trauma
		• Rituals to return the wandering spirit to the body

Illness as the result of magical forces	• The evil eye	• As with loss of spirit, rituals to return the wandering spirit to the body • Charms or amulets meant to ward off the evil eye or other curses

Data from: Juckett J. Cross-cultural medicine. *Am Fam Physician*. 2005;72(11):2267-2274; Lipson JG, Dibble SL. *Culture and Clinical Care*. San Francisco, CA: UCSF Nursing Press; 2005.

into the 1800s, and some practices have regained popularity among followers of the New Age movement. It is not uncommon for immigrants, and the children of immigrants, to practice a blend of Western and traditional health practices. They may alternate between their traditional healer and their Western medical provider.

Two folk medicine practices that you should recognize are "cupping" and "coining," because they may be easily misinterpreted as signs of physical abuse.[27] These practices are discussed in more detail in Chapter 44, *Pediatric Emergencies*. An important part of your history taking is to ask if any traditional healing practices have been used.

Another area of traditional folk medicine is the use of herbal medications. Many pharmaceuticals in everyday use were derived from older folk remedies. These herbal medications include aspirin from willow bark or birch bark, which is used to reduce pain or fever, and quinine from the cinchona tree, which is used to treat malaria. The use of traditional remedies is widespread, and an awareness of what the patient is taking is essential. Many herbal medications have significant pharmacologic effects that may be a source of the patient's symptoms or interact with other prescribed medications.

Patients may also be taking medications brought from their native country or supplied by family members back home. These medications often have different brand or generic names than their North American equivalents, or they may not be approved for use in the United States. The best practice is to collect all of the patient's medications (over the counter, prescribed, herbal, and those from foreign pharmacies) and bring them to the hospital with the patient so they can be identified, and so that the receiving staff are aware of everything the patient is taking.

Finally, consider that some patients may not share their family's or culture's background beliefs and, therefore, may disagree with family members regarding their condition and treatment. Always remain sensitive to the patient's individual religious, cultural, and sociologic beliefs.

Language Interpretation

Probably the most significant communication challenge that may arise with members of other cultures is lack of a common language. This challenge makes it difficult, if not impossible, to perform a good history and assessment. Language interpretation is vital when caring for a patient who speaks a different language, including people with hearing impairment who use sign language.

Unless you are fluent in the other language, it is always best to use a qualified interpreter. Health facilities are legally required to provide interpretation services, and patients in the prehospital setting deserve the same service level. Obtaining qualified medical interpretation is more challenging in the field, but it is possible. **TABLE 5-4** lists the types of interpretation services that may be available to you. When dealing with a patient who speaks another language, you should always assume you are missing something important in your history and assessment, and act accordingly.

TABLE 5-4 Language Interpretation Resources

Option	Advantages	Disadvantages
Interpreters provided by the hospital or dispatch center	• Qualified medical interpreters • May be available by telephone or radio	• Not present with you in the field • Selection of languages may be limited • Hours of availability may be limited
Other responders as interpreters (other EMS personnel, firefighters, law enforcement, etc)	• Easy access	• May or may not be fluent, or may not have knowledge of medical terminology • May be unable to accompany the patient to the hospital
Interpretation services via telephone	• Easy access from anywhere • Qualified medical interpreters	• Requires telephone access • Usually involves a subscription or other fee
Electronic translation applications (smartphones, etc)	• Easy access from tablet or smartphone • Many are inexpensive	• Not specific to medical interpretation • May not meet legal requirements
Family members or friends as interpreters	• Often present with the patient at scene • Patient may be more comfortable with a family member or friend	• May have limited fluency • May have limited understanding of questions being asked or of medical concepts • Accuracy of interpretation may be questionable (eg, they may edit what the patient says or give their own opinion, not what the patient has said)
Minors acting as interpreters	• Immediately available • May have good bilingual ability	• Seldom a good idea • May have limited fluency • Often will have limited understanding • Accuracy of interpretation may be questionable • Ethics of using young children in this role are questionable

Abbreviation: EMS, emergency medical services

YOU are the Paramedic SUMMARY

1. As a paramedic in the EMS system, how will you be notified about the incident's location and nature?

A call for emergency medical assistance will be placed through 9-1-1 to the PSAP, where a dispatcher will obtain the information and direct the appropriate resources (you) to the scene.

2. What will the dispatcher be doing while you are en route to the call?

The dispatcher will obtain more information from the caller and provide any necessary prearrival medical instructions to the caller. The dispatcher will update the ambulance crew with any new information.

3. How will you communicate with the other responders and agencies involved in the emergency response?

Communication between responders will use the emergency communications system, which may make use of radio, cellular devices, or computer terminals. The most common method of on-scene communications is a simplex channel using portable and mobile radios.

4. How will you initiate communication with this patient?

As soon as is reasonably possible, begin by introducing yourself. This introduction does not entail any special social skills or societal standards. For example, say: "Good morning, my name is Mark. I am a paramedic with the fire department. What is your name?" This simple exchange offers comfort and promotes a feeling of togetherness and goodwill.

Be sure you make eye contact and maintain it. This action reinforces trust and honesty. It also allows you to evaluate the patient's neurologic status, because certain conditions can cause an altered mental status that is evident through the person's gaze. A vague, far-off stare may suggest the presence of physical issues or substance abuse. The eyes may also signal agitation, hostility, or potential for violence.

5. Is the television noise a consideration in your assessment?

Sometimes, even with the best communication techniques, it is difficult to communicate with the patient. External factors such as noise, disruptive scenes, language barriers, and sensory impairment can make communication difficult. In this situation, the noise of the television may interfere with effective communication with the patient. Resist the urge to walk over and simply turn it off. Whenever possible, ask permission before moving furniture or turning off appliances. The respect you demonstrate will go a long way toward improving overall communications with your patient.

6. What does it mean to "get on the same level as the patient"? What is the importance of this action?

If no threat is evident, then physically get on the same level as the patient. This practice means placing yourself in a position where the patient will not have to look up at you; it promotes trust and alleviates anxiety. This technique is beneficial when dealing with children. In essence, you are demonstrating a stance of equality through physical orientation.

7. How can you address the problem of a family member answering questions for the patient?

If this type of problem occurs, do not become irritated with the family member. This specific method of communication may work well for this couple because the patient has a hearing impairment. You have several options available in such a case. You can politely ask the family member to allow the patient to speak so you can hear their voice. You can also ask the family member to perform another function, such as gathering medications, which will allow you to speak one-on-one with the patient. Whatever you choose to do, do it tactfully.

8. Give some examples of effective communication techniques for people with hearing impairment.

Differing levels of hearing impairment exist, ranging from minimal deficits to total deafness. Do not yell, because the patient may not have hearing impairment. Take your cues from family members. In this case, Mrs. Smith leaned close to the patient's left ear and spoke to him. Alternatively, position yourself so the patient can clearly see you; speak slowly and clearly to the patient. Many people who are deaf or hard of hearing can read lips and facial expressions. You might also try writing down your questions and allowing the patient to write the answers. It may be necessary to utilize an American Sign Language interpreter when working with people who are deaf.

YOU are the Paramedic SUMMARY continued

9. How can your body language affect your assessment of this patient?

Avoid a closed posture (such as crossing your arms) because this type of body language sends negative signals. Be mindful of your facial expressions and gestures. Do not frown or smirk at the patient's answers. Rolling your eyes at your partner is also not appropriate because it is rude and could provoke a fight from a patient with a behavioral issue. Maintain constant, nonjudgmental eye contact. Demonstrate patience to the patient. Use open-handed gestures to demonstrate openness.

10. How could you have prevented the patient's reaction to the nasal cannula?

It can be frightening when someone reaches over your face with a piece of equipment. You told the patient, "It is just a cannula." Does the patient know what a cannula is and what it is designed to do? Before touching a patient, you need to educate and communicate what you are trying to do for a patient. Explain what an oxygen cannula does, how it is worn, and how it will help before placing it on the patient's face. The same is true for any item you place on the patient.

EMS Patient Care Report (PCR)

Date: 07-01-22	**Incident No.:** 876	**Nature of Call:** General medical	**Location:** 450 Maple Street

Dispatched: 0810	**En Route:** 0812	**At Scene:** 0816	**Transport:** 0836	**At Hospital:** 0845	**In Service:** 0855

Patient Information

Age: 86 **Sex:** M **Weight (in kg [lb]):** 59 kg (130 lb)	**Allergies:** NKDA **Medications:** Numerous—see attached list **Past Medical History:** Pancreatic cancer, A-fib **Chief Complaint:** General weakness

Vital Signs

Time: 0821	**BP:** 110/66	**Pulse:** 76	**Respirations:** 14	**Spo_2:** 93% on room air
Time: 0826	**BP:** 110/64	**Pulse:** 78	**Respirations:** 14	**Spo_2:** 98% on 4 L/min NC
Time:	**BP:**	**Pulse:**	**Respirations:**	**Spo_2:**

EMS Treatment (circle all that apply)

Oxygen @ __4__ L/min via (circle one): **(NC)** **NRM** **Bag-mask device**		**Assisted Ventilation**	**Airway Adjunct**	**CPR**
Defibrillation	**Bleeding Control**	**Bandaging**	**Splinting**	**Other:**

Narrative

Pt is an 86-year-old man with a history of cancer who reports general weakness and difficulty breathing for the past 2–3 days. Pt states his physician changed a cardiac medication within the last week and pt believes this may be causing the weakness, but he does not know the medication's name. Pt is alert and oriented ×4, sitting in a recliner. Breath sounds are equal but diminished in all fields, with no wheezing. Pt denies chest pain, dizziness, and nausea/vomiting. Cardiac monitor shows A-fib. Extensive medication list attached to this report. Pt placed on 4 L/min O_2 NC before transport. Pt lifted from recliner to stretcher and secured. Medical control report to Dr. Brown, no orders. Pt transported without change to Regional Hospital. Report to Shari, RN, on arrival.
End of report

Prep Kit

Ready for Review

- To fulfill your role as a paramedic, you must be able to communicate rapidly, efficiently, and effectively when responding to an emergency call.
- During an EMS call, the phases of communication include notification, information gathering, dispatch, response, potential prearrival instructions for the caller, communication during on-scene care, transport, and communication with medical control or the receiving facility while en route.
- Dispatchers communicate with people who call 9-1-1 in an emergency, and with the EMS responders being sent to the scene. The dispatcher identifies the patient's exact location, the telephone number, the nature of the emergency, and specific information about the patient's condition and emergency, such as the types of vehicles involved in a motor vehicle crash or hazards at the scene.
- Dispatchers are also responsible for monitoring communications with the ambulance, coordinating communications with medical control and other agencies, and recording when the call's various phases occurred.
- Emergency medical dispatch requires special training that teaches dispatchers to provide basic medical instructions to emergency callers over the phone. Updates resulting from this prearrival care can be communicated to the EMS crew while they are en route.
- Radio is one of the main methods of communication in EMS. The most commonly used bands for medical communications are the VHF and UHF bands. The higher the frequency, the less interference there is, but the shorter the transmission range will be.
- Systems used for radio transmissions include simplex, duplex, and multiplex.
  - Simplex operates on one frequency and allows the transmission to go one way.
  - Duplex utilizes two paired frequencies, which may allow simultaneous transmission and reception or the use of repeaters to boost range.
  - Multiplex allows for the transmission of multiple data streams simultaneously.
- An EMS communications system consists of a base station, mobile and portable transceivers, repeaters, and a backup communications system.
- Digital trunked radio systems utilize sophisticated computer systems to manage frequency and channel use for multiple users, and permit communication among a wide range of users.
- Interoperability is the capability of radio communications systems to communicate with each other and with equipment from different manufacturers and systems.
- The FCC controls radio frequency allocation and licensing in the United States. It also establishes technical standards for radio equipment, establishes and enforces rules and regulations for radio equipment operation, and monitors transmissions. Frequencies assigned for medical purposes are to be used strictly for that purpose.
- Cell phones are becoming more common in EMS communications systems. Many newer cell phones (smartphones) have built-in GPS systems, which aid the enhanced 9-1-1 operating system in determining exactly where the call is being made.
- Biotelemetry (or telemetry) is used to transmit patient data to a remote terminal. In EMS, it is most often used to transmit 12-lead ECGs. This technology can help diagnose STEMI and aid medical control or you in making the appropriate treatment and destination decisions.
- Keep radio communication clear, accurate, and concise. One of the main goals is clarity. Use the International Radiotelephony Phonetic Alphabet to clarify spellings as necessary.
- Remember that your words can be heard by anyone who is listening to the radio

Prep Kit continued

communication. Keep your communications professional at all times. Do not transmit a patient's name or personal information over the radio, as that would violate the HIPAA privacy rules.

- Most EMS systems use clear text or plain language in radio communications, but some still use radio codes. If your agency uses codes, learn them and use them correctly.
- When you report medical information, include the destination facility and ETA; patient's age and sex; chief complaint; brief history; medications and important allergies; anything the physician needs to know about the patient's past medical history relative to the current situation, including major underlying medical conditions; level of consciousness and degree of distress; mental status; vital signs; physical findings in head-to-toe order; ECG findings; treatment; and response to treatment.
- Many of the calls you will run as a paramedic will take you into people's homes, day and night, and in the most private moments of their lives. Try to see every invitation into the home of someone else as a personal honor in a time and place where no one else would be welcome. Give your patients your undivided attention.
- Active listening is repeating the key parts of a patient's responses to questions. It helps confirm the information the patient is providing and can clear up any misunderstanding.
- As a therapeutic communicator, your challenge is to convey calm, genuine concern for someone you have never met.
- When you first meet a patient, introduce yourself and ask for the patient's name. This technique communicates your respect.
- Patient modesty matters, no matter how acute the medical condition. If the patient is not personally sensitive to it, then family members most certainly are.
- When you need to know how patients feel, try asking open-ended questions—questions that do not have a yes or no answer, and that do not give patients specific options from which to choose. When you are trying to find specific facts (eg, a medical history), use closed-ended or direct questions.
- If you sense that patients are trying to put something into words but are having trouble forming their response, be patient. Do not say anything at all for a few seconds. Let them talk.
- If you have tried clarification and are still not sure what patients are trying to tell you, it sometimes helps to vocalize what you think they have said and invite them to correct you.
- Nonverbal communication can be as powerful as words.
- Direct eye contact generally communicates honesty and concern, but this technique may not be expected in some cultures.
- Posture is important. Try to position your eyes at the same level or below the level of the patient's eyes.
- Some people do not like to be touched at all. To others, touch offers a valuable assurance that someone cares about them. Try gently touching the patient on a neutral part of the body, such as a shoulder or arm, especially when trying to reassure someone or reduce fear.
- Hostile or angry patients may present a threat to you and others. Always approach with caution and maintain eye contact. Do not interview hostile or potentially violent patients or bystanders by yourself.
- Do not presume that older people will pose special communication challenges relative to younger people, just because of their age.
- Children can pose treatment and communication challenges to even the most experienced EMS personnel. Minimize your movements, lower your voice, and touch pediatric patients as gently as you can. Try keeping your eye level with or below the child's eye level by sitting on the floor and placing the child on the cot or on a parent or caregiver's lap.

Prep Kit continued

- When you encounter a patient who has trouble communicating, remember that family members or primary caregivers who know these patients well can facilitate your efforts. They can also help you alleviate the patient's fear and anxiety.
- Interacting with people of cultures different from your own can be challenging. Learn about the different cultural groups that exist in your service area. It is considered respectful if you make an effort to learn about another person's language and culture.
- Manners, hand gestures, and body language may differ among cultures. Remember that another person's culture may have different rules for polite behavior than your own.
- As an EMS provider, you may encounter traditional or folk medicine practices that seem strange to you. If you do not understand a particular practice, consider the possibility that the patient or family may be trying to manage the illness using traditional health practices from their native culture.
- Make use of qualified medical interpreters whenever possible for patients who speak a different language. Be cautious when using family members to interpret, and avoid using young children as interpreters unless no other option is available.

Vital Vocabulary

automatic crash notification (ACN) Specialized onboard computer systems in motor vehicles that automatically send telemetry data to a monitoring station in the event of a crash, which then relays the data to emergency responders; also called advanced automatic crash notification.

base station A radio at a fixed location (ie, hospital or dispatch center) consisting of a transmitter, receiver, and antenna.

biotelemetry Transmission of physiologic data, such as an electrocardiogram, from the patient to a distant point of reception (commonly known as telemetry in EMS).

cell phones Wireless telephones that communicate via radio waves with the telephone system through an interconnected network of repeater stations called cells.

clear text Using regular language (plain English) and accepted terms to enhance clarity of communication, rather than using ten-codes or other code systems.

closed-ended question A question that is specific and focused, requiring either a yes or no answer, or an answer chosen from specific options; this type of question is helpful for patients who report shortness of breath.

computer-assisted dispatch (CAD) Linked dispatch center computer consoles and vehicle-mounted mobile data terminals.

crew resource management (CRM) An operational practice designed to enhance communication and teamwork, and to thereby reduce preventable errors.

cultural competence An understanding of the predominant cultures that exist in the geographic area in which the paramedic provides patient care.

culture The system of beliefs, attitudes, and behaviors that are learned and shared by members of a group.

digital radio The transmission of information via radio waves using native digital (computer) data or analog (voice) signals that have been converted to a digital signal and compressed.

dispatch To send to a specific destination or to send on a task.

duplex Radio system using paired frequencies to permit the use of remote repeaters or simultaneous transmission and reception.

emergency medical dispatch (EMD) A program specifically designed to meet the unique needs

Prep Kit continued

of emergency medical services response and of callers reporting a medical emergency, including first aid instructions given by specially trained dispatchers to callers over the telephone while an ambulance is en route to the call.

encoded radio signals Embedded signals that allow multiple users to share frequencies and repeaters.

enhanced 9-1-1 systems Emergency communications systems that collect information about 9-1-1 calls from the telephone network, such as the caller's phone number and location, and display this information on the computer dispatch terminal.

ethnocentrism Viewing other cultures based solely on the standards and values of one's own culture; a belief in the inherent superiority of one's own culture or ethnic group.

Federal Communications Commission (FCC) The independent government agency that regulates interstate and international communications by radio, television, wire, satellite and cable in all 50 states, the District of Columbia, and US territories.

frequency The number of oscillations (or cycles) per second of a radio signal.

geographic information system (GIS) Technology that uses global positioning system and other data to (1) track and predict ambulance response times, (2) determine the distance to the closest trauma center or other hospitals from specific locations, (3) track the frequency of motor vehicle crashes and the severity of injuries from different geographic locations, (4) determine the location of emergency helipads, and (5) provide other information useful in EMS system operations and planning.

hertz (Hz) Unit of measure of a frequency equal to 1 cycle per second; 1 million Hz equals one megahertz and 1,000 megahertz equals one gigahertz.

interoperability Public safety communications systems that are compatible across all local, tribal, state, and federal agencies.

landline Communications system linked by wires, usually in reference to a conventional telephone system.

medical priority dispatch system (MPDS) A dispatch system using a specific format to indicate the nature of the emergency (EMD protocol) and its priority (determinant level/number).

multiplex Simultaneous transmission of multiple data streams, most often voice and electrocardiogram signals.

mutual aid Agreements with neighboring or regional jurisdictions to back up each other in the event of a large-scale incident.

narrow band Reassignment of frequencies by the Federal Communications Commission to a 12.5 megahertz spacing, now required for all EMS and public safety radio systems.

noise Interference in a radio signal.

off-line medical control Patient care orders in the form of protocols or standing orders that do not require direct contact with the medical control physician.

online medical control Patient care orders provided directly to the paramedic by the medical control physician by radio or telephone.

open-ended question A question that does not have a yes or no answer, and that does not give the patient specific options from which to choose.

pervasive developmental disorders (PDDs) A group of disorders that cause delays in many areas of childhood development, such as the development of skills to communicate and interact socially, and may include repetitive body movements and difficulty with changes in routine; include autism and Asperger syndrome, among others.

public safety answering point (PSAP) The location to which 9-1-1 calls are routed, which may or may not serve as the dispatch center.

radio dead spots Areas where mobile or portable radios are unable to communicate with a repeater or each other.

Prep Kit continued

remote terminal A terminal that receives transmissions of telemetry and voice from the field and transmits messages back, usually through the base station.

repeater Remote radio transceiver that receives radio signals and rebroadcasts them at a higher power, extending the range of a radio communications system.

simplex Radio communication using a single frequency.

situation, background, assessment, and recommendation (SBAR) A structured patient report format designed to convey important information in a concise manner.

squelch Filtering system to block out background noise, but still allow radio signals to be heard.

telemedicine Computer-based system permitting real-time two-way transmission of sound, video, vital signs, ECG tracings, and other diagnostic data between the paramedic and medical control physician.

ten-code A radio code system using the number 10 plus another number. No longer used in many EMS systems.

therapeutic communication Communicating with the patient using specific strategies to encourage the patient to express ideas and feelings, and to convey respect and acceptance.

transceivers Radios containing both a transmitter and a receiver; two-way radios.

trunked radio systems Computerized sharing of radio frequencies by multiple units, agencies, or systems.

ultra high frequency (UHF) band The portion of the radio frequency spectrum between 300 and 3,000 megahertz.

universal timeout A planned pause before the beginning of a procedure that improves safety and communication among all personnel, and helps prevent human errors.

very high frequency (VHF) band The portion of the radio frequency spectrum between 30 and 300 megahertz.

References

1. Communicate. *Merriam-Webster: Dictionary and Thesaurus*. http://www.merriam-webster.com. Accessed January 29, 2021.
2. Trembley AL, Page D. EMS improves with crew resource management training. *J Emerg Med Serv.* https://www.jems.com/patient-care/ems-improves-with-crew-resource-management-training/. Published April 6, 2015. Accessed January 29, 2021.
3. Page D. New psychomotor exam for nationally registered paramedics begins in January. *J Emerg Med Serv.* https://www.jems.com/training/new-psychomotor-exam-for-nationally-registered-paramedics-begins-in-january/#:~:text=New%20Psychomotor%20Exam%20for%20Nationally%20Registered%20Paramedics%20Begins%20in%20January,-David%20Page%2C%20MS&text=Beginning%20January%202017%2C%20candidates,new%20and%20improved%20psychomotor%20exam. Published September 30, 2016. Accessed January 29, 2021.
4. APCO International. *Minimum Training Standards for Public Safety Telecommunicators.* APCO ANS 3.103.2.2015. https://www.apcointl.org/download/minimum-training-standards-for-public-safety-telecommunicators-3/?wpdmdl=6288. Accessed January 29, 2021.
5. Wilson MJ. *The ARRL Operating Manual*. 9th ed. Newington, CT: Amateur Radio Relay League; 2007:2-1–4-28.
6. U.S. Fire Administration, Federal Emergency Management Agency. *Voice Radio Communications Guide for the Fire Service: June 2016.* https://www.usfa.fema.gov/downloads/pdf/publications/Voice_Radio_Communications_Guide_for_the_Fire_Service.pdf. Accessed January 29, 2021.
7. Federal Communications Commission. Narrowbanding overview. https://www.fcc.gov/narrowbanding-overview. Updated February 3, 2016. Accessed January 29, 2021.
8. Office of Emergency Communications, US Department of Homeland Security. *National Interoperability Field Operations Guide, Version 1.4.* https://www.dhs.gov/xlibrary/assets/nifog-v1-4-resized-for-pda-viewing.pdf. January 2011. Accessed January 29, 2021.
9. US Department of Homeland Security. Statement of requirements for public safety wireless communications and interoperability. The SAFECOM Program. Version 1.1. https://www.npstc.org/documents/SRSoR_V11_030606.pdf. Published January 26, 2006. Accessed January 29, 2021.

Prep Kit continued

10. APCO Project 25 Steering Committee. APCO Project 25 statement of requirements. http://project25.org/images/stories/ptig/15-009_12131211_Approved_P25_SoR_12-11-13.pdf. Published December 11, 2013. Accessed January 29, 2021.
11. LeBlanc C. Three additional EMS employees terminated over Facebook posts. https://www.ems1.com/ems-management/articles/3-additional-ems-employees-terminated-over-facebook-posts-ye4HNJVr8fIg4akZ/. Published July 19, 2016. Accessed February 19, 2021.
12. Wang SC, Kohoyda-Inglis CJ, MacWilliams JB, et al. Results of first field test of telemetry based injury severity prediction. Abstract presented at 24th International Technical Conference on the Enhanced Safety of Vehicles (ESV). Gothenburg, Sweden: June 8–11, 2015.
13. Amateur Radio Relay League. Two flavors of amateur radio emergency operation. http://www.arrl.org/ares-races-faq. Accessed January 29, 2021.
14. Grigoriev AI, Orlov OI. Telemedicine and spaceflight. *Aviat Space Environ Med*. 2002;73(7):688-693.
15. Grose T. Speed is the drug. *Newsweek*. http://www.newsweek.com/2014/05/02/speed-drug-248536.html. Published April 24, 2014. Accessed March 18, 2016.
16. Rao A, Kardouh Y, Darda S, et al. Impact of the prehospital ECG on door-to-balloon time in ST elevation myocardial infarction. *Catheter Cardiovasc Interv*. 2010;75(2):174-178. doi:10.1002/ccd.22257.
17. American Heart Association. Opportunities to improve STEMI systems of care. https://www.heart.org/en/professional/quality-improvement/mission-lifeline/opportunities-to-improve-stemi-systems-of-care. Reviewed June 29, 2018. Accessed February 19, 2021.
18. Bashford C. Telemedicine today: part 1—getting started. *EMSWorld*. https://www.emsworld.com/article/12184039/telemedicine-today-part-1-getting-started. Published March 18, 2016. Accessed January 29, 2021.
19. Sierra Wireless. The "firstnet-ready" mobile office: top considerations for connecting first responders [White paper]. http://www.jems.com/whitepapers/2015/12/the-firstnet-ready-mobile-office-top-considerations-for-connecting-first-responders.whitepaperpdf.render.pdf. Published November 10, 2015. Accessed January 29, 2021.
20. e-CFR Title 47, Chapter 1, Subchapter D, Part 90, Subpart B, §90.15. Electronic Code of Federal Regulations. US Government Publishing Office.ecfr.gov/cgi-bin/text-idx?SID=b41258b0691d3b0b98a9ff13931e8597&mc=true&node=pt47.5.90&rgn=div5#se47.5.90_115. Accessed January 29, 2021.
21. Federal Emergency Management Agency. NIMS and use of plain language [FEMA publication no. NA: 023-06]. https://www.fema.gov/pdf/emergency/nims/plain_lang.pdf. Updated December 19, 2006. Accessed January 29, 2021.
22. Harrington JW. Surgical time outs in a combat zone. *AORN J*. 2009;89(3):535-537.
23. American College of Emergency Physicians. Transfer of patient care between EMS providers and receiving facilities [Policy statement]. *Ann Emerg Med*. 2013;63(4):503. doi:10.1016/j.annemergmed.2013.12.023.
24. SBAR toolkit. Institute for Healthcare Improvement. http://www.ihi.org/resources/Pages/Tools/SBARToolkit.aspx. Accessed January 29, 2021.
25. Masters R. Preventing invisible wounds. *EMSWorld*. https://www.emsworld.com/article/12223916/preventing-invisible-wounds. Published August 1, 2016. Accessed January 29, 2021.
26. Beyene Y. Ethiopians and Eritreans. In: Lipson JG, Dibble SL, eds. *Culture and Clinical Care*. San Francisco, CA: UCSF Nursing Press; 2008:163-176.
27. Galanti G-A. *Caring for Patients from Different Cultures*. 5th ed. Philadelphia, PA: University of Pennsylvania Press; 2014.

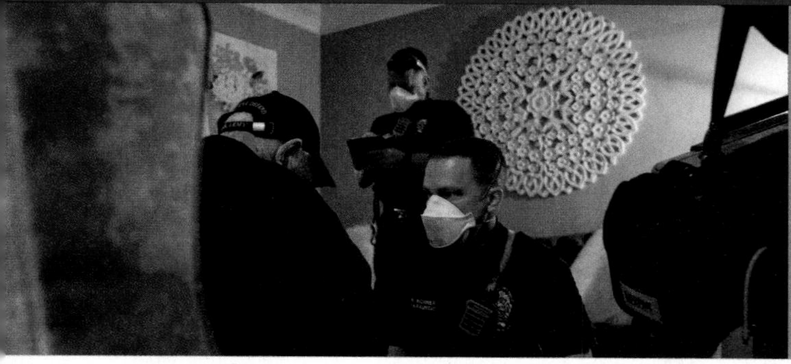

Chapter 6

Documentation

NATIONAL EMS EDUCATION STANDARD COMPETENCIES

Preparatory

Integrates comprehensive knowledge of EMS systems, the safety/well-being of the paramedic, and medical/legal and ethical issues, which is intended to improve the health of EMS personnel, patients, and the community.

Documentation

- Recording patient findings (pp 207, 209–210, 218–221)
- Principles of medical documentation and report writing (pp 221–222)

KNOWLEDGE OBJECTIVES

1. Explain the legal implications of the patient care report (PCR). (p 207)
2. Discuss the implications of the Health Insurance Portability and Accountability Act of 1996 as they relate to documentation. (p 207)
3. Describe the purposes of documentation. (pp 207–209)
4. Compare handwritten PCRs with electronic PCRs, and discuss the pros and cons of each type. (pp 209–210)
5. Identify the information required in a PCR, including standard items that must be documented for every emergency call. (pp 210–211)
6. Discuss the process for documenting transfer of care and care before arrival. (pp 211–212)
7. Discuss the process for documenting refusal of care, including the legal implications. (pp 212–213)
8. Discuss state and/or local reporting requirements for special circumstances, including workplace injuries and illnesses, multiple-casualty incidents, occupational exposures, cases of alleged abuse or neglect, and involvement of on-scene physicians or other agencies. (pp 213–217)
9. Discuss various formats for the narrative portion of the PCR. (pp 218–221)
10. Discuss why it is essential that documentation be accurate, legible, and professional. (pp 222–224)
11. Explain the procedure to follow should an error occur during or after creating a PCR. (pp 224–225)
12. Discuss the consequences of intentional falsification of documentation. (p 225)
13. Discuss why it is important to accurately document incident times. (p 226)

SKILLS OBJECTIVES

1. Demonstrate completion of a PCR. (pp 214–216)

Introduction

Although documentation may not be the first item that comes to mind when you are thinking of pursuing a career in emergency medical services (EMS), it is an integral part of the patient care process. Thorough documentation pulls together the run for all parties involved. The adage, "No job is finished until the paperwork is done," is especially true in EMS. Your report, most commonly referred to as the **patient care report (PCR)** or sometimes called the prehospital care report, is the only written record of the events that transpired during the call for service. Writing an effective, accurate, and proper PCR is one of the most important skills you will learn as a paramedic. The PCR is the legal record for the call, and it will become part of the patient's medical record and the patient's emergency department (ED) chart at the receiving hospital. A complete PCR will not only allow other health care providers to obtain information about what happened from the start of the call to its conclusion, but also guide future patient care via research and quality assurance **FIGURE 6-1**. As a paramedic, you must be able to create a PCR thoroughly and efficiently.

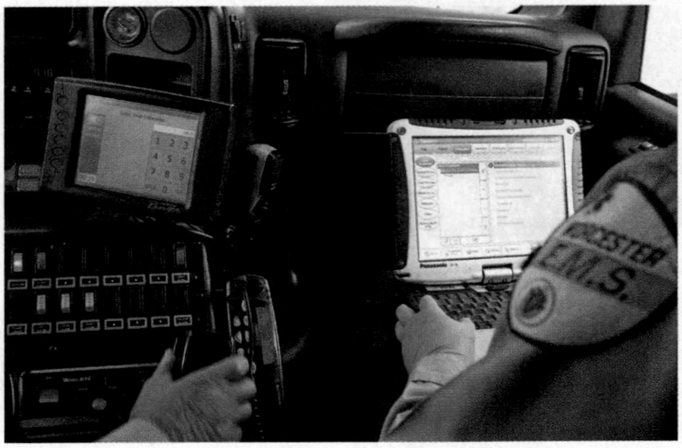

FIGURE 6-1 Electronic patient care reports, or ePCRs, shown here, are the standard in EMS documentation.

You need to know what constitutes a PCR, what information must be included, who might read the PCR, when the PCR must be completed, and what terminology may be used. The information in your report may be categorized as either objective or subjective. **Objective information** includes measurable signs that you observe and record (eg, pulse rate, respiratory rate, blood pressure). **Subjective information** includes information that is told to you, but that cannot be seen (eg, symptoms that patients describe, degree of pain, nausea). When you write your PCR, try to use the patient's own words as much as possible. Place quotation marks around any direct statements; for example, "The patient rates the pain an '8' on a 0 to 10 scale." You must record both objective *and* subjective information and the details of patient care for every call.

The PCR needs to be complete, accurate, and legible because it can provide the basis of your defense if legal proceedings arise after the call. The PCR is vital to your service or agency for many other reasons, including facilitating quality care, continuity of care, and billing to insurance providers. Your report should paint a picture of the entire call that is accurate and clear to the reader.

YOU are the Paramedic

PART 1

Your unit has been dispatched to a single-vehicle collision involving a pole near the county courthouse at approximately 1300 hours on a weekday. On arrival, you ensure the scene is safe before you exit the ambulance. The vehicle appears to have light damage to the front bumper and hood. You don your personal protective equipment and approach the vehicle. As you walk up, a man opens the vehicle's door and attempts unsuccessfully to stand up. The man falls back down on the seat and exclaims in a loud, slurred voice, "I need my lawyer." You look past the patient into the passenger compartment and see that the airbags have deployed.

1. What is your first consideration in regard to this patient?
2. What is your first consideration in regard to the scene?

Legal Implications of a PCR

Although you may include subjective information from the patient in your report (such as statements they make about symptoms), do not include any personal bias or your opinions. For example, avoid subjective statements such as "The patient was drunk and out of control." Instead, use objective statements such as "The patient had an altered mental status and stated he had 'eight beers' today." Poorly written, inappropriately documented PCRs could have adverse implications both for patient care and for your career. Omissions or errors in your report could lead to further errors in care. Improper and inadequate reports also could result in litigation, loss of your job or position, a negative reflection on your reputation as an EMS professional, and more.

The US court system has found paramedics guilty of neglect based on failure to perform patient exams and submit completed paperwork. In one such example, a crew responded to a motor vehicle crash scene, and the patient declined medical transport after a brief discussion with the paramedics. The crew cleared the scene without evaluating the patient. Later, the paramedics were called back for the same patient, who had collapsed at the scene. The paramedics claimed that they owed no duty to act because they never initiated patient care. The judge did not accept this claim and found the paramedics to be negligent. Assuming the providers conducted a proper patient assessment, its documentation would have offered evidence to support their claim. Even if the patient had refused any contact by the paramedics, they should have documented the refusal to help defend why they were unable to assess the patient.

Your report should be complete, well written, legible, and professional, no matter what your particular writing style is. In addition, it should serve as your sole source of information about the call. Perhaps long after the call is over, the PCR may be used in legal proceedings against you or someone else. In some cases, it may be your only defense against a complaint about a call: if you accurately document what happened, then you will have tangible evidence of your conduct and what transpired on the call. Your memory may not serve you well 5 to 7 years from now, but your written report will remain as the only record of why you performed a specific procedure or why you administered a particular medication to a patient. If it is well written, it will jog your memory and provide a clear picture of the call's events to all who read it. In addition, you must use correct spelling, proper grammar, and accurate terminology in your report, as discussed in Chapter 7, *Medical Terminology*. Improper documentation could result in patient care errors and put your professional character at risk if the report is called into question. The consequences of poor documentation are discussed later in this chapter.

The Health Insurance Portability and Accountability Act (HIPAA) outlines ramifications related to patient care reporting. Refer to Chapter 4, *Medical, Legal, and Ethical Issues*, for a discussion of HIPAA.

Words of Wisdom

HIPAA requires that reasonable administrative, technical, and physical safeguards be in place to protect patient information. If you are unsure whether the equipment you may be using is safeguarded, seek advice from your organization's administrators.

Documentation and Communication

To help protect patient information, do not leave paper PCRs or assessment cards on counters or any other area that is not secured. Always sign out of any computer systems that you may be using to create your ePCR after completing it. Many agencies provide lockboxes where completed paper PCRs should be placed.

Purposes of Documentation

Continuity of Care

The PCR serves as a record of the patient's condition on your arrival at the scene, the care provided, any changes in the patient's condition en route, and the patient's condition on arrival at the hospital. You must document the incident as clearly as possible because the PCR will help other health care providers at the hospital understand the particular emergency and assessments and treatments performed thus far. Accurate reporting helps paint a picture of the environment where you found the patient, along with the mechanism of injury (MOI) or nature of illness (NOI), and ultimately leads to better patient care.

Minimum Requirements and Billing

Billing and administration are significant reasons why your PCR needs to be accurate and complete. Most EMS agencies bill for services to recover the costs of providing patient care. For complete and accurate revenue recovery, you must document all procedures performed and obtain appropriate **medical necessity** signatures (where required). Medicare, a national insurance program, establishes the standards for medical necessity. **TABLE 6-1** identifies some of the significant findings that are required to show that the patient needed to be transported by an ambulance rather than by other means of transportation.

Be as specific as you can in the narrative portion of your PCR (the section that allows for free-form writing). Include information such as the quadrant in which the patient had abdominal pain, what supplies you used, what rhythm the cardiac monitor showed, and if the patient had a diabetes-related condition, whether it was hypoglycemia or hyperglycemia. Some insurance companies will deny charges for anything that is not documented in the narrative statement. (Narrative writing is discussed later in this chapter.)

Especially in the case of private or scheduled transports, you need to document why a patient may have needed emergency care to ensure your service's billing information will result in payment from the responsible insurer, agency, or private payer. You must be accurate and complete in your documentation so that time is not spent correcting the documentation, thus delaying billing processing. You will often be trained by your agency and its billing company about what additional forms you need to complete as part of each EMS response. For all calls, completing the billing paperwork and supplying the most accurate and defensible information to the EMS agency are necessary parts of the call.

TABLE 6-1 Examples of Significant Findings That Indicate Medical Necessity for Ambulance Transport

The following conditions must be met to be considered eligible for Medicare emergent ambulance service (December 2017):

- Patient is transported by an approved supplier of ambulance services.
- Patient is experiencing an illness or injury that contraindicates transport by other means.

The following examples constitute medical necessity:

- Patient is transported in an emergency situation (eg, as a result of an accident, injury, or acute illness).
- Patient requires restraint to prevent injury to themselves or others.
- Patient is unconscious or in shock.
- Patient is experiencing signs and symptoms of acute respiratory distress or cardiac distress such as shortness of breath or chest pain.
- Patient is experiencing signs and symptoms that indicate the possibility of acute stroke.
- Patient must remain immobile because of a fracture or the possibility of a fracture.
- Patient was confined to a bed before and after ambulance transport.
- Patient requires emergency treatment while being transported (eg, oxygen therapy, intravenous therapy).
- Patient has uncontrollable hemorrhage.

Data from: Local Coverage Determination (LCD): Ambulance Services (Ground Ambulance) (L35162). Centers for Medicare & Medicaid Services. https://www.cms.gov/medicare-coverage-database/details/lcd-details.aspx?LCDId=35162. Accessed July 13, 2021.

EMS Research

Just as billing has become necessary in EMS, so has research. Collectively, EMS providers' proper documentation results in compiled data that are reviewed by researchers, who then use those data to justify innovative, life-saving techniques, as mentioned in Chapter 1, *EMS Systems*. Many states now require EMS agencies to submit data to the state EMS office to verify call volumes and skills used. These data may include the number of calls to which an agency responds, the types of calls, care provided, and patient outcomes, when known. Such patient care data collection can lead to improvement of the EMS system as a whole.

The National Emergency Medical Services Information System (NEMSIS) stores standardized

EMS data from each state. This central repository assists states in collecting comparable data elements, so that the entire nation can benefit from research and use the trends indicated in the data for future curriculum development. NEMSIS aims to define EMS care by collecting data to improve patient care, identifying equipment needs, and defining a standard of care across the nation.

Incident Review and Quality Assurance

On occasion, PCRs may be requested for medical audits and other educational activities. Run reviews or sessions in which peers and other medical professionals review PCRs for adherence to local protocols, quality assurance, and quality monitoring should occur on a regular basis. These peer review sessions support a healthy quality assurance process and allow the reviewers to learn from others' patient care techniques. Your reports may also be used to determine the number of times you have performed a specific skill, such as medication administration or oral intubation. Always accurately document all skills attempted and performed during patient care.

Documentation and Communication

EMS agencies and departments should have a process to ensure that all reports are well written and a quality assurance program to ensure that no discrepancies exist between what was written in the PCR and what actually occurred on the call.

Types of PCRs

Electronic documentation has become the standard in EMS. Although some services still use paper documentation, you will most likely document your emergency calls and other reports electronically. The many benefits of electronic documentation are discussed later in this section. Perhaps the most significant benefit is the ability to share electronic data, not only between the facilities and personnel involved in a patient's care, thereby improving continuity and efficiency, but also among state and national databases to improve national data collection and further the advancement of evidence-based practice.

Many PCR designs exist throughout the United States, ranging from half-page notes to complete and thorough reports. EMS patient care reporting has evolved over the years because the field of medicine has recognized the necessity for information about the patient's condition and interventions performed in the field. Some services have developed PCRs that nearly eliminate the narrative section and replace the space with either checkboxes or dropdown menus with predetermined terms. You may encounter some reports with hundreds of checkboxes that allow you to mark every action you took. The problem with this format is that it increases the risk of errors—your eyes may become overwhelmed by so many checkboxes that you accidentally select the wrong box. Regardless of what form of patient reporting your service uses, you must document the correct information.

Many PCR designs exist that capture data using checkboxes, but it is only necessary for legal reasons to document your care once. Everything necessary relating to the patient's care and treatment must be captured in the PCR, but documenting it more than once, known as **double documentation**, can lead to errors and cause the report to be questioned by the court. Remember that report writing should be precise, but concise. Unfortunately, a small amount of double documentation may be necessary due to your agency's software and the need for insurance reimbursement. Be aware of this danger when double documenting and take extra care when proofreading your report. Make sure you know and understand your agency's policy in this regard.

In most areas of the United States, paper reporting has become a thing of the past because it duplicates other work in the health care system. Handwritten reports must be entered into an electronic system to fulfill EMS data collection requirements, either by health care agencies or by outsourcing to third-party companies. Along with the additional data entry needs, a paper system requires space to store the records, possibly for a lengthy period depending on state laws. The final reason for the shift away from paper reporting systems is error reduction. Too often, poor penmanship and spelling mistakes lead to medical errors related to medication doses and orders; an electronic system minimizes these errors. However, unless your ambulance carries a printer, you will most likely use a written refusal form when it is necessary to obtain a patient's signature. You should then leave a copy of the refusal form with the patient. Patient refusals are discussed later in this chapter.

Many companies have created and now market a variety of ePCR options. These services range from the scanning of paper forms to the creation of computer-based programs and applications for desktops, laptops, tablets, and smartphones that allow for more accurate and legible reports **FIGURE 6-2**.

Modern data systems can incorporate data from many different sources, such as multiple facilities. This feature aligns with the significant effort on the part of hospitals and physicians to improve the quality of cardiac, stroke, and diabetic care, and improve the success of resuscitation efforts. Such cutting-edge systems will ultimately include EMS documentation so that the PCR contains both information from the field and data collected in the hospitals or facilities where the patient was treated. The result will be one comprehensive record of the care the patient received.

Electronic documentation systems should be NEMSIS-compliant to ensure that data can be shared on a national level. As mentioned, data submission to NEMSIS is essential for EMS research, and to assess and improve EMS care throughout the country. NEMSIS aims to facilitate the submission of EMS data from all states, and part of that process involves implementing electronic documentation systems in all states. Today, most states and territories of the United States are either submitting electronic data to NEMSIS or actively working toward achieving this goal soon.

Documentation for Every EMS Call

Every EMS call requires documentation. The **minimum data set** is the clinical assessment standard information that must be documented on every emergency call according to the Medicare and Medicaid rules, and per the National Highway Traffic Safety Administration as input to the national data system. The minimum data set is divided into two sections: run data and patient data. Run data consist of such information as incident times,

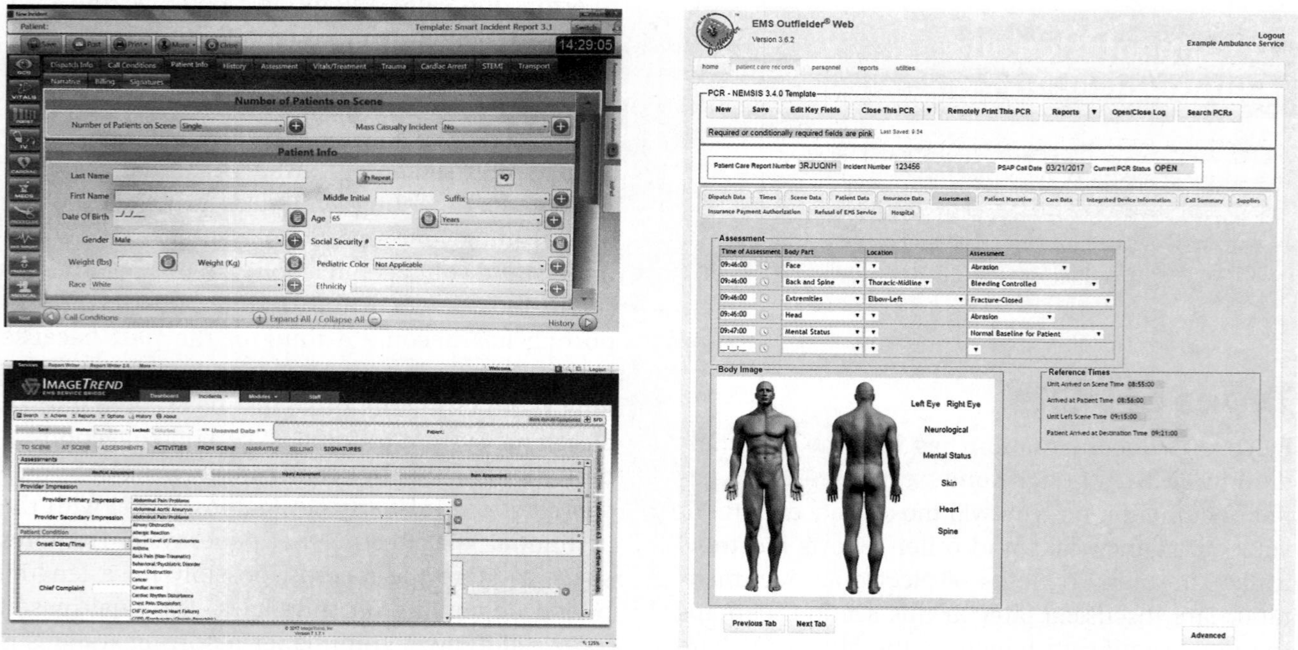

FIGURE 6-2 Several software programs exist for creating electronic patient care reports, allowing EMS personnel to clearly document details of each call.

Courtesy of Rhonda Hunt; Courtesy of Jim Emerton; © Inspironix, Inc. Used with permission.

locations, responding units, and crew members' names working at the incident. Patient data include the following items:

- Chief complaint
- Level of consciousness (according to the AVPU [Awake and alert, responsive to Verbal stimuli, responsive to Pain, Unresponsive] scale) or mental status
- Vital signs
- Assessment
- Patient demographics (age, sex, ethnic background)

The PCR should document your objective observations of the scene, the treatments provided, the effects of those treatments, and any changes in the patient's condition during the emergency call **FIGURE 6-3**. Your objective observations of the scene need to reflect such factors as the patient's living conditions, the MOI in a motor vehicle crash, or other concerns that you might have but do not meet the reporting criteria. Depending on the type of your transport service, you may need to differentiate the treatments between those that were scheduled, such as in a transfer transport, and those that were unexpected and became necessary because of changes in the patient's condition.

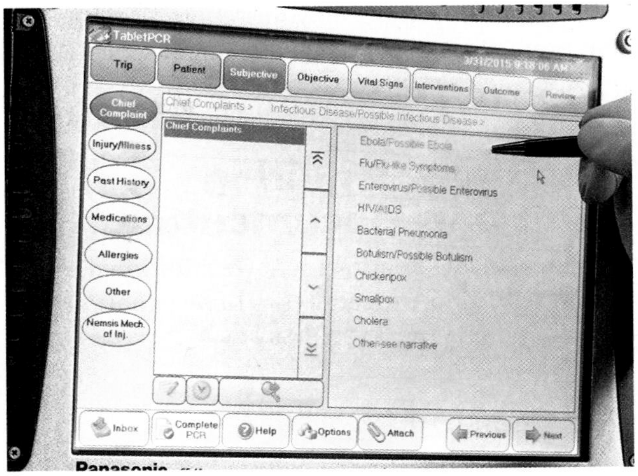

FIGURE 6-3 The minimum data set includes patient information and administrative information.

Transfer of Care

As the need for medical care continues to grow and begins to exceed the available services, EMS personnel are seeing overwhelmed EDs and often find themselves leaving patients in hallways waiting to be seen by hospital providers. In your PCR, you must be able to show in whose care you left the patient; otherwise, you could face allegations of abandonment (as discussed in Chapter 4, *Medical, Legal, and Ethical Issues*). Some agencies require signatures from physicians or nurses to verify that the patient was left with a medical professional with a higher training level. Another situation that may require you to document a transfer of care is when you hand over your patient to another agency, such as an air medical team.

Words of Wisdom

To reduce medicolegal risk, including avoiding abandonment charges, be sure your report includes to whom your handoff report was given and when it was given. Know your local policies regarding who can receive a handoff report and, if a signature is required, who is authorized to sign it.

Care Before Arrival

More emergency dispatch centers are shifting to **emergency medical dispatch (EMD)**, which is a sophisticated system that assists dispatchers in selecting appropriate units to respond to a particular call for assistance and provides callers with vital instructions until the arrival of EMS crews. You may encounter such cases in your response area. It is essential not only to obtain the information from the patient or caller about what care they have received before your arrival, but also to document such findings. For example, suppose a person calls 9-1-1 and tells the dispatcher at an EMD center that they are experiencing chest pain. After detailed questioning, the dispatcher may have the patient chew 324 mg of aspirin. If you fail to obtain information about this treatment from the patient, then that information will not be relayed to the hospital via your PCR. As a result, the patient could accidentally receive another dose of the same medication, increasing the risk of complications.

You may also encounter off-duty health care providers and/or laypeople providing emergency care prior to EMS arrival. Be sure to include their names and procedures in your report, with specific notations that this emergency medical care was provided before your arrival.

Situations Requiring Additional Documentation

Certain special situations require additional or different reporting procedures. These situations are discussed in the next sections.

Refusal of Care

Legal aspects of patient care were discussed in Chapter 4, *Medical, Legal, and Ethical Issues*, but this section covers the necessary documentation in more depth. With the increase in malpractice lawsuits, refusal of care is both one of the most challenging patient care documentation elements and one of the most important. Competent adult patients have the right to refuse medical care or to consent to treatment. Know and understand the rights of your patients. Familiarize yourself with your state's applicable laws about patient care and who has the right to refuse such care. For a person to refuse care, the decision must be based on the patient's sufficient knowledge of their situation.

Your most important job is to ensure the patient is fully informed about the current situation, the right to receive or refuse medical care, and the consequences of a refusal of care. Explain in detail the potential consequences of refusing medical care when it may be warranted, including the possibility of death. You must convey this information in a language that the person understands, and then document it on the PCR. In some agencies, the EMS provider will have a witness observe the patient's reading of the refusal statement and then ask the patient to initial the statement, followed by a signature on the refusal section of the PCR. This process is not merely geared toward getting the patient to sign the refusal section. That is, the refusal documentation should clearly show the process you went through, how it was documented, and who witnessed it.

If you must transport a patient against their wishes, it is imperative that you thoroughly document your reasoning for doing so. You must document by what means the patient was transported against their will, as well as whether the patient was restrained, coached verbally, or in some other way coerced. Consider asking medical control to talk to the patient to see if they can provide a different perspective (some services require this consultation).

YOU are the Paramedic

PART 2

The engine company that was dispatched with you arrives on scene, and they park their vehicle to ensure scene safety. Your crew directs the engine company to ensure the crashed vehicle is secure while you and your partner attempt to speak to the patient. The patient yells at you to leave him alone. Your partner taps your shoulder and asks you if you smell alcohol; you reply that you do. She also points to an empty vodka bottle on the floor of the vehicle. The patient yells, "You don't know who I am, do you? You're going to pay!" You hear a bystander say, "Isn't that Assemblyman Taylor?"

Recording Time:	0 Minutes
Appearance	Awake
Level of consciousness	Alert
Airway	Open
Breathing	Adequate
Circulation	Appears normal

3. Why is it unacceptable to document the patient's appearance as "drunk" on a PCR?

4. Would it be acceptable to document that the patient is "yelling" for the breathing description on a PCR?

Unresponsive patients may be treated under implied consent. Be familiar with your state's laws regarding the age of consent, care of minors, emancipated minors, and people with mental or cognitive impairments, such as mental illness or the effects of drug or alcohol use. Above all else, you need to confirm that you have made every reasonable effort to ensure the patient's welfare and best interests.

If the person refusing care has an obvious injury or medical condition that requires immediate medical attention, involve online medical control for further guidance and assistance. If you disagree with the refusal, your agency should have a protocol or policy in place to guide your next steps; for example, contact your supervisor, involve law enforcement, or involve medical control. If you make contact with any of those parties, document it on the PCR, including the events that transpired.

It is essential that you have a witness to the refusal process to ensure that the patient has sufficient decisional capacity to make an informed choice. If the patient refuses to sign the refusal form, the witness should also be present at that time. Document the observations of the witness, and include the patient's name and contact information as well.

Perform or attempt a complete medical history and patient assessment when possible and practical. This process includes obtaining a full set of baseline vital signs. If a patient refuses to allow such an assessment, document this refusal carefully on the PCR. Be sure to evaluate the patient's mental status using the AVPU scale. You may consider a person's mental status to be impaired if the person makes nonsensical statements or is not oriented to person, place, or time. Such an impairment can result from an injury, a medical condition (such as electrolyte imbalance or hypoglycemia), mental illness, or drug or alcohol use.

Always politely and tactfully explain to patients that they have the right to change their minds and may contact EMS again later. Such an exchange of information should be witnessed and documented with signatures. Include identifying information such as phone numbers of the witnesses involved, who frequently may be law enforcement personnel or others at the scene. Clearly document the emergency medical care that you intended to provide if the patient had not refused care. You should also document in whose care you left the patient, such as self, law enforcement personnel, or a family member.

Also, make sure that you have proposed all potential methods of care, including alternative options, even if they are not your first choice of treatment. For example, you could suggest that the patient be taken to the hospital for further care by a family member. Although that situation may not be ideal, the patient will ultimately be seen at the hospital. Always encourage transport via ambulance because a patient's condition can change at any time, and without medical personnel available to intervene immediately, the change could have serious consequences.

Sometimes, patients may agree to transport but refuse a particular procedure, such as intravenous therapy or immobilization. In such cases, handle the refusal of the specific procedure(s) as if it is a complete refusal of care. Include an explanation of any associated risks and complications of refusal, a signature from the patient acknowledging refusal of a portion of care, and a witness's signature. Ensure complete and accurate documentation **FIGURE 6-4**.

TABLE 6-2 provides a reasonable list of items to include when documenting a refusal of care in the PCR.

Documentation and Communication

During your patient assessment, consider speech pattern, gait, ability to repeat back instructions, and other observations that may have a bearing on the person's decision-making capacity.

Workplace Injuries and Illnesses

With the growing budgetary restrictions in many workplaces, a paramedic, rather than a traditional nurse, often provides medical care. According to the Occupational Safety and Health Administration (OSHA) guidelines, workplace injuries must be logged. Institutions may also have specific forms and requirements for documenting workplace injuries. Many injuries are minor, requiring only basic first aid and thus do not require an OSHA record; however, the employer may still require local documentation. When you document a workplace injury or illness, be sure to record what precautions

Patient Name: Smith, John A.()

EMS Agency Name: *eMEDS Testing/Demo Service
EMS Agency Number: 18551-DA

MD: Patient Refusal Form

Section 1: Medical Capacity

1.a. Disoriented to Person?: No

1.c. Disoriented to Time?: No

1.b. Disoriented to Place?: No

1.d. Disoriented to Situation?: No

2. Altered level of consciousness?: No

3.a. Alcohol or drug ingestion by history or exam with slurred speech?: No

3.b. Alcohol or drug ingestion by history or exam with unsteady gait?: No

4. Patient does not understand the nature of illness and potential bad outcome?: No

Section 1: At Risk Criteria

5.Adult.a. Abnormal vitals signs for adult: Pulse greater than 120 or less than 60?: No

5.Adult.b. Abnormal vitals signs for adult: systolic BP less than 90?: No

5.Adult.c. Abnormal vitals signs for adult: Respirations greater than 30 or less than 10?: No

5.Ped.a. Abnormal vitals signs for minor/pediatric: Age inappropriate HR or: Not a Minor/Pediatric

5.Ped.b. Abnormal vitals signs for minor/pediatric: Age inappropriate RR or: Not a Minor/Pediatric

5.Ped.c. Abnormal vitals signs for minor/pediatric: Age inappropriate BP?: Not a Minor/Pediatric

6. Serious chief complaint (chest pain, SOB, syncope)?: No

7. Head injury with history of loss of consciousness?: No

Incident Number: 123456

Crew Member Completing this Report: User, Demo (DemoUser653)
EMS Unit Call Sign: A391

Current Date: 05/25/2021 15:54

FIGURE 6-4 A sample refusal of care form. A competent adult patient has the right to refuse medical treatment, but it is essential that you fully inform the patient of the potential consequences.

Patient Name: Smith, John A.()

EMS Agency Name: *eMEDS Testing/Demo Service
EMS Agency Number: 18551-DA

8. Significant MOI or high suspicon of injury?: No

9. For minor/pediatric patients: ALTE, significiant past medical history, or suspected intenti: Not a Minor/Pediatric

10. Provider impression is that the patient requires hospital evaluation: Yes - Consult

Section 2: For Providers

1. Did you perform an assessment (including exam) on this patient?: Yes

If yes to #1, skip to #3

2. If unable to examine, did you attempt vital signs?:

3. Did you attempt to convince the patient or guardian to accept transport?: Yes

4. Did you contact medical direction for patient still refusing service?: Yes

Section 3: (Check All That Apply

Initial Disposition (Check all that apply): EXAM: Patient Refused; TRANSPORT: Patient Refused; TREATMENT: Patient Refused

Interventions (Check all that apply): Attempt to Convince Patient; Contact Medical Direction

Facility Contacted for Medical Direction: St Elsewhere ED

Final Disposition: EXAM: Patient Accepted; TRANSPORT: Patient Refused; TREATMENT: Patient Accepted

Section 4: MUST COMPLETE

Incident Number: 123456

Crew Member Completing this Report: User, Demo (DemoUser653)
EMS Unit Call Sign: A391

Current Date: 05/25/2021 15:54

FIGURE 6-4 *(continued)*

Patient Name: Smith, John A.()

EMS Agency Name: *eMEDS Testing/Demo Service
EMS Agency Number: 18551-DA

Provide in the patient's own words why they refused the above care/service:: Patient reports that despite the damage to his vehicle, he has only a small laceration on his finger and no other symptoms. He eventually agreed to allow EMS to evaluate him and provide a bandage for a small finger laceration on his right index finger. He agreed to follow-up with his primary doctor later today. When offered transport to the hospital, he indicated "No thanks, I will be fine." Discussed plan with Dr. Smith at St Elsewhere ED; he agrees with follow-up for laceration care.

Signatures

Incident Number: 123456

Crew Member Completing this Report: User, Demo (DemoUser653)
EMS Unit Call Sign: A391

Current Date: 05/25/2021 15:54

FIGURE 6-4 *(continued)*

TABLE 6-2 Components of a Thorough Patient Refusal Document
Evidence the patient is able to make a rational, informed decision.
Documentation of complete assessment. If the patient refuses care or does not allow a complete assessment, document that the patient did not allow for proper assessment and document whatever assessments were completed.
Discussion with the patient as to what care/transportation you would like to provide.
Discussion with the patient about what may happen if EMS is not allowed to provide care or transportation. (You should list these consequences clearly and include the possibility of severe illness/injury or death if care or transportation is refused.)
Discussion with family members/friends/bystanders to encourage the patient to allow care.
Discussion with medical direction according to the local protocol.
Discussion with the patient regarding other alternatives (eg, seeing a family physician, having a family member drive the patient to the hospital).
Discussion with the patient regarding the willingness of EMS to return if the patient changes their mind.
Signatures: Have a family member, police officer, or bystander sign the form as a witness. If the patient refuses to sign the refusal form, have a family member, police officer, or bystander sign the form verifying that the patient refused to sign.

were taken and what protective equipment was being worn by the person involved. Because companies can be fined heavily for safety violations, proper documentation is essential from both the employer's and OSHA's perspectives. Note that reporting regulations vary from state to state. Familiarize yourself with the requirements of your state. As a paramedic, you may also perform medical monitoring for hazardous materials teams, may respond to workplace injuries of other public employees, or may experience an on-the-job injury or illness yourself, which you will need to appropriately document and report to supervisors to receive workers' compensation.

Special Circumstances

The documentation requirements of some circumstances that you will encounter can be puzzling. Examples of these situations include multiple-casualty incidents (MCIs), occupational exposures, cases of alleged abuse or neglect, and instances when a physician arrives or is already present on the scene of a call. Each of these situations may require specialized forms per your state or local agency, so become familiar with these local forms of documentation and the requirements for their use.

During an MCI, the patient load can easily overwhelm providers and, in the best interest of patient care, documentation often occurs initially on triage tags. Do not wait until an MCI occurs to become familiar with triage tags. Learn where they are stored, the information needed on the tags, and situations that may warrant their use in your agency or department. Triage tags and procedures are discussed in Chapter 48, *Incident Management and Mass-Casualty Incidents*. Each emergency responder needs to complete the tags to supply as much information as possible. When the time comes to transport the patient, the ambulance crew should complete a PCR on each patient. Although the information contained in the PCR will be limited, it is still imperative to complete this report to the best of your ability.

During your work as a paramedic, you will inevitably be exposed to body fluids or other potentially toxic or infectious agents. If your barrier devices fail or do not offer enough protection, then complete an occupational exposure report. In states where it is now legal to use marijuana for medical or recreational purposes, some agencies consider marijuana smoke to be an occupational exposure. If you are exposed to marijuana smoke on a call, then include this information in your narrative report. Because each agency or state creates its own forms for these exposures, you must familiarize yourself with the requirements. If you treat and/or transport a coworker for an occupational exposure, complete a full PCR along with the occupational exposure form.

You may encounter additional specialized documentation when you are called to scenes of alleged neglect or abuse. Supply as much detail as possible about these circumstances, because your initial findings may later be the focus of a criminal investigation. Some providers do not document their suspicions of abuse and neglect for fear of **slander** (a false verbal statement that injures a person's good name) allegations from either the patient or the abuser. Best practice is to document your objective findings and allow the legal system to investigate and make the ultimate determination of abuse or neglect.

When a physician (from any specialty) arrives or is present on the scene of your call, the physician may have authority under the local protocol to interject with patient care and give directives. Once a physician begins care that is beyond the paramedic's scope, most protocols require that the physician accompany the patient to the hospital to avoid being accused of abandonment. When you complete your documentation of such a run, document all physicians' orders and actions.

Also document the use of mutual aid services such as helicopters, specialized rescue teams, and other agencies called in to assist with the incident. Document unusual occurrences as well, including the need to secure the patient with restraining devices for safe transport. If you summon lift assistance or a specialty vehicle for lifting a heavy patient or have an extended scene time because of a prolonged extrication, then clearly document this information to explain why something out of the ordinary occurred. If severe weather conditions delay your response, document this information as well.

Another special circumstance that requires appropriate documentation, as defined by medical control and your state laws, is drawing of a blood sample as evidence for law enforcement personnel who have a driver suspected of being under the influence in their custody. Always follow the policy of your medical director in these circumstances.

Community paramedicine programs are increasing in number across the United States. Paramedics in these programs may need to provide documentation beyond that typically included under the prehospital model. If you operate within such a program, then ensure you understand and follow your state and local guidelines.

Finally, EMS providers are increasingly being permitted to use controlled substances to treat patients. As a paramedic, you are responsible for the security and accountability of these medications, if you carry them on your unit. Most services require a double-signature system when a controlled substance is checked, used, discarded, or replaced. In your PCR, document the date and time, the amount of substance used versus the amount wasted, the patient to whom it was given, and by whom it was given, along with any specialized accountability forms your agency uses.

Completing a PCR

EMS documentation is a required and necessary element of patient care. Just as you take pride in your patient care skills, you should take pride in your documentation skills. Now that you have been given an overview of the various aspects of the PCR along with special situations to document, you will learn how to complete the PCR.

PCR Narrative

As mentioned earlier, the PCR contains both check-boxes and a narrative portion. The narrative portion should be a detailed segment explaining the specific elements of the call. It should be written in a format accepted by your agency and should be accurate and complete. Merely writing "Followed ACLS protocols" may not be sufficient documentation for your agency or medical director. Instead, record specifics of the call, such as "The patient was intubated with a 7.5 ET tube and ventilatory assistance provided with supplementary oxygen at 15 L/min. Bilateral breath sounds and chest rise confirmed ET tube placement before securing the ET tube at the mark of 22 at the teeth. The end-tidal CO_2 detector and pulse oximeter were placed immediately, and their readings were SpO_2 94% and $ETCO_2$ 35 mm Hg." (Always be sure to clarify which is which.) Also, some services require attaching a copy of the reading(s) to the documentation; you may wish to do this. **TABLE 6-3** provides guidelines on how to write the narrative portion of your report.

In the narrative section, document any medical control orders and/or medical advice that you received. In some EMS systems, you must also document items such as consultations, orders requested or received from medical control, and any refusal situations in which medical control has been consulted. Simply writing "See refusal on back" is not an effective method of patient care documentation.

Many methods for narrative documentation exist, but your EMS agency or medical director may prefer a specific method to be used when documenting PCRs. Be familiar with the approved methods and all required elements for report writing for your agency. Examples of narrative writing styles for PCRs include the following options:

- **Chronological order.** This method allows you to explain the call in a story format from start (time of the initial dispatch) to finish (completion of the call) **FIGURE 6-5**.
- **SOAP method**: Subjective information, Objective information, Assessment, and Plan (for treatment). This simple and logical method allows you to document various aspects of the patient care encounter **FIGURE 6-6**.
- **CHARTE method**: Chief complaint, History (this includes the history of the event as well as the patient's medical history), Assessment, Treatment, Transport, and Exceptions. This approach is similar to the SOAP method, but allows you to break down the narrative into

YOU are the Paramedic

PART 3

You and your partner attempt to reason with the patient, asking him to allow you to assess for injuries. The patient tries to push you away and says in a slurred voice, "Keep your hands off me! I have rights!" You contact your dispatcher to confirm that law enforcement officers are en route to your location.

Recording Time: 5 Minutes	
Respirations	Unable to measure; appear adequate, approximately 20 to 24 breaths/min
Pulse	Unable to measure
Skin	Unable to measure; appears normal color
Blood pressure	Unable to measure
Oxygen saturation (SpO_2)	Unable to measure
Pupils	Unable to measure

5. How should you document that the patient has directed you to "keep your hands off," as well as account for your inability to obtain the patient's vital signs?

6. Does this patient have the right to refuse treatment?

TABLE 6-3 How to Write a Narrative

Topic	Items to Include
Standard precautions	State which precautions you used and why.
Scene safety	Did you have to make your scene safe? If so, state what you did and why you did it. Did this step create a delay in patient care?
MOI/NOI	Simply state. Example: "motor vehicle crash" or "difficulty breathing."
Number of patients	Record only when more than one patient is present. Example: "This is patient 2 of 3."
Additional resources	Did you call for help? If so, then state why, at what time, and what time the help arrived. Was transport delayed?
Cervical spine	State whether you applied manual stabilization or spinal motion restriction. You may want to include the reason why. Example: "Because of significant MOI . . ."
Initial general impression	Simply state, if not already documented on the PCR.
LOC	Report LOC, any changes in LOC, and at what time changes occurred.
Chief complaint	Note and quote pertinent statements made by the patient and/or bystanders, including any pertinent negatives. Example: "Patient denies chest pain . . ."
Life threats	List all interventions and how the patient responded. Example: "Assisted ventilations with bag-mask and oxygen (15 L/min) at 20 breaths/min with no change in LOC."
ABCDE	Document what you found, and any interventions performed.
Oxygen	Record whether you administered oxygen, how you applied it, and how much you administered.
Primary survey, patient history, secondary assessment, or reassessment	State the type of assessment you used and any pertinent findings. Example: "Secondary assessment revealed unequal pupils, crepitus to right ribs, and an apparent closed fracture of the left tibia." Note the time each assessment was made and the findings.
SAMPLE/OPQRST	Note and quote any pertinent answers.
Vital signs	Record the times when you took the patient's vital signs and the findings. (Your service may want you to record vital signs in the narrative portion, as well as other places in the PCR.)
Medical direction	Quote any orders given to you by medical control, and state who gave them.
Management of secondary injuries/treat for shock	Report all interventions, at what time they were completed, and how the patient responded.

Abbreviations: ABCDE, Airway, Breathing, Circulation, Disability, and Exposure; LOC, level of consciousness; MOI, mechanism of injury; NOI, nature of illness; OPQRST, Onset, Provocation/palliation, Quality, Region/radiation, Severity, Timing; PCR, patient care report; SAMPLE, Signs and symptoms, Allergies, Medications, Past pertinent medical history, Last oral intake, Events leading up to the illness or injury

Reprinted with permission. Courtesy of Jay C. Keefauver.

logical sections similar to those used in the patient assessment **FIGURE 6-7**.

- **Body systems/parts approach.** In this format, your assessment of each body system is documented from head to toe. This method of report writing may be challenging to apply in EMS and may be too time-consuming for paramedics.

Regardless of which style of narrative report writing you and your service agree on, make sure that you follow it routinely. If you switch from one format to another or attempt to change formats during report writing, then you may forget certain elements or essential details.

Proper grammar and spelling are essential when writing reports. Consider carrying a pocket

Squad called to residence for ill man. On arrival found an alert and oriented 78 yo man sitting on the couch reporting CP. Pt sts this began approximately 30 min prior when he was mowing the lawn. Pt denies any radiation of the pain and rates it at a "7" out of 10 on pain scale. Pt has a known cardiac history with an MI 2 years prior. Pt is compliant with all meds as listed above. Pt denies any SOB or N/V with this episode. V/S stable, lungs CTA, Spo_2 93% RA, Skin pale/warm/dry to touch, PERRLA 4 mm, GCS 15. Pt placed on O_2 @ 15 L/min via NRB. Monitor showed RSR @ 88 bpm without ectopy.
IV of NS was established in L AC with 18 g @ TKO (medic 785). 4 × 81 mg ASA were given PO @ 1501 (medic 785). Pt was given 1 SL 0.4 mg nitro @ 1503 with relief down to a "4" on scale (medic 785). V/S still stable. Secondary exam showed negative new findings. Med control contacted with negative orders. Left pt in care of ED staff with report in room 7.

FIGURE 6-5 Example of a narrative written in chronological order.

Note: In this example, "(medic 785)" identifies which provider performed the intervention. The provider's initials may also be used. It is important to document who performed the procedure, because the person who is writing the narrative may not have been the crew member who performed the procedure or administered the medication.

(S) Called to scene for 78 yo man complaining of chest pain. Pt states pain began approximately 30 min prior to arrival when he was mowing the lawn. Pt denies any radiation of pain. States pain is "7" out of 10 on pain scale. Pt has known cardiac hx with an MI 2 yrs prior. Pt denies SOB or N/V. Pt has no allergies and is compliant with all meds listed above.

(O) U/A found Pt sitting on the couch. Pt alert and oriented with NARD and strong radial pulse. Pt calm and cooperative. Skin: Pale/warm/dry. Pupils PERRLA 4 mm, GSC 15. Lungs CTA. No noted JVD. Abd soft and nontender. PMS × 4. Secondary exam unremarkable.

(A) Possible MI.

(P) Primary, secondary Hx, V/S as listed above. Assisted pt to cot. Cardiac monitor: showed RSR @ 88 bpm without ectopy. IV: NS 18 g in L AC @ TKO (BW); Spo_2 93% RA, O_2 @ 15 L/min via NRB 100%; 4 × 81 mg ASA given PO, 1 SL 0.4 mg nitro (BW) pain down to "4". Transported to ______. Pt care transferred to ED with report.

FIGURE 6-6 Example of a narrative written with the SOAP method.

(C) 78 yo man complaining of chest pain without radiation. Pt sts pain is a "7" out of 10 on pain scale.

(H) Pt has a known cardiac history with an MI 2 years prior.

(A) Pt denies any SOB or nausea/vomiting with this episode. Vital signs stable, lungs clear to auscultation, Spo_2 93% RA, skin pale/warm/dry to touch, PERRLA 4 mm, GCS 15. Monitor showed RSR @ 88 bpm without ectopy.

(R) Pt placed on O_2 @ 15 L/min via NRB. IV of NS was established in L AC with 18 g @ TKO (medic 785). 4 × 81 mg ASA were given PO @ 1501 (medic 785). Pt was given 1 SL 0.4 mg nitro @ 1503 (medic 785).

(T) Pt improved during transport, pain went down to a "4" on the scale, V/S remained stable, and patient care was transferred to ED staff.

(E) None.

FIGURE 6-7 Example of a narrative written with the CHARTE method.

guide, reference manual, or medical terminology text or using an app on your smartphone to avoid spelling errors.

When you write your PCR, be sure to document any **pertinent negatives**—a record of negative findings that warrant no medical care or intervention but indicate that a thorough exam and history were performed. For example, your narrative might say, "The patient denies any shortness of breath with his chest pain, and denies any radiation of the chest pain to other parts of the body." This statement indicates that you obtained the information about chest pain and inquired about shortness of breath and radiation of the pain.

The inclusion of pertinent spoken accounts given by your patient and others on scene may be essential to the continuum of patient care. If you reference any spoken accounts made by the patient or others in your PCR, then be sure to indicate who made the statement and place exact words in quotation marks. Pertinent spoken accounts may include statements about the patient's behavior, MOI, and safety-related information such as weapons use. It can also be helpful to list information that may prove useful to criminal investigators as part of their investigation, disposition of valuables, admissions of suicidal intentions made by a patient, and any first aid interventions provided by bystanders before EMS arrival.

Elements of a Properly Written PCR

The accuracy of documentation depends on the completeness and precision of the report. You must provide all information, such as incident times and narrative information. Complete all sections of the report, even if a section did not apply to the call. For example, if your PCR contains checkboxes for specific information for cardiac arrest calls but the call you are documenting did not involve a cardiac arrest, then note that fact on the report in a manner approved by your agency. Merely leaving the checkboxes blank may raise questions about the completeness of the report.

When you handwrite a report, write legibly in ink. The color of ink used may be determined by your EMS agency. Standard ink colors—black and blue—are most commonly selected for this purpose. Handwriting, especially in the report's narrative portion, needs to be neat and easily read by others. In addition, take great care not to contaminate your written reports with any liquids found in the field. Place all your completed reports in a secure location agreed on by you and your partner that protects the patient's privacy, until they can be secured in the proper place at your EMS agency office or headquarters.

The PCR needs to be timely, even in EMS systems with high call volumes. If you respond to multiple calls without accurately completing PCRs before proceeding to the next call, then you may forget details and/or omit important information. Even worse, you may record inaccurate information. Your EMS agency should allow you a reasonable amount of time to complete your reports, replenish supplies, and clean and disinfect the vehicle before returning it to service. Many paramedics use assessment cards during their calls to take notes, and use the electrocardiographic (ECG) monitor to note times and vital signs. They then complete the PCR after the call, rather than on the bumpy ride to the ED. Set aside time at the hospital to neatly complete all documentation.

If you do not have enough time to complete the full PCR while at the hospital, then you must still leave a written record with the patient. In these cases, most EMS systems will have a drop report or transfer report **FIGURE 6-8**. These single-page, abbreviated forms are used as a memory aid during an EMS call. If you cannot remain at the hospital to complete the PCR, then copy these documents and leave them with the nurse or physician. Some states require that copies of written reports (or electronic records) be supplied to the receiving facility or hospital within a specific time frame, such as 24 hours. Know the applicable laws and requirements of your state and EMS system. In some systems, EMS providers fax the completed form to the ED because the hospital has a secure fax location that meets HIPAA requirements.

As mentioned previously, all PCRs should be free of jargon, slang, and personal opinions. Be sure that your documentation is not libelous. **Libel** is a false statement in written form that could be harmful to a person's current or future reputation. Document true and accurate statements only. If your narrative includes quotes from bystanders or statements made by the patient, then be sure to indicate who made them and place the exact words in quotation marks on the report.

Carefully review all reports before submitting them to the receiving medical facility and to your EMS agency. Always review your PCR for completeness, accuracy, and proper grammar, spelling, medical terminology, and abbreviations. Your goal is to file a complete, accurate, professional, and legible report.

Too often, the importance of report writing and documentation in EMS is ignored. Always

Maryland Institute for Emergency Medical Services Systems

Short Form Patient Information Sheet

Jurisdiction: ______ **Date:** ______
Incident # ______ **Time Arrived at Hospital:** ______
Unit #: ______
Age: ______ **DOB:** ______ **Wt:** ______ **Kg** **Gender:** ☐M ☐F
Priority: ☐ 1 ☐ 2 ☐ 3 ☐ 4 **Trauma Category:** ☐ A ☐ B ☐ C ☐ D
Patient's Name: ______
Patient's Address: ______
City: ______ **State:** ______
Point of Contact: ______ **Phone Number:** ______
Chief Complaint: ______
Time of Onset: ______ **Past Medical History: (DNR/MOLST ☐ A1 ☐ A2 ☐ B)**
Cardiac ☐ CHF ☐ Hypertension ☐ Seizure ☐ Diabetes ☐ COPD ☐ Asthma ☐
Other: ______
Current Meds: ______
Allergies: Latex ☐ Penicillin/Ceph ☐ Sulfa ☐ Other: ______

Assessments

Vitals	**Respiration** (Left / Right)	**Skin**	**GCS**
Time: ______	☐ Clear ☐	☐ Warm	Eyes (4): ______
Temperature ______	☐ Rales ☐	☐ Hot	Motor (6): ______
B/P: ______ / ______	☐ Labored ☐	☐ Cool	Verbal (5): ______
Pulse: ______	☐ Stridor ☐	☐ Dry	**TOTAL:** ______
Respirations: ______	☐ Rhonchi ☐	☐ Clammy	**Pupils**
SAO2: ______ %	☐ Wheezes ☐	☐ Diaphoretic	☐ PERRL
Capnography: ______	☐ Decreased ☐	☐ Cyanotic	☐ Unequal
Carbon Monoxide: ______	☐ Agonal ☐		☐ Fixed/Dilated
Repeat Vitals	☐ Absent ☐		**Neuro**
Time: ______	**Pulse**		☐ A ☐ V
B/P: ______ / ______	☐ Regular ☐ Irregular		☐ P ☐ U
Pulse: ______	☐ JVD ☐ Peripheral Edema		
Respirations: ______	Cap Refill: ______ seconds		
SAO2: ______ %			
Capnography: ______			
Carbon Monoxide: ______			

Assessment

Procedures

Cardiac Rhythm:	**Cincinnati Stroke Scale** *Normal/Abnormal*
Perform 12 Lead Yes ☐ No ☐ 12	Facial Droop Normal ☐ Abnormal ☐
Lead Transmit Yes ☐ No ☐	Arm Drift Normal ☐ Abnormal ☐
Glucometer:	Speech Normal ☐ Abnormal ☐
	Last Known Well Time/Date: ______
☐ IV1 ☐ IV2 Time Started ______	**Los Angeles Motor Scale (LAMS)**
☐ IO ☐ EJ	*Facial Droop*: Absent 0, Present 1 — *Grip Strength*: Normal 0, Weak Grip 1, No Grip 2
Amount Infused:	*Arm Drift*: Absent 0, Drifts Down 1, Falls Rapidly 2 — Score: ______
CPR Performed Yes ☐ No ☐	**Oxygen**
ROSC Yes ☐ No ☐	☐ NRB Mask ☐ King Airway
Induced Hypothermia Yes ☐ No ☐	☐ Nasal Cannula ☐ CPAP
	☐ NPA/OPA ☐ NDT
	☐ BVM ☐ Ventilator
	☐ ET ☐ NT ☐ NGT
	☐ Easy Tube

Treatment:

Jurisdictional Additions:

Print Clinician Name: ______

rev. 05.05.2021

FIGURE 6-8 Prehospital notepad/drop report (transfer report).

remember that the report that you write reflects directly on you. Remember, your call is incomplete until you have completed the documentation process.

Documentation and Communication

Remember to document problems encountered when responding to or during the call (eg, an infectious disease exposure, a delayed response, a conflict at the scene with family or other response agencies, an MCI, an injury to an EMS provider that happened while providing care to the patient).

Consequences of Poor Documentation

Inappropriate, inaccurate, and insufficient documentation can adversely affect the quality of care received by patients after their arrival at the hospital. For example, imagine that you administered a breathing treatment en route to the hospital but forgot to document the medication, procedure, and administration time. The hospital would not be aware of the administered medication, and the patient could be inappropriately treated because you failed to document the care you provided. By documenting what the patient or family members tell you and your findings from examining the patient, you enhance patient care quality. For example, do not forget to document the specific time that a suspected stroke patient was last seen to be "normal" by family members; this information is vital in determining the window of time in which treatment using fibrinolytics may be appropriate. As another example, if hospital personnel know that a patient has a seizure disorder or that a patient who has had transient ischemic attacks in the past had symptoms of stroke en route to the hospital, then they can more effectively plan for proper care.

As mentioned previously, the legal implications of documentation can be significant. Poorly written, inaccurate, or illegible reports might lead a judge or jury to decide in the plaintiff's favor if litigation arises after the call. Conversely, a lawyer may decide not to pursue a case when the documentation reveals a correctly written and well-documented report.

The following is an example that illustrates the importance of neat and accurate documentation. The EMS agency in a town was being sued for allegedly providing inappropriate care to a patient with a spine injury. During the discovery phase of the lawsuit, the town's attorney decided to settle the case out of court based on the fact that the PCR was sloppy (because sloppy documentation implies sloppy care) and incomplete (because the providers did not clearly document whether distal pulses and motor and sensory functions were assessed *before and after* patient immobilization).

Another example of poor documentation occurred in a case where a 15-year-old boy was involved in a motor vehicle crash and the paramedic crew had to secure his airway because of head trauma. The patient was transferred to a trauma center, where the ED physician found the patient to be extubated. The patient survived but sustained a significant brain injury. The family sued the paramedic crew, claiming that their son experienced hypoxic brain damage caused by the failed intubation, rather than by the significant head trauma. The crew testified that they had used continuous capnography to confirm a secured airway throughout transport, but failed to document these readings in their narrative. Although it was likely that the extubation occurred while the patient was being moved to the exam bed in the ED, the crew's failure to document their readings resulted in a favorable

YOU are the Paramedic

PART 4

When law enforcement officers arrive on scene, the patient yells, "Great! Officers, arrest these people. They're harassing me!" One officer tells the patient to relax and do what the EMS crew asks, saying, "All they are trying to do is make sure you're OK." The officer asks the patient, "Have you been drinking today?" The patient replies, "I only had a few at lunch . . . that's all. I'm just fine." The officer asks for, and receives, the patient's driver's license. He says to the patient, "I'm sure you are aware, Assemblyman Taylor, that there are laws you have to obey and it would look much better to your constituents if you cooperated. Going to the hospital in an ambulance is much better than in a police car." The patient agrees, and you can finally assess the patient and prepare for transport.

Recording Time: 15 Minutes	
Respirations	16 breaths/min with adequate tidal volume
Pulse	100 beats/min, strong and regular
Skin	Warm, dry, normal color
Blood pressure	130/80 mm Hg
Oxygen saturation (Spo_2)	97% on ambient air
Pupils	Pupils Equal, Round, and Reactive to Light and Accommodation (PERRLA)

7. Is it essential to document the interaction between the patient and law enforcement officers when no patient care is involved?

8. What is the legal basis for determining whether a patient is competent to refuse care?

ruling for the family. The agency lost a significant monetary amount as a result.

Poor documentation skills can also affect your reputation as a paramedic. Poorly written, inappropriate, or inaccurate reports might make others question the care you provided. In contrast, a well-written report can suggest organizational skills, knowledge of patient conditions and needs, and respect for organizational policies and procedures. Part of being a good paramedic is completing the paperwork and reports as required. If you find it difficult to write reports, then take additional classes on this subject or study report writing skills to enhance your abilities. Your agency or service might have an educational program to assist you with such education and training.

Errors and Falsification

Although you should make every attempt to create an accurate and legible initial report, on some occasions it may be necessary to revise or correct your initial PCR. If a report must be revised or corrected, then note the revised report's date and time and the purpose for writing the revision or making the correction. Never discard or destroy the original PCR.

Only the person who wrote the original report can revise it. Additions or notations added by others after completing the report may raise questions about the authenticity of the report and your agency's confidentiality practices. Routine administrative report handling and reviews are necessary for entering information into computer databases, billing for services, and quality assurance monitoring. At no time should administrative activities involve altering or rewriting the report or portions of it.

If you make an error when handwriting your report, place a single horizontal line through the error and initial and date the line, preferably in a different color ink. Write the corrected information next to it **FIGURE 6-9**. Do not erase information, scribble through errors, or use correction fluid or tape. Remember, the PCR is a legal document.

If you discover an error after submitting an ePCR, most systems will allow for amendments but will prevent erasure in a completed document. Refer to the operating directions for instructions on how to amend the original ePCR. If it is not possible to electronically change the report, then print a copy of the ePCR and follow the same procedure used for a written document. When it is possible to make corrections electronically, keep in mind that the system records a so-called change history, even though the end product does not show it. Therefore, once a run has been posted, you must document

FIGURE 6-9 If you make a mistake while handwriting your report, the proper way to correct it is to draw a single horizontal line through the error, initial it, and write the correct information next to it.

SAFETY

In 1999, the Institute of Medicine's (IOM) *To Err Is Human* report noted that almost 100,000 Americans die each year secondary to medical errors, making this the eighth leading cause of death in the United States. The major revelation in this report was that failures or errors in care were frequently not results of individual behavior or decisions, but rather were often related to intrinsic processes of care in the health care system. Thus, the IOM suggested, efforts to improve safety should focus on improving process errors rather than targeting people. Slowly, over time, the idea of "system failure" rather than "human error" has gained credence. Organizations such as the National Quality Forum, the Institute for Healthcare Improvement, the Agency for Healthcare Research and Quality, and others are invested in decreasing the frequency of medical errors. The critical nature of their efforts is clear: An analysis published in 2016 suggests that medical errors may now be the third leading cause of death, annually claiming some 251,000 lives in the United States.[1]

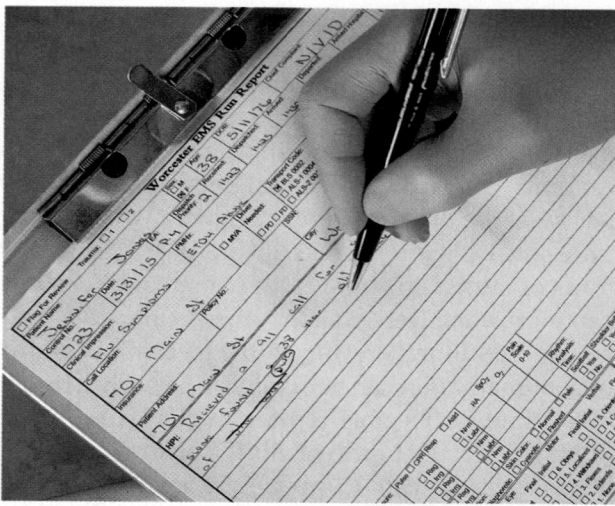

SAFETY

It is widely believed that near-miss events are subtsantially underreported. A **near miss** is an unplanned event that did not cause an injury, illness, or damage, but had the potential to do so. Often staff will not report these events for fear of discipline, a perceived lack of support or caring by supervisors, or belief that it is unnecessary to report the incident if no patient harm occurred. In fact, near-miss events are among the most important to report because they allow the organization to analyze its processes and improve safety. Moreover, talking about near misses can be easier for staff because there are fewer liability concerns when no one was actually harmed.

SAFETY

The EMS Voluntary Event Notification Tool (EVENT) is an anonymous, nonpunitive, and confidential system launched by the National Association of Emergency Medical Technicians (NAEMT) in 2012. Its goal is to identify flawed processes and systems that require improvement.

why any amendments to an ePCR were made. Most ePCR systems keep a record of who made an alteration to the report and when it was made.

If you forgot to include important information, then you may need to write an addendum to your original report. You may also need to write an addendum if you are asked to write statements of events related to quality assurance or risk management and to answer complaints. In your addendum, note that it was added to your original report and explain the reason for the late entry. Include the date of entry, the time of entry, and your signature.

Supplemental narratives may also be needed if additional information becomes available after the original report has been written. Document such reports with the date, the time, the reason for the added information, and your signature. Some EMS agencies use a supplemental report to write lengthy information when the original report's space is limited. Follow the policies of your service for using supplemental reports and the procedures for writing them. Regardless of when the supplemental reports are added, they should be attached in some way to the original report for record-keeping purposes.

As part of your role, you may be required to obtain and document billing information for the service(s) provided. It is critical that you understand the sensitive and confidential nature of such information and the laws and regulations pertaining to billing and documentation security under HIPAA. EMS agencies should take care not to add information provided by billing clerks or others after the report has been submitted, as doing so might violate local, state, or federal laws. If you have additional information to document after handing in the form, follow your agency's policy regarding whether a supplementary form is needed. Always be honest and thorough in your documentation process.

Lost reports are associated with substantial legal implications for paramedics, EMS agencies and departments, and medical directors. Remember, you are responsible for ensuring that your reports are completed and turned in as required by policy or procedure. (Do not keep copies of your reports. If you need to document numbers of procedures or ages of patients for your paramedic internship, follow your training center's specific policy.) If lost reports are an ongoing concern for an agency or provider, then they should take steps to correct the problem. Attempting to recreate PCRs is irresponsible, and sometimes even illegal. Also, record keeping may be a legal requirement in your state, and the time allowed for the submission of reports may be specified in state regulations.

Documentation and Communication

Reports should be written such that professionals at all levels who will have access to your report, whether your medical director or the administrative office clerk billing for the service provided, can read them and understand exactly what transpired on the EMS call. If your report does not paint a clear picture of what happened, then it is not written well. Remember, your report is a reflection of your actions and your professionalism.

Documenting Incident Times

Accurate timekeeping is essential to all EMS operations. The role of timekeeper for the overall incident falls to dispatchers. When it comes to the on-scene procedures, however, you must keep track of time during your documentation. Compare your times with those of the dispatcher to ensure accuracy and proper timekeeping, and ensure that your and your dispatcher's clocks are synchronized. For example, if your ECG monitor reports or documentation times are not synchronized with those of the dispatcher, then this discrepancy could create a controversy in the courtroom.

In particular, it is crucial that you track and document the following incident times:

1. **Time of call.** Time when the call for help is placed or requested.
2. **Time of dispatch.** Time when call is toned or alerted for a response.
3. **Time of arrival at the scene.** Time when EMS unit arrives on scene.
4. **Time with patient.** Time recorded when patient contact is made, which may not be the same as time of arrival. For example, when responding to a patient on the 17th floor of a high-rise building, you should include the time it takes to physically get to the patient.
5. **Time of medication administration.** Time when medications are administered for adherence to protocols and patient's response. Example: 1 × 0.4 mg of nitroglycerin was given SL at 1804 without relief [medic 785].
6. **Time of medical procedure.** Time when a procedure is conducted on the patient, such as when vital signs are taken, when a patient is intubated, or when a child is delivered. Example: Pt was intubated with a 7.5 Fr ET tube with confirmation of absent epigastric sounds, clear bilateral lung sounds in all fields, and a waveform capnography reading of 35 mm Hg at 1807 by medic 785.
7. **Time of departure from scene.** Time recorded when EMS unit leaves the scene.
8. **Time of arrival at medical facility.** Time when arriving at the medical facility (if a patient is transported).
9. **Time of transfer of care.** Time when care was transferred to another health care professional at the receiving facility (if a patient is transported).
10. **Time back in service.** Time when EMS unit and crew are ready for return to service.

It is standard procedure to use 24-hour (military) time in EMS documentation. This format ensures that each time is unique; for example, 1:00 AM cannot be confused with 1:00 PM. Military times are shown in **TABLE 6-4**.

TABLE 6-4 Military Time

Standard Time	Military Time	Standard Time	Military Time
Midnight	0000	Noon	1200
1:00 AM	0100	1:00 PM	1300
2:00 AM	0200	2:00 PM	1400
3:00 AM	0300	3:00 PM	1500
4:00 AM	0400	4:00 PM	1600
5:00 AM	0500	5:00 PM	1700
6:00 AM	0600	6:00 PM	1800
7:00 AM	0700	7:00 PM	1900
8:00 AM	0800	8:00 PM	2000
9:00 AM	0900	9:00 PM	2100
10:00 AM	1000	10:00 PM	2200
11:00 AM	1100	11:00 PM	2300

YOU are the Paramedic SUMMARY

1. What is your first consideration in regard to this patient?

The patient is not well enough to stand up when he attempts to exit the vehicle under his own power and appears to have inadequate balance. At this point, you do not know whether the patient has been drinking. The patient's behavior could potentially result from medical conditions such as diabetes, an allergic reaction, or cardiac insufficiency. Trauma may also be present. The patient may have struck his head, which could be affecting his balance. He may also have something as simple as a foot injury that is painful to stand on. Slurred speech may be caused by loose teeth or dentures from the crash. Do not assume a patient has been drinking. You must obtain more information to make the determination.

2. What is your first consideration in regard to the scene?

Although the vehicle's visible damage appears to be minor, hazards ranging from leaking fluids to sharp, torn metal may still be present. Because of these potential hazards, you must wear personal protective equipment to ensure your safety, even if the scene initially appears to be safe. The county courthouse would be a busy place at 1300 hours on a weekday, and you should be concerned with traffic control as well as crowd control. Ensure that law enforcement personnel have been dispatched to the incident.

3. Why is it unacceptable to document the patient's appearance as "drunk" on a PCR?

Document only the facts. Do not describe the situation according to your first suspicions, such as describing the patient as "Awake and appears drunk." Subjective statements such as this may come back to haunt you in a courtroom as you try to define how you determined the patient was "drunk." Include objective findings, such as "has an altered mental status" or "smells of alcohol." Perform a thorough assessment before determining whether a patient is intoxicated.

4. Would it be acceptable to document that the patient is "yelling" for the breathing description on a PCR?

The patient is obviously breathing because he is attempting to extricate himself from the vehicle. You do not have the other points of direct assessment to determine respiratory rate, rhythm, and quality. You are directly witnessing the patient yelling, which is an accurate description of your initial observation, so you could document this.

5. How should you document that the patient has directed you to "keep your hands off," as well as account for your inability to obtain the patient's vital signs?

Use the patient's own words as much as possible. It would be acceptable to write, "When attempting to approach the patient to begin an assessment, the patient stated, 'Keep your hands off of me.' We were unable to assess pulse, respiration, blood pressure, pupils, Spo_2 level, or skin signs other than visually until after the intervention of law enforcement." Review Chapter 4, *Medical, Legal, and Ethical Issues*, for information on the concepts of patient consent and refusal.

6. Does this patient have the right to refuse treatment?

The patient is exhibiting signs associated with being intoxicated. The patient told the officer that he had had a few drinks at lunch. You also saw an empty bottle of alcohol on the floor of the vehicle. Because the patient's decision-making ability has been impaired, you should not accept a refusal request. You also need to further assess the patient's mental status (orientation to person, place, and time, and observations such as speech and gait).

7. Is it important to document the interaction between the patient and law enforcement officers when no patient care involved?

You must document the interaction between the law enforcement officer and the patient. State laws usually allow officers to detain people if they are a "danger to themselves or others." Review the rights of law enforcement officers in relation to patients for your area. In this case, the officer appealed to the patient's sense of self to convince him of the better of two courses of action, so detaining the patient was not necessary. When you document an interaction between law enforcement personnel and a patient, make sure to document the officer's name, badge number, and agency on your form. This information will help you and your agency if you should need more information on the call.

YOU are the Paramedic SUMMARY continued

8. What is the legal basis for determining whether a patient is competent to refuse care?

As a paramedic, you should be familiar with the laws of your state regarding the age of consent, care of minors, emancipated minors, and people with mental or cognitive impairments, such as mental illness or the effects of drug or alcohol use. Above all else, you need to ensure that every reasonable effort has been made for the patient's welfare and best interests. Do not assume the patient is "just drunk," and always provide the highest level of care.

EMS Patient Care Report (PCR)

Date: 06-01-22	**Incident No.:** 890	**Nature of Call:** MVC		**Location:** 200 First Street	
Dispatched: 1300	**En Route:** 1301	**At Scene:** 1305	**Transport:** 1335	**At Hospital:** 1345	**In Service:** 1355

Patient Information

Age: 60 **Sex:** M **Weight (in kg [lb]):** 113 kg (250 lb)	**Allergies:** NKDA **Medications:** None **Past Medical History:** None **Chief Complaint:** MVC

Vital Signs

Time: 1320	**BP:** 130/80	**Pulse:** 100	**Respirations:** 16	**Spo_2:** 97%
Time:	**BP:**	**Pulse:**	**Respirations:**	**Spo_2:**
Time:	**BP:**	**Pulse:**	**Respirations:**	**Spo_2:**

EMS Treatment (circle all that apply)

Oxygen @ _____ L/min via (circle one): **NC NRM Bag-mask device**		**Assisted Ventilation**	**Airway Adjunct**	**CPR**
Defibrillation	**Bleeding Control**	**Bandaging**	**Splinting**	**Other:**

Narrative

Arrived on scene to find a single-vehicle collision involving a pole in front of the county courthouse. On exiting our unit, we witnessed a man open the driver's door of the vehicle involved in the crash and attempt to exit the vehicle without assistance. He could not keep his balance and sat back down on the driver's seat. Once we approached the vehicle, we determined that the airbag system had deployed on impact. There was minimal visible damage to the front of the vehicle. Pt contact was made with a 60 yo male who was awake but disoriented. When attempting assessment of pt's BP, pulse, respiration, and Spo_2 level, the pt, in slurred speech, stated, "I need my lawyer" and "Keep your hands off me." The pt exhibited signs associated with being intoxicated. Open empty vodka bottle was visible on the floor of the vehicle. Confirmed that law enforcement was en route. Officer B. D. Smith, Badge 1345, Downtown Police Dept, and Officer R. H. Jenkins, Badge 1429, also from Downtown, arrived to assist. Officer Smith convinced the pt to allow our assessment, treatment, immobilization, and transport without further incident. This accounts for the initial delay in obtaining vital signs on this pt. Pt was cooperative and his condition remained unchanged during transport. V/S stable as listed, Spo_2 97% RA, lungs CTA, skin normal color/warm/dry to touch, PERRLA. Primary survey and secondary assessment findings were unremarkable. Downtown Hospital med control was contacted with negative orders. Pt was transported and verbal report given to Shelley RN on pt transfer.

End of report

Prep Kit

Ready for Review

- For each EMS call, you must complete a formal written report before leaving the hospital. This action is a vital part of providing emergency medical care and ensuring the continuity of patient care. This information guarantees the proper transfer of responsibility, complies with health departments and law enforcement agencies' requirements, and fulfills administrative needs.
- Your written or electronic patient care report (PCR) serves as a legal record. It should be complete, well written, legible, and professional.
- Your report may be used in legal proceedings against you or someone else, and it is the only record of the care you provided and why.
- When you document what a patient said, use the patient's actual words and enclose them in quotation marks.
- Billing and administration are significant reasons why your PCR needs to be accurate and complete. Be sure to document all procedures performed, and obtain the appropriate medical necessity signature (where required).
- The PCR may be handwritten or electronically written. Either way, it will include a checklist and a narrative portion. The report should be objective, accurate, and neat; this reflects good patient care.
- If a patient refuses care, then ensure that you have obtained vital signs and a complete history, fully inform the patient of the situation, involve medical control if needed, and thoroughly document the refusal of care. Also document in whose care the patient was left.
- Special situations that may require filling out different or additional forms include injuries that occur in the workplace, mass-casualty incidents, exposure to potentially infectious diseases, cases that involve alleged abuse or neglect, transfer of care to an on-scene physician, interfacility transports, calls involving controlled substances, cancelled emergency calls, and calls involving other agencies. Reporting regulations vary from state to state, and you should familiarize yourself with your state's requirements.
- Many methods exist for recording the narrative in your PCR. Options include the chronological method, the SOAP method, the CHARTE method, and the body systems approach.
- The PCR needs to be filled out promptly. Make sure to complete it immediately after the call.
- If you must revise or correct your PCR, note the date, time, and purpose of the correction. Use your system's protocol for amending electronic reports. If you must correct a handwritten report, then place a single, horizontal line through the error and write the correct information next to it. Write down what did or did not happen and the steps that were taken to correct the situation.
- Inaccurate or insufficient documentation could lead to subsequent health care providers providing inappropriate care to the patient. It could also be detrimental for you if a lawsuit is initiated and negatively affect your reputation.
- Accurate timekeeping is essential to all EMS operations. The use of 24-hour time (military time) is standard in EMS documentation.

Prep Kit continued

Vital Vocabulary

CHARTE method A narrative writing method that allows the narrative to be broken down into logical sections similar to the steps of the patient assessment; components include chief complaint, history (ie, history of the event as well as patient medical history), assessment, treatment, transport, and exceptions.

double documentation The act of documenting the care and treatment provided at an incident more than once, which increases the risk of errors and inconsistencies.

emergency medical dispatch (EMD) A system that assists dispatchers in selecting appropriate units to respond to a particular call for assistance and provides callers with vital instructions until the arrival of EMS crews.

libel A false statement in written form that could be harmful to a person's current or future reputation.

medical necessity A standard used by Medicare to determine whether a patient's condition requires ambulance transport in a particular situation.

minimum data set The mandatory clinical assessment standard information that must be documented on every emergency call, as determined by Medicare and Medicaid, and per the National Highway Traffic Safety Administration for the purpose of informing the national data system.

near miss An unplanned event that did not cause an injury, illness, or damage, but had the potential to do so.

objective information Information that is observable and measurable, such as a patient's blood pressure.

patient care report (PCR) A legal document used to record all patient care activities during an incident; a handwritten or electronic report that describes the nature of the patient's injuries or illness at the scene and the treatment provided; also known as the prehospital care report.

pertinent negatives A record of negative findings that warrant no medical care or intervention, but which show evidence of the thoroughness of the patient exam and history.

slander A false verbal statement that injures a person's good name.

SOAP method A narrative writing method in which information is organized into four categories: Subjective information, Objective information, Assessment, and Plan (for treatment).

subjective information Information that is obtained from the patient but cannot be seen, such as the symptoms a patient describes.

Reference

1. Makary MA, Daniel M. Medical error—the third leading cause of death in the US. *BMJ* 2016;353:i2139.

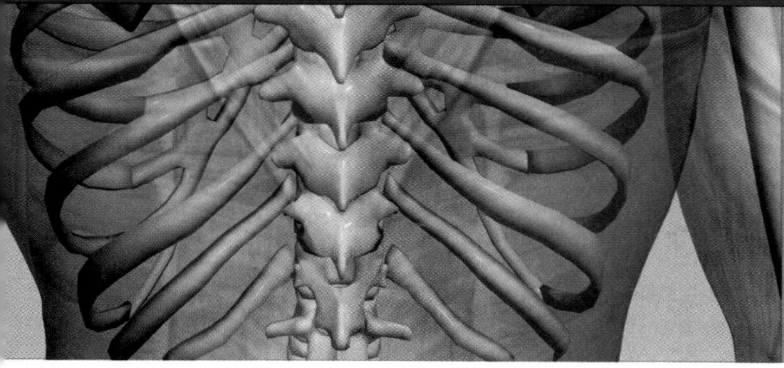

Chapter 7

Medical Terminology

NATIONAL EMS EDUCATION STANDARD COMPETENCIES

Medical Terminology

Uses foundational anatomic and medical terms and abbreviations in written and oral communication with colleagues and other health care professionals.

KNOWLEDGE OBJECTIVES

1. Explain the purpose of medical terminology and the importance of being familiar with it. (p 232)
2. Explain the Greek and Latin origins of medical terms. (pp 233–234)
3. Define medical eponyms, homonyms, antonyms, and synonyms; give examples of each. (pp 233, 239–240)
4. Recognize word roots, combining forms, prefixes, and suffixes; give examples of each. (pp 234–237)
5. Describe how compound words are created and how the plural is formed when using medical terminology; give examples of each. (p 239)
6. Describe the anatomic position and explain why it is used. (pp 240–241)
7. Identify the three planes of the human body. (p 241)
8. List medical terms associated with regional anatomy. (p 241)
9. Explain the importance of using accurate medical terminology for direction, movement, and position in your documentation and other communication. (pp 243–246)
10. Describe the topography of the abdominal region, including the four abdominal quadrants and the nine abdominal regions. (pp 246–247)
11. Identify specialized prefixes used to indicate position, direction, and location. (p 236)
12. Define specific terms used to indicate the patient's position on the scene or before transport: prone, supine, Fowler position, and recovery (left lateral recumbent) position. (pp 247–248)
13. Interpret standard, widely accepted medical abbreviations, acronyms, and symbols. (pp 248–249)
14. Identify error-prone medical abbreviations, acronyms, and symbols. (p 250)
15. Know appropriate terminology related to pharmacology. (pp 251–261)

SKILLS OBJECTIVES

There are no skills objectives for this chapter.

Introduction

As a paramedic, you must develop a strong working knowledge of medical terminology, the international language of medicine and health care. Medical terminology is used to describe and record every aspect of patient care, including medical history, assessment results, treatment, and outcomes. The language of medicine is derived primarily from Greek and Latin terms. If you understand the origin of medical terms (words), the components (parts), and the guidelines for forming words, you will be able to identify and use medical terminology correctly and communicate effectively with other health care providers.

Consider what could happen if you, as a paramedic, used medical terminology incorrectly:

- A term used incorrectly in a radio report or documented improperly in the patient care report (PCR) could lead to the patient being given an ineffective or even harmful treatment at the hospital.
- Patients could lose trust in the paramedic's ability to care appropriately for them.

Your comprehension of key terms, acronyms, symbols, and abbreviations is vital for effective communication and documentation. Understanding medical terminology requires you to break down each word into its components and to have a good working knowledge of those parts. Learn the established and accepted medical terms and abbreviations for your local area. Some EMS systems have specific lists of approved medical abbreviations and terms you must use.

Words of Wisdom

Never use a medical term if you are uncertain of its meaning. If you cannot remember *femur*, it is better to say *thigh bone* than to risk using an incorrect term.

The more extensive your vocabulary is, the more competent you will appear to the rest of the medical community and the better the patient care you will be able to provide. In addition to accepted terminology, you will undoubtedly hear some common slang terms used in EMS, such as *boarding* a patient for transport or *bagging* or *tubing* the patient during airway management. Download a medical terminology app or carry a field guide or documentation handbook, so you can quickly and easily look up any unfamiliar terms without memorizing page after page of terms **FIGURE 7-1**.

YOU are the Paramedic

PART 1

You and your partner are dispatched to a local elementary school to help a person who has fallen. On arrival, you are directed to the playground, where a young boy is lying beneath a set of playground climbing bars on his left side, curled into a fetal position, sniffling and holding his abdomen. His second-grade teacher, Miss Hawthorne, tells you he fell from the top, approximately 5 feet (1.5 m), and has a bump on the right side of his head just above his eye. She says she has been trying to keep him still and has not let him try to get up.

Recording Time: 0 Minutes	
Appearance	Awake
Level of consciousness	Alert
Airway	Open
Breathing	Adequate
Circulation	Appears normal

1. What is the correct medical term for the position in which the child is lying?

2. How can knowledge of medical terminology assist in your documentation of care for this patient?

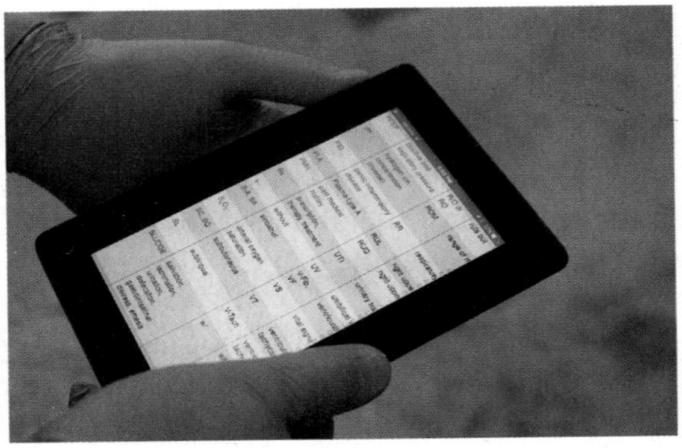

FIGURE 7-1 Medical terminology apps are an excellent resource to reference terms while working in the field.

Origins of Medical Words

Understanding the origins of medical terms helps you decipher their meaning. As noted earlier, most medical terms have Greek or Latin origins **TABLE 7-1**. In general, medical terms that refer to disease, diagnosis, and treatment are derived from Greek words. Words that refer to anatomic structures are usually derived from Latin words. The original word and its meaning are often quite interesting. For example, the word *muscle* comes from the Latin word for mouse, because the movement of a muscle under the skin was thought to resemble the scampering of a mouse. The word *coccyx*, indicating the lower end of the spine, originated from the Greek word for cuckoo; this structure resembles a cuckoo's bill.

Eponyms

The language used in medicine also comes from eponyms and terms that have resulted from advances in modern medicine, such as *fiberoptic* and *pacemaker*. An **eponym** is the name of a disease, device, procedure, or drug based on the person who invented, discovered, or first described it. You use eponyms every day and may not even be aware of where they originated. For example, the diesel engine is named for its German inventor, Rudolf Diesel. Medical eponyms sometimes appear in the possessive form (such as Hodgkin's disease) and sometimes not (Hodgkin disease). (Note: This text does not include the possessive form.) Eponyms often include the name of the physician or surgeon who discovered, described, developed, identified, or invented a particular anatomic part or region, physiologic function or process, disease or syndrome, diagnostic or surgical procedure, treatment protocol, or instrument. Here are some examples:

- Alzheimer disease
- Apgar score
- Babinski reflex
- Cesarean section

SAFETY

One type of medication error involves prescribing and dispensing look-alike, sound-alike (LASA) medications (eg, magnesium sulfate [$MgSO_4$] and morphine [MS and MSO_4]). The Joint Commission recommends focusing on prescription legibility through improved handwriting or the use of electronic prescriptions. Other solutions include physically separating LASA medications into different storage areas and using tall-man or mixed-case lettering to emphasize the differences in drug names (eg, DOPamine versus DoBUTamine).

TABLE 7-1 Selected Medical Terms With Greek or Latin Origins

Greek	Disease	Latin	Anatomic
burs/o	bursitis	dors/o, dors/i	back/dorsal
cholecyst/o	cholecystitis	faci/o	face/facioplegic
gloss/o	glossitis	lingua	tongue/linguistic
hepat/ic	hepatitis	mamm/o	breast/ mammogram
nephr/o	nephritis	ren	kidney/renal

- Cheyne-Stokes respirations
- Crohn disease
- Foley catheter
- Guillain-Barré syndrome
- Levine sign
- Marfan syndrome
- McBurney point

Words of Wisdom

Thorough knowledge of anatomy and an understanding of the context in which each term is typically used can help you determine (and spell) the correct word to use in a given situation.

Medical Term Components

When you encounter a new word, break it up into its parts. Some medical terms are quite long, consisting of three or four parts. If you know each part's meaning, you can combine the definitions to determine the broader meaning of the word. Medical terms are composed of distinct parts that perform specific functions:

- **Word root**. The foundation of the term
- **Prefix**. The portion that appears before the word root
- **Suffix**. The portion that appears after the word root
- **Combining form**. A word root, prefix, or suffix with an added vowel that links one or more word roots to another component of a term

The meaning of each part and the manner in which the parts come together determine the word's meaning. Changing or deleting any portion of a term can significantly alter its content.

Beyond the discussion that follows, a set of master tables at the end of this chapter list medical terminology, including prefixes, suffixes, word roots, and abbreviations, that you will often use in your work.

Word Roots

The word root, sometimes referred to as the *root word,* is the body of a word. It establishes the word's basic meaning. Some word roots are complete words by themselves; others are not. For example, the word root *cell* is itself a complete word, but the word root *cephal* is not a complete word until it is joined with other word parts (eg, cephalic, cephalopod). Further, the same word root may have different meanings in different fields of study. You may have to consider the context of a word before assigning its meaning.

In the medical field, it is important to understand the word roots relating to color, as these terms are used frequently to describe patient presentation and many other key concepts. **TABLE 7-2** lists some common word roots relating to color.

Prefixes

Prefixes are often found in everyday language (for instance, *auto*pilot, *sub*marine, *tri*cycle), and they are common in medical and scientific terminology. A prefix appears at the beginning of a word and generally describes the location or intensity of the word root that follows. Not all medical terms have prefixes.

A prefix does not change the meaning of the word root, but it does change the meaning of the medical term by describing the what, how, why, or when of the root. For example, *cutaneous* means skin, regardless of what precedes it. The prefix *sub-* means below; therefore, *subcutaneous* means below the skin. Another word, *apnea,* which means without breath, can easily be understood when you know it is formed from the prefix *a-*, which means without or lack of, and the word root *-pnea,* which means breath.

Many prefixes are used to indicate the number of sides, limbs, or sensory organs affected (monocular vision, for example). Other numerical prefixes are used to specify time, such as octogenarian (a person between 80 and 89 years of age), or to indicate quantities that are uncountable (semicomatose, for instance). Common numerical prefixes are listed in **TABLE 7-3**.

Specialized prefixes are used to specify position, direction, or location. Among other functions, these prefixes can do the following:

- Describe movement of the body or something within it, such as a blood clot or tumor metastasis
- Indicate the location of an organ, foreign body, or mass

TABLE 7-2 Word Roots That Describe Color

Root	Definition	Example	Definition
alb-, albin/o	white	albinism	Condition in which a person's skin, hair, and eyes lack pigmentation (white hair, very pale skin, and a nonpigmented iris)
chlor/o	green	chlorophyll	Green pigment in leaves that is necessary for the plant to carry out photosynthesis
cirrh/o	yellow-orange	cirrhosis	Inflammation of an organ, such as cirrhosis of the liver, which causes yellow-orange pigmentation of the skin
cyan/o	blue	cyanosis	Blue skin discoloration
erythr/o	red	erythrocyte	Red blood cell that contains hemoglobin to carry oxygen
jaund/o	yellow	jaundice	Yellow skin and sclerae
leuk/o	white	leukocyte	White blood cell that fights infection
melan/o	black	melena	Black, tarry stool caused by upper gastrointestinal bleeding
poli/o	gray	poliomyelitis	Acute viral disease that attacks the gray matter of the brain
purpur/i	purple	purpura	Purple areas of the skin or mucous membranes measuring between 4 and 10 mm in diameter; smaller areas are called *petechiae*
xanth/o	yellow	xanthoma	Skin condition in which yellow-colored cholesterol deposits build up under the skin surface

TABLE 7-3 Common Numerical Prefixes

Prefix	Meaning	Example
mono-, uni-	one	monochromatic (having one color), unilateral (affecting one side of the body)
bi-, di-	two, double, twice	bilateral (pertaining to both sides of the body), dioxide (an oxide that contains two oxygen atoms)
tri-	three	tricuspid (a tooth with three cusps or points, heart valve with three cusps)
quad-, quadri-, tetra-	four	quadriplegia (paralysis of all four extremities), tetralogy of Fallot (a congenital anomaly involving four anatomic abnormalities of the heart)
quint-	five	quintipara (a woman who has had five pregnancies resulting in five live births)
diplo-	double or in pairs	diplopia (double vision)
nulli-	none	nullipara (a woman who has never given birth)
primi-	first	primigravida (a woman pregnant for the first time)
multi-	many	multipara (a woman who has given birth to more than one child)
semi-	half; part	semipermeable (partly permeable)
hemi-	half; one-sided	hemiplegia (weakness on one side of the body)
ambi-	both	ambidextrous (able to use the right and left hands equally well)
pan-	all, entire	pandemic (a disease outbreak occurring over a wide geographic area)

- Describe a surgical procedure and the medical instrument used to perform it
- Refer to the direction of radiation or ultrasound waves used in diagnosis or treatment

Common prefixes used in medical terminology for specifying position, direction, or location are shown in **TABLE 7-4**.

Suffixes

A *suffix* is a component added to the end of a word root. It changes or adds to the word's meaning or provides further definition. In medical terminology, a suffix usually specifies a procedure, condition, disease, or part of speech. For example, the suffix *-ase* indicates an enzyme. Lipase (*lip-*, which means

TABLE 7-4 Selected Prefixes Specifying Position, Direction, or Location

Prefix	Definition	Example
ab-	away from	abduction (away from the midline of the body, or a specified point of reference)
ad-	to, toward	adduction (toward the midline of the body)
ante-, pre-	before, in front of	antepartum (the period before childbirth), precancerous (abnormal cells or a condition that may develop into cancer if untreated)
circum-, peri-	around, about	circumferential burn (a burn around an entire area such as the arm, chest, and abdomen), pericardium (sac around the heart)
contra-	against, opposite	contralateral (pertaining to the opposite side)
de-	down, from, remove	debride (to remove contaminants from a wound to enhance healing)
ecto-, ex-, exo-, extra-	outside, without, away from	ectopic pregnancy (pregnancy where the embryo develops outside of the uterus), extraneous (existing or belonging outside the organism)
en-, endo-	within, inside	endoscope (a lighted instrument used to view structures within the body)
epi-	above, upon, on	epigastric (above the stomach)
hyper-	above, excessive	hyperglycemia (excessive blood glucose)
hypo-, infra-, sub-	beneath, under, below normal	hypothermia (below normal temperature), infrascapular (below the scapula), subcutaneous (under the skin)
inter-	between	intercostal (between the ribs)
intra-	inside, within	intrauterine (within the uterus)
ipsi-	same	ipsilateral (on or affecting the same side)
para-	near, adjacent, apart from, abnormal	parathyroid (adjacent to the thyroid)
per-	through, by	percutaneous (through the skin)
retro-	behind	retroperitoneal (area behind the peritoneum)
sub-	under, below	subclavian (below the clavicle)
supra-	upper, above	suprasternal notch (above the sternum)
trans-	across, through, beyond	transurethral (across or through the urethra)

fat, plus -*ase*) is an enzyme that digests fats. Gastritis, which means inflammation of the stomach, is a combination of the word root *gastr-*, which means stomach, and the suffix -*itis*, which means inflammation. Suffixes can change the medical term to a noun or adjective as needed. Examples of suffixes related to symptoms or diagnoses are shown in **TABLE 7-5**.

Combining Forms and Vowels

Some word roots, prefixes, and suffixes cannot combine with other word forms without help **TABLE 7-6**. A combining form is a word root, prefix, or suffix with an added vowel, known as a **combining vowel**. The most commonly used combining vowel is *o*. Combining vowels make pronunciation easier and

TABLE 7-5 Selected Suffixes Related to Symptoms or Diagnoses

Suffix	Definition	Example
-edema	swelling	lymphedema (swelling caused by the buildup of lymph fluid in the body)
-emesis	vomiting	hematemesis (vomiting of blood)
-genic	causing	carcinogenic (cancer causing)
-oid	resembling	mucoid (involving or resembling mucus)
-penia	deficiency	leukopenia (deficiency of white blood cells)
-spasm	sudden involuntary movements such as twitching, cramping, or contraction	bronchospasm (abnormal contraction of bronchial smooth muscle)

YOU are the Paramedic

PART 2

After briefly speaking with the teacher, you kneel to get at eye level with the child. "Hi, I'm a paramedic, and we're here to take care of you. My partner, Matt, is going to hold your head still while we talk for a minute. Does your head or your tummy hurt?"

The child says his name is Tommy and his stomach hurts more than his head does. He is alert and oriented to person, place, time, and event. His respiratory rate is 22 breaths/min and normal, and his radial pulse is strong and regular, with a rate of 104 beats/min. He says he has been dizzy all morning, and it made him fall. Miss Hawthorne tells you that Tommy has type 1 diabetes. The school nurse arrives and indicates that his mother reported that his glucose level was 183 mg/dL when he arrived at school this morning. The nurse also states that he is not allergic to any medications.

Recording Time:	3 Minutes
Respirations	22 breaths/min
Pulse	104 beats/min
Skin	Pale, cool, dry
Oxygen saturation (Spo_2)	98%
Pupils	Pupils Equal, Round, and Reactive to Light and Accommodation (PERRLA)

3. Why would you want to avoid using medical terminology when talking to this patient?
4. What are the correct medical terms to describe Tommy's mental status and blood glucose level?
5. How would you document that the patient has no medication allergies?

TABLE 7-6 Selected Combining Forms

Combining Form	Meaning	Combining Form	Meaning
arthr/a	joint	pelv/i	pelvis
cardi/o	heart	rhabd/a	rod-shaped
carp/o	wrist	thorac/o	chest, thorax
cephal/o	head	thyr/o	thyroid gland
chol/e	bile	trache/o	trachea
chrondr/i	cartilage	ureter/o	ureter
cyst/a	bladder	vas/o	vessel
gloss/o	tongue	vesic/o	bladder, blister
nas/o	nose	viscer/o	viscera
ot/o	ear		

aid the formation of new, more complex terms. In this chapter, a combining form can be recognized by a diagonal slash before an ending vowel. For example, in *osteopathic,* the first word root is *osteon* (Greek for bone). The *n* is dropped and the combining vowel *o* added to create the combining form *oste/o.* Thus, adding the *o* facilitates the addition of a second combining form, *-pathy* (from the word root *patho-,* meaning disease).

Consider another example. The word root *gastr-,* which means stomach, cannot combine gracefully with *megaly,* which means enlargement. The resulting term, gastrmegaly, would be awkward to pronounce and would have an odd spelling. A hyphen at the end of a word root indicates that *gastr-* is not a complete word. Adding a vowel to it—in this case, an *o*—solves the problem. *Gastr/o* + *megaly* makes *gastromegaly,* or enlargement of the stomach. If the suffix begins with a vowel, a combining vowel is unnecessary. For example, *gastr-* + *-ic* = *gastric.* No additional letters are needed to form the word.

When adding combining vowels to root words, follow these guidelines:

- Use a combining vowel before a suffix that begins with a consonant (eg, *cyt/o* + *logy*).
- Use a combining vowel to join other root words (eg, *gastr/o/enteritis*).
- Do not use a combining vowel before a suffix that begins with a vowel (eg, *gastritis,* not *gastroitis*).

Some other examples of combining forms and vowels include these terms:

- *cardi* + *o* + *logy* = cardiology (study of the heart)
- *neur* + *o* + *logy* = neurology (study of the nervous system)

Plural Endings

Certain rules apply when changing a medical term from singular to plural. In most cases, as with other English words, the plural is formed simply by adding an *-s* to the singular word. *Lung* becomes *lungs,* for instance. However, for other medical terms, forming the plural is more complicated:

Singular words ending in *-a* change to *-ae* in the plural.
- Example: *vertebra* becomes *vertebrae*

Singular words ending in *-is* change to *-es* in the plural.
- Example: *diagnosis* becomes *diagnoses*

Singular words ending in *-ex* or *-ix* change to *-ices.*
- Example: *apex* becomes *apices*

Singular words ending in *-on* or *-um* change to *-a.*
- Examples: *ganglion* becomes *ganglia; ovum* becomes *ova*

Singular words ending in *-us* change to *-i.*
- Example: *bronchus* becomes *bronchi*

Compound Words

Some medical terms contain more than one word root; they are called **compound words**. In compound words, each word root retains its basic meaning. Simple examples of compound words containing two word roots are *electrocardiogram* and *thermometer*. A more complicated example is *osteoarthritis*. The combining form *oste/o* comes from the word root *ost-*, meaning bone; the word root *arthr-* means joint or joints; and the suffix *-itis* means inflammation. Therefore, the combined word *osteoarthritis* means inflammation of the bone joints.

Homonyms

Incorrect pronunciation of medical terms can lead to misdiagnosis or other serious medical errors. Correct pronunciation and spelling are essential with certain words known as **homonyms**, which are two or more words that are spelled and/or pronounced the same way but have different meanings **TABLE 7-7**.

Antonyms

Different word parts perform different functions. **Antonyms** are pairs of word roots, prefixes, or suffixes with the opposite meaning of another word **TABLE 7-8**.

Synonyms

Synonyms are pairs of word roots, prefixes, or suffixes with the same, or almost the same, meaning. For example, the prefixes of the words

TABLE 7-7 Selected Homonyms Used in Medical Terminology

Homonym	Meaning
basal	forming, or related to, a bottom layer or base
basil	an herb
dysphagia	difficulty eating or swallowing
dysphasia	difficulty speaking
foul	offensive to the senses; an action contrary to the rules of a sport
fowl	bird
humerus	long bone of the upper arm
humorous	funny
ileum	last anatomic portion of the small intestine
ilium	largest bone of the pelvis
pail	bucket
pale	having little color
palate	roof of the mouth
palette	artist's paint board
pleural	serous membranes covering the lungs and lining the thoracic cavity
plural	more than one
sight	vision
site	location, place, position
vial	small container, usually made of glass, often used to store liquids
vile	unpleasant, disgusting
wheal	slightly raised skin area that is redder or paler than the surrounding skin
wheel	round object made of hard material that can revolve on an axle

TABLE 7-8 Selected Antonyms Used in Medical Terminology

Word Part and Meaning		Opposite Word Part and Meaning	
ad-	toward	ab-	away from
bio-	life	necro-	death
brady-	fast	tachy-	slow
dextro-	right	sinistr/o	left
eu-	good, normal	mal-, dys-	bad, difficult, painful, abnormal
hyper-	above, excessive	hypo-	beneath, under, below normal
pre-	before	post-	after, behind

pneumonologist and pulmonologist both mean lung, yet these words are not interchangeable. The reasons for this are more historical than logical; the term *pneumonologist* simply has not gained acceptance, but the term *pulmonologist* has. **TABLE 7-9** shows more synonyms you are likely to encounter in your work.

In medical terminology, we can often use a single word to express a concept that might otherwise require many words of explanation. For example, you can say "arthritis" faster than you can say "inflammation of the joint." In the next section, we take a more in-depth look at commonly used medical terms and their meanings.

Topographic Anatomy

The body's surface has many superficial visible features that serve as guides or landmarks indicating the structures that lie beneath them. These features make up the body's topography (from the Greek word *topos*, meaning place, and *-graphy*, meaning description). Familiarize yourself with these living landmarks—the body's **topographic anatomy**—so that you can perform a thorough assessment.

To describe topography accurately, you must imagine the body in a fixed position, known as the **anatomic position**: The person is standing, facing you, arms at the sides, with the palms of the hands

TABLE 7-9 Selected Synonyms Used in Medical Terminology

Word Part and Meaning		Similar Word Part and Meaning	
angi/o	vessel (as in angiogram)	vas/o	vessel (as in vascular)
cardi/o	heart (as in cardiology)	coron/o	heart (as in coronary)
mammo/o	breast (as in mammogram)	mast/o	breast (as in mastectomy)
nephr/o	kidney (as in nephritis)	ren/o	kidney (as in renal)
pulmon/o	lung (as in pulmonologist)	pneum/o	lung (as in pneumonia)

YOU are the Paramedic

PART 3

You explain to Tommy that your partner is going to hold his head still and you are going to roll him over onto his back so you can check where it hurts. You observe a golf ball–size hematoma and a small laceration just above his right eye. Bleeding is controlled, and the patient's pupils are equal and reactive. His abdomen is very tender on the right side just below his ribs, and bruising is present. He denies pain in any other area. Tommy tells you he took his insulin this morning and ate breakfast before school.

Recording Time: 8 Minutes	
Respiration	22 breaths/min
Pulse	108 beats/min
Skin	Pale, cool, dry
Oxygen saturation (Spo_2)	99%
Pupils	PERRLA

6. Describe the position of the patient's head injury.

7. What is the abbreviation for the abdominal quadrant that is tender to the touch?

Words of Wisdom

There is only one anatomic position. Don't confuse this with the patient's position—prone or supine, for instance—or with patient positioning, such as the Fowler position.

facing forward, so the thumbs point away from the body. This position serves as a shared reference point, so the meanings of the various directional terms stay constant, regardless of the patient's actual body position or movement. For example, suppose a person reports pain in his arm and you need to document it. Whose left or right do you use? To be consistent, health care providers use the *patient's* left and right in the anatomic position as their reference point.

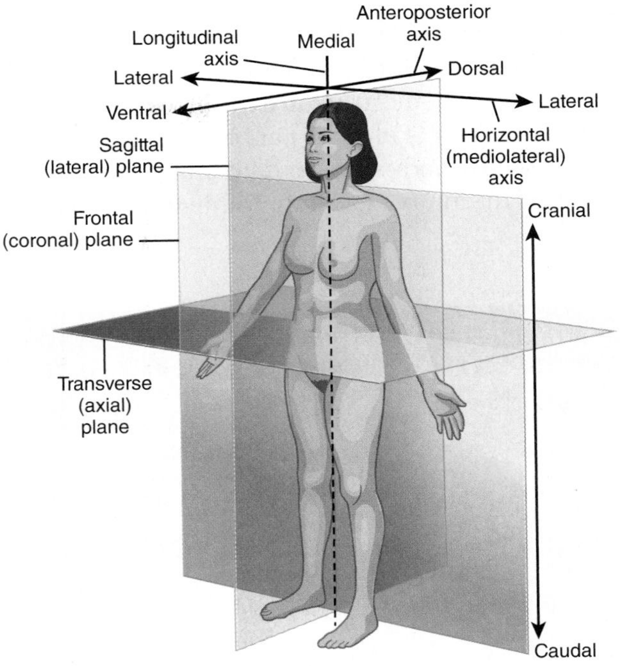

FIGURE 7-2 Planes and axes of the body.

Anatomic Planes and Axes of the Body

An anatomic plane of the body is an imaginary flat surface—imagine sheets of glass slicing through the body, dividing it horizontally and vertically into sections **FIGURE 7-2**. An *axis* is an imaginary line that divides the body equally and creates a point of rotation. Think of it as a skewer or pole through the middle of an object. The body can be divided along three main axes to create the following planes:

1. **Coronal (frontal) plane**. Imagine a sheet of glass (the plane) slicing the body vertically, from ear to ear, dividing it into front (ventral) and back (dorsal) portions. We call this the coronal plane—a term that is easy to remember, because corona means head.
2. **Transverse (axial) plane**. Now imagine a plane passing horizontally through the body at the waist, creating top and bottom portions. This slice is referred to as the transverse plane.
3. **Sagittal (lateral) plane**. Finally, imagine that we divide the body vertically again, but this time slicing it from front to back. This is the sagittal plane. *Sagitta* (Latin for arrow) describes how the straight line of this plane divides the body into left and right portions. A sagittal plane might or might not go through the midline of the body. If it does, it is called the **midsagittal plane (midline)** and divides the body into equal left and right halves. Your nose and navel are found along this imaginary line. Other sagittal planes lie parallel to the midline.

The body can be divided along three axes:

1. The **anteroposterior axis** runs perpendicular to the coronal plane.
2. The **longitudinal axis** runs perpendicular to the transverse plane.
3. The **horizontal axis**, also called the mediolateral axis, runs perpendicular to the sagittal plane.

These planes and axes help you to identify the location of internal structures and understand the relationships between and among the organs **TABLE 7-10**.

A **cross section** is taken by slicing across an object, perpendicular to its long axis, as you would do if you wanted to count the rings in a tree trunk. A **longitudinal section**, in contrast, is a view of an object cut along its long axis. In medicine, this slicing is often imaginary or can be accomplished with a camera or a beam of radiation, rather than a scalpel.

Specific Structures of the Body

In addition to using planes and topographic landmarks, many body structures have specific names. When a person is injured, paramedics rely on anatomic planes, body surfaces, and imaginary lines to describe the injury's location. Familiarizing yourself with these body regions will not only help you communicate with other professionals, but also help you break down other terms, because many of them are used as root words. For example, sternocleidomastoid is a combination of *sterno-*, *cleido-*, and *-mastoid*, which refer to the sternum, clavicle, and mastoid process, respectively. If you understand those roots, you will be able to locate the origin and insertion of this large neck muscle. **TABLE 7-11** lists combining forms associated with specific body structures.

TABLE 7-10 Anatomic Planes of the Body

Plane of the Body	Description
Coronal (frontal)	Front and back
Transverse (axial)	Top and bottom
Sagittal (lateral) • Midsagittal (midline)	Left and right (divides the body at any point on or parallel to the midline) • Left and right (divides the body into equal left and right halves)

Body Cavities

The human body contains several cavities, which in turn contain various organs and other structures. These cavities can be grouped into dorsal cavities, which are more posterior, and ventral cavities, which are anterior. The dorsal cavities include the cranial cavity (contains the brain) and the spinal cavity (surrounds the spinal cord). The ventral cavities include the thoracic cavity (encloses the heart, lungs, and great vessels), the abdominal cavity

TABLE 7-11 Combining Forms Associated With Specific Body Structures

Combining Form	Meaning	Combining Form	Meaning
abdomen/o	abdomen	cardi/o, card/o, coron/o	heart
acr/o	extremities (arms, legs)	carp/o	wrist bones
adip/o	fat	caud/o	tail
adren/o, adrenal/o	adrenal glands	cephal/o	toward or pertaining to the head
aort/o	aorta	cerebell/o	cerebellum
append/o, appendic/o	appendix	cerebr/o	brain, cerebrum
arthr/o, articul/o	joint	cervic/o	neck, cervix
aur/o, auricul/o, ot/o	ear	cholecyst/o	gallbladder
axill/o	axilla, armpit	clav/i, clavicul/o, cleid/o	clavicle, collarbone
blephar/o	eyelid	col/o	colon, large intestine
brachi/o	arm, upper arm	crani/o	cranium or skull
bronch/o	bronchus	cutane/o, derm/a, derm/o, dermat/o	skin
bucc/o	cheek	cyst/o	bladder, sac
calcane/o	calcaneus, heel bone	dactyl/o	digit (toes, fingers)

Combining Form	Meaning	Combining Form	Meaning
encephal/o	brain	ocul/o, ophthalm/o	eye
enter/o	small intestine	olecran/o	elbow
epitheli/o	epithelium	or/o, stomat/o	mouth
femor/o	femur, thigh	oste/o	bone
fibul/o	fibula	patell/o	patella, kneecap
gastr/o	stomach	pector/o	chest
glute/o	buttock	ped/o	foot
hem/o, hemat/o	blood	phalang/o	phalanges, finger or toe bones
hepat/o	liver	pharyng/o	pharynx
hist/o	tissue	pleur/o	pleura
humer/o	humerus	pod/o	foot
inguin/o	groin	proct/o	anus, rectum
laryng/o	larynx	pulm/o, pulmon/o, pneumon/o	lung
lumb/o	lumbar, lower back	pub/o	pubic bone, genital region
lymph/o	lymph	somat/o	body
mamm/o, mast/o	breast	spin/o	spine
metacarp/o	metacarpals, hand bones	tars/o	tarsals, ankle bones
metatars/o	metatarsals, foot bones	thorac/o	chest
muscul/o, my/o	muscle	umbilic/o	umbilicus, navel
nas/o, rhin/o	nose	vascul/o	blood vessel
nephr/o, ren/o	kidney	vertebr/o	vertebrae
neur/o	nerve	viscer/o	internal organ

(holds several digestive and endocrine organs), and the pelvic cavity (contains many digestive organs and the female reproductive organs). The abdominal and pelvic cavities can be referred to together as the abdominopelvic cavity **FIGURE 7-3**. The retroperitoneal cavity is separate from and lies posterior (dorsal) to the abdominal cavity and contains different organs, most notably the kidneys.

Directional Terms

Directional terms used in the study of anatomy describe relative positions of body parts and imaginary anatomic divisions. When you discuss, describe, or document the location of pain or injury, it is essential to use the correct directional terms **FIGURE 7-4**. **TABLE 7-12** provides the basic terms used in medicine. Since every direction has an opposite—above and below, front and behind, and so on—directional terms in medicine tend to occur in pairs.

Superior and Inferior

The **superior** portion of any body part is the portion above or closest to the head from a specific reference point. The body part closest to the feet is the

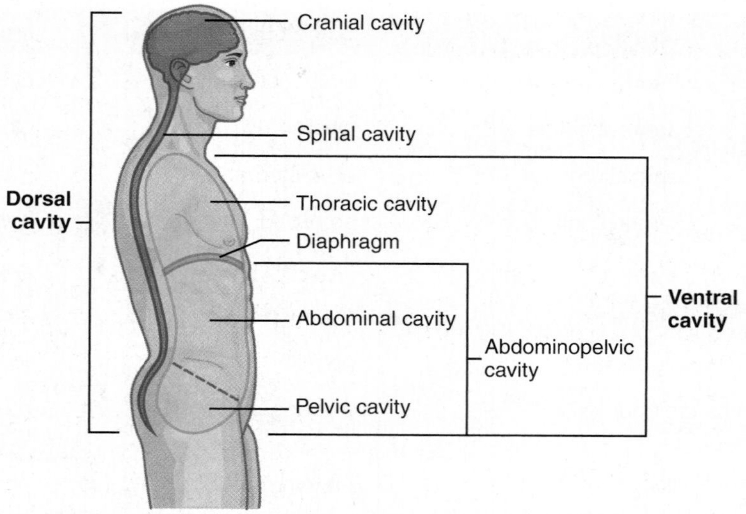

FIGURE 7-3 Body cavities.

TABLE 7-12 Common Directional Terms

Common Term	Directional Term	Definition
Right and left	Right Left	Patient's right Patient's left
Top and bottom	Superior Inferior	Closest to the head Closest to the feet
Middle and side	Medial Lateral	Closest to the midline Farthest from the midline
Closest and farthest	Proximal Distal	Closest to the point of attachment Farthest from the point of attachment
In and out	Superficial Deep	Closest to the surface of the skin Farther inside the body
Front and back	Anterior (ventral) Posterior (dorsal)	Front of the body Back of the body

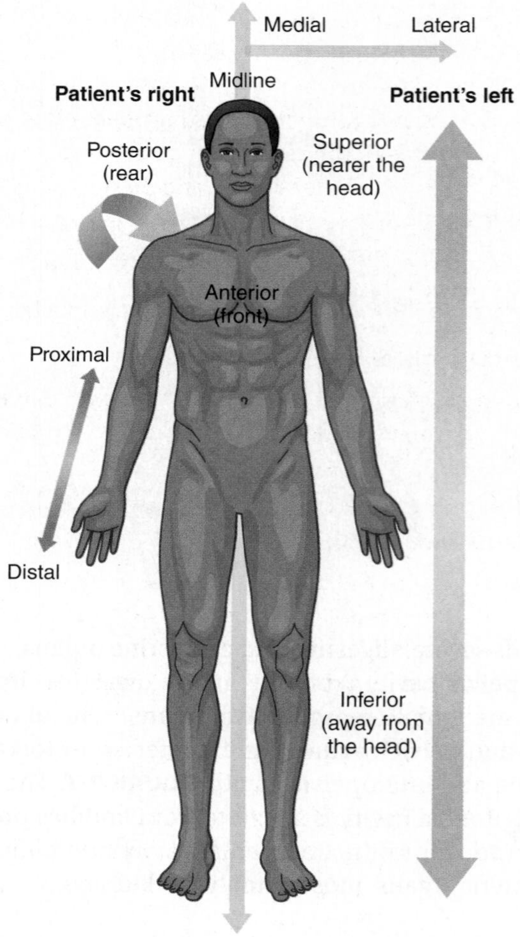

FIGURE 7-4 Directional terms indicate distance and direction from the midline.

inferior portion. These terms are used to describe the relationship of one structure to another. For example, the knee is superior to the foot and inferior to the pelvis.

Lateral and Medial

Parts of the body that lie farther from the midline are described as **lateral** (outer). The parts that lie closer to the midline are described as **medial** (inner). For example, the knee has medial (inner) and lateral (outer) aspects (surfaces).

Proximal and Distal

It is sometimes useful to describe a portion of an extremity relative to its distance from the body's midline. **Proximal** describes structures that are closer to the body. For example, a fracture of the proximal humerus would involve the end of the bone that is closest to the shoulder. **Distal** indicates structures that are farther from the trunk—that is, nearer to the free end of the extremity. Using our previous example, a fracture of the distal humerus involves the end of the bone farther from the body (adjacent to the elbow). You can use these terms to describe the relationship of one structure to another. For example, the elbow is distal to the shoulder and proximal to the wrist and hand.

Superficial and Deep

Superficial means closer to or on the surface of the skin. **Deep** means farther inside the body and away from the skin.

Anterior and Posterior

Anterior refers to the belly side of the body. Another term for anterior is **ventral**. **Posterior** refers to the spinal side of the body, including the back of the hand (recall, the palms face forward when the body is in the anatomic position). Another term for posterior is **dorsal**. In human medicine, the terms anterior and posterior are used more frequently than the terms ventral and dorsal, which are more common in the veterinary and zoologic sciences.

Palmar and Plantar

The front region of the hand is referred to as the palm or **palmar** or volar surface. The bottom of the foot is referred to as the **plantar** or volar surface.

Apex

The **apex** (the plural is *apices* or *apexes*) is the tip of a structure. For example, the heart's apex is the bottom (inferior portion) of the ventricles in the left side of the chest.

Movement and Positional Terms

From the simplest grasp to the most graceful ballet step, all body movements can be broken down into a series of simple components and described with specific terms. As with the terms describing anatomic location and direction, an accepted set of terms describes body movement. These are particularly useful in explaining the mechanism of injury.

Range of motion is the full distance that a joint can be moved. In the anatomic position, moving the distal point of an extremity toward the trunk is usually called **flexion**. For example, flexion of the elbow brings the hand closer to the shoulder, flexion of the knee brings the foot up to the buttocks, and flexion of the fingers forms the hand into a fist.

In some instances, specific terms are used to clarify movement, such as in the foot. Dorsiflexion is movement of the foot toward the dorsal aspect, while plantar flexion describes movement toward the sole. **Extension** is the return of a body part from a flexed position to the anatomic position. In the anatomic position, all extremities are in extension. **Abduction** of an extremity moves it away from the midline. **Adduction** moves the extremity toward the midline **FIGURE 7-5**. A patient's neck can be in one of several positions when the patient is lying supine **FIGURE 7-6**.

The prefix *hyper-* is often added to the terms *flexion* or *extension* to indicate a mechanism of injury. *Hyper-* indicates that the normal range of

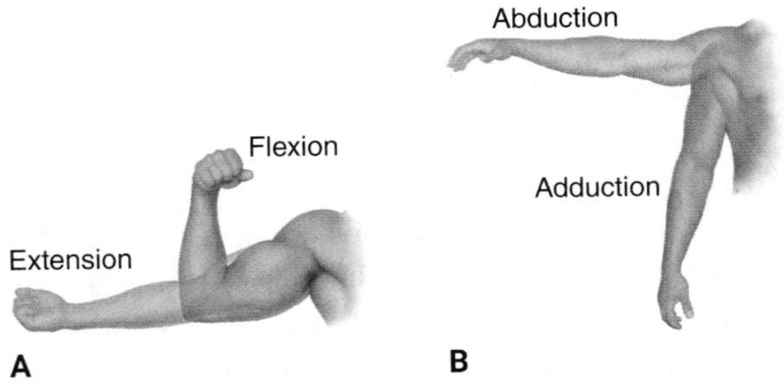

FIGURE 7-5 A. Flexion and extension. **B.** Abduction and adduction.

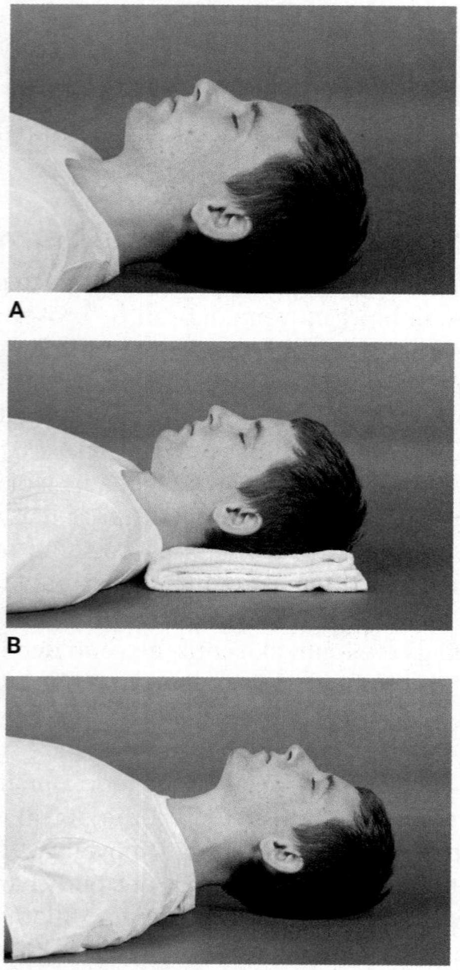

A B C

FIGURE 7-6 Positions of the neck in a patient found in a supine position. **A.** Neutral. **B.** Flexed. **C.** Extended.

motion for the particular joint was maximized or even exceeded, possibly resulting in injury. **Hyperflexion** refers to a body part that was flexed to the maximum level or even beyond the normal range of motion. **Hyperextension** refers to extension of a body part to the maximum level or even beyond the normal range of motion. An example of a hyperextension injury is one that occurs when a person falls on an outstretched hand, resulting in a distal radius fracture. A hyperflexion injury of the back can occur while bending. Wrist injuries can also be described using the terms **supination** and **pronation**. Turning the palms upward (toward the sky) constitutes supination of the forearm. Turning the palms downward (toward the ground) pronates the forearm.

Documentation and Communication

Use the correct anatomic terminology in your PCR. It makes the report more useful to hospital personnel and enhances your professional image as a paramedic.

Internal rotation means turning the anterior portion of an extremity toward the midline. The lower extremity is internally rotated when the toes are turned inward. **External rotation** means turning an extremity away from the midline. Often, when you are comparing an injured extremity with the uninjured extremity, you will note rotational deformities. A hip can be dislocated anteriorly or posteriorly. In an anterior hip dislocation, the foot is externally rotated and the head of the femur is palpable in the inguinal area (the lower lateral regions of the abdomen and groin). In the more common posterior hip dislocation, the knee and foot are usually flexed and internally rotated. The term *rotation* also can be applied to the spine. The spine is rotated when it twists on its axis. Placing the chin on the shoulder rotates the cervical spine.

Other Directional Terms

A body part or condition that appears on both sides of the midline is said to be **bilateral**. For example, the eyes, ears, hands, and feet are bilateral structures, as are structures inside the body, such as the lungs and kidneys. Structures that appear on only one side of the body are said to be **unilateral**. For example, the spleen is found only on the left side of the body, and the liver is predominantly on the right side. The terms unilateral and bilateral can also describe the location of pain, numbness, itching, or other phenomena (eg, pain on one side of the body is unilateral pain). You may also use the terms ipsilateral and contralateral. The term **ipsilateral** refers to the same side of the body. A patient having a stroke in the right hemisphere of the brain will usually have facial drooping ipsilaterally, in this case on the right side. **Contralateral** refers to the opposite side of the body. The same patient would have hemiplegia on the contralateral, or the opposite, side from the area of brain injury.

As part of your assessment process, you will palpate the abdomen and report your findings. To do so, you must be able to describe the exact location of areas of the abdomen. The abdominal cavity is divided into four equal parts called **quadrants**: the right upper quadrant (RUQ), left upper quadrant (LUQ), right lower quadrant (RLQ), and left lower quadrant (LLQ). The quadrants are formed from two lines intersecting at the umbilicus **FIGURE 7-7**. Pain or injury in a given quadrant usually arises from or involves the organs in that quadrant. Again, remember that right and left refer to the patient's right and left, not yours.

To describe location even more specifically, the abdomen can also be divided into nine regions **FIGURE 7-8**.

Position of the Patient

You will use specific terms to describe the patient's position on the scene or when you are ready to transport the patient to the emergency department **FIGURE 7-9**.

Prone and Supine

The body is in the **prone** position when lying facedown; it is **supine** when lying faceup.

Fowler Position

The **Fowler position** was named after an American surgeon, George R. Fowler, at the end of the nineteenth century. Dr. Fowler placed his patients in a sitting position with their heads elevated to a 90° angle to help them breathe more easily and to control their airway. A patient who is sitting straight up, with the knees either bent or straight, is described as being in the Fowler position. A patient in the semi-Fowler position is sitting with the back at a 45° angle. This position is generally a position of comfort for patients who do not need spinal motion restriction.

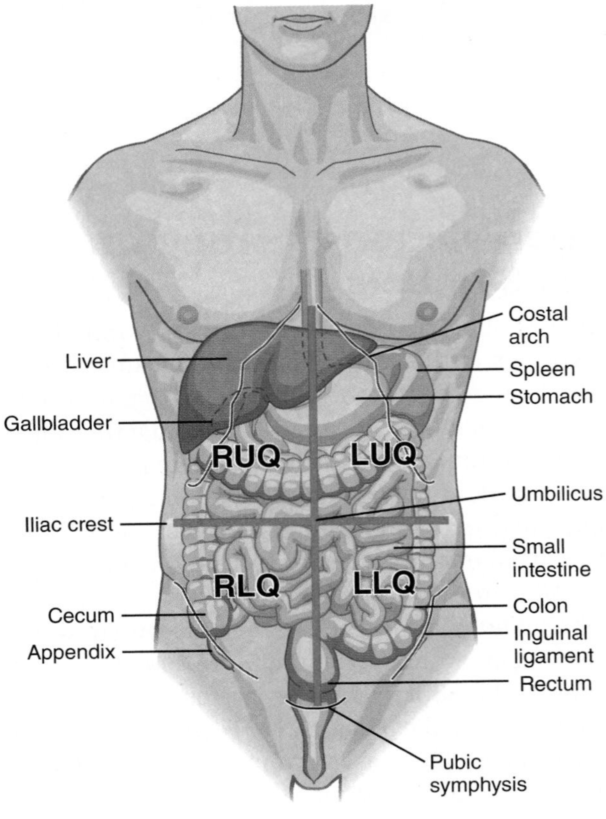

FIGURE 7-7 The abdomen is divided into four quadrants: RUQ, right upper quadrant; LUQ, left upper quadrant; RLQ, right lower quadrant; and LLQ, left lower quadrant.

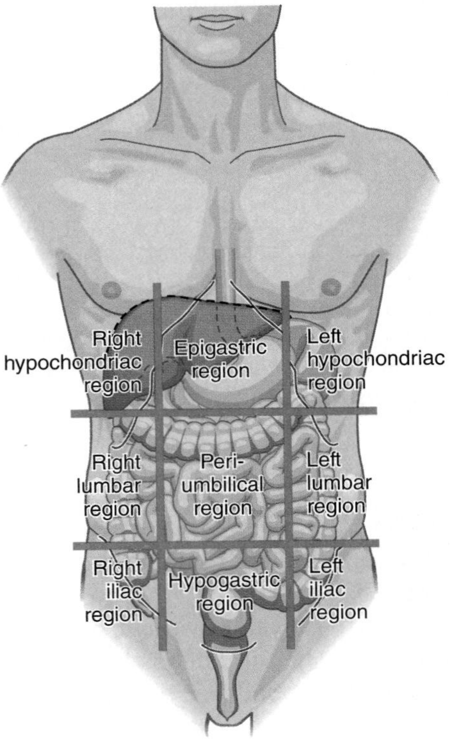

FIGURE 7-8 Abdominal regions.

Data from: Shier DN, Butler JL, Lewis R. *Hole's Essentials of Human Anatomy and Physiology,* 10th ed. New York: McGraw-Hill Higher Education; 2009.

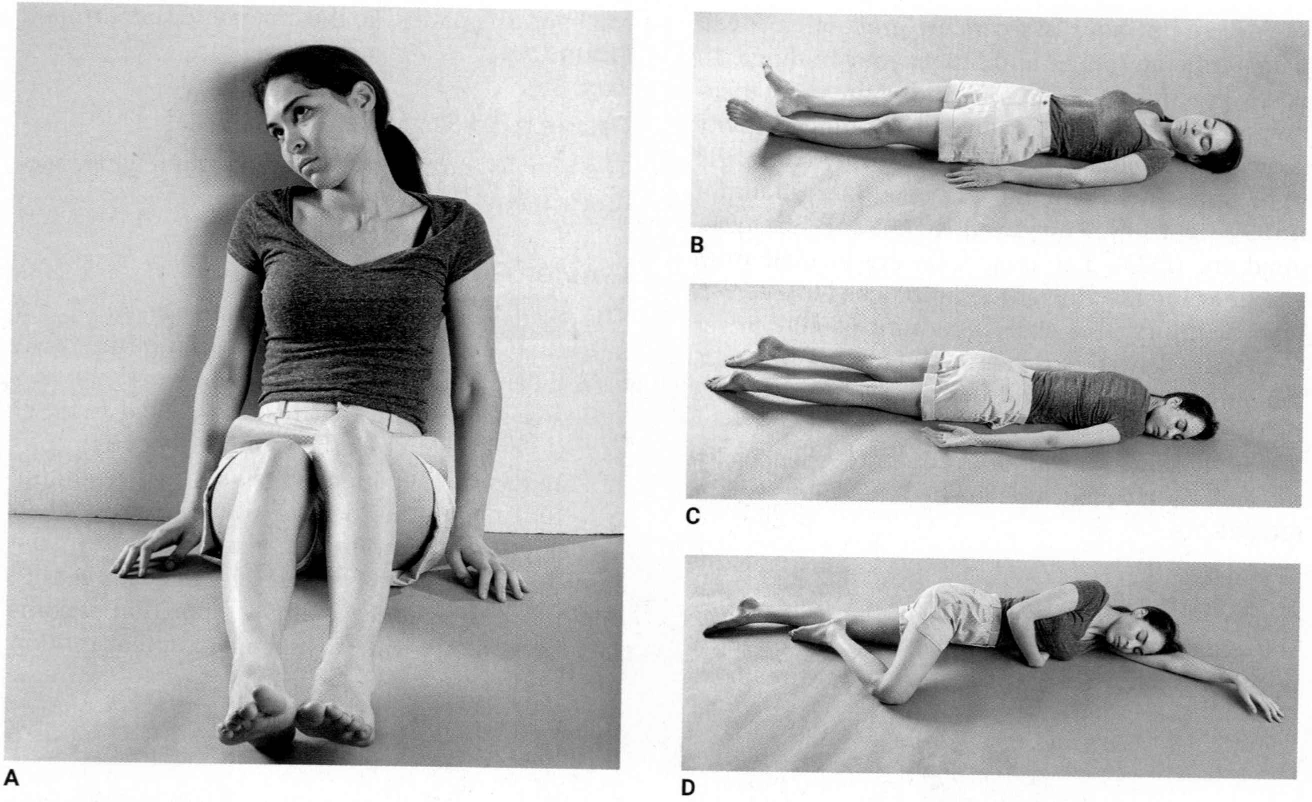

FIGURE 7-9 Patient positions. **A.** Fowler position. **B.** Supine. **C.** Prone. **D.** Recovery (left lateral recumbent) position.

> **Words of Wisdom**
>
> In addition to medical terminology, the population of a specific geographic area can have its own slang or regional jargon. Familiarize yourself with this language to improve your communication when responding to calls in these locations. For example, in the South many older adults refer to diabetes as "the sugars" and hypertension as "high blood."

Recovery Position

The recovery position helps maintain a clear airway in an unresponsive patient. In this position, the patient is lying on the left side, with the head resting on the bottom arm. The top knee is bent, angling the front of the patient's body slightly toward the floor or ground. This position, also referred to as the *left lateral recumbent position,* helps prevent aspiration of vomitus. The recovery position is discussed in greater detail in Chapter 16, *Airway Management.*

Abbreviations, Acronyms, and Symbols

Medical abbreviations, acronyms, and symbols are a type of shorthand used to communicate in health care. They evolve for the same reason that we abbreviate words in text messages and chats: they allow us to communicate faster. However, in patient care, it is important not to trade speed for accuracy. Use only commonly understood acronyms and abbreviations to minimize misinterpretation and errors.

All acronyms are abbreviations, but not all abbreviations are acronyms. When you shorten a word using an abbreviation, you pronounce each letter of the abbreviation separately. For example, emergency medical technician is abbreviated EMT, pronounced "E–M–T." Acronyms form shortened words from the initials of several words to produce a new word. Acronyms and other abbreviations are sometimes combined to shorten a phrase. For example, the acronym for Urban Search and Rescue, USAR, is pronounced "U-sar."

SAFETY

Be careful with look-alike, sound-alike drug names. Pay close attention to labels to ensure you accurately write down the names. Some common mistakes are listed here. Each drug is different, yet their names can be confused because of similar spelling and/or pronunciation:

- Zantac – Xanax
- Toradol – Tegretol
- Clonazepam – Lorazepam
- Alprazolam – Lorazepam
- Amiodarone – Amrinone
- Celebrex – Celexa
- Sinequan – Singulair
- Prozac – Prilosec

An abbreviation is still considered an acronym if it is pronounced as a word, even if the word formed is not part of the English language. An example is HIPAA, short for Health Insurance Portability and Accountability Act, a law that protects patients' privacy. This abbreviation is classified as an acronym because it is pronounced "hippa," not spelled out letter by letter. In contrast, DEA, which is an abbreviation for the US Drug Enforcement Agency, is not considered an acronym because it is spelled out as "D-E-A," rather than pronounced "dia."

Medical Abbreviations

Abbreviations take the place of the words they represent, with the goal of shortening patient care notes or other documentation. Some acronyms have become a standard part of the English language. For example, ASAP stands for "as soon as possible," but is commonly spoken as its own word. Medical abbreviations can be handy for documentation purposes, but you must ensure they are consistent with those approved for use in your EMS system.

YOU are the Paramedic

PART 4

"Well, Tommy, we need to take you to the hospital so they can check that bump on your head and find out why your tummy hurts. Matt and I are going to put you on a board with some seat belts and fix it so your head doesn't move. Don't worry, it won't hurt, and we'll be right here with you. Miss Hawthorne called your mom and dad, and they're going to meet us at the hospital."

After applying a cervical collar and securing Tommy on a backboard with straps and a cervical immobilization device, he is loaded onto the stretcher and into the ambulance. You place him on the cardiac monitor, which shows a sinus rhythm at 98 beats/min. His blood pressure is 96/54 mm Hg and respirations are 18 breaths/min, but his skin is pale, cool, and clammy to touch. Tommy's breath sounds are clear and equal, and his oxygen saturation (Spo_2) is 96%. You apply a small bandage to his forehead and reassess his abdomen. You note that it is still very tender to the touch and appears slightly discolored.

Recording Time: 13 Minutes	
Respiration	18 breaths/min, normal
Pulse	98 beats/min
Skin	Pale, cool, clammy
Blood pressure	96/54 mm Hg
Oxygen saturation (Spo_2)	96%
Pupils	PERRLA

8. Why is knowledge of anatomy pertinent when assessing and treating this patient?

9. What is the medical term for clammy skin?

10. What is the medical term for a phenomenon (such as pain, swelling, or a rash) affecting both sides of the body?

Error-Prone Abbreviations

The Joint Commission and the Institute for Safe Medication Practices (ISMP) have each published a do not use list of abbreviations they believe to be especially prone to misinterpretation.[1,2] Serious errors can occur when an abbreviation is not interpreted as intended. For example, HS on a prescription can mean either hour of sleep (meaning that the medication should be taken at bedtime) or half-strength. To avoid such errors, some agencies limit the use of abbreviations or do not allow abbreviations at all.

Trailing Zeros and Naked Decimals

Another common problem area concerns *trailing zeros* and *naked decimals.* Avoid using trailing zeros after a decimal point. For example, 5.0 mg may be read as 50 mg if the decimal is not seen. The same is true if a leading zero is left off before a decimal. If 0.5 mg is written without the leading zero as .5 mg, it may be mistaken for 5 mg if the decimal is not seen. Always leave off trailing zeros after the decimal, but include leading zeros before the decimal to avoid errors.

Symbols

Like abbreviations, symbols are sometimes used as a shortcut in documentation and other communication. It is important that you use only symbols that are widely understood and accepted **TABLE 7-13**.

To better ensure patient safety, some abbreviations should not be used at all. For example, because morphine sulfate (MS or MSO_4) and magnesium sulfate ($MgSO_4$) can be mistaken for each other, the complete drug name should always be spelled out.

Each EMS system should also keep a list of medical abbreviations approved for reporting and documentation purposes. Learn which abbreviations are acceptable in your service area before you use them in a report. For example, some agencies do not use SOB as an abbreviation for shortness of breath. When in doubt, write out the term in full. Accuracy, neatness, and completeness reflect a professional writing style.

YOU are the Paramedic

PART 5

You cover Tommy with a blanket and start an intravenous (IV) line in the back of his left hand, using a 20-gauge catheter to infuse normal saline at a rate of 10 drops per minute. You also assess his blood glucose level, which is now 147 mg/dL.

You and your crew transport the patient to a pediatric trauma center, where Tommy's parents are waiting, and give a verbal report to the receiving staff. Then you sit down in the EMS office to write your report while Matt cleans and restocks the ambulance.

Recording Time: 18 Minutes	
Respiration	20 breaths/min
Pulse	98 beats/min
Skin	Pale, cool, clammy
Blood pressure	98/60 mm Hg
Oxygen saturation (Spo_2)	99%
Pupils	PERRLA
Blood glucose level	147 mg/dL

Medical Terminology Related to Pharmacology

As a paramedic, you must be familiar with terminology related to medications and medication administration, such as common metric conversions used in drug calculation **TABLE 7-14**, and common medical abbreviations related to pharmacology **TABLE 7-15**.

Master Tables

TABLE 7-16 and **TABLE 7-17** provide reference lists of prefixes, suffixes, combining forms, and abbreviations.

TABLE 7-13 Common Symbols

°	degrees	/	per
1°	first, first degree, primary	±	plus or minus
2°	second, second degree, secondary	≠	not equal
↑	increase(d)	>	greater than
↓	decrease(d)	<	less than
Ⓡ	right	≥	greater than or equal to
Ⓛ	left	≤	less than or equal to
α	alpha	?	questionable, possible
β	beta	Δ	change
Ø	null or none	–	negative
~, ≈	approximately	♀	female
N	normal	♂	male
×2	times two		

TABLE 7-14 Metric Conversions Used in Drug Calculation

Weight		**Temperature**	
1 kilogram (kg)	2.2 pounds (lb) 1,000 grams (g)	37° Celsius (°C)	98.6° Fahrenheit (°F)
1 gram (g)	1,000 milligrams (mg)	**Length**	
1 milligram (mg)	1,000 micrograms	1 centimeter (cm)	0.39 inch (in.) 10 millimeters (mm)
Volume		100 centimeters (cm)	1 meter (m)
1 liter (L)	1,000 milliliters (mL)		

TABLE 7-15 Selected Medical Abbreviations Associated With Pharmacology

Abbreviation	Meaning	Abbreviation	Meaning
ac	before meals	LR	lactated Ringer (solution)
amp	ampule	max	maximum
bid/b.i.d./BID	twice daily	MDI	metered-dose inhaler
caps	capsules	mEq	milliequivalent
elix	elixir	mg	milligram
ET	endotracheal	mL	milliliter
fl, fld	fluid	NS	normal saline
g	gram	NSAID	nonsteroidal anti-inflammatory drug
gtt	drop(s)	NTE	not to exceed
h, hr	hour	OTC	over-the-counter
HHN	handheld nebulizer	oz	ounce
IM	intramuscular	PR	per the rectum
IV	intravenous	PRN	as needed
IVP	intravenous push	RL	Ringer lactate (solution)
IVPB	intravenous piggyback	Rx	prescription
kg	kilogram	stat	immediately
KO	keep open	SVN	small-volume nebulizer
KVO	keep vein open	tab	tablet
L	liter	tid/t.i.d./TID	three times a day
lb	pound	TKO	to keep open

TABLE 7-16 Selected Prefixes, Suffixes, and Combining Forms Used in Medical Terminology

Word Part	Meaning	Word Part	Meaning
a-, an-	without, lack of	adip/o, adipos/o	fat
ab-	away from	-al	pertaining to
abdomin/o	abdomen	-algia	pain
-ac	pertaining to	-alysis	breaking down
ac-	toward	-an	pertaining to
acous/o	hearing	an-	not, without
-ad, ad-	toward	ana-	up, apart, away
aden/o	gland	andr/o	male

Word Part	Meaning	Word Part	Meaning
angi/o	vessel	-crine	secrete
ante-	before, forward, in front of	-cyst	sac
anter/o	front	cyst/o	bladder or any fluid-containing sac
anti-	against, opposed to	cyt/o	cell
aort/o	aorta	-cyte	cell
-apheresis	removal	de-	down from, lack of
apo-	separate, away from	dia-	through, across, complete
aqua-	water	dis-	bad, abnormal, not, opposite of
-ar	pertaining to	dors/o, dors/i	back
-arche	beginning	dur/o	hard, tough
arteri/o	artery	-eal	pertaining to
-ary	pertaining to	-ectasis	dilation or distention of a tubular structure
-ase	enzyme	-ectomy	surgical removal of, cutting out
-ation	process of	electr/o	electricity
atri/o	atrium	-emia	blood-related condition
auto-	self	end-, end/o	within
bas/o	base, bottom	-ent	pertaining to
bi/o	life	enter/o	small intestines, intestines
-blast	immature cell	epi-	upon, on, above
blephar/o	eyelid	esthesi/o	feeling, sensation, perception
brady-	slow	ex-	out
calculi/o	calculus, stone	foramin/o	foramen, hole
carcin/o	cancer	fract-	break
-cardia	condition of the heart	-genic	causing
-cele	herniation, protrusion	ger/o	old age
-centesis	procedure in which an organ or body cavity is punctured	gest-	carry, produce
-ceps	heads	gluc/o, glyc/o	sugar
cili/o	tiny hairs	-gnosis	knowledge
cleid/o	clavicle	-gram	record (as in written documentation or results of a study)
coagul/o	clotting	-graph	record or the instrument used to create the record
cost/o	pertaining to a rib	gravid/o	pregnancy, gestation

(continues)

TABLE 7-16 Selected Prefixes, Suffixes, and Combining Forms Used in Medical Terminology (continued)

Word Part	Meaning	Word Part	Meaning
-gravida	pregnancy, gestation	mening/o	meninges
gyn/e, gynec/o	female, woman	micro-	small
hemi-	half	my/o	muscle
herni/o	hernia	myel/o	spinal cord, bone marrow
heter/o	other, different	narc/o	sleep
hiat/o	opening	nas/o	nose
home/o, hom/o	same	neo-	new
hydr/o	water, fluid	nephr/o	kidney
hyster/o	uterus	neur/o	nerve
-iasis	presence of, condition	noct/i	night
-ic, -itic	pertaining to	nuch/o	neck
-igo	condition	-oid	resembling
infer/o	downward	olig/o	little, scanty
is/o	equal	-oma	tumor, mass
-ismus	spasm	oophor/o	ovary
-itis	inflammation	-opia, -opsia	condition related to vision
-kine, -kinesis	movement	orch/o, orchi/o, orchid/o	testis, testicle
lacrim/o	tear	or/o	mouth, oral cavity
lact/o	milk	orth/o	upright, straight
-lapse	fall	-osis	disease process (see also -sis)
later/o	side	oss/i, osse/o, oste/o	bone
-lepsy	seizure	-ous	pertaining to
lith/o	stone, calculus	-ostomy	surgical creation of an opening, or hole
log/o	study	-otomy	surgical incision
lys/o	break down, dissolve	ov/i, ov/o, ovari/o, ovul/o	ovum, egg
-lysis	break down, dissolve	pan-	all
macro-	large	par-	near, beside
-malacia	softening	-para	delivery
medi/o	middle	para-	by the side of, abnormal
-megaly	enlargement	path/o	disease

Word Part	Meaning	Word Part	Meaning
-pathy	disease process or a system for treating disease	salping/o	tube
-pause	stop, end	scler/o	hard; also the sclera of the eye
-penia	deficiency	-scope	instrument for examination
peri-	around	-scopy	examination with an instrument
phag/o	eat, ingest, swallow	sebac/o, seb/o	sebum, oil
pharmac/o	medication	sept/o	septum, wall, partition; also refers to the number seven
phas/o	speech	septic/o	infection
phleb/o	vein	ser/o	serum
-phobia	irrational fear	sin/o, sinus/o	sinus, cavity, channel, or hollow space
-physis	growth	-sis	process, action, or condition
pil/o	hair	spir/o	breathing
-plasia	form, develop	-stalsis	contraction
-plasty	surgical formation, as in plastic or reconstructive surgery	-stasis	slowing or stopping of the normal flow of a fluid, such as blood
-plegia	paralysis	-stenosis	narrowing
-pnea	breathing	steth/o	chest
poly-	many, excessive, frequent	tax/o	order, arrangement of
poster/o	after, behind	therm/o	temperature
pro-	before, in front of	tox/o, toxic/o	poison
proct/o	rectum and anus	-trophy	nutrition
prurit/o	itching	-ule	small
pseud/o	false	-ure	condition
psych/o	mind	ur/o	urinary system, urine
-ptosis	drooping, falling	-uria	urinary condition
ptyal/o	saliva	vag/o	vagus nerve
pur-, py/o	pus	valv/o, valvul/o	valve
pyel/o	kidney, renal pelvis	ventr/o	belly side
pyr/o	fever, fire	xen/o	foreign (material)
-rrhage, -rrhagia	abnormal or excessive flow or discharge	xer/o	dry
-rrhaphy	suture of; repair of	zygom/o, zygomat/o	zygoma, cheekbone
-rrhea	flow, discharge		

TABLE 7-17 Common Abbreviations in Medical Terminology[a]

Abbreviation	Meaning	Abbreviation	Meaning
A&P	anatomy and physiology	ARDS	adult respiratory distress syndrome
ā	before	ASA	aspirin (acetylsalicylic acid)
AAA	abdominal aortic aneurysm	ASCVD	atherosclerotic cardiovascular disease
abd	abdomen	ASHD	arteriosclerotic or atherosclerotic heart disease
ABCDE	airway, breathing, circulation, disability, and exposure	AV	atrioventricular
AC	antecubital (fossa)	BBB	bundle branch block
ACE	angiotensin-converting enzyme	BGL	blood glucose level
ACLS	advanced cardiac life support	BKA	below-the-knee amputation
ACS	acute coronary syndrome	BM	bowel movement
ADL	activities of daily living	BMD	bag-mask device
ad lib	as desired	BMI	body mass index
AED	automated external defibrillator	BMV	bag-mask ventilation
AF, A-fib, Afib, AFib	atrial fibrillation	BP, B/P	blood pressure
AICD	automatic implantable cardioverter-defibrillator	BPM	beats per minute
AIDS	acquired immunodeficiency syndrome	BS	blood sugar, breath sounds, bowel sounds, bachelor of science (degree)
AIS	acute ischemic stroke	BSA	body surface area
AK	above the knee	BVM	bag-valve-mask
AKA	above-the-knee amputation	bx, Bx	biopsy
ALTE	apparent life-threatening event	c̄	with
AMA	against medical advice	°C	degrees Celsius (centigrade)
amb	ambulatory	CA	cancer, carcinoma, cardiac arrest, chronologic age, coronary artery, cold agglutinin
AMI	acute myocardial infarction	CABDE	circulation, airway, breathing, disability, and exposure
AMS	altered mental status	CABG	coronary artery bypass graft
ant	anterior	CAD	coronary artery disease
AO × 4, A/O × 4, A&O × 4	alert and oriented to person, place, time, and event	CBC	complete blood cell count
AP	anteroposterior (front-to-back), action potential, angina pectoris, anterior pituitary, arterial pressure	CC, C/C	chief complaint

Abbreviation	Meaning	Abbreviation	Meaning
CCU	coronary care unit or critical care unit	DM	diabetes mellitus
C diff	*Clostridioides difficile, Clostridium difficile*	DNR	do not resuscitate
CHD	coronary heart disease	DOA	dead on arrival
CID	cervical immobilization device	DOB	date of birth
CKD	chronic kidney disease	DOD	date of death
cm	centimeter	DOE	dyspnea on exertion
CNS	central nervous system	DON	director of nursing
c/o	complaining of	DPT	diphtheria and tetanus toxoids and pertussis vaccine, doctor of physical therapy
CO	cardiac output, carbon monoxide	DSD	dry sterile dressing
CO_2	carbon dioxide	DtaP	diphtheria and tetanus toxoids and acellular pertussis vaccine
COLD	chronic obstructive lung disease	DTP	diphtheria and tetanus toxoids and pertussis vaccine
COPD	chronic obstructive pulmonary disease	DTs	delirium tremens
COVID-19	coronavirus disease-2019 (novel coronavirus)	DVT	deep vein thrombosis
CP	chest pain, chemically pure, cerebral palsy	Dx	diagnosis
CPAP	continuous positive airway pressure	EBL	estimated blood loss
CPR	cardiopulmonary resuscitation	ECG	electrocardiogram, electrocardiograph, electrocardiography
CR	capillary refill	ED	emergency department, erectile dysfunction
CRNA	certified registered nurse anesthetist	EDC	estimated date of confinement
CRT	capillary refill time, cathode ray tube	EDD	expected (estimated) date of delivery
CSF	cerebrospinal fluid	EEG	electroencephalogram
CVA	cerebrovascular accident	EF	ejection fraction
CVD	cardiovascular disease	EKG	electrocardiogram (the "K" comes from the German word *Elektrokardiogramm*)
DBP	diastolic blood pressure	ENT	ears, nose, and throat
dL	deciliter	EOC	Emergency Operations Center

(continues)

TABLE 7-17 Common Abbreviations in Medical Terminology[a] (continued)

Abbreviation	Meaning	Abbreviation	Meaning
ER	emergency room	HF	heart failure
ESRD	end-stage renal disease	HH	hiatal hernia
ETA	estimated time of arrival	HIV	human immunodeficiency virus
$ETCO_2$	end-tidal carbon dioxide	H_2O	water
ETOH	ethyl alcohol	HPI	history of present illness
ETT	endotracheal tube	HPV	human papillomavirus
°F	degrees Fahrenheit	HR	heart rate
FIO_2	fraction of inspired oxygen	HTN	hypertension
FBS	fasting blood sugar	Hx	history
Fe	iron	I&O	intake and output
FHR	fetal heart rate	ICP	intracranial pressure
FHx	family history	ICS	incident command system, intercostal space
fx	fracture	ICU	intensive care unit
GB	gallbladder	IDDM	insulin-dependent diabetes mellitus
GCS	Glasgow Coma Scale	IHCA	in-hospital cardiac arrest
GERD	gastroesophageal reflux disease	IHD	ischemic heart disease
GI	gastrointestinal	IMS	incident management system
GSW	gunshot wound	IO	intraosseous
GTT	glucose tolerance test	IPPB	intermittent positive pressure breathing
GU	genitourinary	IPPV	intermittent positive pressure ventilation
GYN, gyn	gynecology	IUD	intrauterine (contraceptive) device
H&P	history and physical	JVD	jugular venous distention
H/A	headache	KED	Kendrick Extrication Device
Hb, Hgb	hemoglobin	lac, LAC	laceration
HBP	high blood pressure	LE	lower extremity, left eye, lupus erythematosus
HAV	hepatitis A virus	LLL	left lower lobe (of the lung)
HBV	hepatitis B virus	LLQ	left lower quadrant (of the abdomen)
HCV	hepatitis C virus	L/M, LPM	liters per minute
HCVD	hypertensive cardiovascular disease	LMP	last menstrual period
HD	heart disease	LOC	level of consciousness, loss of consciousness
LOM	loss of motion	NKDA	no known drug allergies

Abbreviation	Meaning	Abbreviation	Meaning
LSB	long spine board	NOI	nature of illness
LUL	left upper lobe (of the lung)	NPA	nasopharyngeal airway
LUQ	left upper quadrant (of the abdomen)	NRB, NRBM	nonrebreathing mask
LVAD	left ventricular assist device	NSR	normal sinus rhythm
MACE	major adverse cardiovascular events	NSTEMI	non–ST-segment elevation myocardial infarction
MAE	moves all extremities	NTG	nitroglycerin
MAEW	moves all extremities well	N/V, N&V	nausea and vomiting
MI	myocardial infarction	N/V/D	nausea, vomiting, and diarrhea
MICU	mobile intensive care unit; medical intensive care unit	O_2	oxygen
min	minute	OB	obstetrics
mm	millimeter	OBS	organic brain syndrome
mm Hg	millimeters of mercury	OD	overdose, right eye, optical density, outside diameter, doctor of optometry
MOI	mechanism of injury	OHCA	out-of-hospital cardiac arrest
MRI	magnetic resonance imaging	OP	outpatient
MRSA	methicillin-resistant *Staphylococcus aureus*	OPA	oropharyngeal airway
MVA	motor vehicle accident	OR	operating room
MVC	motor vehicle crash	OSA	obstructive sleep apnea
MVP	mitral valve prolapse	p̄	after
NA, N/A	not applicable, not available	PAD	peripheral artery disease
NAD	no apparent distress, no appreciable disease	pc	after meals
NARD	no apparent respiratory distress	PCI	percutaneous coronary intervention
NC	nasal cannula	P_{CO_2}	partial pressure of carbon dioxide
NG	nasogastric (tube)	PDR	*Prescriber's Digital Reference* (formerly called *Physicians' Desk Reference*)
NICU	neonatal intensive care unit	PE	pulmonary embolism, physical examination
NIDDM	non–insulin-dependent diabetes mellitus	PEARL, PERL	pupils equal and reactive to light
NKA	no known allergies	PEARLA	pupils equal and reactive to light and accommodation

(continues)

TABLE 7-17 Common Abbreviations in Medical Terminology[a] (continued)

Abbreviation	Meaning	Abbreviation	Meaning
PEARRL	pupils equal and round, regular in size, react to light	ROM	range of motion, rupture of membranes
ped, peds	pediatric	RUL	right upper lobe (of the lung)
PEEP	positive end-expiratory pressure	RUQ	right upper quadrant (of the abdomen)
PERRL	pupils equal, round, and reactive to light	s̄	without
PERRLA	pupils equal, round, and reactive to light and accommodation	SAH	subarachnoid hemorrhage
PID	pelvic inflammatory disease	Sao_2	oxygen saturation
PMH	past medical history	SARS	severe acute respiratory syndrome
PND	paroxysmal nocturnal dyspnea	SBP	systolic blood pressure
PO	postoperative, post op	SCA	sudden cardiac arrest
psi	pounds per square inch	SCD	sudden cardiac death
PSVT	paroxysmal supraventricular tachycardia	SICU	surgical intensive care unit
pt	patient	SIDS	sudden infant death syndrome
PT	physical therapy, prothrombin time	SL	sublingual
PTA	prior to admission, plasma thromboplastin antecedent	SOB	shortness of breath
PTT	partial thromboplastin time	Spo_2	saturation of peripheral oxygen
PVC	premature ventricular complex, polyvinyl chloride	S/S, S&S	signs and symptoms
PVD	peripheral vascular disease	STE	ST-segment elevation
q̄	every	STEMI	ST-segment elevation myocardial infarction
RA	rheumatoid arthritis, right atrium	STI	sexually transmitted infection
RAD	reactive airway disease, right axis deviation	SUID	sudden unexpected infant death
RBC	red blood cell	SVN	small-volume nebulizer
Rh	Rhesus blood factor, rhodium	SVT	supraventricular tachycardia
RLL	right lower lobe (of the lung)	sym, Sx	symptoms
RLQ	right lower quadrant (of the abdomen)	T	temperature
RML	right middle lobe (of the lung)	TB	tuberculosis
RN	registered nurse	TBA	to be admitted, to be announced
R/O	rule out	tech	technician, technologist

Abbreviation	Meaning	Abbreviation	Meaning
TIA	transient ischemic attack	VT, Vtach	ventricular tachycardia
Tx	treatment	W/	with
UA, U/A	urinalysis	WBC	white blood cell
UE	upper extremity	WMD	weapon of mass destruction
URI	upper respiratory infection	WNL	within normal limits
UTI	urinary tract infection	W/O	without
VF, V fib, VFib	ventricular fibrillation	wt	weight
VRE	vancomycin-resistant enterococcus	yo; y.o.; y/o	year old
VS	vital signs	$\bar{x}$	except

[a] Sometimes abbreviations are written with periods (for example, abd.), and sometimes different capitalization might be used and might convey a different meaning. Not all possible meanings for each abbreviation are given in this table. Unless you are certain about the meaning, ask the person who used the abbreviation and do not use it yourself.

YOU are the Paramadic SUMMARY

1. What is the correct medical term for the position in which the child is lying?

He is lying on his left side, which is the recovery position, also called the left lateral recumbent position.

2. How can knowledge of medical terminology assist in your documentation of care for this patient?

Medical terminology is the language of medicine and health care. As a paramedic, you should have a good understanding of medical terminology and be able to identify and use terms correctly. This knowledge enables you to communicate effectively with other health care providers and ensures you use accurate and concise documentation, resulting in better continuity of care.

3. Why would you want to avoid using medical terminology when talking to this patient?

Patients, especially children, are rarely familiar with medical terminology. Therefore, using medical terms during a patient interview may lead to misunderstanding and a lack of pertinent information. When you talk with patients, use everyday terms to improve the likelihood of communicating clearly. As a paramedic, you must also be familiar with terms and phrases that are common in the geographic area in which you work.

4. What are the correct medical terms to describe Tommy's mental status and blood glucose level?

His mental status is documented as AO × 4 because he is alert to person, place, time, and event. The appropriate term for a high blood glucose level is hyperglycemia. It is formed from the prefix *hyper-* (excessive) + the combining form *glyc/o* (glucose) + the suffix *-emia* (pertaining to the blood).

5. How would you document that the patient has no medication allergies?

The correct abbreviation for no known drug allergies is NKDA.

6. Describe the position of the patient's head injury.

His injury is on the right side of his forehead, just above his eye. Since superior is the term for above and orbit is the eye socket, it would be documented as superior to the right orbit. You could also use ® to replace the directional term *right* in your documentation.

7. What is the abbreviation for the abdominal quadrant that is tender to the touch?

The abdomen is divided into quadrants by two imaginary lines intersecting at the umbilicus. Tommy reports having pain in the upper quadrant on the right side. The abbreviation is RUQ.

YOU are the Paramedic SUMMARY continued

8. Why is knowledge of anatomy pertinent when assessing and treating this patient?

Familiarity with the structures and functions of the body's systems enables you to better assess a patient and predict potential complications resulting from occult injuries (those not visible to the eye). In this instance, if you know which organs are located in the RUQ, you can predict possible injuries, which allows for a greater index of suspicion and results in more appropriate treatment and transport to the proper facility.

9. What is the medical term for clammy skin?

The term for clammy skin associated with signs of shock is *diaphoresis*.

10. What is the medical term for a phenomenon (such as pain, swelling, or a rash) affecting both sides of the body?

Many body structures are bilateral, and certain medical conditions tend to occur either unilaterally or bilaterally. A phenomenon affecting or appearing on both sides of the midline is said to be bilateral.

EMS Patient Care Report (PCR)

Date: 4-20-22	**Incident No.:** 050109	**Nature of Call:** Fall	**Location:** 184 Primary Way

Dispatched: 0935	**En Route:** 0936	**At Scene:** 0942	**Transport:** 0957	**At Hospital:** 1009	**In Service:** 1017

Patient Information

Age: 8 **Sex:** M **Weight (in kg [lb]):** 25 kg (56 lb)	**Allergies:** NKDA **Medications:** Insulin **Past Medical History:** IDDM **Chief Complaint:** Fall

Vital Signs

Time: 0945	**BP:**	**Pulse:** 104	**Respirations:** 22	**Spo_2:** 98%
Time: 0950	**BP:**	**Pulse:** 108	**Respirations:** 22	**Spo_2:** 99%
Time: 0955	**BP:** 96/54	**Pulse:** 98	**Respirations:** 18	**Spo_2:** 96%
Time: 1000	**BP:** 98/60	**Pulse:** 98	**Respirations:** 20	**Spo_2:** 99%

EMS Treatment (circle all that apply)

Oxygen @ ____ L/min via (circle one): **NC NRM Bag-mask device**		**Assisted Ventilation**	**Airway Adjunct**	**CPR**
Defibrillation	**Bleeding Control**	**Bandaging:** Hematoma Ⓡ forehead (circled)	**Splinting**	**Other:** Spinal motion restriction (circled)

Narrative

9-1-1 dispatch for a male pt who fell. On arrival at the scene, found the pt, an 8 y/o male, lying Ⓛ lat recumbent in fetal position and holding abdomen; comforted by teacher. Teacher states pt fell about 5 ft from top of playground equipment and has not been moved. Pt AO × 4, c/o pain in RUQ. Presents with a golf ball–size hematoma superior to the Ⓡ orbit c̄ small lac—bleeding controlled. Pt states he has been "dizzy" this morning, causing his fall. PERRLA, slightly tachycardic and tachypneic. Hx—IDDM, for which he takes insulin and has NKDA. Teacher states blood glucose level was 183 mg/dL on arrival this a.m. Pt states he ate and took insulin this a.m. Further assessment of pt's abd revealed that it was soft, but very tender to palpation of RUQ, with discoloration of area. Patient fully c-spine immobilized on LSB c̄ c-collar and CID and loaded into ambulance for transport to the pediatric trauma center. En route, VS reassessed and noted above, BS clear and equal bilaterally, skin pale, cool, and diaphoretic, glucose 147 mg/dL. Pt covered to maintain warmth, head wound bandaged, placed on cardiac monitor showing sinus rhythm Ⓢ ectopy, and 20 g IV Ⓛ AC fossa c̄ NS TKO. Reassessment of abd finds ↑ tenderness and darker discoloration. Met pt's parents and transferred pt care to receiving hospital without incident. Verbal report given to Mary RN. Written report completed and ambulance cleaned and restocked. Departed the hospital and returned to service.

End of report

Prep Kit

Ready for Review

- Knowledge of medical terminology is essential for health care team members to communicate effectively and document calls.
- You must be able to identify superficial landmarks of the body. These landmarks indicate which structures lie underneath the skin, so you can perform an accurate patient assessment.
- Understanding how terms are formed and the definitions for the various parts of a medical term will help you determine the meaning of an unknown term.
- To strengthen your grasp of medical terminology, become familiar with commonly used medical eponyms, homonyms, and antonyms, as well as symbols and terms used in pharmacology.
- A prefix is the part of a term that appears at the beginning of a word. It generally describes the location and intensity of the word root that follows.
- A suffix is placed at the end of a word to change the original meaning. In medical terminology, a suffix usually indicates a procedure, condition, disease, or part of speech.
- The word root is the foundation of the term. It establishes the basic meaning of the word.
- A combining vowel is the part of a term that connects a word root to a suffix or other word root to make it easier to pronounce.
- Prefixes can also indicate numbers or direction. Word roots can also describe color.
- Compound words are words that contain more than one word root.
- To make some terms plural, *-s* is added to the term. Other terms use other plural forms.
- Patient position refers to the position the patient is in when you arrive on scene. Patient positions include prone, supine, and Fowler.
- Anatomic position assumes the person is standing, facing you, arms at the sides, with the palms of the hands facing forward. Anatomic planes of the body include coronal (frontal), transverse (axial), and sagittal (lateral).
- Directional terms indicate distance and direction from the midline. These include right, left, superior, inferior, lateral, medial, proximal, distal, superficial, deep, ventral, dorsal, anterior, posterior, palmar, plantar, and apex.
- Terms related to movement and position include flexion, extension, adduction, abduction, supination, pronation, and rotation.
- Other directional terms relate to a position on one or both sides of the body. Such terms include bilateral, unilateral, ipsilateral, and contralateral.
- The concept of quadrants is useful in medical terminology. The abdomen is commonly divided into quadrants to help specify an area of pain or injury.
- Abbreviations, acronyms, and symbols are used as shorthand to communicate and document concisely. To avoid potentially dangerous misinterpretation of your documentation, ensure you use only abbreviations that are commonly understood in your system; avoid using abbreviations that are not recommended.

Vital Vocabulary

abduction Movement of a limb away from the midline.

adduction Movement of a limb toward the midline.

anatomic position The position of reference, in which the patient stands facing you, arms at the side, with the palms of the hands facing forward.

Prep Kit continued

anterior The front surface of the body; the side facing you in the anatomic position.

anteroposterior axis The axis that runs perpendicular to the coronal plane.

antonyms Pairs of word roots, prefixes, or suffixes that have opposite meanings.

apex The pointed extremity of a conical structure.

bilateral In anatomy, a body part or condition that appears on both sides of the midline.

combining form A word root, prefix, or suffix followed by a vowel.

combining vowel The vowel used to combine two word roots or a word root and a prefix or suffix.

compound words Words containing more than one word root.

contralateral On the opposite side of the body.

coronal (frontal) plane An imaginary plane in which the body is cut into front and back portions.

cross section The product of slicing an object crosswise, perpendicular to its long axis.

deep Farther inside the body and away from the skin.

distal Farther from the trunk and nearer to the free end of the extremity.

dorsal The posterior surface of the body, including the back of the hand.

eponym The name of a disease, device, procedure, or drug that is based on the person who invented, discovered, or first described it.

extension The straightening of a joint.

external rotation Rotating an extremity at its joint away from the midline.

flexion The bending of a joint.

Fowler position A sitting position, with the head elevated at a 90° angle (sitting straight upright).

homonyms Words that sound alike but are spelled differently and have different meanings.

horizontal axis The axis that runs perpendicular to the sagittal plane; also called the mediolateral axis.

hyperextension Maximum extension or extension beyond the normal range of motion.

hyperflexion Maximum flexion or flexion beyond the normal range of motion.

inferior Below or closer to the feet.

internal rotation Rotating the anterior surface of an extremity toward the midline.

ipsilateral On the same side of the body.

lateral In anatomy, parts of the body that lie farther from the midline.

longitudinal axis The axis that runs perpendicular to the transverse plane.

longitudinal section The view of an object cut along its long axis.

medial Closer to the midline.

midsagittal plane (midline) An imaginary vertical line drawn from the middle of the forehead through the nose and the umbilicus (navel) to the floor.

palmar The forward-facing part of the hand in the anatomic position.

plantar The sole or bottom surface of the foot.

posterior In anatomy, the body's back surface; the side away from you in the standard anatomic position.

prefix Part of a term that appears before a word root, changing the meaning of the term.

pronation Turning the palms downward (toward the ground).

prone Lying flat, facedown.

proximal Closer to the trunk.

quadrants The four sections of the abdominal cavity shown by two imaginary lines intersecting at the umbilicus, dividing the abdomen into four equal areas.

range of motion The full distance that a joint can be moved.

Prep Kit continued

sagittal (lateral) plane A plane of the body that passes vertically from front to back, dividing the body into left and right portions.

suffix The part of a term that comes after the word root, at the end of the term.

superficial Closer to or on the surface of the skin.

superior Above or closer to the head.

supination Turning the palms upward (toward the sky).

supine Lying faceup.

synonyms Pairs of word roots, prefixes, or suffixes that have the same or almost the same meaning.

topographic anatomy Superficial landmarks of the body that serve as guides to the structures that lie beneath them.

transverse (axial) plane An imaginary plane passing horizontally through the body at the waist, dividing it into top and bottom halves.

unilateral Occurring or appearing on only one side of the body.

ventral The anterior surface of the body.

word root The foundation of a word; establishes the basic meaning of a word.

References

1. List of error-prone abbreviations, symbols, and designations. Institute for Safe Medication Practices website. https://www.ismp.org/recommendations/error-prone-abbreviations-list. Accessed March 4, 2020.
2. Official "do not use" list. The Joint Commission website. https://www.jointcommission.org/facts_about_do_not_use_list/. Updated August 2020. Accessed March 4, 2020.

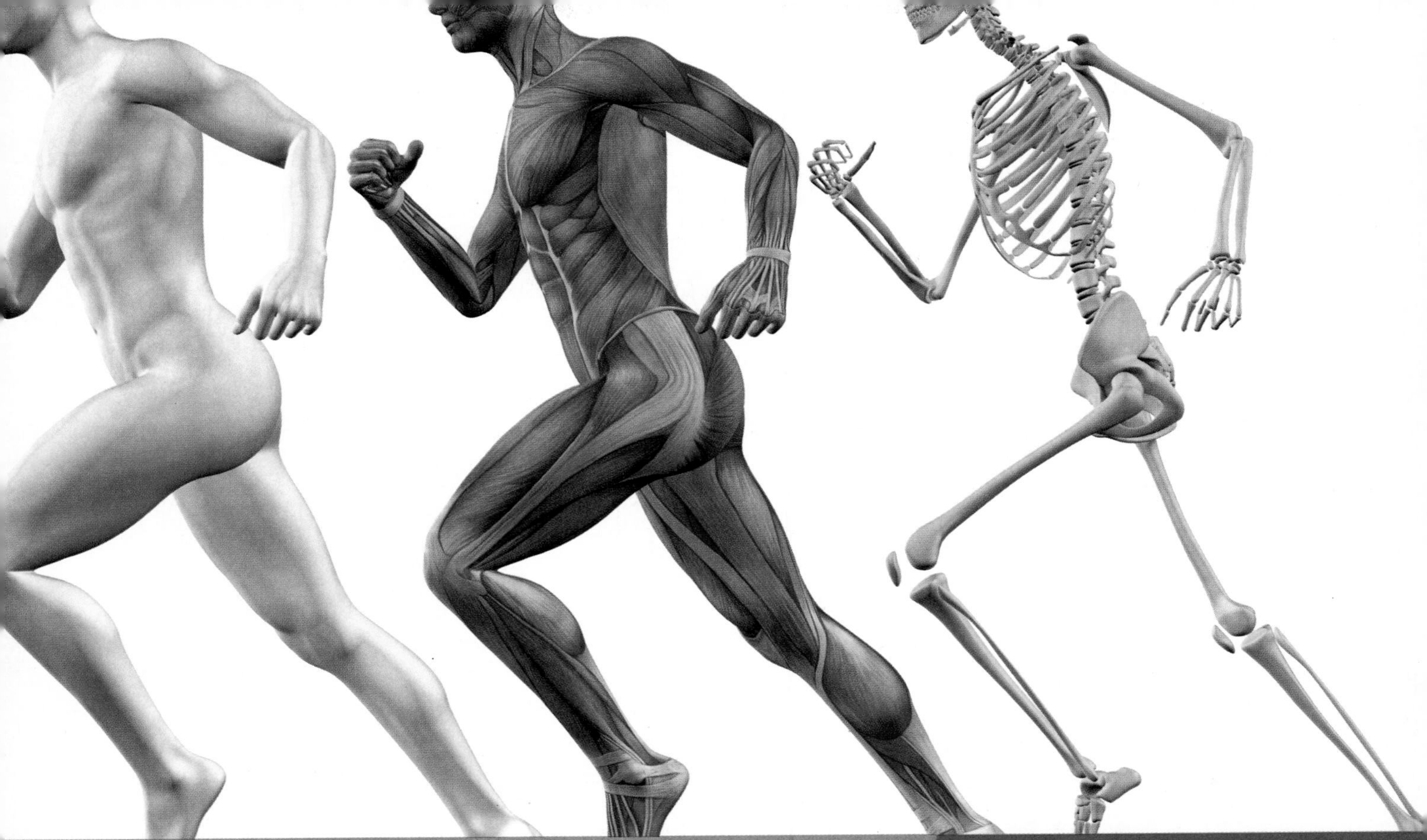

The Human Body and Human Systems

VOLUME 1

SECTION

2

Chapter 8

Anatomy and Physiology

NATIONAL EMS EDUCATION STANDARD COMPETENCIES

Anatomy and Physiology

Integrates a complex depth and comprehensive breadth of knowledge of the anatomy and physiology of all human systems.

KNOWLEDGE OBJECTIVES

1. Discuss the characteristics shared by all living things. (p 271)
2. Describe the levels of organization in the body, from the least complex to the most complex. (p 272)
3. Discuss the body's chemical composition, including key substances: carbohydrates, proteins, lipids, nucleic acids, trace elements, and enzymes. (pp 273–279)
4. Discuss the atomic composition of the body, including chemical bonds and chemical reactions. (pp 272–280)
5. Explain the concept of fluid balance, including the purpose and mechanisms for maintaining homeostasis. (pp 280–282)
6. Differentiate between anabolism and catabolism. (p 280)
7. Describe the components of the cell, including the function of cellular structures. (pp 283–287)
8. Discuss the life cycle of a cell, including interphase, mitosis, cytokinesis, and differentiation. (pp 288–289)
9. Discuss aerobic and anaerobic cellular metabolism. (pp 290–291)
10. Identify the major fluid compartments of the body. (pp 291–292)
11. Discuss cell transport mechanisms, including diffusion, facilitated diffusion, osmosis, and active transport. (pp 292–296)
12. Define *isotonic, hypotonic,* and *hypertonic*. (pp 294–296)
13. Describe the types of tissues found in the body, including epithelial tissue, connective tissue, muscle tissue, neural tissue, and membranes. (pp 296–304)
14. Discuss how the body maintains homeostasis. (pp 304–306)
15. Describe the anatomy and physiology of the integumentary system, including its function, layers of the skin, and other structures present in the skin. (pp 308–311)
16. Discuss the components of the skeletal system, including types of bones. (pp 311–312)
17. Describe the characteristics and composition of bones, including long bone architecture. (pp 312–313)
18. Discuss bone formation, growth, and related hormones. (pp 314–315)
19. Discuss the classifications and types of joints. (pp 315–318)
20. List the sections of the spine. (pp 324–326)
21. Discuss the anatomy and physiology of the muscular system, including gross and

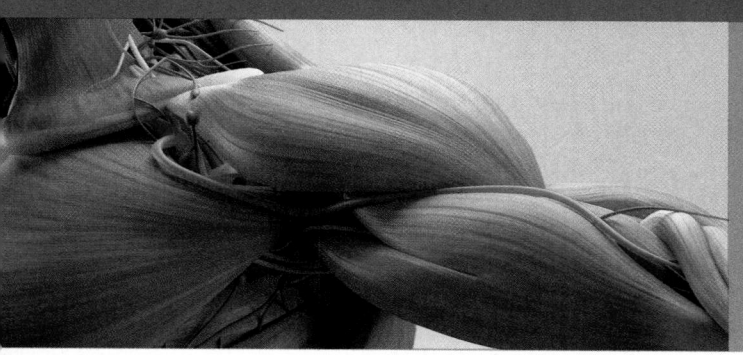

microscopic anatomy, actions of muscles, contraction of skeletal muscle fibers, and major muscles of the body. (pp 334–340)
22. List the divisions and subdivisions of the nervous system. (pp 340–341)
23. Describe the structures involved in the conduction of electrical impulses between the brain and the rest of the body. (pp 341–344)
24. List the structures of the central nervous system and their functions. (pp 345–356)
25. Define the terms *cerebral perfusion pressure* and *pulse pressure*. (p 347)
26. Describe the components of the subdivisions of the peripheral nervous system. (pp 356–368)
27. Describe the sensory function of the nervous system, including types of pain. (pp 368–376)
28. Describe the basic anatomy of the sense organs and explain how they function. (pp 370–376)
29. Discuss the anatomy and physiology of the endocrine system, including endocrine and exocrine glands, chemistry of hormones, regulation of hormone secretion, and the roles of hormones in various processes in the body. (pp 376–387)
30. Discuss the anatomy and physiology of the circulatory system, including the composition and function of blood, the heart, the blood vessels, and the blood groups. (pp 387–396)
31. Discuss the concepts of cardiac output, stroke volume, preload, afterload, and systemic vascular resistance. (pp 396–399)
32. Discuss the Frank-Starling mechanism. (pp 398–399)
33. Discuss the anatomy and physiology of the lymphatic and immune systems, including their primary structures. (pp 411–413)
34. Discuss the anatomy and physiology of the respiratory system, including the structure and function of the nasal cavities, pharynx, larynx, trachea, bronchial tree, alveoli, lungs, and pulmonary capillaries. (pp 413–423)
35. Discuss the lung volumes and dead space. (pp 423–424)
36. Differentiate between ventilation, oxygenation, and respiration. (pp 424–429)
37. Describe the process of gas exchange in the alveoli. (pp 429–430)
38. Explain how oxygen and carbon dioxide are transported in the blood. (pp 428–430)
39. Discuss the mechanisms that regulate breathing. (pp 430–432)
40. Describe the concept of hypoxic drive. (p 432)
41. Explain how the level of carbon dioxide in the blood and the pH of blood relate to ventilation. (pp 432–434)
42. Explain the anatomy and physiology of the digestive system, including its general function, organs and structures involved in digestion, and the process of digestion. (pp 434–445)
43. Describe the anatomy and physiology of the urinary system, including its components, general function, the process of urine formation, and the role of the kidneys in regulating electrolyte balance, acid–base balance, and blood pressure. (pp 445–451)
44. Discuss the anatomy and physiology of the reproductive system, including hormones and structures involved in reproduction, spermatogenesis and oogenesis, and the menstrual cycle. (pp 451–461)

SKILLS OBJECTIVES

There are no skills objectives for this chapter.

Introduction

Knowledge of anatomy and physiology is fundamental to the education of any health care provider and is paramount for successful practice as a paramedic. In every patient encounter, you will call on your knowledge of anatomy and physiology to help you understand the patient's presentation, anticipate or understand the suspected disease process, and make decisions about the care you will provide. A strong foundation of anatomy and physiology is also required to help you fully understand the concepts you will learn in many other chapters of this text, including those related to patient assessment, pharmacology, and specific disease processes.

Anatomy is the study of the structure and makeup of the organism. This knowledge can be divided into gross anatomy, which studies organs and their location in the body, and microscopic anatomy, which studies the tissue and cellular components that cannot be seen with the naked eye.

Physiology is the study of the processes and functions of the body. These systems, operating simultaneously and relying on myriad interactions, all work to maintain a state of balance in which organs and systems can function effectively, known as **homeostasis**. Maintaining homeostasis means the body has the range of temperature, acid–base balance, gas and mineral concentrations, and other conditions necessary for normal life processes to function correctly. Adding the prefix *patho-*, meaning "disease," to the word *physiology* forms the term *pathophysiology*, which is the study of how body functions change and react when the body encounters disease or when homeostasis is otherwise disturbed. See Chapter 9, *Pathophysiology*, for more information.

Characteristics of Life

To understand the design and function of the body, it is beneficial to consider the following characteristics, which are shared by all living things:

- **Absorption.** The ability to take in or soak up materials through various membranes, such as absorbing material through the digestive tract.
- **Circulation.** The ability to transport substances throughout the body via body fluids.
- **Digestion.** The ability to convert food sources into simpler compounds.
- **Excretion.** The ability to expel waste materials.
- **Growth.** The ability to increase in size.
- **Movement.** The ability of the organism to move locations, change position, or move internal structures.
- **Reproduction.** The ability to create new cells, such as in cellular reproduction, or the ability to create new organisms, such as offspring.
- **Respiration.** The ability to use food sources in combination with oxygen to release the energy contained within those sources into the environment.
- **Responsiveness.** The ability to react to internal and external stimuli.

Organizational Structure

To achieve the functions listed previously, the body is organized to ensure the organism works as a whole. This is one of the most important concepts to understand in anatomy and physiology; in fact, the term *organism* comes from *organize* + *-ism*, which indicates that organization is crucial in the body.[1] The levels of organization progress from the simplest (chemical) to the most complex (body as a whole). The six basic units of organization are presented in **TABLE 8-1**.

Chemical Level

Chemical changes within cells influence body functions and the status of the structures of the body. Chemicals of the body include water, **proteins**, **carbohydrates**, **lipids**, **nucleic acids**, and salts, as well as those ingested in the form of foods, drinks, and medications.

Matter, Elements, and Atoms

Mass is a physical property that determines the weight of an object based on the gravitational pull of the earth. Matter includes liquids, gases, and solids

YOU are the Paramedic

PART 1

You and your crew are dispatched to a "truck versus motorcycle" collision on a two-lane highway. On arrival, you learn that a ¾-ton pickup truck was stationary in the left turn lane waiting for traffic to clear. A motorcycle with a single rider was moving toward the truck at highway speed in the opposite lane of traffic when it drifted across the yellow line and struck the truck in the center of the front bumper. The collision caused the truck to be deformed. The motorcyclist was ejected and collided with the truck's windshield, after which the rider rolled to the ground.

1. What anatomic areas of the motorcyclist's body may be injured as a result of this collision?
2. Which anatomic areas of the motorcyclist's body may have life-threatening injuries in this scenario?

TABLE 8-1 Levels of Organization in the Human Body

Level	Description
Chemical	The chemical level consists of atoms and molecules. Atoms are small particles that form the building blocks of matter, which is anything (liquids, gases, and solids) that takes up space and has weight. A molecule is formed when two or more atoms unite through their electron structures.
Cellular	The cellular level is made up of cells, which are the basic living units of structure and function in the human organism. Each cell in the body has a specific purpose or function.
Tissue	**Tissues** are created when several cells with common functions join to form a structure. For example, many muscle cells join to create **muscle tissue**.
Organ	Organs are created when several types of tissue join to perform a function. For example, the heart contains muscle tissue as well as epithelial and nervous tissues.
Organ system	Organ systems are created when several organs combine to perform a common function. For example, the digestive system includes several organs, each of which has a role in breaking down food into components the body can utilize.
Organism	The organism, or human (as in our study of human anatomy), is the combination of all lower levels of organization working together to ensure survival.

both inside and outside of the human body. All living and nonliving matter is made up of elements, which are the simplest form of matter. Elements cannot be broken down into two or more different substances. For example, carbon, hydrogen, oxygen, and nitrogen are elements that make up 96% of a human's body weight. **TABLE 8-2** lists the major and trace elements required by the human body.

Atomic Structure

The characteristics of living and nonliving objects result from the atoms they contain. Atoms are the smallest units of an element, which vary in size, mass (or atomic weight), and how they combine and interact with other atoms. By forming chemical bonds, atoms can combine and interact with other atoms that are not similar to them.

Atoms are composed of particles that include the proton, which carries a positive charge; the electron, which carries a negative charge; and the neutron, which is neutral. An atom that has the same number of protons and electrons has no net charge; that is, it is neither positive nor negative. Protons and neutrons, which are similar in size and mass, are located in the atom's **nucleus**. The mass of an atom is determined mostly by the number of protons and neutrons in its nucleus. The mass of a larger object, such as the human body, is the sum of the masses of all of its atoms.

Electrons orbit the nucleus of an atom at high speed, forming a spherical electron cloud. Atoms normally contain equal numbers of protons and electrons. The number of protons in an atom is known as its atomic number. Thus, hydrogen (H), the simplest atom, has one proton, giving it the atomic number 1, whereas magnesium, with 12 protons, has the atomic number 12.

The atomic weight of an atom of an element equals the number of protons and neutrons in its nucleus. For example, oxygen (O) has eight protons and eight neutrons, so its atomic weight is 16. Atoms with nuclei containing the same number of protons, but different numbers of neutrons, are known as isotopes.

Chemical Bonds

Atoms can bond with other atoms by forming chemical bonds that result from interactions between their electrons. During this process, the atoms may gain, lose, or share electrons. Chemically inactive atoms are known as *inert* atoms. An example of a chemical that is made up of inert atoms is helium.

An atom that gains or loses electrons carries an electrical charge. Electrically charged atoms or groups of atoms are known as **ions**. Ions with a positive charge ($^+$) are *cations*, and those with a negative charge ($^-$) are *anions*. When electrons are transferred or shared between atoms, chemical bonds

TABLE 8-2 Elements of the Human Body

Major Elements (totaling 99.9%)	Percentage in the Body
Oxygen (O)	65%
Carbon (C)	18.5%
Hydrogen (H)	9.5%
Nitrogen (N)	3.2%
Calcium (Ca)	1.5%
Phosphorus (P)	1%
Potassium (K)	0.4%
Sulfur (S)	0.3%
Chlorine (Cl)	0.2%
Sodium (Na)	0.2%
Magnesium (Mg)	0.1%
Trace Elements (totaling 0.1%)	
Chromium (Cr)	
Cobalt (Co)	
Copper (Cu)	
Fluorine (F)	
Iodine (I)	
Iron (Fe)	
Manganese (Mn)	
Zinc (Zn)	

are formed that hold the atoms together, thereby forming a molecule. An **ionic bond** is a chemical bond formed from the attraction between two oppositely charged ions. For example, sodium chloride (table salt) is created when sodium forms an ionic bond with chlorine.

A covalent bond occurs when atoms are bonded to form molecules by sharing electrons. Some covalent bonds do not share electrons equally, resulting in a *polar molecule*—one that has an uneven distribution of charges. Polar molecules have equal numbers of protons and electrons, but one end of the molecule is slightly negative whereas the other end is slightly positive. An example of a polar molecule is water, which is formed from two hydrogen and one oxygen atoms. A peptide bond, which is another type of covalent bond, is discussed in relation to proteins later in this chapter.

A hydrogen bond is a chemical bond formed between a hydrogen atom and a negatively charged atom such as oxygen, nitrogen, or fluorine. Hydrogen bonds are important in protein and nucleic acid structure, and form between polar regions of different parts of a single, large molecule.

A molecular formula represents the numbers and types of atoms in a molecule. The molecular formula for water is H_2O, signifying that it consists of two atoms of hydrogen and one atom of oxygen. Structural formulas are used to signify how atoms are joined and arranged inside molecules. Single lines represent single bonds, and double lines represent double bonds. When structural formulas are represented in three-dimensional models, different colors are used to show different types of atoms.

Compounds

A **compound** is a substance that can be broken down into the two or more elements contained within it. Examples of compounds include water, table sugar, baking soda, alcohol (ie, as used in beverages), natural gas, and most medicinal drugs. A molecule of a compound includes specific types and numbers of atoms. For example, as noted earlier, water consists of two hydrogen atoms and one oxygen atom. When two hydrogen atoms bind with two oxygen atoms, they form hydrogen peroxide instead of water.

A **mineral** is a naturally occurring, inorganic element. Minerals are used in the chemical reactions that occur in the body and are necessary to sustain normal cell function. Humans obtain minerals from plant foods or from animals that have eaten plants. Minerals are most highly concentrated in the bones and teeth. Minerals are classified as *macrominerals* (also called macronutrients, trace minerals, or trace elements) when the daily dietary requirement for them is 100 milligrams (mg) or more; they are classified as *microminerals* when the body needs less than 100 mg daily. Examples of macrominerals include calcium, magnesium, and phosphorus. Chromium, copper, iodine, iron, selenium, and zinc are examples of microminerals.

Organic Compounds

Organic compounds contain the element carbon. Many organic molecules are made up of long chains of carbon atoms linked by covalent bonds. The carbon atoms usually form additional covalent bonds with hydrogen or oxygen atoms and, less commonly, form covalent bonds with nitrogen, phosphorus, sulfur, or other elements.

Organic compounds that occur in living organisms are called *biochemical compounds.* Biochemical compounds are essential for many of the chemical reactions necessary to sustain life. They include carbohydrates, proteins, lipids, vitamins, and nucleic acids.

Carbohydrates

Carbohydrates (saccharides) are sugars or starches. These compounds are composed of carbon, hydrogen, and oxygen. Energy from carbohydrates is used chiefly to power cellular processes.

Types of carbohydrates include **monosaccharides** (simple sugars), **oligosaccharides** (simple sugars consisting of 2 to 10 monosaccharides), disaccharides (double sugars), and **polysaccharides** (complex sugars). Glucose (dextrose), an important simple sugar, is normally found in the blood (the fluid that moves within the cardiovascular system). Fructose, found in fruit juices and honey, and galactose, found in milk and dairy products, are also simple sugars. **Enzymes** in the liver (the largest internal organ in the body) convert fructose and galactose into glucose, which is the form of carbohydrate most commonly oxidized for use as cellular fuel. Ribose and deoxyribose are simple sugars used in the manufacture of ribonucleic acid (RNA) and **deoxyribonucleic acid (DNA)**, which provide the so-called blueprint of the cell.

Disaccharides must be broken down into monosaccharides before they can be absorbed and used by the cells of the human body. Examples of disaccharides include sucrose (table sugar), maltose (malt sugar), and lactose (milk sugar).

Plant starch, animal starch, and cellulose are examples of polysaccharides, which consist of long chains of monosaccharides linked together. Sources of plant starch include potatoes, rice, and peas. **Glycogen**, or animal starch, is the main polysaccharide in the body and is the form in which glucose (sugar) is stored in the human body, primarily in the liver and skeletal muscle. Cellulose is a complex carbohydrate that cannot be digested by humans. It provides bulk (fiber, or roughage) that helps the muscular digestive system walls push food through its tubes.

Proteins

Proteins are the most abundant of the body's organic compounds. All proteins contain carbon, oxygen, hydrogen, and nitrogen. Many proteins also contain sulfur, iron, zinc, and magnesium, and some include phosphorus.

Proteins found in the body include enzymes, plasma proteins, muscle components (actin and myosin), hormones, and antibodies. **Hormones** are substances formed in tiny amounts by one specialized organ or group of cells and then carried to another organ or group of cells in the same organism to perform regulatory functions; thus, they act as chemical messengers. *Antibodies* (also called immunoglobulins) are proteins that detect and destroy foreign substances. After digestion breaks down proteins into amino acids, they may also supply energy. These amino acids are transported to the liver, where they undergo deamination—that is, the loss of their nitrogen-containing portions. The remnants react to form the waste urea, which is excreted in the urine. Other types of proteins include structural proteins such as collagen, a twisted rope-like protein that gives strength to ligaments and **connective tissues**, and keratin, which functions to prevent water loss through the skin. Proteins of the **cell membrane** (cell wall) may serve as receptors and carriers for specific molecules.

Twenty-one different amino acids make up the proteins found in humans and most other living organisms. Protein molecules consisting of amino acids held together by peptide bonds are called **peptides**. A **polypeptide** is formed from many amino acids bound into a chain. Polypeptides usually have specialized functions. When a polypeptide contains more than 100 molecules, it is considered a protein. Certain protein molecules have more than one polypeptide.

An adult human's body can synthesize all except nine of the required amino acids. Essential amino acids are required for proper growth and tissue repair, but the body cannot produce them on its own; therefore, these amino acids must be obtained from dietary sources. Nonessential amino acids are produced by the liver, so they are not considered part of the dietary requirements. Complete proteins (found in milk, meats, and eggs) contain adequate amounts of the essential amino acids. Incomplete proteins (such as those found in corn) have too little tryptophan and lysine to maintain human tissues or support growth and development.

A partially complete protein (such as gliadin, found in wheat) does not have enough lysine to promote growth, but does have enough to maintain life.

Lipids

Lipids are composed of carbon, hydrogen, and oxygen. Many lipids also contain nitrogen and phosphorus. Although lipids are not soluble in water, they may dissolve in other lipids, oils, ether, chloroform, or alcohol.

The most common lipids in the body are triglycerides, **phospholipids**, and steroids (a group that includes cholesterol) **TABLE 8-3**. Triglycerides (fats) are made up of glycerol and fatty acids. The most common lipids found in the diet, they are found in both plant- and animal-based foods. Fats that have a liquid consistency at room temperature are often called oils. **Prostaglandins** are derivatives of an essential fatty acid and are widely distributed in cells throughout the body.

Saturated fats are found mostly in meats, eggs, milk, animal fat (lard), palm oil, and coconut oil. These fats, when consumed in excessive amounts, are a risk factor for cardiovascular disease. Unsaturated fats are present in nuts, seeds, and plant oils. Monounsaturated fats—the healthiest type of fats—are found in olive, peanut, and canola oils. Cholesterol is found in animal products, including liver, egg yolk, whole milk, butter, cheese, and meats. It is not present in foods of plant origin.

Lipids have many functions, but mostly they supply energy to the body. Triglyceride molecules must first undergo hydrolysis (breakdown in the presence of water) before they can release their energy. Via this process, fatty acids and glycerol are released, absorbed, and transported in lymph and blood to the tissues. Some fatty acid portions react to form molecules of acetyl coenzyme A by means of reactions known as *beta oxidation*. Excess amounts of this coenzyme are converted into ketone bodies such as acetone, but can be converted back to their original form if necessary.

The liver uses free fatty acids to synthesize triglycerides, phospholipids, and lipoproteins. However, the liver cannot synthesize some essential fatty acids. For example, linoleic acid (necessary for phospholipid synthesis, cell membrane formation, and transport of lipids) is an essential fatty acid found in corn, cottonseed, and soy oils.

Lipids are less dense than proteins; therefore, the proportion of lipids in a lipoprotein increases as the density of the particle decreases. The reverse is also true. Very low-density lipoproteins have a relatively high concentration of triglycerides. Low-density lipoproteins have a relatively high concentration of cholesterol. High-density lipoproteins have a relatively high concentration of proteins.

The liver controls the level of cholesterol in the body. It synthesizes cholesterol, releases it into the bloodstream, and removes it from the bloodstream to be excreted via bile or to produce bile salts. Although cholesterol does not create energy, it does provide structural materials for cell membranes, and it contributes to the production of certain sex hormones and adrenal hormones.

Triglycerides are stored in adipose tissue (fat tissue) and may be hydrolyzed (broken down) into free fatty acids and glycerol when blood lipid concentration drops, such as during fasting. Lipid functions are shown in **TABLE 8-4**.

TABLE 8-3 Types of Lipids

Type	Examples
Lipids	• Phospholipids • Steroids (eg, cholesterol, bile salts, adrenocortical hormones, sex hormones) • Triglycerides
Lipoid substances	• Fat-soluble vitamins • Lipoproteins • Prostaglandins

Vitamins

Vitamins are organic compounds that are required for normal metabolism. Metabolism may be generally defined as the chemical changes that occur within cells that are necessary to maintain life. Body cells cannot synthesize adequate amounts of vitamins, so they must come from foods. Vitamins are classified by their solubility. Fat-soluble vitamins include A, D, E, and K. Water-soluble vitamins include the B vitamin group and vitamin C.

Bile salts in the small intestine promote the absorption of fat-soluble vitamins. Because these bile salts accumulate in various tissues, their intake must be controlled. For example, when too much vitamin A is consumed, the body receives too much beta-carotene, and the skin may appear orange in color. **TABLE 8-5** describes the fat-soluble vitamins.

TABLE 8-4 Functions of Lipids

Lipid Type	Function
Lipids	
Triglycerides	Long-term energy storage; protection and insulation of body organs
Phospholipids	Essential component of cell membranes
Steroids	
Cholesterol	Helps stabilize cell membranes; necessary for many reactions within the cell
Bile salts	Assist in fat digestion and absorption
Lipid hormones	Sex hormones secreted by **ovaries** and testes; adrenocortical hormones influence blood pressure and fluid volume
Lipoid Substances	
Fat-soluble vitamins	Assist in regulation of biologic processes
Prostaglandins	Help regulate inflammation and tissue repair; regulate effects of several hormones; stimulate smooth muscle; inhibit gastric secretion; influence blood pressure; affect platelet aggregation (clumping)
Lipoproteins	Assist in transportation of fatty acids to and from cells

TABLE 8-5 Fat-Soluble Vitamins

Vitamin	Sources	Characteristics	Functions
A	Liver, fish, whole milk, butter, eggs, leafy green vegetables, yellow and orange vegetables, and fruits	Several forms; synthesized from carotenes; stored in the liver; stable in heat, acids, and bases; unstable in light	Necessary for synthesis of visual pigments, mucoproteins, and mucopolysaccharides; for normal development of bones and teeth; and for maintenance of epithelial cells
D	Produced when skin is exposed to ultraviolet light; also found in milk, egg yolk, fish liver oils, and fortified foods	A group of steroids; resistant to heat, oxidation, acids, and bases; stored in the liver, skin, brain, spleen, and bones	Promotes absorption of calcium and phosphorus, as well as development of teeth and bones
E	Oils from cereal seeds, salad oils, margarine, shortenings, fruits, nuts, and vegetables	A group of compounds; resistant to heat and visible light; unstable in the presence of oxygen and ultraviolet light; stored in muscles and adipose tissue	An antioxidant; prevents oxidation of vitamin A and polyunsaturated fatty acids; may help maintain stability of cell membranes
K	Leafy green vegetables, egg yolk, pork liver, soybean oil, tomatoes, and cauliflower	Occurs in several forms; resistant to heat, but destroyed by acids, bases, and light; stored in the liver	Required for synthesis of prothrombin, which functions in blood clotting

The water-soluble vitamins include the B vitamins and vitamin C. The B vitamins, which consist of compounds essential for normal metabolism, help to oxidize carbohydrates, lipids, and proteins. The B vitamins are often present together in foods; hence, they are referred to as the vitamin B complex. Cooking and food processing destroy some of these vitamins. Vitamin C (ascorbic acid) is one of the least stable vitamins. It is found in many plant foods, and it is necessary for the body to produce collagen, convert folacin to folinic acid, and metabolize certain amino acids. Vitamin C also promotes synthesis of hormones from cholesterol and is vital for iron absorption.

Nucleic Acids

Nucleic acids are large organic molecules (macromolecules) formed by joining many smaller molecules (nucleotides). Nucleic acids carry genetic information or form structures within cells. They contain carbon, hydrogen, oxygen, nitrogen, and phosphorus. Nucleic acids are found in all living things, cells, and viruses.

Nucleic acid molecules are of two types: DNA and RNA. DNA, the genetic material of the cell, is arranged in hereditary units called genes. This genetic information is stored in the genetic code, which specifies the structure and function of the organism. For example, the DNA in your cells determines your inherited characteristics, including hair color, eye color, and blood type. DNA molecules encode the information needed to build proteins. By directing structural protein synthesis, DNA controls the shape and physical characteristics of the human body.

RNA plays an essential role in the process of manufacturing proteins, which relies on the information provided by DNA. Human cells have three types of RNA: (1) messenger RNA, (2) transfer RNA, and (3) ribosomal RNA.

Important structural differences distinguish RNA from DNA. An RNA molecule consists of a single chain of nucleotides, whereas a DNA molecule consists of a pair of nucleotide chains **FIGURE 8-1**. The two DNA strands twist around each other in a double helix that resembles a spiral staircase.

Inorganic Compounds

Inorganic compounds are necessary for fluid balance and for transporting materials through cell membranes. **Fluid balance** is the process of maintaining homeostasis through equal intake of fluids (water taken into the body) and output of fluids (water excreted from the body). Inorganic substances in body cells include oxygen, carbon dioxide, compounds known as salts, and water. The most abundant compound in the human body is water, which accounts for nearly two-thirds of body weight. A **solute** is a dissolved substance. Because solutes dissolved in water are more likely to react with each other as they break down into smaller particles, most metabolic reactions occur in water. In the blood, the watery (aqueous) portion carries vital substances such as oxygen, salts, sugars, and vitamins to and from the digestive tract, respiratory tract, and the cells.

Oxygen enters the body through the respiratory organs, and it is transported in the blood. The red blood cells (RBCs), also known as erythrocytes, carry the largest amount of oxygen to the tissues. **Organelles** are structures inside the cells that use oxygen to release energy from **nutrients** such as glucose and drive cellular metabolic activities. Carbon dioxide is an inorganic compound produced as a waste product when some metabolic processes release energy. Carbon dioxide is exhaled via the lungs, the two primary organs of breathing.

Salts are compounds composed of oppositely charged ions that are abundant in tissues and fluids. Many ions required by the body are supplied in the form of salts. Salt ions are important for transporting substances to and from the cells, as well as for muscle contractions and nerve impulse conduction. **TABLE 8-6** summarizes the common inorganic substances found in the body's cells.

Chemical Reactions

Chemical substances can be altered by chemical reactions that form and break chemical bonds. Nerve, muscle, and blood cells are specialized to carry out distinctive chemical reactions; however, every type of cell performs certain basic chemical reactions—namely, the buildup and breakdown of carbohydrates, lipids, nucleic acids, and proteins.

Enzymes are among the most important of all the body's proteins because they catalyze the reactions that sustain life. *Catalysts* are chemical substances that speed up the rate of a chemical reaction without being consumed in the process.

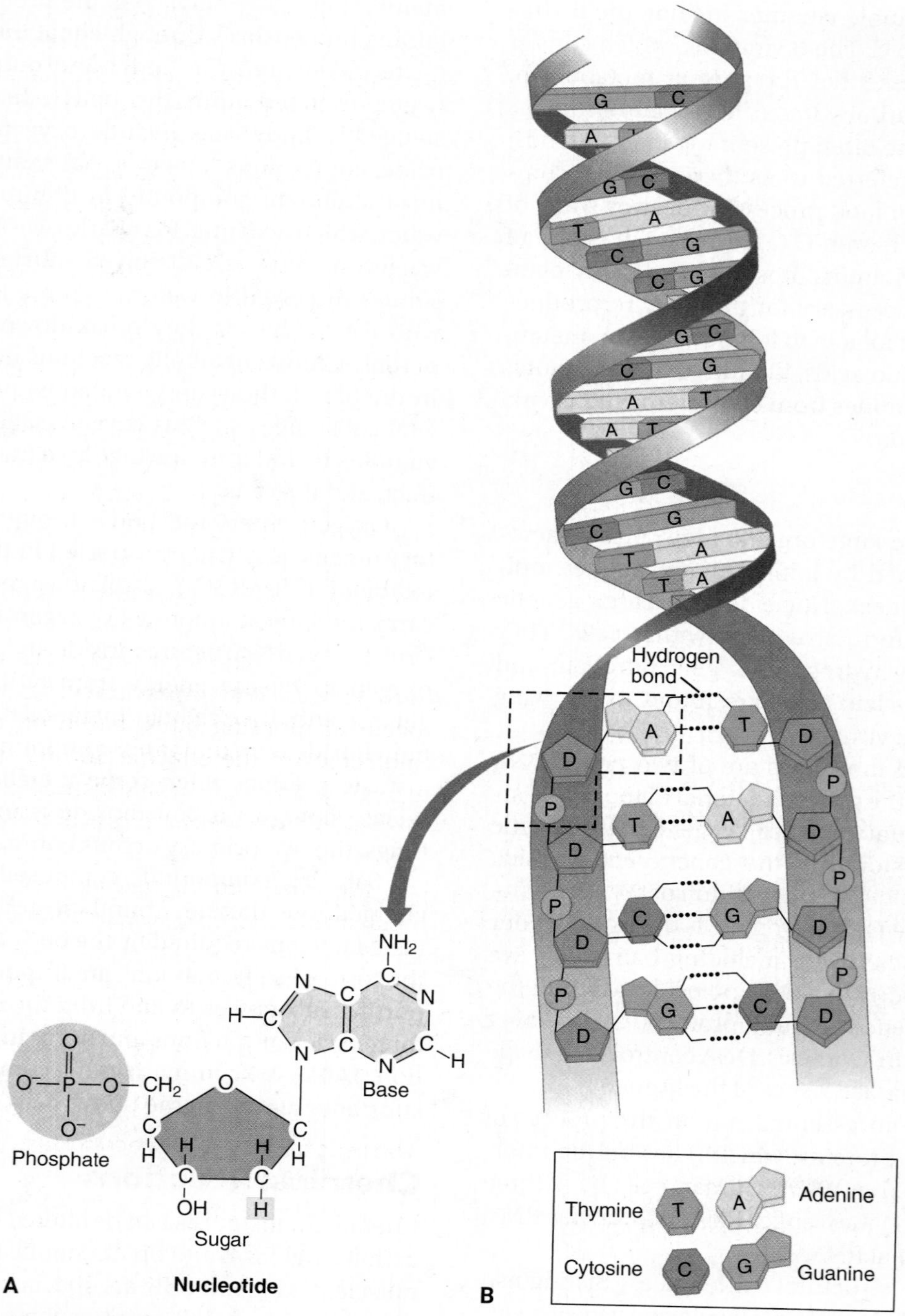

FIGURE 8-1 DNA. **A.** Nucleotide. **B.** The spiral staircase structure of DNA.

A cell manufactures an enzyme molecule to promote a specific reaction. Enzyme molecules that are not used in the reactions they catalyze are recycled.

Specific enzymes facilitate nearly every chemical reaction that occurs in the human body. For example, enzymes assist in the digestion of food, drug metabolism, protein formation, and many other types of reactions. Enzymes make metabolic reactions possible inside cells by controlling temperature conditions that otherwise would be too tepid for reactions to occur. They also promote chemical reactions by lowering the amount of activation

TABLE 8-6 Inorganic Substances in Cells

Molecule or Ion	Function
Carbon dioxide molecules	Metabolic waste product; forms carbonic acid via reaction with water
Oxygen molecules	Used for energy release from glucose molecules
Water molecules	Major component of body fluids, biochemical reactions, chemical transport, and temperature regulation
Bicarbonate ions	Assist in acid–base balance
Calcium ions	Used in bone development, muscle contraction, and blood clotting
Carbonate ions	Used in formation of bone tissue
Chloride ions	Assists in maintaining water balance
Magnesium ions	Used in formation of bone tissue and certain metabolic processes
Phosphate ions	Used in adenosine triphosphate, nucleic acid, and other vital substance synthesis; necessary for formation of bone tissue and to maintain cell membrane polarization
Potassium ions	Used in cell membrane polarization
Sodium ions	Used in cell membrane polarization and maintenance of water balance
Sulfate ions	Assist in cell membrane polarization

energy needed for metabolic reactions, which speeds up the rates of the reactions through a process known as catalysis.

Each enzyme acts on a substrate, which is a particular chemical affected by the enzyme. Enzymes are often named after their substrates, using the suffix *-ase*. For example, a lipid is broken down to glycerol or other alcohols with the help of an enzyme called lipase. Another enzyme, called catalase, facilitates the breakdown of hydrogen peroxide into water and oxygen. Hydrogen peroxide is a toxic substance that results from certain metabolic reactions.

Every cell holds hundreds of enzymes, each of which recognizes its specific substrates. Enzyme molecules have three-dimensional shapes (conformations) that allow them to identify their substrates. The coiled and twisted polypeptide chain of each enzyme specifically fits the shape of its substrate. The active site of an enzyme molecule combines with portions of its substrate molecules temporarily to form an enzyme-substrate complex. When such enzyme-substrate complexes are formed, some chemical bonds within the substrates become distorted or strained. As a result, less energy is required to carry out the reaction, and the enzyme is then released as it was originally configured. These reactions are often reversible. Sometimes, the same enzyme catalyzes the reaction in both forward and reverse directions. Reactions may occur at differing rates, based on the number of molecules in the enzyme and its substrate. Some enzymes process a few substrate molecules every second, whereas others can process thousands in the same length of time.

Enzymes can change because of exposure to heat, electricity, chemicals, radiation, or fluids that have extreme pH levels. Many enzymes are inactive at 45°C (111°F), and most of them are denatured at 55°C (131°F). Denaturation is a process that changes some of the structures of the enzyme. Poisons such as potassium cyanide denature enzymes to achieve their effects. This process stops the cells from being able to release energy from nutrient molecules.

Some enzymes must combine with a nonprotein component if they are to become active. These nonprotein components, which are referred to as cofactors, may consist of the ion of an element (eg, calcium, magnesium, copper, iron, or zinc). Cofactors may also be small, nonprotein, organic molecules called coenzymes. The human body converts many vitamins into essential coenzymes. An example is coenzyme A, which is involved in **cellular respiration** (discussed later in this chapter).

Chemical reactions are represented by chemical equations, which indicate the number and type of molecules involved in the reaction. Four types of chemical reactions are essential to physiology: synthesis reactions, decomposition reactions, exchange reactions, and reversible reactions.

Synthesis Reactions

Chemical reactions change the bonds between atoms, molecules, and ions to generate new chemical combinations. A synthesis reaction occurs when two or more reactants (atoms) bond to form a more complex product or structure. The formation of water from hydrogen and oxygen molecules is a synthesis reaction. Synthesis always involves the formation of new chemical bonds, whether the reactants are atoms or molecules. Synthesis also requires energy, and it is important for the growth and repair of tissues. A synthesis reaction is represented as follows:

$$A + B \rightarrow AB$$

Decomposition Reactions

A decomposition reaction occurs when bonds within a reactant molecule break, forming simpler molecules, or separate atoms or ions. For example, a typical meal contains molecules of sugars, proteins, and fats that are too large and too complex to be absorbed and used by the body in their original form. Decomposition reactions in the digestive tract break down these molecules into smaller fragments before absorption of the nutrients begins. A decomposition reaction is symbolized as follows:

$$AB \rightarrow A + B$$

Exchange Reactions

In an exchange reaction, two substances are decomposed and synthesized to produce new compounds. An example of an exchange reaction is the reaction of an acid with a base, which forms water and a salt. An exchange reaction is symbolized as follows:

$$AB + CD \rightarrow AD + CB$$

Reversible Reactions

In a reversible reaction, the products of the reaction can change back into the original reactants. These reactions can proceed in opposite directions, depending on the relative proportions of reactants and products, as well as how much energy is available. Many important biologic reactions are freely reversible.

A reversible reaction is typically represented using a double-sided arrow, as shown here:

$$H_2O + CO_2 \leftrightarrow H_2CO_3$$

Double arrows ($\leftrightarrows$), also called bidirectional harpoons, technically are considered the proper symbol for reversible reactions. However, the double-sided arrow ($\leftrightarrow$) is commonly used in online documents because it is easier to code.

Cellular Metabolism

Within the structural hierarchy of the human body, the functions of the tissues, organs, and organ systems depend on the functions of individual cells. Thus, cells are constantly breaking down substances and building substances necessary for the survival of the organism. Because of metabolism, organisms grow, maintain body functions, release or store energy, produce and eliminate waste, digest nutrients, and destroy toxins. These reactions alter a substance's chemical nature and allow the organism to maintain a state of homeostasis.

Metabolic processes include both catabolism and anabolism. In **catabolism**, chemical reactions break down larger molecules into smaller ones that the body can use for its own needs. Energy is released during catabolism that is eventually converted to **adenosine triphosphate (ATP)**, the powerful energy source of the body that is used to drive chemical reactions. Catabolism occurs continuously to differing degrees. Excessive catabolism leads to the wasting of tissues.

In contrast to catabolism, **anabolism** is the process of building larger substances from smaller substances, such as building proteins from amino acids. Anabolic reactions generally require energy in the form of ATP. When a person is healthy and has adequate nutrition, the body uses simple nutrients (eg, amino acids, fats, and glucose) to build the basic chemicals that support cellular functioning and sustain life. Cellular metabolism is discussed in more detail later in this chapter.

Electrolytes

Electrolytes are substances that release ions in water. The body's ability to perform normal functions, such as nerve impulse transmission, depends on the presence of appropriate amounts of these substances. When electrolytes dissolve in water, the negative and positive ends of water molecules cause their ions to separate and interact with water molecules instead of each other. The resulting solution contains electrically charged particles (ions) that will conduct electricity.

A **solution** is a mixture of two substances: (1) a **solvent**, which is the fluid that does the dissolving or the substance that contains the dissolved components, and (2) a solute, which is the dissolved particles contained in the solvent. Water in the body serves as the universal solvent, dissolving a variety of solutes. These solutes can be classified as electrolytes or nonelectrolytes.

The unit of measurement for electrolytes is the milliequivalent (mEq); it represents the chemical combining power of the ion and is based on the number of available ionic charges in an electrolyte solution. One mEq of any cation reacts completely with 1 mEq of any anion. For example, sodium (Na^+) is a singly charged (monovalent) cation, and chloride (Cl^-) is a singly charged anion. Thus, 1 mEq of Na^+ will react with 1 mEq of Cl^- to form NaCl, which is table salt. Calcium (Ca^{+2}) has two positive charges (bivalent); thus, the Ca^{+2} ion represents 2 mEq and reacts completely with 2 mEq of a singly charged anion.

The primary cations in the body are sodium, potassium, calcium, and magnesium.

- **Sodium.** Sodium (Na^+) is the principal extracellular cation and the most significant solute in determining total body water and water distribution in the body's intravascular and interstitial fluid compartments. Its role in maintaining adequate cellular perfusion gives rise to the saying, "Where sodium goes, water follows."
- **Potassium.** About 98% of all the body's potassium (K^+) is found inside the body's cells, making it the principal intracellular cation. Potassium plays a significant role in neuromuscular function and in the conversion of glucose into glycogen. Cellular potassium levels are regulated by insulin. The presence of insulin and epinephrine helps the **sodium-potassium pump** operate (discussed later in this chapter). Hypokalemia, which is a low potassium level in the serum, or blood **plasma**, can lead to decreased skeletal muscle function, gastrointestinal (GI) disturbances, and alterations in cardiac function. High potassium levels in the serum (hyperkalemia) can lead to hyperstimulation of neural cell transmission, resulting in cardiac arrest.
- **Calcium.** Calcium (Ca^{+2}) is the principal cation needed for bone growth. It also plays a vital role in the functioning of heart muscle, nerves, and cell membranes and is necessary for proper blood clotting. Low serum calcium levels (hypocalcemia) can lead to overstimulation of nerve cells. High serum calcium levels (hypercalcemia) can lead to decreased stimulation of nerve cells.
- **Magnesium.** Magnesium (Mg^{+2}) has an essential role as a coenzyme in the metabolism of proteins and carbohydrates. In addition, it acts like calcium in controlling neuromuscular irritability.

The primary anions in the body are bicarbonate, chloride, and phosphate.

- **Bicarbonate.** Bicarbonate (HCO_3^-) levels are a determining factor in metabolic acidosis and alkalosis in the body (discussed next). Bicarbonate is the primary buffer used in circulating all body fluids.
- **Chloride.** Chloride (Cl^-) primarily regulates the pH level of the stomach. It also regulates extracellular fluid levels.
- **Phosphorus.** Phosphorus (P) is an essential component in ATP.

Acids, Bases, and the pH Scale

Acids are electrolytes that release hydrogen ions in water. An example of an acid is hydrochloric acid, which is made up of hydrogen (H^+) and chloride (Cl^-) ions. A *base*, or alkali, is an electrolyte that releases ions that bond with hydrogen ions. An example of a base is sodium hydroxide (NaOH), which is composed of sodium (Na^+), oxygen, and hydrogen ions. The oxygen and hydrogen atoms, held together by a covalent bond, form hydroxide (OH^-). The acidity or basicity (alkalinity) of a solution is determined by the amount of free hydrogen in the solution. In body fluids, the concentrations of hydrogen and hydroxide ions greatly affect chemical reactions. These reactions control certain physiologic functions, such as blood pressure (BP) and breathing rates.

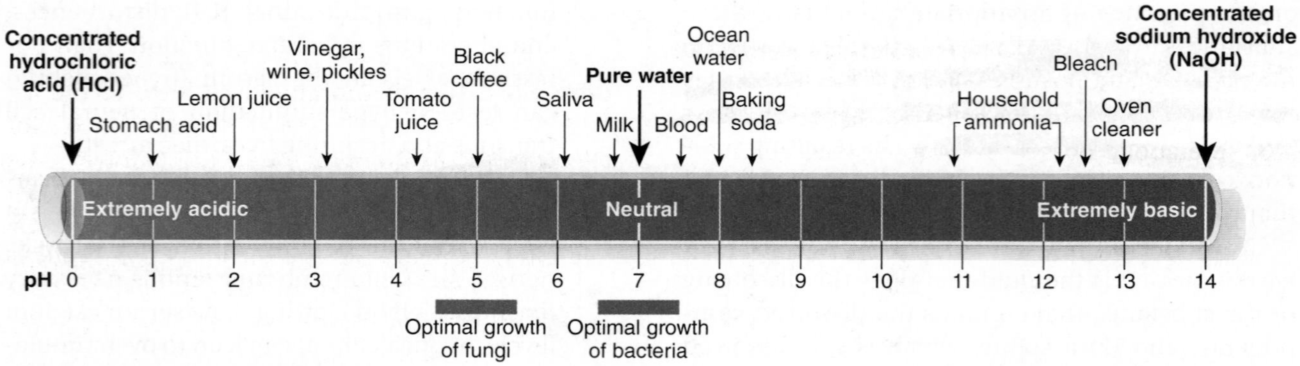

FIGURE 8-2 The pH scale.

The hydrogen ion concentration in body fluids is expressed in a mathematical shorthand based on concentrations calculated in moles per liter (where a mole represents a certain amount of solute in a solution). Hydrogen ion concentrations can also be measured by **pH**; the pH of a solution indicates its acidity or alkalinity. The pH scale ranges from 0 to 14, with 7 being the midpoint (meaning the solution has equal numbers of hydrogen and hydroxide ions) **FIGURE 8-2**. Pure water has a pH of 7, and this midpoint is considered neutral (neither acidic nor alkaline). Milk is an example of a slightly acidic solution owing to its lactic acid concentration. A pH of less than 7 is considered acidic, meaning the substance has more hydrogen ions than hydroxide ions. A pH of more than 7 is considered basic, also known as alkaline, meaning the substance has more hydroxide ions than hydrogen ions. Any solution with a very high pH (such as liquid drain cleaner, which can have a pH approaching 14) is considered a strong base. In contrast, any solution with a very low pH (such as stomach acid, with a pH ranging from 1.5 to 3.5) is considered a very strong acid.

Normally, the human body is slightly alkaline, with a pH between 7.35 and 7.45. Abnormal fluctuations in pH can damage cells and tissues, change the shapes of proteins, and alter cellular functions. **Acidosis** is an abnormal physiologic state caused by blood pH that is lower than 7.35. If blood pH falls below 7, then coma may result. **Alkalosis** results from blood pH that is higher than 7.45. If blood pH rises above 7.8, then it generally causes uncontrollable and sustained skeletal muscle contractions.

The body relies on its buffer systems to maintain its delicate acid–base balance. *Buffers* are molecules or compounds that limit changes in pH by neutralizing excessive acids or bases. In the absence of buffers, the rapid buildup of acid can cause an abrupt change in pH. Buffers regulate changes in pH to avoid such swift changes. For example, bone acts as a buffer by absorbing excess acids and bases and by releasing calcium into the bloodstream.

The ability of weak acids to bond weakly to H^+ ions makes them ideal buffers because they can readily accept or donate H^+ ions, depending on the body's needs. Buffer systems include proteins, phosphate ions, and bicarbonate (HCO_3^-). Because acid production is the major challenge to pH homeostasis, most physiologic buffers combine with H^+. Protein buffering refers to the fact that charged proteins in the cells can accept or donate hydrogen ions, thereby helping to regulate acid–base balance by moving hydrogen into or out of the blood.

Cellular Level

As discussed previously, cells are the basic functional unit of the body. The body's cells vary in shape and function. Over time cells mature, or differentiate. Through this process of **differentiation**, cells become specialized to perform a specific function. For example, some cells make hair, other cells are involved in storing memory, and others help to move your eyes as you read this page. Cells with a common job are grouped closely together into tissues. Groups of tissues that all perform interrelated jobs form organs. A series of organs working together make up the body systems that are discussed in this chapter.

Cells perform the following seven general functions:

1. Movement (muscle cells)
2. **Conductivity** (nerve cells)
3. Metabolic absorption (kidney and intestinal cells)
4. Secretion (mucous gland cells)
5. Excretion (all cells)
6. Respiration (all cells)
7. Reproduction (most cells)

Cell Structure

The human body contains two general classes of cells. Sex cells (also called germ cells or reproductive cells) are discussed in more detail later in this chapter. Somatic cells (derived from the term *soma*, meaning "body") include all the other cells in the human body. This section focuses on somatic cells.

Cells are highly organized structures surrounded by a cell membrane, also called the cytoplasmic membrane or plasma membrane **FIGURE 8-3**. Numerous structures with specific functions are found within the cell; collectively, these structures are called organelles. Inside the cell, the organelles are suspended within a substance called the **cytoplasm**. Most of the cells of the body also contain a nucleus. Genetic material is stored in the nucleus, allowing for the cell's reproduction and new cell growth.

Cell Membrane

The cell membrane encloses the cytoplasm and its organelles. This membrane gives form to the cell and is where most cellular activity takes place. Molecules in the cell membrane create pathways that allow signals outside the cell to be detected and transmitted inside. When cells form tissues, the cell membrane assists in their interconnection by adhering each cell to other cells. The membrane of each cell is extremely thin and delicate, and is able to stretch to differing degrees. Tiny folds on the surface help the cell to increase its surface area.

The cell membrane is composed of a bilayer (two layers), which consists of phosphate and fat molecules called phospholipids. This bilayer forms a fluidlike framework for the membrane **FIGURE 8-4**. The membrane also forms the outer border of the cell and separates the interior of the cell from the fluid surrounding the cell. Any substances within this membrane are termed *intracellular*, and substances outside this membrane are termed *extracellular*.

In addition to providing physical isolation between the intracellular and extracellular compartments, one of the primary functions of the cell membrane is to regulate the transfer of substances in and out of the cell. Depending on their structure, cell membranes can be either differentially

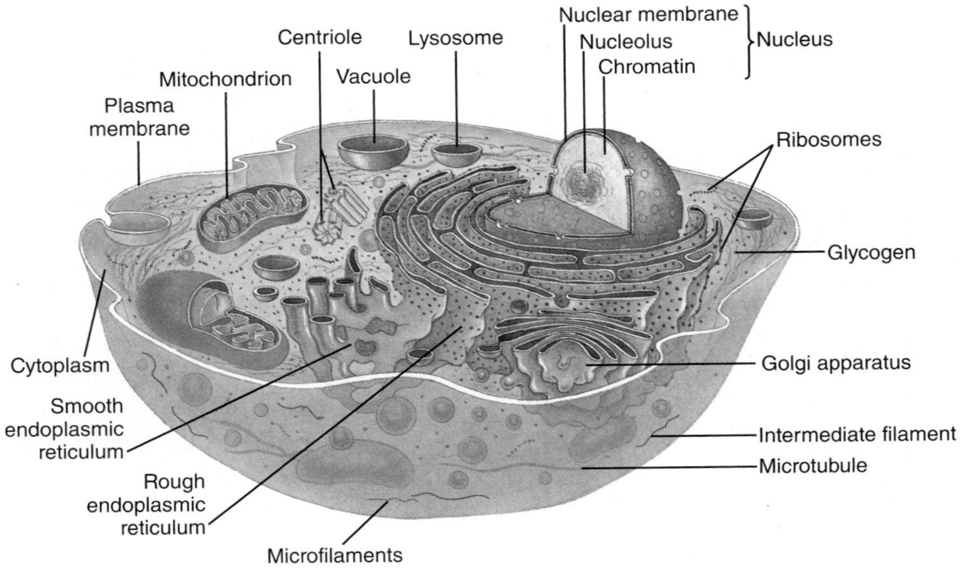

FIGURE 8-3 Cell structure. The cell is divided into nuclear and cytoplasmic compartments. The cytoplasm is packed with organelles.

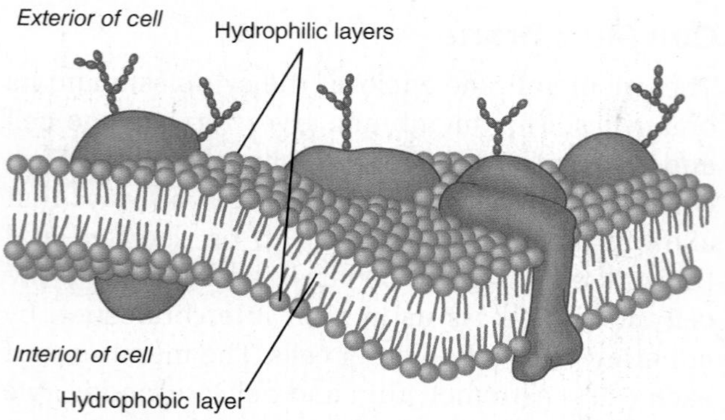

FIGURE 8-4 The phospholipid bilayer.

permeable or **semipermeable**. A semipermeable membrane allows certain elements to pass through while not allowing others to do so. In some instances, and often depending on various factors, only certain substances can enter or leave each cell (a condition known as selective permeability). You can visualize the design of the cell membrane as a series of balloons, with their strings tied together and the balloons facing outward. The balloons represent the phosphate molecules, and the strings represent the lipid molecules. The phosphate molecules attract water, and the lipid molecules repel water, which results in a selectively permeable membrane in which oxygen, carbon dioxide, alcohol, and other substances that are soluble in lipids can freely pass through the membrane. However, water and other substances such as amino acids, proteins, nucleic acids, certain ions, and sugars are unable to pass through the membrane itself. The transport of substances in and out of the cell is discussed in more detail later in this chapter.

The cell membrane also has several proteins, known as membrane proteins, embedded and floating within it. These proteins serve the following functions:

- **Channel proteins.** Channel proteins act as a pore through the membrane that allows the passive passage of substances into the intracellular compartment. As an example, consider how water enters and leaves the cell. As previously mentioned, water is unable to cross through the membrane itself; however, because of the amount of channel proteins that allow the passage of water, it can essentially freely enter and exit the cell. Another category of channel proteins are gated ion channels, which open and close at specific times and generally allow only specific substances to pass through. Calcium, for example, passes through the calcium channels, and sodium passes through the sodium channels. Both are examples of voltage-gated ion channels. Some medications that you will administer (eg, calcium channel blockers and sodium channel blockers) cause a dramatic effect on cellular function by altering transport through membrane channel proteins.
- **Enzyme receptors.** Enzyme receptors act as sites where enzymes can bind. Binding occurs inside the cell, and the enzyme acts as a catalyst for a reaction to occur in the cell itself.
- **Proteins that act as receptor sites.** These proteins have their binding site on the outside of the cell membrane. The majority of these receptor sites are specific to certain molecules; when the correct molecule binds to the receptor site, a change in cellular function occurs. Such changes are crucial to the proper function of the cell; however, as a paramedic, you will also use these sites for therapeutic purposes. For example, administering a narcotic or narcotic antagonist results in the medication binding to narcotic receptor sites.
- **Identifier proteins.** These proteins identify the cell as part of a particular organism. The immune system uses this identification to determine "self" from "nonself" as part of its defense against outside invaders.
- **Carrier proteins.** These proteins bind to substances and transport them across the cell membrane, which is generally an active process. For example, the sodium-potassium pump moves sodium out of the cell and potassium into the cell.

In addition, some membrane proteins attach to the cytoskeleton of the cell and help determine its shape. Other membrane proteins adhere to the membrane proteins of adjacent cells, thereby forming tissues.

Cytoplasm

The cytoplasm is the fluidlike material in which the organelles of the cell are suspended. It lies between the cell membrane and the nucleus. The fluid

> **Words of Wisdom**
>
> Fatty compounds (such as those found in the cell membrane) are chemically neutral (uncharged), whereas electrolytes (such as sodium and potassium) are water based (charged). Thus, a charged molecule has to travel through a special pathway to permeate a cell membrane. These transport channels—the so-called ion channels—consist of protein-lined pores (openings) specifically sized for each substance (eg, calcium, potassium). Local anesthetics (such as lidocaine) and antidysrhythmic drugs (such as amiodarone) exert their effects by blocking ion channels.

contained within the nucleus is the *nucleoplasm.* The cytoplasm usually appears clear with scattered specks, though more powerful magnification reveals that it contains membranous networks, protein frameworks, and a cytoskeleton (cell skeleton).

Cytosol is the fluid portion of cytoplasm; it contains mostly water, as well as glucose, amino acids, fatty acids, ions, lipids, proteins, ATP, and waste products. Many of the chemical reactions necessary for life take place within the cytoplasm. One of the most important of these reactions is glycolysis, the first step in cellular respiration.

Organelles

The organelles within the cytoplasm work like miniature factories within the cell to perform specific functions related to cell structure, growth, maintenance, and metabolism. The following organelles have specific actions that help the cell to carry out its activities:

- **Centrioles.** Cell division requires a pair of centrioles, which are cylindrical structures made up of short microtubules. During cell division, the centrioles form the spindle-shaped structure needed for movement of DNA strands. Cardiac muscle cells, skeletal muscle cells, mature RBCs, and typical **neurons** (nerve cells) have no centrioles; therefore, these cells are incapable of dividing. The centrosome is the cytoplasm surrounding the centrioles. Microtubules of the cytoskeleton usually begin at the centrosome and radiate through the cytoplasm.
- **Cilia and flagella.** These structures extend from certain cell surfaces. Cilia are hairlike extensions, which move in a coordinated sweeping motion to propel fluids over the surface of tissues. They are found on cells lining both the respiratory and reproductive tracts. The cells that line the respiratory tract have a large number of cilia that act to move particles that have been inhaled and trapped in the **mucus** into the **oropharynx**, where they can be either swallowed or expelled. Whereas cilia move substances other than cells, flagella, which are longer than cilia, propel the cells to which they are attached. In humans, a flagellum appears as the tail of a sperm cell.
- **Ribosomes.** Ribosomes are made of complex strands of macromolecules of protein and RNA.[2,3] Ribosome chains create the framework for the genetic blueprint and the synthesis of proteins. Ribosomes may be found either floating freely within the cytoplasm or attached to the endoplasmic reticulum. Because their functions involve the formation of proteins, ribosomes are often called the protein factories of the cell.
- **Endoplasmic reticulum (ER).** The ER is a chain of canals and sacs that wind through the cytoplasm and connect the nuclear membrane to the cell membrane. The ER moves substances and proteins through the cell. It also plays a part in the detoxification process. The ER is identified as either smooth or rough based on the presence or absence of ribosomes on its surface **FIGURE 8-5**. The smooth ER lacks ribosomes, and can synthesize phospholipids and cholesterol, which are needed for the growth and maintenance of the cell membrane. The rough ER has ribosomes on its surface, and is found in cells that produce proteins to be excreted for use outside the cell. Both free and fixed ribosomes synthesize proteins based on instructions from messenger RNA. After creating proteins, the ribosomes transfer the proteins into the rough ER for transport to the Golgi apparatus, where they will be further processed.
- **Golgi apparatus.** Also called the Golgi complex, this organelle consists of a stack of several flattened sacs. These pancakelike structures are hollow, with cavities called cisternae inside

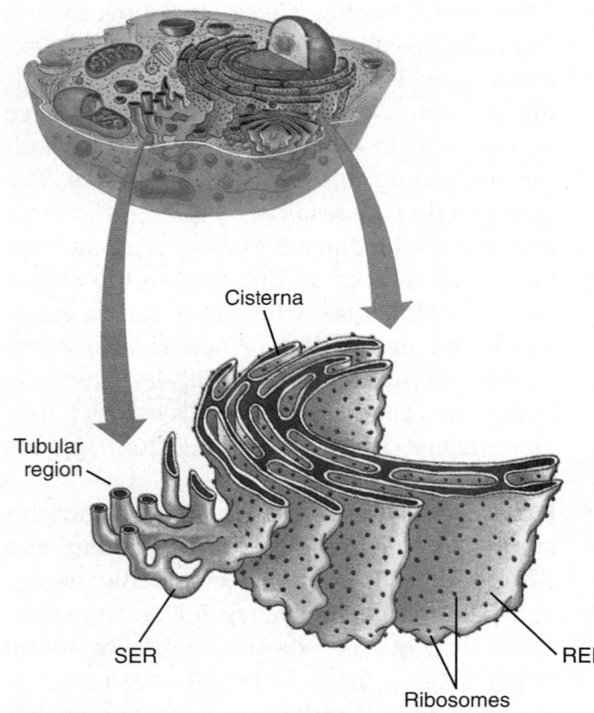

FIGURE 8-5 Rough endoplasmic reticulum (RER) with fixed ribosomes on its outer surface.

Abbreviation: SER, smooth endoplasmic reticulum

them. The Golgi apparatus deals primarily with proteins synthesized on the ribosomes. One end of this organelle is specialized to receive glycoproteins and then modify them by removing or adding sugar molecules. The Golgi apparatus has three main functions: (1) concentrating and packaging secretions (such as hormones or enzymes) for their release out of the cell, (2) packaging special enzymes inside vesicles for use in the cytosol, and (3) renewing or modifying the cell membrane. Mucus is an example of a Golgi apparatus product.

- **Lysosomes.** These tiny sacs perform "housekeeping" tasks within the cell. The enzymes contained within these structures help digest nucleic acids, fats, proteins, polysaccharides, and lipids. Certain white blood cells (WBCs, or leukocytes) have large amounts of lysosomes that contain enzymes designed to digest bacteria. Lysosomes also digest nonfunctional organelles.
- **Microfilaments.** The smallest of the cytoskeletal elements, microfilaments are composed of two proteins, actin and myosin. They are typically found in muscle cells. Microfilaments enable cell movement and contraction via interaction with actin and myosin. This process can also change the shape of the entire cell.
- **Mitochondria.** The so-called power plants of the cell and the body, mitochondria are the site of aerobic respiration. Aerobic respiration results in the creation of ATP, which serves as a source of energy throughout the body. The number of mitochondria (singular, *mitochondrion*) in a particular cell varies based on the cell's energy demands. The liver, kidneys, and muscles have many mitochondria in their cells because they use ATP at a high rate. Two membranes surround a mitochondrion: The outer membrane gives the organelle its shape, and the inner membrane creates several folds called cristae. These two membranes are important in cellular respiration. Mitochondria contain their own DNA, albeit in a more primitive form than that found within the cell's nucleus.
- **Peroxisomes.** These sacs contain enzymes that speed up many biochemical reactions. They are abundant in the liver and kidney cells, and their diverse actions include the synthesis of bile acids, detoxification of hydrogen peroxide or alcohol, and breakdown of lipids and biochemicals.
- **Thick filaments.** These organelles are relatively massive bundles of subunits composed of the protein myosin. Thick filaments appear in muscle cells only, where they interact with actin filaments to produce powerful contractions.
- **Vesicles.** Also known as vacuoles, these sacs are formed when part of a cell membrane folds inward, establishing a bubblelike structure within the cytoplasm. They transport a wide variety of substances inside the cell (endocytotic vesicles) and to the exterior of the cell (exocytotic vesicles).

Nucleus

The nucleus is usually a large structure located near the center of a typical cell. The nuclear membrane surrounds the nucleus. This membrane (similar to the cell membrane) encases the nucleoplasm. Within the nucleoplasm are specialized structures that carry the genetic material that the cell uses for reproduction. This material serves as a blueprint for the cell's function. DNA resides on threads of chromatin, which are tangles of **chromosomes** that contain thousands of genes.

The nucleus also contains a suborganelle called the nucleolus, which is nonmembranous. The nucleolus is densely packed with RNA and surrounded by chromatin. RNA is responsible for ribosome production. After their creation, ribosomes pass through pores in the nuclear envelope (the outer boundary between nucleus and rest of the cell) to the ER for protein synthesis. Recall that RNA and DNA are the so-called blueprints of the cell. Because of this function, the products, appearance, reproduction, and all other aspects of the cell are controlled by the nucleus. Cells without a nucleus, such as RBCs, have a limited life span.

TABLE 8-7 summarizes cell structures and function.

TABLE 8-7 Cell Structures and Function

Location	Cell Structure	Function
Nucleus • Control center of the cell • Stores genetic information • Responsible for cell reproduction	Chromatin	Long, slender threads on which DNA is present; during cell division or replication, the chromatin coils to form chromosomes that contain genes
	Nuclear membrane	Composed of two layers and surrounds the nucleus; contains pores (openings) for transport of materials; controls movement of material into and out of the nucleus
	Nucleolus	Small, spherical structure that has a high concentration of RNA and is the site of ribosome formation
Cytoplasm • Clear, sticky, fluidlike material found outside the nucleus but within the cell membrane that surrounds, supports, and protects organelles • Medium through which nutrients and waste move	Centrioles	Tiny cylinders that help separate the chromosomes during mitosis (cell division)
	Cytoskeleton	Protein rods that provide intracellular shape and support and aid movement of materials into and out of cells
	Endoplasmic reticulum (ER)	Membranous channels that serve as the transport system of the cell through the cytoplasm; rough ER contains ribosomes where protein is synthesized; smooth ER is the site of steroid, phospholipid, and fatty acid synthesis; smooth ER in liver cells breaks down alcohol and some drugs, such as amphetamines
	Golgi apparatus	Membranous structures that resemble a stack of pancakes; found near the nucleus and serve to package and export proteins
	Lysosomes	Small, round structures that perform "housekeeping" tasks within the cell, digesting cell waste through powerful enzymes
	Mitochondria	Fluid-filled sacs that serve as the so-called power plants of the cell and carry on cellular respiration, converting energy in nutrients to ATP
	Ribosomes	Small granules of RNA that, when fully assembled, function as miniature protein factories
	Vesicles	Tiny membranous sacs used for storage and transport of cellular products and digestion of the metabolic waste of the cell
Surface • Encloses the cytoplasm and forms the outer boundary of the cell	Plasma membrane	Provides support and protection; the plasma membrane is selectively permeable, allowing some substances to enter and leave the cell while not allowing other substances to cross

Abbreviations: ATP, adenosine triphosphate; DNA, deoxyribonucleic acid; RNA, ribonucleic acid

Life Cycle of the Cell

The life cycle of the cell is regulated via stimulation from hormones or growth factors. Disruption of this cycle can affect the health of the body. Most human cells divide between 40 to 60 times before they die. The life cycle of a cell includes the following four steps:

1. **Interphase.** The cell obtains nutrients to grow and duplicate.
2. **Cell division (mitosis).** The nucleus divides.
3. **Cytoplasmic division (cytokinesis).** The cytoplasm divides.
4. **Differentiation.** The cell becomes specialized.

Interphase

A cell must grow and duplicate most of its contents before it can actively divide. *Interphase* describes this period of preparation for division. The cell manufactures new living material during interphase by duplicating membranes, lysosomes, mitochondria, and ribosomes. The cell also replicates its own genetic material.

Cell Division and Cytoplasmic Division

The two types of cell division are meiosis and mitosis/cytokinesis. **Meiosis** is cell division that occurs in the production of eggs (**oocytes**) and sperm. During meiosis, the number of chromosomes is reduced by one-half, from 46 to 23. When a sperm joins with an egg and fertilization occurs, the resulting cell will have 46 chromosomes, having received 23 from the sperm and 23 from the egg.

In the rest of the body, cell numbers are increased by **mitosis**, the division of the nucleus of a cell, and cytokinesis, the division of the cytoplasm of a cell. The nucleus must divide precisely so the new cell can make an accurate copy of the DNA. Most human body cells, except for sex cells and RBCs, reproduce by mitosis.

In this continuous process of division and multiplication, one cell divides to become two new cells that are identical to the original cell (the two cells are referred to as daughter cells). Many cells of the body reproduce in this fashion throughout life (eg, skin cells). Other cells divide only in the fetus, with their replication eventually stopping near birth (eg, nerve and skeletal cells).

Mitosis proceeds through four stages **FIGURE 8-6**:

1. **Prophase.** The two new centriole pairs move to opposite ends of the cell. The chromatin

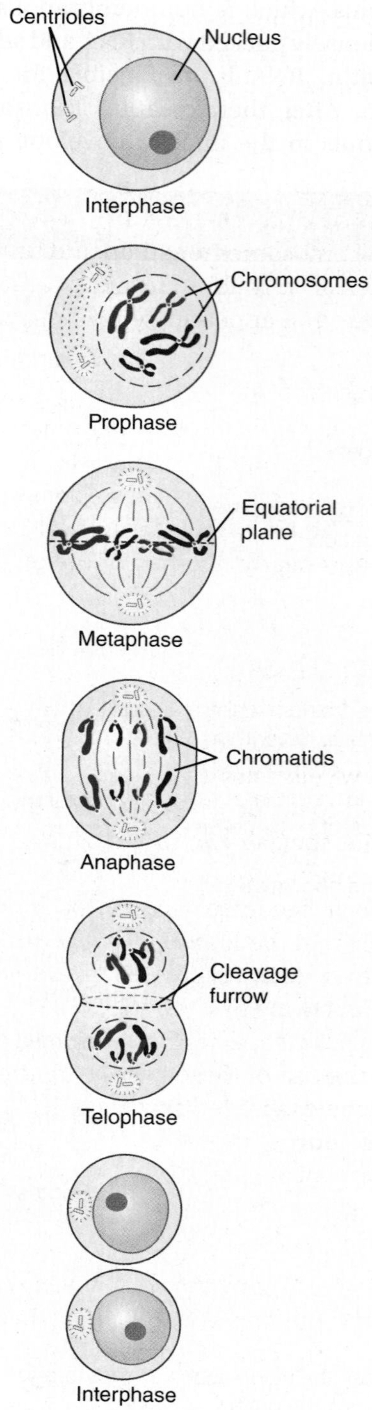

FIGURE 8-6 Mitosis and cell division.

becomes shorter and thicker. Spindle fibers develop, whereas the nucleolus and nuclear membrane disappear.

2. **Metaphase.** The chromosomes line up near the middle portion of the cell, between the centrioles, and spindle fibers attach to them.
3. **Anaphase.** The central areas of each chromosome, called centromeres, are pulled apart to become individual chromosomes, and move toward opposite ends of the cell.
4. **Telophase.** The spindle fibers disappear and the chromosomes lengthen and unwind, with a nuclear envelope forming around them and nucleoli appearing in each newly formed nucleus.

Cytoplasmic division (cytokinesis) begins during anaphase, when the cell membrane constricts down the middle portion of the cell. This process continues through telophase to divide the cytoplasm. The two newly formed nuclei are then separated and nearly one-half of the organelles are distributed into each new cell.

Differentiation

As discussed previously, differentiation—that is, the process of specialization of a cell—makes each cell unique. New cells must be generated for growth and tissue repair to occur. **Stem cells** can divide repeatedly without specializing. They can divide into two identical daughter cells or can divide so that one daughter cell becomes partially specialized (progenitor cells). In the human body, all differentiated cell types are ultimately created from stem and progenitor cells. Owing to stem cells' ability to turn into multiple types of specialized cells, researchers are exploring the use of these cells in treating diseases such as diabetes, heart disease, stroke, macular degeneration, burns, osteoarthritis, and rheumatoid arthritis, as well as spinal injuries.

Cell Division and Cancer

Cell division and growth usually occur at approximately the same rate as cell death. However, when cell division and growth occur at a higher rate than the cell death rate, tissues become enlarged. A **neoplasm** (tumor) is a mass of tissue produced by abnormal cell growth and division. A tumor is *benign* when it remains within the epithelium (a capsule made of connective tissue). A benign tumor seldom becomes life threatening and can usually be surgically removed if it affects tissue function.

In contrast, a *malignant* tumor spreads into surrounding tissues in a process called invasion. Malignancy often occurs when a normal gene mutates; such mutated genes are called oncogenes. In the disease known as cancer, the mutations disrupt normal cell growth. The malignant cells may escape the tumor of origin (the primary tumor or primary neoplasm) and invade other organs or tissue, resulting in secondary tumors. This process—metastasis—is not easily controlled. Usually, tumor cells are daughter cells of just one malignant cell. Cancer often begins where stem cells divide, because the more frequently chromosomes are copied for cell division, the greater the chance of errors in the DNA copying process, leading to mutations in the new cells.

Cancer cells change shape as they grow, such that they gradually resemble normal cells less and less. If tumor cells penetrate blood vessels, then they circulate throughout the body. If tumor cells enter the **lymphatic system**, then they build up in **lymph nodes**. The presence of tumor cells stimulates the growth of new blood vessels wherever the cells situate themselves. The blood carried by these new vessels supplies the cells with more nutrients, accelerating their growth and further metastasis.

As metastasis increases, organ function changes. Cancer cells grow and multiply by taking nutrients and space from normal cells, causing weight loss in most patients with cancer as the normal cells deteriorate. Death may occur when cancer cells compress vital organs or replace healthy cells in vital organs.

Cellular Signaling

To work collectively as a cohesive unit, cells must be able to communicate with other cells and within individual cells. How cells communicate electrochemically is called intercellular communication or cellular signaling. Cellular signaling is used to maintain homeostasis, fight infection, reproduce, and perform other normal functions. Alterations in signals also can lead to dysfunction. Indeed, some tumors and cancers are believed to result from disruptions in this process. Cellular signaling is discussed in more detail later in this chapter.

Cellular Respiration

Almost all metabolic functions require energy. The primary source of energy for the cells is a six-carbon sugar, glucose ($C_6H_{12}O_6$). The use of glucose by the cell is called oxidation, and this process results in carbon dioxide (CO_2), water (H_2O), and the high-energy molecule ATP. ATP is the true source of cellular energy because of the high-energy bonds contained between its phosphate molecules. When needed for cellular function, these bonds are broken to release their stored energy. Although a large amount of energy is contained in these bonds and released by breaking them, glucose actually has the potential to release even more energy. If glucose molecules were to be broken down in one step, then a considerable loss of energy to heat would occur, with minimal ATP production. To maximize the number of molecules of ATP created for each molecule of glucose, however, cellular respiration occurs in three stages.

Glycolysis

As the first step in cellular respiration, **glycolysis** occurs in the cytoplasm. Glycolysis is an *anaerobic* process, meaning it does not require oxygen **FIGURE 8-7**. After the glucose molecule moves into the cell, two phosphate molecules, gained from breaking two ATP molecules, immediately attach to it in separate steps. This process prevents both the glucose from leaving the cells and the glucose concentration inside the cells from becoming higher than the concentration outside the cells. It also prepares the glucose molecule for further breakdown. Next, a series of complex steps occur to break down the glucose molecule into its final product, two molecules of pyruvic acid. During this phase of cellular respiration, two molecules of pyruvic acid and four ATP molecules are formed. However, recall that two ATP molecules were broken down in the early steps of this process; therefore, the net result of glycolysis is two molecules of pyruvic acid and two molecules of ATP. This process is an inefficient use of glucose, but fortunately, it does not end here.

Krebs Cycle

The second step in cellular respiration is the Krebs cycle, also known as the **citric acid cycle** (tricarboxylic

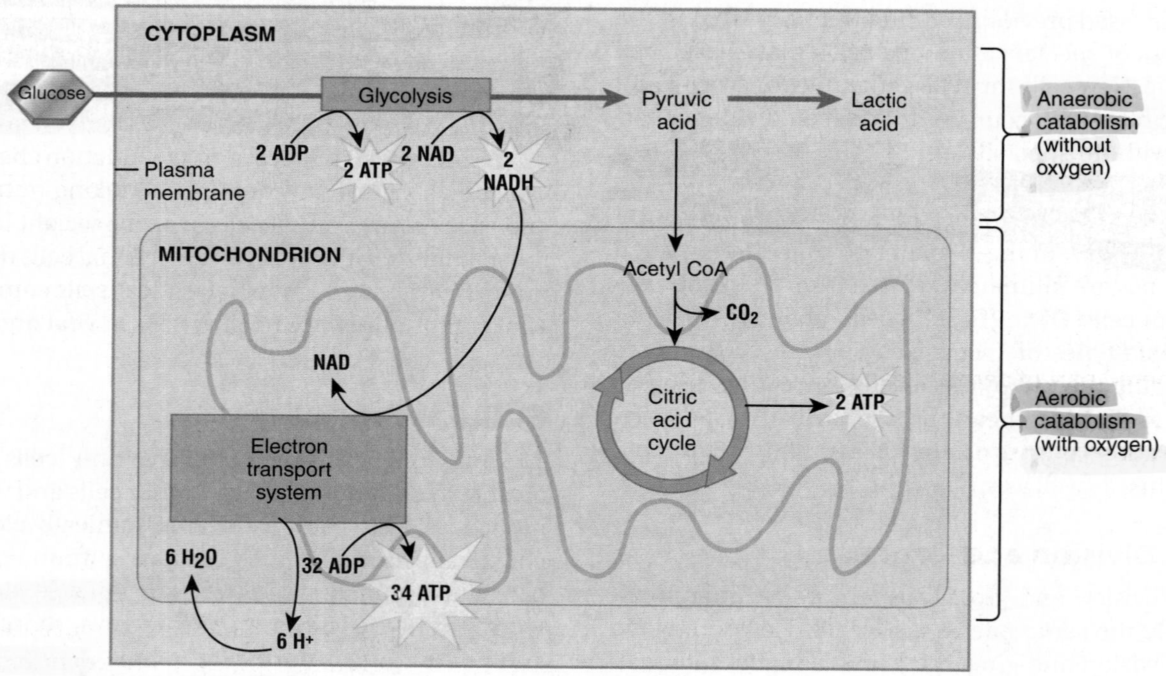

FIGURE 8-7 During anaerobic metabolism, which occurs in the cytoplasm, the breakdown of glucose results in lactic acid. During aerobic metabolism, which occurs in the mitochondrion, the breakdown of glucose results in carbon dioxide, water, and adenosine triphosphate (ATP).

Abbreviations: ADP, adenosine diphosphate; CoA, coenzyme A; NAD, nicotinamide adenine dinucleotide; NADH, reduced nicotinamide adenine dinucleotide acid cycle). The key to this stage in the breakdown of glucose is the presence or absence of oxygen: The Krebs cycle occurs only in the presence of oxygen (**aerobic metabolism**) (see Figure 8-7). Within the matrix (the nonliving material that separates cells in the connective tissue) of the mitochondria, the pyruvic acid formed during glycolysis undergoes a complex series of steps that produce several products, including three carbon dioxide molecules and one molecule of ATP. Because two molecules of pyruvic acid are produced during glycolysis, the Krebs cycle occurs twice for each molecule of glucose that is oxidized. Therefore, the result of the Krebs cycle is six molecules of carbon dioxide (this principle is vital in the concept of capnography) and two molecules of ATP for every glucose molecule.

To summarize ATP production thus far in cellular respiration, four ATP molecules have been produced—two from glycolysis and two from the Krebs cycle. Meanwhile, only a minimal amount of energy has been gained from the original glucose molecule.

Electron Transport System

The final step in the oxidation of glucose involves the electron transport chain, which occurs on the inner cristae of the mitochondria. During this step, the production of ATP takes place. Several other products are created in addition to the ATP and carbon dioxide molecules produced during glycolysis and the Krebs cycle. After moving to the inner cristae, these products transfer their electrons during a series of reactions that ultimately produces 34 molecules of ATP. Because the electron transport system depends on the Krebs cycle, this process is considered part of aerobic respiration.

Results of Cellular Respiration

At the completion of all steps of cellular respiration, 38 molecules of ATP have been produced: 2 molecules from glycolysis and 36 molecules from aerobic respiration (2 from the Krebs cycle and 34 from the electron transport system). Although this result represents an efficient use of the energy contained in one molecule of glucose, it is not 100% efficient because some energy loss occurs in the form of heat.

Aerobic Versus Anaerobic Respiration

As described previously, the presence of oxygen is crucial to the efficient oxidation of glucose by the cells. When oxygen is present, most of the respiration that takes place is aerobic (see Figure 8-7). However, respiration can also occur in the absence of oxygen (anaerobic respiration). In this situation, glycolysis occurs as it normally would. However, because of the absence of oxygen, pyruvic acid cannot be oxidized in the Krebs cycle. As a result, the pyruvic acid quickly converts to **lactic acid**. Excessive anaerobic respiration can result in *lactic acidosis.* This condition occurs in situations such as shock, in which sufficient oxygen is unavailable to the cells. Fortunately, when oxygen is restored to the cells, lactic acid is converted back to pyruvic acid, and aerobic respiration can resume.

It is often said that anaerobic respiration *starts* during a lack of oxygen; however, a more accurate statement is that aerobic respiration *stops* during a lack of oxygen because anaerobic respiration (glycolysis) is the first step in cellular respiration, regardless of the presence of oxygen. However, anaerobic respiration is a highly inefficient use of glucose by itself, resulting in a net gain of only 2 ATP molecules compared with a gain of 38 molecules of ATP when both anaerobic and aerobic respiration occur.

Words of Wisdom

When cells function by using oxygen, they use aerobic and anaerobic components of metabolism. They generate large amounts of ATP (cellular energy) and produce carbon dioxide and water as wastes. When cells function without using oxygen, they use purely **anaerobic metabolism**. They generate small amounts of ATP (cellular energy) and produce lactic acid as waste.

Body Fluid Composition

Specific parameters must be maintained for the cells, tissues, organs, and organ systems to perform their functions efficiently. These parameters include the amount, distribution, and movement of body fluids; electrolyte balance; and the number of hydrogen ions, or acid–base balance.

The most prevalent fluid in the human body is water, which is an essential part of all the chemical reactions that regularly occur in the body. Water also serves as a transport medium for nutrients, hormones, and waste materials. The total amount

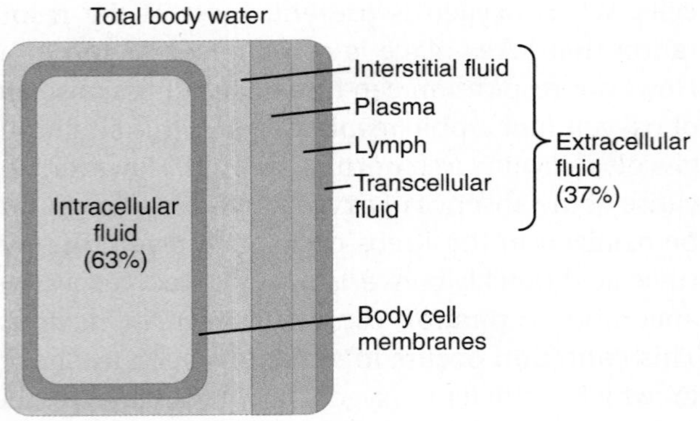

FIGURE 8-8 Cell membranes separate intracellular and extracellular fluids.

of fluid in the body at any given time is referred to as **total body water (TBW)**. TBW constitutes about 60% of the weight of a healthy adult male and is made up of **intracellular fluid (ICF)** and **extracellular fluid (ECF)**. Cell membranes separate the intracellular and ECF compartments. ICF consists of fluid found within the cells. This intracellular compartment contains about 63% of TBW, and the extracellular compartment contains the remaining 37% of TBW **FIGURE 8-8**. ICF contains large amounts of potassium, magnesium, and phosphate ions. In contrast, ECF contains large amounts of sodium, chloride, and bicarbonate ions plus nutrients for the cells, such as oxygen, glucose, fatty acids, and amino acids.[4] ECF also contains waste products to be excreted by the lungs (carbon dioxide) and kidneys (other cellular waste).

At birth, the total percentage of fluid in the body (about 75% to 80%) is higher than the corresponding percentage in an adult, with proportionately more ECF being present in adults. This percentage decreases during the first year of life. Infants lose body water for physiologic reasons as they adjust to their new environment outside the womb. This age group is at an increased risk for adverse consequences of excessive fluid losses (dehydration) because of their greater metabolic rate and higher body surface area. By the time the child reaches adolescence, the TBW drops to about 60%, or normal adult values. This trend continues throughout a person's life. As the body ages and the amount of muscle mass and adipose tissue changes, the TBW decreases because muscle mass is composed of more water than is found in adipose tissue, which repels water. Infants are also at risk for deadly consequences from fluid and electrolyte imbalances.

The ECF is composed of **interstitial fluid**, plasma, lymph, and **transcellular fluid**. The intravascular component is the fluid contained within the chambers of the heart and the blood vessels. *Blood volume* refers to the total volume of the intravascular compartment. About 3 L of the total blood volume is blood plasma, referred to as the plasma volume. The remaining 2.5 L consists of RBCs, WBCs, and **platelets** (thrombocytes), which make up the formed elements of the blood. Most of the ECF is composed of interstitial found outside the intravascular compartment, where it bathes the nonblood cells of the body.[5] The walls of capillaries separate the intravascular and interstitial compartments. Transcellular fluid is found in spaces that are surrounded by epithelial cells, such as the **synovial fluid** within joints (formed where two bones come in contact) and the clear, watery **cerebrospinal fluid (CSF)** that surrounds the brain and spinal cord (discussed later in this chapter).[5]

Cellular Transport Mechanisms

Preserving the delicate balance among the fluid compartments of the body is essential to maintain homeostasis. Under normal conditions, the total volume of water in the body and its distribution in the body compartments remain relatively constant, even though the amount of water that enters and is excreted from the body each day fluctuates.

The fluids in the body exist as a solution of dissolved elements and water. Recall that the cell membrane is semipermeable, allowing lipid-soluble substances to move into and out of the cell freely while not allowing water-soluble substances to cross the membrane. However, to sustain life, both types of substances must be allowed to enter and exit the cell.

Water and electrolytes move among the body's fluid compartments according to some basic chemical and biologic principles. One governing principle is that unequal concentrations on different sides of a cell membrane will move to balance themselves equally on both sides of the membrane. Balance across a cell membrane has two components: (1) the balance of compounds (eg, water and electrolytes) on either side of the cell membrane, and (2) the balance of charges [the positive ($^+$) or negative (⁻) charges carried on the atoms] on either side of the cell membrane.

When concentrations of charges or compounds are greater on one side of the cell membrane than on the other side, the imbalance creates a gradient. The natural tendency for materials is to flow from an area of higher concentration to one of lower concentration, establishing a *concentration gradient.* The concentration gradient is the difference in concentrations of a substance on either side of a semipermeable membrane. Gradients are categorized according to the type of material that flows down them: Chemical compounds flow down chemical gradients, whereas electrical currents flow down electrical gradients. The process of flowing down a gradient depends on whether the cell membrane will allow the material to pass through it. Certain compounds can travel freely across the cell membrane (a kinetically favorable situation that requires little energy). Others require **active transport** across the membrane because of the size of the compound or because of an incompatible charge. Active transport is discussed in more detail later in this chapter.

Each of the compartments of the body is separated by a membrane. **Osmotic pressure** is the pressure exerted by the concentration of the solutes in a given space to stop the flow of solvent across a semipermeable membrane. The osmotic pressure of a solution, or the ability to affect water movement, is *osmolality*. It is expressed in osmoles or milliosmoles per kilogram of water. Generally, the amount of water in each compartment is tightly regulated to maintain the osmolality of TBW in equilibrium. The body uses several mechanisms to accomplish a balanced osmolality in each of the compartments.

Diffusion

Diffusion is the process in which particles move from an area of higher concentration to an area of lower concentration along a concentration gradient until equilibrium is achieved **FIGURE 8-9**. Because diffusion does not require energy, it is considered a passive transport mechanism. Diffusion of both solids and gases can occur within the human body. By moving some of the solute from one side of the membrane to the other, the body reduces or eliminates the concentration gradient and creates balance as much as possible. As discussed previously, this natural tendency of the body is referred to as moving with the concentration gradient. Complete elimination of concentration gradients is impossible because ions and molecules are always in motion in a random pattern. However, the net change is close to zero. This process is how the body can move some nutrients and waste products into and out of the cell. With gases, the molecules are spread farther apart, and the diffusion rate depends on the weight of the gas.

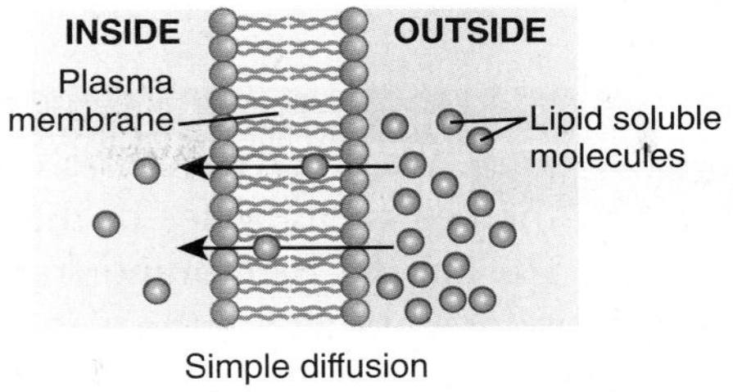

FIGURE 8-9 Diffusion.

To visualize diffusion, imagine that too many people show up for a theater performance. The theater manager decides to open another seating area to accommodate the crowd. Patrons (charges or compounds) are concentrated in a small area (the cell) outside the door (the cell membrane) leading to the new seating area. When the theater manager opens the door, patrons can move through it (selective cell membrane permeability) from the congested area (down a concentration gradient). The patrons spread themselves out evenly (diffuse) throughout the total area, with some choosing to stay behind in the original seating area as others move into the new area until all patrons have an equal amount of room.

Substances that can freely cross the cell membrane, such as oxygen and carbon dioxide, move by the process of diffusion in the human body. For example, blood returning to the lungs from the body has a high concentration of carbon dioxide and a low concentration of oxygen. The lungs, however, have a high concentration of oxygen and a low concentration of carbon dioxide. As blood passes through the pulmonary vasculature, carbon dioxide leaves the blood and enters the lungs until an equal amount of carbon dioxide is present in both. By the same process, oxygen leaves the lungs and enters the blood until an equal amount of oxygen is present in both. As a result of this principle, the amount of expired carbon dioxide is nearly equal to the amount of carbon dioxide in arterial blood.

Filtration

Filtration is the process commonly used by the kidneys to clean blood. Water carries dissolved compounds across the cell membranes of the tubules of the kidney. The tubule membrane traps these dissolved compounds but allows the water to pass through. This process cleans the blood of wastes and removes the trapped compounds from circulation, so that they can be flushed out of the body. The antidiuretic hormone (ADH) prevents water loss from the kidneys by causing its reabsorption into the tubules.

Facilitated Diffusion

It is sometimes necessary to move molecules across a membrane, even when those molecules cannot use diffusion or must move against the concentration gradient. In these situations, the movement occurs by either active transport or facilitated diffusion.

Active transport is used to move substances against the concentration gradient or toward the side with a higher concentration. Just as it sounds, this type of transport requires the use of energy by the cell, but it is faster than diffusion. Active transport is similar to operating a motor vehicle, in that the vehicle can roll down a hill in neutral gear without the engine being on, but the vehicle has to be running and in gear to go uphill.

Facilitated diffusion is a passive transport mechanism similar to diffusion, in that it involves particles moving from an area of higher concentration to an area of lower concentration. However, in this type of diffusion, the molecule entering the cell cannot enter without the assistance of a carrier protein. During facilitated diffusion, the substance needed in the cell binds with the carrier protein, and one of two processes occurs: The molecule–carrier protein combination may be lipid soluble and pass through the cytoplasmic membrane, or the two may enter the cell through a membrane protein. This step is possible because of the new shape of the carrier-molecule combination or because the combination of the two can attach to a binding site in the membrane protein **FIGURE 8-10**. The membrane protein then changes shape to allow passage of the carrier-molecule combination into the cell. After the carrier protein enters in the cell, it breaks off from the molecule and returns to the surface of the membrane, where it is free to transport other molecules into the cell.

Glucose, for example, enters the cell by this facilitated diffusion process. Glucose is not lipid soluble, so it cannot cross the cell membrane; it is also too large a molecule to cross through the membrane proteins. By attaching to a carrier protein, glucose is able to enter the cell. Insulin is a hormone responsible for regulating the speed with which carrier proteins move glucose into cells.

Osmosis

Osmosis is the movement of a solvent, such as water, from an area of low solute concentration to one of high concentration through a selectively permeable membrane. Osmosis is another passive transport mechanism; however, unlike diffusion, the particles themselves do not move in osmosis.

Recall that solutions contain both a liquid (solvent) and particles suspended in the liquid (solutes). The primary solvent in the body is water, considered the universal solvent. Within this solvent are several solutes: electrolytes, such as sodium and potassium; and molecules, such as glucose. Water can generally move without much difficulty between the different body compartments because the membranes that separate the compartments are permeable to water. The cell membrane is considered semipermeable because it also is selectively permeable to certain solutes **FIGURE 8-11**. Selective permeability is accomplished through pores in the membrane that block or permit entry based on the molecule's size, shape, or electrical charge. The body tries to maintain an equal solute concentration on each side of the membrane. An **isotonic solution** is one in which an equal concentration of solutes and water is present on either side of a semipermeable membrane.

For example, if a solution on one side of a membrane has 25 sodium ions and 100 water molecules (25% solution), and a solution on the other side of the membrane has 50 sodium ions and 100 water molecules (50% solution), then the water will move from the area of lower solute concentration to the area of higher solute concentration in an effort to achieve an equal concentration on both sides of the membrane. In this example, the result will be 25 sodium molecules and 66 water molecules on one side (37%), and 50 sodium molecules and 134 water molecules on the other (37%).

The concentration of a solution, or its ability to draw or give water, is described as its tonicity

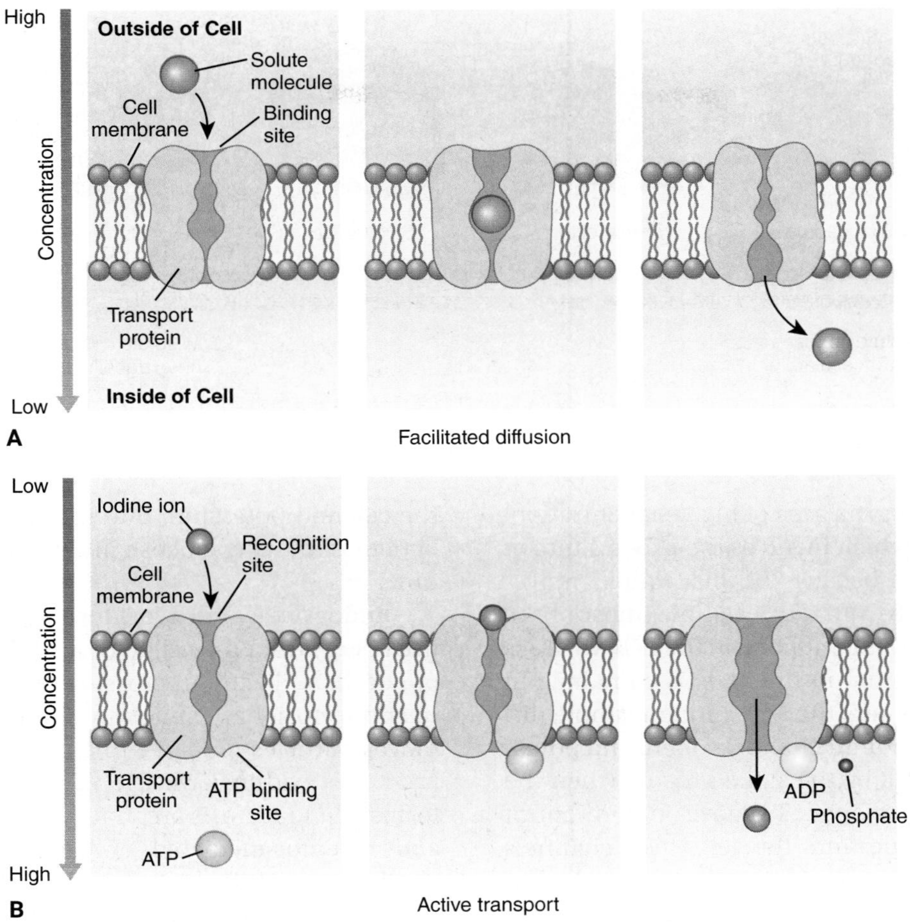

FIGURE 8-10 A. Facilitated diffusion involves particles moving from an area of higher concentration toward an area of lower concentration with the assistance of a protein. **B.** Active transport uses energy from adenosine triphosphate (ATP) to open a pathway for compounds to move against a concentration gradient.

Abbreviation: ADP, adenosine diphosphate

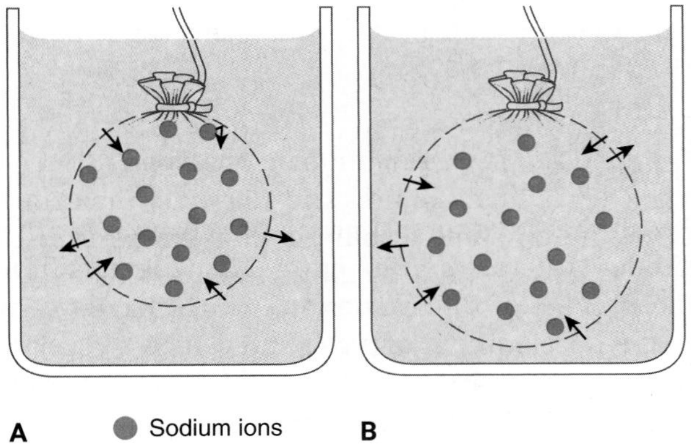

FIGURE 8-11 A. An example of osmosis occurs when a permeable bag of salt water is immersed in a solution of pure water. **B.** Water moves into the bag (toward the area with lower water concentration), equalizing the concentrations on each side of the membrane.

FIGURE 8-12, and the difference in concentrations from one side of a selectively permeable membrane to the other is the osmotic gradient. The degree of difference between the two concentrations determines how much osmotic pressure is present and how quickly the two concentrations will tend to equalize. A solution with a higher solute concentration compared with another solution is **hypertonic**, and a solution with a lower solute concentration is **hypotonic**. If too much water moves out of a cell, then the cell shrinks abnormally, a process known as crenation. If too much water enters a cell, then it will swell and burst, a process known as lysis.

Active Transport

As discussed previously, in some situations, ions and molecules must be transported from an area of

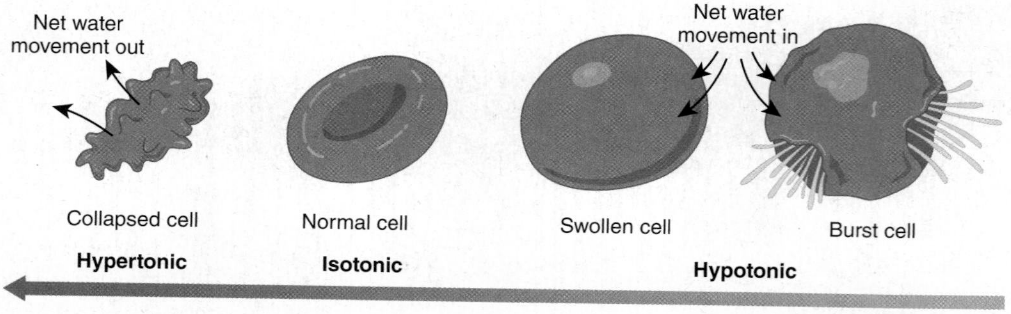

FIGURE 8-12 Tonicity.

low concentration to an area of high concentration. Active transport, which involves the expenditure of energy, is required because of this "uphill" movement (see Figure 8-10B). For example, most of the sodium in the body is contained in the ECF, whereas most of the potassium in the body is contained in the ICF. Sodium enters the cell through simple diffusion when the sodium channels open, and potassium leaves the cell by the same process when the potassium channels open. To move sodium out of the cell or potassium into the cell, these channels cannot simply be opened again because a higher concentration of sodium on the outside and potassium on the inside is always present. An active transport process—the sodium-potassium pump—must be used to move these ions against their concentration gradient. Like facilitated diffusion, this process uses a system in which the particle being moved binds with a carrier protein. However, unlike facilitated diffusion, this binding requires the use of energy. After the particle is bound, it is transported through the membrane and then released. Although active transport demands a high energy expenditure, its benefits outweigh the initial use of ATP as an energy source. Pumping sodium out of the cell and potassium into the cell has the added benefit of moving glucose into the cell at the same time.

> **Words of Wisdom**
>
> The sodium-potassium pump continuously removes three sodium ions from the cell for every two potassium ions that are moved back into the cell. If this pump is impaired because of insufficient potassium in the body, then sodium builds up and causes the cells to swell.

Endocytosis and exocytosis are processes that use energy from the cell to move substances into or out of the cell without crossing the cell membrane. In endocytosis, a secretion from the cell membrane moves particles too large to enter the cell by other processes within a vesicle of the cell. The three forms of endocytosis are pinocytosis, phagocytosis, and receptor-mediated endocytosis. **Pinocytosis** ("cell drinking") is the transport of droplets of ECF into the cell membrane. In **phagocytosis** ("cell eating"), a cell surrounds a foreign particle and engulfs it. Receptor-mediated endocytosis involves the movement of specific kinds of particles into the cell, with protein molecules extending through part of the cell membrane to the outer surface. The opposite process to endocytosis is exocytosis, in which a substance stored in a vesicle is secreted from the cell. Cellular transport mechanisms are summarized in **TABLE 8-8**.

Tissue Level

Recall that a tissue is a group of cells that share a similar structure and function. Tissue results from the process of differentiation, which occurs early in the development of a cell and causes the cell to become specialized for a specific purpose. For example, a cell can become specialized as a cardiac cell or a bone cell. When stem cells undergo mitosis, one daughter cell remains an undifferentiated stem cell, whereas the other differentiates and takes on the characteristics of a particular tissue.

TABLE 8-8 Cellular Transport Mechanisms

Mechanism	Movement
Diffusion	The movement of a solvent, such as water, from an area of low solute concentration to one of high concentration through a selectively permeable membrane to equalize the solute concentration on both sides of the membrane
Filtration	The movement of water and a dissolved substance from an area of high pressure to an area of low pressure
Facilitated diffusion	Assistance of the passage of a substance from an area of higher concentration to an area of lower concentration by a transport (helper) molecule within the membrane
Osmosis	The movement of a solvent, such as water, from an area of low solute concentration to one of high concentration through a selectively permeable membrane to equalize the solute concentration on both sides of the membrane
Active transport	Movement via transport molecules, or pumps, that require energy to move substances from an area of low concentration to an area of high concentration

The human body is primarily made up of four types of tissue that are classified by their shape, structure, and function: epithelial, connective, muscle, and nervous tissues. **Epithelial tissues** cover body surfaces, cover and line internal organs, and make up the glands. Connective tissues are widely distributed throughout the body, fill the internal spaces, and function to bind, support, and protect body structures. Muscle tissues are specialized for contraction and include the skeletal muscles, the heart, and the muscular walls of hollow organs. Skeletal muscles are attached to bones and are used for movement of the body. **Nervous tissues** carry information from one part of the body to another via electrical impulses; they are found in the brain, spinal cord, and nerves.

Words of Wisdom

Epithelial tissue is able to repair itself (regenerate) quickly if injured.

Epithelial Tissues

Epithelial tissue covers most of the surfaces of the body (both external and internal surfaces) and the interior of hollow organs. It is composed of many cells that fit tightly together, forming a continuous layer of cells with little or no intercellular material (material between the cells). Epithelial tissue has two surfaces. Because it forms coverings and linings, one surface of the tissue is typically unattached and exposed either to the outside (eg, outer surface of the skin, inner lining of the mouth) or internally to an open space (eg, intestinal lining). On the side opposite the free surface (ie, the undersurface), the cells are attached to a basement membrane, a very thin layer of tissue that anchors the epithelium to the underlying structure, such as connective tissue. Because epithelial tissue is generally avascular (ie, it has no blood supply of its own), it receives oxygen and nutrients by diffusion from the blood vessels that supply the underlying connective tissues. Glands are secretory structures derived from epithelia.

Epithelia perform four essential functions:

1. **Physical protection.** Epithelia protect exposed and internal surfaces from abrasion, dehydration, and destruction from biologic or chemical agents.
2. **Permeability.** Any substance entering or leaving the body must cross an epithelium, so the epithelia control permeability. Some epithelia are relatively impermeable, whereas others are crossed easily by compounds of various sizes. In response to stimuli, the epithelial barrier may be modified and regulated. Hormones can affect ion and nutrient transport through epithelial cells. Physical stress can also alter the structure and properties of these tissues. An example is the formation of calluses on the hands after repeated manual labor.
3. **Sensation.** Most epithelia are sensitive to stimulation because they have a large supply of sensory nerves.
4. **Specialized secretions.** Epithelial cells that produce secretions are called gland cells,

and individual cells of this type are scattered among other types of cells in an epithelium. Most or all of the epithelial cells in a glandular epithelium produce secretions, which are either discharged onto the surface of the epithelium or released into the surrounding interstitial fluid and blood.

Epithelial tissue can be divided into groups according to its microscopic shape and the number of layers in the tissue **TABLE 8-9**. It is classified by shape as squamous (flat, thin, and scalelike), cuboidal (cubed), columnar (taller than wide), or transitional **FIGURE 8-13**. Transitional cells, which are typically found in the **urinary system**, can stretch

TABLE 8-9 Types of Epithelial Tissue

Type	Description	Function	Location
Simple squamous	Single layer of thin, flat cells	Permit diffusion of oxygen and carbon dioxide between alveolar air and blood	Alveoli of lungs
		Absorption by diffusion, filtration, and osmosis	Lines walls of capillaries and lymphatic vessels
		Filtration of water and electrolytes	Kidneys
Simple cuboidal	Single layer of cells that are as wide as they are tall (cube-shaped)	Absorption of water and electrolytes	Lines kidney tubules
		Secretion of enzymes and hormones	Lines the ovary surface, ducts of some glands (salivary glands, thyroid gland, pancreas)
Simple columnar	Single layer of cells that are taller than they are wide; some cells are equipped with cilia	Protection; secretion of digestive enzymes; absorption of nutrients	Lines stomach and intestines
		Moves particles of dust and other foreign material away from lungs by means of cilia	Lines parts of respiratory tract
Pseudostratified columnar	Single layer of cells of differing heights, some of which do not reach the unattached surface	Protection; secretion of mucus	Lines trachea and most of upper respiratory passages; lines male urethra
		Moves egg toward uterus	Lining of fallopian tubes
Stratified squamous	Multiple cell layers	Protection	Outer layer of skin; surface lining of mouth, esophagus, vagina, and anus
Stratified cuboidal	Typically two layers of cubelike cells	Protection	Linings of larger mammary gland ducts, sweat gland ducts, salivary glands
Stratified columnar	Multiple cell layers	Protection; secretion	Part of male urethra, parts of pharynx, and large ducts of some glands
Transitional	Cells appear simple when stretched and appear stratified when unstretched	Protection; stretch and change appearance	Inner urinary bladder lining, linings of ureters, and part of urethra

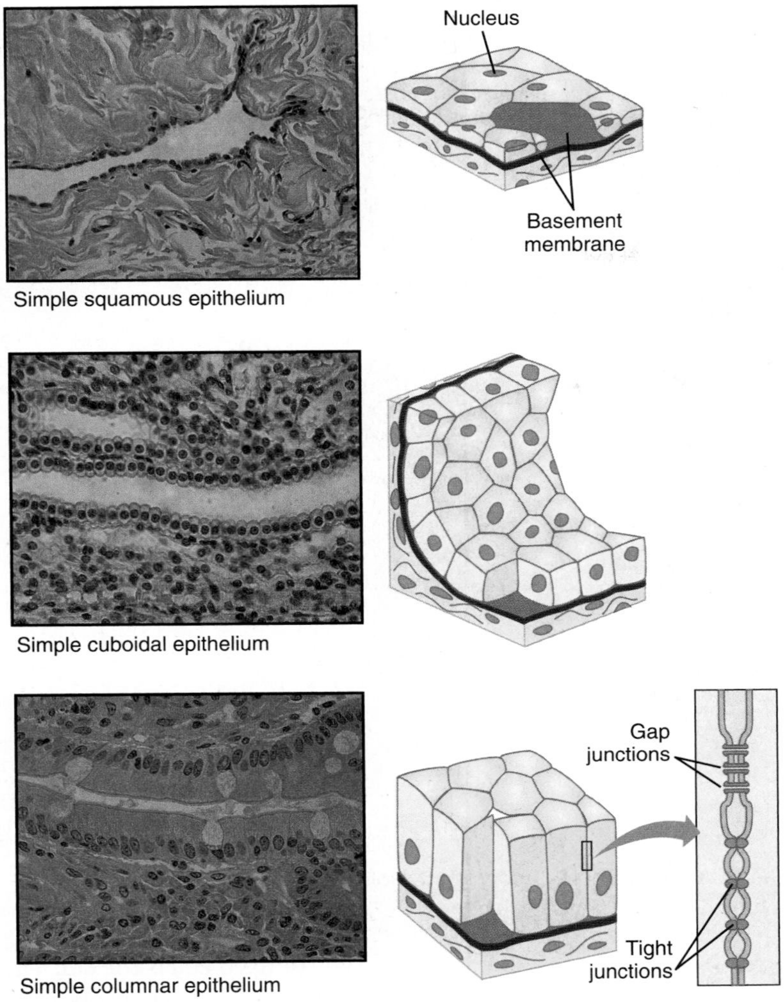

FIGURE 8-13 Shapes of some types of epithelial cells.

Micrographs: © Donna Beer Stolz, PhD, Center for Biologic Imaging, University of Pittsburgh Medical School; **illustrations:** © Jones & Bartlett Learning.

and change their appearance to look like any of the other three types. Epithelial tissue can also be classified according to the number of layers. *Simple epithelium* is composed of a single layer of cells; *stratified epithelium* is composed of two or more layers; and *pseudostratified epithelium* is made up of epithelium that appears to have multiple layers but does not. The pseudostratified ("falsely stratified") impression occurs because the cells are irregularly shaped, and their nuclei appear at different levels in the tissue, giving the impression of multiple layers.

Epithelial tissue is sometimes subdivided into membranous epithelium and glandular epithelium. Membranous epithelium covers the body; lines the pleural, pericardial, and peritoneal cavities; lines the respiratory, digestive, and genitourinary tracts; and lines the blood and lymphatic vessels. Glandular epithelium consists of specialized cells that produce and secrete substances into ducts or body fluids. It is usually found in **exocrine glands** (which have ducts that open onto surfaces or into the digestive tract) or in **endocrine glands** (which have no ducts and secrete into tissue fluid or blood). The three types of exocrine glands are merocrine, apocrine, and holocrine **FIGURE 8-14**. Merocrine glands release fluid by exocytosis. Apocrine glands lose parts of their cell bodies during secretion. Holocrine glands release entire cells that disintegrate to release secretions.

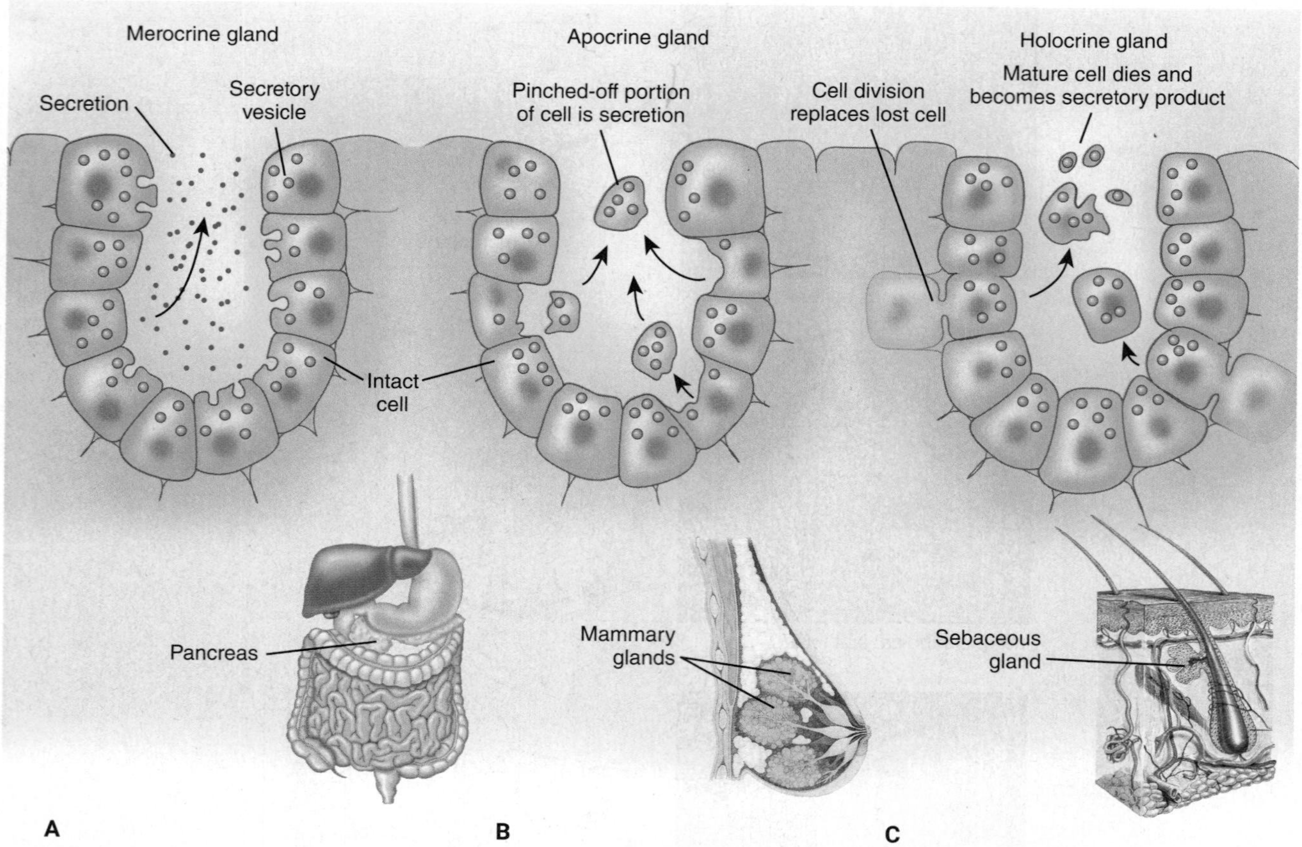

FIGURE 8-14 Exocrine glands. **A.** Merocrine. **B.** Apocrine. **C.** Holocrine.

Connective Tissues

Connective tissue is both the most abundant type of body tissue and the most widely distributed. These tissues bind body structures, provide support and protection, create frameworks, fill body spaces, store fat, produce blood cells, transport fluids and dissolved materials, repair damaged tissues, and protect the body from infection.

Unlike the cells of epithelial tissue, which fit tightly together, the cells in connective tissue are separated from each other by the matrix. This intercellular substance serves as the cement that gives the connective tissue its basic characteristics (connection of tissue). Although cells make up the majority of epithelial tissue, the matrix usually accounts for the majority of connective tissue.

Most connective tissue cells divide, have a good blood supply, and require large amounts of nourishment. They include bone, cartilage, and fat. Connective tissues contain different types of cells, including those that are fixed or wandering. The most common type of fixed cell is the star-shaped fibroblast, which produces fibers via protein secretion into the extracellular matrix. **TABLE 8-10** summarizes the major cells and tissue fibers of connective tissue.

Fibroblasts produce three types of connective tissue fibers:

1. **Collagenous fibers**. Essential for body parts that hold structures together (ie, ligaments, which connect bone to bone, and tendons, which connect muscle to bone). Collagenous fibers are also called dense connective tissue or white fibers.
2. **Elastic fibers.** Common in body parts that are often stretched, such as the vocal cords. They are composed of a protein called elastin, and are also called yellow fibers.
3. **Reticular fibers.** Form delicate supporting networks in the spleen and other tissues.

Other types of cells found in connective tissue include mast cells, macrophages, adipocytes, and melanocytes. **Mast cells** are distributed throughout

TABLE 8-10 Connective Tissue Cells and Tissue Fibers

Tissue Cell Type	Action
Fibroblasts	Produce fibers
Macrophages	Engulf and devour unwanted microorganisms
Mast cells	Secrete histamine and heparin
Tissue Fiber Type	**Action**
Collagenous	Bind structures together with high tensile strength
Elastic	Ease of stretching
Reticular	Form delicate support networks

connective tissues, usually near blood vessels, and release both heparin (to prevent blood clotting) and histamine (for inflammatory and allergic response). **Macrophages** are responsible for phagocytosis. Adipocytes (fat cells) store body fat. Melanocytes are specialized cells in the deeper epithelium that are responsible for producing the pigment **melanin**, which gives skin its color.

Classifications of Connective Tissues

Connective tissues are classified based on their physical properties **FIGURE 8-15**. The three general categories of connective tissue are connective tissue proper, supporting connective tissues, and fluid connective tissues:

1. Connective tissue proper includes those connective tissues with many types of cells and

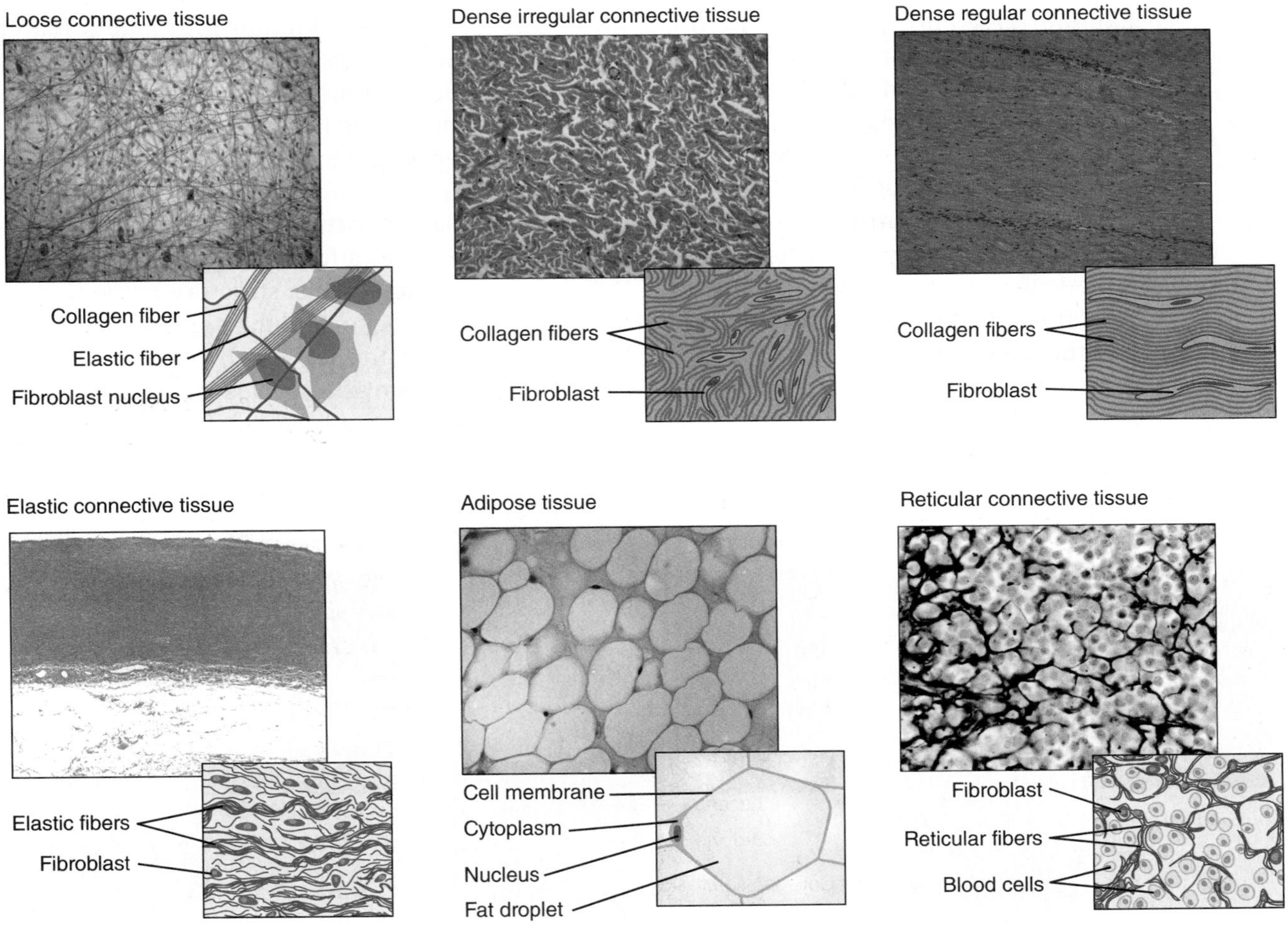

FIGURE 8-15 Types of typical connective tissues.

extracellular fibers in a syrupy ground substance. Ground substance gives the skin resistance to compression. These tissues are further divided into dense connective tissue and loose connective tissue.

- Dense connective tissue is composed of bundles of strong, white, collagenous fibers in parallel rows. Tendons are composed of this type of tissue; they are relatively strong and inelastic. Dense connective tissue also exists in the eyeballs and deep skin layers. This type of tissue is repaired very slowly because it has a poor blood supply.
- Loose connective tissue includes adipose tissue, areolar tissue, and reticular connective tissue. Adipose tissue lies beneath the skin, between muscles, around the kidneys, behind the eyes, in certain membranes of the abdomen, on the surface of the heart, and around some joints. It functions as a cushion for these body parts. Adipose tissue is also important for storing energy in fat molecules (triglycerides). **Areolar tissue** binds skin to underlying organs, fills in spaces between muscles, supports other tissues, holds body fluids, defends against infection, and stores nutrients as fat. It is found beneath most layers of the epithelium. Reticular connective tissue helps to create a framework inside internal organs such as the spleen and liver.

2. Supporting connective tissue differs from connective tissue proper in that it has a less diverse cell population and a matrix that contains many more densely packaged fibers. This tissue protects soft tissues and some or all of the weight of the body. The two types of supporting connective tissue are cartilage and bone.

- Cartilage is a tough but flexible connective tissue that protects the body from excessive tension and compression. It is composed of cells called chondrocytes, which are distributed in a somewhat rigid matrix. The exact makeup of cartilage varies depending on its location and function in the body. Cartilage is harder than dense connective tissue but softer than bone. It also lacks nerve fibers. A covering called the perichondrium provides the needed nutrients to cartilage via diffusion. Because it has a limited supply of blood vessels, cartilage heals very slowly. There are three major types of cartilage **FIGURE 8-16**:
  - **Hyaline cartilage.** This type of cartilage is smooth and firm and is found on the ends of bones in many joints, in the soft portion of the nose, and in the supporting rings of the respiratory passages. The most common type of cartilage, it is important for bone growth.
  - **Elastic cartilage.** This flexible cartilage provides a framework for the **epiglottis** (a thin, flaplike structure at the root of the tongue) and the pinna (the external part of the ear).
  - **Fibrocartilage.** This tough form of cartilage absorbs shock in the intervertebral disks of the spinal column, in the

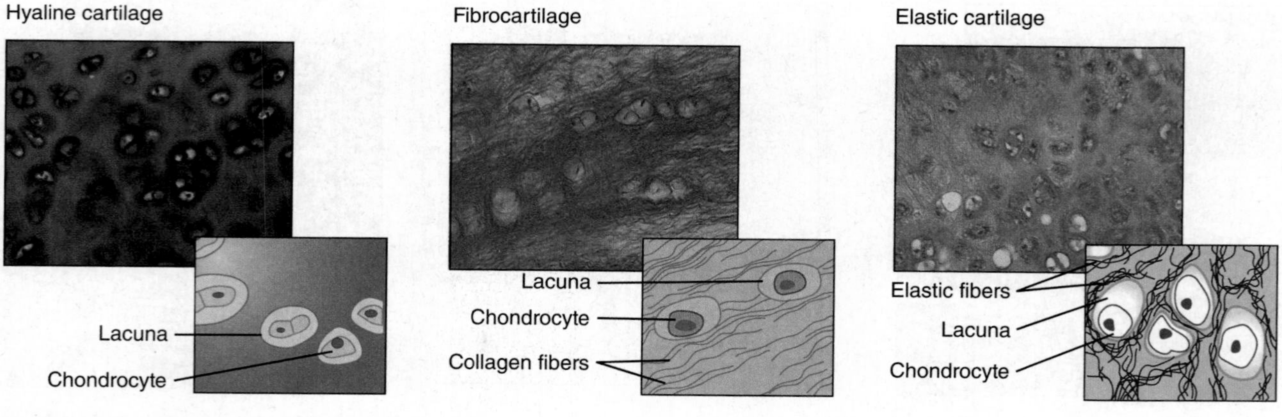

FIGURE 8-16 Types of cartilage.

spongy cartilages of the knees, and in the pelvic girdle (bony pelvis).

- Bone is the most rigid type of connective tissue and establishes the framework of the body. It consists of a matrix of connective tissue, blood vessels, and minerals (particularly calcium and phosphorus). Bones are classified according to their shape. Bone tissue is also classified as either cancellous (spongy) or compact (solid). **Bone marrow** is the soft tissue that fills the inside of bones, and is where production of RBCs, platelets, and most WBCs takes place.

3. Blood is classified as connective tissue because the matrix (the RBCs, WBCs, and platelets between the cells) is liquid (mainly water). This matrix allows the transportation of nutrients, oxygen, and waste products. Lymph forms as interstitial fluid enters lymphatic vessels, which return lymph to the cardiovascular system. Unlike other connective tissues, blood and lymph do not connect structures or provide any mechanical support.

Muscle Tissues

Muscle tissue is contractile tissue. It is the basis of movement of the body. Muscle tissue is specialized to contract forcefully (shorten). This tissue is classified by its anatomic location (skeletal, smooth, and cardiac) and function **TABLE 8-11**.

1. **Skeletal muscle tissue**. Also called voluntary muscle tissue because its use is usually under conscious control. This tissue is connected to the skeletal framework of the body by tendons. Skeletal muscle is sometimes referred to as striated muscle because it contains long, threadlike cells with light and dark markings, called striations, that are visible under a microscope **FIGURE 8-17**. This appearance results from alternating dark, thick bands of myosin and light, thin bands of actin. Skeletal muscle also contains several nuclei per cell. This tissue moves the head, trunk, and limbs,

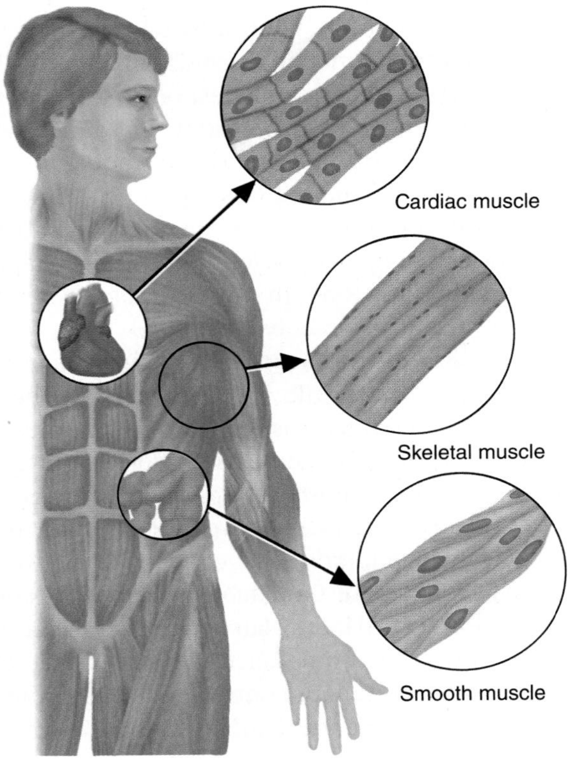

FIGURE 8-17 The three types of muscle are cardiac, skeletal, and smooth.

TABLE 8-11 Types of Muscle

Type	Control	Striations	Location	Purpose
Skeletal muscle (voluntary muscle)	Voluntary	Yes	Attached to bone	Produce movement
Smooth muscle (nonstriated involuntary muscles or unstriated muscle)	Involuntary	No	In the walls of hollow internal structures and blood vessels	Various: some organ functions, pupil contraction, changes in blood vessel diameter, gland duct operation, hair movement
Cardiac muscle (myocardium)	Involuntary	Yes	Heart	Pump blood

allowing all voluntary movements in these body areas. Injury to skeletal muscle can result in considerable bleeding because of its rich blood supply.

2. **Smooth muscle tissue.** Also called nonstriated involuntary muscles or unstriated muscles. Smooth muscle tissue is composed of elongated, spindle-shaped cells and is found in hollow internal organ walls (eg, intestines, stomach, blood vessels, uterus). In most cases, smooth muscle cannot be controlled by conscious effort. Its main functions include constricting the lumen of blood vessels in response to the body's needs, aiding in the breakdown and digestion of food, moving fluid through the body, and assisting in eliminating waste products. Smooth muscle fibers are shorter than striated fibers, and have only one nucleus per spindle-shaped fiber. Because smooth muscle cells can divide, they regenerate after being injured.
3. **Cardiac muscle tissue.** Also called myocardium; the thick, contractile middle layer of the heart wall. Cardiac muscle is similar to skeletal muscle in that it is striated, but has a different structure from skeletal muscle. Cardiac cells generally have one nucleus, but occasionally have two nuclei. In addition, the connection between cells is different: Cardiac cells form tight connections called intercalated disks. Cardiac muscle also differs from skeletal muscle in that it is not under conscious control, but rather is completely involuntary. Cardiac muscle relies on pacemaker cells or nodes of tissue in the heart's conduction system to stimulate contraction.

> **Words of Wisdom**
>
> Muscles are supplied by a rich collection of blood vessels and nerves. Loss of proper blood supply or loss of innervation (ie, the nerve supply of an organ or body part) results in muscle wasting, or atrophy. In patients with permanent nerve injuries or poor distal circulation, muscle atrophy is often observed and may be a clue to an underlying disease process.

Nervous Tissues

The nervous tissue of the body can conduct electrical impulses that allow communication between body structures and control body functions. Nervous tissues contain two basic types of cells: (1) neurons and (2) several kinds of supporting cells, collectively called neuroglia, or glial cells. Nervous tissues are found in the brain, peripheral nerves, and spinal cord; the basic cells of these tissues are the neurons. Neurons are the basic structure of neural tissue. When interconnected, neurons act as conduits that send signals to and from other neurons, muscles, and glands and receive sensory information from the outside world.

Neuroglia are the supporting cells of nervous tissue that are crucial to neuronal functioning. The functions of neuroglia include nourishment, protection, and insulation. They also phagocytize other cells and help in communications between cells.

Types of Membranes

Membranes form a barrier or an interface. Epithelial membranes are thin structures made up of epithelium and underlying connective tissue. They cover body surfaces and line body cavities. The body contains four types of membranes **TABLE 8-12**:

1. **Serous membrane.** Lines body cavities that lack openings to the outside of the body, such as the thoracic, abdominal, and pelvic cavities. Serous membranes consist of two layers. The parietal membrane adheres to the cavity wall, and the visceral membrane adheres to the organ. Serous membranes secrete serous fluid, which lubricates membrane surfaces.
2. **Mucous membrane.** Lines body cavities that open to the outside of the body, including the nose and mouth, as well as digestive, respiratory, urinary, and reproductive tubes. Mucous membranes contain goblet cells that secrete mucus.
3. **Cutaneous membrane.** The skin, which covers the body surface.
4. **Synovial membrane.** Forms an incomplete lining within the cavities of the synovial joints. It is entirely made up of connective tissues.

Homeostasis

As discussed previously, adaptive responses to various stimuli allow the cells and tissues to respond and function within their respective environments, in a constant effort to preserve a degree of stability or equilibrium. This process is known as homeostasis (from the Greek words for "same"

TABLE 8-12 Membranes of the Body

Membrane Type	Name	Location
Cutaneous	Skin	All exterior surfaces of the body
	Periosteum	Surrounds mature bone
	Perichondrium	Surrounds developing bone
Mucous	Oral mucosa	Soft, mucus-producing membranes lining the nose and mouth
Serous	Visceral pleura	Inner lining covering the lungs
	Parietal pleura	Outer lining separating the visceral pleura and the interior of the chest wall
	Pericardium	Surrounds the heart
	Peritoneum	Surrounds the abdominal organs
	Meninges	Coverings between the brain and skull
Synovial	Knee capsule	Surrounds the synovial fluid contained in the knee joint

and "steady"); it is also called the dynamic steady state. Physiologic cell turnover refers to the process in which older cells are eliminated and replaced by newer cells. This process occurs via apoptosis, which is normal cell death. Apoptosis is genetically programmed into the cell as a part of normal development, organogenesis (formation of organs and organ systems), immune function, and tissue growth. It has a normal role in aging, early development, menses, lactating breast tissue, thymus involution, and RBC turnover. Appropriate cell turnover is one component of homeostasis; for example, it allows damaged cells to be replaced so that proper tissue function can continue.

Homeostasis in the body is possible because normal regulatory systems are counterbalanced by counterregulatory systems. In other words, for every cell, tissue, or organ that performs one function, at least one component performs the opposing function. Other homeostatic mechanisms include the control of internal body temperature despite fluctuations in the external temperature, the regulation of pH and acid–base balance in the body, and the balance of water or hydration in the cells and overall body.

Regulatory systems communicate within the body, mainly at the cellular level. Recall that cells communicate electrochemically through cellular signaling, in which they release molecules (ie, hormones) that bind to protein receptors on the cell surface. This signaling triggers chemical reactions in the receptor cells that initiate a biologic action. When the action has been completed, the opposing system is alerted to discontinue the action through a process called feedback inhibition or **negative feedback** **FIGURE 8-18**.

The thermostat mechanism in a home is a good example of a feedback mechanism. In the middle of the winter, heat loss continually occurs through drafty windows, doors, and poorly insulated areas such as the roof or walls. The thermostat detects decreases in temperature and signals the furnace to produce heat to rewarm the house. After the temperature has risen to a certain point, the thermostat gives negative feedback to the furnace, causing it to shut down to prevent overheating. This feedback process keeps the temperature of the house within a selected range **FIGURE 8-19**. Similarly, the body constantly generates heat through cellular processes. Five primary mechanisms help the body reduce excess temperature or eliminate heat: (1) convection, (2) conduction, (3) radiation, (4) evaporation, and (5) respiration. In short, the thermostat of the body balances the generation of heat with the elimination of heat.

The human body also maintains homeostasis by balancing what it takes in with what it puts out. For example, the body takes in chemicals and electrolytes, food, and water. It uses the nutrients, proteins, sugars, and oxygen from these inputs, and then eliminates the unnecessary chemicals and by-products through respiration (carbon dioxide), sweating (excess liquids), urination, and defecation (feces). **FIGURE 8-20** illustrates this normal balance.

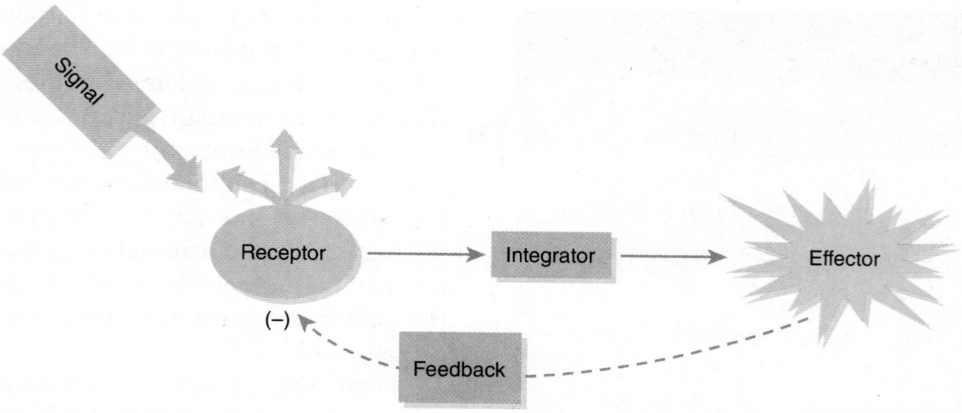

FIGURE 8-18 Most cellular communication (cellular signaling) includes a component of negative feedback in which the product of a reaction returns information about its own manufacture, thereby stopping its own production.

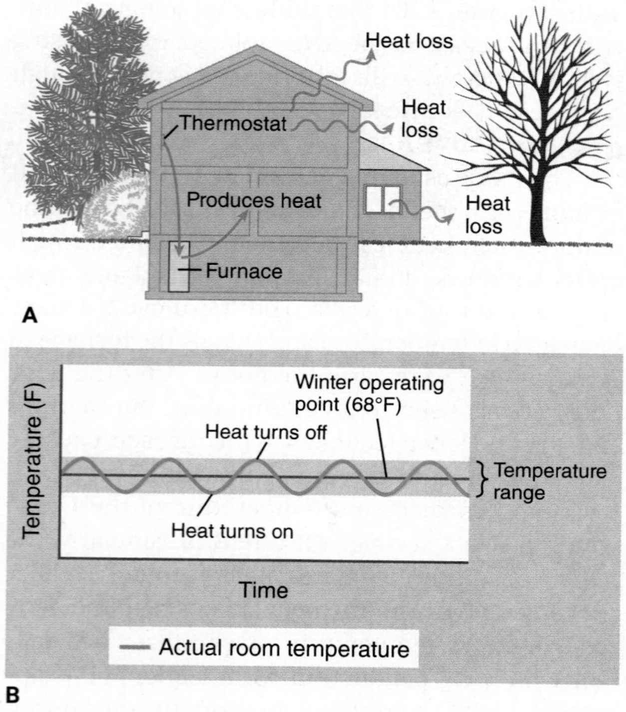

FIGURE 8-19 Homeostasis and the house. **A.** Heat is maintained in a house by a furnace, which compensates for heat loss. The thermostat monitors the internal temperature and switches the furnace on and off in response to temperature changes. **B.** A hypothetical temperature graph showing temperature fluctuation around the set point.

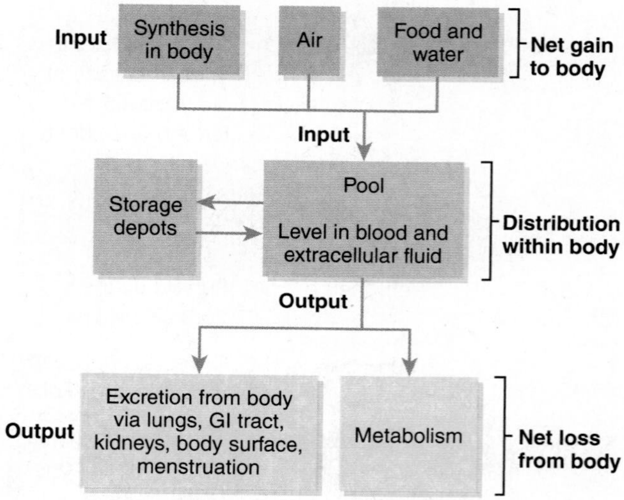

FIGURE 8-20 Generalized view of the homeostatic system. Inputs and outputs are balanced to maintain more-or-less constant chemical and physical parameters.

When normal cellular signaling is interrupted, disease occurs. The counterregulatory mechanisms of the body are rendered ineffective, and its regulatory systems begin to operate autonomously. The system stops providing critical negative feedback, but instead gives unopposed positive feedback.

Organ Systems

Recall that an organ is composed of at least two kinds of tissue that are organized to perform a more complex task than a single tissue can. An organ system comprises at least two kinds of organs that are organized to perform a more complex task than a single organ can. The 12 major organ systems of the body are the integumentary, skeletal, muscular, nervous, endocrine, circulatory, lymphatic, immune, respiratory, digestive, urinary, and reproductive systems **FIGURE 8-21**.

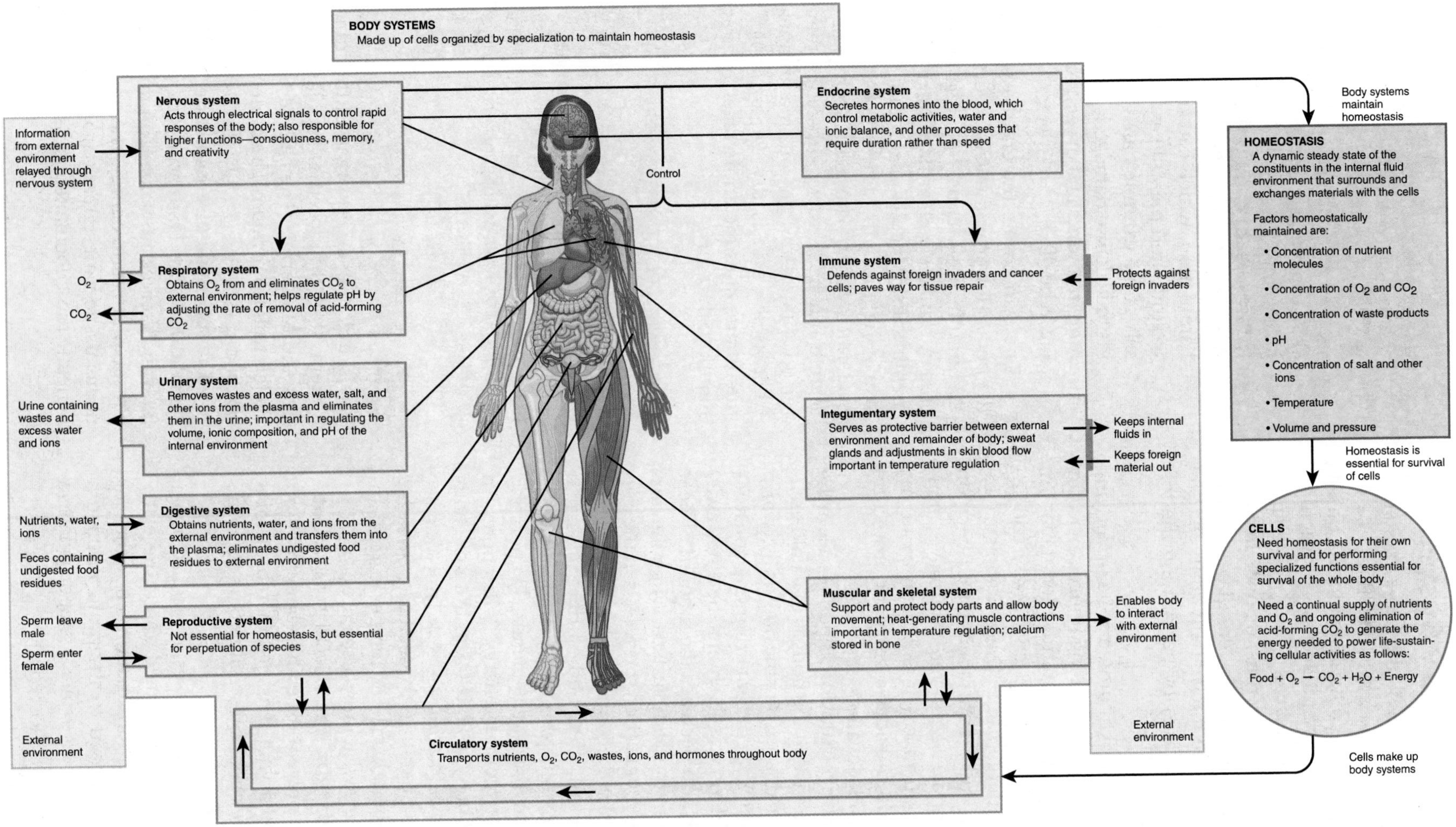

FIGURE 8-21 Systems of the body.

The Integumentary System

The **integumentary system** is the largest system in the human body and serves as the interface between the body and the outside world. It consists of the skin (integument) and accessory structures, such as hair, nails, **sebaceous glands** (oil glands), and **sweat glands** (sudoriferous, or odor forming, glands). The integumentary system plays a crucial role in maintaining the internal environment in a steady state (homeostasis) by performing the following functions:

- **Protection.** The skin protects the underlying tissue from injury, including injury caused by temperature extremes, ultraviolet radiation, mechanical forces, toxic chemicals, and invading microorganisms. These organisms are everywhere and are routinely found lying on the skin surface. However, they never penetrate the skin unless it is broken by injury; thus, the skin provides a constant protection against outside invaders.
- **Temperature regulation.** Blood vessels in the skin constrict when the body is in a cold environment and dilate when the body is in a warm environment. In a cold environment, constriction of the blood vessels shunts the blood away from the skin to decrease the amount of heat radiated from the body surface. When the outside environment is hot, the vessels in the skin dilate, the skin becomes flushed or red, and heat radiates from the body surface. Also, in a hot environment, sweat is secreted to the skin surface from the sweat glands. Evaporation of the sweat requires energy. This energy, in the form of body heat, is taken from the body during the evaporation process, which causes the body temperature to decrease. Sweating alone will not reduce body temperature; evaporation of the sweat must also occur.
- **Fluid regulation.** The skin acts as a watertight seal to prevent excessive water loss from the body and drying of tissues, thereby helping maintain the chemical stability of the internal environment.
- **Sensation.** The skin serves as a sense organ, keeping the brain informed about the external environment. Information from the environment is carried to the brain through a rich supply of **sensory nerves** that originate in the skin. Nerve endings that lie in the skin are adapted to perceive and transmit information about heat, cold, external pressure, pain, and the body's position in space. The skin thus recognizes any changes in the environment. The skin also reacts to pressure, pain, and pleasurable stimuli.
- **Inflammatory response.** The integument responds to injuries and wounds with inflammation, which causes redness, increased warmth, and painful swelling. The blood vessels of the wounded area dilate and allow fluids to leak into damaged tissues. This provides more nutrients and oxygen to the tissues, aiding in healing.

The skin covers the entire external surface of the body. However, the various orifices—including the mouth, nose, anus, and vagina—are not covered by skin. Instead, orifices are lined with mucous membranes. Mucous membranes are similar to skin in that they provide a protective barrier against bacterial invasion. They differ from skin in that they secrete mucus, a sticky substance that lubricates the openings. Thus, mucous membranes are moist, whereas the skin is dry. For example, a mucous membrane lines the entire digestive tract from the mouth to the anus.

Words of Wisdom

If the skin sustains considerable damage, it may leave the body vulnerable to bacterial invasion, temperature instability, and major disturbances of fluid balance. This is precisely what happens when an injury results in an opening in the skin.

Skin

The skin is the largest organ of the integumentary system. It is composed of two layers, the epidermis and the dermis. The cells of the epidermis are sealed to form a watertight protective covering for the body.

The subcutaneous tissue layer lies beneath the skin **FIGURE 8-22**. This tissue is composed largely of fat, which serves as an insulator for the body and as a reservoir to store energy. The amount of subcutaneous tissue varies greatly from person to person. Beneath the subcutaneous tissue lie the muscles

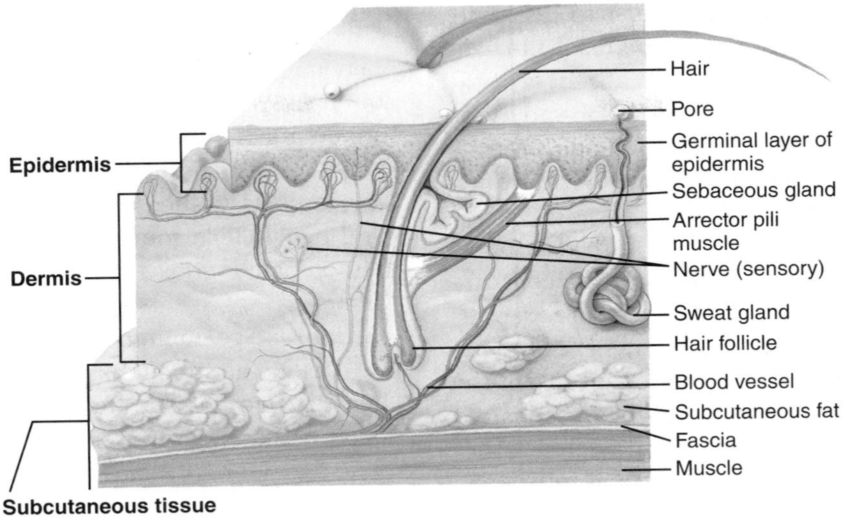

FIGURE 8-22 The skin has two principal layers: the epidermis and the dermis. Below the skin is a layer of subcutaneous tissue.

and the skeleton. The subcutaneous layer helps to anchor the skin to the structures below. As a person ages, the loss of the subcutaneous layer causes the skin to have limited support. This process is why wrinkles form in the skin.

Epidermis

The epidermis, the outermost layer of the skin, varies in thickness in different body areas. On the soles of the feet, the back, and the scalp, it is quite thick. In contrast, the epidermis is only two or three cell layers thick in other areas of the body.

The epidermis is composed of several layers of cells, which can be separated into two regions. The outermost layer of the epidermis, the **stratum corneum**, consists of dead cells in which the cytoplasm has been replaced with keratin. Keratin is a tough, waterproof substance that provides further protection to the underlying tissues from light, heat, microorganisms, some chemicals, and minor trauma. Because cells of the stratum corneum are dead, they are constantly shed and replaced by new cells that move up through the layers of the epidermis.

The innermost epidermal layer, known as the germinal layer, the stratum germinativum, or the stratum basale, is the only location in the epidermis in which the cells can undergo mitosis. New cells produced in this layer work their way up through the layers of the epidermis until they are eventually keratinized, become part of the stratum corneum, and are shed. The ability to reproduce skin cells allows the epidermis to repair itself if injured, providing further protection against injury and infection.

The germinal layer also contains melanocytes, which produce melanin. The darkness of a person's skin is directly proportional to the amount of melanin present.

Dermis

The dermis lies below the epidermis. These two layers are joined together by the dermal-epidermal junction. One cause of blisters is injury to this junction. The dermal layer is much thicker than the epidermis. It mainly consists of connective tissue containing both collagen and elastin fibers, which connect the cells. The collagenous fibers are tough fibers that give the skin resiliency. The elastin fibers give the skin its ability to stretch and (usually) spring back to its normal contour.

The dermis is subdivided into two layers: the papillary layer and the reticular layer. The vasculature inside the papillary dermis serves two functions: It provides nutrients to the epidermis, which does not have its own blood supply, and it aids in **thermoregulation** (the process of maintaining homeostasis). Dilation of these vessels increases blood flow to the skin, allowing heat to dissipate. Conversely, blood vessel constriction results in heat retention. The size and presence (or absence) of oxygen in these blood vessels cause color variations such as redness or cyanosis. The reticular layer is made of dense, irregular connective tissue, which provides strength and elasticity.

Macrophages and **lymphocytes** are also found within the dermal layer. Both types of cells are part of the inflammatory process and are responsible for combating microorganisms that breach the epidermal layer. After a pathogen enters the dermis, macrophages and lymphocytes destroy the invading microorganism and signal other cells to migrate into the area. Physical injury will trigger mast cells to release granules into the surrounding tissue (degranulate) and produce special chemical mediators. The result is increased blood flow to the affected area, manifested as redness and warmth.

The dermis contains the following specialized structures:

- **Nerve endings.** These structures mediate the senses of touch, temperature, pressure, and pain.
- **Blood vessels.** These structures carry oxygen and nutrients to the skin and remove carbon dioxide and metabolic waste products. Cutaneous blood vessels also have a crucial role in regulating body temperature by altering the volume of blood that flows from the warm core of the body to its cooler surface.
- **Sweat glands.** These glands produce sweat, which they discharge through ducts passing to the surface of the skin.
- **Hair follicles.** These small, tubelike structures produce hair and enclose the hair roots. Each follicle contains a single hair. Attached to the hair follicle is a small muscle that, on contraction, causes the follicle to assume a more vertical position. Hairs in each part of the body have definite periods of growth, after which they are shed and replaced.
- **Sebaceous glands.** These glands, located at the neck of each hair follicle, are a specialized secretory mechanism that produce an oily substance (sebum). The secretions of the sebaceous glands empty into the hair follicles and from there, reach the surface of the skin.

Fascia

Between the dermis and the underlying muscle and bone is a thick layer of connective tissue known as subcutaneous tissue, or the superficial **fascia**. This subcutaneous tissue is composed of adipose tissue and areolar tissue. Blood vessels, **lymph vessels**, and hair follicle roots are also found in this layer. The subcutaneous tissue insulates, protects, and stores energy in the form of fat. Subcutaneous injections are given in this layer.

Below the subcutaneous tissue is a thick, dense layer of fibrous tissue known as the **deep fascia**. The deep fascia is composed of tough bands of tissue that surround muscles and other internal structures. It supports and protects underlying structures from injury. Muscles and bones are found below this layer.

Accessory Structures

The accessory structures of the integumentary system include hair, nails, and sebaceous and sweat glands.

Hair

The main function of hair is protection from physical injury, the sun, and the entry of dust and other particles into the eyes and nose. Hair goes through stages of growth and rest, and it is nourished by the blood vessels that provide nutrients and oxygen to the skin.

Hair growth begins in a hair follicle. Within each follicle is a small cluster of cells known as the hair papilla. The growth of hair begins in this cluster of cells, which is hidden in the follicle. Over time, the cells move upward to become keratinized and form the hair's shaft. Each follicle is surrounded by arrector pili, a smooth muscle responsible for goose bumps (the pulling upward of the hair and downward of the skin in response to cold, fear, or excitement).

Words of Wisdom

Evaluate a patient's nails for color, shape, attachment, and presence of indentations to obtain valuable information during the physical exam.

Nails

Nails protect the ends of the fingers and toes. They consist of a nail plate above a skin surface called the nail bed. The part of the nail plate that grows most actively is covered by a white, crescent-moon-shaped lunula, where epithelial cells divide and become keratinized. The nail cells push forward over the nail bed, causing the nail to continually grow outward. The nail of the middle finger grows fastest, whereas the nail of the thumb grows slowest.

Glands

Two types of glands are located under the skin: sebaceous and sweat glands. As discussed previously, sebaceous glands are found in the dermis and secrete oil (sebum) in the hair follicle shaft and the skin. Sebum prevents excessive drying of the skin and hair, prevents water loss, and keeps the skin pliable. It also protects the skin from some forms of bacteria.

The two types of sweat glands are merocrine and apocrine glands. Merocrine (eccrine) glands are the predominant type of sweat glands and are present at birth. These glands, which open directly to the body's surface, are found on the forehead, neck, back, and upper lip, although the palms and soles have the most of these glands. When the body temperature rises, these glands produce sweat, which is composed of water and salts. The evaporation of this water from the skin surface is one of the body's major mechanisms for shedding excess heat. Apocrine glands open into hair follicles, including in and around the genitalia, axillae, and anus. These glands secrete an organic substance (which is odorless until acted on by surface bacteria) into the hair follicles.

> **Words of Wisdom**
>
> The skin is affected by the process of aging and environmental exposure. With age, a loss of skin elasticity occurs. In addition, sebaceous glands produce less oil, the epidermis and subcutaneous layers become thinner, and skin cells are replaced at a slower rate. Exposure to ultraviolet light can cause pigment changes, loss of skin elasticity, thickening of the skin, and skin cancer.

Both mammary glands and ceruminous glands are modified sweat glands. Mammary glands, found in the breasts, secrete milk. Ceruminous glands, located in the external auditory canal of the ear, secrete cerumen (earwax). Cerumen is an oily, sticky substance that traps foreign material.

The Skeletal System

The skeleton is the integrated structure formed by the 206 bones of the body. The skeletal system has the following functions:

1. **Support.** The skeletal system provides a rigid framework and bears the weight of the body.
2. **Leverage.** Many muscles of the body attach to various locations on the skeletal system, which provides movement through leverage of the attachment sites.
3. **Protection.** The skeletal system protects the internal structures of the body.
4. **Storage.** The matrix that gives the bone its strength is composed of calcium phosphate material. This combination of minerals is stored in a usable form of bone. In addition, bone serves as a storage location for yellow bone marrow, which is an inactive, fatty bone marrow that stores lipids.
5. **Maintenance of calcium levels.** Calcium is the main element the various bones cells use to create a hard and resilient structure. Bones act as a reservoir from which calcium can be withdrawn and deposited. When the concentration of calcium in the blood and tissue fluid falls too low, **parathyroid hormone (PTH)** stimulates the release of calcium from bones. When the concentration of calcium is too high, the thyroid gland secretes the hormone calcitonin, which inhibits the removal of calcium from bone.
6. **Blood cell production.** Cavities within the bones contain red marrow—the substance responsible for making RBCs, WBCs, and platelets. The location of red marrow varies with age. However, after the age of 4 years, blood cell production is limited to the ribs, sternum (breastbone), **pelvis**, skull, spinal column, and proximal ends of the humerus and femur (thighbone). The production of blood cells in the bone marrow is referred to as *hematopoiesis* (discussed later in this chapter).

The skeleton consists of two distinct portions: the **axial skeleton** and the **appendicular skeleton**. The axial skeleton is composed of the bones of the central part, or axis, of the body; its divisions include the skull, thoracic cage, and vertebral column (spine). The skull is composed of the **cranium** (the vaultlike portion of the skull behind and above the face), basilar skull, face, and inner ear. The spine is composed of 33 irregular bones known as the spinal vertebrae. Moving anteriorly, the thorax (thoracic cavity) is formed by the sternum and 12 pairs of ribs. The appendicular skeleton is made up of the shoulder girdle, the pelvic girdle, and the bones of the upper and lower extremities.

Bones constitute the primary structure of the skeletal system. Cartilage, tendons, and ligaments are essential connective tissues that work with bones to provide the supportive framework of the skeleton.

The cartilage covering the ends of the bones where they form joints is known as articular cartilage. These pieces of connective tissue provide cushioning and allow the bones to move smoothly against each other.

Tendons are specialized tough cords or bands of dense, white connective tissue that connect muscles to bones. Ligaments are tough white bands of tissue that connect bones to each other. Tendons and ligaments are composed of densely packed fibers of collagen. A sprain occurs when the bone ends partially or temporarily dislocate and the supporting ligaments are partially stretched or torn.

Words of Wisdom

Collagenous fibers in bone lend flexible strength to the bone, much like reinforcing rods embedded in a concrete structure. The mineral components of the bone supply strength for bearing weight, much like concrete does in a structure. Bone without the necessary amount of mineral is flexible; bone without enough collagen is extremely brittle.

When a muscle contracts, tendon pulls on bone, resulting in motion at the joint, the point where two or more bones come together, allowing movement to occur. A strain, or muscle pull, occurs when a muscle is stretched or torn. A strain results in pain, swelling, and bruising of surrounding soft tissues. No ligament or joint damage occurs with a strain. Sprains and strains are graded based on their severity and findings during the physical exam.

Characteristics and Composition of Bones

Bones are classified based on their shape. *Long bones* are found in limbs; they are longer than they are wide. They have a body (called a shaft) and two ends that permit movement at joints. These bones have attachment points for muscles, which allow the mechanical basis of movement. The humerus, ulna, radius, femur, tibia (shinbone), and fibula are good examples of long bones. Even some bones that we may consider "short" are actually classified as long bones because of their shape and function; examples include the phalanges (which make up the fingers and toes), **metacarpals** (which form the bony portion of the hand), and metatarsals (which form the arches of the feet)

Short bones are nearly as wide as they are long and are found only in the wrists and feet. Short bones assist with fine movements in several anatomic planes and are compact and strong.

Flat bones are thin, broad bones that usually protect and encase vital organs. They are often curved to help form walls of cavities. The sternum, ribs, scapulae, and certain skull bones are examples of flat bones.

Irregular bones have unique shapes and functions that are designed to perform a specific function. These bones include the mandible (lower jaw), many facial bones, and the bones that make up the vertebrae in the spine and pelvis. Sesamoid bones, which are generally considered a type of irregular bone, are sometimes grouped into a separate category of their own. Sesamoid bones, such as the patella (kneecap), develop in certain tendons to protect the tendons from excessive wear where they cross major joints. Sesamoid bones are so named because they resemble the size and shape of a sesame seed.

Special Populations

Fractures are common in older people because of a decrease in bone mineral density. The result is weak bones.

Typical Long Bone Architecture

All types of bone share common characteristics despite the differences in their shape. The long bones are used as an example for this description. Bones are composed of two layers: compact (solid or cortical) bone and spongy bone (also called cancellous bone or trabecular bone) **FIGURE 8-23**. Compact bone is mostly solid, with few spaces, and contains a central space called the marrow cavity or marrow canal. Cancellous bone consists of a lacy network of bony rods called trabeculae. The trabeculae are oriented along the lines of stress to increase the weight-bearing capacity of the long bones.

Words of Wisdom

In adults, most bone marrow in the extremities' long bones contains adipose tissue and is called yellow marrow. The bones of the axial skeleton and girdles contain red marrow, where most RBCs are manufactured.

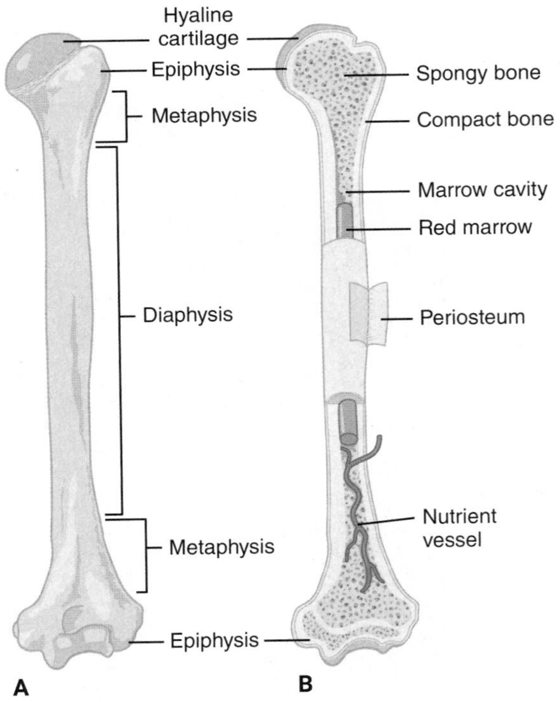

FIGURE 8-23 The components of the long bone. **A.** Illustration of the humerus. Notice the long shaft and dilated ends. **B.** Longitudinal section of the humerus showing compact bone, spongy bone, and marrow.

The long bone is divided into three regions: the diaphysis, the epiphysis, and the metaphysis. The **diaphysis**, or shaft of a long bone, is composed of compact bone tissue. Although long bones look solid, the diaphysis is actually a hollow tube that serves to lighten the bone while maintaining its strength. The hollow area within the diaphysis is the medullary canal. It is lined with a thin membrane called the endosteum, which contains specialized cells that are important in forming and repairing bone. The medullary canal contains blood vessels and yellow bone marrow.

At each end of the diaphysis is the epiphysis. This area is made of spongy bone, which is composed of several thin plates of bone with spaces between them that contain the red marrow and also serve to lighten the bone.

Between and joining the diaphysis and epiphysis is the metaphysis. When bones are lengthening during childhood and adolescence, this region contains the physis, also called the **epiphyseal plate** or growth plate. The physis is made up of cartilage that is replaced by bone as it lengthens. After a person reaches adulthood, the growth plate closes and the mature adult bone is complete.

Covering the end of the epiphysis is a thin, slick layer of cartilage called the articular cartilage. The term *articulate*, or *articulation*, refers to where structures come together. Articular cartilage absorbs shock and reduces friction between bones, allowing them to move smoothly and efficiently.

The periosteum is a double layer of connective tissue that lines the outer surface of the entire bone except for areas covered by articular cartilage. The periosteum contains a rich supply of blood vessels, lymphatic vessels, nerves, bone cells, and elastic fibers. Pain results when the periosteum is disrupted (such as with a fracture). An extensive network of Haversian canals and Volkmann canals supply nutrients and remove waste products from the bone. Blood vessels, lymphatic vessels, and nerves originating in the periosteum enter the compact bone through the horizontal Volkmann canals. After entering the bone, they join with the Haversian canals, which run along the length of the bone, and provide blood and nerve supply to the entire bone. A bone stripped of its periosteum will ultimately die, just as the heart muscle dies when the arteries supplying the muscle become blocked.

Bone Formation and Growth

Bone (osseous tissue) is a type of connective tissue that is composed of bone cells and matrix. Three main types of cells are found in bone. **Osteoblasts** form bone and maintain the strength of existing bone. **Osteoclasts** break down and reabsorb bone. **Osteocytes** are mature osteoblasts found in lacunae (small cavities or chambers) within the bony matrix. Osteocytes, which are connected together by long, threadlike extensions of the osteocyte cytoplasm, move nutrients and waste through the matrix of the bone. Osteoclasts produce enzymes that cause bone minerals to dissolve, releasing calcium and phosphate into the bloodstream.

Bones begin to form in utero during the first 6 weeks after fertilization. Intramembranous bones originate between layers of connective tissues and have a sheetlike appearance. Examples of intramembranous bones are the flat, broad bones of the skull. These bones emerge when unspecialized connective tissues form at the sites where future bones will be developed. Osteoblasts are then produced, depositing bony matrix around them. When extracellular matrix has surrounded the osteoblasts, they are termed osteocytes. The surrounding membranous tissues begin to form the periosteum, or membrane that lines the surface of all bones. Inside the periosteum, the osteoblasts form a compact bone layer over the new spongy bone.

Endochondral bones begin as cartilaginous masses that are eventually replaced by bone tissue. These bones develop from hyaline cartilage that is shaped similarly to the bones they will become. They grow rapidly at first, and then begin to change in appearance. When spongy bone begins to replace the original cartilage, a primary ossification center is created, with bone tissue developing outward toward the ends of the structure. Eventually, secondary ossification centers will appear in the epiphyses, forming more spongy bone.

During the first 6 weeks of fetal development, the skeleton is cartilaginous. The bones increase greatly in size as the fetus develops, and then throughout childhood **FIGURE 8-24**. Bone growth continues through adolescence. The process of replacing other tissues with bone, which involves the deposition of calcium salts, is called **ossification**.

Osteogenesis is the formation of bone. Long bones initially consist of hyaline cartilage, which is

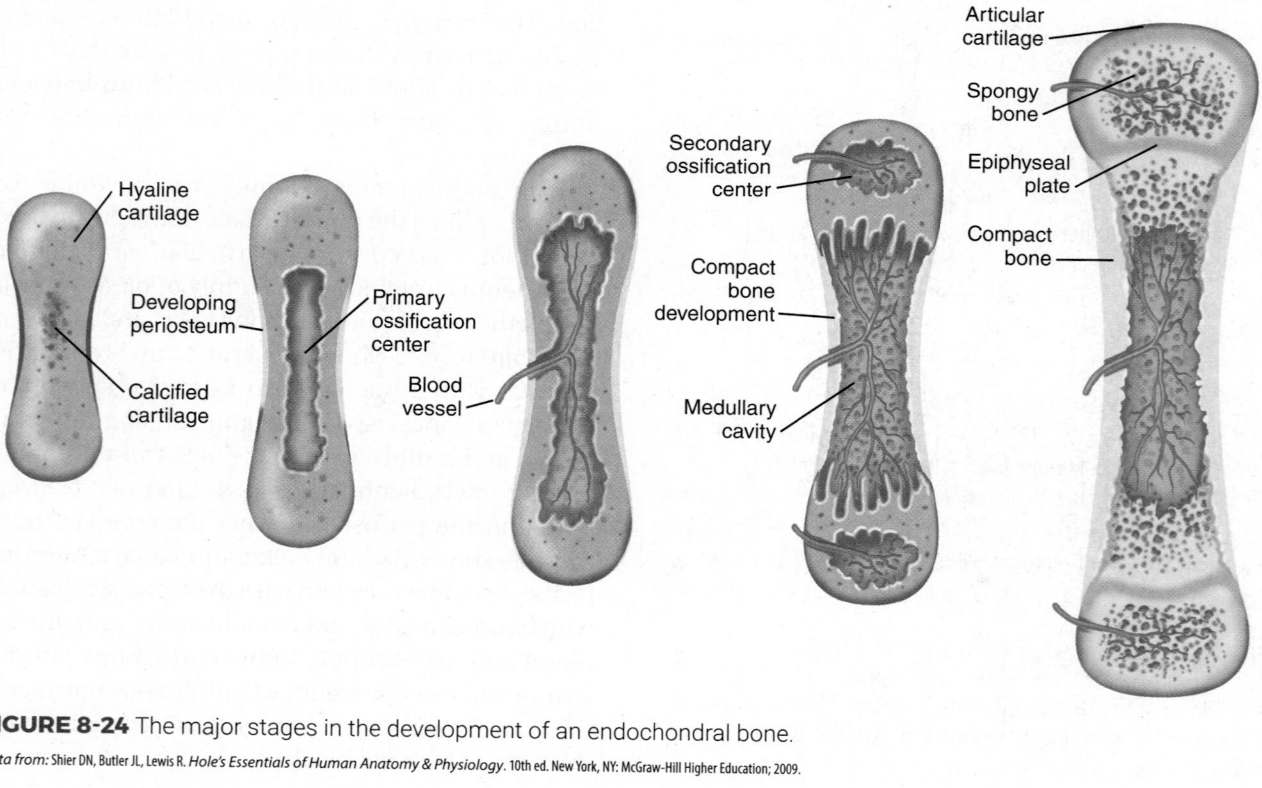

FIGURE 8-24 The major stages in the development of an endochondral bone.

Data from: Shier DN, Butler JL, Lewis R. *Hole's Essentials of Human Anatomy & Physiology*. 10th ed. New York, NY: McGraw-Hill Higher Education; 2009.

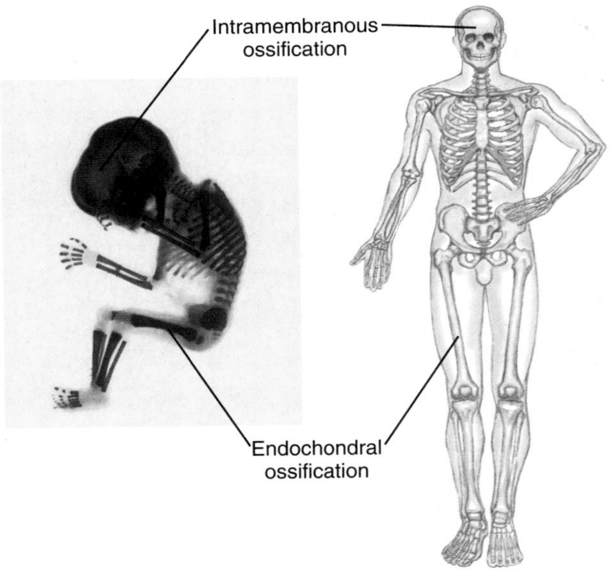

FIGURE 8-25 Intramembranous ossification results in the development of flat bones. Endochondral ossification results in the production of long bones.

A: © Ralph Hutchings/Visuals Unlimited; B: © Jones & Bartlett Learning.

later replaced by bony tissue that becomes compact bone. This process begins with the diaphysis and ends with the epiphyses of each long bone. Most bones of the body develop through this process, which is called endochondral ossification.

In contrast, flat bones develop from connective tissue membranes that are replaced by spongy bone, and then compact bone. This process is called intramembranous ossification. In infants, **fontanelles** (so-called soft spots) are sheets of tough connective tissue between the flat bones of the skull; they soften and expand during childbirth and are gradually replaced as the bones of the skull fuse together **FIGURE 8-25**.

Lengthwise bone growth occurs at the epiphyseal plate, a thin layer of cartilage that lies between the epiphyses and metaphyses, until the epiphyseal plate closes. Growth of long bones depends on good nutrition and the actions of several hormones, including human growth hormone. Other hormones involved in long bone growth include thyroid hormone, **estrogen**, and **testosterone** **TABLE 8-13**. After the epiphyseal plate closes, the long bones can no longer grow **FIGURE 8-26**. Length of bone is balanced by increased bone width. Osteoblast and osteoclast activity is balanced in the body so that bones grow with uniformity.

TABLE 8-13 Hormones Involved in Bone Growth and Maintenance
• Human growth hormone • Thyroxine • Insulin • Parathyroid hormone • Calcitonin • Estrogen • Testosterone

Bone development, growth, and repair are influenced by heredity, nutrition, hormones, and exercise. Vitamin D is required for the absorption of calcium in the small intestine. Without it, calcium is not absorbed well, leading to softening bones and potentially causing deformity. Growth hormone from the **pituitary gland** (an endocrine gland responsible for directly or indirectly affecting all body functions) stimulates cell division in the epiphyseal plates, and sex hormones stimulate ossification of these plates. Exercise stresses the bones, stimulating them to become thickened and strong.

Joints

Recall that wherever long bones come in contact, a joint (articulation) is formed. A joint consists of the ends of the bones that make up the joint and the surrounding connecting and supporting tissue. Joints typically allow movement of the extremities that rigid bone would not allow. Another essential function of joints is to allow **proprioception**, the awareness of motion and position of a body part. Most joints in the body are named by combining the names of the two bones that form that joint. For example, the sternoclavicular joint is the articulation between the sternum and clavicle (collarbone).

Types of Joints

Anatomists classify joints according to structure. The structural classification of a joint is determined by the type of soft tissue that connects the bones of a joint (eg, fibrous, cartilaginous, synovial) **TABLE 8-14** **FIGURE 8-27**.

Physiologists classify joints according to function (the type and degree of movement it allows). Functionally, joints fall into three categories: synarthroses, amphiarthroses, and diarthroses.

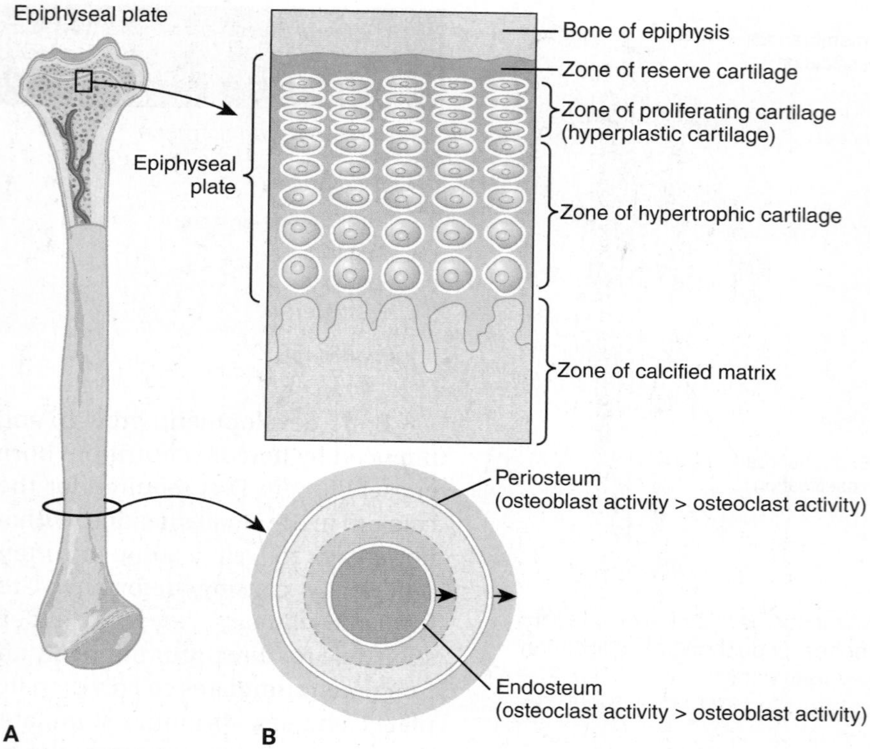

FIGURE 8-26 A. Lengthwise growth occurs at the epiphyseal plate until individuals reach skeletal maturity (typically around age 14 years in girls and age 17 years in boys) and the epiphyseal plate closes, becoming the epiphyseal line. **B.** Growth in a bone's diameter involves altered rates of osteoclast and osteoblast activity at the periosteum and endosteum.

TABLE 8-14 Structural and Functional Classifications of Joints

Structural Name	Functional Name	Type	Description	Example
Fibrous joints	Synarthroses (no movement)	Gomphosis	Fibrous connection with peg-in-hole–shaped bones	Between teeth and mandible; between teeth and maxilla
		Suture	Fibrous connections and interlocking projections	Between skull bones
		Syndesmosis	Bones united by a strong membrane or by interosseous ligaments	Between distal tibia and fibula; between radius and ulna
Cartilaginous joints	Amphiarthroses (little movement)	Symphysis	Connections via a fibrocartilage pad	Symphysis pubis of pelvis; joints formed by intervertebral disks
		Synchondrosis	Bones united by hyaline cartilage	Between the ribs and costal cartilages of rib cage
Synovial joints	Diarthroses (free movement)	(no subcategories)	Complex joint in a joint cavity with synovial fluid	Numerous (wrist, elbow, shoulder, hip, ankle); subdivided according to range of movement

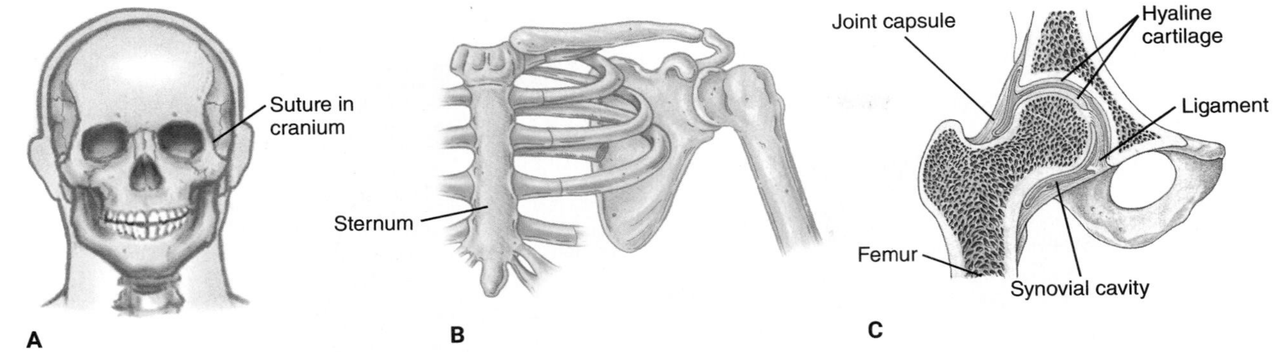

FIGURE 8-27 Types of joints. **A.** Fibrous. **B.** Cartilaginous. **C.** Synovial.

Synarthroses are separated by a thin layer of fibrous connective tissue and are immovable. They include joints such as the gomphosis, suture, and syndesmosis. The temporary joints formed in the growth plates in the long bones of children are examples of synchondroses. Amphiarthroses are connected by a cartilaginous disk, hyaline cartilage, or a fibrocartilage pad and are slightly movable. They include joints such as the symphysis and synchondrosis. Diarthroses are freely movable; they include the synovial joints.

The 230 joints in the human body are summarized as follows:

- **Fibrous joints**. Lying between bones that closely contact each other, fibrous joints are joined by thin, dense connective tissue. An example of a fibrous joint is a suture between flat bones of the skull. No real movement takes place in most fibrous joints, making them synarthrotic in classification. Those with limited movement (amphiarthrotic) include the joint between the distal tibia and fibula.
- **Cartilaginous joints**. Also called amphiarthroses, these joints allow for minimal movement between the bones. The soft tissue that unites the bones of a cartilaginous joint consists of either hyaline cartilage (synchondroses) or fibrocartilage (symphyses). The pubic symphysis and the joints connecting the ribs to the sternum are examples of this type of joint.
- **Synovial joints.** These diarthrotic joints are the most mobile and complex joints of the body. Articular cartilage covers each end of the opposing bones, which reduces the friction created by movement of the bone ends and absorbs vibrations and shocks. The bones of a synovial joint are connected by a **joint capsule**, which encloses a joint cavity. The joint capsule is an extension of the periosteum and insulates the joint from surrounding tissues **FIGURE 8-28 FIGURE 8-29**. The joint capsule is made up of an outer layer of fibrous connective tissue and an inner synovial membrane layer. The synovial membrane secretes synovial fluid into the joint cavity, which lubricates and nourishes the inner surfaces of the joint. Because cartilage is avascular, the synovial membrane also removes waste products, microorganisms, and debris. The articulating bones of the joint are held in place by strong ligaments, which add support. Because the ligaments are flexible, they allow movement; at the same time, they are strong enough to resist dislocation. Although synovial joint ligaments are usually located outside of the joint capsule, they are sometimes found inside it. The cruciate ligaments of the knee joint are examples of ligaments that are found within the joint capsule. Ligaments found outside the joint capsule may be completely independent of the capsule or attached to the capsule's outer layer. Examples of synovial joints include the ball-and-socket, hinge, pivot, condyloid, saddle, and gliding

Words of Wisdom

A joint that is virtually surrounded by tough, thick ligaments has little motion. A joint such as the shoulder, with few ligaments, is free to move in almost any direction—and will, as a result, be more susceptible to dislocation.

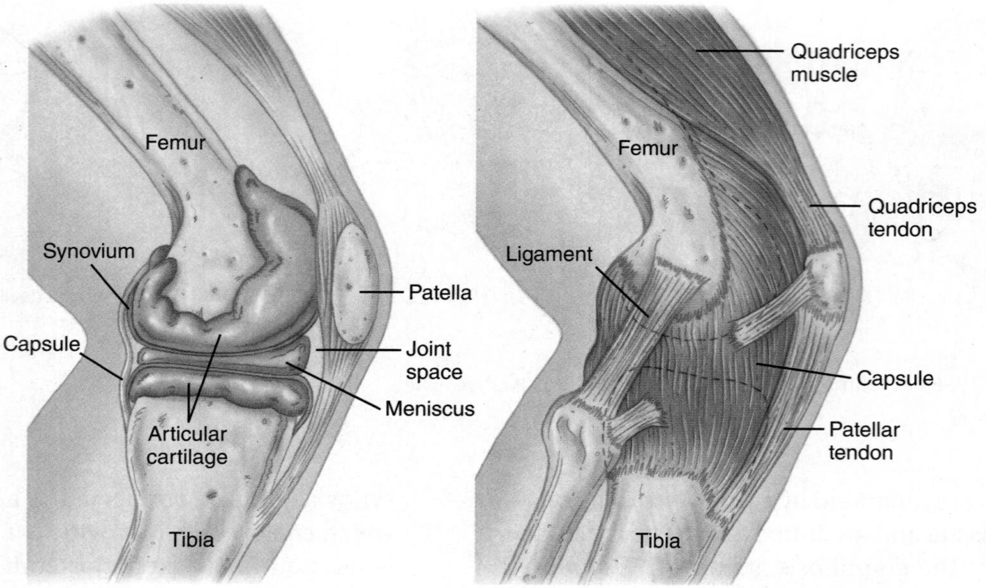

FIGURE 8-28 A synovial joint consists of bone ends, the fibrous joint capsule, the synovial membrane, and ligaments. The degree to which a synovial joint can move is determined by how the ligaments hold the bone ends and by the configuration of the bones themselves.

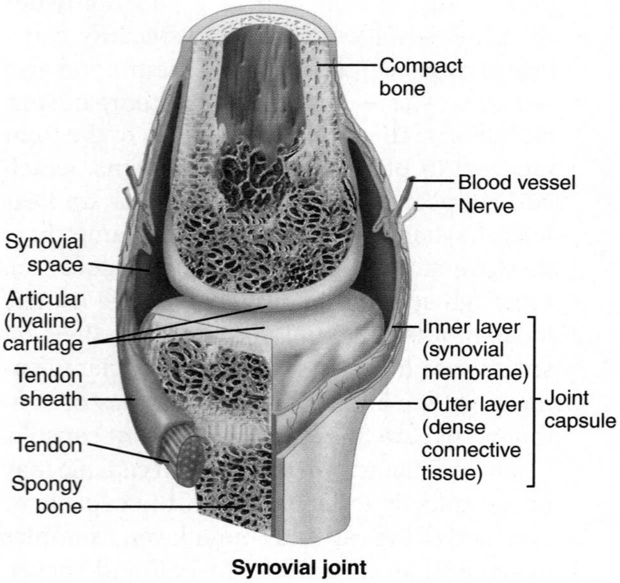

FIGURE 8-29 A synovial joint.

joints **FIGURE 8-30 TABLE 8-15**. Some synovial joints have shock-absorbing fibrocartilage pads called menisci. They may also have fluid-filled sacs called bursae, commonly located between tendons and underlying bony prominences, such as in the knee or elbow.

Bursa

A **bursa** is a small, padlike sac or cavity filled with a small amount of fluid that helps reduce the amount of friction between a tendon and a bone or between a tendon and a ligament. A bursa is usually located near a joint. Examples include the olecranon bursa of the elbow and the prepatellar bursa of the knee. Bursitis is inflammation of a bursa.

Axial Skeleton

The axial skeleton is composed of the skull, thoracic cage, and vertebral column. The brain lies within the skull. The heart, lungs, and great vessels are enclosed in the thorax (thoracic cavity), which is part of the torso. Much of the liver and spleen are protected by the lower ribs. The spinal cord is contained within and protected by a bony spinal canal formed by the vertebrae. It connects the brain to skeletal muscle, skin, and other structures by means of the spinal nerves. Thirty-one pairs of **spinal nerves** attach to the spinal cord and communicate with structures primarily located in the neck, trunk, and extremities.[6]

Skull

At the top of the axial skeleton is the skull, consisting of 28 bones organized into three anatomic groups:

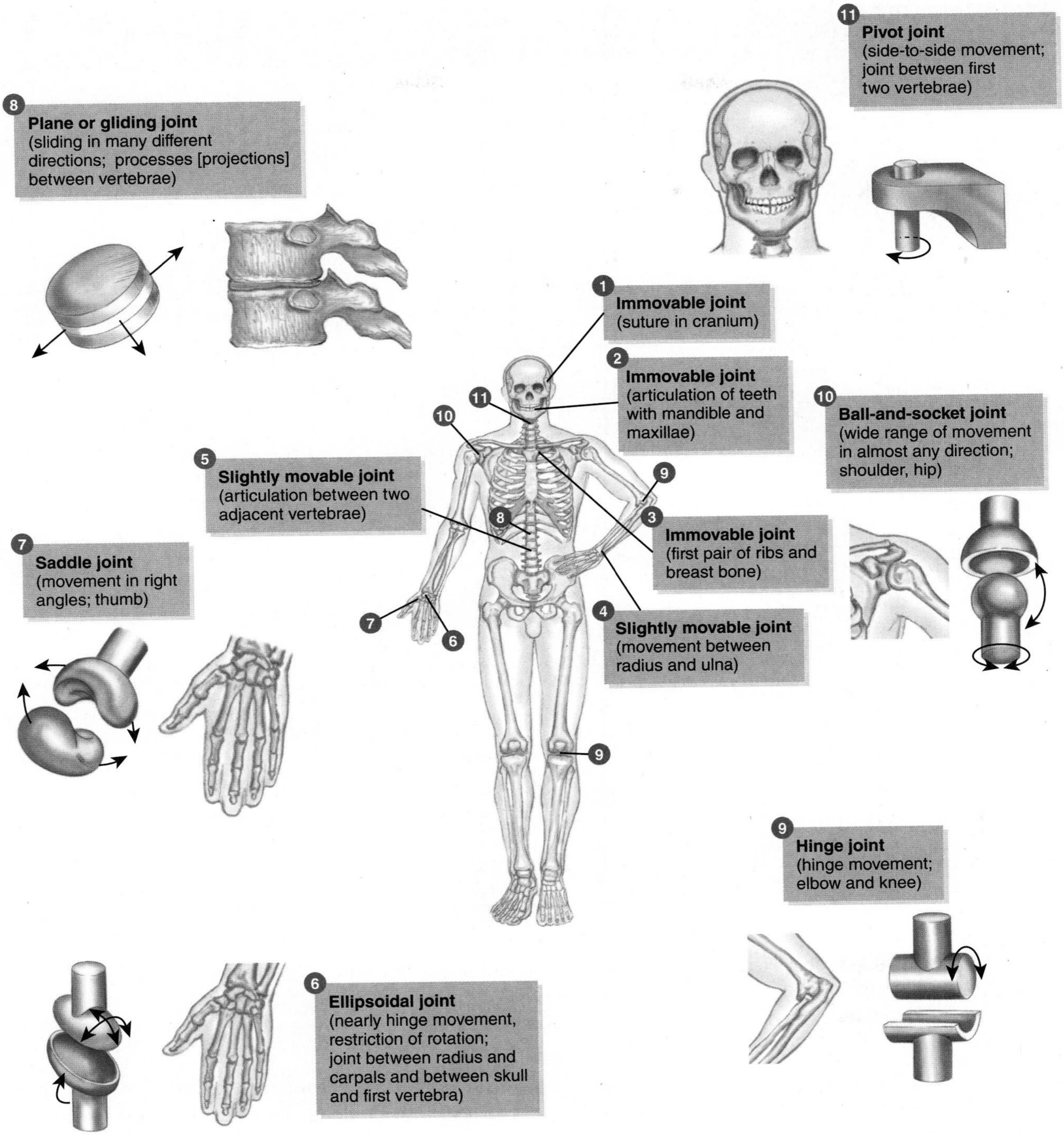

FIGURE 8-30 Types of joints in the body.

the auditory ossicles, cranium, and face **FIGURE 8-31**. The six auditory ossicles (three on each side of the head) function in hearing and are located deep within cavities of the temporal bone. The remaining 22 bones constitute the cranium and the face.

Auditory Ossicles

Found within the middle ear are the ossicles, three tiny auditory bones responsible for converting the sound waves collected by the eardrum into pressure waves that are transmitted to the **cochlea**, a bony

TABLE 8-15 Types of Synovial Joints

Type	Movement	Example
Ball-and-socket	Flexion, extension, abduction, adduction, and rotation	Shoulder and hip joints
Hinge	Flexion, extension, pronation, supination	Elbow and knee joints
Pivot	Rotation	Atlantoaxial joint; proximal ends of radius and ulna (elbow joint)
Condyloid (ellipsoidal)	Flexion, extension, abduction, adduction; no rotation	Metacarpophalangeal joints (knuckles); temporomandibular joint (jaw)
Saddle	Flexion, extension, abduction, adduction; limited rotation	Carpometacarpal joint (thumb)
Gliding (plane)	Sliding motion without rotation	Intercarpal joints (wrist); intertarsal joints (ankle)

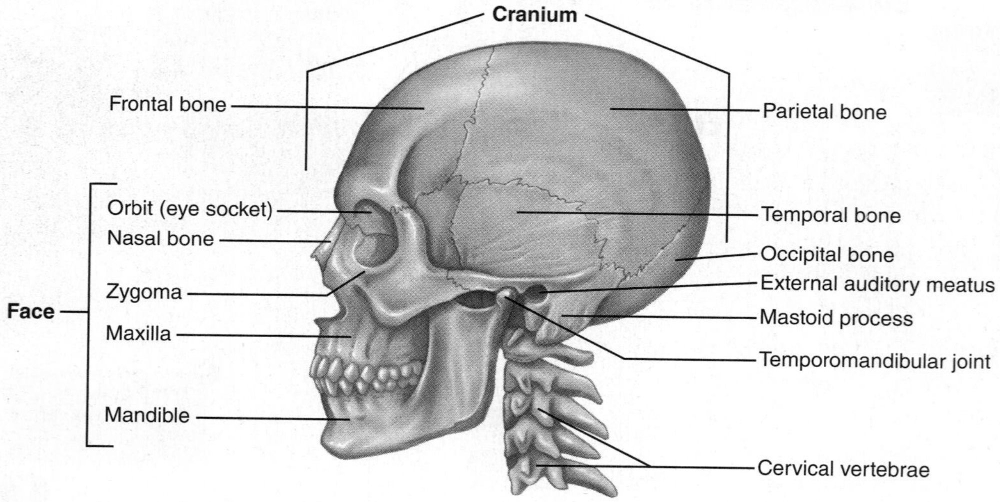

FIGURE 8-31 The skull consists of 28 bones organized into three anatomic groups: the auditory ossicles (not shown here), cranium, and face.

structure resembling a tiny snail shell. These ossicles are called the hammer (malleus), anvil (incus), and stirrup (stapes) based on their shapes.

Cranium

The dome-shaped roof of the skull, the **cranial vault**, surrounds and protects the upper portion of the brain. Together, eight bones form the cranial vault: two parietal bones, two temporal bones, and the frontal, occipital, sphenoid, and ethmoid bones **FIGURE 8-32**. The frontal bone forms the forehead and the roof of the bony sockets that contain the eyeballs. The parietal and temporal bones are considered paired bones because one is found on each side of the skull. The parietal bones form the roof and upper part of the sides of the cranium. The temporal bones form the lower sides and base of the cranium. At the base of the temporal bone is a cone-shaped section of bone known as the mastoid process. This area is an important site for the attachment of various muscles. The occipital bone forms the back and base of the skull

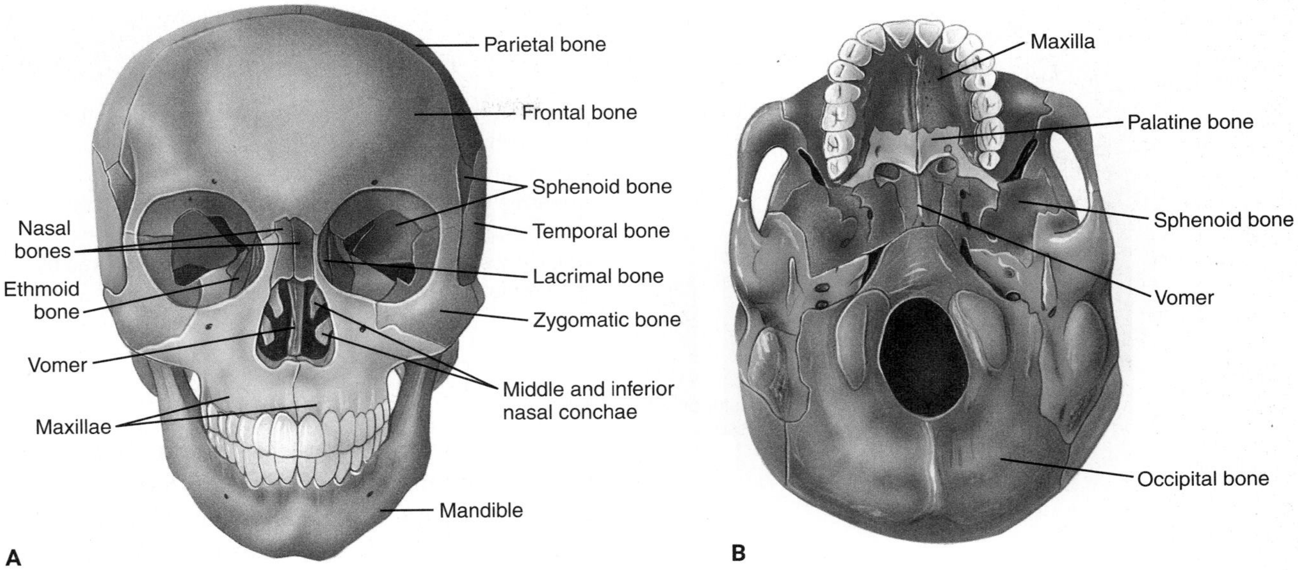

FIGURE 8-32 The skull and its components. **A.** Anterior view. **B.** Inferior view.

and joins the parietal and temporal bones. The *foramen magnum* is the opening in the occipital bone at the base of the skull through which the spinal cord passes. The sphenoid bone is a bat-shaped bone that joins with the frontal, occipital, and ethmoid bones and forms part of the skull base. The thin ethmoid bone contains many small holes. It forms part of the **orbits** (cone-shaped depressions that enclose and protect the eyes) and supports the nasal cavity (the chamber inside the nose that lies between the floor of the cranium and the roof of the mouth).

The skull bones are connected at special joints known as **sutures** **FIGURE 8-33**. The paired parietal bones join together at the sagittal suture; they abut the frontal bone at the coronal suture. The occipital bone attaches to the parietal bones at the lambdoid suture. As discussed previously, fibrous tissues called fontanelles link the sutures in infants. The tissue felt through the fontanelles are layers of the scalp and thick membranes overlying the brain. Under normal conditions, the brain may not be felt through the fontanelles. By the time a child reaches 18 months of age, the sutures should have solidified and the fontanelles closed.

Viewed from above, the floor of the interior of the skull is divided into three compartments: anterior fossa, middle fossa, and posterior fossa **FIGURE 8-34**. The crista galli forms a prominent bony ridge in the center of the anterior fossa and is the point of attachment of the meninges, the membranes that surround the brain. On either side of the crista galli is the **cribriform plate** of the ethmoid bone. This horizontal bone is perforated with numerous openings (foramina) that allow for the passage of the olfactory nerves from the nasal cavity.

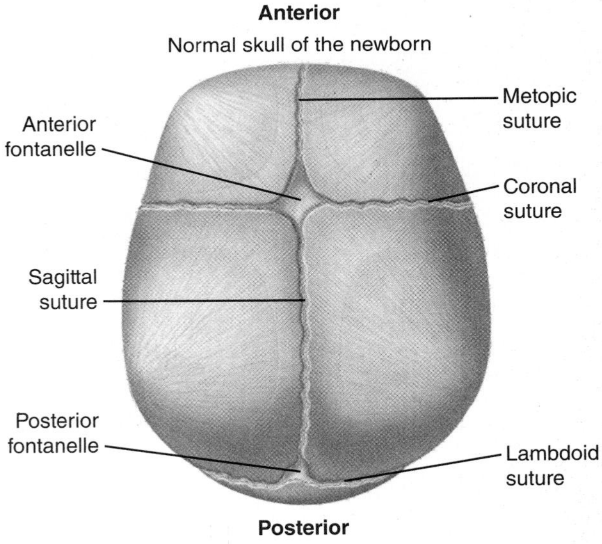

FIGURE 8-33 The sutures of the skull of a newborn.

When the mandible is removed, the base of the skull appears amazingly complex, with numerous

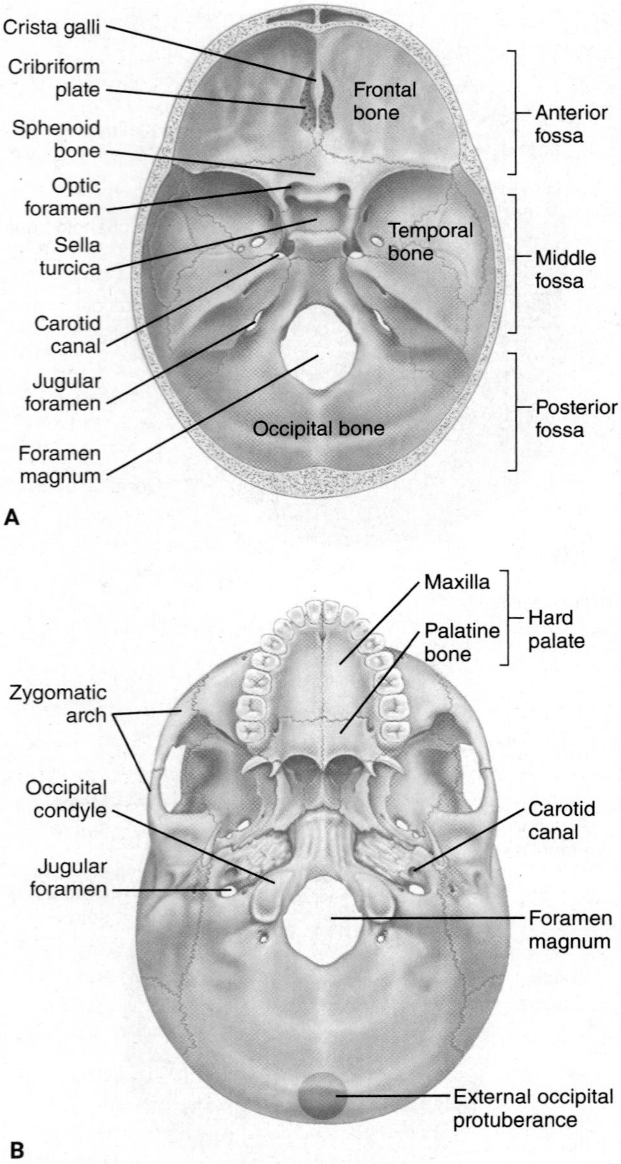

FIGURE 8-34 A. The floor of the cranial vault and its anatomy. **B.** The base of the skull from below.

foramina visible (see Figure 8-34B). The occipital condyles on the occipital bone, which are the points of articulation (connection) between the skull and the vertebral column, lie on either side of the foramen magnum. Portions of the maxilla and palatine bone, the irregularly shaped bone in the posterior nasal cavity, form the **hard palate**, the bony, anterior part of the **palate** (roof of the mouth). The zygomatic arch is the bone that extends along the front of the skull below the orbit.

Words of Wisdom

A blow to the eye may result in a fracture of the floor of the orbit, called a blowout fracture. The orbits are extremely thin and break easily, resulting in transmission of forces away from the eyeball itself to the bone. Blood and fat may then leak into the maxillary sinus below. **Sinuses** are cavities formed by the cranial bones.

Face

The facial bones consist of 14 separate bones that form the structure of the face. These bones protect the eyes, nose, and tongue and provide attachment points for the muscles that allow chewing. They are relatively thin but protect the entrances to the digestive system and the respiratory system. The 14 facial bones include the paired maxillae, a single mandible (the only freely moving bone in the skull), paired zygomatic bones, paired palatine bones, paired nasal bones, paired lacrimal bones, a single vomer bone, and paired inferior nasal conchae bones. Both the frontal and ethmoid bones contribute to the cranial vault and face.

The facial portion of the cranium contains two orbits. In addition to the eyeball and muscles that move it, each orbit contains blood vessels, nerves, and fat. The frontal, sphenoid, zygomatic, maxilla, lacrimal, ethmoid, and palatine bones each form portions of the orbits.

The right and left upper jawbones (maxillae) are located between the orbits and upper teeth and help form the following parts of the face: the upper face, infratemporal region, orbital floor, lateral wall of the nasal cavity, floor of the nasal cavity, and roof of the oral cavity. In the condition known as cleft palate, the right and left maxillae do not join before birth. The lower jaw consists of the body of the mandible anteriorly and the ramus of the mandible posteriorly. The body and ramus meet posteriorly to form the angle of the mandible. The only facial bone capable of movement, the mandible joins the skull in the area of the temporal bone, forming the temporomandibular joint on each side of the skull. The zygoma (cheekbone) forms the anterior wall of the infratemporal area and the lateral wall of the orbit. The zygoma meets the lateral skull to form the zygomatic arch, which lends shape to the cheeks.

The palatine bones help form the lateral wall and floor of the nasal cavity, the oral cavity (posterior third of the hard palate), and a small portion of the posterior wall of the orbit. The nasal bones help form part of the bony bridge of the external nose, the lateral wall of the nasal cavity, and a small part of the bony nasal septum. The lacrimal bones form the medial wall of the orbits and the lateral wall of the nasal cavity. The vomer is a thin, flat bone that forms a large part of the bony nasal septum. The inferior conchae help form the lateral wall of the nasal cavity and part of the maxillary sinus. The external portion of the nose is mostly cartilage.

The **paranasal sinuses** are hollow, air-filled spaces that help reduce the weight of the skull and provide voice resonance. They are located around the nasal cavity and drain into it **FIGURE 8-35**. There are four pairs of paranasal sinuses: ethmoid sinuses within the ethmoid bone, frontal sinuses within the frontal bone, maxillary sinuses within the right and left maxillae (the largest of paranasal sinuses), and sphenoid sinuses within the body of the sphenoid bone. The paranasal sinuses are lined with epithelium. The cilia within this epithelium move in a synchronized beating pattern toward the anterior portion of the nasal cavity. Tiny goblet cells in the epithelium secrete a sticky mucus substance onto the cilia, which traps contaminants as they enter the nasal cavity. The cilia then move the mucus toward the front of the nasal cavity, where the mucus is removed by blowing the nose or moved down to the throat where it can enter into the digestive system. During sleep, this mucus may flow backward (postnasal drip).

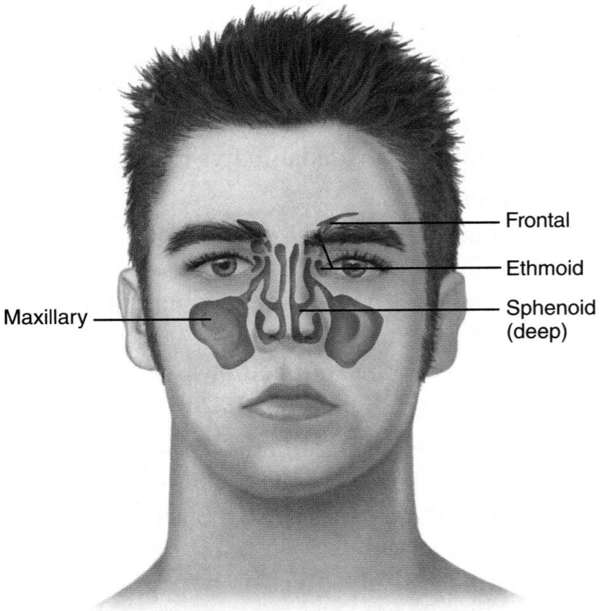

FIGURE 8-35 The paranasal sinuses.

Words of Wisdom

Sinusitis is a relatively common inflammation of the paranasal sinuses. Sinusitis may range in severity from a simple upper respiratory tract infection consisting of headache and nasal drainage to a potentially life-threatening brain infection, depending on the extent of infection and which sinuses are affected.

The **hyoid bone** is a horseshoe-shaped bone that "floats" beneath the mandible, with the open end of the horseshoe pointed posteriorly. Every bone in the body articulates with at least one other bone, except the hyoid bone. Although the hyoid is not part of the skull, it is attached to the skull by muscles and ligaments. It anchors the tongue and is a point of attachment for many important neck and tongue muscles. If the hyoid bone is damaged by a blow to the anterior neck, then the patient may have a hoarse and low-volume voice because of airway swelling.

The nerves that provide facial sensory and motor control are discussed later in this chapter.

Neck

The neck contains many important structures. It is supported by the cervical spine, which comprises the first seven vertebrae in the spinal column. The spinal cord exits the foramen magnum and lies within the spinal canal formed by the vertebrae. The upper part of the esophagus (which helps transport food from the mouth to the stomach) and the trachea (windpipe) lie in the midline of the neck. The carotid arteries are found on either side of the trachea, along with jugular veins and several nerves.

Several useful landmarks can be palpated and seen in the neck **FIGURE 8-36**. The most obvious is the firm prominence in the center of the

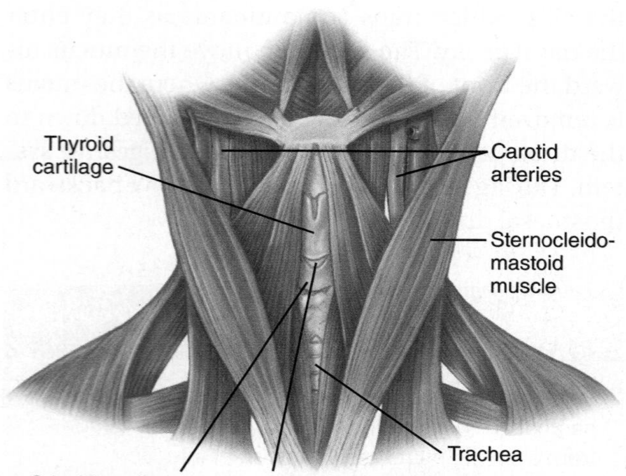

FIGURE 8-36 The principal structures of the neck include the trachea, along with many blood vessels, muscles, and nerves.

anterior surface commonly known as the Adam's apple. Specifically, this shield-shaped prominence is the upper part of the **thyroid cartilage**. It is more prominent in men than in women. The lower portion is the **cricoid cartilage**, a firm ridge of cartilage inferior to the thyroid cartilage, which is somewhat more difficult to palpate. The **cricothyroid membrane** is a soft depression made up of a thin sheet of connective tissue (fascia) that joins the thyroid and cricoid cartilages in the midline of the neck. The cricothyroid membrane is covered at this point only by skin.

Inferior to the **larynx** (voice box), several additional firm ridges are palpable in the anterior midline. These ridges are the cartilage rings of the trachea. The trachea connects the larynx with the main air passages of the lungs (the bronchi). The thyroid gland lies on either side of the lower larynx and the upper trachea. Unless this gland is enlarged, it is usually not palpable.

Pulsations of the carotid arteries are easily palpable in a groove about 0.5 inch (1 cm) lateral to the larynx. Lying immediately adjacent to these arteries, but not palpable, are the internal jugular veins and several important nerves. The sternocleidomastoid muscles, which allow head movement, are found lateral to these vessels and nerves. These muscles originate from the mastoid process of the cranium and insert into the medial border of each clavicle and the sternum at the base of the neck.

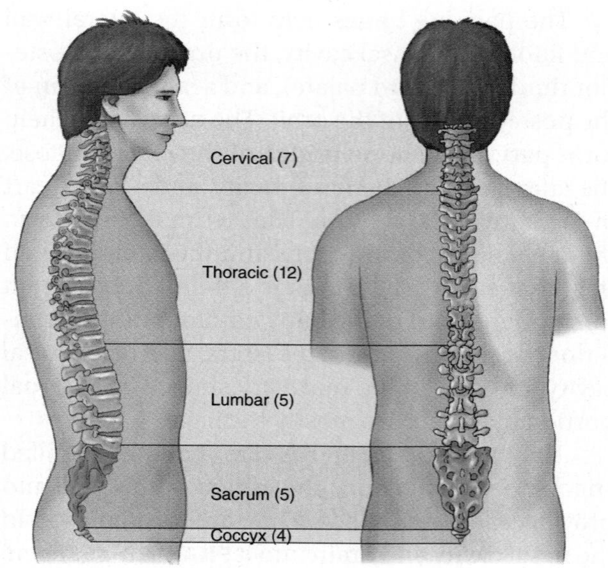

FIGURE 8-37 The spinal column consists of 33 bones, which can be organized into five sections. Each vertebra is numbered and referred to by a letter corresponding to the section of the spine where it is located (eg, the fifth thoracic vertebra is referred to as T5).

Vertebral Column

The spinal cord is encased by the vertebral column (spine), which consists of 33 vertebrae. The vertebrae articulate to form the vertebral column, which is the major structural component of the axial skeleton. Both ligaments and muscle stabilize these skeletal components. Together, these components support and protect neural elements while allowing for fluid movement and an erect stature.

Vertebrae are divided into five regions:

- 7 cervical
- 12 thoracic
- 5 lumbar
- 5 sacral (fused together in adults to form the sacrum)
- 4 coccygeal (fused together in adults to form the coccyx, or tailbone) **FIGURE 8-37**

Each vertebra is identified by its region (eg, cervical, thoracic) and then given a number. Thus the first vertebra is cervical 1, or C1. Starting at C1 and following the spinal column inferiorly, each vertebra gets progressively larger than the previous one because each vertebra must support more weight than the bone above it. The fifth lumbar vertebra is the largest, after which the sacral and coccygeal

Words of Wisdom

Various types of spinal curvatures may be identified in patients. Lordosis is an exaggeration of lumbar curvature, creating a swayback appearance; kyphosis is an exaggeration of thoracic curvature, causing a humpback appearance; and scoliosis is an abnormal lateral curvature of the spine. As a paramedic, you must be familiar with these conditions because they can affect breathing, immobilization, and other aspects of the patient's condition or care.

vertebrae get progressively smaller until they reach the most distal coccygeal vertebrae, the tailbone. The spinal column has four curves to add strength, assist in balance, and prevent injury: two curve posteriorly (cervical and lumbar curvatures) and two curve anteriorly (thoracic and sacral curvatures).

The five sections of spine, from top down, are as follows:

- **Cervical spine.** The first seven vertebrae (C1 through C7) in the neck form the cervical spine. The skull rests on the first cervical vertebra and articulates with it. The first and second cervical vertebrae—named the **atlas** and the **axis**, respectively—are highly specialized, providing support for the head and permitting it to articulate with the spinal column **FIGURE 8-38**.

  The atlas articulates with the occipital condyles at the base of the skull at the atlanto-occipital joint, permitting the head to nod and rotate left to right. The axis has an upward projection called the odontoid process. The atlas sits on this process, which acts as a pivot point and allows head rotation.
- **Thoracic spine.** The next 12 vertebrae make up the thoracic spine. One pair of ribs is attached to each thoracic vertebra. In addition to the supporting muscles and ligaments found in the vertebral column, the thoracic spine is further stabilized by rib attachments. The spinous processes are slightly larger; these bony projections serve as attachment points for muscles that hold the upper body erect and assist with movement of the thoracic cavity during breathing.
- **Lumbar spine.** The lumbar spine includes the five largest bones in the vertebral column, and is integral in carrying a large portion of the upper body weight. This area of the spine is especially susceptible to injury because of its weight-bearing capacity.
- **Sacrum.** The five sacral vertebrae are fused to form one bone. The sacrum is joined to the iliac hip bones with strong ligaments at the **sacroiliac joints** to form the pelvis.
- **Coccyx.** The last four vertebrae, which are also fused, form the coccyx.

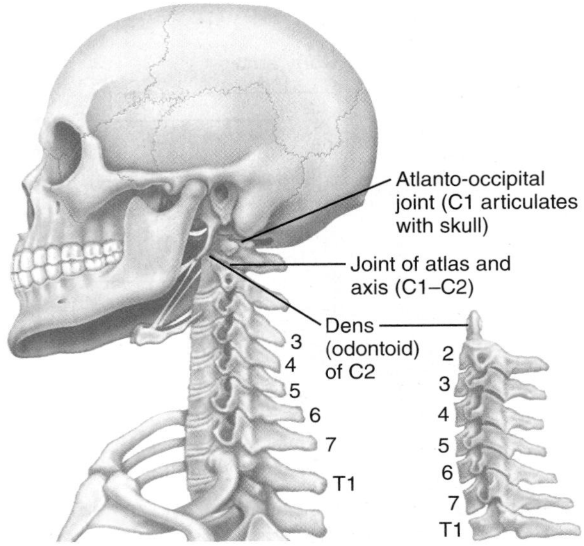

FIGURE 8-38 The cervical vertebrae.

With the exception of C1, each vertebra has a vertebral body, which consists of an inner, thick, round anterior portion that is the spine's weight-bearing component that provides support and stability **FIGURE 8-39**. The posterior, or rear-facing, side of a vertebra is the vertebral arch (also called the bony arch, posterior arch, or dorsal arch). The vertebral arch comprises a spinous process and a thin plate of bone called the lamina between each transverse process and spinous process. When you feel the spine's midline, you are feeling the spinous process; the vertebral column is also called the spine for this reason. The vertebral arch serves as a connection point for muscles and ligaments, allows movement by acting as a lever for muscles, and is the site of interlocking articulation between multiple vertebrae. The thoracic vertebrae also articulate with the ribs at the vertebral arch. Together, the vertebral body and vertebral arch form a space called the vertebral

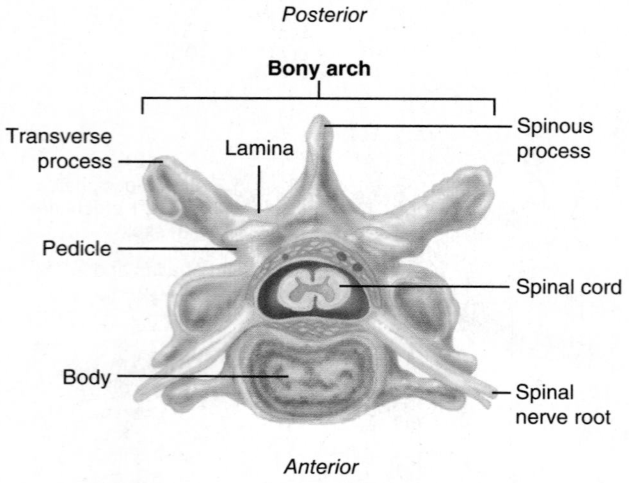

FIGURE 8-39 A general representation of the human vertebra. Vertebrae in different sections of the spinal column vary in shape. The space through which the spinal cord passes is the canal, and the space through which a nerve root passes is a foramen.

foramen. When all vertebrae are aligned, this space creates a large canal running the spinal column's length. The spinal cord, spinal nerve roots, meninges, and many vessels are housed within this canal, and are protected by the vertebrae and intervertebral disks.

Words of Wisdom

As the body ages, loss of water content occurs in the intervertebral disks, causing them to become thinner. This process results in the height loss associated with aging. Stress on the vertebral column may cause a disk to herniate into the spinal canal, resulting in a spinal cord injury or a nerve root injury. Nerves can also be injured at the peripheral level (anywhere outside the spinal cord), a condition called peripheral nerve injury.

The pedicle is a short, thick bony projection that connects the vertebral body to the transverse process of the vertebra. Each pedicle joins with a lamina. The articular process is a bony structure that projects outward from the vertebra. The transverse spinous processes comprise the junction of each pedicle and the lamina on each side of a vertebra. They project laterally and posteriorly and form points of attachments for muscles and ligaments. The posterior spinous process is formed by the fusion of the posterior lamina and serves as an attachment site for muscles and ligaments.

A cartilaginous cushion, called an intervertebral disk, rests between most vertebrae; it provides padding and space for flexibility. There is no disk between the occiput and C1, or between C1 and C2.[7] The space created by these disks allows spinal nerves to exit the spinal cord. These spinal nerves allow control over the periphery of the body.

The ligaments and intervertebral disks allow some motion so the trunk can bend forward (flex) and back (extend), and they allow for rotation and lateral movement. However, they also limit motion of the vertebrae so the spinal cord will not be injured. An injury to the spine may damage parts of the spinal cord and its nerves that may not be protected by the vertebrae. As a paramedic, you must use extreme caution in caring for a patient with a suspected spinal injury to prevent secondary damage to these structures.

Thorax

The thorax (chest) consists of a bony cage overlying some of the most vital organs in the human body. The dimensions of the thorax are defined posteriorly by the thoracic vertebrae and ribs, inferiorly by the **diaphragm** (a specialized skeletal muscle), anteriorly and laterally by the ribs, and superiorly by the thoracic inlet **FIGURE 8-40**.

Words of Wisdom

The thorax's dimensions are of great importance in the physical assessment of the patient. Although the thoracic cavity extends to the 12th rib posteriorly, the diaphragm attaches to the lower six ribs of the anterior thoracic cage. With the movement of the diaphragm during breathing, the size and dimensions of the thoracic cavity will vary, which could in tum affect organs or cavities (thoracic versus abdominal) in patients with a blunt or penetrating injury.

The bony structures of the thorax include the sternum, clavicle, scapula, thoracic vertebrae, and 12 pairs of ribs. The sternum is a dagger-shaped bone located in the chest's midline. It consists of the superior manubrium (handle), central sternal body (blade), and inferior xiphoid process

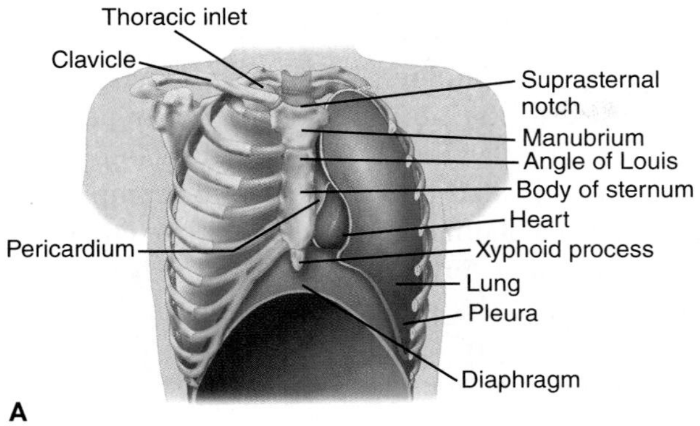

A

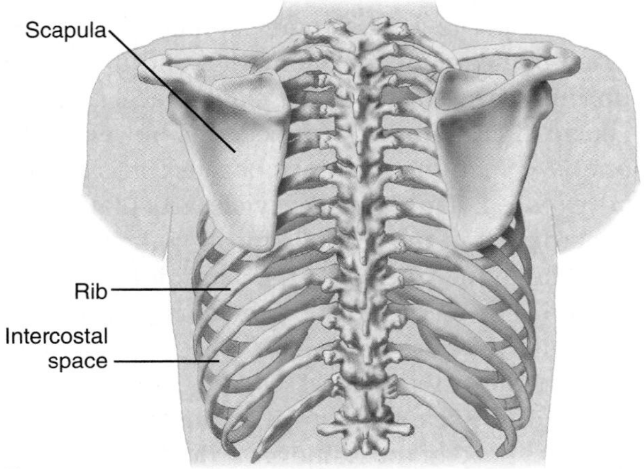

B

FIGURE 8-40 The thorax. **A.** Anterior view. **B.** Posterior view.

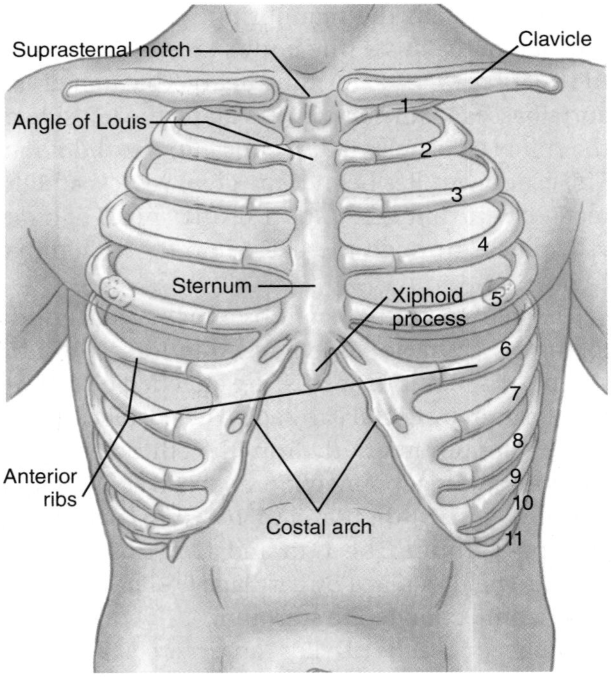

A

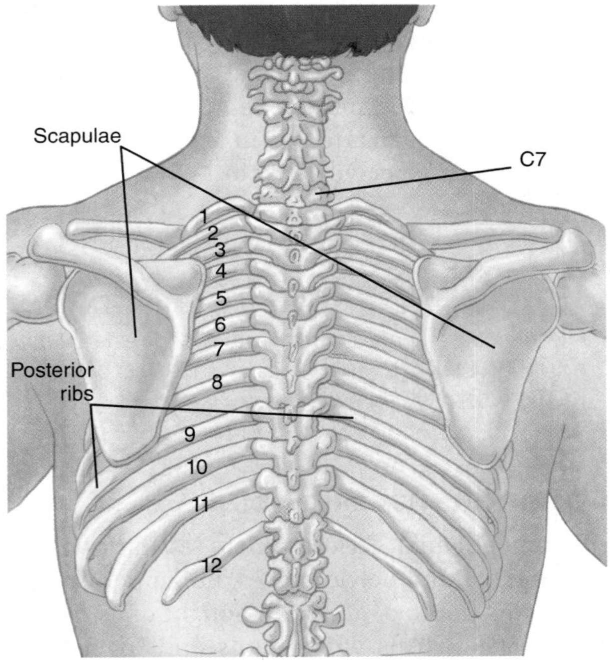

B

FIGURE 8-41 The rib cage. **A.** Anterior view. **B.** Posterior view.

(blunt tip) **FIGURE 8-41**. The space superior to the manubrium is the **suprasternal notch** (also known as the jugular notch), and the junction of the manubrium and sternal body is the **angle of Louis** (also called the sternal angle or manubriosternal junction).

The central region of the thorax is the **mediastinum**, which contains the heart, great vessels, part of the esophagus, lymphatic channels, trachea, primary bronchi, and paired vagus and phrenic nerves. Anteriorly, the lungs extend down to the surface of the diaphragm at the level of the xiphoid process. Posteriorly, the lungs extend farther inferiorly to the surface of the diaphragm at the level of the 12th thoracic vertebra.

The heart lies immediately behind the sternum (retrosternal). It extends from the second to sixth ribs anteriorly and from the fifth to eighth thoracic vertebrae posteriorly. The heart's inferior border extends into the left side of the chest. Diseased hearts may be larger or smaller than normal. The major blood vessels that travel to and from the heart also lie in the chest cavity. On the right side of the spinal column, the superior and inferior venae cavae carry blood to the heart.

Just beneath the manubrium of the sternum, the arch of the **aorta** (the body's largest artery) and the **pulmonary artery** exit the heart. The arch of the aorta passes to the left and lies along the left side of the spinal column as it descends into the abdomen. The esophagus lies behind the great vessels and directly on the anterior aspect of the spinal column as it passes through the chest into the abdominal cavity.

Each of the 12 pairs of ribs attaches posteriorly to the 12 thoracic vertebrae. Anteriorly, the first seven pairs of ribs (true ribs) are attached directly to the sternum by costal cartilage. The costal cartilage then continues inferiorly from the 7th rib and provides an indirect connection between the anterior portions of the 8th, 9th, and 10th ribs (false ribs) and the sternum. The 11th and 12th ribs (floating ribs) are held in place by cartilage and have no anterior connection to the sternum.

Between each rib lies an intercostal space. These spaces are numbered according to the rib superior to the space—for example, the space between the second and third ribs is the second intercostal space. The intercostal spaces house the intercostal muscles and the neurovascular bundle, which consists of an artery, vein, and nerve that run on the bottom aspect of each rib.

Words of Wisdom

The intercostal spaces are important landmarks when you report the anatomic location of injuries and when you perform procedures.

Appendicular Skeleton

The appendicular skeleton includes the bones of the shoulder and pelvic girdles, the upper extremities (arms [more commonly thought of as the upper arms], forearms, wrist, hands, and fingers), and the lower extremities (thighs, legs, ankles, instep, and toes).

Words of Wisdom

The clavicle is one of the most commonly fractured bones in the body, whereas the scapula is extremely difficult to fracture.

Shoulder and Upper Extremity

The scapula (shoulder blade) is a flat, triangular bone held to the rib cage posteriorly by powerful thoracic muscles that buffer it against injury. The scapula is divided into two posterior components by a sharp diagonal ridge (or spine); the end of the scapular spine forms the **acromion process**. The acromion process protects the shoulder joint and provides a site of attachment for the clavicle and various shoulder muscles. Important muscles of the shoulder, including those of the rotator cuff, originate here.

The clavicle is a slender, S-shaped bone attached by ligaments at the medial end to the manubrium of the sternum. The clavicle acts as a strut to keep the shoulder propped up; however, this bone is vulnerable to injury because it is slender and exposed. The lateral clavicle articulates with the acromion of the scapula, forming the acromioclavicular joint. Anterior to the acromion process is a fingerlike projection called the coracoid process, which also provides an area for muscle attachment. Between these two processes is a saucer-shaped portion of the scapula known as the glenoid fossa, where the head of the humerus articulates.

Together, the scapula and clavicle form the pectoral girdle (shoulder girdle), which serves as a point of attachment for the upper extremities to the axial skeleton **FIGURE 8-42**. The upper extremity joins the shoulder girdle at the glenohumeral (shoulder) joint, which is a ball-and-socket joint.

The proximal portion of the humerus, which is the second largest bone in the human body, has a head that articulates with the scapula **FIGURE 8-43**. On this proximal portion of the humerus are two small extensions off either side of the bone (tubercles). These tubercles serve as muscular attachments for the shoulder joint. The distal end of the humerus articulates with the proximal ends of the radius and ulna (forearm bones) to form the hinged elbow joint. Several ligaments connect the humerus, radius, and ulna at the elbow joint, and a fluid-filled bursa cushions and protects the joint posteriorly.

The forearm extends from elbow to wrist. The radius lies on the thumb side of the forearm. The proximal portion of the radius is the radial head. The distal portion contains a small bony protrusion, the styloid process, to which some of the ligaments of the wrist are attached. Distally, the ulna

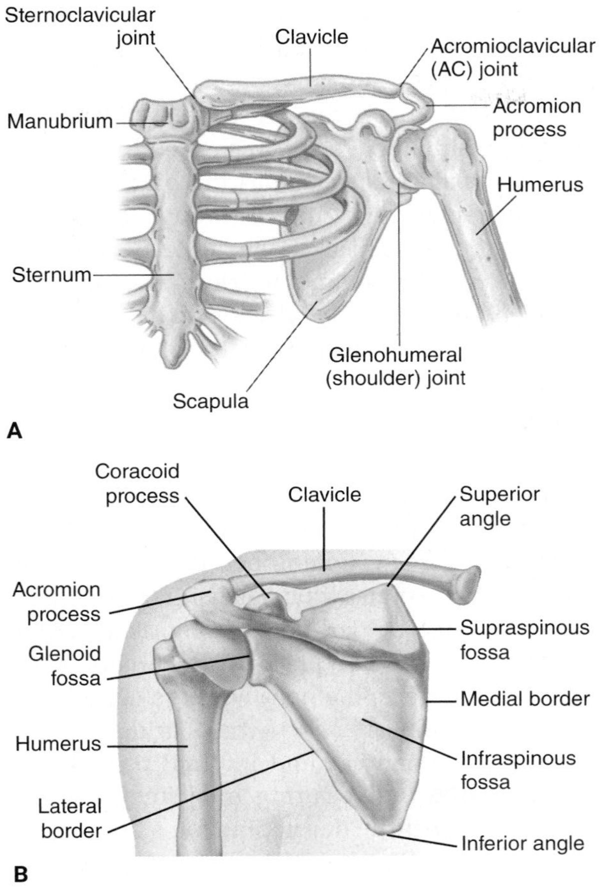

FIGURE 8-42 The pectoral (shoulder) girdle. **A.** Anterior view, including clavicle. **B.** Posterior view, including the scapula.

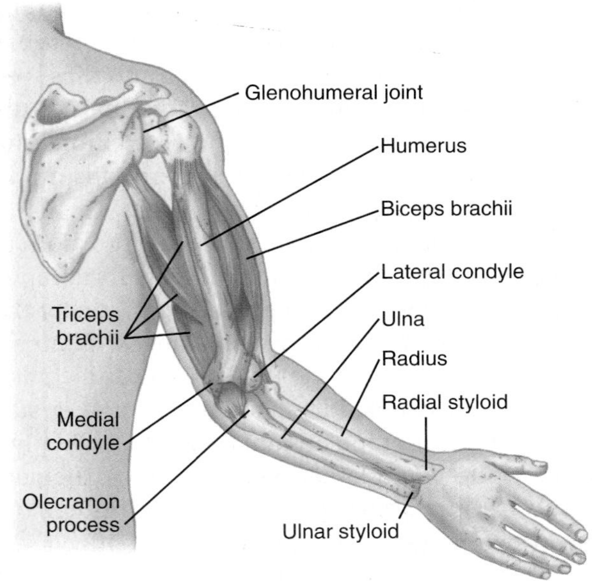

FIGURE 8-43 The upper arm contains the humerus; the forearm contains the radius and ulna.

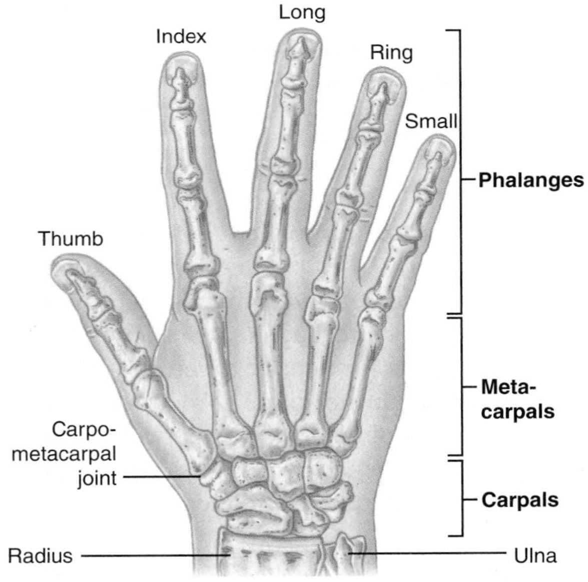

FIGURE 8-44 The principal bones in the wrist and hand include the carpals, metacarpals, and phalanges.

is narrow and is found on the little-finger side of the forearm. It serves as the pivot around which the radius turns at the wrist to rotate the palm upward (supination) or downward (pronation). The proximal end of the ulna has a large, blunt bony process (olecranon process), which forms the tip of the elbow. Lateral to this process, the proximal end of the radius articulates with the humerus. The distal end of the radius articulates with the irregularly shaped **carpal bones** of the wrist. The distal end of the ulna articulates directly to the radius.

The carpal bones of the wrist are arranged in two rows **FIGURE 8-44**: The proximal row contains, from radial to ulnar, the scaphoid (carpal navicular), lunate, and triquetrum bones, and the distal row contains the trapezium, trapezoid, capitate, and hamate bones. The pisiform is a sesamoid bone located just palmar to the triquetrum and although listed with the proximal row is not involved with motion of the proximal row. The carpal tunnel is formed by the space bounded by the trapezium and hamate dorsally and the flexor retinaculum, a sheath of tough connective tissue that forms the roof of the carpal tunnel, on the palmar side. Tendons, nerves, and blood vessels lie within the carpal tunnel. Structures within the carpal tunnel include the long flexor tendon to the fingers and the median nerve, which supplies sensory and motor function to the radial half of the palm. Carpal bones, especially the scaphoid, are vulnerable to fracture when a person falls on an outstretched hand.

Five metacarpals form the bony portion of the hand. The phalanges in the fingers form hinge joints. Each finger has three phalanges, except the thumb, which has only two phalanges. The carpometacarpal joint of the thumb is a **saddle joint**, consisting of two saddle-shaped articulating surfaces that are oriented at right angles to each other so that the complementary surfaces articulate with each other. Movement in these joints can occur in two planes. Arthritis commonly affects the carpometacarpal joint, resulting in stiffness and deformity.

Words of Wisdom

Here is a tip to help remember which bones are carpals (hand bones) and which bones are tarsals (foot bones): "I steer my CAR (pal) with hands and walk through TAR (sal) with my feet."

Innervation of the upper extremities arises from the brachial plexus. **Plexuses** are areas where spinal nerves come together and transmit their impulses to areas of the body through a common nerve. The brachial plexus is formed by a network of nerves that originate from the spinal cord at the C5 to T1 levels. The fibers of these nerves network with one another to form five distinct nerves: axillary, radial, musculocutaneous, ulnar, and median.

Words of Wisdom

Pay attention to the spelling of medical terminology to prevent misunderstandings. Even though *ilium* and *ileum* are pronounced the same way, they refer to two different parts of the body.

- The *ilium* is one of the bony prominences of the pelvis.
- The *ileum* is the lower three-fifths of the small intestine.

The blood supply to the upper extremity originates from the subclavian artery. When the subclavian artery reaches the axilla, it is referred to as the axillary artery. After giving off several branches that supply the shoulder region with blood, the artery leaves the axilla and becomes the brachial artery. After the brachial artery passes through the elbow, it divides into the radial artery and ulnar artery. In the hand, the radial and ulnar arteries form superficial and deep arcades of blood vessels that branch to form the arteries of each finger, the digital arteries.

Pelvis and Lower Extremity

The pelvis is a ring formed anteriorly from the fusion of the ilium, ischium, and pubis bones on either side of the body to form the right and left innominate bones during early adulthood. Posteriorly, these two innominate bones articulate with the sacrum to form the pelvic ring. The pelvis supports the weight of the trunk, serves as a place of attachment for the thighs, and protects the pelvic cavity's organs—the intestines, **urinary bladder** (where urine is stored before its elimination), and internal reproductive organs **FIGURE 8-45**. During pregnancy, the pelvic bones protect the developing fetus and provide a passageway through which the newborn passes during delivery. The two innominate bones articulate anteriorly at the symphysis pubis and posteriorly with the sacrum at the sacroiliac joints. An extensive nerve and vascular supply travels along either side of the pelvis to the lower extremities.

Words of Wisdom

The femoral neck is a common site for hip fractures, especially in the older population.

The lower extremity is made up of the thigh, knee, leg, ankle, foot, and toes **FIGURE 8-46**. The femur is the longest and one of the strongest bones in the body. It articulates proximally in the ball-and-socket joint of the pelvis and distally in the hinge joint of the knee. The femoral head is the ball-shaped part that fits into the **acetabulum**, a cup-shaped structure formed by the coxal bones. The femoral head is connected to the shaft, or long tubular portion of the femur, by the femoral neck and intertrochanteric region. The proximal portion

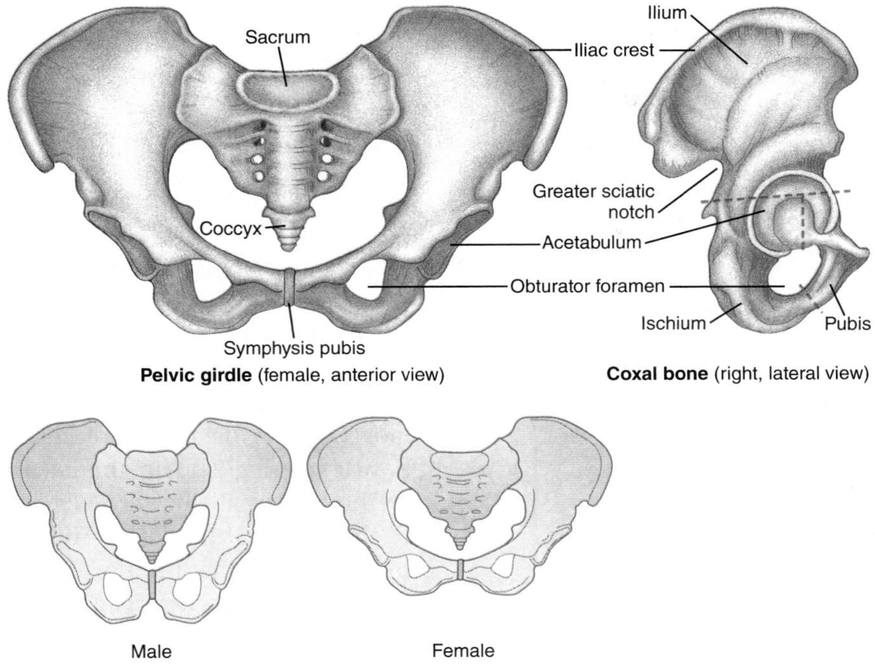

FIGURE 8-45 The pelvic girdle.

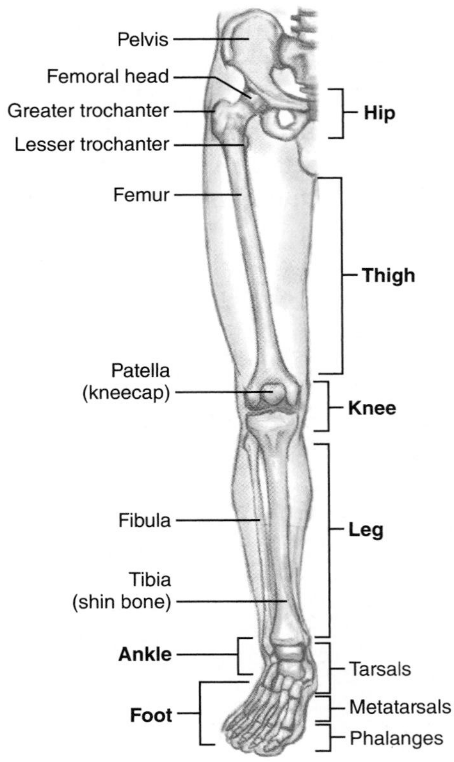

FIGURE 8-46 The principal parts of the lower extremity: the femur, femoral head, greater and lesser trochanters, patella, tibia, and fibula.

of the femur has two separate points of muscular attachment: the greater trochanter and the lesser trochanter **FIGURE 8-47**. The greater trochanter arises lateral to the juncture of the neck and shaft and is clinically considered part of the hip. Several ligaments and muscle tendons provide integrity to the hip joint. The articular capsule is supported by strong ligaments, which support much of the weight of the body.

At the distal end of the femur, the lateral and medial condyles articulate with the proximal tibia at the knee **FIGURE 8-48**. These are important sites of muscle and ligament attachment. The patella lies within the major anterior tendon of the thigh muscles and articulates with the femur. The knee joint is traditionally classified as a hinge joint and is unusual because it contains ligaments within the joint. Thick, crescent-shaped articular disks (menisci) cover the margins of the tibia to cushion the articular surface. The anterior cruciate ligament, which extends between the tibia and the femur, prevents abnormal anterior movement (hyperextension) of the tibia. The posterior cruciate ligament prevents abnormal posterior displacement of the tibia. Several tendons, as well as collateral ligaments, lend further strength to the knee joint. Several fluid-filled bursae surround the knee.

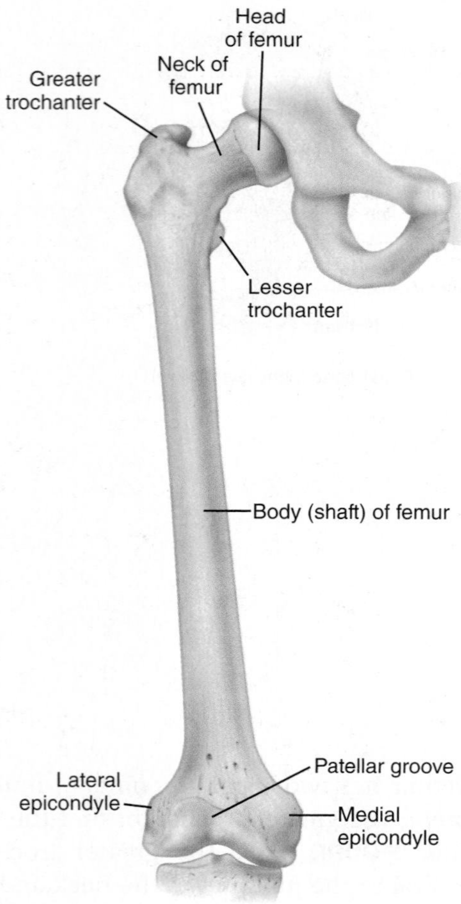

FIGURE 8-47 The femur.

Words of Wisdom

The tibial tuberosity is an important landmark for you to identify before inserting an intraosseous (IO) needle into the tibia.

The two bones of the lower leg are the tibia and fibula. The tibia is the longer and thicker of the two bones and is located on the anteromedial side of the leg. It is vulnerable to direct blows and can be felt just beneath the skin. Proximally, the tibia articulates with the distal femur and is the weight-bearing bone of the leg. The flat medial and lateral condyles of the proximal tibia articulate with the condyles of the femur at the knee. The tibial tuberosity is a projection on the anterior surface of the proximal tibia that serves as an attachment point for the quadriceps muscle. Distally, the tibia forms the medial malleolus, which is the medial side of the ankle joint. The fibula is a long, slender bone that is much smaller than the tibia. It does not bear any weight, and does not articulate directly with the femur, but rather with the tibia at the head. An enlargement of the distal end of the fibula forms the lateral wall of the ankle joint, the lateral malleolus.

The foot (tarsus) is made up of seven bones called tarsals. The largest of these bones is the **calcaneus** (heel bone). The talus articulates with

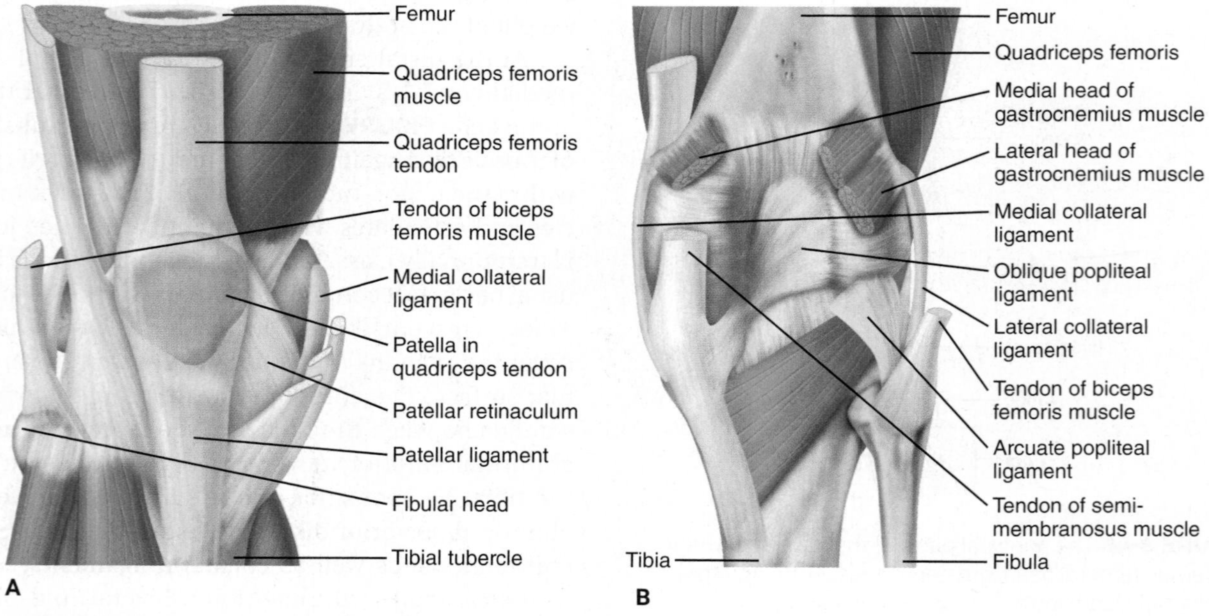

FIGURE 8-48 The knee. **A.** Anterior view. **B.** Posterior view.

the tibia and fibula to form the ankle **FIGURE 8-49**. The ankle bones are arranged so that the talus forms a hinge with the lower portion of the tibia and fibula.

The calcaneus lies inferior and lateral to the talus, providing additional support to it. This bone is vulnerable to injury when a person falls from a height and lands on the feet. A fibrous capsule surrounds the ankle joint; the medial and lateral portions are thickened to form ligaments. Movements of the ankle and posterior foot include dorsiflexion and plantar flexion, as well as limited inversion and eversion.

The metatarsals and phalanges of the foot are arranged much like the bones of the hand. The toes have three phalanges each, except the big toe, which has two phalanges. The ball of the foot is the junction between the metatarsals and the phalanges.

Innervation of the lower extremities is provided by the lumbar and lumbosacral plexuses, which are formed by the spinal nerves that originate from L1 to S4. The networking of nerves within these two plexuses leads to the formation of multiple distinct nerves, including the sciatic nerve—which branches in the popliteal fossa to form the peroneal and tibial nerves—and the femoral nerve.

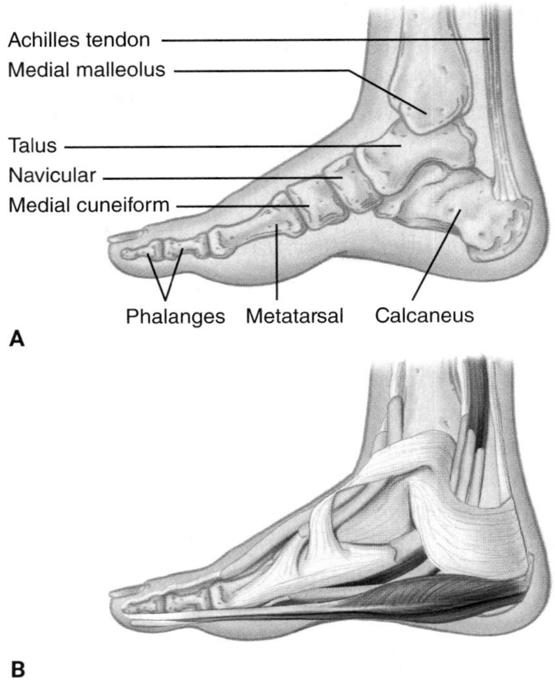

FIGURE 8-49 A. The surface landmarks of the foot: the talus, calcaneus, and phalanges. **B.** Soft tissues of the ankle.

YOU are the Paramedic

PART 2

The motorcycle rider is lying facedown on the pavement next to the front driver's door of the pickup truck. He is unresponsive. You apply manual cervical spine stabilization and, with assistance, log roll the patient onto his back. You immediately note the patient appears pale and sweaty. His upper front teeth have been knocked out and his eyes are swollen shut. You find the patient has a rapid pulse and his breathing is rapid and shallow. He has a large abrasion in the middle of his left chest just below the clavicle. He has deformity and a large laceration on the lower right leg immediately above the inner ankle bone.

Recording Time: 3 Minutes	
Appearance	Found prone on pavement; minimal bleeding from right leg laceration
Level of consciousness	Unresponsive
Airway	Open; fresh blood in mouth
Breathing	24 breaths/min, shallow
Circulation	118 beats/min

3. Given the broken upper teeth and facial swelling, what body structures may have been injured?

4. What is the best way to describe the location of the injury on the left chest?

5. What is the best way to describe the location of the deformity and injury on the right leg?

The blood supply of the lower extremity originates from the external iliac artery. When the external iliac artery reaches the leg, it becomes the femoral artery. When it reaches the knee, the femoral artery turns posteriorly and laterally and is referred to as the popliteal artery. The popliteal artery divides into the anterior and posterior tibial arteries. The anterior tibial artery travels along the anterior and lateral surface of the tibia until it reaches the ankle, where it proceeds along the dorsal surface of the foot toward the great toe and becomes the dorsalis pedis artery. The posterior tibial artery travels along the posterior aspect of the tibia until it reaches the ankle, where it follows a path just behind the medial malleolus until it reaches the plantar aspect of the foot. Within the foot, arcades of arteries supply the various structures with blood and give off branches that form the digital arteries of the toes.

The Musculoskeletal System

The term **musculoskeletal** refers to the bones and voluntary muscles of the body. Muscles are a form of tissue that allows body movement. The musculoskeletal system contains more than 600 muscles. Important functions of the musculoskeletal system are movement and maintenance of posture, joint stability, and production of heat.

> **Words of Wisdom**
>
> Approximately 40% to 50% of normal body weight is skeletal muscle, because it has a high water content. In addition, because skeletal muscle has a high metabolic rate and a high demand for energy and oxygen, it has a very rich blood supply, which causes it to bleed extensively when injured.

Skeletal muscle, so named because it attaches to the skeleton, forms the major muscle mass of the body. As discussed previously, other types of muscle outside of the musculoskeletal system include smooth muscle and cardiac muscle. Skeletal muscle is also called voluntary muscle because all skeletal muscle is under direct voluntary control of the brain and can be stimulated to contract or relax at will. Movements of the body, such as waving or walking, result from skeletal muscle contraction or relaxation. Usually, a specific motion is the result of several muscles contracting and relaxing simultaneously.

Skeletal muscle includes all of the muscles attached to the skeleton and forms the bulk of the tissue of the arms and legs. It is also found along the spine and buttocks. By maintaining a state of partial contraction, this type of muscle allows the body to maintain its posture and to sit or stand. Skeletal muscle varies greatly in size and shape, from thin strands to the large thigh and back muscles. It also constitutes the muscles of the tongue, **soft palate**, scalp, pharynx, upper esophagus, and eye.

Skeletal muscle cells possess the following properties that relate to their functions:

- **Excitability.** The ability to receive and respond to a stimulus
- **Contractility.** The ability to shorten (contract)
- **Extensibility.** The ability to stretch (extend)
- **Elasticity.** The ability to rebound—that is, to resume the original shape and length after contraction

Components of Connective Tissue

A skeletal muscle is considered an organ of the muscular system, whose function is to contract and create a pulling force. Skeletal muscles are made up of hundreds of skeletal muscle cells bundled together to form muscle fibers, which are surrounded by a delicate sheath of connective tissue called the endomysium. The endomysium is where the metabolic exchanges between muscle fibers and capillaries take place.[8] Muscle fibers are arranged in bundles called fascicles, which provide a conduit for blood vessels and nerves. Each fascicle is covered with a layer of connective tissue called the perimysium, which holds the fascicles together. The entire skeletal muscle is sheathed in a tough covering of connective tissue called the epimysium. The epimysium, perimysium, and endomysium are continuous with one another. Recall that muscles are separated by muscular fascia or deep fascia, located outside the epimysium, which merges with the tissue of the tendon. The many layers of connective tissue that enclose and separate skeletal muscles allow for a great deal of independent movement by these muscles.

Muscle Attachments

Skeletal muscles form attachments to other structures either directly or indirectly. For example, a direct attachment is formed when extensions of the epimysium merge with the periosteum of a bone.

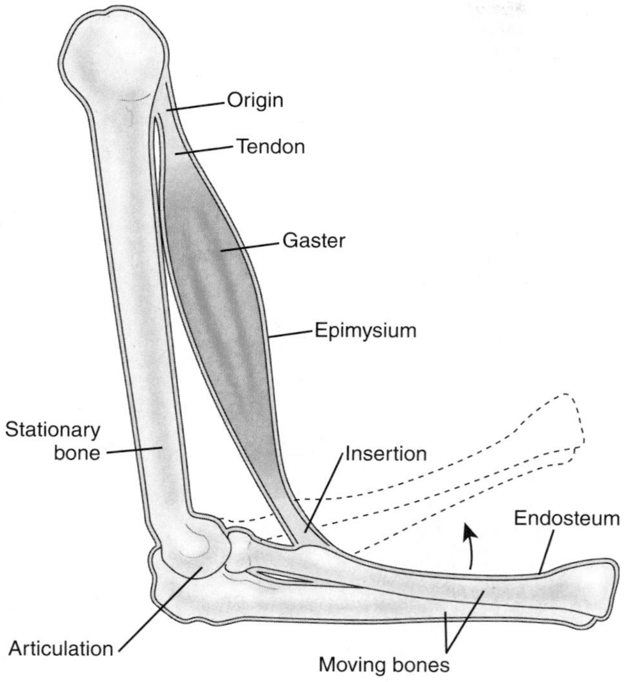

FIGURE 8-50 The parts of a muscle. The actual origin of the muscle shown is in the scapula. The origin on the humerus is shown for clarity.

When extensions of epimysium form tendons, an indirect attachment is made. Tendons cross joints to create a pulling force between two bones when a muscle contracts.

One end of a skeletal muscle—the **origin**—usually is fastened to a relatively immovable part at a movable joint **FIGURE 8-50**. The other end—the **insertion**—connects to a movable part on the other side of the joint. As contraction occurs, the insertion is pulled toward the origin. More than one origin or insertion may be present, such as in the biceps brachii muscle of the arm. When this muscle contracts, the insertion is pulled toward its origin, which causes the forearm to flex at the elbow. The head of a muscle is the part closest to its origin.

Muscle Function

Skeletal muscles usually function in groups, with the nervous system stimulating the desired muscles to perform the intended function. A muscle that contracts to provide most of the desired movement is called a prime mover or agonist. Other muscles, known as synergists, work with a prime mover to make its action more effective. For example, when you bend your elbow, the agonist muscles are the biceps, whereas the brachialis functions as a synergist.

Other muscles act as antagonists to the prime movers, causing movement in the opposite direction. In the preceding example, the triceps would be an antagonist to the biceps. Smooth body movement depends on antagonists relaxing while prime movers contract. Muscles may work together or opposite each other to control various movements. **FIGURE 8-51** and **TABLE 8-16** identify the major muscles, their locations, and their functions.

Muscle Fibers

A skeletal muscle fiber is a single cell that contracts in response to stimulation and relaxes when stimulation ceases. These fibers are thin, elongated cylinders with rounded ends. The cell membrane of a muscle cell is called the sarcolemma, and the cytoplasm of a muscle cell is called the sarcoplasm. Sarcoplasmic reticulum, a special type of smooth endoplasmic reticulum that is found in smooth and striated muscle fibers, stores and releases calcium ions. Each muscle fiber is made up of long, cylindrical, threadlike myofibrils that are arranged parallel to each other. Myofibrils, in turn, are made up of contractile units called sarcomeres. Thus, muscles are considered to be collections of sarcomeres.

Sarcomeres are made up of myofilaments that are formed by threads of contractile proteins. Four types of proteins are found in myofilaments: **actin**, **myosin**, **troponin**, and **tropomyosin**. Myosin molecules consist of two protein strands with globe-shaped cross-bridges that project outward. Groups of many myosin molecules make up a myosin filament.

Actin molecules are globe-shaped and have a binding site that attaches to myosin cross-bridges. Groups of many actin molecules twist in double strands (helixes) to form an actin filament, which includes troponin and tropomyosin. When the muscle is at rest, the binding sites on the actin molecules are covered by tropomyosin molecules held in place by troponin molecules. A noncontractile protein called **titin** (connectin) is found in sarcomeres of cardiac and skeletal muscle. Titin is essential for the alignment of the thick myosin filaments in the sarcomere. *Dystrophin*, another noncontractile protein, holds the thin actin filaments to the sarcolemma and contributes to muscle fiber strength. Dystrophin deficiency has been established as one

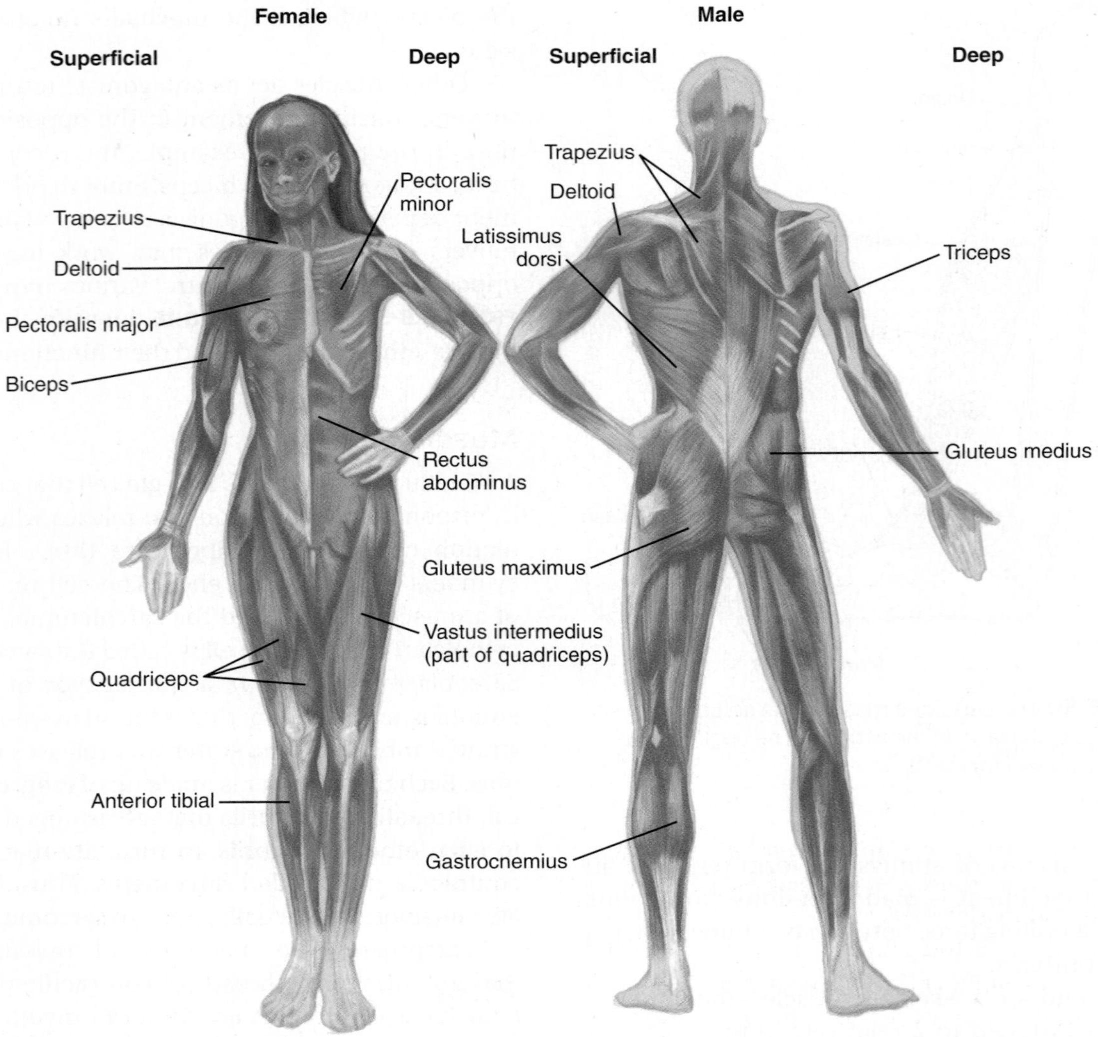

FIGURE 8-51 The major muscle groups.

TABLE 8-16 Location and Function of Major Muscles

Name of Muscle	Origin	Function
Biceps	Anterior, humerus	Flexes elbow
Triceps	Posterior, humerus	Extends elbow
Pectoralis	Anterior, thorax	Flexes and rotates arm
Latissimus dorsi	Posterior, thorax	Extends and rotates arm
Rectus abdominis	Anterior, abdomen	Flexes and rotates spine
Tibialis anterior	Anterior, tibia	Points toes toward head
Gastrocnemius	Posterior, tibia	Points toes away from head
Quadriceps (four separate muscles)	Anterior, femur	Extends knee
Biceps femoris	Posterior, femur	Flexes knee
Gluteus (three separate muscles)	Posterior, pelvis	Extends and rotates leg

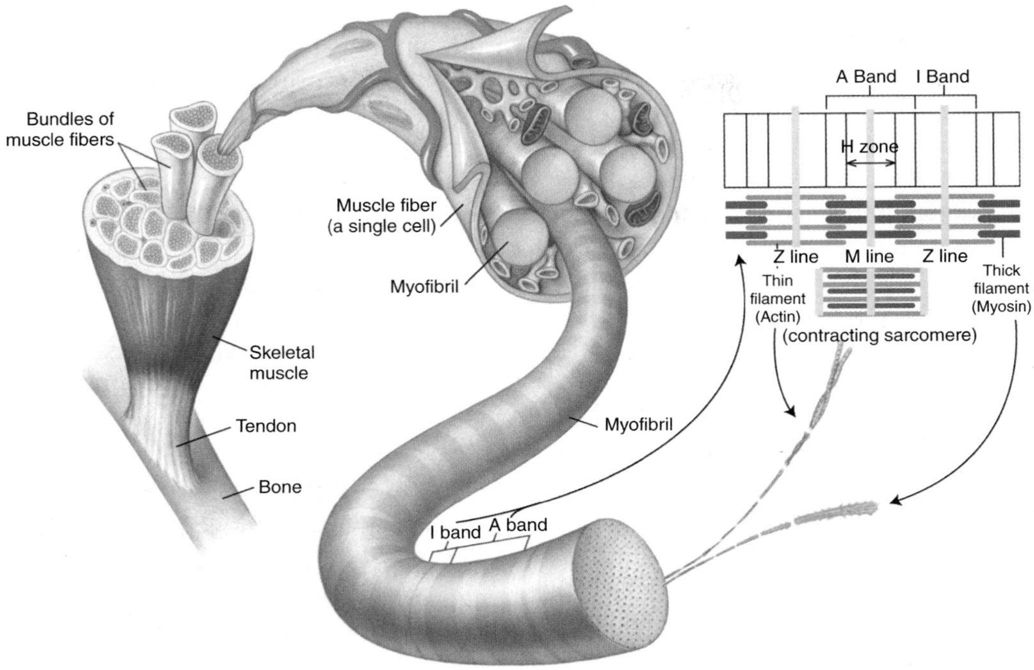

FIGURE 8-52 Details of the contractile machinery of a muscle cell.

cause of muscular dystrophy, a group of genetically transmitted conditions that cause progressive weakness and loss of muscle mass.

The overlap of thick and thin filaments creates striations in skeletal and cardiac muscle, which are the source of the name striated muscle. The striation pattern of skeletal muscle fibers contains two main parts. The light bands (I bands) consist of thin filaments of actin attached to Z lines. The dark bands (A bands) consist of thick filaments of myosin that overlap thin filaments of actin. A central region (H zone) is composed of thick filaments, with a thickened area (M line) made up of proteins holding them in place. Sarcomeres extend from one Z line to another Z line, as shown in **FIGURE 8-52**.

Inside the sarcoplasm of a muscle fiber, a network of channels surrounds each myofibril. These membranous channels form the sarcoplasmic reticulum. Other membranous channels, called transverse tubules (T-tubules), extend inward and pass through the fiber. These tubules open to the outside of the muscle fiber and contain ECF. Each tubule lies between enlarged structures called cisternae, near the point where the actin and myosin filaments overlap. Together, the sarcoplasmic reticulum and T-tubules activate muscle contraction when stimulated.

To understand how muscles move, you must understand how they are stimulated, which is discussed in detail later in this chapter.

Muscle Contraction

A **motor nerve** is made up of many nerve cells called **motor neurons**. A motor unit is a group of muscle fibers innervated by one motor neuron. When stimulated, the motor unit contracts as a whole. A steady contraction occurs throughout the muscle because motor neuron axons are present throughout the fleshy part of the muscle (muscle belly). The impulse that stimulates muscle contraction enters the muscle fibers at the **neuromuscular junction**. There, the muscle fibers of the motor unit create the motor

Words of Wisdom

Myasthenia gravis is an autoimmune disorder in which the immune system attacks the ACh receptors on the motor end plate, resulting in muscular weakness or failure. A myasthenic crisis is a life-threatening presentation of this disorder, in which weakness of respiratory muscles can lead to respiratory failure or arrest.

end plate, which contains receptors for the neurotransmitter **acetylcholine (ACh)**. ACh stimulates skeletal muscle to contract.

The impulse that causes contraction of skeletal muscle is transmitted through motor neurons as a nerve impulse. These impulses, known as **action potentials**, are transmitted from one cell to another in the nervous system, causing each successive cell in the chain to fire. **Depolarization** is the process by which cells activate in response to action potentials.

When the cell is at rest, ions are actively transported into and out of the cell to create an electrochemical gradient across the cell membrane, resulting in a **polarized** state. When the release of a neurotransmitter activates the cell, proteins in the cell wall open rapidly, allowing a rapid influx of ions that equalizes charges on either side of the cell wall. When charges are equal, the cell has depolarized, and the protein channels close. Then begins the process of **repolarization**, which again creates the electrochemical gradient so the cell can fire again.

Words of Wisdom

Muscle contraction requires energy. This energy is derived from glucose metabolism and results in lactic acid production (lactate). Lactic acid, in turn, is converted into carbon dioxide and water, through a process that requires oxygen. For that reason, vigorous muscular activity is often followed by an increased ventilatory rate, which increases both delivery of oxygen to, and removal of carbon dioxide from, tissues.

ACh is synthesized in the cytoplasm of motor neurons and released into the synaptic clefts between motor neuron axons and motor end plates. It diffuses rapidly, binding to specific protein receptors in the muscle fiber membrane, and increasing permeability to sodium. These charged particles stimulate a muscle impulse that passes in many directions over the muscle fiber membrane. Eventually, this impulse reaches the sarcoplasmic reticulum.

The sarcoplasmic reticulum has a high calcium ion concentration, and it responds to the impulse by making cisternae membranes more permeable, diffusing calcium into the sarcoplasm. Calcium binds to troponin in the thin filaments, causing tropomyosin molecules to shift, thereby exposing the binding sites on the actin molecules. Because actin and myosin are chemically attracted to each other, the heads of the myosin molecules bind to the exposed actin molecules, creating cross-bridges. The actin and myosin filaments pull themselves toward each other, thereby shortening their length and causing contraction. Because the actin "slides" over the myosin during this process, this is known as the **sliding filament theory** of muscle contraction **FIGURE 8-53**. The cycle repeats as long as there is enough ATP for energy and muscular stimulation occurs.

Muscle Tone

Skeletal muscles cause unique movements based on which type of joint they attach to and where the attachment points are located. Muscle tone is the amount of tension present in a muscle at any given point in time. It is the result of a constant state of partial contractions in the body. While some motor units contract, others relax. Muscle tone in skeletal muscles helps maintain balance and body position. In the maintenance of posture, muscle tone allows the head to stay upright and the back to remain straight.

Words of Wisdom

In smooth muscle, tone maintains the size of blood vessels and aids in digestion.

Muscle Relaxation

Muscle relaxation is caused by the decomposition of ACh via the enzyme **acetylcholinesterase**. This process prevents a single nerve impulse from stimulating the muscle fiber continuously. When the stimulus ceases, calcium ions are transported back to the sarcoplasmic reticulum. Without calcium, the actin and myosin linkages break, and the muscle relaxes.

Energy Sources

Muscular contraction requires ATP and continues as long as ACh is released. Muscle fibers have just enough ATP for short-term contraction. ATP must

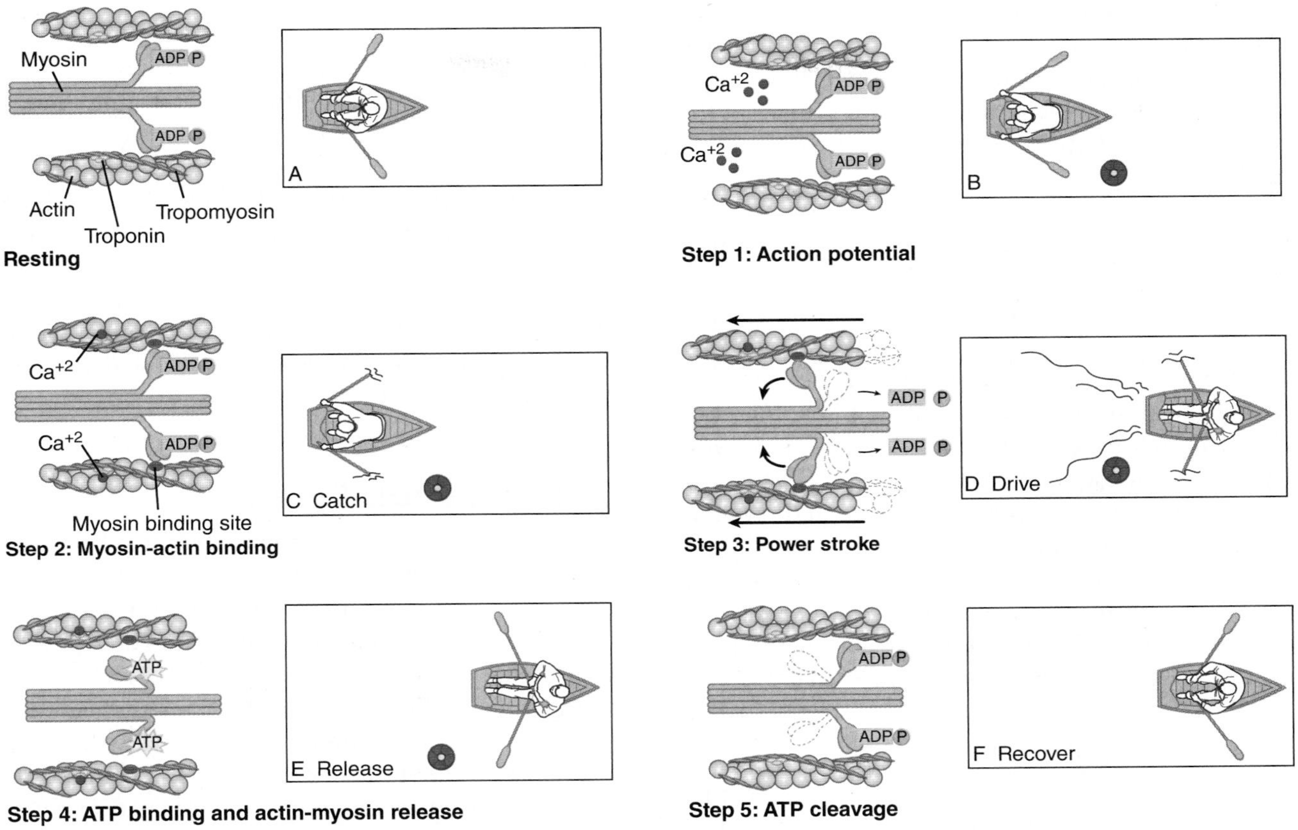

FIGURE 8-53 The sliding filament theory describes how muscle fibers contract.

Abbreviations: ADP, adenosine diphosphate; ATP, adenosine triphosphate

be regenerated when fibers are active, using existing ATP molecules in the cells. ATP is regenerated from adenosine diphosphate (ADP) and phosphate. Creatine phosphate is an organic compound in muscle tissue that can store and provide energy for muscle contraction in the form of high-energy phosphate bonds. Creatine phosphate is between four and six times more abundant in muscle fibers than ATP is; however, it does not directly supply energy. Instead, it stores excess energy from the mitochondria in its phosphate bonds.

> **Words of Wisdom**
>
> Skeletal muscles are profoundly affected by the amount of training and work to which they are subjected. Unused muscles tend to atrophy (shrink or waste away), whereas physical training promotes hypertrophy (increase in size).

When ATP breaks down, energy from creatine phosphate is transferred to ADP molecules to convert them back into ATP. Creatine phosphate stores are exhausted rapidly when muscles are active; therefore, the muscles use cellular respiration of glucose as energy to synthesize ATP.

Oxygen Use and Debt

Oxygen is required for the breakdown of glucose in mitochondria. RBCs carry oxygen, bound to hemoglobin molecules. **Hemoglobin** is the pigment that makes blood appear red. One hemoglobin molecule reversibly binds with four oxygen molecules. The pigment **myoglobin** is synthesized in the muscles and gives skeletal muscles their red-brown color. Myoglobin can also combine with oxygen and temporarily store it to reduce muscular requirements for continuous blood supply during contraction.

When skeletal muscles are used for 1 minute or longer, anaerobic respiration is required for energy.

In one type of anaerobic respiration, glucose is broken down via glycolysis to yield pyruvic acid, which reacts by producing lactic acid. Recall that lactic acid can accumulate in muscles, but diffuses in the bloodstream, where it is synthesized into glucose in the liver.

When a person exercises strenuously, oxygen is mainly used to synthesize ATP. As the amount of lactic acid in the body increases, an oxygen debt develops. Oxygen debt is equivalent to the amount of oxygen that liver cells require to convert lactic acid into glucose, as well as the amount needed by muscle cells to restore ATP and creatine phosphate levels. It may take several hours for the body to convert lactic acid back into glucose.

Muscles may experience a change in their metabolic activity as a person's exercise levels change. For example, increased exercise raises the muscles' capacity to perform glycolysis. Aerobic exercise increases the muscles' capacity for aerobic respiration. This process is summarized in **TABLE 8-17**.

Muscle Fatigue

Prolonged exercise may cause a muscle to become unable to contract. This condition, called fatigue, may also occur because of interruption of muscular blood supply, or occasionally a lack of ACh in motor neuron axons. The accumulation of lactic acid is the usual cause of muscular fatigue. As lactic acid lowers pH levels, muscle fibers cannot respond to stimulation. When a muscle becomes fatigued and cramps, it experiences a sustained, involuntary contraction. Though not fully understood, muscle cramps appear to be caused by changes in the ECF surrounding muscle fibers and motor neurons.

Heat Production

Muscles need a great deal of energy to contract. This energy is delivered in the form of ATP. The energy required for muscular contraction is released by the breakdown of ATP (breaking of bonds). One of the by-products of this breakdown is heat, which is used to maintain a normal body temperature. If the body temperature drops below a set point, then the nervous system stimulates the muscles to start shivering (a form of rapid contractions). Shivering, in turn, generates heat used to elevate body temperature.

The Nervous System

The **nervous system** is perhaps the most complex organ system within the human body. It is composed of two major structures—the brain and spinal cord—and thousands of nerves that allow every part of the body to communicate. This system is responsible for fundamental functions such as controlling breathing, pulse rate, and BP. However, the true complexity of the nervous system becomes evident when we consider higher-level functions such as reading a book, enjoying music, having a discussion with a friend, and watching television. All of these activities require the brain to engage memory, thought, intelligence, and understanding.

The main functions of the nervous system include the following:

- Monitoring of internal and external environments
- Integration of sensory information
- Coordination of voluntary and involuntary responses

TABLE 8-17 Changes in Muscular Metabolism

Type of Exercise	Pathway Needed	Production of ATP	Result
Low to moderate intensity: blood flow provides enough oxygen for the needs of the cell	Glycolysis, which leads to formation of pyruvic acid and aerobic respiration	For skeletal muscle, 36 molecules of ATP per 1 glucose molecule	Exhalation of carbon dioxide
High intensity: oxygen supply is not enough for the needs of the cell	Glycolysis, which leads to formation of lactic acid	2 molecules of ATP per 1 molecule of glucose	Buildup of lactic acid

Abbreviation: ATP, adenosine triphosphate

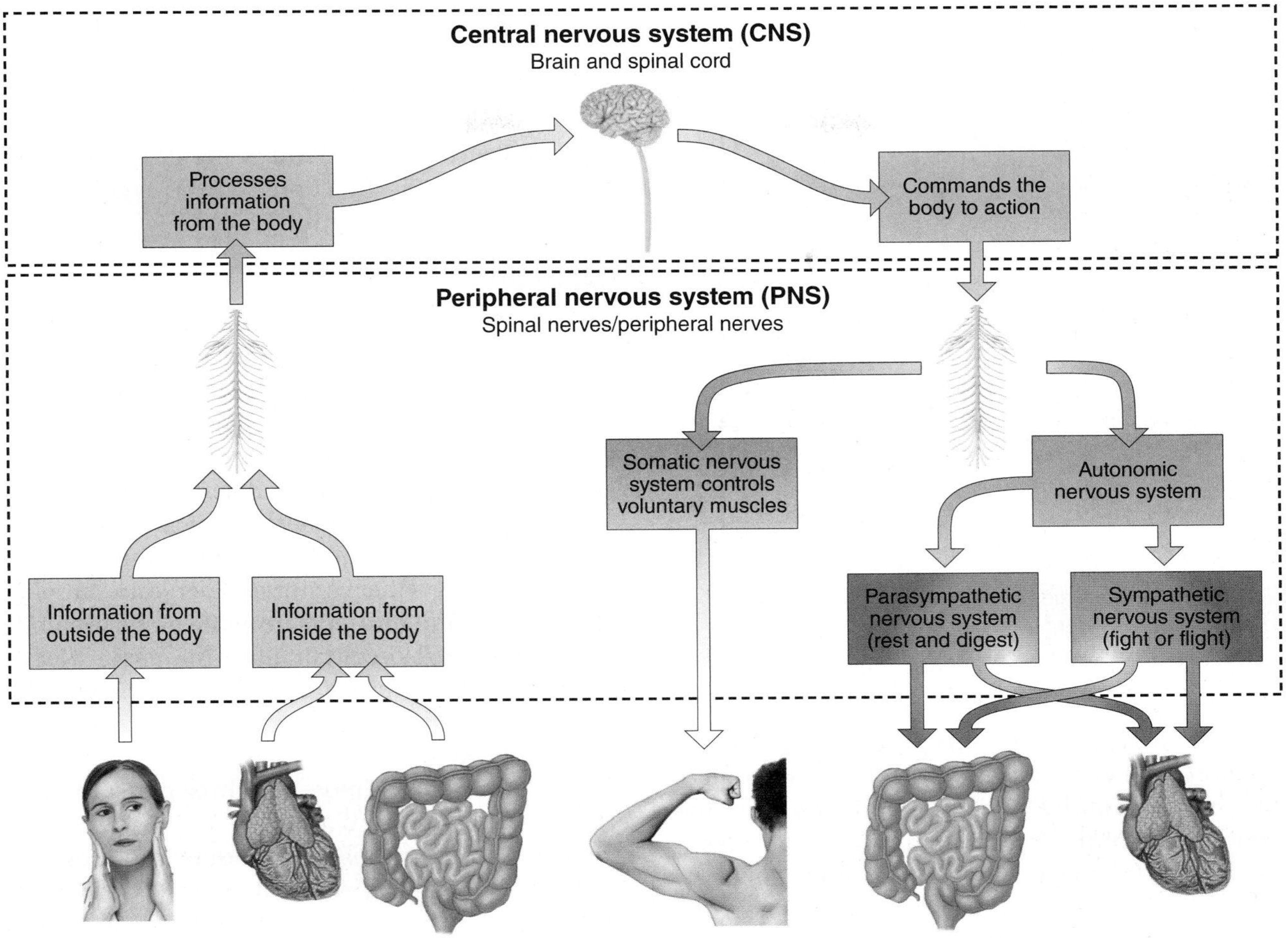

FIGURE 8-54 Organization of the nervous system. The brain and spinal cord work together to process information in the form of signals generated in response to stimuli from inside and outside the body. The peripheral nervous system commands the body to act, and the autonomic nervous system oversees involuntary responses.

The primary structures of the nervous system are divided into two main categories: the **central nervous system (CNS)** and the **peripheral nervous system (PNS)**. The CNS is responsible for thought, perception, feeling, and autonomic body functions. The PNS consists of the somatic nervous system and autonomic nervous system. The **somatic nervous system** regulates activities over which the person has voluntary control, such as walking, talking, and writing. The **autonomic nervous system (ANS)** controls the many body functions that occur without voluntary control—for example, digestion, dilation and constriction of blood vessels, sweating, the fight-or-flight response, and all other involuntary actions necessary for essential body functions. Thus, the nervous system as a whole can be divided anatomically into the CNS and PNS and functionally into somatic (voluntary) and autonomic (involuntary) components **FIGURE 8-54**.

Neurons and Impulse Transmission

The nervous system is composed of specialized tissue that conducts electrical impulses between the brain and the rest of the body. Recall that neural tissue contains two basic types of cells: neuroglia and neurons.

Neuroglia

Neuroglia are supporting cells that form about one-half the mass of the brain.[9] They perform the

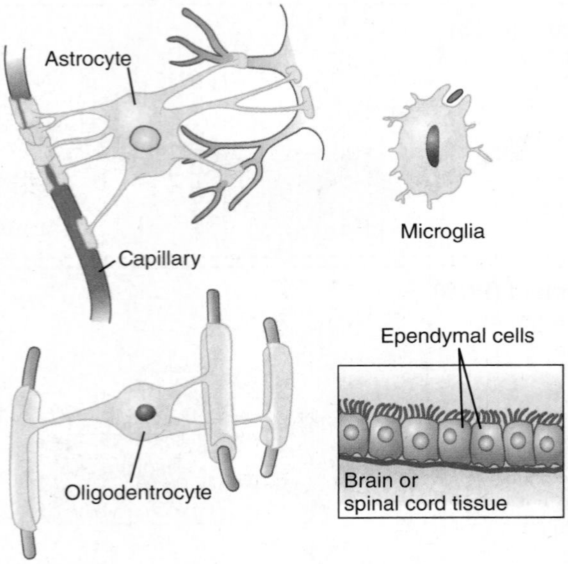

FIGURE 8-55 Examples of the neuroglia found in the central nervous system.

following basic functions: (1) provide a supporting skeleton for neural tissue, (2) isolate and protect the cell membranes of neurons, (3) regulate the composition of interstitial fluid, (4) defend neural tissue from pathogens, and (5) aid in the repair of injury. Neuroglia can divide, whereas most neurons cannot. Types of neuroglia include the following **FIGURE 8-55**:

- **Astrocytes.** Found in the CNS, these cells are the most numerous type of neuroglia. They attach to neurons and blood capillaries of the brain and provide nourishment to neurons by picking up glucose from the blood, converting it to lactic acid, and passing it to the neurons to which they are connected.[10] Astrocytes form tight sheaths around the brain capillaries and participate in recycling some neurotransmitter substances after their release.
- **Ependymal cells.** Found in the CNS, these cells line fluid-filled cavities, such as the ventricular system of the brain. Some ependymal cells secrete CSF; others have cilia that serve to circulate fluid within the cavities they line.
- **Microglial cells.** Found throughout the CNS, these cells phagocytize bacterial cells and cellular debris.
- **Oligodendrocytes.** Found in the CNS, these cells help hold nerve fibers together and form insulating myelin sheaths around axons within the brain and spinal cord.
- **Schwann cells.** Found in the PNS, these cells manufacture myelin.
- **Satellite cells.** Found in the PNS, these cells have similar functions to the astrocytes in the CNS.[9]

Neurons

To understand how muscles move, you must first understand how they are stimulated. Neurons, which are nerve cells, are the fundamental elements of the nervous system and are present throughout the body. Groups of nerve cells are bundled together to form nerve fibers. Groups of nerve fibers are bundled together to form a nerve, which connects the nervous system with body parts or organs.

The neurons that comprise a nerve are supplied with oxygen and nutrients from the bloodstream by blood vessels also contained in the nerve. Nerves are, in essence, information highways. Impulses travel to and from the brain and spinal cord along these highways.

Neurons are composed of three parts: the dendrites, cell body, and axon. **Dendrites** are short, branchlike projections that conduct impulses from nearby cells toward the cell body. Essential cell functions, such as energy production and waste removal, are performed within the nucleus of the cell body. After being conducted through the cell body, the impulse exits the neuron through the axon. An **axon** is another projection that sends the signal from the cell body to target tissues or other neurons **FIGURE 8-56**. Neurons may have dozens of dendrites but usually have only one axon. An axon is long and highly branched, allowing it to link with many other cells.

The axon may or may not be wrapped in myelin, a mixture of proteins and lipids manufactured by oligodendrocytes in the CNS and by Schwann cells in the PNS. Myelin is white, an appearance that leads to the term **white matter**. Myelinated axons form the white matter in the brain, the **brainstem** (which connects the brain and spinal cord), and the spinal cord. Myelin allows the cell to transmit its signal consistently, without "shorting out" or losing electricity to surrounding fluids and tissues. It also increases the speed of conduction. Gaps between the myelinated regions are called nodes of Ranvier **FIGURE 8-57**. These nodes speed impulse

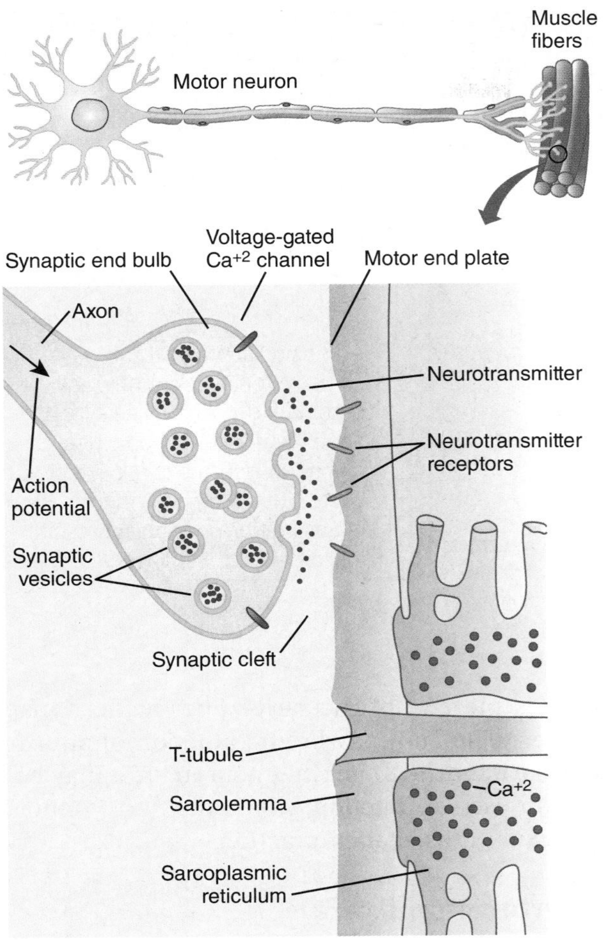

FIGURE 8-56 A synapse or neuroeffector junction.

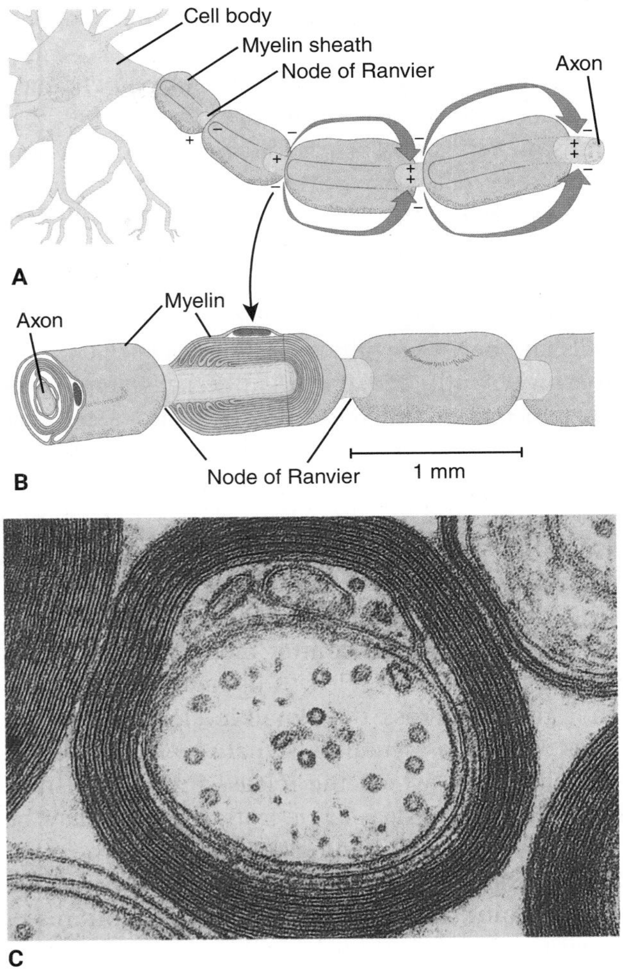

FIGURE 8-57 A myelinated nerve. **A.** The myelin sheath allows impulses to jump from node to node, greatly accelerating the rate of transmission. **B.** The node of Ranvier. **C.** A transmission electron micrograph shows a cross section of an axon with a myelin sheath.

transmission through the axon because impulses cannot travel through insulating myelin, but rather jump from node to node as they travel along the axon (saltatory conduction). Axons without myelin sheaths are termed gray matter. Because these axons lack the myelin sheath, impulses travel more slowly through them than they do in white matter. The axon terminal is the portion of the axon where neurotransmitters are manufactured.

Nerve cells are classified by the direction in which they transmit impulses. Afferent (sensory) nerves carry impulses from sensory receptors in the internal organs and skin to the brain and spinal cord. Efferent (motor) nerves carry impulses from the CNS to organs, muscles, and glands. Interneurons carry impulses from sensory neurons to motor neurons.

Synapses and Synaptic Transmission

Dendrites and axons of adjacent nerve cells are not in physical contact with each other, but rather are separated by a small gap called a **synapse**. This slight gap between each cell allows for a far greater level of fine control than if each cell were in direct contact with the next. A synapse is made up of three main parts. The first part is the presynaptic plasma membrane (or terminal), which is the membrane on the signal-passing side of the synapse. The second part is the **synaptic cleft** (synaptic gap), which is a small, fluid-filled space (see Figure 8-56). The third part is the postsynaptic plasma membrane, which is the membrane on the signal-receiving side of the synapse.

Two types of synapses are distinguished: chemical and electrical. Most neurons use **neurotransmitters** to transmit their signal across the synapse to other neurons. Because a synapse may exist between a neuron and a muscle or between a neuron and a gland, neurotransmitters also may be used to transmit a nerve signal across the synapse to muscle or gland cells. Electrical synapses occur between cardiac muscle cells and between some smooth muscle cells where the presynaptic and postsynaptic cell membranes are joined by channels called gap junctions. Because gap junctions can pass electric current, nerve impulses can spread rapidly to neighboring cells.

At the end of the axon of the presynaptic (signal-passing) neuron are tiny bulges called synaptic knobs or synaptic terminals. Within each synaptic knob are many small sacs called **synaptic vesicles** containing neurotransmitter molecules. When the presynaptic neuron releases its neurotransmitters, they diffuse across the synaptic cleft to receptor sites on the postsynaptic (signal-receiving) plasma membrane, to which the released neurotransmitters bind. The released neurotransmitter may be either excitatory (initiating an impulse on the postsynaptic side) or inhibitory (stopping the impulse at that point). As a paramedic, you may administer a variety of medications to enhance, slow, or even stop these neurotransmissions.

The following process details how the transmission of nervous impulses occurs. When the cell is at its resting potential, greater concentrations of extracellular sodium and intracellular potassium are available. The cell also contains the negatively charged chloride ion, whose presence results in a relative negative charge inside the cell compared with the outside. As with muscle cells, depolarization of nerve cells results from the opening of the sodium channels and influx of sodium into the cell. This influx creates a positive charge, causing an action potential inside the cell. A wave of depolarization sweeps along the nerve fiber as each cell depolarizes when stimulated by the previous neuron. Repolarization occurs as potassium leaves the cell in an attempt to restore the negative charge inside the cell. Repolarization is complete when the sodium-potassium pump restores sodium and potassium to their original balance within the cell. As the depolarization wave continues, it eventually reaches the end of the nerve fiber at the synaptic cleft. The end may be the junction of an axon and the dendrite of another neuron, or it may be a neuromuscular junction, where the nerve impulse stimulates muscular contraction.

TABLE 8-18 Examples of Neurotransmitters

Category	Examples
Amino acids	Gamma aminobutyric acid (GABA), glutamate, glycine
Biogenic amines	Dopamine, epinephrine, histamine, norepinephrine, serotonin
Choline esters	Acetylcholine (ACh)
Neuropeptides	Adrenocorticotropin, cholecystokinin, dynorphins, endorphins, enkephalins, glucose-dependent insulinotropic peptide, glucagon, neurotensin, oxytocin, secretin, substance P, thyrotropin-releasing hormone, vasopressin, vasoactive intestinal peptide

Neurotransmitters

Many neurotransmitters are present within the brain and throughout the body. These substances are grouped into the following categories: amino acids, biogenic amines, choline esters, and neuropeptides **TABLE 8-18**.

Neurotransmitters of the somatic nervous system include ACh; neurotransmitters of the ANS include ACh and **norepinephrine**; and neurotransmitters of the CNS include dopamine, serotonin, and gamma aminobutyric acid, among others. After the neurotransmitter is released from the presynaptic (signal-passing) terminal, it binds with receptor sites on the postsynaptic (signal-receiving) membrane, triggering an impulse that is propagated in the manner previously described. The neurotransmitters are quickly deactivated by substances such as acetylcholinesterase (which breaks down ACh) and monoamine oxidase (which breaks down monoamines such as norepinephrine). After being broken down, these substances are reabsorbed by vesicles in the presynaptic terminal, where neurotransmitters are re-created.

Central Nervous System

As discussed previously, the CNS consists of the brain and spinal cord. This part of the nervous system is responsible for integration and coordination of sensory information and motor responses.

Protection

Because CNS structures can be easily damaged with potentially devastating results, the body has four protective mechanisms in place to protect it: bone, meninges, CSF, and the blood–brain barrier. The brain has an additional protective layer called the scalp.

Scalp

The scalp consists of the following layers, given in descending order:

- Skin, with hair.
- Subcutaneous tissue, which contains major scalp veins that bleed profusely when lacerated.
- Galea aponeurotica, a tendon expansion that connects the frontal and occipital muscles of the cranium.
- Loose connective tissue (alveolar tissue) that is easily stripped from the layer beneath in so-called scalping injuries. The looseness of the alveolar layer also provides room for blood to build up between the scalp and skull bone after blunt trauma.
- Periosteum, the dense fibrous membrane covering the surface of bones.

Bone

Bone provides physical protection for the CNS. The brain is protected from mechanical injury by the cranium, and the vertebral column protects the spinal cord.

Meninges

The **meninges** form a covering over the brain and spinal cord. The meninges are composed of three distinct connective tissue layers: the **dura mater**, arachnoid, and **pia mater** **FIGURE 8-58**. In common usage, the term *mater* is often dropped, so the three layers are referred to simply as dura, arachnoid, and pia.

The dura is the outermost, thickest, and toughest of the three layers (*dura mater* means "tough mother" in Latin). It has two layers: a parietal (outer) layer and a visceral (inner; from the Greek *viscera*, meaning "guts") layer. The parietal layer tightly adheres to the cranial vault and serves as periosteum for the skull's inner surface, whereas the visceral layer lies over the CNS. In some areas of the CNS, the parietal and visceral layers of the dura are fused.

The dura has two projections. The falx cerebri is a vertical projection that separates the two hemispheres of the brain. The tentorium cerebelli, or **tentorium**, is a horizontal projection of the dura that separates the cerebellum from the cerebrum. The temporal lobes are positioned on an opening in the tentorium (tentorial notch, or tentorial incisura). This opening allows passage of the midbrain and oculomotor nerves. These structures play an important role in increased intracranial pressure (ICP) and brain herniation.

Above the dura is a potential space referred to as the epidural space. The meningeal arteries run in the periosteal layer of the dura. If one of these vessels becomes injured, such as with an injury to the skull, bleeding can occur between the dura and skull, opening up the potential epidural space and causing an epidural hematoma.

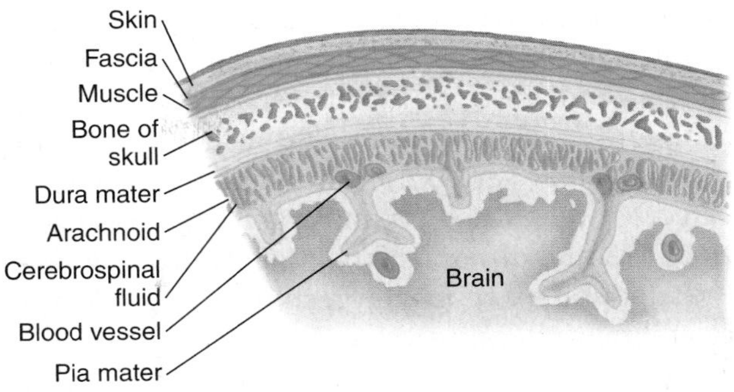

FIGURE 8-58 The meninges.

> **Words of Wisdom**
>
> A tip to help you remember the names of the meningeal layers is to think of them as a PAD from the inside out, as follows:
>
> **P** Pia mater (innermost layer)
> **A** Arachnoid (middle layer)
> **D** Dura mater (outermost layer)

The arachnoid, the second meningeal layer, is semitransparent, thin, delicate, and weblike (the Greek word *arachne* means "spider's web"). The dura and arachnoid layers end at the level of the second sacral vertebra.[11] The subdural space, located between the dura and arachnoid, contains a small amount of serous fluid. Collection of blood in the subdural space, usually resulting from tearing of a cerebral vein, causes a subdural hematoma.

The innermost meningeal layer, the pia mater ("tender mother" in Latin), is delicate and tightly adheres to the CNS. The pia that adheres to the brain contains a network of small blood vessels; the pia that surrounds the spinal cord is less vascular. The **subarachnoid space**, located between the arachnoid and pia, contains a vast network of cerebral arteries and veins running through it that are held against the pia by sheets and strands of connective tissue before penetrating the brain.[12]

Cerebrospinal Fluid

The brain contains four hollow, fluid-filled cavities called ventricles. Each cerebral hemisphere contains a lateral ventricle, which communicates with the third ventricle located in the diencephalon, which in turn communicates with the fourth ventricle of the pons and medulla oblongata in the brainstem.

Each ventricle houses a specialized spongelike structure called the **choroid plexus**. CSF is secreted within the brain by the choroid plexuses. The choroid plexus is the so-called kidney of the brain because it stabilizes the composition of CSF, just as the kidney stabilizes the composition of blood plasma.[13]

Words of Wisdom

Whereas the protective qualities of the blood–brain barrier are generally beneficial, they can present a problem when the delivery of therapeutic medications is needed to treat conditions such as Alzheimer disease, multiple sclerosis, and CNS infections and cancers. Medications are sometimes administered directly into the subarachnoid space (intrathecal injection) to enhance the delivery of the drug into the brain, bypassing the blood–brain barrier. The development of techniques to open the blood–brain barrier and therapeutic agents with improved barrier penetrability are areas of ongoing research.

The cerebral ventricles are linked by small openings that allow CSF to flow easily among them. CSF circulates through the ventricles and then leaves the fourth ventricle through three openings to flow through the subarachnoid spaces of the brain and spinal cord, where it eventually enters the venous blood system. The meninges float in CSF.

The total volume of CSF in adults is about 155 mL; 30 mL is found within the cerebral ventricles and about 125 mL in the subarachnoid space.[14] CSF is constantly produced and reabsorbed, with the total amount of CSF being replaced every 6 to 8 hours.[15] CSF must be produced and reabsorbed at the same rate to maintain a relatively constant pressure within the skull. Excess CSF is eliminated through the venous sinuses located in the folds of the dura in the cranium.

Words of Wisdom

Because the brain, CSF, and blood are enclosed within the bony cranium and the relatively inelastic dura, an increase in the size (volume) of the brain or any increase in the amount of CSF or blood can lead to a marked increase in pressure within the system (that is, ICP) unless there is a corresponding decrease in the volume of one of the other components. Increased ICP can disrupt brain **perfusion** (circulation of blood within an organ or tissue) and function. The many possible causes of increased ICP include bleeding into the brain, fluid around the brain, swelling within the brain secondary to injury, increased pressure within the brain because of a mass (eg, tumor), increased CSF production, and an obstruction to the flow or absorption of CSF.

Because the brain and spinal cord essentially float in CSF, one of this fluid's main functions is to absorb outside forces that might otherwise be transmitted to the CNS, causing damage there. The CSF also plays a role in delivering nutrients, eliminating waste products, and maintaining a constant ionic environment.

Blood–Brain Barrier

The brain needs a stable chemical environment for its optimal functioning. The endothelial cells that line capillaries in many parts of the body have openings between them that enable passage of substances by diffusion. In contrast, the endothelial cells in the walls of the capillaries leading to the brain form tight junctions. Extensions of astrocytes (one type of neuroglia) wrap around these capillaries to provide additional protection. This combination of tight junctions and astrocyte extensions forms the (**blood–brain barrier**) between the blood within the brain capillaries and the ECF in brain tissue. Substances can pass through the barrier only by diffusion or active transport, rather than between cells. Water-soluble substances such as water, glucose, and essential amino acids pass easily. Likewise, most lipid-soluble molecules (eg, alcohol) and gases (eg, oxygen, carbon dioxide, and volatile anesthetics) can diffuse easily across the barrier. In contrast, substances that may be damaging to CNS function, such as bacteria, viruses, and many pharmaceuticals, are normally not permitted to cross the blood–brain barrier. However, this barrier may be compromised by diseases such as encephalitis, multiple sclerosis, stroke, or tumors.

Brain

The **brain** is the primary organ of the nervous system. At birth, the typical brain contains about 100 billion nerve cells, and this number declines with age. Each neuron may have thousands or tens of thousands of synapses. The brain occupies 80% of the cranial vault and is the control center for nearly all body functions. The remaining intracranial contents include cerebral blood (12%) and CSF (8%).

The brain accounts for only 2% of total body weight, yet it is the most metabolically active and perfusion-sensitive organ in the body. The brain must receive a constant supply of oxygen and nutrients, such as glucose, to function properly. It receives about 15% of the *cardiac output* (CO), defined as the amount of blood pumped by the ventricles in 1 minute. It also metabolizes 25% of the body's glucose (approximately 60 mg/min) and consumes 20% of the total body oxygen (45 to 50 L/min). Because the brain has no effective means of storing oxygen or glucose, it is sensitive to decreases in glucose, oxygen, and blood flow through it. As a result, the brain continually manipulates the physiology as needed to guarantee that a ready supply of oxygen and glucose is available. If the blood supply to the brain is disrupted, the patient may experience changes in mental status and vital signs.

The brain consists of four primary areas: the cerebrum, diencephalon, brainstem, and cerebellum

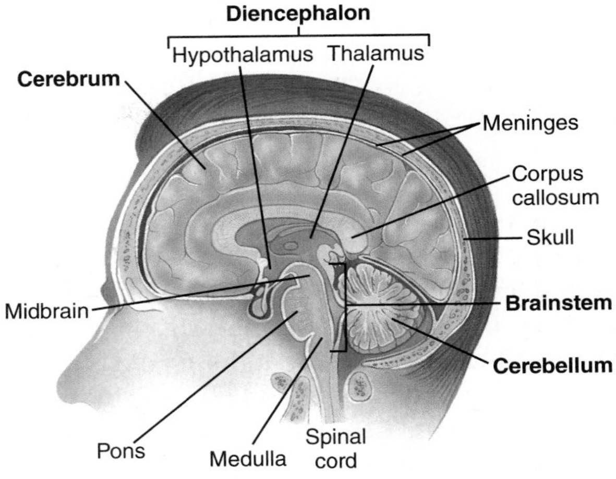

FIGURE 8-59 The major structures and landmarks of the brain.

FIGURE 8-59. The brain and much of the spinal cord receive their arterial blood supply through the internal carotid arteries and vertebral arteries. The vertebral arteries form the basilar artery. Branches of the internal carotid arteries and basilar artery form a circle of arteries at the base of the brain called the circle of Willis. The internal carotid arteries provide about 80% of the blood supply to the brain, supplying most of the cerebrum and much of the diencephalon. The vertebral system provides the remaining 20%, supplying the brainstem and cerebellum, as well as parts of the diencephalon, spinal cord, and occipital and temporal lobes.

Venous drainage of the brain occurs through a series of superficial and deep veins that contain no valves. These vessels empty into venous sinuses located in the folds of the dura and into a network of veins around the base of the brain. These veins empty, in turn, into the internal jugular veins at the base of the skull and ultimately join the general circulation.

Cerebral Blood Flow

Blood flow through the brain (cerebral blood flow) depends on cerebral perfusion pressure. **Cerebral perfusion pressure (CPP)** is the pressure of the blood filling the arteries of the brain. CPP is calculated as the difference between the mean arterial pressure (MAP) and ICP:

$$CPP = MAP - ICP$$

Pulse pressure is the difference between the systolic BP and the diastolic BP. MAP is an indicator of how well the brain is being supplied with nutrients, such as oxygen and glucose. It can be closely approximated by adding the diastolic blood pressure (DBP) plus one-third of the pulse pressure (PP):

$$MAP = DBP + 1/3\ PP$$

The normal ICP is between 5 mm Hg and 15 mm Hg, and the normal MAP is between 85 mm Hg and 95 mm Hg. This results in a normal CPP in the range of 70 mm Hg to 90 mm Hg. The brain receives sufficient blood flow at these pressures, with adequate levels of oxygen and glucose, to meet its metabolic needs. Cerebral blood flow (CBF) and therefore CPP are affected by the diameter of the vessels in the brain.

Autoregulation is the mechanism by which the brain regulates the diameter of the vessels within the brain (and therefore CBF) in response to a wide range of MAP measurements. Adequate CBF occurs when the CPP is between 60 mm Hg and 160 mm Hg. CPP of less than 60 mm Hg results in inadequate brain perfusion, whereas pressures greater than 160 mm Hg result in hypertensive encephalopathy. Increased ICP disrupts autoregulation by decreasing CPP based on the mathematical formula given earlier. As CPP decreases, blood vessels within the brain dilate, increasing the blood volume in the brain. As a result, ICP increases. This further decreases CPP, which leads to further cerebral vasodilation, and so on.

The body's responses to combat increasing ICP have been described as the Monro-Kellie doctrine. Recall that the cranial vault is a rigid, nondistensible box that is filled by the brain, CSF, and cerebral blood. In response to an expanding intracranial mass, the body attempts to regulate ICP by expelling CSF and venous blood out of the cranial vault, creating more space for the mass. Keeping ICP within normal limits during the early stages of an expanding mass can result in subtle signs and symptoms that may be easily missed unless the paramedic maintains a high index of suspicion. As with all compensatory mechanisms, there is a limit to the effectiveness of the brain's efforts to mitigate increased ICP. At the point where no additional CSF or venous blood can be expelled, ICP will increase exponentially.

After ICP begins to rise, the body attempts to maintain CPP by increasing MAP. This process is evidenced by not only an increased BP (both systolic and diastolic), but also a widening pulse pressure.

Other factors can also interfere with CPP. For example, too much carbon dioxide in the blood causes cerebral vasodilation, resulting in increased cerebral blood volume, which leads to increased ICP, and so on. Hypotension results in a decreased MAP, which causes a decrease in CPP. As stated previously, when the MAP drops to 60 mm Hg or less, CBF begins to decrease. This decrease leads to cerebral vasodilation, and the cycle repeats itself.

When swelling or bleeding occurs in the brain, the brain sends out signals requesting more oxygen. This process triggers a vicious cycle: The more blood that enters the brain, the more oxygen it requires, resulting in increased swelling. If ICP gets too high, then brain tissue has nowhere to go except through the tentorium incisura, foramen magnum, or both.

Cerebrum

The **cerebrum** is the largest part of the brain, making up about three-fourths of the volume of the brain. The surface of the cerebrum is composed of a thin layer of folded gray matter known as the **cerebral cortex**. White matter lies just beneath the gray matter and makes up the bulk of the cerebrum. Additional areas of gray matter called **basal ganglia** or basal nuclei are scattered throughout the white matter with connections to other areas of the CNS, including the cerebral cortex, cerebellum, and thalamus. The basal ganglia are involved in control of the body's motor tone, automatic movements (eg, swallowing saliva, blinking), and specific body movement sequences associated with skeletal muscle activity (eg, arms swinging alternating with legs during walking). The basal ganglia may also play a role in thinking and learning.

The cerebral cortex folds onto itself, forming ridges called gyri that maximize surface area. Gyri are separated by grooves that are called sulci, if they are shallow, or fissures, if they are deep. Although the cerebrum is partially divided into right and left hemispheres by the longitudinal fissure, a large band of white matter called the **corpus callosum** provides a communication pathway between them.

Each cerebral hemisphere can be subdivided into five lobes: insula, frontal, temporal, parietal, and occipital. Four of the lobes have the same name as the skull bone that lies over the lobe (ie, frontal, parietal, occipital, and temporal) **FIGURE 8-60**.

The insula, also called the central lobe or island of Reil, is covered by parts of the frontal, parietal, and temporal lobes in the lateral fissure. **TABLE 8-19** summarizes the primary functions of each lobe.

The frontal lobe extends from the anterior cerebrum to roughly halfway to the rear of the brain. This area regulates many important functions, including speech, abstract thinking, and personality. The temporal lobe lies behind and inferior to the frontal lobe. Here, impulses from the ears are received and then processed into sounds. One portion of the temporal lobe, the Wernicke area, is the center of the brain that is responsible for understanding speech. The parietal lobe lies directly above the temporal lobe. This area also manages functions related to speech. In addition, the sense of body positioning (proprioception) is regulated within the parietal lobe. When you raise your arm above your head, you know its location because of activity in the parietal lobe. The most posterior portion of the cerebrum is the occipital lobe. The primary function of this lobe is to process optic nerve information and form the sense of sight (discussed later in this chapter).

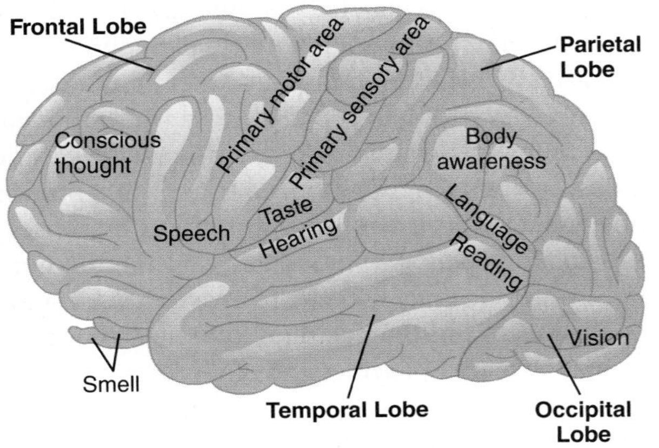

FIGURE 8-60 The cerebral cortex. Four of the lobes of the brain and the primary functions of those lobes are shown. The fifth lobe, the insula, is hidden.

The three distinct areas of the cerebral cortex are the motor area, sensory area, and association area. The motor area of the cerebral cortex is located in the frontal lobes (except for the anterior portion) and can be divided into two portions. Just in front of the division of the frontal lobe and parietal lobe is a small strip known as the primary motor center (motor strip). This area provides impulses for

TABLE 8-19 Functions of the Cerebral Lobes

Cerebral Lobe	Function
Frontal	Higher cognitive functions (eg, ability to form concepts, plan, problem-solve, reason, judge); voluntary motor function; expressive language (verbal and written); long-term memory storage; sexual behavior; and emotions (eg, aggression, motivation, impulse control, and mood)
Insula	Processes information from receptors in the skin and internal organs, including perception of temperature, itch, pain, taste, hunger, thirst, and sense of body position in space; assists in motor function, regulation of homeostasis, and social emotions (eg, lust and disgust, pride and humiliation, gratitude and resentment, self-confidence and embarrassment, trust and distrust, truthfulness and deception, guilt and atonement)
Occipital	Processes and perceives visual information; responsible for color vision, spatial perception, recognition of movement, and linking images from the eyes with experiences, images, and knowledge stored in memory
Parietal	Processes information from sensory receptors in the skin and joints, including perception of pain, temperature, and vibration; processes and integrates information related to sight, sound, and taste; determines shapes, sizes, and distances; determines right from left; responsible for the ability to perform mathematical calculations and recognize and manipulate numbers as well as the ability to process language and understand speech
Temporal	Processes higher-order visual information (eg, facial recognition); speech comprehension; memory formation and retrieval; processes, perceives, and integrates memories and sensations of taste, smell, sound, sight, and touch

precise muscular control of voluntary muscles. Impulses from the motor strip are conducted down the spinal cord to the muscles of the body. Specific portions of the motor strip are responsible for certain areas of the body. Just anterior to the motor strip is the premotor area. The premotor area is responsible for muscular coordination. As an example of how the motor and premotor areas work together, imagine the decision to turn the page of a book. After you make the decision, the premotor area determines which muscles must be used and transmits that information to the motor strip. The motor strip then transmits impulses by way of the spinal cord to specific muscles of your arm and hand, allowing you to turn the page.

The Broca region, located in the inferior left frontal lobe just anterior to the motor cortex, is responsible for muscular actions associated with speech. Patients who have damage to this area may have expressive aphasia. Patients with this condition can understand what they hear and know what they want to say, but have difficulty producing language. They may speak slowly with long pauses between words, use incorrect or imprecise words, or say something that does not resemble a sentence.

Words of Wisdom

Damage to the Wernicke area can result in receptive aphasia. Patients with this condition can usually speak normally, but have difficulty understanding written and spoken words. As a result, they often use nonsense words when speaking and may not recognize that the words they are saying are not appropriate to the situation.

The primary sensory area is a strip that lies just posterior to the motor strip. However, sensory areas are also distributed across the cerebral cortex. These areas receive sensory stimuli from the body and interpret what they mean or which actions are needed to respond to the stimuli. For example, the primary sensory area receives sensations from the skin. Other sensory areas contained in the visual cortex of the occipital lobe interpret visual stimuli.

The Wernicke area is located at the junction of the temporal and parietal lobes. The sensory area for speech recognition, it allows comprehension and understanding of speech. The Broca region and Wernicke area are physically connected and work together to allow verbal communication.

The association areas of the cerebral cortex are located in the anterior frontal lobe as well as in the lateral portions of the temporal, occipital, and parietal lobes. These areas are responsible for analyzing and interpreting sensory information the brain receives and allowing effective interaction with the environment. The association areas of the frontal lobes deal with judgment, concentration, abstract thought, and problem solving. Areas within the parietal lobes are used in understanding speech and choosing words to express emotions. The temporal lobe association areas interpret complex sensory information such as when reading, visual memory, and understanding speech. The visual association area is located in the occipital lobe near the visual cortex. This area provides the ability to analyze visual patterns and combine visual information with other sensory information.

Words of Wisdom

One of the major roles of the diencephalon is to filter out unnecessary information before it reaches the cerebral cortex. For example, the diencephalon keeps you from having to think about shifting your weight on a chair when it becomes uncomfortable. Instead, signals of pressure or pain sent through peripheral nerves initially stop in the diencephalon, which dispatches the command for you to switch positions slightly without being conscious of doing so.

Diencephalon

The **diencephalon** is located above the brainstem and between the cerebral hemispheres **FIGURE 8-61**. It is composed of several structures: the epithalamus, thalamus, hypothalamus, and subthalamus.

The epithalamus is the uppermost portion of the diencephalon. It contains the **pineal gland**, which synthesizes melatonin, a hormone associated with the body's sleep-wake cycle. The **thalamus** is the sensory switchboard, receiving and relaying sensory information (except the sense of smell) to the sensory cortex for processing. The thalamus is located deep inside the brain and makes up 80% of the diencephalon.[9] The **hypothalamus** is located inferior to the thalamus and plays a key role in

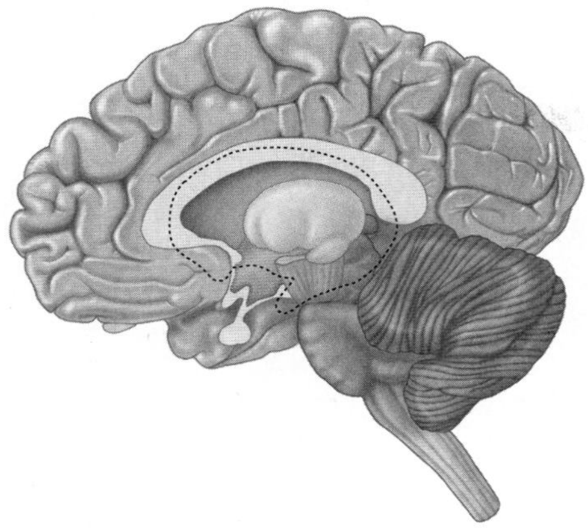

FIGURE 8-61 The diencephalon.

the emotions and sexuality of the body through the limbic system. The hypothalamus also contains the temperature regulatory centers of the body, controls the pituitary gland, and is the site of integration for the nervous and endocrine systems **TABLE 8-20**. The subthalamus controls motor functions. A lesion in the subthalamus is characterized by involuntary but violent flinging movements of limbs on one side of the body.

TABLE 8-20 Functions of the Hypothalamus

Function/ Regulation	Description
Autonomic	Regulates involuntary body functions, including activity of cardiac muscle, smooth muscles, and glands
Eating and drinking	Promotes and inhibits eating through hunger and satiety centers; promotes drinking through thirst
Emotional	Regulates psychosomatic illness, stress-related conditions, fear, and rage; exerts emotional influence over body functions
Endocrine	Regulates pituitary gland secretions and affects metabolism and sexual development and functions
Muscular	Stimulates shivering in some muscles; controls muscles responsible for swallowing
Sleep	Regulates responses to the sleep-wake cycle in coordination with other areas of the brain
Temperature	Regulates temperature through sweat to promote heat loss and through shivering to promote heat generation

Body Temperature. By tradition, temperature is one of the most common factors measured when assessing the body. Heat is a by-product of many cellular and chemical processes, so it follows that presence of body heat is one of the most basic signs of life. Many cells and enzymes require that the body temperature be strictly regulated to allow certain processes to function. As discussed previously, this process of maintaining homeostasis of temperature is known as thermoregulation.

The body's average temperature is maintained through a balance of gains and losses. Skeletal muscle generates heat with each contraction. The process of digesting food, with its innumerable decomposition reactions, also generates heat. (The **calorie** is a measure of the heat that may be produced from a given amount of food, rather than the food's nutritional value. The technical term for this unit of heat is a **kilocalorie**.) These processes are controlled partly by the secretion of thyroxine, which has many functions, including regulating body temperature. These processes can also be influenced by activation of the sympathetic nervous system.

The body also has means for releasing heat. The simplest of these mechanisms can be seen when a person exercises in warm atmospheres: The pulse quickens, circulating more blood to the periphery, where it can give off heat through the skin; the skin itself begins to perspire, which amplifies heat loss through evaporation; and respirations accelerate, which exchanges warmed air for cooler air with each breath. Inhibition of digestion and other mechanisms of heat generation also contribute to net heat loss.

The commonly accepted average body temperature is 98.6°F (37°C). However, the reality is that a "normal" body temperature can fall within a wide range, from 97°F to 99°F (36.1°C to 37.2°C).

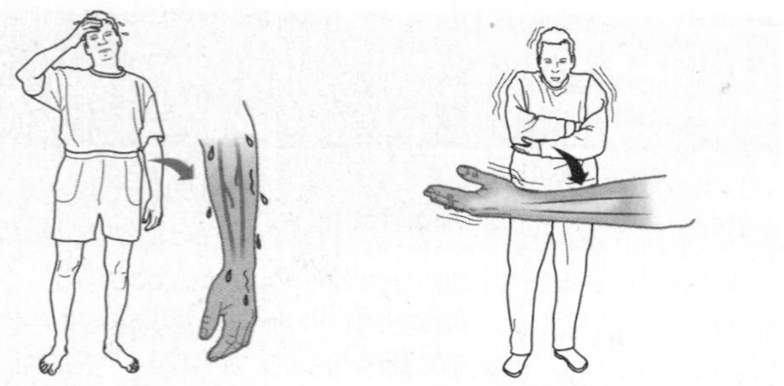
Hot Environment
• Hypothalamus stimulated
• Blood vessels dilate, maximizing heat loss from skin
• Body sweats, causing evaporation and cooling
Body temperature *decreases*
Cold Environment
• Hypothalamus stimulated
• Blood vessels constrict, minimizing heat loss from skin
• Muscles shiver, generating heat
Body temperature *increases*

FIGURE 8-62 The hypothalamus notes a rise or fall in core body temperature and elicits responses to regulate it.

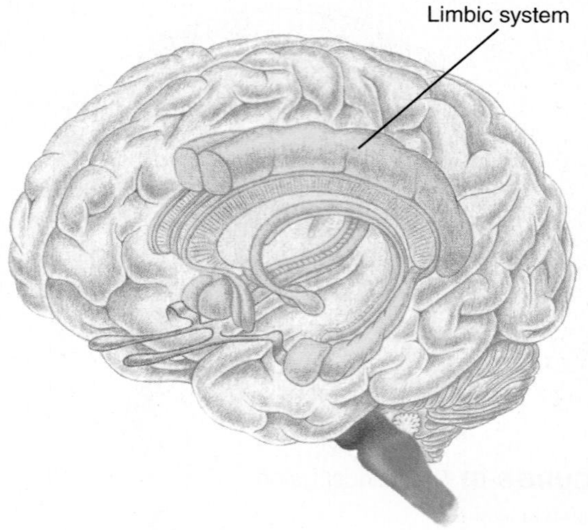
Limbic system

FIGURE 8-63 The limbic system.

A person's body temperature is usually lower in the morning and increases during the day. Moreover, body temperature can vary slightly from person to person as well as based on other conditions without causing any adverse effect on the body; therefore, these variances are not necessarily considered abnormal or pathologic. Body temperature regulation begins in the hypothalamus, which acts similar to a thermostat in activating the mechanisms for increasing or decreasing body temperature **FIGURE 8-62**.

In many disease processes, the hypothalamus is influenced to raise the body temperature. A fever is present when the target body temperature is more than 1°F (0.6°C) above the patient's "normal" temperature. Although the usefulness of fever is a matter of debate, it is known that a fever increases metabolism and activity of phagocytes, which may aid in the destruction and removal of infectious organisms. In most patients, a fever of only a few degrees above normal is generally not harmful, other than creating the characteristic body aches and fatigue that make it so uncomfortable. This fact, combined with the theory that fever may actually be beneficial in the healing process, makes treatment of mild fevers controversial. However, moderate fevers that persist for significant periods can cause or exacerbate other symptoms and effects of illness, such as dehydration. High fevers can cause febrile seizures in children and, if they persist, have the potential to cause long-term CNS damage in both children and adults. For this reason, moderate to high fevers are usually treated with antipyretics such as acetaminophen or ibuprofen, and dangerously high fevers are sometimes treated with active cooling measures.

Limbic System. The limbic system is the so-called emotional brain, or the feeling and reacting brain. It comprises several structures beneath the cerebral cortex with connections to other parts of the brain, including the thalamus, hypothalamus, and frontal and temporal lobes of the cerebrum **FIGURE 8-63**.

The limbic system is involved in the generation, integration, and control of emotions, and connects these emotions with behavioral responses (eg, anger, rage, fear, surprise, sadness, anxiety, tension).[16] In addition, this system is important in motivation, learning, and transition of information from short- to long-term memory. The limbic system is also closely linked to functions necessary for self-preservation, particularly in response to emotional stimuli.

Brainstem

Recall that the brainstem connects the brain to the spinal cord. Its name reflects that the brain appears to be sitting on this portion of the CNS much as a plant sits on its stem. The brainstem lies deep within the cranium and is the best-protected part of the CNS. It is responsible for many of the essential functions the body requires to survive (vegetative functions).

Street Smarts

Paramedics will learn, sometimes the hard way, that not every patient screaming obscenities at them is actually mad, especially a patient who may have sustained a blow to the frontal portion of the skull.

The limbic system constantly generates emotional impulses (raw emotions), which are filtered by anterior portions of the frontal lobe (conscience or judgment). Inhibition of the frontal lobe can stop this filtering process and allow these raw emotions to be displayed. These emotional outbursts may present in many ways, including verbal or physical aggression, choice of language, or behavior the individual would not normally display.

In cases of head injury, protect the patient and yourself and try to understand where those raw emotions could be coming from.

The brainstem is permeated by a group of specialized neurons that are collectively called the **reticular activating system (RAS)** or reticular formation. More of a network than a structure, the RAS is a mixture of gray and white matter and extends from the spinal cord into the diencephalon. Sensory axons from many different sources, particularly the cranial nerves, send impulses into the RAS. The **cranial nerves** are 12 pairs of peripheral nerves that are associated with the brain and innervate structures primarily in the head.

The RAS filters and then sends impulses that excite the cerebrum and keep the body awake. Consciousness is maintained by the interaction of the RAS and the cerebral cortex. Disruption of this interaction, or loss of the connection between the RAS and the cerebral cortex, results in an altered level of consciousness.

The divisions of the brainstem are the midbrain, pons, and medulla (see Figure 8-59). The **midbrain** (mesencephalon) is the most superior portion of the brainstem. It contains reflex centers for pupillary reflexes and eye movements. The midbrain is also involved in coordinating motor activity and muscular tone, and serves as a relay for impulses from the cerebral cortex to the pons and spinal cord.

The **pons** is the middle portion of the brainstem and serves as a relay of both afferent (ascending) nerve fibers and efferent (descending) nerve fibers. The pons plays a role in the body's arousal and sleep cycles and contains respiratory centers that, along with the medulla, control movements associated with breathing.

The **medulla oblongata** is the inferior part of the brainstem. It is continuous with the spinal cord at the foramen magnum. The medulla contains three vital centers that are crucial for survival: the cardiac center, vasomotor center, and respiratory center. The cardiac center is responsible for altering the heart rate (HR; the number of cardiac contractions per minute—in other words, the pulse rate) and the strength of cardiac contractions to meet the body's demands. The vasomotor (vessel muscle) center regulates the diameter of blood vessels, thereby regulating BP. The respiratory center works with the pons to regulate the rhythm of breathing. The medulla also contains centers responsible for coughing, sneezing, vomiting, swallowing, and hiccupping.

The ascending and descending nerve fibers that connect the brain and spinal cord pass through the medulla. About three-fourths of the descending (motor) fibers leave the cerebral cortex, descend through the pons, cross sides in the medulla (ie, right fibers move to the left side, and vice versa), and extend down the spinal cord. As a result, the motor area of the left cerebral hemisphere controls motor movement on the right side of the body, and vice versa. Approximately one-fourth of the descending motor fibers leave the cerebral cortex and descend through the pons, but do not cross over or decussate in the medulla, continuing down the same side of the spinal cord from which they came and connecting with motor neurons in the spinal cord.

Words of Wisdom

In the brainstem, most nerves cross from one side to the other. Motor and sensory nerves on the left side of the brain, for example, serve the right side of the body. This is why a person who has had a stroke or trauma in one hemisphere has nerve deficits on the opposite side of the body. Because cranial nerves do not cross over, their function will be affected on the same side of the face as the injury or stroke.

Cerebellum

The **cerebellum** is the second largest part of the human brain and is similar in size and shape to two large walnuts (see Figure 8-59). It is located inferior to the occipital lobes of the cerebrum and is involved in both fine (small muscle groups) and gross (major muscle groups) muscle coordination. The cerebellum is responsible for interpreting movement and correcting any movements that interfere with coordination and body position. To accomplish this, it depends on information received from the sensory and motor cortexes. The cerebellum determines the direction, force, and duration of the movement and sends this information back to the motor cortex. The jerky tremors of patients with Parkinson disease are an example of cerebellar dysfunction.

Spinal Cord

Recall that the spinal cord is the part of the CNS that connects the brain to skeletal muscle, skin, and other structures through the spinal nerves. The spinal cord leaves the skull through the foramen magnum and extends through the spinal column **FIGURE 8-64**. It is encased within the vertebral canal, which also contains blood vessels, a cushion of adipose tissue, meninges, and CSF. The vertebrae and their associated ligaments provide additional protection for the cord. In most adults, the spinal cord ends at L2; however, in some patients, the spinal cord may end as high as the disk between the T11 and T12 vertebrae or as low as the L3 vertebra. The end of the spinal cord is known as the conus medullaris. A group of spinal nerves then continues to travel through the remainder of the spinal column. Known as the cauda equina, this collection of nerve roots, found just below the level of the conus medullaris, is not part of the spinal cord or even the CNS.

The spinal cord has many long, stringlike strands running through it. Two grooves, the anterior median fissure and posterior median sulcus, incompletely divide the spinal cord into symmetric halves. Each half is further divided into three longitudinal columns (anterior, lateral, and posterior) that run the cord's length. Within each column are bundles of nerve fibers (tracts) with similar functions. These tracts are either ascending or descending, and each carries specific signals. Ascending tracts transmit impulses and sensations from the body to the brain, whereas descending tracts transmit motor impulses from the brain to the body.

The spinal cord contains a central canal through which CSF flows, that extends the spinal cord's entire length **FIGURE 8-65**. The central canal is surrounded by gray and white matter. The cord's gray matter, which is primarily responsible for motor function, is rich in nerve cell bodies that form longitudinal columns (horns) along the cord. When cut transversely, these columns form a characteristic butterfly or H shape in the central regions of the cord. The anterior portions of the letter H are *anterior horns*, the posterior areas are *posterior horns*,

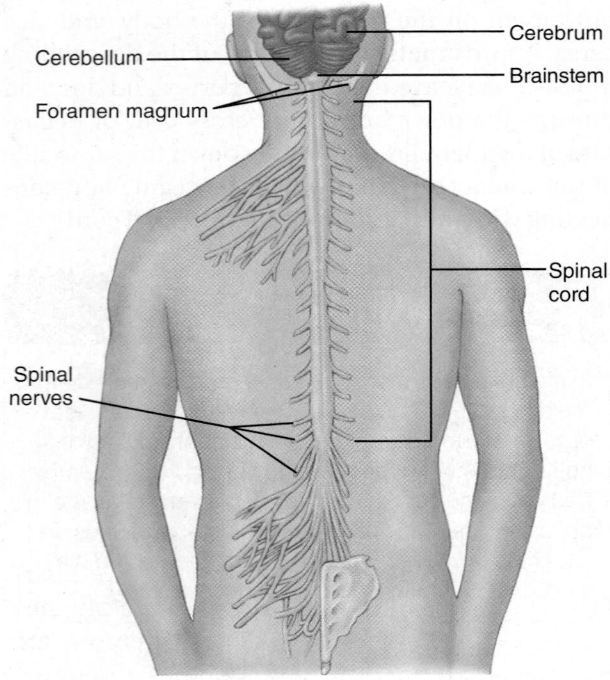

FIGURE 8-64 The spinal cord exits the skull at the foramen magnum and extends down to the level of the second lumbar vertebra in most adults.

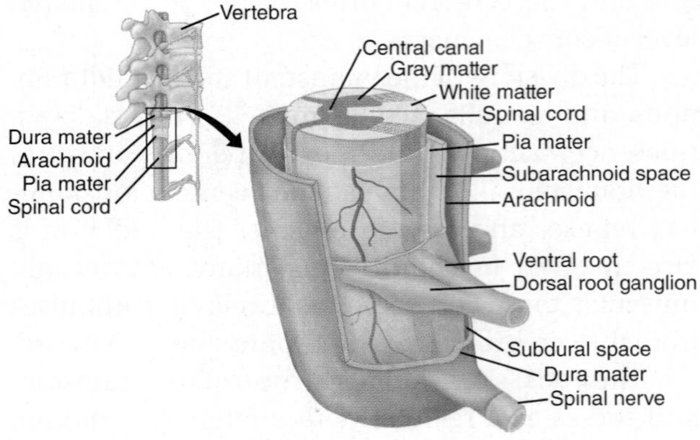

FIGURE 8-65 Components of the spinal cord. The meninges enclose the brain and spinal cord.

and *lateral horns* (found only in thoracic region and upper two or three lumbar nerve roots) are located between the anterior and posterior horns.

The white matter of the spinal cord is rich in axons. The white matter is divided by the gray matter into three longitudinal columns on each side, known as anterior, lateral, and posterior funiculi (Latin *funiculus*, meaning "string") or white columns. Lateral and posterior white matter both return sensory signals from the body to the brain, whereas anterior white matter, like gray matter, carries motor signals to the body. The funiculi contain ascending and descending tracts that are often named according to their points of origin and termination. The ascending spinal cord tracts and their functions are described as follows:

- **Fasciculus gracilis and fasciculus cuneatus.** The posterior funiculi, also referred to as the *posterior column–medial lemniscus system*, contains the fasciculus gracilis and fasciculus cuneatus tracts. These tracts conduct sensations necessary for discrimination, such as light touch, deep pressure, vibration, proprioception, and recognition of objects by touch (stereognosis). The tracts travel the same side of the spinal cord as the impulses they receive and do not cross to the opposite side of the body until they reach the medulla. Although this process does result in the right brain sensing impulses from the left body and the left brain sensing impulses from the right body, in the setting of injury to these tracts, the physical deficits will be ipsilateral (on the same side as the injury).
- **Spinothalamic tracts.** The anterior spinothalamic tract and lateral spinothalamic tract lie within the anterior and lateral funiculi, respectively. Although these two tracts represent a cruder system than the posterior funiculi, they transmit certain sensations. The anterior spinothalamic tract transmits crude touch and pressure, whereas the lateral spinothalamic tract transmits pain and temperature sensations. These tracts travel on the opposite side of the body relative to the impulses they receive. This process results in the right brain sensing impulses from the left body, and vice versa. Moreover, if an injury to one of these tracts occurs, physical deficits will be contralateral (on the opposite side of the injury).
- **Spinocerebellar tracts.** The spinocerebellar tracts are found near the lateral funiculi and include both posterior and anterior tracts. The fibers of the posterior spinocerebellar tract are uncrossed and are more numerous than the anterior spinocerebellar tract fibers. The posterior spinocerebellar tract transmits sensations associated with motor function, equilibrium, proprioception, muscle tone, and limb movement. The fibers of the anterior spinocerebellar tract are mostly crossed (although some fibers do remain uncrossed) and receive less information than the fibers of the posterior tract. The anterior tract is stimulated by motor signals arriving from the brain through the corticospinal tracts and from internal motor pattern generators in the cord itself. The main function of the anterior tract is to provide feedback to the brain that motor signals have arrived to the anterior horns of the gray matter. In the setting of a lesion or injury to one of the spinocerebellar tracts, physical deficits will be ipsilateral.

The descending spinal cord tracts originate in the brain and convey impulses to various muscle groups by inhibiting or exciting spinal activity.[17] A motor neuron that originates in the motor cortex of the cerebrum and travels down in a descending white matter tract is called an upper motor neuron. Upper motor neurons can impact movement only through the lower motor neurons. Lower motor neurons originate in the spinal cord, extend into the PNS, and transmit impulses directly to muscles to effect movement. Upper motor neurons begin and end within the CNS; in contrast, lower motor neurons are found in both the CNS and PNS. Because the lower motor neurons and their fibers (axons) constitute the only connection between the spinal cord and skeletal muscles, they are considered the final common pathway to muscles. This principle of the final common pathway is important to understand the differences between upper and lower motor neuron diseases and injuries, and the differences between their physical findings and prognoses. For example, when upper motor neurons are injured, the injury results in initial flaccid (floppy) paralysis with a loss of tendon reflexes, which is followed by partial recovery (typically including spasticity with abnormally brisk reflexes [hyperreflexia]) over an extended period.[17] In contrast, when lower motor neurons supplying a muscle are destroyed or interruption of their axons occurs, the injury results in paralysis or weakness of that muscle.

Functions of the descending spinal cord tracts are described as follows:

- **Corticospinal tracts.** The corticospinal tracts (pyramidal tracts) originate in the cerebral cortex (with most arising from the frontal lobe area of the cerebrum) and descend through the anterior and lateral funiculi toward the spinal cord. Most of the corticospinal tract fibers cross to the side of the body to which they transmit impulses at the level of the medulla, becoming the lateral corticospinal tract. Those fibers that do not cross at the level of the medulla continue down the same side of the cord as the side of the brain they originated in, becoming the anterior corticospinal tract. However, the anterior corticospinal tract fibers also cross to the side of the body contralateral to their origination in the brain. This process generally occurs in the neck or upper thoracic region. Both tracts transmit motor impulses from the cortex to the spinal nerves, where they are distributed to the voluntary muscles. Most of the corticospinal tract's fibers terminate at interneurons near the gray matter of the spinal cord. However, those fibers that are responsible for the fine motor function of the fingers and hands terminate directly on the anterior horn(s) of the gray matter, allowing fine motor control. When these tracts are injured, physical findings such as loss of motor control occur on the ipsilateral side as the injury.
- **Extrapyramidal tracts.** Although the corticospinal tracts are primarily responsible for voluntary movement, additional tracts play a role in motor activity. Often called the *extrapyramidal system,* the extrapyramidal tracts are not well defined and lie outside the pyramidal system. They are responsible for some degree of movement and posture that is not under control of the pyramidal system, as well as control of the sweat glands.
- **Reticulospinal tracts.** The lateral reticulospinal tract is located in the lateral funiculi. Most of these fibers cross at the level of the medulla, but a few do not. The medial reticulospinal tract is contained in the anterior funiculi, and these fibers do not cross to the opposite side of the body after they leave the brain. These tracts transmit impulses to the body that control muscular tone and the activity of the sweat glands.
- **Rubrospinal tracts.** On leaving the brain, these tracts immediately cross to the opposite side of the body and travel down the lateral funiculi. Their primary function is to transmit impulses from the brain that control muscle coordination and posture.

Important spinal tracts are summarized in **TABLE 8-21**.

> **Words of Wisdom**
>
> Compression of a spinal nerve as it passes through the intervertebral foramen can result in symptoms such as tingling, numbness, muscle weakness, reduced reflexes, and radiating pain. This condition is often called radiculopathy or, generically, sciatica.

Peripheral Nervous System

To respond effectively to its surrounding environment, the CNS needs input from structures outside it, and a means to send its output to the body's smooth muscle, cardiac muscle, skeletal muscle, and glands. This process is accomplished by using the PNS, which is responsible for communication between the CNS and the rest of the body.

As discussed previously, the PNS is functionally divided into two divisions: the somatic division and the visceral division. The somatic division is mainly involved with sensing and responding to information from the external environment. The skin, joints, tendons, and skeletal muscle are innervated by somatic nerve fibers (both sensory and motor). In contrast, the body's internal environment is monitored and controlled by the visceral (autonomic) division of the PNS. Visceral fibers carry afferent information from body organs to the CNS and provide efferent control of smooth muscle, cardiac muscle, and glands.[6]

Spinal Nerves

A spinal nerve attaches to the lateral surface of the spinal cord by two roots: a posterior (dorsal) root and an anterior (ventral) root. The nerve root is either sensory or motor. The posterior root contains afferent

TABLE 8-21 Major Spinal Tracts

Name	Function	Comments
Ascending Tracts (Transmit Impulses and Sensations From the Body to the Brain)		
Anterior spinothalamic	Conveys light touch and pressure, tickle, and itch sensations on opposite side	In the setting of lesion or injury, physical deficits will be contralateral.
Fasciculi gracilis and cuneatus	Proprioception, vibration, light touch, deep pressure, two-point discrimination, and stereognosis	In the setting of lesion or injury, physical deficits will be ipsilateral. The fasciculus cuneatus carries impulses from the upper body; the fasciculus gracilis carries impulses from the lower body.
Lateral spinothalamic	Conveys pain and temperature sensations on opposite side	In the setting of lesion or injury, physical deficits will be contralateral.
Spinocerebellar	Transmit sensations to the cerebellum associated with motor function, equilibrium, proprioception, muscle tone, and limb movement	In the setting of lesion or injury, physical deficits will be ipsilateral.
Descending Tracts (Transmit Motor Impulses From the Brain to the Body)		
Anterior corticospinal (pyramidal)	Voluntary motor commands on same side of the body	In the setting of lesion or injury, physical deficits will be ipsilateral.
Lateral corticospinal (crossed pyramidal)	Voluntary motor commands on the opposite side of the body	In the setting of lesion or injury, physical deficits will be contralateral.
Reticulospinal (extrapyramidal)	Maintain posture during movement	In the setting of lesion or injury, physical deficits will be ipsilateral.
Rubrospinal (extrapyramidal)	Muscle coordination and posture	In the setting of lesion or injury, physical deficits will be contralateral.

nerve fibers that conduct sensory information to the spinal cord. The cell bodies of peripheral neurons are often grouped into clusters called *ganglia* (singular, *ganglion*). The anterior root contains efferent nerves that conduct motor impulses to the body.

The spinal nerves are named for the vertebra at which they exit the spinal column: cervical (8), thoracic (12), lumbar (5), sacral (5), and coccygeal spinal nerves (1). The first seven cervical spine nerves exit above their respective cervical vertebrae. The eighth cervical nerve exits between C7 and T1 (ie, inferior to C7). All spinal nerves below the eighth cervical nerve exit below their respective vertebrae.

The eight cervical roots perform different functions in the scalp, neck, shoulders, and arms. The 12 thoracic nerve roots have varied functions: The upper thoracic nerves supply the chest muscles that help in breathing and coughing, whereas the lower thoracic nerves provide abdominal muscle control and contain nerves of the sympathetic nervous system. The five lumbar nerve roots supply hip flexors and leg muscles and provide sensation to the legs. The five sacral nerves provide for bowel and bladder control, sexual function, and sensation in the posterior legs and rectum (lowermost end of the colon). The coccyx has a single nerve root.

Plexuses

Recall that spinal nerves combine in five areas of the body to form networks (plexuses) where spinal nerve roots come together and transmit their impulses to areas of the body through a common nerve. This principle allows several spinal nerves to control one area of the body. In essence, a plexus in the body acts like an electrical junction box that distributes wires to different parts of a house.

The five main plexuses in the body are the cervical plexus, brachial plexus, lumbar plexus, sacral plexus, and coccygeal plexus **FIGURE 8-66**. The cervical plexus innervates the neck, back of the head, upper shoulders, and diaphragm. The brachial plexus supplies the lower shoulders, arms, and hands. The lumbar plexus innervates muscle and skin in the lower trunk and lower extremities. The sacral plexus supplies the buttocks, posterior thigh muscles, and leg and foot muscles. The coccygeal plexus supplies the perineum. Damage to these areas can result in widespread neurologic deficits such as pain, weakness, and sensation loss, because many nerves will be affected.

Words of Wisdom

The lumbar and sacral plexuses are often considered together as the lumbosacral plexus because of overlap between their nerve fibers.

Dermatomes

A myotome is a region of skeletal muscle innervated by a single spinal nerve. Sensory spinal nerves carry sensory information from a specific area of skin on the surface of the body. These areas, known as **dermatomes**, correspond to specific spinal nerves at various levels **FIGURE 8-67**. You must become

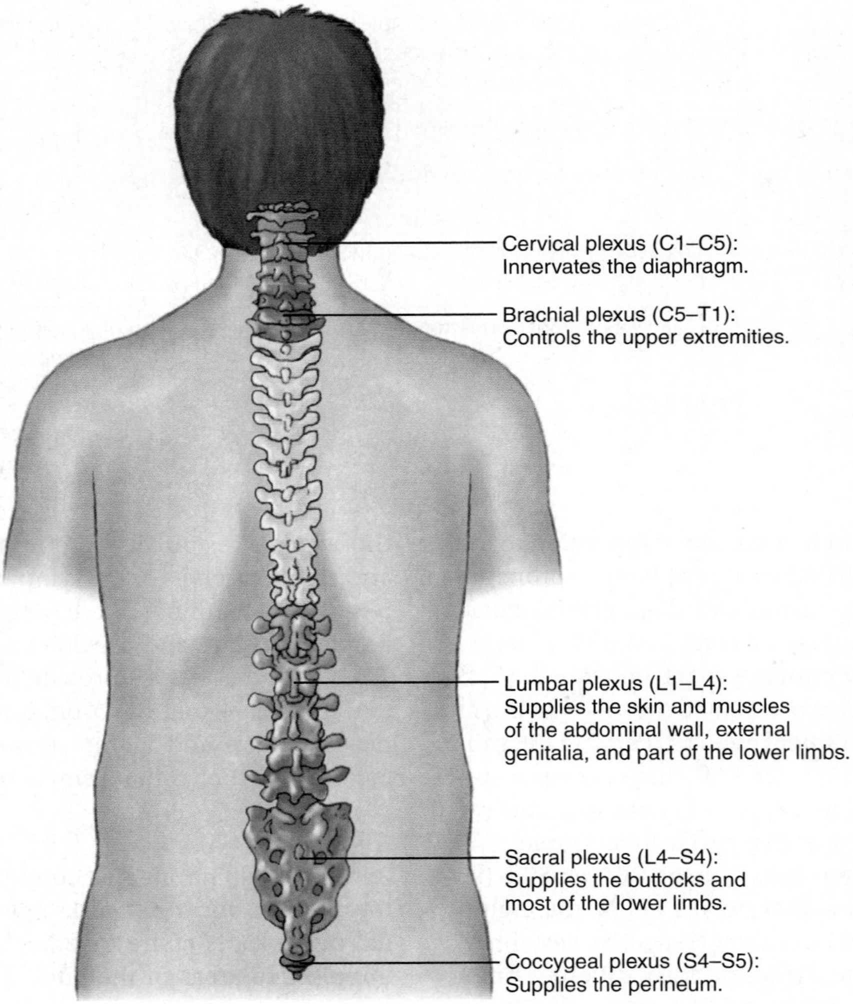

FIGURE 8-66 Nerve roots originating from groups of vertebrae along the spine converge in plexuses, allowing them to function as a group.

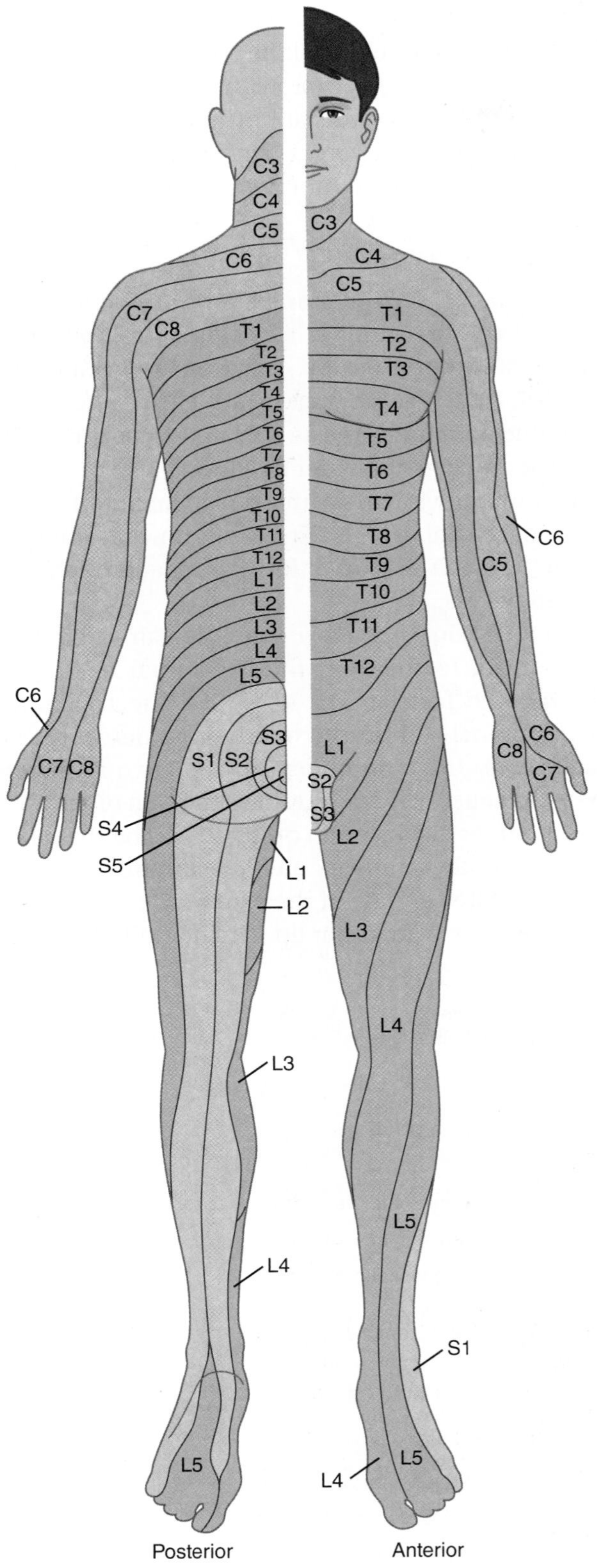

FIGURE 8-67 Dermatome map showing the association between spinal nerves and cutaneous areas of the body.

familiar with the dermatomes throughout the body to better understand the presentation of a patient's symptoms if the spinal cord is injured. Keep in mind that anatomic variations are possible, be aware that dermatomal areas overlap, and recognize that the relationship between dermatomes and vertebral levels is an approximation because spinal cord length may vary among patients.[18]

Spinal cord injuries generally do not result in a lack of function to a specific part of the body (eg, numbness and tingling from the knee down); rather, some impairment of motor and sensory skills is found along the path of specific dermatomes. An injury may be isolated to one dermatome, or an injury may begin along that dermatome and continue distally. Injured nerves manifest as motor impairment, sensory impairment, or both. Musculoskeletal injuries often lead to neurovascular bundle impairment, which is seen with a loss of circulation as well as motor and sensory function distal to the injury site.

Reflexes

The spinal cord contains the main reflex centers of the body. A **reflex arc** is a sensory message that reaches the spinal cord and meets with a motor nerve to cause an action; the reflex action occurs without the message first having to reach the brain to voluntarily cause the action.[19] Components of a reflex arc generally include a sensory receptor, an afferent neuron, one or more interneurons, an efferent neuron, and an effector organ (eg, skeletal muscle, gland).

An example of a simple reflex arc is the patellar reflex (knee-jerk reflex). When the tendon is stretched, such as with a collapsing knee when walking, the reflex is to straighten the knee to avoid a fall. If this process required involvement of the brain, then the fall would likely occur before the conscious thought of straightening the knee could occur. In this example, while the tendon is stretched, sensory impulses travel along afferent axons to the posterior root ganglia. This impulse is then transmitted through an interneuron that determines the motor response to the sensory impulse. From that point, the impulse travels by efferent axons to the skeletal muscles.

A flexor reflex (flexor-withdrawal reflex) involves many interneurons. It is initiated by receptors in the skin, occurring in response to a tactile, painful, or noxious stimulus. For example, after accidentally touching a hand to something hot or sharp, you automatically flex the muscles of the affected limb, thereby withdrawing the hand from the area. The term *withdrawal reflex* may be more appropriate because extensor muscles are sometimes used in this response. For example, because flexion would drive the thigh into a painful stimulus that was applied to its anterior surface, the appropriate withdrawal response uses the extensor muscles of the affected limb.

Stroking the skin with a firm object elicits a superficial reflex (cutaneous reflex), causing the muscles to contract. The plantar reflex is an example of a superficial reflex that is used to detect corticospinal tract dysfunction. It is assessed by stroking the lateral aspect of the sole of the foot from the heel forward with a firm object, such as the examiner's gloved thumb or end of a reflex hammer. In patients older than 2 years, the normal response to this stimulus is curling under of all the toes (plantar flexion). Extension of the great toe with or without fanning of the other toes is an abnormal response called *Babinski reflex* or *Babinski sign* and is generally an indication of upper motor neuron dysfunction.

Words of Wisdom

Assessment of reflexes can provide the examiner with useful information about the integrity of peripheral nerves and specific areas of the spinal cord and the presence or absence of upper motor neuron dysfunction such as spinal cord injury or brain injury.

Cranial Nerves

Recall that 12 pairs of cranial nerves arise from the base of the brain. All but two pairs, the olfactory nerves and optic nerves, exit from the brainstem **FIGURE 8-68**. Cranial nerves are either referred to by name or abbreviated as CN I, II, and so forth. The number reflects the order in which they connect to the brain, moving from anterior to posterior. Some pairs of cranial nerves transmit motor information, some transmit sensory information, and others are mixed nerves.

Two major nerves provide sensory and motor control to the face: the trigeminal nerve (CN V) and the facial nerve (CN VII). The trigeminal nerve branches into the ophthalmic nerve, maxillary nerve, and mandibular nerve. The ophthalmic nerve (a sensory nerve) supplies the skin of the forehead, upper eyelid, and conjunctiva. The maxillary nerve (another sensory nerve) supplies the skin on the posterior part of the side of the nose, lower eyelid, cheek, and upper lip. The mandibular nerve

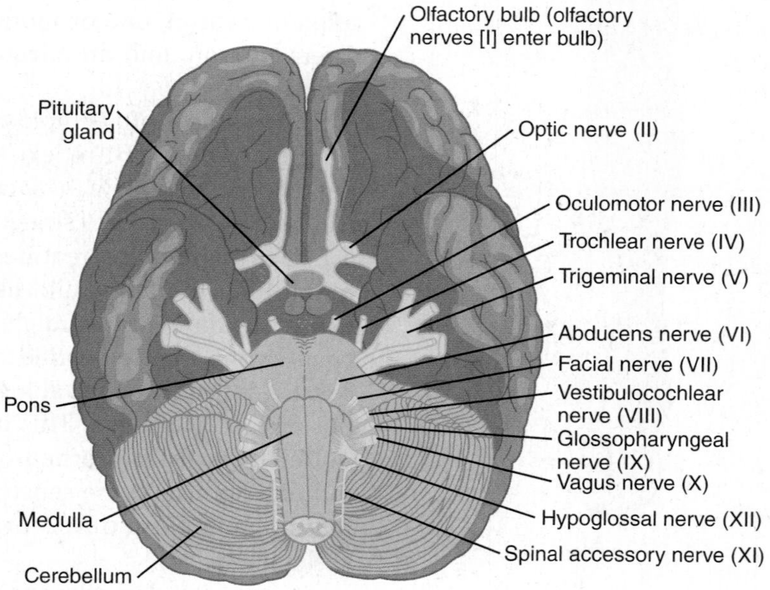

FIGURE 8-68 The 12 cranial nerves.

TABLE 8-22 Cranial Nerves

Number	Name	Type	Function
I	Olfactory	Sensory	Reception and interpretation of smell
II	Optic	Sensory	Sense of sight
III	Oculomotor	Motor	Eye movement; elevation of upper eyelids; regulation of pupil size
IV	Trochlear	Motor	Movement of eyeball in a downward, inward direction
V	Trigeminal	Mixed	Jaw clenching and chewing movements; corneal reflex; sensations (touch, pain) in face, cornea, scalp, and teeth
VI	Abducens	Motor	Movement of eyeball in a lateral direction
VII	Facial	Mixed	Facial expressions; secretion of saliva and tears; blinking; sensation of taste on anterior two-thirds of tongue (sweet, salty)
VIII	Vestibulocochlear	Sensory	Sense of hearing and balance
IX	Glossopharyngeal	Mixed	Swallowing movements; secretion of saliva; sensation of taste on posterior one-third of tongue (bitter, sour); prevents aspiration as part of the gag reflex
X	Vagus	Mixed	Swallowing; part of the gag reflex; sensation behind ear; innervation of pharynx and epiglottis; parasympathetic innervation of organs of thorax and abdomen
XI	Accessory	Motor	Movement of shoulders; turning of head
XII	Hypoglossal	Motor	Movement of tongue muscles for speech and swallowing

(a sensory and motor nerve) supplies the muscles of chewing (mastication) and skin of the lower lip, chin, temporal region, and part of the external ear. The facial nerve supplies the muscles of facial expression.

Blood supply to the face is provided primarily through the external carotid artery, which branches into the temporal, mandibular, and maxillary arteries. Because the face is highly vascular, it tends to bleed heavily when injured.

A summary of the cranial nerves is shown in **TABLE 8-22**.

Autonomic Nervous System

The ANS is the part of the PNS that is not under voluntary control. Its two main branches are the sympathetic and parasympathetic divisions. Most structures innervated by the ANS are innervated by both sympathetic and parasympathetic fibers. In contrast, most blood vessels, the spleen, and the piloerector muscles are examples of structures that are solely innervated by the sympathetic division.[20]

Recall that with a neuromuscular junction, the target (effector) tissue, a skeletal muscle fiber, is innervated by a single motor neuron **FIGURE 8-69**. Axons of motor neurons course directly to skeletal muscles. ACh receptors are localized on the motor end plate. In contrast, autonomic pathways, which are used to innervate organs, vessels, or glands, require two neurons: preganglionic (synonymous with presynaptic) neurons and postganglionic (synonymous with postsynaptic) neurons **FIGURE 8-70**. **TABLE 8-23** compares the somatic nervous system and the ANS.

The cell body of preganglionic (signal-passing) neurons is located within a root of the spinal cord or within some cranial nerves exiting the brainstem. Axons of preganglionic neurons exit the CNS and pass out to the periphery to synapse with autonomic ganglia, which function as relay centers; thus, the CNS and PNS connect at the autonomic ganglia.

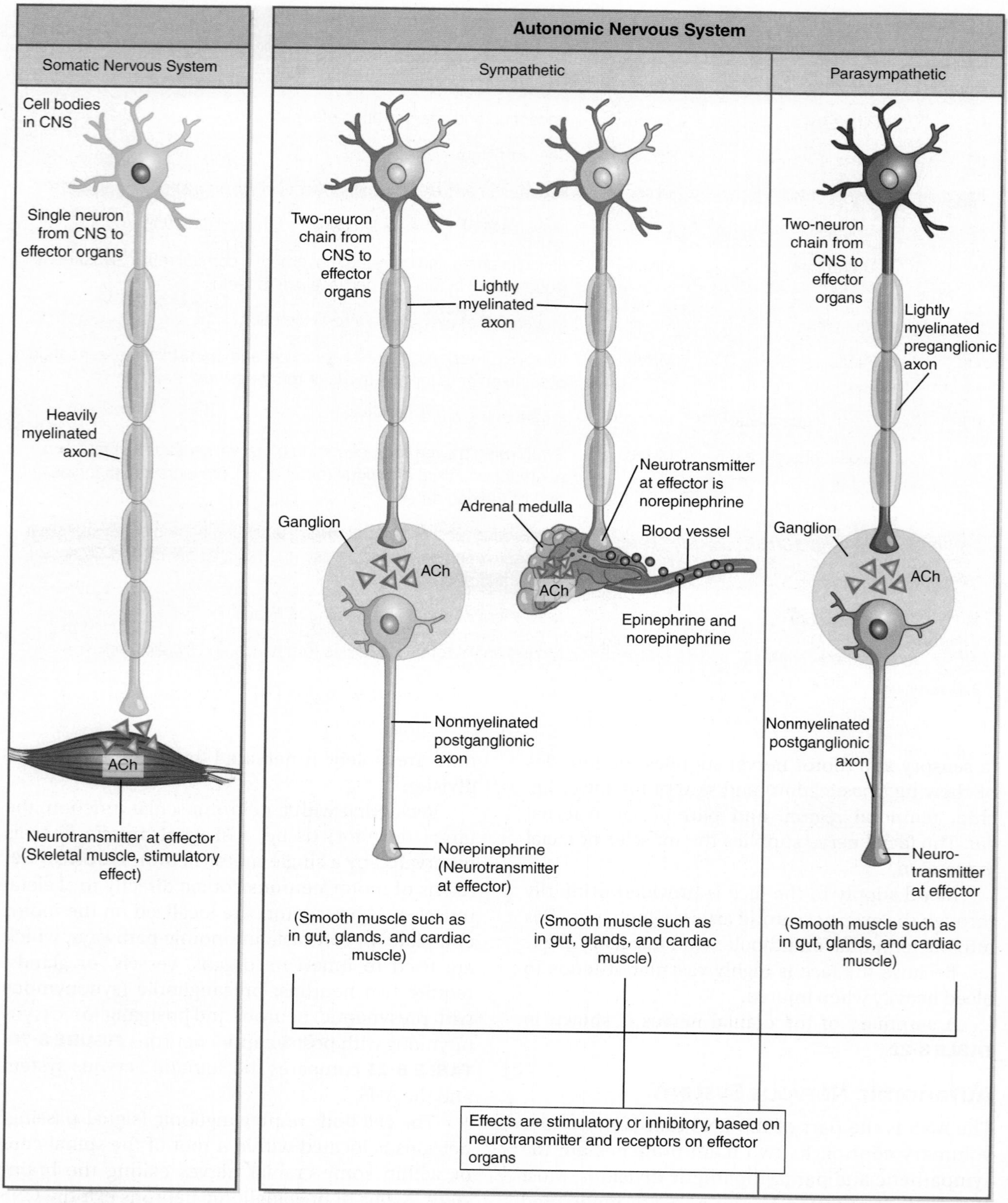

FIGURE 8-69 Neurons and neurotransmitters of the somatic nervous system and autonomic nervous system.

Abbreviations: ACh, acetylcholine; CNS, central nervous system

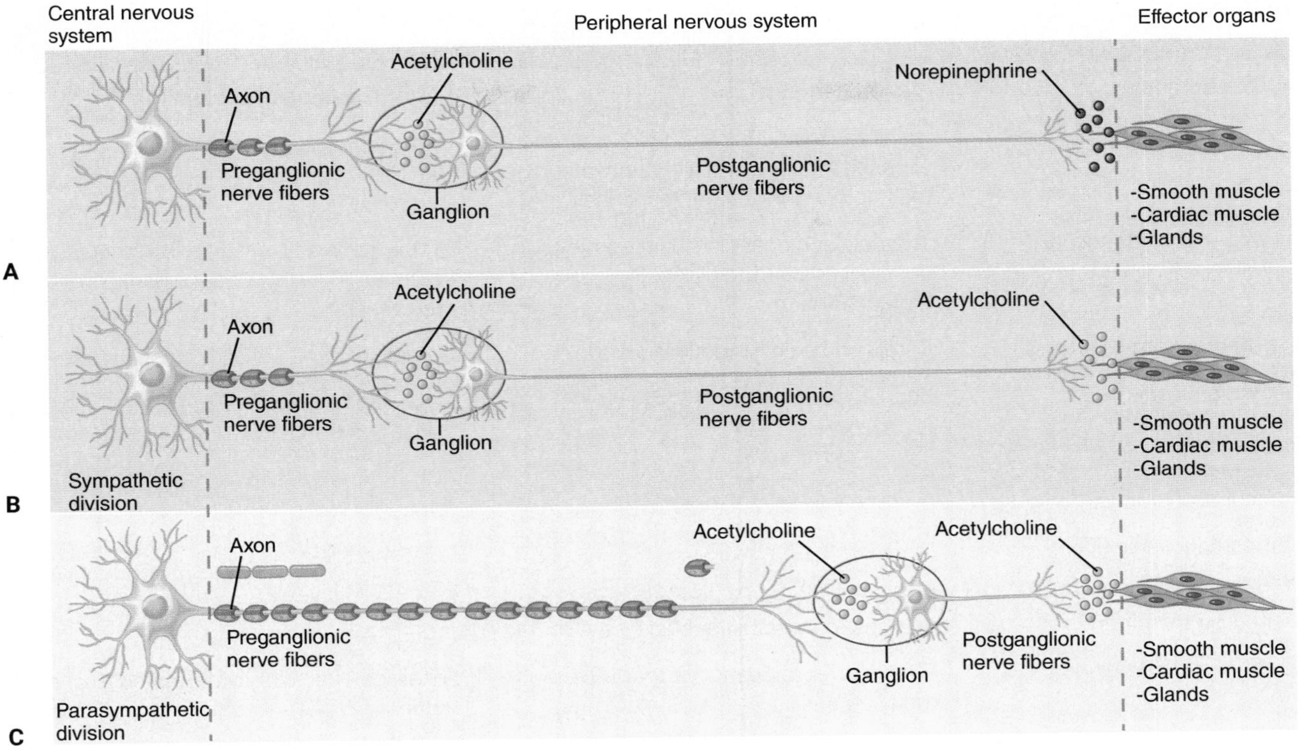

FIGURE 8-70 All preganglionic fibers secrete ACh. **A.** Sympathetic preganglionic fibers are short. Sympathetic postganglionic fibers are relatively long; most are adrenergic because they secrete norepinephrine and stimulate alpha or beta receptors in effector cells. **B.** Sympathetic postganglionic fibers that innervate sweat glands are cholinergic because they secrete acetylcholine (ACh) and stimulate muscarinic receptors in effector cells. **C.** Parasympathetic preganglionic fibers are relatively long, whereas parasympathetic postganglionic fibers are short. All parasympathetic fibers are cholinergic. Postganglionic fibers stimulate muscarinic receptors in effector cells.

TABLE 8-23 Somatic Nervous System Versus Autonomic Nervous System

Characteristic	Somatic Nervous System	Autonomic Nervous System
Control	Usually voluntary	Usually involuntary
Target (effector) organ	Skeletal muscle	Smooth muscle, cardiac muscle, glands
Pathway	Single motor neuron and skeletal muscle fiber	Two neurons: a preganglionic neuron and a postganglionic neuron
Location of cell bodies	Cell body of motor neuron located in the CNS	Cell body of preganglionic neuron located in the CNS
Synaptic location	Axon synapses with skeletal muscle	Preganglionic axons synapse with postganglionic neurons at autonomic ganglia; postganglionic neurons synapse with effector organs
Neurotransmitter	ACh	Preganglionic: ACh; postganglionic: ACh or norepinephrine
Effect on target cells	Excitatory	Excitatory or inhibitory

Abbreviations: ACh, acetylcholine; CNS, central nervous system

TABLE 8-24 Autonomic Nervous System: Sympathetic Versus Parasympathetic Divisions

Characteristic	Sympathetic Division	Parasympathetic Division
General functions	Mobilizes the body for activity and, when exposed to a stressful situation, prepares the body's fight-or-flight response	Conserves energy and maintains organ function
Origin of preganglionic nerve cell bodies	Thoracic and upper lumbar segments of spinal cord (T1 to L2 or L3); thoracolumbar	Cranial nerves III, VII, IX, and X and sacral segments S2 to S4 of the spinal cord; craniosacral
Effector (target) organs	Cardiac muscle, smooth muscle, glands	Cardiac muscle, smooth muscle, glands
Preganglionic fibers	Short, located near the CNS	Relatively long, located near the structures they innervate
Preganglionic neurotransmitter	ACh	ACh
Postganglionic fibers	Long	Relatively short
Postganglionic neurotransmitter	Primarily norepinephrine; postganglionic neurons to sweat glands release ACh	ACh
Effects of stimulation	Effects often widespread; may affect many organs	Localized effects; may be limited to one organ

Abbreviations: ACh, acetylcholine; CNS, central nervous system

The axons of postganglionic (signal-receiving) neurons travel from the autonomic ganglia to the desired structure to which they provide innervation. Typically, the sympathetic division has a larger number of postganglionic neurons associated with each preganglionic fiber than does the parasympathetic division.

For physiologic action at the target organ to occur, preganglionic neurons must first send an impulse to the ganglia and then from the ganglia to the postganglionic neurons. Recall that these neurons are not physically connected; instead, they meet at the synaptic cleft. Each nerve impulse that is conducted along the nerve generates an action potential and the chemical discharge of a neurotransmitter. When preganglionic neurons release their neurotransmitters, they diffuse across the synaptic cleft and interact with specific receptor sites on the dendrites and cell body of postganglionic neurons or on cells of the target (effector) organ. This process causes either another nerve impulse or a physiologic action at the effector organ.

Nerves are traditionally classified by the chemical transmitters that they contain; those containing norepinephrine are **adrenergic**, whereas those containing ACh are **cholinergic**. The term *cholinergic* also refers to other structures or functions that are related to ACh. For instance, cholinergic receptors are proteins in cell membranes that react with ACh and cause cells to respond in a characteristic way (eg, muscles contract, glands secrete).[20] Similarly, the term *adrenergic* refers to structures or functions that are related to norepinephrine and epinephrine (adrenaline). **TABLE 8-24** summarizes the characteristics of the sympathetic and parasympathetic divisions of the ANS.

Sympathetic Division

The sympathetic division of the ANS mobilizes the body for activity **FIGURE 8-71**. In particular, when exposed to a stressful situation, the sympathetic division initiates the body's fight-or-flight response. This response is characterized by diversion of blood from the skin and GI tract to the brain, heart, and skeletal muscles; increased mental activity and alertness; increased blood glucose concentration; increased HR and arterial pressure; dilation of the bronchial tree; sweating of the skin; pupil dilation; and slowing of digestion and urination.

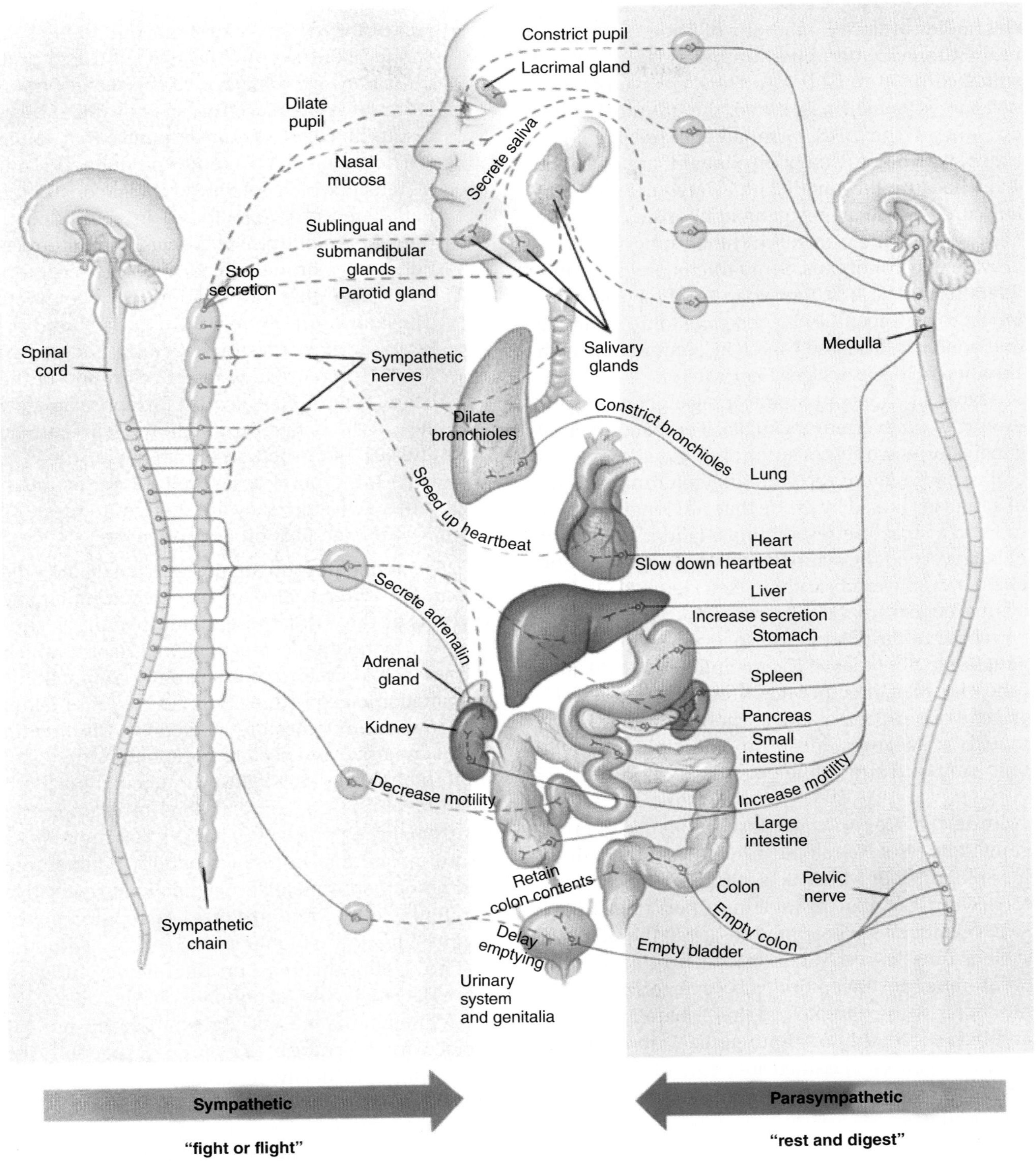

FIGURE 8-71 Comparison of the divisions of the autonomic nervous system.

Sympathetic Nerve Fibers. Preganglionic neuron cell bodies of the sympathetic division are located in the thoracic and upper lumbar segments of the spinal cord (T1 to L2 or L3). Thus, the sympathetic division is sometimes called the thoracolumbar division of the ANS. Sympathetic preganglionic axons, which are usually myelinated, are relatively short because the ganglia are located near the spinal cord, but their postganglionic axons are long because they must travel to the periphery and innervate effector organs. Sympathetic preganglionic fibers release ACh at the synapse, which then acts on nicotinic receptors in postganglionic neurons; this action is discussed later in conjunction with cholinergic receptors (see Figure 8-70).

Most of the sympathetic preganglionic axons extend to paravertebral ganglia. The paravertebral ganglia form two sets of autonomic ganglia, one lateral to each side of the vertebral column. Each set of ganglia is linked by axons that run longitudinally to form a structure resembling a ladder or a chain of beads called the sympathetic trunk, sympathetic chain, or paravertebral chain (see Figure 8-71). The sympathetic trunk extends from the second cervical vertebrae to the level of the coccyx. The long postganglionic fibers leave the sympathetic trunk and innervate their effector organs (heart, blood vessels, visceral organs, and glands), where they relay information at synapses. Most sympathetic postganglionic axons are unmyelinated.

Adrenergic Receptors. Most sympathetic postganglionic fibers release the neurotransmitter norepinephrine, which acts on adrenergic receptors. Sympathetic postganglionic fibers that supply sweat glands and some blood vessels in the skin and skeletal muscles use ACh as their neurotransmitter.

Adrenergic receptors are categorized into five main types: alpha-1, alpha-2, beta-1, beta-2, and beta-3. In addition, both alpha-1 and alpha-2 receptors can be classified into sets of three subtypes.[21] Stimulation of these receptors has the following effects:

- Alpha-1 receptors primarily cause vasoconstriction (narrowing of the blood vessels).
- Alpha-2 receptors generally cause smooth muscle contraction, inhibition of insulin release, induction of glucagon release, and suppression of further norepinephrine release.
- Beta-1 receptors are found in the heart and kidneys. Stimulation of these sites in the heart results in an increase in HR (positive chronotropy), an increase in the strength of cardiac contraction (positive inotropy) and, ultimately, irritability of cardiac cells. Stimulation of beta-1 receptor sites in the kidneys results in release of **renin** into the blood. Renin is a hormone that promotes production of angiotensin, which is a powerful vasoconstrictor.
- Beta-2 receptors are found in several locations in the body. In the lungs, their stimulation causes bronchodilation. These receptors also cause mild vasodilation; **glycogenolysis** (breakdown of glycogen to glucose); and relaxation of the intestines, bladder, and uterus. Beta-2 receptors have also been found in the heart, where they account for approximately 20% of the beta receptors in the left ventricle and 40% of the beta receptors in the atria.[22]
- Beta-3 receptors are localized in fat cells. When activated, they are thought to promote lipolysis and heat production in fat.

The inner portion of the adrenal gland, the *adrenal medulla,* is also a part of the sympathetic division of the ANS. The adrenal medulla is supplied by sympathetic preganglionic axons, which release ACh as their neurotransmitter. Sympathetic preganglionic axons directly innervate chromaffin cells found within the adrenal medulla. Chromaffin cells synthesize and secrete norepinephrine (20%) and epinephrine (80%) into the circulation. Both norepinephrine and **epinephrine** are examples of **catecholamines** that is, substances that function as neurotransmitters, hormones, or both. Epinephrine and norepinephrine are broken down into inactive compounds by the enzymes catechol-*O*-methyltransferase and monoamine oxidase, with the by-products of this reaction then being reused to make new molecules of norepinephrine.

All sympathetic neurotransmitters do not interact with adrenergic receptors in precisely the same way. Specifically, norepinephrine stimulates alpha-1, alpha-2, beta-1, and beta-3 receptors[21] and has minimal beta-2 receptor activity.[20] Epinephrine stimulates all types of alpha and beta receptors about equally.[21] Adrenergic receptors are summarized in **TABLE 8-25**.

Parasympathetic Division

The parasympathetic division of the ANS is responsible for conserving energy and maintaining organ function, while counterbalancing the sympathetic

TABLE 8-25 Adrenergic Receptors

Receptor Type	Location	Effects of Stimulation
Alpha-1	Bladder sphincters	Constriction
	Eye	Contraction of radial muscle of iris causes increased pupil size
	GI sphincters	Constriction
	Male reproductive organs	Ejaculation
	Peripheral small arteries and arterioles	Constriction
	Smooth muscle of GI system	Inhibits movement
	Urethral sphincter	Contraction
	Vascular smooth muscle	Constriction
Alpha-2	Pancreatic enzymes and insulin	Inhibits release
	Presynaptic nerve terminals in PNS	Inhibits norepinephrine release
	Smooth muscle of GI system	Inhibits motility
Beta-1	Adipose tissue	Lipolysis
	Heart	Increased rate and force of contraction
	Kidneys	Release of renin
Beta-2	Arterioles of heart, lungs, skeletal muscle	Dilation
	Bronchi	Dilation
	Ciliary muscle of eye	Relaxation
	Liver	Increased glycogenolysis and gluconeogenesis
	Pancreas	Increased release of glucagon
	Uterus	Relaxation
Beta-3	Adipose tissue; brown adipose tissue	Promote lipolysis (adipose tissue) and heat production (brown adipose tissue)

Abbreviations: GI, gastrointestinal; PNS, peripheral nervous system

division (see Figure 8-71). The parasympathetic division handles the "rest-and-digest" response of the ANS, which controls functions such as digestion, growth, healing, and removal of toxins.

Parasympathetic Nerve Fibers. Preganglionic neuron cell bodies of the parasympathetic division are located in the nuclei of cranial nerves III, VII, IX, and X, and in sacral segments S2 to S4 of the spinal cord; hence, the parasympathetic division is also called the craniosacral division of the ANS. Cranial nerves III (oculomotor), VII (facial), IX (glossopharyngeal), and X (vagus) innervate structures in the head and neck, and in the thoracic and abdominal cavities. Think of the two vagus nerves as the superhighways of parasympathetic function: They account for 90% of all preganglionic parasympathetic fibers in the body.[9] The vagus nerves supply the heart, tracheobronchial tree, liver, spleen, kidney, and entire GI tract except for the distal part of the colon.[20] The sacral division of the parasympathetic system forms the pelvic nerve, which innervates a portion of the GI tract and pelvic organs, including the bladder and reproductive organs. A small number of blood vessels also receive parasympathetic innervation.

Parasympathetic preganglionic fibers join with autonomic ganglia near the organ that will be innervated. The short postganglionic fibers leave the autonomic ganglion and innervate the target organ. Parasympathetic preganglionic fibers release ACh, which then stimulates nicotinic receptors in postganglionic neurons (see Figure 8-70). Parasympathetic postganglionic fibers release ACh, which then acts on muscarinic receptors.

Cholinergic Receptors. Two main types of cholinergic receptors are found in the parasympathetic division of the ANS: nicotinic and muscarinic receptors. These receptors received their names when scientists observed their responsiveness to nicotine (commonly found in cigarettes) and muscarine (found in mushrooms). Nicotinic receptors are found on skeletal muscle, cells of the adrenal medulla, and cell bodies of all postganglionic neurons of the parasympathetic and sympathetic divisions of the ANS.

Five subtypes of muscarinic receptors have been identified (M_1 to M_5). M_1 receptors are generally located in autonomic ganglia, M_2 receptors are located in the heart, and M_3 receptors are found in many glands and smooth muscles. Although the locations of M_4 and M_5 receptors are less certain, all five types of muscarinic receptors are known to be present in the CNS.[21] Some muscarinic receptors are found on sympathetic preganglionic neurons and inhibit the release of norepinephrine. Others are located on parasympathetic preganglionic neurons and, when stimulated, inhibit the further release of ACh.

Some of the effects of muscarinic receptors are facilitated by specific second messenger systems. A second messenger (biochemical messenger) is a molecule that relays signals from a receptor on the surface of a cell to target molecules in the cell's nucleus or internal fluid where a physiologic action is to take place. Second messengers can greatly amplify the strength of the signal received from the receptor.

When ACh binds to nicotinic receptors, an excitatory response occurs. When it binds with muscarinic receptors, the result may be either excitation or inhibition, depending on the target tissues in which the receptors are found. By interacting with these receptors, ACh causes a physiologic response. Once bound with its receptor, it must be broken down to make way for a new ACh molecule. As noted earlier, acetylcholinesterase is the enzyme that breaks down ACh into smaller molecules. The by-products from this reaction are recycled to make new molecules of ACh.

Enteric Division

The third division of the ANS, the **enteric nervous system (ENS)**, is embedded in the lining of the digestive system. The ENS contains millions of neurons, distributed in many thousands of small ganglia. Most of these ganglia are found in the myenteric and submucosal plexuses, which are interconnected networks of ganglia. Connections between the ENS and CNS are made via the vagus and pelvic nerves and sympathetic pathways.[23] Because the ENS includes efferent neurons, afferent neurons, and interneurons, coordinated and purposeful GI function can continue independently even after its connections with the CNS are severed. The ENS releases many different neurotransmitters, including nitric oxide, ACh, norepinephrine, serotonin, ATP, and several peptides.

The myenteric plexus receives its messages from the vagus nerve. This plexus extends from the upper esophagus to the internal anal sphincter.[23] The myenteric plexus controls the tone and intensity of muscle contractions of the intestinal wall. The submucosal plexus is primarily responsible for absorption, secretion, and mucosal blood flow.

Sensory Function

Sensation is an awareness of a body state or condition that results from stimulation of sensory receptors that respond to specific internal or external stimuli. Through the sensation process, the PNS can collect and relay information about the body and external environment. These messages are generated and transmitted by thousands of **sensory receptors** that monitor conditions within or outside the body. Although receptors are capable of monitoring for more than one type of sensation, they often become specialized for one specific or a few related sensations.

Sensory receptors convert the energy of a stimulus into action potentials, which are then transmitted along an afferent nerve fiber to the CNS. After these action potentials reach the CNS, they are routed to the specific center responsible for interpreting that stimulus, where the message is processed and is brought to conscious thought through perception. Perception is an automatic response that is generated through reflexes or other mechanisms, or else the message is discarded as unimportant. The intensity of the stimulus is determined by how many nerve endings are activated, how frequently action potentials are created and propagated, and how many messages are received by the CNS. However, through adaptation, the CNS may temporarily or permanently reduce sensitivity to a particular stimulus. For example, when you walk into a crowded restaurant, the noise of bustling wait staff and dozens of conversations being held over background music may initially strike you as loud and may rise to your consciousness so that you might even mention it to the rest of your party. However, over the next several minutes, the cerebral cortex adjusts to that level of noise, and after that, the noise level may not enter your thoughts again until you walk out of the restaurant into a much quieter environment.

The perception that a stimulus is still present after the stimulus has been removed is called an afterimage. The spots of light you see after glancing at the sun or after a camera flash are examples of afterimages.

General Senses

The general senses of pain, temperature, touch, pressure, and position are the means by which the body gathers information from its environment. Sensory receptors for the general senses are widely distributed throughout many tissues of the head and body. Somatic general senses are those that provide sensory information about the body and environment. Visceral general senses supply information about the body's internal organs.

Pain and Temperature

Pain receptors, or nociceptors, have nerve endings that are sensitive to mechanical, thermal, electrical, or chemical stimuli that could damage the body. Temperature receptors, or thermoreceptors, are nerve endings that respond to heat. The sensations of pain and temperature are related because their receptors overlap, they are conveyed by the same types of fibers in the PNS, and they use the same pathways in the CNS.[14]

Visceral pain is deep pain caused by activation of pain receptors in internal areas of the body that are enclosed within a cavity, such as the chest, abdomen, or pelvis. Visceral sensory nerve fibers travel with autonomic nerves to communicate with the CNS. Visceral pain is poorly localized and generally described as cramping, burning, or gnawing. It often is accompanied by sweating, restlessness, nausea, vomiting, perspiration, and pallor. The patient may move about to relieve the discomfort.

Somatic pain is caused by activation of pain receptors in the body's superficial tissues, such as the skin, bones, muscles, and joints. Compared to visceral pain, somatic pain is generally more intense and more precisely localized. The discomfort accompanying acute appendicitis is an example of both visceral and somatic pain associated with the GI system. In early acute appendicitis, the patient typically reports vague abdominal pain in the area around the umbilicus (visceral pain). As the inflammation spreads, the patient can localize the pain in the right lower quadrant of the abdomen (somatic pain).

Referred pain is pain perceived as occurring in one part of the body other than its actual source. This type of pain frequently occurs with GI disorders. For example, pain from gallbladder disease often is described as, or accompanied by, pain in the right shoulder. Similarly, when the heart muscle lacks sufficient oxygen to meet the body's demand, pain is often felt in the chest wall, left arm, and left jaw.

Phantom pain may occur secondary to damage to a peripheral nerve. This type of pain may be present after a limb amputation in some patients. For example, the patient may report cramping, squeezing, shooting, or burning pain in the foot of a limb that no longer exists.

Peripheral and central thermoreceptors are integrated with the CNS, enabling heat loss and heat production to be balanced while maintaining the core body temperature within relatively normal limits.[24] Peripheral thermoreceptors that are present on the surface of the body relay information to the hypothalamus about the ambient temperature. These receptors are most numerous on the face, lips, and fingers and least numerous on the surface of the trunk. Temperature extremes stimulate pain receptors. Information from thermoreceptors on the skin also travels to the cerebral cortex, enabling conscious awareness of the environmental temperature. Core thermoreceptors that are present in the brain and spinal cord are monitored by the hypothalamus, which adjusts the body's rate of heat production and dissipation as needed, such as during exercise.[24]

Touch and Pressure

Mechanoreceptors (stretch sensors) monitor for changes in physical properties. Among them are tactile receptors that sense touch, proprioceptors responsible for tracking position in space, and **baroreceptors** that measure changes in pressure. Tactile receptors are mechanoreceptors that are located in the skin. Some mechanoreceptors are sensitive to light touch, whereas others are stimulated by heavy pressure.

Baroreceptors play a vital role in many autonomic functions. The most important of these may be measuring the so-called stretch produced in the great vessels. The ANS uses this information to regulate various cardiovascular functions so as to maintain sufficient CO. Similarly, **chemoreceptors** measure the content of various chemicals in the body and/or bloodstream. For example, by sending messages about the amount of carbon dioxide present in the body, the ANS can regulate the rate and depth of breathing to ensure proper levels.

Proprioception

Proprioceptors are found in joint capsules, skeletal muscles, and tendons.[14] They provide information about body limb position, muscle stretch, and movement. This information is used by the cerebellum to coordinate motor functions and by the cerebral cortex for conscious awareness of the position of body parts.

Special Senses

The special senses, which serve as the body's first line of protection against environmental hazards, are integrated with the CNS by means of the cranial nerves. Sensory receptors for the special senses of smell, taste, sight, hearing, and balance are localized in a particular area.

Olfaction

The sense of smell, formally called olfaction, is controlled by the first cranial nerve (CN I) and by nerve fibers that lie in the upper part of the nasal cavity. Olfactory chemoreceptor cells are nerve cells that allow people to perceive smells. One end of the olfactory cell has dendrites that identify chemical stimuli, and the other end has an axon that projects directly into the brain. The dendrites of the olfactory neurons extend from the olfactory bulb (in the brain) to the upper part of the nasal cavity **FIGURE 8-72**.

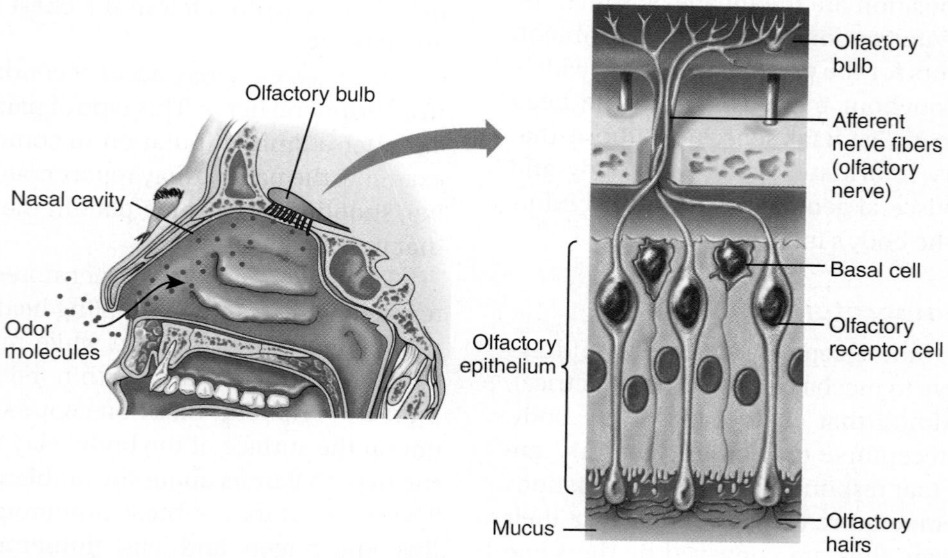

FIGURE 8-72 Location and structure of olfactory cells.

Olfactory cells respond to chemicals dissolved in the mucus covering these cells. Those chemicals may eventually reach a threshold level, often as a result of sniffing to introduce more airflow and therefore more of the substance to be smelled. At that point, the chemicals bind with proteins in the olfactory receptors and cause a change in membrane permeability, which in turn creates an action potential. The resulting impulses travel through the olfactory nerves to the olfactory centers in the brain, which interpret these impulses as odors.

Words of Wisdom

Unlike the signals for the other senses, olfactory signals are transmitted directly to the cerebral cortex without first being filtered by the thalamus. This process creates a close connection to the emotional centers in the brain, and is why you can often recall a feeling or mood associated with a smell even before you remember from where you recognize it.

The sense of smell is also important in helping you decipher the taste signals sent by the taste buds. You have probably noticed that when your sense of smell is diminished, such as when you have a cold, foods that normally have mild flavors may have none at all, and others require a much stronger taste stimulus to trigger a response.

Gustation

The senses of smell and taste (gustation) work together to enable you to distinguish among foods. Taste receptor cells are not neurons, but rather modified epithelial cells that synapse onto the axons of sensory neurons that communicate with the CNS.[25] Taste receptors respond to four primary taste sensations: sweet, salty, sour, and bitter. An additional sensation called umami is often included for non-Western diets. Taste is sensed by taste buds located in small elevations called papillae **FIGURE 8-73**. One taste bud contains 50 to 150 chemoreceptors.[25] Most people have 2,000 to 5,000 taste buds, although the number can range from 500 to 20,000.[25]

The facial nerve (CN VII) supplies taste buds on the anterior two-thirds of the tongue, the glossopharyngeal nerve (CN IX) supplies taste buds on the posterior one-third of the tongue, and the vagus nerve (CN X) supplies a few taste buds in the larynx and upper esophagus.[14] Dissolved chemicals from the food or beverage introduced into the mouth combine with specific receptors and cause an action potential that is transmitted to the thalamus for further processing.

Sight

The sense of sight is controlled by the second cranial nerve (CN II). It is facilitated by the eyes, accessory

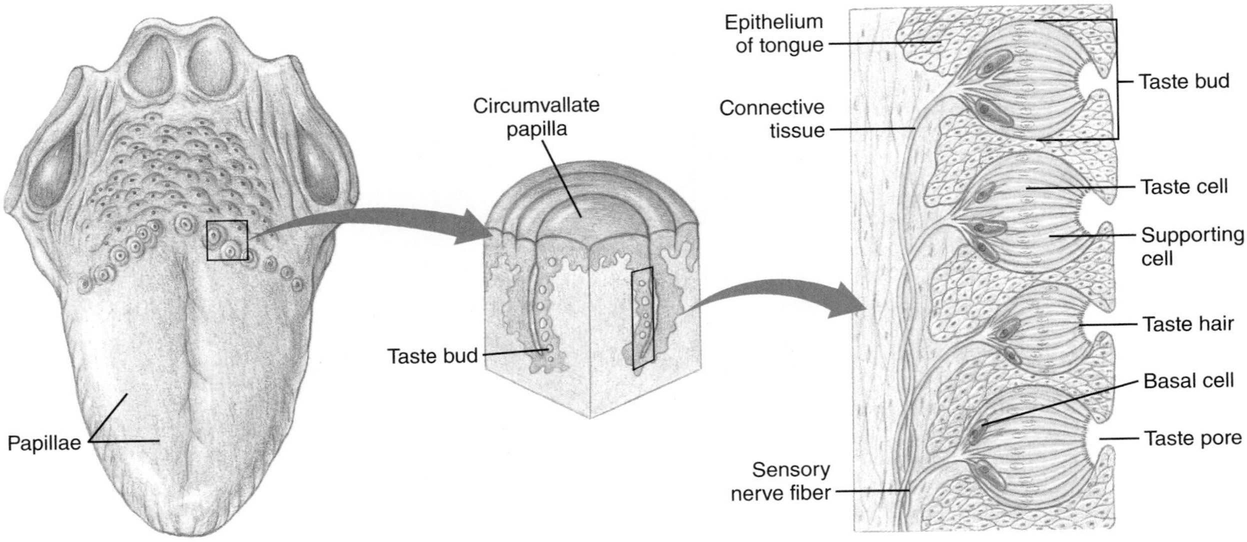

FIGURE 8-73 The taste buds of the tongue.

structures, optic nerve, and tracts that conduct impulses to the brain. Recall that each eyeball is recessed into a small frontal skull cavity called the orbit. The eye has two major components: an optical part to gather and focus light and to form an image, and a neural part (retina) to convert the optical image into a neural code.[25] The eye distinguishes two aspects of light: brightness (luminance) and wavelength (color).

The Eye. The eyeball, or globe, is the source of the information the brain processes into pictures **FIGURE 8-74**. It is imperfectly round and fills the space of the orbit, along with the external muscles and a layer of orbital fat that provides cushioning and support. The lens, suspensory ligaments, and ciliary body form a partition that divides the eyeball's interior into an anterior cavity and a posterior cavity. The posterior cavity, which is located between the lens and retina, is filled with **vitreous humor**, a jellylike fluid that helps the globe maintain its shape without distorting light. It also helps hold the retina in place against the wall of the eye.

The iris divides the anterior cavity of the eye into anterior and posterior chambers. The anterior chamber is the portion of the globe between the iris and cornea; the posterior chamber is the portion of the globe between the iris and lens.[9] Both chambers of the anterior cavity are filled with **aqueous humor**, a clear, watery fluid that maintains intraocular pressure, provides nutrients to the inner surface of the eye, and helps to bend light.[26] Aqueous humor is continuously being formed and reabsorbed. Therefore, if loss of aqueous humor occurs through a penetrating injury to the eye, it will gradually be replenished. The aqueous humor circulates through the pupil and drains into the venous system by the canal of Schlemm, a thin-walled vein extending around the eye. **Glaucoma** is a common cause of blindness resulting from blockage of the outflow of aqueous humor, which leads to an increase in intraocular pressure. A persistent increase in intraocular pressure can permanently destroy optic nerve fibers.

The globe is controlled and directed within the orbit by six **extrinsic muscles** attached to the globe's exterior. The oculomotor (CN III), trochlear (CN IV), and abducens (CN VI) nerves provide the motor nerve supply to these six muscles. CN III also supplies the muscles of the upper eyelid and the sphincter of the pupil and ciliary muscle.

As light passes into the globe, it enters a series of transparent structures that create a **refracting system** responsible for miniaturizing and focusing the image onto specialized nerve endings in the eye. This process is accomplished through redirecting, or refracting, light as it passes through media of different densities. A classic demonstration of this concept occurs when you attempt to retrieve an object from shallow water—for example, retrieving an item from the ocean at the beach. Because the light

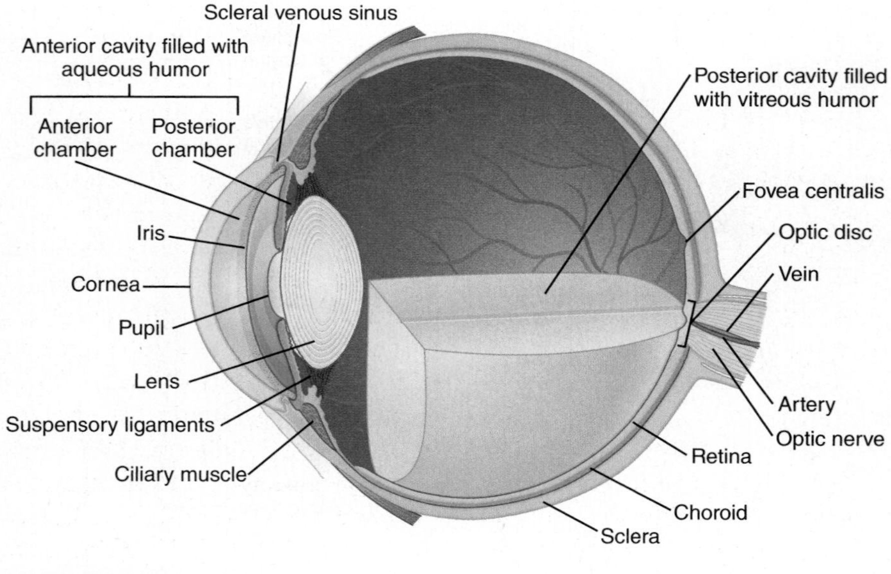

FIGURE 8-74 The eye.

is refracted, putting your hand exactly where you see the object will result in a failed attempt to grab the object: The direction of the light changes as it goes from water to air, leading to a misperception of the actual position of the object in space.

The **lens** is a transparent, biconvex elastic disc suspended by ligaments that are attached to ciliary muscles. Contraction and relaxation of the ciliary muscles change the shape of the lens (making it either more rounded or flatter), which affects how light rays entering the eye are refracted, or bent. By altering the shape and thickness of the lens, the eye can bring an image into focus. **Accommodation** refers to the lens's ability to change its shape to focus on a close object. When light rays entering the eye are not refracted at the correct angle, they do not focus on the retina, resulting in visual defects such as farsightedness (hyperopia) and nearsightedness (myopia). **Hyperopia** occurs when light rays focus behind the retina because the distance between the lens and the retina is too short. **Myopia** occurs when light rays converge and focus in front of the retina because the eyeball is too elongated. In **astigmatism**, irregularities in the shape of the lens create visual defects because parts of the image are out of focus when other parts are in focus. Prescription eyeglasses or contact lenses are used to treat errors of refraction. The increased difficulty in focusing that occurs with aging is called **presbyopia**, although debate exists as to the actual mechanism. Although the lens is normally transparent, it can develop **cataracts**, which can cause varying levels of obstruction ranging from a light film covering the lens to complete obstruction.

The walls of the globe are composed of three layers of connective tissue—the fibrous tunic, vascular tunic, and nervous tunic—with the lens suspended inside them. The outermost layer, the fibrous tunic, is continuous with the dura mater. It consists of the sclera and cornea. The **sclera** is the firm, opaque, white outer layer of the eye. It is nonvascular and helps maintain the shape of the eye. The sclera continues posteriorly as the sheath of the optic nerve. It also serves as an attachment for the extrinsic muscles that move the eye. The **cornea** is an avascular, transparent structure that permits light through to the eye's interior. The cornea is sensitive to pain and is nourished by the aqueous humor.

The middle layer, the vascular tunic, is aptly named because it contains blood vessels that supply the eye tissues, as well as lymph vessels and the intrinsic eye muscles. It is composed of the iris, ciliary body, and choroid. This vascular layer is the primary route through which blood vessels and nerves (other than the optic nerve) travel within the wall of the eye. The iris is the colored (pigmented) part of the eye. It consists of a ring of smooth muscle that surrounds the pupil, which regulates the amount of light entering the eye. The pupil is not a structure itself; instead, its boundaries are simply empty space left by the changing size of the iris. Light enters through the pupil, and the iris controls the size (diameter) of the pupil. The **ciliary body** supports the ciliary muscles that control the curvature of the lens through a ring of fibers called the suspensory ligament. The parasympathetic fibers of CN III supply the ciliary muscles. The **choroid** is a thin, vascular membrane of venous and arterial capillaries covering the posterior two-thirds of the eyeball. It supports the outer layers of the retina and contains pigment that absorbs stray light.

The innermost layer of the globe, the nervous tunic, contains the **retina**, which consists of an outer pigmented area and an inner sensory layer that responds to light. Light passes through eye structures in this order: cornea, aqueous humor, lens, vitreous humor, and then the entire layer of the retina.[9] The retina receives light impulses and converts them to nerve signals, which are conducted to the brain by the optic nerve. The optic nerve transmits the image to the brain, where it is converted into conscious images in the visual cortex. The retina is part of the CNS, receiving oxygen and nutrients from the choroid plexus and retinal blood vessels. Notably, the retina is the only place where the brain's circulatory system can be viewed directly with an ophthalmoscope.[27]

The sensory part of the retina contains photoreceptor cells (rods and cones), which convert light energy into electrical signals. Photoreceptor cells, which are supplied by capillaries from the choroid, relay impulses to the optic nerve. **Cones** are used for day and color vision, and **rods** are used for night vision. Each of the three kinds of cones is sensitive to a different color: red, green, or blue. Rods and cones transmit information through intermediary cells that synapse with the ganglia cells whose axons form the optic nerve. The point where these nerves penetrate the posterior globe to form the base of the optic nerve is a structure known as the optic disk. The optic disk contains no rods or cones, so it creates a blind spot in the visual field of each eye. As image-related signals follow the optic nerve toward the CNS, they pass through the **optic chiasm**, where about one-half of the nerve fibers from each eye cross over to the opposite side of the brain.

Words of Wisdom

An absence of one or more of the color-sensitive pigments in the retina's cone cells results in color blindness. For example, an individual whose cones lack red pigment cannot distinguish between red and green (the most common form of color blindness). Sometimes all cone cell pigments are present but one cell type functions abnormally, detecting a different color than normal.

The vision centers on each side of the brain interpret information separately but then combine those signals to create one image that the brain "sees." This merging of two images into one is known as **binocular vision**. Binocular vision creates depth perception when both eyes can focus on the same target. However, in **strabismus**, there is a loss of depth perception and overlapping or doubled images because the eyes fail to coordinate their movement and may become crossed or separated. The opposite condition is also possible. In *amblyopia* ("lazy eye"), the eyes may be oriented correctly but one fails to send adequate signals to the vision centers, which also causes a loss of depth perception and poor-quality images.

The fovea centralis is located in the center of the retina. It lies in the visual axis, which is a line passing from the center of the eye's visual field through the center of the lens. The fovea has a higher concentration of cones than any area of the retina and is the point of the most acute vision (eg, sharpest visual acuity and acute color vision). The **macula** is the area that surrounds the fovea. It is relatively free of blood vessels and has a high concentration of cones. Many photoreceptor cells in the macula contain yellow pigment.

Two types of vision exist: central and peripheral. Central vision aids in visualizing objects directly in front of you and is processed by the macula. The remainder of the retina processes peripheral vision, allowing visualization of lateral objects while looking forward.

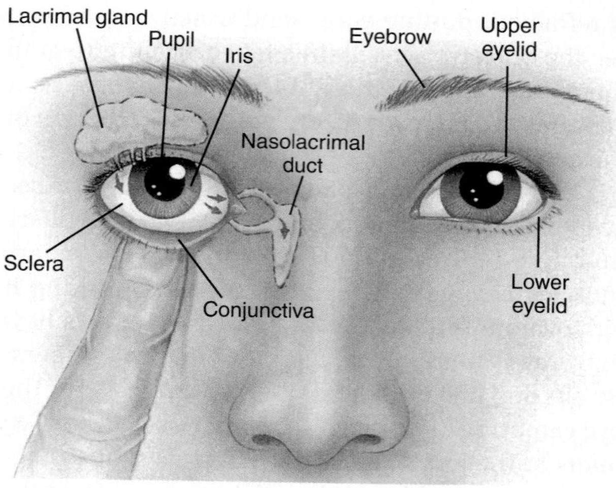

FIGURE 8-75 The accessory structures of the eye include the eyebrows, eyelids, conjunctivae, and lacrimal glands.

Accessory Structures. The accessory structures of the eye protect, lubricate, move, and aid in the function of the eye. These structures include the eyebrows, eyelids, **conjunctivae**, and **lacrimal glands** (tear glands) **FIGURE 8-75**.

The eyebrows protect the eyes by providing shade and preventing perspiration and foreign material (eg, sweat, dust) from entering the eye from above. The eyelids protect the eyes from foreign objects. Blinking lubricates the eyes by spreading tears over the surface of the eye. The medial canthus is the site of union of the upper and lower eyelids near the nose; the lateral canthus is the site of union of the upper and lower eyelids away from the nose. The eyelashes help prevent small particles from falling into the eye when it is open.

The conjunctivae are a layer of soft mucous membranes lining the inside of the eyelid that cushion and allow smooth movement of the globe. **Conjunctivitis** is an inflammation of the conjunctiva. Bacterial conjunctivitis (pink eye) is a common eye infection that results in inflammation and pain.

The lacrimal gland is one of a pair of glands situated superior and lateral to the eyeball. It makes lacrimal fluid (tears). This watery, slightly alkaline secretion consists of tears and saline that moistens the conjunctiva. Lacrimal fluid also contains enzymes that help protect the eye from protein material (eg, bacteria). The act of blinking, whether voluntary or involuntary, uses tears to sweep debris, bacteria, or other material from the surface of the eye. Excess fluid collects at the medial corner of the eye and drains into the nasal cavity through the nasolacrimal duct. The nasolacrimal duct is a superficial structure on the outer lateral aspects of the nose. Superficial lacerations to this area can disrupt these ducts, which can result in lifelong complications with the drainage of tears.

Hearing and Balance

The organs of hearing are divided into three portions: external, middle, and inner ear **FIGURE 8-76**. The external and middle ear are involved in hearing only. The inner ear functions in both hearing and balance, which occur by way of the vestibulocochlear cranial nerve (CN VIII). CN VIII arises from the brainstem and supplies the inner ear, which lies within the temporal bone. Inside the temporal bone, this nerve divides into a cochlear portion that goes to the cochlea, where it carries information about sound, and a vestibular portion that goes to the semicircular canals, where it conveys impulses concerned with balance, position, and movement of the head.

The external ear includes the auricle (**pinna**) and the external auditory canal (external auditory meatus). Recall that the pinna is a cartilage formation that is covered with skin and protects the ear. The external canal is lined by hair and ceruminous glands, which produce cerumen (earwax). The external ear conducts sound to the tympanic membrane, or eardrum. This thin membrane separates the ear canal from the middle ear. Vibration of the tympanic membrane ultimately results in movement of the fluids of the inner ear.

The middle ear is an air-filled chamber within the temporal bone. As discussed previously, the middle ear contains the auditory ossicles. The malleus, incus, and stapes articulate with each other to transmit sound waves to the cochlea. The **eustachian tube** joins the middle ear cavity to the nasopharynx. This tube is normally closed, but it opens during swallowing or yawning, allowing air to enter the middle ear. This process allows pressure to equalize on both sides of the tympanic membrane. The medial end of the stapes is attached to another membrane, the **oval window**, which separates the middle ear from the entrance to the cochlea. Sound is amplified by the middle ear and transmitted through this membrane to the delicate structures of the inner ear, which are filled with fluid. The movement of fluid within this enclosed space is made possible by the round window, which allows the fluid to move in minute amounts as it flexes out of the canal.

The fluid-filled inner ear holds the sensory organs for hearing and balance. The inner ear is composed of a group of canals called the labyrinth.

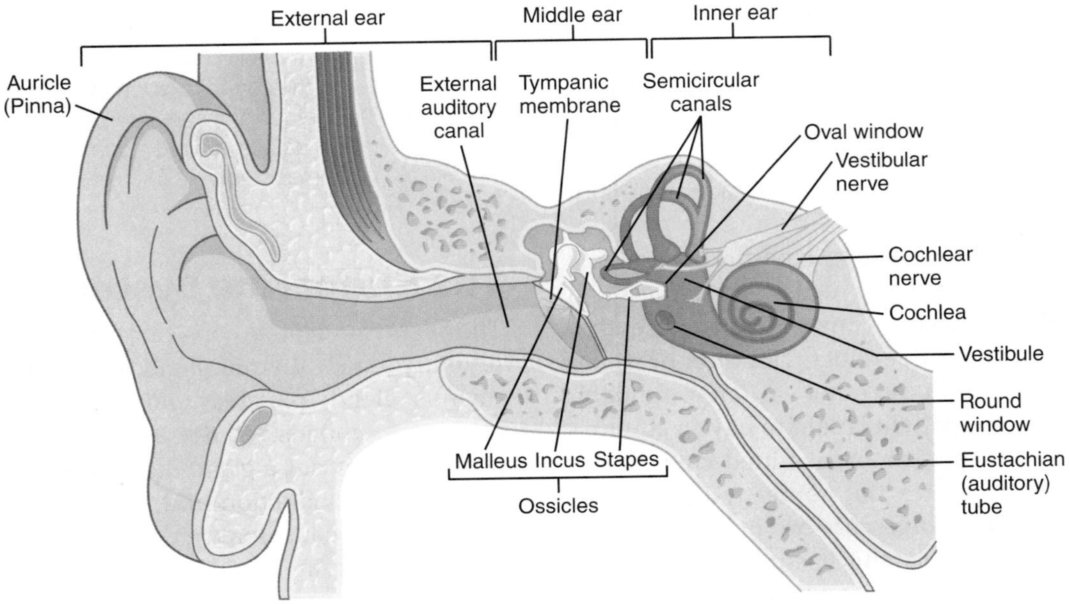

FIGURE 8-76 The ear.

A series of sacs and tubes make up the membranous labyrinth, which contains a thick fluid, called **endolymph**, that is similar to ICF. Auditory and vestibular receptor cells (hair cells) are located in the walls of this labyrinth. Some of these hair cells respond to sound, others to head movement, and still others to head position. The membranous labyrinth is suspended within the **bony labyrinth**, a cavity in the temporal bone. The bony and membranous labyrinths are separated by a fluid called **perilymph**, which is similar to CSF.

Sound waves are conducted through the inner ear by endolymph and perilymph. The bony labyrinth is separated into three areas: the vestibule, cochlea, and semicircular canals. The vestibule, which is the space or cavity that serves as the entrance to the inner ear, leads directly to the cochlea. The semicircular canals, which are three bony fluid-filled loops, are involved in balance. The utricle and saccule are two membranous expansions located within the vestibule. The cochlea contains the organ of hearing, the **organ of Corti**, which contains many hair cells. Permanent damage to the cochlea can result from exposure to high-intensity sounds, such as those produced by subway trains, jet engines, chain saws, and ambulance sirens.

The auricle of the external ear is designed to collect sound waves directed toward the tympanic membrane. When sound waves cause this membrane to vibrate, the vibration is transmitted to the middle ear, causing the ossicles to vibrate. This vibration, in turn, results in movement of fluids in the inner ear. Motion of these fluids stimulates hair cells, which then stimulate the nerve endings of CN VIII, relaying this information to the brain for interpretation.

Any condition that results in partial or complete loss of hearing is known as deafness. Deafness can result from many causes. If any of the structures that normally transmit, or conduct, vibration of sound from the outer ear to the inner ear fail to function properly, then the patient is said to have a conductive deafness. If sound is transmitted correctly by the physical structures but some dysfunction or malformation of the organ of Corti or receptor cells is present, then the patient has a nerve deafness. In the least-common case, nerve impulses may reach the auditory centers of the brain appropriately, but the brain may have a damaged ability to interpret those signals. Patients with this condition are said to have central deafness.

The inner ear is also home to the vestibular system, which consists of a pair of fluid-filled sacs known as **otoliths** and three more fluid-filled, looping passageways known as semicircular canals. These formations do not affect hearing, but rather are used by the CNS to collect information about movement and orientation in space. The semicircular canals use fluid movement to sense rotational movement in each of three planes. The saccule gathers information from its mass of fluid to capture linear movements, while the utricle monitors the degree of head tilt. By processing all of these sensations simultaneously, the vestibular system keeps you upright and aware of your position in space (proprioception).

Words of Wisdom

The nervous system is like a telephone system that communicates through a complex system of hard wires. This system works well for crisis management and in situations requiring quick fixes or corrections. However, when long-term management is required, the endocrine system starts to work. The hard wiring of the nervous system reaches only a percentage of the body, whereas the endocrine system and its hormones reach every cell of the body. Thus, the endocrine system can achieve a level of cellular control that is not possible with the nervous system, even though hormonal control is relatively slow compared with the control exerted by the nervous system. The nervous and endocrine systems of the body operate in parallel toward a common goal: maintaining homeostasis.

The Endocrine System

The **endocrine system** consists of the hypothalamus, pituitary gland, thyroid gland, parathyroid glands, thymus gland, pancreas, adrenal glands, pineal gland, and gonads **FIGURE 8-77**. Although the hypothalamus is not a gland, its endocrine functions include the production and release of hormones; therefore, it is considered a neuroendocrine organ.[9]

The endocrine glands send hormones throughout the body to maintain homeostasis. Through its hormones, the endocrine system regulates many metabolic functions of the body. Some hormones

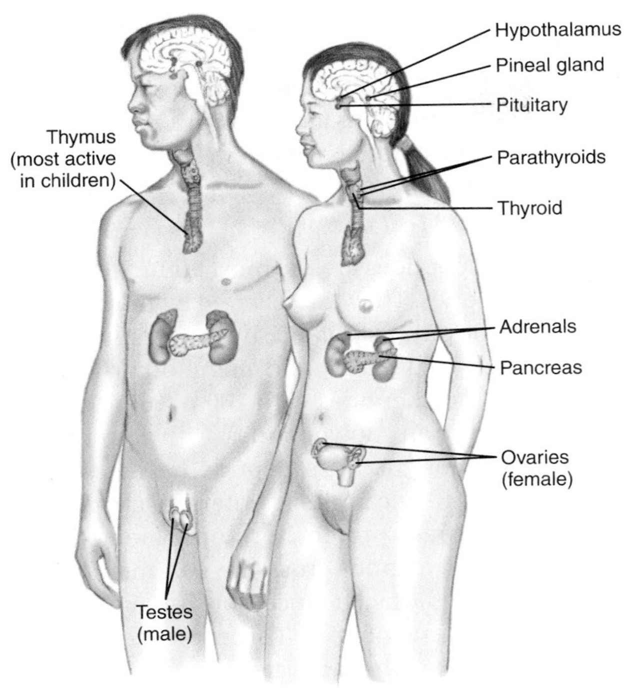

FIGURE 8-77 The endocrine system uses various glands to deliver chemical messages to organ systems throughout the body.

may affect tissues in only one body system; other hormones may have target tissues in many body systems.

The endocrine glands secrete hormones directly into interstitial fluid and then into the circulatory system without the use of ducts. These hormones are then distributed to the entire body, where they affect the activity of other cells. The exocrine glands contain ducts and release their chemical products through those ducts directly to the site where they are to be used. For example, the lacrimal glands produce lacrimal secretions that are deposited directly onto the eye by the lacrimal ducts; these secretions bathe the eye with nutrients and protect it. Some cells and tissues outside the endocrine system also produce hormones; they are discussed later in this chapter.

Intercellular Communication

The human body is a complex organism composed of multiple interconnected systems. To function effectively, these body systems must be regulated and coordinated down to the cellular level. Cells from within a body system and between body systems must interact to achieve this level of coordination. The means by which cells communicate is called intercellular communication or cellular signaling.

The body uses many different chemical messengers (signaling molecules) to relay information to neighboring or distant cells and maintain homeostasis. Examples of chemical messengers include neurotransmitters, hormones, ions, growth factors, and products of cellular metabolism. Most chemical messengers act on specific receptors on target cells that, once activated, trigger a series of secondary events that mediate the response of target cells to that stimulus.[28]

In a few special situations, cells with similar functions may communicate through direct or contact-dependent communication. For direct communication to occur, cells must share extensive physical contact. Some cells possess gap junctions that enable adjacent cells to connect to them. Recall that gap junctions function as electrical connections and permit the exchange of nutrients, metabolites, ions, and small molecules.

You have learned that the nervous system relies on neurotransmitters for nerve cells to communicate, a form of intercellular communication called synaptic communication or synaptic transmission. After their release into the synapse between nerve cells, neurotransmitters quickly trigger receptors on the next neuron. Neurotransmitters are rapidly broken down and reabsorbed for future use. Because the nervous system is located throughout the entire body, this form of intercellular communication can transmit messages over long distances in short order.

In endocrine communication, glands or specialized cells secrete an endocrine hormone into the blood that then circulates throughout the body, allowing it to influence tissues distant from the hormone's site of manufacture. Different body systems have target cells containing receptors that are activated by specific hormones floating in the bloodstream. After these cells have been activated, they exhibit preprogrammed responses that regulate essential body functions. Most hormones have antagonizing hormones that act to balance, or buffer, each other. For example, consider two competing hormones, insulin and glucagon. Through complex mechanisms, insulin acts to lower blood glucose levels, whereas glucagon acts to raise blood glucose levels. In this manner, the body is better able to achieve homeostasis.

Another form of intercellular communication is known as paracrine communication. Paracrine hormones are chemical messengers that are released into the circulation by one type of cell and act on a neighboring cell of a different type. They are usually taken up by target cells or rapidly broken down by enzymes. The release of ACh at the neuromuscular junction is an example of paracrine signaling.[28] In contrast to paracrine hormones, autocrine hormones are chemical messengers that are released into the circulation and affect the function of the same cells that produced them or cells of the same type. Cytokines are peptides that are released into the ECF and can function as autocrine, paracrine, or endocrine hormones.

Hormones

Hormones are manufactured in endocrine glands within the body and are released directly into the circulatory system, instead of into ducts. From there, they travel to specific target cells, which have receptors that carry out a complex set of instructions and actions when exposed to the specific hormone for which they are designed. These target cells can exist anywhere in the body. Hormones' effects on an individual cell are more gradual and have a longer duration than the effects related to the nervous system. Each target cell has specific receptor sites on the cell membrane, or inside the cell, to which the specific hormone can attach or bind. These receptors have two main functions: (1) to recognize and bind to their particular hormones and (2) to initiate an appropriate signal. After the hormone has attached to the cell's receptor site, the message to alter cellular function is delivered.

Many cells contain multiple receptors and act as targets for several hormones—or for molecules introduced into the body as therapy. *Agonists* are molecules that bind to a cell's receptor and trigger a response by that cell; they produce some kind of action or biologic effect. **Antagonists** are molecules that bind to a cell's receptor and block the action of agonists, thereby preventing a biologic response. Hormone antagonists are widely used as drugs.

Chemistry of Hormones

The endocrine system is composed of several glands spread throughout the body that are not physically connected. Each gland is responsible for creating specific hormones that generate specific responses in specific target cells. The three general classes of hormones are proteins and polypeptides, amine hormones, and steroid hormones.

Proteins and Polypeptides

Proteins and peptides are the most abundant of the body's hormones. They are secreted by the anterior and posterior pituitary gland, hypothalamus, pancreas, parathyroid gland, and many other tissues. Proteins are polypeptides with 100 or more amino acids; peptides are polypeptides with fewer than 100 amino acids. Because peptide hormones are water soluble, they can easily enter the circulatory system. In contrast, protein hormones are not lipid soluble, so they cannot cross the cell membrane. These hormones attach to receptor sites on the surface of the cell membrane. This process creates a reaction in the cell that activates a second messenger in the cell, such as cyclic adenosine monophosphate (cyclic AMP). The activation of the second messenger then starts a chain of events resulting in cellular change. For example, this series of events may lead to changes in cellular membrane permeability, changes in cell shape, or an increase or decrease in cellular production.

Insulin and epinephrine are examples of protein hormones that are often administered as medications. Insulin binds with the cell membrane and causes an increase in the absorption of glucose. Epinephrine binds with alpha and beta receptors, causing vasoconstriction, bronchodilation, increased HR, and other effects specific to these receptors.

Amine Hormones

Amine hormones that are derivatives of the amino acid tyrosine are secreted by the adrenal medullae and the thyroid gland. Examples of amine hormones include dopamine, epinephrine, and norepinephrine. Serotonin is an amine hormone made from tryptophan by endocrine cells located within the mucosa of the gut.

Steroid Hormones

Steroid hormones, which are derivatives of cholesterol, are secreted by the adrenal cortex, ovaries, and testes (also called testicles or gonads). Examples of steroid hormones include aldosterone, cortisol, progesterone, and testosterone. Because steroid hormones are lipid soluble, they can readily cross the cell membrane and act on receptors within the cell. Once inside the cell, they combine with a protein receptor to form a steroid-protein complex. This complex enters the nucleus, where it triggers the cell to create proteins used as enzymes.

Regulation of Hormones

Hormones operate within feedback systems (either positive or negative) to maintain an optimal internal operating environment in the body. Hormone release is regulated by a variety of chemical factors, other hormonal factors, and neural control. Endocrine regulation, through negative feedback, is the most important method by which hormonal secretion is maintained within a physiologic range.

One example of this negative feedback mechanism is the release of epinephrine from the adrenal medulla in response to stress. When stress stimulates the body's neural regulation by means of the sympathetic nervous system, the adrenal medulla releases epinephrine into the bloodstream to help the body respond to this stimulus. When the stressor is removed, nervous system stimulation decreases and less epinephrine is released.

With positive feedback mechanisms, one effect leads to or causes another effect. Normal positive feedback mechanisms in the body include the clotting cascade and childbirth. However, positive feedback mechanisms also can occur in harmful situations. In decompensated shock, lack of perfusion to the tissues leads to failure of the cardiac and vasomotor centers, which leads to decreased HR and decreased vasoconstriction. This then leads to further decreases in perfusion, which further depress the body's ability to combat the shock, thereby creating a vicious circle.

Prostaglandins

Recall that prostaglandins (PGs) are derivatives of an essential fatty acid. Although PGs are not hormones, they are mentioned here because they have effects similar to those of hormones. PGs are sometimes called tissue hormones because their effects are usually localized on or near the cell in which the PG is made. At least 16 different PGs exist, and their effects are of short duration.

Examples of changes caused by PGs include changes in capillary permeability, smooth muscle tone, platelet aggregation (clumping), endocrine and exocrine functions, and the inflammatory process (including the development of fever and pain). Several PGs produced in the kidneys cause vasodilation of arterioles. In uterine smooth muscle, PGs increase the intracellular concentration of calcium, thereby increasing uterine contractility. Although some PGs functions are beneficial to the body, PG synthesis has also been implicated in the mechanisms underlying cardiovascular disease, cancer, and inflammatory diseases.[28] Nonsteroidal anti-inflammatory drugs (eg, aspirin, ibuprofen) inhibit the synthesis of PGs.

Leukotrienes and thromboxanes are examples of fatty acid compounds that are tissue hormones similar to PGs. Their effects are localized but potent. Leukotrienes play an important role in the body's inflammatory response. Thromboxane A_2 is a short-lived compound that can cause platelet clumping and constrict small blood vessels.[28]

Hypothalamus

The human body regulates itself by communicating at the cellular level through the nervous and endocrine systems. The hypothalamus links these two systems. Recall that the hypothalamus is located deep in the cerebrum of the brain. This brain structure contains cells that function both as nerve cells and as glandular cells. The neuron functions of these cells receive input from the ANS, including feedback from the body's self-monitoring system.

Information processed by the hypothalamus includes reports on BP, HR, body temperature, and blood glucose levels. Some of the hypothalamic neural cells pass this information on to the CNS, some of these neural cells conduct impulses to the posterior pituitary gland, and some of the hypothalamic glandular cells produce and release hormones that target tissues in the anterior and posterior lobes of the pituitary gland. These hormones (known as regulatory hormones) direct the pituitary gland to increase or decrease its production of hormones that coordinate body systems **TABLE 8-26**.

Hormones that are secreted by neurons into the circulating blood and that influence the function of target cells in another location in the body are called neuroendocrine hormones. The hypothalamus contains neuroendocrine cells whose axons terminate in the posterior pituitary gland.

TABLE 8-26 Hormones of the Hypothalamus

Hormone	Target Site	Effect
Corticotropin-releasing hormone (CRH)	Anterior pituitary	Stimulates release of adrenocorticotropic hormone
Growth hormone–releasing hormone (GHRH)	Anterior pituitary	Stimulates release of growth hormone
Growth hormone–inhibiting hormone (GHIH)	Anterior pituitary	Inhibits release of growth hormone
Gonadotropin-releasing hormone (GnRH)	Anterior pituitary	Stimulates release of luteinizing hormone and follicle-stimulating hormone
Prolactin-inhibiting hormone (PIH)	Anterior pituitary	Inhibits release of prolactin
Prolactin-releasing hormone (PRH)	Anterior pituitary	Stimulates release of prolactin
Thyroid-releasing hormone (TRH)	Anterior pituitary	Stimulates release of thyroid-stimulating hormone

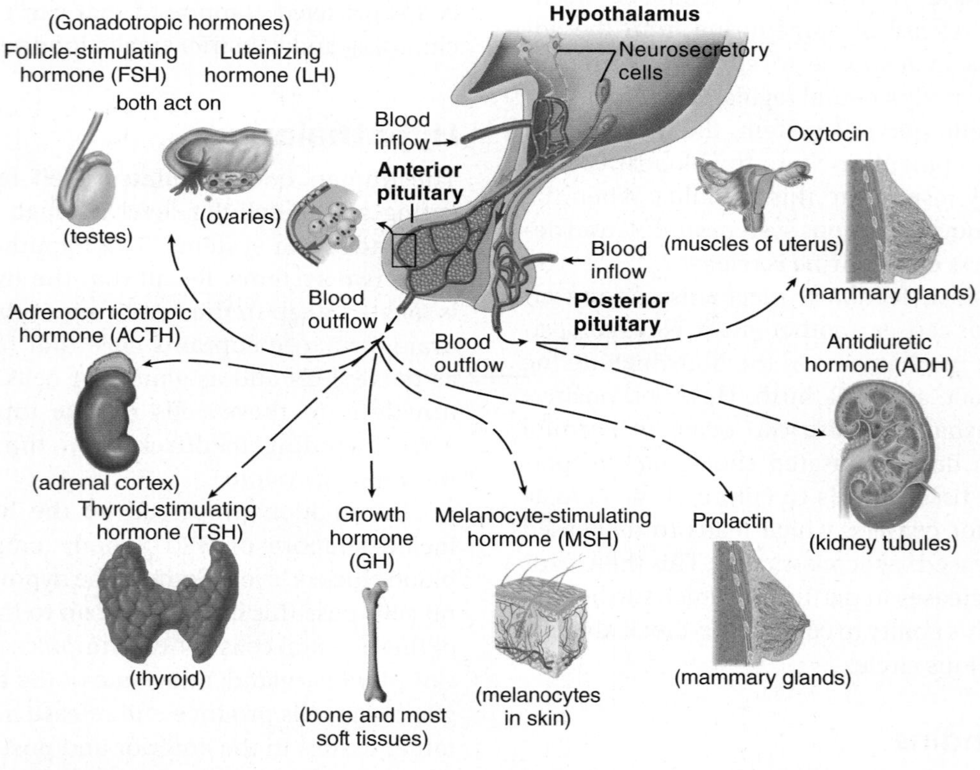

FIGURE 8-78 The pituitary gland secretes hormones from its anterior and posterior lobes.

Pituitary Gland

The pituitary gland (hypophysis) is often referred to as the master gland because its secretions control the secretions of other endocrine glands within the body. A small gland, about the size of a grape, the pituitary gland is found just inferior to the hypothalamus inside a depression in the sphenoid bone. It rests just above the roof of the mouth and connects to the hypothalamus by a thin piece of tissue called the pituitary stalk. The pituitary is divided into an anterior lobe and a posterior lobe **FIGURE 8-78**.

The anterior lobe is controlled by hormones released from the hypothalamus. Because this lobe is not physically connected to the hypothalamus, these hormones are released into circulation and absorbed in the anterior lobe by small blood vessels called the hypothalamic-hypophysial portal veins. When the anterior lobe is stimulated by the hypothalamus, endocrine cells within this structure produce several hormones. Some of the hormones released by the anterior lobe of the pituitary gland do not directly affect body systems, but instead stimulate other glands to release hormones that regulate body functions. The hormones released by the anterior lobe of the pituitary gland are shown in **TABLE 8-27**. Release of these hormones stops (is inhibited) when the hypothalamus releases the appropriate inhibitory hormone.

The posterior lobe of the pituitary gland contains the distal ends of some hypothalamic neurons. These hypothalamic neurons produce hormones but do not release them directly into the bloodstream. Instead, axons originating in the hypothalamus extend directly into the posterior lobe of the pituitary gland, where they are stored in secretory vesicles. These hormones are then secreted into the bloodstream when stimulated by nerve impulses from the hypothalamus. The hormones released in the posterior lobe include ADH and oxytocin. ADH, also called arginine vasopressin, increases reabsorption of water into the bloodstream. In the absence of ADH, an individual may develop diabetes insipidus, in which the kidneys pass copious amounts of water because they are not told to retain it. Arginine vasopressin also acts as a peripheral vasoconstrictor. Oxytocin stimulates milk release and smooth muscle contractions of the uterine wall, prompting fetal delivery.

Thyroid Gland

The large gland at the base of the neck is the **thyroid gland**. The thyroid affects almost every organ in the body, including the nervous, cardiovascular, and GI systems; reproductive organs; and skin, hair, and nails. Its proper functioning is critical for normal metabolism.

The thyroid gland consists of two lobes that are connected by a narrow band of tissue, and is covered by a capsule of connective tissue with secretory parts called follicles. It is filled with a clear

TABLE 8-27 Hormones of the Pituitary Gland

Hormone	Target Site	Effect
Pituitary Gland, Anterior		
Adrenocorticotropic hormone (ACTH)	Adrenal cortex	Stimulates release of steroidal hormones by the adrenal cortex
Follicle-stimulating hormone (FSH)	Ovaries or testes	Stimulates development of ovum or sperm
Growth hormone (GH)	All cells, but especially growth cells	Stimulates cell growth and replication, especially in skeletal muscles and cartilage
Luteinizing hormone (LH)	Ovaries or testes	Stimulates release of hormones by the ovaries or testes
Prolactin	Mammary glands	Stimulates production and release of milk
Thyroid-stimulating hormone (TSH)	Thyroid	Stimulates release of thyroid hormones
Pituitary Gland, Posterior		
Antidiuretic hormone (ADH)	Kidneys	Stimulates increased reabsorption of water into bloodstream
Oxytocin	Uterus and breasts of women	Stimulates uterine contractions and milk release

TABLE 8-28 Hormones of the Thyroid Gland

Hormone	Target Site	Effect
Calcitonin	Bone	Works in conjunction with parathyroid hormone to maintain homeostasis of calcium; increases storage of calcium in bone, thereby lowering blood calcium levels
Triiodothyronine (T_3)	All cells	Stimulates cellular metabolism
Thyroxine (T_4)	All cells	Stimulates cellular metabolism

TABLE 8-29 Hormones of the Parathyroid Gland

Hormone	Target Site	Effect
Parathyroid hormone (PTH)	Bones, intestines, kidneys	Stimulates calcium release from bones, calcium uptake from intestinal tract, and calcium reabsorption in kidneys, leading to a net increase in blood calcium levels

substance called colloid, which stores hormones produced by the follicles. The two main hormones of the thyroid gland, triiodothyronine (T_3) and thyroxine (also known as tetraiodothyronine or T_4), are produced in the thyroid follicles **TABLE 8-28**. Of the two thyroid hormones, T_3 is the more potent, though it is present in the circulation in much smaller quantities than T_4.

Thyroid-stimulating hormone (TSH), which is released by the pituitary gland, causes the thyroid gland to release T_3 and T_4. Collectively, the thyroid hormones regulate metabolism of carbohydrates, lipids, and proteins, determining the body's **basal metabolic rate** (the rate at which nutrients are consumed in the body). Increasing the body's metabolic rate increases oxygen consumption and heat production. Thyroid hormones are required for growth, development, and nervous system maturation.

Because iodine is essential to form normal quantities of thyroid hormones, the thyroid follicles use iodine absorbed through the digestive tract. Without proper dietary iodine intake, thyroxine cannot be produced, and the person's physical and mental growth is diminished.

The thyroid gland also secretes calcitonin, although it is produced by its extrafollicular cells rather than by its follicular cells. Calcitonin, in conjunction with PTH, regulates concentrations of calcium in body fluids. This hormone is secreted directly into the bloodstream when the thyroid detects high calcium levels in ECF. Calcitonin travels to the bones, where it stimulates bone-building cells to absorb the excess calcium. It also stimulates the kidneys to absorb and excrete excess calcium.

Parathyroid Glands

The **parathyroid glands** are embedded in the posterior portion of each thyroid lobe. They produce and secrete PTH, which maintains normal calcium levels in the blood and normal neuromuscular function **TABLE 8-29**. The effects of PTH are opposite to those of calcitonin. Parathyroid hormone is secreted when calcium blood levels are low. It stimulates bone-dissolving cells to break down bone and release calcium into the bloodstream. In the kidneys, PTH decreases the amount of calcium released in the urine.

Thymus Gland

The **thymus** is located in the mediastinum, just behind the sternum. A soft gland, it consists of two lobes that are enclosed in a connective tissue capsule. The thymus functions to help the immune system identify and destroy foreign intruders. During infancy and early childhood, an individual's thymus is large. It diminishes in size as the person reaches adulthood.

The thymus, which is often associated with the lymphatic system, releases several hormones that are together called thymosin **TABLE 8-30**. Thymosin promotes the maturation of **T lymphocytes** (T cells), the WBCs primarily responsible for immunity. **Immunity** refers to the body's ability to protect itself from acquiring a disease.

Pancreas

The **pancreas** is located partially in the retroperitoneal space behind the stomach (see Figure 8-77). This slender organ has both endocrine and exocrine functions **TABLE 8-31**. Approximately 99% of the pancreatic volume consists of exocrine gland cells called pancreatic acini. These cells connect to ducts that deposit an alkaline, enzyme-rich fluid required for the digestion of lipids, carbohydrates, and proteins directly into the digestive tract. The remainder of the pancreas is composed of clusters of endocrine cells, which form islet cells called the **islets of Langerhans**. These groups of cells within the pancreas act like "an organ within an organ." Four types of cells are found in the islets of Langerhans: (1) alpha cells, which produce glucagon; (2) beta cells, which produce insulin; (3) delta cells, which produce somatostatin; and (4) F cells, which produce pancreatic polypeptide. Somatostatin is identical to growth hormone–inhibiting hormone released by the hypothalamus. Somatostatin also decreases the motility of the digestive system and decreases absorption and secretion in the digestive system.

Insulin and glucagon work in opposition to each other and play an important role in maintaining a proper blood glucose balance. Recall that these two hormones form a negative feedback system: When the level of one rises, the level of the other declines.

As blood glucose levels in the body rise, parasympathetic stimulation causes insulin release into the bloodstream. This release promotes the movement of glucose from the bloodstream into the cells. (Brain cells, however, do not depend on insulin to help move glucose from the bloodstream into the cells.) Insulin also prompts the liver to convert circulating glucose into glycogen. All of these actions work to reduce the blood glucose level. In addition, insulin increases amino acid absorption, protein synthesis, and triglyceride synthesis and inhibits glucagon release.

TABLE 8-30 Hormones of the Thymus Gland

Hormone	Target Site	Effect
Thymosin	WBCs	Promotes the development and maturation of lymphocytes (WBCs involved in immunity)

Abbreviation: WBCs, white blood cells

TABLE 8-31 Hormones of the Pancreas

Hormone	Target Site	Effect
Glucagon	All cells, but primarily in liver, muscle, and fat	Excreted when blood glucose level is low (hypoglycemia); increases conversion of glycogen to glucose (glycogenolysis)
Insulin	All cells, but primarily in liver, muscle, and fat	Excreted when blood glucose is high (hyperglycemia); increases conversion of glucose to glycogen; assists glucose across cell membrane
Pancreatic polypeptide	Gallbladder; pancreatic exocrine glands	Inhibits gallbladder contraction; regulates some pancreatic enzymes
Somatostatin (identical to growth hormone–inhibiting hormone)	Alpha and beta cells in the pancreas	Excreted with increased levels of insulin and glucagon; decreases secretion of insulin and glycogen; slows the absorption of nutrients

Conversely, when blood glucose levels begin to decrease, sympathetic stimulation triggers the release of glucagon into the bloodstream, which inhibits the release of insulin. Glucagon causes the liver and skeletal muscles to convert glycogen back into glucose, a process known as glycogenolysis. In addition, glucagon increases the breakdown of fats into fatty acids and body proteins into amino acids for conversion by the liver into glucose. This production of glucose in the liver is called **gluconeogenesis**. Depending on the body's metabolic needs, free fatty acids and glycerol may be metabolized directly or converted to ketones. In small amounts, ketone production is normal. In disease states, such as diabetic ketoacidosis, increased plasma glucagon concentrations and unopposed glucagon activity lead to excessive production, which may potentially harm the patient.

The body uses glycogen for energy when blood glucose levels may not be high. Glycogen is also stored in skeletal muscle cells in a lesser amount that is not readily available for systemic use.

Somatostatin inhibits both insulin and glucagon production. By inhibiting the release of both of these hormones, the body can avert wide swings in blood glucose levels as insulin and glucagon exert their opposing effects.

Adrenal Glands

The **adrenal glands** are located on each side of the body on the superior aspect of each kidney. Each adrenal gland is a yellow, pyramid-shaped gland composed of two distinct layers. The outer cortex surrounds the inner medulla **FIGURE 8-79**. The **adrenal cortex** is made up of endocrine tissue. However, like the hypothalamus, the adrenal medulla contains cells that function both as neural cells and as endocrine cells. The cortex and the medulla manufacture and secrete different hormones.

The adrenal medulla interacts closely with the sympathetic division of the ANS. When stimulated by sympathetic neurons, the medullar cells release epinephrine and norepinephrine. Instead of being secreted near an organ and acting as neurotransmitters, these catecholamines are released into the bloodstream and act as hormones that cause an increase in cardiac activity, vasoconstriction, and glycogenolysis, which are all key components in the body's fight-or-flight response.

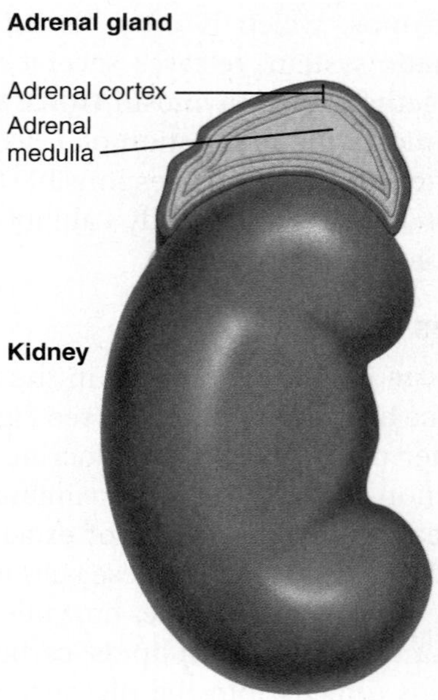

FIGURE 8-79 The adrenal glands sit on top of the kidney and consist of the adrenal medulla and adrenal cortex.

The adrenal cortex is composed of three zones (layers) of secreting cells, each of which releases different steroidal hormones known as **corticosteroids** (adrenocortical steroids). Corticosteroids, which are synthesized from cholesterol, are essential to life. Cells of the innermost zone secrete small amounts of glucocorticoids and gonadocorticoids (sex hormones). The middle zone makes up most of the adrenal cortex and secretes glucocorticoids. Cells of the outer zone secrete mineralocorticoids. Mineralocorticoids are important in regulating mineral salts (electrolytes) in the ECF, particularly sodium and potassium. Collectively, these corticosteroids assist in the regulation of blood glucose levels, promote the peripheral use of lipids, stimulate the kidneys to reabsorb sodium, and exert anti-inflammatory effects.

During times of stress, the hypothalamus secretes a hormone that stimulates the anterior pituitary to release **adrenocorticotropic hormone (ACTH)**. ACTH targets the adrenal cortex and causes it to secrete cortisol, a glucocorticoid. **Cortisol** influences protein and fat metabolism, inhibits protein synthesis, promotes fatty acid release, and stimulates the liver to synthesize glucose from noncarbohydrates. Cortisol helps balance blood glucose and is controlled by negative feedback; stress plays an

TABLE 8-32 Hormones of the Adrenal Gland

Hormone	Target Site	Effect
Adrenal Gland, Cortex		
Cortisol (glucocorticoid)	Most cells	Stimulates release of amino acids from skeletal muscles, lipids from adipose tissue, and glucose and glycogen from liver (mimics effects of glucagon); anti-inflammatory effects
Aldosterone (mineralocorticoid)	Kidneys, blood	Increases renal reabsorption of sodium and water (more so in the presence of antidiuretic hormone) and increases urinary loss of potassium; net increase in blood volume
Estrogen	Most cells	Stimulates development of secondary sexual characteristics
Progesterone	Uterus	Stimulates uterine changes in preparation for gestation
Testosterone	Most cells	Stimulates development of secondary sexual characteristics
Adrenal Gland, Medulla		
Epinephrine	Muscle, liver, cardiovascular system	Stimulates cardiac activity; increases vasoconstriction; stimulates glycogenolysis; raises blood glucose levels
Norepinephrine	Muscle, liver, cardiovascular system	Stimulates vasoconstriction

important part in triggering cortisol release. Cortisol also helps regulate the immune response by decreasing histamine response, which results in lessened swelling, as well as protecting healthy tissues from unnecessary lysosome activation.

If the body experiences a drop in BP or volume, a decrease in sodium, or an increase in potassium, then the adrenal cortex is stimulated to secrete **aldosterone**, a mineralocorticoid. Aldosterone helps the kidneys to balance sodium and potassium, and stimulates water retention via the process of osmosis. This mechanism is an excellent example of the complex interplay of multiple hormones found in many areas of the body. In this instance, if blood sodium decreases or blood potassium increases, the adrenal cortex secretes renin. The renin stimulates an increase in angiotensin I, which is then converted into angiotensin II. The presence of increased levels of angiotensin II stimulates the production of aldosterone, as well as several other endocrine functions that help preserve water balance and improve perfusion. Stimuli from many systems can also produce this reaction. Because of this multitude of interactions, the endocrine system is constantly adjusting to maintain homeostasis and is quite complex. The hormones produced by the adrenal gland are summarized in **TABLE 8-32**.

Gonads

In both males and females, the primary functions of the gonads are to promote sexual maturation to puberty and fulfill any subsequent reproductive needs. In males, the gonads, or testes, are located in the scrotum. Cells of the testes produce male hormones known as *androgens*. The most prominent of these hormones is testosterone. Testosterone promotes healthy sperm production, determines secondary male sex characteristics (eg, deepening of the voice, growth of facial and pubic hair), and stimulates growth. Testosterone has also been shown to affect muscle production and aggressive behavioral responses.

In females, the gonads are the ovaries, which are located inside the pelvic cavity on either side of the uterus. The anterior pituitary gland directs the actions of the ovaries through the release of

TABLE 8-33 Hormones of the Gonads

Hormone	Target Site	Effect
Estrogen	Most cells, but primarily those in the female reproductive system	Stimulates development of secondary sexual characteristics; involved in pregnancy; regulation of menstrual cycle
Progesterone	Uterus	Stimulates uterine changes in preparation for gestation; regulation of menstrual cycle; prevents maturation of additional egg during ovulation
Testosterone	Most cells, but primarily those in the male reproductive system	Stimulates development of secondary sexual characteristics

follicle-stimulating hormone (FSH) and luteinizing hormone (LH). The ovaries produce estrogen, progesterone, and a small amount of testosterone. Estrogen promotes follicular maturation (egg development) before ovulation, secondary sex characteristics (eg, enlargement of the breasts, uterine enlargement, fat deposits in the hips and thighs, development of hair under the arms and in the pubic area), and associated behaviors. **Progesterone** prepares the uterus for implantation of the fertilized egg. During pregnancy, progesterone ensures that the uterine wall maintains functionality and prepares the mammary glands for activity. The gonad hormones are summarized in **TABLE 8-33**.

TABLE 8-34 Hormones of the Pineal Gland

Hormone	Target Site	Effect
Melatonin	Specific nervous system tissues	Regulates sleep-wake cycle

Pineal Gland

The pineal gland is located in the posterior end of the third ventricle of the brain. It synthesizes and secretes melatonin **TABLE 8-34**, a hormone that

YOU are the Paramedic

PART 3

While in transit to the hospital, you begin your rapid exam of the patient. When you assess his chest, you feel instability and a grating sensation on palpation of the anterior chest. You observe that the chest does not rise and fall equally. It is extremely difficult to obtain breath sounds because of noise from traffic and running diesel engines.

Recording Time: 5 Minutes	
Respirations	24 breaths/min, shallow
Pulse	120 beats/min
Skin	Pale, moist, and warm
Blood pressure	106/70 mm Hg
Oxygen saturation (Spo_2)	90% on room air; ventilations assisted with a bag-mask device
Pupils	Pupils Equal, Round, and Reactive to Light and Accommodation (PERRLA)

6. What is the obvious injury you find to the patient's chest?

7. What are the potential hidden injuries you should consider?

affects sleep-wake patterns and seasonal functions (behavior patterns that occur in mammals, such as the mating season).

The Circulatory System

The **circulatory system** (also called the cardiovascular system) includes the heart and a complex arrangement of connected tubes, including the arteries, arterioles, capillaries, venules, and veins **FIGURE 8-80**. The circulatory system, which is entirely closed, includes two circuits: the systemic circulation (travels throughout the body) and the **pulmonary circulation** (travels only between the heart and lungs). The systemic circulation carries oxygen-rich blood from the left ventricle through the body and back to the right atrium. As blood passes through the tissues and organs in the systemic circulation, it gives up oxygen and nutrients and absorbs cellular wastes and carbon dioxide. The cellular wastes are eliminated as blood passes through the liver and kidneys. The pulmonary circulation carries oxygen-poor blood from the right ventricle through the lungs and back to the left atrium. In the pulmonary circulation, blood is refreshed with oxygen and gives up carbon dioxide as it passes through the lungs.

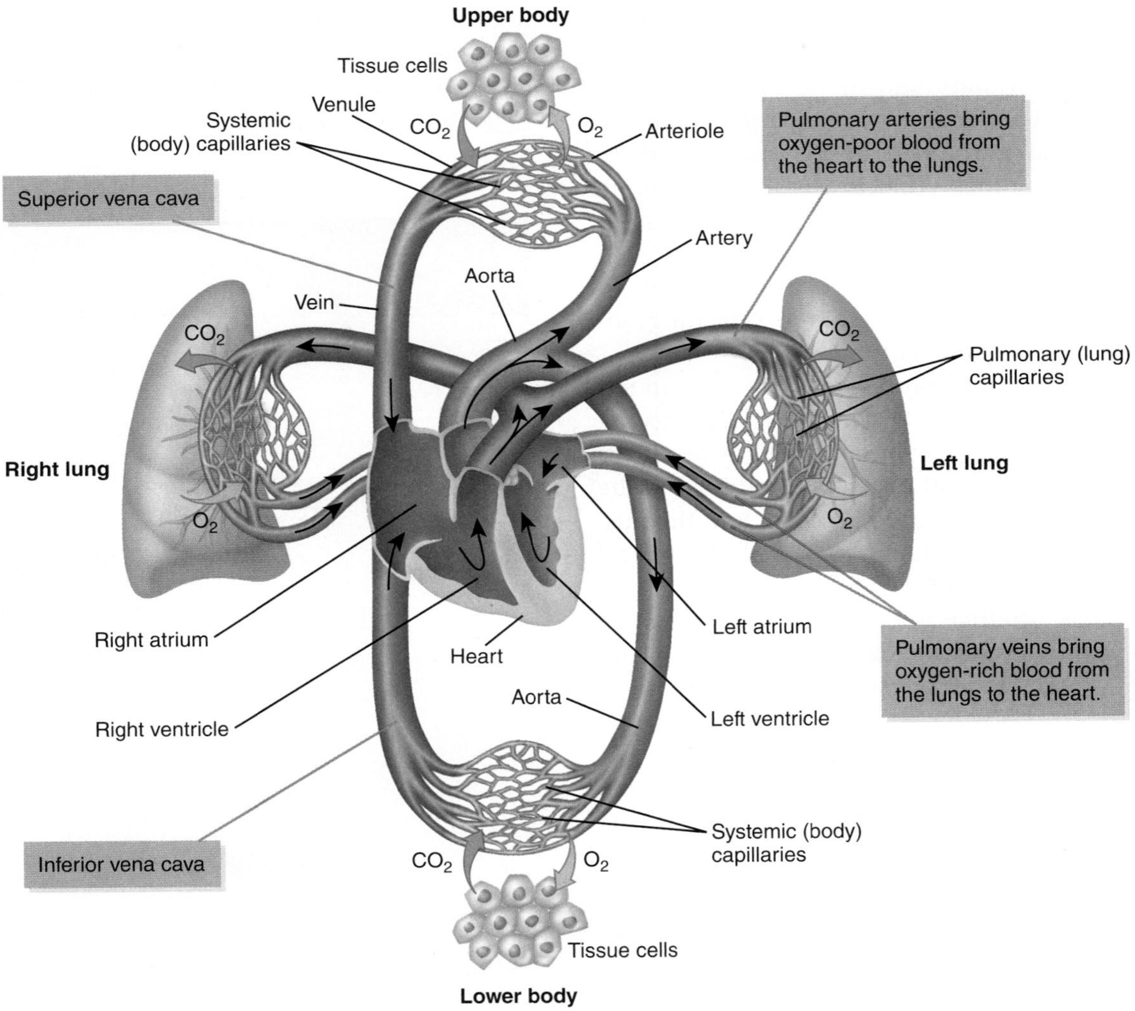

FIGURE 8-80 The circulatory system includes the heart, arteries, veins, and interconnecting capillaries. The capillaries are the smallest vessels and connect venules and arterioles. At the center of the system, and providing its driving force, is the heart. Blood circulates through the body under pressure generated by the two sides of the heart.

The vasculature, which is a system of blood vessels, provides the body's internal piping. It is responsible for bringing nutrients (eg, oxygen, carbohydrates, proteins, and fats) to cells and transporting waste products (eg, carbon dioxide, nitrogen waste products) away for elimination. Blood also plays a key role in regulating temperature and fluid balance in the body and helps protect the body from pathogens. The heart works as a pump that provides the force needed to move blood around the body.

Blood

As mentioned previously, hematopoiesis is the process of blood cell formation. The **hematopoietic system** comprises the blood components and the organs involved in their development and production. The primary site of hematopoietic cell production is bone marrow. Secondary hematopoietic organs that participate in this process include the lymphoid tissues—that is, the thymus, lymph nodes, and spleen. The spleen is involved with filtering and breaking down RBCs, assists with production of lymphocytes (one type of white blood cell), and has an important role in providing homeostasis and infection control.

Two types of hematopoietic tissue are found in the body: myeloid and lymphoid. Myeloid tissue is mainly found in bone marrow; it produces RBCs, WBCs, and blood platelets. Lymphoid tissue is found in the lymph nodes, spleen, and thymus. This type of tissue is home to lymphocytes and other cells derived from them, such as **plasma cells**. Plasma cells produce antibodies (immunoglobulins) to destroy **antigens** (proteins recognized by the immune system) or antigen-containing particles.

Functions of Blood

Sometimes called "the fluid of life," blood performs five functions:

- **Respiratory.** Transports oxygen from the lungs to the tissues and carbon dioxide from the tissues to the lungs.
- **Nutritional.** Carries nutrients (glucose, proteins, and fats) from the digestive tract to cells throughout the body.
- **Excretory.** Ferries waste products of metabolism from the cells where they are produced to the excretory organs.
- **Regulatory.** Transports hormones to their target organs and transmits excess internal heat to the surface of the body to be dissipated.
- **Defensive.** Carries defensive cells and antibodies, which protect the body against foreign organisms.

Blood Composition

Blood is primarily composed of plasma (55%) and formed cellular elements (45%). Plasma is the liquid portion of blood in which the formed elements of blood are suspended. It accounts for the major portion of whole blood. The formed elements are a mixture of RBCs, WBCs, and platelets. Human adult male bodies contain about 70 mL/kg, or about 5 L, of blood, whereas female bodies contain about 65 mL/kg. **TABLE 8-35** outlines the major functions of the blood components.

TABLE 8-35 Major Functions of Blood Components

Component	Function
Basophils	Inflammatory response; release histamine and heparin
Chemicals within the plasma	Control (buffer) pH
Eosinophils	Help control allergic reactions and inflammation; release enzymes that weaken or destroy parasites
Red blood cells (RBCs; erythrocytes)	Oxygen transport (hemoglobin)
Lymphocytes	Immune response
Monocytes	Phagocytize pathogens and cellular debris
Neutrophils	Immune defenses; find and phagocytize bacteria
Plasma	Transport of carbon dioxide, waste, and nutrients
Platelets (thrombocytes)	Control blood loss from disrupted vessels; begin clotting (coagulation) process

Plasma

Plasma is made up of the following substances **FIGURE 8-81**:

- **Water.** Constitutes 92% of plasma. Water enters the plasma from the digestive tract, from fluids between cells, and as a by-product of metabolism.
- **Proteins.** Constitute 7% of the plasma.
  - **Albumins.** Make up the majority of the plasma proteins. Albumins function mainly to regulate oncotic pressure, and thereby control movement of water into and out of the circulation.
  - **Globulins.** Antibodies made by the liver that represent approximately 36% of the plasma proteins. The gamma globulins, which are produced in the lymphatic tissue, include proteins that act as antibodies in the immune system.
  - **Fibrinogen.** Important for blood clotting; makes up approximately 4% of the plasma proteins.
- **Gases**
  - **Oxygen.** Little oxygen is dissolved in the plasma; almost all oxygen is bound to hemoglobin.
  - **Carbon dioxide.** Transported as bicarbonate in the plasma.
  - **Nitrogen.** Dissolved within the plasma; the air that you breathe is mostly nitrogen.
- **Electrolytes.** Calcium, sodium, potassium, and chloride are examples of electrolytes in plasma.
- **Nutrients, vitamins, and hormones.** Glucose, amino acids, fatty acids, and glycerol together with mineral salts and vitamins are used by body cells for energy, heat, and production of other blood components and body secretions.
- **Wastes.** Carbon dioxide from tissue metabolism is carried to the lungs for elimination. Waste products of protein metabolism such as urea, uric acid, and creatinine are formed in the liver and transported by the blood to the kidneys for elimination.

Hematopoietic Stem Cells

Hematopoiesis starts with a common stem cell that can change into many different types of cells. Through a series of transformations, most of which begin in the bone marrow in mature humans, a type of stem cell specific to the circulatory system, known as a hematocytoblast, forms and begins the process of maturation. Through multiple changes and stages, the hematocytoblasts gradually differentiate into one of the blood components discussed further in this chapter. Some become normoblasts

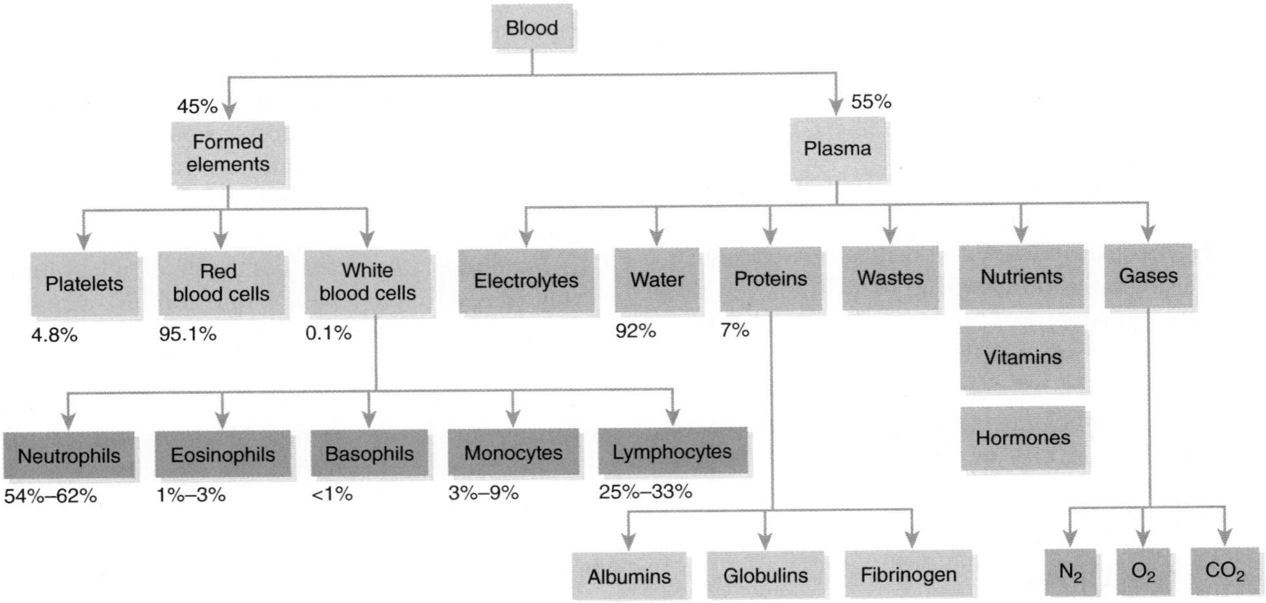

FIGURE 8-81 Composition of blood.

and eventually mature into reticulocytes, precursors to RBCs. Other hematocytoblasts follow a different path to become other formed elements.

Red Blood Cells

Recall that RBCs carry oxygen to the tissues. These disc-shaped cells are the most numerous of the formed elements. An average human has between 4.2 and 5.8 million RBCs per cubic millimeter of blood. RBCs are unable to move on their own, but flowing plasma passively propels them throughout the body. RBCs contain hemoglobin, which gives them their red color. Each hemoglobin molecule is capable of binding up to four gaseous molecules, most often oxygen. The RBCs carry this oxygen to end organs, where it diffuses into tissues.

Erythropoiesis is the ongoing process by which RBCs are made. Erythropoietin, a hormone produced mainly by the kidneys, stimulates RBC production by stem cells within bone marrow. The RBCs may take 5 days to mature and have an average life span of 120 days. Those cells destined for destruction decompose in the spleen and other tissues rich in macrophages. (Recall that macrophages protect the body against infection.) The body "recycles" some hemoglobin components from the discarded RBCs, such as the protein, globin, and iron. The part of hemoglobin that is not recycled is converted to **bilirubin**, a waste product that undergoes further metabolism in the liver. Normally, a chemical derivative of bilirubin, urobilinogen, is excreted in stool and in urine.

The following laboratory tests are commonly performed on blood:

- **RBC count.** Measures the number of RBCs in a sample of blood.
- **Hemoglobin level.** Identifies the amount of hemoglobin found within the RBCs.
- **Measurement of hematocrit.** Gives the overall proportion of RBCs in the blood. The patient's blood is considered balanced (even if the numbers are too high or low) if the hemoglobin level is one-third of the hematocrit value and the RBC count is one-third of the hemoglobin level.

White Blood Cells

The structure of WBCs allows for their movement through the capillary walls and into the tissues. The total WBC count averages between 4,500 and 10,000 cells/mm^3 in a healthy person, but becomes elevated during an inflammatory response, immune response, or both.

WBCs are derived from stem cells. The various types of WBCs have different functions—for example, phagocytosis, production of antibodies, secretion of heparin and histamine, and secretion of other chemokines. The life span of WBCs generally ranges from 13 to 20 days. After this time, they are destroyed in the lymphatic system. Most WBCs are motile and leave the blood vessels by a process known as **diapedesis** to move toward the tissue where they are needed most.

The specific types of WBCs are named according to their appearance in a stained preparation of blood. In general, granulocytes have large cytoplasmic granules that are easily seen with a simple light microscope; *agranulocytes* are WBCs that lack these granules. The three types of granulocytes are neutrophils, eosinophils, and basophils. The two types of agranulocytes are monocytes and lymphocytes.

Neutrophils are normally the most common type of granulocyte in the blood. Neutrophils spend their short lives (usually a day or less) circulating in blood and tissues. Because neutrophils are widely dispersed in the body and are highly specialized for finding and destroying bacteria, they are a primary defense against bacterial infection. These cells are also a major component of the inflammatory response.

Eosinophils release substances that damage or kill parasitic invaders. They also have a major role in mediating the allergic response. Eosinophils release chemotactic factors, substances that cause cells to migrate into an area and that can trigger severe bronchospasm.

Basophils, the least common of all granulocytes, play a role in both allergic and inflammatory reactions. When activated, these cells release histamine and heparin. **Histamine** dilates blood vessels, speeds blood flow to injured tissue, and makes blood vessels more permeable so that neutrophils, clotting proteins, and other blood components can enter connective tissues more quickly.[29] The release of *heparin*, a substance that inhibits blood clotting, enhances the mobility of other WBCs in the area.[29]

Monocytes are one of the first lines of defense in the inflammatory process. In response to infection, these cells migrate out of the blood vessels and into the tissues, where they differentiate into macrophages. Macrophages function primarily as scavengers, engulfing microbes and digesting them during phagocytosis.

Lymphocytes are the smallest of the granulocytes. Although most lymphocytes are found in lymphoid tissues, many are found in circulating lymph and blood as well. Two major types exist: T lymphocytes and **B lymphocytes** (B cells). T lymphocytes, which are formed in the thymus, mainly work to rid the body of bacteria and viruses that enter the body through direct invasion. B lymphocytes, which are formed in the bone marrow, mainly work to rid the body of bacterial and viral organisms by producing antibodies.

Platelets

As you have learned, platelets (thrombocytes) are a vital component in forming clots or coagulation. Platelet production is mainly controlled by thrombopoietin, a protein hormone that is related to erythropoietin. Cells in the liver and kidneys secrete thrombopoietin at a constant rate. Approximately two-thirds of the total platelets circulate in the blood, and the remaining one-third are stored in the spleen's blood vessels. Platelets circulate in the blood for about 7 to 10 days.

> **Words of Wisdom**
>
> Any process that interferes with the activation or continuation of the clotting cascade or hemostasis is known as a coagulopathy. Coagulopathies are bleeding disorders that can lead to heavy or prolonged bleeding.

Normal Hemostasis

Following injury to a blood vessel wall, a predictable series of events takes place, resulting in **hemostasis** (cessation of bleeding) and formation of the final blood clot. The coagulation process is a complex set of events involving platelets, clotting proteins in the plasma (clotting factors), other proteins, and calcium. Most of the clotting factors are produced in the liver, where vitamin K is required for their formation.

The immediate physiologic response to bleeding is vasoconstriction, which clamps down and cuts off blood flow at the affected site. Locally, vasoconstrictors such as thromboxane are released. Should the bleeding prove to be a significant threat to homeostasis, the adrenal glands release epinephrine (a potent vasoconstrictor), leading to systemic vasoconstriction. The secondary response to hemorrhage is platelet plugging. Recall that platelets are cellular fragments that stick to collagen and become activated. Collagen is found within the deep membranes of blood vessels, and a cut or rupture exposes it to the platelets within the circulation. The first platelets to be activated release chemicals that cause aggregation (clumping) of additional platelets at the injury site. This process of coagulation involves about a dozen clotting factors that become activated when the body is injured. Each of these factors requires the presence and activation of the preceding factor to work.

Activated platelets express a surface protein that stimulates the **clotting cascade** (coagulation cascade), the set of interactions that ultimately lead to the formation of a clot **FIGURE 8-82**. These steps are typically organized into extrinsic and intrinsic pathways that converge into a common pathway. The extrinsic pathway (tissue factor pathway) is triggered by damage to the tissues, which then release clotting factors. These factors react with other clotting factors and calcium, with the final product of their reactions being tissue **thromboplastin**. The intrinsic pathway (contact activation pathway) is activated when damaged platelets release clotting factors. These factors also react with other clotting factors and calcium, with the final product being platelet thromboplastin. The extrinsic and intrinsic pathways work in parallel—that is, at the same time. The tissue thromboplastin and platelet thromboplastin produced via these processes eventually meet in the common pathway, where they convert **prothrombin** (produced by the liver) to its active form, **thrombin**. Thrombin, in turn, acts on fibrinogen, another blood protein that is also produced by the liver. When activated, fibrinogen is converted to fibrin. **Fibrin** takes the form of long, branching fibers that produce a weblike network in the damaged blood vessel wall. It binds to the mass of platelets, forming a plug that stops blood flow to the tissue. Calcium acts as a binding agent in this plug, holding fibrin fibers close together to form the meshwork of the clot.

After the bleeding has stopped and the injured vessel is healed, plasma proteins break down the

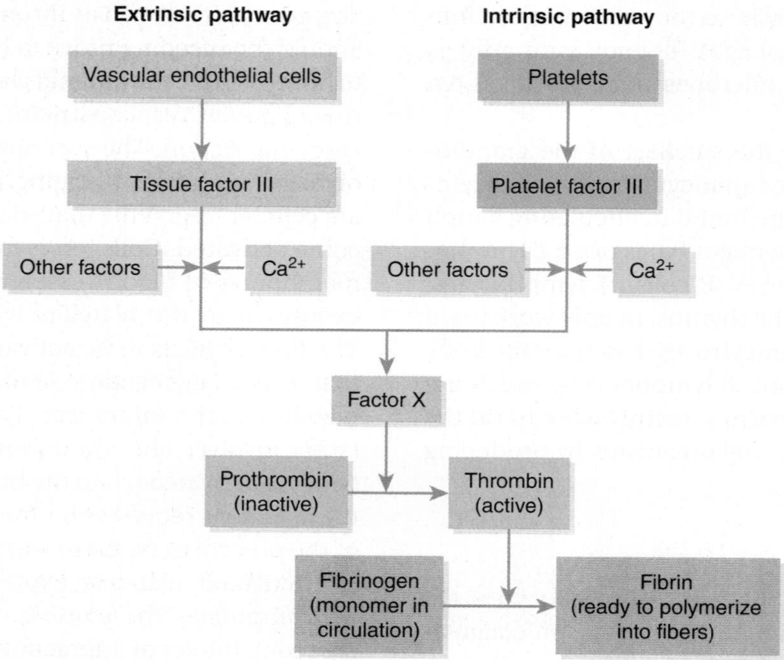

FIGURE 8-82 The clotting cascade. The extrinsic and intrinsic pathways merge into the final common pathway, whose end product is fibrin.

fibrin fibers of the clot into fragments. During the clot-dissolving portion of coagulation, which is called fibrinolysis, the enzyme plasminogen is converted to **plasmin**, which dissolves the fibrin fibers of the clot.

ABO and Rh Blood Groups

RBCs contain antigens on their surface. Within the plasma are antibodies, which react with these antigens. To ensure compatibility and prevent medical complications during blood component replacement, people are classified as having one of four blood types based on the presence or absence of these specific antigens. This process of classification is referred to as blood typing, or determining the ABO blood group. In the **ABO system**, the RBC classification types are O, A, B, and AB, which indicate the antigens found in the plasma membrane **TABLE 8-36**.

TABLE 8-36 ABO Blood Groups

Blood Type	Antigen	Antibody	Potential Donor
A	A	Anti-B	A, O
B	B	Anti-A	B, O
AB	A and B	Neither antibody	AB, A, B, O
O	Neither antigen	Anti-A and anti-B	O

Type A blood contains RBCs with type A surface antigens and plasma containing type B antibodies; type B blood contains type B surface antigens and plasma containing type A antibodies. Type AB blood contains both types of antigens but the plasma contains no ABO antibodies. Type O contains neither A nor B antigens, but does contain both A and B plasma antibodies. A person's blood type determines which type of blood they may receive in a blood transfusion.

Type O blood, because it has no ABO antigens, can be given to anyone; thus, a person with type O blood is known as a universal donor. A person with type AB blood can receive blood from any donor without having an ABO reaction because type AB blood has no ABO antibodies; thus, the person is known as a universal recipient.

Blood contains a secondary antigen, known as the Rh antigen (the name signifies that the antigen was first discovered in rhesus monkeys). The Rh blood group consists of several antigens, with D being the most prevalent. The Rh antigen D (**Rh factor**), determines whether an immune response will occur as a result of a blood transfusion. A person with the Rh factor present in the blood is considered Rh-positive; Rh-negative means that the antigen is not present. Unlike the case with the ABO antigens, human plasma does not normally contain Rh antibodies. In consequence, a person with Rh-negative blood must first be exposed to Rh-positive blood to develop antibodies to the Rh antigen. The same is true for a person with Rh-positive blood. Rh antibodies are produced within about 2 weeks of exposure, then remain in the blood. The second time the person is exposed to the Rh antigen, a severe reaction may occur.

Another situation in which the Rh blood group may present a problem is in pregnancy. For example, suppose an Rh-negative mother is exposed to the Rh-positive blood of her unborn child during pregnancy, birth, miscarriage, or abortion. As a result of this exposure, the woman's immune system will develop antibodies to the Rh antigens, though they generally do not create an issue during the first pregnancy. However, in subsequent pregnancies, if the unborn child has Rh-positive blood, then the mother's immune system will launch an attack against the RBCs of the fetus. This incompatibility can be addressed through treatment provided at the time of delivery. For this to be possible, prenatal testing of the mother's blood is necessary.

Heart

The driving force behind the cardiovascular system is the heart **FIGURE 8-83**. This remarkable pump sits in the chest, above the diaphragm, behind and slightly left of the lower sternum. The tip of the heart is the apex, and the top of the heart is its base. The base lies at about the area of the second intercostal space, and the apex (bottom) lies at about the fifth intercostal space near or a little medial to the mid-clavicular line. The heart is not much larger than a person's fist and weighs about 9 ounces (between 250 and 300 g). Despite its relatively small size, the heart is strong enough to circulate 7,000 L to 9,000 L of blood around the body every day!

The large vessels that carry blood to the heart include the superior and inferior venae cavae (vessels that return venous blood from the upper and lower parts of the body to the right atrium), and the pulmonary veins (vessels that return oxygenated

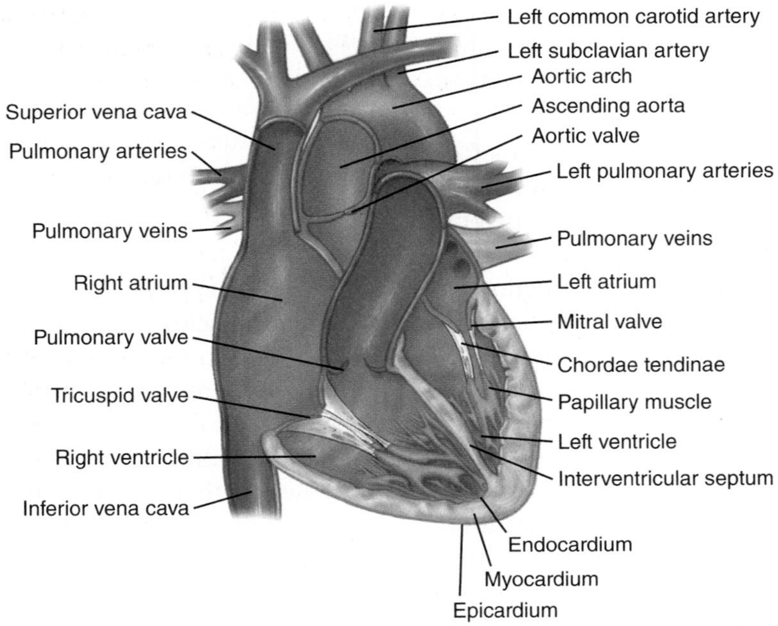

FIGURE 8-83 Anatomy of the heart.

blood from the lungs to the left atrium). The large vessels that carry blood away from the heart include the aorta (which delivers blood from the left ventricle to the body) and the pulmonary arteries (which deliver unoxygenated blood from the right ventricle to the lungs).

Heart Wall

The **pericardium** (pericardial sac) is a thick, fibrous membrane that surrounds the heart. The pericardium anchors the heart within the mediastinum and prevents overdistention of the heart. It has an outer, fibrous membrane (parietal), and an inner membrane (visceral). The fibrous pericardium is made of dense connective tissue. This tissue is attached to the central diaphragm, posterior sternum, vertebral column, and large blood vessels connected to the heart. An inner, double-layered visceral pericardium covers the heart as well. At the base of the heart, the visceral pericardium folds back to become the parietal pericardium. Between the parietal and visceral layers is the pericardial cavity, which contains a small volume of serous fluid (about 5 mL) that reduces friction between the pericardial membranes as the heart moves within them.

The wall of the heart consists of three layers **FIGURE 8-84**:

- The **epicardium** protects the heart by reducing friction. This layer, which is the visceral portion of the pericardium on the surface of the heart, consists of connective tissue and some deep adipose tissue.
- The myocardium is the middle layer of the heart wall found between the epicardium and endocardium. Recall that the thick myocardium is made mostly of cardiac muscle tissue and is responsible for cardiac contraction and efficient ejection of blood from the heart. The myocardium has a large capillary supply to meet the heart's oxygen demands; most areas of the myocardium have a 1:1 ratio of capillaries to muscle cells.
- The **endocardium** comprises epithelium and connective tissue containing many elastic and collagenous fibers. This surface is smooth so that blood flow and platelets are not disrupted as they pass through the heart. This lining is continuous with the innermost lining of the blood vessels of the body.

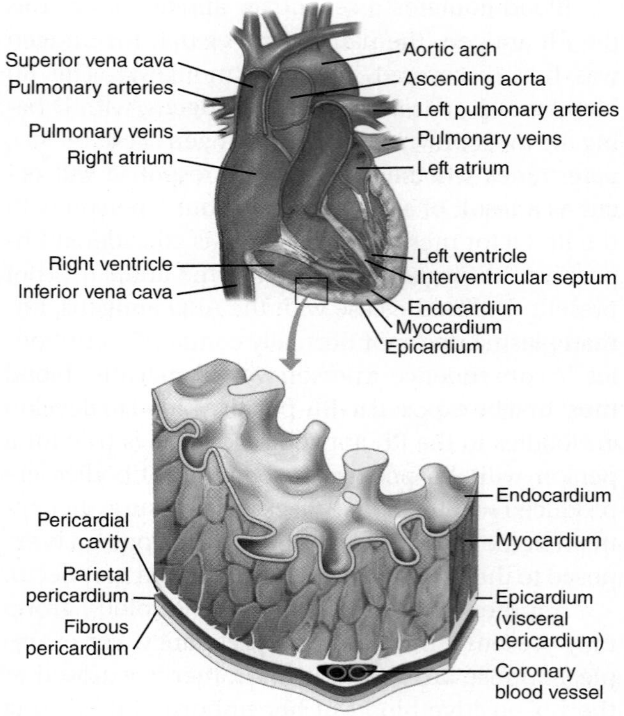

FIGURE 8-84 The three layers of the heart are the epicardium, myocardium, and endocardium.

Heart Chambers

The normal human heart consists of four chambers: two receiving chambers called **atria** and two pumping chambers called ventricles (see Figure 8-83). The heart is divided into right and left halves by a tough piece of tissue called the septum. The interatrial septum separates the two atria; a thicker wall, the interventricular septum, separates the right and left ventricles.

Cardiac Muscle

Cardiac muscle is unique to the heart. However, just like other muscles, its contraction occurs when calcium interferes with troponin and tropomyosin, allowing actin and myosin fibers to create cross links that pull against each other to contract (shorten).

Recall that cardiac muscle fibers are long, branching cells that fit together tightly at intercalated disks. The arrangement of these tight-fitting junctions gives an appearance of a syncytium; in other words, it resembles a network of cells with no separation between individual cells. The intercalated disks fit together and form gap junctions. By taking advantage of these gap junctions, an electrical impulse can be quickly conducted throughout the wall of a heart chamber. This characteristic allows the walls of both atria (and, likewise, the walls of both ventricles) to contract almost at the same time. The heart consists of two sets of chambers: atrial and ventricular.

Heart Valves

The heart has four valves: two **atrioventricular (AV) valves** and two **semilunar (SL) valves** **FIGURE 8-85**. The AV valves separate the atria from the ventricles. The right AV valve is the **tricuspid valve**, and the left AV valve is the **mitral valve** (bicuspid valve). These valves direct blood flow between the chambers as well as prevent backward flow during ventricular contraction (regurgitation). Fibrous bands of tissue called **chordae tendineae** are attached to each part, or cusp, of the valve. Attached to the chordae tendineae and endocardium of the ventricles are **papillary muscles**. During ventricular contraction (ventricular systole), the AV valves are closed because of increased pressure in the chamber. The papillary muscles also contract during ventricular systole, providing counterpressure to the cusps of the AV valves. This pressure prevents the AV valves from "blowing out" or being forced open into the atria. During ventricular relaxation (ventricular diastole), the papillary muscles relax and the AV valves open due to the force of blood flowing down from the atria to the ventricles.

The SL valves separate the ventricles and their associated great vessels. Each of these valves has three cusps. The right SL valve, also called the **pulmonic valve**, separates the right ventricle and the pulmonary trunk. The SL valve on the left. also known as the **aortic valve**, separates the left ventricle from the aorta. These valves have no tendon or muscular support. Moreover, their functioning solely relies on the relative pressure differences between the ventricles and great vessels they separate. When the ventricle contracts, the pressure in the ventricle exceeds the pressure in the pulmonary trunk; this causes the valve to open, allowing blood to enter the great vessel. When the pressure in the great vessel exceeds the pressure of the ventricle, the valve closes.

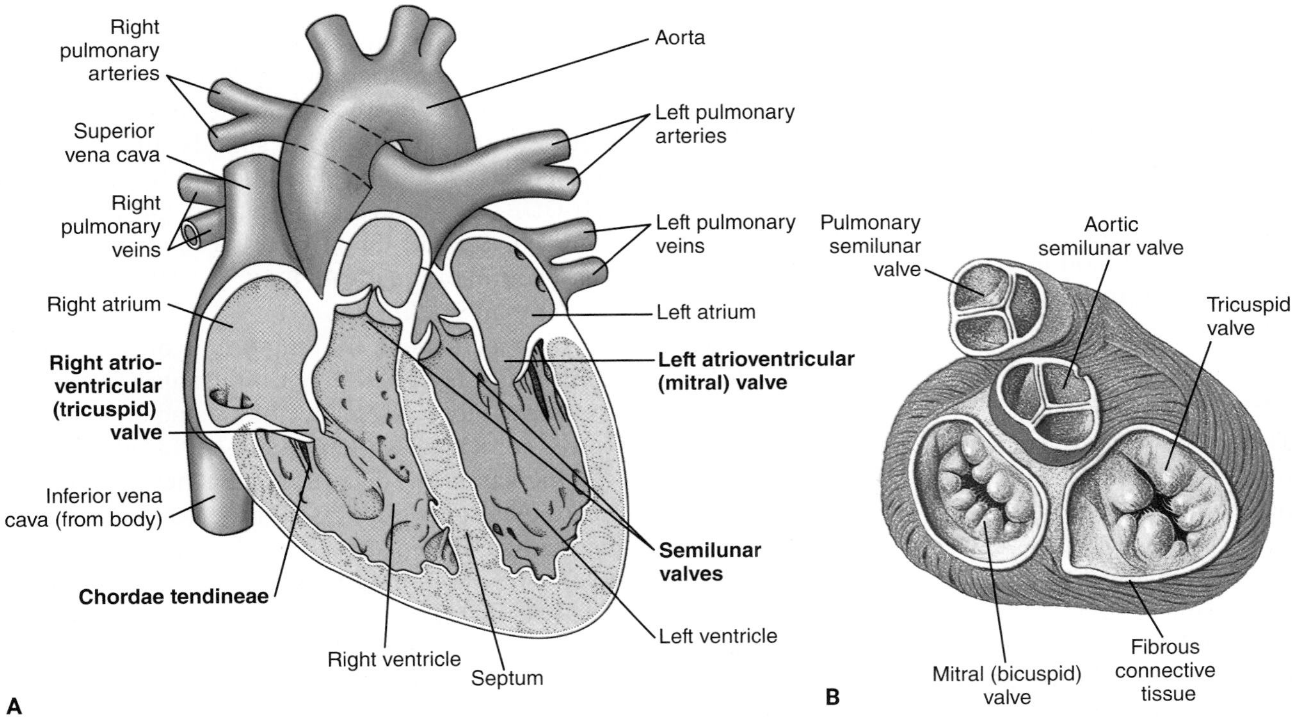

FIGURE 8-85 A. Heart valves. **B.** Cross section of heart valves.

Blood Flow Through the Cardiovascular System

The body's total blood volume can be divided as follows: systemic circulation (85%), pulmonary circulation (about 10%), and heart chambers (about 5%).[30] Blood enters the right atrium by way of the superior and inferior venae cavae and the coronary sinus (the venous drain for the coronary circulation). Approximately 70% to 80% of this blood flows passively from the right atrium through the tricuspid valve and into the right ventricle. The remaining 20% to 30% is forced into the right ventricle during atrial contraction (atrial kick). The right ventricle expels the blood through the pulmonic valve into the pulmonary trunk. The pulmonary trunk divides into a right and left pulmonary artery, each of which carries blood to one lung (pulmonary circulation; see Figure 8-80).

Blood flows through the pulmonary arteries to the lungs. Blood that is low in oxygen passes through the pulmonary capillaries. There it comes in direct contact with the alveolar-capillary membrane, where oxygen and carbon dioxide are exchanged. The newly oxygenated blood then flows into the **pulmonary veins**. The left atrium receives this oxygenated blood from the lungs via the four pulmonary veins (two from the right lung and two from the left lung). Again, 70% to 80% of the blood moves passively from the left atrium into the left ventricle through the mitral valve. The remaining 20% to 30% of the blood is forced into the ventricle through the atrial kick. With contraction of the left ventricle, blood is ejected through the aortic valve to the aorta. Blood is then distributed throughout the body (systemic circulation) through the aorta and its branches.

Cardiac Cycle

The **cardiac cycle** refers to a repetitive pumping process that includes all the events associated with blood flow through the heart. This cycle includes two phases for each heart chamber: systole and diastole. *Systole* is the period during which the chamber is contracting and blood is being ejected. The atria and ventricles each have a distinct systolic phase. **Diastole** is the period of relaxation during which the chambers are allowed to fill. The atria and ventricles each have a distinct diastolic phase. The myocardium receives its fresh supply of oxygenated blood from the coronary arteries during ventricular diastole. The cardiac cycle depends on the ability of the cardiac muscle to contract and on the condition of the conduction system of the heart. The efficiency of the heart as a pump may be affected by abnormalities of the cardiac muscle, valves, or conduction system.

During the cardiac cycle, pressure within each heart chamber rises in systole and falls in diastole. The valves of the heart ensure that blood flows in the proper direction and prevent backflow. Blood flows from one heart chamber to another if the pressure in the current chamber is greater than the pressure in the next. This pressure relationship depends on careful timing of contractions. The conduction system of the heart provides the necessary timing of events between atrial and ventricular systole.

Think of the heart as a two-sided pump. The low-pressure right side is responsible for pulmonary circulation, and the high-pressure left side is responsible for systemic circulation. Importantly, though, the atria and ventricles function together. As both atria undergo systole, the ventricles are in diastole; conversely, as both ventricles undergo systole, the atria are in diastole.

Heart Sounds

Heart sounds are created by the contraction and relaxation of the heart and the flow of blood. These sounds can be heard during auscultation with a stethoscope. Normal heart sounds are often described as sounding like "lub-DUB, lub-DUB, lub-DUB. . . ." The "lub" is called the first heart sound or S_1, and the "DUB" is called the second heart sound or S_2 **FIGURE 8-86**. S_2 ("DUB") is often louder than S_1 ("lub").

S_1 occurs near the beginning of ventricular contraction (systole), when the tricuspid and mitral valves close. Normally, the closing of these two valves coincides as the pressure within the ventricles increases. Any delay in closing these two valves, heard as a split sound, is considered abnormal. S_2 occurs near the end of ventricular contraction (systole), when the pulmonary and aortic valves close. The two valves can close simultaneously or with a slight delay between them under normal physiologic circumstances.

Two other heart sounds, S_3 and S_4, are not usually heard in people with normal heart sounds **FIGURE 8-87**. S_3 is a soft, low-pitched heart sound

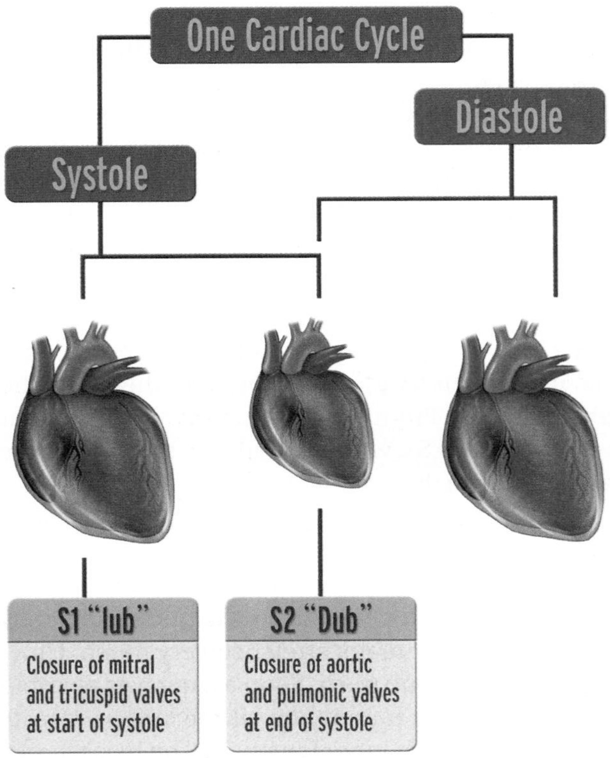

FIGURE 8-86 The normal S_1 and S_2 heart sounds

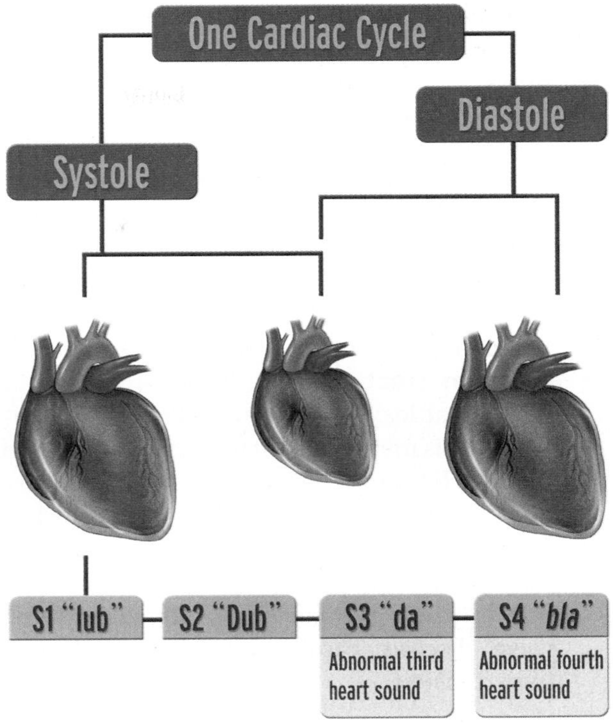

FIGURE 8-87 The abnormal S_3 and S_4 heart sounds.

that occurs about one-third of the way through ventricular diastole. It is caused by vibrations of the ventricular walls, resulting from the rapid filling period of the ventricle during the beginning of diastole. When an S_3 sound is present, the heart beat cycle is described as sounding like "lub-DUB-da." S_3 is sometimes present in healthy children and in young adults. When this heart sound is heard in older adults, it is often associated with abnormally increased filling pressures in the atria secondary to moderate to severe heart failure.

S_4 is a medium-pitched heart sound that occurs immediately before the normal S_1 sound. When an S_4 sound is present, the heart contraction cycle sounds like "bla-lub-DUB." This heart sound represents either decreased stretching (compliance) of the left ventricle or increased pressure in the atria, and is almost always a signal of an abnormality in the heart.

Other sounds, all abnormal, may be heard when you auscultate the heart and great vessels. Some of these sounds are easy to auscultate; others may require years of experience to identify. These sounds include murmurs, bruits, ejection clicks, and opening snaps. A **murmur** is an abnormal whooshing sound heard over the heart that indicates turbulent blood flow through the heart valves. Although many murmurs are functional (benign) and often go away, several are characteristic of heart disease. A **bruit** is an abnormal whooshing sound heard over a main blood vessel that indicates turbulent blood flow within the blood vessel. A bruit often indicates localized atherosclerotic disease (plaque formation in the arteries). Both ejection clicks and opening snaps indicate abnormal cardiac valve function. They occur at different times in the cardiac cycle, depending on which valve is diseased. Although these sounds are clinically significant, most of them are fleeting and difficult to hear.

Cardiac Output

It is necessary to learn the following technical terms to understand how the heart functions as a pump:

- **Cardiac output (CO).** The amount of blood that is pumped by the ventricles in 1 minute. The left and right ventricles are approximately equal in interior size, so they have relatively equivalent outputs. Normal CO for an average adult is 5 to 6 L/min.

- **Stroke volume (SV).** The amount of blood pumped out by either ventricle in a single cardiac contraction (heartbeat). Normally, the SV is between 60 and 100 mL for a healthy adult, but the heart has considerable capacity and can easily increase SV by at least 50%.
- **Heart rate (HR).** The number of cardiac contractions per minute (pulse rate). The normal HR for an adult at rest is 60 to 100 beats/min.
- **Ejection fraction (EF).** The percentage of blood that leaves the heart each time it contracts. This measurement is usually taken from only the left ventricle because it is the primary pump for the heart. The left ventricular EF has a normal range of 55% to 70% in an adult, but may be lower if the heart sustains some type of damage (eg, myocardial infarction, heart valve disease, cardiomyopathy, or chronic hypertension).

The heart must be able to increase its output several times over in response to changes in the body's demand for oxygen. For example, the heart's oxygen demand is increased during exercise and decreased during sleep. CO is a function of both the SV and the HR. This relationship is mathematically expressed as follows:

$$CO = SV \times HR$$

For example, if SV is 70 mL and HR is 80 beats/min, CO would be 70 mL × 80 beats/min, or 5,600 mL/min (5.6 L/min). This equation indicates that the heart can increase its output by increasing its SV, increasing its rate, or both. Factors that influence SV, HR, or both will affect CO and, therefore, oxygen delivery (perfusion) to tissue.

SV is influenced by preload, afterload, and the contractile state (contraction or relaxation) of the myocardium. **Preload** (end-diastolic volume) is the volume of blood in the ventricle at the end of diastole and primarily reflects venous return (the amount of blood returned to the heart).[31] **Afterload** is the force against which the ventricles must contract to eject blood. Afterload is influenced by arterial BP, arterial distensibility (the stretching ability of the arteries), and arterial resistance. The greater the afterload, the harder the ventricle must work to pump the blood.

The heart has several ways of increasing SV. One characteristic of cardiac muscle is that when it is stretched, it contracts with greater force, up to a limit—a property called the *Frank-Starling mechanism,* or Starling's law. If an increased blood volume is returned from the systemic veins to the right side of the heart or from the pulmonary veins to the left side of the heart, then the muscle surrounding the cardiac chambers must stretch to accommodate this larger volume. The more the cardiac muscle stretches, the greater the force of its contraction, the more completely it empties, and, therefore, the greater the SV. From the CO equation, it is clear that any increase in SV, with HR held constant, will cause an increase in the overall CO.

To visualize this relationship, think of a latex balloon. If you blow up the balloon a bit and then let the air escape, the air exits slowly and with little force. This outcome reflects that the elastic walls of the balloon were not stretched very much. However, if you blow up the balloon as much as possible without popping it and then let the air out, it exits quickly and much more forcefully. The heart works the same way. If the walls are stretched a bit, then a small amount of blood is released. If the walls are stretched a great deal, then a large amount of blood is released.

As mentioned earlier, the pressure under which a ventricle fills (preload) is influenced by the volume of blood returned by the veins to the heart. In situations of increased oxygen demand, the body returns more blood to the heart (preload increases), and CO consequently increases through the Frank-Starling mechanism. In a diseased heart, the same mechanism is used to achieve a normal resting CO (which explains why some diseased hearts become enlarged).

The heart can also vary the degree of contraction of its muscle without changing the stretch on the muscle—a property called contractility. Changes in contractility may be induced by medications that have a positive or negative **inotropic effect** (*inotropic* means "affecting the contractility of muscle tissue"). The ventricles are never completely emptied of blood with any single heartbeat. However, if the heart squeezes into a tighter ball when it contracts, then a larger percentage of ventricular blood will be ejected, thereby increasing SV and overall CO. The nervous system regulates the contractility of the heart from heartbeat to heartbeat. When the body requires increased CO, the nerves signal that myocardial contractility should increase, thereby augmenting SV.

The heart can also increase its CO, given a constant SV, by increasing the number of contractions per minute—that is, by increasing the HR. Increasing the rate of contraction is known as a positive **chronotropic effect**.

The Frank-Starling mechanism is an intrinsic property of heart muscle, meaning that it is not under nervous system control. By contrast, contractility and changes in the HR are regulated by the nervous system.

Blood Pressure

Blood pressure is the pressure that the blood exerts against the walls of the arteries as it passes through them. As mentioned earlier, systole and diastole are the phases in the cardiac cycle in which the left ventricle contracts and relaxes, respectively. The pulsed forceful ejection of blood from the left ventricle of the heart into the aorta is transmitted through the arteries as a pulsatile pressure wave. This pressure wave keeps the blood moving through the body.

Measuring BP is one method to evaluate the effectiveness of CO. BP is a function of both CO and **systemic vascular resistance** (the resistance to blood flow within all blood vessels except the pulmonary vessels). The resistance to the flow of blood is determined by the diameter of the blood vessel and the tone (the normal state of balanced tension in body tissues) of the vascular musculature. A dilated (widened) vessel offers less resistance to blood flow, whereas a constricted (narrowed) vessel offers more resistance to this flow.

Coronary Circulation

Like all cells in the body, myocardial cells require an uninterrupted supply of oxygen and nutrients. However, cardiac oxygen demand is particularly unrelenting because the heart never stops to rest (at least, not without catastrophic consequences). To support this ever-present demand, the heart needs a reliable blood supply. Oxygenated blood reaches the heart through the coronary arteries **FIGURE 8-88**, which branch off the aorta at the coronary ostia, located just above the leaflets of the aortic valve. The coronary arteries are the first vessels that receive blood after left ventricular contraction.

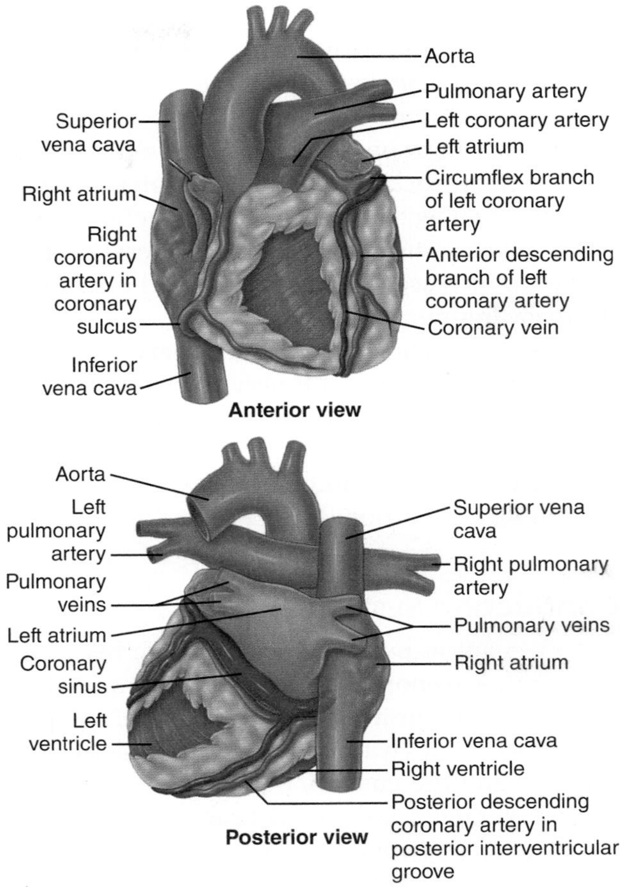

FIGURE 8-88 The two main coronary arteries and their branches supply the heart with blood.

Because the coronary arteries are compressed during ventricular systole, they fill only during ventricular diastole.

The two main coronary arteries are the left and right coronary arteries. The left main coronary artery is the largest and shortest of the myocardial blood vessels. It rapidly divides into the **left anterior descending artery** and the **circumflex coronary artery**, both of which branch widely to supply the more muscular left ventricle of the heart along with the interventricular septum and part of the right ventricle. The **right coronary artery** travels between the right atrium and right ventricle through the AV groove. Branches of this artery supply blood to the right atrium and ventricle walls, a portion of the inferior part of the left ventricle, and portions of the conduction system.

The numerous connections (anastomoses) between the arterioles of the various coronary arteries allow for the development of alternative routes of blood flow. In the early stages of coronary heart disease, the inside diameter of the coronary arteries begins to narrow as plaque is deposited on the vessel walls. In response to the decreased ability to perfuse the myocardium, additional blood vessels form that connect arterioles originating from other blood vessels. The result of this *collateral circulation* is an increase in oxygenated blood delivery to the myocardium.

The arteries and the main coronary vein cross the heart in a groove (coronary sulcus) that separates the atria from the ventricles. Venous blood empties into the **coronary sinus**, a large vessel in the posterior part of the coronary sulcus, which in turn ends in the right atrium of the heart.

Conduction System

The mechanical pumping action of the heart can occur only in response to an electrical stimulus. This impulse causes the heart to beat via a set of complex chemical changes within the myocardial cells. Both the CNS and the endocrine system can influence the rate, strength, and speed of contraction.

In general, cardiac cells have either a mechanical (contractile) function or an electrical (pacemaker) function. Myocardial cells (working cells) contain contractile filaments. When these cells are electrically stimulated, the contractile filaments slide together, and the myocardial cell contracts. These myocardial cells form the thin, muscular layer of the atrial walls and the thicker muscular layer of the ventricular walls (the myocardium). These cells do not normally generate electrical impulses on their own. Pacemaker cells (conducting cells) are specialized cells of the electrical system of the heart that are responsible for spontaneously generating and conducting electrical impulses. Myocardial cells respond to impulses from the pacemaker cells by contracting.

Cardiac cells demonstrate four essential properties that help the heart to function as an efficient machine: (1) automaticity, (2) excitability, (3) conductivity, and (4) contractility. **Automaticity** is the ability of cardiac pacemaker cells to create an electrical impulse without being stimulated from another source. As discussed previously, excitability refers to the ability of cardiac muscle cells to respond to a stimulus. Conductivity enables a cardiac cell to receive an electrical impulse and pass it on to an adjoining cardiac cell. Contractility refers to the ability of myocardial cells to shorten in response to an impulse, which results in contraction.

Pacemakers of the Heart

The cardiac conduction system consists of six parts: the sinoatrial (SA) node, atrioventricular (AV) node, bundle of His, right and left bundle branches, and Purkinje fibers **FIGURE 8-89**.

The **sinoatrial (SA) node**, a mass of specialized tissue located high in the right atrium, is the normal site of origin of the electrical impulse. Cells of the SA node can reach threshold on their own, enabling them to initiate impulses through the myocardium, which stimulate contraction of cardiac muscle fibers. Because it creates these impulses more frequently than other sites in the heart, the SA node is the most common natural pacemaker. The impulse then travels to the **atrioventricular (AV) node**. The AV node is a group of cells composed of thin fibers, which is located in the floor of the right atrium immediately behind the tricuspid valve and near the opening of the coronary sinus. The AV node delays the impulse, allowing atrial systole to occur before ventricular systole starts.

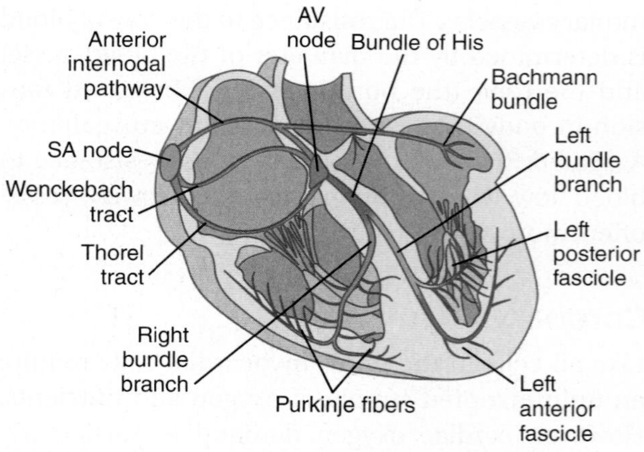

FIGURE 8-89 The electrical conduction system of the heart. Impulses originating in the sinoatrial (SA) node spread through the atria and along the internodal pathways to the atrioventricular (AV) node. The impulses travel from the AV node down the bundle of His and the right and left bundle branches and into the Purkinje network of the ventricles. Note that the Bachmann bundle is an interatrial pathway that initiates depolarization of the left atrium.

After passing through the AV node, the impulse enters the **bundle of His**, which is located in the upper portion of the interventricular septum. From there, it proceeds rapidly to the right and left bundle branches. The right bundle branch innervates the right ventricle. The left bundle branch spreads the electrical impulse to the interventricular septum and left ventricle, the walls of which are thicker and more muscular than the right ventricle. The right and left bundle branches divide into increasingly smaller branches, and finally into a fibrous network called the **Purkinje fibers**. The impulse spreads out, via the Purkinje fibers, first to the left myocardium, and then to the right ventricular myocardium, resulting in ventricular contraction or systole.

Regulation of Heart Function

The sympathetic division of the ANS innervates the heart through cardiac nerves. Branches of the vagus nerves provide parasympathetic innervation. Networks of these sympathetic and parasympathetic fibers form cardiac plexuses near the arch of the aorta. From the cardiac plexuses, fibers course along the base of the heart on the surface of the great vessels and are distributed to the various heart chambers.[32] The fibers then penetrate the myocardium, usually along the right and left coronary arteries. Although most of the fibers terminate in the SA node, some end in the AV node and in the atrial myocardium. A few parasympathetic fibers extend to the ventricles.

Stimulation of sympathetic (accelerator) nerves results in an increased force of contraction and increased HR. Increases in HR shorten all phases of the cardiac cycle. When the length of time for ventricular relaxation is shortened, less time is available for the ventricles to fill adequately with blood. Stimulation of parasympathetic (inhibitory) nerve fibers slows the discharge rate of the SA node, slows conduction through the AV node, decreases the strength of atrial contraction, and can cause a small decrease in the force of ventricular contraction.

Other factors that influence HR include electrolyte and hormone levels, metabolic rate, medications, stress, anxiety, fear, and body temperature.

Blood Vessels and Circulation

The vasculature is a closed system of vessels that distributes blood from the heart to the body's tissues and returns blood from the tissues to the heart (see Figure 8-80). It can be divided into the following components: (1) the arterial system, which takes blood from the heart and distributes it to the tissues; (2) the venous system, which returns blood from the tissues to the heart; and (3) the microcirculation, where nutrients and cellular waste products are exchanged between the blood and tissues.

Blood vessels are composed of different layers of elastic tissue and smooth muscle called tunics. The innermost layer is the **tunica intima**, or endothelium **FIGURE 8-90**. It is composed of a single layer of epithelial cells and provides almost no resistance to blood flow. The middle layer, the **tunica media**, is composed of elastic connective tissue and smooth muscle cells that support the vessel walls. The smooth muscle tissue of this layer is innervated by nerve fibers of the ANS, which can alter the diameter of the lumen of the vessel. The outermost layer of blood vessels is the **tunica adventitia**, which is composed of nerves and connective tissue that contains elastic and collagenous fibers. The collagenous fibers of the tunica adventitia help hold the vessel open and are the means by which the vessel attaches to nearby body tissues. Tiny blood vessels called the vasa vasorum extend from the tunica adventitia to the tunica media, providing the blood supply for the tissues of the vessel wall. The opening within the blood vessel is called the lumen.

Although each blood vessel may hold only a small amount of blood, the total volume of all vessels in the body forms a large container when considered as a whole. The size of this container is dynamic; that is, it changes in response to conditions present within and outside of the body. For example, if the body becomes moderately or severely dehydrated, then the amount of circulating blood volume falls. If the total volume of the circulatory system (the container) were to remain constant during this scenario, then the patient's SV, BP, and CO could decrease significantly. The blood vessels receive constant feedback from the ANS to prevent this undesirable outcome. If baroreceptors in the central circulation detect a decrease in pressure, then the blood vessels constrict to shrink the size of the container proportionally. These adjustments are coordinated by a wide array of feedback mechanisms, which collectively act to maintain homeostasis. In some cases, the ANS also changes the distribution of blood by constricting peripheral blood vessels to a greater degree than the blood

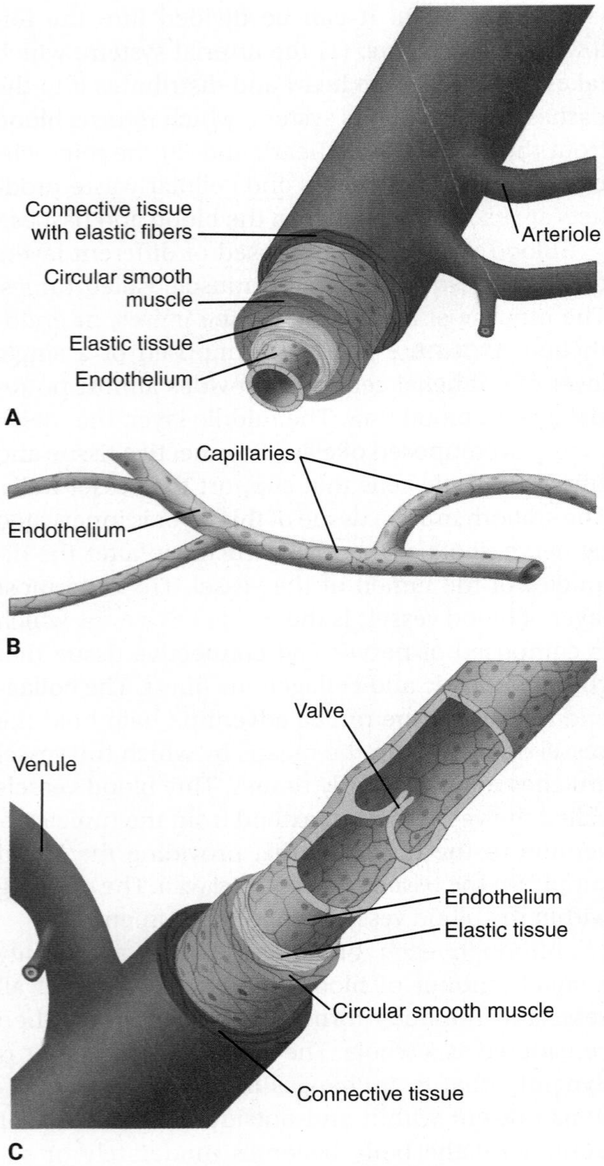

FIGURE 8-90 The walls of the blood vessels are composed of three layers of tissue: the endothelium (tunica intima), elastic tissue (tunica media), and connective tissue (tunica adventitia). **A.** Artery. **B.** Capillary. **C.** Vein.

vessels supplying the vital organs. This process, known as shunting, is a sign of shock.

Arterial System

The arteries make up the body's distribution system **FIGURE 8-91**. The aorta is the largest artery of the body, and its branches deliver blood to all body organs and tissues. The aorta has three main regions: (1) the ascending aorta, (2) the aortic arch, and the (3) descending aorta. The *ascending aorta* originates from the base of the heart and terminates by becoming the arch of the aorta. The aorta curves posteriorly and to the left at the level of the second costal cartilage and forms the segment called the *aortic arch*. The aortic arch descends to vertebral level T4 and continues inferiorly as the **descending aorta**. The descending aorta is named according to its location within the body cavities. The thoracic aorta is the portion of the descending aorta that extends from the aortic arch to the diaphragm. The thoracic aorta ends by passing through the diaphragm to become the abdominal aorta at about vertebral level T12. The main divisions of the aorta and its principal branches are shown in **TABLE 8-37**.

Conducting arteries are large arteries that arise from the aorta and its main branches. Because their function is to transport blood under high pressure to the tissues, these vessels are equipped with more elastic tissue and less smooth muscle, allowing them to stretch under great pressures and quickly return to their original shape. Examples of large arteries include the aorta and the brachiocephalic, common carotid, common iliac, and subclavian arteries. The elasticity of large arteries helps to reduce the heart's workload. If these arteries were rigid rather than elastic, then the pressure would rise dramatically during systole. This increased pressure would require the ventricles to pump against increased afterload, thereby increasing the work of the heart. In reality, as blood is ejected into these vessels, they distend, which reduces the resultant increase in systolic BP, and thus the work of the heart.[32]

Medium and small arteries are called distributing arteries or muscular arteries. These arteries supply individual organs and larger amounts of smooth muscle, which gives the body the ability to adjust blood flow. Examples include the brachial, gastric, and superior mesenteric arteries.

The smallest of the arteries are arterioles (resistance vessels). The strong muscular walls of these vessels act as stopcocks through which blood is released into the capillaries.

The Head and Neck

The brachiocephalic artery is the first vessel to branch from the aortic arch. It is relatively short and rapidly divides into the right common carotid

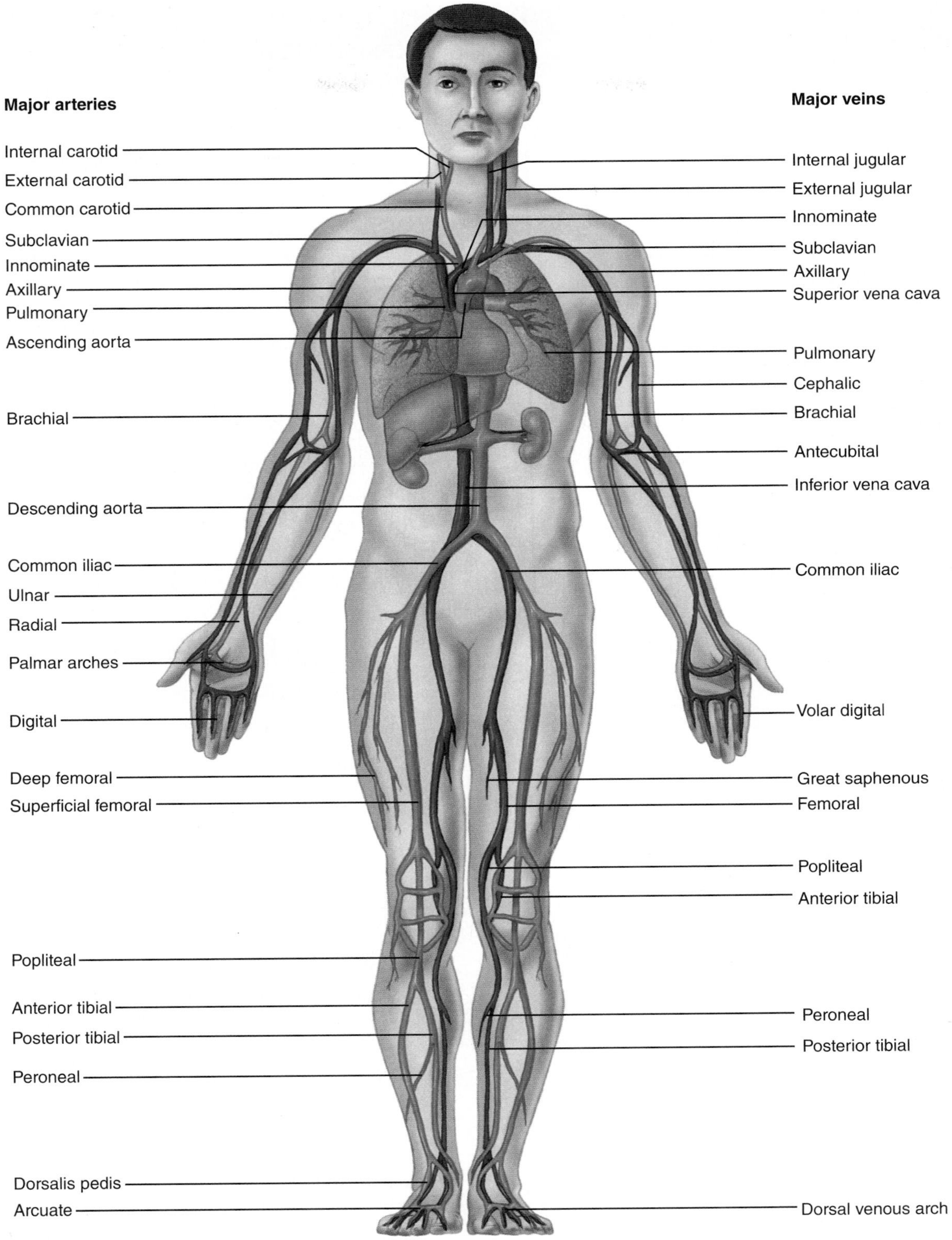
Major arteries
Internal carotid
External carotid
Common carotid
Subclavian
Innominate
Axillary
Pulmonary
Ascending aorta
Brachial
Descending aorta
Common iliac
Ulnar
Radial
Palmar arches
Digital
Deep femoral
Superficial femoral
Popliteal
Anterior tibial
Posterior tibial
Peroneal
Dorsalis pedis
Arcuate
Major veins
Internal jugular
External jugular
Innominate
Subclavian
Axillary
Superior vena cava
Pulmonary
Cephalic
Brachial
Antecubital
Inferior vena cava
Common iliac
Volar digital
Great saphenous
Femoral
Popliteal
Anterior tibial
Peroneal
Posterior tibial
Dorsal venous arch

FIGURE 8-91 The major arteries and veins.

TABLE 8-37 Major Arteries

Branch of the Aorta	Artery	Area Supplied
Ascending	Right and left coronary arteries	Myocardium
Aortic arch	Brachiocephalic (innominate)	Head and neck, shoulder, upper extremity
	Common carotid	Head and neck
	Subclavian	Head and upper extremity
Descending (Thoracic)		
Visceral branches	Supply the organs contained within the thorax	
	Bronchial	Bronchi of lungs
	Esophageal	Esophagus
Parietal branches	Supply the wall of the thoracic cavity	
	Posterior intercostal	Intercostal muscles, lateral rib cage
	Subcostal	Chest wall
	Superior phrenic	Superior surface of diaphragm
Descending (Abdominal)		
Visceral branches	Supply the organs contained within the abdomen	
	Celiac trunk	Esophagus, liver, pancreas, spleen, stomach
	Inferior mesenteric	Descending colon, rectum
	Middle suprarenal arteries	Adrenal gland
	Ovarian	Ovary, fallopian tube, ureter
	Renal	Kidney
	Superior mesenteric	Colon, pancreas, small intestine
	Testicular	Testis, ureter
Parietal branches	Supply the walls of the abdomen	
	Common iliac	Pelvis, lower extremity
	Inferior phrenic	Inferior surface of diaphragm, adrenal gland
	Lumbar	Back muscles, lumbar vertebrae
	Median sacral	Sacrum

artery and right subclavian artery. The carotid arteries transport blood to the head and neck, whereas the subclavian arteries transport blood to the upper extremities.

Each common carotid artery branches at the angle of the mandible into the internal and external carotid arteries. This point of division is called the carotid bifurcation. A slight dilation at this bifurcation, the carotid sinus, contains structures that are important in regulating BP. Branches of the external carotid artery supply blood to the face, nose, and mouth. The internal carotid arteries, together with the vertebral arteries (branches of the subclavian arteries), supply blood to the brain **FIGURE 8-92**.

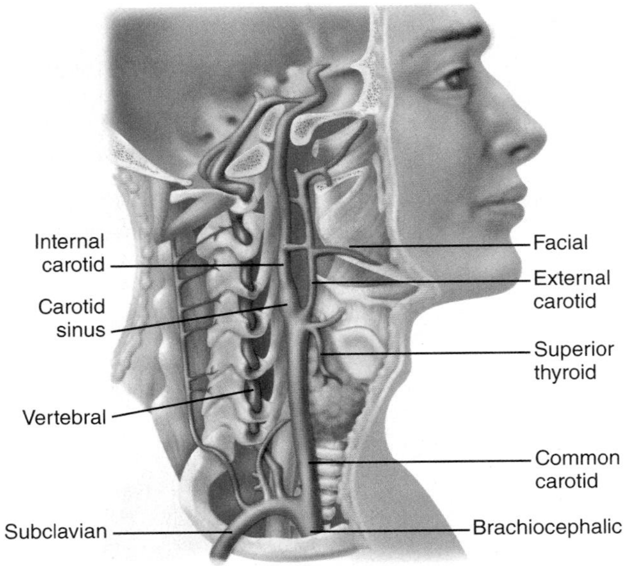

FIGURE 8-92 The arteries of the head and neck.

The Upper Extremity

The subclavian artery supplies blood to the brain, neck, anterior chest wall, and shoulder. Shortly after its point of origin, the subclavian artery gives rise to the vertebral arteries. The subclavian system then continues from the thorax into the upper extremity. It becomes the axillary artery at the shoulder joint, then the brachial artery below the head of the humerus. The brachial artery divides into the ulnar and radial arteries **FIGURE 8-93**.

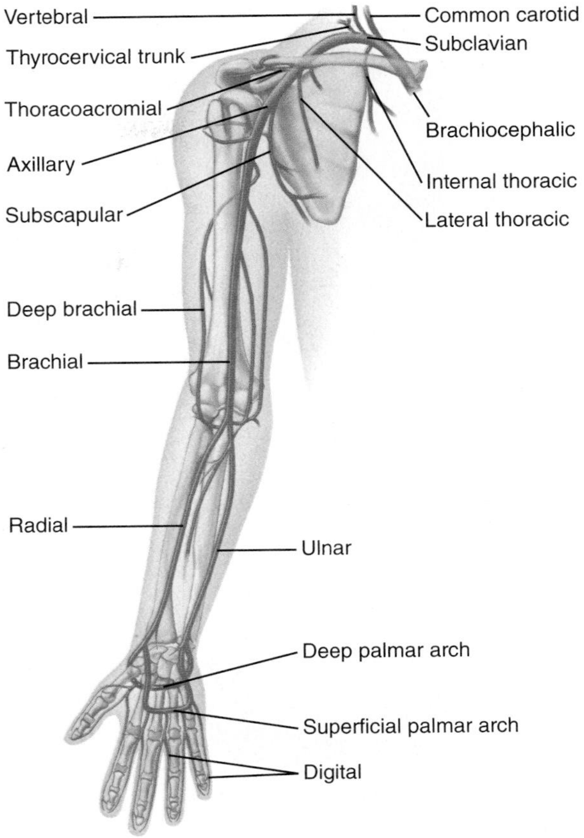

FIGURE 8-93 The arteries of the upper extremity.

The Thoracic Aorta

Two branches of arteries make up the thoracic aorta: the visceral arteries and the parietal arteries. The visceral arteries supply blood to the thoracic organs, and the parietal arteries supply blood to the thoracic wall.

The intercostal arteries run along the ribs and provide circulation to the chest wall. These arteries branch into the anterior and posterior intercostal arteries. The anterior intercostal arteries originate as branches of the subclavian system; the posterior intercostal arteries arise directly from the aorta. Visceral branches of the thoracic aorta supply the bronchial arteries in the lungs and the esophageal arteries.

The Abdominal Aorta

Like their thoracic counterparts, the branches of the abdominal aorta are divided into visceral and parietal portions. The visceral arteries are subdivided into paired and nonpaired arteries: The three major unpaired branches are the celiac trunk, superior mesenteric, and inferior mesenteric arteries **FIGURE 8-94**. The celiac trunk supplies blood to the esophagus, stomach, duodenum, spleen, liver, and pancreas **FIGURE 8-95**. The superior mesenteric artery and its branches supply blood to the pancreas, small intestine, and colon. The inferior mesenteric artery and its branches supply blood to the descending colon and rectum. The paired branches of the visceral abdominal aorta supply blood to the kidneys, adrenal gland, and gonads. The parietal branches supply blood to the diaphragm and abdominal wall.

The Pelvis and Lower Extremity

At the level of the fifth lumbar vertebra, the aorta divides into the two common iliac arteries. These arteries further divide into the internal iliac arteries, which supply blood to the pelvis, and the

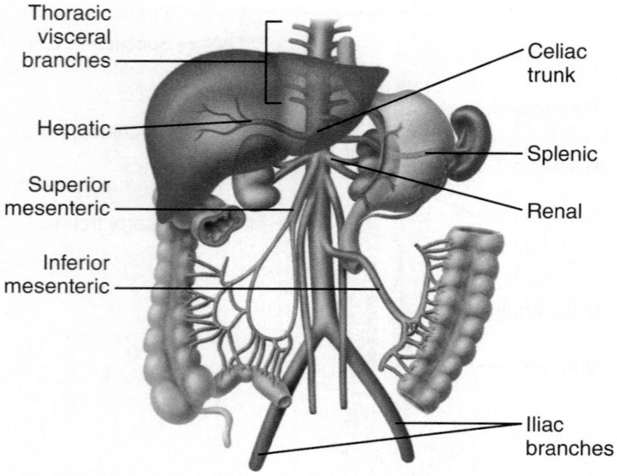

FIGURE 8-94 The branches of the abdominal aorta.

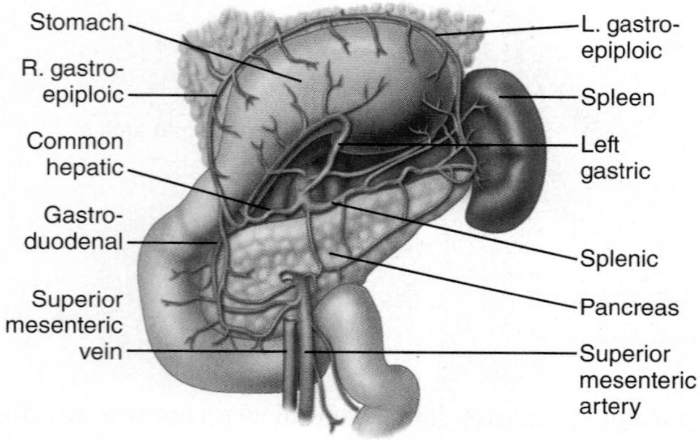

FIGURE 8-95 The celiac trunk and superior mesenteric vessels.

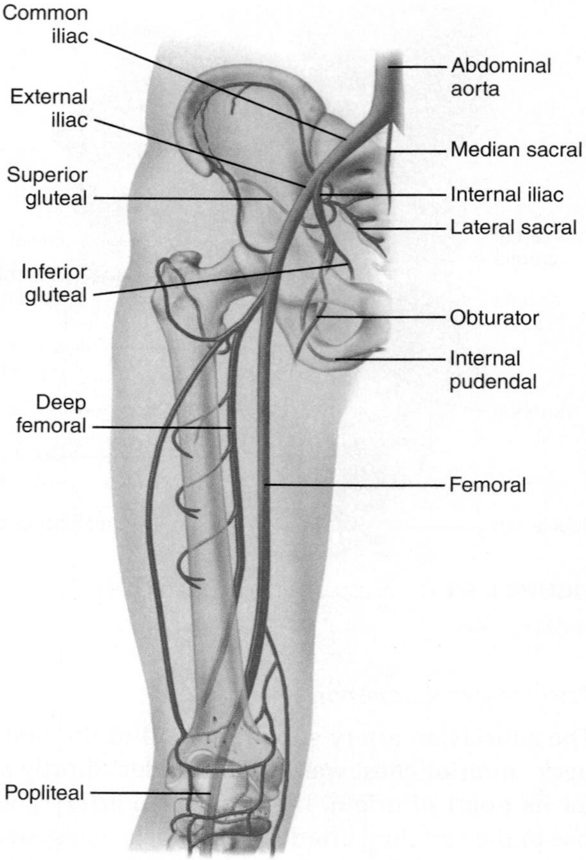

FIGURE 8-96 The arteries of the pelvis and thigh.

external iliac arteries, which enter the lower extremity **FIGURE 8-96**. The internal iliac artery sends out visceral branches to the rectum, vagina, uterus, and ovary. Parietal branches supply blood to the sacrum, gluteal muscles of the buttocks region, pubic region, rectum, external genitalia, and proximal thigh.

Like the vessels of the upper extremity, the vessels of the lower extremity form a continuum. The external iliac arteries become the femoral arteries. Each femoral artery supplies blood to the thigh, external genitalia, anterior abdominal wall, and knee. The femoral artery becomes the popliteal artery in the lower thigh. Each popliteal artery then branches into the anterior tibial, posterior tibial, and peroneal arteries. At the foot, the anterior tibial artery becomes the dorsalis pedis artery. Plantar arteries arise from the posterior tibial artery and subdivide into digital branches that supply blood to the toes **FIGURE 8-97**.

Venous System

In essence, the venous system acts as a collection system (see Figure 8-91). Venules, the smallest of the venous vessels, have very little smooth muscle in their middle layer. Venules are called capacitance (storage) vessels because they are capable of holding large amounts of blood. Because 70% of the body's blood is contained in the venous system, the veins are able to adjust the blood volume returning to the heart (preload) so that the needs of the body can be met when cardiac output is altered, such as in shock.[32] Venous blood flow depends on skeletal muscle action, respiratory movements, and gravity. Medium and large veins have valves within them

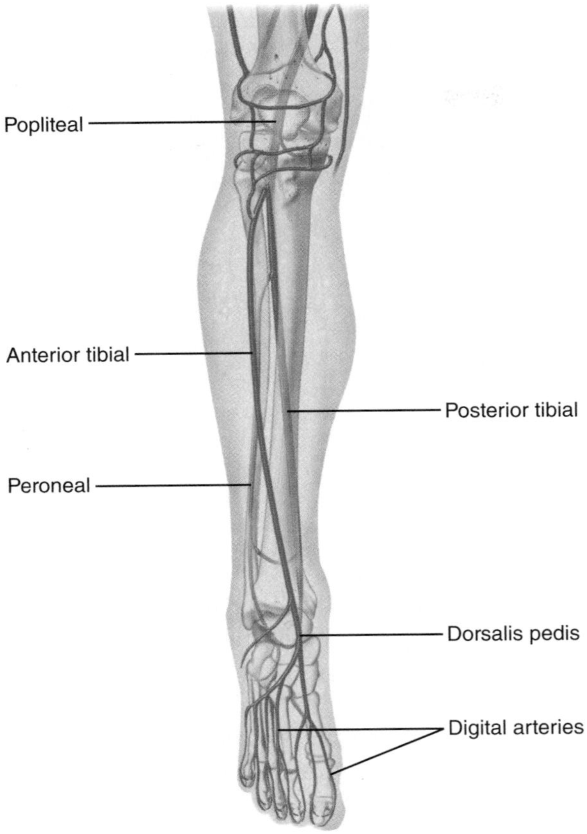

FIGURE 8-97 The arteries of the lower extremity.

TABLE 8-38 Major Veins

Vein	Areas Drained
Veins That Empty Into the Superior Vena Cava	
Azygos	Bronchi, esophagus, mediastinum, pericardium, posterior wall of thorax and abdomen
Brachiocephalic (innominate)	Head, neck, upper extremity
External jugular	Muscles and skin of face, neck, and scalp
Internal jugular	Brain, skull
Subclavian	Mammary glands, upper extremity
Veins That Empty Into the Inferior Vena Cava	
Common iliac	Lower extremities
Hepatic	Liver
Ovarian	Ovaries
Renal	Kidneys
Testicular	Testes

that prevent a backward flow of blood. Veins of the arms and legs have more valves than other veins of the body, preventing the backflow of blood in response to gravity.

The venules gradually increase in thickness and become medium-size vessels. As they approach the heart, veins become progressively larger. The two largest veins of the body are the superior vena cava and inferior vena cava, which empty into the right atrium. In the pulmonary circulation, the pulmonary veins transport oxygenated blood from the lungs to the heart's left atrium. From the systemic circulation, veins transport blood with a reduced oxygen content from the body tissues to the heart's right atrium. The major veins of the body and the areas they drain of blood are shown in **TABLE 8-38**.

The Head and Neck

The two major veins that drain the head and neck of blood are the external and internal jugular veins. The external jugular vein is more superficial and often is visible immediately beneath the skin. It primarily drains the posterior head and neck. The internal jugular vein drains the cranial vault as well as the anterior portion of the head, face, and neck. Spaces between the membranes surrounding the brain form venous sinuses; these sinuses are the primary means of venous drainage from the brain and feed into the internal jugular vein.

The external and internal jugular veins join the subclavian veins (the proximal part of the main vein of the arm) to form the brachiocephalic veins, which drain into the superior vena cava **FIGURE 8-98**.

The Upper Extremity

The veins of the upper extremity vary somewhat from person to person **FIGURE 8-99**. The names of the veins of the hands, wrists, and forearm follow the arteries of the same name. In the upper forearm, these veins combine to form the basilic vein and the cephalic vein, the major veins of the arm. The basilic and cephalic veins combine to form the axillary vein, which drains into the subclavian vein.

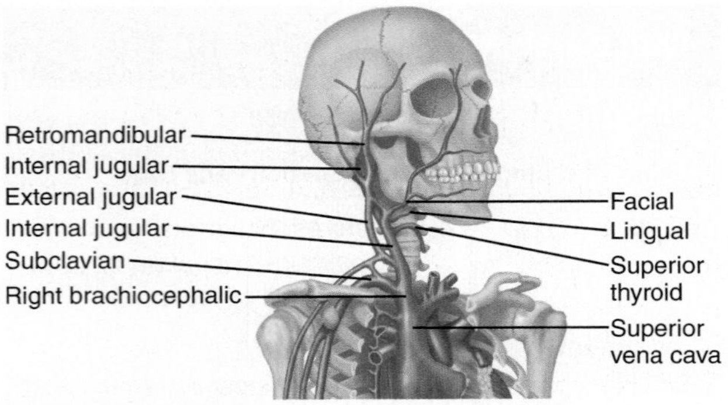

FIGURE 8-98 The veins of the head and neck.

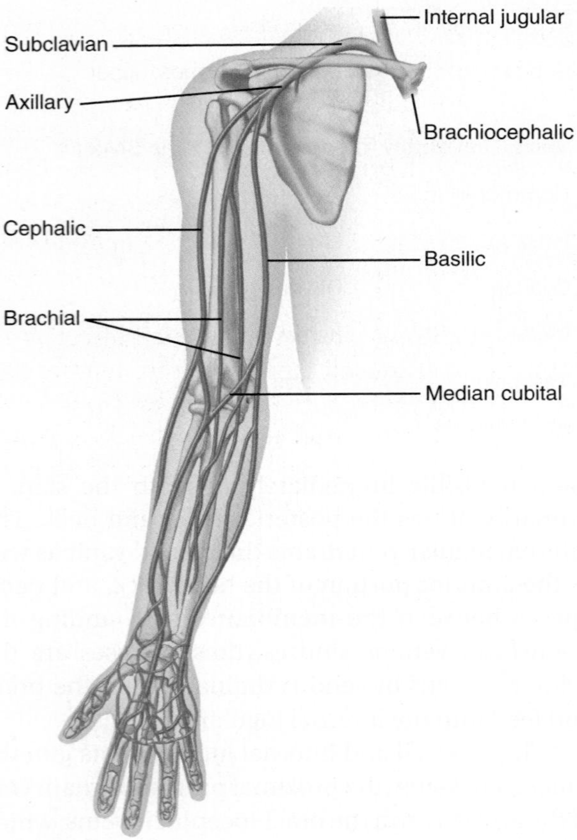

FIGURE 8-99 The veins of the upper extremity.

The Thorax

In the thorax, venous drainage begins at the anterior and posterior intercostal veins. The intercostal veins empty into the azygos vein on the right side of the thorax and into the hemiazygos vein on the left side. These veins, and the right and left brachiocephalic veins, provide the major source of flow into the superior vena cava.

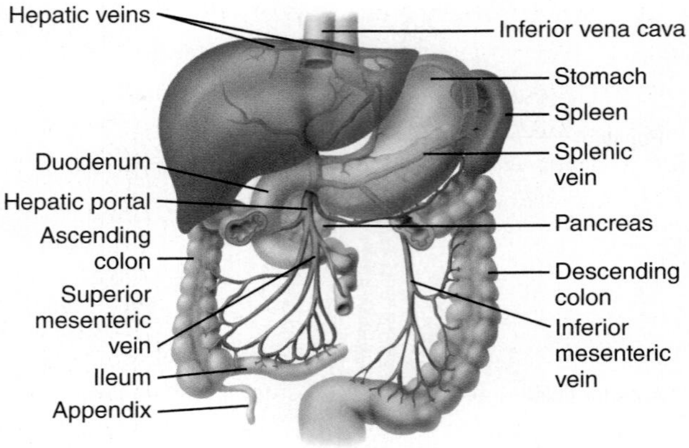

FIGURE 8-100 The hepatic portal system.

The Abdomen and Pelvis

Ultimately, all venous drainage from the lower part of the body passes through the inferior vena cava. The inferior vena cava returns deoxygenated blood from the lower parts of the body to the right atrium for **oxygenation**, the process of loading oxygen molecules onto hemoglobin molecules in the bloodstream. Within the abdominal and pelvic cavities, veins of the same name accompany the major arteries, providing venous drainage from structures including the kidney, adrenal glands, gonads, and diaphragm. The internal iliac veins drain the pelvis, and the external iliac veins drain the lower limbs. The internal and external iliac veins combine in the pelvis, forming the common iliac veins, which then combine to form the inferior vena cava.

Hepatic Portal Circulation

The **hepatic portal system** is a specialized part of the venous system that carries capillary blood rich in digestive nutrients from the digestive organs to the liver. Venous blood from most abdominal organs is returned directly to the inferior vena cava. However, venous blood from the gallbladder, intestines, pancreas, spleen, and stomach first enters the hepatic portal system before being transported to the liver and then to the inferior vena cava **FIGURE 8-100**. The portal system encompasses the passage of blood returning from the digestive tract through two sets of capillaries before it returns to the heart—first the capillaries of the abdominal organs, and then the liver capillaries. The hepatic portal vein collects blood from capillaries in the abdominal organs, enters the liver, and ultimately ends as a capillary bed, where the liver extracts needed nutrients from the blood and stores others. Hepatic veins drain the capillary beds of the hepatic portal vein. The hepatic veins return blood to the inferior vena cava, which empties into the right atrium of the heart

The Lower Extremity

The longest vein in the body is the great saphenous vein, which drains the foot, leg, and thigh. The saphenous vein originates over the dorsal and medial sides of the foot, ascends along the medial side of the leg and thigh, and empties into the femoral vein, which then drains into the external iliac vein. Laterally, the small saphenous vein helps drain the leg and lateral side of the foot. The veins of the feet also drain into the anterior and posterior tibial veins, which accompany their respective arteries, uniting at the knee to form the popliteal vein. The popliteal vein ascends through the thigh, becoming the femoral vein **FIGURE 8-101**.

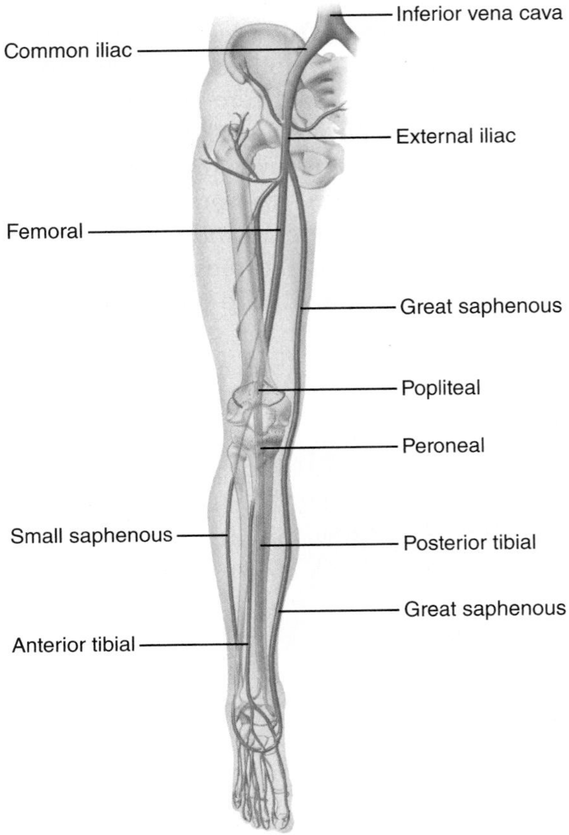

FIGURE 8-101 The veins of the lower extremity.

Microcirculation

The microcirculation is the portion of the vasculature consisting of the arterioles, capillaries, and venules **FIGURE 8-102**. Essentially, it acts as a diffusion and filtration system. The most important functions of the microcirculation are the transport of nutrients to the tissues and the removal of cellular waste.[33]

Arterioles are the major resistance vessels. Their smooth muscle lining allows them to alter their diameter, thereby directing and regulating blood flow into the capillaries. Thus, the arterioles can alter blood flow in each tissue in response to its specific needs.

Capillaries form connections between arterioles and venules in most body tissues. The capillary walls are very thin and contain pores, which permit the exchange of gases, water, nutrients, electrolytes, hormones, and waste products between the blood and the interstitial fluid that bathes the tissue cells. Pores are absent in cerebral capillaries, where the blood–brain barrier blocks the entry of many small molecules.[32]

In some tissues, arterioles branch directly into capillaries and control blood flow through the capillary bed (network of capillaries) by constricting or dilating. In other tissues, arterioles branch into smaller arterioles (metarterioles). Metarterioles are short, connecting vessels that can either directly

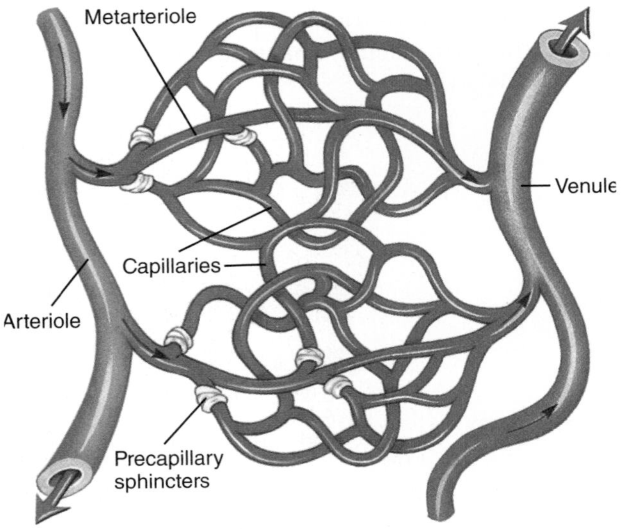

FIGURE 8-102 The microcirculation is the portion of the vasculature consisting of the arterioles, capillaries, and venules.

link to capillaries or bypass the capillary bed and connect to venules. The proximal ends of metarterioles are encircled by a small cuff of smooth muscle called a **precapillary sphincter**. These sphincters function as regulatory valves, controlling blood flow into the capillary bed. Metarterioles are partially lined with smooth muscle, enabling them to adjust their diameter.

Metarterioles and precapillary sphincters are not found in all tissues. Where metarterioles and precapillary sphincters are present, they are in close contact with the tissues they serve and are responsive to their needs. For example, precapillary sphincters constrict and reduce blood flow, or relax and increase blood flow, in each area depending on local tissue oxygen requirements and the concentrations of nutrients, end products of metabolism, and hydrogen ions. The intermittent contraction and relaxation of the arterioles, metarterioles, precapillary sphincters, and some small arteries is called vasomotion.[32]

In some tissues of the body, a direct connection exists between arteries and veins. These connections, called arteriovenous anastomoses, serve to shunt blood away from the capillary bed and route it from small arterioles directly into small venules of the tissue in need of oxygen and nutrients. Examples of sites where arteriovenous anastomoses can be found include the skin (eg, hands, feet, nose, ear, lips) and the mucosa of the nose and gut.

Capillary Filtration

The exchange of nutrients and waste products between the intravascular space and the intracellular space is crucial to survival. Most of these substances, including oxygen and carbon dioxide, pass between these spaces through diffusion, facilitated diffusion, and osmosis. However, other substances rely on the process of capillary filtration to perform this exchange. Capillary filtration depends on three factors: (1) capillary membrane permeability, (2) arterial hydrostatic pressure, and (3) venous oncotic pressure.

All capillaries do not share the same membrane permeability. For example, the liver capillaries are permeable, enabling plasma proteins (such as albumin) to pass through them easily. In contrast, the capillaries of skeletal muscle contain few pores. Permeability is also not uniform along the length of a capillary. The precapillary side is arterial and the postcapillary side is venous **FIGURE 8-103**. The venous ends of the capillary are more permeable than the arterial ends, and permeability is greatest in the venules, probably because of the greater number of pores in these areas.[32]

The movement of water between the plasma in the intravascular compartment and the **interstitial space** (the space between the cells) is driven by pressure differences. This pressure occurs at the capillary level by filtration. Recall that filtration is the movement of fluid from **intravascular fluid**, which is under high pressure, to interstitial fluid, which generally is under lower pressure.

The two main forces at work inside the capillary are hydrostatic pressure and oncotic pressure. **Hydrostatic pressure** is the pressure exerted by a liquid and occurs when blood moves through the

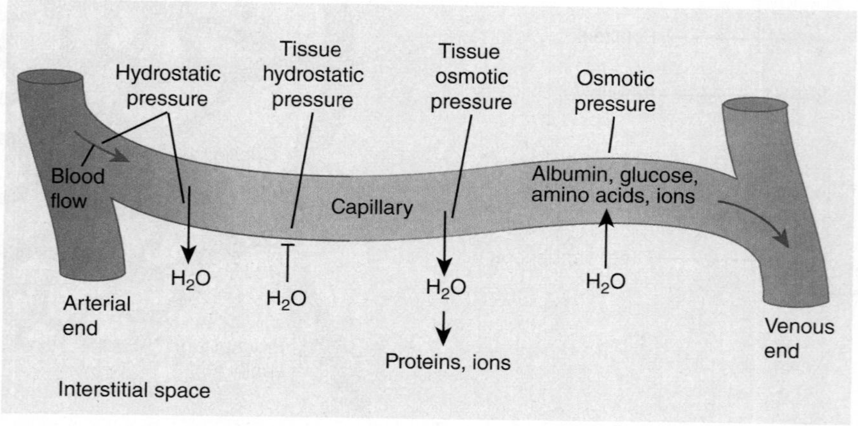

FIGURE 8-103 Movement of water into and out of capillaries is a result of four separate forces.

artery at relatively high pressures. In the vascular system, hydrostatic pressure is the pressure generated in vessels by the heart's contraction (ie, BP), gravity, and other forces. When blood meets the capillary walls, the fluid pressure pushes against the walls to force fluid out of the capillary. The opposing force is **oncotic pressure**, a form of osmotic pressure exerted by proteins in the blood plasma that usually acts to pull water into the circulatory system. These proteins tend to make the blood thicker. This thickness means that more water is present outside the capillary than inside relative to the interstitial space. Diffusion occurs as a result of this imbalance, with water seeking to move into the capillary.

The precapillary and postcapillary sphincters help maintain the delicate balance of pressure gradients. This process, called net filtration, is described by Starling's law: Net filtration is equal to the combined forces favoring filtration (ie, capillary hydrostatic pressure and interstitial oncotic pressure) minus the combined forces opposing filtration (ie, plasma oncotic pressure and interstitial hydrostatic pressure).

FIGURE 8-104 shows the entire process of capillary filtration. As illustrated in the figure, blood flows into the arterial side of the capillary. Plasma is trying to enter the capillary from the interstitial space, but the hydrostatic pressure on the arterial side of the capillary is higher, so plasma, carrying nutrients, leaves the capillary and enters the interstitial space. The hydrostatic pressure is greatly diminished by the time the fluid reaches the venous side of the capillary because the effort of pushing the fluid out of the capillary decreased its force. This decrease in pressure is beneficial because now oncotic pressure can push fluid into the capillary; plasma, carrying all of the wastes from the cells, enters the venous side of the capillary. These wastes are then carried away.

The Lymphatic System

The lymphatic system is considered part of the circulatory system. This system has three primary functions:

- **Removal of excess fluid from tissues of the body and recovery of fluid needed to maintain the proper balance of water.** Lymph is drained from the tissues and returned to the venous side of the vascular system.
- **Production and circulation of lymphocytes.** Lymphocytes are produced within lymphoid organs, which provide a significant portion of the body's immune function.
- **Distribution of various products that are unable to enter the bloodstream directly.** These products include nutrients and some hormones.

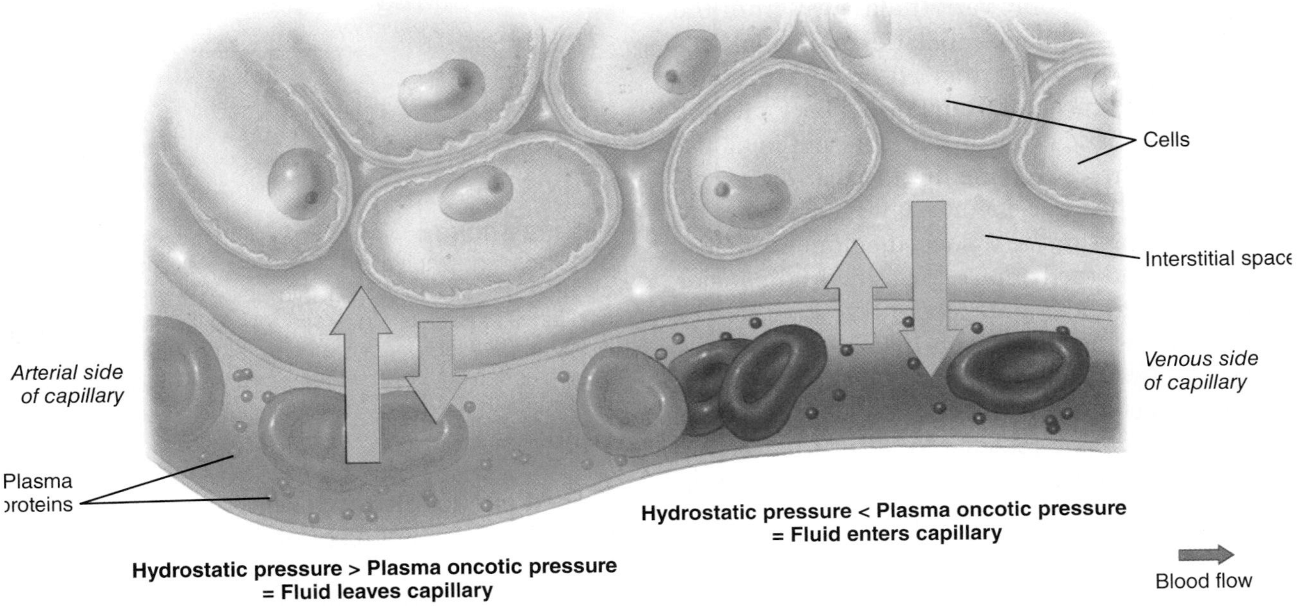

FIGURE 8-104 Fluid movement from capillaries to interstitial space and back.

The lymphatic system transports lymph by passive circulation. Recall that **lymph** is a thin, plasma-like fluid formed from interstitial or ECF that bathes the body's tissues. Lymphatic capillaries pick up the lymph and drain it into larger vessels. Lymph circulates throughout the body in thin-walled lymph vessels that travel close to the major arteries and veins **FIGURE 8-105**. Like veins, lymphatic vessels contain valves that limit backflow. Foreign material such as debris or bacteria is filtered from the lymph in the lymph nodes, a series of round or bean-shaped structures that are interspersed along the course of the lymph vessels. From the lymph nodes, the lymph returns to the main circulatory system via the **thoracic duct**, one of the two great lymph vessels. The thoracic duct collects lymph from the lower body, left side of head and neck, and left arm. It returns lymph to the central circulation by connecting with the left subclavian vein. The right lymphatic duct collects lymph from the right arm, right side of thorax, and right side of the head and neck. This duct returns lymph to the central circulation connecting with the right subclavian vein. Various body dynamics, such as changes in respiratory pressure, muscular contractions, and movement of organs surrounding lymphatic vessels, combine to move lymph through the lymphatic system.

Lymphatic Vessels

Lymphatic vessels only carry fluid away from the tissues. In the lymphatic capillaries, epithelial cells contain one-way valves that allow fluid to enter the vessel but prevent it from flowing back into the tissues. Lymphatic capillaries are present in all tissues except the CNS, bone marrow, cartilage, epidermis, and cornea. Generally, fluid flows from the blood capillaries to the tissues, then out of the tissue spaces into the lymph capillaries. In the major blood capillary beds of the body, the internal hydrostatic pressure allows a normal and continuous leak of a total of 3 to 4 mL/min of fluid into the interstitial spaces. The lymphatic vessel must absorb this excess fluid and return it to the central venous circulation to prevent the tissues from becoming edematous (swollen).

Thymus

The thymus is located in the thorax, anterior to the aorta and posterior to the upper sternum. It is divided into lobules by inward-extending connective tissues. The lobules contain large amounts of lymphocytes, including primarily inactive thymocytes, which formed from stem cells in the bone marrow and settled in the thymus. Some thymocytes mature into T lymphocytes, which leave the

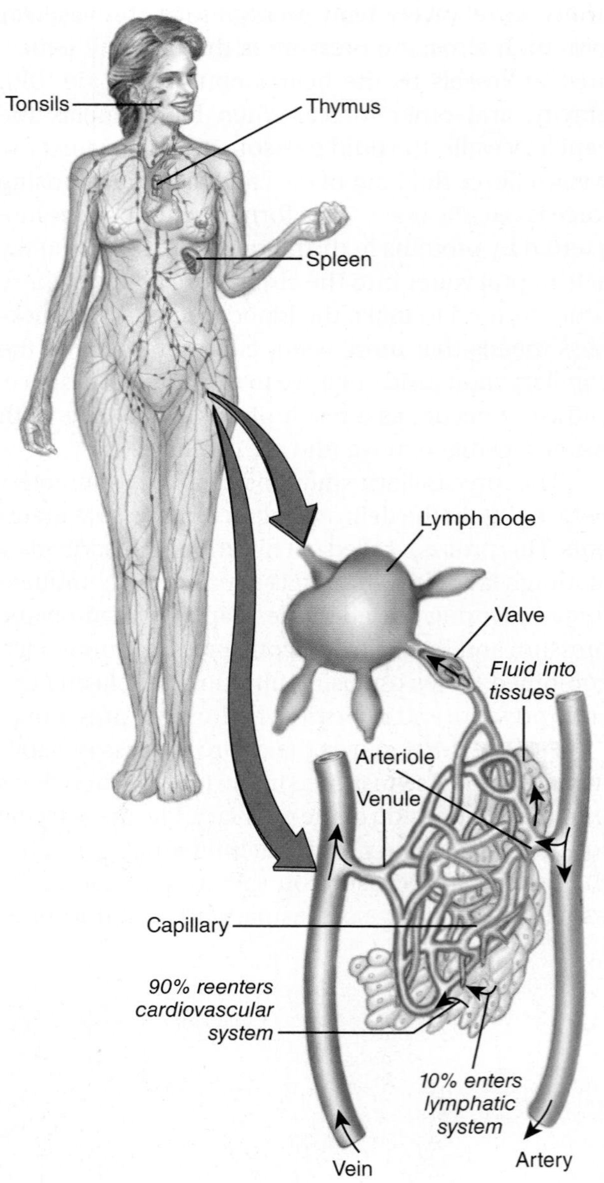

FIGURE 8-105 The lymphatic system consists of vessels that transport lymph and excess tissue fluid back to the circulatory system. Lymph is picked up by lymphatic capillaries that drain into larger vessels. Like the veins, the lymphatic vessels contain valves that prohibit backflow. Lymph nodes are interspersed along the vessels and filter the lymph.

thymus after 3 weeks and provide immunity in the body. Thymosin, a hormone secreted by the epithelial cells of the thymus, causes T lymphocytes to mature.

Spleen

The spleen is located in the upper left abdominal cavity, inferior to the diaphragm and posterior and lateral to the stomach. The body's largest lymphatic organ, it resembles a large, subdivided lymph node. The spleen contains the largest amount of lymphatic tissue in an adult's body. It differs from lymph nodes in that its venous sinuses are filled with blood, rather than lymph.

Two types of tissues are found inside the splenic lobules. White pulp is present throughout the spleen in small "islands," made up of splenic nodules containing many lymphocytes. The remainder of the lobules are filled with red pulp, which contains many RBCs, lymphocytes, and macrophages. The blood capillaries of the red pulp are highly permeable, so RBCs can easily squeeze through the capillary walls to enter the venous sinuses. If older RBCs become damaged during this process, macrophages inside the splenic sinuses engulf them. Via the action of macrophages and lymphocytes, the spleen filters blood similarly to how lymph nodes filter lymph.

Words of Wisdom

The spleen is susceptible to injury during rapid deceleration or compression and may be punctured if the overlying left lower ribs are fractured.

Immune System

The human body has multiple defense mechanisms that work together to provide immunity, which is defined as the ability to fight disease, illness, and infection. An infection may be caused by the presence and multiplication of a disease-causing agent (pathogen), which can be a virus, bacterium, fungus, or protozoan.

The immune system has two anatomic components: lymphoid tissues and cells that are responsible for the immune response. Lymphoid tissues are distributed throughout the body. The two primary lymphoid tissues are bone marrow and the thymus gland. Bone marrow is specialized soft tissue found within bone. Red bone marrow, which is widespread in children's bones and is found in some adult bones (in the sternum and ribs), is essential for forming mature blood cells. Red bone marrow produces B lymphocytes. Meanwhile, T lymphocytes originate from precursor cells in the bone marrow, leave the bone marrow, and mature in the thymus gland.

Clusters of lymphoid tissue, which are collectively called mucosa-associated lymphoid tissue, are found in the skin and the respiratory, urinary, GI, and reproductive tracts. Lymphoid tissues contain immune cells that can intercept pathogens before they reach the general circulation. The tonsils are perhaps the best known type of mucosa-associated lymphoid tissue. Unencapsulated lymphoid tissue is particularly prominent in the GI tract. Called the gut-associated lymphoid tissue, this tissue lies just under the inner lining of the esophagus and intestines.

The salivary glands (accessory organs of the digestive system) and the lacrimal glands play a role in the immune system as well: They produce an antibody, secretory immunoglobulin A, that bathes mucous membranes. Thus, saliva contains antibodies that fight pathogens that enter the mouth, and tears contain antibodies that fight pathogens that enter the eye. Secretory immunoglobulin A is also found in the mammary glands. Although secretory immunoglobulins play an important role in immunity, the primary cells of the immune system are the WBCs, which were discussed earlier in this chapter. Immunity and the immune response are discussed in detail in Chapter 9, *Pathophysiology*.

The Respiratory System

The cells of the body must have energy to function. This energy is produced through a series of complicated steps that require oxygen. The primary function of the **respiratory system** is to bring oxygen into the body and eliminate carbon dioxide. This system also provides nonspecific defenses against disease, helps control pH, and permits vocalization. The respiratory system is composed of the following parts:

- The respiratory tract, a series of passages through which air moves to and from the exchange surfaces
- The **respiratory membrane**, where gas exchange takes place (oxygen is picked up in the

bloodstream and carbon dioxide is eliminated through the lungs)

- The lungs, which allow the mechanical movement of air to and from the respiratory membrane
- The diaphragm, the muscles of the chest wall, and the **accessory muscles** of breathing, which permit normal respiratory movement, and the nerves from the brain and spinal cord to those muscles

The airway is separated into upper and lower structures, which can be distinguished based on their location above or below the **glottis** or glottic opening (the vocal cords and the opening between them) **FIGURE 8-106**.[34] Thus, the upper airway includes respiratory structures in the head and neck, while the lower airway includes respiratory structures in the chest.

Upper Airway

Structures of the upper airway include the nose, mouth, tongue, jaw, oral cavity, larynx, and **pharynx**. The primary functions of the upper airway are to warm, filter, and humidify air as it enters the body

Words of Wisdom

Any trauma to the nasal passages, such as improper or overly aggressive placement of airway devices, may result in profuse bleeding from the posterior nasal cavity. Bleeding from this area cannot be controlled by direct pressure. Extrinsic factors (such as cocaine use) can also damage the delicate nasal passages or the nasal septum. See Chapter 16, *Airway Management*, for more information.

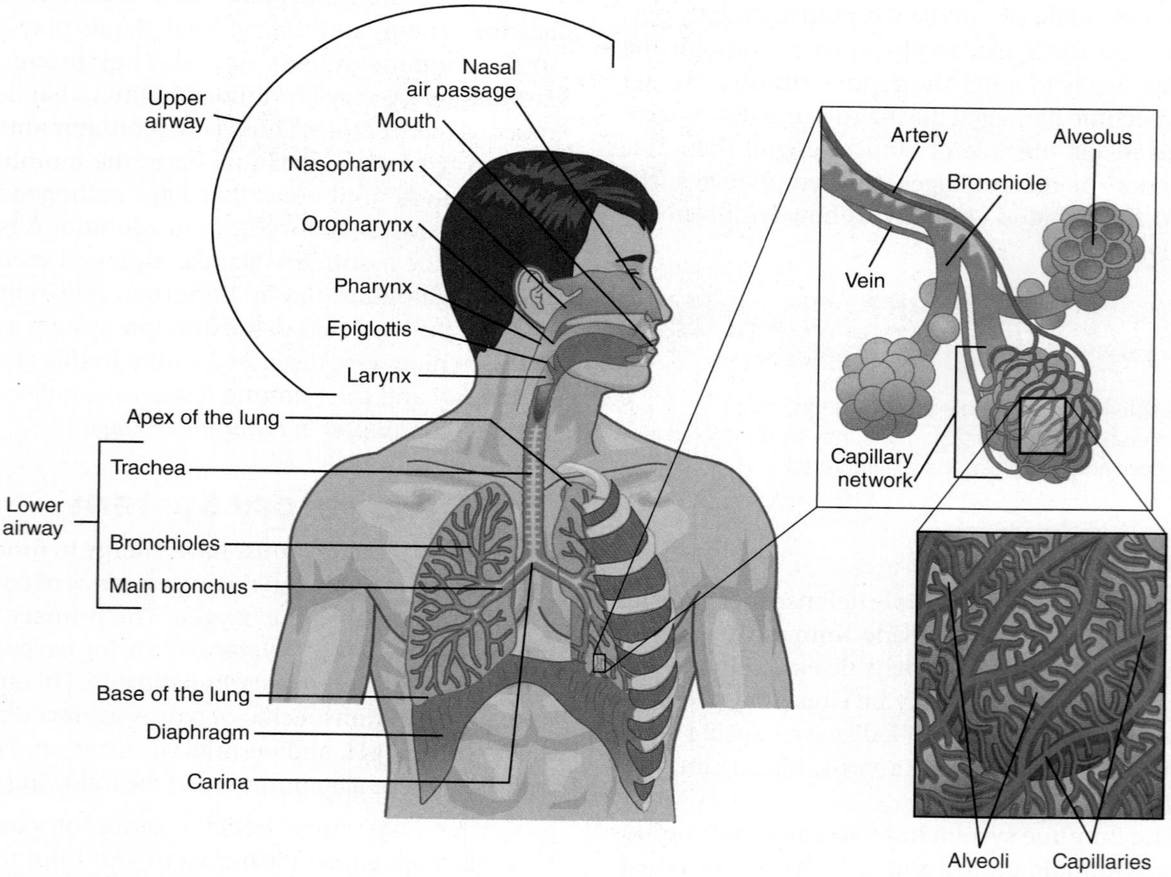

FIGURE 8-106 The respiratory system consists of all structures of the body that contribute to the process of breathing.

through the nose and mouth so that by the time it reaches the trachea, it is at body temperature and fully humidified. Humidification is accomplished as the air picks up moisture from the soft tissues of the airway.

The entrance to the respiratory tract begins at the nasal and oral cavities. The area between the nasal cavity and the larynx and posterior to the oral cavity is referred to as the pharynx. The pharynx (throat), which extends from the base of the skull to the level of the sixth cervical vertebrae, allows passage of air to the lower airway and food to the esophagus. It is divided into three regions for anatomic purposes, although no physical structures separate these areas.

Nasopharynx

On **inhalation** (the active, muscular part of breathing), air normally enters the body through the nose. It passes into the **nasopharynx**, which extends from the back of the nasal cavity to the level of the soft palate. Recall that the palate is the roof of the oral cavity and separates the nasal cavity from the oral cavity. The hard palate, which is the anterior portion of the palate, is supported by bone (primarily the maxillary bone) **FIGURE 8-107**. The posterior portion is called the soft palate because it consists of mucous membrane, muscular fibers, and mucous glands and has no bony support. The palatoglossal arch, the posterior border of the oral cavity,

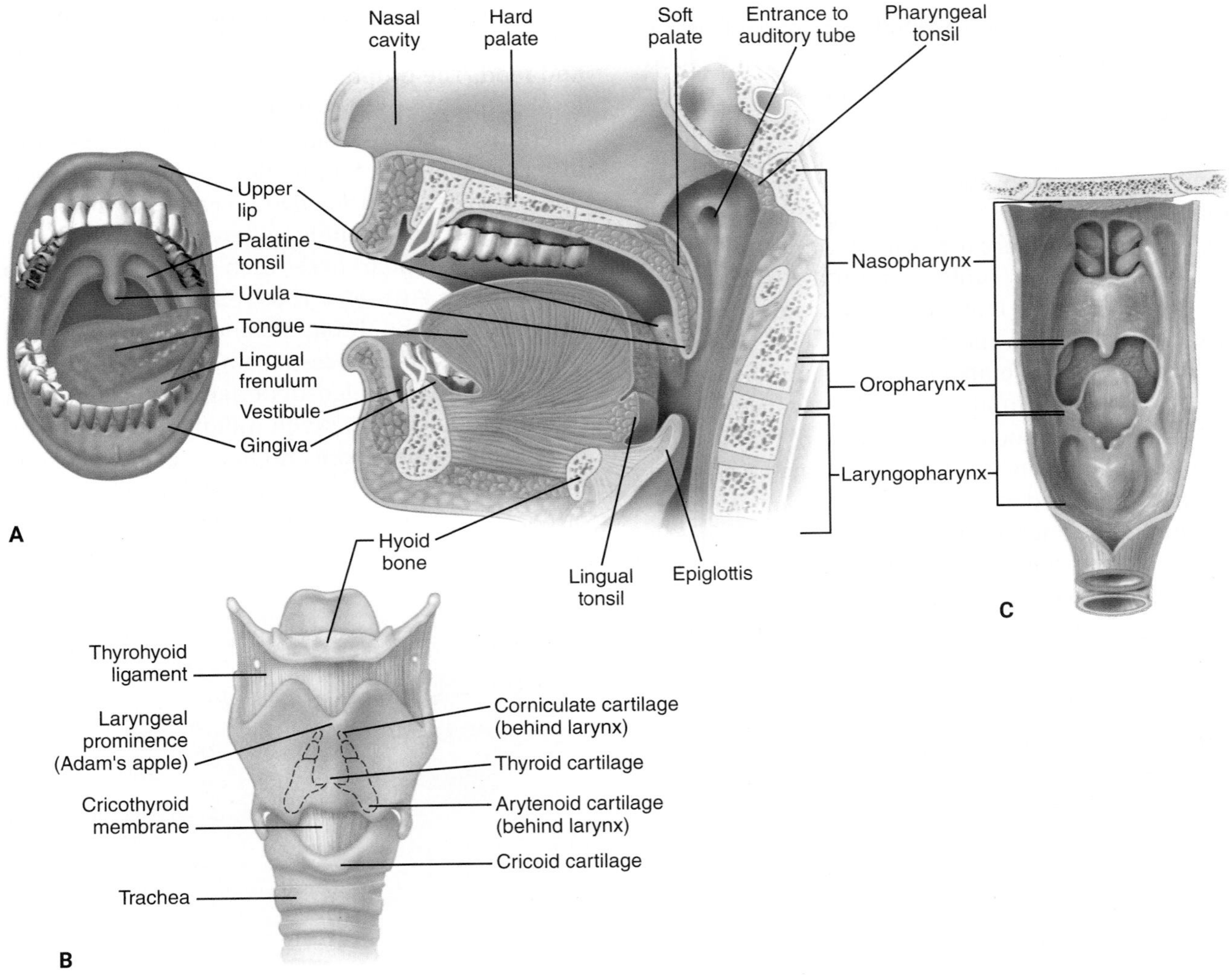

FIGURE 8-107 A. The oral cavity. **B.** The larynx. **C.** The pharynx.

is an extension of the soft palate. The uvula, a small, fleshy tissue structure that resembles a punching bag, projects downward from the posterior part of the soft palate and extends into the palatoglossal arch. When swallowing, muscles elevate the soft palate so that it touches the posterior wall of the pharynx, sealing off the nasopharynx from the oropharynx.

The entire nasal cavity is lined with a ciliated mucous membrane that keeps contaminants such as dust and other small particles out of the respiratory tract. During illness, the body produces additional mucus to trap potentially infectious agents. This mucous membrane is extremely delicate and has a rich blood supply. Olfactory receptors located in the epithelium in the nasal cavity are responsible for recognizing odors.

The nasopharynx is divided into two passages by the nasal septum, a rigid partition with a rich blood supply. It is composed of the ethmoid and vomer bones and cartilage. Normally, the nasal septum is in the midline of the nose. In some people, the septum may be deviated to one side or the other—a condition that becomes important when contemplating insertion of a nasal airway device. Three bony shelves (turbinates) protrude from the lateral walls of the nasal cavity and extend into the nasal passageway, parallel to the nasal floor. The turbinates increase the surface area of the nasal mucosa and cause turbulence in airflow, making inhaled particles stick to the mucus-coated walls of the nostrils. This combination of vascular supply and turbulence warms, filters, and humidifies the air as it is inhaled.

Along the lateral walls of the nasal passageway are numerous openings that extend into the frontal and maxillary sinuses. The sinuses lessen the weight of the skull, give resonance to a person's voice, and prevent contaminants from entering the respiratory tract. These cavities also act as tributaries for fluid to and from the eustachian tubes and tear ducts. Because the sinuses help trap particles, they are a common source of infection.

Eustachian tubes (auditory tubes) are passages from the inner ear that allow drainage of fluid as well as equalization of pressure that may occur behind the tympanic membrane. Because these tubes are connected to nasal passages, which may contain bacteria, infections can migrate to the middle ear through these tubes, especially in toddlers. The back of the nasal cavity opens into the oropharynx.

Words of Wisdom

Because of their closeness to underlying brain structures and the thin nature of the bones forming the sinuses, fractures of the bones that comprise the sinuses may cause CSF to leak from the nose (cerebrospinal rhinorrhea) or the ears (cerebrospinal otorrhea). CSF may drain from the posterior nasopharynx down the throat in some patients, causing a salty taste in the mouth.

Oropharynx

The oropharynx is the portion of the pharynx visible within the mouth (see Figure 8-107). Whereas the nasopharynx is a passageway for air only, the oropharynx functions as a passageway for both air and food. The oropharynx begins superiorly at the level of the soft palate and extends to the epiglottis inferiorly.[34] The posterior pharynx has a rich supply of sensitive nerves. Stimulation of this area triggers the **gag reflex**, a protective mechanism that initiates coughing or retching to prevent aspiration.

The palatopharyngeal arch is the entrance to the pharynx **FIGURE 8-108**. Associated structures in the back of the throat include the tonsils. These lymphatic tissues are responsible for filtering bacteria and other foreign materials, especially from the mouth and nose. When inflamed and swollen, the tonsils become sore and may make swallowing difficult. Two sets of tonsils are located on each side of the throat. The palatine tonsils are located just

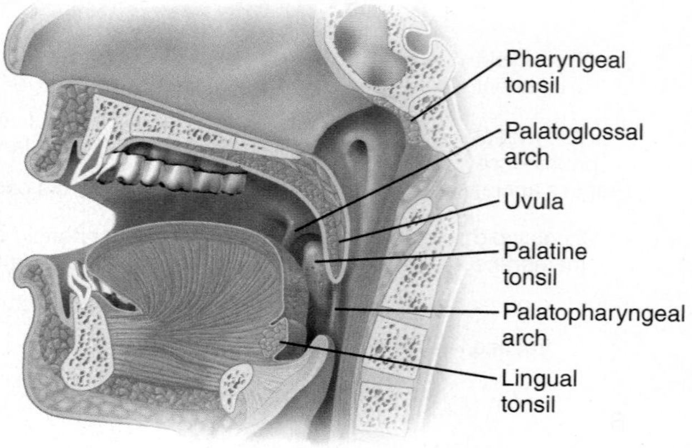

FIGURE 8-108 The tonsils.

behind the walls of the palatoglossal arch, anterior to the palatopharyngeal arch. The *adenoids,* also called the pharyngeal tonsils, are located on the upper rear wall of the oral cavity near the opening of the eustachian tubes. The adenoids, when inflamed, can present an increased risk of ear infection during childhood because they may block drainage exiting the tube. The lingual tonsils are found at the base of the tongue.

Within the mouth are several structures that have relevance to the airway—namely, the teeth and tongue. Adults who have retained all their teeth typically have 32 teeth. Teeth provide a supporting structure for the oral cavity and aid in digestion by chewing food.

> **Words of Wisdom**
>
> The 32 adult teeth are embedded in the gums in such a manner that significant force is required to dislodge them. However, trauma of lesser severity may result in fracture or avulsion of teeth, potentially obstructing the upper airway or causing aspiration of tooth fragments into the lungs.

The tongue, a muscular structure in the floor of the mouth, is the primary organ of taste; it is also important in the formation of speech and in the chewing and swallowing of food. The tongue is attached at the mandible and hyoid bone. The hyoid bone is buried in the soft tissues behind the chin. As mentioned earlier, it is unique in that it does not articulate with any other bones. Serving as a primary anchor of the tongue, the hyoid bone is also the point of attachment for several ligaments that support the trachea and larynx.

> **Words of Wisdom**
>
> The tongue tends to fall back and block the posterior pharynx when the mandible relaxes. In fact, the tongue is the most common cause of anatomic upper airway obstruction in an unresponsive patient.

Laryngopharynx

The laryngopharynx (hypopharynx) functions in respiration and digestion and extends from the epiglottis to the top of the esophagus. It is the shortest of the three divisions of the pharynx. The laryngopharynx opens into the larynx anteriorly and the esophagus posteriorly.

Two passageways are located at the bottom of the pharynx: the esophagus behind and the trachea (windpipe) in front. Food and liquids enter the pharynx and pass into the esophagus, which carries them to the stomach. Air and other gases enter the trachea and go to the lungs. The epiglottis protects the opening of the trachea. The epiglottis is attached inferiorly to the thyroid cartilage. The superior portion of the epiglottis is movable, flexing up and down when swallowing. The epiglottis serves as a gatekeeper, covering the opening into the larynx during swallowing so that ingested materials enter the esophagus, thereby preventing the passage of foreign matter into the trachea.

> **Words of Wisdom**
>
> The epiglottis is an important landmark when you perform orotracheal intubation with a straight laryngoscope blade. The epiglottis must be lifted out of the way so you can visualize and pass an endotracheal tube between the vocal cords. More of an anatomic landmark than an actual structure, the vallecula (which means "little valley") is a depression (or pocket) between the base of the tongue and the epiglottis. The vallecula is an important landmark when you intubate a patient with a curved laryngoscope blade.

Recall that the vocal cords (white bands of tough tissue) and the opening between them are collectively called the glottis or the glottic opening.[34] At rest, the vocal cords are partially separated; that is, the glottis is partially open. During forceful inhalation, the vocal cords open widely to provide minimum resistance to air flow.

> **Words of Wisdom**
>
> When the airway is stimulated, such as during aspiration of foreign material or in a submersion incident, defensive reflexes cause spasmodic closure of the vocal cords (laryngospasm), which seals off the airway. This reflex normally lasts a few seconds. Persistent laryngospasm can threaten airway patency by preventing ventilation (the mechanical process of moving air into and out of the lungs) altogether.

Larynx

Serving as a bridge extending from approximately the fourth through the sixth cervical levels, the larynx joins the pharynx to the trachea. It marks where the upper airway ends and the lower airway begins. The larynx has three purposes: (1) to facilitate the passage of air; (2) as a sphincter, to prevent foreign solids and liquids from entering the lungs; (3) and to produce speech.

> **Words of Wisdom**
>
> Be aware of other associated structures in proximity to the larynx. Specifically, the thyroid gland is a bow tie–shaped gland that lies across the trachea just inferior to the cricoid cartilage. Several blood vessels, including the carotid arteries, jugular veins, and several vessels branching off these arteries, run alongside the trachea as well as across it.

The larynx comprises an outer cage of nine cartilages that protect and support the vocal cords (see Figure 8-107). Muscles and ligaments connect these cartilages. The largest of the laryngeal cartilages, the thyroid cartilage, forms the anterior part of the larynx. It is usually identifiable externally as the Adam's apple. The glottic opening is located directly behind the thyroid cartilage.

The superior border of the glottis is the epiglottis **FIGURE 8-109**. At the inferior border of the glottic opening are the corniculate and cuneiform cartilages, which appear as bumps just below the glottis. The pyramid-shaped **arytenoid cartilages** form the posterior attachment of the vocal cords; they are valuable guides for endotracheal intubation. The vestibular folds (false vocal cords) and the true vocal cords are found within the larynx. The vocal folds move to the sides of the larynx during inhalation, allowing air to pass freely. A person is able to produce sound during exhalation (the passive part of the breathing process) by controlling the distance between these folds, which vibrate when air is forced through them.

The piriform fossae are two pockets of tissue on the lateral borders of the larynx. Airway devices are occasionally inadvertently inserted into these pockets, resulting in a tenting of the skin under the jaw.

Directly inferior to the thyroid cartilage is the cricoid cartilage, which forms the lowest portion of the larynx (see Figure 8-107). Considered the first cartilage to begin the trachea, it is a complete ring of cartilage—unlike the other cartilages in the larynx, which are C-shaped rings on the posterior surface. The gaps in these C-shaped rings permit the esophagus, which lies behind the trachea, to bulge forward as food moves to the stomach.

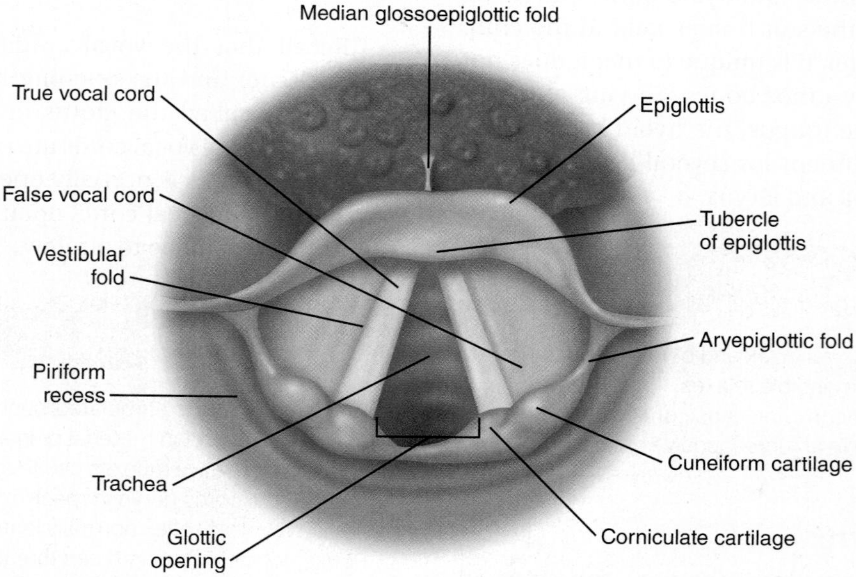

FIGURE 8-109 The glottis and surrounding structures.

Located between the thyroid and cricoid cartilage is the cricothyroid membrane (see Figure 8-107). This membrane does not contain many blood vessels and is covered only by skin and minimal subcutaneous tissue. It is a potential site for performing a cricothyrotomy (an incision through the skin and cricothyroid membrane to relieve difficulty breathing caused by an airway obstruction) if the airway cannot be secured with an advanced airway device.

Lower Airway

Below the glottis is the lower airway. The structures of the lower airway include the trachea, bronchial tree, **alveoli** (tiny sacs of tissue where gas exchange takes place), and lungs. The connective tissue, small airways, and alveoli are collectively referred to as the lung parenchyma. The lower airway is where gas exchange occurs. Functionally, oxygen diffuses from the alveoli into the pulmonary capillaries, while carbon dioxide diffuses in the opposite direction.

Trachea

Recall that the trachea is the air passage that connects the larynx to the lungs. Structurally, the trachea is composed of C-shaped cartilaginous rings that support its anterior and lateral walls. The area between the tracheal cartilages consists of connective tissue and smooth muscle that allow the diameter of the trachea to change as needed. These rings protect the trachea and prevent it from collapsing.

The trachea lies anterior to the esophagus and bifurcates (branches) into two primary bronchi, called the main stem bronchi (right and left). The point at which this bifurcation occurs is called the **carina** **FIGURE 8-110**. An external landmark for the carina is the junction of the body and manubrium of the sternum, referred to as the angle of Louis.

The trachea is lined with columnar epithelial tissue and goblet cells. Goblet cells also line the airways. These cells produce mucus that blankets the entire lining of the conducting airways. The mucus covers the cilia, forming a two-layer blanket that

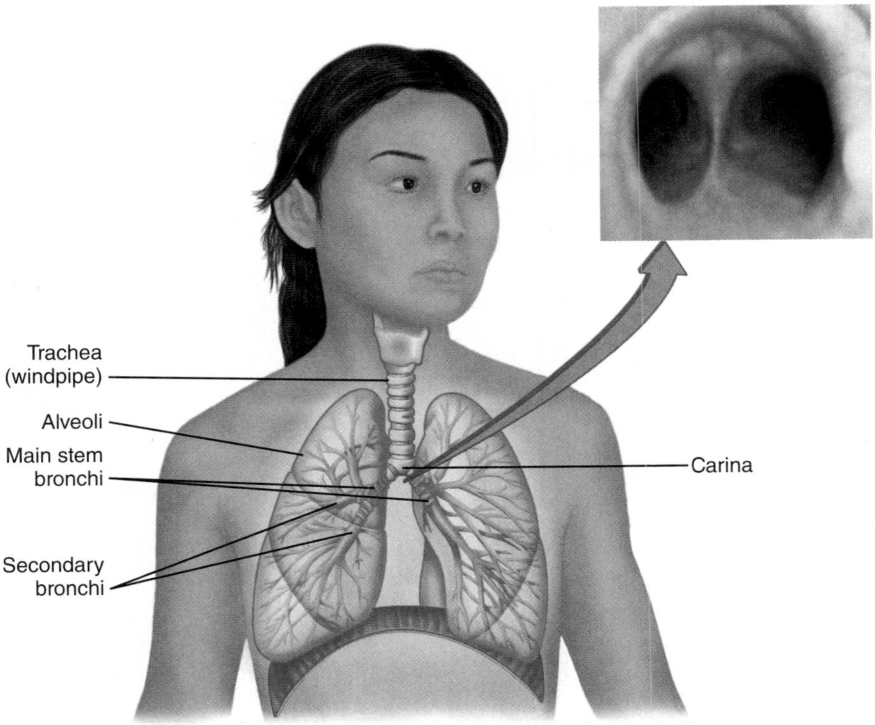

FIGURE 8-110 The point of bifurcation of the right and left primary (main stem) bronchi is at the carina. In an adult, this location is at roughly the fifth intercostal space.

Words of Wisdom

The carina is an important anatomic landmark because the tip of an endotracheal tube is often documented on radiographic study in relation to the carina.

is thick on the surface (gel layer) and thin and watery next to the cilia (sol layer). The thick gel layer floats over the sol layer. In a healthy person, cilia constantly push this gel layer up and out of the airway **FIGURE 8-111**. As the cilia beat, they reach out into the gel layer, pushing it up and toward the glottis. On the return stroke, the cilia collapse into the sol layer, so that they do not pull the gel layer back down. In this manner, the cilia slowly move the entire gel layer up and out of the tracheobronchial tree, where it is swallowed or expectorated.

Bronchial Tree

The right and left primary bronchi divide into secondary (lobar) bronchi (one for each lobe of the lung). In turn, the secondary bronchi divide into tertiary (segmental) bronchi and continue to subdivide into smaller and smaller bronchi, finally becoming bronchioles. Each bronchus directs air into its respective lung. The right primary bronchus is shorter and wider than the left primary bronchus, and leaves the carina at a less-acute angle than the left does. Like the trachea, the bronchi are lined with ciliated epithelial cells and goblet cells to prevent the inhalation of foreign particles.

The progressively branching pulmonary airways are referred to by generation numbers, where generation zero is the trachea, the first-generation airways are the right and left primary bronchi, and so on **FIGURE 8-112**. Approximately 23 generations of airways are present in the human body.[35] As the airway passages become smaller, their generation number increases and the amount of cilia, number of mucus-secreting cells, presence of submucosal glands, and amount of cartilage in airway walls all gradually decrease, so that smooth muscle and elastic fibers become more prominent.[35] Bronchi possess cartilage (up to about the 10th generation) whereas bronchioles (beginning about the 11th generation) lack cartilage. Because bronchioles lack cartilaginous support, they are especially

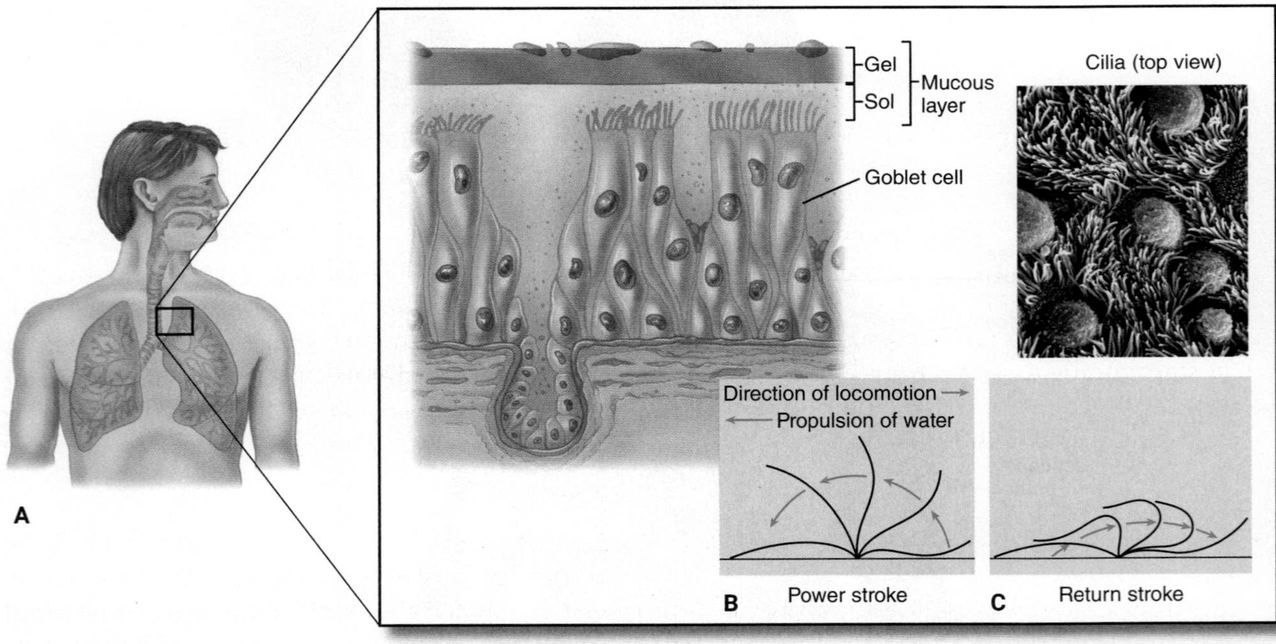

FIGURE 8-111 Cilia line the larger airways of the respiratory tract **(A)**. Their regular pattern of movement between the gel and sol layers of mucus helps move foreign material out of the tracheobronchial tree **(B** and **C)**.

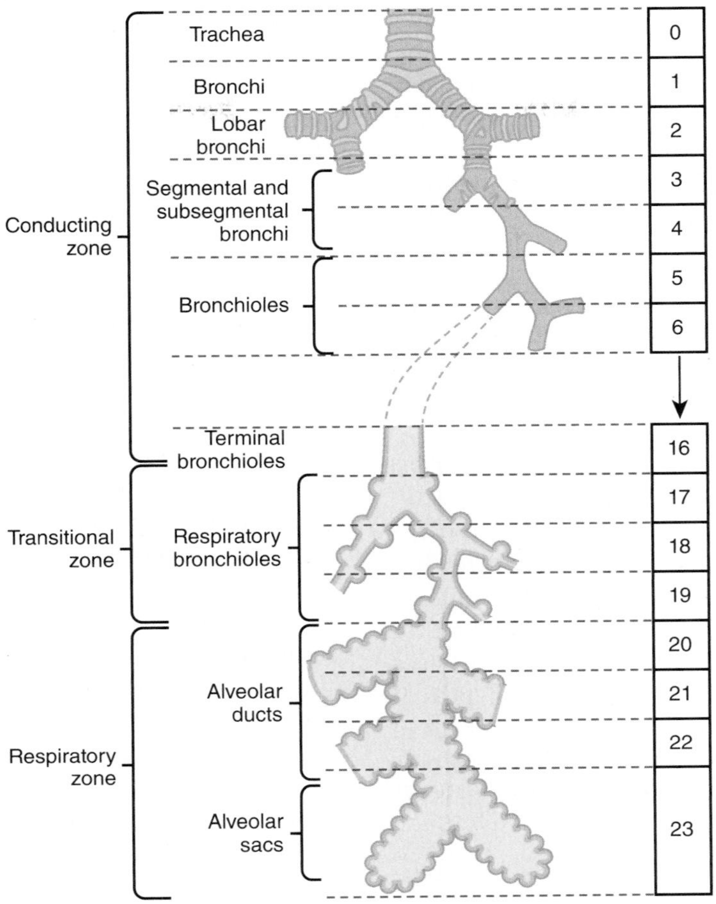

FIGURE 8-112 The first 16 generations of the lower airway are conducting airways. Transitional airways (generations 17 through 19) consist of respiratory bronchioles that lead into the airways that make up the respiratory zone (generations 20 through 23), where gas exchange occurs.

susceptible to collapse during expiration. They can maintain an open lumen only because the pressure surrounding them may be more negative than the pressure inside them, and because of the outward pull of surrounding tissues.[35] Terminal bronchioles are present at about the 16th generation and are distinguished by being the smallest airways without alveoli.[36] The conducting airways, which move air to those areas of the lung that participate in gas exchange, begin at the nose and lips and end at the terminal bronchioles.[35]

Respiratory bronchioles (generations 17 to 19) make up the transitional airways (also called the transitional zone). The respiratory bronchioles participate in gas exchange over at least part of their surface and contain an increasing number of alveolar ducts (generations 20 to 22) that direct air into the alveoli (generation 23).[35] Generations 20 through 23 are referred to as the respiratory zone of the lung. The respiratory bronchioles, the alveolar ducts, and the alveoli are considered the respiratory, or gas-exchanging, units of the lungs.[36]

Alveoli

Each alveolar duct ends in alveoli. As an analogy, you can think of alveoli as small balloons at the end of a straw. Each alveolus is composed of multiple alveoli, whose very thin walls consist of a single layer of epithelial tissue and elastic fibers. These walls become thinner as they expand, making diffusion of oxygen and carbon dioxide possible. The elastic fibers allow the alveolus to expand and recoil during breathing.

A network of capillaries surrounds each alveolus. The thin alveolocapillary membrane, which lies between the alveolus and the capillary, consists of only one cell layer. Respiratory exchange between the lung and blood vessels occurs in the alveoli at this membrane.

Alveoli are made up of two types of cells:

- Type I alveolar cells (pneumocytes) are almost empty, allowing for better gas exchange. They lack cellular components that would permit them to reproduce.
- Type II pneumocytes can make new type I cells and also produce **surfactant**, a slippery substance that reduces surface tension and helps keep the alveoli expanded. Each alveolus has several type II pneumocytes. When alveoli are damaged by infection, cigarette smoking, or other trauma, their ability to repair themselves correlates directly to the number of type II cells that remain. After all of the type II cells in an alveolus have been destroyed, the alveolus cannot make new cells or surfactant and is essentially dead.

Alveoli function best when they are kept partially inflated. Remember the balloon analogy: Blowing up a balloon takes a lot of pressure. Once the balloon is partially inflated, however, it is much easier to inflate it the rest of the way. The same is true of alveoli. By reducing the surface tension of the alveoli, surfactant makes it easier for them to expand. When surfactant is washed out of the alveoli, as may occur in pulmonary edema, submersion incidents, or severe shock, they are much more likely to collapse.

Collapsed, fluid-filled, or pus-filled alveoli do not participate in gas exchange. Instead, these alveoli contribute to a shunt, in which blood from the right side of the heart bypasses the alveoli and returns to the left side of the heart in an unoxygenated state, perhaps resulting in hypoxemia. Conditions related to ventilation, perfusion, or both can prevent oxygen from reaching the bloodstream.

Lungs

The lungs are two large, paired structures located within the pleural cavities. These organs are attached to the heart by the pulmonary trunk (arterial) and pulmonary veins. The point of entry for bronchial vessels, bronchi, and nerves in each lung is the hilum. The base of each lung rests on the diaphragm, and its apex extends approximately 1 inch (2.5 cm) above each clavicle. The apex of the left lung is slightly more superior than that of the right. Significantly more blood is circulated to the lung bases compared with the lung apices. Because humans are upright, gravity-dependent creatures, most infections and pathologic conditions occur at the base of the lung.

The right lung is divided into three lobes: upper, middle, and lower. The left lung has only two lobes, one upper and one lower. The left lung also has a notch where the heart lies (the cardiac notch). Each lobe of the lung is composed of separated lobules; these lobules can be surgically removed, leaving the rest of the lung intact.

The right and left pleural cavities are separate compartments on either side of the mediastinum.[37] Each pleural cavity encloses a lung and its associated bronchial tree and vessels, nerves, and lymphatics.[37] Each lung is contained within a double-layered serous membrane called the **pleura**. The **visceral pleura** is tightly attached to the lung surface. At the hilum, the visceral pleura is continuous with the **parietal pleura**, which lines the wall of the thorax. The parietal pleura is attached to the interior of the mediastinum, superior surface of the diaphragm, and inner surface of the rib cage. This design is important in the physiology of breathing.

The parietal pleura contains blood vessels that are believed to produce a filtrate of plasma called pleural fluid.[35] The visceral pleura contains lymphatic vessels that drain pleural fluid from the pleural space.[35] The **pleural space** is a potential space between the visceral and parietal pleura **FIGURE 8-113**. Normally, this space contains only a small amount (about 2 teaspoons [10 mL]) of pleural fluid, which separates the parietal and visceral pleurae.[35] The surface tension caused by the fluid between the two pleural layers causes the layers to stick together. As a result, when the parietal pleura moves with the chest wall, it takes the visceral pleura with it, expanding the lungs. The pleural fluid also allows the lungs to move with minimal friction. Think of the pleural layers and the fluid between them as analogous to two pieces of glass separated by a thin film of water. Because of the surface tension between the membranes and the fluid, the

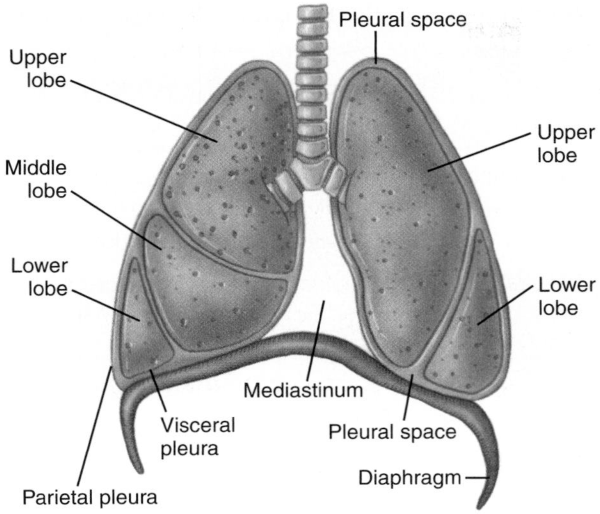

FIGURE 8-113 The pleura lining the chest wall and covering the lungs is an essential part of the breathing mechanism. The pleural space is not an actual space until blood or air leaks into it, causing the pleural surfaces to separate.

layers glide easily over each other but can be pulled apart only with difficulty.[38]

Pleural fluid occasionally becomes infected, causing irritation of the surface of the lung with respiratory movement; this condition is known as pleuritis or pleurisy. Under certain disease conditions or following trauma, the pleural space can also fill with fluid, air (pneumothorax), or blood (hemothorax).

As you have learned, the lungs receive blood in two ways. Deoxygenated blood flows from the right ventricle via the pulmonary arteries. This blood flows through pulmonary capillaries, is reoxygenated at the alveoli, and then returns to the heart via the pulmonary veins. In addition, bronchial arteries branch off of the thoracic aorta and supply the lung tissues themselves with blood. Deoxygenated blood returns to the heart via the bronchial veins. Peripherally in the lungs, venous blood from the bronchi enters the pulmonary veins, returning with oxygenated blood from the alveoli.

Lung Volumes

A substantial amount of air can be moved within the respiratory system. **FIGURE 8-114** shows the typical lung volumes. An adult man has a total lung capacity of 6,000 mL (equivalent to three 2-liter bottles of soda). An adult woman has about one-third less total capacity because the lung size is smaller.

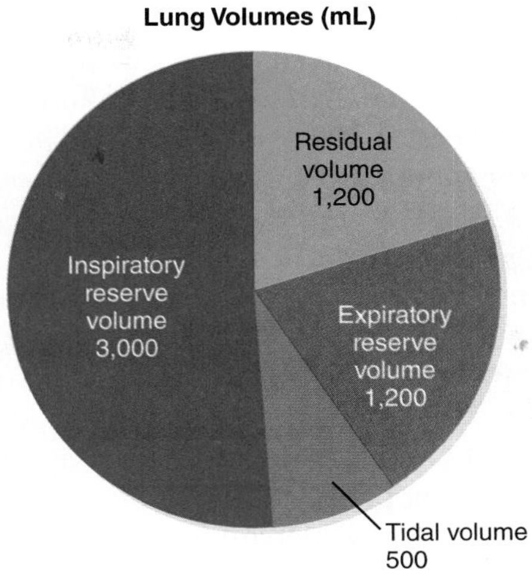

FIGURE 8-114 Lung volumes.

As you are reading this book, the amount of your air movement is about 500 mL (unless you just finished exercising). This measurement is called **tidal volume**; it is the amount of air that moves into or out of the lungs during a single breath. **Inspiratory reserve volume** is the additional amount of air that can be inhaled after the normal tidal volume has been reached. The average person can inhale an additional 3,000 mL of air when needed in times of physiologic stress. Conversely, **expiratory reserve volume** is the additional amount of air that can be exhaled after the normal tidal volume is expelled. The average person can exhale an additional 1,200 mL of air when needed in times of physiologic stress. The **residual volume** is the amount of air that remains in the lungs after maximal exhalation, where it serves to prevent alveolar collapse (atelectasis) by keeping the alveoli slightly inflated. The residual volume is 1,200 mL in the average person. Some loss of residual volume occurs when a person is hit in the chest and has the "wind knocked out" of them. **Vital capacity** is the amount of air moved in and out of the lungs with maximum inspiration (inhalation) and expiration (exhalation).

When you assist a patient's breathing, you move air in and out of the lungs. To do so, you will use a bag-mask device—a large bag filled with air that, when squeezed, pushes air out one end. The typical device holds approximately 1,000 to 1,200 mL of air.

Note that although a person's resting tidal volume is 500 mL, you need to use a bag-mask device that provides more than twice that volume because of dead space. *Anatomic dead space* is the portion of the respiratory system that has no alveoli and, therefore, where little or no exchange of gas between air and blood occurs. The mouth, trachea, bronchi, and bronchioles are all considered anatomic dead space. When you ventilate a patient with any device, you create more dead space. Gas must first fill the device before it can be moved into the patient.

Typically, anatomic dead space is approximately 1 mL per pound of ideal body weight. Thus, a 150-pound (68-kg) person has about 150 mL of anatomic dead space. If this patient took an average breath (tidal volume) of 700 mL, then about 550 mL would participate in ventilation at the alveolar level; the other 150 mL would fill the conducting airways, and would never be exposed to blood flow. If the same patient were to have a tidal volume of 500 mL, then only 350 mL would participate in ventilation, because 150 mL would be stuck in the tubes.

Physiologic dead space is a function of the number of damaged alveoli that cannot participate in gas exchange. Unlike anatomic dead space, which is fairly constant among patients, physiologic dead space varies widely based on medical history and exposure to toxins that damage alveoli, among other factors. Physiologic dead space is the anatomic dead space plus the amount of space occupied by damaged alveoli and can be as much as 1 to 2 L in volume.

Words of Wisdom

Although physiologic dead space cannot be measured in the prehospital setting, you must keep this principle in mind and apply it to an individual's history and presentation when determining ventilation effectiveness.

One of the critical determinants of ventilation's effectiveness is the amount of air moved in and out of the respiratory system in 1 minute, known as the **minute volume**. Calculating the minute volume helps you to determine how deeply a patient is breathing.

$$\text{Minute volume} = \text{Respiratory rate} \times \text{Tidal volume}$$

TABLE 8-39 Ventilation, Oxygenation, and Respiration

Function	Definition
Oxygenation	The process of loading oxygen molecules onto hemoglobin molecules in the bloodstream
Respiration	The actual exchange of oxygen and carbon dioxide in the alveoli and the tissues of the body
Ventilation	The physical act of moving air into and out of the lungs

Ventilation

The respiratory and cardiovascular systems work together to ensure that a constant supply of oxygen and nutrients is delivered to every cell in the body and that carbon dioxide and other waste products are removed from every cell. If one of these systems becomes compromised, then oxygen delivery will be ineffective and cellular death may occur.

Ventilation is the mechanical process of moving air into and out of the lungs. The two separate phases of ventilation are inhalation (inspiration) and exhalation (expiration) **TABLE 8-39**. Each combination of inhalation and exhalation is a *respiratory cycle*. Essential to this process is a change in pressures within the thoracic cavity that allow the passive flow of air into and out of the lungs.

The lungs have no muscle tissue, so they cannot move on their own. Thus, they need the help of other structures to be able to expand and contract during inhalation; that is, their ability to function properly depends on the movement of the chest and supporting structures. These structures include the thorax, thoracic cage (chest cage), diaphragm, intercostal muscles, and accessory muscles. The intercostal nerves innervate muscles of the chest wall.

Recall that the diaphragm is connected to the sternum anteriorly, the ribs laterally, and the vertebrae posteriorly. The diaphragm is innervated by the phrenic nerves, which arise from the third through fifth cervical nerve roots (hence the phrase, "C3 to C5 keep the diaphragm alive"). The diaphragm functions as both a voluntary (skeletal) and an involuntary (smooth) muscle. It acts as a voluntary muscle when you take a deep breath, cough, or hold your breath. However, unlike other skeletal or voluntary muscles, the diaphragm also performs an automatic function, so that breathing continues during sleep and at all other times. Even though you can hold your breath or temporarily breathe faster or slower, you cannot continue these variations in breathing pattern indefinitely. When the concentration of carbon dioxide rises in the blood, the autonomic regulation of breathing resumes under control of the brainstem. Therefore, although the diaphragm looks like voluntary skeletal muscle and is attached to the skeleton, it behaves, for the most part, like an involuntary muscle.

Words of Wisdom

The process of breathing is typically easy and requires little muscular effort. Now imagine breathing through a straw, when suddenly the diameter of the straw decreases. The smaller the diameter of the straw, the more effort you will have to exert to move air. As the resistance in the airway increases, you begin to use more muscle groups—namely, your abdominal and pectoral muscles—to assist the diaphragm in moving air.

Inhalation is governed by **Boyle's law**, which states that the pressure of a gas is inversely proportional to its volume. The air pressure outside the body—atmospheric pressure—is normally higher than the air pressure within the thorax. During inhalation, the diaphragm and external intercostal muscles between the ribs contract. When the diaphragm contracts, it moves down slightly, enlarging the thoracic cage from top to bottom. When the external intercostal muscles contract, they move the ribs up and out. These actions combine to enlarge the chest cavity in all dimensions. Pressure in the thorax then falls, becoming lower than the atmospheric pressure, which creates a slight vacuum. This vacuum pulls air in through the trachea, causing the lungs to fill, a process called **negative-pressure ventilation**. The alveoli inflate, allowing gases such as oxygen and carbon dioxide to move from an area of higher pressure to an area of lower pressure (diffusion) until the pressures are equal. In this way, oxygen moves from the alveoli into the pulmonary capillaries, while carbon dioxide moves into the alveoli for removal from the body. The combined actions of these muscles enlarge the thorax in all dimensions. Maximum inhalation occurs when the diaphragm and intercostal muscles are contracted and the lungs fill with air. When the air pressure inside the thorax equals the air pressure outside the body, air stops moving and inhalation stops. The diaphragm and inspiratory muscles relax, allowing the chest to recoil. As these muscles relax, all dimensions of the thorax decrease, and the ribs and muscles assume their normal resting position. When the chest cavity volume decreases, air in the lungs is compressed into a smaller space, such that the pressure there is greater than the atmospheric pressure. *Intrapulmonic pressure* (the pressure within the lungs and airways) is increased, and air is pushed out through the trachea.

Words of Wisdom

Normal breathing involves negative intrathoracic pressure and pulling air into lungs (negative-pressure ventilation). Negative intrathoracic pressure cannot be created when a patient has ineffective chest movement (such as with reduced tidal volume) or no chest movement (as in apnea). When this occurs, the only way to move air into the lungs is by positive-pressure ventilation, the forcing of air into the lungs. Positive pressure can be created with a bag-mask device, pocket face mask, or mechanical ventilation device.

Exhalation is normally a passive process, which means that it does not typically require muscular effort. If more forceful exhalation is required, then the posterior internal intercostal muscles contract, pulling the ribs and sternum downward and inward to further increase the pressure in the lungs. Exhalation ends when the *intrapleural pressure* (the pressure between the pleura of the lungs) is equal to the atmospheric pressure, at which point air stops flowing from the lungs to the outside. At the equilibration point, all pressures in the respiratory system are exactly equal to atmospheric pressure except the intrapleural pressure. Intrapleural pressure stays just slightly negative as the visceral pleura is pulled inward by the tendency of the lungs to collapse and the parietal pleura is pulled outward by its adhesion to the chest wall.

It may help you to understand the ventilation process if you think of the thoracic cage as a bell jar

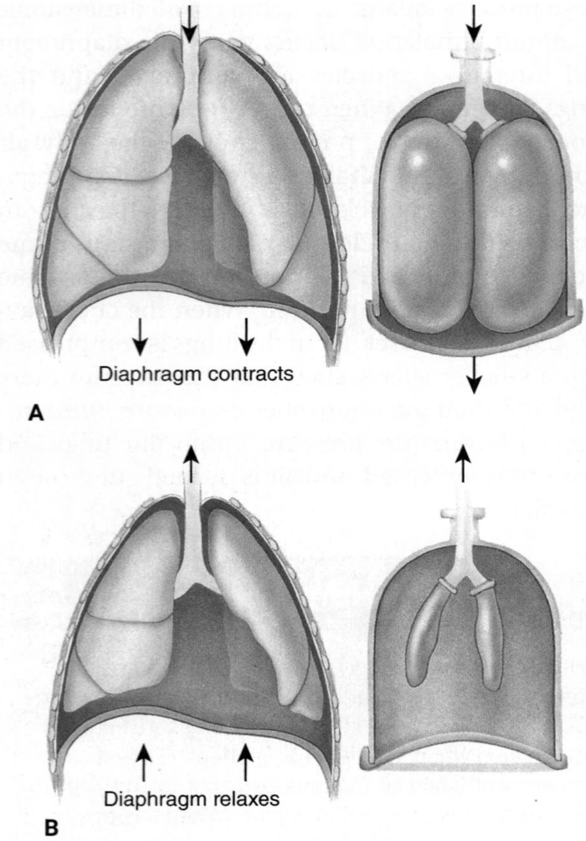

FIGURE 8-115 The mechanism of ventilation can be illustrated by a bell jar. **A.** Inhalation and chest expansion, anatomic (left) and bell jar (right). **B.** Exhalation and chest contraction, anatomic (left) and bell jar (right).

in which balloons are suspended **FIGURE 8-115**. In this example, the balloons are the lungs. The base of the jar is the diaphragm, which moves up and down slightly with each breath. The ribs, which are the sides of the jar, maintain the shape of the chest. The only opening into the jar is a small tube at the top, similar to the trachea. During inhalation, the bottom of the jar moves down slightly, causing a decrease in pressure in the jar and creating a slight vacuum. As a result, the balloons fill with air.

The accessory muscles are not generally active during quiet breathing **TABLE 8-40**. When greater amounts of air must be moved, such as during exercise or illness, these muscles (some of which are innervated by cranial nerves) can be recruited to cause more dramatic pressure changes. The intercostal muscles attach each rib to the ribs above it. These muscles allow the ribs to be pulled up and out, expanding the thoracic cavity and allowing more air to be taken in. Accessory muscles of the neck and back and elsewhere, such as the shoulder girdle, can also help open up the thorax.

TABLE 8-40 Muscles of Breathing

Ventilatory Phase	Role	Muscles
Inhalation	Primary	Diaphragm External intercostal muscles
	Accessory	Latissimus dorsi (lower back) Pectoralis major (anterior chest) Scalene muscles (neck) Serratus anterior (anterior chest) Sternocleidomastoid (neck) Trapezius (upper back)
Exhalation	Primary	External oblique muscles (abdomen) Internal intercostal muscles (chest) Internal oblique muscles (abdomen) Rectus abdominis (abdomen)
	Accessory	Latissimus dorsi (lower back)

Words of Wisdom

Ventilation and respiration are different processes, although these terms are often used interchangeably. *Ventilation*, the mechanical movement of air into and out of the lungs, is often misnamed *respiration*, which is the exchange of gases during cellular metabolism. Similarly, assessment of a patient's respiratory rate is an assessment of their ventilatory rate, or the number of times air is inhaled and exhaled per minute.[39]

Oxygenation

Recall that oxygenation is the process of loading oxygen molecules onto hemoglobin molecules in the bloodstream. Adequate oxygenation is required for internal respiration, but it does not guarantee that internal respiration is taking place. Oxygenation requires that the air used for ventilation contain an adequate percentage of oxygen. Whereas oxygenation cannot occur without ventilation, ventilation is possible without oxygenation. Ventilation without oxygenation may occur in places where the oxygen level in the air has been depleted, such as in mines and confined spaces. Oxygenation can also be impeded when other gases—for example, carbon monoxide—prevent oxygen from binding to hemoglobin.

Ventilation without adequate oxygenation also occurs in climbers who ascend too quickly to an altitude with inadequate atmospheric pressure. At high altitudes, the percentage of oxygen in the air remains the same (approximately 21%), but the atmospheric pressure makes it difficult to bring sufficient amounts of oxygen into the body.

The **fraction of inspired oxygen (Fio_2)** is the percentage of oxygen in inhaled air. The Fio_2 increases when supplemental oxygen is given to a patient and is commonly documented as a decimal number. For example, a person breathing room air, which contains about 21% oxygen, would be documented as having an Fio_2 of 0.21.

Oxyhemoglobin Dissociation Curve

Hemoglobin is an iron-containing molecule that has a great affinity for oxygen molecules. **Oxyhemoglobin** is hemoglobin that has oxygen molecules bound to it. Approximately 95% of the protein in an RBC is hemoglobin. Recall that one hemoglobin molecule reversibly binds with four oxygen molecules. Oxygen saturation (expressed as Spo_2 if measured by pulse oximetry and as Sao_2 if measured in arterial blood gases) is proportional to the amount of oxygen dissolved in the plasma component of the blood (Pao_2). The relationship between Pao_2 and Sao_2/Spo_2 is represented by the oxyhemoglobin dissociation curve **FIGURE 8-116**. Under normal conditions (Pao_2 = 105 mm Hg), the Spo_2/Sao_2 level is about 98%.

While the term *deoxygenated* is often used to describe the venous blood returning to the heart during circulation, this blood is not completely devoid of oxygen. Some oxygen remains bound to hemoglobin because the respiratory system's ability to supply oxygen to the rest of the body exceeds the demand in normal resting conditions. When

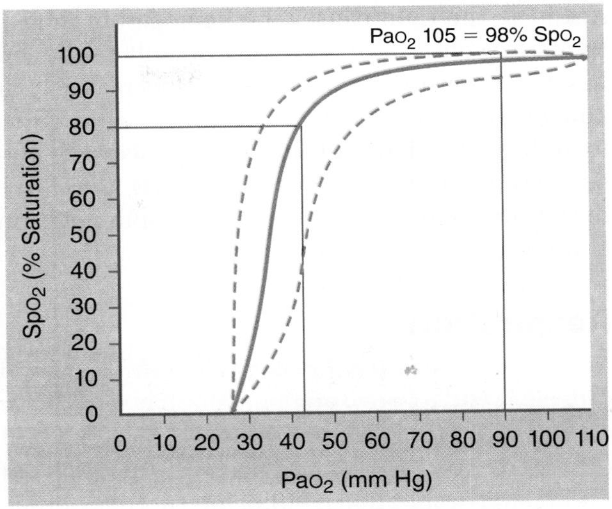

FIGURE 8-116 The oxyhemoglobin dissociation curve. Shifts are represented by dotted lines.

metabolism increases, however, the demand for oxygen increases and venous blood contains less oxygen. As blood is circulated to the tissue level, the Pao_2 begins to drop. At this point, the hemoglobin releases its oxygen molecules to make them available for cellular respiration.

In response to changes in metabolism, hemoglobin changes how tightly it holds onto oxygen. More oxygen molecules are released as the acidity of the blood increases (when pH decreases). This change results in a shift in position of the oxyhemoglobin dissociation curve. Various other conditions can also shift the entire curve to the left or right.

Words of Wisdom

Physiologic dead space is an example of a *ventilation/perfusion mismatch*. This situation occurs when an area of the lung is either ventilated but not perfused or perfused but not ventilated. In the case of ventilaton without perfusion, oxygen is in the alveoli but no blood flow can pick up the oxygen; in the case perfusion without ventilation, blood flow to the alveoli is present but no oxygen is available at that location to be absorbed. With both types of ventilation/perfusion mismatch (lack of oxygen or lack of blood flow), the outcome is a *right-to-left shunt*. In essence, the unoxygenated blood from the right atrium is returning to the left atrium in an unoxygenated state.

A shift to the right causes the hemoglobin to give up its oxygen faster and earlier; a shift to the left has the opposite effect. Acidosis (decreased pH) and increased carbon dioxide levels cause the curve to shift to the right. Alkalosis (increased pH) and decreased carbon dioxide levels cause the curve to shift to the left, so that the hemoglobin holds on to more oxygen.

Respiration

Respiration is the exchange of gases between a living organism and its environment. Human respiration provides oxygen to the body while removing carbon dioxide as one of the chief metabolic by-products of the system. Respiration is either internal or external.

External Respiration

External (pulmonary) respiration is the exchange of gases between the alveoli of the lungs and the RBCs traveling through the pulmonary capillaries **FIGURE 8-117**. Fresh air that is inspired into the lungs contains approximately 21% oxygen, 78% nitrogen, and small amounts of other gases. As this air reaches the alveoli, it comes into contact with surfactant, which reduces surface tension within the alveoli and keeps them expanded; this expansion facilitates the exchange of oxygen and carbon dioxide.

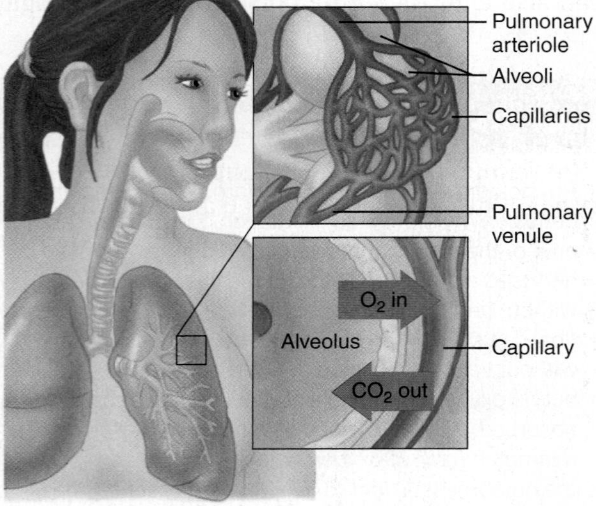

FIGURE 8-117 External (pulmonary) respiration.

> **Words of Wisdom**
>
> Although adequate ventilation is necessary for external respiration to occur, it does not guarantee that external respiration is being achieved.

After oxygen crosses the alveolar membrane, it is bound to hemoglobin. Hemoglobin molecules that are low in oxygen concentration are pumped from the right side of the heart into the capillaries of the pulmonary circulation. The capillaries surrounding the alveoli contain high concentrations of oxygen (from inspired air). The hemoglobin molecules pick up fresh oxygen as it crosses the alveolar membrane and transport it back to the left side of the heart, where it is pumped out to the rest of the body. Under normal conditions, 96% to 100% of the hemoglobin receptors contain oxygen.

Internal Respiration

Once in the bloodstream, gases are exchanged between blood cells and tissues through internal (cellular) respiration **FIGURE 8-118**. Without an intact cardiovascular system, internal respiration cannot occur.

Recall that in the presence of oxygen, the mitochondria of the cells convert glucose into energy through aerobic metabolism (aerobic respiration). Energy in the form of ATP is produced through the Krebs cycle and oxidative phosphorylation, which

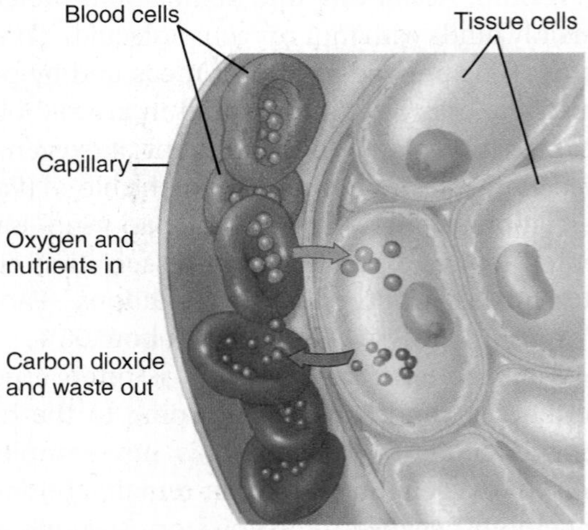

FIGURE 8-118 Internal (cellular) respiration.

is the process by which the liberated energy (via oxidation of metabolites) is used to synthesize ATP. Together, these chemical processes yield nearly 40 molecules of energy-rich ATP for each molecule of glucose metabolized. Without adequate oxygen, the cells do not completely convert glucose into energy, and lactic acid and other toxins build up in the cell. This process, which is called anaerobic metabolism (anaerobic respiration), cannot meet the metabolic demands of the cell. Another intracellular process, glycolysis, also contributes to the production of ATP and does not require oxygen. Glycolysis results in less production of ATP, but does produce lactic acid waste products and toxins. If anaerobic metabolism is not corrected, then the cells will eventually die. Adequate perfusion and ventilation must be present to support sufficient ATP production and, therefore, aerobic internal respiration. Although perfusion and ventilation are necessary for internal respiration, they do not guarantee that aerobic internal respiration will occur.

When the mitochondria within each cell use oxygen to convert glucose to energy, carbon dioxide—the main waste product—builds up in the cell. Carbon dioxide is then transported through the circulatory system and back to the lungs for exhalation.

In the absence of oxygen, anaerobic metabolism creates a series of events that will eventually result in cellular death. Initially, cells become hypoxic. Later, as stores of glucose are depleted, lactic acid, which is the by-product of glycolysis, accumulates in the cells. The increasingly acidic environment destroys cellular proteins, in turn leading to cellular death.

Role of Diffusion

The process of oxygen transfer from air into the capillaries in the alveoli involves diffusion. Several concepts are useful in understanding this process.

Partial pressure is a term used to describe the amount of gas in air or dissolved in liquid, such as the blood. It is governed by **Henry's law**, which states that the amount of a gas in a solution varies directly with the partial pressure of a gas over a solution. In other words, as the pressure of a gas over a liquid decreases, the amount of gas dissolved in that liquid will also decrease. As more pressure is applied over the liquid, more gas can be dissolved in the liquid. In practical terms, Henry's law means that molecules of a gas can be dissolved in a liquid and remain in the liquid as long as the liquid is in a pressurized, closed container (eg, the cardiovascular system). Partial pressure is measured in millimeters of mercury (mm Hg); 1 mm Hg is equivalent to 1 torr (symbol: Torr). Note that the partial pressure of a gas is not the same as its concentration.

When multiple gases are present, each gas exerts a pressure. When several gases are contained within the same space, their partial pressures can be measured. Four main gases are found in Earth's atmosphere: nitrogen, oxygen, water vapor, and carbon dioxide. The average total pressure exerted by the gases composing the atmosphere is sufficient to elevate a column of mercury (Hg) 760 mm. Therefore, at sea level the total atmospheric pressure is 760 Torr.

Inspired air is a mixture of 78% nitrogen, 21% oxygen, 0.04% carbon dioxide, and a nominal amount of other gases exerting a pressure of 760 mm Hg at sea level. Each gas represents a portion of the air mixture, so it exerts a partial pressure. The sum of the partial pressures is equal to the total pressure of the mixture. Because gases are lipid soluble, they freely cross the cell membrane and move by diffusion. The partial pressures of the air mixture are responsible for its diffusion across cell membranes. In the healthy lung, the normal partial pressure of oxygen (Pao_2) in arterial blood is 80 to 100 Torr and the normal partial pressure of carbon dioxide ($Paco_2$) in arterial blood is 35 to 45 Torr.

In the venous blood returning to the lungs, carbon dioxide exerts a high partial pressure and oxygen exerts a low partial pressure, in contrast to the high partial pressure of oxygen and low partial pressure of carbon dioxide in arterial blood in the lungs. As a result, carbon dioxide diffuses out of the venous blood into the lungs **FIGURE 8-119**. Oxygen diffuses out of the alveoli and into the arterial blood, where about 97% of oxygen combines with the hemoglobin molecule of the RBC for transport.

Arterial blood that reaches the tissues has a high partial pressure of oxygen and a low partial pressure of carbon dioxide. When this blood reaches the capillaries, oxygen diffuses out of the arterial blood and into the interstitial fluid (and eventually into the ICF), whereas carbon dioxide diffuses out of the interstitial fluid and into the venous blood.

Unlike oxygen, which is transported by hemoglobin, carbon dioxide is transported by one of

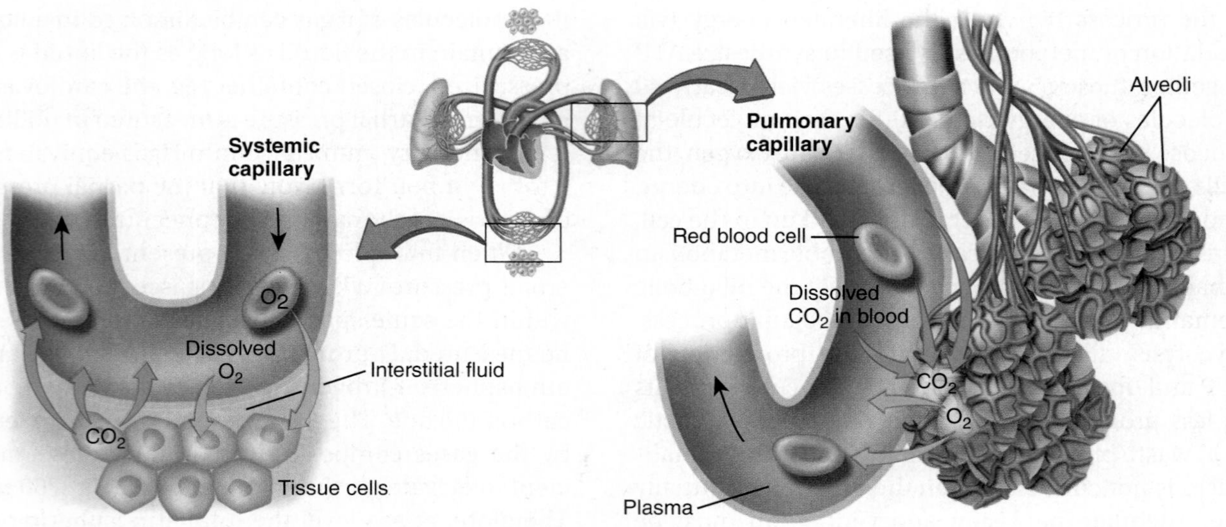

FIGURE 8-119 In the lungs' capillaries, oxygen passes from the blood to the tissue cells, and carbon dioxide and waste pass from the tissue cells to the blood. Diffusion occurs when molecules move from an area of higher concentration to an area of lower concentration.

three methods by the venous blood: dissolved in the blood, attached to the hemoglobin, or in the form of bicarbonate ions, which are created when carbon dioxide combines with water. The carbon dioxide that is attached to the hemoglobin attaches to amino groups, whereas oxygen attaches to iron atoms. Given their different points of attachment, the two molecules may both be carried at the same time and do not need to compete for binding sites on the hemoglobin.

Control of Breathing

The body's need for oxygen is dynamic; it is constantly changing. The respiratory system must be able to accommodate the perpetual changes in oxygen demand by altering the rate and depth of ventilation. These changes are regulated primarily by the pH of the CSF, which is directly related to the amount of carbon dioxide dissolved in the plasma portion of the blood ($Paco_2$). The regulation of ventilation involves a complex series of receptors and feedback loops that sense gas concentrations in the body fluids and send messages to the respiratory centers in the brain to adjust the rate and depth of ventilation accordingly.

Neural Control of Ventilation

Breathing is largely an involuntary mechanism, although it can be consciously altered for a short period. Involuntary breathing is controlled by the respiratory centers of the brainstem (the medulla and pons), which relay impulses through nerves to the inspiratory and expiratory muscles, causing them to contract and relax. Voluntary breathing is necessary for activities such as speaking, singing, holding one's breath, laughing, and blowing up a balloon. With voluntary breathing, control begins in the motor cortex of the cerebrum. Impulses travel down the corticospinal tracts to integrating centers in the spinal cord, thereby bypassing the brainstem.[34]

The control system that regulates involuntary breathing is made up of three components:

- **Control center.** The control center consists of three pairs of respiratory centers in the reticular formation of the medulla oblongata and pons; there is one of each on the right and left sides of the brainstem.[34] These respiratory centers are the **ventral respiratory group (VRG)** and the **dorsal respiratory group (DRG)** of the medulla and the **pontine respiratory group (PRG)** located in the pons (formerly called the pneumotaxic center) **FIGURE 8-120**.
- **Effectors.** The effectors are the respiratory muscles, whose activity is directed by the respiratory centers, resulting in muscle contraction and relaxation.
- **Sensors.** Sensors include central chemoreceptors in the medulla (which respond to changes

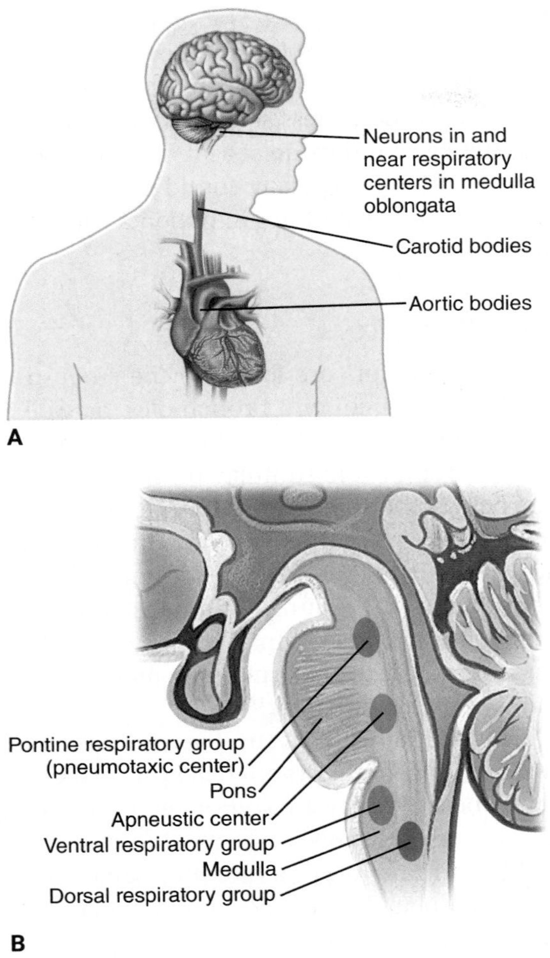

FIGURE 8-120 Important structures in the regulation of ventilation. **A.** Chemoreceptor locations. **B.** Respiratory centers.

in $P\text{CO}_2$ and pH); peripheral chemoreceptors in the carotid and aortic bodies (which respond to changes in $P\text{O}_2$, $P\text{CO}_2$, and pH); mechanoreceptors (which are located in the chest wall and lungs, lung stretch receptors, and skin thermoreceptors); proprioceptors in muscles, tendons, and joints;[40] and irritant receptors in the trachea and large airways.

The VRG is a network of inspiratory and expiratory motor neurons with nuclei located in the ventral portion of the medulla. The rhythm of normal, quiet breathing results from alternating patterns of stimulation and inhibition of the motor neurons that innervate the diaphragm (the phrenic nerves) and external intercostal muscles (the intercostal nerves). During inhalation, inspiratory neurons of the VRG send impulses by way of these motor nerves, resulting in contraction of the diaphragm and external intercostals, enlargement of the thoracic cage, and the inhalation of air. As the activity of the inspiratory neurons declines, the expiratory neurons fire. Signals are sent to the internal intercostal and abdominal muscles, the inspiratory muscles relax, the lungs recoil, and air is exhaled from the lungs. As the activity of the expiratory neurons decreases, the inspiratory neurons resume firing, and the cycle repeats.

The DRG, also located in the medulla, functions as an integration center. It receives input from several sources, including the PRG, glossopharyngeal (CN IX) and vagus (CN X) nerves,[41] central chemoreceptors in the medulla, and peripheral chemoreceptors.[34] The DRG signals the VRG to alter the rhythm and depth of ventilation to restore homeostasis.

The PRG receives input from the cerebral cortex, the hypothalamus, and the limbic system and communicates information to both the VRG and DRG.[34] Although the respiratory centers of the medulla can generate a basic respiratory rhythm, the PRG influences and modifies the ventilatory rate and depth established by the medullary centers.[40] For example, the PRG is thought to smooth the transition between each phase of the ventilatory cycle and alter breathing by making each breath shorter and shallower or longer and deeper, depending on the body's needs. The **apneustic center** of the pons is thought to work with the PRG to regulate the length and depth of inspiration.[42]

Chemical Control of Ventilation

The goal of the respiratory system is to keep the blood's concentrations of oxygen and carbon dioxide and its acid–base balance within narrow ranges. The body has several receptors that monitor variables and provide feedback to the respiratory centers, which then prompts them to adjust the rate and depth of breathing based on the body's needs. These chemoreceptors have important effects on ventilatory rate and depth.

Chemoreceptors that constantly monitor the chemical composition of body fluids are located throughout the body to provide feedback on many metabolic processes. Both central and peripheral chemoreceptors affect respiratory function (see Figure 8-120).

Central chemoreceptors, located in the medulla, respond to changes in carbon dioxide and pH of the CSF. Any changes noted in the Pco_2 of arterial blood are quickly reflected in the pH level of the CSF. The acidity of the CSF is an indirect measure of the amount of carbon dioxide in arterial blood because the carbon dioxide in the blood readily diffuses across the blood–brain barrier and combines with water to form carbonic acid. When this carbonic acid dissociates, the pH drops as the hydrogen ion concentration increases. An increase in the acidity of the CSF triggers the central chemoreceptors to increase the rate and depth of breathing to blow off excess carbon dioxide building up in the body. Conversely, when pH levels of the CSF become more alkaline because of low levels of Pco_2 in the blood, the ventilatory rate decreases.

Peripheral chemoreceptors in the carotid bodies and aortic bodies respond to changes in Po_2, Pco_2, and pH. These receptors sense tiny changes in the carbon dioxide level and send signals to the respiratory center via the cranial nerves. The carotid bodies send signals to the brainstem via the glossopharyngeal nerve (CN IX), whereas chemoreceptors in the aortic arch communicate by way of the vagus nerve (CN X).

When serum carbon dioxide or hydrogen ion levels increase because of a medical condition or traumatic injury involving the respiratory system, chemoreceptors stimulate the respiratory control centers in the medulla to increase the ventilatory rate, so as to remove more carbon dioxide or acid from the body.

Hypoxic Drive

Patients with chronic obstructive pulmonary disease (COPD), such as emphysema and chronic bronchitis, have difficulty eliminating carbon dioxide through exhalation; therefore, they always have higher blood levels of carbon dioxide. This persistently high level can potentially alter their primary respiratory drive, which is based on increased arterial carbon dioxide levels and the pH of the CSF. The theory is that the respiratory centers in the brain gradually accommodate elevated carbon dioxide levels. In patients with end-stage COPD, the body uses a backup system to control breathing. The current theory is that this secondary control, called **hypoxic drive**, stimulates breathing when the arterial oxygen level falls. However, the nerves in the brain, walls of the aorta, and carotid arteries that act as oxygen sensors (chemoreceptors) are easily satisfied with a minimal oxygen level. Therefore, hypoxic drive is much less sensitive and less powerful than the carbon dioxide sensors in the brainstem. Hypoxic drive is typically found in patients with end-stage COPD, and not in patients with a recent diagnosis of COPD.

Lung Receptors

Mechanoreceptors are found in the smooth muscles of the bronchi and bronchioles, as well as in the visceral pleura.[34] When the lungs inflate, these stretch receptors are stimulated, with nerve signals then being sent to the respiratory centers by the vagus nerve to inhibit inspiration. This reflex, called the **Hering-Breuer reflex**, is designed to prevent overinflation of the lungs in a conscious, spontaneously breathing person. Because this reflex also increases ventilatory frequency, it maintains a constant alveolar ventilation.[41]

The epithelial cells in the airway's mucous membranes contain irritant receptors, which are so named because they are stimulated by smoke, pollen, dust, excess mucus, chemical fumes, and cold air. When irritant receptors are stimulated, the vagus nerve conducts the signals to the brainstem, which then signals the respiratory and bronchial muscles, triggering protective reflexes such as coughing, bronchoconstriction, or shallow breathing.[34]

Buffer Systems

Recall that a buffer is a substance that can absorb or donate hydrogen ions. Buffers absorb hydrogen ions when they are in excess and donate hydrogen ions when they are depleted. In this way, **buffer systems** act as rapid defenses against acid–base changes, providing almost immediate protection against changes in the hydrogen ion concentration of the ECF. Problems occur when the amount of acid in circulation is too great for the buffer system to accommodate. To grasp this concept, imagine the buffer system as a bucket that contains the acid in the body **FIGURE 8-121**. Like a bucket, the buffer system can hold only a certain amount before it overflows.

Three primary buffer systems help the body maintain pH within the optimal range: (1) the circulating bicarbonate buffer component, (2) the

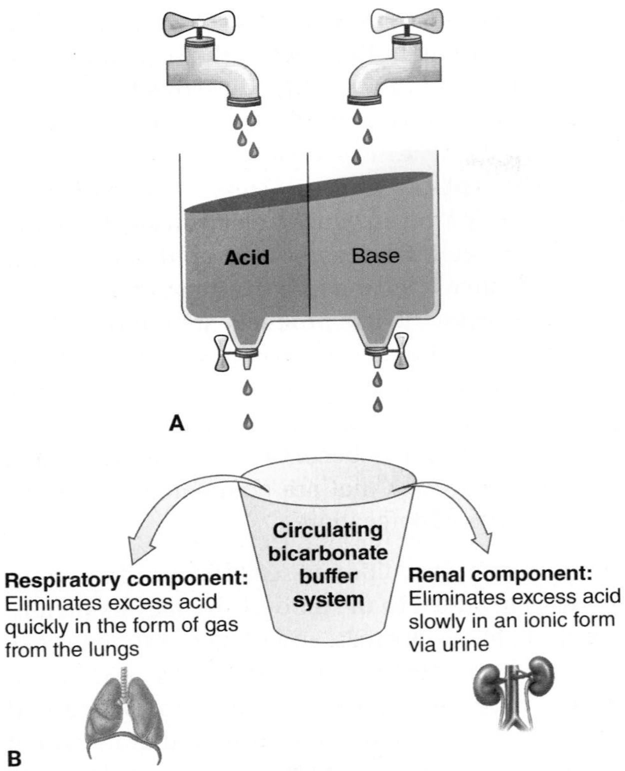
Acid
Base
A
Circulating bicarbonate buffer system
Respiratory component: Eliminates excess acid quickly in the form of gas from the lungs
Renal component: Eliminates excess acid slowly in an ionic form via urine
B

FIGURE 8-121 Buffer systems. **A.** As acid or base levels fluctuate, the body must work to ensure that acid–base balance is maintained. **B.** The respiratory component and the renal component are two systems for eliminating excess acid.

respiratory system, and (3) the renal system. The body's fastest means of restoring acid–base balance is the so-called blood buffer—the bicarbonate content of ICF and ECF. When an excessive level of acid builds up, it is eliminated through the respiratory system, when carbon dioxide is expelled from the lungs. Conversely, slowing the rate of breathing encourages the retention of carbon dioxide. The renal system regulates pH by filtering out hydrogen and retaining bicarbonate when necessary, or vice versa.

Circulating Bicarbonate Buffer Component. During cellular metabolism, large amounts of carbon dioxide are produced as a waste product. Most of this carbon dioxide is stored in ICF and ECF in the form of bicarbonate, the body's most important buffer system. This system is like a bucket that holds and neutralizes excess acid.

In the bicarbonate buffer system, excess acid (H^+) combines with bicarbonate (HCO_3^-) to form carbonic acid ($H_2CO_3^-$). This compound rapidly dissociates into water and carbon dioxide, which is then exhaled. Because the acid is eliminated in the form of water and carbon dioxide, the total pH does not change significantly. A similar process occurs with the production of metabolic base (bicarbonate).

Carbonic acid is a weak acid that can give up an extra hydrogen ion to once again form a bicarbonate ion. The extra hydrogen ion from this reaction is then converted during metabolism into compounds that are easily expelled from the body, thereby eliminating excess acid.

Respiratory Buffer Component. Aside from the circulating bicarbonate buffer component, the fastest way the body can eliminate excess hydrogen ions is to create water and carbon dioxide, which can be expelled as gases from the lungs.

Carbonic acid is created when carbon dioxide combines with circulating water in the blood. Chemoreceptors in the brain sense the rising level of carbonic acid and signal the respiratory centers to increase the ventilatory rate to reduce the amount of circulating carbon dioxide. Although the respiratory buffer reacts within minutes, it responds much more slowly than the circulating bicarbonate buffer component.

Acidosis can develop because of abnormal ventilatory function, including a breathing rate that is too fast or too slow, labored breathing, or shallow breathing (reduced tidal volume). At the other end of the acid–base spectrum, alkalosis can develop if the ventilatory rate is too high or the volume too large.

Renal Buffer Component. The kidneys monitor hydrogen and bicarbonate levels in the tubules of nephrons as part of their effort to maintain pH. However, the renal buffer component responds more slowly to an increasing acid level than the bicarbonate and respiratory buffer components. Indeed, it could take hours or even days for the renal buffer system to restore the body's pH to normal.

When the blood contains high levels of carbonic acid, the kidneys respond by excreting more hydrogen ions and breaking down carbonic acid into carbon dioxide and water. In the tubule cell, the carbon dioxide is reabsorbed; a new bicarbonate ion is formed and diffuses through peritubular capillaries into the blood. Reabsorbed bicarbonate is neutralized by reabsorbed sodium ions, which are exchanged for hydrogen ions excreted in the urine. When the blood contains low levels of carbonic acid, the kidneys excrete fewer hydrogen ions and more bicarbonate.

Control of Ventilation by Other Factors

Multiple other factors influence the control of ventilatory rates. Factors such as elevated body temperature, CNS stimulants, pain, emotion, hypoxia, and acidosis cause an increased ventilatory rate. Sleep, decreased metabolic states, and CNS depressants, including alcohol, decrease the ventilatory rate.

The Digestive System

The digestive system comprises two major divisions: (1) the alimentary canal and (2) the accessory digestive organs. The alimentary canal, which consists of a series of muscular tubes, is specialized along its length for the sequential processing of food.[43] Collectively, these tubes are designed to move food and liquid from its entrance into the body (typically the mouth) to its elimination from the body through the anus. The GI tract is the portion of the alimentary canal that consists of the stomach and intestines. The accessory digestive organs produce and secrete enzymes and juices essential in the digestive process.

The digestive system is responsible for six processes:

1. **Ingestion.** This process brings material into the digestive tract via the mouth.
2. **Mechanical processing.** Materials are crushed and broken into smaller fragments, making them easier to move through the digestive tract; enzymes begin to attack the particles during chewing, while the teeth and tongue are used to tear and mash food. Additional mechanical processing is provided by the mixing motions of the stomach and intestines.
3. **Digestion.** The chemical breakdown of food material creates smaller fragments that can be absorbed into the circulatory system. Simple molecules (eg, glucose) are absorbed intact, whereas more complex molecules (eg, polysaccharides, proteins, triglycerides) must first be broken down before they can be absorbed.
4. **Secretion.** The release of water, acids, enzymes, and buffers aids in the breakdown and digestion of food in the digestive tract. These secretions come from both the digestive tract and the accessory organs.
5. **Absorption.** Organic substrates (molecules acted on by enzymes), electrolytes, vitamins, and water move across the epithelium of the digestive tract and into the interstitial fluid.
6. **Excretion.** Waste products are removed from the body fluids via secretions from the digestive tract and glandular organs. After mixing with residue that cannot be digested, these waste products become *feces*, the undigested food particles that are eliminated during the process of defecation.

In succession, different secretions, primarily enzymes, are added to the food by the salivary glands, stomach, liver, pancreas, and small intestine to convert food into basic sugars, fatty acids, and amino acids. These basic products of digestion are carried across the wall of the intestine and transported through the portal vein to the liver. In the liver, the products are processed further and either stored or transported to the heart through veins draining the liver. The heart then pumps the blood with these nutrients throughout the arteries to the capillaries, where the nutrients pass through the capillary walls to nourish the body's individual cells.

The alimentary canal extends from the mouth to the anus. It includes the mouth, pharynx, esophagus, stomach, intestines, rectum, and anus. The walls of the alimentary canal consist of four layers, which are specialized in certain regions for particular functions **FIGURE 8-122**:

- **Mucosa (mucous membrane).** Surface epithelium, underlying connective tissue, and a small amount of smooth muscle. It is folded in some regions, with projections extending into the lumen that increase its absorptive surface. The mucosa carries out secretion and absorption.
- **Submucosa.** Loose connective tissue with glands, blood vessels, lymphatic vessels, and nerves. It nourishes surrounding tissues and carries away absorbed materials.
- **Muscular layer.** Produces movements of the tube. This layer is made of two smooth muscle tissue coats: Circular fibers of the inner coat

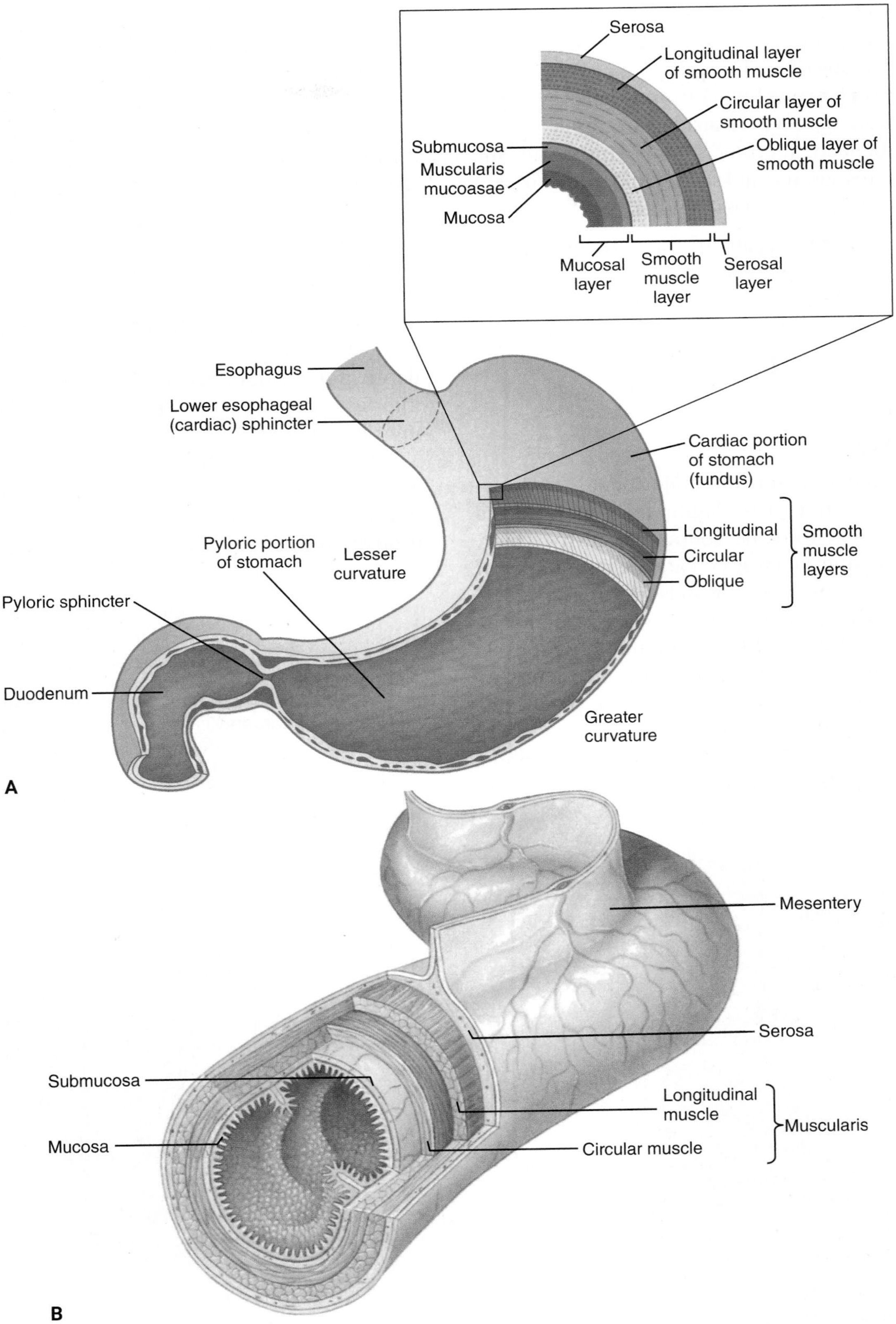

FIGURE 8-122 The layers of the alimentary canal. **A.** Layers of the stomach. **B.** Layers of the intestines.

encircle the tube, causing contraction, and longitudinal fibers run lengthwise, causing shortening of the tube.
- **Serosa (serous layer).** Composed of a visceral peritoneum on the outside and connective tissue beneath. It protects underlying tissues and secretes serous fluid so that abdominal organs slide freely against each other.

The accessory organs of the alimentary canal include the teeth, tongue, salivary glands, liver, gallbladder, and pancreas. The secretions from these accessory organs empty via ducts into the digestive tract. The organs of the digestive system are found within the abdomen.

Abdomen

The abdomen contains the major organs of digestion and excretion. The diaphragm separates the thoracic cavity from the abdominal cavity. Thick, muscular abdominal walls create the boundaries of this space anteriorly and posteriorly. Inferiorly, the abdomen is separated from the pelvis by an imaginary plane that extends from the pubic symphysis through the sacrum **FIGURE 8-123**. Some organs may lie in both the abdomen and the pelvis, depending on the patient's posture.

The simplest and most common method of describing the portions of the abdomen is by quadrants—that is, by envisioning four equal areas formed by two imaginary lines that intersect at right angles at the umbilicus. On the anterior abdominal wall, the quadrants formed in this way are the right upper quadrant (RUQ), the right lower quadrant (RLQ), the left lower quadrant (LLQ), and the left upper quadrant (LUQ) **FIGURE 8-124**. The area around the umbilicus is the periumbilical area.

In the RUQ, the major organs are the liver, the gallbladder, and a portion of the colon and small intestine. Most of the liver lies in this quadrant, almost entirely under the protection of the 8th to 12th ribs. The liver fills the entire anteroposterior depth of the abdomen in the RUQ. In consequence, injuries in this area are frequently associated with injuries of the liver.

In the LUQ, the principal organs are the stomach, the spleen, and a portion of the colon and small intestine. The spleen is almost entirely under the protection of the left rib cage, whereas the stomach

Words of Wisdom

The solid organs of the abdomen include the liver, spleen, pancreas, and kidneys. The hollow organs of the abdomen include the stomach, gallbladder, urinary bladder, and small and large intestines.

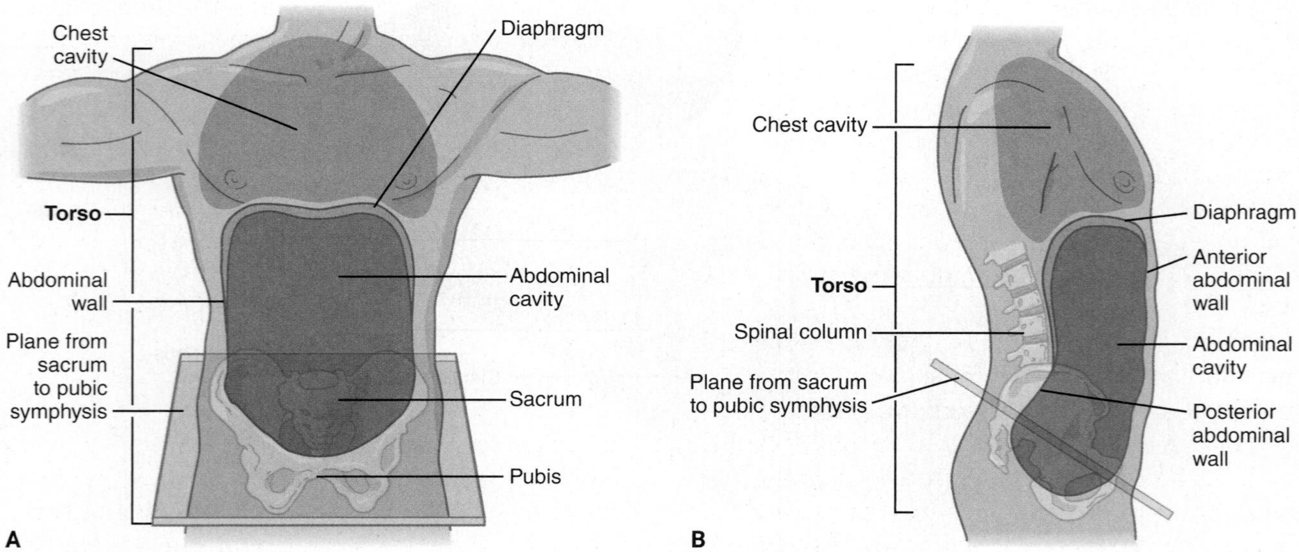

FIGURE 8-123 The boundaries of the abdomen are the anterior and posterior abdominal cavity walls, the diaphragm, and an imaginary plane from the pubic symphysis to the sacrum. **A.** Anterior view. **B.** Lateral view.

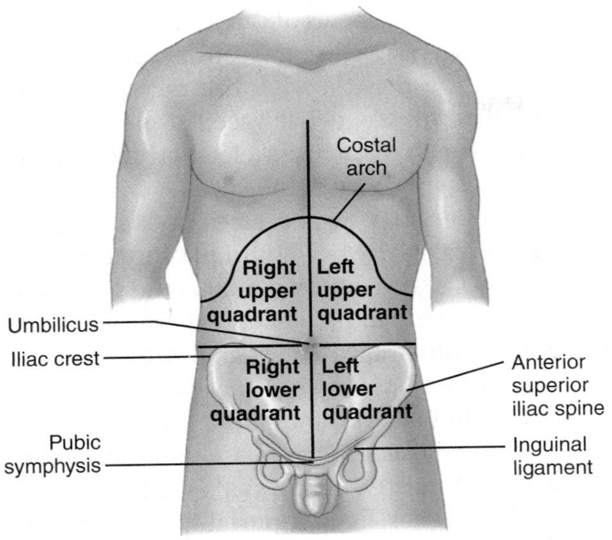

FIGURE 8-124 The four abdominal quadrants.

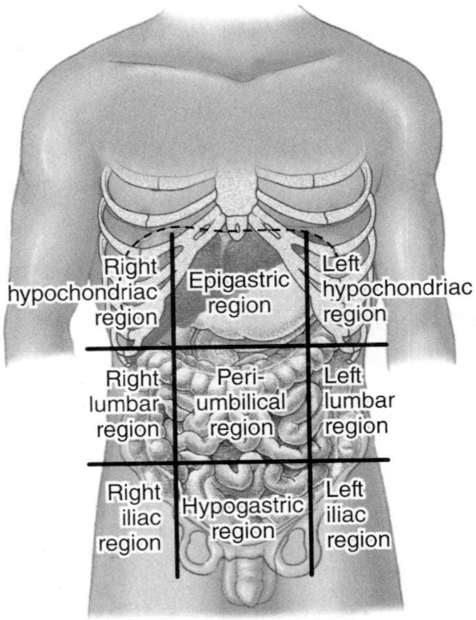

FIGURE 8-125 The nine abdominal regions.

may sag down into the LLQ when full. The spleen lies in the lateral and posterior portion of the LLQ, under the diaphragm and immediately in front of the 9th to 11th ribs. The spleen is frequently injured, especially when these ribs are fractured.

The RLQ contains two portions of the large intestine: the cecum, the first portion into which the small intestine (ileum) opens, and the ascending colon. The *appendix* is a small, tubular structure (about 3 to 4 inches [8 to 10 cm] long) that is effectively a small pouch attached to the lower border of the cecum. This structure is thought to contain nonpathogenic (ie, "good") intestinal bacteria that can migrate into the colon and restore balance if the bacterial balance within the colon becomes disrupted because of antibiotic use, infection, or diarrheal illness. The appendix may easily become obstructed, resulting in inflammation and infection. The descending and sigmoid portions of the colon lie in the LLQ.

Several organs lie in more than one quadrant. The small intestine, for example, occupies the central part of the abdomen around the umbilicus, and parts of it lie in all four quadrants. The pancreas lies just behind the abdominal cavity on the posterior abdominal wall in both upper quadrants. The large intestine also traverses the abdomen, beginning in the RLQ and ending in the LLQ as it passes through all four quadrants. The urinary bladder is located just behind the pubic symphysis in the middle of the abdomen, so it lies in both lower quadrants as well as in the pelvis. Less commonly, the abdomen and pelvis can be divided into nine sections to assist in describing the location of abdominal organs, pain, incisions, or scars **FIGURE 8-125**.

Most intra-abdominal structures are covered by a large, moist, continuous sheet of serous membrane called the **peritoneum**. The peritoneum is composed of two parts: the parietal peritoneum, which lines the walls of the abdominal cavity, and the visceral peritoneum, which covers the organs within the abdominal cavity. The potential space between these two layers is known as the peritoneal cavity. Organs in the abdominopelvic cavity are located either inside the peritoneum (intraperitoneal) or behind the peritoneum (retroperitoneal) **FIGURE 8-126**. The upper peritoneal cavity, also known as the thoracoabdominal component of the abdomen, is covered by the lower part of the thorax. The diaphragm, liver, spleen, stomach, gallbladder, and transverse colon are located here. The lower peritoneal cavity contains the small bowel, sigmoid colon, parts of the descending and ascending colon, and, in women, the internal reproductive organs. The retroperitoneal space contains the abdominal aorta, inferior vena cava, pancreas, kidneys, adrenal glands, **ureters** (tubes that carry urine from the kidneys to the bladder), most of the duodenum, and the posterior aspects of the descending and ascending colon, as well as the retroperitoneal components of the pelvic cavity. The rectum, ureters, bladder, iliac vessels, pelvic vascular plexus, major vascular structures, pelvic skeletal structures, and reproductive organs lie in the pelvis.

The abdominal organs are suspended within the abdominal cavity by folds of peritoneum called mesentery. The mesentery contains the nerves, arteries, veins, and lymph vessels that supply the intestines and other intra-abdominal structures.

Finally, the abdomen includes many vital blood vessels, including the abdominal aorta, superior and inferior mesenteric vessels, renal artery, gonadal arteries, gastric artery, splenic artery, hepatic artery, iliac arteries, hepatic portal system, and inferior vena cava **FIGURE 8-127**.

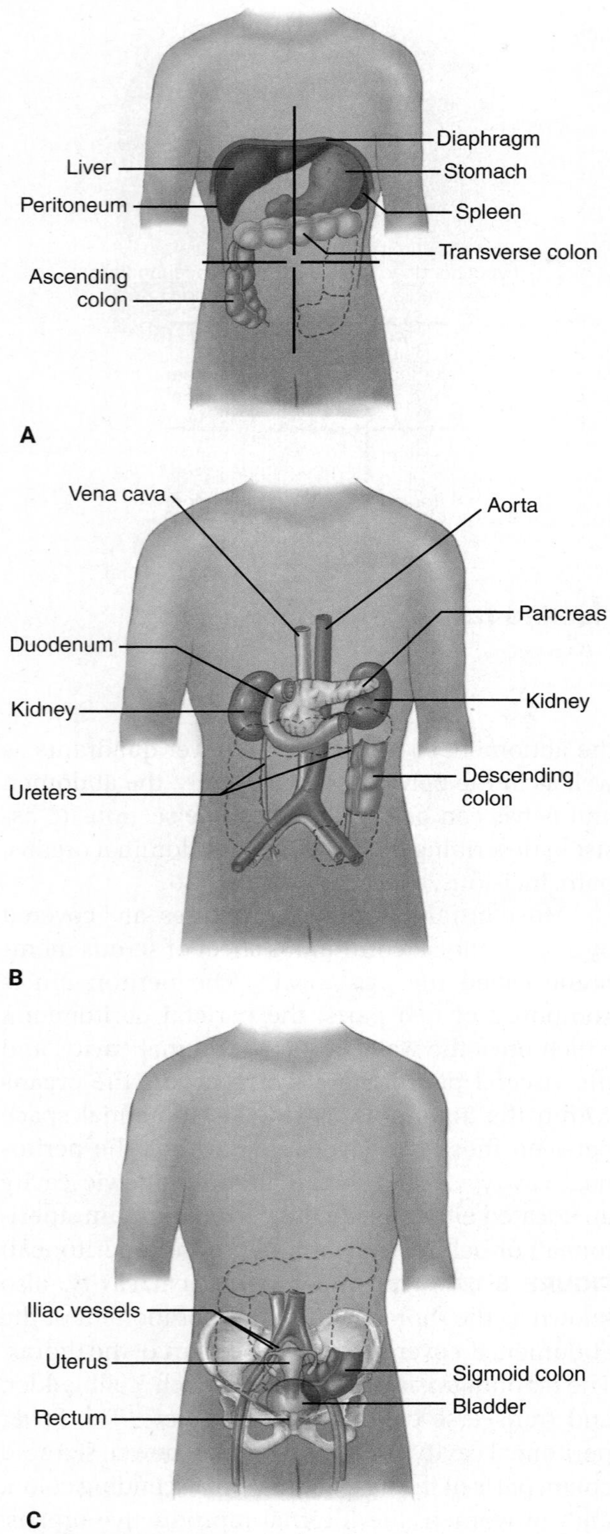

FIGURE 8-126 Different organs of the abdomen are contained in the peritoneum **(A)**, the retroperitoneal space **(B)**, and the pelvis **(C)**.

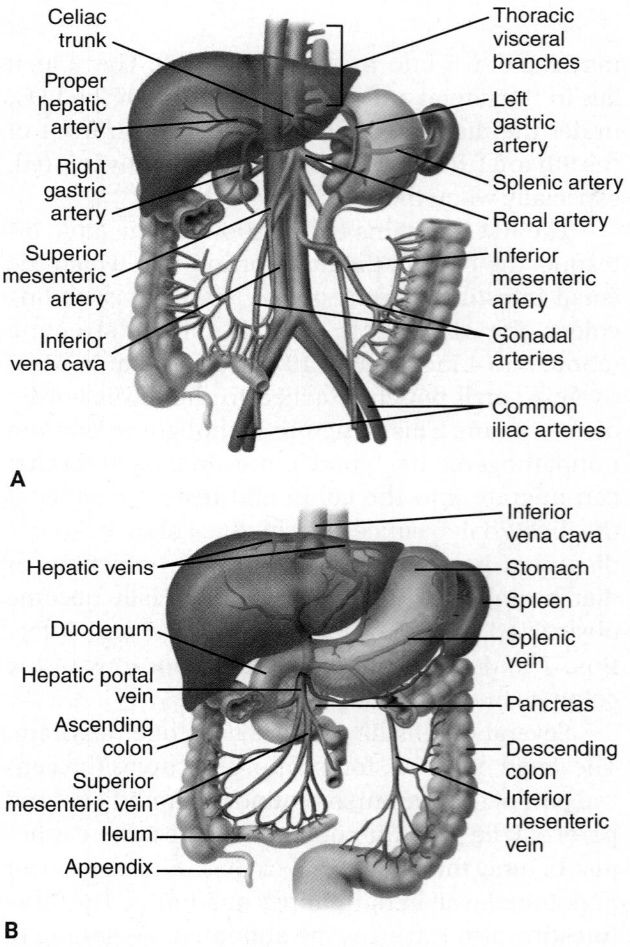

FIGURE 8-127 A. Arteries of the abdomen. **B.** Veins of the abdomen.

Oral Cavity

The first part of the digestive system is the oral cavity (mouth). The mouth consists of the lips, cheeks, gums, teeth, and tongue. A mucous membrane lines the mouth. The hard and soft palates form the roof of the mouth. The hard palate is a bony plate lying anteriorly; the soft palate is a fold of mucous membrane and muscle that extends posteriorly from the hard palate into the throat. The soft palate is designed to hold food that is being chewed within the mouth and to help initiate swallowing. The cheeks make up the lateral walls of the oral cavity. The floor of the oral cavity is formed mainly of soft tissues, such as the tongue.

Digestion begins in the mouth with mastication, or the chewing of food by the teeth. The hypoglossal (CN XII), glossopharyngeal (CN IX), trigeminal (CN V), and facial (CN VII) nerves supply the mouth and its structures. The hypoglossal nerve provides motor function to the muscles of the tongue. The glossopharyngeal nerve provides taste sensation to the posterior portions of the tongue and carries parasympathetic fibers to the salivary glands on each side of the face. The mandibular branch of the trigeminal nerve provides motor innervation to the muscles of mastication. In addition to supplying motor activity to all muscles of facial expression, the facial nerve provides the sense of taste to the anterior two-thirds of the tongue and cutaneous sensations to the tongue and palate.

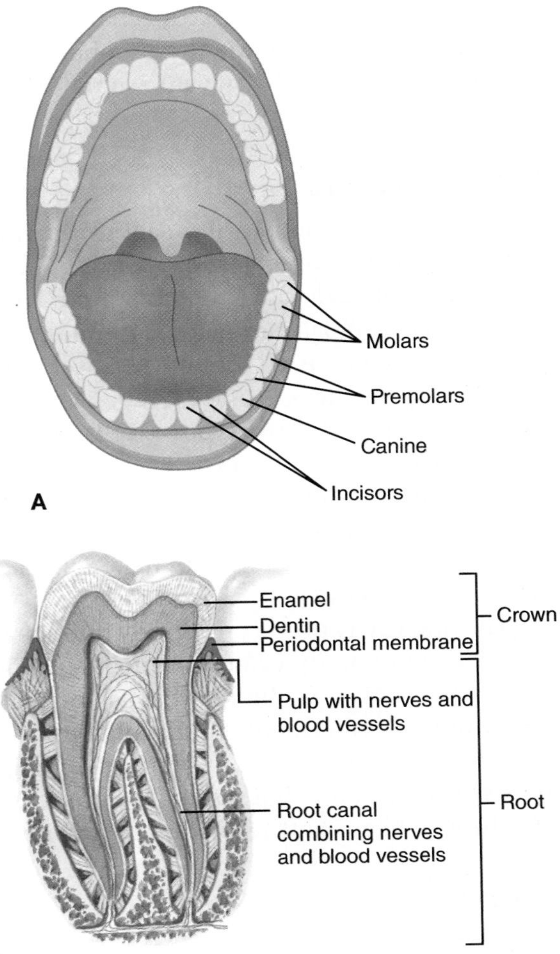

FIGURE 8-128 The teeth of the adult mouth. **A.** The incisors are used for biting. The canines are used for tearing food. The premolars and molars are used for grinding and crushing. **B.** Each tooth contains nerves and blood vessels.

Teeth

Recall that the normal adult mouth contains 32 permanent teeth. Loss of the primary or deciduous teeth occurs during childhood, with the permanent teeth then replacing them. The adult teeth are distributed about the maxillary and mandibular arches. The teeth on each side of the arch are mirror images of each other and form four quadrants: right upper, left upper, right lower, and left lower. Each quadrant contains one central incisor, one lateral incisor, one canine, two premolars, and three molars **FIGURE 8-128**. The third molars (wisdom teeth) do not appear until late adolescence.

The top portion of the tooth, external to the gum, is the crown, which contains one or more cusps. Below the crown lie the neck and the root. The pulp cavity fills the tooth's center; it contains blood vessels, nerves, and specialized connective tissue, called pulp. Dentin and enamel surround the pulp cavity and protect the tooth from damage. Dentin, which forms the principal mass of the tooth, is much denser and stronger than bone. The bony sockets for the teeth found in the mandible and maxilla are called alveoli. The ridges between the teeth, known as alveolar ridges, are covered by the gingiva, or gums, which consist of thickened connective tissue and epithelium. Teeth are attached to the alveolar bone by a periodontal membrane.

Your front teeth are mainly used to tear or cut the food. While chewing, the food is worked toward the back of the mouth, where the flat surfaces of the molars crush and grind the food into a more easily swallowed consistency. This mechanical activity eases food's passage down the esophagus during swallowing and helps to prevent aspiration of food into the lungs.

Salivary Glands

As mentioned previously, the salivary glands are accessory organs of digestion. During mastication, food is mixed with secretions from the salivary glands. Two salivary glands are found under the tongue, one on each side of the lower jaw, and one inside each cheek **FIGURE 8-129**. Each of these glands is composed of two types of cells: serous and mucous. The serous cells produce amylase, a salivary enzyme that begins the digestive process of starchy food material. The mucous cells produce mucus that binds and lubricates material placed in the mouth, such as food.

The oral cavity opens posteriorly into the pharynx. The oropharynx extends vertically from the back of the mouth to the esophagus and trachea. An automatic movement of the pharynx during swallowing lifts the larynx to permit the epiglottis to close over it so that liquids and solids are moved into the esophagus and away from the trachea.

Esophagus

Starting from the pharynx, the esophagus proceeds distally through the chest cavity, passes through the diaphragm, and terminates at the stomach. The esophagus is a hollow tube approximately 10 inches (25 cm) long and surrounded by smooth muscle. Although it helps transport food from the mouth to the stomach, it cannot absorb nutrients. The esophagus typically lies collapsed in on itself, like a dry fire hose. This deflated position allows air to flow easily into the lungs, rather than into the stomach. However, the esophagus dilates when food or liquid travels through it.

The esophagus lies posterior to the trachea. It begins to the right of the aorta and then passes anterior to the aorta as it traverses inferiorly to end at the stomach. Intertwined around the esophagus are veins that drain into another, more complex series of veins that ultimately converge to form the portal vein. The portal vein transports venous blood from the GI tract directly to the liver for processing of the nutrients that have been absorbed during the digestive process.

The esophagus propels material into the stomach by a series of wavelike contractions called **peristalsis**. Peristalsis is not limited to the esophagus; it is responsible for movement throughout the entire GI tract.

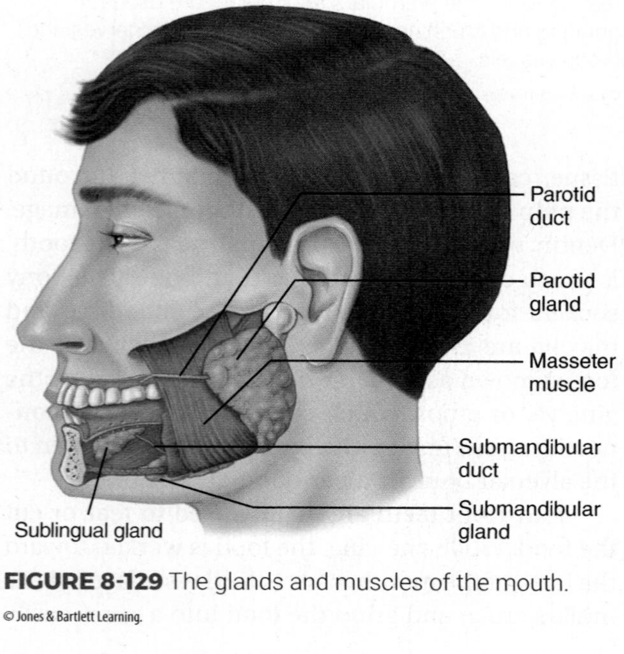

FIGURE 8-129 The glands and muscles of the mouth.

Stomach

The stomach is an intraperitoneal hollow organ that lies just inferior to the diaphragm in the LUQ of the abdomen. It is partially covered by the left lobe of the liver and largely protected by the lower left ribs. The stomach is concave (lesser curvature) on its right side, and convex (greater curvature) on its left side. The entrance into the stomach is surrounded by the cardiac sphincter, which controls the movement of material into this organ. When empty, the stomach is relatively small, but it can stretch to many times its normal size to accommodate meals. The principal function of the stomach is to receive food in large quantities intermittently, store it, and provide for its movement into the small intestine in small amounts.

The fundus of the stomach (its uppermost part) can adapt to varying amounts of food. This part is also where gas bubbles rise to, particularly after a meal. The body is the largest part of the stomach and serves primarily as the storage area for ingested food and liquid. The lower part of the stomach, known as the antrum, is somewhat funnel-shaped.

Words of Wisdom

The duodenum is the last section of the upper GI system. The jejunum is the first part of the lower GI system.

Its narrow end connects to the pyloric canal, which empties into the duodenum.

The stomach wall is composed of three layers (see Figure 8-122). The external layer, the longitudinal muscle, is continuous with the longitudinal muscle of the esophagus. The middle, or circular layer, is the strongest of the three layers; it completely covers the stomach. This circular muscle becomes significantly thicker where it forms the pyloric sphincter. The inner layer, or oblique layer, is the strongest in the fundus region and becomes progressively weaker toward the pylorus (a circumferential muscle at the end of the stomach that acts as a valve).

Blood is supplied to the stomach via the celiac trunk, which branches from the abdominal portion of the aorta. Blood from the stomach is returned to the venous system via the portal vein, which carries blood to the liver. The nerve supply is provided by the sympathetic (celiac or solar plexus) and parasympathetic (vagus nerve or CN X) divisions of the ANS.

The stomach contains acid that assists in the digestive process. The gastric juice secreted in the stomach consists of a mixture of water, hydrochloric acid (strong enough to dissolve metal, with a pH of 1.5 to 3), organic substances (mucus, pepsin, and protein), and electrolytes (potassium, sodium, bicarbonate, sulfate, and phosphate). As food enters the stomach, hydrochloric acid is secreted, which helps to break down the food. The stomach contracts to help mix the acid with the food more evenly, churning the acid and food mixture together until a relatively smooth consistency is achieved. The resulting substance is called chyme. The stomach expels chyme through the pyloric sphincter and into the duodenum, the first part of the small intestine.

Small Intestine

The small intestine is the major hollow organ of the abdomen. The cells lining the small intestine produce enzymes and mucus to aid in digestion. Enzymes from the pancreas and the small intestine carry out the final processes of digestion. More than 90% of the products of digestion (amino acids, fatty acids, and simple sugars), together with water, ingested vitamins, and minerals, are absorbed across the wall of the lower end of the small intestine into veins to be transported to the liver.

The small intestine is composed of the duodenum, jejunum, and ileum. The duodenum, which is 9 to 11 inches (23 to 28 cm) long, is the part of the small intestine that receives food from the stomach. It forms a C-shaped curve around the head of the pancreas. The duodenal bulb is the widest part of the small intestine. As contents pass through the stomach, they move through the pylorus, which acts as a valve between the stomach and the duodenum. The duodenum connects the pancreas, liver, and gallbladder to the digestive system **FIGURE 8-130**.

The jejunum, a major site of nutrient absorption, and the ileum together measure more than 20 feet (6 m), on average, and make up the rest of the small intestine. The ileum, an area of decreased nutrient absorption, is where chyme is prepared for entry into the large intestine.

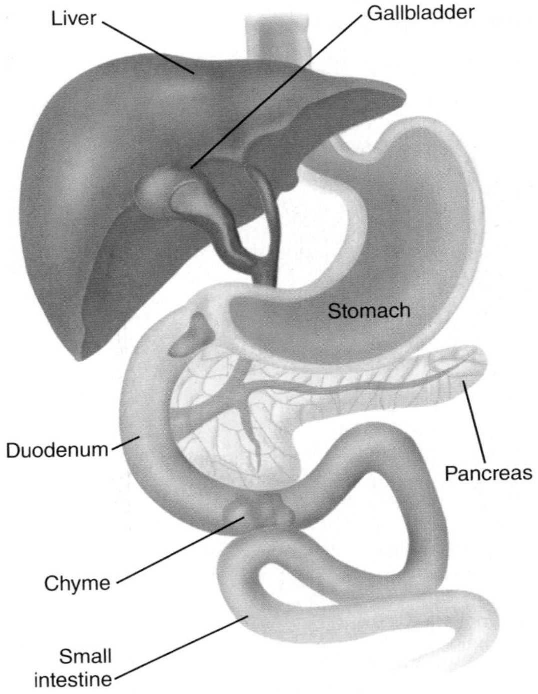

FIGURE 8-130 The duodenum connects the pancreas, liver, and gallbladder to the digestive system.

In the small intestine, water-soluble and fat-soluble vitamins are absorbed by diffusion into the bloodstream. The small intestine also produces enzymes that work with pancreatic enzymes to turn chyme into substances that can be directly absorbed into the bloodstream through the capillaries on its surface. Blood enriched with these energy molecules exits the intestinal circulation and flows to the liver, where fat and protein metabolism occur. The blood then leaves the liver and enters the subclavian vessels.

Large Intestine

The large intestine, which is about 5 feet (2 m) long, encircles the outer border of the abdomen around the small intestine. Its primary role is to complete the absorption of water, although most water will have already been absorbed in the small intestine. This osmotic function of the colon helps to solidify stool. Intestinal flora (normal bacteria) synthesize some vitamins, such as folic acid, vitamin K, riboflavin, and nicotinic acid. Cellulose, which is indigestible by humans, moves through the small intestine with little change and provides bulk to the large intestine's contents.

The first segment of the large intestine is the cecum and its accessory structure, the appendix **FIGURE 8-131**. The ileocecal valve joins the ileum to the cecum. The appendix opens into the cecum in the RLQ of the abdomen. Rising up from the cecum is the ascending colon. It attaches to the transverse colon, which runs from right to left. A 90° turn occurs, and the descending colon begins. The sigmoid colon then takes an S-shaped turn. Feces travel through the descending colon, then progress to the sigmoid colon and then through the rectum, which joins the anal canal, to exit the body by the anus. The anus contains two **sphincters**, the internal and external. The internal anal sphincter (under autonomic control) has stretch receptors that give the sensation of the need to defecate. The external anal sphincter (under voluntary control) allows a controlled bowel movement.

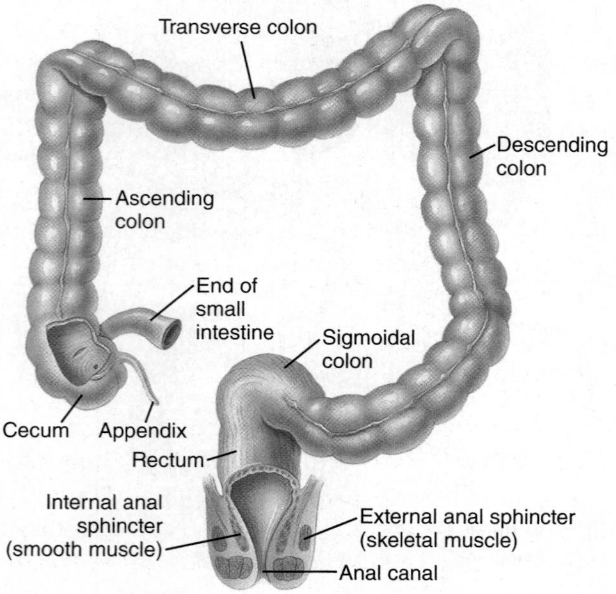

FIGURE 8-131 The large intestine.

Peristaltic waves happen in the large intestine only two or three times per day. During these waves, the intestinal walls constrict vigorously (mass movements) to force contents toward the rectum. These movements usually follow a meal, but irritations of the intestinal mucosa may also cause them.

TABLE 8-41 summarizes the organs and functions of the digestive system.

Accessory Organs

The liver, gallbladder, and pancreas are considered part of the digestive system because they are involved in the digestion of food and elimination of waste.

Liver

As noted earlier, the liver takes up most of the area immediately beneath the diaphragm in the RUQ and extends into the LUQ of the abdomen. This complex organ has many functions. It is responsible for the maintenance of blood glucose. It detoxifies the blood by removing drugs and other poisonous substances such as ammonia, which it converts into urea, to be excreted in urine. The liver is also responsible for manufacturing plasma proteins (albumin, fibrinogen, and globulins) and clotting factors, which allow the body to seal off damaged vessels to prevent blood loss. Finally, it plays a role in regulating fats. As old RBCs enter the liver, they are broken down into bile, which is necessary to decompose ingested fats. The liver also produces cholesterol and proteins that carry fats through the body to ultimately drain into the small intestine.

TABLE 8-41 Functions of the Digestive Organs

Organ/Structure	Function
Mouth	Mechanically breaks down food; begins chemical breakdown of food with saliva
Esophagus	Moves food from the mouth to the stomach; provides muscular and vascular structure
Stomach	Performs mechanical and chemical breakdown of food (food in, chyme out)
Small intestine	Major site for chemical breakdown of food; major site of absorption of water, fat, proteins, carbohydrates, and vitamins
Large intestine	Absorption of water; formation of feces; bacterial digestion of food
Rectum/anus	Controls release of feces
Accessory Organs	
Liver	Produces bile; assists with metabolism of carbohydrates, proteins, and fat; stores and manufactures vitamins; responsible for detoxification of blood and elimination of waste
Gallbladder	Stores bile
Pancreas	Exocrine: produces enzymes for protein, carbohydrate, and fat breakdown within the duodenum Endocrine: produces insulin, glucagon, and somatostatin

The liver is a highly vascular organ through which 100% of the body's blood circulates. Its vascular supply has two sources: the hepatic artery and the portal vein. The liver receives its blood and nutrient supply from the circulatory system through the hepatic artery. The portal vein is composed of a group of vessels that originate from the digestive system. These vessels ensure that all nutrients absorbed from the intestinal tract are first detoxified in the liver before being released into the general venous circulation (known as the first-pass effect).

Gallbladder

The liver is connected to the intestine by the bile ducts. The gallbladder is an outpouching from the bile ducts that serves as a reservoir and concentrating organ for bile produced in the liver. Together, the bile ducts and the gallbladder form the biliary system. The gallbladder is connected to the common bile duct via the cystic duct. Bile is expelled through the common bile duct into the duodenum. The presence of food in the duodenum triggers a contraction of the gallbladder to empty it. The sphincter of Oddi, found at the end of the common bile duct, regulates the movement of bile into the duodenum. The liver connects to the common bile duct via the hepatic duct.

Pancreas

Recall that the pancreas performs both endocrine and exocrine functions. Its endocrine functions include the synthesis of glucagon, insulin, and somatostatin. Both glucagon and insulin are critical in maintaining blood glucose levels. The exocrine functions include production of pancreatic digestive juices (pancreatic amylase, trypsin, chymotrypsin, and carboxypeptidase), which aid in the digestion of carbohydrates, fats, proteins, and nucleic acids. Pancreatic amylase, for example, continues the digestion of starchy material begun in the mouth. The pancreatic duct expels these substances at its junction with the duodenum, which is located next to the opening of the common bile duct.

Digestion and Absorption of Nutrients

Throughout this discussion of human anatomy and physiology, we have emphasized that numerous chemical and biologic processes run continuously as long as the organism is alive, and some continue even after the organism has died. *Metabolism* is the sum of all of these reactions. Lay people use this term to describe the rate at which the body processes food. For example, someone with a so-called high metabolism burns more calories at rest than someone with a low metabolism. These terms are simplistic but essentially true, because a large part of the body's resting metabolism is devoted to the intake, processing, and use of nutrients, the substances that fuel the "engine" of each individual cell. Recall that the correct term for the rate at which nutrients are consumed in the body is the basal metabolic rate.

The body obtains nutrients through a variety of processes, but the most common are through inhalation (oxygen) and ingestion (food). The various systems of the body break down these substances into usable forms. As discussed previously, nutrients include carbohydrates, lipids, proteins, vitamins, minerals, and water. Macronutrients are those nutrients required in large amounts (carbohydrates, lipids, and proteins); they provide energy and have other specific functions. Micronutrients are the nutrients required in much smaller amounts (vitamins and minerals); they do not directly provide energy, but facilitate biochemical reactions that extract energy from macronutrients. Essential nutrients are those that human cells cannot synthesize (such as certain amino acids).

A calorie is the amount of heat needed to raise the temperature of 1 gram of water by 1°C. As discussed previously, the kilocalorie is used to measure food energy and is typically referred to simply as a calorie in the nutritional setting. Cellular oxidation causes the following calorie releases:

- 1 gram of carbohydrate yields about 4 calories.
- 1 gram of protein yields about 4 calories.
- 1 gram of fat yields about 9 calories.

Digestion breaks down nutrients so they can be absorbed and transported via the bloodstream. If the amounts of nutrients are more abundant than the body's needs, then some nutrients can be stored (eg, lipids are stored as fatty tissue). In this way, the body can prepare itself for times when nutrients are not plentiful and draw on those reserves. In other cases, however, excesses cannot be stored and are simply excreted through elimination of waste. When the amount of nutrients and energy consumed by the body exceeds the amount available in the diet, body structures may be metabolized to sustain life.

Typical meals contain carbohydrates, lipids, proteins, water, electrolytes, and vitamins. The digestive system handles each of these components differently. Digestion involves breaking down large organic molecules before absorption can occur. Water, electrolytes, and vitamins can be absorbed without preliminary breakdown, but may require special transport mechanisms.

Energy from carbohydrates is primarily used to power cellular processes. Digestion breaks carbohydrates down into monosaccharides (which include fructose, galactose, and glucose) for easy absorption.

YOU are the Paramedic

PART 4

Your physical exam of the patient's abdomen reveals rigidity throughout both lower quadrants. When you press on his pelvis, you feel instability and grinding. The patient remains unresponsive during your assessment.

Recording Time: 10 Minutes	
Respirations	24 breaths/min, shallow
Pulse	118 beats/min
Skin	Pale, moist, and warm
Blood pressure	102/66 mm Hg
Oxygen saturation (Spo_2)	97% (assisted with a bag-mask device)
Pupils	PERRLA

8. What structures are located in the lower abdominal quadrants?

9. What might the instability of the pelvis indicate?

Liver enzymes convert fructose and galactose into glucose, which is the form of carbohydrate most commonly oxidized for use as cellular fuel.

Although many cells get their energy by oxidizing fatty acids, neurons require a continuous supply of glucose to survive. In fact, the nervous system can be seriously impaired by a lack of glucose. When sufficient carbohydrates are not consumed, the liver may convert amino acids (from proteins) into glucose.

Some excess glucose is converted to glycogen, which is stored in the liver and muscles. Glucose can be rapidly mobilized from glycogen, but only a certain amount of glycogen can be stored. Excess glucose is usually converted into fat and stored in adipose tissue. For energy, the body first metabolizes glucose, then glycogen into glucose, and lastly, fats and proteins. Proteins supply essential amino acids and provide nitrogen and other elements.

The Urinary System

The urinary system controls the discharge of certain waste materials filtered from the blood by the kidneys. In the urinary system, the kidneys are solid organs; the ureters, bladder, and **urethra** (through which urine is expelled) are hollow organs **FIGURE 8-132**. The main functions of the urinary system are to (1) control fluid balance in the body, (2) filter and eliminate wastes, and (3) control pH balance.

Kidneys

The body has two bean-shaped kidneys, which are located on either side of the spine between the 12th thoracic vertebra and the 3rd lumbar vertebra. The right kidney is positioned lower than the left to make room for the liver. Both kidneys are located between the back muscles and the peritoneum. They are positioned within the retroperitoneal space, which is behind and outside the peritoneal cavity.

The kidneys help maintain homeostasis by regulating the ECF's composition, pH, and volume. This process is accomplished by removing metabolic wastes from the blood and diluting them with water and electrolytes. It results in the formation of urine, which the kidneys excrete. The other vital functions of the kidneys include the following:

- **Regulating water and electrolytes.** Water and electrolyte excretion must be matched to water and electrolyte intake to achieve homeostasis. The kidneys alter their filtration and excretion rates to match the body's intake of water and electrolytes.
- **Regulating acid–base balance.** The renal system functions as a compensatory mechanism for maintaining acid–base balance. This system is the slowest method for returning the pH to a normal range; it sometimes takes days to accomplish the task. The kidneys regulate the pH by monitoring the elimination of hydrogen and the reabsorption of bicarbonate in the tubules of **nephrons** (the kidneys' urine-producing units). If the body is too acidic, then it will increase the amount of hydrogen eliminated in the urine and recover bicarbonate. If not enough hydrogen is present (alkalosis), then the kidneys will retain hydrogen and eliminate bicarbonate. The renal system can also eliminate hydrogen if ammonia (NH_3) is present. The kidneys combine ammonia with a hydrogen ion to create ammonium (NH_4^+). This substance is easily excreted in the urine, thereby decreasing the acidity of the body.
- **Excreting waste products and foreign chemicals.** The kidneys are the primary means of eliminating waste products generated by metabolism, including urea, creatinine, uric acid, and bilirubin (from the breakdown of hemoglobin). They also eliminate other foreign chemicals ingested or produced by the body such as toxins, food additives, and medications.
- **Secreting hormones.** Erythropoietin (EPO) and calcitriol are hormones secreted by the kidneys. EPO acts on bone marrow to increase production of RBCs. Calcitriol, the active form of vitamin D, promotes calcium absorption from food and mobilizes calcium from bones to the blood. Renin is a hormone formed in the kidney that initiates the eventual formation of angiotensin II, which is discussed in the next section.
- **Regulating arterial BP.** The kidneys primarily regulate BP by excreting large amounts of sodium and water. However, over a short period, the kidneys exert control over arterial BP through the renin-angiotensin-aldosterone mechanism. This mechanism involves secretion of renin, which then leads to the formation

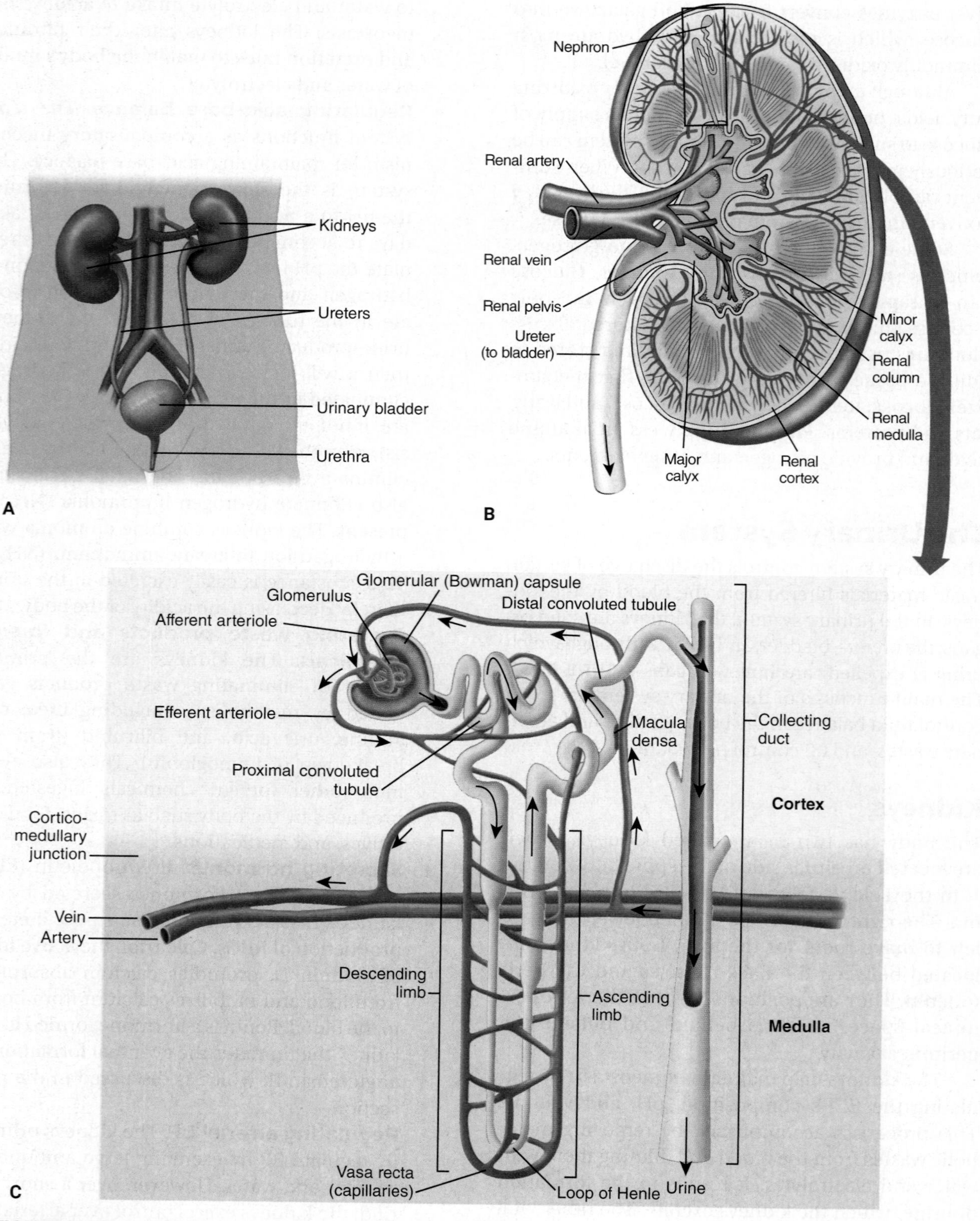

FIGURE 8-132 The urinary system. **A.** Anterior view showing the relationship of the kidneys, ureters, urinary bladder, and urethra. **B.** Cross-section of the human kidney showing its structures and blood flow through it. **C.** Blood flow through a nephron.

of angiotensin II, a powerful vasoconstrictor. This is an important concept, especially when you consider a patient in shock. When a patient goes into shock, the kidneys respond by producing renin. Renin combines with angiotensinogen to produce angiotensin I. In the lungs, angiotensin-converting enzyme converts angiotensin I to angiotensin II, which constricts the peripheral arteries as a compensatory mechanism to maintain the patient's BP. In addition, angiotensin II stimulates the production of aldosterone. Aldosterone, produced by the adrenal glands, exerts an effect on the kidneys by increasing reabsorption of sodium into the circulatory system. As sodium is reabsorbed, so is water, thereby maintaining the circulating fluid volume. ADH is produced by the hypothalamus and released by the posterior pituitary. Increases in ADH cause decreased elimination of water, whereas decreases in ADH cause increased elimination of water.

- **Producing new glucose.** During prolonged fasting, the kidneys produce new glucose from amino acids and other chemicals. This gluconeogenesis is comparable to that carried out in the liver when the individual has gone without food for a long time.

A fibrous capsule envelops the kidney and protects it against infection. Surrounding this capsule is a fatty mass of adipose tissue, which cushions the kidney and holds it in place in the abdomen. A layer of dense fibrous connective tissue called the renal fascia anchors the kidney to the abdominal wall.

The internal anatomy of each kidney can be divided into three distinct areas: (1) the renal cortex, (2) the renal medulla, and (3) the renal pelvis (see Figure 8-132). The lighter-colored, outer layer of the kidney, closest to the fibrous capsule, is the **renal cortex**. The **renal medulla**, the middle layer, forms cone-shaped areas called renal pyramids (parallel bundles of urine-collecting tubules). Renal columns, which are inward extensions of the renal cortex, separate these renal pyramids. The renal pyramids point toward the **renal pelvis**, which collects urine and forms the upper portion of the ureter. The edges of the renal pelvis, called calyces, collect urine. The major and minor calyces branch off the renal pelvis and connect with the renal pyramids to receive the urine that drains from the collecting tubules. This arrangement has been said to resemble several strands of uncooked spaghetti (the collecting tubules) sitting in a thimble (the papilla, or tip, of the renal pelvis). The collected urine flows through the renal pelvis and into the ureter on its way to the bladder.

Approximately one-fourth of the body's systemic cardiac output flows through the kidney each minute. Blood ejected from the heart flows from the abdominal aorta into the kidney by way of the renal artery. Each kidney has a medial indentation (known as the hilus) through which the renal artery, vein, lymphatic vessels, and nerves enter and leave. After entering the kidney at the hilus, the renal artery branches several times to become the afferent arteriole. The afferent arteriole quickly branches into a tuft of capillaries called a glomerulus, the main filter of the kidney. From the glomerulus, the blood enters the efferent arteriole, which branches into the peritubular capillaries, where tubular reabsorption occurs. This secondary set of capillaries is unique to the kidney; no other organ in the body has two distinct capillary beds. The capillaries then merge, forming venules and veins, until the renal vein leaves the hilus, carrying the cleansed blood to the inferior vena cava.

Nephrons

Nephrons (found in the cortex) filter the blood, collect excreted water and waste products, and reabsorb water, nutrients, and electrolytes. Each normal adult kidney contains more than 1 million nephrons. Blood flow to the kidneys is supplied by the renal arteries, which divide into arterioles and capillaries.

The nephron contains the glomerulus; the glomerular capsule (Bowman capsule), which surrounds the glomerulus; the proximal convoluted tubule (PCT); the loop of Henle; and the distal convoluted tubule (DCT), which connects with the collecting tubules of the kidney. The glomerulus and glomerular capsule compose the **renal corpuscle**. Blood enters the glomerulus by an afferent arteriole and leaves by an efferent arteriole. Pores in the walls of the capillaries in the glomerulus allow the blood to be filtered. Filtered water and wastes (filtrate) flow from the glomerular capsule through the **renal tubules**.

The glomerular capsule is a double-layered cup in which the inner layer infiltrates and surrounds

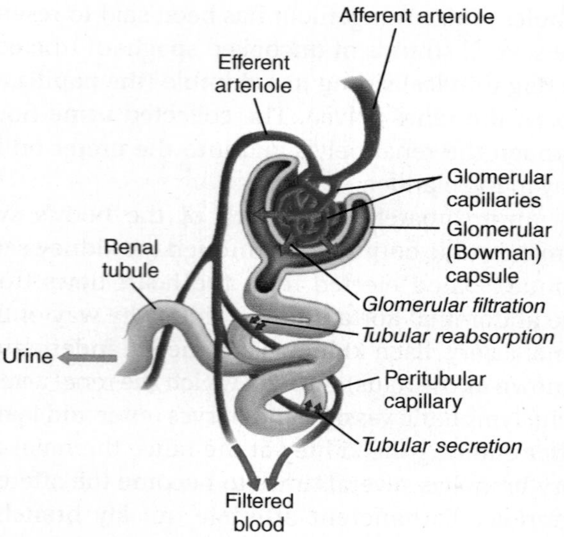

FIGURE 8-133 The glomerulus of the kidneys. The nephron carries out three blood-filtering processes: glomerular filtration, tubular reabsorption, and tubular secretion.

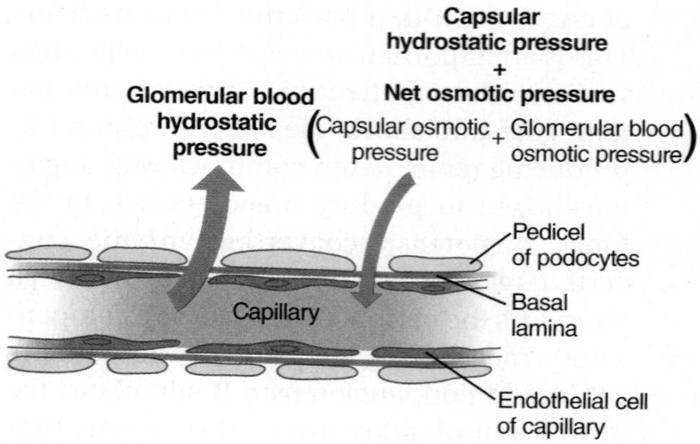

FIGURE 8-134 The presence of an efferent arteriole results in a high glomerular (blood) hydrostatic pressure. This pressure exceeds the sum of the pressures that oppose fluid movement through the glomerular filtration membrane. Filtration is the outcome of this balance of pressures.

the capillaries of the glomerulus. Special cells in the inner membrane called podocytes wrap around the capillaries in the glomerulus, forming filtration slits. The filtrate passes through these slits, across the filtration membrane, and into the capsule. In this manner, the filtration membrane prevents large molecules, such as proteins, from entering the glomerular capsule **FIGURE 8-133**.

Imagine watering your garden with an open-ended hose. If you place your finger over one-half of the opening of the hose, then the same amount of water must now pass through half the space. As a result, the pressure increases and you can spray water farther. The same effect occurs at the glomerulus. As blood moves from the relatively large afferent arteriole into the smaller capillaries of the glomerulus, the pressure increases. This effect, along with the smaller diameter of the efferent arteriole, causes the pressure in the glomerulus to rise enough to force the filtrate from the blood into the glomerular capsule **FIGURE 8-134**.

The amount of filtrate produced, called the glomerular filtration rate, is maintained at a relatively constant rate of 125 mL/min in healthy adults. Initially, the filtrate contains everything that can pass through the filtration membrane: salts, minerals, glucose, water, and metabolic wastes. As the filtrate passes through the rest of the nephron, **tubular reabsorption** and **tubular secretion** convert the filtrate into urine **FIGURE 8-135**. As the fluid passes through the PCT, the cells lining the PCT remove all organic nutrients and plasma proteins, as well as some ions, from the filtrate. These compounds are deposited in the interstitial fluid surrounding the

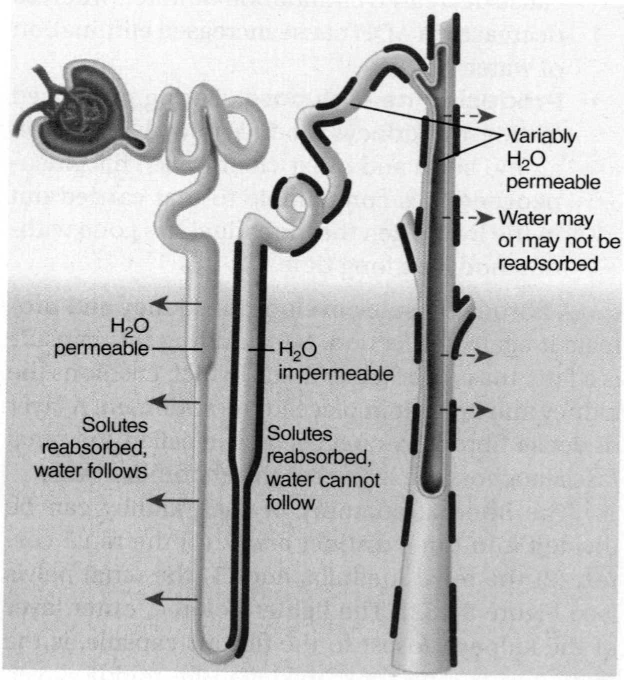

FIGURE 8-135 A single nephron and the tubular reabsorption of water.

PCT. As these solutes accumulate, their concentration in the surrounding fluid becomes higher than that in the filtrate. Water will then move from the filtrate by osmosis. The fluid and nutrients in the interstitial fluid, in turn, move into the peritubular capillaries around the PCT. This process reestablishes the homeostatic balance in the blood and reduces the volume of the tubular filtrate.

Additional reabsorption of water and electrolytes occurs in the loop of Henle. The loop of Henle has two sections: the descending limb, which extends toward the medulla, and the ascending limb, which stretches toward the cortex. The cells in the descending limb are permeable to water, but impermeable to sodium and chloride ions; the cells in the ascending limb are permeable to sodium and chloride ions, but impermeable to water. As a consequence, when the sodium and chloride ions move out of the ascending limb, they increase the solute concentration of the fluid surrounding the descending limb. Water moves by osmosis from the descending limb into the surrounding tissue and eventually into the vasa recta, a series of peritubular capillaries surrounding the loop of Henle. This countercurrent multiplier process allows the body to produce either concentrated or diluted urine, depending on its needs.

After leaving the loop of Henle, the fluid enters the DCT. At this point, approximately 80% of the water and 85% of the solutes originally forced out of the glomerulus have been reabsorbed. As the urine passes through the DCT and the collecting ducts to which it is attached (both of which are impermeable to solutes), its composition undergoes its final adjustments. Ions are actively secreted or reabsorbed, and the body alters the permeability of the DCT and collecting ducts to water as necessary, depending on the body's homeostatic needs. These adjustments to the final composition of the urine facilitate the removal of metabolic wastes while maintaining the body's fluid-electrolyte balance.

A structure called the juxtaglomerular apparatus is formed at the site where the efferent arteriole comes in contact with the DCT. The pressure-sensitive cells in the efferent arteriole (juxtaglomerular cells) monitor the BP. The cells in the DCT (macula densa cells) are sensitive to chemical changes and monitor the concentration of the filtrate in the DCT. When triggered by changes in the BP or the filtrate content, the juxtaglomerular cells release renin. As noted earlier, renin stimulates an increase in angiotensin I, which is then converted into angiotensin II. The presence of increased levels of angiotensin II, in turn, stimulates production of aldosterone.

The final adjustments to the urine composition at the DCT and collecting duct are controlled primarily by two hormones: ADH and aldosterone. Neurons in the hypothalamus monitor the solute concentration of the blood. When it increases (eg, because sweating or decreased fluid intake), ADH is released into the bloodstream. This hormone travels to the DCT and collecting ducts, increasing the permeability of these structures to water. Water subsequently leaves the DCT and collecting ducts, and reenters the bloodstream. As the solute concentration returns to normal, secretion of ADH will stop.

Aldosterone increases the rate of active reabsorption of sodium and chloride ions into the blood; a corresponding increase occurs in the rate of water reabsorption. This hormone also decreases reabsorption of potassium ions, resulting in excess potassium being secreted in urine.

Other hormones also influence the retention or secretion of various substances. For example, PTH causes a decrease in the amount of calcium excreted in urine. **Atrial natriuretic peptide** is a hormone produced by the atria when they are distended by increased blood volume. This hormone inhibits the absorption of water and sodium in the renal tubules, thereby increasing elimination of water.

Urea is an end product of amino acid catabolism, and its plasma concentration reflects the amount of protein in the diet. Urea filters into the renal tubule. Approximately 80% of urea is reabsorbed, while the remainder is excreted in urine. Uric acid is a result of metabolism of certain organic bases in nucleic acids. Active transport reabsorbs most of the uric acid present in the glomerular filtrate.

The composition of urine reflects the water volume and the amount of solutes that the kidneys must eliminate or retain to maintain homeostasis. Urine is approximately 95% water, and usually contains urea and uric acid. It is slightly heavier than water, with a specific gravity of 1.003 to 1.035. Its pH is usually close to neutral, but can vary widely depending on many factors—not the least of which is what the patient has eaten. Urine can be clear to straw-colored, but a darker color usually indicates a higher concentration of solutes caused by dehydration or some other malady. This fluid may also contain traces of amino acids and electrolytes.

Urine production varies between 0.6 and 2.5 L per day. Urine production of 50 to 60 mL/h is considered normal, whereas output of less than 30 mL/h (or approximately 0.5 mL/kg/h) is suggestive of renal failure.

Ureters

After urine enters the collecting ducts (the renal pyramids of the medulla), it passes through the minor calyx, into the major calyx, and then into the renal pelvis. From there, the urine is drained from each kidney through thin-walled muscular tubes called ureters. These tubes are about 12 inches (30 cm) in length. Urine moves out of the kidney by peristaltic contractions that begin inside the kidney and minor and major calyces. These contractions continue in the renal pelvis and propel urine along the ureters toward the urinary bladder.

Urinary Bladder

The urinary bladder is a hollow, muscular sac surrounded by smooth muscle. This organ is responsible for storing urine before it is eliminated from the body. Most of the bladder rests in the anterior abdominal cavity, but its dome sits in the posterior abdominal cavity, (retroperitoneum), along with the ureters and kidneys. When empty, the bladder collapses and the muscular walls fold over onto themselves. In contrast, as urine accumulates, the bladder expands and becomes pear-shaped. The stretching of the bladder walls ultimately stimulates nerve impulses to produce the micturition reflex. This spinal reflex causes contraction of the bladder's smooth muscle, which in turn produces the urge to void as pressure is exerted on the internal urinary sphincter. Normally, the brain controls this urge, keeping the external urinary sphincter contracted until conditions are favorable for urination. At this point, inhibition of the external urinary sphincter is reduced and the urine passes from the urinary bladder into the urethra.

Urethra

The urinary bladder and urethra make up the lower urinary tract. The beginning of the urethra sits at the inferior aspect of the bladder. In males, the urethra passes from the anterior base of the bladder through the penis. In females, the urethra opens in front of the vagina. The female urethra (2 inches [5 cm]) is shorter than the male urethra (8 inches [20 cm]) **FIGURE 8-136**.

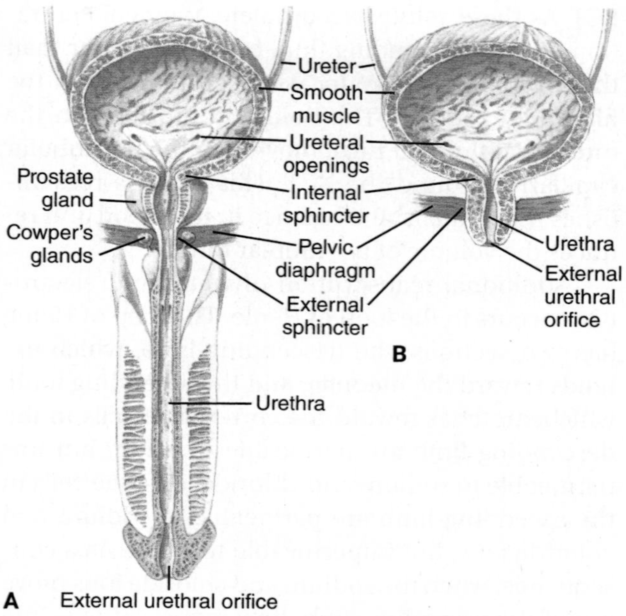

FIGURE 8-136 Comparison of the urethra in males **(A)** and females **(B)**.

The male urethra is divided into three regions:

- **Prostatic urethra.** This region begins at the bladder and extends through the prostate gland.
- **Membranous urethra.** This region extends from the prostate gland through the abdominal wall and into the penis.
- **Spongy (penile) urethra.** This region passes through the penis to the external urethral opening.

Fluid Balance

Certain mechanisms in the body maintain the balance between what is taken in and what is excreted—including fluids. For example, when the fluid volume drops, the pituitary gland secretes ADH **FIGURE 8-137**. ADH causes the kidney tubules to reabsorb more water into the blood and excrete less urine, allowing fluid volume in the body to build up. Thirst also regulates fluid intake. The sensation of thirst occurs when body fluids become

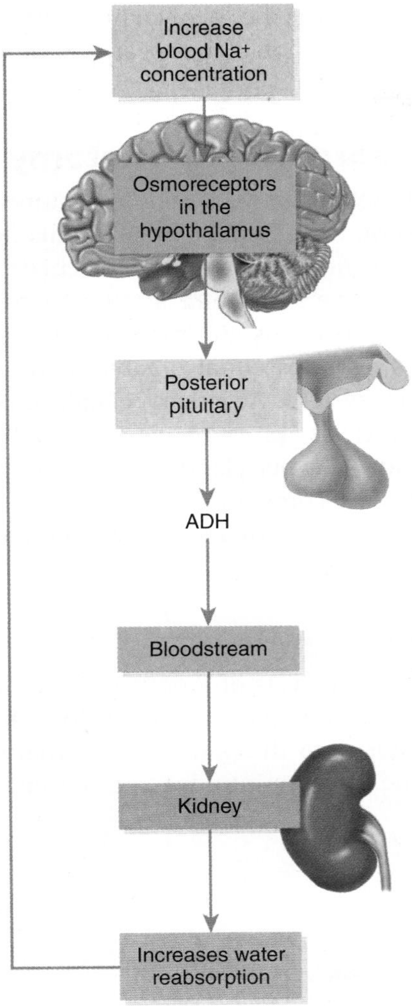

FIGURE 8-137 The role of antidiuretic hormone (ADH) in regulating fluid levels.

decreased, stimulating a person to take in more fluids. Conversely, when too many fluids enter the body, thirst decreases, the kidneys are activated, and more urine is excreted, eliminating the excess fluid.

Maintaining the proper balance of fluids and electrolytes within the body is necessary for life. A person's body can become depleted of fluids and electrolytes for several reasons, including severe burns or dehydration. When necessary, the body can maintain fluid balance by shifting water from one compartment to another. Water moves in response to osmotic forces as well as hormonal stimuli such as ADH. By moving unequal amounts of electrolytes into and out of the cells, it is also possible for the body to balance other properties of ICF.

TABLE 8-42 Major Mechanisms for Fluid Homeostasis

- Antidiuretic hormone (ADH)
- Thirst
- Kidneys
- Water shifts

For a patient whose fluids or electrolytes are depleted, rapid restoration of fluid balance may mean the difference between life and death **TABLE 8-42**.

The Reproductive System

The **reproductive system** controls the reproductive processes by which life is created. The male and female reproductive systems contain organs and glands that create sex cells and transport them to areas where fertilization can occur. Although the male and female reproductive systems are functionally very different, the first step in reproduction for each is to produce sex cells (also called gametes)—that is, cells specially created to combine with a partner's cells to create a new organism. Male gametes are called sperm; female gametes are called oocytes, or eggs.

Gametes are described as **haploid cells** because they carry genetic instructions via 23 individual chromosomes. When sex cells from a man and a woman unite during fertilization, the chromosomes from each partner unite with their corresponding chromosome from the opposite gamete, called a **homologous chromosome**, to form 23 pairs of chromosomes, for a total of 46 chromosomes. This first fertilized cell, from which all other body cells are created, is known as the zygote. It, and all other cells besides the gametes, are described as **diploid cells** because they carry two of each of the 23 chromosomes—one from the father and one from the mother. Among these, 22 chromosomes are **autosomes**, which have a corresponding homologous chromosome in both men and women. The 23rd chromosome pair is made up of **sex chromosomes**—one X chromosome, which both men and women have, and either a second copy of the X chromosome or a Y chromosome. If the 23rd pair in the zygote is XX, then the organism will be biologically female; if it is XY, then it will be biologically a male.

It is crucial to understand how critical these chromosomes are and how far-reaching their effects can be on the developing organism. Chromosomes contain the entire sequence of genetic information the organism will have throughout its entire life (unless some artificial change is effected). This genetic information contains the instructions for every structure and process in the body. Chromosomes also contain sequences that determine or influence various characteristics such as hair color, skin color, body composition, height, and predisposition to certain diseases. These traits are determined through the action of dominant and recessive **alleles** of the same gene. For example, the allele that contains instructions for red hair color is recessive. If it is paired with an allele from the other parent that is dominant, then the cell is said to be heterozygous, and hair color will be dictated by the dominant allele (the allele for red hair will be overridden by the dominant allele). If, however, it is paired with another "redhead" allele, then the cell is said to be homozygous, and the new organism's hair color will be red. The arrangement of genes and their characteristics is known as the person's **genotype**, whereas the set of characteristics that results from expression of those genes is known as the **phenotype**.

Male Reproductive Anatomy

The male reproductive system structures include the scrotum, testes, epididymis, ductus deferentia (also called the vas deferentia), ejaculatory ducts, urethra, and penis **FIGURE 8-138**. The two testes, in which sperm cells and male sex hormones are formed, are the essential organs of the male reproductive system. Accessory glands include the seminal vesicles, prostate gland, and bulbourethral glands (Cowper glands). The scrotum, penis, and spermatic cords are supporting structures. In males, the urethra is shared by the reproductive and urinary systems.

Scrotum

The **scrotum** consists of a pouch of skin and subcutaneous tissue that extends below the abdomen, posterior to the penis. An internal partition divides the scrotum into two compartments, each

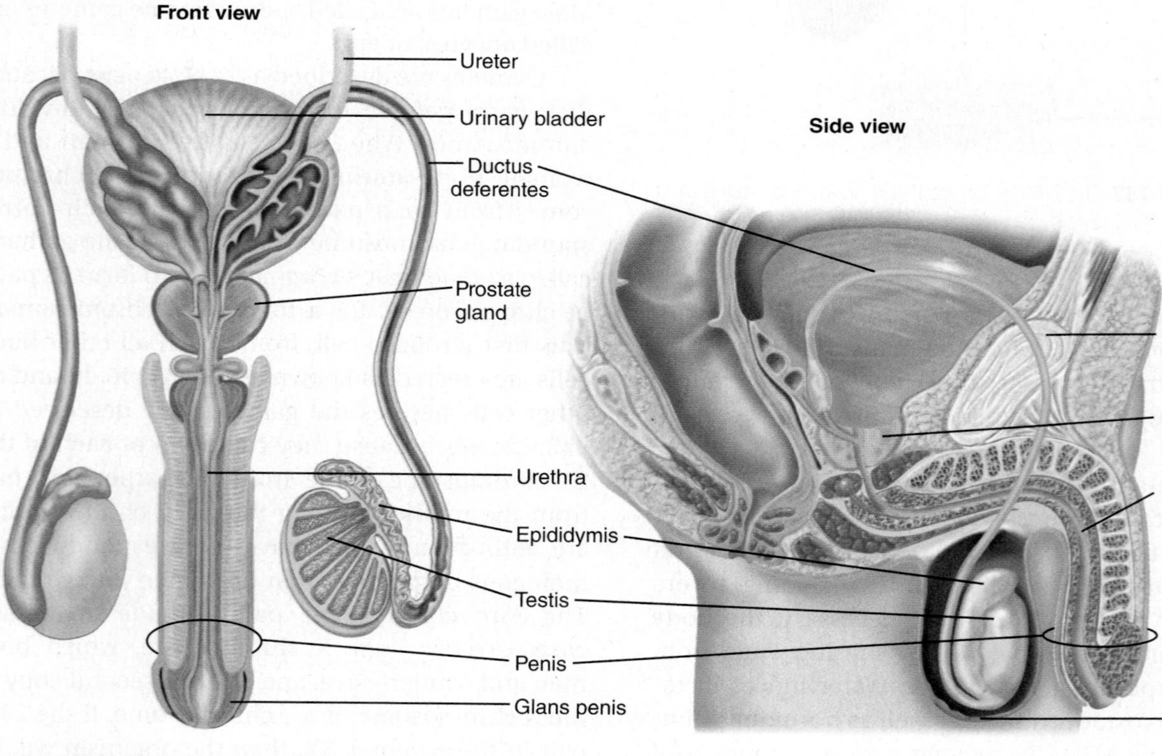

FIGURE 8-138 The male reproductive system.

enclosing a testis. This partition protects each testis from possible infection from the other. Generally, the left testis is suspended lower than the right so the two are not compressed against each other between the thighs.[44] Each testis is also enclosed in a serous membrane so that it moves smoothly inside the scrotum.

The cremaster and dartos muscles of the scrotum react to temperature changes. When environmental temperatures are cold, the scrotum contracts and wrinkles, moving the testes closer to the pelvic cavity to absorb heat. When it is warmer outside, the scrotum relaxes and hangs loosely to ensure that the testes are approximately 3°F to 4°F (1.7°C to 2.2°C) cooler than body temperature. This cooler temperature provides a better environment for production and survival of the sperm cells.

Testes

The testes, or testicles, are considered part of the endocrine system because they produce testosterone, as well as part of the male reproductive system because they produce sperm. Between 2 months before birth and shortly thereafter, oval-shaped testes typically descend from the pelvis into the scrotum. This descent occurs through the inguinal canal, an opening in the abdominal wall.

A testicular artery, which arises from the abdominal aorta just below the renal artery, supplies blood to each testis. The testes are served by the sympathetic and parasympathetic divisions of the ANS. In the testes, the ductus deferens, testicular artery and vein, lymphatic vessels, and nerve fibers compose the spermatic cord, which passes through the inguinal canal.

A tough, fibrous, white capsule surrounds each testis. This tissue extends inward, forming a partition that divides each testis into about 250 to 300 lobules. Each lobule contains up to four highly coiled seminiferous tubules. These four tubules merge to form a straight tubule that leads to a tubular network called the rete testis. Efferent ductules connect the rete testis to the epididymis. Sperm cells are produced in the seminiferous tubules.

Between the seminiferous tubules are interstitial cells that secrete testosterone. Testosterone enlarges the testes and accessory reproductive organs, and triggers the development of the male secondary sex characteristics during puberty. These characteristics include the following:

- Increased body hair on the face, chest, armpits, and pubic region
- Decreased hair growth on the scalp (varies by individual)
- Enlargement of the larynx and thickening of the vocal folds, which lower the pitch of the voice
- Thickening of the skin
- Increased muscular growth, broadening of the shoulders, and narrowing of the waist
- Thickening and strengthening of the bones

Testosterone also increases cellular metabolism and the production of RBCs. The more testosterone that is received by the interstitial cells, the greater the speed at which the male secondary sex characteristics develop. A period in a man's life known as the male climacteric marks a decrease in testosterone level and a decline in sexual function.

Spermatogenesis

At puberty, testosterone levels increase and spermatozoa production begins. Each mature sperm cell appears like a tiny tadpole. It has a flattened head, a cylinder-shaped body, and a long tail **FIGURE 8-139**.

Spermatogenesis is the process by which sperm cells are formed. In a male embryo, spermatogenic cells (also called spermatogonia) are

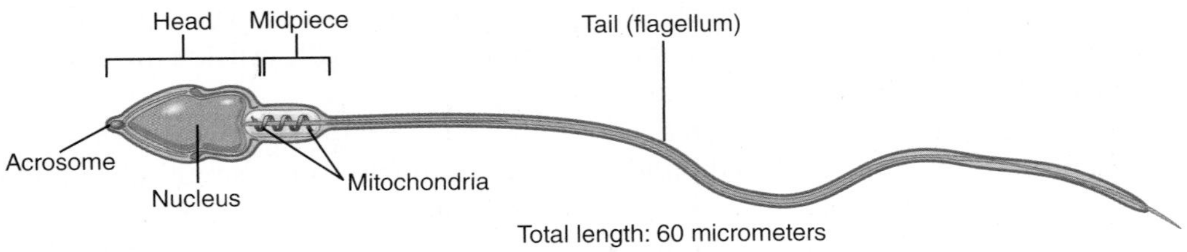

FIGURE 8-139 The mature sperm cell.

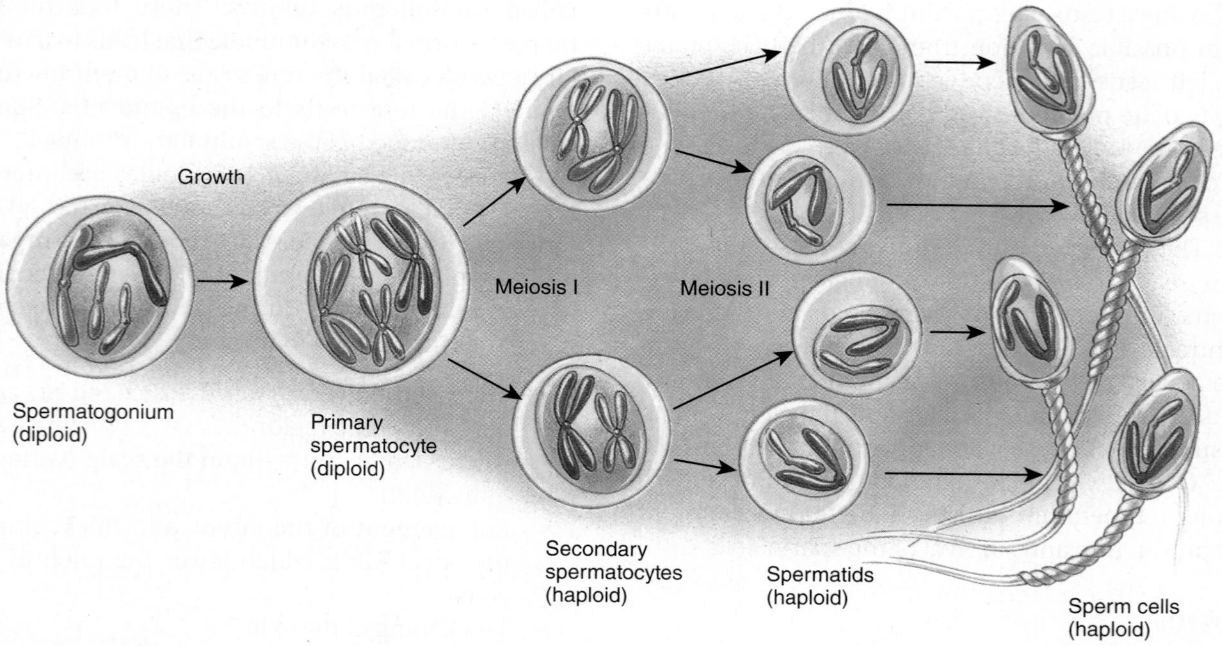

FIGURE 8-140 Meiosis.

undifferentiated and contain 46 chromosomes. During embryonic development, the spermatogonia undergo mitosis, creating two daughter cells. One of these is a new "type A" spermatogonium that maintains the supply of undifferentiated cells; the other is a "type B" spermatogonium that enlarges to become a primary spermatocyte.

During puberty, primary spermatocytes reproduce via meiosis, a type of cell division that includes first and second meiotic divisions. This process differs in important ways from mitosis, the process by which most body cells divide. Meiosis I (the first division) separates chromosome pairs that are homologous, meaning they are matched "gene for gene." This does not mean the genes are identical; in fact, genes may vary because of hereditary factors. Each homologous chromosome is replicated before meiosis I occurs, so it consists of two complete DNA strands (chromatids). These attach at areas called centromeres, and carry all the genetic information associated with that specific chromosome. Each of the four daughter cells produced has one-half as many chromosomes as a typical diploid body cell.

In meiosis II, the chromatids in one member of each homologous pair separate. This produces other haploid cells (with one set of chromosomes), in which the chromosomes are no longer present in replicated form. In essence, meiosis II causes each of the chromatids to become an independent chromosome. Each primary spermatocyte divides into two secondary spermatocytes; these divide again to form two spermatids, which mature. Thus, for each primary spermatocyte that undergoes meiosis, four sperm cells, with 23 chromosomes in each of their nuclei, are formed **FIGURE 8-140**. In the final phase of spermatogenesis, called spermiogenesis, each spermatid matures into a single sperm or *spermatozoon.*[45]

Spermatic Ducts

Sperm cells must first pass through a series of ducts before they reach the outside of the body. Sperm travel from the seminiferous tubules to the rete testes, to the efferent ductules, to the epididymis, to the ductus deferens, to the ejaculatory ducts, to the urethra, and finally outside the body.[46]

Efferent Ductules

Efferent ductules are small tubes that carry sperm produced in the seminiferous tubules through the rete testis to reach the epididymis. These small ducts have clusters of ciliated cells that help move sperm through them.

Epididymis

Sperm cells mature in the epididymis. This tightly coiled tube is connected to the posterior border of the testis. Each epididymis lies along the top of and descends behind the testis, and then courses upward to become the vas deferens. The epididymis can be felt through the skin of the scrotum.

The epididymis stores and protects spermatozoa and aids in their maturation. Immature sperm cells are nonmotile when they reach the epididymis, so rhythmic peristaltic contractions are needed to move them through the duct as they mature. It takes about 20 days for sperm to travel from the head and body of the epididymis to the tail. On reaching the tail, the sperm are stored and remain viable for 40 to 60 days.[46] Once mature, sperm cells can move independently to fertilize egg cells, but usually do not "swim" until after ejaculation. Sperm that are not ejaculated disintegrate and are picked up by the epididymal blood vessels for reabsorption.

Ductus Deferens and Ejaculatory Duct

At the tail of each epididymis, the sperm duct turns 180° and becomes the ductus deferentia. These muscular tubes pass upward along the medial side of the testes, through the spermatic cord and inguinal canal, and into the pelvic cavity. They end behind the urinary bladder, joining just outside the prostate gland with the duct of a seminal vesicle. This forms a short ejaculatory duct, passing through the prostate gland to empty into the urethra.

Male Accessory Glands

The seminal vesicles are a pair of saclike structures that attach to the ductus deferentia near the base of the urinary bladder. They have glandular tissue linings that contribute nearly 60% of semen volume (the fluid that the male urethra conveys to the outside of the body during ejaculation). The seminal vesicles secrete a thick, yellow fluid, which contains fructose and other carbohydrates that provide energy for sperm cells, a protein that helps semen stick to the vaginal walls, and PGs that stimulate muscular contractions within the female reproductive organs. These contractions aid the movement of sperm cells toward the egg cell. The secretions of the seminal vesicles are discharged into the ejaculatory duct at emission (when peristaltic contractions are occurring in the vas deferens, seminal vesicles, and prostate gland). The sympathetic division of the ANS controls these contractions.

The prostate gland surrounds the proximal portion of the urethra, slightly inferior to the urinary bladder. It is composed of glandular tissue that produces a thin, white fluid that enhances the motility of sperm and a muscular portion that contracts during ejaculation to prevent urine flow. Prostatic fluid is alkaline, which helps to protect sperm from the acidic environment of the vagina.[46]

The bulbourethral glands lie inferior to the prostate gland and are surrounded by the fibers of the external urethral sphincter muscle. A short duct connects these glands with the penile portion of the urethra. During sexual arousal, a mucuslike, alkaline fluid is secreted that counteracts the acid present in the male urethra and female vagina. This fluid also lubricates the end of the penis to prepare for sexual intercourse.

Semen is made up of prostatic fluid (about 30%), seminal vesicle fluid (60%), and sperm (10%).[44] Semen has an alkaline pH between 7.2 and 8.0 and includes PGs and nutrients.[45] Between 2 and 5 mL of semen is released at one time, containing between 20 and 150 million sperm per milliliter.[45] Sperm cells begin to swim as they mix with accessory gland secretions. They acquire the ability to fertilize a female egg cell once they are inside the female reproductive tract.

Penis

The **penis** is cylindrical in shape, and conveys urine and semen through the urethra. When erect, it stiffens and enlarges, enabling insertion into the vagina during sexual intercourse. The penis is divided into three regions: the root, body, and glans. The root of the penis is the fixed portion that attaches the penis to the body wall. The shaft (or body) of the penis is the tubular, movable portion of the organ. It contains three columns of erectile tissue **FIGURE 8-141**. Dense connective tissue surrounds each column in a capsule. The penis is enclosed by a layer of connective tissue, a thin layer of subcutaneous tissue, and skin.

The glans penis is the expanded distal end of the penis that surrounds the external urethral orifice. This structure covers the ends of the corpora cavernosa and opens as the external urethral orifice. Skin in this area is thin and hairless, with sensory receptors for sexual stimulation. Boys are born with

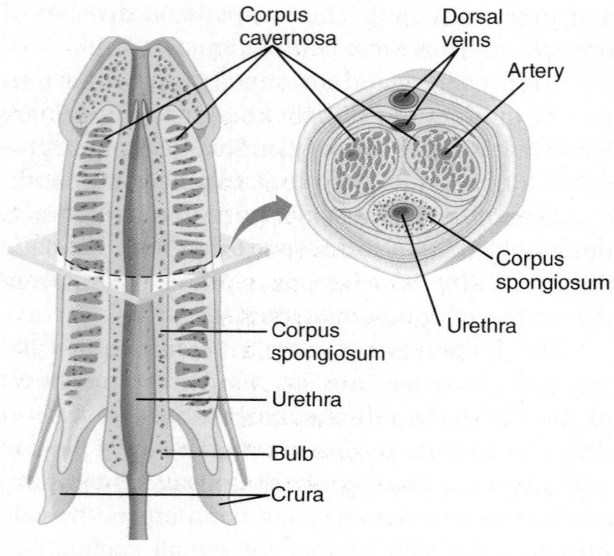

FIGURE 8-141 The penis.

a loose fold of skin called the foreskin (prepuce) that extends to cover the glans, as a sheath. It is often removed soon after birth in a surgical procedure called circumcision.

When sexual arousal occurs, parasympathetic nerve fibers trigger local release of nitric oxide. This release results in relaxation of smooth muscle in the walls of the penile blood vessels and dilation of local arterioles leading into the penis. As the erectile tissue expands with blood, the penis swells and elongates to produce an erection.

Physiologic and emotional release, known as an orgasm, is the culmination of sexual stimulation. Male orgasm is accompanied by emission and ejaculation. During emission, sperm cells from the testes, along with secretions of the prostate gland and seminal vesicles, are moved into the urethra. Emission occurs as a result of sympathetic nerve impulses that stimulate peristaltic contractions in the testicular ducts, epididymides, ductus deferentia, and ejaculatory ducts. Other sympathetic impulses simultaneously cause rhythmic contractions of the seminal vesicles and prostate gland. The urethra fills with semen as sensory impulses pass into the sacral portion of the spinal cord. Somatic motor impulses are then transmitted to certain skeletal muscles, causing rhythmic contractions of the penile erectile columns. This process increases pressure inside the erectile tissues, helping to force semen through the urethra and ultimately outside of the body (ejaculation).

TABLE 8-43 Male Reproductive Structures

Structure	Function
Scrotum	Regulates the temperature of the testes by enclosing and protecting them
Testis	Interstitial cells produce and secrete sex hormones; seminiferous tubules produce sperm cells
Epididymis	Stores and protects spermatozoa and aids in their maturation
Ductus deferens	Transfers sperm cells to the ejaculatory duct
Seminal vesicle	Secretes fluid containing carbohydrates that provide energy for sperm cells, a protein that helps semen stick to the vaginal walls, and prostaglandins that stimulate muscular contractions within the female reproductive organs
Prostate gland	Secretes an alkaline fluid that helps protect sperm from the acidic environment of the vagina
Bulbourethral gland	Secretes fluid into the penile urethra that counteracts the acid present in the male urethra and female vagina
Penis	Copulatory organ that surrounds the urethra and introduces semen into the female vagina; also part of the urinary system.

Fluid from the bulbourethral glands is expelled first during emission and ejaculation, followed by fluid from the prostate gland, passage of sperm cells, and lastly fluid from the seminal vesicles. After ejaculation, the arteries of the erectile tissue immediately constrict. Smooth muscles in the vascular spaces contract partially, and veins of the penis carry away excess blood, gradually returning the penis to its flaccid state.

TABLE 8-43 summarizes the functions of the male reproductive structures.

Female Reproductive Anatomy

The female reproductive organs consist of two ovaries, two uterine (fallopian) tubes, the uterus (womb), **cervix**, vagina (birth canal), mammary glands, and external genitalia **FIGURE 8-142**. The

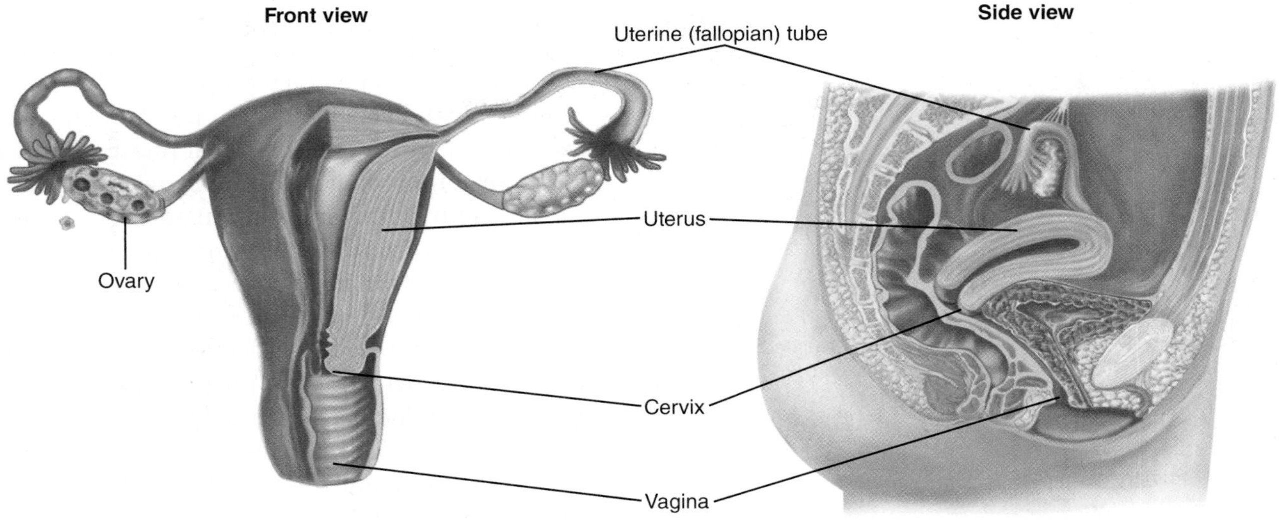

FIGURE 8-142 The female reproductive system.

ovaries are considered the essential organs of the female reproductive system because they produce the female gametes. The uterine tubes, uterus, vagina, mammary glands, and external genitalia are considered accessory organs.

Ovaries

The ovaries are solid structures that are roughly the size and shape of an unshelled almond. They are positioned in the lateral wall of the pelvic cavity in shallow depressions on each side of the uterus. The ovaries perform three main functions: (1) production of immature female gametes (oocytes), (2) secretion of female sex hormones (including estrogens and progestins), and (3) secretion of inhibin.

The ovaries are suspended in the pelvic cavity by ligaments. They receive their blood supply from the ovarian artery, which runs alongside the ovarian ligament, and the ovarian branch of the uterine artery. Each ovary has an outer cortex and an inner portion called the ovarian medulla. Within the cortex are small follicles. Each follicle contains an oocyte, the female germ cell. Each month, during the menstrual cycle, about 20 of these follicles begin the process of maturation, but only a single follicle ultimately matures and releases an ovum. The remaining follicles die off and are reabsorbed by the body.

Oogenesis

During fetal development, diploid (46 chromosomes) germ cells in the ovaries differentiate into oogonia—that is, cells that have the potential to develop into ova. Although many oogonia die, those that survive enter a growth phase, enlarge, and become primary oocytes. The primary oocytes begin to undergo meiosis early in their development in the fetus, but then the process stops and does not restart until puberty.

Oogenesis is the process of oocyte formation, which begins at puberty under the influence of FSH. Some primary oocytes continue meiosis during this time, with each primary oocyte producing two daughter cells: a secondary oocyte and a first polar body **FIGURE 8-143**. The secondary oocyte is large and contains 23 chromosomes, cytoplasm, and organelles. The first polar body is small, containing 23 chromosomes but lacking cytoplasm and organelles. The large secondary oocyte can be fertilized by a sperm cell. Because the first polar body is not a functional oocyte, it degenerates and dies. If fertilization of the secondary oocyte occurs, then it divides unequally, producing a tiny second polar body and a large fertilized egg cell (zygote). If fertilization does not occur, then the secondary oocyte deteriorates and is expelled from the uterus, along with its second polar body, during menstruation.

The Menstrual Cycle

Also called the menses, period, or menstrual cycle, **menstruation** is the cyclic and periodic vaginal discharge of 25 to 65 mL of blood, epithelial cells, mucus, and tissue. The duration of this cycle differs

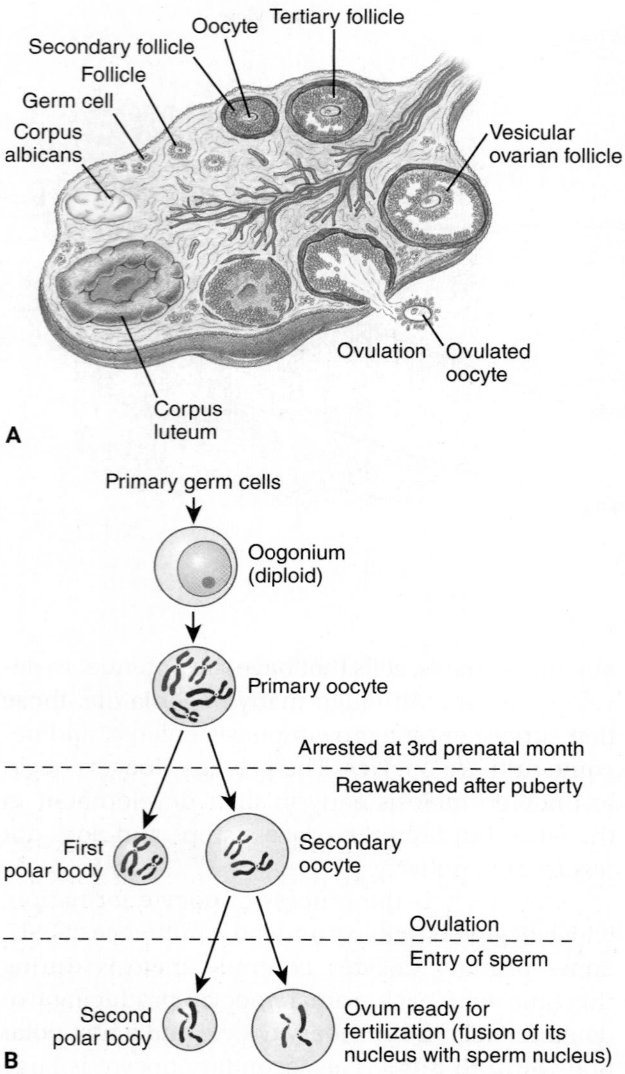

FIGURE 8-143 Ovarian follicle development and oogenesis. **A.** Secretion from the ovary. **B.** Differentiation of the oocyte.

from woman to woman, ranging from an average of 24 days to 35 days. The onset of first menses, when a girl reaches childbearing age, is called **menarche**. Depending on genetics, socioeconomic factors, and individual health, this event may occur anywhere between the ages of 11 and 14 years. The last menses, when a woman has reached the end of childbearing age, is called **menopause** or the female climacteric. The advent of menopause typically begins between the ages of 40 and 50 years, and is signaled by menstrual cycles becoming less frequent.

The menstrual cycle comprises two phases: the ovarian cycle (ovarian changes) and the uterine cycle (changes in the uterus). The ovarian and uterine cycles are linked, such that events in the ovarian cycle affect those in the uterine cycle.

The ovarian cycle is divided into the follicular phase (days 1 to 13) and the luteal phase (days 14 to 28). Secretion of gonadotropin-releasing factor from the hypothalamus stimulates the release of FSH and LH from the anterior pituitary gland. FSH stimulates ovarian follicles to develop and to secrete estrogen and some progesterone. LH stimulates some ovarian cells to secrete hormones such as testosterone, which is then used to produce estrogen. As the follicular phase of the menstrual cycle progresses, peak levels of estrogen and LH cause the mature ovarian follicle to rupture and release its oocyte, a process called **ovulation**. The term *ovum* (plural: *ova*) is used to describe the egg after ovulation has occurred.

The luteal phase of the ovarian cycle occurs during days 14 to 28. This is the time from when the oocyte is released from the ovary (ovulation) until the first day of menstruation. LH continues to be excreted throughout the ovarian cycle and subsequent pregnancy, should it occur. After the egg has been released, what is left of the follicle becomes the corpus luteum, which in turn secretes estrogen, progesterone, and inhibin. All three hormones inhibit secretion of FSH from the anterior pituitary gland, thereby preventing the further development of follicles. If the egg is fertilized, then the corpus luteum will continue to secrete hormones to support the pregnancy for 90 days. If fertilization does not occur, then the corpus luteum gradually shrinks, turns white, stops secreting hormones, and is absorbed into the tissue of the ovary.

The uterine cycle is divided into the proliferative phase (days 5 to 14) and the secretory phase (days 15 to 28). The proliferative phase spans from the time after menstruation and until the next ovulation occurs. During this phase, in response to estrogen released by the follicle, the uterine lining (endometrium) increases in thickness in preparation to receive a fertilized oocyte. The secretory phase spans from the time after ovulation until menstruation. During this phase, the uterine lining continues to thicken. After ovulation, the corpus luteum mainly secretes progesterone, which stimulates glands in the uterine lining to secrete glycogen, a nutritional source for a fertilized egg. If fertilization does not occur, then estrogen and

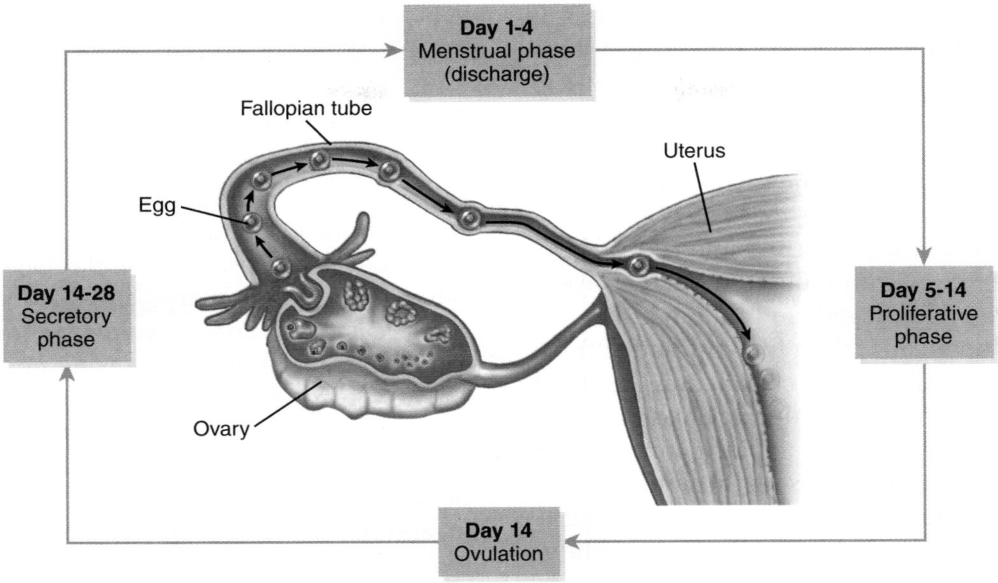

FIGURE 8-144 The menstrual cycle, based on an average 28-day cycle. The length of the cycle and the number of days in each phase vary from woman to woman, but generally fall within a range of 24 to 35 days.

progesterone levels decrease and the thick lining of the uterus is shed from the woman's body. With a 28-day cycle, the menstrual phase (discharge) lasts about 5 days **FIGURE 8-144**.

The female body undergoes many major changes during pregnancy, including development of the placenta, the umbilical cord, and, of course, the fetus. These changes, as well as fetal circulation, fetal respiration, stages of labor, and physiologic changes in the infant after birth, are covered in Chapter 42, *Obstetrics*, and in Chapter 43, *Neonatal Care*.

Uterine Tubes

The uterine tubes (fallopian tubes or oviducts) open near the ovaries, and are each about 4 inches (10 cm) long. They pass medially to the uterus, penetrate its wall, and open into the uterine cavity. Normally, one uterine tube is associated with each ovary. When the oocyte is released, it travels through the fallopian tube to the uterus. The fertilization of the oocyte by a sperm usually occurs when the oocyte is inside the fallopian tube. The fertilized oocyte then continues to the uterus, where it develops into an embryo (the early stage of the fetus) and implants into the uterine wall.

Each uterine tube extends out laterally from the uterus, terminating just short of an ovary. The proximal end of each fallopian tube is very thick and narrow and connects to the uterus itself. Each uterine tube is composed of three layers of tissue. The outer layer consists of a serous membrane that protects the tubes. The middle layer is made of smooth muscle that contracts to help move the ovum through the tube and into the uterus. The innermost layer contains secretory cells and cilia that also move the ovum along and may play a part in providing nutrition to the ovum.

When an ovary releases an egg, the ciliary motion in these layers sweeps the egg into the uterine tube. Smooth muscle contractions and the inner mucosa move the ovum through the tube to the uterus. If the egg encounters a sperm cell along the way, then it may become fertilized. Fertilization can occur at any time within about a 24-hour window after ovulation.

Uterus

The uterus (womb) is the organ where the embryo grows. The contractions of the uterus during labor ultimately help to push the newborn, placenta, and membranes through the birth canal at delivery. A hollow and muscular organ, the uterus is shaped slightly like an inverted pear. It is located in the anterior pelvic cavity and lies between the urinary bladder and the rectum. The dome-shaped top of the uterus is the fundus. Below the dome, the uterus begins to taper and narrow, forming the body. The narrowest portion of the uterus (the cervix) opens into the vagina. The interior of the body of the uterus is known as the uterine cavity, and the interior of the cervix is called the **cervical canal**.

The uterine wall is thick, containing three layers of tissue: the perimetrium (outer protective layer), myometrium (middle layer), and endometrium (inner lining). The myometrium is composed of three layers of muscle fibers; the contractions of these muscles help expel the fetus during childbirth. The endometrium is a mucous membrane composed of two layers; the layer innermost to the uterine cavity is shed during menstruation. As the follicle starts developing and pumping out estrogen, the endometrium is stimulated to increase its thickness in preparation for the reception and future growth of a fertilized egg.

Vagina

The vagina is a distensible muscular structure lined with mucous membranes. It extends from the cervix to the outside of the body. The vagina has the following physiologic functions: (1) serves as a passageway for the elimination of menstrual fluids, (2) receives the penis during sexual intercourse, (3) holds the spermatozoa before their passage into the uterus, and (4) serves as the passageway for childbirth.

The interior of the vagina is acidic owing to the breakdown of glycogen (found in large amounts in the vaginal mucosa), which creates a low-pH environment that inhibits bacterial growth. This acidity, while beneficial to the female body, is injurious to sperm cells. Semen, however, is alkaline in nature and has antibacterial properties. The alkalinity of seminal fluid neutralizes the acidity of the vagina, allowing the sperm cells to survive and fertilize the ovum.

Just inside the lower vagina are two tiny openings that lead to the Bartholin glands. These glands secrete mucus that acts as a lubricant during intercourse. Before first sexual intercourse, the vaginal orifice is protected by the hymen. This membrane, which is made up of connective tissue and epithelium, forms a border around the vaginal orifice, partially enclosing it. It has a central opening that allows uterine and vaginal secretions to pass to the outside of the body.

Breasts and Mammary Glands

The breasts, located above the pectoralis major muscles, extend from the second to the sixth ribs, from the sternum to the axillae. Each breast is mainly composed of adipose tissue and collagen. The main purpose of the mammary glands—a series of modified sweat glands housed within the breasts—is lactation (milk secretion) to provide nourishment to the newborn. Milk is carried to the surface of each breast through lactiferous ducts that terminate in a nipple. The nipple of the breast is surrounded by a darker-pigmented area called the areola. Prolactin, an anterior pituitary hormone, stimulates milk production. Oxytocin, a hormone released by the posterior pituitary, stimulates ejection of milk into the ducts of the mammary glands.

External Genitalia

The female external genitalia, collectively called the vulva or pudendum, are the structures seen from the outside of the body **FIGURE 8-145**. The anatomic landmark known as the mons pubis is a rounded pad of adipose tissue that overlies the symphysis pubis, located anterior to the urethral and vaginal openings. Coarse, dark hair normally appears here in early puberty, becoming sparser later in life with the advent of menopause. The **labia majora** and **labia minora**, described as "lips," surround and protect the vaginal opening as well as the more anterior opening of the urethra. The labia majora are covered with pubic hair, whereas the labia minora are not. The area between the vaginal opening and the anus is called the perineum. The clitoris is located

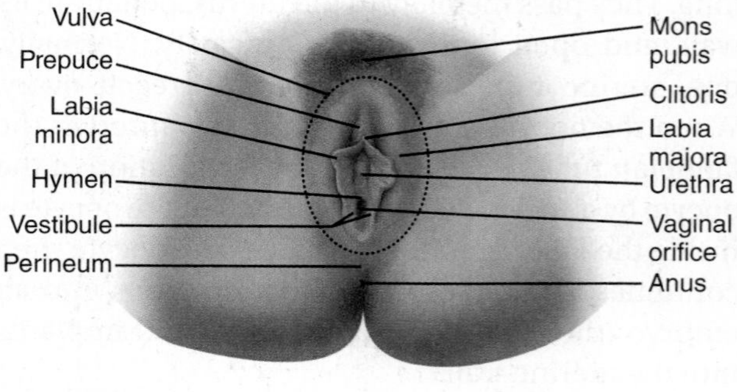

FIGURE 8-145 The female external genitalia.

at the anterior junction of the labia minora, just below a layer of skin called the prepuce. A small, cylindrical mass of erectile tissue and nerves, the clitoris is similar to the glans penis of the male.

Between the labia minora is a cleft referred to as the **vestibule**. Located within the vestibule is the urethral opening (orifice), the vaginal opening, and the hymen. One vestibular gland lies on each side of the vaginal opening. The urethra, which leads to the bladder, allows for passage of urine. The length of the urethra in females averages about 2 inches (5 cm). This short length is one reason why women are more susceptible to urinary tract infections and bladder infections than are men.

The erectile tissues of the clitoris and vaginal entrance respond to sexual stimulation. Parasympathetic nerve impulses release nitric oxide to dilate the erectile tissues, increase blood flow, and swell the tissues. In addition, the vagina expands and elongates. If sexual stimulation is sufficiently intense, then parasympathetic impulses cause the vestibular glands to secrete mucus into the vestibule, moistening and lubricating the surrounding tissues and lower vagina. This facilitates insertion of the penis. The clitoris responds to local stimulation, culminating in an orgasm if stimulation is sufficient. Just before orgasm, the outer third of the vagina becomes engorged with blood. This increases friction on the penis, with orgasm initiating reflexes directed by the sacral and lumbar spinal cord. The muscles of the perineum and walls of both the uterus and uterine tubes contract rhythmically. This contraction helps transport sperm through the female reproductive tract toward the upper uterine tubes.

TABLE 8-44 summarizes the functions of the female reproductive structures.

TABLE 8-44 Female Reproductive Structures

Structure	Function
Ovary (ovaries)	The female reproductive organ that produces oocytes and sex hormones
Uterine (fallopian) tubes	Transports secondary oocytes in the direction of the uterus; fertilization occurs here, with the developing embryo conveyed to the uterus
Uterus	The muscular organ of the female reproductive tract, in which implantation, placenta formation, and fetal development occur
Vagina	Transports uterine secretions to outside of the body, receives the erect penis during intercourse; the fully developed fetus passes through the vagina during normal delivery
Labia majora	Protects and encloses the external reproductive organs
Labia minora	Protects the openings of the vagina and urethra
Clitoris	Gives pleasurable sensations during sexual stimulation
Vestibule	Contains the vaginal and urethral openings
Vestibular glands	Moisten and lubricate the vestibule with a secretion

YOU are the Paramedic SUMMARY

1. What anatomic areas of the motorcyclist's body may be injured as a result of this collision?

Possible areas of injury include the face, skull, brain, thoracic cavity, pelvis, limbs, and spine.

2. Which anatomic areas of the motorcyclist's body may have life-threatening injuries in this scenario?

Areas of the body that may potentially have life-threatening injuries include the brain, airway, pelvis, femur, and mediastinum.

3. Given the broken upper teeth and facial swelling, what body structures may have been injured?

Structures that may have been injured include the maxilla (upper jaw) and zygomas (cheekbones).

4. What is the best way to describe the location of the injury on the left chest?

The patient has an injury to the superior chest at the left midclavicular line.

YOU are the Paramedic SUMMARY continued

5. What is the best way to describe the location of the deformity and injury on the right leg?

The patient has a deformity and a laceration just proximal to the right medial malleolus.

6. What is the obvious injury you find to the patient's chest?

The patient has an injury to the left anterior ribs.

7. What are the potential hidden injuries you should consider?

Because there is obvious injury to the patient's chest, you must also suspect internal injuries to the underlying structures, such as the heart and great vessels, and abdominal organs. In addition, the findings of unequal chest rise and fall, as well as a grating sensation, indicate that the patient has a substantial injury.

8. What structures are located in the lower abdominal quadrants?

The large and small intestine, bladder, and (in women) ovaries and uterus are located in the lower abdominal quadrants.

9. What might the instability of the pelvis indicate?

This finding suggests a pelvic fracture and the potential for significant internal bleeding. Knowledge of anatomy, physiology, and signs/symptoms of internal injury will be key to treating this patient.

EMS Patient Care Report (PCR)

Date: 04-02-22	**Incident No.:** 245	**Nature of Call:** MVC		**Location:** N/B I-95 @ county line	
Dispatched: 1430	**En Route:** 1430	**At Scene:** 1440	**Transport:** 1450	**At Hospital:** 1507	**In Service:** 1515

Patient Information

Age: 22 **Sex:** M **Weight (in kg [lb]):** 91 kg (200 lb)	**Allergies:** Unknown **Medications:** Unknown **Past Medical History:** Unknown **Chief Complaint:** Unresponsive from MVC

Vital Signs

Time: 1443	**BP:** Not yet obtained	**Pulse:** 118	**Respirations:** 24	**Spo_2:** Not yet obtained
Time: 1445	**BP:** 106/70	**Pulse:** 120	**Respirations:** 24	**Spo_2:** 90% (ambient air)
Time: 1453	**BP:** 102/66	**Pulse:** 118	**Respirations:** 24	**Spo_2:** 97% (assisted with bag-mask device)

EMS Treatment (circle all that apply)

Oxygen @ 15 L/min via (circle one): **NC NRM (Bag-mask device)**		**(Assisted Ventilation)**	**Airway Adjunct**	**CPR**
Defibrillation	**Bleeding Control**	**Bandaging**	**Splinting**	**Other:**

Narrative

Crew dispatched to truck versus motorcycle crash. While traveling at highway speeds, motorcycle struck front bumper of a stationary pickup, pushing truck back 10 feet (3 m). Motorcyclist was ejected from bike, collided with truck windshield, then rolled to the ground. On arrival, found pt unresponsive, lying prone on the pavement. Pt's spine manually stabilized immediately and logrolled into supine position. Pt immobilized per protocol. Physical exam revealed missing upper front teeth with dried blood present, bilateral swelling of the orbital tissue, and an abrasion to superior chest at left midclavicular line. Instability and grating of anterior chest noted on palpation. Unequal chest rise and fall. Bilateral rigidity of lower abdominal quadrants. Palpation of pelvis revealed instability and grinding. Deformity and laceration present just proximal to the right medial malleolus. Pt remains unresponsive. Vital signs as noted above. Ventilations assisted with bag-mask device. Pt condition remained unchanged during transport to Regional Trauma Center. Reported on arrival to Dr. Warren.

End of report

Prep Kit

Ready for Review

- To care for your patients properly, you must have a thorough understanding of human anatomy and physiology, as well as homeostasis, so you can assess the patient's condition and communicate with hospital personnel and other health care providers.
- To achieve the functions necessary for life, the body is organized by levels. From least complex to most complex, these levels of organization are as follows: chemical, cellular, tissue, organ, organ system, and the organism as a whole.
- If you understand the basics of chemistry, then your understanding of anatomy and physiology will be improved. Chemical changes within cells influence body functions and the status of the body's structures.
- Chemicals can basically be divided into two main groups: organic and inorganic. Organic substances include carbohydrates, lipids, proteins, and nucleic acids. Inorganic substances in body cells include oxygen, carbon dioxide, salts, and water.
- Enzymes are often involved in the chemical reactions that occur in the body. These reactions alter the chemical nature of a chemical substance, in an effort to maintain homeostasis.
- Through the body's functions, individual cells are supplied with nutrients and use them in various processes. As a result of cellular metabolism, organisms grow, maintain body functions, release or store energy, produce and eliminate waste, digest nutrients, or destroy toxins.
- Body functions also often require electrolytes. Important ions for body functions include sodium, potassium, calcium, magnesium, bicarbonate, chloride, and phosphorus.
- Another important concept related to homeostasis is acid–base balance. Abnormal fluctuations in pH level can cause damage to cells, tissues, and proteins. The buffer system of the body helps neutralize excessive acids or bases.
- Cells are the foundation of the human body. Cells with a common job grow close to each other and form tissues. Groups of tissues that all perform interrelated jobs form organs.
- The life cycle of a cell is regulated via stimulation from hormones or growth factors. This cycle includes stages known as interphase, cell division or mitosis, cytoplasmic division, and differentiation. Cell division and growth that occur at a rate higher than cell death leads to cancer. Tumors can be benign or malignant.
- Cellular respiration is a process that releases energy from organic compounds. It proceeds through three stages: glycolysis, the Krebs cycle, and the electron transport chain. The end result is formation of adenosine triphosphate molecules, in which energy is stored.
- Cell transport mechanisms, which determine how materials enter and exit cells, contribute to maintenance of fluid quantity and distribution. Several mechanisms, such as diffusion, filtration, osmosis, facilitated diffusion, osmosis, active transport, endocytosis, and exocytosis, allow material to pass through the cell wall.
- The human body is primarily made up of four major types of tissues: epithelial, connective, muscle, and nervous tissues. Tissue results from differentiation, the process by which a cell becomes specialized for a specific purpose.
- Membranes form a barrier or an interface. The four types of membranes are serous membranes, mucous membranes, cutaneous membranes, and synovial membranes.
- Homeostasis is the adaptive process by which cells and tissues respond to preserve the body's equilibrium. Cellular signaling—electrochemical communication between cells—triggers the chemical reactions needed to maintain homeostasis. Feedback occurs to stop the reaction once it is no longer needed.
- Organ systems include the integumentary, skeletal, muscular, nervous, endocrine, circulatory, lymphatic, immune, respiratory, digestive, urinary, and genital systems.
- The integumentary system, which serves as the interface between the body and the

Prep Kit continued

outside world, includes the skin, hair, nails, sebaceous glands, and sweat glands. Its functions include protection, temperature regulation, fluid regulation, sensation, and inflammatory response.

- The skin is divided into two parts: the superficial epidermis, which is composed of several layers of cells (including the germinal layer and the stratum corneal layer), and the deeper dermis, which contains specialized skin structures such as sweat glands, sebaceous (oil) glands, nails, hair follicles, blood vessels, and specialized nerve endings.
- Subcutaneous tissue is found below the skin and is composed largely of fat. It serves as an insulator for the body and as a reservoir to store energy, and also helps to anchor the skin to the structures beneath it.
- The skeleton gives the body its recognizable human form through a collection of bones, ligaments, tendons, and cartilage. Functions of the skeletal system include support, leverage, protection, storage, maintenance of calcium levels, and blood cell production.
- Bones are classified according to their shape, as long bones, short bones, flat bones, and irregular bones. The bones increase greatly in size as the fetus develops and throughout adolescence.
- A joint is where two bones come into contact. Joints are classified as immovable (synarthrotic), slightly movable (amphiarthrotic), or freely movable (diarthrotic). Most joints allow motion (knee, hip, elbow), and some bones fuse at joints to form a solid, immobile, bony structure (skull). The 230 joints in the human body are categorized as fibrous, cartilaginous, or synovial.
- The axial skeleton forms the body's foundation on which the arms and legs are hung. The appendicular skeleton consists of the arms and legs, their connection points, and the pelvis.
- The five sections of the spine are the cervical spine, thoracic spine, lumbar spine, sacrum, and coccyx.
- Contraction and relaxation of the musculoskeletal system gives the body its ability to move. Skeletal muscle, so named because it attaches to the bones of the skeleton, forms the major muscle mass of the body. It is also called voluntary muscle, because all skeletal muscle is under direct voluntary control.
- The nervous system is perhaps the most complex organ system within the human body. It consists of the brain, spinal cord, and nerves.
- The nervous system is responsible for fundamental functions such as controlling breathing, HR, and BP. This system also allows the performance of higher-level activities, such as memory, understanding, and thought.
- The nervous system is divided into the central nervous system (CNS) and the peripheral nervous system (PNS). The CNS includes the brain and spinal cord. The somatic nervous system is the part of the PNS that regulates activities over which there is voluntary control, such as walking, talking, and writing. The autonomic nervous system (ANS) is the part of the PNS that controls the many body functions that occur without voluntary control, such as digestion, dilation and constriction of blood vessels, and sweating.
- The ANS is split into two areas. The sympathetic nervous system is responsible for the fight-or-flight response, and the parasympathetic nervous system is responsible for conserving energy and maintaining organ function, including digestion, growth, healing, and the removal of toxins.
- The endocrine system is made up of various glands located throughout the body. Major endocrine glands include the pituitary gland, thyroid gland, parathyroid glands, adrenal glands, pancreas, thymus gland, and reproductive glands.
- The hypothalamus serves as the communication center between the nervous and endocrine systems.
- Endocrine glands help regulate metabolism, control chemical reactions, transport

Prep Kit continued

substances, regulate water and electrolyte balances, and aid in reproduction, growth, and development.

- The circulatory system is a complex arrangement of connected tubes, including the arteries, arterioles, capillaries, venules, and veins.
- Blood consists of plasma and formed elements or cells that are suspended in the plasma. These cells include red blood cells (erythrocytes), white blood cells (leukocytes), and platelets (thrombocytes).
- Blood has many functions, including fighting infection, transporting oxygen and carbon dioxide, controlling pH, transporting wastes and nutrients, and clotting.
- Cardiac muscle has the property of automaticity; it can generate and conduct electricity without influence from the brain.
- The cardiac cycle begins with myocardial contraction and concludes at the beginning of the next contraction. Contraction of the heart results in pressure changes within the cardiac chambers, resulting in movement of blood from areas of high pressure to areas of low pressure.
- The pressure in the aorta against which the left ventricle must pump blood is called the afterload. The greater the afterload, the harder it is for the ventricle to eject blood into the aorta, which reduces the stroke volume (the amount of blood ejected per contraction).
- Cardiac output is the amount of blood pumped through the circulatory system in 1 minute; it is expressed in liters per minute (L/min). The cardiac output equals the HR multiplied by the stroke volume.
- Increased venous return to the heart stretches the ventricles, resulting in increased cardiac contractility. This relationship is known as the Frank-Starling mechanism.
- The lymphatic system helps maintain fluid balance in the body, fight infection by producing and circulating lymphocytes, and distribute various products that are unable to enter the bloodstream directly (eg, nutrients and some hormones). The spleen is the body's largest lymphatic organ.
- The immune system is composed of lymphoid tissues and cells involved in immune response. The body's defense mechanisms work together to resist disease, illness, and infection.
- The respiratory system consists of all structures of the body that contribute to the process of breathing. It includes the nose, mouth, throat, larynx, trachea, bronchi, and bronchioles. This system also includes the lungs, diaphragm, muscles of the chest wall, and accessory muscles of breathing.
- The primary function of the respiratory system is to conduct respiration. Oxygen is essential for the body to function. Gas exchange of oxygen into blood and carbon dioxide out of blood occurs in the alveoli of the lungs via diffusion.
- The respiratory center in the brainstem controls breathing. Nerves in this area sense the level of carbon dioxide in the blood and spinal fluid. The brain adjusts breathing as needed if the level of carbon dioxide or oxygen in the arterial blood is either too high or too low.
- Increases in the level of carbon dioxide in the blood ($Paco_2$) cause decreased pH levels in the respiratory center, which triggers an increase in ventilation. Decreases in $Paco_2$ result in increased pH levels in the respiratory center and a decrease in ventilation.
- The hypoxic drive is a backup system that the body uses to control respiration. Areas in the brain, walls of the aorta, and carotid arteries act as oxygen sensors and stimulate breathing if the oxygen level falls.
- The digestive system functions consist of a series of steps, which include ingestion, mechanical processing, digestion, secretion, absorption, and excretion.
- The alimentary canal extends from the mouth to the anus. It includes the mouth, pharynx, esophagus, stomach, small intestine, large intestine, rectum, and anus. The accessory organs of the alimentary canal include the teeth,

Prep Kit continued

tongue, salivary glands, liver, gallbladder, and pancreas.
- The main functions of the urinary system are to control fluid balance in the body, to filter and eliminate wastes, and to control pH balance.
- In the urinary system, the kidneys are solid organs; the ureters, bladder, and urethra are hollow organs.
- The kidneys rid the blood of toxic waste products and control its balance of water and salt.
- The male and female reproductive systems contain organs and glands that create sex cells and transport these gametes to areas where fertilization can occur.
- Chromosomes contain the entire sequence of genetic information the organism will have throughout its entire life. This genetic information contains the instructions for every structure and process in the body. Genes also contain sequences that will determine or influence various characteristics such as hair color, skin color, body composition, height, and predisposition to certain diseases.
- The male's primary sex organs (gonads) consist of two testes, in which sperm cells and male sex hormones are formed. The testes are considered part of both the endocrine and male reproductive systems because they produce testosterone (a hormone) and sperm.
- Testosterone enlarges the testes and accessory reproductive organs, and promotes development of the male secondary sex characteristics during puberty. These characteristics include an increased amount of body hair; enlargement of the larynx and thickening of vocal folds, which lowers the pitch of the voice; thickening of the skin; increased muscular growth; and thickening and strengthening of bones.
- The female reproductive organs produce and maintain oocytes (eggs), which are the female sex cells.
- The female's primary sex organs (gonads) are the two ovaries, which reproduce female sex cells and sex hormones.
- In nonpregnant females, the ovaries are the main source of estrogens, and they secrete increasing amounts of estrogens beginning at puberty. These hormones stimulate enlargement of accessory sex organs and develop and maintain the female secondary sex characteristics, including development of breasts and mammary gland systems.
- The female reproductive cycle involves regular, recurring changes in the uterine lining as well as menstrual bleeding (menses).

Vital Vocabulary

ABO system The commonly used blood classification system, based on the antigens present or absent in the blood.

accessory muscles The muscles not normally used during quiet breathing; examples include the sternocleidomastoid muscles of the neck, the chest pectoralis major muscles, and the abdominal muscles.

accommodation The ability of the lens of the eye to change its shape to focus on a close object.

acetabulum The socket formed by the coxal (hip) bone into which the ball-shaped femoral head fits snugly.

acetylcholine (ACh) A neurotransmitter released at synapses within the autonomic nervous system and by motor neurons to stimulate skeletal muscle contraction.

acetylcholinesterase An enzyme found in the central nervous system, in red blood cells, and in motor endplates of skeletal muscle that causes the decomposition of acetylcholine.

acidosis A pathologic condition resulting from the accumulation of acids in the body (blood pH less than 7.35).

acids Molecules that can give up a hydrogen ion, and therefore increase the concentration of hydrogen ions in a water solution.

acromion process The tip of the shoulder and the site of attachment for the clavicle and various shoulder muscles.

Prep Kit continued

actin A contractile protein found in the thin filaments of skeletal muscle cells.

action potentials Sequences of changes in the membrane potential that occur when an excitable cell (neuron or muscle) is stimulated.

active transport A method used to move compounds across a cell membrane to create or maintain an imbalance of charges, usually against a concentration gradient and requiring the expenditure of energy.

adaptation The temporary or permanent reduction of sensitivity to a particular stimulus.

adenosine triphosphate (ATP) The nucleotide formed from the metabolism of nutrients in the cell; involved in energy metabolism; used to store energy.

adrenal cortex The outer layer of the adrenal gland; it produces hormones that are important in regulating the water and salt balance of the body.

adrenal glands Paired endocrine glands located on top of the kidneys, which release epinephrine and norepinephrine when stimulated by the sympathetic nervous system; each adrenal gland consists of an inner adrenal medulla and an adrenal cortex.

adrenergic Having the characteristics of the sympathetic division of the autonomic nervous system.

adrenocorticotropic hormone (ACTH) Hormone that targets the adrenal cortex and causes it to secrete cortisol (a glucocorticoid).

aerobic metabolism Metabolism that can proceed only in the presence of oxygen.

afterimage The perception that a stimulus is still present after the stimulus has been removed.

afterload The pressure in the aorta against which the left ventricle must pump blood.

albumins The smallest of plasma proteins; they make up approximately 60% of the plasma proteins and are responsible for the oncotic pressure in the vasculature, thereby controlling the movement of water into and out of the circulation.

aldosterone Hormone responsible for the reabsorption of sodium and water from the kidney tubules.

alkalosis A pathologic condition resulting from the accumulation of bases in the body (blood pH greater than 7.45).

alleles Variant forms of a gene, which can be identical or slightly different in a sequence of deoxyribonucleic acid.

alveoli The air sacs of the lungs in which the exchange of oxygen and carbon dioxide takes place; also, the bony sockets for the teeth that reside in the mandible and maxilla (singular, *alveolus*).

anabolism The building of larger substances from smaller substances, such as the building of proteins from amino acids.

anaerobic metabolism Metabolism that occurs in the absence of oxygen.

anatomy The study of the structure of an organism and its parts.

angle of Louis A prominence of the sternum that indicates the point where the second rib joins the sternum; also called the sternal angle or manubriosternal junction.

antagonists Molecules that block the ability of a given chemical to bind to its receptor, preventing a biologic response.

antigens Proteins, polysaccharides, glycoproteins, or glycolipids commonly found on the surfaces of red blood cells that stimulate an immune system response and cause formation of antibodies; cells learn to recognize antigens as either "self" or "nonself" (foreign).

aorta The principal artery leaving the left side of the heart and carrying freshly oxygenated blood to the body; the largest artery in the body.

aortic valve The semilunar valve that regulates blood flow from the left ventricle to the aorta.

apneustic center A portion of the pons that is thought to work with the pontine respiratory group to regulate the length and depth of inspiration.

Prep Kit continued

appendicular skeleton The portion of the skeletal system made up of the upper extremities, shoulder girdle, pelvic girdle, and lower extremities.

aqueous humor Watery fluid filling the anterior eye cavity; its quantity determines the intraocular pressure, which is critical to sight.

areolar tissue A type of loose connective tissue that binds skin to underlying organs and fills in spaces between muscles.

arytenoid cartilages Six paired cartilages stacked on top of each other in the larynx.

astigmatism Condition where parts of the image are out of focus and others are in focus; caused by irregularities in the shape of the eye lens.

atlas The first cervical vertebra (C1), which provides support for the head.

atria The two upper chambers of the heart (singular, *atrium*).

atrial natriuretic peptide Hormone produced by the atria when they are distended by increased blood volume; it inhibits the absorption of water and sodium in the renal tubules, thereby increasing the elimination of water.

atrioventricular (AV) node A group of cells that conduct an electrical impulse through the heart; located in the floor of the right atrium immediately behind the tricuspid valve and near the opening of the coronary sinus.

atrioventricular (AV) valves The mitral and tricuspid valves, through which blood flows on its way from the atria to the ventricles.

automaticity Ability of cardiac pacemaker cells to initiate an electrical impulse spontaneously without being stimulated from another source (such as a nerve).

autonomic nervous system (ANS) A subdivision of the nervous system that controls primarily involuntary body functions; composed of the sympathetic and parasympathetic nervous systems.

autosomes The chromosomes that do not carry genes that determine sex.

axial skeleton The portion of the skeleton made up of the skull, thoracic cage, and vertebral column.

axis An imaginary line joining the positive and negative electrodes of a lead; also the second cervical vertebra.

axon Long, slender extension of a neuron (nerve cell) that conducts electrical impulses away from the nerve cell body to adjacent cells.

B lymphocytes Lymphocytes that exist in the blood, and are abundant in the lymph nodes, bone marrow, intestinal lining, and spleen; also called B cells.

baroreceptors Nerve endings that are stimulated by pressure changes, including increased arterial blood pressure; they are located in the aortic arch and carotid sinuses.

basal ganglia Structures located deep within the cerebrum, diencephalon, and midbrain that have an important role in coordination of motor movements and posture.

basal metabolic rate The rate at which nutrients are consumed in the body.

basophils White blood cells that contain histamine granules and other substances that are released during inflammatory and allergic responses.

bilirubin A waste product of red blood cell destruction that undergoes further metabolism in the liver.

binocular vision The merging of two images into one.

blood–brain barrier A layer of tightly adhered cells that protects the brain and spinal cord from exposure to medications, toxins, and infectious particles.

bone marrow Soft tissue that fills the inside of bones and is the site of production of red blood cells, platelets, and most white blood cells.

bony labyrinth The collection of hollows in the bone of the inner ear that provide protection to the structures of the inner ear from damage and from extraneous stimulation.

Prep Kit continued

Boyle's law Gas law that demonstrates that as pressure increases, volume decreases; at a constant temperature, the volume of a gas is inversely proportional to its pressure (if the pressure on a gas is doubled, then its volume is halved); written as $PV = k$, where P = pressure, V = volume, and k = a constant.

brain The part of the central nervous system located within the cranium; contains billions of neurons that serve a variety of functions, including consciousness, perception, control of reactions to the environment, emotional responses, and judgment.

brainstem The area of the brain between the spinal cord and the cerebrum that contains the midbrain, pons, and medulla; controls functions that are necessary for life, such as breathing.

bruit Abnormal whooshing sounds indicating turbulent blood flow within a narrowed blood vessel, usually heard in the carotid arteries.

buffer systems Fast-acting defenses against acid–base changes, which provide almost immediate protection against changes in the hydrogen ion concentration of extracellular fluid.

bundle of His The portion of the conduction system of the heart located in the upper portion of the interventricular septum that conducts an electrical impulse from the atrioventricular junction to the right and left bundle branches.

bursa A small, padlike sac or cavity filled with a small amount of synovial fluid that helps reduce the amount of friction between a tendon and a bone or between a tendon and a ligament, usually located near a joint.

calcaneus The heel bone; the largest of the tarsal bones.

calorie The amount of heat needed to raise the temperature of 1 gram of water by 1°C; the amount of energy that can be obtained from the nutrients taken in through the diet; also called a kilocalorie.

carbohydrates Substances (including sugars and starches) that provide much of the energy required by the body's cells and help build cell structures.

cardiac cycle The repetitive pumping process that begins with the onset of cardiac muscle contraction and ends just before the beginning of the next contraction; each cycle consists of ventricular contraction (systole) and relaxation (diastole).

carina The point of bifurcation of the right and left primary (main stem) bronchi.

carpal bones The eight small bones of the wrist.

cartilaginous joints Joints connected by hyaline cartilage, or fibrocartilage, such as the joints that separate the vertebrae.

catabolism The breakdown of larger molecules into smaller ones.

cataracts Clouding of the lenses of the eyes or their surrounding transparent membranes.

catecholamines Amine substances such as dopamine, epinephrine, and norepinephrine that function as neurotransmitters, hormones, or both.

cell membrane The cell wall; a selectively permeable layer that surrounds the intracellular contents and controls movement of substances into and out of the cell; also called the cytoplasmic membrane or plasma membrane.

cellular respiration A biochemical process resulting in the production of energy in the form of adenosine triphosphate.

central nervous system (CNS) The brain and spinal cord.

cerebellum Area of the brain involved in fine and gross muscle coordination; responsible for interpretation of actual movement and correction of any movements that interfere with coordination and the body's position.

cerebral cortex The outer covering of gray matter that covers the cerebral hemispheres; regulates voluntary skeletal movement and plays an important role in the individual's level of awareness.

cerebral perfusion pressure (CPP) Pressure inside the cerebral arteries and an indicator of brain perfusion; calculated by subtracting intracranial pressure from mean arterial pressure.

Prep Kit continued

cerebrospinal fluid (CSF) Fluid produced in the ventricles of the brain that flows in the subarachnoid space and bathes the meninges.

cerebrum The largest part of the brain; made up of several lobes that control movement, hearing, balance, speech, visual perception, emotions, and personality; divided into right and left hemispheres; also called gray matter.

cervical canal The interior of the cervix.

cervix The lower one-third or neck of the uterus.

chemoreceptors Sense organs that monitor the levels of oxygen and carbon dioxide and the pH of cerebrospinal fluid and blood; they provide feedback to the respiratory centers to modify the rate and depth of breathing based on the body's needs at any given time.

cholinergic Having the characteristics of the parasympathetic division of the autonomic nervous system; also refers to other structures or functions that are related to acetylcholine.

chordae tendineae Thin bands of fibrous tissue that attach to the atrioventricular valves in the heart and prevent them from inverting.

choroid The vascular, pigmented middle layer of the eye wall.

choroid plexus Group of specialized cells in the ventricles of the brain; filters blood through cerebral capillaries to create cerebrospinal fluid.

chromosomes Structures formed from condensed fibers and protein of deoxyribonucleic acid; these threadlike structures are found in the nucleus of the cells.

chronotropic effect Related to the effect of the rate of contraction of the heart.

ciliary body The structure associated with the choroid layer of the eye that secretes aqueous humor and contains the ciliary muscle.

circulatory system The complex arrangement of connected tubes, including the arteries, arterioles, capillaries, venules, and veins, that moves blood, oxygen, nutrients, carbon dioxide, and cellular waste throughout the body.

circumflex coronary artery One of two branches of the left main coronary artery.

citric acid cycle A sequence of enzymatic reactions involving the metabolism of carbon chains of glucose, fatty acids, and amino acids to yield carbon dioxide, water, and high-energy phosphate bonds; also known as the Krebs cycle or tricarboxylic acid cycle.

clotting cascade A set of interactions that lead to the formation of a fibrin clot; also called the coagulation cascade.

cochlea The portion of the inner ear that has hearing receptors.

compound A substance that can be broken down into the two or more elements contained within it.

conductivity The property that allows a cardiac cell to receive an electrical impulse and pass it on to an adjoining cardiac cell.

cones One of the two kinds of photoreceptors within the retina that can distinguish colors; it requires a greater amount of light to activate and create an image.

conjunctivae The membranous coverings on the anterior surface of the eye, and which also line the eyelids.

conjunctivitis Inflammation of the conjunctiva.

connective tissues Tissues that bind, support, protect, frame, and fill body structures; they also store fat, produce blood cells, repair tissues, and protect against infection.

contractility The ability of myocardial cells to shorten in response to an impulse, which results in contraction.

cornea The transparent tissue layer in front of the pupil and iris of the eye.

coronary sinus Venous drain for the coronary circulation into the right atrium.

corpus callosum A deep bridge of nerve fibers connecting the brain hemispheres.

corticosteroids Any of several steroids secreted by the adrenal gland.

Prep Kit continued

cortisol A glucocorticoid released by the middle adrenal cortex that influences protein and fat metabolism and stimulates synthesis of glucose from noncarbohydrates.

cranial nerves The 12 pairs of nerves that arise from the base of the brain.

cranial vault The bones that encase and protect the brain, including the parietal, temporal, frontal, occipital, sphenoid, and ethmoid bones; the roof of the skull (cranium).

cranium The area of the head above the ears and eyes; the part of the skull that houses the brain.

cribriform plate A horizontal bone perforated with numerous openings for the passage of the olfactory nerve filaments from the nasal cavity.

cricoid cartilage A firm ridge of cartilage that forms the lower part of the larynx; the first ring of the trachea and the only upper airway structure that forms a complete ring; also called the cricoid ring.

cricothyroid membrane A thin sheet of fascia located between the thyroid and cricoid cartilage that is relatively avascular and contains few nerves; the site for emergency access to the airway.

cytoplasm The gellike material that fills out a cell and in which the organelles are suspended; it makes up most of the volume of the cell.

deep fascia A dense layer of fibrous tissue below the subcutaneous tissue; composed of tough bands of tissue that surround muscles and other internal structures.

dendrites Branchlike projections of nerve cells that receive impulses or sensory information from nearby cells and conduct impulses toward the nerve cell body.

deoxyribonucleic acid (DNA) Specialized structure within the cell that carries genetic material for reproduction.

depolarization In response to an action potential, the rapid movement of electrolytes across a cell membrane that changes the overall charge of the cell. This rapid shifting of electrolytes and cellular charges is the main catalyst for muscle contractions and neural transmissions.

dermatomes Areas of the skin supplied by specific sensory spinal nerves.

descending aorta The portion of the aorta that extends through the thorax and abdomen into the pelvis.

diapedesis A process whereby leukocytes move through the wall of a capillary and out to the tissues where they are needed most.

diaphragm Large skeletal muscle that plays a major role in breathing and separates the chest cavity from the abdominal cavity.

diaphysis The shaft of a long bone.

diastole Phase of the cardiac cycle in which the atria and ventricles relax between contractions and blood enters these chambers.

diencephalon Portion of the brain between the brainstem and cerebrum; contains the epithalamus, the thalamus, the hypothalamus, and the subthalamus.

differentiation The process of specialization of a cell.

diffusion The process of particles moving from an area of higher concentration to an area of lower concentration along a concentration gradient until equilibrium is achieved.

digestion The chemical breakdown of food material into smaller fragments that can be absorbed into the circulatory system.

diploid cells Cells that carry two of each of the 23 chromosomes—one from the father and one from the mother.

dorsal respiratory group (DRG) The portion of the medulla oblongata that functions as a respiratory integration center; it receives input from several sources including the pontine respiratory group, the glossopharyngeal and vagus nerves, central chemoreceptors in the medulla, and peripheral chemoreceptors.

Prep Kit continued

dura mater The outermost of the three meninges that enclose the brain and spinal cord; the toughest meningeal layer.

electrolytes Salt or acid substances that become ionic conductors when dissolved in a solvent (such as water); chemicals dissolved in the blood.

endocardium The thin membrane lining the inside of the heart.

endocrine glands Glands that have no ducts and secrete directly into tissue fluid or blood.

endocrine system The complex message and control system that integrates many body functions, including the release of hormones.

endolymph A fluid containing nerve receptors that resides inside the membranous labyrinth. Sound waves converted into pressure waves are transmitted through this fluid to the auditory nerves.

enteric nervous system (ENS) The subdivision of the autonomic nervous system that controls the digestive system.

enzymes Substances designed to speed up the rate of specific biochemical reactions.

eosinophils Leukocytes that may play a role following infection in various areas in the body.

epicardium The layer of the serous pericardium that lies closely against the heart; also called the visceral pericardium.

epiglottis A thin, flaplike structure that allows air to pass into the trachea but prevents food and liquid from entering it.

epinephrine A hormone produced by the adrenal medulla that has a vital role in the function of the sympathetic division of the autonomic nervous system; mediates the fight-or-flight response; also called adrenaline.

epiphyseal plate The growth plate of a long bone; a major site of bone development during childhood; also called the physis.

epithelial tissues Body tissues that cover organs, form the inner lining of cavities, and line hollow organs.

estrogen Hormone released from the ovaries that stimulates the uterine lining during the menstrual cycle.

eustachian tube A branch of the internal auditory canal that connects the middle ear to the oropharynx.

excitability The ability of cardiac muscle cells to respond to an electrical, chemical, or mechanical stimulus.

exhalation The passive part of the breathing process in which the diaphragm and the intercostal muscles relax, forcing air out of the lungs.

exocrine glands Glands that secrete chemicals into ducts that open onto a surface for elimination.

expiratory reserve volume The amount of air that can be exhaled following a normal exhalation; average volume is about 1,200 mL.

extracellular fluid (ECF) Fluid outside of the cell, which contains most of the body's supply of sodium; accounts for 15% to 20% of body weight.

extrinsic muscles In the eye, these are the six muscles that attach to the exterior of the globe and are controlled by the cranial nerves.

fascia A sheet or band of tough fibrous connective tissue that covers, supports, and separates muscles, and that also covers arteries, veins, tendons, and ligaments.

fibrin A white, insoluble protein formed by the action of thrombin on fibrinogen during the blood clotting process; forms the matrix of a blood clot.

fibrinogen A plasma protein that is important for blood clotting.

fibrous joints Joints that lie between bones that closely contact each other, and are joined by thin, dense connective tissue.

filtration The movement of fluid from intravascular fluid under high pressure to interstitial fluid, which is generally under lower pressure.

fluid balance The process of maintaining homeostasis through equal intake (water taken into

Prep Kit continued

the body) and output (water excreted from the body) of fluids.

fontanelles The soft spots in the skull of a newborn and infant where the sutures of the skull have not yet grown together.

fraction of inspired oxygen (FIO_2) The percentage of oxygen in inhaled air.

gag reflex A normal neural reflex elicited by touching the soft palate or posterior pharynx; it leads to symmetric elevation of the palate, retraction of the tongue, and contraction of the pharyngeal muscles.

general senses Sensations monitored throughout the body by receptors scattered throughout many different tissues.

genotype The arrangement of a person's genes and their characteristics is based on the combination of alleles, for one gene or many.

glaucoma A disease of the eye caused by an increase in intraocular pressure; when severe enough, it may damage the optic nerve and potentially cause permanent loss of vision.

globulins Antibodies made by the liver or lymphatic tissues that represent approximately 36% of the plasma proteins.

glottis The true vocal cords and the opening between them.

gluconeogenesis A process that stimulates both the liver and the kidneys to produce glucose from noncarbohydrate molecules.

glycogen A long polymer from which glucose is converted in the liver (animal starch).

glycogenolysis The breakdown of glycogen to glucose.

glycolysis Process by which glucose and other sugars are broken down to yield lactic acid (anaerobic glycolysis) or pyruvic acid (aerobic glycolysis). The breakdown releases energy in the form of adenosine triphosphate.

haploid cells Cells that carry genetic instructions via 23 individual chromosomes.

hard palate The anterior portion of the palate that is supported by bone (primarily the maxillary bone).

hematocrit A measure of the relative percentage of blood cells (mainly erythrocytes) in a given volume of whole blood.

hematopoietic system The blood components and the organs involved in their development and production.

hemoglobin An iron-containing pigment found in red blood cells that carries oxygen to the cells from the lungs and carbon dioxide away from the cells to the lungs.

hemostasis The stoppage of bleeding; it involves the steps of blood vessel spasm, platelet plug formation, and blood clotting.

Henry's law A gas law that states that the amount of a gas in a solution varies directly with the partial pressure of a gas over a solution.

hepatic portal system A specialized part of the venous system that carries blood from the digestive tract to the liver and then to the inferior vena cava.

Hering-Breuer reflex A protective mechanism that terminates inhalation, thereby preventing overexpansion of the lungs.

histamine A substance found in large amounts in basophils that increases tissue inflammation.

homeostasis A tendency toward constancy or stability in the body's internal environment; processes that balance the supply and demand of the body's needs.

homologous chromosome A chromosome of the same numbered pair from the opposite parent.

hormones Substances that are produced in one tissue or organ and are released into the blood and carried to other (target) organs, where they act to produce a specific response.

hydrostatic pressure The pressure of water against the walls of its container.

hyoid bone A small, horseshoe-shaped bone to which the jaw, tongue, epiglottis, and thyroid cartilage attach.

Prep Kit continued

hyperopia Farsighted; the ability to see distant objects, combined with difficulty focusing on objects close.

hypertonic Concentration of solute is higher compared with another solution.

hypothalamus An area of the diencephalon that is the primary link between the endocrine system and the nervous system; responsible for control of many body functions, including heart rate, digestion, sexual development, temperature regulation, emotion, hunger, thirst, and regulation of the sleep cycle.

hypotonic Concentration of solute is lower compared with another solution.

hypoxic drive A situation in which a person's stimulus to breathe comes from a decrease in Pao_2 rather than the normal stimulus, an increase in $Paco_2$.

immunity The body's ability to protect itself from acquiring a disease.

inhalation The active process of moving air into the lungs; also called inspiration; also a route of medication delivery.

inotropic effect The effect on the contractility of muscle tissue, especially cardiac muscle.

insertion A movable part of the body to which a skeletal muscle is fastened at a movable joint; its action opposes that at the origin.

inspiratory reserve volume The additional amount of air that can be inhaled after the normal tidal volume has been reached.

integumentary system The largest organ system in the body, consisting of the skin and accessory structures (eg, hair, nails, glands).

interstitial fluid The fluid located outside of the blood vessels in the spaces between the body's cells.

interstitial space The space in between the cells.

intracellular fluid (ICF) Fluid within cells in which most of the body's supply of potassium is contained; accounts for 40% to 45% of body weight.

intravascular fluid Fluid outside cells but inside the circulatory system; the majority of it consists of plasma, the fluid component of blood.

ionic bond A chemical bond in which oppositely charged ions attract each other.

ions Atoms that have become positively or negatively charged, by either giving up or acquiring an electron.

islets of Langerhans Groups of cells located in the pancreas that produce insulin, glucagon, somatostatin, and pancreatic polypeptide.

isotonic solution A solution containing an equal concentration of solutes and water on either side of a semipermeable membrane. In this case, water does not shift across the membrane, and no change in cell shape occurs.

joint capsule A saclike envelope that encloses the cavity of a synovial joint.

kilocalorie The amount of energy that can be obtained from the nutrients taken in through the diet; typically referred to simply as a calorie in the nutritional setting.

labia majora Two prominent, rounded folds of skin lateral to the labia minora of the female external genitalia.

labia minora A pair of skin folds in the female external genitalia that border the vestibule.

lacrimal glands The glands that produce fluids to keep the eye moist; also called tear glands.

lactic acid A metabolic end product of the breakdown of glucose that accumulates when metabolism proceeds in the absence of oxygen.

larynx A complete structure formed by the epiglottis, thyroid cartilage, cricoid cartilage, arytenoid cartilage, corniculate cartilage, and cuneiform cartilage; also called the voice box.

left anterior descending artery One of the two branches of the left main coronary artery that supplies blood to the left ventricle and other areas of the heart.

lens The transparent disc within the eye that refracts light to focus images on the retina.

Prep Kit continued

lipids Fats, fatlike substances (cholesterol and phospholipids), and oils that supply energy for body processes and building of certain structures.

lymph A thin liquid formed from interstitial fluid that flows through the lymphatic vessels and lymph nodes; it aids in immune response and debris removal.

lymph nodes Round or bean-shaped structures interspersed along the course of the lymph vessels, which filter the lymph and serve as a source of lymphocytes.

lymph vessels Unidirectional, thin-walled vessels through which lymph circulates in the body; they travel close to the major veins.

lymphatic system A network of capillaries, vessels, ducts, nodes, and organs that helps to maintain the body's fluid environment by producing lymph and transporting it through the body.

lymphocytes White blood cells that have an important role in immunity.

macrophages Large cells, usually derived from monocytes, that are specialized for phagocytosis; they kill pathogens, absorb foreign materials, and slow infections and infectious agents.

macula A yellow depression in the retina where acute vision arises; also known as the macula lutea.

mast cells Cells located in connective tissues to which antibodies, formed in response to allergens, attach; the cells burst and release chemical mediators in response to an antigen-antibody reaction.

mediastinum The space between the lungs, in the center of the chest, that contains the heart, great vessels, part of the esophagus, lymphatic channels, trachea, primary bronchi, and paired vagus and phrenic nerves.

medulla oblongata Inferior part of the brainstem that is continuous inferiorly with the spinal cord; serves as a conduction pathway for the ascending and descending nerve tracts; responsible for maintenance of basic life functions, such as heart rate and breathing.

meiosis A type of cell division that occurs in the production of eggs and sperm.

melanin The pigment that gives skin its color.

menarche The first menstrual cycle; the onset of menses.

meninges A set of three tough membranes—the dura mater, arachnoid, and pia mater—that enclose the entire brain and spinal cord.

menopause The period during which a woman's reproductive cycle ceases; also called the female climacteric.

menstruation Cyclical shedding of the endometrial lining.

metacarpals The five bones that form the palm and back of the hand.

midbrain The most superior portion of the brainstem; it works with the pons to route information from higher within the brain to the spinal cord, and vice versa.

mineral An inorganic element essential for human metabolism.

minute volume The amount of air that moves in and out of the lungs per minute minus the dead space; also called minute ventilation.

mitosis The division of chromosomes in a cell nucleus.

mitral valve The atrioventricular valve in the heart, which separates the left atrium from the left ventricle.

monocytes White blood cells that mature in the blood and then travel to the tissues, where they differentiate into macrophages; function primarily as scavengers for the tissues.

monosaccharides The simplest carbohydrate molecules.

motor nerve Nerve that carries information from the central nervous system to the muscles of the body.

Prep Kit continued

motor neurons Nerve cells that transmit instructions from the central nervous system to end organs; also known as efferent neurons.

mucous membrane The lining of body cavities and passages that communicates directly or indirectly with the environment outside the body.

mucus The opaque, sticky secretion of mucous membranes that lubricates the body openings.

murmur An abnormal heart sound, heard as a "whooshing," indicating turbulent blood flow within the heart.

muscle tissue Contractile tissue consisting of filaments of actin and myosin, which slide past each other, shortening cells.

musculoskeletal The bones and voluntary muscles of the body.

myocardium The middle, thickest layer of the heart; it contains the cardiac muscle fibers that cause contraction of the heart, as well as the conduction system and blood supply.

myoglobin A pigment synthesized in the muscles that gives skeletal muscles their red-brown color.

myopia Nearsighted; the ability to see objects nearby combined with difficulty seeing objects far away.

myosin A contractile protein found in the thick filaments of skeletal muscle cells.

nasopharynx The part of the pharynx that lies above the level of the palate.

negative feedback The concept that once the desired effect of a process has been achieved, further action is inhibited until it is needed again; also called feedback inhibition.

negative-pressure ventilation Drawing of air into the lungs; airflow from a region of higher pressure (outside the body) to a region of lower pressure (the lungs); occurs during normal breathing.

neoplasm A mass of tissue produced by abnormal cell growth and division that may be malignant (cancerous) or benign.

nephrons The functional (urine-producing) units of the kidneys.

nervous system The system that controls virtually all activities of the body, both voluntary and involuntary.

nervous tissues Tissues composed of neurons and neuroglia.

neuroglia Supporting cells that provide a supporting skeleton for neural tissues, isolate and protect the cell membranes of neurons, regulate the composition of interstitial fluid, defend neural tissues from pathogens, and aid in the repair of injury.

neuromuscular junction The connection between a motor neuron and a muscle fiber.

neurons The basic nerve cells of the nervous system, which contain a nucleus within a cell body and one or more processes extending from the cell body; masses of these cells form nervous tissue.

neurotransmitters Chemicals released from one nerve that crosses the synaptic cleft to reach a receptor.

neutrophils One of the three types of granulocytes; these cells have multilobed nuclei that resemble a string of baseballs held together by a thin strand of thread; they destroy bacteria, antigen-antibody complexes, and foreign matter.

norepinephrine A naturally occurring catecholamine that functions as a neurotransmitter and adrenal hormone; it is synthesized by the adrenal medulla, the peripheral sympathetic nerves, and the central nervous system, and produces vasoconstriction through its alpha-stimulator properties. It is also available as a drug that is sometimes used in the treatment of severe hypotension.

nucleic acids Large organic molecules, or macromolecules, that carry genetic information or form structures within cells; they include deoxyribonucleic acid and ribonucleic acid.

nucleus In the context of the cell, a cellular organelle that contains the genetic information; it controls the function and structure of a cell.

Prep Kit continued

In the context of an atom, the central portion of an atom that contains protons and neutrons.

nutrients Substances that provide nourishment for growth such as carbohydrates, lipids, proteins, vitamins, minerals, and water.

oligosaccharides Simple sugars composed of 2 to 10 monosaccharides.

oncotic pressure The pressure of water to move, typically into the capillary, as the result of the presence of plasma proteins.

oocytes Immature female sex cells produced in the ovary that may develop by meiosis into ova (eggs).

oogenesis The process of egg cell formation, which begins at puberty.

optic chiasm Location where approximately one-half of the nerve fibers from each eye cross over to the opposite side of the brain.

orbits Eye sockets of the skull.

organ of Corti The organ that is the primary receptor for sound; made up of thousands of individual cilia, each with its own associated nerve.

organelles Structures within cells that have specialized functions.

origin A relatively immovable part of the body where a skeletal muscle is fastened at a movable joint; its action opposes that of an insertion.

oropharynx A tubular structure that extends vertically from the back of the mouth to the esophagus and trachea.

osmosis The movement of a solvent, such as water, from an area of low solute concentration to one of high concentration through a selectively permeable membrane to equalize concentrations of a solute on both sides of the membrane.

osmotic pressure The pressure exerted by the concentration of the solutes in a given space to stop the flow of solvent across a semipermeable membrane.

ossification The formation of bone by osteoblasts.

osteoblasts Cells involved in the formation of bony tissue.

osteoclasts Macrophages of the bone surface that dissolve the matrix and return minerals to the extracellular fluid.

osteocytes Mature bone cells.

otoliths A pair of fluid-filled sacs within the inner ear that are used by the central nervous system to collect information about movement and orientation in space.

oval window The opening between the stapes and inner ear.

ovaries Female glands that produce sex hormones and ova (eggs).

ovulation Midcycle release of an ovum during the menstrual cycle.

oxygenation The process of loading oxygen molecules onto hemoglobin molecules in the bloodstream.

oxyhemoglobin Hemoglobin to which oxygen molecules are bound.

palate The roof of the nasal cavity; separates the nasal cavity from the oral cavity.

pancreas An organ with both endocrine and exocrine functions; it is a major source of digestive enzymes and produces the hormone insulin.

papillary muscles Muscles attached to the chordae tendineae of the atrioventricular heart valves and the ventricular muscle of the heart.

paranasal sinuses The sinuses, or hollowed sections of bone in the front of the head, which are lined with mucous membrane and drain into the nasal cavity; the frontal, ethmoid, sphenoid, and maxillary sinuses.

parathyroid glands Four glands that are embedded in the posterior portion of each lobe of the thyroid; they produce and secrete parathyroid hormone.

parathyroid hormone (PTH) Hormone produced and secreted by the parathyroid glands; it maintains normal levels of calcium in the blood and supports normal neuromuscular function.

Prep Kit continued

parietal pleura The lining of the pleural cavity, which is attached tightly to the interior of the chest cage.

partial pressure The pressure exerted by an individual gas in a mixture.

pelvis The attachment of the lower extremities to the body, consisting of the sacrum and two pelvic bones.

penis The cylindrical male sex organ; it conveys urine and semen through the urethra.

peptides Protein molecules consisting of amino acids held together by peptide bonds.

perception Becoming aware of or understanding something using the senses.

perfusion The circulation of oxygenated blood within an organ or tissue in adequate amounts to meet the cells' current needs.

pericardium In the heart, a thin, double-layered membrane made up of the fibrous pericardium and serous pericardium.

perilymph Fluid within the bony labyrinth that surrounds and protects the membranous labyrinth while allowing transmission of pressure waves caused by sound.

peripheral nervous system (PNS) The part of the nervous system that consists of 31 pairs of spinal nerves and 12 pairs of cranial nerves, which are responsible for communication between the central nervous system and the rest of the body. It includes sensory nerves, motor nerves, and connecting nerves.

peristalsis The wavelike contraction of smooth muscle by which the ureters or other tubular organs propel their contents along their length.

peritoneum The double-layered serous membrane that lines the abdominal cavity and covers the organs located in the abdominopelvic cavity.

pH A measure of the acidity or alkalinity of a solution.

phagocytosis A form of endocytosis in which a cell surrounds a foreign particle and engulfs it.

phantom pain A sensation of pain in a part of the body that is no longer present.

pharynx The area between the nasal cavity and the larynx, located posterior to the oral cavity; the throat.

phenotype The appearance, health condition, or other characteristics associated with a particular genotype.

phospholipids Lipid molecules that make up the cell membrane.

physiology The study of the processes and functions of the living organism.

pia mater The innermost of the three meninges that enclose the brain and spinal cord; it rests directly on the brain and spinal cord.

pineal gland A gland in the brain that synthesizes and secretes melatonin, a hormone that affects patterns of sleep and wakefulness.

pinna The external ear; the cartilage formation that protects the ear and collects sounds into the ear canal, while allowing some perception of the direction from which the sound comes; also called the auricle.

pinocytosis A form of endocytosis in which the cell membrane sinks inward and ingests droplets of extracellular fluid.

pituitary gland An endocrine gland responsible for directly or indirectly affecting all body functions; also called the hypophysis.

plasma A watery, yellow fluid that carries the blood cells and nutrients and transports cellular waste material to the organs of excretion.

plasma cells Cells that produce antibodies (immunoglobulins) to destroy antigens or antigen-containing particles; formed from divided and differentiated B cells.

plasmin A naturally occurring enzyme that dissolves the fibrin fibers in blood clots; usually present in the body in its inactive form, plasminogen.

platelets Formed elements of the blood that function in blood clotting; also called thrombocytes.

Prep Kit continued

pleura The serous membranes covering the lungs and lining the thoracic cavity.

pleural space The potential space between the parietal pleura and the visceral pleura.

plexuses Clusters of nerve roots that permit peripheral nerve roots to rejoin and function as a group.

polarized A condition in which active transport of ions into and out of the resting cell creates an electrochemical gradient across the cell membrane.

polypeptide A peptide formed from many amino acids bound into a chain. When it has more than 100 molecules, it is considered to be a protein.

polysaccharides Complex carbohydrates that contain many simple joined sugar units, such as plant starch. Some, such as cellulose, cannot be broken down for nutrition in humans but play important roles in digestion.

pons Area of the brainstem that contains the sleep and respiratory centers for the body and that, along with the medulla, controls breathing.

pontine respiratory group (PRG) A portion of the pons that communicates information to both the ventral and dorsal respiratory groups; it is thought to smooth the transition between each phase of the ventilatory cycle and alter breathing by making each breath shorter and shallower or longer and deeper, depending on the body's needs.

precapillary sphincter Smooth muscle located at the entrance to a capillary; responsive to local tissue needs.

preload The volume of blood in the ventricle at the end of diastole; it is primarily a reflection of venous return (the blood returned to the heart).

presbyopia The increased difficulty in focusing on objects that occurs with aging.

progesterone A female hormone released from the ovaries that promotes changes in the uterus during the reproductive cycle, affects the mammary glands, and helps regulate gonadotropin secretion.

proprioception The awareness of motion and position of a body part.

prostaglandins Lipids made from arachidonic acid that usually act more locally than hormones, are very potent, stimulate hormone secretions, and help to regulate blood pressure.

proteins Large peptides created from amino acids; they include enzymes, plasma proteins, muscle components (actin and myosin), hormones, and antibodies.

prothrombin A protein made in the liver and released into the blood, where it is converted into thrombin during the process of blood clotting.

pulmonary artery One of two arteries that carry deoxygenated blood from the right ventricle to the lungs.

pulmonary circulation The flow of blood from the right ventricle through the pulmonary arteries and all of their branches and capillaries in the lungs, and back to the left atrium through the venules and pulmonary veins; also called the lesser circulation.

pulmonary veins The four veins that return oxygenated blood from the lungs to the left atrium of the heart.

pulmonic valve The semilunar valve that regulates blood flow between the right ventricle and the pulmonary artery; also called the pulmonary semilunar valve.

pulse pressure The difference between the systolic and diastolic blood pressures.

Purkinje fibers A system of fibers in the ventricles that conducts the excitation impulse from the bundle branches to the myocardium.

referred pain Pain that feels as if it is originating from a body part other than the site being stimulated.

reflex arc A sensory message that reaches the spinal cord and meets with a motor nerve to cause an action; the reflex action occurs without the message first having to reach the brain to voluntarily cause the action.

Prep Kit continued

refracting system A series of transparent structures within the eye that redirect light as it passes through media of different densities.

renal corpuscle The initial blood-filtering component of the nephron.

renal cortex The outer portion of each kidney; it forms renal columns and has tiny tubules associated with the nephrons.

renal medulla The inner portion of each kidney; it is made of conical renal pyramids, and has striations.

renal pelvis A cone-shaped collecting area that connects the ureter and the kidney.

renal tubules Portions of the nephron containing the tubular fluid that has been filtered through the glomerulus.

renin A hormone produced by cells in the juxtaglomerular apparatus when the blood pressure is low.

repolarization The process by which ions move across the cell membrane to return the cell to a polarized state.

reproductive system The system in males and females that controls the reproductive processes via organs and glands that create sex cells and transport them to areas where fertilization can occur.

residual volume The amount of air remaining in the lungs and airway passages that is unable to be expelled after a maximal forced exhalation.

respiration The exchange of gases between a living organism and its environment.

respiratory membrane The site where gas exchange takes place; at this point of contact, oxygen is picked up in the bloodstream and carbon dioxide is eliminated through the lungs.

respiratory system All the structures of the body that contribute to the process of breathing, consisting of the upper and lower airways and their component parts.

reticular activating system (RAS) Group of specialized neurons in the brainstem; involved in sleep-wake cycles; maintains consciousness.

retina The inner layer of the eye wall, including the visual receptors.

Rh factor An antigen found on the red blood cells of most people; when a woman without this protein is impregnated by a man with this protein, the woman's body can create antibodies against the protein that then attack future pregnancies.

right coronary artery Blood vessel that provides oxygenated blood to the right side of the heart muscle.

rods One of two types of photoreceptors of the retina that are sensitive to light, but do not discriminate colors; they produce a picture that is somewhat less focused and essentially black and white.

sacroiliac joints The points of attachment of the ilium to the sacrum.

saddle joint Two saddle-shaped articulating surfaces oriented at right angles to each other so that complementary surfaces articulate with each other; an example is found in the thumb.

Schwann cells Neuroglial cells in the peripheral nervous system that form a myelin sheath around axons.

sclera The white, fibrous outer layer of the eyeball.

scrotum A pouch of skin and subcutaneous tissue hanging from the lower abdominal region, posterior to the penis.

sebaceous glands Glands that produce an oily substance called sebum, which is discharged along the shafts of the hairs.

semilunar (SL) valves The aortic and pulmonic valves, which are shaped like half-moons and separate the heart from the aorta and pulmonary arteries.

semipermeable Property of the cell membrane that describes the ability to allow certain elements to pass through while blocking the passage of others.

sensory nerves The nerves that carry sensations of touch, taste, heat, cold, pain, and other

Prep Kit continued

modalities from the body to the central nervous system.

sensory receptors Structures located in the dermis that initiate nerve impulses that can reach the individual's conscious awareness.

sex chromosomes The X and Y chromosomes, which determine sex.

sinoatrial (SA) node The normal site of the origin of electrical impulses; located high in the right atrium, it is the natural pacemaker of the heart.

sinuses Cavities formed by the cranial bones that trap contaminants from entering the respiratory tract and act as tributaries for fluid to and from the eustachian tubes and tear ducts.

skeletal muscle tissue Voluntary muscle tissue attached to bones and composed of long, threadlike cells that have light and dark striations.

sliding filament theory An explanation of the action of muscle contraction focusing on how sarcomeres shorten, with thick and thin filaments sliding past each other toward the center of the sarcomere from both ends.

sodium-potassium pump The mechanism by which the cell brings in two potassium ions and releases three sodium ions.

soft palate The posterior portion of the palate, which is made up of mucous membrane, muscular fibers, and mucous glands; it is so named because it has no bony support.

solute The dissolved particles contained in a solvent.

solution A mixture of a solvent and a solute.

solvent The fluid that dissolves a solute, or the substance in which a solute is dissolved or mixed.

somatic nervous system The part of the nervous system that regulates activities over which there is voluntary control.

somatic pain Pain caused by the activation of pain receptors in the body's superficial tissues, such as the skin, bones, muscles, and joints; compared to visceral pain, it is generally more intense and more precisely localized.

spermatogenesis The process by which sperm cells are formed.

sphincters Muscles arranged in circles that are able to decrease the diameter of tubes. Examples are found within the rectum, bladder, and blood vessels.

spinal nerves The 31 pairs of nerves that originate from the spinal cord and exit the spine on either side between vertebrae; each has a sensory root and a motor root, and is responsible for sending and receiving sensory and motor messages to and from the central nervous system from a portion of the body.

stem cells Cells that retain the ability to divide repeatedly without specializing, and that allow for continual growth and renewal.

strabismus Loss of perception of depth and overlapping or doubled images.

stratum corneum The outermost or dead layer of the skin.

stroke volume (SV) The volume of blood pumped forward with each ventricular contraction.

subarachnoid space The space located between the pia mater and the arachnoid membrane.

suprasternal notch The indentation formed by the superior border of the manubrium and the clavicles, which is often used as a landmark for procedures such as subclavian vein access; also known as the jugular notch.

surfactant A liquid protein substance that coats the alveoli in the lungs, decreases alveolar surface tension, and keeps the alveoli expanded; a low level in a premature infant contributes to respiratory distress syndrome.

sutures Seams that occur only between the bones of the skull; they are a type of fibrous joint.

sweat glands The glands that secrete sweat, which are located in the dermal layer of the skin.

synapse A functional connection where neurons communicate with other cells.

synaptic cleft The space between neurons; also called the synaptic gap.

Prep Kit continued

synaptic vesicles Small sacs that contain neurotransmitters.

synovial fluid The fluid secreted by synovial membranes that lubricates synovial joints.

synovial joints Complex joints that allow free movement of the component bones and are lubricated with synovial fluid.

synovial membrane The lining of a joint that secretes synovial fluid into the joint space.

systemic vascular resistance The resistance that blood must overcome to be able to move within the blood vessels; related to the amount of dilation or constriction in the blood vessel.

T lymphocytes Lymphocytes that interact directly with antigens, producing the cellular immune response; they also stimulate the B lymphocytes to produce antibodies; also called T cells.

tentorium A horizontal projection of the dura that separates the cerebellum from the cerebrum.

testosterone The most important male sex hormone (androgen).

thalamus Structure of the diencephalon that acts as the sensory switchboard of the brain, through which almost all signals travel on their way in or out of the brain.

thermoregulation The process by which the body maintains temperature through a combination of heat gain by metabolic processes and muscular movement and heat loss through breathing, evaporation, conduction, convection, and perspiration.

thoracic duct One of two great lymph vessels; it empties into the superior vena cava.

thrombin An enzyme that causes the conversion of fibrinogen to fibrin, which binds to a platelet plug, forming a final mature clot.

thromboplastin A chemical that stimulates blood clotting.

thymus A lymphatic organ located in the thorax that is important in early immunity; it shrinks with age and is eventually replaced by other types of tissue.

thyroid cartilage A firm prominence of cartilage that forms the upper part of the larynx; the Adam's apple.

thyroid gland A large endocrine gland located at the base of the neck; it produces and excretes hormones that influence growth, development, and metabolism.

tidal volume The amount of air moved in and out of the lungs in one relaxed breath; approximately 500 mL for an adult.

tissues Groups of cells that share a similar structure and function.

titin A noncontractile protein found in sarcomeres of cardiac and skeletal muscle.

total body water (TBW) Total amount of fluid in the human body; accounts for approximately 60% of the weight of a healthy adult male; divided into various compartments within the body.

transcellular fluid Fluid classified as extracellular, but which is formed from the transport activities of cells. Examples include cerebrospinal fluid, bladder urine, aqueous humor, and synovial fluid of the joints.

tricuspid valve The atrioventricular valve that separates the right atrium from the right ventricle.

tropomyosin An actin-binding protein that regulates muscle contraction and other actin-related mechanical functions of the body.

troponin A regulatory protein in the actin filaments of skeletal and cardiac muscle that attaches to tropomyosin.

tubular reabsorption The process that moves substances from the tubular fluid into the blood, within the peritubular capillary.

tubular secretion The process that moves substances from the blood in the peritubular capillary into the renal tubule.

tunica adventitia The outer layer of tissue of a blood vessel wall, composed of elastic and fibrous connective tissue.

Prep Kit continued

tunica intima The smooth, thin, inner lining of a blood vessel.

tunica media The middle, thickest layer of tissue of a blood vessel wall, composed of elastic tissue and smooth muscle cells that allow the vessel to expand or contract in response to changes in blood pressure and tissue demand.

ureters Small, hollow tubes that carry urine from the kidneys to the bladder.

urethra The canal that conveys urine from the bladder to outside the body.

urinary bladder A sac behind the pubic symphysis made of smooth muscle that collects and stores urine.

urinary system The organs that control the discharge of certain waste materials filtered from the blood and excreted as urine.

uterus A muscular, inverted pear-shaped organ that lies situated between the urinary bladder and the rectum.

ventilation The mechanical process of moving air into and out of the lungs in two separate phases: inhalation (inspiration) and exhalation (expiration).

ventral respiratory group (VRG) An area of the medulla oblongata that can cause inspiration or expiration depending on which motor neurons are stimulated.

vestibule The structure into which the vagina opens posteriorly, and into which the female urethra opens in the midline; also, the central part of the labyrinth of the ear, behind the cochlea and in front of the semicircular canals.

visceral pain Deep pain caused by activation of pain receptors in internal areas of the body that are enclosed within a cavity, such as the chest, abdomen, or pelvis.

visceral pleura The lining of the pleural cavity, which adheres tightly to the surface of the lung.

vital capacity The amount of air moved in and out of the lungs with maximum inspiration and exhalation.

vitamins Organic compounds required for normal metabolism.

vitreous humor A jellylike fluid filling the posterior eye cavity that helps the globe maintain its shape without distorting light.

white matter Bundles of myelinated nerves.

References

1. Online Entymology Dictionary. © 2001-2006 Douglas Harper. https://www.etymonline.com/word/organism#etymonline_v_7141. Accessed April 16, 2021.
2. Moini J. Cells. In: *Anatomy and Physiology for Health Professionals*. 2nd ed. Burlington, MA: Jones & Bartlett Learning; 2016:45-66.
3. Patton KT, Thibodeau GA. Cell structure. In: *Anatomy & Physiology*. 10th ed. St. Louis, MO: Elsevier; 2019:75-97.
4. Hall JE, Hall ME. Functional organization of the human body and control of the "internal environment." In: Hall JE, ed. *Guyton and Hall Textbook of Medical Physiology*. 14th ed. Philadelphia, PA: Elsevier; 2021:3-10.
5. Aronson PS, Boron WF, Boulpaep, EL. Transport of solutes and water. In: Boron WF, Boulpaep EL, eds. *Medical Physiology: A Cellular and Molecular Approach*. 3rd ed. Philadelphia, PA: Elsevier; 2017:102-140.
6. Darby SA. General anatomy of the spinal cord. In: Cramer GD, Darby SA, eds. *Clinical Anatomy of the Spine, Spinal Cord, and ANS*. 3rd ed. St. Louis, MO: Mosby; 2014;65-97.
7. Cramer GD. General characteristics of the spine. In: Cramer GD, Darby SA, eds. *Clinical Anatomy of the Spine, Spinal Cord, and ANS*. 3rd ed. St. Louis, MO: Mosby; 2014;15-64.
8. Hunter SK, Senefeld JW, Neumann DA. Muscle: The primary stabilizer and mover of the skeletal system. In: *Kinesiology of the Musculoskeletal System: Foundations for Rehabilitation*. 3rd ed. St. Louis, MO: Elsevier; 2017:48-76.
9. Moini J. Control and coordination. In: *Anatomy and Physiology for Health Professionals*. 2nd ed. Burlington, MA: Jones & Bartlett Learning; 2016:223-346.
10. Patton KT, Thibodeau GA. Nervous system cells. In: *Anthony's Textbook of Anatomy & Physiology*. 21st ed. St. Louis, MO: Elsevier; 2019:389-407.
11. Jenkins DB. The back. In: *Hollinshead's Functional Anatomy of the Limbs and Back*. 9th ed. St. Louis, MO: Saunders; 2009:204-237.
12. Vanderah TW, Gould DJ. Meningeal coverings of the brain and spinal cord. In: *Nolte's The Human Brain: An*

Prep Kit continued

Introduction to Its Functional Anatomy. 7th ed. Philadelphia, PA: Elsevier; 2016:84-102.

13. Ransom BR. The neuronal microenvironment. In: Boron WF, Boulpaep EL, eds. *Medical Physiology: A Cellular and Molecular Approach.* 3rd ed. Philadelphia, PA: Elsevier; 2017:275-294.
14. Rubinson K, Lang EJ. The nervous system. In: Koeppen BM; Stanton BA, eds. *Berne & Levy Physiology.* 7th ed. Philadelphia, PA: Elsevier; 2018:51-240.
15. Privitera MD, Zakaria T, Khatri R. Nervous system. In: Kaplan LA, Pesce AJ, eds. *Clinical Chemistry: Theory, Analysis, Correlation.* 5th ed. New York, NY: Mosby; 2009:904-928.
16. Braun K. The prefrontal-limbic system: development, neuroanatomy, function, and implications for socioemotional development. *Clin Perinatol.* 2011;38(4):685-702.
17. Ball JW, Dains JE, Flynn JA, et al. Neurologic system. In: Ball JW, Dains JE, Flynn JA, et al, eds. *Seidel's Guide to Physical Examination: An Interprofessional Approach.* 9th ed. St. Louis, MO: Elsevier; 2019:567-606.
18. Darby SA, Frysztak RJ. Neuroanatomy of the spinal cord. In: Cramer GD, Darby SA, eds. *Clinical Anatomy of the Spine, Spinal Cord, and ANS.* 3rd ed. St. Louis, MO: Mosby; 2014;341-412.
19. Brand RW, Isselhard DE. Nervous system. In: Brand RW, Isselhard DE, eds. *Anatomy of Orofacial Structures: A Comprehensive Approach.* 8th ed. St. Louis, MO: Elsevier; 2018:356-367.
20. Glick DB. The autonomic nervous system. In: Miller RD, Cohen NH, Eriksson LI, et al, eds. *Miller's Anesthesia.* 8th ed. Philadelphia, PA: Saunders; 2015:346-386.
21. Wecker L, Theobald RJ Jr. Introduction to the autonomic nervous system. In: Wecker L, Taylor DA, Theobald RJ Jr, eds. *Brody's Human Pharmacology: Mechanism-Based Therapeutics.* 6th ed. Philadelphia, PA: Mosby; 2019:54-63.
22. Bers DM, Borlaug BA, Hasenfuss G. Mechanisms of cardiac contraction and relaxation. In: Zipes DP, Libby P, Bonow RO, et al, eds. *Braunwald's Heart Disease: A Textbook of Cardiovascular Medicine.* 11th ed. Philadelphia, PA: Elsevier; 2019:418-440.
23. Furness JB, Callaghan BP, Rivera LR, Cho HJ. The enteric nervous system and gastrointestinal innervation: integrated local and central control. *Adv Exp Med Biol.* 2014;817:39-71.
24. Morrison SF. Regulation of body temperature. In: Boron WF, Boulpaep EL, eds. *Medical Physiology: A Cellular and Molecular Approach.* 3rd ed. Philadelphia, PA: Elsevier; 2017:1193-1203.
25. Connors BW. Sensory transduction. In: Boron WF, Boulpaep EL, eds. *Medical Physiology: A Cellular and Molecular Approach.* 3rd ed. Philadelphia, PA: Elsevier; 2017:353-389.
26. Rizzo DC. The nervous system: The brain, cranial nerves, autonomic nervous system, and the special senses. In: *Fundamentals of Anatomy and Physiology.* 4th ed. Boston, MA: Cengage Learning; 2016:250-277.
27. Page CP, Curtis MJ, Walker, MJ, Hoffman BB. Drugs and the eye. In: *Integrated Pharmacology*. 3rd ed. Philadelphia, PA: Mosby; 2006:545-562.
28. Cantley L. Signal transduction. In: Boron WF, Boulpaep EL, eds. *Medical Physiology: A Cellular and Molecular Approach.* 3rd ed. Philadelphia, PA: Elsevier; 2017:47-72.
29. Saladin KS. The circulatory system: blood. In: *Anatomy & Physiology: The Unity of Form and Function.* 7th ed. New York, NY: McGraw-Hill Education; 2015:672-707.
30. Boulpaep EL. Arteries and veins. In: Boron WF, Boulpaep EL, eds. *Medical Physiology: A Cellular and Molecular Approach.* 3rd ed. Philadelphia, PA: Elsevier; 2017:447-460.
31. Lohr NL, Benjamin IJ. Structure and function of the normal heart and blood vessels. In: Benjamin IJ, Griggs RC, Wing EJ, Fitz JG, eds. *Andreoli and Carpenter's Cecil Essentials of Medicine.* 9th ed. Philadelphia, PA: Saunders; 2016:16-21.
32. Pappano AJ. The cardiovascular system. In: Koeppen BM, Stanton BA, eds. *Berne & Levy Physiology.* 7th ed. Philadelphia, PA: Elsevier; 2018:300-432.
33. Hall JE, Hall ME. The microcirculation and lymphatic system. In: Hall JE, ed. *Guyton and Hall Textbook of Medical Physiology.* 14th ed. Philadelphia, PA: Elsevier; 2021:193-201.
34. Saladin KS. The respiratory system. In: *Anatomy & Physiology: The Unity of Form and Function.* 7th ed. New York, NY: McGraw-Hill Education; 2015:848-888.
35. Boron WF. Organization of the respiratory system. In: Boron WF, Boulpaep EL, eds. *Medical Physiology: A Cellular and Molecular Approach.* 3rd ed. Philadelphia, PA: Elsevier; 2017:590-605.
36. Cloutier MM, Thrall RS. The respiratory system. In: Koeppen BM, Stanton BA, eds. *Berne & Levy Physiology.* 7th ed. Philadelphia, PA: Elsevier; 2018:433-510.
37. Drake RL, Vogl AW, Mitchell AW. Thorax. In: *Gray's Basic Anatomy.* Philadelphia, PA: Churchill Livingstone; 2012:57-132.
38. Waugh A, Grant A. The respiratory system. In: *Ross and Wilson Anatomy and Physiology in Health and Illness.* 12th ed. Edinburgh, UK: Churchill Livingstone; 2014:242-273.
39. Brashers VL. Structure and function of the pulmonary system. In: McCance KL, Huether SE, Brashers VL, Rote NS, eds. *Pathophysiology: The Biologic Basis for Disease in Adults and Children* 8th ed. St. Louis, MO: Elsevier; 2019:1143-1162.
40. Spyer KM, Gourine AV. Chemosensory pathways in the brainstem controlling cardiorespiratory activity. *Philos Trans R Soc Lond B Biol Sci.* 2009;364(1529):2603-2610.

Prep Kit continued

41. Boron WF. Mechanics of ventilation. In: Boron WF, Boulpaep EL, eds. *Medical Physiology: A Cellular and Molecular Approach*. 3rd ed. Philadelphia, PA: Elsevier; 2017:606-627.
42. Corne S, Bshouty Z. Basic principles of control of breathing. *Respir Care Clin North Am*. 2005;11(2):147-172.
43. Binder HJ. Organization of the gastrointestinal system. In: Boron WF, Boulpaep EL, eds. *Medical Physiology: A Cellular and Molecular Approach*.3rd ed. Philadelphia, PA: Elsevier; 2017:852-862.
44. Saladin KS. The male reproductive system. In: *Anatomy & Physiology: The Unity of Form and Function*. 7th ed. New York, NY: McGraw-Hill Education; 2015:1028-1057.
45. Moini J. Reproductive system. In: *Anatomy and Physiology for Health Professionals*. 2nd ed. Burlington, MA: Jones & Bartlett Learning; 2016:553-584.
46. Roiger D, Bullock NJ. The male reproductive system. In: *Anatomy, Physiology, & Disease: Foundations for the Health Professions*. New York, NY: McGraw-Hill Education; 2014:592-621.

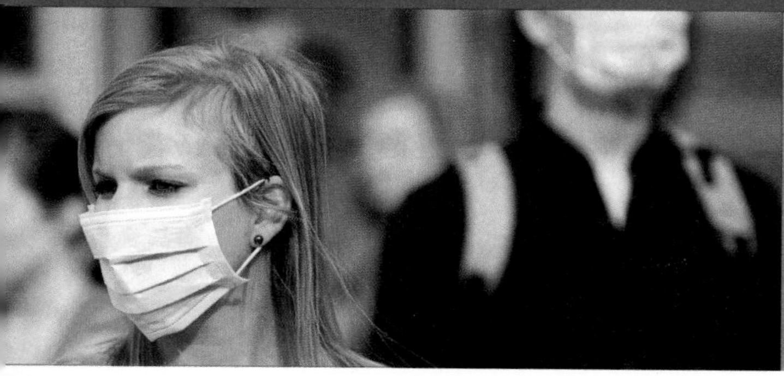

Chapter 9

Pathophysiology

NATIONAL EMS EDUCATION STANDARD COMPETENCIES

Pathophysiology

Integrates comprehensive knowledge of pathophysiology of major human systems.

KNOWLEDGE OBJECTIVES

1. Define pathophysiology, including its role in diagnosing and treating disease. (p 488)
2. Compare atrophy, hypertrophy, hyperplasia, dysplasia, and metaplasia as means of cellular adaptation. (p 488)
3. List factors that can affect or upset homeostasis. (pp 489–490)
4. Explain the causes, clinical manifestations, assessment, and management of edema. (pp 490–491)
5. Discuss types of fluid deficits and potential resulting complications. (p 491)
6. Explain the physiologic consequences of electrolyte imbalances in sodium, potassium, calcium, phosphate, and magnesium. (pp 491–494)
7. Compare respiratory acidosis, respiratory alkalosis, metabolic acidosis, and metabolic alkalosis. (pp 495–498)
8. Outline how cellular injury occurs in patients with hypoxia, chemical exposures, infection (sepsis), immunologic exposures (hypersensitivity reactions), inflammatory conditions, genetic disorders, nutritional imbalances, physical damage (mechanical injury), and other harmful exposures, such as extremes of hot and cold. (pp 498–503)
9. Explain the concept of apoptosis. (p 503)
10. Define perfusion, including the physiologic consequences of hypoperfusion. (pp 504–505)
11. Analyze the mechanisms by which the body compensates for hypoperfusion. (pp 504–505)
12. Discuss the causes of central and peripheral shock, including cardiogenic, obstructive, hypovolemic, and distributive shock. (pp 505–508)
13. Explain how to manage a patient in shock. (pp 508–509)
14. Describe multiple organ dysfunction syndrome. (pp 509–510)
15. Examine the body's three defense mechanisms against pathogens: anatomic barriers, the immune response, and the inflammatory response. (pp 510–523)
16. Explain how plasma protein systems—the complement system, the coagulation (clotting) system, and the kinin system—modulate the inflammatory response. (pp 519–520)
17. Compare wound healing by primary intention with wound healing by secondary intention. (pp 521–523)
18. Outline each of the four types of hypersensitivity reactions and mechanisms for immunologic injury. (pp 524–526)
19. List several autoimmune reactions. (pp 526–527)

20. Compare inherited and acquired immunodeficiencies. (pp 527–529)
21. Analyze the controllable and uncontrollable risk factors that intersect to cause disease. (pp 529–530)
22. Outline how incidence, prevalence, morbidity, and mortality data are used to analyze disease risk. (p 530)
23. Recognize autosomal dominant and autosomal recessive patterns of inheritance. (pp 530–532)
24. Analyze risk factors for cancer and cardiovascular disease. (pp 533–537)
25. Describe how hematologic disorders occur. (pp 534–535)
26. Name common renal, gastrointestinal, and neuromuscular disorders. (pp 537–540)
27. List the stages of the general adaptation syndrome and explore the relationship between stress and disease. (pp 541–544)

SKILLS OBJECTIVES

There are no skills objectives for this chapter.

Introduction

The human body is made up of cells, tissues, and organs, which collectively function in a constantly changing microenvironment. The study of the origin, growth, structure, behavior, and reproduction of living organisms is known as *biology*. **Pathophysiology** is the study of the physiology of altered functioning in the presence of disease. This term is derived from the Greek words *pathos*, meaning "suffering," and *physis*, meaning "form." When the structure and function in cells, tissues, and organs break down in response to stressors and the body can no longer maintain homeostasis, disease may result. Determining the origin of a disease process often helps paramedics choose the best approach to patient evaluation and initial treatment.

To understand disease processes, you must understand the ways disease alters the structure and function of cells. We begin this chapter by reviewing the changes that affect cells, disrupt the body's ability to maintain homeostasis, and lead to disease. Next, we consider how inflammation and shock influence the development of disease. We also discuss the role of immunity and defense mechanisms in protecting the human body from disease. We conclude with a discussion on the effects genetics and stress have in disease development.

Adaptations in Cells and Tissues

When exposed to adverse conditions, cells undergo a process of adaptation to guard against injury. In some situations, the cells change permanently; in others, the structure or function of the cells changes only temporarily.

Atrophy is a decrease in cell size due to a loss of subcellular components, which in turn leads to a decrease in the size of the tissue and organ. The actual number of cells remains unchanged. The decreased size represents an attempt to cope with a new steady state in the setting of less-than-favorable conditions or a lack of use. For example, the muscle mass of a casted, immobilized limb shrinks as a result of disuse atrophy.

Hypertrophy is an increase in the size of the cells due to synthesis of more subcellular components, which in turn leads to an increase in tissue and organ size. For example, the heart's left ventricle may hypertrophy due to chronic high resistance pressures from hypertension (elevated blood pressure [BP]).

Hyperplasia is an increase in the actual number of cells in an organ or tissue, usually resulting in an increase in the size of the organ or tissue. For example, a callus represents hyperplasia of the keratinized layer of the epidermis of the foot in response to increased friction or trauma.

Dysplasia is an alteration of the size, shape, and organization of cells. It is most often found in epithelial cells with irregular, atypical changes in response to chronic irritation or inflammation. For example, the development of cervical dysplasia in women is strongly associated with exposure to specific human papillomaviruses.

Metaplasia refers to the reversible cellular adaptation in which one adult cell type is replaced by another adult cell type. For example, in squamous metaplasia, the ciliated epithelium in the airways of smokers may be replaced by metaplastic epithelium.

Disturbances in Fluid Balance

The human body is composed primarily of water, so all biochemical reactions that take place within the body occur in an aqueous environment. Given this fact, changes in fluid and electrolyte balance that disrupt homeostasis can cause or exacerbate various disease processes. The result may be an emergent condition.

Homeostasis can be upset in several ways, such as via excessive output or input of fluids. Profuse sweating can cause dehydration, while excessive salt intake can contribute to hypertension.[1] Not drinking enough water can also alter homeostasis. In fact, a person deprived of water for 3 days or more may die.

The degree of fluid imbalance required to compromise homeostasis and cause illness depends on the patient's size, age, and any underlying medical conditions. In healthy adults, loss of more than 30% of total body fluid generally produces symptoms. By comparison, in a small child, symptoms may

Special Populations

The total volume of water in the body as a percentage of body weight—also called simply the total body water—varies by age and body composition throughout the life span. At birth, a healthy, term neonate has about 80% total body water; however, this percentage decreases with age **FIGURE 9-1**. After several weeks, an infant's total body water drops to about 70%.[2] In childhood, the total body water as a percentage of body weight falls to around 60%. Adults have 50% to 60% total body water, but water may constitute only 45% of body weight in older adults. Therefore, dehydration can be a serious concern in older adults. Dehydration also poses a concern in the pediatric population. Despite having higher total body water content than adults do, infants are at higher risk of dehydration due to their increased rate of fluid loss during disease and pathologic states.

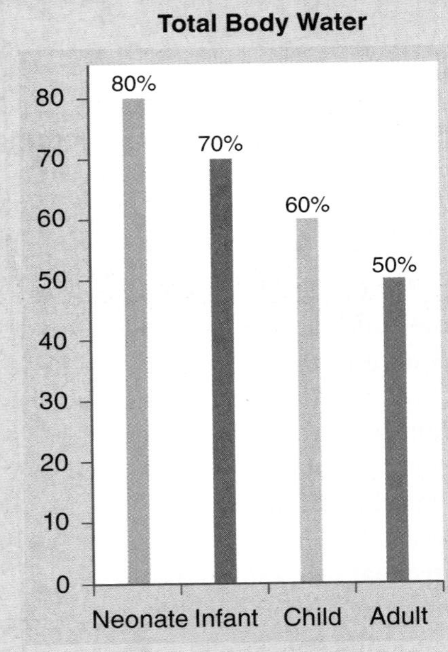

FIGURE 9-1 Average total water volume in the body, by age.

YOU are the Paramedic

PART 1

You and your partner are dispatched to a single-family residence to assist a 72-year-old man who is having difficulty breathing. On arrival, a neighbor greets you at the door. She tells you the resident of the home—your patient—lives alone, has had numerous heart attacks, and is not doing well. As you approach him, you assess his surroundings. You observe a large number of used facial tissues on the side table, along with an array of prescription medication bottles. The patient is sitting upright in a chair. He is wearing a nasal cannula attached to a home oxygen unit. He can speak only a few words at a time. He says he cannot breathe, and you note that he presents with pallor: an unhealthy pale appearance.

1. What is your general impression of the patient?
2. What can you learn about the patient from his surroundings?

appear with a loss of only 10% to 15% of total body fluid. In such cases, fluid therapy is a fundamental step in resuscitation.

Words of Wisdom

A hypertonic solution has a relatively higher osmotic pressure (that is, it contains more solute) than does the interstitial fluid or the fluid within and surrounding the brain. Administering a hypertonic solution such as mannitol, sodium bicarbonate, or hypertonic saline can cause excess fluid to drain from the tissues and into the blood and can decrease swelling in the brain.

Edema

Edema is swelling caused by excessive fluid that becomes trapped in the body tissues **FIGURE 9-2**. Edema may have several causes. One possible cause is increased capillary hydrostatic pressure, which may be associated with any of the following conditions:

- Arteriolar dilation (eg, from allergic reactions or inflammation)
- Venous obstruction (eg, hepatic obstruction, heart failure, or thrombophlebitis)
- Increased vascular volume, as occurs in patients with heart failure
- An increased level of adrenocortical hormones
- Premenstrual sodium retention
- Pregnancy
- Environmental heat stress
- The effects of gravity from prolonged standing

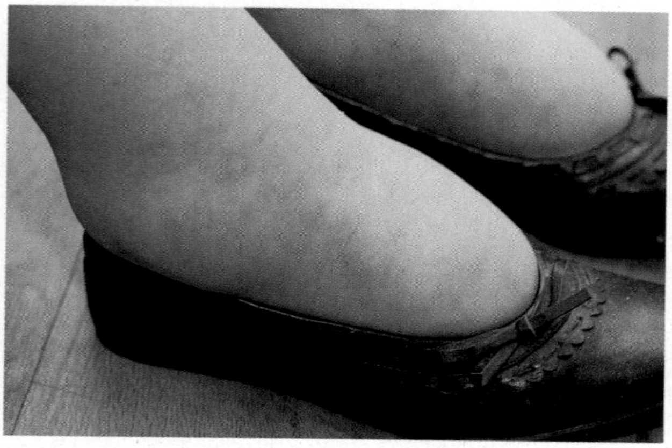

FIGURE 9-2 Edema is an excessive amount of fluid in the interstitial space.

Decreased colloidal osmotic pressure in the capillaries, another possible cause of edema, can be associated with various processes:

- Decreased production of plasma proteins, such as occurs in starvation and in patients with liver disease or severe protein deficiency
- Increased loss of plasma proteins attributable to protein-losing kidney diseases, extensive burns, or other causes

Obstruction of lymphatic vessels can also cause edema. Such obstruction can be associated with infection, lymphatic disease, or removal of lymphatic structures (eg, removal of lymph nodes during mastectomy can cause upper-extremity edema). When lymph vessels become blocked, the amount of fluid exiting through the arterial end of the capillaries is not equal to the amount of fluid being returned to the venous side. Consequently, more fluid leaves the arterial side, where the mean forces favoring outward movement are slightly higher. The lymphatic system picks up this additional fluid.

Severe edema, then, may be caused by long-standing lymphatic obstruction. Peripheral edema (as in the ankles and feet) is the most common form. If a person cannot get out of bed for an extended period, then edema may occur in the sacral area (sacral edema). *Ascites,* the abnormal accumulation of fluid in the peritoneal cavity, is also a type of edema.

The clinical manifestations of edema may be local or generalized. Patients with cardiac disease may have pulmonary edema, or edema may occur after submersion, narcotic overdose, or high-altitude pulmonary edema (HAPE). Patients with acute pulmonary edema have an excessive amount of fluid in their lungs. This excess fluid impairs oxygen diffusion into the pulmonary capillaries, leaving the patient hypoxic and severely short of breath.

As a paramedic, you must perform an in-depth physical assessment that includes auscultation of breath sounds, evaluation for pedal and sacral edema and jugular venous distention, electrocardiography (ECG), and obtaining vital signs. It is essential to determine a patient's medical history and current and past medications and to perform a thorough exam. Often, treatment is dictated by the patient's chief complaint and presenting problem. The definitive treatment of edema depends on the underlying medical condition that caused it. Possible interventions may include continuous positive airway pressure (CPAP), supplemental oxygen, positional therapy, nitrates, and diuretics.

> **Words of Wisdom**
>
> When you eat a bag of potato chips, you ingest a large quantity of salt. Acutely, the body responds by holding on to water; consequently, urine output temporarily declines. In healthy people, the kidneys and other regulatory mechanisms return both sodium and water levels to normal homeostatic balance.

Isotonic Fluid Deficit

An isotonic fluid deficit is a decrease in extracellular fluid with proportionate losses of sodium and water (decreased total body sodium); it is the most common form of fluid loss. Common causes of such deficits include vomiting, diarrhea, loss of plasma or whole blood (eg, burns, hemorrhage), use of loop diuretics, fever, decreased oral fluid intake, and excessive sweating. Excessive sweating or the combination of increased physical exertion with other comorbidities may complicate fluid loss and cause additional problems. In contrast, an isotonic fluid excess is a proportionate increase of sodium and water in extracellular fluid (increased total body sodium); common causes of this imbalance include heart failure, cirrhosis, renal failure, steroids, and excessive sodium intake. The concept of tonicity is discussed in more detail in Chapter 8, *Anatomy and Physiology*.

The manifestations of these conditions depend on the serum sodium level. When the body becomes dehydrated, orthostatic hypotension and decreased urine output (**oliguria**) often occur. When the sodium level is very high (>160 mEq/L), the patient is at risk of delirium and coma.

Electrolyte Imbalances

Sodium

Sodium, an element essential to the human body, is found primarily in the blood and fluid outside the cells. It regulates fluid balance, total fluid volume, and BP by controlling the movement of water across cellular membranes. It also facilitates muscle contraction and nerve impulse transmission. A blood test can determine the level of serum sodium (Na^+); the normal range is 136 to 142 mEq/L.[3]

A *hypertonic fluid deficit* occurs when the body loses water without a proportionate loss of sodium—in other words, there is a relative water loss. This condition, called **hypernatremia**, is clinically defined as a serum sodium level of a minimum of 143 mEq/L. A fluid deficit with hypernatremia can result from diabetic ketoacidosis, diabetes insipidus, high protein intake, or severe diarrhea. Fluid excess with hypernatremia can result from the administration of hypertonic sodium solutions. Signs and symptoms of hypernatremia include thirst, irritability, restlessness, weakness, edema, and elevated BP.

A *hypotonic fluid deficit* occurs when sodium is lost from the body without a proportionate water loss, resulting in a relative water excess. This deficit causes **hyponatremia**, which is characterized by a maximal serum sodium level of 135 mEq/L. A fluid deficit with hyponatremia can result from vomiting, diarrhea, prolonged sweating, or thiazide diuretic use. Fluid excess with hyponatremia can result from heart failure, cirrhosis, or renal failure, and a normal fluid volume with hyponatremia can be caused by syndrome of inappropriate antidiuretic hormone (SIADH). Signs and symptoms of hyponatremia include fatigue, loss of appetite, nausea, muscle cramps, weakness, abdominal discomfort or cramps, headache, confusion, seizures, and decreased BP.

Clinical findings typically depend not only on the absolute sodium level, but also on when the abnormality developed. People who become hyponatremic over a period of days tend to have fewer symptoms than people in whom the abnormality develops acutely. See Chapter 39, *Environmental Emergencies*, for additional discussion of hyponatremia.

Potassium

Potassium (K^+), the major intracellular cation, is crucial to many cellular functions, including neuromuscular control; regulating skeletal, smooth, and cardiac muscles; regulating acid–base balance; facilitating intracellular enzyme reactions; and maintaining intracellular osmolarity. The normal serum level of potassium ranges from 3.5 to 5.0 mEq/L.[3]

Hypokalemia is a decreased serum potassium level. Common causes of this electrolyte imbalance include the following:

- Decreased dietary potassium intake and absorption
- Decreased shift of potassium into the cells as a result of insulin administration, alkalosis, or beta-adrenergic stimulation, such as with epinephrine
- Renal potassium loss, such as with increased aldosterone activity or diuretic use
- Extrarenal potassium loss, such as with vomiting, diarrhea, or laxative use

Fatigue, muscle weakness, and cramps are the most frequent symptoms of mild to moderate hypokalemia. If the potassium level dips below 2.5 mEq/L, then the patient may experience ascending paralysis that begins in the legs and moves to the arms, hyporeflexia, and sustained muscle contraction (tetany). Acute hypokalemia can be treated with intravenous (IV) potassium supplementation in the hospital setting.

Hyperkalemia is an elevated serum potassium level. Common causes of this condition include the following:

- Decreased excretion (from renal failure or from medications that inhibit potassium excretion [spironolactone, angiotensin-converting enzyme inhibitors, nonsteroidal anti-inflammatory drugs])
- Shifts of potassium from within the cell (as occurs with burns, crush injuries, metabolic acidosis, and insulin deficiency)
- Excessive dietary potassium intake

An elevated potassium level interferes with normal neuromuscular function, leading to fatigue, nausea, muscle weakness, abnormal sensations (paresthesias), and, rarely, ascending paralysis. ECG changes and cardiac dysrhythmias typically precede these signs.

Words of Wisdom

While ECG changes may increase your index of suspicion for a given pathology, it is impossible to diagnose an electrolyte imbalance based entirely on findings from a cardiac monitor.

Calcium

Calcium is essential for muscle contraction, blood clotting, nerve impulse transmission, and the secretion of many hormones and chemicals. Nearly all (98%) of the body's calcium (Ca^{+2}) is found in the bones and teeth. This element lends strength and stability to the collagen and ground substance that form the matrix of the skeletal system. Calcium enters the body through the gastrointestinal (GI) tract. Its absorption from the intestine is aided by vitamin D **FIGURE 9-3**, which is manufactured largely by the body in a complex process that begins with exposure of the skin to sunlight. Calcium is then stored in bone tissue and ultimately excreted by the kidney. The normal level of serum calcium ranges from 8.2 to 10.2 mg/dL.[3]

Hypocalcemia, a decreased serum calcium level, can be caused by the following conditions:

- Decreased calcium intake or absorption (as in malabsorption and vitamin D deficit)
- Increased calcium loss (as in alcoholism and diuretic therapy)
- Endocrine disease (eg, hypoparathyroidism)
- Sepsis

Signs and symptoms of hypocalcemia stem from the increased excitation of the neuromuscular and cardiovascular systems. Skeletal muscle spasms can cause cramps or sustained muscle contraction (tetany). Laryngospasms with stridor can obstruct the airway. Seizures can occur, as can paresthesias affecting the lips and extremities. Cardiac dysrhythmias may be observed on the ECG.

Hypercalcemia is an increased serum calcium level. Selected causes of this imbalance are listed here:

- Increased calcium intake or absorption (such as with excessive antacid ingestion)
- Endocrine disorders (eg, primary hyperparathyroidism, adrenal insufficiency)
- Neoplasms (cancers)
- Miscellaneous causes (eg, use of diuretics, sarcoidosis)

The signs and symptoms associated with hypercalcemia are sometimes vague and can include fatigue, weakness, nausea, constipation, and frequent urination (**polyuria**). In severe cases, patients may exhibit stupor, coma, or renal failure. Treatment of

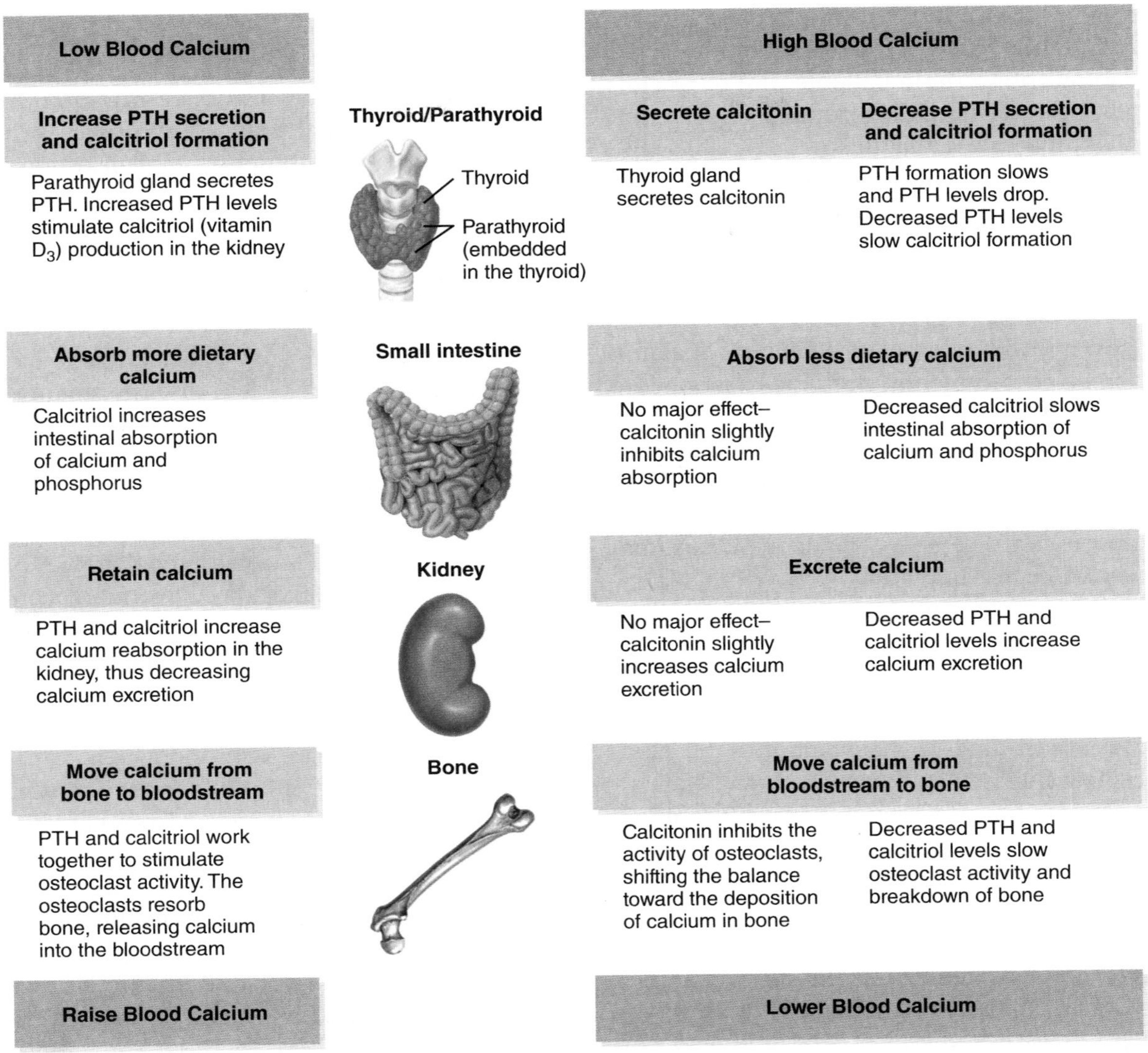

Low Blood Calcium
High Blood Calcium
Increase PTH secretion and calcitriol formation
Parathyroid gland secretes PTH. Increased PTH levels stimulate calcitriol (vitamin D3) production in the kidney
Thyroid/Parathyroid
Thyroid
Parathyroid (embedded in the thyroid)
Secrete calcitonin
Thyroid gland secretes calcitonin
Decrease PTH secretion and calcitriol formation
PTH formation slows and PTH levels drop. Decreased PTH levels slow calcitriol formation
Absorb more dietary calcium
Calcitriol increases intestinal absorption of calcium and phosphorus
Small intestine
Absorb less dietary calcium
No major effect– calcitonin slightly inhibits calcium absorption
Decreased calcitriol slows intestinal absorption of calcium and phosphorus
Retain calcium
PTH and calcitriol increase calcium reabsorption in the kidney, thus decreasing calcium excretion
Kidney
Excrete calcium
No major effect– calcitonin slightly increases calcium excretion
Decreased PTH and calcitriol levels increase calcium excretion
Move calcium from bone to bloodstream
PTH and calcitriol work together to stimulate osteoclast activity. The osteoclasts resorb bone, releasing calcium into the bloodstream
Bone
Move calcium from bloodstream to bone
Calcitonin inhibits the activity of osteoclasts, shifting the balance toward the deposition of calcium in bone
Decreased PTH and calcitriol levels slow osteoclast activity and breakdown of bone
Raise Blood Calcium
Lower Blood Calcium

FIGURE 9-3 Regulation of the blood calcium level. Calcitonin inhibits reabsorption of Ca^{+2} from bone, thereby helping to lower the level of Ca^{+2} in the blood. In a patient with a prolonged calcium elevation or deficiency, the action of parathyroid hormone (PTH) is the most powerful hormonal mechanism for maintaining a normal blood calcium level.

hypercalcemia focuses on addressing the underlying cause.

Phosphate

Phosphate (PO_4^{-3}), which is primarily an intracellular anion, is essential for the formation of bone and teeth, cellular energy metabolism, regulation of blood and urinary pH, and muscle and nerve functions. Phosphate levels are regulated by the same mechanisms that regulate calcium.

Hypophosphatemia is a decrease in the level of serum phosphate. Its causes include the following conditions:

- Decreased supply or absorption, as can occur in starvation, malabsorption, or blocked absorption (eg, with use of aluminum-containing antacids)
- Excessive loss of phosphate in patients with hyperparathyroidism, hyperthyroidism, or alcoholism

- Intracellular shift of phosphorus (eg, after administering glucose, anabolic steroids, or oral contraceptives, or in patients with respiratory alkalosis or salicylate poisoning)
- Electrolyte abnormalities (eg, hypercalcemia and hypomagnesemia)
- Abnormal loss of nutrients followed by inadequate replenishment, as can occur in patients with diabetic ketoacidosis or chronic alcoholism

Signs and symptoms of hypophosphatemia can include altered mental status, loss of appetite, dysrhythmias, hypotension, and muscle weakness. Acute, severe hypophosphatemia can lead to tremors, paresthesias, seizures, coma, acute blood disorders, and increased susceptibility to infection. The breakdown of muscle fibers (rhabdomyolysis) may also occur. Hospital treatment involves oral replenishment in mild to moderate cases and IV phosphate replacement in severe cases.

Hyperphosphatemia, an increased serum phosphate level, has many possible causes:

- Massive loading of phosphate into the extracellular fluid
  - Excessive use of vitamin D, laxatives, or enemas containing phosphate
  - IV phosphate supplements
  - Chemotherapy
  - Metabolic acidosis
- Decreased excretion into the urine (such as in renal failure and hypoparathyroidism, and with excessive administration of growth hormone [which results in acromegaly])

Signs and symptoms of hyperphosphatemia vary widely but may include tremor, paresthesia, hyperreflexia (overactive reflexes), confusion, seizures, muscle weakness, decreased mental status, coma, hypotension, heart failure, or a prolonged QT interval.[4-6] The normal range for serum phosphate is 2.3 to 4.7 mg/dL.[3]

Magnesium

Magnesium (Mg^{+2}) is the second most abundant intracellular cation, after potassium. It has a vital role in muscle contraction. Approximately 50% of the body's magnesium is stored in the bones, 49% in other body cells, and the remaining 1% in the extracellular fluid. The normal range of serum magnesium is 1.3 to 2.1 mEq/L.[3]

Hypomagnesemia, a decreased serum magnesium level, has several possible causes:

- Diminished magnesium absorption or intake (as occurs in alcohol use disorder, decreased dietary consumption, malabsorption, or malnutrition)
- Increased renal loss of magnesium (related to thiazide diuretic use, chronic kidney disease, primary aldosteronism, hypercalcemia, or genetic diseases)
- Increased GI loss of magnesium (related to diarrhea, vomiting, celiac disease, inflammatory bowel disease, or proton pump inhibitor use)
- Miscellaneous causes, such as insulin administration and pancreatitis

Weakness and muscle cramps are common symptoms of this electrolyte imbalance. A person with hypomagnesemia may have marked neuromuscular and central nervous system (CNS) hyperirritability, with tremors, jerking, insomnia, and personality changes. Hypertension, tachycardia, or ventricular dysrhythmias may occur, and confusion and disorientation can be pronounced.

Hypermagnesemia is an increased serum magnesium level. It usually results from kidney insufficiency, in which the body is unable to excrete magnesium taken in from food or drugs, especially antacids and laxatives. Symptoms include muscle weakness, decreased deep tendon reflexes, altered mental status, and cardiac dysrhythmias. Respiratory muscle paralysis and cardiac arrest are possible as well.

TABLE 9-1 summarizes the major electrolytes of the body.

TABLE 9-1 Major Electrolytes

Electrolyte	Symbol	Normal Serum Level
Sodium	Na	135–147 mEq/L
Chloride	Cl^-	95–107 mEq/L
Potassium	K^+	3.5–5.2 mEq/L
Bicarbonate	HCO_3^-	19–25 mEq/L
Calcium	Ca^{+2}	8.8–10.3 mg/dL
Magnesium	Mg^{+2}	1.6–2.4 mEq/L

Data from: Laboratory values. Global RPH website. https://globalrph.com/laboratory-values/. Updated October 10, 2017. Accessed October 7, 2021.

Disturbances of Acid–Base Balance

Recall that pH represents the concentration of hydrogen ions (H^+) in a solution. In other words, it is a measure of the acidity or alkalinity of a solution. There is an inverse relationship between pH and H^+ ion concentration: The lower the pH, the higher the acidity. The concept of pH is discussed in more detail in Chapter 8, *Anatomy and Physiology*.

In the human body, maintaining pH within a narrow range is vital. Acids and bases neutralize each other; therefore, they must remain in balance for the body to preserve homeostasis. Many patient issues you encounter as a paramedic will involve acid–base balance/imbalance. For example, a patient hyperventilating from pain may have a resulting alkalosis (pH greater than 7.45), whereas a patient in diabetic ketoacidosis will experience an underlying acidosis (pH less than 7.35).

Acidosis is an increase in extracellular H^+ ions; **alkalosis** is a decrease in extracellular H^+ ions.

$$\downarrow \text{pH means} \uparrow H^+ \text{ concentration} = \text{Acidosis}$$

$$\uparrow \text{pH means} \downarrow H^+ \text{ concentration} = \text{Alkalosis}$$

Disturbances of acid–base balance are associated with disturbances of potassium balance, in part because of the kidney transport system that moves H^+ and K^+ in opposite directions. In acidosis, the kidneys excrete H^+ and resorb K^+. Conversely, in alkalosis, the kidneys resorb H^+ and excrete K^+. In addition, Ca^{+2} ions shift out of the cell in response to an influx of hydrogen ions.

Types of Acid–Base Imbalance

Acid–base disorders are associated with four main clinical presentations: respiratory acidosis, respiratory alkalosis, metabolic acidosis, and metabolic alkalosis. Fluctuations in the bicarbonate level in the body cause metabolic acidosis or alkalosis, whereas respiratory disorders cause respiratory acidosis or alkalosis. When the body's buffering systems cannot immediately correct an acid–base imbalance, compensatory mechanisms respond to help restore the normal balance. (Buffering systems are discussed in Chapter 8, *Anatomy and Physiology*.) For example, respiratory alkalosis may occur as a compensatory response to metabolic acidosis. Thus, patient treatment may involve managing more than one acid–base imbalance.

Respiratory Acidosis

The following equation demonstrates how a diminished rate of respiration can precipitate acidosis:

$$\downarrow \text{Respiration} \rightarrow \uparrow CO_2 + H_2O \rightarrow \uparrow H_2CO_3 \rightarrow \text{Acidosis}$$

Respiratory acidosis is always related to hypoventilation. Decreased lung tidal volume reduces the amount of CO_2 that is exhaled, causing hypercapnia (increased CO_2) and increased levels of circulating carbonic acid. Because the acidosis is linked to inadequate breathing, the renal buffer system is initiated as a compensatory mechanism, conserving bicarbonate ions and eliminating H^+ ions to rebalance the increased acid level.

Some causes of respiratory acidosis include the following:

- CNS depression (eg, stroke, infection, opioids, sedatives, alcohol, hypoxic brain damage)
- Upper airway disease (eg, aspiration, laryngospasm, obstructive sleep apnea, airway obstruction)
- Pulmonary disease (eg, asthma, chronic obstructive pulmonary disease [COPD], acute respiratory distress syndrome, pneumonia, pulmonary edema)
- Miscellaneous causes (eg, muscular dystrophy, multiple sclerosis, obesity hypoventilation syndrome, closed head injury, chest trauma, respiratory or cardiac arrest)

Hypoventilation associated with any of these conditions can devolve quickly into an overwhelming, life-threatening acidosis, making it impossible for the renal system to compensate in time to accomplish a pH shift.

Signs and symptoms of respiratory acidosis depend on the speed of onset and the severity of CO_2 retention. Examples may include the following:

- Systemic or cerebral vasodilation (or both)
- Headache, light-headedness, restlessness
- Warm, flushed skin[7]
- CNS depression
- Nausea and vomiting

Tachypnea is usually present as a compensatory mechanism to correct the existing hypoventilation.

However, **bradypnea** (slow respiratory rate) may be present if CNS depression is the cause of the respiratory acidosis, or it may develop as the patient tires, suggesting imminent respiratory failure.

COPD gradually destroys lung tissue and inhibits oxygen and carbon dioxide exchange, eventually resulting in respiratory acidosis **FIGURE 9-4**. In patients with this kind of pulmonary disease, the normal stimulus for gas exchange is absent. Carbon dioxide retention leads to an increasing level of carbonic acid. Chemoreceptors eventually become unable to detect the presence of metabolic acids.

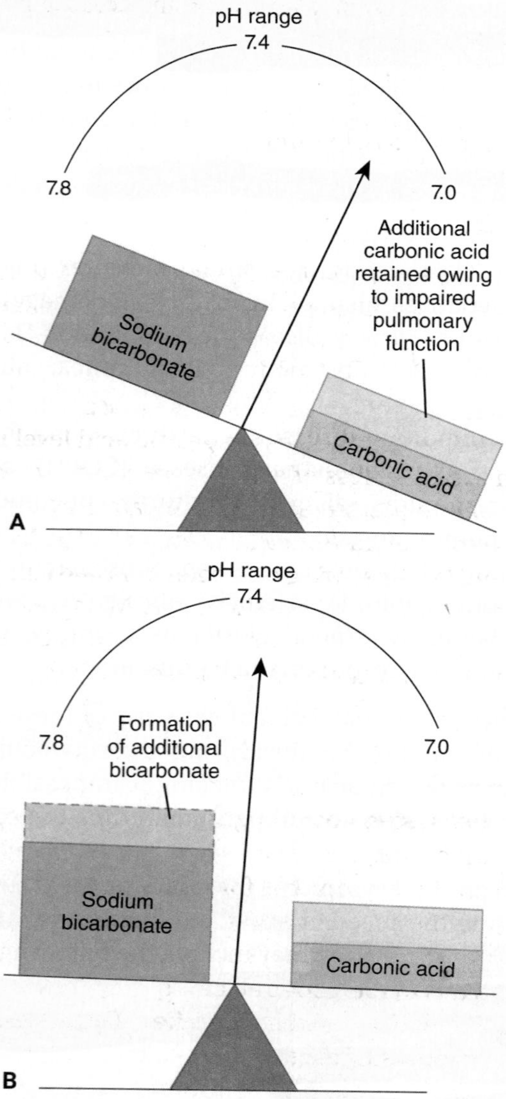

FIGURE 9-4 A. Derangement of acid–base balance in respiratory acidosis. **B.** Compensation by formation of additional bicarbonate.

As a result, the only remaining breathing stimulus is the hypoxic drive, which stimulates breathing by sensing a decreased oxygen level in the blood.

The slow onset of this form of respiratory acidosis in patients with COPD makes it survivable. The renal system slowly moderates the acidosis, preventing the life-threatening cardiac dysrhythmias often associated with acute acidosis.

> **Words of Wisdom**
>
> Compensatory mechanisms for pH imbalances bring the pH closer to normal. Whereas respiratory compensation (acidosis or alkalosis) occurs rapidly and relatively predictably, metabolic compensation, if it occurs at all, takes hours or days to present. Acute compensation is never complete. In contrast, chronic compensation, such as occurs in patients with COPD, often returns the pH to normal.

Respiratory Alkalosis

The following equation demonstrates how an increased respiratory rate can produce alkalosis:

$$\uparrow \text{Rate of respiration} \rightarrow \downarrow CO_2 + H_2O \rightarrow \downarrow H_2CO_3 \rightarrow \text{Alkalosis}$$

Respiratory alkalosis is associated with conditions that result in hyperventilation. Over time, an increased respiratory rate decreases the amount of CO_2 circulating in the body. In respiratory alkalosis, the CO_2 level in the blood drops, which reduces the level of circulating carbonic acid. The renal system then begins to retain H^+ ions and eliminate bicarbonate ions to rebalance the depleted acid level. At the same time, H^+ ions begin to shift from the extracellular fluid compartment to the intracellular fluid.

Hyperventilation and respiratory alkalosis may be caused by the following factors:

- Medications (eg, salicylate intoxication, caffeine)
- CNS stimulation (eg, fever, pain, anxiety disorder, panic disorder)
- Pulmonary causes (eg, asthma, pneumonia, pulmonary edema, pulmonary embolism, pneumothorax, acute respiratory distress syndrome)
- Miscellaneous causes (eg, overzealous bag-mask ventilation, carbon monoxide poisoning, heart failure, liver failure, pregnancy, high altitude, heat exposure, sepsis, trauma)

Signs and symptoms of respiratory alkalosis include the following:

- Light-headedness
- Carpopedal spasm
- Paresthesias of the lips, face, extremities
- Chest tightness, palpitations
- Vertigo
- Blurred vision

Metabolic Acidosis

The following equation demonstrates how an increased carbonic acid level can produce metabolic acidosis:

$$\uparrow H_2CO_3 \rightarrow \uparrow H^+ + HCO_3^- \rightarrow \text{Acidosis}$$

Any acidosis unrelated to the respiratory system is considered metabolic. An increased breathing rate (tachypnea) represents the body's attempt to restore acid–base balance by eliminating excess CO_2 through the respiratory system. For example, patients with diabetic ketoacidosis often present with Kussmaul respirations (deep, closely spaced, sighing breaths), in which the body hyperventilates in an attempt to blow off CO_2 and correct the acidosis. The kidneys attempt to compensate for the acidosis by retaining bicarbonate ions and eliminating hydrogen ions in the urine.

Causes of metabolic acidosis include the following:

- **Lactic acidosis.** Lactic acidosis is the product of anaerobic cellular respiration, which occurs when tissues and organs are inadequately perfused, as in shock and cardiac arrest.
- **Ketoacidosis.** Ketoacidosis is associated with insulin deficiency or cell desensitization to insulin. When they are unable to use glucose for energy, cells begin metabolizing fatty acids. Extremely acidic compounds called ketones are the by-products of this alternative metabolism pathway. Alcoholic ketoacidosis can result from an alcoholic binge with vomiting combined with inadequate food intake or from ingesting an excessive amount of ethyl alcohol.
- **GI losses.** Because diarrhea causes a loss of bicarbonate from the body, it can precipitate metabolic acidosis, particularly in children.
- **Ingestion of some drugs or toxins.** Ingestion of large doses of aspirin can directly stimulate the respiratory centers of the brain, producing tachypnea. This rapid breathing then leads to respiratory alkalosis, and initiation of renal compensatory mechanisms leads to metabolic acidosis. Inhaling toluene or ingesting methanol (wood alcohol), ethylene glycol (antifreeze), or paraldehyde can also induce metabolic acidosis.

The clinical presentation of metabolic acidosis depends on its severity. Possible signs and symptoms include the following:

- Headache, drowsiness (progressing to confusion and coma with increasing acidosis)
- Loss of appetite
- Tachypnea
- Nausea and vomiting
- Cardiac dysrhythmias

Metabolic Alkalosis

The following equation demonstrates how a decreased H^+ ion concentration can produce alkalosis:

$$\downarrow H^+ \rightarrow \downarrow H_2CO_3 \rightarrow \text{Alkalosis}$$

Metabolic alkalosis occurs when increased urine output or a decreased gastric acid level leads to an excessive loss of acid. The respiratory system attempts to restore acid–base balance by slowing the respiratory rate and retaining CO_2. The kidneys respond by conserving hydrogen ions and eliminating bicarbonate ions in the urine. Metabolic alkalosis is rarely an acute condition, but it is common among chronically ill patients, especially those who require nasogastric suctioning.

Several factors associated with upper GI losses can lead to metabolic alkalosis:

- **Excessive vomiting.** Illness or an eating disorder, such as anorexia nervosa or bulimia, can be responsible for upper GI acid loss. Expelling a great deal of acid from the stomach can trigger a complex metabolic pathway that leads to metabolic alkalosis.
- **Excessive water intake.** Drinking large amounts of water during vigorous exercise dilutes the stomach acid and stimulates the small intestine to prepare for incoming food from the stomach. An outpouring of strongly alkaline digestive enzymes into the lower GI tract exacerbates any existing acid–base imbalance.

- **Nasogastric suctioning.** Removal of contents directly from the GI tract eliminates acids from the body, resulting in alkalosis.
- **Excessive use of alkaline substances.** Metabolic alkalosis can stem from excessive reliance on antacids or similar alkaline substances. This possibility is important to remember when assessing a patient who reports having self-medicated for hours or days with over-the-counter antacids. Another cause of excessive intake of bases is the overzealous administration of sodium bicarbonate during resuscitation. Administering liberal amounts of sodium bicarbonate into the circulatory system can dramatically alter the serum pH level.

Words of Wisdom

The word pale, as used in this text, may apply to any patient whose skin presentation suggests reduced blood flow or oxygenation. The skin color produced by pallor depends largely on the patient's baseline skin color. In all patients, however, the mucous membranes inside the inner lower eyelid and the oral mucosa will have a pink coloration in healthy patients, regardless of baseline skin color; thus, a white or pale appearance of these areas in any patient suggests reduced blood flow or oxygenation.

Signs and symptoms of metabolic alkalosis may include light-headedness, confusion, paresthesias, muscle tremors and cramps, and possibly cardiac dysrhythmias.

Cellular Injury

The manifestations of cellular injury or death depend on how many and which types of cells are damaged. Various processes may cause cellular injury:

- Hypoxia (lack of oxygen)
- Ischemia (lack of blood supply)
- Chemical injury
- Infectious injury
- Immunologic (hypersensitivity) injury
- Physical damage (mechanical injury)
- Inflammatory injury

Manifestations of cellular injury occur at the microscopic (structural) and functional levels. Common microscopic abnormalities (eg, cardiac cell **necrosis** [a process in which the cell breaks down] as a result of long-standing hypoxemia) include cell swelling, rupture of cell membranes or nuclear membranes, and breakdown of nuclear material such as chromosomes **FIGURE 9-5**. This kind of cellular damage often distorts the cell's shape and disrupts its function. Functional disturbances may include inefficient oxygen utilization, intracellular acidosis, toxic waste accumulation, and derangement of nutrient metabolization.

YOU are the Paramedic

PART 2

You ask your partner to obtain a baseline oxygen saturation level and baseline vital signs, including waveform capnography. While she is setting up her equipment, you ask the patient about his past medical history. With great difficulty, he replies, "Heart failure."

Recording Time: 1 Minute	
Appearance	Awake, in distress, anxious
Level of consciousness	Alert (oriented to person, place, and day)
Airway	Open
Breathing	Accelerated rate; accessory muscle use; productive cough
Circulation	Weak radial pulses; moist, pale, cool skin

3. How does the recruitment of accessory muscles facilitate breathing?
4. How might the productive cough help you identify the source of the patient's breathing difficulty?

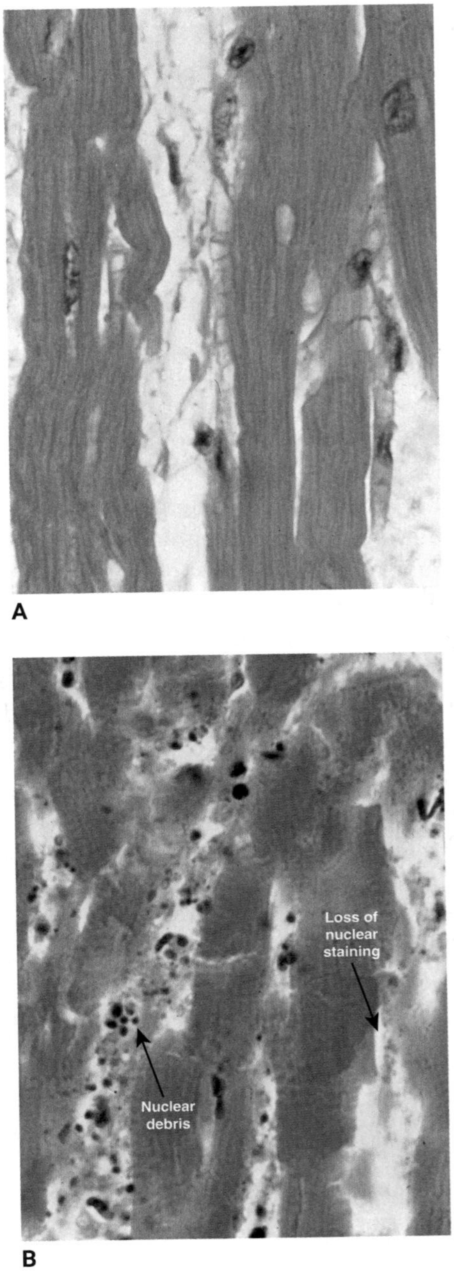

FIGURE 9-5 Comparison of normal cardiac muscle fibers **(A)** to necrotic cardiac fibers **(B)**. Note the fragmentation of fibers, loss of nuclear staining, and fragmented bits of nuclear debris. Cellular injury causes swelling, resulting in nuclear membrane rupture and breakdown of the nuclear material (original magnification ×400).

From: An Introduction to Human Disease, 7th ed. Photo courtesy of Leonard V. Crowley, MD, Century College.

Changes in individual cells often affect the entire organism. In some cases, the changes are associated with only minor systemic abnormalities, such as fever. At other times, such as when renal failure occurs, entire organ systems collapse and the patient's condition becomes critical. Because all body systems are ultimately connected, dysfunction in one system inevitably affects the function of other systems, upsetting the homeostatic balance on which the body depends to sustain life.

Words of Wisdom

The fatty compounds of which the cell membrane is composed are chemically neutral (uncharged); however, electrolytes (ie, sodium, potassium) are dissolved in water and therefore carry a charge. Charged molecules must travel along special pathways to permeate a cell membrane. Such transport channels (the ion channels) consist of protein-lined pores specifically sized to accommodate a given substance (ie, calcium, potassium). Lidocaine and other local anesthetics, and antidysrhythmic drugs such as amiodarone, exert nerve-blocking effects on these ion channels.

With proper treatment, cellular injury can be repaired up to a point; however, when irreversible injury occurs, no treatment will help. In that case, cell death is followed by necrosis. The cell membrane becomes abnormally permeable, allowing an influx of electrolytes and fluids. Then the cell and its organelles swell, and lysosomes release enzymes that destroy intracellular components. These processes occur during and after cell death.

Hypoxic Injury

Hypoxic injury is a common—and often deadly—cause of cellular injury. It may result from decreased amounts of oxygen in the air or loss of hemoglobin function (eg, carbon monoxide poisoning), a decreased number of red blood cells (as from bleeding), disease of the respiratory or cardiovascular system (eg, COPD), or loss of cytochromes (mitochondrial proteins that convert oxygen to adenosine triphosphate [ATP], a process seen in cyanide poisoning).

Although hypoxia has deleterious effects on cells, the damage does not stop there. Cells that are hypoxic for more than a few seconds produce mediators (substances) that may damage areas near or far from the initial area of damage in the body. The result is a positive feedback cycle in which mediators lead to more cell damage, which leads to more hypoxia, which leads to further mediator production, and so forth.

The earliest and most dangerous mediators produced by cells in response to hypoxia are **free radicals**. A free radical molecule is missing one electron in its outer shell. The presence of this odd, unpaired electron causes chemical instability as free radicals randomly attack cells and membranes in an attempt to steal back the missing electron. The result is widespread and potentially deadly tissue damage.

Chemical Injury

Various chemicals, including poisons, lead, carbon monoxide, ethanol, and pharmacologic agents, may injure and ultimately destroy cells. Commonly encountered poisons include cyanide and pesticides. Cyanide induces cell hypoxia by blocking oxidative phosphorylation in the mitochondria and preventing the metabolism of oxygen. Pesticides block an enzyme, acetylcholinesterase, thereby preventing proper transmission of nerve impulses.

Long-term ingestion of lead, which can happen when young children chew on windowsills covered with lead-based paint or inhale renovation dust containing lead (lead-based paint was last sold in the United States in 1978), leads to brain injury and neurologic dysfunction. The ability of lead to substitute for calcium (molecules of lead and calcium are a similar size) is a common factor in many of its toxic actions.

Carbon monoxide binds to hemoglobin more readily than does oxygen, preventing adequate oxygenation of the tissues. A low-level exposure to carbon monoxide causes nausea, vomiting, and headache. A higher level of carbon monoxide exposure can be fatal in less than 2 hours.[7]

At lower doses, ethanol, as found in drinking alcohol, causes inebriation. Higher doses produce severe CNS depression and hypoventilation, sometimes precipitating cardiovascular collapse.

Some pharmacologic agents produce toxic products when the agents are metabolized in the body, especially in overdose conditions. For example, excessive doses of acetaminophen (Tylenol) can poison the liver and sometimes be fatal.

Infectious Injury

Infectious injury to cells occurs as a result of an invasion of the body by bacteria, fungi, viruses, or other pathogens. Bacteria may cause injury either by acting directly on cells or by producing toxins. Viruses often initiate an inflammatory response that leads to cell damage and patient symptoms.

Virulence measures the disease-causing ability of a microorganism. The pathogenicity of any particular microorganism is a function of its ability to reproduce and cause disease within the human body. In particular, the growth and survival of bacteria in the body depend on the effectiveness of the body's defense mechanisms and on the bacteria's ability to resist those mechanisms. A depressed immune system is less capable of fighting off microorganisms that the body perceives as harmful; populations with weaker immune systems include newborn infants, older adults, people with diabetes, and people with cancer or other chronic diseases.

Bacteria

Many bacteria have a capsule that protects them from ingestion and destruction by **phagocytes**—white blood cells that engulf and consume foreign material such as microorganisms and cellular debris **FIGURE 9-6**. However, not all bacteria are encapsulated, and some of these bacteria may stubbornly resist destruction, resulting in the phagocytes transporting them throughout the body.

Bacteria can be categorized based on the results of Gram staining. In Gram staining, a dried, fixed suspension of bacteria, prepared on a microscopic slide, is stained first with a purple dye and then with an iodine solution. Next, the slide is decolorized with alcohol or another solvent; it is then stained with a red dye. Bacteria that resist decolorization and retain the purple stain are called **gram-positive** bacteria. In contrast, those that have been decolorized and accept the red counterstain are termed **gram-negative** bacteria. Gram-positive bacteria have thick cell walls composed of many layers of peptidoglycan (amino acids and glucose); in contrast, the cell walls of gram-negative bacteria consist primarily of lipids. The pathogenic qualities of gram-negative bacteria (which include the microorganism that causes bubonic plague) make them especially problematic for humans.

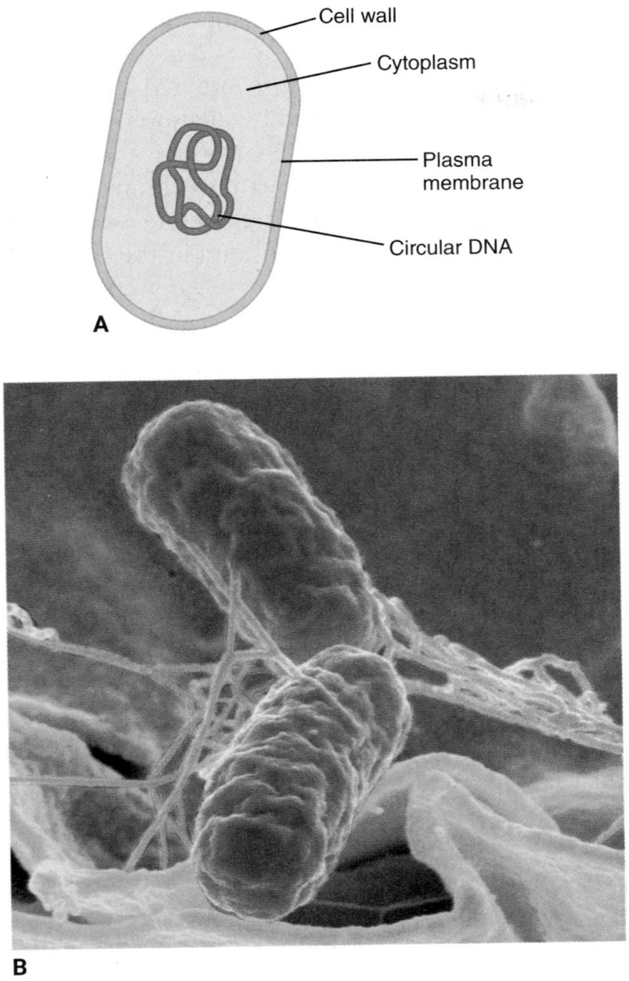

FIGURE 9-6 General structure of a bacterium. **A.** Bacteria come in many shapes and sizes, but all have a circular strand of deoxyribonucleic acid (DNA), cytoplasm, and a plasma membrane. A cell wall surrounds the membrane in many bacteria. **B.** An electron micrograph of *Salmonella* bacteria. Many bacteria have a capsule that protects them from ingestion and destruction by phagocytes.

A: © Jones & Bartlett Learning; B: Courtesy of Rocky Mountain Laboratory, National Institute of Allergy and Infectious Diseases, National Institutes of Health.

Bacteria also produce exotoxins or endotoxins—substances such as enzymes or toxins—that can injure or destroy cells. Staphylococci, streptococci, and *Clostridium tetani,* for example, secrete exotoxins into the medium surrounding the cell. Exotoxins are produced within the cell and then released into surrounding tissues or fluids (blood or lymph). The actions of these poisonous substances vary; for example, neurotoxins damage nervous tissue, enterotoxins affect the tissues of the GI tract, and cytotoxins damage various host tissues. Inactive exotoxins are sometimes used as the basis for vaccines.

Endotoxins are lipopolysaccharides that are part of the cell walls of gram-negative bacteria. Endotoxins cause inflammation, fever, chills, and malaise, as well as affect vascular tone. When large amounts of endotoxins are present in the body, the patient may experience septic shock. Endotoxins remain active even after the bacteria are destroyed, which may be one reason why the effects of antibiotics are delayed in patients with such infections.

When cells are injured, circulating white blood cells are attracted to the site of injury. These white blood cells release endogenous **pyrogens**, which then result in a fever. Indeed, the body's most common reaction to the presence of bacteria is inflammation. Some bacteria can produce hypersensitivity reactions. The presence of bacteria in the blood is called bacteremia; septicemia (sepsis) is a systemic disease, which may be life threatening, caused by the proliferation of microorganisms (or related toxins) in the blood.

Viruses

Viruses are among the most common causes of afflictions. These intracellular parasites take over the metabolic processes of the host cell and use the cell to help them replicate. A virus consists of a nucleic acid core of RNA or DNA. Surrounding the viral core is a protein coat known as the capsid, which protects the virus from phagocytosis. Some viruses have an additional protective coat known as the envelope.

The replication of a virus occurs inside the host cell, because viruses do not have organelles. Viral infection of a host cell leads to a decreased synthesis of macromolecules vital to the host cell. Unlike bacteria, however, viruses do not produce exotoxins or endotoxins. Instead, viruses induce pathology by disrupting the normal metabolic processes, but are protected from antibiotics because they live and replicate inside the host cell and effectively hide from the medication.

A symbiotic relationship may exist between a virus and normal cells that allows the virus to persist without causing an active infection. Viruses such as the human immunodeficiency virus (HIV) can elicit a strong immune response, rapidly producing an irreversible, lethal injury in susceptible cells.

Immunologic and Inflammatory Injury

Inflammation is a protective response occurring in the presence of cellular injury, including trauma, infection, and hypoxia. Infection is characterized by an invasion of microorganisms that causes cell or tissue injury, which leads to an inflammatory response. The inflammatory response can be triggered by an agent that is physical (heat or cold), chemical (eg, concentrated acid or alkali or another caustic chemical), or microbiologic (eg, bacterium or virus). The inflammatory response is characterized by both local and systemic effects, as shown in **FIGURE 9-7** and discussed in detail later in this chapter.

Local effects consist of dilation (expansion) of blood vessels and increased vascular permeability. Leukocytes (white blood cells) are attracted to the site of injury. These cells adhere to the endothelium of the small blood vessels, exert force to break through the cell walls, and migrate to the area of tissue damage. The characteristic signs of inflammation are heat, redness, tenderness, swelling, and pain. The increased warmth and redness of the inflamed tissues are caused by dilation of capillaries and slowing of blood flow through the vessels. Swelling occurs because the extravasation (leakage) of plasma from the dilated and more permeable vessels increases the fluid volume in the inflamed tissue. The tenderness and pain are secondary to irritation of sensory nerve endings at the site of the inflammatory process.

If the inflammatory process is severe, then systemic effects will become evident. The person feels ill, and the temperature is elevated. The bone marrow accelerates its production of leukocytes so the number of leukocytes circulating in the bloodstream increases, a process called **leukocytosis**. The liver produces and releases a variety of acute-phase proteins into the bloodstream in response to tissue injury or inflammation; these proteins help protect the body from the tissue injury caused by the inflammation. The best known of these proteins, C-reactive protein, is often measured to monitor the activity of diseases characterized by tissue inflammation.

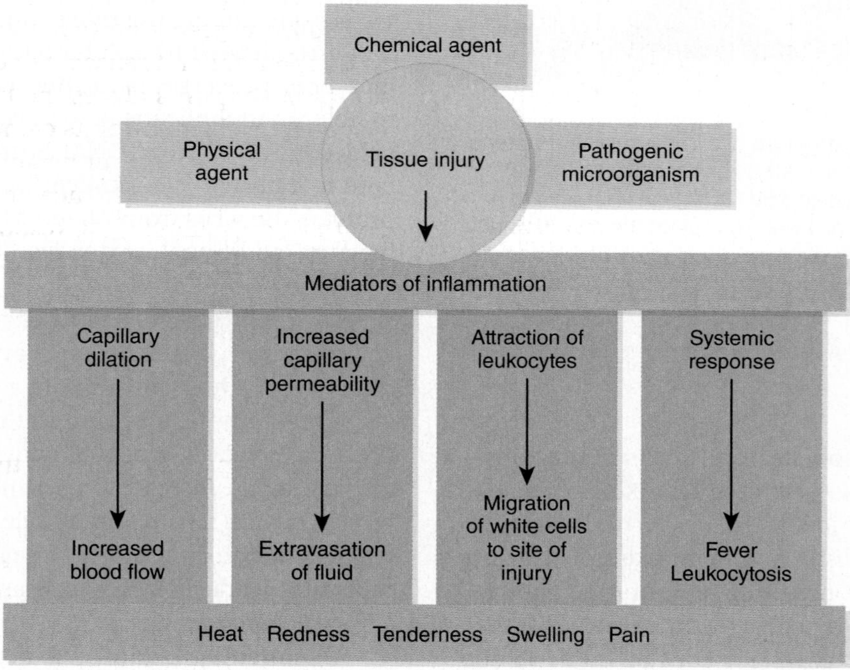

FIGURE 9-7 Local and systemic effects of tissue injury caused by various agents.

The outcome of an inflammation depends on the amount of tissue damage. If the inflammation is mild, then it soon subsides, and the tissues return to normal. If the inflammatory process is severe, tissue is destroyed to some extent and must be repaired. During healing, damaged cells are replaced, and the framework of the injured tissue is repaired as an ingrowth of cells produces connective-tissue fibers and new blood vessels. Scar tissue replaces large areas of tissue destruction. Sometimes, the scarring after a severe inflammation is so severe that function is seriously disturbed in the affected tissue.

Cellular membranes may be injured when they come in direct contact with the cellular and chemical components of the immune or inflammatory process, such as phagocytes (neutrophils and macrophages), histamine, antibodies, and lymphokines. In such a case, potassium leaks out of the damaged cell and water flows inward, causing the cell to swell. The nuclear envelope, organelle membranes, and cell membrane may rupture, resulting in cell death. The degree of swelling and chance of membrane rupture depend on the severity of the immune and inflammatory responses.

Injurious Genetic Factors

Genetic factors that may damage cells include chromosomal disorders, premature development of atherosclerosis, and, sometimes, obesity. An abnormal gene may develop in a person in one of three ways: by mutation of the gene during meiosis, which affects the newly formed fetus; by heredity; or due to other causes later in life. In trisomy 21 (Down syndrome), the child is born with an extra chromosome 21. Rheumatoid arthritis has a genetic link as well.

Injurious Nutritional Imbalances

Good nutrition is required to maintain good health and assist the cells in fighting disease. Nutritional imbalances that can injure cells and the organism as a whole include obesity, malnutrition, vitamin excess or deficiency, and mineral excess or deficiency. These conditions can lead to alterations in physical growth, mental and intellectual retardation, and even death.

Injurious Physical Agents or Conditions

Physical agents, such as heat, cold, and radiation, may also cause cell injury (eg, burns, frostbite, radiation sickness, tumors). The degree of cell injury that results is determined by the agent's strength and the length of exposure.

Apoptosis

Apoptosis is normal cell death. It is unique because it is genetically programmed into the cell as a part of normal development, organogenesis, immune function, and tissue growth. This process has a normal role in aging, early development, menses, lactating breast tissue, thymus involution, and red blood cell turnover.

During apoptosis, cells exhibit characteristic nuclear changes, and they typically die in well-defined clusters rather than in a random manner. The molecular mechanism underlying apoptosis involves the activation of genes that encode for proteins known as caspases (*c*ysteine-*aspa*rtic prote*ases*). The production of these proteins essentially leads to cell suicide. Unlike in the case of cell death from disease processes, proteins and DNA undergo controlled degradation that allows their remnants to be taken up and reused by neighboring cells. In this way, apoptosis allows the body to eliminate a cell but recycle many of its components. Pathologically, areas that have undergone apoptotic death do not show any evidence of inflammation. In contrast, an inflammatory response is typically observed when cells undergo necrosis from hypoxia or cellular toxins.

Apoptosis can be activated prematurely by pathologic factors such as cell injury. This premature stimulation, which occurs in some forms of heart failure, causes early cell death. Another example of pathologic apoptosis is the death of hepatocytes (liver cells) in patients with viral hepatitis, yellow fever, and other viral diseases. The dying cells form lumps of chromatin known as Councilman bodies. Inhibition of the normal course of apoptosis allows for destructive cellular proliferation, such as in cancer and rheumatoid arthritis (uncontrolled synovial tissue proliferation). **FIGURE 9-8** illustrates the process by which cancerous cells develop from normal cells.

Abnormal Cell Death

If the injury leading to cellular degeneration is of sufficient intensity and duration, then irreversible cell injury leads to cell death. Necrosis (tissue death) is the result of the morphologic changes that occur following cell death in living tissues. It is classified as either simple or derived.

Simple necrosis refers to areas of necrosis where the gross and microscopic tissue and some of the cells are recognizable. This tissue death may be caused by acute ischemia, acute toxicity (eg, from heavy metals), or direct physical injury (eg, from caustic chemicals and burns).

Derived necrosis includes caseation necrosis, dry gangrene, fat necrosis, and liquefaction necrosis. Caseation necrosis is manifested by the loss of all features of the tissue and cells, so they come to resemble cheese when viewed through a microscope. Dry gangrene results from invasion and putrefaction of necrotic tissue, after the blood supply is compromised and the tissue undergoes coagulation necrosis. Fat necrosis results from the destruction of fat cells, usually by enzymes (eg, pancreatic proteases, lipases). Liquefaction necrosis results from coagulation necrosis followed by conversion of tissues into a liquid form and invasion by putrefying bacteria that multiply in a warm moist environment; the bacteria produce lytic enzymes and gas.

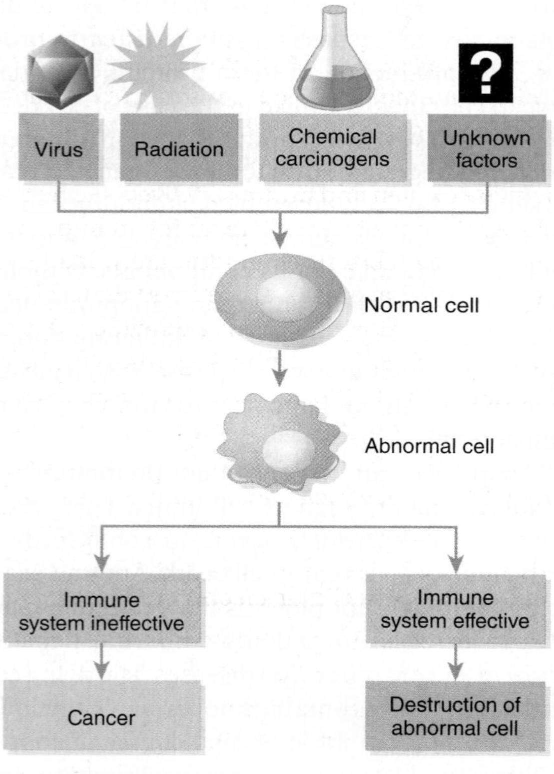

FIGURE 9-8 The onset of cancer. Viruses and other factors induce a normal cell to become abnormal. When the immune system is working effectively, it destroys the abnormal cells, so no cancer develops. When abnormal cells evade the immune system, they form a tumor and may become a spreading cancer.

Hypoperfusion

Perfusion is defined as the delivery of oxygen and nutrients and removal of wastes from the cells, organs, and tissues by the circulatory system. Adequate circulation is dependent on a pumping heart, intact vascular system, and an appropriate amount of oxygen-carrying blood. A deficiency in any of these areas will cause problems with perfusion. **Hypoperfusion** occurs when the level of tissue perfusion decreases below normal. It is important to evaluate a patient's level of organ perfusion during emergency medical care, especially in diagnosing shock. See Chapter 41, *Management and Resuscitation of the Critical Patient*, for further discussion of shock.

Shock has various causes. Whatever the cause, blood pressure ultimately falls. The decrease in BP stimulates baroreceptors located in the carotid sinus and aortic arch, in turn stimulating the cardiovascular control center contained in the medulla. This process increases sympathetic activity to the heart and vessels to compensate for the decrease in pressure. Signs of compensated and decompensated (hypotensive) shock appear in **TABLE 9-2**.

In response to hypoperfusion, the body releases catecholamines (epinephrine and norepinephrine), which increase the strength of cardiac contraction (positive inotropy), the pulse rate, vasoconstriction and, consequently, systemic vascular resistance. In addition, the renin-angiotensin-aldosterone system (RAAS) is activated, and the pituitary gland releases antidiuretic hormone. Together, these actions trigger salt and water retention and peripheral vasoconstriction, thereby increasing the amount of fluid in the vascular space and improving BP and cardiac output. Depending on the severity of the insult, various amounts of fluid will shift from the interstitial tissues into the vascular compartment. The spleen also releases some of the red blood cells

TABLE 9-2 Signs and Symptoms of Compensated and Decompensated Hypoperfusion (Shock)

Compensated Shock	Decompensated Shock
Agitation, anxiety, restlessness	Altered mental status (verbal to unresponsive)
Sense of impending doom	Hypotension
Weak, rapid (thready) pulse	Labored or irregular breathing
Clammy (cool, moist) skin	Thready or absent peripheral pulses
Pallor with cyanotic lips	Ashen, mottled, or cyanotic skin
Shortness of breath	Dilated pupils
Nausea, vomiting	Diminished urine output (oliguria)
Delayed capillary refill time in infants and children	Impending cardiac arrest
Thirst	
Normal blood pressure	

that are normally sequestered there, which augments the oxygen-carrying capacity of the blood.

The overall effect of these initial compensatory mechanisms is to increase the preload (venous return), stroke volume, and heart rate to ensure adequate cardiac output. The result is usually an increase in cardiac output and myocardial oxygen demand.

If hypoperfusion persists, myocardial stress will increase. Eventually, the above-normal compensatory mechanisms can no longer keep up with the increased oxygen demand. Myocardial function then worsens, manifested as decreased cardiac output and ejection fraction. Tissue perfusion decreases, leading to impaired cell metabolism. Often, the BP decreases, especially in patients with progressive hypoperfusion. Fluid may leak from the blood vessels, causing systemic and pulmonary edema. At this point, other signs of hypoperfusion may also be present, such as dyspnea, dusky skin, low BP, oliguria, and impaired mentation. Postcapillary sphincters eventually relax as hydrogen ion levels reach a certain threshold and microclots are then released into the circulation.

As mentioned in previous sections, capillaries normally leak plasma into the tissues through the forces of hydrostatic pressure. Nearby cells are bathed in this oxygen- and nutrient-rich fluid. In times of profound hypotension, blood flow through the capillary membrane decreases and this hydrostatic push fails. Pre- and postcapillary sphincters are positioned around the capillary to regulate flow through the capillary. Postcapillary sphincters contract when capillary blood flows diminishes, blocking the outflow of blood from the capillary in an attempt to increase the flow of plasma across the capillary membrane. The consequent pooling of blood in the capillaries produces mottled skin.

Shock is an abnormal state associated with inadequate oxygen and nutrient delivery to the metabolic apparatus of the cell, resulting in impairment of cellular metabolism and, ultimately, inadequate perfusion of vital organs. Once a certain level of tissue hypoperfusion has been reached, cell damage proceeds in a similar manner regardless of the type of initial insult. Impairment of cellular metabolism prevents the body from properly using oxygen and glucose at the cellular level. Cells revert to anaerobic metabolism, which causes increased lactic acid production and metabolic acidosis, decreased oxygen affinity for hemoglobin, decreased ATP production, changes in cellular electrolyte levels, cellular edema, and release of lysosomal enzymes. Glucose impairment raises the level of blood glucose as catecholamines and cortisol are released. In addition, fat breakdown (lipolysis) with ketone formation may occur.

Documentation and Communication

The terms *shock* and *hypoperfusion* are often used interchangeably; however, they are not synonymous. Localized hypoperfusion, such as from arterial occlusion, is not shock.

Types of Shock

Shock can occur due to inadequacy of the central circulation (the heart and the great vessels) or the peripheral circulation (the remaining vessels, including the microscopic circulation—that is, arterioles, venules, and capillaries). (The anatomy of the circulatory system is illustrated in Chapter 8, *Anatomy and Physiology.*) With a "mechanistic approach," two types of shock are distinguished: central and peripheral. **Central shock** includes cardiogenic shock and obstructive shock; **peripheral shock** includes hypovolemic shock and distributive shock. The following sections provide an overview of types of shock. These topics are also discussed in Chapter 31, *Bleeding,* and Chapter 41, *Management and Resuscitation of the Critical Patient.*

Central Shock

Cardiogenic Shock

Cardiogenic shock occurs when the heart cannot circulate enough blood to maintain adequate peripheral oxygen delivery. In ischemic heart disease, this condition occurs when there is a loss of 40% or more of functioning myocardium. The most common cause of cardiogenic shock is myocardial infarction, as a single event or by cumulative damage. Other forms of cardiac dysfunction may also precipitate cardiogenic shock, such as a large ventricular septal defect or hemodynamically significant dysrhythmias. See Chapter 18, *Cardiovascular Emergencies,* for further discussion of cardiogenic shock.

Obstructive Shock

Obstructive shock occurs when blood flow becomes blocked in the heart or great vessels. In **pericardial tamponade** **FIGURE 9-9**, diastolic filling of the right and left ventricles of the heart is impaired due to significant amounts of fluid in the pericardial sac surrounding the heart. Decreased ventricular filling associated with pericardial tamponade leads to a decrease in cardiac output. Aortic dissection leads to a false lumen (aortic opening), with loss of normal blood flow **FIGURE 9-10**. A left atrial tumor may obstruct flow between the atrium and the ventricle and decrease cardiac output. Obstruction of the superior or inferior vena cava (vena cava syndrome) decreases cardiac output by decreasing venous return. A large pulmonary embolus (blood clot in the lung) or a tension pneumothorax (lung collapse) may prevent adequate blood flow to the lungs, resulting in inadequate venous return to the left side of the heart.

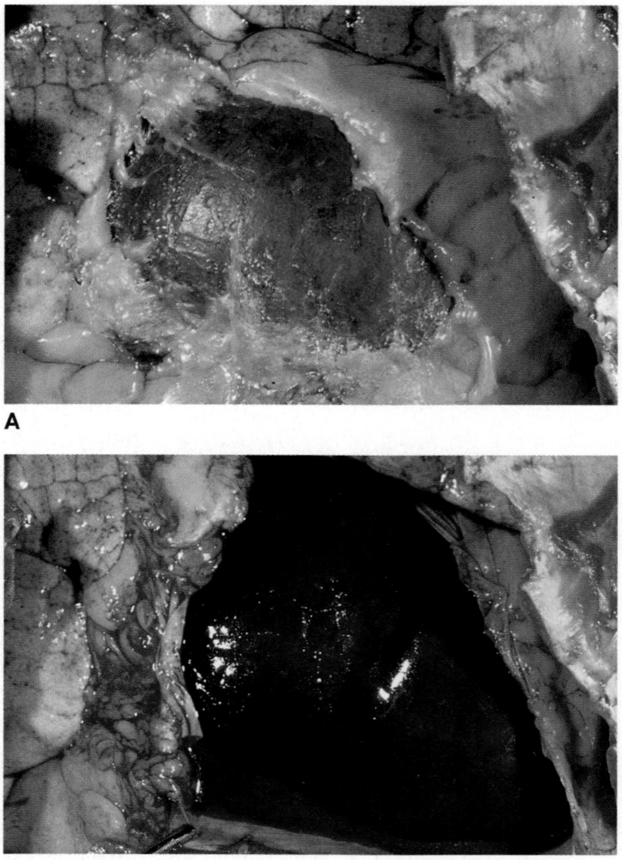

A

B

FIGURE 9-9 Cardiac tamponade following myocardial rupture. **A.** Distended pericardial sac. **B.** Pericardial sac opened, showing clotted blood surrounding the heart, which compressed the heart and prevented filling of the right ventricle in diastole.

> **Words of Wisdom**
>
> Neurogenic shock can involve bradycardia if the injury occurs in the high thoracic region because of disruption in the sympathetic autonomic pathway. Cardiogenic shock can involve bradycardia when myocardial infarction is the cause and the electrophysiologic pathway is disrupted.

Peripheral Shock

Hypovolemic Shock

In **hypovolemic shock**, the circulating blood volume is insufficient to deliver adequate oxygen and nutrients to the body. Two types of hypovolemic

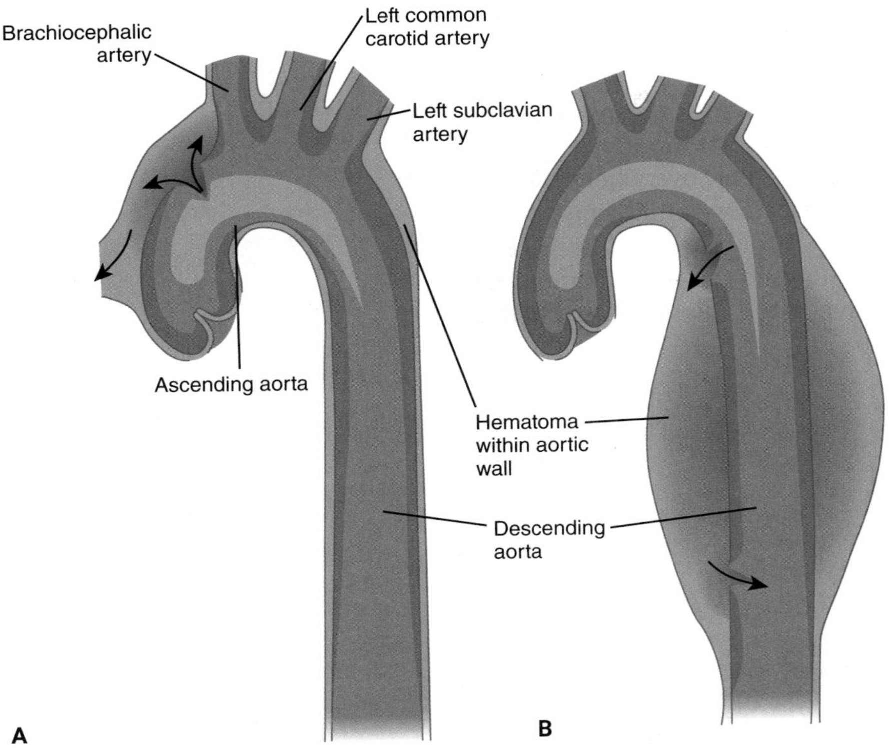

FIGURE 9-10 Sites of thoracic aortic dissection. **A.** A tear in the ascending aorta causes proximal and distal dissection. **B.** A tear in the descending aorta may cause extensive distal dissection.

shock—exogenous and endogenous—are possible, depending on where the fluid loss occurs. The most common cause of exogenous hypovolemic shock is external bleeding (ie, from an open wound), but this condition may also result from loss of plasma volume caused by diarrhea or vomiting. Endogenous hypovolemic shock occurs when the fluid loss is contained within the body.

Distributive Shock

Distributive shock occurs when there is widespread dilation of the resistance vessels (small arterioles), the capacitance vessels (small venules), or both. The circulating blood volume then pools in the expanded vascular beds, and tissue perfusion decreases. The three most common types of distributive shock are anaphylactic shock, septic shock, and neurogenic shock.

Anaphylactic shock (also called anaphylaxis) occurs when histamine and other vasodilator proteins are released following exposure to an **allergen** (any substance that causes a hypersensitivity reaction). Anaphylactic shock is also accompanied by wheezing and **urticaria** (hives). The result is widespread vasodilation that causes distributive shock and leaking of blood vessels. As fluid leaks out of the blood vessels and into the interstitial spaces, it produces intravascular hypovolemia.

Words of Wisdom

In anaphylaxis, interstitial fluid may cause significant swelling. In some cases, this swelling may occlude the upper airway, resulting in a life-threatening condition manifesting as the adventitious sound of stridor. Recurrent large areas of subcutaneous edema of sudden onset, usually disappearing within 24 hours, are called angioedema. This condition is seen frequently as a result of allergy to food or drugs, such as angiotensin-converting enzyme (ACE) inhibitors.

Septic shock results from widespread infection, usually bacterial. Complex interactions occur between the bacterial invader and the body's defense systems. Initially, the body's defense mechanisms may keep the infection at bay. If the normal immune mechanisms become overwhelmed, the body produces many substances that cause vasodilation and decreased cardiac output. If this condition is left untreated, then the result is multiple organ dysfunction syndrome (discussed later) and often death.

> **Words of Wisdom**
>
> Typically, the earliest signs of shock are restlessness and anxiety (related to hypoxia). The patient looks scared!

Neurogenic shock usually results from spinal cord injury. It leads to loss of normal sympathetic nervous system tone and vasodilation **FIGURE 9-11**. Patients often have fluid-refractory hypotension due to the degree of vasodilation.

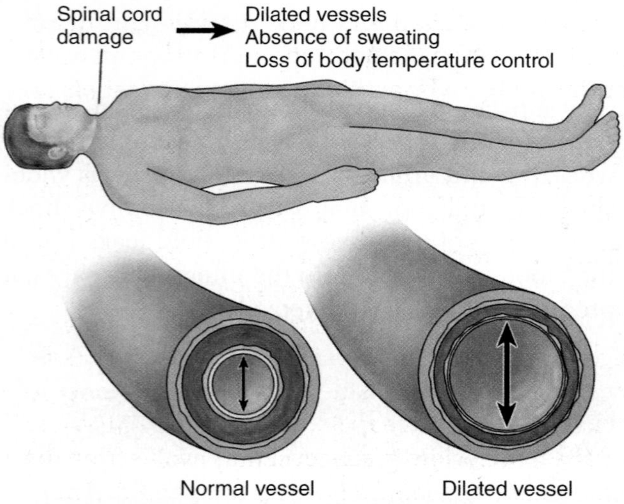

FIGURE 9-11 Damage to the spinal cord can cause significant injury to the part of the nervous system that controls the size and muscle tone of blood vessels. If the smooth muscle in the blood vessels is cut off from its impulses to contract, then the vessels dilate widely, increasing the size and capacity of the vascular system. The blood in the body can no longer fill the enlarged vessels, which results in inadequate perfusion and neurogenic shock.

Management of Shock

Most types of shock are characterized by reduced cardiac output, circulatory insufficiency, and rapid heartbeat. Although low BP is classically associated with shock, it is a late sign, especially in children.

> **Words of Wisdom**
>
> A possible exception to the standard use of IV fluid therapy to treat shock is hypovolemic shock caused by ongoing bleeding. Permissive hypotension, in which the provider attempts to achieve an appropriate mental status and adequate peripheral pulses, may be safer than attempting restoration of normotension, which may aggravate ongoing bleeding. When hypovolemic shock is treated with IV fluids rather than blood transfusion, the IV fluids given do not have the same oxygen-carrying capacity as blood products. In essence, fluid resuscitation sufficient to restore normotension in these patients thins out the blood in the circulatory system and decreases the blood's oxygen-carrying capacity.
>
> As always, follow your local protocols. Monitoring end-tidal carbon dioxide ($ETCO_2$) levels is also beneficial in developing target outcomes for patients in shock.

Clinically, determining the presence or absence of shock requires you to evaluate the presence and volume of the peripheral pulses and assess end-organ perfusion and function. Strength of the peripheral pulses is related to stroke volume of the heart and pulse pressures. Peripheral pulses should be readily palpable if the person is not in shock, although cold environments or obesity may compromise the presence or strength of these pulses. Normal skin perfusion is indicated by warm, dry extremities, fingers, and toes that are not altered from the patient's baseline color; in contrast, a slow, delayed, or prolonged **capillary refill time** indicates shock (although this technique is more reliable in children). Mottling, pallor, peripheral or central cyanosis, and delayed capillary refill may signal the presence of shock, whereas altered mental status indicates inadequate brain tissue perfusion.

To test the capillary refill time, briefly squeeze the toenail or fingernail, and then observe the time it takes for color to return. A normal capillary refill time is less than 2 seconds after blanching of the toe or finger, whereas a person in shock may have a capillary refill time of more than 2 seconds.

Measuring $ETCO_2$ levels may also be useful to the astute clinician. While $ETCO_2$ monitoring provides valuable information regarding the patient's respiratory and ventilatory status, you can also interpret the effectiveness of perfusion in the patient based on changes in capnography and capnometry. Carbon dioxide is one of the by-products of cellular metabolism, so a decreasing $ETCO_2$ level is an early indicator of shock. A low $ETCO_2$ level combined with other signs and symptoms of shock such as hypotension and altered mental status are ominous clinical findings.

Treatment of shock primarily addresses the underlying condition. See Chapter 31, *Bleeding*, for further discussion of preventing shock by controlling bleeding.

Multiple Organ Dysfunction Syndrome

Multiple organ dysfunction syndrome (MODS), first described in 1975, is a progressive condition that occurs in some critically ill patients. It is characterized by the concurrent failure of two or more organs or organ systems that were initially unharmed by the acute disorder or injury that caused the patient's current illness. Six organ systems are surveyed in diagnosing MODS: respiratory, hepatic, renal, hematologic, neurologic, and cardiovascular. Each system is assigned a score to determine the patient's overall risk. For example, the Glasgow Coma Scale score is used to score the patient's neurologic system function. While MODS may begin in one physiologic system, the disease process often progresses in a cyclical manner, including multiple organ systems and complicating factors throughout its course.

The overall mortality rate for MODS varies widely depending on the underlying etiology and ensuing diagnosis and treatment. Despite the inevitability its name suggests, this condition is often reversible, particularly in patients who were healthy before the physiologic insult occurred.[8] Nevertheless, MODS is a major cause of death following sepsis, trauma, and burn injuries, with mortality rates as high as 70% in patients with these injuries.[8]

Primary MODS is a direct result of an insult, such as a pulmonary contusion from striking the chest on the steering wheel during a motor vehicle crash. Secondary MODS is a slower, more progressive organ dysfunction.

MODS occurs when injury or infection (septic shock) triggers a massive systemic immune, inflammatory, and coagulation response accompanied by endotoxin release. Overactivating the complement system further increases inflammation and cellular damage. Vascular endothelial damage triggers overactivation of the coagulation system, which leads to uncontrolled coagulation in the venules and arterioles. This coagulation, in turn, causes microvascular thrombus formation and tissue ischemia. In addition, MODS activates the kallikrein-kinin system, stimulating the release of bradykinin, a potent vasodilator. Kallikrein is an inactive enzyme of the pancreas. When it becomes activated, it can dilate blood vessels, influence BP, modulate salt and water excretion by the kidneys, and influence cardiac remodeling after acute myocardial infarction (AMI). Bradykinin increases vascular permeability, dilates blood vessels, contracts smooth muscle, and causes pain when injected into the skin. Vasodilation leads to tissue hypoperfusion and may also contribute to hypotension.

The net outcome of the activation of these systems is maldistribution of systemic and organ blood flow. Often the body attempts to compensate for this problem by accelerating tissue metabolism. The result is an imbalance in oxygen supply and demand that causes tissue hypoxia, initiating a cascade of ill effects including tissue hypoperfusion, exhaustion of the cells' fuel supply (ATP), metabolic failure, lysosome breakdown, anaerobic metabolism and acidosis, and impaired cellular function.

Typically, MODS develops hours or days following resuscitation. Its signs and symptoms include hypotension, insufficient tissue perfusion, uncontrollable bleeding (coagulopathy), and multisystem organ failure. A low-grade fever may evolve from the inflammatory response, tachycardia, and dyspnea. Patients may also be difficult to oxygenate because of acute lung injury and acute respiratory distress syndrome.

During a 14- to 21-day period, renal and liver failure can develop in patients with MODS, along with collapse of the GI and immune systems. The kidneys depend on adequate perfusion pressure to carry out their tasks. Once the mean arterial pressure drops, the kidneys stop functioning. When this happens, many patients require continuous bedside dialysis.

The liver is a complex organ with a key role in excreting wastes and toxins. Adequate liver function is also essential for the synthesis of blood proteins and coagulation proteins, as well as the storage of glycogen, iron, and vitamins. Unfortunately, there are no definitive treatments for liver failure. Instead, treatment focuses on minimizing the effects of liver damage.

The brain, adrenal glands, and heart are also affected early in MODS. The level of consciousness deteriorates quickly in patients in hypoxic states, but it declines precipitously in patients with MODS. Cerebral hypoxia and subsequent ischemia can cause permanent deficits as a result of anoxic brain injury.

Perhaps the heart is affected more than any other organ in a patient with MODS. As the heart struggles to maintain arterial perfusion pressure, it too becomes hypoxic. Hypotension cannot be controlled despite the administration of fluids and vasopressors. Compensatory tachycardia consumes even more oxygen, and dysrhythmias such as bradycardia, ventricular tachycardia, and ventricular fibrillation develop. Cardiovascular collapse and death typically occur within days to weeks of the initial insult.

The Body's Self-Defense Mechanisms

The **immune system** includes all structures and processes associated with the body's defense against foreign substances and disease-causing agents. The body has three lines of defense: anatomic barriers, the inflammatory response, and the immune response.

Anatomic Barriers

Several anatomic barriers decrease the chances of foreign substances invading the body. The skin serves as a major deterrent. Hairs in the upper respiratory tract (the nose) and the lining of the lower respiratory tract (cilia-covered epithelial cells) also help repel foreign matter, especially small particles, and some bacteria. Acid in the stomach prevents many infectious agents from entering the body via the GI tract.

Immune Response

The **immune response** is the body's defense reaction to any substance it recognizes as foreign. This response is often directed toward invading microbes, such as bacteria or viruses. It is also triggered by foreign bodies, such as a splinter, and

YOU are the Paramedic

PART 3

Your partner is preparing to switch from high-flow oxygen to CPAP, assessing the patient's vital signs, placing the cardiac monitor, and setting up an IV line. You auscultate lung sounds and hear little air movement. You hear coarse crackles (rales) bilaterally in all fields. The patient coughs, and you notice pink, foamy sputum. You ask your partner to assess the medications on the side table while you establish the IV line.

Recording Time: 2 Minutes	
Respirations	22 breaths/min; shallow
Pulse	110 beats/min
Skin	Cool, moist, and pale
Blood pressure	140/90 mm Hg
Oxygen saturation (Spo_2)	89% before CPAP
Pupils	Pupils Equal, Round, and Reactive to Light and Accomodation (PERRLA)

5. On the basis of what you know about physiology, what is causing the pink, foamy sputum?

6. How do you account for the decreased Spo_2 level?

even abnormal cell growths, such as tumors. The immune response involves only one type of white blood cell: lymphocytes.

The body's immune system cannot destroy all invaders. In some cases, the best compromise the body can reach is controlling the damage and keeping the invader from spreading. Often, the immune system succeeds in preventing severe disease following infection. When the normal systems become overwhelmed or fail, serious disease occurs.

The body responds to different kinds of immune challenges in remarkably similar ways. Although the details depend on the particular challenge, the basic pattern is the same: The innate response starts first and is then reinforced by the more specific acquired response. These two pathways are interconnected.

Consider what happens when bacteria enter the body. If the bacteria are not encapsulated, then macrophages immediately begin to ingest these microorganisms. If the bacteria are encapsulated, then antibodies (opsonins) must coat the capsule before it can be ingested by phagocytes.

Components of the cell wall then activate the complement system. Some components of the activated complement system, termed **chemotaxins**, attract leukocytes from the circulation to help fight the infection. The complement cascade ends with the formation of a set of proteins called the **membrane attack complex**. These molecules insert themselves into the bacterial membrane, weakening those areas in the membrane. Ions and water then enter the cell through the weakened areas, leading to lysis of the bacterium (a chemical process that does not involve immune cells).

If antibodies to the bacteria are already present in the body, then these antibodies will assist the innate response by acting as opsonins and neutralizing bacterial toxins. Although it often takes several days, memory B cells attracted to the infection site will be activated if a recognized antigen is encountered. If the infection is new to the body—that is, preexisting antibodies are not present—then B cells will be activated. Helper T cells and cytokines are then released, antibodies are produced, and memory B and T cells are formed.

TABLE 9-3 describes the types of immune system cells.

Characteristics of the Immune Response

The native and acquired immune responses protect the body from infectious agents such as viruses and bacteria and from foreign substances that have gained access to the body through the skin or the lining of internal organs.

Natural immunity, also called native immunity, is a nonspecific cellular and humoral (antibody) response that operates as the first line of defense against pathogens. Most natural immunity is associated with the initial inflammatory response.

Acquired immunity (also called adaptive immunity) is a highly specific, inducible, discriminatory method by which armies of cells respond to an immune stimulant, such that the immune system will never fail to recognize the same stimulant when it is subsequently encountered, even years later. This mechanism is activated when the body is exposed to a foreign substance or disease and produces antibodies to the invader. Passively acquired immunity is the receipt of preformed antibodies to fight or prevent infection. Examples of passively acquired immunity include the transplacental passage of antibodies and the passage of antibodies in colostrum (the mother's initial breast milk to her infant), which protects the infant until their immune system matures sufficiently to take over. The injection of immunoglobulin (a concentrated form of antibodies obtained from donors) is also a form of passively acquired immunity.

The primary (initial) immune response takes place during the first exposure to an **antigen** (a foreign substance; a neoantigen is an antigen associated with cancerous cells). This encounter may not produce any clinical symptoms. Sometimes, the body's initial response is to produce an antibody that triggers symptoms on subsequent exposures. The secondary (amnestic) immune response occurs with reexposure to the foreign substance. The body has already developed a memory, of sorts, for that substance, so a more rapid and vigorous reaction occurs when the body encounters it again.

An **antibody** binds a specific antigen so the complex can attach itself to specialized immune cells that ingest the complex to destroy it or release biologic mediators such as histamine to induce an allergic or inflammatory response. The specific features

TABLE 9-3 Immune System Cells

Type of Cell	Description
Basophils	A type of white blood cell that releases histamine during inflammation.
Eosinophils	A type of white blood cell that phagocytizes the antigen–antibody complex; attacks parasites.
Neutrophils	A type of white blood cell that phagocytizes bacteria.
Monocytes	A type of white blood cell that phagocytizes bacteria, dead cells, and cellular debris.
Lymphocytes	A type of white blood cell involved in immune protection; attacks cells directly or produces antibodies.
Macrophages	White blood cells within tissues; produced by differentiation of monocytes. Functions include phagocytosis and stimulating lymphocytes and other immune cells to respond to pathogens; one of the first lines of defense in the inflammatory process.
Mast cells	Cells found in the connective tissues, beneath the skin, in the gastrointestinal mucosa, and in the mucosal membranes of the respiratory system. Functions relate to allergic reactions, immunity, and wound healing.
Plasma cells	White blood cells that develop from B cells and produce large volumes of specific antibodies.
B cells (B lymphocytes)	Cells that mature in the bone marrow, where they differentiate into either memory cells or immunoglobulin-secreting (antibody) cells. Functions include eliminating bacteria, neutralizing bacterial toxins, preventing viral reinfection, and producing immediate inflammatory response.
Helper B cells	A type of regulator cell that activates B cells to produce antibodies.
Memory B cells	A type of B cell that aids in the quick response to subsequent exposures to an antigen; these cells recall the antigen as foreign. They rapidly produce antibodies.
T cells (T lymphocytes)	Cells that are produced in the bone marrow and mature in the thymus. Two major types work to destroy antigens—regulator cells and effector cells.
Killer T cells	A type of T cell that destroys cells infected with viruses by releasing lymphokines that destroy cell walls; also called cytotoxic or effector cells.

of the antigen–antibody interaction depend on the foreign substance involved **FIGURE 9-12**.

An **immunogen** is an antigen capable of generating an immune response. Thus, an immunogen is an antigen, but an antigen is not necessarily an immunogen. Antigens and immunogens can be categorized by size. Proteins, polysaccharides, and nucleic acids are larger, whereas amino acids, monosaccharides, and fatty acids are smaller. A **hapten** is a substance that normally does not stimulate an immune response but that can be combined with an antigen and, later, initiate a specific antibody response on its own.

Humoral Immune Response

In **humoral immunity**, B cell lymphocytes produce antibodies called immunoglobulins, which recognize a specific antigen and then react with it **FIGURE 9-13**. This differs from cell-mediated immunity (discussed later), in which macrophages and T cells attack and destroy pathogens or foreign substances.

B Lymphocytes

Like all blood cells, B cells are born in the bone marrow, where they are descended from stem cells. The clonal selection theory holds that each B cell makes antibodies that have only one type of antigen-binding region and, therefore, are specific for a particular antigen, known as the cognate antigen. Antibodies are found on the surface of B cells, where they can recognize the presence of their cognate antigens. When a B cell recognizes the cognate antigen, it proliferates to make more identical

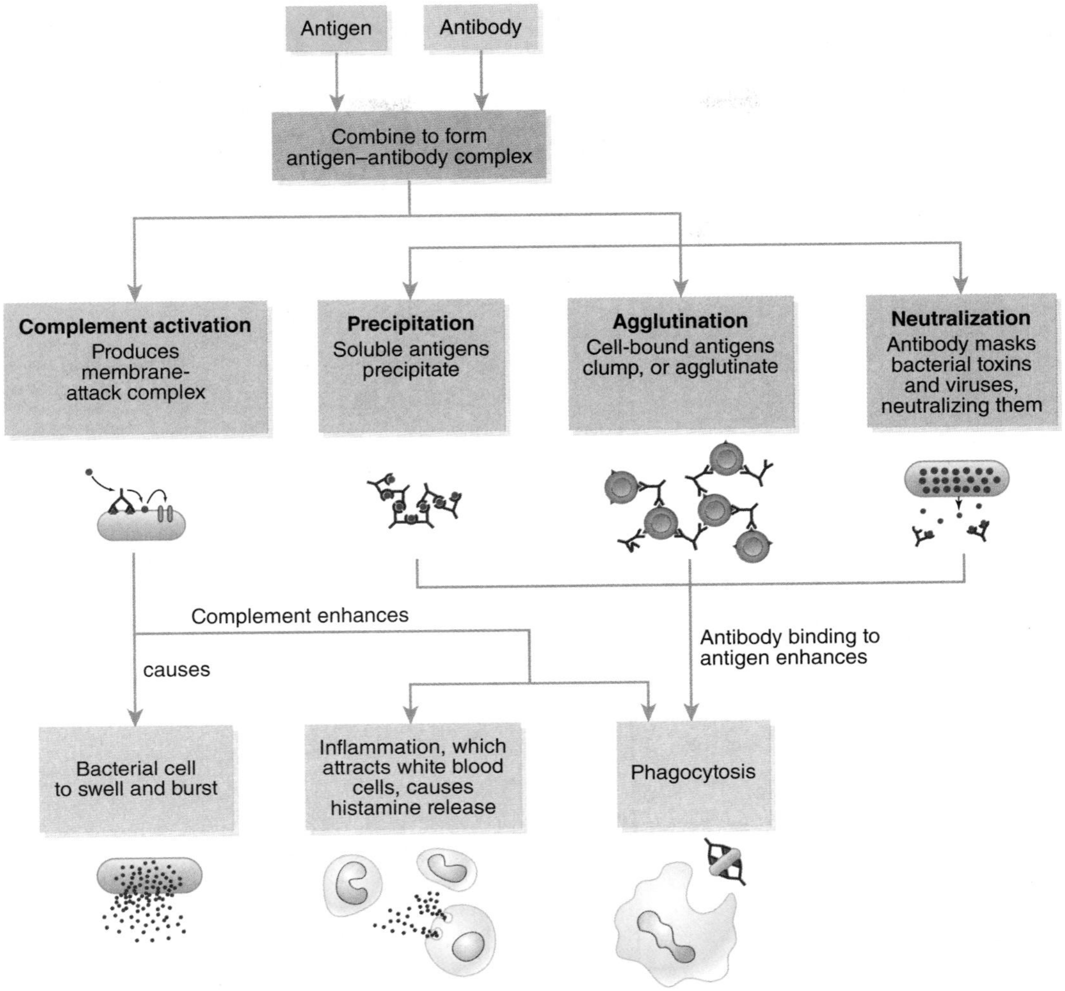

FIGURE 9-12 How antibodies work.

B cells exponentially; each of the new cells can make antibodies that recognize the same antigen.

For B cells to produce antibodies, those cells must first be activated. The most common way this occurs is via **helper T cells** **FIGURE 9-14**:

1. A macrophage engulfs the antigen via phagocytosis. It digests the antigen, pushing the discarded particles to the cell surface. These remnants interact with the B cell and a helper T cell.
2. The antigen binds to the B cell and the helper T cell, activating both.
3. The activated helper T cell secretes a lymphokine, a substance that stimulates the B cells to produce a clone. A clone is a group of identical cells formed from the same parent cell. The clone comprises two types of identical cells with different functions: plasma cells, which make the antibodies, and memory cells, which "remember" the initial encounter with the antigen. B cells produce many such clones, called polyclonal antibodies. It is also possible for monoclonal antibodies to be created. These highly specific antibodies are used in laboratory research and in some cancer therapies, but are not particularly relevant to paramedic field practice.

The human body distinguishes between foreign substances and its own cells and tissues by means of the major histocompatibility complex, a group of genes located on a single chromosome that permits a person who is capable of generating an immune

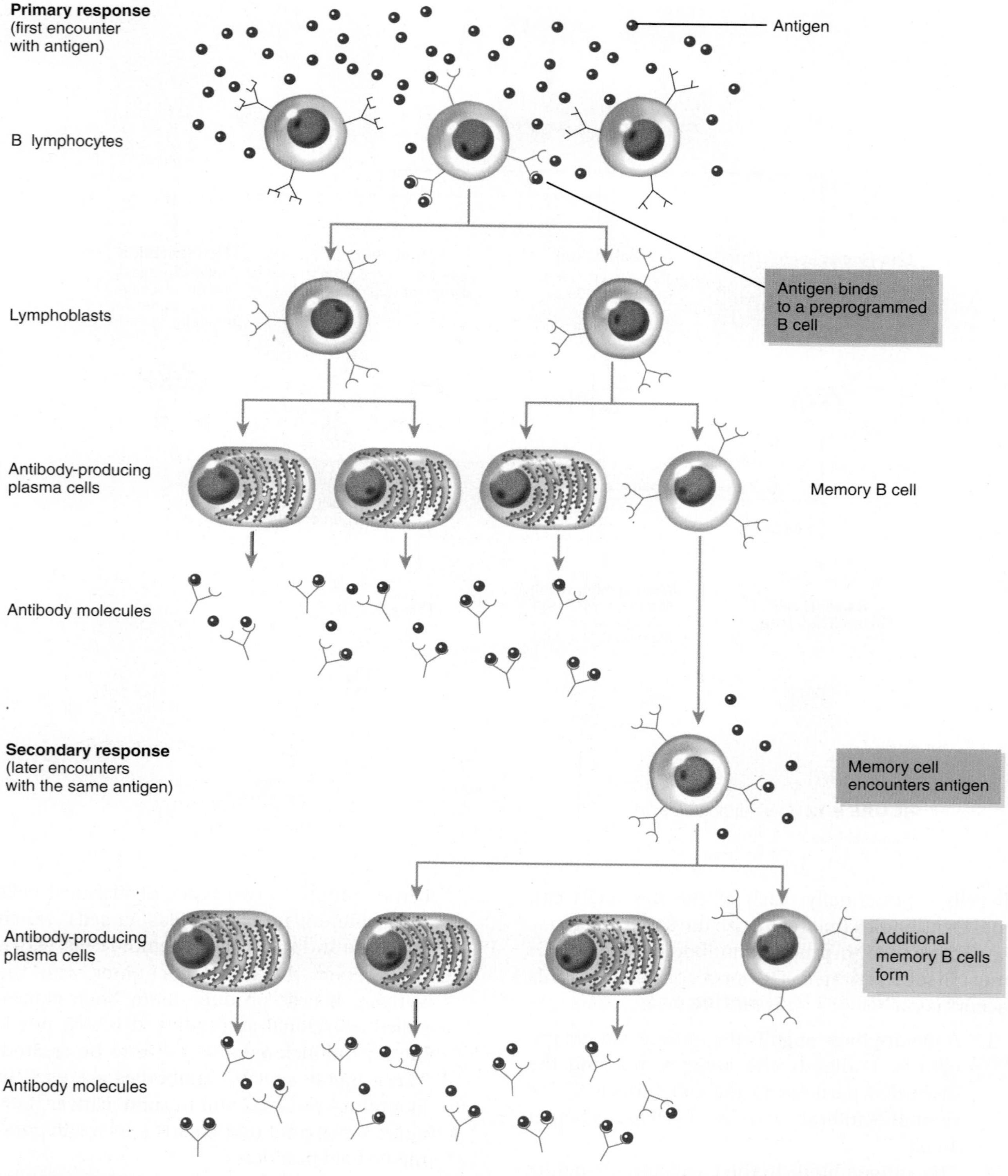

FIGURE 9-13 B cell activation. Immunocompetent B cells are stimulated by the presence of an antigen, producing an intermediate cell, the lymphoblast. The lymphoblasts divide, producing plasma cells and some memory B cells. Memory B cells respond to subsequent antigen encroachment, yielding a rapid secondary response.

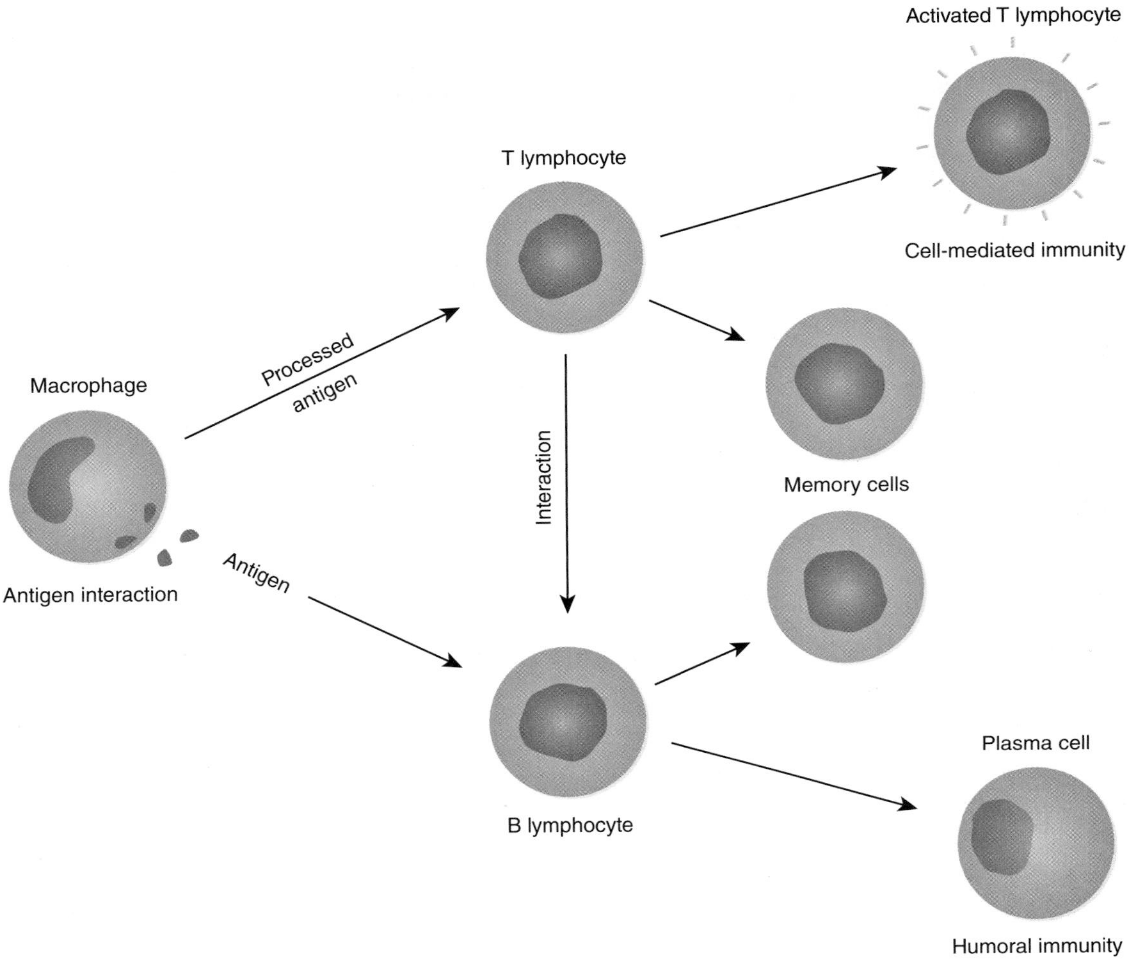

FIGURE 9-14 Interaction of cell-mediated and humoral immunity. A macrophage presents processed antigen fragments to the T lymphocyte. The B lymphocyte processes the intact antigen and displays fragments of the same antigen on its cell membrane. The T lymphocyte, which has responded to the same antigen, stimulates the B lymphocyte to proliferate, mature into plasma cells, and make antibodies.

response to distinguish *self* from *nonself* (namely, what is foreign). The human leukocyte antigen gene complex is the human major histocompatibility complex and is present in all nucleated human cells. It encodes for numerous antigens that are unique to a person. When the immune system encounters these particular antigens, it recognizes them as self, and no immune response occurs.

Immunoglobulins

The antibodies secreted by B cells are called **immunoglobulins** (this text uses the terms *immunoglobulins* and *antibodies* interchangeably, unless otherwise stated). These Y-shaped proteins consist of a crystallizable fragment (Fc) portion and two antigen-binding fragment (Fab) regions that bind only a specific antigen. The basic antibody molecule has four chains linked into a Y shape. Each side of the Y is identical, with one light chain attached to one heavy chain **FIGURE 9-15**. The two arms, or Fab regions, contain antigen-binding sites. The stem, or Fc region, interacts with other antibodies or receptors on immune cells. For example, mast cells are studded with immunoglobulin E (IgE) receptors that bind and carry IgE antibodies. When an antigen binds to one of these IgE antibodies, the mast cell is stimulated to release histamine granules. It makes sense, then, that IgE antibodies are associated with allergy **FIGURE 9-16**.

Antigens on antibodies are classified into three main categories: isotypic, allotypic, and idiotypic.

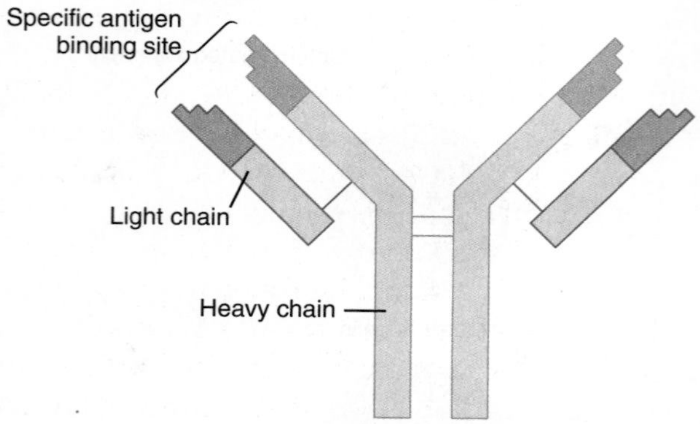

FIGURE 9-15 Structure of an immunoglobulin molecule.

An isotypic antigenic marker occurs in all members of a subclass of an immunoglobulin class. An allotypic antigenic marker is found on some members of a subclass of an immunoglobulin class, but not all of them. An idiotypic antigenic determinant is a unique structure that is created on the light and heavy chains of an immunoglobulin molecule. Some of these structures are involved in immune regulation.

Most antibodies are found in the plasma. In fact, antibodies make up approximately 20% of the plasma proteins in a healthy person. Antibodies make antigens more visible to the immune system in three ways:

- Antibodies act as opsonins. In **opsonization**, an antibody coats an antigen to facilitate its recognition by immune cells. Antibodies are not toxic themselves, but they label antigens so other immune cells will attack them.

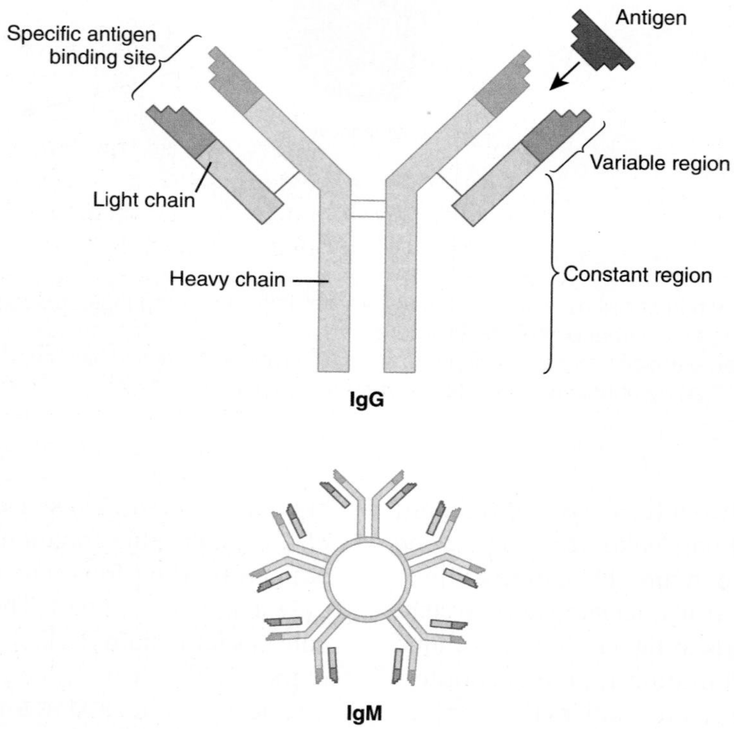

FIGURE 9-16 General structure of an antibody. Note that immunoglobulin G (IgG) is a monomer; it is one molecule. Immunoglobulin M (IgM) is a pentamer; it is a cluster of five antibodies and effectively combines with foreign antigens. The antigen fits exactly into the antigen-binding site; if it did not, it would not be able to bind there. Antigen-binding sites have different structures depending on the antigen to which they are designed to bind.

- Antibodies cause antigens to clump (precipitate, also known as agglutinate) for easier phagocytosis.
- Antibodies bind to and inactivate some toxins produced by bacteria. Macrophages can then ingest and destroy the inactivated toxins.

Antibodies are divided into five general classes of immunoglobulins **TABLE 9-4**. Fetal immunity is a passively acquired immunity that is derived primarily from maternal immunoglobulin G (IgG) and immunoglobulin M (IgM) antibodies. As a fertilized ovum grows, its peripheral cells differentiate into a group of cells called the trophoblast. The trophoblast forms the placenta and other structures that will support and nourish the embryo. The pregnant woman's immunity passes through the trophoblast. In fact, the umbilical cord's blood cells contain immunologic properties and have been used in medical treatment, which is a reason why some people decide to store their children's umbilical cord blood. In paramedicine, it is important to recognize that the umbilical cord contains immunologic properties because when cutting the umbilical cord, the position of the newborn is important. In addition, the paramedic should ensure the newborn is not held too high or too low relative to the mother; otherwise, the newborn could have a loss or gain of excess blood and, therefore, immunity. Following delivery, the antibodies that were passed to the fetus persist until the neonate's own B cells take over. A substantial number of antibodies are also transferred through breast milk, which is one of many reasons that many experts favor breastfeeding.

TABLE 9-4 General Classes of Immunoglobulins

Class	Description
IgG	The most common immunoglobulin. Accounts for 75% of the antibodies in the blood. Found in lymph, synovial fluid, peritoneal fluid, cerebrospinal fluid, and breast milk. IgG is the only immunoglobulin that crosses the placenta, giving infants immunity during the first few months of life.
IgA	Accounts for 15% of the antibodies in the blood. Also found in tears, saliva, respiratory tract secretions, and the stomach. IgA combines with a protein in the mucosa and defends body surfaces against invading microorganisms.
IgM	Accounts for 5% to 10% of the antibodies in the blood and is the dominant antibody in ABO (blood type) incompatibilities. IgM is the initial antibody formed in most infections.
IgE	Accounts for less than 1% of the antibodies in the blood and is associated with allergic reactions. When mast cell receptors combine with IgE and antigen, the mast cells degranulate and release chemical mediators such as histamine.
IgD	Accounts for less than 1% of the antibodies in the blood. The physiologic role of IgD is unclear.

Abbreviation: Ig, immunoglobulin

Cell-Mediated Immune Response

Cell-mediated immunity is characterized by the formation of a population of lymphocytes that can attack and destroy foreign material. It is the main defense against viruses, fungi, parasites, and some bacteria. Cell-mediated immunity is the mechanism by which the body rejects transplanted organs and eliminates the abnormal cells that sometimes arise spontaneously in cell division.

In cell-mediated immunity, T cell lymphocytes recognize antigens and contribute to the immune response in two major ways: (1) by secreting cytokines that attract other cells or (2) by becoming cytotoxic and killing infected or abnormal cells. There are five subgroups of T cells:

1. **Killer T cells.** Killer T cells (also called cytotoxic T cells) destroy the antigen. They help rid the body of cells that have been infected by viruses and cells that have been transformed into cancer cells. Killer T cells are also responsible for the rejection of tissue and organ grafts.
2. **Helper T cells.** Helper T cells activate many immune cells, including B cells and other T cells (also called T4 or $CD4^+$ cells).
3. **Suppressor T cells.** Suppressor T cells (also called T8 or $CD8^+$ cells) suppress the activity of other lymphocytes so they do not destroy normal tissue.

4. **Memory T cells.** Memory T cells remember the reaction for the next time it is needed.
5. **Lymphokine-producing cells.** Secreted by lymphocytes, these cells work to damage cells; for example, lymphokines destroy cells that have been infected with a virus.

During the cell-mediated response, macrophages ingest pathogens. When a macrophage digests a pathogen, it releases small particles of antigen. This antigen pushes its way to the macrophage surface, where it is recognized by specific T cells. Other T cells, such as helper T cells and killer T cells, then bind to the antigen and macrophage, destroying the invader.

Special Populations

T cell and B cell function is often deficient in older adults. Depressed lymphocyte function is accompanied by a decrease in macrophage activity. As a result of this aging-related change in their immune system, older adults are more susceptible to infections and recover slowly. In addition, older adults have an increased level of **autoantibodies** (antibodies directed against the self), which partly explains why older adults are susceptible to autoimmune disease.

Inflammatory Response

The **inflammatory response** is a response of the tissues of the body to irritation or injury. It is characterized by pain, swelling, redness, and heat. White blood cells of various types are a major component of this response.

Although they often occur simultaneously, the inflammatory reaction and the immune response are independent processes. That is, inflammation can be present without activation of the immune response, and vice versa. Inflammation is a dynamic process that, once initiated, triggers a complex cascade involving local and systemic events. The two most common causes of inflammation are infection (eg, bacterial or viral) and injury.

Acute Inflammation

The acute inflammatory response involves both vascular and cellular components. Initially, the arterioles constrict in an attempt to limit blood loss, but then dilate, allowing an influx of blood under increased pressure. This process increases the intravascular pressure and causes the blood vessel to expand; as in a balloon that is being inflated, the vessel walls become thinner. The higher pressure combined with increased vessel wall permeability causes fluid to leak into the interstitial spaces (edema). When enough fluid has escaped into the surrounding area and the intravascular pressure has been released, the vessel wall contracts and the flow slows, leading to pooling of blood in the capillaries.

A variety of blood cells participate in tissue inflammatory reactions: white blood cells (leukocytes), platelets, mast cells, and plasma cells (B lymphocytes that create antibodies). Specific cell types include neutrophils, monocytes, lymphocytes, eosinophils, basophils, and activated platelets. Chemical mediators, primarily produced by the mast cells, account for the vascular and cellular events that occur during the acute inflammatory response. Cell-derived mediators include histamine, arachidonic acid derivatives, and cytokines such as interleukins and tumor necrosis factor.

Words of Wisdom

Corticosteroids can decrease the initial inflammatory response, which is a necessary part of wound healing. However, as immunosuppressants, corticosteroids also increase the risk of wound infection. This consideration is important in patients with diabetes because development of such infections in this population is common.

Mast Cells

Mast cells have a major role in inflammation. During inflammation, mast cells degranulate and release a variety of substances. The primary stimuli for the degranulation of mast cells during the inflammatory response are physical injury (trauma), chemical agents (eg, bacterial toxins), and immunologic substances (eg, interaction of an antigen and an IgE antibody).

After degranulation, mast cells release **vasoactive amines**. The most important of these substances, **histamine** and **serotonin**, increase vascular permeability, cause vasodilation, and can lead to bronchoconstriction, nausea, and vomiting.

Because histamine is a preformed vasodepressor amine stored in mast cells, it can be released quickly, so its actions are seen early in the inflammatory response. Mast cells also synthesize chemotactic factors that attract neutrophils (neutrophil chemotactic factor) and eosinophils (eosinophilic chemotactic factor).

Mast cells also synthesize leukotrienes. **Leukotrienes**—also known as slow-reacting substances of anaphylaxis—are a family of biologically active compounds derived from arachidonic acid. The clinically important leukotrienes participate in host defense reactions and pathophysiologic conditions that paramedics commonly see in the field, such as immediate hypersensitivity and inflammation. Leukotrienes have potent actions on many parts of the body, including the cardiovascular, pulmonary, immune, and central nervous systems, as well as the GI tract.

Leukotrienes are primarily endogenous mediators of inflammation. They contribute to the signs and symptoms seen in acute inflammatory responses, including responses resulting from the interaction of allergens with IgE antibodies on mast cells. Certain leukotrienes are bronchoconstrictors, stimulate airway mucus secretion, and are very effective at increasing the permeability of postcapillary venules (including those in the bronchial circulation), thereby causing plasma protein exudation (oozing out of the tissue) and edema. Some leukotrienes may also promote eosinophil migration into the airways of animals and people with asthma, and increase bronchial hyperresponsiveness through an action on sensory nerves.

Finally, mast cells synthesize **prostaglandins**. These substances, which are derived from arachidonic acid, comprise a group of about 20 lipids that are composed of modified fatty acids attached to a five-member ring. Prostaglandins are found in many vertebrate tissues, where they act as messengers in reproduction, the inflammatory response to infection, and pain perception. Aspirin and nonsteroidal anti-inflammatory drugs inhibit prostaglandin synthesis, leading to reduced inflammation and pain.

Plasma Protein Systems

Some plasma-derived mediators modulate the inflammatory process. Called plasma protein systems, they include the complement system, the coagulation (clotting) system, and the kinin system. The interaction of these systems is vital to a normal inflammatory response. Each system consists of a cascade of biochemical reactions. As one compound is produced, it catalyzes the formation of the next compound, much like knocking over a line of dominoes.

- **Complement system.** The **complement system** is a group of plasma proteins that attract white blood cells to sites of inflammation, activate white blood cells, and directly destroy cells. The central compound in this complement cascade, called complement component 3 (C3), is produced by one of the two complement pathways: the classic pathway or the alternative pathway. The classic pathway starts when an antigen–antibody complex binds to a complement component 1q (C1q); activation of this pathway is dependent on the presence of antibodies. The alternative pathway can be triggered by bacterial toxins and does not require antibodies for its activation.

  Regardless of which pathway is taken, the main products are the same: C3b, anaphylatoxins, and the membrane attack complex. C3b coats bacteria, making it easier for macrophages to engulf them. Anaphylatoxins (C3a, C4a, and C5a) stimulate smooth-muscle contraction and increase vascular permeability by stimulating the release of histamine from mast cells and platelets. The membrane attack complex is a set of complement proteins (C5b, C6, C7, C8, and C9) that bind together to form a hollow tube, much like a short straw, that can puncture the plasma membrane of a cell. In this way, transmembrane channels are formed that allow ions, water, and other small molecules to pass through the cell membrane, resulting in loss of cellular osmolarity and death of the cell.
- **Coagulation system.** The **coagulation system** serves a vital role in the formation of blood clots in blood vessels. Inflammation triggers the coagulation cascade, initiating a complex series of reactions that encourage fibrin formation. **Fibrin** is a protein that polymerizes (bonds) to form the fibrous component of a blood clot. The various coagulation factors are counterbalanced by a variety of inhibitors, so that the coagulation remains restricted to one

area. Simultaneously, the **fibrinolysis cascade** is activated to dissolve the fibrin and create fibrin split products (ie, fragments of the dissolving clot).

- **Kinin system.** The **kinin system** leads to the formation of the vasoactive protein bradykinin from kallikrein. Kallikrein is an enzyme that is normally found in blood plasma, urine, and body tissue in an inactive state. When it becomes activated, it can dilate blood vessels, influence BP, modulate salt and water excretion by the kidneys, and influence cardiac remodeling after AMI. Bradykinin increases vascular permeability, dilates blood vessels, contracts smooth muscle, and causes pain when injected into the skin.

  The kinin system is spurred into action by the activation of Hageman factor (coagulation factor XII). (**TABLE 9-5** lists the various coagulation factors.) In addition to its role in the kinin system, Hageman factor participates in the clotting, fibrinolytic, and complement cascades. Its activators include bacterial lipopolysaccharides and endotoxin. Activated factor XII triggers the intrinsic clotting cascade, a series of reactions that is initiated when blood is exposed to collagen or other substances. For example, when a blood vessel is cut, the skin cells are damaged and the blood comes in contact with collagen. The extrinsic clotting cascade is activated by substances released from injured cells when tissue damage occurs.

Cellular Components of Inflammation

The goal for the cellular components of the acute inflammatory response is for inflammatory cells—namely, **polymorphonuclear neutrophils (PMNs)**—to arrive at the sites in the tissue where they are

TABLE 9-5 Coagulation Factors

Factor Number	Name	Description
I	Fibrinogen	Protein synthesized in the liver; converted into fibrin in stage 3
II	Prothrombin	Protein synthesized in the liver (requires vitamin K); converted into thrombin in stage 2
III	Tissue thromboplastin	Released from damaged tissue; required in extrinsic stage 1
IV	Calcium ions	Required throughout the entire clotting sequence
V	Proaccelerin (labile factor)	Protein synthesized in the liver; required to form prothrombin activator in intrinsic and extrinsic stage 1
VII	Serum prothrombin conversion accelerator (stable factor, proconvertin)	Protein synthesized in the liver (requires vitamin K); functions in extrinsic stage 1
VIII	Antihemophilic factor (antihemophilic globulin)	Protein synthesized in the liver; required for intrinsic stage 1
IX	Plasma thromboplastin component	Protein synthesized in the liver (requires vitamin K); required for intrinsic stage 1
X	Stuart factor (Stuart-Prower factor)	Protein synthesized in the liver (requires vitamin K); required to form prothrombin activator in intrinsic and extrinsic stage 1
XI	Plasma thromboplastin antecedent	Protein synthesized in the liver; required for intrinsic stage 1
XII	Hageman factor	Protein required for intrinsic stage 1
XIII	Fibrin-stabilizing factor	Protein required to stabilize the fibrin strands in stage 3

needed. This process involves two major stages: an intravascular phase and an extravascular phase. During the intravascular phase, leukocytes move to the sides of blood vessels and attach to the endothelial cells. During the extravascular phase, leukocytes travel to the site of inflammation and kill organisms. The cellular events follow this sequence **FIGURE 9-17**:

1. **Margination**. Loss of fluid from the blood vessels into the inflamed or infected tissue gives the blood that remains in the vessels increased viscosity, which slows blood flow and produces stasis. PMNs, which usually travel toward the center of the vessel, settle toward the sides as the blood flow slows. As stasis develops, leukocytes also move (marginate) toward the sides of the vessels, where they bump into the endothelial cells and bind to them. Stress can lead to demargination of some white blood cells, which stimulates the bone marrow to produce more, in turn increasing the white blood cell count.
2. **Activation**. Mediators of inflammation trigger the appearance of selectins and integrins on the surfaces of endothelial cells and PMNs, respectively.
3. **Adhesion**. PMNs attach to endothelial cells, as mediated by selectins and integrins.
4. **Transmigration (diapedesis)**. The PMNs permeate the vessel wall, passing into the interstitial space.
5. **Chemotaxis**. The PMNs move toward the site of inflammation in response to chemotactic factors released by bacteria or formed from activated complement, chemokines, or arachidonic acid derivatives (such as leukotrienes) in response to cell injury.

Cellular Products of Inflammation

Cytokines are products of cells that affect the function of other cells. They include interleukins, interferons, monokines, and lymphokines, as well as some other factors. Monocytes release monokines, and lymphocytes release lymphokines.

Interleukins include IL-1 (interleukin-1) and IL-2 (interleukin-2), which attract white blood cells to the sites of injury and bacterial invasion. **Interferon** is a protein produced by cells when viruses invade them. This cytokine is released into the bloodstream or intercellular fluid to induce healthy cells to manufacture an enzyme that counters the infection.

Lymphokines stimulate leukocytes. Macrophage-activating factor stimulates macrophages to help engulf and destroy foreign substances. Migration inhibitory factor keeps white blood cells at the site of infection or injury until they can perform their designated task.

Injury Resolution and Repair

Normal wound healing involves four steps—repair of damaged tissue, removal of inflammatory debris, restoration of tissues to a normal state, and regeneration of cells. Healing after tissue injury or loss caused by inflammation depends on the type of cells that make up the affected organ. Labile cells divide continuously, so organs derived from these cells (such as skin and intestinal mucosa) heal completely. Stable cells, such as those found in the liver and kidney, are replaced by regeneration of the remaining cells, which are stimulated to enter mitosis. Permanent cells, such as nerve cells and cardiac myocytes, cannot be replaced; scar tissue is laid down instead. However, research is being done on the use of stem cells to replace damaged nerve cells.

Wounds may heal by either primary or secondary intention. Healing by primary intention occurs in clean wounds with opposed margins (such as clean surgical wounds or surgically debrided wounds). First, blood fills the defect and coagulates, forming a scab—a meshlike structure composed of fibrin and fibronectin. If the inflammatory process was severe, tissue may have been destroyed and require repair. Next, macrophages remove cellular debris and secrete growth factors. These growth factors stimulate angiogenesis and growth of fibroblasts, encouraging the formation of granulation tissue. The epithelium then regenerates, covering the surface defect. Deposition of collagen produces fibrous union. By the end of the first week, 10% of the preinjury strength is regained. Scar maturation occurs as collagen cross-linking takes place. By the end of 3 months, 80% of the normal tensile strength of the tissue has been restored.

Healing by secondary intention occurs in large, gaping wounds. Wounds that heal by secondary intention have a more pronounced and prolonged inflammatory phase, causing the neutrophils to persist for days. They also have more abundant

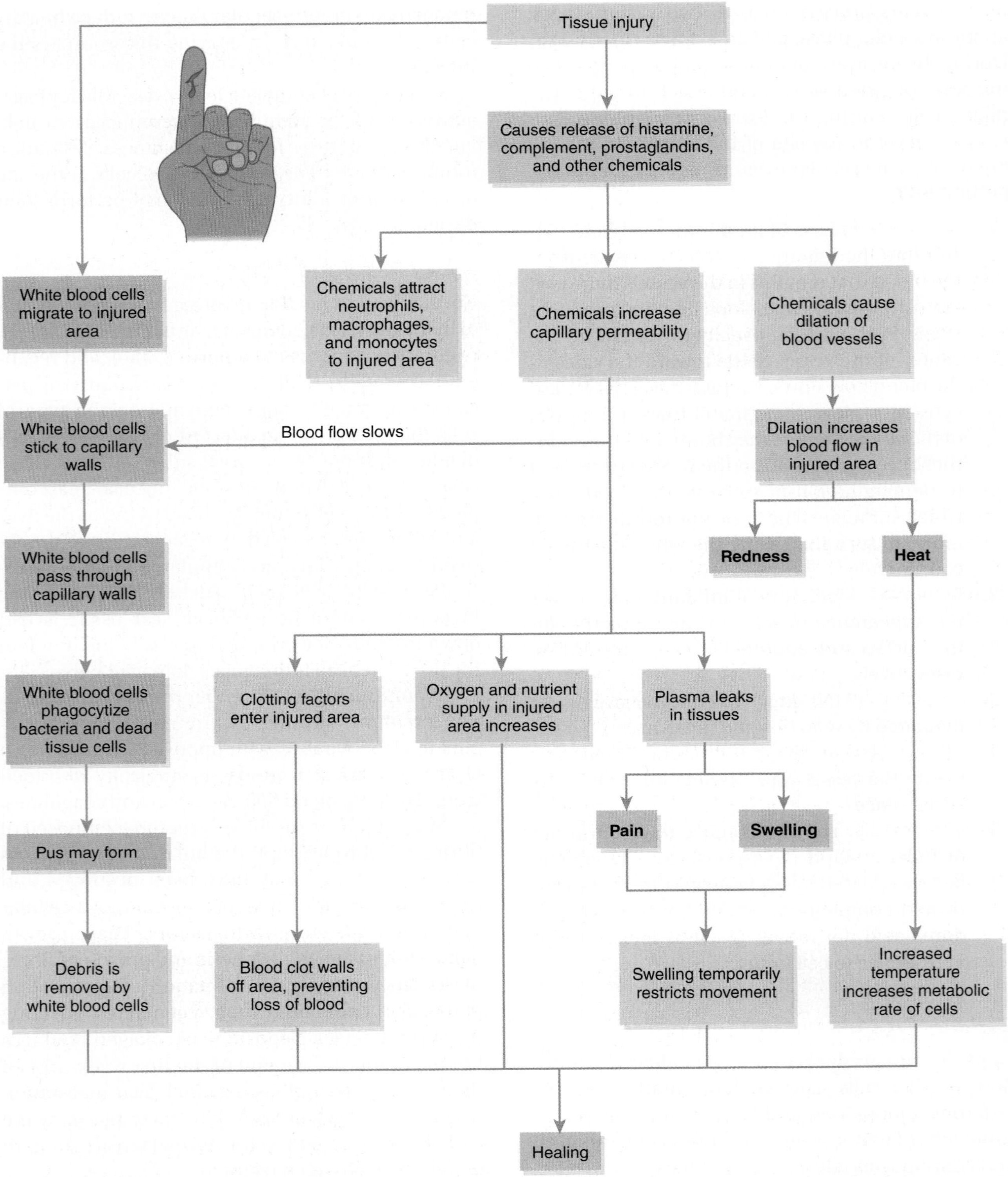

FIGURE 9-17 The inflammatory response.

granulation tissue. Wound contraction is mediated by myofibroblasts, which help to draw the margins of the wound closer to each other as time passes. Note that if infection is present, methods to promote secondary intention may be used, but the wound will not heal if the infection persists.

Dysfunctional Wound Healing

Factors that can lead to dysfunctional wound healing may be local or systemic. Local factors include infection, which diverts the body's healing efforts to fighting off the cause of the infection; an inadequate blood supply (as in diabetes) that produces tissue hypoxia, which slows wound healing and may promote infection; and foreign bodies in the wound, which stimulate acute and chronic inflammation, both of which interfere with wound healing.

Several systemic factors may also influence wound healing. Collagen is necessary for wound healing, but inadequate nutritional intake can lead to insufficient collagen levels, which in turn can lead to inadequate scar formation and suppression of the immune system. Anything that interferes with epithelialization—the process in which epithelial cells migrate upward and repair the wounded area along with the platelet-formed scab that protects the wound from the outside world—will prevent proper wound healing. *Wound contraction* is the process during which the size of the wound becomes smaller, as part of healing. Anything that interferes with wound contraction can also prevent healing.

Additional systemic factors that may disrupt wound healing include hematologic abnormalities, because proper wound healing requires adequate numbers of white blood cells. Patients who have impaired bone marrow stores of white blood cells are susceptible to infection and their wounds often heal more slowly. Diabetes and acquired immunodeficiency syndrome (AIDS) affect the cells of the immune system, which have a direct role in wound healing, and increase the likelihood of wound infection. Corticosteroids suppress the initial inflammatory response required for the proper formation of scar tissue and increase the risk of wound infection by slowing the immune system response.

Finally, if a wound separates—for example, from stress—this will slow the healing process. In such a case, healing needs to start over, at least to some extent.

Special Populations

Neonates and older adults often have relative impairment of their immune systems, potentially slowing their inflammatory responses. Consequently, signs of inflammation may be more subtle in these populations. In addition, wound healing often takes longer in these groups, especially in older patients. The immune system is not fully developed until a child is between 2 and 3 years old; therefore, you must be aggressive and thorough when you treat fever in younger children. Many experts recommend hospital admission for a temperature greater than 100.4°F (38°C) in a child younger than 3 months.

Chronic Inflammatory Responses

Chronic inflammatory responses are usually caused by an unsuccessful acute inflammatory response to a foreign body, a persistent infection, or the presence of an antigen. They are associated with formation of an infiltrate (pus) containing monocytes and lymphocytes and usually involve tissue destruction and repair (or scar formation). The vascular events are similar to those that take place in acute inflammation but also include the growth of new blood vessels, a process known as **angiogenesis**.

Variances in Immunity and Inflammation

Hypersensitivity

Hypersensitivity is any response of the body to any substance to which a patient has increased sensitivity. It is a generic term covering a variety of reactions. **Allergy** is a hypersensitivity reaction to the presence of an agent (allergen). **Autoimmunity** is the production of antibodies or T cells that work against the tissues of one's own body, producing hypersensitivity reactions or autoimmune disease (as in systemic lupus erythematosus [SLE]). **Isoimmunity** is the formation of T cells or antibodies directed against the antigens on another person's cells (typically after the transplantation of an organ or tissues). A blood transfusion reaction is an example of an isoimmune reaction to another person's red blood cells. The destruction of cells by antibodies or T cells may be an autoimmune or an isoimmune reaction.

Transient neonatal diseases refer to diseases that are present at birth but eventually resolve. Some examples include transient neonatal hyperglycemia, transient neonatal myasthenia gravis, and transient neonatal neutropenia. Transient neonatal diseases occur due to pathogenic immunoglobulins passing from the pregnant woman to the fetus during pregnancy. In some cases, the disease can become permanent, such as if pathogenic immunoglobulins develop in the infant.

Types of Hypersensitivity Reactions

A hypersensitivity reaction may be immediate, occurring within seconds to minutes, or delayed, occurring hours to days after exposure to an antigen. The speed of symptom evolution depends on the antigen and the type of response the body mounts against it. Hypersensitivity reactions are typically classified based on how the immune system caused the injury. **TABLE 9-6** describes the four types of injuries.

Type I: Immediate Hypersensitivity Reactions

A type I hypersensitivity reaction is an acute reaction that occurs in response to a stimulus, such as a bee sting, penicillin, or shellfish. The mechanism involves interaction between the stimulus (antigen) and a preformed antibody of the IgE type. At first exposure to a specific antigen, specific IgE antibodies bind to mast cells via the nonspecific region (Fc) portion. On secondary exposure to the same antigen, these bound antibodies are cross-linked by the antigen, resulting in degranulation of the mast cell and release of histamine and other mediators **FIGURE 9-18**. The released histamine feeds back on mast cells and eosinophils, leading to the release of additional histamine and other mediators. The severity of the symptoms that develop in a particular patient depends on the extent of mediator release.

The degree of severity of hypersensitivity reactions varies from severe, life-threatening reactions, such as anaphylaxis, to milder reactions, such as allergic rhinitis (edema and irritation of the nasal mucosa), bronchial asthma (bronchial constriction, mucus production, and airway inflammation), wheal and flare (such as an insect bite leading to vasodilation and swelling), and mild food allergy (leading to diarrhea, GI distress, and vomiting). A propensity toward type I reactions may be diagnosed through skin tests (such as the patch test and scratch test) and other laboratory procedures (ie, measurement of specific IgE antibody levels). Treatment focuses on avoiding the antigen, but desensitizing injections may be helpful in severe cases.

TABLE 9-6 Mechanisms of Immunologic Injury

Type	Mechanism	Examples
I: Immediate hypersensitivity reactions	IgE antibodies fix to mast cells and basophils. Later contact with a sensitizing antigen triggers mediator release and clinical manifestations.	Localized response: hay fever, food allergy Systemic response: bee sting, penicillin, anaphylaxis
II: Cytotoxic hypersensitivity reactions	Antibody binds to cell or tissue antigen, and a complement is activated, which damages the cell, causes inflammation, and promotes destruction of the antibody-coated cell by phagocytosis.	Autoimmune hemolytic anemia Blood transfusion reactions Rh hemolytic disease Some types of glomerulonephritis
III: Immune complex disease	Circulating antigen–antibody complexes form, which activate complement and cause inflammatory reaction.	Some types of glomerulonephritis Lupus erythematosus Rheumatoid arthritis
IV: Delayed (cell-mediated) hypersensitivity	Sensitized (delayed hypersensitivity) T cells release lymphokines, which attract macrophages and other inflammatory cells.	Tuberculosis Fungal and parasitic infections Contact dermatitis

Abbreviation: IgE, immunoglobulin E

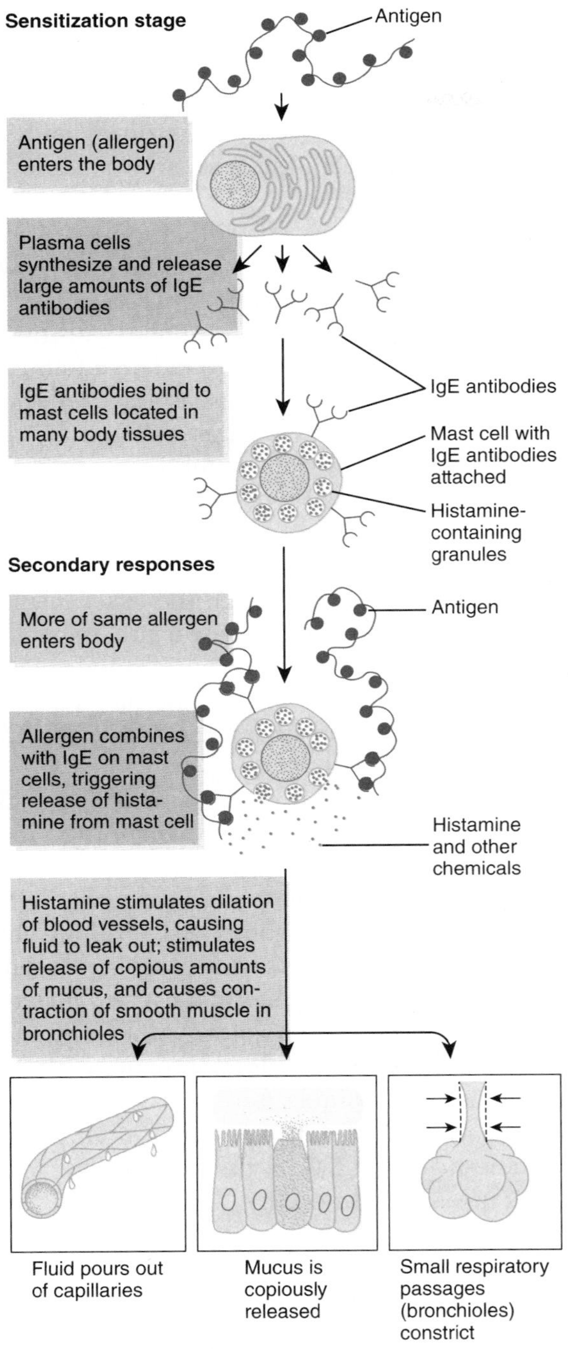
Sensitization stage
Antigen
Antigen (allergen) enters the body
Plasma cells synthesize and release large amounts of IgE antibodies
IgE antibodies bind to mast cells located in many body tissues
IgE antibodies
Mast cell with IgE antibodies attached
Histamine-containing granules
Secondary responses
More of same allergen enters body
Antigen
Allergen combines with IgE on mast cells, triggering release of histamine from mast cell
Histamine and other chemicals
Histamine stimulates dilation of blood vessels, causing fluid to leak out; stimulates release of copious amounts of mucus, and causes contraction of smooth muscle in bronchioles
Fluid pours out of capillaries
Mucus is copiously released
Small respiratory passages (bronchioles) constrict

FIGURE 9-18 Type I allergic reaction. The antigen stimulates the production of massive amounts of immunoglobulin E (IgE), a type of antibody produced by plasma cells, which then attaches to mast cells. This is a sensitization stage. When the antigen enters the body again, it binds to the IgE antibodies on the mast cells, triggering a massive release of histamine and other chemicals. Histamine causes blood vessels to dilate and become leaky, and promotes increased production of mucus in the respiratory tract. Mast cell degranulation may also cause bronchospasm in some people.

It is impossible to predict the severity of any given reaction. A person who has had a severe reaction in the past is at an increased risk for another one with subsequent antigen exposures. Always assume an IgE-mediated reaction could rapidly become a life-threatening event. These reactions need to be treated quickly in the field, and most prehospital providers are trained to administer epinephrine by using an epinephrine auto-injector or by giving a subcutaneous injection.

Type II: Cytotoxic Hypersensitivity

Type II hypersensitivity reactions are cytotoxic (cell destructive) and classically involve the combination of IgG or IgM antibodies with antigens on the cell membrane. Cells are lysed (destroyed) by complement fixation or by other antibodies. This process also destroys many of the body's healthy cells. Histamine release from mast cells is not involved, and IgG-mediated allergic responses occur within a few hours of antigen exposure. Examples of IgG-mediated responses include transfusion reactions and newborn hemolytic disease.

Type III: Tissue Injury Caused by Immune Complexes

Type III hypersensitivity responses involve primarily IgG antibodies that form immune complexes with antigen to recruit phagocytic cells, such as neutrophils, to a site where they can release inflammatory cytokines. Because histamine release from mast cells is not involved, IgG-mediated allergic responses occur within a few hours of antigen exposure. Reactions may be either systemic or localized.

The systemic form, called **serum sickness**, results from a large, single exposure to an antigen, such as horse antibody serum. Antigen–antibody complexes formed in the bloodstream are then deposited in sites around the body, most notably in the kidney, with resultant inflammatory reactions (such as serum sickness from penicillin). Signs and symptoms of serum sickness may include fever, malaise, rashes, joint aches, lymphadenopathy, and splenomegaly.

The localized form of a type III response is called an Arthus reaction. Arthus reactions consist of a circumscribed area of vascular inflammation (**vasculitis**). An example of an Arthus reaction is farmer's lung, a type of hypersensitivity pneumonitis reaction in the lung caused by inhalation of moldy hay dust.

Type IV: Delayed (Cell-Mediated) Hypersensitivity

Type IV allergic responses, also known as cell-mediated hypersensitivity, are primarily mediated by soluble molecules released by specifically activated T cells. These reactions are classified into two subtypes: delayed hypersensitivity and cell-mediated cytotoxicity.

Delayed hypersensitivity involves lymphocytes and macrophages. T cells respond to an antigen and activate CD4 (helper T cell) lymphocytes. These lymphocytes release mediators that are designed to destroy the foreign substance. An example of a delayed hypersensitivity response is contact hypersensitivity to poison ivy.

Cell-mediated cytotoxicity involves only sensitized T cells (CD8 lymphocytes or **killer T cells**). These cells kill the antigen-bearing target cells rather than activating the CD4 lymphocytes to do so. Examples include the body's response to viral infections, tumor immune surveillance, and the mechanism by which transplant rejection occurs.

Targets of Hypersensitivity Reactions

The immune system targets different molecules, depending on the type of hypersensitivity reaction. In allergic reactions, the target is an antigen or allergen. Allergens are substances that cause a hypersensitivity reaction, such as those listed in **TABLE 9-7**.

TABLE 9-7 Allergens That Can Cause Hypersensitivity Reactions

Type	Examples
Inhalants	Pollen, dust, smoke, fungi, plastic, odors
Food	Eggs, dairy, wheat, chocolate, strawberries
Drugs	Aspirin, antibiotics, serums, codeine
Infectious agents	Bacteria, viruses, fungi, animal parasites
Contactants	Animals, plants, metals, chemicals
Physical agents	Light, pressure, radiation, heat and cold

Autoimmune Reactions

In autoimmune reactions, the target is the person's own tissues. For reasons that are unclear, normal tolerance of "self" tissues breaks down and the immune system treats the body's own tissues as foreign.

Graves disease is an autoimmune disease caused by thyroid-stimulating or thyroid-growth immunoglobulins. These antibodies activate receptors for thyroid-stimulating hormone, causing increased activity by the thyroid gland. In addition to hyperthyroidism, Graves disease is associated with characteristic eye changes (lid retraction, stare, and exophthalmos [protrusion of the eyes]) and skin changes (pretibial myxedema: localized edematous skin in the pretibial area).

Type 1 diabetes mellitus is also considered an autoimmune disease. Although the exact insult is unknown (but is suspected to be a viral infection), some agent stimulates the body to produce autoantibodies against beta cells in the pancreas that produce insulin. The result is a deficiency of insulin and, therefore, diabetes.

Rheumatoid arthritis is a chronic systemic disease that affects the entire body. One of the most common forms of arthritis, it is characterized by inflammation of the synovium (the connective tissue membrane lining the joint) with resulting pain, stiffness, warmth, redness, and swelling. Inflammatory cells release enzymes that cause damage to bone and cartilage. The involved joint can lose its shape and alignment, resulting in pain and loss of movement. Rheumatoid arthritis is associated with the formation of rheumatoid factor, that is, IgM antibodies to tissue IgG. In the joints, the synovial membrane is thickened due to infiltration of inflammatory cells (lymphocytes).

Myasthenia gravis is an acquired autoimmune disease that is characterized by an autoimmune attack on the nerve-muscle junction. The circulating autoantibodies cause abnormal muscle fatigability. They typically affect the smallest motor units first, such as the extraocular muscles, producing ptosis (droopy eyelid) and diplopia (double vision). Other muscles may be involved as well, leading to problems such as difficulty swallowing (dysphagia). Characteristically, repeated contraction of the affected muscles makes the symptoms worse. Two-thirds of people with myasthenia gravis have thymic abnormalities, with the most common being thymic hyperplasia. A minority of people have a tumor of the thymus, called a thymoma.

Neutropenia refers to a decrease in circulating neutrophils. Neutrophils are usually the first immune cells to arrive at the scene of an infection, where they scavenge pathogenic microorganisms so infection cannot spread. Once the neutrophils are fully used up, they die and become part of the yellow wound drainage (pus). When a patient has neutropenia, an insufficient neutrophil level decreases the body's ability to fight infection. Isoimmune neutropenia refers to this condition in a neonate. It develops when a pregnant woman produces antibodies against neutrophils, which then cross the placenta and cause neutropenia in the fetus.

Idiopathic thrombocytopenic purpura (ITP), also known as immune thrombocytopenic purpura, is a blood disorder in which antibodies form to blood platelets and cause their destruction. Thrombocytopenia describes a decrease in blood platelets; purpura is purple areas of the skin and mucous membranes (such as the lining of the mouth) where bleeding has occurred as a result of decreased numbers of platelets or ineffective platelets. Some cases of ITP are caused by certain types of medications, whereas others are associated with infection, pregnancy, or immune disorders such as SLE.[9] Approximately one-half of all cases are classified as idiopathic, meaning their cause is unknown.

Bleeding is the main symptom of ITP and can include bruising and tiny red dots on the skin or mucous membranes. In some cases, bleeding from the nose, gums, and digestive or urinary tracts may occur. Rarely, patients may have bleeding within the brain.

Treatment of idiopathic ITP is based on the severity of the symptoms and the patient's platelet count. In some cases, no therapy is needed. In most cases, drugs that alter the immune system's attack on the platelets are prescribed, such as corticosteroids (eg, prednisone) and IV infusions of immunoglobulin. Another treatment that usually increases the number of platelets is removal of the spleen, the organ that destroys antibody-coated platelets.

SLE is a chronic autoimmune disease with many manifestations, but whose cause is not known. In SLE, the body's immune system is directed against the body's tissues. Although this disease is more common in young women, it can occur in either sex at any age. The production of autoantibodies leads to formation of immune complexes, which can then be deposited in the glomeruli, skin, lungs, synovium, and mesothelium, among other places. Symptoms include arthritis, a red rash over the nose and cheeks, fatigue, weakness, fever, and photosensitivity. Glomerulonephritis (kidney disease), pericarditis, anemia, and neuritis may develop. In addition, many people with SLE have renal complications from overproduction or underproduction of a hormone, as described in **TABLE 9-8**.

Immune Deficiencies

Immunodeficiency is an abnormal condition in which some part of the body's immune system is inadequate, so that resistance to infectious diseases is decreased. It may be congenital or acquired.

TABLE 9-8 Effects of Inappropriate Hormone Production

Hormone	Gland	Underproduction	Overproduction
Growth hormone (GH)	Anterior pituitary	Pituitary dwarfism	Acromegaly
Antidiuretic hormone (ADH)	Posterior pituitary	Diabetes insipidus	Syndrome of inappropriate antidiuretic hormone (SIADH)
Thyroxine (T_4), triiodothyronine (T_3)	Thyroid	Myxedema coma	Graves disease
Parathyroid hormone (PTH)	Parathyroid	Hyperparathyroidism	Hypothyroidism
Cortisol	Adrenal	Addison disease	Cushing disease
Insulin	Pancreas	Diabetes mellitus	

Congenital Immunodeficiencies

Patients with severe combined immunodeficiency disease (SCID) have defects that involve lymphoid stem cells. Consequently, T cells (cellular immunity) and B cells (humoral immunity) are affected. Patients with SCID are at risk for infection with all types of organisms—bacteria, mycobacteria, fungi, viruses, parasites, and prions. There are two forms of this disease, both of which are inherited.

X-linked agammaglobulinemia (XLA) is one of the most common forms of inherited primary immunodeficiency and occurs predominantly in males. XLA results in a decrease in the level of mature B cells,[10] which results in a decreased ability to produce antibodies, and therefore decreased ability to effectively protect against bacteria and viruses.[10,11]

This process results in a markedly decreased level of all immunoglobulins and of mature B lymphocytes; however, T lymphocytes function normally. Recurrent pyrogenic infections develop, but patients have no problems with fungal and viral infections because their cell-mediated immunity is unaffected. These infections first emerge in affected infants at about 6 months of age, when the level of maternal immunoglobulin has decreased.

Isolated deficiency of IgA is probably the most common form of immunodeficiency. This disease results from blocking of the terminal differentiation of B lymphocytes. Most patients are asymptomatic, but some may experience chronic sinus infections. Patients also have an increased incidence of autoimmune disease.

Acquired Immunodeficiencies

Any nutritional deficiency can hamper normal immune function and the inflammatory response. Nutritional deficiencies may depress bone marrow function and diminish white blood cell development. A lack of protein in the diet, for example, decreases the liver's ability to manufacture inflammatory mediators and plasma proteins.

The stress of trauma can also cause immunodeficiency. Other contributors to this condition may include hypoperfusion or shock, mediator production, damage to vital organs, and the decreased nutrition occurring during trauma states.

Medications most often cause iatrogenic (treatment-induced) immunodeficiency. For example, corticosteroids, whether taken orally or inhaled, suppress the immune system. This immune system suppression is often of therapeutic benefit. However, in a small number of patients, the immunosuppression leads to other diseases, such as tuberculosis. Because of the potential adverse effects of corticosteroids, physicians are usually cautious

YOU are the Paramedic

PART 4

Your partner reports that all of the patient's medication bottles are out of date and empty. You ask the patient about this issue, and he states he does not have the means necessary to buy the medications. When you look at the list of medications, you find one for a diuretic. Your cardiac monitor indicates a sinus tachycardia matching the pulse rate. No ectopy is noted. The $ETCO_2$ waveform appears appropriate in shape and reads 36 mm Hg.

Recording Time: 7 Minutes	
Respirations	24 breaths/min; shallow
Pulse	114 beats/min
Skin	Cool, pale, and moist
Blood pressure	138/88 mm Hg
Oxygen saturation (Spo_2)	92% with CPAP administration
Pupils	PERRLA

7. Why would a diuretic be prescribed for a patient with heart failure?

8. Why would this patient have a normal or slightly high BP?

about prescribing this therapy for a prolonged period. In addition, idiosyncratic reactions to antibiotics may cause bone marrow suppression. Bone marrow suppression in cancer is often a direct side effect of chemotherapy, rather than a true idiosyncratic reaction.

Physical or mental stress has been shown to decrease white blood cell and lymphocyte function. It may also lead to decreased production of various antibodies.

AIDS is an immunodeficiency disease caused by HIV, an RNA retrovirus. HIV binds to the CD4 surface protein of helper T cells, infects these cells, and kills them. The destruction of the cells causes decreased humoral and cell-mediated reactions.

Treatment of Immunodeficiencies

Replacement therapy is available for immunodeficiencies such as common variable immunodeficiency. IV gamma globulin has been used as a therapy for many immunologic disorders of the nervous system, especially myasthenia gravis and inflammatory neuropathies, with considerable success. Bone marrow transplantation may restore immune competence in patients with acquired causes of immunodeficiency, such as following chemotherapy to treat cancer. Transfusion is another form of replacement therapy for immunodeficiencies. In the future, gene therapy may be useful to treat congenital and acquired causes of immunodeficiency.

Factors That Cause Disease

A variety of genetic, environmental, age-related, and sex-associated factors can cause or contribute to disease. Genetic factors are present at birth and are passed on through a person's genes to future generations. Environmental factors include microorganisms, immunologic vulnerabilities, personal habits and lifestyle, exposure to chemicals and other toxins, the physical environment, and the psychosocial environment. Family violence, for example, might be a key factor in causing depression or substance abuse, perhaps even years after it occurs. A sedentary lifestyle and a high-fat diet can contribute to obesity, diabetes, heart disease, stroke, and other diseases.

Disease can also have anatomic causes. For example, malrotation of the colon is a condition in which the colon does not form properly, resulting in partial blockage. Another example is degenerative diseases of the spine; as intervertebral disks age, they may degenerate to the extent that the patient experiences pain due to nerve compression. *Aortic stenosis* is a condition in which the aortic valve becomes very tight and narrowed, resulting in chest pain from decreased perfusion of the coronary arteries or heart failure.

Finally, an immunologic reaction may result in disease. An example is exposure to an agent that triggers an abnormal immune response against myelin, leading to the development of multiple sclerosis.

Controllable Versus Uncontrollable Risk Factors

Some uncontrollable factors, such as genetics and race, influence disease development, but many other factors can be controlled. For example, behaviors such as smoking, drinking alcohol, inadequate nutrition (excessive fat, salt, and sugar intake or insufficient intake of protein, fruits, vegetables, and fiber), lack of physical activity, and stress can be modified.

Age-Related Risk

The risk of a particular disease often depends on a person's age. For example, newborns are at greater risk of certain diseases because their immune systems are not fully developed (see Chapter 43, *Neonatal Care*). Teenagers are at high risk of injury due to trauma and illicit drug and alcohol use. The risk of having cancer, heart disease, stroke, and Alzheimer disease increases with age (see Chapter 45, *Geriatric Emergencies*).

Sex-Associated Factors

In some cases, sex is related to the risk of having a certain disease. Note that a person's physical sex and gender are not necessarily the same. In this discussion, we are referring to a person's genetic sex; for example, a person born with an XY sex chromosome is genetically and physically male, even if the person's gender is female.

Some diseases (eg, AMI) present differently in women compared with men. For example, the hormones found in premenopausal women have been shown to have protective benefits in major head trauma and certain cardiac conditions.

Finally, genetic disorders are related to a person's sex when the defective gene is located on a sex chromosome. Most sex-linked disorders are X linked. X-linked disorders may be either recessive or dominant. Because females have two X chromosomes, those with a defective X gene may not have the disorder; if the disorder is recessive, the X chromosome without the defect will mask the defective X chromosome. Men with a defective X gene will always be affected because they have only one X chromosome, so the defect cannot be masked.

Analysis of Disease Risk

Analyzing disease risk involves considering both disease rates and disease risk factors (causal and noncausal). Risk factors that can directly cause a disease to develop are called causal risk factors. For example, *Mycobacterium tuberculosis* is a causal risk factor for a person becoming infected with tuberculosis. Risk factors that are associated with risk for a disease but are not a direct cause of that disease are called *noncausal risk factors.* For example, poverty is a noncausal risk factor for tuberculosis.

All studies of a disease should consider the incidence, prevalence, morbidity, and mortality of the disease. The **incidence** is the number of new cases of a disease in a population (eg, six cases of West Nile virus infection were identified in the county). **Prevalence** refers to the number of cases of a disease or condition in a particular population within a particular period (eg, last year, more than 100,000 patients had this disease). **Morbidity** refers to the presence of disease or to the incidence or prevalence of a disease. **Mortality** is most often discussed as the mortality rate, which is the number of deaths from a disease in a given population, expressed as a proportion (eg, 1 in 50 affected people in the United States). **TABLE 9-9** illustrates how the concepts of incidence, prevalence, morbidity, and mortality might be expressed, using statistics for diabetes as an example.

Interaction of Risk Factors

Risk factors, age, and sex differences often interact to affect the likelihood of a person having a disease. For example, suppose a person has a genetic tendency toward coronary artery disease; the risk of myocardial infarction or sudden death is higher in this person even if they exercise regularly and have no other risk factors. A person who smokes heavily but has no other risk factors may have a similarly elevated risk. **TABLE 9-10** shows the interplay of various risk factors in causing respiratory disease.

Common Familial Diseases and Associated Risk Factors

The terms *genetic risk* and *familial tendency* are often used interchangeably. A true genetic risk is one that is passed through generations by inheritance of a gene. In contrast, with a familial tendency, diseases seem to cluster in family groups even though there is no evidence of heritable gene-associated abnormalities.

TABLE 9-11 lists some of the traits and diseases carried on human chromosomes. An **autosomal recessive** pattern of inheritance involves genes located on autosomes (ie, any chromosome other than sex chromosomes). A person needs to inherit

TABLE 9-9 Incidence, Prevalence, Morbidity, and Mortality Rates of Diabetes in the United States

Term	Example
Incidence	Every year, 1.5 million Americans are newly diagnosed with type 1 or type 2 diabetes. In 2015, an additional 88 million Americans age 18 years and older were newly categorized as prediabetic.
Prevalence	In 2018, 10.5% of the total US population (adults and children) had diabetes.
Mortality rate	In 2017, diabetes was responsible for or a key contributor to the deaths of 270,702 people.
Financial cost	In 2017, Americans spent $237 billion treating diagnosed diabetes, and the disease cost the US economy another $90 billion in reduced productivity.

Data from: Centers for Disease Control and Prevention. *National Diabetes Statistics Report, 2020.* Atlanta, GA: US Department of Health and Human Services; 2020. https://www.cdc.gov/diabetes/data/statistics/statistics-report.html. Accessed July 28, 2020; American Diabetes Association. Statistics about diabetes. http://www.diabetes.org/diabetes-basics/statistics/. Accessed July 28, 2020.

TABLE 9-10 Common Respiratory Diseases

Disease	Pathology and/or Symptoms	Causes and Possible Contributing Causes
Emphysema	Breakdown of alveoli, shortness of breath	Smoking Air pollution Possible genetic susceptibility Exacerbated by obesity
Chronic bronchitis	Cough, shortness of breath	Smoking Air pollution Possible genetic susceptibility Exacerbated by obesity
Acute bronchitis	Inflammation of the bronchi; coughing up yellow mucus; shortness of breath	Many viruses and bacteria Possible genetic susceptibility Smoking Exacerbated by obesity
Sinusitis	Inflammation of the sinuses; characterized by mucus discharge, blocked nasal passages, and headache	Many viruses and bacteria Poor general health
Laryngitis	Inflammation of larynx and vocal cords, sore throat, hoarseness, mucus buildup, and cough	Many viruses and bacteria Poor general health
Pneumonia	Inflammation of the lungs, ranging from mild to severe; cough and fever, shortness of breath at rest, chills, sweating, chest pain, blood-tinged mucus	Bacteria, viruses, fungi, or inhalation of irritating gases Lack of physical activity
Asthma	Constriction of bronchioles, mucus buildup in bronchioles, periodic wheezing, difficulty breathing	Allergy to pollen, certain foods, food additives, dander (dead skin cells and other debris shed by dogs, cats, or birds) Physical activity (exercise-induced asthma) Probable genetic link

TABLE 9-11 Traits and Diseases Carried on Human Chromosomes

Trait or Disease	Result
Autosomal Recessive	
Albinism	Lack of pigment in eyes, skin, and hair
Cystic fibrosis	Pancreatic failure, mucus buildup in lungs
Sickle cell anemia	Abnormal hemoglobin characterized by sickle-shaped red blood cells that obstruct vital capillaries
Tay-Sachs disease	Improper metabolism of gangliosides in nerve cells
Phenylketonuria	Accumulation of phenylalanine in blood; causes mental retardation
Attached earlobe	Earlobe attached to skin of the neck
Hyperextensible thumb	Thumb bends past a 45° angle

(continues)

TABLE 9-11 Traits and Diseases Carried on Human Chromosomes (continued)

Trait or Disease	Result
Autosomal Dominant	
Achondroplasia	Dwarfism resulting from a defect in the epiphyseal plates that interferes with the formation of long bones
Marfan syndrome	Defect of connective tissue resulting in excessive growth and a high risk of aortic rupture
Widow's peak	Hairline coming to a point on the forehead
Huntington disease	Progressive deterioration of the nervous system beginning in a person's late 20s or early 30s; causes mental deterioration and early death
Brachydactyly	Disfiguration of hands, shortened fingers
Freckles	Permanent aggregations of melanin in the skin

two copies of a particular form of a gene to show that trait. A parent who carries the gene for an autosomal recessive trait but does not display the trait has a 25% chance of passing the inherited condition to their child if the other parent is also a carrier for the trait. If both parents have the inherited condition, then all of their children will have the condition. Hemochromatosis, which causes the accumulation of too much iron in the body, has an autosomal recessive pattern of inheritance: a person must inherit a copy of the hemochromatosis gene from each parent for the disease to manifest.

In **autosomal dominant** inheritance, a person needs to inherit only one copy of a particular form of a gene to show that trait; it does not matter which form of the gene is inherited from the other parent. A parent has at least a 50% chance of passing on an autosomal dominant inherited condition to their child. Familial adenomatous polyposis, which places people at extremely high risk for colorectal (colon) cancer, has an autosomal dominant pattern of inheritance.

Immunologic Disorders

Immunologic diseases are caused by hyperactivity or hypoactivity of the immune system. Most immunologic diseases that exhibit familial tendencies involve an overactive immune system (eg, allergies, asthma, rheumatic fever). Significant overlap often exists among causative factors, including the person's environment.

Special Populations

Rheumatic fever is an inflammatory disease that occurs primarily in children. This disease results from a delayed reaction to an untreated streptococcal infection of the upper respiratory tract (such as strep throat). Symptoms, which appear several weeks after the acute infection, may include fever, abdominal pain, vomiting, arthritis, palpitations, and chest pain. Recurrent episodes of rheumatic fever may cause permanent myocardial damage, especially to the cardiac valves. A family history of acute rheumatic fever may predispose a person to the disease.

Allergies are acquired following initial exposure to an allergen. Repeated exposures then cause the immune system to react to the allergen **FIGURE 9-19**. Although the clinical presentation varies, it usually includes swelling and itching, runny nose, coughing, sneezing, wheezing, and nasal congestion. A person who has an allergic tendency is said to be **atopic**. Environmental conditions may also increase a person's susceptibility to an allergic reaction.

Asthma is a chronic inflammatory condition of the lower airway resulting in intermittent wheezing and excess mucus production. Viral infections precipitate nearly 60% of asthma attacks, allergies account for another 20%, and stress and emotions cause the remainder. In addition to the familial component, chromosomal differences in certain patients may enhance their susceptibility to asthma.

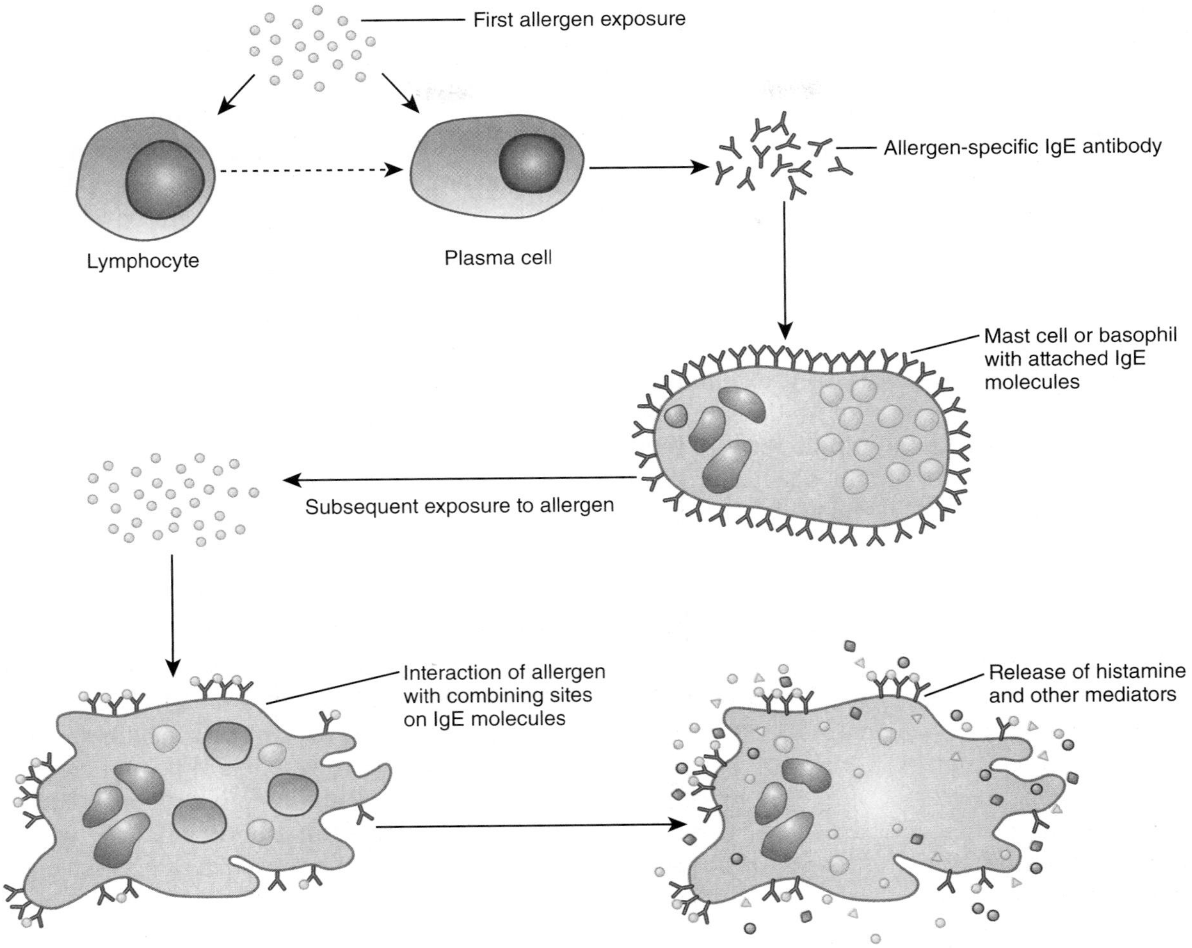

FIGURE 9-19 Pathogenesis of allergy. The first exposure to an allergen induces formation of specific IgE antibodies in susceptible patients; these antibodies bind to mast cells and basophils. Subsequent exposure to the same allergen leads to antigen–antibody interaction by activating memory cells, liberating histamine and other mediators from mast cells and basophils. These mediators induce allergic manifestations.

Cancer

Cancer describes the pathology associated with malignant growths (neoplasms) in various anatomic areas of the human body. Essentially, all cancers are inappropriate tissue growth due to unregulated cellular division. Mutations in DNA sometimes affect the genes that control cell division. The more mutations, the more aggressive the cancer's growth will be and the more difficult it is to regain control of those cells. The prognosis often depends on the extent of the cancer's spread (metastasis) and the effectiveness of treatment.

A major risk factor associated with lung cancer is cigarette smoking. Research has identified eight alterations in the genetic material of lung cancers that suggest a genetic tendency to develop the disease. Other predisposing factors include exposure to asbestos, coal products, and other industrial and chemical products. Symptoms include cough, difficulty breathing, blood-tinged sputum, and repeated infections. Treatment depends on the type, site, and extent of the cancer and may include surgery, chemotherapy, and/or radiotherapy.

Breast cancer is the most common type of cancer among women. The American Cancer Society reported 316,120 new cases of breast cancer in the United States in 2017 and 40,610 deaths from breast cancer.[12] Women whose first-degree relatives (ie, parent, sister, or daughter) have breast cancer are more likely to have the disease. Risk varies with the age at which the affected relative was diagnosed: The younger the age at occurrence, the greater the risk posed to relatives. Approximately 5% to 10% of patients with breast cancer have a pattern of autosomal dominant inheritance, in which cancer predisposition is transmitted from generation to generation.[13] This susceptibility may be inherited through either the mother's or the father's side of the family.

Early symptoms of breast cancer are usually detected by the woman during breast self-examination and include a small, painless lump, thick or dimpled skin, or a change in the nipple **FIGURE 9-20**. Later symptoms include nipple discharge, pain, and swollen lymph glands in the axilla. Treatment depends on the location, size, and metastasis of the tumor.

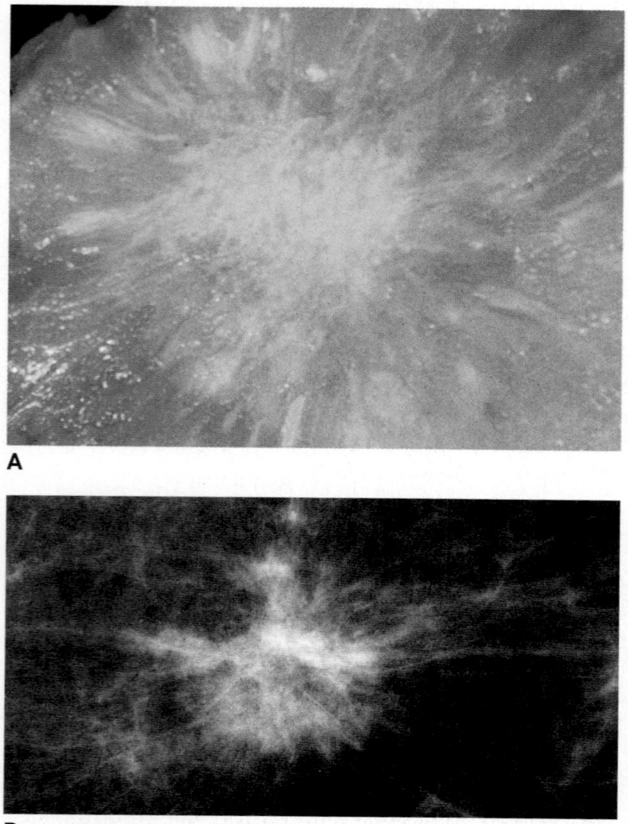

A

B

FIGURE 9-20 Breast carcinoma. **A.** Cross-section of breast biopsy specimen. The tumor appears as a firm mass with poorly defined edges that infiltrate the surrounding fatty breast tissue. **B.** Appearance of breast carcinoma in a mammogram. The tumor appears as a white area with infiltrating margins.

Colorectal cancer is the third most common type of cancer in men and women. In 2021, the American Cancer Society reports an expected 149,500 new cases and an estimated 52,980 deaths from colorectal cancer in the United States.[14] Relatives of people diagnosed with colorectal cancer are more likely to have the disease themselves, and parents can pass on to their children changes in certain genes that can lead to colorectal cancer. Symptoms may be minimal, consisting only of small amounts of blood in the stool. Treatment involves surgery and sometimes chemotherapy. Periodic rectal examinations and colonoscopy are recommended for adults age 45 years and older to detect the disease at an early stage.[14]

Endocrine Disorders

Diabetes mellitus is one of the most significant endocrine diseases. This chronic disorder of metabolism is associated with partial insulin secretion or total lack of insulin secretion by the pancreas, which affects the body's ability to use glucose. Symptoms include excessive thirst and urination, weight abnormalities, and the presence of excessive glucose in the urine and the blood.

Type 1 diabetes is also known as insulin-dependent diabetes mellitus (or ketoacidosis-prone diabetes) because patients need exogenous insulin to survive. Type 2 diabetes is called non–insulin-dependent diabetes (or non–ketoacidosis-prone diabetes), even though many people with type 2 diabetes require exogenous insulin injections. Both forms have a hereditary predisposition. Type 1 diabetes has no known cure (other than pancreas transplantation) at the present time; type 2 diabetes can occasionally be brought under control with weight loss, regular physical activity, and medications.

Hematologic Disorders

Hemolytic anemia is characterized by increased destruction of red blood cells. This disorder has several causes, such as an Rh factor blood transfusion reaction (which would most likely occur in the neonate population), a disorder of the immune system, and exposure to bacterial toxins or chemicals such as benzene. **FIGURE 9-21** depicts how the body handles iron. Hemolytic anemia following an

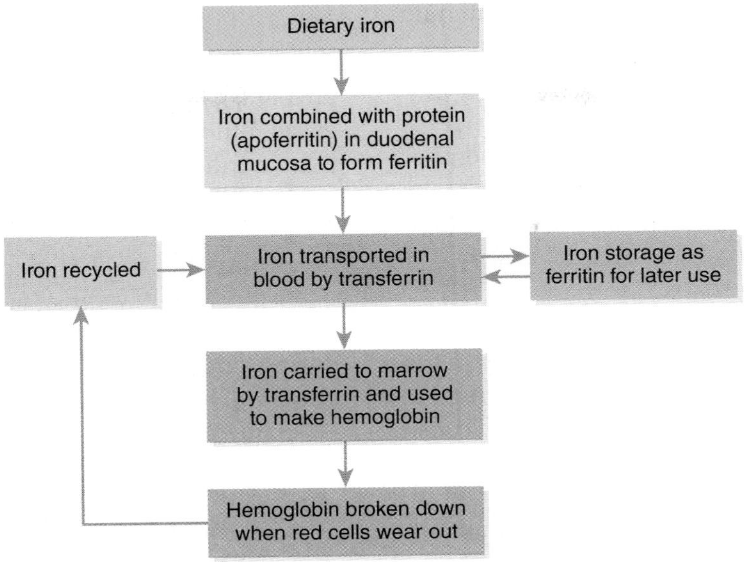

FIGURE 9-21 Iron uptake, transport, storage, and utilization for hemoglobin synthesis. Most of the iron used for hemoglobin synthesis is recycled from worn-out red blood cells. Chronic blood loss removes iron-containing cells from the circulation, and the iron contained in the red blood cells can no longer be recycled to make hemoglobin, leading to iron-deficiency anemia.

aspirin overdose or penicillin administration is rare; it is much more common, albeit still rare, with sulfa drugs used to treat urinary tract infections, such as the trimethoprim-sulfamethoxazole combination (known as Septra and Bactrim). An inherited enzyme deficiency (glucose-6-phosphatase dehydrogenase deficiency) markedly increases a person's susceptibility to sulfa drug–induced hemolytic anemia.

Hemophilia is an inherited disorder characterized by excessive bleeding. It is a sex-linked condition, occurring predominantly in males, and is passed from asymptomatic mothers to sons.[15] In this disorder, one of the blood-clotting proteins (usually factor VIII) necessary for normal blood coagulation is missing or is present in abnormally low amounts. Patients experience greater-than-usual blood loss in dental extractions and following simple injuries. They may also have bleeding into joints and, rarely, into the brain. Treatment consists of administration of the missing blood-clotting factors.

Hemochromatosis is an inherited (autosomal recessive) disease in which the body absorbs more iron than it needs. The excess iron is stored in various organs, including the liver, kidneys, and pancreas. Hemochromatosis can lead to diabetes, heart disease, liver disease, arthritis, impotence, and a bronzed skin color. These symptoms can be avoided by regularly drawing blood (phlebotomy).

Cardiovascular Disorders

Several cardiovascular disorders are known to follow specific patterns of inheritance. Still others have strong familial tendencies (such as coronary heart disease).

Long QT Syndrome

Long QT syndrome is a cardiac conduction system abnormality characterized by prolongation of the QT interval on the ECG. Because most cases of long QT syndrome are inherited in an autosomal dominant manner, all first-degree relatives of affected people must be screened. Sometimes these syndromes are associated with congenital hearing loss, hypertrophic cardiomyopathy, or mitral valve prolapse (MVP). Patients are at risk for palpitations and ventricular dysrhythmias, especially torsades de pointes. Many patients are asymptomatic until they have a dysrhythmia that causes syncope or sudden death. Always consider syncope under the following conditions to be due to a life-threatening dysrhythmia until proven otherwise:

- Exercise-induced syncope
- Syncope associated with chest pain
- A history of syncope in a close family member (ie, parent, sibling, or child)
- Syncope associated with startle (eg, loud noises such as phones or alarm clocks)

Cardiomyopathy

Cardiomyopathy is a general term for diseases of the myocardium (heart muscle) that ultimately progress to heart failure, AMI, or death. These diseases cause the heart muscle to become thin, flabby, dilated, or enlarged. One variant, known as hypertrophic cardiomyopathy, is genetically autosomal dominant. The main feature of hypertrophic cardiomyopathy is an excessive thickening of the heart muscle (hypertrophy means to thicken or grow excessively) **FIGURE 9-22**. In addition, microscopic examination of the heart muscle shows that it is abnormal. Patients may have shortness of breath, chest pains, palpitations, or syncope; sudden cardiac death is also possible. Beta blockers are an effective treatment in some patients. Others require surgery or an implantable cardiac defibrillator, which is designed to deliver a shock to the heart to restore its normal rhythm.

Mitral Valve Prolapse

Also referred to as a floppy mitral valve, MVP is relatively common. A familial tendency toward MVP exists, but the condition is usually associated with other cardiovascular conditions. In MVP, the mitral valve leaflets balloon into the left atrium during systole. Although this condition is often benign and asymptomatic, some patients have chest pain, fatigue, dizziness, dyspnea, or palpitations. Generally, the only physical finding is a clicking sound heard during cardiac auscultation. A small number of patients will have cardiac dysrhythmias.

Sometimes MVP leads to mitral regurgitation (also called mitral insufficiency), in which a large amount of blood leaks backward through the defective valve. Mitral regurgitation can lead to thickening or enlargement of the heart wall, due to the extra pumping of the heart needed to make up for the backflow of blood. It sometimes causes people to feel tired or short of breath. Mitral regurgitation usually can be treated with medication, but some people need surgery to repair or replace the defective valve.

Coronary Heart Disease

Coronary heart disease, often called coronary artery disease, is caused by impaired circulation to the heart. Typically, patients have occluded coronary

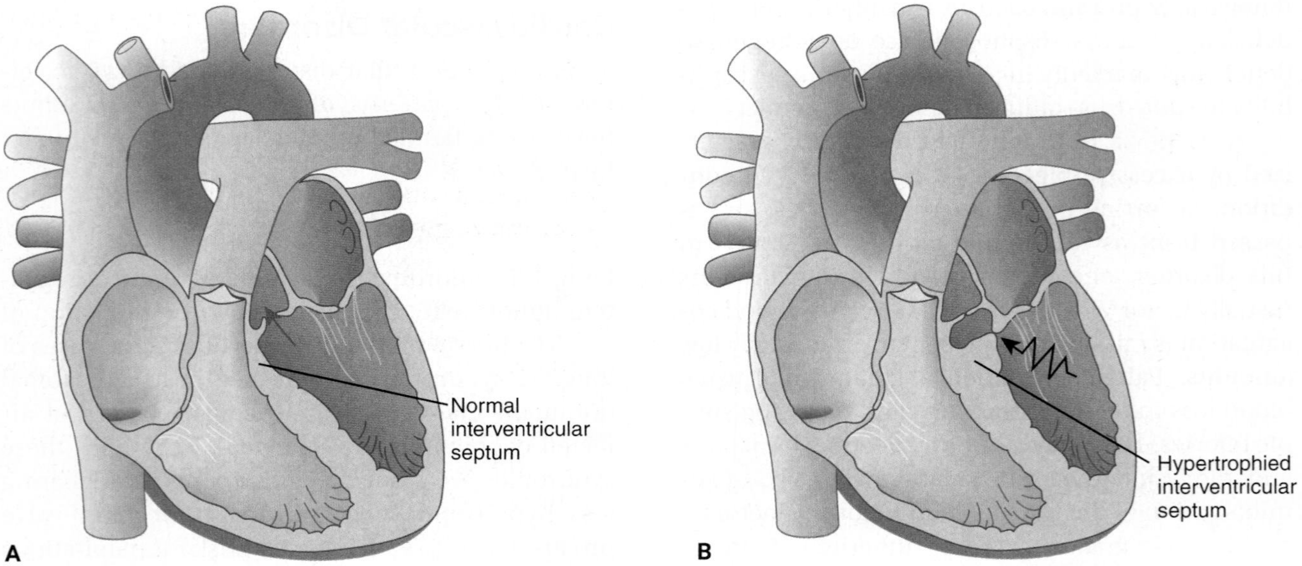

FIGURE 9-22 Comparison of normal cardiac function with malfunction characteristic of hypertrophic cardiomyopathy.
A. Normal heart, illustrating the unobstructed flow of blood from the left ventricle into the aorta during ventricular systole.
B. Hypertrophic cardiomyopathy, illustrating obstruction to the outflow of blood from the left ventricle by the hypertrophied septum, which impinges on the anterior leaflet of the mitral valve.

arteries from atherosclerotic plaque buildup. The effects can range from ischemia to infarction and necrosis (death) of the myocardium. Almost one-half of all cardiovascular deaths are caused by coronary heart disease.[16] This condition has a familial tendency; significant risk factors for coronary artery disease development include having a father who had an AMI or died suddenly younger than 55 years or having a mother who had an AMI or died suddenly younger than 65 years. Other risk factors include hypercholesterolemia, cigarette smoking, hypertension, age (as age increases, the risk for coronary heart disease increases), and diabetes.

Hypercholesterolemia is an elevation of the blood cholesterol level. The blood cholesterol level is divided into two portions: high-density lipoprotein (HDL; "good cholesterol") and low-density lipoprotein (LDL; "bad cholesterol"). Even though a patient might have a normal total cholesterol level, the presence of an abnormally low level of HDL and/or an elevation of LDL increases the risk of coronary heart disease.

Hypertension and Stroke

Hypertension (high BP) is associated with an increased risk of coronary artery disease and is also strongly associated with an increased risk of stroke. Risk factors for developing hypertension can be categorized as genetic or lifestyle-related. They include age (as age increases, the risk increases), race (more common in African Americans), sex (men are more likely to experience hypertension), family history, obesity or being overweight, sedentary lifestyle, tobacco use, diet (too much salt, too little potassium, too little vitamin D, too much alcohol), and stress.

Stroke risk factors are also either genetic or lifestyle related. They include age (adults 55 years or older are at increased risk), race (more common in African Americans, Hispanics, and American Indian/Alaska Natives), sex (men are more likely to have a stroke), family history, obesity or being overweight, sedentary lifestyle, hypertension, hypercholesterolemia, tobacco use, diabetes, cardiovascular disease, using birth control pills or hormone therapies, and excessive alcohol consumption.

Renal Disorders

Gout

Gout is an abnormal accumulation of uric acid due to a defect in metabolism. As a result of this defect, uric acid accumulates in the blood and joints, causing pain and swelling of the joints, especially the big toe. Often, the patient has fever and chills. Gout is more common among men than women and usually has a genetic basis. If left untreated, gout causes destructive tissue changes in the joints and kidneys. Treatment includes diet and medications to reduce inflammation and to increase the excretion of uric acid or decrease its formation.

Kidney Stones

Kidney stones are small masses of uric acid or calcium salts that can form in any part of the urinary system (kidney, ureter, or urinary bladder). There are four main types of stones:

- **Calcium oxalate.** This type of kidney stone is the most common and is created when calcium combines with oxalate in the urine. Inadequate calcium and fluid intake, as well other conditions, may contribute to their formation.
- **Uric acid.** This type of kidney stone is also common and is association with consumption of foods such as organ meats and shellfish that have high concentrations of purines. High purine intake leads to a higher production of monosodium urate, which can cause stones to form in the kidneys. Occurrence of these stones tends to run in families.
- **Struvite.** These stones are less common and are caused by infections in the upper urinary tract.
- **Cystine.** These stones are rare and tend to run in families.

Kidney stones may cause severe pain, nausea, and vomiting when the body attempts to pass them. Although most stones are small, occasionally they become large enough to adopt the internal contours of the kidney **FIGURE 9-23**. Researchers have found a gene that causes the intestines to absorb too much calcium, which can lead to the formation of kidney stones. Uric acid stones also often have a genetic basis. Some are small enough to pass in the urine, with or without pain; others must be removed surgically.

GI Disorders

Malabsorption Disorders

Malabsorption disorders are caused by defects in the function of the bowel wall that prevent

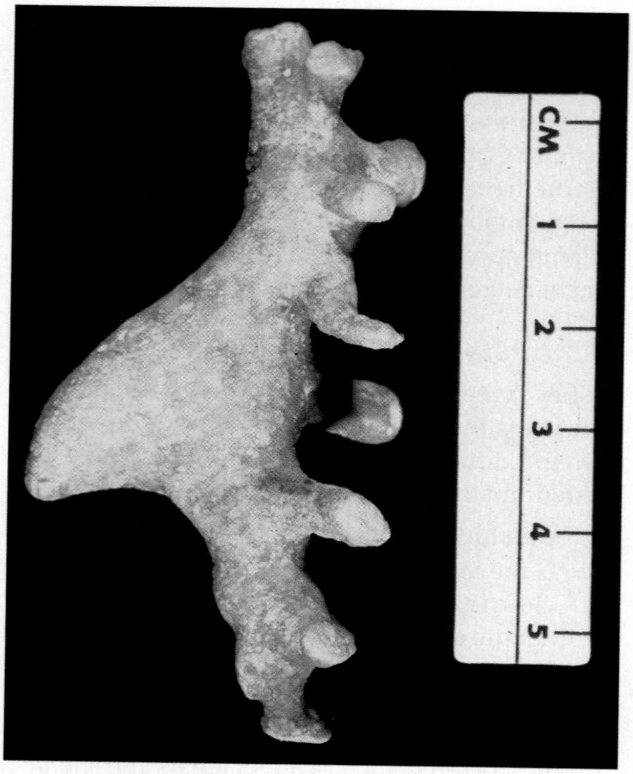

FIGURE 9-23 Large staghorn-shaped kidney stone.

Courtesy of Leonard V. Crowley, MD, Century College.

adequate nutrient absorption. The result is a complex of symptoms, including loss of appetite, bloating, weight loss, muscle pain, and stools with high fat content. Diarrhea, which may be bloody, may also be a prominent symptom.

Lactose intolerance is caused by a defect or deficiency of the enzyme lactase, resulting in an inability to digest lactose (milk sugar). Symptoms include bloating, flatulence, abdominal discomfort, nausea, and diarrhea after ingesting dairy or dairy products.

Ulcerative colitis is a serious chronic inflammatory disease of the large intestine and rectum. This disease, which shows a familial tendency, is characterized by recurrent episodes of abdominal pain, fever, chills, and profuse diarrhea, with stools containing pus, blood, and mucus. Treatment consists of anti-inflammatory agents, including corticosteroids. Patients with severe cases may require surgery to remove parts of the intestinal tract. Patients are at increased risk for the development of colorectal cancer.

Crohn disease is a chronic inflammatory condition that affects one or more areas of the GI tract, from the mouth to the anus, but that most often affects the terminal portion of the small intestine. Although its exact cause is unknown, possible causes include bacterial, viral, allergic, autoimmune, and undetermined gene abnormalities. Manifestations of Crohn disease primarily depend on the anatomic area involved, the extent of the disease, and the presence of complications. Symptoms include frequent episodes of diarrhea, abdominal pain, nausea, fever, weakness, and weight loss. Management involves nutrition therapy, anti-inflammatory agents, antibiotics, and sometimes surgery to remove the damaged portion of the bowel, fistulas, or scar tissue.

Peptic Ulcer Disease

Peptic ulcer disease is characterized by circumscribed erosions (ulcerations) of the mucous membrane lining of the GI tract—specifically, in the esophagus, stomach, duodenum, or jejunum. Peptic ulcers may be associated with excess acid production or a breakdown in the normal mechanisms protecting the mucous membranes. Although this disease seems to have a genetic component, a major contributor to its development is infection with the bacterium *Helicobacter pylori*; the observed familial patterns seem to be due to shared infections with *H pylori*. Symptoms include gnawing pain, which is often worse when the stomach is empty, after the person eats certain foods, or when the person is under stress. Treatment includes avoiding irritants such as tobacco, alcohol, and certain foods, antibiotics, and medications to decrease acidity. In refractory cases, surgery may be necessary.

Gallstones

Gallstones (choleliths) are stonelike masses in the gallbladder or its ducts caused by precipitation of substances contained in bile, such as cholesterol and bilirubin. Factors that contribute to the formation of gallstones include abnormalities in the composition of bile, or stasis of bile. Gallstones may initially be asymptomatic but later cause symptoms when they obstruct the flow of bile. They may cause inflammation of the gallbladder. Small stones that pass into the common duct can produce indigestion and biliary colic. Biliary colic pain has a sudden onset, increases steadily, and is usually located in the upper right quadrant or the epigastric area and may be referred to the back. Larger stones may cause jaundice (yellow skin and sclerae).

Obesity

Obesity is an unhealthy accumulation of body fat; it is often defined as a body mass index (BMI) greater than or equal to 30 kg/m^2. This is a good general guideline, except in cases where body weight does not correlate to excess fat—for example, in very muscular people. The Centers for Disease Control and Prevention (CDC) further defines obesity as follows:

- Class 1: BMI of 30 kg/m^2 to less than 35 kg/m^2
- Class 2: BMI 35 kg/m^2 to less than 40 kg/m^2
- Class 3: BMI of 40 kg/m^2 or higher

Health risks increase with each increase in class.

The CDC would term class 3 obesity as **morbid obesity**. Morbid obesity includes all of the health risks associated with obesity, but it also makes essential functions such as walking or breathing difficult.

People who are overweight are also at increased risk for disease, although the risk is not as high as for those who are obese. **Overweight** is defined as a BMI of 25 to 29.9 kg/m^2.[17]

In recent decades, obesity has become an epidemic among adults and children in the United States. Almost 75% of adults aged 20 and older in the United States have obesity or are overweight. More than 50% of children and adolescents in the United States are obese.[18]

Obesity has many deleterious effects, both medical and social. Health risks associated with obesity include hypertension, hyperlipidemia, cardiovascular disease, glucose intolerance, insulin resistance, diabetes, gallbladder disease, infertility, and cancer of the endometrium, breast, prostate, and colon. Social and psychological effects of obesity include depression, anxiety, shame, rejection, and discrimination in various environments, including school and the workplace.

Although some people likely have a genetic predisposition to obesity, the roles of specific genes in its development have yet to be determined. Behavioral and environmental factors are better known. Behavioral factors that contribute to obesity include choosing a sedentary lifestyle, overeating, and eating high-calorie, low-nutritional-value foods, such as fast food and soda. A person's community or work environment may also make it difficult to choose to be physically active or to eat properly. For example, a lack of sidewalks in a community would contribute to the risk of community members becoming obese. Large portion sizes offered by restaurants contribute to a lack of understanding of a proper portion size. Finally, watching television and engaging with technological media may take time away from physical activity and encourage unhealthy product consumption. Because people tend to snack while watching TV or using a computer, they may consume unnecessary additional calories.

Neuromuscular Disorders

Although environmental contributions are highly likely, certain neuromuscular disorders have a familial and genetic basis. The next few sections present several of the better known and more worrisome disorders in this category.

Huntington Disease

Huntington disease (also called Huntington chorea) is a hereditary condition (autosomal dominant). It is characterized by progressive chorea (involuntary rapid, jerky motions) and mental deterioration, leading to dementia. Symptoms usually first appear in the third or fourth decade of life and progress to death, often within 15 years.

Muscular Dystrophy

Muscular dystrophy is a generic term for a group of hereditary diseases of the muscular system characterized by weakness and wasting of groups of skeletal muscles, leading to increasing disability. The various forms differ in age of onset, rate of progression, and mode of genetic transmission. Duchenne muscular dystrophy is a sex-linked recessive disease (affecting only males); symptoms first appear around the age of 4 years. Progressive wasting of leg and pelvic muscles produces a waddling gait and abnormal curvature of the spine. Usually by age 12, the person becomes unable to walk and begins to use a wheelchair. No known treatment exists, and the person often dies, most often of a heart disorder, by age 20.

Multiple Sclerosis

Multiple sclerosis is a progressive disease in which the myelin sheath surrounding the nerve fibers of the brain and spinal cord become damaged.[19] Although this disease is not directly inherited, some patients have a familial predisposition, suggesting a genetic influence on susceptibility. Multiple sclerosis usually appears in early adulthood and progresses slowly, with periods of remission and exacerbation. Early symptoms include abnormal sensations in the face or extremities, weakness, and visual disturbances (such as double vision), which progress to ataxia (lack of coordination), abnormal reflexes, tremors, difficulty in urination, and difficulty in walking. Depression is also common. No specific treatment or cure has been developed, but corticosteroids and other drugs are used to treat symptoms.

Special Populations

Never assume that new or worsening confusion in an older adult is due solely to Alzheimer disease, without first considering potentially correctable causes such as new medications, infections, or myocardial infarction. An apparent emotional, psychological, or behavioral disorder may have an organic cause, especially in the older adult population.

Alzheimer Disease

Alzheimer disease is characterized by cortical atrophy and loss of neurons in the frontal and temporal lobes of the brain; in addition, as the brain ventricles become enlarged, a loss of brain tissue occurs. More than 5.8 million Americans are currently living with Alzheimer disease.[20] Histologic changes in the brain of a person with Alzheimer disease include neurofibrillary tangles and senile plaques **FIGURE 9-24**. Studies of the genetics of inherited early-onset Alzheimer disease have been linked to mutations on three genes.

Alzheimer disease is progressive. Early in its progression, it is characterized by memory loss, lack of spontaneity, subtle personality changes, and disorientation to time and date. Over time, it may progress to include impaired cognition and abstract thinking, restlessness and agitation, wandering, inability to carry out activities of daily living, impaired judgment, and inappropriate social behavior. Advanced Alzheimer disease involves indifference to food, inability to communicate, urinary and fecal incontinence, and seizures.

Psychiatric Disorders

Some common psychiatric disorders seem to have a familial and perhaps even genetic component. Two of the most important are schizophrenia and bipolar disorder.

Schizophrenia

Schizophrenia comprises a group of mental disorders characterized by gross distortions of reality (psychoses), withdrawal from social contacts, and disturbances of thought, language, perception, and emotional response. Its symptoms are highly varied, but may include apathy, catatonia or excessive

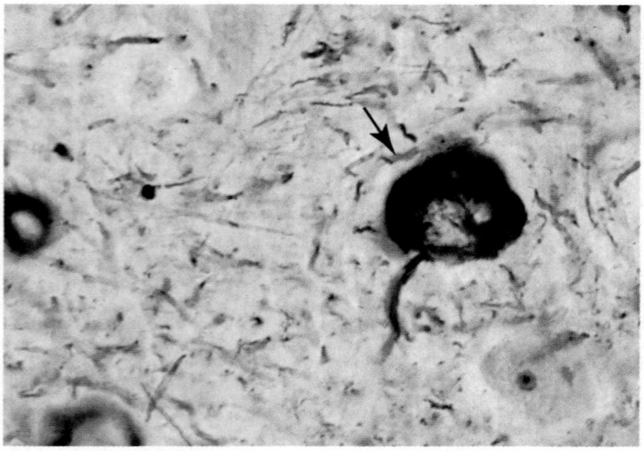

A

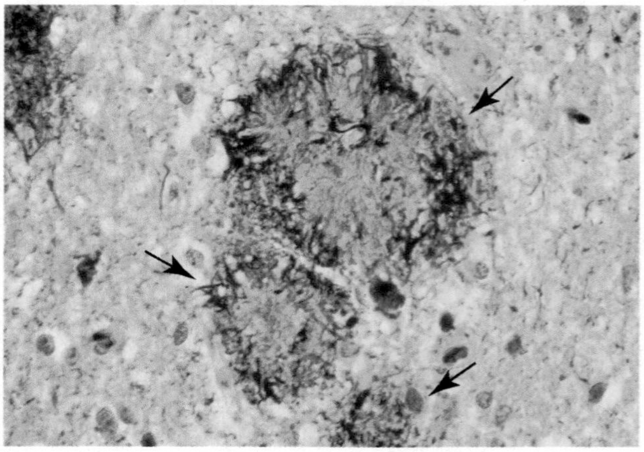

B

FIGURE 9-24 Alzheimer disease. **A.** Thickened neurofilaments encircle and obscure the nuclei of nerve cells (arrow), forming a neurofibrillary tangle (original magnification, ×400). **B.** Three senile plaques (arrows) composed of broken masses of thickened neurofilaments (original magnification, ×100).

Courtesy of Leonard V. Crowley, MD, Century College.

activity, bizarre actions, hallucinations, delusions, and rambling speech. Although the cause of schizophrenia has not been identified, a combination of hereditary or genetic predisposing factors is likely to play a role in most cases.

Bipolar Disorder

Bipolar disorder (formerly known as manic-depressive disorder or manic-depressive psychosis) is a mental disorder characterized by episodes of mania and depression. One or the other phase may be dominant at any given time, the phases may alternate, or aspects of both phases may be present at once. An estimated 4.4% of US adults experience bipolar disorder at some time in their lives.[21,22] The higher rates of bipolar disorder among relatives, identical twins, and biologic parents versus adoptive parents have been cited as evidence of the role of genetics in this disorder. Treatment consists of psychotherapy plus antidepressants and tranquilizers.

Stress and Disease

Stress is the medical term for a wide range of strong external stimuli, physiologic and psychological, that can cause a physiologic response. Physiologic stress is defined as a change that makes it necessary for the body's cells to adapt. **FIGURE 9-25** shows the series of events that occur when the body responds to a stimulus or stressor. Three concepts related to physiologic stress include the stressor itself, its effect in the body, and the body's response to the stress.

The brain and CNS constantly interact with a person's consciousness. Research has shown a strong connection between the human psyche and brain physiology. When a person experiences stress, the body's defense mechanisms are activated. Usually, the stress response is appropriate and beneficial. However, an unchecked stress response can have deleterious outcomes, including chemical dependency, heart attack, stroke, depression, headache, and abdominal pain.

General Adaptation Syndrome

General adaptation syndrome, a term introduced by Austrian endocrinologist Hans Selye in the 1920s, comprises the three-stage reaction to stressors, whether physical (such as injury) and emotional (such as loss of a loved one).

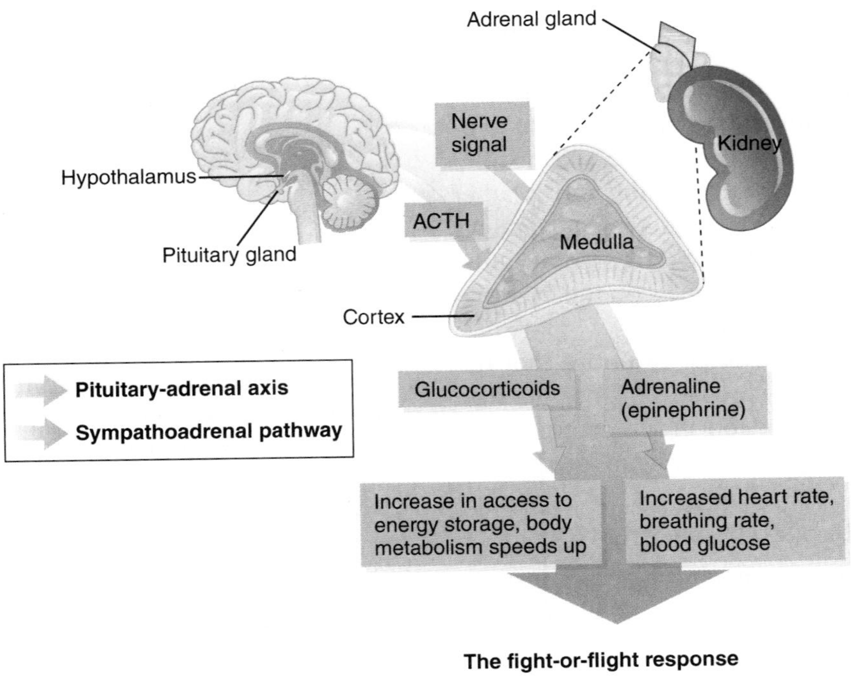

FIGURE 9-25 Physiologic response to stress.

Abbreviation: ACTH, adrenocorticotropic hormone

Stage 1: Alarm

The body reacts to stress first by releasing catecholamines, chemical compounds derived from the amino acid tyrosine that act as hormones or neurotransmitters. These substances are produced mainly from the adrenal medulla and the postganglionic fibers of the sympathetic nervous system. Catecholamines are soluble, so they circulate in the body dissolved in blood. The most abundant catecholamines are epinephrine (adrenaline), norepinephrine (noradrenaline), and dopamine. Adrenaline acts as a neurotransmitter in the CNS and as a hormone in the blood. Noradrenaline is primarily a neurotransmitter of the peripheral sympathetic nervous system, but is also present in the blood (mostly through spillover from the synapses of the sympathetic system).

As shown in Figure 9-25, stress causes the sympathetic nervous system to be stimulated. When the body senses stress, the brain causes the adrenal medulla of the endocrine system to send catecholamines (the hormones epinephrine and norepinephrine) that activate the sympathetic nervous system by binding to **receptor** sites. In the sympathetic nervous system, binding to (activation of) alpha and beta receptors allows certain responses to be activated and a predictable sequence of responses occurs. Activation of alpha receptors results in vasoconstriction, whereas activation of beta receptors results in increased heart rate, increased force of contraction, and increased conduction velocity. Beyond those cardiac effects of catecholamines, other physiologic effects include an increase in respiratory rate, decreased blood flow to the skin, smooth-muscle constriction, and various effects on the liver that increase the body's use of glucose.

Normally, the fight-or-flight response that occurs in the alarm reaction prepares the body to deal with stress. When activated too often, however, it can weaken the immune system, leading to infection.

Stage 2: Resistance or Adaptation

During stage 2, the resistance or adaptation stage, the body adapts to stressors. It does so primarily by stimulating the adrenal gland to secrete two types of corticosteroid hormones that increase the blood glucose level and maintain BP: glucocorticoids and mineralocorticoids. The most significant glucocorticoid in the body is cortisol, which controls carbohydrate, fat, and protein metabolism. Cortisol also has potent anti-inflammatory actions. Mineralocorticoids (predominantly aldosterone) control electrolyte and water levels in the body, mainly by promoting sodium retention by the kidneys.

During times of stress, the hypothalamus secretes a hormone that stimulates the anterior pituitary to release adrenocorticotropic hormone (ACTH) **FIGURE 9-26**. ACTH targets the adrenal cortex, resulting in cortisol secretion. Cortisol, in turn, stimulates body cells to increase their energy production in response to increased stressors; it increases serum glucose levels and impairs the use of glucose by peripheral tissues. In addition, cortisol decreases protein reserves and permits mobilization of fatty acids by epinephrine and growth hormone. It reduces inflammation when inflammation has served its purpose; therefore, it has a role in wound healing. Although cortisol increases red blood cell production and affects electrolyte levels, it also decreases the size of lymphoid tissue. Since the lymphatic system has an essential role in immunity, this may explain why stress and disease are linked.

Endorphins are neurotransmitters released during times of stress. These hormones help reduce pain and stress by activating opiate receptor sites. In essence, they produce a type of analgesia.

Additional hormones affected by stress include growth hormone, prolactin, and testosterone. Growth factor is a hormone that promotes cell and tissue growth and repair. In the context of stress, growth factor levels are reduced. Since the presence of growth factor correlates with the body's ability to heal, this means that there is a reduced ability to heal when the body is under chronic stress.

Prolactin is a hormone that stimulates breast milk production. It is also believed to play a role in the immune system. In times of stress, prolactin levels increase. Research suggests that prolactin levels increase more in people with ineffective coping mechanisms.

There is a direct link between levels of cortisol (the primary stress hormone) and levels of testosterone: When cortisol levels are high, testosterone levels are reduced. When the body is not under stress, testosterone levels are protected from cortisol by an enzyme. In the presence of stress, however, cortisol levels are too high for the enzyme to sufficiently handle them. As a result, the excess cortisol causes testosterone levels to decrease.

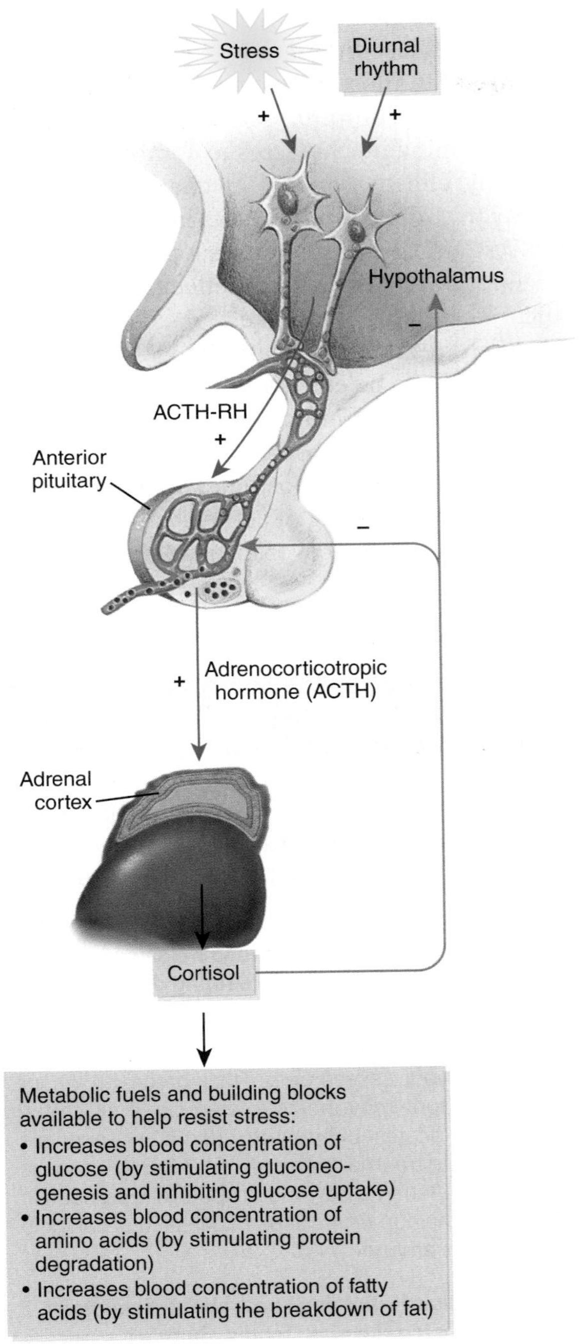

FIGURE 9-26 Stress triggers secretion of adrenocorticotropic hormone, which results in cortisol secretion.

It was once believed that elevated testosterone levels were linked to a suppressed immune system. More recent research suggests that testosterone may be related to the distribution of white blood cells in the body. It is theorized that in times of stress, white blood cells are sent to the skin to protect against wound infection. In the context of chronic stress, this would mean fewer white blood cells are present in other parts of the body on a regular basis, making those parts more susceptible to infection.

Cortisol levels and the sympathetic nervous system return to normal during the resistance or adaptation stage, causing fight-or-flight symptoms to disappear. Continuation of stress and accompanying corticosteroid release, however, eventually lead to fatigue, lapses in concentration, irritability, lethargy, depression, and a depressed immune system.

Stage 3: Exhaustion

After a long period of stress, the person enters the exhaustion stage. The adrenal glands become depleted, decreasing the blood glucose level, which results in decreased stress tolerance, progressive mental and physical exhaustion, illness, and collapse. At this point, the body's immune system is compromised, significantly reducing a person's ability to resist disease. Heart attack, high BP, or severe infection may result.

Effects of Chronic Stress

The **hypothalamic-pituitary-adrenal axis** is a major part of the neuroendocrine system that controls reactions to stress. The hypothalamic-pituitary-adrenal axis triggers a set of interactions among the glands, hormones, and parts of the midbrain that mediate the general adaptation syndrome. Continued stress, however, leads to loss of these normal control mechanisms. As a result, the adrenals continue to produce cortisol, which exhausts the stress mechanism and leads to fatigue and depression. Cortisol also interferes with serotonin activity, furthering the depressive effect.

A consistently high cortisol level suppresses the immune system by increasing production of interleukin-6, an immune system messenger. Research indicates that stress and depression have negative effects on the immune system. Reduced immunity makes the body more susceptible to everything from colds and flu to cancer. For example, the incidence of serious illness, including cancer, is significantly higher among people whose spouse has died during the past year.

Although severe, prolonged stress does not cause death directly, it does cause the body to lose its ability to fight disease in its effort to manage the stress. Stress also encourages the body to release fat and cholesterol into the bloodstream, which in turn block the arteries and can eventually cause a heart attack or stroke. Many people start drinking alcohol to excess to combat their stress. Other diseases and conditions related to chronic stress include depression, headaches, insomnia, ulcers, diuresis, acne, diabetes mellitus, rheumatoid arthritis, and asthma. The variety in this list shows that stress affects most every organ system in the body.

Ultimately, though, a person's reaction to stressful events correlates to elevation or reduction in hormone levels. Therefore, coping mechanisms play a role in the physiologic stress response. A healthy person who experiences stress may manage that stress with minimal adverse effects on the immune system if the person has effective coping mechanisms. In contrast, ineffective coping mechanisms will have deleterious effects on immune status. These effects will be worst in those patients whose immune systems are already compromised and who do not have adequate coping mechanisms to combat the stress. Conversely, effective coping mechanisms can go a long way toward helping patients improve their immune system's response. Finally, a person's outlook has been shown to relate to the effectiveness of their medical treatment: Much like a placebo effect, if a patient believes that the treatment will be effective, it is more likely to be effective.

Fortunately, this immune suppression process can be corrected with psychotherapy, medication, or any number of other positive influences that restore hope and a feeling of self-esteem. The ability of human beings to recover from adversity is quite remarkable.

YOU are the Paramedic SUMMARY

1. What is your general impression of the patient?

The patient is in obvious respiratory distress because he cannot speak complete sentences without taking a breath. This finding is significant because it indicates there is not enough oxygen available in the patient's body to allow him to speak effectively.

2. What can you learn about the patient from his surroundings?

The scene assessment gives numerous indications that the patient has a significant medical history. The first significant finding is that you were met at the door by a neighbor. The neighbor tells you the patient has had medical issues and lives alone. Once you enter the residence, you observe multiple prescription medication bottles and an abundance of used facial tissues on the side table. These items need to be investigated further. The patient is also wearing a nasal cannula attached to a home oxygen unit, which indicates a preexisting respiratory condition.

3. How does the recruitment of accessory muscles facilitate breathing?

As you have learned, the act of breathing relies on positive and negative pressures. The chest and other related muscles expand and contract to create these pressures. When the act of breathing becomes difficult, accessory muscles assist with the mechanical aspect of breathing. The nasal passages will flare to provide as much space as possible to increase airflow into the airways. The musculature in the chest will work visibly harder to move the chest wall and diaphragm to create the pressure gradient necessary for breathing. Sitting upright aligns the airway to decrease the amount of pressure needed within the chest.

4. How might the productive cough help you identify the source of the patient's breathing difficulty?

The productive cough could indicate many disease processes. The color of the sputum is of particular interest in your assessment. Thick green, brown, or yellow sputum may indicate infection. Pink, frothy sputum indicates pulmonary edema. Hemoptysis may indicate trauma or carcinoma. After you assess the color, determine how much sputum is present. In this case, the numerous used facial tissues can help indicate the amount.

5. On the basis of what you know about physiology, what is causing the pink, foamy sputum?

Pink, foamy sputum is an indication of pulmonary edema, which in this case may be a sign of exacerbation of heart failure. If the heart's left ventricle is not pumping effectively, then blood backs up in the system. This backup causes an increase in pressure within the pulmonary vasculature. The increased pressure forces fluid through the alveolar membranes and into the alveoli. Blood will enter the alveoli through the alveolar membranes in small amounts, producing a pink rather than red appearance of the sputum. The froth comes from the additional fluid being exposed to the air in the patient's lungs and airways.

YOU are the Paramedic SUMMARY continued

6. How do you account for the decreased Spo_2 level?

In this case, the patient has a decreased surface area for oxygen exchange due to pulmonary edema. Less surface area means less oxygen will "saturate" the cells, which in turn will be read by the pulse oximeter as a decrease in saturation. It is important to note that the saturation amount shown on the electronic device represents any gas that is saturating the cells. Oxygen is one of many gases that can affect the reading. In addition, saturation levels may be compromised by the patient's lack of circulation.

7. Why would a diuretic be prescribed for a patient with heart failure?

If a patient has heart failure, then the heart is not pumping blood effectively. This causes a backup within the circulatory system, which causes fluid to build up in the pulmonary vasculature. A diuretic helps eliminate some of the fluid from the system and lessens the workload on the heart. Most diuretics work on the kidneys to eliminate water and electrolytes. The elimination moves fluid from the extracellular space to the intravascular space, transporting it out of the body. The goal is to reduce the cardiac preload, which will reduce the amount of work the cardiac system has to do and reduce the fluid backup.

8. Why would this patient have a normal or slightly high BP?

In patients with heart failure, the heart is working harder to pump fluid volume. According to the Starling law, increased venous return to the heart increases cardiac preload. The heart muscle stretches in response to the increased amount of fluid. The heart muscle will then contract with greater force—up to a point—to expel the fluid. This accounts for a normal or higher-than-normal BP, as the body is trying to compensate for a lack of the heart's muscular ability.

EMS Patient Care Report (PCR)					
Date: 08-01-21	**Incident No.:** 1234	**Nature of Call:** Difficulty breathing		**Location:** 420 Beach Street	
Dispatched: 2041	**En Route:** 2041	**At Scene:** 2045	**Transport:** 2052	**At Hospital:** 2107	**In Service:** 2120
Patient Information					
Age: 72 **Sex:** M **Weight (in kg [lb]):** 80.2 kg (177 lb)			**Allergies:** NKDA **Medications:** Numerous **Past Medical History:** Heart failure **Chief Complaint:** Difficulty breathing		

Vital Signs				
Time: 2047	**BP:** 140/90	**Pulse:** 110	**Respirations:** 22	**Spo_2:** 89%
Time: 2052	**BP:** 138/88	**Pulse:** 114	**Respirations:** 24	**Spo_2:** 92%
Time:	**BP:**	**Pulse:**	**Respirations:**	**Spo_2:**
EMS Treatment (circle all that apply)				
Oxygen @ 15 L/min via (circle one): **NC (NRM) Bag-mask device**		**Assisted Ventilation**	**Airway Adjunct**	**CPR**
Defibrillation	**Bleeding Control**	**Bandaging**	**Splinting**	**(Other: CPAP)**

Narrative

Arrived to find a 72 y/o man being attended by his neighbor. Pt lives alone in this residence. Pt alert (oriented to person, place, and day). Pt unable to speak in complete sentences due to respiratory effort. Pt states he has not been compliant with his meds. Pt states he has a history of "heart failure" and is on home O_2 at 2 L/min via cannula. Coarse crackles heard in all fields. Pt has productive cough with pink foamy sputum. O_2 via NRM applied initially at 15 L/min and then switched over to CPAP on scene and throughout transport. IV line of NS established TKO, ECG shows sinus tach @114, no ectopy noted. $ETCO_2$ waveform appears appropriate in shape and reads 36 mm Hg. Treatment per local protocol, radio report during transport, and verbal report to Halifax Health on arrival. Pt transferred to room A-20.

End of report

Prep Kit

Ready for Review

- Pathophysiology is the study of the physiology of altered functioning in the presence of disease.
- Pathophysiology in the cellular environment includes disturbances in fluid balance and electrolyte imbalances. These various imbalances can upset homeostasis and may result in or contribute to emergency conditions.
- Cellular injury is caused by factors such as hypoxia, ischemia, chemical injury, infectious injury, immunologic injury, inflammatory injury, and physical damage such as from radiation, and adverse conditions such as extreme cold.
- When cells are exposed to adverse conditions, they undergo a process of adaptation to guard against injury. Examples of adaptation include atrophy, hypertrophy, hyperplasia, dysplasia, and metaplasia.
- Inflammatory response is characterized by both local and systemic effects. Local effects consist of dilation (expansion) of blood vessels and increased vascular permeability. If the inflammatory process is severe, then systemic effects such as fever become evident. The outcome of inflammation depends on how much tissue damage has occurred.
- Immunologic diseases occur because of hyperactivity or hypoactivity of the immune system. Allergies are acquired following initial exposure to an allergen; repeated exposures then cause the immune system to react to the allergen.
- Perfusion is the delivery of oxygen and nutrients and removal of wastes from the cells, organs, and tissues by the circulatory system. Hypoperfusion occurs when the level of tissue perfusion decreases below normal.
- Shock is an abnormal state associated with inadequate oxygen and nutrient delivery to the metabolic apparatus of the cell, resulting in an impairment of cellular metabolism and, ultimately, inadequate perfusion of vital organs.
- Central shock consists of cardiogenic shock and obstructive shock. Cardiogenic shock occurs when the heart cannot circulate enough blood to maintain adequate peripheral oxygen delivery. Obstructive shock occurs when blood flow within the heart or great vessels (aorta and pulmonary vein) becomes blocked.
- Peripheral shock includes hypovolemic shock and distributive shock. In hypovolemic shock, the circulating blood volume is insufficient to deliver adequate oxygen and nutrients to the body's cells. Distributive shock occurs when there is widespread dilation of the resistance vessels (small arterioles), the capacitance vessels (small venules), or both.
- Multiple organ dysfunction syndrome (MODS) occurs in acutely ill patients; it is characterized by the concurrent failure of two or more organs or organ systems that were initially unharmed by the acute disorder or injury that caused the patient's current illness. Six organ systems are surveyed in diagnosing MODS: respiratory, hepatic, renal, hematologic, neurologic, and cardiovascular.
- The immune system includes all of the structures and processes associated with the body's defense against foreign substances and disease-causing agents.
- The body has three lines of defense: anatomic barriers, the inflammatory response, and the immune response.
- There are two general types of immune response: natural and acquired.
- Immunity may be humoral or cell mediated.
- Important white blood cells in the immune system include neutrophils, eosinophils, basophils, monocytes, and lymphocytes. Other important cells of the immune system include macrophages, mast cells, plasma cells, B cells, and T cells.
- The antibodies secreted by B cells are called immunoglobulins. Antibodies make antigens more visible to the immune system in three ways: by acting as opsonins, by making

Prep Kit continued

antigens clump, and by inactivating bacterial toxins.

- The inflammatory response is a response of the tissues of the body to irritation or injury. It is characterized by pain, swelling, redness, and heat.
- The two most common causes of inflammation are infection (such as bacterial or viral) and injury.
- The plasma protein systems that modulate the inflammatory process include the complement system, the coagulation (clotting) system, and the kinin system.
- Cytokines are products of cells that affect the function of other cells; they include interleukins, lymphokines, and interferons.
- Chronic inflammatory responses are usually caused by an unsuccessful acute inflammatory response to a foreign body, a persistent infection, or the presence of an antigen.
- Normal wound healing involves four steps: repairing the damaged tissue, removing the inflammatory debris, restoring the tissue to a normal state, and regenerating cells.
- Wounds may heal by primary or secondary intention. Healing by primary intention occurs in clean wounds with opposed margins. Wounds that heal by secondary intention have a more pronounced and prolonged inflammatory phase and more abundant granulation tissue.
- Hypersensitivity is the body's response to any substance to which a patient has increased sensitivity; it is a generic term that encompasses a variety of reactions. A hypersensitivity reaction may be immediate, occurring within seconds to minutes, or delayed, occurring hours to days after exposure to an antigen.
- Hypersensitivity reactions may be classified as type I, immediate hypersensitivity; type II, cytotoxic hypersensitivity reactions; type III, immune complex disease; and type IV, delayed (cell-mediated) hypersensitivity.
- Immunodeficiency may be congenital or acquired.
- Age-related and sex-associated factors interact with a combination of genetic and environmental factors, anatomic causes, or immunologic reactions to cause disease.
- Analyzing disease risk involves consideration of disease rates (incidence, prevalence, morbidity, and mortality) and controllable and uncontrollable disease risk factors (causal and noncausal). These risk factors, age, and sex differences interact to influence a person's level of risk.
- A true genetic risk is passed through generations by inheritance of a gene. In contrast, with a familial tendency, diseases seem to cluster in family groups despite lack of evidence for heritable gene-associated abnormalities. In autosomal dominant inheritance, a person needs to inherit only one copy of a particular form of a gene to show the trait. In autosomal recessive inheritance, the person must inherit two copies of a particular form of a gene to show the trait.
- Although severe, prolonged stress does not cause death directly, it does cause the body to lose its ability to fight disease to manage the stress. Effective coping mechanisms can go a long way toward helping a patient improve the immune system's response.
- The general adaptation syndrome describes the body's short- and long-term reactions to stress.
- Stress causes stimulation of the sympathetic nervous system. This occurs through the release of catecholamines that bind to alpha and beta receptor sites, resulting in effects that are collectively described as the fight-or-flight response.
- Stress also causes secretion of cortisol, which has many useful effects, such as increasing serum glucose levels, decreasing protein reserves, and permitting mobilization of fatty acids. However, continuous secretion of cortisol has deleterious effects on the body.

Prep Kit continued

Vital Vocabulary

acidosis An increase in extracellular H^+ ions; a blood pH of less than 7.35.

acquired immunity The immunity that occurs when the body is exposed to a foreign substance or disease and produces antibodies to the invader; also called acquired immunity.

activation In the inflammatory response, the stage in which mediators of inflammation trigger the appearance of selectins and integrins on the surfaces of endothelial cells and polymorphonuclear neutrophils, respectively.

adhesion In the inflammatory response, the stage characterized by attachment of polymorphonuclear neutrophils to endothelial cells, mediated by selectins and integrins.

alcoholic ketoacidosis A metabolic acidotic state that manifests because of inadequate nutritional habits associated with chronic alcohol abuse. The liver and body experience inadequate fuel reserves of glycogen and, therefore, have to switch to fatty acid metabolism.

alkalosis A decrease in extracellular H^+ ions; a blood pH greater than 7.45.

allergen Any substance that causes a hypersensitivity reaction.

allergy A hypersensitivity reaction to the presence of an agent (allergen).

anaphylactic shock A severe hypersensitivity reaction that involves bronchoconstriction and cardiovascular collapse; also called anaphylaxis.

angiogenesis The growth of new blood vessels.

antibody A protein secreted by certain immune cells that bind antigens to make them more visible to the immune system.

antigen A foreign substance recognized by the immune system.

apoptosis Normal cell death.

asthma A chronic inflammatory lower airway condition resulting in intermittent wheezing and excess mucus production.

atopic An allergic tendency.

atrophy A decrease in cell size due to a loss of subcellular components.

autoantibodies Antibodies directed against the self.

autoimmunity The production of antibodies or T cells that work against the tissues of one's own body, producing hypersensitivity reactions or autoimmune disease.

autosomal dominant A pattern of inheritance that involves genes located on autosomes (any chromosome other than sex chromosomes). Inheritance of only one copy of a particular form of a gene is needed to show the trait.

autosomal recessive A pattern of inheritance that involves genes located on autosomes (any chromosome other than sex chromosomes). Inheritance of two copies of a particular form of a gene is needed to show the trait.

bradypnea A slow respiratory rate.

capillary refill time A test performed on the fingernails or toenails that involves briefly squeezing the toenail or fingernail and evaluating the time it takes for the color to return.

cardiogenic shock A condition caused by loss of 40% or more of the functioning myocardium; the heart cannot circulate enough blood to maintain adequate peripheral oxygen delivery.

carpopedal spasm A contorted position in which the fingers or toes flex in a clawlike manner; may result from hyperventilation or hypocalcemia.

cell-mediated immunity The immune process by which T cell lymphocytes (1) recognize antigens and then secrete cytokines (specifically lymphokines) that attract other cells or (2) become cytotoxic cells themselves and kill infected or abnormal cells.

central shock A type of shock caused by central pump failure, including cardiogenic shock and obstructive shock.

Prep Kit continued

chemotaxins Components of the activated complement system that attract leukocytes from the circulation to help fight infections.

chemotaxis The movement of polymorphonuclear neutrophils toward the site of inflammation in response to chemotactic factors released by bacteria or formed from activated complement, chemokines, or arachidonic acid derivatives (such as leukotrienes) in response to cell injury.

coagulation system A system that serves a vital role in the formation of blood clots in blood vessels. Inflammation triggers the coagulation cascade, initiating a complex series of reactions that encourage fibrin formation.

complement system A group of plasma proteins that attract white blood cells to sites of inflammation, activate white blood cells, and directly destroy cells.

cytokines The products of cells that affect the function of other cells.

distributive shock A type of shock caused by widespread dilation of the resistance vessels (small arterioles), the capacitance vessels (small venules), or both.

dysplasia An alteration in the size, shape, and organization of cells.

edema Swelling caused by excessive fluid trapped in the body tissues.

fibrin The protein that polymerizes (bonds) to form the fibrous component of a blood clot.

fibrinolysis cascade The breakdown of fibrin in blood clots and the prevention of the polymerization of fibrin into new clots.

free radicals Molecules that are missing one electron in their outer shell.

gallstones Stonelike masses in the gallbladder or its ducts caused by precipitation of substances contained in bile, such as cholesterol and bilirubin; also known as choleliths.

general adaptation syndrome A three-stage reaction to stressors, either physical (such as injury) or emotional (such as loss of a loved one). The stages include alarm, resistance or adaptation, and exhaustion.

gram-negative A reaction of bacteria to a Gram stain in which the bacteria do not retain the dark purple stain; such bacteria have cell walls that consist largely of lipids, and have pathogenic qualities that make them especially problematic for humans.

gram-positive A reaction of bacteria to a Gram stain in which the bacteria retain the dark purple stain; such bacteria have thick cell walls composed of many layers peptidoglycan (amino acids and glucose).

hapten A substance that normally does not stimulate an immune response but can be combined with an antigen and, at a later time, initiate a specific antibody response on its own.

helper T cells A type of T lymphocyte that is involved in cell-mediated and antibody-mediated immune responses; it secretes cytokines that stimulate the B cells and other T cells.

hemochromatosis An inherited (autosomal recessive) disease in which the body absorbs more iron than it needs, which it then stores in the liver, kidneys, and pancreas.

hemolytic anemia A disease characterized by increased destruction of the red blood cells. This disorder has several causes, such as an Rh factor blood transfusion reaction (most likely to occur in the neonate population), a disorder of the immune system, and exposure to bacterial toxins or chemicals such as benzene.

hemophilia An inherited sex-linked disorder characterized by excessive bleeding.

histamine A vasoactive amine that increases vascular permeability, causes vasodilation, and can cause bronchoconstriction, nausea, and vomiting.

humoral immunity A type of immunity in which B cell lymphocytes produce antibodies called immunoglobulins, which recognize a specific antigen and then react with it.

Prep Kit continued

hypercalcemia An increased serum calcium level.

hypercholesterolemia An elevated blood cholesterol level.

hyperkalemia An elevated serum potassium level.

hypermagnesemia An increased serum magnesium level.

hypernatremia A serum sodium level greater than or equal to 143 mEq/L.

hyperphosphatemia An increased serum phosphate level.

hyperplasia An increase in the actual number of cells in an organ or tissue, usually resulting in an increase in the size of the organ or tissue.

hypersensitivity A generic term for responses of the body to a substance to which a patient has increased sensitivity.

hypertrophy An increase in the size of the cells due to synthesis of more subcellular components, which in turn leads to an increase in tissue and organ size.

hypocalcemia A decreased serum calcium level.

hypokalemia A decreased serum potassium level.

hypomagnesemia A decreased serum magnesium level.

hyponatremia A serum sodium level that is less than or equal to 135 mEq/L.

hypoperfusion A condition that occurs when the level of tissue perfusion decreases below normal.

hypophosphatemia A decreased serum phosphate level.

hypothalamic-pituitary-adrenal axis A major part of the neuroendocrine system that controls reactions to stress; the mechanism for a set of interactions among glands, hormones, and parts of the midbrain that mediate the general adaptation syndrome.

hypovolemic shock A type of shock that occurs when the circulating blood volume is insufficient to deliver adequate oxygen and nutrients to the body.

immune response The body's defense reaction to any substance it recognizes as foreign.

immune system The body system that includes all of the structures and processes associated with the body's defense against foreign substances and disease-causing agents.

immunodeficiency An abnormal condition in which some part of the body's immune system is inadequate, and, consequently, resistance to infectious disease is decreased.

immunogen An antigen capable of generating an immune response.

immunoglobulins Antibodies secreted by B cells.

incidence The number of new cases of a disease in a population.

inflammatory response A reaction by tissues of the body to irritation or injury, characterized by pain, swelling, redness, and heat.

interferon A protein produced by cells in response to viral invasion that is released into the bloodstream or intercellular fluid to induce healthy cells to manufacture an enzyme that counters the infection.

interleukins Chemical substances that attract white blood cells to the sites of injury and bacterial invasions.

isoimmunity The formation of antibodies or T cells that are directed against the antigens on another person's cells (typically after the transplantation of an organ or tissues).

ketoacidosis An acidotic state created by the production of ketones via fat metabolism.

ketones Acidic by-products of fat metabolism.

killer T cells The cells released during a type IV allergic reaction that kill antigen-bearing target cells.

kinin system A group of polypeptides that mediate inflammatory responses by stimulating visceral smooth muscle and relaxing vascular smooth muscle to produce vasodilation.

lactic acidosis The product of anaerobic cellular respiration, which occurs when tissues and

Prep Kit continued

organs are inadequately perfused, as in shock and cardiac arrest.

leukocytosis An increased number of leukocytes in the blood, often due to inflammation.

leukotrienes Arachidonic acid metabolites that function as chemical mediators of inflammation; also known as slow-reacting substances of anaphylaxis.

lymphokines Cytokines released by lymphocytes, including many of the interleukins, gamma interferon, tumor necrosis factor beta, and chemokines.

margination In the inflammatory response, the stage in which the loss of fluid from blood vessels into the inflamed or infected tissue increases the viscosity of the blood remaining in the vessels, which slows the flow of blood and produces stasis.

membrane attack complex Molecules that insert themselves into the bacterial membrane, weakening those areas in the membrane.

metabolic acidosis A pathologic condition characterized by a blood pH of less than 7.35 and caused by an accumulation of acids in the body from a metabolic cause.

metabolic alkalosis A pathologic condition characterized by a blood pH of greater than 7.45 and caused by an accumulation of bases in the body from a metabolic cause.

metaplasia A reversible, cellular adaptation in which one adult cell type is replaced by another adult cell type.

morbidity The presence of disease or the incidence or prevalence of a disease.

morbid obesity An excessively unhealthy accumulation of body fat, defined as a body mass index greater than or equal to 40 kg/m^2.

mortality The number of deaths from a disease in each population.

multiple organ dysfunction syndrome (MODS) A grave but sometimes reversible condition in a critically ill patient, characterized by the concurrent failure of two or more organs or organ systems that were initially unharmed by the acute disorder or injury that caused the patient's current illness.

natural immunity A nonspecific cellular and humoral (antibody) response that operates as the body's first line of defense against pathogens; also called native immunity.

necrosis The death of tissue, usually caused by a cessation of the blood supply.

neurogenic shock A type of shock that usually results from spinal cord injury; loss of normal sympathetic nervous system tone and vasodilation occur.

obesity An unhealthy accumulation of body fat; a body mass index of greater than or equal to 30 kg/m^2.

obstructive shock A type of shock that occurs when blood flow becomes blocked in the heart or great vessels.

oliguria Decreased urine output.

opsonization The process by which an antibody coats an antigen to facilitate its recognition by immune cells.

overweight An unhealthy accumulation of body fat; a body mass index of 25 to 29.9 kg/m^2.

pathophysiology The study of the physiology of altered functioning in the presence of disease.

perfusion The delivery of oxygen and nutrients and removal of wastes from the cells, organs, and tissues by the circulatory system.

pericardial tamponade The impairment of diastolic filling of the right and left ventricles due to significant amounts of fluid in the pericardial sac surrounding the heart, leading to a decrease in the cardiac output.

peripheral shock Shock caused by peripheral circulatory abnormalities; includes hypovolemic shock and distributive shock.

phagocytes White blood cells that engulf and consume foreign material such as microorganisms and cellular debris.

Prep Kit continued

polymorphonuclear neutrophils (PMNs) A type of white blood cell formed by bone marrow tissue that has a nucleus consisting of several parts or lobes connected by fine strands.

polyuria Frequent and plentiful urination.

prevalence The number of cases of a disease or condition in a particular population within a particular period.

prostaglandins A group of lipids that act as chemical messengers in reproduction, the inflammatory response to infection, and pain perception.

pyrogens Chemicals or proteins that travel to the brain, where they affect the hypothalamus and stimulate a rise in the body's core temperature.

receptor A specialized area in tissue that initiates certain actions after specific stimulation.

respiratory acidosis A pathologic condition characterized by a blood pH of less than 7.35 and caused by an accumulation of acids in the body from a respiratory cause.

respiratory alkalosis A pathologic condition characterized by a blood pH of greater than 7.45 and caused by an accumulation of bases in the body from a respiratory cause.

septic shock A type of shock that occurs as a result of widespread infection, usually bacterial; if left untreated, the result is multiple organ dysfunction syndrome and often death.

serotonin A vasoactive amine that increases vascular permeability, causes vasodilation, and can cause bronchoconstriction, nausea, and vomiting.

serum sickness A condition in which antigen–antibody complexes formed in the bloodstream become deposited in sites around the body, most notably the kidneys, resulting in inflammatory reactions there.

transmigration (diapedesis) In the inflammatory response, the stage in which polymorphonuclear neutrophils permeate the vessel wall, passing into the interstitial space.

urticaria Multiple small, raised areas on the skin that may be one of the warning signs of impending anaphylaxis; also known as hives.

vasculitis An inflammation of the blood vessels.

vasoactive amines Substances such as histamine and serotonin that increase vascular permeability, cause vasodilation, and can cause bronchoconstriction, nausea, and vomiting.

virulence A measure of the disease-causing ability of a microorganism.

References

1. He F, Li J, MacGregor GA. Effect of longer term modest salt reduction on blood pressure: Cochrane systematic review and meta-analysis of randomised trials. *BMJ.* 2013;346:f1325.
2. Friis-Hansen BJ, Holiday M, Stapleton T, Wallace WM. Total body water in children. *Pediatrics*. 1951;7(3):321-327.
3. Fontanarosa PB, Christiansen S. Units of measure. Table 2: selected laboratory tests, with reference ranges and conversion factors. In: American Medical Association, ed. *AMA Manual of Style: A Guide for Authors and Editors*. 11th ed. New York, NY: Oxford University Press; 2020:798-815.
4. Paz J, West M, Panasci, K, Greenwood, K. *Acute Care Handbook for Physical Therapists.* 5th ed. St. Louis, MO: Elsevier; 2020.
5. Speakman E. *Body Fluids and Electrolytes: A Programmed Presentation.* 8th ed. St. Louis, MO: Elsevier/Mosby; 2002.
6. Stipanuk MH, Caudill M. *Biochemical, Physiological, and Molecular Aspects of Human Nutrition.* 4th ed. St. Louis, MO: Elsevier; 2019.
7. Rose JJ, Wang L, Xu Q, et al. Carbon monoxide poisoning: pathogenesis, management and future directions of therapy. *Am J Resp Crit Care.* October 18, 2016. [Epub ahead of print]. doi:10.1164/rccm.201606-1275CI.
8. Schmidt H, Müller-Werdan U, Hoffmann T, et al. Autonomic dysfunction predicts mortality in patients with multiple organ dysfunction syndrome of different age groups. *Crit Care Med.* 2005;33(9):1994-2002.
9. Mayo Clinic Staff. Diseases and conditions: lupus: symptoms & causes. Mayo Foundation for Medical Education

Prep Kit continued

and Research. https://www.mayoclinic.org/diseases-conditions/lupus/symptoms-causes/syc-20365789. Accessed February 19, 2021.

10. MedlinePlus. X-linked agammaglobulinemia. https://medlineplus.gov/genetics/condition/x-linked-agammaglobulinemia/. Accessed February 19, 2021.
11. American Academy of Allergy, Asthma, and Immunology. X-linked agammaglobulinemia (XLA). https://www.aaaai.org/conditions-and-treatments/conditions-dictionary/x-linked-agammaglobulinemia-(xla). Accessed February 19, 2021.
12. Breast cancer facts and figures, 2017–2018. American Cancer Society website. https://www.cancer.org/content/dam/cancer-org/research/cancer-facts-and-statistics/breast-cancer-facts-and-figures/breast-cancer-facts-and-figures-2017-2018.pdf. Published 2017. Accessed August 18, 2021.
13. Howlader N, Noone AM, Krapcho M, et al., eds. *SEER Cancer Statistics Review, 1975–2017*. Bethesda, MD: National Cancer Institute. https://seer.cancer.gov/csr/1975_2017/. Based on November 2019 SEER data submission; posted April 2020. Accessed February 19, 2021.
14. American Cancer Society. *Cancer Facts and Figures 2021*. Atlanta, GA: American Cancer Society; 2021. https://www.cancer.org/content/dam/CRC/PDF/Public/8604.00.pdf. Accessed February 19, 2021.
15. National Hemophilia Foundation. Hemophilia A. https://www.hemophilia.org/bleeding-disorders-a-z/types/hemophilia-a. Accessed February 19, 2021.
16. CDC WONDER Online Database. Underlying cause of death 1999–2019. Centers for Disease Control and Prevention website. Underlying cause of death 1999–2013 on CDC WONDER Online Database, released 2015. Data are from the Multiple Cause of Death Files, 1999–2013, as compiled from data provided by the 57 vital statistics jurisdictions through the Vital Statistics Cooperative Program. Reviewed March 11, 2021. Accessed April 30, 2021.
17. Defining adult overweight and obesity. Centers for Disease Control and Prevention website. https://www.cdc.gov/obesity/adult/defining.html. Reviewed March 3, 2021. Accessed May 4, 2021.
18. Obesity and overweight. Centers for Disease Control and Prevention website. https://www.cdc.gov/nchs/fastats/obesity-overweight.htm. Page last reviewed January 11, 2021. Accessed February 23, 2021.
19. National Multiple Sclerosis Society. What Is MS? https://www.nationalmssociety.org/What-is-MS. Accessed February 19, 2021.
20. Alzheimer's Foundation of America. About Alzheimer's disease and dementia. https://alzfdn.org/caregiving-resources/about-alzheimers-disease-and-dementia/. Copyright 2019. Accessed February 19, 2021.
21. Depression and Bipolar Support Alliance. Bipolar disorder statistics. https://www.dbsalliance.org/education/bipolar-disorder/bipolar-disorder-statistics/. Accessed February 19, 2021.
22. National Institute of Mental Health website. https://www.nimh.nih.gov/health/statistics/bipolar-disorder.shtml. Last updated November 2017. Accessed February 23, 2021.

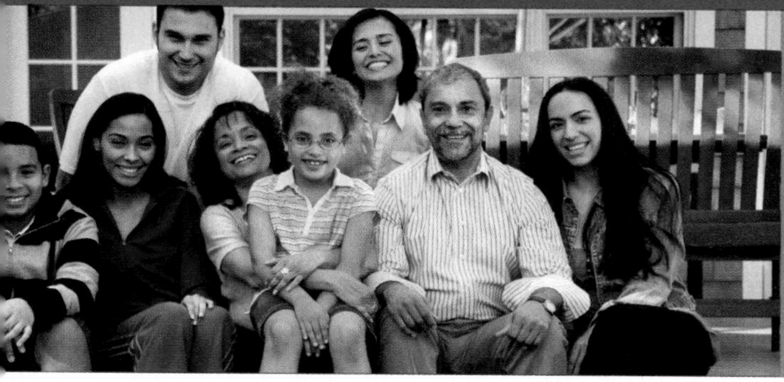

Chapter 10

Life Span Development

NATIONAL EMS EDUCATION STANDARD COMPETENCIES

Life Span Development

Integrates comprehensive knowledge of life span development.

KNOWLEDGE OBJECTIVES

1. Know the terms used to designate the following developmental stages of life: infants, toddlers and preschoolers, school-age children, adolescents (teenagers), early adults, middle adults, and late adults. (pp 555–574)
2. Describe the major physiologic and psychosocial characteristics of an infant's life. (pp 556–561)
3. Describe the major physiologic and psychosocial characteristics of a toddler's and preschooler's life. (pp 561–564)
4. Describe the major physiologic and psychosocial characteristics of a school-age child's life. (pp 564–565)
5. Describe the major physiologic and psychosocial characteristics of an adolescent's life. (pp 565–567)
6. Describe the major physiologic and psychosocial characteristics of an early adult's life. (p 567)
7. Describe the major physiologic and psychosocial characteristics of a middle adult's life. (pp 568–569)
8. Describe the major physiologic and psychosocial characteristics of a late adult's life. (pp 569–574)

SKILLS OBJECTIVES

There are no skills objectives for this chapter.

Introduction

One of the most interesting things about humans is that people evolve over the life span. As a paramedic, you must be aware of the obvious and subtle changes that humans undergo physically and mentally at various stages of life, and understand how these changes may affect your approach to patient care.

Infants

As any parent or caregiver can attest, **infants** develop at an astonishing rate **FIGURE 10-1**. In medicine, an

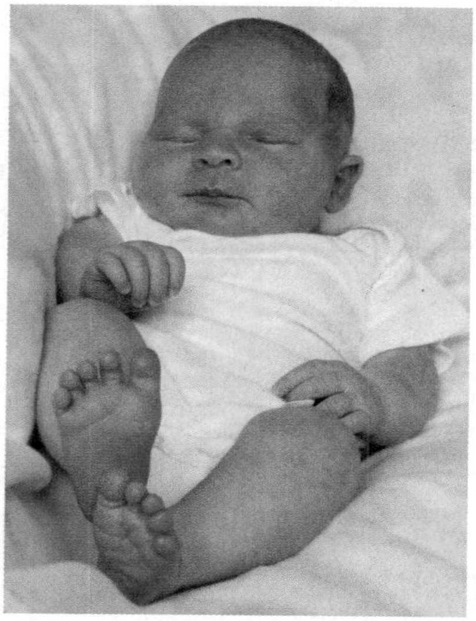

FIGURE 10-1 An infant.

infant is defined as a baby who is age 1 month to 1 year. Babies younger than age 1 month are categorized as either newborns or neonates depending on their age, and are covered in detail in Chapter 43, *Neonatal Care.*

Infants both grow and develop. Growth is defined as an increase in size, while development represents increased function or mastery of skills.[1]

Physical Changes

Vital Signs

Normal ranges of vital signs for various age groups are outlined in Chapter 11, *Patient Assessment,* and Chapter 44, *Pediatric Emergencies.* The younger the person, the faster the pulse rate and respirations. An awake neonate's pulse rate typically ranges from 100 to 205 beats/min, and their respiratory rate ranges between 30 and 60 breaths/min. Typically, tidal volume in infants is about 6 to 8 mL/kg and the oxygen saturation level is 94% or greater. Blood glucose level is normally 45 mg/dL or greater at birth, then increases to 60 mg/dL or greater from age 1 month on.[2]

In children, blood pressure (BP) often directly corresponds to the patient's weight, so it typically increases with age. At birth, an infant's systolic BP is usually in the range of 67 to 84 mm Hg. By age 1 year, systolic BP is in the range of 72 to 104 mm Hg.

Weight

A newborn at term usually weighs around 7.5 pounds (3.4 kg) at birth.[3] In the first week after birth, infants may lose 10% to 12% of their birth weight due to fluid loss and limited nutritional intake. By the second week of life, however, infants usually gain weight. From this point forward, infants grow at a rate of about 1 ounce (30 g) per day, doubling their weight by age 6 months and tripling it by age 1 year.[3]

Words of Wisdom

Infants often land headfirst when they fall because an infant's head accounts for a much larger percentage of the body weight than the head of an adult does. Also, most infants cannot stretch out their arms in time to cushion or slow their fall. Keep this point in mind when you assess an infant for potential head, neck, and spine injuries.

YOU are the Paramedic

PART 1

Your unit is dispatched to a private residence for a 3-year-old girl who has fallen in the backyard. The dispatcher advises that the child was running and fell, striking her head on a wooden deck. The dispatcher states that the child is crying audibly over the phone. As you arrive in front of the residence, the father comes toward your vehicle to meet you, carrying the child in his arms. The child appears to be vigorously struggling to be set down and is crying loudly.

1. What is your first concern at this scene?

2. Which stage of development describes a 3-year-old child, and how will this information affect your assessment?

Cardiovascular System

Before birth, fetal circulation occurs through the placenta. Just after birth, physiologic changes occur in the cardiovascular system that allow independent circulation via the newborn's own vasculature. This process is covered in detail in Chapter 43, *Neonatal Care.*

Pulmonary System

Prior to an infant's first breath, the lungs have never been inflated. An infant's first breath is therefore forceful—it has to be! An infant's first breath results from chemical, mechanical, thermal, and sensory triggers.[4]

Young infants are primarily "nose breathers" for the first several months of their lives.[5,6] Infants younger than 6 months are particularly prone to nasal congestion, which can cause viral upper respiratory infections. If you respond to a call for an infant who is choking, always make sure the infant's nasal passages are clear and unobstructed by mucus.

The rib cages of infants are less rigid than those of older people. The diaphragm is the newborn's major respiratory muscle. Because the intercostal muscles are not well developed, you will typically observe the abdomen bulge with each inspiration ("belly breathers"), but see little thoracic expansion.[6] Because of the immaturity of the accessory muscles, the infant can quickly become fatigued.

Words of Wisdom

When you count respirations in an infant, you may choose to count the number of times the abdomen rises instead of concentrating solely on chest rise.

Fluid and heat loss occur through exhalation. Thus, the rapid respiratory rate of infants can lead to significant heat and fluid loss. Keep infants warm, and monitor them for signs of dehydration.

An infant's airway differs from an adult's airway in many ways. Notably, the infant's tongue is larger in proportion to the oral cavity, and the airway is proportionally shorter and narrower. As a result, an infant's airway can be occluded more easily than the airway in older children or adults. An infant also has fewer alveoli in the lungs, which decreases the surface area available for gas exchange.

When you provide bag-mask ventilations to an infant, be aware that an infant's lungs are fragile. Ventilations that are delivered with excessive force or excessive volume can result in trauma from pressure, known as **barotrauma** **FIGURE 10-2**. It is imperative to use a bag-mask device that is the correct size for the patient **FIGURE 10-3**.

Renal System

Newborns and infants can easily become dehydrated. Newborn kidneys are less able than adult kidneys to concentrate urine and excrete water.

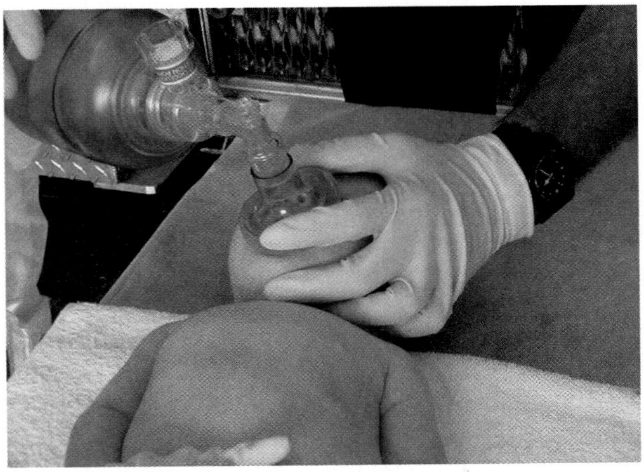

FIGURE 10-2 An infant's lungs are fragile. Use caution when providing bag-mask ventilations to avoid barotrauma.

Courtesy of Marianne Gausche-Hill, MD, FACEP, FAAP.

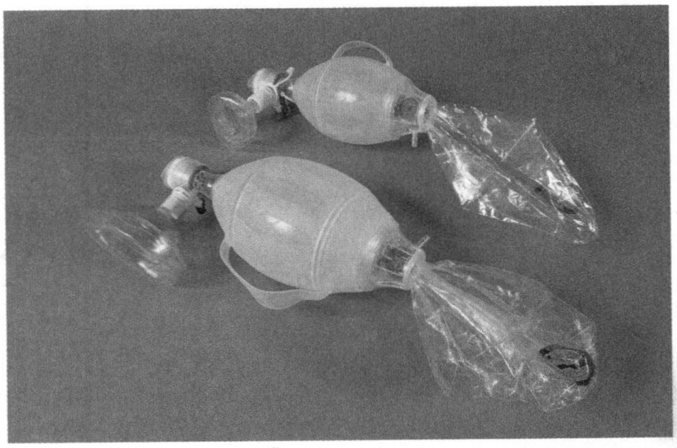

FIGURE 10-3 Child (left) and newborn/neonatal (right) bag-mask devices. Use the appropriate size for your patient.

Thus, when they experience dehydration, newborns and infants cannot compensate to the same extent adults can.[7] Also, an infant's urine consists mainly of water, which can cause the child to develop electrolyte imbalances.

Immune System

While in the womb, infants receive antibodies from the maternal blood. For the first year of life, the infant maintains some of the mother's immunities, and so has naturally acquired passive immunities. Infants can also receive antibodies via breastfeeding, further bolstering their immune systems.

Nervous System

Although an infant's nervous system is developed at birth, its evolution continues after birth. For example, a newborn lacks the ability to localize and isolate a particular response to sensation. An infant's brainstem and spinal column are present and functioning, but memory and fine motor coordination are not yet fully developed. Also, the ability to control body temperature is limited in members of this age group.[7]

An infant is born with certain reflexes. The cranial nerves control these necessary reflexes, such as the blinking, sucking, and gag reflexes. The **Moro reflex** (startle reflex) occurs when an infant is caught off guard by something or someone; the infant opens arms wide, spreads the fingers, and seems to grab at things. A **palmar grasp** occurs when an object is placed into the infant's palm; the infant will close the fingers around the object. The **rooting reflex** occurs when something touches an infant's cheek; the infant will instinctively turn the head toward the touch. In conjunction with the **sucking reflex**, which occurs when an infant's lips are stroked, these reflexes are often tested during feeding.

An infant's **fontanelles** (soft spots) are sheets of tough connective tissue between the flat bones of the skull that soften and expand when the newborn passes through the birth canal **FIGURE 10-4**. The fontanelles are gradually replaced as the bones of the skull fuse together and form suture joints by age 2 years. The fontanelles play a key role in your assessment of an infant. An anterior fontanelle that is sunken may be a sign of dehydration.

Perhaps the neurologic development in infants that is of most interest to parents and/or caregivers is the development of a sleep pattern. The sleep pattern evolves through a combination of central nervous system (CNS) development and parental efforts. Most infants develop the ability to sleep for 5 hours by age 3 months, but some do not develop this until age 1 year.[1] A concern related to infant sleep is sudden infant death syndrome (SIDS); this is discussed in Chapter 44, *Pediatric Emergencies.*

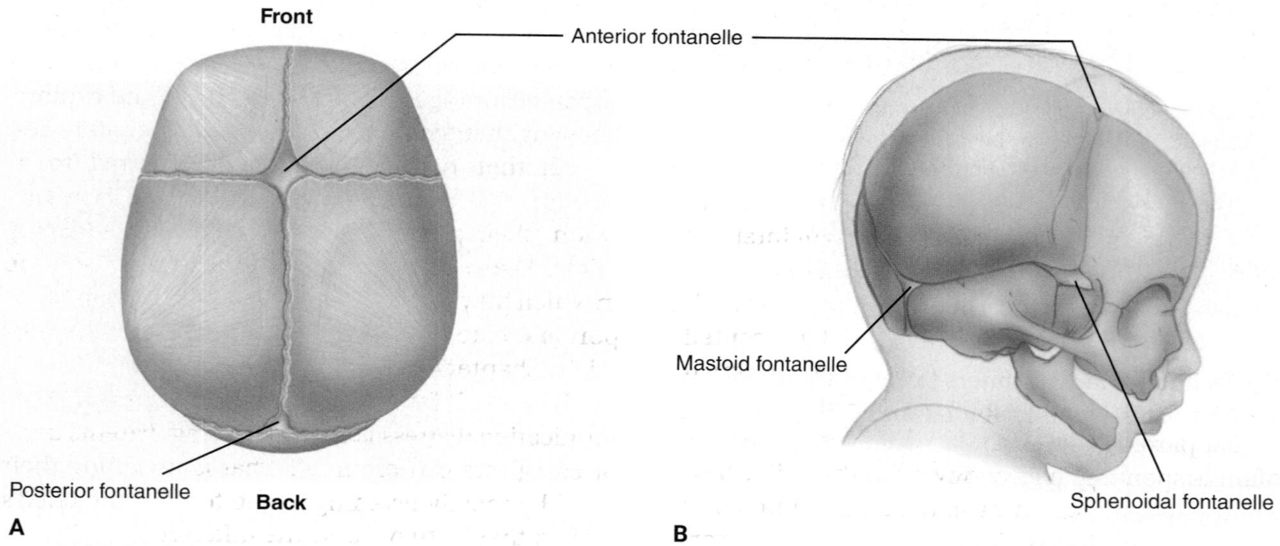

FIGURE 10-4 The fontanelles. **A.** Superior view. **B.** Lateral view.

Musculoskeletal System

Growth plates (epiphyseal plates) are located on either end of a long bone and are the centers where longitudinal bone growth occurs. Growth charts are used to track an infant's or child's growth; they provide percentiles comparing the child's growth with the expected growth of an average infant or child of that age.

Teeth

Teething (ie, when teeth erupt or break through the gums) often starts between the ages of 4 and 7 months and can be a challenge to both parents and infants. As with many life changes, this time frame is an estimate: Some infants will have teeth erupt as early as 1 month, and some may have to wait as long as 1 year. Teeth usually erupt in a predetermined order, and a child should have a full set by the age of 3 years. The child will usually keep this set of "baby teeth" until around the age of 6 years, when permanent teeth start to come in.

Words of Wisdom

Infants are oral explorers, meaning everything they find goes into their mouths. Airway obstructions from foreign bodies can occur as a result of them exploring their world. When you are called for breathing difficulty in an infant, especially as the child becomes mobile, remember to look closely at the airway for obstructions.

TABLE 10-1 Psychosocial Characteristics at Various Ages

Age (in months)	Noticeable Characteristics
2	Recognizes familiar faces; tracks objects with the eyes
3	Brings objects to the mouth; smiles and frowns
4	Reaches out to people; drools
5	Sleeps through the night; recognizes family from strangers
6	Teething begins; sits upright in a chair; speaks one-syllable words
7	Afraid of strangers; has mood swings
8	Responds to "no"; sits upright alone; plays peek-a-boo
9	Pulls self up; places objects in mouth to explore them
10	Responds to own name; crawls efficiently
11	Starts to walk without help; frustrated with restrictions
12	Knows own name; can walk

Psychosocial Changes

An infant's psychosocial development begins at birth and continues to evolve as the infant interacts with and reacts to the environment. Parents and/or caregivers are often concerned about whether their child's development matches the socially accepted norms. **TABLE 10-1** outlines typical ages at which major psychosocial changes are noticed.

For parents, one key to having a happy, healthy infant is spending quality time with the child. Nevertheless, infants often have their own timetables as to when they will become attached to their parents and other family members. **Bonding**, or the formation of a close, personal relationship, is usually based on a **secure attachment**. A secure attachment occurs when infants understand that parents and/or caregivers will respond to their needs. This realization encourages infants to reach out and explore, knowing that their parents will provide a safety net.

Another type of attachment, referred to as **anxious avoidant attachment**, is observed in infants whom their parents and/or caregivers repeatedly reject. These children develop an isolated lifestyle in which they do not have to depend on others' support and care. Child neglect is covered in more detail in Chapter 44, *Pediatric Emergencies*.

In most infants, the primary method of communicating distress is through crying. Parents and/or caregivers can often tell what is upsetting their child by merely listening to the tone of the child's crying; that is, they know the difference between a basic cry (which conveys hunger, discomfort, frustration, or sleepiness) and one that conveys anger or pain. Infants occasionally make another distinct cry—an alarming, distressed cry. This cry may be heard when an unexpected event occurs, causing a **situational crisis** (a crisis caused by a specific set of circumstances) for the infant.

Infants who have bonded well with their parents and/or caregivers and have good relationships will usually respond predictably when a situational crisis occurs. The most prevalent example of a situational crisis is being separated from the parent and/or caregiver. Separation anxiety is common in older infants. The normal reaction peaks between the ages of 10 and 18 months, and involves clingy behavior and fear of unfamiliar places and people. An infant's reaction to a situational crisis is classified into the following three phases:

- The **protest phase** can start immediately and usually lasts about a week. It is easily recognized by loud crying, irritability, restlessness, and rejection of other caregivers' efforts.
- The **despair phase** follows, which is characterized by the monotonous wailing indicating that the infant begins to believe the situation will not change.
- **Withdrawal** eventually occurs, and the infant becomes almost apathetic and appears bored by their surroundings.

As infants become accustomed to their homes and families, they begin to need the security of a predictable environment. If an infant's environment is too unpredictable, then the infant may despair and become withdrawn, which may lead to problems in the development of trust. **Trust and mistrust** refers to the developmental stage that spans from birth to about 18 months of age. Most infants desire that their worlds be planned, organized, and routine. If the infant perceives that the parents and/or caregivers will provide this predictable environment, the infant gains trust in them. The opposite also holds true: If an infant perceives that the parents and/or caregivers will not provide an organized and routine environment, then the infant may develop behavioral problems.

Infants respond well to **scaffolding**, an instructional technique in which a person builds on what has already been learned. As a student, you can also benefit from this technique! For example, the basic assessment skills that you learned in your emergency medical technician course will now be used as building blocks for the advanced assessments taught in this paramedic course.

Temperament

With regard to temperament (behavioral style), children are classified as being easy, difficult, or slow to warm up to their surroundings and lifestyles. Easy children are characterized by the relative ease by which they adapt. Their body functions work properly, they have low-intensity reactions, and they accept new surroundings well. Difficult children usually have intense reactions, and they do not acclimate to new surroundings well. Children who are slow to warm up usually have low-intensity reactions, but generally exhibit negative moods.

As a paramedic, it can be helpful to adjust your approach according to the patient's developmental stage. Useful techniques include having the parent or caregiver hold the infant and allowing the infant to hold a toy **FIGURE 10-5**. In fact, you may complete your physical assessment of an infant with the infant in the parent's or caregiver's arms—unless the child is in respiratory failure, in need of spinal

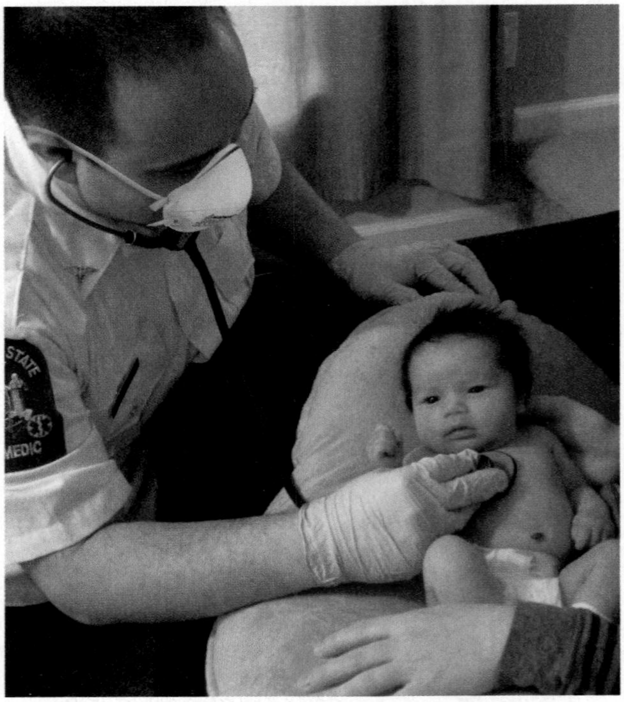

FIGURE 10-5 Have the parent or caregiver hold the infant while you perform your assessment and treatment, if possible.

motion restriction, or has a reduced level of consciousness. You may also distract the child and save the most challenging part of the assessment and treatment for last.

> **Words of Wisdom**
>
> If the parent or caregiver who is holding the sick or injured child is upset, they may create a stressful environment for the child, who will react to the parent's distress. This can make your assessment more difficult. If another parent or family member who is calmer is available, consider having them hold the sick or injured child if the situation allows.

Toddlers and Preschoolers

Physical Changes

In **toddlers** (ages 1 to 2 years **FIGURE 10-6**) and **preschoolers** (ages 3 to 5 years **FIGURE 10-7**), the pulse rates and respiratory rates are slower than in infants, whereas the systolic BP is higher (approximately 100 mm Hg). In addition, the rate of weight gain should level off in these children.

A toddler's cardiovascular system is not dramatically different from that of an adult. A toddler's lungs continue to develop more bronchioles and alveoli. Although toddlers and preschoolers have more lung tissue, they do not have well-developed lung musculature, which prevents them from sustaining deep or rapid respirations for an extended time.

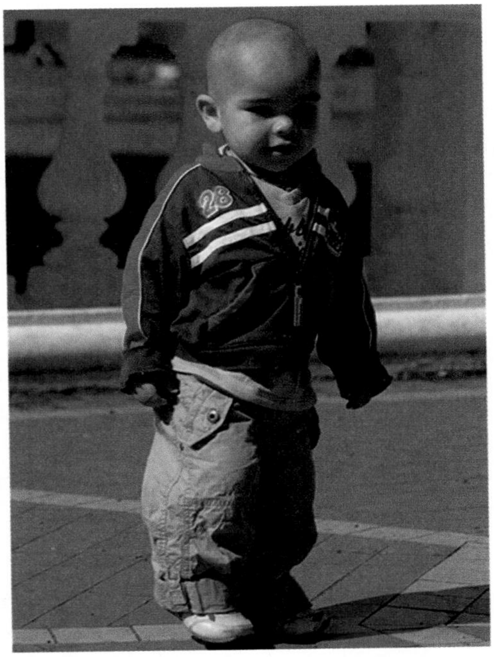

FIGURE 10-6 A toddler.

YOU are the Paramedic

PART 2

You and your partner convince the mother and father to sit down on the front steps of the residence rather than immediately climb up into your vehicle. You ask the child her name and she buries her face in her father's chest. The mother tells you her name is Juliet. The father tries to forcefully turn Juliet so she will face you, and the child clings to him even harder and cries louder.

Recording Time: 2 Minutes	
Appearance	Actively moving and crying
Level of consciousness	Conscious and agitated
Airway	Open
Breathing	Loud crying
Circulation	Adequate

3. Why is Juliet clinging to her father and turning away from you?

4. What are some of the measures you can take to alleviate the child's distress?

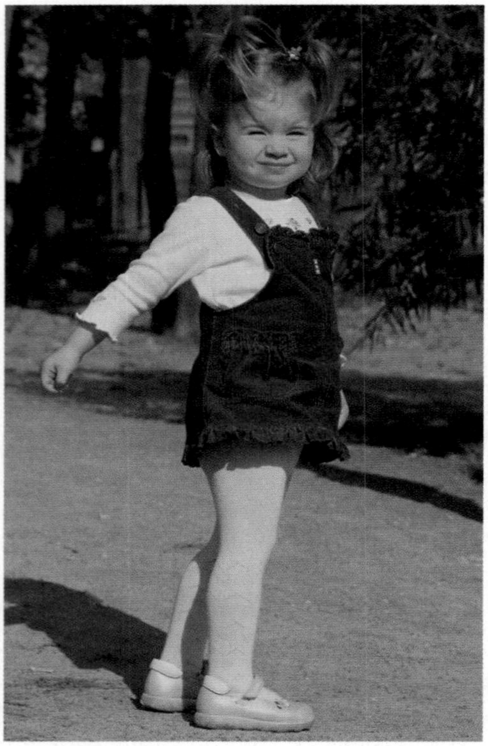

FIGURE 10-7 A preschooler.

© Maxim Bolotnikov/Shutterstock.

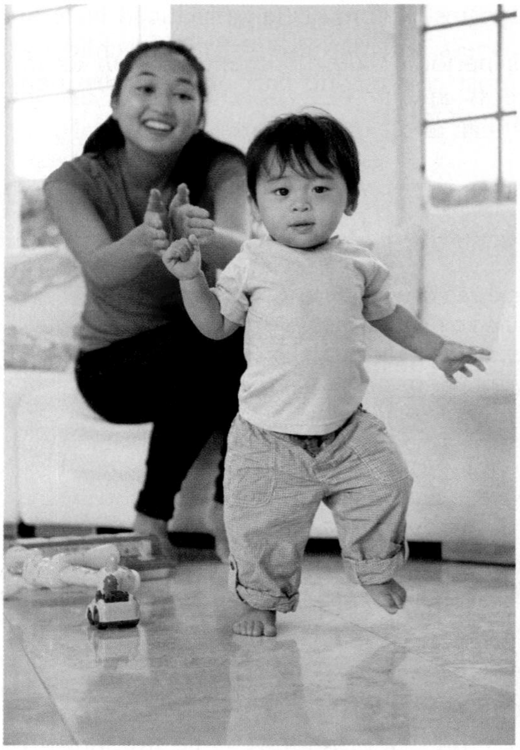

FIGURE 10-8 Toddlers learn to walk, one of the major milestones in life.

© monkeybusinessimages/iStock/Getty.

The loss of passive immunity in the immune system is perhaps the most readily apparent developmental change at this stage of human life. Toddlers and preschoolers often develop common colds, which may manifest as gastrointestinal distress or upper respiratory tract infections. As toddlers spend more time around playmates and classmates, they acquire their own immunity as the body is exposed to various pathogens.

Neuromuscular growth also makes considerable progress at this age. Toddlers and preschoolers spend a great deal of time finding out exactly how to use their nervous system and the muscles it controls by walking, running, jumping, and playing catch **FIGURE 10-8**. By age 3 years, bone density and muscle mass increase to become more like those of an adult. Watching children play as they age from 1 to 5 years demonstrates how they move from gross motor activities (grabbing an object with the full palm) to fine motor activities (picking up a crayon). By the end of this stage, a preschooler will have a brain that weighs 90% of its final adult weight. In addition, all of this playing places stress on the muscles and bones. Consequently, muscle mass increases, as does bone density.

This stage also features the renal system's continued development and perhaps the most anticipated event of this stage of life: toilet training! Physiologically, toddlers develop bowel control before bladder control.[1] Toddlers have the neuromuscular control needed for bladder control and can feel when the bladder is full by 12 to 15 months of age. On average, the 18-month-old child can control the muscles to delay excretion for a short time. However, the child may not be psychologically ready to do so until 18 to 30 months of age. There might not be any greater satisfaction for a child of this age than to run up to the parents and tell them, "I'm a big kid now—I used the potty!"

Other developments that continue during this time frame include the continued emergence of baby teeth; teething can be painful and accompanied by fever. In addition, parents and/or caregivers and toddlers are enthralled with sensory development (ie, tickling).

Psychosocial Changes

This period of development is often exciting for parents and/or caregivers. Toddlers are learning to speak and express themselves, thereby taking a major step toward independence. At the same time, toddlers are very attached to their parents and feel safe with them. As mentioned previously, separation anxiety peaks between 10 and 18 months of age. It is fascinating to watch a child struggle through the conflict of wanting to play independently, yet also wanting to be protected.

Children understand language long before they begin to speak. Language acquisition occurs in phases, beginning with speaking one or two words at age 1 year, and achieving basic language mastery at 36 months of age.[1] From ages 2 to 5, the number of words in a spoken sentence typically equals the child's age; in other words, at age 3, a toddler speaks three-word sentences.[3] Refinement of language skills continues throughout childhood. By the age of 3 or 4 years, most children can use and understand full sentences. As they progress through this stage of their life, they will transition from using language to communicate what they want to using language creatively and playfully.

This period is also when toddlers begin to interact with other children and start to play games. Playing games teaches control, obedience, and even competitiveness. A great deal of learning and development occur when children watch their peers during group outings, such as playdates. Of course, behavior observed on television and the Internet can be learned as well, which is why some parents and/or caregivers limit their children's viewing choices or the amount of time they devote to these activities. During this developmental phase, children also learn to recognize sexual differences by observing their role models and siblings.

As with infants, it is essential to include the parent or caregiver when working with a toddler or preschooler. Position yourself at the child's level so that you are making eye contact. Explain to the child what you plan to do before you do it, and allow the child to make choices when possible. As with infants, save the most difficult part of the assessment and treatment for last.

Another tip: Do not try to reason with young children about why a procedure (eg, establishing an intravenous [IV] line) has to be done. Explain it briefly using words they can understand, then do it! Often the psychological experience can be worse than the physical one if you give a child too much time to worry about a minor procedure. Never lie to the patient. If a child asks if an IV will hurt, answer honestly: "Yes, it will feel like a pinch for a second." If you lie to a child, that child will not trust you for the rest of your assessment or treatment, and your rapport will be gone.

Street Smarts

When you interact with very young patients, try to keep their routines the same by keeping family and familiar items nearby.

With toddlers and preschoolers, you might try to "break the ice" by giving them a teddy bear and explaining what you are going to do by showing them on the teddy bear. Such children may be able to understand by show-and-tell more clearly than by listening to a verbal description. Be sure that the toy has no removable parts, and store it in a clean plastic bag between calls.

Documentation and Communication

When you document your assessment of an infant or young child, it is often best to avoid the struggle of obtaining a BP with a stable patient. Simply documenting breath sounds, an apical pulse, work of breathing, and the child's interactions with the surroundings can more than adequately describe the patient's condition.

Parenting Styles

A child's development is affected by the parenting style employed by the child's parents. Although parenting is a complex behavior, and one that is rarely well defined in any particular individual, four idealized approaches may be examined.

An **authoritarian** parenting style demands absolute obedience from a child, no matter what the situation. This parenting style shows no regard for the child's personal freedoms; for example, a child may be punished for simply questioning a parent.

Children who are raised in this manner often develop self-esteem problems; girls are more likely to become shy and boys are more likely to become argumentative or hostile.

Authoritative parenting is based on respect for parental authority and balance with the child's individual freedom. These parents regularly respond to the personal needs of the child. They set rules and enforce them fairly; however, they believe that children need certain freedoms and attempt to maintain a balance between the two. This style can allow children to develop into adults who are independent, well socialized, and easygoing.

Permissive parenting does not impose many rules, if any, on the child. The child is in control, and the parent takes a tolerant approach to the child's behavior, including socially unacceptable behaviors. Permissive parenting is classified into two subcategories: indifferent and indulgent. The former style describes parents who just do not care; the latter style describes excessively lenient parents. Permissive parents rarely, if ever, punish their children, so their children may grow up to be considered spoiled. These children often become adults who are immature and irresponsible, and who lack self-control.

Uninvolved (neglectful) parenting forces children to raise themselves. The parents are not involved in the child's life and rarely know where the child is or what the child is doing. There are often few or even no rules for the child to follow, and the child is not accountable to anyone. This style of parenting is not always the parent's deliberate choice. Factors in the parent's life such as a mental health or substance use disorder, or even the need to work to provide income, can contribute to uninvolved parenting. The child who is raised with this parenting style often has impulsive behavior, performs poorly in school, and suffers from depression.

Divorce

Almost one-half of all marriages in the United States end in divorce.[8] No matter what stage of life a child is in, a divorce will profoundly affect that child. Children naturally question if the divorce was their fault, may wonder what they could have done to prevent it, and experience pain from the changes in their environment. Many parents respond to their children's feelings and needs together. Through this kind of ongoing partnership, they assure their children that although they will experience some changes in their lives, they will always have parents who love them very much. As long as both parents maintain their children as their priority, most children adapt relatively easily to the social changes that a divorce brings on a family.

School-Age Children

Physical Changes

School-age children are those age 6 to 12 years. A school-age child's vital signs and body gradually approach those observed in adulthood **FIGURE 10-9**. Obvious physical traits and body function changes become apparent during this developmental phase, as most children grow about 5.5 to 7.7 pounds (2.5 to 3.5 kg) and 2 inches (5 cm) each year.[1] Brain function develops further in both hemispheres, and permanent teeth come in during this period. Also, the onset of puberty may begin in elementary school-age children and has been documented at age 10 years or younger.

Psychosocial Changes

Children engage in a great deal of psychosocial growth during the school years, though the pace of development varies from child to child.

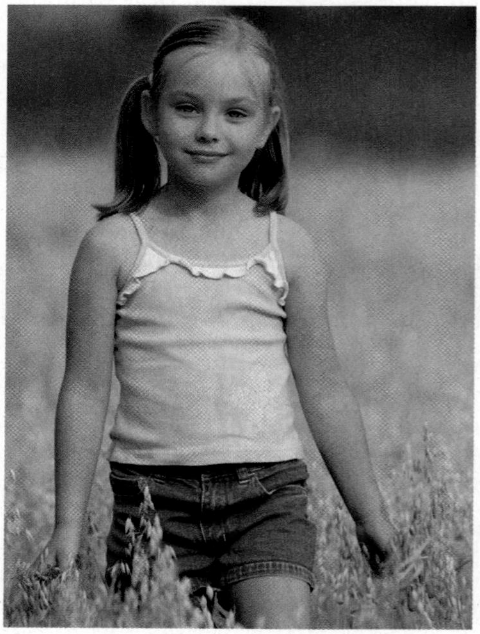

FIGURE 10-9 A school-age child.

Parents as a whole do not devote as much time to their children during this phase. Nevertheless, it is at this critical time in human development that children learn various types of reasoning. In **preconventional reasoning**, children act almost purely to avoid punishment and to get what they want. In **conventional reasoning**, they look for approval from their peers and society. In **postconventional reasoning**, children make decisions guided by their conscience.

During the school-age years, children begin to develop their **self-concept** and **self-esteem**. Self-concept is a person's perception of themself; self-esteem is how a person feels about themself and about how they fit in with peers.

When you are working with a school-age child, use the same techniques you would use with a preschooler; that is, position yourself at the child's level, explain what you plan to do, and give choices when possible. Always be honest about what you are doing. For example, if a procedure might hurt, then say so to your patient. The biggest issue with school-age children is trust. You have to earn it quickly through open and honest communication, and you must never lose it through lies or sneaky maneuvers. If you are direct with them and remain assertive, then school-age children will respond well most of the time.

Adolescents (Teenagers)

Physical Changes

The vital signs of **adolescents** (children ages 13 through 18 years) begin to level off within the adult ranges, with a systolic BP between 110 and 131 mm Hg, a pulse rate between 60 and 100 beats/min, and respirations in the range of 12 to 20 breaths/min **FIGURE 10-10**.

Adolescence is also the phase of life when humans experience a rapid, 2- to 3-year growth spurt (ie, an increase in muscle and bone growth) as well as changes in blood chemistry. Growth begins with the hands and feet, then moves to the long bones of the extremities, and finishes with growth of the torso. As a whole, boys experience this stage of development later in life than girls do. However, when this period of growth has finished, boys are generally taller and physically stronger than girls. Muscle mass and bone density are nearly at adult levels.

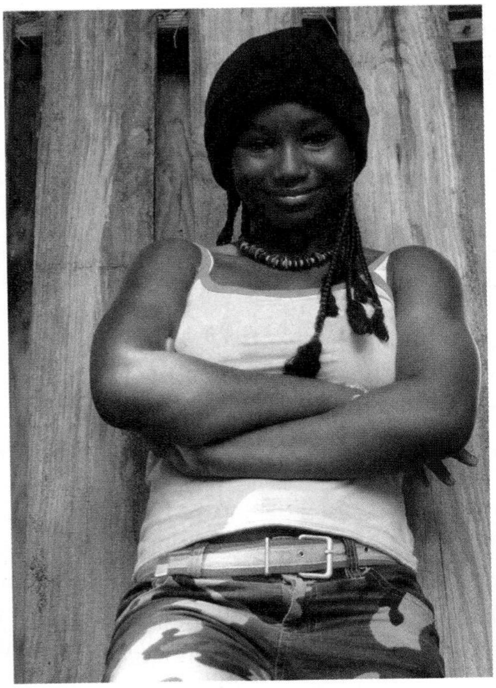

FIGURE 10-10 An adolescent.

An important change during this phase of life is the maturation of the human reproductive system. Secondary sexual development begins during adolescence, along with enlargement of the external sex organs. Pubic hair and axillary hair begin to appear. Voices start to change in range and depth. In girls, the breasts and thighs increase in size as adipose tissue is deposited there. Traditionally, menstruation has been considered to begin during this time; however, **menarche** (the first menstrual bleeding) is starting to occur at increasingly younger ages, such that many girls now begin menstruation before becoming a teenager.

Another key development in girls is the release of follicle-stimulating hormone and luteinizing hormone, both of which increase estrogen and progesterone production. In contrast, the hormone gonadotropin is secreted in boys and results in the production of testosterone. Acne can occur due to hormonal changes.

These changes in the endocrine and reproductive systems provide the platform for reproduction. By the middle of adolescence, boys are able to produce sufficient sperm and girls are able to develop eggs, which allows reproduction to take place.

Psychosocial Changes

Adolescents and their families often deal with conflict, as teenagers try to gain control of their lives from their parents. Privacy becomes an issue among adolescents, their siblings, and their parents. Self-consciousness also increases. Adolescents may struggle to create their own identities—to define who they are, for example, by dressing in a particular clothing style to fit their personalities **FIGURE 10-11**. Adolescents use the feedback from their family and peers to help create their adult images. Adolescents are often caught between two worlds: They want to be treated like adults, yet cared for like younger children.

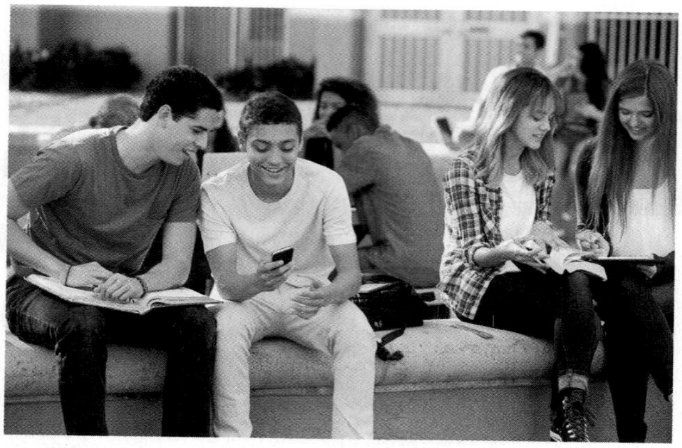

FIGURE 10-11 Adolescents want to fit in and may struggle to create their identities.

Rebellious behavior can be part of an adolescent trying to find their own identity. Adolescents continually compare themselves with their peers, which makes peer pressure a significant factor in an adolescent's psychological growth. Antisocial behavior peaks during the eighth or ninth grade. Adolescence is also a time when eating disorders may develop, as teenagers become obsessed with body image. Self-destructive behaviors such as smoking, drinking alcohol, and experimenting with drugs may begin as well. Although these behaviors can be troubling to parents, adolescents are trying to determine if they are ready to take control of their own lives. An adolescent's struggle toward independence may include setbacks, some of which can be devastating. Patience and support from family and friends are essential in assisting an adolescent's transition into adulthood.

Adolescents may also show greater interest in sexual relations. Many are fixated on their public

YOU are the Paramedic

PART 3

Your partner asks the mother what Juliet's favorite item is and she answers, "Her pink blanket." Your partner asks the mother to retrieve the blanket and to show her where the fall occurred. The mother agrees, and both enter the residence. The father is still struggling with the child. You ask him to loosen his embrace and allow the child to pick her position of comfort. At that point, your partner and the mother return with the child's blanket. Your partner sits down on the ground, slightly lower than the child, and offers her the blanket. Juliet takes the blanket from her and appears to calm down considerably. You carefully begin your assessment.

Recording Time: 7 Minutes	
Respirations	Crying
Pulse	130 beats/min
Skin	Hot, dry, flushed
Blood pressure	Unable to obtain
Oxygen saturation (Spo_2)	Unable to obtain
Pupils	Pupils Equal, Round, and Reactive to Light and Accommodation (PERRLA)

5. Measurement of Spo_2 level and BP requires equipment. How can you gain the child's trust to use your equipment?

6. What is the expected normal range for a 3-year-old child's pulse rate and respiratory rate?

FIGURE 10-12 Try to interview adolescent patients in private, if possible.

images and are terrified of being embarrassed. At this age, adolescents develop a code of personal ethics, based partly on the parents' ethics and values and partly on the influence of their own environment. During this tumultuous time, adolescents are at a higher risk than other populations for suicide and depression.

When you work with adolescents, be respectful and discreet. Remember, privacy is important to adolescents. If possible, have your partner speak with the parent in a separate area while you talk with the patient **FIGURE 10-12**. This may make the adolescent more comfortable and provide you more accurate answers than you would receive in a parent's presence.

Street Smarts

It is best to ask adolescents certain questions in total privacy, where they feel they can answer without constraint. Also be considerate when clothing removal is necessary for treatment, and remember that this population can be particularly self-conscious about their body. As with any patient, keep any exposed skin covered for privacy.

Early Adults

Physical Changes

Early adults range in age from 19 to 40 years **FIGURE 10-13**. Their vital signs do not vary significantly from those seen throughout adulthood. The pulse rate ranges from 60 to 100 beats/min, the respiratory rate is in the range of 12 to 20 breaths/min, and the systolic BP is between 90 and 140 mm Hg.

FIGURE 10-13 An early adult.

From age 19 years to just a little after age 25 years, the human body should function at its optimal level. After this point, the discs in the spine begin to settle, and height can sometimes be affected, causing a "shrinking." Fatty tissue increases, which leads to weight gain. Muscle strength decreases, and the reflexes slow.

Psychosocial Changes

During this period, humans strive to create a place for themselves in the world, and many do everything they can to "settle down." As early adults struggle to find stability in their careers, job stress increases. Along with this natural tendency to settle come the experiences of romantic and affectionate love. Childbirth is most common in this age group. Despite all of this stress and change, this age group enjoys one of the more stable life periods. People in early adulthood generally experience fewer psychological conditions related to well-being.

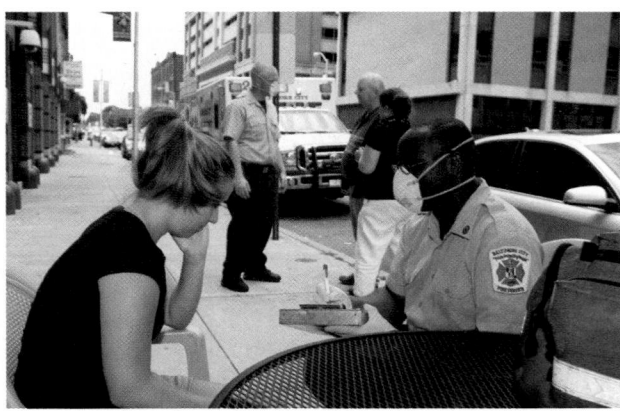

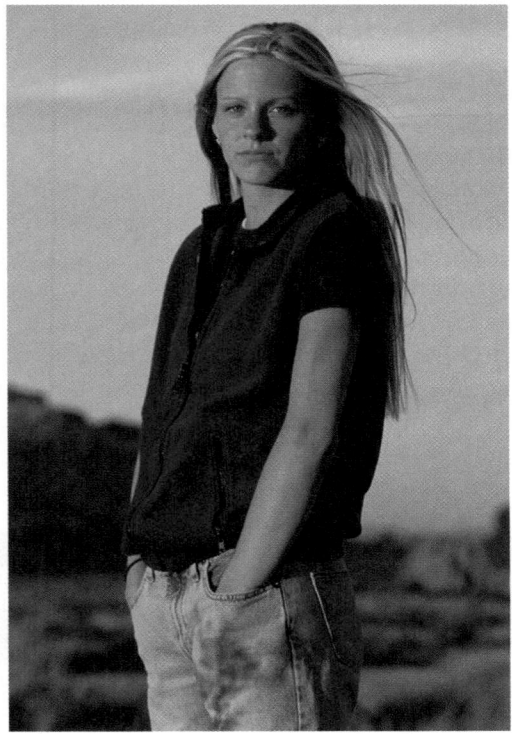

Middle Adults

Physical Changes

Middle adults range in age from 41 to 60 years **FIGURE 10-14**. Even though the body is still functioning at a high level, this age group is vulnerable to vision and hearing loss and other varying degrees of degradation. Cardiovascular health also becomes an issue for many people in this age group. Cardiac output (the amount of blood circulated each minute) decreases, while cholesterol levels increase, leading to higher incidences of cardiovascular disease. Owing to the less efficient metabolism, it becomes more difficult for middle adults to control their weight. Middle adults also experience a greater incidence of cancer.

In women, **menopause**—the cessation of menstruation—begins in the late 40s or early 50s. This change can result in both the loss of bone density and the development of cardiovascular disease. Subsequently, these women are at a higher risk for fractures and cardiac conditions.

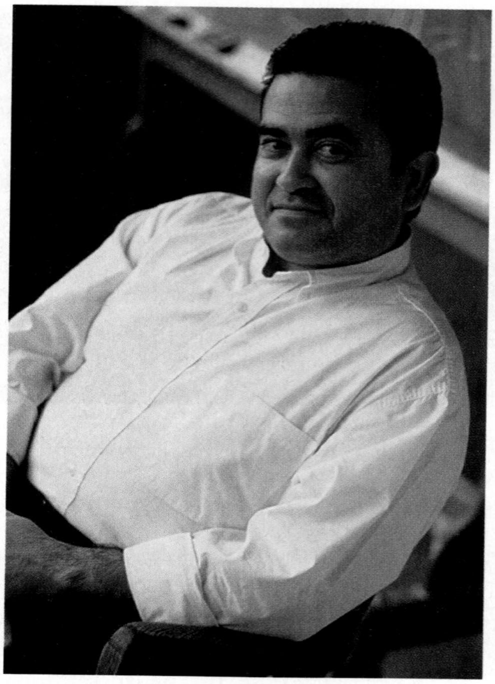

FIGURE 10-14 A middle adult.

Psychosocial Changes

Middle adults tend to focus on achieving their life's goals, as they realize that they are past the halfway point in human life expectancy (discussed next). After years of nurturing and living with children, parents must readjust their lifestyle as their children leave the home, a phenomenon commonly called the empty nest syndrome. Finances may become a worrisome issue, as people plan for retirement while still managing everyday financial demands.

YOU are the Paramedic

PART 4

You and your partner are slowly gaining the trust of your patient. You are able to see a 0.5-inch (1-cm) laceration on the child's forehead with a corresponding abrasion and hematoma. The wound is not actively bleeding.

Recording Time: 17 Minutes	
Respirations	20 breaths/min
Pulse	118 beats/min
Skin	Hot, dry, normal color
Blood pressure	Unable to obtain
Oxygen saturation (Spo_2)	99% on room air
Pupils	PERRLA

7. You need to bandage your patient's laceration. Offer some ideas to make this process more acceptable to the patient.

8. How should you transport this patient?

During this time, people often view crises as challenges to be overcome rather than as threats to be avoided.

Late Adults

Physical Changes

Late adults include those ages 61 years and older **FIGURE 10-15**. **Life expectancy** is constantly changing, so what is considered the "end of life" period continues to be revised. When the first edition of this text was printed in 1979, human life expectancy at birth in the United States was about 73 years. It is now about 77 years.[9]

Later in life, vital signs depend on the patient's overall health, medical conditions, and medications taken. Today's late adults are staying active longer than their ancestors did. Thanks to medical advances, they can often overcome numerous medical conditions, but may need multiple medications to do so **FIGURE 10-16**.

Cardiovascular System

Cardiac function declines with age consequent to anatomic and physiologic changes that are largely related to **atherosclerosis**. In this disorder, which most commonly affects the coronary vessels, cholesterol and calcium build up inside the walls of blood vessels and form plaque. The accumulation of plaque eventually leads to partial or complete blockage of blood flow. Atherosclerosis can also contribute to development of an **aneurysm**, or weakening and bulging of the blood vessel wall; an aneurysm may potentially rupture if it is subjected to high stretching forces. Many people older than 65 years have atherosclerotic disease.

Words of Wisdom

Just like the wiring and plumbing in your homes, the body's wiring (nervous system) and plumbing (arteries, veins, heart, and lungs) begin to break down over time.

Other age-related changes typically include a decrease in pulse rate, a decline in cardiac output, and an inability to elevate cardiac output to match the body's demands. These changes translate into a heart that is less able to respond to exercise or disease (eg, with an increased pulse rate). In the event of a life-threatening illness, the body typically needs to increase the pulse rate to ensure adequate BP. Because heart muscle may be weakened with age, an increase in the pulse rate can cause damage to the heart itself.

The vascular system also becomes stiff in older adults. In turn, the diastolic BP increases with age. The left ventricle must then work harder to move blood effectively, so it becomes thicker. A loss of elasticity occurs. The thickening and stiffening of the left ventricle hinder filling in the ventricle, thereby decreasing cardiac output. Similar

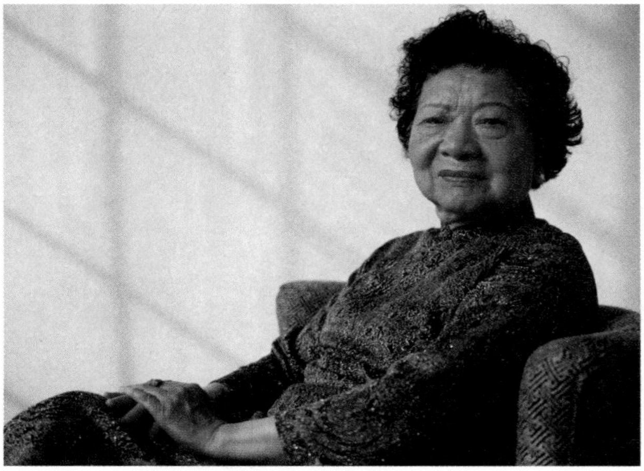

FIGURE 10-15 A late adult.

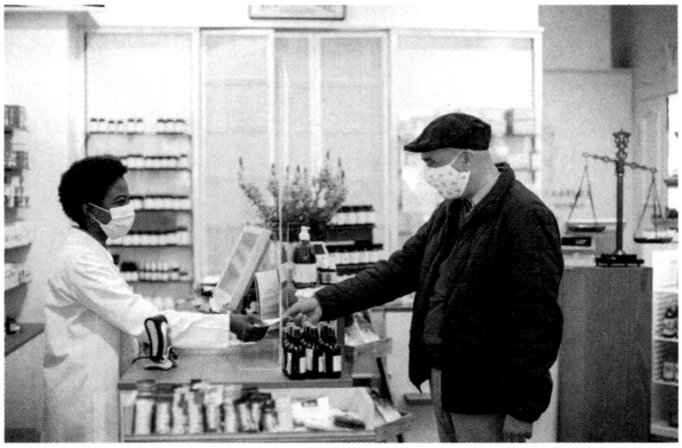

FIGURE 10-16 Older people are often prescribed multiple medications to help them stay active.

stiffening occurs in the heart valves, which may impede normal blood flow into and out of the heart. As the blood passes through these stiffened valves, a heart murmur may be heard, even in the absence of disease. In some individuals, decreases in elastin and collagen in blood vessel walls reduce the peripheral vessels' elasticity by as much as 70%. Compensating for these BP changes can be challenge because the stiffened vessels are less able to distend and contract.

Blood cells are also affected by aging. These cells originate from within the bone marrow. As a person ages, more of the bone marrow becomes replaced with fatty tissue, which decreases the bones' ability to manufacture more blood cells when needed. Although the fatty tissue typically does not pose a problem by itself, if an older person sustains trauma, then the body's ability to produce blood cells to replace those lost from the injury is diminished. Finally, functional blood volume gradually declines over time.

Respiratory System

In late adults, the size of the airway increases and the surface area of the alveoli decreases. Metabolic changes cause the lungs' natural elasticity to decrease, forcing people to increasingly rely on their intercostal muscles to breathe. In addition, the chest becomes more rigid because of calcification of the ribs to the sternum, which exacerbates any breathing difficulties. As the lungs' elasticity decreases, the overall strength of the intercostal muscles and diaphragm decreases as well. Collectively, these factors turn breathing into a more labor-intensive process in older people. As with all of the physical changes related to aging, these respiratory system changes are often gradual and go unnoticed until a severe, life-threatening condition occurs. An older person will then have less respiratory reserve to maintain adequate breathing.

You might think that a rigid chest would be more protective, but this rigidity actually makes the chest more fragile. Overall, the bone structure of late adults is weakened. Instead of the chest being able to bend and give if struck, the chest's calcified bony structure may fracture.

Within the mouth and nose, there is a gradual loss of the mechanisms that protect the upper airway. This loss leads to a decreased ability to clear secretions and decreased cough and gag reflexes. The number of cilia that line the airways also diminish with age, which results in decreased sensation to foreign objects, such as dust or smoke, and less responsiveness when structures of the airway are innervated. With a lessened ability to maintain upper airway function, aspiration and obstruction become more likely.

When a younger patient inhales, the airway maintains its shape, allowing air to enter. As the smooth muscles of the lower airway weaken with age, strong inhalation can make the walls of the airway collapse inward and cause inspiratory wheezing **FIGURE 10-17**. These collapsing airways result in low flow rates, because less air can move through the smaller airways, and air trapping, because air does not completely exit the alveoli (incomplete expiration).

In older adults, vital capacity (the volume of air moved during the deepest inspiration and expiration) is significantly decreased as compared with that noted in young adulthood. Factors contributing to this decline include loss of respiratory muscle mass, increased stiffness of the thoracic cage, and decreased surface area available for the exchange of air.

In addition to the decreases in vital capacity, residual volume (the amount of air left in the lungs after expiration of the maximum possible amount of air) increases with age. Consequently, stagnant air remains in the alveoli and hampers gas exchange. This effect can produce **hypercapnia** (increased carbon dioxide in the bloodstream) and acidosis, even when the person is at rest.

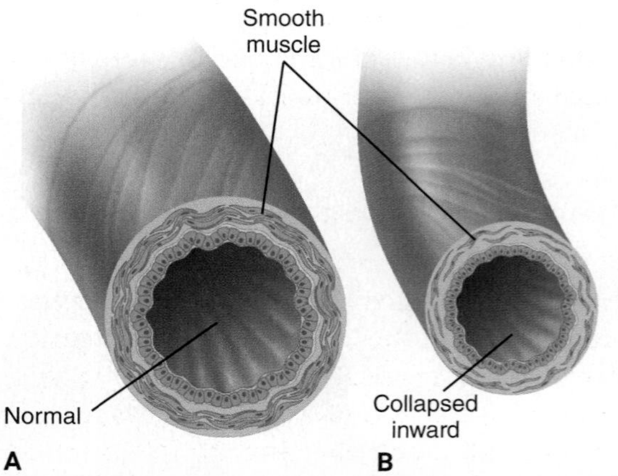

FIGURE 10-17 A. Healthy muscle in a younger patient's airway helps maintain the open airway during the pressures of inhalation. **B.** Muscle weakening with age can lead to airway collapse that may produce wheezing.

Words of Wisdom

When ventilating a late adult, keep in mind that the tidal volume you give the patient may not be the same amount needed to ventilate a younger person. Use only enough force to achieve gentle chest rise and fall, and feel for resistance during ventilation.

Endocrine System

As with other systems of the body, the function of the endocrine system gradually declines with age. As people get older, they tend to slow their physical activity. Unfortunately, many people do not decrease their food intake. When a person gains weight, more insulin is needed to control the body's metabolism and blood glucose (sugar) level. However, insulin production and glucose metabolism gradually decrease, so late adults are more prone to the development of diabetes mellitus. Changes in a late adult's mental status may also reflect changes in the blood glucose level.

The reproductive systems of both men and women change with age. Men can produce sperm long into their 80s, but the rigidity of the penis tends to decrease over time. It is unclear whether this decrease is due to aging itself or other conditions such as cardiovascular disease. During menopause, decreased production of regulating hormones results in atrophy of women's reproductive organs. The uterus and vagina both decrease in size. Hormone production for both sexes gradually decreases as people age. Note that while sexual desire may diminish with age, it does not cease.

Renal and Gastrointestinal Systems

In the kidneys, both structural and functional changes occur in the late adult. The mass and filtration function of the kidneys decrease significantly between the ages of 20 and 90 years. Hardening of the blood vessels supplying the kidneys slows blood flow through them, affecting the rate at which the glomeruli can filter blood in the kidney's **nephrons**. This decreased blood supply causes more abnormal glomeruli to be present as a person ages. Aging kidneys respond less efficiently to hemodynamic stress (ie, stress related to the circulation of blood) and to fluid and electrolyte imbalances. In turn, the body's ability to eliminate wastes diminishes, as does its ability to conserve fluids when needed.

Changes in gastrointestinal function may inhibit nutritional intake and utilization in older adults, resulting in vitamin and mineral deficiencies. In the mouth, for example, the taste buds' sensitivity to salty and sweet sensations decreases. Teeth become weaker during this phase of life, making it more difficult for late adults to chew certain foods. Wear and tear of the teeth increases the risk for decay, while receding gums increase the risk for oral and cardiac disease. The secretion of saliva decreases, which reduces the body's ability to process complex carbohydrates. Gastric motility (movement of the gastrointestinal system and the contents within it) slows with age because of the loss of intestinal tract neurons, which can lead older adults to experience an early sensation of fullness or feel constipated. Likewise, gastric acid secretion diminishes. Blood flow in the vessels supplying the mesentery (membranes that connect organs to the abdominal wall) may drop by as much as 50%, decreasing the intestines' ability to extract nutrients from digested food.

Gallstones become increasingly common with age, and anal sphincter changes reduce elasticity and can produce fecal incontinence. Bowel movements are often a great concern to patients in this age group. Many patients keep meticulous track of their bowel movements and can become concerned if they do not have a bowel movement for a day or two. Although this situation does not necessarily constitute a medical emergency, it can still be a valid fear for the patient. Ask about bowel habits during the interview, and remember that patients have the right to define their own emergency.

Street Smarts

Late adults may have a beloved pet as their primary companion, which can present an obstacle when it comes to convincing these patients that they need to be transported for further care. To allay patients' fears about their pet's welfare, identify animal resources in your area that can either watch the pet in the home or kennel the pet while the patient receives care in the hospital.

Nervous System

Nervous system changes can result in the most debilitating of age-related ailments. In the CNS, the brain weight may shrink 10% to 20% by age 80 years.[10] A selective loss of 5% to 50% of neurons occurs, and the surviving neurons shrink in size. The frontal lobe may lose as many as 20% of its synapses (the junctions between neurons) over the course of a person's life. Motor and sensory neural networks become slower and less responsive. The metabolic rate in the older adult's brain does not change, however, and oxygen consumption remains constant throughout life.

One natural consequence of aging is a change in sleep patterns. For example, instead of sleeping through the night, older people may nap during the day and stay up late at night. The sleep cycle may move into a biphasic (two-phase) sleep cycle; for example, individuals may sleep from 0100 hours to 0600 hours and nap from 1200 hours to 1500 hours.

The brain, which is surrounded by the meninges, takes up almost all of the space in the skull. Cerebrospinal fluid protects the brain inside these membranes. Unfortunately, age-related shrinkage creates a void between the brain and the outermost layer of the meninges, which provides room for the brain to move when stressed. This shrinkage also stretches the bridging veins that return blood from inside the brain to the dura mater. If trauma moves the brain forcibly, then the bridging veins can tear and bleed **FIGURE 10-18**. Bleeding can empty into this void, resulting in a subdural hematoma, which may go unnoticed for some time in this age group. Increased intracranial pressure is required for signs of head trauma to be present; the intracranial pressure will not rise—and, therefore, its signs will not be present—until the void has been filled and pressurized. (For more information, see Chapter 35, *Head and Spine Trauma*.)

Functioning of the peripheral nervous system also slows with age. Consequently, sensation becomes diminished and may be misinterpreted. The ability to know where the body is in space (proprioception) can be hampered, and increased reaction times can cause longer delays between stimulation and motion. The resulting slowdown in reflexes and decreased kinesthetic sense (awareness of the position and movement of body parts) may contribute to increased incidence of falls and trauma in older adults. With aging, nerve endings deteriorate, and the skin's ability to sense the surroundings dwindles. Hot, cold, sharp, and wet items can all create dangerous situations for late adults because both reaction time and pain perception are diminished in this population.

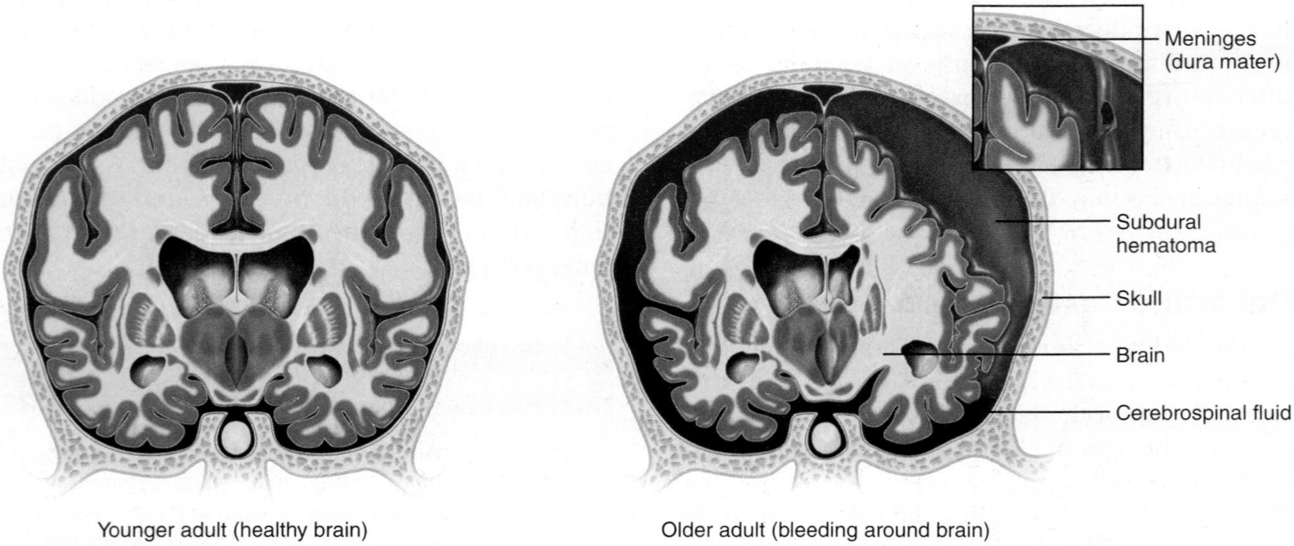

FIGURE 10-18 Age-related atrophy or shrinkage of the brain results in a space between the brain and its cover, the dura mater. Bleeding into this area can occur more easily from trauma because veins are stretched. Because of the additional space, bleeding in an older adult's brain does not always produce immediate signs of increased intracranial pressure.

Sensory Changes

In addition to a diminished sensation of touch, the other senses are affected by aging. Often it is assumed that older people are hard of hearing and have difficulty seeing. In all late adults, changes occur that diminish the effectiveness of the eyes and ears; however, most can still hear well and are able to see clearly. They may need eyeglasses or hearing aids, but it is simply wrong to assume that every older patient is deaf and nearly blind.

Pupillary reaction and ocular movements become more restricted with age. The pupils are generally smaller in older patients, and the opacity of the lens of the eye diminishes visual acuity and makes the pupils sluggish when responding to light. Visual distortions are also common in older people. Age-related thickening of the lens makes it harder for the eye to focus, especially at close range. Peripheral fields of vision narrow, and a greater sensitivity to glare constricts the visual field.

Hearing loss is about four times more common than loss of vision in late adults. Changes in several hearing-related structures may lead to a loss of high-frequency hearing, or even deafness.

Finally, loss of taste bud sensation and a decline in olfactory (sense of smell) perception are normal occurrences in late adults. Unfortunately, these changes make eating less pleasurable, contributing to many older people's lack of adequate nutrition.

Special Populations

When you need to transport a patient who uses glasses or hearing aids, try to locate those items and bring them with you to the hospital, because the patient will need them for interactions with the hospital staff. If applicable and time permits, also consider bringing the patient's dentures, if not already in place.

Psychosocial Changes

As a paramedic, you should treasure your opportunities to spend time with and communicate with late adults. Many of them have amazing stories and experiences to share, yet younger people often take them for granted. Older people have a great amount of wisdom to share, and they may need to be reminded of their worth. Indeed, until about 5 years before death, most late-stage adults retain high brain function. In the 5 years preceding death, however, mental function is presumed to decline, a theory referred to as the **terminal drop hypothesis**.

As the geriatric population continues to grow, we as a society are responsible for seeking out unique ways to accommodate their needs during their last 20 to 40 years of life. Many older people live at home. They may have the assistance of family, friends, or home health care providers, but most are relatively healthy, active, and independent. In addition, the number of assisted-living communities is growing across the United States. These facilities allow older adults to live in campus-based communities with people of similar age, while enjoying the privacy of their own apartment and the security of nursing care, maintenance, and food preparation, if desired **FIGURE 10-19**. Unfortunately, these facilities can be expensive.

Most people deal with financial issues throughout their lives, and few things in life produce more worry and stress than money problems. Late adults, in particular, may constantly worry about the rising costs of health care and are often forced to make decisions such as whether to pay for groceries or their medications. Today, many single women in the United States who are age 60 years or older live at or below the poverty level.[11,12] This thorny problem remains unresolved.

One of the important issues that older people need to face is their own mortality. The fact is that everyone dies. For most younger people, this concept is an intellectual exercise with a distant

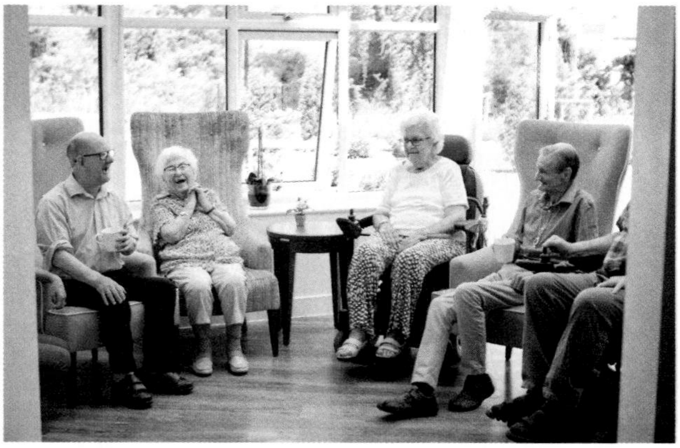

FIGURE 10-19 Many older adults live in assisted-living facilities.

connection to reality. For late adults, it can be difficult to watch as their friends, relatives, and companions grow older and die, leaving them seemingly alone. Late adults may feel that they lack purpose or worry about being a burden to their families as their health declines and they are no longer able to take care of themselves. Isolation and depression are challenges for far too many older people.

Nevertheless, many older people are happy and actively participating in life. With adequate financial resources and a support system of family and friends, older people in their 80s and beyond can enjoy life and continue to feel productive.

Words of Wisdom

Know what resources your community has to offer late adults. The health care provider's goal should be to help late adults remain in their home, versus being relocated to an assisted-living or nursing home, as long as they are not at excessive risk in that setting. Work within your community to identify older persons who need such services as home visits, companion programs for social interaction, or simple home repairs.

YOU are the Paramedic SUMMARY

1. What is your first concern at this scene?

Because the family is actively moving toward your vehicle, scene safety is the primary concern. The mother and father may try to open the vehicle doors to get their daughter inside for your emergency medical care. A fall or other unintended injury could occur as a result. Remember, in this case you have three patients to care for until you can gain control of the situation.

2. Which stage of development describes a 3-year-old child, and how will this information affect your assessment?

You should suspect bone injuries in this patient. By age 3 years, bone density and muscle mass increase to become more like those of an adult. On impact, children of this age are less flexible because they have less cartilage and fat storage.

3. Why is Juliet clinging to her father and turning away from you?

Fear of strangers is especially pronounced in toddlers and preschoolers. Juliet has also had an interruption in her typical routine and a loss of control over her environment. She may be sensing her parents' sense of urgency, reinforcing the thought, "Something is really wrong here." These issues must all be overcome to ensure the successful treatment of this child.

4. What are some of the measures you can take to alleviate the child's distress?

Gaining the trust of the father and mother is paramount to gain the toddler's trust. After you gain their support, approach the toddler in a calm, friendly manner. If you can find a favorite toy or object that will usually comfort the child, then use it. In this case, Juliet prefers her pink blanket. The father is actively forcing his daughter to turn around and face you. Toddlers look for their parents and/or caregivers to protect them from harm, not to hurt them. Allowing the toddler to move as she wishes (as long as her condition permits that freedom) is preferred rather than physically forcing her into a position.

5. Measurement of Spo_2 level and BP requires equipment. How can you gain the child's trust to use your equipment?

Unfamiliar equipment can be especially frightening for a child. Any item that attaches to the child may present a problem. One of the best methods to overcome the child's fear is to show the equipment to the child. Show Juliet what the equipment is and how it is used, and let her touch it before using it (if her condition allows). If any part of your exam or treatment will hurt, then never lie and say it will not. If you lie, it will eliminate the patient's trust that you have so carefully built.

YOU are the Paramedic SUMMARY continued

6. What is the expected normal range for a 3-year-old child's pulse rate and respiratory rate?

A normal pulse rate for an awake toddler ranges from 80 to 120 beats/min. A normal respiratory rate ranges from 20 to 28 breaths/min.

7. You need to bandage your patient's laceration. Offer some ideas to make this process more acceptable to the patient.

As mentioned earlier, it is essential to explain what you plan to do before you do it. In this case, you need to bandage a laceration on the toddler's forehead. Ask the parents to assist you with the bandaging (her condition permitting). Allow the child to hold a toy or other special item during bandaging so the situation will be less scary.

8. How should you transport this patient?

Most EMS providers have a policy on family members accompanying patients to the hospital; make sure you are familiar with this policy. Younger children have a strong fear of being left alone or of being taken away from their family. It is preferable to have one of the parents ride in the patient compartment with the child for their comfort. This practice is only advisable if the family member can be properly seated with an acceptable automotive restraint firmly fastened.

EMS Patient Care Report (PCR)

Date: 05-01-22	**Incident No.:** 0909	**Nature of Call:** Fall		**Location:** 215 Shady Glen Way	
Dispatched: 1400	**En Route:** 1400	**At Scene:** 1407	**Transport:** 1429	**At Hospital:** 1449	**In Service:** 1459

Patient Information

Age: 3 years **Sex:** F **Weight (in kg [lb]):** 13.6 kg (30 lb)	**Allergies:** Family denies **Medications:** Family denies **Past Medical History:** Family denies **Chief Complaint:** Lac & abrasion to forehead

Vital Signs

Time: 1414	**BP:** Unable to obtain	**Pulse:** 130	**Respirations:** Crying	**Spo_2:** Unable to obtain
Time: 1424	**BP:** Unable to obtain	**Pulse:** 118	**Respirations:** 20	**Spo_2:** 99% room air

EMS Treatment (circle all that apply)

Oxygen @ ____ L/min via (circle one): **NC NRM Bag-mask device**		**Assisted Ventilation**	**Airway Adjunct**	**CPR**
Defibrillation	**Bleeding Control**	**Bandaging** (circled)	**Splinting**	**Other:**

Narrative

Arrived in front of residence to find father carrying 3-year-old girl to this unit. Mother also present. Child appeared to be actively resisting the father, who was trying to hold her. Family asked to move from roadway to front steps of residence. Father allowed to hold the child, who was actively crying. Mother stated child was running in backyard when she fell forward, striking her head on the deck. Assessment showed 0.5-inch (1-cm) lac approx 1 inch (2.5 cm) superior to right eye, with corresponding hematoma and abrasion around lac. Pt initially resisted attempts at assessment but was able to be calmed. Lac bandaged with assistance from family. Transported to Children's Hospital with further calming during transport. Father allowed per policy in pt compartment with seat belts in place. Report to Jim RN on arrival at Children's Hospital.

End of report

Prep Kit

Ready for Review

- The developmental stages of life include the following: infants, toddlers and preschoolers, school-age children, adolescents (teenagers), early adults, middle adults, and late adults.
- Each developmental stage is marked by different physical and psychosocial changes and characteristics.
- Infants (ages 1 month to 1 year) develop at a startling rate, experiencing specific developmental milestones during every month of the first year of life.
- Two important points regarding an infant's airway are that an infant's tongue can more easily occlude the airway, and the infant's lungs are fragile.
- An infant's primary means of communication is crying. With regard to temperament, children are classified as being easy, difficult, or slow to warm up to their surroundings and lifestyles.
- The vital signs of toddlers (ages 1 to 2 years) and preschoolers (ages 3 to 5 years) differ somewhat from those of infants.
- Toddlers and preschoolers learn to speak and express themselves. Toddlers have the neuromuscular control needed for bladder control and can feel when the bladder is full by 12 to 15 months of age; however, the child may not be psychologically ready for potty training until 18 to 30 months of age.
- A child's development is affected by the parenting style employed by the caregivers. Types of parenting styles include authoritarian, authoritative, permissive, and uninvolved. No matter what stage of life a child is in, a divorce will profoundly affect that child.
- From ages 6 to 12 years, the school-age child's vital signs and body gradually approach those observed in adulthood.
- School-age children develop self-concept, self-esteem, and reasoning abilities. They also experience the emergence of their permanent teeth.
- The vital signs of adolescents (ages 13 through 18 years) begin to level off within the adult ranges.
- Adolescents (teenagers) undergo significant reproductive development. They also focus on creating their self-images and are self-conscious. Some may engage in self-destructive behavior.
- Vital signs do not vary greatly through adulthood; however, the vital signs of late adults do differ depending on the individual's health.
- Early adults (ages 19 to 40 years) focus on work and family. The body typically functions at an optimal level, and lifelong habits are developed.
- Middle adults (ages 41 to 60 years) focus on achieving life goals. During this stage, medical conditions such as diabetes, hypertension, and cancer become more common.
- Late adults (ages 61 years and older) undergo significant physical changes. They also focus on their mortality. Suicide and depression are concerns in this age group.

Vital Vocabulary

adolescents People who are 13 through 18 years of age.

aneurysm A swelling or enlargement of part of a blood vessel, resulting from weakening of the vessel wall.

anxious avoidant attachment A bond formed between an infant and the parent or caregiver in which the infant is repeatedly rejected and develops an isolated lifestyle that does not depend on the support and care of others.

atherosclerosis A disorder in which cholesterol and calcium build up inside the walls of the blood vessels, forming plaque, which eventually leads to partial or complete blockage of blood flow.

Prep Kit continued

authoritarian A parenting style that demands absolute obedience.

authoritative A parenting style that balances parental authority with the child's freedom by setting and enforcing rules, but also allowing the child to have some freedom.

barotrauma Trauma resulting from increased pressure; for example, from too much pressure in the lungs.

bonding The formation of a close, personal relationship.

conventional reasoning A type of reasoning in which a child looks for approval from peers and society.

despair phase The second phase of an infant's response to a situational crisis; characterized by monotonous wailing.

early adults People who are 19 to 40 years of age.

fontanelles Sheets of tough connective tissue between the flat bones of the skull that soften and expand when the newborn passes through the birth canal; they are gradually replaced as the bones of the skull fuse together and form suture joints by age 2 years; also called soft spots.

growth plates Structures located on either end of long bones, which are the centers of longitudinal bone growth during childhood.

hypercapnia Increased carbon dioxide levels in the bloodstream.

infants Babies from age 1 month to 1 year.

late adults People who are 61 years of age or older.

life expectancy The average number of years a person can be expected to live.

menarche A female's first menstrual period.

menopause The cessation of menstruation, which begins in a woman's late 40s or early 50s, and which marks the end of the reproductive years.

middle adults People who are 41 to 60 years of age.

Moro reflex A reflex in which an infant opens the arms wide, spreads the fingers, and seems to grab at things when caught off guard.

nephrons The basic filtering units in the kidneys.

palmar grasp An infant reflex that occurs when something is placed in the infant's palm, and the infant grasps the object.

permissive A parenting style in which the parent does not impose many rules, if any, on the child; two subcategories include indifferent and indulgent.

postconventional reasoning A type of reasoning in which a child makes decisions guided by the child's conscience.

preconventional reasoning A type of reasoning in which a child acts almost purely to avoid punishment and to get what the child wants.

preschoolers Children ages 3 to 5 years.

protest phase An infant's initial response to a situational crisis; characterized by loud crying.

rooting reflex A reflex that occurs when something touches an infant's cheek, and the infant instinctively turns the head toward the touch.

scaffolding An instructional technique that builds on what has already been learned.

school-age children Children ages 6 to 12 years.

secure attachment A bond formed between an infant and the parent or caregiver, in which the infant understands that parents and/or caregivers will be responsive to the infant's needs and provide care when help is needed.

self-concept A person's perception of oneself.

self-esteem How people feel about themselves and how they fit in with peers.

situational crisis A crisis caused by a specific set of circumstances.

sucking reflex A reflex in which an infant starts sucking when the lips are stroked.

terminal drop hypothesis The theory that a person's mental function declines in the last 5 years of life.

Prep Kit continued

toddlers Children ages 1 to 3 years.

trust and mistrust A phrase that refers to a stage of development from birth to about 18 months of age, during which infants learn to trust their parents and/or caregivers if their world is planned, organized, and routine.

withdrawal In the context of infant behavior, the final phase of an infant's response to a situational crisis; characterized by apathy and boredom.

References

1. Leifer G, Fleck E. *Growth and Development Across the Lifespan: A Health Promotion Focus.* 2nd ed. St. Louis, MO: Saunders; 2013:94-211.
2. Newborn (infant) vital signs pediatric nursing. RegisteredNurseRN.com website. https://www.registerednursern.com/newborn-infant-vital-signs-pediatric-nursing/. Accessed February 2, 2021.
3. Kliegman RM, St Geme JW, Blum NJ, et al. *Nelson Textbook of Pediatrics.* 21st ed. Philadelphia, PA: Elsevier; 2020:128-146.
4. Blackburn S. *Maternal, Fetal, and Neonatal Physiology: A Clinical Perspective*. 5th ed. St. Louis, MO: Elsevier; 2020:297-350.
5. Jarvis C. *Physical Examination and Health Assessment.* 7th ed. St. Louis, MO: Elsevier; 2016:413-458.
6. Duderstadt K. *Pediatric Physical Examination: An Illustrated Handbook.* 3rd ed. St. Louis, MO: Elsevier; 2019:132-150.
7. Hazinski MF. *Nursing Care of the Critically Ill Child.* 3rd ed. St. Louis, MO: Mosby; 2012:1-18.
8. Marriage and Divorce. Centers for Disease Control and Prevention website. https://www.cdc.gov/nchs/fastats/marriage-divorce.htm. Updated May 5, 2020. Accessed March 4, 2021.
9. Life expectancy and healthy life expectancy: data by country. World Health Organization website. https://apps.who.int/gho/data/node.main.688. Updated December 4, 2020. Accessed May 21, 2021.
10. Balter M. The incredible shrinking human brain. *Science.* https://www.sciencemag.org/news/2011/07/incredible-shrinking-human-brain. Published July 25, 2011. Accessed March 4, 2021.
11. Munnell AH. Why are so many older women poor? Just the facts on retirement issues. Center for Retirement Research at Boston College. https://crr.bc.edu/wp-content/uploads/2004/04/jtf_10%20.pdf. April 2004. Accessed February 2, 2021.
12. Weiss L. Unmarried women hit hard by poverty. Center for American Progress. https://www.americanprogress.org/issues/women/news/2009/09/10/6683/unmarried-women-hit-hard-by-poverty/. Published September 10, 2009. Accessed February 2, 2021.

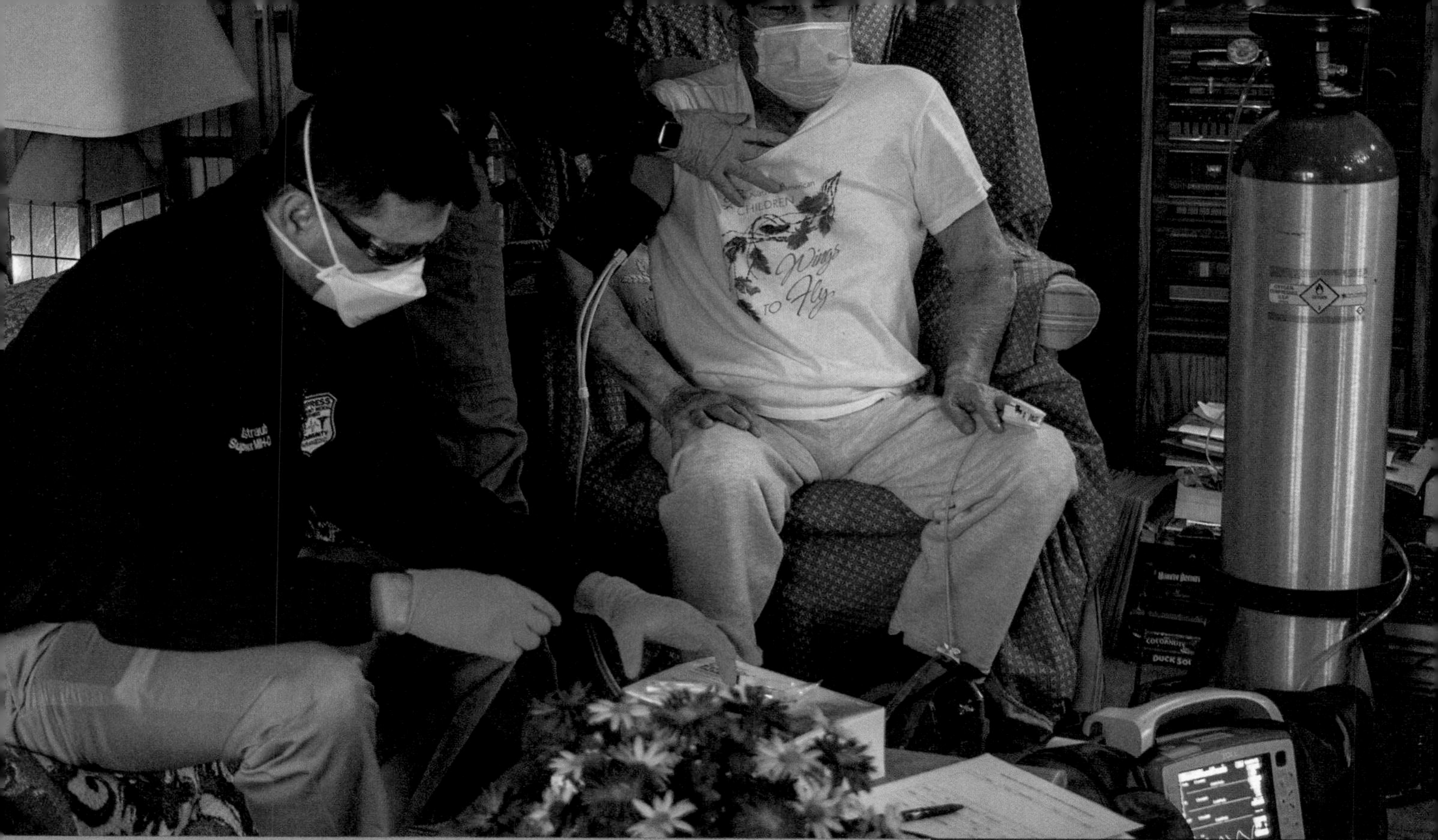

Patient Assessment

VOLUME 1

SECTION

3

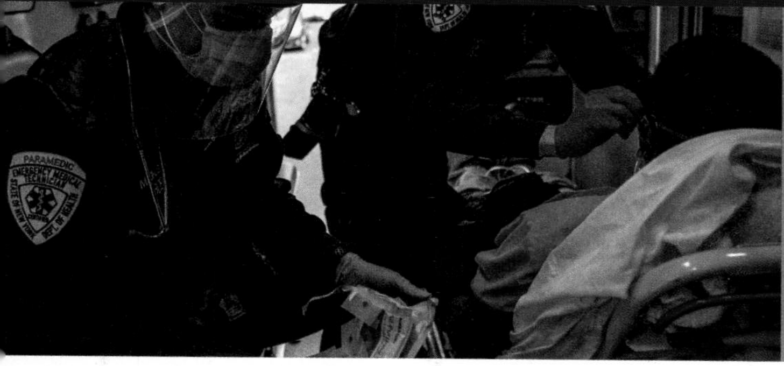

Chapter 11

Patient Assessment

NATIONAL EMS EDUCATION STANDARD COMPETENCIES

Assessment

Integrate scene and patient assessment findings with your knowledge of epidemiology and pathophysiology to form a field impression. Use clinical reasoning to develop a list of differential diagnoses, modify the assessment, and formulate a treatment plan.

Scene Size-up

- Scene safety (pp 588–592)
- Scene management (p 588)
  - Impact of the environment on patient care (p 590)
  - Addressing hazards (pp 589–592)
  - Violence (pp 589–591)
  - Need for additional or specialized resources (pp 592–593)
  - Standard precautions (p 593)
  - Multiple patient situations (pp 590–592)

Primary Survey

- Primary survey for all patient situations:
  - Initial general impression (pp 595–596)
  - Level of consciousness (p 595)
  - ABCDEs (pp 596–602)
  - Identifying life threats (pp 602–603)
  - Assessment of vital functions (pp 602–603)
- Begin interventions needed to preserve life (p 595)
- Integration of treatment/procedures needed to preserve life (pp 595–596)

History Taking

- Determining the chief complaint (pp 604–605)
- Investigation of the chief complaint (pp 619–620)
- Mechanism of injury/nature of illness (pp 592–593)
- Past medical history (pp 622–623)
- Associated signs and symptoms (pp 626–628)
- Pertinent negatives (p 626)
- Components of the patient history (pp 619–623)
- Interviewing techniques (pp 604–611)
- How to integrate therapeutic communication techniques and adapt the line of inquiry based on findings and presentation (pp 606–608)

Secondary Assessment

- Performing a rapid full-body scan (pp 632–633)
- Focused assessment of pain (pp 641–644)
- Assessment of vital signs (pp 634–639)
- Techniques of physical examination (pp 631–634, 640, 641)
- Respiratory system (pp 658–662)
  - Presence of breath sounds (pp 660–662)
- Cardiovascular system (pp 662–666)
- Neurologic system (pp 682–687)
- Musculoskeletal system (pp 672–676)

Techniques of physical examination for all major
- Body systems (pp 626–628)
- Anatomic regions (pp 649–655)

Assessment of:
- Lung sounds (pp 657–662)

Monitoring Devices
- Obtaining and using information from patient monitoring devices including (but not limited to):
  - Pulse oximetry (pp 637–639)
  - Noninvasive blood pressure (pp 690–691)
  - Blood glucose determination (pp 689–690)
  - Continuous ECG monitoring (p 691)
  - 12-lead ECG interpretation (p 690)
  - Carbon dioxide monitoring (pp 690–691)
  - Basic blood chemistry (pp 691–692)

Reassessment
- How and when to reassess patients (p 693)
- How and when to perform a reassessment for all patient situations (p 693)

Medicine
Integrates assessment findings with principles of epidemiology and pathophysiology to formulate a field impression and implement a comprehensive treatment/disposition plan for a patient with a medical complaint.

Medical Overview
Assessment and management of a:
- Medical complaint (pp 584, 587, 595, 604, 619–620, 695)

Pathophysiology, assessment, and management of medical complaints to include:
- Transport mode (pp 602–603, 694–695)
- Destination decisions (pp 587, 602–603, 694–695)

KNOWLEDGE OBJECTIVES
1. Name the components of the patient assessment process; include the most important determination made by paramedics. (pp 584–585)
2. Explain how to determine the mechanism of injury (MOI) or nature of illness (NOI) at an emergency medical scene; include why it is essential to differentiate trauma patients from medical patients. (pp 592–593)
3. Discuss possible hazards that may be present at an emergency medical scene, ways to recognize them, and precautions to protect personal safety. (p 593)
4. List the minimum standard precautions EMS personnel should follow and the personal protective equipment that should be worn at an emergency medical scene; include examples of when additional precautions would be appropriate. (p 593)
5. Describe the principal goals of the primary survey process. (p 594)
6. Describe how a general impression of a patient is formed as part of the primary survey; include why this step is critical to patient management. (pp 595–596)
7. Recall how to identify life threats by inspecting and palpating for open and closed findings during the primary survey. (p 594)
8. Explain how to assess the airway status in responsive and unresponsive patients; include examples of possible signs and causes of airway obstruction in each case, and the appropriate response by paramedics. (pp 596–597)
9. Explain how to assess a patient's breathing status; include key information paramedics must obtain during this process and the care required for patients with adequate and inadequate breathing. (pp 597–598)
10. Explain how to assess a patient's circulatory status; include the different methods to obtain a pulse and appropriate management depending on the patient's status. (pp 598–599)
11. Explain how to assess a patient's skin using color, temperature, and condition (CTC); include examples of normal and abnormal findings for diverse groups, and how this information relates to the patient's status. (pp 599–600)
12. Determine the priority of patient care and transport at an emergency scene; include examples of conditions that necessitate immediate transport. (pp 602–603)
13. Identify the MOIs most likely to produce life-threatening injuries. (pp 623–626)
14. Discuss the process of obtaining a patient history; include the purpose and the initial approach to a patient. (pp 604–605)

15. Give examples of different techniques paramedics may use to obtain full and accurate information from patients during the history-taking process. (pp 605–608)
16. Discuss challenges paramedics may face when obtaining a patient history in which sensitive information must be collected; include strategies to facilitate such situations. (pp 608–610)
17. Understand the unique challenges that arise during history taking involving pediatric and geriatric patients. (pp 617–619)
18. Identify the elements of the history to be obtained from responsive medical patients, from family or bystanders in the case of unresponsive medical patients, and from trauma patients. (pp 619–626)
19. Recognize which aspects of the body systems should be covered during the history-taking process. (pp 626–628)
20. Apply clinical reasoning, based on the results of the primary survey and patient history, to form a differential diagnosis. (p 629)
21. Explain the purpose of performing a secondary assessment; include physical exam techniques, and equipment used in the secondary assessment. (pp 630–641)
22. Name the devices used to monitor a patient's medical condition during the secondary assessment and reassessment. (pp 689–692)
23. Explain the importance of assessing a patient's mental status; include examples of different methods used to assess alertness, responsiveness, and orientation. (pp 645–647)
24. Explain general (systemic) conditions considered during the secondary assessment; include examples of what the secondary assessment should include based on a patient's chief complaint. (pp 630, 641–644, 649–655, 657–666, 671, 672, 682–687)
25. Describe normal and abnormal lung sounds heard during auscultation. (pp 657–662)
26. Explain the importance of performing patient reassessment; include reassessing mental status and ABCDE as well as reassessing transport priority and any interventions applied. (pp 693–695)

SKILLS OBJECTIVES

1. Demonstrate how to evaluate and document a patient's orientation and status. (pp 595–596)
2. Demonstrate how to assess a patient's airway and breathing, and correctly obtain information on respiratory rate, rhythm, quality/character, and depth. (pp 596–598)
3. Demonstrate how to assess a patient's circulation by evaluating pulses and assessing skin CTC. (pp 598–600)
4. Demonstrate how to perform a rapid full-body scan. (pp 632–633, Skill Drill 11-1)
5. Demonstrate how to perform percussion as an assessment technique. (p 634, Skill Drill 11-2)
6. Demonstrate how to compare the patient's serial vital signs with baseline measurements to identify trends in the patient's status. (pp 634–635)
7. Demonstrate how to perform a full-body exam for patients with potentially serious—and potentially hidden—injuries. (pp 641–644, Skill Drill 11-3)
8. Demonstrate how to assess a patient's blood glucose level using a glucometer. (p 646, Skill Drill 11-4)
9. Demonstrate how to examine a patient's head, assessing for open and closed findings. (p 651, Skill Drill 11-5)
10. Demonstrate how to perform a general eye exam. (p 653, Skill Drill 11-6)
11. Demonstrate how to examine a patient's neck for injury. (p 656, Skill Drill 11-7)
12. Demonstrate how to examine a patient's chest and auscultate the lung fields. (pp 658–659, Skill Drill 11-8)
13. Demonstrate how to auscultate heart sounds. (p 664)
14. Demonstrate how to obtain a patient's orthostatic vital signs to assess the extent of any internal bleeding. (pp 667–668)
15. Demonstrate how to examine a patient's abdomen, including inspection, auscultation, percussion, and palpation techniques. (p 668, Skill Drill 11-9)
16. Demonstrate how to examine a patient's musculoskeletal system. (pp 673–674, Skill Drill 11-10)
17. Demonstrate how to examine a patient's peripheral vascular system, including the upper and lower extremities. (p 678, Skill Drill 11-11)

18. Demonstrate how to examine and palpate a patient's spine for abnormalities, and evaluate range of motion. (p 681, Skill Drill 11-12)
19. Demonstrate how to perform a neurologic exam, including using the COASTMAP mnemonic and AVPU scale to test for patient responsiveness. (p 685, Skill Drill 11-13)
20. Demonstrate how to evaluate deep tendon reflexes and score the patient's responses. (p 686, Skill Drill 11-14)

Introduction

As a paramedic, one of the most important skills you will develop is the ability to assess a patient. Assessment combines a number of steps: assessing the scene, obtaining the patient's **chief complaint** (the reason the patient, or others, called for help) and medical history, and performing a secondary assessment (physical exam). One of the most encouraging things about your patient assessment skills is *there is no limit to how good they can be.* In the hospital setting, physicians and nurses are able to use additional tools (eg, radiography, ultrasonography, and lab test results) to help them develop a diagnosis. However, most paramedics do not have these resources available and must rely on their ability to obtain an accurate patient history, perform a systematic physical exam, and use available diagnostic tools (eg, cardiac monitor, capnography, and glucometry) wisely.

To the patient, the entire assessment process should appear seamless. To the provider, the process usually unfolds by integrating questions and answers into a physical exam. What varies from patient to patient is the number and types of questions that must be asked and the extent to which the patient should be examined before a "working diagnosis" is reached. Your **differential diagnosis** is the list of possible diagnoses based on the patient assessment findings. The **working diagnosis** is the one diagnosis from the differential list on which you are basing your treatment plan. It is important for you to develop experience in prioritizing patients, since some patients must be evaluated quickly and transported immediately to the facility best equipped to handle their suspected condition (eg, life-threatening trauma, stroke, heart attack). The entire patient assessment process should be organized and thorough yet be flexible because of the varied environments where patients are found.

Aside from the **primary survey**, which focuses on identifying and addressing life threats, the sequence of the remaining components of the patient history and secondary assessment is flexible. In other words, you can perform most of your assessment and physical exam in the order that is in the patient's best interest *once the primary survey has been completed and life threats addressed.*

A key to making your prehospital practice successful is developing and cultivating your own assessment style and overall strategy for evaluating and providing patient care in the unique and varied circumstances encountered in the field. Within the parameters of applicable standards of care, you can add personal touches, such as deciding which gear to take with you on a given call or choosing to kneel, sit, or stand while you interview a particular patient.

YOU are the Paramedic

PART 1

You are working the night shift, and your unit is dispatched for a "man down" in a questionable part of town. The dispatcher says he has no further information because the call was relayed from a third party. Your unit is the first on the scene. You see a man lying on his left side on the sidewalk in front of an abandoned strip mall. There appears to be no one else around. Your partner turns on the scene lights, and you see what appears to be blood near the man on the sidewalk.

1. What is your first concern at this scene?
2. How will you address this concern?

Patient Assessment

Scene Size-up

Ensure scene safety
Determine mechanism of injury/nature of illness
Take standard precautions
Determine number of patients
Consider additional/specialized resources

↓

Primary Assessment*

Form a general impression

Assess

- Responsiveness/level of consciousness

Assess and treat

- Airway
- Breathing
- Circulation

Also assess

- Disability
- Exposure

Identify

- Chief complaint/life threats (treat)
- Priority of patient care
- Transport decision

↓

History Taking

History of present illness (OPQRST)
Past medical history (SAMPLE)

↓

Secondary Assessment

Is the patient's condition medical or trauma?

Assess

- Baseline vital signs
- Monitoring devices (as appropriate)

Systematic physical exam

- Full-body exam or rapid full-body scan
- Focused on injury
- Based on body system (respiratory, cardiovascular, neurologic, reproductive, etc)

↓

Reassessment

- Repeat the primary assessment
- Obtain vital signs
- Reassess the chief complaint
- Recheck interventions
- Identify and treat changes in the patient's condition

Reassess patient

- Unstable patients: every 5 minutes
- Stable patients: every 15 minutes

***Note:** The primary survey usually follows an ABCDE sequence (Airway, Breathing, Circulation, Disability, Exposure), but if the patient appears lifeless or has severe external bleeding, use a CABDE sequence (Circulation, Airway, Breathing, Disability, Exposure).

Remember, your overall job as a paramedic is to quickly identify your patient's problem(s), set care priorities, develop a patient care plan, and quickly and efficiently execute it.

Words of Wisdom

The acronym SOAP sums up the general approach to assessment. That is, you acquire **S**ubjective information from an interview (symptoms), as well as observe and measure **O**bjective information (signs), and compare the data with your previous experiences to arrive at an **A**ssessment of what you believe is wrong (differential diagnosis), so you can **P**lan the most appropriate treatment for your working diagnosis.

Sick Versus Not Sick

The most important assessment skill for you to acquire, and one that comes only from much experience, is quickly determining whether the patient is *sick* or *not sick*. This quick, early assessment is based on the chief complaint, respiration, pulse, mental status, and skin color, temperature, and condition (CTC). Together, these items reflect the overall performance of the patient's respiratory, cardiovascular, and neurologic systems. These three critical systems balance the body like a three-legged stool. Together they support the body. However, if you kick out one leg, such as the respiratory system, then the other two systems will only momentarily support the body before all systems collapse. For trauma patients, the mechanism of injury (MOI) and obvious signs of trauma should be factored in as well.

If the patient is sick, the next step is to determine how sick. On one end of the sickness scale is a patient with a miserable sinus infection. Is the patient sick? Yes. Is this a life-threatening event? Probably not. On the other end of the scale is a patient with blue lips who is drenched in sweat and struggles to answer your questions, but is so short of breath that only one- or two-word sentences are possible. Is this patient sick? Yes. Is this a life-threatening event? Based on these signs and symptoms, the answer is yes.

Every time you assess a patient, you must *qualify* whether that patient is sick or not sick. Then you must *quantify* how sick the patient is (ie, a patient in respiratory distress is considered to be "sick" and the use of accessory muscles of breathing and retractions indicate the sickness is "severe"). Once you have done so, you are in a position to decide what, if any, care must be provided at the scene, versus in the ambulance en route to the hospital.

Establishing a Field Impression

More often than not, you will form your **field impression** based on the patient's history and chief complaint. A field impression is an initial summary of the patient's condition based on the clinical presentation and the exclusion of other possible causes based on the differential diagnoses. You must be able to obtain quality information from patients with differing cognitive abilities and educational, cultural, and ethnic backgrounds, some of whom may be impaired by alcohol or drugs.

Being good at patient assessment is like being a good detective. As you interview the patient, sift through the information you obtain to glean clues throughout the process. On that basis, ask more questions relevant to the patient's chief complaint. Your questions about current medications may yield nothing important, for example, yet your next line of questioning may yield a wealth of pertinent information about medical history. Just as a veteran detective methodically collects and analyzes clues to crack a case, you must also follow a similar process to deliver the best care to your patient.

In time, every paramedic develops their own assessment style. As you develop this essential job skill, it is critical to think of patient assessment as a fluid process. As a patient interview unfolds, be able to change the sequence of your questioning as the situation or the patient's condition dictates. Develop a feel for when to expand your questioning to focus on important information. Of course, your style must be based on sound medical practice, keeping in mind that (1) how you learn and how you practice technical skills as a student will carry over to how you deliver care and perform technical skills in the field, and (2) there is a psychomotor examination, including assessment, that students must pass, which follows a relatively prescriptive format.

Is This a Medical Emergency or Trauma?

Just as hospitals are organized into medical and surgical units, there are two basic patient classifications in prehospital care: medical and trauma. For patients with medical conditions, your priorities are to identify the chief complaint and sift carefully through the medical history for clues to the patient's current condition. In contrast, trauma calls generally result from unexpected events. When trauma is the primary culprit, a patient's medical history is often less relevant to your care plan, and the specific destination may be significant. For example, some trauma patients can be stabilized only under the "bright lights and cold steel" of a surgical suite. Other patients may require specific destinations for treatment, such as a patient with ST-segment elevation myocardial infarction (STEMI), a patient with burns, a patient who experienced cardiac arrest with return of spontaneous circulation (ROSC), or a patient who experienced a stroke: Each of these patients needs transport to a specialty care center. Prioritizing and determining the appropriate destination for critical trauma patients is discussed in detail in Chapter 30, *Trauma Systems and Mechanism of Injury.*

That said, never forget that medical events can cause trauma. For example, a patient with diabetes who takes insulin may crash their vehicle if they miss breakfast, causing a subsequent drop in their blood glucose level. Likewise, traumatic events can produce medical conditions. For example, the stress of an assault might trigger breathing difficulties in a patient with asthma. In other words, sometimes what seems obvious turns out not to be the whole story. For example, you may be called to a nursing home, where an elderly man was found on the floor with an "obvious" fracture of his right hip. It is essential to look beyond this obvious deformity and determine how he ended up on the floor. A twist, snap, and fall is different from passing out and waking up on the floor, which might indicate a dysrhythmia caused the syncopal episode. Keep your mind open to the varied patient care scenarios you may encounter in your practice so you are mentally ready to respond to each patient's needs. Remember, any given call may be 100% trauma, 100% medical, or any combination of the two. As a medical professional, you must look beyond the obvious and consider a list of conditions that could account for the patient's illness, referred to as the differential diagnosis.

Patient Assessment

Scene Size-up

- Ensure scene safety
- Determine mechanism of injury/nature of illness
- Take standard precautions
- Determine number of patients
- Consider additional/specialized resources

↓

Primary Assessment

↓

History Taking

↓

Secondary Assessment

↓

Reassessment

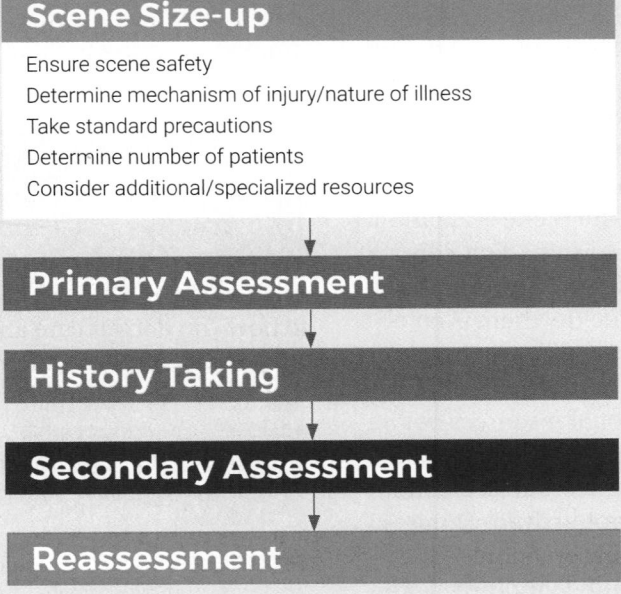

Scene Size-up

Dynamic scene management begins by assessing the scene itself, a process known as **scene size-up**. Regardless of when or where you respond to an emergency call, before initiating any patient care, the first step is to evaluate the overall scene safety and stability. Look for any threats to you, your rescue team, the patient, and any friends, family, or bystanders. Additionally, ensure you have safe and secure access into the scene for your team and their equipment, and ready scene egress as well. Last, consider any special resources you may need, such as a hazardous materials team or police support, and get them headed in your direction. Remember, the sooner you call for help, the sooner it will arrive.

If you do not take a few moments to evaluate the scene and address safety issues, you and/or your partner could join the list of casualties. An injured paramedic simply adds to the rescue team's burden and subtracts from the available resources.

The success of the overall coordination of any incident can be greatly affected by your ability to perform an adequate scene size-up. This step sets the tone for the remainder of an incident. Without this early assessment, the scene is likely to be chaotic and patient care will suffer.

Scene Safety: A Dynamic Process

The main focus of your size-up is the safety and well-being of your emergency medical services (EMS) team and any other emergency responders. Ask yourself, "Is it safe for me and my team to enter this scene and approach the patient?" To answer that question, use a wide-angle lens for scene evaluation. If you determine it is safe, establish patient contact and proceed with your assessment. However, if the scene does not appear to be safe (ie, there is an obvious danger present), or if it is unclear whether it is safe (ie, danger may be present), then either secure the scene or call in additional resources before you begin patient care. Remember, it may become necessary to exit an unsafe or uncertain scene until law enforcement personnel have arrived. Doing so is not abandonment, it is self-preservation!

Scene and environmental conditions can change rapidly, so maintaining vigilance is an important concept to understand for all EMS personnel. The EMS occupation is dangerous, and every effort should be made to reduce the potential for injuries or fatalities. According to the National Institute for Occupational Safety and Health (NIOSH), 21,500 on-the-job injuries occurred among EMS personnel in 2019,[1] constituting an injury rate that is three times greater than that for the general workforce; moreover, members of the EMS industry experience three times the lost workday rate of all private-industry workers. Common causes of injuries include body mechanics (eg, patient lifting); exposures to harmful substances; slips, trips, and falls; motor vehicle incidents; and violence/assault.[2]

Crash and rescue scenes often include multiple threats and extrication hazards, such as unstable vehicles, leaking fuel, jagged metal and broken glass, fire or explosion hazards, downed power lines, and hazardous materials **FIGURE 11-1**. In addition, just conducting EMS and rescue operations on an active roadway poses a hazard. Many motorists are distracted by trying to view the incident scene as they

SAFETY

Ensuring scene safety is a dynamic process requiring constant reassessment. This process, which in the past was often thought of simply as a task to be "checked off" at the start of the encounter, should not be undervalued.

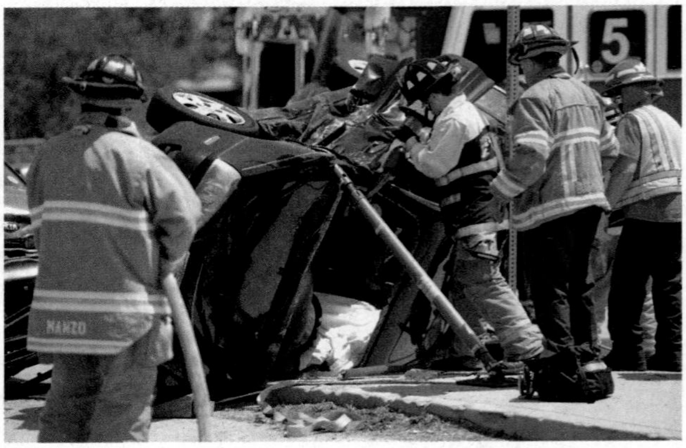

FIGURE 11-1 Crash scenes pose many threats to you, your partners, and the patient.

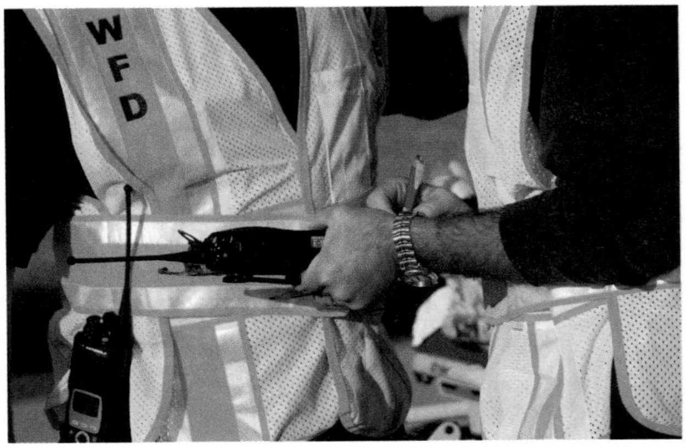

FIGURE 11-2 Wear a certified high-visibility public safety vest when working on any roadway.

pass, commonly referred to as "rubbernecking." These drivers may not be alert to EMS personnel in the roadway. Therefore, even at incidents where there appears to be limited danger involved in the extrication process, the threat of another motorist disrupting your scene is always possible. When working next to a public roadway, wear, at a minimum, an American National Standards Institute (ANSI/ISEA) 107 or 207 certified high-visibility public safety vest **FIGURE 11-2**. National Fire Protection Association (NFPA) 1901, 2009 edition, requires one traffic vest for each seating position. This vest must have a five-point breakaway feature. Wearing a vest gives you adequate visibility while minimizing interference with your other clothing and equipment. In addition, several manufacturers offer specialty gloves, coats, and boots with reflective properties. It is always better to be overly safe than to not be safe enough.

Another major consideration is access and egress. You and your team must safely gain access to the scene and the patient, and then safely exit with the patient. If the scene cannot be secured to your standards, consider making a snatch and grab. That is, make a quick entry to find the patient, provide the *absolute least* amount of care that will allow the patient to be moved safely, and make a quick exit with the patient to a more secure, stable location (ie, your ambulance).

In all cases, establish a safe perimeter to keep bystanders out of harm's way. At some point, scene tape or barricades may be required. Initially, though, scene security is usually established simply with personnel assigned that task. Without that perimeter, allowing bystanders uncontrolled entry into an emergency scene can quickly cause chaos, greatly complicating your call, hindering patient care, and increasing the likelihood of injury to patients, bystanders, and EMS personnel.

Arriving at a scene with hazards and multiple patients can become overwhelming to you and your EMS team. Formulate a basic plan with your team and visually scan the scene, if possible, before exiting your vehicle. This promotes better coordination of patient care and early identification of the need for additional resources. For example, when you arrive at the scene of a motor vehicle crash (MVC), you may notice multiple patients in potentially unstable vehicles. In addition, the incident may have occurred at a busy intersection, with multiple motor vehicles still driving past the scene. It may be apparent that the fire department, specialized rescue, and police will be needed. Fire department and rescue personnel can help stabilize vehicles and extricate patients, while law enforcement personnel can control traffic and investigate the crash. In addition, since multiple patients are involved, this would be a good time to request additional ambulances as needed.

Toxic substances are found at many scenes. From the cleaning products found in almost every home to the countless chemicals used in industry and manufacturing facilities, always be alert for the presence of toxic substances. Be wary of working in environments in which the atmosphere itself is toxic. Smoke is the by-product of incomplete combustion that can contain toxins, pathogens, and carcinogens. Having proper body and respiratory protection is a must before entering such a scene and initiating patient care **FIGURE 11-3**.

All too often, EMS personnel are the first to arrive (sometimes unknowingly) at a crime scene. Do not think of crime scenes in the past tense, because there is always a possibility that more violence may occur. Under ideal circumstances, when EMS personnel are dispatched to a possible crime scene, law enforcement personnel should enter and secure the scene first. For example, dispatch might receive a call for an injured person; on arrival, EMS responders might discover that the patient has a gunshot wound. Request law enforcement assistance immediately, because it is nearly impossible for you and

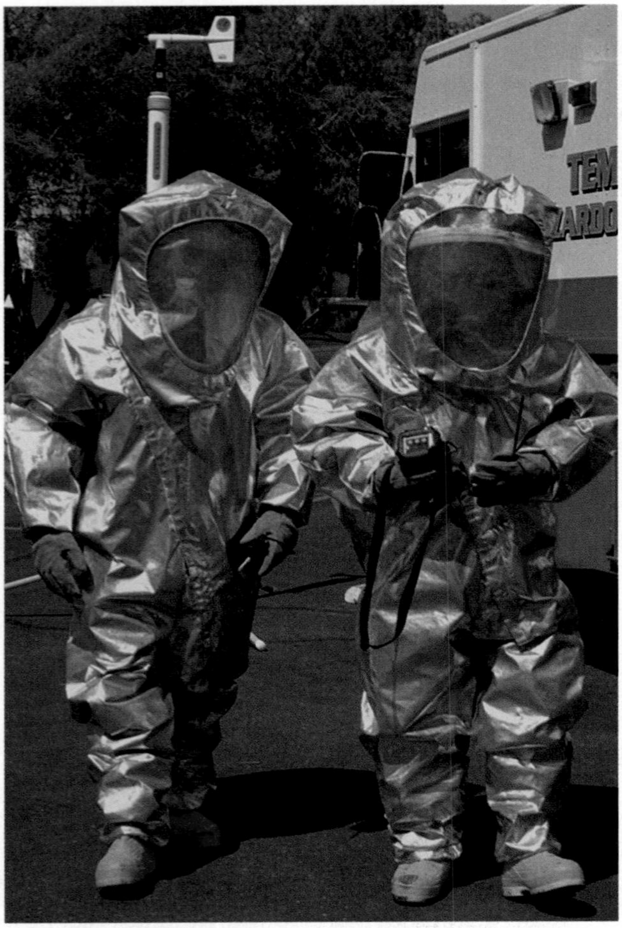

FIGURE 11-3 Scenes involving toxic substances may require specifically trained rescuers with extra protective equipment.

Courtesy of Tempe Fire Department.

your partner to control such a scene and care for the patient at the same time **FIGURE 11-4**. Such a scene must be considered unsecured because a perpetrator could return.

When faced with an unstable scene or one that is beginning to deteriorate (for instance, a crowd is becoming progressively louder or more unruly, or making aggressive gestures or threats), consider retreating to your rig until the scene has been secured and deemed safe. If you believe you can maneuver safely and remove the patient from the scene with you, then do so, but remember that making such an attempt is a judgment call. In making this judgment, you must draw on all of the information you have gleaned through constant situational awareness.

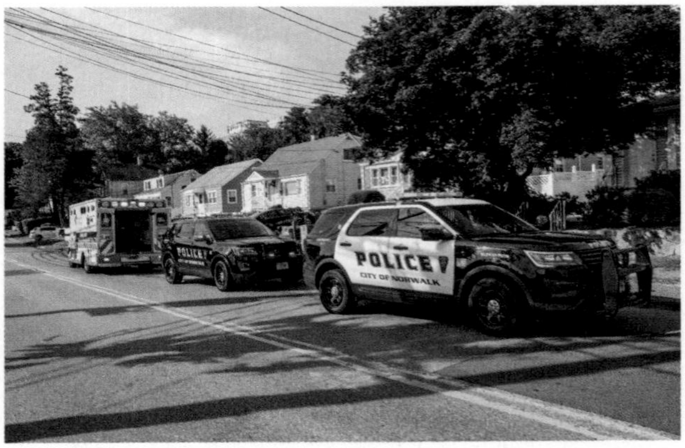

FIGURE 11-4 After you request law enforcement support, wait in your vehicle at a safe distance.

© Miro Vrlik Photography/Shutterstock.

When dispatched to a scene where the potential for violence is high, you and your partner must formulate a plan of escape should the scene become unsafe. When you arrive, park your vehicle away from the scene, lock it, and refrain from entering the scene until law enforcement personnel have secured the area.[3] From the moment you arrive in your vehicle, carefully and thoroughly survey the scene to look for clues that indicate a potential for violence. In addition to the threat from bystanders, the risk of a patient becoming aggressive is always present, particularly when cocaine or methamphetamine is involved. With the increase in manufacture and misuse of methamphetamines, EMS personnel are seeing a growing number of patients who are at the tail end of multiple sleepless days fueled by meth. Such people are often paranoid, emotionally unstable, and almost always armed, making them a far more serious threat than an average patient with a non–drug-induced behavioral emergency. In addition, methamphetamine and crack users are at high risk of experiencing excited or agitated delirium. **Delirium** is characterized by a sudden acute change in mental status, secondary to some significant underlying factor/incident. Such patients may present in a blind rage and be almost uncontrollable. Never hesitate to call for law enforcement assistance in managing any patient who may become violent. Further information about violent patients and sedation is provided in Chapter 29, *Psychiatric Emergencies*.

Other scene risks relate to the scene's physical environment. Unstable surfaces are everyday occurrences in the field. In some parts of the United States, snow- or ice-covered surfaces can persist for 4 months of the year. Rain occurs most everywhere. The longer a patient is exposed to wind and rain, the more likely it is that hypothermia will become a factor. Of course, a hot asphalt highway is not a good place for a patient, either. When the environment is unfriendly: perform the primary survey, address life threats, and move the patient into the controlled environment of your ambulance as quickly as possible.

In addition, most of the country has terrain issues ranging from hills to mountains to sandy beaches. Thus, working on unstable surfaces is an inevitable part of prehospital medicine **FIGURE 11-5**. Take the time to make all of your patient lifts and moves as safe and controlled as possible. Focusing on this aspect of your practice will go a long way toward preventing falls and injuries.

Also, consider the stability of the structures around you and the threat of a secondary collapse. If you have any doubt about the structural integrity of any scene, leave the area, establish a safe perimeter, and request additional resources to secure the scene.

Once the safety of EMS personnel has been established, patient and bystander safety are the next priority. If the scene becomes unsafe for EMS personnel at any time, it also becomes unsafe for the patient. Therefore, the first step is to minimize the likelihood that any such hazard could injure EMS personnel or the patient. If you cannot do so, move the patient to a safe area, as long as taking this action does not place you, your partner, or other responders at unreasonable risk. Next, consider bystanders' safety. Many bystanders attempt to help during an emergency; always remember they are probably not trained to handle EMS equipment or treat or manage illnesses or injuries. If a bystander happens to be a health care provider by profession, it is best to follow the policy of your service or regional medical control to determine what role they should take.

Establish a perimeter or barrier around the emergency scene to prevent bystanders and media from entering. Today, almost everyone carries a cell phone with a camera, and often inappropriate videos are published to social media before you even know it. It may be best to isolate the patient or bystanders to facilitate appropriate patient care or to establish a safer environment. If the scene becomes unsafe for bystanders, have them removed from the scene immediately with the help of law enforcement.

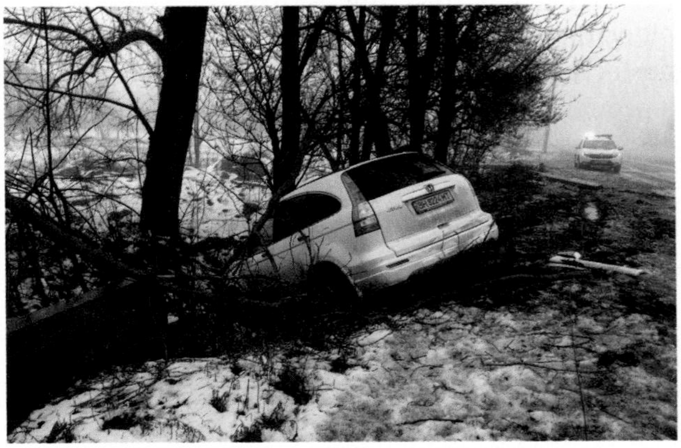

FIGURE 11-5 At times, you may need a team to carry patients out of areas with unstable terrain.

Mechanism of Injury or Nature of Illness

Most calls to 9-1-1 will be for a medical emergency or some form of trauma. Remember, a call for an injured man could prove to be for a man who fell and injured himself due to a low blood glucose level. Similarly, a trauma victim may have crashed her vehicle when she passed out because of an abnormal heart rhythm. Prudent paramedics keep their minds open to multiple possibilities when figuring out what is going on with patients. Failure to do so leads to tunnel vision and poor patient care.

The **mechanism of injury (MOI)** is how a traumatic injury occurs; it comprises the forces that act on the body to cause injury. Assess and evaluate the MOI to help you predict the likelihood that certain injuries have occurred and estimate their severity. The patterns of injury sustained in traumatic events are discussed in detail in Chapter 30, *Trauma Systems and Mechanism of Injury*.

On medical calls, quickly determine why EMS personnel were requested from the patient (family, friends, or bystanders). The **nature of illness (NOI)** is the general type of illness a patient is experiencing.

At this point in the call, if there is more than one patient or if the patient is morbidly obese (so that multiple responders or a specialty unit is needed to lift the patient from the scene), then you may need to request those resources. If multiple patients have similar symptoms or complaints on a medical call, consider carbon monoxide poisoning (or contact with some other noxious agent) or food poisoning as prime candidates. Irrespective of the cause of the problem, the presence of multiple patients means that they must be triaged to determine which additional resources you need and how you will allocate them.

Likewise, when multiple patients require care at a trauma scene, you must triage them. Identify the number of patients and estimate the severity of their injuries. Then request enough additional resources to support the responders already at the scene (eg, additional EMS, fire, police, specialty rescue, public utilities, or hazardous materials personnel). Listen for clues in the dispatch information, such as the number of patients and bystanders and any hazards identified; this information might lead you to request additional resources sooner or to activate the incident command system (ICS) if necessary. Consider calling in law enforcement early if protecting the patient or securing the scene from bystanders is necessary. Do not underestimate the value of surplus. Remember, you can always cancel the extra help if it is not needed. This concept is easily remembered by the expression, "Do not undersell overkill!"

Be familiar with the various specialized resources available to you. These specialized agencies use specific equipment to ensure their safety when carrying out their operations. Chemical and biologic suits, specialized extrication equipment, dry suits, and ascent or descent gear may be needed at a given scene. Only specifically trained responders may participate in these rescue operations.

The process of scene size-up must be completed quickly. Once you have analyzed the dispatch information, evaluated the overall scene safety, donned appropriate personal protective equipment (PPE), determined the MOI or NOI, and summoned additional help, you are ready to begin assessment of the patient. If the responding crew can manage the situation without further assistance, assess the need for manual stabilization and proceed with patient care. Based on the scene size-up and MOI, EMS personnel may need to ensure they provide manual stabilization on reaching the patient.

Throughout this text, the terms *manual stabilization, spinal immobilization,* and *spinal motion restriction (SMR)* are used. Regardless of the terminology used, providers should keep in mind that applying a cervical collar and backboarding do not completely immobilize the spine. The same is likely true with all forms of splinting. This text uses terms like *manual stabilization* and *spinal immobilization* to represent the *intended consequence* of these actions. Indications for manual stabilization and spinal immobilization are covered in Chapter 35, *Head and Spine Trauma.*

Standard Precautions

To reemphasize the point made earlier, your first and foremost concern on any call is to ensure your safety and that of your team. After all, you cannot help the patient if you become injured. Suppose you contract an infectious disease because you neglected to take standard precautions. You would then miss time from work. In the worst-case scenario, you might contract a career-ending or life-threatening disease.

Any patient with whom you come in contact should be considered potentially infectious. Diseases do not discriminate; they can be found in suburban children and urban children, older adults in residential homes or nursing homes, and prosperous business professionals as well as homeless people. Standard precautions were developed to ensure that health care workers would treat all patients the same way: as potentially infectious.

Wear properly fitting gloves on every call. If blood or other fluids could splash or spray, wear eye protection. When inhaled particles are a risk, wear a proper-size and fitted respirator (high-efficiency

Words of Wisdom

Remember to change your gloves between patients to prevent any possible contamination. Immediately wash your hands or use an alcohol-based hand sanitizer/rub every time you remove or change your gloves.[4] Handwashing is the best way to prevent transmission of most diseases.

particulate air [HEPA] or N95). In some cases, a gown may also be indicated. Always take the steps necessary to protect yourself on calls. When in doubt, it is always better to err on the side of caution. Infection control is covered in depth in Chapter 2, *Workforce Safety and Wellness*.

Also, consider other hazards involved in patient care and take necessary precautions to protect yourself. PPE includes clothing or specialized equipment that provides some protection from substances that may pose a health or safety risk. It includes items like steel-toe boots to protect your feet and toes, leather gloves, a helmet, heat-resistant outerwear, and self-contained breathing apparatus.

SAFETY

In addition to scene safety, patient safety has become a central topic in EMS. The Health and Medicine Division (HMD) of the National Academies of Sciences, Engineering, and Medicine defines patient safety as "freedom from accidental injury," while the National Patient Safety Foundation defines its goal as the "avoidance, prevention, and amelioration of adverse outcomes or injuries stemming from the process of care." **Patient safety** is defined as the reduction of risk of unnecessary harm associated with EMS care to an acceptable minimum that is defined by the limits of the best available medical evidence, equipment, technology, and human skill.

Patient Assessment

Scene Size-up

↓

Primary Assessment*

Form a general impression

Assess

- Responsiveness/level of consciousness

Assess and treat

- Airway
- Breathing
- Circulation

Also assess

- Disability
- Exposure

Identify

- Chief complaint/life threats (treat)
- Priority of patient care
- Transport decision

↓

History Taking

↓

Secondary Assessment

↓

Reassessment

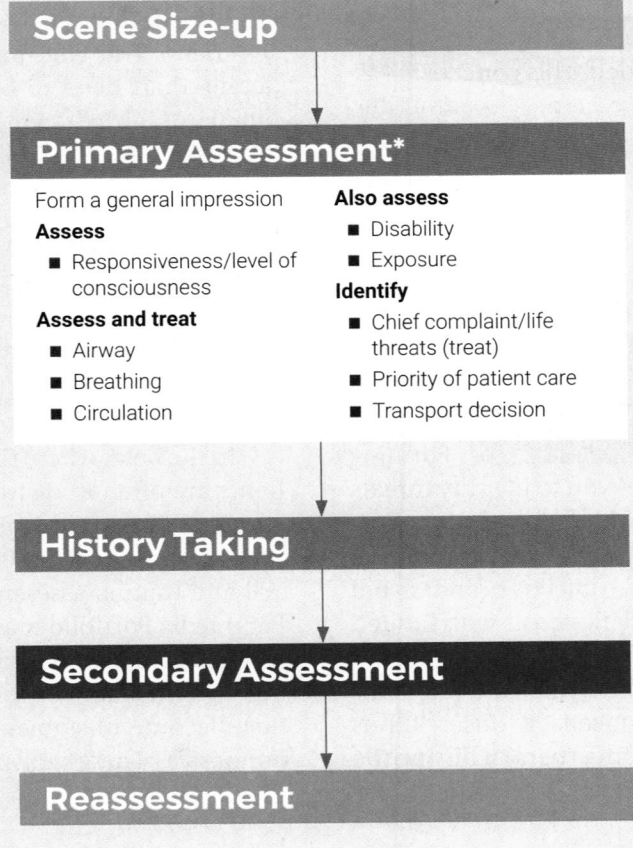

Primary Survey

Examination Techniques

Before we discuss the primary survey, we highlight three important examination techniques that you can use during your assessment. You may use these during the primary survey or the secondary assessment, depending on the urgency of the patient's condition.

- **Inspection**. Inspection is simply looking over the patient and noting any abnormalities or asymmetry (eg, swelling, deformity, or discoloration) that may indicate soft-tissue injuries.
- **Palpation**. Palpation is the process of touching to feel for abnormalities (eg, swelling or deformities). At times, palpation is gentle, but a firm touch will help you to identify areas where the patient has pain or tenderness. Your fingertips are well suited for detecting texture and consistency, while the back of your hand is better at noting skin temperature.
- **Auscultation**. Auscultation is listening to sounds within the body (eg, lung, heart, bowel, and blood pressure [BP]) using a stethoscope.

Form a General Impression

The primary survey can be the most intense portion of the assessment process because it focuses on identifying and managing life-threatening problems. In the first 60 to 90 seconds, as you look at, talk with, and touch the patient, you form a **general impression**, which is your overall initial impression that determines the priority for patient care; based on the patient's surroundings, MOI, signs and symptoms, and the chief complaint. Forming a general impression enables you to identify threats to the ABCDE (Airway, Breathing, Circulation, Disability, and Exposure). As additional information becomes available, remain objective and avoid tunnel vision: making a field diagnosis with limited clinical information.

Each of us, without even trying or being conscious of doing so, makes dozens of observations about the appearance of another person during the first few seconds of an encounter; for example, we note whether the person is sitting or standing, overweight or thin, smiling or frowning, dressed neatly or unkempt. When assessing a patient, you must make similar observations, but in a much more conscious, objective, and systematic manner. Look for specific clues to give you an immediate sense of the situation's seriousness. A patient who gasps, "I just . . . can't . . . catch . . . my breath," is clearly very sick. An even more obvious example of a priority is a patient who reports thoracic pain after being stabbed in the chest.

An important note regarding the National Registry Paramedic Portfolio follows. You will be tested on this information should you choose to pursue National Registration. The assessment format described in this section is designed for sick or injured patients. In some situations, patients may have no complaints and may not be in any distress. Those patients may be given a "well-patient exam," which is more comprehensive than the medical or trauma exams and takes more time. In the National Registry Paramedic Portfolio, there is a form for a lab session involving the comprehensive normal adult physical assessment. The well-patient exam includes more details than need to be obtained during prehospital care in the streets. For example, the general impression for the well-patient exam includes the patient's appearance, whether the patient speaks when approached, facial expression, skin color, eye contact, weight estimated in kilograms, work of breathing, posture, ease of movement, odors of body or breath, dress, hygiene, and grooming. Performing these assessments during an emergency call could take time that would be better spent providing lifesaving care and transportation.

In the field, where time is of the essence and patients are often in distress, use the assessment format presented in this chapter, which is consistent with National Registry Paramedic Portfolio for medical and trauma assessment. The National Registry Paramedic Portfolio is available at nremt.org.

The goal here is to answer two questions: (1) Is this patient stable or unstable, and if stable, might they become unstable? and (2) Is this patient sick or not sick? These questions take a slightly different form in trauma: (1) Is this patient hurt? and (2) If so, how seriously?

Whether the call is for a medical or trauma patient, question 1 is a qualification and, question 2 is a quantification. "Is this patient sick?" requires a yes or no answer, whereas "How sick is this patient?" attempts to rate the severity of the situation. With time and experience, you will be able to answer both questions and form your general impression within that 60- to 90-second window.

Mental status is often one of the primary indicators of how sick a patient is. Changes in level of consciousness (LOC) may provide a first clue to an alteration in patient condition. Thus, establish a baseline as soon as you encounter the patient. As you assess mental status in a trauma patient, decide whether to implement spinal immobilization procedures. Other considerations for mental status include observing the patient's speech (quality, rate, volume, articulation of words, fluency), mood, orientation (to person, place, and time), memory (short term, long term). These are discussed further in this chapter under secondary assessment.

Once you have established the severity of the patient's complaint, determine your care priorities, develop a care plan, and put it into action. If the primary problem seems to be a traumatic injury, identify and evaluate the MOI. If the primary problem seems to be medical, identify the NOI. Identify the age and sex of the patient, because this information may change how the patient presents. For example, an older woman having a heart attack might have no chest pain, whereas an older man with the same condition may have severe chest pain. Likewise, a school-age girl will often be more emotionally mature than a same-age boy, changing how each child answers your questions and reacts to the emergency itself.

Information gleaned from the primary survey is crucial to the patient's overall outcome. Treat life threats as you find them and decide what additional care is needed, what must be done on scene versus en route, when to initiate transport, and which facility is most appropriate given the patient's unique needs.

Words of Wisdom

The primary survey consists of GI, MS, ABCDE (or CABDE), and priority decision.

To be specific, first form a general impression (GI) of the patient, then quickly determine the patient's mental status (MS) using the AVPU scale (discussed next). Then, assess and manage life threats found in the ABC order. The exception to this is when the patient looks lifeless or has life-threatening external bleeding, in which case follow the CAB or XABC order, respectively. If the patient has no pulse, begin chest compressions. If the patient has life-threatening bleeding, apply a tourniquet immediately.

The DE portion of the acronym reminds you that disability and exposure are important because they help identify all potentially life-threatening injuries. It is important to assess disability and to expose the patient, then cover up the patient. The treatment of airway, breathing, and circulation threats to life are emphasized because they must be managed within seconds. Remember, "When seconds count, your treatment can't be minutes away." This sums up the importance of assessing and managing life threats identified during the primary survey.

A patient's mental status is initially assessed using the **AVPU** scale:

A *Alert* (responds appropriately; further define mental status as follows)
Alert and Oriented × *4* = Person, place, time, and event
Alert and Oriented × *3* = Person, place, and time
Alert and Oriented × *2* = Person and place
Alert and Oriented × *1* = Person only

V Responsive to *verbal* stimuli

P Responsive to *pain*

U *Unresponsive*

With the AVPU scale, mental status can be assessed by determining whether the patient is **alert and oriented (A × O)** in four areas: person, place, time, and event. Regarding orientation to time, if the patient knows the correct day but is unsure about the time, then this could indicate disorientation.

Similarly, if the patient knows the time but is unsure of the day, month, or year, then this also indicates disorientation. Therefore, ask the day, month, and year if you suspect disorientation, and document the patient's responses in your patient care report (PCR/ePCR).

When patients exhibit mental status changes, they remain awake but become disoriented. Generally, patients first become disoriented to events. Then they forget the time, and then they forget where they are. Forgetting who they are is the last orientation lost.

Describing how a patient is acting is more helpful than simply documenting the patient's level of responsiveness. For example, you may describe a patient as "alert and cooperative," or "awake and combative," or even "awake but slow to respond to questions."

As you classify the response to stimuli, grade the patient according to their best response you elicit. For example, a patient passed out on the street who moans in response to a loud shout from you would score a "V" on the AVPU scale. Responding to tactile stimuli (eg, pinching the nail bed, twisting the skin of the forearm, pinching the muscle mass above the clavicle) would earn a "P." Is it an appropriate response (ie, withdrawal from the pain source) or does it merely represent neurologic posturing (ie, decorticate posturing [flexing the arms and extending the legs] or decerebrate posturing [extension of both arms and legs])? No response to verbal or tactile stimuli would be classified as "U." A mental status of "U" means you applied painful stimuli and received no response.

Assess the Airway

Assess the patient's airway status by focusing on two questions: Is the airway open and patent? If it is open, is it likely to remain so? Immediate life threats may be caused by the tongue, foreign body airway obstruction, liquids, and anatomic (crush/swelling) obstruction. For air to be drawn into the lungs, the airway must be properly positioned and unobstructed (anatomically open). Responsive patients who are talking or crying give you a clue about the adequacy of their airway. If you hear sonorous breath sounds (snoring respirations), think "position problem": The sounds are most likely caused by partial airway obstruction by the tongue. If you hear gurgling or bubbling sounds, think "suction": There are most likely fluids (ie, blood, mucus, or vomit) in the mouth or posterior pharynx.

As you consider airway management options, move from simple to complex. The easiest problem to solve is head position. No equipment is required and this position can be improved quickly. In the case of obstruction, such as by food, use basic life support (BLS) procedures (eg, chest compressions/abdominal thrusts) to clear the obstruction. Suctioning takes longer, because of the need to set up and use the equipment, and is more complicated than repositioning the patient. In addition, suctioning for too long may create new problems, such as hypoxia and bradycardia secondary to vagal stimulation.

The possibility of a spine injury (or lack thereof) drives the decision of which technique to initially use to open the airway: head tilt–chin lift maneuver in medical patients or jaw-thrust maneuver in trauma patients.

Special Populations

If you perform the head tilt–chin lift maneuver, remember the anatomic differences among the various age groups. Ensure you do not create an airway obstruction by improperly positioning the head. Infants and young children do not have well-developed cartilaginous rings to provide tracheal support, as adults do. Thus, a child's trachea is easily collapsed or occluded as the head position changes.

If a mechanical means is required to keep the airway open, you must choose an airway adjunct. If you opt to place an oropharyngeal airway (OPA) or nasopharyngeal airway (NPA), you must retrieve the equipment, select the correct size for the patient, and then insert the airway. This procedure takes time, so always bring all the equipment needed for a primary survey to the patient's side.

If you determine the patient cannot maintain their airway and you cannot maintain it by any other means, use a more invasive technique, such as endotracheal intubation or a rescue airway (eg, King LT, i-gel, laryngeal mask airway), as discussed in Chapter 16, *Airway Management*.

Assess Breathing

Assess a patient's breathing in the same way regardless of their age. Focus on two key questions: First, is the patient breathing? If no, then you have to breathe for the patient. Second, if the patient is breathing, is the breathing adequate? Examples of life threats to breathing include open pneumothorax, tension pneumothorax, flail chest, and inadequate minute volume.

Expose the chest and inspect for injuries. If you locate a flail segment, then ensure adequate ventilations and support them as needed. If you locate a sucking chest wound, then seal it with a three-sided occlusive dressing, oxygenate, and ventilate the patient as needed. If a patient shows signs of respiratory failure or shock and has diminished or absent breath sounds on one side of the chest, then consider the possibility of a tension pneumothorax. Needle decompression of the chest should be performed, if indicated.

The amount of air moved in and out of the lungs each minute is the best measure of breathing adequacy. This is called the *minute volume* and is calculated by multiplying the respiratory rate by the tidal volume (ie, the volume of air inspired with each inhaled breath), as explained in detail in Chapter 16, *Airway Management*. For example, an adult patient breathing slowly and deeply, at 12 breaths/min and 500 mL/breath, has a minute volume of 6,000 mL. A patient breathing faster and in a shallow manner, at a rate of 24 breaths/min and 250 mL/breath, would also have a minute volume of 6,000 mL. On a per-minute basis, the volumes of these two patients are identical, even though the second patient is breathing twice as fast as the first patient. As a general rule, a breathing rate of *greater* than 24 breaths/min is considered too fast for an adult patient. Likewise, a breathing rate of 8 breaths/min is considered too slow. In both cases, prompt treatment needs to be initiated, albeit more urgently with the patient breathing at 8 breaths/min versus 24 breaths/min.

Besides assessing tidal volume, note the patient's breathing rate and the work of breathing (ie, respiratory effort). Signs of increased work of breathing may include the use of accessory muscles, chest retractions, restlessness, and leaning forward to inhale. Assess for chest rise and fall, note the symmetry of the chest wall, and observe the depth and rhythm of respirations (eg, regular, irregular, periodic). Auscultate lung sounds, noting their presence and clarity, as well as any abnormal sounds. Alternate from side to side and compare your findings. During the primary survey, the type of lung sounds a patient has is as important as noting whether they are present and equal. If the breathing assessment reveals hypoxia or inadequate ventilations, then it is important to begin correcting these problems by utilizing supplemental oxygen and/or positive-pressure ventilation as needed.

Assess Circulation

Assess circulation by performing a full-body scan. Look for major hemorrhage or other life-threatening injuries, check for a pulse, and evaluate the skin. In some cases, blood loss can occur very rapidly, quickly leading to shock, exsanguination, or even death. Signs of blood loss include active bleeding from wounds and other evidence of bleeding, such as blood on the patient's clothing or pooled nearby. Profuse bleeding from a large vein is characterized by steady blood flow. Bleeding from an artery is characterized by spurting blood. Of course, if the patient already has significant blood loss, then their systolic BP will have dropped, and blood will be ejected less forcefully. In contrast, if a major artery has been severed, exsanguination can occur in minutes.

When you evaluate an unresponsive patient, scan for blood by quickly and lightly running your gloved hands from head to toe, pausing periodically to see if your gloves are bloody. Immediately control all life-threatening external bleeding. If an extremity is hemorrhaging, it is appropriate to immediately apply a tourniquet. The tourniquet should be applied in less than 30 seconds to address arterial bleeding.[5] In a responsive patient, this step should come before assessing the patient's pulse, airway, or breathing. More information about applying tourniquets and controlling blood loss is discussed in Chapter 31, *Bleeding*.

Words of Wisdom

Use the ABCDE mnemonic when approaching the patient (Airway, Breathing, Circulation, Disability, and Exposure). This mnemonic is sometimes adjusted during the primary survey in two scenarios. First, when life-threatening bleeding is present, the sequence may be described as XABCDE, where X represents eXsanguination (life-threatening bleeding). Second, when the patient appears lifeless and is in suspected cardiac arrest, the sequence is described as CABDE to prioritize circulation.

Assessing the pulse involves a rapid check of the rate, quality, and rhythm of the heartbeat. To palpate the pulse, gently compress an artery against a bony prominence, which allows you to feel the pressure wave generated by the heart's contraction. In responsive adults and children, the pulse is best palpated at the radial artery; in unresponsive patients, it is most readily assessed at the carotid artery. Use the tips of your index and middle fingers to palpate the pulse. In responsive and unresponsive infants, palpate the pulse at the brachial artery. In any patient, if you cannot find a pulse, begin chest compressions.

For most patients, it is best to count the pulses felt in 30 seconds and then multiply by 2 to obtain the per-minute rate. A pulse that is weak and difficult to palpate, irregular, or extremely slow should be palpated and counted for 1 full minute. In resting adults, the normal pulse rate is between 60 and 100 beats/min. People who are physically fit may have a resting rate in the high 40s, whereas people who are out of shape might have a resting pulse rate of perhaps 112 beats/min. In general for adults, a rate of less than 60 beats/min is considered slow and is referred to as *bradycardia*. A rate higher than 100 beats/min is considered fast and is referred to as *tachycardia*.

Compare the strength and quality of the central and peripheral pulses. Assess the quality or strength of the pulse to evaluate cardiac output. A normal pulse is easily felt, as if a strong wave were passing beneath your fingertips. A weak pulse is difficult to feel, and a thready pulse is one that is weak and fast. A patient with hypertension will produce a more forceful pulse than usual, a so-called bounding pulse. A weak central pulse may indicate hypotensive shock (discussed in Chapter 41, *Management and Resuscitation of the Critical Patient*). A peripheral pulse that is difficult to find, weak, or irregular suggests poor peripheral perfusion and may be a sign of shock, hemorrhage, or a cardiac dysrhythmia.

Note the pulse's rhythm. A normal rhythm is regular, like a ticking clock. If some beats come early or late or are skipped, the pulse is considered irregular. Although many cardiac dysrhythmias are not life threatening, an irregular pulse can indicate a serious condition. As such, consider all patients who have an irregular pulse and are symptomatic (eg, short of breath, weak, excessive sweating) to be at risk of deterioration until proven otherwise. Report your findings by describing the pulse's rate, quality, and rhythm. For example, you might say, "Patient's pulse is 72, strong, and regular" or "Pulse is 138, thready, and irregular."

As part of this phase of the primary survey, assess the patient's skin for CTC. Collectively, these criteria provide insights into the patient's overall **perfusion**. To assess the warmth and moisture of the patient's skin, use the back of your hand, as it tends to be more sensitive than your palm **FIGURE 11-6**.

The color of the skin **TABLE 11-1**, especially in light-skinned patients, reflects the circulation status immediately beneath the skin, including oxygen saturation of the blood. In people of color, changes may not be readily evident in the skin but may be assessed by closely examining the mucous membranes (eg, lips or conjunctivae). When the blood vessels supplying the skin are fully dilated in a light-skinned person, the skin becomes warm and

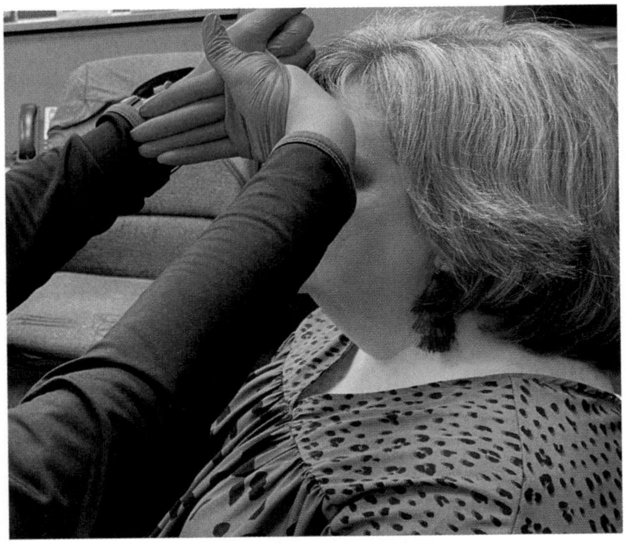

FIGURE 11-6 Assessing the skin CTC: color, temperature and condition. Use the back of the hand to assess the temperature and moisture of the skin.

Courtesy of Rhonda Hunt.

pink. When the blood vessels supplying the skin constrict or cardiac output drops, the skin becomes paler or mottled and cool. If the patient does not receive enough oxygen (eg, a narcotic overdose may cause respiration as slow as 4 breaths/min), the blood will desaturate as the oxygen level drops. The skin will then turn a dusky gray or blue, a condition described as **cyanosis**. In a patient whose baseline skin tone is dark, poor circulation will manifest as blue or mottled skin coloration. **Pallor**, or paleness, occurs if arterial blood flow ceases to part of the body (eg, owing to a blood clot or massive bleeding). Hypothermia will also result in pallor as the body shunts blood to the core and away from the extremities.

Skin temperature rises as peripheral blood vessels dilate; it falls as vessels constrict. Fever and a high environmental temperature usually stimulate vasodilation, whereas shock elicits vasoconstriction. Normal skin is moderately warm and dry and does not feel "oily." The dryness or moisture of the skin is primarily determined by the sympathetic nervous system (SNS). Stimulation of the SNS, as occurs in shock or with any other severe stress or pain, causes intense or excessive sweating (**diaphoresis**). Depression of the SNS, as occurs when the thoracic or lumbar spine is injured, can cause the affected skin to become abnormally dry and cool **TABLE 11-2**.

TABLE 11-1 Inspection of the Skin

Skin Color	Possible Cause
Red (flushed)	Fever Hypertension Superficial burns Allergic reaction Alcohol intake Carbon monoxide poisoning (late sign)
White (pallor)	Excessive blood loss Anaphylaxis Hypoglycemia Anxiety
Blue (cyanosis)	Hypoxemia, oxygen desaturation
Mottled	Cardiovascular embarrassment (as in shock), disseminated intravascular coagulopathy
Jaundice	Liver dysfunction

Special Populations

Capillary refill time (CRT) is included as part of the assessment of children in many pediatric training programs as a tool to evaluate the child's cardiovascular status. Because of variability in peripheral perfusion, use of nail polish, and hand hygiene, many physicians and nurses view capillary refill in adults as a less reliable proxy for peripheral perfusion than it is in children. Delayed capillary refill can actually be normal in some adults. Capillary refill is discussed in Chapter 44, *Pediatric Emergencies*.

TABLE 11-2 Skin Palpation

Skin Condition	Possible Cause
Hot, dry	Excessive body heat (heatstroke)
Hot, wet	Reaction to increased internal or external temperature
Warm, dry	Fever
Cool, dry	Exposure to cold
Cool, wet	Shock

Evidence-Based Medicine

A 2015 study found that CRT was 2 seconds or less when measured on the finger in healthy children and older infants, but may extend to 4 seconds when measured on the chest or foot. Study results revealed that CRT is an important "red flag" for identifying children with serious illness; that is, finding an abnormal CRT increases the likelihood of a serious outcome, including death and dehydration. However, a normal CRT does not make a serious outcome less likely. Therefore, a normal CRT should not be used to rule out serious illness in children.[6]

Restoring Circulation

If a patient has inadequate circulation, take immediate action to restore or improve circulation, control severe bleeding, and improve oxygen delivery to the tissues. Remember to follow standard precautions, which may specify gloves, protective eyewear, and use of a barrier device for ventilation. Prolonged impaired circulation is devastating because it deprives the body's cells of oxygen, which is necessary for normal cell functioning.

The apparent absence of a palpable pulse in a responsive patient indicates low cardiac output, not cardiac arrest. However, if you cannot detect a pulse in an unresponsive adult, immediately begin chest compressions and obtain and apply a defibrillator (either automated external defibrillator [AED] or manual). Although patients with traumatic cardiac arrest will probably require intravenous (IV) fluid therapy for blood loss, certain medications will be needed to treat the cardiac arrest itself. Identify the patient's cardiac rhythm with a cardiac monitor/defibrillator to enable you to administer the most appropriate medication. Cardiopulmonary resuscitation (CPR) and control of bleeding are intended to maintain circulation. Oxygen delivery is improved by administering supplemental oxygen. Patients with impaired circulation should receive high-flow oxygen via a nonrebreathing mask or assisted ventilation to improve oxygen delivery at the cellular level. CPR and defibrillation procedures are discussed in Chapter 18, *Cardiovascular Emergencies.*

Words of Wisdom

Research from military operations has shown that most combat wounds occur in the extremities, and 7% of battlefield deaths could be prevented with properly applied tourniquets.[7,8] One reason that wounds typically occur to the extremities in the combat setting is that soldiers wear body armor and helmets to protect their head and chest areas. Further, they are more likely to encounter diffuse MOIs, such as improvised explosive devices. The common characteristic of these combat wounds tends to be the high-velocity penetrating MOI. In the civilian setting, an analogous MOI is a gunshot wound. Most (58%) gunshot wounds to civilians are to the head or chest, with only 20% occurring in the extremities.[9] Thus, the survivability of this MOI is much lower in the civilian setting.

Remember, only a few medical conditions cause sudden death: airway obstruction, respiratory arrest, cardiac arrest, and severe bleeding. Often (but certainly not always) these conditions are reversible; however, to reverse them, you must be able to recognize them quickly and take immediate steps to correct them. This is the purpose of the primary survey!

Assess the Patient for Disability

Once you have examined the patient's airway, breathing, and circulation and addressed any life-threatening conditions, perform a brief neurologic evaluation. A mini-neurologic exam includes the AVPU scale, pupils (eg, size, equality, reactivity to light), a quick assessment for neurologic deficits, and the **Glasgow Coma Scale (GCS)**. The GCS is the most commonly used, reliable, and consistent method of assessing mental status and neurologic function. It assigns a point value (score) for eye opening, verbal response, and motor response; these values are added for a total score **TABLE 11-3**. While it may take slightly longer to perform than the AVPU scale, calculating a GCS score provides much greater insight into the patient's overall neurologic function. When you report and record your findings, be sure to include the score for each GCS category, not just a cumulative score.

To illustrate how the GCS works, let's walk through a sample scenario. You encounter an older man who tracks you with his eyes as you enter his room. As you speak with him, you note that his verbal response is disoriented, even though he follows your commands. His GCS values would be 4, 4, and 6, for a total score of 14. By comparison, if he opened his eyes only to pain, moaned as his only verbal response, and withdrew to pain, then he would be assigned GCS values of 2, 2, and 4, for a total score of 8.

Finally, as part of your brief neurologic evaluation, assess for any gross neurologic deficits by having the patient carefully move all extremities to pinpoint any motor deficits. Assess bilaterally for motor strength or weakness by asking the patient to move each extremity against the resistance of your hands. Assess grip strength by having the patient squeeze two of your fingers bilaterally and simultaneously so that any unilateral neurologic deficits will be obvious. Quickly assess for any loss of sensation by touching the distal portions of the extremities with a blunt or sharp object to assess for gross sensory defects.

Expose, Then Cover

As you physically examine the patient, visually inspect each area to ensure an accurate and thorough assessment. Although not every patient needs to

TABLE 11-3 Glasgow Coma Scale

Eye Opening		Best Verbal Response		Best Motor Response	
Spontaneous	4	Oriented conversation	5	Follows commands	6
To verbal command	3	Disoriented conversation	4	Localizes pain	5
To pain	2	Nonsensical speech	3	Withdraws to pain	4
No response	1	Unintelligible sounds	2	Abnormal flexion	3
		No response	1	Abnormal extension	2
				No response	1

Scores:

15: Indicates no neurologic disabilities

13–14: Mild dysfunction

9–12: Moderate to severe dysfunction

8 or less: Severe dysfunction (The lowest possible score is 3.)

be completely exposed for appropriate assessment to occur, it is important to keep in mind that you cannot assess what you cannot see. Therefore, adequate exposure of each area being examined is essential to the physical exam process. When you are finished, cover up the patient to respect their privacy and to maintain body heat.

Words of Wisdom

When a patient is a high priority and there is no time for a complete secondary assessment on scene, perform a rapid full-body scan (sometimes called a rapid full-body sweep) before applying a cervical collar on the patient. The rapid full-body scan is discussed in the Secondary Assessment section later in this chapter.

SAFETY

A National Academy of Science report, *Crossing the Quality Chasm: A New Health System for the 21st Century*, identified six quality aims that health care should embrace:[10,11]

- **Safety.** Avoid injuries to patients from care intended to help them.
- **Timeliness.** Reduce waits and sometimes harmful delays for both those who receive care and those who give care.
- **Effectiveness.** Provide services based on scientific knowledge to all who could benefit, and refrain from providing services to those not likely to benefit.
- **Efficiency.** Avoid waste, including waste of equipment, supplies, ideas, and energy.
- **Equity.** Provide care that does not vary in quality because of personal characteristics (ie, sex, ethnicity, geographic location, and socioeconomic status).
- **Patient centeredness.** Provide care that is respectful of and responsive to individual patient preferences, needs, and values, and ensure that patient values guide all clinical decisions.

Make a Transport Decision

As noted previously, early in the assessment process, identify priority patients who will benefit from limited scene time and rapid transport. Priority patients are typically deemed to be in either an unstable or potentially unstable condition and need definitive care that cannot be accomplished in the field.

Patients in stable condition are generally deemed not to be high-priority cases. These patients, while injured or ill, are not necessarily in critical (unstable) condition and therefore do not require expedient transport.

In transporting patients to the hospital, safety should always be of the utmost importance. With a priority patient, expedite transport, doing only what is absolutely necessary at the scene and handling everything else en route (eg, appropriate patient history gathering, secondary assessment, and reassessment). The following is a list of priority patients:

- **Patients receiving CPR, in respiratory arrest, or being given life-sustaining ventilatory/circulatory support.**
- **Poor general impression.** The patient is in obvious distress and does not look well.
- **Unresponsive.** Unresponsiveness is never a good sign and typically points to a patient in serious or critical condition who may not be able to protect their airway.
- **Responsive but does not or cannot follow commands.** Altered mentation is another poor sign; the question you must answer is exactly how bad the patient's condition is, especially if there is a possible traumatic brain injury.
- **Difficulty breathing.** Breathing difficulty is one of the most common chief complaints in prehospital care. Patients having difficulty breathing are in trouble; those who are working to breathe are in much bigger trouble.
- **Hypoxia that fails to correct rapidly** (within 1 to 2 minutes of field intervention).
- **Hypoperfusion or shock.** Without question, hypoperfusion or shock is an obvious sign of a high-risk patient. A weak or absent peripheral pulse, sustained tachycardia, and skin that is paler than baseline, cool, and wet all point to a very ill patient.
- **Complicated childbirth.** If any part of the neonate other than the newborn's head (a shoulder or foot, for example) presents from the birth canal, the situation is unlikely to be managed successfully in the field setting.
- **Chest pain with a systolic BP of less than 100 mm Hg.** Especially in the context of

tachycardia, this sign may indicate shock or cardiac compromise and a high-risk patient in unstable condition.

- **Suspected acute myocardial infarction (AMI) with electrocardiogram (ECG) showing STEMI.** This patient must be managed quickly and taken to the most appropriate cardiac center in your region, since "time is muscle."
- **Suspected stroke.** When signs and symptoms of a stroke are identified, it is important to establish the last time the patient was seen "normal" and begin transport to a stroke center.
- **Uncontrolled bleeding.** Whether internal or external, such bleeding is a serious life threat.
- **Severe pain anywhere.** Any person with severe pain, especially enough to wake the patient up from sleeping, should be considered a priority patient.
- **Multiple injuries (including severe burns).** Whereas a patient may have multiple minor injuries that by themselves are not serious, several small problems can add up to one large problem.
- **Abdominal injuries.** Consider any signs or symptoms of abdominal injury as serious and indicative of a high-priority patient in unstable condition.
- **Severe hypertension.** Patients can be in a hypertensive crisis or having a stroke.
- **Inability to move** any part of the body.
- **Apparent life-threatening event (ALTE).** An episode characterized by a combination of apnea (central or obstructive), color change (cyanotic, pallid, erythematous, or plethoric), change in muscle tone (usually diminished), and choking or gagging.

YOU are the Paramedic

PART 2

You immediately request law enforcement personnel to respond to the scene and advise the dispatcher of what you see. You use the public address (PA) system to say to the patient, "If you can hear me, wave at me." The patient gestures in your direction. Law enforcement personnel arrive with two patrol cars. The officers approach the patient, and then motion for you to come to them. The first officer informs you the patient has been stabbed in the chest. The patient's shirt is bloody, but you cannot see a knife or other implement that may have been used as a weapon. The patient looks up at you but says nothing when you ask him what happened.

Recording Time: 3 Minutes	
Appearance	Awake
Level of consciousness	"V" verbal
Airway	Open and clear
Breathing	Adequate
Circulation	Adequate
Disability	Equal strength in four extremities
Exposure	A single injury to chest; blanket applied

3. What is your general impression of this patient?
4. What is your next step in assessing this patient?

Patient Assessment

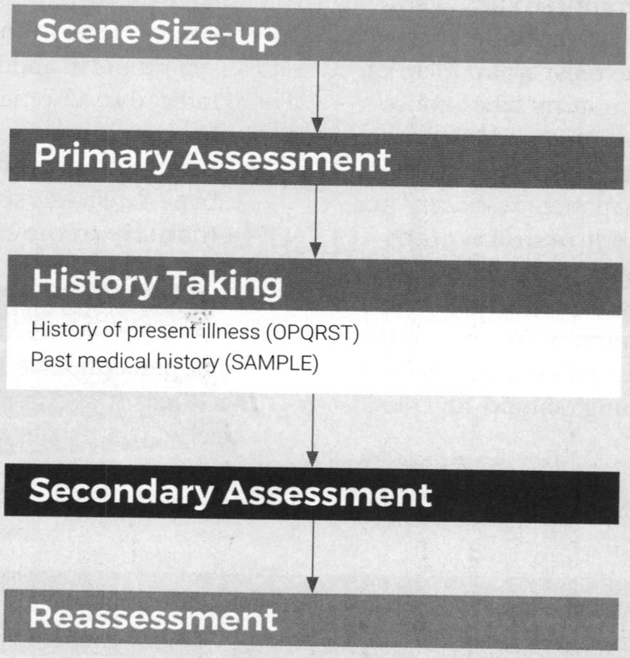

Street Smarts

A good provider can gather data about the patient's current medical conditions and the patient's medical history. Gathering data is not always as easy as it sounds. Your ability to communicate in a friendly and compassionate manner is essential. You must determine how reliable the patient is in their ability to provide an accurate medical history. If the patient is unable to provide a reliable history for some reason, you must find a caregiver or bystander who can speak to the patient's medical issues. For example, a patient involved in a high-speed MVC may not be able to provide an accurate history because of alterations in mental status from a head injury. Similarly, a patient under the influence of alcohol or other drugs may not be in a state of mind to provide a reliable history.

History Taking

Purpose

The purpose of obtaining a **patient history** (the patient's chief complaint, present symptoms, and previous illnesses) is to gain information about the patient and learn about the events surrounding the incident. Your goal is to obtain a clear and accurate patient history of the immediate event and pertinent past medical history (discussed in detail later in the chapter), noting details to help you distinguish life threats from nonemergency complaints. When pertinent, expanded details about the patient history can help narrow down your differential diagnosis.

As a general rule, open-ended questions typically yield more information, as they allow patients to respond in their own words with various answers. Closed-ended questions, answered "yes or no," yield valuable information but little detail. Avoid asking leading questions because they may take the patient down an irrelevant information pathway. At times you must ask very direct questions, such as with a depressed patient: "Have you had thoughts about hurting yourself or committing suicide?"

Ensure your questions are age appropriate and education appropriate. Also, be patient. Ask a question and then wait for the answer. Rushing your patient along almost guarantees you won't capture the information you want and need. During the assessment process, you may even find time to do some patient teaching, for example, "You may want to consider using a week-at-a-time pill box to help you keep up with your medications."

Street Smarts

How you approach an interview can make or break a therapeutic relationship. Patients must know you are interested in their well-being as a whole and not simply their condition or injury. Learn to listen carefully to what patients say without interrupting them and before initiating a physical examination. More often than not, the cause of the patient's symptoms can be determined from the patient's own words, with the physical examination and diagnostic tests simply confirming the suspected cause or differential diagnosis. It has often been said, "patients don't care how much you know until they know how much you care."

Patient Information

Several components collectively make up the patient history. On most calls, the two most important pieces of patient history you must obtain are the patient's name and chief complaint. After that, you can obtain the rest of the patient history in whatever order is most convenient and conducive to good patient care.

Techniques for History Taking

Your Appearance and Demeanor

Every time you care for a patient, you must first establish a professional relationship. In most cases, this is a short-term relationship, often less than 90 minutes, lasting only until you provide your handoff report and turn over the patient to the emergency department (ED) staff.

Although time is short, you will want to leave a positive impression in the communication you establish with all involved. When you first meet your patients, they should be looking at a clean, neat, health care provider. Maintain good personal hygiene and grooming, and wear professional, clean, and wrinkle-free attire **FIGURE 11-7**. Your patients will likely form a good first impression of you if you look professional. By comparison, if you look unprofessional, it may be difficult for your patients to trust that they will receive competent care. Remember, this perception is in the eyes of the patient, not the eyes of the provider. In many communities, most patients are older adults, who may have more traditional views than you. Gaining the trust of your patients is an important aspect of care.

Along with your appearance, be aware of your demeanor. On every call, your attitude is on display. If you are unhappy, you may look sad. Remember, your facial expressions and body language send powerful messages. If you have come to believe that calls to 9-1-1 must meet *your* expectations, *you are wrong.* If patients think a problem is serious enough to merit a call to 9-1-1, you have an obligation to treat those patients and their complaints accordingly—professionally and to the best of your ability.

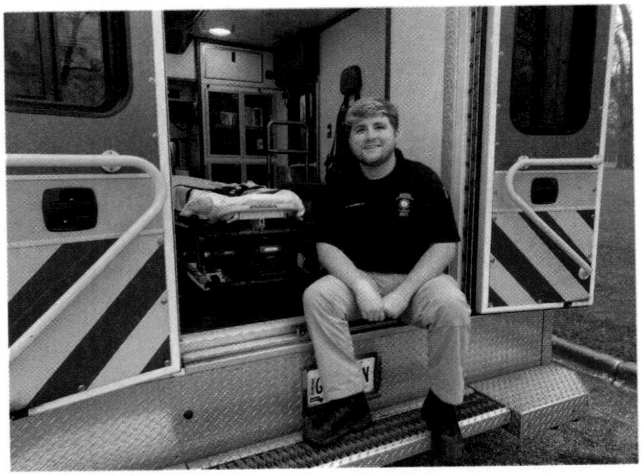

FIGURE 11-7 Your appearance should be professional and your demeanor positive and friendly.

Courtesy of Rhonda Hunt.

> **Street Smarts**
>
> Remember, if you are wearing PPE, including a mask, patients and others on scene cannot see your smile! Other indicators, such as word choice, vocal inflections, and body language, will need to convey your good intentions.

Note Taking

As you begin to gather information, let the patient know you will be asking several questions and while they are answering, you or your partner will be taking notes. This lets patients know they are not being ignored and that the information being provided is important enough to write down **FIGURE 11-8**.

With this approach, remember to make eye contact with the patient. Too often, EMS personnel reel off a list of questions to their patients to fill in all the blanks on a PCR. Do not bury your nose in a tablet computer or clipboard! If possible, position yourself at the patient's eye level. Maintain good eye contact and pay attention.

Communication Techniques

Introducing Yourself and Addressing the Patient Introduce yourself to your patient, tell them you are a paramedic, and offer the name of your service. Introduce your partner as well. Then ask the patient their name and how they would like to be addressed. Err on the side of formality, using Mr, Miss, Mrs, or Ms. There is a world of difference between Mr. John Markham (formal), John (more casual), or Johnnie (really casual). Your patient will say, "Call me Johnnie," if that is what he prefers. Addressing patients by a name they prefer is professional, but until you know their preferred name, assuming formality is respectful and will help establish better rapport than being too familiar.

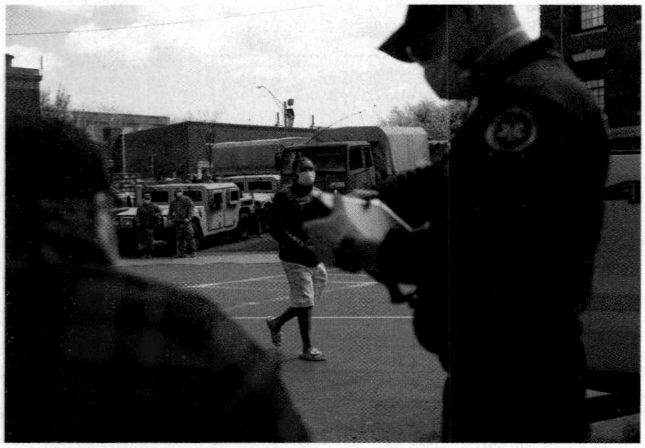

FIGURE 11-8 You may want to take notes on an assessment card or directly into your tablet during the patient history.

> **Street Smarts**
>
> Be sure to use the name or pronoun (Mr, Ms, Sir, Madam) the patient prefers, or, better yet, simply use their name as they introduce themselves. Every patient you care for deserves to be treated with compassion and respect.

Avoid catch-all nicknames like "pal," "buddy," "sport," "chief," "dude," "friend," "honey," "sweetie, "cutie," and "darling." You can bog down the process of obtaining a patient history by demeaning the patient and treating them unprofessionally. Using casual nicknames can also be problematic when there are cultural differences. Certain terms have negative connotations in some cultures. Become familiar with the cultural groups in your service area and with issues that could lead to misunderstanding. It is helpful for paramedics to develop "**cultural intelligence**": the ability to function effectively across various cultural contexts, interacting with people of all nationalities and getting along with those of all ethnic, political, and even generational differences.

Asking About Feelings Asking about a patient's feelings is one of the most difficult conversations you may have as a paramedic. But as part of obtaining a good health history, ask if a patient is tired, depressed, or having any number of feelings that are most easily dealt with by denial.

Keep any unpleasant sights, sounds, and smells from disturbing a patient who is feeling bad. You can also validate your patient's feelings: "This is a tough situation." That type of response is empathy in action. Do your best to continuously attend to the patient's psychological needs throughout the call. It is a challenging part of your job, but such needs can profoundly affect a person's physical health.

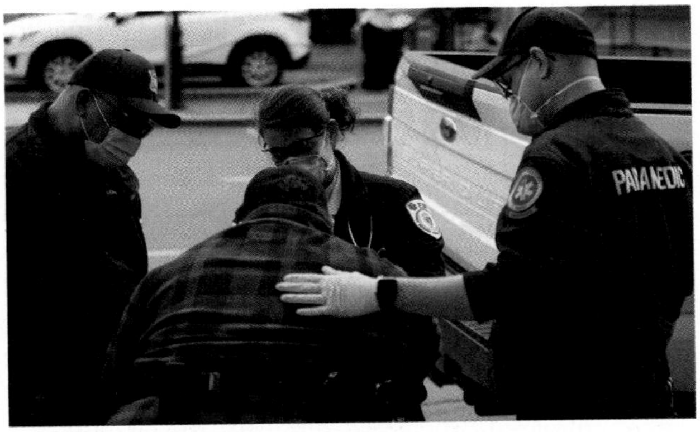

FIGURE 11-9 Be as empathetic as possible if a patient conveys sad or tragic information.

Communicating Empathy Empathy is an underlying quality of compassionate care. It is often described as one step further than sympathy. Empathy is a psychological gift that allows you to feel what the patient is feeling; it is the ability to put yourself in their shoes. Sometimes as you gather the patient history, you will hear sad or even tragic information from patients. Do not hesitate to communicate your feelings and address the emotional effect of what you have heard **FIGURE 11-9**. Empathy can help you set the patient on the path to healing, no matter the diagnosis.

Street Smarts

Compassionate care demonstrates an awareness of the patient's suffering and your wish to relieve it. A compassionate statement, such as "I could see how this chest pain would make you worried about having a heart attack," shows the patient that you can identify with them as another human being. Such mutual understanding allows the patient to feel comfortable revealing information to you and often helps improve patient satisfaction with the encounter. But be aware that patients can sometimes misconstrue sympathetic statements as insincere gestures of comfort. Genuine sympathy can be challenging to express unless you have personally experienced what the patient is encountering. Providing compassionate responses to patient concerns is an art that can only be learned with time, observation, and practice.

While being empathetic with your questioning, it is important to remain effective. Do not ask, "Are you okay?" This is the most tempting of all yes or no questions! Instead, ask for facts first, and then follow up. When asked, for example, most people would deny they feel exhausted, frazzled, scared, or depressed. After all, the patient met you only a few minutes ago. Establish that you are a caring health professional by asking a series of "safe" questions about physical health before asking about mental health conditions.

Offering Reassurance With that positive demeanor also comes the temptation to reassure your patients, sometimes inappropriately. Be cautious about what you tell your patients so you do not make promises you cannot keep.

For example, you may be tempted to reassure a metal worker who caught his wedding ring on a piece of metal that a few stitches are all that is needed for treatment. In reality, many circumferential finger cuts can result in an amputation. Imagine how much distress you will cause your patient when he arrives at the ED and receives news that is not so positive.

In addition, if your reassurance is inappropriate, then the patient could choose not to share quite as much information as they might have under other circumstances, leaving you with less information rather than more.

Sometimes, however, it is appropriate to offer some reassurance. When an unexpected event occurs, it can overwhelm people emotionally. Patients and their family members, along with their friends and neighbors, can suddenly find themselves under extreme levels of stress as a result of the emergency situation. Just as some people react with anger and hostility to a stressful situation, others cry when they are overcome by sadness, happiness, fear, or anxiety. Patience and some soothing words, such as "We're here to take care of you now," go a long way.

Fortunately, the presence of EMS arriving on the scene often exerts a calming effect. During your career, you will be surprised at how often you hear someone say "Thank goodness, the paramedics are here!" the moment you walk through the door. Collectively, your calm demeanor and patient approach; appropriate touch, such as a hand on the shoulder; and a quiet, "I'm in control now" tone of voice will help a person stop crying and allow you to begin your assessment and care.

Reading Nonverbal Cues Remain alert for nonverbal signs of distress. Pain, psychological distress, and fear often register in body movements and facial expressions. As you work in the field as a student, you will learn how to read patients' many nonverbal cues. The paramedics you work with will help you decipher them, as will experienced caregivers in the ED and at the hospital.

One of the most critical elements of the interview process is being a *great listener*, and a big part of being a great listener is being a *patient listener*. For many reasons, a patient can be slow to respond. Do not let a period of silence make you uneasy. Maybe the person didn't hear your question, didn't understand you, is afraid to answer, is trying to recall distant details related to the question you just asked, or is trying to decide if they trust you enough to reply truthfully or at all. Ask and then wait. Give patients time to think before they answer; otherwise, a patient may become silent if you display a lack of sensitivity. If you cannot determine the cause of a patient's silence, consider whether your manner could be responsible and adjust your approach.

Throughout the assessment process, look for nonverbal communication, such as changes in facial expression, heavy sighs, or aggressive gestures (ie, finger pointing, clenched fist), any of which can affect your information processing.

When you communicate with patients, be poised and confident, with a positive demeanor. Keep in mind that any information you fail to obtain could be the information you need to treat the patient.

Encouraging Dialogue You will make patient care decisions based on the answers to your questions, combined with data from your diagnostics. Certain approaches and conversation techniques can improve the volume and quality of information you obtain during the patient interview. These techniques are summarized in **TABLE 11-4** and discussed further in Chapter 5, *Communications*.

Avoiding Medical Terminology Remember to speak in layperson's terms, not in the language of medicine. Patients with no background in medicine will generally use nonmedical terms to answer your assessment questions. Do not try to impress patients with medical terminology. Simple phrases will be much more readily understood by patients, especially those with developmental challenges and those whose primary language is different from yours. On the one hand, asking someone, "Do you think you're having an attack of unstable angina?" may get you little more than a blank stare in return. On the other hand, asking, "Are you having chest pain?" may get you just the information you need to proceed with patient care.

Match your terminology to the patient's level of knowledge and understanding. While a patient who is an ED nurse or a retired surgeon will understand medical terminology, a patient who speaks little English may need focused and straightforward communication.

Documentation and Communication

As you move through your assessment, use open-ended questions whenever you can. If possible, avoid asking questions that can be answered only with a "yes or no," but ask the patient a closed-ended question if that is what the situation requires. Avoid leading questions, which are phrased in a way that suggests your opinion, rather than encouraging the patient to give an answer based on their observations. Examples of leading questions are "Do you think this is a cardiac emergency?" or "Is the pain in your chest a dull ache? Does it radiate behind your sternum and into your jaw?" You do not want to put words into patients' mouths or ideas into their heads. Either give them a choice of answers to choose from or simply ask them to describe in their own words how they feel. Many patients, particularly older adults, are eager to please and will give the answer they think the interviewer wants to hear. Asking leading questions may lead to the wrong diagnosis and hinder patient care.

Dealing With Sensitive Topics

The **social history** is not typically gathered in the prehospital arena. However, it provides valuable information regarding the patient's overall health

TABLE 11-4 Communication Techniques

Technique	Meaning	Examples
Facilitation	Encourage your patient to feel open to give you any information you need.	Pay attention. Make eye contact. Repeat key information from the patient's answers. Nod your head. Use phrases such as: "That's helpful." "Anything else you can think of?" "Please go on."
Reflection	Pause to consider something significant your patient has told you.	Patient: "I couldn't catch my breath." You: "That's very helpful. Hold on a second, and let me think about that for a moment."
Clarification	Ask for more information when some aspect of the patient history is vague or unclear to you.	You: "What's going on today, Mrs. Hendrickson?" Patient: "Oh, I don't know. I'm just . . . well, I'm just not feeling like myself." You: "I'm sorry. Could you try to be a little more specific? If you could give me some details, it'll help me figure out what's going on with you today." Patient: "I'm always full of energy first thing in the morning, but I'm so weak right now that I couldn't even take Princess outside."
Confrontation	Make your patient aware that you perceive an inconsistency between their behavior (or the information they are giving you) and the actual scene or your exam/diagnostic findings.	Use a direct approach. For example, with a patient who has chronic depression, ask whether they are contemplating suicide and, if so, if they have a plan. Remain professional and nonjudgmental, but direct.
Interpretation	Infer the cause of the patient's distress, then asking the patient if you are right.	Maintain a diplomatic approach. Use the phrase: "So, if I understand you correctly . . ."

status and helps to identify risk factors for various disease processes. Examples of social history components include tobacco use, alcohol and drug use, sexual behavior, diet, travel history, housing environment, and occupation.

Obtaining a History of Alcohol and Drug Misuse According to the National Highway and Traffic Safety Administration (NHTSA), in 2016 there were 10,497 fatalities in motor vehicle traffic crashes involving a driver with a known blood alcohol content (BAC) of 0.08 g/dL or higher.[12] This number represents 28% of total traffic fatalities for that year in the United States.

Alcohol can mask any number of signs and symptoms, including pain. When a patient who experienced a significant traumatic event denies neck or back pain, and you smell what you believe to be alcohol on the patient's breath, or if the patient's behavior raises your suspicion of alcohol or drug use, perform manual stabilization of the neck.

The patient may offer an unreliable history of pain, alcohol consumption, or drug use. People who misuse drugs or alcohol routinely understate the amount if asked how much they have consumed. Experienced paramedics say the typical answer to how many drinks a person has had is "a couple" even when the person's behavior and the physical signs indicate the person has had many more. People who regularly misuse drugs or alcohol become adept at hiding the signs and symptoms from their friends, family, and workplace associates, and at denying there is a problem. Such denial can go on for years.

With intoxication also comes a decrease in patience; as the patient tries to explain things to you, their hostility or anger can escalate faster than if they were not intoxicated. A common scenario involving this type of behavior occurs at minor MVCs, when an intoxicated driver wants to get back into their vehicle and continue driving. The patient's behavior can become explosive. In such cases, do not aggravate the patient. Your ability to be patient and diplomatic is paramount in such dangerous situations. Dealing with intoxicated people can be frustrating for you and can stand in the way of your best efforts to care for the health of your patients; however, remain objective and nonjudgmental. Remember, you are there to help.

Words of Wisdom

A patient may be unable to provide an accurate history for various reasons (eg, altered mental status [AMS], intoxication). A patient's information may also not be reliable because the patient cannot remember, does not trust the provider, or is not motivated to assist the provider. Judge the reliability of your source of information at the end of your evaluation, not at the beginning. If you determine the reliability of the information at the beginning, then you may not accurately listen to the history and may miss vital information.

Alcohol is a legal drug. Marijuana is now also legal in many states. If a patient is using other substances to "get high," either the substances themselves or how they are used (ie, huffing paint fumes) is most likely illegal. The fear of punishment might lead patients to deny use. Let the patient know you are a medical provider, and anything they tell you will be kept in confidence to the extent the law allows. Do your best to win your patient's trust because you need accurate information to provide proper treatment.

Keep your best professional attitude as you work with patients you suspect of having used drugs or alcohol. Never judge your patients by their appearance or behavior. An unkempt homeless person might be in desperate need of assessment and immediate care for head trauma or hypoglycemia, rather than for alcoholism. Remember, no one calls EMS to be judged!

Taking a Sexual History The social history may include information regarding sexual behavior. Discussing sexual activity is an uncomfortable topic, even for seasoned paramedics. Use caution and tact as you ascertain this information; few patient encounters require a detailed sexual history. However, for some patients, obtaining a sexual history is essential. For instance, a woman in her 20s with left lower quadrant pain and a missed menstrual cycle could have an ectopic pregnancy, a potentially life-threatening emergency. A sexual history of this patient will be an important aspect of the overall patient assessment. Interview the patient in a setting that is as private as possible. Remember, patients of all ages are hesitant to share private or embarrassing information. Ensure your patients feel so secure with you they will give you the information you need.

Special Populations

Some preteens may be confused when asked about their sexual activities. Be direct and avoid using questions like "Are you sexually active?" Some young people may think "active" means "often."

Several factors may influence patients to be less than forthcoming about their sexual history. Having a religious upbringing, wanting to conform with cultural or societal mores, and having engaged in sexual practices outside the "perceived mainstream" may inhibit a patient from giving an accurate sexual history. You may need to ask patients if they have ever been tested for human immunodeficiency virus (HIV), acquired immunodeficiency syndrome (AIDS), or hepatitis, or in some cases, if the patient has male or female genitalia. Do not interject any opinions or biases about presentation, appearance, or behavior. Their lives are not your lives, just as your lives are not theirs. Today, more patients are open about being transgender.

Domestic Violence and Sexual Assault or Rape

As a paramedic, you are required to report a case if you have reason to suspect physical abuse or domestic violence. Although it would be inappropriate for you to accuse someone of abuse at the scene, never hesitate to call for law enforcement personnel if you have reason to believe abuse has occurred. Police can help stabilize the scene, provide another set of professional eyes, and, if necessary, take someone into custody.

> **Words of Wisdom**
>
> If you find yourself suddenly in a dangerous position and your partner is unaware of it, use a predetermined code word to alert them. For example, one inconspicuous code is to use the name of something in your emergency vehicle: "Could you get the drug box?" Your partner should know that this code means there is danger and that they should summon law enforcement personnel.

Some clues may lead you to suspect domestic violence. Injuries inconsistent with the information you are being given are common in such cases, as are multiple injuries in various stages of healing. Unspoken messages may be given by the family's behavior. You may notice the fearful posture of the woman at the kitchen table as her husband or significant other stands over her and answers your questions for her. If an injured family member does not give you information but waits for someone else to speak up, that may be a clue that the injured family member is being repressed. You can suggest that the significant other, who is doing all the talking, go to the ambulance to help with the stretcher. The moment the door shuts, you may receive valuable information, such as "My husband is beating me, and I'm scared to death. You have got to get me out of here before he kills me or one of our kids." *Immediately* request law enforcement personnel if anything resembling this situation occurs.

Emergency scenes involving domestic violence are some of the most dangerous for EMS and law enforcement personnel alike. Do not even think of handling them without law enforcement personnel on hand.

In sexual assault or rape cases, handle all clothing per local protocol, and bag it with any other evidence (use paper bags rather than plastic). Sexual assault and rape have devastating psychological effects. Be supportive, caring, and nonjudgmental during your care. Ideally, have an EMS provider of the same sex care for the person who has been assaulted.

Handling Physical Attraction to Patients

It is not unusual for clinicians and patients to be attracted to each other. Although these feelings are normal, it is *never* appropriate for a clinician to act on them. If a patient becomes seductive or makes sexual advances, politely but firmly explain that your relationship is professional rather than personal. Should this occur, try to keep your partner, a member of law enforcement, or a family member in the room with you at all times to witness any events that occur, and as a support person to help the patient recognize that their behavior is inappropriate. Make certain that you do not cross the line that separates personal from professional behavior, and do not allow the patient to cross that line either.

Ensuring Confidentiality

As a paramedic, you have a duty to maintain the confidentiality of the patient's information; this topic is discussed in more detail in Chapter 4, *Medical, Legal, and Ethical Issues*. The Health Insurance Portability and Accountability Act (HIPAA) and state laws govern the disclosure of patient information. Be familiar with the relevant laws. Also, show the patient that you respect the confidentiality of their medical information to help build rapport and contribute to a favorable overall patient care experience.

Protecting the Patient's Privacy

Interview patients in a private setting. Most people do not want to admit to having bad habits, such as smoking or drug/alcohol misuse. If a patient seems reluctant to divulge such information, perhaps out of fear of prosecution, you must be persistent enough to obtain it. Do not hesitate to ask nonessential personnel to leave the room or at least to step back, because you will frequently find yourself asking patients personal or intimate questions to elicit necessary information. If the setting makes a patient feel threatened or uncomfortable, they may choose not to answer your questions, or may answer inaccurately. Privacy is usually readily available in your office (the ambulance) should you need to move the patient to get a clearer medical history. Ensuring the patient's privacy, confidentiality, and comfort level goes a long way toward establishing positive patient rapport and encouraging more honest, open communication.

Gathering Information From Third Parties

Some patients might not be able to give you any or much information, in which case you may have to turn to their family and friends for assistance. It is important to document the sources of such information in your record. Although you need the information to help the patient, be aware that the further you go from the primary source, the greater the chance the information will contain inaccuracies. As when working with interpreters, family and friends often function as filters for information. They may be able to describe the patient's chief complaint, history of the present illness, past medical history, and possibly current health status.

> **Words of Wisdom**
>
> Patients' medications, their living conditions, and their physician's name can often give clues about their medical history. For example, insulin means the patient has diabetes, and an oxygen tank and nebulizer in their home probably denotes chronic obstructive pulmonary disease (COPD). The name of a specialist physician, such as an oncologist or a psychiatrist, may indicate the patient is being treated for cancer or mental illness, respectively.

Remember, you cannot reveal medical information about your patients to their family, so forming your questions will be difficult. However, obtaining information about your patient is critical, so work with people who can help your patients.

Law enforcement personnel and bystanders can also be valuable sources of information. Never forget that the best source of information is your patient. Answers provided by others may be less accurate, and therefore less helpful.

If emergency medical responders are already on scene, find out what information they have already obtained and the results of any care they provided, such as whether any bleeding has been controlled or oxygen administered. Ask if the patient's medications have been obtained (prescriptions, over-the-counter [OTC] medications, recreational drugs, and supplements). Gather this information to save time and avoid asking the same questions again.

Many day-to-day patient contacts in EMS are routine transfers from assisted living or extended care facilities to the hospital and back. Take a few moments to review the transfer paperwork. Learn the patient's medical history so you will be prepared to provide care should your planned routine transfer take an unexpected turn.

Keep in mind the importance of evaluating your sources of information for reliability. Although medical records in a transfer packet from an extended care or other health care facility should be assumed to be reasonably accurate, the reliability of individual caregivers' documentation inevitably varies. You are ultimately responsible for patient care decisions, so ensure you work with information that is as accurate as possible.

Cultural Competence

To communicate effectively, you must strive to understand inherent differences among all people. Only then can you adjust your efforts to accommodate and overcome cultural barriers.

> **Street Smarts**
>
> The most common communication barriers are those related to race, ethnicity, age, sex, language, education, religion, geography, and economic status. The collection of all these characteristics can be termed "culture." However, culture and ethnicity are *not* the same thing, although a person's culture may be affected by their ethnicity.

You cannot treat your patients effectively if you use your own culture as your only reference. EMS personnel cannot impose their own morality on their patients. Take time to understand other cultures, especially the cultures prevalent in your service area. This knowledge is essential and helps you communicate effectively when treating patients who have different cultural backgrounds than yours. Culture has an effect on our modern society in many ways. Cultural beliefs can affect many medical decisions and treatment plans. For example, some cultures believe evil spirits may cause illness. When treating a patient who believes an evil spirit caused an illness, do not dismiss this belief and fear. Be compassionate. Your approach will ensure communication is kept open to maintain continuity of care.

Street Smarts

There is a fine line between cultural competence and stereotyping. Cultural awareness involves sensitivity to the possibility that the other person's beliefs, values, and experiences differ from your own. This sensitivity is a starting place toward recognizing differences between yourself and the other person; it is *not* an assumption that such differences exist. Assumptions are the basis of stereotyping, which is a conclusion drawn about another person based on incomplete, typically superficial information. While cultural competence is a key step toward more fully understanding your patient, which will allow you to provide more effective and compassionate care, stereotyping is a dangerous mental shortcut that may lead you to make incorrect assumptions about your patient and thereby deliver inappropriate care.

It is important to note that efforts toward cultural competence, such as intercultural training, must be done carefully and in a manner that does not inadvertently reify cultural stereotypes.[13]

Dietary practices and family relationships must also be considered during patient care. For example, in some cultures, people may eat certain foods that may not be healthy, making them more susceptible to diabetes and heart disease. When you have the opportunity, making recommendations about healthy eating choices can improve the entire family's health.

In cultures with an identified leader in the household who makes most decisions regarding diet and medical care, it is important to establish a good relationship with that person to help facilitate patient care.

With regard to health care, certain cultures and religions do not believe in administering vaccinations and medications for disease prevention and treatment. Some of these groups object to the transfusion of blood products, no matter how serious the illness. For this reason, always gain consent before administering any medication to a patient. Remember, as long as the patient is a mentally competent adult, they may refuse treatment of any kind; however, if the patient is a child, the parents do not have the right to deny lifesaving interventions on cultural or religious grounds. If in doubt, consult medical control.

A person's economic status may relate to their overall physical health. People with low incomes have fewer financial resources to maintain good health. You must provide the best possible care for all patients regardless of income or ability to pay.

Classes and seminars are available that focus on handling cultural differences. What do all of these classes and seminars actually teach? In a word, respect. You may not get everything right when you encounter a person from another culture, but your communication efforts must reflect your respect, which makes a positive impression. Remember that manners are important. Use phrases such as "Yes, sir," "No, ma'am," "Thank you," "Please," "Would you," "Could you," and "May I." If at any time you notice that the patient seems to have become embarrassed or uncomfortable, adjust your approach, if possible, to help maintain the patient's dignity.

Facilitating Cross-Cultural Communication

The world is home to many groups of people who do not speak the primary language of the countries in which they live. But when they are sick, you want to provide the best possible care for all your patients **FIGURE 11-10**.

Documentation and Communication

Medical terms and jargon often do not translate well, such as "ECG leads," "CAT scan," "JAWS," and "stool."

The first person to look to for help is an interpreter: someone who speaks both your language and the patient's language. (If there are large groups of people who speak one language in your service

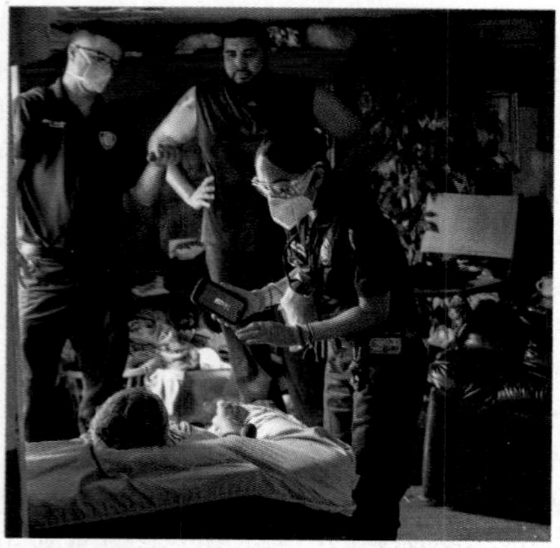

FIGURE 11-10 You will work with people of other cultures, which may require using an interpreter.

area, it would be wise to learn how to ask for an interpreter in that other language.) However, using an interpreter comes with inherent risks because, ultimately, an interpreter acts as a filter. How a question is phrased can make a world of difference; therefore, it is best to ask closed-ended questions that yield short answers. For example, you might ask, "Are you having trouble breathing?" The tradeoff is that these types of questions do not yield a large amount of information; however, if you ask thoughtful questions and wait for the patient's reply, you will be able to extract the information you need to provide care. Last, take a moment to remind the interpreter that they should not share this private information about the patient with anyone else.

Often, the only person available to interpret will be the patient's child, as children absorb a new language quickly in their schools. However, if you can find someone older and not so intimately attached to the patient, then they would be a better choice for obtaining a good patient history. Keep your questions as straightforward as possible, and do your best not to scare a child. Your agency may use video remote interpreting, a service that uses an electronic device, such as a computer tablet, to quickly connect providers with an interpreter via both audio and video. The video component enables greater accuracy when communicating with a non-English speaker and also enables communication with individuals who are deaf or hard of hearing.[14]

Maintaining patient confidentiality should be considered when selecting an appropriate interpreter. For this reason, using a certified medical interpreter is preferred. Certified interpreters are trained to understand medical terminology and are also aware of patient confidentiality laws. Confidentiality may become a potential problem when choosing a family member or a bystander to interpret. The patient may not want certain medical information divulged through an interpreter. Therefore, every attempt should be made to find a qualified medical interpreter to ensure the patient's rights are not violated. Realistically, finding a medical interpreter in the field may not be practical, but it should be considered.

Do not let a few broken words of yours be a substitute for an interpreter's services. Also, simply speaking louder during your questioning will not overcome a language barrier.

Finally, remember that manners, hand gestures, and body language have different meanings in different cultures. Develop a communication style free of mannerisms or gestures that could be misinterpreted or have culture-specific meanings.

Special Challenges in History Taking

Dealing With Talkative or Reserved Patients

Another challenge you are likely to face is patients who talk too much or not enough. You will need to help some patients filter the information they offer. For example, they may want to tell you about every cold and splinter they have ever had. Some people learn to talk endlessly to socialize, but you must consider possible clinical reasons for the chattiness. Recovering from a fight-or-flight situation, consuming a triple espresso 15 minutes ago, or taking an illegal drug (eg, cocaine, crack, or methamphetamine) might be the reason.

Whatever the cause, the first requirement in caring for a talkative patient is, once again, to remain patient. Give the patient free rein for several minutes. When patients are given free rein, most will talk for less than 2 minutes. During the first couple of minutes, you will typically gain most of the valuable information you will need. Try not to interrupt them unless it is necessary to clarify something that was said. If the patient continues to talk for longer, or if what they are saying is simply incomprehensible, then try interrupting to clarify a piece of information. This allows you to quickly summarize what you have just heard.

Other patients will offer very little information or take you so literally that it may obscure your assessment. For example, if you ask a patient, "Do you have any heart problems," such a person might say, "No." However, when you open this patient's shirt, you find a scar running down the middle of the chest from open-heart surgery. You reply, "I thought you said you didn't have any heart problems." The patient replies: "I don't have any heart problems. I did a few years ago, but they fixed the damaged valve." With reserved patients, it is essential to ask open-ended questions since they are unlikely to volunteer additional information.

Words of Wisdom

A common cause of anxiety is hypoxia (low oxygen levels in the blood). The patient may be sweaty and restless and become agitated easily. Hypoxia is often misinterpreted as anxiety or panic.

Handling Patients With Anxiety

Although you may not want to believe it, you may be a cause for many of your patients being overly anxious. No matter how much the public loves to watch emergencies on television, it is frightening to see an ambulance, fire engine, or law enforcement vehicle pull up and stop in front of your house. Expect patients to be somewhat anxious initially, but then to calm down shortly after your arrival. If not, consider other possibilities. For example, high anxiety is an early sign of physiologic shock, which must be treated immediately. Alternatively, a patient could be hiding something, such as physical abuse or illegal drug use.

Talking to Patients With Depression Unlike most other health care providers, paramedics see people when an illness or traumatic event just occurred. As a result, their patients are uniquely vulnerable and uniquely demanding. Try your best to develop empathy for all of your patients.

If a patient doesn't have an apparent medical condition, consider the possibility that they might be depressed and that a mental health condition referral might be needed. Depression is a common reason for seeking medical attention. For example, if a patient seems sad, restless, and irritable; has sleep or eating disruptions; says they have low energy; or has pain for which you cannot find a source, consider that your patient might be depressed.

There are two basic types of depression: situational and chronic. Situational depression describes a normal reaction to a stressful event, such as a job loss, divorce, or death of a loved one. Chronic depression is ongoing and has no apparent cause.

Most people with situational depression can eventually accept what has happened and begin to get on with their lives. Others develop chronic depression. Either form of depression can lead to harmful behavior, including suicide. Ask about your patient's feelings to assess suicide risk. If the patient admits to having had thoughts about taking their own life, follow your protocol to ensure this patient is connected to a mental health professional.

Earlier chapters discussed ways of becoming knowledgeable about the various resources that may help your patients.

Dealing Safely With Anger and Hostility

Frequently, you will find yourself the target of patients' and family members' frustrations, which may manifest as anger or hostility. Such reactions to unfairness and harsh realities are normal. Do not take these situations personally; instead, take them professionally.

Special Populations

Most patients are older than the paramedics taking care of them. They may feel threatened by strange "youngsters" telling them what is best for them. Listen and be respectful to these older patients. Without talking down to them or becoming impatient, explain what you are doing and why. Patients may not know what is in their best interest, and a calm, courteous explanation may put them at ease.

A valuable coping skill is not to get angry yourself. When you are in control of your anger, you can work to calm the situation. Be attentive to changes in body language, such as threatening gestures or an escalating volume of conversation or, worse yet, having a heated dialog melt down into an outright yelling match. When people are angry or hostile, the worst thing you can do is to get angry yourself.

Establishing a safe and secure scene is your first order of business on any call. If you cannot calm the patient or family members, it is time to call for law enforcement personnel. If someone is hostile, you might need to tell the person directly that if they continue to shout, you won't feel safe enough to provide care and will have to seek law enforcement assistance before you can resume. However, if the patient or the family members are already angry, then telling them police are on the way will not suddenly make them happy. In the worst-case scenario, you may have to withdraw to the safety of your emergency vehicle and wait for law enforcement personnel to arrive.

If the hostile person suddenly leaves the room, especially in the middle of the conversation, then you or your partner should consider that a threat, as the person may be going to obtain a weapon and potentially come back and shoot you, your partner, and maybe the patient. If law enforcement has not yet arrived, then it may be best to retreat to a safe location until they arrive.

Clarifying a Confusing History or Unusual Behavior

Paramedics sometimes find that the patient's history given at the scene is different from the history the patient gives to a physician in the hospital ED. Sometimes, information is so different that it seems as if this is an entirely different patient. Patients may be too frightened or embarrassed to give particular information to a paramedic, but they will give a physician vital information by telephone.

The human brain is an impressive organ, but it may malfunction for many reasons. Confusing behavior is often related to a lack of glucose or oxygen, two fuels that are essential for brain function, although it cannot store either of them. Many other possibilities could account for a patient's confusing behavior, such as a toxic environment, a cerebrovascular accident (stroke), or a transient ischemic attack (TIA). Also, consider the possibility of mental illness or drug-induced delirium. In addition, organic causes such as Alzheimer disease, other forms of dementia, or a brain tumor can contribute to discrepancies.

Treating Patients With Sensory or Developmental Challenges

Limited Education or Intellectual Challenges

Never, ever presume you will not be able to obtain a history directly from the patient. Some patients will not know much about the health care system or its specialized vocabulary. Other patients will be developmentally challenged. Assume you can get at least some worthwhile history from all patients. Assume it is your job to keep asking questions differently until you get the answers you need.

> **Words of Wisdom**
>
> Never, never, never assume it is impossible to talk to a patient until you have tried.

With a skillful question-and-answer approach (and patience), you can frequently obtain adequate information from patients with limited education or intellectual capabilities. However, be alert for omissions or partial answers to your questions. These patients may not know or be able to recall the information you are requesting. For patients with severe mental challenges, you may need to get information from family members, friends, or another caregiver.

Hearing Loss, Low Vision, or Blindness Another interesting challenge relates to working with patients with hearing or vision loss. Hearing loss can range from a slight loss to total deafness. For patients with only minimal loss, such as older people, speaking slowly and slightly louder may be all that is necessary. For people with more severe hearing loss, you may want to let them wear your stethoscope as you hold the bell and speak to them. If you do this, clean the earpieces before you offer them to the patient and put them back on.

> **Words of Wisdom**
>
> After completing a paramedic program, two of the best investments in continuing education you can make for your future are learning conversational Spanish and learning sign language.

Many patients with varying degrees of low vision are self-sufficient and live independently. When interacting with a patient who is blind or has low vision, first and foremost announce yourself, giving the patient your identity and your reason for being there. If you pull up a chair to sit next to a patient with low vision or blindness, remember to put it back exactly where you found it; the same is true if furniture has to be moved to provide access or egress. People who are blind have arranged their living environments in the way they want it so that they can get around with remarkable ease. Ensure you leave things the way you found them.

Once you move the patient to the ambulance, they are in a foreign environment and require assistance from EMS personnel for transport and an orderly transition into the ED. Inform the person what you are doing and the location of the transport vehicle at all times (eg, "We'll be at the hospital in about 10 minutes" or "We're arriving at the hospital, and we will be wheeling you off the ambulance and into the ED in just a minute").

Managing Age-Related Considerations

Pediatric Patients

Most of the pediatric problems encountered in the field are respiratory or fluid related. Just a day or two of vomiting or diarrhea can put a small child at high risk. In a trauma scenario, pediatric patients are top-heavy, so they are more likely to fall and strike their heads, especially in vehicle-versus-pedestrian incidents. A full discussion of pediatric assessment appears in Chapter 44, *Pediatric Emergencies*. The initial approach to any pediatric patient should be similar to that for an adult, with a few exceptions. Always begin with a scene size-up; forming a general impression; and assessing and treating life-threatening conditions affecting airway, breathing, or circulation. However, there are differences in the overall interaction you will have with the pediatric patient and their parents.

Obtaining an accurate **history of the present illness**, which is a narrative detail of the symptoms that the patient is experiencing, can be complex in the pediatric population. Whereas every effort should be made to include the child in the history-taking process, the most accurate and complete history will come from a parent or a responsible caregiver. Typically, parents are familiar with their children's habits and demeanor and know when something is wrong. Therefore, listen when a parent shows concern and tells you their child is not acting appropriately.

Many times parents call for EMS out of fear for the welfare of their child. It is vital for you as the health care provider to understand the parents'

YOU are the Paramedic

PART 3

You immediately determine that the patient has the potential to deteriorate quickly. Your partner pulls the stretcher out of the ambulance with the help of a police officer. Meanwhile, you determine that the patient is responsive and disoriented. You cut off the patient's shirt and find an approximate 1-inch (2.5-cm) penetration on the left side of the chest, just inferior to the center of the clavicle. The wound has stopped bleeding. You apply a three-sided occlusive dressing. The patient is breathing rapidly and appears to be very restless.

Recording Time: 5 Minutes	
Respiration	28 breaths/min, shallow
Pulse	122 beats/min, weak
Skin	Cool, paler than baseline color, clammy
Blood pressure	90/64 mm Hg
Oxygen saturation (Spo_2)	93% on room air
Pupils	Pupils Equal, Round, and Reactive to Light and Accommodation (PERRLA)

5. On the basis of your assessment of ABCDE, what is your first priority in the care of this patient?

6. Can you determine the transport priority of this patient at this point?

fears and to continue to ascertain and investigate those concerns in more detail. For instance, a febrile seizure in a pediatric patient is a fairly common entity encountered by EMS personnel and a relatively benign condition; however, it can be a frightening, emotionally traumatic event for a new parent. Parents want to know what is wrong with their child and will typically seek out Internet sources for answers. The problem with this approach is that it leaves a great deal to the imagination, and online sources are not always credible. Therefore, a parent of a child experiencing a febrile seizure is probably not just thinking about the immediate event, but is also worried about all possible causes of a seizure (ie, bleeding into the brain, a brain tumor, or cancer), when in reality it may be a benign condition. Be aware of these fears and consider them when caring for parents or other legal guardians.

As you obtain information from a parent or caregiver, pay attention to the relationship between this person and the child. Typically, sick children cling to the parent or caregiver and are reluctant to allow a paramedic to examine them or remove them from the parent's arms. However, a child who readily allows you to remove them from the parent for examination should raise your concern that the child may be seriously ill and should also bring into consideration the possibility of neglect and/or abuse.

In neonates and infants, a maternal health history is important. Ask about the mother's health status during pregnancy; the type of prenatal care provided; use of medications, hormones, and vitamins; and alcohol or drug use during pregnancy. A birth history should also be obtained: Find out the duration of pregnancy, birth location, labor conditions, any delivery complications, whether it was a vaginal or cesarean delivery, condition of the infant at birth, and birth weight. Ask about maternal gestational history and any other pregnancies or children, including stillbirths and any deceased children.

The first month following birth, otherwise known as the neonatal period, is an important part of the pediatric history. Questions should be asked about congenital anomalies, feeding problems, the presence of jaundice, evidence of any illness, and developmental landmarks.

Around age 3 to 5 years, children can provide a history of the current problem. Once in school, the focus of questioning should change based on the child's age. Asking about the child's school performance helps determine whether there are any developmental challenges or intellectual disabilities. Questioning should also focus on the child's dentition, growth, sexual development, illnesses, and immunizations.

If the child is an adolescent, focus more on them than on the parent when obtaining a history. Adolescents struggle for independence and want to be in charge of their bodies. Gather your history from the adolescent to help establish trust and a good rapport. As the line of questioning for an adolescent becomes more private, consider interviewing the patient in a more private location, in the presence of your partner. Focus your questioning on risk-taking behaviors, self-esteem issues, rebelliousness, drug and alcohol use, and sexual activity. Some patients may be reluctant to discuss these issues with you, which is why establishing trust and rapport is so important.

In addition to gathering information about the child, ensure you gather an accurate family medical and recent travel history. More information on the relevance of recent travel history is found in Chapter 27, *Infectious Diseases*.

A review of body systems should also be included in the pediatric history. While every system should be covered, pay special attention to any skin **lesions** (localized areas of skin that do not resemble the area surrounding it); any history of otitis media (inner ear infections); any snoring, mouth breathing, and environmental allergies; and any dental problems.

Geriatric Patients

Geriatric patients can pose different challenges for paramedics. This patient population is increasing and frequently represents the primary customers for EMS. This population has a variety of medical and traumatic conditions not seen in other patients.

With aging often comes decreased sensorium, so complaints of pain are less frequent. Diabetes will add problems of peripheral neuropathy, further diminishing pain sensitivity, as well as eyesight and kidney diseases. Balance and equilibrium problems increase the likelihood of falls. Many older patients are on blood thinners as part of an atrial fibrillation treatment regimen. Even a minor fall may be deadly if blood cannot clot in a timely fashion.

Even if it does, a fall can be lethal for an older adult, as evidenced by the data (see Chapter 45, *Geriatric Emergencies*).

An older adult may have difficulty seeing you or hearing your questions during the patient assessment. If the patient wears eyeglasses or a hearing aid, ensure these aids are available during the interview. You may need to speak more slowly and loudly when treating older patients; however, do not assume that all older adults have difficulty hearing. In addition, it may be helpful to face the patient when asking questions, in case the patient is adept at lip reading to help with communication. This may require removing your mask to speak to the patient. Accommodating these sensory losses can improve the amount and quality of information gathered during the patient assessment.

Words of Wisdom

Any patient taking five or more drugs likely has some form of drug interaction.

Medication compliance is a challenge for any patient, but much more so for older adults. They tend to have multiple chronic medical conditions that can complicate the history-taking process. Multiple chief complaints can make it difficult to distinguish between acute and chronic complaints. For example, suppose a 68-year-old man tells you, "I'm really weak, and it feels like there are butterflies in my chest." First, determine whether these symptoms are related. If you believe they are related, you must identify the origin of the problem to provide appropriate care. In this case, you may want to ask, "Have you had this problem before?" to see if the patient has had problems in the past with tachycardia and weakness.

You also need to prioritize multiple complaints. For example, suppose the patient complains of being dizzy and having pain in her left ankle. You might then ask questions and further determine the two complaints are unrelated. Decide which condition is your priority.

In addition, older adult patients often take many prescription and OTC medications that may contribute to their various complaints, a phenomenon called *polypharmacy*, or that cause **iatrogenic** illnesses. An iatrogenic condition is one caused by medications or other medical treatment and can mask other illnesses that may need immediate medical attention.

Accidental overdoses and adverse drug reactions are common issues with older adults. Gather an accurate medication history, along with current dosages, to assist other health care providers with continued patient care.

Disease symptoms may become less dramatic in an older patient. As the body ages, responses to conditions like shock and pain are often dulled. This can complicate the assessment process because these patients do not always exhibit a "textbook" response to an illness. Their symptoms may be vague and nonspecific, especially in postmenopausal women with AMI. Maintain a high clinical index of suspicion when treating older adults, and always consider the worst-case scenario.

Consider including a functional assessment during the body systems review in the older adult with an apparent disability. This typically includes assessment of mobility at home and in the community, upper extremity function and limitations, and activities of daily living (ADLs). In addition, physicians will typically assess instrumental ADLs (IADLs) when examining older patients. This includes assessing tasks such as getting dressed, bathing, and cooking, and may even extend to areas such as financial management and shopping. Assist in this process by assessing some of these functions in the field; this evaluation should be part of your assessment of patients in both stable and unstable conditions, as time allows.

Responsive Medical Patients

For a responsive patient with a medical condition, you will usually form a working field impression based on information gathered during the history-taking process. The secondary assessment and any diagnostic tests you perform after obtaining the history will help you further pinpoint the problem.

Chief Complaint

Ensure the patient is as comfortable as possible before you start—warm or cool enough, privacy ensured—and that you have gained the patient's confidence and trust. Then ask your patient why they called for your help (chief complaint). The patient's chief complaint is the most serious thing concerning the patient. Ideally, the chief complaint should be recorded in the patient's own words. For example, if the patient says, "My ribs hurt," then you should write "My ribs hurt" in quotation marks as the chief complaint in your documentation. For patients who are unresponsive or otherwise unable to speak, writing their primary medical condition or simply "unresponsive" is generally considered acceptable.

In addition to the patient's name and chief complaint, ask about the *day of the week and location,* to determine if the patient is alert. Next, ask about *events* surrounding the current situation to elaborate on the chief complaint. Your EMS system may require you to collect additional identifying data, such as age, sex, address, and occupation. You will also want to know who called 9-1-1: Did the patient place the call for help, or did a friend, family member, or bystander make the call?

Look for items on the scene or in the home that may help you learn more about the patient's condition. Items such as pill containers and medical jewelry can provide invaluable insights into a patient's underlying conditions. Medical identification devices may take the form of a bracelet, necklace, or wallet card. Such an item is used to identify patients with a history of allergies, certain medical conditions (ie, diabetes, cardiac conditions, pacemaker placement, hypertension, and renal disease), and other conditions that may need to be addressed, such as the existence of an implantable cardioverter defibrillator (ICD).

With a responsive medical patient, some type of pain, discomfort, or body dysfunction ("I haven't had a bowel movement in 4 days") likely prompted the call for help. The complaint may be vague ("I just don't feel right today"). Vague complaints are common among older people. Such complaints challenge you to ask the right questions and be a patient listener as you work to obtain the information you need to make good care decisions **FIGURE 11-11**.

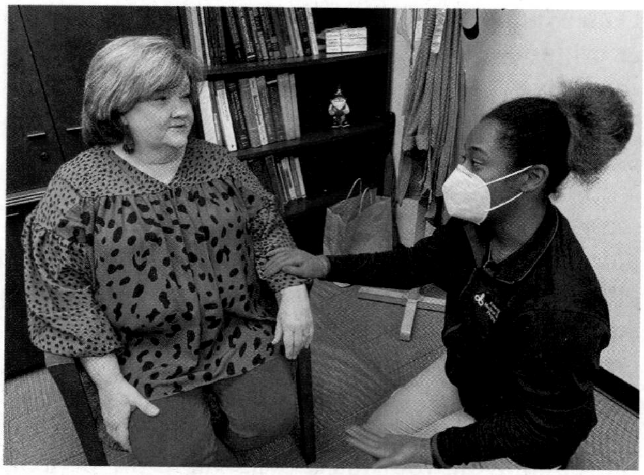

FIGURE 11-11 Be especially patient when obtaining information about a vague complaint.

Courtesy of Rhonda Hunt.

History of the Present Illness

After determining the chief complaint, obtain the history of the present illness. This information should provide you with a clear sequence and chronologic account of the patient's signs and symptoms—specifically, *what happened* and *when.* **Signs** are objective observations or measurements that you make, and **symptoms** are subjective information that the patient tells you.

Be sure to ask about the *region* or location of the pain, including the following questions:

- Where exactly does it hurt?
- Can you point to where it hurts with one finger; is it in a specific area?
- Does the pain stay right there, or does it move or radiate anywhere else?
- If your pain does move or radiate, where does it go?

The OPQRST mnemonic offers a helpful approach to analyzing a patient's chief complaint and obtaining a full, clear, chronologic account of the patient's symptoms. For example, when exploring a complaint of pain, you might ask the following questions:

- **Onset.** What were you doing when the pain started?
- **Provocation/Palliation.**
    - Did the pain start suddenly or come on gradually?
    - Does anything make the pain go away or feel better or worse?
- **Quality.** If you were trying to make me feel the way you do, what would you do to me to give me that same feeling?
- **Region/Radiation/Referral.**
    - Can you point to the place where it hurts?

- Does the pain stay there, or does it go somewhere else?

- **Severity.** On a scale of 0 to 10, with 0 being no pain and 10 being the worst pain you can imagine, how would you rank this pain?[15,16]
- **Time.** How long have you felt this way?

Documentation and Communication

Documenting the pain severity rating is essential. Also, note how distressed the patient appears: mildly, moderately, or severely distressed.

The SAMPLE mnemonic may also be useful in the interview process. It addresses the following issues: Signs and symptoms of current complaint; Allergies; Medications; Pertinent past medical history; Last oral intake; and Events leading up to current injury or illness.

The history of the present illness starts with one of the most open-ended of all medical questions: "What is going on today that made you call 9-1-1?" This or a similar question will get the conversation moving. If the patient's behavior is inappropriate, consider the possibility that it might be due to hypoxia; to a medical cause such as sepsis or stroke, low blood glucose level, or hypothermia; or to a behavioral emergency. Alternatively, the patient may have altered mentation secondary to drug or alcohol ingestion.

One of the more challenging aspects of the history-taking process is pulling together the patient's **current health status**, because it comprises many unrelated pieces of information. However, it often ties together some of the past medical history with the history of the present illness or current event, so it is unquestionably of value to the assessment process. In addition, the patient's current health status focuses on environmental and personal habits of the patient that may influence their general state of health.

Questions that are most helpful to obtain a useful history of the patient's current health status include the following:

- What prescription medicines are you taking? How much and how often? Patients can, and often do, confuse when and how to take their medications; if this is the case, you could be witnessing a drug reaction. As you gain experience as a paramedic, your familiarity with drugs and drugs' effects will give you an idea of the patient's illness. Medications will also give you a clue about mental health conditions or dementia without you needing to antagonize a reluctant patient.
- Do you take any OTC medications, such as aspirin, or supplements, such as herbs or vitamins?
- Are you allergic to anything? Can you describe the reaction you experienced?
- Do you drink beer, wine, or cocktails? How much? How often? If necessary, remind the patient that certain information is necessary to know for you to treat them appropriately.
- Do you smoke? Gather information about quantity of smoking, along with length of time. (This history is typically recorded in "pack years." For example, a patient who smokes one pack of cigarettes per day for 15 years is charted as having a 15 pack-year history. A patient who smokes one-half of a pack of cigarettes per day for 15 years is charted as having a 7.5 pack-year history.)
- Do you take any illicit drugs? (Assure the patient of confidentiality as you make such inquiries, to the extent that the law allows.)
- What did you have to eat yesterday and today?
- Ask about relevant screening tests. For example, for difficulty breathing, ask, "Have you had a chest x-ray lately?"
- Are your immunizations up to date? Have you had a flu shot or pneumococcal or COVID-19 vaccine? Ask about childhood immunizations, too.
- Have you been getting a good night's sleep? Look for maladaptive sleep patterns.
- Do you exercise? How much? How often?
- Ask about specific hazards (ie, cleaners, chemicals, or environmental hazards) that may be present at home or at a worksite, making the patient more vulnerable to injury or illness.
- Regarding safety measures, ask about the use of safety belts, protective eyewear, bicycle helmets, gun locks, medication lockboxes, and outlet covers (if small children are present in the home).
- Do you have a family history of any specific diseases? Conditions that should be evaluated in family members include alcoholism,

anemia, arthritis, cancer, diabetes, drug addiction, epilepsy, headaches, heart disease, hypertension, kidney disease, mental illness, stroke, and tuberculosis.

- Where do you live? What do you like to do at home? Is there anyone in your life whom you might be afraid of? (You might need to assess a difficult home situation, such as failure to thrive.)
- How do you spend your time during the day? The response to this question may help assess the patient's ability to function independently in society.
- Have you had any important experiences recently? Ask about any recent significant life events such as divorce, job changes, or moving to a new home. Even some positive experiences in life, such as weddings, can be stressful to patients.
- Do you have any religious beliefs that would prevent me from administering treatment? Ask about religious preference to ensure you respect the patient's belief systems.
- Are you an optimistic person? (It is essential to get your patient's overall outlook on life to assess for depression or other psychiatric conditions.)
- Have you traveled recently to any countries associated with infectious diseases?

Special Populations

In some cases, a patient's religious beliefs may be relevant, such as if those beliefs pertain directly to medical care. If your patient indicates such beliefs are important, this information should be passed along to ED staff.

Of course, you do not have to obtain every piece of information on this list for every patient. It takes time, practice, and a certain amount of common sense to know the right questions to ask each patient. Decide which of the listed items you want to explore and which you do not. For a sick patient with immediate life threats, you may not have time to explore any of them. For a patient in stable condition who does not appear to be in apparent distress, you may have time and decide to explore all relevant topics.

A brief family medical history helps to establish patterns and risk factors for diseases. If a 35-year-old man with chest pain tells you his father died of a heart attack at age 39, for instance, be concerned this patient could be experiencing a massive heart attack as well. Remember, not every aspect of the family history is necessarily important in the immediate emergent setting. Your goal is to collect information pertinent to the patient's current medical condition.

You may need to ask questions about the patient's occupation, living environment, and travel history to complete the social history. Occupation identification provides information about possible exposure to toxic substances and gives details regarding physical health. The environment in which the patient resides provides details regarding lifestyle and chronic exposures. A travel history may point to the possibility of certain illnesses that are uncommon in the United States. In that case, consider whether any of those illnesses put you at risk of contracting a communicable disease. A travel history is also useful when pulmonary embolism (PE) is suspected. People who have been on long flights are susceptible to developing blood clots from not having moved their lower extremities for extended periods. Anytime a patient presents with an unusual or puzzling illness, obtain a travel history.

Questions about the patient's diet are also part of the patient's social history. It is appropriate to ask about your patient's typical daily food intake, as well as the timing and quantity of food consumption. This information may help you narrow down the list of possible differential diagnoses. For example, patients who do not eat certain foods because of personal, cultural, or religious reasons may experience nutritional deficiencies that are reflected in their symptoms.

Past Medical History

The **past medical history** allows you to learn about any of the patient's pertinent or chronic underlying medical conditions. Some aspects of the past medical history may not seem important now, but obtaining a careful and thorough history will help paint a clear picture of the patient's overall health status. Not only might this help in your assessment, but it will also help maintain the overall continuity of care when other health care providers assume responsibility for the patient in the ED.

The past medical history is frequently linked to the patient's current condition. For example, people with diabetes who do not manage their blood glucose levels may have progressively worsening problems with peripheral circulation, eyesight, wound healing, or kidney function. Likewise, most patients with stable angina will eventually develop unstable angina; at some point, they may experience a heart attack.

The past medical history should include current medications and dosages. While this information may not seem important at the time, it may be quite helpful later. Not only should information about prescription medications be obtained, but any OTC medications, recreational drugs, and herbal/alternative medication therapies or dietary supplements should be identified as well. In addition, any allergies should be documented. This includes allergies to medications and allergies to other substances (eg, food, detergents, pet dander). As you record this information, ask the patient what their reaction is to each specific allergen. This information will be valuable later in the patient care process.

Childhood illnesses and immunizations should be assessed briefly if time allows. This will help you rule in or out various disease processes as you take a history and perform a secondary assessment.

Ask the patient to tell you about any illnesses or conditions for which they are currently being treated by a physician. This information will provide insights and details that may pertain to the current emergent medical condition. For example, suppose the patient reports chest pain. In that case, a past medical history of hypertension, hyperlipidemia, and diabetes is pertinent because each of those conditions is considered an independent risk factor for AMI. Ask the patient about past surgeries. A great way to approach this topic is if you notice a surgical scar in your primary survey, ask the patient how they got it. However, not all surgical scars are noticeable, and some procedures leave no scar. Therefore, ask each patient about past surgeries, including when they occurred.

A history describing past hospitalizations and any disabilities from previous illnesses will help you fine-tune your assessment. A history of hospitalization for COPD, for example, gives you clues as to how advanced or severe the patient's disease might be. A neurologic deficit from a previous traumatic event might obscure the physical exam findings in a patient with suspected stroke; therefore, it is important to ask about previous disabilities.

The patient's emotional affect, which is their expression of emotion or lack thereof, provides insights into the patient's overall mental health and helps you assess their mental status. For example, a patient who has just been involved in an MVC is likely to be upset. However, when a patient appears to have an emotional response that is not typical or appropriate for the current circumstances, consider the possibility of AMS. Ask about any mental health conditions the patient might be having and whether they have ever been hospitalized for a mental health condition. Although it is often difficult for patients and families to admit to mental health conditions, you may get an honest answer if you are matter-of-fact and dignified in asking the question.

As you inquire about past medical history, take time to explore how some of the patient's problems were solved (eg, "It took a couple of breathing treatments before I felt better" or "After my last asthma attack, I had to be intubated and was in the hospital on a ventilator for a week").

Equally important is the situation in which the patient presents with an illness they have never experienced. An acute presentation of a new illness or condition is best considered serious until proven otherwise.

Unresponsive Patients

You start at a disadvantage when you assess an unresponsive patient because your most reliable source of information cannot answer your questions. Owing to this serious limitation, history taking and secondary assessment of an unresponsive patient are much like a trauma assessment. You must rely on a thorough head-to-toe physical exam, plus normal diagnostic tools (pulse oximetry, capnography, cardiac monitor, BP, and glucometer) to acquire the information necessary for patient care (discussed later in the section Secondary Assessment of Unresponsive Patients).

Trauma Patients

As you move into history taking for a trauma patient, quickly revisit all information from the primary survey, including reconsidering the MOI. Collectively, these data may help you identify patients who must be transported quickly to a trauma center. Unresponsiveness can indicate serious injury, usually a traumatic brain injury, even if the MOI does not seem significant. Evidence of a high-energy impact should increase your suspicion for life-threatening injuries **FIGURE 11-12**:[17]

- Falls
  - Adults: greater than 20 feet (6 m; one story is equal to 10 feet, or 3 m)
  - Children: greater than 10 feet (3 m) or two or three times the height of the child
- High-risk MVC
  - Intrusion, including roof: greater than 12 inches (30 cm) into the occupant site; greater than 18 inches (46 cm) into any site
  - Ejection (partial or complete) from a motor vehicle
  - Death in the same passenger compartment
  - Vehicle telemetry data, available in many new vehicles, consistent with a high risk of injury
  - Vehicle versus pedestrian/bicyclist: thrown, run over, or with significant (greater than 20 mph) impact
- Motorcycle or all-terrain vehicle (ATV) crash greater than 20 mph

If the patient is an infant or a child, MOIs that would indicate a high-priority patient include the following **FIGURE 11-13**:

- Fall from more than 10 feet (3 m), or two to three times the child's height

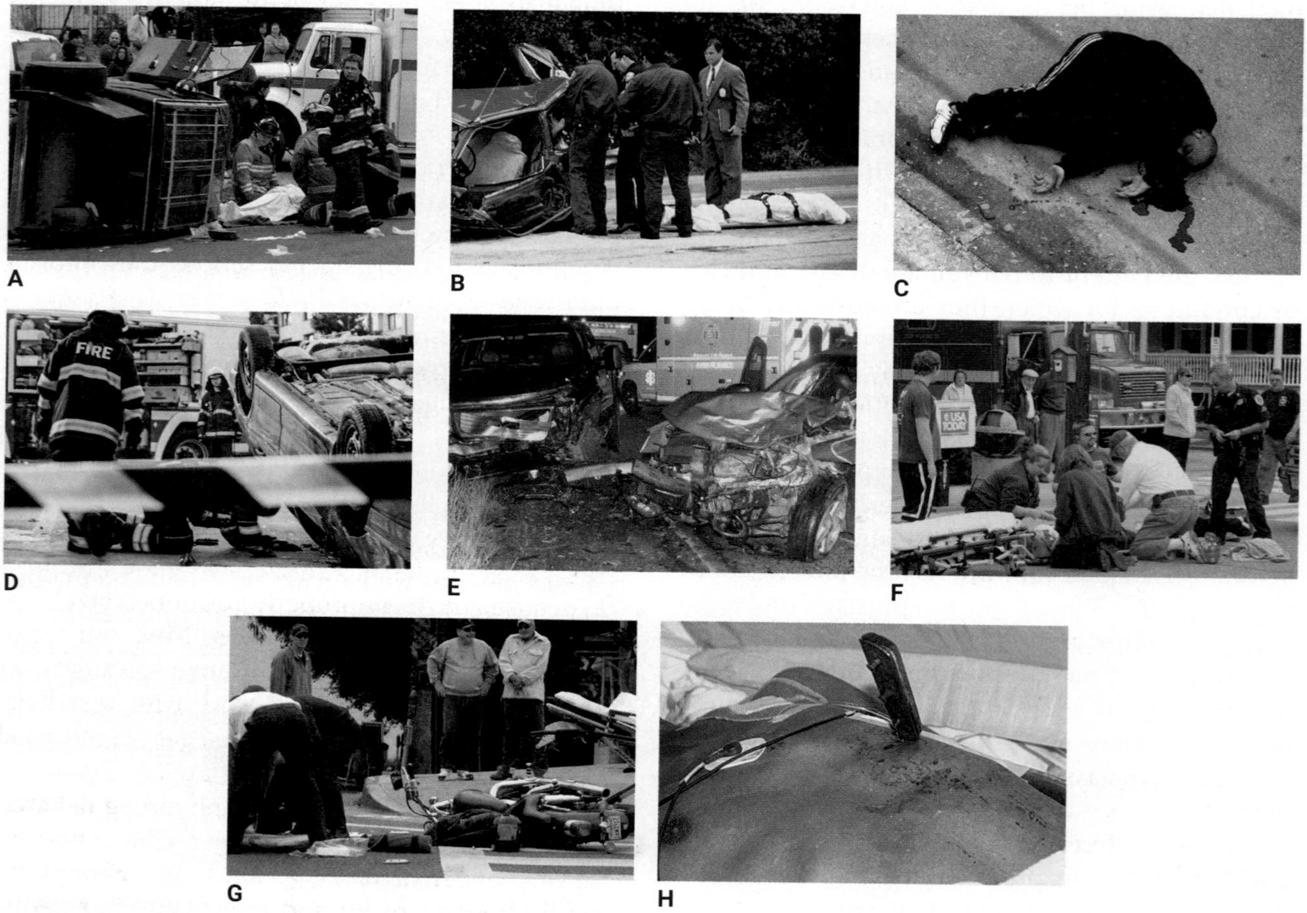

FIGURE 11-12 Significant mechanisms of injury. **A.** Ejection (partial or complete) from any motor vehicle (eg, car, motorcycle, all-terrain vehicle). **B.** Death of another patient in the same passenger compartment. **C.** Adult fall from more than 20 feet (6 m). **D.** Vehicle telemetry data consistent with high-risk injury. **E.** High-speed motor vehicle collision. **F.** Vehicle–pedestrian collision. **G.** Motorcycle crash greater than 20 mph. **H.** Penetrating injuries to head, neck, torso, or extremities.

A: © Enigma/Alamy Stock Photo; **B:** © Corbis/Getty Images; **C:** © Joseph Eid/AFP/Getty Images; **D:** © simonkr/E+/Getty Images; **E:** © Jack Dagley Photography/Shutterstock; **F:** © Larry St. Pierre/Shutterstock; **G:** © micheal ledray/Shutterstock; **H:** © Jones & Bartlett Learning.

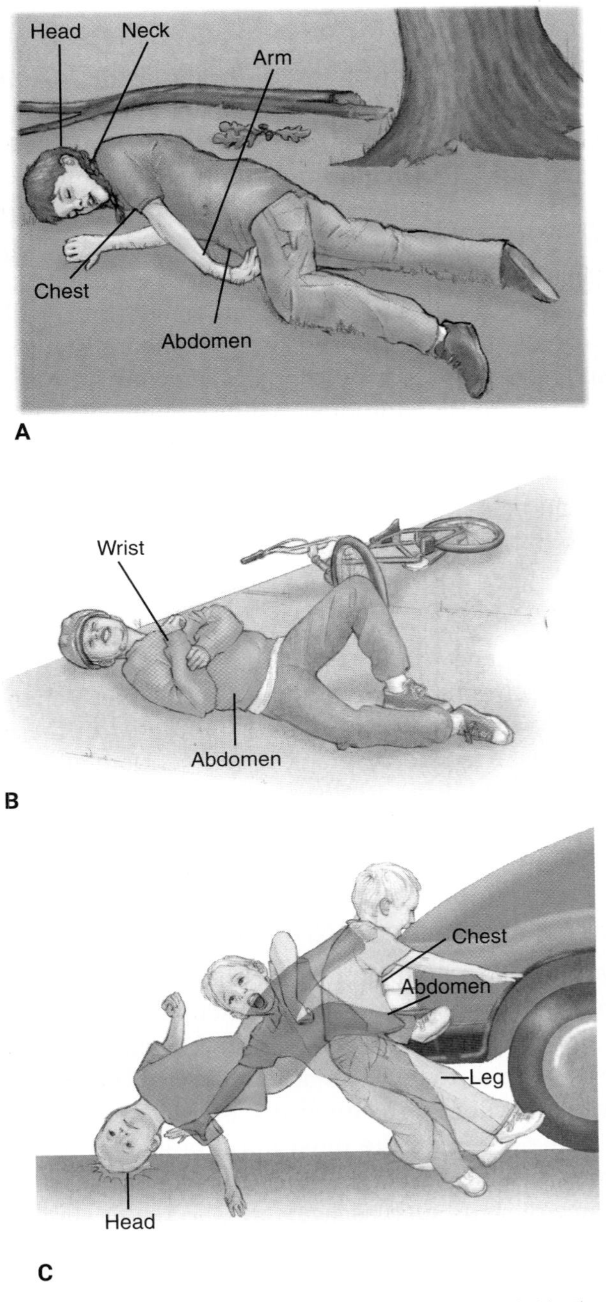

FIGURE 11-13 Significant MOIs for an infant or child. The primary areas of potential injury are labeled. **A.** Falls from more than 10 feet (3 m). **B.** Bicycle collision. **C.** Vehicle–pedestrian collision.

- Fall of less than 10 feet with loss of consciousness
- Bicycle collision
- Medium- to high-speed MVC (25 mph or greater)

In many cases, multiple MOIs come into play during a traumatic event. For example, a lateral collision may leave the patient with a crushed upper arm and pelvic girdle as well as penetrating trauma from a piece of door trim impaled in the chest. Therefore, a patient with any of the previously mentioned mechanisms should immediately raise your index of suspicion.

Words of Wisdom

Two or more serious MOIs markedly increase the likelihood that a patient will sustain a serious or fatal injury.

Seat belts and airbags have significantly reduced the prevalence of death and disability associated with MVCs. At the same time, seat belts and airbags can also cause injury. As you evaluate a patient who was involved in an MVC, look for signs and ask questions to determine whether seat belts and/or airbags were involved. Check the clavicle where the shoulder strap crosses. The clavicle is a small bone, and the subclavian vein and artery run directly beneath it. In shorter patients, a shoulder strap mounted on the B post in a car can ride up across the neck, increasing the risk of soft-tissue and cervical spine injury. Examine the area where the lap belt crosses the pelvic girdle. If the belt is not across the iliac spine but has ridden up over the lower abdomen, a person has an increased risk of organ damage and thoracic or lumbar spine injury. Passengers who tuck the shoulder harness under their arms for comfort and are then involved in rollover crashes are at high risk of death from liver injury caused by the improperly positioned belt.

Airbags have saved countless lives, but many people do not realize that they are a secondary restraint system, designed to work with seat belts to reduce injuries. When the seat belt is not used and a crash occurs, the airbag deploys, momentarily catching the patient. As the airbag deflates, it releases the driver or passenger, who continues moving forward and may go down-and-under (into the dashboard) or up-and-over (into the steering wheel and/or windshield) if they are not restrained by a seat belt. At the scene of any crash with airbag deployment, lift the bag and look beneath it for a bent steering wheel—another possible source of life-threatening internal injuries. During your handoff report at the ED, inform hospital personnel

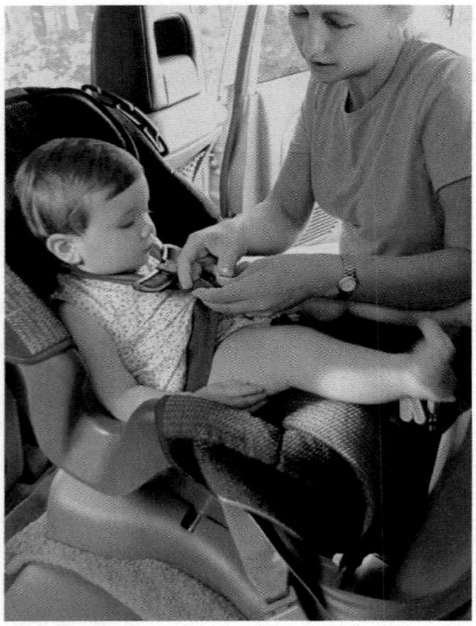

FIGURE 11-14 A child should be correctly positioned in a proper-size and fitted child safety seat in the rear seat of the vehicle.

whether seat belts were used and properly positioned, and whether airbags deployed.

Child safety seats have also saved countless lives **FIGURE 11-14**. If they are improperly installed or positioned in the vehicle, however, they can be rendered useless as a safety device. If the child safety seat comes loose during a crash, the risk of face, head, neck, and spine trauma to the child increases markedly. Similarly, if the child is too large or too small for the seat, it will not provide the intended level of protection.

Most trauma calls involve patients with a single, isolated injury or, on occasion, several minor injuries. In nearly all of these cases, lack of serious or critical injuries is consistent with absence of a significant MOI: A collision on the basketball court results in a sprained ankle; a skater crashes and ends up with a distal radius fracture; a loose piece of metal spins off a lathe in the machine shop, lacerating the machinist's forearm. Patients should not show any sign of systemic involvement (hypotension). If they do, there is more going on than an isolated injury. Continue your assessment to find and correct the more serious injury.

Review of Body Systems

The review of body systems during history taking provides additional information that could help you form an accurate field impression. To collect even more information, many prehospital providers include **pertinent negatives**: an absence or lack of certain signs and symptoms characteristic of particular illnesses. For instance, people experiencing an AMI typically have chest pain. In addition, such patients often report shortness of breath, nausea and/or vomiting, sweating, and syncope. The absence of these additional symptoms tells you just as much as their presence does, helping you form a more accurate field impression. Another example would be a patient who struck their head but "denies any loss of consciousness."

General Symptoms

Many patients present with vague, nonspecific signs and symptoms that tend to be classified as "generalized weakness" and "flulike symptoms." In these patients, it is often difficult to differentiate among various field diagnoses; asking questions about fever, chills, malaise, fatigue, night sweats, and weight variations can help focus on a likely diagnosis.

Skin, Hair, and Nails

Questions about the integumentary system should focus on items like rashes (particularly in pediatric patients), itching or hives, and sweating. This system tends to be one of the most easily forgotten systems when performing the physical exam, yet is actually one of the most important. Symptoms vary because they are subjective, but the significance of signs such as sweating and pallor should not be downplayed. Look for and ask about these conditions because many patients will dismiss such subtle complaints or neglect to communicate them to you.

Musculoskeletal

Issues with the musculoskeletal system tend to be attributed to trauma, but some medical conditions also affect this system. For patients reporting signs and symptoms that could be associated with the musculoskeletal system, ask about joint pain, loss of range of motion (ROM), and any swelling, redness, and localized heat or deformity.

Head and Neck

Multiple structures within the head and neck can affect a patient's overall health status. Pay particular attention to patients experiencing a severe headache or loss of consciousness because these could result in a life-threatening condition.

Eyes and Ears Ask questions regarding the eyes and vision, including visual acuity, blurred vision, **diplopia** (double vision), photophobia (sensitivity to light), pain, and flashes of light seen in the field of vision. Questions about the ears should focus on hearing loss, pain, discharge, tinnitus (ringing), and vertigo (sensation of the room spinning).

Nose, Throat, and Mouth Ask patients about their sense of smell, rhinorrhea (runny nose), obstruction, epistaxis, postnasal discharge, and sinus pain. Questions about the throat and mouth should focus on complaints such as sore throat, bleeding, pain, dental problems, ulcers, and changes in the sense of taste.

Endocrine System

The endocrine system is a complicated network of hormone-secreting glands that help regulate various functions in the human body. Many endocrine system diseases are seen in the field and should be included in your review of systems. Because multiple glands and organs are part of the endocrine system, there is a broad range of questions pertaining to this system. Ask if the patient has ever been told they have an enlarged thyroid gland. While subtle enlargement is typically noticed only with palpation, the patient generally notices excessive enlargement.

Additional endocrine system questions pertain to temperature intolerance, skin changes, swelling of hands and feet, weight changes, polyuria (increased frequency of urination), polydipsia (increased thirst), polyphagia (increased appetite), and any changes in body or facial hair.

Chest and Lungs

Complaints regarding the heart and lungs are common reasons for requesting EMS. A review of systems would not be complete without screening for possible cardiac and respiratory conditions. Always screen patients for dyspnea and chest pain. Other respiratory questions should focus on coughing, wheezing, hemoptysis (coughing up blood), and the presence of active tuberculosis. With regard to coughing, obtain a description of the cough (eg, production of mucus or phlegm). When you question a patient about cardiac complaints, focus initially on whether this is a first-time or recurring event. The next priority will be questions about pain or discomfort. As described earlier, elaborate on the chief complaint using the OPQRST questions. Other questions related to the heart and blood vessels pertain to orthopnea, edema, and past cardiac evaluation and tests.

Hematology and Lymph Nodes

Ask patients about any history of anemia, bruising, or fatigue. Anemia may exacerbate multiple medical conditions that could be seen during an EMS call. Note any bruising, especially when it is atraumatic. This could suggest a clotting disorder that may affect traumatic injuries as well as other medical conditions. Note any bruising that may point toward physical abuse, and report suspected abuse in accordance with state laws.

Tender and enlarged lymph nodes can be seen with conditions ranging from infection to cancer. Many patients encountered by EMS personnel have an infection. Questioning the patient about tender or enlarged lymph nodes can point you toward a possible field impression.

Gastrointestinal

Gastrointestinal (GI) complaints are common reasons for EMS calls. Paramedics must understand GI ailments and ask appropriate questions in the review of systems to help distinguish among various illnesses. Ask patients about appetite, general digestion, food allergies and intolerances, heartburn, any nausea or vomiting, diarrhea, hematemesis (blood in vomit), bowel irregularity, changes in stool (size, shape, smell, or color), flatulence, jaundice, and any past GI evaluations. Pay particular attention to signs and symptoms that point toward active GI bleeding, a life-threatening condition.

Many patients hesitate to offer information about urination. Some people attribute changes in urinary habits to aging, but often such changes are a new finding that could indicate an underlying infection or other problem that should be addressed. Ask about urinary habits or changes in urinary habits, including dysuria (painful urination), increased frequency of urination, urgency (sudden need to urinate), nocturia (waking up in the middle of sleeping to urinate), hematuria (blood in urine), or polyuria (excessive urination). Ask about flank pain and pain in the suprapubic region if you suspect that the chief complaint could represent an underlying urinary problem.

Genitourinary

The genitourinary system (GU) also includes the genitals. As mentioned earlier, patients may not find it easy to discuss their genitals with a stranger. However, medical conditions such as sexually transmitted infections can be serious. Even though this may be an embarrassing topic for both patients and paramedics, ask about any current or history of sexually transmitted infections. Some questions are specific to the male and female sexes. Both male and female sex organs secrete hormones belonging to the endocrine system.

Keep your questions focused. For a woman reporting acute abdominal pain, foul-smelling vaginal discharge, pain on urination, or genital lesions, ask if her menstrual cycle is regular, when she last had her period, and if she has dysmenorrhea (menstrual pain). In addition, ask when she last had sexual intercourse, whether she has had multiple sex partners, what kind of contraception she uses (if any), and whether she has ever been pregnant. Female gynecologic and obstetric conditions are discussed further in Chapter 23, *Gynecologic Emergencies*, and Chapter 42, *Obstetrics*.

When you question male patients, ask about erectile dysfunction, any fluid discharge, and testicular pain. It may seem trivial to the patient, but problems with erectile dysfunction are frequently related to systemic diseases such as hypertension or diabetes. In addition, the medications used to treat many of these conditions can affect the care provided by paramedics, such as not giving nitroglycerin to a patient taking erectile dysfunction drugs like Viagra or Cialis.

For men who report pain on urination, discharge from the penis, or genital lesions, ask when their most recent sexual encounter was and if they use condoms. Ask them to describe the characteristics of any discharge or lesions.

Neurologic

When a patient summons EMS for a neurologic complaint, you must understand the importance of assessing for neurologic pathology. That means asking specific questions during the review of systems that cover or involve the nervous system. For example, ask about a history of seizures or syncope, loss of sensation, weakness in the extremities, paralysis, loss of coordination or memory, and muscle twitches or tremors. In addition, be alert for signs of facial asymmetry, especially when the chief complaint is headache. If you suspect a stroke or a TIA, use a stroke assessment tool per your local protocols. Stroke scales are discussed in detail in Chapter 19, *Neurologic Emergencies*.

Psychiatric

Paramedics are often called to the scene of a behavioral health emergency. Some communities are now dispatching mental health professionals and no longer sending law enforcement personnel to these types of complaints. Because many medical problems can initially present with behavioral symptoms, it is unknown how effective this approach will be. If paramedics are on the scene, they should question patients appropriately to differentiate among the various mental illnesses. Ask the patient about a history of or any current depression, mood changes, difficulty concentrating, anxiety, irritability, sleep disturbances, daytime fatigue, and suicidal or homicidal ideation. This step is essential to deliver appropriate patient care and ensure the safety of yourself, the crew, and the patient.

Critical Thinking

The aim of your assessment should be to figure out the most likely reason for the patient's chief complaint and how best to address it. In Chapter 12, *Critical Thinking and Clinical Decision Making,* you will learn the details of critical thinking. There are five aspects of critical thinking: (1) concept formation, (2) data interpretation, (3) application of principles (guidelines or algorithms), (4) reflection in action (being willing to change course as you interpret the patient's condition), and (5) reflection on action (doing honest and thorough postrun critiques to benefit learning).

Being able to think and perform well under pressure is a big part of becoming a good paramedic. In many ways, critical thinking and decision making are just two more skills you will need to work on, not just while you are a student, but for the rest of your career.

Clinical Reasoning

Clinical reasoning combines your knowledge of anatomy, physiology, and pathophysiology with information about the patient's complaints to direct questioning as you take a history. Note any abnormal symptoms or physical findings, as well as their anatomic location. Pay careful attention to any signs or symptoms inconsistent with your working diagnosis, because they may point you in a different direction. As the patient answers your interview questions, you will begin to analyze the information based on your medical knowledge. Once the history of the chief complaint, history of the present illness, past medical history, and review of systems have been completed, you can begin to develop a differential diagnosis: a working hypothesis of the nature of the problem. Your differential diagnosis is the list of possible causes of the patient's complaint. For example, a patient reports sudden onset of shortness of breath in the absence of trauma. You could begin to refine your differential diagnosis by ruling out myocardial infarction, pulmonary edema, pneumonia, allergy, reactive airway disease, and so on. Part of the history and physical exam is to "rule in or rule out" possible diagnoses in your differential diagnosis. In the preceding example, the patient's shortness of breath began suddenly, and dyspnea is probably not due to pneumonia in a patient with no fever. There is no trauma, so it is unlikely to result from a fractured rib.

Similar to a detective, you can then begin to test this hypothesis to determine whether it holds true. You can accomplish this through further assessment and testing (eg, a 12-lead ECG or a glucose check). The process evolves as you ask different questions based on the patient's answers. This exploration, in turn, helps you focus your physical assessment and narrow down your list of possible field diagnoses even further.

As you develop your differential diagnosis, begin with broad possibilities; that is, decide which body systems might be contributing to the patient's complaint. For instance, chest pain could involve the cardiac, respiratory, or GI systems. This approach helps you avoid tunnel vision, in which you lock into a diagnosis too early, before considering all possibilities and systematically ruling out each one to determine the actual diagnosis.

The physical exam (discussed later in this chapter) is another crucial aspect of clinical reasoning. Tenderness or other specific exam findings help point you toward specific anatomic locations that can tighten up your diagnostic possibilities. Once you identify the possible organ systems involved, use your knowledge of pathophysiology to determine the most likely diagnosis. Once you settle on a working diagnosis, continue your questioning of the patient to help confirm this diagnosis. In addition, reevaluate the overall situation and complaint to ensure you address all patient complaints.

Patient Assessment

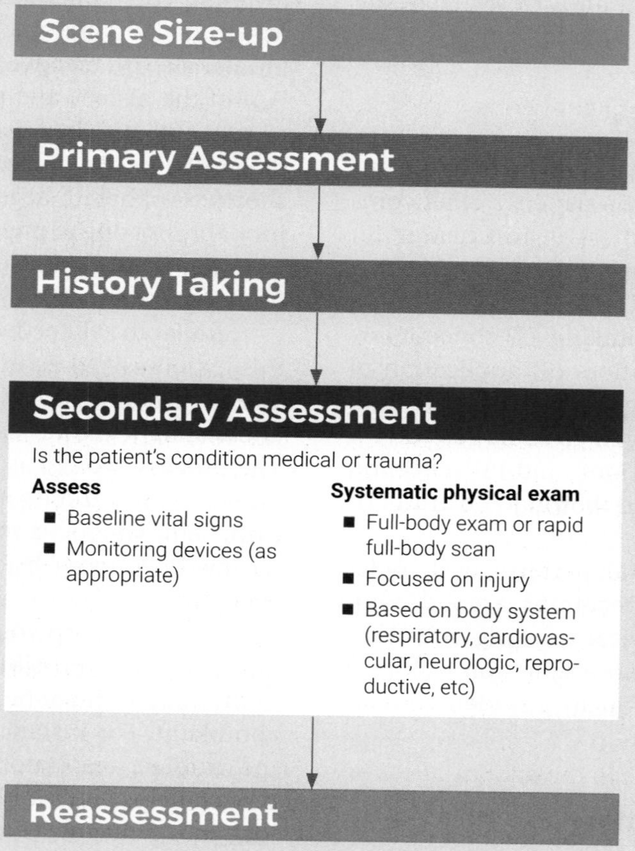

Scene Size-up
Primary Assessment
History Taking
Secondary Assessment
Is the patient's condition medical or trauma?
Assess
Baseline vital signs
Monitoring devices (as appropriate)
Systematic physical exam
Full-body exam or rapid full-body scan
Focused on injury
Based on body system (respiratory, cardiovascular, neurologic, reproductive, etc)
Reassessment

Secondary Assessment

Secondary assessment is the process by which quantifiable, objective (based on fact or observable) information is obtained from a patient about their overall state of health. This information is compared with subjective (observed or perceived by the patient), historical information obtained from the patient. Armed with these two types of information, you can obtain a field impression and develop a differential diagnosis for the patient. While performing an assessment, you may see the patient's condition as a clinical phenomenon; however, a caring and empathetic approach will yield better results and a more accurate evaluation. Likewise, putting forth a professional appearance and demeanor will instill trust and confidence in your abilities as a care provider.

The secondary assessment consists of two elements:

1. Obtaining baseline vital signs that measure overall body function
2. Performing a systematic physical exam such as the full-body exam (also called the head-to-toe survey), a focused exam on a specific injury, or an exam based on the body system identified in the chief complaint (ie, respiratory, cardiovascular, neurologic, reproductive, etc)

Of course, the prehospital setting conditions may determine how the secondary assessment is performed. Sometimes it may be condensed. For example, for an unresponsive medical patient or a trauma patient with a significant MOI, there may be only enough time to perform a rapid full-body scan, as discussed later in this section.

The overall patient assessment helps you determine whether a medical condition exists, so actions can be taken to manage it. However, before you can appreciate abnormalities on examination, you must understand the variety of typical presentations. This knowledge can be learned only through direct, hands-on experience and patient interaction. Thus, every patient encounter represents an opportunity for you to gain experience about the normal human condition.

As you approach the patient, consider the major body systems and their anatomic locations. An understanding of anatomy and physiology will help you tremendously during the assessment and while forming your field impression. For example, as you palpate the chest, it is essential to remember the heart, lungs, great vessels, and esophagus are located in that anatomic region and should be considered when a patient reports pain in that area. In addition, understanding the GI system and the locations of specific organs in the abdominal cavity can help narrow down a differential diagnosis.

As stated earlier, the general approach to examining a patient should be systematic. However, the actual starting point for your exam is determined by several factors, such as the patient's stability, the chief complaint, the history, the patient's ability to communicate, and the potential for unrecognized illness or injury. For example, a patient who reports isolated ankle pain does not necessarily warrant an exam that begins with assessing the head. With that said, a patient with multisystem trauma may require a rapid assessment from head to toe at the beginning of the assessment. Depending on their level of stability, some patients may never get a complete assessment because you will be too busy managing the life-threatening injuries identified in the primary survey. Therefore, not every aspect of the secondary assessment will be completed in every patient. In addition, additional challenges associated with underlying comorbidities (simultaneous existence of two or more chronic conditions found in a patient) may arise when examining a patient. For example, an unresponsive patient involved in an MVC may have an underlying diabetic emergency that contributed to the crash.

Other factors to consider when beginning an exam include the location of the exam, the patient's position and point of view, and the need to maintain professionalism. Always consider your environment and ask yourself if this is the most appropriate environment in which to conduct the exam. Factors such as noise, lighting, and the patient's position might hinder your assessment. In addition, the patient's privacy should *always* be considered, not only because of the need to expose the patient, but also to discourage bystanders from watching, listening, and creating videos of the exam process to post on social media. If necessary and feasible, move the patient to a more private location, such as your office (ambulance), before conducting an in-depth secondary assessment. Remember, the patient is probably going through an emotional and traumatic event.

Your touch during the exam will contribute to the patient's stress level. Explain everything to the patient before performing the exam to help alleviate the patient's stress. This helps you establish a high level of professionalism and shows that you are attentive to the patient's needs. Keep in mind, most people do not care for physical exams, so being kind, professional, and compassionate will go a long way toward calming their anxiety and fears.

Physical Exam of Priority Patients

The physical exam you perform is based on the needs of your patient. If the patient is an unresponsive medical patient or a trauma patient with a significant MOI, then you may not have the time to perform the physical exam traditionally done in the secondary assessment. It may be necessary to do a **rapid full-body scan** (sometimes called a rapid full-body sweep) and get moving to the ED. The rapid full-body scan is a 60- to 90-second nonsystematic review and palpation of the patient's body to identify injuries that must be managed or protected immediately. If there is time to do the traditional head-to-toe physical exam, that should be performed as discussed in the next section.

During the rapid full-body scan, *inspect* the soft tissue, look for open or closed wounds, and *palpate* for pain or tenderness. Evaluate each area of the body for the following:

- **Open:**
  - Abrasions/amputations/avulsions
  - Punctures/penetrations
  - Lacerations
- **Closed:**
  - Deformities or swelling
  - Burns
  - Contusions/crush injuries

Words of Wisdom

When done properly, palpation should not cause harm. Deep palpation is rarely performed by EMS workers, and requires practice and an understanding of when to stop.

To perform a rapid full-body scan of the patient, follow the steps in **SKILL DRILL 11-1**. Remember, this exam should take no longer than 60 to 90 seconds!

Skill Drill 11-1 Performing a Rapid Full-Body Scan

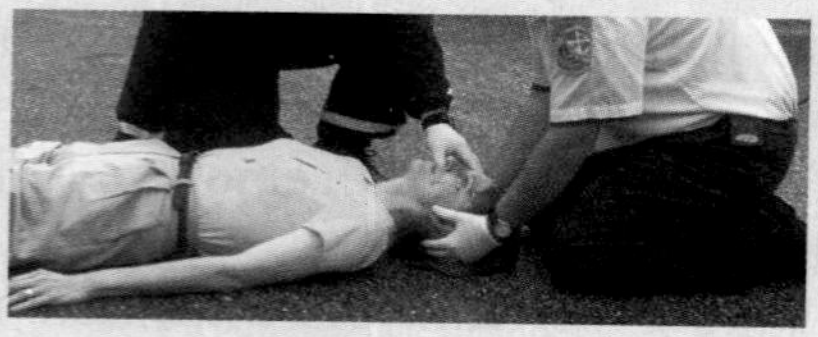

Step 1

Inspect and palpate the head for open/closed findings and crepitus.

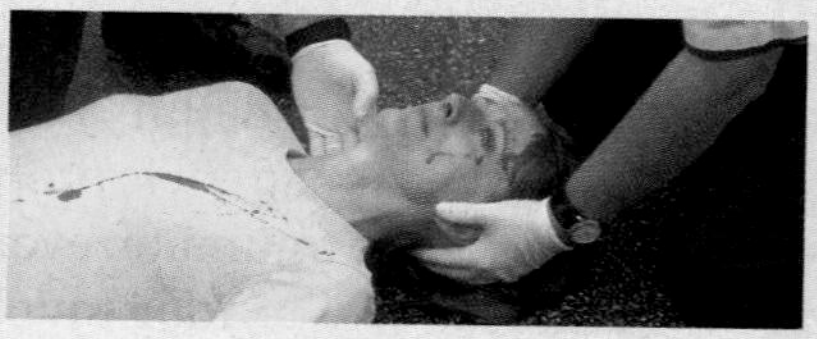

Step 2

Inspect and palpate the neck for open/closed findings, **jugular venous distention (JVD)** (visible bulging of the jugular veins when a patient is in semi-Fowler or full Fowler position), tracheal deviation, and crepitus. In trauma patients, consider applying a cervical spinal immobilization device. It is imperative to assess the neck before covering it with a cervical collar.

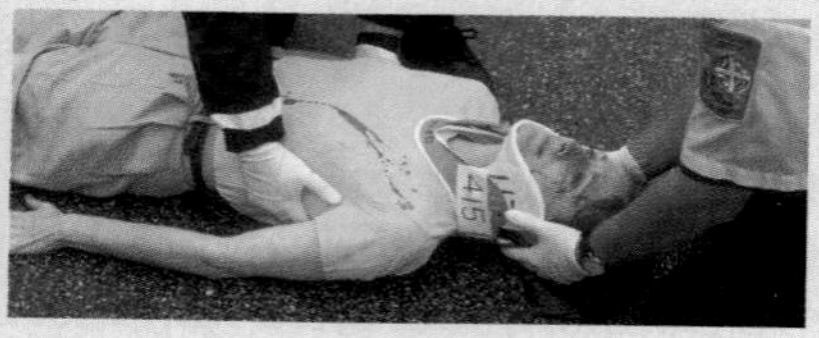

Step 3

Inspect and palpate the chest for open/closed findings, paradoxical motion, and crepitus. Listen to breath sounds on both sides of the patient's chest.

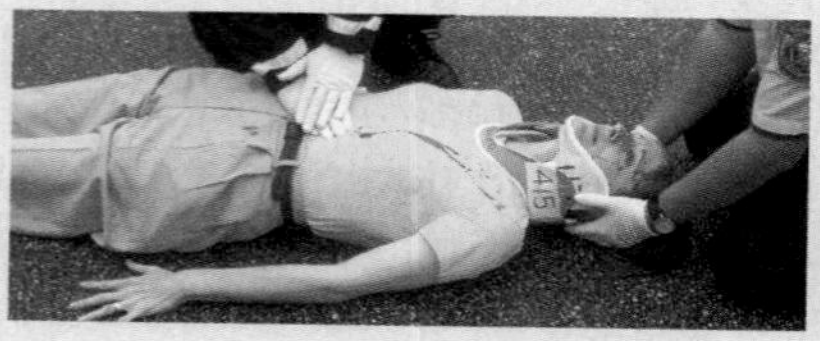

Step 4

Inspect and palpate the abdomen for open/closed findings, rigidity (firm or soft), and distention.

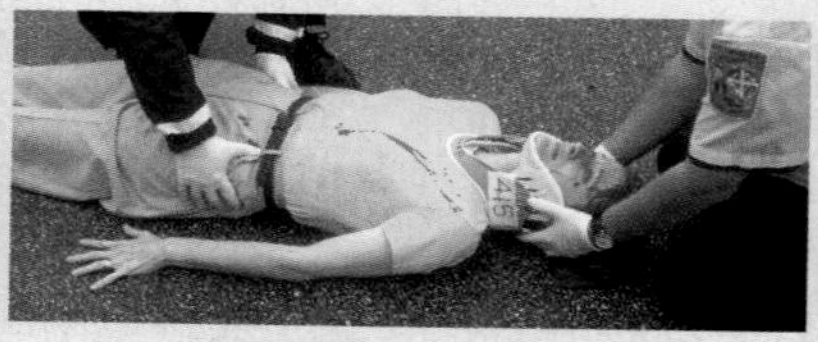

Step 5

Inspect and palpate the pelvis for open/closed findings. If there is no pain, gently compress the pelvis downward and inward to look for tenderness and instability.

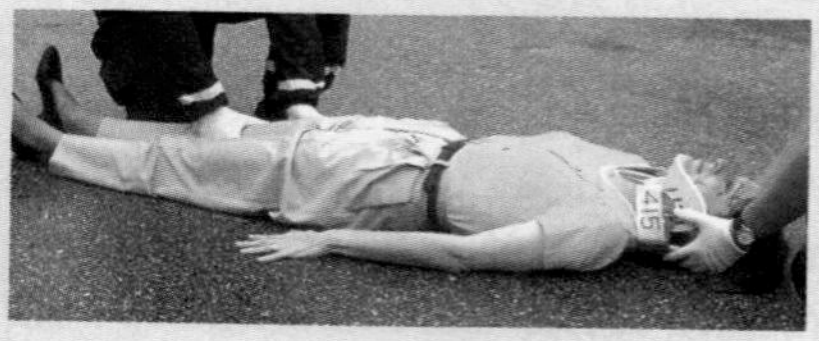

Step 6

Inspect and palpate all four extremities for open/closed findings. Assess bilaterally for distal pulses and motor and sensory functions.

Skill Drill 11-1 Performing a Rapid Full-Body Scan (continued)

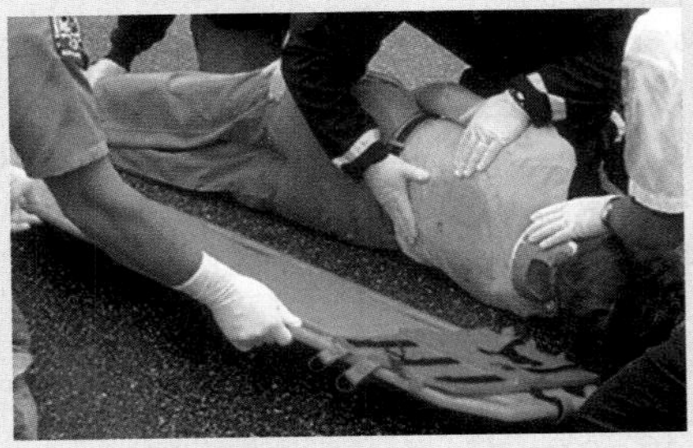

Step 7

Inspect and palpate the back and buttocks for open/closed findings. In all trauma patients, maintain in-line stabilization of the spine while rolling the patient on their uninjured side in one smooth motion. If you place the patient on a backboard, check the back before you finish log rolling the patient onto the board. If you use a scoop stretcher, you won't be able to inspect or palpate the lower thoracic and lumbar spine, but there is a lot less movement.

Assessment Techniques

The techniques of inspection, palpation, auscultation, and percussion allow you to use your physical senses to obtain information and learn about the normal (versus abnormal) functions of a patient's body. Recall that inspection involves looking at the patient, either in general or at a specific area. For example, you might take in a patient's overall appearance from the doorway and then look specifically at the chest wall for abnormalities or deformities **FIGURE 11-15**.

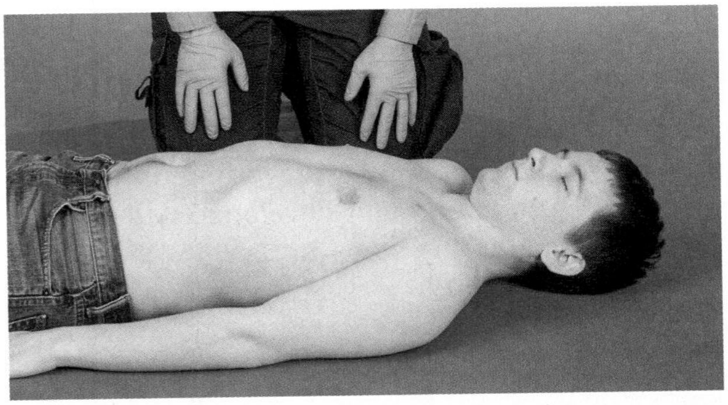

FIGURE 11-15 Physical exam: inspection.

Palpation is touching to obtain information, such as detecting tenderness (eliciting pain), feeling for any deformity, **crepitus** (a grating or grinding sensation or sound made when two pieces of broken bone rub together), mass, or abnormal organ enlargement, and judging pulse quality **FIGURE 11-16**. You will typically use your fingertips to check pulses but will use your palms to sweep across and around the skull, for example, to assess structural integrity as well as to assess for defects (ie, knots or dents). Use the back of your hand to touch a patient's skin for fever assessment because it is more sensitive than your palm.

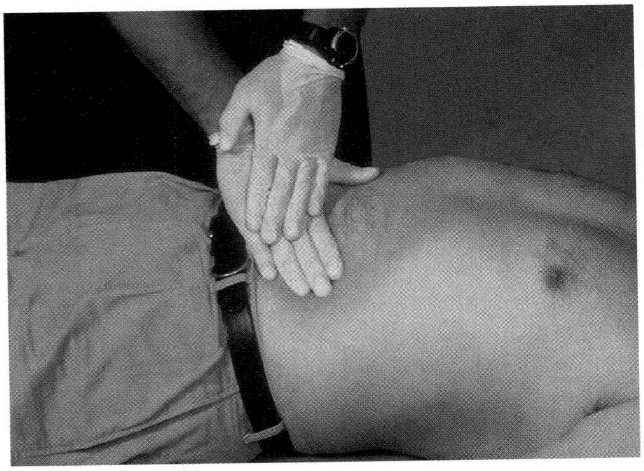

FIGURE 11-16 Physical exam: palpation.

Various palpation techniques are used to examine specific areas. Palpation with the hands and fingertips is typically performed on the chest, abdomen, and extremities. Accomplish this by keeping your hand and forearm on a horizontal plane, with fingers together and flat on the patient, and palpating with a sliding or dipping motion, depending on the area being examined. Palpation with the fingertips may be reserved for examining the distal extremities, the head, and the neck. Use the ulnar surface of the hand when examining the abdomen. Some patients will immediately tense their abdominal muscles during the exam, regardless of whether they have pain. When you use only the ulnar surface of one hand, the exam seems less intrusive to the patient, and the results are more likely to be accurate. Use the dorsal aspect of the hand in the same manner as the ulnar surface. This technique is also used when assessing skin temperature.

Percussion entails gently striking the surface of the body, typically where it overlies various body cavities. This technique allows you to detect changes in the densities of the underlying structures. For example, percussion of a normal lung will yield medium to loud, low-pitched, resonant sounds. Percussion sounds over muscle and bone should be soft, high-pitched, and flat. Percussion sounds over hollow organs such as the intestines are often described as loud, high-pitched, and tympanic (like a drum).

Percussion is a skill that requires a lot of practice to perfect. An internist who performs this skill a dozen times a day becomes competent quickly. By comparison, percussion is rarely done in the field and, as such, is a minimally developed skill for most providers. Follow the steps in **SKILL DRILL 11-2** to perform percussion.

Auscultation is listening to body sounds with a stethoscope. The body generates a variety of high- and low-frequency sounds, both normal and abnormal, that can be detected via auscultation. You can assess bowel sounds via auscultation, as you can lung and heart sounds. Appreciating the presence of and differences in auscultated sounds requires keen attention, a thorough understanding of what "normal" sounds like, and lots of practice.

Vital Signs

Vital signs consist of measuring pulse rate, rhythm, and quality; respiratory rate, rhythm, and quality; BP; temperature; and pulse oximetry. Besides overall patient appearance, vital signs provide the most objective data for determining patient status. Measuring vital signs requires you to use the techniques of auscultation, palpation, and inspection. The first set of vital signs, commonly taken in the secondary assessment, is called the *baseline*. The additional sets of readings, commonly taken during reassessment, are called *serial vital signs*. Reviewing the serial vital signs and comparing the measurements with the

Skill Drill 11-2 Performing Percussion

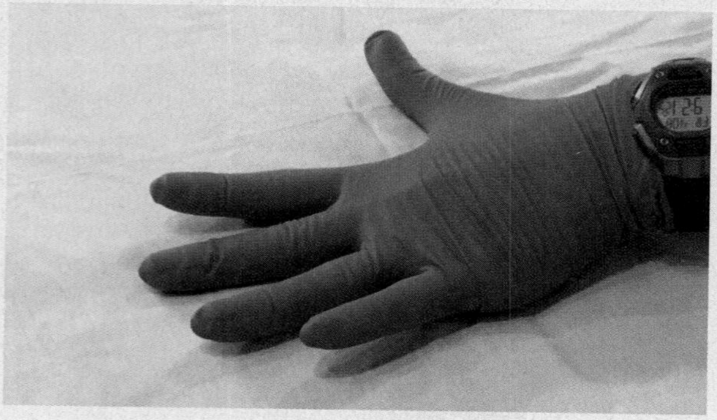

Step 1

Hyperextend your middle finger, and apply firm pressure to the surface to be percussed.

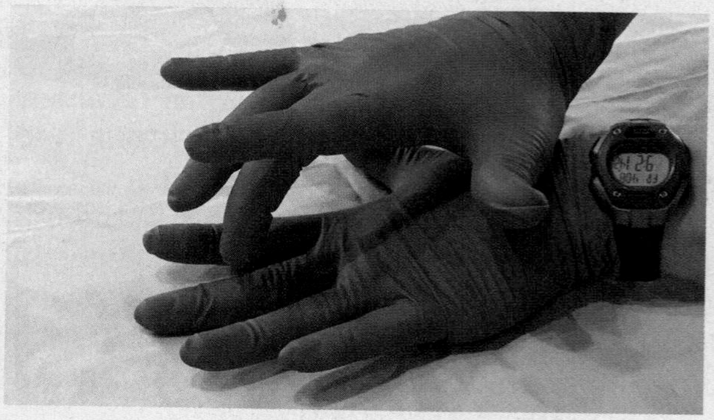

Step 2

Directly strike the middle phalanx of your middle finger with one or two fingertips of your other hand. Apply the same force over each area of the body to accurately compare the sounds produced by percussion.

Special Populations

In pediatric patients, and in adults with irregular breathing, the respiratory rate should be measured for a minimum of 30 seconds, and then multiplied by 2 to obtain the rate per minute.

Assessing the work of breathing in a pediatric patient is one of the single most predictive signs; therefore, when you see a child with excessive work of breathing who begins to show signs of ventilatory fatigue, a physiologic collapse is usually moments away.

Palpating the pulse in an infant often presents a real challenge. Because an infant's neck is often short and fat, and the pulse rate is quite fast, you may have a hard time finding a carotid pulse. Therefore, in infants (younger than 1 year), palpate the brachial artery to assess the pulse.

baseline readings helps you establish trends showing patient improvement or deterioration. This is called *vital signs trending.* Because vital signs can change dramatically over relatively short periods, failing to check them frequently and observe trends, especially in the context of a significantly ill or injured patient, can lead to poor patient care.

Pay strict attention to vital signs, as they measure critically important parameters. Normal limits, as shown in **TABLE 11-5**, can vary, depending on factors such as age and medication use. Interpret readings with those factors in mind.

Pulse

Pulse measurements should assess the rate, presence, location, quality, and regularity of the

TABLE 11-5 Normal Vital Signs at Various Ages

Age	Pulse Rate (beats/min)	Respirations (breaths/min)	BP (mm Hg)	Temperature (°F)
Neonate (0 to 1 month)	Awake: 100 to 205 Asleep: 90 to 160	30 to 60	Systolic: 67 to 84 Diastolic: 35 to 53 Mean arterial pressure: 45 to 60	98 to 100 (37°C to 38°C)
Infant (1 month to 1 year)	Awake: 100 to 180 Asleep: 90 to 160	30 to 53	Systolic: 72 to 104 Diastolic: 37 to 56 Mean arterial pressure: 50 to 62	96.8 to 99.6 (36°C to 37.5°C)
Toddler (1 to 2 years)	Awake: 98 to 140 Asleep: 80 to 120	22 to 37	Systolic: 86 to 106 Diastolic: 42 to 63 Mean arterial pressure: 49 to 62	96.8 to 99.6 (36°C to 37.5°C)
Preschool age (3 to 5 years)	Awake: 80 to 120 Asleep: 65 to 100	20 to 28	Systolic: 89 to 112 Diastolic: 46 to 72 Mean arterial pressure: 58 to 69	98.6 (37°C)
School age (6 to 12 years)	Awake: 75 to 118 Asleep: 58 to 90	18 to 25	Systolic: 97 to 120 Diastolic: 57 to 80 Mean arterial pressure: 66 to 79	98.6 (37°C)
Adolescent (12 to 15 years)	Awake: 60 to 100 Asleep: 50 to 90	12 to 20	Systolic: 110 to 131 Diastolic: 64 to 83 Mean arterial pressure: 73 to 84	98.6 (37°C)
Early adult (18 to 40 years)	60 to 100	12 to 20	Systolic: 90 to 140	98.6 (37°C)
Middle adult (41 to 60 years)	60 to 100	12 to 20	Systolic: 90 to 140	98.6 (37°C)
Older adult (61 years and older)	60 to 100	12 to 20	Systolic: 90 to 140	98.6 (37°C)

Pediatric data from: American Heart Association (AHA). Vital signs in children. In: AHA. *Pediatric Advanced Life Support.* Dallas, TX: AHA; 2020.

heartbeat. Pulses can be obtained at several points in the body, including the radial, brachial, femoral, and carotid arteries **FIGURE 11-17**. As mentioned in the Primary Survey section, when you formally count the pulse rate, time the pulses for a minimum of 30 seconds and then multiply by 2 to obtain the rate per minute.

EMS personnel should compare the proximal and distal pulses during patient evaluation. If the pulse is irregular or slow, it is best to count for a full minute. If you are unable to palpate a radial pulse, reassess for a pulse using the carotid artery.

Although it is appropriate to check for a central pulse in an unresponsive patient, the actual pulse

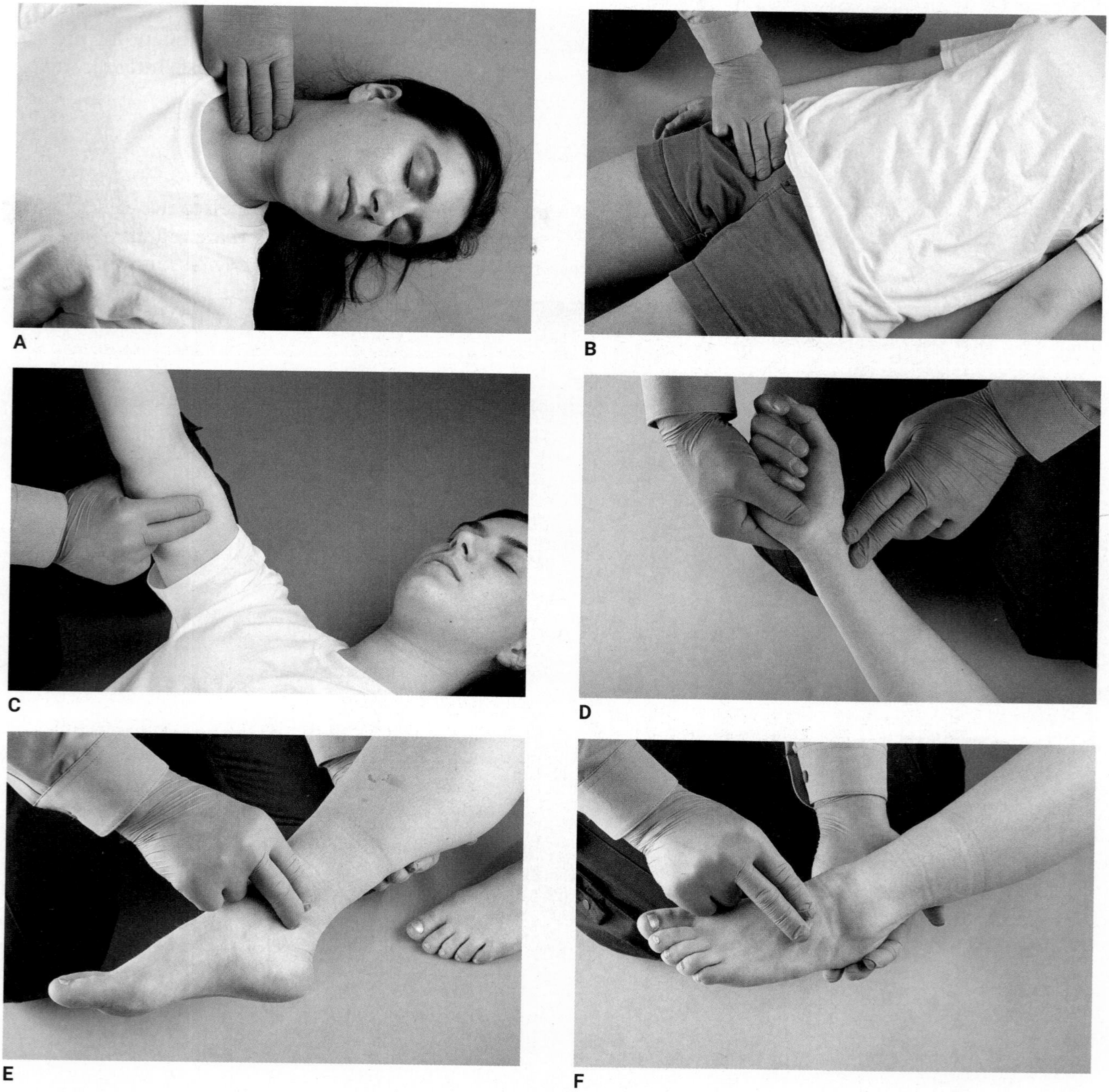

FIGURE 11-17 Common pulse points. **A.** Carotid pulse. **B.** Femoral pulse. **C.** Brachial pulse. **D.** Radial pulse. **E.** Posterior tibial pulse. **F.** Dorsalis pedis pulse.

rate should be counted in a peripheral location that can be palpated. In the responsive patient, determine the respiratory rate while you appear to be checking the pulse; this may decrease patients' tendency to inadvertently alter their breathing pattern or rate when they become aware of being evaluated.

Respiration

The respiratory rate is typically measured by observing the rise and fall of the patient's chest. Overall respiratory effort can be assessed by visualizing portions of the abdominal wall, neck, and face, and by assessing accessory muscle use. Although the absolute respiratory rate is important, the quality of the respiratory effort should be evaluated as well. Learn to recognize pathologic respiratory patterns **TABLE 11-6**. Refer to Chapter 17, *Respiratory Emergencies*, for depictions of these patterns. Similarly, learn to recognize when patients exhibit tripod positioning, accessory muscle use, or retractions. This is especially critical information when assessing pediatric patients.

Blood Pressure

Blood pressure (BP) is the measurement of the force exerted against the walls of the blood vessels. It is commonly measured in a peripheral artery, although it can be obtained essentially anywhere in the circulatory system. BP is a product of cardiac output and peripheral vascular resistance, so it includes two components: systolic pressure and diastolic pressure, reported in millimeters of mercury (mm Hg). **Systolic pressure** is created by the left ventricle while it is contracting (ie, during systole). **Diastolic pressure** is the result of residual pressure in the system while the left ventricle is relaxing (ie, during diastole). Normally, diastolic pressure should not fall to zero, because peripheral vascular resistance in the arteriolar side of the circulatory system should continually provide for a diastolic pressure. The coronary arteries receive blood flow by this mechanism, so a drop in diastolic pressure means less myocardial perfusion.

> **Words of Wisdom**
>
> Many patients exhibit an increase in BP because of the anxiety and stress of an acute injury or illness. Look at the patient and trends in vital signs before concluding BP is truly abnormal.

> **Words of Wisdom**
>
> Whenever possible, avoid taking BP on a painful/injured extremity, on an arm with an arteriovenous shunt or fistula, or on a post-mastectomy side. Doing so can cause pain and/or result in inaccurate readings.

BP must be measured using a cuff appropriate to the patient's size and habitus (physique or body build). The cuff should be one-half to two-thirds the size of the upper arm. Cuffs that are too small or too tight will yield an artificially high pressure; cuffs that are too large or too loose will give inaccurately low results. Although BP should ideally be auscultated, it can be palpated to estimate the systolic pressure; however, this method introduces the potential for error. Periodic inspection of the BP cuff's gauge is necessary because it can lose accuracy and require recalibration or replacement.

Temperature

Many methods can be used to evaluate body temperature. EMS providers have begun to pay more attention to fever than they did in the past due to the COVID-19 pandemic. If you use a device to measure the tympanic membrane temperature to obtain a patient's body temperature, be aware that extrinsic factors may increase or decrease the temperature reading. Ensure that the external auditory canal is free of **cerumen** (ear wax), which can lower the temperature reading. Position the probe in the canal so the infrared beam is aimed at the tympanic membrane; otherwise, the measurement will be invalid. Wait 2 to 3 seconds until the digital temperature reading appears. This method measures core body temperature, which is usually higher, and more accurate, than an oral temperature. The oral temperature is considered a proxy of the actual temperature, which is core body temperature.

Pulse Oximetry

Arterial oxygen saturation determined via **pulse oximetry** (Spo_2) has become part of regular vital

TABLE 11-6 Pathologic Respiratory Patterns

Waveform	Pattern	Description	Causes
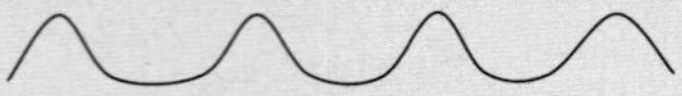	Eupnea	Regular rate and pattern; inspiration and expiration are equal	Normal
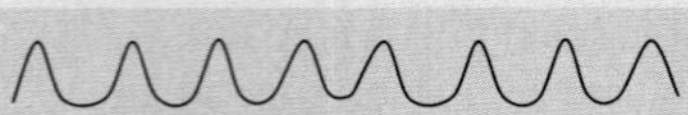	Tachypnea	Excessively rapid and shallow breathing, regular pattern	Stimulants, exercise, excitement, lung disease or other medical cause (ie, anxiety, asthma, choking, chronic obstructive pulmonary disease, heart failure, or pulmonary embolus)
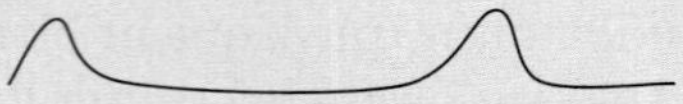	Bradypnea	Decreased respiratory rate, regular pattern	Opioids, sedatives, alcohol, pneumonia, sleep apnea, carbon monoxide exposure, traumatic brain injury
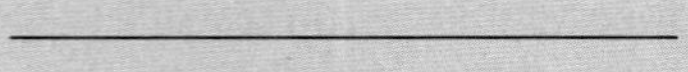	Apnea	Absence of breathing	Severe hypoxia, depressants, head injury, heart attack, irregular heartbeat, metabolic disorders (ie, chemical, mineral, or acid–base imbalance), submersion, stroke
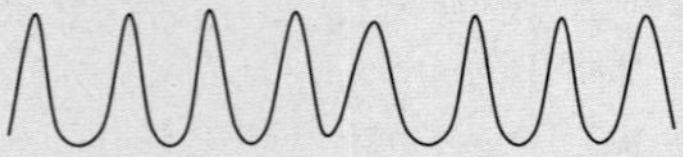	Hyperpnea	Rapid, regular, deep respirations	Stimulants, overdose, exercise
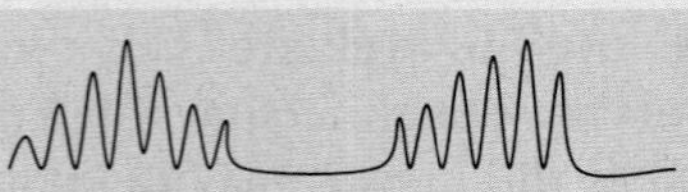	Cheyne-Stokes respirations	Gradual increase in respiratory rate and depth, followed by a gradual decrease with intermittent periods of apnea	Pre-death pattern, brainstem injury, brain herniation syndrome
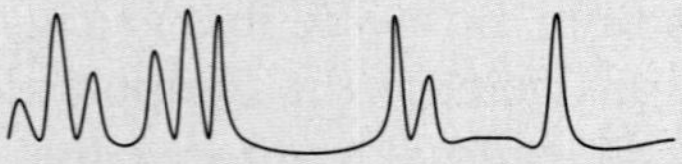	Biot/ataxic respirations	Irregular pattern, rate, and depth of respirations with periods of apnea	Brainstem injury, increased intracranial pressure
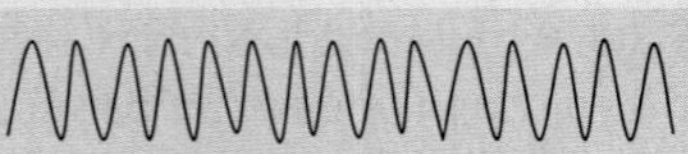	Kussmaul respirations	Deep, gasping respirations (extreme tachypnea and hyperpnea)	Acidosis Diabetic ketoacidosis
	Apneustic respirations	Prolonged inspiratory phase with shortened expiratory phase and bradypnea	Brainstem injury

signs monitoring **FIGURE 11-18**. Typically, administration of supplemental oxygen is a consideration for symptomatic patients (those with signs of hypoxia) who have an Spo_2 of less than 94%. Although pulse oximetry is a valuable tool, it should not be used as an absolute indicator of the need for oxygen therapy. Pulse oximetry measures the percentage of hemoglobin saturation and can be inaccurate in certain situations. You must know the limitations of pulse oximetry to appropriately process

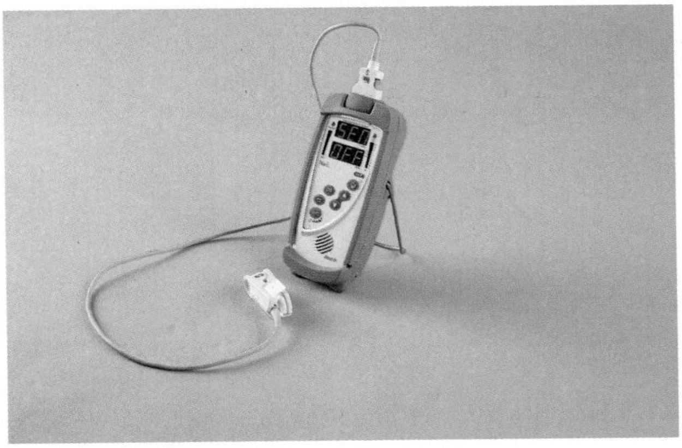

FIGURE 11-18 A pulse oximeter.

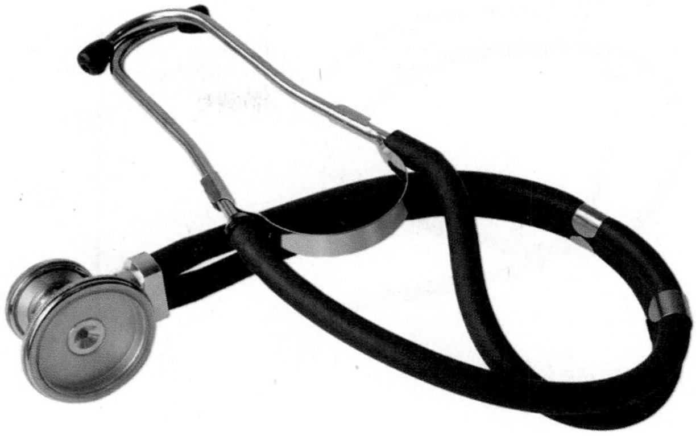

FIGURE 11-19 A stethoscope.

the information it provides. Inaccurate readings may be obtained for a variety of reasons, including hypotension, hypothermia, carbon monoxide poisoning, sickle cell disease, anemia, vascular dyes, patient motion, incorrect placement, and even certain types of nail polish.

Words of Wisdom

Look at the patient, not the number. If the patient looks sick but the pulse oximetry reading is normal, then the patient is still sick.

Equipment Used in the Secondary Assessment

Equipment used to perform the secondary assessment includes a stethoscope, **sphygmomanometer** (ie, BP cuff), pulse oximeter, capnography and glucometry equipment, reflex hammer, reliable light source, gloves, and a sheet or blanket.

Stethoscopes are available in two forms: acoustic and electronic **FIGURE 11-19**. The acoustic stethoscope does not amplify sounds; rather, it simply blocks out ambient noises, allowing you to hear and appreciate the sounds of the body. An electronic stethoscope converts acoustic sound waves into an electronic signal that is then amplified.

Today's acoustic stethoscope, which is the device most commonly seen in the prehospital setting, consists of two earpieces attached to an air-filled tube connected to a chest piece. The chest piece has two sides, a diaphragm (plastic disk) and a bell (hollow cup), either of which can be placed against the patient to sense sounds. The diaphragm is vibrated by the sounds of the body, which are then transmitted up to the stethoscope's earpieces; thus, the diaphragm side is used to pick up higher-frequency sounds. The bell, which usually transmits lower-frequency sounds, senses the sounds directly off the skin of the patient. Some stethoscopes have attenuated diaphragms, meaning they have an outer metal ring and another ring closer to the center of the head. Pushing lightly on the head allows you to listen to one set of sounds while pressing firmly seats the diaphragm against the inner ring, allowing you to hear a different set of sounds.

Words of Wisdom

There are important differences between the bell and the diaphragm of a stethoscope. The cup-shaped bell is used to listen for deep and low-pitched sounds (heart sounds). It is placed lightly on the skin, just enough to form a seal. The flat diaphragm is used to listen for high-pitched sounds (breath, bowel, and normal heart sounds); it is placed firmly on the skin.

A sphygmomanometer, or BP cuff, measures BP **FIGURE 11-20**. The traditional device consists of an inflatable cuff, which occludes blood flow, and a manometer (pressure meter), which is used to determine the pressure in the artery. These two components are connected by tubing. In manual cuffs, a separate tube is attached to an inflation bulb. Bladderless BP cuffs are also available, but they can be uncomfortable against bare skin.

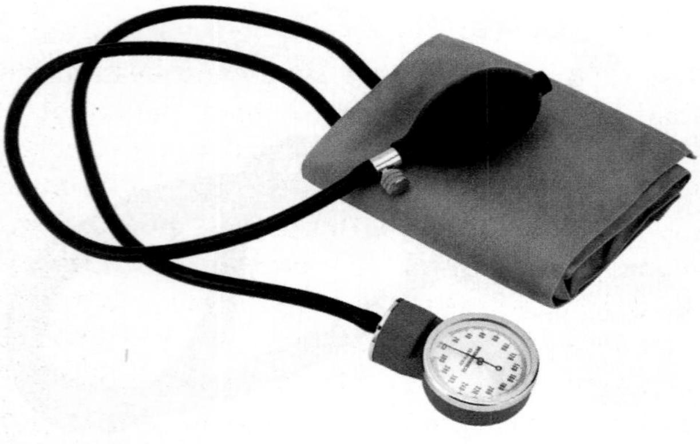

FIGURE 11-20 A sphygmomanometer.

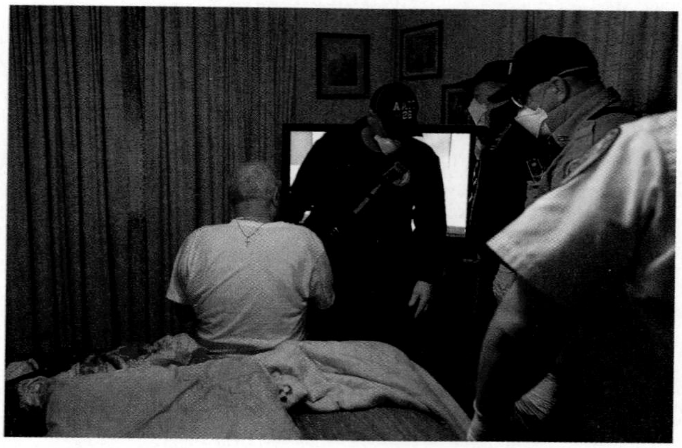

FIGURE 11-21 Get a general impression of the overall situation as you approach the patient.

The **ophthalmoscope** allows you to examine a patient's eyes and view the retina and aqueous fluid. An **otoscope** is used to evaluate a patient's ears. These two devices are rarely used in paramedicine. Chapter 20, *Diseases of the Eyes, Ears, Nose, and Throat,* discusses assessment of these anatomic structures in detail.

Controversies

Ultrasonography, including the focused assessment with sonography in trauma (FAST) exam, represents cutting-edge prehospital medical care. This technology can be used to quickly evaluate patients to decide if they require transport to a trauma center. However, the cost of equipment and training is significant, and many services' medical directors have opted against making this investment pending sufficient research evidence demonstrating prehospital ultrasonography's benefits.[18] Thus, this intervention has not yet become mainstream paramedic practice. Medical directors may choose to train their system's paramedics and authorize protocols for FAST exams, but it is crucial that application of this skill never delay the transport of a trauma patient to the regional trauma center.

The Physical Exam

The physical exam of a patient in the prehospital setting is the most important skill a health care provider can master. Establishing vascular access, administering medications, and performing endotracheal intubation are skills that require extensive practice to achieve proficiency. By comparison, the skills of assessing a patient and interpreting the findings of a physical exam truly separate the accomplished paramedic from the novice. The physical exam consists of a review of systems to determine the nature and extent of the patient's illness or injury.

As soon as you approach the scene, you will have already begun to gather information about the patient's overall presentation **FIGURE 11-21**. A patient lying on the ground on a rainy, cool evening, for instance, should be considered hypothermic until proven otherwise. A quick look at the environment in which patient is found and their general appearance provides a substantial amount of information before you even begin to ask questions.

Look for signs of significant distress, such as mental status changes, anxiousness, labored breathing, difficulty speaking, diaphoresis, obvious pain, obvious deformity, and guarding or splinting of a painful area. It is not uncommon for people experiencing substantial and incapacitating pain to present with a quiet and still affect.

Other aspects that may be readily apparent and worth noting include dress, hygiene, expression, overall size, posture, foul or unusual odors, and overall state of health. As you characterize the patient's overall state, use the appropriate terms to describe the degree of distress: no apparent distress, mild (slight or not harsh), moderate (small or average), acute (very great or bad), and severe (dangerous or difficult to endure). Other acceptable terms to describe the general state of a patient's

Street Smarts

Many technological devices are available to EMS personnel to aid in patient assessment. Although this equipment is considered to have excellent performance, always remember you are assessing a patient, not a machine. Take time to explain what your tools are and why you are using them. This simple action may help lessen a patient's anxiety. Also know how to take measurements manually (eg, BP) before you start relying on machines!

health include chronically ill, frail, feeble, robust, and vigorous.

The secondary assessment should be driven by the information you gathered during the primary survey and the history-taking phase. For a patient who tells you, "I . . . just can't . . . catch my . . . breath," early assessment of breath sounds is a must. If the patient tells you, "My leg feels numb," assessment of pulse, motor function, and sensation in the affected and unaffected extremities is indicated. Exercise good judgment to make the best use of your time. Do not waste time palpating a patient's abdomen or auscultating heart sounds if the patient reports knee pain. In general, the care you provide for a responsive medical patient will be driven by your local protocols in conjunction with your consultation with the base station physician.

The Full-Body Exam

The **full-body exam** is a systematic head-to-toe exam. Like the rapid full-body scan, the full-body exam includes inspection, palpation, and auscultation. It also includes percussion and clearly takes more time to complete. This process aims to identify hidden injuries or other problems you may not have found during the primary survey. Any patient who has sustained a significant MOI, is unresponsive, or is in critical condition should receive this type of exam. An unresponsive patient cannot tell you what's wrong; therefore, this type of exam may give you clues to identify the problem. Based on the severity of the patient's condition, this exam is often performed en route to the ED.

To perform a full-body exam of a patient with no suspected spinal injuries, follow the steps in **SKILL DRILL 11-3**. To perform a full-body exam when the patient has sustained significant trauma, ensure manual stabilization is still in place and follow the steps in Skill Drill 11-3.

A **focused exam**, sometimes called a focused assessment, is generally performed on patients who have sustained insignificant MOIs and on responsive medical patients. This type of exam is based on the chief complaint. The most common complaints from responsive medical patients involve the head, heart, lungs, or abdomen, individually or in combination.

Skill Drill 11-3 Performing the Full-Body Exam

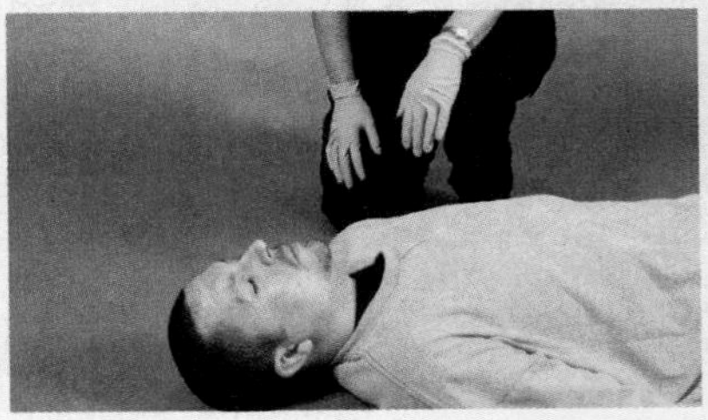

Step 1

Examine the face for obvious lacerations, bruises, fluids, and deformities.

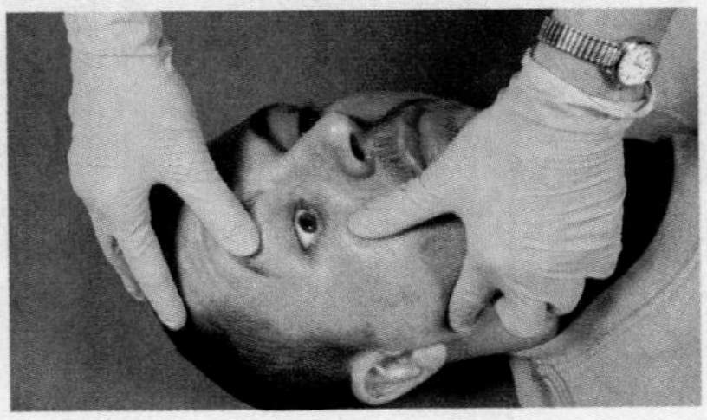

Step 2

Inspect the area around the eyes and eyelids.

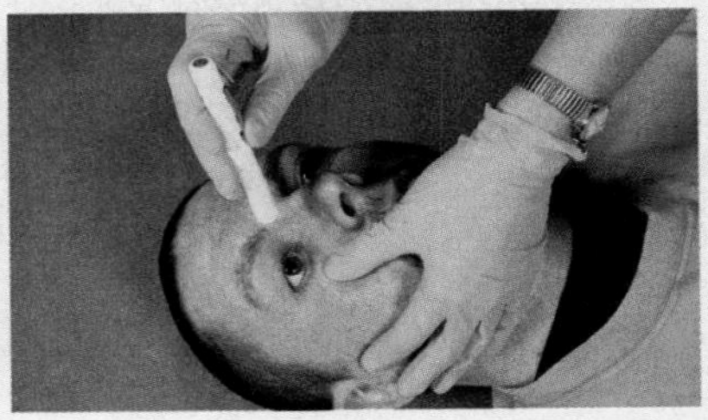

Step 3

Examine the eyes for redness and for contact lenses. Use a penlight to assess the pupils.

(continues)

Skill Drill 11-3 Performing the Full-Body Exam (continued)

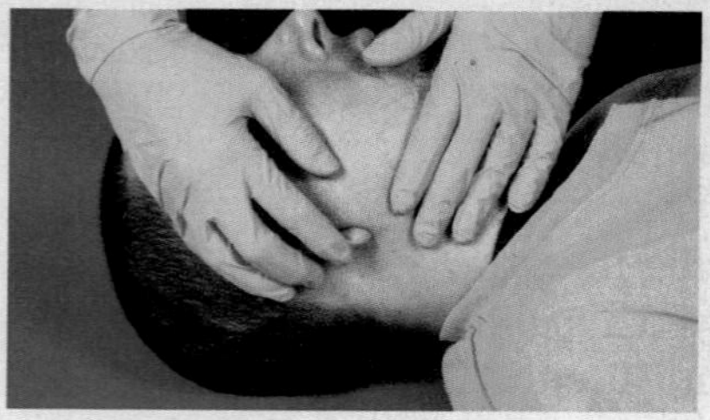

Step 4

Look behind the ears for bruising (Battle sign).

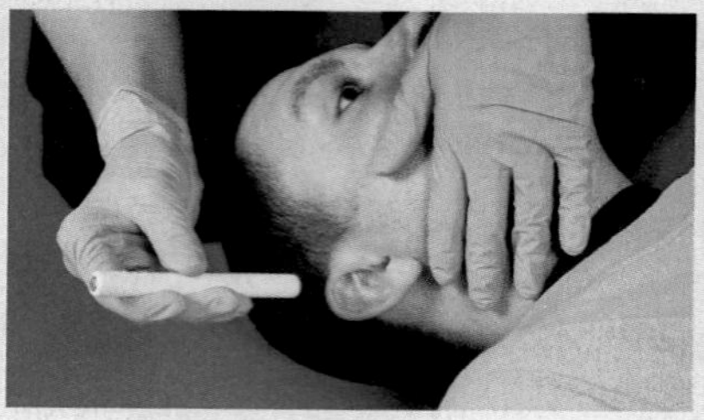

Step 5

Use the penlight to look for drainage of cerebrospinal fluid (CSF) or blood in the ears.

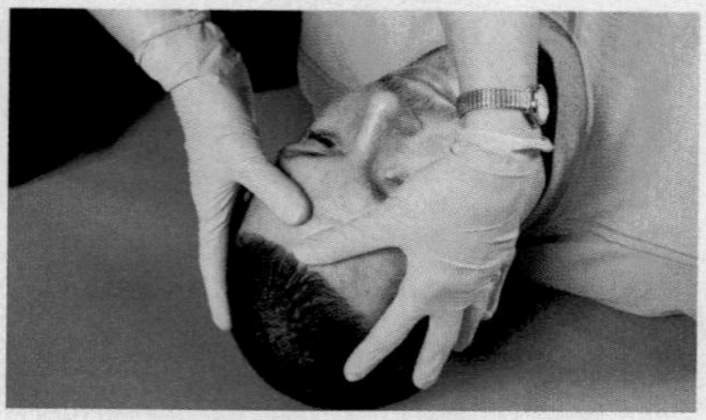

Step 6

Examine the head for bruising and lacerations. Palpate for tenderness, skull depressions, and deformities.

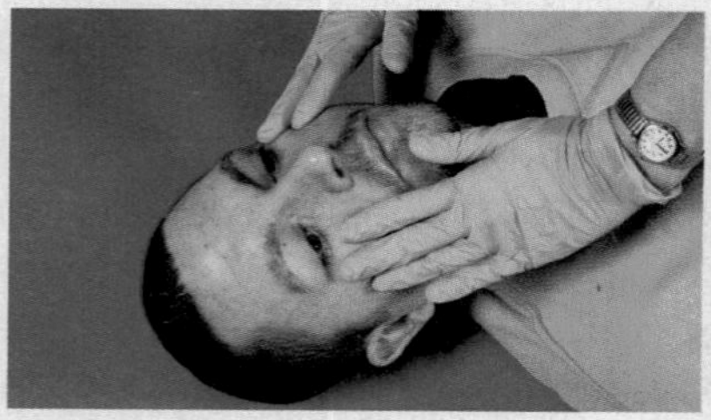

Step 7

Palpate the zygomas for tenderness, symmetry, and instability.

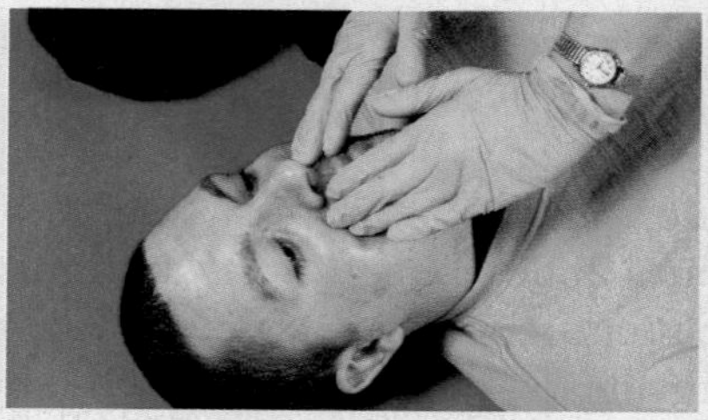

Step 8

Palpate the maxillae.

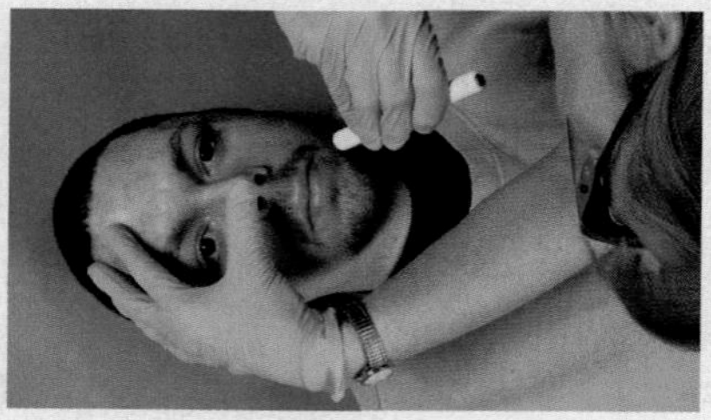

Step 9

Check the nose for blood and drainage.

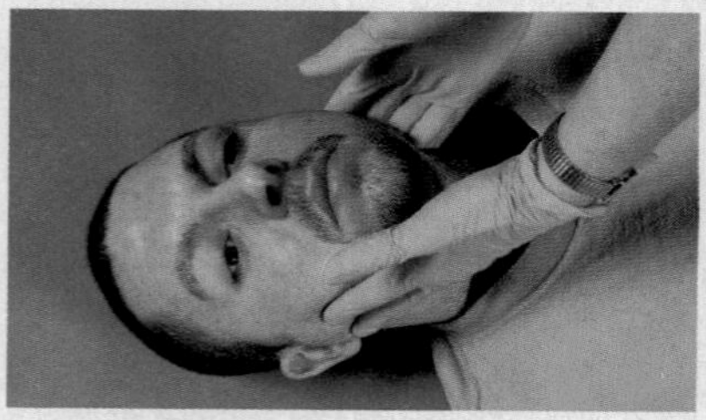

Step 10

Palpate the mandible.

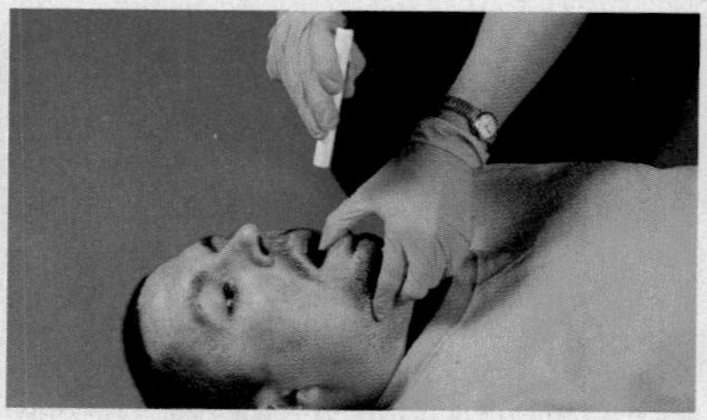

Step 11

Assess the mouth and nose for cyanosis, foreign bodies (including loose or broken teeth or dentures), bleeding, lacerations, and deformities.

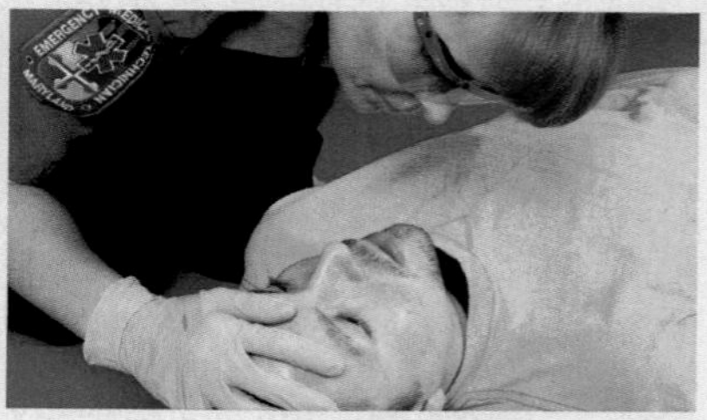

Step 12

Check for unusual odors on the patient's breath.

Skill Drill 11-3 Performing the Full-Body Exam (continued)

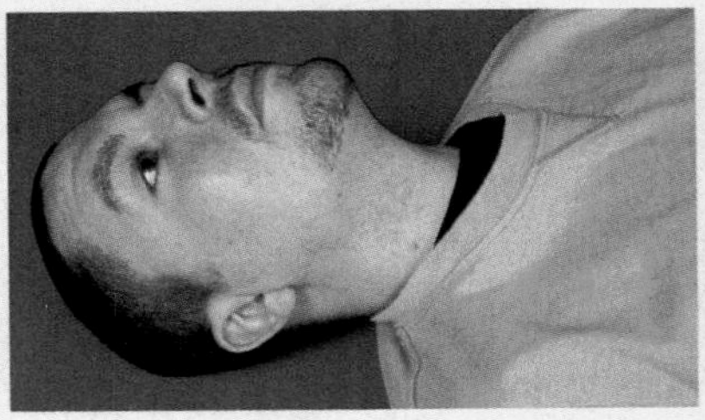

Step 13

Inspect the neck for obvious lacerations, bruises, and deformities. Observe for JVD and palpate for tracheal deviation.

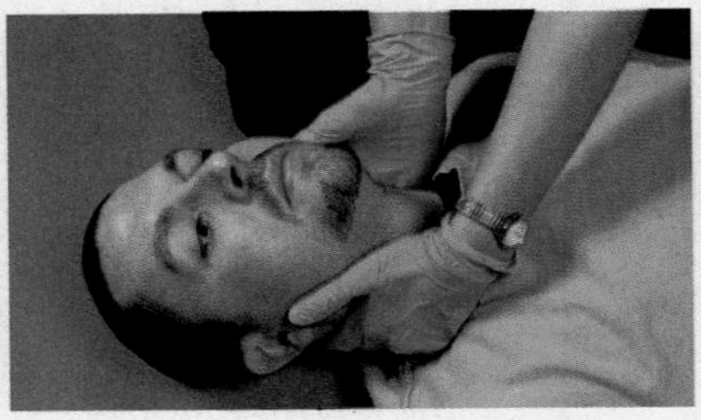

Step 14

Palpate the front and the back of the neck for tenderness and deformity.

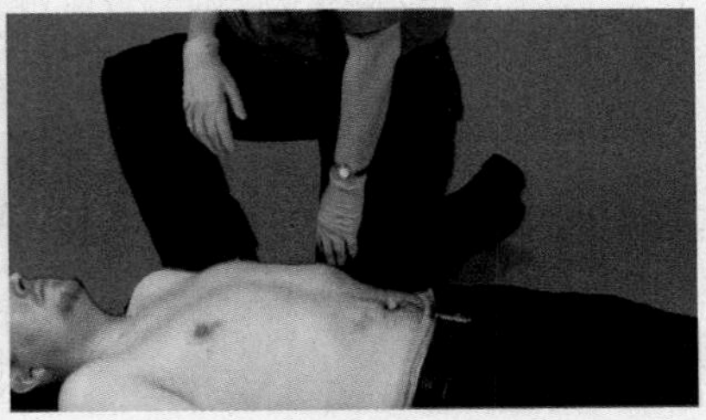

Step 15

Inspect the chest for obvious signs of injury before you begin palpation. Watch for movement of the chest with respiration. Assess the work of breathing.

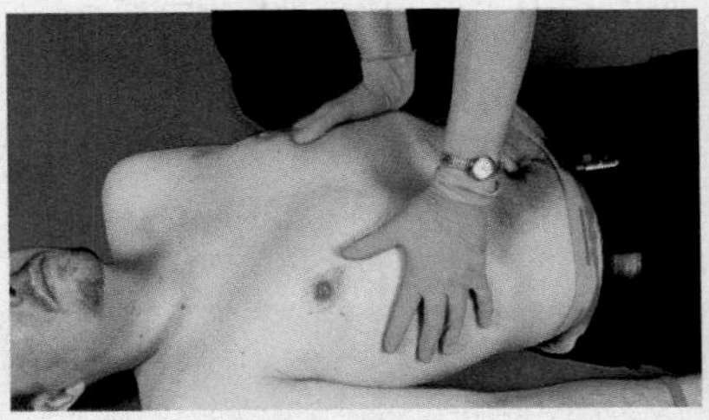

Step 16

Gently palpate over the ribs to assess structural integrity and elicit tenderness. Avoid pressing over obvious bruises and fractures.

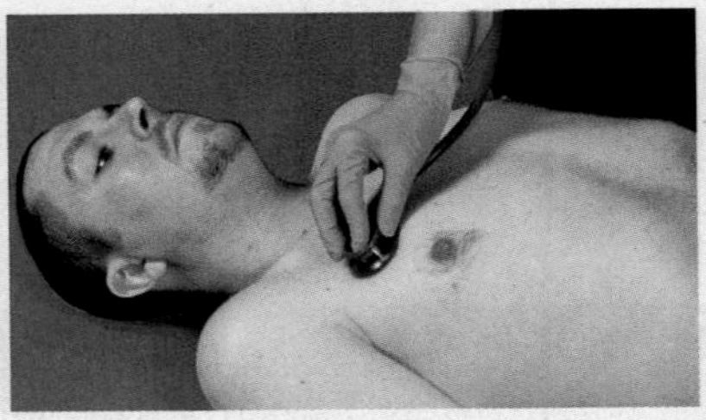

Step 17

Listen for breath sounds over the midaxillary and midclavicular lines—a minimum of four fields if you are checking the anterior chest, and six fields if you are assessing the posterior chest.

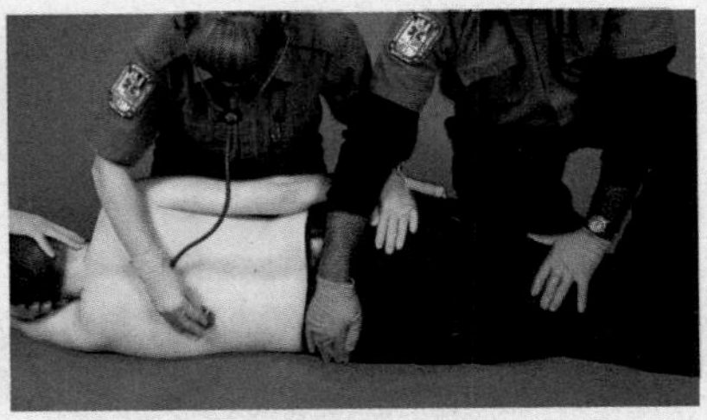

Step 18

Assess the lung bases and apexes. At this point, also assess the back for tenderness and deformities, so that you log roll the patient only once. Remember, if you suspect a spinal cord injury, use spinal precautions as you log roll the patient.

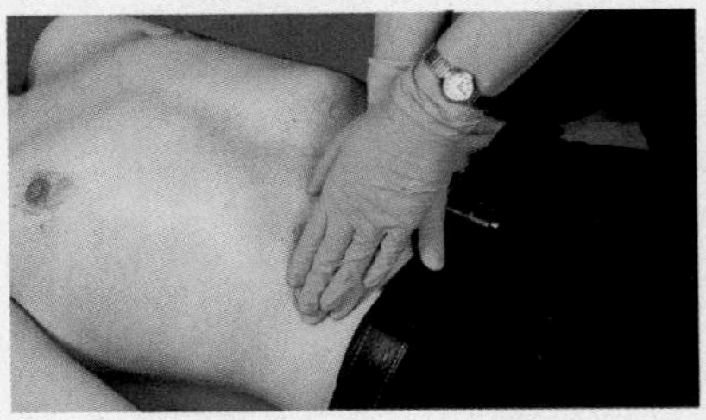

Step 19

Look for obvious laceration, bruising, and deformity of the abdomen and pelvis. Gently palpate the abdomen for tenderness. Palpate the quadrant diagonal from where any pain is located. If the patient indicates their pain is localized to one quadrant, palpate that area last. The contraction of abdominal muscles in response to palpation is seen with underlying conditions such as appendicitis and is described as "guarding." When the contraction persists throughout the abdominal musculature, the abdomen is described as "rigid," a condition seen with severe abdominal inflammation such as peritonitis.

(continues)

Skill Drill 11-3 Performing the Full-Body Exam (continued)

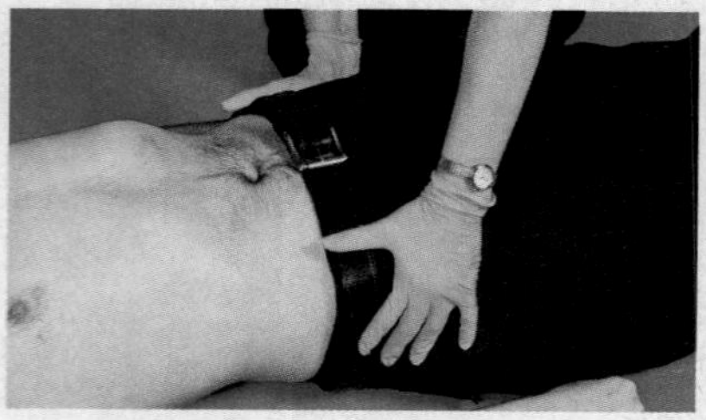

Step 20

Gently compress the pelvis from the sides to assess for tenderness.

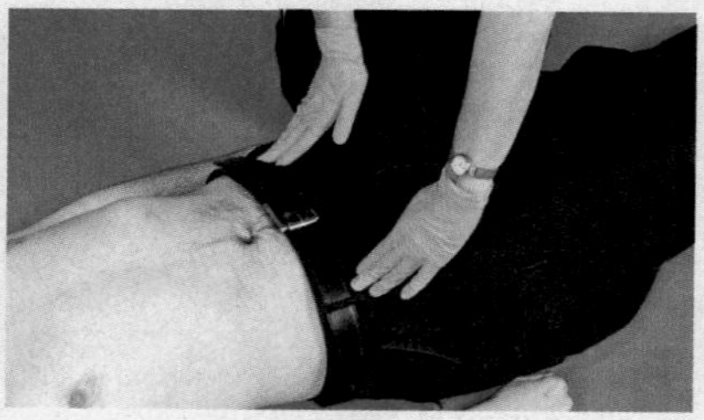

Step 21

Gently press the iliac crests to elicit instability, tenderness, and/or crepitus.

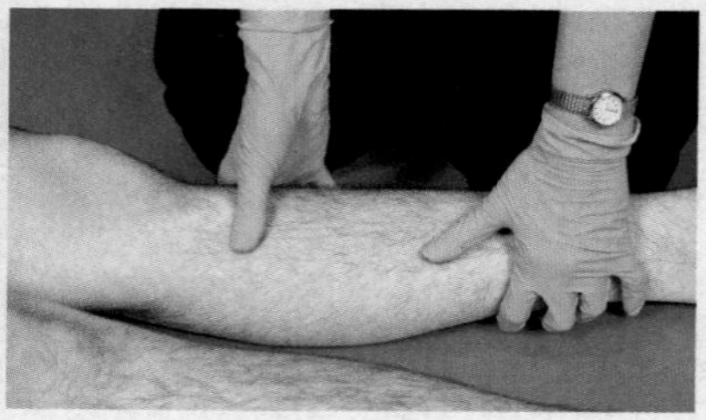

Step 22

Inspect all four extremities for any lacerations, bruises, swelling, deformities, or medical alert jewelry. Also, assess distal pulses and motor and sensory functions in all extremities. Compare the right and left sides whenever possible.

TABLE 11-7 Common Chief Complaints and Focused Exams

Chief Complaint	Focused Exam
Chest pain	Evaluate the skin, pulse, and BP. Look for trauma to the chest, assess the external jugular veins, and listen to breath sounds. Assess for pedal/dependent edema. Obtain a 12-lead ECG.
Abdominal pain	Evaluate the skin, pulse, and BP. Look for trauma to the abdomen, and palpate the abdomen for tenderness or rigidity.
Shortness of breath	Evaluate the skin, pulse, BP, and rate and depth of respiration. Assess for airway obstruction. Listen carefully to breath sounds, and assess for hypoxemia (ie, use pulse oximetry). Assess for pedal/dependent edema. Obtain a 12-lead ECG.
Dizziness	Evaluate the skin, pulse, BP, and adequacy of respiration. Monitor level of consciousness and orientation carefully. Check the head for signs of trauma. Evaluate for signs of stroke (ie, facial droop, slurred speech, and weakness on one side). Check for a history of inner ear problems. Assess blood glucose level. Obtain an ECG.
Any pain associated with bones or joints	Evaluate the skin, pulse, movement, and sensation adjacent and distal to the affected area.

Abbreviations: BP, blood pressure; ECG, electrocardiogram

For example, if a patient reports a headache, carefully and systematically assess the head and/or the neurologic system. In contrast, a patient with an arm laceration may need to have only that arm evaluated. The goal of a focused exam is to focus your attention on the immediate complaint. **TABLE 11-7** gives examples of common chief complaints and corresponding focused exams.

Mental Status

For patients with head-related symptoms (ie, confusion, headache, AMS), assess and palpate the head to look for signs of trauma. Check for facial asymmetry, such as facial droop or other signs of a suspected stroke. Dilated or constricted pupils may indicate recreational drug use, whereas red conjunctivae may suggest drug or alcohol use. Elevated BP often accompanies a headache, possibly secondary to hypertension.

Special Populations

Clearly, a child or infant will respond differently during the mental status exam than an adult would, so the mental status of pediatric patients may be difficult to evaluate. Therefore, a modified assessment should be used for these patients. First, determine whether the child is alert. Even infants should be alert to your presence and should follow you with their eyes (a process called "tracking"). Ask the parent whether the child is behaving normally, particularly concerning alertness. Most children older than 2 years know their names and the names of their parents and siblings. Evaluate mental status in school-age children by asking about holidays, recent school activities, or teachers' names. This issue is addressed in Chapter 44, *Pediatric Emergencies*.

Evaluate a patient's mental status by assessing cognitive function (ability to use reasoning). At a minimum, evaluate the patient's degree of alertness. Use the AVPU scale, as described in the Primary Survey section, to help identify the patient's LOC. Test the patient's blood glucose using a glucometer if there is AMS, especially if the patient has a history of diabetes. The steps for using a glucometer are shown in **SKILL DRILL 11-4**.

You can further assess mental status by considering whether the patient is alert and oriented (A × O) in four areas—person, place, time, and the event itself—and by determining the GCS score, as discussed previously in this chapter. Assessing whether the patient can recall their name tests long-term memory, whereas assessing whether the patient knows where they are and what happened tests short-term memory.

Once the basic mental status has been assessed, conduct a thorough mental status exam, especially in patients experiencing a behavioral emergency. This exam begins by assessing the patient's general appearance, including posture, facial expression, and ability to relax. Does the posture change with discussion topics, activities, or as certain people draw near the patient? A tense posture, restlessness, and fidgeting suggest the patient may be anxious, while a slumped posture and slow movements might indicate underlying depression. Observe the patient's face, both at rest and as they interact with others. Watch for variations in expression with topics of discussion. Are the facial expressions appropriate? A relatively immobile face (ie, a patient who does not blink, or whose face appears to be frozen in a stare) throughout the exam may indicate Parkinson disease.

Note the patient's speech and language patterns. Pay attention to the quantity, rate, volume, articulation, and fluency of speech. Alterations in language suggest an underlying psychiatric or central nervous system (CNS) disease.

Ask the patient about their mood. This is an objective statement similar to the chief complaint. Simply asking, "How do you feel?" may elicit an appropriate response; however, more direct questioning regarding mood might be needed. All patients should be asked about suicidal ideation. Any patient who expresses thoughts of suicide should be evaluated at an appropriate facility.

Assessing the patient's thoughts and perceptions is an important part of the complete mental status exam. Assess the logic, relevance, organization, and coherence of the patient's thoughts simply by listening to their conversation. Listen for irregularities such as abrupt shifting of the conversation from one subject to another, invented or distorted words, and largely incomprehensible speech, which may indicate an underlying disorder such as schizophrenia. The patient's perceptions deal with senses. Ask your patient if they sometimes hear, see, or feel things others do not, even when no one else is there. Patients who answer "yes" to any of these questions may be experiencing hallucinations related to an underlying psychiatric illness or CNS disorder.

Listen for thought content that suggests phobias, obsessions, anxieties, or delusions. Delusions are false, fixed, personal beliefs not shared by most other members of the patient's culture. It is essential that any observations made regarding the patient's thought content be relayed to the ED.

Skill Drill 11-4 Using a Glucometer to Assess Blood Glucose Level

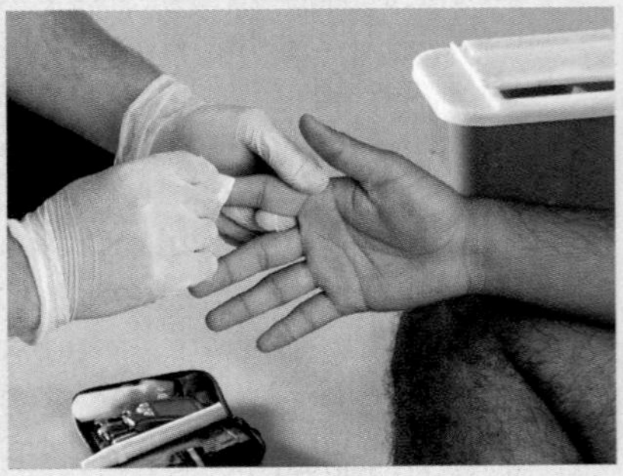

Step 1

Identify the need to obtain a blood glucose level, normal parameters for blood glucose level, contraindications, and possible complications. Take standard precautions. Clearly explain the procedure to the patient. Select, check, and assemble the equipment (glucometer, test strip, needle or spring-loaded puncture device, alcohol prep pads). Turn on the glucometer and insert a test strip. Cleanse the patient's fingertip with an alcohol prep pad.

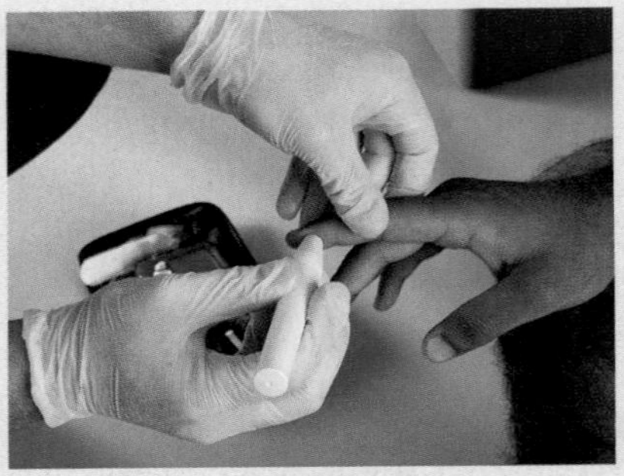

Step 2

Puncture the prepped site with the lancet needle or puncture device, drawing capillary blood.

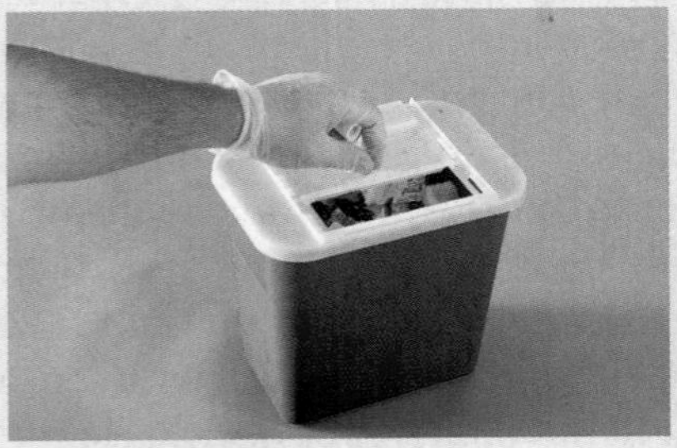

Step 3

Dispose of the lancet needle in a sharps container.

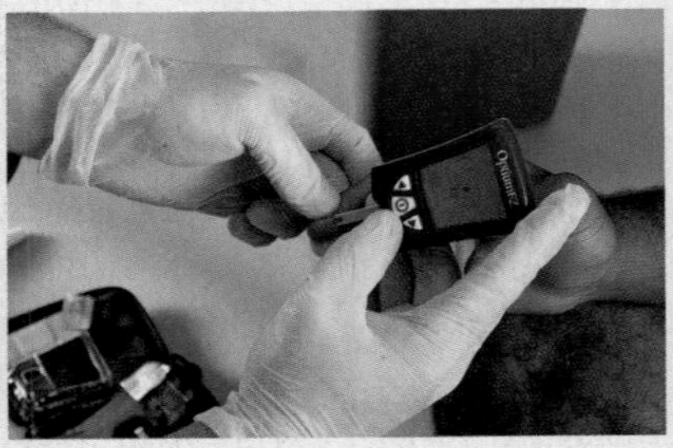

Step 4

Insert the test strip into the glucometer, express a blood sample, transfer it to the test strip, and activate the device per the manufacturer's instructions.

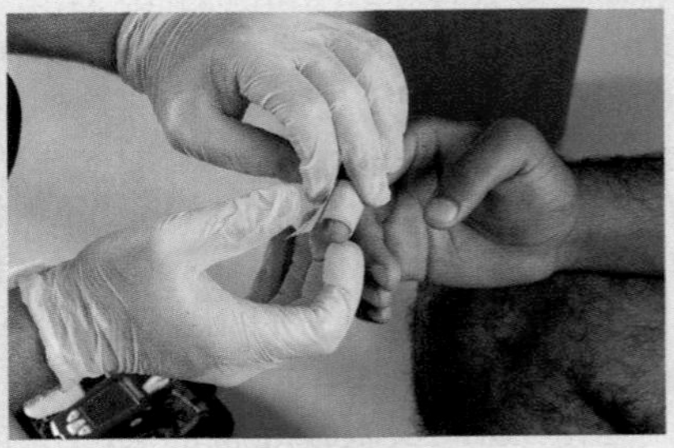

Step 5

Dress the fingertip wound with pressure and an alcohol prep pad, then place a bandage over the puncture site. Record the reading from the glucometer and document it appropriately.

Assess the patient's insight and judgment. Insight shows the patient's awareness of their illness and need for treatment. You can simply ask, "What do you think is wrong?" Some patients may respond by saying, "I'm depressed, and I know I need to get help." This demonstrates that the patient has positive insight into their illness. Other patients may believe it is normal to hear nonexistent voices and feel they do not need treatment. These patients are considered to be lacking insight.

You can usually assess judgment by noting the patient's response to questions about family and interpersonal conflict, jobs, and use of money. For example, you can ask, "Who's going to look after your home while you're in the hospital?" Any inappropriate response may indicate delirium, dementia, a developmental delay, or a psychotic state.

Finally, a complete mental status exam includes further assessing the patient's cognitive function. This assessment is usually not done in the field by paramedics, as this exam might be difficult to interpret without a scoring sheet and adjusted for education level.

Words of Wisdom

In cases of potential head injury, a specific scoring sheet, requiring additional training to implement, is sometimes used. Following this sheet, you would assess the patient's attention, memory, and learning ability. There are several ways to assess the patient's attention: two methods commonly used are *serial 7s* and *spelling backward*. Serial 7s is conducted by having the patient start at 100, subtract 7, and continue subtracting 7. Note the patient's effort, speed, and accuracy. Spelling backward is another way to assess attention. Ask the patient to spell a five-letter word, such as W-O-R-L-D, forward and then backward. Once again, note the patient's effort, speed, and accuracy.

To assess memory, begin by assessing remote memory, such as birthdays, anniversaries, schools attended, and jobs held. It can be difficult to assess the accuracy of remote memory if there is no one available to confirm the patient's answers; thus, this method is not always the most accurate assessment tool. Next, inquire about the patient's recent memory. This could involve the events of the day. For example, ask the patient which medications they took today and what they ate for breakfast. As with the remote memory test, someone must be available to confirm the accuracy of the patient's answers. Finally, assess the patient's memory recall by giving them three or four words to remember, such as *ball, key,* and *lawnmower*. Ask the patient to recite the words 3 to 5 minutes later.

Skin, Hair, and Nails

Skin Perhaps the quickest and most reliable initial way to evaluate a patient's overall degree of distress is to look at the skin. Relatively subtle but serious changes in overall circulation usually manifest early on in the skin's appearance.

In a cold environment, blood vessel constriction shunts blood away from the skin to decrease the amount of heat loss through radiation from the body surface (observed as pallor or mottled skin). When the environment is hot, the blood vessels dilate, the skin becomes flushed or red, and heat loss occurs as it radiates from the body surface. Also, in a hot environment, sweat is secreted by sweat glands and carried to the skin surface by tiny ducts. A loss of energy, in the form of body heat, occurs during the evaporation process, which causes body temperature to fall. Notably, at a humidity level of more than 85%, evaporation does not work.

Special Populations

When assessing skin turgor in an older patient, use the skin of the upper chest. This is a much more reliable indicator than the skin on the extremities.

Examine the skin by both inspection and palpation. Pay careful attention to the skin's CTC: color, temperature, and condition (moisture or texture). Also note **turgor** and any significant lesions or obvious deformities. Look for evidence of diminished perfusion, evaluate for pallor and cyanosis, and be wary of diaphoresis. In patients with dark skin, you will need to rely on the color of the conjunctivae for signs of shock. Reddened or pink skin can be seen in a variety of normal states, but is also evident in states of relative **vasodilation** (flushing). Flushed skin is usually apparent in patients with fever, and it may be seen in patients experiencing an allergic process. Reddened skin should also be considered in the context of superficial burns.

Words of Wisdom

Always be alert for signs of possible abuse or maltreatment as you inspect the skin. Multiple bruises at different stages of healing or even pressure sores should raise concerns about possible physical abuse or neglect, and should be reported. Fingerprint bruises (ie, bruises caused by being grabbed, lifted, or dragged) should always make you suspicious.

Some medical conditions and folk medicine practices may be mistaken for abuse. For example, Mongolian spots are benign and not associated with any conditions or illnesses. Ehlers-Danlos syndrome is a condition associated with cuts, bruises, and scars attributable to the fragility of the patient's skin. Blood disorders such as hemophilia, von Willebrand disease, and leukemia can also cause skin changes similar to those seen in abuse situations.

Examining the skin for changes in perfusion is usually best accomplished in areas in which the epidermis is thinnest, such as the fingernails, lips, and conjunctivae. It is sometimes useful to examine the palms and soles as well. Pallor occurs when red blood cell perfusion to the capillary beds of the skin is poor. You may also be able to detect pallor by looking at the patient's lips or the conjunctivae of the eyes. Pallor is a relatively common finding in seriously ill patients and may indicate severe **vasoconstriction**, as seen in profound anemia, acute cardiovascular events, other shocklike states, and hypothermia. Local areas of blanched, cool, white skin are typical of frostbite.

Words of Wisdom

The word *pale*, as used in this text, may apply to any patient whose skin presentation suggests reduced blood flow or oxygenation. In patients with light skin, pallor typically presents as unusual lightness compared with the person's baseline skin color. In patients with dark skin, pallor may appear as ashen or gray skin on general assessment. In general, the mucous membranes inside the inner lower eyelid and the oral mucosa will have a pink coloration in all healthy patients, regardless of baseline skin color; thus, a white or pale appearance of these areas in any patient suggests reduced blood flow or oxygenation.

Because providers do not necessarily know the patient's baseline skin color, they should consider the observations of friends or family members present at the scene. Simply asking, "Does her skin look like its usual color to you?" may offer useful insight into the patient's condition.

Cyanosis indicates a relative lack of oxygen perfusion, although the number of red blood cells may be adequate to carry any available oxygen. Cyanosis correlates extremely closely with low arterial oxygen saturation. Generally, it can be visualized in the skin, but more specifically in the fingernail beds, face, and lips. Although cyanotic skin is commonly seen in states of oxygen desaturation, it can also be a function of hypothermia, especially in young patients. **Mottling** is a typical finding in states of severe, protracted hypoperfusion and shock and is easily recognized in seriously ill or injured pediatric patients. However, when mottling is seen in a pediatric patient, do not immediately consider the finding "normal." It is important to consider all aspects of the history and physical exam to ensure there is no evidence of hypoperfusion.

Ecchymosis is localized bruising or blood collection within or under the skin. Evaluate large ecchymoses for the possibility of serious underlying soft-tissue, bony, or organ injury. Serious wounds to the head, neck, and torso should also be noted, as well as any evidence of a hemorrhage.

It takes practice to accurately gauge patients' relative perfusion and hydration status. Becoming familiar with the abnormal findings of the skin and mucous membranes is an excellent aid in judging both. Turgor relates directly to hydration. Poor skin turgor is an expression of poorly hydrated skin, with associated **tenting** evident in extreme cases, particularly in young children. Tenting is present when skin slowly retracts, rather than quickly springing back into place, when it is pinched and pulled slightly away from the body. Just a few hours of profuse vomiting and diarrhea can leave an infant seriously dehydrated. Because of normal changes in elastin and connective tissues with advanced age, skin turgor is an insignificant indicator in older adult (geriatric) patients, as is skin that is abnormally dry to the touch.

Pay attention to skin temperature, as it can sometimes prove useful in determining etiologies of different medical conditions (eg, respiratory distress). Sometimes it can help you make a clinical distinction between pneumonia and heart failure accompanied by pulmonary edema.

TABLE 11-8 Abnormal Findings of the Nails

Condition	Findings	Possible Cause
Beau lines	Transverse depressions in nails indicating a period of growth inhibition	Systemic illness, severe infection, or nail injury
Clubbing	The angle between the nail and the nail base approaches or exceeds 180°	Flattening and enlargement of the fingertips is associated with chronic respiratory disease
Psoriasis	Pitting, discoloration, and subungual thickening of the nail	Autoimmune disease
Splinter hemorrhages	Red or brown linear streaks in the nail bed	Bacterial endocarditis or trichinosis
Terry nails	Transverse white bands covering the nail except for the distal tip	Cirrhosis

Examine the skin for lesions. Lesions result from many causes that are often difficult to determine. An accurate description of skin lesions is essential. They may be elevated, flat, or depressed. Lesions may also be categorized as vascular (associated with a blood vessel), infectious, traumatic, or inflammatory. They may result from a localized skin process or represent a manifestation of systemic disease. Examples of common lesions include birthmarks, moles, blisters, ulcers, scars, and warts. Skin lesions may sometimes be the only external evidence of a serious internal injury. Take note of any large areas of ecchymosis, palpable crepitus (palpable fractures), and open wounds. Devastating internal injuries can produce external signs that look relatively benign. Be aware of any body areas hidden by clothing or by devices such as a backboard and head immobilizer. Always visually inspect and manually palpate the patient's back and expose the entire body. Likewise, evaluate the skin for rashes by discreetly examining areas of skin otherwise hidden by clothing.

Hair and Nails Examine the hair by inspection and palpation. In this survey, note the quantity, distribution, and texture of the hair. Recent changes in the growth or loss of hair can indicate an endocrine disorder, such as diabetes, or may be the result of treatment modalities for disease processes, such as chemotherapy or radiation treatment of cancer. Although recent hair loss may be related to a disease process, it can also be normal in older patients.

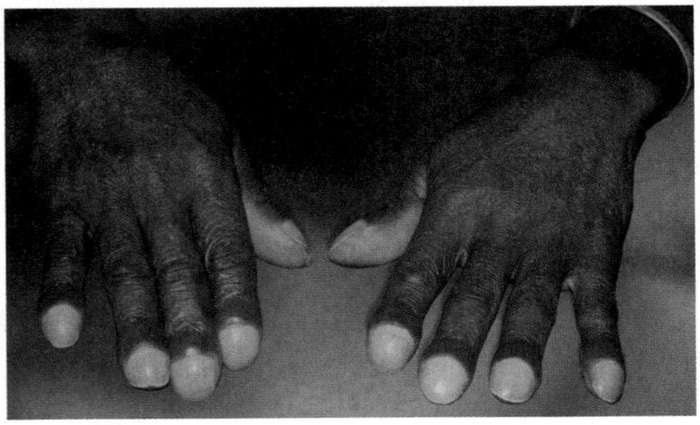

FIGURE 11-22 Clubbing is associated with chronic respiratory disease.

Hair that has been forcibly ripped out often points to an abuse scenario.

Examine the fingernails and toenails to reveal many subtle findings **TABLE 11-8 FIGURE 11-22**. The color, shape, texture, and presence or absence of lesions should all be assessed. The normal nail should be firm and smooth on palpation. Normal changes to the nails with aging include the development of striations and a color change (yellow tint) related to reduction in body calcium. Overly thick nails or nails that have lines running parallel to the finger often suggest a fungal infection.

Head, Eyes, Ears, Nose, and Throat

The head, eyes, ears, nose, and throat (HEENT) exam consists of an evaluation of the head and related structures. It is crucial because the head contains the brain, several sensory organs, and the upper airway anatomy. The eyes are a nervous system structure involving motor pathways (lids, extraocular muscles, pupillary constrictors, corneal blink reflex) and sensory pathways. The ears provide for both hearing and balance control. The nose is a sensory organ involved with the senses of smell and taste; it also plays a vital role in assisting with breathing. The throat consists of the mouth, posterior pharynx, and all the intrinsic structures. This complicated organ simultaneously coordinates many motor and sensory functions, while also coordinating the initial activities of the respiratory and digestive systems.

Head Examine the head by feeling it and inspecting it visually. This step is important in managing (possible) trauma patients, those with AMS, and those who are unresponsive. Inspect and feel the entire cranium for signs of deformity or asymmetry. Do not palpate any depressions; doing so can push bone fragments into the cranial vault or the brain **FIGURE 11-23**. Note any warm, wet areas; they usually represent blood, CSF, or a combination of the two. If you find evidence of external bleeding, attempt to separate the hair manually and irrigate the clot; this should allow you to identify the source of bleeding. Evaluate the skull for any deformity or tenderness. Observe the general shape and contour of the skull. Look for scars or shunts that suggest a history of trauma or problems with the CNS. If you suspect the presence of a cerebral shunt, ask the patient where the shunt was placed and where it drains in the body.

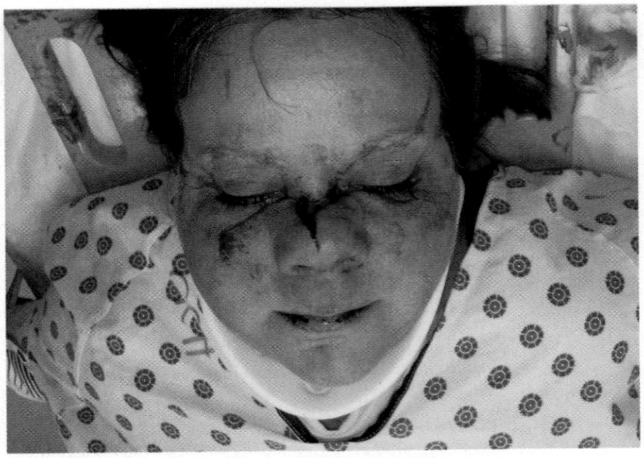

FIGURE 11-23 When examining the head and face, do not palpate any depression in the skin; you could push bone fragments into the cranial vault or brain.

Words of Wisdom

Protecting fragile CNS structures from further damage is vital to the patient's prospects for living a normal life. Lean toward caution and overprotection in assessing and treating possible brain and spinal cord injuries.

As you evaluate the face, assess the color and moisture of the skin, as well as the expression, symmetry, and contour of the face itself. Asymmetry of the face could suggest an underlying nervous system problem, such as a stroke or facial nerve palsy. Also, pay attention to any swelling or apparent areas of injury, and note any signs of respiratory distress. Follow the steps in **SKILL DRILL 11-5** to assess the head.

Eyes The eyes are a tremendously complex sensory organ. They process light stimuli for the brain, so the brain can translate light impulses into visual images. The eyes are a critical link to the CNS, and as such they allow the examiner to more precisely assess the functions of the CNS.

Each eye consists of an anterior chamber and a posterior chamber, which are always assessed in a standardized fashion, from front to back. The outer aspects of the eye are checked first, with deeper structures subsequently evaluated. After you assess the outer eye, assess the patient's **visual acuity**—that is, how well the patient can see,—by examining each eye in isolation. The standard tool for checking visual acuity is the Snellen (E chart) chart **FIGURE 11-24**, although it is not appropriate in the prehospital setting. More appropriate tools in this environment are simple tests, such as light/dark discrimination and finger counting. Reporting on visual acuity must include the distance from which finger counting was measured.

The pupil is a circular opening in the center of the pigmented iris of the eye. The diameter and reactivity of the patient's pupil to light reflect the brain's perfusion status. The pupils are normally round and of approximately equal size; they serve as optical diaphragms, adjusting their size to

Skill Drill 11-5 Assessing the Head

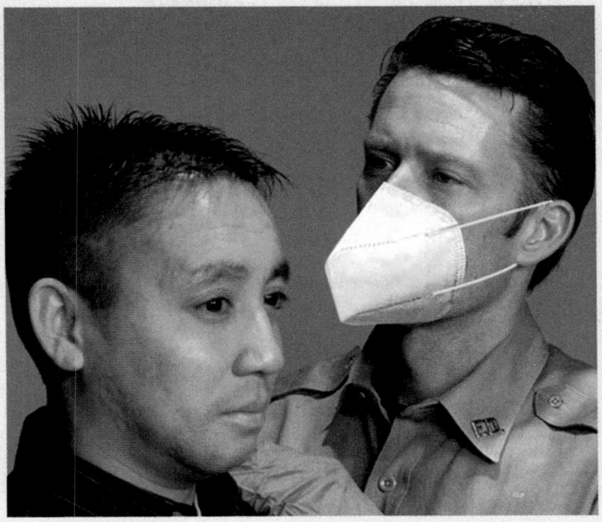

Step 1

Inspect and palpate the head for open/closed findings and crepitus.

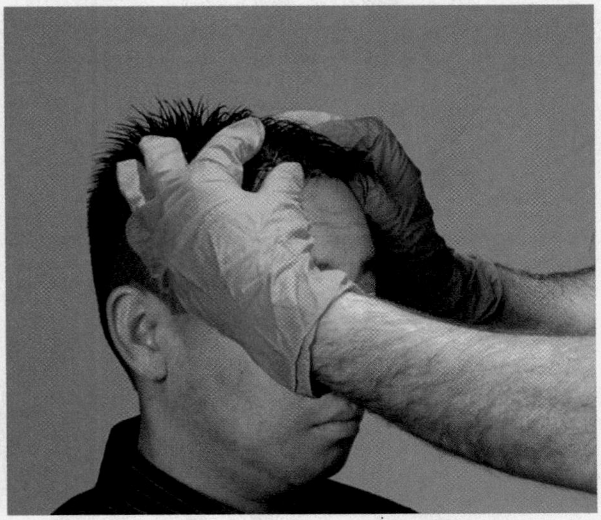

Step 2

Palpate the top and back of the head to locate any subtle abnormalities. Use a systematic approach, going from front to back, to ensure nothing is missed.

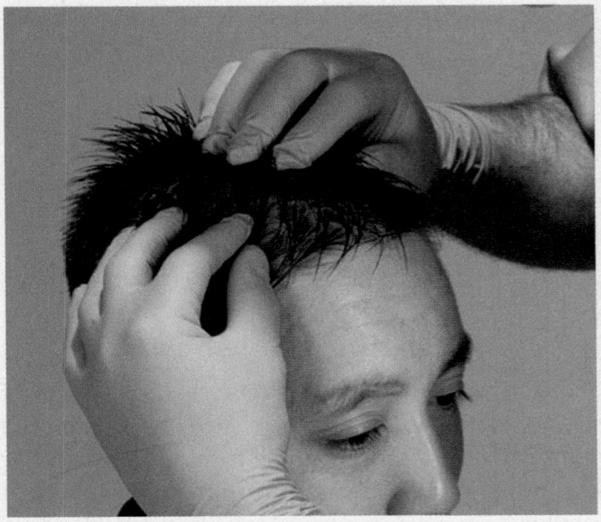

Step 3

Part the hair in several places to examine the condition of the scalp. Identify any lesions beneath the hair.

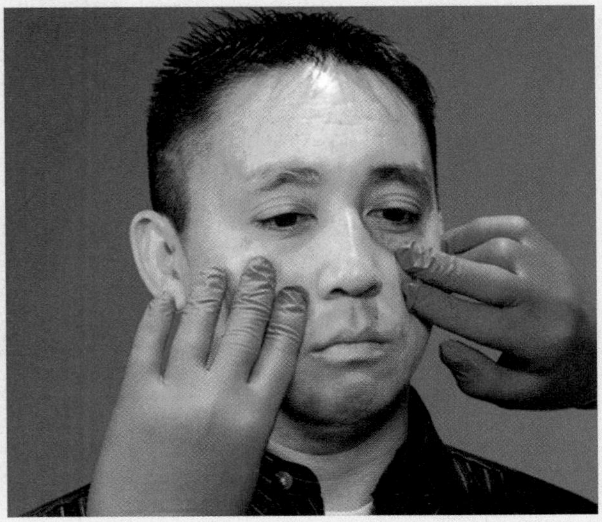

Step 4

Palpate the structure of the face. Note any open/closed findings and crepitus. Pay attention to the condition of the skin, hair distribution, and the shape of the face.

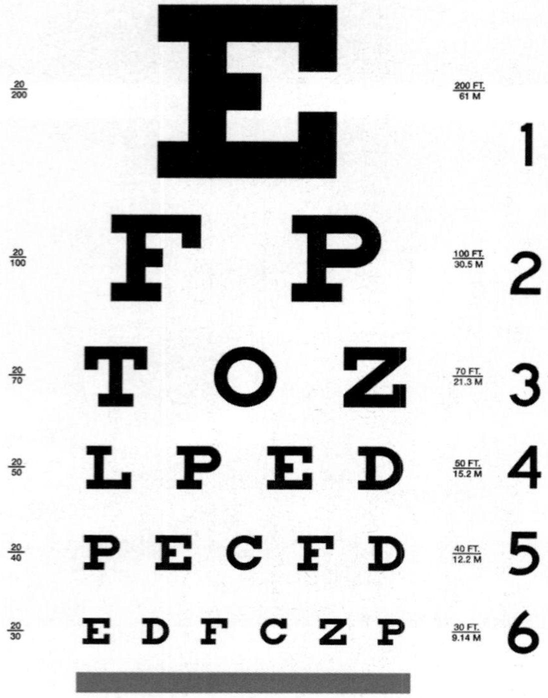

FIGURE 11-24 Because of its size and complexity, the Snellen chart is not a good prehospital tool.

> **Words of Wisdom**
>
> Failure of the eyes to track in a certain direction indicates weakness of an extraocular muscle or dysfunction of the cranial nerve innervating it. Cataracts appear as opaque black areas against the red reflex.

> **Words of Wisdom**
>
> Use of an ophthalmoscope requires frequent practice. This device is not used in the traditional prehospital care setting, but may be used in situations where paramedics have received *significant* additional training and are working in an expanded scope setting.

accommodate available light. The pupils will become fully relaxed and dilated in the absence of light. In normal room light, the pupils appear to be midsize. With high light levels or when a bright light is suddenly introduced, the pupils instantly constrict, allowing less light to enter, thereby protecting the sensitive receptor cells at the back of the eye.

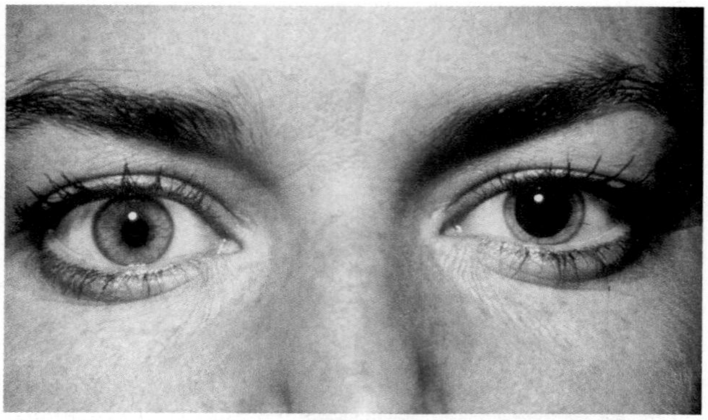

FIGURE 11-25 Asymmetric pupils may be normal or could signify a severe brain injury.

Pupil size is regulated by a series of continuous motor commands that the brain automatically sends through an oculomotor nerve (third cranial nerve) traveling to each eye. For example, when a bright light is introduced into one eye (or higher levels of light enter one eye only), both pupils should constrict equally to the appropriate size for the pupil receiving the most light.

> **Words of Wisdom**
>
> The mnemonic PERRLA (Pupils Equal, Round, and Reactive to Light and Accommodation) is commonly used in both the prehospital and in-hospital settings. Because accommodation is not always tested, or even testable, in the prehospital setting, EMS systems often use the abbreviation PERRL, without the *A* for accommodation. The PERRLA mnemonic is used in this text as a reminder that accommodation may be included in this assessment.

Anisocoria is a condition in which the pupils are asymmetric, differing in size by greater than 1 mm. This condition can be found in up to 30% of the population. It sometimes indicates significant ocular or neurologic pathology, but the condition must be correlated with the patient's overall presentation[19] **FIGURE 11-25**. Topical application of certain medications and substances can also provoke pupillary changes.

Also test muscle movement. Muscles are responsible for physically moving the eyes from side to side and up and down, allowing for seamless binocular vision.

To examine the eye, follow the steps in **SKILL DRILL 11-6**.

Skill Drill 11-6 Examining the Eye

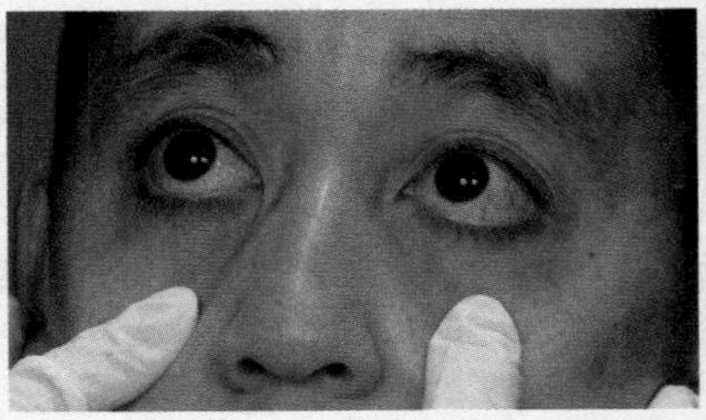

Step 1

Examine the exterior portion of the eye. Carefully inspect and palpate the upper and lower orbits, starting at the nose and working toward the lateral edge. Look for any obvious trauma or deformity. Ask about general problems, including any pain or redness, altered vision, vision loss, diplopia (double vision), photophobia, blurring, discharge, sensitivity to light, and corrective lens use. Note periorbital ecchymosis (raccoon eyes).

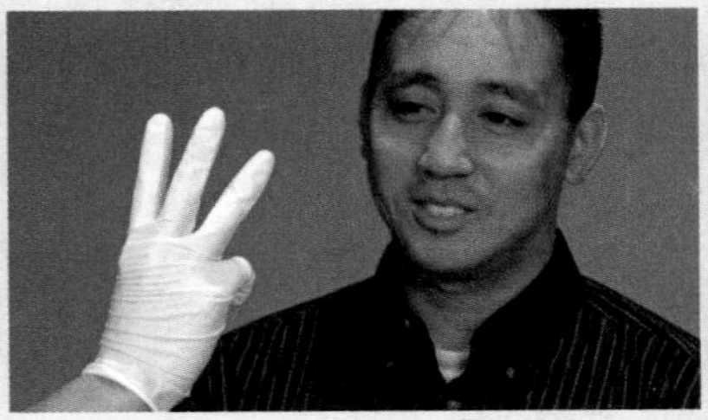

Step 2

Measure visual acuity by having the patient count the number of fingers you are holding up at varying distances (usually 6 feet [2 m], 3 feet [1 m], and 1 foot [0.3 m] away from the patient). Perform this exam on each eye independently. If corrective lenses are normally worn, check visual acuity with the correction in place.

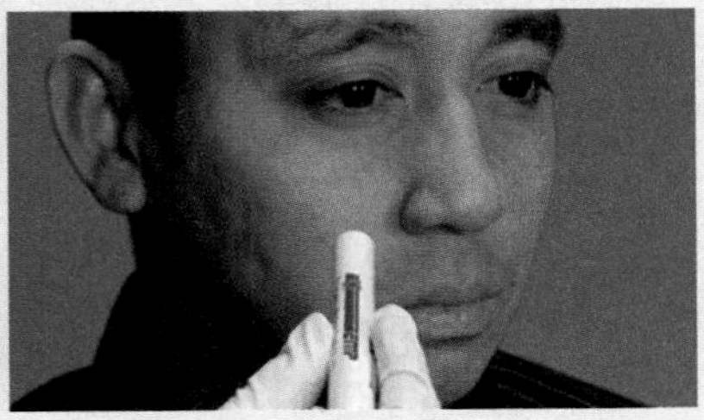

Step 3

Examine the pupils for size (in millimeters), shape, and symmetry. They should be equal. Test the pupils for their reactivity to light in as dark an environment as possible. Both pupils should constrict when exposed to light, and they should be equal in their response.

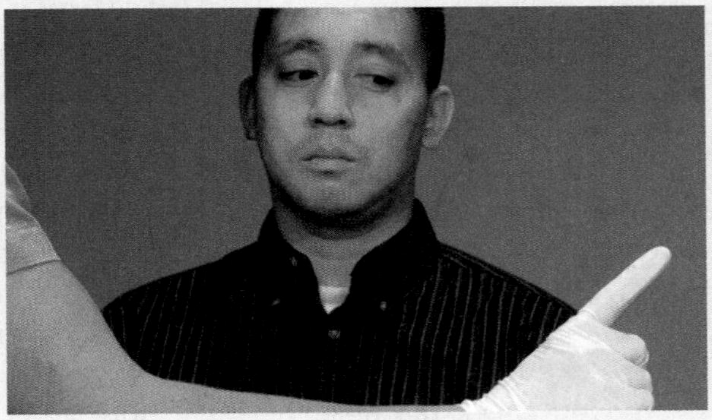

Step 4

Test for cranial nerve function by asking the patient to follow your fingers in a Z or H pattern. The eyes should move smoothly and symmetrically, tracking your finger movement. Evaluate whether the eyes move in sync (conjugate gaze) and whether they can track in all fields (up, down, left, right). Note any abnormal movement of the eyes. A visual field exam assesses the retina's (and therefore the optic nerve's) ability to perceive light. This is done by checking the patient's peripheral vision, examining each eye separately.

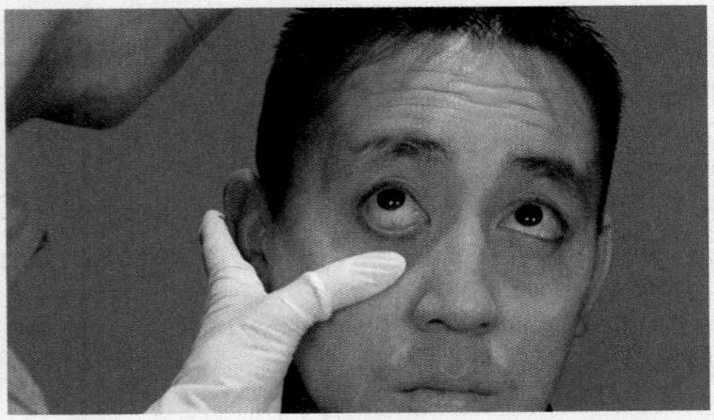

Step 5

Inspect the eyelids, lashes, and tear ducts for evidence of trauma or discharge. Turn up the lids to look for foreign bodies, and inspect the conjunctivae and sclera. The sclera ought to be white, not jaundiced or injected (red). Painless subconjunctival hemorrhage is a common but benign presentation. The conjunctivae should be pink, rather than cyanotic, pale, or overly reddened. The cornea and lens will be difficult to examine without additional assessment tools, although you should note whether the globe is patent in a trauma situation. Next, examine the anterior chamber and iris for clarity, noting any cloudiness or bleeding.

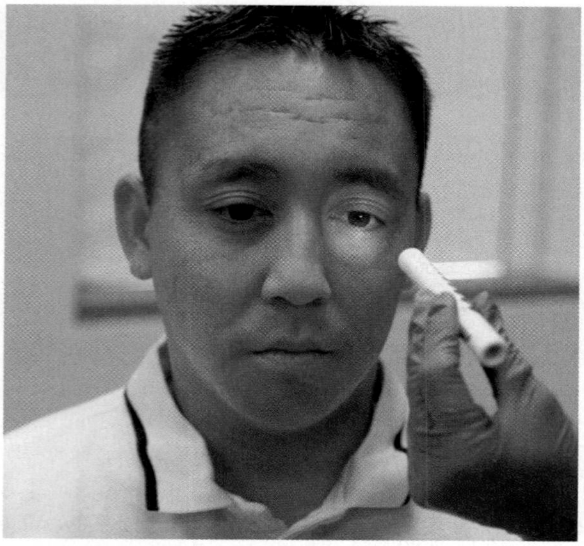

FIGURE 11-26 Penlight eye exam.

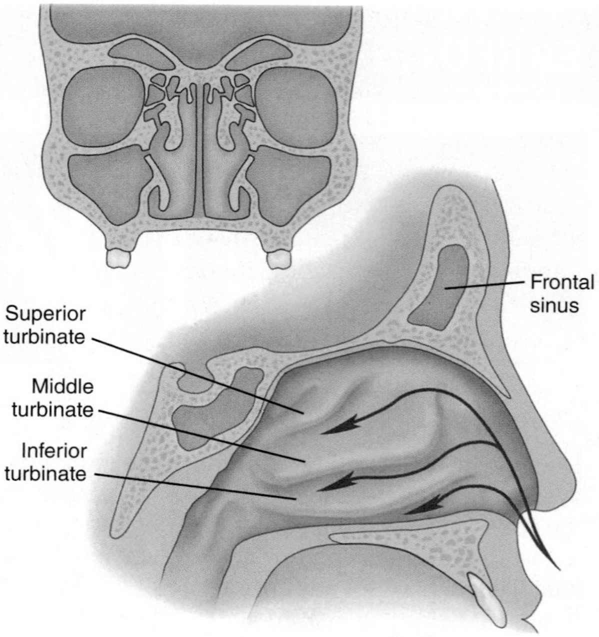

FIGURE 11-27 The nose has two chambers, divided by a septum. Each chamber is composed of layers of bone called turbinates. Above the nose are the frontal sinuses. On either side of the nose are the orbits of the eyes.

After the general eye exam, a more precise penlight exam is typically undertaken **FIGURE 11-26**.

Ears The ear is a sensory organ chiefly involved with hearing and sound perception, but is also intimately involved with balance control. The ear consists of an outer portion, a middle portion, and an inner portion.

Assessing the ears essentially involves checking for new aberrations in hearing perception and inspecting and palpating for wounds, swelling, or drainage (pus, blood, CSF). Often the mastoid process of the skull, which is palpated immediately posterior to the auricle, is assessed for discoloration and tenderness (**Battle sign**).

Words of Wisdom

Following trauma, frank blood or clear, watery drainage (CSF) from the ears or nose suggests a basilar skull fracture.

Nose The nose is a sensory organ involved with smell and taste; it is also part of the respiratory system. As you assess injuries of the nose, it helps to picture the inside of the nose itself **FIGURE 11-27**. The nasal cavity is divided into two sections, or chambers, by the nasal septum, which is made of cartilage. Each nasal chamber contains three layers of bone (turbinates) covered with a moist lining. Both chambers have superior, middle, and inferior turbinates. Air moves through the nasal chambers and is filtered and humidified as it passes over the turbinates during nasal breathing.

As you check the nose, assess it both anteriorly and inferiorly. Look for evidence of asymmetry, deformity, wounds, foreign bodies, discharge or bleeding, and tenderness. Note any evidence of respiratory distress, such as flaring of the nostrils. Inspect the exterior of the nose, looking for color changes, symmetry, and structural abnormalities. The nose should be firm and the nares clear of obstruction. Examine the column of the nose; it should be midline with the face. Inspect the septum for any deviation from midline. The nares should be symmetric. Slight deviation or asymmetry of the nares, septum, and column is a normal finding;

however, gross abnormalities should be noted. Note any drainage or discharge.

Throat Assess the throat by evaluating the mouth, the pharynx, and sometimes the neck. The throat is a conduit for both respiration and digestion, and it is close to numerous vital neurovascular structures.

As part of assessing the patient's overall hydration status, pay close attention to the lips, teeth, oral mucosa, and tongue. In patients who present with markedly AMS, rapidly determine upper airway status; prompt assessment of the throat and upper airway structures is mandatory. Depending on the situation, assess for the presence of a foreign body or **aspiration** in either the throat or lower airway structures. Situations requiring removal of foreign bodies, secretions, or blood can manifest in many types of emergency cases. Always be prepared to assist with clearing the pharynx using manual techniques and suction.

Examine the mouth beginning with the lips, which should be normal color for the patient and free of edema or surface irregularities. Confirm the mouth is symmetric. The gums should be pink, with no lesions or edema. Cyanosis often presents early around the lips. Be alert for this sign! Listen for hoarseness and note any unusual odors.

Inspect the airway for obstructions. Visually inspect the tongue, noting its color, size, and moisture. The tongue should be located at midline, without swelling, and should be moist.

Inspect and palpate the maxilla and the mandible, assessing the integrity and symmetry of both structures. Open the mouth, and look for signs of trauma (eg, cracked or missing teeth, or missing crowns). Check the bite for fit.

Examine the oropharynx, identifying any discoloration or pustules that might indicate an infection. Be alert for any unusual odors on the patient's breath (eg, alcohol, ketones). Check the posterior pharynx for fluids that may need to be suctioned. Inspect the uvula for edema and redness.

The neck is an extraordinarily muscular region, through which many vital structures pass. Its external anatomy includes the jaw, cricothyroid membrane, external jugular veins, thyroid cartilage, suprasternal notch, and cervical spinous processes. As you assess the neck, look for any abnormalities, including those related to symmetry, masses, and venous distention. When a patient is lying supine and sitting up at as much as a 45° angle, the jugular veins are naturally distended in a patient with an adequate blood volume. If JVD is present when the patient is sitting up at more than a 45° angle, then it is a sign of venous system overload or hypertension. JVD can be most readily observed by evaluating the anterolateral aspects of the neck; it can be provoked in a normal person by having the person lie supine and elevate the legs. Note how much distention is present, measured in centimeters from the origin of the jugular vein at the base of the neck to the angle of the jaw. Note the angle of the patient's position relative to a 0° angle (flat) when you take the measurement. Palpate the carotid pulses and note the relative strength of the impulse. Look for any pulsating or expanding mass near the carotid pulse point. Palpate the suprasternal notch to identify any tracheal deviation. Look for a tracheal stoma. These orifices are present in patients who have had a laryngectomy, and the stoma serves as their only means of a patent airway. If one is present, assess to ensure it is free of any obstruction. In these patients, all airway management should focus on the stoma. Have the patient open and close the jaws as you palpate over the temporomandibular joint during your examination of the jaw. Palpate for swollen lymph nodes, which are a sign of infection. Normally, lymph nodes are about the size of peas. When full of infectious material, they can increase to the size of grapes. To examine the neck, follow the steps in **SKILL DRILL 11-7**.

Cervical Spine

The cervical spine is the pathway by which the spinal cord makes its way out of the brain and into the torso, enabling the spinal nerves to reach and innervate the rest of the body **FIGURE 11-28**. It is also the point at which the head connects to the body. The spine is supported by a large muscle mass, as well as multiple tendinous and ligamentous supports. Cervical injury can present in a variety of ways, and the assessment for such injury must be conducted carefully.

Evaluate the patient first for the MOI and then for the presence of pain. Does the patient have AMS, or did a loss of consciousness occur at the

Skill Drill 11-7 Examining the Neck

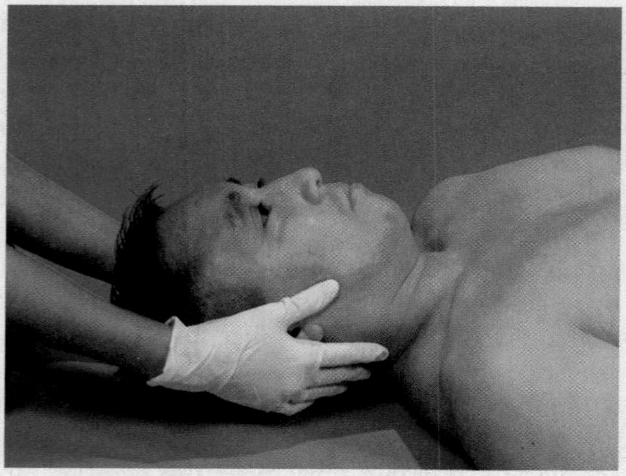

Step 1

If spinal trauma is suspected, take precautions to protect the patient's cervical spine in accordance with your protocol. Assess for usage of accessory muscles during respiration.

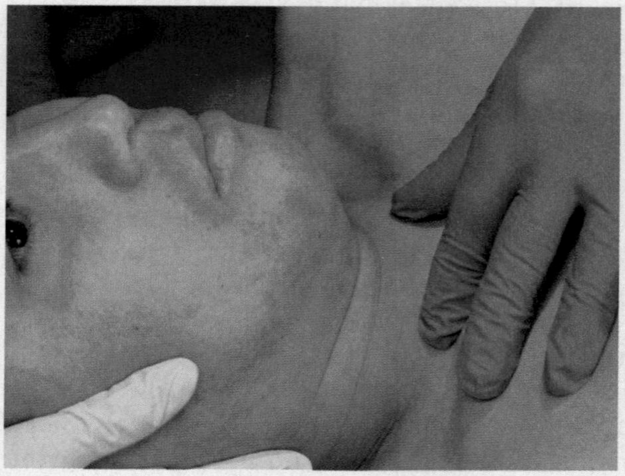

Step 2

Palpate the neck to find any structural abnormalities or subcutaneous air, and to ensure the trachea is midline. Begin at the suprasternal notch and work your way toward the head. Be careful when applying pressure to the area of the carotid arteries, because doing so may stimulate a vagal response.

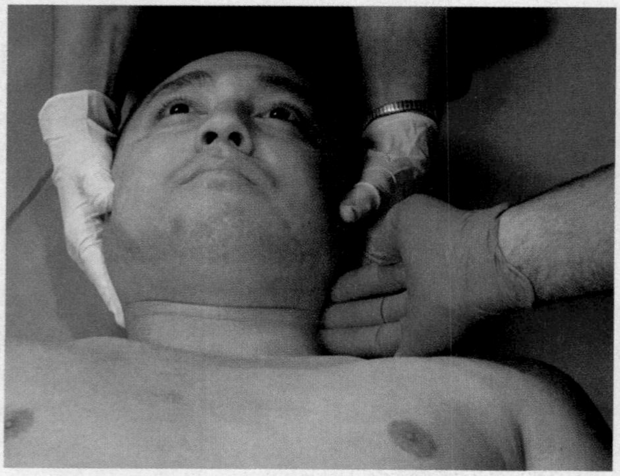

Step 3

Assess the lymph nodes and note any swelling, which may indicate infection.

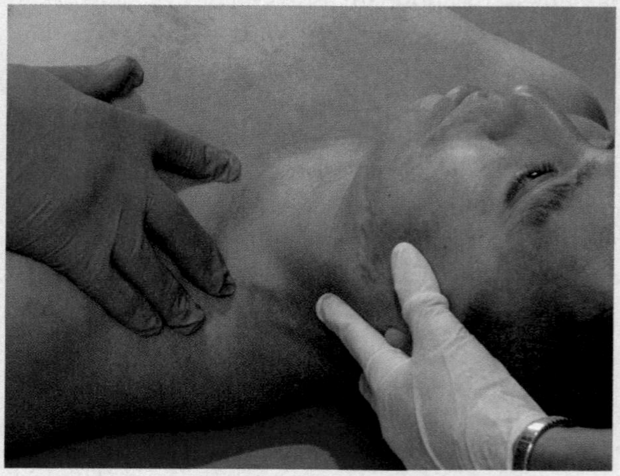

Step 4

Assess the jugular veins for distention, which may indicate a problem with venous return to the heart.

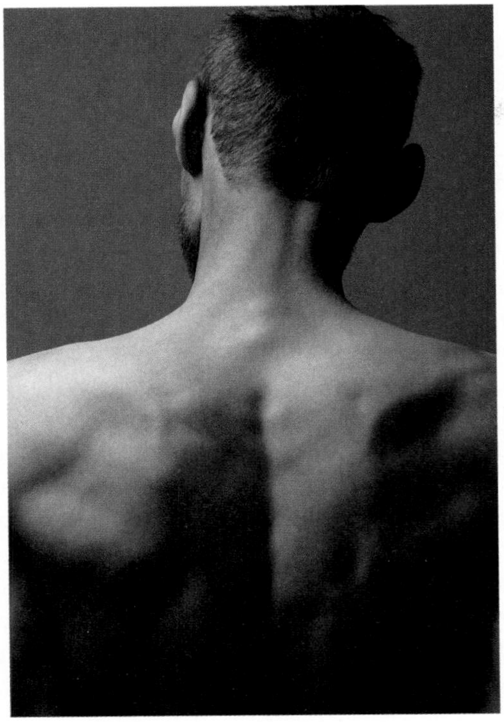

FIGURE 11-28 The cervical spine, as seen from the back of the neck.

time of the event? According to *Prehospital Trauma Life Support*, indications for spinal immobilization include the following:

- Tenderness on palpation of the spinal column
- Complaint of pain in the spine
- AMS (eg, traumatic brain injury, under the influence of ethyl alcohol or intoxicating substances)
- Inability to communicate effectively (eg, extremely young age, language barrier)
- GCS score of less than 15
- Evidence of a distracting injury
- Paralysis or other neurologic deficit or complaint

As you examine the cervical spine, inspect and palpate it, looking for evidence of tenderness and deformity. Pain is the single most reliable indicator of a spine injury or spinal cord injury. Midline posterior tenderness involving the bony spinous processes should always arouse concern. Palpable discomfort over the lateral aspects of the neck usually signals a muscular or ligamentous problem, not an injury to the bony spinal column itself. Any manipulation that results in pain, tenderness, or tingling should prompt you to stop the exam *immediately* and place the patient into a proper-size cervical collar. Any complaint of neck pain in patients who have sustained a significant MOI warrants careful evaluation and, depending on the findings, may warrant stabilization with a cervical collar and backboard depending on your local protocol. Continued assessment of a patient's ROM should take place only when there is no potential for serious injury.

As you evaluate the neck, if there is no complaint of pain, no neurologic abnormalities such as weakness or numbness in the arms or legs, and no midline tenderness, ask the patient to actively move their neck through a ROM. Instruct the patient to stop if they encounter discomfort or any neurologic symptoms. Never move the patient's neck yourself (referred to as *passive motion* because the patient's participation is passive); this could result in spinal cord injury. To check ROM, first have the patient slowly rotate their head from shoulder to shoulder. Then, if there is no pain or discomfort, have the patient extend the head back and flex the head and neck, touching chin to chest. Any discomfort elicited by these maneuvers should prompt you to terminate the exam immediately and protect the patient's spine.

Chest

The chest (or thorax) consists of the superior aspect of the torso, from the base of the neck to the diaphragm, as delineated by the costal arch **FIGURE 11-29**. The chest wall is divided into anterior and posterior portions: the patient's front and back. The back of the chest extends down the patient's back, to the level of the diaphragm posteriorly, which moves up and down with breathing. The chest contains many vital structures, including the lungs and mediastinal elements (heart, great vessels). The chest wall serves as a protective covering for the internal components. It consists of numerous musculoskeletal, vascular, nervous, connective, and lining structures.

Words of Wisdom

The lungs are hyperinflated in patients with chronic emphysema, resulting in hyperresonance where you would expect to hear cardiac dullness.

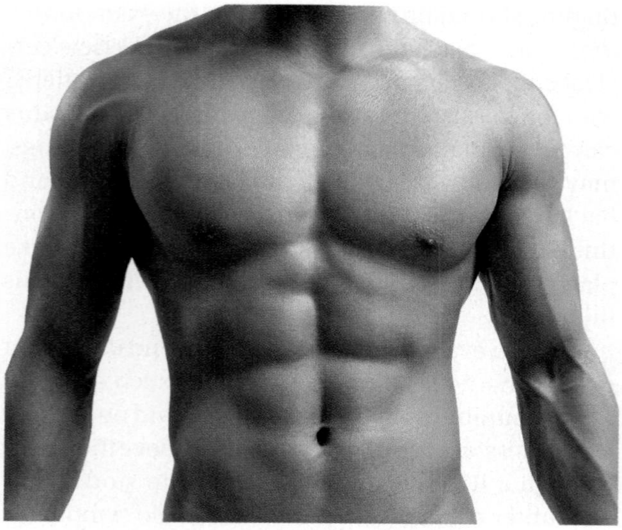

FIGURE 11-29 The chest (thorax) consists of the superior aspect of the torso, from the base of the neck to the diaphragm, as delineated by the costal arch.

Typically, the chest exam proceeds in three phases: The chest wall is checked, a pulmonary evaluation is conducted, and the cardiovascular assessment is performed. The chest must be inspected to assess for deformities in wall patency and to look for external clues of respiratory distress. Expose the chest and begin your assessment, using the techniques of inspection, palpation, percussion, and auscultation. The examination of the posterior chest is the same as the examination of the anterior chest. Follow the steps in **SKILL DRILL 11-8** to examine the chest.

Pay close attention to any signs of abnormal breathing movements (eg, paradoxical or accessory muscle use, impaired or diminished breathing movement) and retractions (ie, suprasternal, sternal, intercostal, or subcostal). Look for signs of ventilatory fatigue, such as decreased mentation or a tired, worn-out appearance that often precedes ventilatory failure and, frequently, respiratory or

Skill Drill 11-8 Examining the Chest

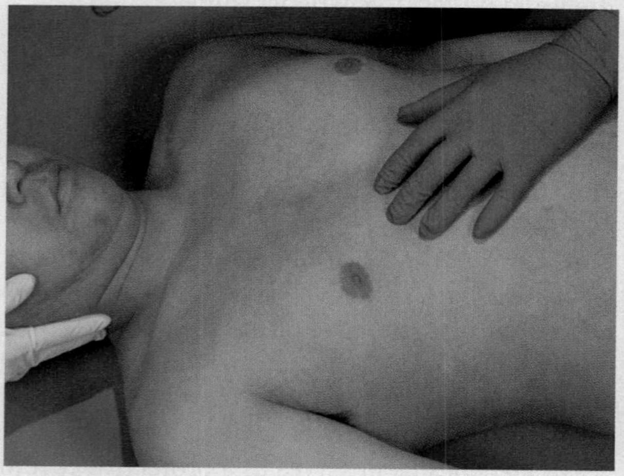

Step 1

Ensure the patient's privacy as best you can. Inspect and palpate the chest for open/closed findings, paradoxical motion, and crepitus. Observe the chest wall for respiratory effort, and document the respiratory rate, depth, and rhythm. If you find any open wounds, dress them appropriately.

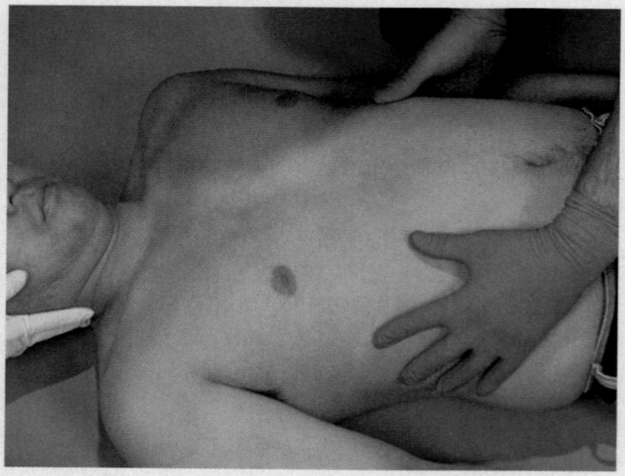

Step 2

Compare the two sides of the chest for symmetry. Note the shape of the patient's chest: It can give you clues to many underlying medical conditions, such as emphysema. Look for any surgical scars, such as a midline "zipper" scar, which may result from a previous cardiac surgery. Palpate the chest to reveal any air under the skin (as occurs in subcutaneous emphysema).

Skill Drill 11-8 Examining the Chest (continued)

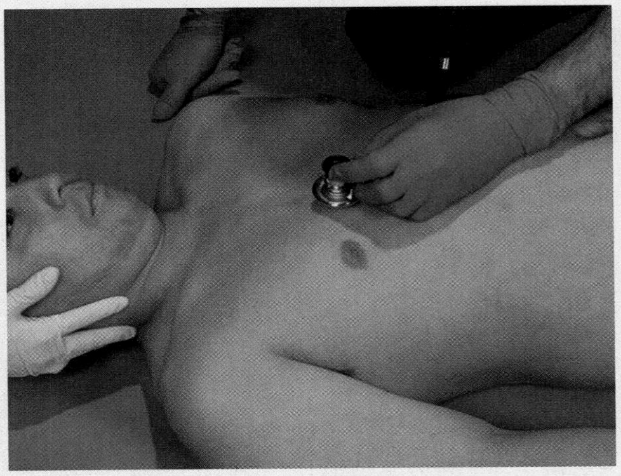

Step 3

Auscultate the lung fields. Note any abnormal lung sounds. Auscultate for heart tones. Always auscultate directly to the patient's skin, not through their clothing. Listening over the fabric will result in breath sounds being muted by the clothing. With each stethoscope placement, listen to at least one full inhalation and exhalation. If the patient is able to cooperate, have them breathe through an open mouth to help emphasize the lung sounds.

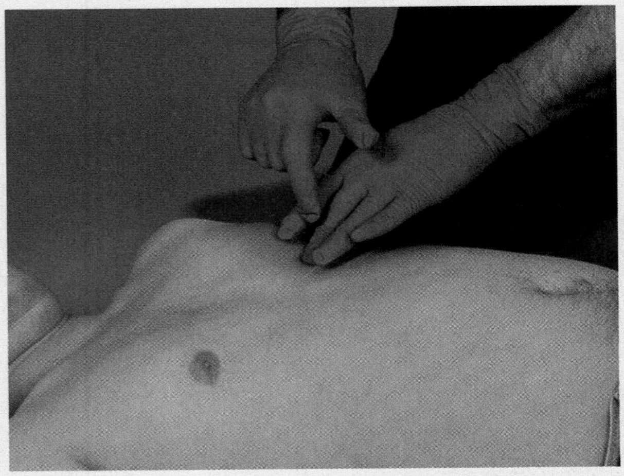

Step 4

Percuss the chest to detect any abnormalities. Repeat the appropriate portions of the exam for the posterior aspect of the thorax.

cardiac arrest. Watch for the appearance of JVD with patients who have respiratory complaints; it may point to pneumothorax or heart failure.

Look for signs of accessory muscle use or retractions, which suggest respiratory distress. Note any chest deformities, such as barrel chest (COPD), flail segments or subcutaneous air (trauma), kyphoscoliosis of the spine (compression fractures), significant bruising, and any suspicious wounds. Remember, flail segments may not be accompanied by paradoxical movement early on, because of the splinting effect of muscle spasms.

Palpate any areas of the chest wall that were initially noted to be abnormal on inspection. Palpation will also enable you to better appreciate respiratory symmetry and expansion, and the overall work of breathing. Although often impractical in the prehospital environment, chest wall percussion can allow for enhanced evaluation of the underlying chest cavity by distinguishing either dullness or hyperresonance.

The lungs have five discrete lobes: The right side contains upper, middle, and lower lobes; the left side contains upper and lower lobes. During your exam, listen over each lobe, comparing from side to side, both anteriorly and posteriorly. To facilitate your auscultatory assessment, have the patient take as deep a breath as they can through an open mouth. Listen to as many portions of the lungs as possible, while avoiding any bony prominences, attached medical equipment, and clothing. You can often hear a patient's breath sounds better from the patient's back; therefore, if the patient's back is accessible, listen there and assess six fields **FIGURE 11-30**. If you have stabilized the patient or if the patient is in a supine position, listen from the front and sides and assess four fields. Always use the best stethoscope available.

Normal breath sounds are clear and quiet during inspiration and expiration and are heard in three areas. **Bronchial sounds**, heard over the trachea, are hollow, tubular sounds with a lower pitch. The inspiration/expiration ratio is 1:3. The normal sounds found in the midchest or in the posterior chest between the scapula are called **bronchovesicular sounds**. They reflect a mix of pitch between the vesicular and bronchial sounds; the inspiration/expiration ratio is 1:1. The soft and

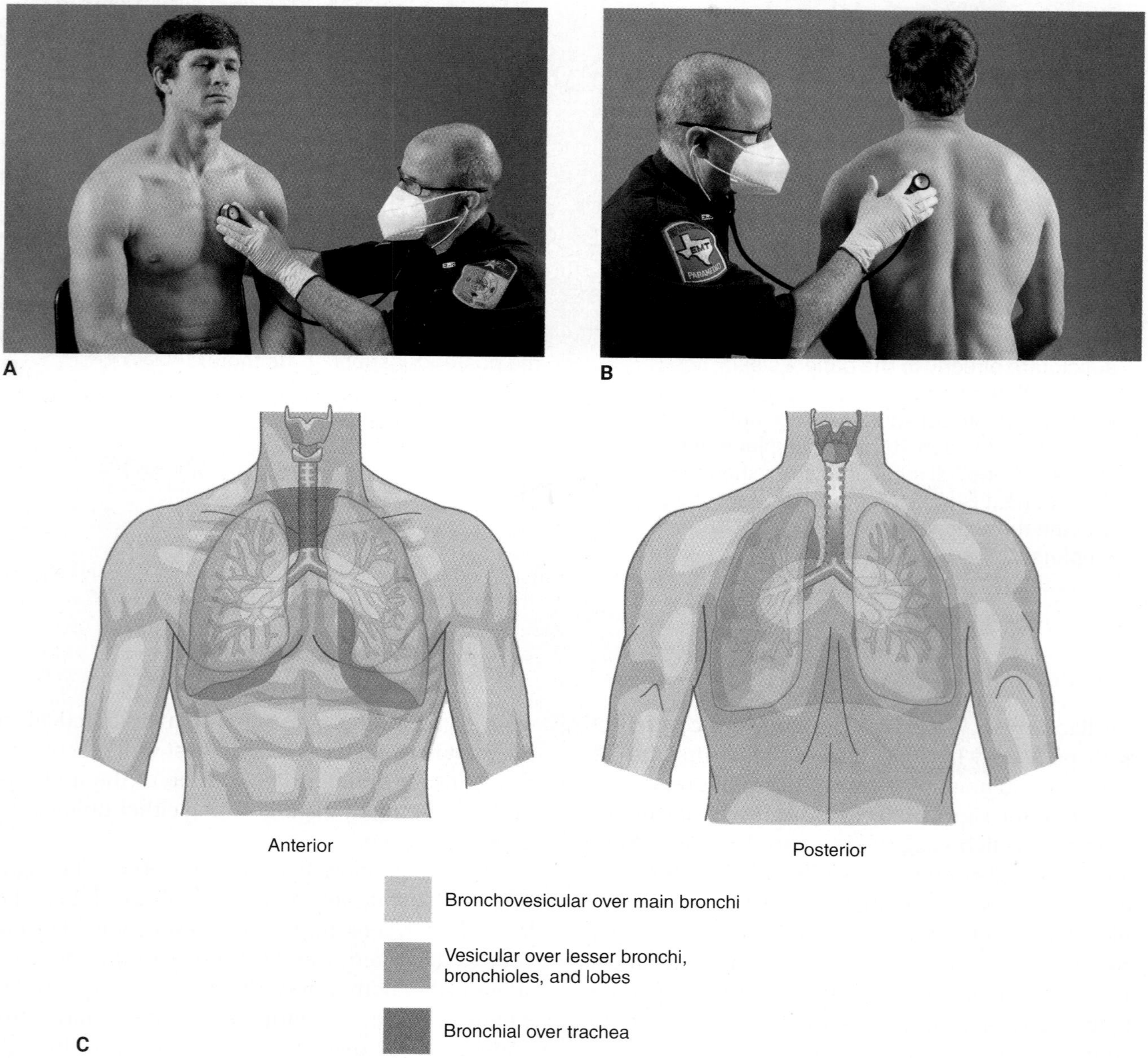

FIGURE 11-30 Locations for auscultating breath sounds: both sides of the chest in multiple lung fields, as shown. **A.** Stethoscope position for auscultating the front of the chest. **B.** Stethoscope position for auscultating the back. **C.** The colors in the illustration correspond to the areas where sounds are heard.

low-pitched sounds normally heard over most of the lung surface, which have a rustling quality during inspiration and a softer sound during expiration, are known as **vesicular sounds**.

For patients with respiratory complaints, assess breath sounds early and often. Pathologic or **adventitious breath sounds** include the following **FIGURE 11-31**:

- **Wheezing breath sounds.** These sounds suggest lower airway obstruction. **Wheezing** is a high-pitched whistling sound that is most prominent on expiration but can be heard on inspiration in sicker patients. If wheezing is unilateral, suspect an aspirated foreign body or infection. If wheezing is bilateral, suspect asthma. Other potential causes include an inhaled irritant, such as chlorine; other, less common lung diseases, such as asbestosis, may also be the problem.
- **Crackles** (also called *rales*). Wet breath sounds may indicate cardiac failure or infection, especially in a young child. Such sounds are often difficult to hear, especially in the back of a moving ambulance. Crackles are characterized as a moist crackling, usually heard on inspiration and expiration. They are produced by oxygen passing through moisture in the bronchoalveolar system or by closed alveoli opening abruptly. Examples of conditions in which crackles may be heard include pneumonia, heart failure, asthma, and restrictive pulmonary diseases.
- **Rhonchi**. Rhonchi, or congested breath sounds, are continuous sounds with a lower pitch and a rattling quality. They indicate fluid in the larger airways. They may indicate the presence of mucus in the lungs, for example, as a result of infection (eg, pneumonia) or inflammation (eg, bronchitis). Expect to hear low-pitched, noisy sounds that are most prominent on expiration. The patient often reports a productive cough associated with these sounds. Aspiration of fluid may also produce rhonchi.
- **Stridor**. Stridor is a brassy crowing sound often heard without a stethoscope. It is caused by narrowing, swelling, or obstruction of the upper airway and may indicate the patient has an

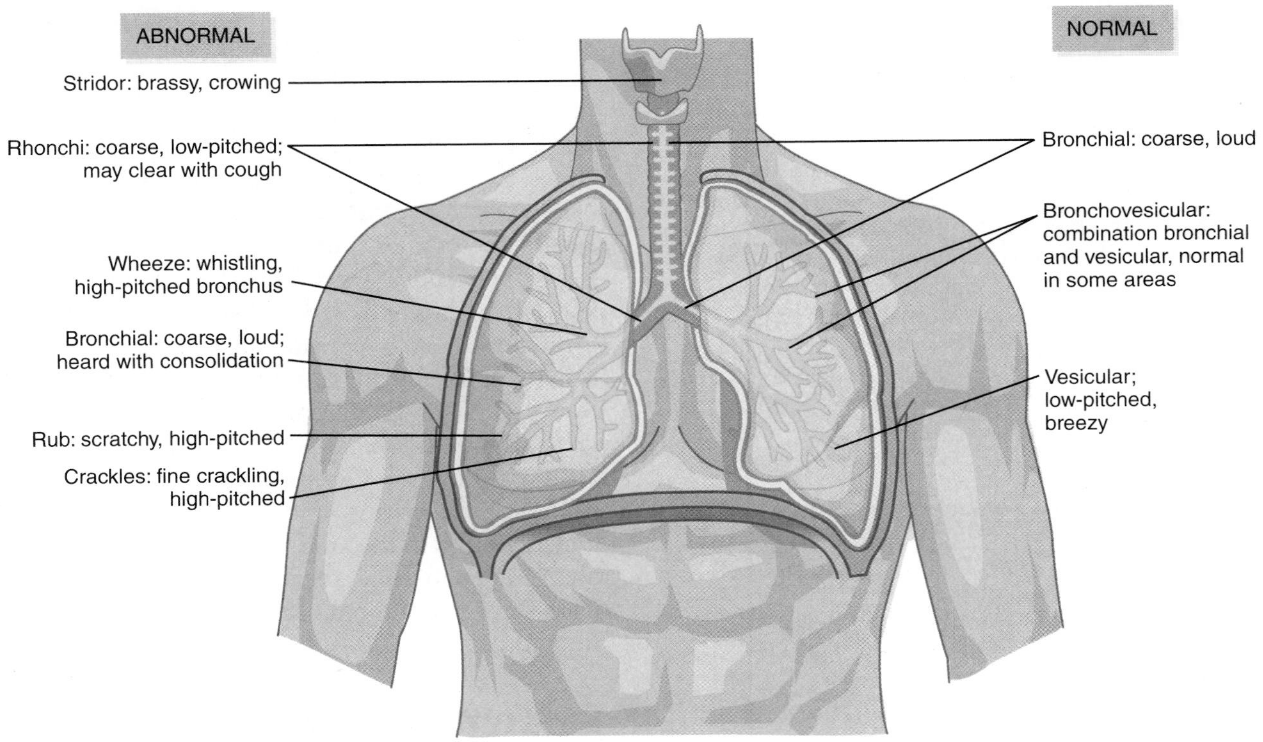

FIGURE 11-31 Locations and descriptions of abnormal (adventitious) breath sounds versus normal breath sounds.

airway obstruction in the neck or upper part of the chest. It is most prominent on inspiration. Stridor may be caused by bacterial epiglottitis, viral croup, swelling from upper airway burns, or a partial foreign body airway obstruction. Stridor often indicates a life-threatening condition, because it equates to an 85% reduction in airway size. The onset of crowing or stridor in the presence of fever or upper respiratory infection should be recognized as a threat to life.
- **Pleural friction rubs**. These squeaking or grating sounds occur when the pleural linings rub together. If this occurs, the pleural layers have lost their lubrication, most commonly because of pleural inflammation. This condition is usually associated with pain on inspiration. The sounds may be heard anytime the chest wall moves; therefore, they can be heard on inspiration, expiration, or both.

Words of Wisdom

One of the most important and perhaps most overlooked aspects of pulmonary assessment is appreciating when breath sounds are diminished or absent. Numerous medical conditions can cause decreased breath sounds, including pneumothorax, hemothorax, pleural effusion, PE, atelectasis/consolidation, exacerbated COPD, status asthmaticus, opiate intoxication, pneumonia, bronchitis, and AMS. You cannot be aware of diminished or absent breath sounds without first developing an appreciation of the wide spectrum of normal presentations that exist. Before going out into the field, spend many hours listening to normal breath sounds so you develop an understanding of what constitutes the many variations of normal breathing. After that, spend time listening to patients with respiratory difficulty, preferably alongside an experienced provider who can point out the significant variations in the presenting abnormalities.

Words of Wisdom

Normal breathing should be quiet and not grossly evident to you. If you can see or hear the patient working hard to breathe, there's a problem.

At times even the most experienced provider has difficulty deciphering the various pathologic lung sounds. In these instances, it might be helpful to describe the sounds rather than attempt to classify them immediately. Ask yourself if the sounds appear to be dry or moist. Moist sounds might suggest pneumonia or pulmonary edema. Are the sounds continuous or intermittent? Continuous sounds suggest a pathologic process, whereas intermittent sounds could be from a partial foreign body obstruction or a reversible process, such as bronchospasm. Define the sounds as coarse or fine. Coarse sounds are louder and harsher and suggest a possible problem in the bronchial tree, whereas fine sounds are quieter and sometimes associated with a lower airway problem.

Decreased breath sounds can be localized to a portion of one lung, or they can encompass the entire chest. When hypoventilation is suspected, take immediate action. Decreased breath sounds typically signal a lack of respiratory excursion or decreased tidal volume. If decreased breath sounds are localized to a specific area, assess transmitted voice sounds to see if there is any increased vocal resonance, which is a sign of consolidation in the lung, suggesting possible pneumonia. Further assessment of increased vocal resonance can be made by testing for **bronchophony**. Place the diaphragm of the stethoscope over the suspected area of consolidation and ask the patient to say "ninety-nine." In healthy lung tissue, the term should sound muffled and indistinct; however, if the sound is loud and clear, this is considered bronchophony and suggests an area of consolidation. A similar test, called **whispered pectoriloquy**, is performed in the same manner, but with the patient whispering "ninety-nine." Once again, a normal response should be muffled and indistinct. A louder and clearer whisper is considered a positive test. Another test for consolidation is **egophony**. With this test, you place the diaphragm over the area of decreased breath sounds and ask the patient to say a drawn-out "*eeee*." A normal response will elicit a muffled long vowel sound. However, if there is any consolidation in the area, the sound will sound like an "A." Keep in mind, these tests require an optimal listening environment, something that is hard to find at an emergency scene.

Cardiovascular System

The cardiovascular system circulates blood throughout the body, an activity that maintains perfusion of the body's tissues. Blood flows through two circuits:

the systemic circulation in the body and the pulmonary circulation in the lungs. The systemic circulation carries oxygen-rich blood from the left ventricle through the body and back to the right atrium. As this blood passes through the tissues and organs, it gives up oxygen and nutrients and absorbs cellular wastes and carbon dioxide. The cellular wastes are, in turn, eliminated as the liver and kidneys filter the blood. The pulmonary circulation carries oxygen-poor blood from the right ventricle through the lungs and back into the left atrium.

The cardiac cycle consists of cardiac relaxation (diastole), filling, and contraction (systole). These mechanical events are coordinated electrically with the heart's pacing and conduction system.

The contraction and relaxation of the heart, combined with the flow of blood, generates characteristic heart sounds during auscultation with a stethoscope. The normal pattern sounds much like this: "lub-DUB, lub-DUB, lub-DUB . . ." The "lub" is referred to as the first heart sound or S_1, and the "DUB" (emphasized because it is often louder) is the second heart sound, or S_2. S_1 represents the closure of the atrioventricular valves, marking the onset of ventricular contraction, or systole. S_2 represents the closure of the semilunar valves, marking the onset of ventricular relaxation, or diastole.

Pathologic heart sounds include S_3 and S_4. The S_3, or third heart sound, is a soft, low-pitched rare sound occurring early in ventricular diastole as the mitral valve opens to allow passive filling of the left ventricle. Although S_3 is sometimes present in healthy young people, it is most commonly associated with abnormally increased filling pressures in the atria secondary to moderate to severe heart failure. S_4, which is considered a "gallop" rhythm, is a low-pitched sound occurring with late diastolic filling of the ventricle due to atrial contraction. S_4 occurs immediately before the normal S_1 sound; it is always abnormal. The S_4 sound represents either decreased stretching (compliance) of the left ventricle or increased pressure in the atria. Events on the right side of the heart usually occur slightly later than those on the left side, creating two discernible sounds, rather than one heart sound. This is known as **splitting**. This most often occurs with

Words of Wisdom

The S_3 sound is associated with heart failure and should be considered abnormal in patients older than age 35.

YOU are the Paramedic

PART 4

Your crew has finished moving the patient onto your stretcher, and you are moving the patient to the ambulance for transport to the trauma center. En route, you plan to start an IV line for fluid administration, oxygenate the patient, and closely monitor his ventilation.

Recording Time: 10 Minutes	
Respirations	28 breaths/min, shallow
Pulse	120 beats/min, weak
Skin	Cool, paler than baseline, clammy
Blood pressure	92/62 mm Hg
Oxygen saturation (Spo_2)	99% on 15 L/min O_2 via nonrebreathing mask
Pupils	PERRLA

7. How can you determine the level of internal damage if you do not have the implement that was used to stab the patient?

8. What is the relevance of past medical history in this case?

S_2 and is a finding during auscultation of the S_2 heart sound. It is caused when the closure of the aortic valve and the closure of the pulmonary valve are not synchronized normally. A split S_2 that does not change with respiration may indicate a serious heart problem and warrants further evaluation.

You can appreciate heart sounds by listening to the chest wall in the parasternal areas superiorly and inferiorly, as well as in the region superior to the left nipple. To auscultate heart sounds, place the patient in a position that will bring the heart closer to the left anterior chest wall, such as sitting up and leaning slightly forward. Place your stethoscope at the fifth intercostal space over the apex of the heart; this should correspond approximately to the mitral valve. **FIGURE 11-32** shows where to place the stethoscope to hear various heart sounds.

Korotkoff sounds are related to a patient's BP. There are five Korotkoff sounds, but only the first and fifth are clinically significant. The sounds are as follows, and occur in this order:

1. Phase I—Clear, faint, tapping sounds that gradually increase in intensity; correlates to systolic contraction.
2. Phase II—Sounds change to a soft *swishing* sound.
3. Phase III—Sounds become crisper again and increase in intensity; softer than tapping sounds in Phase I.
4. Phase IV—Sounds become muffled.
5. Phase V—All sounds disappear; correlates to diastolic pressure.

The second and third Korotkoff sounds have no known clinical significance.

In some patients, between Phases II and III, sounds may disappear briefly. This is referred to as an auscultatory gap.

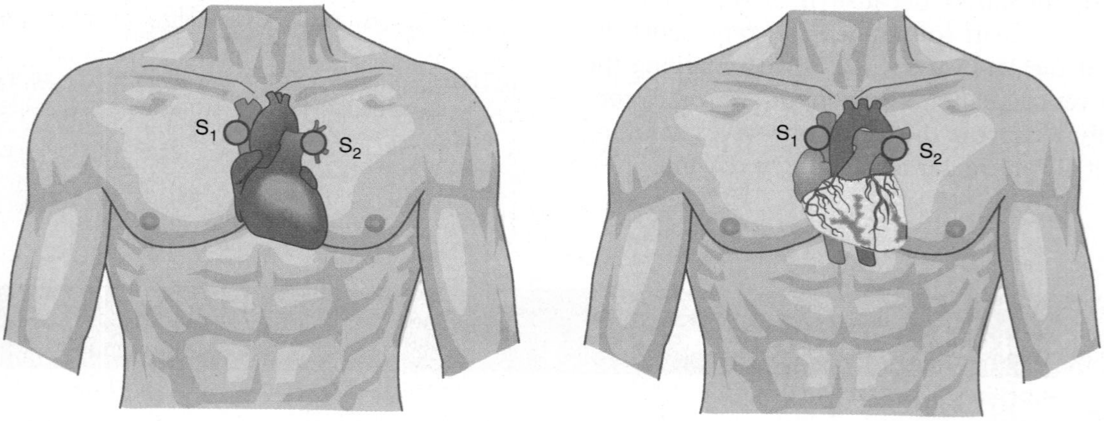

Heart Sound	Represents	Where Heard
S_1	Aortic region—closure of atrioventricular valve	Second to third intercostal space at right sternal border
S_2	Pulmonic region—closure of semilunar valve	Second to third intercostal space at left sternal border
S_3	Tricuspid region	Fourth, fifth, and sixth intercostal space at left sternal border
S_4	Mitral region—closure of mitral valve	Apex of the heart—fifth to sixth intercostal space at left midclavicular line

FIGURE 11-32 Locations for stethoscope placement when auscultating heart sounds. To appreciate the S_2 sound, ask the patient to breathe normally and hold their breath on inhalation. Auscultate the area above the left nipple to listen for S_3 and S_4 heart sounds.

While inspecting and palpating the patient's chest, listen for heart sounds. Feel the chest wall to locate the point of maximum impulse (PMI) and appreciate the apical pulse. Palpate for any **lift** (also called **heave**—the perception of the heart beating very strongly) in the chest wall, suggesting hypertrophy. Be aware of any **thrill** (humming vibration). A palpable thrill suggests an underlying bruit or murmur and warrants further investigation. Listen over the areas in which the cardiac valves are located: The aortic valve is near the second intercostal space, to the right of the sternum. The pulmonic valve lies near the second intercostal space, to the left of the sternum. The tricuspid valve is auscultated over the lower left sternal border. The mitral valve can be assessed over the cardiac apex, lateral to the lower left sternal border near the midclavicular line. Note the intensity of the heart sounds, and listen for S_1, S_2, and any extra sounds and murmurs.

A **bruit** is an abnormal *whooshing* sound that indicates turbulent blood flow moving through a narrowed artery (most significant in the carotid arteries). A **murmur** is an abnormal *whooshing* sound heard over the heart that indicates turbulent blood flow around a cardiac valve. Murmurs are graded according to intensity, from 1 (softest) to 6 (loudest). Many people have normal physiologic murmurs. In some patients, they can represent a degree of pathology, depending on the nature of the underlying condition and the specific anatomy of the valve involved. To fully appreciate the nature and quality of normal heart sounds and murmurs, you must thoroughly practice your listening skills using excellent equipment.

Arterial pulses represent systolic BP. They occur when contraction of the left ventricle and subsequent ejection of blood into the systemic circulation generate a pressure wave, which then travels throughout the arterial system. Arterial pulses are palpable wherever an artery crosses a bony prominence.

Venous pressure tends to be low. In fact, in the normal setting, the pressure in the venae cavae just before blood is received into the right atrium is close to zero. Veins are relatively nonmuscular, thin-walled vessels that do not affect systemic vascular resistance or support systemic BP. Blood flows through the venous system and returns to the heart in part because it is propelled continuously from behind, draining the capillary network. Most venous blood return is a function of the respiratory cycle, propelled by the negative intrathoracic pressure generated at inspiration during normal breathing.

Assess the extremities, particularly the lower extremities, for any sign of venous obstruction or insufficiency. Signs include venous engorgement, palpable edema, swelling, hyperpigmentation, and mild erythema. Patients may report swelling, painful superficial veins, heaviness in the extremities, or changes in skin color.

Occasionally, jugular venous pressure helps you estimate the capacity of the venous system. Anytime you see JVD, determine the location of the venous obstruction that is impeding blood return to the heart. If the patient has penetrating left chest trauma, JVD may indicate cardiac tamponade. If the patient has pedal edema, consider heart failure. Specifically, in right-side heart failure, blood flow into the right atrium tends to be sluggish. Venous capacitance increases in an effort to compensate, which in turn elevates pressure and results in JVD. If you palpate the liver and see significant JVD, this suggests liver disease or inflammation secondary to hepatitis.

In situations involving hypotension, evidence of JVD may be absent, even while the patient is supine. However, hypotensive patients with JVD must be carefully assessed as to the nature of their condition. Depending on the clinical situation, patients with JVD may be experiencing cardiogenic shock or have a ruptured cardiac valve. In the setting of chest trauma, neck vein distention and hypotension may point to a tension pneumothorax or pericardial tamponade.

The ability of the circulatory system to constrict and dilate can diminish markedly as a person ages. Although this limitation varies considerably from patient to patient, an older patient's ability to compensate for a cardiovascular insult may be profoundly curtailed by age-related changes, especially arterial atherosclerosis and diabetes. In addition, many medications that older people routinely take to manage medical conditions such as high BP can impair the body's ability to handle sudden changes in the demand for blood supply (eg, the body wants to increase the pulse rate, but a beta blocker medication won't let it accelerate). By contrast, the vessels of children and young adults are better able to vasoconstrict and increase the pulse rate to compensate for a vascular insult; this compensation mechanism can fool you into believing young patients are less sick than they actually are.

As you examine a patient's cardiovascular system, pay attention to arterial pulses, noting their location, rate, rhythm, and quality. In addition, note the amplitude of the pulses (eg, weak and thready versus strong and bounding). Obtain an accurate BP and repeat this measurement periodically to monitor the patient's hemodynamic stability. Determine whether the patient has a history of hypertension, and if so, note which category of hypertension the patient falls into **TABLE 11-9**. Palpate the carotid arteries and listen to them with the bell of the stethoscope to assess for any bruits (discussed later).

In a patient with a suspected heart problem, assess the pulse for regularity and strength, and examine the skin for signs of hypoperfusion (pallor and cool, moist skin) or oxygen desaturation (cyanosis). If the pulse feels irregular, assess it over 1 minute, rather than for only 30 seconds, to obtain a more accurate measurement of the rate. Listen to breath sounds, since many cardiac conditions are associated with respiratory problems—crackles secondary to pulmonary edema, for instance. Obtain baseline vital signs. Serious hypotension with sustained or progressive tachycardia is common in patients with cardiogenic shock; stay alert for this condition, because it has a mortality rate of more than 80%. Check for JVD, too. It can indicate heart failure, cardiac tamponade, or pneumothorax. Examine the extremities for signs of peripheral edema, which may indicate right-side heart failure.

TABLE 11-9 BP Categories for Adults (2017 American College of Cardiology/American Heart Association Clinical Practice Guidelines)[a]

BP Category[a]	SBP		DBP
Normal	<120 mm Hg	and	<80 mm Hg
Elevated	120–129 mm Hg	and	<80 mm Hg
Hypertension			
Stage 1	130–139 mm Hg	or	80–89 mm Hg
Stage 2	≥140 mm Hg	or	≥90 mm Hg

[a] Individuals with systolic blood pressure (SBP) and diastolic blood pressure (DBP) measurements in two categories should be placed in the higher blood pressure (BP) category.

Reproduced with permission from Whelton PK, Carey RM, Aronow WS, et al. 2017 ACC/AHA/AAPA/ABC/ACPM/AGS/APhA/ASH/ASPC/NMA/PCNA guideline for the prevention, detection, evaluation, and management of high blood pressure in adults: A report of the American College of Cardiology/American Heart Association Task Force on Clinical Practice Guidelines. *J Am Coll Cardiol*. 2018 May 15;71(19):e127-e248. doi:10.1016/j.jacc.2017.11.006.

Abdomen

Because of the large number of organs within the abdomen, the location of those structures, and the complexity of associated medical complaints, the abdomen is easily described by mentally dividing it into four quadrants. The diaphragm is the large, dome-shaped muscle used for respiration at the top of the abdominal cavity, and the pelvis is at the bottom. The quadrants—left upper quadrant (LUQ), right upper quadrant (RUQ), left lower quadrant (LLQ), right lower quadrant (RLQ)—are marked by a set of imaginary perpendicular lines intersecting at the umbilicus, which serves as the central reference point **FIGURE 11-33**.

Alternatively, assess the abdominal organs by dividing the abdomen into nine regions: right hypochondrial, RH; epigastric, E; left hypochondrial, LH; right lumbar, RL; umbilical, U; left lumbar, LL; right iliac, RI; hypogastric, H; and left iliac, LI **FIGURE 11-34**.

Words of Wisdom

Assess all four quadrants of the abdomen for pain/tenderness, rigidity, swelling, guarding, and distention. Begin in an area where the patient has no pain.

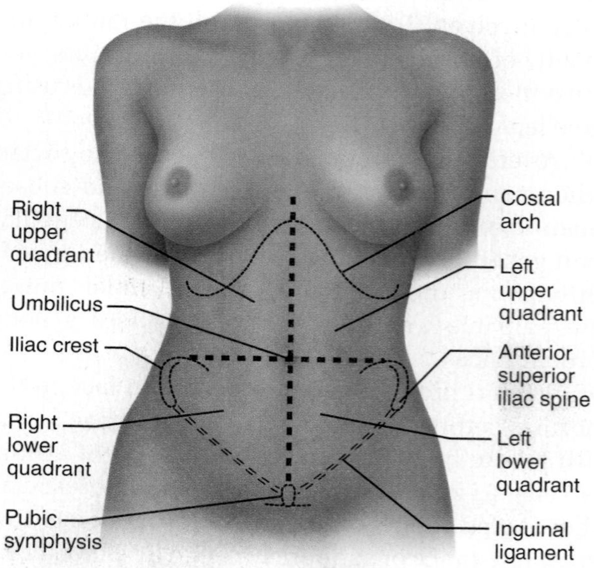

FIGURE 11-33 The abdomen is divided into quadrants by imaginary vertical and horizontal lines that intersect at the umbilicus.

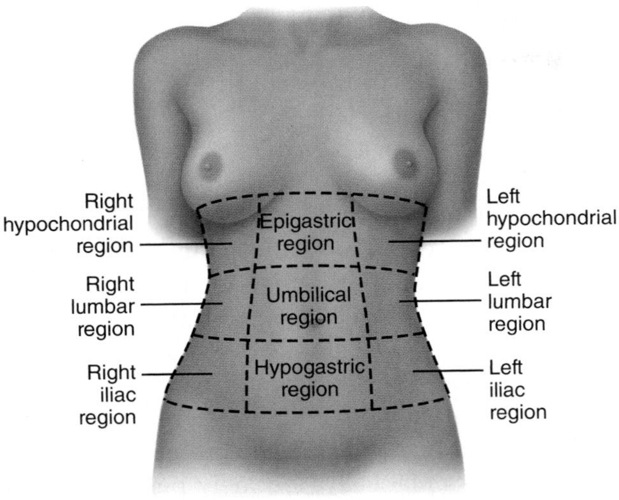

FIGURE 11-34 The abdomen can be divided into nine regions.

The abdomen contains almost all of the organs of digestion, the organs of the GU system, and significant neurovascular structures. The abdominal wall is a relatively thick muscular organ overlying the peritoneum. The peritoneum is a well-defined layer of fascia made up of the parietal peritoneum and visceral peritoneum. Abdominal organs are often characterized as being intraperitoneal or extraperitoneal, depending on their location relative to this layer. Intraperitoneal organs include the stomach, proximal duodenum of the small intestine, pancreas, jejunum, ileum, appendix, cecum, transverse colon, sigmoid colon, proximal rectum, liver, gallbladder, spleen, omentum, and female internal genitalia. Extraperitoneal organs include the mid- and distal duodenum, abdominal aorta, mid- and lower rectum, kidneys, pancreatic tail, adrenal glands, ureters, renal blood vessels, male gonadal blood vessels, ascending colon, descending colon, and urinary bladder.

One of the most challenging complaints for you to assess in the field setting is abdominal pain because it can have multiple causes and often presents with little or no external signs. Three basic mechanisms produce abdominal pain:

- *Visceral pain* occurs when hollow organs are obstructed, thereby stretching the smooth muscle wall, which in turn produces cramping and more diffuse, widespread pain.
- *Inflammation* or irritation of the somatic pain fibers located in the skin, the abdominal wall, and the musculature may produce sharp, localized pain, as in the case of pelvic inflammatory disease (PID) or appendicitis. If gastric contents, blood, or urine enters the peritoneum, it will also produce somatic pain, albeit usually much less localized and more diffuse.
- *Referred pain* occurs when pain originates in a particular organ, but the patient perceives it in a different location. Examples include flank pain associated with kidney stones, inner thigh pain from appendicitis or PID, capsular pain from cholecystitis, and groin pain (waves of pain) from renal colic.

Obtaining baseline vital signs is an integral part of any secondary assessment. The clues obtained from this assessment can help you determine the seriousness of the patient's condition and the function of internal organs. Remember that shock, whether medical- or trauma-related, is seen in different stages. Changes in a patient's BP may be the last piece of evidence you see when shock changes from one level to the next. BP must be sufficient to maintain adequate end-organ perfusion.

Words of Wisdom

The increased intestinal motility that occurs in bowel hyperactivity produces loud, high-pitched, rushing, or tinkling sounds. Hypoactive or absent sounds may follow recent abdominal surgery or in response to peritoneal inflammation.

Normally, baroreceptors in the body sense dropping BP and volume and stimulate a catecholamine and renin–aldosterone response. This, in turn, causes peripheral vasoconstriction, increased pulse rate, and fluid retention, which puts more blood into the core circulation and increases volume and BP. In patients with volume depletion, there is not enough circulating blood to push into the core circulation, especially as they move from a supine position to sitting or standing. **Orthostatic vital signs**, also called the "tilt test," are measurements of a patient's BP and pulse taken in the supine and sitting or standing positions. The results of this test can help you determine the extent of volume depletion and indicate whether the patient needs fluid replacement. The tilt test is generally used for patients with complaints of nausea, vomiting, diarrhea, syncope, and GI problems.

Words of Wisdom

If a patient becomes dizzy when moving from a supine position to a sitting position, do not have them stand up because they will probably pass out.

In some studies, a tilt test or orthostatic change is considered positive when the patient's systolic BP decreases up to 20 mm Hg, diastolic BP increases more than 10 mm Hg (a narrowing pulse pressure), and the pulse rate increases by 20 beats/min. Take vital signs at 1-minute intervals between moving a patient to a new position, and then place the cuff on the same arm in the same location. Document whether the pulse was regular, if the patient is being monitored and there is an attached ECG strip, and whether the patient is experiencing other symptoms. If a fluid bolus for volume replacement is given, repeat the orthostatic assessment after assessing lung sounds.

As you examine a patient's abdomen, be sure to make the patient as comfortable as possible. Sometimes this requires administering pain medication first, which usually helps the patient to be more cooperative and better able to focus with less discomfort. Assess the abdomen with the patient in a supine position. To examine and palpate/percuss over the posterior aspects of the abdomen, however, ask the patient to sit up or log roll the patient into position. Always proceed with abdominal assessment systematically, routinely performing inspection, auscultation, and palpation, as shown in **SKILL DRILL 11-9**.

Skill Drill 11-9 Examining the Abdomen

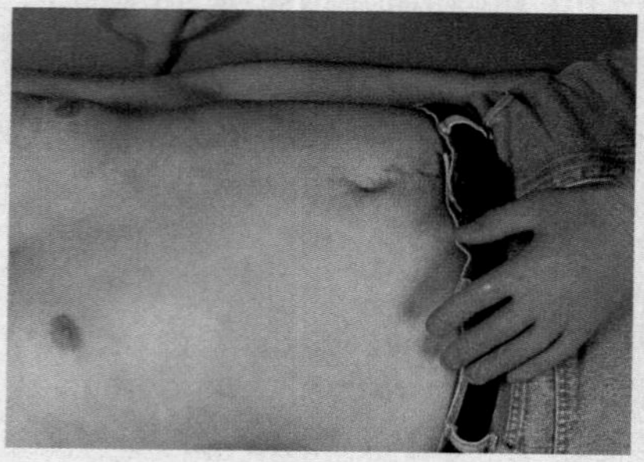

Step 1

Inspect and palpate the abdomen for open/closed findings, rigidity (firmness), tenderness, distention, swelling, or bruising. Look at the skin as well as the contour and overall appearance of the abdominal wall. Note any surgical scars, because they may be clues to an underlying illness, previous trauma, or surgeries. Look for symmetry and distention. Look for a rash or other signs of an allergic reaction. Finally, note any wounds, striae, dilated veins, or generalized distention or localized masses.

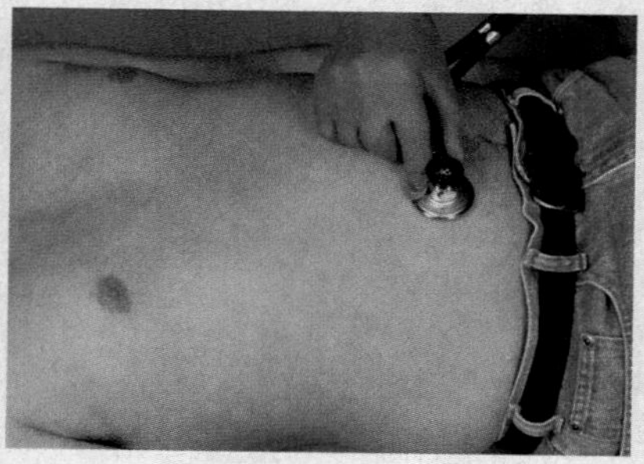

Step 2

Auscultate the abdomen for bowel sounds (if time and noise level permit). Note the presence or absence of bowel sounds. Note the frequency and character of any hyperactive sounds.

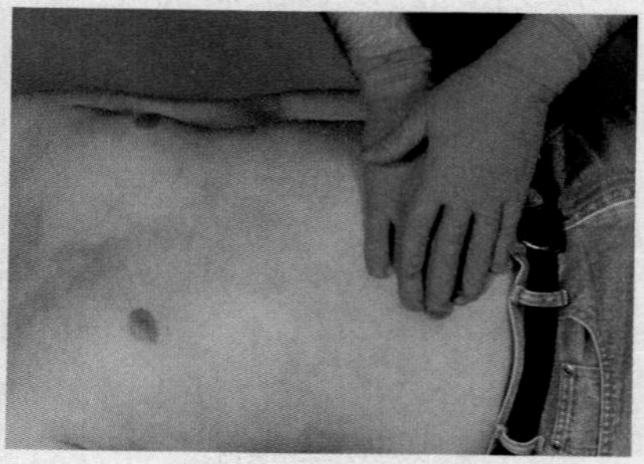

Step 3

Before palpating the abdomen, ask the patient to point to the area of greatest discomfort. Avoid touching that area until last. Systematically palpate the four quadrants of the abdomen, beginning with the quadrant farthest from the patient's complaint. Work slowly, and avoid quick movements. Perform percussion as appropriate. Pay special attention to the patient's expressions because they may yield valuable information.

Words of Wisdom

Restlessness and constant changes of position occur with the colicky pain of gastroenteritis or bowel obstruction. Absolute stillness, resisting any movement, is demonstrated with the pain of peritonitis (inflammation of the peritoneum). Knee flexion, facial grimacing, and rapid/uneven respiration are also signs of pain.

The abdomen can be described as flat, rounded, protuberant (bulging), scaphoid (hollow or boat [skiff] shaped), or pulsatile (pulsing or throbbing). In a normal abdomen, the cavity should appear soft with no tenderness or masses. Any abdominal distention must be distinguished from obesity. An obese patient's abdomen tends to be more protuberant than distended (tense and bloated), and is typically exceptionally pliable.

Some patients may have **ascites**, a collection of fluid within the peritoneal cavity. Ascites is similar to edema, but instead of affecting the interstitial tissues of the legs, it involves the abdomen. The patient's abdomen may appear markedly distended, and a visible or palpable fluid wave may be evident during examination, with shifting dullness noted on percussion. Ascites typically occurs in patients with liver disease, but it can also be associated with a malignancy or even renal or cardiac insufficiency.

Words of Wisdom

Pain on release of pressure is described as rebound tenderness, a reliable sign of peritoneal inflammation, such as that seen in appendicitis. Do not repeatedly check for rebound tenderness since it hurts the patient.

Blue discoloration in the periumbilical area (Cullen sign) or along the flanks (Grey Turner sign) is indicative of intraperitoneal hemorrhage, with two of the more common causes being ruptured ectopic pregnancy and acute pancreatitis.

Abdominal auscultation is part of a routine abdominal exam, although it may have limited utility in the prehospital setting. To hear bowel sounds, the environment must be fairly quiet and the patient must remain still. Take time to ensure an adequate assessment. Sometimes an abnormality is characterized by hyperactivity (increased) or hypoactivity (decreased), rather than a total absence of bowel sounds. Obstruction typically produces a high-pitched or tinkling sound. Differentiating normal from abnormal findings can sometimes be challenging, so practice this skill on many healthy people to develop a full appreciation for the abnormal situations you are likely to encounter.

In addition to auscultating for bowel sounds, use the bell of the stethoscope to listen for any bruits in the abdomen. Recall that bruits are sounds made from turbulent blood flow through the arteries. In the abdominal cavity, listen for bruits over the aorta, right and left renal arteries, and common iliac arteries. Bruits in these areas suggest arterial stenosis or blockage.

Palpation yields the most significant diagnostic information during the abdominal exam: tenderness (elicited pain). A moan, facial grimace, or sudden withdrawal all send the same message: You have touched something or somewhere that causes pain or discomfort. A patient who contracts their abdominal muscles shows guarding. **Guarding** can be either voluntary or involuntary and typically indicates underlying conditions such as appendicitis. Marked persistent contraction throughout the abdominal musculature is described as rigid and often indicates peritonitis. This finding is clinically important and often results in urgent surgical evaluation and intervention.

You may be able to correlate these findings with historical information related to the patient's current illness or situation to determine what's wrong. Tightness or guarding can result from internal bleeding, an inflamed organ, and many other causes. Possible sources of LUQ pain include a ruptured spleen or mononucleosis. Unless it can be ruled out, LUQ pain should always be assumed to be the spleen, since misdiagnosing a ruptured spleen could be fatal. Patients with LLQ abdominal pain, especially if they have a history of constipation, nausea, vomiting, and fever, should be suspected of having diverticulitis. With RLQ abdominal pain, appendicitis is a likely culprit. Generalized abdominal pain in women of childbearing age can be caused by an ectopic pregnancy, a ruptured ovarian cyst, or some other obstetric or gynecologic condition, which can be life threatening.

When appropriate, speak with the patient about the NOI while palpating the abdomen. Palpate each quadrant gently but firmly, and recognize that the patient may respond in many ways. Once an area of tenderness has been localized, attempt to visualize which structures may underlie it, and think about what might be causing the problem. If the patient has penetrating trauma, this step is less of a priority; it is difficult to localize areas damaged with a high-velocity MOI by visualizing and palpating the abdominal wall. Consider any signs or symptoms of abdominal injury as serious and indicative of a high-priority patient in unstable condition. That key information is worth pursuing in your assessment.

Rebound tenderness is rarely checked in the field, primarily because doing so can be painful. It requires slowly pushing down and then rapidly releasing sections of the abdomen. A positive sign (the patient cries out or withdraws) indicates peritoneal irritation. Such irritation may arise when a peritoneal organ becomes inflamed or when a hollow organ ruptures, emptying its contents into the peritoneal cavity. Large-volume bleeding with peritoneal distention may also produce this phenomenon. However, be aware that in trauma cases, solid-organ bleeding does not always cause peritoneal irritation, guarding, and rigidity.

Patients with less discrete (localized), guarded tenderness to palpation may have a more visceral problem. Although this may represent an early manifestation of a serious condition, it can also be associated with various degrees of bowel obstruction, renal colic, biliary colic, or urinary tract infection. The pain is often deep-seated and poorly described by the patient. Cases of colic typically involve a problem with peristalsis, the wave-like contraction motion of a hollow tubular structure such as the small or large intestine, common bile duct, or ureter. A stone may obstruct the tube, for example, or an adhesion or hernia may prevent proper intestinal peristalsis. Some patients will describe the pain as wavelike or waxing and waning. Other lower-abdominal sources of pain and tenderness include GU processes.

As you palpate the abdominal cavity, attempt to palpate the liver, gallbladder, and spleen. To palpate the liver, place your left hand behind the patient, parallel to and supporting the right 11th and 12th ribs and adjacent soft tissues below. Place your right hand on the patient's right abdomen just below the rib cage. Ask the patient to take a deep breath. Try to feel the liver edge as it comes down to meet your fingertips. If you feel it, slightly lighten the pressure of your palpating hand so the liver can slip under your finger pads and you can feel its anterior surface.

Use the same technique to assess the gallbladder. While the gallbladder is typically not palpable, eliciting pain or a sudden gasp indicates possible inflammation. The difference in the technique is that when the patient takes a deep breath, you attempt to move your fingertips under the edge of the liver, rather than palpating its anterior surface. This will bring your fingertips closer to the gallbladder.

The spleen is a very difficult organ to palpate, and you will likely be able to palpate it only if it is inflamed. With your left hand, reach over and around the patient to support and press forward the lower left rib cage and adjacent soft tissue. With your right hand below the left costal margin, press in toward the spleen. Begin palpation low enough that you are below a possible enlarged spleen. Ask the patient to take a deep breath, and try to feel the tip or edge of the spleen as it comes down to meet your fingertips.

Vascular sources can cause significant abdominal pain, most notably aortic aneurysm. Occasionally, a markedly dilated aorta can be seen pulsating in the midline of the upper abdomen. If the patient has an obvious pulsatile mass, do not palpate it. However, if no pulsatile mass is seen, then proceed with abdominal palpation. A ruptured aortic aneurysm also tends to be tender to palpation. Once you suspect an aortic aneurysm, take extreme care to minimize manipulation. The aorta is a retroperitoneal structure, so a lack of obvious findings while assessing the anterior abdomen does not rule out this diagnosis.

Another notable palpable abdominal wall mass is a *hernia*, a localized weakening of the abdominal wall musculature. Occasionally, you might find a hernia in the ventral wall of the abdomen. This is different from a hernia that might be found in the groin. Many of these types of hernias, such as umbilical hernias, are congenital, whereas others are the result of a previous abdominal surgery (incisional hernia). Hernias in the ventral wall are not always visible. If you suspect a hernia but do not see an umbilical or incisional hernia, place the patient in the supine position and ask them to raise their head and shoulders off the table. This maneuver will usually produce the bulge of a hernia. Most of the time, such findings are considered benign in the EMS environment. However, it is a true medical emergency if a section of bowel becomes entrapped and strangled in the hernia. In such cases, the patient's symptoms will include pain, fever, and possibly shock.

Female Genitalia

The female genitalia consist of the ovaries, fallopian tubes, uterus, vagina, and external genitalia. The ovaries lie in the lowermost portion of the abdomen, in the inguinal region, just superior to the inguinal crease. In the nonpregnant state, the uterus is a small structure not palpable on external examination. Chapter 23, *Gynecologic Emergencies*, provides a detailed review and illustrations of the female genitalia.

In general, assessment of female genitalia is performed in a limited and discreet manner. Always keep the patient appropriately draped during the exam. Male paramedics should be assisted by a woman if possible. Reasons to examine the genitalia include concern over life-threatening hemorrhage or when you suspect delivery is imminent in a pregnant patient.

As you assess the abdomen, palpate both the bilateral inguinal and hypogastric regions. If the decision is made to examine the genitalia specifically, limit the exam to inspection only. Pain and tenderness in the fallopian tubes and ovaries can be elicited during patient assessment. Clinically significant causes of this pain include an ectopic pregnancy, complications of third-trimester pregnancy, and ovarian disorders or pelvic infections in nonpregnant patients. In trauma patients where pelvic fracture is a concern, genital bleeding is a possibility, albeit an unlikely one. In the case of injury involving intentional trauma, significant bleeding is possible; if you must intervene in this kind of situation, then preserve any garments and give them to law enforcement personnel as soon as possible. Note the amount and quality of any bleeding, as well as any inflammation, discharge, swelling, or genital lesions.

Male Genitalia

The male reproductive system consists of the testes, reproductive ducts, seminal vesicles, prostate, penis, and urethra **FIGURE 11-35**. The testes are analogous to the ovaries, in that they are the principal organs of reproduction. The testes, which lie outside the torso in a sac (*scrotum*), produce hormones and reproductive cells (sperm). The sperm is then transported from the testes to the pelvis, where it mixes with semen from the seminal vesicles and fluid from the prostate and is released during the process of ejaculation.

As you examine the male genitalia, ensure your partner is present, and perform the exam in a limited and discreet manner. In the prehospital setting, situations requiring assessment of the male genitalia are limited. Always assess the entire abdomen and

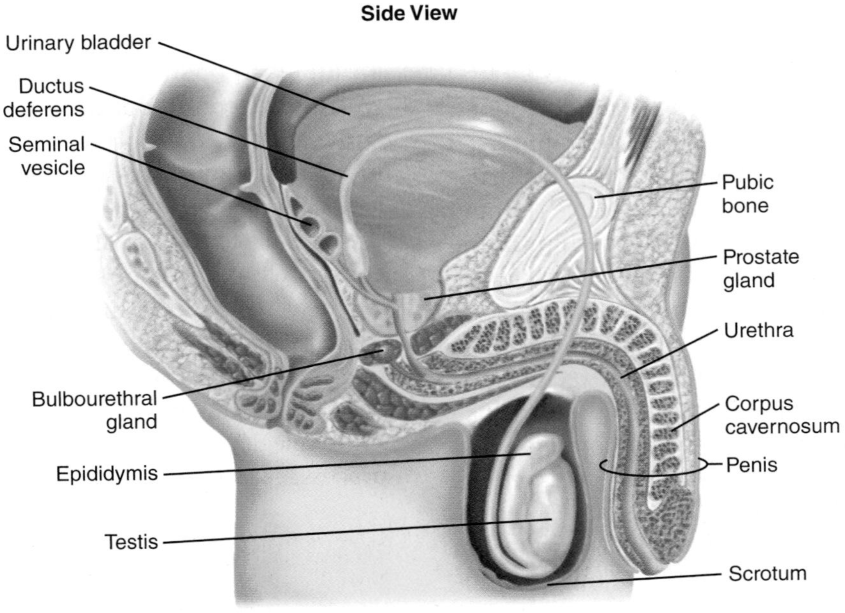

FIGURE 11-35 Male genitalia.

note any pertinent findings, because lower abdominal problems are occasionally referred from the genitalia. For example, patients with testicular torsion or an inguinal hernia sometimes complain of lower abdominal pain but minimal abdominal tenderness. In the case of a trauma patient, assess for the possibility of significant genital bleeding and injury or underlying fracture. Note any inflammation, discharge, swelling, or lesions. Also, priapism is a prolonged erection of the penis, usually resulting from a spinal cord injury. In addition, look for evidence of urinary incontinence, especially in an unresponsive patient. Incontinence in an unresponsive patient may be associated with spinal cord injury or seizure.

Anus

The anus is the distal orifice of the alimentary canal and is often evaluated at the same time as the genitalia. It is examined in only a few circumstances and is always done with the patient appropriately draped and your partner present. With a positive history (eg, rectal bleeding, severe anal pain) or signs or symptoms of trauma, examine the area to assess the need to control bleeding or initiate another intervention (eg, treatment for shock or care of eviscerated parts). The exam usually involves inspection only and occurs with the patient in a laterally recumbent position. Examine the back, posterior buttocks, and perineum, noting obvious bleeding, trauma, lumps, ulcers, inflammation, rash, abrasions, or evidence of fecal incontinence.

Musculoskeletal System

The extremities consist of both soft tissue and bones. Joints are areas where the ends of bones abut each other to form a kind of moving structure. This structure is held together by ligaments, creating a jointed appendage. Each joint has a shock-absorbing lining (the cartilage) and is filled with fluid (synovial fluid). Joints allow the body to perform mechanical work. Indeed, the mechanical process of motion becomes possible when joints are alternately flexed and extended by skeletal (striated) muscles that traverse joints. These skeletal muscles are anchored to bone by tendons. Each muscle is named according to its location and function.

The principal joints of the upper extremities are the shoulder (acromioclavicular and glenohumeral joints), elbow (olecranon), and wrist (radiocarpal). The principal joints of the lower extremities are the hip (acetabulum), knee (patellar), and ankle (tibiotalar).

> **Words of Wisdom**
>
> To assess a patient with a possible shoulder dislocation, position yourself behind the patient and compare the two shoulders. The dislocated side is usually lower than uninjured side.

In older patients, musculoskeletal complaints are common. As joints age, they become more vulnerable to repetitive-motion stress and trauma, and the loss of articular cartilage due to inflammatory or mechanical breakdown leads to osteoarthritis in older adults. These patients are likely to have decreased mobility and ROM secondary to joint and muscle changes. Disruption of the bones, joints, and soft tissues can take various forms, and discomfort or disability may be a manifestation of an acute problem, a chronic problem, or both. In addition to joint changes, muscle mass decreases with age and from a lack of use. Older adults tend to live a more sedentary lifestyle, contributing to these conditions. A common finding when assessing joints is crepitus with movement. Whereas this would be considered an abnormal finding in the younger population, it is a normal variant of aging, typically associated with advanced arthritis.

Common musculoskeletal and soft-tissue injuries include fractures, sprains, strains, dislocations, contusions, hematomas, and open wounds. Fractures may be characterized in many ways. For example, an open fracture is essentially a fracture with direct communication to the body's exterior surface, whereas a closed fracture is associated with intact surrounding skin. On some occasions, what looks like an open fracture is simply an open wound that is close to the site of fracture but not actually in contact with the fracture. Nevertheless, any fracture with a nearby wound should be considered an open fracture until the actual communication between the fracture and the wound is proven to be absent, typically based on results of a surgical exploration.

While fractures always involve a pathologic process, it is important to distinguish a **pathologic**

> **Words of Wisdom**
>
> Point tenderness is the most reliable indicator of an underlying fracture.

fracture from a traumatic fracture. A pathologic fracture occurs when normal forces are applied to abnormal bone structures, producing a fracture. A traumatic fracture occurs when abnormal forces are applied to normal bone structures, producing a fracture. Traumatic fractures usually occur in high-intensity blunt trauma. Pathologic fractures often occur as a result of decreased bone density, such as osteopenia or occult malignancy, and can occur with relatively little application of force.

Examine the skeleton and joints, paying attention to their structure and function. Consider how the joint and associated extremity look and how well they function. Does the extremity look normal and move easily? In particular, note any limitation in ROM, as well as any bony crepitus or pain with motion. Look for evidence of inflammation or injury, such as swelling, tenderness, increased heat, redness, ecchymosis, and decreased function. Also evaluate the joint or extremity for obvious deformity, diminished strength, atrophy, and asymmetry. The musculoskeletal exam should not cause the patient any pain; if pain occurs, it should be considered an abnormal finding. Follow the steps in **SKILL DRILL 11-10** to examine the musculoskeletal system.

Skill Drill 11-10 Examining the Musculoskeletal System

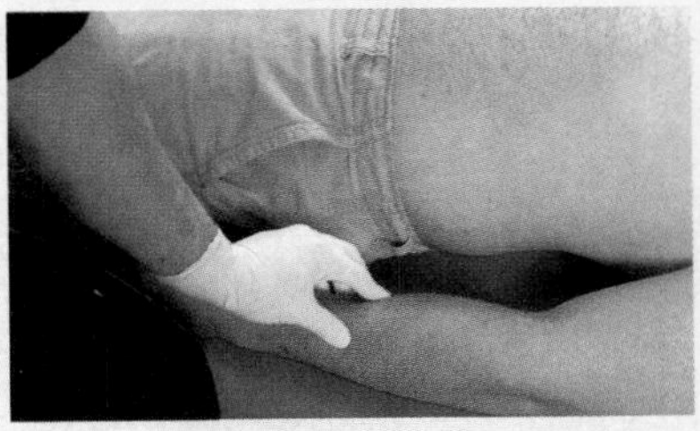

Step 1

Beginning with the upper extremities, inspect the skin overlying the muscles, bones, and joints for soft-tissue damage. Note any deformities or abnormal structures.

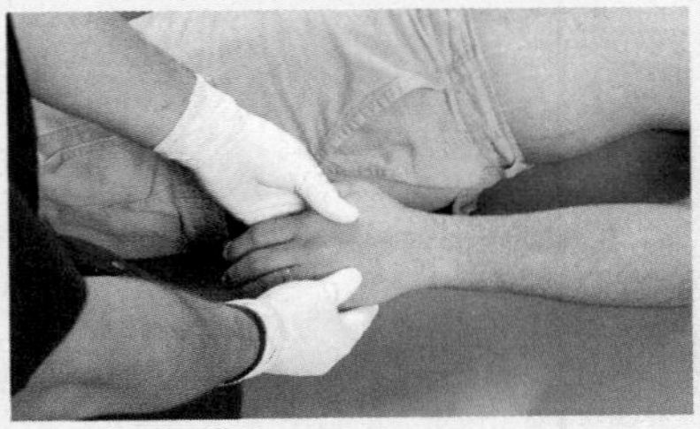

Step 2

Inspect and palpate the hands and the wrists. Note any open/closed findings and crepitus.

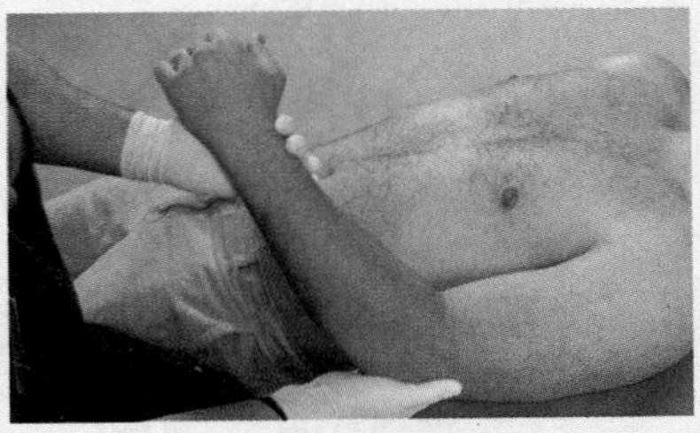

Step 3

Inspect and palpate the elbows. Ask the patient to flex and extend the elbow to establish ROM. Note any abnormalities.

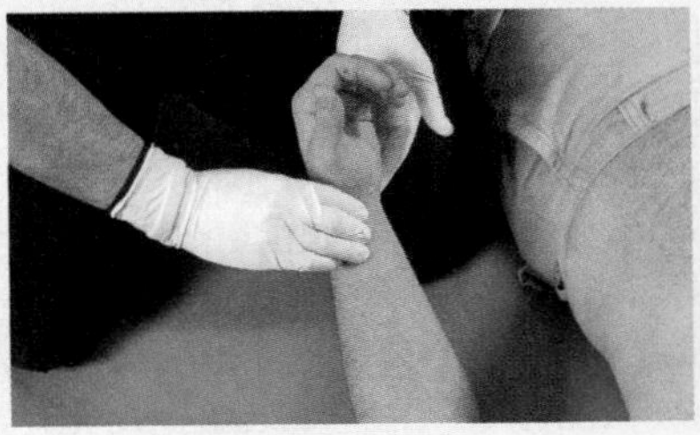

Step 4

Check for adequate distal pulse, motor function, and sensation in each extremity.

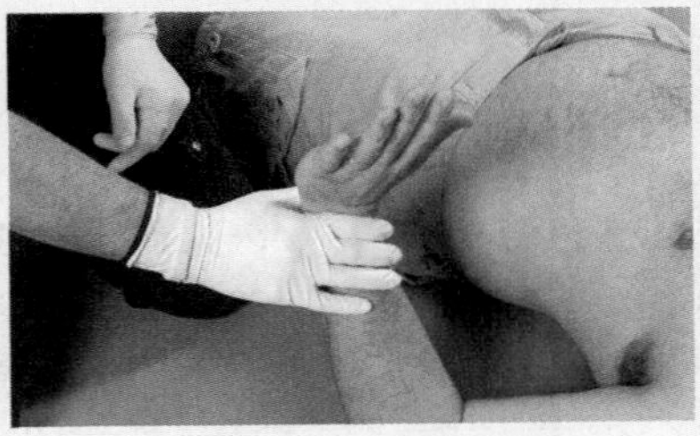

Step 5

Ask the patient to flex and extend the joints of the fingers, hands, and wrist to establish ROM. If the patient experiences any discomfort, immediately stop that portion of the exam.

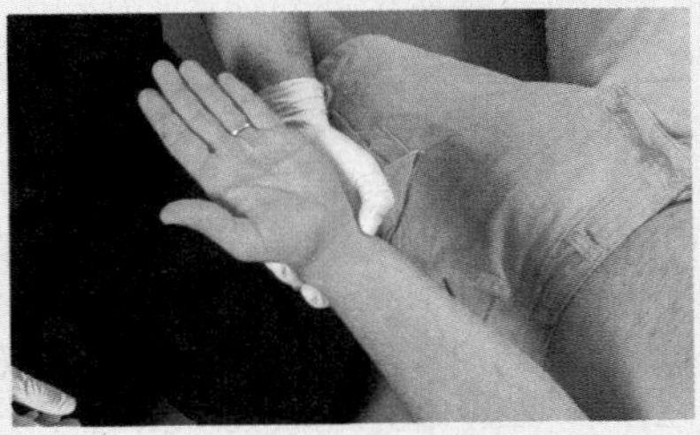

Step 6

While holding the patient's elbow still, ask the patient to turn their hand from the palm-down position to the palm-up position and back again.

(continues)

Skill Drill 11-10 Examining the Musculoskeletal System (continued)

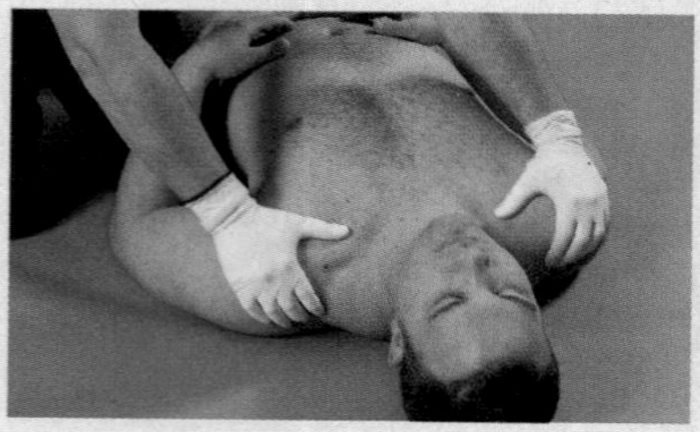

Step 7

Inspect and palpate the shoulders. Ask the patient to shrug the shoulders and raise and extend both arms.

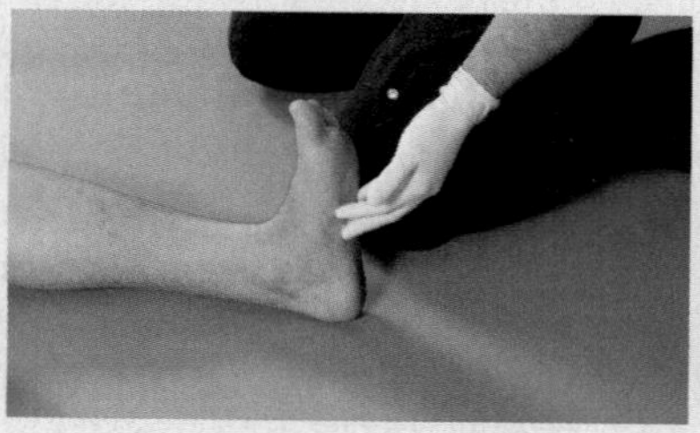

Step 8

Inspect and palpate the bony structures to establish ROM. Ask the patient to point and bend their toes.

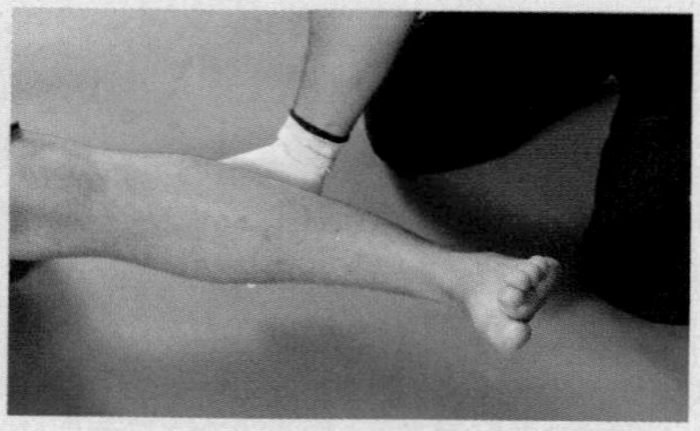

Step 9

Ask the patient to rotate the ankle to check for pain or restricted ROM.

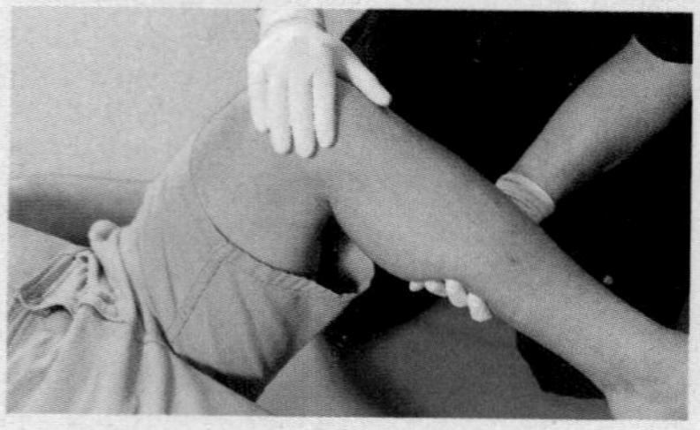

Step 10

Inspect and palpate the knee joints and patella to establish ROM. Ask the patient to bend and straighten both knees.

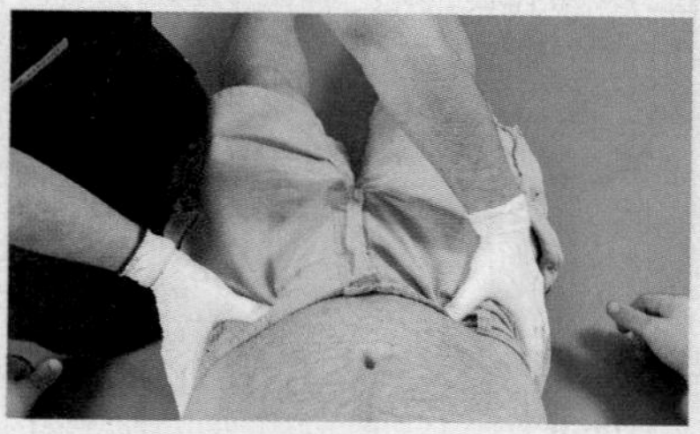

Step 11

Check for structural integrity of the pelvis by applying gentle pressure to the iliac crests, pushing in and then down.

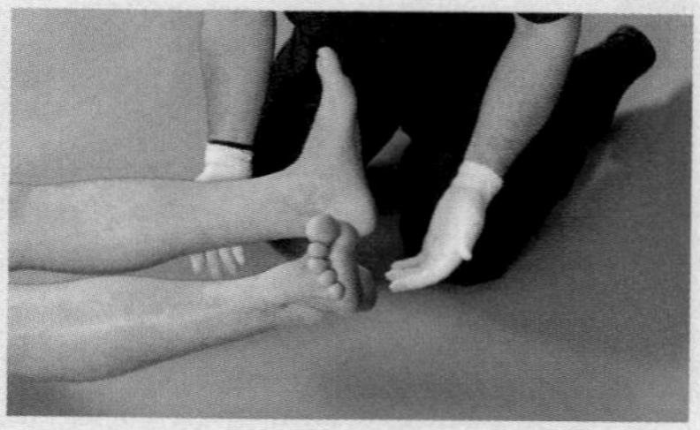

Step 12

Ask the patient to lift both legs, bend at the hip and turn the legs inward and outward. Note any abnormalities.

Often the diagnosis of a problem involving the shoulders and related structures can be made simply by noting the patient's posture at the time of your first contact. For example, a glenohumeral joint dislocation may be manifested as the loss of normal contour of the shoulder, with abnormal squaring of the lateral aspect of the shoulder, and the humeral head visible and/or palpable in the soft tissues of the chest wall, in the subacromial region **FIGURE 11-36**.

Palpate the proximal upper extremity and shoulder. Assess the sternoclavicular joint, acromioclavicular joint, subacromial area, and bicipital groove (origin of the biceps, just distal to the anterior aspect of the humeral head). Note any tenderness, swelling, crepitus, deformity, rotation, or ecchymosis in these areas.

When possible, check ROM by asking the patient to raise their arms to the vertical position, above the head. Next, ask the patient to demonstrate external rotation and abduction by placing both hands behind the neck, with the elbows out to the sides. Finally, perform internal rotation by asking the patient to place both hands behind the lower back.

Evaluate the elbows by performing an overall inspection for gross deformity or abnormal rotation.

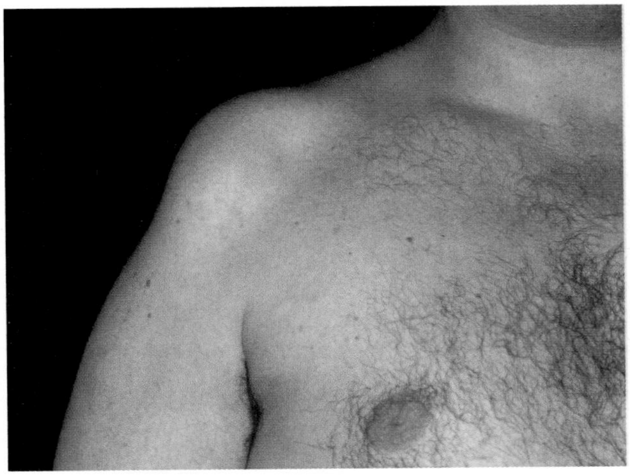

FIGURE 11-36 Abnormal squaring of the shoulder.

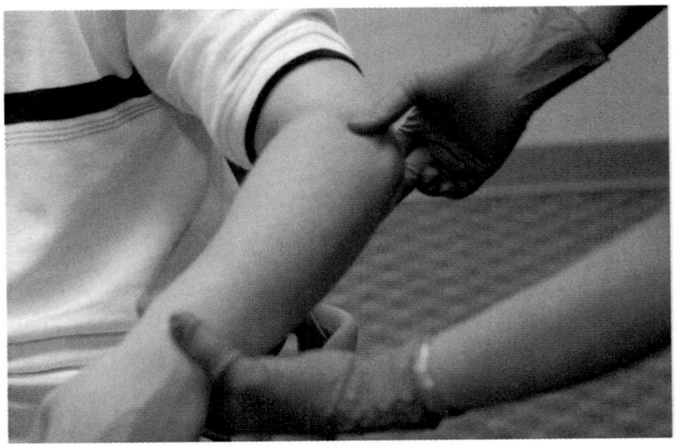

FIGURE 11-37 Palpate the elbow.

Palpate the elbow between the epicondyles and olecranon, and also palpate each epicondyle and the olecranon **FIGURE 11-37**. Note any tenderness, crepitus, swelling, or thickening. Perform ROM testing last because suspicion of significant pathology or fracture of the elbow mandates appropriate immobilization as soon as possible. When testing the elbows, flex and extend them both passively and actively. Then have the patient supinate and pronate the forearms while the elbows are flexed at the patient's sides.

Inspect the hands and wrists for any abnormalities, including swelling, redness, contusions, wounds, nodules, deformities, or atrophy. Palpate the hands, feeling the medial and lateral aspects of each interphalangeal joint on each finger

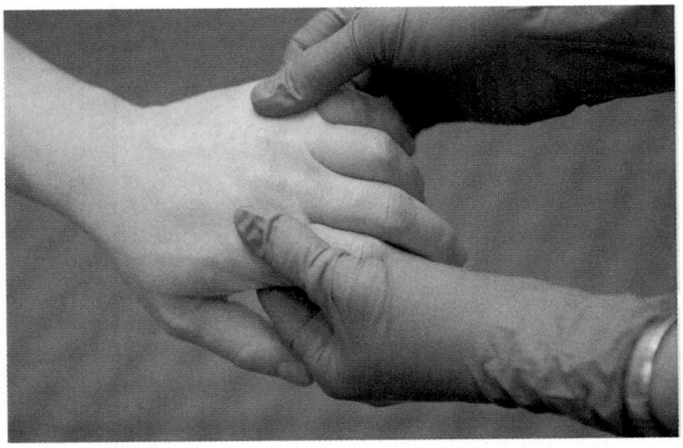

FIGURE 11-38 Palpate the hand and fingers.

FIGURE 11-38. Squeeze the hands, compressing the metacarpophalangeal joints. Palpate the carpal bones of the wrists, noting any areas of swelling, tenderness, or bogginess. Perform ROM evaluations by asking the patient to make fists with both hands, then extend and spread the fingers, then flex and extend the wrists, and finally move the hands laterally and medially, with the palms facing down. At this point, check capillary refill (in pediatric patients), symmetry of radial pulses, and overall limb temperature.

A rapid appreciation of injury or disability involving the lower extremities can be gained by evaluating the patient's ability to walk. Of course, this may not be a practical first approach to assessment in many prehospital cases.

Examine the knees and hips by inspecting the overall alignment and symmetry of the lower extremities **FIGURE 11-39**. Identify any lower extremity deformity, especially shortening and/or rotation, either internal or external; these findings are often evident with an injury to the proximal aspect of the lower extremity or hip joint. In particular, an open-book pelvic fracture, which presents with both feet rotated outward, is a life-threatening injury. Look for evidence of thickening, swelling, or bruising of the thigh. Note any crepitus or palpable tenderness. If possible, test ROM of knees and hips to determine the presence of underlying injury to those structures. Ask the patient to bend each knee and raise the bent knee toward the chest. Assess for rotation and abduction of the hips, both passively and actively. Next, palpate each hip individually

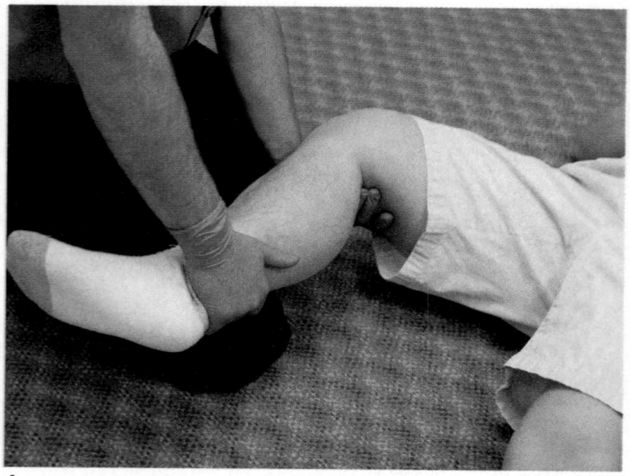
A

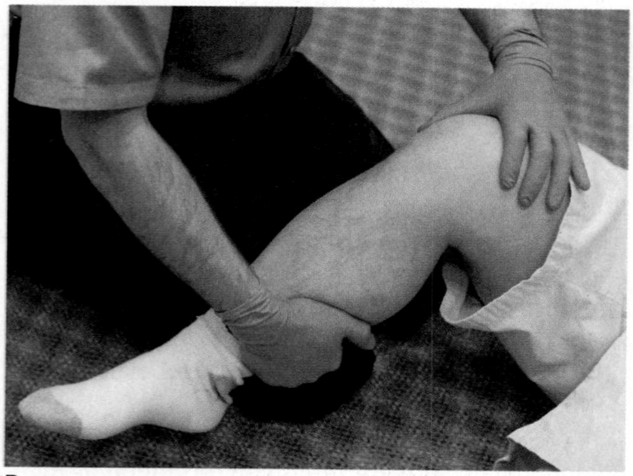
B

FIGURE 11-39 Examination of the lower extremities. **A.** Hip. **B.** Knee.

distal to the inguinal crease and over the anterior, lateral, and posterior aspects. Finally, palpate and gently compress the pelvis downward and then inward.

Examine the ankles and feet, observing all surfaces. Note any wounds, deformities, discolorations, nodules, or swelling. Palpate all aspects of the feet and ankles, noting tenderness, bogginess, swelling, or crepitus. Measure distal pulses over the dorsalis pedis and tibialis posterior, and assess the overall limb temperature. Pulse strength may decrease in older patients, especially those with a history of moderate edema and peripheral vascular disease. Because of the small anatomic size of young pediatric patients, pulses may be difficult to palpate. In this situation, capillary refill will be a more reliable indicator of perfusion (as discussed in Chapter 44, *Pediatric Emergencies*). Assess ROM by having the patient plantar flex, dorsiflex, and invert and evert the ankles and feet. Check the forefoot and toes by inspection, palpation, and ROM testing **FIGURE 11-40**.

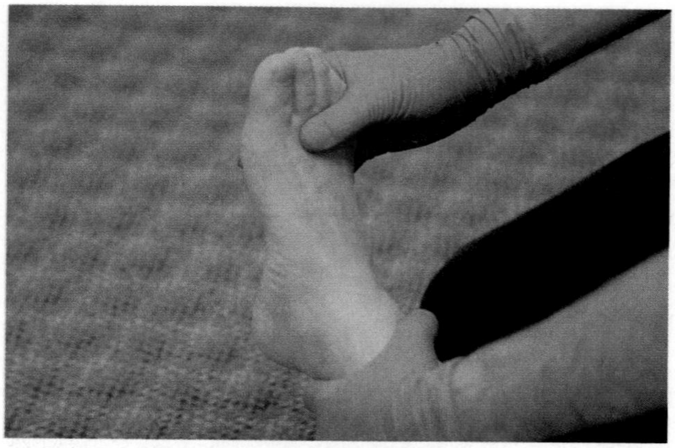
FIGURE 11-40 Inspect the patient's feet.

Peripheral Vascular System

The peripheral vascular system comprises all aspects of the circulatory system except the heart, the great vessels immediately involved with the mediastinum, and the coronary circulation. Thus, it includes all of the body's arteries, veins, arterioles, venules, capillaries, lymphatics, and the respective fluids these structures carry.

Words of Wisdom

Pitting edema 4-point scale:

+1 = 0 to ¼ inch (0 to 0.635 cm)
+2 = ¼ to ½ inch (0.635 to 1.27 cm)
+3 = ½ to 1 inch (1.27 to 2.54 cm)
+4 = > 1 inch (> 2.54 cm)

Words of Wisdom

Bilateral, dependent, pitting edema occurs with systemic conditions such as heart failure and hepatic cirrhosis. Unilateral edema occurs with local conditions such as deep vein occlusion.

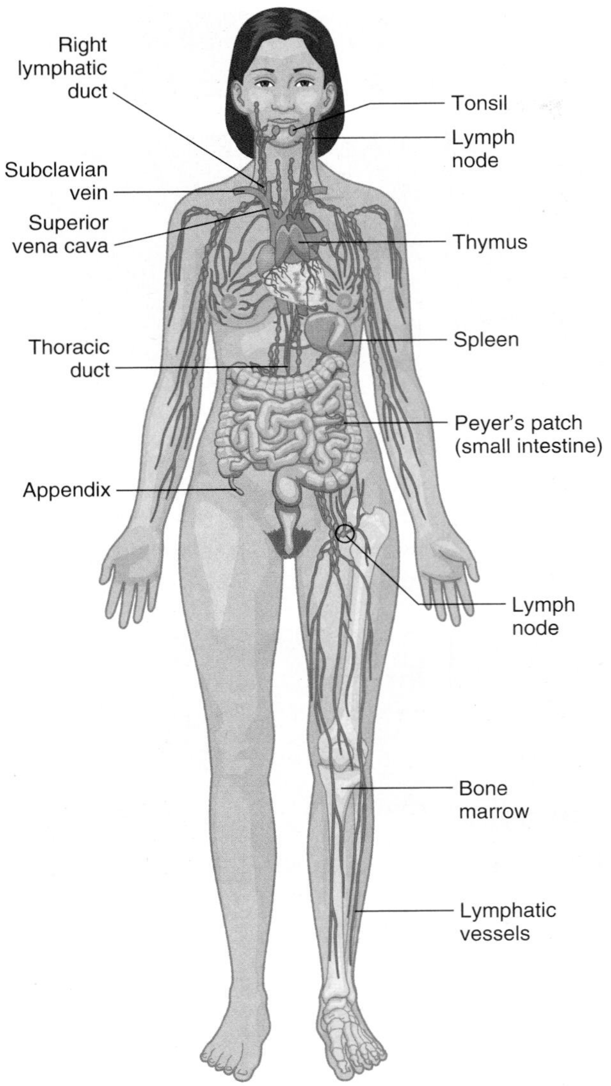

FIGURE 11-41 Lymphatic system.

The lymphatic system is an intricate network of nodes and ducts of various sizes dispersed throughout the body **FIGURE 11-41**. Lymph nodes are larger accumulations of lymphatic tissue, and smaller amounts of lymph are distributed in tissue throughout the body. All lymphatic tissue contains large numbers of immunologically active cells; thus, the lymphatics manage a key function in the body's immune system. The ducts contain a fat-rich fluid known as lymph, which transports materials from the lymph tissue into the central venous circulation via the thoracic ducts.

Perfusion occurs in the peripheral circulation via a network of capillary beds. Blood cells and plasma in close proximity to tissue offload substances required by the cells for proper metabolic functioning and simultaneously transport metabolic wastes out of the tissues for eventual elimination from the body. Impaired functioning of the peripheral vascular system means the capillary beds cannot adequately perfuse tissues and organs, causing significant morbidity and mortality.

Diseases of the peripheral vascular system are often seen in patients with other underlying medical conditions (ie, diabetes, hypertension, dyslipidemia, obesity, and those caused by tobacco use). These disease processes typically damage the smaller-diameter vessels of the peripheral vascular system, resulting in disease of the tissues and organs that depend on those vessels for proper functioning. With age and the advance of these various disease processes, the vasculature can no longer manage rapid changes in perfusion requirements, thereby becoming a source of illness.

As you assess the peripheral vascular system, pay attention to both the upper and lower extremities. Look for signs that indicate either acute or chronic vascular problems. A wide range of disorders, from chronic venous stasis and lymphedema to intermittent claudication (cramp-like pain in the lower legs because of poor circulation or low potassium levels) and acute arterial occlusion, can affect the peripheral vascular system. Peripheral vascular disease can manifest in many forms, depending on the point in the vasculature where the abnormality is located. Carotid artery disease can manifest as a stroke, for example, while arterial embolization involving the mesenteric vessels can cause bowel ischemia and necrosis. In the extremities, involvement of the peripheral vasculature can lead to limb ischemia. Follow the steps in **SKILL DRILL 11-11** to examine the peripheral vascular system.

Inspect the upper extremities from fingertips to shoulders. Note each extremity's relative size, and evaluate it for symmetry by comparing one side with the other. Pay attention to any obvious swelling, unusual venous patterns, skin CTC, and color of the nail beds. If indicated, palpate the epitrochlear and axillary lymph nodes, noting their size, tenderness, mobility, and overlying redness. Palpate the radial pulses simultaneously, and compare them. In situations of unilaterally absent pulses, check proximally over the brachial pulse sites. As you evaluate a limb for ischemia, consider the five

Skill Drill 11-11 Examining the Peripheral Vascular System

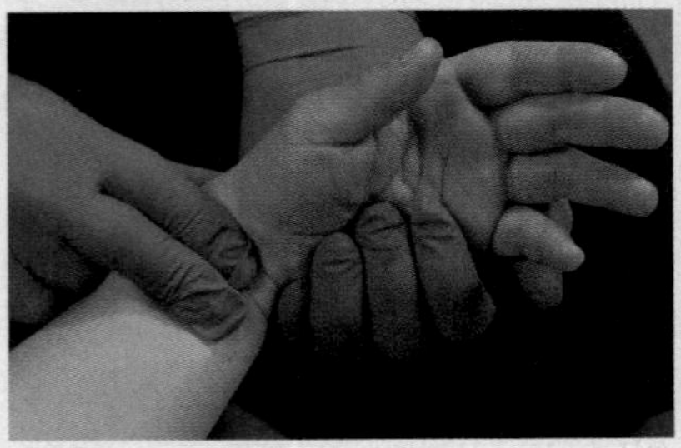

Step 1

As you examine the upper extremities, note any abnormalities in the radial pulse, skin color, temperature, or condition.

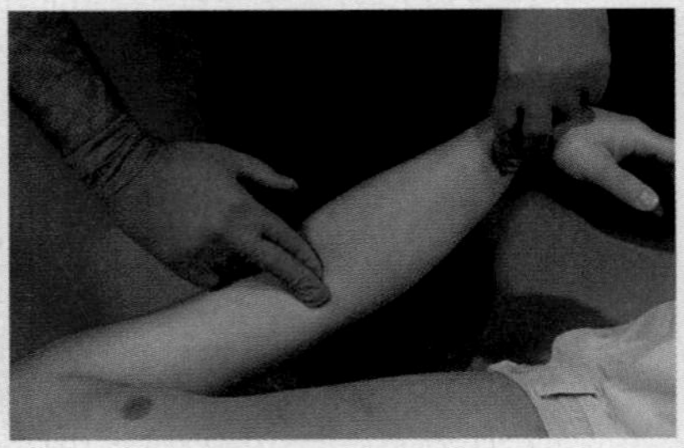

Step 2

If you note abnormalities in the distal pulse, work your way proximally, check those pulse points, and note your findings.

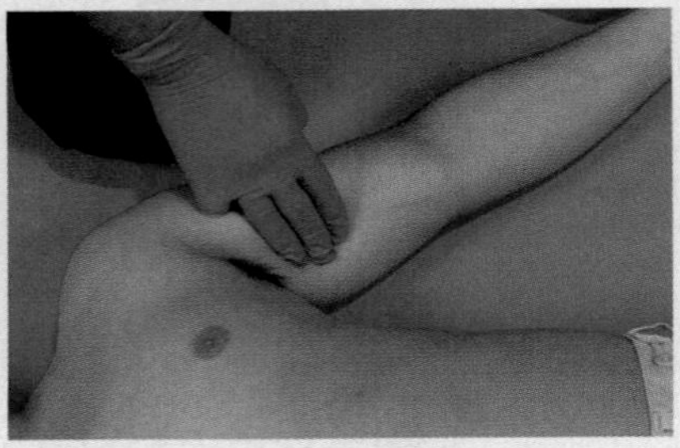

Step 3

Palpate the epitrochlear and brachial nodes of the lymphatic system. Note any swelling or tenderness.

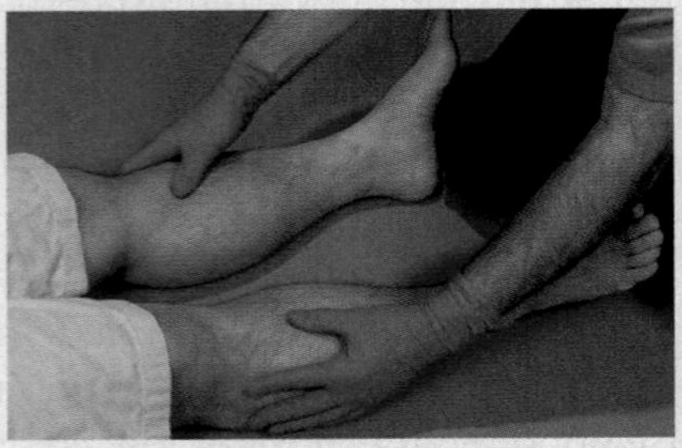

Step 4

Examine the lower extremities, noting any abnormalities in the size and symmetry of the legs. Evaluate the temperature of each leg relative to the rest of the body and to each other.

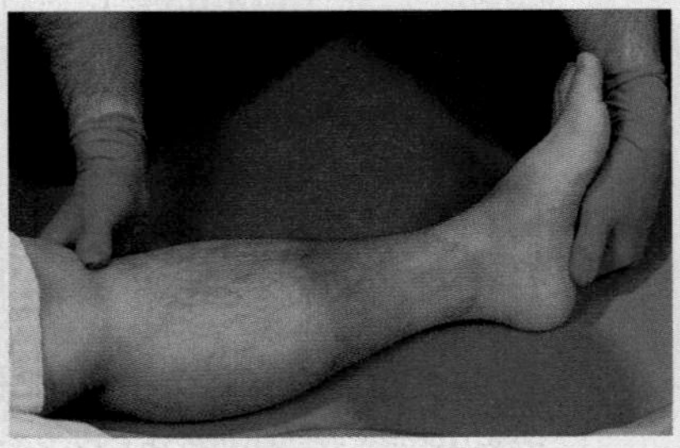

Step 5

Inspect the skin color and condition. Note any abnormal venous patterns or enlargement.

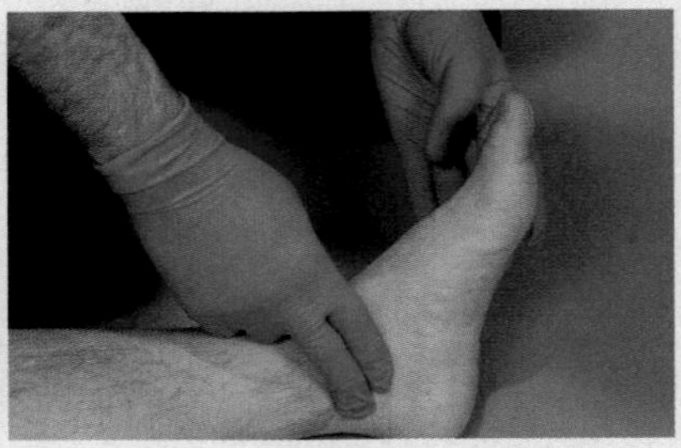

Step 6

Check distal pulses, noting any abnormalities.

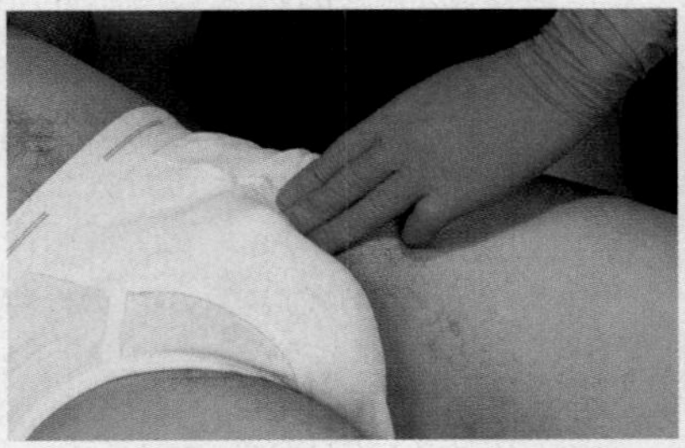

Step 7

Palpate the inguinal nodes for swelling or tenderness.

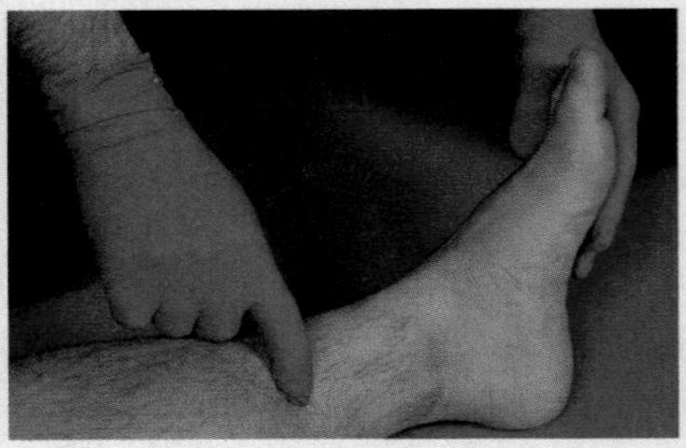

Step 8

Evaluate for pitting edema in the legs and feet.

Ps of acute arterial insufficiency that you learned in EMT training: Pain, Pallor, Paresthesia, Paresis, and Pulselessness. The loss of a palpable pulse is the worst indicator of such a problem because it is considered a late finding.

Proper evaluation of the vascular status of the lower extremities requires the patient to be lying down and draped appropriately. Remove the patient's socks, stockings, and shoes before proceeding with the exam. Inspect the lower extremities from the groin and buttocks to the feet. Always compare the right side with the left side. Look at the size and symmetry of the legs, noting any localized versus generalized swelling. Pay attention to any remarkable superficial venous patterns or venous enlargement. Observe the skin pigmentation, as well as the skin color and texture. **Rubor**, ecchymosis, or pallor may all be encountered in patients with significant vascular insufficiency. Also note the presence of any rashes, scars, or ulcers, and determine whether they are shallow or deep.

Palpate pulses in the lower extremities to assess the arterial circulation. In particular, palpate pulses over the dorsalis pedis and posterior tibialis, and in the femoral regions. The popliteal pulse can also occasionally be appreciated. Note the temperature of the feet and legs and attempt to palpate any edema in the legs. To do so, press your thumb over the dorsum of the foot and anteriorly over the tibias, and hold the thumb with firm, gentle pressure for at least 5 seconds. If indicated, palpate the superficial inguinal lymph nodes, noting their mobility, size, tenderness, and any overlying redness.

Spine

Assessment of the cervical spine was introduced earlier. This section covers the complete assessment of the spine. The spine represents the core of the axillary skeleton. It consists of 33 individual vertebrae, the lower nine of which are fused.

To assess the spine, begin by inspecting the back from both the posterior and lateral aspects. The spine features several curves, representing the cervical, thoracic, and lumbar regions. Some amount of curvature in the spine is normal, however, lordosis and kyphosis are abnormal amounts of spine curvature. **Lordosis** refers to the inward curve of the lumbar spine just above the buttocks. *Exaggerated* lordosis results in swayback **FIGURE 11-42**.

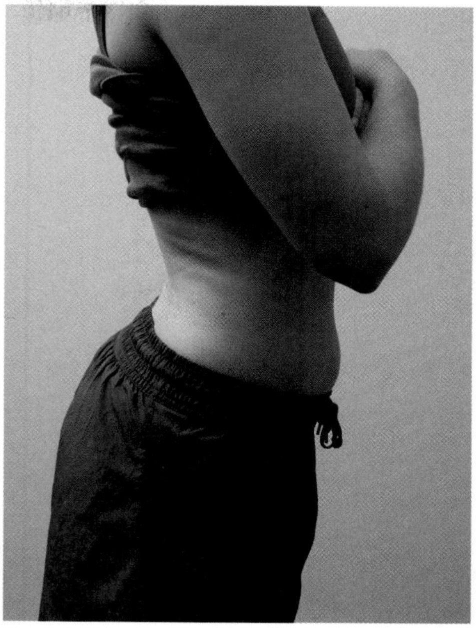

FIGURE 11-42 Lordosis is inward curvature of the lumbar spine just above the buttocks.

Kyphosis refers to the outward curve of the thoracic spine **FIGURE 11-43**. It is frequently exaggerated in older adults because of degenerative joint disease, osteoporosis, and vertebral compression fractures. At its worst, kyphosis can become a source of restrictive lung disease, a form of COPD. **Scoliosis**, a sideways curvature of the spine, is also abnormal **FIGURE 11-44**. As you examine the spine, look for differences in the height of the shoulders as well as differences in the height of the iliac crests of the pelvis. Look at the entire back, noting any wounds or ecchymosis.

> **Words of Wisdom**
>
> Log rolling the patient onto a backboard always gives you a valuable opportunity to quickly inspect and palpate the back for signs of injury. Instruct and position your assistants to facilitate this brief exam.

Palpation of the spine is typically done while the patient is supine, often after they have been log rolled onto one side to facilitate access to the back and placement of a spinal immobilization device. As you palpate the spine, use your thumb to touch each spinous process. This allows you to identify

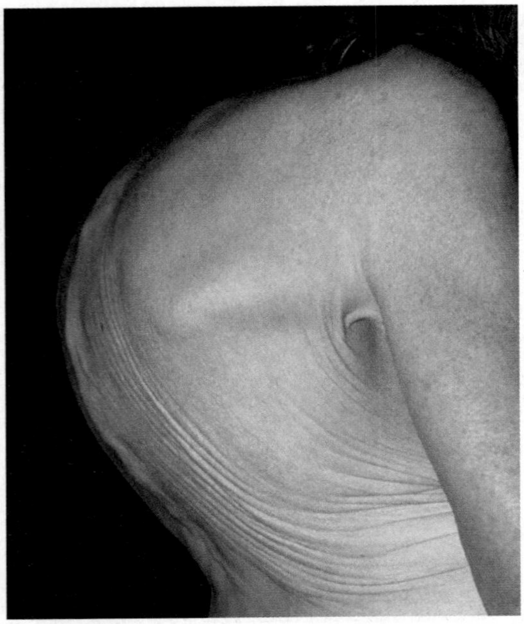

FIGURE 11-43 Kyphosis is outward curvature of the spine; it can be exaggerated in older adults.

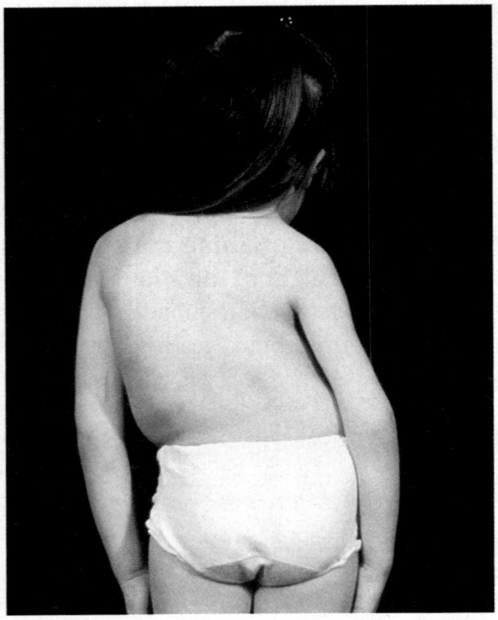

FIGURE 11-44 Scoliosis is the sideways curvature of the spine.

any tenderness, step-off, or crepitus. Step-off occurs in the context of a displaced fracture or a dislocation **FIGURE 11-45**. If you identify any abnormality, promptly institute proper splinting and protective measures per your regional protocols.

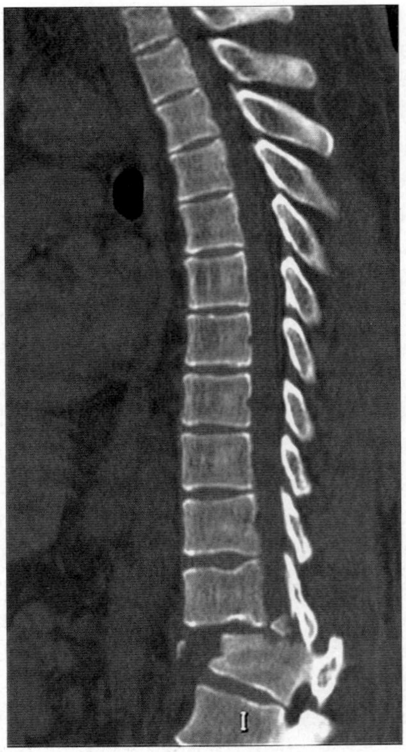

FIGURE 11-45 In the context of a displaced fracture or a dislocation, there may be a step-off when palpating from one vertebra to the next, as shown here.

Check the rest of the back for any other significant findings on palpation. Tap over the costovertebral angles, and palpate the scapulae, paraspinal areas, and base of the neck. Also, check the buttocks. Finally, perform a ROM evaluation. Although this evaluation may be of limited utility in the prehospital setting, it may prove quite helpful in areas that practice selective spinal immobilization. ROM should *never* be done passively. The awake and alert patient will protect themself and will not transect their own spinal cord by actively moving their neck. Conversely, you can do just that. Always ask the patient to move their neck through a comfortable ROM. If at any time during the ROM the patient experiences pain in the spine or tingling in the extremities, immediately stop that phase of the assessment and immobilize the spine per your regional protocols.

During your assessment of the patient's active ROM, pay attention to the smoothness and symmetry of the patient's movement, along with the actual degree of motion elicited or accomplished. Follow the steps in **SKILL DRILL 11-12** to examine the spine.

Skill Drill 11-12 Examining the Spine

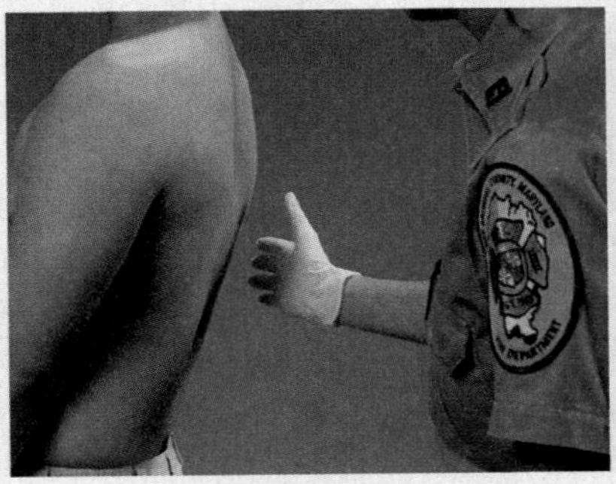

Step 1

Inspect the cervical, thoracic, and lumbar curves for any abnormalities.

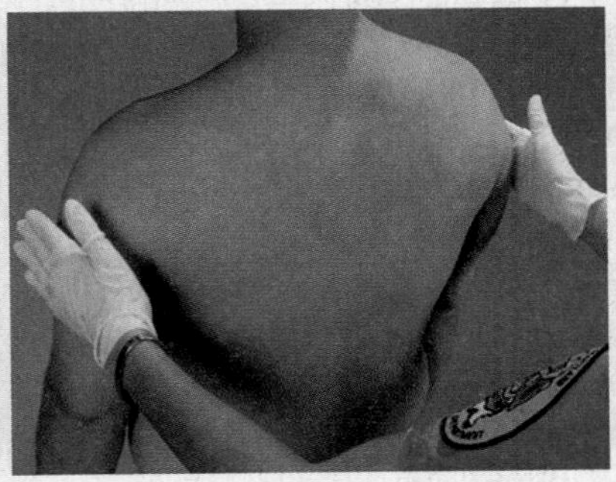

Step 2

Evaluate the height of the shoulders and iliac crests. Differences between one side and the other may indicate abnormal spinal curvature.

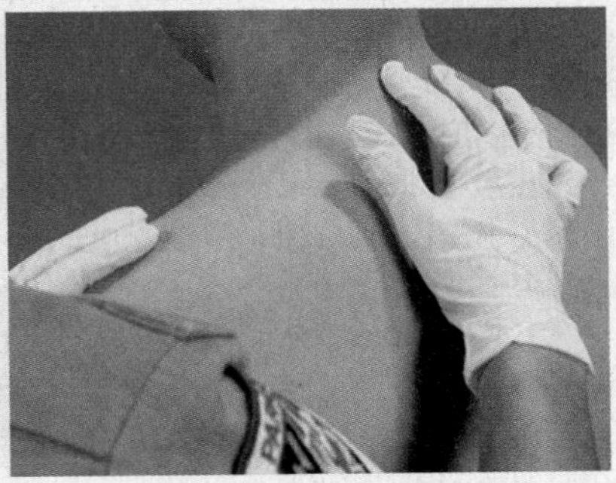

Step 3

Palpate the posterior portion of the cervical spine, noting any point tenderness or structural abnormalities.

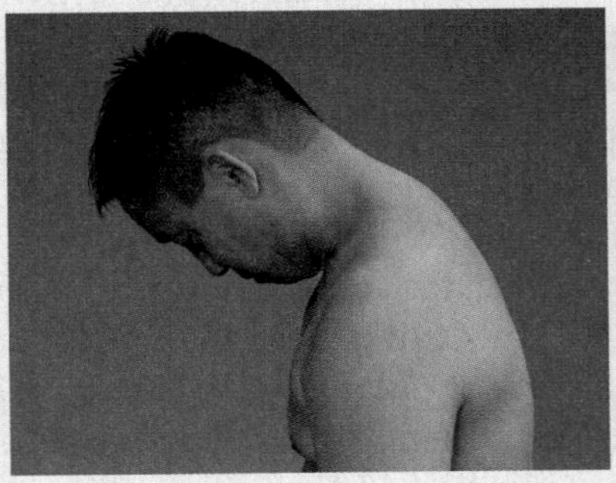

Step 4

In the nontrauma patient, and in the absence of reported pain, ask the patient to move their head forward, backward, and from side to side.

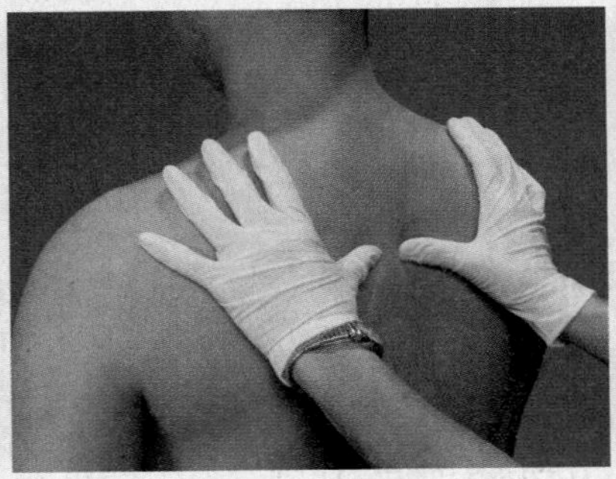

Step 5

Palpate each vertebra with the thumbs.

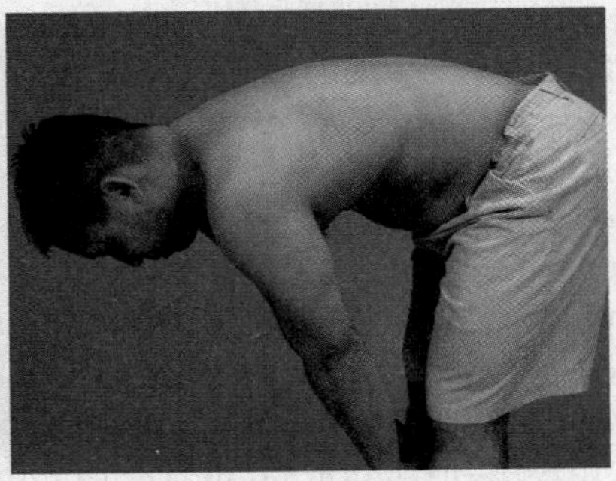

Step 6

In the absence of pain or trauma, ask the patient to bend at the waist in each direction to establish ROM.

Nervous System

The brain is a complex structure with an enormous perfusion requirement, as you learned in Chapter 8, *Anatomy and Physiology*. With the exception of the cranial nerves, all nerves are ultimately channeled to the brain via the spinal cord. The spinal cord plays the role of a large conduit, passing information back and forth along its sensory pathways. Recall that the nervous system is divided into involuntary (autonomic) and voluntary portions, with the autonomic nervous system being further subdivided into the sympathetic and parasympathetic systems.

Reflexes are involuntary motor responses to specific sensory stimuli, such as giving a tap on the knee or stroking the eyelash. The location of what is stimulated determines which muscle will contract reflexively. Spinal reflexes occur when sensory input comes from receptors in the muscles, joints, and skin. The motor response to this stimulation occurs entirely within the spinal cord; no brain processing is required. Other reflexes include the deep tendon reflexes and the superficial and brainstem reflexes. **Primitive reflexes**, including the Babinski, grasping, and sucking signs, are normal findings in infants. In older people, once the long motor pathways of the peripheral nervous system (PNS) have become fully myelinated, these primitive reflexes represent abnormal findings, typical of injury or disconnection between the cerebral cortex and the brainstem.

A Babinski reflex test may be used to check neurologic function. It is accomplished by stimulating the sole of the foot by rubbing it with your thumb or by running a pen or other pointed object along the length of it. In a normal reaction, the great toe will flex. However, *do not* perform a Babinski reflex test on a patient who has lower extremity injuries. Doing so could prompt the patient to pull the leg back, causing pain.

Neurologic Exam The check of the nervous system is one of the most time-consuming elements of the physical exam. Most of the time, performing a complete and thorough neurologic exam will be impossible in the field and would be inappropriate; however, if the patient displays signs and symptoms of a neurologic condition, every attempt should be made to perform relevant portions of the neurologic exam. At a minimum, the neurologic exam should determine the patient's baseline mental status (AVPU), cranial nerve function (pupils, eyes, smile, speech, swallow, shoulder shrug), distal motor function (ability to move), and distal sensory function (ability to feel). It may also test deep tendon reflexes if necessary.

Words of Wisdom

Restlessness is a danger signal!

First, assess the patient's overall mental status. Is the patient awake? If so, is the patient alert, and to what degree? If a change in LOC has occurred, what kind of stimulus does it take to get a response, and to what degree does the patient's mental status improve? In the case of AMS, do you observe any unusual postures? Is there any alteration in physical status (eg, can the patient move successfully and symmetrically)? A detailed explanation of the mental status exam was covered earlier in the chapter. Here is a quick review using the COASTMAP mnemonic:

- **C** **Consciousness.** Along with LOC, note the patient's ability to pay attention and concentrate. Is the patient easily distracted?
- **O** **Orientation.** Ask about the year, season, month, day, and date. Have the patient identify the present location; that is, state, city or town, and specific location. Can the patient recall and describe the current event?
- **A** **Activity.** Does the patient appear anxious or restless? Are they sitting still, scarcely moving at all? Are they making any strange or repetitive motions (possibly because of methamphetamine use)?
- **S** **Speech.** Note the rate, volume, articulation, and intonation of the patient's speech. Does it sound pressured (forced)? Does the speech have a flat, monotonous delivery consistent with depression? Is the speech garbled or slurred (dysarthria)? Garbled or slurred speech has many possible causes, including alcohol or drug impairment, stroke, and traumatic brain injury.
- **T** **Thought.** Listen to the patient's story. What's on their mind? Is the patient making sense? Is there anything unusual about their reasoning? Is the patient expressing apparently false ideas (delusions)? Are voices telling the patient what to do or think (psychosis)? Does the patient report thoughts that people are "out to get me" (paranoia)?
- **M** **Memory.** You can form an impression of the patient's memory by listening to them reconstruct past events. A more precise assessment requires asking a few questions. First, explain to the patient that you would like them to try to remember three words. Then slowly say the names of three unrelated words (eg, *apple, bicycle, sewing machine*). Ask the patient to repeat those words to ensure they have heard and understood them. A few minutes later, ask the patient if they can remember the three words you named before; this tests retention and memory.
- **A** **Affect.** The patient's affect (mood) may be most apparent in their body language. A posture of shoulders drooping and head bent, for

example, conveys depression. Note whether the affect seems appropriate to the situation.

P Perception. Detecting perception disorders may be difficult because patients are often hesitant to answer questions about hallucinations. Sometimes it is helpful to ask the patient, "Do you ever hear things that other people can't hear?"

After assessing the patient's overall mental status, begin the comprehensive neurologic exam. Of course, this exam is not needed in every case. Its details may vary greatly, depending on the nature of the patient's problem. Also, many portions of the neurologic exam may have been completed earlier, during other aspects of the patient assessment. Keep track of your initial findings so you can report them, so they are not needlessly repeated, and so any subsequent changes in mental status can be noted. Are left- and right-side motor and sensory findings symmetric? If not, how do they differ? Does the presenting problem appear to be more of a CNS or a PNS malfunction, or is it secondary to swelling or bone displacement from trauma?

When testing the cranial nerves, several simple maneuvers can be employed to determine the presence and degree of disability **TABLE 11-10**. With practice, the entire cranial nerve examination can

TABLE 11-10 Tests for Cranial Nerve Dysfunction

Cranial Nerve	Function	Assessment Technique
I. Olfactory	Smell	Not usually assessed. Use ammonia or another known scent as an inhalant.
II. Optic	Vision	Place a finger in front of the patient's face. Ask if they can see your finger.
III. Oculomotor	Movement of eye, pupil, and eyelid	Have the patient follow your finger as you move it in an "H" shape. Ask the patient to blink.
IV. Trochlear	Movement of eye	(Tested in the same way as the oculomotor nerve.)
V. Trigeminal	Chewing Pain Temperature Touch of mouth and face	Ask the patient to smile.
VI. Abducens	Movement of eye	(Tested in the same way as the oculomotor nerve.)
VII. Facial	Movement of face Tears Salivation and taste	(Tested in the same way as the trigeminal nerve.)
VIII. Auditory	Hearing and balance	Ask the patient to follow your spoken commands.
IX. Glossopharyngeal and X. Vagus	Glossopharyngeal: Swallowing, taste, and sensations in mouth and pharynx Vagus: Sensation and movement of pharynx, larynx, thorax, and gastrointestinal system	Ask the patient to smile and then swallow.
XI. Accessory	Movement of head and shoulders	Ask the patient to shrug their shoulders; hold both of the patient's shoulders at the same time to assess symmetry.
XII. Hypoglossal	Movement of tongue	Ask the patient to stick out their tongue.

be performed in less than 3 minutes. That said, do not waste time performing this exam if the patient has more pressing needs.

Adequate evaluation of the motor system involves assessing several distinct areas. Although motor activity may represent the localized workings of the musculoskeletal system, the nervous system has an overriding influence on motor activity. Observe the patient's initial posture and body position **FIGURE 11-46** as well as their body position both at rest and with movement, if appropriate. Observe any apparent involuntary movements, and document the quality, rate, rhythm, and amplitude. Determine whether these involuntary movements are related to the patient's posture or activity, and consider whether their presentation includes a component of fatigue or emotion. Make a general assessment of the bulk of the patient's major muscle groups. Compare the sizes of these muscles and the symmetry of their contours. Document associated muscle tone by checking for resistance to passive motion.

The Medical Research Council Manual Muscle Testing scale is a commonly accepted method of evaluating muscle strength. Using this method, the provider grades the patient's strength on a scale of 0 to 5 by assessing the patient's level of effort in using key muscles from the upper and lower extremities:[20]

0. No muscle activation
1. Trace muscle activation, such as a twitch, without achieving full range of motion

FIGURE 11-46 Note the patient's posture and body position.

Courtesy of Rhonda Hunt.

2. Muscle activation with gravity eliminated, achieving full range of motion
3. Muscle activation against gravity, achieving full range of motion
4. Muscle activation against some resistance, achieving full range of motion
5. Muscle activation against examiner's full resistance, achieving full range of motion

Strength is expressed as a ratio, with 5/5 representing normal muscle tone—for example, "strength is 4 over 5 (4/5) in the bilateral upper and lower extremities." When checking strength, be prepared to test for flexion, extension, grip, abduction, adduction, and opposition, depending on the location of the muscle groups involved.

Check coordination as part of the neurologic exam; this assessment tests various nervous system functions, especially those involving cerebellar function. Assess coordination by evaluating a patient's ability to perform rapid alternating movements, point-to-point movements (eg, finger-to-nose and heel-to-shin testing), stance, and gait. Evaluate gait and stance, but only in those patients whose status allows them to be placed safely in a standing position. Note any upper extremity tremors or **pronator drift**. Pronator drift is seen when the patient is asked to hold their arms straight out with palms up and with their eyes shut. The patient should be able to hold the arms in this position for 20 to 30 seconds if the motor pathway is intact; if one of the palms turns downward (pronates) in this time, suspect abnormal function in the opposite brain hemisphere, a sign of shock.

In addition to coordination, test **proprioception**, the patient's awareness of motion and position of a body part. Proprioception is a function of the cerebellum. Loss of proprioception can be seen in medical conditions such as trauma, multiple sclerosis, vitamin B_{12} deficiency, and peripheral neuropathy. Test for proprioception by grasping the patient's great toe, holding it by its sides between your thumb and index finger, and then pulling it away from the other toes. Next, demonstrate for the patient "up" and "down" as you move the patient's toe clearly upward and downward. Then, with the patient's eyes closed, ask for a response of "up" or "down" as you move the large toe.

Of course, it is also helpful to assess the GCS score, as discussed in the Primary Survey section. The steps in **SKILL DRILL 11-13** summarize examination of the nervous system.

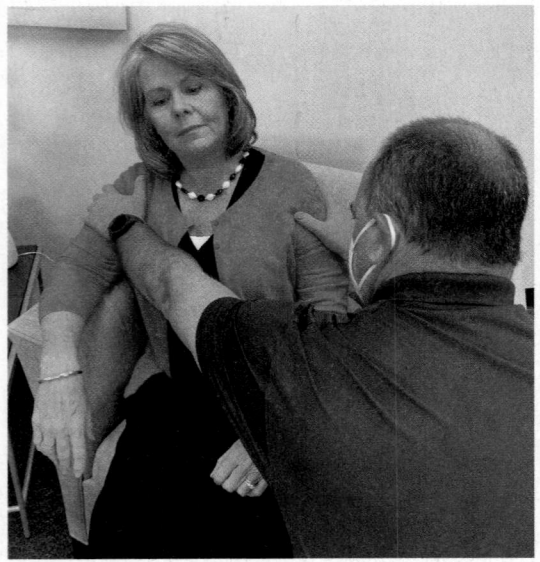

Skill Drill 11-13 Examining the Nervous System

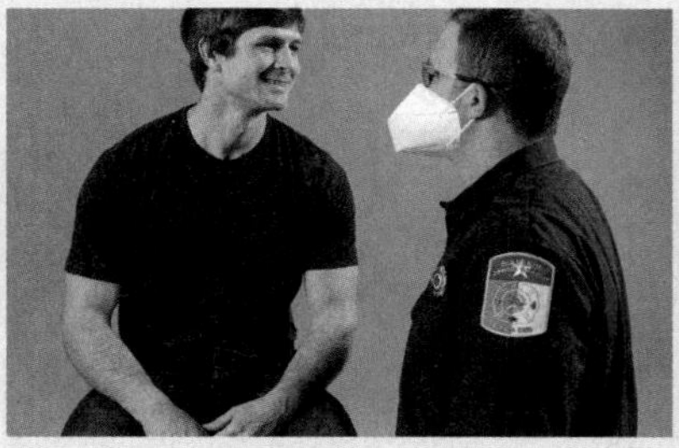

Step 1

Use the AVPU scale to assess the patient's mental status. Note the patient's posture. Evaluate cranial nerve function (see Table 11-10).

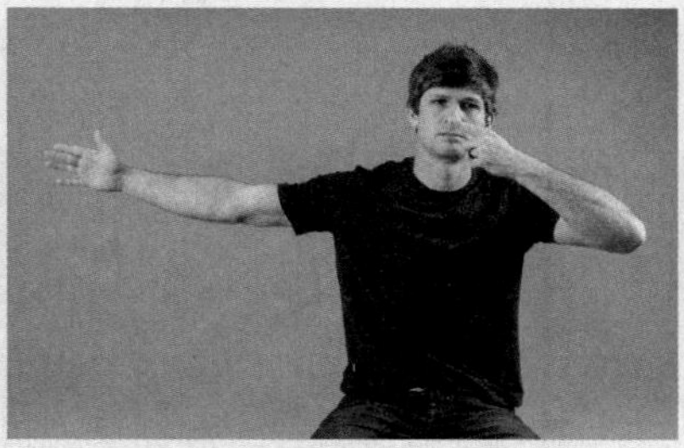

Step 2

Evaluate the patient's coordination by performing the finger-to-nose test using alternating hands.

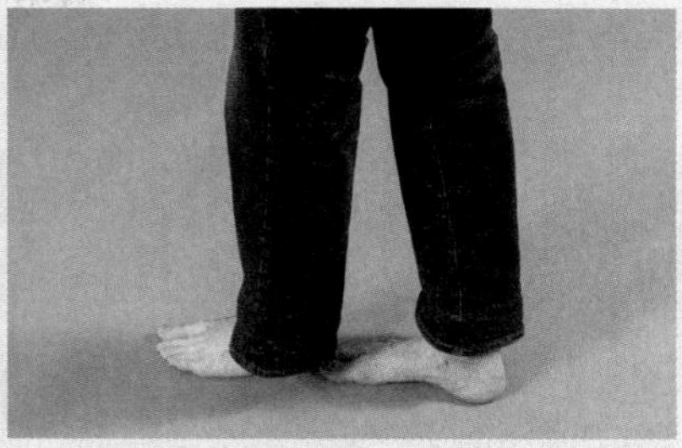

Step 3

If appropriate, test the patient's gait and balance by having them walk heel-to-toe or take a heel-to-shin stance.

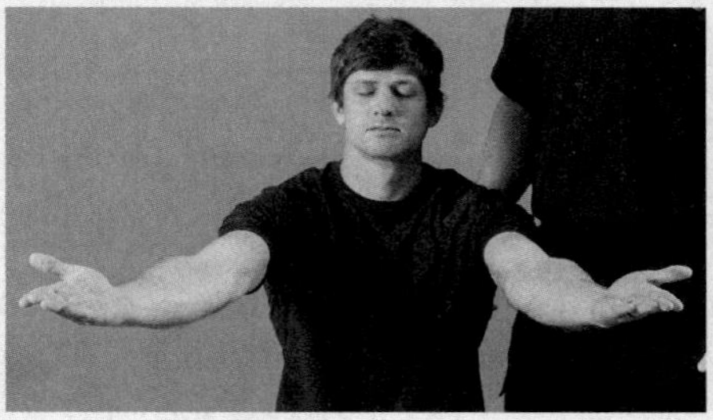

Step 4

Perform the pronator drift test by asking the patient to close their eyes and hold both arms out in front of the body. There should not be a difference in movement on either side.

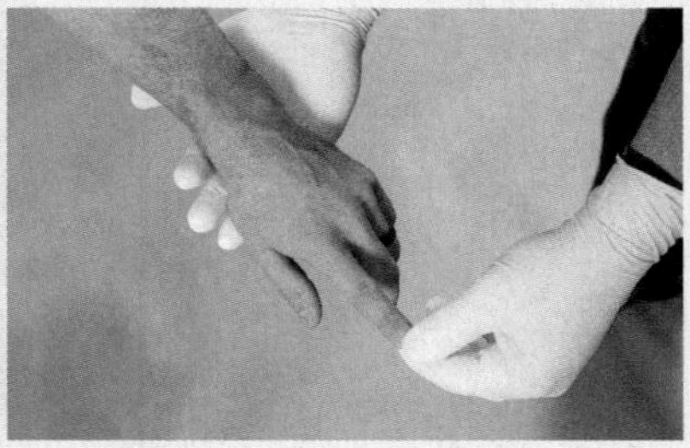

Step 5

Evaluate the patient's sensory function by checking their responses to both gross and light touch. If appropriate, check for deep tendon reflexes.

Just as you use motor function to test nervous system function from the brain to the body, use sensory function to test the nervous system's communication between the body and the brain. Test sensory processes bilaterally, looking for asymmetry and comparing proximal to distal processes. A sensory exam is typically the first evaluation performed when performing the primary survey of a patient who appears to be gravely ill. In this exam, assess both primary and cortical sensory functions. Attempt initial "shake and shout" maneuvers to check for evidence of higher cerebral functioning and determine whether the patient's primary sensory functioning is intact. Typically, these tests look for any response to gross stimuli (such as a loud shout in the face) or more noxious forms (eg, squeezing the nail bed, squeezing two fingers together).

To appropriately assess cortical functioning, the patient's primary functioning must be intact. The brain's primary sensory cortex gathers sensory information and uses it to perform higher-level cortical functions. Therefore, if the primary function is disrupted, any examination of cortical function will be unreliable. However, if primary sensory functioning seems to be intact, proceed with testing the patient's perception of gross versus light touch (the fingers are used; no equipment is required). This test evaluates areas of cortical sensory function. More involved sensory evaluation requires checking sharp versus dull perception and two-point discrimination. Sensation is commonly reported relative to dermatomal location on the body's surface. Dermatomes are areas of the skin that are supplied by a specific sensory nerve.

Follow the steps in **SKILL DRILL 11-14** to evaluate deep tendon reflexes. A method of scoring deep tendon reflexes is covered in **TABLE 11-11**.

Skill Drill 11-14 Evaluating Deep Tendon Reflexes

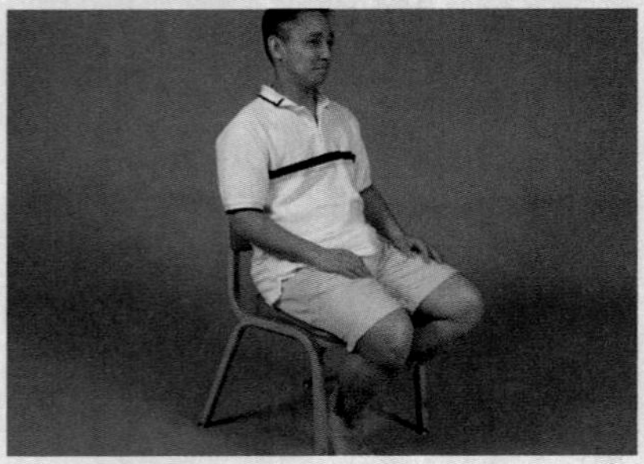

Step 1

Place the patient in a sitting position.

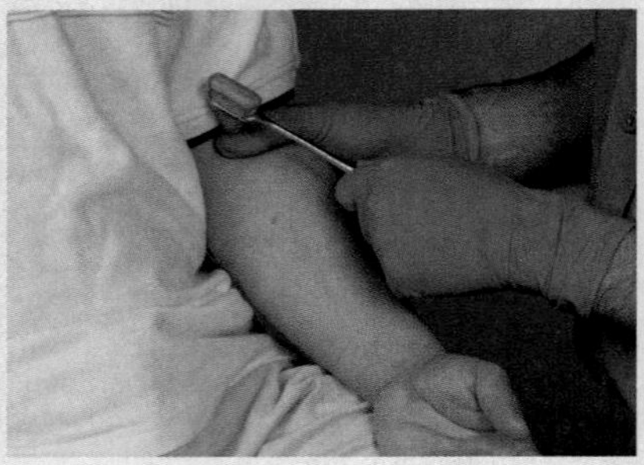

Step 2

Flex the patient's arm at the elbow to a 45° angle. Locate the biceps tendon in the antecubital fossa. Place your thumb over the tendon, with your fingers behind the elbow. Strike your thumb with the reflex hammer and note the flexion of the elbow.

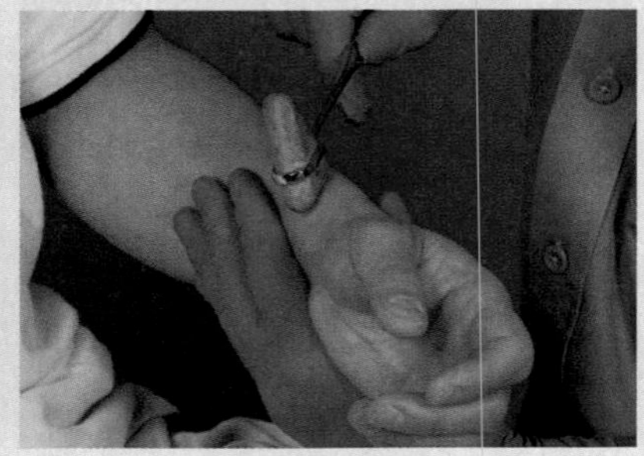

Step 3

With the patient's arm remaining at a 45° angle, rest the patient's forearm on your arm, with the hand slightly pronated. Strike the patient's brachioradialis tendon proximal to the wrist and note the flexion of the elbow.

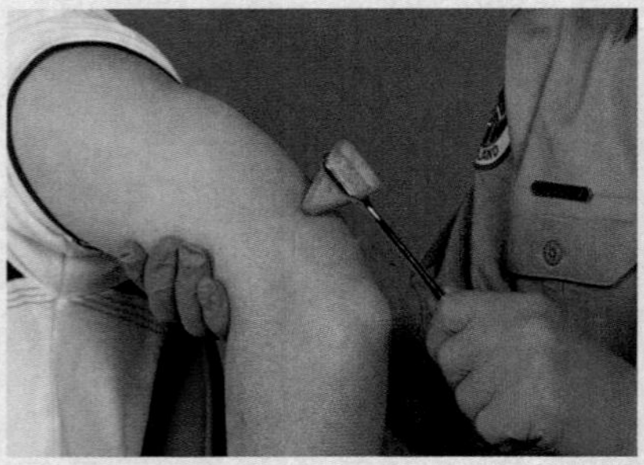

Step 4

Flex the patient's arm at the elbow to a 90° angle, and rest their hand against the body. Locate and strike the triceps tendon, noting contraction of the triceps or extension of the elbow.

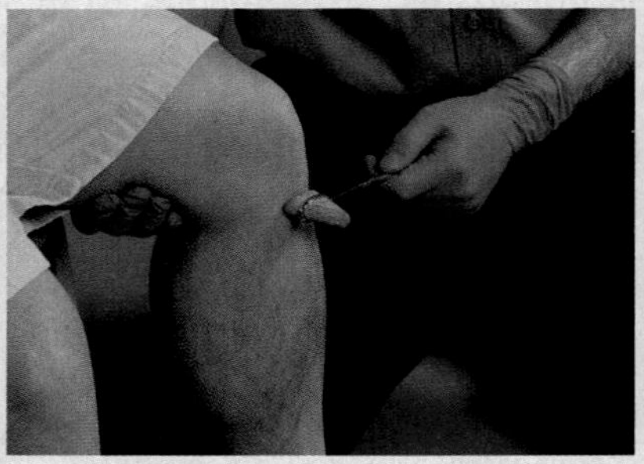

Step 5

Flex the patient's knee to a 90° angle, allowing the leg to dangle. Support the upper leg with your hand and strike the patellar tendon just below the patella. Note the contraction of the quadriceps and the extension of the lower leg.

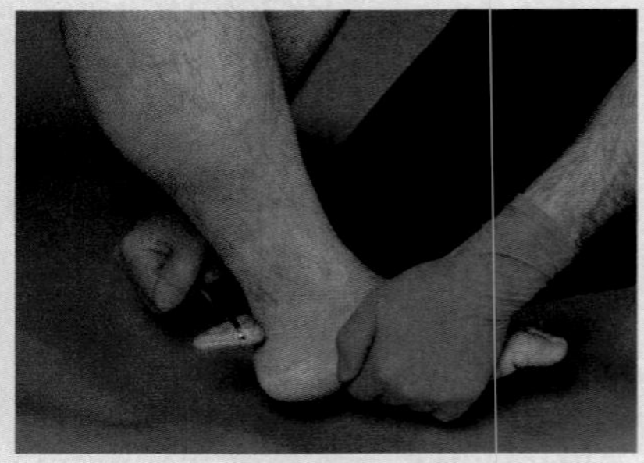

Step 6

With the patient's leg in the same position, hold the heel of the patient's foot in your hand. Strike the Achilles tendon, noting the plantar flexion of the foot.

TABLE 11-11 Scoring Deep Tendon Reflexes

Grade	Deep Tendon Reflex Response
0	No response
1+	Sluggish
2+	Active (expected response)
3+	Slightly hyperactive
4+	Hyperactive

Results of the Neurologic Exam Abnormal findings on the neurologic exam can take a wide variety of forms. Most common are mental status changes that can represent any number of acute or chronic processes, many of which have a non-neurologic origin. Mental status changes are often associated with inadequate perfusion or are encountered as a subtle indicator of early sepsis (which is common among older adults).

When caring for a patient with AMS, distinguishing between delirium and dementia is important. Delirium is an acute change in mental status, secondary to some significant underlying factor and/or incident. **Dementia** is a gradual and pervasive deterioration of cognitive cortical functions, typically secondary to slow progression of a disease such as Alzheimer disease.

Commonly encountered motor abnormalities include facial and extremity strength asymmetry along with difficulty in speaking (expressive **aphasia**). These signs are typical of cerebrovascular disease. Other commonly encountered abnormalities include ataxia, dystonia, seizures, vertigo, visual changes, tinnitus, and tremor. In the setting of trauma, global changes in mental status are more indicative of intracranial mass lesions, whereas decreased extremity motor function may present with proximal versus distal asymmetry and objective **paresthesias** (tingling or sensory changes), which is more consistent with a spinal lesion.

Secondary Assessment of Unresponsive Patients

After completing the primary survey and ruling out trauma, place an unresponsive patient in the recovery position (left lateral recumbent position) to facilitate drainage of vomit, blood, or other fluids and to help prevent aspiration. If spinal trauma is suspected, position the patient in neutral alignment, fitted with a proper-size rigid cervical collar, and implement spinal immobilization procedures per your regional protocol.

> **Words of Wisdom**
>
> Unresponsive patients should always be considered in unstable condition, so rapid transport to the appropriate facility is indicated. Throughout transport, perform reassessment, which includes rechecking ABCDE and reassessing any sign or symptom associated with the patient's chief complaint.

Perform a thorough assessment of the head, neck, chest, abdomen, pelvis, posterior body, and extremities, looking for signs of illness, such as rash or urticaria (hives), fever, unusual or excessive bruising, pulmonary or peripheral edema, and irregular pulse. Follow up your exam with at least two sets of vital signs: one obtained now and another obtained a few minutes after you begin your initial interventions (ie, supplemental oxygen and IV therapy). The first set of readings establishes a baseline (baseline vital signs); the second and additional sets (serial vital signs) provide comparative data to help you evaluate whether the patient's condition is improving, maintaining the status quo, or worsening. If time allows, take additional sets of vital signs to obtain further data, and allow you to map trends such as a steadily accelerating pulse rate. Ensure the vital signs include an auscultated BP, accurate pulse and respiratory rates, and temperature. Recheck breath sounds as well. All unresponsive patients should have their posture assessed. If there is no spontaneous movement, you may need to apply a painful stimulus. If the patient responds normally, they will push the stimulus away or withdraw from it. Abnormal postural responses include decorticate and decerebrate posturing of the trunk and extremities. More information on postural presentations can be found in Chapter 19, *Neurologic Emergencies*.

Secondary Assessment of Trauma Patients

Trauma patients can be classified into two broad groups: patients with an isolated injury and patients with multisystem trauma. From a secondary assessment perspective, the difference is that an isolated injury allows you to focus immediately on the main injury. In contrast, in a patient with multisystem trauma, you should first find all of the various injuries, or as many of them as you reasonably can. Then, prioritize the injuries by severity and plan the order in which you will address them. During the assessment, continually think about how each injury or condition relates to the others. For example, the mortality rate doubles for a patient with a serious traumatic brain injury who has just a single episode of hypotension.[21] In such a case, if you do not recognize and address the hypotension, and the consequent lack of adequate perfusion pressure, this can have a huge, sometimes fatal, effect on the patient.

Words of Wisdom

The salvage of lives takes precedence over the salvage of limbs.

Another important consideration is the high "visibility factor" of many injuries, which sometimes creates a distraction. A compound fracture of the lower leg and ankle, with the foot twisted sideways and jammed under the brake pedal of a vehicle, is not a pretty sight, but it is not life threatening. Because the grossly deformed ankle draws your attention, though, you may miss the early signs and symptoms of shock associated with the more serious but probably invisible internal injuries and bleeding that you cannot see.

Any unresponsive trauma patient with AMS should be considered a high-risk, priority patient requiring immediate transport to a trauma center. This patient may have a traumatic brain injury, stroke, hypoglycemia, or alcohol or drug intoxication. All are serious, possibly lethal circumstances or devastating injuries.

Recall that you will perform the primary survey and, if indicated, a rapid full-body scan for trauma patients. Though there may not always be time for further physical examination of a trauma patient, take advantage of the opportunity to continue the exam if time and the patient's condition do allow for it. Remember, examining a trauma patient *takes lots and lots of practice.*

Before physically examining a trauma patient, ensure the cervical spine is manually immobilized in the neutral position if you suspect a spine injury. Quickly reassess the patient's current mental status, comparing it with baseline readings. Last, revisit your transport decision. If you decide the patient needs immediate transport, perform the rapid full-body scan and do not delay transport to pursue a more thorough examination.

Also, mentally piece together all that you now know about your patient, including the chief complaint, the history of the present event, the medical history, and any information about the patient's current health status. Combine that knowledge with the other information and insights you gained from your various assessments, along with the data from your diagnostics, and you should have more than enough information to make good clinical choices for your patient.

Recording Secondary Assessment Findings

Medical information may be presented in both verbal and written forms. Documentation should always be recorded in an orderly, concise way, without omitting important facts. The information you obtain may then be practically and accurately relayed to the receiving medical staff. In addition, thorough documentation ensures that an accurate accounting of the patient's history before the patient reached the hospital will be legally entered into the formal medical record. Several acceptable formats are currently in use, including electronic records. Use the documentation method that is required by your local protocols.

Secondary assessment requires physical interaction between you and the patient and can be

Street Smarts

Remember the legal and ethical components of assessment:

1. Respect the patient's decision-making autonomy.
2. Be accountable to the patient.
3. Respect the patient's confidentiality and privacy.
4. Obtain consent.
5. Understand and respect advance directives.
6. Document facts accurately and nonjudgmentally.

performed successfully on a patient who cannot communicate. As you record your exam findings, note objective signs, pertinent negatives, and similar relevant information. Objective information is usually recorded in a standard format, in the same order used for the written PCR.

Limits of the Secondary Assessment

As a paramedic, the ability to perform a secondary assessment competently is one of the most valuable skills you can possess. This assessment can, for example, uncover information that the patient is unable or unwilling to share. An accomplished clinician will use this skill in conjunction with the history taking and other diagnostic tools to form an impression and formulate a treatment plan.

Nevertheless, despite the emphasis placed on a comprehensive physical exam, the secondary assessment has some limitations. Even the most experienced provider understands that not everything can be discovered in such an assessment. Learn to keep the total time in the field to a minimum. There is no reason to proceed with a thorough secondary assessment in the field, including an assessment of deep tendon reflexes, when the result will be transport to the ED regardless of the findings. The ED physician will need to repeat the exam. A secondary assessment should rarely take more than a few minutes. Move things along expeditiously, especially if the patient has a priority condition where time is crucial. In the prehospital setting, it is important to remember that evaluation by a trained physician, coupled with laboratory and radiographic studies, is needed for a definitive diagnosis.

Monitoring Devices

Whereas the history-taking and secondary assessment process is the best method for determining a patient's differential diagnosis, certain diagnostic and monitoring devices and laboratory tests are typically used to aid in the assessment process. Although these devices are helpful, they cannot replace a good past medical history and secondary assessment. Avoid the pitfall of relying on monitoring devices and not on the physical exam and patient presentation. Always remember to treat the patient, not the monitor.

Continuous ECG Monitoring

The purpose of continuous ECG monitoring in the prehospital environment is to establish a baseline ECG rhythm and monitor the patient for dynamic changes in cardiac electrical activity.

Patients should be on continuous cardiac monitoring if they present with cardiac signs and symptoms or with signs and symptoms of illnesses that could affect the heart. Many patients' illnesses meet this threshold, which is why paramedics frequently place patients on cardiac monitors as part of their routine advanced life support (ALS) care.

Most ECG monitors designed for the prehospital environment work in the same fashion. The electrodes must be placed correctly to accurately monitor the cardiac rhythm **FIGURE 11-47**. Cardiac rhythm monitoring devices typically use three to five leads. The leads are usually colored and labeled to help with placement. The lead wires are attached to electrodes, which are adhesive disks with a gel center to aid in skin contact. Some manufacturers offer a "diaphoretic" electrode that sticks more effectively to a sweating patient.

Whereas continuous ECG monitoring provides real-time visibility of cardiac electrical activity, it shows you only one aspect of the heart's electrical activity. An ECG tracing gives you limited information about the muscular function of the heart, and it will not always accurately assess the adequacy of the blood supply to the cardiac muscle via the coronary

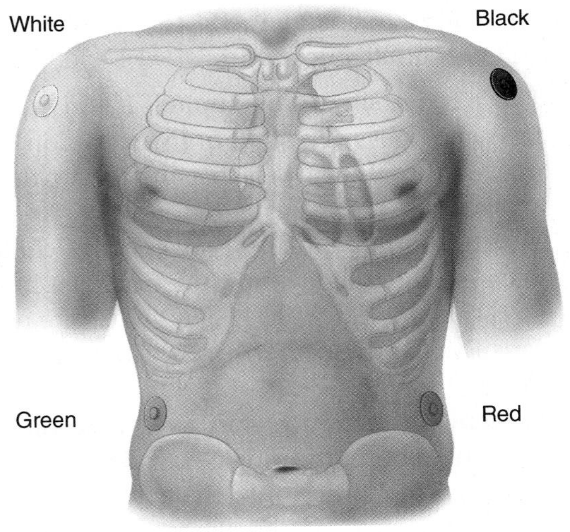

FIGURE 11-47 Four-lead electrode placement.

vessels. The heart is like a light bulb in a socket: The bulb contains everything it needs to function, but it requires a supply of electricity. When a light bulb burns out and stops working, electricity is still flowing to the socket. As long as the switch remains on, the electricity is there whether the bulb works or not. The same principle is true here: There are times when the ECG looks normal, but the heart is nevertheless not functioning properly. More information on ECG interpretation can be found in Chapter 18, *Cardiovascular Emergencies.*

Twelve-Lead ECG Monitoring

For the purposes of rhythm interpretation, a single lead (usually lead II) is often sufficient. However, to localize the site of injury to the heart muscle, you must be able to look at the heart from several angles, which is the purpose of a 12-lead ECG.

The addition of the 12-lead ECG to the paramedic's toolbox has opened the door for more advanced patient care in the field. For example, paramedics can now diagnose AMI in the patient's home. This early recognition allows hospitals to prepare before patients arrive, thereby decreasing the time it takes for patients to receive definitive care. In addition, paramedics in some areas of the United States are performing early intervention in the field by administering fibrinolytics to patients with STEMI or by diverting them to cardiac centers with catheterization labs.

The only way to learn how to take a 12-lead ECG is to practice with the equipment itself. Here are some guidelines to ensure the ECGs you obtain are of the highest quality possible:

- The patient should be supine. If the patient feels shortness of breath in that position, you may elevate the back of the stretcher to about a 30° angle.
- Ensure the patient does not become chilled, because shivering will produce artifact in the ECG tracing. Note that 12-lead ECGs are more sensitive to artifact than are 3-lead monitoring ECGs.
- Prepare the patient's skin as you would for placement of monitoring electrodes.
- Connect the four limb electrodes. Double-check that the correct electrode is on each limb (the "LA" electrode is on the left arm, the "RA" electrode is on the right arm, and so on).

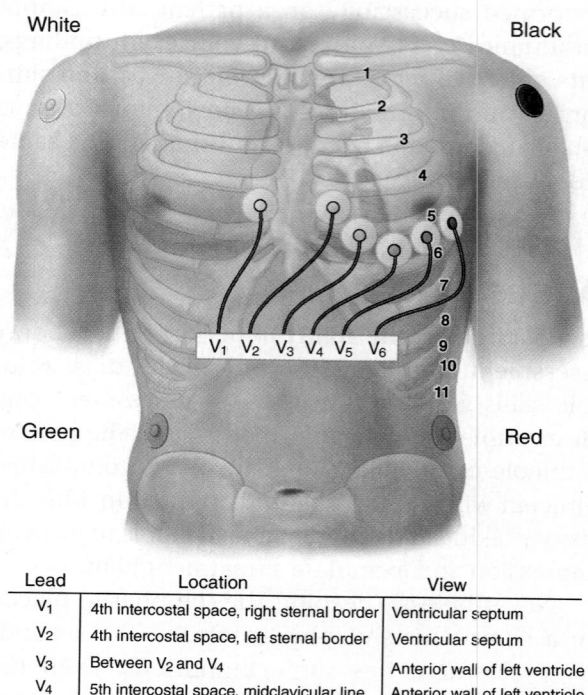

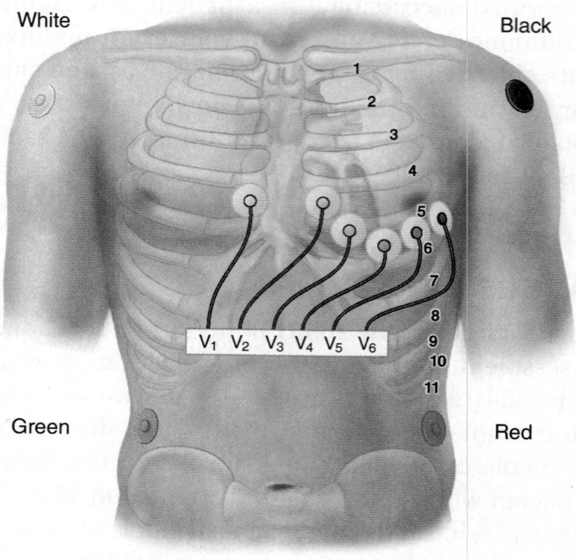

Lead	Location	View
V_1	4th intercostal space, right sternal border	Ventricular septum
V_2	4th intercostal space, left sternal border	Ventricular septum
V_3	Between V_2 and V_4	Anterior wall of left ventricle
V_4	5th intercostal space, midclavicular line	Anterior wall of left ventricle
V_5	Lateral to V_4 at the anterior axillary line	Lateral wall of left ventricle
V_6	Lateral to V_5 at the midaxillary line	Lateral wall of left ventricle

FIGURE 11-48 Twelve-lead electrode placement.

- Connect and apply the precordial leads as indicated in **FIGURE 11-48**.
- Record the ECG.

Interpretation of 12-lead ECGs is discussed in detail in Chapter 18, *Cardiovascular Emergencies.*

Carbon Dioxide Monitoring

Carbon dioxide is a naturally occurring by-product of cellular metabolism in the human body, as you learned in Chapter 8, *Anatomy and Physiology.* As the metabolism responds to stressors, change in carbon dioxide output can be seen and measured. As a paramedic, you must be able to recognize carbon dioxide output in a patient and use that information to determine treatment strategies.

There are two ways in which carbon dioxide is monitored in the field: capnometry and capnography. **Capnometry** typically consists of a disposable or electronic device that provides you with a means of measuring carbon dioxide output. **Capnography** measures carbon dioxide output and provides a waveform based on serial measurements. It is the ECG of ventilation, so to speak. A capnograph is a practical device that is simple to use in the prehospital environment. Whereas the older models were heavy and sometimes difficult to operate, newer devices are user-friendly and easy to interpret. These devices can be used to confirm endotracheal tube placement. In conscious and breathing patients, they can also be used to produce a continuous picture of ventilatory status and alert you to bronchospasm, shock, or acidosis.

Evidence-Based Medicine

The correlation between end-tidal carbon dioxide ($ETCO_2$) and cardiac output has two important implications during CPR. First, the effectiveness of CPR in producing adequate cardiac output can be monitored based on $ETCO_2$ values. Second, abrupt increases in $ETCO_2$ values suggest concomitant increases in cardiac output and are indicative of ROSC.

In intubated patients, the device is placed on the proximal end of the endotracheal tube and then connected to your portable ECG monitor or a separate monitoring device. For breathing patients, a special nasal cannula adapted for collecting carbon dioxide while administering oxygen is used. Although the capnograph has monitoring quality superior to that of the capnometer, it also has limitations. Such devices typically require a minimum airflow to calculate a reading and are sometimes affected by secretions in the tubing. They also require periodic calibration.

The purpose of capnometry is to verify correct endotracheal tube placement. The idea is that the capnometer is placed on the proximal end of an endotracheal tube. If the tube is in the trachea, exhaled carbon dioxide should pass by the sensor and provide information about tube placement.

Capnometry and capnography are discussed in more detail in Chapter 16, *Airway Management.*

Basic Blood Chemistry

A variety of elements found in blood can aid you in deciding between possibilities within the differential diagnosis. Although results from the history taking and secondary assessment are paramount in initially determining the differential diagnosis, sometimes a laboratory result helps to narrow the scope of possibilities.

Glucometer Measuring the blood glucose level of every patient with AMS is a must. It is a relatively easy test to perform and rapidly provides you with information about the patient's level of available glucose. A low glucose level helps you in forming the differential diagnosis for an unresponsive patient. Likewise, a high glucose level in a patient with nausea, vomiting, and abdominal pain may indicate diabetic ketoacidosis.

Blood glucose levels should be assessed in all patients known to have diabetes, all patients who are unresponsive for unknown reasons, and patients with generalized malaise/weakness. In addition, a blood glucose level can be assessed on any patient whom you feel has a poor general impression.

There are generally two ways to obtain a rapid blood glucose reading in the field: from the hub of an IV catheter or from a finger stick. When obtaining a blood sample from an IV catheter, establish IV access as usual, place the test strip against the hub of the catheter before you connect the IV tubing, and allow a drop of blood to touch the test strip. For patients with an IV line already placed, use a lancet needle to obtain a drop of blood. Next, cleanse the site (finger) with antiseptic, and puncture the site with the lancet. Immediately dispose of the needle in a sharps container, and collect a drop of blood on the test strip. When you are finished, place a bandage over the puncture site.

Most glucometers take only a few seconds to produce a reading. Keep in mind that while this is convenient for you, "rapid" does not always equate to "accurate." Glucometers must be calibrated regularly to maintain accuracy. In addition, verify the test strips are correct for the glucometer you are using and have not expired. Finally, ensure you have prepped the site adequately, and that the finger is clean.

Cardiac Biomarkers Cardiac biomarkers are used to assess for cardiac muscle damage. Typically, such blood tests are performed to determine whether the patient has had an AMI. Earlier in this chapter, we covered the use of 12-lead ECGs in the field to help determine whether a STEMI has occurred; however, most heart attacks are known as non-ST-elevation myocardial infarctions (NSTEMIs). These events are typically diagnosed by means of lab results, using cardiac biomarkers; however, several devices are now available to measure these cardiac markers quickly in the field.

In the EMS environment, cardiac biomarkers should be assessed in all patients with a cardiac condition, provided doing so is consistent with your local protocol. They should also be assessed in any patient with signs and symptoms of a stroke. The procedure is similar to obtaining a blood glucose level. However, the accuracy of the test depends on proper calibration of the equipment and use of an appropriate unexpired testing medium (ie, test strips). In addition, understand that it can take several hours for cardiac biomarkers to appear in a patient's blood after an AMI. Therefore, if elevated levels are not seen in the field, you cannot necessarily rule out the possibility that an AMI is taking place. AMI is discussed in greater detail in Chapter 18, *Cardiovascular Emergencies.*

Other Blood Tests With the invention of rapid laboratory testing devices, more EMS systems, particularly those that handle specialty care transports, are beginning to perform basic laboratory tests in the field.

The i-STAT handheld device operates with single-use, disposable i-STAT test cartridges **FIGURE 11-49**. Test cartridges for the i-STAT cover a broad menu of the most commonly performed diagnostic tests, such as those for cardiac markers, lactate, coagulation, blood gases, chemistries and electrolytes, and other hematology studies.

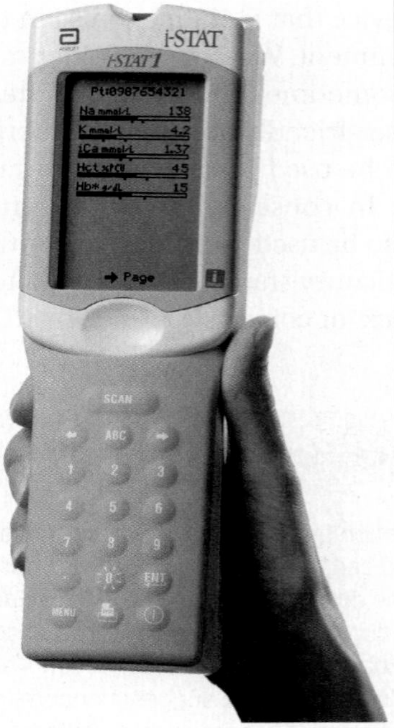

FIGURE 11-49 The i-STAT portable testing device.

Tests such as a basic and complete metabolic profile (CHEM 7 and CHEM 12) reveal the patient's electrolyte status, along with the renal and, sometimes, liver function. The brain natriuretic peptide (BNP) level is typically elevated in a patient experiencing an exacerbation of chronic heart failure. A BNP test helps you to differentiate cardiac versus pulmonary causes of respiratory distress. These tests are not generally used in the field unless you are working in a specialty clinic setting.

Patient Assessment

Scene Size-up

↓

Primary Assessment

↓

History Taking

↓

Secondary Assessment

↓

Reassessment

- Repeat the primary assessment
- Obtain vital signs
- Reassess the chief complaint
- Recheck interventions
- Identify and treat changes in the patient's condition

Reassess patient

- Unstable patients: every 5 minutes
- Stable patients: every 15 minutes

Reassessment

After the primary survey, **reassessment** is the most critical assessment process you will perform. When performing reassessment, reassess ABCDE to ensure you have adequately addressed the chief complaint; obtain another set of vital signs; and close any other patient care loops, such as dressing small wounds and placing ice packs. Reassessment represents a continuous, yet cyclical process you perform throughout transport, right up to the time you turn over patient care to the ED staff. For patients in stable condition, do a reassessment every 15 minutes or so. For patients in unstable condition, make a concerted effort to repeat reassessment every 5 minutes.

Reassessment of the Primary Survey

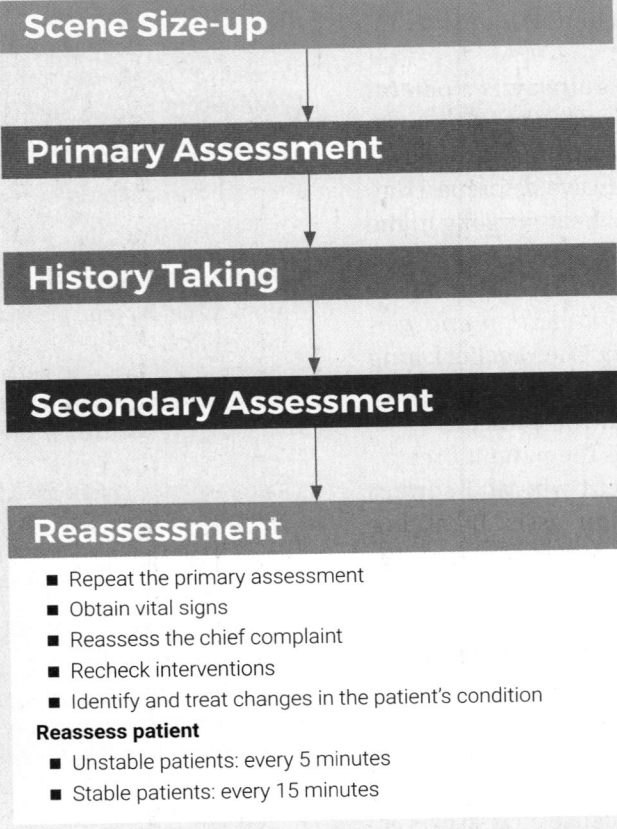

Reassessment combines repetition of the primary survey, reassessment of vital signs and breath sounds, and repetition of the secondary assessment. During the reassessment, continue to evaluate and reevaluate the patient's status and the efficacy of any treatments already administered by comparing serial vital signs. This information indicates which changes have occurred and which critical conditions have been addressed and corrected.

First, compare the patient's LOC with your baseline assessment. Is the LOC changing? If so, how? If mentation is decreasing, can the patient still protect the airway? If you have doubts, consider inserting an advanced airway.

Second, review the patient's airway. Is it patent? Swelling, bleeding, or just a change of position can quickly obstruct the airway, so ensure the airway is properly positioned and dry. Always be prepared to suction, and do not delay if you hear gurgling in the upper airway. It is far better to prevent aspiration than to treat it later. If the airway needs to be secured, *prepare the patient for intubation and perform the procedure immediately.* Then recheck lung sounds and perform oximetry and capnography periodically to confirm correct tube placement.

Third, reassess breathing. Is the patient breathing adequately? If not, figure out why and correct the problem. For hypoventilation, assist breathing with oxygen and a bag-mask device. Correct hypoxia with high-concentration oxygen therapy. For patients with diminished or absent breath sounds, JVD, and progressive dyspnea (signs of pneumothorax), decompress the chest.

Stay alert for signs of ventilatory fatigue, such as a decreasing pulse oximetry reading or a patient who looks increasingly tired. Be especially alert for this possibility in children, because it is a classic sign of impending disaster. Patients of any age who show signs of ventilatory fatigue need to have their airway aggressively managed for them.

Finally, reassess the patient's circulation. Note the overall skin color as an initial gauge of cardiovascular function and hemodynamic status. Think shock if the skin is paler than baseline, cool, and wet; think oxygen desaturation if cyanosis is present; think end-stage shock if mottling is present.

Ensure all bleeding is controlled. If you find blood-soaked dressings, add fresh dressings to the stack and rebandage them in place. Reassess BP, watching closely for signs that the patient is beginning to decompensate.

Reassess the pulse, including its rate, strength, and regularity. Progressive tachycardia may indicate that the patient's problem has not been corrected (the patient is still bleeding, is hypoxic, or is developing cardiogenic shock). In contrast, sustained or progressively worsening bradycardia may reflect rising intracranial pressure (from trauma or a stroke) or end-stage shock.

Special Populations

During a crisis, the responses of children and older adult patients may differ. In turn, you may have to take a different approach to reassessment. Adult patients tend to show signs of deterioration as their condition becomes unstable. Children, however, will decompensate much faster; therefore, frequent reassessment is imperative. Any indication of deteriorating mental status or changes to airway, breathing, or circulation should prompt immediate intervention.

Geriatric patients differ from other adult and pediatric patients in that they may lack appropriate compensatory mechanisms and, therefore, may not show signs of deterioration as their medical condition becomes unstable. In addition, many of these patients have underlying diseases or take medications that mask the relevant assessment findings. For example, a patient who is going into shock would typically demonstrate an increased pulse rate. However, many older adult patients either lack the ability to increase their pulse rate or take medications that regulate the pulse rate. Reassessment of mental status may also prove challenging in this population. For some patients, a seemingly AMS is their baseline behavior; therefore, it becomes difficult to assess whether the patient is improving. Therefore, frequent reassessment is necessary to determine and monitor a patient's overall progress and stability.

Reassessment of Patient Care and Transport Priorities

After reassessing the patient, think about your care plan. Have you addressed all life threats? Do you need to revise your priority list based on what you know? If so, make the change and move on. Conversely, if your plan is working well and you have addressed most or all of the patient's chief complaints, there's no need to revise the care plan.

As you reevaluate your patient care priorities, reassess the transport plan as well. Should routine transport be stepped up to priority? Is the patient's condition worsening to the point that you should consider diverting to a closer facility? Do you need to set up a rendezvous with an air ambulance?

Alternatively, if your patient's condition has improved and stabilized, step down from priority and transport the patient as a routine case, which is clearly the safer choice.

Get another complete set of vital signs, and compare them with the expected outcomes from your therapies. For example, if you administered a 500-mL bolus of normal saline to a patient with GI bleeding, you would expect BP to rise and pulse rate to drop. With any priority patient, even with a short transport, you should obtain three sets of vital signs at a minimum. With most priority patients, you will have four or five sets of vital signs. Thus, you can look for trends or patterns, such as slowing pulse, rising BP, and erratic respiratory patterns that represent the **Cushing reflex**, a grave sign for patients with head trauma. Alternatively, narrowed pulse pressure, muffled heart tones, and JVD are associated with cardiac tamponade (**Beck triad**), usually secondary to penetrating chest trauma.

The last element of the reassessment is to revisit the patient's chief complaint(s) (from the history taking), along with your interventions. Have any complaints improved or resolved? For instance, has the 9 over 10 chest pain improved with the nitroglycerin you administered? Did the second albuterol treatment ease the patient's breathing? Which situations remain unresolved? Worsening situations are especially worrisome because they could indicate an unseen problem or ineffective interventions. With each reassessment, document your findings so the medical record is accurate and complete. Finally, if you haven't reached the receiving facility, begin the process again; that is why it is called *reassessment*.

Words of Wisdom

You cannot recognize narrowing pulse pressures until you have taken two or three sets of BP readings. Multiple checks provide the comparative data you need.

YOU are the Paramedic SUMMARY

1. What is your first concern at this scene?

You do not know at this point what happened to the patient. This may or may not be a crime scene. Either way, the main priority is to ensure the safety and well-being of you and your partner. Consider whether it is safe to enter this scene and approach the patient. Assess and evaluate the scene through a wide-angle lens. If you are in doubt as to whether the scene is safe, then request the appropriate additional resources before you proceed. In this case, the scene safety issue is related to the potential for violence. You are not trained to make this scene safe; therefore, it is mandatory that you request law enforcement prior to exposing yourself to the danger.

2. How will you address this concern?

Request law enforcement personnel immediately in cases that could involve a crime, because it is nearly impossible for you and your partner to control the scene and care for the patient at the same time, and because the perpetrator could return with additional weapons. If you are unsure what to do, protect yourself and your crew before anything else. This may mean staying in the ambulance until law enforcement personnel arrive to secure the scene.

3. What is your general impression of this patient?

You know the patient is responsive and bleeding from a chest wound, but he is not responsive to simple commands. Even with this limited information, you know this patient could deteriorate rapidly into shock and could require rapid transport.

4. What is your next step in assessing this patient?

Changes in LOC may provide the first clue to an alteration in the patient's condition, so establish a baseline as soon as you encounter the patient. As you assess the patient's mental status, if trauma is involved, decide whether you suspect spinal trauma and implement spinal immobilization procedures. The quickest and simplest way to assess the patient's mental status or LOC is to use the AVPU scale.

5. On the basis of your assessment of ABCDE, what is your first priority in the care of this patient?

Airway assessment focuses on two questions: Is the airway open and patent? Is it likely to remain so? If you determine the patient cannot maintain their airway, an OPA or NPA may resolve the problem. However, if you cannot maintain the airway by any other means, use a more invasive technique, such

YOU are the Paramedic SUMMARY continued

as endotracheal intubation. Breathing is proportional and related to airway adequacy. Thus, assessing breathing likewise focuses on two questions: Is the patient breathing? If not, then you have to breathe for the patient. If the patient is breathing, is the breathing adequate? Again, if breathing is not adequate, do what is necessary to support the patient's breathing or consider performing rapid sequence intubation.

6. Can you determine the transport priority of this patient at this point?

Yes. When you have a priority (unstable) patient, expedite transport, doing only what is absolutely necessary at the scene and handling everything else en route, including the appropriate history taking and physical exam. This patient presents with a poor general impression, is responsive but does not or cannot follow commands, and has difficulty breathing because of a penetrating injury to his chest. Based solely on these three criteria, rapid transport of this patient is a priority.

7. How can you determine the level of internal damage if you do not have the implement that was used to stab the patient?

Any chest injury, regardless of the object used, can cause significant internal damage. The chest contains many structures that are vital to life, including the lungs and mediastinal elements (heart, great vessels). The chest (or thorax) consists of the superior aspect of the torso, from the base of the neck to the diaphragm, as delineated by the costal arch. The chest wall is divided into anterior and posterior portions (the patient's front and back). The back of the chest extends down the patient's back, to the level of the diaphragm posteriorly, which tends to move up and down with breathing. The chest wall serves as a protective covering for the internal components. It consists of numerous musculoskeletal, vascular, nervous, connective, and lining structures.

8. What is the relevance of past medical history in this case?

The past medical history allows you to learn about any pertinent or chronic underlying medical conditions the patient may have. Although some aspects of the past medical history may not seem important with this patient, a careful and thorough history will help paint a clear picture of his overall health status. However, he may not be willing or able to give you this information. Rely on what you learned during your patient assessment and inspection as much as possible. Always look for any medical alert jewelry or devices, and note any scars that may indicate prior open heart or chest wall surgery, such as placement of a pacemaker or an ICD.

EMS Patient Care Report (PCR)					
Date: 04-28-22	**Incident No.:** 902	**Nature of Call:** Stabbing		**Location:** 4th Ave/Main St	
Dispatched: 0200	**En Route:** 0201	**At Scene:** 0205	**Transport:** 0215	**At Hospital:** 0225	**In Service:** 0240

Patient Information	
Age: Approx 30 **Sex:** M **Weight (in kg [lb]):** 75 kg (165 lb)	**Allergies:** NKDA **Medications:** Unknown **Past Medical History:** Unknown **Chief Complaint:** 1-inch (2.5 cm) penetrating wound to upper left chest

Vital Signs				
Time: 0210	**BP:** 90/64	**Pulse:** 122	**Respirations:** 28	**Spo_2:** 93% on room air
Time: 0215	**BP:** 92/62	**Pulse:** 120	**Respirations:** 28	**Spo_2:** 99% on 15 L/min
Time: 0220	**BP:** 92/60	**Pulse:** 118	**Respirations:** 26	**Spo_2:** 99% on 15 L/min

YOU are the Paramedic SUMMARY continued

EMS Treatment (circle all that apply)				
Oxygen @ 15 **L/min via (circle one):** **NC** (**NRM**) **Bag-mask device**		**Assisted Ventilation:**	**Airway Adjunct:**	**CPR**
Defibrillation	**Bleeding Control**	**Bandaging**	**Splinting**	(**Other:** Occlusive dressing)

Narrative
Unit 84 dispatched for a man down in front of the strip mall at 4th Avenue & Main Street. This unit arrived to find this pt lying left lateral recumbent on the sidewalk. There appears to be no one else present on the scene. Before exiting the vehicle, scene lights reveal what appears to be blood on the sidewalk near the pt's chest. Because of safety concerns, level of consciousness was assessed via the PA system. Pt demonstrated following commands at that time. PD on scene approximately 1 minute after our arrival. Scene secured for pt assessment and treatment. Pt is an approx. 30-year-old man with a penetrating wound, approx. 1 inch in length just inferior to the center of the left clavicle. Bleeding has stopped. Three-sided occlusive dressing applied. Pt is responsive, responds to commands, but is not verbal. Sensation and motion normal in all extremities; based on the clinical evaluation no spinal immobilization was applied. VS as noted and 15 L/min O_2 via NRM applied. IV NS established with 16ga, right AC. Pt able to maintain his own airway but had increased difficulty breathing on lying supine on the stretcher. Pt transported to the regional trauma center with early notification. Head of the backboard raised 15%, which provided some relief to breathing effort. Pt report given to Dr. Solomon on arrival.
End of report

Prep Kit

Ready for Review

- Patient assessment is the foundation on which quality prehospital care is built and the single most important skill you bring to patient care.
- There are five components in the patient assessment process: scene size-up, primary survey, history taking, secondary assessment, and reassessment.
- The first step of the patient assessment process is the scene size-up, because your first and foremost concern on any call is to ensure your safety and the safety of other EMS personnel.
- During the scene size-up, you also determine MOI or NOI.
- Another important step in protecting yourself is to take standard precautions. Don all necessary PPE before approaching the patient.
- The first step in the primary survey is to form a general impression of the patient's condition. As you approach the patient, note whether they appear to be in stable or unstable condition, and observe the environment for clues.
- During the primary survey, identify threats to ABCDE and address them immediately.
- Assess the patient for disability, then make a transport decision. If the patient has sustained trauma, perform a rapid full-body scan (from the secondary assessment portion of the assessment process) to identify injuries that require care before you immobilize the patient.
- Once the primary survey is completed and all life threats are addressed, move into the history-taking component of assessment.
- Patient history is a primary means of determining the chief complaint in the field; its value depends on your ability to skillfully elicit complete and accurate information.

Prep Kit continued

- Use constructive communications skills as you talk with patients: facilitation, reflection, clarification, empathy, confrontation, interpretation, and direct questions about feelings.
- At times you must ask patients about sensitive topics, such as alcohol or drug misuse, physical abuse or other violence, or sexual history. Be familiar with techniques for successfully interviewing patients about these topics.
- Within your service and with your partner, work on strategies for communicating positively with patients who are silent, overly talkative, anxious, angry or hostile, intoxicated, crying, depressed, or seeking reassurance. Discuss how to determine the chief complaint in a patient with multiple symptoms. Discuss how to remain professional when treating a patient to whom you are physically attracted.
- For responsive medical patients, obtain the past medical history directly from the patient, although certain patients (ie, young children) may need assistance. For responsive medical patients, ask questions about each body system to obtain a thorough picture of the patient's health.
- For unresponsive medical patients and trauma patients, it may be necessary to obtain the medical history from family members or bystanders.
- The first part of a patient's medical history also serves as a good mental status examination: Ask for the patient's name; the date, time, and location; the chief complaint; and the events leading up to the call for EMS.
- After clarifying the history of the present illness, ask the patient about their past medical history, the general state of their health, and any pertinent family history. Ask for a list of the patient's medications and allergies, as part of this questioning.
- Obtaining a medical history from an older adult patient may be challenging. Older patients may have multiple medical conditions, take numerous medications, and have a different patient presentation than younger adults, which can make their emergencies more complex. They may also have sensory losses that require you to adjust your approach to collect necessary information.
- Secondary assessment (also known as head-to-toe physical exam) is the process by which you obtain quantifiable, objective information from a patient about their overall state of health.
- The two types of physical examinations performed during the secondary assessment are the full-body exam and the focused assessment. If the patient has serious life threats, you may not have time to perform a secondary assessment at all. Alternatively, you may focus on the area of the chief complaint first, and then move on to other body systems as time permits.
- Secondary assessment includes obtaining vital signs that measure overall body function, and performing a head-to-toe physical exam that evaluates the function of specific body systems. This exam is done in a sequential manner to ensure every aspect of the body's function is evaluated.
- The techniques of inspection, palpation, percussion, and auscultation allow you to use your physical senses to obtain physical information and understand the normal (versus abnormal) functions of a patient's body.
- Vital signs consist of a measurement of BP; pulse rate, rhythm, and quality; respiratory rate, rhythm, and quality; body temperature; and, pulse oximetry. Other than overall patient appearance, vital signs are some of the most valuable objective data for determining patient status.
- Monitoring devices used by the paramedic include continuous ECG monitoring, 12-lead ECG, carbon dioxide monitoring (capnography and capnometry), blood chemistry analyses, blood glucose monitoring, and cardiac biomarkers, among others.
- Alter your approach to patient assessment when caring for infants and children. If a young

Prep Kit continued

child cannot speak, assess their condition based largely on what you can see and hear. Family members or caregivers may also be able to provide useful information.

- After the primary survey, the reassessment is the single most important assessment process you will perform.
- Reassessment is performed on all patients. It gives you an opportunity to reevaluate the chief complaint and to reassess your interventions to ensure they are still effective. Information from the reassessment may be used to identify and treat changes in the patient's condition.
- A patient in stable condition should be reassessed every 15 minutes, whereas a patient in unstable condition should be reassessed every 5 minutes. A critical patient must be evaluated continuously.

Vital Vocabulary

adventitious breath sounds Abnormal breath sounds, such as wheezing, rhonchi, crackles, stridor, and pleural friction rubs.

alert and oriented (A × O) A determination made when assessing mental status by looking at whether the patient is oriented in four areas: person, place, time, and the event itself. Each element provides information about different aspects of the patient's memory.

anisocoria Unequal pupils with a greater than 1-mm difference.

aphasia The language impairment that affects the production or understanding of speech and the ability to read or write.

apparent life-threatening event (ALTE) An episode characterized by some combination of apnea (central or obstructive), skin color change (cyanotic, pallid, erythematous, or plethoric) change in muscle tone (usually diminished), and choking or gagging.

ascites Abnormal accumulation of fluid in the peritoneal cavity; typically signals liver failure.

aspiration The entry of fluids or solids into the trachea, bronchi, and lungs; the act of drawing material in or out by suction.

auscultation The act of using a stethoscope to listen to sounds within the body.

AVPU A method of assessing mental status by determining whether a patient is Awake and alert, responsive to Verbal stimuli or Pain, or Unresponsive; used principally in the primary survey.

Battle sign Bruising over the mastoid process, which may indicate a basilar skull fracture; also known as retroauricular ecchymosis or raccoon eyes.

Beck triad The combination of a narrowed pulse pressure, muffled heart tones, and jugular venous distention associated with cardiac tamponade; usually caused by penetrating chest trauma.

blood pressure (BP) The measurement of the force exerted against the walls of the blood vessels as the heart contracts and relaxes; it is calculated as the product of cardiac output and peripheral vascular resistance.

bronchial sounds Hollow, tubular, lower-pitched sounds heard over the trachea.

bronchophony A test of decreased breath sounds performed by placing the diaphragm of the stethoscope over the area in question while the patient says "ninety-nine"; a loud, clear sound indicates lung consolidation.

bronchovesicular sounds A combination of the tracheal and vesicular breath sounds; heard where the airways and alveoli are found, in the upper part of the sternum and between the scapulae.

bruit An abnormal *whooshing* sound of turbulent blood flow moving through a narrowed artery; usually heard in the carotid arteries.

Prep Kit continued

capnography The use of a noninvasive diagnostic tool that can quickly and efficiently provide information on a patient's ventilatory and circulatory status with a graphic and digital depiction similar to an electrocardiogram.

capnometry The use of a capnometer, which is a monitoring device used to measure amount of expired carbon dioxide. The reading is usually given as a digital reading.

cerumen Ear wax.

chief complaint The reason the patient is seeking help.

crackles Wet rattling, bubbling, or crackling lung sounds indicative of fluid in the small airways; also known as rales.

crepitus A crackling, grating, or grinding sound often heard when fragments of broken bones rub together.

cultural intelligence Ability to function effectively across various cultural contexts, interacting with people of all nationalities and getting along with those of all ethnic, political, and generational differences.

current health status A composite picture of a number of factors in a patient's life, such as dietary habits, current medications, allergies, exercise, alcohol or tobacco use, recreational drug use, sleep patterns and disorders, and immunizations.

Cushing reflex The combination of a slowing pulse, rising blood pressure, and an erratic respiratory pattern; a grave sign for patients with head trauma or cerebrovascular accident.

cyanosis A blue-gray skin color that is caused by inadequate levels of oxygen in the blood.

delirium An acute confusional state characterized by global impairment of thinking, perception, judgment, and memory.

dementia The gradual and pervasive deterioration or loss of cognitive cortical functions.

diaphoresis Excessive sweating; it is often associated with shock.

diastolic pressure The result of residual pressure in the circulatory system while the left ventricle is relaxing (ie, in diastole).

differential diagnosis The process of weighing the probability of one disease versus other diseases by comparing clinical findings that could account for a patient's illness; also refers to the list of possible conditions considered based on the patient's signs and symptoms.

diplopia Double vision.

ecchymosis Localized bruising or collection of blood within or under the skin.

egophony A test of decreased breath sounds performed by placing the diaphragm of the stethoscope over the area in question while the patient says a drawn-out "ee"; an "A" sound indicates lung consolidation.

field impression A field conclusion about the patient's problem based on the clinical presentation and the exclusion of other possible causes through considering the differential diagnoses.

focused exam A type of physical exam that is typically performed on responsive patients who have sustained an isolated injury; it is based on the chief complaint and focuses on one body system or part.

full-body exam A systematic head-to-toe exam performed during the secondary assessment of a patient who has sustained a significant mechanism of injury, is unresponsive, or is in critical condition.

general impression The overall initial impression that determines the priority of patient care; based on the patient's surroundings, the mechanism of injury, signs and symptoms, and the chief complaint.

Glasgow Coma Scale (GCS) An evaluation tool used to determine level of consciousness by evaluating and assigning point values (scores) for eye opening, verbal response, and motor response, which are then totaled; effective in helping predict patient outcomes.

Prep Kit continued

guarding Contraction of the abdominal muscles indicating peritoneal irritation.

heave The perception that the heart is beating very strongly; felt on palpation of the chest wall, this finding suggests hypertrophy; also called lift.

history of the present illness A narrative detail of the symptoms that a patient is experiencing, usually obtained using the OPQRST mnemonic.

iatrogenic Related to a side effect or complication of medications or other medical treatment.

inspection Looking at the patient, either in general or at a specific area (ie, a patient's overall appearance from the doorway versus looking specifically at the chest wall for abnormalities/deformities).

jugular venous distention (JVD) The visible bulging of the jugular veins when a patient is in semi-Fowler or full Fowler position; indicates inadequate blood movement through the heart and/or lungs.

Korotkoff sounds Sounds related to blood pressure measurement that are heard by stethoscope.

kyphosis Outward curve of the thoracic spine.

lesions Localized areas of the skin that do not resemble the area surrounding them.

lift A sensation felt on palpation of the chest wall, in which the heart beats extremely strongly; suggests hypertrophy; also called heave.

lordosis Inward curve of the lumbar spine just above the buttocks. An exaggerated form results in the condition known as swayback.

mechanism of injury (MOI) The series of events that result in traumatic injuries; the forces that act on the body to cause injury.

mottling A blotchy pattern on the skin; a typical finding in states of severe protracted hypoperfusion and shock.

murmur An abnormal *whooshing* sound heard over the heart that indicates turbulent blood flow around a cardiac valve.

nature of illness (NOI) The general type of illness a patient is apparently experiencing.

ophthalmoscope An instrument used to examine a patient's eyes and view the retina and aqueous fluid; consists of a concave mirror and a battery-powered light that is usually contained in the handle.

orthostatic vital signs Multiple sets of vital signs taken with the patient in different positions. (eg, in supine and sitting or standing positions) to determine the degree of hypovolemia; also called a tilt test.

otoscope An instrument used to examine the ears of a patient; consists of a head and a handle. The head contains an electric light source and a low-power magnifying lens.

pallor Skin coloration that diverges from the patient's baseline skin tone and suggests reduced blood flow or oxygenation.

palpation Physical touching for the purpose of obtaining information (eg, to detect tenderness).

paresthesias Tingling feeling or sensory change.

past medical history Information obtained during the history-taking process, such as the patient's general state of health, childhood and adult diseases, surgeries and hospitalizations, psychiatric and mental illnesses, or traumatic injuries, which may relate to the patient's current condition.

pathologic fracture A fracture that occurs when normal forces are applied to abnormal bone structures.

patient history Information about the patient's chief complaint, present symptoms, and previous illnesses.

patient safety Reduction of the risk of unnecessary harm associated with emergency medical services care to an acceptable minimum, which is defined by the limits of the best available medical evidence, equipment, technology, and human skill.

percussion Gently striking the surface of the body, typically overlying various body cavities, to detect changes in the densities of the underlying structures.

Prep Kit continued

perfusion The circulation of oxygenated blood through the body tissues and vessels.

pertinent negatives The absence of certain signs and symptoms normally expected of specific illnesses or conditions; these findings warrant no medical care or intervention, but demonstrate the thoroughness of the patient exam and history.

pleural friction rubs Squeaking or grating sounds that occur when the pleural linings rub together, which may be heard on inspiration, expiration, or both; commonly caused by inflammation of the pleura.

primary survey The part of the assessment process that focuses on identifying immediate or potential life-threatening conditions so you can initiate lifesaving care.

primitive reflexes Reflex reactions such as Babinski, grasping, and sucking signs normally found in infants.

pronator drift The drifting of one arm downward toward a patient's feet while they hold out their arms, palm side up, with their eyes shut; can be a sign of a stroke.

proprioception The perception of the position and movement of the body or limbs.

pulse The wave of pressure created as the heart contracts and forces blood out the left ventricle and into the major arteries; palpated at a point where an artery passes close to a bone.

pulse oximetry An assessment tool used to measure oxygen saturation of hemoglobin in the capillary beds.

rapid full-body scan A 60- to 90-second nonsystematic review and palpation of the patient's body to identify injuries that must be managed or protected immediately; also called a rapid full-body sweep.

reassessment The portion of the assessment process in which a patient's condition is reevaluated and responses to treatment are assessed.

reflexes Involuntary motor responses to specific sensory stimuli, such as a tap on the knee or stroking the eyelash.

rhonchi Coarse, low-pitched breath sounds heard in patients with chronic mucus in the upper airways.

rigidity A clinically important sign characterized by marked peritoneal irritation and guarding, indicating an injury or illness for which urgent surgical intervention may be required.

rubor Redness; one of the classic signs of inflammation.

scene size-up A step in the patient assessment process involving a quick assessment of the scene and its surroundings to gather information about the overall safety and stability of the scene and the mechanism of injury or nature of illness. This process is carried out before you enter the scene and begin patient care.

scoliosis Sideways curvature of the spine.

secondary assessment The process by which more detailed, quantifiable, objective information is obtained from the patient about their overall state of health.

signs Objective observations that can be seen, heard, felt, smelled, or measured.

social history A subsection of the patient history that provides valuable information regarding the patient's overall health status and helps to identify risk factors for various disease processes; includes items such as tobacco use, alcohol and drug use, sexual behavior, diet, travel history, living environment, and occupation.

sphygmomanometer A device to measure blood pressure; a blood pressure cuff.

splitting In the context of heart sounds, a situation in which events on the right side of the heart occur slightly later than those on the left side, creating two discernible sounds rather than one heart sound.

stridor A harsh, high-pitched respiratory sound produced as air moves past an obstruction within or immediately above the glottic opening; associated with severe upper airway obstruction.

symptoms Subjective information the patient feels, such as pain, discomfort, or other abnormality.

Prep Kit continued

systolic pressure Blood pressure created by the left ventricle as it contracts (ie, in systole).

tenting A condition in which the skin slowly retracts after being pinched and pulled away slightly from the body; a sign of dehydration.

thrill A humming vibration that can be palpated through the chest wall, suggesting an underlying bruit or murmur.

traumatic fracture A fracture that occurs when abnormal forces are applied to normal bone structures.

turgor Loss of skin elasticity.

vasoconstriction Narrowing of the diameter of a blood vessel.

vasodilation Widening of the diameter of a blood vessel.

vesicular sounds Normal breath sounds made by air moving in and out of the alveoli.

visual acuity Determined by the ability or inability to see, and by how far.

wheezing A high-pitched whistling sound that may be heard on inspiration, expiration, or both, indicating air movement through a constricted lower airway, as in asthma.

whispered pectoriloquy A test of decreased breath sounds performed by placing the diaphragm of the stethoscope over the area in question as the patient whispers "ninety-nine"; a loud, clear sound indicates lung consolidation.

working diagnosis The one diagnosis from a differential diagnosis list used as the basis for the patient's treatment plan.

References

1. Emergency medical services workers: injury data. Centers for Disease Control and Prevention website. https://www.cdc.gov/niosh/topics/ems/data.html. Reviewed September 21, 2021. Accessed January 27, 2022.
2. Maguire BJ, Smith S. Injuries and fatalities among emergency medical technicians and paramedics in the United States. *Prehosp Disaster Med*. 2013;28(4):376-382.
3. Reichard AA, Marsh SM, Moore PH. Fatal and nonfatal injuries among emergency medical technicians and paramedics. *Prehosp Emerg Care*. 2011;15(4):511-517.
4. Centers for Disease Control and Prevention. Guideline for hand hygiene in health-care settings: recommendations of the Healthcare Infection Control Practices Advisory Committee and the HICPAC/SHEA/APIC/IDSA Hand Hygiene Task Force. *MMWR*. 2002;51(RR-16).
5. Tourniquet: clinical indications. JointEMS Protocols website. https://www.jointemsprotocols.com/Tourniquet. Accessed January 27, 2022.
6. Fleming S, Gill P, Jones C, et al. The diagnostic value of capillary refill time for detecting serious illness in children: a systematic review and meta-analysis. Huy NT, ed. *PLoS One*. 2015;10(9):e0138155.
7. Kragh JK, Littrel ML, Jones JA, et al. Battle casualty survival with emergency tourniquet use to stop limb bleeding. *J Emerg Med*. 2011;41(6):590-597.
8. Beekley AC, Sebesta JA, Blackbourne LH, et al. Prehospital tourniquet use in Operation Iraqi Freedom: effect on hemorrhage control and outcomes. *J Trauma*. 2008;64(2 suppl):S28-S37.
9. Smith ER, Shapiro G, Sarani B. The profile of wounding in civilian public mass shooting fatalities. *J Trauma Acute Care Surg*. 2016;81(1):86-92.
10. The National Academies of Sciences, Engineering, and Medicine. https://www.nationalacademies.org/hmd/About-HMD.aspx. Accessed January 27, 2022.
11. Institute of Medicine Committee on Quality of Health Care in America. *Crossing the Quality Chasm: A New Health System for the 21st Century*. National Academy of Sciences website. http://www.nationalacademies.org/hmd/~/media/Files/Report%20Files/2001/Crossing-the-Quality-Chasm/Quality%20Chasm%202001%20%20report%20brief.pdf. Published March 2001. Accessed January 27, 2022.
12. Traffic safety facts 2016 data: alcohol-impaired driving. National Highway Traffic Safety Administration website. https://crashstats.nhtsa.dot.gov/Api/Public/ViewPublication/812450. Published October 2017. Accessed January 27, 2022.
13. Buchtel EE. (2014). Cultural sensitivity or cultural stereotyping? Positive and negative effects of a cultural psychology class. *Int J Intercult Relat*. 2014:39;40-52.
14. Molinet J. Northwell equips ambulances with video remote interpreting access. https://www.northwell.edu/center-for-emergency-medical-services/news/the-latest/northwell-equips-ambulances-with-video-remote-interpreting-access-. Published May 22, 2019. Accessed March 4, 2022.

Prep Kit continued

15. Krebs EE, Carey TS, Weinberger M. Accuracy of the pain numeric rating scale as a screening test in primary care. *J Gen Intern Med*. 2007;22(10):1453-1458.
16. Lord B. The assessment of pain in paramedic practice. EMS World website. May 1, 2016. https://www.hmpgloballearningnetwork.com/site/EMSWorld/211793/assessment-pain-paramedic-practice. Accessed January 27, 2022.
17. Sasser SM, Hunt RC, Faul M, et al. Guidelines for field triage of injured patients: recommendations of the National Expert Panel on Field Triage, 2011. Centers for Disease Control and Prevention website. https://www.cdc.gov/mmwr/preview/mmwrhtml/rr6101a1.htm. Accessed January 27, 2022.
18. Taylor J, McLaughlin K, McRae A, et al. Use of prehospital ultrasound in North America: a survey of emergency medical services medical directors. *BMC Emerg Med*. 2014;14:6.
19. What is anisocoria? American Association for Pediatric Ophthalmology and Strabismus website. https://aapos.org/glossary/anisocoria-and-horners-syndrome. Accessed February 27, 2021.
20. Naqvi U, Sherman AI. Muscle strength grading. StatPearls [Internet]. Treasure Island (FL): StatPearls Publishing. https://www.ncbi.nlm.nih.gov/books/NBK436008/. Updated September 2, 2021. Accessed March 4, 2022.
21. Spaite DW, Hu C, Bobrow BJ, et al. The effect of combined out-of-hospital hypotension and hypoxia on mortality in major traumatic brain injury. *Ann Emerg Med*. 2017;69(1):62-72.

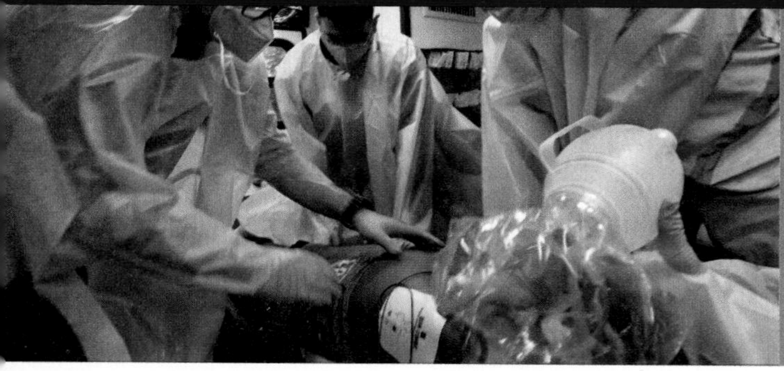

Chapter 12

Critical Thinking and Clinical Decision Making

NATIONAL EMS EDUCATION STANDARD COMPETENCIES

Assessment

Integrate scene and patient assessment findings with knowledge of epidemiology and pathophysiology to form a field impression. This includes developing a list of differential diagnoses through clinical reasoning to modify the assessment and formulate a treatment plan.

KNOWLEDGE OBJECTIVES

1. Describe the four cornerstones of effective paramedic practice. (pp 706–709)
2. Explain the benefits and drawbacks of patient protocols or standing orders and patient care algorithms in the emergency medical services (EMS) system. (p 708)
3. Explain how to distinguish patients with critical life threats from those in serious condition and those with minimal, non–life-threatening injuries. (pp 709–710)
4. Describe the five stages of critical thinking and thought processing in the prehospital setting. (pp 710–715)
5. Describe the Six Rs of clinical decision making. (pp 715–719)

SKILLS OBJECTIVES

There are no skills objectives for this chapter.

Introduction

The most fundamental description of what a paramedic does on a day-to-day basis is as follows: identify problems, set patient care priorities, develop a treatment plan, and execute that plan. Although these steps are crucial, **cookbook medicine**—the practice of blindly following steps without thinking about what you are doing or whether it is working—is not an effective way to practice paramedicine. Effective paramedicine requires you to be a "thinking cook," because many patients present atypically when compared with classic textbook descriptions. To further complicate matters, the prehospital environment is dynamic; you must always maintain situational awareness because scene stability is often an issue that can deteriorate without warning **FIGURE 12-1**. Some paramedics who have worked in a hospital emergency department (ED) say that working in an ED is less chaotic than working in the

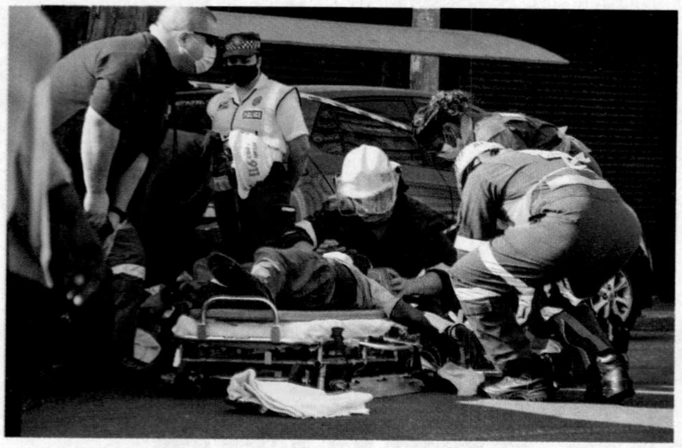

FIGURE 12-1 Your work as a paramedic is rarely done in a quiet, stress-free setting. You will need to master the skill of making decisions in a sometimes chaotic environment.

streets. Most EDs are generally well lit, are located in well-known areas, and usually are safe places for health care professionals to work. That is not always the case when working in the field. Paramedics may encounter patients in many different environments: in the street, on a highway, in an alley, at a crime scene, or in the patient's home, to name a few possibilities. The variety keeps the job fresh and sometimes exciting. As they say, "If you have seen one EMS call, you have seen one EMS call!" Despite the unpredictability of your job, as a paramedic working in the prehospital setting, you are expected to provide quality patient care at scenes that may be stressful and even unstable.

This chapter is divided into two parts, starting with an explanation of critical thinking and concluding with a practical discussion of how you can apply critical thinking skills in the streets. To become a master at critical thinking and clinical decision making, you need to know the cornerstones of thinking processes and the terms that describe them.

Cornerstones of Effective Paramedic Practice

Gathering, Evaluating, and Synthesizing Information

The first cornerstone of your paramedic practice involves gathering, evaluating, and synthesizing (processing) information. Every day, call by call, you will find yourself challenged as you try to obtain information from patients of different age groups and educational backgrounds, with varying abilities to communicate. At times, use of alcohol or drugs, language barriers, or hearing difficulties may impair a patient's ability to respond to your questions, further complicating the patient assessment process.

After you have gathered information, you must assess and evaluate it to formulate a treatment plan (recall the SOAP mnemonic: obtain Subjective and Objective information, make an Assessment, and then Plan for treatment). You need to check the validity of information—often relying on your own judgment and communication skills to do so. For example, you may encounter a patient with a minor sprained ankle who asks for morphine for pain. You may initially think this person is seeking an illicit drug. Another consideration, however, is that your patient may be a health care professional or is knowledgeable about medications and has a low tolerance for pain. Because morphine is not typically a first-line drug for a sprained ankle, you may

YOU are the Paramedic

PART 1

At 1102 hours, you and your partner are dispatched to Winner's Cheerleading Gym for a 15-year-old girl who injured her shoulder during cheerleading practice. On arrival, you ascend to the third floor and see a girl surrounded by people. A coaching staff member is holding the girl's left arm. A second staff member tells you the patient was practicing a pyramid maneuver and was not caught on dismount. The patient fell approximately 8 feet (2.4 m) onto a spring floor with her arms outstretched.

1. Summarize your general impression of this emergency call and what factors may be involved.
2. What is included in your primary survey and initial management steps for this patient?

need to explain to your patient why the drug cannot be administered and offer alternatives. As a thinking paramedic, you must be as objective as possible in your decision-making process.

After you have evaluated the information you obtained from the scene, patient, or a bystander, and determined which information is valid or invalid, you need to **synthesize** this information. To synthesize is to combine several elements, such as history details, into a coherent whole.

Street Smarts

Your professional ethics demand that you consider all possibilities when communicating with a patient. No one calls EMS to be judged! Focus on how you can best meet your patient's needs.

For example, suppose you encounter a 64-year-old man having chest pain. This patient has had type 1 diabetes mellitus since childhood, started smoking in high school, and has had chronic obstructive pulmonary disease (COPD) since his 50s. Synthesis requires that you consider how each element interacts with others, and ultimately how they affect this patient's current condition **FIGURE 12-2**.

Words of Wisdom

After you have established a differential diagnosis, your treatment plan will be determined by patient care protocols or standing orders in the EMS system where you work.

Comorbidity is defined as two or more chronic diseases or conditions present in a patient. In this scenario, the patient has diabetes and COPD. A comorbid condition such as diabetes is directly related to circulatory complications (eg, the development of vascular disease). In addition, in the context of shock, a high blood glucose level can make progressively thickening blood stickier, further worsening the situation. Also, whereas an extremely low blood glucose level may kill someone or result in brain damage quickly, a chronically higher-than-normal blood glucose level takes its toll on every organ and body system. Think about how many people with long-term diabetes you encounter who have vision impairment or amputated fingers or toes from circulation and healing issues. The patient's other comorbid condition, COPD, is a disease of poor gas exchange that frequently results in a combination of hypoxia and hypercapnia. You

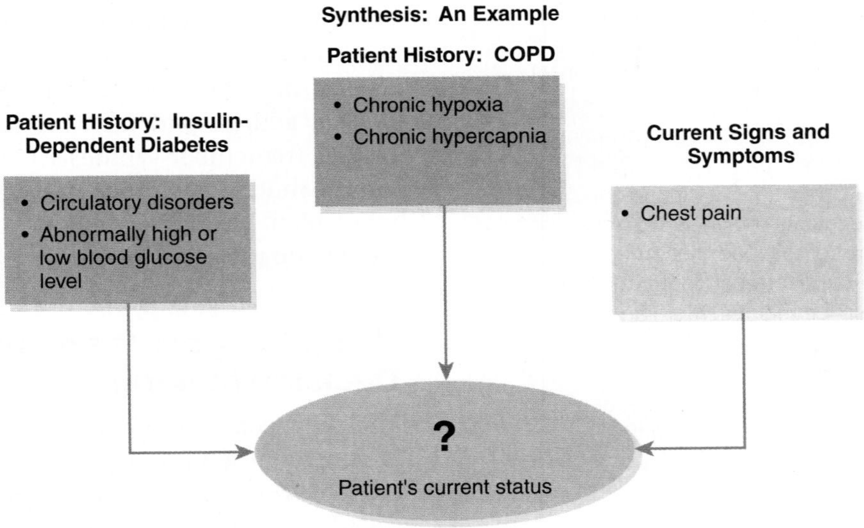

FIGURE 12-2 When you synthesize the patient information you have gathered, assess the relative importance of the patient's medical history (blue boxes) and the signs and symptoms (yellow box). These factors usually affect each other.

Abbreviation: COPD, chronic obstructive pulmonary disease

must consider patient comorbid conditions while you assess his new symptom, onset of chest pain. It is likely that coronary artery disease has caused one or more of the heart muscle vessels to become blocked, causing cells in the patient's heart to begin to necrose, or die. If you take all the information you have gathered and synthesize it, then your conclusion would sound something like this: "I have a patient with diseases of both circulation and gas exchange. There is a possibility that part of his heart is dying because blood vessels are unable to deliver oxygenated blood to a portion of the heart muscle."

You must treat the combined effect of this patient's disease processes to prevent the unperfused section of the heart from dying, which may kill the patient. This is the synthesis part of paramedic practice—taking individual conditions and mentally gluing them together to determine their potential for having a life-threatening effect. In the scenario just described, you should consider the working diagnosis of acute coronary syndrome, a potentially life-threatening condition.

Controversies

A **diagnosis** is the identification of a disease based on its signs and symptoms. The question as to whether prehospital providers diagnose conditions has been debated for years. Some insist that prehospital providers merely treat symptoms and that only physicians can formally diagnose patients' conditions. Others contend that prehospital providers *do* diagnose, even in the absence of sophisticated equipment, using information obtained from the patient's history and physical examination and, when indicated, the results obtained with diagnostic tools and tests (eg, stethoscope, glucometer, pulse oximeter, capnometer, electrocardiograph). The phrase used to describe the patient's diagnosis changes as more information is gathered while providing patient care (eg, field impression, working diagnosis, differential diagnosis) and changes again as patient care is transferred to other health care providers (eg, admitting diagnosis).

Developing and Implementing a Treatment Plan

The second cornerstone of your paramedic practice is your ability to develop and implement a treatment plan. This step is much simpler than analyzing the validity of the information you have gathered. After determining the patient's primary problem by identifying the chief complaint and establishing your working diagnosis, your treatment plan is defined and guided by the patient care protocols or standing orders in the EMS system where you work. Recall that your differential diagnosis is the list of possible diagnoses based on the patient assessment findings. The working diagnosis is a single diagnosis from that differential list on which you are basing your treatment plan.

Protocols or standing orders define the essential clinical standard of care for patients with certain injuries, illnesses, or behavioral conditions, as described in Chapter 1, *EMS Systems*. They further specify performance parameters (ie, what therapies or interventions you can or cannot do without contacting medical control) as well as when you need to contact medical control before providing additional care. Collectively, protocols promote both a standard approach and a standard of quality care as defined by regional, state, or national standards. Protocols also provide parameters for medical control physicians so they do not order treatment with medications beyond your level of training or what is usually carried on your unit.

Unfortunately, protocols, standing orders, and patient care algorithms address only "classic textbook lists" of patient care presentations. As a rule, they do not cover vague patient complaints that do not fit neatly into a clinical description—nor do they address patients with multiple disease etiologies (remember synthesis?). Those patients will require multiple treatment modalities in their treatment plan. Therefore, your next step is to decide what to do to best meet the patient's specific needs.

Using Judgment and Independent Decision Making

The third cornerstone of your paramedic practice is judgment and independent decision making **FIGURE 12-3**. For example, suppose you have been called to a factory where an individual has been injured on the job and suffered a serious gash to the upper part of his leg. You see a substantial amount of blood gushing from the area of his femoral artery with every contraction of his heart. In such a situation, it is in the patient's best interest to delay any

SAFETY

Several studies have examined clinical decision making by EMS personnel and assessed the accuracy of preliminary diagnoses made by paramedics,[1] how paramedics determine medical necessity for transport,[2] appropriate cancellation of advanced life support (ALS) calls, paramedic competence,[3] effectiveness of paramedic scope of practice, and other clinical issues. Collectively, these study results suggest that perhaps EMS providers are being asked to make decisions they are not trained to make. Furthermore, as procedures and tasks have been added to the paramedic scope of practice, a sort of "scope creep" (uncontrolled change) may result in decisions that could harm patients. Although this observation points to an increased potential for error due to increasing demands on EMS providers' skills and decision making, no concrete recommendations have been proposed to deal with this dilemma. Nevertheless, it would seem likely that additional training in complex decision making; low-frequency, high-risk skills; and advanced equipment will be needed, as well as additional real-time support from medical control physicians.

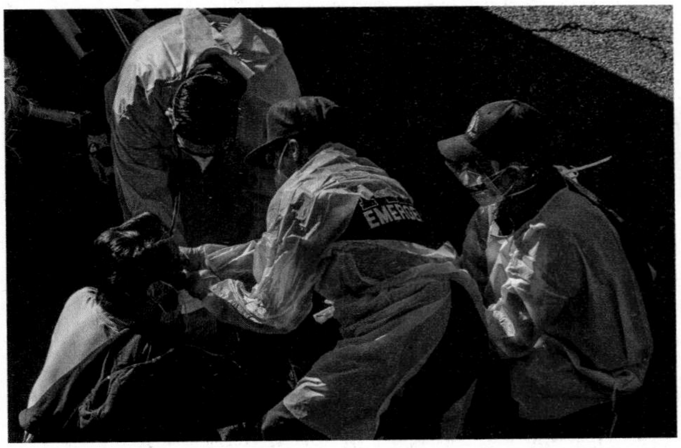

FIGURE 12-3 Every call has its own unique circumstances and challenges. Much of your patient care relies on the use of careful, open-minded decision making.

contact with medical control until you have controlled the bleeding and are en route to the hospital. You must take life-saving action immediately or this patient may die. Even under the best circumstances, if you do not address the bleeding first, this patient may die well before you complete your call with medical control. To save the patient, you must recognize the severed artery as an immediate life threat and apply a tourniquet above the wound and a hemostatic dressing to ensure bleeding control.

Consider another scenario in which you are called for a patient who is in cardiac arrest on her lawn at the mailbox. In such a situation, you would immediately begin high-quality CPR on scene, including defibrillation if indicated. Then, once en route, you would provide ALS care (ie, obtaining intravenous [IV] or intraosseous access, administering vasopressors, and inserting an advanced airway). Now imagine that same patient was instead located in a third-story attic apartment with a small, treacherous exterior stairway as your only access point. Because of the physical environment, you realize it is impossible to quickly and efficiently remove the patient from the apartment for transport to the ED. In this case, you have a decision to make: Either you terminate resuscitation at the scene, or you resuscitate and stabilize the patient before transport.

As circumstances change, so may your treatment plan. However, necessary treatment changes will happen only if you use your critical thinking and decision-making skills to the best of your abilities.

Thinking and Working Under Pressure

The fourth and final cornerstone of your paramedic practice is your ability to think and work under pressure. Imagine that you ring the doorbell at a residence to which you have been dispatched and a hysterical mother opens the door. She hands you a 14-month-old child with cyanosis and apnea who was submerged in the bathtub "for just a minute or two." Your critical thinking tells you the child must start breathing within the next few seconds or cardiac arrest will occur, if it has not yet happened, further decreasing your chance of saving the child's life. Only a combination of knowledge coupled with excellent clinical skills will allow you to avert a patient care disaster: the death of a child. You must be able to work under extreme pressure and think, analyze the situation, and perform quickly and effectively.

The Range of Patient Conditions

A key element of your paramedic practice is being able to quickly determine if the patient is sick or not sick. For patients who are sick, you must be able to quantify how sick they are, which in turn allows you to make the best choices as to the care you provide at the scene and the care you provide in the ambulance while en route. This process becomes more complicated when you have multiple sick or injured patients.

Special Populations

It can be challenging to recognize whether an infant or child is sick or not sick because these patients tend to be "low frequency yet high acuity." In other words, paramedics do not go on many calls for children, but when they do, these tend to be serious calls. To improve your ability, consider taking continuing education courses and reading research articles on pediatrics. Simulation training may also be helpful preparation.

Critical Thinking and Clinical Decision Making

As an EMS provider, you need to understand the processes of thinking and decision making. By having a better understanding of how your thoughts are formed and processed, you can learn to think more effectively. The critical thinking process can be broken down into five stages: concept formation, data interpretation, application of principle, reflection *in* action, and reflection *on* action.

Concept Formation

The first stage of the thought process in prehospital care is gathering information—things you see, hear, smell, or feel and information that you gather by applying your diagnostic tools. This process is called **concept formation.**

Concept formation starts as you arrive at the scene, become situationally aware, and evaluate the scene to ensure the safety of yourself, your crew, and your patient. In the patient assessment process, this step is known as scene size-up. As we have discussed, it is not an isolated act but rather requires maintaining constant awareness throughout the entire encounter. Determine the mechanism of injury (MOI) for trauma, or for a medical call, the nature of the present illness (NOI). How does the patient present? Does the patient appear uncomfortable, frightened, or deathly ill? Assess the patient's level of consciousness (LOC), in part to determine whether the patient can provide you with reliable

YOU are the Paramedic

PART 2

As you talk with the staff member, he tells you he saw the patient fall and reports that only her arm seems injured. He did not witness any trauma to the head or neck. You examine the patient and find that her left arm has an angular deformity in the humerus region. You observe abnormal motion every time she tries to move the arm, and she cannot move it without "really bad" pain. The patient rates her level of pain as 9 on a scale of 0 to 10 but denies having any head, neck, or back pain. You obtain her vital signs while a staff member continues holding her arm. The patient's parents are not on scene, but a staff member tells you they are being contacted. Although the patient is visibly shaken, she is not crying and is answering questions appropriately.

Recording Time: 0 Minutes	
Appearance	Visibly upset, obvious deformity to the arm
Level of consciousness	Alert and oriented
Airway	Open and patent
Breathing	Normal, 22 breaths/min
Circulation	Radial pulse, tachycardic

3. Have you gathered enough data to turn your field impression into a treatment plan?
4. Should you administer pain medication?

information to act on. This initial evaluation of the LOC will also establish a baseline to refer to later as the call progresses and in case the patient's condition changes.

You move further into the information-gathering process as you perform your primary survey, focusing on identification and correction of any immediate threats to the patient's life relative to the ABCDEs (Airway, Breathing, Circulation, Disability, and Exposure). You continue on as you perform a secondary assessment and physical exam and identify the patient's chief complaint. By obtaining a SAMPLE (Signs and symptoms; Allergies; Medications; Pertinent past medical history; Last oral intake; Events leading up to the illness or injury) history, you will be able to gather important information from the patient, including any medications the patient is taking (eg, prescription, over-the-counter, illicit, herbal).

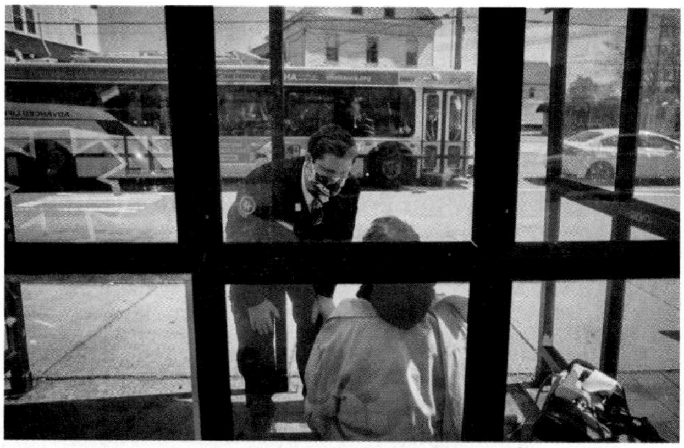

FIGURE 12-4 Take in clues not only from the patient's affect, but also from the surroundings. Assess the entire environment to make sure you fully understand its effect on the patient's condition. This call was for a woman who was weak and dizzy at a bus stop.

Street Smarts

Situational awareness is an essential paramedic skill. It will help you anticipate factors that could disrupt patient care or even lead to physical danger for you and your team. It may prompt a gut feeling that "something just isn't right here." As part of your situational awareness, observe family members for clues. Do they seem worried or nervous? Does calling 9-1-1 seem routine for them? Are they huddled in a corner crying or are they trying to watch their favorite show on television during your assessment?

Be alert for situations that are not what they seem to be.

One of the most important observations you need to judge is your patient's **affect**, or emotional state reflected in physical behavior **FIGURE 12-4**. The affect might not coincide with what the patient tells you. For example, you may treat a patient who presents with manic behavior that can be associated with amphetamine abuse, yet the patient denies any drug use. You might even see drug paraphernalia. You must assess the accuracy of the information you are receiving if it does not match what you are seeing and hearing.

Last, you need to obtain the patient's vital signs and relevant clinical test results by using your primary diagnostic tools (eg, glucometer, pulse oximeter, capnometer, electrocardiogram [ECG] monitor, blood pressure [BP] cuff, and stethoscope).

Data Interpretation

During the second stage of the critical thinking process, you must evaluate all the information you have gathered and form a conclusion, which is called **data interpretation**. To understand how the body works and how it responds when complications arise, you need a solid background in anatomy, physiology, and pathophysiology. Another key element is your level of education and experience. If you have come to your paramedic program as an experienced EMT, then you may have an excellent platform to build on. However, even without that background, applying yourself in your studies will help you meet the challenges of working in EMS. Always feel free to ask questions of your instructors and mentors. The only bad question, generally, is the one that was not asked.

How you think and form conclusions is affected not only by your patients' attitudes but also by your attitude as a health care provider. For example, you should *never* consider a call to be a waste of your time or talent. Furthermore, unprofessional comments, such as "I can't believe you called us for *this*!", show a lack of compassion and interest in providing quality patient care. Having a negative attitude about any patient or patient care situation will almost guarantee that the care you provide will be suboptimal. To maintain the standards of care set by your profession, you must provide the best care you can for every patient you encounter. In fact, many paramedic programs ask their students to pledge the Declaration of Geneva or Code of Ethics statement at their graduation ceremonies.

Application of Principle

In the third stage of the critical thinking process, your field impression becomes your working diagnosis. The key word here is *working*. The working diagnosis is what you tentatively believe to be the problem and the focus of your treatment. Note that your working diagnosis may not always be narrowed down to just one problem; it could include a number of conditions from your differential diagnosis and the conditions for which you are treating the patient.

From this point on, your treatment plan is driven by patient care protocols, or standing orders, in the EMS system where you work.

Reflection *in* Action

In the fourth stage of the critical thinking process, you actively treat the patient while monitoring your interventions' effects. Think of *reflection in action* as *thinking while doing*.

For example, if the patient is having considerable difficulty breathing (Spo_2 level less than 94% combined with obvious signs of hypoxia), then you would administer supplemental oxygen and reassess the patient after a few minutes, asking, "Is it getting any easier for you to breathe?" If the situation does not improve, additional interventions (ie, administering a drug or more aggressive ventilation) may be appropriate. It is essential to periodically check your interventions to see whether they are making the patient feel better. Asking the patient how the treatment is working reassures the patient and indicates that you are concerned and keeping abreast of the situation **FIGURE 12-5**. Reassessment is a vital part of your patient care.

Documentation and Communication

It is essential to document what procedures are done, what medications are given, and the effect the procedure or medication had, if any, on the patient.

FIGURE 12-5 A patient's condition can change rapidly, especially when the person is critically ill or injured. Continually monitor any changes to a patient's condition.

Consider a scenario in which a 58-year-old man has experienced chest pain while moving rocks to landscape his yard. Although he has no history of cardiac disease, he is in the right age group for you to suspect a heart condition. When you ask him if he can pinpoint where the pain seems to be, his fingers curl into a fist (known as the Levine sign) as he points to the location on his chest directly over his heart. His heart could still be the issue, so you continue with assessment and a "rule out myocardial infarction" treatment plan.

You ask if anything makes the pain better or worse, and the patient explains that if he holds his left arm still, the pain goes away. However, with arm movement, the pain becomes severe. This statement is key because you know that the pain associated with a heart attack is not relieved by merely sitting still and not moving an extremity. You now revise your impression and focus your assessment on the possibility of a musculoskeletal injury, and your treatment plan and interventions change accordingly. Prior to obtaining this information, you would likely have given the patient aspirin, nitroglycerin, and perhaps oxygen therapy to enhance oxygen delivery to offset potential infarction of the patient's heart. Instead, you might now consider providing an analgesic for pain relief for an isolated musculoskeletal injury.

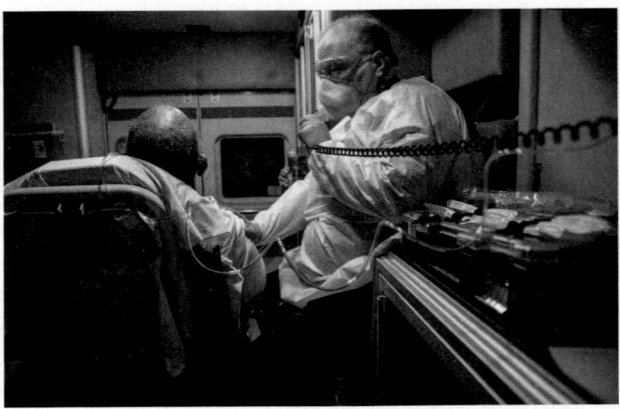

> **Words of Wisdom**
>
> To provide optimal patient care, avoid tunnel vision when determining the cause of a patient's condition. Do not focus only on your general impression. As you gather information, modify your treatment plan according to the additional history acquired and the patient's needs.

One of the key elements of this critical thinking process stage is avoiding **tunnel vision**. Tunnel vision occurs when you focus on or consider only one aspect of a situation without first taking into account all possibilities. Keep an open mind to all potential causes of the patient's current condition. Perhaps this patient is having a heart attack that presents in a manner different from the typical signs and symptoms, so obtain a 12-lead ECG and continually reassess the patient's condition.

> **Words of Wisdom**
>
> Knowing what services your response area offers before you go on a call is crucial to ensure good patient outcomes and service sustainability. Many EDs and EMS systems have become overwhelmed with patient loads and are being used as primary care locations for some individuals, so it is essential to consider the need and appropriate destination for patient transport. Your response area may offer nonemergent services that help patients find resources to aid them when the 9-1-1 call is not a medical or traumatic emergency. Such programs allow "superusers of a system" to be evaluated for service needs such as home health, transport services, food services, and safety issues that may have been identified during the EMS crew's initial response. With the growth of community paramedicine, you may also find yourself attending to a patient who can be treated at home and released based on your local protocols and follow-up services that can be offered.

Reflection *on* Action

The last stage in the critical thinking process occurs after the call is over and commonly encompasses run reviews, run critiques, or debriefings. During this stage, you look back at the call and reflect on how you gathered and processed information and reached your decisions. One of the most challenging aspects of this stage is learning to accept that something went wrong or that better treatment choices could have been made. It is essential to establish an attitude that there is always room for personal and professional improvement. A review of the run is an excellent opportunity to evaluate what might have gone wrong and how you can improve your skills as a paramedic. Do not blame or criticize yourself; just analyze, learn, and move on. Remember, you did not cause the patient's heart attack—genetics, improper nutrition, and a sedentary lifestyle likely played a role.

You will periodically encounter patients with atypical presentations, meaning they do not show

> **SAFETY**
>
> A medical error is an act of omission or commission in planning or execution that contributes or could contribute to an unintended result.[4] Rather than deeming every medical error the result of a single human error, it is necessary to look deeper and see other factors that may have set the stage for failure. Medical errors can be categorized as adverse drug events, wrong-site surgeries, falls, burns, pressure ulcers, and mistaken patient identities. High error rates with serious consequences are most likely to occur in the intensive care unit, operating room, or ED, and during care delivered by paramedics in the field or during critical care transports. They frequently occur during transitions of care, which underscores the importance of proper communication with the ED.
>
> A just culture (beliefs, customs, and acceptable behaviors within an organization) focuses on identifying issues that lead to errors or unsafe behaviors, while still maintaining individual accountability for reckless behavior. It helps distinguish various types of errors, including human error (ie, missteps), at-risk behavior (ie, taking shortcuts), and reckless behavior (ie, ignoring required safety steps). Humans are not perfect, so any human-made system should anticipate some level of error. A mistake or lapse can happen to even the best paramedics. Human error is typically a product of system design and behavioral choices. It therefore should not be viewed as a punishable action, but rather as an opportunity to think critically about, and ultimately improve, the system.

the classic signs and symptoms of a condition. For example, you may see a patient with a neck fracture who has no pain. To make an accurate diagnosis, you must also use all you have learned about communication with patients. For instance, the patient might come from a culture that minimizes the presence of pain, so that the patient hesitates to report this symptom.

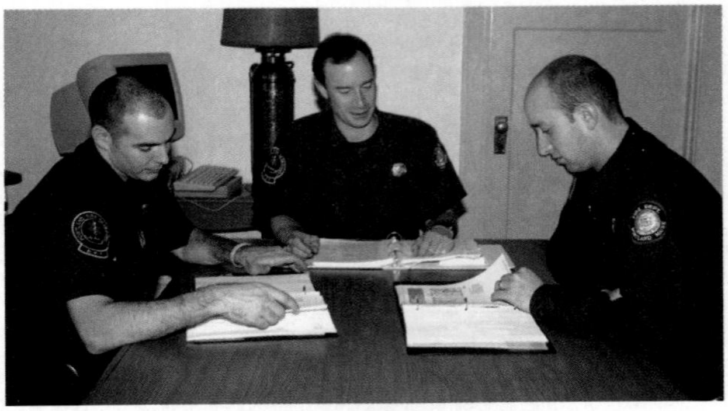

FIGURE 12-6 A formal review, or audit, of your performance can seem intimidating. However, it is also an opportunity for you to gain meaningful feedback and improve as a paramedic, so keep an open mind.

Words of Wisdom

The more you learn, the less you will use the words "always" and "never."

Reflection gives you a chance to continuously improve your thinking and decision-making skills. In turn, your patient care will improve as you become more experienced. Be open to learning, and remember that every run you go on, every class you take, and every run review you attend is another opportunity to improve your skills **FIGURE 12-6**. *Personal and professional growth will not happen if you cannot admit mistakes or are unwilling to continue learning.* The successful completion of the paramedic program is only a starting point in your career as an ALS provider. To provide the best possible care, you must commit to a lifetime of learning. The most important trait for a successful lifetime career in EMS is a genuine desire to continuously improve as a paramedic.

A list of the fundamental elements that contribute to the critical thinking and clinical

YOU are the Paramedic

PART 3

The staff member tells you she has tried calling the parents twice but has not reached them yet. She says she will continue to try. Due to the patient's extreme pain, you decide to call medical control regarding pain medication. You give the physician a report, including the patient's height (5 feet [1.5 m]) and weight (100 lb [45 kg]), and he advises you to administer 5 mg of morphine followed by another 2-mg dose of morphine 10 minutes later. The patient agrees, and you start an IV line and administer 5 mg of morphine.

Recording Time: 5 Minutes	
Respirations	26 breaths/min
Pulse	110 beats/min
Skin	Warm and dry
Blood pressure	110/80 mm Hg before pain medication (morphine) 2 min after morphine administration: 100/50 mm Hg
Oxygen saturation (Spo_2)	100%
Pupils	Pupils Equal, Round, and Reactive to Light and Accommodation (PERRLA)

5. What is your working diagnosis?

6. What effects can be expected from the administration of morphine?

decision-making process follows. As you look over each item, ask yourself, "Do I have this quality already, or do I need to develop it?"

- Adequate knowledge of anatomy, physiology, and pathophysiology
- Ability to gather and organize data and form concepts
- Ability to focus on specific and multiple elements of data
- Ability to identify and deal with **medical ambiguity**—uncertainty regarding the specific cause of the patient's condition (Few calls will follow the "scripts" in your protocols to the letter).
- Skill in differentiating between relevant and irrelevant data
- Ability to analyze and compare similar as well as contrary situations
- Ability to articulate your reasoning and construct arguments

From Theory to Practical Application

Several unique factors come into play with every call. Consider the following scenario:

> You are dispatched to a "car off the road" call, in which a single vehicle with four passengers has spun off a slippery road into a ditch at an estimated speed of 35 miles per hour (mph). Think about how each of the following variables might change how you respond to and manage this call:
>
> - The passengers were not wearing seat belts.
> - The vehicle was traveling at 65 mph and not 35 mph.
> - The vehicle flipped over and is on its roof.
> - It is 20°F (–7°C) outside and the crash location was not discovered for at least an hour.

As you can see from the list, different variables create many possible new outcomes for patients. Likewise, your ability to manage the call and patient care properly becomes more challenging. Even if only a few calls you respond to on a day-to-day basis represent life-threatening emergencies, you must handle every call in the same professional manner and provide the best possible care.

As a paramedic, you must learn to cope with your reactions, such as the effect of the fight-or-flight response, when confronted with extreme medical emergencies (a topic discussed in more detail in Chapter 2, *Workforce Safety and Wellness*). This response can impair your critical thinking skills and diminish your concentration and assessment abilities. One way to counter these negative effects is to improve your mental conditioning and your skill performance. Practice your skills until you can do them instinctively (known as muscle memory) and perform them on command in a skills lab setting. Once you have reached that level of skill mastery, you can quickly draw on these skills in a real-life setting, allowing you to better focus on patient assessment or other decision-making areas.

Facilitate better thinking under pressure by memorizing the following mental checklist for all calls:

1. Take a moment to scan the scene.
2. Take another moment to stop and think.
3. Move forward and make decisions and act on behalf of the patient.
4. Stay calm and in control, and maintain situational awareness.
5. Regularly and continually reevaluate the patient.

Words of Wisdom

Do not be fooled by patients who initially appear uninjured or healthy. Do not hesitate to take a thorough history and perform a complete physical exam as well as another set of vital signs for such patients.

Taking It to the Streets

When you are out on a call, critical thinking can be summed up with the *Six Rs of clinical decision making* **FIGURE 12-7**.

1. Read the Scene

An emergency scene is filled with information readily available to you. This information tells a story that is only available at the scene; it becomes

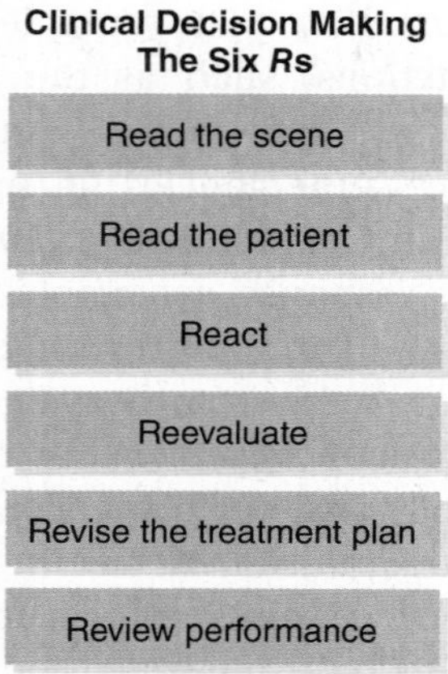

FIGURE 12-7 The Six Rs of clinical decision making.

unavailable the moment you initiate transport to the ED. To effectively read the scene, you must evaluate the following items: (1) the overall safety of the situation, (2) the environmental conditions, (3) the immediate surroundings, (4) any access and egress issues, and (5) the MOI or NOI **FIGURE 12-8**. In particular, when you are considering the MOI, take time to evaluate all aspects of the incident.

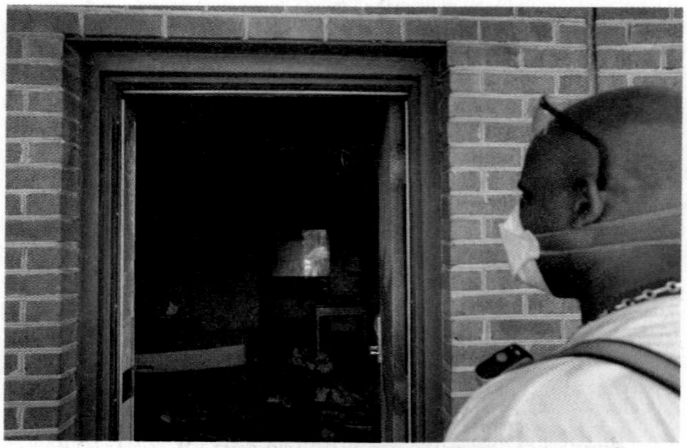

FIGURE 12-8 Although you need to focus on treating patients as soon as possible, always take a moment to take in important information about the scene. An effective scene size-up will help you remain safe and provide quality patient care, as explained in Chapter 11, *Patient Assessment*.

Other issues to consider when you size up the scene include assessing the environment. Is it hot, cold, or wet? Also, are eyewitnesses, friends, or family members available to provide additional information?

YOU are the Paramedic

PART 4

On reassessment, the patient feels less pain and rates it as 5 on the 0 to 10 scale. You proceed to immobilize her arm with a sling. After you and your partner place the patient onto a stretcher and move her to the ambulance, her aunt arrives on scene. You give Aunt Julie a complete report and tell her you will be transporting her niece to the local ED for treatment. You also advise Aunt Julie that you are administering a second dose of morphine. The aunt tells you "No!" and says you should not have given her niece pain medication.

Recording Time: 10 Minutes	
Respirations	18 breaths/min
Pulse	70 beats/min
Skin	Warm and dry
Blood pressure	100/60 mm Hg
Oxygen saturation (Spo_2)	100%
Pupils	PERRLA
ECG	Sinus without ectopy

7. How should you respond to the aunt's statement that pain medication should not have been administered?

8. Did you have the right to give the patient pain medication without a parent present?

2. Read the Patient

One of the greatest skills you can develop is learning to read a patient quickly. As you approach the patient, does the patient see you and visually track you? Offer the patient your gloved hand to shake (or an appropriate gesture based on the person's culture and customs), introduce yourself, and ask why 9-1-1 was called. If the patient takes your hand and answers you appropriately, then you have just determined the patient has a Glasgow Coma Scale score of 15 (spontaneous eye opening, follows commands, appropriate verbal response). Other components of an effective primary survey and history taking include the following:

- **Observe the patient.** What is the patient's LOC and level of comfort or discomfort? Skin color? Position? Work of breathing? Any obvious deformity or asymmetry?
- **Talk to the patient.** Determine the chief complaint. Is this a new condition or the worsening of a preexisting condition? Obtain the medical history and the events leading up to the illness or injury.
- **Touch the patient.** Assess the skin for color, temperature, and condition. Assess the rate, regularity, and strength of the pulse.
- **Auscultate breath sounds.** Confirm the adequacy or inadequacy of breathing and assess the patency of the airway.
- **Identify and correct any life threats** relative to the ABCDEs in the order you find them.
- **Obtain complete and accurate vital signs** **FIGURE 12-9**. For every patient, including those being transported on routine transfers, you must obtain a baseline set of vital signs. Recall that a patient's vital signs are influenced by patient age, underlying physical and medical conditions, and current medications. For patients with serious conditions, two sets of serial vital signs provide comparative data to begin to establish trends. For patients in critical condition, three or more sets of vital signs allow you to assess trends and to reassess whether the patient's condition is stabilizing, improving, or getting worse. If the patient's condition is deteriorating, then obtain multiple sets of vital signs to track the progression.

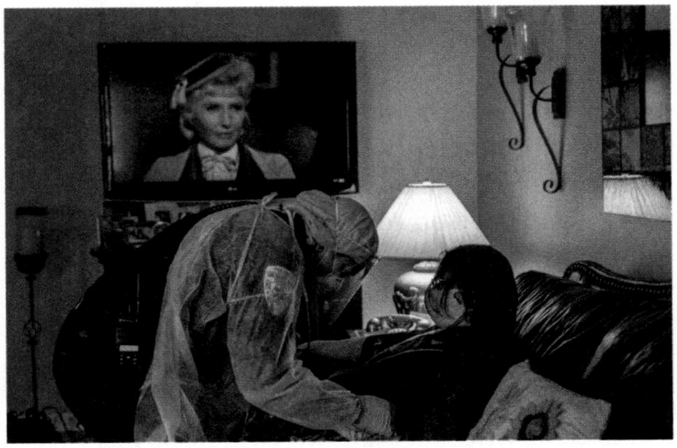

FIGURE 12-9 The more accurate your patient information, the more reliable your diagnosis. Take time to obtain a set of baseline vital signs for every patient.

SAFETY

Effective communication is vital to all members of the patient care team in the aftermath of an adverse patient safety event, such as serious physical or psychological injury. Communicating effectively helps the team navigate competing priorities, overcome issues related to human factors, and reduce error.

A huddle is a communication technique and event that often takes the form of a structured, short meeting in which a patient care team comes together to talk about a patient, procedure, or situation. A huddle can also be called whenever a team needs to regroup and share concerns, discuss resource allocation, anticipate outcomes, and create contingency plans. After a serious adverse event, the team is advised to huddle (as social distancing allows) and discuss the event that occurred, including stabilization of the patient and situation; determine the facts of what happened; mitigate any ongoing harm; address staff safety concerns; secure equipment or materials; and alert others as deemed necessary by the senior staff member leading the huddle. The huddle is critical to ensure that actual events, sequences, and timing are accurately recorded to aid in further analysis and corrective actions related to the situation. It is also the only opportunity to preserve equipment in the actual state it was in when the incident occurred; for example, a problem caused by a faulty ventilator or IV pump cannot be properly analyzed if the settings are changed or the equipment is returned to use.

3. React

As a paramedic, your priority during patient care is to treat any life threats. Next, consider possible causes of the patient's symptoms, and rule certain conditions either in or out as you gather more information and develop your differential diagnosis, and ultimately, a working diagnosis.

If you cannot narrow the differential diagnosis to a working diagnosis by the end of your assessment, then provide care based on the patient's presenting signs and symptoms. You will often care for patients whose conditions cannot be diagnosed until they reach the ED. In fact, some patients are admitted to a critical care unit for further tests and monitoring (eg, to rule out myocardial infarction). Many conditions cannot be treated in the field, so transport to an appropriate facility may be one of the most important aspects of the care you provide. For all these reasons, it is just as essential to determine a treatment plan as it is to treat life threats. This plan must include rapid transport if your analysis of the patient's condition suggests that it is warranted.

4. Reevaluate

As you continue to provide patient care, make certain you follow up on your interventions. Check whether the splint you applied has eased the pain in the patient's injured leg. If you treat a patient with pain medication, then reevaluate their pain level to see if the medication is effective. On challenging calls, it is easy to get into "treatment mode" and focus on doing things while forgetting to follow up on whether what you are doing is actually improving the patient's condition.

As you reassess the patient, take time to add any information you may have gathered from the secondary assessment to the primary survey, such as discovering less obvious problems. For example, you find that the patient has no breath sounds in the upper right lobe secondary to a fractured rib that caused a small pneumothorax. By itself, a small pneumothorax is not an immediate life threat to a relatively healthy person. This patient, however, also has bilateral fractured femurs, substantial blood loss, and a minor head injury. Under those circumstances, a small pneumothorax may complicate matters far more than if it were a single, isolated condition. When you care for patients, especially trauma patients with multiple injuries, you must assess the cumulative effect of all factors as you develop your treatment plan. Your goal is to ensure that you do not overlook anything that should be addressed in the field.

Street Smarts

Dealing With Controversies and Change

For many years, EMS personnel have provided patients with effective prophylactic treatments even though the need for some interventions has not been supported by evidence-based research. Should every trauma patient be immobilized on a backboard? Probably not. Should every unresponsive person be given naloxone? Probably not. Should EMS personnel be aggressive with fluids or limit them? What are the most up-to-date standards, and what happens when the guidelines change but an EMS system lags in implementing those updates?

Stay on top of the research, be aware of the changes that may be coming, and learn the rationale for change. Your medical director (or region) will decide to update the local treatment protocols at the most practical point, recognizing that updates usually involve training. Your agency's leaders will learn the rationale for the changes and help their peers understand and accept them.

Adaptability is a beneficial attitude in EMS. Remember, paramedicine is always evolving, so expect lifelong learning and learn to embrace change!

5. Revise the Treatment Plan

As a thinking paramedic—and no matter how sure you are of the working diagnosis—you must always keep your mind open to other possibilities that might explain the patient's presentation. As the call unfolds and additional information becomes available, be prepared to revise your treatment plan as necessary. By remaining mentally "light on your feet," you position yourself to be receptive to changing presentations or circumstances, which in turn helps you avoid tunnel vision.

6. Review Performance

Again, after a call is over, you have the opportunity to look back and reexamine your work **FIGURE 12-10**. Whether this review occurs in the formal setting of a continuous quality improvement meeting, a post–field code debriefing, or a conversation with your partner back at the station, taking time to critically assess your work allows for real growth opportunities, especially when you may have made a mistake. Although success is satisfying and certainly feels good, it offers few opportunities for growth. However, when you make a mistake, you can learn how to avoid repeating the mistake and how to do better next time. Excellence in prehospital care is the gradual result of you continually striving to improve your performance, which requires that you *always* have an open attitude to learning.

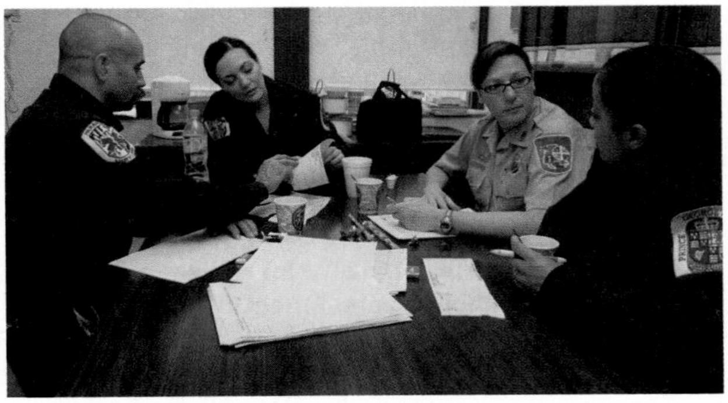

FIGURE 12-10 You can learn something new with every call you run. One of the best ways to review your performance—and to continually learn and improve—is to talk it over with peers.

Being a thinking paramedic will happen only if you choose to work on your critical thinking skills daily, call by call, throughout your career. If you continue to improve the way you think and make decisions, then your patient care will improve as well. Your reward will be excellence in your practice—the ultimate job satisfaction.

YOU are the Paramedic SUMMARY

1. Summarize your general impression of this emergency call and what factors may be involved.

The call was for a child who injured her shoulder during cheerleading practice. On scene, you are told by a staff member that the patient fell 8 feet (2 m) onto a spring floor with her arms outstretched. You realize that you will be caring for a pediatric patient with injuries that may be severe. The process of gathering your general impression based on everything you see, hear, smell, and feel is called concept formation.

2. What is included in your primary survey and initial management steps for this patient?

You need to immediately rule out any injury to the patient's cervical spine, back, or head. Assess the patient's vital signs, including her LOC and ABCDEs. Monitor the patient's respiratory status and administer oxygen if you see any signs of difficulty breathing. Also, ask the patient whether pain medication would help her before immobilizing her arm in a sling. Remember that parental consent must be obtained, if possible, before providing emergency treatment to a minor.

3. Have you gathered enough data to turn your field impression into a treatment plan?

You have enough information to make a treatment plan. The patient has sustained an isolated trauma to her arm. You must complete the following critical actions: immobilize the arm, make the patient comfortable, and transport the patient to a hospital for further treatment.

4. Should you administer pain medication?

You are ethically responsible for making each patient as comfortable as possible. In the absence of parental consent, you may administer medication to pediatric patients to help relieve pain, although this practice varies from jurisdiction to jurisdiction. If a parent or guardian is unavailable to give consent to emergency treatment, then you may undertake emergency treatment to sustain life without consent under the doctrine of implied consent. When in doubt, obtain online guidance from medical control. Know your state laws and local protocols concerning the treatment of minors.

YOU are the Paramedic SUMMARY continued

5. What is your working diagnosis?

You have ruled out multisystem trauma and determined that the patient has an isolated extremity trauma. There is no medical condition associated with the emergency, and the patient denies having any significant medical history or medication allergies. Your treatment includes immobilization of the injury and ensuring the patient's comfort while en route to the hospital.

6. What effects can be expected from the administration of morphine?

Morphine is a common narcotic analgesic that many EMS agencies carry. The effect of morphine differs for each patient. Although pain medication may not eliminate the patient's pain, it will reduce the level of pain. Some benefits to giving pain medication are a more relaxed patient, which will result in positive changes in vital signs and a decreased level of anxiety. Some patients may be allergic to pain medications; any allergies should be established before medication administration. In addition, pain medications sometimes cause adverse effects, such as nausea and/or vomiting. Those effects should be anticipated and patients can be treated with an antiemetic medication.

7. How should you respond to the aunt's statement that pain medication should not have been administered?

Minors present unique issues for the paramedic. Usually, a parent is the legal decision maker for a child; a relative is not a legal decision maker unless the parent has signed legal documents stating otherwise. Recognizing that the relative may have a valid concern, explain that your treatment was authorized by a physician and is standard care. Advise Aunt Julie to contact the patient's parents to discuss her concerns. Remember to stay friendly and do not argue with the family member, as that might unnecessarily escalate the situation.

8. Did you have the right to give the patient pain medication without a parent present?

Under certain circumstances, you do have the right to treat a minor without a parent present. In this situation, you have been given authority by medical control to treat the patient. Often, obtaining consent to treat a child may be difficult. At times, a parent or guardian of a child may not want you to treat the child for various reasons. In such cases, you must respect the parent's (or guardian's) wishes and discuss the medical consequences of that decision. However, you may not withhold care from the patient when the person making this request is not the parent or guardian. As a patient advocate, you need to be aware of the challenges associated with obtaining permission and be prepared to discuss the need for care.

EMS Patient Care Report (PCR)

Date: 04-24-22	**Incident No.:** 110435	**Nature of Call:** Child injured		**Location:** Winner's Cheerleading Gym	
Dispatched: 1102	**En Route:** 1103	**At Scene:** 1105	**Transport:** 1130	**At Hospital:** 1145	**In Service:** 1201

Patient Information

Age: 15 **Sex:** F **Weight (in kg [lb]):** 45 kg (100 lb)	**Allergies:** NKDA **Medications:** None **Past Medical History:** None **Chief Complaint:** Upper arm pain

Vital Signs

Time: 1110	**BP:** 110/80; 2 min after morphine admin, 100/50	**Pulse:** 110	**Respirations:** 26	**Spo_2:** 100%
Time: 1115	**BP:** 100/60	**Pulse:** 70	**Respirations:** 18	**Spo_2:** 100%
Time:	**BP:**	**Pulse:**	**Respirations:**	**Spo_2:**

YOU are the Paramedic SUMMARY continued

EMS Treatment (circle all that apply)				
Oxygen @ _____ L/min via (circle one): **NC NRM Bag-mask device**		**Assisted Ventilation**	**Airway Adjunct**	**CPR**
Defibrillation	**Bleeding Control**	**Bandaging**	**Splinting** (circled)	**Other:**

Narrative
Arrived on scene to find 15-year-old girl in care of coaching staff. Staff states pt was on top of a pyramid performing a cheerleading maneuver and was not caught on dismount. Pt states she fell about 8 feet (2 m) onto her left arm and right arm, with most of the force absorbed by the left arm. The gym floor was on springs and was able to absorb most of the energy of the fall. Pt states she has "really bad" left upper arm pain. Pt denies any head, neck, or back pain. Pt denies any other injury, problem, or pain other than in her left arm. Assessment of pt's arm reveals extreme pain with arm movement. Pt agreed to receive medication for pain. Medical control at Midtown Hospital authorized 5 mg of morphine initially and another 5 mg after 10 minutes if pain is still severe. Hospital staff awaiting our arrival. IV line established in right AC vein with 20-gauge needle, saline well attached, and saline drip started at KVO rate. 5 mg of morphine administered at 1115. Minutes later pt stated pain level changed from 9/10 to 5/10, and pt's arm was immobilized with a sling. Pt was moved to ambulance and reassessed; vital signs taken and noted above. Pt stated pain level was still at 5 after 10 minutes. Pt was given second dose of 5 mg of morphine. Pt's Aunt Julie met us before leaving for hospital and expressed displeasure with EMS giving her niece morphine. EMS reassured aunt that the medical control physician authorized pt treatment and stated that pt was feeling much better and in less pain. Pt transported without further incident. Vital signs monitored and pt's pain decreased from 5 to 4. Pt released to nurse in ED room 4 with report. IV patent and less than 200 mL infused. RN witnessed waste of 6 mg of morphine. Waste form attached to PCR. **End of report**

Prep Kit

Ready for Review

- The first cornerstone of your paramedic practice is having the ability to gather, evaluate, and synthesize (process) information.
  - After you have gathered information, assess and evaluate its validity and the effect it may have on the treatment plan you are developing.
  - After you have evaluated the information you obtained from the scene, the patient, or any bystanders and determined which information is valid, then you need to synthesize that information.
- The second cornerstone of your paramedic practice is developing and implementing a treatment plan.
  - Your treatment plan is almost always defined by the patient care protocols or standing orders in the EMS system where you work.
- The third cornerstone of your paramedic practice is judgment and making independent decisions.
- The fourth and final cornerstone of your paramedic practice is your ability to think and work under pressure.
- The first stage of the thought process in prehospital care is gathering information—things you see, hear, smell, or feel or obtain with your diagnostics. This process leads to concept formation.
  - As part of your primary survey, focus on the identification and correction of any immediate life threats relative to the ABCDEs.
- The second stage of the critical thinking process is data interpretation—evaluating the

Prep Kit continued

information you have gathered and forming a conclusion.

- The third stage of the critical thinking process is application of principle—when your field impression becomes your working diagnosis.
- The fourth stage of the critical thinking process is reflection in action—actively treating the patient while monitoring the effects of your interventions.
- The last stage in the critical thinking process is reflection on action. It occurs after the call is over and is commonly associated with run reviews, run critiques, or debriefings. Look back at the total call and reflect on how you processed all the information you gathered and reached the decisions that you did.
- Use the *Six Rs of clinical decision making* to summarize what must be done on a call:
  - Read the scene.
  - Read the patient.
  - React.
  - Reevaluate.
  - Revise the treatment plan.
  - Review performance.
- Excellence in prehospital care results from a constant effort to improve your practice, which requires that you always have an attitude that is open to learning.

Vital Vocabulary

affect The patient's emotional state as reflected in the patient's physical behavior.

comorbidity The existence of two or more chronic diseases or conditions in a patient.

concept formation Pattern of understanding based on initially obtained information; the first stage of the critical thinking process in prehospital care.

cookbook medicine Blindly following a protocol or algorithm without thinking about what is being done and whether it is working.

data interpretation The process of reaching conclusions based on comparing the patient's presentation with information from your training, education, and past experiences; the second stage of the critical thinking process in prehospital care.

diagnosis The identification of a disease based on its signs and symptoms.

medical ambiguity Vague or unclear aspects of medicine.

synthesize To combine several things, such as history elements, into a coherent whole.

tunnel vision Focusing on or considering only one aspect of a situation without first taking into account all possibilities.

References

1. Koivulahti O, Tommila M, Haavisto E. The accuracy of preliminary diagnoses made by paramedics: a cross-sectional comparative study. *Scand J Trauma Resusc Emerg Med.* 2020;28(70):1-7. doi:10.1186/s13049-020-00761-6.
2. Gratton MC, Ellison SR, Hunt J, Ma OJ. Prospective determination of medical necessity for ambulance transport by paramedics. *Prehosp Emerg Care.* 2003;7(4):466-469.
3. Tavares W, Boet S. On the assessment of paramedic competence: a narrative review with practice implications. *Prehosp Disaster Med.* 2016;31(1):64-73.
4. Grober ED, Bohnen JM. Defining medical error. *Can J Surg.* 2005;48(1):39-44.

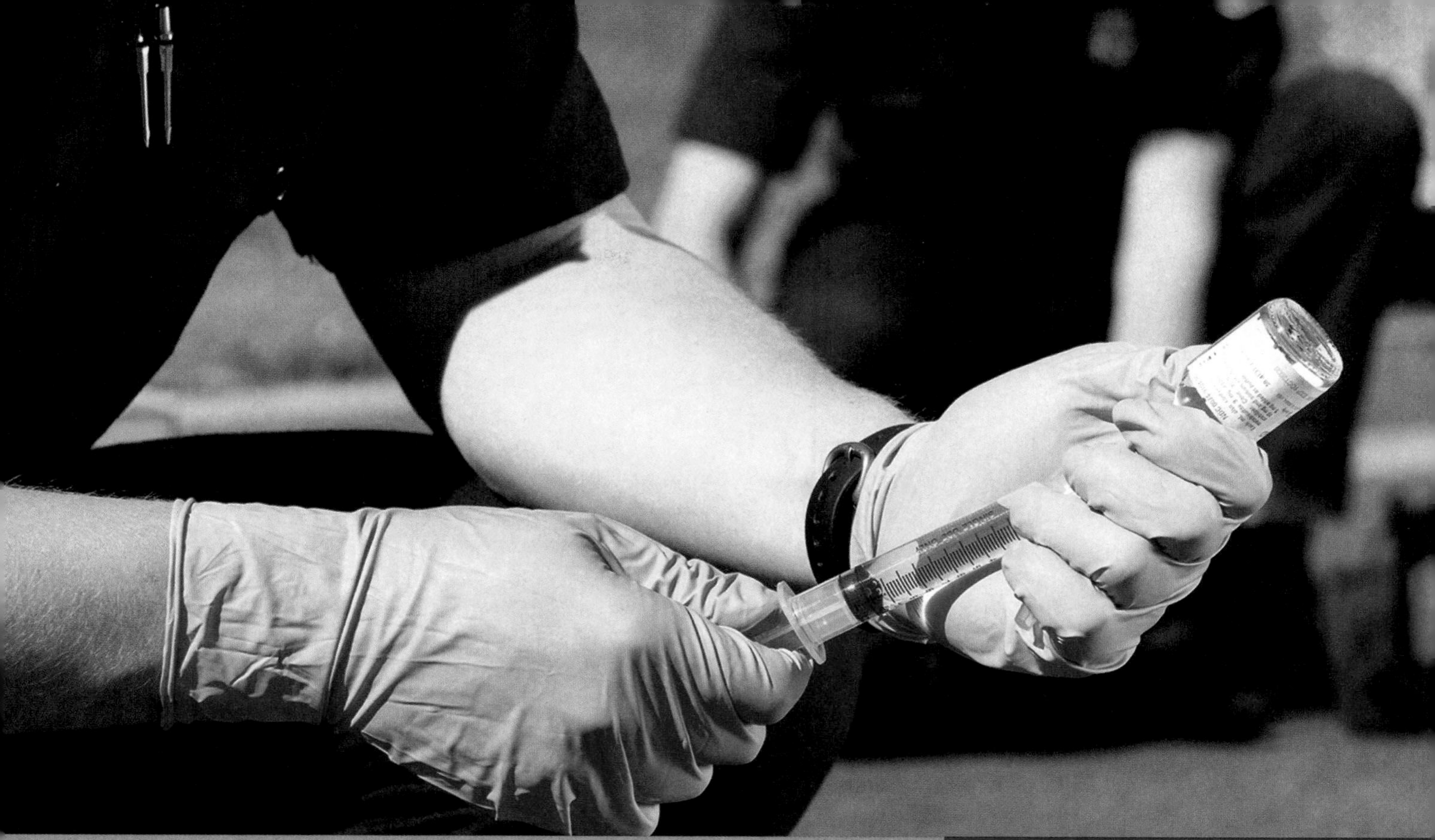

Pharmacology

VOLUME 1

SECTION

4

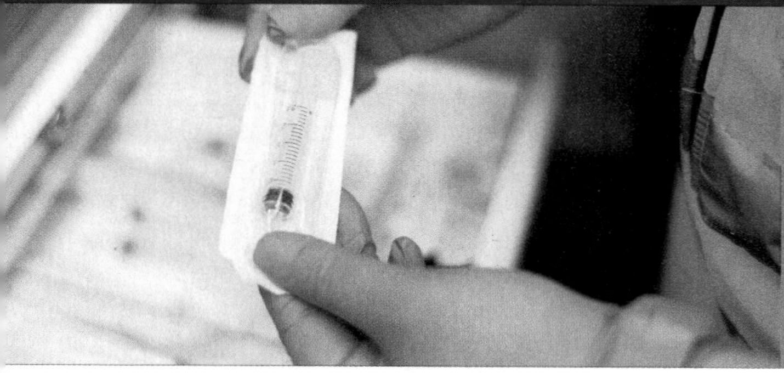

Chapter 13

Principles of Pharmacology

NATIONAL EMS EDUCATION STANDARD COMPETENCIES

Pharmacology

Integrates comprehensive knowledge of pharmacology to formulate a treatment plan intended to mitigate emergencies and improve the overall health of the patient.

Principles of Pharmacology

- Medication safety (pp 732–733)
- Medication legislation (pp 727–728)
- Naming (pp 729–730)
- Classifications (p 732)
- Schedules (pp 727–728)
- Pharmacokinetics (pp 745–747)
- Storage and security (pp 732–733)
- Autonomic pharmacology (p 761)
- Metabolism and excretion (pp 753–755)
- Mechanism of action (p 731)
- Phases of medication activity (pp 733–734)
- Medication response relationships (pp 741–745)
- Medication interactions (p 745)
- Toxicity (pp 745, 784)

Medication Administration

- Routes of administration (pp 747–752)
- Self-administer medication (see Chapter 14, *Medication Administration*)
- Peer-administer medication (see Chapter 14, *Medication Administration*)
- Assist/administer medications to a patient (see Chapter 14, *Medication Administration*)
- Within the scope of practice of the paramedic, administer medications to a patient (see Chapter 14, *Medication Administration*)

KNOWLEDGE OBJECTIVES

1. Explain how pharmacology relates to paramedic clinical practice. (p 726)
2. Describe the regulatory measures affecting medications administered in the prehospital setting. (pp 726–727)
3. Describe how drugs are classified. (pp 727–728)
4. Outline reliable sources of medication information available to paramedics. (pp 728–729)
5. List the components of a medication profile. (p 731)
6. Discuss requirements for medication storage, security, and accountability. (pp 732–733)
7. Describe the pharmacokinetic and pharmacodynamic properties of medications in general. (pp 733–734, 745–747)
8. Identify situations in which medication effects will be altered by the age, sex, weight, and other characteristics of a particular patient. (pp 737–741)
9. Identify steps to reduce the incidence of medication errors and limit the severity of harmful effects associated with medication administration. (pp 755–757)
10. Discuss the prevention, recognition, and management of adverse medication reactions. (pp 742–743)

11. Select the optimal medication and method of medication administration for patients with a particular clinical condition or situation. (pp 747–752)
12. Identify the various classes of medications that influence the sympathetic nervous system. (pp 757–761)
13. List notable classes of medications that may be taken by patients in the prehospital setting. (pp 762–765)
14. Explain the medications likely to be used by patients with respiratory conditions, including what each medication is used for. (pp 767–768)
15. Recognize the medications commonly prescribed to patients with cardiovascular diseases. (pp 768–770)

SKILLS OBJECTIVES

There are no skills objectives for this chapter.

Introduction

Medication administration is a defining element of paramedic clinical practice. When given appropriately, medications have the unique ability to correct or decrease the severity of an illness or injury, treat many life-threatening conditions, and substantially reduce patient discomfort. Conversely, if you administer the incorrect medication, use the incorrect route, select an inappropriate dose, or fail to follow the correct technique for administration, severe and often life-threatening consequences are possible in many situations. This chapter will assist you in minimizing the risks associated with medication administration while providing patients with a large variety of benefits available from pharmacologic interventions.

Throughout this chapter, the terms *medications* and *drugs* are used interchangeably. When commercial medications, illicit drugs, and other chemicals enter the human body, they may share common characteristics and produce similar clinical effects, despite entering the body under vastly different circumstances.

Words of Wisdom

The terms medication and drug are often used interchangeably but have differing meanings. A **medication** refers to a substance used to treat an illness or condition. A **drug**, generally speaking, is any substance that produces a physiologic effect, whether therapeutic or not; when used in a clinical sense, this term is understood to refer to a substance that produces a therapeutic effect when given in the appropriate circumstances and in the appropriate dose. Therefore, every medication is a drug, but not every drug is a medication.

Pharmacology is the scientific study of how various substances interact with or alter the function of living organisms. As a paramedic, you will use the science of pharmacology in various ways, such as when treating patients who already receive medications on an intermittent or long-term basis. You will also encounter patients who are experiencing adverse effects of medications taken at home, so it is crucial to obtain a medication history during the patient assessment. It is also essential to understand pharmacology when administering medications to treat patient symptoms during an EMS response or while treating a patient who has been exposed to a potentially toxic chemical, drug, or medication.

Historical Perspective on Medication Administration

For centuries, chemicals, primarily derived from plants or animals, have been used to cure disease or relieve symptoms. Early Chinese, Mesopotamian, and Egyptian societies used chemical remedies to treat everything from pain to baldness. Diseases were poorly understood, and natural remedies were directed toward relieving various symptoms rather than ending the disease process itself. Formal scientific study of the effects of medication on the body began to emerge during the late 17th century and into the 18th century. Today, the science of pharmacology has evolved into large-scale commercial pharmaceutical production—a highly profitable and tightly regulated industry. Many unique subspecialties, such as genetic manipulation and toxicology, continue to blur the line between pharmacology, medicine, and a variety of other scientific fields. Although the science of pharmacology has evolved into a sophisticated area of health care, certain medications discovered in ancient times are still in use.

The process of medication selection and administration is no longer random or anecdotal as it was in previous centuries. Evidence-based guidelines assist clinicians in using pharmacologic interventions across the spectrum of medical specialties. Medications now undergo extensive testing and numerous clinical trials before their widespread use is permitted. Yet despite the advanced science of pharmacology, adverse reactions to medications remain commonplace.

Medication and Drug Regulation

The United States has implemented a comprehensive system of medication and drug regulation. The first significant regulation was enacted in 1906, with the passage of the Pure Food and Drug Act. As its name implies, this act prohibited altering or mislabeling medications. In 1909, the importing of opium was prohibited under the Opium Exclusion Act. The Harrison Narcotics Act, which restricted the use of various opiates and cocaine, became law in 1914.

Under the Food, Drug, and Cosmetic Act (1938), the US Food and Drug Administration (FDA) was given authority to enforce rules requiring that new drugs be safe and pure. The FDA remains the federal agency responsible for approving new medications and removing unsafe medications from the market. Approval of a new medication typically takes several years, and only a small fraction of medications submitted to the FDA ultimately receive marketing approval. Occasionally, breakthrough medications for life-threatening conditions may receive preferential expedited consideration or emergency approvals (eg, the COVID-19 vaccines). Notably, many medications, once approved and available commercially, are used "off-label"—that is, for a purpose not approved by the FDA, at doses different from the recommended doses, or by a route of administration not approved by the FDA. Off-label use is widespread in health care, but a physician medical director or paramedic may have an increased risk of liability for ill-advised off-label use of a medication that results in a bad outcome for a patient. Medications should be administered off-label only when they are specifically approved for this use by the service's medical director or by agency/regional protocol. The use of intravenous (IV) tranexamic acid in patients who have experienced trauma, discussed later in this chapter, is an example of off-label medication use in EMS.

As an EMS provider, you must be familiar with the rules and regulations implemented under the Controlled Substances Act (also known as the Comprehensive Drug Abuse Prevention and Control Act) of 1970. This act classifies certain medications with the potential of abuse into five categories (schedules), with corresponding security, dispensing, and record-keeping requirements **TABLE 13-1**. The US Drug Enforcement Agency is responsible for enforcing this act.

Schedule I medications may not be prescribed, dispensed, used, or administered for medical use. Marijuana, which is sometimes prescribed for medical purposes, remains a controversial Schedule I controlled substance. Various states permit prescription marijuana for specific medical conditions, and some allow both medical and recreational use.

Paramedics are likely to carry and administer Schedule II medications such as fentanyl

YOU are the Paramedic

PART 1

The communications center dispatches you and your partner to a skilled nursing facility for an 88-year-old woman reported to have altered mental status. Additional dispatch information advises that the patient has a pulse and is breathing, but has a decreased level of consciousness.

1. What medical conditions would you expect to encounter in a skilled nursing facility or long-term care facility?

TABLE 13-1 Classification of Medications Considered Controlled Substances

Schedule	Description	Examples
I	High abuse potential; no recognized medical purpose	Heroin, marijuana (cannabis), LSD, peyote
II	High abuse potential; legitimate medical purpose	• Opioids: codeine, fentanyl (Sublimaze), hydrocodone, hydromorphone (Dilaudid), morphine • Stimulants: amphetamine (Adderall), cocaine, methylphenidate (Ritalin)
III	Lower potential for abuse than Schedule II medications	• Opioids: acetaminophen with codeine (Tylenol with codeine #3) • Nonopioids: anabolic steroids, ketamine
IV	Lower potential for abuse than Schedule III drugs	Alprazolam (Xanax), diazepam (Valium), lorazepam (Ativan)
V	Lower potential for abuse than Schedule IV drugs	Opioid cough medicines

Abbreviation: LSD, lysergic acid diethylamide

(Sublimaze) and morphine sulfate, and Schedule IV medications such as midazolam (Versed), diazepam (Valium), and lorazepam (Ativan). All Schedule II through V medications require locked storage, detailed record keeping, and controlled wasting procedures. State EMS, pharmacy, or law enforcement agencies may impose additional requirements for the security and accountability of these controlled substances.

Words of Wisdom

Maintaining careful accountability of controlled substances can protect both the paramedic and the EMS organization. Failure to adequately control and waste controlled substances may jeopardize your job, your reputation, and your professional certification or licensure.

Sources of Medication

Medications can be derived or manufactured from a variety of sources. Ancient societies used medications isolated from the roots, leaves, seeds, fruit, flowers, or bark of certain plants. Animals, particularly animal endocrine systems, are used as the source of other medications. Minerals represent yet another source of many medications used for a wide variety of clinical conditions. Microorganisms such as bacteria, fungi, and mold also are used for the manufacture of medication. **TABLE 13-2** lists sources of many common medications.

TABLE 13-2 Sources of Medications

Source	Examples
Plant	Atropine, aspirin, digoxin, morphine
Animal	Heparin, antivenom, thyroid preparations, insulin
Microorganism	Streptokinase, numerous antibiotics, dextran
Mineral	Iron, magnesium sulfate, lithium, phosphorus, calcium

Many other medications are either synthetic (made entirely in a laboratory setting) or semisynthetic (made from chemicals derived from plant, animal, or mineral sources that have been chemically modified in a laboratory setting). Genetic engineering is also used to manufacture certain medications that cannot otherwise be obtained from natural sources.

Pharmaceutical companies tightly control the concentration, purity, preservatives, and other ingredients present in medications during the manufacturing process. The *United States Pharmacopeia–National Formulary* ([USP-NF] discussed later) is an excellent source of information regarding the manufacturing details of a particular medication. On the packaging of each medication, you will notice a manufacturing lot number and expiration date.

Forms of Medication

You will manage and administer medications in various forms. The vast majority of medications administered in EMS practice are sterile injectable solutions. These solutions require careful handling and aseptic technique during administration to avoid contamination with microorganisms or other harmful substances. These solutions are supplied in larger IV bags, vials, and ampules, and occasionally in glass bottles (eg, nitroglycerin and ethanol). Other forms of medication are outlined in **TABLE 13-3**.

Medication Management for Paramedics

Medication Names

Every medication in the United States is given three distinct names: a chemical name, a generic or nonproprietary name, and a brand or proprietary name. During their initial development, medications are given a chemical name, which is often long and difficult to pronounce and may contain specific letters or numbers that indicate the medication's chemical composition. The chemical name is rarely used in clinical practice. Sodium bicarbonate, potassium chloride, and some other medications are among the few exceptions in which the chemical name is used in clinical practice. Most medication reference sources used by paramedics do not publish the chemical name or structure of a medication.

Every medication also receives a nonproprietary, or generic, name. The manufacturer proposes

TABLE 13-3 Forms of Medication

Form	Description	Examples
Capsule	Powdered or solid medication enclosed in a dissolvable cylindrical gelatin shell	Acetaminophen (Tylenol), ibuprofen (Motrin), diphenhydramine (Benadryl)
Tablet	Solid medication particles bound into a shape designed to dissolve or be swallowed	Aspirin (ASA), nitroglycerin SL
Powder	Small particles of medication designed to be dissolved or mixed into a solution or liquid	Glucagon, vecuronium (Norcuron)
Droplet	Sterile solution or nonsterile liquid intended for direct administration into the nose or ear	Phenylephrine (Neo-Synephrine, Afrin), tetracaine, naloxone (Narcan)
Parenteral solution	Sterile solution for direct injection into a body cavity, tissue, or organ	Fentanyl (Sublimaze), epinephrine
Skin preparation	Gel, ointment, or paste substance designed to permit transdermal (through the skin) absorption	Nitroglycerin paste, fentanyl (Sublimaze) patch
Suppository	Medication in a wax like material that dissolves in the rectum or other body cavity	Promethazine (Phenergan), acetaminophen (Tylenol)
Liquid	Medication dissolved or suspended in liquid intended for oral consumption	Infant acetaminophen (Tylenol), cough syrup
Inhaler/spray	Medication in gas or fine mist form intended for inhalation and absorption through the lung, airway, or oral tissues	Albuterol (Ventolin), nitroglycerin spray

Abbreviations: ASA, acetylsalicylic acid; SL, sublingual

the generic name, which must be approved by the US Adopted Names Council and the World Health Organization. The generic name is regulated internationally to promote consistency and avoid duplication in drug names. Generic names typically include a "stem" that links them to other medications in the same **drug class** (the grouping to which a medication belongs). Often the stem is found at the end of the name, but it may also appear at the beginning or within the drug name. For example, many benzodiazepine medications, such as midazolam, diazepam, and lorazepam, have the stem "am." The stem "pril" signifies that a medication is a member of the angiotensin-converting enzyme (ACE) inhibitor medication class, such as enalapril (Vasotec), captopril (Capoten), and lisinopril (Prinivil, Zestril). Several other examples of stems exist. In addition to knowing that stems provide information about the class of drugs, you need to know the specific names of and indications for all drugs that you administer.

SAFETY

Do not rely solely on the stem when attempting to determine the medication class to which a drug belongs, because different classes might have the same stem. The names for tricyclic antidepressants, such as amitriptyline (Elavil) and desipramine (Norpramin), have the same stem as the names for some selective serotonin reuptake inhibitors (SSRIs), such as fluoxetine (Prozac) and paroxetine (Paxil). An overdose of a tricyclic antidepressant is often life threatening, whereas an overdose of an SSRI does not typically pose the same risk.

The final type of medication name is the brand name, which is chosen by the manufacturer and approved by the FDA. The brand name does not have the same functional requirements as the generic name, but it must meet certain minimum criteria set by the FDA. Brand names are often selected for marketing purposes. Creative examples are sometimes linked to a particular condition. Metoprolol, a beta adrenergic blocking agent, has the brand name Lopressor, which may be a subtle reference to lowering pressure (of the blood). Oseltamivir has the brand name Tami*flu* and is used to treat in*flu*enza.

The three distinct types of medication names can be illustrated with an example. The following medication is commonly administered by paramedics:

Chemical name: 4-chloro-*N*-furfuryl-5-sulfamoylanthranilic acid
Generic name: furosemide
Brand name: Lasix

Many reference sources now use "tall man" lettering to print the names of certain medications. This approach is intended to avoid confusion of medications with similarly spelled names. The capitalized letters highlight a portion of the name in medications with similar names. Examples include DOBUTamine and DOPamine, and diphenhydrAMINE and dimenhyDRINATE.

SAFETY

Many medication names look and sound the same. Minimize the risk of medication errors by double-checking the medication container label every time you are preparing to administer a medication. Concentrations and packaging may change unexpectedly.

Medication Reference Sources

A vast array of medication reference sources are available to assist you in clinical practice. When selecting a reference source to use or purchase, consider a variety of factors, including the reliability of the reference source; whether the source is printed, electronic, or both; the depth of information needed or provided; accessibility; cost; availability of updates; and size of materials used (if a printed product).

Medication information is typically compiled in a format called a **medication monograph** or medication profile. The details may vary dramatically between reference sources, but the basic structure remains consistent. **TABLE 13-4** highlights common components of medication profiles.

The *USP-NF* and the *Prescriber's Digital Reference* (*PDR*, formerly called the *Physicians' Desk Reference*) provide a wealth of reliable, detailed information about thousands of medications. The information includes graphic diagrams of the

TABLE 13-4 Components of Medication Profiles

Component	Description
Medication names	Sources typically include both the brand name and the generic name. Print sources often alphabetize entries by generic name. Electronic sources can typically be searched by either brand name or generic name.
Category or class of medication	The grouping to which a medication belongs. Medications are grouped according to their characteristics, traits, or primary components.
Use/**indication**	A sign, symptom, or condition that would potentially benefit from a particular medication; the reason for giving a medication.
Mechanism of action (pharmacodynamics)	The way in which a medication produces the intended response.
Pregnancy risk factor	A scale indicating the likelihood of potential harm to the fetus if the medication is administered to a pregnant patient.
Contraindications	Any condition, but especially a disease, that is known to render some particular line of treatment improper or undesirable.
Available forms (how supplied)	The manner in which the manufacturer packages the medication for distribution and sale. Typical methods of packaging are prefilled syringes, vials, or ampules.
Dosage (often differentiated based on age or indication)	The typical or average volume or dose of medication that is to be administered to the patient and the route by which the medication should be introduced to the patient.
Administration and monitoring considerations	Any additional information needed to safely administer the medication and any important parameters that should be observed following administration.
Potential incompatibilities	Problems that may occur when two or more medications are administered together, which could be at the same time, in the same solution, or through the same intravenous tubing or delivery device (nebulizer, syringe, etc).
Adverse effects	Any abnormal or harmful effects caused by exposure to a chemical. An effect may be classified as adverse if it causes functional or anatomic damage, causes irreversible change in the person's homeostasis, or increases the person's susceptibility to other chemical or biologic stress.
Pharmacokinetics	The medication's effects on the body, as described by the following terms: **Onset**. The estimated amount of time it will take for the medication to enter the body/system and begin to take effect. **Peak**. The estimated amount of time it will take for the medication to have its greatest effect on the patient/system. **Duration (of action)**. The estimated amount of time that the medication will have any effect on the patient/system.

Special Populations

Pediatric and older patients often have slower medication absorption and elimination times, necessitating modification of the doses of many drugs administered to these patients. Pregnant patients are limited in terms of the medications they can take because of the potential risk to the fetus.

chemical structure and other specific chemical properties of the medications. Electronic versions of these resources, such as those available through smartphone apps, have improved their accessibility in the field. The earlier printed forms were impractical to use in prehospital settings because of their size and amount of information. Despite the improved form factor, many of the details in these sources are not needed in prehospital settings, making it difficult for paramedics to locate needed information rapidly. The electronic versions of the *USP-NF* and *PDR* may be helpful to EMS educators and administrators developing agency-specific medication protocols or creating training materials.

Manufacturers provide written materials with every package of medication distributed. These "package inserts" are written by the manufacturers and approved by the FDA. Such package inserts include information on **dosing**, route of administration, contraindications, adverse effects, and various other characteristics of a particular medication.

Hospital pharmacies often compile medication information into formularies that are specific to the information needs of the specific hospital. The hospital formulary typically includes much of the same information that is included in the medication package insert, *USP-NF*, or *PDR*, but it is tailored to the needs of prescribers in the hospital. Paramedics in hospital-based or hospital-affiliated EMS systems may have access to the hospital formulary.

You have many other choices for commercially published medication information references. Some resources are specifically geared toward prehospital or critical care transport providers, emphasizing medication selection, dosing, and administration for patient conditions encountered in these settings. Other references focus exclusively on IV medications or emphasize only information needed during hands-on patient care. As mentioned, advancements in portable electronic devices and smartphones mean that many medication references are now accessible electronically, making an entire library of information available within the limited confines of the emergency vehicle. State EMS agencies and individual fire and EMS organizations frequently develop specific protocols or medication formularies, which compile information on approved medications given by paramedics in a particular setting.

Words of Wisdom

Find a pocket-size medication reference source (print or electronic, such as a smartphone app) that works well for you, and always keep it, along with a copy of your regional protocols, with you while on duty.

AHA Classification of Recommendations and Level of Evidence

In most EMS settings, you will follow guidelines established and distributed by the American Heart Association (AHA). These guidelines may be referenced directly, or they may be incorporated into more extensive department or agency policies or protocols. The medications and interventions listed within the AHA guidelines have varying degrees of support from reliable scientific evidence. Chapter 1, *EMS Systems*, discusses the distinction and relationship between a *class* and a *level of evidence*. You can generally infer the level of evidence by the assigned class for a proposed intervention. To provide greater clarity to health care providers regarding the level of evidence, the AHA uses the following system to describe the relative importance of certain medications or interventions[1]:

- *Class I* indicates that strong evidence supports the use of the procedure/medication, the benefit is greater than the risk, and the intervention should be performed or administered.
- *Class IIa* indicates moderate evidence that the benefit is greater than the risk, the intervention is reasonable, and the intervention may be useful.
- *Class IIb* indicates weak evidence that the benefit is greater than the risk; the intervention may be considered.
- *Class III no benefit* indicates the evidence is weak, the benefit equals the risk, and the intervention should not be performed/administered.
- *Class III harm* indicates there is strong evidence that the risk is greater than the benefit, and the intervention should not be performed/administered.

Medication Storage

Medication storage is an essential consideration for paramedics. The uncontrolled prehospital environment is a difficult place to maintain the safety and integrity of medication packages. Medications must be kept in a location that provides adequate protection for medication supplies, yet is convenient enough to allow quick access in emergency situations.

A fundamental concern regarding medication storage is the integrity of the medication container. Medication should be stored in a manner that prevents physical damage to the medication vial, ampule, solution, or tablets. It is often necessary to remove most of the packaging provided by the manufacturer, leaving only the medication container in the vehicle or response bag. Because drug boxes or bags may be dropped accidentally during a call, medication containers should be placed in protective bins or surrounded by enough padding to prevent damage to them during a response or while performing patient care at the scene. Organize medication containers in a manner that facilitates quick, accurate identification of the medication during emergency situations. The needs of individual EMS organizations dictate the type and quantity of medications that are available on a particular response vehicle or in a provider's bag. Carrying excessive medication quantities may make storage difficult or cause unnecessary waste due to expiration. Conversely, having insufficient quantities on hand may undermine patient care or necessitate frequent restocking.

State EMS regulations require that EMS agencies have policies in place that define appropriate storage, maintenance, and replacement of medications and IV fluids. Direct sunlight, extremes of heat and cold, and physical damage to medication containers can hasten the degradation of many medications, making them ineffective or unsafe for use.[2–4] Many EMS agencies use medication heaters, coolers, or refrigerators in their emergency vehicles to control the temperatures at which medications are stored and ensure the safety and integrity of the medications they carry.

Words of Wisdom

Take steps to ensure medications are stored at the proper temperature. Paramedics working in locations subject to extreme temperatures may be administering medications that have reduced effectiveness due to the environment in which they are stored.[5]

Medication Security

Controlled substances (as described in Table 13-1) require additional security, record keeping, and disposal precautions. These medications must be kept in locked storage cabinets or continuously held by an on-duty EMS provider responsible for administration. Disposal of partially used or damaged medication containers requires verification by a witness or return of the damaged or unused portion to the department responsible for dispensing the medication. EMS agencies and individual paramedics are jointly responsible for adhering to all federal, state, and local regulations regarding the security and accountability of controlled substances. These regulations vary slightly from region to region. In general, every last milliliter or milligram of a controlled substance needs to be documented—from ordering, to receipt by the EMS agency, to administration by the EMS provider (or discard as waste). The particular forms and procedures may vary from place to place, but the standard for accountability remains constant.

Controlled substances are often the target of tampering or diversion. Inspect medication vials, ampules, and the like for subtle signs of tampering, which may be as small as a pinhole. Suspect tampering in situations in which appropriate doses of analgesic or sedative medications seem ineffective, especially when patient tolerance is unlikely.

The Physiology of Pharmacology

The purpose of medications is to produce a desired effect in the body, usually in response to a particular illness, injury, or medical condition, but occasionally to prevent a specific harmful situation. As a medication is administered, it begins to alter a function or process within the body. This action is known as **pharmacodynamics**.

Any medication capable of beneficial clinical effects can cause toxic effects when given at an excessive dose. Toxic effects may also occur if a medication is given by an incorrect route or when a delivery device, such as an IV catheter or intraosseous (IO) needle, malfunctions. In other cases, medications may become ineffective when given at an inadequate dose or through the incorrect route. Even in the absence of error, many factors related to the patient, the patient's condition, and the particular medication may cause toxicity or adverse effects.

The human body simultaneously begins the process of **absorption**, **distribution**, possibly **biotransformation**, and, ultimately, **elimination** of a medication or chemical following administration. The body's action on a medication is known as **pharmacokinetics**. You must always consider the principles of pharmacodynamics and pharmacokinetics when deciding whether to administer a particular medication.

Principles of Pharmacodynamics

Research has demonstrated the presence of **receptor** sites in proteins connected to cells throughout the body. Various receptors are activated by **endogenous** chemicals, those occurring naturally within the body, and by the presence of medications and chemicals absorbed into the body. Activation of these receptors produces a specific response by individual cells, tissues, organs, and, ultimately, body systems. When a medication binds with a receptor site, one of four possible actions will occur:

1. Channels permitting the passage of ions (charged particles) in cell walls are opened or closed.
2. A biochemical messenger becomes activated, initiating other chemical reactions within the cell.
3. A normal cell function is prevented.
4. A normal or abnormal function of the cell begins.

For purposes of this chapter, **exogenous** (from outside the body) chemicals will be referred to as medications, even though exposure to chemicals in the environment can cause effects similar to those of medications, including adverse effects. Clandestine methamphetamine laboratories are an excellent example of environmental exposure to a chemical. Law enforcement officers and other emergency responders may experience accidental inhalation or dermal exposure to methamphetamines during an emergency response and demonstrate clinical effects identical to those of people who intentionally abuse these substances. In another example, toddlers who accidentally ingest certain mouse poisons will exhibit clinical effects identical to those experienced following the therapeutic administration of warfarin (Coumadin). The exposure is different from normal therapeutic administration in each of these instances, yet the clinical effects are identical.

Later sections of this chapter will discuss specific medications and chemicals used by paramedics and introduce the properties of various classes of medications pertinent to prehospital care. Chapter 28, *Toxicology*, discusses the adverse properties of commonly abused drugs. Functionally, the distinction between the terms *therapeutic medications*, *exogenous chemicals*, and *illicit drugs* is largely irrelevant. These terms reflect substances that follow similar (and often predictable) patterns when interacting with the body.

Medications are developed to reach and bind with particular receptor sites of target cells. Newer medications are designed to target only specific receptor sites on certain cells to minimize their adverse effects. In contrast, many older medications, including those used by paramedics, affect cells and tissues unrelated to the condition being treated, causing adverse effects throughout the body.

Two types of medications or chemicals directly affect cellular activity by binding with receptor sites on individual cells. **Agonist medications** initiate or alter a cellular activity by attaching to receptor sites, prompting a cell response. **Antagonist medications** prevent endogenous or exogenous agonist chemicals from reaching cell receptor sites and initiating or altering a particular cellular activity **FIGURE 13-1**. Specific notable agonist-antagonist pairs are discussed at various points later in this chapter. For example, opioids such as morphine sulfate and fentanyl are agonist chemicals that cause **analgesia** and respiratory depression. The effects of these chemicals can be reversed by the opioid antagonist naloxone (Narcan).

Agonist Medications

The dose of a particular medication, the route of administration, and many other factors determine the concentration of a medication present at target cell receptor sites. **Affinity** is the ability of a medication to bind with a particular receptor site. Together, medication concentration and affinity determine the number of receptor sites bound by that medication. As noted earlier, agonist medications bind with receptor sites, initiating or altering an action by the cell.

A certain minimum concentration of the agonist medication must be present for cellular activity to be initiated or altered. As the concentration of the medication increases and crosses the **threshold level**, initiation or alteration of cellular activity begins. Increasing concentrations of medication

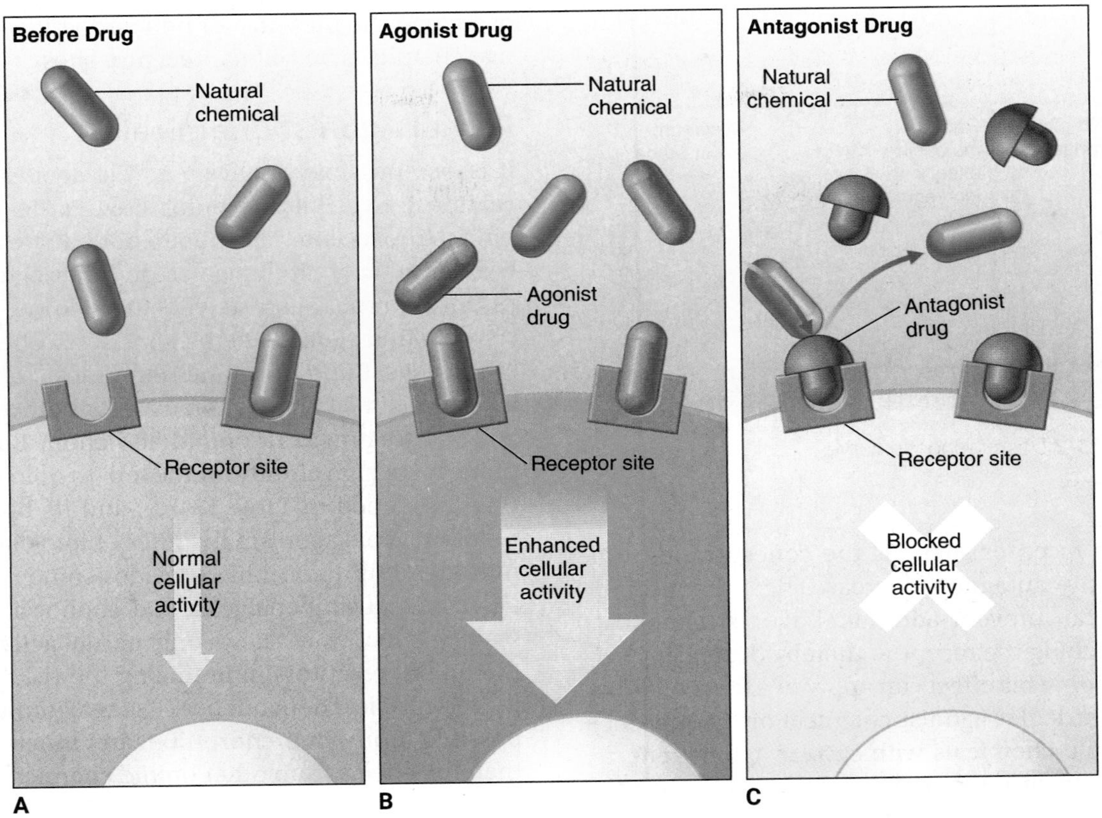

FIGURE 13-1 A. Normally, natural chemicals bind to receptor sites to cause actions. **B.** When an agonist drug is present, it binds to the receptor site and enhances cellular activity. **C.** When an antagonist drug is present, it binds to the receptor site and blocks cellular activity.

cause increased effects until all receptor sites become occupied or the maximum capability of the cell is reached. The concentration of the medication required to initiate a cellular response is known as the medication's **potency**. As the potency of a medication increases, the concentration or dose required for a particular cellular response decreases. Conversely, a higher concentration is required when the potency of a medication is low. The ability to initiate or alter cell activity in a therapeutic or desired manner is referred to as **efficacy**. Once all the cellular receptor sites become bound with the agonist medication, cellular activity plateaus and no increase or further change in activity is possible. At this point, the effect of the medication has peaked, and additional doses or higher concentrations of the medication will not cause additional cellular action. The **dose-response curve** illustrates the relationship between medication dose (or concentration) and efficacy. The relative potency of two different medications causing the same effect can be demonstrated by comparing their dose-response curves. The threshold dose is lower for medications with a higher potency **FIGURE 13-2**.

Antagonist Medications

As mentioned earlier, antagonist medications bind with receptor sites to prevent a cellular response to agonist chemicals. Antagonists may be used to inhibit normal cellular activation by naturally occurring agonist chemicals within the body. Antagonist medications may also be used to treat the harmful agonist effects of exogenous medications or chemicals, possibly following an overdose or a toxic exposure.

Antagonists may be competitive or noncompetitive. **Competitive antagonists** temporarily bind with cellular receptor sites, displacing agonist chemicals. The efficacy of a competitive antagonist medication is directly related to its concentration

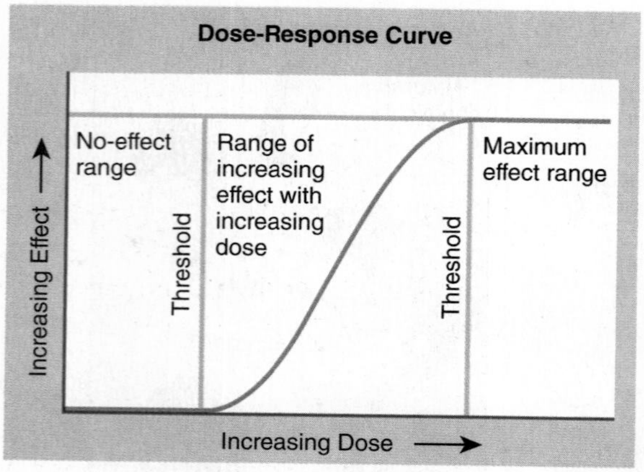

FIGURE 13-2 Dose-response curve.

near the receptor sites. As the concentration of a competitive antagonist increases near the receptor sites, it can prevent additional agonist chemicals from reaching the receptor, thereby decreasing cellular action. This effect can apply to a large quantity of one particular agonist chemical or the presence of multiple chemicals with similar agonist effects. As the concentration of the competitive antagonist decreases (due to elimination of the drug or substance, such as through the kidneys) or when the concentration of agonist chemicals increases, more agonist chemicals can bind with receptor sites and continue or resume cellular activation.

The efficacy of a competitive antagonist medication is also related to the strength of its affinity (ability to bind at a receptor site) compared with the affinity of the agonist chemicals present. Competitive antagonist medications with a lower affinity require a higher concentration to be effective.

Noncompetitive antagonists permanently bind with receptor sites and prevent activation by agonist chemicals. Effects of noncompetitive antagonist medications continue until new receptor sites or new cells are created, which may be a long time after the last dose of antagonist medication was given. Ketamine (discussed later) is a noncompetitive antagonist of the agonist glutamate on *N*-methyl-D-aspartate receptors in the central nervous system (CNS). Effects of ketamine last for only 10 to 15 minutes. Aspirin (also discussed later) is a noncompetitive antagonist that binds to the enzyme cyclooxygenase, causing antiplatelet effects that last up to 10 days when platelets are regenerated. Even increased doses of agonist chemicals will not overcome the presence of noncompetitive antagonist chemicals on cellular receptor sites.

Partial Agonist Chemicals

It is also possible to have a **partial agonist** chemical attach to cellular receptor sites. Partial agonists bind to the receptor site but do not initiate as much cellular activity or change as do other agonists. In essence, partial agonists effectively lower the efficacy of other agonist chemicals that may be present at the cells. Buprenorphine (Buprenex, Subutex) is a partial agonist medication used for both analgesia and the treatment of opioid addiction. Buprenorphine has a high affinity for the mu (μ) opioid receptors (described in Table 13-10), and its binding to them prevents agonism by other opioid chemicals. Although buprenorphine provides some degree of agonism, causing analgesia and euphoria, it has a "ceiling effect" that allows only partial activation of the opioid receptors, minimizing the risk of toxicity and physical dependence. The maximum effects possible from buprenorphine are much weaker than the effects from other opioid chemicals.

Alternative Mechanisms of Drug Action

Some medications can alter cell, tissue, organ, and system function in the body without directly interacting with receptors on individual cells. For example, medications may be engineered to target other sites throughout the body, including microorganisms, lipids, water, and exogenous toxic substances. **Antimicrobials**, such as **antibiotics** and **antifungals**, may be designed to target specific substances present in the cell walls of a particular bacterium or fungus. Other medications, known as **chelating agents**, bind with heavy metals such as lead, mercury, and arsenic in the body and create a compound that can be eliminated. Sodium bicarbonate (discussed in detail later in this chapter), a medication used for a wide variety of medical conditions, breaks down after administration, producing bicarbonate ions. Bicarbonate ions can bind with excess hydrogen ions, raising the pH and decreasing the acidity of various body fluids.

Mannitol (Osmitrol) is a **diuretic** medication, designed to distribute into water in the body, creating **osmotic** changes that alter the distribution of fluids and electrolytes. The resulting diuretic effect draws excess water from certain body tissues, including the brain and eyes, while enhancing urine excretion. Plasma expanders and bulk laxatives target water in the body and alter the distribution of various body fluids.

Electrolyte-based medications such as magnesium, potassium, and calcium change the concentration and distribution of ions in cells and fluids throughout the body, affecting many cell activities. An alteration in the concentration of certain electrolytes at the cellular level affects the ability of various cells to function. Alterations of cell function occur without chemicals directly binding to cell receptor sites.

Factors Affecting Response to Medications

Several factors determine how a particular medication will affect a patient. These factors may influence the choice of medication, dose, route, timing, manner of administration, and monitoring necessary after a patient receives a medication. Even weight-based medication dosing, which is common in the prehospital setting, produces profound differences in how a medication affects an individual patient because of the factors described in the following sections.

Age

The distribution, metabolism, and elimination of medications continue to change throughout the human life span. Therefore, the responses of older adult and pediatric patients to various medications can be much different from the responses seen in adolescents and adults. You may encounter unusual situations that require you to consult with online medical control to adjust the dose of medication for infants, children, and older patients to obtain the desired response.

Medications become distributed into three primary types of body substances (water, lipids or fat, and protein) following administration. The percentage of body fat is lowest in preterm infants, increases significantly in toddlers, decreases through adolescence, and increases in adults, including older adults. The percentage of body water is highest in newborns and steadily decreases throughout the life span. The percentage of body protein varies throughout the life span, generally peaking in preteens, adolescents, and adults. Infants and older adults have the lowest percentage of body protein. If a medication is **water-soluble**, higher weight-based doses must be administered to infants (who have a higher percentage of body water) than to adults and older adults. Fat- and lipid-soluble medications require higher weight-based doses in older adults because of their higher body fat percentage and increased fat distribution.

When treating pediatric or older patients with altered percentages of body water, fat or lipids, and protein, consider performing careful titration of the medication selected rather than simply administering a weight-based bolus. Water-soluble and lipid-soluble medications may require increased initial doses to overcome the dilution that inevitably occurs with their widespread distribution in the body. Older adult patients, for example, generally have a lower percentage of body water. Therefore, water-soluble medications, such as digoxin, will have higher serum levels in older patients than in other patients who weigh the same and are given the same dose. Older adults have less body water for the digoxin to spread into, which leads to a higher concentration of this medication in the body water that is present, particularly in the blood (serum). Older adult patients also generally have a higher percentage of body fat. Lipid-soluble medications such as diazepam initially produce much lower serum levels for a given dose, but they take much longer for the body to eliminate, dramatically prolonging their effects. Without careful monitoring, it can be easy to exceed therapeutic serum levels when administering repeated doses, causing adverse or toxic effects that may persist for hours to days. Information on the solubility of a medication is typically included in its reference materials.

Alteration of metabolism and elimination in pediatric and older patients may prolong the effects of medications or result in higher medication concentrations in various tissues. Medication metabolism in the liver is affected by the **cytochrome P-450 system** (discussed later in this chapter). This system works differently on different types of medications, is extremely variable in infants and children, and shows a functional decline in older adults. Hepatic metabolism is also generally impaired in older adults due to decreases in blood flow to the liver. A decline in liver or kidney function, due to aging or another cause, requires a decrease in the dosage of many medications because their elimination from the body will be impaired.

Patients at extremes of age are disproportionately susceptible to **paradoxical** medication reactions—that is, clinical effects opposite to the intended effects of the medication. For example, sedative medications can produce profound excitement or agitation rather than sedation. Barbiturates can cause unexpected excitement or agitation in older patients. Promethazine (Phenergan), diphenhydramine (Benadryl), chloral hydrate, and various benzodiazepines, such as midazolam, can cause paradoxical excitement or agitation in children. Paradoxical reactions frequently complicate an already delicate clinical situation when patients who need sedation become even more excited, agitated, or combative.

Weight

Many medications used in prehospital care and critical care transport are administered using weight-based dosing. To calculate the recommended dose for the individual patient, a quantity of medication (usually grams, milligrams, micrograms, or milliliters) is multiplied by the patient's weight in kilograms. This method of medication dosing has both advantages and limitations. The major advantage of this method is that the amount of medication administered is proportional to the patient's size. Medication manufacturers and clinicians have already calculated factors affecting absorption, distribution, metabolism, rates of elimination, and desired quantity present at target cells or tissues when giving a particular medication at a weight-based dose. You can use the weight-based formula to determine the appropriate medication dose for patients ranging from preterm neonates to large adults.

Limitations associated with this method include the fact that the patient's weight in kilograms is needed to calculate a weight-based medication dose. A patient's weight must be estimated in emergency situations and, often, converted from pounds to kilograms. Even in controlled settings, health care providers might have difficulty accurately estimating patient weights. One study revealed that a significant portion of health care providers' estimates of patient weight were off by more than 10% to 15%.[6] Patients generally estimate their own weight more accurately than do health care providers. An inaccurate estimate of a patient's weight, depending on the degree of error, could result in administration of an incorrect dose of medication.

Another limitation with weight-based dosing is the risk that multiplication of numbers in the formula during a stressful situation or at an uncontrolled scene may lead to dosing errors. Using a calculator or a preprinted medication dose chart when administering weight-based medications can help reduce these kinds of errors.

Special Populations

Before administering any medication to a pediatric patient, ask the parents whether the child has had a previous reaction, such as a paradoxical reaction.

The weight-based method of dose calculation also does not consider the various alterations in distribution, metabolism, and elimination discussed earlier. Standard data regarding the percentages of body water, fat, and protein at various ages become less reliable as obesity and malnutrition affect patients. Weight-based medication doses can be calculated by using the patient's actual body weight or ideal body weight. For example, lidocaine, an antidysrhythmic medication, is administered based on a patient's actual body weight. In contrast, the cardiac medication digoxin is given based on a patient's ideal body weight. Unfortunately, many reference sources do not provide guidance about whether the patient's actual or ideal body weight should be used for medication dose calculations. The formulas for ideal body weight in adults are as follows:

For men: Ideal weight (kg) = 50 + (2.3 times patient's height in inches over 5 feet)

For women: Ideal weight (kg) = 45.5 + (2.3 times patient's height in inches over 5 feet)

For example, the ideal weight for a 6-foot-tall man is 77.6 kg [50 + (2.3 × 12)], and the ideal weight for a 5-foot, 5-inch woman is 57 kg [45.5 + (2.3 × 5)].

Environment

Both hyperthermia and hypothermia can affect medication absorption, metabolism, and efficacy. Fever causes tachycardia that may increase hepatic blood flow, theoretically increasing the initial metabolism of drugs in the liver and reducing the amount of drug returned to circulation by the liver. Fever also suppresses the function of the cytochrome P-450 system in the liver, which ultimately decreases the rate of metabolism of certain classes of medications. In consequence, individual patient responses may vary from the expected response.

Hypothermia is known to impair the effectiveness of medications used in traditional advanced cardiac life support (ACLS). The 2020 AHA ACLS guidelines state that it may be reasonable to consider the administration of epinephrine during cardiac arrest caused by accidental hypothermia per the standard ACLS algorithm concurrent with rewarming strategies.[7]

Genetic Factors

Be extremely careful when deciding whether to administer medications to patients with specific genetic disorders. Primary pulmonary hypertension, sickle cell disease, and glucose-6-phosphate dehydrogenase deficiency are some notable conditions that require special consideration, and their presence in a patient may rule out the use of certain medications frequently administered by paramedics. Patients with primary pulmonary hypertension may experience acute decompensation when they receive vasopressor medications. Salicylate medications such as aspirin (acetylsalicylic acid) may precipitate **hemolysis** (destruction of red blood cells [RBCs] by disruption of the cell membrane) in patients with glucose-6-phosphate dehydrogenase deficiency. Patients with sickle cell disease require adequate hydration and intravascular fluid volume. Medications that cause diuresis, such as furosemide (Lasix), or vasoconstriction, such as epinephrine or dopamine, may cause or worsen potentially fatal complications of sickle cell disease. Many other genetically linked conditions require careful consideration when administering medications in the prehospital setting.

Subtle genetic variations among individuals may trigger significantly different responses to the same medication. The effects of ACE inhibitors, beta-2 agonists, antipsychotic medications, warfarin, aspirin, and glycoprotein IIb/IIIa inhibitors are all linked to the actions of particular genes. Variations in the expression of these linked genes will cause differing responses to each of these medications or medication groups (along with many others). The profound impact of genetic variations on medication response has prompted the development of a vast array of genetic screening tests specific to certain disease states or medications.

Street Smarts

Patients with genetic disorders and their family members are often excellent sources of information specific to the disorder. You should take advantage of the knowledge of patients and family members about genetic conditions; admitting a lack of knowledge about an unusual genetic condition and treating patients and families as experts on the genetic condition can help build their confidence in you.

Pregnancy

Pregnancy causes an array of physiologic changes in the body, which in turn can significantly affect medication decisions. Cardiac output and intravascular volume increase dramatically during pregnancy, with each rising by about 40% above prepregnancy levels. The **hematocrit** (ie, the percentage of RBCs in the intravascular space) decreases in response to an increase in overall blood plasma volume. Respiratory tidal volume and minute volumes increase, while the inspiratory and expiratory reserve volumes decrease. Gastrointestinal (GI) motility decreases as pregnancy progresses. Renal blood flow and urinary elimination increase, roughly in proportion to cardiac output and intravascular volume. Most endocrine glands undergo some degree of change during pregnancy, leading to emotional instability, altered glucose metabolism, thyroid-generated tachycardia, and other conditions.

Each of these changes can affect the absorption, distribution, or elimination of medications during pregnancy. The stress imposed on the body during pregnancy from these changes can also exacerbate an underlying disease process, potentially threatening the life or health of the patient and fetus. In addition to accounting for alterations in the woman's body during pregnancy, you must consider potential harmful effects on the developing fetus when administering medication to a pregnant patient. To determine whether a specific medication is safe for a pregnant woman and the developing fetus, paramedics should consult the medication's label (ie, the package insert), which provides FDA-approved information on the following topics[8]:

- Pregnancy, including labor and delivery
  - Pregnancy exposure registry
  - Risk summary
  - Clinical considerations
  - Data
- Lactation, including nursing mothers
  - Risk summary
  - Clinical considerations
  - Data
- Reproductive potential effects, for both females and males
  - Pregnancy testing
  - Contraception
  - Infertility

As of 2018, this drug label format officially replaced the FDA's previous risk letter categories (A, B, C, D, and X), which were criticized for providing misleading or insufficient information.

In general, medications and interventions that protect the life and health of the mother are usually in the best interest of the dependent fetus. Most medications given by paramedics do not pose an unacceptable risk to a fetus. Even so, you must consider pregnancy risk implications whenever you are contemplating medication administration to a potentially pregnant patient. Avoid medications known to cause harm to the fetus in all but the most extreme, life-threatening situations for the mother. In situations involving a direct threat to the patient's life, it is often necessary to administer a higher-risk medication to preserve the life of the mother, regardless of the risk to the unborn child. Online medical control physicians can often provide guidance in these difficult situations.

Most commercial reference sources provide the FDA pregnancy risk category for each medication. A medication's pregnancy risk category is also listed within its medication monograph. Aspirin and certain benzodiazepines such as diazepam and midazolam are common prehospital medications known to cause fetal harm.

Special Populations

Treat every female of childbearing age as though she could be pregnant.

Psychosocial Factors

Be aware of the role of psychosocial factors in the effectiveness of medications when selecting and administering medications. Pain, anxiety, and overall discomfort can vary dramatically among individual patients with the same illness or injury. Unlike measurable vital signs and readily observable clinical findings, patients' perceptions of and responses to discomfort are largely subjective. Psychological, cultural, emotional, and situational factors may influence the amount of discomfort reported by patients in relation to the underlying medical condition, patient positioning, environmental stressors, and the interventions you may perform during treatment. You should be alert to verbal and nonverbal cues when assessing for discomfort and administering medications for anxiety, pain, and sedation. Nonverbal cues may be indicated by changes in vital signs, facial expression, posture and movement changes, altered respiratory patterns, tears or crying, and other behaviors. These cues can provide potentially useful information about patient pain, anxiety, or discomfort but can have different meanings to different people, so your interpretation of the cues should be confirmed with the patient.

Medication administration is further complicated by the **placebo effect**. Numerous studies have demonstrated that patients often experience measurable clinical improvement or have unexplained adverse effects after receiving a medication with no pharmacologic properties. Placebos were used commonly in 17th- and 18th-century medical practice, and their use continued until the early 1900s. Pharmacologically inactive medications continue to be used by health care researchers to validate the efficacy or adverse effects of investigational medications by quantifying the placebo effect present in the particular study. The physiologic mechanism of the placebo effect remains under speculation. Pain relief from a placebo may come from endorphins released by the brain in anticipation of pain relief from the placebo. Adverse effects following placebo administration may somehow be linked to negative expectations or anxiety, although the mechanism remains uncertain. The efficacy of a placebo may be related to the timing of administration in relation to pharmacologically active medications.

It may be tempting to exploit the placebo effect by administering inactive substances to a patient as an alternative to pharmacologic treatment.

This practice is demeaning to patients and may lead to discipline or criminal prosecution if the act involves the diversion of controlled substances. Placebo use by paramedics violates ethical principles, deceives patients, and undermines the credibility of the EMS profession.

Types of Medication Responses

Every medication capable of a therapeutic benefit also can potentially have adverse or toxic effects at excessive doses. Even at appropriate doses, many medications produce harmful or undesired effects in susceptible people. You may prevent or minimize adverse effects by properly selecting the correct medication, route, dose, method of administration, and supportive treatment necessary for each patient.

SAFETY

Many types of errors can occur in health care. Perhaps most notable are medication and prescription errors, but other, less common errors include wrong patient identification, transfusion errors, preventable suicides, falls, burns, wrong-side procedures, and errors in the transition of care or handoffs. Types of medical errors are listed in **TABLE 13-5**.

TABLE 13-5 Types of Medical Errors

Error Category	Specific Errors
Diagnostic	Error or delay in diagnosis Failure to employ indicated tests Use of outmoded tests or therapy Failure to act on results of monitoring or testing
Treatment	Error in the performance of an operation, procedure, or test Error in administering the treatment Error in the dose or method of using a drug Avoidable delay in treatment or in responding to an abnormal test Inappropriate care
Preventive	Failure to provide prophylactic treatment Inadequate monitoring or follow-up of treatment
Other	Failure of communication Equipment failure Other system failure

Data from: Kohn LT, Corrigan JM, Donaldson MS, eds. *To Err Is Human: Building a Safer Health System.* Washington, DC: National Academy Press; 2000.

Therapeutic (Desired) Response

Pharmacologic interventions are based on a patient's actual or anticipated illness, injury, presenting complaint, sign, or symptom. This condition should match the use or indication listed on the profile for the specific medication. EMS agencies and organizations often formulate protocols that specify which medications should or can be administered in certain situations. Medical directors may authorize off-label uses (discussed earlier) for approved medications when this use reflects accepted medical practice. When the existing protocols or guidelines do not seem appropriate for a patient's needs, in many EMS systems, you may be able to contact online medical control for advice or authorization for medication administration.

Medication is administered in a dose intended to produce a desired clinical response for the patient. Sometimes this response may be complete resolution of the problem following a single dose of medication. In other cases, you may need to administer multiple doses of the same medication to obtain the desired response. Certain medications require frequent repeated dosing, careful titration, or continuous administration to obtain or maintain the desired response. These medications are capable of demonstrating **cumulative action**, meaning that several smaller doses of a medication produce the same desired clinical effect as a single, larger dose of that same medication. This approach can lead to the same therapeutic benefit while decreasing any risks associated with administering too much of a medication by a single, larger dose. Not every medication or situation allows for cumulative action. For instance, many medications require a minimum threshold concentration to cause a clinical effect. Metabolism and elimination (discussed later) may remove medication molecules before the threshold concentration is reached if the doses are too small or infrequent. The clinical situation and medication choice will determine which manner of medication administration is necessary or optimal.

Adverse Medication Effects

Adverse and toxic effects are important considerations during medication selection and administration. Pharmaceutical researchers and manufacturers attempt to develop medications that target only specific receptor sites on particular types of cells. Unfortunately, the vast number of possible receptor sites within the body makes medications selective (rather than specific) at best. Even medications that bind with a limited group of receptor sites can cause undesired responses in a variety of cells.

The term *side effect* is often used to mean *adverse effect*. Although both terms are typically used to mean harmful or potentially harmful effects, the term *adverse effect* more clearly indicates the possibility of serious consequences. Some side effects can be beneficial; for example, a physician may prescribe a specific antidepressant to treat postmenopausal symptoms, such as "hot flashes," because a positive side effect of the drug was identified. Also, a side effect of a medication can be desirable in certain situations and harmful in others. For example, benzodiazepines are used to treat seizure activity and are known to cause sedation. Sedation may be desirable for a combative patient with a head injury but could also jeopardize the life of the same patient if they are vomiting.

Various sources may also refer to adverse effects as **untoward effects**. Both adverse and untoward effects are clinical changes caused by a medication that are not desired and cause some degree of harm or discomfort to the patient.

SAFETY

The process of a patient receiving a medication is complex and fraught with opportunities for error, including prescribing, dispensing, administering, and monitoring errors. The uncontrolled prehospital environment creates additional challenges for paramedics when administering medications.

Undesired or harmful responses to a medication may be directly related to the intended cellular response or to random activation of unrelated cells throughout the body. Examples of undesired or harmful responses include hypoglycemia after the administration of insulin (exaggerated "therapeutic" effect); profound bradycardia after taking metoprolol, a beta adrenergic antagonist medication (exaggerated therapeutic effect); and an allergic reaction to a medication (not a therapeutic effect). Examples of common adverse effects include nausea, vomiting, sedation, palpitations, hypotension,

YOU are the Paramedic

PART 2

On arrival, you are directed to the patient's room. The nursing staff report that the patient is usually awake, alert, and oriented; however, she was noted to be "not herself" over the past several hours and now looks much worse. The staff also report that the patient was admitted to the skilled nursing facility for complications of diabetes mellitus and was slowly improving until she developed nausea, vomiting, and diarrhea over the past 36 to 48 hours. The patient's temperature was 99.7°F (37.6°C) just before your arrival.

Recording Time: 0 Minutes	
Appearance	Pale skin (Staff confirms her skin tone is pale as compared to its baseline color.)
Level of consciousness	Decreased responsiveness, moaning and incoherent speech, eyes open to deep tactile stimuli
Airway	Patent
Breathing	Clear breath sounds, slightly diminished at bases bilaterally
Circulation	Normal pulse strength, slightly increased heart rate

2. Based on this brief history and physical examination, what problems do you suspect?

3. What additional information would assist you with identifying possible causes of the patient's condition?

hypertension, bradycardia, tachycardia, respiratory depression, and dizziness. Medication reference sources often categorize adverse effects by body system, frequency of occurrence, or severity.

When selecting medications, consider possible adverse effects in relation to the patient's condition. For example, the respiratory depressant properties of opioid analgesics, such as morphine sulfate, are unlikely to adversely affect a patient with burns who is intubated and being mechanically ventilated; however, an immediate threat to life might result if morphine is given to a patient who is becoming fatigued during an asthma attack. Another example of how adverse effects play a role in decision making involves choosing between two or more medications that can be given for the same condition. For example, both ondansetron (Zofran) and promethazine (Phenergan) are antiemetic medications. Promethazine causes significant hemodynamic and electrocardiographic (ECG) changes, which are not known to occur with ondansetron. Ondansetron may prove to be a safer antiemetic medication for patients who are particularly susceptible to the adverse effects associated with promethazine. In general, a medication should be avoided or used with caution in patients who are particularly susceptible to the adverse effects associated with that medication.

Patients with certain chronic medical conditions are generally more susceptible to the adverse effects of medications than are patients without such conditions. Significant cardiovascular disease, diabetes, impaired immune function, and renal failure are more often associated with greater severity or frequency of adverse effects. Many adverse effects of medications directly relate to these conditions; for example, renal failure hinders the capability of the kidneys to eliminate medications properly. In addition, patients with respiratory distress, shock, multiple trauma, or other life-threatening conditions may be unable to tolerate even mild adverse effects. You must use caution when selecting medications for patients with these conditions. You also need to be alert for adverse effects once medications have been given.

Adverse effects may range in severity from changes that are barely perceptible to patients and paramedics to an immediately life-threatening condition requiring aggressive intervention. For example, certain antidepressant medications can cause cardiomyopathy, a disease of the heart muscle. Some antibiotics and antiseizure medications are known to cause **Stevens-Johnson syndrome**, a severe, possibly fatal medication reaction that mimics a burn. Several medications cause anemia (low RBC count) through bone marrow suppression or direct hemolysis.

Adverse effects occasionally occur that are completely unexpected and not previously known to be associated with a particular medication. These **idiosyncratic** medication reactions involve abnormal susceptibility to a medication, possibly because of genetic traits or dysfunction of a metabolic enzyme peculiar to an individual patient.

Therapeutic Index

Pharmaceutical companies and scientists devote intensive efforts to evaluating the safety and effectiveness of a potential medication before it is made available to the public. Animal testing establishes the **median lethal dose (LD_{50})**, which is the weight-based dose of a medication that causes death in 50% of the animals tested. In addition, manufacturers determine the **median toxic dose (TD_{50})** for a particular adverse effect of the medication, which means that 50% of the animals tested had toxic effects at or above this weight-based dose. Human or animal testing also reveals the **median effective dose (ED_{50})** for a particular use or indication of the medication. The relationship between the median effective dose and the median lethal dose or median toxic dose is known as the **therapeutic index**, or therapeutic ratio. If there is a significant difference between the median effective dose and the median toxic dose or median lethal dose, the medication is considered safe or possibly even nontoxic. If the ratio is relatively small, however, careful patient selection, medication use, and medication monitoring are essential. A relatively unsafe medication may be used in clinical practice if it is the only choice for an otherwise fatal medical condition.

Immune-Mediated Medication Response

Medications and substances present in the environment can trigger an exaggerated response from the body's immune system, which is described generally as an allergic reaction. Allergic reactions can range from mild skin changes to multisystem, life-threatening reactions. You may encounter patients with this condition who request EMS assistance or may observe it immediately after administering a medication to a patient for an unrelated condition.

Patients who are genetically predisposed to an allergic reaction must typically have an initial exposure and sensitization to a particular allergen. Following the initial exposure, various components of the body's immune system evolve into antibodies that specifically target this type of allergen. If the patient then has a subsequent exposure to this type of allergen, a potentially massive cascade of immune system activity, known as **anaphylaxis**, begins. In severe cases, this reaction dramatically alters the function of the skin, GI, respiratory, and cardiovascular systems, ultimately manifesting as shock and respiratory failure. Chapter 26, *Immunologic Emergencies,* includes additional discussion of the pathophysiology and management of an immune-mediated medication response.

Patients predisposed to an allergic reaction, anaphylaxis, or other immune-mediated medication response may report previous reactions to medications, latex, foods, or other substances in the environment. Aspirin and antibiotics, most commonly penicillin and sulfa-based antibiotics, are the primary culprits in immune-mediated medication responses. A very small amount of any medication can cause this reaction. An immune-mediated reaction can occur days or weeks after initiating a medication.

Patients may also have a **medication sensitivity** that is not related to an exaggerated immune system response. A mild to severe reaction may occur after the first exposure to a medication or other substance, often presenting with many of the same signs and symptoms as an immune-mediated reaction. The treatment for medication sensitivity is similar to the treatment for an immune-mediated response. Avoid administering medications to patients who have had a serious reaction to the specific medication (or a medication in the same class) unless the adverse effect was clearly dose-related and can be lessened by judicious administration and careful monitoring.

Medication Tolerance

Certain medications are known to have decreased efficacy or potency when taken repeatedly by a patient, a state known as **tolerance**. One theory suggests that tolerance results from a mechanism that reduces the number of cell receptors available for binding with a particular medication, a process known as **down-regulation**. The body compensates for the effects of a medication by increasing the metabolism and/or elimination of the medication, resulting in a decreased concentration of the medication present near receptor sites. In some instances, the desirable effects continue while other unintended or adverse effects decrease. In other situations, adverse effects persist or increase while additional medication is required to achieve the same therapeutic goal.

Repeated exposure to a medication within a particular class, such as opioids or benzodiazepines, can cause a tolerance to other medications in the same class. This phenomenon, known as **cross-tolerance**, becomes problematic when patients use or abuse medications, drugs, or chemicals regularly and then require medications from that class for a legitimate medical purpose. Determining the appropriate dose for these patients can prove quite challenging, and often results in them receiving inadequate or excessive doses of therapeutic medications.

A similar condition, known as **tachyphylaxis**, occurs with certain medications. Giving repeated doses of medication within a short time frame can rapidly cause tolerance, making the medication virtually ineffective. Tachyphylaxis is likely to occur with certain sympathomimetic medications (discussed later) and may occur with other medications that you may administer, such as nitroglycerin and dobutamine.

Words of Wisdom

Do not be afraid to ask the same patient about allergies more than once if multiple medications are being administered.

Words of Wisdom

Consider patient tolerance, IV infiltration or disconnect, or possible medication tampering whenever administration of a controlled substance does not produce the expected clinical effect.

Medication Abuse and Dependence

Certain classes of medications and similar groups of illicit chemicals have serious potential for misuse and abuse. Some people may choose to experience many of the desired clinical effects from medications or chemicals even when they do not have an underlying medical condition or symptom. Patients who receive certain medications for legitimate medical conditions may continue to use these medications long after their initial medical condition has resolved. It is often difficult to determine whether an appropriate medical indication for certain medications continues to exist. In the course of your EMS practice, you are almost certain to encounter patients who misuse or abuse medications, illicit drugs, and other chemicals.

Two distinct groups of medications and chemicals are especially susceptible to misuse and abuse: stimulants and depressants. **Stimulant** chemicals cause a transient increase in physical, mental, or emotional performance. Caffeine, cocaine, and amphetamines are stimulants that have serious potential for misuse or abuse. In general, these medications increase a person's level of consciousness, increase the heart rate, increase blood pressure (BP), and otherwise activate the sympathetic nervous system. The immediate or long-term effects of stimulant medications have the potential to become life threatening.

Depressant medications and chemicals, in contrast to stimulants, reduce CNS and sympathetic nervous system functioning, causing sedation, anxiolysis, respiratory depression, bradycardia, hypotension, and a variety of similar clinical symptoms. Benzodiazepines, alcohol, and opioids are common depressant substances. Toxicity from depressant substances is also potentially life threatening following acute or long-term exposure.

Repeated exposure to certain medications or chemicals causes a patient to experience **habituation**, an abnormal tolerance to the adverse or therapeutic effects associated with a substance. In essence, the body adapts to accommodate the exposure and protect itself from the severity of clinical changes associated with a substance. Prolonged or significant exposure to depressants, stimulants, and other medications and chemicals can cause some degree of **dependence**. Dependence is the physical, emotional, or behavioral need for these substances to maintain a level of "normal" function. When it exists, the person has adapted to the frequent presence of the substance. In the absence of the substance, adverse clinical effects occur. In severe cases, abrupt withdrawal from a substance can precipitate life-threatening clinical changes.

Medication Interactions

Patients receiving multiple medications, drugs, or other chemicals are at risk of an unintended interaction between the various substances, possibly leading to unexpected results. Undesirable medication interactions are referred to as medication **interference**. You should consider the possibility of illicit drugs, over-the-counter and prescribed medications, and herbal remedies interacting with any medication that might be given to a patient. As patients are prescribed a greater number of medications to treat chronic medical conditions, the risk of a medication interaction increases dramatically.

The most obvious concern with medication interactions is incompatibility during administration. When given simultaneously through the same IV tubing, the chemical composition of some medications will change, possibly creating solid particles in the tubing, which then travel into the patient. Other medication combinations will deactivate one or more of the medications, making them ineffective. Medications also require use of the proper IV solution, as some can be mixed only in normal saline or dextrose-containing solutions. Consult a reliable medication reference source before administering multiple medications, especially continuous medication infusions, through the same IV tubing. Notably, sodium bicarbonate and furosemide are two medications used in the prehospital setting that are incompatible with several other common prehospital medications.

A medication can increase the effect, decrease the effect, or alter the effect of another medication within the body. **TABLE 13-6** describes various types of medication interactions.

Principles of Pharmacokinetics

You must carefully consider the pharmacokinetic properties of any medication you are considering administering to a patient. As a medication is administered, the body begins a complex process of

TABLE 13-6 Medication Interactions

Type of Interaction	Description	Example
Addition or summation	Two medications with a similar effect combine to produce an effect equal to the sum of the individual effect of each medication (eg, 1 + 1 = 2).	The antipyretic properties of acetaminophen (Tylenol) and the antipyretic properties of ibuprofen (Motrin, Advil) combine to reduce a fever in patients with fevers that could not be controlled by either medication alone.
Synergism	Two medications with a similar effect combine to produce an effect greater than the sum of the medications' effects.	Patients experience profound sedation when IV opioid medications such as fentanyl (Sublimaze) are given with IV benzodiazepines such as midazolam (Versed), greater than the expected sum of these two medications.
Potentiation	The effect of one medication is greatly enhanced by the presence of another medication, which does not produce the same effect.	Promethazine (Phenergan) is given to increase the effects of codeine or other antitussives (cough suppressants) for more improved relief of cough than is achieved with the antitussive alone.
Altered absorption	The action of one medication increases or decreases the ability of another medication to be absorbed by the body. For example, medications that increase or decrease gastrointestinal pH or motility may increase or decrease the absorption of other medications taken orally.	Famotidine (Pepcid), an H_2 blocker, can reduce absorption of ketoconazole (an antifungal) or certain cephalosporin antibiotics.
Altered metabolism	The action of one medication increases or decreases the metabolism of another medication within the body. For example, many medications (and certain foods) alter the performance of the cytochrome P-450 system in the liver, which is responsible for the metabolism of a variety of other medications.	Fluconazole (Diflucan), an antifungal medication, inhibits the function of cytochrome P-450 enzyme CYP3A4, significantly increasing bleeding risks associated with warfarin (Coumadin), an anticoagulant medication.
Altered distribution	The presence of one medication alters the area available for the distribution of another medication in the body, which becomes important when both medications are bound to the same site, such as plasma proteins. If proteins are already occupied by one medication, toxic levels of the other medication may develop.	The anticonvulsant medication valproic acid (Depakote, Depakene) competes with another anticonvulsant medication, phenytoin (Dilantin), causing potentially increased or decreased serum levels and possibly unpredictable clinical effects.
Altered elimination	Medications may increase or decrease the functioning of the kidneys or other route of elimination, influencing the amount of or duration of effect of another medication in the body.	Ethanol decreases the metabolism of warfarin (Coumadin), which may predispose the patient to bleeding risk.

Type of Interaction	Description	Example
Physiologic (drug) antagonism	Two medications, each producing opposite effects, are present simultaneously, resulting in minimal or no clinical changes.	Sodium nitroprusside (Nipride) and dobutamine (Dobutrex) are often given simultaneously for cardiogenic shock. By itself, dobutamine increases cardiac output, possibly causing an elevated BP. Sodium nitroprusside causes vasodilation and possibly hypotension. When given together, these medications can be titrated to maintain a normal patient BP.
Neutralization	Two medications bind together in the body, creating an inactive substance.	Digoxin-specific antibodies (Digibind, Digifab) are administered to patients with toxicity to the medication digoxin. These medications combine, rendering digoxin molecules inactive.

Abbreviations: BP, blood pressure; H_2, histamine$_2$ receptor antagonist; IV, intravenous

Data from: Schelleman H, Bilker WB, Brensinger CM, et al. Warfarin with fluoroquinolones, sulfonamides, or azole antifungals: interactions and the risk of hospitalization for gastrointestinal bleeding. *Clin Pharmacol Ther.* 2008;84(5):581-588.

moving that medication, possibly altering the medication's structure, and ultimately removing the medication from the body. The medication dose, route of administration, and patient's clinical status will largely determine the duration and effectiveness of the medication (see the section *Principles of Pharmacodynamics*, earlier in this chapter). Actions of absorption, distribution, metabolism, and elimination are discussed in detail in the following text.

The pharmacokinetics section of a medication profile typically states the *onset, peak,* and *duration of effect* for the medication. These values vary by route of administration and may have a broad range, depending on the characteristics of individual patients. The onset and peak of a medication are generally related to absorption and distribution. In particular, a minimum dose or concentration of medication must be present at certain sites in the body for clinical effects to occur (see the earlier section *Principles of Pharmacodynamics*).

The duration of effect is generally related to medication metabolism and elimination. As the amount of a medication found near cell receptors (or other site of action) decreases, the clinical effects caused by the medication begin to decrease and normal function resumes.

If a medication permanently binds with a receptor site or irreversibly alters the function of a cell, the duration of its effect is determined by the body's ability to regenerate cells. In these cases, the duration of effect may be almost entirely unrelated to the dose or concentration of medication present in the body. A single dose of aspirin, for example, is rapidly eliminated by the body, usually within several hours, but can cause an inhibition of platelet activity lasting for 3 to 10 days.

Street Smarts

Communicating the time of onset and peak of a medication to the patient can build trust and credibility.

Routes of Medication Administration

Medication must enter the body to provide a clinical benefit. Thus, you need to select a route of administration capable of delivering an appropriate amount of medication to the correct location within the patient's body. The route of administration is determined by the physical and chemical properties of the medication, the routes of administration available for a specific patient, and how quickly the effects of the medication are needed.

The chosen route of administration determines the percentage of the unchanged medication that reaches the systemic circulation. This percentage, known as **bioavailability**, varies significantly from one medication to another, except when administered by the IV route. Medications administered by the IV route, by definition, have 100% bioavailability. Bioavailability is irrelevant for medications that are sequestered in the GI tract, such as activated charcoal and certain cathartic medications. In contrast, it is a critical consideration for other medications that are poorly absorbed by certain routes or subject to immediate metabolism by the liver before reaching the systemic circulation. Several important groups of medications, such as beta blockers and calcium channel blockers, have a relatively low bioavailability when taken orally. The IV doses of these medications are often lower than the oral doses when given for the same indication. Lidocaine and fentanyl are generally not given orally because of their low bioavailability with this route. Various routes of administration available to paramedics are discussed in the following sections.

Oral, Orogastric Tube, and Nasogastric Tube Administration

Many medications prescribed for chronic medical conditions and several important prehospital medications are administered into the GI system. Use of this route requires that a patient be responsive and able to swallow or have a nasogastric tube or an orogastric tube in place. Aspirin, antipyretic medications, activated charcoal, diphenhydramine, and oral glucose are prehospital medications that may be administered into the GI system. Once administered via this route, medication absorption varies depending on several factors **TABLE 13-7**.

TABLE 13-7 Factors Affecting GI Medication Absorption

Factor	Effects on Medication Absorption
GI motility	Ability of medication to pass through the GI tract into the bloodstream
GI pH	Perfusion of the GI system (may be decreased during systemic trauma or shock)
Presence of food, liquids, or chemicals in the stomach	Injury or bleeding in the GI system (both can alter GI motility, decreasing the time that oral medications can be absorbed)

Abbreviation: GI, gastrointestinal

In addition to these factors, GI medications may be subject to first-pass metabolism. Medication passes from the GI tract into the portal vein, which brings it directly into the liver. Once in the liver, metabolism occurs, altering and potentially inactivating the medication before it ever reaches systemic circulation. This first-pass metabolism can be exploited if it changes a previously inactive medication into an active medication. Codeine, for example, undergoes a significant **first-pass effect** in which a portion of the medication can be converted to morphine, a more potent analgesic, by the liver. Metabolism of a medication may also occur within the GI tract and as the medication enters the bloodstream. Bioavailability of medications given orally or through a nasogastric or an orogastric tube can range from 5% to 100%, depending on the particular medication and the effect of first-pass metabolism. Several cardiac medications, such as metoprolol and verapamil, are subject to significant first-pass metabolism when taken orally. The reduction in bioavailability due to first-pass hepatic metabolism has already been taken into account with oral dosing, explaining why the oral doses are significantly higher than the IV doses of these medications when given for the same purpose. Patients with hepatic (liver) dysfunction are at risk of toxicity when these medications are given orally, even at conventional doses, because the first-pass effect is impaired in these individuals, such that a greater quantity of the medication reaches their systemic circulation.

Endotracheal Administration

ACLS protocols emphasize using the IV or IO routes of medication administration over the endotracheal route. If the endotracheal route is chosen, sources recommend administering at least 2 to 2.5 times the IV dose for medications approved for this route, followed by a 5- to 10-mL flush with sterile water or normal saline.[9] With improved IO techniques and devices, it is likely that the use of the endotracheal route of medication administration will become increasingly limited. However, you may still administer bronchodilators or mucolytic medications in specific critical care settings via the endotracheal route.

Intranasal Administration

With the intranasal route of medication administration, liquid medications are converted into a fine mist that is sprayed into one or both nostrils. Fentanyl, midazolam, and naloxone can be administered using this route, with their resulting effectiveness often being equal to or better than that of the same drugs given by other methods. Medication absorption occurs rapidly through this route, and the bioavailability of intranasal medications appears close to 100% in certain studies. Other studies suggest that this method is superior to the IV and rectal routes of administration. Nasal medication administration can occur almost immediately, without delay for initiating an IV line, especially when IV access is difficult or impossible to obtain. Additionally, nasal administration does not place you at risk for a needlestick injury when treating uncooperative patients.

Intravenous Administration

The IV route remains the preferred method for administering most medications used in the prehospital setting. A small-diameter catheter is inserted into a peripheral or external jugular vein, allowing medications to be administered directly into the systemic circulation. In special situations, you may be permitted to use permanent indwelling venous catheters or large-bore catheters that have already been inserted into central veins by other health care professionals.

The bioavailability of IV medication is 100% by definition. Medications administered by the IV route have an onset of action significantly quicker than the onset of action for medications given orally or through an orogastric or nasogastric tube, often allowing an immediate response or creating the ability to titrate a medication carefully in a rapidly evolving clinical situation.

Several important limitations apply regarding the IV route of medication administration. First, access can be challenging in some groups of patients—specifically, patients who have abused IV drugs, patients in profound shock or with cardiovascular collapse, patients with morbid obesity, and patients with certain chronic medical conditions such as diabetes and renal failure. Second, the IV access procedure can cause pain or infection and is somewhat time consuming. Finally, uncontrolled scenes, environmental extremes, and movement of the transport vehicle make IV access challenging in the prehospital setting. Establishing IV access is discussed further in Chapter 14, *Medication Administration.*

Words of Wisdom

Frequently reassess the IV site for infiltration or tubing disconnect during transport. Confirm that the IV is still working properly during patient turnover, especially if the medication being administered has a high potential to cause an adverse effect.

The infiltration of IV medication into tissues around the blood vessel is a significant concern for paramedics. Certain medication classes, such as **sympathomimetics** and electrolyte solutions, can cause significant pain and tissue damage when they accumulate in surrounding tissues. In extreme cases, tissue death will occur in affected areas, leaving a large area of necrotic tissue or skin.

Intraosseous Administration

The IO route of medication administration provides a viable alternative when IV access cannot be obtained. When this route is used, a needle is inserted through the patient's skin and into the bone. The tip of the needle pierces the hard, outer layer of bone and enters the softer bone marrow. Vascular uptake from the bone marrow provides a reliable route for medications and IV fluids **TABLE 13-8**. Chapter 14, *Medication Administration,* describes the technique for IO access in greater detail.

Any medication or fluid that can be administered by the IV route can also be administered by the IO route. Infusion rates for IO fluids are comparable to IV rates when a pressure bag or mechanical

TABLE 13-8 Veins Used During IO Infusion

Intraosseous Site	Vein
Proximal tibia	Popliteal vein
Femur	Femoral vein
Distal tibia (medial malleolus)	Great saphenous vein
Proximal humerus	Axillary vein
Manubrium (sternum)	Internal mammary and azygos veins

Abbreviation: IO, intraosseous

infusion device is used. The IO devices can generally be left in place for up to 24 hours, allowing for their ongoing use as a medication or fluid administration route until IV access can be obtained.

Administration by the IO route is contraindicated in bones that are fractured. It is also discouraged when patients have bone diseases or a skin infection over a possible insertion site. Newer devices allow IO insertion in a variety of anatomic locations and across the spectrum of patient ages and weights.

Intramuscular Administration

Some medications used in the prehospital setting can be administered by the intramuscular (IM) route. With this administration technique, sterile medication is drawn into a syringe attached to a needle and injected into one of the patient's larger muscles. This route is used when IV access cannot be established or when the clinical situation requires immediate medication administration that cannot wait for IV access. Medications have a bioavailability ranging from 75% to 100% following IM administration. The absorption rate is determined by the accuracy of the injection landmark and the perfusion to the chosen muscle.

As a paramedic, you should use caution when performing an IM injection. Uncooperative patients may move suddenly, placing you or other responders at risk for a contaminated needlestick. Auto-injection devices, such as the EpiPen and DuoDote Auto-Injector, are commercially available, are spring-loaded, and deliver a predetermined quantity of medication. Unfortunately, these devices usually do not retract the needle following administration, which means they present the risk of a contaminated needlestick.

You should confirm that a medication is appropriate for IM use before administering it via this route. Even if a medication is safe for IM use, medication reference sources may indicate that a particular muscle should be used or recommend a specific injection technique. Many medications are safe for IV use but can cause significant injury if given by the IM route. Other medications are indicated only for IM use and will cause complications if given by the IV route.

Subcutaneous Administration

Subcutaneous medication administration is similar to IM administration. In this technique, sterile medication solution is drawn into a syringe attached to a needle. The medication is then injected into various subcutaneous tissue sites throughout the body. The anterior part of the abdomen, just outside the umbilicus, and the skin overlying the triceps muscle are common sites for subcutaneous injection. Compared to IM needles, the needles for subcutaneous administration are shorter and have a smaller diameter. Certain medications may be indicated for subcutaneous use only and should not be given by the IV route, even if a patent IV line is already in place. The slower absorption that occurs through the subcutaneous tissue may prevent adverse cardiovascular effects, as compared with the nearly instantaneous absorption that occurs with IV administration of the medication. Consult advanced life support (ALS) protocols or a reliable medication reference for specific information about the subcutaneous administration of a medication. The techniques for subcutaneous and IM medication administration are discussed in greater detail in Chapter 14, *Medication Administration.*

Dermal and Transdermal Administration

You may encounter patients in the prehospital setting who are receiving medication via the transdermal route. Patches commonly containing nicotine, antiemetics, analgesics, nitroglycerin, or other medications may be placed in various locations on the body. Because transdermal medications may alter a patient's clinical presentation or interfere with the medications you will administer during the EMS response, ask a patient or family member if a transdermal medication patch is in place while obtaining a patient's medication history.

Transdermal patches deliver a relatively constant dose of medication over an extended period. Changes in patient temperature or perfusion may alter medication delivery to the patient, potentially causing significant clinical changes. In addition, transdermal patches often contain a large quantity of medication. If these patches are chewed or ingested, particularly by children, life-threatening toxic effects are possible.

Sublingual Administration

Nitroglycerin is frequently given to patients using the sublingual (SL) route of administration. Nitroglycerin tablets are placed under a patient's tongue or nitroglycerin is sprayed under the patient's tongue, where it is absorbed rapidly by the mucous membranes, resulting in a relatively quick onset of action. The bioavailability of SL nitroglycerin is quite low, so relatively large doses are required when this route is used compared with an IV infusion—close to 100 times larger for initial dosing. Patients must be responsive and alert to receive SL medications. In addition, a lack of moisture or saliva in a patient's mouth may significantly delay the absorption of SL medications. In this case, the spray formulation is preferable over SL tablets. You may also encounter patients receiving certain analgesic medications by lozenges and other medications administered sublingually using lollipops, gums, and orally dissolving tablets.

Inhaled or Nebulized Administration

Some medications may be inhaled or nebulized into the respiratory tract, providing paramedics with a vital route of medication administration. Oxygen is an example of an inhaled prehospital medication. You may also administer or assist patients in administering respiratory medication using a metered-dose inhaler (MDI), typically for asthma or chronic obstructive pulmonary disease (COPD). Activation of the MDI converts the liquid medicine into a gas, allowing the medication to pass into the patient's lungs. When used with a spacer, MDIs are at least as effective as nebulizers for administering bronchodilator medications.

Medication in liquid form may also be nebulized (converted into a fine spray) for administration directly into the respiratory system. With this administration technique, tubing with oxygen or compressed air is attached to a small chamber, creating a mist as the gas passes through the liquid medication. The chamber is attached to a mouthpiece or a mask, allowing patients to receive droplets of medication with each inspired breath. Unfortunately, a portion of the medication is lost during exhalation and during any pauses in patient respiration. Nebulized medications are typically administered to treat bronchospasm or airway edema. Albuterol, levalbuterol (Xopenex), and ipratropium bromide (Atrovent) are nebulized medications available in the prehospital setting. In some instances, you may be instructed to administer other medications by nebulizer. Be aware that nebulized medications have the potential to cause bronchospasm.

Rectal Administration

Certain medications used in the prehospital setting may be administered via the rectal route. The rectal route is preferred over the oral route in several situations—for example, when the patient is unresponsive, having seizures, vomiting, or unable to swallow oral medications. In addition, rectal medications are usually not subject to first-pass metabolism, which decreases the bioavailability of many oral medications. In fact, certain medications administered rectally may have greater than 90% bioavailability. If a medication is administered into the proximal rectum, some level of first-pass effect is still possible. Medications administered into the lower rectum are less likely to have any dose reduction due to the first-pass effect. Whenever possible, medications should be administered into the lower, rather than proximal, rectum. Absorption of rectal medications can be unpredictable, often related to the specific absorption site within the rectum. The rectal dose of a medication is often higher than is the oral or IV dose.

Rectal medications are manufactured in the form of suppositories, a waxlike substance molded into a shape similar to a bullet. The suppository is lubricated and inserted into the patient's rectal cavity. Antiemetics and antipyretic medications are often available in suppository form.

Ophthalmic Administration

EMS systems may approve the administration of medications by the ophthalmic route. In the prehospital setting, the ophthalmic route is generally limited to ocular **anesthetic** agents given to facilitate eye irrigation following a chemical exposure. Although the role of ophthalmic medications in the prehospital setting is generally limited, you should be aware that these medications can cause systemic toxic effects following ophthalmic administration.

Other Methods of Medication Administration

Hemodialysis is one of the rare exceptions in which medications produce beneficial effects outside the patient's body. In this procedure, blood from a patient is pumped through a dialysis machine, where the blood is exposed to a dialysate solution that removes toxins, excess electrolytes, and other chemicals from the blood; the cleansed blood is then returned to the patient. Paramedics working in the prehospital setting are unlikely to use this method of medication administration.

As a paramedic, you may encounter patients receiving medication through a variety of other routes. These methods are not generally used in the prehospital setting and may cause serious or life-threatening complications if employed by untrained personnel. You should not use any unfamiliar catheters, lines, tubes, or other devices for medication or fluid administration unless you have received appropriate training and authorization in their use.

Distribution of Medication

The chemical and physical properties of a medication determine how that medication moves through the body. Many medication-related factors, such as the size of medication molecules, the ability to bind with other substances within the body, and the ability to dissolve in certain body fluids, determine which cells, tissues, and organs a particular medication will reach. Individual patient factors such as fat, water, and protein content also determine how much of a medication is available to cause physiologic changes at a given dose.

The human body has an elaborate system of barriers designed to prevent the introduction of foreign substances into the body and into specific cells, tissues, and organs. Consequently, medication molecules need to pass through various barriers to reach their target sites within the body. To cross these barriers, medication molecules must move through spaces between individual cells or pass directly through the center of individual cells.

The process of **osmosis** is used to enhance the distribution of certain medications, electrolytes, and IV fluids. During osmosis, free water and certain particles such as sodium and potassium can pass through a semipermeable membrane to equalize the concentration of the water and other particles on each side of the membrane. This process allows IV fluids to leave the intravascular space and enter tissues and cells. Osmosis is also one of the mechanisms that the kidneys use to regulate the fluid balance within the body.

Filtration is a process within the body, similar to osmosis, that is used to redistribute water and other particles. Most discussion of filtration within the body focuses on renal sodium and water filtration in the glomerular capillaries. Hydrostatic pressure forces different body fluids against semipermeable membranes, causing the passage of certain substances into an adjacent compartment.

The skin, GI tract, eyes, and urinary tract contain epithelial cells that create a continuous barrier. This barrier prevents the movement of medication molecules between the epithelial cells. To cross the epithelial barrier, the medication molecules must pass directly through cells to enter the body. Small medication molecules that are **nonionic** (uncharged) and **lipophilic** (attracted to fats and lipids) pass easily through cell membranes. In fact, all but the largest lipid-soluble medications can pass easily through cell membranes.

In contrast, larger, **hydrophilic** (attracted to water molecules), and ionic (charged) medication molecules must find another route of entry into cells. When confronted with larger medication molecules, cells use a process called **pinocytosis** to ingest extracellular fluids and their contents. Medication molecules may also bind with carrier proteins for transport into cells. This process of binding with carrier proteins is called **facilitated diffusion** when no energy is expended and is called **active transport** when energy is used to move the molecules against a concentration gradient.

In addition to the epithelial barrier, the human body has capillary barriers near specific tissues. Once inside blood vessels, medication molecules must pass through capillary walls to reach their target cells or other sites. The blood–brain barrier, the blood–placenta barrier, and the blood–testes barrier are all areas where capillary cells form a continuous barrier, preventing medication molecules from passing through openings in capillary walls. These three anatomic barriers prevent various medication molecules from reaching the underlying tissues. Only certain medications can pass through the cell membranes in these areas and enter the adjacent tissues.

Capillaries in the kidney, thyroid, pancreas, and other areas allow medication molecules to pass freely through the capillary walls into the surrounding tissues. Only protein-bound medications have difficulty passing through the capillaries in these areas. The lungs and peritoneum also permit medication molecules to enter and exit easily through the capillary walls.

Plasma protein binding significantly alters the distribution of certain medications within the body. Medication molecules temporarily attach to proteins in the blood plasma. Albumin and other plasma proteins effectively store a quantity of medication largely independent of the concentration of the medication present in the blood or other body tissues. Patient age, nutritional status, and medical condition influence the amount of plasma protein present in the body. As plasma protein levels change or when another medication that binds with plasma proteins is introduced, the concentration of the original medication in blood and body tissues may change significantly.

Protein binding increases the amount of medication needed to produce the desired clinical effect. This reversible process also releases medication as circulating levels of a particular medication begin to fall, leading to a longer duration of action for the medication. A patient can have a therapeutic (safe) level of a protein-bound medication until a second protein-bound medication with greater affinity is administered. The second medication displaces the original medication attached to plasma proteins, causing a dramatic increase in the amount of the original medication present in the circulation and subsequent toxic effects.

Fat tissue is another site of medication distribution that alters the amount of medication available for action within the body. Large quantities of lipophilic medications can be sequestered in the fat tissues of people with obesity. In this case, the medication is released slowly, causing prolonged effects compared with the same dose in people with a lean body composition. As the percentage of body fat increases, the same weight-based dose of a hydrophilic medication results in a higher concentration in the plasma and water throughout the body.

Volume of Distribution

The **volume of distribution** for a medication describes the extent to which a medication will spread within the body. Certain medications do not readily leave the plasma. Other medications spread into the water throughout the body. Still other medications readily bind with bone, teeth, or other tissues, resulting in a relatively low concentration in the blood. The volume of distribution relates the medication dose to the anticipated plasma level of a given medication in a "typical" patient. Medications with a lower volume of distribution are present in higher levels in the plasma at a given dose compared to medications with a higher volume of distribution. Conversely, for medications with a high volume of distribution, a larger total dose is needed to reach a certain level in the plasma than for medications with a lower volume of distribution. It is also possible to estimate the amount of a medication or chemical present in the body by knowing the level of the medication present in the plasma and the known volume of distribution for a particular medication. This value may help explain why a large dose of additional medication may cause only a modest increase in the amount of available medication.

Medication Metabolism

Many medications undergo some degree of chemical change by the body, known as biotransformation. As a medication undergoes biotransformation, it becomes known as a metabolite. Metabolites can be either active or inactive. **Active metabolites** remain capable of some pharmacologic activity, such as altering a cell process or body function. Active metabolites can go from helpful or therapeutic to harmful. **Inactive metabolites** no longer possess the ability to alter a cell process or body function.

Biotransformation has four possible effects on a medication absorbed into the body:

1. An inactive substance can become active, producing desired or unwanted clinical effects (active metabolite).
2. An active medication can be changed into another active medication (active metabolite).
3. An active medication can be completely or partially inactivated (inactive metabolite).
4. A medication can be transformed into a substance (active or inactive metabolite) that is easier for the body to eliminate.

Most biotransformation occurs in the liver. The cytochrome P-450 system in the liver uses a complex, enzyme-based process to alter the chemical structure of a medication or other chemical. Separate pathways within the cytochrome P-450 system are responsible for the metabolism of different medication groups. These pathways can be selectively influenced by other medications, chemicals, and diet choices, altering the metabolism of certain groups of medications. For example, ethanol, oral contraceptives, and grapefruit juice are known to cause potentially life-threatening alterations in the cytochrome P-450 metabolism of certain medications.

The kidneys, skin, lungs, GI tract, and many other body tissues have some ability to cause biotransformation as well. Microorganisms present in the GI tract begin the biotransformation of certain medications taken orally. Biotransformation makes medications and chemicals more water-soluble and easier for the kidneys and other organs to eliminate from the body. Suspect altered medication metabolism in patients with chronic alcoholism, liver disease, or any condition known to affect the liver.

Medication Elimination

Medications and other chemicals are primarily removed from the body by the kidneys. The original medication or its metabolite (the chemical produced following biotransformation) is filtered by the kidneys and excreted into the urine. Several factors influence how quickly the medication is eliminated from the body. Notably, kidney dysfunction or disease impairs the elimination of many substances. Patients with acute or chronic renal failure are at significant risk for toxic effects of medications or metabolic waste products in the body. Renal blood flow, urinary tract obstruction, and alterations in urine pH may all affect the kidneys' ability to remove medication and toxins from the body.

Medications and chemicals in the body follow two distinct patterns of metabolism and elimination: zero-order elimination and first-order elimination. Under **zero-order elimination**, a fixed amount of a substance is removed during a certain period, regardless of the total amount in the body. Ethanol is a classic example of zero-order elimination. Chronic consumption of ethanol increases the liver's ability to metabolize ethanol because of enhanced activation of the cytochrome P-450 system. Despite the increased elimination rate, only a fixed amount of ethanol will be eliminated each hour, regardless of the initial plasma level. The duration of intoxication is directly related to the initial plasma level.

The majority of medications and chemicals undergo **first-order elimination**, in which the plasma levels of the substance directly influence the rate of elimination. In essence, the more substance in the plasma, the more the body works to eliminate the substance. First-order elimination is quantified as

YOU are the Paramedic

PART 3

You give the patient oxygen via a nonrebreathing mask; however, the patient resists keeping the mask in place. One of the staff nurses assists with providing oxygen to the patient while you establish IV access by placing an 18-gauge catheter into the patient's right antecubital space and obtain a blood glucose level. Your partner obtains vital signs and places the patient on the cardiac monitor.

Recording Time: 10 Minutes	
Respirations	22 breaths/min
Pulse	108 beats/min, regular
Skin	Pale, warm, dry
Blood pressure	96/64 mm Hg
Oxygen saturation (Spo_2)	98% on 10 L/min oxygen via nonrebreathing mask
Blood glucose level	132 mg/dL
ECG	Sinus tachycardia with motion artifact

4. Would IV dextrose solution be indicated for this patient?

5. Do the ECG findings assist in identifying the cause of this patient's condition?

the medication's **half-life** on the medication profile. The half-life of a medication is the time needed in an average person for the metabolism or elimination of 50% of the substance in the plasma. It takes much longer than two half-lives to completely eliminate a medication, despite the literal meaning of the term. A medication's half-life can be altered by factors such as disease states, changes in perfusion, and medication interactions. Consider the following example of half-life calculations:

> Patient A has taken an overdose of medication X, which has a half-life of 2 hours. The plasma level of the medication on arrival to the emergency department was 100 mcg/mL. After 2 hours, the plasma level will be 50 mcg/mL. Four hours after arrival, the plasma level will be 25 mcg/mL. After another 2 hours, the plasma level will be 12.5 mcg/mL.

A medication half-life pertains only to the quantity of medication within the body, not necessarily to the clinical effects of the medication. Aspirin, as discussed earlier, has a half-life of only 15 to 20 minutes, but it causes antiplatelet effects that can last for up to 10 days. Adenosine, a medication given in the prehospital setting for tachydysrhythmias, has a half-life of less than 10 seconds, but it may permanently resolve supraventricular tachycardia. The benzodiazepine clonazepam (Klonopin) has a long half-life: 19 to 50 hours in adults. Patients often remain sedated for several days following an intentional overdose.

Physicians and other health care providers attempt to create a steady state when administering certain medications. In other words, they try to administer medications at a dose and frequency that equal the body's elimination rate, resulting in a constant level of medication within the body. A medication steady state is desirable for anticoagulants, antibiotics, antiseizure medications, and some antidysrhythmic medications. You should suspect changes in the steady state of a medication when patients manifest symptoms of an underlying disease (eg, seizures or dysrhythmia) that is usually well controlled by long-term medications.

Smaller amounts of medication, medication metabolites, and other chemicals can be eliminated through other body systems, such as in expired air from the lungs, stool, saliva, breast milk, and perspiration. When given orally, activated charcoal can bind with certain oral toxins (and several chemicals present in the bloodstream) and eliminate them through the GI tract. (Activated charcoal is discussed further in Chapter 28, *Toxicology*.)

Reducing Medication Errors

As a paramedic, you will have the difficult tasks of assessing patients, performing invasive procedures, and administering medications in the uncontrolled prehospital setting. In this environment, the patient history is often limited, inaccurate, or nonexistent. You will not always have the time or resources to carefully evaluate the risks and benefits associated with medications you are considering administering to a patient. Medication decisions are often based on memory and frequently occur in the context of a stressful, life-threatening patient situation. You and other paramedics are constantly at risk for making a cognitive error, such as choosing the wrong medication or dose, or a technical error, such as administering a greater volume of medication than was intended. **TABLE 13-9** lists the rights of medication administration.

TABLE 13-9 The Rights of Medication Administration

Right Patient
Although you will typically treat one patient at a time, sometimes you may have to treat multiple patients. It is essential to confirm the identity of a patient before administering any medication, especially when patients are unresponsive or are unable to communicate (because of extremes of age, altered level of consciousness, or other factors). Always attempt to have the patient confirm their identity verbally, or confirm the identity of the patient yourself through identification devices (eg, a bracelet or ID card), to the extent possible. A critical issue, as identified in the SAMPLE (Signs/symptoms, Allergies, Medications, Pertinent past history, Last oral intake, Events leading to injury or illness) history, is to ensure that the patient does not have allergies to the medication(s) you intend to give **FIGURE 13-3**.

(continues)

TABLE 13-9 The Rights of Medication Administration (continued)
Right Medication and Indication
Administration of the wrong medication is the most common pharmacology-related error. Several factors may lead to "wrong medication" errors, including similar packaging and labeling, similar names and storage practices, and ineffective communication. Always repeat (echo) the medication order, and confirm that the packaging matches the intended order. Avoid using abbreviations, and always recheck the order before administering the medication. Confirm indications and contraindications. Ensure that the medication is appropriate for the patient's medical condition and medical history.
Right Dose
Doses of nearly every medication depend on patient-specific factors (eg, condition, weight, and age). The actual dose needed is often not equal to the amount supplied in an ampule or a prefilled syringe in the prehospital setting. Therefore, you will have to calculate the patient-specific dose. When calculating the correct dose, always recheck your math and, if possible, have your partner recheck and verify the final dose.
Right Route
Many medications can be administered by a variety of routes; the optimal route depends on the patient's condition and the speed with which the medication needs to take effect. Errors can occur when medication doses and routes are confused. For example, IV drip doses can be different from doses for the same medication injected into an IV as a bolus. Another important route-related issue is the patient's condition. If a patient is in profound shock, you must consider how well the medication will be absorbed and distributed to the target tissues. Choosing the right route helps ensure the medication will have the correct effect. Always verify the route of administration.
Right Time
Because all medications take a certain amount of time to take effect and may have the potential to interfere with other medications, you must always follow the recommended guidelines for the proper frequency of medication administration. Evaluate the patient's condition before and after you administer any medication, and document any noted response or change in the patient's condition. Also remember that some medications require a specific administration frequency to maintain a therapeutic level.
Right Patient Education
Patient education should begin as soon as possible. Responsive patients should be informed of any pertinent risks and benefits before medication administration. Involve responsive patients in ongoing evaluation and monitoring by informing them of any important symptoms they may experience or that should be reported.
Right to Refuse
Respect patient autonomy. Patients with decision-making capacity or a surrogate decision maker may refuse medications and other interventions, even if refusing a medication may result in harm. Consult online medical control in any high-risk situation. Make sure the patient is aware of the potential consequences of refusing a medication or treatment.
Right Response and Evaluation
Continually monitor the patient. Observe for desired effects and any possible adverse reactions for any medication administered. Certain medications may require careful monitoring; other medications may require multiple doses to achieve the desired effect.
Right Documentation and Reporting
Because you will almost always transfer care of a patient to other health care providers, it is critical to document in writing the medications administered, the dose, the time when they were administered, and the effects the patient experienced. Whenever possible, communicate this information in writing (on the patient care report) and in a verbal report to the next level of care.

Abbreviation: IV, intravenous

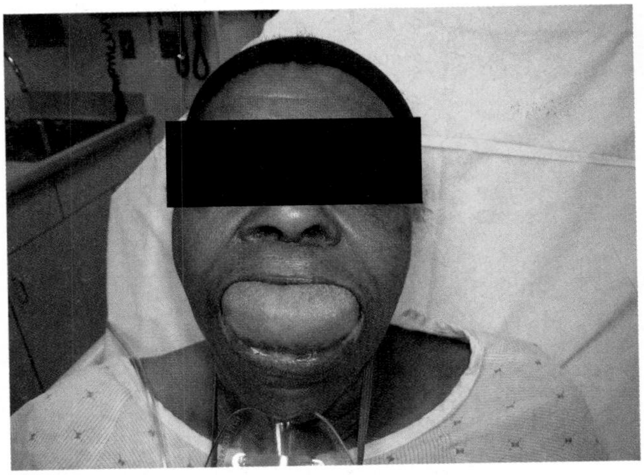

FIGURE 13-3 Angioedema is acute swelling, sometimes of the lips and tongue, that may be caused by an allergic reaction. Some medications cause angioedema after the first or second dose.

Patient safety experts strongly recommend using specific practices to decrease the likelihood of medication errors. Perform a verbal read-back of any orders received from online medical control. The read-back should include the medication, dose, and route. When multiple providers are present, call out the medication name and dose before its administration. Both of these practices allow your colleagues the opportunity to catch potential medication errors before they reach the patient.

Unlabeled syringes pose a significant hazard in health care. Many medications are supplied in vials, requiring that providers draw the medication into a syringe. Because most injectable medications are supplied as a clear liquid, and because the same medication may be supplied in different concentrations, a medication drawn into a syringe may not have any readily noticeable identifying characteristics. Whenever possible, use premade stickers or hand-written labels that indicate at least the medication's name and concentration, even if the medication is intended to be administered immediately. In EMS, workflow is frequently disrupted, which may result in the presence of several syringes on the scene. In addition, there may be a delay between when a medication is drawn into a syringe and when it is actually administered to the patient.

Patient safety experts recommend building an environment where EMS providers feel comfortable reporting errors (and near misses). In these environments, errors are identified/disclosed and evaluated, and system changes are implemented to prevent future occurrences. In this type of environment, often referred to as a "just culture," the focus is on improving systems rather than seeking to punish individuals.

Before transporting a patient to a health care facility, attempt to locate and bring the patient's current home medications with you. Having the medications on hand allows the receiving health care providers to accurately transcribe the various medications, doses, frequency, and other pertinent information, rather than rely on the patient's memory or notes from EMS personnel.

You should use a current, reliable medication reference source whenever you are administering potentially unfamiliar medications or considering an unusual dose or route of administration. To help avoid technical errors, have your partner confirm the volume in a syringe or a weight-based medication calculation. Many health care settings require that two providers check pediatric and high-risk medication calculations. You should also evaluate for a patient medication allergy or hypersensitivity before each medication administration.

The Joint Commission and the Institute for Safe Medication Practices have each developed a list of medication abbreviations that should be considered dangerous in the health care setting. When physicians, paramedics, and other health care providers use these symbols and abbreviations, there is an increased likelihood of a medication error due to miscommunication. Error-prone symbols and abbreviations and medical terms related to pharmacology are discussed in Chapter 7, *Medical Terminology*.

Drugs That Act on the Sympathetic Nervous System

As discussed earlier, receptor sites exist in proteins connected to cells throughout the body. Receptors are activated by chemicals, whether naturally occurring or in the form of a medication. Drugs that influence the sympathetic nervous system are classified according to the receptors with which they interact **TABLE 13-10**.

A drug receptor is comparable to the ignition switch in a car. When the proper key is inserted into the car's ignition and turned, a predictable

TABLE 13-10 Important Receptor Sites Within the Body

Receptor	Agonist Effect
Alpha(α)	• α-1 receptors cause constriction of peripheral small arteries and arterioles, vascular smooth muscle, and bladder and GI sphincters. • α-2 receptors inhibit pancreatic enzyme and insulin release, suppress norepinephrine release, and inhibit GI motility.
Beta (β)	• β-1 receptors (mnemonic: one heart = beta-1) increase heart rate (chronotropic effect), myocardial contractility (inotropic effect), and myocardial conduction (dromotropic effect); they also affect renin secretion. • β-2 receptors (mnemonic: two lungs = beta-2) cause bronchodilation; cause dilation of arterioles of the heart, lungs, and skeletal muscle; inhibit insulin release; increase release of glucagon; and cause relaxation of the intestines, bladder, and uterus. • β-3 receptors increase lipolysis and heat production in fat.
Dopaminergic[a]	Each type of dopamine receptor has a unique function: • D1: memory, attention, impulse control, regulation of renal function, locomotion • D2: locomotion, attention, sleep, memory, learning • D3: cognition, impulse control, attention, sleep • D4: cognition, impulse control, attention, sleep • D5: decision making, cognition, attention, renin secretion
Nicotinic	These receptors allow acetylcholine to stimulate muscle contraction.
Muscarinic	The muscarinic receptors have the following functions: • M1: affect cognition, arousal, gastric acid secretion • M2 (cardiac): decrease heart rate and contractility • M3: stimulate gland secretion and smooth muscle contraction • M4: act on potassium and calcium channels • M5: affect dopamine release
Opioid	• Mu (μ) receptors are the most prominent, with the greatest affinity for both morphine and naloxone (opioid antagonist); stimulation causes analgesia, sedation, mood changes, constricted pupils, respiratory depression, and decreased GI motility. • Delta receptor stimulation causes spinal analgesia, respiratory depression, and decreased GI motility. • Kappa receptor stimulation causes spinal analgesia, sedation, dysphoria, and decreased GI motility.

Abbreviation: GI, gastrointestinal

[a] Bhatia A, Lenchner JR, Saadabadi A. Biochemistry, dopamine receptors. *StatPearls*. https://www.ncbi.nlm.nih.gov/books/NBK538242/. Updated July 26, 2020. Accessed July 5, 2021; and Mishra A, Singh S, Shukla S. Physiological and functional basis of dopamine receptors and their role in neurogenesis: possible implication for Parkinson's disease. *J Exp Neurosci*. 2018;12. doi:10.1177/1179069518779829.

sequence of events follows: The battery sends a current to the starter and the spark plugs, which fire; combustion of gasoline and air occurs; and the engine starts. Although many keys may fit into a specific car's ignition, not every key that fits will turn and start the car, but all that do turn cause the same reaction. Likewise, the organs of the body have several "ignition switches." In the sympathetic nervous system, those switches (receptors), are labeled alpha and beta. Whenever one of those switches is activated by a "key" (a drug or hormone), a predictable sequence of responses occurs.

The heart has only one ignition switch for a beta agent. A beta agonist will increase the heart's rate, force, and **automaticity** (generation of a spontaneous impulse from within). The arteries, by contrast, have receptors for alpha and beta agents. An alpha agonist will turn on the switch that causes **vasoconstriction**; a beta agonist will activate the switch that causes **vasodilation**. Similarly, the lungs

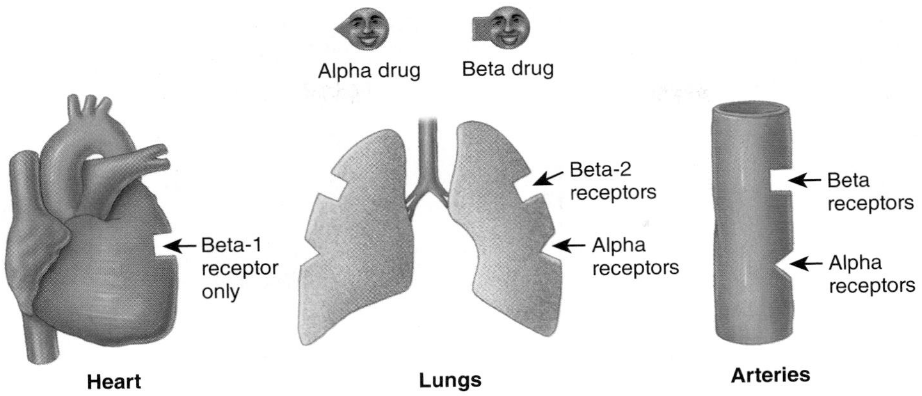

FIGURE 13-4 Receptor sites of the sympathetic nervous system in the heart, lungs, and arteries.

have alpha and beta receptors. Alpha agents do not have much effect on the lungs; at most, they cause minor **bronchoconstriction**. By contrast, beta adrenergic agonists (such as drugs used to treat asthma) trigger significant **bronchodilation**. **FIGURE 13-4** depicts these concepts schematically.

Drugs with alpha or beta properties are called sympathomimetic drugs because they imitate (mimic) the actions of naturally occurring sympathetic chemicals. If you know whether a sympathomimetic drug is an alpha or a beta agent, you can predict the response by the heart, lungs, and arteries. Consider, for example, isoproterenol (Isuprel). It is a pure beta agent. Armed with this knowledge, you can immediately recognize that isoproterenol acts in the manner shown in **FIGURE 13-5**; it stimulates the heart, dilates the bronchi, and dilates the arteries. Phenylephrine (Neo-Synephrine), by contrast, is a pure alpha agent. It has no direct effect on the heart but causes slight bronchoconstriction and marked vasoconstriction **FIGURE 13-6**.

Unfortunately, predicting the effects of a drug is not always so simple. Although isoproterenol and phenylephrine are pure beta and alpha agents, respectively, most other sympathomimetic drugs have varying degrees of alpha and beta activity **FIGURE 13-7**. For example, norepinephrine (Levophed) is chiefly an alpha agent and primarily causes vasoconstriction; however, because it has some beta activity, it will also affect the heart. Epinephrine (Adrenalin) likewise exerts effects on both alpha and beta receptors. When given in small doses, it has a greater affinity for beta receptors, but alpha receptor stimulation predominates when given in larger doses. Norepinephrine and epinephrine are also naturally occurring chemicals of the sympathetic nervous system. Their actions are the same whether they are produced in the body and released

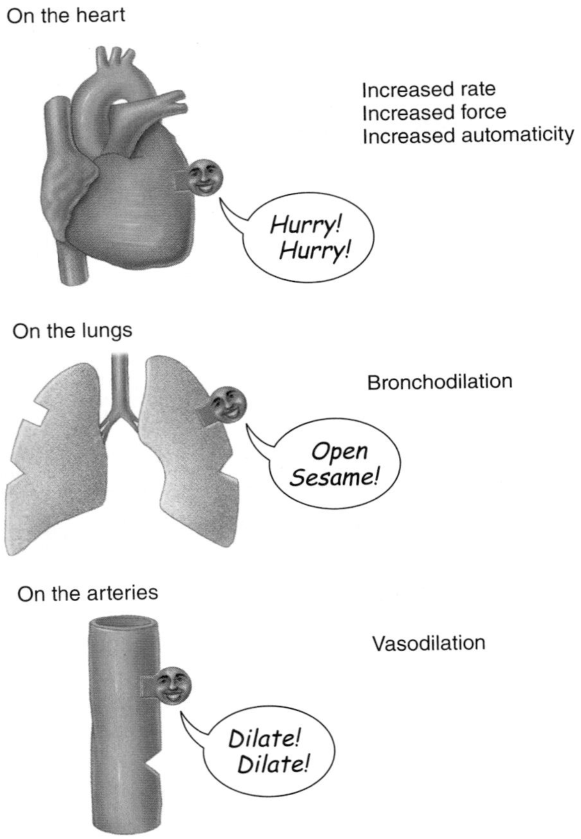

FIGURE 13-5 Beta sympathetic agents increase the rate, force, and automaticity of the heart; dilate the bronchi; and dilate peripheral arteries.

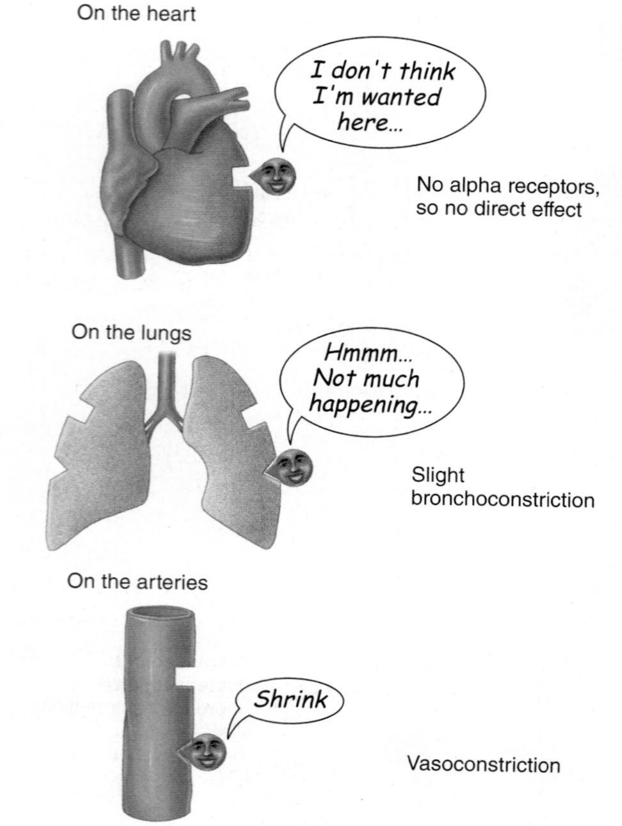

FIGURE 13-6 Alpha agents have no direct effect on the heart; they cause slight bronchoconstriction and marked vasoconstriction.

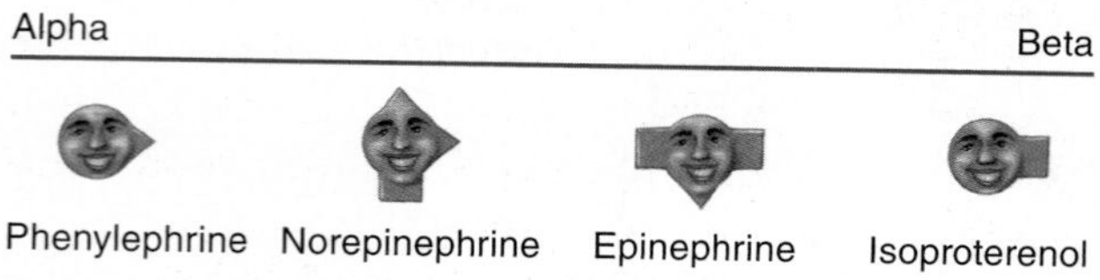

FIGURE 13-7 While some sympathomimetic agents stimulate alpha (phenylephrine) or beta (isoproterenol) receptor sites, others (eg, norepinephrine, epinephrine) exert varying effects on both alpha and beta receptors.

from the nervous system or manufactured in a factory and injected.

Beta sympathetic agents can be classified into two groups based on the subtle differences between the beta receptors in the heart and the lungs. Drugs that act primarily on cardiac beta receptors are called beta-1 adrenergic agonists; those acting chiefly on pulmonary beta receptors are called

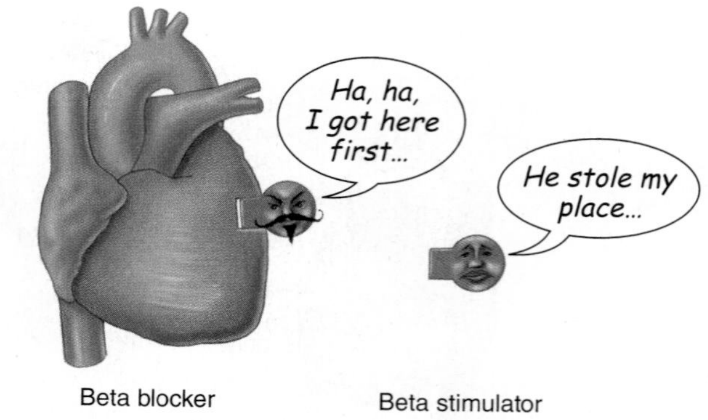

FIGURE 13-8 A sympathetic blocker (antagonist) occupies the receptor site for the stimulating drug (agonist), thereby preventing the stimulating drug from exerting its usual effect.

beta-2 adrenergic agonists. Commonly prescribed bronchodilators (beta-2 adrenergic agonists) include albuterol, formoterol, salbuterol, levalbuterol, and salmeterol.

Another class of drugs that acts on the sympathetic nervous system comprises the sympatholytic or sympathetic blockers. As their name implies, they block the action of sympathetic agents by beating them to the receptor sites and preventing these agents from turning on the ignition. The receptor sites cannot distinguish a blocker from a stimulator until it is too late. With the blocker occupying the receptor site, the stimulating agent cannot access it to turn on the switch **FIGURE 13-8**.

Words of Wisdom

To remember which type of adrenergic agonist (beta-1 or beta-2) acts on which type of beta receptor, ask yourself, "How many hearts do I have?" One heart: beta-1. "How many lungs do I have?" Two lungs: beta-2.

Beta adrenergic blockers occupy beta receptors in the heart, lungs, and arteries, and elsewhere in the body. Thus, beta agents, whether released from sympathetic nerve endings or given intravenously, cannot exert their full effects when a beta blocker such as propranolol (Inderal) or metoprolol (Lopressor) has been administered previously **FIGURE 13-9**.

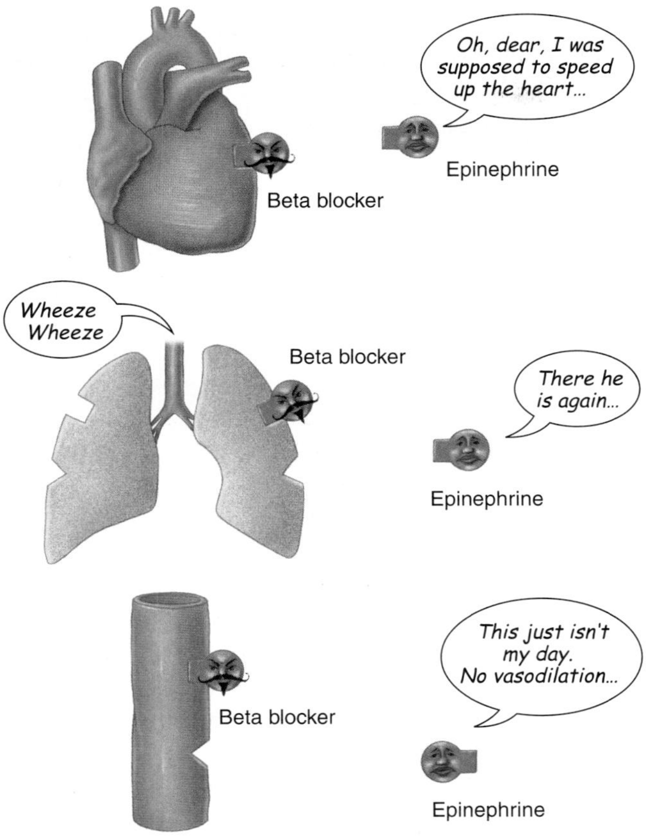

FIGURE 13-9 By occupying beta receptor sites, the beta blocker prevents epinephrine from exerting its usual effects on the heart, lungs, and blood vessels.

> **Words of Wisdom**
>
> The indications for the major autonomic stimulating and blocking agents can be deduced once you know the properties of the drugs and how they interact with the autonomic nervous system.

Important Medications in the Prehospital Setting

As a paramedic, you must understand the indications and limitations of several important groups of medications. The following sections provide an overview of the medications and medication groups used to treat medical conditions primarily affecting specific body systems. Many of these medication groups have indications for a wide range of medical conditions, including outside the context of a particular body system **TABLE 13-11**.

Medications Used in Airway Management

In certain EMS systems, you may be permitted to use a variety of medications for airway management. Rapid sequence intubation and medication-facilitated airway placement are controversial procedures in the prehospital setting and are not permitted in all locations. In these procedures, sedative medications with or without chemical paralytic medications are used to secure an artificial airway in patients with an intact gag reflex and some degree of responsiveness. When patients become adequately sedated, the gag reflex disappears and trismus or other facial muscle tension ceases following the correct use and sequence of airway medication. If performed correctly, patients have no awareness or memory of the procedure.

Sedative-Hypnotic Agents Used in Airway Management

Etomidate (Amidate) and ketamine (Ketalar) are two ultra-short-acting sedative medications used to facilitate airway placement. Etomidate works as a single-dose profound sedative and is preferred because of its minimal effect on BP and other hemodynamic parameters. Its short duration of action is usually desirable for airway procedures, but the patient will need to be promptly resedated with an alternative sedative medication during or immediately after inserting the airway device.

Ketamine is another possible adjunct to airway placement. It has a chemical composition similar to phencyclidine (PCP) and causes profound dissociation and general anesthesia. Ketamine can maintain the BP and heart rate, but raises intracranial pressure, making it less than optimal for patients with head injury who require airway placement. This medication causes some degree of bronchodilation, which is potentially helpful in patients with asthma or COPD who require airway placement for respiratory failure. Some providers and settings are using ketamine to control refractory pain or delirium unresponsive to other medications. Check with your medical director on their thoughts about this medication.

TABLE 13-11 Notable Medication Groups Affecting Prehospital Patient Care

Medication Class	Common Indications or Purposes	Primary Body System Affected	Examples
Alkalinizing agents	Increase serum or urine pH	Renal	Sodium bicarbonate
Alkylating agents	Group of cancer medications that attack the DNA of cancer cells, causing cell death	Varied	Cisplatin, cyclophosphamide (Cytoxan), ifosfamide (Ifex)
Antacids	Neutralize excess acids present in the stomach	GI	Sucralfate (Carafate), aluminum salts, calcium carbonate
Anthelmintics	Treat intestinal parasites	GI	Mebendazole (Vermox)
Antibiotics	Treat bacterial infection	Varied	Penicillin, ciprofloxacin (Cipro)
Anticoagulants	Reduce efficacy of clotting factors present in the blood	Hematologic	Heparin, warfarin (Coumadin)
Antidiarrheals	Decrease GI motility, alter GI secretion activity	GI	Loperamide (Imodium), diphenoxylate-atropine combination (Lomotil)
Antidysrhythmics	Prevent or control various cardiac dysrhythmias	Cardiovascular	Lidocaine, amiodarone (Cordarone)
Antiemetics	Treat or prevent nausea and vomiting	GI, CNS	Promethazine (Phenergan), ondansetron (Zofran)
Antiflatulents	Prevent or treat excess intestinal gas	GI	Simethicone, lactase
Antifungals	Treat fungal infections	Varied	Fluconazole (Diflucan), ketoconazole (Nizoral)
Antiglaucoma agents (usually eyedrops)	Treat glaucoma	Varied	Brinzolamide (Azopt), bimatoprost (Lumigan)
Antihistamines	Block histamine receptors, dry mucous membranes, inhibit immune response in allergic reactions	Varied	Diphenhydramine (Benadryl), loratadine (Claritin)
Antihyperlipidemics	Decrease blood cholesterol, sequester cholesterol chemicals in bile	Hematologic, cardiovascular	Cholestyramine (Questran), colesevelam (Welchol)
Antimetabolites	Cancer medications that mimic normal substances within a cell, disrupt cell metabolism, and kill cancer cells	Varied	Methotrexate (Rheumatrex, Trexall) 5-fluorouracil (5-FU, Adrucil)
Antiparasitic agents	Treat parasitic infections	Varied	Nitazoxanide (Alinia)
Antipsychotics	Treat psychoses, including schizophrenia	Sympathetic nervous system	Haloperidol (Haldol), olanzapine (Zyprexa)

Medication Class	Common Indications or Purposes	Primary Body System Affected	Examples
Antitumor antibiotics	Antibiotic medications (as described earlier) that have the additional ability to target and kill certain cancer cells	Varied	Doxorubicin (Adriamycin), mitomycin (Mutamycin)
Antivirals	Treat viral infections	Varied	Acyclovir (Zovirax), famciclovir (Famvir)
Barbiturates	Reduce or prevent seizures, provide sedation	CNS	Phenobarbital
Benzodiazepines	Treat anxiety and seizures, provide sedation	CNS	Lorazepam (Ativan), diazepam (Valium), oxazepam (Serax)
Beta agonists	Bronchodilation	Respiratory	Albuterol, levalbuterol (Xopenex)
Beta blocking agents	Reduce heart rate and BP	Cardiovascular	Metoprolol (Lopressor), atenolol (Tenormin)
Calcium channel blockers	Reduce heart rate and BP	Cardiovascular	Diltiazem (Cardizem), verapamil (Calan)
Cardiac glycosides	Decrease heart rate and improve contractility	Cardiovascular	Digoxin (Lanoxin)
Chemotherapeutic agents	Treat cancer or malignancy	Varied	Vincristine (Oncovin, Vincasar), cisplatin (Platinol)
Cholesterol synthesis inhibitors	Prevent cholesterol conversion in the liver	GI	Atorvastatin (Lipitor), simvastatin (Zocor)
Cholinergics	Activate secretory glands in eyes and GI tract; improve muscle weakness in myasthenia gravis	Parasympathetic nervous system	Pilocarpine (Isopto); pyridostigmine (Mestinon)
Corticosteroids	Decrease inflammation; immunosuppressant; replace or augment function of the adrenal cortex (see glucocorticoids and mineralocorticoids entries)	Endocrine and immune	Prednisone, dexamethasone (Decadron)
Cough suppressants	Decrease bronchial irritation causing cough	CNS	Codeine, dextromethorphan
Digestants	Enhance digestion of food; may include supplemental pancreatic enzymes	GI	Glutamine
Diuretics	Promote excretion of urine; relieve fluid overload	Renal	Mannitol (Osmitrol), furosemide (Lasix)
Fibrinolytics	Dissolve clots present in blood vessels or vascular access devices	Hematologic	Tissue plasminogen activator (tPA), tenecteplase (TNKase)

(continues)

TABLE 13-11 Notable Medication Groups Affecting Prehospital Patient Care (continued)

Medication Class	Common Indications or Purposes	Primary Body System Affected	Examples
Glucocorticoids	Replacement or maintenance therapy, treat systemic inflammation, numerous other uses	Endocrine and immune	Hydrocortisone, beclomethasone (Beconase)
Glycoprotein IIb/IIIa inhibitors	Deactivate proteins involved in platelet aggregation	Hematologic	Tirofiban (Aggrastat), eptifibatide (Integrilin)
$Histamine_2$ receptor antagonists	Block histamine receptors, including those responsible for gastric acid secretion	GI and immune	Famotidine (Pepcid)
Hormone replacement drugs	Replace hormones; improve bone density that has decreased due to aging and hormone loss; replace or augment function of impaired pituitary or thyroid glands	Endocrine	Estrogen, progesterone, levothyroxine (Synthroid), testosterone, recombinant human growth hormone
Immunomodulators	Inhibit or enhance functioning of the immune system	Immune	Interferon, levamisole (Ergamisol)
Immunosuppressants	Prevent rejection of transplanted organs and tissues; treat rheumatoid arthritis	Immune	Cyclosporine (Gengraf), tacrolimus (Prograf)
Insulin	Positive inotropic effects, allows cellular glucose uptake, treat hyperkalemia	Endocrine	Insulin (Humalog, Humulin)
Laxatives	Increase GI motility	GI	Bisacodyl (Dulcolax), docusate (Colace)
Mineralocorticoids	Promote sodium and water retention	Endocrine and immune	Fludrocortisone (Florinef)
Mucolytics	Assist with elimination of mucus in the respiratory tract	Pulmonary	Acetylcysteine (Mucomyst)
Mydriatics	Dilate pupils for ocular diagnostic and treatment procedures	Ocular and parasympathetic nervous system	Cyclopentolate (Cyclogyl)
Nasal decongestants	Decrease upper airway mucus secretion	Sympathetic nervous system	Pseudoephedrine (Sudafed), phenylephrine (Neo-Synephrine)
Neuromuscular blocking agents	Provide chemical paralysis in intubated and ventilated patients	Peripheral nervous system and musculoskeletal	Succinylcholine (Anectine), rocuronium (Zemuron)
Nonsteroidal anti-inflammatory drugs	Treat pain and inflammation	Endocrine	Ibuprofen (Motrin, Advil), ketorolac (Toradol), indomethacin (Indocin)
Opioid analgesics	Relieve pain and relieve or suppress cough	CNS	Morphine, oxycodone

Medication Class	Common Indications or Purposes	Primary Body System Affected	Examples
Oral contraceptives	Prevent conception (pregnancy)	Endocrine and genitourinary	Estrogen, progesterone
Oral hypoglycemic agents	Treat type 2 diabetes mellitus	Endocrine	Glyburide (Diabeta), metformin (Glucophage), glipizide (Glucotrol)
Phosphodiesterase inhibitors	Treat erectile dysfunction	Cardiovascular	Sildenafil (Viagra), tadalafil (Cialis)
Plant alkaloids	Cancer medications derived from plants	Varied	Vincristine (Vincasar), etoposide (Toposar)
Platelet inhibitors	Decrease platelet aggregation in patients at risk of thrombus formation	Hematologic	Aspirin, clopidogrel (Plavix)
Protein pump inhibitors	Suppress activity of parietal cell acid secretion	GI	Omeprazole (Prilosec), esomeprazole (Nexium)
Selective serotonin reuptake inhibitors	Treat depression, anxiety, and related conditions	CNS	Paroxetine (Paxil), sertraline (Zoloft)
Sympathomimetics	Increase BP, heart rate, and cardiac output; constrict blood vessels	Cardiovascular	Epinephrine (Adrenalin), phenylephrine (Neo-Synephrine)
Tocolytics	Decrease or eliminate uterine contractions during preterm labor	Endocrine and genitourinary	Magnesium sulfate
Tricyclic antidepressants	Treat depression, neuropathy, and chronic pain syndromes	CNS	Amitriptyline (Elavil), doxepin, desipramine (Norpramin)
Xanthines	Bronchodilation	Respiratory	Theophylline (Uniphyl)

Abbreviations: BP, blood pressure; CNS, central nervous system; GI, gastrointestinal

Benzodiazepines

Benzodiazepine medications are widely used in the prehospital setting, including diazepam, lorazepam, and midazolam. Patients may be prescribed other benzodiazepines such as clonazepam and temazepam (Restoril) for use on a long-term basis. Benzodiazepines have potent antiseizure, anxiolytic, and sedative properties, making them desirable in many situations. These agents can be used as the primary sedative for airway placement procedures, but high doses are generally required to achieve adequate sedation. At high doses, benzodiazepines cause hypotension, which will further complicate the condition of a patient with shock or multiple trauma. Thus, these medications are best used for maintenance sedation following airway placement.

Benzodiazepines provide some degree of seizure protection in patients with head injuries. Active seizures can be treated initially with IV, IM, intranasal, and rectal administration of these medications. Lower doses may also be helpful to reduce anxiety, although this use is not approved in all EMS systems.

All three benzodiazepine medications used in prehospital practice (ie, diazepam, lorazepam, and midazolam) are classified as pregnancy class D, which means they have demonstrated potential harm to the fetus. These medications should be administered to pregnant patients only during life-threatening situations when no safer alternative medications are available.

Chemical Paralytic Agents

Two classes of chemical paralytic agents (depolarizing and nondepolarizing) may be used in the prehospital setting. These medications provide muscle relaxation that facilitates airway device placement and prevents patient-ventilator asynchrony during mechanical ventilation. Paralytic agents allow better visualization of airway structures than when only sedative medications are used. The class of chemical paralytic agent used largely influences the onset and duration of muscle relaxation.

Under normal circumstances, nerve cells release acetylcholine (ACh), which binds to nicotinic receptor sites on muscle cells, causing muscle contraction. Chemical paralytic (neuromuscular blocking) medications bind with nicotinic receptor sites on muscle cells, antagonizing (preventing activation by) ACh **FIGURE 13-10**.

Succinylcholine (Anectine) is a **competitive depolarizing** paralytic agent. It reaches the neuromuscular junction, binds with nicotinic receptors on muscles, causes a transient activation known as **fasciculation**, and prevents additional activation by ACh. Many health care providers prefer succinylcholine because of its rapid onset (within 60 seconds) and relatively brief duration of effect (4 to 6 minutes). Malignant hyperthermia is a rare but immediately life-threatening, adverse reaction to succinylcholine; it is characterized by severe hyperthermia (elevated temperature), muscle rigidity, and metabolic acidosis. Other anesthetic agents also can cause this disorder. Patients able to communicate should be screened for personal or family reactions to anesthesia before you administer succinylcholine to them.

Words of Wisdom

Because of the serious adverse reactions that may potentially occur with succinylcholine administration, many clinicians prefer to use other neuromuscular blocking agents, even if the other agents have a significantly longer duration of action.

Several **nondepolarizing** paralytic agents are used in the prehospital or critical care transport setting. Nondepolarizing agents compete with ACh at nicotinic receptor sites. They occupy (but do not activate) these receptor sites, thereby preventing their activation by ACh. Members of this drug class generally have a longer duration than succinylcholine and fewer adverse effects. Rocuronium

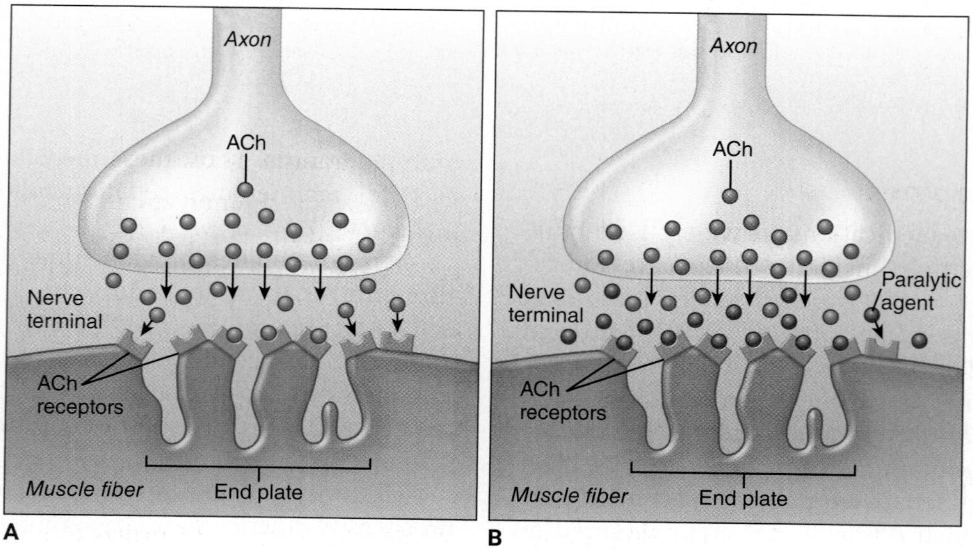

FIGURE 13-10 Chemical paralytic medications bind with nicotinic receptor sites on muscle cells, antagonizing acetylcholine (ACh). **A.** Normal function of nerve cells, in which ACh binds to its receptors. **B.** Effect of chemical paralytic medication, in which ACh receptors are blocked.

(Zemuron) has the most rapid onset combined with a shorter duration (30 to 60 minutes), making it an appropriate nondepolarizing agent for the placement of airway devices in emergency situations. Vecuronium (Norcuron) may also be administered either as an adjunct or as a sole chemical paralytic agent for emergency airway procedures. It has a shorter duration of action (20 to 35 minutes) than rocuronium.

Depolarizing and nondepolarizing chemical paralytic agents create an immediate threat to life if they are administered by paramedics who cannot secure an artificial airway. Paramedics authorized to administer these medications must be proficient with bag-mask ventilation and skilled with the placement of backup "rescue" airway devices, as discussed in Chapter 16, *Airway Management*. If you are not able to oxygenate and ventilate a patient adequately following administration of a chemical paralytic agent, potentially fatal complications are likely.

Other Airway Medications

Paramedics in certain EMS systems may use medications to treat upper airway edema in patients who are responsive and spontaneously breathing. Specifically, corticosteroid, vasoconstrictor, and bronchodilator medications may be administered when upper airway edema is present. These medications are discussed later in this chapter.

Medications Used in Respiratory Management

Effective respiration requires adequate oxygenation and ventilation. Respiratory emergencies can be a primary complaint or the manifestation of a disease process in another body system. Medication groups discussed in this section relate to primary respiratory conditions such as asthma and COPD.

Beta Agonist Medications

Beta adrenergic agonist medications remain the primary treatment for acute bronchospasm associated with asthma, COPD, and other conditions. When activated by beta-2 agonist medications, beta-2 receptor sites on bronchial smooth muscle cause muscle relaxation and bronchodilation. Paramedics can administer a variety of beta-2 agonists to patients experiencing bronchospasm.

Beta agonist medications can be selective, targeting only beta-2 receptor sites, or nonselective, affecting both beta-1 and beta-2 receptor sites. Despite their advertised selectivity, many beta-2 agonist medications actually demonstrate some degree of beta-1 activation. Thus, you must carefully monitor for adverse cardiovascular effects whenever you administer beta agonist medications.

Albuterol (Ventolin, Proventil) is a commonly used selective beta-2 agonist. This medication is typically nebulized or administered using an MDI for the emergency treatment of bronchospasm. Albuterol may cause varying degrees of tachycardia, especially during prolonged administration. It can promote cellular uptake of potassium, making it a potential temporary treatment for hyperkalemia until definitive potassium removal occurs. Levalbuterol is structurally similar to albuterol, without many of the reported beta-1 effects.

Mucokinetic and Bronchodilator Medications

Paramedics may supplement beta agonist medications with ipratropium bromide or a similar medication when treating patients with bronchospasm or reactive airway disease. Ipratropium bromide is a short-acting antimuscarinic agent, which means that it antagonizes muscarinic receptors, causing bronchodilation and decreased mucus in the upper and lower airways. Cardiovascular effects from ipratropium are usually limited because of its poor systemic absorption.

Corticosteroids

Many respiratory emergencies involve some degree of airway inflammation. In the prehospital setting, corticosteroid medications are administered to reduce airway inflammation and, ultimately, improve oxygenation and ventilation. These medications significantly reduce the severity of respiratory compromise from asthma, COPD, allergic reactions, and other causes of airway inflammation. Methylprednisolone (Solu-Medrol), dexamethasone (Decadron), and prednisone are administered in some prehospital systems. Corticosteroid medications have immunosuppressant properties and can alter an array of endocrine functions. These medications have many contraindications and adverse effects, so EMS systems may limit or restrict their use by paramedics. If you are permitted to administer these medications, you must take care to evaluate the potential risks and benefits for each patient.

Leukotriene Receptor Antagonists

Patients with asthma have an overproduction of chemicals called leukotrienes. Leukotrienes bind to receptor sites within the lungs, causing powerful bronchoconstriction as well as inflammatory, mucus-promoting, and vascular permeability effects. They are reported to be exponentially more potent at causing bronchoconstriction than histamines. Leukotriene receptor antagonist medications, such as montelukast (Singulair) and zafirlukast (Accolate), are taken by patients with asthma and certain allergies on a long-term basis. These medications are intended to provide long-term symptom relief, and are not used to treat emergent episodes of bronchospasm and inflammation.

Medications Affecting the Cardiovascular System

The cardiovascular system is divided into three functional components: the pump (heart), the plumbing (arteries, veins, and capillaries), and the blood. Many medications are used to affect one or more of these components. Blood products and medications affecting the functions of the blood are discussed separately in other chapters. Antidysrhythmic medications specifically target cells within the heart to resolve a dysrhythmia or suppress **ectopic foci** (sites of electrical impulse generation other than normal pacemaker cells). Many antidysrhythmic medications affect cells in other parts of the cardiovascular system or throughout the body. Still other cardiovascular medications alter the activity of the heart or change the tone of blood vessels.

Several of the medications discussed in this section are not generally used in the prehospital setting. However, you may encounter them during interfacility transport or while responding to an emergency in a health care setting outside of a hospital.

Antidysrhythmic Medications

A variety of medications have the ability to improve or correct abnormalities in a patient's cardiac rhythm. Many of the medications used to treat cardiac dysrhythmias also have a similar ability to cause cardiac dysrhythmias and produce a large number of adverse effects in patients receiving these medications. Given this potential for a negative outcome, you must carefully consider the risks and benefits of administering a particular medication in the context of an individual patient. In many cases, you will benefit from the expert guidance of a physician through online medical control when treating patients in hemodynamically stable condition with a cardiac dysrhythmia.

Medications used to treat cardiac dysrhythmias are grouped into four classes using the **Vaughan-Williams classification** scheme. This classification scheme is based on mechanism of action rather than on specific medication groups. Certain medications have a mechanism of action that places them in more than one class. Adenosine (Adenocard) is a medication used to treat certain cardiac dysrhythmias but is not included in the Vaughan-Williams classification.

A brief overview of cardiac cellular activity is essential to understanding the action of antidysrhythmic medications. There are five phases of cardiac cell activity, numbered 0 through 4. The cardiac cycle begins at phase 4. During phase 4, cardiac cells are at rest, waiting for the generation of a spontaneous impulse from within (automaticity) or transfer of an impulse from an adjacent cardiac cell. This period coincides with diastole of the heart.

Phase 0 begins when a cardiac muscle cell receives an impulse. Sodium ions rapidly enter the cell through sodium channels in the cardiac cell. Calcium, entering more slowly through calcium channels, causes the release of calcium for muscle contraction. **Depolarization** occurs, altering the electrical charge present in the cell, and contraction begins **FIGURE 13-11**.

During phase 1, sodium channels close while potassium exits the cell. During phase 2, sodium and calcium slowly enter the cell, while potassium continues to leave the cell. During phase 3, calcium channels slowly close and calcium leaves the cell while potassium channels open, enabling the rapid movement of potassium out of the cell. Repolarization, which began during phase 2, is complete at the end of phase 3.

Throughout phases 0, 1, and 2 and up to the middle of phase 3, no additional depolarization may occur because of external stimuli. This protection

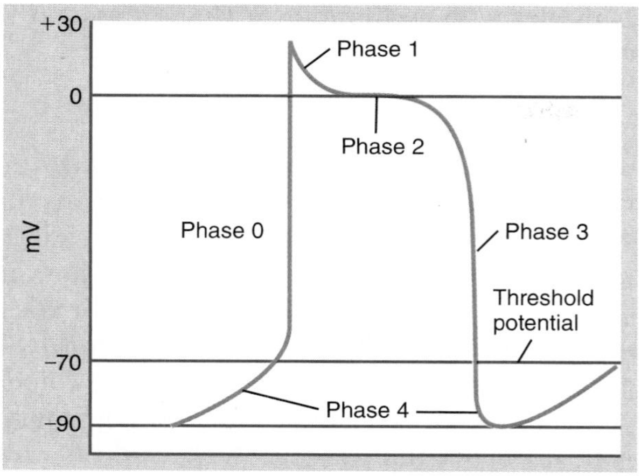

FIGURE 13-11 Action potential in a cardiac muscle cell.

Reproduced from *12-Lead ECG: The Art of Interpretation*, courtesy of Tomas B. Garcia, MD.

limits the potential maximum heart rate by ensuring that a certain amount of time elapses between myocardial contractions. This period is known as the **absolute refractory period** or effective refractory period. Immediately following the absolute (effective) refractory period, there is a brief window of time in which an unusually powerful stimulus can initiate depolarization, known as the **relative refractory period**.

It is also possible for nonpacemaker cells to initiate electrical activity spontaneously. During periods of cellular hypoxia, certain ion channels become altered. These changes permit calcium (instead of sodium) to initiate depolarization, resulting in the ectopic beats that frequently accompany myocardial ischemia.

Class I Antidysrhythmic Medications

Class I antidysrhythmic medications slow the movement of sodium through channels in certain cardiac cells. Procainamide (Pronestyl), for example, is a class IA medication that can suppress activity of ectopic foci and slow conduction velocity. This mechanism has the potential to prolong the QRS and QT intervals. Procainamide is an effective treatment for a variety of atrial and ventricular dysrhythmias but requires careful administration and monitoring.

Lidocaine is a class IB antidysrhythmic medication that blocks sodium channels in the Purkinje fibers and ventricles, effectively resolving various ventricular dysrhythmias and suppressing ectopic foci. This medication is also used as a local anesthetic during soft-tissue repair and as an adjunct to sedation in patients who are at risk of increased intracranial pressure during intubation attempts. Lidocaine has numerous significant medication interactions and should be used with caution in patients with liver or kidney disease.

Class II Antidysrhythmic Medications/ Beta Adrenergic Blocking Agents

Beta adrenergic blocking agents (beta blockers) constitute the second major class of antidysrhythmic agents. Beta blockers competitively inhibit catecholamine (epinephrine and norepinephrine) activation of beta receptor sites. At therapeutic doses, certain beta blockers are capable of some beta-1 selectivity, affecting heart rate, contractility, or cardiac conduction velocity, without substantial impact on beta-2 receptors in the lungs. This selectivity is lost when higher doses or nonselective beta blockers are administered. Toxic effects from beta blockers typically include bradycardia, hypotension, conduction delays, and a variety of other cardiovascular effects.

Beta blockers should be used with extreme caution in patients with reactive airway disease because of the potential for beta-2 antagonism causing bronchospasm. Beta blockers may also cause conduction abnormalities or significant hypotension when given simultaneously with calcium channel blockers. Carefully monitor the patient's BP, heart rate, and cardiac rhythm during and after administration of a beta blocker.

Class III Antidysrhythmic Medications

Class III antidysrhythmic medications increase the duration of phases 1, 2, and 3 of the cardiac cycle. By extending the cellular action potential, these medications prolong the absolute refractory period, thereby treating atrial or ventricular tachycardias. With some class III medications, the degree of prolongation of the action potential is inversely proportional to the baseline heart rate, essentially making these medications less effective for treating extremely rapid heart rates while dramatically decreasing relatively slower baseline heart rates.

Amiodarone (Cordarone) is a class III antidysrhythmic medication that is useful for treating atrial and ventricular dysrhythmias. This agent is administered by the IV route in the prehospital or critical care setting and can be continued orally for long-term maintenance. Amiodarone becomes widely distributed throughout the body, potentially causing a wide range of adverse effects. In addition to severe adverse cardiovascular effects, it causes various life-threatening pulmonary conditions in up to 10.7% of patients.[10] Patients typically develop pulmonary complications after several months on oral amiodarone; however, these complications can occur at any point during treatment.

Sotalol (Betapace) is another class III medication that you may encounter in the prehospital setting. This medication is often taken orally by patients for either ventricular or atrial dysrhythmias. It can be used intravenously for termination of ventricular tachycardia.

Class IV Antidysrhythmic Medications/ Calcium Channel Blockers

Calcium channel blockers have many potential uses in the prehospital setting. These medications can be used for reducing BP and controlling the heart rate and may increase myocardial oxygen delivery during periods of ischemia. In addition, these medications may be used to inhibit uterine contractions during preterm labor, for long-term management of migraines, and for the treatment of cardiomyopathy.

Calcium channel blockers displace calcium at certain receptor sites or enter smooth muscle cells in place of calcium. This action relaxes smooth muscle present in the heart, blood vessels, GI tract, and uterus. Calcium channel blockers slow conduction through the atrioventricular node, decrease the automaticity of ectopic foci within the heart, and decrease the velocity of cardiac contraction. Cardiac workload and oxygen consumption are decreased by lowering peripheral vascular resistance (afterload) while simultaneously reducing cardiac output.

Verapamil (Calan) and diltiazem (Cardizem) are two calcium channel blockers commonly used in prehospital and critical care transport settings. In most cases, these medications are used to control the heart rate in stable patients with a narrow QRS tachycardia or to control the ventricular rate in patients with atrial fibrillation or atrial flutter without preexcitation. Diltiazem appears to have less effect on BP, making it more desirable for patients at risk for hypotension. Both medications are administered by the IV route over at least 2 minutes with continuous ECG and frequent BP monitoring.

Adenosine

Adenosine is the only member of the fifth (unnamed) class of antidysrhythmic medications that is used routinely in the prehospital setting. It has a rapid onset of action, a brief duration of action, and a half-life of less than 10 seconds. Adenosine can be used to treat most stable, regular, narrow-QRS tachycardias, including those involving AV nodal reentry. It may be considered for treating patients with unstable narrow-QRS tachycardias while preparing for cardioversion, or used to assist in diagnosis when the origin or pattern cannot be determined on an ECG because of an unusually fast heart rate.

Patients and health care providers alike often experience similar levels of anxiety during the 5- to 15-second pause in electrical and mechanical cardiac activity caused by adenosine. Run a continuous paper ECG recording whenever you administer adenosine. Doing so will assist you and other health care providers in identifying the patient's dysrhythmia if conversion with adenosine proves unsuccessful.

Additional Cardiovascular Medications

Alpha Adrenergic Receptor Antagonists

Alpha adrenergic receptor antagonists (alpha blockers) prevent endogenous catecholamines from reaching alpha receptors, primarily in the smooth muscle of blood vessels. In general, these medications lower BP (particularly diastolic) and decrease systemic vascular resistance. Nonselective blockade of alpha-2 receptors causes a "reflex" tachycardia by allowing increased norepinephrine secretion from the sympathetic nervous system.

Patients taking alpha blocking medications at home are frequently susceptible to orthostatic hypotension (hypotension related to sudden position changes) and tachycardia. Alpha adrenergic receptor antagonists are prescribed for patients with hypertension, an enlarged prostate gland, and glaucoma. Alpha receptor antagonism also occurs frequently as a seemingly unrelated adverse effect of other medications.

It is conceivable that you might administer one of three alpha adrenergic medications in the prehospital or critical care transport setting. Clonidine (Catapres) is a primarily alpha-2 receptor agonist, which is often given orally for emergency treatment of hypertension. By activating alpha-2 receptors, clonidine suppresses the release of norepinephrine, a potent vasoconstrictor, causing vasodilation.

You may also administer phentolamine (Regitine). Catecholamines and sympathomimetics (discussed later) can cause profound tissue necrosis if **extravasation** (seepage of blood and medication into the tissue surrounding the blood vessel) occurs during their administration through a peripheral IV line. When extravasation occurs, blood vessels in the skin and soft tissue constrict, cutting off blood flow to cells in the affected area. Phentolamine can be delivered by subcutaneous injection to reverse vasoconstriction in affected soft tissue, thereby preventing tissue death.

Finally, you may administer labetalol (Trandate), an unusual medication with a combination of alpha-1, beta-1, and beta-2 antagonism properties. This agent is administered in emergency settings for hypertension. The IV form has a far greater effect on beta-1 and beta-2 receptors than it has on alpha-1 receptors. Patients who are at risk for unopposed alpha stimulation, such as those with a pheochromocytoma or cocaine overdose, should receive another alpha adrenergic antagonist before receiving labetalol for a hypertensive emergency. In this case, a declining cardiac output from the beta-1 antagonism prompts the secretion of endogenous catecholamines, causing potentially uncontrolled hypertension.

Angiotensin-Converting Enzyme Inhibitors

The medications known as ACE inhibitors alter the function of the renin-angiotensin system in the body. This system causes vasoconstriction and fluid retention in response to hypotension or hypoperfusion. When the conversion of angiotensin I to angiotensin II is altered by the use of ACE inhibitor medications, a variety of clinically beneficial effects occur. BP is reduced and cardiac afterload is decreased without significantly altering cardiac output or causing an increased heart rate. ACE inhibitors are useful for treating hypertension, cardiomyopathy, and heart failure. In addition, they protect kidney function in certain groups of people susceptible to those conditions.

Patients taking ACE inhibitors may experience a chronic dry cough, which is thought to be linked to an accumulation of chemicals from the now-altered renin-angiotensin system. Some may experience sudden, life-threatening angioedema: swelling of the mouth, face, and airway as a result of a rapid increase in subdermal and submucosal vascular permeability. When this type of angioedema occurs, the usual treatments such as epinephrine and antihistamines are not as effective. You should expect to provide close monitoring and supportive treatment or, in severe situations, prepare for an extremely difficult endotracheal intubation.

Some EMS systems may use ACE inhibitors as part of their patient care, particularly enalapril (Vasotec). You should follow your local protocols regarding indications and administration for this agent, and be aware of important contraindications if enalapril or another ACE inhibitor is used in your EMS system.

Anticholinergic Medications

Anticholinergic medications are used in prehospital and other health care settings for several important clinical purposes. The parasympathetic and sympathetic nervous systems continually respond to internal and external stimuli by releasing various biochemicals. These chemicals enhance or suppress the function of many tissues, organs, and body systems. Throughout the day, activity of either the sympathetic nervous system or the parasympathetic nervous system will predominate, depending on the body's perceived needs. The sympathetic nervous system predominates in responding to stress, releasing catecholamines to improve cardiovascular performance, enhance respiration, and retain body water. As the stressful stimulus disappears, the parasympathetic nervous system predominates again, allowing vital functions such as rest, digestion, and urination to resume.

The vagus nerve (cranial nerve X) is a major component of the parasympathetic nervous system. This nerve controls parasympathetic stimulation of receptor sites in the heart, lungs, and digestive system and throughout the chest and abdomen. The vagus nerve releases ACh, which acts on muscarinic-2 receptors in the heart to decrease heart rate and contractility and cardiac conduction velocity. Excessive activation of muscarinic-2 receptors in the heart by ACh causes bradycardia and conduction delays. Excessive activation of other muscarinic receptors causes increased salivation, bronchoconstriction, pulmonary secretions, vomiting, emesis, diarrhea, tearing, and a vast array of unwanted clinical effects. Many of these symptoms are present in patients who are exposed to acetylcholinesterase inhibitors in pesticides and nerve agents, which permits excessive release of ACh and leads to elevated ACh levels in the body. Atropine sulfate is used in prehospital and other health care settings to treat many **cholinergic** symptoms associated with excessive release of ACh.

Atropine is considered a competitive muscarinic receptor antagonist. Its effectiveness is largely related to its concentration at receptor sites compared with ACh. When ACh levels increase dramatically due to inhibition of **acetylcholinesterase** (the enzyme that breaks down ACh), massive doses of atropine may be required.

Atropine is used for the treatment of bradycardia when vagal (vagus nerve) stimulation of muscarinic-2 receptors is suspected. This medication may be administered empirically to exclude the possibility of vagal stimulation during episodes of bradycardia with an unidentified cause. When atropine is administered for bradycardia, ACh activation of muscarinic-2 receptors is prevented, allowing the underlying sympathetic stimulation to predominate. Atropine is unlikely to be effective for the treatment of bradycardia caused by blocked cardiac conduction, such as occurs with second- and third-degree atrioventricular blocks.

Notably, atropine is used before airway manipulation, especially in children. Laryngoscopy can stimulate the vagus nerve, causing ACh-induced bradycardia. In addition to preventing bradycardia, atropine can suppress the release of saliva and other secretions in the patient's airway.

Finally, atropine is the life-saving antidote for acetylcholinesterase inhibitor toxicity. When patients are exposed to pesticides and nerve agents, this medication is continuously administered until the patient's respiratory and hemodynamic status improves, regardless of the total dose required. Emergency vehicle and hospital atropine supplies can be quickly exhausted following severe exposures, especially when an incident involves multiple patients. Atropine does not bind with nicotinic receptors; consequently, it will not improve muscle weakness, fasciculations, or paralysis from cholinergic poisoning.

Catecholamines and Sympathomimetics

Catecholamines are naturally occurring chemicals in the body that stimulate receptor sites in the sympathetic nervous system. These chemicals contain two structures: the catechol group and the monoamine group. Endogenous catecholamines include epinephrine, norepinephrine, and dopamine. These chemicals stimulate alpha, beta, and dopaminergic receptor sites, causing the "fight-or-flight" response to stressful stimuli. These three chemicals are manufactured commercially for administration to patients with certain medical conditions. Catecholamines are rapidly metabolized by monoamine oxidase and catechol-*O*-methyltransferase (an enzyme), resulting in a brief duration of action after administration. You may encounter certain catecholamine and sympathomimetic medications in the prehospital setting. Other medications in this category may be encountered during critical care transport.

Sympathomimetic chemicals are not found naturally within the body. These synthetic chemicals mimic naturally occurring catecholamines, activating receptor sites in the sympathetic nervous system. Various amphetamines, albuterol, phenylephrine, and cocaine have sympathomimetic properties. Sympathomimetic medications do not undergo the same metabolism as catecholamines, so they have a longer duration of action following their administration.

Epinephrine (Adrenalin), also known as adrenaline (note the similarity with the brand name), is a catecholamine that stimulates alpha, beta-1, and beta-2 receptor sites. It can be administered via the IV, IO, IM, subcutaneous, endotracheal, and nebulized routes, depending on the clinical situation and the type of medication access available. Epinephrine, like many catecholamines and sympathomimetic chemicals, can dramatically increase the cardiac workload and myocardial oxygen demand. These medications should be used with extreme caution in patients with myocardial ischemia, cardiomyopathy, or cardiogenic shock.

Norepinephrine is another naturally occurring catecholamine that stimulates beta-1 and alpha receptor sites. Its vasoconstrictor (alpha) effects are usually greater than its cardiac (beta-1) effects. Conditions that involve loss of vasomotor tone, such as sepsis, neurogenic shock, and anaphylactic shock, are the primary indications for norepinephrine, owing to its effects in restoring intravascular volume. Norepinephrine is administered by continuous IV infusion and titrated according to patient response. Like other vasopressor medications, it has the potential to cause tissue necrosis if extravasation occurs during IV administration. Frequent assessment of the IV site is imperative if norepinephrine is being administered through a peripheral IV site. Paramedics who have been appropriately trained should ideally administer norepinephrine and other vasoconstrictor medications through a central venous catheter when available.

Dopamine (Intropin) is frequently used for hypotension refractory to volume resuscitation. The dose of this agent is determined based on a weight-based infusion calculation, typically using units of micrograms per kilogram per minute, and it is administered via an infusion pump. The clinical effects of dopamine vary depending on the dose being administered.

Dobutamine is a synthetically manufactured catecholamine that is similar to dopamine. It activates beta-1 and, to a lesser degree, beta-2 and alpha receptor sites. Dobutamine may slightly increase heart rate, while providing a significant improvement in inotropic effects (force of cardiac contraction). When used for the treatment of cardiogenic shock, this agent is frequently combined with an IV vasodilator medication to increase the inotropic effects and decrease afterload, resulting in improved cardiac output. In a hospital or critical care transport setting, dobutamine is administered with an infusion pump and careful cardiac and hemodynamic monitoring is performed.

Milrinone (Primacor) is an agent that can be given either orally or intravenously for the treatment of heart failure. It has the ability to increase cardiac contractility while simultaneously causing dilation of systemic arteries and veins. Although this combination improves cardiac output, it increases patient mortality when milrinone is used on a long-term basis.

Phenylephrine is a synthetic, almost pure, alpha agonist medication. As a paramedic, you may use phenylephrine as a mucosal vasoconstrictor during artificial airway placement.

Digitalis Preparations

Digitalis preparations are prescribed for treatment of chronic heart failure or certain rapid atrial dysrhythmias (eg, rapid atrial flutter, atrial fibrillation, and supraventricular dysrhythmias). Digitalis acts by increasing the strength of cardiac contractions, thereby improving cardiac output and slowing conduction through the atrioventricular junction (such as in atrial fibrillation or flutter), allowing fewer impulses to be conducted to the ventricles and thereby slowing the overall heart rate. Patients may experience a wide variety of signs and symptoms as an adverse reaction to digitalis preparations, including loss of appetite, nausea, vomiting, headache, blurred vision, yellow vision, or various cardiac dysrhythmias. *Virtually any cardiac dysrhythmia may be caused by the toxic effects of digitalis*, so it is important to ask all patients with disturbances in cardiac rhythm whether they are taking digitalis.

Patients taking digitalis are sensitive to calcium preparations, and are highly sensitive to a decline in serum potassium levels. Therefore, you must exercise caution when giving agents that might reduce the body's potassium stores, such as diuretics or large quantities of sodium bicarbonate. Commonly used digitalis preparations include digoxin (Lanoxin) and digitoxin (Crystodigin).

> **Words of Wisdom**
>
> **Antianginal Agents**
>
> Three major classes of drugs are used to relieve the pain of angina: nitrates, beta blockers, and calcium channel blockers. All of them work exclusively or primarily on the demand side of the oxygen supply-demand equation; that is, all of them diminish, in one way or another, myocardial oxygen demand.

Direct Vasodilator Medications

Various direct vasodilator medications are used for the management of uncontrolled hypertension, heart failure, myocardial infarction, cardiac ischemia, and cardiogenic shock. These medications act on arteries, veins, or both, causing vascular smooth muscle relaxation and vasodilation. These medications have the potential to reduce cardiac preload and afterload and pulmonary vascular resistance.

Nitroglycerin (Nitro-Bid, Nitrostat) is a direct vasodilator that is administered for a variety of cardiovascular conditions. Nitroglycerin primarily dilates veins and coronary arteries, decreasing cardiac preload, reducing myocardial oxygen demand, and improving coronary circulation. Some clinicians recommend obtaining a 15-lead ECG (12-lead ECG with additional evaluation for ischemia of the right side of the heart) before initiating treatment with nitroglycerin. Right-side myocardial infarction requires an adequate preload to maintain adequate cardiac output, which may be compromised by the administration of nitroglycerin.

Because SL nitroglycerin tablets are susceptible to degradation, they must be stored in a closed, light-protected container. However, nitroglycerin binds with the plastic of containers and IV fluids or tubing, so glass bottles should be used for IV administration as safety and availability permit. The use of nitroglycerin should be avoided in patients taking phosphodiesterase-5 inhibitors used for erectile dysfunction, such as sildenafil (Viagra) and tadalafil (Cialis) **FIGURE 13-12**. When combined, nitroglycerin and phosphodiesterase-5 inhibitors may cause severe, refractory hypotension.

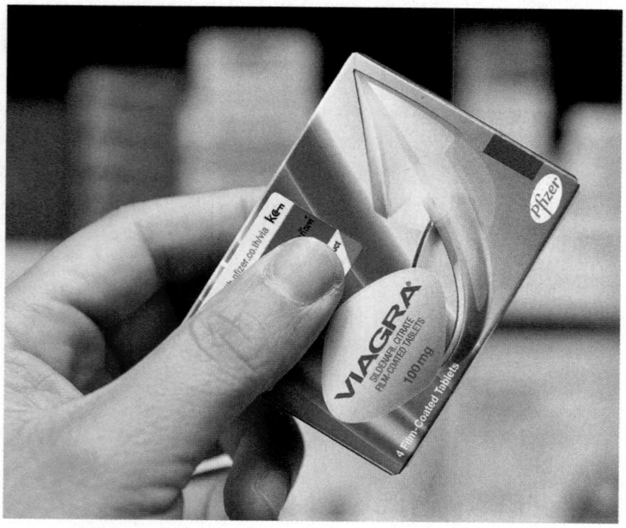

FIGURE 13-12 Administration of nitroglycerin in patients who have taken erectile dysfunction medication within certain time frames is contraindicated.

Sodium nitroprusside (Nipride) is a potent IV vasodilator, affecting the smooth muscle of veins and arteries. It is frequently used in conjunction with inotropic medications for the management of cardiogenic shock. Sodium nitroprusside is also used for malignant hypertension and in situations where intentional hypotension is desired, such as with an unstable vascular aneurysm. The IV infusion rates can be adjusted to maintain optimal BP and cardiac output. Sodium nitroprusside is metabolized into cyanide and thiocyanate, which can cause toxicity during a prolonged infusion. When it is administered in the critical care transport setting, you should ask the sending facility staff or provider about obtaining plasma cyanide and thiocyanate levels before your departure with the patient.

Hydralazine (Apresoline) is a direct vasodilator that you may administer in patients with pregnancy-induced hypertension. This medication dilates arterioles, lowering pulmonary and systemic vascular resistance.

A subgroup of patients with idiopathic pulmonary artery hypertension may be dependent on life-sustaining, continuous infusions of epoprostenol (Flolan). This medication is a potent vasodilator, impacting both pulmonary and systemic blood vessels. Additionally, epoprostenol inhibits platelet aggregation, which likely decreases the prevalence or severity of pulmonary thrombus (blood clot) formation. Patients who are on continuous epoprostenol infusions often have compact infusion pumps and long-term IV access in place, typically a peripherally inserted central catheter or similar device. EMS assistance may be requested in case of an unexpected failure of either the infusion device or IV access. EMS systems may provide protocols for paramedics to assist with administration of a patient's own epoprostenol; however, this medication is not typically administered to patients for the first time in the prehospital setting. Adverse effects include tachycardia, palpitations, dysrhythmia, bleeding, and flushing. You should consult with online medical control if considering adjustments to the continuous infusion rate. In most cases, paramedic involvement will be limited to reestablishing IV access and troubleshooting the infusion pump, unless a concurrent medical condition is present.

Diuretic Medications

Paramedics administer diuretic medications to correct volume overload, manage heart failure, and improve respiration in patients experiencing pulmonary edema. Diuretic medications also have the potential to preserve kidney function when large quantities of by-products from cellular destruction, such as from muscle breakdown or blood cell hemolysis, are released. These agents are used to eliminate certain toxins from the body and to promote the excretion of excess electrolytes. **TABLE 13-12** lists commonly prescribed diuretic medications.

Furosemide is a diuretic medication used in the prehospital setting. People may also take furosemide on a long-term basis for the management of hypertension, heart failure, liver disease, or kidney dysfunction. Furosemide is generally administered for treatment of pulmonary edema, often related to cardiac dysfunction. Careful consideration is necessary before administering furosemide to patients with hemodynamic instability and known electrolyte disturbances.

Mannitol is an osmotic diuretic that may or may not be available for use by paramedics. In critical care settings, this medication is used to decrease intracranial pressure associated with cerebral edema. Osmotic diuretics can target specific body tissues, removing excess water from the brain and eyes. Osmotic pressure gradients also draw water out of selected body tissues and through the kidneys to maintain urine flow when the kidneys risk becoming clogged with cellular by-products. Many electrolyte disturbances are possible following mannitol administration. Prolonged mannitol infusions have been known to cause a paradoxical increase in intracranial pressure.

Words of Wisdom

Contact online medical control if you encounter a patient in the community who is receiving an infusion of a medication you are not accustomed to administering.

Antihypertensive Agents

As the name implies, antihypertensive agents are used to treat hypertension. Many of the diuretic agents just mentioned are also used as antihypertensives or in combination with antihypertensives for a synergistic effect. Similarly, beta blockers are used in the treatment of hypertension.

It is often difficult to regulate the dosage of antihypertensive medications so that the patient's BP is lowered enough but not too much. As a consequence, some patients taking these agents may have symptoms of hypotension, including weakness and dizziness. Many will experience a feeling of dizziness with a change in position, such as when moving from a recumbent to a sitting or standing position; this phenomenon is termed orthostatic hypotension. Every patient taking antihypertensive drugs, therefore, should have their BP checked in the recumbent and sitting positions to detect orthostatic hypotension. **TABLE 13-13** lists commonly prescribed antihypertensive agents.

TABLE 13-12 Commonly Prescribed Diuretics

Category	Generic Name (Trade Name)
Loop diuretics: disrupt sodium reabsorption in the thick ascending limb in the loop of Henle within the kidneys	Furosemide (Lasix) Bumetanide (Bumex) Torsemide (Demadex)
Potassium-sparing diuretics: impair sodium reabsorption in the cortical collecting tubule of the kidney	Spironolactone (Aldactone) Triamterene (Dyrenium)
Thiazide diuretics: inhibit sodium transport within the distal tubule of the kidney	Chlorothiazide (Diuril) Hydrochlorothiazide Metolazone (Diulo, Zaroxolyn)
Vasodilators/nitrates	Hydralazine (Apresoline)
Combination drugs	Hydrochlorothiazide and spironolactone (Aldactazide) Triamterene and hydrochlorothiazide (Dyazide, Maxzide)

© Jones & Bartlett Learning.

TABLE 13-13 Commonly Prescribed Antihypertensive Agents

Category	Generic Name (Trade Name)
Nonselective beta blockers (have both beta-1 and beta-2 effects)	Labetalol (Normodyne, Trandate) Propranolol (Inderal)
Angiotensin-converting enzyme inhibitors (The generic drug names in this class of medications end in -pril)	Benazepril (Lotensin) Captopril (Capoten) Enalapril (Vasotec) Fosinopril (Monopril) Lisinopril (Prinivil, Zestril) Quinapril (Accupril) Ramipril (Altace)
Alpha agonist	Clonidine (Catapres) Methyldopa (Aldomet)
Alpha blocker	Prazosin (Aldomet)
Other antihypertensive	Reserpine (Sandril, Ser-Ap-Es, Serpasil)

© Jones & Bartlett Learning.

TABLE 13-14 Other Medications Prescribed to Treat or Prevent Heart Disease

Category	Generic Name (Trade Name)
Angiotensin II receptor blockers (The generic drug names in this class of medications end in -sartan)	Losartan (Cozaar); valsartan (Diovan); irbesartan (Avapro); candesartan (Atacand)
Cholesterol-lowering drugs	Statins: lovastatin (Altoprev, Mevacor); fluvastatin (Lescol); pravastatin (Pravachol); atorvastatin (Lipitor); simvastatin (Zocor) Niacins: nicotinic acid (Niacor); extended-release niacin (Niaspan) Bile acid resins: colestipol (Colestid); cholestyramine (Questran); colesevelam (Welchol) Fibrates: clofibrate (Atromid); gemfibrozil (Lopid); fenofibrate (Tricor)
Vasodilators	Isosorbide dinitrate[a] (Dilatrate-SR, Iso-Bid, Isonate, Isordil, Isotrate, Sorbitrate); isosorbide mononitrate (Imdur); hydralazine[a] (Apresoline)

[a]Isosorbide dinitrate and hydralazine are given together.

© Jones & Bartlett Learning.

Other Cardiac Medications

In addition to those discussed thus far, **TABLE 13-14** lists medications that may be prescribed for patients with cardiac conditions.

Blood Products and Medications Affecting the Blood

In the body, blood acts as the primary transport mechanism for oxygen, carbon dioxide, nutrients, waste products, biochemicals, and medications. Health care providers have the ability to manipulate or enhance many characteristics of the blood for therapeutic clinical purposes. In certain situations, they will want to suppress the blood's clotting ability to enhance circulation or mitigate the effects of hypoperfusion. In other cases, they will need to augment the blood's oxygen-carrying or clotting ability when these functions become impaired. A variety of medications affecting the blood are used in the prehospital and critical care transport settings. In addition, many EMS systems allow paramedics to initiate or monitor the administration of various blood products in appropriate clinical situations.

Blood Product Administration

The average adult has approximately 5 L of blood, constituting about 7% to 8% of body weight. Blood is roughly 55% plasma. Because such a high percentage of plasma is water (92%), water makes up approximately 50% of the total intravascular volume. RBCs account for approximately 45% of the blood volume. Many chemicals, cells, proteins, and hormones make up the remainder of blood composition. Trauma and a vast array of medical conditions can alter the total amount, composition, or performance of the blood. Health care providers, including paramedics, may administer several different blood products to correct these abnormalities. Patients receive transfusions of specific components of the blood that are diminished or have impaired function. Administration of whole blood is being studied and reintroduced into some EMS systems.[11]

Blood components may be unmatched, type-specific to a particular patient, or cross-matched to a particular recipient. Type-specific blood products can be used as soon as the decision has been made and the recipient patient's blood type is known, but they are associated with a somewhat greater risk of an adverse, potentially life-threatening transfusion reaction. Cross-matched blood has a decreased risk of transfusion reaction but requires a blood sample from the patient, followed by careful analysis of this sample in the blood bank before the blood product can be released for administration to the patient.

In the prehospital setting, you will most likely use unmatched blood, possibly carried by air-medical crews or sent to the scene of a prolonged extrication where a patient has a profound hemorrhage and will remain entrapped for a long period. Unmatched blood is almost always type O, Rh-negative (O negative). (Rh is the antigen responsible for hemolytic disease of the newborn.) Type O-negative blood products can theoretically be administered to patients with any blood type, although other proteins and chemicals in the blood product may cause a transfusion reaction.

During interfacility patient transports, you may face the dilemma of deciding whether to administer unmatched, type O-negative blood products or to delay transport to obtain type-specific or cross-matched blood products. The stability of the patient's clinical condition and the duration of anticipated delays for blood typing or cross-matching often make the decision obvious. In the absence of a clear choice, consult online medical control and/or the sending physician, as they are valuable resources for guidance.

Recently, low-titer group O whole blood (LTOWB) has started to be used in the prehospital setting.[11] LTOWB is blood collected from a single donor and tested for levels of specific immunoglobulins that can cause the patient to have a transfusion reaction. Research has shown that the presence or absence of the Rhesus antigen (the Rh factor) is not a significant factor when resuscitating patients with hemorrhagic shock. Advantages related to the use of LTOWB include rapid administration of blood, fewer additives and anticoagulants, and reduced likelihood of human error. The primary disadvantage is its short shelf life.[12]

Blood products require careful patient monitoring during their administration, as many types of transfusion-related reactions are possible. Any paramedic who is expected to initiate or monitor blood product transfusions should be able to

YOU are the Paramedic

PART 4

As you prepare to transport, a 250-mL normal saline fluid bolus is infusing from a 1-L bag through 10-gtt tubing. The patient remains on oxygen, and her cardiac rhythm remains unchanged. The nursing staff provide the following additional information on this patient:

- Allergies:
  - Penicillin
  - "Sulfa" medications
- Scheduled/daily medications:
  - Metformin
  - Aspirin, once daily
  - Lisinopril
  - Atorvastatin
  - Vitamin C
  - Folate
- As-needed medications:
  - Acetaminophen
  - Diphenhydramine
  - Metoclopramide
  - Ondansetron
  - Promethazine
  - Docusate

6. Does the patient's allergy and medication list add any possible causes of her current condition?

7. Which medications on this list, if any, should be used with particular caution in older patients?

recognize and manage potential transfusion reactions during transport. In addition to pulse rate and BP monitoring, temperature should be reassessed frequently during transport. If an indwelling urinary catheter is present, you should monitor for changes in urine color that may indicate a life-threatening hemolytic transfusion reaction.

Most blood products require special filtered IV tubing for their administration. This tubing may become clogged during massive blood product transfusions. In addition, certain IV fluids are incompatible with blood products when combined in the same IV tubing. Normal saline is the preferred IV fluid for Y-site tubing administration during blood product transfusions.

Packed Red Blood Cells

Packed RBCs (PRBCs) can be administered by paramedics to correct anemia resulting from blood loss, inadequate RBC production, or the massive destruction of circulating RBCs, known as hemolysis. Patients without a concurrent serious medical condition may compensate well for profound anemia that has developed during weeks to months. When blood cell loss occurs suddenly from trauma, hemorrhage, or hemolysis, however, patients are far less able to compensate. In general, the rate of administration of PRBCs should be proportional to the rate of blood cell loss.

A unit of PRBCs contains approximately 225 to 250 mL of concentrated RBCs, along with a preservative. Administration of 1 U of PRBCs will increase the hematocrit value, the percentage of RBCs in the blood, by roughly 3% (or less with continued RBC loss). In children and infants, a patient-specific volume of PRBCs is administered. Patients at risk for volume overload, such as those with renal failure or heart failure, require slow PRBC administration and careful monitoring of fluid volume and respiratory status.

Typically, PRBCs are administered over no longer than 4 hours per unit. In patients in critical condition, PRBCs can be administered rapidly through a commercial pressure infuser-warmer or by using pressure bags. You should use the largest IV catheter possible. In adults, at least a 20-gauge IV catheter should be used, preferably an 18-gauge or larger. Patients with trauma and hemorrhage should have adequate IV fluid resuscitation before or concurrently with PRBC administration. For blood cells, type AB is the universal recipient and type O is the universal donor.

Units of PRBCs usually contain a citrate-based preservative. Hypocalcemia may develop as the citrate binds with calcium in the body. During massive PRBC transfusions, you should monitor for signs of hypocalcemia, such as tetany and a prolonged QT interval on the ECG tracing.

Patients receiving PRBCs are also at risk for hyperkalemia. If PRBCs are stored for a long period or if hemolysis occurs during PRBC administration, large amounts of intracellular potassium are released. In severe situations, hyperkalemia can be life threatening. Peaked T waves on the ECG tracing are highly suggestive of hyperkalemia.

Fresh Frozen Plasma

Impaired blood clotting can be treated by the administration of fresh frozen plasma (FFP). Because FFP contains many clotting factors, it is often given following trauma, hemorrhage, warfarin toxicity, disseminated intravascular coagulation, and other conditions. Whenever large volumes of other blood components (such as PRBCs) are administered, FFP should also be used. The FFP must be compatible with a patient's blood type but does not need to be Rh compatible.

In general, units of FFP have the same volume as units of PRBCs (ie, 225–250 mL). These units require adequate defrosting before administration. FFP is used for replacement of clotting factors, not volume expansion. Volume expansion is usually best accomplished with IV fluids and PRBC transfusion. Some medical centers and EMS agencies have started using liquid plasma, also known as never-frozen plasma, which has superior stability and efficacy to FFP.[13]

Cryoprecipitate is a blood product that contains a concentrated assortment of blood clotting factors, without the additional volume present in FFP. It is unlikely that you will administer cryoprecipitate in the prehospital setting. Type AB plasma and cryoprecipitate can be given to patients with any blood type.

Platelets

Paramedics and other health care providers administer platelets to correct thrombocytopenia, a low platelet level in the blood. Thrombocytopenia can be caused by trauma, hemorrhage, and various chronic medical conditions, as well as by certain anticoagulant medications. Patients may also have a normal level of platelets that are dysfunctional because of a clotting disorder or antiplatelet medication. Platelets must be blood type and Rh compatible.

Medications That Alter Blood Performance

Blood platelets combine with clotting or coagulation chemicals in the bloodstream to terminate bleeding when a blood vessel ruptures. This complicated process is essential for human survival. Indeed, without this process, spontaneous bleeding would readily occur and otherwise minor trauma would cause death from exsanguination. When blood clotting occurs in a blood vessel, a thrombus (blood clot) is created. This thrombus can occlude the blood vessel, jeopardizing dependent cells, tissues, and organs. During prehospital care and interfacility transport, you may administer or monitor several important medications that alter the blood's ability to form a thrombus, with the aim of preventing or limiting the injury to vital organs such as the heart and lungs.

Tranexamic Acid

Tranexamic acid (Lysteda) has emerged as a powerful medication intervention to promote blood clotting and reduce mortality in trauma patients with severe bleeding. This medication is being used by many trauma centers, by the military, and in an increasing number of EMS settings. International Trauma Life Support has supported the use of tranexamic acid in the management of traumatic hemorrhage with the approval of medical control.[14]

In patients who experience trauma, the process of blood clot formation begins in response to their injury and bleeding. This clot formation is often coupled with *hyperfibrinolysis*, resulting in the rapid dissolving of new blood clots. Left unchecked, hyperfibrinolysis leads to dramatically increased mortality of trauma patients. Tranexamic acid is a commercial preparation of lysine, an amino acid in the body responsible for preventing the breakdown of fibrin clots. When administered within 3 hours of the traumatic event, tranexamic acid significantly decreases patient mortality from excessive bleeding; after 3 hours, complications increase.[15]

Anticoagulant Medications

Anticoagulant medications impair the function of clotting or coagulation chemicals in the bloodstream. Human blood contains a balance of substances that promote the formation of blood clots or are capable of dissolving blood clots. This balance permits the termination of bleeding while simultaneously allowing blood clots to dissolve once blood vessel integrity is restored. Anticoagulant medications enhance the function of substances in the blood that inhibit clot formation. These medications prevent the formation of new blood clots and the growth of existing clots, but they do not dissolve existing blood clots.

Heparin and enoxaparin (Lovenox) are frequently used anticoagulant medications that enhance antithrombin III to inhibit blood coagulation. Both medications are used to treat or prevent acute coronary syndrome, deep vein thrombosis, and pulmonary embolus. These medications are not generally initiated in the prehospital setting, although it is conceivable that paramedics in remote locations or ambitious EMS systems might administer these medications in specific clinical situations. Both heparin and enoxaparin have the potential to cause bleeding, thrombocytopenia, and a variety of other adverse effects.

You may also encounter patients who are taking fondaparinux (Arixtra), another anticoagulant medication. Fondaparinux is typically administered to prevent deep vein thrombosis, to treat thrombosis, or during the period immediately following an ST-elevation myocardial infarction to prevent reinfarction.

Warfarin (Coumadin) is a commonly used anticoagulant medication that patients take orally on a short- or long-term basis for treatment or prevention of blood clots. Warfarin works by preventing the production of four different blood clotting factors that use vitamin K. Patients are at risk of life-threatening bleeding when warfarin levels are not adequately controlled, following trauma, or when any other hemorrhage occurs. Certain foods, alcohol, and a variety of medications can increase the effects of this medication. In addition, a wide variety of physiologic conditions can predispose patients taking warfarin to severe bleeding. Warfarin levels are inferred by blood prothrombin time (PT) and international normalized ratio (INR) levels. During interfacility and critical care transports, the patient's PT and/or INR values are essential to understanding the severity of the patient's situation and should be included in the handoff report to the receiving facility's personnel.

Several treatment options are available if patients taking warfarin develop severe bleeding or require emergent surgery. The risk of hemorrhage must be weighed against the risks associated with reversing the protective effects from warfarin. In many instances, providers will attempt to control bleeding without completely reversing the warfarin. This decision usually requires specialty consultation and thoughtful deliberation among providers.

Antiplatelet Medications

Platelets perform an essential role in blood clotting and thrombus formation. Both oral and IV antiplatelet medications can be used to reduce platelet aggregation (clumping), thereby preventing new thrombus formation or the extension of an existing thrombus. **TABLE 13-15** lists commonly prescribed anticoagulant and antiplatelet agents.

Aspirin is an oral antiplatelet medication that is used extensively for the treatment and prevention of thrombus formation. It is administered in the prehospital setting for treatment of acute coronary syndrome, which is often suspected in patients reporting chest pain. Aspirin is also indicated for the treatment of a stroke once the presence of hemorrhage has been reliably excluded.

When indicated, aspirin is crushed or chewed before swallowing, promoting rapid GI absorption. This medication is rapidly eliminated by the body, but its antiplatelet effects persist until all affected platelets are replaced, which may take up to 10 days. Patients may claim an aspirin allergy based on GI upset. You should ask about the specific circumstances when a patient reports an aspirin allergy or sensitivity and aspirin is otherwise clinically indicated.

Clopidogrel (Plavix) and ticlopidine (Ticlid) are other oral antiplatelet medications that paramedics may administer as an aspirin alternative. These medications inhibit platelet aggregation by a mechanism different from that of aspirin. Clopidogrel has been shown to be superior to aspirin in certain clinical situations. Ticlopidine has several serious adverse effects that limit its role in prehospital and long-term treatment. Aspirin, clopidogrel, and ticlopidine may cause various types of bleeding in patients, depending on the medication, dose, or combination.[16,17]

You may encounter various glycoprotein IIb/IIIa inhibitor medications during interfacility transports. Abciximab (ReoPro), tirofiban (Aggrastat), and eptifibatide (Integrilin) provide potent platelet inhibition in a manner more effective than that of the oral antiplatelet medications. These medications are administered by an IV infusion, which is often continued during interfacility transport to a tertiary cardiac care center. Bleeding and thrombocytopenia are adverse effects observed in roughly 5% to 7% of patients receiving these medications.[18]

TABLE 13-15 Commonly Prescribed Anticoagulant and Antiplatelet Agents

Category	Generic Name (Trade Name)
Antiplatelet agents	Clopidogrel (Plavix); ticlopidine (Ticlid); aspirin; prasugrel (Effient)
Coumarin anticoagulants	Warfarin (Coumadin)
Direct thrombin inhibitors	Dabigatran (Pradaxa)
Factor Xa inhibitors	Rivaroxaban (Xarelto); apixaban (Eliquis); edoxaban (Savaysa)

Fibrinolytic Drugs

Fibrinolytic drugs (eg, Activase) dissolve blood clots in arteries and veins. These medications are administered for the emergency treatment of acute myocardial infarction and stroke. In addition, fibrinolytics are sometimes administered in lower doses to open vascular catheters that have become occluded by a presumed blood clot.

Fibrinolytics have a serious potential to cause life-threatening hemorrhage. Careful patient selection and exclusion are essential before these medications are administered. Any condition suggestive of blood clot formation elsewhere in the body, such as recent trauma or surgery, is likely to rule out the use of fibrinolytics in a patient. In addition, numerous other absolute and relative contraindications to fibrinolytic therapy exist.

Fibrinolytics remain valuable in remote locations and smaller community hospitals but have a limited role in the treatment of acute myocardial infarction when interventional cardiology services are readily available. Many hospitals have developed rapid diagnostic and treatment procedures to optimize the effectiveness of fibrinolytics for patients with acute ischemic stroke.

Avoid multiple IV attempts and unnecessary trauma in any patient who is a likely candidate for fibrinolytics. A careful determination of the time of onset of symptoms will influence the decision about whether fibrinolytics will be administered. You should not unnecessarily delay patient transport; these medications are indicated only within a short period after the onset of symptoms. Prolonged prehospital time may preclude the administration of fibrinolytics.

Medications Used for Neurologic Conditions

As a paramedic, you may encounter and treat a large number of patients with neurologic complaints and conditions. Pain accompanies the vast majority of traumatic injuries and is a common symptom associated with many medical conditions. Seizure activity is another event that frequently triggers EMS activation. Many patients encountered by EMS would benefit clinically from the treatment of anxiety or the administration of sedative medications.

Paramedics rely heavily on opioid medications for analgesia (treatment of pain) in the prehospital setting. These medications are effective in eliminating or reducing pain caused by a variety of conditions. You will likely also need to administer naloxone, a powerful reversal agent for patients who have received dangerous amounts of opioid chemicals.

Benzodiazepine medications (discussed earlier in the *Medications Used in Airway Management* section) are the primary treatment modality for persistent seizure activity. These medications also work well for sedation and the treatment of anxiety.

Opioid Analgesic Medications

Paramedics administer medications that stimulate opioid receptors in the body to relieve or prevent pain associated with an injury, medical condition, or medically related procedure or movement. The human body contains at least seven types of opioid receptors in the CNS, peripheral nervous system, and GI tract. Medications used by paramedics act on mu opioid receptor sites. Natural endorphins also stimulate (activate) mu receptor sites, causing analgesia, euphoria, constricted pupils, respiratory depression, and decreased GI motility. Opioid medications are also known to suppress the cough reflex, which can be either a desirable or an adverse clinical effect depending on the situation.

Opioid chemicals, medications, and illicit drugs are known for causing tolerance, cross-tolerance, and addiction. Patients who receive opioid substances on a long-term basis often require unusually high doses of opioid medications for relief of pain from an acute illness or injury. They may also experience severe withdrawal symptoms if opioid reversal is required following an error during treatment.

Opioid medications can cause profound sedation, respiratory depression, and apnea when excessive doses are administered. Other adverse effects may include hypotension, bradycardia, palpitations, dysrhythmias, and noncardiogenic pulmonary edema. The severity or likelihood of adverse effects varies significantly among the different opioid medications.

SAFETY

The potential for medication errors in the EMS environment is enhanced by issues such as packaging and labeling changes. Unfortunately, in recent years, EMS agencies have been dramatically affected by medication manufacturing shortages (eg, shortages in $D_{50}W$ [50% dextrose in water], sodium bicarbonate, epinephrine, dopamine, morphine sulfate, ondansetron, and glucagon). As substitutes for the unavailable medications, agencies may use medications with which paramedics are less familiar, medications from different manufacturers that use different labeling or packaging, and medications that have different dosing regimens. In a high-pressure, uncontrolled environment, such as the back of a moving ambulance with a patient who is decompensating or going into cardiac arrest, errors can easily occur.

> **Words of Wisdom**
>
> Consider carrying a magnifying glass to read the small print on labels (eg, concentration, expiration date). The zoom function of a cell phone's camera can also be used for this purpose.

Of the opioid medications, paramedics administer morphine sulfate or fentanyl most commonly in the prehospital setting. Meperidine (Demerol), hydromorphone (Dilaudid), and newer synthetic opioids may be used in selected EMS or critical care transport settings. Depending on the medication chosen, paramedics may use the IV, IM, or intranasal route of administration.

Morphine sulfate is used frequently in EMS. In addition to the aforementioned adverse effects, this medication is known to cause nausea or vomiting in up to 60% of patients.[19] Always use extreme caution when administering morphine to patients who are unable to protect their airway. Patients with an altered level of consciousness and patients secured to a backboard may experience a life-threatening airway obstruction if vomiting occurs after administration of this opioid. Morphine may also prompt a histamine release that causes pruritus (itching), flushing, and diaphoresis. These symptoms are often inaccurately described as an allergic reaction.

Fentanyl is gaining popularity as an opioid analgesic in the prehospital setting. It is generally not as likely to result in hypotension, making it the preferred analgesic for patients in critical or unstable condition. Fentanyl also does not have the same risk of nausea and histamine release that morphine has, and it can be administered intranasally.

Opioid Antagonist Medication

Naloxone is a powerful opioid receptor antagonist that is used by paramedics and other health care providers to reverse the effects of excessive opioid chemicals in the body. Naloxone competes with opioid chemicals at opioid receptor sites, causing a complete or partial reversal of the clinical effects of opioids. Its efficacy is dose-dependent. Large doses are often required to reverse the effects of potent opioid chemicals. In addition, the duration of naloxone's effects in the body is less than that of many opioid chemicals. Recurrent toxic effects are a risk when naloxone is eliminated more rapidly than the opioid chemicals in the body. Severe opioid overdose situations require repeated administration or continuous IV infusion of naloxone.

When administering naloxone to patients who receive opioids on a long-term basis, administer only enough to correct life-threatening conditions such as respiratory depression and airway compromise. Complete opioid reversal is likely to cause severe withdrawal symptoms, endangering both the patient and the health care providers treating that patient.

Phenytoin and Fosphenytoin

Phenytoin (Dilantin) and fosphenytoin (Cerebyx) are administered to prevent seizure activity. Patients may receive either of these medications on a long-term basis for control of a seizure disorder. You may also encounter these medications while performing an interfacility transport of patients with a head injury, intracranial hemorrhage, or status epilepticus. Both medications decrease the potential for seizure activity by altering sodium channels, limiting cellular sodium in portions of the CNS.

Medications Affecting the GI System

Paramedics administer two major groups of medications that affect the GI system. Histamine$_2$ receptor antagonists are used to reduce the acid in the stomach and GI tract and also augment other medications used in the treatment of allergic reactions. Antiemetic agents are given to prevent and treat nausea and vomiting.

Histamine$_2$ Receptor Antagonists

Histamine$_2$ receptor antagonist medications (H_2 blockers) decrease acid secretion in the stomach. You may encounter patients who take H_2 blockers for short-term and episodic treatment of acid-related GI conditions. These medications are also administered in emergency settings to offset histamine release during an immune-mediated medication reaction or other type of allergic reaction. H_2 blockers prevent histamine from stimulating receptor sites on parietal cells in the stomach. This reduces acid secretion, protecting against ulcers, GI bleeding, acid-aspiration pneumonitis, and a variety of other related conditions. Cimetidine (Tagamet) and famotidine (Pepcid) are two H_2 blockers available for oral and IV administration.

Antiemetic Medications

Several types of antiemetic medications are available for use in the prehospital setting. Some patients may activate EMS with a primary complaint of nausea or vomiting. In other cases, nausea and vomiting are symptoms associated with primary events such as head injury, pregnancy, overdose, and myocardial ischemia. Beyond the obvious discomfort associated with nausea and vomiting, vomiting may dramatically worsen many serious medical conditions. Protracted vomiting may cause a Mallory-Weiss tear (a tear in the mucous membrane of the lower part of the esophagus or the upper part of the stomach), leading to GI bleeding. Vomiting can also raise intracranial and intraocular pressure, adversely affecting patients with head or eye injuries. In addition, vomiting can cause pulmonary aspiration in patients with an inadequately protected airway because of a decreased level of consciousness or positioning (such as being secured to a backboard or lying supine). Vomiting with aspiration of activated charcoal, administered following a toxic exposure, is often lethal. Patients with epiglottitis, peritonsillar abscess, or other airway disease may have increased edema due to vomiting. You are strongly encouraged to use antiemetic medications to prevent nausea and vomiting in at-risk patients.

Phenothiazine medications have both antiemetic and antipsychotic properties. These medications activate dopaminergic receptors in the brain, releasing hormones that depress the reticular activating system of the brain, and, ultimately, inhibit emesis. Promethazine (Phenergan, Promethegan, Phenadoz) and prochlorperazine (Compazine) are phenothiazine antiemetic medications used in various health care settings; both are available in oral and IV preparations. Promethazine is notorious for causing tissue injury during IV administration. Prochlorperazine is known for causing hypotension if administered rapidly through an IV line. **Dystonic** reactions are also possible with these medications, causing unusual muscle activity and significant patient discomfort. Dystonic reactions can be treated with IV diphenhydramine. Many other adverse effects are possible as well.

Metoclopramide (Reglan) is an antiemetic that may be available in the prehospital setting. This agent increases GI motility by enhancing the effects of ACh at receptor sites in the upper GI tract. Increased GI motility promotes gastric emptying, an effect that is useful in a variety of clinical situations. Metoclopramide can be administered orally, by slow IV injection, and by IV infusion. Dystonic reactions are also a possible adverse effect of metoclopramide and are again treated with IV diphenhydramine.

Antiemetic medications that antagonize the 5-hydroxytryptamine$_3$ (5-HT_3) receptor sites have experienced a recent surge in popularity. The 5-HT_3 receptors are present in the brain and GI tract, and they have a prominent role in activation of the vomiting center of the brain. Medications with the ability to occupy these receptor sites prevent certain (but not all) mechanisms that induce vomiting. For example, 5-HT_3 antagonists do not prevent vomiting related to motion sickness.

Ondansetron (Zofran), granisetron (Kytril), and dolasetron (Anzemet) are 5-HT_3 receptor antagonists that are available in oral and IV preparations for clinical use. Certain 5-HT_3 medications are now available in orally dissolving tablets. This preparation may eliminate the need for starting an IV line in patients who are actively vomiting but not showing signs of dehydration. Adverse effects are minimal but include the potential for QT prolongation shown on an ECG tracing.

Octreotide

You may encounter octreotide (Sandostatin) during interfacility transport of certain patients. Octreotide is not routinely administered in the prehospital setting. This medication is a synthetic version of somatostatin, a hormone that inhibits serotonin release, causing decreased secretion of insulin, glucagon, growth hormones, and various other chemicals. Octreotide has many potential uses. You may be requested to monitor an IV octreotide infusion during interfacility transport of a patient with bleeding esophageal varices. Octreotide decreases blood flow through esophageal blood vessels, reducing bleeding until definitive treatment can be provided. You should carefully monitor patients receiving this medication for a wide array of adverse effects, including bradycardia and chest pain related to octreotide.

Miscellaneous Medications Used in the Prehospital Setting

Certain medications are used widely in the prehospital setting but do not belong to one of the medication classes previously discussed. You should expect to use these medications in a variety of clinical situations. Additional dosing and administration information is available in Chapter 15, *Emergency Medications.*

Acetaminophen

Acetaminophen (Tylenol, APAP) is a medication with antipyretic (fever reduction) and mild analgesic properties. Paramedics and other EMS providers may administer acetaminophen as an adjunct to other analgesic medications, to reduce discomfort by treating fever symptoms, or to prevent febrile seizures in pediatric patients. Acetaminophen is not indicated for hyperthermia related to the toxic effects of medications or environmental exposure.

Acetaminophen is available as a tablet and capsule, liquid, and rectal suppository. At least two liquid concentrations are available, which may lead to dose calculation errors if you do not confirm the concentration before administration. Oral administration should be avoided in patients who are at high risk for seizures or airway compromise.

Adverse effects are rare when this medication is given at therapeutic doses. Toxicity from acetaminophen overdose is insidious and often mismanaged by health care providers. Elevated acetaminophen levels can cause severe, potentially fatal liver damage. Toxicity is determined by patient history and evaluation of a serum acetaminophen level, calculated according to the likely time of overdose. Once toxicity has been determined, many providers continue to mistakenly associate toxicity with serum acetaminophen levels. Liver damage will continue to occur from the presence of a harmful metabolite, rather than from the acetaminophen itself.

Calcium Preparations

In the prehospital setting, IV calcium has many potentially life-saving uses. It can be used for all of the following purposes:

- As an antidote to calcium channel blocker overdose
- To treat magnesium (sulfate) toxicity
- To prevent dysrhythmia during severe hyperkalemia
- For calcium repletion in patients with hypocalcemia
- For calcium restoration after hydrofluoric acid exposure
- As a pretreatment to prevent hypotension associated with IV verapamil administration

Calcium is not indicated for routine use during cardiac arrest resuscitation.

Typically, IV calcium is available as calcium chloride or calcium gluconate. Calcium chloride contains approximately three times the amount of elemental calcium per gram that is found in calcium gluconate. Both medications are known to be extremely irritating to blood vessels and should be diluted for slow IV infusion whenever possible. Carefully monitor IV catheter sites to avoid extravasation. Avoid subcutaneous or IM administration and assess for incompatibility when administering these agents simultaneously with other medications. Precipitation in IV tubing has been known to occur.

Dextrose

IV dextrose solution is administered to patients with known or presumptive hypoglycemia. In most cases, hypoglycemia is diagnosed with a handheld glucometer, now available on most ALS ambulances. When a glucometer is not immediately available, various clinical clues, such as a known history of diabetes, concurrent ethanol intoxication, and altered mental status, will prompt an astute paramedic to suspect hypoglycemia.

Once hypoglycemia is diagnosed, dextrose solution is administered through a large-bore IV catheter while the IV site is continually observed for signs of infiltration. Extravasation of IV dextrose can cause tissue destruction and edema. You should confirm IV placement with an adequate flush or free-flowing IV fluid before administering dextrose.

Rebound hypoglycemia is possible following dextrose administration. You should continue to monitor a patient's clinical status and blood glucose level following this treatment.

Diphenhydramine

EMS providers frequently use diphenhydramine for a variety of clinical situations. This competitive histamine-1 receptor antagonist prevents receptor activation by histamine released during various medical conditions. Diphenhydramine has a wide range of potential uses in the prehospital setting:

- Treatment of anaphylaxis in conjunction with other medications and interventions
- Sole treatment of mild allergic or immune-mediated medication reactions
- Mild sedative
- Mild antitussive (cough suppressant)
- Treatment of dystonic reaction or extrapyramidal symptoms
- Treatment of pruritus from an unknown cause
- Drying of the mucous membranes in patients with symptomatic rhinorrhea

Paramedics most commonly administer diphenhydramine by the IV or IM route. Oral capsule, tablet, and liquid preparations are also available commercially and are routinely taken by many people to treat minor conditions, such as seasonal allergies. Adverse effects from therapeutic doses of diphenhydramine are usually limited to mild sedation, palpitations, and anxiety. These symptoms become more significant if excessive amounts of diphenhydramine are administered in error. Profound toxicity and death are possible following large overdoses.

Glucagon

Glucagon (GlucaGen) is another medication with a variety of potential uses in the prehospital setting. This naturally occurring peptide hormone, which is secreted by the pancreas, is also manufactured commercially for the treatment of certain medical conditions.

As a paramedic, you may use glucagon for the treatment of hypoglycemia. Glucagon converts glycogen stores in the liver to circulating blood glucose, which can be used by various cells. This medication is useful if you are unable to initiate IV access in patients with diabetes who would otherwise be given IV glucose (dextrose). Patients who are combative because of moderate hypoglycemia and unresponsive patients without IV access are also likely candidates for receiving glucagon by the IM route. Glucose production takes 5 to 20 minutes following IV administration of glucagon and 30 minutes following IM administration. Blood glucose levels remain increased for only a limited time after glucagon is administered. Be sure to continually monitor for a return of hypoglycemia. An IV dextrose solution remains the preferred treatment for patients with hypoglycemia.

Glucagon is also used to increase heart rate and contractility following a beta adrenergic antagonist (beta blocker) overdose. It produces positive chronotropic and inotropic effects without directly activating beta-1 receptors. In addition, glucagon is used in the treatment of severe calcium channel blocker overdoses to reverse myocardial depression.

You may also administer glucagon to patients who present with a foreign body or large food particle lodged in the esophagus. Glucagon relaxes the smooth muscle in the GI tract, which may potentially allow the object to pass into the stomach for digestion. Glucagon should typically be administered for this purpose only after consultation with online medical control.

Ketorolac

Certain EMS systems use ketorolac (Toradol) as an alternative or adjunct to opioid analgesic medications. Ketorolac is a nonsteroidal anti-inflammatory drug (NSAID) that inhibits prostaglandin synthesis, treating both pain and inflammation. It is typically administered via the IV or IM route, although oral forms are available. GI irritation and headache are the most common adverse effects. Ketorolac is also known to cause pain at the injection site. Avoid this medication or use it with caution in any patient known to be susceptible to GI bleeding or a similar disorder. Some surgeons have been concerned that ketorolac can inhibit bone healing. An increasing body of evidence shows this fear is unfounded.[20]

Magnesium Sulfate

Magnesium sulfate is an IV electrolyte medication with several important clinical indications:

- Emergency treatment of torsades de pointes or similar ventricular dysrhythmia
- Correction of known or presumptive hypomagnesemia, a common condition in patients who are malnourished or consume ethanol on a long-term basis
- Prevention or treatment of seizures in pregnant patients with preeclampsia or eclampsia
- Adjunctive treatment with bronchodilators and other treatments for severe, refractory asthma

Magnesium sulfate replaces magnesium deficiencies in the body. Magnesium is essential for the movement of other electrolytes such as sodium, calcium, and potassium through channels of cell membranes. Hypomagnesemia causes seizure activity and cardiac dysrhythmias. As magnesium sulfate is administered, it decreases the excitability of cell membranes and slows conduction through the atrioventricular node, prolonging conduction time.

Magnesium sulfate acts to relax various smooth muscle tissues. Its clinical effects on smooth muscle are most notable in the lower airways, causing bronchodilation, and in the uterus, causing tocolysis. Respiratory depression, decreased muscle tone, and loss of deep tendon reflexes are possible from excessive doses of magnesium sulfate. Toxic effects from this medication are treated by discontinuing the infusion and administering an IV calcium preparation.

Sodium Bicarbonate

Sodium bicarbonate is an alkalinizing agent used in the prehospital and other health care settings. It is administered for the following purposes:

- Raise the blood pH in patients with a severe metabolic acidosis.
- Stabilize profound hyperkalemia in an emergency situation.
- Provide cardiac cell membrane stabilization following tricyclic antidepressant overdose.
- Promote urinary excretion of salicylate chemicals and certain tissue waste products.
- Replace bicarbonate lost due to various medical conditions.

Sodium bicarbonate can be administered by rapid IV push or added to IV fluids for intermittent or continuous infusion. You should evaluate for potential incompatibility when it is administered in the same IV tubing as other prehospital medications, especially calcium preparations and catecholamines. Patients receiving sodium bicarbonate should be monitored for changes in electrolyte and blood pH levels. Giving excessive amounts of this agent can cause fluid volume overload, alkalosis, numerous electrolyte abnormalities, and cerebral and pulmonary edema. In many cases, sodium bicarbonate is titrated to maintain a desired arterial or urinary pH value.

Tetracaine

Tetracaine, a mild ophthalmic anesthetic, is used when inserting the Morgan lens into an eye, to facilitate flushing the eyes. This procedure is discussed in Chapter 20, *Diseases of the Eyes, Ears, Nose, and Throat.*

Thiamine

Thiamine is a commercial medication preparation of vitamin B_1. Paramedics administer it to correct a presumptive thiamine deficiency before dextrose administration in patients who are malnourished or who consume alcohol on a long-term basis. Thiamine deficiency can cause Wernicke encephalopathy, a neurologic disorder, which may be exacerbated by the sudden administration of IV dextrose. Thiamine is administered by the IV or deep IM route. Toxic and adverse effects are unlikely when therapeutic doses are administered.

YOU are the Paramedic SUMMARY

1. What medical conditions would you expect to encounter in a skilled nursing facility or long-term care facility?

A vast array of medical conditions may be present in patients living in a skilled nursing facility or long-term care facility. Many medical interventions that were previously performed only in hospitals and rehabilitation facilities are now commonplace in skilled nursing facilities and long-term care facilities—for example, IV therapy, dialysis, complex wound care, and orthopaedic treatment. Dementia is the most common reason for skilled nursing facility placement. Other conditions, such as stroke (cerebrovascular accident), heart failure, Parkinson disease, osteoarthritis, and complications from diabetes mellitus, are also common in these patients.

YOU are the Paramedic SUMMARY continued

2. Based on this brief history and physical examination, what problems do you suspect?

This brief history and physical examination cannot exclude any of the possible causes or conditions that the patient may have.

3. What additional information would assist you with identifying possible causes of the patient's condition?

Vital signs, blood glucose level, physical examination, thorough history of the present illness, and a medication list would be helpful in identifying possible causes of this patient's altered mental status.

4. Would IV dextrose solution be indicated for this patient?

IV dextrose solution is not indicated for this patient. Normal blood glucose levels range from 70 to 99 mg/dL. This patient has a blood glucose level of 132 mg/dL and would be considered hyperglycemic. It is unlikely that this patient would benefit from IV dextrose solutions. Additionally, administration of dextrose solution could worsen other possible causes of altered mental status in older patients.

5. Do the electrocardiogram (ECG) findings assist in identifying the cause of this patient's condition?

The ECG tracing reveals sinus tachycardia. This finding indicates a state of physiologic stress on the body, but it is not specific enough to identify the cause of this patient's condition. Sinus tachycardia typically represents an increased catecholamine release from a wide variety of causes, such as exercise or physical exertion, fever, hypovolemia, shock, sepsis, pain, anxiety, hypoxia, or anemia, among numerous other possible causes. Many potential causes of altered mental status in older patients cause sinus tachycardia. It is not diagnostic in this scenario.

6. Does the patient's allergy and medication list add any possible causes of her current condition?

This patient is currently receiving 12 different medications on either a regularly scheduled or an as-needed basis. While certain medications on this patient's profile are relatively benign, other medications on her profile are extremely likely to alter many body organs, systems, and function. Medication interactions and medication side effects are frequently implicated as the cause of altered mental status in older patients. Medication toxicity, medication side effects, and medication interactions should be evaluated whenever searching for causes of altered mental status, particularly in older patients.

7. Which medications on this list, if any, should be used with particular caution in older patients?

Both promethazine (Phenergan) and metoclopramide (Reglan) require caution when used in older patients. Each of these medications can cause a number of serious cardiovascular and neurologic symptoms. Neurologic symptoms range from mild drowsiness to serious reactions, such as seizures and hallucinations. Promethazine is notorious for causing bizarre and unpredictable responses in older patients, including paradoxical excitation rather than sedation.

EMS Patient Care Report (PCR)					
Date: 7-23-22	**Incident No.:** 2056	**Nature of Call:** Altered mental status		**Location:** 1 Goldenbridge Lane	
Dispatched: 1510	**En Route:** 1511	**At Scene:** 1516	**Transport:** 1545	**At Hospital:** 1600	**In Service:** 1615
Patient Information					
Age: 88 **Sex:** F **Weight (in kg [lb]):** 60 kg (133 lb)			**Allergies:** Penicillin, sulfa medications **Medications:** Metformin, aspirin QD, lisinopril, atorvastatin, vitamin C, folate **Past Medical History:** Diabetes mellitus, nausea and vomiting **Chief Complaint:** Altered mental status		

YOU are the Paramedic SUMMARY continued

Vital Signs				
Time: 1521	**BP:** 96/64	**Pulse:** 108	**Respirations:** 22	**Spo_2:** 98% on O_2
Time: 1531	**BP:** 104/68	**Pulse:** 106	**Respirations:** 22	**Spo_2:** 99% on O_2
Time: 1541	**BP:** 112/72	**Pulse:** 104	**Respirations:** 20	**Spo_2:** 99% on O_2
Time: 1551	**BP:** 114/76	**Pulse:** 98	**Respirations:** 20	**Spo_2:** 98% on O_2

EMS Treatment (circle all that apply)				
Oxygen @ 10 L/min via (circle one): **NC (NRM) Bag-mask device**		**Assisted Ventilation**	**Airway Adjunct**	**CPR**
Defibrillation	**Bleeding Control**	**Bandaging**	**Splinting**	(**Other:** Cardiac monitoring)

Narrative

On arrival, found 88-year-old woman in bed with decreased responsiveness, moaning and incoherent speech, eyes open to deep tactile stimuli. Pt admitted for complications of diabetes mellitus. Pt developed nausea, vomiting, and diarrhea over past 36 to 48 hours. Pt noted to be "not herself." Pt temp. 99.7°F (37.6°C) just prior to arrival. Pt given 100% O_2 via nonrebreathing mask. Blood glucose checked, with a result of 132 mg/dL. Pt vitals taken and noted above. Slightly elevated pulse noted, and cardiac monitor applied. ECG tracing shows sinus tachycardia. Started IV in the right antecubital space with an 18-gauge catheter. Normal saline bag hung with 10-drop set at KVO rate. Pt placed on stretcher and vitals taken. Pt transported to Memorial Hospital without further changes. Report given to RN in room 4; IV patent and rhythm shown on the monitor.

End of report

Prep Kit

Ready for Review

- Although the science of pharmacology has evolved into a sophisticated area of health care, certain medications discovered in ancient times are still in use.
- Paramedics need to be familiar with the rules and regulations implemented under the Controlled Substances Act (also known as the Comprehensive Drug Abuse Prevention and Control Act) of 1970.
- Schedule I medications may not be prescribed, dispensed, used, or administered for medical use.
- All Schedule II through V medications require locked storage, significant record keeping, and controlled waste-disposal procedures.
- Every medication in the United States is given three distinct names:
  - Chemical name
  - Generic name
  - Brand name
- Reference sources, such as the *United States Pharmacopeia–National Formulary* and the *Prescriber's Digital Reference*, provide details about thousands of medications.
- Direct sunlight, extremes of heat and cold, and physical damage to medication containers can make medications ineffective or unsafe for use.
- As a medication is administered, it begins to alter a function or process in the body. This action is known as pharmacodynamics.

Prep Kit continued

- Medications are developed to reach and bind with particular receptor sites of target cells. Alpha and beta receptors include alpha-1 (vasoconstriction), alpha-2 (insulin restriction, glucagon secretion, inhibition of norepinephrine release), beta-1 (cardiac effects), and beta-2 (smooth muscle relaxation and bronchodilation).
- Newer medications are designed to target only very specific receptor sites on certain cells in an attempt to minimize side effects.
- A wide variety of factors, including the patient's genetic makeup, determine how a particular medication will affect a patient and may influence the choice of medication, dose, route, timing, manner of administration, and monitoring necessary after a patient receives a medication.
- The terms *side effect* and *adverse effect* are often used interchangeably, but adverse effect is usually meant in prehospital settings. Adverse effects are undesired or harmful responses to a medication.
- The relationship between the median effective dose and the median lethal dose or median toxic dose is known as the therapeutic index or therapeutic ratio.
- Repeated exposure to a medication within a particular class has the potential to cause a tolerance affecting other medications in the same class.
- Patients receiving multiple medications, drugs, or other chemicals are at risk of an unintended interaction between the various substances, possibly with unexpected results.
- As a medication is administered, the body begins a complex process of moving the medication, possibly altering the structure of the medication, and ultimately removing the medication from the body. The medication dose, route of administration, and clinical status of a patient will largely determine the duration of action and effectiveness of the medication.
- Many medication factors, such as the size of medication molecules, the ability to bind with other substances in the body, and the ability to dissolve in certain body fluids, determine which cells, tissues, and organs a particular medication will reach.
- Biotransformation is a process that has four possible effects on a medication absorbed into the body:
  - Can become active, producing wanted or unwanted clinical effects
  - Can be changed into another active medication
  - Can become completely or partially inactivated
  - Can be transformed into a substance that is easier for the body to eliminate
- Paramedics are constantly at risk for a cognitive error (such as choosing the wrong medication or dose) or a technical error (such as administering more volume of medication than intended).
- The rights of medication administration include the following considerations:
  - Right patient
  - Right medication and indication
  - Right dose
  - Right route
  - Right time
  - Right patient education
  - Right to refuse
  - Right response and evaluation
  - Right documentation and reporting
- Medications that influence the sympathetic nervous system are classified according to the receptors with which they interact—alpha or beta.
- Medications and medication groups often used in the prehospital setting include medications used for airway and respiratory management; medications used to manage conditions affecting the cardiovascular, gastrointestinal, and neurologic systems; and blood products and medications used to manage conditions affecting the blood.

Prep Kit continued

Vital Vocabulary

absolute refractory period The early phase of cardiac repolarization, during which the heart muscle cannot be stimulated to depolarize; also known as the effective refractory period.

absorption The process by which the molecules of a substance are moved from the site of entry or administration into systemic circulation.

acetylcholinesterase An enzyme that breaks down acetylcholine.

active metabolites Medications that have undergone biotransformation and are able to alter a cellular process or body function.

active transport The process of molecules binding with carrier proteins when energy is used to move the molecules against a concentration gradient.

adverse effects Abnormal or harmful effects to an organism caused by exposure to a chemical; indicated by some result such as death, a change in food or water consumption, altered body and organ weights, altered enzyme levels, or visible illness.

affinity The ability of a medication to bind with a particular receptor site.

agonist medications A group of medications that initiates or alters a cellular activity by attaching to receptor sites, prompting a cellular response.

analgesia The state of being insensible to pain while still conscious.

anaphylaxis An extreme systemic form of an allergic reaction involving two or more body systems.

anesthetic A medication that causes the inability to feel sensation.

antagonist medications A group of medications that prevent endogenous or exogenous agonist chemicals from reaching cell receptor sites and initiating or altering a particular cellular activity.

antibiotics Medications used to fight infection by killing the microorganisms or preventing their multiplication to allow the body's immune system to overcome them.

antifungals Medications used to treat fungal infections.

antimicrobials Medications used to kill or suppress the growth of microorganisms.

automaticity A state in which cardiac cells are at rest, waiting for the generation of a spontaneous impulse from within.

bioavailability The percentage of the unchanged medication that reaches systemic circulation.

biotransformation A process with four possible effects on a medication absorbed into the body: (1) An inactive substance can become active, capable of producing desired or unwanted clinical effects. (2) An active medication can be changed into another active medication. (3) An active medication may be completely or partially inactivated. (4) A medication is transformed into a substance (active or inactive) that is easier for the body to eliminate.

bronchoconstriction Narrowing of the bronchial tubes.

bronchodilation Widening of the bronchial tubes.

chelating agents Medications that bind with heavy metals in the body and create a compound that can be eliminated; used in cases of ingestion or poisoning.

cholinergic A term used to describe the fibers in the parasympathetic nervous system that release a chemical called acetylcholine.

competitive antagonists Medications that temporarily bind with cellular receptor sites, displacing agonist chemicals.

competitive depolarizing A term used to describe paralytic agents that act at the neuromuscular junction by binding with nicotinic receptors on muscles, causing fasciculations and preventing additional activation by acetylcholine.

contraindications Any conditions, especially any diseases, that render some particular line of treatment improper or undesirable.

cross-tolerance A process in which repeated exposure to a medication within a particular class

Prep Kit continued

causes a tolerance that may be "transferred" to other medications in the same class.

cumulative action Several smaller doses of a particular medication capable of producing the same clinical effects as a single larger dose of that same medication.

cytochrome P-450 system A hemoprotein involved in the detoxification of many drugs.

dependence The physical, behavioral, or emotional need for a medication or chemical to maintain "normal" physiologic function.

depolarization The process of discharging resting cardiac muscle fibers by an electric impulse that causes them to contract.

depressant A chemical or medication that decreases the performance of the central nervous system or sympathetic nervous system.

digitalis preparations Drugs used in the treatment of heart failure and certain atrial dysrhythmias.

distribution The movement and transportation of a medication throughout the bloodstream to tissues and cells and, ultimately, to its target receptor.

diuretic A chemical that increases urinary output.

dose-response curve A graphic illustration of the response of a drug according to the dose administered.

dosing The specified amount of a medication to be given at specific intervals.

down-regulation The process in which a mechanism reducing available cell receptors for a particular medication results in tolerance.

drug A substance that has some therapeutic effect (such as reducing inflammation, fighting bacteria, or producing euphoria) when given in the appropriate circumstances and in the appropriate dose.

drug class The grouping to which a medication belongs. Medications are grouped according to their characteristics, traits, or primary components.

duration (of action) In a pharmacologic context, the time a medication concentration can be expected to remain above the minimum level needed to provide the intended action.

dystonic Pertaining to voluntary muscle movements that are distorted or impaired because of abnormal muscle tone.

ectopic foci Sites of generation of electrical impulses other than normal pacemaker cells.

efficacy In a pharmacologic context, the ability of a medication to produce the desired effect.

elimination In a pharmacologic context, the removal of a medication or its by-products from the body.

endogenous Originating from within the organism (body).

exogenous Originating outside the organism (body).

extravasation Seepage of blood and medication into the tissue surrounding the blood vessel.

facilitated diffusion The process of medication molecules binding with carrier proteins when no energy is expended.

fasciculation Brief, uncoordinated, visible twitching of small muscle groups; may be caused by the administration of a depolarizing neuromuscular blocking agent (namely, succinylcholine).

filtration Use of hydrostatic pressure to force water or dissolved particles through a semipermeable membrane.

first-order elimination The process in which the rate of elimination is directly influenced by plasma levels of a substance.

first-pass effect The alteration of a medication via metabolism within the gastrointestinal tract before it reaches systemic circulation.

habituation An unusual tolerance to the therapeutic and adverse clinical effects of a medication or chemical.

half-life The time needed in an average person for metabolism or elimination of 50% of a substance in the plasma.

Prep Kit continued

hematocrit The percentage of red blood cells in a blood sample.

hemolysis The destruction of red blood cells by disruption of the cell membrane.

hydrophilic Attracted to water molecules.

idiosyncratic In a pharmacologic context, abnormal susceptibility to a medication, possibly due to genetic traits or dysfunction of a metabolic enzyme, that is peculiar to an individual patient (and usually unexplained).

inactive metabolites Medications that have undergone biotransformation and are no longer able to alter a cell process or body function; not pharmacologically active.

indication A circumstance that points to or shows the cause, pathology, treatment, or issue of an attack of disease; that which points out; that which serves as a guide or warning.

interference A situation in which one medication or chemical taken by a patient undermines the effectiveness of another medication taken by or administered to a patient.

lipophilic Attracted to fats and lipids.

mechanism of action The way in which a medication produces the intended response.

median effective dose (ED_{50}) The weight-based dose of a medication that was effective in 50% of the humans and animals tested.

median lethal dose (LD_{50}) The weight-based dose of a medication that caused death in 50% of the animals tested.

median toxic dose (TD_{50}) The weight-based dose of a medication that demonstrated toxicity in 50% of the animals tested.

medication A substance used to treat an illness or condition.

medication monograph A document that gives detailed information about drugs, such as their indications and uses, dosing information, precautions, contraindications, and adverse effects.

medication sensitivity A mild to severe reaction after the first exposure to a medication or other substance, which often features many of the same signs and symptoms as an immune-mediated reaction.

noncompetitive antagonists Medications that permanently bind with receptor sites and prevent activation by agonist chemicals.

nondepolarizing A term used to describe drugs that produce muscle relaxation by interfering with impulses between the nerve ending and the muscle receptor.

nonionic Uncharged.

onset The time needed for the concentration of the medication at the target tissue to reach the minimum effective level.

orthostatic hypotension A fall in blood pressure when changing to a standing position.

osmosis The movement of a solvent, such as water, from an area of low solute concentration to one of high concentration through a selectively permeable membrane to equalize concentrations of a solute on both sides of the membrane.

osmotic Characterized by the movement of a solvent, such as water, across a semipermeable membrane (eg, the cell wall) from an area of lower solute concentration to an area of higher concentration.

paradoxical Opposite from expected.

partial agonist A chemical that binds to the receptor site but does not initiate as much cellular activity or change as other agonists do; lowers the efficacy of other agonist chemicals present at the cells.

peak In a pharmacologic context, the point of maximum effect of a drug.

pharmacodynamics The biochemical and physiologic effects and mechanism of action of a medication in the body.

pharmacokinetics The activity of medications in the body over time, such as absorption, distribution, and elimination.

Prep Kit continued

pharmacology The scientific study of how various substances interact with or alter the function of living organisms.

pinocytosis A process by which cells ingest the extracellular fluid and its contents.

placebo effect In a pharmacologic context, the positive and negative effects of an inactive medication on a person that are related to the person's expectations and other factors.

plasma protein binding A process in which medication molecules temporarily attach to proteins in the blood plasma, significantly altering medication distribution in the body.

potency The relationship between the desired response of a medication and the dose required to achieve the response.

receptor A specialized area in tissues that initiates certain actions after specific stimulation.

relative refractory period The period in the cell-firing cycle at which it is possible but difficult to restimulate the cell to fire another impulse.

Stevens-Johnson syndrome A severe, possibly fatal reaction that mimics a burn; may be due to a medication.

stimulant A medication or chemical that temporarily enhances central nervous system and sympathetic nervous system functioning.

sympathomimetics Medications administered to stimulate the sympathetic nervous system.

tachyphylaxis A condition in which repeated doses of medication within a short period rapidly cause tolerance, making the medication virtually ineffective.

therapeutic index The relationship between the median effective dose and the median lethal dose or median toxic dose; also known as the therapeutic ratio.

threshold level In a pharmacologic context, the concentration of medication at which initiation or alteration of cellular activity begins.

tolerance A condition that develops following repeated use by a patient of a medication that results in decreased efficacy or potency.

untoward effects Clinical changes caused by a medication that cause harm or discomfort to a patient; also known as adverse effects.

vasoconstriction Narrowing of the diameter of a blood vessel.

vasodilation Widening of the diameter of a blood vessel.

Vaughan-Williams classification A classification scheme for medications based on the mechanism of action rather than on specific medication groups.

volume of distribution The extent to which a medication will spread within the body.

water-soluble A property that indicates a material can be dissolved in water.

zero-order elimination A process in which a fixed amount of a substance is removed during a certain period, regardless of the total amount in the body.

References

1. Applying class of recommendations and level of evidence to clinical strategies, interventions, treatments, or diagnostic testing in patient care. American Heart Association website. https://cpr.heart.org/en/resuscitation-science/cpr-and-ecc-guidelines/tables/applying-class-of-recommendation-and-level-of-evidence. Updated May 2019. Accessed July 5, 2021.
2. Brown LH, Bailey LC, Medwick T, Okeke CC, Krumperman K, Tran CD. Medication storage on US ambulances: a prospective multi-center observational study. *Pharm Forum.* 2003;29:540-547.
3. Gammon DL, Su S, Roger Huckfeldt R, et al. Alteration in prehospital drug concentration after thermal exposure. *Am J Emerg Med.* 2008;26(5):566-573.
4. McMullan JT, Pinnawin A, Jones E, et al. The 60-day temperature-dependent degradation of midazolam and lorazepam in the prehospital environment. *Prehosp Emerg Care.* 2013;17(1):1-7.
5. Madden JF, O'Connor RE, Evans J. The range of medication storage temperatures in aeromedical emergency medical services. *Prehosp Emerg Care.* 1999;3(1):27-30.

Prep Kit continued

6. Lin BW, Yoshida D, Quin J, Strehlow M. A better way to estimate adult patients' weights. *Am J Emerg Med*. 2009;27(9):1060-1064.
7. Panchal AR, Bartos JA, Cabañas JG, et al. Part 3: Adult basic and advanced life support: 2020 American Heart Association guidelines for cardiopulmonary resuscitation and emergency cardiovascular care. *Circulation*. 2020;142(16 suppl 2):S366-S468.
8. FDA pregnancy categories. Drugs.com website. https://www.drugs.com/pregnancy-categories.html. Accessed July 5, 2021.
9. Pozner CN. Advanced cardiac life support (ACLS) in adults. UpToDate website. https://www.uptodate.com/contents/advanced-cardiac-life-support-acls-in-adults?topicKey=EM%2F278&elapsedTimeMs=6&view=print&displayedView=full#. Updated April 1, 2021. Accessed May 11, 2021.
10. Patterson SJ, Oliphant CS, Self TH. Amiodarone-induced lung disease *Consultant*. 2014;54(3):207-208.
11. Ebrom C, Manifold C, Schaefer R. Resident eagle: whole blood in the rural EMA environment. EMS World website. https://www.emsworld.com/article/1224535/resident-eagle-whole-blood-rural-ems-environment. Published July 2020. Accessed May 11, 2021.
12. Arefleva CAL, Chen B, Redman TT, et al. The use of low-titer group O whole blood in emergency medicine. Emergency Medicine Residents' Association website. https://www.emra.org/emresident/article/group-o-whole-blood/. Published October 17, 2018. Accessed May 11, 2021.
13. Matijevic N, Wang YW, Cotton BA, et al. Better hemostatic profiles of never-frozen liquid plasma compared with thawed fresh frozen plasma. *J Trauma Acute Care Surg*. 2013;74(1):84-91.
14. Napolitano LM. Prehospital tranexamic acid: what is the current evidence? *Trauma Surg Acute Care Open*. 2017;2(1):e000056. https://doi.org/10.1177/14604086211001163.
15. Napolitano LM, Cohen MJ, Cotton BA, et al. Tranexamic acid in trauma: how should we use it. *J Trauma Acute Care Surg*. 2013;74(6):1575-1586.
16. Bucchiara BL, Messe SR. Antithrombotic therapy for the secondary prevention of ischemic stroke. UpToDate website. https://www.uptodate.com/contents/antithrombotic-therapy-for-the-secondary-prevention-of-ischemic-stroke/. Updated April 26, 2021. Accessed May 11, 2021.
17. Bhatt DL, Fox KAA, Hacke W, et al. Clopidogrel and aspirin versus aspirin alone for the prevention of atherothrombotic events. *N Engl J Med*. 2006;354(16):1706-1717.
18. Anondo Stangi P, Lewis S. Review of currently available GP IIb/IIIa inhibitors and their role in peripheral vascular interventions. *Semin Intervent Radiol*. 2010;27(4):412-421.
19. Smith HS, Smith JM, Seidner P. Opioid-induced nausea and vomiting. *Ann Palliat Med*. 2012;1(2):121-129.
20. McDonald E, Winters B, Nicholson K, et al. Effect of postoperative ketorolac administration on bone healing in ankle fracture surgery. *Foot Ankle Int*. 2018;39(10):1135-1140.

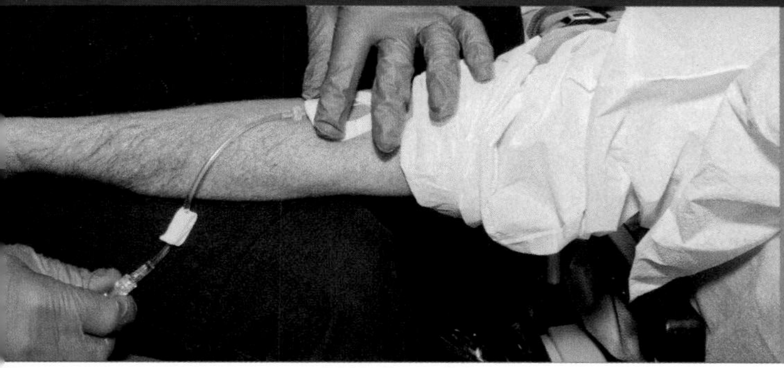

Chapter 14

Medication Administration

NATIONAL EMS EDUCATION STANDARD COMPETENCIES

Pharmacology

Integrates comprehensive knowledge of pharmacology to formulate a treatment plan intended to mitigate emergencies and improve the overall health of the patient.

Medication Administration

- Routes of administration (see Chapter 13, *Principles of Pharmacology*)
- Self-administer medication (p 871)
- Peer-administer medication (p 871)
- Assist/administer medications to a patient (pp 798, 834–841, 843–875)
- Within the scope of practice of the paramedic, administer medications to a patient (pp 798, 834–841, 843–875)

KNOWLEDGE OBJECTIVES

1. Describe the role of medical direction in medication administration. (p 798)
2. Discuss the benefits of performing a Medication Administration Cross-Check (MACC) before administering a medication. (p 799)
3. Explain the importance of properly documenting medication administration. (p 798)
4. Discuss paramedics' responsibilities related to security of medications stocked on the ambulance. (p 799)
5. Explain the differences between aseptic, clean, and sterile techniques. (p 800)
6. Describe the use of standard precautions related to medication administration. (p 801)
7. Discuss the signs and symptoms that can occur with changes in the body's fluid status. (pp 801–803)
8. List commonly used intravenous (IV) fluid compositions and types of IV solutions. (pp 803–806)
9. Discuss the techniques for performing IV therapy. (pp 806–821)
10. Discuss the factors to consider when choosing an IV solution. (p 807)
11. Discuss the factors to consider when choosing an administration set. (pp 808–809)
12. Discuss the factors to consider when choosing an IV site. (pp 809–812)
13. List the types of IV catheters. (p 847)
14. Describe special considerations when performing IV therapy on a pediatric or older adult patient. (pp 820–821)
15. List the factors to check if the IV flow rate is incorrect. (p 821)
16. Describe complications that can occur as a result of IV therapy. (pp 821–825)
17. Discuss transport considerations for a patient undergoing a blood transfusion. (p 827)
18. Discuss the advantages, disadvantages, and techniques for establishing an intraosseous (IO) line. (pp 827–834)

19. List the types of IO devices available. (pp 829–831)
20. Discuss the potential complications of IO infusion. (pp 831–834)
21. Discuss the systems of weights and measures used when administering medication. (pp 837–840)
22. Explain the principles of drug dose calculations, including desired dose, concentration on hand, volume on hand, volume to administer, and IV drip rate. (pp 839–843)
23. Discuss the advantages, disadvantages, and techniques of oral medication administration. (pp 843–844)
24. Discuss the advantages, disadvantages, and techniques of rectal medication administration. (pp 844–845)
25. Discuss the advantages, disadvantages, and techniques of intradermal medication administration. (pp 852–853)
26. Discuss the advantages, disadvantages, and techniques of subcutaneous medication administration. (pp 853–854)
27. Discuss the advantages, disadvantages, and techniques of intramuscular medication administration. (pp 855–857)
28. Discuss the advantages, disadvantages, and techniques of IV medication administration. (pp 857–864)
29. Discuss the advantages, disadvantages, and techniques of IO medication administration. (pp 864–865)
30. Discuss the advantages, disadvantages, and techniques of transdermal medication administration. (pp 865–867)
31. Discuss the advantages, disadvantages, and techniques of sublingual medication administration. (p 867)
32. Discuss other methods of medication administration, including the buccal, ocular, and aural routes. (pp 867–869)
33. Discuss the advantages, disadvantages, and techniques of intranasal medication administration. (p 869)
34. Discuss the advantages, disadvantages, and techniques of inhaled medication administration. (pp 869–875)
35. Discuss the rates at which medication is absorbed through various routes. (p 878)

SKILLS OBJECTIVES

1. Demonstrate how to spike an IV bag. (p 815)
2. Demonstrate how to obtain vascular access. (pp 815–817, Skill Drill 14-1)
3. Demonstrate how to obtain a blood sample. (pp 825–827)
4. Demonstrate how to gain IO access. (pp 832–833, Skill Drill 14-2)
5. Demonstrate how to administer oral medication to a patient. (pp 843–844)
6. Demonstrate how to administer medication via a gastric tube. (p 844)
7. Demonstrate how to draw medication from an ampule. (pp 848–849, Skill Drill 14-3)
8. Demonstrate how to draw medication from a vial. (pp 850–851, Skill Drill 14-4)
9. Demonstrate how to administer a subcutaneous medication to a patient. (p 854, Skill Drill 14-5)
10. Demonstrate how to administer an intramuscular medication to a patient. (pp 856–857, Skill Drill 14-6)
11. Demonstrate how to administer a medication via the IV bolus route. (p 858, Skill Drill 14-7)
12. Demonstrate how to administer a medication via IV piggyback. (pp 861–863, Skill Drill 14-8)
13. Demonstrate how to perform an IO infusion. (pp 865–866, Skill Drill 14-9)
14. Demonstrate how to administer a sublingual medication to a patient. (p 868, Skill Drill 14-10)
15. Demonstrate how to administer an intranasal medication to a patient. (p 870, Skill Drill 14-11)
16. Demonstrate how to assist a patient with a metered-dose inhaler. (p 872, Skill Drill 14-12)
17. Demonstrate how to assist a patient with a small-volume nebulizer. (p 874, Skill Drill 14-13)
18. Demonstrate how to access nontunneling and implanted vascular access devices. (pp 875–878)

Introduction

Your paramedic education will provide you with knowledge of anatomy and physiology, pathophysiology, and the effects that pharmacologic treatments have on patients. It is your responsibility to administer the appropriate medications and the appropriate dosage when needed, and to determine the most effective route by which to administer them. Always remember that any procedure that you perform, including medication administration, must be approved by a medical director through either established protocols or online medical direction.

Vascular access is often needed in emergency medicine for hemodynamically unstable patients who need intravenous (IV) fluids, various medications, or both. Several techniques are used to gain vascular access in the prehospital setting, including cannulation of a peripheral extremity vein, external jugular (EJ) vein cannulation, intraosseous (IO) access, and long-term vascular access devices (VADs). **Cannulation** is the insertion of a catheter into a body cavity, duct, or vessel to allow for fluid flow. The survival of critically ill or injured patients often depends on your ability to obtain vascular access quickly and effectively. Because these procedures are invasive, you must be proficient in performing them. Significant harm to the patient can result from use of improper technique,

SAFETY

One concept that contributes to an effective safety culture is the high-reliability organization (HRO).[1,2] The airline and nuclear power industries, which are populated with many HROs, share some common traits. For example, all HROs are preoccupied with failure, and each organization's culture well understands that failures will inevitably occur. However, HROs focus on managing these failures, so that a failure does not reach the customer (the patient, in the health care industry). This drive has led to the redundancy in training, equipment, and maintenance seen in the airline industry. Both the airlines and nuclear power plants recognize that a person or piece of equipment may fail, so they have put considerable effort into ensuring a single failure does not cause a catastrophic event (ie, plane crash, nuclear meltdown). In health care, an HRO would focus on double checks (eg, cross-checking a medication being administered) and other systems to ensure a single failure, which is inevitable, does not lead to patient harm.

YOU are the Paramedic

PART 1

You respond to a private residence for a call concerning a 26-year-old man who experienced a syncopal episode. On your arrival, the patient states that he had a sudden onset of palpitations while in the bathroom and felt dizzy. He lowered himself to the ground before briefly losing consciousness. The patient reports that the palpitations are still present, but he denies chest discomfort or dyspnea. Your primary survey reveals no immediate life threats. As your partner applies the cardiac monitor and obtains a baseline set of vital signs, you note a rapid, irregular pulse.

Recording Time: 1 Minute	
Appearance	Warm and moist skin
Level of consciousness	Alert (oriented to person, place, time, and event)
Airway	Spontaneously patent
Breathing	20 breaths/min, nonlabored
Circulation	Strong, rapid, irregular radial pulse

1. Given this scenario, what route of delivery do you anticipate using to administer medications? What are the advantages of this route?
2. What aspects of the patient history are important to consider before administering any medication to this patient?

insufficient knowledge of the medications being administered, or both.

This chapter discusses the various types of IV solutions used in the prehospital setting and IV/IO therapy techniques. It describes the mathematic principles used in pharmacology, and for calculating medication doses: those given as a **bolus** (a single dose, usually administered by the IV route) and as maintenance infusion. Paramedics administer medications in different forms. The chapter concludes with a discussion of routes for administering medications.

Medical Direction

Several points related to medical direction, specifically for medication administration, are important to highlight here (medical direction is discussed in depth in Chapter 1, *EMS Systems*). For example, your medical director may require you to make contact with medical control before you perform specific procedures (eg, administering certain opioids). When requesting orders from online medical control, be confident and detailed. Gather all patient information before contacting medical control. You should be able to paint a picture of the patient to the physician and demonstrate the need for the medication you are requesting.

Local policies and procedures are designed to guide you in specific situations. The principles of crew resource management, discussed in Chapter 5, *Communications*, and Chapter 40, *Responding to the Field Code*, suggest you should use any resources available to help reduce cognitive load. Therefore, if you are not confident about a drug dose, indication, contraindication, or any other aspect of medication administration, then you should use your protocols, a drug formulary, a flip guide, a smartphone or tablet application, or any other available resource. Beyond the resources available on your response unit, consider medical control for assistance. Online medical control is not just an authority to be consulted for the approval of medications that are outside of your protocols. You can also access medical control for general consultation of treatment modalities with which you are not confident. *If you have any doubt regarding the correct action, then consult medical control!*

Ensuring Correct and Safe Medication Administration

You must ensure that the medications you deliver are administered accurately and safely. Medication errors are an issue throughout health care. Paramedics administer medications based on standing orders or online medical direction, but actual oversight in the moment of administration is minimal. This is why the emergency medical services (EMS) system must develop tools to mitigate errors arising from human factors, and why paramedics must make a conscious effort to use these tools.

The danger of something going wrong when you are administering a drug, such as administering the incorrect drug or the incorrect dose of a drug, can also be minimized by using a tool to verify the drug dose, name, route, rate of administration, indication for administration, contraindications, drug **concentration**, and volume to be administered.[3] Never guess what the physician has ordered. When in doubt, ask for clarification. The rights of medication administration should always be followed; they are discussed in Chapter 13, *Principles of Pharmacology*.

Documenting medication administration is extremely important. You must list the dose administered, name of the medication, route, rate, time of administration, who administered the drug, who helped perform the medication check, and the patient's response. The dose should be listed by the total quantity administered at that time, the units of measure for that drug, and the volume administered to the patient. Verify the spelling of the drug name; this is where medication errors commonly occur. The rate should be documented in reference to a bolus, infusion, or other administration method.

Local Drug Distribution System

Before responding to an EMS call, you must ensure all equipment on the emergency vehicle is fully functional; this verification occurs during your check of the vehicle at the beginning of your shift. All medications must be checked to ensure they are not expired or damaged, and are readily available in the right quantity. You must be thoroughly familiar

Words of Wisdom

Wichita-Sedgwick County EMS System in Kansas developed a tool known as Medication Administration Cross-Check (MACC) **FIGURE 14-1**.[4] This tool uses crew resource management principles by requiring a process for verification for every medication every time. In addition, the tool uses job aids to help reduce cognitive load and ensure the process is completed each time a medication is administered.

Because EMS systems vary in configuration—for example, a paramedic working with a basic life support (BLS) provider—the MACC tool is designed to work with all provider levels. Although BLS providers may lack familiarity with all medications, they can verify quantities, medication names, expiration dates, and other information. More importantly, the second provider, regardless of certification level, acts as a sounding board for the first provider. This practice forces the first provider to validate the medication administration. Some providers may catch the error as they read it back to themselves. Others may catch it when the second provider asks them to repeat something that did not sound right. Sometimes the second provider can catch the error and bring it to the first provider's attention. Although the MACC tool will not eliminate all medication errors, its proper use can significantly reduce the number of medication errors.

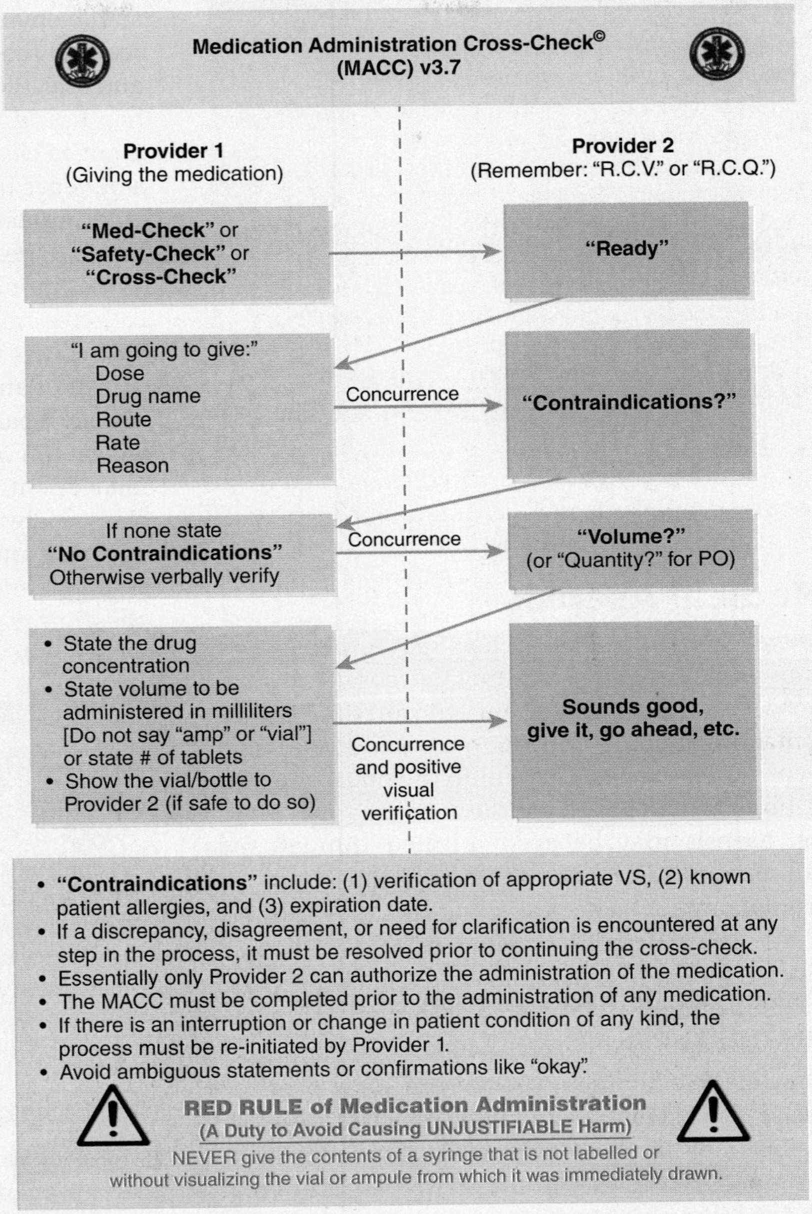

FIGURE 14-1 Medication Administration Cross-Check job aid.

Reproduced from: Misasi P, Braithwaite S. *The Medication Administration Cross-Check (MACC) User's Manual.* Wichita-Sedgwick County EMS System; March 2012. https://kansasemstransition.files.wordpress.com/2012/08/macc-user-manual-v2-0.pdf. Accessed May 27, 2021.

with the system used to exchange and replace outdated or damaged drugs in your EMS system.

You are also responsible for the documentation and security of all controlled substances carried on your vehicle, including accounting for all controlled substances that were wasted (ie, residual medication that was not administered to the patient). Follow the specific policies and procedures of your local drug distribution, security, and accountability system.

Documentation and Communication

In addition to the normal documentation of a medication given, you will need to follow your medical director's policy on documenting any "wasted" medication. For example, if you administer a controlled substance (eg, morphine, midazolam [Versed], fentanyl [Sublimaze, Duragesic]), then document the amount of medication that you gave to the patient and the amount of medication that you wasted (did not give to the patient). Have your partner, a nurse or physician from the receiving facility, or your supervisor witness (actually see) you wasting the medication. Both of you should sign the form documenting the disposal of the wasted medication.

Medical Asepsis

Medical asepsis is the practice of preventing contamination from pathogens by using **aseptic technique**. This cleansing method is intended to prevent contamination of a site when you are performing an invasive procedure such as starting an IV line or administering a medication. Medical asepsis may be accomplished through the use of sterilization of equipment, antiseptics, or disinfectants.

Clean Technique Versus Sterile Technique

Some of the equipment you will use in the field has been sterilized for patient safety. For example, some medications have been packaged using **sterile** technique. Sterile technique refers to the destruction of all living organisms and is achieved through the application of heat, gas, or chemicals.

To create a sterile field, multiple pieces of sterile equipment must be used and rules must be followed. You will need to wear a mask and sterile sleeves or a gown that covers you from the wrist to 2 inches (5 cm) proximal to the elbow. In addition, you must don appropriate-size sterile gloves, which are identified using numeric sizes rather than "small" to "extra large" sizing. Place sterile drapes around the procedural area; anything below the drapes should be considered nonsterile. Only sterile items and personnel may enter the sterile field to ensure that the area remains sterile.

Because it may not be feasible to maintain a sterile environment in the field, you must practice medical asepsis to reduce the risk of contamination and infection. Examples of medical asepsis include handwashing, wearing gloves, and keeping equipment as clean as possible. For example, the site on a patient's hand that has been cleaned with iodine, chlorhexidene, or alcohol before starting an IV line is said to be "medically clean."

If you open an IV catheter package and the IV catheter inadvertently falls to the ground or otherwise comes in contact with a contaminated surface, discard it and obtain a new IV catheter. If you have already cleaned the injection port on the IV tubing where you intend to inject a medication but then inadvertently touch the cleaned injection port, recleanse the port before injecting the medication. You must always make a conscious effort to prevent contamination, whether handling equipment, supplies, or the patient.

Words of Wisdom

In addition to ensuring medications have not expired or become contaminated, you must ensure medications are kept at the recommended temperatures while stored in your emergency vehicle. Some medications become inactive in extreme heat or cold conditions. The package insert for each medication will provide this information.

Antiseptics and Disinfectants

Antiseptics are used to cleanse an area before performing an invasive procedure such as IV therapy or medication administration. Even though antiseptics are capable of destroying pathogens, they are not toxic to living tissues. Isopropyl alcohol (rubbing alcohol), iodine, and 2% chlorhexidine gluconate (ChloraPrep) are the antiseptics you will most often use in the field.

Disinfectants, in contrast to antiseptics, are toxic to living tissues; therefore, you should never use them on a patient. Use disinfectants only on nonliving objects such as the inside of the ambulance, laryngoscope blades, and other nondisposable equipment.

Standard Precautions and Contaminated Equipment Disposal

The first rule of standard precautions is to treat any body fluid as being potentially infectious. Chapter 2, *Workforce Safety and Wellness*, discusses these principles in detail.

Disposal of Contaminated Equipment

After an IV catheter or needle has penetrated a patient's skin, it is contaminated. Accidental needlesticks are becoming less common thanks to standard precautions and safety-conscious needle designs, but they remain a leading cause of disease transmission in the health care setting.[5] Always handle contaminated equipment carefully and dispose of it immediately and properly. **Sharps** include IV, intramuscular (IM), and subcutaneous needles and catheters, scalpels, broken ampules or vials, and anything else that can penetrate or lacerate the skin.

Immediately dispose of all sharps in a puncture-proof sharps container that bears a biohazard logo **FIGURE 14-2**. Sharps containers should be readily accessible to minimize the time spent handling needles, catheters, and other sharps **FIGURE 14-3**. In addition, you should include a smaller sharps container in your jump kit or drug box to allow for immediate disposal of sharps while not in the emergency vehicle. **TABLE 14-1** lists some safe practices that will minimize your risk of an inadvertent needlestick.

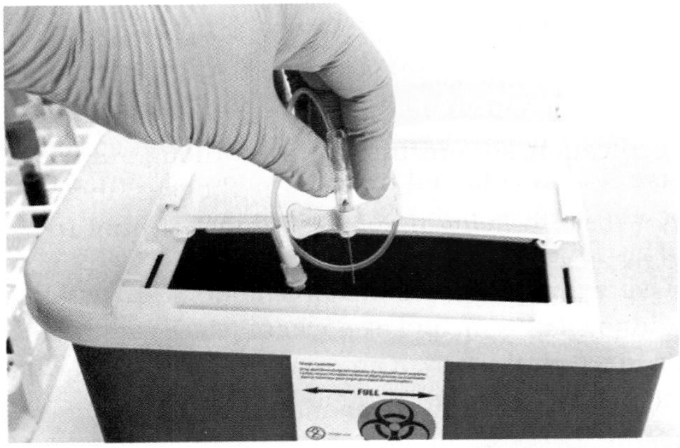

FIGURE 14-2 Always dispose of sharp objects or blood-filled items in a puncture-proof sharps container.

Cellular Fluid Composition and Status

Body Fluid Composition

The human body is composed mostly of water, which provides the environment where the chemical reactions necessary for life take place, as described in Chapter 8, *Anatomy and Physiology*. The healthy body maintains a delicate balance between intake and output of fluids and electrolytes, ensuring the internal environment remains relatively constant. However, the ill or injured body may be unable to maintain homeostasis, and excesses or deficits of fluids and electrolytes may occur. As a paramedic, you need to know when IV fluids

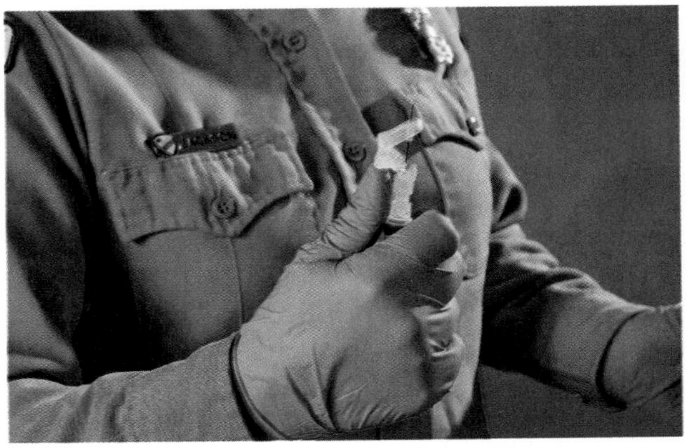

A

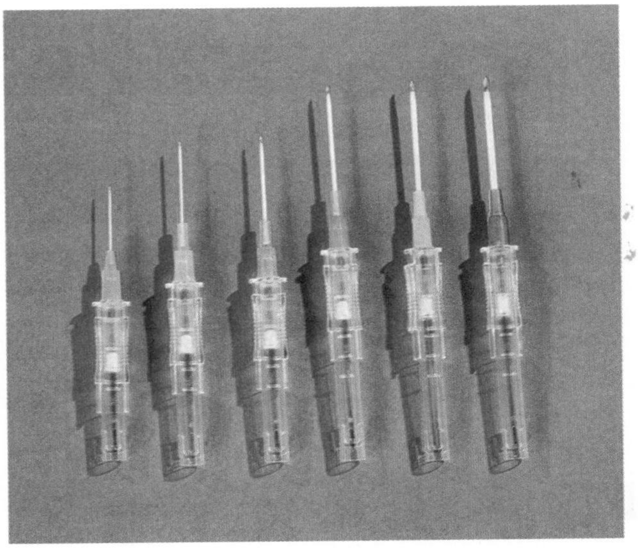

B

FIGURE 14-3 Safety hypodermic needle **(A)** and safety intravenous catheters **(B)**.

TABLE 14-1 Minimizing Your Risk of a Needlestick

Use blunt-tip needles when drawing medication from vials or infusing medications directly into an IV solution.
Use a needleless delivery system so the needle "recaps" itself, which will greatly reduce the risk of a needlestick.
Immediately dispose of all sharps in a puncture-proof sharps container. *Do not* drop the sharps on the floor for later disposal, and *do not* attempt to recap a needle and syringe before placing it in the sharps container. Even if you use a needle or IV line that automatically retracts, you still must discard it in a sharps container.
When possible, perform invasive procedures at the scene. If the patient's condition warrants starting an IV line or administering a medication en route to the hospital, then *use extreme caution*. Although most paramedics become proficient at starting IV lines in the back of a moving ambulance, it may be necessary to have your partner briefly stop the ambulance, especially if you are traveling over rough terrain.
Recap needles *only* as an absolute last resort. If you must recap a needle, then use the one-handed technique: Place the needle cover on a stationary surface, then slide the needle with one hand—into the needle cap.

Abbreviation: IV, intravenous

are indicated, which kinds of fluids are required in different situations, and when IV fluids can be dangerous.

A healthy person loses approximately 2 to 2.5 L of fluid daily through urine output, through the lungs (exhalation), and through the skin. These losses are replaced by intake of fluids and by nutrients that are partially converted to water in their metabolism. In illness, abnormal states of hydration may occur where intake and output are no longer in balance.

Dehydration

Dehydration is defined as inadequate total systemic fluid volume. It is usually a chronic condition of young and older patients and may take days to manifest. As fluid loss occurs from the vascular compartment, the body reacts by shifting interstitial fluid into the vascular area; fluid also shifts from the intracellular to the extracellular compartments. The result of these fluid movements is a total systemic fluid deficit.

Signs and symptoms of dehydration include altered level of consciousness, orthostatic hypotension, tachypnea, dry mucous membranes, decreased urine output, tachycardia, poor skin turgor, and flushed, dry skin. Causes of dehydration include diarrhea, vomiting, gastrointestinal drainage, infections, metabolic disorders such as diabetic ketoacidosis, hemorrhage, environmental emergencies, a high-caffeine diet, and insufficient fluid intake.

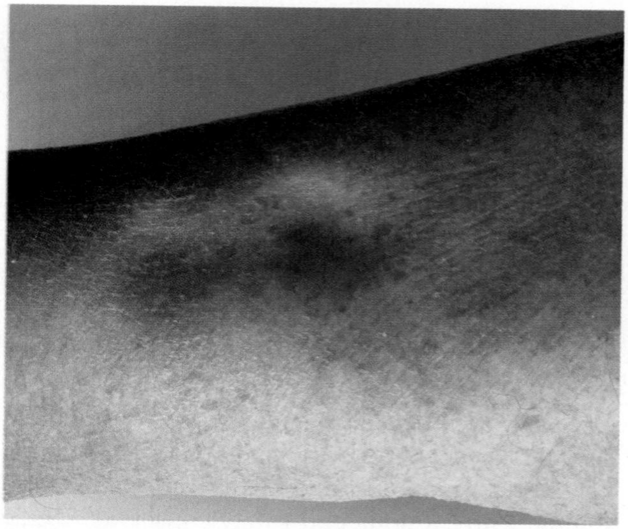

FIGURE 14-4 One sign of fluid backup is pitting edema, shown in this patient. Pitting edema occurs when the skin is pressed with a finger and an indentation remains after removing the finger, as seen here.

Overhydration

When the body's total systemic fluid volume increases, **overhydration** occurs. Fluid fills the vascular compartment, filters into the interstitial compartment, and is forced from the engorged interstitial compartment into the intracellular compartment. This fluid backup can lead to death **FIGURE 14-4**. Overhydration may occur in patients with impaired kidney function, and also when health care professionals administer an amount of fluid beyond what the body can excrete. Neonates (children younger than 1 month) are also more likely to experience overhydration because their kidneys are not yet fully developed.

Signs and symptoms of overhydration include shortness of breath, puffy eyelids, edema, polyuria, moist crackles (formerly called rales), and acute weight gain. Causes of overhydration include unmonitored IV lines (in pediatric patients), kidney failure, water intoxication in endurance sports, and prolonged hypoventilation.

Words of Wisdom

The cardinal sign of overhydration is edema.

IV Fluid Composition

The use of IV fluids can significantly alter the patient's condition and facilitate patient treatment. Each bag of IV solution must be sterile and safe; therefore, each bag of IV solution is individually sterilized **FIGURE 14-5**.

Human plasma contains a variety of electrolytes, as discussed in Chapter 9, *Pathophysiology*. The compounds and ions dissolved in IV solutions are identical to those found in the body, although their concentrations may vary. **TABLE 14-2** lists the electrolyte composition of various IV fluids.

Sodium is used as the benchmark to calculate a solution's tonicity. The concentration of sodium in the cells of the body is approximately 0.9%. Therefore, altering the concentration of sodium in the IV solution can move the water into or out of any fluid compartment in the body.

When selecting the appropriate IV solution for a patient, it is vital to understand how electrolytes operate. A patient's electrolyte levels can become altered as a result of excessive vomiting, diarrhea, dietary issues, medications (taken regularly or administered by the EMS crew), blood loss, or a variety of other injuries. Understanding the role of each electrolyte, and the clinical presentation you may encounter if a patient has too much or not enough of an electrolyte, will help you select the appropriate IV solution.

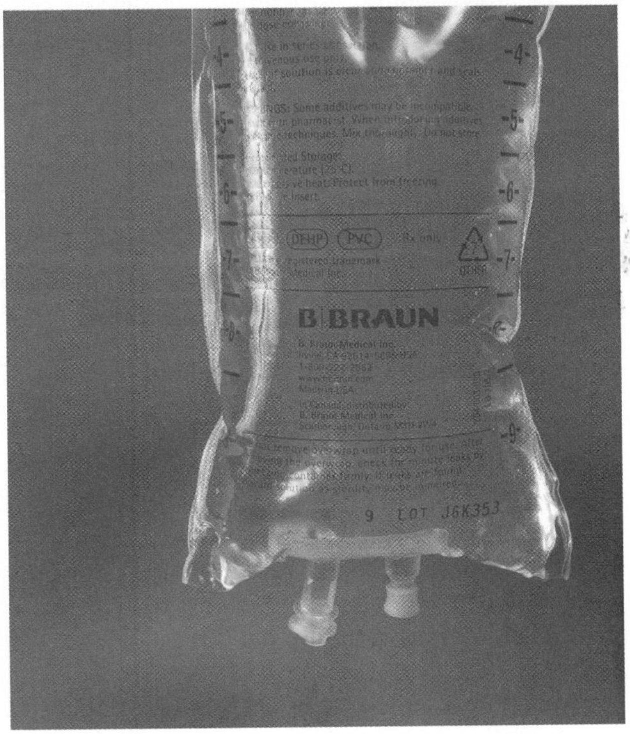

FIGURE 14-5 Each bag of intravenous solution must be sterile, leak-free, clear, and not expired.

TABLE 14-2 Electrolyte Composition of Intravenous Fluids

Fluid	Sodium (Na) mEq/L	Chloride (Cl) mEq/L	Potassium (K) mEq/L	Calcium (Ca) mEq/L	Magnesium (Mg) mEq/L
Human plasma	135–145	95–105	3.5–5	8–10.5	1.5–2.5
0.45% sodium chloride	77	77	0	0	0
0.9% sodium chloride	154	154	0	0	0
3.0% sodium chloride	513	513	0	0	0
Lactated Ringer	130	109	4	3	0

Types of IV Solutions

Based on their dissolved components, or makeup, IV solutions are categorized as either crystalloid or colloid. Based on their tonicity, they are also categorized as isotonic, hypotonic, or hypertonic. IV fluids use combinations of these solutions to create the desired effects inside the body.

Crystalloid Solutions

Crystalloid solutions are dissolved crystals (eg, salts or sugars) in water. The ability of these fluids to cross membranes and alter fluid levels makes them the best choice for prehospital care of injured patients who need body fluid replacement. When you use an **isotonic crystalloid solution** for fluid replacement to support blood pressure (BP) after blood loss, the goal is to administer enough fluid to maintain perfusion and continue to provide oxygenated red blood cells to the heart, brain, and lungs. In the past, the recommended replacement rule has typically been 3 mL of isotonic crystalloid solution to replace 1 mL of patient blood. This amount was recommended because approximately two-thirds of the infused isotonic crystalloid solution will leave the vascular spaces in about 1 hour. However, it is now more commonly acknowledged that with significant blood loss, the optimal replacement fluid is ideally as near to whole blood as possible, beginning with administration of packed red blood cells and plasma at a ratio of 1:1 or 1:2.

When you replace volume loss in a patient, it is imperative to remember that crystalloid solutions do not carry oxygen. Fluid boluses should be administered as appropriate based on the working diagnosis to maintain perfusion but not to restore BP to the patient's normal level. Increasing BP too much with IV solutions not only dilutes remaining blood volume, thereby decreasing the proportion of hemoglobin in this volume, but in the case of hemorrhagic shock, may also increase internal bleeding by interfering with **hemostasis**, the body's internal blood-clotting mechanism. BP should be titrated to 90 mm Hg systolic in adults, unless otherwise noted by local protocol.[6]

> **Words of Wisdom**
>
> In patients who experience trauma, isotonic crystalloid solutions such as normal saline and lactated Ringer (LR) solution replace volume loss but do not carry oxygen. Replace volume loss to maintain perfusion, but recognize the need for blood product administration and surgery. Fluid resuscitation should not take precedence over rapid transport.

Colloid Solutions

Colloid solutions contain molecules (usually proteins) that are too large to pass through the capillary membranes and, therefore, remain in the vascular system. These large protein molecules give colloid solutions a high osmolarity. As a result, they draw fluid from the interstitial and intracellular compartments into the vascular compartments. Colloid solutions work well in reducing edema (eg, pulmonary or cerebral edema) while expanding the vascular compartment. If they are not administered in a controlled setting, however, they can also cause dramatic fluid shifts and place the patient in considerable danger. For this reason, along with their short duration of action and low cost-to-benefit ratio in the prehospital setting, colloids are rarely used in prehospital medicine but may be seen in interfacility transports. Examples of colloid solutions include albumin, dextran, Plasmanate, and hetastarch (Hespan).

Solution Tonicity

As mentioned earlier, IV solutions are also categorized by their tonicity. There are three categories related to tonicity:

- *Isotonic:* 0.9% sodium chloride (normal saline), LR
- *Hypotonic:* 5% dextrose in water (**D_5W**) (considered isotonic, but becomes hypotonic when administered)
- *Hypertonic:* 3% saline, blood products, albumin

The effects of osmotic pressure on a cell are referred to as the tonicity of the solution. Tonicity is the concentration of sodium in a solution and the movement of water in relation to the sodium levels inside and outside the cell:

- An **isotonic solution** has the same concentration of sodium as does the cell. In this case, water does not shift and no change in cell shape occurs.

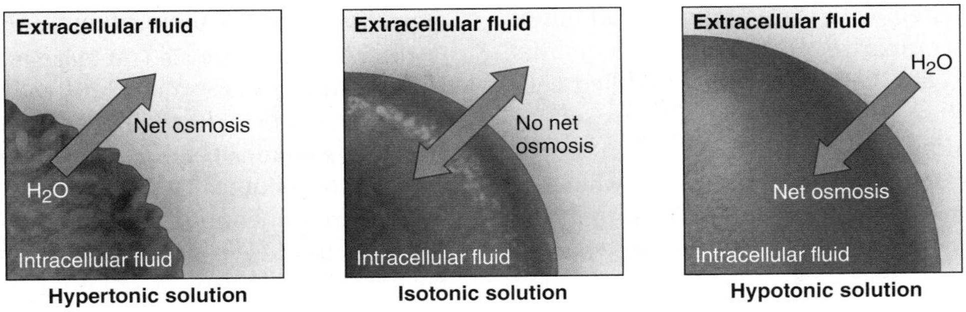

FIGURE 14-6 Fluid movement with hypertonic, isotonic, and hypotonic solutions.

- A **hypertonic solution** has a greater sodium concentration than does the cell. Water is drawn out of the cell, and the cell may collapse from the increased extracellular osmotic pressure.
- A **hypotonic solution** has a lower sodium concentration than does the cell. Water flows into the cell, causing it to swell and possibly burst from the increased intracellular osmotic pressure.

Fluid movement across a cell membrane resulting from hypertonic, isotonic, and hypotonic solutions is illustrated in **FIGURE 14-6**. IV fluids introduced into the circulatory system can affect the tonicity of the extracellular fluid, resulting in serious consequences unless care is used.

Isotonic Solutions

Isotonic solutions such as **normal saline** (0.9% sodium chloride) have almost the same **osmolarity** (concentration of sodium) as serum and other body fluids. Consequently, isotonic solutions expand the contents of the intravascular compartment without shifting fluid to or from other compartments or changing cell shape, an important consideration when you are caring for hypotensive or hypovolemic patients. When administering isotonic solutions, you must be careful to avoid fluid overload. Patients with hypertension and heart failure are at greatest risk of this problem.

Lactated Ringer (LR) solution is generally used in the field for patients who have significant blood loss. As its name implies, it contains lactate, which is metabolized in the liver to form bicarbonate, the key buffer that combats the intracellular acidosis associated with severe blood loss. LR solution should not be given to patients with liver problems because they cannot metabolize the lactate. This isotonic solution has not shown an overwhelming benefit over normal saline for fluid resuscitation. LR is contraindicated during blood product transfusions because the calcium binds to the **anticoagulants** added to transfused blood, creating a possible blood clot. LR is also contraindicated in patients receiving mannitol, methylprednisolone, nitroglycerin, nitroprusside, norepinephrine, procainamide, and propranolol infusions.

D_5W (5% dextrose in water) is a unique type of isotonic solution. As long as it remains in the bag, it is considered an isotonic solution. Once administered, however, the dextrose is quickly metabolized, and the solution becomes hypotonic. D_5W is rarely administered by itself; that is, it is usually administered while you are preparing medication infusions such as dopamine (Intropin) or amiodarone (Cordarone).

> **Words of Wisdom**
>
> When treating patients with hypertension and heart failure, administer fluids cautiously. Frequent reassessment of lung sounds and work of breathing can prevent the patient from developing fluid overload.

Hypotonic Solutions

A hypotonic solution has a lower concentration of sodium (osmolarity) than the cell's serum. When this fluid enters the vascular compartment, it begins diluting the serum. Soon, the serum's osmolarity is less than that of the interstitial fluid, and water is pulled out of the vascular compartment and into the interstitial fluid compartment. Eventually, this process is repeated, with water being pulled out of the interstitial compartment and into the interstitial compartment cells. Ultimately, the overfilled cells will swell and possibly burst from the increased intracellular osmotic pressure.

Hypotonic solutions hydrate the cells while depleting the vascular compartment. They may be needed for a patient who is receiving dialysis when diuretic therapy dehydrates the cells. Solutions such as hypotonic saline may be used to treat hyperglycemic conditions such as diabetic ketoacidosis, in which high serum glucose levels draw fluid out of the cells and into the vascular and interstitial compartments.

Hypotonic solutions can cause a sudden shift of fluid from the intravascular space to the cells, leading to cardiovascular collapse and increased intracranial pressure from shifting fluid into the brain cells. For example, giving D_5W for an extended period can increase intracranial pressure. This makes hypotonic solutions dangerous for patients with stroke or any head trauma. Administering these solutions to patients with burns, trauma, malnutrition, or liver disease is also hazardous because these patients are at risk for developing **third spacing**, an abnormal fluid shift into the body's serous linings.

One hypotonic solution you may see is 0.45% sodium chloride, commonly referred to as half-normal saline. It is rarely administered in the prehospital setting, but may be infusing during interfacility transports of patients who have normal sodium levels but need fluid replenishment.

Hypertonic Solutions

A hypertonic solution has an osmolarity higher than that of serum, meaning that the solution has a higher **ionic concentration** than serum and pulls fluid and electrolytes from the intracellular and interstitial compartments into the intravascular compartment. The danger is that the cells may collapse from the increased extracellular osmotic pressure. Hypertonic solutions shift body fluids into the vascular spaces and help stabilize BP, increase urine output, and reduce edema. These fluids are rarely used in the prehospital setting but are commonly encountered during interfacility transports. The high electrolyte concentration of hypertonic solutions may be used for a variety of problems.

Often the term "hypertonic" is used to refer to solutions that contain high concentrations of proteins. These proteins have the same effect on fluid as sodium. Careful monitoring is needed to guard against fluid overload when you are administering hypertonic fluids, especially with patients who have impaired heart or kidney function. Also, hypertonic solutions should not be given to patients with diabetic ketoacidosis or others at risk of cellular dehydration.

You may encounter the hypertonic solution 3% sodium chloride in your EMS protocols for interfacility transport. Due to the fluid shifts that occur due to sodium movements, 3% sodium chloride is administered to patients with severe traumatic brain injuries. It is used as a temporizing measure to draw out fluid and reduce intracranial pressure until the patient can be taken into neurosurgery.

Oxygen-Carrying Solutions

The best fluid to replace blood loss is whole blood. Unlike the crystalloid and colloid solutions, whole blood contains hemoglobin, which carries oxygen to the body's cells. On occasion (eg, aeromedical transports, multiple-casualty incidents), O-negative blood (the universally compatible blood type) may be administered outside a hospital setting. However, because of its refrigeration requirements and other storage issues, general use of whole blood is impractical in the prehospital setting.

Research is ongoing to find a synthetic blood substitute. Perfluorocarbon (PFC) blood substitutes are synthetic products derived from chemicals containing fluorine and carbon. PFCs can dissolve large amounts of gases, such as oxygen, but must be emulsified before administration to patients because they do not mix with blood. Although early clinical trials of these products showed promise, later clinical trials were discontinued because patients receiving PFCs showed a higher risk of adverse effects than those receiving donor blood. As of June 2020, clinical trials of hemoglobin-based oxygen carriers were halted because of safety concerns.[7] No oxygen-carrying blood substitutes are approved for use by the US Food and Drug Administration to date.

IV Techniques and Administration

Intravenous (IV) means "within a vein." **Intravenous therapy** involves cannulation of a vein with a catheter to access the patient's vascular system. It is one of many invasive techniques you will perform as a paramedic. **Peripheral vein cannulation** involves cannulating veins of the periphery: that is, veins that can be seen and/or palpated (eg, veins of the hand, arm, or lower extremity and the EJ vein).

A crucial point to remember about IV therapy is that you must keep the IV equipment sterile. Forethought and attention to detail will help prevent mental and procedural errors while starting the IV line. One way to ensure proper technique is to develop a routine for how you assemble the appropriate equipment.

Assembling Your Equipment

To avoid delays and IV site contamination, gather and prepare all your equipment before you attempt to start an IV line. In some cases, the patient's condition may make full preparation difficult, in which case working as a team becomes critical. The members of your own crew, by anticipating your needs, often can assemble the needed IV equipment. Although procedures may vary from service to service, most services prepackage supplies in their IV kit. Some variation of the following equipment will be available **FIGURE 14-7**:

- Latex-free tourniquet
- Antiseptic wipes or applicators
- Gauze pads
- Tape or adhesive bandage
- Transparent polyurethane dressing
- Appropriate-size IV catheter
- IV extension set
- A saline flush
- IV fluid and administration set appropriate for the patient's condition
- Sharps container

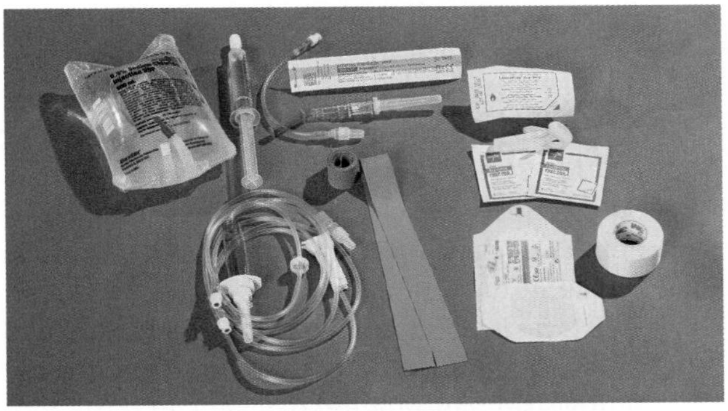

FIGURE 14-7 Intravenous equipment.

Choosing an IV Solution

When you are choosing the most appropriate IV solution, you must identify the needs of the patient. Ask yourself the following questions:

- Is the patient's condition critical?
- Is the patient's condition stable?
- Does the patient need fluid replacement?
- Will the patient need medications?
- Does the patient have any preexisting conditions (eg, kidney failure) that may preclude or change the standard IV therapy choice?

In the prehospital setting, the choice of IV solution is usually limited to two isotonic crystalloids: normal saline and LR solution. D_5W is often reserved for administering medication because dextrose has the potential to alter fluid and electrolyte levels in the body.

Each IV solution bag is wrapped in a protective sterile plastic bag and is guaranteed to remain sterile until the posted expiration date. Once the protective wrap is torn and removed, the IV solution must be used within 24 hours. Each IV bag has two ports: an injection port for medication and an **access port** for connecting the administration set. A removable pigtail protects the sterile access port. Once this pigtail is removed, the bag must be used immediately or discarded.

IV solution bags come in several different fluid volumes **FIGURE 14-8**. Volumes commonly used in

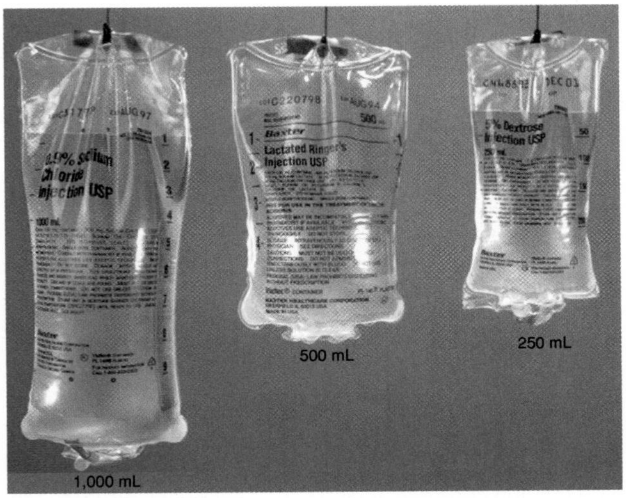

FIGURE 14-8 Intravenous solution bags come in several different fluid volumes.

hospitals are 1,000, 500, 250, 100, and 50 mL; the more common prehospital volumes are 1,000 and 500 mL. The smaller volumes (250 and 100 mL) typically contain D_5W or saline and are used for mixing and administering maintenance medication infusions.

Choosing an Administration Set

An **administration set** moves fluid from the IV bag into the patient's vascular system. IV administration sets are sterile as long as they remain in their protective packaging. Each set contains a **piercing spike** protected by a plastic cover. Once this spike is exposed and the cap's seal is broken, the set must be used immediately or discarded.

On most drip sets, a number on the package indicates the number of drops it takes for 1 milliliter of fluid to pass through the orifice and into the **drip chamber** **FIGURE 14-9**. Administration sets come in two primary sizes: microdrip and macrodrip. **Microdrip sets** allow 60 **gtt** (drops) per milliliter (mL) to pass through the needlelike orifice inside the drip chamber. They are ideal for medication administration or pediatric fluid delivery because it is easy to control their fluid flow. **Macrodrip sets** allow 10 or 15 gtt/mL to pass through a large opening between the piercing spike and the drip chamber. They are best used for rapid fluid replacement. Some drip sets allow the provider to dial the desired drip rate in; those allow the provider to adjust the drip rate to 10, 15, or 60 drops.

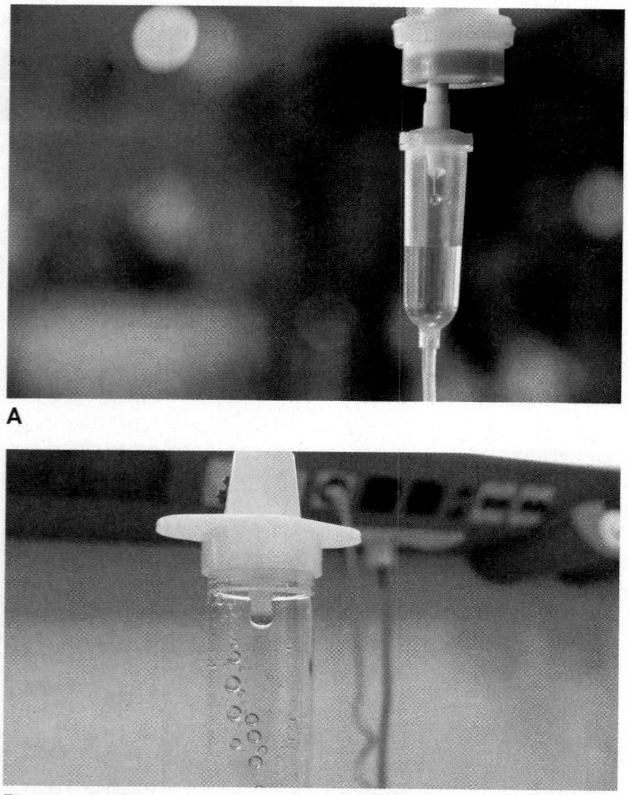

FIGURE 14-9 An intravenous administration drip set's packaging contains a number referring to the number of drops it takes for 1 mL of fluid to pass through the orifice into the drip chamber. A microdrip set **(A)** and a macrodrip set **(B)** are shown here.

Preparing an Administration Set

After choosing the IV administration set and the IV solution bag, verify the solution's expiration date and check the solution's clarity. Then, prepare to spike the bag with the administration set. The steps for spiking the bag are as follows:

1. Take standard precautions. Ensure you have the proper solution, the solution is clear and has not expired, and the protective tail port covers are in place.
2. Ensure you have chosen the correct administration set drip rating, the tubing is not tangled, and protective covers are present on both ends, and check that the flow clamp is up almost to the drip chamber and closed.
3. Remove the protective covering found on the end of the IV bag while maintaining sterility. This bag should still be sealed at this point and will not leak until the piercing spike punctures this port. While maintaining sterility, remove the protective cover from the piercing spike (remember, this spike is sterile and sharp!) and slide the spike into the IV bag port until it is seated against the bag **FIGURE 14-10**.
4. Squeeze the drip chamber to the fill line on the chamber, then run fluid into the line to flush the air out of the tubing.
5. Twist the protective cover of the opposite end of the IV tubing to allow air to escape. Do not remove this cover yet; the cover keeps the tubing end sterile until it is needed. Let the fluid

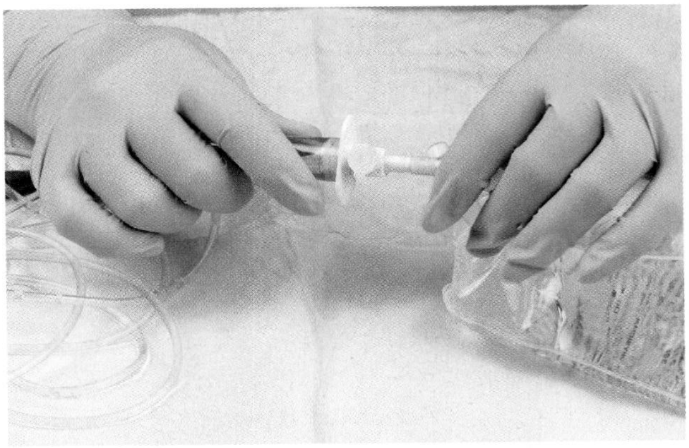

FIGURE 14-10 Spiking the intravenous solution bag.

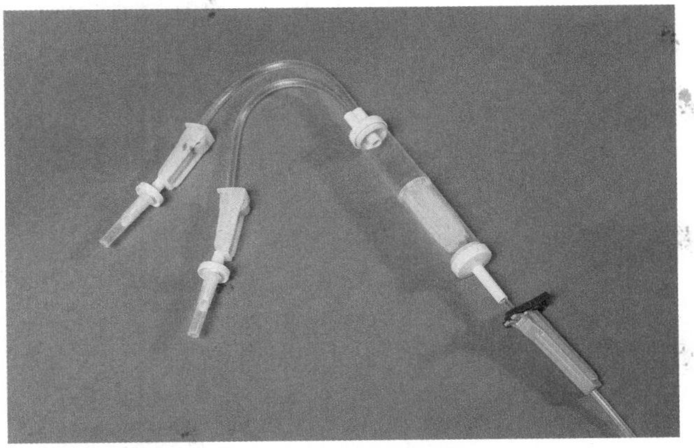

FIGURE 14-11 Most blood sets contain dual piercing spikes that allow two bags of fluid to be used at the same time for the same patient.

flow until air bubbles are removed from the line, then either turn the roller clamp wheel to stop the flow or set the drip rate per the required dose.

6. Next, go back and check the drip chamber; it should be only half-filled. The fluid level must be visible to calculate drip rates. If the fluid level is too low, squeeze the chamber until it fills. If the chamber is too full, with the roller clamp in the off position, invert the bag and the chamber and squeeze the chamber to empty the fluid back into the bag. Hang the bag in an appropriate location, where the end of the IV tubing is easily accessible.

Other Administration Sets

Blood tubing is a macrodrip administration set that is designed to facilitate rapid fluid replacement by manual infusion of multiple IV bags or IV and blood replacement combinations. Most blood tubing administration sets contain dual piercing spikes that allow two fluid bags to be used simultaneously for the same patient **FIGURE 14-11**. The central drip chamber has a special filter designed to filter the blood during transfusions.

Adequate fluid control for pediatric patients and certain older adult patients is essential. A microdrip set called a **Volutrol** (also called a Burettrol or burette) allows you to fill a 100- or 200-mL calibrated drip chamber with a specific amount of fluid and administer only that amount, which helps to avoid inadvertent fluid overload. This type of set is commonly used in pediatric patients. A proximal roller clamp enables you to shut off the Volutrol drip chamber from the IV bag. If the patient needs additional fluids, you can simply open the proximal roller clamp and fill the Volutrol with more fluid.

Choosing an IV Site

It is important to select the most appropriate vein for IV catheter insertion. Common sites for IV catheter insertion are shown in **FIGURE 14-12**. Avoid areas of the vein that contain valves and bifurcations, because a catheter will not pass through these areas easily and the needle may cause damage there. Valves can be recognized as small bumps located in the vein. Bifurcations are points where one vein may split into two. Use the following criteria to select a vein:

- Locate the vein section with the straightest appearance **FIGURE 14-13**.
- Choose a vein that has a firm, round appearance or is springy when palpated.
- Avoid areas where the vein crosses over joints.
- Avoid edematous, injured, infected, or paralyzed extremities and any extremity with a dialysis fistula or on the side where a mastectomy was performed.

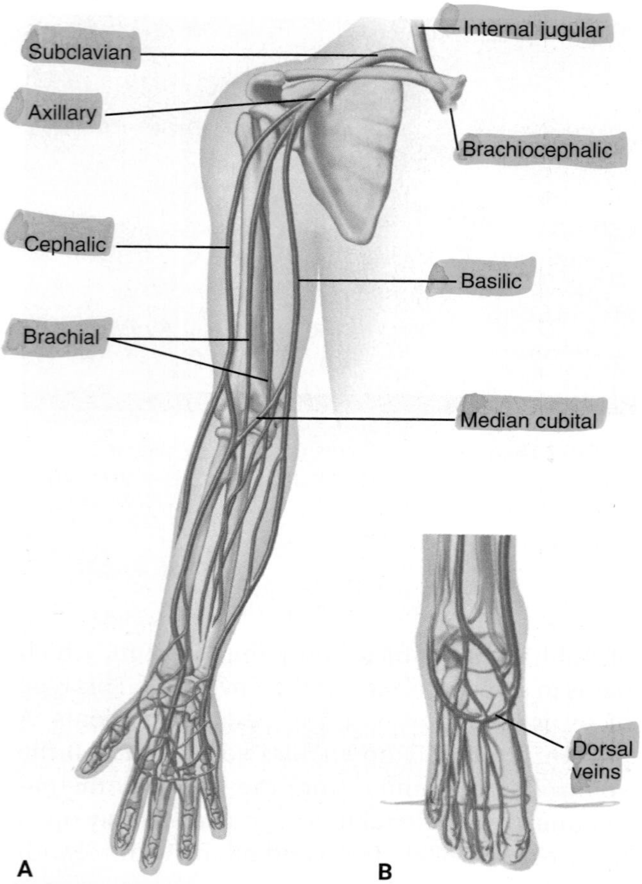

FIGURE 14-12 A. Commonly used intravenous (IV) sites in the upper extremity include the brachial and cephalic veins in the proximal arm, the radial and ulnar veins in the distal arm, the antecubital veins that lie anterior to the elbow, and the dorsal veins of the hands. **B.** Commonly used IV sites in the lower extremity include the dorsal veins of the feet.

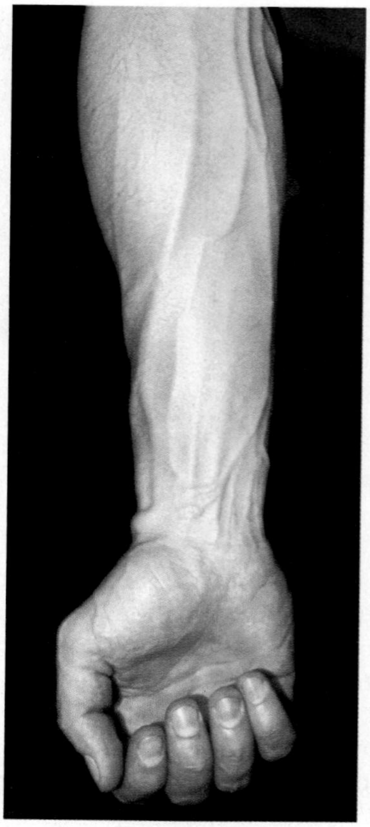

FIGURE 14-13 Look for veins that are relatively straight and spring back when palpated.

Words of Wisdom

As a general rule, you should start distally and work your way up the patient's extremity when starting an IV line. For patients who need rapid fluid replacement, are in cardiac arrest, or are otherwise hemodynamically unstable, use a readily available site such as the antecubital vein. Unlike other extremity veins (eg, hand, forearm), this vein is usually visible and easier to palpate. Also consider cannulating an EJ vein or obtaining IO access in the leg or humerus.

If IV therapy is being given for a life-threatening illness or injury, the choice of administration site is often limited to the areas that remain open during hypoperfusion. Otherwise, limit IV access to the more distal areas of the extremities: *Start distally; work proximally.* If the most distal site ruptures or infiltrates, then you can move up the extremity to the next appropriate site. Because failed cannulation creates the possibility of leakage into the surrounding tissues, any fluid introduced immediately below an open wound has the potential to enter the tissue and cause damage.

Large, protruding arm veins can be deceiving in terms of their ease of cannulation. Often these bulging veins will roll from side to side during a cannulation attempt, causing you to miss the vein. A remedy is to apply manual traction to the vein to lock it into position and then be sure not to insert the IV needle too deeply. Traction techniques differ depending on the location chosen for cannulation. Hold hand veins in place by pulling the skin over the vein taut with the thumb of your free hand as you flex the patient's hand **FIGURE 14-14**. Stabilize

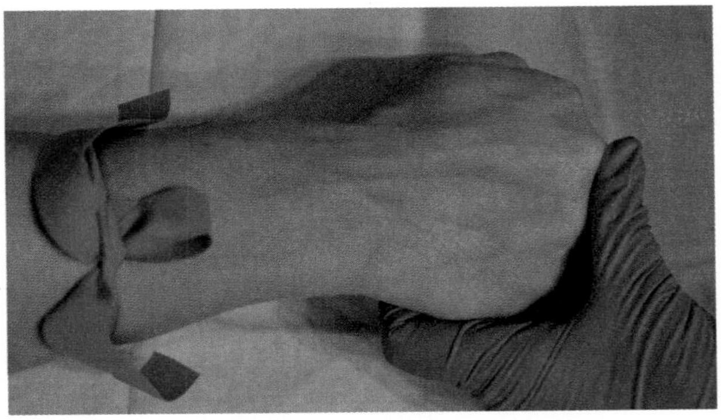

FIGURE 14-14 Hold hand veins in place by pulling the skin over the vein taut with the thumb of your free hand as you flex the patient's hand.

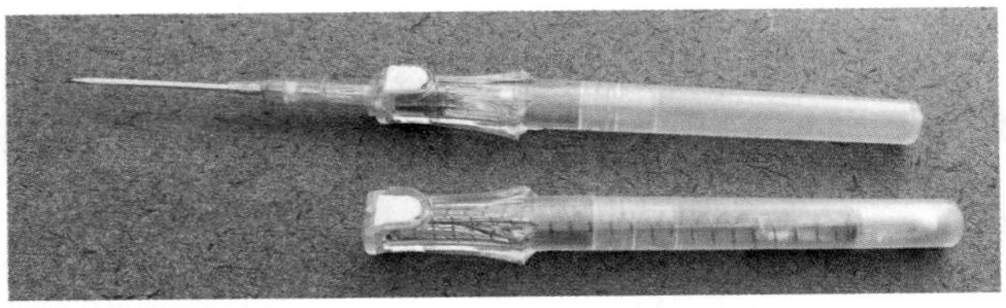

FIGURE 14-15 An over-the-needle catheter (needle plus catheter) and safety shield. The top catheter is shown before needle retraction, and the lower catheter is shown after retraction.

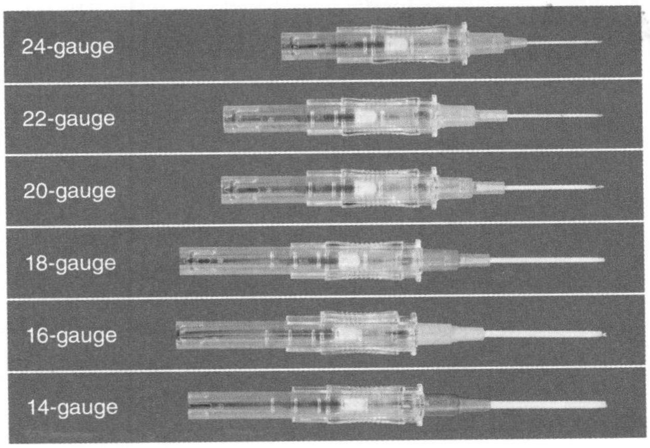

FIGURE 14-16 Note the difference in the catheters' sizes.

wrist veins by flexing the wrist and pulling the skin taut over the vein. Applying lateral traction to the vein with your free hand can stabilize veins in the forearm and **antecubital** areas. Stabilizing and cannulating the EJ vein requires a different approach (discussed later in this chapter).

The patient's opinion should also be considered when selecting an IV site because the patient may know an IV location that has worked in the past and be able to identify historically problematic sites. Avoid attempts to insert an IV in an extremity if it shows signs of trauma or infection. Also, pay careful attention to areas of the vein that have **track marks**; they are usually a sign of sclerosis caused by frequent cannulation or puncture of the vein (eg, from IV drug misuse).

Hospitals prefer that IV lines be located in nonarticulating areas such as the top of the hand or forearm. This preference may be considered if you anticipate a long emergency department (ED), intensive care unit (ICU), or medical/surgical unit stay for a patient. Otherwise, the hospital may reestablish your IV line in a more desirable position. If there is injury to a hand or other part of the extremity, apply the IV line to the other arm so it will not be in the way of definitive care. However, in critical situations, you may be unable to take these issues into consideration.

Some protocols allow IV cannulation of leg veins. However, use caution when you are cannulating veins in these areas because they can place the patient at greater risk of **venous thrombosis** and subsequent **pulmonary embolism**.

Choosing an IV Catheter

Catheter selection should reflect the purpose of the IV line, the patient's age, and the location for the IV line. The types most commonly used in the prehospital setting are over-the-needle catheters and butterfly catheters. An **over-the-needle catheter** **FIGURE 14-15** is a Teflon catheter inserted *over* a hollow needle (eg, Angiocath, Terumo, Jelco). Over-the-needle catheters use automatic needle retraction after insertion to decrease the risk of accidental injury from a **contaminated stick**: an event in which a paramedic punctures the skin with the same catheter used to cannulate the patient's vein. Needle retraction is usually accomplished with a locking slide mechanism or a spring-loaded slide mechanism.

Over-the-needle catheters sizes are determined by their diameter, which is referred to as the **gauge** **FIGURE 14-16**. The smaller the catheter's gauge, the larger its diameter and the greater the flow rate can be. Thus, a 14-gauge catheter has a larger diameter than a 22-gauge catheter; 14-gauge is the largest, and 27-gauge is the smallest. The larger the diameter, the more fluid that can be delivered through the catheter. The most common lengths are 1¼ inch (3 cm) and 2¼ inch (6 cm). While 10- and 12-gauge catheters do exist, they are not typically used by EMS providers for vascular access. Their presence in the prehospital realm is reserved for needle decompression.

Select the largest-diameter catheter that will fit the vein you have chosen or that will be the most appropriate and comfortable for the patient. An 18- or 20-gauge catheter is usually a good size for adults. Metacarpal veins of the hand can usually accommodate 18- or 20-gauge catheters. Generally, an 18-gauge catheter should be used when the patient requires fluid replacement (eg, for patients in hypovolemic shock).

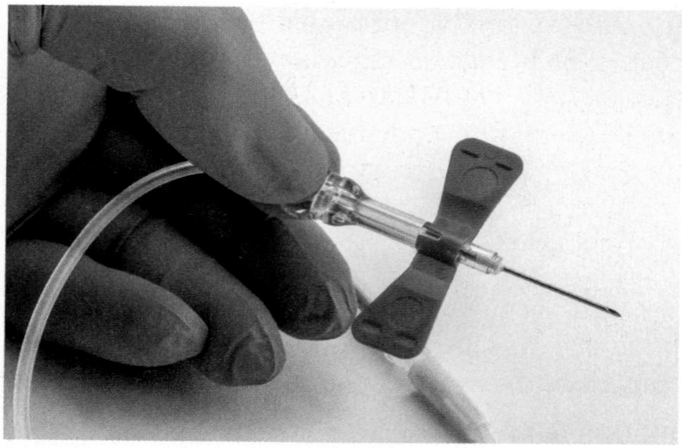

FIGURE 14-17 The wings of a butterfly catheter facilitate handling.

Words of Wisdom

Typically, hospitals prefer to have an 18-gauge catheter or larger available if providers need to administer blood products or IV contrast agents (a dye administered to improve the view during radiologic studies). However, do not waste time trying to establish an IV line of that size if you do not see a vein that will accommodate it. It is possible that if you establish vascular access using a 22-gauge catheter, this may be sufficient until the hospital can insert a larger-gauge catheter. If the hospital providers are unable to obtain a larger-gauge vascular access, then they can still use the smaller-gauge peripheral IV line (which was established before the patient's arrival at the hospital) for blood transfusions or other management needs. Ultimately, you should obtain the best vascular access you can in your current situation without prolonging scene time.

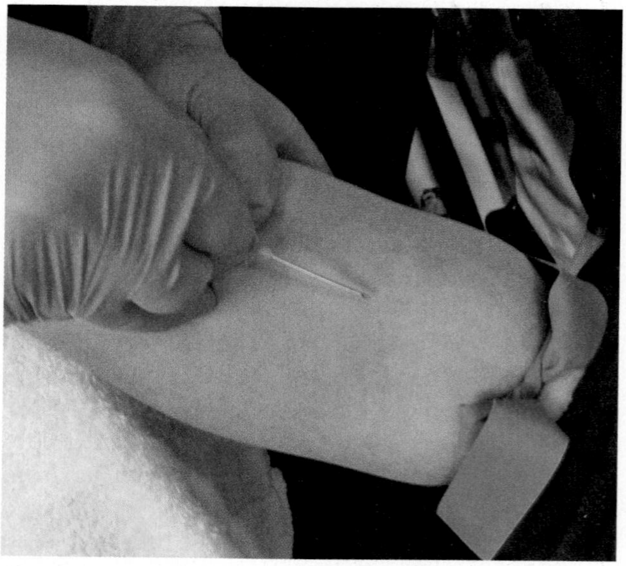

FIGURE 14-18 Keep the beveled side of the catheter up when inserting the needle in a vein.

A **butterfly catheter** is a hollow, stainless steel needle with two plastic wings to facilitate its handling **FIGURE 14-17**. These catheters are most commonly employed in phlebotomy, but are sometimes used for IV placement in scalp veins for pediatric patients. An intracatheter is a tube that enters the bloodstream with the puncturing needle. It can be used in the hospital setting for medication administration, blood samples, and hemodynamic monitoring. Although once used in the prehospital setting, these devices are rarely used in this setting today.

Inserting the IV Catheter

Each paramedic has a unique technique to insert an IV line, and you should observe many different techniques to determine what works best for you. Two considerations, however, apply to *any* technique:

1. Keep the beveled side of the catheter up when you are inserting the needle in a vein **FIGURE 14-18**.
2. Maintain adequate traction on the vein during cannulation.

A latex-free IV tourniquet that looks like a long, flat, 1-inch-wide (3-cm-wide) rubber band is often packaged in IV start kits. Apply the constricting band about 4 to 8 inches (10 to 20 cm) above the intended venipuncture site to allow blood to fill the veins. This technique allows vascular pressure to engorge the veins with blood below the band. The band should be snug enough to diminish venous flow but should not hamper arterial flow. The constricting band should be left in place only long enough to complete the IV insertion, obtain blood samples (if needed), and attach the line. *Do not leave the constricting band in place while you assemble the IV equipment*; doing so can cause the vein to overfill, resulting in a hematoma during venipuncture. Some patients have fragile skin and veins. The use of a constricting band or an aggressive approach to IV access in these individuals can cause the patient's skin to tear or the intended vein to "blow."

Constricting bands can be challenging to manage, especially when you are wearing gloves. You should develop a technique that will allow you to release the constricting band with a small tug on one end.

At times, visualizing or palpating IV sites may be difficult. In such cases, providers may choose to replace the constricting bands with another device that may apply more pressure, such as a BP cuff or a larger-diameter and thicker band known as a **Penrose drain**.

Because receiving facilities often have specific requirements regarding which solutions used while starting a field IV constitute aseptic technique, providers should try to discover those preferences ahead of time. After selecting an insertion site, cleanse the site according to your local or agency protocols. Do not touch the site after it has been prepped. If you contaminate the site, then you will need to clean it again. While maintaining sterility, remove the IV needle and catheter from the IV start kit. Inspect the needle for burrs or other imperfections. If none are present, loosen the catheter hub with a twisting motion to break the seal. Conversely, if you see an imperfection, discard the IV needle and catheter in a sharps container and select another. Take care not to move the catheter up and down the shaft: Doing so can tear the catheter on the needle tip, risking a catheter shear and subsequent catheter embolism.

Words of Wisdom

Once a catheter has been advanced over a needle, never, never, never pull it back!

Words of Wisdom

Agency preferences for cleansing an IV site vary. Most recommend cleansing the site starting from the center and moving outward in a circular motion. Some recommend a back-and-forth motion over a wide area for 30 seconds, and still others recommend a horizontal, then vertical, then circular pattern before performing a venipuncture. In all cases, once the area has been cleansed, do not touch the site. Follow your agency's protocols.

Apply gentle downward or lateral traction on the skin over the vein (**distal traction**) with your free hand while holding the catheter, bevel side up, in your dominant hand. Use caution as you apply traction to avoid collapsing the vein. Distal traction will stabilize the vein and keep it from "rolling" as you insert the needle. Begin by establishing an insertion angle of about 35° to 45° **FIGURE 14-19**. Tell the patient they are about to feel a stick, and then advance the catheter through the skin until the vein is pierced. You should feel a "pop" as the needle enters the vein and see a splash of blood in the catheter's **flash chamber**. Immediately drop the angle down to about 15° and advance the catheter a few more centimeters to ensure the catheter sheath is in the vein. Slide the sheath off the needle and into the vein until the hub touches the skin; do not advance the catheter too far because it can puncture the other side of the vein. After it is fully advanced, apply pressure just proximal to the end of the catheter to occlude the vein. Remove the needle, activate the shielding device, and dispose of the needle in a sharps container. Remove the protective cap from the IV tubing and attach it to the catheter hub while maintaining sterility. Release the constricting band and then ensure that the line is patent by opening the flow clamp and allowing fluid to flow for a brief period before securing the IV tubing and setting the flow rate.

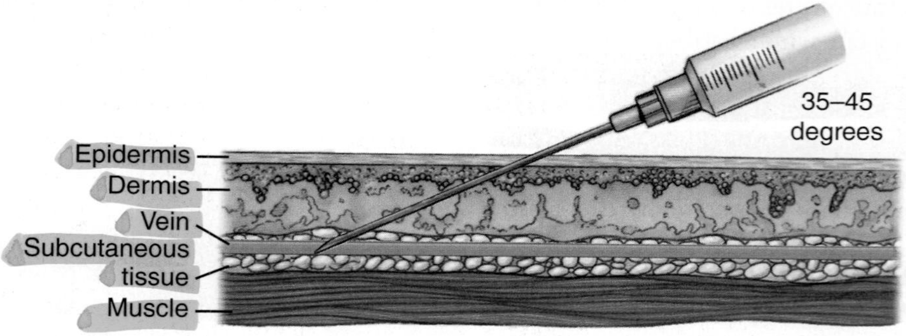

FIGURE 14-19 Intravenous needle insertion. Upon entering the vein, immediately drop the angle to about 15° and advance the catheter a few more centimeters to ensure the catheter sheath is in the vein.

> **Words of Wisdom**
>
> Iodine can help make veins more visible by changing the ambient light reflection. This technique is particularly beneficial in people with dark skin.[8,9] As with any patient, ensure the patient is not allergic to iodine before using it.

Vein Identification Assistive Devices

Several devices are available that can help visualize a patient's vasculature when the provider is faced with a challenging IV start. Examples include near-infrared technology devices, ultrasonographically guided devices, and portable vein transilluminators. Of these options, transillumination devices are currently the most economically feasible in the prehospital setting. Because procedures may vary from one device to another, be sure to follow the manufacturer's recommendations.

Securing the Line

Once the catheter is in position and the contents of the IV bag are flowing properly, you must secure the IV line. A transparent polyurethane dressing, usually packaged within commercial IV start kits, is applied directly over the IV insertion site to minimize the risk of dislodgement and infection. **FIGURE 14-20**. When using tape, tear it before starting the IV line because you will need one

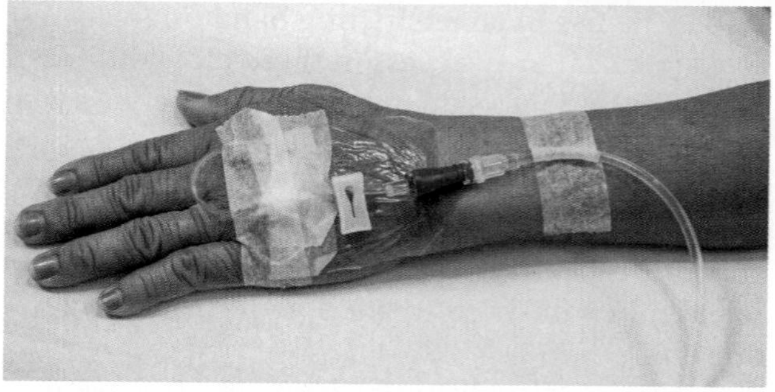

FIGURE 14-20 Secure the catheter and intravenous tubing to the patient.

> **Words of Wisdom**
>
> Helpful IV hints:
>
> - Allow the patient's arm to hang off the stretcher.
> - Pat or rub the area, without being too firm. If this is done too vigorously, then it can initiate a vasoconstriction reflex.[8]
> - Apply wrapped chemical heat packs for about 60 seconds.
> - If you meet resistance from a valve, then elevate the extremity.
> - After two misses, let your partner try. (You are having a bad day!)
> - Try sticking without a constricting band if the IV line keeps infiltrating.
> - Never pull the catheter back over the needle. You could shear off the tip of the catheter and cause this plastic tip to become an embolus.
> - The more IV insertions you perform, the more proficient you will become.

Documentation and Communication

To document the establishment of an IV line, you need to include the following information:

1. The gauge of the needle
2. The IV attempts versus successes
3. The site (eg, left forearm, left EJ)
4. The type of fluid you are administering
5. The rate at which the fluid is running

For example, if you initiated an IV line in the left antecubital fossa on your first attempt with an 18-gauge catheter and are infusing normal saline at a rate of 120 mL per hour, the documentation should appear as follows:

18g IV × 1 in left AC with NS @ 120 mL/h by Medic 785

hand to stabilize the site while you apply the tape. Double back the tubing to create a loop that will act as a shock absorber if the line is pulled accidentally. Avoid circumferential taping around any extremity because it may impair circulation. If the tubing needs to be secured circumferentially because the patient is attempting to pull the line, then consider wrapping the extremity and tubing with roller gauze.

To establish vascular access, follow the steps in **SKILL DRILL 14-1**.

Changing an IV Bag

You may have to change the IV bag for some patients, particularly those requiring larger volumes of IV fluid (ie, hypovolemic shock). Do not allow an IV fluid bag to become *completely* depleted of fluid.

Skill Drill 14-1 Obtaining Vascular Access

NR Skill

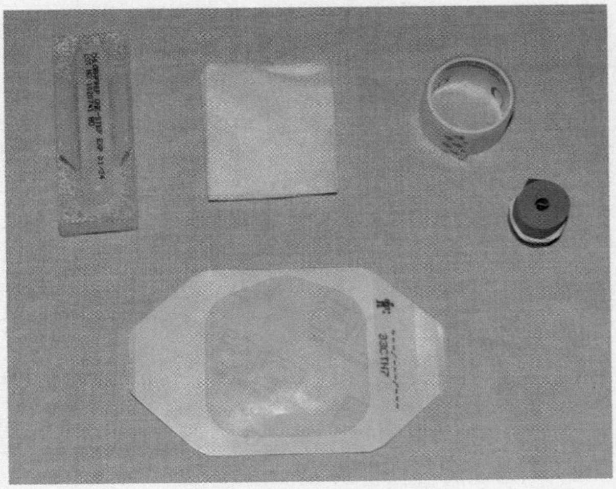

Step 1

Explain the procedure to the patient. Assemble the supplies needed for the venipuncture; tear the tape needed to secure the site; open antiseptic swabs, gauze pads, occlusive dressing, and anything else needed for vascular access per local protocol. Choose the appropriate fluid and drip set for the patient's condition.

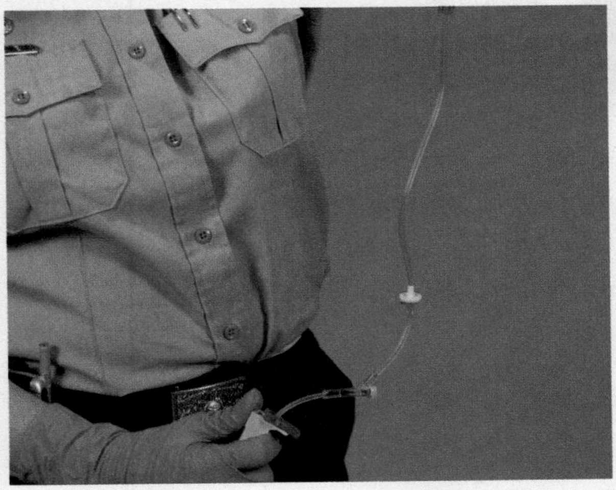

Step 2

Examine the bag for clarity and ensure the fluid has not expired. While maintaining sterility, remove the protective covers on the drip chamber and IV bag tail port. Without touching the piercing spike, spike the IV bag and then turn the bag upright. Squeeze the drip chamber and fill it halfway. Open the roller clamp, and flush or "bleed" the fluid through the tubing to remove air. Close the clamp after flushing the line.

(continues)

NR Skill

Skill Drill 14-1 Obtaining Vascular Access (continued)

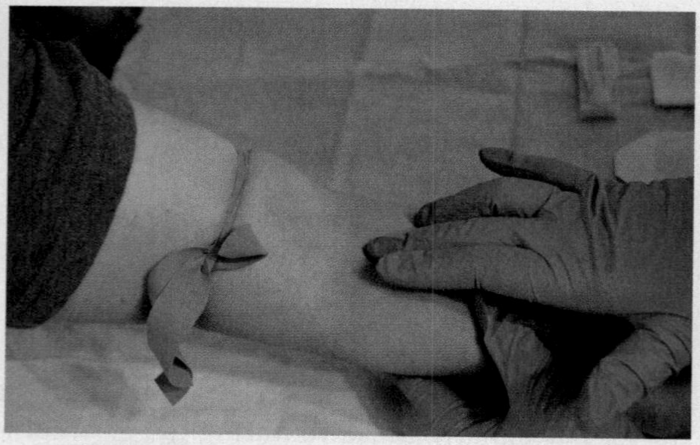

Step 3

Take standard precautions and locate a potential site for cannulation. Apply the constricting band above the intended IV site and then palpate and identify a suitable vein. Cleanse the area using aseptic technique.

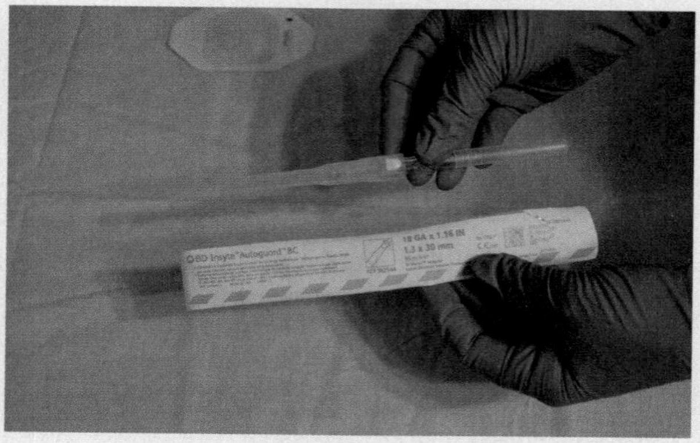

Step 4

Remove an appropriate-size catheter from its packaging and examine it for imperfections. Discard the catheter if you discover any flaws. Loosen the catheter hub by using a twisting motion to break the seal.

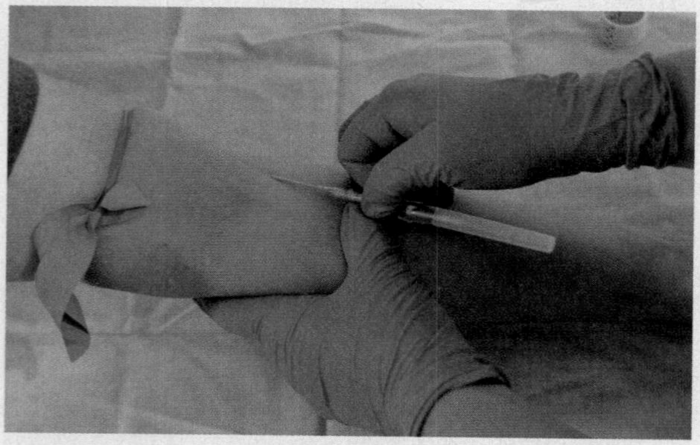

Step 5

Advise the patient to expect a needlestick. While applying distal traction at the site with one hand, insert the catheter with the bevel up at an angle of approximately 35° to 45°. Feel for a "pop" as the stylet enters the vein and observe for "flashback" as blood enters the catheter. Lower the stylet and gently advance the catheter an additional ⅛ to ¼ inch (0.3 to 0.6 cm).

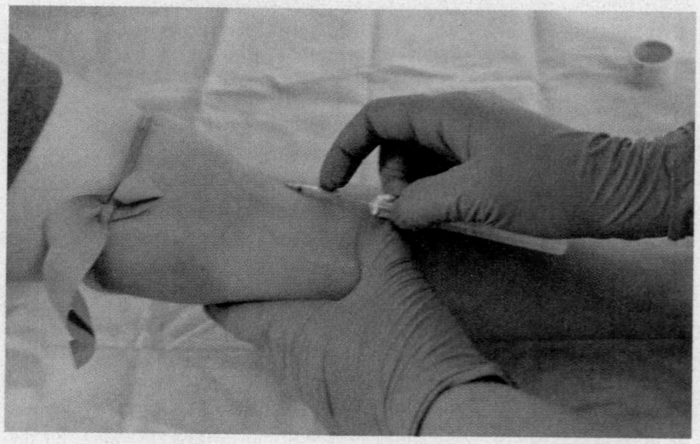

Step 6

Stabilize the needle and slide the catheter off the needle until the hub touches the skin.

NR Skill

Skill Drill 14-1 Obtaining Vascular Access (continued)

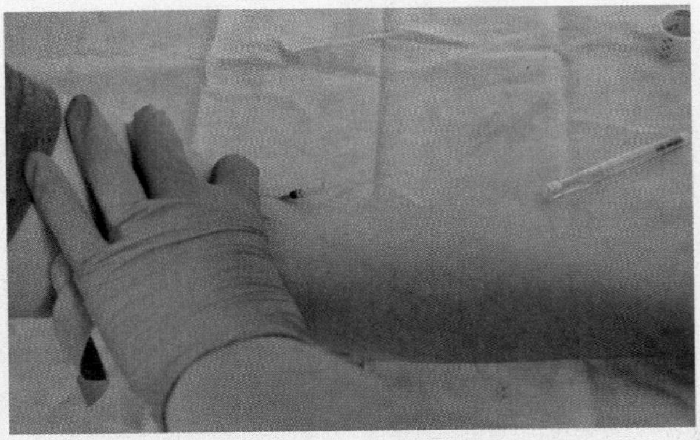

Step 7

Apply pressure over the end of the catheter proximal to the insertion site to prevent blood from leaking from the vein while removing the needle. Remove the needle and immediately dispose of it in the proper container.

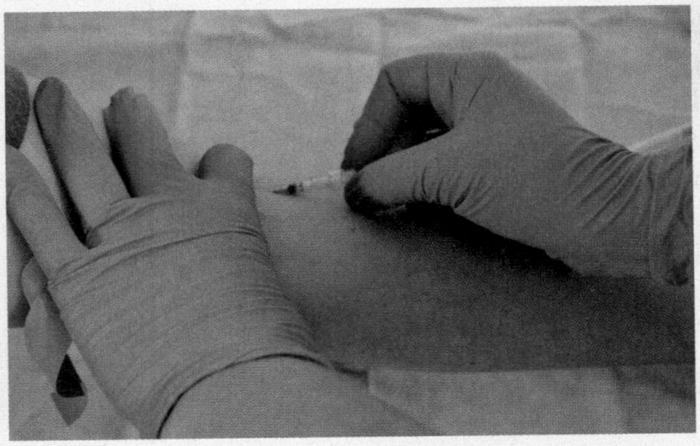

Step 8

Connect the IV line and release the constricting band.

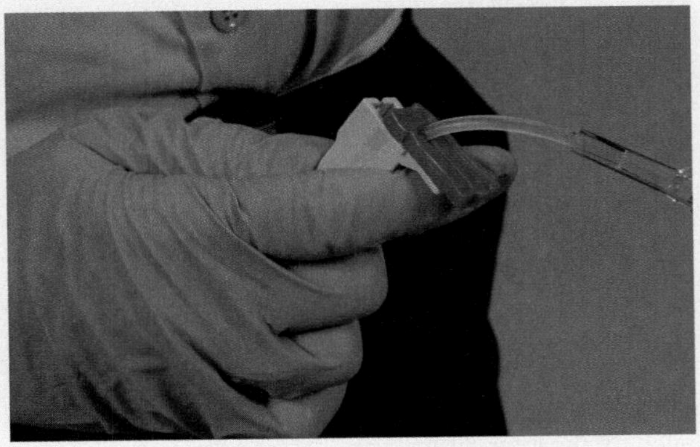

Step 9

Slowly open the IV line to ensure the IV is patent. Observe for any swelling or **infiltration** (the escape of fluid into the surrounding tissue, causing a localized area of edema) around the IV site. If the site is patent, adjust the flow rate as appropriate. If the fluid does not flow, check whether the constricting band has been released. If infiltration is noted, immediately stop the infusion and remove the catheter while holding pressure over the site with gauze pads to prevent bleeding.

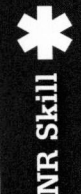

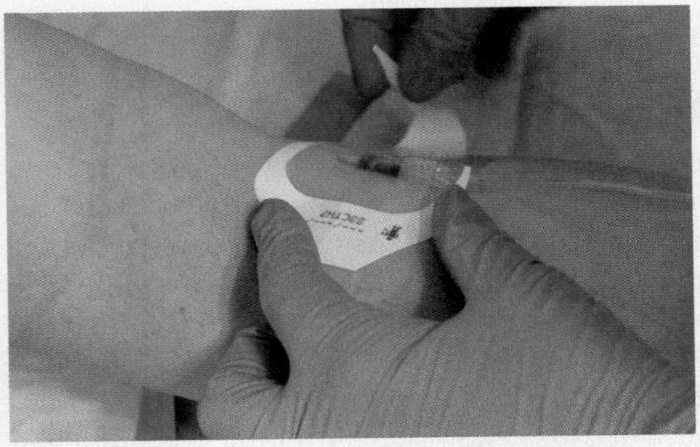

Step 10

Secure the catheter and IV tubing with tape or a commercial device. Assess the patient for indications of a therapeutic response or signs of an adverse reaction.

Change the bag when approximately 25 mL of fluid is left.

Like the initial setup of the IV bag and administration set, replacing the IV bag requires use of sterile technique. If the equipment becomes contaminated, then replace it with new equipment. Always ensure some fluid remains in the drip chamber and tubing of the set. This simple action will prevent air from entering the patient's vein.

The steps for changing an IV fluid bag are as follows:

1. Stop the flow of fluid from the depleted bag by closing the roller clamp.
2. Prepare the new IV bag by removing the pigtail from the piercing spike port. Inspect the new bag of IV fluid for clarity and discoloration; also ensure it has not expired.
3. Remove the piercing spike from the depleted bag and insert it into the port on the new bag. *Do not touch the piercing spike of the administration set.*
4. Ensure the drip chamber is appropriately filled, and then open the roller clamp and adjust the fluid rate accordingly.

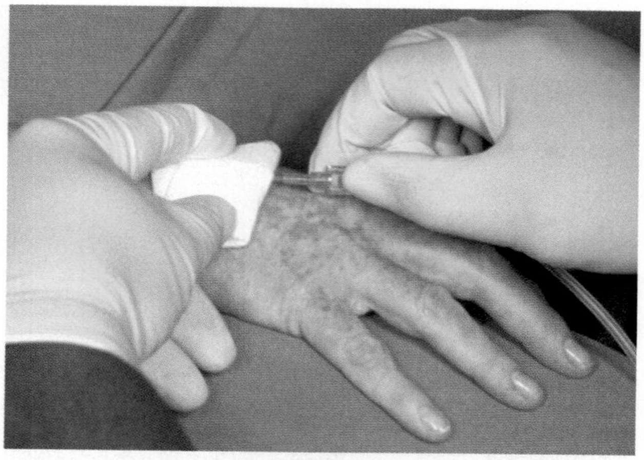

FIGURE 14-21 When removing a catheter and intravenous line, gently pull them straight out without twisting and then apply pressure to control bleeding.

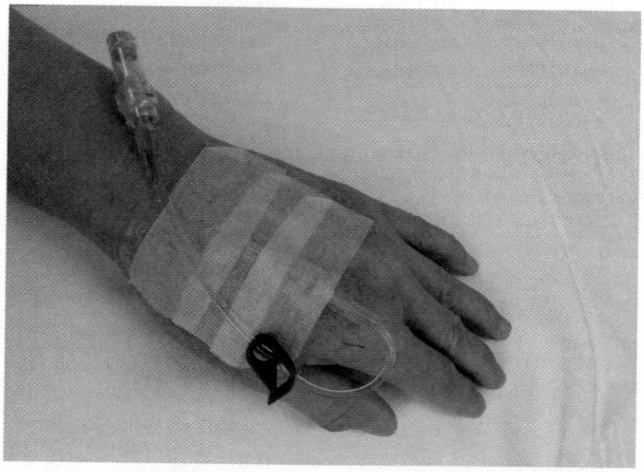

FIGURE 14-22 A saline lock is a vascular access device used for the intermittent intravenous administration of fluids or medications.

Discontinuing the IV Line

To discontinue the IV line, shut off the flow from the IV with the roller clamp. Gently peel the tape back toward the IV site. As you get closer to the site and the catheter, stabilize the catheter while you loosen the remaining tape holding the catheter in place. Do not remove the IV tubing from the hub of the catheter. Fold a 4 × 4–inch (10 × 10–cm) piece of gauze and place it over the site, holding it down while you pull back on the hub of the catheter. Gently pull the catheter and the IV line from the patient's vein while applying pressure to control bleeding **FIGURE 14-21**. After maintaining direct pressure for a minute or so, apply a bandage or tape the gauze in place.

Alternative IV Sites and Techniques

Saline Locks

Saline locks (buff caps) are a way to maintain an active IV site without running fluids through the vein. A saline lock consists of a male Luer-lock connector that attaches to the hub of an IV catheter and a female Luer-lock connector that can connect to syringes for medication administration or to an IV administration set. Saline locks are used primarily for patients who do not need additional fluids but who may need intermittent IV fluids or medications (eg, antibiotics). A saline lock is attached to the end of an IV catheter and filled with approximately 2 mL of normal saline to keep blood from clotting at the end of the catheter **FIGURE 14-22**. Because this is a sealed-access site, the saline remains in the port without entering the vein, thereby preventing clotting.

EJ Vein Cannulation

The external jugular (EJ) vein **FIGURE 14-23** runs downward and obliquely backward behind the angle of the jaw until it pierces the deep fascia of the neck just above the middle of the clavicle. It ends in the subclavian vein, where valves retard the backflow of blood. The EJ vein is fairly large and usually easy to cannulate; however, because it lies so near the skin's surface, it tends to roll if not appropriately anchored during cannulation. This vein is also located near other vessels (eg, the carotid artery) that may be damaged during cannulation.

You should exhaust all other means of cannulating a peripheral vein (ie, in the arm or hand) before attempting cannulation of the EJ vein. Although it is a "peripheral" vein, cannulation of this vein is associated with significantly more risks—namely, inadvertent puncture of the carotid artery, a *rapidly* expanding hematoma (an accumulation of blood in the tissues surrounding an IV site) if infiltration occurs, and air embolism.

Follow these steps to cannulate the EJ vein:

1. Place the patient in a supine, head-down position to fill the jugular vein. Turn the patient's head to the side opposite the intended venipuncture site. ***Always** feel carefully for a pulse before cannulating an EJ vein. It is imperative not to pierce the carotid artery.*

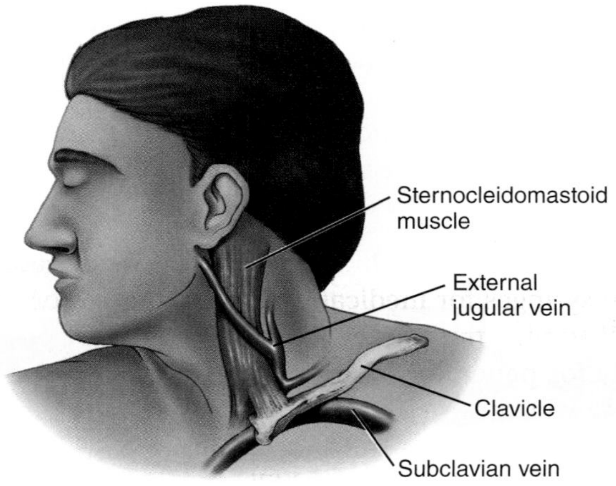

FIGURE 14-23 Anatomy of the external jugular vein.

2. Appropriately cleanse the venipuncture site.
3. Occlude the jugular vein with your finger, distal to the catheter insertion site; this causes the vessel to distend, allowing it to become more visible and easier to cannulate.
4. Align the catheter in the direction of the vein, with the point aimed toward the shoulder on the side of the venipuncture **FIGURE 14-24**.
5. Make the puncture midway between the angle of the jaw and the midclavicular line. Stabilize the vein by placing a finger lightly on top of it just above the clavicle.
6. Proceed as described for cannulation of a peripheral vein. *Do not let air enter the catheter once it is in the vein.* Patients can draw in as much as 10% of their tidal volume through an open EJ vein, causing a large air embolism.
7. Tape the line securely, but do *not* put circumferential dressings around the neck.

Special Populations

IV Therapy Considerations for Special Populations

Pediatric IV Therapy Highlights	Geriatric IV Therapy Highlights
• Use smaller-gauge catheters or butterfly needles for peripheral IV access due to the smaller vasculature. • IV catheters and tubing may need additional gauze to secure them from being pulled out by the patient. • Arm boards or splints may be needed to help secure the lines. • Access may be obtained in other locations such as scalp veins or umbilical veins.	• Use smaller-gauge catheters to increase comfort and reduce the risk of extravasation. • Distal traction is needed due to increased skin elasticity, but should be applied carefully. Aggressive traction can cause skin tears. • Slower flow rates should be considered to reduce the possibility of rupturing a vein or causing complications from fluid overload. • Avoid smaller, spider veins, which are not likely to tolerate insertion of a catheter.

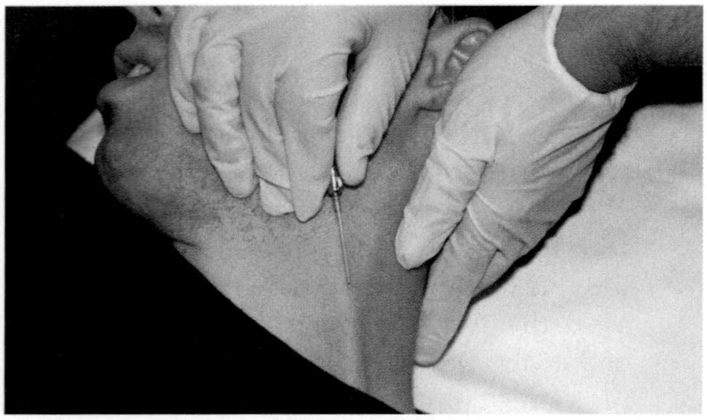

FIGURE 14-24 Cannulation of the external jugular vein.

Courtesy of Rhonda Hunt.

Pediatric IV Therapy Considerations

The same IV solutions and equipment can be used on pediatric patients as on adults, with a few exceptions.

Catheters

If you are using over-the-needle catheters to start a pediatric IV line, then the 20-, 22-, 24-, or 26-gauge catheters are the best choices for insertions. Butterfly catheters can be used in pediatric patients and placed in the same locations as over-the-needle catheters and in visible scalp veins.

IV Locations

When starting an IV line, explain what you are doing to both the child and the parent. A parent can become as stressed as a child, so take time to thoroughly explain the procedure.

The younger the pediatric patient, the fewer choices you have for IV sites. Hand veins are painful and difficult to manage in younger pediatric patients, but remain the location of choice for starting peripheral IV lines. In some cases, the best choice is an antecubital vein with full arm immobilization to avoid dislodging the IV line. Protecting the IV site is crucial and may require immobilizing the site before cannulation with an arm board. While securing the site, ensure the catheter hub and tubing connection are covered with a clear dressing so they can be continually assessed. Consider wrapping the tubing and catheter with roller gauze if there is a fear of the child pulling the catheter out. Do not wrap them so tightly that it impedes circulation or fluid flow in the tubing.

One of the better techniques for starting pediatric IV lines is to use a penlight to illuminate the veins on the back of the hand. Shine the light through the palm side of the hand to illuminate the veins on the backside of the hand. Be sure not to burn the patient with the penlight (although this is unlikely). Once you have located a suitable site, slightly graze the surface of the hand with your fingernail so you can find the location after you turn off the penlight. Proceed with the IV insertion, using the mark you created as a guide.

Although scalp veins are usually readily visible in children younger than 18 months, they can be challenging to cannulate and secure because of the child's head shape and the presence of hair. Scalp vein cannulation is often aesthetically unpleasant for both the child and the parents and can produce apprehension in both simply because of the location. When you are securing a scalp vein, tape a paper cup over the site to avoid applying any direct pressure to the butterfly catheter. Pressure may cause the needle to puncture the other side of the vein and let fluids escape into the tissues (extravasation). In the field, IO access is generally chosen over scalp vein cannulation to obtain vascular access in pediatric patients.

Older Adult IV Therapy Considerations

Smaller catheters may be preferable with older patients unless rapid fluid replacement is needed. Some medications commonly used by older patients tend to increase the fragility of their already frail skin and veins. Often, simply puncturing the vein will cause a large hematoma. The use of tape can lead to skin damage, so be careful when establishing IV lines in older patients. Consider using alternative options such as paper tape or commercial devices that reduce the risk of skin damage.

Catheters

Try using the smaller catheters (such as 20, 22, or 24 gauge) because they may be more comfortable for the older adult patient and can reduce the risk of extravasation.

IV Sets

Be careful when using macrodrips because they can allow rapid infusion of fluids, which may lead

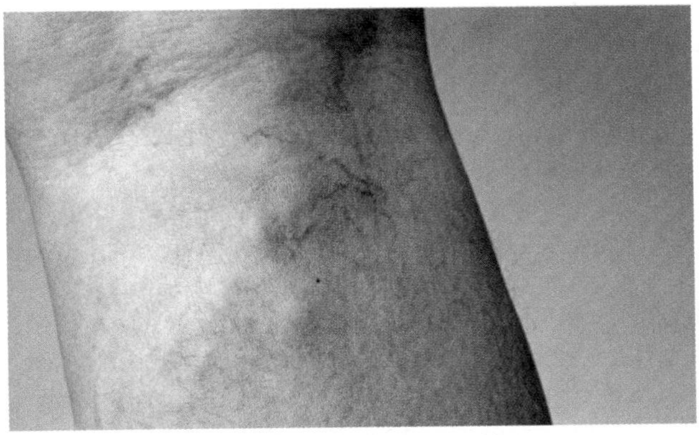

FIGURE 14-25 Avoid small spidery veins and varicose veins when you are looking for an intravenous site.

to edema if they are not monitored closely. With both older and pediatric patients, fluid overload is a potentially serious concern. For this reason, you should monitor fluid administration carefully in both groups.

Locations

In choosing an IV site, you should consider the possibility of poor vein elasticity. One of the consequences of aging is a loss of elasticity in the body tissues. Veins become sclerosed, making them brittle. Certain medications, such as prednisone, can also affect the structure of the vein, making the veins of older patients even more fragile and easily ruptured. Avoid inserting an IV line in small spidery veins that weave back and forth **FIGURE 14-25** because they may rupture easily. Likewise, do not use **varicose veins**; although they often appear to be ideal choices for IV starts, they are almost completely closed off and allow very little circulation.

Factors Affecting IV Flow Rates

Several factors can influence the flow rate of an IV line. For example, if the IV bag is not hung high enough, the flow rate will not be sufficient. Perform the following checks after completing IV administration and whenever a flow problem occurs:

- **Check the IV fluid.** Thick, viscous fluids such as blood products and colloid solutions infuse slowly and may be diluted to help speed delivery. Cold fluids run more slowly than warm fluids. If possible, warm IV fluids before administering them in a cold environment.
- **Check the administration set.** Macrodrips are used for rapid fluid delivery; microdrips deliver a more controlled flow.
- **Check the height of the IV bag.** The IV bag must be hung high enough to overcome gravity. Hang it as high as possible. The closer it is to the patient, the slower the infusion rate will be. If the IV bag falls below the level of the patient, then the IV line will begin to draw blood out of the vein.
- **Check the type of catheter used.** The larger the diameter of the catheter (the smaller the number [a 14-gauge catheter has a larger diameter than a 20-gauge catheter]), the faster fluid can be delivered.
- **Check the constricting band.** Do not leave the constricting band on the patient's arm after establishing the IV line.
- **Check the entire line to ensure it is not clamped at any point.** Occasionally, the roller clamp or the clamp from an extension set is left closed.
- **Check the positioning of the IV line.** The problem with the IV line may be positional, requiring you to ask the patient to keep the arm straight, place gauze underneath the catheter hub, or manipulate the line into position in another fashion.

Potential Complications of IV Therapy

Problems associated with IV therapy can be categorized as local or systemic complications. Local complications include problems at or near the catheter insertion site. **Systemic complications** affect the vascular system or multiple body systems.

Local Complications

Most local complications require you to discontinue the IV and reestablish the IV line in the opposite extremity or in a more proximal location on the same extremity with new equipment. Examples of local complications include infiltration; catheter occlusion; venous spasm; phlebitis and thrombophlebitis; hematoma; nerve, tendon, or ligament damage; and arterial puncture.

Infiltration

Infiltration is the escape of fluid into the surrounding tissue, which causes a localized area of edema. Extravasation is the actual (unintentional) escape or leakage of an irritating agent (a vesicant) from a vessel, which causes blistering within the surrounding tissue. Possible causes of both infiltration and extravasation include the following:

- Dislodgement of the catheter from the vein
- Puncture of the distal vein wall during venipuncture
- Leakage of solution into the surrounding tissue from the cannula's insertion site
- Poorly secured line
- Poor vein or site selection
- Irritating solution or medication that inflames the wall of the vein and causes it to weaken
- Improper cannula size
- High delivery rate or pressure of the solution or medication

Signs and symptoms of infiltration include swelling at the site (with or without pain), sluggish or absent flow rate, continued IV flow after occlusion of the vein above the insertion site, absence of backflow of blood into the tubing when the clamp is fully opened and the solution is lowered below the site, and patient reports of tightness, burning, and pain around the IV site.

If infiltration or extravasation occurs, stop the infusion, remove the catheter, and reestablish the IV line in another site with new equipment. Be sure to document and report this condition when arriving at the receiving facility, especially if medication was in the IV bag (eg, dopamine, epinephrine, norepinephrine). At the receiving facility, a drug that reverses vasoconstriction (namely, phentolamine) can quickly be injected into the area where the infiltration/extravasation occurred, restoring blood flow there.

Catheter Occlusion

Occlusion is the physical blockage of a vein or catheter. If the flow rate is insufficient to keep fluid moving out of the catheter tip such that blood enters the catheter, then a clot may form and occlude the flow. The first sign of occlusion is a decreasing drip rate or the presence of blood in the IV tubing. When an IV line is placed in a positional site, fluid flows at different rates depending on the position of the catheter within the vein; these differences can produce occlusions. Occlusion may also develop if the IV bag nears empty and the patient's BP overcomes the flow, causing fluid backup in the line.

Do not attempt to flush a catheter to clear an occlusion. Using force to clear a catheter occlusion can release the occluding substance into the vascular system, potentially creating an embolus. If a catheter occlusion is suspected, remove the catheter, assess the integrity of the catheter, and apply a dry, sterile dressing to the site.

Venous Spasm

Venous spasm may be caused by a severe reaction following administration of irritating medications or fluids, cold fluids, or blood. Examples of irritating fluids include substances with a high or low pH, and dextrose solutions with concentrations higher than 12.5%. Signs and symptoms include a sluggish or stopped infusion rate when the clamp is open, severe pain from the site radiating up the extremity, blanching of the skin over the site, and redness over and around the site. If a venous spasm occurs, slow the infusion rate until the spasm subsides. Remove the catheter if the spasm persists.

Phlebitis and Thrombophlebitis

Phlebitis, or vein inflammation, may result from the administration of irritating IV solutions or medications (chemical phlebitis), injury to the vein's lining by the catheter (mechanical phlebitis), or infection (bacterial phlebitis). Patients who experience phlebitis typically report pain and tenderness along the affected vein. In addition, you may observe redness and swelling at the site, and the affected area may feel warm. If signs of phlebitis develop, discontinue the IV line and save the equipment for later analysis. Reestablish the IV line in the other extremity with new equipment.

Thrombophlebitis (inflammation of a vein related to a thrombus [blood clot]) may occur in association with venous cannulation. Thrombophlebitis is commonly encountered in patients who misuse drugs and in patients receiving long-term IV therapy in a hospital or hospice setting or with vein-irritating solutions (eg, dextrose solutions or hypertonic solutions of any sort). Signs and symptoms may include a slowed or stopped infusion rate, an aching or burning sensation at the infusion site, warm and red skin around the site, swelling of the extremity, and throbbing pain in the limb. These signs generally do not appear until after several hours of IV therapy, so you are unlikely to see a new-onset case of thrombophlebitis in the field setting except during an interhospital transport of a patient with an established IV line. If you suspect thrombophlebitis, stop the infusion and discontinue the IV at that site. Warm compresses applied to the site may provide some relief.

Hematoma

A hematoma is an accumulation of blood in the tissues surrounding an IV site, often resulting from the advancement of the needle entirely through the vein or inadequate application of pressure to prevent leakage of blood from the vein when the needle is removed. Signs and symptoms include bruising over and around the insertion site, pain at the site, swelling and hardness at the insertion site, inability to flush the IV line, and inability to advance the cannula completely into the vein during insertion **FIGURE 14-26**. Patients with a history of vascular diseases (including diabetes) and patients taking certain medications (eg, corticosteroids or a blood thinner such as warfarin [Coumadin]) or drinking alcohol can have a predisposition to vein rupture or to hematoma development with IV insertion.

If a hematoma develops while you are attempting to insert a catheter, then stop and apply direct pressure to help minimize bleeding. If a hematoma develops after successful catheter insertion, then evaluate both the IV flow and the hematoma. If the hematoma appears to be controlled and the flow is not affected, then monitor the IV site and leave the line in place. If a hematoma develops as a result of discontinuing the IV line, then apply direct pressure with a gauze pad to the site.

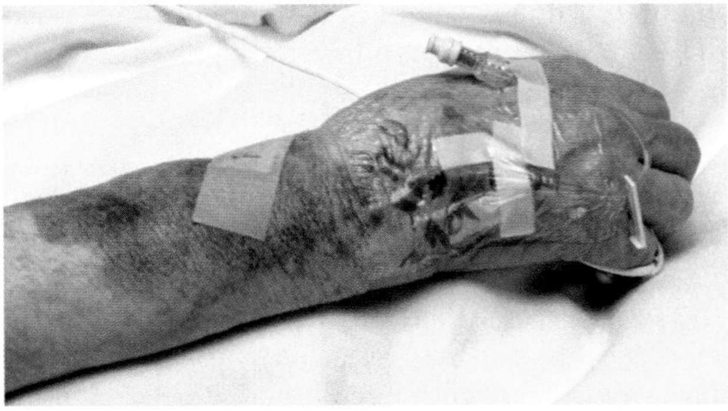

FIGURE 14-26 Hematomas can be caused by the improper removal of a catheter that results in pooling of blood around the intravenous site, leading to tenderness and pain.

Courtesy of Rhonda Hunt.

Nerve, Tendon, or Ligament Damage

Nerve, tendon, or ligament damage may occur as a result of improper venipuncture technique, improper identification of anatomic structures around the IV site, improper securing and stabilization of the cannula and line after insertion, or extravasation of the solution. Selecting an IV site located near joints increases the risk for injury to these structures. When this type of injury occurs, signs and symptoms include sudden and severe shooting pain, tingling, numbness, loss of sensation, and loss of movement. Immediately remove the catheter and select another IV site.

Arterial Puncture

You may accidentally puncture the wrong blood vessel if the vein selected for cannulation lies near an artery. The risk of arterial puncture is especially high when cannulating an EJ vein, so you should use extreme care in such cases. If you insert a catheter into an artery by mistake, then bright red blood will spurt back through the catheter. The blood's color and its flow characteristics will alert you to your error. Moreover, patients with extremely high BP levels may have a rapid backflow into the bag. Carefully evaluate the incident, the landmarks, and the patient. Immediately withdraw the catheter, and apply direct pressure over the puncture site for at least 5 minutes or until bleeding stops.

Words of Wisdom

To minimize the risk of an inadvertent arterial puncture, always check for a pulse in any vessel you intend to cannulate. Under normal circumstances, veins are found near the skin surface and arteries lie much deeper. On occasion, an anatomic anomaly is present and the vessels are transposed, resulting in an artery having a superficial position.

Systemic Complications

Systemic complications usually involve other body systems and can be life-threatening. If the IV line is established and patent in a patient experiencing a systemic complication, then do not remove it because it may be needed for treatment. Potential systemic complications include allergic reactions, pyrogenic reactions, circulatory overload and speed shock, air embolus, vasovagal reactions, and catheter shear.

Allergic Reactions

An allergic reaction can occur as a response to the IV solution, its preservatives, or medications. The patient may have an allergy to the cannula, antiseptic preparation, or tape. Signs and symptoms can range from mild to severe and can affect several body systems. They may develop rapidly or gradually, and their occurrence may be delayed until hours after the allergen has been administered. The patient may experience chills, fever, hives, itching, and shortness of breath, with or without wheezing. If an allergic reaction occurs, stop the infusion, discontinue the IV at that site, and select another IV site.

Pyrogenic Reactions

Pyrogens are foreign proteins capable of producing fever. The presence of pyrogens in the infusion solution or administration set may induce a **pyrogenic reaction**, which is characterized by an abrupt temperature elevation (as high as 106°F [41.1°C]) with severe chills, backache, headache, weakness, nausea, and vomiting. Occasionally, vascular collapse occurs, accompanied by all the signs and symptoms of shock. The reaction usually begins within 30 minutes after the IV infusion has been started.

If you observe *any* signs of such a reaction—for example, if the patient reports a headache or backache after you have started running fluids—*stop the infusion immediately!* Start a new IV line in the other arm with a *fresh infusion solution*, and remove the first IV line. If the patient shows signs of shock, treat as you would any other case of shock.

Pyrogenic reactions can be largely avoided by carefully inspecting the IV bag before use. If the bag has any leaks or if the fluid looks cloudy or discolored, then select another bag and discard the bag in question.

Circulatory Overload and Speed Shock

Circulatory overload can occur when an excessive fluid volume is administered and can lead to pulmonary edema, particularly when the patient has cardiac, pulmonary, or renal dysfunction; patients with these types of dysfunction do not easily tolerate any additional demands from increased circulatory volume. The most common cause of circulatory overload related to IV therapy in the prehospital setting is failure to readjust the drip rate after flushing an IV line immediately after insertion.

Circulatory overload signs and symptoms include anxiety, dyspnea, crackles, cough, jugular vein distention, a bounding pulse, and hypertension. If signs and symptoms of circulatory overload develop, slow the IV rate to keep the vein open and diligently monitor the IV infusion rate. Place the patient in a semi-Fowler position (if not contraindicated) to ease respiratory distress. Administer oxygen if signs of hypoxia are present, and monitor vital signs and breathing adequacy. Consider the use of continuous positive airway pressure (CPAP) to push fluid out of the alveoli, if indicated, and transport the patient quickly.

Speed shock occurs when a medication or solution is rapidly introduced into the circulation, such as during IV bolus therapy. Notably, circulatory overload relates to the *volume* of a solution administered, whereas speed shock, as its name implies, reflects the *rate* at which a substance is administered. Signs and symptoms of speed shock include dizziness, facial flushing, anxiety, pounding headache, chills, dyspnea, tachycardia, and possible cardiac arrest. If signs and symptoms of speed shock develop, stop the infusion or medication. Ensure that the IV line is patent in case medications need to be administered. Monitor vital signs closely and provide supportive care.

Special Populations

Always monitor the IV line to ensure the proper drip rate. If an IV delivery device (eg, Volutrol, Buretrol, infusion pump) is available, consider using it for patients who are at risk for circulatory overload.

Air Embolus

An air embolism occurs when air enters the bloodstream. Air can enter the circulation during IV catheter insertion (usually in a central vein), when the tubing is disconnected to replace a solution, or when a container of solution runs dry. Although IV bags are designed to collapse as they empty to help prevent this problem, this collapse does not always occur. Air introduced into the venous circulation can travel back to the right heart and impede blood flow through the heart, resulting in shock. Signs and symptoms of air embolism include sudden hypotension; pallor leading to cyanosis; cool and clammy skin; weak, thready, rapid pulse; chest, shoulder, and low back pain; a diminished level of consciousness; and respiratory arrest.

If you suspect an air embolism, immediately position the patient on the left side with the head down to trap any air inside the right atrium or right ventricle. Administer 100% oxygen, and rapidly transport the patient to the closest appropriate facility. Be prepared to assist ventilations if the patient experiences inadequate breathing.

Vasovagal Reactions

Vasovagal syncope (also known as "vagaling down") can occur when a patient's body overreacts to a specific trigger, such as the sight of blood or needles. On exposure to the trigger, the venous vasculature dilates, leading to a drop in BP, decreased blood flow to the brain, and a brief loss of consciousness (syncope). Before fainting, the patient may have sweaty palms and describe feeling warm, nauseated, dizzy, or light-headed. In addition, patients may appear pale and diaphoretic.

Symptoms usually quickly resolve when the patient is positioned supine and adequate cerebral blood flow is restored. If symptoms persist, administer oxygen if there is evidence of hypoxia, monitor vital signs, establish an IV line in case fluid resuscitation is needed, provide supportive care, and transport.

Catheter Shear

Catheter shear occurs when part of the catheter is pinched against the needle, and the needle slices through the catheter, creating a free-floating fragment. The catheter fragment can then travel through the circulatory system and possibly end up in the pulmonary circulation, causing a pulmonary embolus. IV catheters are radiopaque (ie, they appear white on a radiograph) to aid in diagnosing this type of problem.

Signs and symptoms of catheter shear include sudden, severe pain at the site and/or a reduced or absent blood return when checking catheter placement. If the catheter fragment does not travel away from the initial site, the patient may be asymptomatic. If it lodges in a heart chamber or the pulmonary circulation, the patient may experience sudden dyspnea, hypotension, tachycardia, chest pain, cyanosis, and/or a loss of consciousness. Treatment involves surgical removal of the catheter fragment.

If you suspect a catheter shear, then place the patient in a left lateral recumbent position with the legs down and the head elevated to try to keep the catheter remnant out of the pulmonary circulation. Because the patient will need continued IV access, try to obtain an IV site in the other extremity, and transport.

Obtaining Blood Samples

If blood samples are needed for laboratory analysis (usually at the hospital's request) you should obtain them at the same time you start the IV line. If you have difficulty drawing blood, however, then stop this effort and finish establishing the IV line. While providers in some critical care transport settings may obtain arterial blood samples as well, the paramedic scope of practice is generally limited to obtaining venous blood samples.

To obtain blood samples when you are starting an IV line, you will need the following equipment:

- A 15- or 20-mL syringe
- An 18- or 20-gauge needle
- Self-sealing blood tubes

The blood-tube tops usually come in red, blue, green, and lavender colors, and the tubes should be filled in that order **FIGURE 14-27**. Use the following mnemonic to help you remember the order for filling the tubes: **R**ed **B**lood **G**ives **L**ife. The *red*-topped tube contains clot activator in plastic tubes (not glass tubes) and is used for serum-based tests. The *blue*-topped tube contains citrate, a reversible anticoagulant; citrate binds calcium, which is required for blood clotting. This blood sample is used for coagulation assays such as prothrombin time, partial thromboplastin time, and international normalized ratio. The *green*-topped tube (plasma separator tube) contains heparin and is used for some plasma-based determinations. Finally, the *lavender*-topped tube contains the anticoagulant

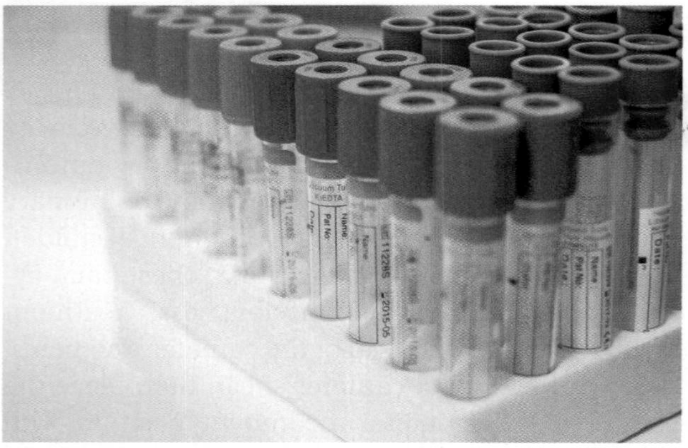

FIGURE 14-27 Self-sealing blood tubes usually come with red, blue, green, and lavender tops, and should be filled in that order.

© Manop Boonjumnian/Shutterstock.

EDTA (ethylenediaminetetraacetic acid) and is used for blood counts (eg, red blood cell, hematocrit, white blood cell, and platelet counts).

After the IV catheter is in place, occlude the catheter and remove the constricting band. Attach a 15- or 20-mL syringe to the hub of the IV catheter and draw the necessary amount of blood. Do not aggressively pull back on the plunger of the syringe. Too much pressure can cause hemolysis, which will make the sample useless. *Do not leave the constricting band on while drawing blood with the syringe; doing so may cause waste products to build up in the blood and could skew laboratory test results.* Detach the syringe after the required amount of blood has been obtained, attach the IV tubing, and begin the infusion. Attach an 18- or 20-gauge needle to the syringe, fill the blood tubes with the necessary amount of blood, and immediately dispose of the syringe and needle in an appropriate sharps container. *Exercise extreme caution when you are filling blood tubes with this technique; you are handling a "live" needle!*

If IV therapy is not indicated but blood samples are required, obtain them by using a cylindrical device that attaches to an 18- or 20-gauge sampling needle (a **Vacutainer** **FIGURE 14-28**). The blood tubes are inserted into the Vacutainer after the needle to which it is attached has entered the vein. To obtain blood using a Vacutainer, follow these steps:

1. Apply a constricting band and locate a suitable vein—typically, the antecubital vein. Take standard precautions.

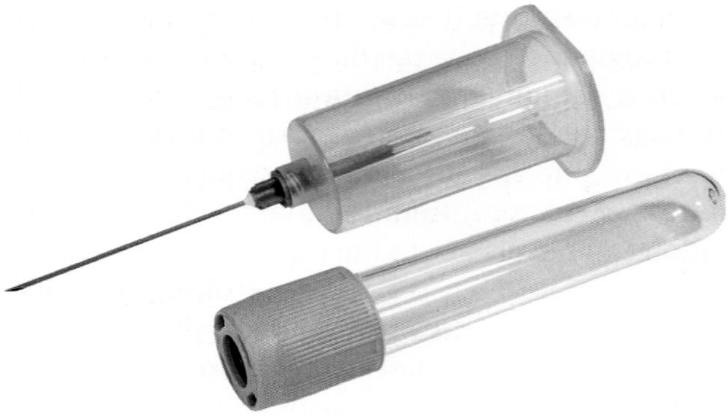

FIGURE 14-28 A Vacutainer is used when IV therapy is not indicated but blood samples are required.

9 ~UserGI15632523/iStock/Getty Images Plus/Getty Images.

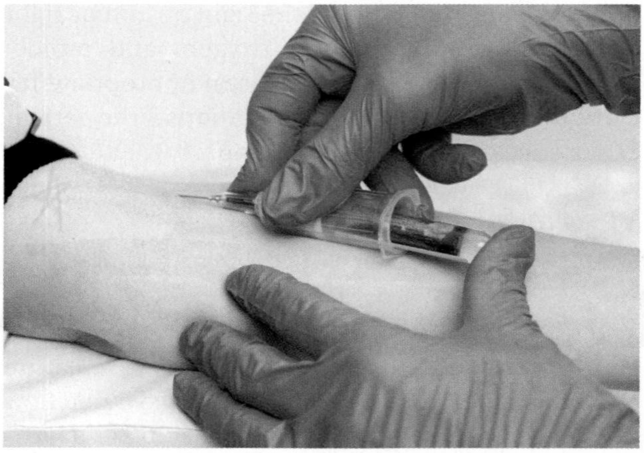

FIGURE 14-29 Obtaining blood samples with a Vacutainer.

© Dmitry Naumov/Shutterstock.

2. Cleanse the site.
3. Insert the needle (already attached to the Vacutainer) into the vein.
4. Remove the constricting band, and insert blood tubes into the Vacutainer to obtain the necessary amount of blood **FIGURE 14-29**.
5. Remove the needle from the vein, and apply direct pressure.
6. Dispose of the needle in a puncture-proof sharps container.
7. Label all the tubes with the patient's name, the date, the time, and your name with your credentials as soon as possible to avoid mixing the tubes with those of another patient.

Once the blood tubes have been filled, gently turn them back and forth several times to mix the anticoagulant and blood evenly. The exception is the red-topped tube, which is intended to separate the serum from the other blood components. Avoid shaking this tube after the blood has clotted, because the motion may destroy the sample.

For blood tubes to be viable for testing, they must be at least three-fourths full. Follow local protocols for the types of blood tubes to fill.

SAFETY

Incorrect patient identification is a potentially serious problem in health care that can lead to medication administration errors. Practice recommendations to help avoid this error include always using multiple patient identifiers. For example, providers administering medications should always use two patient identifiers (ie, name and date of birth). This is particularly important for EMS crews picking up a patient for an interfacility transport. While the 9-1-1 EMS call for a single patient yields one obvious patient in most cases, it is entirely possible for a crew to pick up the wrong patient at a hospital or health care facility and transport that patient to the wrong location.

Blood Transfusions

Some states allow paramedics to transport patients receiving blood and blood products in the interfacility or aeromedical setting. In most cases, the blood infusion will be initiated at a transferring facility prior to arrival and the EMS providers will continue that infusion. Preparation for such transports involving blood transfusion can be time consuming because of the amount of data that must be gathered, checked, and rechecked prior to transport.

Blood type is identified by obtaining a type and crossmatch from the patient's bloodwork. After obtaining the patient's blood type, the facility will place a bracelet on the patient that identifies the blood type. Anytime the bag of blood is changed or care is transferred, the blood being transfused or about to be transfused must be checked against the patient's bracelet and verified by two advanced life support (ALS) providers. These providers can be a paramedic and a nurse, or two paramedics, depending on local, regional, or state regulations. This verification includes the following information:

- The patient's complete name
- The patient's medical record number
- The product being transfused
- The unit number of the product being transfused
- ABO and Rh type of the product
- The expiration date of the unit

In emergency medical settings, the patient's ABO blood type and Rh factor may not be known. In these cases, the hospital will have type O blood available for transfusion. If your crew is expected to switch out units during the transport, then verify the ABO type and Rh factor before leaving the transferring hospital, even if you have two ALS providers on the transporting crew. This ensures you do not accidentally accept a unit that will not be usable. Any blood accepted must be used within 4 hours or returned to the blood bank.

Anytime you accept a transport involving a blood transfusion, ensure the patient has at least one available vascular site that does not have blood running. If a transfusion reaction occurs, any IV lines that have blood transfusing should be discontinued.

When blood is being transfused, it is administered through special tubing that has a filter designed to retain blood clots; it is also mixed with normal saline. Vital signs should be obtained before transport of a patient undergoing a blood transfusion begins, with those data being compared with previous vital signs to identify trends of patient improvement or decline. Vital signs must be assessed every 5 minutes after any additional units of blood are exchanged. When new units are added, you should closely monitor the patient for signs of a transfusion reaction, such as headache, change in mental status, flushing of the skin, nausea and vomiting, difficulty breathing, chills, tachycardia, hypotension, and fever. Save the bag of blood and the tubing because they must be returned to the blood bank for analysis. Transfusion reactions are discussed in more detail in Chapter 25, *Hematologic Emergencies*.

Intraosseous Infusion

Intraosseous (IO) means "within the bone." **Intraosseous infusion** is a technique of administering fluids, blood and blood products, and medications into the **intraosseous space** of the proximal tibia, humeral head, or sternum.

Long bones, such as the tibia, consist of a shaft (**diaphysis**), the ends (**epiphyses**), and the growth

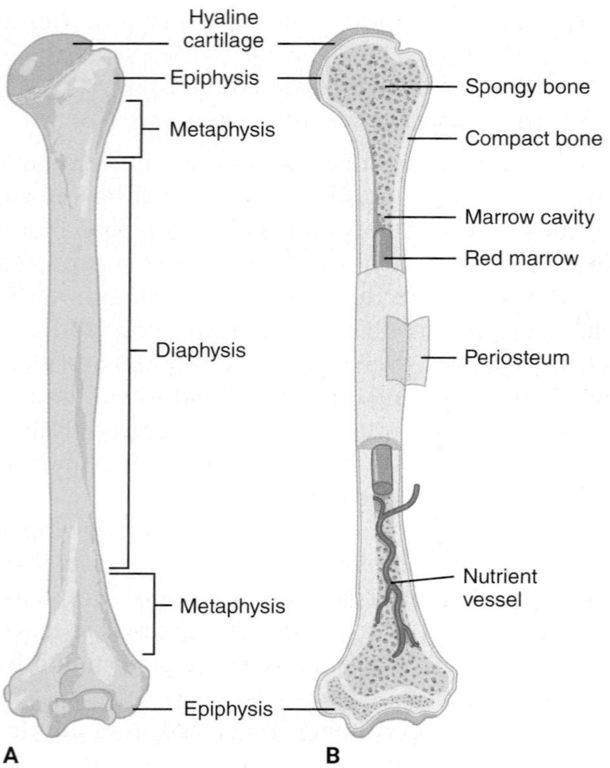

FIGURE 14-30 The components of a long bone.
A. The humerus. Note the long shaft and dilated ends.
B. Longitudinal section of the humerus showing compact bone, cancellous (spongy) bone, and marrow.

plate (**epiphyseal plate**) **FIGURE 14-30**. The IO space collectively comprises the spongy cancellous bone of the epiphyses and the medullary cavity of the diaphysis. Its vasculature drains into the central circulation by a network of venous sinuses and canals.

When a patient is in shock, cardiac arrest, or an otherwise hemodynamically compromised condition, the peripheral veins often collapse, making IV access extremely difficult, if not impossible. However, the IO space remains patent, unless the patient has sustained trauma to its bony structure (eg, a fracture). For this reason, the IO space is commonly referred to as a "noncollapsible vein." It quickly absorbs IV fluids and medications and rapidly gets them to the central circulation—as rapidly as is possible with the IV route. Anything that can be given via the IV route—crystalloids, medications, and blood and blood products—can be given via the IO route.

IO infusion is indicated when you cannot obtain IV access in a critically ill or injured patient—for

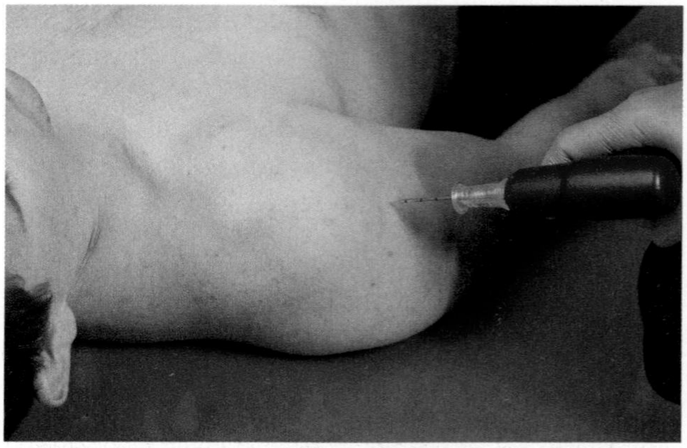

FIGURE 14-31 The humeral site for intraosseous insertion.

example, because of profound shock, cardiac arrest, or status epilepticus. Generally, you should attempt to obtain peripheral IV access before seeking IO access, but this may vary depending on the local protocol and the patient's condition.

IO Sites

Three sites you will commonly use for IO insertion are the sternum, humerus, and proximal tibia. The technique for performing IO infusion requires proper identification of the anatomic landmark in each case.

To locate the humeral IO site, you will need to manipulate the patient's arm and palpate the humeral head **FIGURE 14-31**. Begin by placing the patient's hand over the abdomen, which causes an internal rotation of the humeral head. Place the ulnar aspect of one of your hands vertically over the axilla near the humeral head that will be used for insertion. Place the ulnar aspect of your other hand laterally along the midline of the upper portion of the patient's humerus. Place your thumbs together, palpating up the surgical neck to the humeral head. Appropriate needle selection and stabilization are crucial to use this site successfully.

Identify the sternal IO site by palpating the sternal notch and using the IO device's adhesive target **FIGURE 14-32**. The sternal site has an extremely rapid flow rate. The device's insertion location is near the chest compression landmarks; however, the device does not impede chest compressions.

The flat bone of the proximal tibia is located medial to the tibial tuberosity, the bony protuberance just below the knee. It is necessary to feel the

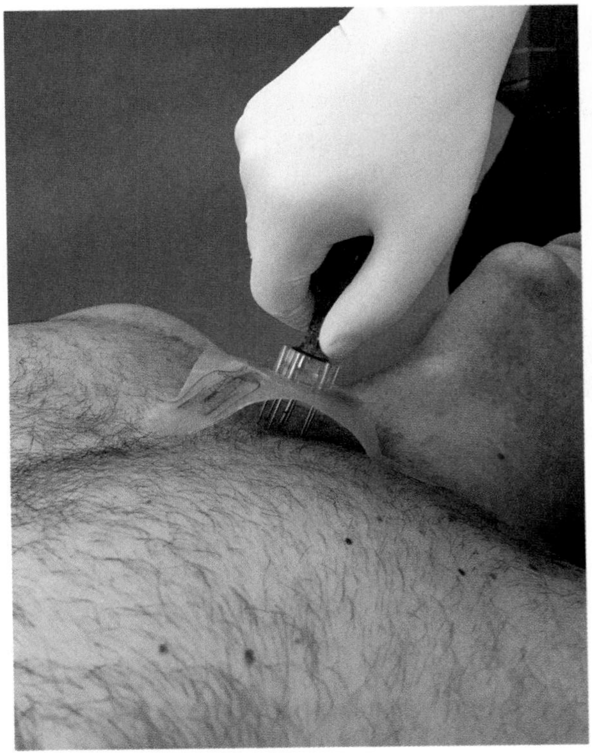

FIGURE 14-32 The sternal site for intraosseous insertion.

Courtesy of Stephen J. Rahm, NRP.

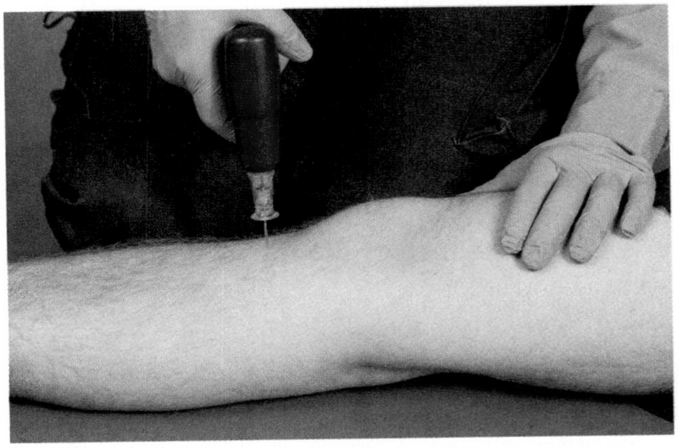

FIGURE 14-33 The proximal tibia site for intraosseous insertion in adults.

© Jones & Bartlett Learning.

leg to differentiate between the first and second landmarks (these cannot be seen; they must be felt). To locate the proximal tibia IO site, palpate the tibial tuberosity, then palpate 0.8 inch (2 cm) medially. This is the IO site for adult patients **FIGURE 14-33**. For pediatric patients, palpate 0.4 to 0.8 inch (1 to 2 cm) distally to avoid the epiphyseal plate.

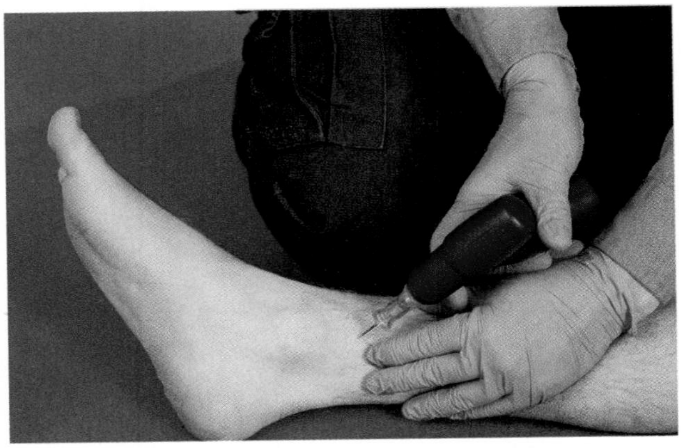

FIGURE 14-34 The distal tibia site for intraosseous insertion in adults.

© Jones & Bartlett Learning.

For the distal tibia IO site, use palpation as well. First, identify the medial malleolus. Then, palpate 0.8 to 1.2 inches (2 to 3 cm) above that site **FIGURE 14-34**. For pediatric patients, you should palpate 0.4 to 0.8 inch (1 to 2 cm) above the medial malleolus.

Equipment for IO Infusion

Several products may be used for placing an IO needle into the IO space: manually inserted IO needles, the FAST1, the EZ-IO, the Bone Injection Gun (BIG), and the New Intraosseous (NIO) device. Use of these devices requires specialized training and thorough familiarity with each device's features, functionality, and clinical application. If your EMS system uses any of these devices, then follow local protocols regarding their application.

Manually inserted IO needles (ie, Jamshedi needle, Cook needle) were the original devices used for establishing IO access in children and continue to be used in the prehospital setting. They consist of a solid boring needle (**trocar**) that is inserted through a sharpened hollow needle **FIGURE 14-35**. The IO needle is pushed into the bone with a screwing, twisting action. Once the needle pops through the bone, the solid needle is removed, leaving the hollow steel needle in place. The IV tubing is then attached to this catheter.

Fluid does not flow as rapidly through an IO needle as it does through an IV line. For this reason, crystalloid boluses should be given by the IO route with a syringe in children and a **pressure infuser**

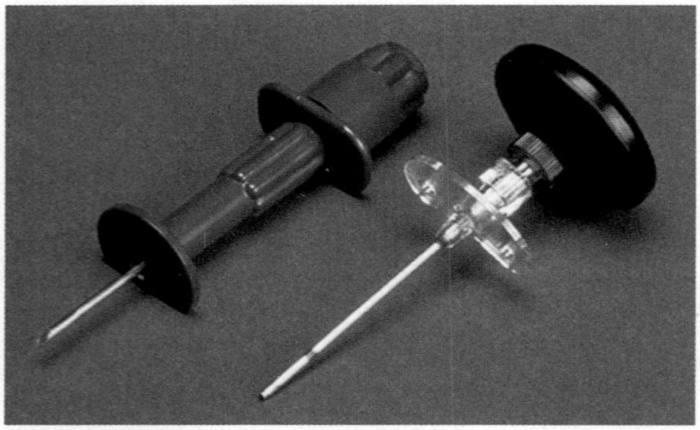

FIGURE 14-35 Manually inserted intraosseous needles.

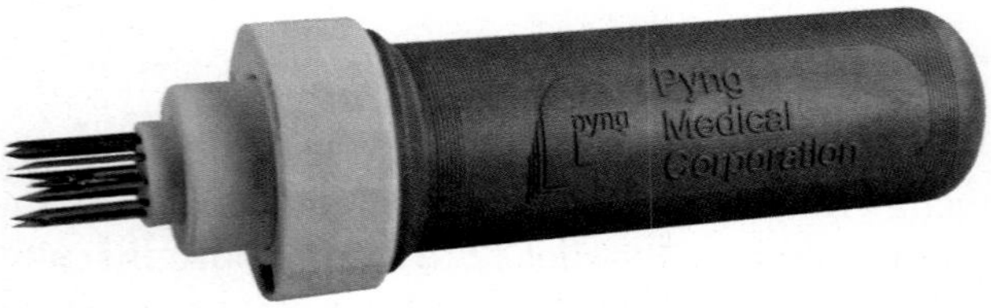

FIGURE 14-36 The FAST1 intraosseous insertion device.

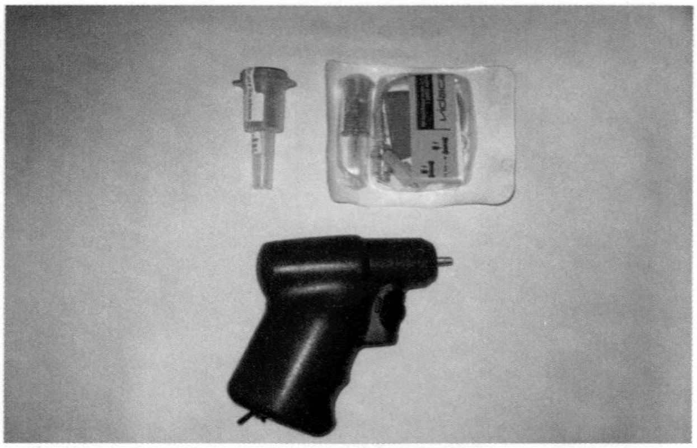

FIGURE 14-37 The EZ-IO vascular access system features a handheld battery-powered driver, to which an intraosseous needle is attached.

device (a sleeve placed around the IV bag and inflated to force fluid from the IV bag) in adults.

Manually inserted IO needles are long, rest at a 90° angle to the bone, and are easily dislodged. Careful stabilization is critical for these lines to maintain adequate flow. Stabilize the IO needle in the same manner that you would any impaled object.

FAST Devices

The **FAST devices** (First Access for Shock and Trauma) were the first IO devices approved for use in patients age 12 years and older. They include four design elements that allow for IO placement in the sternum: an infusion tube and subcutaneous portal, an introducer, a target/strain relief patch, and a protective dome **FIGURE 14-36**. Despite this positioning, FAST devices can be used during cardiac arrest. While chest compressions can continue simultaneously with FAST IO placement, use of mechanical CPR devices must be paused while the FAST device is being inserted. Mechanical CPR can continue once the FAST device is stabilized.

The FAST1 is the original sternal IO device, consisting of a 14-gauge infusion tube and 10 stabilization needles. The target device is shaped to line up with the sternal notch, minimizing the margin for error. The FAST1 device is completely manual (no batteries required).

The FAST Responder (FASTR) is an updated device with many components already assembled, expediting the insertion process. This device has a safety lock that must be removed before its insertion. The FASTR requires only 32 pounds (15 kg) of pressure for insertion. If your EMS system uses these sternal IOs, you should familiarize yourself with both devices.

Both the FAST1 and FASTR devices are designed to remain in place for a maximum of 24 hours. To remove either device, firmly grasp the insertion tube and pull steadily until the device is dislodged. Use one continuous motion during its removal; avoid starting and stopping.

EZ-IO Device

The **EZ-IO** features a handheld battery-powered driver that is used to insert an IO needle into the proximal or distal tibia of adults and children and into the humeral head in adults when IV access is difficult or impossible to obtain **FIGURE 14-37**. The battery-powered driver of the EZ-IO is the same in all of these devices, but different sizes of needles are available. Follow the manufacturer's instructions regarding appropriate needle size selection.

To remove an EZ-IO, use a 10-mL syringe. Attach the syringe to the IO's Luer lock, twist the syringe clockwise, and pull the device out in one swift motion.

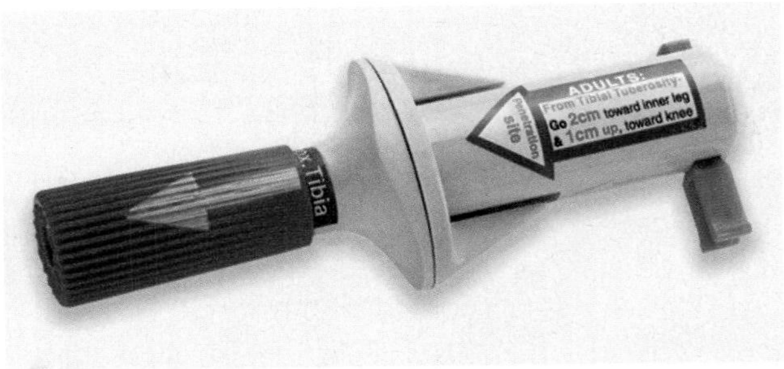

FIGURE 14-38 The Bone Injection Gun (BIG).

Courtesy of PerSys Medical.

Bone Injection Gun Device

The **Bone Injection Gun (BIG)** is a spring-loaded device that is used to insert an IO needle into the proximal tibia of adult and pediatric patients and into the humeral head in adults **FIGURE 14-38**. It comes in an adult size and a pediatric size. Although both versions offer the same operational features, the insertion depth is different for the adult and pediatric devices.

The safety lock of the BIG serves as the stabilization device once the device has been inserted. When you are ready to remove the device, use the stabilization device as the removal tool. Place the wider side of the removal tool over the connection port. Pull the device out in one swift motion while grasping the removal tool.

New Intraosseous Device

The **New Intraosseous (NIO) device** is placed in the proximal tibia of an adult patient to provide IO access **FIGURE 14-39**. The humeral head is an alternative site for this device. This spring-loaded device contains neither a drill nor a battery. It is inserted by unlocking a safety cap. Then, while applying downward pressure with the dominant hand, the fingers of the provider's other hand pull the trigger wings up to deploy the device. The NIO device is then pulled up in a rotating motion while the needle stabilizer is held against the skin. Once the introducing trocar is removed, any Luer-lock tubing can be attached.

A pediatric version, NIO Pediatric (NIO-P), is approved for patients 3 to 12 years of age. This device has an adjustable dial, allowing the provider to adjust it based on the patient's age or the bone's depth (if excessive girth for the age is anticipated). At the time of this writing, the NIO-P is approved for placement in the proximal tibia only.

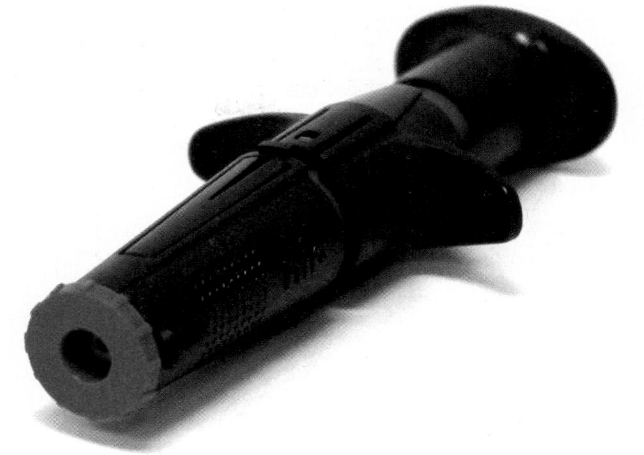

FIGURE 14-39 The New Intraosseous (NIO) device.

Courtesy of PerSys Medical.

Performing IO Infusion

Follow these steps to perform IO infusion using an EZ-IO device **SKILL DRILL 14-2**.

Potential Complications of IO Infusion

If the proper technique is used (ie, proper anatomic landmark identification, aseptic technique), then IO infusion is associated with a relatively low complication rate. However, the same potential complications associated with IV therapy can occur with IO infusion, as well as several others unique to this infusion method.

Infiltration can occur when the IO needle does not enter the IO space, but rather rests outside the bone (because the bone was missed completely or is fractured). In such a case, IV fluid will collect in the soft tissues. The risk of infiltration can be reduced by using the proper insertion technique: *Insert the IO needle at a 90° angle to the bone.* Suspect infiltration if the infusion does not run freely or if the site, especially the posterior aspect of the leg, rapidly becomes edematous. If this occurs, then discontinue the infusion immediately and reattempt insertion in the opposite leg. Undetected infiltration could result in compartment syndrome, which can lead to vascular compromise and even loss of the leg.

Osteomyelitis is inflammation of the bone and muscle caused by an infection. Osteomyelitis can occur as a result of IO insertion, but is rare.

NR Skill

Skill Drill 14-2 Gaining IO Access With an EZ-IO Device

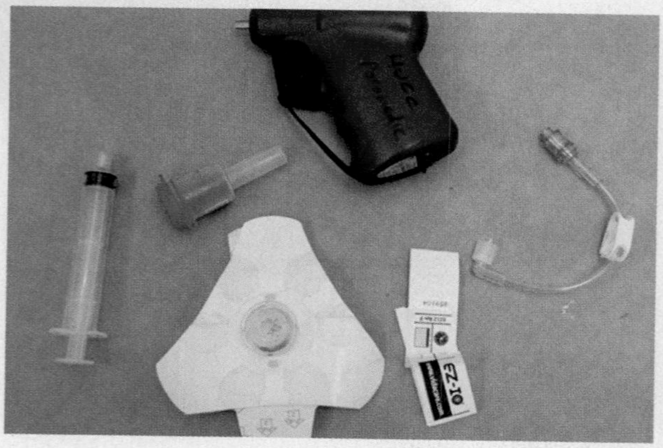

Step 1

Assemble the supplies needed for the procedure, including an IO needle, syringe, saline, extension set, and bulky or stabilizer dressings; tear the tape needed to secure the site, open antiseptic swabs, gauze pads, occlusive dressing, stabilizer dressing, and anything else needed for IO access per local protocol. A three-way stopcock may also be used to facilitate easier fluid administration. Choose the appropriate fluid for the patient's condition. Examine the bag for clarity, ensuring that no particles are floating in the fluid, and confirm that the fluid is not expired. Select a drip set appropriate for the patient's condition, and attach it to the fluid. Prepare the syringe and attach the extension tubing to the end of the IV set.

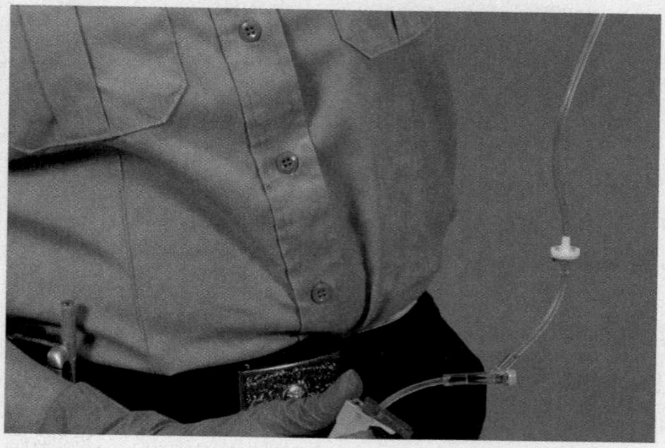

Step 2

While maintaining sterility, remove the protective covers on the drip chamber and IV bag tail port. Without touching the piercing spike, spike the IV bag and then turn the bag upright. Squeeze the drip chamber and fill it halfway. Open the roller clamp, and flush or "bleed" the fluid through the tubing to remove air. Close the clamp after flushing the line. Take standard precautions before making contact with the patient.

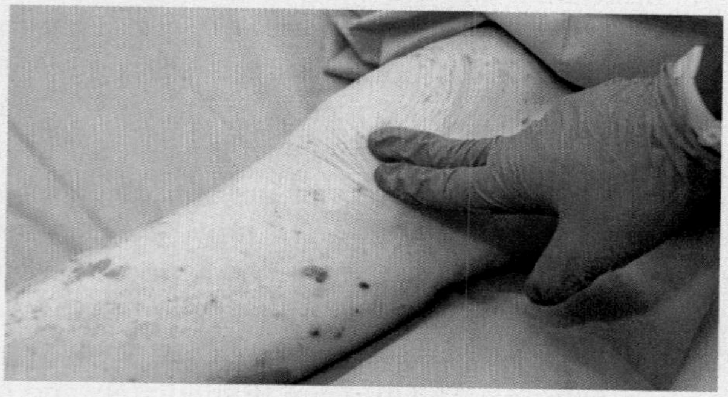

Step 3

Identify the proper anatomic site for IO puncture. Palpate the landmarks and then prepare the site. The tibia may be accessed only with the EZ-IO and the BIG devices. Humeral placement is typically reserved for adults when using the EZ-IO or the BIG devices.

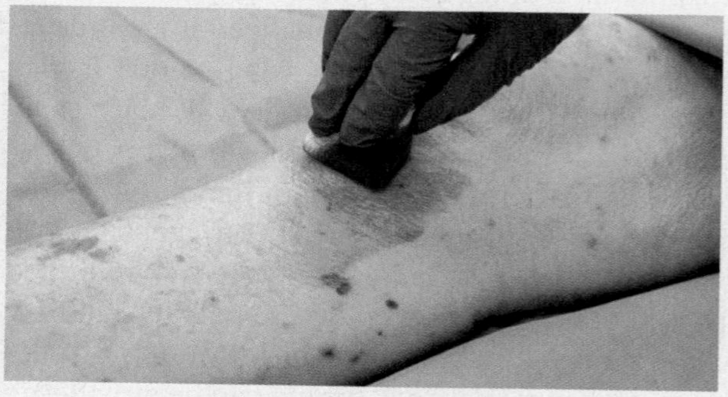

Step 4

Cleanse the site using aseptic technique.

Skill Drill 14-2 Gaining IO Access With an EZ-IO Device (continued)

NR Skill

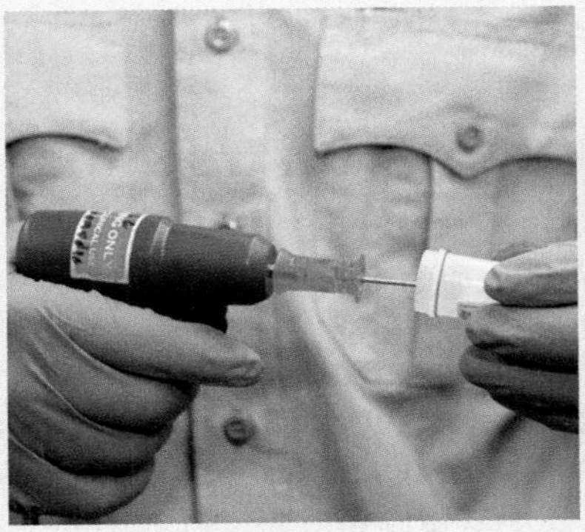

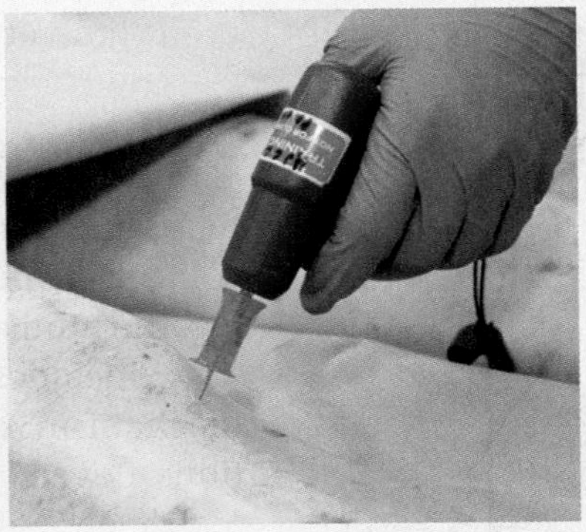

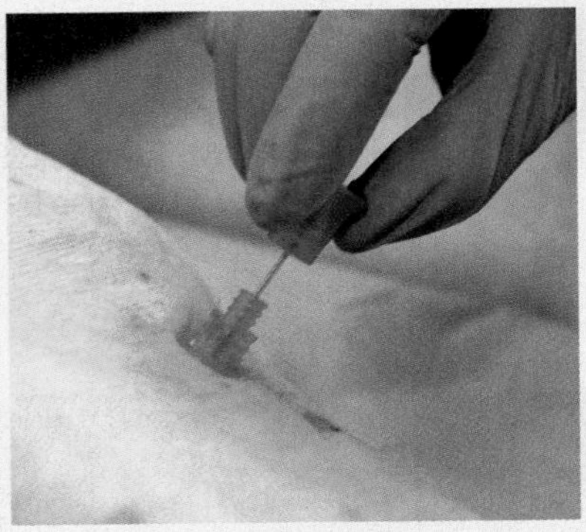

Step 5

Attach the needle to the EZ-IO gun and remove the protective cover. Examine the needle. If you find any imperfections, discard the needle and select another one.

Step 6

Perform the IO puncture by first stabilizing the tibia, then placing a folded towel under the knee, and finally holding the extremity in a manner to keep your fingers away from the site of puncture (eg, if accessing the tibia, do not hold the leg in the palm and perform the IO puncture directly above the hand). For humeral placement, continue to apply pressure on the anterior and inferior aspects of the humerus.

Insert the needle at a 90° angle to the insertion site. Advance the needle with a twisting motion until a "pop" is felt or less resistance is noted.

Step 7

Remove the stylet from the catheter and dispose of the stylet in a sharps container.

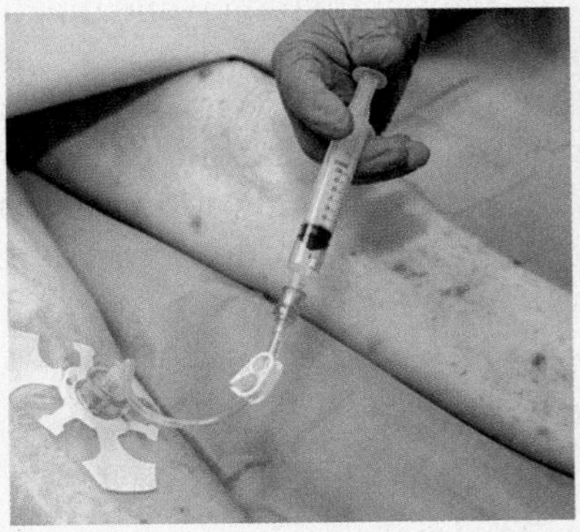

Step 8

Attach the syringe and extension set to the IO needle. Pull back on the syringe to aspirate blood and particles of bone marrow to ensure proper placement. The absence of marrow does not mean the access failed. Responsive patients should receive 1% lidocaine before infusion of fluids begins. Slowly inject saline while observing for signs of infiltration. Stop the infusion immediately if infiltration is noted. It is possible to fracture the bone during insertion of the IO needle. If this happens, then remove the IO needle and switch to another insertion site.

If no signs of infiltration are present, connect the administration set and adjust the flow rate as appropriate. Secure the needle with tape, and support it with a bulky or stabilizer dressing. Be careful not to tape around the entire circumference of the extremity, as doing so could impair circulation and potentially result in compartment syndrome. Assess the patient for a therapeutic response or signs of an adverse reaction.

Words of Wisdom

With the exception of the FAST1 sternal IO device, all IO devices (manual, spring-loaded, and battery-powered) are primarily used to insert an IO needle into the IO space of the proximal tibia, distal tibia, or humeral head. However, other anatomic locations, such as the distal femur, may also be acceptable locations for IO needle insertion.

Documentation and Communication

When you start an IV line to administer a medication, set the flow rate just slow enough to keep the vein patent. This slow flow rate can be documented as KVO (keep vein open), or TKO (to keep open).

Failure to identify the proper anatomic landmark can damage the growth plate, potentially resulting in long-term bone growth abnormalities in children.

If your insertion technique is too forceful, or if you use an IO needle that is too large for the patient's age or size, then fractures can occur. Through-and-through insertion occurs when the IO needle passes through *both* sides of the bone. To avoid this problem, stop inserting the needle when you feel a pop. If you feel a "pop, pop," then you have likely passed the needle through both sides of the bone. If either fracture or through-and-through insertion occurs, remove the needle and attempt insertion on the opposite extremity.

A pulmonary embolism can occur if the IO insertion causes bone, fat, or marrow particles to enter the systemic circulation and lodge in a pulmonary artery. You should suspect a pulmonary embolism if the patient experiences acute shortness of breath, pleuritic chest pain, and cyanosis.

Contraindications to IO Infusion

Cannulation of a peripheral vein remains the preferred route for administering IV fluids and medications. If a functional IV line is available in pediatric or adult patients, IO cannulation is *not* indicated. Other contraindications to IO cannulation and infusion include fracture of the bone intended for IO cannulation, osteoporosis, **osteogenesis imperfecta** (a congenital disease resulting in fragile bones), bilateral knee replacements, and a prosthetic limb at the IO site.

Medication Administration

Before administering any medication to a patient, you must understand how the medication will affect the human body both negatively and positively. This includes familiarity with the medication's mechanism of action, indications, contraindications, adverse effects, routes of administration, pediatric and adult doses, and antidotes (if available) for adverse reactions.

The first rule of medicine is *primum non nocere*: "first, do no harm." For example, administering a drug, such as atropine, to an *asymptomatic* patient could result in undesirable tachycardia and potential hemodynamic compromise. As a result, you could cause harm to a patient who otherwise did not need the drug. Therefore, it is paramount for you to ensure a particular drug is clearly indicated to treat the patient's condition.

You must also have an understanding of basic math for pharmacology to calculate the appropriate medication dose. This section begins with a review of basic mathematic principles as they apply to pharmacology and concludes with the various methods of medication administration.

Drug doses and flow rate calculations are often sources of confusion for many prehospital personnel, yet they are skills you will frequently use in the field and during your initial training while practicing at skill stations. You must learn to quickly and accurately calculate medication doses. Disastrous results, including death, may be the outcome if you administer an inappropriate medication or dose, administer it by the incorrect route, or give the medication too rapidly or too slowly.

Mathematic Principles Used in Pharmacology

Mathematics Review

This section discusses the use of fractions, percentages, and decimals. Basic math skills are imperative for paramedics to appropriately administer medications.

Understanding fractions is vital in formula calculation. Fractions represent a portion of a whole number. They are expressed as a numerator (the top number representing the portion available) over the denominator (representing the total quantity). For example, if you have four EMS units available and one of them is dispatched to an emergency, then one-fourth (¼) of your units are occupied. Think of fractions as the numerator divided by the denominator. For example, ¼ is the same as 1 ÷ 4.

Decimals distinguish numbers that are greater than zero from numbers that are smaller than zero. Whole numbers appear to the left side of the decimal point, and fractions of numbers on the right. Fractions can be easily converted to decimals by dividing the numerator by the denominator. For example, when administering atropine to an adult patient with bradycardia, you would give ½ of 1 milligram. Dividing 1 by 2, you would get 0.5 mg (1 ÷ 2 = 0.5).

Dividing or multiplying by 10 is simple when you remember the following method. If you are dividing a number by 10, then simply move the decimal point to the left. If you are multiplying a number by 10, then simply move the decimal point to the right. In other words, if you are dividing the number 20 by 10, moving the decimal point one space to the left results in 2, which is the correct answer. The following examples show this method.

Multiplication problem: 20 × 10

Step 1: Place the decimal point:

20.0

Step 2: To multiply by 10, move the decimal point one space to the right:

200.0

→

The answer is 200.

Division problem: 20 ÷ 10

Step 1: Place the decimal point:

20.0

Step 2: To divide by 10, move the decimal point one space to the left:

2.00

←

The answer is 2.

Percentages indicate a part of 100 and are denoted by the % symbol. Percentages can be represented as a fraction with the denominator being 100; for example, 21% = 21/100. Decimals can also easily be turned into percentages by moving the decimal point over two places (0.21 is equal to 21%).

The Metric System

The **metric system** is a measurement system based on multiples of 10 (ie, a decimal system) **FIGURE 14-40**. It is used to measure length, volume, and weight, which are represented as follows:

- Meter (m): The basic unit of length
- Liter (L): The basic unit of volume
- Gram (g): The basic unit of mass (weight)

In the metric system, prefixes indicate the fraction of the base being used. Commonly used

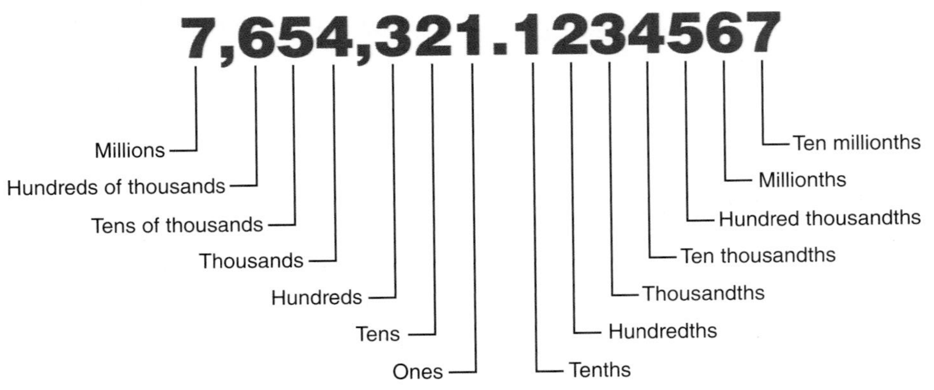

FIGURE 14-40 Decimal scale.

prefixes, from smallest to largest, include the following:

- *micro-* = 0.000001
- *milli-* = 0.001
- *centi-* = 0.01
- *kilo-* = 1,000.0

Medications are supplied in a variety of weights and volumes, and you will be required to convert those weights to volumes to administer the appropriate doses of medications to patients. **TABLE 14-3** lists the metric units of weight and volume.

To administer the appropriate dose of a medication to a patient, you must be able to convert larger units of weight to smaller ones (for example, grams to milligrams) and larger units of volume to smaller ones (for example, liters to milliliters). Conversely, you must be able to convert smaller units of weight to larger ones (for example, milligrams to grams) and smaller units of volume to larger ones (for example, milliliters to liters).

Words of Wisdom

Carry a calculator, EMS field guide, or pocket infusion charts, or use a smartphone app to assist you in converting pounds to kilograms or when calculating a drug dosage.

TABLE 14-3 Metric Units

Unit	Equivalent
Weight (smallest to largest)	
1 mcg	0.001 mg
1 mg	1,000 mcg
1 g	1,000 mg
1 kg	1,000 g
Volume (smallest to largest)	
1 mL	1 cc[a]
100 mL	1 dL
1,000 mL	1 L

[a]Cubic centimeters (cc) is a unit also used to represent milliliters (mL); therefore, 1 cc is the same as 1 mL (1 cc = 1 mL).

Drugs are packaged in different units of weight and volume. However, the weight (for example, micrograms, milligrams, and grams) and volume (for example, milliliters) of the drug to be administered usually accounts for only a small portion of the total amount of its packaged form. For example, a physician may order 50 mg of a drug for a patient, but the drug is packaged in grams. Therefore, you must be able to convert grams to milligrams and then determine how much volume is required to achieve the desired dose. (**Desired dose** refers to the amount of a drug that the physician orders, or the protocol dictates, you to give to a patient).

Volume Conversion

In the prehospital setting, you will usually deal with only two measurements of volume: milliliters and liters. Because 1 L equals 1,000 mL, simply divide or multiply by 1,000 or move the decimal point three places to the left or right to convert between these units.

When you are converting milliliters to liters, divide the smaller unit of volume by 1,000 *or* simply move the decimal point three places to the left, as demonstrated in the following example:

Example 1

Converting 500 mL of normal saline to liters (500 mL = *x* L)

500 mL ÷ 1,000 = 0.5 L *or* 500. = 0.5 L normal saline
←

Conversely, when you are converting liters to milliliters, multiply L by 1,000 *or* simply move the decimal point three places to the right, as demonstrated in the following example:

Example 1

Converting 1.5 L of LR solution to milliliters (1.5 L = *x* mL)

1.5 L × 1,000 = 1,500 mL *or* 1.500 = 1,500 mL
→

Example 2

Converting 25 L of LR solution to milliliters (25 L = *x* mL)

25 L × 1,000 = 25,000 mL *or* 25.000 = 25,000 mL
→

Weight Conversion

Converting units of weight is simply a matter of multiplying or dividing by 1,000 *or* moving the decimal point three places to the right or left.

To convert a larger unit of weight to a smaller one, *multiply* the larger unit of weight by 1,000 *or* move the decimal point three places to the *right*, as demonstrated in the following examples:

Example 1

Converting 25 g of dextrose to milligrams ($25 \text{ g} = x \text{ mg}$)

$$25 \text{ g} \times 1{,}000 = 25{,}000 \text{ mg } \textit{or } 25.000 = 25{,}000 \text{ mg}$$

$$\longrightarrow$$

Example 2

Converting 0.15 mg of fentanyl to micrograms ($0.15 \text{ mg} = x \text{ mcg}$)

$$0.15 \text{ mg} \times 1{,}000 = 150 \text{ mcg } \textit{or } 0.150 = 150 \text{ mcg}$$

$$\longrightarrow$$

Conversely, to convert a smaller unit of weight to a larger unit when the difference is 1,000 (such as mg to g or mcg to mg), divide the mg by 1,000 *or* simply move the decimal point three places to the left, as demonstrated in the following examples. Remember, 1 g equals 1,000 mg and 1 mg equals 1,000 mcg.

Example 1

Converting 200 mcg of fentanyl to milligrams ($200 \text{ mcg} = x \text{ mg}$)

$$200 \text{ mcg} \div 1{,}000 = 0.2 \text{ mg } \textit{or } 200. = 0.2 \text{ mg}$$

$$\longleftarrow$$

Example 2

Converting 250 mg of dextrose to grams ($250 \text{ mg} = x \text{ g}$)

$$250 \text{ mg} \div 1{,}000 = 0.25 \text{ g } \textit{or } 250. = 0.25 \text{ g}$$

$$\longleftarrow$$

Words of Wisdom

One teaspoon is approximately 5 mL, and 1 tablespoon is approximately 15 mL. One cup is approximately 240 mL. Drops vary based on the diameter of the dropper. These measurements may be useful to remember if you need to calculate the exact amount of a patient's medication.

Converting Pounds to Kilograms

Most likely your patients will not be able to tell you how much they weigh in kilograms (kg). However, you can easily convert a patient's weight in pounds to kilograms. This information will frequently be available during interfacility transports. For patients who do not know their weight in pounds or who are unresponsive and unable to provide you with this information, you must perform the following steps:

1. Estimate the patient's weight in pounds (lb).
2. Convert pounds to kilograms (kg).

Although many of the drugs given in emergency medicine are administered in a standard dose (eg, 1 mg of epinephrine), others are administered based on the patient's weight in kilograms (eg, 1 to 1.5 mg/kg of lidocaine). In addition, most drugs administered to pediatric patients are based on their weight in kilograms.

Two formulas can be used to convert pounds to kilograms. Use whichever one is easiest for you to remember.

For example, when converting a 170-pound man's weight to kilograms, the formula would be as follows:

Formula 1

Divide the patient's weight in pounds by 2.2 ($1 \text{ kg} = 2.2 \text{ lb}$)

$$170 \text{ lb} \div 2.2 = 77.27 \text{ kg}$$

Because the value following the decimal point in this example is less than 0.5, you may round the patient's weight in kilograms to 77. If the value after the decimal point in the first example had been greater than 0.5, then you would round up the weight in kilograms to 78. Although this may seem negligible, it is good practice to administer the *most* appropriate amount of the drug to the patient.

Here are some additional examples of this formula's use:

$$250 \text{ lb} \div 2.2 = 113.64 \text{ kg}$$
$$479.6 \text{ lb} \div 2.2 = 218 \text{ kg}$$
$$6.6 \text{ lb} \div 2.2 = 3 \text{ kg}$$
$$30 \text{ lb} \div 2.2 = 14.09 \text{ kg}$$
$$68 \text{ lb} \div 2.2 = 30.91 \text{ kg}$$

Formula 2

Divide the patient's weight in pounds by 2 and subtract 10% of that number

For example, when converting a 120-pound woman's weight to kilograms, the formula would be as follows:

Example 1

Converting a 120-pound woman's weight to kilograms

Step 1: $120 \text{ lb} \div 2 = 60$

Step 2: $60 \text{ lb} \times 10\% = 6$

Step 3: $60 - 6 = 54 \text{ kg}$

Note: This formula provides an approximate weight rather than an exact conversion.

Temperature Conversion

The Fahrenheit and Celsius (or centigrade) temperature scales are commonly used to measure temperature. On the **Celsius scale**, water freezes at 0° and boils at 100°. On the **Fahrenheit scale**, water freezes at 32° and boils at 212°. Normal body temperature is 98.6° Fahrenheit (37° Celsius). Values on each of these scales can easily be interconverted by using the following equations:

- To convert Fahrenheit to Celsius: Subtract 32, then multiply by 0.555 (5/9)

Fahrenheit → Celsius
$98.6°\text{F} - 32 \times 0.555 = 36.9\ (37°\text{C})$

- To convert Celsius to Fahrenheit: Multiply by 1.8 (9/5), then add 32

Celsius → Fahrenheit
$37°\text{C} \times 1.8 + 32 = 98.6°\text{F}$

Examples

Fahrenheit → Celsius
$104.2°\text{F} - 32 \times 0.555 = 40.1°\text{C}$
$100.9°\text{F} - 32 \times 0.555 = 38.2°\text{C}$
$92.4°\text{F} - 32 \times 0.555 = 33.5°\text{C}$

Celsius → Fahrenheit
$37.9°\text{C} \times 1.8 + 32 = 100.2°\text{F}$
$38.6°\text{C} \times 1.8 + 32 = 101.4°\text{F}$
$32.2°\text{C} \times 1.8 + 32 = 90°\text{F}$

YOU are the Paramedic

PART 2

You have completed a secondary assessment and obtained vital signs. The patient denies any chronic medical conditions and says he has never experienced anything like this before. He takes no medications and has no known drug allergies. The cardiac monitor has been applied, and you note that the patient is currently in atrial fibrillation with a rapid ventricular response. You contact medical control and provide a brief report. The physician asks you to administer diltiazem 0.25 mg/kg IV push over 2 minutes; he would like a target heart rate of less than 110 beats/min. The patient weighs 231 pounds (105 kg). Your diltiazem comes prepackaged in a syringe with 30 mg/5 mL.

Recording Time: 5 Minutes	
Respirations	20 breaths/min
Pulse	180 beats/min, irregular
Skin	Warm and dry
Blood pressure	134/90 mm Hg
Oxygen saturation (Spo_2)	99%
Pupils	Pupils Equal, Round, Reactive to Light and Accommodation (PERRLA)
ECG	Atrial fibrillation with a rapid ventricular response

3. What information must you and your partner be sure to communicate to one another as you are preparing to administer this medication?

4. Why is it prudent to contact medical control in this scenario to discuss patient care options?

5. What dose will you administer to the patient? Given the supplied medication, what volume will you administer?

Calculating Medication Doses

Multiple formulas are available for calculating medication doses. This chapter focuses on those formulas that most students find easy to understand. For other calculation formulas, you should consult with your instructor. The method of drug dose calculation demonstrated in this chapter is based on the following three factors:

- Desired dose
- Concentration of the drug available (dose on hand)
- Volume to be administered

> **Documentation and Communication**
>
> To prevent errors when you are documenting decimals, write 0.2 mg or 2 mg instead of .2 mg or 2.0 mg, which could easily be mistaken for 2 mg or 20 mg, respectively.

Desired Dose

The desired dose (ie, the drug order) is the amount of a drug that the physician orders, or the protocol dictates, you to give to a patient. It may be expressed as a standard dose (eg, 5 mg of diazepam [Valium], 25 g of 50% dextrose) or as a specific number of micrograms, milligrams, or grams per kilogram of body weight (eg, 1 to 1.5 mg/kg of lidocaine [Xylocaine]).

Drug Concentrations

After receiving a drug order (desired dose), you must determine how much of the drug you have available. In other words, you must know its concentration—the total weight (micrograms, milligrams, or grams) of the drug contained in a specific amount of volume (milliliters or liters). Sometimes this information is printed on the label of the drug container (eg, Drug X at a concentration of 5 mg/mL); other containers may list the total weight and total volume of the drug separately (eg, 8 mg of morphine sulfate in 2 mL). The following examples identify some common prepackaged drug concentrations:

- Lidocaine, 100 mg/10 mL
- Epinephrine, 1 mg/10 mL (1:10,000)
- Furosemide, 40 mg/4 mL
- Adenosine, 6 mg/2 mL
- 50% dextrose, 25 g/50 mL
- Fentanyl, 100 mcg/1 mL
- Naloxone, 2 mg/2 mL

In the preceding examples, notice that the drugs are contained in different volumes of solution. This is your **volume on hand**. *To administer a drug, you must know the weight of the drug that is present in **1 mL**.* This information will tell you the concentration of the drug that you have on hand. The formula for calculating this is as follows:

$$\text{Total weight of the drug} \div \text{Total volume in milliliters} = \text{Weight per milliliter}$$

By using this formula, you can easily calculate how much of the drug is contained in each milliliter.

Examples

Amiodarone, 150 mg/3 mL

$$150 \text{ mg (total weight)} \div 3 \text{ mL (total volume)} = 50 \text{ mg/mL}$$

Ondansetron, 4 mg/2 mL

$$4 \text{ mg} \div 2 \text{ mL} = 2 \text{ mg/mL}$$

Epinephrine, 1 mg/10 mL

$$1 \text{ mg} \div 10 \text{ mL} = 0.1 \text{ mg/mL}$$

Thiamine, 100 mg/2 mL

$$100 \text{ mg} \div 2 \text{ mL} = 50 \text{ mg/mL}$$

Things become slightly more complex when the label of the drug lists the drug concentration as a percentage: for example, "1% lidocaine (Xylocaine)." What *percentage* means in terms of drug concentration is the number of *grams present in*

> **Words of Wisdom**
>
> If the physician orders a specific number of milliliters to be administered per hour (mL/h), then a quick and easy way to calculate the number of drops per minute (gtt/min) with a 60-gtt set is to divide the number of milliliters per hour:
>
> - By 6, if using a macrodrip that provides 10 gtt/mL
> - By 4, if using a macrodrip that provides 15 gtt/mL
> - By 1, if using a microdrip set that provides 60 gtt/mL

100 mL. Thus, 1% lidocaine (Xylocaine) contains 1 g of drug in every 100 mL (1 dL). By dividing the numerator and denominator by 100, you will arrive at a concentration of 10 mg/mL:

$$\frac{1\text{ g}}{100\text{ mL}} = \frac{1{,}000\text{ mg}}{100\text{ mL}} = 10\text{ mg/mL}$$

Volume to Be Administered

After determining the concentration of the drug present in each milliliter, you must calculate how much volume is needed to give the amount of the drug ordered (desired dose). Use the following formula to calculate the volume to be administered:

Desired dose (mg) ÷ Concentration of drug on hand (mg/mL) = Volume to be administered

Example 1

According to your protocols, you should administer 5 mg of midazolam (Versed) for a patient who is having a seizure. You have a vial of midazolam that contains 10 mg in 5 mL. How many milliliters of midazolam must you give to achieve the ordered dose of 5 mg?

Step 1: Determine the concentration (in mg/mL).

10 mg ÷ 5 mL = 2 mg/mL (concentration)

Step 2: Determine how much volume to administer.

5 mg (desired dose) ÷ 2 mg/mL (concentration) = 2.5 mL

Example 2

Your protocols dictate that you administer 12.5 g of dextrose to a patient with hypoglycemia. You have a prefilled syringe of 50% dextrose containing 25 g in 50 mL. How many milliliters of dextrose will you give?

Step 1: Determine the concentration (in g/mL).

25 g ÷ 50 mL = 0.5 g/mL (concentration)

Step 2: Determine how much volume to administer.

12.5 g (desired dose) ÷ 0.5 g/mL (concentration) = 25 mL

Example 3

You are treating a patient who has nausea and feels as if she is going to vomit. Your protocol says you can administer 4 mg of ondansetron (Zofran). Ondansetron is packaged in a vial of 4 mg in 2 mL.

Step 1: Determine the concentration (in g/mL).

4 mg ÷ 2 mL = 2 mg/mL (concentration)

Step 2: Determine how much volume to administer.

4 mg (desired dose) ÷ 2 mg/mL (concentration) = 2 mL

Example 4

For a patient in cardiac arrest, your protocols allow you to administer 300 mg of amiodarone (Cordarone) as an antidysrhythmic after epinephrine or vasopressin when ventricular fibrillation or ventricular tachycardia is present. Amiodarone is packaged as 150 mg in 3 mL.

Step 1: Determine the concentration (in g/mL).

150 mg ÷ 3 mL = 50 mg/mL (concentration)

Step 2: Determine how much volume to administer.

300 mg (desired dose) ÷ 50 mg/mL (concentration) = 6 mL

Weight-Based Drug Doses

As mentioned earlier, some medication doses are based on the patient's weight in kilograms. Determining the appropriate dose for the patient requires simply adding one step to the previously discussed formula: conversion of the patient's weight in pounds to kilograms. Remember, 1 kg = 2.2 pounds.

Example 1

A 7-year-old girl requires 0.02 mg/kg of atropine to treat symptomatic bradycardia. You have a prefilled syringe of atropine containing 1 mg in 10 mL. The child's mother tells you the child weighs 60 pounds. How many milligrams will you give to this child (ie, what is the desired dose)? How much volume will you give to achieve the required dose?

Step 1: Convert the child's weight in pounds to kilograms.

Formula 1: 60 lb ÷ 2.2 = 27.2 kg (round to 27 kg)
Formula 2: 60 lb ÷ 2 − 10% = 27 kg

Step 2: Determine the desired dose.

0.02 mg/kg × 27 kg = 0.54 mg (round to 0.5 mg [desired dose])

Step 3: Determine the concentration.

1 mg ÷ 10 mL = 0.1 mg/mL (concentration)

Step 4: Determine how much volume to administer.

0.5 mg (desired dose) ÷ 0.1 mg/mL (concentration) = 5 mL

Example 2

You are caring for a patient with excited delirium. Your protocol suggests you can administer 1 to 2 mg IV or 3 to 4 mg/kg IM of ketamine. The patient weighs 110 pounds and you are unable to obtain vascular access. The ketamine is packaged in a vial of 500 mg in 10 mL.

Step 1: Convert the patient's weight in pounds to kilograms.

Formula 1: 110 lb ÷ 2.2 = 50 kg

Step 2: Determine the desired dose.

3 mg/kg × 50 kg = 150 mg

Step 3: Determine the concentration.

500 mg ÷ 10 mL = 50 mg/mL (concentration)

Step 4: Determine how much volume to administer.

150 mg (desired dose) ÷ 50 mg/mL (concentration) = 3 mL

Calculating Fluid Infusion Rates

Once an IV or IO catheter is in place, you need to adjust the flow rate according to the patient's clinical condition or as dictated by medical control. To do so, you must know the following information:

- The volume to be infused
- The period over which it is to be infused
- The properties of the administration set you are using; that is, how many drops per milliliter (gtt/mL) it delivers

By knowing in advance the volume to be infused, the period over which it will be infused, and the properties of the administration set, you can calculate the flow rate.

For example, suppose the physician orders 1 L (1,000 mL) of normal saline to be infused in 4 hours, and the macrodrip administration set provides 10 gtt/mL:

$$\frac{\text{Volume to be infused} \times \text{gtt/mL of administration set}}{\text{Total time of infusion in minutes}} = \text{gtt/min}$$

Information:

Total volume to be infused	=	1,000 mL
gtt/mL of the administration set	=	10
Time of infusion (in minutes)	=	4 h × 60 min/h = 240 min

Calculation:

$$\frac{1{,}000 \text{ mL} \times 10 \text{ gtt/mL}}{240 \text{ minutes}} = \text{approximately } 42 \text{ gtt/min}$$

Calculating the Dose and Rate for a Medication Infusion

Non–Weight-Based Medication Infusions

Following the administration of certain drugs, you may need to begin a continuous infusion to maintain a therapeutic blood level of the drug and prevent a recurrence of the condition. Medication infusions are usually ordered to be administered over a specified period, usually per minute.

To calculate a continuous medication infusion that is not based on the patient's weight, you must know the following information in advance:

- The desired dose (mcg/min or mg/min)
- The properties of the administration set you are using (eg, microdrip [60 gtt/mL])
- Will you be using an infusion pump? (Mechanical infusion pumps are discussed later in this chapter.)

You will use the same formula to calculate a drug dose as previously discussed. Then, however, you will calculate the desired dose to be administered continuously: usually a certain number of micrograms (mcg) or milligrams (mg) per minute.

For example, suppose you have just administered 75 mg of lidocaine to a patient in cardiac arrest, after which time the patient converts to a perfusing rhythm. Medical control then orders you to begin a continuous lidocaine infusion at 2 mg/min. You must determine at how many drops per minute (gtt/min) to set the IV drip rate to deliver the 2 mg/min desired dose. To do so, you will add a certain amount of lidocaine into a bag of IV fluid. In this example, 2 g (2,000 mg) of lidocaine will be added to a 500-mL bag of normal saline, a common combination. The formula to calculate the continuous infusion rate is as follows:

Step 1: Determine the concentration.

2 g (2,000 mg) of lidocaine ÷ 500 mL of normal saline = 4 mg/mL (concentration)

Step 2: Determine the amount of volume to infuse per minute (mL/min).

For this calculation, you must recall the desired dose—in this case, 2 mg/min.

To determine the number of mL/min, you perform the following calculation:

$$\frac{2\text{ mg (desired dose)}}{\text{min}} \times \frac{1\text{ mL}}{4\text{ mg}} = \begin{matrix}0.5\text{ mL/min}\\ \text{(concentration)}\end{matrix}$$

Step 3: Determine how many drops per minute (gtt/min) at which to set the IV flow rate.

For this calculation, you must know the number of drops per milliliter (gtt/mL) that your IV administration set delivers: a microdrip (60 gtt/mL) or a macrodrip (10 or 15 gtt/mL). For a microdrip administration set (typically used when administering a continuous medication infusion), the number of drops per minute for the IV flow rate would be calculated as follows:

0.5 mL/min × 60 gtt/mL = 30 gtt/min

Weight-Based Medication Infusions

Some continuous medication infusions are based on the patient's weight in kilograms. Dopamine (Intropin), for example, is typically administered in a range of 5 to 20 mcg/kg/min. By using the previously discussed formula and factoring in the patient's weight in kilograms to determine the desired dose, you will calculate the IV drip rate for a 70-kg patient who requires a continuous dopamine infusion at 5 mcg/kg/min. In this example, 800 mg of dopamine will be added to a 500-mL bag of normal saline—a common combination.

Example 1

Step 1: Determine the desired dose.

5 mcg/kg/min × 70 kg = 350 mcg/min (desired dose)

Step 2: Determine the concentration.

800 mg (800,000 mcg) of dopamine ÷ 500 mL of normal saline = 1.6 mg/mL (concentration)

The caveat here is that dopamine is administered in *micrograms,* not milligrams. Therefore, you must convert the 1.6 mg/mL concentration to mcg/mL. Recall that to convert a larger unit of weight to a smaller one, you must multiply it by the correct factor or move the decimal to the right. In this case, you must multiply by 1,000 *or* move the decimal point three places to the *right*; in other words, 1.6 mg is equal to *1,600 mcg.*

Step 3: Determine the amount of volume to infuse per minute (mL/min).

Again, you must recall the desired dose: in this case, 350 mcg/min. The calculation continues as follows to determine the number of mL/min:

350 mcg/min (desired dose) ÷ 1,600 mcg/mL (concentration) = 0.22 mL/min

Step 4: Determine how many drops per minute (gtt/min) at which to set the IV flow rate.

Again, you must know the properties of the administration set you are using. In this example, you will use the microdrip set (60 gtt/mL). The number of drops per minute for the IV flow rate would be calculated as follows:

$$\frac{0.22\text{ mL}}{\text{min}} \times \frac{60\text{ gtt}}{\text{mL}} = \begin{matrix}13.2\text{ gtt/min}\\ \text{(round to 13 gtt/min)}\end{matrix}$$

Dobutamine (Dobutrex) is usually administered with an IV pump, so calculating the gtt is rarely needed for this medication. However, paramedics will see this medication in use during interfacility transports, so the following calculation focuses on dobutamine.

Example 2

Dobutamine is commonly administered during interfacility transports for cardiogenic shock. The dose is generally 2 to 20 mcg/kg/min. For this example, you are transferring a 60-kg patient who is on a drip of 10 mcg/kg/min. The dobutamine is packaged as 250 mg in a 500-mL bag.

Step 1: Calculate the desired dose.

$$10 \text{ mcg/kg/min} \times 60 \text{ kg} = 600 \text{ mcg/min (desired dose)}$$

Step 2: Calculate the concentration. The first step in calculating the concentration is to convert the units from mg to mcg.

$$250 \text{ mg} \times \frac{1{,}000 \text{ mcg}}{\text{mg}} = 250{,}000 \text{ mcg}$$

$$250{,}000 \text{ mcg} \div 500 \text{ mL} = 500 \text{ mcg/mL (concentration)}$$

Step 3: Calculate the amount of volume to infuse per minute (mL/min).

$$600 \text{ mcg/min (desired dose)} \div 500 \text{ mcg/mL (concentration)} = 1.2 \text{ mL/min}$$

Step 4: Calculate how many drops per minute (gtt/min) at which to set the IV flow rate.

$$1.2 \text{ mL/min} \times 60 \text{ gtt/mL} = 72 \text{ gtt/min}$$

Pediatric Drug Doses

Several methods may be used to determine the appropriate dose of medication for a pediatric patient. Examples of these methods include length-based resuscitation tape measures, pediatric wheel charts, EMS field guides with tables or charts specific to pediatric patients, and smartphone apps. Most drugs used in pediatric emergency medicine are based on the child's weight in kilograms. Except for the smaller doses and volumes, the calculations for pediatric drug dosing and medication infusions are the same as they are for adults.

Words of Wisdom

The child's caregiver will often know the patient's weight. This information can facilitate calculating drug dosages.

Enteral Medication Administration

Enteral medications, also referred to as alimentary medications, are given through some portion of the digestive or intestinal tract. They include medications that are administered orally, through a feeding tube, or rectally.

Oral Medication Administration

Most patients take their daily medications at home by the oral (per os [PO]) route. Forms of solid and liquid oral medications include capsules, timed-release capsules, lozenges, pills, tablets, elixirs, emulsions, suspensions, and syrups **FIGURE 14-41**.

Drugs taken by mouth are absorbed at a slow rate from the stomach and intestines, usually between 30 and 90 minutes. Because their absorption is slower, it may be necessary for prehospital providers to administer oral medications early in the patient's care.

To prepare for giving oral medications, gather the appropriate equipment for the form of medication you are administering. Examples include a small medicine cup, a medicine dropper, a teaspoon, an oral syringe, or a nipple. Check for indications, contraindications, and precautions, and review the rights of medication administration before giving any medication.

Follow these steps when administering an oral medication **FIGURE 14-42**:

1. Take standard precautions.
2. Determine the need for the medication based on the patient's presentation.
3. Obtain a history, including any drug allergies.
4. Follow standing orders, or contact medical control for permission.
5. Check the medication to ensure it is the right medication, it is not cloudy or discolored, and its expiration date has not passed.

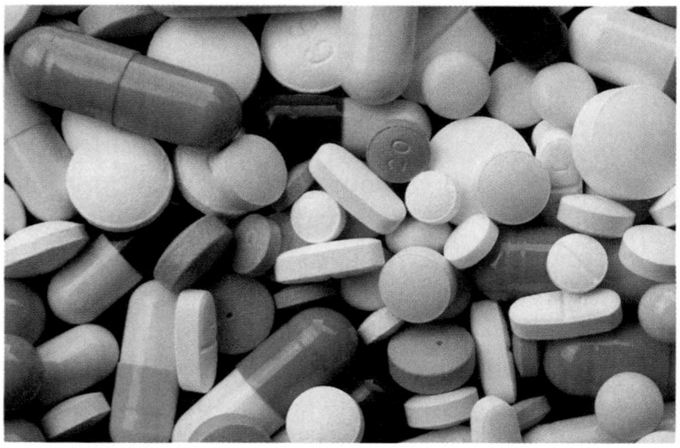

FIGURE 14-41 Oral medications enter the bloodstream through the digestive system.

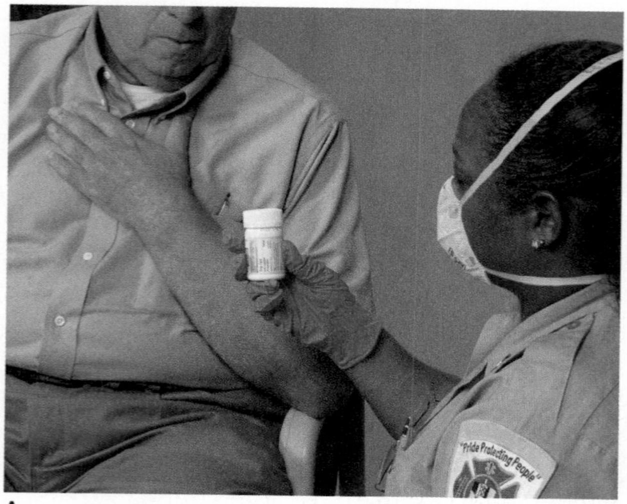

A

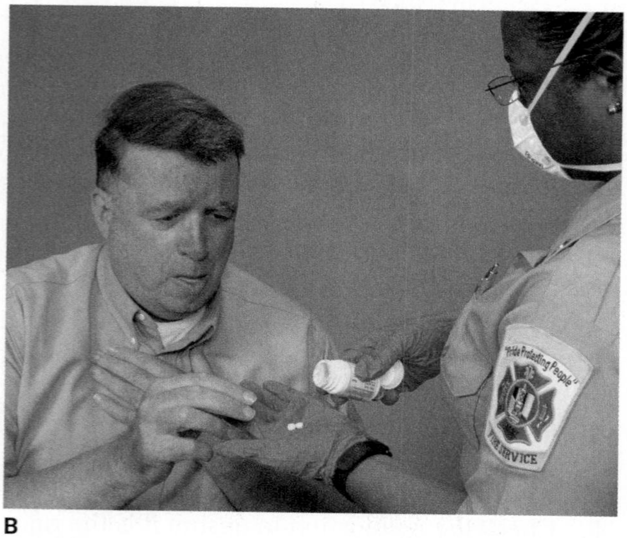

B

FIGURE 14-42 Administering an oral medication. **A.** Check the medication and its expiration date. **B.** Have the patient take the medication. Provide a glass or cup of water if necessary.

6. Determine the appropriate dose. If using a liquid medication, pour the desired amount into a calibrated cup or withdraw the appropriate amount into a syringe or dropper. If administering a solid medication (eg, pill, tablet, capsule), pour the appropriate amount into the bottle's lid and then place it in the patient's hand.
7. Instruct the patient to swallow the medication with water, if administering a pill or tablet.
8. Monitor the patient's condition, and document the medication given, route, time of administration, and patient's response.

You may need to calculate the number of pills, capsules, or tablets to give. For oral medications, the concentration is readily available on the bottle's label. For example, for a patient experiencing an exacerbation of chronic obstructive pulmonary disease, your protocols may call for 60 mg of oral prednisone. The concentration is labeled as 20 mg/tablet.

Calculation:

60 mg (desired dose) ÷ 20-mg tablets (concentration) = 3 tablets

Orogastric and Nasogastric Tube Medication Administration

Gastric tubes (orogastric or nasogastric) are occasionally inserted in the prehospital setting to decompress the stomach, perform gastric lavage, or establish a route for enteral medication administration, although use of this route for medication administration in the field is rare. Some services may allow paramedics to administer activated charcoal by gastric tube for toxic ingestion when oral activated charcoal is contraindicated. Gastric tubes are also commonly present during interfacility transports. The solution most commonly administered through gastric tubes during interfacility transports is liquid nutrition for tube feeding. If your EMS service permits medication administration through an orogastric or nasogastric tube, you should receive in-service training from your medical director regarding these procedures. Chapter 16, *Airway Management*, describes the insertion of orogastric and nasogastric tubes.

Rectal Medication Administration

Certain drugs may be administered rectally if you are unable to establish IV or IO access. For example, in the field, diazepam (Valium) may be administered rectally (per rectum [PR]) in patients having a seizure because IV access can be challenging to obtain in such cases. Medication absorption via this route is rapid and predictable because the rectal mucosa is highly vascular **FIGURE 14-43**. Rectal medications have a rapid onset of action because they are not digested before being absorbed by the body's vasculature and, therefore, skip the first-pass metabolism.

You might be asked to administer specific antiemetic medications that are available in **suppository** form (eg, promethazine [Phenergan]) under certain circumstances. A suppository is a drug mixed

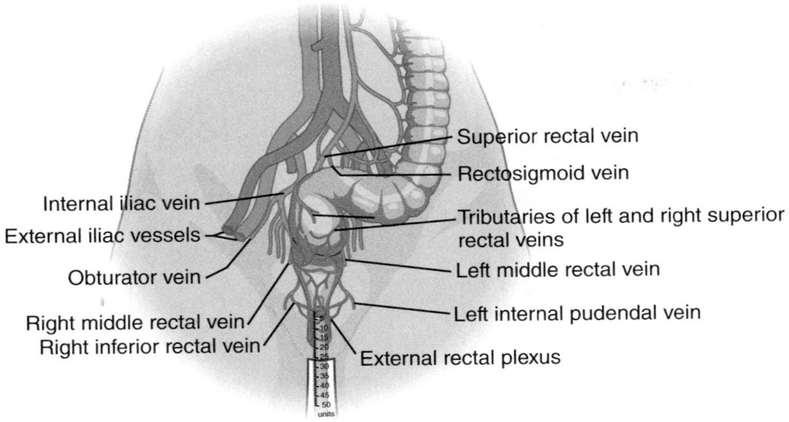

FIGURE 14-43 The rectal mucosa is highly vascular. It rapidly and predictably absorbs medications.

in a firm base that melts at body temperature and is shaped to fit the rectum. In the clinical setting, medications are sometimes administered via an **enema**, a liquid solution that is administered into the rectum, such as for imaging studies of the gastrointestinal tract.

Follow these steps to administer a drug via the rectal route:

1. Take standard precautions.
2. Determine the need for the medication based on the patient's presentation.
3. Obtain a history, including any drug allergies.
4. Follow standing orders, or contact medical control for permission.
5. Determine the appropriate dose, and check that the medication is the right medication, there is no cloudiness or discoloration, and the expiration date has not passed.
6. Use a water-soluble gel for lubrication when you insert a suppository. Insert the suppository into the rectum approximately 1 to 1.5 inches (3 to 4 cm) while instructing the patient to relax and not to bear down.
7. For medications in liquid form, some modifications are needed. You may use a nasopharyngeal airway, a small endotracheal (ET) tube **FIGURE 14-44**, an 18-gauge IV catheter without a needle, or a commercial device as your delivery device.
   - Lubricate the end of the delivery device with a water-soluble gel, and gently insert it approximately 1 to 1.5 inches (3 to 4 cm) into the rectum.

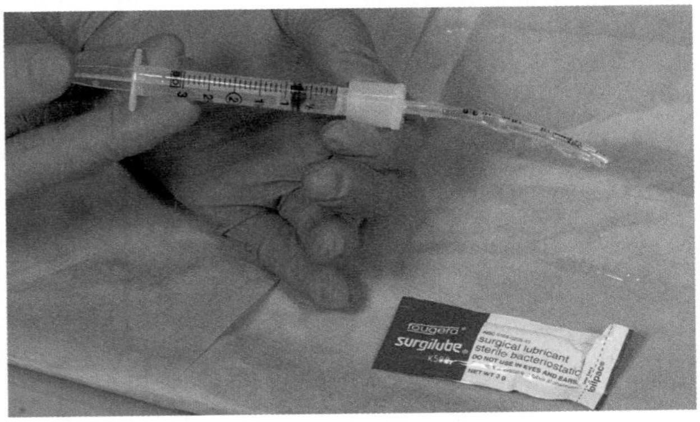

FIGURE 14-44 A syringe attached to a pediatric endotracheal tube can be used for rectal medication administration in a child.

   - Instruct the patient to relax and not to bear down, if possible.
   - With a *needleless* syringe, gently push the medication through the tube.
   - Once the medication has been delivered, remove and dispose of the tube or syringe in an appropriate container.
8. Monitor the patient's condition, and document the medication given, route, time of administration, and patient's response.

Parenteral Medication Administration

The **parenteral route** refers to any route other than the gastrointestinal tract. Parenteral routes for medication administration include the intradermal,

Words of Wisdom

Diazepam (Valium) is available for rectal administration in a specifically designed container, marketed under the name Diastat. The distal end of the container is tapered, which facilitates its insertion into the rectum. This feature eliminates the need for syringes or other methods of injecting the medication into the rectum. Diazepam is a commonly prescribed medication for children with seizures.

SAFETY

Whenever you use a needle to draw up medication from an ampule or vial, to avoid sticking yourself, hold the syringe against your palm with the needle pointing up and draw the ampule or vial down onto the needle using the thumb and forefinger of the palm the syringe is braced against. This technique is especially beneficial if you are in a moving ambulance.

subcutaneous, IM, IV, IO, and percutaneous routes. Compared with enterally administered medications (eg, oral, gastric tube), parenterally administered medications are absorbed into the central circulation more quickly and at a more predictable rate, so they achieve their therapeutic effects faster. Of the various parenteral drug routes, IV administration is the route most commonly used in the prehospital setting and generally is the quickest way to get medication into the central circulation.

Syringes and Needles

A variety of needles and syringes are used for administering parenteral medications. Many syringes come prepackaged with a needle already attached. In other cases, the needles and syringes are packaged separately. Syringes consist of a plunger, body or barrel, flange, and tip **FIGURE 14-45**. To maintain sterility, do not touch the tip of the syringe, the shaft of the plunger, or the inside of the barrel. Handle a

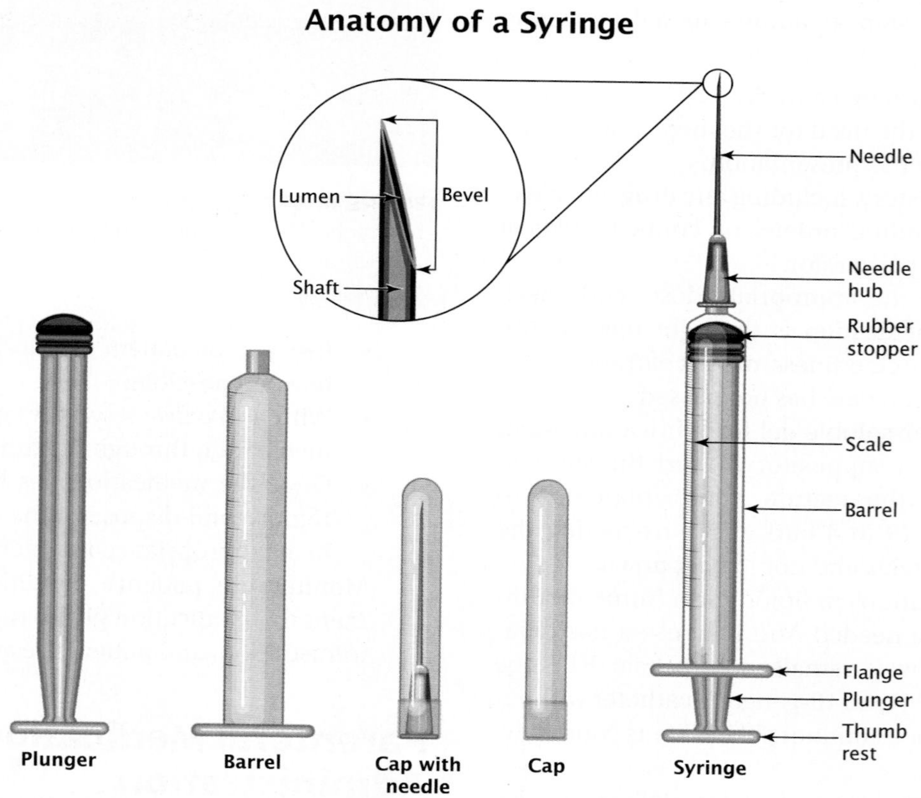

FIGURE 14-45 A syringe consists of a plunger, body or barrel, flange, and tip.

syringe by the outside of the barrel and the handle of the plunger.

Syringe capacities vary from 1 to 60 mL; the 3-mL syringe is commonly used for injections. Syringe selection is based on the volume of medication that you will administer **FIGURE 14-46**. Most syringes are marked with calibration lines on one side of the barrel. Each small line reflects milliliters or fractions of 1 milliliter, depending on the syringe's capacity. The larger the syringe capacity, the greater the interval between the calibration lines. When measuring a medication dose with a syringe, read the calibration from the top ring of the plunger.

When choosing a syringe, the device's capacity and whether its calibration scale is appropriate for the dosage to be given are the primary considerations. To select a syringe with an appropriate capacity, identify how many calibrations it shows in each milliliter. Small-capacity syringes have two scales: One scale typically has calibrations in increments of tenths (or hundredths) of 1 milliliter; the other scale is calibrated in minims. A tuberculin (TB) syringe is used to measure doses of 1 mL or less. Because its calibrations are in hundredths, a TB syringe is often used for measuring pediatric dosages. A 3-mL syringe has calibrations in increments of tenths of 1 milliliter. In addition, 5-, 6-, 10-, and 12-mL syringes have calibrations in increments of 0.2 mL. Calibrations on a 20-mL syringe are in 1-mL increments.

Hypodermic needles have three parts: the hub, shaft, and bevel. The hub is the plastic piece that houses the needle and fits onto a syringe. The shaft (also called the cannula) is the length of the needle. The needle shaft connects to the hub. The bevel is the slanted tip at the end of the needle. The opening within the bevel is called the lumen. Needles are packaged with a plastic shield covering them to maintain sterility. When preparing a needle and syringe for injection, you can handle the hub of the needle to ensure a tight fit on the syringe. However, to maintain sterility, you must not touch either the shaft or the bevel of the needle.

Needle lengths for standard injections vary from $\frac{3}{8}$ inch (0.9 cm) to 2 inches (5 cm). As with IV catheters, the needle gauge refers to the diameter: The smaller the number, the larger the diameter. Common needle gauges range from 18 to 26. The needle gauge used depends on the route of parenteral medication administration. Smaller-gauge needles, for example, are used for subcutaneous injections, whereas larger-gauge needles are used for IM and IV injections.

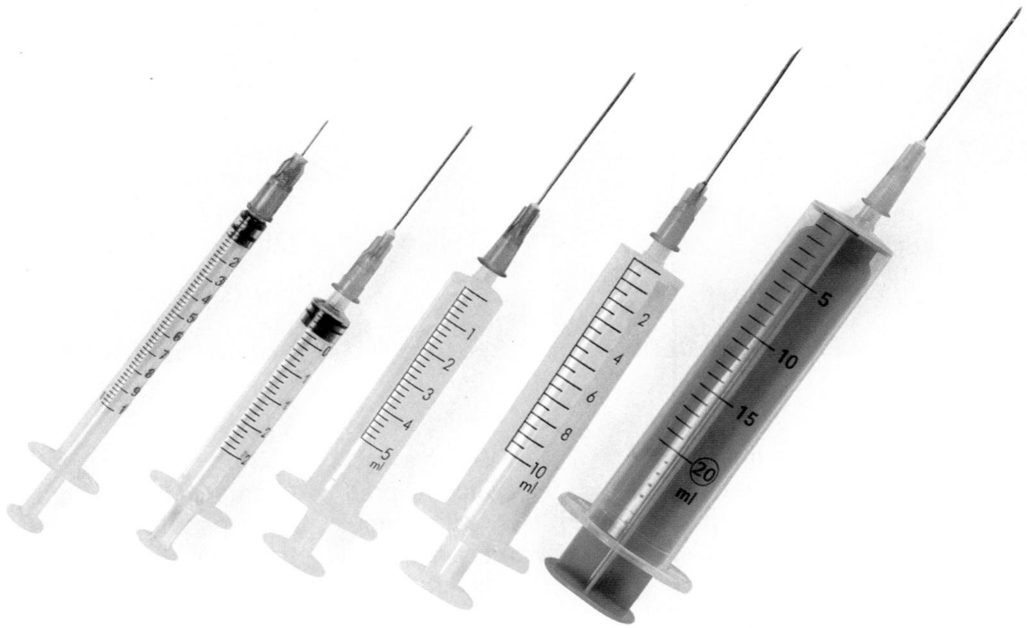

FIGURE 14-46 Syringes are available in various capacities and may be packaged with or without a needle.

Packaging of Parenteral Medications

Medications for injection may be packaged in ampules, vials, or prefilled syringes.

Ampules

Ampules are breakable sterile glass containers that are designed to carry a single dose of medication **FIGURE 14-47**. They may contain as little as 1 mL or as much as 10 mL, depending on the medication.

When you are drawing a medication from an ampule, follow the steps in **SKILL DRILL 14-3**.

Vials

Vials are small glass or plastic bottles with a rubber-stopper top; they may contain single or multiple doses of a medication **FIGURE 14-48**. When you are using a vial of medication, you must first determine how much of the drug you will need and how many doses are present in the vial.

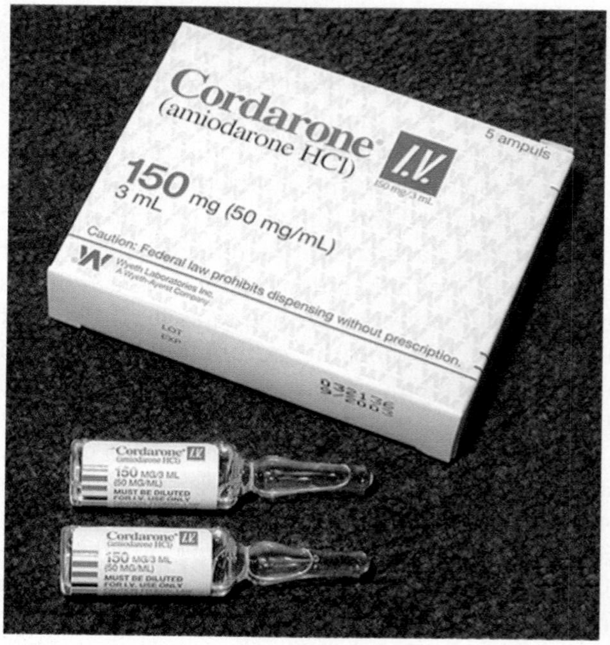

FIGURE 14-47 Medication stored in ampules.

Skill Drill 14-3 Drawing Medication From an Ampule

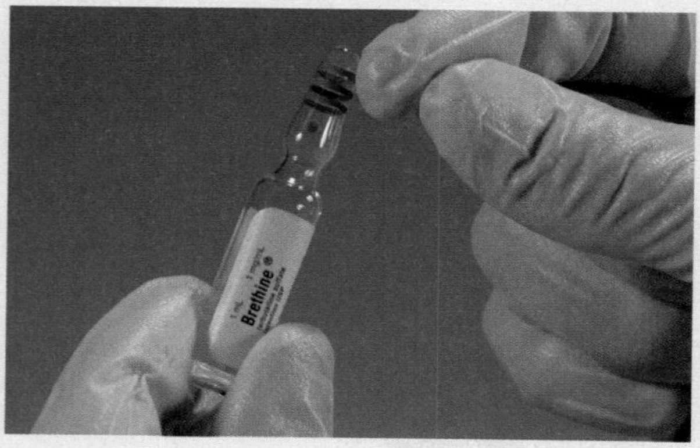

Step 1

Check the medication to ensure that it is the correct drug and concentration, that it is not cloudy or discolored, and that the expiration date has not passed. Ensure that the ampule is not cracked or chipped.

Shake the medication into the base of the ampule. If some of the drug remains stuck in the neck, then gently thump or tap the stem. Alternatively, gently swirl the ampule to displace the medication contents from the top of the container.

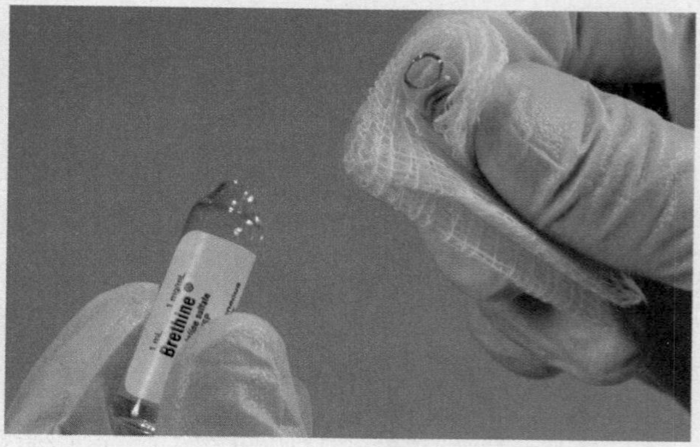

Step 2

Using a 4 × 4–inch (10 × 10–cm) gauze pad, an alcohol prep, or an ampule breaker, grasp the neck of the ampule and snap it off where the ampule is scored in a direction away from you. If the ampule is not scored and you attempt to break it, some sharp edges may be present. Drop the stem in the sharps container.

Skill Drill 14-3 Drawing Medication From an Ampule (continued)

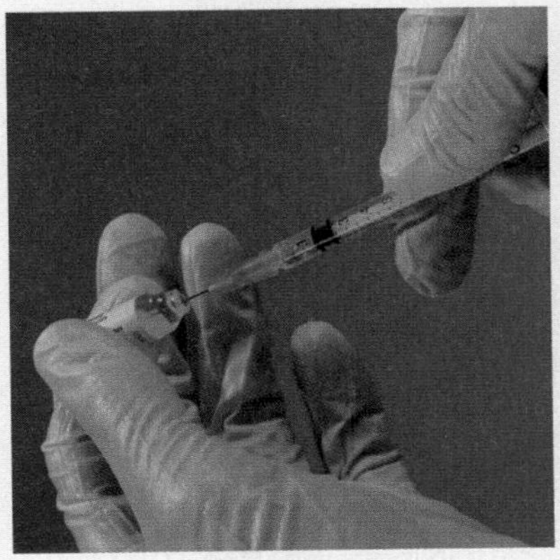

Step 3

Attach a filter needle to the syringe. With the syringe and filter needle in one hand, insert the needle into the ampule without touching the outer sides or rim of the ampule. Draw the solution into the syringe, and dispose of the ampule in the sharps container.

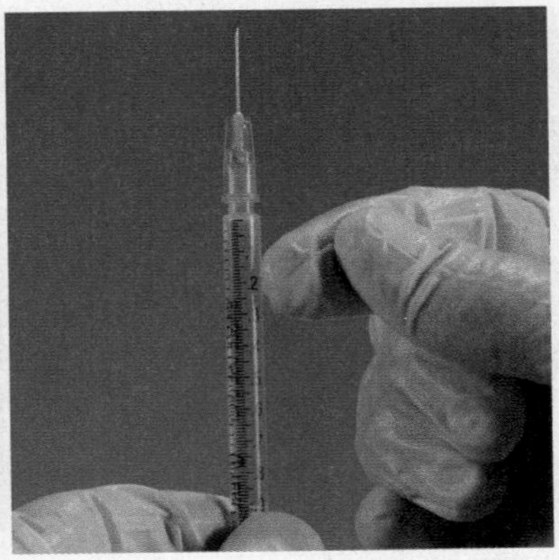

Step 4

Hold the syringe with the needle pointing up, and gently tap the barrel to loosen the air trapped inside and cause it to rise.

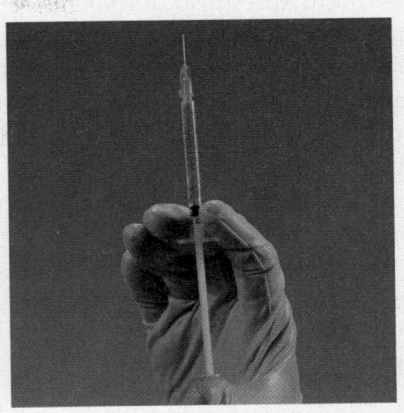

Step 5

Press gently on the plunger to dispel any air bubbles. Recap the needle using the one-handed method. Dispose of the needle in the sharps container and attach a standard hypodermic needle to the syringe, if necessary, to administer the medication.

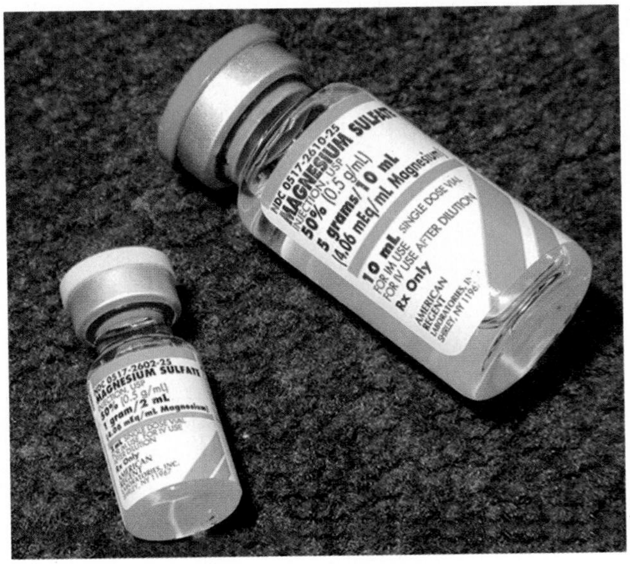

FIGURE 14-48 Vials (single [left] and multiple dose).

When withdrawing contents from a vial, clean the vial's top with alcohol before withdrawing the medication. For a single-dose vial, you may draw up the entire amount in the vial. For multiple-dose vials, you should draw up only the amount needed. Remember, once you remove the cover from a vial, it is no longer sterile. If you need a second dose, remember to clean the vial's top with alcohol.

Some medications that are stored in vials may need to be reconstituted, such as methylprednisolone sodium succinate (Solu-Medrol) and glucagon. Glucagon is stored in two vials: one containing the powdered form of the drug and the other containing sterile water. **Drug reconstitution** involves removing the sterile water (or provided **diluent**) from its vial and injecting it into the vial that contains the powder, thereby making a solution for injection. To reconstitute the contents from two vials, draw the fluid out of the first vial and inject it into the vial that contains the powder. Shake the vial vigorously, unless contraindicated, to mix the medication before drawing out the contents for administration.

Methylprednisolone sodium succinate is stored in a **Mix-o-Vial**, a single vial divided into two compartments by a rubber stopper **FIGURE 14-49**. To reconstitute a drug that is contained in a Mix-o-Vial, squeeze the two vials together; this action releases the center stopper and allows the contents to mix. Then, shake the vial vigorously to mix the contents before drawing out the medication.

When you are drawing medication from a vial, follow the steps in **SKILL DRILL 14-4**.

Prefilled Syringes

Prefilled syringes are packaged in tamper-proof boxes. Two types of prefilled syringes exist: those that are separated into a glass drug cartridge and a syringe **FIGURE 14-50**, and preassembled prefilled syringes **FIGURE 14-51**. These syringes are designed for ease of use. After all, it is much easier and quicker to use a prefilled syringe when you are treating a patient in cardiac arrest than it is to draw

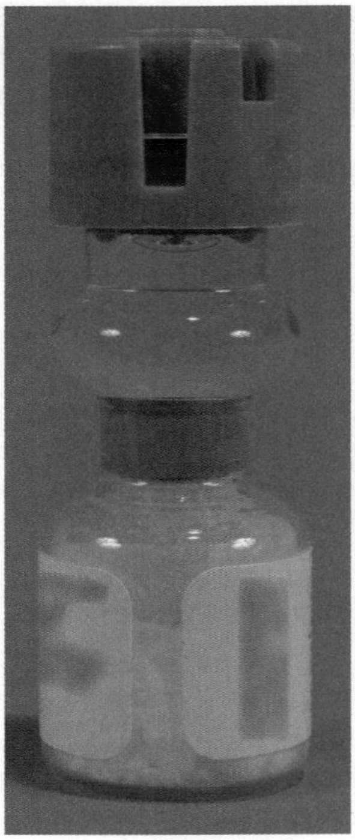

FIGURE 14-49 A Mix-o-Vial.

Skill Drill 14-4 Drawing Medication From a Vial

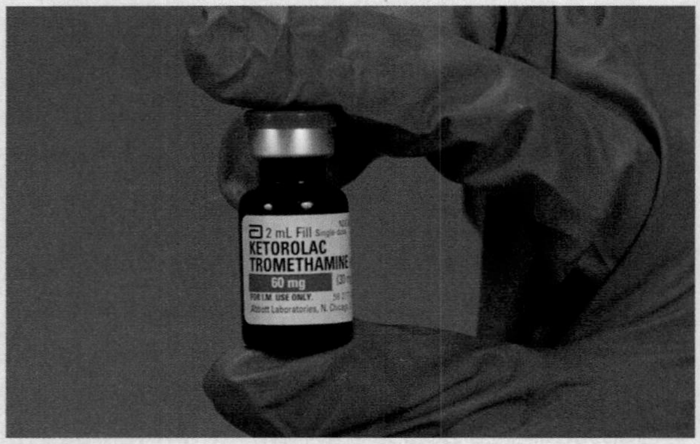

Step 1

Check the medication to ensure that it is the correct drug and concentration, that it is not cloudy or discolored, and that the expiration date has not passed. Remove the sterile cover, or clean the vial's rubber stopper with alcohol if the vial was previously opened.

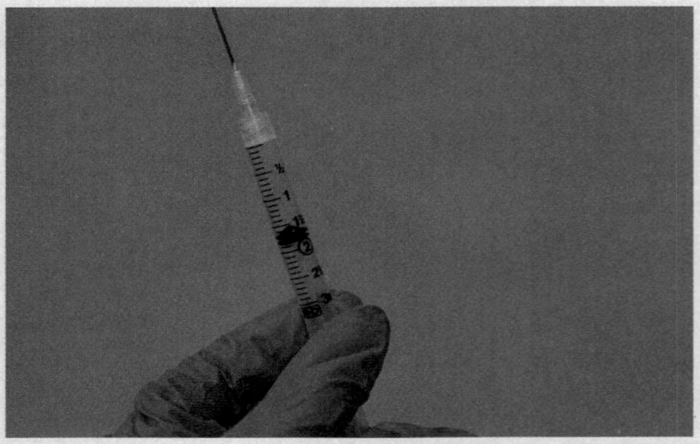

Step 2

Determine the amount of medication that you will need, and draw that amount of air into the syringe. Allow a little extra room to expel some air while removing air bubbles.

Skill Drill 14-4 Drawing Medication From a Vial (continued)

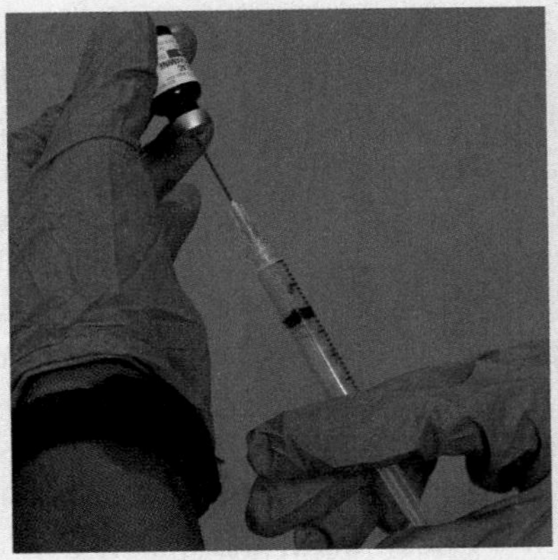

Step 3

Invert the vial, clean the rubber stopper with an alcohol prep, and insert the needle through the rubber stopper into the medication. Unless the vial is a single-use vial, expel the air in the syringe into the vial and then withdraw the amount of medication needed.

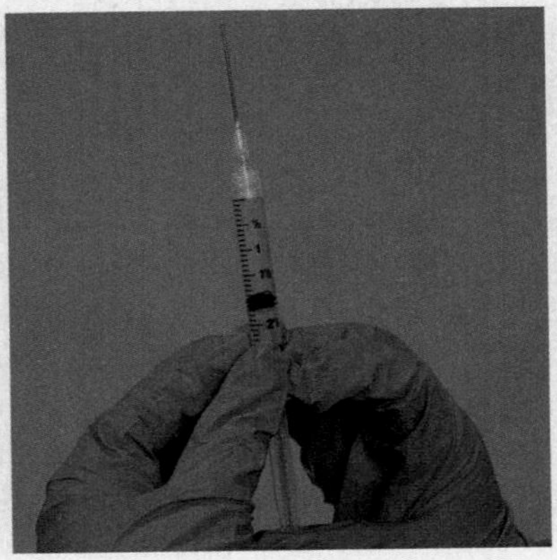

Step 4

Once you have the correct amount of medication in the syringe, withdraw the needle from the vial and expel any air in the syringe.

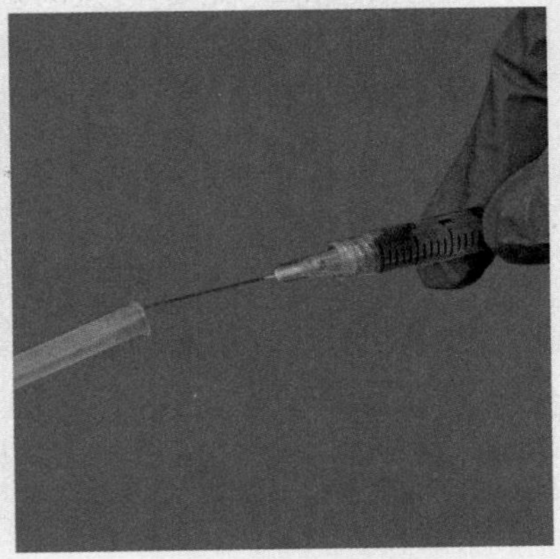

Step 5

Recap the needle using the one-handed method. Label the syringe if the medication is not immediately administered to the patient.

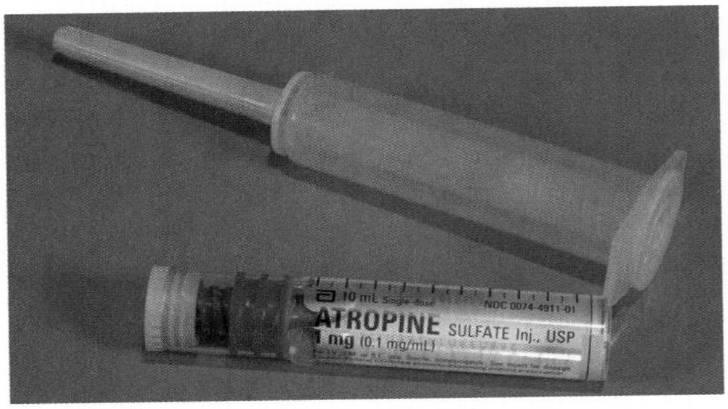

FIGURE 14-50 Two-part prefilled syringes are separated into a glass drug cartridge and a syringe (for example, Bristojet).

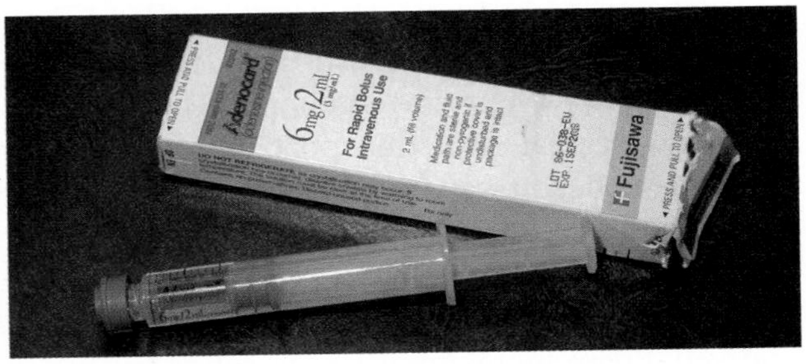

FIGURE 14-51 Preassembled prefilled syringe.

up each individual dose. Be careful when using the drug cartridge and syringe systems: Both pieces of the assembly may contain sharps and should be disposed of properly. In cases where the device is too large to fit into a standard sharps container, it should be handled with care and disposed of either at the receiving facility's larger sharps container or at the station in a larger sharps container.

To assemble the two-part prefilled syringe, pop the yellow caps off of the syringe and the drug cartridge, insert the drug cartridge into the barrel of the syringe, and screw them together. Remove the needle cover, and expel air in the manner previously

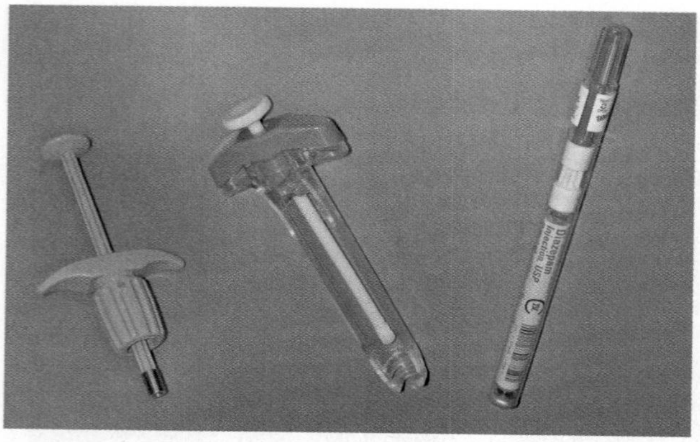

FIGURE 14-52 Reusable syringes (left). Disposable medication cartridge (right).

described. Follow the steps for the route by which the medication is to be given.

Single-dose disposable medication cartridges that are inserted into a reusable syringe are also available. These syringes are commonly referred to by their brand names: Tubex, Aboject, and Carpuject syringes **FIGURE 14-52**.

Push-Dose Pressors

Some vasopressors are available for administration in a small bolus format. These medications are generally reserved for patients with transient hypotension or for EMS systems with short transport times. Epinephrine and phenylephrine (Neosynephrine) are currently available in push-dose format. While push-dose phenylephrine is generally seen in ICUs, EDs, and critical care transport, push-dose epinephrine is becoming a popular substitute for dopamine in many EMS systems.

Generally speaking, to use push-dose epinephrine, you must mix the appropriate concentration yourself. Begin by taking a 10-mL saline flush and wasting 1 mL. Use a blunt-tip needle and draw out 0.1 mg (1 mL) from an epinephrine 1:10,000 (0.1 mg/mL) prefilled syringe. This gives you a concentration of 0.1 mg or 100 mcg in 10 mL. The typical dosing is 10 to 20 mcg every 2 to 5 minutes as needed or until an infusion is initiated.

Intradermal Medication Administration

Intradermal injections involve administering a small amount of medication, typically less than 1 mL, into the dermal layer, just beneath the epidermis. The technique involves using a 1-mL syringe (eg, a tuberculin syringe) and a 25- to 27-gauge, ⅜- to 1-inch (0.9- to 3-cm) needle.

When selecting a site for an intradermal injection, you should avoid areas that contain superficial blood vessels to minimize the risk of systemic medication absorption. Because of their high visibility and relative lack of hair, the anatomic locations most commonly used for intradermal injections are the anterior forearm and upper back.

Medications administered intradermally have a slow rate of absorption; minimal to no systemic distribution occurs. Thus, the medication remains locally collected at the site of the injection. Unless you are anesthetizing the skin before establishing an IV line, you will rarely use the intradermal route to administer medications in the prehospital setting. Instead, these injections are typically given in a physician's office or in the hospital to test a patient for allergies or to perform a PPD (purified protein derivative) skin test for tuberculosis.

Follow these steps to administer a medication via the intradermal route:

1. Take standard precautions. Determine the need for the medication based on the patient's presentation. Obtain a history, including any drug allergies and vital signs. Follow standing orders, or contact medical control for permission.
2. Check the medication to ensure that it is the correct one, that it is not cloudy or discolored, and that the expiration date has not passed, and determine the appropriate amount to give for the correct dose.
3. Advise the patient of potential discomfort while explaining the procedure. Assemble and check the equipment needed: alcohol preps and a 1-mL syringe with a 25- to 27-gauge, ⅜- or 1-inch (0.9- to 3-cm) needle. Draw up the correct dose of medication.
4. Cleanse the area for administration using aseptic technique. Pull the skin taut with your nondominant hand and insert the needle at a 10° to 15° angle with the bevel up **FIGURE 14-53**.
5. Slowly inject the medication while observing for the formation of a wheal, or small bump, which indicates the medication is collecting

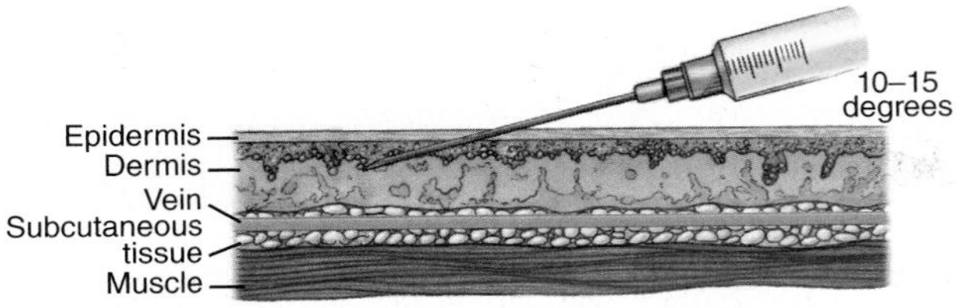

FIGURE 14-53 Intradermal needle insertion.

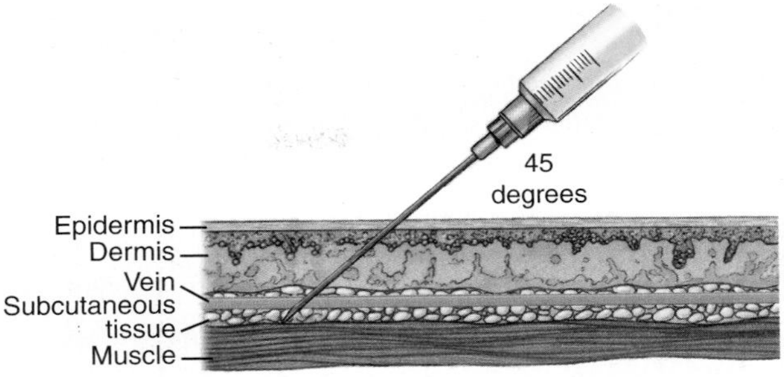

FIGURE 14-54 A subcutaneous injection delivers medication below the dermis and above the muscle.

in the intradermal tissue. If a wheal does not form, the medication is being injected into the subcutaneous tissue.

6. Remove the needle and immediately dispose of it and the syringe in a sharps container.
7. Monitor the patient's condition, and document the medication given, route, administration time, and patient's response.

Subcutaneous Medication Administration

Subcutaneous injections are given into the loose connective tissue between the dermis and the muscle layer using a 24- to 26-gauge 0.5- to 1-inch (1- to 3-cm) needle **FIGURE 14-54**. In adults, the needle is inserted at a 45° angle into the subcutaneous tissue. In contrast, the needle is usually inserted at a 90° angle in a child, although some providers insert the needle at a 45° angle if the child has little subcutaneous tissue. Volumes of a drug administered subcutaneously are usually 2 mL or less in adults and 0.5 to 1 mL in children. Common sites for subcutaneous injections—in both adults and children—include the upper arms, anterior thighs, and the abdomen **FIGURE 14-55**. Patients who take insulin injections usually vary the sites to accommodate the frequent (usually daily) injections they require.

The subcutaneous route should not be used to give medications that are irritating to the tissues or are not water soluble. Absorption may be rapid or slow depending on the water solubility of the drug and blood flow to the injection site. Medications should not be given by this route if the patient shows signs of shock or if the tissue at the selected site is swollen or burned.

Follow the steps in **SKILL DRILL 14-5** to administer a medication via the subcutaneous route.

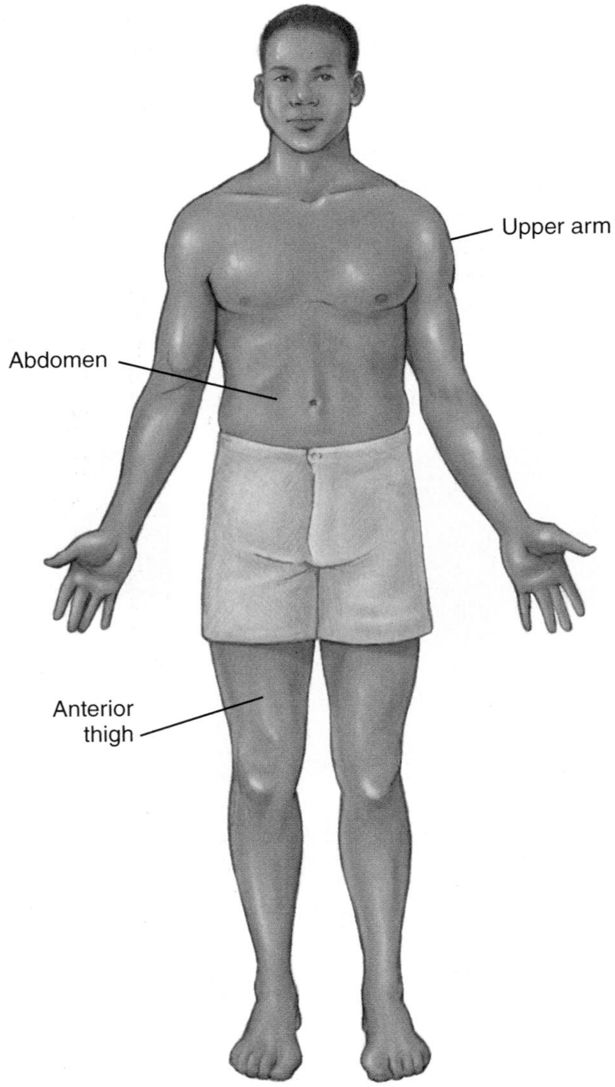

FIGURE 14-55 Common sites for subcutaneous injections.

NR Skill

Skill Drill 14-5 Administering Medication via the Subcutaneous Route

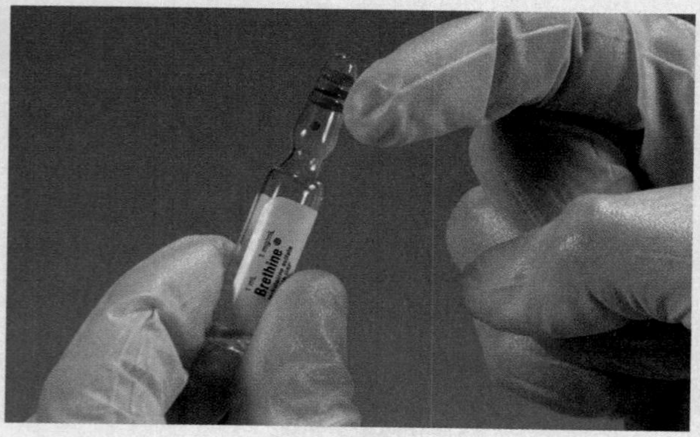

Step 1

Take standard precautions. Determine the need for the medication based on the patient's presentation. Obtain a history, including any drug allergies and vital signs. Follow standing orders, or contact medical control for permission. Check the medication to ensure that it is the correct one, that it is not cloudy or discolored, and that the expiration date has not passed, and determine the appropriate amount and concentration for the correct dose.

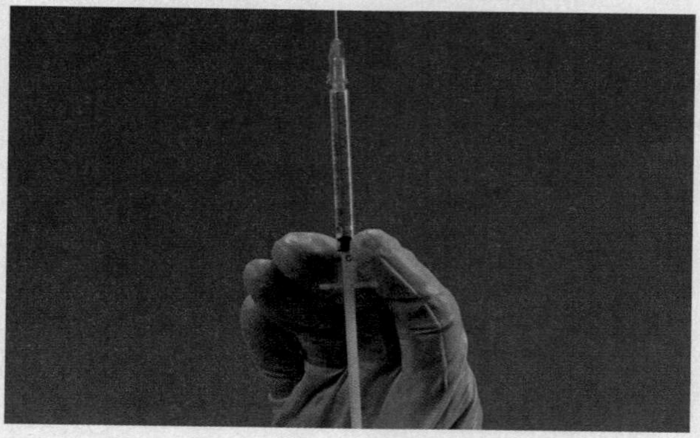

Step 2

Advise the patient of potential discomfort while explaining the procedure.

Assemble and check the equipment needed: alcohol preps and a 3-mL syringe with a 24- to 26-gauge needle. Draw up the correct dose of medication and dispel air while maintaining sterility.

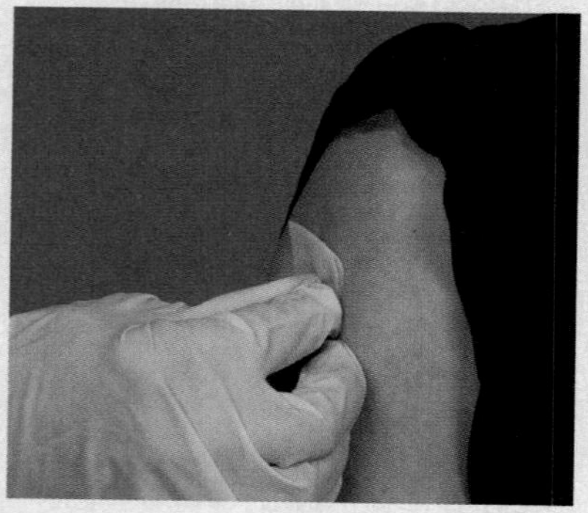

Step 3

Cleanse the area for the administration (usually the upper arm or thigh) using aseptic technique.

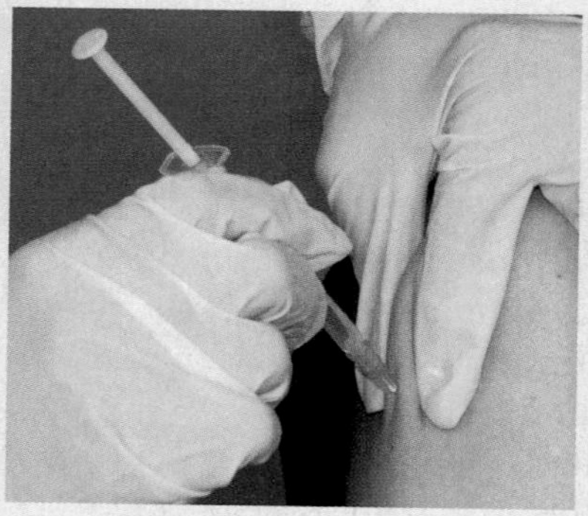

Step 4

Pinch the skin surrounding the area to lift the subcutaneous tissue away from the muscle, advise the patient of a stick, and insert the needle at a 45° angle. Inject the medication, remove the needle, and release the skin. Immediately dispose of the needle and syringe in a sharps container.

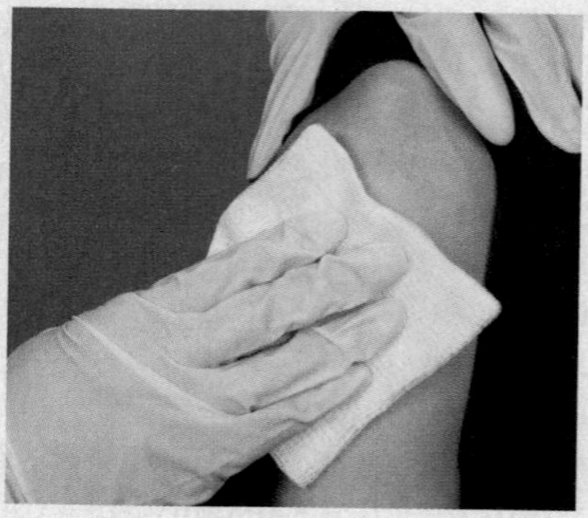

Step 5

To disperse the medication through the tissue, rub the area in a circular motion with your gloved hand (unless contraindicated for the specific medication). Properly store any unused medication. Monitor the patient's condition, and document the medication given, route, administration time, and patient's response.

IM Medication Administration

Intramuscular (IM) injections are given by inserting a needle through the dermis and subcutaneous tissue and into the muscle layer **FIGURE 14-56**. This route is used when a medication cannot be given orally, a more rapid onset of action is desired, or the drug is too irritating to be given subcutaneously. Medications given by the IM route are absorbed more rapidly than those given subcutaneously because more blood flows to muscles than to the subcutaneous tissue layer.

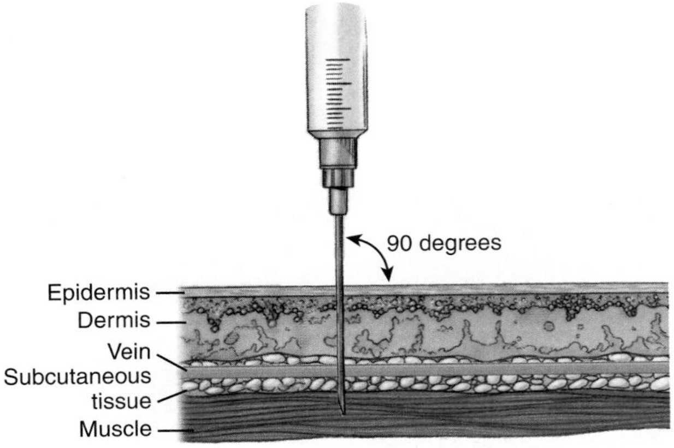

FIGURE 14-56 An intramuscular injection delivers medication below the dermis and subcutaneous layer and into the muscle.

When selecting a needle for an IM injection, the needle must be of sufficient length to reach the middle of the muscle. The gauge of the needle used depends on the thickness of the medication injected. In general, a 19- to 23-gauge needle is used for an IM injection. A 1- to 2-inch (4- to 5-cm) needle is used for most adults: A 1-inch needle may be used for a thin adult, and a 2-inch needle may be necessary for a heavy adult. The needle is inserted at a 90° angle into the muscle.

Multiple sites can be used for an IM injection. When selecting an appropriate site, the thickness and volume of the medication to be given must be considered. The maximal volume of medication that can be given by the IM route varies by the injection site selected. In an adult, as much as 5 mL can be given in some sites. In a child, as much as 2 mL can be given depending on the site chosen. Because IM injections have the potential to damage nerves due to the depth of the injection, it is important to choose the appropriate site. Anatomic sites commonly used for IM injections for adults and children include the following **FIGURE 14-57**:

- **Vastus lateralis muscle**—the large muscle on the lateral side of the thigh.

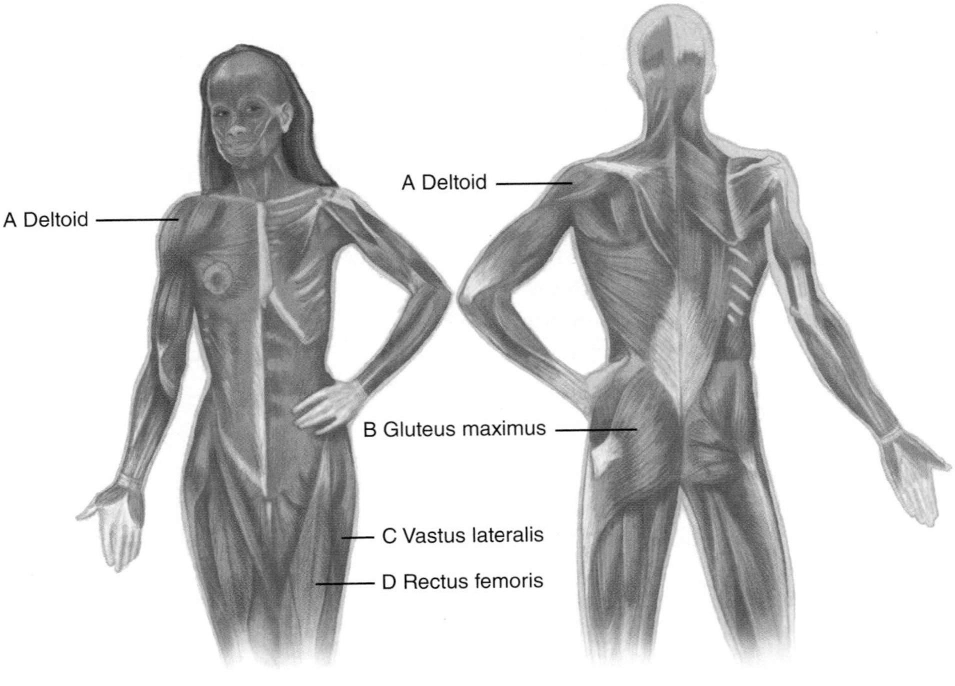

FIGURE 14-57 Common sites for intramuscular injections. **A.** Deltoid muscle. **B.** Gluteal area. **C.** Vastus lateralis muscle. **D.** Rectus femoris muscle.

- **Rectus femoris muscle**—the large muscle on the anterior side of the thigh.
- **Gluteal area**—the buttocks, specifically the upper lateral aspect of either side. When injecting into the gluteal area, you should use the upper, outer quadrant to avoid the sciatic nerve.
- **Deltoid muscle**—the muscle of the upper arm that covers the prominence of the shoulder. The site for injection is approximately 1.5 to 2 inches (4 to 5 cm) below the acromion process on the lateral side.

Follow the steps in **SKILL DRILL 14-6** to administer a medication via the IM route.

Words of Wisdom

Effective absorption of medications administered by the subcutaneous and IM routes requires adequate peripheral perfusion, which is clearly not present in patients who are in profound shock or cardiac arrest. Therefore, subcutaneous and IM injections should not be given to patients with inadequate perfusion unless no other options exist.

Subcutaneous and IM injections also should not be given into skin that is hardened; bruised, red, or otherwise discolored; or stained.

NR Skill

Skill Drill 14-6 Administering Medication via the IM Route

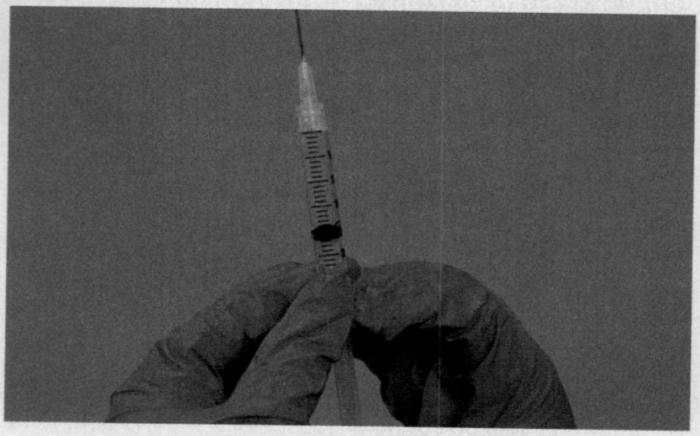

Step 1

Take standard precautions. Determine the need for the medication based on the patient's presentation. Obtain a history, including any drug allergies and vital signs. Follow standing orders, or contact medical control for permission. Check the medication to ensure that it is the correct one, that it is not cloudy or discolored, and that the expiration date has not passed, and determine the appropriate amount and concentration for the correct dose.

Advise the patient of potential discomfort while explaining the procedure. Assemble and check the equipment needed: alcohol preps and a 3- to 5-mL syringe with a 21-gauge, 1- or 2-inch (4- or 5-cm) needle. Draw up the correct dose of medication and dispel air while maintaining sterility.

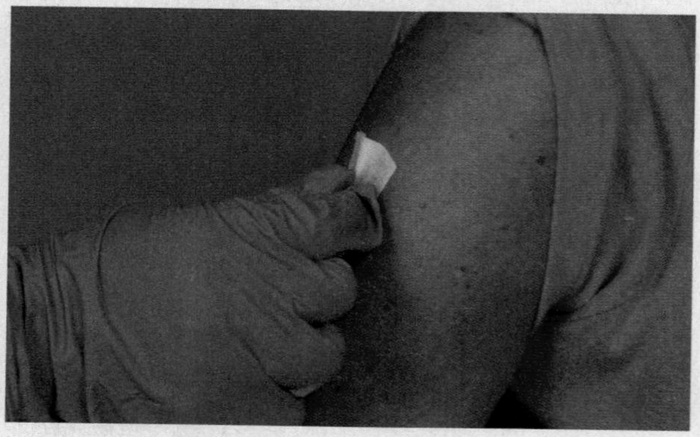

Step 2

Cleanse the area for administration (usually the upper arm or the hip) using aseptic technique.

Skill Drill 14-6 Administering Medication via the IM Route (continued)

NR Skill

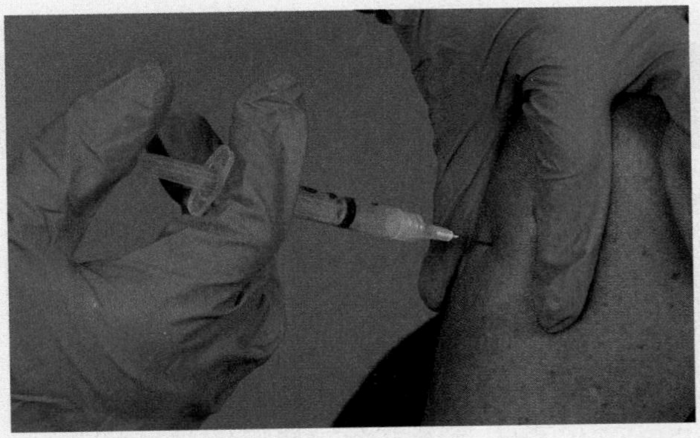

Step 3

Stretch the skin over the cleansed area, advise the patient of a stick, and insert the needle at a 90° angle. Pull back on the plunger to aspirate for blood. The presence of blood in the syringe indicates you may have entered a blood vessel. In such a case, remove the needle, and hold pressure over the site. Discard the syringe and needle in a sharps container. Prepare a new syringe and needle, and select another site. If there is no blood in the syringe, then inject the medication and remove the needle.

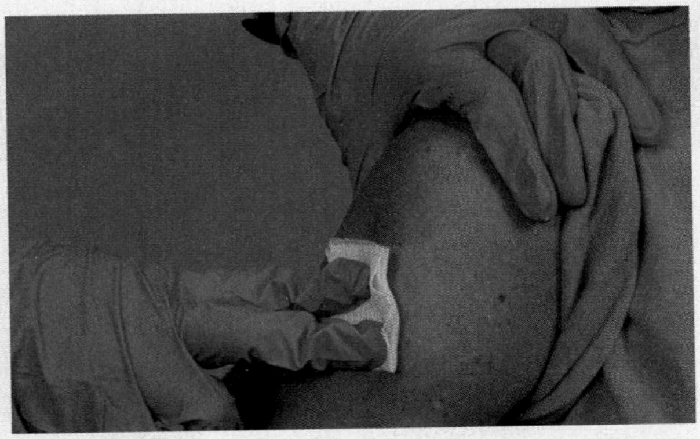

Step 4

Immediately dispose of the needle and syringe in the sharps container. Store any unused medication properly. Monitor the patient's condition, and document the medication given, route, administration time, and patient's response.

IV Bolus Medication Administration

IV bolus drugs are administered by direct injection with a needle and syringe into an established peripheral IV line, thereby delivering the drug directly into the circulatory system. This is the fastest route of medication administration because it bypasses most barriers to drug absorption—but that also means there is no room for error with IV administration.

Needleless systems are used to provide protection against needlesticks during IV administration of medication. When you are using a needleless system, the syringe screws into the injection port of the administration set (IV tubing). If a needleless port is punctured with a needle, the system will leak, requiring you to switch out the administration set for a new one. In a critical situation where time does not allow you to switch out the drip set, you can provide a "temporary patch" on the system by placing a syringe filled with saline on the needleless port.

Recall that a bolus is a single dose, usually given by the IV route. When given in one mass, it may consist of a small or large quantity of a drug and can be given rapidly or slowly, depending on the drug. Some medications, such as lidocaine and amiodarone, require an initial bolus and then may need a continuous IV infusion to maintain a therapeutic level of the drug. Some medications can have devastating effects if administered too rapidly. For example, promethazine can cause an extreme burning sensation if administered too quickly.

Other medications may be ineffective if they are administered too slowly. For example, adenosine has a half-life of 10 seconds and will be ineffective if it does not reach the heart in that time frame.

Follow the steps in **SKILL DRILL 14-7** when you are administering a medication via the IV bolus route.

As discussed earlier in this chapter, saline locks are used for patients who do not require IV fluid

NR Skill

Skill Drill 14-7 Administering Medication via the IV Bolus Route

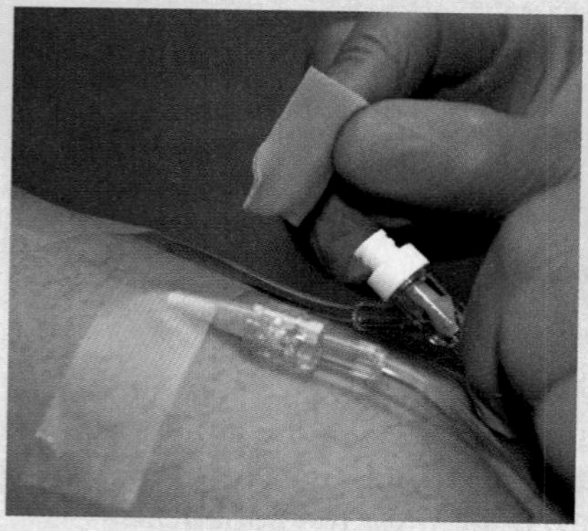

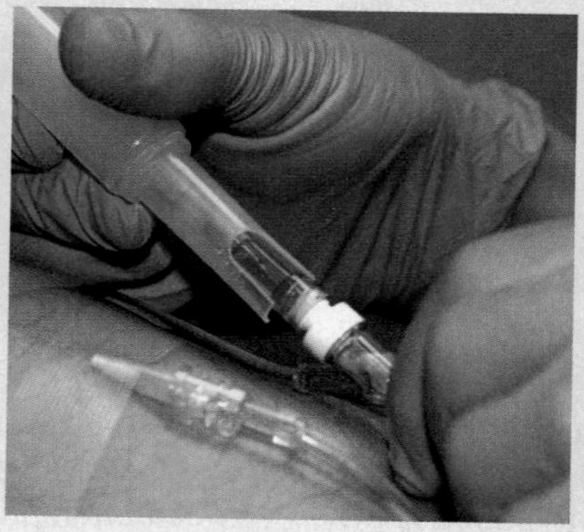

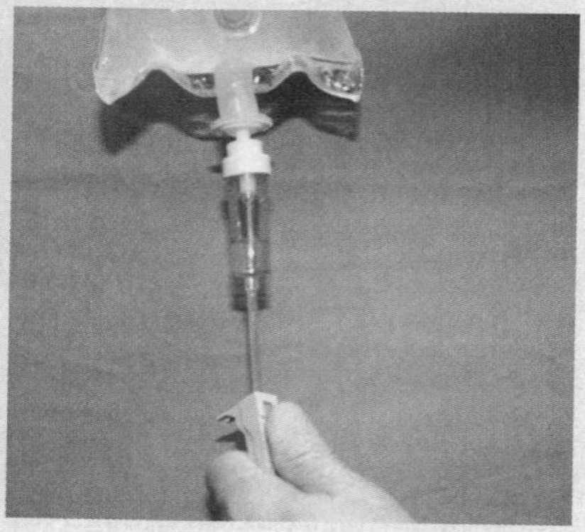

Step 1

Take standard precautions. Determine the need for the medication based on the patient's presentation. Obtain a history, including any drug allergies and vital signs. Follow standing orders, or contact medical control for permission. Check the medication to ensure that it is the correct one, that it is not cloudy or discolored, and that the expiration date has not passed, and determine the appropriate amount and concentration for the correct dose.

Explain the procedure to the patient and the need for the medication. Assemble the needed equipment, and draw up the medication. Expel any air in the syringe. Draw up 20 mL of normal saline to use as a flush for the medication.

Cleanse the injection port with alcohol, or remove the protective cap if using a needleless system.

Step 2

Insert the needle into the port, and pinch off the IV tubing proximal to the administration port. Failure to shut off the line will result in the medication taking the pathway of least resistance—that is, it will flow into the bag instead of into the patient.

Administer the correct dose of the medication at the appropriate rate. Some medications must be administered quickly, whereas others must be pushed slowly to prevent adverse effects.

Step 3

Place the needle and syringe into the sharps container.

Unclamp the IV line to flush the medication into the vein. Allow it to run briefly wide open, or flush with a 20-mL bolus of normal saline. Readjust the IV flow rate to the original setting. Properly store and label any unused medication. Monitor the patient's condition, and document the medication given, route, time of administration, and patient's response.

boluses but may need medication therapy. Follow these steps to administer a medication through a saline lock:

1. Take standard precautions. Determine the need for the medication based on the patient's presentation. Obtain a history, including any drug allergies and vital signs. Follow standing orders, or contact medical control for permission.
2. Check the medication to ensure that it is the correct one, that it is not cloudy or discolored, and that the expiration date has not passed, and determine the appropriate amount and concentration for the correct dose.
3. Explain the procedure to the patient and the need for the medication. Assemble the needed equipment, and draw up the medication. Draw up 20 mL of normal saline to use as a flush for the medication.
4. Cleanse the injection port with alcohol, or remove the protective cap if using the needleless system. Insert the needle into the port while holding it carefully, or screw the syringe onto the port. Clamp off the IV tubing proximally to prevent backflow into the IV solution.
5. Pull back slightly on the syringe plunger, and observe for blood return. If blood appears, then slowly inject the medication, watching for infiltration. If resistance is felt, or if the patient reports any discomfort, then discontinue administration immediately. A new site will need to be established in such a case.
6. Place the needle and syringe into the sharps container. Clean the port, and insert the needle with the syringe containing the flush. Flush the saline lock, and place the needle in the sharps container. Store any unused medication properly.

Words of Wisdom

Medications used for maintenance infusions (eg, dopamine) commonly come in premixed and prepackaged forms, eliminating the need to calculate and draw up the appropriate amount of medication to add to the bag. However, you must still be aware of the concentration (eg, mcg/mL or mg/mL) of the drug in the premixed solution and the appropriate maintenance infusion rate.

YOU are the Paramedic

PART 3

Vascular access has been obtained with an 18-gauge IV needle in the patient's right forearm. The IV line is patent and flushes easily. Your partner connects a 1-L bag of normal saline to the IV line, and the flow rate is set to KVO. Shortly after administering the dose of diltiazem as ordered, the rhythm on the cardiac monitor changes to a sinus rhythm. You contact medical control to provide an update of the patient's condition. The physician asks you to begin a maintenance infusion of diltiazem at 5 mg/h. You have a premixed bag of diltiazem with 30 mg/100 mL and a microdrip administration set.

Recording Time:	10 Minutes
Respirations	18 breaths/min
Pulse	90 beats/min
Skin	Warm and dry
Blood pressure	126/78 mm Hg
Oxygen saturation (Spo_2)	100%
Pupils	PERRLA
ECG	Sinus rhythm

6. Why would it be preferable to use an IV pump for a maintenance infusion of a medication?

7. What is the appropriate flow rate to administer the maintenance infusion of diltiazem?

7. Monitor the patient's condition, and document the medication given, route, time of administration, and patient's response.

Adding Medication to an IV Bag

Certain medications are added to the IV solution itself to be administered as a maintenance infusion—for example, dopamine, lidocaine, and epinephrine. All of these medications require careful titration to achieve the desired effect.

The steps for adding medication to an IV bag are as follows:

1. Check the fluid in the IV bag for clarity or discoloration, and ensure the expiration date has not passed.
2. Check the medication name on the ampule, vial, or prefilled syringe, and then check the concentration of the drug it contains (eg, mcg/mL or mg/mL).
3. Compute the volume of the drug to be added to the IV bag, and draw up that amount in a syringe (if a prefilled syringe is used, note the proportion of the volume of the syringe required).
4. Cleanse the medication injection port on the IV bag with an alcohol swab.
5. Inject the desired volume of medication into the IV bag by puncturing the rubber stopper on the medication injection port **FIGURE 14-58**.
6. Withdraw the needle, and dispose of the needle and syringe in the sharps container. Agitate the IV bag gently to ensure the medication added is well mixed in the solution.

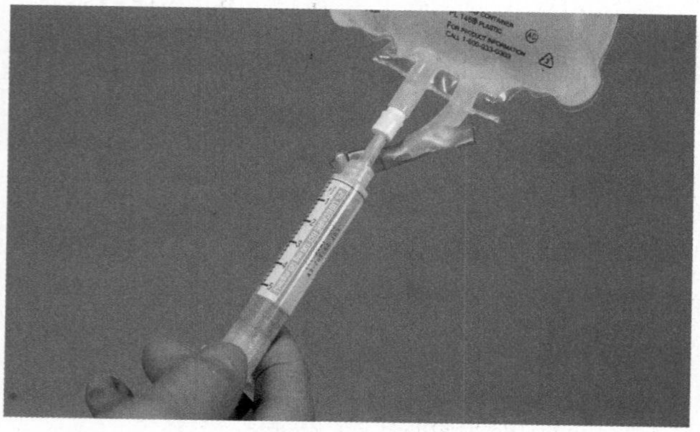

FIGURE 14-58 Adding medication to an intravenous bag.

7. Label the IV bag; on a piece of tape, write the name of the medication added, the amount added, the concentration of medication in the IV bag (eg, mcg/mL or mg/mL), the date and time, and your name.
8. Attach the IV administration set, and prepare the IV bag as discussed earlier in this chapter.

Words of Wisdom

Infusion pumps are the standard of care for any medication infusion. As a clinician and patient advocate, you must advocate for their use within the prehospital realm.

IV Piggyback

The IV administration set that is connected directly to the hub of the IV catheter is referred to as the primary line. This line is generally used to administer an isotonic solution. Saline is the preferred isotonic solution because it mixes with all medications used in the prehospital and interfacility transfer settings. When you are performing a continuous infusion, take the distal end of the drip set that is attached to the mixed medication and connect it to a port on the primary line. The line that is connected to the continuous infusion is referred to as a "piggyback" or secondary line. Multiple lines can be piggybacked onto a primary IV line. When multiple lines are present on a patient, it is important to label each line. This will ensure that when medications are administered en route, no medication interactions occur.

Follow the steps in **SKILL DRILL 14-8** to perform IV piggyback infusion.

IV Infusion Pumps

When you are administering a medication maintenance infusion for which the rate of the medication's administration over time is critical, the standard of care within the medical community is to use an IV **infusion pump**, a mechanical device that infuses a precise volume that is programmed by the clinician **FIGURE 14-59**. The use of microdrip sets to time infusions is not used in any other area of medicine due to the propensity for medication errors and the variability in drip rate depending on bag height, movement, and other factors. An infusion pump

Skill Drill 14-8 Administering a Medication via IV Piggyback Infusion

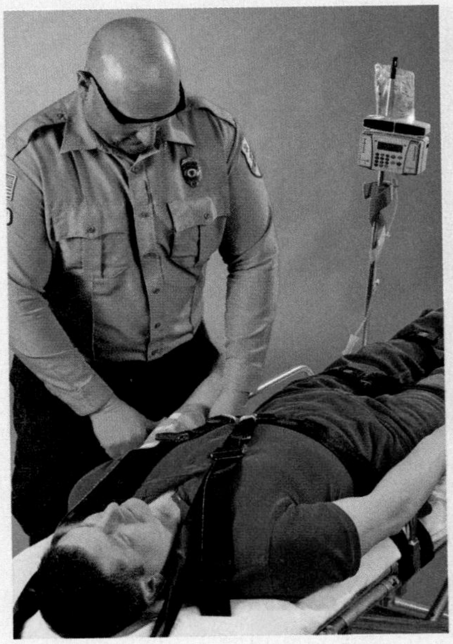

Step 1

Take standard precautions. Ensure the established IV line is patent.

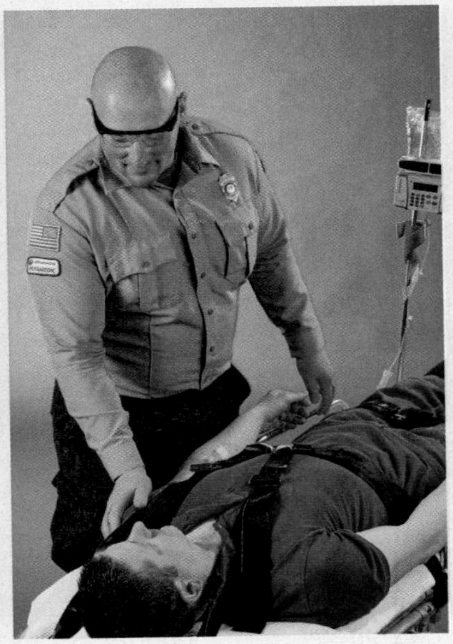

Step 2

Determine the need for the medication based on the patient's presentation. Obtain a history, including any drug allergies and vital signs. Follow standing orders, or contact medical control for permission. Identify the concentration, then determine the appropriate dose and rate of the infusion. Check the medication to ensure that it is the correct one, that it is not cloudy or discolored, and that the expiration date has not passed, and determine the appropriate amount and concentration for the correct dose. Explain the procedure to the patient and/or parent and the need for the medication.

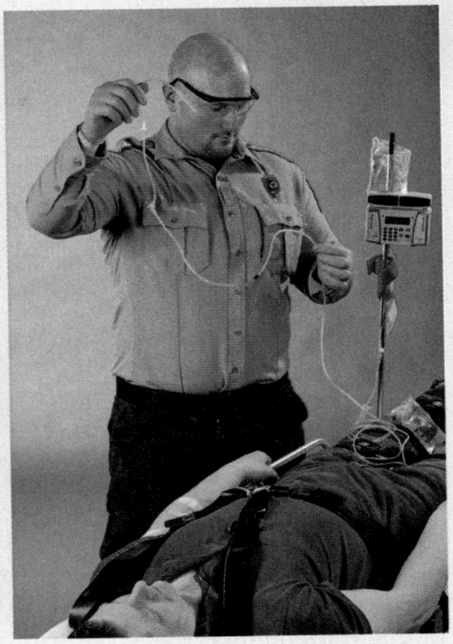

Step 3

Assemble the needed equipment. Ensure you have the proper IV solution, and that it is clear, sterile, and not expired. Ensure you have the correct administration set and correct drip rating. Check for tangling and confirm that the protective covers are on the ends. The flow clamp should be closed.

(continues)

NR Skill

Skill Drill 14-8 Administering a Medication via IV Piggyback Infusion (continued)

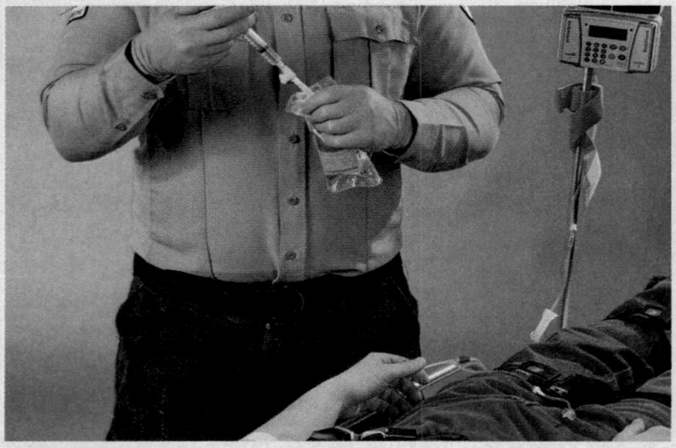

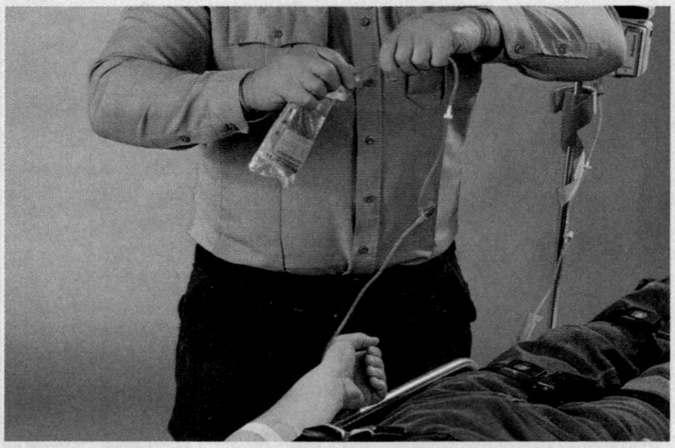

Step 4

Cleanse the injection port of the secondary IV bag (into which the medication will be infused) with alcohol. Inject the medication into the second IV bag and then place the syringe into the sharps container. Gently swirl the IV bag to mix the injected medication into the solution.

Note: Drawing up medications may not be necessary if the manufacturer attaches the medication to the second IV bag (as is the case with IV antibiotics, some antidysrhythmics, and certain other medications).

Step 5

Remove the protective cover on the secondary IV bag. Insert the tubing spike into the second IV bag tail port. Turn the bag containing the medication upright. Squeeze the drip chamber until it is half full. Maintain sterility.

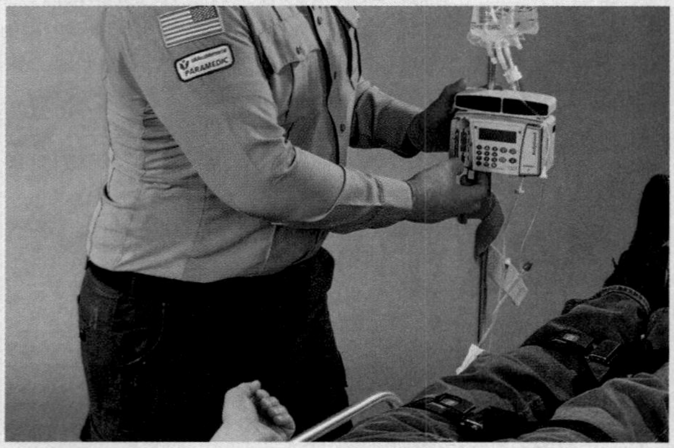

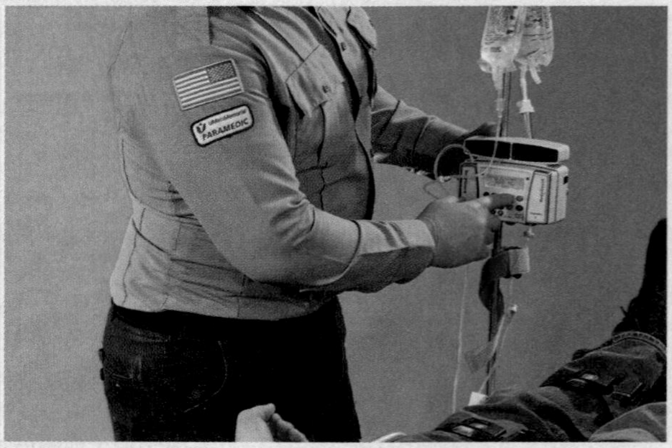

Step 6

Unclamp the line from the secondary IV bag to dispel air from it, or utilize the infusion pump to accomplish this step. Maintain sterility. While removing the air, try to minimize the loss of fluid. Clamp the line after all air bubbles have been removed.

Step 7

If applicable, program the IV infusion pump with the appropriate dose and rate. Place the cartridge from the secondary IV bag in the pump.

NR Skill

Skill Drill 14-8 Administering a Medication via IV Piggyback Infusion (continued)

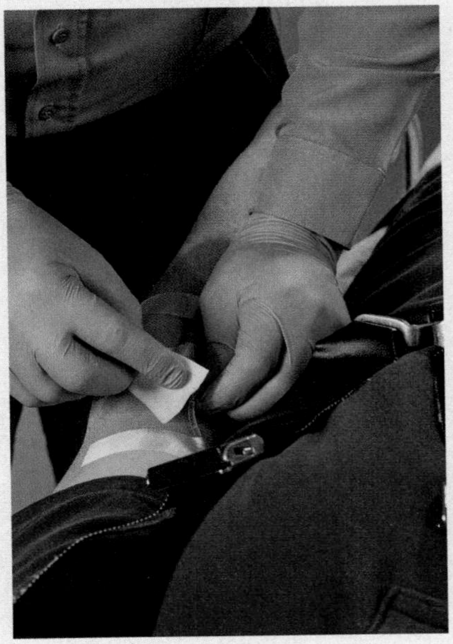

Step 8

Cleanse a port on the primary IV line. Attach the distal end of the secondary IV line to a port on the primary IV line. Begin the flow and ensure that the rate is appropriate. Maintain sterility.

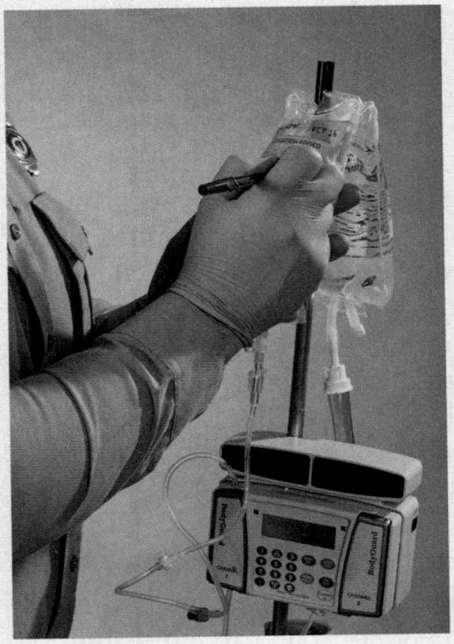

Step 9

Label the secondary IV bag. Monitor the patient's condition, and document the medication given, route, concentration, dose, date time, and your initials. Document the patient's response to the medication.

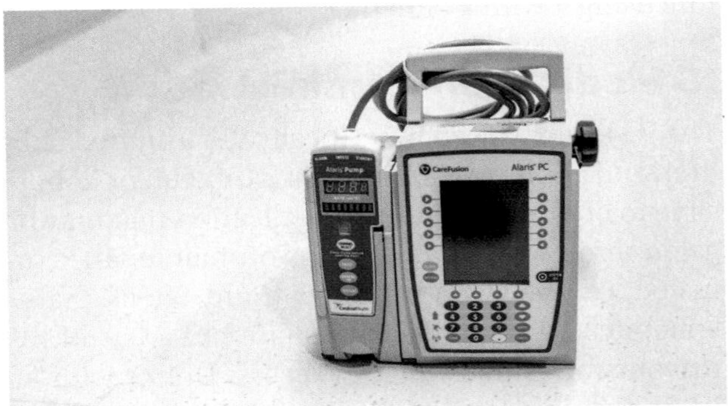

FIGURE 14-59 Intravenous infusion pump.

can also be used to deliver IV fluid maintenance infusions in children and older patients to minimize the risk of a "runaway IV" and subsequent circulatory overload.

IV infusion pumps are widely used both in the hospital and during interfacility transports. In addition, they are sometimes used in the prehospital setting. IV infusion pumps have both advantages and disadvantages. Notably, they reliably deliver medication at the rate set within the pump, and they calculate the amount of fluid that has been infused and the amount of fluid remaining. Because of the lack of uniformity among pumps made by various manufacturers, you need to become familiar with the pumps used by your service.

Pumps can pose problems during patient transport because air can become trapped in the lines, which is detected by the pumps. When air is detected, the pump stops the infusion and an alarm sounds. This can become problematic during transport when the ambulance travels over potholes, makes hard turns, and is exposed to other applied forces.

IV infusion pumps deliver fluids or medications via positive pressure. Although delivery of medications in this manner can result in infiltration of a vein, most infusion pumps are equipped with an alarm that indicates a change in the flow pressure. Other common safety features include alarms that alert you to the presence of occlusion (eg, air in the tubing) or depletion of the medication supply. The tubing for IV infusion pumps is specific to the manufacturer and model and is usually incompatible with other infusion pumps.

You should become familiar with some of the terminology related to infusion pumps. Pumps may have multiple chambers that can hold multiple medications. Each chamber can calculate the rate of administration for one medication. If the medication lines outnumber the available chambers, then it may be necessary to administer an isotonic fluid based on gravity only. In this situation, the gtt/min flow rate for the isotonic line must be set manually instead of being set by the pump. The rate is always established in milliliters per hour. Some IV pumps may be linked to medication databases that will calculate the medication rate based on the desired dose and the patient's weight as necessary.

The volume to be infused is the amount of solution remaining to be infused. For example, if you were infusing 100 mL of amiodarone and 25 mL has already been administered, then 75 mL is your volume to be infused. The volume infused is the amount of solution that has already been administered, 25 mL in the preceding example. If your infusion pump does not perform medication calculations, then the following steps can help you determine the rate at which to set the pump.

Example

Nitroglycerin drips are commonly administered interfacility medications for patients with acute coronary syndrome and are being established in the prehospital setting in some areas. The doses range from 5 to 50 mcg/min. This calculation will start at 5 mcg/min. You have 25 mg in 250 mL.

Step 1: Determine the concentration.

$$25 \text{ mg} \times \frac{1{,}000 \text{ mcg}}{\text{mg}} = 250{,}000 \text{ mcg}$$

$$25{,}000 \text{ mcg} \div 250 \text{ mL} = 100 \text{ mcg/mL}$$
(concentration)

Step 2: Determine the amount of volume to infuse per minute (mL/min).

For this calculation, you must recall the desired dose: in this case, 5 mcg/min. To determine the number of mL/min, you perform the following calculation:

5 mcg/min (desired dose) ÷ 100 mcg/mL (concentration) = 0.05 mL/min

Step 3: Determine the rate and volume to be infused.

The rate can be established by multiplying the mL/min by 60.

$$\frac{0.5 \text{ mL}}{\text{min}} \times \frac{60 \text{ min}}{\text{h}} = 3 \text{ mL/h}$$

The volume to be infused for nitroglycerin as packaged in this example is 250 mL, unless otherwise requested by medical control. Therefore, infuse this volume at 3 mL/h until it is administered, or until you arrive at the receiving facility.

IV infusion pumps come in a variety of configurations. You should be familiar with the basic concepts discussed in this section but seek individual training on the specific infusion pump(s) you will use in practice. In addition, become familiar with the tubing, cartridges, and basic way to navigate the pump and ensure your comfort with the device before using it with a patient.

IO Medication Administration

The IO route is used for critically ill or injured children and adults when IV access is difficult or impossible to obtain. Any fluid or medication that may be given through an IV line, bolus or maintenance infusion, can be given by the IO route. Shock, status epilepticus, and cardiac arrest are but a few of the reasons for establishing IO access. Unlike with an IV line, fluid does not flow well into the bone because of resistance; therefore, it is necessary to use a large syringe to infuse the fluid via the IO route.

A pressure infuser device, a sleeve placed around the IV bag and inflated to force fluid from the IV bag, should be used when infusing IO fluids in adults.

Complications of using the IO route are similar to those associated with the IV route. Along with the complications discussed earlier in this chapter, compartment syndrome may potentially occur if fluid leaks outside the bone and into the osteofascial compartment.

Follow the steps in **SKILL DRILL 14-9** to administer a medication via the IO route.

Percutaneous Medication Administration

With **percutaneous** routes of administration, medications are applied to and absorbed through the skin and mucous membranes. Because percutaneously administered medications bypass the gastrointestinal (GI) tract, their absorption is more predictable. Percutaneous routes of medication administration include the transdermal, sublingual, buccal, ocular, aural, and nasal routes.

Transdermal Medication Administration

Transdermal medications are applied topically; that is, on the surface of the body. Ordinarily, intact skin is an effective barrier to medication absorption. However, some medications have been specifically prepared to cross that barrier at a slow steady rate, so the transdermal route is useful for the sustained release of certain medications.

Skill Drill 14-9 Administering Medication via the IO Route

NR Skill

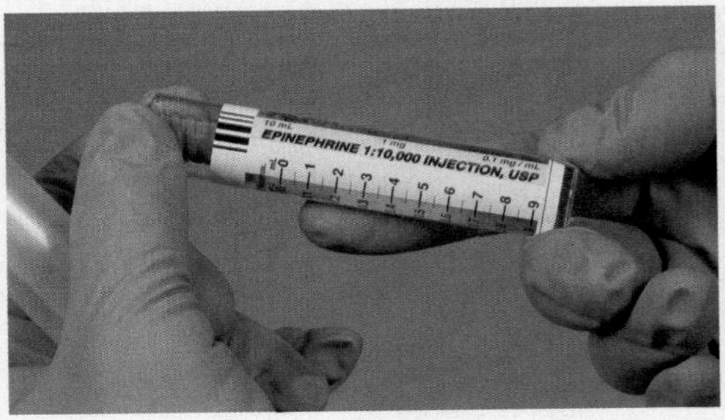

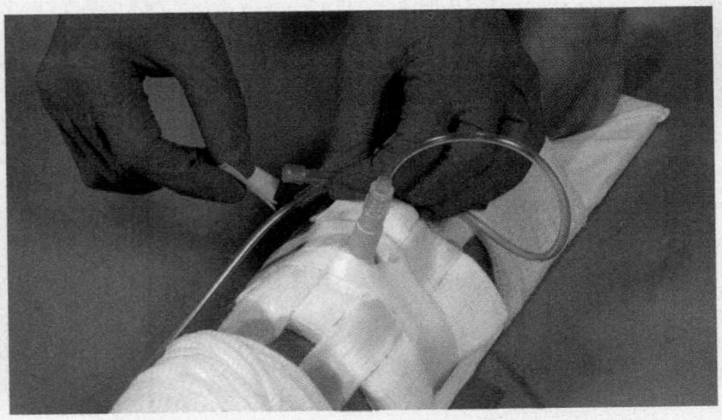

Step 1

Take standard precautions. Determine the need for the medication based on the patient's presentation. Obtain a history, including any drug allergies and vital signs. Follow standing orders, or contact medical control for permission. Check the medication to ensure that it is the correct one, that it is not cloudy or discolored, and that the expiration date has not passed, and determine the appropriate amount and concentration for the correct dose. Explain the procedure to the patient and/or parent and the need for the medication.

Assemble the needed equipment and draw up the medication. Also draw up 20 mL of normal saline for a flush.

Step 2

Cleanse the injection port of the extension tubing with alcohol, or remove the protective cap if using a needleless system.

(continues)

NR Skill

Skill Drill 14-9 Administering Medication via the IO Route (continued)

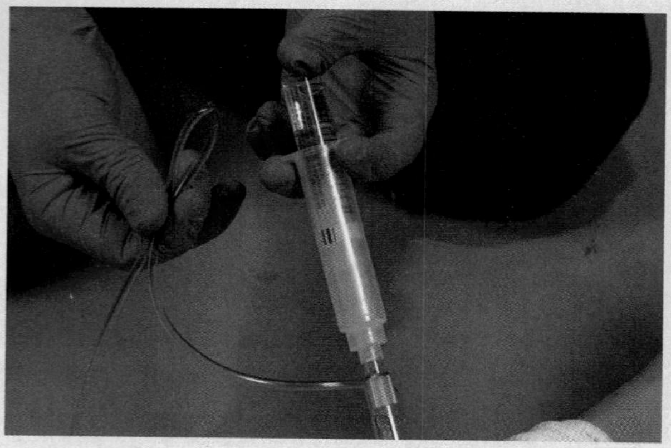

Step 3

Insert the needle into the port, and clamp off the IV tubing proximal to the administration port. This is usually managed with a three-way stopcock. Failure to shut off the line will result in the medication taking the pathway of least resistance: that is, it will flow into the bag instead of into the patient.

Administer the correct dose of the medication at the proper push rate. Some medications must be administered quickly, whereas others must be pushed slowly to prevent adverse effects.

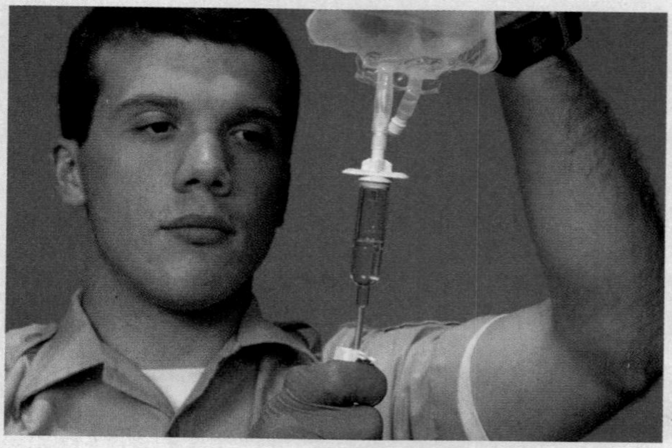

Step 4

Place the needle and syringe into the sharps container. Unclamp the IV line to flush the medication into the site. Flush with at least a 20-mL bolus of normal saline. Readjust the IV flow rate to the original setting. Store any unused medication properly.

Monitor the patient's condition, and document the medication given, route, time of administration, and response of the patient.

Nitroglycerin, estrogen, nicotine, and analgesic patches, for example, are applied to the skin and release medications over a specified period. Creams, lotions, and pastes (eg, nitroglycerin paste, corticosteroid cream) are also transdermally administered medications.

Factors that can increase the speed of transdermal absorption include administration of too much of the medication (ie, inadvertent or intentional overdose) and thin or nonintact skin. Conversely, decreased speed of transdermal absorption can be caused by factors such as thick skin, scar tissue in the area to which the medication is applied, and peripheral vascular disease.

Some transdermal medications, such as nitroglycerin paste, may be applied in the prehospital setting. Usually though, providers will be assisting patients with their own transdermal patches. If your service uses nitroglycerin or another transdermal medication, then you will perform the following steps:

1. Take standard precautions. Determine the need for the medication based on the patient's presentation. Obtain a history, including any drug allergies and vital signs. Follow standing orders, or contact medical control for permission. Check the medication patch or cream to ensure that it is the correct one and that the expiration date has not passed, and determine the appropriate amount for the correct dose.

2. Explain the procedure to the patient and the need for the medication. Clean and dry the area of the skin where the medication will be applied.
3. Apply the medication to the area per the manufacturer's specifications.
4. Monitor the patient's condition, and document the medication given, route, time of administration, and patient's response.

Words of Wisdom

During assessment of a patient, look for transdermal medication patches, especially opioid and nitroglycerin patches. If the patient is already in a hemodynamically unstable condition, then opioids and nitroglycerin may complicate the clinical picture.

Do not, under any circumstances, administer or in any other manner come in contact with transdermal medications without taking the proper standard precautions. Because these medications are designed to be absorbed through the skin, they can easily be absorbed through ungloved hands.

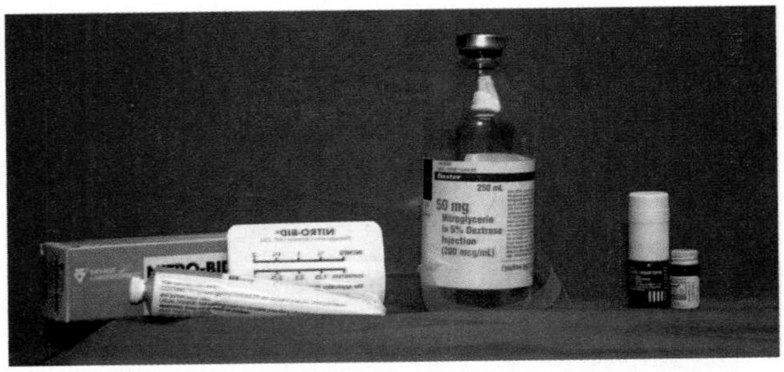

FIGURE 14-60 Nitroglycerin is often given sublingually as a spray or a tablet. It is also available as a transdermal patch or paste and can be administered as an intravenous drip.

Words of Wisdom

If using a spray medication dispenser, then spray it once or twice away from the patient and the crew prior to administration. Doing so will ensure the dispenser is primed and that the patient will receive the full dose of the medication. Also, as with transdermal medications, use proper standard precautions because nitroglycerin can be absorbed through your hands.

Sublingual Medication Administration

The **sublingual** (under the tongue) region is highly vascular, so medications given via the sublingual route are rapidly absorbed. Sublingually administered medications, relative to enterally administered medications, get into the circulation much faster. Nitroglycerin (spray or tablet) is a medication that is most commonly administered via the sublingual route **FIGURE 14-60**.

Medications may also be *injected* into the network of veins (venous plexus) under the tongue (basically this is another form of IV injection). This technique is especially useful for giving opioid antagonists to patients who have overdosed on heroin because finding a suitable vein in such patients may be nearly impossible.

To administer a sublingual medication, follow the steps in **SKILL DRILL 14-10**.

Buccal Medication Administration

The **buccal** region, which is also highly vascular, lies in between the cheek and gums. Most medications administered via the buccal route are in the form of tablets or gels. Glucose is one of the few medications that may be administered buccally in the prehospital setting.

To administer a medication via the buccal route, follow these steps:

1. Take standard precautions. Determine the need for the medication based on the patient's presentation. Obtain a history, including any drug allergies and vital signs. Follow standing orders, or contact medical control for permission.
2. Check the medication to ensure that it is the correct one and that its expiration date has not passed, and determine the appropriate amount for the correct dose. Explain the procedure to the patient and the need for the medication.
3. Place the medication in between the patient's cheek and gum, or ask the patient to do so. Advise the patient not to chew or swallow the tablet, but to let it dissolve slowly.
4. Monitor the patient's condition, and document the medication given, route, administration time, and patient's response.

Skill Drill 14-10 Administering Medication via the Sublingual Route

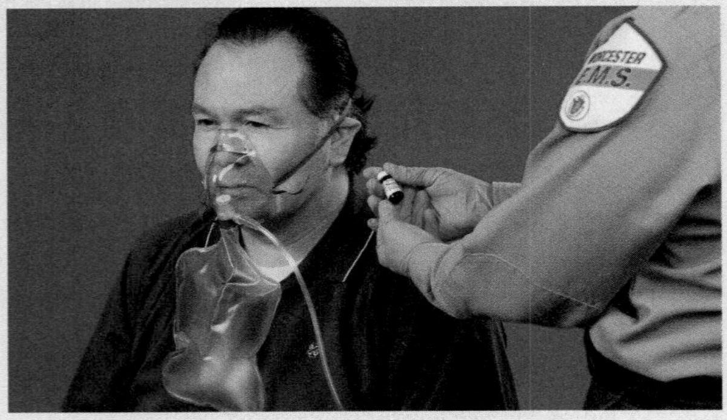

Step 1

Take standard precautions. Determine the need for the medication based on the patient's presentation. Obtain a history, including any drug allergies and vital signs. Follow standing orders, or contact medical control for permission. Check the medication to ensure that it is the correct one, its expiration date has not passed, and determine the appropriate amount for the correct dose.

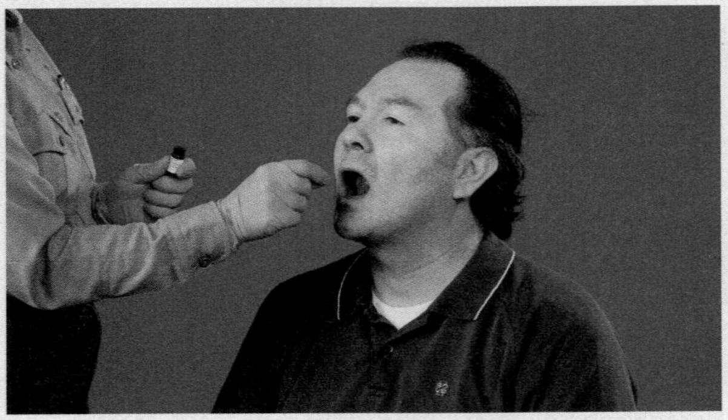

Step 2

Ask the patient to rinse the mouth with a little water if the mucous membranes are dry. Explain the procedure, and ask the patient to lift the tongue. Place the tablet or spray the dose under the tongue, or ask the patient to do so. Advise the patient not to chew or swallow the tablet, but to let it dissolve slowly. Monitor the patient's condition, and document the medication given, route, administration time, and patient's response.

Ocular Medication Administration

Drops or ointments are commonly administered via the **ocular** route **FIGURE 14-61**. Ocular medications are typically administered for pain relief, allergies, drying of the eyes, or infections. Other than assisting a patient with an ocular medication or irrigating a patient's eyes following a toxic exposure, medication administration via the ocular route is rare in the prehospital setting.

In some prehospital systems, providers use bottles to squeeze out the prescribed amount of drops into the eye. A commercial device known as the Morgan lens can also be used to administer some ophthalmic medications, particularly local anesthetics. This device uses a proprietary lens that connects to an IV drop set and IV fluids. While it is used predominantly for irrigation, some medications may be used in or with the Morgan lens. The Morgan lens is discussed in Chapter 20, *Diseases of the Eyes, Ears, Nose, and Throat.*

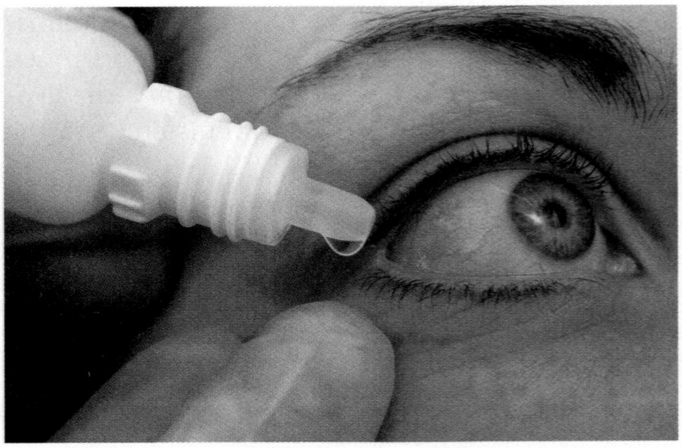

FIGURE 14-61 The ocular route.

If a patient asks you to assist with ocular medication administration, follow these steps:

1. Take standard precautions. If administering a prescribed medication, confirm the medication is prescribed to the patient.

2. Place the patient in a supine position, or have the patient place the head back and look up.
3. *Without touching the eyeball,* expose the conjunctiva by gently pulling down on the lower eyelid.
4. Administer the required amount of medication on the conjunctival sac by using an eye dropper. Do not apply the medication directly on the eyeball. Advise the patient to close the eyes for 1 to 2 minutes.
5. Document the medication name, route, dose, and administration time. Monitor the patient's condition and response.

Aural Medication Administration

Certain medications—mainly antibiotics, analgesics, and earwax removal preparations—are administered via the mucous membranes of the **aural** (ear) canal. As is the case for the ocular route, the aural route is rarely, if ever, used in the prehospital setting.

If the patient asks you to assist in administering an aural medication, follow these steps:

1. Take standard precautions and confirm the medication is prescribed to the patient.
2. Place the patient on the side with the affected ear facing up. Expose the ear canal by pulling the ear up and back (adults) or down and back (infants and children).
3. Administer the medication in the appropriate dose with a medicine dropper.
4. Document the medication name, route, dose, and administration time. Monitor the patient's condition and response.

Intranasal Medication Administration

Intranasal (within the nose) medications include nasal sprays to relieve congestion or solutions to moisten the nasal mucosa. In recent years, this route of medication administration has become more popular in the prehospital setting. Intranasally administered medications are rapidly absorbed, providing a more rapid onset of action than IM injections. For example, some studies suggest that intranasal fentanyl has an equal onset and duration to IV morphine.

Administration of emergency medications via the intranasal route is performed with a **mucosal atomizer device (MAD)** **FIGURE 14-62**. The MAD attaches to a syringe and allows you to spray (atomize) select medications into the nasal mucosa.

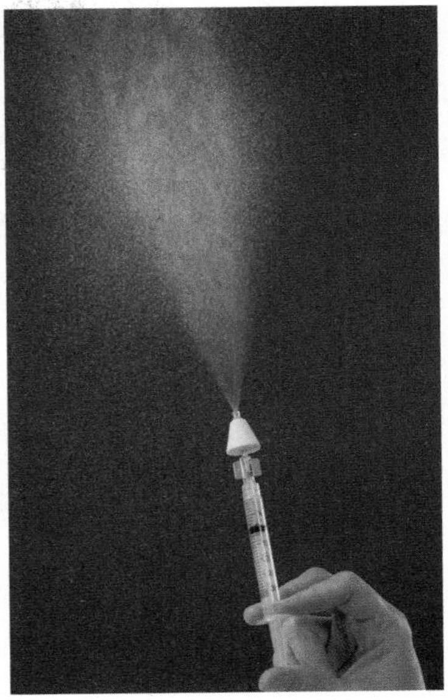

FIGURE 14-62 Mucosal atomizer device.

Courtesy of Telelex Inc.

Owing to the molecular structure of drugs, only a few emergency medications can be given intranasally, including naloxone (Narcan), midazolam (Versed), glucagon (GlucaGen), ketorolac (Toradol), flumazenil (Romazicon), and fentanyl citrate. Typically, intranasal medications require 2 to 2.5 times the dose of IV medications. Follow the local protocol, or consult with medical control about the appropriate doses of these medications and any other medications that may be administered intranasally.

To administer a medication via the intranasal route, follow the steps in **SKILL DRILL 14-11**.

Medications Administered by the Inhalation Route

Nebulizer and Metered-Dose Inhaler

Many medications used in the treatment of respiratory emergencies are administered via the **inhalation** route. The most common inhaled medication is oxygen. In addition, beta-2 agonist bronchodilators (eg, albuterol [Ventolin, Proventil]) are often administered in the prehospital setting for patients experiencing respiratory distress caused by certain obstructive airway diseases. Other medications,

Skill Drill 14-11 Administering Medication via the Intranasal Route

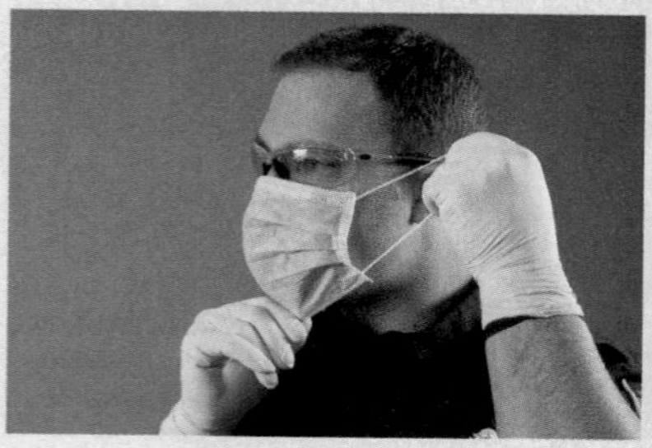

Step 1

Take standard precautions. Determine the need for the medication based on the patient's presentation. Obtain a history, including any drug allergies and vital signs. Assemble and collect the needed equipment, including the MAD. Follow standing orders, or contact medical control for permission. Check the medication to ensure that it is the correct one, that it is not cloudy or discolored, and that the expiration date has not passed.

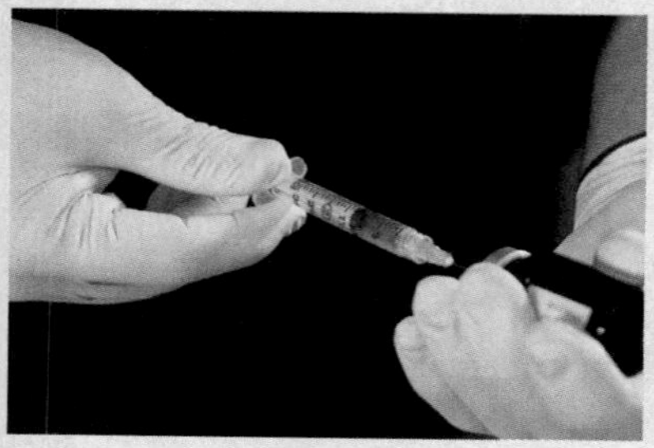

Step 2

Draw up the appropriate dose of medication in the syringe, dispel air, and reconfirm the correct medication. Dispose of the needle properly.

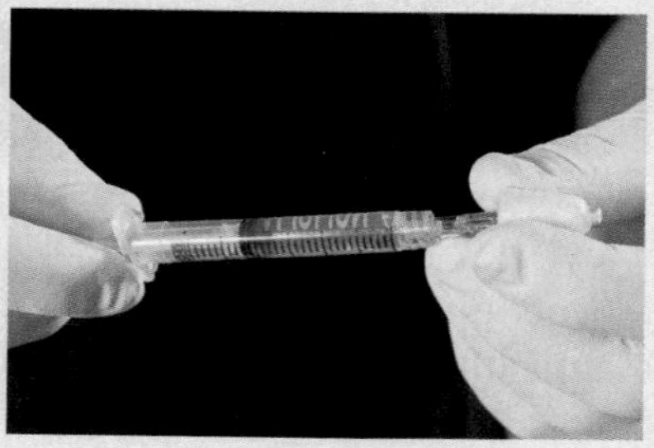

Step 3

Attach the MAD to the syringe, maintaining sterility.

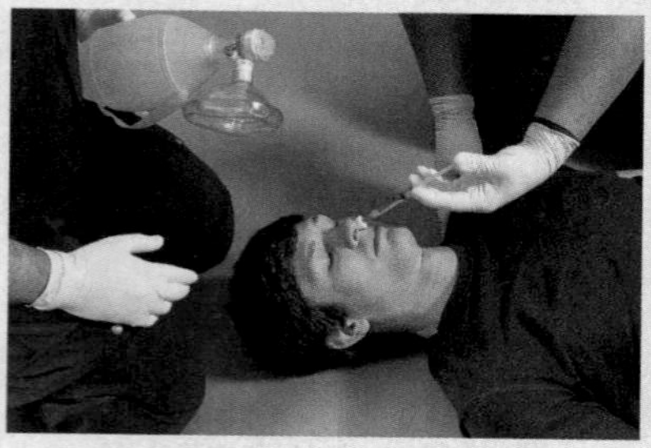

Step 4

Explain the procedure to the patient (or to a relative if the patient is unresponsive) and the need for the medication. Stop ventilation of the patient if necessary; remove any masks. Insert the MAD into the larger and less deviated or less obstructed nostril. Quickly spray the medication dose into a nostril.

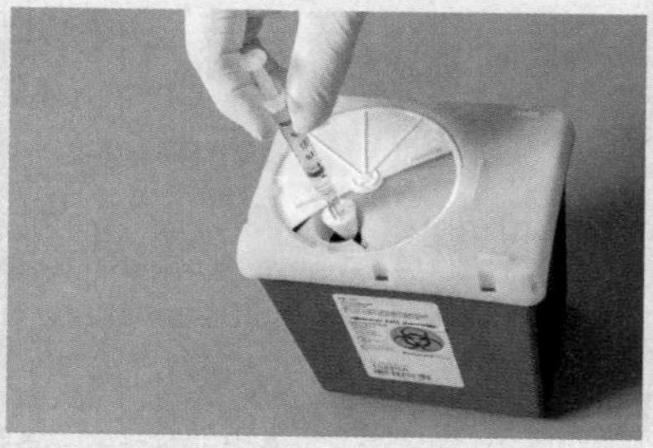

Step 5

Dispose of the MAD and syringe in the appropriate container.

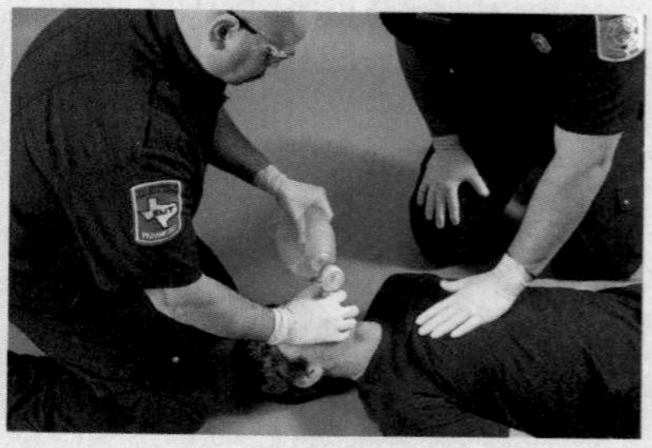

Step 6

Monitor the patient's condition. Document the medication given, route, time of administration, and patient's response.

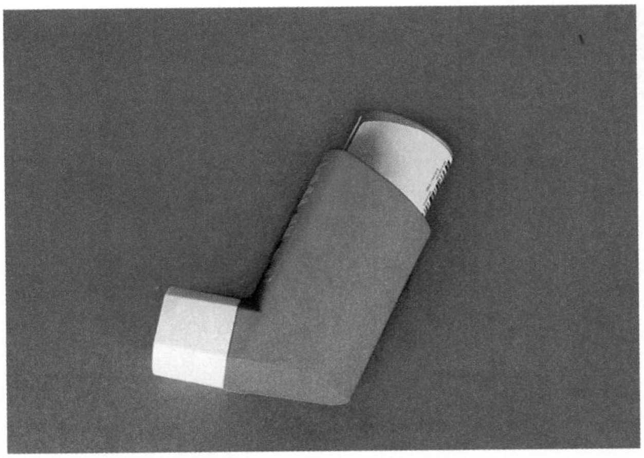

FIGURE 14-63 Some medications are inhaled into the lungs with a metered-dose inhaler so that they can be absorbed quickly into the bloodstream.

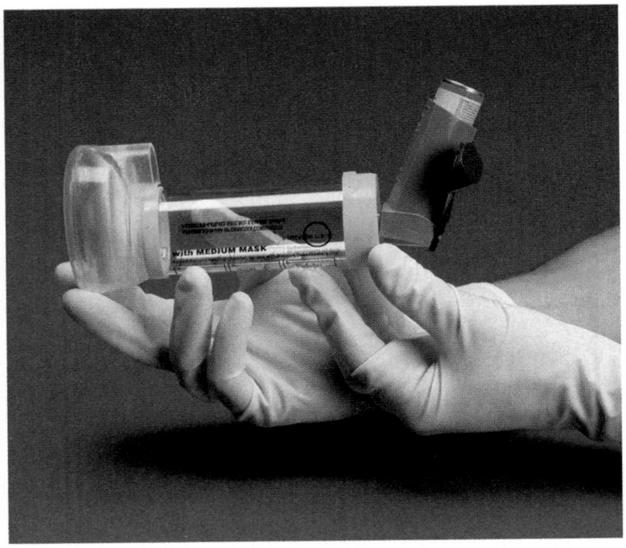

A

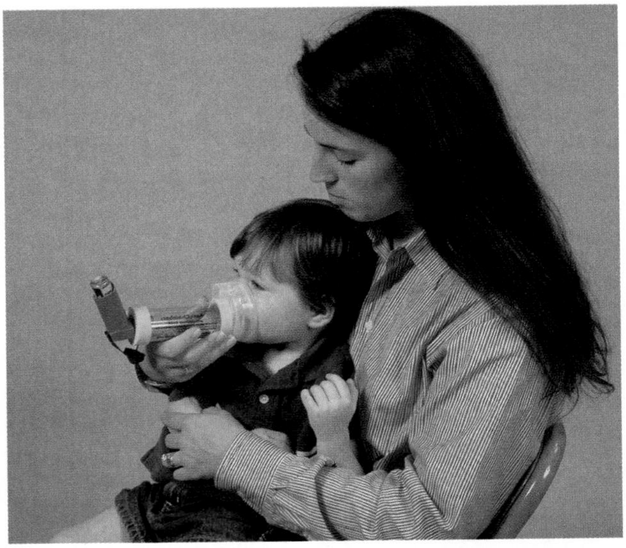

B

FIGURE 14-64 A. In children, a metered-dose inhaler and spacer can be used with or without a mask. **B.** Children as young as 6 months can use a mask and spacer device.

such as ipratropium bromide (Atrovent), an anticholinergic bronchodilator, are also administered via the inhalation route. Check your drug reference guide or the package insert for the indications, contraindications, and precautions before giving any of these medications.

A patient with a history of respiratory problems will usually have a **metered-dose inhaler (MDI)** to use regularly or as needed **FIGURE 14-63**. MDIs are usually administered by the patient using the patient's own prescribed medications, but paramedics must know how to administer drugs via this route because they may assist the patient with administration. Medications administered by an MDI can be delivered through a mouthpiece held by the patient or by a mask, with or without a spacer device, for young children and patients who cannot hold the mouthpiece **FIGURE 14-64**.

Follow the steps in **SKILL DRILL 14-12** to help a patient self-administer medication from an inhaler.

Liquid bronchodilators may be aerosolized in a **nebulizer** for inhalation for patients with more severe problems. Small-volume nebulizers (also called handheld nebulizers) are the most commonly used method of administering inhaled medications in the prehospital setting **FIGURE 14-65**. Oxygen or a compressed air source is connected to the nebulizer to produce the aerosolized mist.

Some nebulizers have been adapted to have child-friendly shapes and images to facilitate their use by pediatric patients. They may allow for blow-by administration to help the patient tolerate the medication. Other medication delivery devices

Words of Wisdom

MDIs are also called HFAs, after the propellant hydrofluoroalkane, which is now used instead of chlorofluorocarbons in these devices; however, MDI is more likely to be the term familiar to patients. More frequently, patients may refer to their MDIs as their "puffers."

Skill Drill 14-12 Assisting a Patient With a Metered-Dose Inhaler

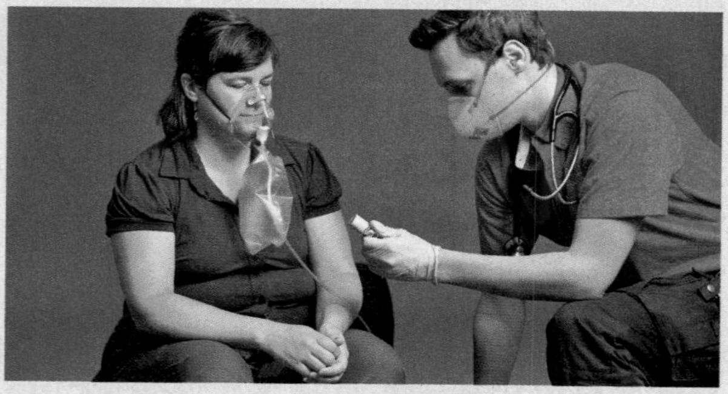

Step 1

Take standard precautions. (Because the patient could cough during this procedure, many services suggest the provider wear eye protection.) Obtain an order from medical control or follow the local protocol. Assemble the needed equipment. Ensure that you have the right medication, right patient, right dose, and right route, and that the medication is not expired.

Ensure the patient is alert enough to use the inhaler. Check whether the patient has already taken any doses. Obtain baseline breath sounds for comparison after a few minutes of inhaler use. Ensure the inhaler is at room temperature or warmer.

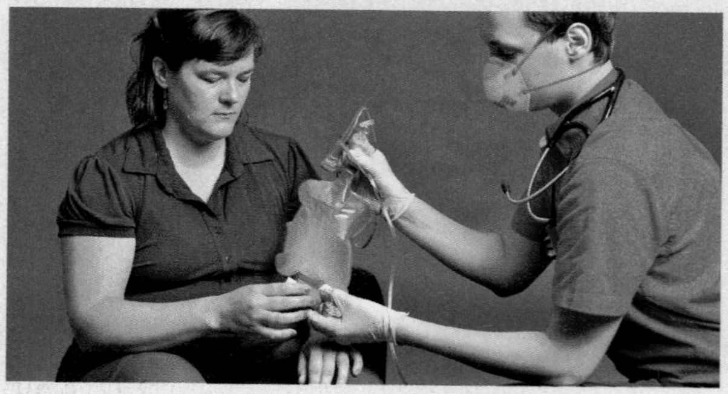

Step 2

Shake the inhaler vigorously several times. Stop administering supplemental oxygen and remove any mask from the patient's face. Ask the patient to exhale deeply and, before inhaling, to put their lips around the opening of the inhaler.

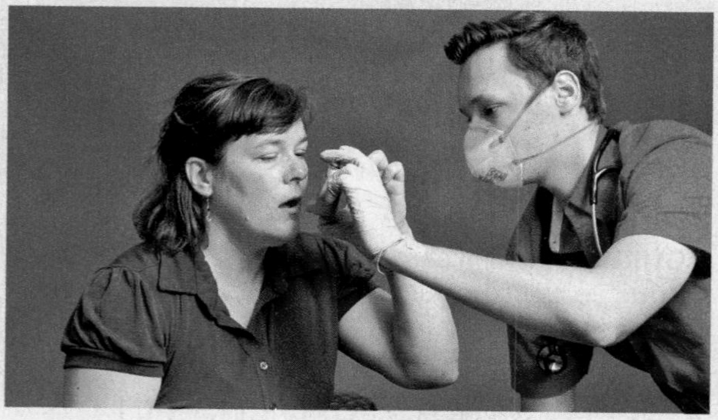

Step 3

If the patient has a spacer, then attach it to allow more effective use of the medication. Have the patient depress the handheld inhaler and begin to inhale deeply. Instruct the patient to not breathe for as long as comfortable to help the lungs absorb the medication.

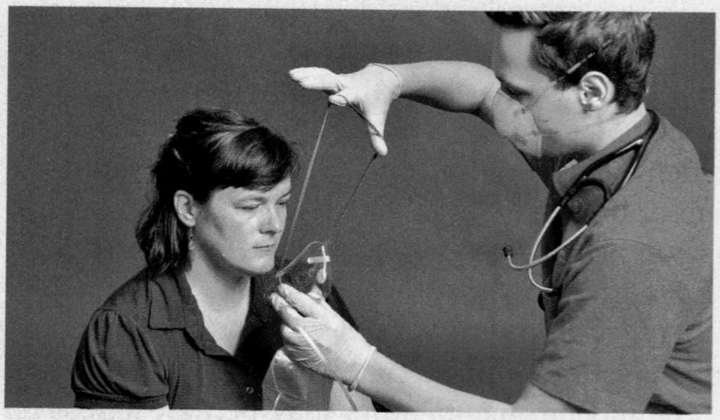

Step 4

Continue administering supplemental oxygen. Allow the patient to breathe a few times, then give the second dose per direction from medical control or according to the local protocol. Monitor the patient's condition, and document the medication given, route, administration time, and patient's response.

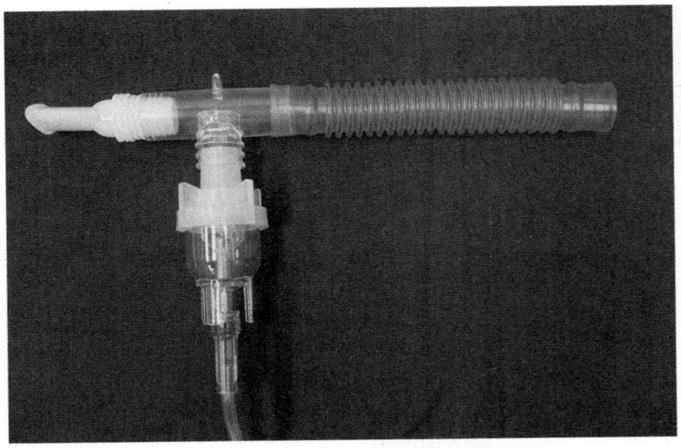

FIGURE 14-65 A small-volume nebulizer is used to deliver medications via aerosolized mist.

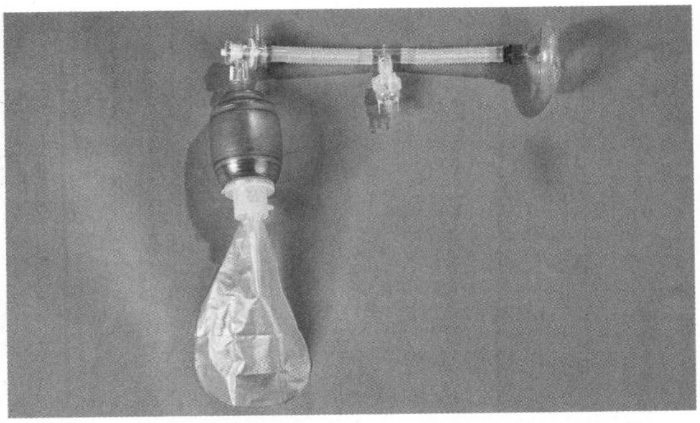

FIGURE 14-66 A nebulizer can be attached to a bag-mask device and administered through the mask.

include a nebulizer mask, which does not require the patient to hold the device. Some adapters have been designed to allow providers to administer nebulized medications to intubated patients with each ventilation **FIGURE 14-66**. These devices may also be adapted for use with CPAP masks **FIGURE 14-67**.

Follow the steps in **SKILL DRILL 14-13** to administer a medication via a small-volume nebulizer.

Controversies

In the past, nebulizers were considered the preferred method of administering beta agonist medications for the treatment of asthma attacks. Recent studies, however, have shown that MDIs, especially when used with spacing devices, are at least as effective as nebulizers and have several distinct advantages[10,11]:

- MDIs are more convenient than nebulizers. They do not require any setup time or a source of compressed gas.
- MDIs are more reliable than nebulizers. With a nebulizer, one cannot be certain that the patient is getting the full dose of the drug. MDIs deliver a more consistent amount of the aerosolized drug.
- Because most people with asthma use MDIs at home, using the MDI in an emergency provides an excellent opportunity to educate the patient on proper use of the device. Studies have shown that more than one-half of patients using MDIs at home employ an incorrect and ineffective technique. Showing a patient the correct technique and demonstrating its effectiveness can improve the outcome of subsequent asthma attacks.

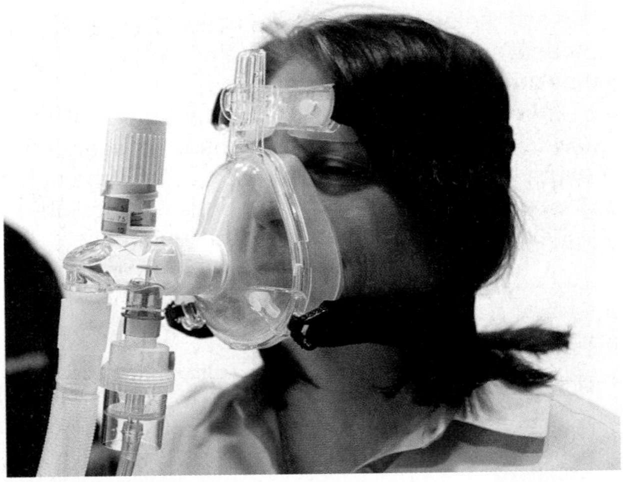

FIGURE 14-67 A nebulized medication being administered through a continuous positive airway pressure (CPAP) mask.

Some patients with respiratory emergencies may be breathing inadequately (ie, inadequate tidal volume, fast or slow respiratory rate) and will not be able to effectively inhale beta agonist medications into the lungs via either a nebulizer or an MDI. In such a case, you can utilize a small-volume nebulizer in-line with the assistive device. If the patient is intubated, assist with bag-mask ventilation or use of a ventilator by placing a short piece of corrugated tubing, separated by a T piece, to connect the nebulizer. When using CPAP, be aware that most manufacturers provide a nebulizer that is designed to work with their device. The nebulizer should be placed between the assistive device and the mask,

NR Skill

Skill Drill 14-13 Administering a Medication via a Small-Volume Nebulizer

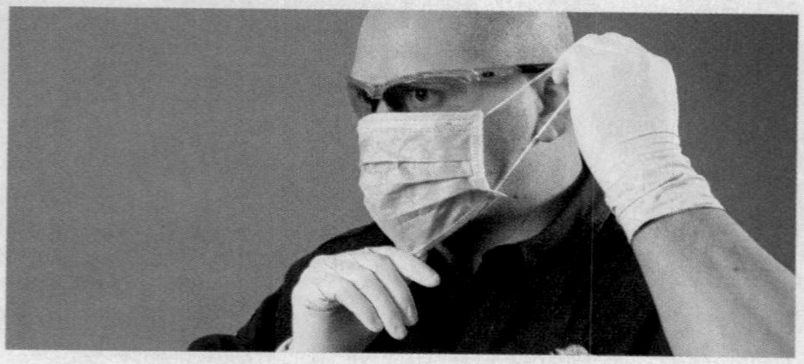

Step 1

Take standard precautions. Determine the need for an inhaled bronchodilator based on the patient's presentation. Obtain a history, including any drug allergies and vital signs.

Follow standing orders, or contact medical control for permission. Check the medication and its expiration date. Make sure that you have the right medication and that it is not cloudy or discolored. Assemble and check the needed equipment.

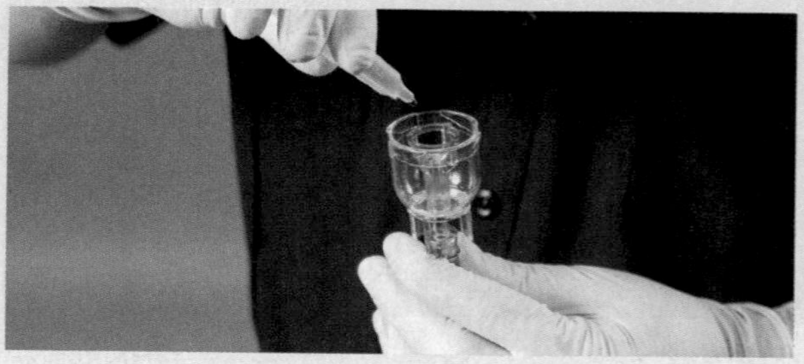

Step 2

If the medication is provided in a premixed package, add it to the bowl of the nebulizer. If it is not premixed, add the medication to the bowl and mix it with the specified amount of normal saline, usually 2.5 to 3 mL.

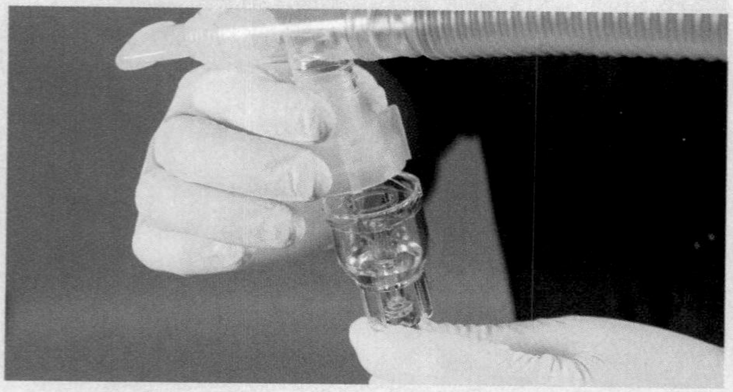

Step 3

Connect the T piece with the mouthpiece to the top of the bowl, or the mask to the bowl, and connect it to the oxygen tubing.

Set the flowmeter at 6 L/min to produce a steady mist. Remove the oxygen mask from the patient if oxygen is being administered.

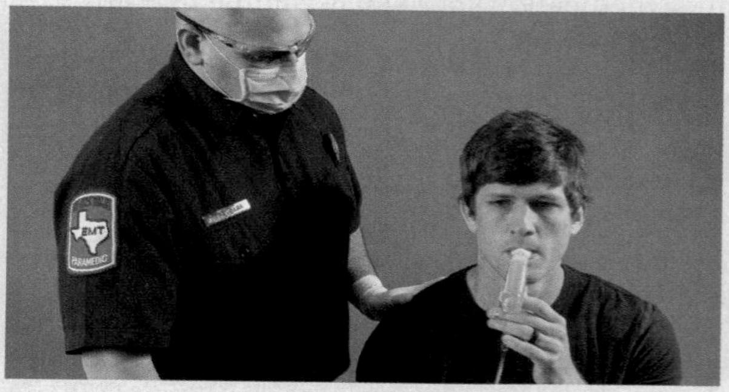

Step 4

With the handheld nebulizer in position, instruct the patient on the proper way to breathe. Have the patient breathe as deeply as possible and wait for 3 to 5 seconds before exhaling. Continue to coach the patient as needed.

Monitor the patient's condition, and document the medication given, route, time of administration, and patient response to the medication.

Cardiac monitoring is essential when administering a beta agonist. If cardiac dysrhythmias are noted, then stop administering the medication, treat the patient according to current resuscitation guidelines, and contact medical control.

or between the device and the ET tube if the patient is intubated, with a separate oxygen line connected to the nebulizer.

Controversies

ET Medication Administration

If IV or IO access is unavailable, then certain resuscitative medications can be administered via the ET tube. Absorption rates for medications given by this route are poor, however, so you should use other, more effective routes before attempting medication administration through an ET tube. The optimal ET dose of most medications is unknown, but the usual dose given by the ET route is 2 to 2.5 times the recommended IV dose for the medication to become adequately dispersed throughout the tracheobronchial tree.[12] When use of this route is necessary, the medications that can be administered via the ET tube can be remembered with the mnemonic LEAN (or LANE): Lidocaine, Epinephrine, Atropine, and Naloxone (Narcan).[12] As always, check your local protocols before administration.

Long-Term Vascular Access Devices

In some situations, IV access is imperative but proves difficult to obtain. Some of these patients may have a long-term VAD inserted and be receiving an antibiotic regimen or chemotherapy, or undergoing regular blood draws for chronic disorders, hemodialysis, or treatment for other acute or chronic illnesses. These patients will be upfront about their medical device and will generally request that you not insert a peripheral line.

Words of Wisdom

Long-term VADs should never be used routinely by prehospital providers. If your EMS agency permits you to access these devices, it is imperative that you seek regular training on how to access and properly use them.

If you encounter patients with long-term VADs, you will observe that there are two general types: nontunneling and implanted. Most protocols allow the use of these VADs only during critical events. These devices are usually preserved with heparin to prevent clotting.

Nontunneling VADs

Nontunneling vascular access devices are inserted by direct venipuncture through the skin directly into a selected vein. The most common types of these devices encountered in the prehospital and interfacility settings are peripheral inserted central catheters (PICCs), midline catheters, and central venous catheters (CVCs).

PICCs are often used for long-term medication administration, chemotherapy, frequent venous sampling, and total parenteral nutrition. These catheters may have a single, double, or triple lumen. They are generally inserted by designated PICC nurses, who receive specific training on their insertion. The insertion point is usually at the antecubital vein, while the distal end of the PICC usually sits at the superior vena cava and is verified by a radiograph. PICCs may be left in place for 6 to 8 weeks. Some patients may have their PICC accessed by family or home health care providers on a regular basis.

Midline catheters are also inserted at the antecubital vein. However, unlike a PICC, the distal end of the midline catheter rests at the proximal end of the extremity. These VADs can generally be used for approximately 4 weeks, but may also be used for shorter medication therapies and venous therapies.

CVCs are generally inserted in emergent situations by physicians into the subclavian, femoral, or internal jugular vein. They are used for emergent medication administration, fluid resuscitation, blood administration, or blood sampling. Generally large-bore catheters, they may sit near the vena cava.

The steps for accessing a nontunneling VAD are as follows:

1. Use aseptic technique. Prepare all of the appropriate equipment: empty 10- to 20-mL syringe (nothing less than a 10-mL syringe should be used), 10-mL normal saline flush, sterile gloves, alcohol prep, 10-gtt administration set, 500 mL normal saline.

   Ensure all lumens are clamped. Air embolism is a serious risk with these patients because many of these devices go directly into the vena cava. That is why central lines must be clamped whenever they are not in use.

   Use an antiseptic swab to cleanse the lumen that will be used **FIGURE 14-68A**.

2. Attach the empty syringe and withdraw a minimum of 10 mL of blood from the lumen. Discard this syringe immediately into the sharps container. Do not withdraw too forcefully. If you meet some resistance, then gently flush and withdraw. Ask the patient to turn the head in the opposite direction of the central line **FIGURE 14-68B**.
3. After you have withdrawn the 10 mL of blood, attach the 10-mL syringe filled with normal saline and slowly administer it **FIGURE 14-68C**.
4. Attach the prepared IV drip set and set it up for a rate of at least 10 mL/h. Depending on the size of the catheter, you can infuse medications at a rate of 125 to 250 mL/h. The line must be running continuously because heparin is not available. Administer IV medications through the attached IV drip set. Monitor the patient's condition, and document the medication given, route, administration time, and patient's response **FIGURE 14-68D**.

Implanted VADs

Implanted vascular access devices are implanted surgically, sutured under the skin. These devices are palpable outside the skin but are not exposed to the outside environment. The VAD consists of a self-sealing core inserted in a stainless steel, titanium, or plastic shell connected to a catheter that runs into the superior vena cava. These devices can only be accessed with a Huber needle that is non-coring and has a mild angle. They can be used for long-term medication administration, total

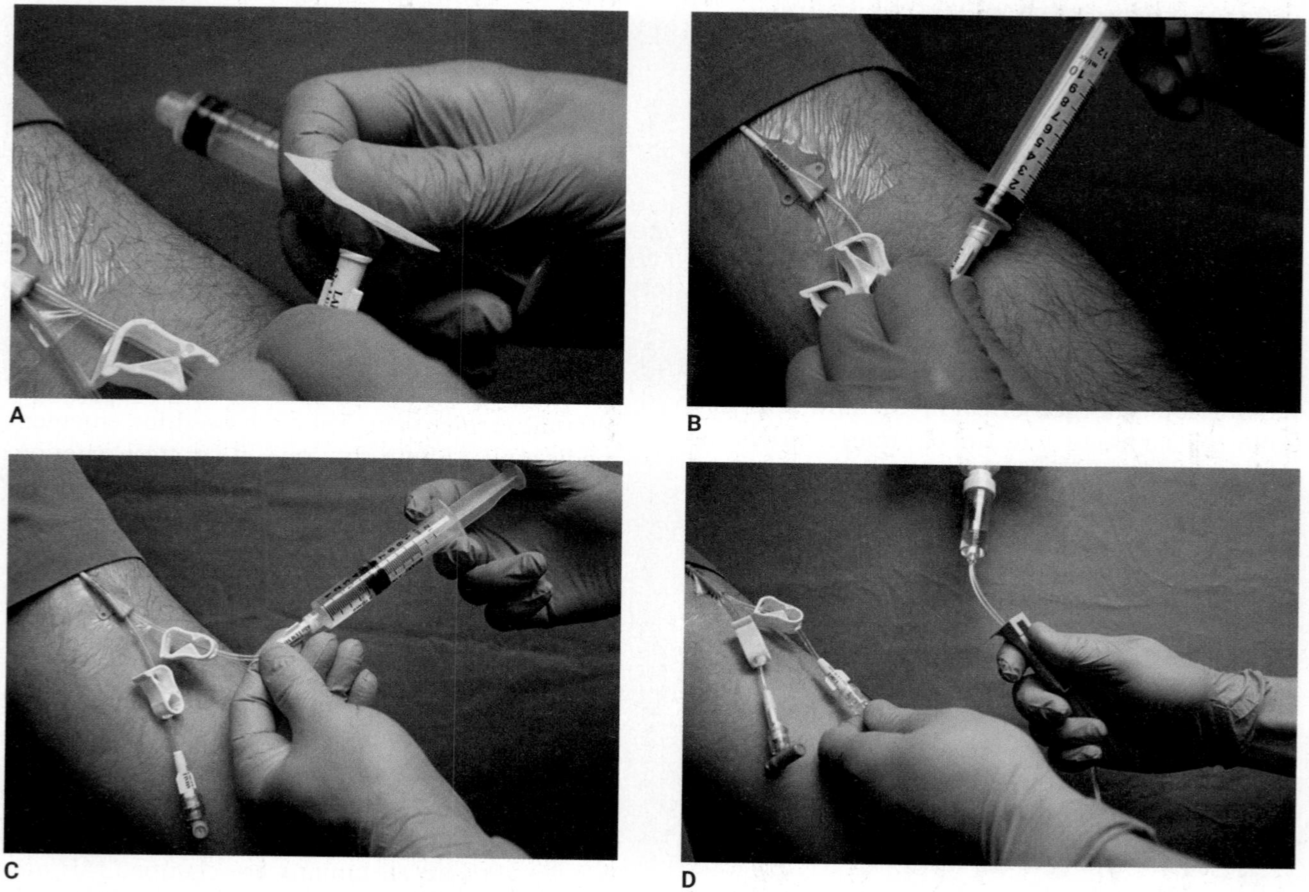

FIGURE 14-68 Accessing a nontunneling device. Using aseptic technique, the general steps include preparing the equipment **(A)**, attaching the empty syringe and withdrawing blood **(B)**, attaching the syringe filled with normal saline and administering it **(C)**, and attaching the intravenous drip set and administering medications **(D)**.

parenteral nutrition, chemotherapy, blood products, or venous blood sampling.

Arteriovenous (AV) fistulas are used for a variety of disorders. They are created by connecting a vein and an artery. To treat patients with kidney failure, hemodialysis uses AV fistulas to dialyze the blood. AV fistulas are also used for plasmapheresis in patients with various disorders, such as myasthenia gravis and Guillain-Barré syndrome. However, these VADs require a unique skill set to access and generally should not be accessed by paramedics.

Accessing an implanted VAD is not in the scope of paramedic practice in most places; special training and medical authorization are required to perform this skill. The steps for accessing such as device are summarized as follows:

1. Use aseptic technique. Prepare all necessary equipment: Huber needle, empty 10- to 20-mL syringe (nothing less than a 10-mL syringe should be used), 10-mL normal saline flush, sterile gloves, chlorhexidine or betadine, 10-gtt administration set, 500 mL normal saline.
2. Identify the site in the upper part of the chest. Stabilize it between the thumb and index finger of your nondominant hand.
3. Clean the site with chlorhexidine. If the patient has an allergy to this chemical, then clean the site with betadine **FIGURE 14-69A**.

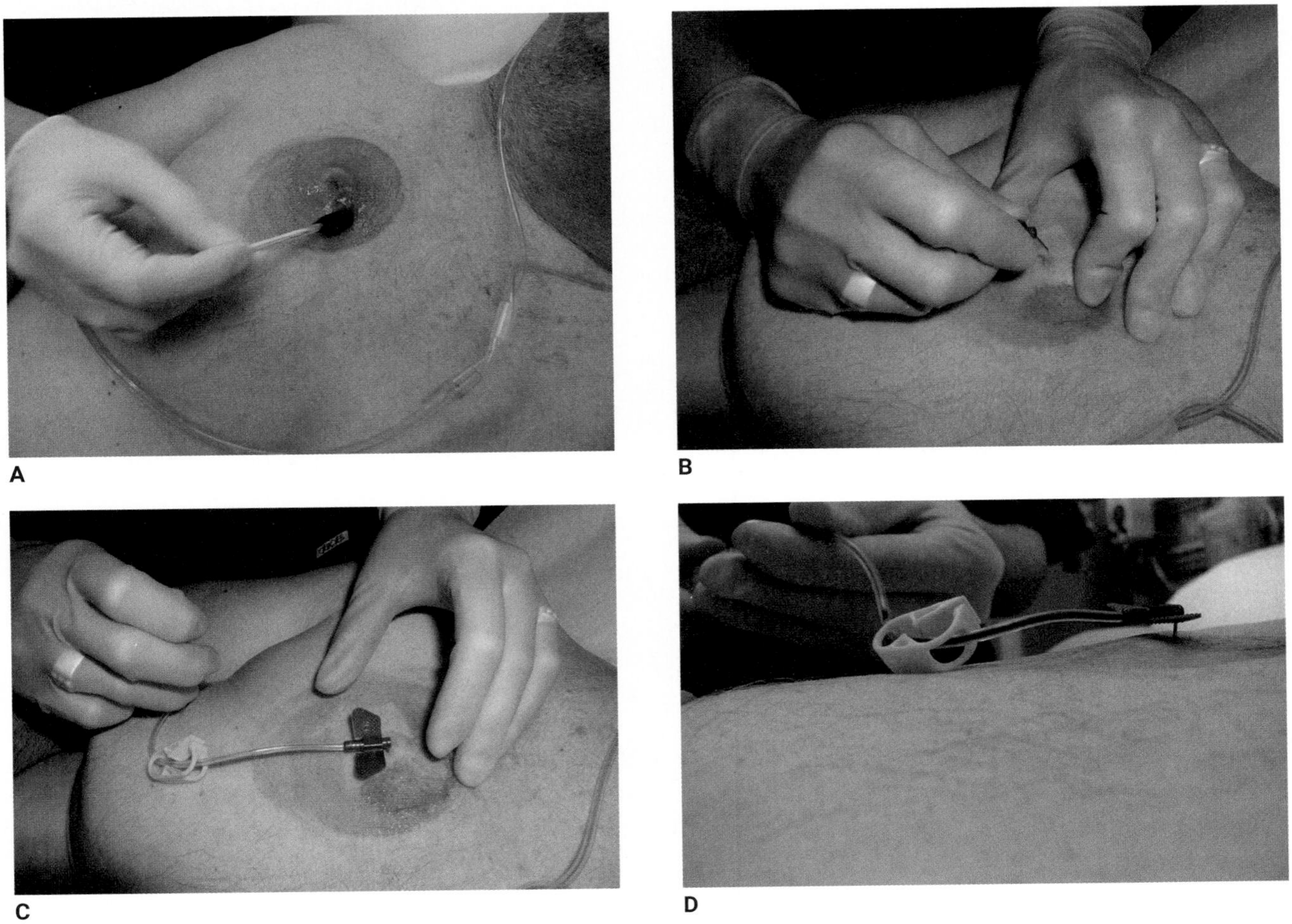

FIGURE 14-69 Accessing an implanted vascular access device. Using aseptic technique, the general steps include identifying and cleaning the site **(A)**, stretching the skin over the site **(B)**, inserting the Huber needle at a 90° angle **(C)**, withdrawing at least 10 mL of blood **(D)**, discarding it, flushing with 10 mL normal saline, attaching the administration set, and administering medications directly into the medication port.

4. Apply pressure around the edges of the port to stretch the skin over the injection site **FIGURE 14-69B**.
5. While stabilizing the device, insert the Huber needle at a 90° angle **FIGURE 14-69C**.
6. Withdraw at least 10 mL of blood from the needleless extension set **FIGURE 14-69D**. Discard it immediately.
7. Flush the set with the 10-mL normal saline flush. Attach the 10-gtt IV administration set.
8. Administer medications directly into the drop set medication port.
9. Monitor the patient's condition, and document the medication given, route, administration time, and patient's response.

The presence of a central line implies that the patient has a significant medical history that should be investigated and that standard IV access may be challenging to obtain. Accessing these devices is risky and requires proper training. The use of aseptic technique is imperative, considering that many VADs sit inside the superior vena cava. These devices are all preserved with heparin, which is why providers must withdraw at least 10 mL of blood from the device. Because EMS providers do not routinely carry heparin, they must keep the IV administration set minimally at a KVO/TKO rate to prevent clots from forming.

Words of Wisdom

When you are accessing multiple-lumen devices, you should always attempt to access the largest lumen first. If the lumens are the same diameter, then you should access the distal lumen. The lumen that should be used will generally be marked by the number "1."

Rates of Medication Absorption

The speed at which a drug is absorbed is directly related to the route by which it is given. Obviously, drugs injected directly into the bloodstream via IV or IO injections gain access to the central circulation the fastest. Oral medications take longer to achieve their therapeutic effects because they must first be absorbed through the GI tract. **TABLE 14-4** summarizes the various medication routes and their rates of absorption. Specific medications are covered in detail in the Chapter 15, *Emergency Medications*.

TABLE 14-4 Medication Routes and Rates of Absorption

Route of Administration	Onset of Action[a]
Intraosseous	30–60 s
Intravenous	30–60 s
Endotracheal	2–3 min
Inhalation	2–3 min
Nasal mucosal atomization	3–5 min
Sublingual	3–5 min
Intramuscular injection	10–20 min
Subcutaneous injection	15–30 min
Rectal	5–30 min
Oral	30–90 min
Topical	Minutes to hours

[a]In a healthy person with adequate perfusion.

Data from: Verma P, Thakur AS, Deshmukh K, et al. Routes of drug administration. *Int J Pharm Sci Res.* 2010;1(1):54-59. http://www.technicaljournalsonline.com/ijpsr/VOL%20I/IJPSR%20VOL%20I%20ISSUE%20I%20JULY%20SEPTEMBER%202010/IJPSR%20VOL%20I%20ISSUE%20I%20Article%208.pdf. Accessed February 16, 2017.

YOU are the Paramedic SUMMARY

1. Given this scenario, what route of delivery do you anticipate using to administer medications? What are the advantages of this route?

Given this patient's presentation, you should anticipate giving medications through the IV route. The sudden onset of symptoms suggests some sort of acute cardiac event, possibly involving a dysrhythmia. IV administration will allow for reliable and quick absorption of the medications in the body. Subcutaneous or IM administration of medications to a patient experiencing a cardiac event may be unreliable due to the patient's perfusion status.

2. What aspects of the patient history are important to consider prior to administering any medication to this patient?

Remember the rights of medication administration, discussed in Chapter 13, *Principles of Pharmacology*. Verify the drug dose, name, route, rate of administration, indication, contraindications, drug concentration, and volume to be administered. While interviewing the patient, determine which medications (or home remedies) the patient is taking and whether the patient has any known drug allergies.

3. What information must you and your partner be sure to communicate to one another as you are preparing to administer this medication?

The MACC method of confirming specific details regarding medication administration is a useful way to minimize the risk of a medication error. During this preadministration check, communication with your partner should involve, at a minimum, details regarding the dose, volume to be administered, indication, and contraindications.

4. Why is it prudent to contact medical control in this scenario to discuss patient care options?

Medical control can serve as an invaluable resource while you are in the field. Establishing a line of communication with online medical control early in a call may assist you in reducing the cognitive load and reducing the potential of making a dosing or judgment error. When discussing patient care with the physician, make sure you are confident and detailed in the information that you provide.

5. What dose will you administer to the patient? Given the supplied medication, what volume will you administer?

The desired dose in this case is 26.25 mg, which is calculated as follows:

$$\frac{0.25 \text{ mg}}{1 \text{ kg}} \times 105 \text{ kg} = 26.25 \text{ mg}$$

The drug concentration is 30 mg in 5 mL of fluid. Therefore, the volume to be administered is calculated as follows:

$$26.25 \text{ mg} \div \frac{30 \text{ mg}}{5 \text{ mL}} = 26.25 \cancel{\text{mg}} \times \frac{\overset{1}{\cancel{5}} \text{ mL}}{30 \underset{6}{\cancel{\text{mg}}}} = 4.375 \text{ mL}$$

Because the order is 26.25 mg and the concentration is 30 mg in 5 mL, there is 6 mg/mL. Therefore, the initial administration of medication is 4.375 mL of diltiazem.

6. Why would it be preferable to use an IV pump for a maintenance infusion of a medication?

IV infusion pumps are the standard of care within the medical community. Although they are not available on every ambulance, you should still recognize that their use would be appropriate if they are available. A mechanical device that infuses a precise volume programmed by the paramedic is preferred over the use of a microdrip set. There is a high propensity for errors in IV flow rates, and therefore a high risk of errors in medication dosing, when using microdrip sets. IV infusion pumps are not vulnerable to variability in drip rate based on bag height, movement, and other factors.

7. What is the appropriate flow rate to administer the maintenance infusion of diltiazem?

You have a premixed bag with 30 mg/100 mL. The infusion is calculated to provide 5 mg/h. First, calculate the concentration:

$$30 \text{ mg} \div 100 \text{ mL} = 0.3 \text{ mg/mL (concentration)}$$

Second, determine the amount of volume to infuse per hour (mL/h):

$$\frac{5 \text{ mg}}{1 \text{ h}} \text{ (desired dose)} \div \frac{0.3 \text{ mg}}{1 \text{ mL}} \text{ (concentration)} = 16.67 \text{ mL/h}$$

YOU are the Paramedic SUMMARY continued

Last, determine the amount of volume to infuse per minute. The rate can be established by dividing the mL/h by 60:

$$\frac{16.67\ \text{mL}}{1\ \text{h}} \times \frac{1\ \text{h}}{60\ \text{min}} = 0.28\ \text{mL/min}$$

Using a microdrip set (60 gtt/mL), you would administer 16.67 gtt/min to achieve a rate of 0.28 mL/min:

$$\frac{0.28\ \text{mL}}{1\ \text{min}} \times \frac{60\ \text{gtt}}{1\ \text{mL}} = 16.67\ \text{gtt/min}$$

Medication calculations like this one help illustrate the importance of understanding the math behind drug administration. As a tip, recall that when using a microdrip set (60 gtt/mL), gtt/min is equal to mL/h. Infusing the diltiazem at a rate of 16.67 gtt/min using a microdrip set will give an administration rate of 16.67 mL/h and achieve the goal of 5 mg/h. However, as described in the previous question, it would be preferable to use a pump for this infusion to ensure that the proper amount of medication and proper volume are administered.

EMS Patient Care Report (PCR)

Date: 08-01-22	**Incident No.:** 1232	**Nature of Call:** Cardiac		**Location:** 247 Pine Street	
Dispatched: 1115	**En Route:** 1116	**At Scene:** 1119	**Transport:** 1137	**At Hospital:** 1207	**In Service:** 1219

Patient Information

Age: 26 **Sex:** M **Weight (in kg [lb]):** 105 kg (231 lb)	**Allergies:** NKDA **Medications:** None **Past Medical History:** None **Chief Complaint:** Palpitations; syncopal episode

Vital Signs

Time: 1120	**BP:** N/A	**Pulse:** N/A	**Respirations:** 20	**Spo_2:** N/A
Time: 1124	**BP:** 134/90	**Pulse:** 180	**Respirations:** 20	**Spo_2:** 99%
Time: 1129	**BP:** 126/78	**Pulse:** 90	**Respirations:** 18	**Spo_2:** 100%
Time:	**BP:**	**Pulse:**	**Respirations:**	**Spo_2:**

EMS Treatment (circle all that apply)

Oxygen @ __ L/min via (circle one): **NC NRM Bag-mask device**		**Assisted Ventilation**	**Airway Adjunct**	**CPR**
Defibrillation	**Bleeding Control**	**Bandaging**	**Splinting**	**Other:**

Narrative

EMS arrived on scene to find 26-year-old male complaining of the sudden onset of palpitations. Pt called 9-1-1 before sitting down on the ground because he felt weak. Pt suffered a syncopal episode and had regained consciousness on EMS arrival. Pt was found awake, alert, and oriented to person, place, time, and event. Pt complained of palpitations. Pt denied having any chest pain or dyspnea. Pt also reported that he no longer feels dizzy or weak but could still feel the palpitations. Pt has no medical history and takes no medications. Pt was found to be in atrial fibrillation with a rapid ventricular response. Online medical direction was obtained with Dr. Adams at Beauregard Hospital. Per Dr. Adams, 0.25 mg/kg of diltiazem (26.25 mg) given IV bolus over 2 minutes. Pt converted to sinus rhythm. Pt reported no complaints. Per Dr. Adams, maintenance infusion of diltiazem initiated at 5 mg/h. Pt transported to Beauregard Hospital without any acute changes. Pt turned over to Dr. Adams in Room 5 in the ED with report to RN.

End of report

Prep Kit

Ready for Review

- Vascular access is often needed in emergency medicine for patients in hemodynamically unstable condition and in need of intravenous (IV) fluids, various medications, or both.
- It is your responsibility to ensure the medications you deliver are administered correctly and safely. Medication errors are an issue throughout health care. To minimize the danger of incorrect medication administration, you should use a tool to verify the drug dose, name, route, rate of administration, indication for administration, contraindications, drug concentration, and volume to be administered.
- Documenting medication administration is extremely important. You must list the dose administered, name of the drug, route, rate, time of administration, who administered the drug, who helped perform the medication check, and the patient's response.
- Maintaining and securing medication supplies on the ambulance are part of a paramedic's role. Follow the specific policies and procedures established by your local drug distribution, security, and accountability system.
- Use aseptic technique when you are performing any invasive procedure to minimize the risk of patient contamination. Always take standard precautions when performing an invasive procedure to maximize your own safety, and dispose of all equipment properly.
- An ill or injured body may be unable to maintain homeostasis, resulting in an excess or deficit of fluids or electrolytes. Understanding the workings of the intracellular and extracellular chemicals and charges will provide you with a better foundation for understanding why different types of IV solutions are administered for different conditions.
- Crystalloid IV solutions are the best choice for injured patients who need fluid replacement. Colloid solutions work well to reduce edema while expanding the vascular compartment.
- A solution can be isotonic, hypotonic, or hypertonic. Isotonic solutions, such as normal saline, have almost the same osmolarity as serum and other body fluids. Lactated Ringer solution is an isotonic solution often used in the prehospital setting for patients who have significant blood loss.
- Hypotonic solutions may be needed for a patient receiving dialysis or for a patient with diabetic ketoacidosis. Hypertonic solutions may be administered to patients with severe traumatic brain injuries.
- Techniques for gaining vascular access include cannulation of a peripheral extremity vein, cannulation of the external jugular vein, and cannulation of the intraosseous (IO) space. Although the ultimate goal when obtaining vascular access is to be able to administer fluids and medications, each of these techniques requires a different approach and must be practiced frequently for initial and ongoing proficiency.
- Several different IV administration sets exist, and you must know which one is most appropriate for a given patient's condition. Microdrip sets (60 gtt/mL) are commonly used for medication infusions. Macrodrip sets (10 or 15 gtt/mL) are used when the patient requires IV fluid boluses to treat dehydration, hypovolemic shock, and other states of hemodynamic instability.
- You must consider two factors when choosing an IV catheter: gauge and length. The larger the gauge (the smaller the number) and the shorter the length, the more fluid that can be infused through it. Over-the-needle catheters are the IV catheters most commonly used in the prehospital setting.
- Cannulation of a peripheral extremity vein is the preferred initial means of establishing vascular access. If it is unsuccessful and the patient is critically ill or injured, proceed with IO cannulation without delay. External jugular vein cannulation is usually attempted only after all other techniques of gaining vascular access have failed.
- The IO space, which acts like a sponge, quickly absorbs fluids and medications and rapidly transports them to the central circulation. Although peripheral veins often collapse

Prep Kit continued

when a patient is in shock or cardiac arrest, the IO space tends to remain patent. Thus IO cannulation and infusion may be life-saving measures if peripheral venous access is not possible. Any fluid or medication that can be administered via the IV route can be administered via the IO route and can travel to the central circulation just as rapidly.

- You must be thoroughly familiar with the equipment you are using when performing IO cannulation. Follow the local protocols and attend in-service training to develop expertise with the specific equipment used for IO cannulation in your EMS system.
- Potential complications of IV therapy include local and systemic reactions. After administering any medication, always monitor the patient for any reaction or improvement.
- You may be asked to obtain a blood sample: for example, for analysis at the receiving facility. Obtain blood samples at the same time you start an IV line.
- Sometimes you may transport a patient who is undergoing a blood transfusion. When receiving such a patient, ensure at least one vascular site is available that is not transfusing blood.
- Good math skills and a thorough understanding of the metric system are imperative to providing the right doses of drugs to your patients. Administering the incorrect drug, using the incorrect route, or giving the incorrect dose can have disastrous effects.
- As a paramedic, you must be familiar with the various routes of medication administration, including the proper use of equipment and proper anatomic locations for administration via each route.
- Parenteral routes are those that do not pass through the GI tract; they include the intradermal, subcutaneous, intramuscular, IV, IO, and percutaneous routes. Enteral routes are those that pass through any portion of the GI tract (oral, sublingual, gastric tube).
- The IV and IO routes are the fastest routes of medication administration.
- IV medication can be administered as a bolus (single dose) or via piggyback (a secondary IV line connected to a port on the primary infusion line).
- The standard of care when administering a maintenance infusion is to use an electromechanical infusion pump. An infusion pump delivers fluid at a set rate and calculates the amount of fluid infused, as well as the remaining amount. You are most likely to encounter an infusion pump during an interfacility transport.
- When in doubt, always follow local protocols or contact medical control as needed for direction when you are administering a medication. *Never make a hasty critical decision.*

Vital Vocabulary

access port A sealed hub on an administration set designed to provide sterile access to the intravenous fluid.

administration set Tubing that connects to the intravenous bag access port and the catheter to deliver intravenous fluid.

ampules Small glass containers that are sealed and whose contents are sterilized.

antecubital The anterior aspect of the elbow.

anticoagulants Substances that prevent blood from clotting.

antiseptics Chemicals used to cleanse an area before performing an invasive procedure, such as starting an intravenous line; they are not toxic to living tissues. Examples include chlorhexidine, isopropyl alcohol, and iodine.

aseptic technique A method of cleansing used to prevent contamination of a site from pathogens when you are performing an invasive procedure, such as starting an intravenous line.

aural Pertaining to the ear.

blood tubing A special type of macrodrip administration set designed to facilitate rapid fluid

Prep Kit continued

replacement by manual infusion of multiple intravenous bags or intravenous–blood replacement combinations.

bolus "In one mass"; in medication administration, a single dose given by the intravenous or intraosseous route; may be a small or large quantity of the drug.

Bone Injection Gun (BIG) A spring-loaded device that is used for inserting an intraosseous needle into the proximal tibia in adult and pediatric patients.

buccal Between the cheek and gums.

butterfly catheter A rigid, hollow, venous cannulation device identified by its plastic "wings" that act as anchoring points for securing the catheter.

cannulation The insertion of a catheter into a body cavity, duct, or vessel to allow for fluid flow.

catheter shear An event in which a needle is reinserted into the catheter and slices through the catheter, creating a free-floating segment.

Celsius scale A scale for measuring temperature, where water freezes at 0° and boils at 100°.

colloid solutions Solutions that contain molecules (usually proteins) that are too large to pass out of the capillary membranes and, therefore, remain in the vascular compartment.

concentration The total weight of a drug contained in a specific volume of liquid.

contaminated stick The puncturing of an emergency care provider's skin with a needle or catheter that was used on a patient.

crystalloid solutions Solutions of dissolved crystals (eg, salts or sugars) in water; contain compounds that quickly dissociate in solution.

D_5W An intravenous solution made up of 5% dextrose in water.

dehydration Depletion of the body's systemic fluid volume.

desired dose The amount of a drug that the physician orders for a patient; the drug order.

diaphysis The shaft of a long bone.

diluent A solution (usually water or normal saline) used for diluting a medication.

disinfectants Chemicals used on nonliving objects to kill organisms; they are toxic to living tissues.

distal traction Gentle downward or lateral traction on the skin.

drip chamber The area of the administration set where fluid accumulates so that the tubing remains filled with fluid.

drug reconstitution Injecting sterile water or saline from one vial into another vial containing a powdered form of the drug.

enema A fluid solution, possibly containing supplemental medications, that can be administered rectally to aid in a variety of gastrointestinal complications.

enteral medications Medication administration that involves the medication passing through a portion of the gastrointestinal tract.

epiphyseal plate The growth plate of a bone; a major site of bone development during childhood.

epiphyses The ends of a long bone.

external jugular (EJ) vein Large neck vein that is lateral to the carotid artery.

EZ-IO A handheld, battery-powered driver to which a special intraosseous needle is attached; used for insertion of the intraosseous needle into the proximal tibia of children and adults.

Fahrenheit scale A scale for measuring temperature, where water freezes at 32° and boils at 212°.

FAST devices First Access for Shock and Trauma devices; manual sternal intraosseous devices used in patients age 12 and older; include an infusion tube, subcutaneous portal, an introducer, a target/strain relief patch, and a protective dome.

flash chamber The area of an intravenous catheter that fills with blood to help indicate when a vein is cannulated.

gastric tubes Tubes that are commonly inserted in patients in the prehospital setting to decompress the stomach; can also be used to administer certain enteral medications.

Prep Kit continued

gauge The internal diameter of an intravenous catheter or needle.

gtt A unit of measure that indicates drops.

hematoma An accumulation of blood in the tissues beneath the skin; a potential complication of intravenous therapy.

hemostasis The body's natural blood-clotting mechanism.

hypertonic solution A solution that has a greater concentration of sodium than does the cell; the increased osmotic pressure can draw out water from the cell and cause it to collapse.

hypotonic solution A solution that has a lower concentration of sodium than does the cell; the increased osmotic pressure lets water flow into the cell, causing it to swell and possibly burst.

implanted vascular access devices Devices that are implanted in surgery, sutured under the skin, for the purpose of long-term medication administration, total parenteral nutrition, chemotherapy, blood product administration, and venous blood sampling; an arteriovenous fistula is an example.

infiltration The escape of fluid into the surrounding tissue; the result of vein perforation during intravenous cannulation.

infusion pump A mechanical device that infuses a precise intravenous volume programmed by the clinician.

inhalation Breathing into the lungs; a medication delivery route.

intradermal The layer of the dermis, just beneath the epidermis; a medication delivery route.

intramuscular (IM) Into a muscle; a medication delivery route.

intranasal Within the nose.

intraosseous (IO) Within the bone.

intraosseous infusion A technique of administering fluids, blood and blood products, and medications into the intraosseous space of a long bone, usually the proximal tibia.

intraosseous space The spongy cancellous bone of the epiphyses and the medullary cavity of the diaphysis, collectively.

intravenous (IV) Within a vein.

intravenous therapy Cannulation of a vein with an intravenous catheter to access the patient's vascular system.

ionic concentration The amount of charged particles found in a particular area.

isotonic crystalloid solution An intravenous solution that does not cause a fluid shift into or out of the cell; examples include normal saline and lactated Ringer solution.

isotonic solution A solution that has the same concentration of sodium as does the cell. Its presence does not cause water to shift, so no change in cell shape occurs.

lactated Ringer (LR) solution A sterile, isotonic, crystalloid solution containing specified amounts of calcium chloride, potassium chloride, sodium chloride, and sodium lactate in water.

macrodrip sets Administration sets named for the large orifice between the piercing spike and the drip chamber; they allow for rapid fluid flow into the vascular system; the maximum flow rate is 10 or 15 gtt/mL, depending on the manufacturer.

medical asepsis The practice of preventing contamination of the patient by using aseptic technique.

metered-dose inhaler (MDI) A pressurized canister that delivers a specific dose of a medication; commonly used for beta agonist bronchodilators.

metric system A measurement system based on multiples of 10 (ie, a decimal system) that is used for the measurement of length, weight, and volume.

microdrip sets Administration sets named for the small needlelike orifice between the piercing spike and the drip chamber; they allow for carefully controlled fluid flow and are ideally suited for medication administration; the maximum flow rate is 60 gtt/mL.

Mix-o-Vial A single vial divided into two compartments by a rubber stopper; methylprednisolone sodium succinate (Solu-Medrol) is stored this way.

mucosal atomizer device (MAD) A device that attaches to the end of a syringe that is used to

Prep Kit continued

spray (atomize) certain medications via the intranasal route.

nebulizer A device for producing a fine spray or mist that is used to deliver inhaled medications.

New Intraosseous (NIO) device A spring-loaded device that contains neither a drill nor a battery; used for inserting an intraosseous needle into the proximal tibia of an adult patient.

nontunneling vascular access devices Devices that have been inserted by direct venipuncture through the skin directly into a selected vein, for the purpose of long-term medication administration, total parenteral nutrition, chemotherapy, and venous blood sampling; peripheral inserted central catheters and central venous catheters are examples.

normal saline A solution of 0.9% sodium chloride; an isotonic crystalloid.

ocular Pertaining to the eye.

osmolarity The ability to influence the movement of water across a semipermeable membrane.

osteogenesis imperfecta A congenital bone disease that results in fragile bones.

osteomyelitis Inflammation of the bone and muscle caused by infection.

overhydration An increase in the body's systemic fluid volume.

over-the-needle catheter A Teflon (plastic) catheter inserted over a hollow needle.

parenteral route A route of medication administration that involves any route other than the gastrointestinal tract.

Penrose drain A type of surgical drain often used as a constricting band.

percutaneous Through the skin or mucous membrane.

peripheral vein cannulation A technique in which a cannula (tube) is inserted into veins of the peripheral areas—that is, veins that can be seen and/or palpated. Examples of peripheral veins include those of the hand, arm, and lower extremity and the external jugular vein.

piercing spike The hard, sharpened plastic spike on the end of the administration set designed to pierce the sterile membrane of the intravenous bag.

prefilled syringes Medication syringes that are prepackaged and prepared with a specific concentration.

pressure infuser device A sleeve that is placed around the intravenous bag and inflated to force fluid to flow from the intravenous bag and into the tubing.

pulmonary embolism A blood clot or foreign matter trapped within the pulmonary circulation.

pyrogenic reaction A reaction characterized by an abrupt temperature elevation (as high as 106°F [41°C]) with severe chills, backache, headache, weakness, nausea, and vomiting; a potential complication of intravenous or intraosseous therapy.

saline locks Special types of intravenous devices that eliminate the need to hang a bag of intravenous fluid; also called a buff cap or INT (intermittent); commonly used for patients who do not require fluid boluses but may require medication therapy.

sharps Any contaminated item that can cause injury; includes intravenous needles and catheters, broken ampules or vials, or anything else that can penetrate or lacerate the skin.

sterile Devoid of all living organisms; achieved by using heat, gas, or chemicals.

subcutaneous Into the tissue between the skin and muscle; a medication delivery route.

sublingual Under the tongue; a medication delivery route.

suppository A drug mixed in a firm base that melts at body temperature and is shaped to fit the rectum.

systemic complications Reactions that affect systems of the body.

third spacing The shifting of fluid into the tissues, creating edema.

Prep Kit continued

thrombophlebitis Inflammation of a vein related to a thrombus (blood clot).

track marks The visible scars from repeated cannulation of a vein; commonly associated with illicit drug use.

transdermal Across the skin; a medication delivery route.

trocar A solid boring needle.

Vacutainer A cylindrical device that attaches to an 18- or 20-gauge sampling needle; accommodates self-sealing blood tubes when blood samples are being obtained.

varicose veins Veins on the leg that are large, twisted, and ropelike and can cause pain, swelling, or itching.

venous thrombosis The development of a stationary blood clot in the venous circulation.

vials Small glass or plastic bottles that contain medication; may contain single or multiple doses.

volume on hand The amount of fluid you have on hand, such as the amount of fluid in an intravenous bag or the amount of fluid in a vial of medication.

Volutrol A special type of microdrip set that features a 100- or 200-mL calibrated drip chamber; used for fluid regulation in patients susceptible to circulatory overload, such as pediatric and older patients; also called a Buretrol.

References

1. Hines S, Luna, K, Lofthus J, et al. *Becoming a High Reliability Organization: Operational Advice for Hospital Leaders*. (Prepared by the Lewin Group under Contract No. 290-04-0011.) AHRQ Publication No. 08-0022. Rockville, MD: Agency for Healthcare Research and Quality; April 2008.
2. Chassin MR, Loeb JM. High-reliability health care: getting there from here. The Joint Commission. *Milbank Q*. 2013;91(3):459-490.
3. National Highway Traffic Safety Administration. Patient safety in emergency medical services: roundtable report and recommendations. www.nhtsa.gov/people/injury/ems/archive/patient_safetyems/patientsafety02.doc. Published October 2002. Accessed June 7, 2021.
4. Misasi P, Braithwaite S. *The Medication Administration Cross-Check© (MACC) User's Manual*. Wichita-Sedgwick County EMS System; 2012. https://kansasemstransition.files.wordpress.com/2012/08/macc-user-manual-v2-0.pdf. Accessed June 7, 2021.
5. King KC, Strony R. Needlestick. *StatPearls*. https://www.ncbi.nlm.nih.gov/books/NBK493147/. Updated January 20, 2021. Accessed July 13, 2021.
6. National Association of Emergency Medical Technicians. *Advanced Medical Life Support*. 2nd ed. Burlington, MA: Jones & Bartlett Learning; 2017:159.
7. Alayash AI. Evaluating the safety and efficacy of hemoglobin-based blood substitutes. US Food and Drug Administration website. https://www.fda.gov/vaccines-blood-biologics/biologics-research-projects/evaluating-safety-and-efficacy-hemoglobin-based-blood-substitutes. Published June 26, 2020. Accessed July 13, 2021.
8. Cantor-Peled G, Halak M, Ovadia-Blechman Z. Peripheral vein locating techniques. *Imaging Med.* 2016;8(3). http://www.openaccessjournals.com/articles/peripheral-vein-locating-techniques.html. Accessed June 7, 2021.
9. Mbamalu D, Banerjee A. Methods of obtaining peripheral venous access in difficult situations. *Postgrad Med J*. 1999;75(886):459-462.
10. Hess D. Delivery of inhaled medication in adults. UpToDate website. https://www.uptodate.com/contents/delivery-of-inhaled-medication-in-adults/print. Updated December 18, 2020. Accessed July 13, 2021.
11. Smith C, Goldman RD. Nebulizers versus pressurized metered-dose inhalers in preschool children with wheezing. *Can Fam Physician*. 2012;58(5):528-530.
12. Link MS, Berkow LC, Kudenchuk PJ, et al. Part 7: adult advanced cardiovascular life support: 2015 American Heart Association Guidelines Update for Cardiopulmonary Resuscitation and Emergency Cardiovascular Care. *Circulation*. 2015;132(18 suppl 2):S444-S464.

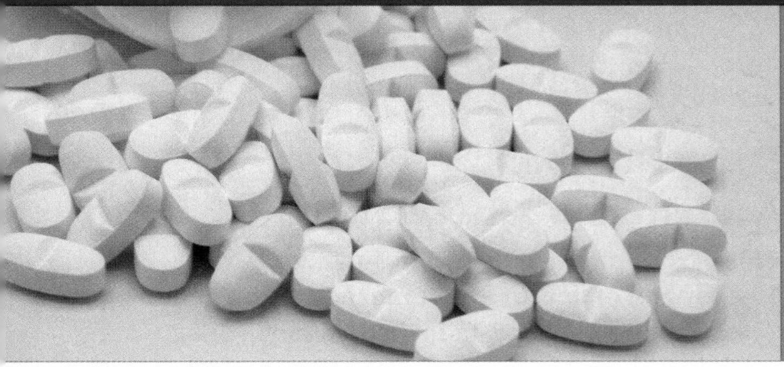

Chapter 15

Emergency Medications

NATIONAL EMS EDUCATION STANDARD COMPETENCIES

Pharmacology

Integrates comprehensive knowledge of pharmacology to formulate a treatment plan intended to mitigate emergencies and improve the patient's overall health.

Emergency Medications

- Actions (pp 888, 890–951)
- Indications (pp 888, 890–951)
- Contraindications (pp 888, 890–951)
- Adverse reactions/side effects (pp 888, 890–951)
- Interactions (pp 888, 890–951)
- Routes of administration (pp 888, 890–951)
- Dosages for the medications administered (pp 888, 890–951)
- Effects (pp 888, 890–951)
- Complications (pp 888, 890–951)

KNOWLEDGE OBJECTIVES

1. Explain the common elements of a drug profile. (p 888)
2. Define the abbreviations used in drug profiles. (p 889)
3. Give the generic and trade names, actions, indications, contraindications, adverse effects, interactions, routes of administration, and doses of medications that may be administered by the paramedic as dictated by state protocols and local medical direction. (pp 888–951)
4. Give the generic and trade names, actions, indications, contraindications, adverse effects, interactions, routes of administration, and doses of intravenous fluids that may be administered by the paramedic as dictated by state protocols and local medical direction. (pp 947–951)

SKILLS OBJECTIVES

There are no skills objectives for this chapter.

Pharmacology Formulary

The formulary provided in this chapter provides a reference for paramedic students as they progress through their education. Recall that "tall man" lettering is sometimes used to avoid confusion of medications with similar spellings.[1] With tall man lettering, capitalization draws attention to the letters that differentiate one medication's name from similar names, as described in Chapter 13, *Principles of Pharmacology*. The drug profiles included in this chapter use tall man lettering, as guided by the Food and Drug Administration,[1] to help reduce medication-related errors.

Current recommendations from multiple resources are referenced throughout these drug profiles. The emergency medications commonly used by paramedics are broken down into the following components, listed in this order:

Generic Name (Trade Name[s])
Class
Mechanism of action
Indications
Contraindications
Adverse reactions/side effects
Drug interactions
Dosage and administration *Adult:*____ *Pediatric:*______
Duration of action *Onset:*________ *Peak effect:*______ *Duration:*______
Special considerations

Medications that are often used in health care delivery but not typically administered by paramedics, including those that patients may be taking for chronic conditions, are presented using a similar but less detailed format. Although paramedics will not carry or administer these medications, they need to understand how these medications affect their patients and the treatment they are providing.

The abbreviations used in the drug profiles that follow are listed in **TABLE 15-1**. It is important to remember that state and regional EMS systems have the right to include other medications in their own formularies, and that the indications for these medications may not be covered in this formulary. Always follow your local protocols.

Drug Profiles

Acetaminophen (Tylenol)

Class Nonopioid analgesic, antipyretic.

Mechanism of action Exact mechanism of action has not been fully established; it may work peripherally to block pain impulse generation and inhibit prostaglandin synthesis in the CNS leading to its analgesic and antipyretic effects.

Indications Pain control, fever control.

Contraindications Known hypersensitivity, severe active liver disease.

Adverse reactions/side effects Nausea, upper abdominal pain, skin rash, itching, loss of appetite; overdose can cause hepatotoxicity.

Drug interactions Increased effect with caffeine; decreased effect with antacids, anticholinergics, carbamazepine, phenytoin. Alcohol may increase hepatotoxicity risk.

Dosage and administration *Adult*:[2] Give 15 mg/kg orally; maximum dose is 1 g. *Pediatric*: Febrile seizures:[2] Give 15 mg/kg; maximum dose is 650 mg; PR/IV/IO (if unable to swallow) or orally if able to swallow.

Duration of action *Onset*: 10 to 30 minutes. *Peak effect*: 30 to 60 minutes. *Duration*: 4 to 6 hours.

Special considerations Pregnancy safety: Category B. Although its analgesic and antipyretic properties are similar to those of NSAIDs, acetaminophen does not have significant anti-inflammatory or antiplatelet effects. Acetaminophen is often combined with scheduled drugs and OTC allergy medications, cough and cold medications, sleep medications, pain relievers, and other products. Since 2011, the FDA has limited the acetaminophen dose to 325 mg when combined with other drugs because of the potential for harm caused with high doses or long-term use.[3] Document pain severity using a scale of 0 to 10 before and after administration and on arrival at the receiving facility.[2]

AcetaZOLAMIDE (Diamox, Diamox Sequels)

Class Carbonic anhydrase inhibitor, diuretic.

Mechanism of action Inhibits hydrogen ion excretion in the renal tubules, increasing sodium, potassium, bicarbonate, and water excretion and producing alkaline diuresis.

TABLE 15-1 Abbreviations Used in Formulary Drug Profiles

Abbreviation	Term	Abbreviation	Term
ACE	angiotensin-converting enzyme	IO	intraosseous
ACS	acute coronary syndrome	IV	intravenous
AF	atrial fibrillation	MAOI	monoamine oxidase inhibitor
AMI	acute myocardial infarction	MAP	mean arterial pressure
AMS	acute mountain sickness	MDI	metered-dose inhaler
ARDS	acute respiratory distress syndrome	MI	myocardial infarction
ASA	acetylsalicylic acid	MOI	mechanism of injury
AV	atrioventricular	NG	nasogastric
BP	blood pressure	NSAID	nonsteroidal anti-inflammatory drug
CAD	coronary artery disease	NSTEMI	non-ST-segment elevation myocardial infarction
CNS	central nervous system	NTG	nitroglycerin
COPD	chronic obstructive pulmonary disease	OTC	over the counter
COVID-19	coronavirus disease 2019	PAC	premature atrial complex
CPR	cardiopulmonary resuscitation	PCI	percutaneous coronary intervention
CVA	cerebrovascular accident	PE	pulmonary embolism
D_5W	dextrose 5% in water (numeral depends on percentage of dextrose)	PEA	pulseless electrical activity
DBP	diastolic blood pressure	PR	per the rectum
DVT	deep vein thrombosis	PSVT	paroxysmal supraventricular tachycardia
ECG	electrocardiogram	PTCA	percutaneous transluminal coronary angioplasty
ET	endotracheal	PVC	premature ventricular complex
ETT	endotracheal tube	RSI	rapid sequence intubation
FDA	US Food and Drug Administration	RV	right ventricular
GABA	gamma-aminobutyric acid	SBP	systolic blood pressure
GERD	gastroesophageal reflux disease	SL	sublingual
GI	gastrointestinal	SNRI	serotonin-norepinephrine reuptake inhibitor
GP IIb/IIIa	glycoprotein IIb/IIIa	SSRI	selective serotonin reuptake inhibitor
H_1/H_2	histamine H_1/H_2 receptor	STEMI	ST-segment elevation myocardial infarction
HACE	high-altitude cerebral edema	SVT	supraventricular tachycardia
HAPE	high-altitude pulmonary edema	TCA	tricyclic antidepressant
HIV	human immunodeficiency virus	TdP	torsades de pointes
ICP	intracranial pressure	TKO	to keep open
IM	intramuscular	VF	ventricular fibrillation
IN	intranasal	VT	ventricular tachycardia

Indications AMS (treatment and prophylaxis), prevention of HACE.

Contraindications Hypersensitivity to acetaZOLAMIDE or sulfa, known hypokalemia, known hyponatremia, renal dysfunction, liver dysfunction. Should not be used for the treatment of HAPE.[4]

Adverse reactions/side effects Fluid and electrolyte imbalance, metabolic acidosis, seizures, nausea, vomiting, anorexia, orthostatic hypotension.

Drug interactions Increased risk of severe acidosis and CNS toxicity with high-dose aspirin. Use caution with diuretics, anticonvulsants. May potentiate the effects of hypoglycemics. Increased risk of renal calculus formation with sodium bicarbonate administration.

Dosage and administration (regular-release tablets) *Adult*: Treatment of AMS: 250 mg orally every 12 hours is recommended by clinical practice guidelines.[4,5] *Pediatric*: Treatment of AMS: 2.5 mg/kg orally every 12 hours (maximum: 250 mg/dose) is recommended by clinical practice guidelines.[4,5]

Duration of action (regular-release tablets) *Onset*: 1 to 1.5 hours. *Peak effect*: 2 to 4 hours. *Duration*: 4 to 12 hours.

Special considerations Pregnancy safety: Category C. AcetaZOLAMIDE can be used at the dosages specified for AMS treatment as an *adjunct* to dexamethasone in HACE treatment, but dexamethasone remains the primary treatment for HACE.[4]

Acetic Acid (vinegar)

Class Otic anti-infective, irrigating solution.

Mechanism of action Otic solution provides an acidic medium during irrigation of the ear that minimizes bacterial and fungal promulgation; may stabilize nematocyst discharge in jellyfish found outside the United States, thereby decreasing pain.[2]

Indications Otitis externa, pain control for envenomation by jellyfish from outside the United States.[2]

Contraindications Hypersensitivity, perforated tympanic membranes, may increase nematocyst discharge for US jellyfish and should be used only outside the United States.[2]

Adverse reactions/side effects Skin irritation, sensitivity, stinging sensation.

Drug interactions None currently identified.

Dosage and administration *Adult and pediatric*: For otic administration, position the patient on the side with the affected ear uppermost, instill 4 to 6 drops into the external ear, and repeat every 2 to 3 hours. For jellyfish stings outside the United States, rinse the area with vinegar (4% to 6% acetic acid) for 30 seconds to limit the discharge of unfired nematocysts remaining on the skin.

Duration of action *Onset*: 5 minutes. *Peak effect*: 45 to 90 minutes. *Duration*: 2 to 3 hours.

Special considerations Pregnancy safety: Category C. Safety and efficacy of acetic acid otic solution has not been established in children younger than 3 years.[5] Several treatment approaches for jellyfish stings, including the topical use of acetic acid, are based on weak scientific evidence and require further study.

Acetylcysteine (Mucomyst, Acetadote)

Class Acetaminophen antidote.

Mechanism of action Restores glutathione concentrations within the liver. Glutathione, an antioxidant, has many actions in the body, including detoxifying substances.

Indications Acetaminophen overdose.

Contraindications Known hypersensitivity, acute asthma.

Adverse reactions/side effects Urticaria, flushing, rash, itching, angioedema, nausea, vomiting, bronchospasm, wheezing, respiratory distress, tachycardia, hypotension.

Drug interactions Nitroglycerin.

Dosage and administration *Adult and pediatric*: Acetaminophen overdose:[2] Loading dose 150 mg/kg IV, mix in 200 mL of D_5W and infuse over 1 hour. Then give 50 mg/kg IV in 500 mL D_5W and infuse over 4 hours. If IV access is not available, give acetylcysteine 140 mg/kg orally.

Duration of action *Onset*: 1 minute. *Peak effect*: 5 to 15 minutes. *Duration*: 100 minutes.

Special considerations Pregnancy safety: Category B. Use cautiously in pregnant and breastfeeding women and only if clearly indicated. When given IV, acetylcysteine can cause anaphylactoid-type reactions (eg, rash, itching, angioedema, bronchospasm, hypotension), usually following the first dose. Reactions may be more common in patients with a history of asthma or reactive airway disease. Reactions can be minimized by ensuring that the medication is infused over 1 hour. Acetylcysteine smells like rotten eggs because of its sulfur content.

Activated Charcoal (Insta-Char, Actidose-Aqua, Liqui-Char)

Class Adsorbent, antidote.

Mechanism of action Adsorbs ingested toxic substances from the GI tract, thereby preventing their systemic absorption.

Indications Most oral poisonings and medication overdoses in the alert patient; can be used after evacuation of poisons.

Contraindications Known hypersensitivity, unprotected airway (beware of aspiration), absence of a gag reflex, ileus, intestinal obstruction; do not use after ingestion of petroleum distillates, hydrocarbons, heavy metals, acids or alkalis (corrosives), alcohols, iron, lithium, solvents. Use caution in patients experiencing abdominal pain of unknown origin or a known GI obstruction.

Adverse reactions/side effects Emesis (if aspirated from emesis or a misplaced NG tube, can induce a fatal form of pneumonitis), constipation, black stools, diarrhea, bowel obstruction.

Drug interactions Bonds with and generally inactivates whatever it is mixed with (eg, syrup of ipecac); moderate interactions with acetylcysteine, citalopram, digoxin, dyphylline, methotrexate, and theophylline.

Dosage and administration *Adult and pediatric older than 1 year*: 25 to 100 g orally or via NG tube. *Pediatric younger than 1 year*: 1 g/kg orally or via NG tube.

Duration of action *Onset*: Immediate. *Peak effect*: Depends on GI function. *Duration*: Will act until excreted.

Special considerations Pregnancy safety: Category C. Shake vigorously before use because separation occurs while it is being stored. Before administering in cases of acetaminophen overdose, contact medical direction because charcoal has moderate interactions with acetylcysteine, an antidote used for acetaminophen overdose. Charcoal aspiration can produce a situation in which management of the patient's airway is nearly impossible; therefore, do not administer activated charcoal to any patient who may have a worsening mental status without first protecting their airway.[2] Activated charcoal is no longer used in some EMS systems, but paramedics may still encounter it.

Adenosine (Adenocard)

Class Antidysrhythmic.

Mechanism of action Short-acting drug that slows conduction through the AV node; can restore sinus rhythm in patients with SVT and terminate regular tachycardias caused by reentrant AV nodal pathways.

Indications First-line drug for most forms of stable, regular, narrow-complex SVT, including those involving AV nodal reentry. May be considered for unstable narrow-complex reentry tachycardia while preparing for cardioversion. Can be used diagnostically for stable, regular, monomorphic wide-complex tachycardia.

Contraindications Known hypersensitivity. Second- or third-degree AV block or sick sinus syndrome or other sinus node disease unless a functioning artificial pacemaker is present; poison- or drug-induced tachycardia. Use with caution in patients with a history of seizure disorder.[5] May induce bronchospasm in a patient with bronchoconstrictive or bronchospastic lung disease (asthma, COPD).

Adverse reactions/side effects Generally transient and of short duration because of adenosine's short half-life; flushing, sweating, dizziness, nervousness, paresthesia, hypotension, feeling of impending doom, severe bronchospasm in patients with asthma. A brief period of most any dysrhythmia, including asystole, may occur during pharmacologic conversion.[6]

Drug interactions Additive effects are possible if used in combination with beta blockers. Methylxanthines (caffeine and theophylline-like drugs) block the actions of adenosine. Dipyridamole (Persantine) potentiates the effect of adenosine. Carbamazepine (Tegretol) may potentiate the AV node blocking effect of adenosine. Nicotine can enhance adenosine's cardiovascular effects; an increase in angina-like chest discomfort or heart rate, or a decrease in BP may be observed.[5]

Dosage and administration *Adult*:[2,7] Give a 6-mg rapid IV/IO bolus over 1 to 3 seconds injected into the IV port as close to the heart as possible, followed by a 10-mL saline flush. If no conversion occurs after 1 to 2 minutes, administer a 12-mg rapid IV/IO bolus over 1 to 3 seconds. May repeat the 12-mg dose once if needed if no conversion occurs after 1 to 2 minutes. Maximum total dosage is 30 mg. Reduce the dose by one-half in patients taking dipyridamole (Persantine) or carbamazepine (Tegretol), in those with transplanted hearts (the transplanted heart is supersensitive to adenosine), or if given via a central IV line.[5] *Pediatric*: [2,7] Initial dose 0.1 mg/kg rapid IV/IO push over 1 to 3 seconds (maximum first dose, 6 mg), followed by a 5- to 10-mL saline flush. Second dose 0.2 mg/kg rapid IV/IO push (maximum second dose, 12 mg) followed by a 5- to 10-mL saline flush.

Duration of action *Onset*: Seconds. *Peak effect*: Seconds. *Duration*: 10 seconds.

Special considerations Pregnancy safety: Category C. Use in pregnant women only if clearly indicated. Continuously monitor the ECG and record a rhythm strip during administration. Ineffective in converting AF, atrial flutter, or VT. Should not be administered for hemodynamically unstable, irregularly irregular, or polymorphic wide-complex tachycardias.

Albuterol (Proventil, Ventolin, Proair, Accuneb)

Class Sympathomimetic, bronchodilator, short-acting beta-2 adrenergic agonist.

Mechanism of action Selective beta-2 adrenergic agonist that causes bronchial smooth muscle relaxation and inhibits mediator release from mast cells.

Indications Treatment and prevention of bronchospasm in patients with reversible obstructive airway disease, treatment of inhaled airway/respiratory irritant agents, and hyperkalemia treatment.

Contraindications Known hypersensitivity; dysrhythmias, especially those caused by digitalis. Synergistic with other sympathomimetics.

Adverse reactions/side effects Often dose-related; include tremors, headaches, nervousness, dizziness, dysrhythmias, chest discomfort, palpitations, nausea/vomiting, and dry mouth.

Drug interactions Additive effects with TCAs, MAOIs, other sympathomimetics. Beta blockers may inhibit pulmonary effects, decreasing effectiveness. May potentiate hypokalemia caused by diuretics.

Dosage and administration *Adult*: Respiratory distress: 2.5 to 5 mg via nebulizer or 1 to 2 inhalations (90 to 180 mcg) by MDI. Respiratory distress with signs of bronchospasm:[2] Give 5 mg via nebulizer or 6 puffs via MDI; repeat this dose with unlimited frequency for ongoing distress. Hyperkalemia:[2] Give 5 mg via nebulizer. *Pediatric*: Mild to moderate asthma, anaphylaxis, hyperkalemia:[7] Using MDI: 4 to 8 puffs as needed every 20 minutes with a spacer. If using a nebulizer and the patient weighs less than 20 kg, give 2.5 mg/dose, or if the patient weighs more than 20 kg, give 5 mg/dose, every 20 minutes. Respiratory distress with signs of bronchospasm:[2] Give 5 mg via nebulizer or 6 puffs via MDI; repeat at this dose with unlimited frequency for ongoing distress.

Duration of action *Onset*: 5 to 15 minutes. *Peak effect*: 30 minutes to 2 hours. *Duration*: 3 to 6 hours.

Special considerations Pregnancy safety: Category C. May precipitate angina pectoris and dysrhythmias. Patients may need to be coached on proper use of the MDI, particularly one with a spacer. Current evidence does not demonstrate a benefit in using albuterol for bronchiolitis.[2]

Commonly Prescribed and OTC Medications

Alprazolam (Xanax)

Class Benzodiazepine, sedative-hypnotic, anticonvulsant; Schedule IV drug.

Indications Anxiety, panic disorder, depression.

Contraindications Known hypersensitivity, respiratory depression, acute alcohol intoxication, psychotic reactions, recent use of respiratory depressants, acute narrow-angle glaucoma.

Adverse reactions/side effects Dizziness, drowsiness, fatigue, CNS depression, headache, difficulty concentrating, changes in sex drive, weight changes.

Drug interactions May precipitate CNS depression if taken with alcohol or other CNS depressants. Grapefruit increases alprazolam levels, and green tea decreases alprazolam effects.

Special considerations Can cause fetal abnormalities and should not be used in pregnancy. Should not be taken while breastfeeding.

Amiodarone (Cordarone, Pacerone)

Class Antidysrhythmic (Class III).

Mechanism of action Blocks sodium, potassium, and calcium channels; prolongs the action potential's duration and delays repolarization; decreases AV conduction and sinoatrial (SA) node function.

Indications Cardiac arrest resulting from VF or pulseless VT after CPR, defibrillation, and epinephrine; stable, regular narrow-complex tachycardia if the rhythm persists despite vagal maneuvers or adenosine or the tachycardia is recurrent; to control the ventricular rate in AF with a rapid ventricular response without pre-excitation; stable wide-complex tachycardia; stable monomorphic VT; polymorphic VT with a normal QT interval.

Contraindications Known hypersensitivity, iodine hypersensitivity (iodine is incorporated in amiodarone's chemical structure),[5] cardiogenic shock, second- or third-degree AV block, or sick sinus syndrome or other sinus node disease unless a functioning artificial pacemaker is present.

Adverse reactions/side effects Hypotension, heart failure, worsening of dysrhythmias, prolonged QT interval, bradycardia, AV block, dizziness, fatigue, cough, progressive dyspnea, nausea, vomiting, burning at the IV site, Stevens-Johnson syndrome.

Drug interactions May increase the effects of digoxin, disopyramide, fentanyl, lidocaine, procainamide, quinidine, or warfarin. Cimetidine may increase amiodarone levels. Use with beta blockers or calcium channel blockers may potentiate bradycardia, sinus arrest, and AV blocks. Persistent use of echinacea can potentiate amiodarone's hepatotoxic effects.[8]

Dosage and administration *Adult*: VF/pulseless VT:[2,7] Initial dose 300 mg IV/IO push. Second dose (if needed) 150 mg IV/IO push. Other indications: Loading dose of 150 mg IV/IO over 10 minutes; may repeat every 10 minutes if needed. After conversion, follow with an infusion of 10 to 50 mg/h over 24 hours.[2] Maximum cumulative dose: 2.2 g IV/IO per 24 hours. *Pediatric*: Refractory VF/pulseless VT: [7] Give 5 mg/kg IV/IO bolus. Can repeat the 5 mg/kg IV/IO bolus up to a total dose of 15 mg/kg IV per 24 hours (2.2 g in adolescents) per 24 hours. Maximum single dose: 300 mg. Poor perfusing ventricular or atrial dysrhythmias:[7] Loading dose 5 mg/kg IV/IO over 20 to 60 minutes (maximum single dose: 300 mg); can repeat to a maximum dose of 15 mg/kg IV per 24 hours (2.2 g in adolescents).

Duration of action *Onset*: 2 hours. *Peak effect*: 3 to 7 hours. *Duration*: Variable.

Special considerations Pregnancy safety: Category D. Drug may cause fetal harm. Fetal risk and maternal benefit should be considered in the emergency setting. Lactating women should not breastfeed following use. May worsen or precipitate new dysrhythmias. Monitor the patient for hypotension and increasing PR and QT intervals. Dosage may change per the most current International Liaison Committee on Resuscitation (ILCOR) recommendations.

Antibiotics

Antibiotics are medications used to kill bacteria or inhibit their growth and replication. They are often classified by their chemical structure or spectrum of activity. Common antibiotics are listed in **TABLE 15-2**.

TABLE 15-2 Common Antibiotics

Aminoglycosides	
Examples	gentamycin (Garamycin), neomycin (Mycifradin), streptomycin (Streptomycin), tobramycin (Tobrex, Nebcin)
Action	Inhibit protein synthesis by binding to ribosomes, causing bacterial cell death.
Indications	Vary depending on the drug. Severe infections of the abdomen and urinary tract, bacteremia, pneumonia, endocarditis prophylaxis, tularemia, plague, bone and joint infections.
Contraindications	Known hypersensitivity. Use with caution in patients with electrolyte imbalance, dehydration, renal disease, neuromuscular disorders (myasthenia gravis, parkinsonism), hearing impairment, and older adults.
Adverse reactions/ side effects	Headache, fever, rash, nausea, vomiting, anemia, superinfection (a secondary infection that occurs when the body flora is disturbed), kidney dysfunction, and inner ear toxicity that can lead to vestibular and auditory dysfunction.
Drug interactions	Acute neuromuscular blockade can occur if used with anesthetic drugs and can enhance other neuromuscular-blocking drugs. Increases risk of ototoxicity with loop diuretics. Increased risk of nephrotoxicity if taken with NSAIDs, diuretics, cephalosporins, and antifungals.
Special considerations	Narrow therapeutic index. Most aminoglycosides are poorly absorbed from the GI tract and are only given parenterally. Neomycin is associated with the most nephrotoxicity; streptomycin is the least nephrotoxic.
Cephalosporins	
Examples	cefazolin (Ancef, Kefzol), cephalexin (Keflex), cefuroxime (Kefurox, Zinacef), cefuroxime axetil (Ceftin), ceftriaxone (Rocephin)
Action	Kill bacteria by preventing the formation of the bacterial cell wall.
Indications	Vary depending on the drug. Uses include skin and soft-tissue infections, perioperative surgical prophylaxis, strep throat, upper respiratory tract infections (sinusitis, otitis media), pneumonia, meningitis, urinary tract infections, streptococcal endocarditis, gonorrhea, severe Lyme disease, and sepsis.
Contraindications	Known hypersensitivity to cephalosporins.
Adverse reactions/ side effects	Nausea, vomiting, diarrhea, dizziness, increased blood clotting time with large doses, oral thrush, anal or vaginal yeast. Severe adverse reactions include anaphylaxis, angioedema, seizures, and *Clostridioides difficile*–associated diarrhea.
Drug interactions	Vary depending on the drug. Some cephalosporins decrease oral contraceptive effectiveness and increase bleeding risk if taken with anticoagulants or salicylates.
Special considerations	Some patients allergic to penicillin could be allergic to a cephalosporin. Unless contraindicated, patients are typically advised to ingest buttermilk, yogurt, or an acidophilus supplement to prevent superinfection of the intestinal flora.[a]
Macrolides and Lincosamines	
Examples	azithromycin (Zithromax), clarithromycin (Biaxin), clindamycin (Cleocin), erythromycin (E-mycin), lincomycin (Lincocin)
Action	Interfere with protein synthesis in bacterial cells, inhibiting bacterial growth and reproduction.

Indications	Vary depending on the drug, but common uses include otitis media, tonsillitis, duodenal ulcer caused by *Helicobacter pylori*, sepsis, endocarditis and other cardiac infections, sexually transmitted infections, diphtheria, osteomyelitis, upper and lower respiratory tract infections, and skin and soft-tissue infections.
Contraindications	Hypersensitivity to macrolide antibiotics. Some macrolides should not be taken during pregnancy. Use with caution in patients with cardiac disease or other conditions that may increase the risk of QT prolongation, including cardiac dysrhythmias, congenital long QT syndrome, heart failure, MI, hypertension, CAD, hypomagnesemia, hypokalemia, and hypocalcemia, or in patients receiving medications known to prolong the QT interval or cause electrolyte imbalances.[b] Macrolides are associated with myasthenia gravis exacerbations.
Adverse reactions/ side effects	Nausea, vomiting, dry skin, erythema, pruritis, headache, abdominal pain and cramping, *C difficile* infection, colitis, liver dysfunction, superinfection. Azithromycin is associated with prolonged QT interval, liver damage.
Drug interactions	Extensive. Can increase serum levels of theophylline, carbamazepine, and warfarin. Hepatotoxicity can occur when erythromycin and azithromycin are taken in high doses with other hepatotoxic drugs, such as phenothiazines, sulfonamides, or acetaminophen.[a] Should not be taken with some antihistamines or statins. Azithromycin increases the effects of digoxin and warfarin, and decreases the effects of penicillins and clindamycin. Simultaneous use of clindamycin with neuromuscular blockers may prolong neuromuscular blockade. Increased risk of sudden cardiac death when erythromycin is given concurrently with verapamil or diltiazem.[a]
Special considerations	Azithromycin has been associated with an increased risk of cardiovascular death.[b]
Penicillins	
Examples	amoxicillin (Amoxil), amoxicillin-clavulanic acid (Augmentin), ampicillin (Omnipen), methicillin (Staphcillin), penicillin G (Bicillin), penicillin V (Pen-Veek), ticarcillin (Ticar)
Action	Kill bacteria by preventing the formation of the bacterial cell wall.
Indications	Vary depending on the drug. Typical uses include otitis media; sinusitis; respiratory, skin, and urinary tract infections. Some penicillins are used to treat anthrax, meningitis, diphtheria, osteomyelitis, syphilis, pericarditis, endocarditis, and severe staphylococcal infections.
Contraindications	Known hypersensitivity to penicillin; dosage adjustment for patients with liver disease or end-stage renal disease.
Adverse reactions/ side effects	Superinfection (oral thrush, anal or vaginal yeast), anorexia, nausea, vomiting, diarrhea. Rash with mild to moderate reaction. Laryngeal edema, bronchoconstriction with stridor, hypotension with severe allergic reaction.
Drug interactions	Vary depending on the drug. Some penicillins decrease oral contraceptive effectiveness and have decreased effects when taken with tetracycline, erythromycin, acidic fruits, and juices. Increased risk of bleeding with oral anticoagulants.
Special considerations	Rash can appear a week after starting therapy. Some patients who are allergic to penicillin could be allergic to a cephalosporin. Individuals with a history of asthma, eczema, or hay fever may be at increased risk of developing a serious allergic reaction to penicillins.

(continues)

TABLE 15-2 Common Antibiotics (continued)

Quinolones and Fluoroquinolones	
Examples	ciprofloxacin (Cipro), levofloxacin (Levaquin), moxifloxacin (Avelox), ofloxacin (Floxin)
Action	Kill bacteria by inhibiting bacterial enzymes needed to replicate the bacterial DNA, thereby preventing the bacteria from multiplying.
Indications	Vary depending on the drug, but uses include UTIs, septicemia and intra-abdominal infections, joint and bone infections, upper and lower respiratory infections (sinusitis, pneumonia, bronchitis), soft-tissue and skin infections, typhoid fever, anthrax, bacterial gastroenteritis, pelvic inflammatory disease, and urethral and gynecologic infections.
Contraindications	Known hypersensitivity. Vary depending on the drug. Pregnancy, breastfeeding. Risk of worsening symptoms for patients with myasthenia gravis. Avoid simultaneous administration with drugs that prolong the QT interval.
Adverse reactions/ side effects	Nausea, vomiting, diarrhea, headache, skin rash, QT prolongation, seizures, hallucinations, angioedema, photosensitivity, hypoglycemia (including risk of hypoglycemic coma), and tendon, muscle, or joint pain, usually involving the knee, elbow, or shoulder; potential for irreversible peripheral neuropathy.
Drug interactions	Extensive. Interactions with NSAIDs, theophylline, TCAs, and corticosteroids, among others. May lower insulin requirements.
Special considerations	In 2018, the FDA required that mental health side effects be listed separately from other CNS side effects in the labeling for all fluoroquinolones and reflect disturbances in attention, disorientation, agitation, nervousness, memory impairment, and delirium.
Sulfonamides	
Examples	silver sulfADIAZINE (Silvadene), sulfADIAZINE (Sulfadiazine), sulfasalazine (Sulfasalazine, Azulfidine), trimethoprim-sulfamethoxazole (Bactrim, Septra)
Action	Inhibit the ability of bacteria to produce a form of folic acid that is necessary to make DNA and proteins, preventing the bacteria from multiplying.
Indications	Vary depending on the drug, but uses include some types of bacterial pneumonia, UTIs, and some protozoal infections.
Contraindications	Known hypersensitivity. Pregnancy (especially third trimester), nursing mothers, infants younger than 2 months.
Adverse reactions/ side effects	Dizziness, headache, lethargy, diarrhea, anorexia, nausea, vomiting, skin rash, hives, photosensitivity, liver damage, urinary crystal formation, leukopenia, anemia, thrombocytopenia.
Drug interactions	Increased bleeding risk with warfarin. Can increase blood levels of digoxin and lead to digoxin toxicity. Hyperkalemia may occur when sulfamethoxazole is taken with an ACE inhibitor. May lower insulin requirements.
Special considerations	Patients receiving sulfonamides should avoid excessive exposure to sunlight. Adequate hydration is essential to prevent urinary crystal formation.
Tetracyclines	
Examples	doxycycline (Doxy, Vibramycin), minocycline (Minocin), tetracycline (Sumycin)
Action	Inhibit protein synthesis in bacterial cells, hindering their growth and reproduction.

Indications	Vary depending on the drug, but typically used to treat infections of the urinary tract, respiratory tract, and skin. Also used in the treatment of chlamydia, gonorrhea, moderately severe acne, rosacea, anthrax, cholera, plague, typhus, Rocky Mountain spotted fever, and *Helicobacter pylori*.
Contraindications	Known hypersensitivity. Vary depending on the drug, Avoid in pregnancy or if breastfeeding (can impair bone development in infants). Most tetracyclines should be avoided in patients with liver disease, kidney disease, or lupus.
Adverse reactions/ side effects	Superinfection (oral thrush, anal or vaginal yeast), photosensitivity, diarrhea, nausea, vomiting, abdominal pain, rash, headache, dizziness.
Drug interactions	Numerous. Should not be taken with magnesium- and aluminum-containing antacid preparations, milk products containing calcium, or iron-containing drugs. Some tetracyclines may increase the effects of digoxin and warfarin. St. John's wort may increase photosensitivity risk.
Special considerations	Patients receiving tetracyclines should avoid excessive exposure to sunlight. Can cause permanent discoloration of the teeth if used in patients younger than 8 years.

Abbreviations: ACE, angiotensin-converting enzyme; CAD, coronary artery disease; CNS, central nervous system; DNA, deoxyribonucleic acid; FDA, US Food and Drug Administration; GI, gastrointestinal; MI, myocardial infarction; NSAIDs, nonsteroid anti-inflammatory drugs; TCAs, tricyclic antidepressants; UTIs, urinary tract infections

[a] McCuistion LE, DiMaggio KV, Winton MB, Yeager JJ. *Pharmacology: A Patient-Centered Nursing Process Approach*, 10th ed. St. Louis, MO: Elsevier; 2021.

[b] Prescriber's Digital Reference [homepage]. https://www.pdr.net/. Accessed July 16, 2021.

Anticoagulants

Anticoagulants prevent the formation of new clots but do not dissolve existing clots. Some of these medications require regular coagulation monitoring to prevent excessive anticoagulation, and patients taking them are typically advised to wear medical identification. Common anticoagulants are listed in **TABLE 15-3**.

TABLE 15-3 Common Anticoagulants

Apixaban (Eliquis)	
Indications	DVT, PE, stroke and systemic embolism prophylaxis.
Contraindications	Known hypersensitivity, active pathologic bleeding.
Adverse reactions/side effects	Syncope, rash, bleeding, hematoma, stroke, anaphylactoid reactions.
Drug interactions	Several. Increased risk of bleeding if used with other drugs that affect coagulation (eg, aspirin and other antiplatelet drugs, other anticoagulants, fibrinolytic agents, SSRIs, SNRIs, and NSAIDs), increased bleeding risk if used with amiodarone, additive bleeding may occur if given in combination with garlic, ginkgo, grapefruit, grapefruit juice, or green tea.
Special considerations	Direct factor Xa inhibitor. This medication does not require routine coagulation monitoring.
Dabigatran (Pradaxa)	
Indications	DVT, PE, stroke and systemic embolism prophylaxis.
Contraindications	Hypersensitivity, prosthetic heart valves, active pathologic bleeding, renal failure or impairment, dialysis.

(continues)

TABLE 15-3 Common Anticoagulants (continued)

Adverse reactions/side effects	Itching, hives, rash, abdominal pain, angioedema, stroke, bleeding, gastritis, anaphylaxis, anaphylactoid reactions.
Drug interactions	Increased risk of bleeding if used with other drugs that affect coagulation (eg, aspirin and other antiplatelet drugs, other anticoagulants, fibrinolytic agents, SSRIs, SNRIs, and NSAIDs); increased bleeding risk if used with amiodarone or verapamil; additive bleeding may occur if given in combination with garlic, ginger, ginkgo, grapefruit juice, or green tea. St. John's wort can reduce effectiveness.
Special considerations	Thrombin inhibitor. This medication does not require routine coagulation monitoring.
Enoxaparin (Lovenox)	
Indications	Prophylaxis and treatment of DVT, PE; treatment of ACS.
Contraindications	Known hypersensitivity to enoxaparin, heparin, or pork products; active major bleeding; thrombocytopenia.
Adverse reactions/side effects	Diarrhea, nausea, anemia, AF, heart failure, intracranial hemorrhage, pneumonia.
Drug interactions	Additive risk for bleeding if given in combination with other agents that affect hemostasis (eg, aspirin and other antiplatelet drugs, other anticoagulants, fibrinolytic agents, SSRIs, SNRIs, and NSAIDs), some penicillins.
Special considerations	Low-molecular-weight heparin. Use cautiously in pregnant women with threatened abortion, and monitor all pregnant women for potential bleeding. Do not administer medication from a multidose vial to pregnant women due to the benzyl alcohol content. Dose adjustments are needed for patients with renal dysfunction.
Heparin Sodium	
Indications	AMI, prophylaxis and treatment of thromboembolic disorders (eg, PE and DVT).
Contraindications	Known hypersensitivity; active bleeding, severe hypertension, bleeding tendencies, or severe thrombocytopenia; recent intracranial, intraspinal, or eye surgery.
Adverse reactions/side effects	Pain, anaphylaxis, shock, hematuria, GI bleeding, hemorrhage, thrombocytopenia, bruising.
Drug interactions	Additive risk for bleeding if given in combination with other agents that affect hemostasis (eg, aspirin and other antiplatelet drugs, other anticoagulants, fibrinolytic agents, SSRIs, SNRIs, and NSAIDs), some penicillins. Decreased effect with NTG.
Special considerations	Requires regular coagulation monitoring to prevent excessive anticoagulation. If heparin is used with fibrinolytic therapy, obtain a blood sample for control of partial thromboplastin time before heparin administration. If the patient experiences uncontrollable bleeding, the reversal agent is protamine.
Rivaroxaban (Xarelto)	
Indications	Prophylaxis and treatment of DVT, PE, and stroke.
Contraindications	Known hypersensitivity, bleeding, moderate or severe hepatic disease, renal failure, renal impairment.
Adverse reactions/side effects	Abdominal and back pain, dizziness, itching, insomnia, fatigue, syncope, angioedema, anaphylaxis, GI bleeding, intracranial bleeding.

Drug interactions	May increase bleeding when taken with other medications that affect coagulation (eg, aspirin and other antiplatelet drugs, other anticoagulants, fibrinolytic agents, SSRIs, SNRIs, and NSAIDs). Increased bleeding may occur when taken with garlic, ginger, ginkgo, grapefruit juice, and green tea. St. John's wort can reduce effectiveness.
Special considerations	Direct factor Xa inhibitor. This medication does not require routine coagulation monitoring.
Warfarin (Coumadin, Jantoven)	
Indications	Prevention and treatment of thromboembolic disease.
Contraindications	Known hypersensitivity. Because warfarin can cause major or fatal bleeding, its use is contraindicated in patients with conditions in which warfarin therapy may result in uncontrolled bleeding.[a]
Adverse reactions/side effects	Chills, headache, vomiting, nausea, fatigue, pallor, dizziness, itching, hives, syncope, bleeding, hypotension.
Drug interactions	Numerous. Additive risk for bleeding if given in combination with other agents that affect hemostasis (eg, aspirin and other antiplatelet drugs, other anticoagulants, fibrinolytic agents, SSRIs, SNRIs, and NSAIDs). Amiodarone and cimetidine are among the many medications that can potentiate warfarin's effects. Alfalfa, dong quai, fish oils, ginger, ginkgo, ginseng, green tea (contains vitamin K), milk thistle, saw palmetto, soy, and St. John's wort can influence (either increase or decrease) effectiveness.
Special considerations	Vitamin K antagonist. Because of its narrow therapeutic range, it requires frequent coagulation monitoring. Patients should avoid sudden dietary changes in their intake of foods and beverages rich in vitamin K. Examples include green tea, beef liver, and large amounts of green, leafy vegetables (eg, broccoli, brussels sprouts, cabbage, kale, lettuce, spinach).

Abbreviations: ACS, acute coronary syndrome; AF, atrial fibrillation; AMI, acute myocardial infarction; DVT, deep vein thrombosis; GI, gastrointestinal; NSAIDs, nonsteroidal anti-inflammatory drugs; NTG, nitroglycerin; PE, pulmonary embolism; SNRIs, serotonin-norepinephrine reuptake inhibitors; SSRIs, selective serotonin reuptake inhibitors

[a] Prescriber's Digital Reference [homepage]. https://www.pdr.net/. Accessed July 16, 2021.

Commonly Prescribed and OTC Medications

Antidepressant Agents

Antidepressants are prescribed to treat clinical depression, obsessive-compulsive disorder, generalized anxiety disorder, and posttraumatic stress syndrome. Several categories of antidepressants exist that differ primarily in their specific sites of action and the neurotransmitter(s) affecting the brain. Most antidepressants work by increasing levels of serotonin, norepinephrine, or dopamine within the brain. The FDA requires that the labels of all antidepressants have black box warnings indicating an increased risk of suicidal ideation in children, adolescents, and young adults.

Many of these drugs have the potential to cause an adverse reaction called serotonin syndrome. Serotonin syndrome can occur when an antidepressant is used alone or in combination with other drugs that affect serotonin levels (ie, serotonergic drugs). Serotonin syndrome typically includes signs and symptoms in three major categories: (1) altered mental status (agitation, anxiety, disorientation, restlessness), (2) neuromuscular abnormalities (tremors, hyperreflexia, motor weakness or muscle rigidity), and (3) autonomic dysfunction (hypertension, tachycardia, flushed skin, shivering, vomiting, dysrhythmias). Common antidepressants are listed in **TABLE 15-4**.

TABLE 15-4 Common Antidepressant Agents

Monoamine Oxidase Inhibitors (MAOIs)	
Examples	isocarboxazid (Marplan), phenelzine (Nardil), tranylcypromine (Parnate); selegiline (Emsam)
Action	Inhibit the action of monoamine oxidase, an enzyme responsible for breaking down the neurotransmitters norepinephrine, serotonin, dopamine, and tyramine in the brain. This action results in increased levels of these neurotransmitters. Selegiline is a selective inhibitor that mainly breaks down dopamine, thereby increasing dopamine levels.
Indications	Vary by drug but can include anxiety, major depressive disorder, Parkinson disease (selegiline is used as an adjunct to therapy with levodopa).
Contraindications	Known hypersensitivity, severe liver and kidney impairment, severe or frequent headache, uncontrolled hypertension, cardiovascular diseases, cerebrovascular diseases.
Adverse reactions/side effects	Dry mouth, nausea, diarrhea, constipation, hallucinations, agitation, insomnia, dizziness or lightheadedness, hyperhidrosis (phenelzine), sexual dysfunction. If a transdermal patch is used, a skin reaction may occur at the patch site.
Drug interactions	Increased risk of serotonin syndrome if used with serotonergic drugs or St. John's wort.
Special considerations	Patients taking MAOIs have an increased sensitivity to sympathomimetics, such as epinephrine. Selegiline is administered via a transdermal patch for depression and orally for Parkinson disease. Patients taking oral MAOIs must maintain a tyramine-restricted diet. Consuming foods or beverages containing tyramine while taking an MAOI can cause a sudden increase in BP, potentially triggering a cerebral hemorrhage. Aged cheeses, dried fruits, avocados, bananas, alcoholic beverages (especially beer containing yeast and red wine), fava beans, and salami are examples of the many foods containing high tyramine levels.
Serotonin-Norepinephrine Reuptake Inhibitors (SNRIs)	
Examples	desvenlafaxine (Pristiq), duloxetine (Cymbalta), levomilnacipran (Fetzima), venlafaxine (Effexor XR)
Action	Block reabsorption of serotonin and norepinephrine into nerve cells in the brain, thereby increasing serotonin and norepinephrine levels.
Indications	Vary by drug but can include chronic pain, diabetic neuropathy, fibromyalgia, generalized anxiety disorder, major depressive disorder (second-line therapy), obsessive-compulsive disorder (venlafaxine), panic disorder, posttraumatic stress disorder (venlafaxine), social anxiety disorder (venlafaxine), stress incontinence in women (duloxetine).
Contraindications	Known hypersensitivity, MAOI therapy, uncontrolled hypertension, uncontrolled narrow-angle glaucoma. Use with caution in pregnancy, breastfeeding, children, cardiovascular disease, renal or live dysfunction, seizures, electrolyte disorders, hyperthyroidism.
Adverse reactions/side effects	Serotonin syndrome, dry mouth, insomnia, nightmares, nausea, dose-dependent hypertension, orthostatic hypotension, seizures, tachycardia, urinary retention.
Drug interactions	Potential additive risk for bleeding if given in combination with other agents that affect hemostasis (eg, aspirin and other antiplatelet drugs, anticoagulants, fibrinolytic agents, SSRIs, and NSAIDs). Hypotension is possible if combined with alcohol and CNS depressants. Increased risk of serotonin syndrome if used with serotonergic drugs or St. John's wort.
Special considerations	Can increase cholesterol and triglycerides. BP should be well controlled before starting SNRI therapy. Risk of hypertensive emergency if taken with MAOIs.

Selective Serotonin Reuptake Inhibitors (SSRIs)	
Examples	citalopram (Celexa), escitalopram (Lexapro), fluoxetine (Prozac), paroxetine (Paxil, Pexeva), sertraline (Zoloft)
Action	Block serotonin reabsorption nerve cells, thereby increasing serotonin levels; do not block dopamine or norepinephrine reabsorption.
Indications	Vary by drug but can include eating disorders, gambling disorder, generalized anxiety disorder, irritable bowel syndrome, major depressive disorder (first-line therapy), obsessive-compulsive disorder, panic disorder, posttraumatic stress disorder, premature ejaculation, social anxiety disorder.
Contraindications	Known hypersensitivity, MAOI therapy, bleeding disorders (eg, hemophilia). Use with caution in pregnancy, breastfeeding, alcohol use disorder, anticoagulant therapy, seizures, CAD, dysrhythmias, thyroid disease.
Adverse reactions/side effects	Serotonin syndrome, dry mouth, blurred vision, sleep disturbances, sweating, agitation, headache, weight gain, sexual dysfunction.
Drug interactions	Potential additive risk for bleeding if given in combination with other agents that affect hemostasis (eg, aspirin and other antiplatelet drugs, anticoagulants, fibrinolytic agents, SNRIs, and NSAIDs). Increased risk of serotonin syndrome if used with serotonergic drugs or St. John's wort. Grapefruit and grapefruit juice can result in possible toxicity with some SSRIs.
Special considerations	Fewer side effects than TCAs.
Tricyclic Antidepressants (TCAs)	
Examples	amitriptyline (Elavil), doxepin (Silenor), desipramine (Norpramin), imipramine (Tofranil), nortriptyline (Pamelor)
Action	Block reabsorption of serotonin and norepinephrine, leading to increased concentrations of these neurotransmitters in the brain; also block histamine and cholinergic receptors.
Indications	Vary by drug; in addition to depression, some are used to treat eating disorders, postherpetic neuralgia, and migraine prophylaxis.
Contraindications	Known hypersensitivity; use with caution in patients with seizure disorders (TCAs lower the seizure threshold).
Adverse reactions/side effects	Anticholinergic effects (dry mouth, constipation, urinary hesitancy or retention, tachycardia, blurred vision), nausea, vomiting, drowsiness, weakness, nightmares, headaches, paresthesias, sexual dysfunction, excessive sweating, changes in appetite or weight, confusion, unsteadiness, cardiotoxicity (eg, prolonged QRS complex and QT interval, dysrhythmias).
Drug interactions	Severe hypertension can result if used with sympathomimetics. Carbamazepine and barbiturates decrease effects; increased effects with quinidine, protease inhibitors, SSRIs, cimetidine, traMADol. Increased risk of serotonin syndrome if used with serotonergic drugs or St. John's wort. Increased sedative effects with alcohol, hypnotics, sedatives, and barbiturates.
Special considerations	Can cause blood disorders, so close monitoring of blood cell counts is necessary, in addition to routine monitoring to determine if serum levels are within therapeutic range.
Atypical Agents	
Examples	buPROPion (Wellbutrin SR, Wellbutrin XL), mirtazapine (Remeron), traZODone (Oleptro), vilazodone (Viibryd), vortioxetine (Brintellix)

(continues)

TABLE 15-4 Common Antidepressant Agents (continued)	
Action	Affect serotonin, norepinephrine, dopamine, and possibly glutamate neurotransmission.
Indications	Vary by drug but can include major depressive disorder, insomnia, and nicotine use disorder (buPROPion).
Contraindications	Known hypersensitivity; seizures and eating disorders (buPROPion).
Adverse reactions/side effects	Nausea, sedation, dizziness, dry mouth, headache, orthostatic hypotension, tachycardia/palpitations (buPROPion), priapism (traZODone).
Drug interactions	Increased risk of serotonin syndrome if used with serotonergic drugs or St. John's wort.
Special considerations	Atypical agents do not fit well into the other antidepressant categories. Some of these medications can increase cholesterol and triglyceride levels, others can cause weight gain, and some cause weight loss.

Abbreviations: BP, blood pressure; CAD, coronary artery disease; CNS, central nervous system; NSAIDs, nonsteroidal anti-inflammatory drugs

Commonly Prescribed and OTC Medications

Antiplatelet Agents

Antiplatelet drugs suppress platelet aggregation and are used to prevent arterial thrombosis.

Common antiplatelet agents are listed in **TABLE 15-5**.

TABLE 15-5 Common Antiplatelet Agents	
Clopidogrel (Plavix)	
Indications[a]	STEMI or moderate- to high-risk NSTEMI, including patients receiving fibrinolysis; substitute for aspirin if suspected ACS and patient cannot take aspirin; prevention of thromboembolic events in AF.
Contraindications	Known hypersensitivity, severe liver impairment, any active bleeding such as peptic ulcer or intracranial hemorrhage.
Adverse reactions/side effects	Abdominal pain, GI hemorrhage, dizziness, headaches, indigestion, bruising, rash, itching, bleeding at puncture sites.
Drug interactions	Interferes with metabolism of phenytoin, warfarin, NSAIDs, calcium channel blockers, morphine, and amiodarone. May increase bleeding when taken with other medications that affect coagulation (eg, aspirin and other antiplatelet drugs, anticoagulants, fibrinolytic agents, SSRIs, SNRIs, and NSAIDs). Bleeding may be increased if taken with garlic, ginger, ginkgo, or green tea.
Special considerations	Often given with other anticoagulants (heparin, eptifibatide) in ACS. No reversal agent is currently available. If excessive bleeding is encountered in a patient on clopidogrel, prompt platelet transfusions are indicated.
Dipyridamole (Persantine), Dipyridamole/Aspirin (Aggrenox)	
Indications	Arterial thromboembolism prophylaxis (eg, AMI prophylaxis, valvular heart disease, TIA).
Contraindications	Hypersensitivity.

Adverse reactions/side effects	Headache, dizziness, nausea, abdominal pain, dyspnea, flushing, chest discomfort, fatigue, bleeding, arthralgia.
Drug interactions	Potential additive risk for bleeding if given in combination with other agents that affect hemostasis (eg, aspirin and other antiplatelet drugs, anticoagulants, fibrinolytic agents, SSRIs, SNRIs, and NSAIDs), adenosine effects are potentiated by dipyridamole; additive bleeding may occur if given in combination with garlic or ginkgo.
Special considerations	IV dipyridamole is an adjunct to myocardial perfusion imaging in patients unable to perform an exercise stress test.[b] Produces peripheral vasodilation that can worsen hypotension.

Abbreviations: ACS, acute coronary syndrome; AF, atrial fibrillation; AMI, acute myocardial infarction; GI, gastrointestinal; IV, intravenous; NSAIDs, nonsteroidal anti-inflammatory drugs; NSTEMI, non-ST-segment elevation myocardial infarction; SNRIs, serotonin-norepinephrine reuptake inhibitors; SSRIs, selective serotonin reuptake inhibitors; STEMI, ST-segment elevation myocardial infraction; TIA, transient ischemic attack

[a] American Heart Association. *2020 Handbook of Emergency Cardiovascular Care for Healthcare Providers*. Dallas, TX: American Heart Association; 2020.

[b] Prescriber's Digital Reference [homepage]. https://www.pdr.net/. Accessed July 16, 2021.

Aspirin (Acetylsalicylic Acid)

Class Platelet inhibitor, NSAID, anti-inflammatory agent.

Mechanism of action Prevents thromboxane A_2 formation, which causes platelets to clump together (aggregate) and form plugs that cause obstruction or constriction; has antipyretic and analgesic properties.

Indications New-onset chest discomfort suggestive of ACS.

Contraindications Hypersensitivity to ASA or NSAIDs (ASA-associated hypersensitivity reactions include ASA-induced urticaria or ASA-intolerant asthma); bleeding disorders including ulcers, hemophilia, hemorrhagic diathesis, hemorrhoids, thrombocytopenia, and ulcerative colitis; hemolytic anemia from pyruvate kinase (PK) and glucose-6-phosphate dehydrogenase (G6PD) deficiency; lactating mothers.[2]

Adverse reactions/side effects Anaphylaxis, bronchospasm/wheezing in allergic patients, GI bleeding, epigastric distress, nausea, vomiting, heartburn, Reye syndrome.

Drug interactions Increased risk of bleeding with anticoagulants and other NSAIDs, diminished effects of ACE inhibitors and loop diuretics. Antacids reduce ASA absorption. Increased risk of hypoglycemia occurs with administration of oral hypoglycemic drugs; effects are decreased by corticosteroids. Increased bleeding can occur when ASA is taken with herbs such as dong quai, feverfew, garlic, ginger, ginkgo, Korean ginseng, and saw palmetto because these herbs interfere with platelet aggregation.[3]

Dosage and administration *Adult*: 162 mg to 325 mg orally. Chewing is preferable to swallowing if the ASA tablet is not enteric coated. *Pediatric*: Not recommended.

Duration of action *Onset*: 15 to 30 minutes. *Peak effect*: 1 to 2 hours. *Duration*: 4 to 6 hours.

Special considerations Pregnancy safety: Category D. Use of NSAIDs around 20 weeks or later in pregnancy may cause rare but serious kidney problems in an unborn baby and can lead to low levels of amniotic fluid surrounding the baby and possible complications. The FDA recommends limiting NSAIDs between 20 to 30 weeks of pregnancy and avoiding use after 30 weeks. If NSAID treatment is determined to be necessary during pregnancy, limit use to the lowest effective dose and the shortest duration possible.[9]

If there are no contraindications, non–enteric-coated, chewable aspirin should be given as soon as possible to all patients with a suspected ACS after symptom onset.

Atropine Sulfate

Class Anticholinergic agent.

Mechanism of action Inhibits acetylcholine at postganglionic parasympathetic neuroeffector sites; increases heart rate in symptomatic bradydysrhythmias; reverses muscarinic effects of cholinergic poisoning.

Indications Hemodynamically unstable bradycardia, acetylcholinesterase inhibitor poisoning (carbamates, nerve agents, organophosphates), RSI in pediatrics, beta blocker or calcium channel blocker overdose.

Contraindications Known hypersensitivity; relative contraindications include narrow-angle glaucoma, GI obstruction, severe ulcerative colitis, toxic megacolon, bladder outlet obstruction, myasthenia gravis, hemorrhage with cardiovascular instability, thyrotoxicosis.[2]

Adverse reactions/side effects Drowsiness; confusion; headache; palpitations; dysrhythmias; nausea; vomiting; pupil dilation; dry mouth/nose/skin; blurred vision; urinary retention; constipation; flushed, hot, dry skin.

Drug interactions Potential adverse effects when administered with digitalis, cholinergics, physostigmine. Effects enhanced by antihistamines, procainamide, quinidine, antipsychotics, benzodiazepines, and antidepressants.

Dosage and administration *Adult*: Symptomatic bradycardia:[5,10] Give 0.5 to 1 mg IV/IO every 3 to 5 minutes as needed, to a maximum dose of 3 mg. Acetylcholinesterase inhibitor poisoning:[7] Extremely large doses (2 to 4 mg or higher) may be needed. *Pediatric*:[7] Symptomatic bradycardia: 0.02 mg/kg IV/IO. Maximum single dose: 0.5 mg. Maximum total dose for a child is: 1 mg; for an adolescent it is 3 mg. ET dose: 0.04 to 0.06 mg/kg. Acetylcholinesterase inhibitor poisoning: Child younger than 12 years: 0.05 mg/kg initially, then repeat and double the dose every 5 minutes until muscarinic symptoms reverse. Child 12 years and older: 1 mg IV/IO initially, then repeat and double the dose every 5 minutes until muscarinic symptoms reverse. RSI: IV/IO: 0.01 to 0.02 mg/kg (maximum dose: 0.5 mg). IM: 0.02 mg/kg.

Duration of action *Onset*: Immediate. *Peak effect*: 2 to 4 minutes. *Duration*: 2 to 4 hours.

Special considerations Pregnancy safety: Category C. Paradoxical bradycardia can occur with doses lower than 0.1 mg. Ineffective in hypothermic bradycardia; may be ineffective in patients who have undergone heart transplantation or in infranodal AV blocks. Use with caution in the presence of myocardial ischemia because atropine increases myocardial oxygen demand.[7]

Benzocaine Spray (Hurricane)

Class Topical anesthetic.

Mechanism of action Prevents impulse transmission along sensory nerve fibers and at nerve endings.

Indications Used as a topical anesthetic (eg, larynx, mouth, trachea, nasal cavity) to facilitate passage of diagnostic and treatment devices. Suppresses the pharyngeal and tracheal gag reflex.

Contraindications Hypersensitivity to benzocaine or other "caine" anesthetics.

Adverse reactions/side effects Signs of methemoglobinemia include pale, gray- or blue-colored skin, lips, and nail beds; headache, light-headedness, shortness of breath; anxiety, fatigue, and tachycardia.

Drug interactions Rare and sometimes fatal cases of methemoglobinemia have been reported with the use of topical or oromucosal benzocaine products. Nitrites and nitrates may induce methemoglobin formation additive to that formed by benzocaine products.[5]

Dosage and administration *Adult*: 0.5- to 1-second spray; repeat as needed. *Pediatric*: 0.25- to 0.5-second spray; repeat as needed.

Duration of action *Onset*: Immediate. *Peak effect*: Less than 5 minutes. *Duration*: 15 to 20 minutes.

Special considerations Pregnancy safety: Category C. The amount of benzocaine contained in a single spray varies among different manufacturers. Use in the mouth and throat can result in potentially dangerous methemoglobin levels. In some cases, methemoglobinemia was reported after a single benzocaine spray; in others, methemoglobinemia resulted after excessive amounts were applied.

Beta Blocking Agents

Beta blocker drugs antagonize the effects of epinephrine on beta adrenergic receptors. Some beta blockers are selective, while others are nonselective. Beta-1 selective blockers, such as atenolol

(Tenormin) and metoprolol (Lopressor), are also called cardioselective beta blockers. Their use results in slowing of the heart rate and force of contraction. Because they primarily block beta-1 receptor sites, they are generally considered safer for use in patients with lung diseases. Nonselective beta blockers, such as propranolol (Inderal), antagonize both beta-1 and beta-2 receptors, resulting in a decrease in heart rate and force of contraction and causing some degree of bronchoconstriction. Nonselective beta blockers are contraindicated in patients with asthma and should be used with caution in patients with COPD.[3] Common beta blockers are listed in **TABLE 15-6**.

TABLE 15-6 Beta Blockers

Examples	atenolol (Tenormin), esmolol (Brevibloc), labetalol (Normodyne, Trandate), metoprolol (Lopressor, Toprol XL), propranolol (Inderal)
Action	Decreases heart rate, conduction velocity, myocardial contractility, and cardiac output. Used to control ventricular response in SVT (PSVT, AF, atrial flutter). Labetalol causes BP reduction without reflex tachycardia; total peripheral resistance is reduced without a significant change in cardiac output.
Indications	• To reduce myocardial ischemia and damage in patients with AMI and elevated heart rate, BP, or both.[a] • Conversion to sinus rhythm or to a slow ventricular rate (or both) in supraventricular tachydysrhythmias (reentry SVT, AF, or atrial flutter) if no signs of heart failure.[a] • Hypertrophic cardiomyopathy. • Noncardiovascular conditions including anxiety, essential tremor, glaucoma, and migraine. • Labetalol is recommended as emergency antihypertensive therapy for hemorrhagic and acute ischemic stroke,[a] and severe hypertension (SBP greater than 160 mm Hg or DBP greater than 110 mm Hg) lasting more than 15 minutes with associated preeclampsia symptoms.[b]
Contraindications	Hypersensitivity; heart failure, cardiogenic shock. Should not be taken by pregnant women or women suspected of being pregnant or during breastfeeding. Relative contraindications include PR interval longer than 0.24 second, second- or third-degree heart block, active asthma, reactive airway disease, severe bradycardia, SBP less than 100 mm Hg.[a] Propranolol is contraindicated, and other beta blockers are relatively contraindicated, in cocaine-induced ACS.[a]
Adverse reactions/ side effects	Dizziness, weakness, fatigue, drowsiness, bronchospasm, cold hands and feet, bradycardia, AV conduction delays, hypotension, heart failure, possible erectile dysfunction.
Drug interactions	Concurrent administration with IV calcium channel blockers can cause severe hypotension and bradycardia/heart block.[a] May potentiate antihypertensive effects when given to patients taking calcium channel blockers or MAOIs. Catecholamine-depleting drugs may potentiate hypotension. May decrease the effects of sympathomimetic drugs. May alter the effectiveness of insulin or oral hypoglycemic agents. Signs of hypoglycemia may be masked (eg, tachycardia). Antihypertensives, alcohol, or nitrates may augment hypotensive effects.
Special considerations	Carefully monitor the patient's BP, heart rate, and ECG during and after administration. ACE inhibitors have largely replaced the use of beta blockers in the management of chronic hypertension. Labetalol should always be administered with the patient in the supine position.

Abbreviations: ACE, angiotensin-converting enzyme; ACS, acute coronary syndrome; AF, atrial fibrillation; AMI, acute myocardial infarction; AV, atrioventricular; BP, blood pressure; DBP, diastolic blood pressure; ECG, electrocardiogram; IV, intravenous; MAOIs, monoamine oxidase inhibitors; PSVT, paroxysmal supraventricular tachycardia; SBP, systolic blood pressure; SVT, supraventricular tachycardia

[a] American Heart Association. *2020 Handbook of Emergency Cardiovascular Care for Healthcare Providers*. Dallas, TX: American Heart Association; 2020.

[b] Prescriber's Digital Reference [homepage]. https://www.pdr.net/. Accessed July 16, 2021.

Bumetanide (Bumex)

Class Loop diuretic.

Mechanism of action A potent loop diuretic with a rapid onset and short duration of action. Inhibits the reabsorption of sodium and chloride in the ascending limb of the loop of Henle.

Indications Pulmonary edema, heart failure.

Contraindications Hypersensitivity to bumetanide, furosemide, or sulfonamides; hypovolemia, anuria, acid–base imbalance, electrolyte imbalance, hepatic coma. Use with caution in patients with hepatic cirrhosis, ascites, or diabetes.

Adverse reactions/side effects Dehydration, dizziness, headache, hypotension, ECG changes due to electrolyte depletion, nausea/vomiting, itching (in patients with liver disease), fatigue.

Drug interactions NSAIDs reduce the effects of diuretics. May increase blood levels of lithium, increasing risk of lithium poisoning. Antihypertensives can cause further hypotension.

Dosage and administration *Adult*: 0.5 to 1 mg IV slowly over 1 to 2 minutes or IM. *Pediatric*: Not recommended for children younger than 12 years as there is limited information on safety, efficacy, and dosage in children. Consult medical direction.

Duration of action *Onset*: Immediate. *Peak effect*: 15 to 30 minutes. *Duration*: 3 to 6 hours.

Special considerations Pregnancy safety: Category C. Use cautiously in pregnant women. Not recommended for use by breastfeeding women. Bumetanide does not have the vasodilatory effects of furosemide. Diuretic potency is about 40 times greater than furosemide.[5]

Calcium Chloride

Class Electrolyte.

Mechanism of action Mineral component of bones and teeth; cofactor in enzymatic reactions and affects the secretory activity of endocrine and exocrine glands; essential for neurotransmission, blood clotting, and contraction of cardiac, smooth, and skeletal muscles.

Indications Hypocalcemia, hyperkalemia, beta blocker and calcium channel blocker toxicity, antidote for magnesium sulfate overdose.

Contraindications Known hypersensitivity, digoxin toxicity, hypercalcemia, suspected severe hypokalemia.

Adverse reactions/side effects Syncope, bradycardia, asystole, hypotension, nausea, vomiting, metallic taste with rapid injection, tissue necrosis at injection site, coronary and cerebral artery spasm.

Drug interactions May increase ventricular irritability and precipitate digitalis toxicity in patients taking digoxin. Potentiated by thiazide diuretics. May antagonize the effects of calcium channel blockers. Incompatible with most all medications; flush the IV/IO line before and after its administration.

Dosage and administration *Adult*: Calcium channel blocker overdose and hyperkalemia:[6,7] Give 500 to 1,000 mg slow IV/IO push over 5 minutes. May repeat as needed. *Pediatric*:[7] Calcium channel blocker overdose, hypocalcemia, and hyperkalemia: 20 mg/kg slow IV/IO push. Maximum dose: 1 g (10 mL).[6] May repeat the dose if documented or suspected clinical indication persists.

Duration of action *Onset*: 1 to 3 minutes. *Peak effect*: Variable. *Duration*: 20 to 30 minutes but may persist for 4 hours (dose-dependent).

Special considerations Pregnancy safety: Category C. Calcium chloride contains three times more elemental calcium than calcium gluconate does. Constant ECG and vital sign monitoring are essential. In children, calcium gluconate is preferred for calcium channel blocker overdose because calcium chloride is associated with an increased risk of tissue damage.[2] Central venous administration is the preferred route in pediatric patients, if available. Monitor the IV site carefully; local infiltration can result in severe tissue necrosis and sloughing. Do not administer by either the IM or subcutaneous routes because this medication is highly irritating to tissues.

Calcium Gluconate

Class Electrolyte.

Mechanism of action Mineral component of bones and teeth; cofactor in enzymatic reactions and affects the secretory activity of endocrine and exocrine glands; essential for neurotransmission, blood clotting, and contraction of cardiac, smooth, and skeletal muscles.

Indications Topical use in hydrofluoric acid burn management,[2] hypocalcemia, hyperkalemia, beta blocker and calcium channel blocker toxicity.

Contraindications Known hypersensitivity, digoxin toxicity, hypercalcemia, suspected severe hypokalemia.

Adverse reactions/side effects Syncope, cardiac arrest, dysrhythmias, hypotension, asystole, peripheral vasodilation, nausea, vomiting, metallic taste, tissue necrosis at injection site, coronary and cerebral artery spasm.

Drug interactions May cause severe bradycardia in patients taking digitalis. May antagonize the effects of calcium channel blockers. Incompatible with most medications; flush the IV/IO line before and after its administration.

Dosage and administration *Adult*: Calcium channel blocker overdose and hyperkalemia:[6,7] Give 1.5 to 3 g (15 to 30 mL of 10% solution) slow IV/IO push over 5 minutes. *Pediatric*:[7] Calcium channel blocker overdose, hypocalcemia, and hyperkalemia: 60 mg/kg slow IV/IO push over 10 minutes. May repeat if documented or suspected clinical indication persists. *Adult and pediatric*: Hydrofluoric acid burn management: Apply generous amounts of calcium gluconate topical gel to the exposed burned skin areas, leave in place for at least 20 minutes, and reassess.[2,11] If commercially manufactured calcium gluconate gel is not available, a topical calcium gluconate gel preparation can be made by combining 150 mL (5 ounces) of a sterile water-soluble gel (eg, Surgilube or KY jelly) with one of the following: 35 mL of calcium gluconate 10% solution, 10 g of calcium gluconate tablets (eg, Tums), or 3.5 g of calcium gluconate powder.[2]

Duration of action *Onset*: 1 to 3 minutes. *Peak effect*: Immediate. *Duration*: 30 minutes to 2 hours.

Special considerations Pregnancy safety: Category C. Constant ECG and vital signs monitoring are essential. In children, calcium gluconate is preferred for calcium channel blocker overdose because calcium chloride is associated with an increased risk of tissue damage.[2] Central venous administration is the preferred route in pediatrics, if available. Monitor the IV site carefully; local infiltration can result in severe tissue necrosis and sloughing. Do not administer by either the IM or subcutaneous routes because this medication is highly irritating to tissues.

Cimetidine (Tagamet)

Class Antiulcer, H_2 blocker.

Mechanism of action Blocks the effects of histamine at H_2 receptors of gastric parietal cells, leading to a reduction of gastric acid volume and gastric acidity.

Indications Gastric or duodenal ulcers, GERD, as an adjunct in treating hives and/or itching in patients experiencing an allergic reaction that does not respond to an H_1 blocker alone (eg, diphenhydrAMINE).

Contraindications Known hypersensitivity to cimetidine or other H_2 blockers.

Adverse reactions/side effects Headache, dizziness, diarrhea, muscle aches, skin rashes, fatigue.

Drug interactions Inhibition of specific liver enzymes may result in increased plasma levels of certain drugs, including warfarin-type anticoagulants, TCAs, Class I antidysrhythmics, calcium channel blockers, diazepam, phenytoin, theophylline, propranolol, and metoprolol.

Dosage and administration[5] *Adult*: 400 mg orally four times daily; maximum is 1,200 mg/day for most indications. *Pediatric:* Use is not recommended unless the anticipated benefits outweigh the potential risk; 20 to 40 mg/kg per day orally in divided doses; maximum is 40 mg/kg per day for most indications.

Duration of action *Onset*: 60 minutes. *Peak effect*: 45 to 90 minutes. *Duration*: 4 to 5 hours.

Special considerations Pregnancy safety: Category B. Can be given orally or IV in conjunction with diphenhydrAMINE for urticaria.

Dexamethasone Sodium Phosphate (Decadron)

Class Corticosteroid, adrenal glucocorticoid, anti-inflammatory agent.

Mechanism of action Suppresses acute and chronic inflammation; immunosuppressive effects.

Indications Anaphylaxis, acute exacerbation of bronchial asthma, AMS, HACE, spinal cord injury, croup, elevated ICP (prevention and treatment), as an adjunct in the treatment of shock, COVID-19 with severe respiratory symptoms.

Contraindications Documented hypersensitivity, systemic fungal infection, preterm infants.

Adverse reactions/side effects Headache, restlessness, nervousness, increased appetite, insomnia, sodium and water retention. None from a single dose.

Drug interactions Many. Simultaneous use with ASA and NSAIDs increases the risk of GI bleeding and ulceration. Concurrent use with diuretics increases potassium loss and can result in hypokalemia. Echinacea may reduce its effectiveness.

Dosage and administration *Adult*: AMS treatment:[2,4] Give 4 mg IM, IV, or orally every 6 hours until symptoms resolve. HACE:[2,4] Give 8 mg IM, IV, or orally, followed by 4 mg IM, IV, or orally every 6 hours until symptoms resolve. Bronchospasm:[2] Give 0.6 mg/kg IM, IV, or orally (maximum dose 16 mg). *Pediatric*: AMS, HACE treatment:[2,4] Give 0.15 mg/kg IM, IV, or orally every 6 hours; maximum: 4 mg/dose. For croup:[2,7] Give 0.6 mg/kg orally, IM, IV, or IO given once; maximum dose: 16 mg. For asthma:[7] Give 0.6 mg/kg IM, IV, or IO every 24 hours (maximum dose: 16 mg).

Duration of action *Onset*: 4 to 8 hours. *Peak effect*: 6 to 12 hours. *Duration*: 24 to 72 hours.

Special considerations Pregnancy safety: Category C. Use cautiously in breastfeeding women. Administer IV/IO doses slowly. Steroids can mask infection because they suppress both the immune and inflammatory systems. Can increase blood glucose levels, so antidiabetic drug dosages may need to be adjusted. If available, hydrocortisone succinate is preferred over methylPREDNISolone and dexamethasone for patients with adrenal insufficiency because of its dual glucocorticoid and mineralocorticoid effects.[2] High doses of glucocorticoids or prolonged use can result in many adverse reactions and side effects. Dexamethasone should not be used for AMS or HACE *prevention* in children.[5]

Dextrose

Class Carbohydrate, glucose-elevating agent.

Mechanism of action Rapidly increases serum glucose levels. Short-term osmotic diuresis.

Indications Hypoglycemia, acutely altered mental status, coma of unknown origin, seizure of unknown origin, status epilepticus.

Contraindications Documented hypersensitivity, hyperglycemia, severe dehydration, anuria, diabetic coma, intracranial or intraspinal hemorrhage, glucose-galactose malabsorption syndrome.

Adverse reactions/side effects Cerebral hemorrhage; cerebral ischemia; warmth, pain, burning, or phlebitis from IV infusion.

Drug interactions Sodium bicarbonate, warfarin (Coumadin).

Dosage and administration *Adult*:[2] Give 25 g of $D_{10}W$ to $D_{50}W$ IV (50 mL of $D_{50}W$, or 100 mL of $D_{25}W$, or 250 mL of $D_{10}W$). May be repeated as necessary until mental status improves or maximum field dosage is reached. *Pediatric*:[2] Give 0.5 to 1 g/kg of $D_{10}W$ to $D_{25}W$ slow IV/IO push (2 to 4 mL/kg of $D_{25}W$, or 4 to 8 mL/kg of 12.5% dextrose, or 5 to 10 mL/kg of $D_{10}W$). May be repeated as necessary until mental status improves or maximum field dosage is reached. *Neonates and infants*: 0.2 g/kg, followed by 5 mL/kg/h $D_{10}W$ IV/IO infusion.[7]

Duration of action *Onset*: Less than 1 minute. *Peak effect*: Variable. *Duration*: Variable.

Special considerations Pregnancy safety: Category C. Draw blood to determine the patient's glucose level before administering. Document reassessment of vital signs and mental status after administration. For children younger than 8 years, a dextrose concentration of no more than 25% should be used.[2] For neonates and infants younger than 1 month, a dextrose concentration of no more than 10% to 12.5% should be used (their vasculature is extremely sensitive to high concentrations).[2] May induce acute thiamine deficiency (Wernicke-Korsakoff syndrome) in malnourished patients and those with chronic alcoholism. For adults with signs of alcohol abuse or malnutrition, administer thiamine (if available) before giving dextrose (if consistent with local protocols). Extravasation may lead to tissue necrosis; use a large vein for administration, and monitor the site closely. Immediately stop administration if extravasation occurs; document it, and notify the receiving facility staff. Do not administer to patients with known stroke unless hypoglycemia is documented.

Diazepam (Valium, Diastat AcuDial)

Class Benzodiazepine, anticonvulsant, anxiolytic, sedative, skeletal muscle relaxant; Schedule IV drug.

Mechanism of action Appears to act on part of the limbic system, as well as on the thalamus and hypothalamus, to induce a calming effect; inhibits GABA receptors in the CNS, reducing neuron excitability; raises the seizure threshold; induces amnesia and sedation.

Indications Uncontrolled shivering associated with hyperthermia/heat exposure, active seizures, chemical restraint, acetylcholinesterase inhibitor poisoning (carbamates, nerve agents, organophosphates).

Contraindications Documented hypersensitivity, neurologic or respiratory depression, narrow-angle glaucoma, myasthenia gravis, head injury.

Adverse reactions/side effects Dizziness, drowsiness, confusion, headache, respiratory depression, hiccups, hypotension, reflex tachycardia, nausea, vomiting, muscle weakness, ataxia, thrombosis, phlebitis.

Drug interactions Incompatible with most drugs and fluids. Concomitant use with other CNS depressants may cause respiratory depression, hypotension, profound sedation, and death. When given orally, milk thistle may decrease diazepam effectiveness, and grapefruit juice can significantly increase serum concentrations. Motherwort can potentiate the sedative effects and may result in coma.[8]

Dosage and administration *Adult*: Shivering associated with hyperthermia/heat exposure:[2] Give 2 mg IV/IO; may repeat once in 5 minutes. Chemical restraint:[2] Give 5 mg IV or 10 mg IM. *Pediatric*: Seizure activity:[2] Give 0.1 mg/kg slow IV or IO; maximum: 4 mg. Shivering associated with hyperthermia/heat exposure:[2] Give 0.1 mg/kg IV/IO: maximum single dose: 2.5 mg. May repeat once for maximum total dose of 5 mg IV/IO *or* 0.5 mg/kg PR (maximum single dose: 10 mg). May repeat PR dose once for maximum total dose of 20 mg. Chemical restraint:[2] Give 0.05 to 0.1 mg/kg IV (maximum dose: 5 mg) or 0.1 to 0.2 mg/kg IM (maximum dose: 10 mg).

Duration of action *Onset*: 2 to 5 minutes IV; 15 to 30 minutes IM. *Peak effect*: 15 minutes IV, 30 to 45 minutes IM. *Duration*: 15 to 60 minutes IV and IM.

Special considerations Pregnancy safety: Category D. Consider decreasing dose by 50% in patients older than 60 years. Convulsive Antidote Nerve Agent (CANA) is a commercially available auto-injector containing 10 mg of diazepam.[2] In cases of an acetylcholinesterase inhibitor agent exposure, administration of diazepam or midazolam is preferred over lorazepam because of their more rapid onset of action.[2]

Commonly Prescribed and OTC Medications

Digoxin (Lanoxin)

Class Inotropic agent, cardiac glycoside, antidysrhythmic.

Indications Heart failure, alternative drug for reentry SVT, ventricular rate control in atrial flutter and AF.

Contraindications Known hypersensitivity, VF, VT, digitalis toxicity. Hypokalemia, hypomagnesemia, and hypercalcemia potentiate digitalis toxicity.

Adverse reactions/side effects Nausea, vomiting, anorexia (early signs of toxicity), fatigue, headache, blurred yellow or green vision, seizures, confusion, dysrhythmias, skin rash.

Drug interactions Amiodarone, verapamil, and quinidine may increase serum digoxin concentrations. Concurrent use of digoxin and verapamil may lead to severe AV block. Diuretics may potentiate cardiac toxicity. St. John's wort can reduce the effects of digoxin effectiveness, and licorice can potentiate its effects.

Special considerations Digoxin can prolong the PR interval and cause ST-segment changes on the ECG; careful cardiac monitoring is essential. Calcium channel blockers or beta blockers are generally preferred for heart rate control in patients with AF; adenosine is preferred to treat reentry SVT. Cardioversion should be avoided if a patient is taking digoxin, but if the situation is life-threatening, use a lower-energy dose (10 to 20 joules).[7]

Diltiazem (Cardizem, Dilacor, Diltiaz)

Class Calcium channel blocker, antidysrhythmic (Class IV), antianginal agent.

Mechanism of action Inhibits extracellular calcium ion influx across membranes of myocardial cells and vascular smooth muscle cells, resulting in inhibition of cardiac and vascular smooth muscle contraction and thereby dilating the main coronary and systemic arteries; no effect on serum calcium concentrations; substantial inhibitory effects on the cardiac conduction system, acting principally at the AV node, with some effects at the SA node.[2] Less-negative inotropic effects than verapamil.

Indications Stable narrow-QRS tachycardia if the rhythm persists despite vagal maneuvers or administration of adenosine, or if the tachycardia is recurrent; to control the ventricular rate in patients with AF or atrial flutter without preexcitation.[6]

Contraindications Known hypersensitivity, hypotension, cardiogenic shock, wide-complex tachycardia (may lead to hemodynamic deterioration and VF), second- or third-degree AV block or sick sinus syndrome or other sinus node disease unless a functioning artificial pacemaker is present, poison- or drug-induced tachycardia, AF or atrial flutter when associated with an accessory bypass tract (eg, Wolff-Parkinson-White syndrome or Lown-Ganong-Levine syndrome). Avoid use in patients with left ventricular systolic dysfunction or decompensated heart failure.[5] Use with extreme caution in patients taking oral beta blockers.[7]

Adverse reactions/side effects Dizziness, weakness, headache, dyspnea, dysrhythmias including cardiac arrest, heart failure, peripheral edema, hypotension, syncope, chest pain, nausea, vomiting, dry mouth.

Drug interactions Use with caution in patients taking medications that affect cardiac contractility. Simultaneous use with IV beta blockers can result in decreased cardiac contractility, bradycardia (including AV blocks), and severe hypotension. Increased risk of sudden cardiac death when given concurrently with erythromycin.[3]

Dosage and administration *Adult*:[7] Initial dose: 15 to 20 mg (0.25 mg/kg) IV/IO slowly over 2 minutes. After 15 minutes, a second bolus of 20 to 25 mg (0.35 mg/kg) IV/IO can be given slowly over 2 minutes if the initial response was inadequate. For patients older than age 65, the recommended maximum initial dose of diltiazem is 10 mg IV/IO and the maximum second dose is 20 mg IV/IO.[2] Maintenance infusion: 5 to 15 mg/h titrated to a physiologically appropriate heart rate. *Pediatric*: Not recommended.

Duration of action *Onset*: 2 to 5 minutes. *Peak effect*: Usually within 7 minutes. *Duration*: 1 to 3 hours.

Special considerations Pregnancy safety: Category C. Dysrhythmias may be observed during pharmacologic conversion. Carefully monitor BP and ECG before, during, and after administration.

DiphenhydrAMINE (Benadryl)

Class Antihistamine (H_1 blocker).

Mechanism of action Blocks H_1 receptors in the respiratory tract, blood vessels, and GI smooth muscle; reverses extrapyramidal reactions.

Indications Symptomatic allergic reactions, symptomatic dystonia, extrapyramidal signs or symptoms caused by phenothiazines, antiemetic, chemical restraint.

Contraindications Known hypersensitivity, newborns and premature infants, breastfeeding. Use with caution in patients with severe vomiting, asthma, narrow-angle glaucoma, benign prostatic hypertrophy, or alcohol intoxication. Use is controversial in patients with lower respiratory tract disease (eg, acute asthma).[2]

Adverse reactions/side effects Drowsiness, sedation, seizures, dizziness, headache, blurred vision, wheezing, thickening of bronchial secretions, palpitations, hypotension, dysrhythmias, dry mouth, diarrhea, nausea, vomiting. Hallucinations, confusion, and paradoxical CNS excitation can occur in children.

Drug interactions Potentiates the effects of alcohol and other CNS depressants. MAOIs prolong and intensify the anticholinergic (drying) effects of diphenhydrAMINE.

Dosage and administration *Adult*:[2] Urticaria or pruritus, anaphylaxis, or allergic reaction: Give 1 mg/kg up to maximum 50-mg dose IM, IV, or orally. IV route is preferred in severe shock. Antiemetic:[2] 12.5 to 25 mg IV/IM or orally. Dystonic/extrapyramidal symptoms: 25 to 50 mg IV/IM. *Pediatric*:[2] Urticaria or pruritus, anaphylaxis, or allergic reaction:[2] Give 1 mg/kg up to maximum 50-mg dose IM, IV, or orally. IV route is preferred in severe shock. Antiemetic: Older than age 2 and weight greater than 12 kg: 0.1 mg/kg IV (maximum: 25 mg). Dystonic/extrapyramidal symptoms: Give 1 to 1.25 mg/kg IV/IO or IM; maximum single dose: 25 mg. Chemical restraint: Give 1 mg/kg IM/IV or orally; maximum dose: 25 mg.

Duration of action *Onset*: 10 to 15 minutes. *Peak effect*: 1 hour. *Duration*: 6 to 8 hours.

Special considerations Pregnancy safety: Category B. Increases the effectiveness of epinephrine and is often used in conjunction with it, as in anaphylaxis. Any H_2-blocking antihistamine (eg, famotidine, cimetidine) can be given orally or IV in conjunction with diphenhydrAMINE for urticaria.[2]

DOBUTamine Hydrochloride (Dobutrex)

Class Adrenergic, inotropic agent.

Mechanism of action Synthetic catecholamine that primarily stimulates beta-1 receptors, with minor stimulation of beta-2 and alpha-1 receptors. Increases myocardial contractility and stroke volume, resulting in increased cardiac output with modest chronotropic effects. Increases renal blood flow secondary to increased cardiac output.

Indications Heart failure with a SBP of 70 to 100 mm Hg and no signs of shock.[7]

Contraindications Known hypersensitivity, suspected or known poison/drug-induced shock, SBP less than 100 mm Hg and signs of shock,[7] idiopathic hypertrophic subaortic stenosis.

Adverse reactions/side effects Headache, dyspnea, tachycardia, hypertension, chest pain, dysrhythmias, nausea, vomiting.

Drug interactions Incompatible with sodium bicarbonate and furosemide. Beta blockers may blunt the inotropic effects.

Dosage and administration *Adult*: IV infusion at 2 to 20 mcg/kg/min titrated to desired effect.[7] *Pediatric*: IV infusion at 2 to 20 mcg/kg/min titrated to desired effect.

Duration of action *Onset*: 2 minutes. *Peak effect*: 10 minutes. *Duration*: 1 to 2 minutes after infusion discontinued.

Special considerations Pregnancy safety: Category B. Monitor BP closely; hemodynamic monitoring recommended. Titrate dose to maintain a heart rate increase of no greater than 10% of baseline. May increase infarct size in patients with MI. May precipitate or exacerbate ventricular ectopy. Older patients may have a significantly decreased response. Patients may become hypotensive from the vasodilatory effect.

DOPamine Hydrochloride (Intropin)

Class Endogenous catecholamine, adrenergic, vasopressor, inotropic agent.

Mechanism of action Immediate metabolic precursor to norepinephrine with mixed alpha adrenergic, beta adrenergic, and dopaminergic effects that are dose-dependent. At doses of 1 to 2 mcg/kg/min, causes vasodilation in the renal, mesenteric, coronary, and intracerebral vascular beds that is thought to result from stimulation of dopamine receptors.[12] At doses of 2 to 10 mcg/kg/min, DOPamine stimulates beta-1 receptors, increasing myocardial contractility and enhancing cardiac impulse conduction. At infusion rates of 10 to 20 mcg/kg/min, DOPamine stimulates alpha receptors, resulting in vasoconstriction, increased systemic vascular resistance, and a rise in BP. Vasoconstriction occurs first in the skeletal muscle vascular beds, but is evident in the renal and mesenteric vessels with increasing doses.[12] At dosages greater than 20 mcg/kg/min, alpha stimulation predominates, and resultant vasoconstriction may compromise circulation in the limbs.[12]

Indications Refractory cardiogenic or distributive shock, hypotension with low cardiac output states, second-line drug for symptomatic bradycardia.

Contraindications Known hypersensitivity, hypovolemia, pheochromocytoma, uncorrected tachydysrhythmias, VF.

Adverse reactions/side effects Headache, anxiety, dyspnea, dysrhythmias, hypotension, hypertension, palpitations, chest pain, dyspnea, nausea, vomiting.

Drug interactions Inactivated in alkaline solutions (sodium bicarbonate). MAOIs prolong and potentiate effects. TCAs may potentiate cardiovascular effects. Beta blockers antagonize cardiac effects. When administered with phenytoin, may cause hypotension, bradycardia, and seizures. Simultaneous use of vasopressor may result in severe hypertension.

Dosage and administration *Adult*:[7] IV/IO infusion at 5 to 20 mcg/kg/min, slowly titrated to patient response. *Pediatric*: Safety and effectiveness in children have not been established.[12]

Duration of action *Onset*: Within 5 minutes. *Peak effect*: 5 to 10 minutes. *Duration*: Less than 10 minutes.

Special considerations Pregnancy safety: Category C. Correct hypovolemia before administering. Should be administered by infusion pump. Extravasation may cause necrosis and sloughing of surrounding tissue. Slow or stop the infusion if tachydysrhythmias or increased ventricular ectopy is observed (follow the local protocol). Sudden cessation of infusion can result in significant hypotension. Research suggests that patients in cardiogenic or septic shock who are treated with norepinephrine have a lower mortality rate than those treated with DOPamine.[2]

Droperidol (Inapsine)

Class Antiemetic, antipsychotic.

Mechanism of action Produces marked tranquilization and sedation; reduces motor activity and anxiety; also possesses adrenergic-blocking, antifibrillatory, antihistaminic, and anticonvulsive properties.[2]

Indications Chemical restraint, acute delirium or psychosis.

Contraindications Known hypersensitivity; known or suspected prolonged QT interval, including patients with congenital long QT syndrome. Use with extreme caution in patients with bradycardia, cardiac disease, concurrent MAOI therapy, or use of Class I and Class III antidysrhythmics or other drugs that prolong the QT interval and cause electrolyte disturbances because of its adverse cardiovascular effects (ie, QT prolongation, hypotension, tachycardia, and TdP).[2]

Adverse reactions/side effects QT interval prolongation, VT, TdP, cardiac arrest, mild to moderate hypotension, hypertension, tachycardia, dizziness, drowsiness, restlessness, anxiety, dysphoria, hyperactivity, hallucinations, extrapyramidal symptoms (when used for extended periods).

Drug interactions Potentiates CNS depressants, reduces pressor effect of epinephrine.

Dosage and administration *Adult*: Chemical restraint:[2] Give 2.5 mg slow IV *or* 5 mg IM. *Pediatric*: Not routinely recommended.

Duration of action *Onset*: 3 to 10 minutes IV/IM. *Peak effect*: 30 minutes IV/IM. *Duration*: 2 to 4 hours IV/IM.

Special considerations Pregnancy safety: Category C. Cases of QT prolongation and/or TdP have occurred in patients with no known risk factors for QT prolongation; some cases have been fatal. Closely monitor vital signs and ECG. Monitor the QT interval with a 12-lead ECG if feasible. Document the QT interval and relay findings to the receiving facility staff.[2]

Epinephrine (Adrenalin, EpiPen, AsthmaNefrin)

Class Sympathomimetic, sympathetic (alpha/beta adrenergic) agonist.

Mechanism of action Catecholamine with strong alpha adrenergic, strong beta-1, and moderate beta-2 effects. Effects of alpha stimulation result in systemic vasoconstriction, increasing peripheral vascular resistance. Effects of beta-1 stimulation result in increases in heart rate, myocardial contractility, cardiac output, and myocardial oxygen demand. Effects of beta-2 stimulation result in bronchial smooth muscle relaxation. Secondary relaxation effect on the smooth muscle of the stomach, intestine, uterus, and urinary bladder.[2]

Indications Cardiac arrest, bradycardia, shock, anaphylaxis, severe refractory wheezing (IM), croup/bronchiolitis (nebulized).

Contraindications Known hypersensitivity, coronary insufficiency, cardiac dilation.[2] Relative contraindications include uncontrolled hypertension, hypothermia, pulmonary edema, myocardial ischemia, hypovolemic shock.

Adverse reactions/side effects Nervousness, restlessness, headache, tremor, dysrhythmias, chest pain, increased myocardial oxygen demand, hypertension, palpitations, nausea, vomiting.

Drug interactions Potentiates other sympathomimetics. Deactivated by alkaline solutions (sodium bicarbonate). MAOIs and antidepressants may potentiate its effects. Beta blockers may blunt its effects.

Dosage and administration *Adult*: Anaphylaxis:[2] Give 0.3 mg IM in the anterolateral thigh (1 mg/mL may be administered from a vial or vial auto-injector, if available). If signs of anaphylaxis persist, additional epinephrine can be administered every 5 to 15 minutes at the same IM dose. If respiratory distress with wheezing is present, consider giving nebulized albuterol and/or 5 mL of 1 mg/mL epinephrine nebulized. If stridor is present, consider 5 mL of 1 mg/mL epinephrine nebulized. Consider an epinephrine IV infusion (0.5 mcg/kg/min) when cardiovascular collapse is present despite repeated epinephrine IM doses and at least 60 mL/kg isotonic fluid boluses. Severe bronchoconstriction with impending respiratory failure:[2] Give 0.01 mg/kg of 1 mg/mL IM; maximum dose: 0.3 mg (should only be given as adjunctive therapy when there are no clinical signs of improvement). Profound bradycardia with signs of hemodynamic instability:[2] IV/IO infusion of 0.02 to 0.2 mcg/kg/min titrated to a mean arterial pressure greater than 65 mm Hg or IV/IO push dose 10 to 20 mcg boluses (1 to 2 mL) every 2 minutes titrated to a mean arterial pressure greater than 65 mm Hg. Prepare an epinephrine push dose by adding 1 mL of 0.1 mg/mL epinephrine to 9 mL of normal saline (NS); results in 10 mcg/mL concentration. Shock unresponsive to IV fluids, or cardiogenic shock with signs of fluid overload:[2] IV/IO infusion 0.05 to 0.3 mcg/kg/min. Cardiac arrest:[7] Give 1 mg (0.1 mg/mL) IV/IO every 3 to 5 minutes during resuscitation. Follow each dose with a 20-mL flush and elevate arm for 10 to 20 seconds after dose. ET: 2 to 2.5 mg diluted in 10 mL NS. *Pediatric*: Anaphylaxis:[2] If weight is less than 25 kg: Give 0.15 mg IM in the anterolateral thigh; if weight is 25 kg or more, give 0.3 mg IM in the anterolateral thigh (1 mg/mL may be administered from a vial or vial auto-injector, if available). If signs of anaphylaxis persist, additional epinephrine can be administered every 5 to 15 minutes at the same IM dose. If respiratory distress with wheezing is present, consider giving nebulized albuterol and/or 5 mL of 1 mg/mL epinephrine nebulized. If stridor is present, consider 5 mL of 1 mg/mL epinephrine nebulized. Consider an epinephrine IV infusion (0.5 mcg/kg/min) when cardiovascular collapse is present despite repeated epinephrine IM doses and at least 60 mL/kg isotonic fluid boluses. Profound bradycardia with signs of hemodynamic instability:[2] IV/IO push dose 0.01 mg/kg (0.1 mL/kg), every 3 to 5 minutes; maximum single dose: 10 mcg (1 mL) titrated to a mean arterial pressure greater than 65 mm Hg. Prepare an epinephrine push dose as previously described. Cardiac arrest:[7] Give 0.01 mg/kg (0.1 mg/mL) IV/IO every 3 to 5 minutes during arrest. Maximum single dose: 1 mg. ET: 0.1 mg/kg (1 mg/mL) every 3 to 5 minutes of arrest until IV/IO access is achieved, then begin with first IV dose. *Neonates*: Bradycardia:[13] Give 0.01 to 0.03 mg/kg (0.1 mg/mL) IV/IO, followed by 0.5 mL to 1 mL NS. Consider giving 0.05 to 0.1 mg/kg (0.1 mg/mL) ET until IV access can be obtained. Dosing may be repeated every 3 to 5 minutes if the heart rate remains less than 60 beats/min.

Duration of action *Onset*: Less than 2 minutes IV, 3 to 10 minutes IM. *Peak effect*: Less than 5 minutes IV, 20 minutes IM. *Duration*: 5 to 10 minutes IV, 20 to 30 minutes IM.

Special considerations Pregnancy safety: Category C. Contraindicated for patients in active labor. Carefully document the dosage, concentration, route, and time of epinephrine administration and the patient's response to each dose. Administer epinephrine as soon as possible in cardiac arrest associated with PEA or asystole.[6] Consider reducing the dose of epinephrine in patients taking MAOIs, per your local protocols.

Etomidate (Amidate)

Class Nonbarbiturate hypnotic, anesthesia induction agent.

Mechanism of action Ultra-short-acting hypnotic that produces rapid sedation with minimal cardiovascular or respiratory depression.[7]

Indications Premedication for medication-facilitated intubation or procedural sedation.

Contraindications Known hypersensitivity, labor/delivery, or septic shock (particularly in children).

Adverse reactions/side effects Apnea of short duration, respiratory depression, hypoventilation, hyperventilation, nystagmus, dysrhythmias, hypotension, hypertension, nausea, vomiting, transient involuntary skeletal muscle movement, pain at injection site.

Drug interactions Effects may be enhanced when given with other CNS depressants.

Dosage and administration *Adult*: Procedural sedation:[7] Give 0.2 to 0.4 mg/kg IV over 30 to 60 seconds (typical adult dose is 20 mg). *Pediatric*: Procedural sedation:[7] Give 0.2 to 0.4 mg/kg IV/IO over 30 to 60 seconds; maximum 20 mg/dose.

Duration of action *Onset*: 30 to 60 seconds. *Peak effect*: 1 minute. *Duration*: 5 to 10 minutes.

Special considerations Pregnancy safety: Category C. Use caution, weighing fetal risk and maternal benefit in pregnant and breastfeeding women. No analgesic properties. Avoid administration into small veins because the solution is highly irritating. Carefully monitor vital signs. Etomidate can suppress adrenal gland production of steroid hormones and cortisol after a single dose, temporarily causing gland failure. Consider decreasing the dose in older patients and patients with cardiac conditions.

Famotidine (Pepcid)

Class Antiulcer, H_2 blocker.

Mechanism of action Inhibits the volume and concentration of gastric secretions.

Indications GI ulcer, suspected upper GI bleeding, GERD, as an adjunct in the treatment of urticaria and/or pruritus in patients experiencing an allergic reaction that does not respond to an H_1 blocker alone (eg, diphenhydrAMINE).

Contraindications Known hypersensitivity to famotidine or other H_2 blockers.

Adverse reactions/side effects Constipation, diarrhea, rhabdomyolysis, seizures, pneumonia, agitation, vomiting, headache, dizziness, vitamin B_{12} deficiency; prolonged QT interval has been reported in patients with moderate to severe renal impairment. Confusion, hallucinations, disorientation, agitation, and seizures have been reported in older adults.

Drug interactions Decreased absorption of iron; decreased effects of ketoconazole, naproxen, pseudoephedrine; increased action of metformin.

Dosage and administration *Adult*: 20 mg IV, 20 mg orally twice daily. *Pediatric*: 0.25 mg/kg/dose every 12 hours IV (maximum 20 mg/dose), 0.5 mg/kg orally (maximum 40 mg/dose).

Duration of action *Onset*: 60 minutes. *Peak effect*: 1 to 3 hours. *Duration*: 10 to 12 hours.

Special considerations Pregnancy safety: Category B. More potent H_2 blocker with fewer adverse effects and drug interactions and a longer duration of action than cimetidine.[3] Can be given orally or IV in conjunction with diphenhydrAMINE for urticaria.

Fentanyl Citrate (Sublimaze)

Class Opioid analgesic; synthetic opioid; Schedule II drug.

Mechanism of action Binds to opioid receptors, producing analgesia, euphoria, respiratory depression, and sedation.

Indications Pain management, anesthesia adjunct, severe respiratory distress (palliative care).

Contraindications Known hypersensitivity; patients who have taken an MAOI during the previous 14 days. Administer with caution to patients with a Glasgow Coma Scale (GCS) score less than 15, hypotension, hypoxia after maximal supplemental oxygen therapy, or signs of hypoventilation.

Adverse reactions/side effects Confusion, paradoxical excitation, delirium, drowsiness, CNS depression, sedation, respiratory depression, apnea, dyspnea, dysrhythmias, hypotension, syncope, nausea, vomiting, abdominal pain, dehydration, fatigue.

Drug interactions Increased respiratory depressant effects when given with other CNS depressants.

Dosage and administration *Adult:*[2] Severe respiratory distress (palliative care): 25 mcg mixed in 2 mL saline nebulized. Moderate discomfort: 1 mcg/kg IM/IN (maximum initial dose: 100 mcg; maximum total dose: 200 mcg). Severe to excruciating discomfort: 1 mcg/kg IV/IO (maximum initial dose: 100 mcg; maximum total dose: 200 mcg). *Pediatric:*[2] Moderate discomfort: 1 mcg/kg IM/IN (maximum initial dose: 100 mcg; maximum total dose: 200 mcg). Severe to excruciating discomfort: 1 mcg/kg IV/IO (maximum initial dose: 100 mcg; maximum total dose: 200 mcg).

Duration of action *Onset*: Immediate. *Peak effect*: 3 to 5 minutes. *Duration*: 30 to 60 minutes.

Special considerations Pregnancy safety: Category C. Fentanyl is 50 to 100 times more potent than morphine and is legally manufactured in injectable and oral liquid, tablet, and transdermal (worn as a patch) forms; however, much of the fentanyl adulterating the heroin supply is illegal fentanyl analogs such as acetyl fentanyl.[2] Patients who experience opioid overdose from fentanyl or fentanyl analogs may rapidly exhibit chest wall rigidity and require positive end-expiratory pressure, in addition to multiple and/or larger doses of naloxone, to achieve adequate ventilation.[2] Document pain severity using a scale of 0 to 10 before and after administration and on arrival at the receiving facility.[2]

Fibrinolytic Agents

Fibrinolytics are administered to dissolve blood clots and restore blood flow in conditions such as AMI, acute ischemic stroke, and pulmonary embolism. They can be given with other agents to maintain vessel patency after the clot is dissolved. Fibrinolytics are listed in **TABLE 15-7**.

Commonly Prescribed and OTC Medications

Furosemide (Lasix)

Class Loop diuretic.

Indications Heart failure, hypertension.

Contraindications Hypersensitivity to furosemide or sulfonamide medications, hypovolemia, anuria, hepatic coma, suspected electrolyte imbalances.

Adverse reactions/side effects Dizziness, headache, ECG changes, blurred vision, orthostatic hypotension, dysrhythmias, nausea, vomiting, diarrhea, dry mouth; may exacerbate hypovolemia and hypokalemia, tinnitus, hyperglycemia (due to hemoconcentration).

Drug interactions Lithium toxicity may be potentiated by sodium depletion. Digitalis toxicity may be potentiated by potassium depletion.

Special considerations Pregnancy safety: Category C. Ototoxicity may occur if too high a dose is taken or if the patient has severe kidney dysfunction.

Glucagon (GlucaGen)

Class Hyperglycemic agent, pancreatic hormone, insulin antagonist.

Mechanism of action Increases blood glucose level by stimulating the breakdown of stored glycogen to glucose (glycogenolysis) and inhibiting the synthesis of glycogen from glucose (glycogenesis). Unknown mechanism of stabilizing cardiac rhythm in beta blocker overdose. Minimal positive inotropic and chronotropic responses. Decreases GI motility and secretions.

Indications Altered mental status when hypoglycemia is suspected. Antidote for symptomatic bradycardia caused by beta blocker or calcium channel blocker overdoses.

Contraindications Known hypersensitivity, pheochromocytoma, hyperglycemia, insulinoma.

Adverse reactions/side effects Dizziness, headache, hypotension, tachycardia, nausea, vomiting, rebound hypoglycemia.

TABLE 15-7 Fibrinolytic Agents

Examples	alteplase (recombinant tissue plasminogen activator [rTPA], Activase), reteplase (Retavase), tenecteplase (TNKase)
Action	Activate fibrin-bound plasminogen at the clot site, converting plasminogen to plasmin. Plasmin degrades fibrinogen, prothrombin, and other clotting factors and digests the clot's fibrin strands, restoring perfusion.
Indications	Acute ischemic stroke (alteplase is the only fibrinolytic agent approved for this indication), AMI in adults, massive PE.
Contraindications	Known hypersensitivity. See the fibrinolytic checklist in Chapter 18, *Cardiovascular Emergencies*.
Adverse reactions/ side effects	Intracranial bleeding, headache, reperfusion dysrhythmias, chest pain, palpitations, hypotension, GI bleeding, nausea, vomiting, abdominal pain, itching, hives, flushing, bronchospasm.
Drug interactions	Additive risk for bleeding if given in combination with other agents that affect hemostasis (eg, aspirin and other antiplatelet drugs, anticoagulants, glycoprotein IIb/IIIa antagonists, SSRIs, SNRIs, and NSAIDs). Increased bleeding risk with feverfew, garlic, ginger, ginkgo, green tea, and omega-3 fatty acids. Tenecteplase is incompatible with dextrose solutions.
Special considerations	Establish two peripheral IV lines and use one line exclusively for fibrinolytic administration.[a] Closely monitor vital signs and observe for bleeding. Only administer with an infusion pump. Due to the risk of severe spontaneous bleeding, invasive procedures (eg, injections, NG tube insertion, or nasotracheal intubation) should be avoided. Sites used for invasive procedures already performed should be assessed regularly.

Abbreviations: AMI, acute myocardial infarction; GI, gastrointestinal; IV, intravenous; NG, nasogastric; NSAIDs, nonsteroidal anti-inflammatory drugs; PE, pulmonary embolism; SNRIs, serotonin-norepinephrine reuptake inhibitors; SSRIs, selective serotonin reuptake inhibitors

[a]American Heart Association. *2020 Handbook of Emergency Cardiovascular Care for Healthcare Providers*. Dallas, TX: American Heart Association; 2020.

Drug interactions Incompatible in solution with most other substances. No significant drug interactions with other emergency medications.

Dosage and administration *Adult:*[2] Hypoglycemia: Give 1 mg IM/IN. May repeat dose until symptoms have resolved. Calcium channel blocker or beta blocker overdose: Give 5 mg slowly via IV push; can repeat in 5 to 10 minutes for a total dose of 10 mg. *Pediatric:*[5] Hypoglycemia: Give 1 mg IM/IN if weight is 20 kg or greater (or age is 5 years or older); 0.5 mg IM/IN if weight is less than 20 kg or age is younger than 5 years. Calcium channel blocker or beta blocker overdose: Give 1 mg slowly via IV push (25 to 40 kg) every 5 minutes as necessary. Give 0.5 mg slowly via IV push (less than 25 kg) every 5 minutes as necessary.

Duration of action *Onset*: 1 minute. *Peak effect*: 5 to 20 minutes. *Duration*: 60 to 90 minutes.

Special considerations Pregnancy safety: Category B. Use in pregnancy only if clearly indicated. Not recommended for use in lactating women. Ineffective if glycogen stores are depleted. Document reassessment of vital signs and mental status after administration.

Glucose, Oral (Insta-Glucose)

Class Hyperglycemic, carbohydrate.

Mechanism of action After absorption in the GI tract, glucose becomes distributed to the tissues, increasing circulating blood glucose levels.

Indications Conscious patients with suspected hypoglycemia.

Contraindications Known hypersensitivity, decreased level of consciousness, nausea, vomiting.

Adverse reactions/side effects Nausea, vomiting.

Drug interactions None.

Dosage and administration[2] *Adult*: 25 g orally in patients with an intact gag reflex and ability to manage their secretions. *Pediatric*: 0.5 to 1 g/kg orally (maximum dose: 25 g) in patients with an intact gag reflex and ability to manage their secretions.

Duration of action *Onset*: 10 minutes. *Peak effect*: Variable. *Duration*: Variable.

Special considerations Must be swallowed. Glucose is not absorbed sublingually or buccally. Check a glucometer reading before administering oral glucose and repeat the reading at least 10 minutes after administration. Nausea and vomiting are common after administration. Document reassessment of vital signs and mental status after administration.

Glycoprotein IIb/IIIa Inhibitors

Glycoprotein (GP) IIb/IIIa inhibitors block the binding of fibrinogen to glycoprotein IIb/IIIa receptors on the surfaces of platelets, thereby inhibiting platelet aggregation. **TABLE 15-8** lists commonly used GP IIb/IIIa inhibitors.

Haloperidol (Haldol)

Class Tranquilizer, antipsychotic.

Mechanism of action Antagonizes dopamine-1 and dopamine-2 receptors in the brain; depresses the reticular activating system and inhibits release of hypothalamic and hypophyseal hormones.[2]

Indications Acute psychotic episodes or agitated/violent behavior refractory to nonpharmacologic interventions, anxiety (palliative care).

Contraindications Documented hypersensitivity, severe CNS depression (including coma), neuroleptic malignant syndrome, poorly controlled seizure disorder, Parkinson disease, agitation secondary to shock and hypoxia.

Adverse reactions/side effects Seizures, sedation, confusion, restlessness, extrapyramidal reactions, dystonia, respiratory depression, hypotension, tachycardia, orthostatic hypotension, constipation, dry mouth, nausea, vomiting, drooling, blurred vision. Risk of QT interval prolongation, TdP, and sudden death from off-label IV administration of higher than the recommended dose.[2]

TABLE 15-8 Glycoprotein IIb/IIIa Inhibitors

Examples	eptifibatide (Integrilin), tirofiban (Aggrastat)
Indications	Prevention of thrombosis in patients undergoing PCI, high-risk unstable angina and NSTEMI.
Contraindications	Known hypersensitivity to any component of the product. Active internal bleeding or bleeding disorder in past 30 days, platelet count less than 150,000/mm^3, hypersensitivity to and concomitant use of another glycoprotein IIb/IIIa inhibitor, surgical procedure or trauma within 1 month, history of intracranial hemorrhage or other bleeding.[a]
Adverse reactions/ side effects	Dizziness, pain, sweating, bradydysrhythmia, abdominal pain, major hemorrhage (cerebrovascular, pulmonary), hypotension, injection site pain, anaphylaxis, thrombocytopenia.
Drug interactions	Additive risk for bleeding if given in combination with other agents that affect hemostasis (eg, aspirin and other antiplatelet drugs, anticoagulants, fibrinolytic agents, SSRIs, SNRIs, and NSAIDs).
Special considerations	Infusion pump required. Avoid invasive procedures (eg, IV starts, injections, NG tube, or nasotracheal intubation) because of risk of severe spontaneous bleeding. Abciximab (ReoPro), another glycoprotein IIb/IIIa inhibitor, is no longer available in the United States.

Abbreviations: IV, intravenous; NG, nasogastric; NSAIDs, nonsteroidal anti-inflammatory drugs; NSTEMI, non-ST-segment elevation myocardial infarction; PCI, percutaneous coronary intervention; SNRIs, serotonin-norepinephrine reuptake inhibitors; SSRIs, selective serotonin reuptake inhibitors

[a]American Heart Association. *2020 Handbook of Emergency Cardiovascular Care for Healthcare Providers*. Dallas, TX: American Heart Association; 2020.

Drug interactions Enhanced CNS depression and hypotension in combination with alcohol. Additive effect with antihypertensive medications. Antagonizes amphetamines and epinephrine. Other CNS depressants may potentiate its effects.

Dosage and administration (Limited data available; optimal dose not established) *Adult*: Chemical restraint:[2] Give 5 mg IV or 10 mg IM. Anxiety (palliative care):[2] Give 5 mg IV. *Pediatric*: Chemical restraint:[2] Ages 6 to 12 years: 1 to 3 mg IM (maximum dose: 0.15 mg/kg).

Duration of action *Onset*: 5 to 10 minutes IV, 10 to 20 minutes IM. *Peak effect*: 30 to 45 minutes. *Duration*: Variable (generally 12 to 24 hours).

Special considerations Pregnancy safety: Category C. Use during pregnancy only if the maternal benefit outweighs the fetal risk, especially during the third trimester. Continuous cardiac monitoring is required if administering IV. Monitor the QT interval with a 12-lead ECG if feasible. Document the QT interval and relay the findings to the receiving facility staff.[2]

Helium Gas Mixture (Heliox)

Class Medical gas.

Mechanism of action Reduces airflow resistance within the bronchial tree in patients with obstructive lung disease; may also reduce the work of breathing and improve pulmonary gas exchange efficiency.[14]

Indications Persistent or severe bronchospasm in non-intubated patients with obstructive airway disease or pediatric patients with croup unresponsive to all other evidence-based medical interventions.[2]

Contraindications None.[2]

Adverse reactions/side effects May reduce the effectiveness of coughing.

Drug interactions Unknown.

Dosage and administration *Adult and pediatric*: Normoxic patients usually are given a mixture of 80% helium and 20% oxygen using a well-fitting nonrebreathing mask with a reservoir bag; hypoxemic patients are given 70% helium and 30% oxygen or 60% helium and 40% oxygen.[15] Ensure the reservoir bag is filled with the helium/oxygen mixture before placing the mask on the patient. After applying the mask, ensure that the reservoir does not collapse by more than one-third during inspiration. If it does, increase the flow.[15]

Duration of action *Onset*: Immediate. *Peak effect*: Minutes. *Duration*: Eliminated within a few breaths.

Special considerations Pregnancy safety: Not classified. The lower the helium percentage, the less effective Heliox is in reducing the patient's work of breathing.[15] Closely monitor the patient's work of breathing during administration. Heliox should not be routinely administered to children with respiratory distress.

HydrALAZINE (Apresoline)

Class Antihypertensive, vasodilator.

Mechanism of action Relaxes arteriolar, but not venous, smooth muscle. Thought to interfere with calcium movement in vascular smooth muscle, which is responsible for vasoconstriction, resulting in lower BP.

Indications Pregnancy-induced hypertension (SBP greater than 160 mm Hg or DBP greater than 110 mm Hg) lasting more than 15 minutes, with associated preeclampsia symptoms.[2]

Contraindications Known hypersensitivity, CAD, mitral valve rheumatic heart disease. Use with caution in patients with stroke, known renal disease, or hypotension.

Adverse reactions/side effects Headache, nausea, flushing, hypotension, palpitations, tachycardia, dizziness, and angina (results of sympathetic stimulation). Paresthesias, numbness, and tingling may also occur.

Drug interactions MAOIs; synergistic effects if given simultaneously with other antihypertensives. NSAIDs may diminish the antihypertensive effects.

Dosage and administration *Adult*: 5 mg IV; may repeat 10 mg after 20 minutes for persistent severe hypertension with preeclampsia symptoms (goal is to reduce MAP by 20% to 25%).[2] *Pediatric*: Not usually indicated in the prehospital setting.

Duration of action *Onset*: 5 to 20 minutes. *Peak effect*: 10 to 80 minutes. *Duration*: 2 to 12 hours.

Special considerations Pregnancy safety: Category C. Not recommended for long-term use during pregnancy. Usually lowers DBP more than SBP.[3]

Hydrocortisone Sodium Succinate (Solu-Cortef)

Class Corticosteroid, adrenal glucocorticoid.

Mechanism of action Anti-inflammatory; immunosuppressive with salt-retaining actions.

Indications Shock with history of adrenal insufficiency or long-term steroid dependence: anaphylaxis, asthma, and COPD.

Contraindications Known hypersensitivity, systemic fungal infections, premature infants (contains benzyl alcohol, which is associated with "fatal gasping syndrome," characterized by CNS depression, metabolic acidosis, and gasping respirations).

Adverse reactions/side effects Headache, vertigo, heart failure, hypertension, fluid retention, nausea.

Drug interactions Simultaneous use with ASA and NSAIDs increases the risk of GI bleeding and ulceration. Concurrent use with diuretics increases potassium loss and can result in hypokalemia.

Dosage and administration *Adult:*[2] Give 2 mg/kg IV/IM (maximum dose: 100 mg). IM administration preferred. *Pediatric:* Consult medical direction.

Duration of action *Onset*: 1 hour. *Peak effect*: Variable. *Duration*: 8 to 12 hours.

Special considerations Pregnancy safety: Category C. Use with caution in pregnant and breastfeeding women. Steroids can mask infection because they suppress both the immune and inflammatory systems. Can increase blood glucose levels, so antidiabetic drug dosages may need to be adjusted. High doses of glucocorticoids or prolonged use can result in many adverse reactions and side effects. If available, hydrocortisone succinate is preferred over methylPREDNISolone and dexamethasone for the patient with adrenal insufficiency because of its dual glucocorticoid and mineralocorticoid effects.[2] Patients with adrenal insufficiency may have an emergency dose of hydrocortisone available that can be administered IV or IM.[2]

HYDROmorphone (Dilaudid)

Class Synthetic opioid analgesic; Schedule II drug.

Mechanism of action Opioid agonist-analgesic of opioid receptors; inhibits ascending pain pathways, thereby altering the response to pain; increases the pain threshold; produces analgesia, respiratory depression, and sedation.[2]

Indications Management of acute moderate to severe pain.

Contraindications Known hypersensitivity, MAOI use during the previous 14 days, GI obstruction. Administer with caution in older adults; in patients with a GCS score less than 15; and in patients with hypotension, hypoxia after maximal supplemental oxygen therapy, signs of hypoventilation, head injury, or concomitant use of CNS depressants.

Adverse reactions/side effects Dizziness, drowsiness, headache, weakness, hypotension, syncope, apnea.

Drug interactions MAOIs, SSRIs; concurrent use with other CNS depressants can induce severe respiratory and/or CNS depression.

Dosage and administration *Adult and pediatric:*[2] Give 0.015 mg/kg IM, IV, or IO. Maximum initial dose: 2 mg; maximum cumulative dose: 4 mg.

Duration of action *Onset*: Variable IM; 5 minutes IV, 15 to 30 minutes oral. *Peak effect*: Variable IM; 10 to 20 minutes IV, 30 to 60 minutes oral. *Duration*: 2 to 3 hours.

Special considerations Pregnancy safety: Category C. Use with caution during pregnancy, weighing the fetal risk against the maternal benefit. Reportedly 5 to 7 times more potent than morphine, with a shorter duration of analgesia.[16] Respiratory depression is managed with naloxone. Document pain severity using a scale of 0 to 10 before and after administration and on arrival at the receiving facility.[2]

Hydroxocobalamin (Cyanokit)

Class Antidote, cyanide poisoning adjunct.

Mechanism of action A synthetic, injectable form of vitamin B_{12} (cobalamin) that binds with cyanide to form nontoxic cyanocobalamin, preventing its toxic effects; excreted renally.

Indications Known or suspected cyanide poisoning.

Contraindications Documented hypersensitivity.

Adverse reactions/side effects Hypertension, allergic reactions, GI bleeding, nausea, vomiting, dyspepsia, dyspnea, dizziness, headache, injection site reactions.

Drug interactions Do not administer in the same IV line with diazepam, DOBUTamine, DOPamine, fentanyl, NTG, propofol, sodium nitrite, or sodium thiosulfate.

Dosage and administration[2] Each 5 g vial of hydroxocobalamin for injection must be reconstituted with 200 mL of lactated Ringer solution, NS, or D_5W (25 mg/mL). *Adult*: Initial dose 5 g administered over 15 minutes at a rate of 10 to 15 mL/min. Maximum single dose: 5 g. An additional 5 g dose may be given with medical consultation. *Pediatric*: Give 70 mg/kg IV at a rate of 10 to 15 mL/min. Maximum single dose: 5 g.

Duration of action *Onset*: Rapid. *Peak effect*: 8 to 10 minutes. *Duration*: Varies.

Special considerations Pregnancy safety: Category C. May cause fetal harm, although the cyanide poisoning risk may outweigh the fetal risk. Breastfeeding should stop following medication administration. Preferred agent in known or suspected cyanide poisoning.[2] Have a high index of suspicion for cyanide poisoning in a patient with a depressed GCS score, respiratory difficulty, and cardiovascular collapse in the setting of an enclosed-space fire.[2] Reassess the patient's airway, oxygenation, and hydration during administration. Administration causes discoloration of the skin and urine, rendering pulse oximetry values inaccurate. Because it interferes with some diagnostic blood tests, it is best to perform prehospital phlebotomy before administering this medication.[2] The use of hydroxocobalamin is replacing the cyanide antidote kit because of its ease of use and presumed superior safety in carbon monoxide–poisoned fire victims. It also does not cause methemoglobinemia and is less hemodynamically destabilizing.

Ibuprofen (Advil, Motrin)

Class NSAID, nonopioid analgesic.

Mechanism of action Inhibits prostaglandin synthesis, thereby reducing swelling, pain, and fever.

Indications Acute pain management, antipyretic.

Contraindications Known ASA/NSAID hypersensitivity, ASA-sensitive asthma, significant renal function impairment, pregnancy, known peptic ulcer disease, active intracranial hemorrhage or GI bleeding, thrombocytopenia, coagulation defects, proven or suspected necrotizing enterocolitis, perioperative pain in the setting of coronary artery bypass graft surgery.

Adverse reactions/side effects Headache, dizziness, drowsiness, fatigue, restless sleep, thirst, sweating, tingling or numbness in hands and feet, tinnitus, blurred vision and eye irritation, fluid retention, nausea, vomiting, frequent urination.

Drug interactions Additive risk for bleeding if given in combination with other agents that affect hemostasis (eg, ASA and other antiplatelet drugs, anticoagulants, SSRIs, SNRIs, and other NSAIDs). Alfalfa, anise, and bilberry may enhance adverse effects. May diminish the antihypertensive effect of HydrALAZINE. May diminish the diuretic effect of loop, thiazide, and thiazide-like diuretics. TCAs may enhance the NSAID antiplatelet effects. May increase bleeding time in patients taking anticoagulants.

Dosage and administration *Adult*:[2] Give 10 mg/kg orally for patients older than 6 months (maximum dose: 800 mg). *Pediatric*: Febrile seizures:[2] Give 10 mg/kg orally, if able to swallow; maximum dose: 600 mg.

Duration of action *Onset*: 30 to 60 minutes. *Peak effect*: 1 to 2 hours. *Duration*: 6 to 8 hours.

Special considerations NSAIDs can increase the risk of heart attack or stroke in patients with or without heart disease or risk factors for heart disease.[17] There is also an increased risk of heart failure with NSAID use.

Commonly Prescribed and OTC Medications

Insulin

Class Antidiabetic, hormone.

Indications Diabetic ketoacidosis or other hyperglycemic state, hyperkalemia (insulin and D_{50} are used together to hyperkalemia), nonketotic hyperosmolar coma.

Contraindications Hypersensitivity, hypoglycemia, hypokalemia.

Adverse reactions/side effects Weakness, fatigue, confusion, headache, seizure, coma, tachycardia, nausea, hypokalemia, hypoglycemia, diaphoresis, itching, swelling, redness.

Drug interactions Incompatible in solution with all other drugs. Glucocorticoids and immunosuppressants may increase insulin requirements. Some antibiotics (eg, fluoroquinolones, sulfonamides) may lower insulin requirements. Insulin dosing adjustments may be necessary if the patient is taking beta blockers. Alcohol and salicylates may potentiate insulin effects.

Special considerations Not used in the emergency prehospital setting, but may be administered by paramedics during interfacility transports. Dosages vary widely depending on the patient's blood glucose level, food intake, indication, and insulin type. The most rapid absorption occurs if insulin is injected in the abdominal wall; the next most rapid absorption if injected in the arm; and the slowest absorption if injected into the thigh.

Ipratropium Bromide (Atrovent)

Class Anticholinergic, bronchodilator, short-acting antimuscarinic agent.

Mechanism of action Antagonizes the action of acetylcholine on bronchial smooth muscle, resulting in bronchodilation.

Indications Persistent bronchospasm, COPD exacerbation, toxic inhalation (in conjunction with albuterol).

Contraindications Hypersensitivity to ipratropium, atropine, alkaloids, or peanuts. Use with caution in patients with urinary retention, narrow-angle glaucoma, cardiovascular disease, or hypertension.

Adverse reactions/side effects Headache, dizziness, nervousness, tremor, dyspnea, worsening COPD symptoms, hypertension, tachycardia, palpitations, flushing, MI, dry mouth, nausea, vomiting, GI distress.

Drug interactions Potential for additive anticholinergic effects when administered with other antimuscarinic or anticholinergic medications.

Dosage and administration *Adult and pediatric:*[2] Give 0.5 mg nebulized, up to three doses, in conjunction with albuterol.

Duration of action *Onset*: 5 to 15 minutes. *Peak effect*: 1.5 to 2 hours. *Duration*: 4 to 6 hours.

Special considerations Pregnancy safety: Category B. Shake well before use. Ipratropium bromide and other anticholinergic agents should not be given to children with bronchiolitis in the prehospital setting.[2]

Isopropyl Alcohol

Class Secondary alcohol.

Mechanism of action In addition to its role as an antiseptic, may be used as an antiemetic.[2] Although its mechanism of action as an antiemetic is not certain, isopropyl alcohol may influence neurotransmission at several sites that activate the chemoreceptor trigger zone.[18]

Indications Nausea and vomiting.

Contraindications None.

Adverse reactions/side effects None in adults.

Drug interactions None.

Dosage and administration *Adult:*[2] Allow the patient to inhale the vapor from an isopropyl alcohol wipe three times every 15 minutes as tolerated. *Pediatric*: Consult medical direction regarding use in this patient population.

Duration of action *Onset*: Within 10 minutes. *Peak effect*: Variable. *Duration*: Variable.

Special considerations None.

Ketamine (Ketalar)

Class Analgesic, general anesthetic, dissociative anesthetic; Schedule III drug.

Mechanism of action Blocks pain receptors and minimizes spinal cord activity, affecting the brain's association pathways between the thalamus and the limbic system.

Indications Procedural sedation, management of agitated or violent behavior, pain control.

Contraindications Known hypersensitivity, infants younger than 3 months of age, pregnancy, angina, heart failure, symptomatic hyperthyroidism, known or suspected schizophrenia, conditions where hypertension would be hazardous to the patient's care. Use with caution in any patient with the potential for increased ICP, including those with head trauma, intracranial mass lesions, intracranial bleeding, or hydrocephalus.[5]

Adverse reactions/side effects Hypertension, hallucinations, nausea/vomiting, nystagmus, bronchodilation, tachycardia, increased secretions, hypersalivation, laryngospasm, respiratory depression, mild to moderate elevations in BP and heart rate.

Drug interactions Ketamine may enhance the CNS depressant effects of alcohol, cannabis, opioids, barbiturates, and nondepolarizing neuromuscular blockers (eg, pancuronium, rocuronium, vecuronium). St. John's wort can reduce its effectiveness.

Dosage and administration *Adults:* Procedural sedation:[7] Give 1 to 2 mg/kg IV push over 1 to 2 minutes. Pain control:[2] Moderate discomfort: 0.5 mg/kg IN (maximum initial dose: 55 mg; maximum total dose: 100 mg). Severe to excruciating discomfort: 0.25 mg/kg IM/IV/IO (maximum initial dose: 25 mg; maximum total dose: 100 mg). Chemical restraint:[2] Give 2 mg/kg IV or 4 mg/kg IM. *Pediatric*: Procedural sedation:[7] Give 1 to 2 mg/kg IV/IO push over 1 to 2 minutes. Chemical restraint:[2] Give 1 mg/kg IV or 3 mg/kg IM.

Duration of action *Onset*: 30 seconds. *Peak effect*: 30 seconds to 5 minutes. *Duration*: 10 to 15 minutes.

Special considerations Pregnancy safety: Category N (not classified). Contraindicated for use during pregnancy or by breastfeeding women. Ketamine is referred to as a dissociative anesthetic because the patient may remain conscious but be insensitive to pain and experience short-term amnesia. Its chemical makeup is similar to that of phencyclidine (PCP), but it is shorter acting and less toxic.[2] Some patients may experience an emergence reaction (eg, dream-like state, confusion, vivid imagery, excitement, hallucinations, delirium, irrational behavior) after the full duration of the medication's effect, which may last a few hours.

Ketorolac Tromethamine (Toradol)

Class NSAID, nonopioid analgesic.

Mechanism of action Potent analgesic that inhibits prostaglandin synthesis; does not have any sedative or anxiolytic properties.

Indications Acute management of moderate to severe pain.

Contraindications NSAID or ASA allergy; ASA-sensitive asthma; renal insufficiency; pregnancy; known peptic ulcer disease; hypotension (due to renal toxicity); women who are in active labor or breastfeeding; significant renal impairment, particularly when associated with volume depletion; previous or current GI bleeding; intracranial bleeding; coagulation defects; patients at high risk of bleeding. Use with caution in older patients due to a higher risk of renal and fatal GI adverse reactions.

Adverse reactions/side effects Drowsiness, dizziness, headache, sedation, bronchospasm, dyspnea, edema, vasodilation, hypotension, hypertension, GI bleeding, diarrhea, dyspepsia, nausea.

Drug interactions May increase bleeding time in patients taking anticoagulants. TCAs may enhance the NSAID antiplatelet effects.

Dosage and administration[2] (one-time dose only) *Adult*: Moderate discomfort: 30 mg IM in adults who are not pregnant. Severe to excruciating discomfort: 15 mg IV in adults who are not pregnant. *Geriatric*: Moderate discomfort: 1 mg/kg IM (maximum dose: 30 mg). *Pediatric (2 to 16 years)*: Moderate discomfort: 1 mg/kg IM (maximum dose: 30 mg). Severe to excruciating discomfort *(2 to 16 years)*: 0.5 mg/kg IV (maximum dose: 15 mg). Febrile seizures: 1 mg/kg IV (maximum dose: 15 mg) if unable to swallow.

Duration of action *Onset*: 10 minutes. *Peak effect*: 1 to 2 hours. *Duration*: 2 to 6 hours.

Special considerations Pregnancy safety: Category C. Contraindicated for use during pregnancy. Use caution if pain is possibly from a traumatic source. Document pain severity using a scale of 0 to 10 before and after administration and on arrival at the receiving facility.[2]

Levalbuterol (Xopenex)

Class Sympathomimetic, bronchodilator, short-acting beta-2 adrenergic agonist.

Mechanism of action Stimulates beta-2 receptors resulting in smooth muscle relaxation of the bronchial tree and peripheral vasculature.

Indications Treatment of acute bronchospasm in patients with reversible obstructive airway disease (COPD/asthma). Bronchospasm prophylaxis in patients with asthma.

Contraindications Known hypersensitivity to the drug, other sympathomimetics, or peanuts; MAOI use within 14 days. Angioedema, tachydysrhythmias, and severe cardiac disease. Avoid administration with other drugs that prolong the QT interval (eg, amiodarone, chlorproMAZINE, droperidol, haloperidol, sotalol, macrolides, fluoroquinolones, procainamide, promethazine). Use with caution in patients with cardiac dysrhythmias and cardiovascular disorders.

Adverse reactions/side effects Headache, anxiety, dizziness, restlessness, hallucinations, throat irritation, tachycardia, hypertension, hypotension, dysrhythmias, angina, nausea, vomiting, dyspepsia, tremors, hypokalemia, hyperglycemia.

Drug interactions Increased actions of bronchodilators, TCAs, MAOIs, and other adrenergic drugs. Increased risk of QT prolongation when administered with other QT-prolonging drugs.

Dosage and administration *Adult*: 1.25 mg in 3 mL NS administered by nebulizer over 5 to 15 minutes and repeated as necessary. *Pediatric*: 0.63 to 1.25 mg in 3 mL NS administered by nebulizer over 5 to 15 minutes and repeated as necessary.

Duration of action *Onset*: 5 to 15 minutes. *Peak effect*: 60 to 90 minutes. *Duration*: 6 to 8 hours.

Special considerations Pregnancy safety: Category C.

Lidocaine Hydrochloride (Xylocaine)

Class Antidysrhythmic (Class Ib), anesthetic.

Mechanism of action *Cardiac*: Combines with fast sodium channels, thereby inhibiting recovery after repolarization, and decreasing myocardial excitability and conduction velocity.[2] *Local anesthetic*: Inhibits ion transport across the neuronal membrane, blocking conduction of normal nerve impulses. *RSI*: May decrease ICP response during laryngoscopy.[7]

Indications Alternative to amiodarone in patients with cardiac arrest from VT, VF; stable monomorphic VT; or stable polymorphic VT with normal baseline QT interval when ischemia is treated and electrolyte balance is corrected. Can be used for stable polymorphic VT with baseline QT interval prolongation if TdP is suspected.[7] Also used as a local anesthetic for various procedures, including intubation and IO infusions.

Contraindications Hypersensitivity to lidocaine or amide-type local anesthetics, second- or third-degree AV block in the absence of an artificial pacemaker, Stokes-Adams syndrome, wide-complex ventricular escape beats with bradycardia, Wolff-Parkinson-White Syndrome.[2] Prophylactic use in AMI is contraindicated.[7]

Adverse reactions/side effects Drowsiness, confusion, seizures, slurred speech, hypotension, dysrhythmias, cardiac arrest, nausea, vomiting.

Drug interactions Apnea induced with succinylcholine may be prolonged by high doses of lidocaine. Cardiac depression may occur in conjunction with administration of IV phenytoin. Procainamide may exacerbate the CNS effects. Metabolic clearance is decreased in patients with liver disease and patients taking beta blockers.

Dosage and administration *Adult*: Cardiac arrest (pulseless VT/VF):[7] Initial dose: 1 to 1.5 mg/kg IV/IO. Repeat dose: 0.5 to 0.75 mg/kg IV/IO repeated in 5 to 10 minutes. Maximum total dose: 3 mg/kg. Maintenance infusion: 1 to 4 mg/min. Stable VT and stable regular wide-complex tachycardia: Initial dose: 1 to 1.5 mg/kg IV/IO. Repeat dose: 0.5 to 0.75 mg/kg IV/IO repeated in 5 to 10 minutes. Maximum total dose: 3 mg/kg. Maintenance infusion: 1 to 4 mg/min. Local anesthetic dose varies depending on the procedure and anatomic location. If IO access is to be used for a conscious patient, consider the use of 0.5 mg/kg of lidocaine 0.1 mg/mL slow push through the IO needle to a maximum of 40 mg to mitigate pain from IO medication administration.[2] *Pediatric*:[7] IV/IO dose: 1 mg/kg IV/IO push. Maintenance IV/IO infusion: 20 to 50 mcg/kg/min. Repeat bolus dose (1 mg/kg) if infusion started more than 15 minutes after initial bolus dose. ET dose: 2 to 3 mg/kg. *RSI*: 1 to 2 mg/kg IV/IO. Local anesthetic dose varies depending on the procedure and anatomic location.

Duration of action *Onset*: 1 to 5 minutes. *Peak effect*: 5 to 10 minutes. *Duration*: 10 to 20 minutes.

Special considerations Pregnancy safety: Category B. Reduce the maintenance infusion in the presence of impaired liver function or left ventricular dysfunction.[7] Discontinue the infusion immediately if signs of toxicity develop.

Lorazepam (Ativan)

Class Benzodiazepine, sedative-hypnotic, anticonvulsant; Schedule IV drug.

Mechanism of action Anxiolytic, anticonvulsant, and sedative effect; suppresses propagation of seizure activity produced by foci in the cortex, thalamus, and limbic areas; inhibits GABA receptors in the CNS, reducing neuron excitability.

Indications Uncontrolled shivering associated with hyperthermia/heat exposure, active seizures, anxiety/sedation, chemical restraint.

Contraindications Documented hypersensitivity, neurologic or respiratory depression, acute narrow-angle glaucoma, sleep apnea, shock, suspected drug abuse.

Adverse reactions/side effects Dizziness, drowsiness, CNS depression, headache, sedation, respiratory depression, apnea, hypotension, bradycardia.

Drug interactions Concomitant use with other CNS depressants may cause respiratory depression, hypotension, profound sedation, and death. Individuals taking passionflower or St. John's wort may experience hand tremors, dizziness, and muscular fatigue. Motherwort can potentiate the sedative effects and may result in coma.[8]

Dosage and administration When given IV/IO, must be diluted with an equal volume of sterile water or sterile saline. *Adult*: Anxiety/sedation: 0.1 mg/kg IV slowly over 2 minutes (maximum single dose: 4 mg); 4 mg IM. Shivering associated with hyperthermia/heat exposure:[2] Give 1 mg IV/IO, may repeat once in 5 minutes; or 2 mg IM, may repeat once in 10 minutes. Chemical restraint:[2] Give 2 mg IV or 4 mg IM. *Pediatric*: Seizures:[2] If vascular access is present, 0.1 mg/kg IV/IO slowly over 2 minutes (maximum single dose: 4 mg). Shivering associated with hyperthermia/heat exposure:[2] Give 0.1 mg/kg IV/IM/IO (maximum single dose: 1 mg). Chemical restraint:[2] Give 0.05 mg/kg IV (maximum dose: 2 mg) or 0.05 mg/kg IM (maximum dose: 4 mg).

Duration of action *Onset*: 2 to 5 minutes IV; 15 to 30 minutes IM. *Peak effect*: Less than 15 minutes IV, 2 to 3 hours IM. *Duration*: 6 to 8 hours IV/IM.

Special considerations Pregnancy safety: Category D. Fetal risk and maternal benefit should be considered before using lorazepam. Monitor respiratory rate and BP during administration. Have advanced airway equipment readily available. Consider decreasing the dose by 50% in patients older than 60 years.

Magnesium Sulfate

Class Electrolyte, Class V antidysrhythmic.

Mechanism of action Depresses the CNS, blocks peripheral neuromuscular transmission, and produces anticonvulsant effects; decreases the amount of acetylcholine released at the end-plate by motor nerve impulses, slows the rate of SA node impulse formation in the myocardium, and prolongs conduction time.[2] Promotes calcium, potassium, and sodium movement in and out of cells and stabilizes excitable membranes.[2] Induces uterine relaxation. Can cause bronchodilation after beta agonists and anticholinergics have been administered.

Indications Management of TdP, severe bronchoconstriction with impending respiratory failure, seizure during the third trimester of pregnancy or in the postpartum patient.[2]

Contraindications Known hypersensitivity, heart block, myocardial damage, diabetic coma, hypermagnesemia, hypercalcemia. Use with caution in patients with known renal insufficiency.

Adverse reactions/side effects Drowsiness, CNS depression, respiratory depression, respiratory tract paralysis, vasodilation, possible hypotension and bradycardia with rapid administration, decreased deep tendon reflexes.

Drug interactions May enhance the effects of other CNS depressants. Serious changes in overall cardiac function may occur with cardiac glycosides.

Dosage and administration *Adult*: Severe hypertension (SBP greater than 160 mm Hg or DBP greater than 110 mm Hg) lasting more than 15 minutes with associated preeclampsia symptoms:[2] Give 4 g of a 20% solution IV/IO over 20 minutes, followed by 1 g/h IV/IO, if available. Seizure activity associated with pregnancy greater than 20 weeks' gestation:[2] Give 4 g of a 50% solution IV/IO over 10 to 20 minutes, followed by 1 g/h IV/IO, if available. Contact medical direction for additional orders if seizure persists despite the initial dose of magnesium sulfate. Cardiac arrest due to hypomagnesemia or TdP: [7] Give 1 to 2 g (2 to 4 mL of 50% solution diluted in 50 to 100 mL of D_5W or NS over 5 to 60 minutes) IV/IO. TdP with pulse or AMI with hypomagnesemia:[7] Loading dose of 1 to 2 g in 50 to 100 mL of D_5W or NS over 5 to 60 minutes IV. Follow with 0.5 to 1 g/h IV (titrate dose to control TdP). Status asthmaticus: Give 1 to 2 g IV over 15 to 30 minutes. Severe bronchoconstriction/impending respiratory failure:[2] Give 40 mg/kg IV over 10 to 15 minutes; maximum dose: 2 g. *Pediatric*:[7] Pulseless VT with TdP: 25 to 50 mg/kg IV/IO bolus of a 50% solution. Maximum dose: 2 g. TdP with pulses or hypomagnesemia: 25 to 50 mg/kg IV/IO of a 50% solution over 10 to 20 minutes. Maximum dose: 2 g. Status asthmaticus: 25 to 50 mg/kg IV/IO of a 50% solution over 15 to 30 minutes. Maximum dose: 2 g.

Duration of action *Onset*: IV/IO: immediate. *Peak effect*: Variable. *Duration*: IV/IO: 30 minutes.

Special considerations Pregnancy safety: Category D. Due to confirmed evidence of human fetal risk, must be used cautiously, although its administration may be justified. Magnesium toxicity signs include hypotension followed by a loss of deep tendon reflexes, somnolence or slurred speech, respiratory paralysis, and, ultimately, cardiac arrest.[2] To treat magnesium toxicity, stop the magnesium infusion, give calcium gluconate 1 g IV in cases of impending respiratory arrest, and support the patient's ventilatory effort.[2] Do not abbreviate magnesium sulfate; spell it out to avoid confusion with morphine sulfate.

Mannitol (Osmitrol)

Class Osmotic diuretic.

Mechanism of action Promotes the movement of fluid from the intracellular space to the extracellular space. Decreases cerebral edema and ICP. Promotes urinary excretion of toxins.

Indications Reduction of ICP in managing neurologic emergencies; promotes diuresis for excretion of toxic substances and metabolites.

Contraindications Known hypersensitivity, hypotension, pulmonary edema or severe pulmonary congestion, electrolyte abnormalities, severe dehydration, intracranial bleeding, heart failure. Use with caution in patients with impaired renal function (fluid overload can result).

Adverse reactions/side effects Headache, confusion, blurred vision, tachycardia, chest pain, heart failure, hypotension/hypertension, hypokalemia/hyperkalemia, hyponatremia/hypernatremia, nausea, vomiting, masking or worsening dehydration, rebound increases in ICP, injection site reaction.

Drug interactions Many. May precipitate digitalis toxicity when given concurrently. Avoid use of other diuretics in combination with mannitol, if possible. Concomitant administration may potentiate mannitol's renal toxicity. Avoid use with salicylates and NSAIDs (increases risk of renal failure). Use with nitrates can cause hypotension.

Dosage and administration *Adult*:[7] Give 0.5 to 1 g/kg IV infusion over 5 to 10 minutes through an in-line filter. Additional doses of 0.25 to 2 g/kg can be given every 4 to 6 hours as needed. *Pediatric*: Consult medical direction.

Duration of action *Onset*: 1 to 3 hours for diuretic effect; 15 minutes for reduction of ICP. *Peak effect*: Variable. *Duration*: 4 to 6 hours for diuretic effect; 3 to 8 hours for reduction of ICP.

Special considerations Pregnancy safety: Category C. May crystallize at low temperatures; store at room temperature. Usage and dosages in emergency care are controversial. Be sure to have ventilatory support available.

Meperidine Hydrochloride (Demerol)

Class Opioid analgesic; synthetic opioid; Schedule II drug.

Mechanism of action Synthetic opioid analgesic whose effects on the CNS and smooth muscle organs are similar to those of morphine; primarily acts as an analgesic and a sedative.

Indications Analgesia for moderate to severe pain.

Contraindications Known hypersensitivity, diarrhea caused by poisoning, patients who have taken an MAOI during the previous 14 days, during labor or delivery of a premature infant. Administer with caution to patients with a GCS score less than 15, hypotension, hypoxia after maximal supplemental oxygen therapy, or signs of hypoventilation. Decrease the dose for patients with hepatic or renal insufficiency.

Adverse reactions/side effects Seizures, confusion, sedation, headache, hallucinations, increased ICP, respiratory depression, apnea, hypotension, orthostatic hypotension, syncope, dysrhythmias, nausea, vomiting, constipation, sweating.

Drug interactions Additive CNS depression with TCAs, alcohol, or other CNS depressants.

Dosage and administration *Adult*: 50 to 100 mg IM; 25 to 50 mg slowly IV/IO. *Pediatric:* Not recommended.

Duration of action *Onset*: 10 to 15 minutes IM, within 1 minute IV. *Peak effect*: Within 60 minutes IM, 5 to 7 minutes IV. *Duration*: 2 to 4 hours IV.

Special considerations Pregnancy safety: Category C. Use with caution in patients with asthma and COPD. May aggravate seizures in patients with known convulsive disorders. Has a shorter duration of action than morphine. Effects are reversible with naloxone. Document pain severity using a scale of 0 to 10 before and after administration and on arrival at the receiving facility.[2]

MethylPREDNISolone Sodium Succinate (Solu-Medrol)

Class Corticosteroid, synthetic glucocorticoid, anti-inflammatory agent.

Mechanism of action Highly potent synthetic glucocorticoid that suppresses acute and chronic inflammation; potentiates vascular smooth muscle relaxation by beta adrenergic agonists; has few to no mineralocorticoid properties.

Indications Allergic reaction, anaphylaxis, acute bronchospastic disease management, shock with a history of adrenal insufficiency or long-term steroid dependence.

Contraindications Known hypersensitivity, serious untreated infections, premature infants. Use with caution in patients with GI bleeding, heart failure, hypertension, recent AMI, renal disease, seizure disorder, Cushing disease.

Adverse reactions/side effects Depression, euphoria, headache, restlessness, seizure, increased ICP, hypertension, heart failure, nausea, vomiting, peptic ulcer, fluid retention, hypernatremia, hyperkalemia.

Drug interactions Hypoglycemic responses to insulin and hypoglycemic agents may be blunted.

Dosage and administration *Adult*: Bronchospasm:[2] Give 2 mg/kg IV/IO/IM; maximum dose: 125 mg. Shock with history of adrenal insufficiency or long-term steroid dependence:[2] Give 2 mg/kg IV; maximum dose: 125 mg. *Pediatric*:[7] For status asthmaticus, anaphylaxis: 2 mg/kg IV/IO/IM loading dose; maximum dose: 60 mg. Maintenance dose: 0.5 mg/kg IV every 6 hours or 1 mg/kg IV every 12 hours up to 120 mg/day.

Duration of action *Onset*: 1 to 2 hours. *Peak effect*: Variable. *Duration*: 8 to 24 hours.

Special considerations Pregnancy safety: Category C. Crosses the placenta and may cause fetal harm. Use with caution in pregnant and breastfeeding women, weighing the potential risks and benefits. Steroids can mask infection because they suppress both the immune and inflammatory systems. Can increase blood glucose levels, so antidiabetic drug dosages may need to be adjusted. If available, hydrocortisone succinate is preferred over methylPREDNISolone and dexamethasone for patients with adrenal insufficiency because of its dual glucocorticoid and mineralocorticoid effects.[2] High doses of glucocorticoids or prolonged use can result in many adverse reactions and side effects.

Metoclopramide (Reglan)

Class Antiemetic, direct-acting cholinergic agonist, prokinetic agent.

Mechanism of action Blocks dopamine receptors (at high doses) and serotonin receptors in the chemoreceptor trigger zone of the CNS; sensitizes tissues to acetylcholine; increases upper GI motility but not secretions; increases lower esophageal sphincter tone.

Indications Nausea, vomiting.

Contraindications Known hypersensitivity to metoclopramide or procainamide; GI hemorrhage, mechanical obstruction, or perforation; history of seizures, tardive dyskinesia, or a dystonic reaction; pheochromocytoma; Parkinson disease; administration with other drugs that can cause extrapyramidal symptoms (eg, phenothiazines, butyrophenones).

Adverse reactions/side effects Nausea, vomiting, headache, fatigue, rash, dystonic reaction, confusion, AV block, bradycardia, hallucinations, laryngospasm.

Drug interactions Increased sedation risk when used with CNS depressants, antihistamines, anticholinergics, MAOIs. May decrease the effects of dopamine agonists. Can increase the rate or extent of ASA absorption because of accelerated gastric emptying.

Dosage and administration[2] *Adult*: 10 mg IV/IM. *Pediatric*: Older than age 2 and weight greater than 12 kg: 0.1 mg/kg IM or 0.1 mg/kg IV; may repeat once in 20 to 30 minutes if no relief (maximum 10 mg/dose IV).

Duration of action *Onset*: 1 to 3 minutes (IV), 30 to 60 minutes. *Peak effect*: Immediate (IV). *Duration*: 1 to 2 hours.

Special considerations Pregnancy safety: Category B. Geriatric patients should receive the lowest dose that is effective; older adults are at greater risk for adverse effects such as tardive dyskinesia, confusion or oversedation, and parkinsonian-like adverse effects.[5]

Midazolam Hydrochloride (Versed)

Class Benzodiazepine, anticonvulsant, antianxiety agent, anxiolytic, sedative-hypnotic; Schedule IV drug.

Mechanism of action Inhibits GABA receptors in the CNS, thereby reducing neuron excitability and causing sedative, anxiolytic, amnesic, and hypnotic effects.

Indications Uncontrolled shivering associated with hyperthermia/heat exposure, active seizures, chemical restraint, severe respiratory distress (palliative care), sedation for medical procedures (eg, intubation, ventilated patients, cardioversion), poisoning/overdose care.

Contraindications Documented hypersensitivity, neurologic or respiratory depression, acute narrow-angle glaucoma, sleep apnea, shock, alcohol intoxication, overdose, depressed vital signs. Concomitant use with barbiturates, alcohol, opioids, or other CNS depressants.

Adverse reactions/side effects Headache, somnolence, respiratory depression, respiratory arrest, hypotension, cardiac arrest, nausea, vomiting, pain at the injection site.

Drug interactions Concomitant use with other CNS depressants may cause respiratory depression, hypotension, profound sedation, and death. Motherwort can potentiate midazolam's sedative effects and may result in coma.[8] St. John's wort and green tea can reduce its effectiveness. Mango and grapefruit juice may potentiate its effects.

Dosage and administration *Adult*: Shivering associated with hyperthermia/heat exposure:[2] Give 2.5 mg IV/IN/IO, may repeat once in 5 minutes; or 5 mg IM, may repeat once in 10 minutes. Seizures:[2] If vascular access is available, 0.1 mg/kg IV/IO slowly over 2 minutes (maximum single dose: 4 mg); if vascular access is not available, 0.2 mg/kg (maximum: 10 mg) IM (preferred) or IN. Chemical restraint:[2] Give 5 mg IV or 5 mg IM or 5 mg IN. Severe respiratory distress (palliative care):[2] Give 2 to 5 mg IV. Procedural sedation:[7] Give 0.1 to 0.3 mg/kg IV (maximum single dose: 10 mg). Poisoning/overdose care:[2] Give 0.1 mg/kg in 2-mg increments via slow IV push over 1 to 2 minutes (maximum single dose: 5 mg). *Pediatric*: Shivering associated with hyperthermia/heat exposure:[2] Give 0.1 mg/kg IV/IO or 0.2 mg/kg IN/IM (maximum single dose: 1 mg). A 5 mg/mL concentration is recommended for IN/IM administration. Seizures:[2] If vascular access is available, 0.1 mg/kg IV/IO slowly over 2 minutes (maximum single dose: 4 mg); if vascular access is not available, 0.2 mg/kg (maximum; 10 mg) IM (preferred) or IN. Chemical restraint:[2] Give 0.05 to 0.1 mg/kg IV (maximum dose: 5 mg) or 0.1 to 0.15 mg/kg IM (maximum dose: 5 mg) or 0.3 mg/kg IN (maximum dose: 5 mg). Poisoning/overdose care:[2] Give 0.1 mg/kg in 2-mg increments via slow IV push over 1 to 2 minutes (maximum single dose: 5 mg) or 0.2 mg/kg IN (maximum single dose: 4 mg).

Duration of action *Onset*: Immediate IV/IN, 15 minutes IM. *Peak effect*: 3 to 5 minutes IV/

IN, 30 to 60 minutes IM. *Duration*: Less than 2 hours IV/IN, 1 to 6 hours IM.

Special considerations Pregnancy safety: Category D. Fetal risk and maternal benefit should be considered before emergent administration. Breastfeeding women should not continue breastfeeding following administration. Requires careful monitoring of respiratory and cardiac function. Reduce the dose by 50% in patients older than 60 years. Evidence supports the use of midazolam IM as an intervention that is at least as safe and effective as IV lorazepam for prehospital seizure cessation.[2] In cases of an acetylcholinesterase inhibitor agent exposure, administration of diazepam or midazolam is preferred over lorazepam because of their more rapid onset of action.[2]

Milrinone (Primacor)

Class Inotrope.

Mechanism of action Increases myocardial contractility; has a direct dilating effect on vascular smooth muscle; does not possess beta adrenergic properties.

Indications[7] Heart failure in postoperative cardiovascular surgical patients, shock with high systemic vascular resistance.

Contraindications Known hypersensitivity. Reduce the dose in patients with renal dysfunction.

Adverse reactions/side effects Headache, nausea, vomiting, hypotension (particularly in volume-depleted patients), hypokalemia, bronchospasm, SVT, ventricular dysrhythmias.

Drug interactions Synergistic with catecholamines.

Dosage and administration Consult medical direction or follow the dosing ordered by the sending physician.

Duration of action *Onset*: 5 to 15 minutes. *Peak effect*: Unknown. *Duration*: 3 to 6 hours.

Special considerations Pregnancy safety: Category C. Hemodynamic monitoring is required. Closely monitor BP and heart rate.

Morphine Sulfate (Roxanol, MS Contin)

Class Opioid analgesic; Schedule II drug.

Mechanism of action Alleviates pain through CNS action. Suppresses the fear and anxiety centers in the brain. Depresses brainstem respiratory centers. Increases peripheral venous capacitance and decreases venous return. Decreases preload and afterload, which decreases myocardial oxygen demand.

Indications Management of acute pain.

Contraindications Known hypersensitivity, patients who have taken an MAOI during the previous 14 days, paralytic ileus, toxin-mediated diarrhea, heart failure due to chronic lung disease, head injuries, brain tumors, delirium tremens, seizure disorders, during labor when premature birth is anticipated, acute or severe bronchial asthma, upper airway obstruction. Administer with caution to patients with a GCS score less than 15, hypotension, hypoxia after maximal supplemental oxygen therapy, or signs of hypoventilation.

Adverse reactions/side effects Confusion, sedation, headache, CNS depression, respiratory depression, apnea, bronchospasm, dyspnea, hypotension, orthostatic hypotension, syncope, bradycardia, tachycardia, nausea, vomiting, dry mouth.

Drug interactions Additive effects with other CNS depressants. MAOIs may cause paradoxical excitation.

Dosage and administration *Adult*: Moderate discomfort:[2] Give 0.1 mg/kg IM (maximum dose: 15 mg). Severe to excruciating discomfort:[2] Give 0.1 mg/kg slow IV/IO (maximum dose: 10 mg). STEMI:[7] Initial dose: 2 to 4 mg slow IV (over 1 to 5 minutes). Repeat dose: 2 to 8 mg at 5- to 15-minute intervals. NSTEMI/unstable angina:[7] Give 1 to 5 mg slow IV push only if symptoms are not relieved by nitrates, provided additional therapy is used to manage the underlying ischemia. *Pediatric*: 0.1 to 0.2 mg/kg per dose IV/IO/IM (maximum dose: 5 mg).

Duration of action *Onset*: Immediate. *Peak effect*: 20 minutes. *Duration*: 2 to 4 hours.

Special considerations Pregnancy safety: Category C. Use with caution in pregnancy, weighing the risks and benefits carefully. Use cautiously in breastfeeding women. Morphine rapidly crosses the placenta. Safety in neonates has not been established. Use with caution in older patients, those with asthma, and those susceptible to CNS depression. The effects are reversible with naloxone. Document pain severity using a scale of 0 to 10 before and after administration and on arrival at the receiving facility.[2] Do not abbreviate morphine sulfate; spell it out to avoid confusion with magnesium sulfate.

Naloxone Hydrochloride (Narcan, EVZIO)

Class Opioid antagonist, opioid reversal agent, antidote.

Mechanism of action Competitive inhibition at opioid receptor sites. Reverses respiratory depression and sedation secondary to opioids.

Indications Complete or partial reversal of CNS and respiratory depression induced by opioids or synthetic opioids.

Contraindications Known hypersensitivity or allergy. Use with caution in opioid-dependent patients. Use with caution in neonates of opioid-addicted mothers.

Adverse reactions/side effects Restlessness, seizures, dyspnea, pulmonary edema, hypotension with rapid administration, hypertension, dysrhythmias, diaphoresis, nausea, vomiting, withdrawal symptoms in opioid-addicted patients.

Drug interactions Incompatible with bisulfite and alkaline solutions.

Dosage and administration *Adult:*[2] Initial dose 0.4 to 2 mg IV/IO/IM/ET tube or up to a dose of 4 mg IN. *Pediatric:*[2] Initial dose 0.1 mg/kg IV/IO/IM/IN/ET tube; maximum dose: 2 mg IV/IM/ET tube; maximum dose: 4 mg IN.

Duration of action *Onset:* Less than 2 minutes, IV; 2 to 10 minutes IM/IN. *Peak effect:* Less than 2 minutes, IV; 2 to 10 minutes IM/IN. *Duration:* 20 to 120 minutes, IV/IM/IN.

Special considerations Pregnancy safety: Category C. The half-life of naloxone is often shorter than the half-life of opioids; repeat dosing may be required. In patients with cardiac arrest, naloxone is generally not beneficial. Begin interventions to support the patient's airway, breathing, and circulation before giving naloxone and provide ongoing airway support as needed until the patient has adequate respiratory effort.[2] Administration can be titrated until adequate respiratory effort is achieved if given with a syringe IV, IM, IN, or ET tube.[2] When administered IN using a needleless syringe, divide doses equally to give a maximum of 1 mL per nostril.[2] Administration can result in the sudden onset of opioid withdrawal (agitation, tachycardia, pulmonary edema, nausea, vomiting, and, in neonates, seizures).[2] Very high naloxone doses may be required when managing novel opioid (eg, fentanyl) overdoses. If naloxone was administered to the patient before EMS arrival, obtain information on the dose and route through which it was administered and, if possible, bring the devices containing the dispensed naloxone with the patient along with all other medications on scene.[2]

NIFEdipine (Procardia, Adalat, Nifedical)

Class Calcium channel blocker.

Mechanism of action Inhibits movement of calcium ions across cell membranes; inhibits cardiac and vascular smooth muscle contraction, thereby dilating the main coronary and systemic arteries, reducing preload and afterload, and reducing myocardial oxygen demand; does not prolong AV nodal conduction.

Indications HAPE prevention and treatment,[4] pregnancy-induced hypertension (SBP greater than 160 mm Hg or DBP greater than 110 mm Hg) lasting more than 15 minutes with associated preeclampsia symptoms.[2]

Contraindications Known hypersensitivity to NIFEdipine or other calcium channel blockers; cardiogenic shock; immediate-release preparation (sublingually or orally) for urgent or emergent hypertension.

Adverse reactions/side effects Headache, dizziness, nervousness, weakness, mood changes, dyspnea, cough, wheezing, heart failure, MI, ventricular dysrhythmias, hypotension, syncope, nausea, abdominal discomfort, diarrhea.

Drug interactions Beta blockers may potentiate NIFEdipine's effects. Effects of theophylline may be increased. Antihypertensives may potentiate the hypotensive effects.

Dosage and administration *Adult:* HAPE prevention and treatment:[4] Give 30 mg of the extended-release preparation orally every 12 hours or 20 mg of the extended-release preparation orally every 8 hours. Pregnancy-induced hypertension:[2] Give 10 mg orally. May repeat 10 to 20 mg orally every 20 minutes, twice, for persistent, severe hypertension with preeclampsia symptoms. Goal is to reduce MAP by 20% to 25%. *Pediatric:* Data are unavailable.

Duration of action *Onset*: 15 to 30 minutes. *Peak effect*: 1 to 3 hours. *Duration*: 6 to 8 hours.

Special considerations Pregnancy safety: Category C. Can be used for HAPE treatment when descent is impossible or delayed and reliable access to supplemental oxygen or portable hyperbaric therapy is unavailable.[4] Hypotension is less common when the extended-release preparation is used but may develop when NIFEdipine is given to patients with intravascular volume depletion.[4] Reassess vital signs every 10 minutes during transport.

Nitroglycerin (Nitrostat, Nitrolingual Pumpspray, NitroQuick, Nitro-Bid, Tridil)

Class Vasodilator, nitrate, antianginal.

Mechanism of action Smooth muscle relaxant, which acts on the vasculature, bronchial, uterine, and intestinal smooth muscle. Dilates peripheral arterioles and veins. Reduces peripheral vascular resistance, preload, and afterload, decreasing the heart's workload and myocardial oxygen demand.

Indications Ischemic-type chest pain, acute and symptomatic hypertension, heart failure, pulmonary edema.

Contraindications Known hypersensitivity, hypotension (SBP less than 90 mm Hg or 30 mm Hg or more below baseline), hypovolemia, intracranial bleeding or head injury, pericardial tamponade, severe bradycardia or tachycardia, RV infarction, previous administration of sildenafil (Viagra) or vardenafil (Levitra) within 24 hours or tadalafil (Cialis) within 48 hours. Use with caution in patients with hepatic disease, anemia, diabetes mellitus, pregnancy, or breastfeeding.

Adverse reactions/side effects Headache, dizziness, weakness, reflex tachycardia, syncope, hypotension, nausea, vomiting, dry mouth, muscle twitching, diaphoresis.

Drug interactions Increased hypotensive effect with alcohol, beta blockers, calcium channel blockers, antihypertensives, benzodiazepines, phenothiazines, and other vasodilators. Incompatible with other drugs given IV. Hawthorn increases NTG levels.[3]

Dosage and administration *Adult*:[7] SL: 0.3 to 0.4 mg; may repeat in 3 to 5 minutes to a maximum of 3 doses. Spray: 1 or 2 sprays; may repeat in 3 to 5 minutes to a maximum of 3 doses. NTG IV: 12.5 to 25 mcg bolus (if no SL or spray is given), then begin 10 mcg/min infusion; increase by 10 mcg/min every 3 to 5 minutes until symptom response or desired effect. Maximum dose: 200 mcg/min. *Pediatric*: Not recommended.

Duration of action *Onset*: 1 to 3 minutes. *Peak effect*: 5 to 10 minutes. *Duration*: 20 to 30 minutes SL, 1 to 10 minutes after discontinuation of IV infusion.

Special considerations Pregnancy safety: Category C. Has been used safely during pregnancy. Use cautiously with breastfeeding women and monitor infants for adverse effects. Hypotension is more common in older patients. If a 12-lead ECG shows an inferior wall infarct, rule out RV infarction via right-side 12-lead ECG before administering NTG. NTG decomposes when exposed to light or heat, so it must be kept in airtight containers. IV NTG must be administered only with an infusion pump direct from the bottle with a vented IV set and non–polyvinyl chloride tubing. The active ingredient may have stinging effect when administered.

Nitroprusside (Nitropress)

Class Antihypertensive, vasodilator.

Mechanism of action Arterial and venous vasodilator that reduces afterload, resulting in decreased BP and increased cardiac output.

Indications Heart failure, acute and symptomatic hypertension.

Contraindications Known hypersensitivity, hypotension, decreased cerebral perfusion, heart failure with reduced peripheral vascular resistance.

Adverse reactions/side effects Confusion, restlessness, flushing, dizziness, headache, palpitations, dysrhythmias, hypotension, methemoglobinemia, cerebrovasodilation leading to increased ICP.

Drug interactions Additive effects with ganglionic blocking agents, general anesthetics, other antihypertensives, and sympathomimetics.

Dosage and administration Consult medical direction or follow the dosing ordered by the sending physician.

Duration of action *Onset*: Immediate. *Peak effect*: Rapid. *Duration*: 1 to 10 minutes.

Special considerations Pregnancy safety: Category C. Use with caution during pregnancy. Contraindicated for use in breastfeeding women. Light sensitive; keep the drug reservoir and tube covered with an opaque material. Can cause cyanide toxicity.

Nitrous Oxide 50:50 (Nitronox)

Class Gaseous analgesic and anesthetic.

Mechanism of action Exact mechanism is unknown; the analgesic action is thought to occur by potentiating the release of endogenous endorphins that react with opioid receptors in the CNS and alter the pain threshold.

Indications Analgesia in the patient who is capable of self-administering this medication.[2]

Contraindications Known hypersensitivity, impaired level of consciousness, head injury, inability to follow or comply with instructions, decompression illness (nitrogen narcosis, air embolism), significant respiratory compromise, suspected abnormal air-filled cavities (eg, pneumothorax, bowel obstruction, air embolism), maxillofacial trauma or facial burns (can interfere with self-administration).[19] Relative contraindications include stroke history, hypotension, pregnancy, known cardiac conditions, and known vitamin B_{12} deficiency.[2]

Adverse reactions/side effects Light-headedness, headache, dizziness, confusion, nausea, vomiting, hallucinations.

Drug interactions Can potentiate the effects of CNS depressants (eg, opioids, sedatives, hypnotics, alcohol).

Dosage and administration *Adult*: Self-administered. Assess the patient's ability to self-administer after the initial dose. *Pediatric*: Same as adult.

Duration of action *Onset*: 2 to 5 minutes. *Peak effect*: 2 to 5 minutes. *Duration*: 2 to 5 minutes.

Special considerations Pregnancy safety: Category C. Some EMS agencies prohibit use of nitrous oxide inside ambulances because of the risk of rescuer exposure, opting to use it only outdoors, on scene, or inside the patient's home.[19] Nitrous oxide is nonflammable and nonexplosive. It is ineffective in 20% of the population. Document pain severity using a scale of 0 to 10 before and after administration and on arrival at the receiving facility.[2]

Norepinephrine Bitartrate (Levophed, Levarterenol)

Class Sympathomimetic, vasopressor.

Mechanism of action Acts predominantly on alpha adrenergic receptors to produce constriction of resistance and capacitance vessels, thereby increasing systemic BP and coronary artery blood flow; also acts on beta-1 receptors. In relatively lower doses, the cardiac-stimulant effect of norepinephrine predominates; with larger doses, the vasoconstrictor effect predominates.[5]

Indications First-line vasopressor in neurogenic shock,[2] hypotension unresponsive to IV/IO fluid resuscitation.

Contraindications Known hypersensitivity; hypotension caused by hypovolemia; pregnancy (relative).

Adverse reactions/side effects Headache; anxiety, dizziness, restlessness, dyspnea; hypertension, dysrhythmias, chest pain, peripheral cyanosis, cardiac arrest; nausea, vomiting; urinary retention, renal failure; tissue necrosis from extravasation; decreased blood flow to the GI tract, kidneys, skeletal muscle, and skin.

Drug interactions TCAs can markedly increase response to pressors. Concomitant use of sympathomimetics may result in additive cardiovascular effects, such as increased BP and heart rate. Alpha adrenergic effects can be blocked during concurrent administration of phenothiazines. Inactivated by alkaline solutions.

Dosage and administration *Adult*:[7] 0.1 to 0.5 mcg/kg/min IV/IO infusion titrated to effect.[2] *Pediatric*:[7] Begin at 0.05 to 0.1 mcg/kg/min IV infusion; adjust rate to achieve desired change in BP and systemic perfusion. Maximum infusion rate: 2 mcg/kg/min.

Duration of action *Onset*: Immediate. *Peak effect*: Less than 1 minute. *Duration*: 1 to 2 minutes.

Special considerations Pregnancy safety: Category C. May cause fetal anoxia when used in pregnancy. Correct hypovolemia before administering. Use an infusion pump and administer through a large, stable vein to avoid extravasation and tissue necrosis. Close monitoring of the IV/IO site and vital signs is essential. Drug- or poison-induced hypotension may require higher doses to achieve adequate perfusion. Research shows that patients in cardiogenic or septic shock treated with norepinephrine have a lower mortality rate than those treated with DOPamine.[2]

Octreotide (Sandostatin)

Class Synthetic hormone, antidiarrheal.

Mechanism of action Mimics the actions of the naturally occurring hormone, somatostatin, decreasing visceral blood flow and inhibiting the release of serotonin, gastrin, vasoactive intestinal peptide, secretin, motilin, and pancreatic polypeptide.

Indications Treatment of active GI bleeding during transport.

Contraindications Known hypersensitivity.

Adverse reactions/side effects Nausea, vomiting, bloating, dizziness, headache, dysrhythmias, pain and irritation at the injection site.

Drug interactions Decreases cycloSPORINE levels.

Dosage and administration Consult medical direction or follow the dosing ordered by the sending physician.

Duration of action *Onset*: 30 minutes. *Peak effect*: 30 minutes. *Duration*: Up to 12 hours.

Special considerations Pregnancy safety: Category B.

Olanzapine (Zyprexa)

Class Second-generation antipsychotic, antimanic agent.

Mechanism of action Exact mechanism has not been determined; may act through a combination of dopamine and serotonin type 2 receptor site antagonism.

Indications Agitated or violent patients experiencing a behavioral emergency; chemical restraint.

Contraindications Documented hypersensitivity. Use with caution in patients who have engaged in strenuous exercise, have dehydration or heat exposure, or are taking medications with anticholinergic effects; impaired core body temperature regulation may occur. Use with caution in patients with a history of seizures or urinary retention.

Adverse reactions/side effects Drowsiness, dry mouth, difficulty speaking, slurred speech, unsteady gait, headache, depression, insomnia, extrapyramidal symptoms (dose-dependent).

Drug interactions Many. Additive effects with alcohol and other CNS depressants. Concurrent use of IM/IV benzodiazepines and olanzapine IM is not recommended, as fatalities have been reported.[2] Ginkgo may potentiate olanzapine's effects.

Dosage and administration[2] *Adult*: Chemical restraint: 10 mg IM. *Pediatric*: Limited data are available for pediatric use. Chemical restraint: Ages 6 to 11 years: 5 mg IM. Ages 12 to 18 years: 10 mg IM.

Duration of action *Onset*: 15 to 30 minutes IM. *Peak effect*: 15 to 45 minutes IM. *Duration*: Variable.

Special considerations Pregnancy safety: Category C. Patients are at risk for severe sedation (including coma) or delirium after each injection, and must be observed for at least 3 hours in a registered facility with ready access to emergency response services.[2] Patients are at significant risk of severe sedation when olanzapine is administered concomitantly with benzodiazepines or to patients taking benzodiazepines.[2]

Ondansetron Hydrochloride (Zofran, Zofran ODT, Zuplenz)

Class Selective serotonin receptor (5-HT_3) antagonist, antiemetic.

Mechanism of action Blocks the action of serotonin, a natural substance that causes nausea and vomiting. Does not affect dopamine receptors, so it does not cause extrapyramidal symptoms.[2]

Indications Prevention and control of nausea or vomiting.

Contraindications Known hypersensitivity to ondansetron or other 5-HT_3 receptor antagonists, known or suspected long QT syndrome, coadministration with apomorphine (the combination is reported to cause profound hypotension and loss of consciousness).

Adverse reactions/side effects Headache, malaise, syncope, wheezing, bronchospasm, dysrhythmias (eg, bradycardia, SVT, VT, PVCs, AF, second-degree AV block), ECG changes (eg, dose-dependent QT prolongation, ST-segment depression), palpitations, constipation, diarrhea, hives, skin rash, serotonin syndrome.

Drug interactions Many. Avoid administration with other drugs that prolong the QT interval (eg, amiodarone, chlorproMAZINE, droperidol, haloperidol, levalbuterol, sotalol, macrolides, fluoroquinolones, procainamide, promethazine). Serotonin syndrome can occur with simultaneous use of several drugs (eg, fentanyl, morphine).

Dosage and administration[2] *Adult*: Antiemetic: 4 mg IV/SL or orally or 4 mg SL of the orally disintegrating tablet formulation. Vomiting associated with AMS: 4 mg IV, SL, or orally every 6 hours. Stimulant poisoning/overdose: 8 mg *slow* IV over 2 to 5 minutes or 4 to 8 mg IM or 8 mg orally disintegrating tablet. *Pediatric*: Ages 6 months to 14 years: Antiemetic: 0.15 mg/kg IV or orally; maximum dose: 4 mg.

Duration of action *Onset*: 30 minutes. *Peak effect*: 1.3 hours (oral), 10 minutes (IV). *Duration*: 3 to 6 hours.

Special considerations Pregnancy safety: Category B. While ondansetron has not been adequately studied in pregnancy to determine its safety in this population, it remains a treatment option for hyperemesis gravidarum in pregnant patients.[2] ECG monitoring is recommended for patients who have electrolyte abnormalities, heart failure, or bradydysrhythmias, or who are also receiving other medications that cause QT prolongation.[2] Ondansetron is the preferred antiemetic in children but can be sedating in very young children.[2]

Commonly Prescribed and OTC Medications

Oral Antidiabetic (Hypoglycemic) Drugs

Oral antidiabetic drugs, also called oral hypoglycemics, are used in conjunction with lifestyle modifications (eg, diet, weight reduction, exercise) to help control serum glucose levels in individuals with type 2 diabetes. Patients with type 2 diabetes have some degree of insulin secretion by the pancreas. All oral antidiabetic agents are contraindicated during pregnancy (including gestational diabetes) and breastfeeding. Fasting blood sugar, pre-meal blood sugar, and hemoglobin A1c levels are periodically measured to assess treatment effectiveness. Patients taking oral antidiabetic drugs are advised to carry medical identification indicating that they have diabetes, the medication taken, and dosage. **TABLE 15-9** lists common oral antidiabetic drugs.

TABLE 15-9 Oral Antidiabetic Agents

Alpha-Glucosidase Inhibitors	
Examples	Acarbose (Precose), miglitol (Glycet)
Action	Inhibit enzymes found in the cells lining the small intestine that convert dietary starch and other complex carbohydrates into simple sugars that can be absorbed, thereby slowing glucose absorption after meals. Intestinal bacteria break down undigested carbohydrates that reach the colon into intestinal gas.
Contraindications	Known hypersensitivity, pregnancy, breastfeeding, diabetic ketoacidosis, cirrhosis, severe renal failure, any preexisting intestinal condition (eg, inflammatory bowel disease, colonic ulceration, bowel obstruction, intestinal disorders of absorption or digestion).

(continues)

TABLE 15-9 Oral Antidiabetic Agents (continued)

Adverse reactions/ side effects	Flatulence, diarrhea, abdominal discomfort.
Drug interactions	Acarbose may increase warfarin absorption. Acarbose and miglitol may decrease digoxin effectiveness. Miglitol decreases the effectiveness of propranolol.
Special considerations	When taken alone, alpha-glucosidase inhibitors do not cause hypoglycemia; however, hypoglycemia is a risk when drugs of this class are combined with other diabetes medications (eg, sulfonylureas, insulin, meglitinides).
Biguanides	
Examples	Metformin (Glucophage)
Action	Decreases the amount of glucose produced by the liver, decreases GI glucose absorption, slows the conversion of carbohydrates into sugar, and increases target cell insulin sensitivity.
Contraindications	Known hypersensitivity, pregnancy, breastfeeding, metabolic acidosis, Class III/IV heart failure, severe liver failure, alcoholism, renal failure, radiologic contrast study within 48 hours.
Adverse reactions/ side effects	Metallic taste in the mouth, mild anorexia, nausea, abdominal discomfort, diarrhea, flatulence, reduced vitamin B_{12} absorption, lactic acidosis (rare).
Drug interactions	Increased cardiovascular risk if used with sulfonylureas. Potential drug interaction exists between metformin and cimetidine, which can increase metformin blood levels.
Special considerations	Unlike other oral antidiabetic agents, does not produce hypoglycemia or hyperglycemia. Generally considered the drug of choice in patients with type 2 diabetes. Must be temporarily discontinued before administering iodinated contrast medium or major surgery to reduce the risk of lactic acidosis.
Meglitinides	
Examples	Nateglinide (Starlix), repaglinide (Prandin)
Action	Lower blood glucose by stimulating insulin release from pancreatic beta cells.
Contraindications	Known hypersensitivity, pregnancy, breastfeeding, severe renal or liver failure.
Adverse reactions/ side effects	Hypoglycemia, weight gain, hepatotoxicity (rare).
Drug interactions	Increased risk of hypoglycemia if used with sulfonylureas.
Special considerations	Often used in obese patients with type 2 diabetes because it promotes weight stabilization or even modest weight reduction. Repaglinide can be used alone or in combination with metformin.
Sulfonylureas	
Examples	First generation: acetoHEXAMIDE (Dymelor), chlorproPAMIDE (Diabinese), TOLAZamide (Tolinase), TOLBUTamide (Orinase) Second generation: glyBURIDE (Micronase), glipiZIDE (Glucotrol), glimepiride (Amaryl)
Action	Stimulate insulin release from beta cells in the pancreas; may improve insulin resistance in peripheral target tissues (muscle fat).

Contraindications	Known hypersensitivity, sulfonamide allergy, pregnancy, breastfeeding, type 1 diabetes, obesity, diabetic ketoacidosis, severe liver or kidney failure. May exacerbate cardiovascular diseases. Some sulfonylureas should be avoided in patients with impaired renal function and used with caution in older adults.
Adverse reactions/ side effects	Syncope, dizziness, nervousness, depression, insomnia, pain, paresthesia, drowsiness, headache, diaphoresis, itching, hypoglycemia, weight gain, diarrhea, flatulence, vomiting, hematologic changes.
Drug interactions	Can potentiate hypoglycemia if used with beta blockers, aspirin, oral anticoagulants, MAOIs, atypical antipsychotics, salicylates, sulfonamides, antacids, cimetidine, or clofibrate, among others. May enhance hyperglycemia if used with oral contraceptives, thiazide diuretics, glucocorticoids, phenothiazines, or anticonvulsants. Green tea may potentiate hypoglycemia with some sulfonylureas.[3]
Special considerations	All sulfonylureas have been associated with weight gain. This class of oral antidiabetic agents is associated with more cardiovascular complications than metformin and has the highest risk of producing hypoglycemia. Second-generation sulfonylureas are more potent and given in much lower doses than the first-generation drugs. Ingesting alcohol while taking sulfonylureas can result in a reaction that includes flushing, headache, sweating, nausea, vomiting, and weakness.[3]
Thiazolidinediones (also called glitazones)	
Examples	Pioglitazone (Actos), rosiglitazone (Avandia)
Action	Reduce insulin resistance by acting on specific receptors in muscle, fat, and the liver to increase the use of glucose and decrease glucose production.
Contraindications	Known hypersensitivity, pregnancy, breastfeeding, liver failure, class III/IV heart failure (use with caution in patients with lesser degrees of heart failure). Pioglitazone is contraindicated if the patient has active bladder cancer and should be used with caution if there is a history of bladder cancer. Use with caution in patients with eye disease.
Adverse reactions/ side effects	Edema, hypoglycemia, cardiac failure, headache, myalgia, sinusitis, pharyngitis, osteoporosis, weight gain.
Drug interactions	Concomitant use of insulin appears to increase the risk of heart failure. Pregabalin (Lyrica) may potentiate fluid retention.
Special considerations	Thiazolidinediones tend to cause weight gain. Rosiglitazone has been associated with increased cardiovascular complications, including AMI. When taken alone, thiazolidinediones do not have a high risk of causing hypoglycemia; however, hypoglycemia is a risk when drugs of this class are combined with other diabetes medications (eg, sulfonylureas, insulin).

Abbreviations: AMI, acute myocardial infarction; GI, gastrointestinal; MAOIs, monoamine oxidase inhibitors

Oxygen

Class Naturally occurring atmospheric gas.

Mechanism of action Reverses hypoxemia.

Indications Any suspected cardiopulmonary emergency (eg, shock, sepsis, major trauma, respiratory arrest, cardiac arrest and postresuscitation, anaphylaxis, carbon monoxide and cyanide poisonings), complaints of shortness of breath and ischemic chest discomfort, all other causes of decreased tissue oxygenation.

Contraindications Observe closely when using with patients who have pulmonary conditions that are known to be dependent on hypoxic respiratory drive (very rare).[7]

Adverse reactions/side effects Decreased level of consciousness (patients with COPD), decreased respiratory drive in patients with COPD, dry mucous membranes.

Drug interactions None.

Dosage and administration *Adult*: Respiratory and cardiac arrest and carbon monoxide poisoning:

100%. After a return of spontaneous circulation, target an SpO_2 of 92% to 98%.[7] For most patients who are not in respiratory or cardiac arrest, target an SpO_2 of 95% to 98%. ACS: Target an SpO_2 of 90%.[7] AMS, HACE, HAPE: Target an SpO_2 higher than 90%.[4] *Pediatric*: Respiratory and cardiac arrest: 100%. After a return of spontaneous circulation, target an SpO_2 of 94% to 99%.[7]

Duration of action *Onset*: Immediate. *Peak effect*: Not applicable. *Duration*: Less than 2 minutes.

Special considerations Be familiar with liter flow rates and each type of delivery device used.

Oxymetazoline (Afrin, Dristan 12-Hour, Vicks Sinus-12 Hour)

Class Intranasal decongestant, vasoconstrictor, topical sympathomimetic.

Mechanism of action Stimulates alpha adrenergic receptors in the arterioles of the nasal mucosa to produce vasoconstriction.

Indications Epistaxis in a patient experiencing facial trauma.

Contraindications Known hypersensitivity, severe hypertension.

Adverse reactions/side effects Rebound nasal congestion, nasal mucosa irritation.

Drug interactions May diminish the vasoconstricting effects of alpha-1 agonists. May enhance the hypertensive effects of sympathomimetics.

Dosage and administration *Adult*: 2 to 3 sprays in each nare. *Pediatric*: 1 to 2 sprays in each nare.

Duration of action *Onset*: Immediate. *Peak effect*: 5 minutes. *Duration*: Up to 5 hours.

Special considerations Pregnancy safety: Category B.

Oxytocin (Pitocin)

Class Pituitary hormone, uterine vasoconstrictor.

Mechanism of action Binds to oxytocin receptor sites on the surface of uterine smooth muscle, increasing the force and frequency of uterine contractions. Causes dilation of vascular smooth muscle, thereby increasing renal, coronary, and cerebral blood flow.

Indications Postpartum hemorrhage due to uterine atony after infant and placental delivery.

Contraindications Known hypersensitivity, presence of a remaining fetus, unfavorable fetal position, anticipated nonvaginal delivery, fetal distress when delivery is not imminent, prolonged use in severe toxemia.

Adverse reactions/side effects Coma, seizures, anxiety, hypotension, dysrhythmias, nausea, vomiting, anaphylaxis, painful uterine contractions, electrolyte disturbances, maternal intracranial hemorrhage.

Drug interactions Can cause severe, persistent hypertension if administered with vasopressors. Synergistic effect with black cohosh, cotton root, squaw vine, and cinnamon.[3]

Dosage and administration *Adult*: IM administration: 10 units IM after delivery of placenta. IV/IO administration: Mix 10 to 40 units in 1,000 mL of a compatible IV solution infused at 10 to 15 drops/min, titrated to the severity of bleeding and uterine response. *Pediatric*: Not applicable.

Duration of action *Onset*: 3 to 5 minutes IM, within 1 minute IV/IO. *Peak effect*: 40 minutes IM, unknown IV/IO. *Duration*: 2 to 3 hours IM, 1 hour after IV/IO infusion is stopped.

Special considerations Pregnancy safety: Category C. Closely monitor vital signs, including fetal heart rate and uterine tone.

Pancuronium Bromide (Pavulon)

Class Nondepolarizing neuromuscular blocking agent, cholinergic receptor antagonist.

Mechanism of action Binds to the receptor for acetylcholine at the neuromuscular junction. Skeletal muscle relaxation proceeds in a predictable order, starting with muscles associated with fine movements (eg, eyes, face, neck), followed by muscles of the limbs, chest, and abdomen, and then the diaphragm; muscle tone returns in the reverse order.[5]

Indications Adjunct to provide skeletal muscle relaxation and facilitate tracheal intubation and ventilation.

Contraindications Known hypersensitivity to pancuronium or a bromide hypersensitivity, inability to control the airway and/or support ventilation with oxygen and positive pressure, neuromuscular disease (eg, myasthenia gravis), hepatic or renal failure. Use with extreme caution in patients with pulmonary disease, such as COPD.

Adverse reactions/side effects Bronchospasm, angioedema, hypotension, edema, tachycardia, flushing, weakness, hypersalivation, itching, hives, prolonged neuromuscular block. Risk of respiratory depression due to relaxation of the intercostal muscles and diaphragm.[5]

Drug interactions Calcium channel blockers may prolong neuromuscular blockade. Positive chronotropic drugs may potentiate tachycardia. Although adequate sedation and analgesia must accompany neuromuscular blocker use, coadministration of opioids may enhance neuromuscular blockade and produce an increased degree of respiratory depression, hypotension, or sedation.[5]

Dosage and administration *Adult*:[5] Give 0.06 to 0.1 mg/kg via slow IV initially, followed by incremental doses of 0.01 mg/kg at 25- to 60-minute intervals as needed to maintain muscle relaxation. *Pediatric*: Consult medical direction.

Duration of action *Onset*: 2 to 3 minutes. *Peak effect*: Paralysis in 4 minutes. *Duration*: 35 to 45 minutes.

Special considerations Pregnancy safety: Category C. Pancuronium does not provide sedation or analgesia and will not stop neuronal seizure activity. If the patient is conscious, explain the effect of the medication before administration. Always sedate the patient before administering pancuronium. Intubation and ventilatory support must be readily available; monitor the patient carefully. Doses should be calculated based on ideal body weight. Anaphylactic and anaphylactoid-type adverse reactions, including fatalities, have been reported in association with neuromuscular blocker use.

Phenylephrine (Neo-Synephrine)

Class Adrenergic, alpha agonist, nasal vasoconstrictor.

Mechanism of action Stimulates alpha adrenergic receptors in the arterioles of the nasal mucosa to produce vasoconstriction.

Indications Epistaxis; to reduce bleeding during nasotracheal intubation.

Contraindications Known hypersensitivity. Use with extreme caution in geriatric patients with preexisting cardiovascular disease.

Adverse reactions/side effects Tremors, palpitations, hypertension.

Drug interactions Exaggerated adrenergic effects if given with, or up to 21 days after, MAOI administration. Hypertensive effects may be potentiated by TCAs, guanethidine, methyldopa, and atropine-like drugs.

Dosage and administration *Adult*: Two sprays in the selected nare before nasotracheal tube insertion.

Duration of action *Onset*: Seconds. *Peak effect*: 30 minutes. *Duration*: 30 minutes to 4 hours.

Special considerations Pregnancy safety: Category C. Each bottle is for single-patient use.

Commonly Prescribed and OTC Medications

Phenytoin (Dilantin)

Class Anticonvulsant.

Indications Prophylaxis and treatment of major motor seizures.

Contraindications Known hypersensitivity, pregnancy, breastfeeding, sinus bradycardia, second- and third-degree heart block, Stokes-Adams syndrome. Should be used with caution in any patient with cardiac disease (eg, cardiac dysrhythmias, heart failure, CAD) because symptoms may be potentiated or exacerbated.

Adverse reactions/side effects Ataxia, agitation, dizziness, headache, drowsiness, CNS depression, respiratory depression, hypotension, dysrhythmias, nausea, vomiting, altered taste, rash, Stevens-Johnson syndrome, nystagmus.

Drug interactions Numerous. Serum phenytoin levels are increased by anticoagulants, cimetidine, sulfonamides, and salicylates. Metabolism is increased by chronic alcohol use. Cardiac depressant effects are increased by lidocaine, propranolol, and other beta blockers. Precipitation may occur when mixed with D_5W. Incompatible with many solutions and medications.

Special considerations Pregnancy safety: Category D.

Potassium Iodide (Pima Syrup, SSKI, ThyroSafe, ThyroShield)

Class Antidote.

Mechanism of action Potassium iodide (KI) can help block radioactive iodine from being absorbed by the thyroid gland, thereby protecting this gland from radiation injury and reducing the risk of thyroid cancer. It does not keep radioactive iodine from entering the body and cannot reverse the health effects caused by radioactive iodine once the thyroid is damaged.[20] The protection against radioactive iodine provided by KI depends on the time after contamination, the rate of KI absorption, and the dose of radioactive iodine.[20]

Indications Environmental radiation emergency to block uptake of radioactive iodine isotopes in the thyroid and reduce thyroid cancer risk.[2]

Contraindications Known iodine hypersensitivity (although an allergy to radiocontrast media, contact dermatitis from iodine-containing antibacterial agents, or allergy to seafood should not be considered evidence of KI allergy), hyperthyroidism, respiratory failure.[2]

Adverse reactions/side effects Skin rash, salivary gland swelling, "iodism" (eg, metallic taste, severe headache, blurred vision, burning mouth and throat, sore teeth and gums, head cold symptoms).

Drug interactions Use with caution in patients taking drugs that may increase serum potassium levels, such as ACE inhibitors. NSAIDs may cause potassium retention.

Dosage and administration Consult medical direction.

Duration of action *Onset*: Data unavailable. *Peak effect*: Data unavailable. *Duration*: Each dose has a duration of action of about 24 hours.

Special considerations Pregnancy safety: Category D. EMS providers may be asked to assist public health agencies in distributing and administering potassium iodide in a mass-casualty incident involving radiation release or exposure.[2] Adults older than 40 years should not take KI unless public health or emergency management officials acknowledge that contamination with a very large dose of radioactive iodine is expected. Adults older than 40 years have the lowest chance of developing thyroid cancer or thyroid injury after contamination with radioactive iodine, and those older than 40 years are more likely to have allergic reactions to or adverse effects from KI.[20]

Pralidoxime (2-PAM, Protopam)

Class Cholinesterase reactivator, antidote.

Mechanism of action Binds to organophosphates and breaks their alkyl phosphate–cholinesterase bonds to restore the activity of acetylcholinesterase.[2]

Indications Antidote in treating poisoning by organophosphate pesticides and related nerve gases (eg, tabun, sarin, soman).

Contraindications Known hypersensitivity; reduce the dose in patients with impaired renal function, older adults with hypertension, and patients with myasthenia gravis.

Adverse reactions/side effects Dizziness, drowsiness, headache, neuromuscular blockade, seizure, laryngospasm, hyperventilation, apnea, tachycardia, cardiac arrest, nausea, muscle rigidity, muscle weakness, rash, pain at injection site. Especially in geriatric patients, excessive doses of pralidoxime chloride may cause severe systolic and diastolic hypertension, neuromuscular weakness, headache, tachycardia, and visual impairment.[2] An overdose of pralidoxime chloride may cause profound neuromuscular weakness and subsequent respiratory depression in children.[2]

Drug interactions Avoid using pralidoxime concurrently with succinylcholine, morphine, aminophylline, theophylline, and other respiratory depressants, including barbiturates, opioid analgesics, and sedative-hypnotics.

Dosage and administration Consult with medical direction; dosage recommendations vary depending on the degree of exposure and patient age and weight. Pralidoxime chloride may be provided in a single-dose vial, prefilled syringes, or auto-injectors.[2] Commercially available auto-injectors contain 600 mg of pralidoxime chloride.

Duration of action *Onset*: Minutes. *Peak effect*: 10 to 20 minutes IM, 5 to 15 minutes IV. *Duration*: Variable.

Special considerations Pregnancy safety: Category C. Slow IV infusion prevents tachycardia, laryngospasm, and muscle rigidity. Consider drawing a blood sample before administration for the hospital to run pretreatment levels. A dose of pralidoxime chloride should be administered shortly after the nerve agent or organophosphate poisoning exposure, as it has a minimal clinical effect if administration is delayed.[2] Cardiac monitoring should be considered in all cases of severe organophosphate poisoning.

Commonly Prescribed and OTC Medications

PredniSONE (Rayos)

Class Adrenal glucocorticoid, synthetic corticosteroid.

Indications Asthma, COPD.

Contraindications Known hypersensitivity, systemic fungal infections.

Adverse reactions/side effects Fluid and sodium retention, weight gain, nausea, diarrhea, increased appetite, increased blood glucose, mood changes.

Drug interactions Simultaneous use with ASA and NSAIDs increases risk of GI bleeding and ulceration. Concurrent use with digoxin increases risk of dysrhythmias. Simultaneous use with diuretics increases potassium loss and can result in hypokalemia. PredniSONE level is decreased with use of ephedra.[3]

Special considerations Steroids can mask infection because they suppress both the immune and inflammatory systems. PredniSONE can increase blood glucose levels, so antidiabetic drug dosages may need to be adjusted. High doses of glucocorticoids or prolonged use can result in many adverse reactions and side effects. The pediatric formulation is often a suspension, prednisoLONE.

Procainamide Hydrochloride (Pronestyl)

Class Class Ia antidysrhythmic.

Mechanism of action[2] Inhibits recovery after repolarization, resulting in decreased myocardial excitability and conduction velocity. Direct membrane depressant that decreases conduction velocity, prolongs the refractory period, decreases automaticity, and reduces repolarization abnormalities.

Indications[7] Stable monomorphic VT with normal QT interval, reentry SVT uncontrolled by vagal maneuvers and adenosine if BP is stable, stable wide-complex tachycardia of unknown origin, AF with a rapid ventricular rate in patients with Wolff-Parkinson-White syndrome.

Contraindications Known hypersensitivity to procainamide or other ingredients, TdP, second- and third-degree heart AV block (without functioning artificial pacemaker), systemic lupus erythematosus, preexisting QT prolongation, digitalis toxicity, TCA overdose. Administer with caution to patients with asthma or digitalis-induced dysrhythmias, myasthenia gravis, or cardiac, hepatic, or renal insufficiency.

Adverse reactions/side effects Can induce or worsen cardiac dysrhythmias, anorexia, nausea, vomiting, confusion, seizures, severe hypotension, and widening of PR, QRS, and QT intervals.

Drug interactions Additive effect with other antidysrhythmic agents. Use with beta agonists may be associated with adverse cardiovascular effects, including QT interval prolongation.[5]

Dosage and administration *Adult*:[7] Recurrent VF/pulseless VT: 20 mg/min slow IV infusion until the dysrhythmia is suppressed. Maximum total dose: 17 mg/kg. In urgent situations, up to 50 mg/min may be administered, up to a total dose of 17 mg/kg. Other indications: 20 mg/min slow IV infusion until any one of the following occurs: dysrhythmia suppression, hypotension, QRS widens by more than 50% of its pretreatment width, or a total dose of 17 mg/kg has been given. Maintenance infusion: 1 to 4 mg/min (diluted in D_5W or NS). In the presence of cardiac, hepatic, or renal dysfunction, reduce the maximum total dose to 12 mg/kg and the maintenance infusion to 1 to 2 mg/min. *Pediatric*: Not recommended in the prehospital setting.

Duration of action *Onset*: 10 to 30 minutes. *Peak effect*: Variable. *Duration*: 3 to 6 hours.

Special considerations Pregnancy safety: Category C. Hypotension may occur with rapid infusion.

Prochlorperazine (Compazine)

Class Antiemetic, first-generation (typical) antipsychotic, phenothiazine.

Mechanism of action Exerts its antiemetic effect by depressing the brain's chemoreceptor trigger zone; also has moderate anticholinergic and alpha adrenergic receptor blocking effects. Alpha-1 adrenergic receptor blockade produces sedation, muscle relaxation, and cardiovascular effects (eg, hypotension, reflex tachycardia, minor ECG pattern changes).[5]

Indications Nausea and vomiting.

Contraindications Documented hypersensitivity to phenothiazines, concurrent use of large amounts of CNS depressants leading to sedation, concomitant use of anticholinergic medications, preexisting cardiac conduction abnormalities, poorly controlled seizure disorder, narrow-angle glaucoma, prostatic hypertrophy, past or current history of tardive dyskinesia, subcortical brain damage, pediatric surgery, children younger than age 2 years.

Adverse reactions/side effects Drowsiness, dizziness, headache, blurred vision, tachycardia, hypotension, prolonged QT interval, extrapyramidal symptoms.

Drug interactions Increased risk of respiratory depression when used with other medications that cause respiratory depression.

Dosage and administration[2] *Adult*: 5 to 10 mg IV/IM. *Pediatric*: Older than age 2 years and weight greater than 12 kg: 0.1 mg/kg slow IV or deep IM; maximum dose: 10 mg.

Duration of action *Onset*: 10 to 20 minutes IM, rapid IV. *Peak effect*: 30 to 60 minutes IV. *Duration*: 3 to 4 hours IM/IV.

Special considerations Pregnancy safety: Category C. Use during pregnancy only if the potential maternal benefit outweighs the fetal risk. Contraindicated for use in breastfeeding women. The label carries an FDA black box warning for children younger than age 2 years.

Promethazine Hydrochloride (Phenergan)

Class Phenothiazine, antiemetic, antihistamine.

Mechanism of action H_1 receptor antagonist; blocks the action (but not the release) of histamine; possesses sedative, antimotion, antiemetic, and anticholinergic activity; potentiates the effects of opioids to induce analgesia.

Indications Nausea and vomiting.

Contraindications Known hypersensitivity to promethazine or other phenothiazines, concurrent use of large amounts of CNS depressants, Reye syndrome, lower respiratory symptoms (eg, asthma), children younger than 2 years (risk of developing potentially fatal respiratory depression). Use with caution, if at all, in patients with a history of sleep apnea, acute or chronic respiratory impairment, or seizure disorders.

Adverse reactions/side effects Headache, dizziness, drowsiness, confusion, restlessness, wheezing, chest tightness, thickening of bronchial secretions, palpitations, bradycardia, reflex tachycardia, QT prolongation, postural hypotension, diarrhea, nausea, vomiting.

Drug interactions Additive with other CNS depressants, increased extrapyramidal effects with MAOIs.

Dosage and administration *Adult*: 12.5 to 25 mg deep IM. *Pediatric:* Older than age 2 years*:* 0.25 to 0.5 mg/kg deep IM.

Duration of action *Onset*: 20 minutes. *Peak effect*: 30 to 60 minutes. *Duration*: 4 to 6 hours.

Special considerations Pregnancy safety: Category C. Use with caution in pregnant women. Contraindicated for use in breastfeeding women. Convulsions and sudden death have been reported when used with children. Do not administer if haloperidol or droperidol will be or has been given (all of these medications increase QT prolongation).[2] Monitor the QT interval with a 12-lead ECG if feasible. Document the QT interval and relay the findings to the receiving facility staff.[2] The recommended route of administration is by deep IM injection because cases of severe tissue injury, including gangrene requiring amputation, have occurred following IV administration of promethazine.

Proparacaine Ophthalmic (Alcaine, Ophthaine)

Class Topical ophthalmic anesthetic.

Mechanism of action Produces local anesthesia by blocking sodium ion channels, thereby stopping cellular depolarization and preventing the action potential development of nerve impulses at the ophthalmic pain nerve cell membrane.

Indications Induction of topical anesthesia before eye irrigation in the management of a chemical injury to the eye.

Contraindications Known hypersensitivity, known or suspected trauma that may have resulted in intraocular injury. Use with caution in patients with cardiac disease or hyperthyroidism.

Adverse reactions/side effects Temporary stinging, burning, and conjunctival redness.

Drug interactions Data unavailable.

Dosage and administration *Adult and pediatric*: 1 to 2 drops in the affected eye(s).

Duration of action *Onset*: 15 to 60 seconds. *Peak effect*: 30 to 120 seconds. *Duration*: 10 to 20 minutes.

Special considerations Pregnancy safety: Category C. Each bottle is for single-patient use. The corneal epithelium may become dry during use because the blink reflex is temporarily lost. Instruct the patient not to rub, touch, or wipe the affected eye because the affected eye will be insensitive to touch for as long as 20 minutes after use.

Propofol (Diprivan)

Class Short-acting general anesthetic, sedative-hypnotic.

Mechanism of action Produces a rapid and brief state of general anesthesia.

Indications Maintenance of sedation in mechanically ventilated patients.

Contraindications Hypovolemia; known sensitivities, including to soybean oil, peanuts, and eggs.

Adverse reactions/side effects Seizure, apnea, dysrhythmias, hypotension (especially in a patient with inadequate vascular volume), hypertension, rash, itching, injection site reactions (eg, burning, stinging, pain), involuntary muscle movement.

Drug interactions Increased anesthetic or sedative effects when combined with alcohol, antihistamines, opioids, and combinations of opioids and sedatives. Avoid mixing with medications that cannot pass through lipids. Simultaneous use with fentanyl can cause profound bradycardia in pediatric patients.

Dosage and administration Consult medical direction or follow the dosing ordered by the sending physician.

Duration of action *Onset*: Less than 1 minute. *Peak effect*: 1 minute. *Duration*: As long as the infusion is running.

Special considerations Pregnancy safety: Category B. Contraindicated in pregnant and breastfeeding women due to potential fetal and infant respiratory depression. Propofol has no analgesic properties. Use with caution in patients with difficult airways; have emergency airway equipment readily available. Avoid rapid administration in older patients to avoid hypotension and airway obstruction. Carefully monitor vital signs and oxygenation. Use a large, stable vein to avoid injection site pain. Infusions may need to be increased during transport because noxious stimuli may arouse patients.

Commonly Prescribed and OTC Medications

Proton Pump Inhibitors

Proton pump inhibitors block the hydrogen/potassium ATPase enzyme system (ie, the gastric proton pump) in the stomach wall, inhibiting the final stage of gastric acid production and limiting the amount of acid produced. **TABLE 15-10** lists common proton pump inhibitors.

Rocuronium Bromide (Zemuron)

Class Nondepolarizing neuromuscular blocking agent, cholinergic receptor antagonist.

Mechanism of action Antagonizes acetylcholine at the motor endplate, producing skeletal muscle paralysis.

TABLE 15-10 Proton Pump Inhibitors

Examples	esomeprazole (Nexium), lansoprazole (Prevacid), omeprazole (Prilosec)
Indications	Prevention and treatment of gastric acid–related disorders, including peptic ulcers, duodenal ulcers, reflux esophagitis, and GERD. May also be used in combination with antibiotics for the treatment of *Helicobacter pylori* infection.
Contraindications	Known hypersensitivity, liver disease, gastric cancer, vitamin B_{12} deficiency, hypomagnesemia, long QT syndrome. Use with caution in patients with bone fractures, osteoporosis, or systemic lupus erythematosus.
Adverse reactions/ side effects	Headache, diarrhea, nausea, vomiting, abdominal pain, constipation, dizziness, iron and vitamin B_{12} deficiency. May increase the risk of *Clostridioides difficile* infection.
Drug interactions	Several, but vary depending on the drug. Use with caution in patients on antiplatelet drugs, iron salts, or digoxin. Ginkgo, St. John's wort, and licorice may decrease the serum level of omeprazole.[a]
Special considerations	Proton pump inhibitors tend to inhibit gastric acid secretion up to 90% more than the H_2 blockers.[a] An infusion pump is required when the medication is administered by continuous IV infusion.

Abbreviations: GERD, gastroesophageal reflex disease; H_2, histamine; IV, intravenous

[a] McCuistion LE, DiMaggio KV, Winton MB, Yeager JJ. *Pharmacology: A Patient-Centered Nursing Process Approach*, 10th ed. St. Louis, MO: Elsevier; 2021.

Indications Adjunct to provide skeletal muscle relaxation and facilitate tracheal intubation and ventilation.

Contraindications Known hypersensitivity to rocuronium or a bromide hypersensitivity, inability to control the airway or support ventilation with oxygen and positive pressure, neuromuscular disease (eg, myasthenia gravis). Use with caution in patients with heart and liver disease.

Adverse reactions/side effects Transient hypotension and hypertension, dose-related tachycardia, nausea, vomiting, injection site edema, hiccups, itching, wheezing, residual muscle weakness.

Drug interactions Additive effects if administered with or following an opioid, sedative, or anesthetic agent.

Dosage and administration *Adult*: 0.6 to 1.2 mg/kg IV/IO. *Pediatric*:[7] Older than 3 months: 0.6 to 1.2 mg/kg IV/IO.

Duration of action *Onset*: 30 to 60 seconds. *Peak effect*: 1 to 3 minutes. *Duration*: 30 to 60 minutes.

Special considerations Pregnancy safety: Category C. Rocuronium does not provide sedation or analgesia and will not stop neuronal seizure activity. If the patient is conscious, explain the effect of the medication before administering it. Always sedate the patient before administering rocuronium. Intubation and ventilatory support must be readily available; monitor the patient carefully. Doses should be calculated based on ideal body weight. Pulse rate and cardiac output are increased with use of rocuronium. Decrease doses for patients with renal disease. Anaphylactic and anaphylactoid-type adverse reactions, including fatalities, have been reported in association with neuromuscular blocker use.

Sildenafil (Revatio, Viagra)

Class Phosphodiesterase-5 enzyme inhibitor.

Mechanism of action Inhibits phosphodiesterase enzyme 5 in lung tissue, which results in relaxation of pulmonary vascular smooth muscle cells and subsequent vasodilation of the pulmonary vasculature.[5]

Indications HAPE prevention.[4]

Contraindications Known hypersensitivity, coadministration with nitrates, significant cardiovascular disease.

Adverse reactions/side effects Headache, nasal congestion, flushing, epistaxis, erythema, diarrhea, skin rash, tinnitus.

Drug interactions Can potentiate the hypotensive effects of nitrates, alpha blockers, antihypertensives, or alcohol. Increased risk of side effects when taken with grapefruit juice and grapefruit products.

Dosage and administration: *Adult:* HAPE prevention:[4] Give 50 mg orally every 8 hours. *Pediatric:* Data unavailable.

Duration of action *Onset*: 20 minutes. *Peak effect*: 30 to 120 minutes. *Duration*: 4 hours.

Special considerations Pregnancy safety: Category B.

Sodium Bicarbonate

Class Systemic hydrogen ion buffer, alkalizing agent.

Mechanism of action Reacts with hydrogen ions to form water and carbon dioxide, correcting metabolic acidosis. Increases blood and urinary pH by releasing a bicarbonate ion, which in turn neutralizes hydrogen ion concentrations.

Indications Management of cardiac arrest in which either hyperkalemia or TCA overdose is suspected, QRS prolongation in known or suspected TCA overdose, crush syndrome.

Contraindications Documented hypersensitivity, known metabolic or respiratory alkalosis, hypokalemia, hypernatremia, hypocalcemia. Use with caution in patients with heart failure and renal disease due to high sodium concentration it produces.

Adverse reactions/side effects Electrolyte imbalance, heart failure, and pulmonary edema (secondary to sodium overload); tremors, twitching, and seizures caused by alkalosis.

Drug interactions Increases the effects of amphetamines. Decreases the effects of benzodiazepines and TCAs. May deactivate sympathomimetics.

Dosage and administration *Adult*:[7] 1 mEq/kg slow IV/IO push. *Pediatric*:[7] 1 mEq/kg slow IV/IO push (4.2% concentration recommended for infants younger than 1 month). Consult medical direction for repeat dosing orders.

Duration of action *Onset*: Seconds. *Peak effect*: Less than 15 minutes. *Duration*: 1 to 2 hours.

Special considerations Pregnancy safety: Category C. Monitor the patient closely for signs and symptoms of fluid overload. Because the buffering action produces carbon dioxide, ensure the patient has adequate airway and ventilatory support. May precipitate or inactivate other medications; flush the IV line well before and after injecting sodium bicarbonate. Extravasation may lead to tissue sloughing, cellulitis, and necrosis at the injection site.

Sodium Thiosulfate (Nithiodote)

Class Cyanide antidote.

Mechanism of action Converts cyanide to the less toxic thiocyanate, which is then excreted in the urine.

Indications Known or suspected cyanide poisoning.

Contraindications Documented hypersensitivity.

Adverse reactions/side effects Diarrhea.

Drug interactions None.

Dosage and administration[2] *Adult*: 12.5 g (50 mL of 25% solution) IV/IO slow push over 10 minutes. *Pediatric*: 0.5 g/kg slow IV/IO (2 mL/kg of 25% solution).

Duration of action *Onset*: 2 to 10 minutes. *Peak effect*: Varies. *Duration*: 30 minutes to 2 hours.

Special considerations Pregnancy safety: Category C. Hydroxocobalamin is the only agent that is considered safe for treating cyanide poisoning in the pregnant patient.[2]

Commonly Prescribed and OTC Medications

Statins

Statins, also known as HMG-CoA (β-hydroxy β-methylglutaryl–coenzyme A) reductase inhibitors, belong to the antihyperlipidemic drug class. They decrease the concentrations of serum cholesterol and triglycerides, decrease low-density lipoprotein (LDL) cholesterol, and slightly increase high-density lipoprotein (HDL) cholesterol. These medications have proved useful in decreasing the risk of CAD and stroke. Common statins are listed in **TABLE 15-11**.

TABLE 15-11 Statins

Examples	atorvastatin (Lipitor), fluvastatin (Lescol), lovastatin (Altoprev), pravastatin (Pravachol), rosuvastatin (Crestor), simvastatin (Zocor)
Indications	To decrease cholesterol levels and serum lipids, especially LDL and triglycerides.
Contraindications	Known hypersensitivity, pregnant patients, breastfeeding, active or chronic liver disease.
Adverse reactions/ side effects	Headache, nausea, hyperglycemia, blurred vision, fatigue, muscle and joint aches, insomnia; some can cause erectile dysfunction.
Drug interactions	Increased risk of muscle injury when used with fibrates (cholesterol-lowering drugs), large doses of niacin, ranolazine (used to treat angina), and colchicine (used to treat gout). Statins increase the effects of warfarin. Amiodarone and verapamil increase the blood levels of some statins. Grapefruit and grapefruit products can reduce the effectiveness of statins.
Special considerations	Patients taking warfarin and a statin require close coagulation monitoring.

Abbreviation: LDL, low-density lipoprotein

Succinylcholine Chloride (Anectine)

Class Depolarizing neuromuscular blocker; skeletal muscle relaxant.

Mechanism of action Ultra-short-acting depolarizing skeletal muscle relaxant that mimics acetylcholine. It binds with the cholinergic receptors on the motor endplate, producing a phase 1 block manifested by muscle fasciculations.

Indications Adjunct to provide skeletal muscle relaxation and facilitate tracheal intubation and ventilation.

Contraindications Known hypersensitivity, inability to control the airway or support ventilation with oxygen and positive pressure, renal failure, muscular dystrophy and other neuromuscular diseases, paraplegia/quadriplegia, penetrating eye injuries (increases intraocular pressure), prolonged immobilization, stroke with residual motor dysfunction, history of malignant hyperthermia. Acute injury after multisystem trauma, major burns, known or suspected hyperkalemia, or extensive muscle injury that may result in hyperkalemia. Use with caution if a difficult airway is anticipated.

Adverse reactions/side effects Apnea, respiratory depression, dysrhythmias, cardiac arrest, excessive salivation, prolonged muscle rigidity, rhabdomyolysis, malignant hyperthermia, hyperkalemia (trauma patients); increased intracranial, intraocular, and intragastric pressure.

Drug interactions Coadministration with CNS depressants may cause profound sedation, coma, respiratory depression, hypotension, or death. Oxytocin, beta blockers, and organophosphates may potentiate its effects. Diazepam may reduce its duration of action.

Dosage and administration *Adult:*[7] Give 1 to 1.5 mg/kg rapid IV. *Pediatric:*[7] Give 1 to 1.5 mg/kg for children, 2 mg/kg for infants.

Duration of action *Onset*: 45 to 60 seconds. *Peak effect*: 1 to 3 minutes. *Duration*: 4 to 6 minutes.

Special considerations Pregnancy safety: Category C. Doses should be calculated based on ideal body weight. If the patient is conscious, explain the effects of the drug before administration. Appropriate sedation and analgesia should be provided to any conscious patient before initiating neuromuscular blockade. Time management is crucial. Postintubation sedation and analgesia should be readily available.

Tadalafil (Cialis, Adcirca)

Class Phosphodiesterase-5 enzyme inhibitor.

Mechanism of action Inhibits phosphodiesterase enzyme 5 in lung tissue, which results in relaxation of pulmonary vascular smooth muscle cells and subsequent vasodilation of the pulmonary vasculature.[5]

Indications HAPE prevention.[4]
Contraindications Known hypersensitivity, coadministration with nitrates, Stevens-Johnson syndrome, exfoliative dermatitis.
Adverse reactions/side effects Headache, nasal congestion, back pain, flushing, epistaxis, erythema, diarrhea, skin rash, tinnitus.
Drug interactions Can potentiate the hypotensive effects of nitrates, alpha blockers, antihypertensives, or alcohol. Increased risk of side effects when taken with grapefruit juice and grapefruit products.
Dosage and administration *Adult:* HAPE prevention:[4] Give 10 mg orally twice daily. *Pediatric:* Data unavailable.
Duration of action *Onset*: 30 to 45 minutes. *Peak effect*: 2 hours. *Duration*: Up to 36 hours.
Special considerations Pregnancy safety: Category B.

Tetracaine Ophthalmic Solution (Pontocaine)

Class Topical ophthalmic anesthetic.
Mechanism of action Produces local anesthesia by blocking sodium ion channels, thereby stopping cellular depolarization and preventing the action potential development of nerve impulses at the ophthalmic pain nerve cell membrane.
Indications Induction of topical anesthesia before eye irrigation in the management of a chemical injury to the eye.
Contraindications Known hypersensitivity, known or suspected trauma that may have resulted in intraocular injury.
Adverse reactions/side effects Blurry vision, transient stinging, burning, and conjunctival redness.
Drug interactions Monitor closely for methemoglobinemia signs if coadministered with methemoglobin-inducing drugs (eg, acetaminophen, NTG, nitroprusside).
Dosage and administration *Adult and pediatric*: 1 to 2 drops in the affected eye(s).
Duration of action *Onset*: Immediate. *Peak effect*: 15 to 30 seconds. *Duration*: 10 to 20 minutes.
Special considerations Pregnancy safety: Not classified. Each bottle is for single-patient use. Instruct the patient not to rub, touch, or wipe the affected eye because the affected eye will be insensitive to touch for as long as 20 minutes after use.

Thiamine Hydrochloride (Vitamin B_1)

Class Vitamin.
Mechanism of action Combines with adenosine triphosphate to form thiamine pyrophosphate, a coenzyme essential for carbohydrate metabolism.
Indications Adjunctive therapy that should precede the administration of dextrose 50% or glucagon in an adult patient if alcoholism or malnourishment is suspected.
Contraindications Known hypersensitivity.
Adverse reactions/side effects Vasodilation, hypotension, weakness (usually a result of too-rapid IV injection), sweating, itching, hives, nausea, feeling of warmth.
Drug interactions Unstable in alkaline solutions.
Dosage and administration *Adult*: 100 mg as a very slow IV/IO bolus over 5 minutes or 100 mg deep IM. *Pediatric*: Consult medical direction.
Duration of action *Onset*: Hours. *Peak effect*: 3 to 5 days. *Duration*: Data unavailable.
Special considerations Pregnancy safety: Category A.

Tranexamic Acid (Cyklokapron, Lysteda)

Class Hemostatic agent, antifibrinolytic agent, plasminogen inhibitor.
Mechanism of action Inhibits the activation of plasminogen, thereby reducing the conversion of plasminogen to plasmin (which breaks down fibrin clots, fibrinogen, and other plasma proteins). By hindering fibrin's breakdown, clotting factors and circulating platelet plugs can form a seal (fibrin clot) and reduce bleeding.
Indications Blunt or penetrating trauma less than 3 hours from onset with hemodynamic compromise, bleeding.
Contraindications Known hypersensitivity; mechanism of injury more than 3 hours prior to EMS care; subarachnoid hemorrhage; history of PE, DVT, or other thromboembolic disorder. Reduce the dose in patients with renal insufficiency.
Adverse reactions/side effects Fatigue, headache, dizziness, abdominal and back pain, joint pain,

musculoskeletal pain, anemia. Rapid infusion may cause hypotension. May increase the risk of thromboembolic disorders.

Drug interactions Hormonal contraceptives and clotting factor complexes increase the risk of thromboembolic disorders.

Dosage and administration *Adult*: 1 g IV infusion over 10 minutes. *Pediatric*: Not recommended.

Duration of action *Onset*: Unknown. *Peak effect*: Unknown. *Duration*: 7 to 8 hours.

Special considerations Pregnancy safety: Category B. Use in pregnant and breastfeeding women should be clearly indicated. Must be mixed into an infusion bag, typically 100 mL of NS.

Vecuronium Bromide (Norcuron)

Class Nondepolarizing neuromuscular blocking agent, cholinergic receptor antagonist.

Mechanism of action Neuromuscular agent with an intermediate duration of action that competes with acetylcholine for receptors at the motor endplate, resulting in neuromuscular blockade.

Indications Adjunct to provide skeletal muscle relaxation and facilitate tracheal intubation and ventilation.

Contraindications Known hypersensitivity to vecuronium or a bromide hypersensitivity, inability to control the airway or support ventilation with oxygen and positive pressure, neuromuscular disease (eg, myasthenia gravis), acute narrow-angle glaucoma, penetrating eye injuries, newborns, hepatic or renal failure.

Adverse reactions/side effects Hypersensitivity reactions associated with histamine release (eg, bronchospasm, flushing, erythema, acute urticaria, hypotension, tachycardia), itching, weakness, prolonged neuromuscular blockade, excessive salivation.

Drug interactions Additive effects if administered with or following an opioid, sedative, or anesthetic agent.

Dosage and administration *Adult*: 0.08 to 0.1 mg/kg IV push over 1 minute. Maintenance dose within 20 to 45 minutes: 0.01 to 0.015 mg/kg IV push every 12 to 15 minutes as needed to maintain muscle relaxation. *Pediatric*:[7] 0.1 to 0.3 mg/kg IV/IO.

Duration of action *Onset*: 3 to 5 minutes. *Peak effect*: Varies. *Duration*: 20 to 35 minutes.

Special considerations Pregnancy safety: Category C. Vecuronium does not provide sedation or analgesia and will not stop neuronal seizure activity. If the patient is conscious, explain the effect of the medication before administering it. Always sedate the patient before administration of vecuronium. Intubation and ventilatory support must be readily available; monitor the patient carefully. Doses should be calculated based on ideal body weight. Decrease doses for patients with renal disease. Anaphylactic and anaphylactoid-type adverse reactions, including fatalities, have been reported in association with neuromuscular blocker use.

Verapamil Hydrochloride (Isoptin, Calan)

Class Calcium channel blocker.

Mechanism of action Slows AV node conduction, shortens the refractory period of accessory pathways, and acts as a negative inotrope and vasodilator.[6]

Indications Stable narrow-QRS tachycardia if the rhythm persists despite vagal maneuvers or adenosine or if the tachycardia is recurrent; to control the ventricular rate in patients with AF or atrial flutter without preexcitation.[6]

Contraindications Known hypersensitivity; Wolff-Parkinson-White syndrome, Lown-Ganong-Levine syndrome; second- or third-degree AV block, sick sinus syndrome, or other sinus node disease unless a functioning artificial pacemaker is present; hypotension, cardiogenic shock, severe left ventricular dysfunction, wide-complex tachycardias; children younger than age 12 months. Use with extreme caution in patients receiving oral beta blockers.[7]

Adverse reactions/side effects Dizziness, headache, dysrhythmias, nausea, vomiting; can decrease myocardial contractility, resulting in peripheral vasodilation and hypotension.

Drug interactions Increases the serum concentration of digoxin. Simultaneous administration with IV beta blockers can produce severe hypotension. Antihypertensives may potentiate the hypotensive effects. May potentiate the activity of depolarizing and nondepolarizing neuromuscular blocking agents. Increased risk of sudden cardiac death when given concurrently with erythromycin.[3] St. John's wort can reduce its effectiveness.

Dosage and administration *Adult*:[7] 2.5 to 5 mg IV bolus over 2 minutes (3 minutes in older patients). Repeat dose of 5 to 10 mg may be given every 15 to 30 minutes to a maximum total dose of 20 mg. Alternative dosing: 5 mg IV bolus every 15 minutes to a total dose of 30 mg. *Pediatric*: Consult medical direction.

Duration of action *Onset*: 2 to 5 minutes. *Peak effect*: Variable. *Duration*: 10 to 20 minutes.

Special considerations Pregnancy safety: Category C. Carefully monitor BP, heart rate, and ECG before, during, and after administration. AV block or asystole may occur because of slowed AV conduction.

Ziprasidone (Geodon)

Class Second-generation antipsychotic.

Mechanism of action Blocks synaptic reabsorption of serotonin and norepinephrine, binds to alpha adrenergic receptors, dopamine receptors, and serotonin receptors.

Indications[2] For the management of agitated or violent patients experiencing a behavioral emergency, anxiety (palliative care).

Contraindications Known hypersensitivity, history of QT prolongation, use of any drugs that prolong the QT interval, recent AMI, uncompensated heart failure. Use with caution in patients with impaired renal function.

Adverse reactions/side effects Dizziness, headache, extrapyramidal symptoms, orthostatic hypotension, suicide attempt, bradycardia, prolonged QT interval.

Drug interactions Avoid simultaneous administration with drugs that prolong the QT interval (eg, sotalol, quinidine, other Class Ia and III antidysrhythmics, droperidol, dolasetron). CNS depressants increase its effects.

Dosage and administration[2] *Adult*: Chemical restraint: 10 mg IM. Anxiety (palliative care): 20 mg IM. *Pediatric*: Limited data available for pediatric use. Chemical restraint: Ages 6 to 11 years: 5 mg IM. Age 12 to 18 years: 10 mg IM.

Duration of action *Onset*: 10 minutes IM. *Peak effect*: 60 minutes. *Duration*: Unknown.

Special considerations Pregnancy safety: Category C. Use during the third trimester is associated with extrapyramidal symptoms in the fetus. Use during pregnancy should be clearly indicated after weighing the fetal risks and maternal benefits. Monitor the QT interval with a 12-lead ECG if feasible. Document the QT interval and relay the findings to the receiving facility staff.

IV Solutions (Colloids and Crystalloids)

Colloids expand plasma volume by taking advantage of colloidal osmotic pressure. These solutions are most often used in patients in hypovolemic shock states.

Crystalloids are substances in solution that can diffuse through the intravascular compartment. Crystalloid solutions are used for electrolyte replacement, as a route for medication, and for short-term intravascular volume expansion.

Albumin (Albumarc, Albutein, Flexbumin)

Class Colloid, blood modifier agent, volume expander.

Mechanism of action Oncotically similar to human plasma; causes the body to shift approximately 3.5 times the amount administered into the intravascular space.

Indications Hypovolemia.

Contraindications Hypersensitivity, patients at risk of hypervolemia. Use with caution in patients with renal insufficiency or anemia.

Adverse reactions/side effects Nausea, vomiting, itching, hives, abdominal pain, angioedema, dysrhythmias, bronchospasm.

Drug interactions None currently identified.

Dosage and administration Infusion rate is adjusted to the patient's requirements.

Duration of action *Onset*: 15 to 30 minutes. *Peak effect*: Unknown. *Duration*: 24 hours.

Special considerations Pregnancy safety: Category C. Administered with 0.9% NS, D_5W, or sodium lactate.

Evidence-Based Medicine

In 2022, the National Association of State EMS Officials, in conjunction with the National Association of EMS Physicians and the American College of Emergency Physicians, led a project to develop evidence-based guidelines for the pharmacologic management of acute pain in the prehospital setting. The purpose of these guidelines is to ensure safe, effective pain management for all prehospital patients by establishing standards that can be objectively interpreted and followed; this objective framework helps guard against the biases and health disparities that have been documented in studies on administration of pain medications in the emergency department, such as the disproportionate administration of pain medications to White versus non-White patients.[21] Recognizing that EMS medical directors and EMS clinicians have several effective options for the management of moderate to severe pain, the panel made the following recommendations:[21]

1. IN fentanyl is recommended over IV/IM opioids to treat moderate to severe pain in pediatric patients before IV access or in whom IV access is not recommended (strong recommendation, low certainty of evidence). Either IN fentanyl or IV opioids is conditionally recommended once IV access is established (conditional recommendation, low certainty of evidence).
2. IV acetaminophen is suggested over IV opioids alone for the initial management of moderate to severe pain in the prehospital setting if IV acetaminophen is available, affordable, and easy to administer (conditional recommendation, low certainty of evidence).
3. IV NSAIDs or IV opioids are suggested for the initial management of moderate to severe pain in the prehospital setting (conditional recommendation, moderate certainty of evidence).
4. IV NSAIDs are suggested over IV acetaminophen for the initial management of moderate to severe pain in the prehospital setting. Additionally, either oral NSAIDs or oral acetaminophen is recommended for the initial management of pain in the prehospital setting if an oral analgesic is considered (conditional recommendation, low certainty of evidence).
5. Either IV ketamine or IV NSAIDs are recommended for the initial management of moderate to severe pain in the prehospital setting (conditional recommendation, moderate certainty of evidence).
6. Either IV ketamine or IV opioids are suggested for the initial management of moderate to severe pain in the prehospital setting (conditional recommendation, very low certainty of evidence).
7. If opioids are selected for pain management, either IV morphine or IV fentanyl is suggested to treat moderate to severe pain in the prehospital setting (conditional recommendation, low certainty of evidence).
8. Weight-based IV opioid administration alone, versus the combination of weight-based IV opioid plus weight-based IV ketamine, is suggested for the initial management of moderate to severe pain in the prehospital setting (conditional recommendation, very low certainty of evidence).
9. No recommendation was made in comparing the combination of an IV opioid plus IV ketamine, versus IV ketamine alone, for the initial management of moderate to severe pain in the prehospital setting. Evidence for this comparison is uncertain and incomplete.
10. No recommendation was made in comparing nitrous oxide to IV opioids for the initial management of moderate to severe pain in the prehospital setting. Evidence for this comparison is uncertain and incomplete.

Bacteriostatic Water

Class Diluent or solvent.

Mechanism of action Works as a solvent or dilutional agent.

Indications Used for diluting or dissolving drugs for IV, IM, or subcutaneous injections based on the drug manufacturer's recommendations.

Contraindications Hypersensitivity to benzyl alcohol due to use as a preservative.

Adverse reactions/side effects None noted if used according to the manufacturer's recommendations.

Drug interactions None noted.

Dosage and administration According to the drug manufacturer's recommendations.

Duration of action Not applicable.

Special considerations Pregnancy category: C. Due to the presence of a benzyl alcohol additive, other dilutional agents should be used if available. Solution should be made approximately isotonic before use.

Dextran

Class Artificial colloid.

Mechanism of action A sugar-containing colloid used as an intravascular volume expander. Remains in the intravascular compartment for approximately 12 hours. Increases intravascular volume by attracting water from other fluid compartments by virtue of its colloid osmotic pressure.

Indications Hypovolemic shock.

Contraindications Known hypersensitivity to the drug; heart failure, renal failure, or known bleeding disorders.

Adverse reactions/side effects Rash, itching, dyspnea, chest tightness, mild hypotension. The incidence of these side effects is very low, and reactions are generally mild. Increased bleeding time has also been reported due to the interference of dextran with platelet function.

Drug interactions Should not be administered to patients receiving anticoagulants because it significantly slows blood clotting.

Dosage and administration Titrate according to the patient's physiologic response.

Duration of action 8 to 12 hours.

Special considerations In the management of burn shock, it is essential to follow standard fluid resuscitation regimens to prevent possible circulatory overload.

Hetastarch (Hespan)

Class Artificial colloid.

Mechanism of action A starch-containing colloid used as an intravascular volume expander. Following administration, the plasma volume is expanded slightly more than the volume of hetastarch administered; this effect has been observed for up to 24 to 36 hours. Hetastarch increases intravascular volume by virtue of its colloid osmotic pressure.

Indications Hypovolemic shock, especially burn shock; septic shock.

Contraindications No significant contraindications when used in the management of life-threatening hypovolemic states.

Adverse reactions/side effects Nausea, vomiting, mild febrile reactions, chills, itching, urticaria; rare severe anaphylactic reactions have been reported.

Drug interactions Should not be administered to patients who are receiving anticoagulants. Patients allergic to corn may be allergic to hetastarch.

Dosage and administration Titrated according to the patient's physiologic response.

Duration of action 24 to 36 hours.

Special considerations Pregnancy safety: Category C.

Lactated Ringer (Hartmann) Solution

Class Isotonic crystalloid solution.

Mechanism of action Replaces water and electrolytes.

Indications Hypovolemic shock; keep open IV, hypoperfusion.

Contraindications Heart failure or renal failure. Avoid use in patients with crush injuries/compartment syndrome because lactated Ringer solution contains potassium.[2]

Adverse reactions/side effects Rare with therapeutic dosages.

Drug interactions Few in the emergency setting.

Dosage and administration Hypovolemic shock; titrate according to the patient's physiologic response. Hypoperfusion: 20 mL/kg IV/IO over 15 minutes; repeat as needed for ongoing hypoperfusion.[2]

Duration of action Short-term therapy.

Special considerations None.

Plasma Protein Fraction (Plasmanate)

Class Natural colloid.

Mechanism of action Protein-containing colloid that remains in the intravascular compartment. Increases intravascular volume by attracting water from other fluid compartments by virtue of its colloid osmotic pressure.

Indications Hypovolemic shock, especially burn shock; hypoproteinemia (low-protein states).

Contraindications No significant contraindications when used to treat life-threatening hypovolemic states.

Adverse reactions/side effects Chills, fever, hives, nausea, vomiting.

Drug interactions Solutions should not be mixed with or administered through the same administration sets as other IV fluids.

Dosage and administration Titrate according to the patient's hemodynamic response. In the management of shock secondary to bums, the physician's orders regarding the administration rate must be closely followed. Standard formulas for IV fluid administration have been developed, and the medical control physician will use these to determine the correct rate of IV administration.

Duration of action 24 to 36 hours.

Special considerations Do not use if the solution is cloudy or if sedimentation is seen.

Total Parenteral Nutrition (TPN; varies based on mixture)

Class Electrolyte, nutrition.

Mechanism of action Replenishes electrolytes and nutrients.

Indications Ordered and customized to each patient based on needs identified from lab work.

Contraindications Vary based on the specific mixture.

Adverse reactions/side effects Vary based on the specific mixture.

Drug interactions Vary based on the specific mixture.

Dosage and administration Vary based on the specific mixture.

5% Dextrose in Water

Class Hypotonic dextrose-containing solution.

Mechanism of action Provides nutrients in the form of dextrose as well as free water.

Indications IV access for emergency drugs; dilution of concentrated drugs for IV infusion.

Contraindications Should not be used as a fluid replacement for hypovolemic states.

Adverse reactions/side effects Rare with therapeutic dosages.

Drug interactions Should not be used with phenytoin (Dilantin) or amrinone (Inocor).

Dosage and administration Usually administered through a minidrip (60 drops/mL) set at a TKO rate.

Duration of action Short-term therapy.

Special considerations D_5W should not be administered simultaneously with blood through the same IV administration set because of the possibility of hemolysis.

10% Dextrose in Water

Class Hypertonic dextrose-containing solution.

Mechanism of action Provides nutrients in the form of dextrose as well as free water.

Indications Neonatal resuscitation, hypoglycemia.

Contraindications Should not be used as a fluid replacement for hypovolemic states.

Adverse reactions/side effects Rare with therapeutic dosages.

Drug interactions Should not be used with phenytoin (Dilantin) or amrinone (Inocor).

Dosage and administration Infusion rate is usually dependent on the patient's condition.

Duration of action Short-term therapy.

Special considerations None.

0.9% Sodium Chloride (Normal Saline)

Class Isotonic crystalloid solution.

Mechanism of action Replaces water and electrolytes.

Indications Heat-related problems (heat exhaustion, heatstroke), freshwater drowning, hypovolemia, diabetic ketoacidosis, keep open IV.

Contraindications Avoid in patients with history of heart failure or renal failure because circulatory overload can be easily induced.

Adverse reactions/side effects Rare with therapeutic dosages.

Drug interactions Few in the emergency setting.

Dosage and administration Infusion rate will depend on the specific situation being treated.

Duration of action Short-term therapy.

Special considerations None.

0.45% Sodium Chloride

Class Hypotonic crystalloid solution.

Mechanism of action Replaces free water and electrolytes.

Indications Patients with diminished renal or cardiovascular function for whom rapid rehydration is not indicated.

Contraindications Cases in which rapid rehydration is indicated.
Adverse reactions/side effects Rare with therapeutic dosages.
Drug interactions Few in the emergency setting.
Dosage and administration The specific situation and patient condition will dictate the rate at which one-half normal saline is administered.
Duration of action Short-term therapy.
Special considerations None.

3% Sodium Chloride (Hypertonic Saline)

Class Hypertonic crystalloid solution.
Mechanism of action Osmotic effect allows fluid to cross the blood–brain barrier, reducing the amount of fluid in the cranial cavity and decreasing the ICP.
Indications Traumatic brain injuries, fluid resuscitation in severe sepsis, hyponatremia.
Contraindications Hypotension. Use with caution in pediatric patients because their sodium levels shift rapidly. Rapid increases can cause significant neurologic complications.
Adverse reactions/side effects Increases sodium levels, seizures, neurologic deficits.
Drug interactions None currently identified.
Dosage and administration Infusion rate will depend on the specific situation being treated.
Duration of action *Onset*: Rapid. *Peak effect*: Unknown. *Duration*: Unknown.
Special considerations Should be administered through a central line due to its high osmolarity and tonicity.

5% Dextrose in 0.45% Sodium Chloride

Class Hypertonic dextrose-containing crystalloid solution.
Mechanism of action Replaces free water and electrolytes and provides nutrients in the form of dextrose.
Indications Heat exhaustion, diabetic disorders; KVO solution in patients with impaired renal or cardiovascular function.
Contraindications Should not be used when rapid fluid resuscitation is indicated.
Adverse reactions/side effects Rare with therapeutic dosages.
Drug interactions Should not be used with phenytoin (Dilantin) or amrinone (Inocor).
Dosage and administration Infusion rate will depend on the specific situation being treated.
Duration of action Short-term therapy.
Special considerations None.

5% Dextrose in 0.9% Sodium Chloride

Class Hypertonic dextrose-containing crystalloid solution.
Mechanism of action Replaces free water and electrolytes and provides nutrients in the form of dextrose.
Indications Heat-related disorders, freshwater drowning, hypovolemia, peritonitis.
Contraindications Should not be administered to patients with impaired cardiac or renal function.
Adverse reactions/side effects Rare with therapeutic dosages.
Drug interactions Should not be used with phenytoin (Dilantin) or amrinone (Inocor).
Dosage and administration Infusion rate will depend on the specific situation being treated.
Duration of action Short-term therapy.
Special considerations None.

5% Dextrose in Lactated Ringer Solution

Class Hypertonic dextrose-containing crystalloid solution.
Mechanism of action Replaces water and electrolytes and provides nutrients in the form of dextrose.
Indications Hypovolemic shock, hemorrhagic shock, some instances of acidosis.
Contraindications Should not be administered to patients with decreased renal or cardiovascular function.
Adverse reactions/side effects Rare with therapeutic dosages.
Drug interactions Should not be used with phenytoin (Dilantin) or amrinone (Inocor).
Dosage and administration Infusion rate will depend on the specific situation being treated.
Duration of action Short-term therapy.
Special considerations None.

Prep Kit

Ready for Review

- Tall man lettering is sometimes used to avoid confusion of medication names with similar spellings. Capitalization draws attention to the letters that differentiate one medication's name from similar names.
- Common elements of a drug profile include the medication's generic name, trade name(s), class, mechanism of action, indications, contraindications, adverse reactions/side effects, drug interactions, dosage and administration (adult and pediatric), duration of action (onset, peak effect, duration), and special considerations.

References

1. FDA name differentiation project. US Food and Drug Administration website. https://www.fda.gov/drugs/medication-errors-related-cder-regulated-drug-products/fda-name-differentiation-project. Updated April 28, 2020. Accessed July 16, 2021.
2. *National Model EMS Clinical Guidelines: Version 2.2*. National Association of State EMS Officials website. https://nasemso.org/wp-content/uploads/National-Model-EMS-Clinical-Guidelines-2017-PDF-Version-2.2.pdf. Published January 2019. Accessed July 16, 2021.
3. McCuistion LE, DiMaggio KV, Winton MB, Yeager JJ. *Pharmacology: A Patient-Centered Nursing Process Approach*. 10th ed. St. Louis, MO: Elsevier; 2021.
4. Luks AM, Auerbach PS, Freer L, et al. Wilderness Medical Society clinical practice guidelines for the prevention and treatment of acute altitude illness: 2019 update. *Wilderness Environ Med*. 2019;30(4):S3-S18.
5. Prescriber's Digital Reference [homepage]. https://www.pdr.net/. Accessed July 16, 2021.
6. Panchal AR, Bartos JA, Cabañas JG, et al. Part 3: adult basic and advanced life support: 2020 American Heart Association guidelines for cardiopulmonary resuscitation and emergency cardiovascular care. *Circulation*. 2020;142(16 suppl 2):S366-S468.
7. American Heart Association. *2020 Handbook of Emergency Cardiovascular Care for Healthcare Providers*. Dallas, TX: American Heart Association; 2020.
8. Tachjian A, Maria V, Jahangir A. Use of herbal products and potential interactions in patients with cardiovascular diseases. *J Am Coll Cardiol*. 2010;55(6):515-525.
9. FDA recommends avoiding use of NSAIDs in pregnancy at 20 weeks or later because they can result in low amniotic fluid. US Food and Drug Administration website. https://www.fda.gov/drugs/drug-safety-and-availability/fda-recommends-avoiding-use-nsaids-pregnancy-20-weeks-or-later-because-they-can-result-low-amniotic. Updated November 11, 2020. Accessed July 16, 2021.
10. Kusumoto FM, Schoenfeld MH, Barrett C, et al. 2018 ACC/AHA/HRS guideline on the evaluation and management of patients with bradycardia and cardiac conduction delay. *Circulation*. 140(8);e382-e482:2018. https://doi.org/10.1161/CIR.0000000000000628.
11. McKee D, Thoma A, Bailey K, Fish J. A review of hydrofluoric acid burn management. *Plast Surg*. 2014;22(2):95-98.
12. US National Library of Medicine. Dopamine hydrochloride and dextrose. DailyMed website. https://dailymed.nlm.nih.gov/dailymed/drugInfo.cfm?setid=cb97d4a0-89ed-407c-a763-209386b6f75c. Updated November 11, 2020. Accessed July 16, 2021.
13. Aziz K, Lee HC, Escobedo MB, et al. Part 5: neonatal resuscitation: 2020 American Heart Association guidelines for cardiopulmonary resuscitation and emergency cardiovascular care. *Circulation*. 2020;142(16 suppl 2):S524-S550.
14. Hashemian SM, Fallahian F. The use of Heliox in critical care. *Int J Crit Illn Inj Sci*. 2014;4(2):138-142.
15. Sills JR. Oxygen and medical gas therapy. In *The Comprehensive Respiratory Therapist Exam Review*. 7th ed. St. Louis, MO: Elsevier; 2020:193-224.
16. Kumar MG, Lin S. Hydromorphone in the management of cancer-related pain: an update on routes of administration and dosage forms. *J Pharmacy Pharm Sci*. 2007;10(4):504-518.
17. FDA Drug Safety Communication. FDA strengthens warning that non-aspirin nonsteroidal anti-inflammatory drugs (NSAIDs) can cause heart attacks or strokes. US Food and Drug Administration website. https://www.fda.gov/drugs/drug-safety-and-availability/fda-drug-safety-communication-fda-strengthens-warning-non-aspirin-nonsteroidal-anti-inflammatory. Published July 9, 2015. Accessed July 16, 2021.
18. Pellegrini J, DeLoge J, Bennett J, Kelly J. Comparison of inhalation of isopropyl alcohol vs promethazine in the treatment of postoperative nausea and vomiting (PONV) in patients identified as at high risk for developing PONV. *AANA J*. 2009;77(4):293-299.
19. Oglesbee S. Using nitrous oxide to manage pain. *JEMS*. 39(4). https://www.jems.com/patient-care/using-nitrous-oxide-manage-pain/. Published April 1, 2014. Accessed July 16, 2021.
20. Radiation emergencies: potassium iodide (KI). Centers for Disease Control and Prevention website. https://www.cdc.gov/nceh/radiation/emergencies/ki.htm. Reviewed April 4, 2018. Accessed July 16, 2021.

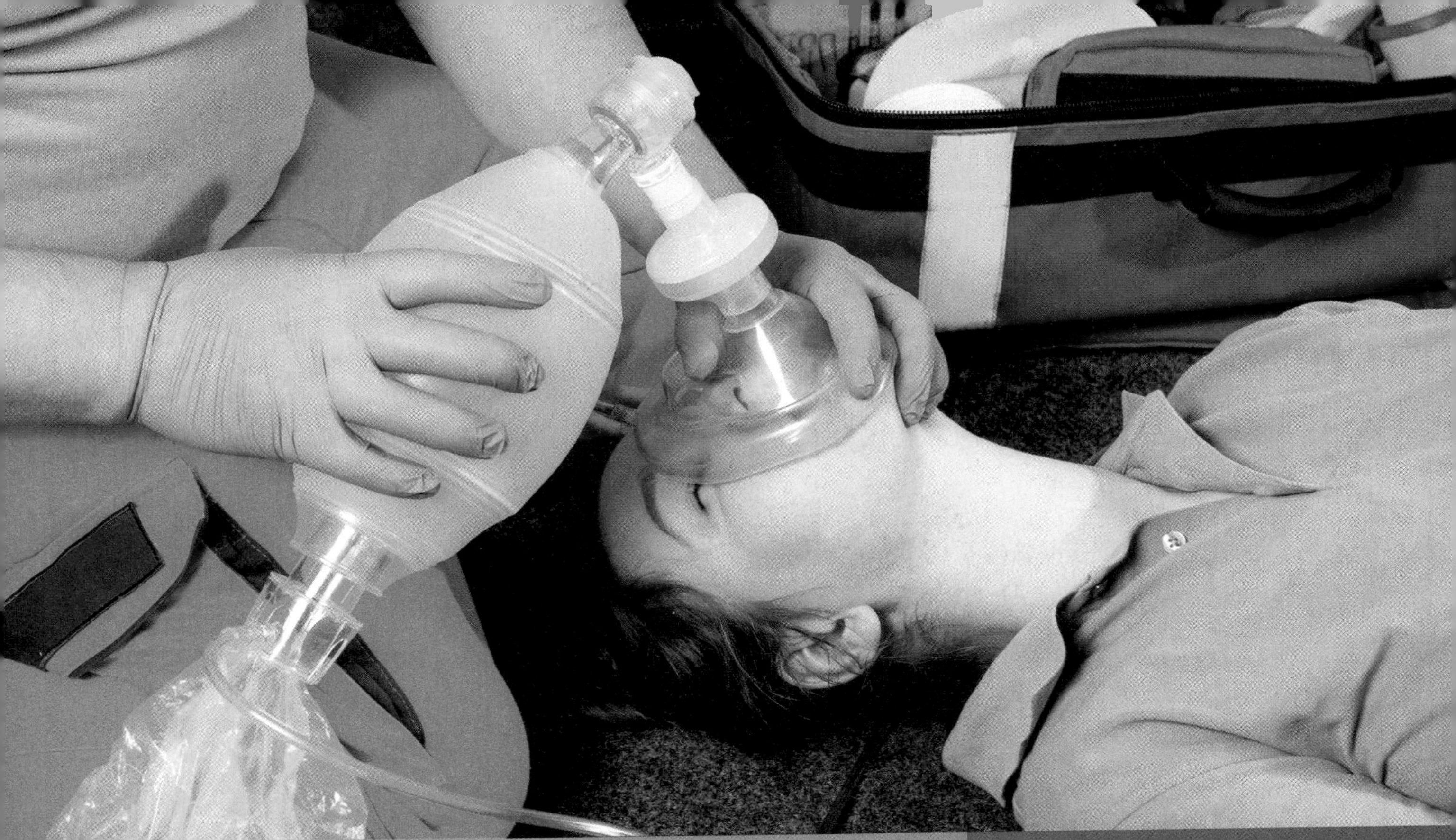

Airway Management

VOLUME 1

Section

5

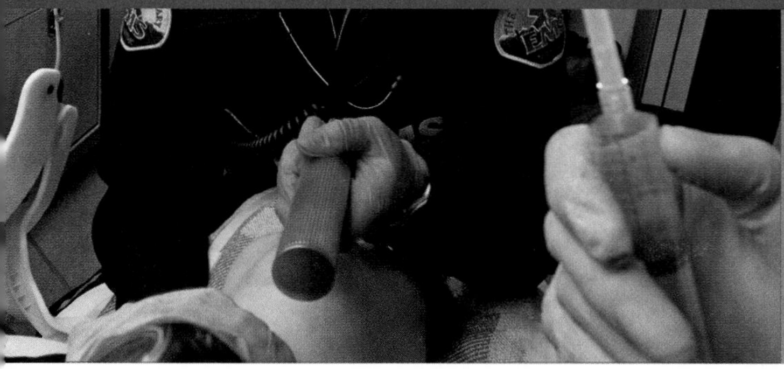

Chapter 16

Airway Management

NATIONAL EMS EDUCATION STANDARD COMPETENCIES

Airway Management, Respiration, and Artificial Ventilation

Integrates complex knowledge of anatomy, physiology, and pathophysiology into the assessment to develop and implement a treatment plan with the goal of ensuring a patent airway, adequate mechanical ventilation, and respiration for patients of all ages.

Airway Management

- Airway anatomy (pp 959–961)
- Airway assessment (pp 967–972)
- Techniques of ensuring a patent airway (p 967)

Respiration

- Anatomy of the respiratory system (p 961)
- Physiology and pathophysiology of respiration (pp 961–966)
  - Pulmonary ventilation (pp 963–964)
  - Oxygenation (pp 961, 972–979)
  - Respiration (pp 961–966)
    - External (p 961)
    - Internal (p 961)
    - Cellular (p 961)
- Assessment and management of adequate and inadequate respiration (pp 967–972, 994–1010)
- Supplemental oxygen therapy (pp 994–997)

Artificial Ventilation

Assessment and management of adequate and inadequate ventilation

- Artificial ventilation (pp 1001–1003)
- Minute ventilation (p 962)
- Alveolar ventilation (pp 978–979)
- Effect of artificial ventilation on cardiac output (p 966)

KNOWLEDGE OBJECTIVES

1. Review the anatomy of the respiratory system, including the major structures of the upper and lower airway. (pp 959–961)
2. Discuss the physiology of breathing, including ventilation, oxygenation, and respiration. (p 961)
3. Describe factors related to the pathophysiology of respiration, including ventilation–perfusion ratio mismatch, hypoventilation, hyperventilation, and circulatory compromise. (pp 961–966)
4. Describe factors related to ventilation, including partial pressure and volumes. (pp 963–964)
5. Explain positive-pressure ventilation versus negative-pressure ventilation. (pp 1000–1001)
6. Discuss acid–base imbalance, specifically respiratory acidosis and respiratory alkalosis. (pp 965–966)
7. Explain how to assess for a patent airway. (p 967)
8. List the signs of adequate breathing. (p 967)
9. List the signs of inadequate breathing. (pp 967–969)

10. Describe the five abnormal breathing patterns to recognize when assessing a patient's breathing. (p 969)
11. Explain how to assess a patient's breath sounds. (pp 969–972)
12. Explain how to assess for adequate and inadequate respiration, including the use of pulse oximetry. (pp 972–974)
13. Discuss the methods for end-tidal carbon dioxide assessment, including its importance. (pp 975–980)
14. Explain the use of the recovery position to maintain a clear airway. (p 981)
15. Describe how to perform the head tilt–chin lift maneuver. (p 982)
16. Describe how to perform the jaw-thrust maneuver. (pp 982–983)
17. Describe how to perform the tongue-jaw lift maneuver. (p 983)
18. Describe the importance and techniques of suctioning. (pp 985–986)
19. Explain how to measure and insert an oropharyngeal (oral) airway. (pp 986–987)
20. Explain how to measure and insert a nasopharyngeal (nasal) airway. (pp 987–989)
21. Describe the causes of foreign body airway obstruction. (pp 989–990)
22. Describe the management of mild and severe foreign body airway obstruction in an adult, a child, and an infant. (pp 990–992)
23. Describe the importance of giving supplemental oxygen to patients who are hypoxic. (p 994)
24. Describe the basics of how oxygen is stored and the various hazards associated with its use. (pp 994–995)
25. Explain how to use a nonrebreathing mask, including the oxygen flow requirements for its use. (pp 997–998)
26. Describe the indications for using a nasal cannula rather than a nonrebreathing mask. (p 998)
27. Describe the indications for using a humidifier during supplemental oxygen therapy. (p 999)
28. Explain how to perform mouth-to-mask ventilation. (pp 1002–1003)
29. Describe the assessment and care of a patient with apnea. (p 1008)
30. Describe the use of a one- and two-person bag-mask device. (pp 1003–1006)
31. Describe the signs associated with adequate and inadequate artificial ventilation. (p 1006)
32. Discuss automatic transport ventilators and how to use them. (pp 1007–1008)
33. Describe the indications, contraindications, and complications of using continuous positive airway pressure (CPAP). (pp 1008–1010)
34. Explain the considerations surrounding gastric distention, including how to perform nasogastric and orogastric decompression. (pp 1010–1015)
35. Discuss airway management considerations for patients with a laryngectomy, tracheostomy, or stoma. (pp 1016–1020)
36. List the advanced airway devices and techniques available for use by paramedics. (p 1022)
37. Discuss methods used to predict the difficult airway. (pp 1022–1025)
38. Describe the advantages, disadvantages, and equipment used when performing endotracheal (ET) intubation. (pp 1025–1027)
39. Explain how to determine correct ET tube size. (p 1025)
40. List factors to consider when determining correct laryngoscope blade size. (p 1027)
41. Discuss the indications and contraindications of orotracheal intubation. (p 1027)
42. List the methods available for confirming correct ET tube placement and the advantages and disadvantages of each method. (p 1034)
43. Describe how to secure an ET tube. (pp 1034–1035)
44. Discuss the indications, contraindications, advantages, disadvantages, and complications of nasotracheal intubation. (pp 1039–1043)
45. Explain what to do when intubation fails. (p 1047)
46. Explain how to perform tracheobronchial suctioning. (pp 1047–1048)
47. Discuss considerations related to field extubation. (pp 1048–1050)
48. List possible pharmacologic adjuncts to airway management and ventilation, including both sedatives and neuromuscular blocking

agents used for emergency intubation. (pp 1050–1053)

49. Discuss the procedure for performing rapid sequence intubation. (pp 1054–1056)
50. Discuss King LT airway devices, including how they work, their indications, contraindications, and complications, and the procedure for insertion. (pp 1057–1058)
51. Discuss the laryngeal mask airway, including how it works, its indications, contraindications, and complications, and the procedure for insertion. (pp 1060–1061)
52. Discuss the i-gel supraglottic airway device, including how it works and the procedure for insertion. (pp 1062–1064)
53. Discuss the indications, contraindications, advantages, disadvantages, and complications of performing surgical cricothyrotomy. (pp 1066–1068)
54. Discuss the indications, contraindications, advantages, disadvantages, and complications of performing needle cricothyrotomy. (p 1072)

SKILLS OBJECTIVES

1. Demonstrate how to use pulse oximetry. (pp 973–974)
2. Demonstrate how to position an unresponsive patient. (p 981)
3. Demonstrate how to place a patient in the recovery position. (p 981)
4. Demonstrate how to perform the head tilt–chin lift maneuver. (p 982)
5. Demonstrate how to perform the jaw-thrust maneuver. (pp 982–983)
6. Demonstrate how to perform the tongue-jaw lift maneuver. (p 983)
7. Demonstrate how to operate a suction unit. (pp 983–985)
8. Demonstrate how to suction a patient's airway. (pp 985–986)
9. Demonstrate how to insert an oropharyngeal (oral) airway. (p 987)
10. Demonstrate how to insert an oropharyngeal airway using a tongue depressor. (p 987)
11. Demonstrate how to insert a nasopharyngeal (nasal) airway. (p 989)
12. Demonstrate how to use Magill forceps to remove an object that is in the airway. (p 993, Skill Drill 16-1)
13. Demonstrate how to place an oxygen cylinder into service. (pp 996–997)
14. Demonstrate how to use partial and nonrebreathing masks to provide supplemental oxygen therapy to patients. (pp 997–998)
15. Demonstrate how to use a Venturi mask to provide supplemental oxygen therapy to patients. (p 999)
16. Demonstrate how to use a humidifier to provide supplemental oxygen therapy to patients. (p 999)
17. Demonstrate mouth-to-mask ventilation. (p 1003)
18. Demonstrate how to assist a patient with ventilations using the bag-mask device for one and two rescuers. (pp 1005–1006)
19. Demonstrate how to use an automatic transport ventilator to assist in delivering artificial ventilation to patients. (p 1007)
20. Demonstrate how to use CPAP. (p 1011, Skill Drill 16-2)
21. Demonstrate how to insert a nasogastric tube. (pp 1013–1014, Skill Drill 16-3)
22. Demonstrate how to insert an orogastric tube. (p 1015, Skill Drill 16-4)
23. Demonstrate how to suction a stoma. (p 1017, Skill Drill 16-5)
24. Demonstrate ventilation through a stoma using a resuscitation mask. (pp 1018–1019, Skill Drill 16-6)
25. Demonstrate bag-mask device-to-stoma ventilation. (p 1019, Skill Drill 16-7)
26. Demonstrate how to replace a dislodged tracheostomy tube. (p 1021, Skill Drill 16-8)
27. Demonstrate the entire procedure for orotracheal intubation using direct laryngoscopy. (pp 1036–1038, Skill Drill 16-9)
28. Demonstrate how to secure an ET tube. (pp 1034–1035)
29. Demonstrate the entire procedure for orotracheal intubation using video laryngoscopy. (pp 1040–1041, Skill Drill 16-10)
30. Demonstrate how to perform blind nasotracheal intubation. (pp 1045–1046, Skill Drill 16-11)

31. Discuss how to perform face-to-face intubation. (pp 1044–1047)
32. Demonstrate how to perform tracheobronchial suctioning. (pp 1048–1049, Skill Drill 16-12)
33. Demonstrate how to perform rapid sequence intubation. (pp 1054–1056)
34. Demonstrate insertion of the King LT airway. (p 1059, Skill Drill 16-13)
35. Demonstrate insertion of the laryngeal mask airway. (pp 1062–1063, Skill Drill 16-14)
36. Demonstrate insertion of the i-gel airway. (pp 1064–1065, Skill Drill 16-15)
37. Demonstrate how to perform a surgical cricothyrotomy. (pp 1070–1071, Skill Drill 16-16)
38. Demonstrate how to perform needle cricothyrotomy and translaryngeal catheter ventilation. (pp 1073–1075, Skill Drill 16-17)

Introduction

Establishing and maintaining a **patent** (open) airway and ensuring effective oxygenation and ventilation are vital aspects of effective patient care. Attempting to stabilize the condition of a patient whose airway is compromised is futile. The human body needs a constant oxygen supply to carry out the physiologic processes necessary to sustain life; the airway is where it all begins. Few situations will cause such acute deterioration and death more rapidly than airway and/or ventilation compromise. To preserve life, the airway must remain patent at all times, regardless of the situation.

The function of the respiratory system is simple: It brings in oxygen and eliminates carbon dioxide (the primary waste product of oxygen **metabolism**, the chemical processes that provide the cells with energy from nutrients). If this process is interrupted, then vital organs of the body will not function properly. For example, brain cells can survive for only 6 minutes or so without oxygen before permanent damage occurs.

Failure to manage the airway and improper management of the airway are major causes of preventable death in the prehospital setting. The basic airway management techniques learned in initial EMT education are among the most crucial skills for you as a paramedic. Failure to use basic airway techniques, improper performance of the techniques (ie, improper bag-mask seal or improper airway positioning), a rush to use advanced interventions, and failure to reassess the patient's condition may all increase mortality and morbidity. Therefore, a large portion of this chapter is dedicated to the reinforcement of basic airway management skills. As a paramedic, you must understand the importance of early detection of airway conditions, rapid and effective interventions to remedy those conditions, and continual reassessment of a patient with airway or breathing compromise.

This chapter begins with a review of anatomy as it relates to the procedures of airway management, followed by a discussion of the processes of ventilation, oxygenation, and respiration. A basic-to-advanced approach, just as airway management is typically performed in the field, is followed to emphasize the importance of securing a patent airway and ensuring adequate ventilation, oxygenation, and respiration. The chapter then describes the techniques of opening and maintaining a patent airway, recognizing and treating airway obstructions, assessing a patient's ventilation and oxygenation status, administering supplemental oxygen,

YOU are the Paramedic

PART 1

At 2125 hours, you are dispatched to a residence for a 67-year-old man experiencing respiratory distress. You and your paramedic partner proceed to the scene; your response time is approximately 5 minutes. All fire units are currently working a structure fire and are unable to respond to assist.

1. What is the difference between respiratory distress and respiratory failure?

2. Is it possible for a patient to ventilate, but not oxygenate? Why or why not?

and providing ventilatory assistance. With a responsive patient, you may not need to open the airway manually, but rather simply provide supplemental oxygen. Even so, you must remember the order in which steps should be performed, bypassing steps that do not apply to the particular situation. Finally, advanced techniques, including advanced airway devices and procedures, are discussed in detail.

Review of Airway Anatomy

To effectively manage a patient's airway, you must identify the key anatomic structures and understand how those structures may need to be manipulated when inserting various airway devices. The following section provides a brief review of airway anatomy. A detailed discussion of airway and respiratory anatomy and physiology is found in Chapter 8, *Anatomy and Physiology*.

Upper Airway

Anatomically, the upper airway includes all structures above the glottic opening (glottis), which is the space between the vocal cords. Therefore, when you perform skills such as endotracheal (ET) intubation, you must identify the upper airway anatomy while you advance the **laryngoscope** blade in the patient's mouth **FIGURE 16-1A**. ET intubation is discussed in detail later in this chapter.

The tongue is the first and largest anatomic structure that must be manipulated when managing a patient's airway, because it tends to fall back into the posterior pharynx of an unresponsive patient. At the base of the tongue, the uvula extends from the soft palate in the posterior oral cavity; manipulation of the uvula is usually unnecessary, although the uvula is an important anatomic landmark to identify as you proceed to the posterior pharynx. The uvula helps prevent food you eat from going up your nose. It also can trigger a gag reflex when stimulated. Some patients may have had their uvula removed, as it is not an essential structure.

The pharynx is a muscular tube that extends from the nose and mouth to the level of the esophagus and trachea; it is composed of the nasopharynx, the oropharynx, and the laryngopharynx (also called the hypopharynx). The laryngopharynx is the lowest portion of the pharynx; it opens into the larynx anteriorly, and into the esophagus posteriorly **FIGURE 16-1B**.

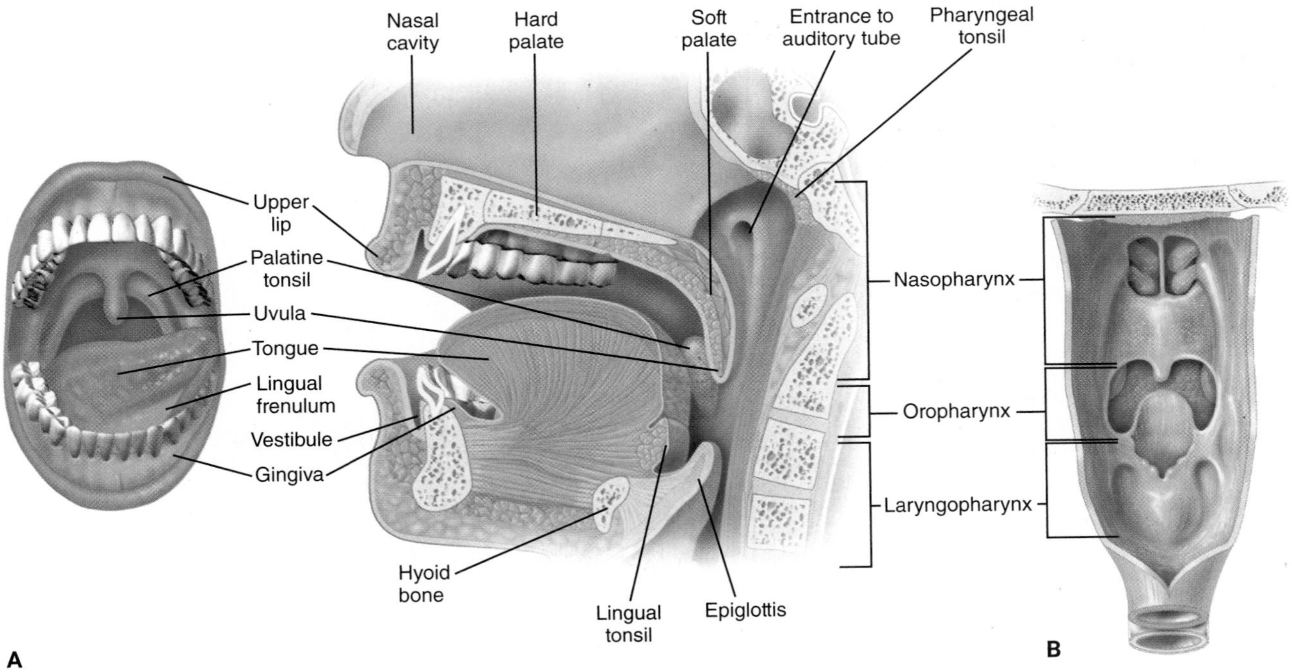

FIGURE 16-1 A. The oral cavity. **B.** The pharynx.

Lower Airway

The lower airway extends from the glottis to the pulmonary capillary membrane. The larynx is a complex structure formed by many independent cartilaginous structures. It marks where the upper airway ends and the lower airway begins **FIGURE 16-2**.

The thyroid cartilage is a shield-shaped structure that is palpable on the anterior neck. The superior part of the thyroid cartilage forms a V shape called the thyroid notch. The laryngeal prominence, known as the Adam's apple, is immediately inferior to the thyroid notch. The Adam's apple is more prominent in men than in women, and it can be difficult to palpate in patients with obesity or patients with short necks. The thyroid cartilage is suspended from the hyoid bone by the thyrohyoid ligaments and is located directly anterior to the glottic opening and vocal cords.

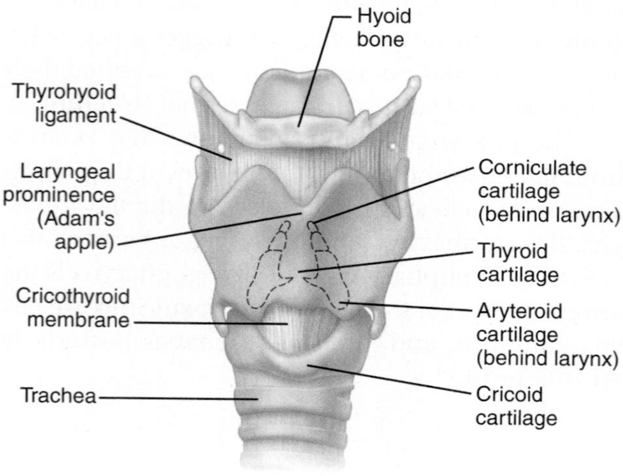

FIGURE 16-2 The larynx.

The cricoid cartilage, or cricoid ring, lies inferior to the thyroid cartilage; it forms the lowest portion of the larynx and is the only circumferential ring of the trachea (the other tracheal rings are semicircular). The cricoid ring is more prominent in females than in males.

The cricothyroid membrane is located between the thyroid and cricoid cartilages; it is the site where providers may obtain emergency surgical and nonsurgical access to the airway (cricothyrotomy). Because it is bordered laterally and inferiorly by the highly vascular thyroid gland, you must locate the anatomic landmarks carefully when accessing the airway via the cricothyroid membrane.

The glottis is the narrowest portion of the adult airway **FIGURE 16-3**. The vocal cords are located at the lateral borders of the glottis. The **epiglottis** (a leaf-shaped cartilaginous structure that closes over the trachea during swallowing) is located at the superior border of the glottis. When you perform ET intubation, you must visualize the epiglottis, glottis, and vocal cords before inserting the ET tube.

Just beyond the vocal cords, the trachea immediately descends into the thoracic cavity; it is not a

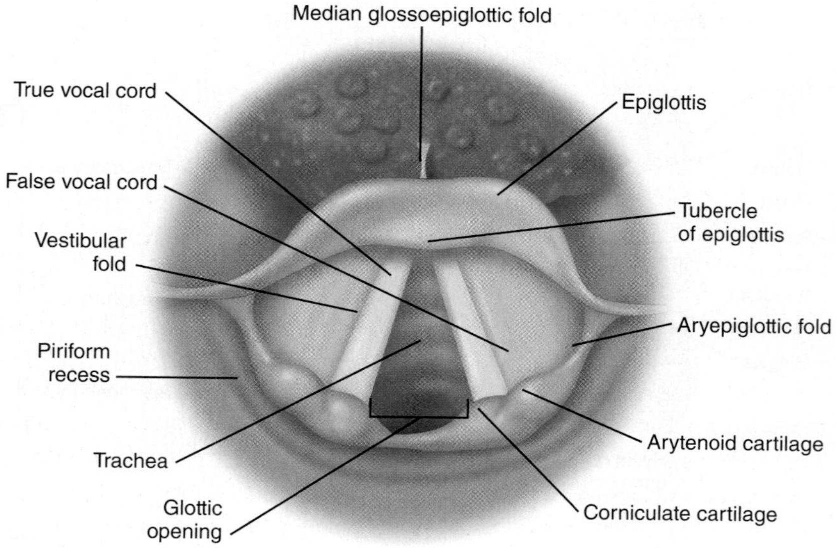

FIGURE 16-3 The glottis and its surrounding structures.

TABLE 16-1 Ventilation, Oxygenation, and Respiration

Function	Definition
Ventilation	The physical act of moving air into and out of the lungs
Oxygenation	The process of loading oxygen molecules onto hemoglobin molecules in the bloodstream
Respiration	The exchange of oxygen and carbon dioxide in the alveoli and the tissues of the body

straight tube. This information is critical when you prepare an ET tube and place it into the trachea.

Ventilation, Oxygenation, and Respiration

The respiratory and cardiovascular systems work together to ensure that a constant supply of oxygen and nutrients is delivered to every cell in the body and that carbon dioxide and other waste products are removed from every cell **TABLE 16-1**.

Ventilation is the physical act of moving air in and out of the lungs. The active, muscular part of ventilation is called inhalation. Exhalation, unlike inhalation, is a passive process and does not normally require muscular effort.

Oxygenation is the process of loading oxygen molecules onto **hemoglobin** molecules in the bloodstream. For oxygenation to occur, the percentage of oxygen inhaled during ventilation, or the fraction of inspired oxygen (FIO_2), must be adequate. Although oxygenation cannot occur without ventilation, ventilation is possible without oxygenation.

Respiration is the process of exchanging oxygen and carbon dioxide. External respiration (pulmonary respiration) is the process of exchanging oxygen and carbon dioxide between the alveoli and the blood in the pulmonary capillaries **FIGURE 16-4**. Internal respiration (cellular respiration) is the exchange of oxygen and carbon dioxide between the systemic circulation and the cells of the body **FIGURE 16-5**. Adequate oxygenation is required for respiration; however, it does not guarantee that respiration is taking place.

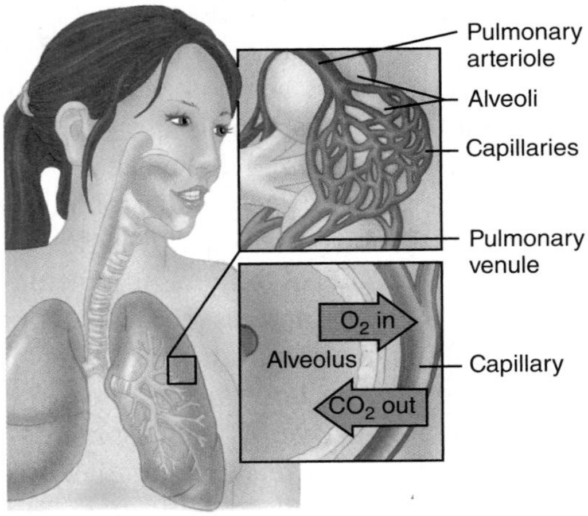

FIGURE 16-4 External (pulmonary) respiration.

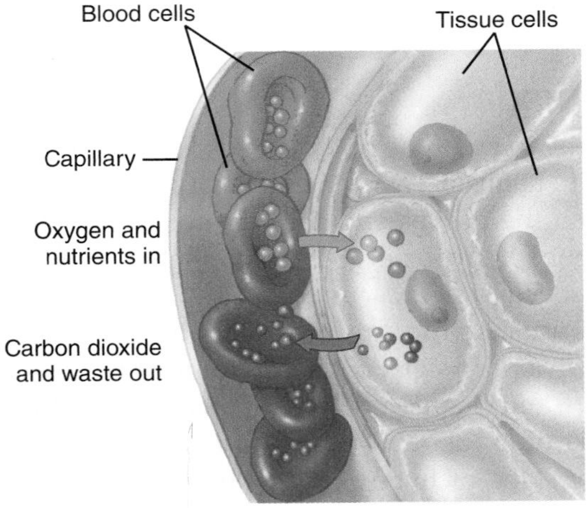

FIGURE 16-5 Internal (cellular) respiration.

Pathophysiology of Respiration

Multiple conditions can inhibit the body's ability to effectively provide oxygen to the cells. Disruptions of pulmonary ventilation, oxygenation, and respiration will cause immediate effects within the body. As a paramedic, you must recognize these conditions quickly and correct them immediately. It is essential to distinguish a primary ventilation problem from a primary oxygenation or respiration problem. For example, an overdose of a central nervous system (CNS) depressant drug (ie, opioid, barbiturate) suppresses the rate and depth (tidal volume) of breathing and causes, at least initially, a ventilation problem. If ventilation is impaired, then adequate oxygen will not be taken into the lungs and distributed to the cells and tissues of the body. By contrast, a person trapped in a place devoid of oxygen may develop an oxygenation problem first; this individual may be ventilating but is not breathing in adequate amounts of oxygen. As a result, oxygen delivery to the cells and tissues will be compromised, resulting in a respiration problem.

Every cell in the body needs a constant supply of oxygen to survive. Whereas some tissues are more resilient than others, eventually all cells will die if deprived of oxygen **FIGURE 16-6**. To provide adequate amounts of oxygen to the body's tissues, external respiration and perfusion (circulation of blood within an organ or tissue in adequate amounts to meet the current needs of the cells) must take place.

Hypoxia

Failure to meet the body's needs for oxygen may result in hypoxia. **Hypoxia** is a dangerous condition in which the tissues and cells do not receive enough oxygen. If hypoxia goes uncorrected, then death may occur quickly.

Patients who are breathing inadequately will show varying signs and symptoms of hypoxia. The onset and degree of tissue damage caused by hypoxia often depend on the quality of ventilations. Early signs of hypoxia include restlessness, irritability, apprehension, tachycardia, and anxiety. Late signs include changes in mental status, a weak (thready) pulse, and **cyanosis**, a blue or purple skin color. (Recall that for patients with dark skin, cyanosis may be easier to appreciate by assessing the mucous membranes [lips, gums, inner eyelids] and nail beds.) Responsive patients often report feeling short of breath (**dyspnea**) and may be unable to speak in complete sentences. You should administer supplemental oxygen to a patient with respiratory distress before signs and symptoms of hypoxia appear.

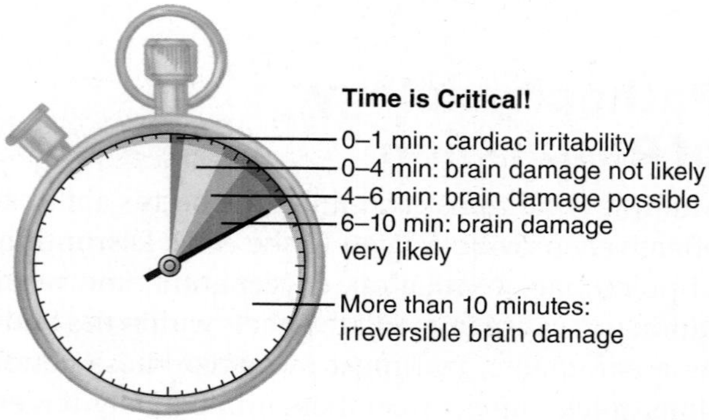
Time is Critical!
0–1 min: cardiac irritability
0–4 min: brain damage not likely
4–6 min: brain damage possible
6–10 min: brain damage very likely
More than 10 minutes: irreversible brain damage

FIGURE 16-6 Cells need a constant supply of oxygen to survive. Some cells (ie, brain cells) may be severely or permanently damaged after only 4 to 6 minutes without oxygen.

Ventilation–Perfusion Ratio and Mismatch

The lungs have a functional role in placing ambient (room) air in close proximity to circulating blood, thereby permitting gas exchange to occur by simple diffusion. Air and blood flow must be directed to the same place at the same time to accomplish this task. In other words, ventilation and perfusion must be matched. A failure to match ventilation and perfusion, or **$\dot{V}/\dot{Q}$ mismatch**, contributes to most abnormalities in oxygen and carbon dioxide exchange.

In most people, the normal resting minute ventilation is approximately 6 L/min. About one-third of this volume fills dead space; therefore, resting alveolar volume is approximately 4 L/min. However, pulmonary artery blood flow is approximately 5 L/min, yielding an overall ratio of ventilation to perfusion of 4:5 L/min, or 0.8 L/min. Because neither ventilation nor perfusion is distributed equally, both are distributed to dependent regions of the lungs at rest. However, an increase in gravity-dependent flow is more marked with perfusion (blood) than with ventilation (air). Hence, the ventilation-to-perfusion ratio is highest at the apex (top) of the lung and lowest at the base (bottom).

When ventilation is compromised but perfusion continues, blood passes over some alveolar membranes without gas exchange occurring; therefore, not all alveoli will be enriched with oxygen. The result is a lack of oxygen diffusing across the membrane and into the circulatory system. Along the same lines, carbon dioxide is unable to diffuse across the membrane and is recirculated into the bloodstream. This condition results in a $\dot{V}/\dot{Q}$ mismatch and could lead to severe hypoxia if the cause of the $\dot{V}/\dot{Q}$ mismatch is not recognized and treated.

Similar problems can occur when perfusion across the alveolar membrane is disrupted. Even though the alveoli are filled with fresh oxygen, a disruption in blood flow does not allow for the optimal exchange of gases across the membrane. The result of inadequate perfusion is less oxygen absorption in the bloodstream and less carbon dioxide removal. This $\dot{V}/\dot{Q}$ mismatch can also lead to hypoxia, and the patient needs immediate intervention to prevent further damage or death.

Factors Affecting Ventilation

Maintaining a patent airway is critical for the provision of oxygen to the tissues of the body. Many intrinsic (internal) and extrinsic (external) factors can cause airway obstruction. Intrinsic conditions such as infection, allergic reactions, and unresponsiveness (possibly leading to airway obstruction by the tongue) can significantly restrict the ability to maintain a patent airway. Swelling from infections and allergic reactions can be fatal if not aggressively managed with medications and, possibly, advanced airway management techniques. The tongue is the most common airway obstruction in an unresponsive patient. This airway obstruction, while easily corrected, can result in hypoxia and hinder adequate tissue perfusion. Snoring respirations and an improper head and/or neck position are good indicators that the tongue may be obstructing the airway. Prompt correction of this obstruction is necessary for adequate ventilation and oxygenation.

Some factors affecting pulmonary ventilation are not necessarily directly part of the respiratory system. The central and peripheral nervous systems have key roles in the regulation of breathing. Interruptions in these systems can have drastic effects on the ability to breathe effectively. Medications that depress the CNS (ie, opioids and benzodiazepines), if taken in excess, will lower the respiratory rate and reduce the tidal volume, which then lead to decreases in alveolar volume and overall minute volume. As a result, the amount of carbon dioxide in the respiratory and circulatory systems increases, resulting in an overall increase in the carbon dioxide content of the blood.

Trauma to the head and spinal cord can also interrupt the nervous system's control of ventilation, resulting in decreased respiratory function and even failure. Neuromuscular disorders, such as muscular dystrophy and poliomyelitis, can also affect the ability of the nervous system to control breathing. Muscular dystrophy causes degeneration of muscle fibers, slow motor development, and loss of muscle contractility. Curvature of the spine is also likely in patients with muscular dystrophy and can impair pulmonary function. Polio is a viral neuromuscular disorder that can affect the nerves, including those that regulate ventilation and result in paralysis. Neuromuscular blocking agents (paralytics), such as those used to facilitate intubation, effectively paralyze a patient and induce apnea (discussed later in this chapter).

Patients with allergic reactions might have a potential airway obstruction due to swelling (angioedema) and a decrease in pulmonary ventilation from bronchoconstriction. As the bronchioles constrict, air must move through smaller lumens; the constraint on air movement results in decreased ventilation. Bronchoconstriction is also associated with conditions such as chronic obstructive pulmonary disease (COPD) and asthma.

Extrinsic factors affecting pulmonary ventilation can include trauma and foreign body airway obstruction. Trauma to the airway or chest requires immediate evaluation and intervention. Blunt or penetrating trauma and burns can disrupt airflow through the trachea and into the lungs, quickly resulting in oxygenation deficiencies. In addition, trauma to the chest wall can result in structural damage to the thorax, leading to inadequate pulmonary ventilation. For example, a patient with numerous rib fractures or a flail chest may purposely breathe shallowly to alleviate the pain caused by the injury. This practice, called respiratory splinting, can result in decreased pulmonary ventilation. Proper ventilatory support is crucial to good outcomes for patients with such injuries or conditions.

If production of carbon dioxide exceeds the body's ability to eliminate this gas by ventilation, then the partial pressure of carbon dioxide ($Paco_2$) rises, resulting in **hypoventilation** (slow and/or shallow breathing). Theoretically, hypoventilation can occur in two ways: Either carbon dioxide production can exceed the body's ability to eliminate it, or carbon dioxide elimination can be depressed to the extent that it no longer keeps up with normal metabolism.

At the other extreme is **hyperventilation** (rapid and/or deep breathing), which occurs when carbon dioxide elimination exceeds carbon dioxide production. For example, a patient experiencing an anxiety attack tends to breathe very deeply and rapidly, so carbon dioxide is eliminated at a rate faster than the body produces it. The level of carbon dioxide in the blood then falls below normal, and the patient experiences symptoms such as dizziness and numbness or tingling in the face and extremities.

Hypoventilation and hyperventilation sometimes represent the body's attempt to compensate for various abnormal conditions. For example, if the pH of the blood is too high (alkalosis), the patient's breathing may become slow and/or shallow in an attempt to retain carbon dioxide (and therefore, hydrogen ions [H^+]) in an attempt to decrease the pH. Conversely, hyperventilation could be a compensatory response of the body to a decrease in the pH of the blood (acidosis), such as what occurs with hyperglycemic ketoacidosis or aspirin overdose.

In addition to the factors discussed thus far, decreases or increases in minute volume can lead to abnormal carbon dioxide levels in the blood **TABLE 16-2**. A decrease in the minute volume decreases carbon dioxide elimination, resulting in a buildup of carbon dioxide in the blood (**hypercapnia**). Conversely, an increase in the minute volume increases carbon dioxide elimination, which lowers the carbon dioxide content of the blood (**hypocapnia**).

Factors Affecting Oxygenation and Respiration

External elements in the environment can affect the overall process of respiration. For proper respiration to occur at the cellular level, oxygenation and perfusion (processes affected by internal factors) must function efficiently.

External Factors

Adequate respiration requires proper ventilation and oxygenation. External factors such as the atmospheric pressure and the partial pressure of oxygen (Pao_2) in the ambient air have key roles in the overall process of respiration. At high altitudes, the percentage of oxygen remains the same, but the partial pressure decreases because the total atmospheric pressure decreases. The low Pao_2 can make it difficult to impossible to adequately oxygenate the tissues, thus interrupting internal respiration. In addition, closed environments, such as mines and trenches, may have decreased levels of ambient oxygen, resulting in poor oxygenation and respiration.

Carbon monoxide, along with other toxic gases, displaces oxygen in the environment and makes proper oxygenation and respiration difficult. In particular, carbon monoxide has a much greater affinity for hemoglobin than does oxygen (250 times more). Thus, the attachment of carbon monoxide molecules to the hemoglobin molecules, which forms carboxyhemoglobin (COHb), inhibits the proper transport of oxygen to the tissues and can cause false pulse oximetry readings. Pulse oximetry is discussed in detail later in this chapter.

TABLE 16-2 Carbon Dioxide Balance

	Hypoventilation	Hyperventilation
Minute volume	↓	↑
CO_2 elimination	↓	↑
$Paco_2$	↑ (hypercapnia)	↓ (hypocapnia)

Abbreviations: CO2, carbon dioxide; Paco2, partial pressure of carbon dioxide

Internal Factors

Conditions that reduce the surface area for gas exchange also decrease the body's oxygen supply, leading to inadequate tissue perfusion. In addition, medical conditions such as pneumonia, pulmonary edema, and COPD may also result in a disturbance of cellular metabolism. These conditions decrease the surface area of the alveoli by damaging the alveoli or by leading to an accumulation of fluid in the lungs.

Nonfunctional alveoli create a barrier to the diffusion of oxygen and carbon dioxide. As a result, blood entering the lungs from the right side of the heart bypasses the alveoli and returns to the left side of the heart in an unoxygenated state, a condition called **intrapulmonary shunting**.

Patients who are submerged in water and patients with pulmonary edema may have fluid in their alveoli. This accumulation of fluid inhibits adequate gas exchange at the alveolar membrane and results in decreased oxygenation and respiration. In addition, exposure to certain environmental conditions (eg, high altitudes) or occupational hazards (eg, epoxy resins) can cause fluid to accumulate in the alveoli over time, leading to an overall decrease in respiration. These conditions can result in anaerobic respiration and an increase in lactic acid accumulation. The excess lactic acid in the blood lowers the pH and can result in numerous life-threatening conditions, such as cardiac dysrhythmias, coma, and shock.

Other conditions that affect the cells of the body include hypoglycemia, hormonal imbalances, and infection. As oxygen and glucose levels decrease, the body cannot maintain a homeostatic balance with regard to energy production. If the metabolic needs of the body cannot be met, then cellular death is likely. Infection also increases the body's metabolic needs and disrupts homeostasis (the tendency toward stability in the body's internal environment). If the disruption in homeostasis is not corrected, then the cells will die as well. If levels of the hormone insulin decrease in the body, then the cellular uptake of glucose will decrease. Without sufficient glucose, the cells will metabolize fatty acids, resulting in ketoacidosis, a form of metabolic acidosis.

Circulatory Compromise

The circulatory system must function efficiently for respiration to occur. When the circulatory system is compromised, perfusion becomes inadequate, and the body's oxygen demands will not be met.

Obstruction of blood flow to individual cells and tissues is typically related to trauma emergencies. Conditions that you may encounter in trauma patients include simple or tension pneumothorax, open pneumothorax (sucking chest wound), hemothorax, hemopneumothorax, and pulmonary embolism. These conditions inhibit gas exchange at the tissue level because of their adverse effects on the respiratory and circulatory systems. In addition, conditions such as heart failure and cardiac tamponade inhibit the ability of the heart to effectively pump oxygenated blood to the tissues.

Both blood loss and anemia (a deficiency of red blood cells) reduce the oxygen-carrying ability of the blood. Without sufficient circulating red blood cells, not enough hemoglobin molecules are available to bind with oxygen.

When the body is in a state of shock, oxygen is not delivered to the cells efficiently. Hemorrhagic shock (a form of hypovolemic shock) is a decrease in blood volume caused by internal or external bleeding; it leads to inadequate oxygen delivery to the body's tissues. In contrast, vasodilatory shock is not caused by a decrease in blood volume, but rather by an increase in the size of the blood vessels. As the diameter of the blood vessels increases, the blood pressure (BP) decreases and blood flow diminishes; oxygen is not effectively delivered to the tissues. Both forms of shock result in poor tissue perfusion that leads to anaerobic metabolism. You should aggressively treat any patient suspected of being in shock to prevent further interruptions in tissue perfusion.

Acid–Base Balance

Hypoventilation and hyperventilation, along with hypoxia, can cause disruptions in the acid–base balance in the body that may lead to rapid clinical deterioration and death. Both the respiratory system and the renal system have roles in maintaining homeostasis. Homeostasis requires a balance between the acids and bases, among other body systems.

When an excess of acid is present in the body, the fastest way to eliminate it is through the respiratory system. Excess acid can be expelled as carbon dioxide from the lungs by increasing the respiratory output. Conversely, slowing respirations will increase the level of carbon dioxide. The renal system regulates pH by filtering out more (or retaining) hydrogen ions and retaining (or filtering out) bicarbonate when needed. Therefore, the fastest way the body can eliminate excess H^+ ions is to create water and carbon dioxide, which are then expelled as gases from the lungs.

Anything that inhibits respiratory function can lead to acid retention and acidosis. Acidosis quickly develops any time a patient is in respiratory distress or is unable to breathe, and can develop as a result of abnormal respiratory function (ie, with bradypnea, labored breathing, or shallow breathing [reduced tidal volume]). Alkalosis can develop if the respiratory rate is too high (or the volume too much).

Acid–base disorders have four main clinical presentations:

- **Respiratory acidosis**
- **Respiratory alkalosis**
- Metabolic acidosis
- Metabolic alkalosis

Fluctuations in pH due to the amount of bicarbonate available in the body result in metabolic acidosis or alkalosis. Fluctuations in pH due to respiratory disorders that result in excess carbon

Words of Wisdom

The Effects of Ventilation on Cardiac Output

During normal breathing, the negative pressure created by each breath increases the venous return of blood to the heart. Just as negative intrathoracic pressure draws air into the chest cavity through the airway (**negative-pressure ventilation**), the same pressure draws venous blood back to the heart from the upper body (via the superior vena cava) and lower body (via the inferior vena cava).

When patients are transitioned from negative-pressure ventilation to **positive-pressure ventilation** (the forcing of air into the lungs [ie, bag-mask ventilation]), they lose this stimulus for venous return, and some patients may experience decreased cardiac output and hypotension as a result. The increased intrathoracic pressure caused by positive-pressure ventilation creates a pressure gradient against which the heart must pump. This process increases the **afterload** (the amount of resistance against which the ventricle must contract), which can further decrease cardiac output. The greater the pressure used to ventilate an apneic or a hypoventilating patient, the greater the decrease in **preload** (the volume of blood in the heart at the end of diastole), which occurs when the heart is literally squeezed by increased intrathoracic pressure.

Patients who are hypotensive, in shock, or are otherwise hemodynamically unstable may experience profound changes in BP because of the hemodynamic effects of positive-pressure ventilation. The best way to minimize this complication is to ventilate the patient for 1 second, with just enough force to cause visible chest rise, and to avoid ventilating the patient too fast. Positive- and negative-pressure ventilation are discussed in more detail later in this chapter.

dioxide retention or elimination result in respiratory acidosis or alkalosis, respectively. The focus here is on respiratory acidosis and respiratory alkalosis.

Acid–base disorders that are not immediately correctable by the body's buffering systems cause the body to initiate compensatory responses to help return levels to normal. For example, metabolic acidosis may create respiratory alkalosis as a compensatory response. Patient care often involves treating more than one form of acid–base imbalance.

Street Smarts

You must know *how* to perform a required airway procedure and *why* you are performing this particular procedure. Understanding why a procedure is performed enables you to select the right intervention at the right time. Knowledge of respiratory anatomy, physiology, and pathophysiology is crucial in this determination.

YOU are the Paramedic

PART 2

You arrive at the scene, enter the residence, and find the patient sitting in a chair in his living room. He is in a tripod position, is in obvious distress, and is anxious. His skin is diaphoretic. Your partner prepares to administer supplemental oxygen to the patient as you begin your primary assessment.

Recording Time: 1 Minute	
Appearance	Obvious respiratory distress, facial cyanosis; diaphoretic
Level of consciousness	Conscious and alert, but anxious
Airway	Patent
Breathing	Labored
Circulation	Radial pulse, rapid and strong; lips and gums appear gray (patient has dark skin)

3. How does oxygenation differ from respiration?
4. What are some clinical signs of inadequate breathing?

Patient Assessment: Airway Evaluation

The importance of carefully assessing a patient's airway and ventilatory status cannot be overemphasized. In the field, you will encounter patients with a variety of airway conditions. Some of these conditions are easily corrected; others require aggressive management. The emergency medical care you provide to a patient with an airway or ventilation problem is only as good as the assessment you perform.

Assessing Airway Patency

When presented with a patient who is experiencing a respiratory problem, first determine if the airway is patent. An adult who is responsive, alert, and able to speak in complete sentences with a normal voice has no immediate airway problem. However, because this status can rapidly change, remain vigilant.

An unresponsive patient is considered to have a compromised airway until careful assessment rules that out. Signs of airway compromise in an unresponsive patient include snoring (caused by partial airway obstruction by the tongue), vomitus (stomach contents) draining from the mouth, and a gurgling sound heard during breathing (which indicates secretions in the airway). Pooling of secretions in the patient's mouth is a clear indicator of a markedly depressed or absent gag reflex. The **gag reflex** is a spastic pharyngeal and esophageal reflex triggered by stimulating the uvula or posterior pharynx; it prevents foreign bodies from entering the trachea. The absence of a gag reflex significantly increases the risk of aspiration.

Recognizing Adequate Breathing

Normal breathing in an adult at rest is characterized by a rate between 12 and 20 breaths/min **TABLE 16-3** with adequate depth (tidal volume), a regular pattern of inhalation and exhalation, and clear and equal breath sounds bilaterally. Breathing at rest should appear effortless, and changes in rate and regularity should be subtle (not obvious).

TABLE 16-3 Normal Respiratory Rate Ranges

Age	Range (breaths/min)
Adults	12 to 20
Children	12 to 37
Infants (ages 1 month to 1 year)	30 to 53

Adult range adapted from National Association of State EMS Officials (NASEMSO). *National Model EMS Clinical Guidelines: Version 2.2.* NASEMSO website. https://nasemso.org/wp-content/uploads/National-Model-EMS-Clinical-Guidelines-2017-PDF-Version-2.2.pdf. Published January 2019. Accessed July 16, 2021; Pediatric ranges adapted from American Association of Critical-Care Nurses, American Heart Association. *PALS: Vital Signs in Children.* Dallas, TX: American Heart Association; 2020.

Recognizing Inadequate Breathing

Any patient you encounter, especially one with a respiratory complaint, should be assessed for breathing adequacy. The fact that a patient is breathing does not guarantee that the patient is breathing adequately. *Generally speaking, if you can see or hear a patient breathe, then a problem exists.*

Words of Wisdom

Hypoxemia is defined as a low oxygen level in arterial blood. Hypoxia, as discussed earlier, is a deficiency of oxygen at the tissue and cellular levels. Although these terms are often used interchangeably, they are different processes. Hypoxemia can often be reversed by administering supplemental oxygen, whereas hypoxia requires more aggressive oxygenation and, in some cases, ventilatory support. Left untreated, hypoxia will lead to **anoxia**: a lack of oxygen that results in tissue and cellular death.

An adult patient who presents with respiratory distress and is breathing at a rate of less than 12 breaths/min or more than 20 breaths/min must be evaluated for other signs of inadequate ventilation, such as shallow breathing (reduced tidal volume), an irregular pattern of breathing, altered mentation, and **adventitious** (abnormal) breath sounds. Cyanosis is a clear indicator of a low blood oxygen content; however, you may not encounter it as an early sign.

Patients with respiratory distress often compensate with preferential positioning, such as an upright sniffing position (in which the patient is sitting up, with the head moved forward until the earlobes are on the same vertical plane as the manubrium of the sternum) or a tripod position (in which the patient is sitting up and leaning forward with elbows bent). Patients experiencing respiratory distress will avoid a supine position because it worsens their breathing difficulties.

There are numerous potential causes of respiratory distress and inadequate ventilation, including severe infection (sepsis), trauma, brainstem injury, a noxious (poisonous) or oxygen-poor environment, and renal failure. Respiratory distress may result from an upper and/or lower airway obstruction, respiratory muscle impairment (eg, spinal cord injury), or CNS impairment (eg, head injury, drug overdose).

If a patient's airway is not patent or breathing is absent or inadequate, then all therapies you may attempt will prove futile. Proper airway management involves (in this order) opening the airway, clearing the airway, assessing breathing, and providing the appropriate intervention or interventions.

Evaluation of a patient with a respiratory complaint includes visual observations, auscultation, and palpation. Use visual techniques at first sight of the patient, literally from the door as you enter the room. Determine answers to the following questions when you assess a patient with respiratory distress:

- How is the patient positioned? In a tripod position (elbows out)?
- Is the patient experiencing **orthopnea** (positional dyspnea)?
- Is chest rise and fall adequate (adequate tidal volume)?
- Is the patient gasping for air (air hunger)?
- What is the skin color? How does this color compare with the patient's baseline color? Is the skin moist or clammy (diaphoretic)?
- Do you see flaring of the nostrils?
- Is the patient breathing through pursed lips?
- Do you note any **retractions** (skin pulling between and around the ribs during inhalation):
  - Intercostal?
  - At the suprasternal notch?
  - At the supraclavicular fossa?
  - Subcostal?
- Is the patient using accessory muscles to breathe?
- Is the patient's chest wall moving symmetrically? (**Asymmetric chest wall movement**, when one side of the chest moves less than the other, indicates that airflow into one lung is decreased.)
- Is the patient taking a series of quick breaths, followed by a prolonged exhalation phase?

A patient with inadequate ventilation may appear to be working hard to breathe (labored breathing). Labored breathing requires effort and may involve the use of accessory muscles. **Accessory muscles** include the sternocleidomastoid muscles (neck muscles), the pectoralis major muscles, and the abdominal muscles. These muscles are not used during normal breathing.

The following signs indicate inadequate ventilation in adults:

- Respiratory rate of fewer than 12 breaths/min or more than 20 breaths/min in the presence of dyspnea
- Irregular respiratory rhythm, such as taking a series of deep breaths followed by periods of apnea
- Diminished, absent, or noisy auscultated breath sounds
- Abdominal breathing
- Reduced flow of exhaled air at the nose and mouth
- Unequal or inadequate chest expansion, resulting in reduced tidal volume
- Increased effort of breathing (use of accessory muscles)
- Shallow depth of breathing (reduced tidal volume)
- Skin that is paler than baseline color, cyanotic, cool, moist (clammy), or mottled
- Retractions
- Staccato speech patterns (one- or two-word dyspnea)

When assessing a patient with respiratory distress, consider the external environment (ie, high altitude and enclosed spaces), which can be associated with impaired oxygenation. Ensure your personal safety if the environment is unsafe.

Feel for air movement at the patient's nose and mouth. Observe the chest for symmetry, and note any **paradoxical motion**: the inward movement of a chest segment during inhalation and the outward movement of the chest during exhalation, opposite of normal chest movements, which are an indication of a flail chest. Assess for **pulsus paradoxus**, a clinical finding in which the systolic BP drops more than 10 mm Hg during inhalation. A change in pulse quality, or even the disappearance of a pulse during inhalation, may also be detected. Pulsus paradoxus is generally seen in patients with decompensating COPD, severe pericardial tamponade, or other conditions that cause an increase in intrathoracic pressure (eg, tension pneumothorax, severe asthma attack).

A history of the present illness is a vital part of assessing a patient with respiratory distress. Ask the following questions to determine the evolution of the current problem:

- Was the onset of the problem sudden or gradual?
  - Some people may perceive respiratory distress that occurred 2 days earlier as arising gradually when, in fact, the onset was sudden; the patient may just have waited 2 days before calling for help.
- Is any cause or "trigger" of the event known?
  - Asthma is commonly exacerbated by stress, cold weather, or environmental allergens.
  - A foreign body airway obstruction is commonly preceded by a sudden onset of difficulty in breathing during a meal or, in children, while playing with small toys or other objects.
- What is the duration (is the problem constant or recurrent)?
- Does anything alleviate or exacerbate the problem?
- Are any other associated symptoms present, such as a productive cough (if yes, then what color is the sputum?), chest pain or pressure, or fever?
- Were any interventions attempted before the arrival of EMS?
- Has the patient been evaluated by a physician or admitted to the hospital for this condition in the past? If so, then what was the diagnosis?
  - Determine specifically whether the patient was hospitalized or seen in the emergency department (ED) and then released. If the patient was hospitalized, then ask whether the admission was to an intensive care unit (ICU) or a regular, unmonitored floor. A condition that warranted admission to an ICU is clinically significant.
- Is the patient currently taking any medications?
  - Do not simply ask which medications were taken today. Instead, determine the overall compliance by asking whether the patient has been taking the medications as prescribed. Ask, "Have you been able to take all of your pills as directed?" "Has anything stopped you from taking your pills as directed, such as running out of some of the pills?" "Is something bothering you about taking a certain pill?" Verify this information by looking at the prescription dates on the medication bottles and by reading the prescription directions.
  - Ask whether the patient has had any changes in current prescriptions, such as a new medication or changes in the prescribing directions of an existing medication.
- Does the patient have any risk factors that could cause or exacerbate the condition (eg, alcohol or illicit drug use, cigarette smoking, an inadequate diet)?

Evaluate the patient for protective reflexes of the airway. These reflexes include coughing, sneezing, and gagging. A patient whose cough mechanism is suppressed, whether by drugs, pain, trauma, or any other cause, is at serious risk of aspirating foreign material. Sneezing is usually elicited by irritation of the nasal cavity.

Sighing is a slow, deep inhalation followed by a prolonged and sometimes audible exhalation. Sighing periodically hyperinflates the lungs, thereby reexpanding atelectatic (collapsed) alveoli. The average person sighs about once per minute. Hiccupping is a sudden inhalation, caused by spasmodic contraction of the diaphragm, cut short by closure of the glottis. Hiccupping serves no physiologic purpose, although persistent hiccups may be clinically significant.

Patients with serious injuries or illnesses may present with changes in their respiratory patterns. **TABLE 16-4** identifies various abnormal respiratory patterns and their causes.

Assessment of Breath Sounds

While you are assessing the patient's breathing, auscultate the breath sounds with a stethoscope. Breath sounds should be clear and equal on both sides of the chest (bilaterally), anteriorly, and posteriorly. Compare each apex (top) of the lung with the opposite apex, and each base (bottom) of the lung with the opposite base.

Breath sounds are created as air moves through the tracheobronchial tree. The size of the airway

TABLE 16-4 Abnormal Respiratory Patterns

Cheyne-Stokes respirations	Gradually increasing rate and depth of respirations, followed by a gradual decrease of respirations with intermittent periods of apnea; associated with brainstem insult **FIGURE 16-7**.
Kussmaul respirations	Deep, rapid respirations; seen in patients with diabetic ketoacidosis.
Biot (ataxic) respirations	Irregular pattern, rate, and depth of breathing with intermittent periods of apnea; results from increased intracranial pressure.
Apneustic respirations	Prolonged, gasping inhalation, followed by extremely short, ineffective exhalation; associated with brainstem insult.
Agonal gasps	Slow, shallow, irregular, or occasional gasping breaths; result from cerebral anoxia. Agonal gasps may be seen shortly after the heart has stopped but the brain continues to send signals to the muscles of respiration.
Central neurogenic hyperventilation	Tachypneic hyperpnea; rapid, deep respirations caused by increased intracranial pressure or direct brain injury; drives the carbon dioxide level down and the pH up, resulting in respiratory alkalosis.

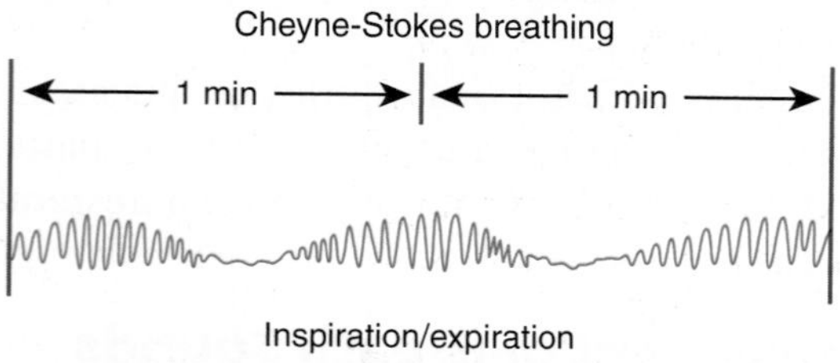

FIGURE 16-7 Cheyne-Stokes breathing shows a crescendo-decrescendo pattern of respirations followed by periods of apnea.

determines the type of sound that will be produced. Significant differences in adult, child, and infant airways exist, resulting in differences in breath sounds. The trachea and bronchi have large diameters; therefore, the sound produced is higher pitched and is heard during inspiration and expiration. Breath sounds are heard over the majority of the chest, representing airflow into the alveoli. **Tracheal breath sounds**, also called bronchial breath sounds, are heard by placing the stethoscope diaphragm over the trachea or over the sternum. Assess breath sounds for duration, pitch, and intensity. **Vesicular breath sounds** are softer, muffled sounds and have been described as "wind blowing through the trees." The expiratory phase is barely audible. **Bronchovesicular sounds** are a combination of the two and are heard in locations where airways and alveoli are found: the upper part of the sternum and between the scapulae. Locations for these sounds are shown in **FIGURE 16-8. FIGURE 16-9** describes the normal breath sounds. Assess bronchovesicular sounds for duration, pitch, and intensity.

Duration refers to the length of time for the inspiratory and expiratory phases of the breath. Normally, expiration is twice as long as inspiration. This relationship is expressed as the **inspiratory/expiratory (I/E) ratio**; a normal I/E ratio is 1:2. When a patient's lower airway is obstructed and the patient has difficulty getting air out (as occurs with asthma), the expiratory phase is prolonged and may be four to five times as long as inspiration. In the case of a patient with asthma, the I/E ratio would be 1:4 or 1:5. In a patient with tachypnea, the expiratory phase is short and approaches that of inspiration; the I/E ratio may be 1:1.

Pitch is described as the intensity of sound that is higher or lower than normal, such as in stridor or wheezing (discussed later in this section). The sound intensity depends on airflow rate, constancy of flow throughout inspiration, patient position, and the site selected for auscultation. Thickness of the chest wall may affect the intensity. Less-intense sounds are said to be diminished. A common error in assessing the intensity of breath sounds occurs when auscultation is performed over the patient's clothing. Always auscultate directly on the patient's skin.

Sounds that might be classified as normal but are present in an unexpected area can indicate an abnormal condition. For example, tracheal sounds in areas that should produce vesicular sounds may indicate pneumonia.

Adventitious (abnormal) breath sounds are usually classified as either continuous or discontinuous.

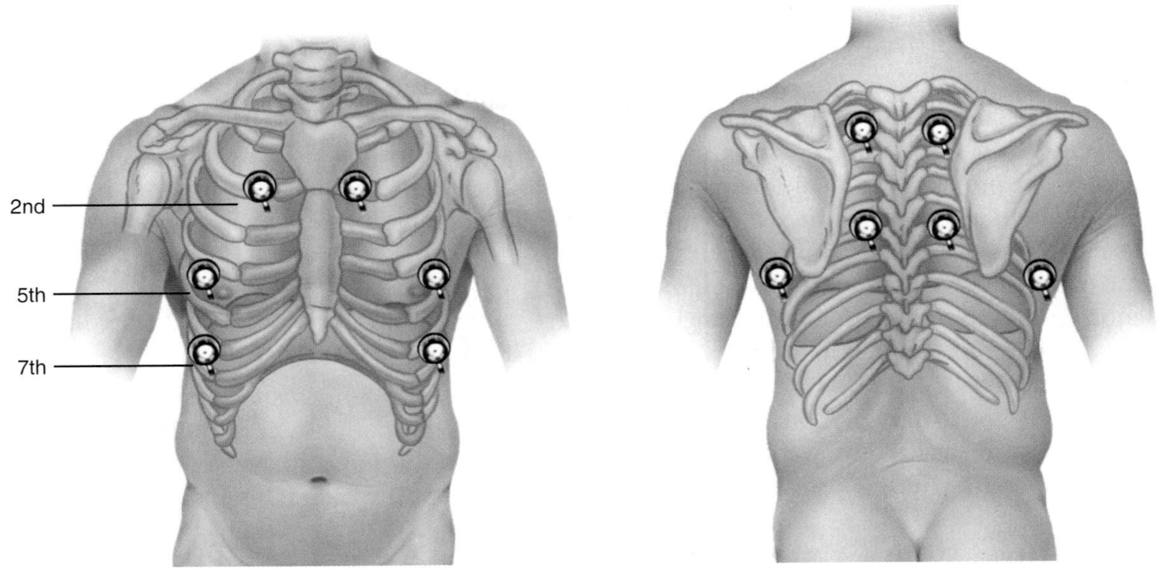

FIGURE 16-8 Common sites of auscultation include the second, fifth, and seventh intercostal spaces as shown.

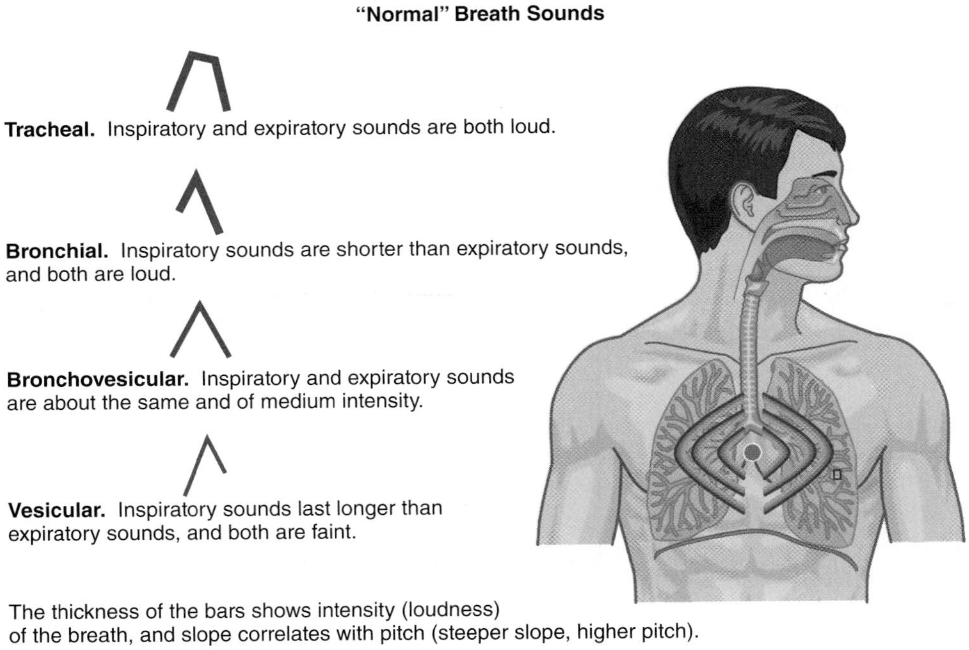

"Normal" Breath Sounds
Tracheal. Inspiratory and expiratory sounds are both loud.
Bronchial. Inspiratory sounds are shorter than expiratory sounds, and both are loud.
Bronchovesicular. Inspiratory and expiratory sounds are about the same and of medium intensity.
Vesicular. Inspiratory sounds last longer than expiratory sounds, and both are faint.
The thickness of the bars shows intensity (loudness) of the breath, and slope correlates with pitch (steeper slope, higher pitch).

FIGURE 16-9 Normal breath sounds are heard over different parts of the chest. Breath sounds become softer away from the largest airways. The character during inspiration versus expiration also changes.

Wheezing is a continuous sound as air flows through a constricted lower airway, such as with asthma or bronchiolitis. This high-pitched sound may be heard on inspiration, expiration, or both. **Rhonchi** are also continuous sounds, although they are low-pitched; they indicate mucus or fluid in the larger lower airways (ie, in pulmonary edema and bronchitis).

Crackles (formerly known as rales) occur when airflow causes mucus or fluid in the airways to move into the smaller lower airways. The crackles tend to clear with coughing. These sounds may also be heard when collapsed airways or alveoli pop open. Crackles are classified as discontinuous sounds and may occur either early or late in the inspiratory cycle. Early inspiratory crackles usually occur when larger, proximal bronchi open and are common in patients with COPD; they tend not to clear with coughing. Late inspiratory crackles occur when peripheral alveoli and airways pop open and are more common in dependent lung regions. These sounds are often heard in patients with reduced lung volumes.

Stridor results from foreign body aspiration, infection, swelling, disease, or trauma within or immediately above the glottic opening. This loud, high-pitched sound is typically heard during the inspiration phase. A **pleural friction rub** results from inflammation that causes the pleurae to thicken. The pleural space can decrease as a result, allowing the surfaces of the visceral and parietal pleurae to rub together. This decrease often creates stabbing pain with breathing or any movement of the thorax.

Words of Wisdom

When you auscultate breath sounds emergently (for example, when confirming proper ET tube placement, ruling in (or ruling out) a pneumothorax, or confirming adequate positive-pressure ventilation) auscultate bilaterally at the third or fourth intercostal space in the midaxillary line. Immediate corrective action is needed if breath sounds are absent altogether or if they are unilaterally diminished or absent.

Quantifying Ventilation and Oxygenation

In addition to your visual and hands-on assessments of the patient with an airway or breathing problem, you may apply several methods and devices to quantify (that is, assign a numeric value to) ventilation and oxygenation.

Pulse Oximetry

Pulse oximetry is a simple, rapid, safe, and noninvasive method of measuring, minute by minute, how well a person's hemoglobin is saturated.

A **pulse oximeter** measures the percentage of saturated hemoglobin in the arterial blood **FIGURE 16-10**. Under normal circumstances, hemoglobin is saturated with oxygen (Spo_2). In pulse oximetry, a sensor probe is clipped to the patient's

YOU are the Paramedic

PART 3

Despite high-flow oxygen via nonrebreathing mask, the patient remains hypoxemic, cyanotic, and in severe distress. Further assessment reveals coarse crackles bilaterally on auscultation of his chest. The patient tells you, in broken sentences, that he has "heart problems" but has not seen his cardiologist in almost 2 years. Your partner applies the cardiac monitor and obtains baseline vital signs.

Recording Time: 4 Minutes	
Respirations	28 breaths/min; labored
Pulse	120 beats/min; strong and regular
Skin	Lips and gums appear gray
Blood pressure	176/96 mm Hg
Oxygen saturation (Spo_2)	76%
Pupils	PERRLA (Pupils Equal, Round, and Reactive to Light and Accomodation; in this case, reactive, equal, and slightly dilated)
$ETCO_2$	60 mm Hg
ECG	Sinus tachycardia

5. What underlying problem do you suspect is impairing this patient's ability to oxygenate?

6. Based on the patient's current clinical status, how should you proceed with your treatment?

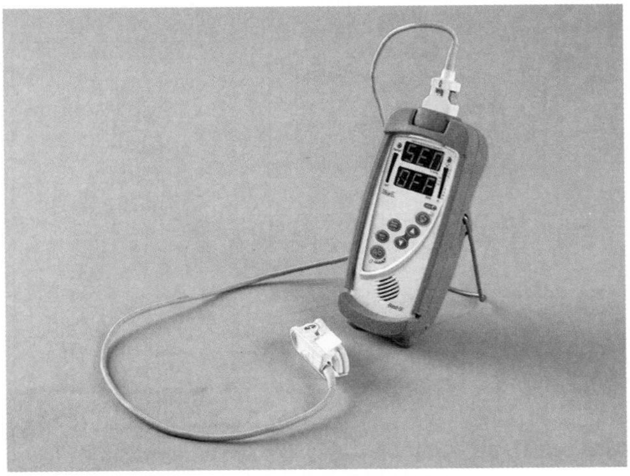

FIGURE 16-10 Pulse oximetry is a noninvasive method of assessing arterial hemoglobin saturation.

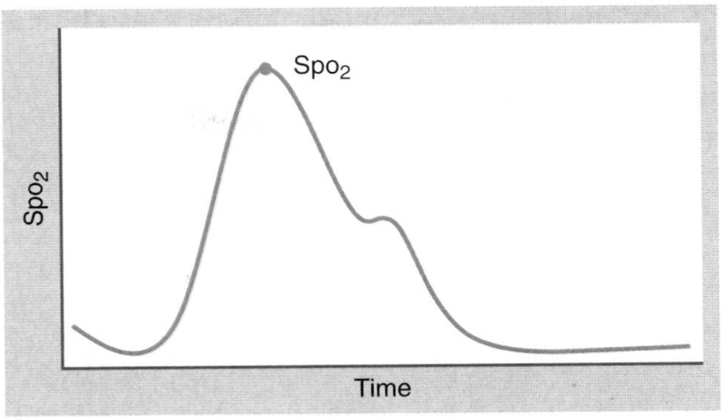

FIGURE 16-11 The characteristic shape of the pulse oximeter waveform confirms that the device is properly sensing.

finger or earlobe; this probe uses a light-emitting diode to transmit light through the vascular bed to a light-sensing detector. The amount of light transmitted across the vascular bed depends on the proportion of hemoglobin that is saturated with oxygen. Pulse oximeters are designed to assess only pulsating blood vessels to ensure that the instrument measures arterial (not venous) oxygen saturation. As a consequence, pulse oximeters also measure the patient's pulse.

One way to check the functioning of a pulse oximeter is to compare the pulse reading it provides with your own measurement of the patient's pulse by palpation. When you use the pulse oximeter that is attached to the cardiac monitor/defibrillator, you can select the option of viewing the Spo_2 waveform to confirm the device is properly sensing **FIGURE 16-11**. Refer to the manufacturer's instructions.

A normally oxygenated, normally perfused person should have an Spo_2 level of greater than 95% while breathing room air. A reading of less than 95% in a nonsmoker suggests hypoxemia; a reading of less than 90% accompanied by respiratory distress signals a need for aggressive oxygen therapy.

Situations in which pulse oximeters may be useful in prehospital emergency medical care include the following:

- **Monitoring the oxygenation status of a patient during an intubation attempt or during suctioning.** The low-saturation alarm on the pulse oximeter can signal that you should abort the intubation attempt and ventilate the patient.
- **Identifying deterioration in the condition of a trauma patient.** In a patient with multiple trauma, signs of a developing tension pneumothorax may not become evident until the condition is advanced. A declining Spo_2 level can alert you to a problem and prompt a search for its cause.
- **Identifying deterioration in the condition of a patient with cardiac disease.** Pulse oximetry may enable early identification of patients who are experiencing heart failure in the wake of acute myocardial infarction.
- **Identifying high-risk patients with respiratory conditions.** For example, pulse oximetry may identify patients with asthma who are having serious attacks or patients with emphysema who are in severe decompensation.
- **Assessing vascular status in orthopaedic trauma.** Pulse oximetry is routinely performed when assessing a fractured extremity to evaluate circulation distal to the fracture. Loss of a pulse means that the limb is in jeopardy and may require urgent action in the field if transport time is long. A pulse oximeter clipped to a finger or toe on a broken limb might provide critical information about the ongoing circulation to the limb.

The usefulness of a pulse oximeter depends on its ability to provide accurate information. A pulse oximeter that gives a reading of 99% when the patient is actually severely hypoxemic will not provide helpful information and could lead to inadequate or erroneous interventions. Be aware of circumstances that might produce erroneous readings:

- **Bright ambient light** may enter the spectrophotometer of the pulse oximeter and create an incorrect reading. Protect the sensor clip by covering it with a towel or aluminum foil.
- **Patient motion** can confuse the pulse oximeter. The device may mistake the motion for arterial pulsation and read the oxygen saturation level from a vein rather than an artery.
- **Poor perfusion** makes it difficult for the pulse oximeter to sense a pulse and therefore to generate a reading. Poor perfusion occurs in states such as shock, cardiac arrest, and cold exposure. If the vessels in a patient's limbs are constricted and the limbs are cold, then it may be necessary to place the pulse oximeter clip on the earlobe or nose.
- **Nail polish** will prevent the sensor from working properly. Carry disposable acetone (nail polish remover) swabs to quickly remove nail polish.
- **Venous pulsations** may occur in some patients with right-side heart failure due to the systemic backup of blood. If a vein is pulsating, then the pulse oximeter may regard it as an artery and measure venous oxygen saturation.
- **Abnormal hemoglobin** (eg, as in carbon monoxide poisoning) may produce a falsely normal Spo_2 level.

The two types of hemoglobin normally found are **oxyhemoglobin (Hbo_2)**, hemoglobin that is loaded with oxygen, and **reduced hemoglobin**, hemoglobin from which oxygen has been released to the cells. However, in the presence of **methemoglobin (metHb)** (a compound formed by oxidation of the iron on the hemoglobin) and **carboxyhemoglobin (COHb)** (hemoglobin loaded with carbon monoxide), normal Spo_2 values may be observed, even though the body is not receiving sufficient oxygen. As mentioned previously, carbon monoxide binds to hemoglobin 250 times more readily than oxygen does. A **carbon monoxide oximeter**, also called a carbon monoxide monitor, is a device that measures absorption at several wavelengths to distinguish Hbo_2 from COHb and determines the level of Hbo_2 saturation (the percentage of oxygenated Hb compared with the total amount of hemoglobin) including COHb, metHb, Hbo_2, and reduced Hb **FIGURE 16-12**. When a patient presents with carbon monoxide poisoning, the carbon monoxide oximeter will detect this Hb, expressed as Spco, and will report a markedly reduced Hbo_2 saturation. Remember, do not make treatment decisions based solely on pulse oximetry, and be aware of its limitations.

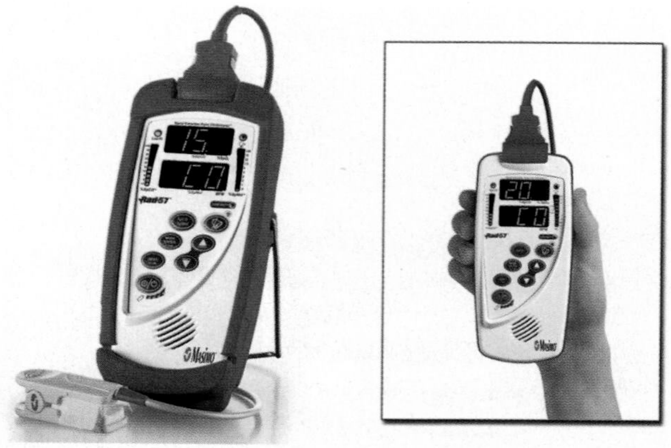

FIGURE 16-12 A carbon monoxide oximeter has the ability to distinguish oxyhemoglobin from carboxyhemoglobin.

The Masimo Rad-ST Pulse CO-Oximeter courtesy of Masimo Corporation (www.masimo.com).

Words of Wisdom

When in doubt, look at the patient!

Always correlate the information provided by the pulse oximeter (or any other device) with clinical observations. If the patient is turning blue and struggling to breathe, then you should ignore the pulse oximeter reading that suggests the patient is adequately oxygenated.

Peak Expiratory Flow Measurement

In patients with certain reactive airway diseases (such as asthma), you can evaluate bronchoconstriction by measuring the peak rate of a forceful exhalation with a peak expiratory flowmeter **FIGURE 16-13**. An increasing **peak expiratory flow** suggests that the patient is responding to treatment (ie, inhaled bronchodilators). A decreasing peak expiratory flow may be an early indication that the patient's condition is deteriorating.

Peak expiratory flow varies based on sex, height, and age. Healthy adults have a peak expiratory flow

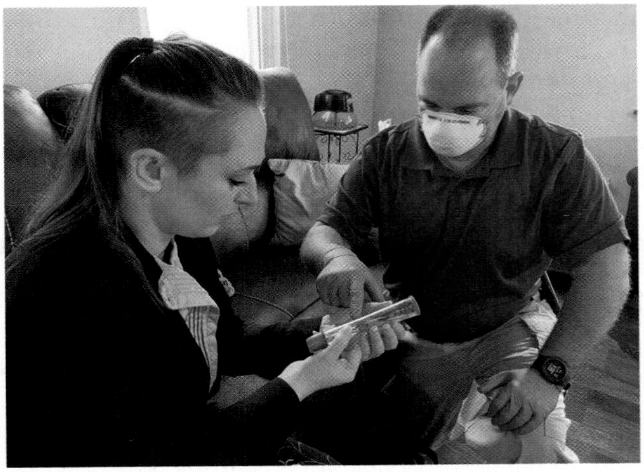

FIGURE 16-13 Peak expiratory flowmeters are used to quantify the degree of bronchoconstriction.

Courtesy of Rhonda Hunt.

TABLE 16-5 Normal Arterial Blood Gas Values

pH	7.35 to 7.45
Pao_2	80 to 100 mm Hg
$Paco_2$	35 to 45 mm Hg
Hco_3^-	21 to 28 mEq/L
Base (excess or deficit)	−2 to 3 mEq/L
Sao_2	>95%

Abbreviations: Hco_3^-, concentration of bicarbonate ions; $Paco_2$, partial pressure of carbon dioxide; Pao_2, partial pressure of oxygen; Sao_2, oxygen saturation

Data from: Fontanarosa PB, Christiansen S. Units of measure. Table 2: selected laboratory tests, with reference ranges and conversion factors. In: American Medical Association, ed. *AMA Manual of Style: A Guide for Authors and Editors.* 10th ed. New York, NY: Oxford University Press; 2007:798-815.

rate of 350 to 750 mL. To assess peak expiratory flow, place the patient in a seated position with legs dangling. Assemble the flowmeter and ensure that it reads zero. Ask the patient to take a deep breath, place the mouthpiece in the mouth, and exhale as forcefully as possible (ensure no air leaks around the device or comes from the patient's nose). Perform the test three times and take the best peak flow rate of the three readings.

Arterial Blood Gas Analysis

Paramedics are not typically trained to obtain arterial blood specimens and do not carry the equipment needed to analyze the patient's blood. As a result, you will rely on noninvasive methods of assessing ventilation and oxygenation (eg, pulse oximetry, capnography/capnometry).

Analysis of arterial blood gases (ABGs) provides the most comprehensive quantitative information about the respiratory system. In this procedure, blood is obtained from a superficial artery, such as the radial or femoral artery. The blood is then analyzed for pH, $Paco_2$, Pao_2, Hco_3^- (concentration of bicarbonate ions), base excess (indicating acidosis or alkalosis), and Sao_2 levels. Normal ABG values are summarized in **TABLE 16-5**.

With ABG measurements, the pH and Hco_3^- values are used to evaluate the patient's acid–base status. The $Paco_2$ value is an indicator of the effectiveness of ventilation. The Pao_2 and Sao_2 values are indicators of oxygenation. To maintain normal ABG values, a balance between alveolar volume and perfusion of the alveolar capillaries must be maintained.

End-Tidal Carbon Dioxide Assessment

Carbon dioxide can be described as the "smoke of metabolism." The body uses oxygen to metabolize the fuel (glucose) and makes carbon dioxide as its by-product. With oxygen present, aerobic metabolism creates 38 molecules of ATP (adenosine triphosphate, or "energy") from each glucose molecule. Without oxygen present, anaerobic metabolism produces only 2 ATP molecules from each molecule of glucose. As long as oxygen is delivered to the cells and tissues, the production of carbon dioxide continues. A helpful analogy is a motor vehicle engine: As long as gasoline continues to burn, exhaust is produced. In the human body, carbon dioxide is the exhaust.

End-tidal carbon dioxide ($ETCO_2$) is the maximal amount of carbon dioxide that leaves the body at the end of exhalation. A normal $ETCO_2$ level is 35 to 45 mm Hg.

$ETCO_2$ assessment has many applications in emergency medicine, and several abnormal processes can be identified using it. For example, it can provide information regarding ventilation adequacy and is the recommended method of monitoring the initial and ongoing placement of an advanced airway device. Capnography can also indicate the adequacy of perfusion, the effectiveness of chest compressions, and the return of spontaneous circulation (ROSC). This information can be obtained because blood must circulate through the lungs for carbon dioxide to be exhaled and measured.

Quantifying Ventilation With $ETCO_2$

Even if adequate carbon dioxide is produced at the cellular level and returned to the lungs, the patient with inadequate ventilation may not effectively eliminate this carbon dioxide through breathing. As a result, the paramedic would expect to observe an increased (greater than 45 mm Hg) $ETCO_2$ reading. For example, in an opioid overdose, the central problem is inadequate ventilation. The patient continues to make carbon dioxide at the cellular level, but it cannot be adequately eliminated from the body via the respiratory system because the patient's breathing is depressed.

In contrast, if a patient is perfusing adequately and making sufficient carbon dioxide at the cellular level, a fast respiratory rate (hyperventilation) can cause carbon dioxide to be eliminated via the respiratory system faster than it is produced in the cells. This condition will result in a low (less than 35 mm Hg) $ETCO_2$ reading.

Because carbon dioxide rapidly equilibrates in the alveolar gases, the carbon dioxide concentration in exhaled gases, particularly the gases present at the end of exhalation, closely approximates the arterial $Paco_2$ level, which normally ranges between 35 and 45 mm Hg. Typically, the $ETCO_2$ level is approximately 2 to 5 mm Hg lower than the arterial $Paco_2$ level. Because carbon dioxide is present only in negligible (0.5% or less) concentrations in the esophagus, the use of an $ETCO_2$ detector (quantitative waveform capnography) is a reliable (and essential) method for confirming and monitoring advanced airway placement.

Quantifying Perfusion With $ETCO_2$

If oxygen delivery to the cells and tissues is reduced, such as from blood loss, septic shock, or any condition that causes inadequate tissue perfusion, then less carbon dioxide is produced in the cells and returned to the lungs. As a result, the paramedic would expect to observe a low (less than 35 mm Hg) $ETCO_2$ reading.

If a patient is in cardiac arrest, perfusion ceases altogether and cellular carbon dioxide production stops. If no carbon dioxide is produced in the cells, there is nothing to return to the lungs; therefore, there would be no detectable exhaled carbon dioxide. However, as perfusion is generated by chest compressions, carbon dioxide production (and return to the lungs) resumes, increasing $ETCO_2$. The more effective the chest compressions, the higher the $ETCO_2$ will be. When ROSC occurs, large amounts of carbon dioxide are returned to the lungs, resulting in an *abrupt and sustained* increase in $ETCO_2$.

In a patient in cardiac arrest, a persistently low (less than 10 mm Hg) $ETCO_2$ should be assumed to result from inadequate chest compressions, and immediate corrective action should be taken. However, in a patient in prolonged cardiac arrest, a low $ETCO_2$ despite adequate chest compressions indicates the presence of severe acidosis and minimal carbon dioxide return to the lungs.

$ETCO_2$ Monitors

End-tidal carbon dioxide ($ETCO_2$) monitors detect the presence of carbon dioxide in exhaled air. The types of $ETCO_2$ monitors include digital and digital/waveform devices.

A **capnometer** provides quantitative information, in real time, by displaying a numeric reading of exhaled carbon dioxide levels. It uses a special adapter, which attaches between the advanced airway and ventilation devices **FIGURE 16-14**.

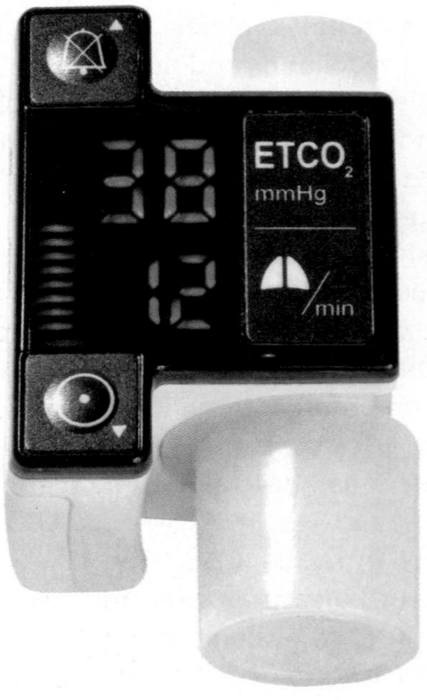

FIGURE 16-14 A capnometer.

A **capnographer** is a device that provides a graphic representation of exhaled carbon dioxide levels. It performs the same function and attaches in the same way as the capnometer. The two types of capnographers are waveform and digital/waveform.

Waveform capnography provides quantitative, real-time information about the patient's exhaled carbon dioxide level. Unlike capnometry, however, waveform capnography displays a graphic waveform. In most cases, portable cardiac monitors/defibrillators provide a numeric reading and a waveform (also called digital/waveform capnography and quantitative waveform capnography).

Waveform capnography can be monitored in spontaneously breathing patients who have an adequate airway by applying a special nasal cannula device to the patient and connecting the sampling line to the cardiac monitor/defibrillator **FIGURE 16-15**. In patients who require positive-pressure ventilation, an in-line adaptor is placed between the bag and mask, the bag and ET tube, or the bag and a supraglottic airway device. The sampling line is then connected to the cardiac monitor/defibrillator **FIGURE 16-16**.

Words of Wisdom

A **colorimetric carbon dioxide detector** provides qualitative information regarding the presence of carbon dioxide in the patient's exhaled breath; that is, it does not assign a numeric value. The colorimetric carbon dioxide detector is attached between the ET tube and ventilation device. The specially treated paper inside the detector should turn from purple to yellow during exhalation, signifying the presence of carbon dioxide. Air exhaled through an ET tube that has been properly placed in the trachea of a patient with adequate perfusion should contain 4% to 5% carbon dioxide, which will cause the paper to turn yellow. If inadvertent esophageal intubation occurs, then a negligible amount (less than 0.5%) of carbon dioxide will be present in the exhaled gas; this amount will cause the paper to remain purple during exhalation.

Several limitations exist with the use of the colorimetric carbon dioxide detector. The device might give a false-positive reading if the patient has carbon dioxide trapped in the stomach from the ingestion of carbonated beverages. Furthermore, the device is sensitive to extremes of temperature and humidity; it may be less reliable if vomitus or other secretions get inside it; and the paper inside the device degrades over time, resulting in a less reliable reading. *The colorimetric carbon dioxide detector should be used **only** when quantitative waveform capnography is not available.*

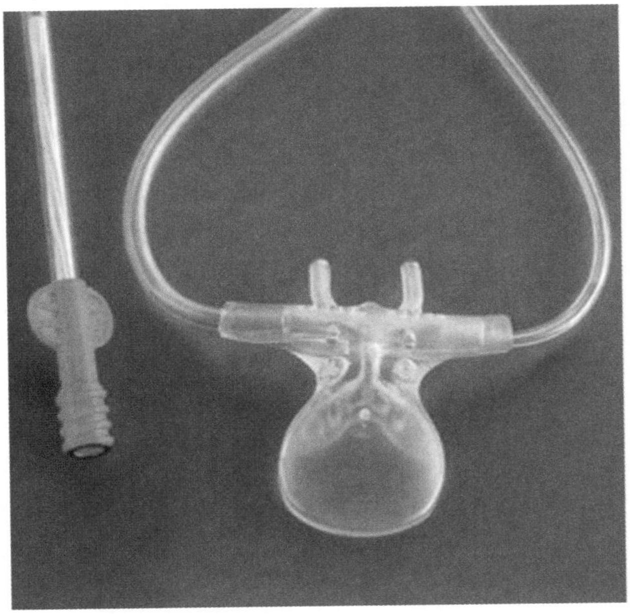

FIGURE 16-15 FilterLine nasal cannula device for monitoring end-tidal carbon dioxide in a spontaneously breathing patient.

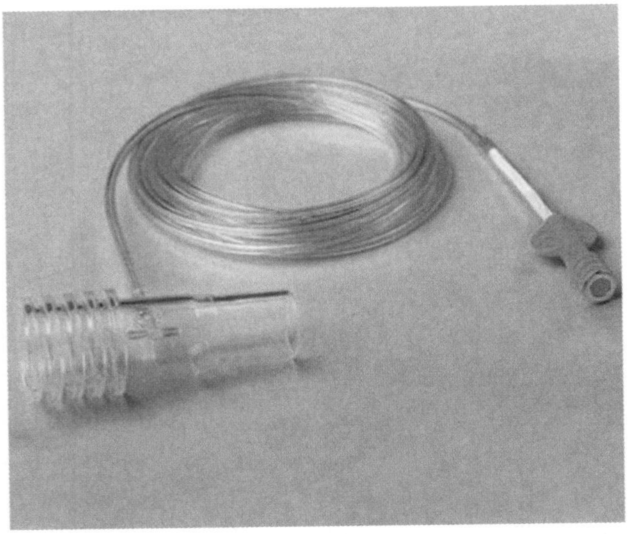

FIGURE 16-16 FilterLine in-line end-tidal carbon dioxide device for use in intubated patients.

Normal Capnographic Waveform

It is important to understand the features of the normal capnographic waveform, including the contour, baseline level, and rate and rise of the carbon dioxide level. A normal waveform has four distinct phases **FIGURE 16-17**. Phase I (A–B), also known as the respiratory baseline, is the initial stage of exhalation; the gas sample consists of dead space gas, which is free of carbon dioxide. Phase II (B–C) is called the expiratory upslope. At point B, alveolar gas mixes with dead space gas, resulting in an abrupt rise in detected carbon dioxide levels. The alveolar plateau is represented by phase III (C–D), and the gas sampled is all alveolar. Point D is the maximal $ETCO_2$ level, the best reflection of the alveolar carbon dioxide level. The height of the waveform at point D correlates with the numeric value of exhaled carbon dioxide, which is also displayed on the cardiac monitor/defibrillator. Fresh gas is introduced during phase IV, the inspiratory downstroke (D–E); this downstroke displaces carbon dioxide, causing the waveform to return to the baseline level of carbon dioxide, approximately 0 mm Hg. The duration (width) of each waveform corresponds to the duration of ventilation, and the space between waveforms corresponds to the patient's respiratory rate.

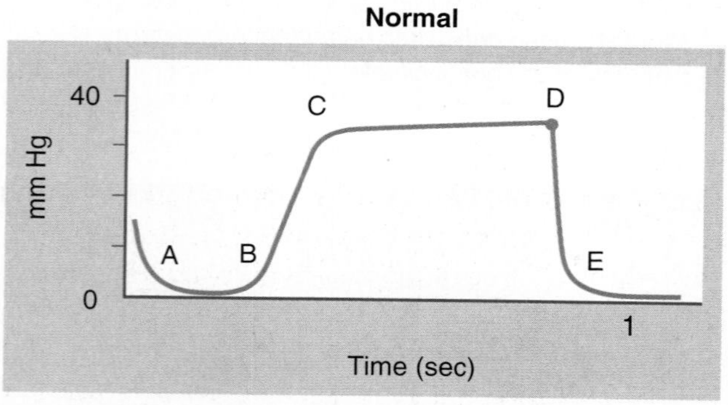

FIGURE 16-17 Normal capnographic waveform with points A through E shown.

Evidence-Based Medicine

Studies of quantitative waveform capnography as a means to verify advanced airway position in patients in cardiac arrest have demonstrated that this technology has high sensitivity and specificity in identifying correct and incorrect airway placement. In addition to clinical assessment, you should regard continuous quantitative waveform capnography as the most reliable method of confirming initial and ongoing advanced airway placement.

Abnormal Capnographic Waveforms

In addition to quantifying the amount of exhaled carbon dioxide, the shape of the capnographic waveform can provide information regarding abnormal breathing processes (eg, hypoventilation, hyperventilation, bronchospasm, rebreathing). You can also recognize inadvertent **extubation** (the process of removing the tube from an intubated patient) by using waveform capnography.

Hypoventilation is a condition in which the production of carbon dioxide exceeds its elimination. Because of the increased carbon dioxide levels (hypercapnia), the capnographic waveforms are tall and the $ETCO_2$ value is correspondingly high (greater than 45 mm Hg). Bradypnea, a common feature of hypoventilation, produces a prolonged alveolar plateau (phase III [C–D]) and longer-than-normal intervals between waveforms **FIGURE 16-18**. Causes of hypoventilation include respiratory depression (ie, opioid overdose) and a ventilatory rate that is too slow in an intubated patient.

Hyperventilation is a condition in which the elimination of carbon dioxide exceeds its production. In this case, the capnographic waveforms are

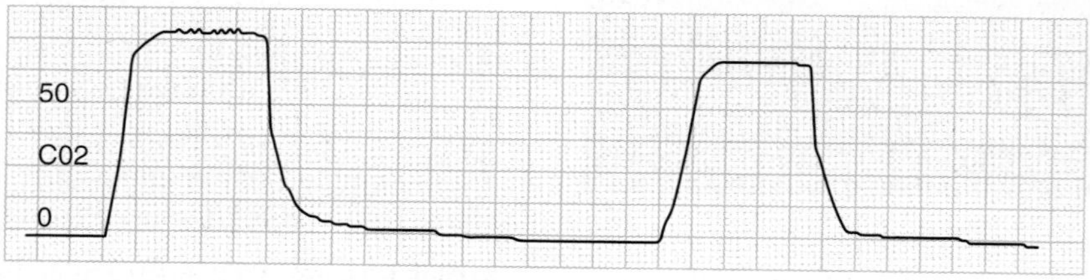

FIGURE 16-18 Capnographic waveforms caused by hypoventilation.

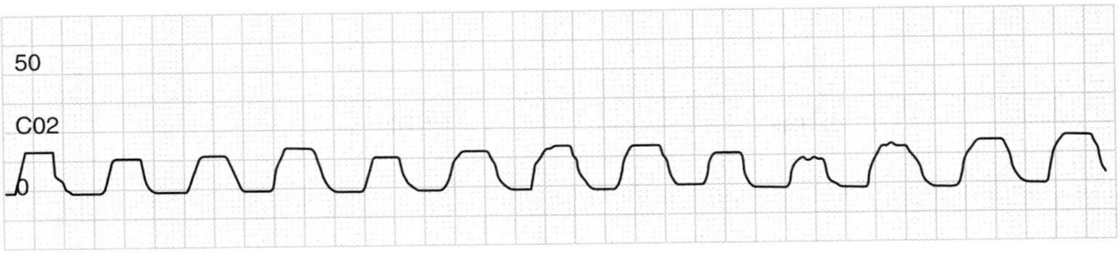

FIGURE 16-19 Capnographic waveforms caused by hyperventilation.

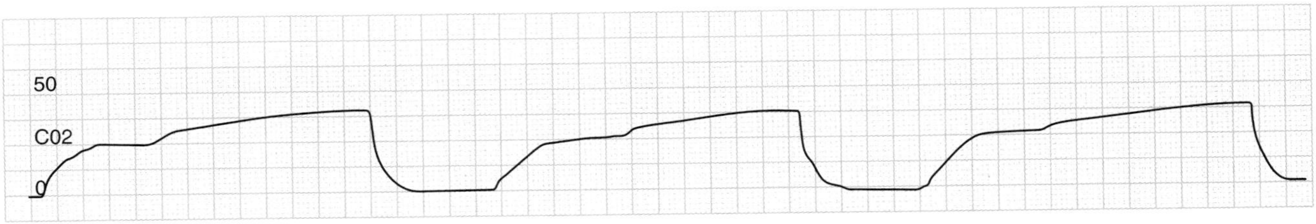

FIGURE 16-20 A shark fin capnographic waveform indicates bronchospasm and incomplete alveolar emptying.

small and the ETCO$_2$ value is correspondingly low (less than 35 mm Hg) because of decreased carbon dioxide levels (hypocapnia). Tachypnea, a clinical sign of hyperventilation, produces a short alveolar plateau (phase III [C–D]) and shorter-than-normal intervals between waveforms **FIGURE 16-19**. The numerous causes of hyperventilation include anxiety/panic attacks, metabolic acidosis, head injury, and pulmonary embolism.

Waveform capnography in the nonintubated patient is an excellent way to assess the severity of asthma, COPD, or any pathologic process that causes pulmonary air trapping; it can also be used to gauge the effectiveness of treatment. The characteristic "shark fin" of bronchospasm appears as a gradual (rather than abrupt) upsloping phase II (B–C); this shape signifies difficulty during the exhalation phase combined with incomplete alveolar emptying **FIGURE 16-20**.

If the patient is rebreathing previously exhaled carbon dioxide, then ETCO$_2$ values increase and the waveforms elevate and never return to the baseline (0 mm Hg) at the end of the inspiratory downstroke (phase IV [D–E]). Causes of rebreathing include inadequate expiratory time, a malfunctioning inspiratory valve on the mechanical ventilator, and an insufficient inspiratory flow rate **FIGURE 16-21**.

If inadvertent extubation occurs, then you would expect to see a complete loss of the capnographic waveform and ETCO$_2$ reading **FIGURE 16-22**.

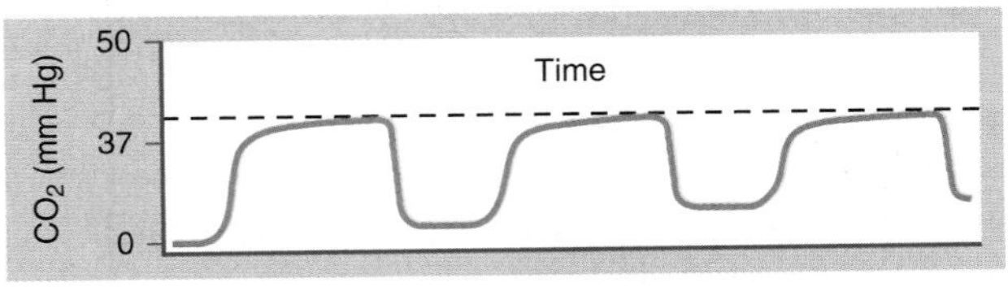

FIGURE 16-21 Capnographic waveforms caused by rebreathing.

This finding requires immediate attention. The numerous methods for confirming proper advanced airway placement are discussed later in this chapter. Although quantitative waveform capnography has shown to be the most reliable method, you should employ all methods of confirmation.

Occasionally, the sampling tubing from the in-line adaptor to the cardiac monitor/defibrillator becomes obstructed with blood or other debris, blocking the flow of gas to the sensor and "zeroing out" the waveform ETCO$_2$ reading. If this complication occurs, then replace the in-line adaptor to restore the waveform and ETCO$_2$ reading.

When you assess the ventilation status of any patient, whether that patient is spontaneously breathing, apneic with a pulse, or pulseless and apneic, it is critical to understand and recognize the causes of increased and decreased ETCO$_2$ levels to make the appropriate adjustments to your treatment **TABLE 16-6**.

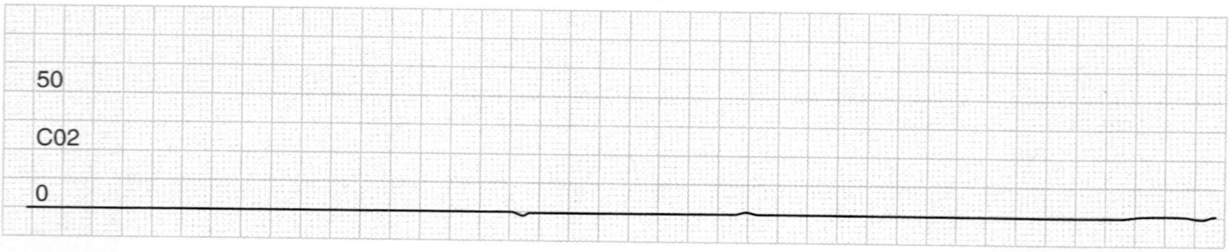

FIGURE 16-22 The complete loss of the capnographic waveform and end-tidal carbon dioxide reading in the intubated patient requires immediate attention.

TABLE 16-6 Causes of Increased and Decreased $ETCO_2$ Levels

	↑ $ETCO_2$	↓ $ETCO_2$
Spontaneously breathing	Hypoventilation	Hyperventilation
Apneic with a pulse	Positive-pressure ventilation is too slow.	Positive-pressure ventilation is too fast.
Apneic and pulseless	Positive-pressure ventilation is too slow. Could indicate ROSC[b]	Misplaced ET tube[a] Decreased CO_2 return to the lungs (prolonged arrest) Chest compressions are of inadequate rate and/or depth. Positive-pressure ventilation is too fast.[c]

Abbreviations: CO_2, carbon dioxide; ET, endotracheal; $ETCO_2$, end-tidal carbon dioxide; ROSC, return of spontaneous circulation

[a] No $ETCO_2$ light-emitting diode reading is displayed, and capnographic waveform is flat.
[b] With ROSC, an abrupt and sustained increase in $ETCO_2$ occurs (typically >40 mm Hg).
[c] In cardiac arrest of short duration.

SAFETY

A consideration related to patient safety is the availability of appropriate equipment that has been properly maintained and checked. For example, intravenous (IV) pumps and ventilators have backup power supplies, and it is critical to ensure that all devices are in good working order with fully charged batteries before initiation of patient care. Waveform capnography is critical for monitoring intubated patients during transport and must be considered a minimum standard of care. Likewise, monitor alarms are critical for monitoring for unexpected changes in the patient's condition. You must correctly set alarm limits and volumes before transport to ensure you are immediately alerted when any parameters move out of range.

Airway Management

Air will reach the lungs only if it travels through the trachea, so a patent airway is essential. Patency is obvious in a responsive patient who is able to talk. However, in a patient with an altered level of consciousness (LOC), the airway is often not patent and you will need to use manual maneuvers to open it. In addition, you may need to use artificial airway adjuncts to assist in maintaining the airway. In a patient with a compromised airway, clearing the airway and maintaining patency is vital. Clearing the airway means removing obstructing material, tissue, or fluids from the nose, mouth, and throat. Maintaining the airway means keeping the airway patent so that air can enter and leave the lungs freely **FIGURE 16-23**.

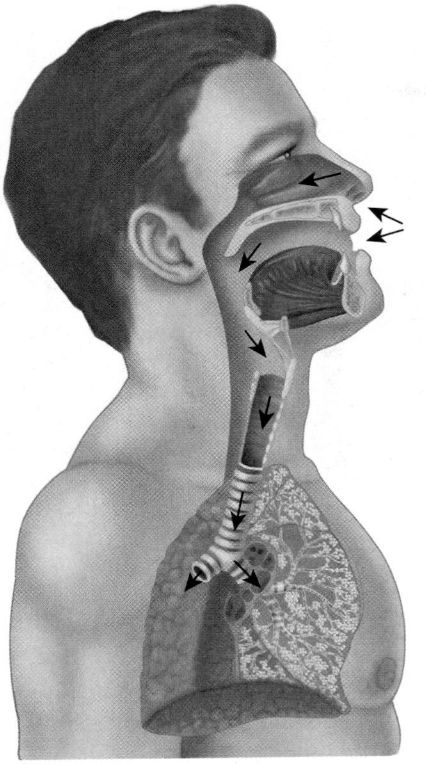

FIGURE 16-23 Air can reach the lungs only if it travels through the trachea. Maintaining the airway means keeping the airway patent so that air can enter and exit the lungs freely.

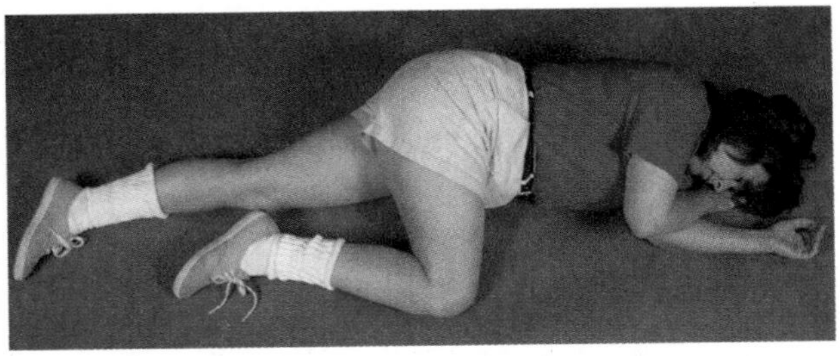

FIGURE 16-24 The recovery position.

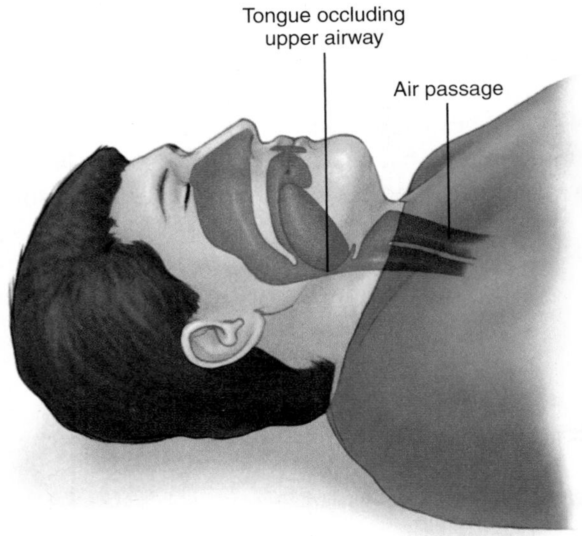

FIGURE 16-25 When the tongue falls back and occludes the posterior pharynx, it may obstruct the airway.

Positioning the Patient

In a perfect world, all patients would present in a supine position, so that you could quickly assess them and intervene without moving them. If an unresponsive patient is found in a prone position, however, then reposition the patient properly so that you can assess the need for ventilations or cardiopulmonary resuscitation (CPR).

To move a patient to a supine position, log roll the person as a unit. After the patient is placed in a supine position, quickly assess for breathing by visualizing the chest for visible movement. Position a patient who is breathing adequately and is not injured in the recovery position. The **recovery position**, which involves placing the patient in a left lateral recumbent position, is indicated if the patient has a decreased LOC; is not suspected of having trauma to the spine, hips, or pelvis; can maintain the airway spontaneously; and is breathing adequately **FIGURE 16-24**.

Manual Airway Maneuvers

If an unresponsive patient has a pulse, but is not breathing or has abnormal breathing (ie, agonal gasps), then you must open the airway manually to provide rescue breathing. As noted earlier, the most common cause of airway obstruction in an unresponsive patient is the tongue **FIGURE 16-25**. To correct this obstruction, manually maneuver the patient's head to propel the tongue forward and open the airway by using the head tilt–chin lift maneuver or the jaw-thrust maneuver (without head tilt).

Head Tilt–Chin Lift Maneuver

Opening the airway can often be done quickly and easily by simply tilting the patient's head back and lifting the chin. This **head tilt–chin lift maneuver** is the preferred technique for opening the airway of a patient who has not sustained cervical spinal trauma. Occasionally, this simple maneuver is all that is required for the patient to resume normal breathing. Consider the following points when using the head tilt–chin lift maneuver:

- **Indications.** An unresponsive patient; a patient with no mechanism for cervical spine injury; or a patient who is unable to protect the airway
- **Contraindications.** A responsive patient or a patient with a possible cervical spine injury
- **Advantages.** No equipment required; is simple, safe, and noninvasive
- **Disadvantages.** May be hazardous to patients with spinal injury; does not protect against aspiration

Evidence-Based Medicine

According to the 2020 Guidelines for CPR and Emergency Cardiovascular Care,[1] the airway should be opened after one of the following circumstances has occurred: The patient is found to be pulseless and 30 chest compressions have been provided, or the patient is found to have a pulse, but is not breathing or has abnormal breathing. To assess for breathing in an unresponsive patient, visualize the chest for obvious movement while simultaneously checking for a pulse; this assessment should take no more than 10 seconds. Chapter 40, *Responding to the Field Code*, covers these topics in detail.

To perform the head tilt–chin lift maneuver, position yourself at the patient's side. Place one hand on the patient's forehead and apply backward pressure with your palm to tilt the patient's head back. This neck extension will propel the tongue forward, away from the posterior pharynx, and open the airway. Place the tips of your other hand's fingers under the lower jaw near the bony part of the chin. Do not compress the soft tissue under the chin because this may push the tongue against the roof of the mouth and block the airway. Lift the chin upward, bringing the entire jaw with it. Do not use your thumb to lift the chin. Lift so that the teeth are nearly brought together, but avoid closing the mouth completely. Continue to hold the forehead to maintain a backward tilt of the head **FIGURE 16-26**.

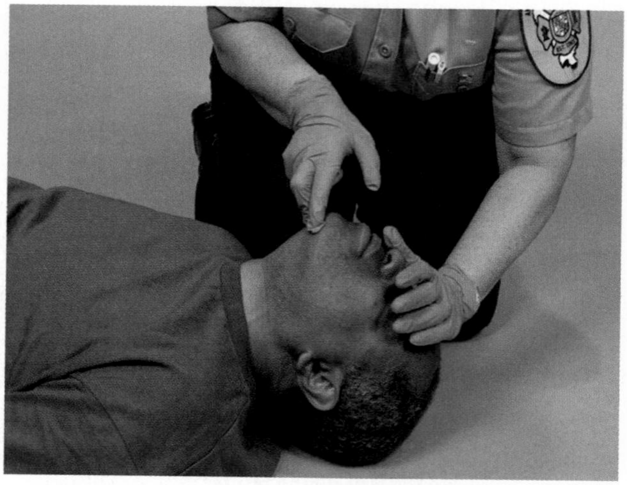

FIGURE 16-26 The head tilt–chin lift maneuver.

Jaw-Thrust Maneuver

If you suspect that the patient has experienced a cervical spine injury, then open the airway with the **jaw-thrust maneuver**. In this technique, you open the airway by placing your fingers behind the angle of the jaw and lifting the jaw forward. As a result, the jaw is displaced forward at the mandibular angle. Consider the following points when using the jaw-thrust maneuver:

- **Indications.** An unresponsive patient; a patient with a possible cervical spine injury; or a patient who is unable to protect the airway.
- **Contraindications.** A responsive patient with resistance to opening the mouth. The jaw-thrust maneuver may be needed in a responsive patient who has sustained a jaw fracture to keep the tongue away from the back of the throat.
- **Advantages.** May be used in patients with cervical spine injury; may be used with a cervical collar in place; no special equipment is required.
- **Disadvantages.** Cannot maintain the jaw-thrust maneuver if the patient becomes responsive or combative; difficult to maintain

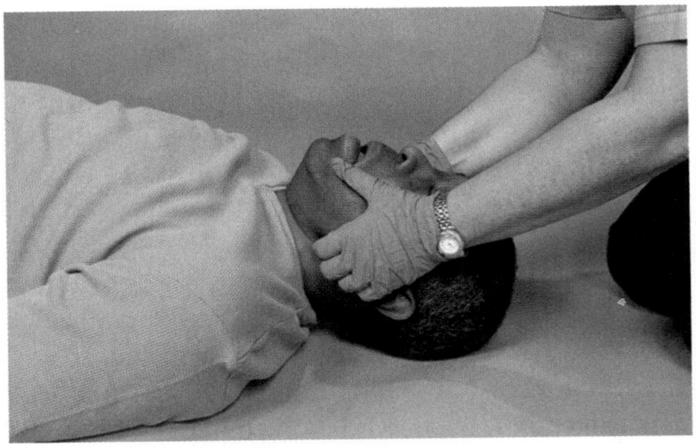

FIGURE 16-27 The jaw-thrust maneuver.

for an extended time; very difficult to use in conjunction with bag-mask ventilation; the thumb must remain in place to maintain jaw displacement; requires a second rescuer for bag-mask ventilation; does not protect against aspiration.

To perform the jaw-thrust maneuver, position yourself at the patient's head. Place the meaty portion of your thumbs on the zygomatic arches, and hook the tips of your index fingers under the angle of the mandible, in the indentation below each ear. While holding the patient's head in a neutral, in-line position, displace the jaw upward and open the patient's mouth with the tips of your thumbs **FIGURE 16-27**. Because opening and maintaining a patent airway is critical, you should carefully perform the head tilt–chin lift maneuver if you are unable to adequately open and maintain the airway using the jaw-thrust maneuver.

Tongue-Jaw Lift Maneuver

The **tongue-jaw lift maneuver** is used more commonly to open a patient's airway for the purpose of suctioning or inserting an oropharyngeal or supraglottic airway. It cannot be used to ventilate a patient because it will not allow for an adequate mask seal on the face.

To perform the tongue-jaw lift maneuver, position yourself at the patient's side. Place the hand closest to the patient's head on the forehead. With the other hand, reach into the patient's mouth and hook your first knuckle under the incisors (front teeth) or gumline. While holding the patient's head and maintaining the hand on the forehead, lift the jaw straight up **FIGURE 16-28**.

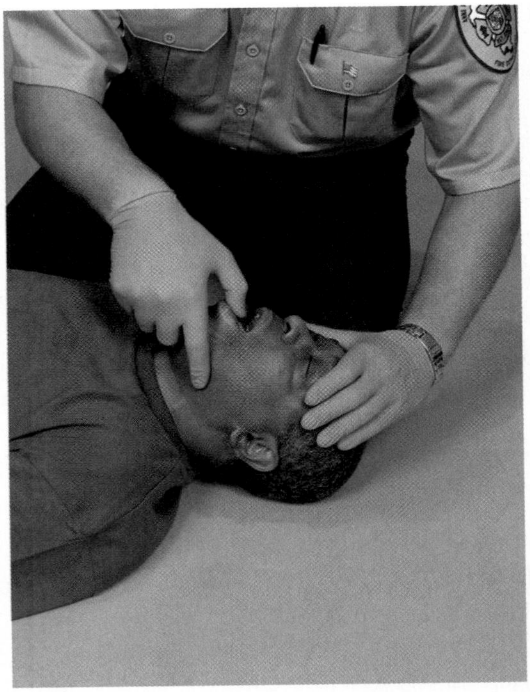

FIGURE 16-28 The tongue-jaw lift maneuver.

Suctioning

When the patient's mouth or throat becomes filled with vomitus, blood, or secretions, a suction apparatus enables you to remove material quickly and efficiently, thereby allowing you to ventilate the patient. Ventilating a patient who has secretions in the mouth will force material into the lungs, resulting in an upper airway obstruction or aspiration. Therefore, if needed, clearing the patient's airway with suction is your next priority after opening the patient's airway with the manual maneuvers previously discussed. Remember: If you hear gurgling, then the patient needs suctioning.

Suctioning Equipment

Ambulances should carry a fixed suction unit (which operates off a vacuum from the engine) and a portable suction unit (battery-operated or hand-powered) **FIGURE 16-29**. Regardless of your location (in the patient's residence, the middle of a field, or the back of the ambulance), you must have quick

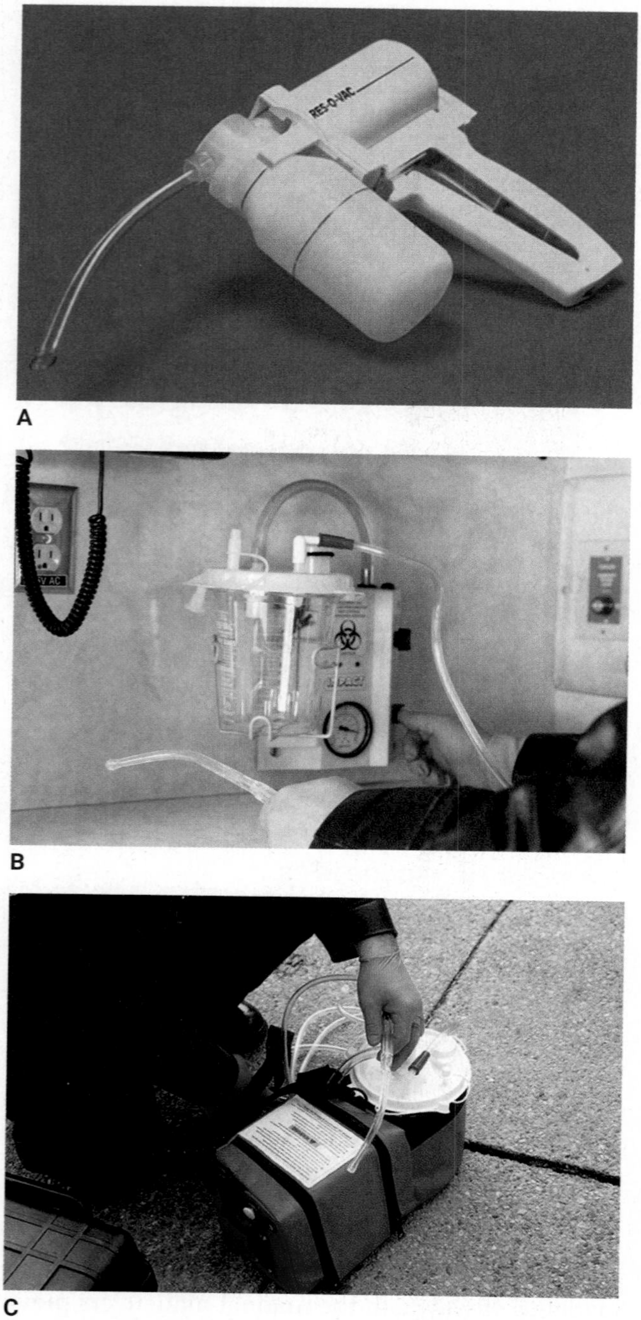

A B C

FIGURE 16-29 Effective suctioning equipment is essential for good airway management. **A.** Hand-operated device. **B.** Fixed unit. **C.** Portable unit.

access to suctioning equipment. It is essential for effective airway management.

Hand-operated suctioning units with disposable canisters are reliable, effective, and relatively inexpensive; they can easily fit into the bag that you carry to the patient's side. Mechanical or vacuum-powered suction units should be capable of generating a vacuum of at least 300 mm Hg within 4 seconds of clamping off the tubing. The amount of suction should be adjustable for use in children and intubated patients. Check the vacuum on the mechanical suction unit at the beginning of every shift by turning on the device, clamping the tubing, and ensuring the pressure gauge registers at least 300 mm Hg. With battery-charged units, ensure that they have fully charged batteries. **TABLE 16-7** lists the advantages and disadvantages of the most common types of suction devices.

Regardless of which type of suction unit you are using, the device must generate enough vacuum pressure to adequately suction the patient's mouth and oropharynx. In addition to the suctioning unit, you should have the following supplies readily accessible at the patient's head:

- Wide-bore, thick-walled, nonkinking tubing
- Plastic, rigid pharyngeal suction tips (tonsil-tip, Yankauer, or DuCanto catheters)
- Nonrigid plastic catheters (French or whistle-tip catheters)
- A nonbreakable, disposable collection bottle
- A supply of water for rinsing the catheters

A suction catheter is a hollow, cylindrical device used to remove fluids and secretions from the patient's airway. A **tonsil-tip catheter** is a good option for suctioning the oropharynx in adults; it may also be used for infants and children. These plastic-tip catheters have a large diameter and are rigid, so they do not collapse. Rigid catheters are capable of suctioning large volumes of fluid rapidly. Tips with a curved contour allow for easy, rapid placement in the oropharynx **FIGURE 16-30**.

Soft plastic, nonrigid catheters, sometimes called French or **whistle-tip catheters**, can be placed in the oropharynx or nasopharynx or down an ET tube. They come in various sizes and have a smaller diameter compared to rigid catheters. Soft catheters are used to suction the nose and liquid secretions in the back of the mouth, and in situations in which a rigid catheter cannot be used, such as for a patient with a stoma **FIGURE 16-31**. (Airway management considerations for such patients are covered later in this chapter.) For example, a rigid catheter could break a tooth in a patient with clenched teeth, whereas a flexible catheter may be

TABLE 16-7 Comparison of Common Suction Devices

Device Type	Advantages	Disadvantages
Hand-powered portable	• Lightweight • Portable • Mechanically simple • Inexpensive	• Limited volume • Manually powered • Body fluid contact • Components not disposable
Oxygen-powered portable	• Lightweight • Small	• Limited suction power • Uses a lot of oxygen for limited suctioning power
Battery-operated portable	• Lightweight • Portable • Excellent suction power • Most problems can be identified and fixed in the field	• More complicated mechanics • May lose battery integrity over time • Some body fluid contact
Mounted vacuum-powered	• Extremely strong vacuum • Adjustable vacuum power • Components are disposable	• Not portable • Body fluid contact • Cannot be fixed in the field • Cannot substitute the power source

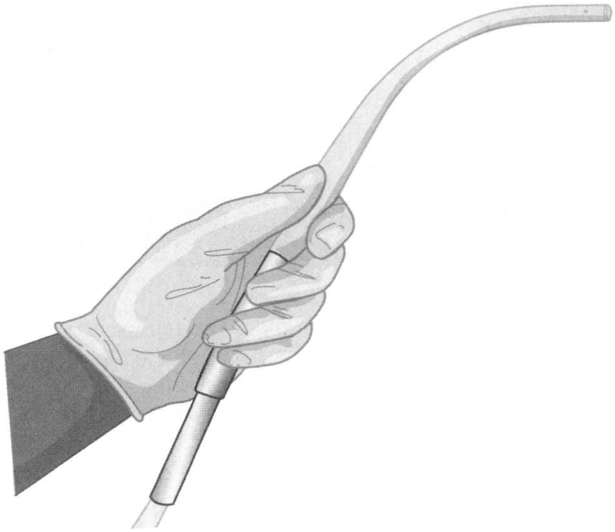

FIGURE 16-30 Large-bore catheters are a good choice for suctioning the oropharynx because they have wide-diameter tips, are rigid, and can remove copious thick secretions and other debris from the airway.

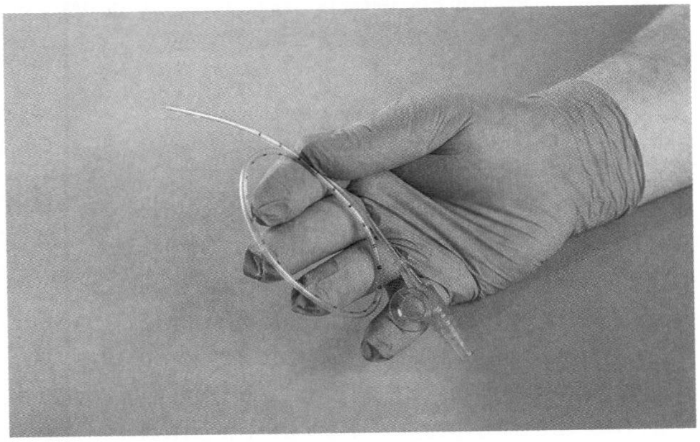

FIGURE 16-31 Whistle-tip (French) catheters are used in situations in which rigid catheters cannot be used, such as when a patient has a stoma or the patient's teeth are clenched. Flexible catheters can also be passed down an endotracheal tube.

worked along the cheeks without causing injury. Suction tubing without the attached catheter facilitates suctioning of large debris in the oropharynx and allows access to the back of the pharynx in a patient with clenched teeth.

Suctioning Techniques

Mortality increases significantly if a patient aspirates; therefore, suctioning the upper airway is critical to avoid this potentially fatal event. Suction the patient's airway until it is clear of liquids or other debris. Remember, ventilating a patient whose airway is full of blood, vomit, or other secretions virtually assures aspiration.

Be careful not to stimulate the back of the throat, especially in a young child or an infant, because this can induce a vagal response and cause bradycardia. After suctioning is complete, continue ventilation and oxygenation.

Soft-tip catheters are best used when passed through an ET tube. Lubricate the catheter with a water-soluble gel when suctioning the nasopharynx. Insert the catheter, and apply suction during extraction of the catheter to clear the airway. After the patient has been suctioned, reevaluate the patency of the airway, and continue to ventilate and oxygenate as needed.

Before inserting any suction catheter into a patient, measure for the proper size: from the corner of the mouth to the earlobe or the angle of the jaw **FIGURE 16-32A**. Never insert a catheter past the base of the tongue because doing so may cause the patient to gag or vomit. Turn the patient's head to the side, or log roll to the side, and insert the suction catheter to the predetermined depth. Apply suction in a circular motion while you withdraw the catheter **FIGURE 16-32B**. Repeat as needed until the airway is clear of secretions.

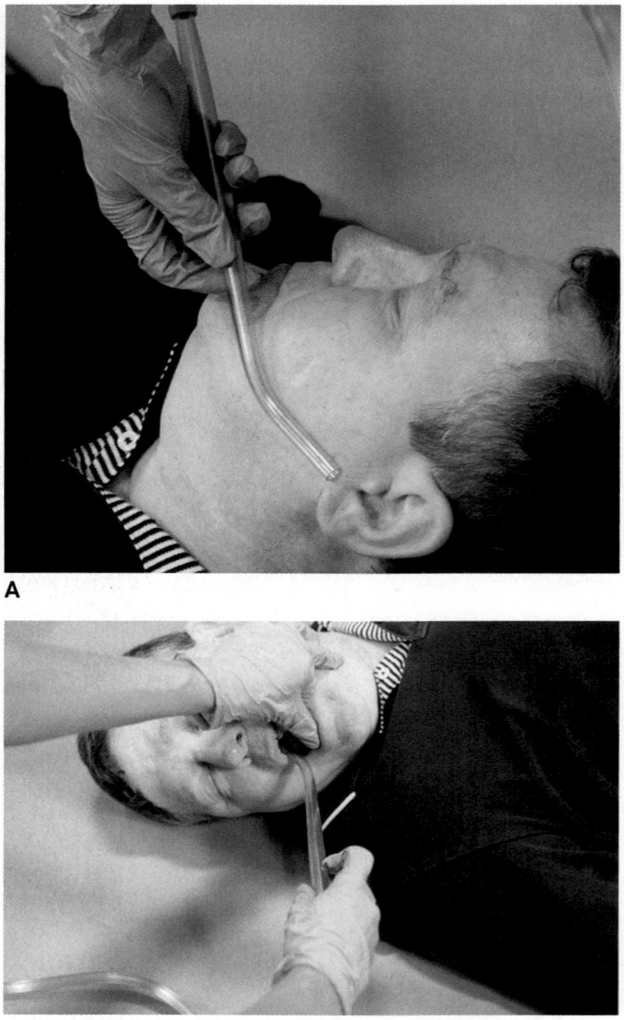

A

B

FIGURE 16-32 A. Measure for the proper-size suction catheter from the corner of the mouth to the earlobe or angle of the jaw. **B.** Apply suction while you are withdrawing the catheter. Repeat as needed until the airway is clear of secretions.

Airway Adjuncts

After manually opening the airway of an unresponsive patient and using suction as needed to clear away any blood or other secretions, you may need to insert an artificial airway adjunct to help maintain airway patency. An artificial airway is not a substitute for proper head positioning: Even after you insert an airway adjunct, you must manually maintain the appropriate position of the patient's head.

Oropharyngeal Airway

The **oropharyngeal (oral) airway** is a curved, hard plastic device that fits over the back of the tongue with the tip in the posterior pharynx **FIGURE 16-33**. It is designed to hold the tongue away from the posterior pharyngeal wall, and its use makes it much easier to ventilate patients with a **bag-mask device** (discussed later in this chapter). The oral airway can also serve as an effective bite block, preventing an intubated patient from biting down on the ET tube.

Promptly insert an oral airway in unresponsive patients (breathing or not) who have no gag reflex. Because its distal end sits in the back of the throat, this device will stimulate gagging and retching in a responsive patient. For that reason, you should use the oral airway only in unresponsive patients without a gag reflex. If the patient gags during insertion of the oral airway, then remove the device immediately and be prepared to suction the oropharynx. Consider the following points when using an oral airway:

- **Indications.** Unresponsive patients and patients with an absent gag reflex
- **Contraindications.** Responsive patients and patients with a gag reflex

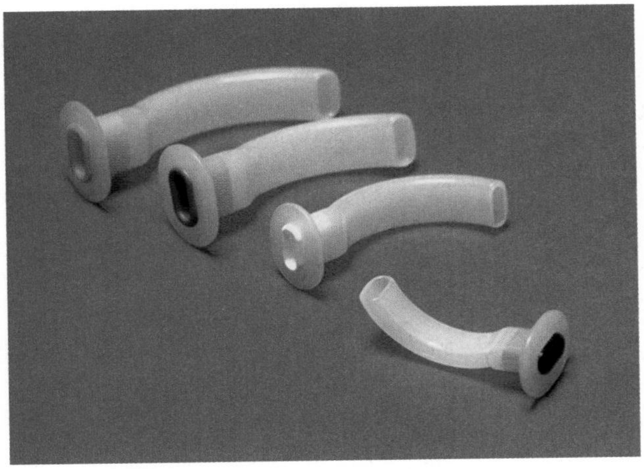

FIGURE 16-33 An oral airway is used for unresponsive patients who have no gag reflex. It keeps the tongue from blocking the airway.

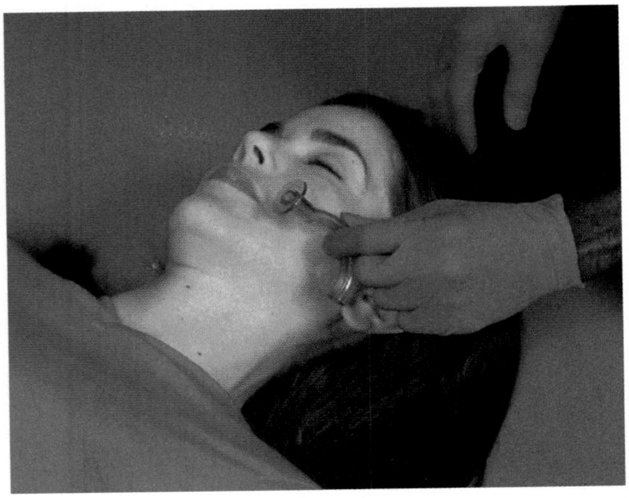

FIGURE 16-34 Size the oral airway by measuring from the corner of the mouth to the earlobe or the angle of the jaw.

- **Advantages.** Noninvasive; easily placed; prevents blockage of the glottis by the tongue
- **Disadvantages.** Does not protect against aspiration
- **Complications.** Unexpected gag may cause vomiting, or improper technique may cause pharyngeal or dental trauma

Words of Wisdom

Many airway management techniques are aerosol-generating procedures. Therefore, it is important to wear an appropriate face mask (ie, an N95 respirator) and protective eyewear or a full-face shield whenever you manage a patient's airway. Body fluids can become aerosolized, and the mucous membranes of your mouth, nose, and eyes can easily come in contact with these contaminants.

If the oral airway is an improper size or inserted incorrectly, it could push the patient's tongue backward into the pharynx, creating an airway obstruction. In addition, rough airway insertion can injure the hard palate, resulting in oral bleeding and creating a risk of vomiting and aspiration. Before inserting an oral airway, suction the oropharynx as needed to ensure that the patient's mouth is clear of blood or other fluids.

To select an oral airway that is the correct size for the patient, measure the distance from the corner of the patient's mouth to the earlobe or the angle of the jaw **FIGURE 16-34**. You can insert the oral airway in one of two ways:

- Open the adult patient's mouth with the cross-finger technique or tongue-jaw lift maneuver, hold the airway upside down with your other hand, and insert the airway in the mouth with the tip facing the hard palate **FIGURE 16-35A**. Advance the oral airway until it reaches the soft palate and then rotate it 180°, allowing it to follow the curvature of the tongue, until the flange rests on the patient's lips **FIGURE 16-35B**.
- Use a tongue blade to depress the adult's or child's tongue, ensuring that the tongue remains forward **FIGURE 16-36A**. Insert the oral airway, with the tip pointing down, and follow the curvature of the tongue until the flange rests on the patient's lips **FIGURE 16-36B**.

Nasopharyngeal Airway

The **nasopharyngeal (nasal) airway** is a soft, rubber tube that is inserted through the nose into the posterior pharynx behind the tongue, thereby allowing passage of air from the nose to the lower airway. Nasal airways are commonly measured using the French (Fr) catheter scale, and range in size from 12 Fr to 36 Fr; the length of the nasal airway depends on its size. A nasal airway is much better tolerated than an oral airway in patients with an

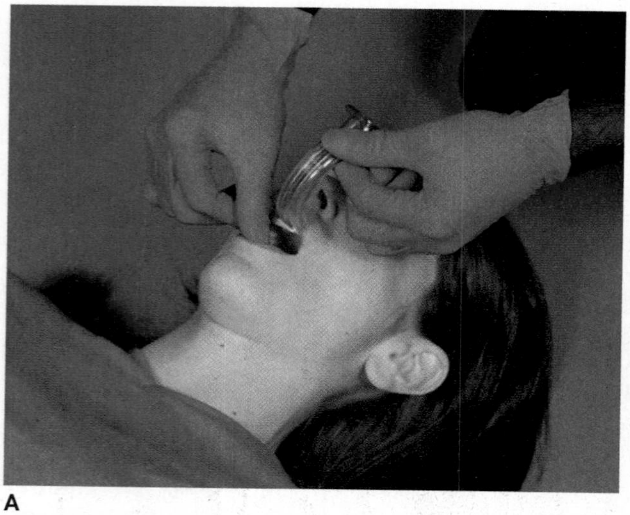

FIGURE 16-35 A. Open the adult patient's airway and insert the airway with the tip facing the hard palate. **B.** Rotate the oral airway 180° after it reaches the soft palate, allowing it to follow the curvature of the tongue, until the flange rests on the patient's lips.

© Jones & Bartlett Learning.

FIGURE 16-36 A. Use a tongue blade to depress the tongue, ensuring that the tongue stays forward. **B.** Insert the oral airway, with the tip pointing down, and allow it to follow the curvature of the tongue until the flange rests on the patient's lips.

© Jones & Bartlett Learning.

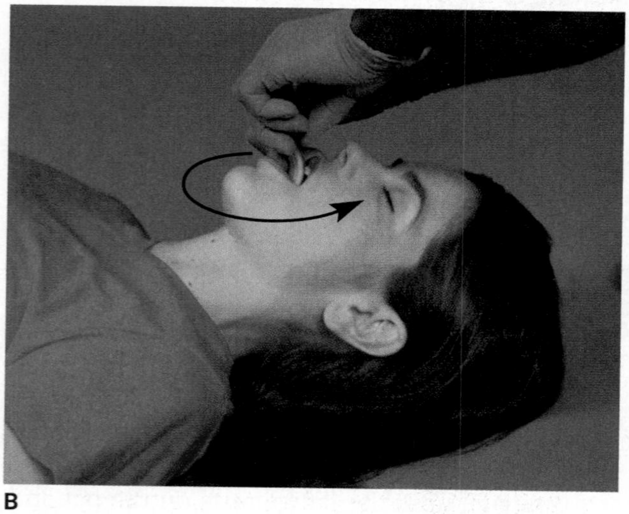

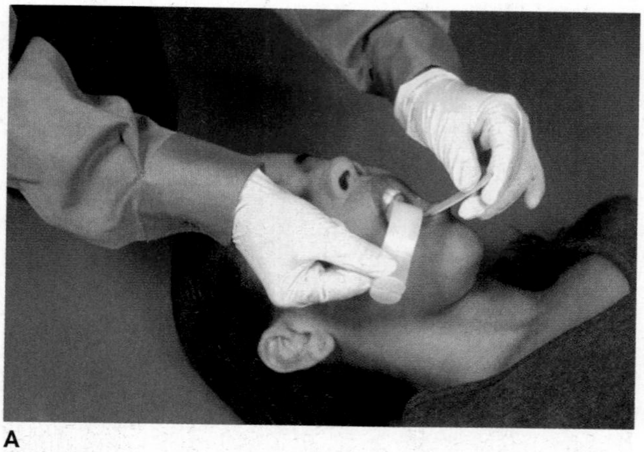

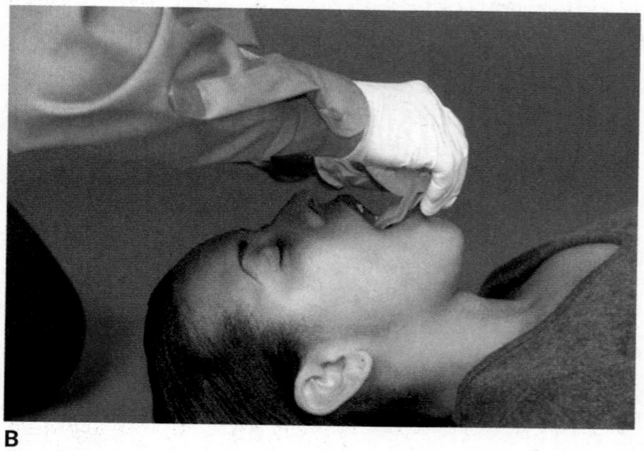

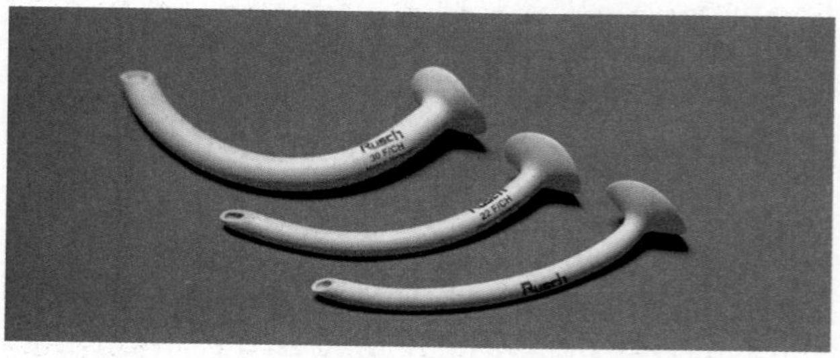

FIGURE 16-37 A nasal airway is better tolerated by patients with an intact gag reflex.

© Jones & Bartlett Learning.

intact gag reflex but an altered LOC **FIGURE 16-37**. Do not use this device if the patient has experienced trauma to the nose or face, or you have reason to suspect a skull fracture (eg, cerebrospinal fluid [CSF] leakage from the nose). Although rare, inserting the airway in such cases may cause it to enter the cranial vault through the hole caused by the fracture.

Insert the nasal airway gently to avoid causing epistaxis (nosebleed). Lubricate the airway with a water-soluble gel, preferably one that contains a local anesthetic, and slide it gently, tip downward, into one nostril. Do not force it. If you meet resistance, then try to pass the airway down the other nostril.

If the nasal airway is too long, then it may obstruct the patient's airway. If the patient becomes intolerant of the nasal airway, then gently remove it from the nasal passage. Although a nasal airway is less likely to cause vomiting than an oral airway is, you should still have suction readily available. Consider the following points when using a nasal airway:

- **Indications.** Unresponsive patients and patients with an altered mental status who have an intact gag reflex
- **Contraindications.** Patient intolerance; presence of facial (specifically, nose) fracture or skull fracture
- **Advantages.** Can be suctioned through; provides a patent airway; can be tolerated by responsive patients; can be safely placed "blindly" (ie, without direct visualization of the airway); no requirement for the mouth to be open
- **Disadvantages.** Improper technique may result in severe bleeding (the resulting epistaxis may be extremely difficult to control); does not protect against aspiration.

Special Populations

In children, using a tongue blade to hold the tongue down while inserting an oral airway is the preferred method. Because the child's hard palate is more fragile than an adult's, rotating the oral airway can lacerate or even fracture the hard palate.

To select a nasal airway that is the correct size for the patient, measure the distance from the tip of the nostril to the earlobe or the angle of the jaw **FIGURE 16-38A**. Insert the prelubricated airway into the larger nostril, with the bevel facing the septum, until the flange rests on the patient's nostril **FIGURE 16-38B**.

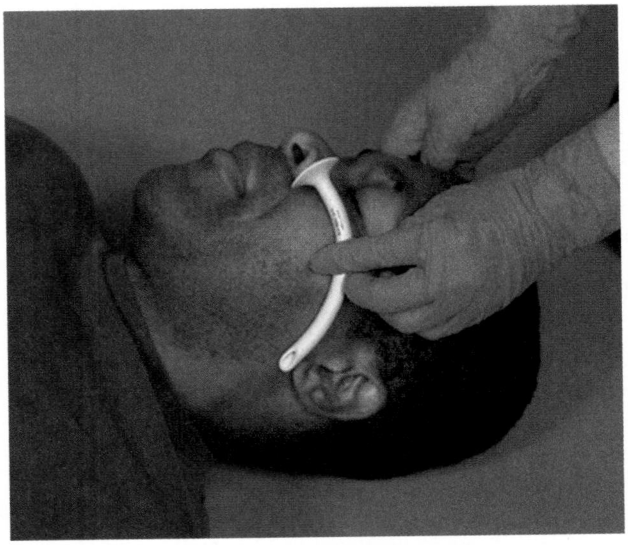

A

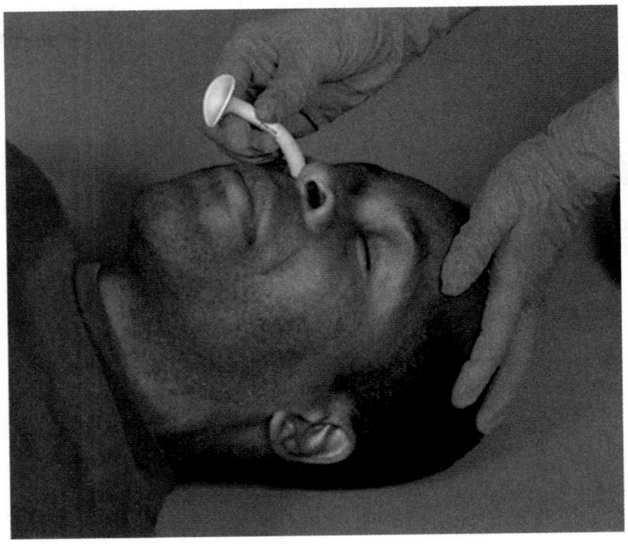

B

FIGURE 16-38 A. Size the nasal airway by measuring from the tip of the nostril to the angle of the jaw or the earlobe. **B.** Insert the nasal airway into the larger nostril, with the bevel facing the septum, until the flange rests on the patient's nostril.

Airway Obstructions

The airway connects the body to the life-giving oxygen in the atmosphere. If the airway becomes obstructed, then this lifeline is cut and the patient dies, often within minutes. As a paramedic, you must recognize the signs of an obstructed airway and immediately take corrective action.

Causes of Airway Obstruction

In an adult, sudden foreign body airway obstruction usually occurs during a meal. In children, it typically occurs while eating or playing with small toys. An otherwise healthy child who presents with a sudden onset of difficulty breathing, especially in the absence of fever, should be suspected of having a foreign body airway obstruction. However, airway obstruction has many other causes, including the tongue, laryngeal edema, laryngeal spasm (laryngospasm), trauma, and aspiration.

When the airway is obstructed because of an infectious process or a severe allergic reaction, repeated attempts to clear the airway as if it were obstructed by a foreign body will be unsuccessful and potentially harmful. These conditions require specific management and prompt transport to an appropriate medical facility. Airway infection is covered in Chapter 17, *Respiratory Emergencies*; allergic reactions are covered in Chapter 26, *Immunologic Emergencies*.

Tongue

In a patient with an altered LOC, the jaw relaxes and the tongue tends to fall back against the posterior wall of the pharynx, blocking the airway. A patient with partial obstruction caused by the tongue will make a snoring sound when breathing (sonorous breathing); a patient whose airway is completely obstructed cannot move any air. Fortunately, airway obstruction by the tongue is simple to correct using a manual maneuver (such as the head tilt–chin lift or jaw-thrust maneuver).

Foreign Body

A significant number of people die of foreign body airway obstructions each year, often as a result of choking on a piece of food. The typical patient is middle-aged or older and wears dentures. The person has usually consumed alcohol, which depresses the body's protective reflexes and adversely affects judgment about how large a piece of food can be prudently placed in the mouth. In addition, people with conditions that decrease their airway reflexes (eg, stroke) are at an increased risk for foreign body airway obstructions.

Signs may include choking, gagging, stridor, dyspnea, **dysphonia** (difficulty speaking), and **aphonia** (inability to speak). Treatment depends on whether the patient is effectively moving air. Techniques for the removal of foreign body airway obstruction are discussed later in this chapter.

Laryngeal Spasm and Edema

A laryngeal spasm (laryngospasm) results in spasmodic closure of the vocal cords, completely occluding the airway. It is often caused by trauma during an overly aggressive intubation attempt or occurs immediately on extubation, especially when the patient has an altered LOC.

Laryngeal edema causes the glottic opening to become extremely narrow or totally closed. Conditions that commonly cause this problem include epiglottitis, anaphylaxis, or inhalation injury (eg, burns to the upper airway).

Airway obstructions caused by laryngeal spasm or edema may be relieved by aggressive ventilation that forces air past the narrowed airway or a forceful upward pull of the jaw in an attempt to reposition the airway. In certain patients, muscle relaxant medications may be effective in relieving laryngeal spasm. Do not let your guard down after the laryngospasm appears to have resolved; resolution of the immediate crisis does not mean that laryngospasm will not recur. Transport the patient to the hospital for evaluation.

Laryngeal Injury

Airway patency depends on good muscle tone to keep the trachea open. Fracture of the larynx increases airway resistance by decreasing airway size due to decreased muscle tone, laryngeal edema, and ventilatory effort. An advanced airway may be required to maintain a patent airway. Penetrating and crush injuries to the larynx can compromise the airway secondary to swelling and bleeding. As with laryngeal fractures, advanced airway management may be required.

Aspiration

As noted earlier, aspiration of blood or other fluid significantly increases mortality. In addition to potentially obstructing the airway, aspiration destroys delicate bronchiolar tissue, introduces pathogens into the lungs, and decreases the patient's ability to ventilate (or be ventilated).

Suction should be readily available for any patient who is unable to maintain their own airway. Always assume that patients who require emergency medical care have a full stomach.

Recognition of an Airway Obstruction

A foreign body lodged in the upper airway can cause a mild (partial) or severe (complete) airway obstruction, depending on the size of the object and its location in the airway. A rapid but careful assessment is required to determine the seriousness of the obstruction, because management of mild versus severe cases differs significantly.

A patient with a mild airway obstruction is responsive and able to exchange air but may show varying degrees of respiratory distress. The patient will usually have noisy respirations and may be coughing, or may wheeze between coughs but not become cyanotic. Patients with a mild airway obstruction should be encouraged to cough and reassured that you are there to help if the obstruction worsens. A forceful cough is the most effective means of dislodging the mild airway obstruction. Attempts to manually remove the object could force it farther down into the airway and cause a severe obstruction. Closely monitor the patient's condition and be prepared to intervene if you see signs of severe airway obstruction.

A patient with a severe airway obstruction typically experiences a sudden inability to breathe or talk. The patient may grasp at the throat (the universal sign of choking) and make frantic, exaggerated attempts to move air **FIGURE 16-39**. A patient with a severe airway obstruction has a weak, ineffective, or absent cough and is in marked respiratory distress; weak inspiratory stridor and cyanosis are often present.

Emergency Medical Care for Foreign Body Airway Obstruction

If a patient with a suspected airway obstruction is responsive, then ask, "Are you choking?" If the patient nods "yes" and cannot speak, then begin treatment immediately. If the obstruction is not promptly cleared, then the amount of oxygen in the blood will decrease dramatically, resulting in severe hypoxia and death. If the obstruction is not resolved, the initially responsive patient will become an unconscious patient with an obstructed airway.

If, after opening the airway, you cannot ventilate the patient (no visible chest rise) or you feel resistance when ventilating (poor lung compliance), then reposition the airway and make another attempt to ventilate the patient. **Lung compliance** is the ability of the alveoli to expand when air is drawn into the lungs during negative-pressure ventilation or pushed into the lungs during positive-pressure ventilation. Poor lung compliance is characterized by increased resistance during ventilation attempts.

If you find large pieces of vomitus, mucus, loose dentures, or blood clots in the airway, then sweep them forward and out of the mouth with your gloved index finger. Blind finger sweeps of the mouth regardless of the patient's age should be avoided and may cause further harm; attempt to remove only foreign bodies that you can see and easily retrieve. After the patient's airway is open, insert your index finger down along the inside of the patient's cheek and into the throat at the base of the tongue, then try to hook the foreign body to dislodge it and maneuver it out of the mouth. Take care not to force the foreign body deeper into the airway. Do not blindly insert any object other than your finger into the patient's mouth to remove a foreign body, because an instrument jammed into the throat can damage the delicate structures of the pharynx and compound the obstruction with

FIGURE 16-39 The universal sign of choking.

Words of Wisdom

Causes of Airway Obstruction

- Relaxation of the tongue in an unresponsive patient
- Foreign objects (eg, food, small toys, balloons, dentures)
- Blood clots, broken teeth, or damaged oral tissue following trauma
- Airway tissue swelling (eg, infection, allergic reaction, inhalation injury)
- Aspirated vomitus

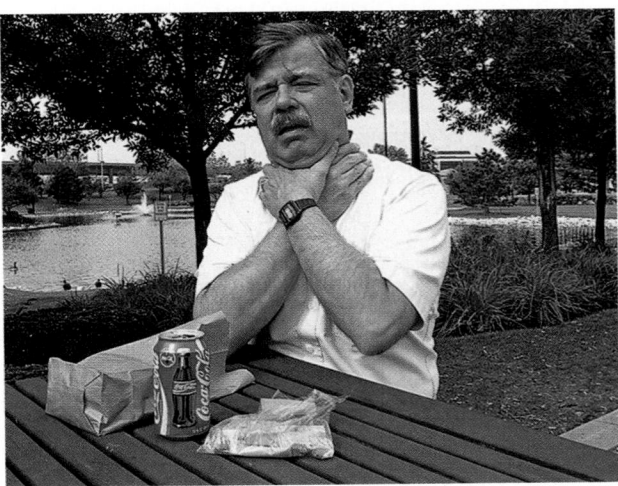

hemorrhage. Use suctioning to clear the airway of secretions as needed. If the patient is in distress, consider administering oxygen, even if the oxygen saturation is greater than 94%, if doing so is consistent with your local protocols.

The **abdominal thrust maneuver** (also called the Heimlich maneuver) is the most effective method of dislodging and forcing a foreign object out of the airway of a responsive adult or child. It aims to create an artificial cough by forcing residual air out of the person's lungs, thereby expelling the object. You should continue to perform the Heimlich maneuver on any responsive child or adult with a severe airway obstruction until the obstructing object is expelled or until the patient becomes unresponsive. If a responsive patient with a severe airway obstruction is in the advanced stages of pregnancy or has morbid obesity, then perform chest thrusts instead of abdominal thrusts.

Controversies

Some organizations have suggested the initial use of back blows in adults with a foreign body airway obstruction and an ineffective cough. However, this recommendation is weak and supported by only low-certainty evidence. Some experts argue against the use of back blows in larger patients due to the simple impracticality of this procedure: The provider can hold an infant with the head downward while giving back blows, allowing gravity to help draw the object out of the airway. In contrast, the provider likely cannot position an adult in an inverted position while giving back blows; thus, if the back blows dislodge the object, gravity may pull it downward, deeper into the airway.

Always follow local protocols and contact medical control for direction when needed.

If the responsive patient with a severe airway obstruction becomes unresponsive, then carefully position the patient supine on the ground and begin chest compressions. Perform 30 chest compressions (15 compressions if two rescuers are present and the patient is an infant or a child), and then open the airway and look in the mouth. Attempt to remove the foreign body only if you can see it. If you are able to retrieve the object, then attempt to ventilate the patient. If you cannot see the object, then resume chest compressions.

Words of Wisdom

Do not blindly insert any instrument, whether improvised or specially designed, into a patient's pharynx. This practice is extremely dangerous!

If you are unable to relieve a severe airway obstruction in an unresponsive patient with the basic techniques previously discussed, then proceed with **direct laryngoscopy** (visualization of the airway with a laryngoscope) for the removal of the foreign body. Insert the laryngoscope blade into the patient's mouth. If you see the foreign body, then carefully remove it from the upper airway with **Magill forceps**, a special type of curved forceps **FIGURE 16-40**. Laryngoscopes and blades are discussed later in this chapter.

To remove an upper airway obstruction with Magill forceps, follow the steps shown in **SKILL DRILL 16-1**.

Words of Wisdom

A patient with a severe upper airway obstruction has very little time before severe hypoxia sets in. If several attempts to relieve the obstruction with basic life support (BLS) methods fail, then proceed with direct laryngoscopy without delay. While you are performing BLS maneuvers, your partner should prepare the laryngoscope, a proper-size laryngoscope blade, and the Magill forceps.

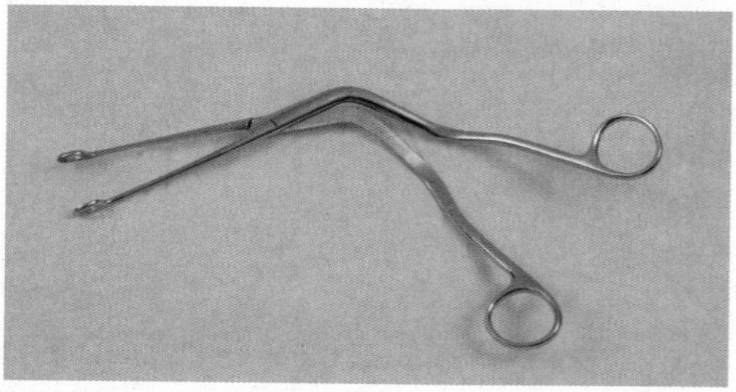

FIGURE 16-40 Magill forceps.

Skill Drill 16-1 Removing an Upper Airway Obstruction With Magill Forceps

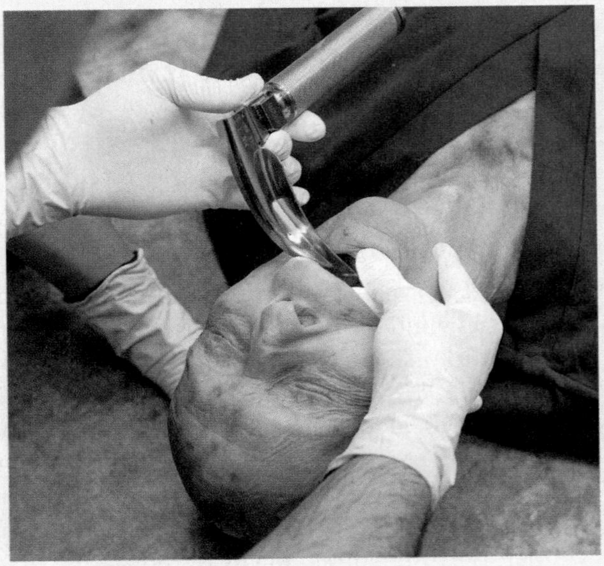

Step 1

With the patient's head in the sniffing position, open the patient's mouth and insert the laryngoscope blade.

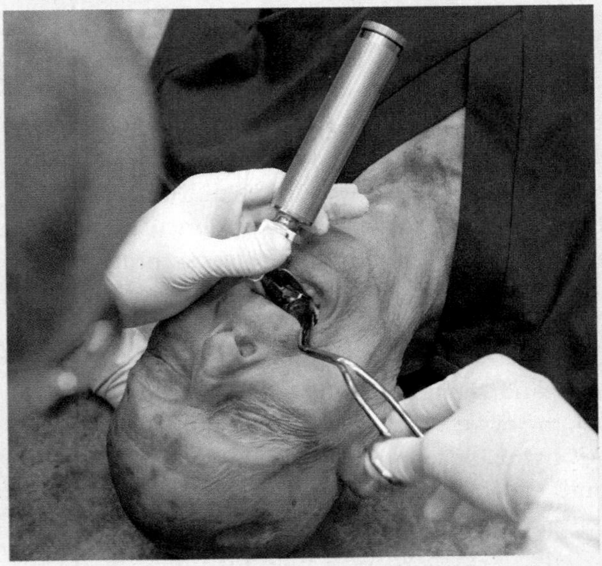

Step 2

Visualize the obstruction and retrieve the object with the Magill forceps.

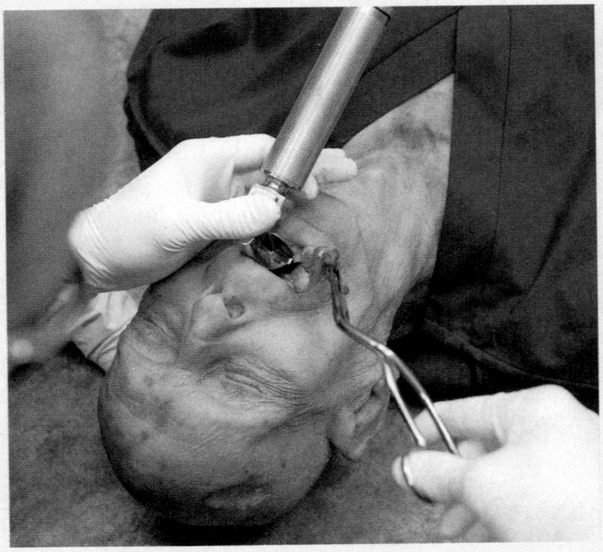

Step 3

Remove the object with the Magill forceps.

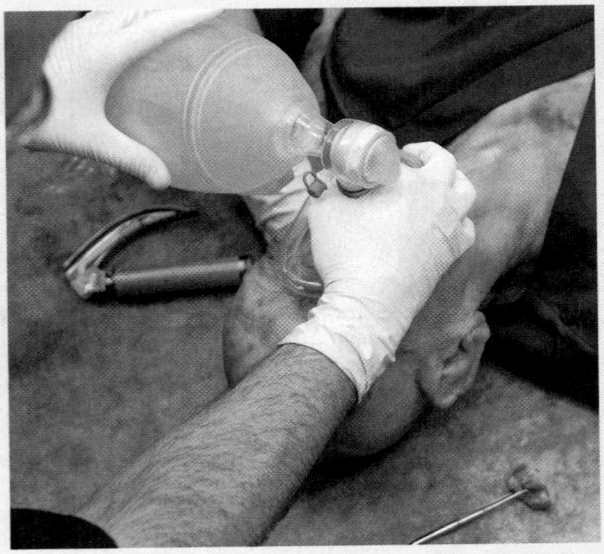

Step 4

Attempt to ventilate the patient.

Supplemental Oxygen Therapy

Supplemental oxygen is indicated for patients with respiratory distress and those with suspected or documented hypoxemia (ie, an oxygen saturation level of 94% or less). In addition, your EMS system protocols may call for supplemental oxygen in other select cases.

Historically, oxygen was administered to patients whose clinical condition did not otherwise indicate its use; that is, no evidence of respiratory compromise, with an oxygen saturation level greater than 94%. Evidence suggests that supplemental oxygen in a well-oxygenated patient may not be indicated because issues such as oxidative stress and hyperoxic injury are of concern. However, the evidence that oxygen is helpful to a patient with hypoxia is profound, so if you doubt the patient's oxygenation status, then administer supplemental oxygen.[1-3]

The oxygen-delivery method must be appropriate for the patient's ventilatory status. Reassess frequently and adjust accordingly based on the patient's clinical condition and adequacy of breathing.

Evidence-Based Medicine

Current guidelines from the American Heart Association state that if the patient is not experiencing respiratory distress and has an oxygen saturation level greater than 94% on room air, then supplemental oxygen is not indicated.[4] Follow your local protocols regarding supplemental oxygen administration.

Oxygen Sources

Oxygen Cylinders

Pure (100%) oxygen is stored in seamless steel or aluminum cylinders. The colors of these cylinders may vary from silver, to chrome, to green, or some combination thereof. Ensure that the cylinder is labeled "medical oxygen." Also, look for letters and numbers stamped on the collar of the cylinder **FIGURE 16-41**. Of particular importance are the month and year stamps, which indicate when the cylinder was last hydrostatically tested.

Oxygen cylinders are available in various sizes. You will most often use the D cylinder, which contains 350 L of oxygen and is typically carried from the ambulance to the patient. The M cylinder

YOU are the Paramedic

PART 4

The patient is extremely restless and agitated, and resists your attempts to apply continuous positive airway pressure (CPAP) therapy. When you reapply oxygen with the nonrebreathing mask, he immediately pulls the mask from his face. Your partner makes a comment about performing rapid sequence intubation (RSI).

Recording Time: 7 Minutes	
Level of consciousness	Conscious, but extremely restless and agitated
Respirations	28 breaths/min; labored
Pulse	140 beats/min; weak and regular
Skin	Lips and gums appear gray
Blood pressure	182/94 mm Hg
Oxygen saturation (Spo_2)	74%
Pupils	PERRLA
$ETCO_2$	63 mm Hg
ECG	Sinus tachycardia

7. Is RSI the best option for the patient at this point? Why or why not?

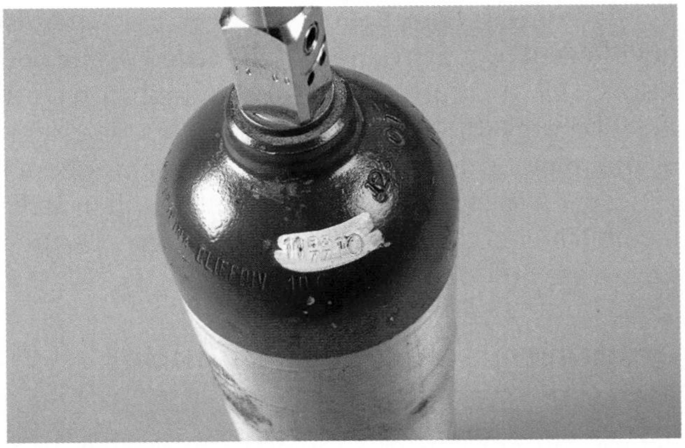

FIGURE 16-41 Oxygen cylinders for medical use have a series of letters and numbers stamped into the metal on the collar of the cylinder.

contains 3,000 L of oxygen and remains on board the ambulance as a main supply tank.

Oxygen delivery is measured in liters per minute (L/min). To prevent running out of oxygen at an inconvenient moment, you should replace an oxygen cylinder with a full one whenever the pressure falls to 200 pounds per square inch (psi) or lower. That level, called the **safe residual pressure**, indicates that it is *unsafe* to continue using the oxygen cylinder. In some EMS systems, the safe residual pressure for an oxygen cylinder is 500 psi. On the basis of the pressure in the oxygen cylinder and the flow rate of oxygen delivery, you can calculate how long the supply of oxygen in the cylinder will last—that is, the tank life **TABLE 16-8**.

Safety Reminders

Any cylinder containing compressed gas under high pressure has the potential, under specific conditions, to exhibit the properties of a rocket. Furthermore, oxygen presents the additional hazard of fire because it supports the combustion process. For these reasons, the following safety precautions are necessary when you are handling oxygen cylinders:

- Keep combustible materials, such as oil and grease, away from contact with the cylinder itself, the regulators, fittings, valves, and tubing.
- Do not permit smoking in any area where oxygen cylinders are in use or on standby.
- Store oxygen cylinders in a cool, well-ventilated area. Do not subject the cylinders to temperatures greater than 125°F (approximately 50°C).

TABLE 16-8 Oxygen Cylinders: Duration of Flow

Formula
(Tank Pressure in psi − 200 psi [the safe residual pressure]) × Cylinder Constant/Flow Rate in L/min = Duration of Flow in min
Cylinder Constant
D = 0.16 G = 2.41 E = 0.28 H = 3.14 M = 1.56 K = 3.14
Steps
Determine the life of an M cylinder that has a pressure of 2,000 psi and a flow rate of 10 L/min.
$\frac{(2{,}000-200)\times 1.56}{10}=\frac{2{,}808}{10}=281\text{ min, or 4 h 41 min}$

Abbreviation: psi, pounds per square inch

- Use an oxygen cylinder only with a safe, properly fitting regulator valve. Regulator valves for one gas should never be modified for use with another gas.
- Close all valves when the cylinder is not in use, even if the tank is empty.
- Secure cylinders so that they will not topple over. In transit, keep them in a proper carrier or rack, or strap them onto the stretcher with the patient.
- When working with an oxygen cylinder, always position yourself to its side. Never place any part of your body over the cylinder valve. A loosely fitting regulator can be blown off the cylinder with sufficient force to cause serious injury.
- Have the cylinder hydrostatically tested every 10 years to ensure it can still sustain the high pressures required. The original test date is stamped onto the cylinder together with its serial number.

Oxygen Regulators and Flowmeters

High-pressure regulators are attached to the cylinder stem to deliver cylinder gas under high pressure. These regulators are used to transfer cylinder gas from one tank to another, such as when you are refilling a portable oxygen cylinder.

The pressure of gas in a full oxygen cylinder is approximately 2,000 psi. Clearly, this is far too much pressure to deliver directly into a patient's airway. Instead, gas flow from an oxygen cylinder to the patient is controlled by a **therapy regulator**, which attaches to the stem of the oxygen cylinder and reduces the high pressure of gas to a safe range (about 50 psi).

Flowmeters, which are usually permanently attached to the therapy regulator, allow the oxygen delivered to the patient to be adjusted within a range of 1 to 25 L/min. The two types of flowmeters most commonly used are the pressure-compensated flowmeter and the Bourdon-gauge flowmeter.

A **pressure-compensated flowmeter** incorporates a float ball within a tapered calibrated tube; this float ball rises or falls based on the gas flow in the tube. The gas flow is controlled by a needle valve located downstream from the float ball. Because this type of flowmeter is affected by gravity, it must remain in an upright position to ensure an accurate flow reading **FIGURE 16-42**. The pressure-compensated flowmeter is most often used with the main oxygen source on the ambulance.

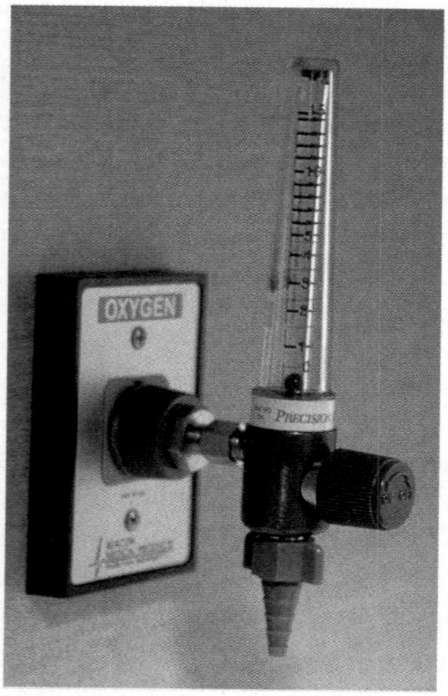

FIGURE 16-42 Pressure-compensated flowmeters contain a float ball that rises or falls based on the gas flow in the tube. It must remain in an upright position to ensure an accurate flow reading.

By contrast, the **Bourdon-gauge flowmeter** is not affected by gravity and can be placed in any position. This pressure gauge is calibrated to record the flow rate **FIGURE 16-43**. The major disadvantage of this type of flowmeter is that it does not compensate for backpressure. As a result, it will usually record a higher flow rate when there is any obstruction to gas flow downstream.

Preparing an Oxygen Cylinder for Use

Before you administer supplemental oxygen, you must prepare the oxygen cylinder and therapy regulator. Inspect the cylinder and its markings, and then remove the plastic seal covering the valve stem opening (if the cylinder was commercially filled). Inspect the opening to ensure that it is free of dirt and other debris. With the tank facing away from yourself and others, use an oxygen wrench to "crack" the cylinder: quickly open and close the valve to ensure that dirt particles and other contaminants are cleared from the valve stem and do not enter the oxygen cylinder.

Attach the regulator/flowmeter to the valve stem, ensuring that the pin-index system is correctly aligned. A metal or plastic O-ring is placed around the oxygen port to optimize the airtight seal between the collar of the regulator and the valve stem. Place the regulator collar over the cylinder valve, with the oxygen port and indexing pins on the side of the valve stem with three holes. Align the regulator so that the oxygen port and the pins

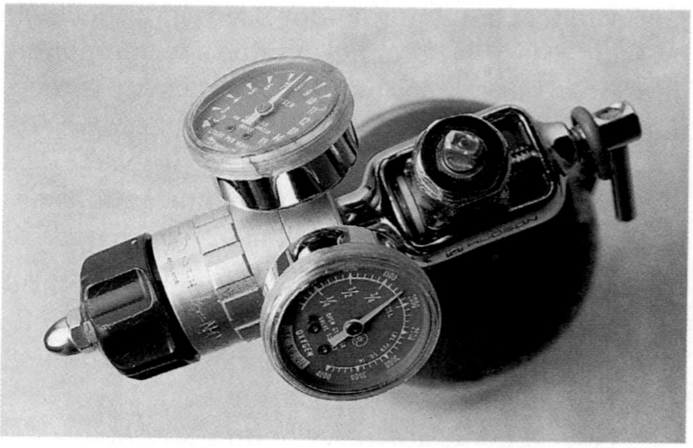

FIGURE 16-43 The Bourdon-gauge flowmeter is not affected by gravity and can be placed in any position.

fit into the correct holes on the valve stem; align the screw bolt on the opposite side with the dimpled depression. Tighten the screw bolt until the regulator is firmly attached to the cylinder. At this point, you should not see any space between the sides of the valve stem and the interior walls of the collar **FIGURE 16-44A**.

With the regulator firmly attached, open the cylinder and read the pressure level on the regulator gauge. A second gauge or selector dial on the flowmeter indicates the oxygen flow rate. Attach the oxygen connective tubing to the "Christmas tree" nipple on the flowmeter, and select the appropriate oxygen flow rate for the patient's clinical status **FIGURE 16-44B**.

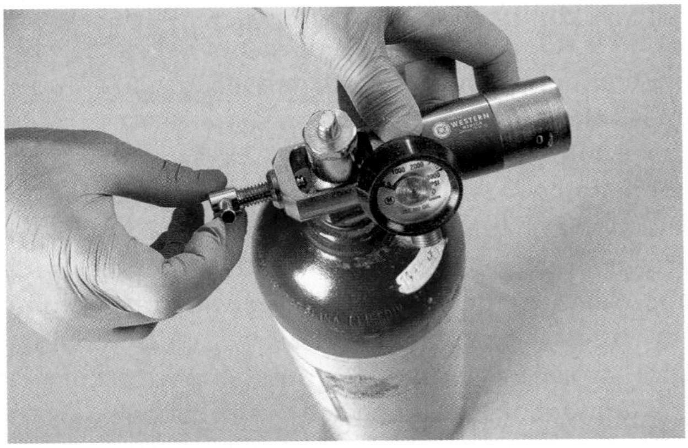

A

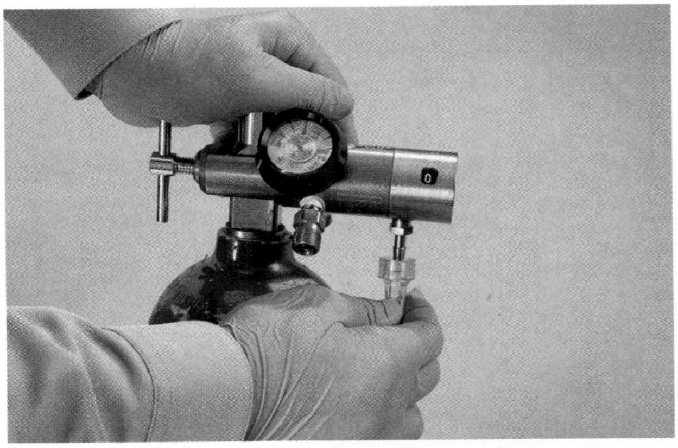

B

FIGURE 16-44 A. Attach the oxygen regulator, ensuring that the pin-indexing system is properly aligned, and tighten the screw bolt until it is secure. **B.** Attach the oxygen-delivery device and select the appropriate flow rate for the patient's clinical status.

Supplemental Oxygen-Delivery Devices

In general, the oxygen-delivery equipment that is used in the prehospital setting is limited to nonrebreathing masks, bag-mask devices, and nasal cannulas, depending on local protocols. However, you may encounter other devices during transports between medical facilities.

Nonrebreathing Mask

The **nonrebreathing mask** is used to administer high-flow oxygen to significantly hypoxemic patients who are otherwise breathing adequately. With a good mask-to-face seal and a flow rate of 15 L/min, it is capable of delivering up to 90% inspired oxygen (FIO_2).

The nonrebreathing mask is a combination mask and reservoir bag system. Oxygen fills a reservoir bag that is attached to the mask by a one-way valve, permitting the patient to inhale from the reservoir bag but not to exhale back into it. The only gas that can enter the reservoir, therefore, is 100% oxygen coming from the oxygen cylinder. Exhaled gas escapes through one-way flapper valves located on the side of the mask **FIGURE 16-45**.

Before you administer oxygen to a patient using a nonrebreathing mask, you must ensure that the reservoir bag is completely filled. The oxygen flow rate is generally adjusted from 12 to 15 L/min to prevent collapse of the bag during inhalation. Use a

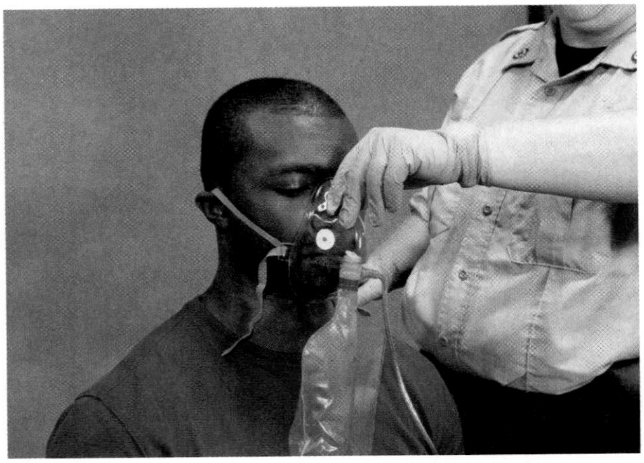

FIGURE 16-45 Nonrebreathing mask.

pediatric nonrebreathing mask, which has a smaller reservoir bag, for infants and small children; they inhale smaller volumes of air.

The nonrebreathing mask is indicated for spontaneously breathing patients who require high-flow oxygen concentrations (ie, patients in shock or with significant hypoxemia) and are breathing adequately (ie, adequate tidal volume and normal rate and regularity). Contraindications include apnea and poor respiratory effort. Because the nonrebreathing mask delivers oxygen passively, the patient's respirations must be of adequate depth to open the one-way valve, thus slightly collapsing the reservoir bag, and drawing air into the lungs. A patient with a marked reduction in tidal volume (shallow breathing) will benefit little, if at all, from a nonrebreathing mask.

Nasal Cannula

The **nasal cannula** delivers oxygen via two small prongs that fit into the patient's nostrils **FIGURE 16-46**. With an oxygen flow rate of 1 to 6 L/min, the nasal cannula can deliver an oxygen concentration of 24% to 44%. Use an oxygen humidifier (discussed later in this section) when giving oxygen via nasal cannula for a prolonged period because it will help prevent mucosal drying and irritation.

The nasal cannula provides low to moderate oxygen enrichment and is most beneficial for patients with mild hypoxemia (oxygen saturation level between 90% and 93%) and for patients who require long-term oxygen therapy (eg, for COPD). It is ineffective if the patient is apneic, has poor respiratory effort, is severely hypoxic, or is a mouth breather. In the prehospital setting, the nasal cannula is primarily used when patients who need oxygen cannot tolerate a nonrebreathing mask or if they require only low concentrations of oxygen to maintain an oxygen saturation level of greater than 94%.

The nasal cannula is generally well tolerated, especially by patients who are claustrophobic and intolerant of an oxygen mask over the face. However, it does not provide high volumes or concentrations of oxygen.

Partial Rebreathing Mask

A **partial rebreathing mask** is similar to the nonrebreathing mask except that it lacks a one-way valve between the mask and the reservoir **FIGURE 16-47**. Consequently, patients rebreathe a small amount of their exhaled air. Room air is not drawn in with inhalation, but residual exhaled air is mixed in the mask and rebreathed.

Contraindications are the same as for the nonrebreathing mask: any patient with apnea or inadequate tidal volume. At flow rates of 6 to 10 L/min, an oxygen concentration of 35% to 60% is possible with these devices. Increasing the oxygen flow rate beyond 10 L/min will not enhance the oxygen concentration, and leakage from the mask around the face decreases the amount of oxygen inhaled by the patient.

Venturi Mask

The **Venturi mask** draws room air into the mask along with the oxygen flow, allowing for the

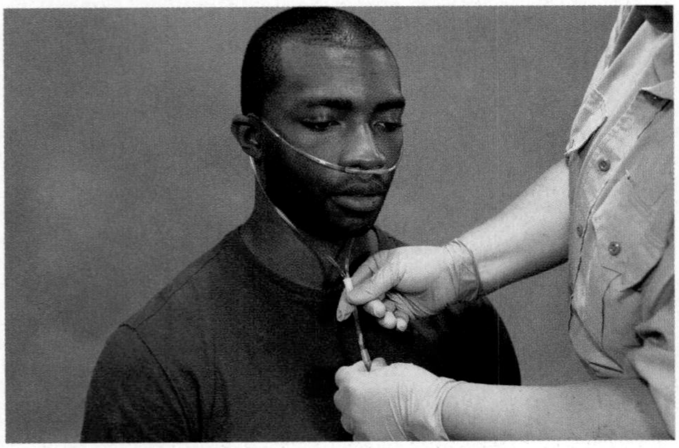

FIGURE 16-46 Nasal cannula.

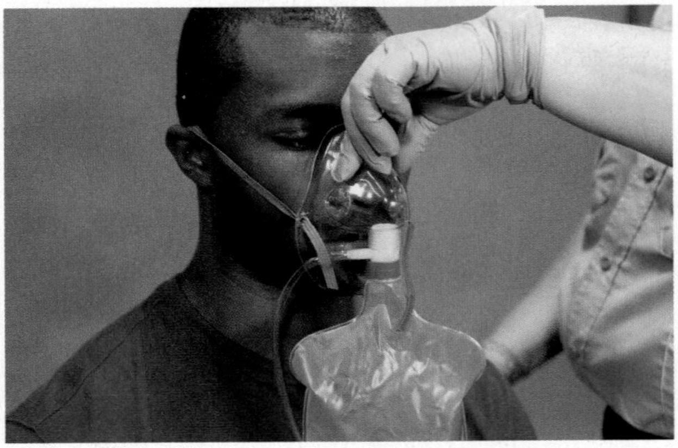

FIGURE 16-47 Partial rebreathing mask.

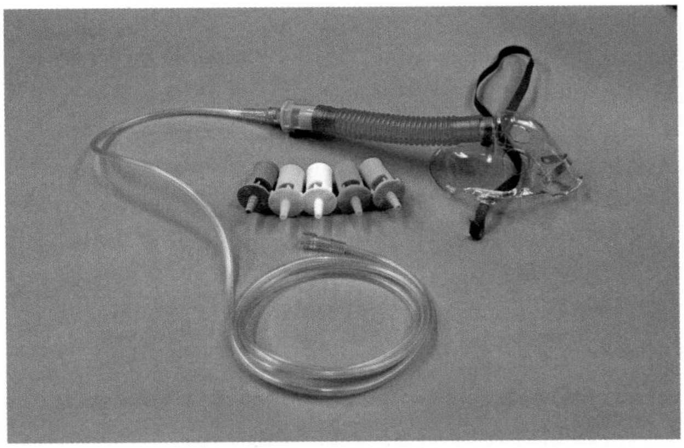

FIGURE 16-48 Venturi mask.

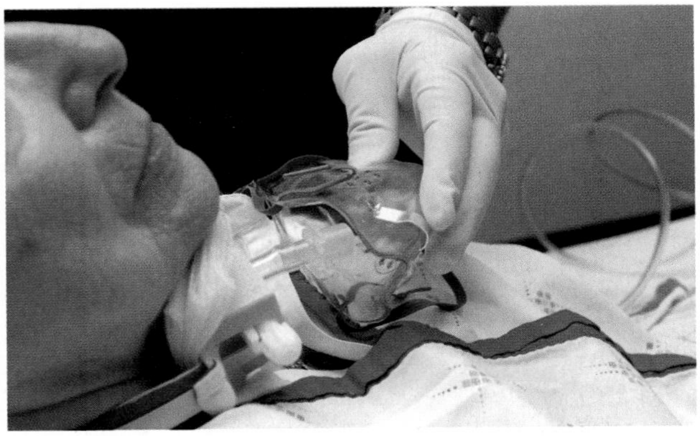

FIGURE 16-49 If a tracheostomy mask is unavailable, then use a face mask instead.

administration of highly specific oxygen concentrations **FIGURE 16-48**. Depending on the adapter used, the Venturi mask can deliver 24%, 28%, 35%, or 40% oxygen. These devices are especially useful in hospital-based care of patients with COPD and other chronic respiratory diseases. They can also benefit patients who require precise oxygen concentrations during long-distance interfacility transports.

Tracheostomy Masks

Patients with tracheostomies do not breathe through the nose and mouth; therefore, a face mask or nasal cannula would be ineffective for providing oxygen to them. Masks designed specifically for patients with tracheostomies cover the tracheostomy hole (stoma) and have a strap that goes around the neck. These masks are usually available in ICUs, where many patients have tracheostomies, and may be unavailable in the emergency setting. If you do not have a tracheostomy mask, then you can improvise by placing a face mask over the stoma. Even though the mask is shaped to fit the face, you can usually get an adequate fit over the patient's neck by adjusting the strap **FIGURE 16-49**.

TABLE 16-9 compares oxygen-delivery devices.

TABLE 16-9 Oxygen-Delivery Devices

Device	Flow Rate	Oxygen Delivered
Nasal cannula	1–6 L/min	24%–44%
Partial rebreathing mask	6–10 L/min	35%–60%
Mouth-to-mask device	15 L/min	Nearly 55%
Nonrebreathing mask	15 L/min	Up to 90%
Bag-mask device with oxygen reservoir	15 L/min	Nearly 100%

Oxygen Humidifier

Oxygen stored in cylinders has zero humidity, and it is not a good idea to deliver dry gases to a patient's airway for long periods. In fact, oxygen that is entirely devoid of moisture will rapidly dry the patient's mucous membranes. An **oxygen humidifier** consists of a small bottle of sterile water through which the oxygen leaving the cylinder becomes moisturized before it reaches the patient **FIGURE 16-50**. Because the humidifier must be kept in an upright position, it is practical only for use with the fixed oxygen unit in the ambulance. In addition, oxygen humidifiers can be a source of infection for the patient. For this reason, you should use a disposable bottle as the humidifier unit.

Ventilatory Support

Obviously, a patient who is not breathing needs artificial ventilation and high-flow supplemental oxygen. Artificial ventilation is among the most

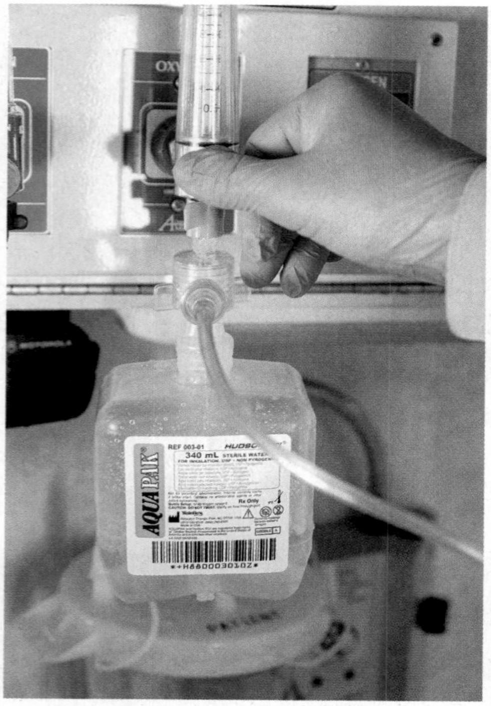

FIGURE 16-50 Administering humidified oxygen is preferred for long-distance transports to avoid drying the patient's mucous membranes.

important skills in EMS at any level. Artificial ventilation is the skill of providing assisted ventilation to a patient who is breathing spontaneously, or of ventilating a patient who is not breathing at all. Artificial ventilation techniques are extremely effective when performed properly. Mastery of these techniques is imperative.

Patients who are breathing inadequately, such as too fast or too slowly with reduced tidal volume (shallow breathing), are often unable to speak in complete sentences. An irregular breathing pattern may also require artificial ventilation to assist in maintaining adequate minute volume. Fast, shallow breathing can be just as dangerous as very slow breathing. Fast, shallow breathing moves air primarily in the larger airway passages (dead space) and does not allow for adequate exchange of oxygen and carbon dioxide in the alveoli. Signs of a depressed mental status and inadequate minute volume are indications for assisted ventilation. In addition, excessive accessory muscle use and fatigue from labored breathing are signs of potential respiratory failure. Patients with these signs need immediate treatment.

Two treatment options are available for patients with severe respiratory distress or respiratory failure: (1) positive-pressure ventilation with a bag-mask device or (2) CPAP or bilevel positive airway pressure (BPAP). The purpose of assisted ventilation is to improve the overall oxygenation and ventilatory status of the patient. CPAP and BPAP are discussed later in this chapter; this section focuses on assisted ventilation with a bag-mask device.

Normal Ventilation Versus Positive-Pressure Ventilation

The act of moving air into and out of the lungs is based on pressure changes within the thoracic cavity. During normal ventilation, the diaphragm contracts and the intercostal muscles expand the chest, generating negative pressure in the chest cavity. This negative pressure draws air into the chest through the mouth/nose and trachea in an attempt to equalize the pressure in the chest with the pressure of the external atmosphere (negative-pressure ventilation). However, positive-pressure ventilation generated by a device, such as a bag-mask device, forces air into the chest cavity from the external environment. It is important to understand the differences between normal ventilation and positive-pressure ventilation because aggressive positive-pressure ventilation can impair a patient's hemodynamics and push air into the stomach **TABLE 16-10**.

The physical act of the chest wall expanding and recoiling during breathing aids the circulatory system in returning blood to the heart. During normal ventilation, the chest wall movement works similarly to a pump. The pressure changes in the thoracic cavity help draw venous blood back to the heart, which improves preload. However, when positive-pressure ventilation is initiated, more air is needed to achieve the same oxygenation and ventilatory effects of normal breathing. This increase in airway wall pressure causes the walls of the chest cavity to push out of their normal anatomic shape, resulting in an increase in intrathoracic pressure. Positive pressure also affects venous return to the heart, which reduces preload. The blood flow is decreased due to the increased intrathoracic pressure. This decreased blood flow results in insufficient venous return to the heart, and as a result,

TABLE 16-10 Normal Ventilation Versus Positive-Pressure Ventilation

	Normal Ventilation	Positive-Pressure Ventilation
Air movement	Air is sucked into the lungs due to the negative intrathoracic pressure created when the diaphragm contracts.	Air is forced into the lungs by means of mechanical ventilation.
Blood movement	Normal breathing facilitates venous return, thereby maintaining preload.	Intrathoracic pressure is increased, which impairs venous return (and preload); as a result, stroke volume and cardiac output are reduced.
Airway wall pressure	Not affected during normal breathing	More volume is required to have the same effects as normal breathing. As a result, the walls are pushed out of their normal anatomic shapes.
Esophageal opening pressure	Not affected during normal breathing	Air is forced into the stomach, causing gastric distention that could result in vomiting and aspiration.
Overventilation	Not typical of normal breathing	Forcing volume and rate results in increased intrathoracic pressure, gastric distention, and decreased cardiac output (hypotension).

the amount of blood pumped out of the heart is reduced.

Therefore, it is *imperative* that you regulate the rate and volume of artificial ventilations to help prevent this drop in cardiac output. Cardiac output is a function of stroke volume multiplied by the pulse rate; stroke volume is the amount of blood ejected by the ventricle in one cardiac cycle. Cardiac output is quantified as the amount of blood ejected by the left ventricle in 1 minute.

Another difference between normal ventilation and positive-pressure ventilation relates to the control of airflow. When a person breathes, air enters the trachea and, generally, not the esophagus. However, the force generated from positive-pressure ventilation allows air to enter not only the trachea, but also the esophagus. Ventilations that are too forceful can open the esophagus (normally a flat tube) and instill air in the stomach. This potential complication, called **gastric distention**, is discussed later in this chapter.

Assisted Ventilation

Follow these steps to assist a conscious patient's ventilations using a bag-mask device. Remember to first explain the procedure to the patient, and take standard precautions (discussed later in this chapter) as needed when managing the patient's airway.

1. Place the mask over the patient's nose and mouth.
2. Squeeze the bag each time the patient inhales, maintaining the same rate as the patient, coaching the patient as needed.
3. After the initial 5 to 10 breaths, slowly adjust the rate and deliver the appropriate tidal volume.
4. Adjust the rate and tidal volume to maintain adequate minute volume.

Artificial Ventilation

Without immediate treatment, patients who are in respiratory arrest will die. The act of breathing for a patient, or artificial ventilation, is a skill that must be practiced frequently and should not be taken lightly. After you determine that a patient is not breathing, begin artificial ventilation immediately. The methods that you may use to provide artificial ventilation include the mouth-to-mask technique and the one- and two-person bag-mask device techniques.

Mouth-to-Mask Ventilation

As you learned in your CPR course, ventilation is routinely performed with a barrier device, such as a mask with a one-way valve or a plastic face shield **FIGURE 16-51**. A barrier device is a protective item that features a plastic barrier placed on a patient's face with a one-way valve to prevent the backflow of secretions, vomitus, and gases. Barrier devices provide you with adequate protection during mouth-to-mask ventilation.

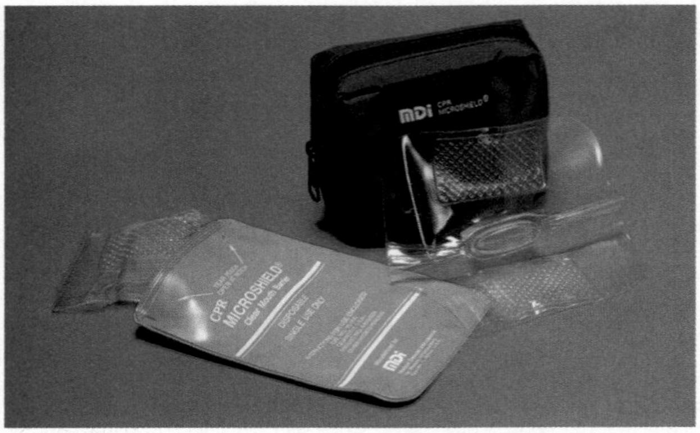

FIGURE 16-51 Plastic face shield.

Mouth-to-mask ventilation (or ventilation using another barrier device) should be performed only if a bag-mask device is unavailable. Advantages of using a mask during ventilation of a patient include placing a physical barrier between your mouth and the patient's mouth. Most masks feature a one-way valve to prevent the provider's exposure to blood and other body fluids. It is also easier to secure an effective seal with a mask because you can use both hands, which enables you to provide adequate tidal volume to the patient.

A mask with an oxygen inlet provides oxygen during mouth-to-mask ventilation to supplement the air from your own lungs. Remember that the gas you exhale contains 16% oxygen, which is adequate to sustain a patient's life for a limited period. With the mouth-to-mask technique, however, the patient receives the additional benefit of significant oxygen enrichment with inspired air: up to 55%. Consider carrying a face mask device with one-way valve in your personal vehicle, in case you encounter an apneic patient while off duty.

The mask may be shaped like a triangle or a doughnut, with the apex (top) placed across the bridge of the nose. The base (bottom) of the mask is

YOU are the Paramedic

PART 5

After administering an appropriate dose of ketamine via the intramuscular route, you find that the patient is less agitated and will now accept CPAP therapy. You reassess his clinical status while your partner retrieves the ambulance stretcher. At this time, you also establish IV access.

Recording Time: 11 Minutes	
Level of consciousness	Conscious, but sedated
Respirations	24 breaths/min; less labored
Pulse	122 beats/min; strong and regular
Skin	Warm and moist; lip and gum color returning to baseline
Blood pressure	176/92 mm Hg
Oxygen saturation (Spo_2)	87%
Pupils	PERRLA
$ETCO_2$	51 mm Hg
ECG	Sinus tachycardia

8. Why is the patient's condition improving, even though you administered sedation?

9. What role does capnography play in assessing a patient's ventilation status?

placed in the groove between the lower lip and the chin. In the center of the mask is a chimney with a 16-mm connector.

Mouth-to-Mask Ventilation Technique

To ventilate a patient using a pocket face mask, open the patient's airway with the head tilt–chin lift or jaw-thrust maneuver. Insert an oral or nasal airway to help maintain airway patency. Connect the one-way valve to the face mask, and place the mask on the patient's face. Ensure the top of the mask is placed over the bridge of the nose and the bottom is between the lower lip and chin. Hold the mask in position by placing your thumbs over the top part of the mask and your index fingers over the bottom half. Grasp the patient's lower jaw with the next three fingers on each hand. Place your thumbs on the dome of the mask, making an airtight seal by applying firm pressure between the thumbs and fingers. Maintain an upward and forward pull on the patient's lower jaw with your fingers to keep the airway open **FIGURE 16-52A**. Exhale slowly over a period of 1 second, just enough to produce visible chest rise, then remove your mouth from the one-way valve and allow the patient to passively exhale **FIGURE 16-52B**.

The effectiveness of ventilation is best determined by watching the patient's chest rise and fall and feeling for resistance of the patient's lungs as they expand. You should also hear and feel air escape as the patient passively exhales. Ensure you provide the correct number of breaths per minute for the patient's age **TABLE 16-11**.

The Bag-Mask Device

With an oxygen flow rate of 15 L/min and an adequate seal, a bag-mask device with an oxygen reservoir can deliver nearly 100% oxygen **FIGURE 16-53**. Most bag-mask devices on the market include modifications or accessories (reservoirs) that permit the delivery of oxygen concentration levels approaching 100%. However, the device can deliver only as much volume as can be squeezed out of the bag by hand. Although the bag-mask device provides less tidal volume than mouth-to-mask ventilation, it delivers oxygen at a much higher concentration.

The bag-mask device is the device most commonly used to ventilate patients in the prehospital setting. An experienced paramedic will be able to provide adequate tidal volume with the bag-mask device. However, its use can be a difficult skill to master, especially if you do not have many opportunities to practice. The mask seal on a medical patient may be difficult to maintain with only one rescuer. Because it takes two hands to perform a jaw-thrust maneuver, it takes two rescuers to use the bag-mask device on a trauma patient unless an advanced airway has already been inserted. The amount of tidal volume and the concentration of oxygen delivered to the patient depend on maintaining the integrity of the mask seal. You should practice this skill frequently by ventilating a manikin with the bag-mask device.

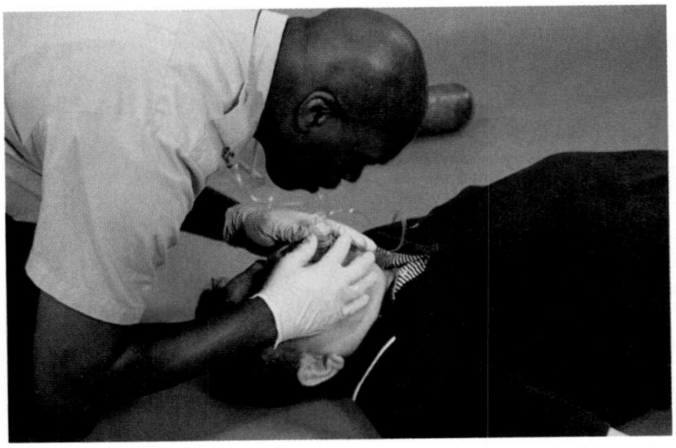

A

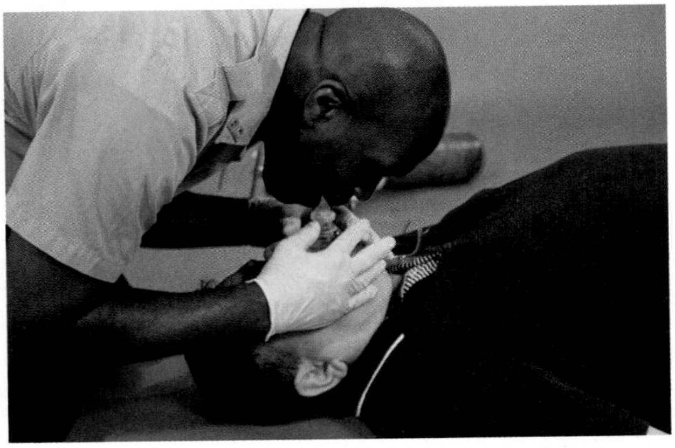

B

FIGURE 16-52 A. Open the patient's airway and properly position the mask on the patient's face. **B.** Deliver each breath over a period of 1 second, observe for chest rise, and allow the patient to passively exhale.

TABLE 16-11 Ventilation Rates by Age

Onset of puberty (12 to 14 years of age) and older	Apneic with a pulse: 1 breath every 6 seconds (10 breaths/min) • With or without an advanced airway in place (eg, ET tube, LMA, i-gel supraglottic airway) Apneic and pulseless (after advanced airway insertion): 1 breath every 6 seconds (10 breaths/min) with continuous chest compressions
Infant (ages 1 month to 1 year) and child (ages 1 year to the onset of puberty)	Inadequate respiratory effort or apneic with a pulse: 1 breath every 2 to 3 seconds (20 to 30 breaths/min) • With or without an advanced airway in place (eg, ET tube, LMA, i-gel supraglottic airway) Apneic and pulseless (after advanced airway insertion): 1 breath every 2 to 3 seconds (20 to 30 breaths/min)

Abbreviations: ET, endotracheal; LMA, laryngeal mask airway

Avoid hyperventilating any patient; hyperventilated lungs may "squeeze" the heart, thus impeding venous return and subsequent cardiac output. Hyperventilation also increases the risks of regurgitation and aspiration.

Data from: Panchal AR, Bartos JA, Cabañas JG, et al. Part 3: adult basic and advanced life support. *Circulation.* 2020;142(suppl 2):S366-S468; Topjian AA, Raymond TT, Atkins D, et al. Part 4: pediatric basic and advanced life support. *Circulation.* 2020;142(suppl 2):S469-S523.

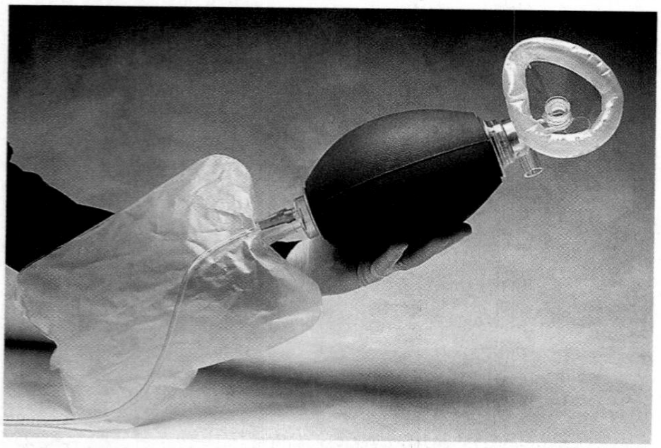

FIGURE 16-53 A bag-mask device with an oxygen reservoir can deliver nearly 100% oxygen if a good seal between the face and mask is maintained and if supplemental oxygen is attached to the device.

Bag-Mask Device Components

All adult bag-mask devices should have the following components and characteristics:

- A disposable, self-inflating bag
- No pop-off valve or, if one is present, then the capability of disabling the pop-off valve
- An outlet valve that is a true nonrebreathing valve
- An oxygen reservoir that permits delivery of a high concentration of oxygen
- A one-way, no-jam inlet valve system that provides an oxygen inlet flow at a maximum of 15 L/min with a standard 15/22-mm fitting for a face mask and an advanced airway (ie, ET tube, laryngeal mask airway [LMA], King LT, i-gel)
- A transparent face mask
- The ability to perform under extreme environmental conditions, including extreme heat and cold

The reservoir bag of an adult bag-mask device usually holds a maximum of 1,200 to 1,600 mL of

SAFETY

Airway management and ventilation procedures often expose providers to blood, vomitus, oral secretions, and aerosolized respiratory droplets. Although blood is the most potentially infectious body fluid, you should exercise great caution to avoid contact with all body fluids. Wear gloves for all airway and ventilation procedures and when handling airway equipment that might have been contaminated with body fluids. To reduce the risk of splashing or aerosolized droplets of body fluid coming in contact with your mouth, nose, and eyes, wear a mask and protective eyewear or a face shield when performing any airway management procedure. When assisting ventilations in the event of a pandemic or when caring for a patient who has a highly contagious disease, place a high-efficiency particulate air (HEPA) viral/bacterial filter between the mask, or advanced airway device, and the bag to reduce the amount of infectious material that becomes airborne. In cases involving significant blood splashing, or if the patient is suspected of having an infectious respiratory infection (eg, SARS-CoV-2 [severe acute respiratory syndrome–coronavirus 2], tuberculosis), you should also wear a protective gown.

gas. The pediatric bag contains 500 to 700 mL, and the infant bag holds 150 to 240 mL.

The volume of air (oxygen) to deliver to the patient is based on one key observation: visible chest rise. A delivered tidal volume of 500 to 600 mL (6 to 7 mL/kg) per breath will produce visible chest rise in most adults. When using a bag-mask device, deliver each breath over a period of 1 second (just enough to produce visible chest rise) at the appropriate rate. Breaths that are given too forcefully or too fast can result in two negative effects: gastric distention (associated with risks of vomiting and aspiration) and decreased venous return to the heart (reducing preload) due to increased intrathoracic pressure.

Improper technique, an ineffective mask-to-face seal, or the presence of gastric distention may cause you to deliver inadequate tidal volume and oxygen. Training and practice are key to ensure proper use of the bag-mask device.

Bag-Mask Device Technique

Whenever possible, you and your partner should work together to provide ventilation with the bag-mask device. One paramedic can maintain a good mask seal by securing the mask to the patient's face with two hands, while the other paramedic squeezes the bag. Ventilation using a bag-mask device is a challenging skill; it may be difficult for you to maintain a proper seal between the mask and the face with one hand while simultaneously squeezing the bag well enough to deliver an adequate volume of air to the patient. As mentioned previously, effective one-person bag-mask ventilation requires considerable practice and experience. Also, performance of this skill depends on having enough personnel to carry out other actions that need to be done simultaneously, such as chest compressions, putting the stretcher in place, or helping to lift the patient onto the stretcher.

Follow these steps to use the two-person bag-mask device technique:

1. Kneel above the patient's head. If possible, your partner should be at the side of the head. Select the proper size of mask.
2. Maintain the patient's neck in a neutral position. Open the airway and suction the oropharynx as needed. Insert an oral or nasal airway to help maintain airway patency.
3. Connect the bag-mask device to supplemental oxygen.
4. Place the mask on the patient's face. Ensure the top is positioned over the bridge of the nose and the bottom is placed in the groove between the lower lip and the chin. If the mask has a large, round cuff around the ventilation port, center the port over the patient's mouth. Inflate (or deflate) the collar to obtain a better fit and seal to the patient's face, if necessary.
5. Bring the lower jaw up to the mask with your last three fingers. This step will help to maintain an open airway. Ensure you do not grab the fleshy part of the patient's neck, as doing so may compress structures and create an airway obstruction. If you think the patient may have a spinal injury, ensure your partner manually stabilizes the cervical spine as you move the lower jaw.
6. Connect the bag to the mask, if you have not already done so.
7. Hold the mask in place while your partner squeezes the bag with two hands until the patient's chest visibly rises **FIGURE 16-54**. If a spinal injury is suspected, stabilize the patient's head and neck with your forearms while maintaining an adequate mask-to-face seal with your hands. Continue squeezing the bag once every 6 seconds for adults and once every 2 to 3 seconds for infants and children.

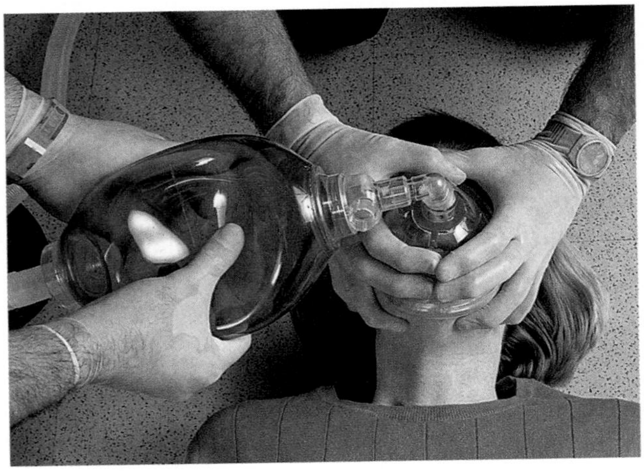

FIGURE 16-54 With two-person bag-mask ventilation, hold the mask in place while your partner squeezes the bag with two hands until the patient's chest visibly rises.

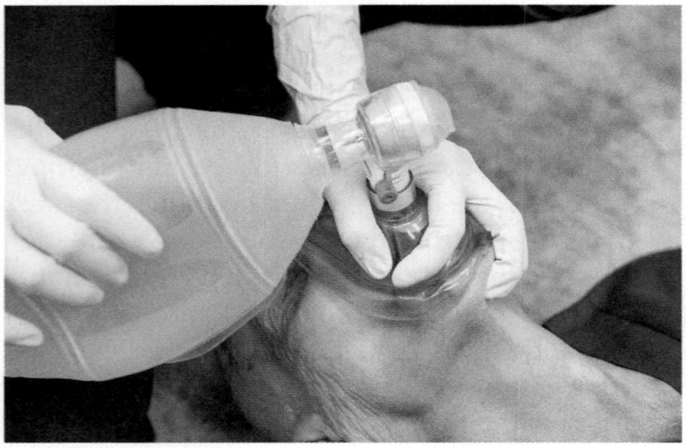

FIGURE 16-55 Maintain the seal of the mask to the face using the EC clamp technique, if you are ventilating the patient by yourself.

8. If you are alone, place your thumb and index finger as high up on the mask as you can to form a C. Maintain the airway by lifting the bony prominence of the chin with your remaining fingers to form an E. Do not push the mask to the patient's face; instead, pull the patient's lower jaw into the mask. This practice, called the EC clamp technique, will maintain an effective mask-to-face seal **FIGURE 16-55**. Use the head tilt–chin lift maneuver to ensure that the airway is open. Squeeze the bag with your other hand in a rhythmic manner once every 6 seconds for adults and once every 2 to 3 seconds for infants and children.
9. Observe for gastric distention, changes in compliance of the bag with ventilations, and either improvement or deterioration of the patient's clinical status.

When using the bag-mask device to assist ventilation, you should squeeze the bag as the patient inhales. Then, for the next 5 to 10 breaths, slowly adjust the rate and tidal volume until an adequate minute volume is achieved.

To assist ventilations of a conscious patient who is breathing too fast (hyperventilation) with reduced tidal volume, first explain the procedure if the patient is coherent. Initially assist ventilations at the rate at which the patient has been breathing, squeezing the bag each time the patient inhales. Then, for the next 5 to 10 breaths, slowly adjust the rate and tidal volume until an adequate minute volume is achieved.

As you are ventilating a patient with a bag-mask device, evaluate the effectiveness of your ventilations. Artificial ventilations are inadequate if the patient's chest does not rise and fall with each ventilation, if you are unable to hear breath sounds when auscultating the chest, if the rate of ventilation is too slow or too fast for the patient's age, or if the pulse rate and/or oxygen saturation level do not improve. If the patient's chest does not rise and fall, you may need to reposition the head or insert an oral and/or nasal airway.

If the patient's stomach, rather than the chest, seems to be rising and falling, reposition the head. In a patient with a possible spinal injury, you should reposition the jaw rather than the head. If too much air is escaping from under the mask, readjust your hands and reposition the mask for a better seal. If the patient's chest still does not rise and fall after you have made these corrections, check for an airway obstruction. If an obstruction is not present, attempt ventilation with another device.

Advanced airway techniques are beneficial when ventilation with basic means is ineffective, the patient has a cervical spine injury, or the patient's condition otherwise warrants them.

Words of Wisdom

Indications That Artificial Ventilation Is Adequate[a]

- Adequate and equal chest rise and fall with ventilation
- Breath sounds can be heard during auscultation of the chest
- Ventilations are given at the appropriate rate:
  - 10 breaths/min for adults
  - 20 to 30 breaths/min for infants and children
- Pulse rate returns to a normal range
- Oxygen saturation level improves

Indications That Artificial Ventilation Is Inadequate

- Minimal or no chest rise and fall
- Breath sounds cannot be heard during auscultation of the chest
- Ventilations given too fast or too slow for patient's age
- Pulse rate does not return to a normal range
- Oxygen saturation level does not improve

[a]In patients who are apneic with a pulse (ie, not in cardiac arrest).

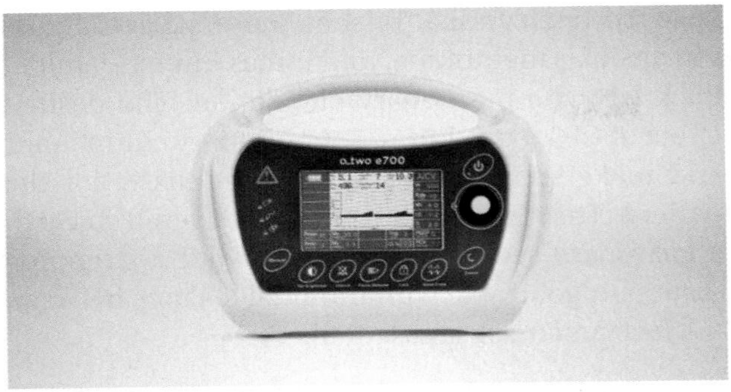

FIGURE 16-56 Automatic transport ventilator.

Used with permission of O-Two Medical Technologies, Inc.

Automatic Transport Ventilators

The **automatic transport ventilator (ATV)** allows the variables of ventilation—ventilatory rate, tidal volume, and peak inspiratory time—to be precisely set; these features allow for consistent ventilation **FIGURE 16-56**. Many types of ATVs are available. Some offer only basic settings; others include more advanced settings and features, such as FIO_2 titration, inspiratory-to-expiratory (I:E) ratio, and positive end-expiratory pressure (PEEP). In addition, different ventilation modes can be set with more sophisticated ATVs, including assist/control (AC), synchronized intermittent mandatory ventilation (SIMV), and pressure support.

In AC mode, the ventilator guarantees a minimum ventilation rate. The patient can breathe over the set rate, but each breath is at the preset tidal volume or pressure. Thus, AC mode controls the work of breathing but allows the patient to set the respiratory rate.

In SIMV mode, a set respiratory rate and volume or pressure are delivered and synchronized with each patient-initiated breath. Each breath is at the patient-initiated volume. The machine will deliver a certain number of mandatory breaths; all other breaths are spontaneous, at the patient's own rate and depth. SIMV mode allows the patient to assume some or most of the work of breathing, depending on the mandatory rate.

Pressure support is a clinician-selected amount of positive pressure used to augment a patient's spontaneous breaths. The pressure overcomes the superimposed resistance of the airway and ventilator circuit and improves lung compliance. This mode of ventilation requires the patient to be able to initiate a breath.

The steps for using the ATV are as follows:

1. Attach the ATV to the wall-mounted oxygen source.
2. Set the ventilatory rate, tidal volume, and peak inspiratory time on the ATV as appropriate for the patient's age and condition. If available and clinically indicated, set the ventilation mode and I:E ratio accordingly.
3. Connect the ATV to the 15/22-mm fitting on the ET tube or other advanced airway device.
4. Auscultate the patient's breath sounds and observe for equal chest rise to ensure adequate ventilation.

Although the ATV lacks the sophisticated controls of a hospital ventilator, it frees your hands to perform other, non–airway-related tasks. However, although the ATV is helpful to paramedics, you must always have a bag-mask device readily available should the ATV malfunction.

The respiratory rate is set at the midpoint or average for the patient's age in most cases. You can estimate tidal volume using a formula based on 6 to 7 mL/kg of ideal body weight, which can be adjusted based on chest rise and the patient's physiologic response. ATVs are considered volume-cycled, rate-controlled ventilators, which means that they deliver a preset volume at a preset ventilatory rate, although this does not guarantee that all of the volume is being delivered to the lungs, unless the patient is intubated. When using the ATV in the intubated patient who is in cardiac arrest, it is critical to set the rate and tidal volume accordingly to reduce the risk of hyperventilation.

Most ATVs are oxygen-powered, although some models may require an external power source. This kind of ventilator generally consumes

Words of Wisdom

An adult's lungs do not increase in size or hold more volume just because of increased body weight. This is why tidal volume with a mechanical ventilator, such as an ATV, is set based on the patient's ideal body weight (IBW)—*not* the actual body weight. Calculate a patient's ideal body weight as follows:

Males: IBW = 50 kg + 2.3 kg for each inch over 5 feet

Females: IBW = 45.5 kg + 2.3 kg for each inch over 5 feet

5 L/min of oxygen, whereas a bag-mask device uses 15 to 25 L/min. In addition, the ATV has a pressure relief valve, which can lead to hypoventilation in patients with inadequate lung compliance, increased airway resistance, or airway obstruction. The possibility of **barotrauma** (trauma resulting from excessive pressure) exists if the pressure relief valve fails or if ventilation is too fast or too forceful.

Continuous Positive Airway Pressure

Continuous positive airway pressure (CPAP) is a noninvasive means of providing ventilatory support for patients experiencing respiratory distress. Many people with obstructive sleep apnea wear a CPAP unit at night to maintain their airway while they sleep **FIGURE 16-57**. The use of CPAP in the prehospital setting has proved to be an excellent adjunct in the treatment of respiratory distress caused by acute pulmonary edema, obstructive lung disease, and acute bronchospasm (such as in asthma), especially when used in conjunction with beta-2 agonists. Typically, many patients with these conditions would be managed with advanced airway techniques, such as ET intubation. Early intervention with CPAP is an alternative means of providing ventilatory assistance and can prevent the need for intubation. Because of the simplicity of the device and its great benefit to patients, CPAP is widely used by paramedics.

CPAP increases pressure in the lungs, opens collapsed alveoli and prevents further alveolar collapse (atelectasis), pushes more oxygen across the alveolar membrane, and forces interstitial fluid back into the pulmonary circulation. The desired effect of CPAP is to improve pulmonary compliance and make spontaneous ventilation easier for the patient. This therapy is typically delivered through a face mask secured to the head with a strapping system. A good seal with minimal leakage between the face and mask is essential.

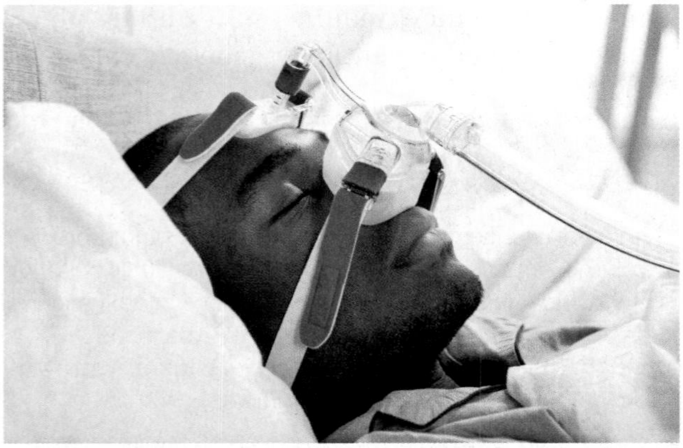

FIGURE 16-57 Many people with sleep apnea wear a CPAP unit at night to maintain their airway while they sleep.

Special Populations

Artificial Ventilation of Pediatric Patients

The flat nasal bridge of pediatric patients makes it more challenging to achieve an effective mask-to-face seal compared with adult patients. In addition, compressing the mask against the pediatric patient's face to improve the mask seal may result in obstruction. The best mask seal is achieved by the two-person bag-mask ventilation technique with jaw displacement.

Use a pediatric bag-mask device with a minimum tidal volume of 450 mL for term neonates and infants. In children (ages 1 year to the onset of puberty [ages 12 to 14 years]), consider the child's size when determining bag size. You may use an adult-size bag-mask device with a volume of 1,500 mL, but a pediatric bag-mask device is preferred. Children older than 12 to 14 years require an adult-size bag-mask device for adequate ventilation. Choose a size that will ensure a proper mask fit. The mask should reach from the bridge of the nose to the cleft of the chin. A length-based resuscitation tape may also be used to estimate the most appropriate size of bag-mask device for pediatric patients who weigh up to 75 pounds (34 kg).

When you are ventilating a pediatric patient, ensure a proper mask seal by using the EC clamp technique (discussed earlier in this chapter). Avoid placing pressure on the soft area under the chin, because this pressure may cause an airway obstruction. In addition, avoid placing pressure on the patient's eyes with the mask. Doing so can stimulate the oculocardiac reflex, which involves decreasing the heart rate and/or BP level. Also, if the mask is positioned too high on the face, it will leak around the orbits.

Deliver each ventilation over 1 second: just enough to produce visible chest rise. Do not overinflate. Deliver one breath every 2 to 3 seconds (20 to 30 breaths/min), allowing adequate time for exhalation. While ventilating, look for adequate chest rise. Auscultate breath sounds at the third or fourth intercostal space on the midaxillary line bilaterally. Also assess for improvements in skin color, pulse rate, oxygen saturation, and $ETCO_2$.

The face mask is fitted with a pressure relief valve that determines the amount of pressure delivered to the patient (such as 5 cm of water [cm H_2O]). This pressure results in a high inspiratory flow and the need to push a pressure valve open with exhalation. Although a great deal of effort is often required to achieve this outcome, especially while the patient is in respiratory distress, many patients improve dramatically when CPAP is applied.

Indications for CPAP

CPAP is indicated for patients experiencing respiratory distress in which their own compensatory mechanisms cannot keep up with their oxygen demands. Although the condition of most patients improves after the application of CPAP, it is important to remember that CPAP is merely treating the symptoms; it is not necessarily treating the underlying pathology.

The following conditions are general indications for using CPAP:

- Patient is alert and able to follow commands
- Obvious signs of moderate to severe respiratory distress (eg, accessory muscle use, tripod position, retractions) from an underlying disease such as heart failure with pulmonary edema, obstructive lung disease (eg, COPD), acute bronchospasm (eg, in acute asthma), and suspected pneumonia
- Respiratory distress after a submersion incident
- Breathing that is so rapid that it affects overall minute volume
- Pulse oximetry reading of less than 90%

Although you should consider these guidelines when assessing the need for CPAP, it is important that you follow your local guidelines and protocols.

Contraindications for CPAP

CPAP can be immensely beneficial to patients experiencing respiratory distress from acute pulmonary edema, acute bronchospasm, and obstructive lung disease; however, at times CPAP is not appropriate.

The following conditions are general contraindications for using CPAP:

- Patient is unresponsive or otherwise unable to follow verbal commands
- Respiratory arrest or agonal respirations
- Patient is unable to speak
- Patient is unable to protect the airway
- Hypoventilation (slow respiratory rate and/or reduced tidal volume)
- Hypotension (systolic BP is less than 90 mm Hg)
- Signs and symptoms of a pneumothorax or chest trauma (either blunt or penetrating)
- Closed head injury
- Facial trauma
- Cardiogenic shock
- Tracheostomy
- Active gastrointestinal bleeding, nausea, or vomiting
- History of recent gastrointestinal surgical procedure
- Patient is unable to sit up
- Inability to properly fit the CPAP system mask and strap
  - Excessive facial hair or dysmorphic facial features can impede your ability to ensure a proper-fitting mask and tight seal.
- Patient cannot tolerate the mask

In addition, always reassess the patient for signs of clinical deterioration and/or respiratory failure. Although CPAP is an excellent tool to assist with ventilation, not all patients will experience improvement in their conditions with use of this device. After signs of respiratory failure become apparent or the patient is no longer able to follow commands, you should remove the CPAP device and initiate positive-pressure ventilation with a bag-mask device attached to high-flow oxygen. In some patients, intubation will be required.

Application of CPAP

Several varieties of CPAP units are available to EMS systems; however, most follow the same general guidelines for use and setup. The CPAP unit typically consists of a generator, a mask, a circuit that contains corrugated tubing, a bacteria filter, and a one-way valve. During the expiratory phase, the patient exhales against a resistance called expiratory positive airway pressure (EPAP), which generates **positive end-expiratory pressure (PEEP)**. Within the CPAP generator, a valve determines the amount of PEEP; however, some CPAP models have PEEP valves that connect separately. Depending on the device, the PEEP is controlled by manually adjusting the PEEP using a manometer or is predetermined by a fixed setting on the PEEP valve. A PEEP of 5 to

10 cm H_2O is generally an acceptable therapeutic range for a patient using CPAP, although it can be adjusted (higher or lower) if necessary. Always consult the operations manual of your particular CPAP device for proper assembly instructions.

Because most CPAP units are powered by oxygen, it is important to have a full cylinder of oxygen available when using CPAP and a backup cylinder. Some CPAP units use a continuous flow of oxygen, whereas others use oxygen on more of a demand basis. Continuously monitor the amount of oxygen available in the cylinder. Some CPAP units will empty a D cylinder in as little as 5 to 10 minutes. Therefore, proper planning for rapid oxygen consumption is necessary when considering applying CPAP. In addition, some of the newer CPAP devices allow you to adjust the F_{IO_2} level. Most CPAP devices are set to deliver a fixed F_{IO_2} level of 30% to 35%; however, some can deliver levels as high as 95%.

Follow the steps shown in **SKILL DRILL 16-2** to use CPAP.

Complications of CPAP

The application and administration of CPAP is a relatively easy process. However, some patients may find CPAP claustrophobic and will resist its application, and many patients will resist the therapy simply because they are already experiencing respiratory distress. As a patient becomes more hypoxic, the application of the mask to the face is sometimes perceived as suffocating, rather than an attempt to help with breathing. It is essential to explain the use of CPAP to patients and coach them through the application process, allowing them to adjust to the situation. Do not force the mask on any patient, as this will create a higher level of anxiety in the patient and increase oxygen demand. Coaching patients to accept CPAP is not always easy; it takes practice and a willingness to work closely with a patient during a difficult time.

Because of the high volume of pressure generated by CPAP, the emergence of a pneumothorax caused by barotrauma is possible. Remain alert to this risk, and continually assess the patient for signs and symptoms of a pneumothorax.

In addition to pneumothoraces, increased pressure in the chest cavity can result in hypotension. As the intrathoracic pressure increases, venous blood returning to the heart (which affects preload) meets resistance from the increased pressure in the chest, which can cause hypotension. Although hypotension is uncommon with lower levels of CPAP, it is essential to continuously monitor the patient's BP.

As with any form of positive-pressure ventilation in the unprotected airway, air may enter the stomach, which increases the risk of aspiration if vomiting occurs.

> **SAFETY**
>
> CPAP systems should be equipped with a viral filter to decrease aerosolized secretion dispersal during exhalation.

Gastric Distention

Any form of artificial ventilation that blows air into the patient's mouth, instead of blowing air directly into the trachea via an ET tube, may lead to inflation of the patient's stomach with air. Gastric distention, defined as inflation of the patient's stomach with air, is especially likely to occur if excessive pressure is used to inflate the lungs, if ventilations are performed too fast or too forcefully, or if the airway is partially obstructed during ventilation attempts. In such cases, the excessive pressure in the airway forces open the esophagus, allowing air to flow into the stomach. Gastric distention occurs most often in children but is common in adults as well.

> **Words of Wisdom**
>
> **Bilevel positive airway pressure (BPAP)**, another form of noninvasive positive-pressure ventilation, is also used to treat patients with obstructive lung disease, acute bronchospasm, and acute pulmonary edema. Whereas CPAP delivers a single pressure (which is most beneficial to the patient during exhalation), BPAP delivers two pressures: a higher inspiratory positive airway pressure (IPAP), which opens the lower airways, and a lower EPAP, which helps keep the lower airways open. Commonly used BPAP settings deliver 10 cm H_2O during inhalation and 5 cm H_2O during exhalation; the difference between the IPAP and the EPAP is called pressure support. The indications, contraindications, and precautions for BPAP are the same as those for CPAP. Follow your EMS system protocols regarding the use of BPAP and the desired IPAP and EPAP settings.

NR Skill

Skill Drill 16-2 Using CPAP

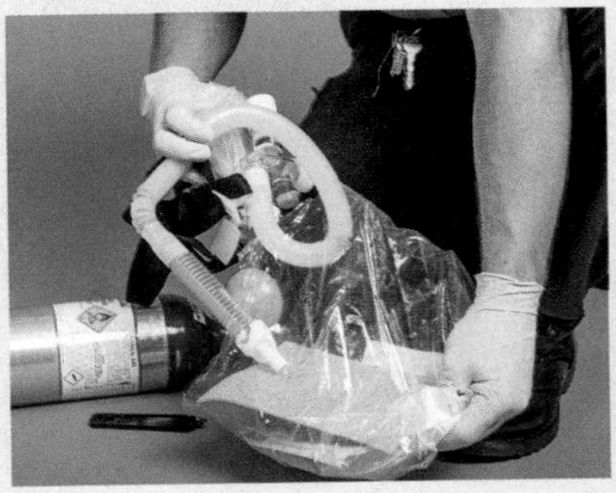

Step 1

Take standard precautions. Assess the patient for indications and contraindications of CPAP. Confirm the patient's BP, and explain the procedure. Check your equipment, then connect the circuit to the CPAP generator.

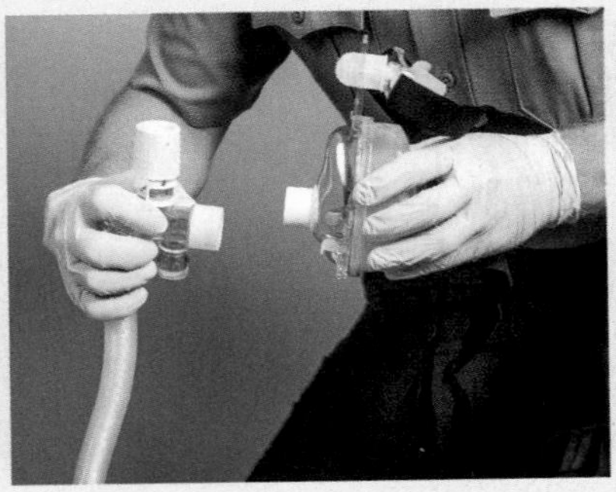

Step 2

Connect the face mask to the circuit tubing. After the system is connected, look for an on/off button or switch (some models have this feature). Confirm the device is powered on and working before you apply CPAP to the patient.

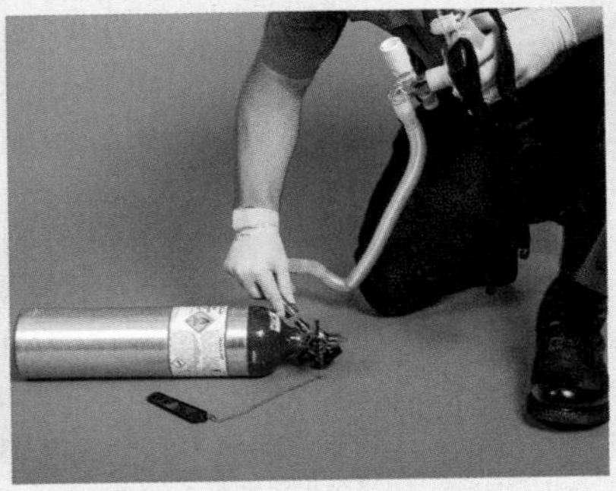

Step 3

Connect the tubing to the oxygen tank.

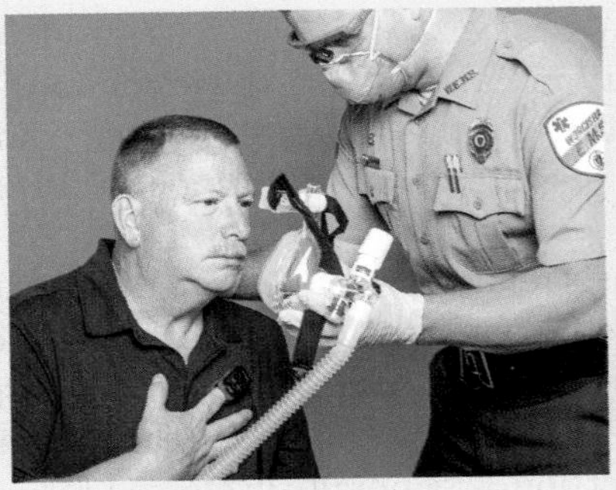

Step 4

Place the patient in a high Fowler position to facilitate breathing, and provide coaching through the initial application of the mask. Place the mask over the patient's nose and mouth, creating the most airtight seal possible. To reduce some of the stress and anxiety associated with the application of CPAP, it may be beneficial to initially allow the patient to hold the mask to the face. Allow the patient to get used to the mask.

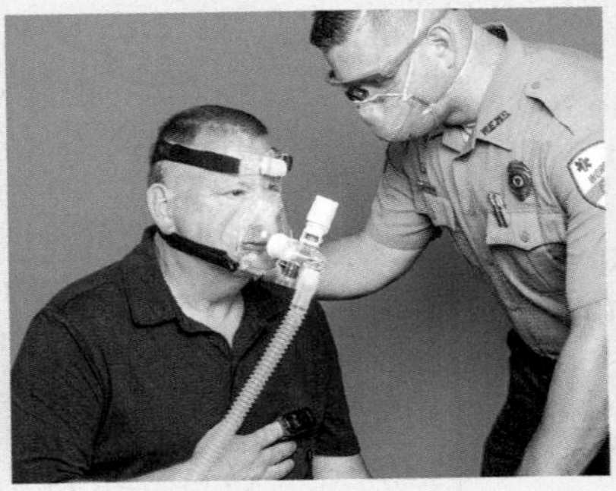

Step 5

After the mask is placed on the face and the patient adjusts to it, use the strapping mechanism to secure the mask to the patient's head. Ensure the seal between the mask and face remains intact. Consult the manufacturer's guidelines for specific strapping instructions.

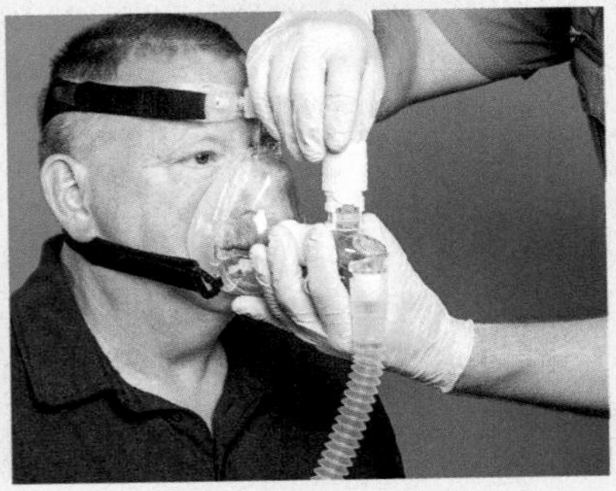

Step 6

Adjust the PEEP valve and the FIO_2 level according to the manufacturer's recommendations to maintain adequate oxygenation and ventilation. With CPAP in place, the patient's oxygenation saturation level should improve, the work of breathing should decrease, and the ability to speak should improve. Constantly reassess the patient for signs of clinical deterioration or complications (ie, pneumothorax, hypotension).

A distended stomach is harmful for at least two reasons. First, it promotes regurgitation of stomach contents, which can lead to aspiration of the stomach contents. Second, a distended stomach pushes the diaphragm upward into the chest, reducing the amount of space in which the lungs can expand.

Signs of gastric distention include an increased diameter of the stomach, an increasingly distended abdomen, and increased resistance to bag-mask ventilations. If you observe these signs, then reassess and reposition the airway as needed and observe the patient's chest for adequate rise and fall as you continue ventilating. In addition, limit ventilation times to 1 second or the time needed to produce adequate chest rise.

Gastric Decompression

Invasive gastric decompression involves inserting a **gastric tube** into the patient's stomach and removing the contents with suction. The gastric tube is an effective tool for removing both air and liquid from the stomach because removal of the stomach contents decreases the pressure on the diaphragm and virtually eliminates the risks of regurgitation and aspiration.

You can insert the gastric tube into the patient's stomach either through the mouth (**orogastric [OG] tube**) or through the nose (**nasogastric [NG] tube**). Consider the use of a gastric tube for any patient who will need positive-pressure ventilation for an extended period, especially if the patient is not intubated. You should also insert an NG or OG tube when gastric distention interferes with ventilations: for example, when children are receiving positive-pressure ventilation or have swallowed large volumes of air because of increased work of breathing.

Use extreme caution when inserting NG and OG tubes in patients with known esophageal diseases (eg, tumors, varices, strictures). Never use NG and OG tubes in patients whose esophagus is not patent. After insertion, ensure the tube has been placed into the stomach. Occasionally, the tube may remain in the esophagus without entering the stomach (supragastric placement) or may have been placed into the trachea.

Nasogastric Tube

An NG tube is inserted through the nose, into the nasopharynx, through the esophagus, and into the stomach **FIGURE 16-58**. When implemented as part of airway management and ventilation, it decompresses the stomach, thereby decreasing pressure on the diaphragm and limiting the risk of regurgitation.

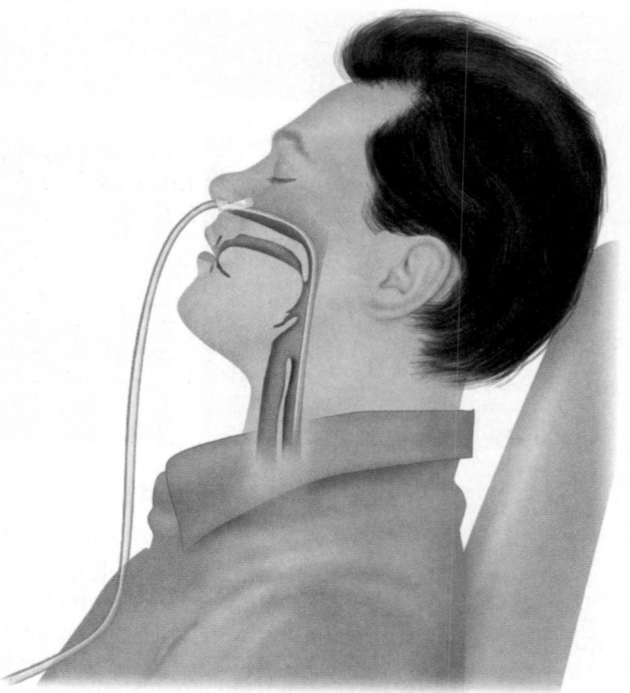

FIGURE 16-58 Nasogastric tube.

The NG tube is relatively well tolerated, even by patients who are responsive. Patients can still talk with an NG tube in place, and, after a few hours, most patients get used to it. For these reasons, the NG route of insertion is generally preferred for responsive patients.

During the insertion of an NG tube, most patients who are responsive will gag and may vomit, even if their gag reflexes are suppressed. In a patient with a decreased LOC, vomiting can seriously threaten the airway.

Insertion of an NG tube in patients with severe facial injuries, particularly midface fractures and skull fractures, is contraindicated. Although such events are rare, the NG tube may be inadvertently inserted through the fracture and into the cranial vault. For patients with these conditions, use the OG route of insertion.

Improper technique during NG tube insertion can cause trauma to the nasal passageways, esophagus, or gastric lining; therefore, use caution and be gentle when inserting the NG tube.

Use of an NG tube in patients who are not intubated may interfere with the mask seal of the bag-mask device. If you cannot effectively ventilate a patient because of severe gastric distention, however, you must balance the benefit of gastric decompression against the risk of a poor mask seal and determine which has a higher priority. Of course, if the patient is unresponsive and requires ET intubation, you can easily pass an ET tube around the NG tube.

The steps of NG tube insertion are shown in **SKILL DRILL 16-3**.

Skill Drill 16-3 Inserting a Nasogastric Tube in a Responsive Patient

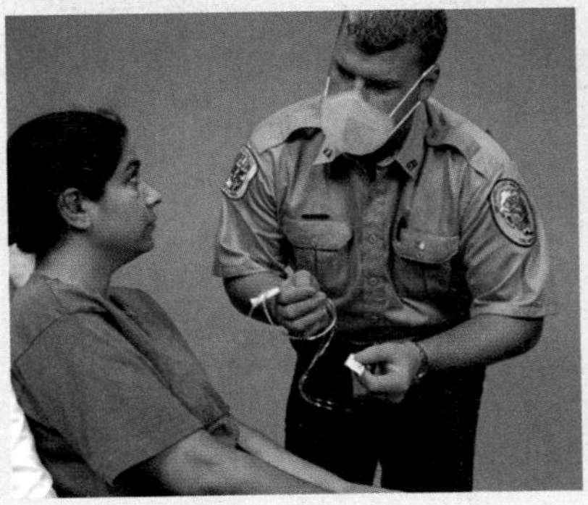

Step 1

Explain the procedure to the patient and provide oxygen, if necessary and possible. Ensure the patient's head is in a neutral or slightly flexed position. Suppress the gag reflex with a topical anesthetic spray.

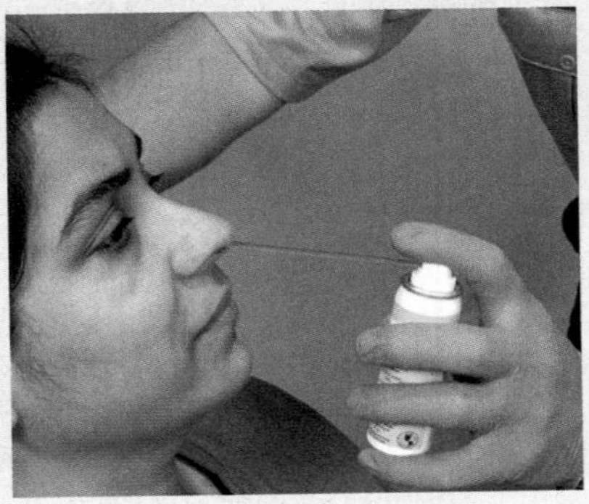

Step 2

Constrict the blood vessels in the nares with a topical alpha agonist, if available.

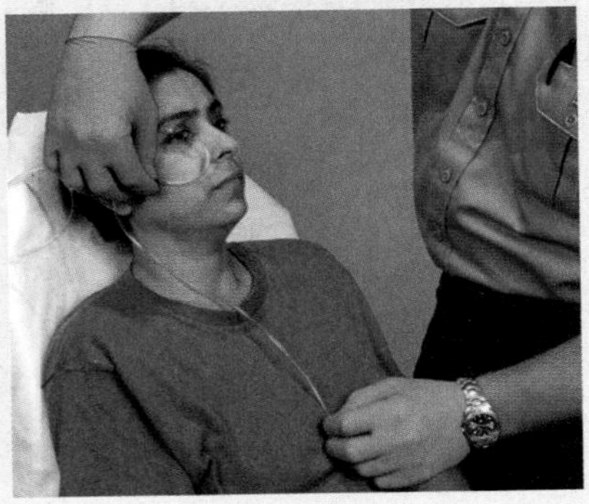

Step 3

Measure the tube for the correct depth of insertion (nose to ear to xiphoid process).

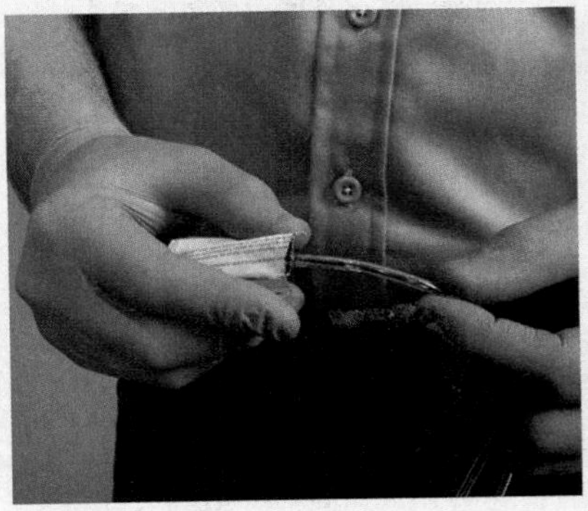

Step 4

Lubricate the tube with a water-soluble gel. Consider administering a topical anesthetic.

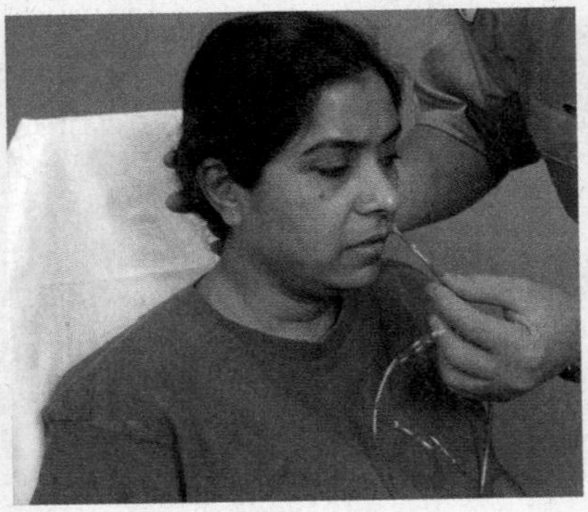

Step 5

Advance the tube gently along the nasal floor.

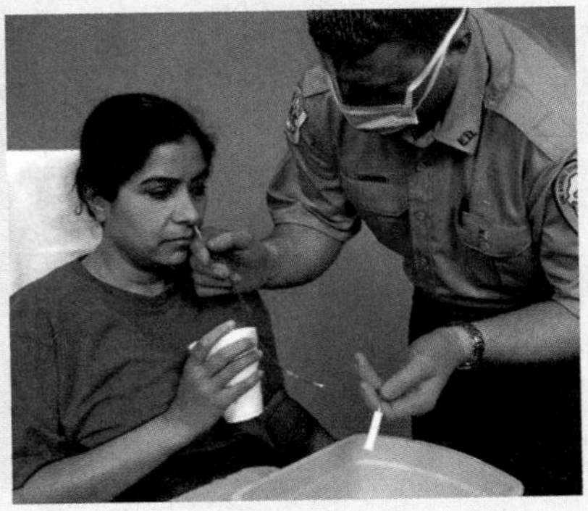

Step 6

Encourage the patient to swallow or drink to facilitate passage of the tube into the esophagus.

(continues)

Skill Drill 16-3 Inserting a Nasogastric Tube in a Responsive Patient (continued)

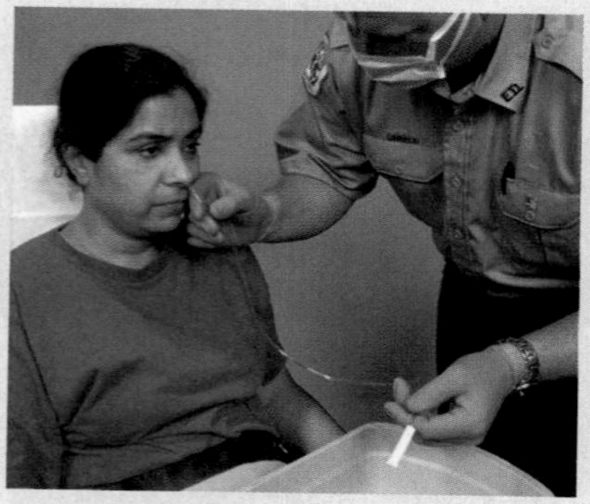

Step 7

Advance the tube into the stomach.

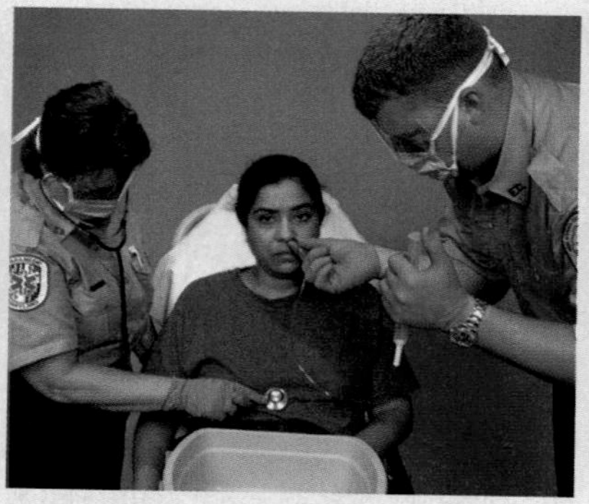

Step 8

Confirm proper placement: Auscultate over the epigastrium while injecting 20 to 30 mL of air into the tube, and/or observe for gastric contents in the tube. There should be no reflux around the tube.

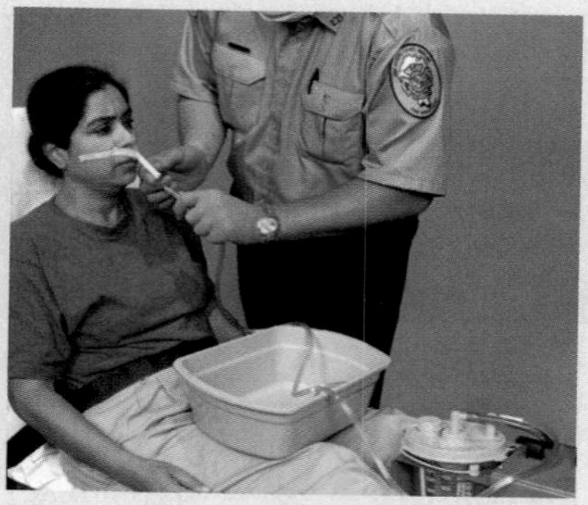

Step 9

Apply suction to the tube to aspirate the stomach contents and secure the tube in place. The blue extension of the gastric tube should remain open to the air.

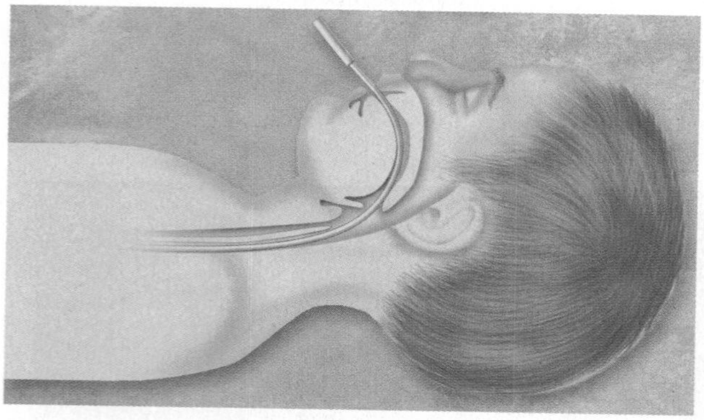

FIGURE 16-59 Orogastric tube.

Words of Wisdom

After you insert an advanced airway device, consider inserting a gastric tube (orally or nasally) if no contraindications to its placement exist. Doing so will maximize your ability to ventilate the patient by removing air that may have entered the stomach from bag-mask ventilation that occurred before you inserted the advanced airway device. A gastric tube is particularly important in submersion incidents (drowning), especially in young children. In these patients, drowning often involves ingesting and inhaling water, which then fills the stomach and lungs.

Orogastric Tube

An OG tube serves the same purpose as an NG tube, but is inserted through the mouth instead of the nose **FIGURE 16-59**. The advantages and disadvantages of the OG tube are essentially the same as those for the NG tube. The major differences are that the OG tube carries no risk of nasal bleeding and is safer in patients with severe facial trauma. In addition, you can use larger tubes, which is helpful if the patient requires gastric lavage. Gastric lavage, also called gastric irrigation, is the process of cleaning out the stomach's contents; it is typically performed in the ED for patients who have ingested toxins.

However, the OG tube is less comfortable for responsive patients, causes gagging much more often, and increases the possibility of vomiting. Responsive patients also tend to bite the tube as it is passed orally. The OG route is generally preferred for patients who are unresponsive without a gag reflex.

The steps of OG tube insertion are shown in **SKILL DRILL 16-4**.

Skill Drill 16-4 Inserting an Orogastric Tube in an Unresponsive Patient

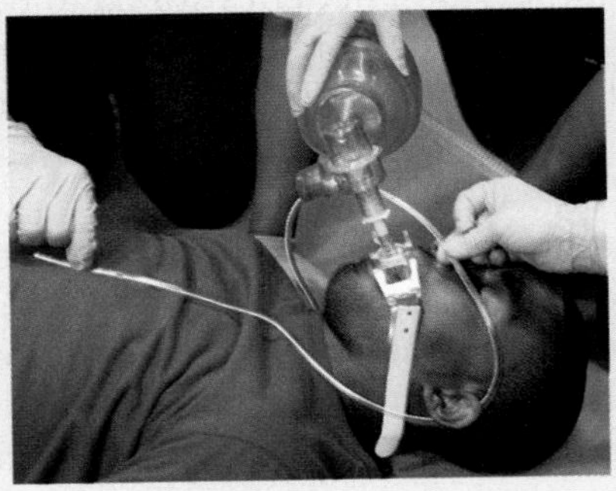

Step 1

Position the patient's head in a neutral or slightly flexed position. Measure the tube for the correct depth of insertion (mouth to ear to xiphoid process).

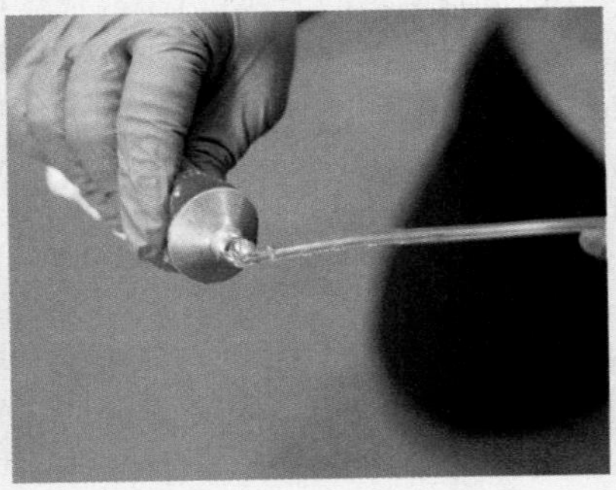

Step 2

Lubricate the tube with a water-soluble gel.

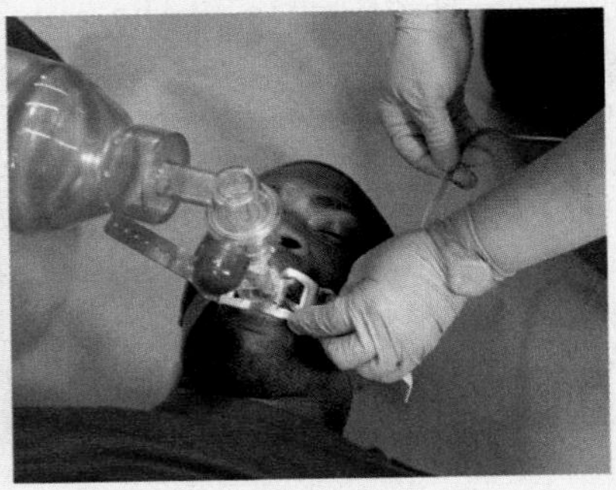

Step 3

Introduce the tube at the midline and advance it gently into the oropharynx. Advance the tube into the stomach.

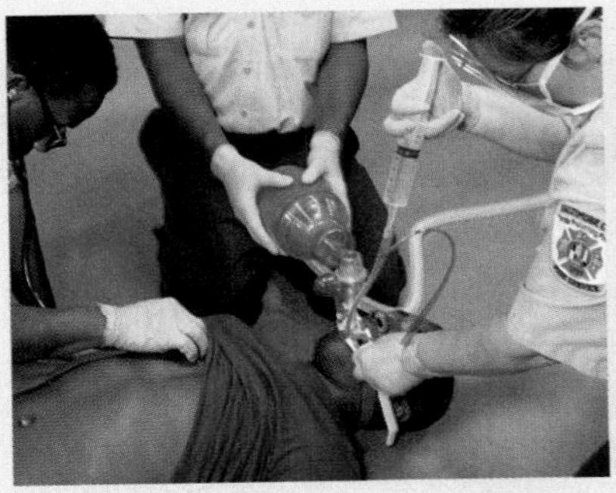

Step 4

Confirm proper placement: Auscultate over the epigastrium while injecting 20 to 30 mL of air and/or observe for gastric contents in the tube. There should be no reflux around the tube. Afterwards, auscultate over the lung fields to confirm the ET tube has not been dislodged.

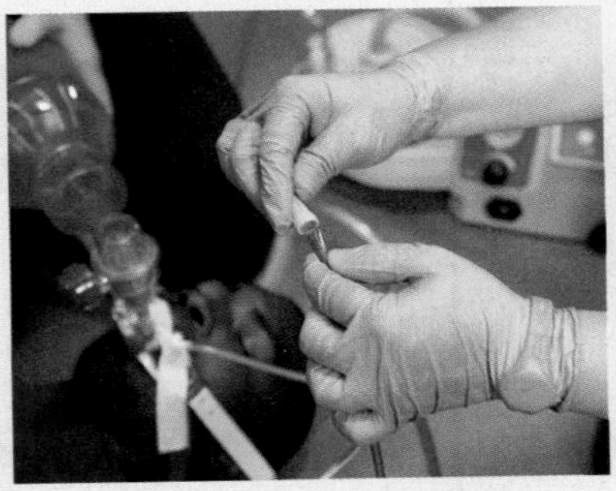

Step 5

Apply suction to the tube to aspirate the stomach contents.

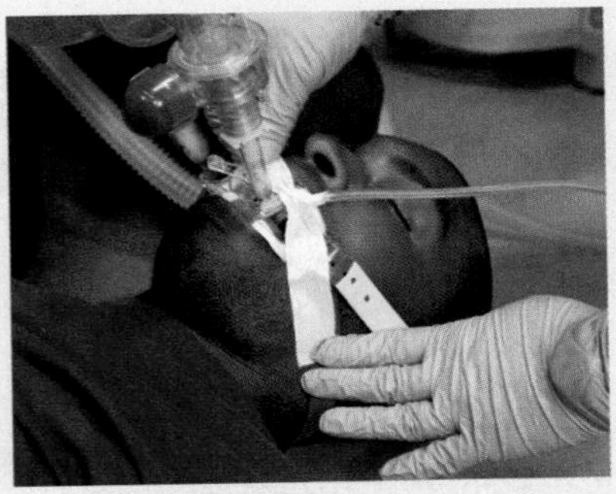

Step 6

Secure the tube in place.

Special Patient Considerations

Laryngectomy, Tracheostomy, Stoma, and Tracheostomy Tubes

A **laryngectomy** is a surgical procedure in which the larynx is removed. This procedure is performed by making a **tracheostomy** (a surgical opening into the trachea), thereby creating a **stoma**, an orifice that connects the trachea to the outside air. The tracheal stoma is located in the midline of the anterior part of the neck, inferior to the cricoid cartilage. Surgical removal of the entire larynx is called **total laryngectomy**. A person who has had this procedure is sometimes known as a laryngectomee, or neck breather, because the person breathes through the stoma in the neck. Because a connection no longer exists between the patient's pharynx and lower airway, you cannot ventilate the patient through the nose and mouth with a bag-mask device or other face mask. The air blown into the mouth or nose can only go down the esophagus into the stomach; it will not reach the lower airway.

A **partial laryngectomy** entails surgical removal of a portion of the larynx. People who have had this procedure are called partial neck breathers, because they breathe through the stoma and the nose or mouth. In practice, you may be unable to tell whether a person has had a total or partial laryngectomy until you attempt artificial ventilation.

Suctioning of a Stoma

You may encounter patients who require suctioning of thick secretions from the stoma. Failure to recognize and identify this need could result in hypoxia. It is common for a patient's stoma to become occluded with mucus plugs. Patients with a laryngectomy have a less efficient cough and, therefore, have difficulty spontaneously clearing the stoma.

You must perform suctioning of the patient's stoma with extreme care, especially if you suspect laryngeal swelling. Even the slightest irritation of the tracheal wall can result in a violent laryngospasm and complete airway closure. Limit suctioning of the stoma to 10 seconds at a time.

The steps for suctioning a stoma are shown in **SKILL DRILL 16-5**.

Ventilation of Patients With a Stoma

Neither the head tilt–chin lift maneuver nor the jaw-thrust maneuver is required for ventilating

YOU are the Paramedic

PART 6

With CPAP therapy continuing, the patient is secured to the stretcher and loaded into the ambulance. You obtain a 12-lead ECG, which does not show any evidence of an acute myocardial infarction. You begin transport to the hospital and reassess the patient's condition.

Recording Time: 15 Minutes	
Level of consciousness	Conscious, but sedated
Respirations	22 breaths/min; slightly labored
Pulse	114 beats/min; strong and regular
Skin	Warm and moist; lip and gum color have returned to baseline
Blood pressure	169/88 mm Hg
Oxygen saturation (Spo_2)	95%
Pupils	PERRLA
$ETCO_2$	46 mm Hg
ECG	Sinus tachycardia

10. How should you proceed with your treatment of this patient?

Skill Drill 16-5 Suctioning of a Stoma

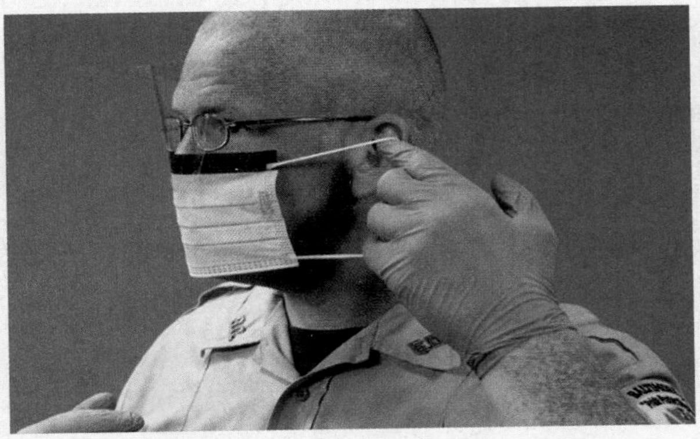

Step 1

Take standard precautions.

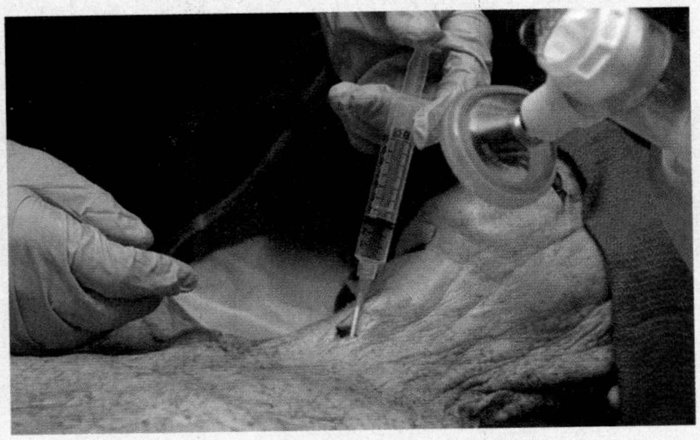

Step 2

Inject 3 mL of sterile saline through the stoma and into the trachea.

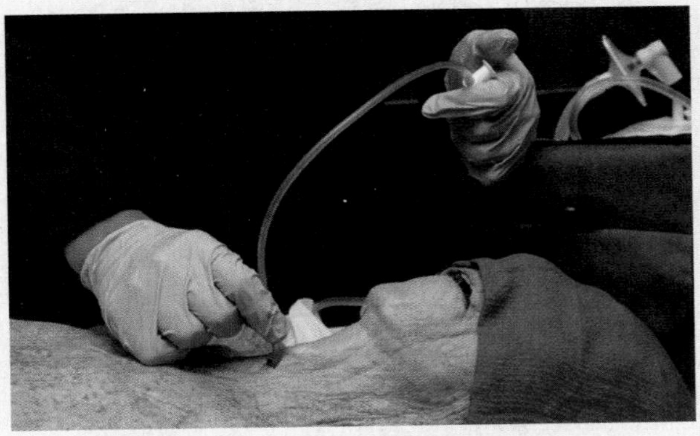

Step 3

Instruct the patient to exhale (if responsive), and insert the catheter without providing suction until resistance is felt (no more than 12 cm).

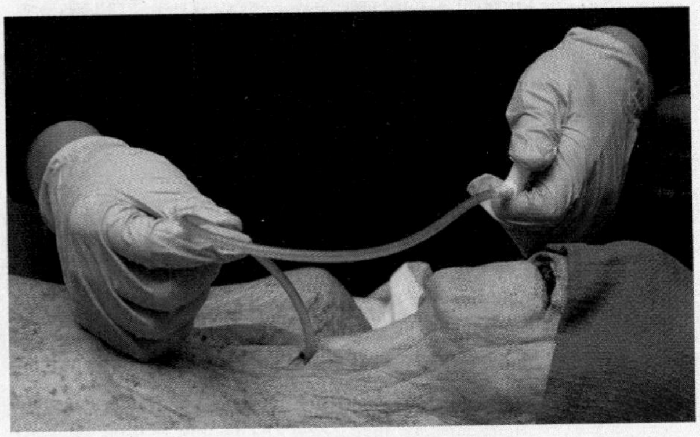

Step 4

Suction while withdrawing the catheter.

a patient with a stoma. If the patient has a stoma and no tracheostomy tube (discussed next) in place, then you can perform ventilations using the mouth-to-stoma (with a resuscitation mask) technique or with a bag-mask device. Regardless of the technique used, you should use an infant- or child-size mask to make an adequate seal over the stoma. Seal the patient's nose and mouth with one hand to prevent leakage of air up the trachea. Release the seal of the patient's mouth and nose following each ventilation, allowing exhalation to occur through the upper airway. Two rescuers are needed to perform bag-mask device-to-stoma ventilations: one to seal the nose and mouth, and the other to squeeze the bag-mask device.

If you are unable to ventilate a patient who has a stoma, try suctioning the stoma and mouth with a soft-tip (French) catheter before providing artificial ventilation through the nose and mouth. Note that this technique will work only if the patient has undergone a partial laryngectomy, not a total laryngectomy. If you seal the stoma during ventilation, then the ability to artificially ventilate the patient in this way may be improved, or it may help to clear any obstructions.

The steps for performing mouth-to-stoma ventilation with a resuscitation mask are shown in **SKILL DRILL 16-6**.

The steps for performing bag-mask device-to-stoma ventilation are shown in **SKILL DRILL 16-7**.

Skill Drill 16-6 Ventilating Through a Stoma Using a Resuscitation Mask

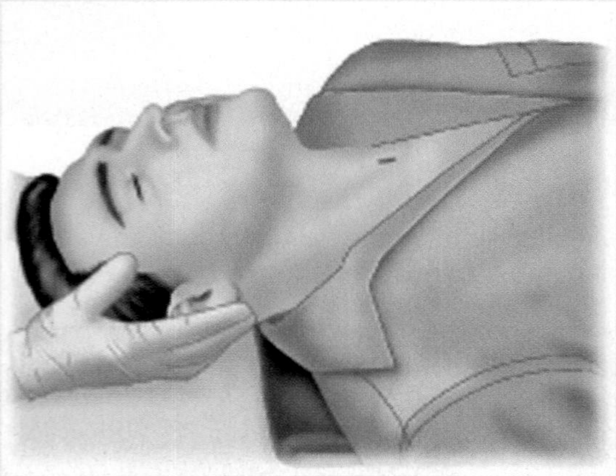

Step 1

Position the patient's head in a neutral position, with the shoulders slightly elevated.

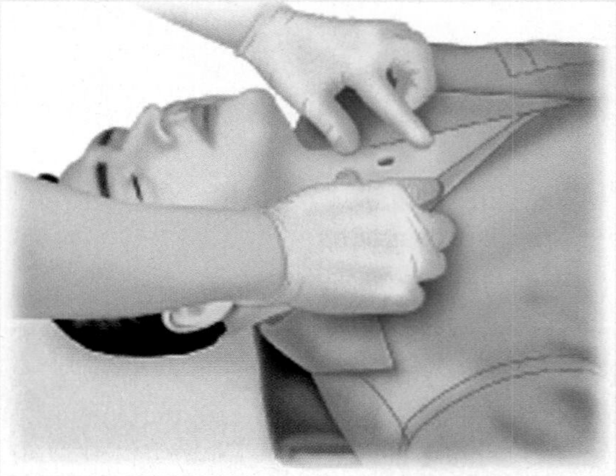

Step 2

Locate and expose the stoma site.

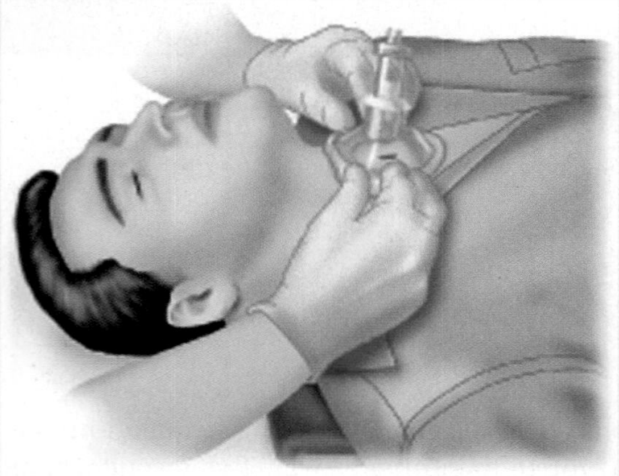

Step 3

Place the resuscitation mask over the stoma, and ensure an adequate seal. For best results, use a pediatric mask.

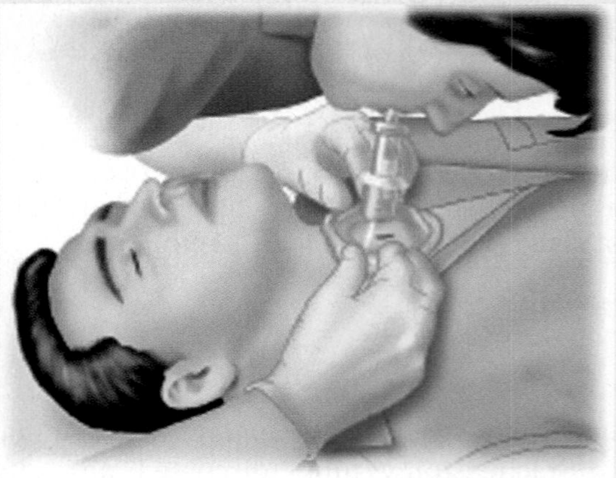

Step 4

Maintain the patient's head in a neutral position, and ventilate the patient by exhaling directly into the resuscitation mask. Assess the patient for adequate ventilation by observing for chest rise and feeling for air leaks around the mask.

Skill Drill 16-6 Ventilating Through a Stoma Using a Resuscitation Mask (continued)

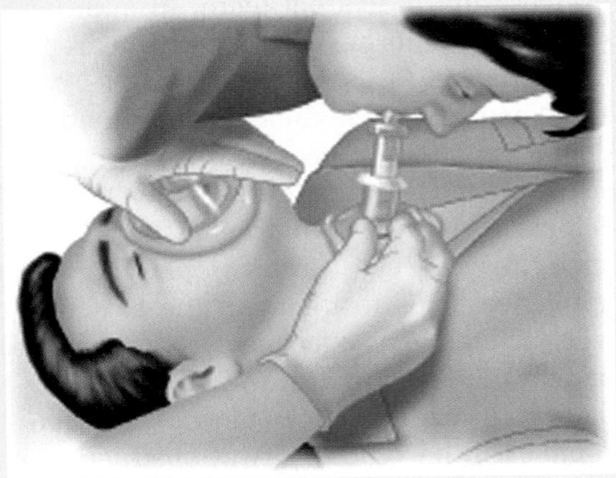

Step 5

If air leakage is evident, seal the patient's mouth and nose and then ventilate.

Skill Drill 16-7 Ventilating Through a Stoma With a Bag-Mask Device

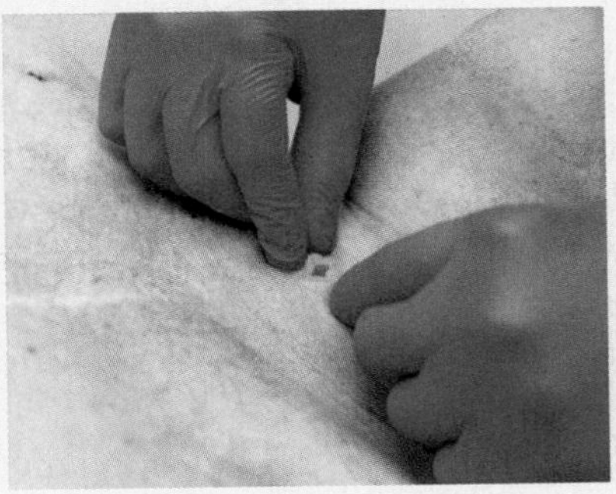

Step 1

With the patient's head in a neutral position, locate and expose the stoma.

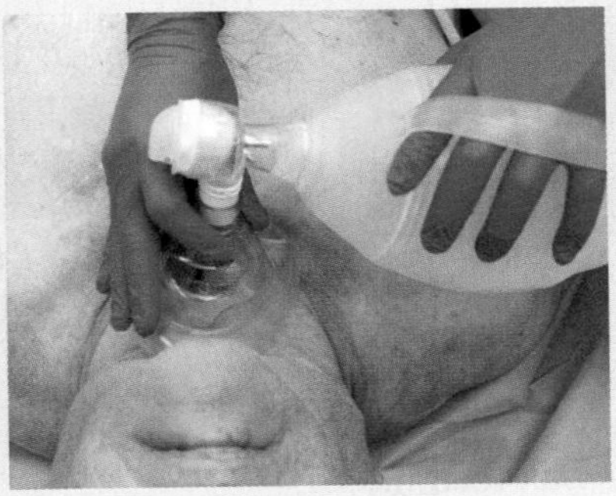

Step 2

Place the bag-mask device (with a pediatric mask) over the stoma, and ensure an adequate seal. Ventilate the patient by squeezing the bag-mask device, and assess for adequate ventilation by observing chest rise and feeling for air leaks. Seal the mouth and nose if air leakage is evident from the upper airway.

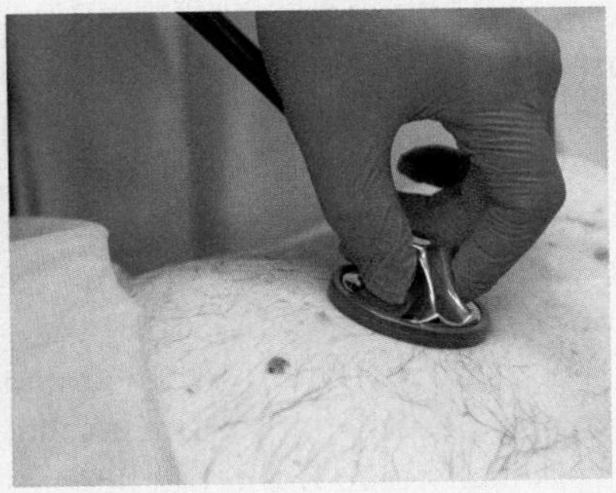

Step 3

Auscultate over the lungs to confirm adequate ventilation.

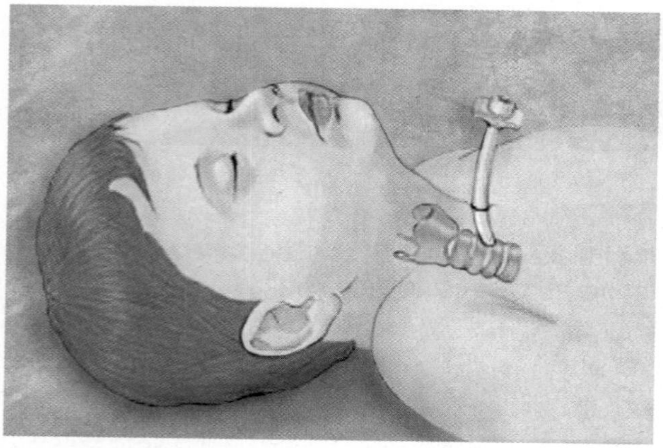

FIGURE 16-60 A tracheostomy tube.

Tracheostomy Tubes

A **tracheostomy tube** is a plastic tube placed within the tracheostomy site (stoma) **FIGURE 16-60**. It requires a 15/22-mm adapter to be compatible with ventilatory devices, such as a mechanical ventilator or bag-mask device. Patients with a tracheostomy tube may receive supplemental oxygen via tubing designed to fit over the tube or by placing an oxygen mask over the tube. Ventilation is accomplished by simply attaching the bag-mask device to the 16-mm adaptor on the tracheostomy tube.

Patients with a tracheostomy tube who experience sudden dyspnea often have thick secretions in the tube. In this case, perform suctioning through the tracheostomy tube as you would through a stoma.

If a tracheostomy tube becomes dislodged, **stenosis** (narrowing) of the stoma may occur; this is especially true if the tracheostomy was recently performed. Stenosis is a potentially life-threatening condition because soft-tissue swelling decreases the diameter of the stoma and impairs the patient's ventilatory ability. In such cases, you may be unable to replace the tracheostomy tube itself and may have to insert an ET tube into the stoma before it becomes totally occluded. Because a patient with a stoma already has a significant underlying pathology (eg, brain injury, chronic respiratory insufficiency), the patient may be less tolerant of even brief periods of hypoxia.

The steps for replacing a dislodged tracheostomy tube are shown in **SKILL DRILL 16-8**.

Dental Appliances

Dental appliances are frequently encountered in the geriatric population. They can take many different forms: dentures (upper, lower, or both), bridges, and individual teeth. In addition, many younger patients have braces, another type of dental appliance.

When you assess the airway of a patient with a dental appliance, especially one who is unresponsive, you must determine whether the appliance is loose or whether it fits well. If the dental appliance fits well, then leave it in place. A well-fitting appliance helps to maintain the structure of the face, facilitating an effective mask-to-face seal if the patient requires mouth-to-mask or bag-mask ventilation. If the appliance is loose, however, then it could easily become an airway obstruction and you should remove it.

If an unresponsive patient has an airway obstruction caused by a dental appliance, perform the usual steps to clear an obstruction, such as chest compressions, direct laryngoscopy, and use of the Magill forceps. If the obstruction is caused by a bridge, then you must take great care when clearing the obstruction; these devices often contain sharp metal ends that can easily lacerate the posterior pharynx or larynx.

Often it is not the dental appliance itself that hinders your ability to manage a patient's airway, but rather attempts to identify and remove the device. Do not become overly concerned with the presence of the dental appliance; instead, concentrate on managing the airway. In addition, the oropharyngeal anatomy may be somewhat distorted by the presence of a dental appliance.

In general, it is best to remove dental appliances (if indicated) before intubating a patient. After the ET tube is in place and has been secured, removal of the dental appliance will be extremely difficult and dangerous because it may cause dislodgement of the tube or inflict unnecessary oropharyngeal trauma.

Facial Trauma

Effectively managing the airway of a patient with facial injuries can be quite challenging **FIGURE 16-61**. Because the face is highly vascular, facial trauma can result in severe tissue swelling and bleeding into the airway. Control bleeding with direct

Skill Drill 16-8 Replacing a Dislodged Tracheostomy Tube With a Temporary ET Tube

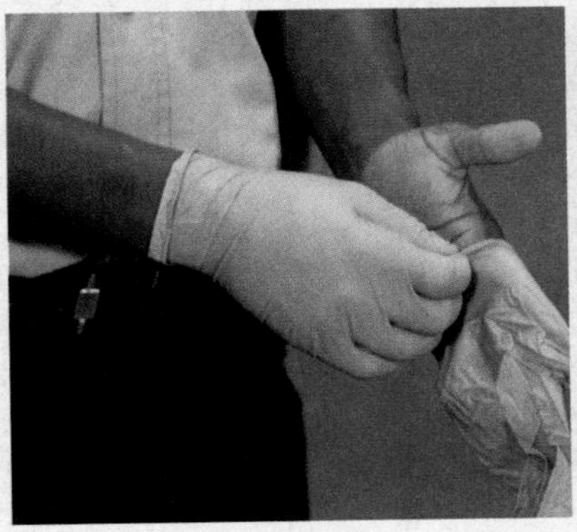

Step 1

Take standard precautions. Assemble the equipment.

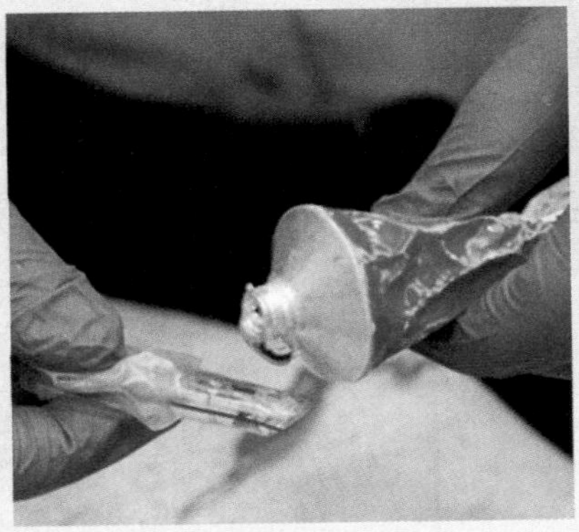

Step 2

Lubricate the same-size tracheostomy tube or an ET tube (at least 5.0 mm) with a water-soluble gel.

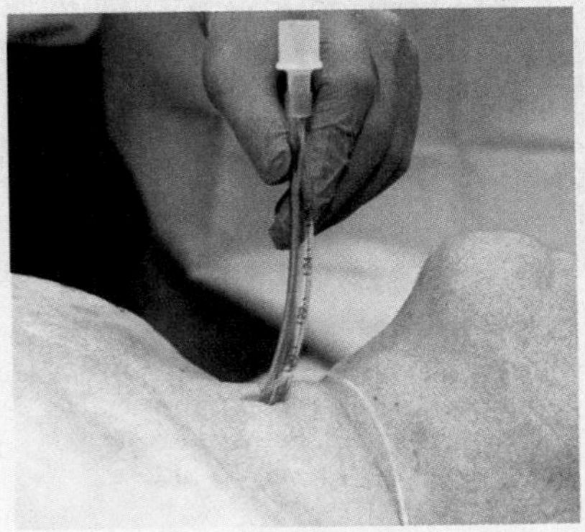

Step 3

Instruct the patient to exhale, and gently insert the tube approximately 0.5 to 0.75 inch (1 to 2 cm) beyond the balloon cuff.

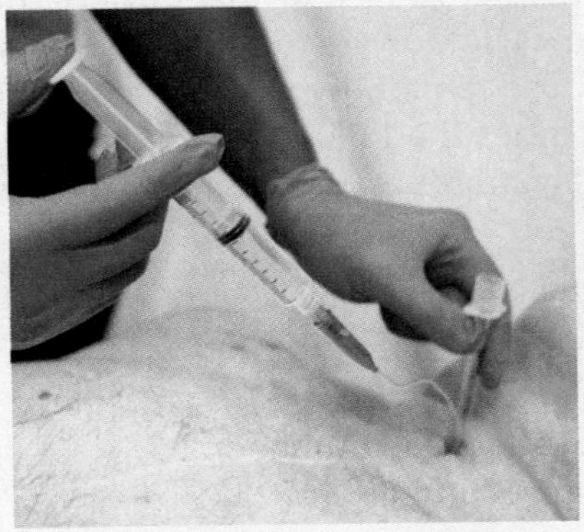

Step 4

Inflate the balloon cuff.

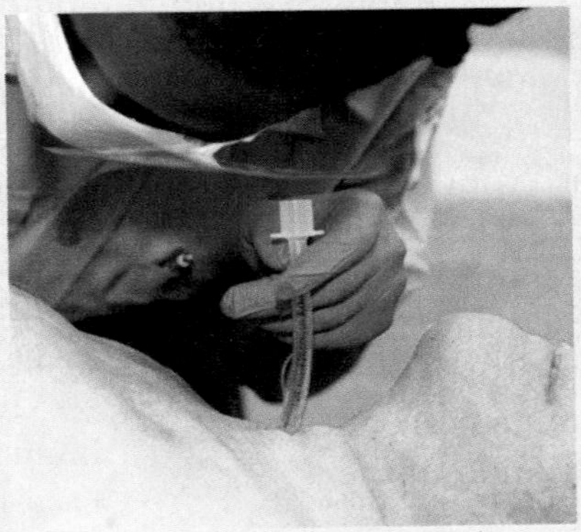

Step 5

Ensure the patient is comfortable, and confirm patency and proper placement of the tube by observing for chest rise, listening for air movement from the tube, and noting the patient's clinical status. Ensure that a false lumen (placement of the tube into the soft tissues of the neck, rather than in the trachea) was not created.

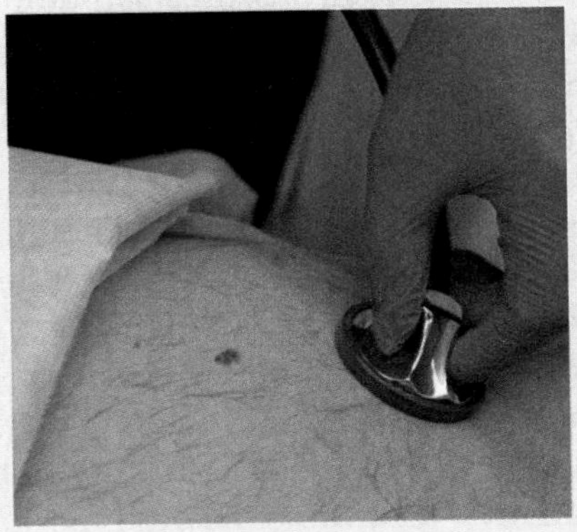

Step 6

Auscultate the lungs to confirm correct tube placement.

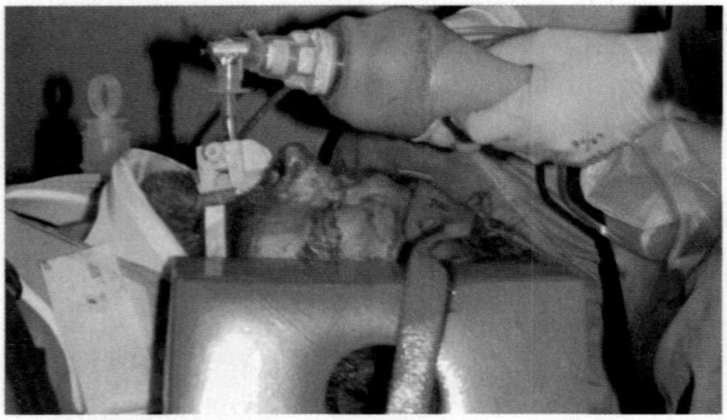

FIGURE 16-61 Airway management can be especially challenging in patients with facial injuries.

pressure, and suction the airway as needed. You may encounter a patient with severe facial trauma who is breathing inadequately and has severe oropharyngeal bleeding; both problems are life threatening. In this situation, you must suction the airway until it is clear and then ventilate the patient. Remember, ventilating a patient whose airway is full of blood virtually assures aspiration. If you cannot control the source of the oropharyngeal bleeding, then perform continuous suctioning and intubate the trachea.

Facial injuries should also increase your index of suspicion for a cervical spine injury. Therefore, when managing the airway, use the jaw-thrust maneuver and keep the patient's head in a neutral, in-line position. ET intubation of a trauma patient is most effectively performed by two paramedics: one who maintains neutral, in-line stabilization of the patient's head while the other performs the intubation. An alternative technique, especially if you are the only paramedic managing the patient's airway, is to stabilize the patient's head in a neutral, in-line position with your thighs and then perform the intubation.

While you are ventilating a patient with facial injuries, stay alert for changes in ventilation compliance or sounds that may indicate laryngeal edema (eg, stridor). If you cannot effectively ventilate or orally intubate a patient with severe facial injuries, then perform a cricothyrotomy (either surgical or needle). Advanced airway management techniques, including ET intubation, supraglottic airway devices, and needle and surgical cricothyrotomy, are discussed next.

Advanced Airway Management

One of the most common mistakes when caring for a patient with respiratory or cardiac arrest is to proceed with advanced airway management too early, forsaking the basic techniques of establishing and maintaining a patent airway in a patient who is already hypoxic. Never abandon the basics of airway management; do not immediately proceed with advanced techniques simply because you can. While the techniques used to manage a patient's airway may vary, the objective is the same: to optimize oxygenation and ventilation.

If attempts to establish and maintain a patent airway and ensure adequate oxygenation and ventilation with the basic techniques and maneuvers are not successful, you should consider advanced airway management. Patients primarily require advanced airway management for two reasons: (1) failure to maintain a patent airway and/or (2) failure to adequately oxygenate and ventilate. Advanced airway management involves the insertion of a number of advanced airway devices that are designed to facilitate adequate oxygenation and ventilation. The remainder of the chapter discusses and illustrates the following advanced airway devices and techniques:

- ET tube
  - Orotracheal intubation
    - Direct laryngoscopy
    - Video laryngoscopy
  - Blind nasotracheal intubation
  - Face-to-face intubation
- King LT airway
- Laryngeal mask airway
- i-gel
- Surgical and needle cricothyrotomy

Predicting the Difficult Airway

As a paramedic, you must decide how to accomplish airway management. Ask yourself, "Can I manage this airway with BLS techniques? Can (or should) I intubate this patient's trachea?" This section discusses the factors to consider when caring for a patient who has a difficult airway.

History is one factor. Anatomic findings that suggest a difficult airway may include congenital abnormalities (ie, dysmorphic face), recent surgeries, trauma, infection, or neoplastic diseases (such as cancer).

A commonly used mnemonic to guide assessment of the difficult airway is LEMON, which stands for:

Look externally
Evaluate 3-3-2
Mallampati classification
Obstruction
Neck mobility

As indicated by the *L* in the mnemonic, simply looking at the patient may indicate the relative difficulty that may be encountered in airway management. Patients with short, thick necks may be difficult to intubate. Morbid obesity significantly complicates intubation. Dental conditions, such as an overbite or "buck" (protruding) teeth, may also make intubation difficult.

The *E* stands for Evaluate 3-3-2. Three anatomic measurements are assessed when using the **3-3-2 rule** **FIGURE 16-62**. The first *3* refers to the mouth opening. Ideally, a patient's mouth should open at least three fingerbreadths (approximately 2 inches [5 cm]). A width of less than three fingerbreadths indicates a potentially difficult airway. Of course, if the patient can open the mouth on command, then you should reconsider your decision to intubate. The second *3* refers to the length of the mandible. At least three fingerbreadths is optimal. This length is measured from the tip of the chin to the hyoid bone. Patients with smaller mandibles have less room for displacement of the tongue and epiglottis, which can make airway management more difficult. Finally, the *2* refers to the distance from the hyoid bone to the thyroid notch; it should be at least two fingerbreadths wide.

The *M* in the LEMON mnemonic stands for Mallampati classification. An anesthesiologist, Seshagiri Rao Mallampati, developed the **Mallampati classification** in 1985 to predict the relative difficulty of intubation **FIGURE 16-63**. This classification notes the oropharyngeal structures visible in an upright, seated patient who is conscious and alert and is able to fully open the mouth. Although this evaluation is an accurate predictor of intubation difficulty, it is of no value in unresponsive patients and in patients who cannot follow commands. *If a patient is cooperative and able to comply with this evaluation, then emergency prehospital intubation is probably not indicated.* However, the evaluation is important because it can provide useful information should intubation become necessary.

Compared with the Mallampati classification, the **Cormack-Lehane classification** has more applicability in an emergent setting. It classifies views obtained by laryngoscopy based on the structures seen **FIGURE 16-64**.

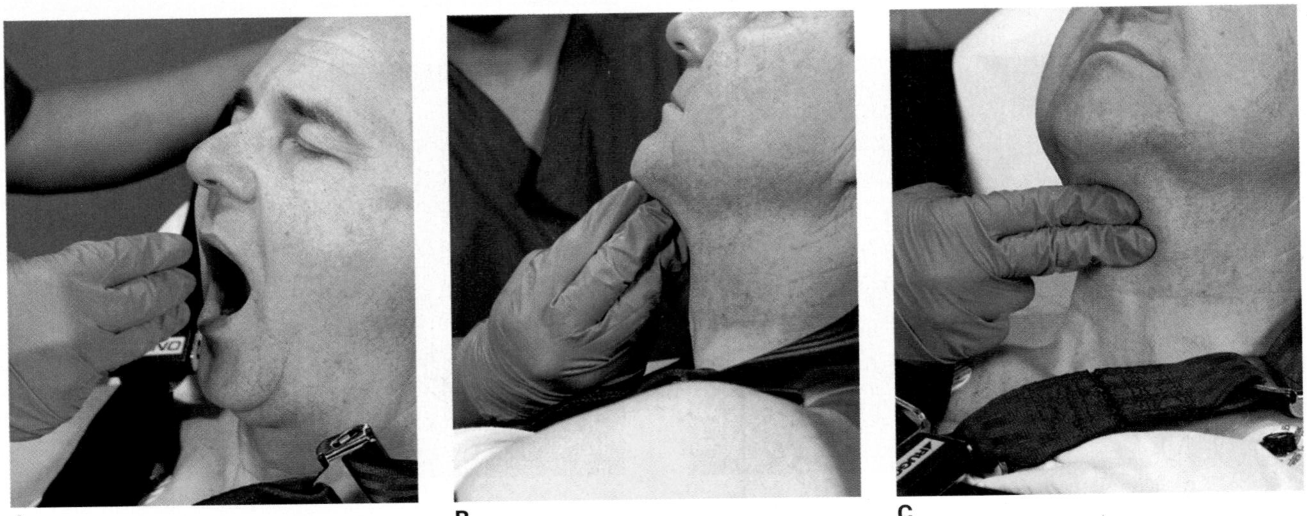

A B C

FIGURE 16-62 The 3-3-2 rule. **A.** The mouth should be at least three fingerbreadths wide when open. **B.** The space from the chin to the hyoid bone should be at least three fingerbreadths wide. **C.** The distance from the hyoid bone to the thyroid notch should be at least two fingerbreadths wide.

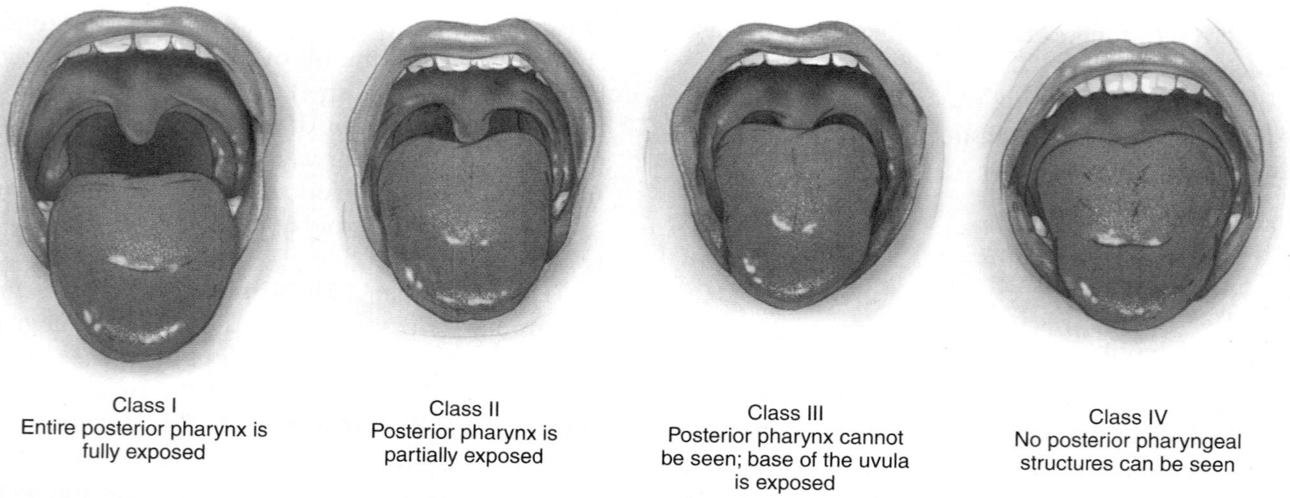
Class I
Entire posterior pharynx is fully exposed
Class II
Posterior pharynx is partially exposed
Class III
Posterior pharynx cannot be seen; base of the uvula is exposed
Class IV
No posterior pharyngeal structures can be seen

FIGURE 16-63 Mallampati classification.

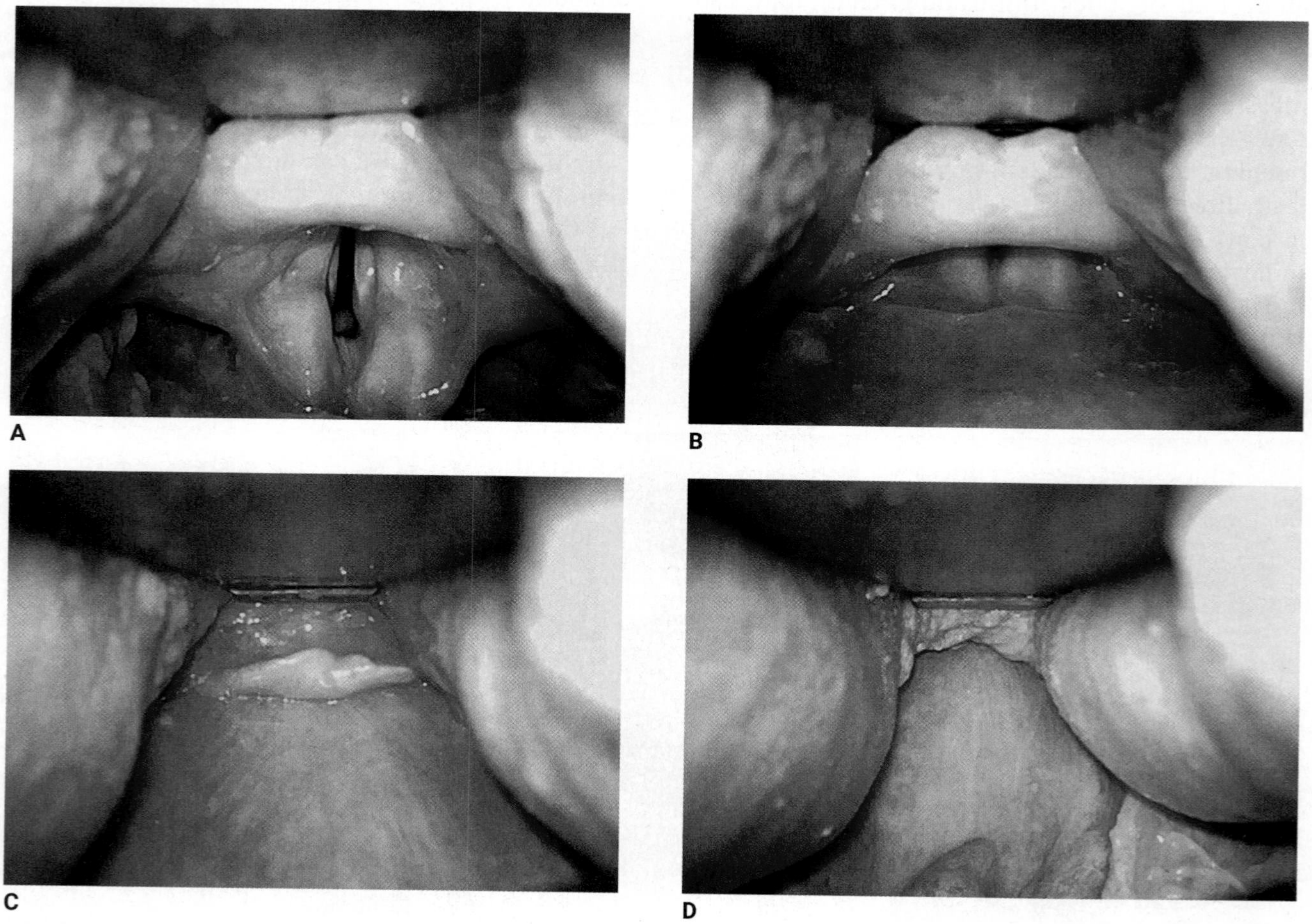
A
B
C
D

FIGURE 16-64 Laryngoscopic views of the airway demonstrating the Cormack-Lehane classification. **A.** Class 1: Full view of the epiglottis, arytenoid cartilage, and vocal cords is available. **B.** Class 2: The epiglottis is in full view, but only a portion of the glottis or arytenoid cartilage can be seen. In a modified system, Class 2a indicates partial view of the glottis, and Class 2b indicates the arytenoids or posterior part of the vocal cords is barely visible. **C.** Class 3: Only the epiglottis can be seen. Neither the glottis nor the arytenoid cartilage is visible. **D.** Class 4: Neither the epiglottis nor the glottis is visible.

The *O* in the mnemonic stands for obstruction. Note anything that might interfere with visualization or ET tube placement. Foreign body obstruction, obesity, hematoma, and masses are all examples of situations that can create a difficult airway.

Finally, the *N* stands for neck mobility. The ideal position for visualization and intubation is the sniffing position (ears aligned with the sternal notch). Neck mobility problems are most commonly associated with trauma patients (due to cervical collars or injury) and older patients (due to osteoporosis or arthritis). An inability to place the patient in the sniffing position can significantly reduce your ability to visualize the airway.

ET Intubation

In **endotracheal (ET) intubation**, an ET tube is passed through the glottic opening and the tube is then sealed with a cuff inflated against the tracheal wall. When the tube is passed into the trachea through the mouth, the procedure is called **orotracheal intubation**. When the tube is passed into the trachea through the nose, the procedure is called **nasotracheal intubation**.

Intubation of the trachea is the only definitive means of achieving complete control of the airway. You need a solid understanding of the basics of this technique when making urgent decisions about when to intubate a patient (or not). Consider the following points when performing ET intubation:

- **Advantages.** Provision of a secure airway and protection against aspiration
- **Disadvantages.** Special equipment required; physiologic functions of the upper airway (warming, filtering, humidifying) are bypassed
- **Complications.** Bleeding; hypoxia; laryngeal swelling; laryngospasm; vocal cord damage; mucosal necrosis; barotrauma

ET Tubes

The basic structure of an **endotracheal (ET) tube** **FIGURE 16-65** includes the proximal end, the tube itself, the cuff and pilot balloon, and the distal tip. The proximal end is equipped with a standard 15/22-mm adapter that allows it to be attached to any ventilation device. It also includes an inflation port with a pilot balloon. The distal cuff is inflated with a syringe attached to this inflation port, which has a one-way valve. The pilot balloon indicates whether the distal cuff is inflated or deflated after the tube has been inserted into the mouth.

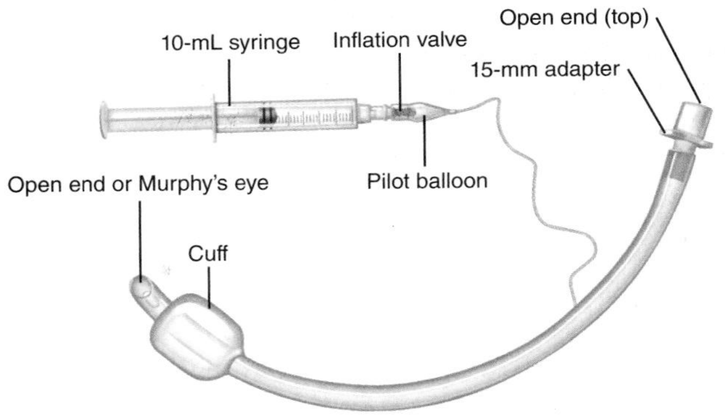

FIGURE 16-65 Endotracheal tube.

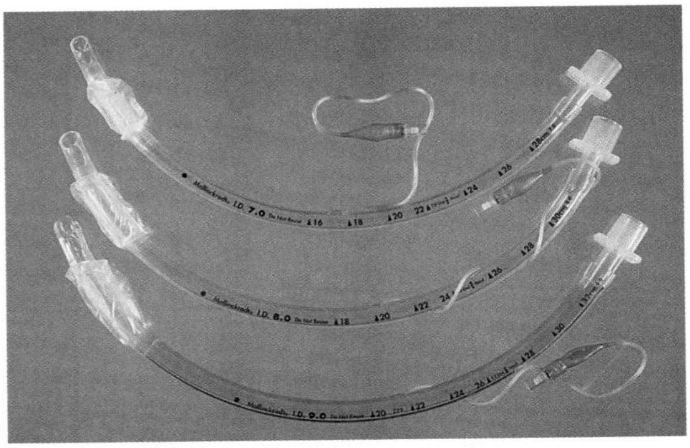

FIGURE 16-66 Endotracheal tubes are available in a variety of sizes.

Centimeter markings along the length of the ET tube provide a measurement of its depth. The distal end of the tube has a beveled tip to facilitate its insertion and an opening on the side called the **Murphy eye**, which enables ventilation to occur even if the tip becomes occluded by blood, mucus, or the tracheal wall.

ET tubes range in size from 2.0 to 10.0 mm in inside diameter, and from 12 to 32 cm in length **FIGURE 16-66**. Sizes ranging from 5.0 to 10.0 mm (inside diameter) are equipped with a distal cuff that, when inflated, makes an airtight seal with the tracheal wall. It is possible to obtain smaller tubes with a cuff to comply with 2020 neonatal guidelines. A tube that is too small for the patient will lead to increased resistance to airflow and difficulty in ventilating. A tube that is too large can be difficult to insert and may cause trauma. Usually, an adult female patient will require a 7.0- to 7.5-mm tube, and an adult male patient will require a 7.5- to 8.0-mm tube.

The **stylet**, a semirigid wire that is inserted into the ET tube to mold and maintain the shape of the tube, enables you to guide the tip of the tube over the arytenoid cartilage and through the vocal cords. Lubricate this device with a water-soluble gel to facilitate its removal, and bend its end to form a gentle "hockey stick" curve. The end of the stylet should rest at least 0.5 inch (1 cm) back from the end of the ET tube; if the stylet protrudes beyond the end of the tube, then it may damage the vocal cords and surrounding structures. Bend the other end of the stylet over the proximal tube connector, so that the stylet cannot slip farther into the tube.

In pediatric patients, use ET tubes ranging in size from 2.5 to 5.0 mm (inside diameter). In children, the funnel-shaped cricoid ring (the narrowest portion of the pediatric airway) forms an anatomic seal with the ET tube, eliminating the need for a distal cuff in most of these patients. The proximal end of the tube still has a 15/22-mm adapter for use with standard ventilation devices, and the distal end has a beveled tip with distal end markings. However, because it lacks a balloon cuff, a pilot balloon is not included.

A number of anatomic clues can help you determine the proper size of ET tube for adults and children. The internal diameter of the nostril is a good approximation of the diameter of the glottic opening. The diameter of the little finger or the size of the thumbnail is also a good approximation of airway size. Because all attempts to predict the ET tube size required for a given patient are estimates, however, you should always have three ET tubes ready: one tube of the size you think will be appropriate, one a size larger, and one a size smaller. A more accurate way to determine tube size in pediatric patients is to use a length-based tape, pediatrics pocket reference card, or other rapidly accessed resource that identifies the tube size based on kilograms of weight and age.

Laryngoscopes and Blades

A laryngoscope is required to perform orotracheal intubation by laryngoscopy: a procedure in which the vocal cords are visualized for placement of the ET tube. The laryngoscope consists of a handle and interchangeable blades **FIGURE 16-67**. The handle contains the power source for the light on the laryngoscope blade. Most laryngoscopes run on disposable batteries, but some are rechargeable. The handle has a bar designed to connect with a notch on the blade **FIGURE 16-68**. When the blade is moved into the perpendicular position, the bright light shines near the tip of the blade. Newer laryngoscopes feature a light source within the handle itself, which attaches to a fiberoptic blade.

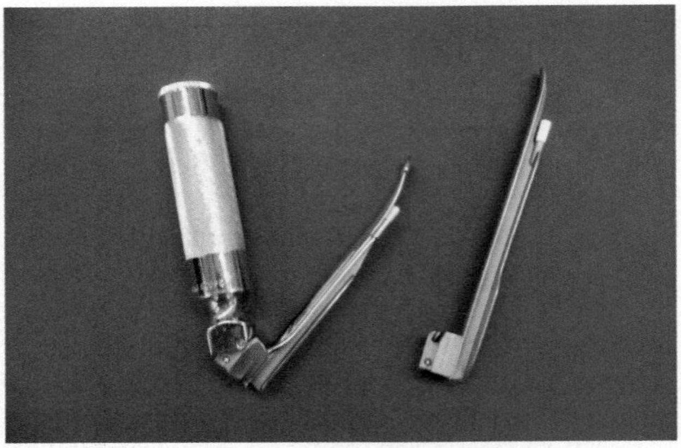

FIGURE 16-67 A laryngoscope with a straight blade.

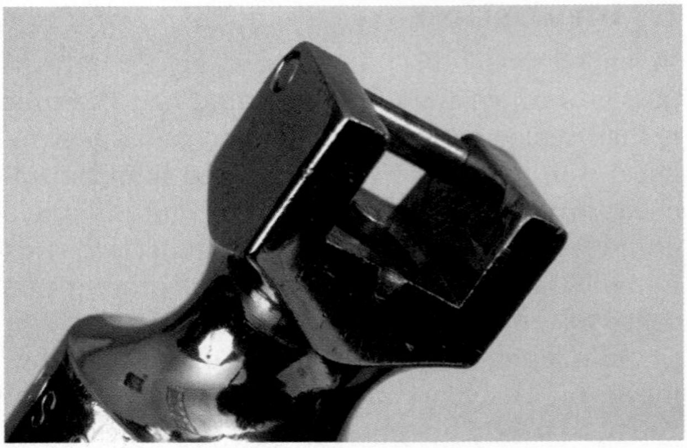

FIGURE 16-68 The handle of the laryngoscope has a bar designed to connect with a notch on the blade.

Laryngoscope blade options include the straight (Miller) blade and the curved (Macintosh) blade. The **straight laryngoscope blade** is designed so that its tip will extend beneath the epiglottis and directly lift it up **FIGURE 16-69**. This is a particularly useful feature in infants and small children, who often have a long, floppy epiglottis that can be difficult to elevate out of the way with a curved blade. In an adult, use of a straight blade requires great care;

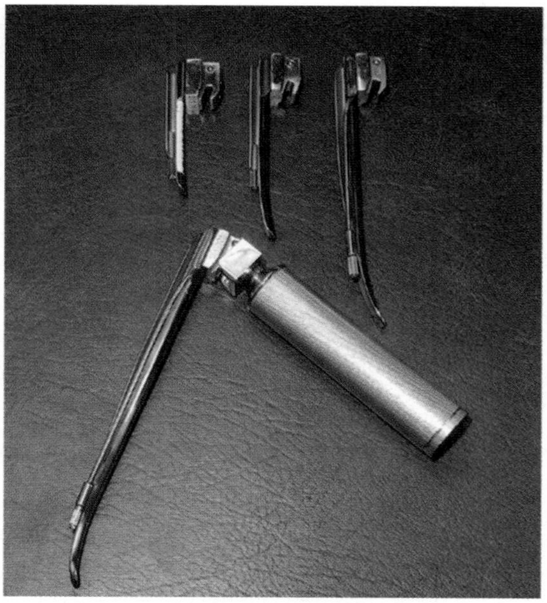

FIGURE 16-69 A laryngoscope and an assortment of straight (Miller) blades.

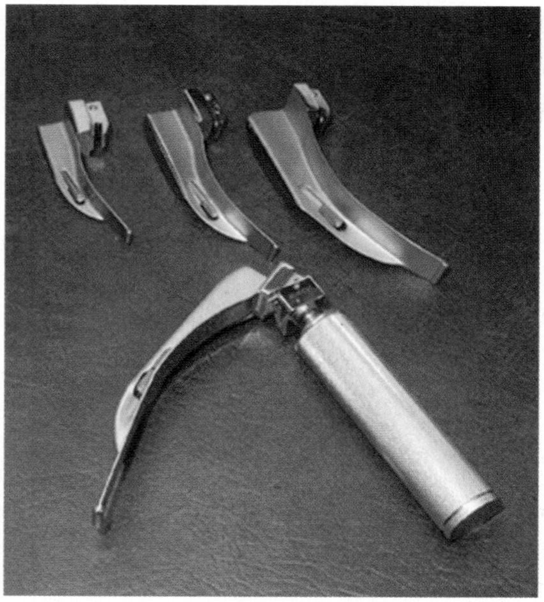

FIGURE 16-70 A laryngoscope and an assortment of curved (Macintosh) blades.

if used improperly and levered across the upper jaw, the straight blade is more likely to damage the patient's teeth. The **curved laryngoscope blade** is less likely to be levered against the teeth by an inexperienced paramedic **FIGURE 16-70**. The direction of the curve conforms to that of the tongue and pharynx, so the blade follows the outline of the pharynx with relative ease. The tip of the curved blade is placed in the vallecula (the space between the epiglottis and the base of the tongue) rather than beneath the epiglottis; it indirectly lifts the epiglottis to expose the vocal cords. During an orotracheal intubation attempt, you should have both curved and straight blades readily available.

Blade sizes range from 0 to 4. Sizes 0, 1, and 2 are appropriate for infants and children, whereas sizes 3 and 4 are considered adult blades. For pediatric patients, blade sizes are often recommended based on the child's age or height. Choose the blade for adults based on your experience and the size of the patient (3 for average-size adults and 4 for larger people).

Orotracheal Intubation by Direct Laryngoscopy

Orotracheal intubation by direct laryngoscopy involves inserting an ET tube through the mouth and into the trachea while directly visualizing the glottic opening with a laryngoscope. The indications and contraindications for orotracheal intubation include the following:

- **Indications**
  - Airway control needed as a result of coma, respiratory arrest, and/or cardiac arrest
  - Ventilatory support before impending respiratory failure
  - Prolonged ventilatory support required
  - Traumatic brain injury
  - Unresponsiveness
  - Impending airway compromise (such as in burns or trauma)
- **Contraindications**
  - An intact gag reflex
  - Inability to open the patient's mouth because of trauma, dislocation of the jaw, or a pathologic condition
  - Inability to see the glottic opening
  - Copious secretions, vomitus, or blood in the airway

TABLE 16-12 summarizes the equipment and preparation required before performing orotracheal intubation. Make a copy of this table and affix it to your intubation kit, so that you can check the kit systematically at the beginning of every shift.

TABLE 16-12 Preparing Equipment for Intubation

Equipment	What to Check, Prepare, and Assemble
Ventilation equipment	Have your partner ventilate the patient while you are assembling, checking, and preparing your equipment. Ensure the patient is being ventilated with 100% oxygen and the pulse oximeter reading is greater than 95%.
ET tube	Select the proper size tube (7.0–7.5 for adult females; 7.5–8.0 for adult males). Inject 10 mL of air into the cuff, and ensure that the cuff holds air. Confirm the 15/22-mm adapter is firmly inserted into the tube. Insert the stylet, and ensure that the tip is proximal to the Murphy eye. Straighten the ET tube completely, and place a slight bend (in the shape of a hockey stick) just proximal to the cuff **FIGURE 16-71**. Increase the angle of the bend as needed to facilitate tube placement through the vocal cords.
Laryngoscope and blades	Have an assortment of blades (straight and curved) available, because some patients are easier to intubate with one than with the other. Confirm the blade you select is free of nicks, which could easily cause soft-tissue trauma to the upper airway. Ensure that the light is bright, white, and steady. The light should be bright enough so that it is uncomfortable to look at directly. It should be white, not yellow or dim. The light should not flicker, especially as the blade is moved on the handle. With older laryngoscope blades, the bulb is screwed into the blade; you must ensure that the bulb is tightly secured to prevent it from being aspirated into the lungs. Modern blades utilize fiberoptics to provide light, and the light source is located in the laryngoscope handle itself; nonetheless, confirm the batteries have enough power to provide sufficient light.
Towels	You may need towels to properly position the patient's head.
Suction	You may need suction to clear the airway of blood or other secretions to obtain an adequate laryngoscopic view of the glottic opening and vocal cords.
Magill forceps	Have Magill forceps available in case you encounter a foreign body obstruction during laryngoscopy.
Confirmation devices	Stethoscope and an $ETCO_2$ detector (use quantitative waveform capnography to confirm initial and ongoing ET tube placement). Use a colorimetric carbon dioxide detector *only* if capnography is not available.
ET tube–securing device	Have the appropriate device readily available to secure the ET tube. A commercial device specifically designed to secure the ET tube is recommended.

Abbreviations: $ETCO_2$, end-tidal carbon dioxide; ET, endotracheal

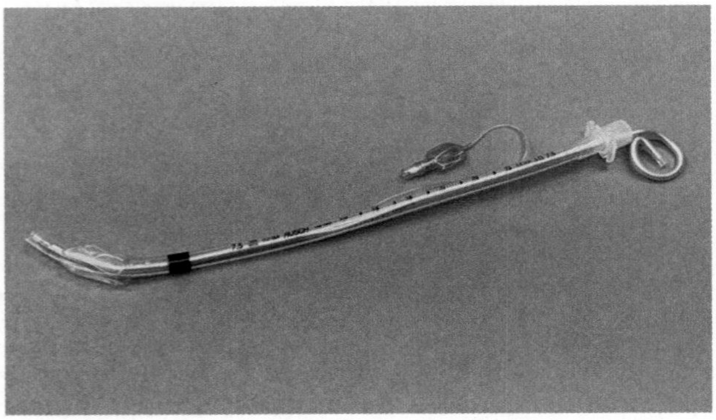

FIGURE 16-71 Prior to use, straighten the endotracheal tube/stylet combination and place a slight bend just proximal to the cuff.

Courtesy of Steve Rahm.

Standard Precautions

As with airway management in general, intubation may expose you to blood, secretions, or aerosolized respiratory droplets. In particular, diseases such as COVID-19 (coronavirus disease 2019) and tuberculosis are spread through respiratory droplets. Therefore, standard precautions during intubation should include an N95 mask, safety glasses and/or a full-face shield, gloves, and, if necessary, a gown.

Preoxygenation

Adequate preoxygenation with a bag-mask device and 100% oxygen is a critical step before intubating a patient. You should preoxygenate an apneic or

Words of Wisdom

Perform ventilations with a bag-mask device and 100% oxygen for at least 2 to 3 minutes before attempting intubation. The patient needs an oxygen reserve to tolerate the period without ventilation that will occur during the insertion of an advanced airway. You also need the time to check your equipment properly.

hypoventilating patient for 2 to 3 minutes. During the intubation attempt, the patient will undergo a period of so-called forced apnea, during which time the patient will not be ventilated. The goal of preoxygenation is to prevent hypoxia from occurring during this time. Unfortunately, you will be unable to perform an extensive preintubation evaluation of the patient (such as obtaining hemoglobin and hematocrit values), and patients who are intubated in the prehospital setting are usually in a physiologically unstable condition.

Monitor the patient's Spo_2 level and achieve as close to 100% saturation as possible during the 2- to 3-minute preoxygenation period. During the intubation attempt, you must continually monitor the Spo_2 level and maintain it at greater than 94%.

The consequences of even brief periods of hypoxia can be disastrous. Do not rely solely on pulse oximetry to quantify a patient's oxygenation status; it can produce falsely high readings, even if the patient is severely hypoxic. Although some sequelae of hypoxia are dramatic and occur immediately, most are subtle and occur gradually. Some of the poor neurologic outcomes following aggressive airway management result from intubation-induced hypoxia, also known as peri-intubation hypoxia.

Words of Wisdom

If the patient has experienced a possible neck injury, then you must place the head in a neutral, in-line position. Do not use the sniffing position or extend the patient's head in any way. Intubation of a trauma patient is most effectively performed by two paramedics.

Positioning the Patient

Successful laryngoscopy will be extremely difficult, if not impossible, without proper positioning of the patient's head. The airway has three axes: oral, tracheal, and pharyngeal. When the head is in a neutral position, these axes are at acute angles, facilitating entry of food into the esophagus rather than into the trachea **FIGURE 16-72**. Although this positioning is advantageous to a conscious, spontaneously breathing person, the angles of these axes make laryngoscopy difficult.

To facilitate visualization of the airway, the three axes must be aligned to the greatest extent possible. This alignment is most effectively achieved by placing the patient in the sniffing position. In most supine patients, the sniffing position can be achieved by elevating the occiput about 1 to 2 inches (2.5 to 5 cm). Elevate the head with folded towels, or have your partner elevate the head, until the earlobes are at the level of the sternum **FIGURE 16-73**. When you use towels, you can easily adjust their thickness by changing the number of folds. For patients with obesity, padding under the head alone may not result in the sniffing position; you may need to add padding under the shoulders and neck as well. To confirm that the patient is in a true sniffing position, view the person from the side to ensure that the earlobes and sternum are on the same horizontal plane.

Laryngoscope Blade Insertion

After you have properly positioned the patient's head and provided preoxygenation, direct your partner to stop ventilating. Position yourself at the top of the patient's head. If the patient is on a

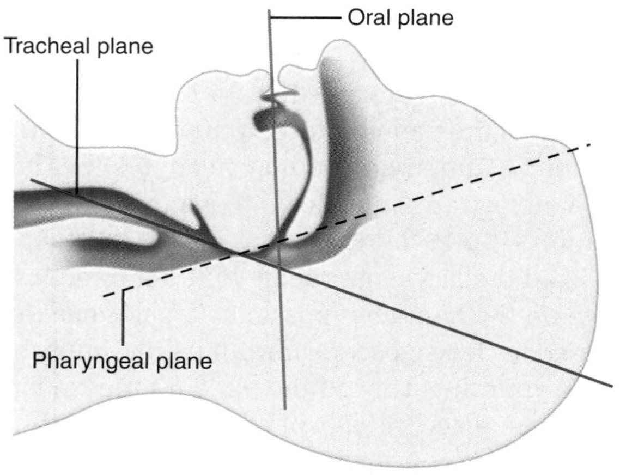

FIGURE 16-72 When the head is in a neutral position, the three axes of the airway (oral, tracheal, and pharyngeal) are at acute angles and make laryngoscopy difficult.

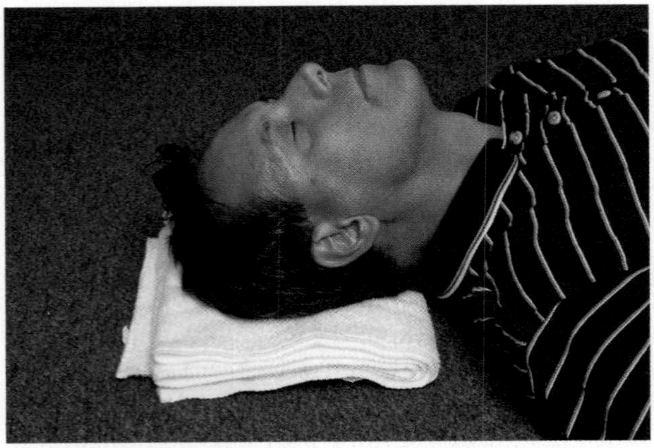

FIGURE 16-73 The sniffing position is achieved by elevating the head until the earlobes are at the level of the sternum.

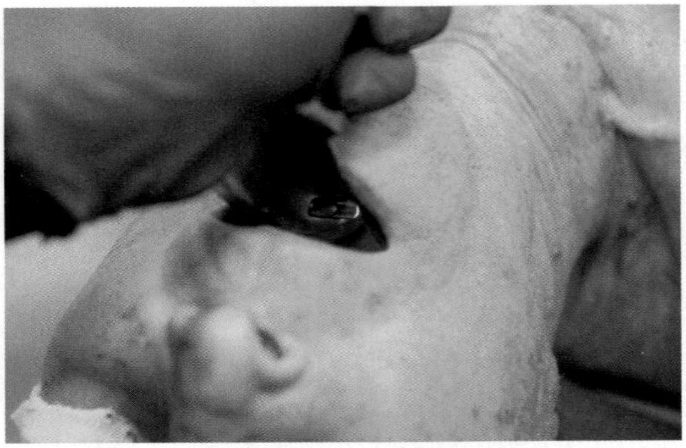

FIGURE 16-75 The tongue is a sticky, amorphous structure that can hinder visualization of the airway. Proper manipulation of the laryngoscope blade in the mouth is critical to controlling the tongue.

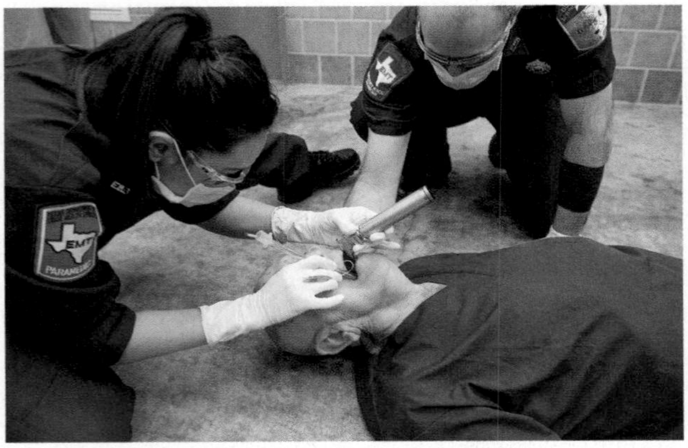

FIGURE 16-74 If the patient is on the floor or ground, then you may need to kneel and lean forward or lie on the floor to get into the proper position.

stretcher, then you can squat to put your head at the level of the patient's face. If the patient is on the floor or ground, then you may need to either kneel and lean forward or lie down to get into the proper position **FIGURE 16-74**.

Hold the laryngoscope in your left hand, as far down on the handle as possible. It is not necessary to grasp the laryngoscope in your palm; simply hold it with your fingertips. If the patient's mouth is not open, then place the side of your right-hand thumb just below the bottom lip and push the mouth open, or "scissor" your thumb and index finger between the molars. As an alternative, you can open the mouth with the tongue-jaw lift maneuver.

Insert the blade into the right side of the patient's mouth. Use the flange of the blade to sweep the tongue gently to the left side of the mouth while moving the blade into the midline. Place the little finger of your left hand under the patient's chin; doing so will help you lift the jaw and will help prevent you from levering the blade back against the patient's teeth. Take care not to catch the patient's lips between the laryngoscope blade and the teeth. Moving the tongue from right to left is a critical step. If you simply insert the blade in the midline, then the tongue will hang over both sides of the blade and all you will see is the tongue **FIGURE 16-75**.

Slowly advance the blade while continuing to sweep the tongue to the left until you identify the uvula; you should now be visualizing the posterior pharynx. Continue advancing the blade until the epiglottis comes into view. *The epiglottis is a critical structure to identify during laryngoscopy.* Gently manipulate the blade until you can see the epiglottis. Do not pry back on the laryngoscope; prying will cause you to use the patient's upper teeth as a fulcrum, resulting in potential breaking and aspiration of teeth **FIGURE 16-76**. Laryngoscopy does *not* require brute force; it is a technique of finesse and simple anatomic manipulation. It is critical to relax when using a laryngoscope; a human's jaw is easy to manipulate, unlike that of a manikin. The correct motion is similar to holding a champagne (flute) glass and offering a toast **FIGURE 16-77**.

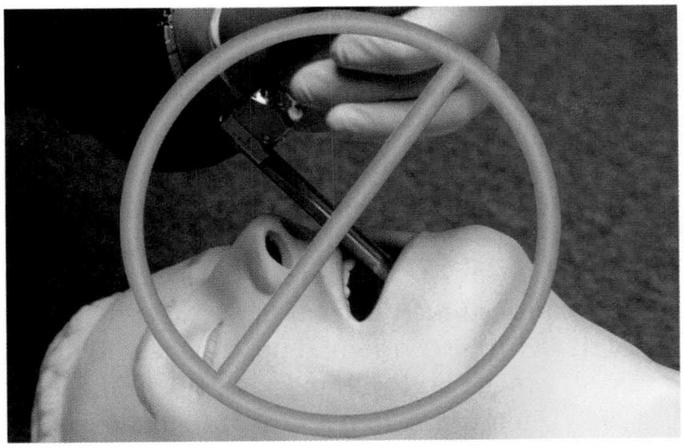

FIGURE 16-76 Avoid prying against the upper teeth with the laryngoscope, which may potentially result in breaking and aspiration of the teeth.

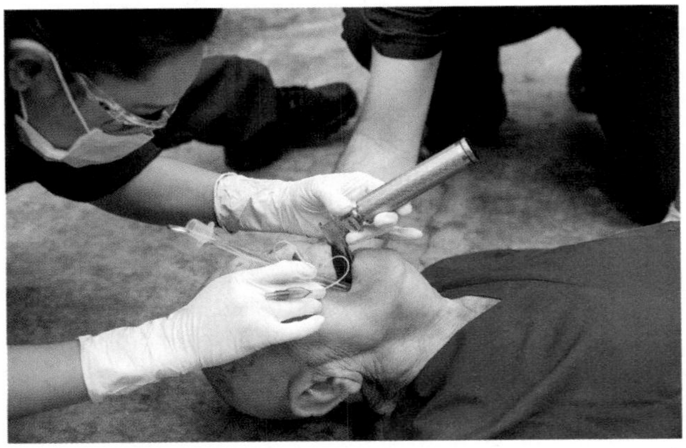

FIGURE 16-77 Relax your arms and gently advance the laryngoscope blade until the anatomy can be visualized.

Visualization of the Glottic Opening

After you identify the epiglottis, place the tip of the curved blade in the vallecular space, which is above the epiglottis. Position the straight blade directly under the epiglottis, then gently lift until the glottic opening comes into full view. You should see the vocal cords and the arytenoid cartilage. The vocal cords are white fibrous bands that lie vertically within the glottic opening. The arytenoid cartilage is located inferiorly on both sides of the glottic opening **FIGURE 16-78**. Identifying these structures enables to you make small adjustments in the position of the blade to ensure maximal visualization of the glottic opening.

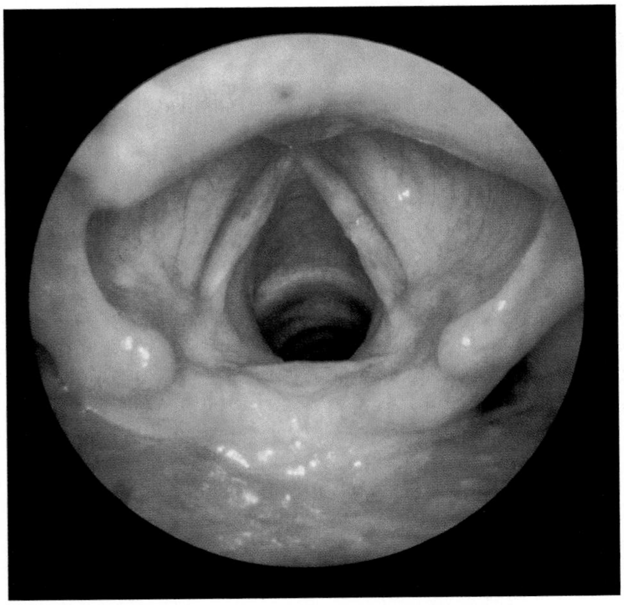

FIGURE 16-78 Laryngoscopic view of the epiglottis, vocal cords (white fibrous bands), and arytenoid cartilage.

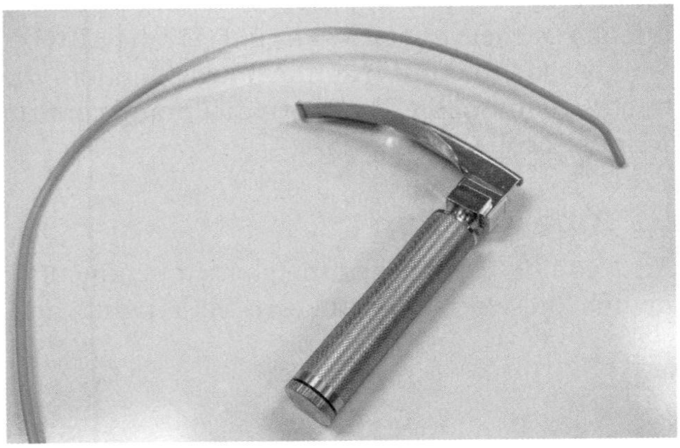

FIGURE 16-79 A gum bougie is shown next to a laryngoscope.

The **gum bougie**, also called an ET tube introducer, is a flexible device that is 0.20 inch (5 mm or 15 Fr) in diameter and about 2 feet (70 cm) long. A 30° bend is found at the distal tip **FIGURE 16-79**. Reusable and disposable versions are available in both adult and pediatric sizes. The bougie is used in epiglottis-only views to facilitate intubation. It can make intubation possible in some difficult situations, especially when your view of the glottic opening is limited. The bougie is rigid enough that it can be easily directed through the glottic opening, yet flexible enough that it does not damage the tracheal walls. Many paramedics routinely use a bougie when intubating patients, even if they have an unobstructed view of the vocal cords.

Words of Wisdom

When you use a gum bougie to facilitate intubation, orienting the tip anteriorly will enable you to feel the tracheal rings. Advance it until you meet resistance, which indicates that the bougie is at the level of the carina. In addition, remember that advancing anything into the trachea beyond the epiglottis requires sterile technique. The risk of introducing an infection with a bougie is a serious consideration, so be careful how you store the device.

The bougie is inserted through the glottic opening under laryngoscopy. The angle at its distal tip facilitates entry into the glottic opening and enables you to "feel" the ridges of the tracheal wall **FIGURE 16-80**. After the bougie is placed deeply into the trachea, it serves as a guide for the ET tube. Simply slide the tube over the bougie and into the trachea. Remove the bougie, ventilate, and confirm proper ET tube placement.

ET Tube Insertion

After you have visualized the glottic opening, pick up the preselected ET tube in your right hand, holding it with two fingers (like a pencil). The lower down you hold the tube, the more control you have over it. Under visualization, insert the tube from the right corner of the patient's mouth.

As you see the tube pass through the vocal cords, rotate the tube to the right and direct the tip of the ET tube downward, allowing it to descend into the trachea. *The trachea is not a straight tube; it descends immediately beyond the vocal cords.* If the tip of the ET tube is oriented up, then it will hit the cricoid cartilage and will not pass. If you meet resistance when trying to pass the tube between the vocal cords, back the tube up slightly and then advance the tube while simultaneously rotating it.

Advance the ET tube until the proximal end of the cuff is 0.5 to 0.75 inch (1 to 2 cm) past the

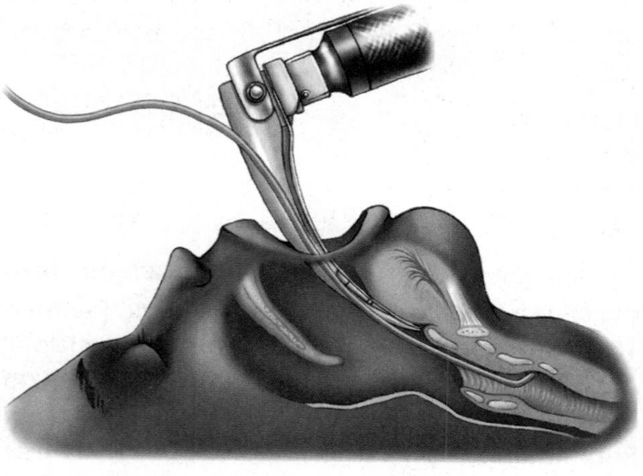

FIGURE 16-80 The angle at the distal tip of the gum bougie facilitates entry into the glottic opening and enables you to feel the tracheal rings.

Words of Wisdom

Improving Your Laryngoscopic View

During laryngoscopy, you (the intubator) can reach around with your right hand and manipulate the larynx (external laryngeal manipulation) while directly observing the effect on your view of the vocal cords. After the view is optimized, an assistant can maintain this laryngeal position as you insert the ET tube with your right hand. This procedure, called **bimanual laryngoscopy**, is an effective method for improving your laryngoscopic view **FIGURE 16-81**.

During external laryngeal manipulation, the intubator (or an assistant) can perform the **BURP maneuver**. In this maneuver, backward, upward, and rightward pressure is applied to the lower third of the thyroid cartilage.

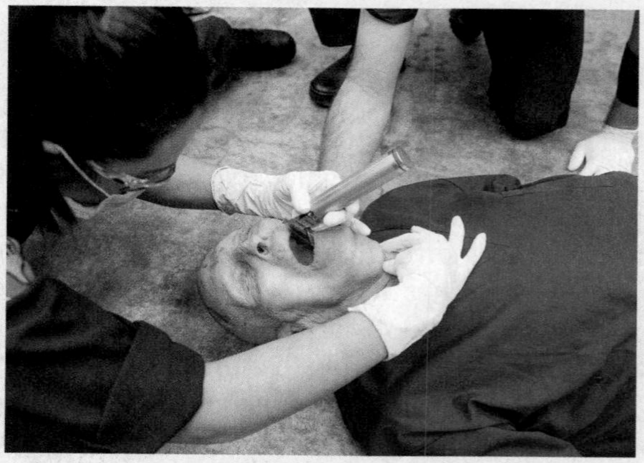

FIGURE 16-81 Bimanual laryngoscopy using external laryngeal manipulation.

vocal cords. You *must* see the tip of the ET tube pass through the vocal cords. If you cannot see the vocal cords, then do not insert the tube! An ET tube inserted blindly down the throat will almost always come to rest in the esophagus, not in the trachea; the only way to be certain that the tube has passed through the vocal cords is to see it pass through the vocal cords. If you take your eye off the tip of the tube (and the vocal cords), even for a second, then you significantly increase the likelihood of intubating the esophagus.

Do not try to pass the ET tube down the barrel of the laryngoscope blade, especially when you are using a straight blade. The laryngoscope blade is not designed as a guide for the tube; it is a tool used only to visualize the glottic opening. Placing the tube down the barrel of the blade will obscure your view of the glottic opening **FIGURE 16-82**.

Ventilation

After you have seen the cuff of the ET tube pass roughly 0.5 to 0.75 inch (1 to 2 cm) beyond the vocal cords, gently remove the blade, anchor the tube securely to the teeth with your right index and/or middle finger, and remove the stylet from the tube. Back out the stylet carefully to avoid extubating the patient. *Removing the stylet without manually securing the tube to the teeth can result in inadvertent extubation.*

Inflate the distal cuff with 5 to 10 mL of air, and then detach the syringe from the inflation port. If the syringe is not removed immediately following inflation of the distal cuff, then air from the cuff may leak back into the syringe, resulting in an inadequate seal between the cuff and the tracheal wall. Avoid inflating the distal cuff with excess pressure, which may cause ischemia or necrosis of the tracheal wall; ultimately, this could lead to tracheal stenosis (narrowing).

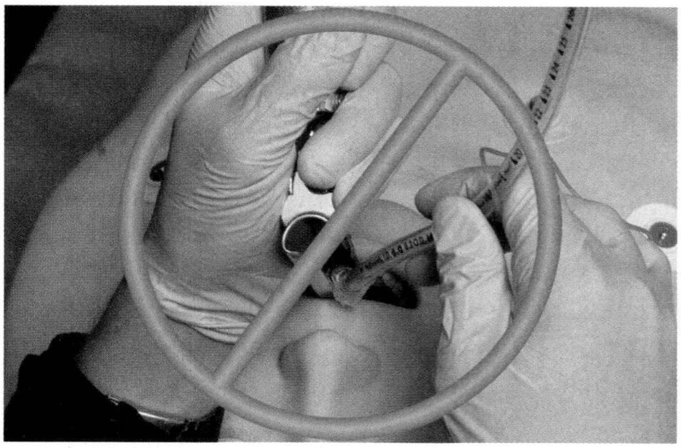

FIGURE 16-82 Avoid placing an endotracheal tube down the barrel of the blade because it obscures your view of the glottic opening.

Words of Wisdom

It should not take longer than 10 to 15 seconds to intubate a patient from the time you insert the laryngoscope into the mouth. Be gentle and work with deliberate speed, but do not be hasty. During the attempt, monitor the patient's oxygen saturation and heart rate. If you cannot successfully intubate the patient in short order, abort the attempt and reoxygenate the patient with 100% oxygen before attempting intubation again. *Do not allow the patient's oxygen saturation to fall below 95% during any intubation attempt!* If the patient is in cardiac arrest, then do not interrupt chest compressions to insert an ET tube. If you cannot intubate a patient with CPR in progress, choose a different airway management strategy.

Note the depth of the ET tube (in centimeters) at the patient's teeth. This observation will enable you and other health care personnel involved in the patient's medical care to determine whether the tube migrated after it was placed. For example, if the depth of the ET tube was initially 20 cm at the teeth but is now 24 cm, then you know that the tube has advanced 4 cm farther into the trachea.

Have your assistant attach the bag-mask device to the ET tube and continue ventilation. Place an in-line capnography monitor, which is attached to the cardiac monitor/defibrillator, between the bag-mask device and the ET tube. While the first ventilations are delivered, look at the patient's chest to ensure that it rises with each ventilation. At the same time, listen with a stethoscope to the stomach over the epigastrium and over both lungs at the third or fourth intercostal space in the midaxillary line. If the ET tube is positioned correctly, you will hear equal breath sounds bilaterally and a quiet epigastrium. However, epigastric sounds may be transmitted to the lungs in patients with obesity or patients with significant gastric distention, leading you to believe that you have inadvertently intubated the esophagus, one of the many reasons that quantitative waveform capnography is essential in these situations.

Continue ventilation as dictated by the patient's age. Recall from Table 16-11 that you should ventilate an apneic adult with a pulse at a rate of 10 breaths/min (one breath every 6 seconds), and an apneic infant or child with a pulse at a rate of 20 to 30 breaths/min (one breath every 2 to 3 seconds). If the patient (adult, child, or infant) is in cardiac arrest, then ventilate at a rate of 10 breaths/min (one breath every 6 seconds).[1,5–7] Do not stop chest compressions to deliver ventilations (asynchronous CPR).

Confirmation of Tube Placement

Visualizing the ET tube passing between the vocal cords is your first and most reliable method of confirming that the tube has entered the trachea; however, you must continue gathering information to assess and monitor the location of the tube. A misplaced tube that goes undetected is a fatal error. You must incorporate multiple assessment findings to make a correct determination of the tube's location.

Auscultation is the next step in confirming proper tube placement. Unequal or absent breath sounds suggest esophageal placement, main stem bronchus placement, pneumothorax, or bronchial obstruction.

Bilaterally absent breath sounds or gurgling over the epigastrium when auscultating during ventilation indicates that you have intubated the esophagus rather than the trachea. If copious vomitus is being emitted from the ET tube, then do not remove it! Instead, inflate the distal cuff, turn the tube to the side, and continue ventilation with a bag-mask device. If vomitus is not being emitted from the ET tube, then remove it and resume bag-mask ventilation. Reoxygenate the patient, be prepared to suction the airway as needed, and consider another attempt at intubation.

If you hear breath sounds only on the right side of the chest, then the ET tube has likely been advanced too far and entered the right main stem bronchus. Follow these steps to reposition the tube:

1. Deflate the distal cuff.
2. Place your stethoscope over the left side of the patient's chest.
3. While ventilation continues, slowly retract the tube while simultaneously listening for breath sounds over the left side of the chest.
4. Stop as soon as you hear bilaterally equal breath sounds.
5. Note the depth of the tube (in centimeters) at the patient's teeth.
6. Reinflate the distal cuff.
7. Secure the tube.
8. Resume ventilations.

If the ET tube has been positioned correctly in the trachea, then it should be easy to compress the bag-mask device, and you should see corresponding chest expansion. Increased resistance (decreased ventilation compliance) during ventilations may indicate gastric distention, esophageal intubation, or tension pneumothorax. Each of these conditions warrants immediate reassessment and corrective action.

Words of Wisdom

If any question arises about the placement or position of the ET tube, you should not hesitate to revisualize the airway and confirm that the tube is still between the vocal cords. Occasionally, the filter line from the capnography adaptor gets occluded by blood or other secretions, blocking the flow of gas into the monitor/defibrillator and causing a loss of the waveform. If this occurs, replace the in-line $ETCO_2$ detector. When you make the clinical decision to intubate a patient, you *must* follow and document a rigorous tube confirmation protocol.

In addition to a clinical assessment (such as auscultating over the epigastrium and over the lung fields bilaterally and assessing for visible chest rise), continuous waveform capnography (discussed earlier in this chapter) is regarded as the most reliable method of confirming and monitoring correct placement of the ET tube. The ideal time to attach the in-line capnography monitor is when the bag-mask device is attached to the ET tube. If waveform capnography is unavailable, you can use a colorimetric $ETCO_2$ detector (also discussed earlier in this chapter), along with a clinical assessment of the patient, to confirm and monitor ET tube placement.

Securing the Tube

The last step in orotracheal intubation by direct laryngoscopy is to secure the ET tube. Inadvertent extubation is relatively common and can be traumatic to the patient. As a paramedic, it can be discouraging to accomplish a difficult intubation, only to have the ET tube slip out of the trachea. Reintubation will almost certainly be even more difficult. Never take your hand off the ET tube before it has been secured with an appropriate device. Even then, it is a good idea to support the tube manually while you ventilate the patient to avoid a sudden jolt from the ventilation device that pulls the tube from the trachea.

Many commercial tube-securing devices are available. Familiarize yourself with the specific device used by your EMS system. The steps for securing an ET tube are as follows:

1. Note the depth of the ET tube (in centimeters) at the patient's upper teeth, or upper gum if teeth are absent.
2. Remove the ventilation device from the ET tube.
3. Position the ET tube in the center of the patient's mouth.
4. Place the securing device over the ET tube. Tighten the screw to secure it in place. Fasten the strap.
5. Reattach the ventilation device, auscultate again over both lungs and over the epigastrium, and note the capnography reading and waveform.

Some commercially manufactured ET tube–securing devices feature a built-in bite block to prevent occlusion of the tube if the patient bites down. If you do not have a commercially manufactured ET tube–securing device available, you can secure the tube in place with tape and insert a bite block or oral airway between the molars to prevent the patient from biting the tube.

Documentation and Communication

On the patient care report, document the means of assessing placement of the ET tube, such as breath sounds, visualization, and waveform capnography findings. Also document the depth of the tube, as noted by the centimeter marking at the patient's teeth. In addition, indicate when correct placement was confirmed and the method(s) by which it was confirmed: at the time the ET tube was placed, any time the patient was moved (ie, from floor to stretcher, loaded into the ambulance), and on arrival at the hospital.

It is also important to minimize head movement in an intubated patient. With a firmly secured tube, the tip can move as much as 2 inches (5 cm)

YOU are the Paramedic

PART 7

During transport, you reassess the patient and note that his clinical status has deteriorated. His respiratory rate has markedly slowed, his breathing has become shallow, and the gray color of his lips and gums is returning. You inform your partner of the status change, and he asks you if you want him to pull over so the patient can be intubated.

Recording Time: 20 Minutes	
Level of consciousness	Responsive to pain only
Respirations	10 breaths/min; labored and shallow
Pulse	122 beats/min; weak and regular
Skin	Cool and moist; lips and gums are gray
Blood pressure	144/76 mm Hg
Oxygen saturation (Spo_2)	79% (with CPAP)
Pupils	PERRLA
$ETCO_2$	58 mm Hg
ECG	Sinus tachycardia

11. How should you adjust your treatment of the patient?

during head flexion and extension. If the patient's head is hyperflexed, then the ET tube can be completely pulled out of the trachea. If the head is hyperextended, then the ET tube could be pushed farther into the trachea, potentially into a main stem bronchus. Keep the patient's head in a neutral position to reduce the likelihood of tube dislodgement during transport. Consider applying head blocks or equivalent measures to minimize head movement.

The steps for orotracheal intubation by direct laryngoscopy are shown in **SKILL DRILL 16-9**.

NR Skill

Skill Drill 16-9 Performing Orotracheal Intubation Using Direct Laryngoscopy

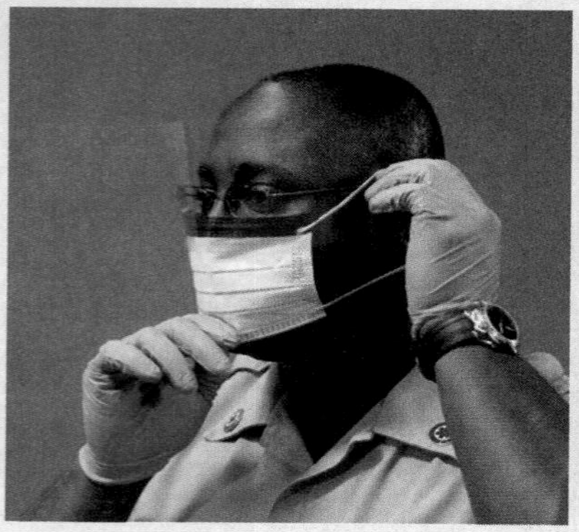

Step 1

Take standard precautions. If you suspect trauma, then maintain manual in-line stabilization of the patient's head.

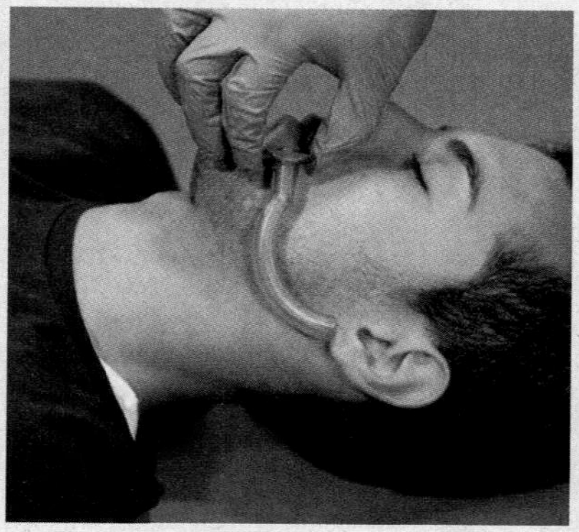

Step 2

Measure for the proper size, and insert an oral airway.

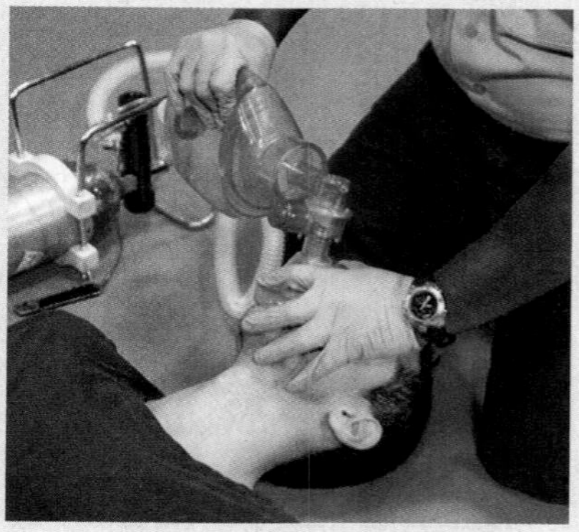

Step 3

Ventilate the patient with a bag-mask device at a rate of 10 breaths/min with sufficient volume to produce chest rise. Preoxygenate the patient for 2 to 3 minutes with 100% oxygen.

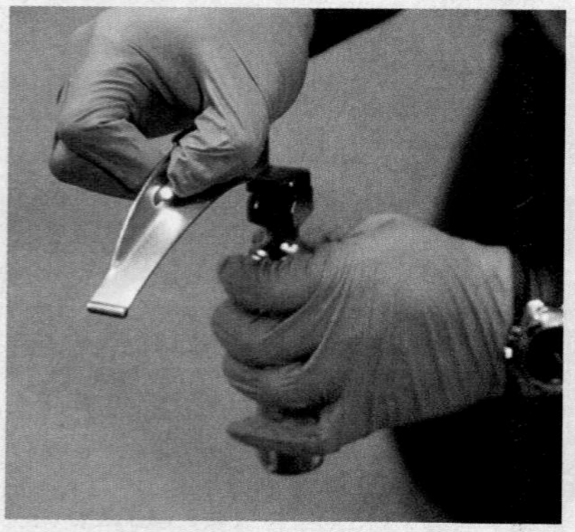

Step 4

Check, prepare, and assemble your equipment.

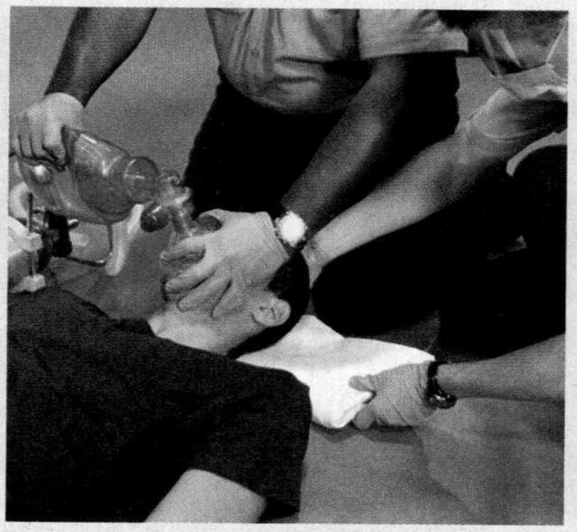

Step 5

Place the patient's head in the sniffing position.

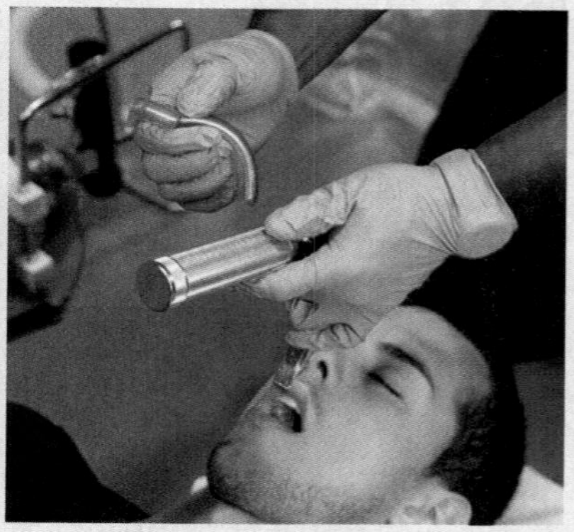

Step 6

Remove the oral airway, then insert the blade into the right side of the patient's mouth, and displace the tongue to the left.

Skill Drill 16-9 Performing Orotracheal Intubation Using Direct Laryngoscopy (continued)

NR Skill

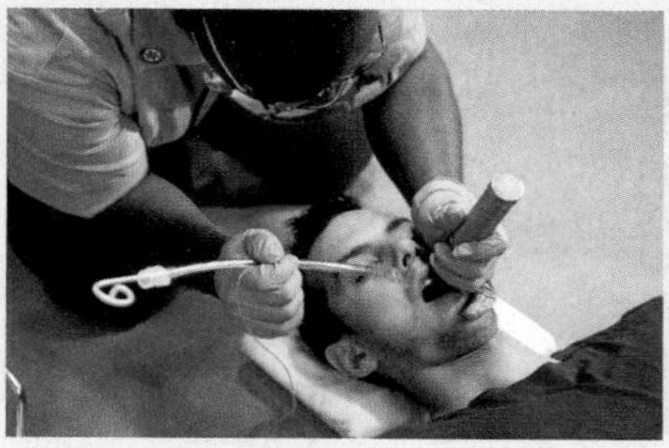

Step 7

Gently lift the long axis of the laryngoscope handle until you can visualize the glottic opening and the vocal cords.

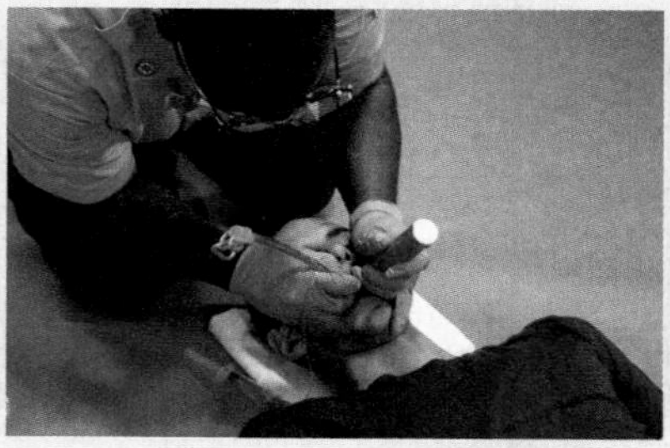

Step 8

Insert the ET tube through the right corner of the mouth.

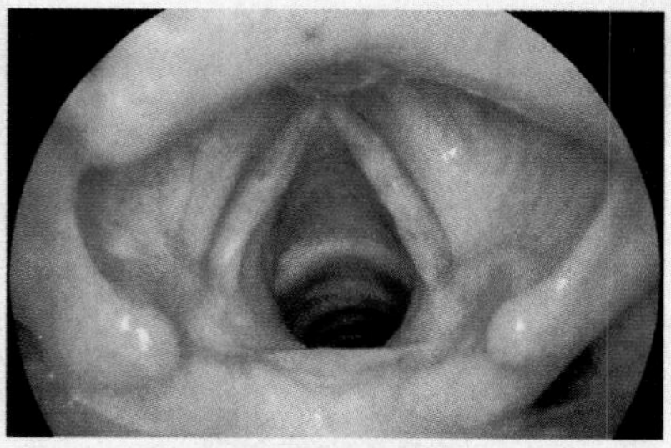

Step 9

Visualize the entry of the ET tube between the vocal cords.

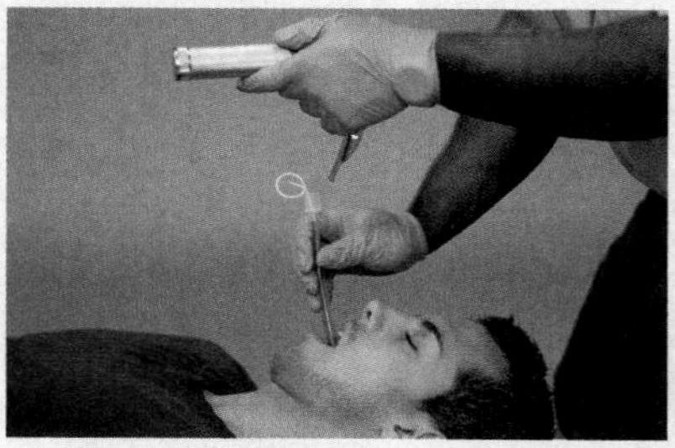

Step 10

Remove the laryngoscope from the patient's mouth.

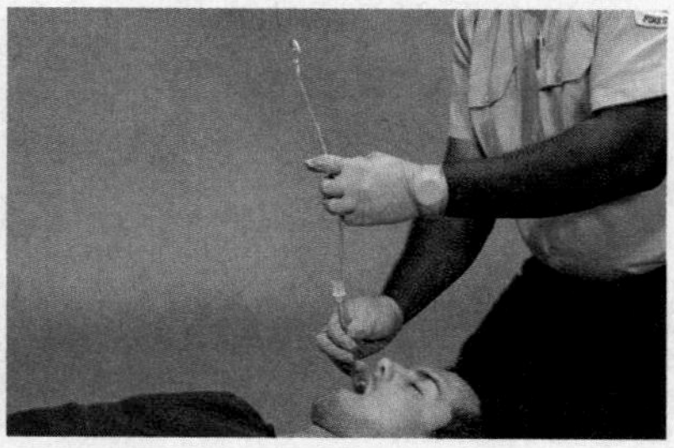

Step 11

Note the depth of the ET tube (in centimeters) at the patient's teeth and remove the stylet from the ET tube.

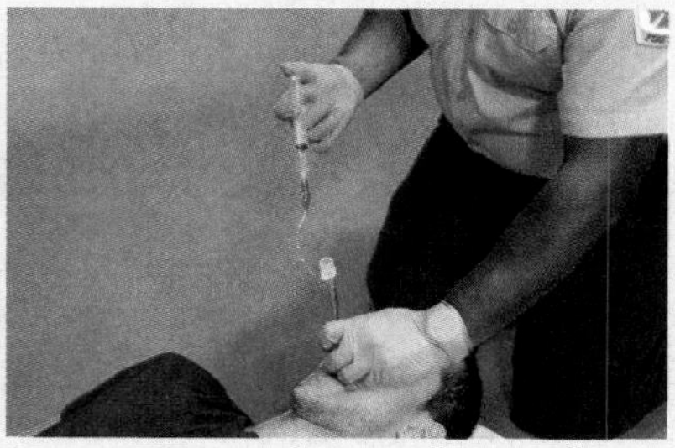

Step 12

Inflate the distal cuff of the ET tube with 5 to 10 mL of air, and immediately detach the syringe from the inflation port.

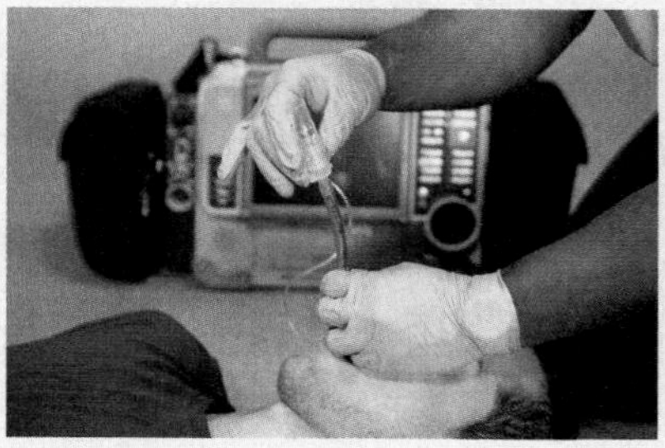

Step 13

Attach the $ETCO_2$ detector (waveform capnography is preferred) to the ET tube.

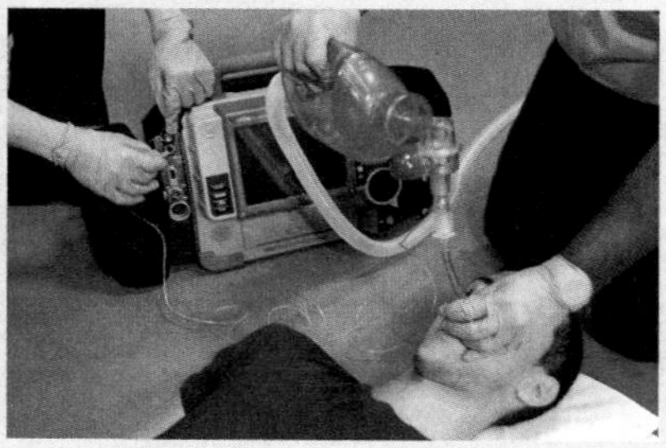

Step 14

Attach the $ETCO_2$ detector to the cardiac monitor/defibrillator and observe for a capnographic waveform and numeric carbon dioxide reading.

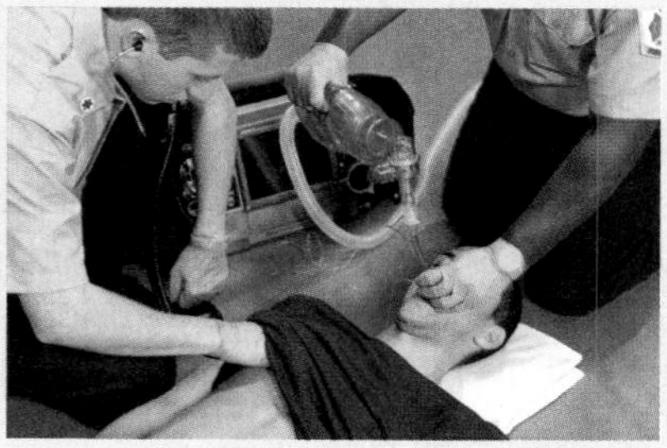

Step 15

Attach the ventilation device and ventilate. Listen over the epigastrium and over both lungs.

(continues)

NR Skill

Skill Drill 16-9 Performing Orotracheal Intubation Using Direct Laryngoscopy (continued)

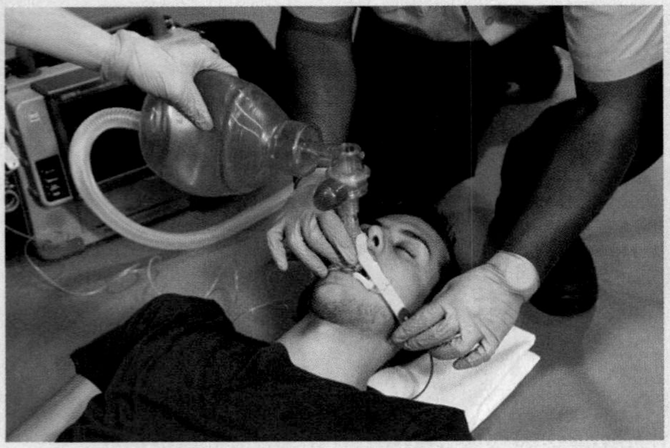

Step 16

Secure the ET tube with a commercial device or tape. Ventilate the patient at the proper rate while monitoring capnography and pulse oximetry.

Orotracheal Intubation by Video Laryngoscopy

Video laryngoscopy is popular in the prehospital and in-hospital settings because it facilitates visualization of the glottic opening and vocal cords, even in patients with the most difficult airways. Instead of trying to visualize the vocal cords around the laryngoscope, as with direct laryngoscopy, you can guide placement of the ET tube with the use of a video monitor. However, video laryngoscopy requires better hand-to-eye coordination than direct laryngoscopy does.

Types of Video Laryngoscopes

Several video laryngoscopes are commercially available. Some have a laryngoscope and separate video monitor **FIGURE 16-83** and **FIGURE 16-84**, and others have the video monitor attached to the laryngoscope itself **FIGURE 16-85**. All video laryngoscopes feature single-use blades of various sizes.

Some video laryngoscopes require displacement of the tongue, such as the McGrath laryngoscope. Others are inserted in the midline of the mouth and simply follow the curvature of the tongue, such as the King Vision **FIGURE 16-86** laryngoscope. The King Vision, a nondisplacing device, also features an optional channeled blade through which the ET tube is placed, thereby avoiding the need for a stylet.

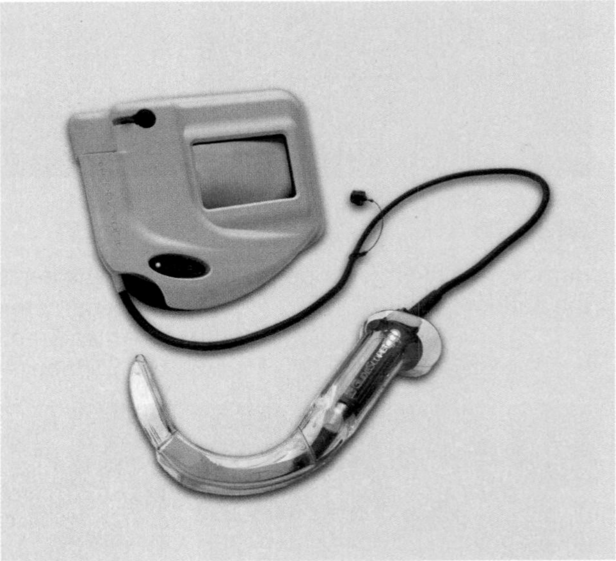

FIGURE 16-83 The GlideScope Ranger video laryngoscope.

Certain video laryngoscopes, such as the McGrath, can allow you to directly visualize the airway structures if the video monitor suddenly stops working.

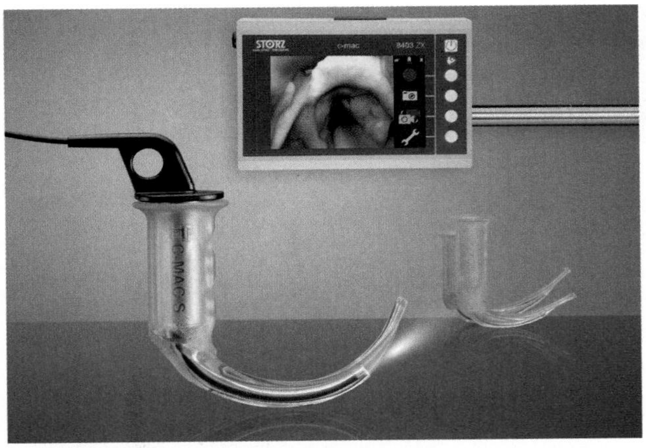

FIGURE 16-84 The C-MAC video laryngoscope.

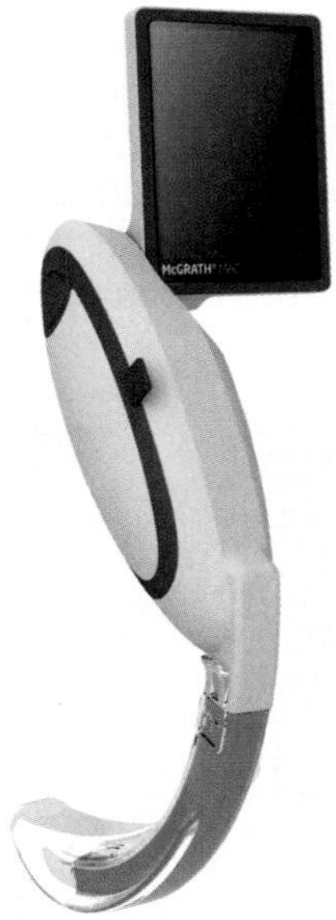

FIGURE 16-85 The McGrath video laryngoscope.

Evidence-Based Medicine

The results of studies comparing direct laryngoscopy and video laryngoscopy are mixed. However, a systematic review of the literature shows that video laryngoscopy leads to higher rates of first-pass success, shorter intubation times, and better overall success when used by less-experienced intubators.[8–10]

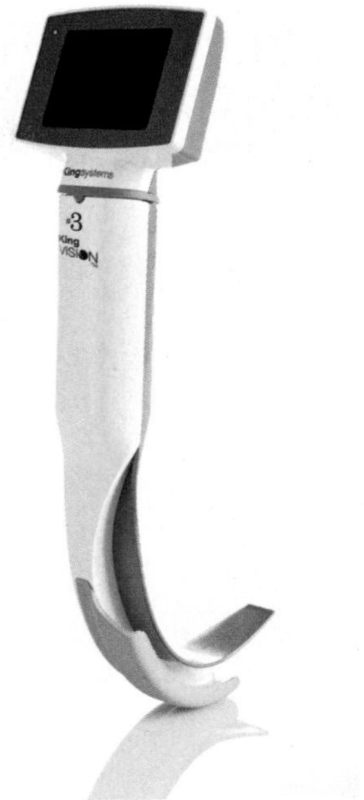

FIGURE 16-86 The King Vision video laryngoscope.

Words of Wisdom

The camera on the video laryngoscope is located on the distal end of the device. You will be unable to obtain a view of the airway anatomy if the camera becomes clouded by secretions. Keep the camera ahead of any secretions, and use suction to remove secretions before you advance the blade.

Video laryngoscopy can be beneficial in a variety of environments. Consult the manufacturer's guidelines for the video laryngoscope used by your service. The steps for orotracheal intubation by video laryngoscopy are shown in **SKILL DRILL 16-10**.

Nasotracheal Intubation

Nasotracheal intubation is the insertion of an ET tube into the trachea through the nose. It is usually performed without directly visualizing the vocal cords, hence the term "blind" nasotracheal intubation.

Blind nasotracheal intubation is an excellent technique for establishing control over the airway in situations in which it is difficult or hazardous to

Skill Drill 16-10 Performing Orotracheal Intubation Using Video Laryngoscopy

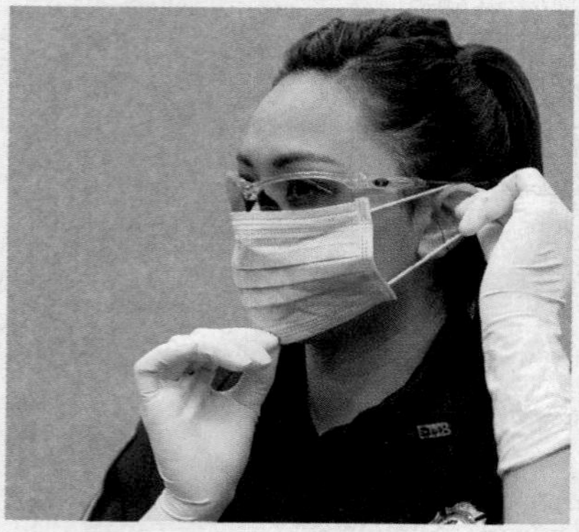

Step 1

Take standard precautions. If you suspect trauma, maintain manual in-line stabilization of the patient's head.

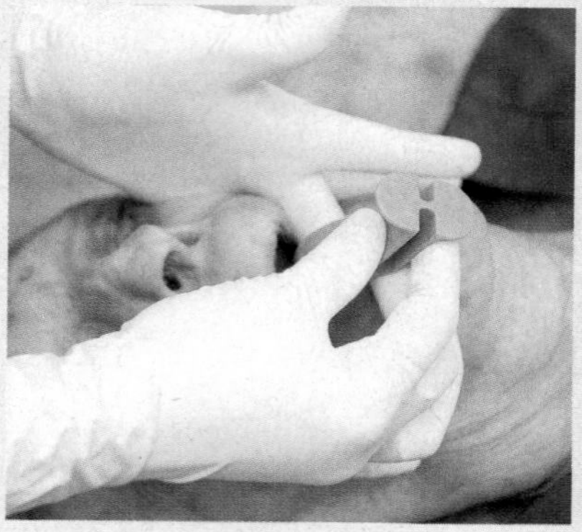

Step 2

Measure for the proper size, and insert an oral airway.

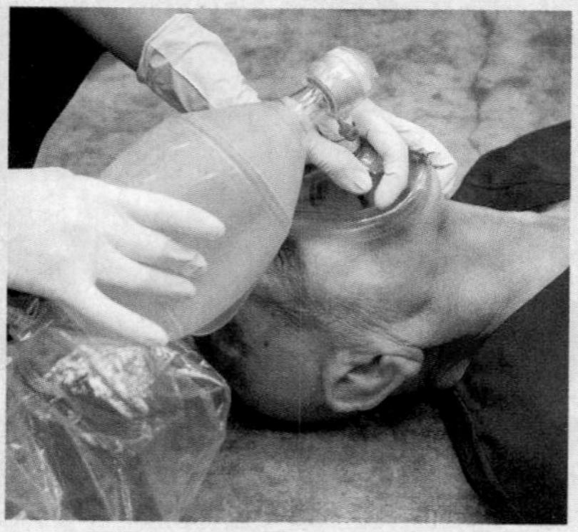

Step 3

Ventilate the patient with a bag-mask device at a rate of 10 breaths/min with sufficient volume to produce chest rise. Preoxygenate the patient for 2 to 3 minutes with 100% oxygen.

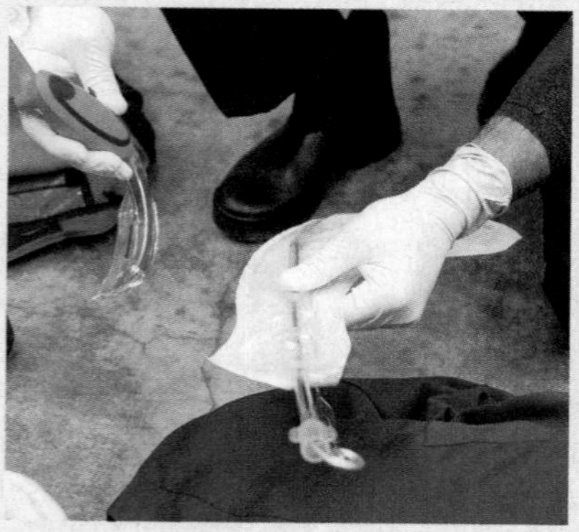

Step 4

Check, prepare, and assemble your equipment. Turn on the video laryngoscope and ensure the light and camera are functioning correctly.

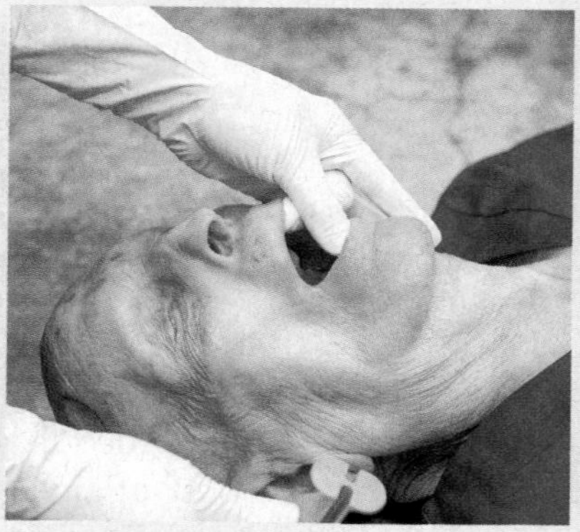

Step 5

Remove the oral airway and place the patient's head in the sniffing position.

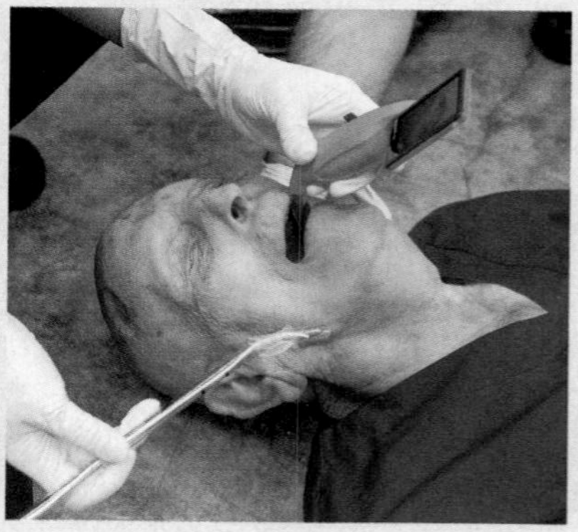

Step 6

Insert the video laryngoscope blade into the right side of the patient's mouth (displacing laryngoscope) or the midline of the mouth (nondisplacing laryngoscope). If using a displacing laryngoscope, sweep the tongue to the left. Visualize the epiglottis, vocal cords, and arytenoid cartilage.

Skill Drill 16-10 Performing Orotracheal Intubation Using Video Laryngoscopy (continued)

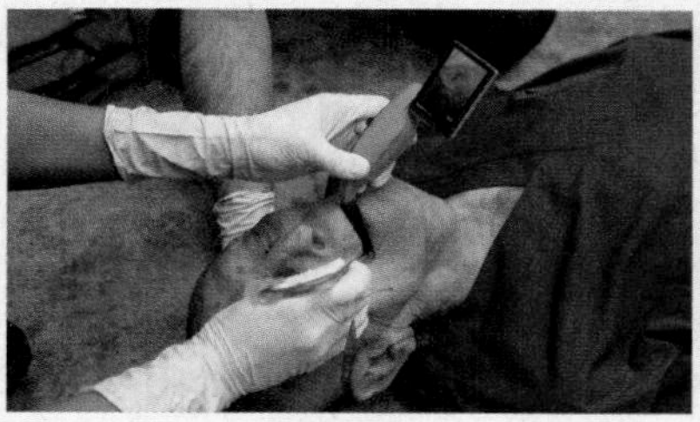

Step 7

Visualize entry of the ET tube between the vocal cords on the video monitor.

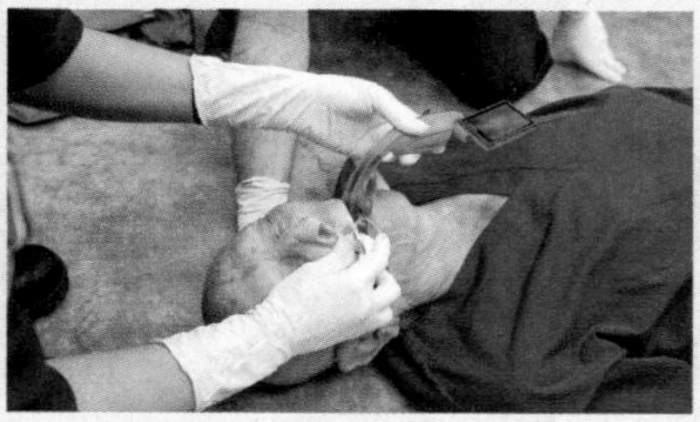

Step 8

Anchor the tube to the patient's teeth with your finger(s) and remove the laryngoscope from the patient's mouth.

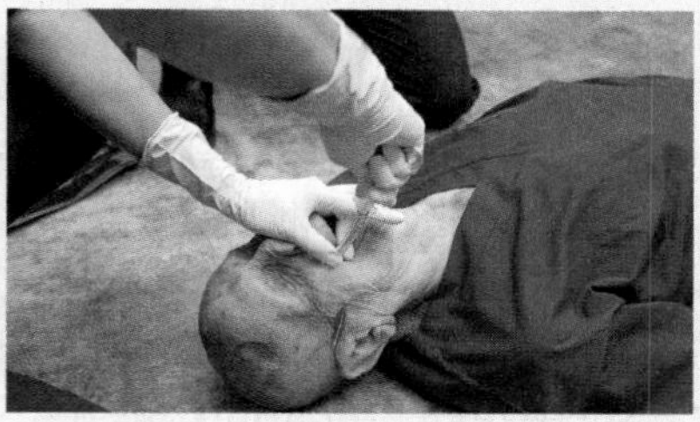

Step 9

Remove the stylet from the ET tube (if used).

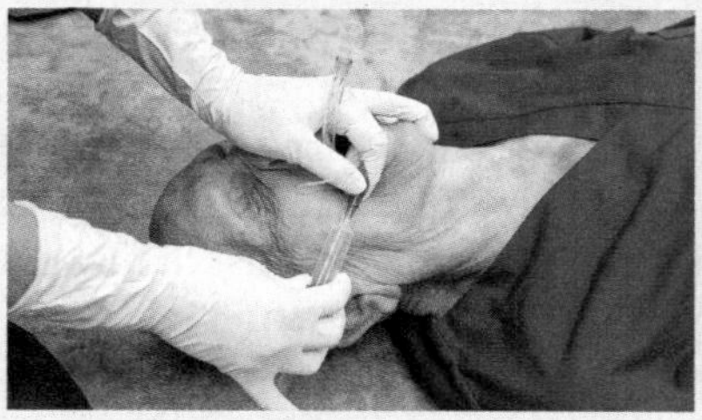

Step 10

Inflate the distal cuff of the ET tube with 5 to 10 mL of air, and immediately detach the syringe from the inflation port.

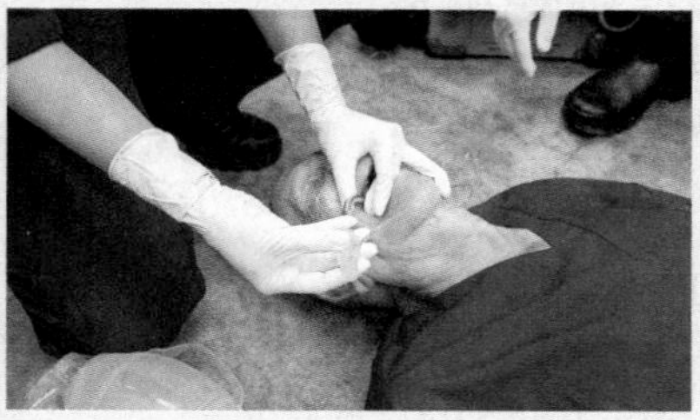

Step 11

Attach the $ETCO_2$ detector (waveform capnography is preferred) to the ET tube.

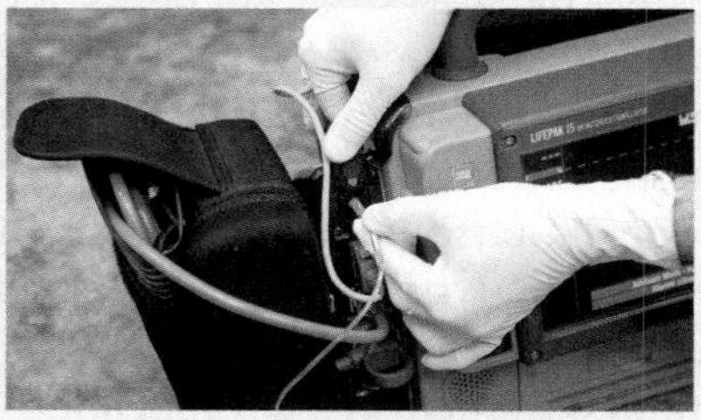

Step 12

Attach the $ETCO_2$ detector to the cardiac monitor/defibrillator and observe for a capnographic waveform and numeric carbon dioxide reading.

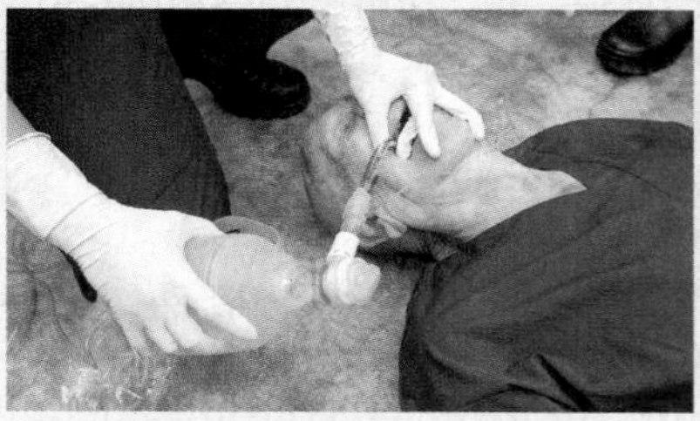

Step 13

Attach the ventilation device and ventilate the patient. Auscultate over the epigastrium and over both lungs.

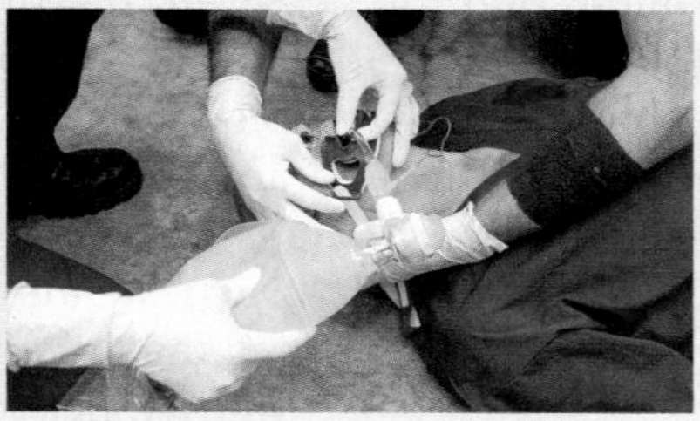

Step 14

Secure the ET tube with a commercial device or tape.

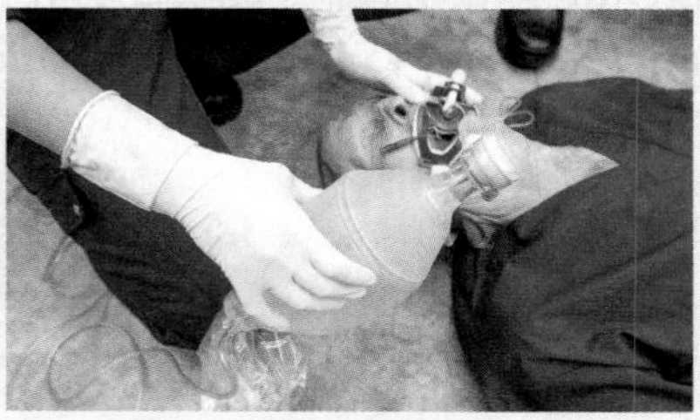

Step 15

Ventilate the patient at the proper rate while monitoring capnography and pulse oximetry.

perform laryngoscopy, or if it is not in the patient's best interest to administer sedatives and other pharmacologic agents to facilitate orotracheal intubation. Because this procedure is performed only on patients with spontaneous breathing, it is less likely to result in hypoxia.

Indications and Contraindications

Nasotracheal intubation is indicated for patients who are breathing spontaneously but require definitive airway management to prevent further deterioration of their condition. Responsive patients and patients with an altered mental status and an intact gag reflex who are in respiratory failure because of conditions such as COPD, asthma, or pulmonary edema are excellent candidates for nasotracheal intubation.

Nasotracheal intubation is contraindicated in apneic patients; these patients should receive orotracheal intubation. This procedure is also contraindicated in patients with head trauma and possible midface fractures, as evidenced by CSF drainage from the nose following a head injury. In patients with these types of injuries, a nasally inserted ET tube may enter the cranial vault and penetrate the brain; although this complication is rare, it is possible. Other contraindications to nasotracheal intubation include anatomic abnormalities, such as a deviated septum or nasal polyps, and frequent cocaine use. Nasal insertion of an ET tube in patients with these contraindications may result in severe epistaxis.

Avoid nasotracheal intubation, if possible, in patients with blood-clotting abnormalities and in patients who take anticoagulation medications (such as warfarin [Coumadin], apixaban [Eliquis], dabigatran [Pradaxa], or rivaroxaban [Xarelto]). These situations also increase the likelihood and severity of epistaxis following insertion of anything in the nose.

Advantages and Disadvantages

The primary advantage of blind nasotracheal intubation is that you can be perform it on patients who are responsive and breathing. This procedure does not require placement of anything in the mouth (such as a laryngoscope), so the nasotracheal route is associated with much less retching and a lower risk of vomiting in patients with an intact gag reflex.

Another major advantage of nasotracheal intubation is that you do not need to use a laryngoscope, which eliminates the risk of trauma to the patient's teeth or soft tissues of the mouth. Because the patient's mouth does not need to be opened, this technique is better suited to patients with limited temporomandibular joint mobility, such as patients with mandibular wiring, mandibular fractures, seizures, or clenched teeth (**trismus**).

Nasotracheal intubation does not require the patient to be placed in a sniffing position, which makes it an ideal technique for intubating patients with a possible spinal injury, unless you suspect a midface fracture. Finally, because the tube is inserted through the nose, the patient cannot bite the tube. The nasotracheal tube can also be secured more easily than a tube that is inserted orally because the nose generally has less secretions than the mouth.

On the downside, because nasotracheal intubation is a blind technique, you cannot use one of the major methods to confirm correct tube placement: visualizing the tube passing through the vocal cords. Confirming proper tube position is critical, regardless of the intubation method used; however, you should be even more diligent when confirming tube placement following nasotracheal intubation.

Complications

Bleeding is complication most commonly associated with nasotracheal intubation. If intubation is successful, then the airway is protected and the risk of aspiration is eliminated. However, severe bleeding can occur, especially with rough technique. Severe bleeding poses an additional threat to an already compromised airway because swallowing blood greatly increases the likelihood of vomiting and subsequent aspiration.

The incidence of bleeding associated with nasotracheal intubation can be reduced by gently inserting the tube into the nostril and lubricating the tip with a water-soluble gel. If available, an anesthetic lubricant containing a vasoconstrictive agent (such as phenylephrine hydrochloride [Neo-Synephrine]) will reduce both patient discomfort and the likelihood and severity of nasal bleeding with this procedure.

Equipment

To perform blind nasotracheal intubation, you use the same equipment as for orotracheal intubation,

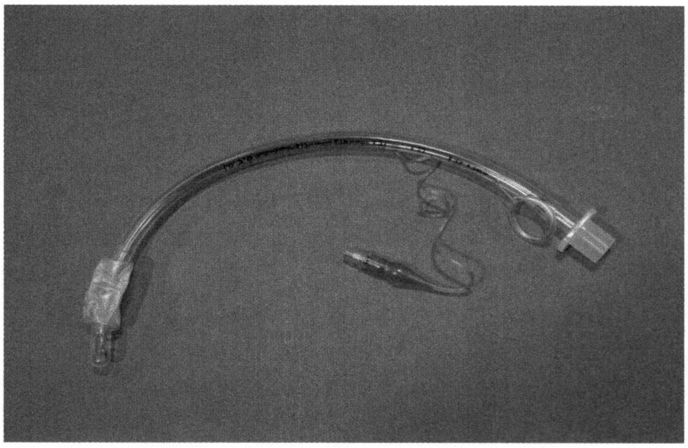

FIGURE 16-87 The Endotrol tube makes nasotracheal intubation safer, easier, and more efficient.

© Jones & Bartlett Learning. Courtesy of MIEMSS.

TABLE 16-13 Devices Used to Determine Maximum Airflow During Nasotracheal Intubation	
Humid-Vent 1	A device that attaches to the 15/22-mm adapter at the end of the ET tube to prevent secretions from being expelled from the tube
Beck Airway Airflow Monitor (BAAM)	A small whistle that attaches to the 15/22-mm adapter and emits a high-pitched sound as air moves in and out of the tube
Stethoscope with head removed	Stethoscope tubing placed in the proximal end (approximately 1 in. [2 to 3 cm]) of the ET tube that enables you to hear air movement without placing your face next to the tube

Abbreviation: ET, endotracheal

© Jones & Bartlett Learning.

minus the laryngoscope and stylet. Standard ET tubes should be 1.0 to 1.5 mm smaller when inserted nasally. When choosing the size of the tube, select one that is slightly smaller than the nostril in which it will be inserted.

Some ET tubes are designed specifically for blind nasotracheal intubation. For example, the Endotrol tube **FIGURE 16-87** is slightly more flexible than a standard ET tube and is equipped with a "trigger" that is attached to a piece of line, which is itself attached to the tip of the tube. Pulling the trigger moves the tip of the tube anteriorly and increases the overall curvature of the tube. This feature replaces the function of the stylet.

The movement of air through the ET tube helps to verify proper tube placement following nasotracheal intubation. A number of devices have been developed that allow you to confirm successful nasotracheal intubation without the need to place your face next to the tube, which increases the risk of contact with contaminants in the patient's exhaled breath **TABLE 16-13**.

Technique for Nasotracheal Intubation

When you perform blind nasotracheal intubation, you use the patient's spontaneous respirations to guide a nasotracheal tube into the trachea and confirm proper placement. The tube is advanced as the patient inhales. At this point, the vocal cords are open at their widest, which facilitates placement of the tube into the trachea.

After preparing your equipment and preoxygenating the patient, insert the tube into the nostril with the bevel facing toward the nasal septum. The right nostril is typically used because the curvature of the tube is in the correct orientation in relation to the bevel. If the right nostril is obstructed or if significant resistance is met, then insert the tube into the left nostril, but rotate the tube 180° as its tip enters the nasopharynx.

The angle of insertion is critical when performing nasotracheal intubation. Aim the tip of the tube straight back toward the ear **FIGURE 16-88**. The goal is to follow the floor of the nasal cavity until the tube enters the nasopharynx. Do not insert the tube with the tip aimed upward toward the eye; doing so can damage the turbinates and cause significant bleeding.

As the tube is advanced into the nasopharynx, you will begin to hear air rushing in and out of the tube as the patient breathes. Your goal is to position the tube just above the glottic opening so that the patient will draw the tube into the trachea during deep inhalation. Manipulate the patient's head to control the position of the tip of the tube. Cup your left hand (if the tube is inserted in the right nostril) under the patient's occiput. Move the patient's head

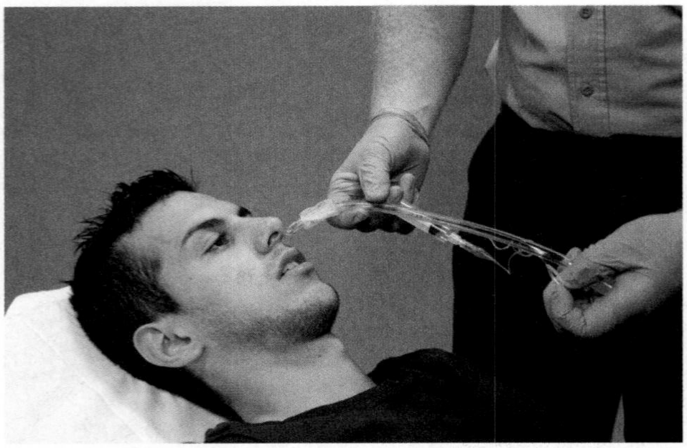

FIGURE 16-88 Aim the tip of the tube straight back toward the ear.

until you find the position that results in the maximum amount of air moving through the tube. At this point, the tube should be positioned just above the glottic opening.

As the patient inhales, the negative pressure created by inhalation facilitates movement of the tube through the glottic opening. Instruct the patient to take a deep breath, and gently advance the tube with the inhalation. Placement of the tube in the trachea will be evidenced by increased air movement through the tube.

If you see a soft-tissue bulge on either side of the airway, then the tube has probably been inserted into the piriform fossa. Hold the patient's head still and slightly withdraw the tube. After maximum airflow is detected, advance the tube on inhalation. If you do not see a soft-tissue bulge and no air is moving through the tube, then the tube has entered the esophagus. Withdraw the tube until you detect airflow, and then extend the patient's head.

Words of Wisdom

During blind nasotracheal intubation, keep a laryngoscope and Magill forceps within easy reach in case the patient becomes apneic during the procedure. In such a case, you can use the Magill forceps to direct the tube through the glottic opening under laryngoscopy.

After the tube has been properly positioned, inflate the distal cuff with the minimum amount of air necessary to achieve an airtight seal. Attach a ventilation device to the tube, and ventilate based on the patient's clinical condition. Because you do not have the benefit of visualizing the tube passing between the vocal cords, confirmation (by multiple techniques) and continuous monitoring of proper tube position are critical. Although the movement of air in and out of the tube during breathing is a good indicator that the tube is placed in the trachea, it is not foolproof. In some cases, only the tip of the nasotracheal tube has passed through the glottic opening; even slight patient movement may then dislodge the tube into the esophagus, which might not be recognized. Movement of the tube can also result in main stem placement.

Clean up any secretions or excess lubricant, and secure the tube with tape. Document the depth of insertion at the nostril, and monitor it frequently to detect movement of the tube. The steps for performing blind nasotracheal intubation are shown in **SKILL DRILL 16-11**.

Face-to-Face Intubation

You may perform intubation with your face at the same level as the patient's face when other positions are not possible; for example, in a motor vehicle crash in which the patient is seated in a tight space and the space above the head cannot be accessed, or when a seated patient suddenly becomes unconscious and apneic. This technique is called **face-to-face intubation**. The procedure is essentially the same as orotracheal intubation using direct laryngoscopy, with the following exceptions:

- The patient's head cannot be placed in the sniffing position. It should be manually stabilized by a second paramedic during the entire procedure.
- The laryngoscope (with a curved [Macintosh] blade) is held in the right hand with the blade facing downward like a hatchet, and the ET tube is held in the left hand. The laryngoscope blade is inserted into the right side of the patient's mouth, the tongue is swept to the patient's left, and the vocal cords are visualized **FIGURE 16-89**.
- After the laryngoscope blade has been placed, you may slightly adjust the patient's head to ensure better visualization by pulling the mandible forward while pressing down.

Skill Drill 16-11 Performing Nasotracheal Intubation

NR Skill

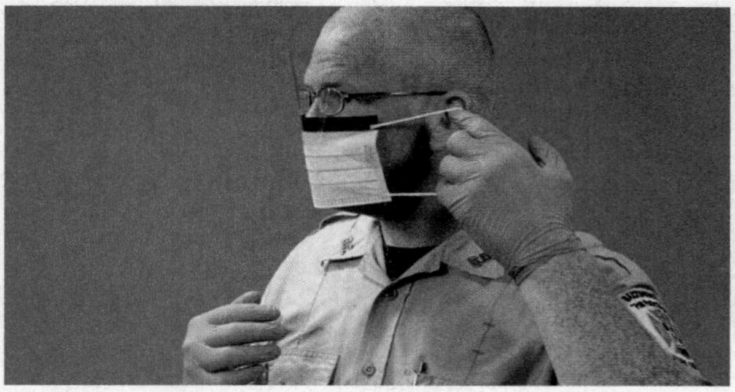

Step 1

Take standard precautions.

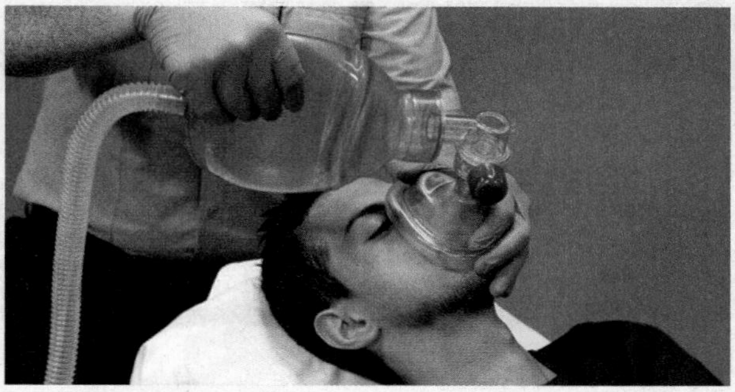

Step 2

Preoxygenate the patient whenever possible with a bag-mask device and 100% oxygen. Auscultate the patient's breath sounds to confirm adequate ventilation.

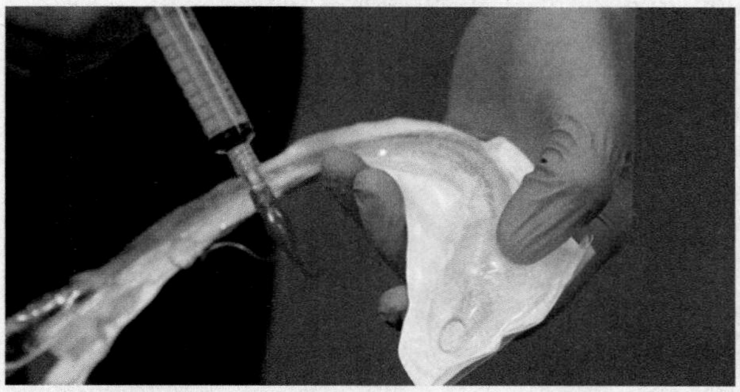

Step 3

Check, prepare, and assemble your equipment.

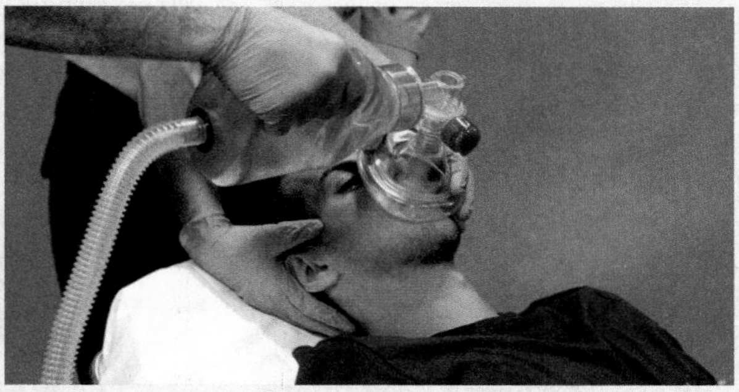

Step 4

Place the patient's head in a neutral position.

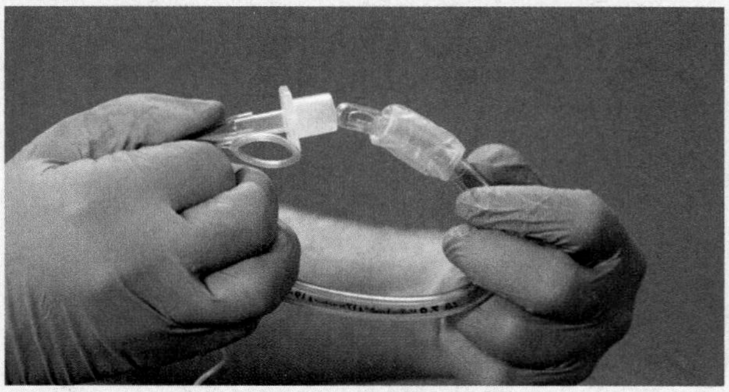

Step 5

Preform the nasotracheal tube by bending it in a circle.

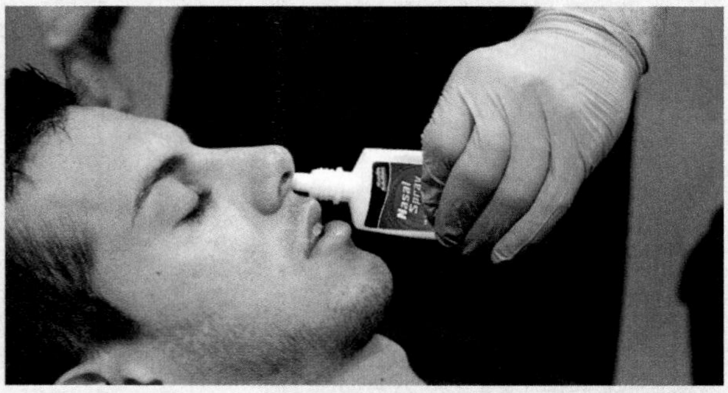

Step 6

Administer nasal spray to cause vasoconstriction of the nasal mucosa.

(continues)

NR Skill

Skill Drill 16-11 Performing Nasotracheal Intubation (continued)

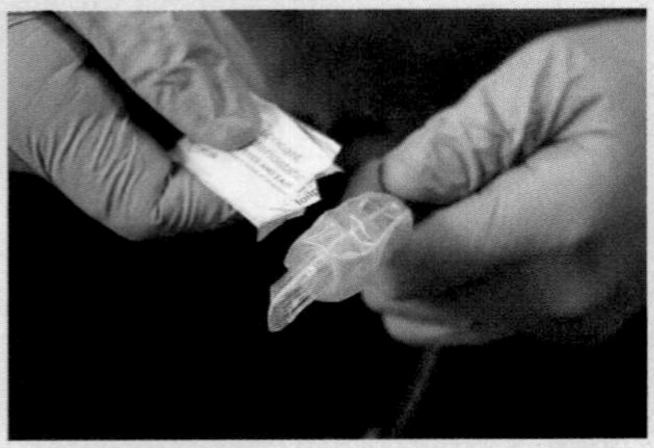

Step 7

Lubricate the tip of the nasotracheal tube with a water-soluble gel.

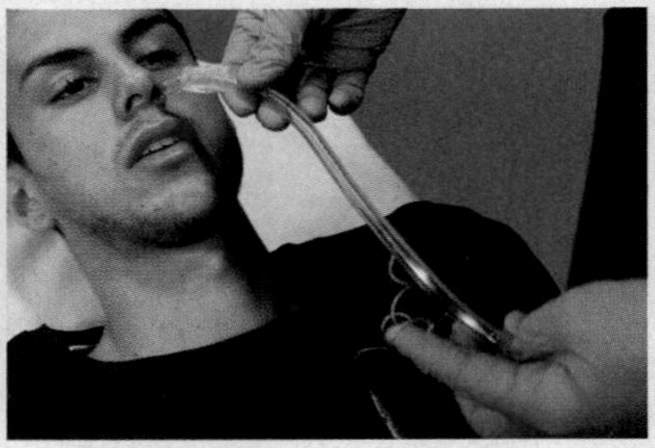

Step 8

Gently insert the nasotracheal tube into the more compliant nostril, with the bevel facing toward the nasal septum, and advance the tube along the nasal floor. Pause to ensure that the tip of the tube is positioned just superior to the vocal cords. Observe for condensation in the tube and note audible breath sounds from the proximal end of the tube.

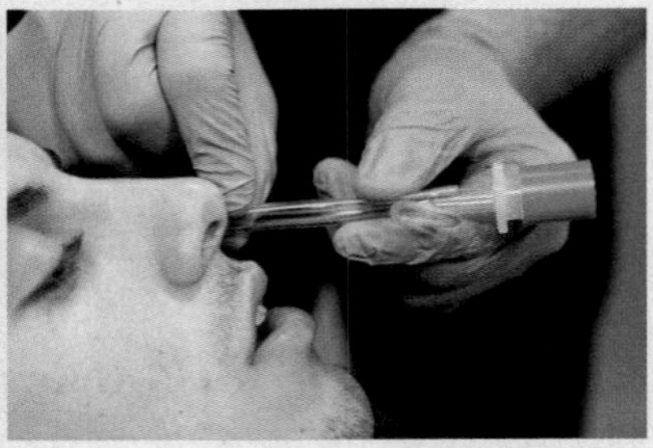

Step 9

Advance the nasotracheal tube through the vocal cords as the patient inhales. The Beck Airway Airflow Monitor (BAAM) device can be helpful in this step. Ensure that the patient is aphonic (unable to speak).

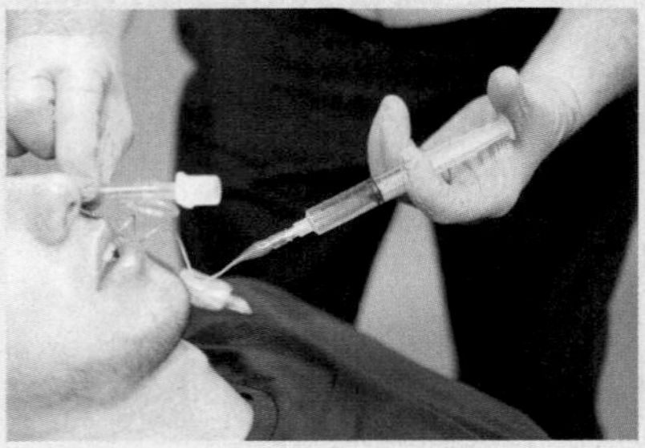

Step 10

Inflate the distal cuff with 5 to 10 mL of air, and immediately detach the syringe.

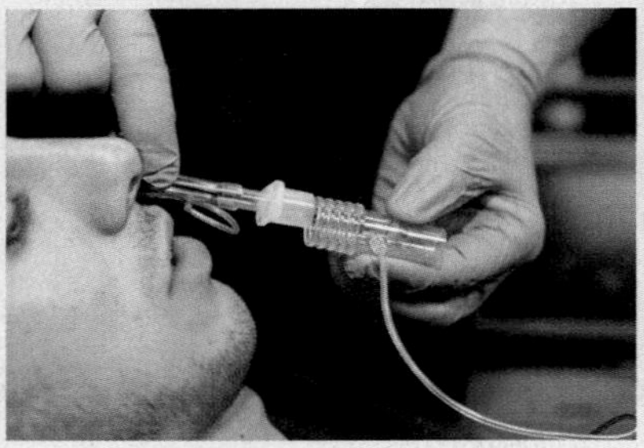

Step 11

Attach the $ETCO_2$ detector (waveform capnography is preferred) to the nasotracheal tube.

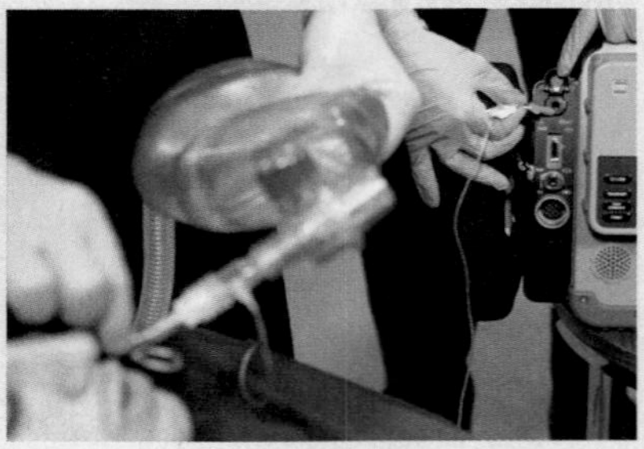

Step 12

Attach the $ETCO_2$ detector to the cardiac monitor/defibrillator.

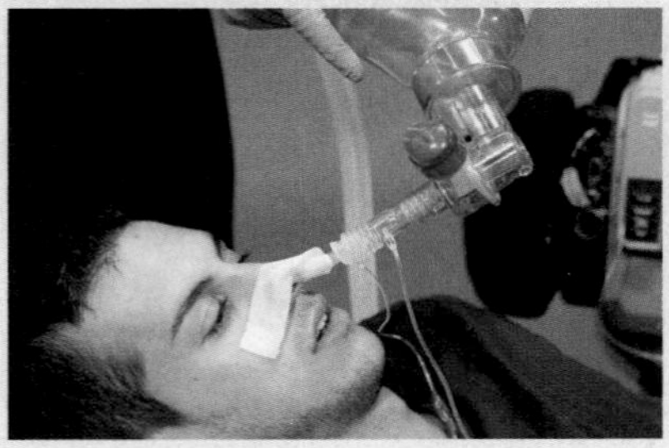

Step 13

Attach the bag-mask device, ventilate the patient, and auscultate over the epigastrium and over both lungs. Ensure proper tube placement with waveform capnography. Secure the nasotracheal tube. Ventilate the patient at the appropriate rate, while monitoring capnography and pulse oximetry.

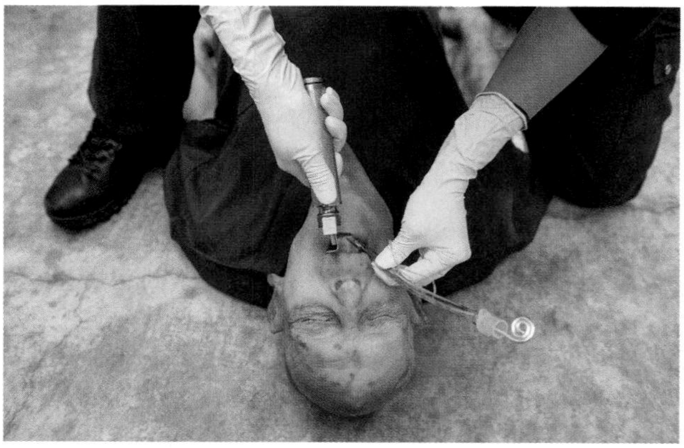

FIGURE 16-89 To perform face-to-face intubation, hold the laryngoscope in your right hand, with the blade facing downward, and hold the endotracheal (ET) tube in your left hand. Insert the blade in the right side of the patient's mouth and sweep the tongue to the patient's left. Adjust the patient's head, if needed, to improve your view and advance the ET tube until the cuff is 0.5 to 0.75 inch (1 to 2 cm) past the vocal cords.

Failed Intubation

A study using data from 40 states demonstrated an overall prehospital ET intubation success rate of 85.3%.[11] At the service and regional levels, intubation success rates should be closely monitored as part of physician-led quality-assurance efforts, because the implications for failed intubation—and, more importantly, an unrecognized esophageal intubation—are significant for the paramedic, the medical director of the EMS agency, and the regional system. In addition, failed intubation can potentially be fatal to the patient.

A "failed airway" is defined as the failure to maintain adequate ventilation and oxygenation, regardless of the technique(s) of airway management being used. Methods to minimize complications associated with airway management have been discussed in this chapter. However, frequently you do not have a choice of methods in the prehospital setting. If permitted by local protocol, consider a surgical airway (ie, cricothyrotomy) in case of a failed airway.

Tracheobronchial Suctioning

Tracheobronchial suctioning involves passing a suction catheter into the ET tube to remove pulmonary secretions. The first rule to remember about performing tracheobronchial suctioning is this: Do not do it if you do not have to! This kind of suctioning requires strict attention to sterile technique, which is nearly impossible to maintain in the prehospital environment. Suctioning the trachea can also cause cardiac dysrhythmias; cardiac arrest has been reported during tracheobronchial suctioning. For these reasons, you should avoid suctioning through an ET tube unless the secretions are so massive that they interfere with ventilation. If you must perform tracheobronchial suctioning, use sterile technique (if possible) and monitor the patient's cardiac rhythm and oxygen saturation during the procedure.

Words of Wisdom

ET Intubation: Points to Remember

- Never attempt ET intubation before the patient has been adequately preoxygenated.
- Assemble and check all equipment before you begin.
- Position is everything! Ensure that the patient's head is in the proper position to align the airway axes.
- Do not rush. Work with deliberate speed.
- Get it right the first time, because the second attempt will likely be more difficult. Remember that it is acceptable to manage the airway with BLS techniques until a more experienced provider is available to insert an advanced airway.
- Confirm the ET tube is in the right place. Take *nothing* for granted.
- Secure the ET tube appropriately. Otherwise, you might soon be trying to reinsert it.
- Even when the ET tube is properly secured, stabilize it with your hand as you ventilate the patient.
- Consider applying head blocks after intubating a patient. Doing so will minimize the amount of head movement and the risk of inadvertent extubation.
- Reconfirm proper ET tube placement after any major patient move (ie, from the ground to the stretcher, after loading into the ambulance, after transferring the patient to the hospital stretcher).
- Perform simple BLS airway maneuvers with an oral airway and/or a nasal airway and a bag-mask device. With good technique, you can provide adequate oxygenation and ventilation. The objective is to ventilate and oxygenate—not intubate.
- Consider using a rescue airway device, such as the King LT, LMA, or i-gel (discussed later in this chapter).

Preoxygenation of the patient is essential before performing tracheobronchial suctioning. Lubricate a soft-tip (whistle-tip) catheter, and ensure maximal preoxygenation. It may be necessary to inject 3 to 5 mL of sterile water down the ET tube to loosen extremely thick pulmonary secretions.

Gently insert the suction catheter down the ET tube until you feel resistance. Apply suction while extracting the catheter, taking care not to exceed 10 seconds of suctioning in an adult. After tracheobronchial suctioning is complete, reattach the ventilation device, continue ventilations, and reassess the patient.

The steps for performing tracheobronchial suctioning are shown in **SKILL DRILL 16-12**.

Field Extubation

As mentioned previously, extubation is the process of removing the ET tube from an intubated patient. Patients are rarely extubated in the prehospital setting. Generally, the only reason to consider

Skill Drill 16-12 Performing Tracheobronchial Suctioning

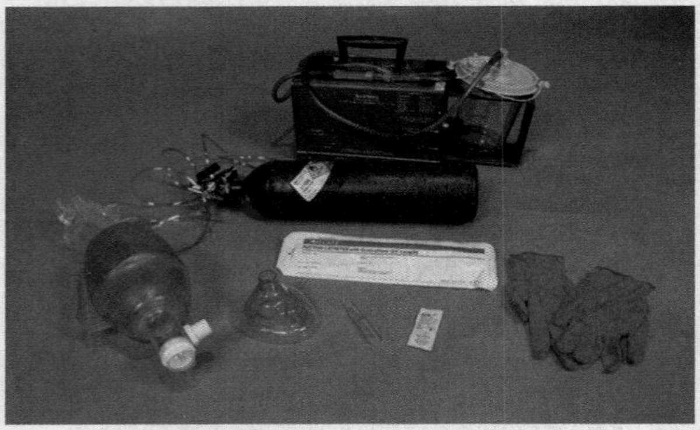

Step 1

Check, prepare, and assemble your equipment.

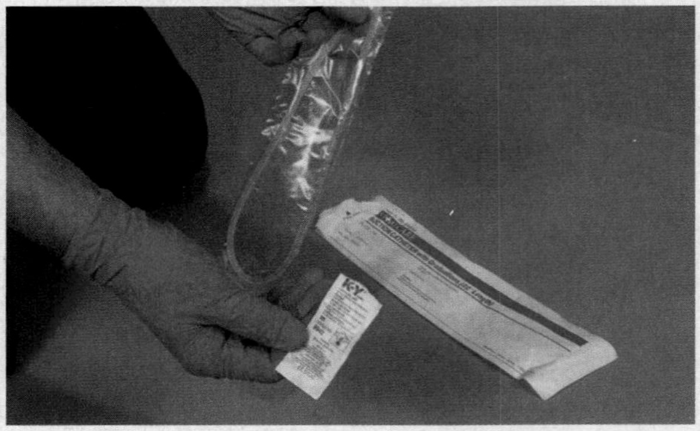

Step 2

Lubricate the suction catheter.

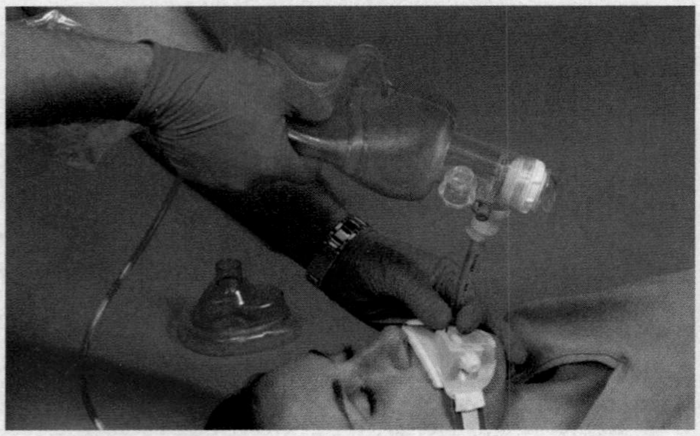

Step 3

Preoxygenate the patient.

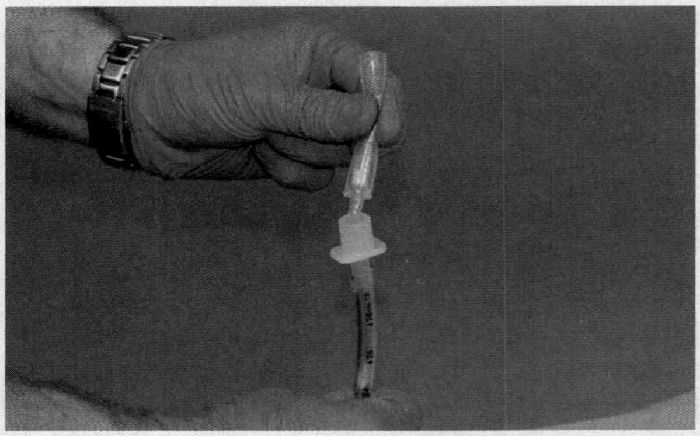

Step 4

Detach the ventilation device. If absolutely necessary to mobilize very thick secretions, consider injecting 3 to 5 mL of sterile water down the ET tube using sterile technique.

Skill Drill 16-12 Performing Tracheobronchial Suctioning (continued)

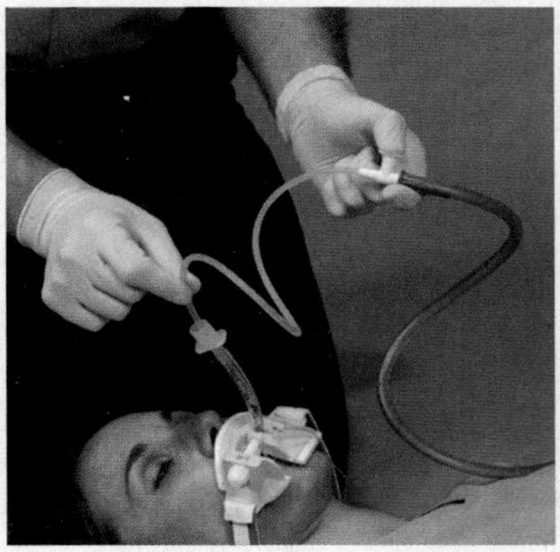

Step 5

Gently insert the catheter into the ET tube until you feel resistance.

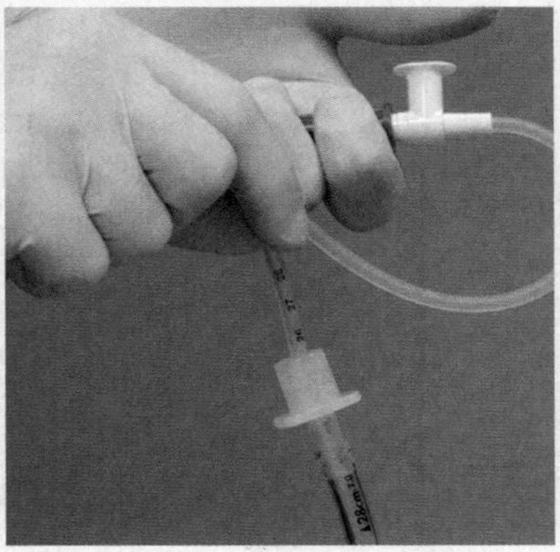

Step 6

Suction in a rotating motion while withdrawing the catheter. Suction for no longer than 10 seconds. Monitor the patient's cardiac rhythm and oxygen saturation level during the procedure.

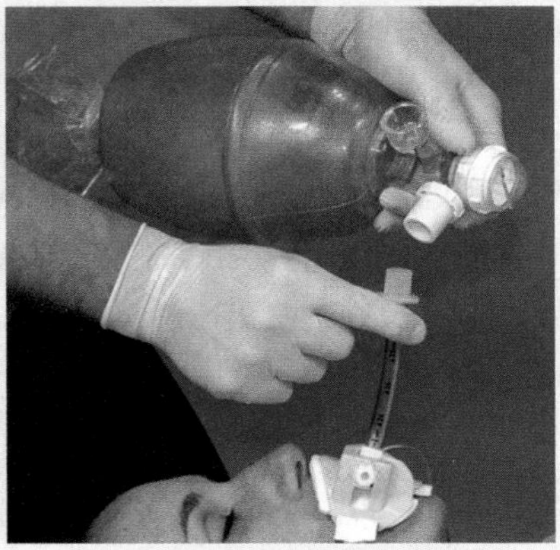

Step 7

Reattach the ventilation device, and resume ventilation and oxygenation.

performing extubation in the field is a patient who is unreasonably intolerant of the ET tube (ie, extremely combative, gagging, or retching). In general, it is safer to sedate the patient rather than remove the ET tube, but sedation (discussed next) may not be an option in all EMS systems or for patients in hemodynamically unstable condition. Before performing field extubation, you should contact medical control or follow locally established protocols.

The most obvious risk associated with extubation is overestimation of the patient's ability to protect the airway. In addition, when extubation is performed on responsive patients, a high risk of laryngospasm exists, and most patients experience some degree of upper airway swelling because of the trauma of having the tube in the trachea. These two facts, along with the ever-present potential for vomiting, can make successful reintubation extremely challenging. If you are not absolutely sure that you can reintubate the patient, then do not remove the ET tube. Instead, sedate the patient. If you used a paralytic drug to facilitate intubation, then consider administering additional doses (if clinically indicated and allowed by local protocol), in conjunction with a sedative. Field extubation is absolutely contraindicated if any risk exists of recurrent respiratory failure or there is uncertainty about a patient's ability to maintain an airway spontaneously.

If field extubation is necessary, then first ensure that the patient is adequately oxygenated. Discuss the procedure with the patient, and explain what you plan to do. If possible, have the patient sit up or lean slightly forward into a safe position should vomiting occur after extubation. Assemble and have available all equipment to suction, ventilate, and reintubate, if necessary. After confirming that the patient remains responsive enough to protect the airway, suction the oropharynx to remove any secretions or debris that may threaten the airway after the tube has been removed. Deflate the distal cuff on the ET tube while the patient begins to exhale so that any accumulated secretions proximal to the cuff will not be aspirated into the lungs. On the next exhalation, remove the tube in one steady motion, following the curvature of the airway. Place a towel or emesis basin in front of the patient's mouth in case vomiting occurs.

Pharmacologic Adjuncts to Airway Management and Ventilation

Pharmacologic agents are used in airway management to decrease the discomfort of intubation, decrease the incidence of complications associated with laryngoscopy and intubation, and facilitate aggressive airway management in patients who need it but are unable to cooperate.

Sedation in Emergency Intubation

Sedation is used in airway management to reduce a patient's anxiety, induce amnesia, and decrease the gag reflex. It is useful for anxious, combative, or agitated patients and for patients who need aggressive airway management but are too responsive to tolerate intubation. When used properly and under the correct circumstances, sedation effectively increases patient compliance and comfort, making definitive airway management easier and safer to perform. When used improperly, however, it can cause further harm.

The complications associated with sedation in airway management are related primarily to undersedation and oversedation. Undersedation can result in inadequate patient cooperation, the complications of gagging (eg, trauma, tachycardia, hypertension, vomiting, and aspiration), and incomplete amnesia of the event. Oversedation can result in uncontrolled general anesthesia, loss of protective airway reflexes, respiratory depression, complete airway collapse, and hypotension.

Words of Wisdom

Hypersensitivity to sedative medications is the primary contraindication to use of these drugs. Obtain an accurate and thorough medical history, to the extent possible, before giving any drug to any patient.

YOU are the Paramedic

PART 8

Your partner calls in your radio report with an estimated time of arrival of 5 minutes. Following your treatment adjustment, you determine that the patient's condition has improved. You continue to assist his breathing with a bag-mask device and deliver him to the ED staff.

Recording Time: 25 Minutes	
Level of consciousness	Responsive to verbal stimuli
Respirations	14 breaths/min (with bag-mask ventilation assistance)
Pulse	100 beats/min; strong and regular
Skin	Baseline color, warm, and moist
Blood pressure	148/80 mm Hg
Oxygen saturation (Spo_2)	97%
Pupils	PERRLA
$ETCO_2$	41 mm Hg
ECG	Sinus tachycardia

12. Why did you determine not to proceed with intubation?

TABLE 16-14 Sedatives Used in Airway Management

Drug Type	Examples
Benzodiazepines: sedative-hypnotic	Diazepam (Valium) Midazolam (Versed)
Dissociative anesthetics	Ketamine (Ketalar)
Opioids: sedative-analgesic	Fentanyl (Sublimaze) Alfentanil (Alfenta)
Non-opioids/ nonbarbiturates: sedative-hypnotic	Etomidate (Amidate)

The level of sedation desired dictates the amount of medication administered. Patients' responses to sedatives are dose-dependent. Follow local protocol or contact medical control to determine the appropriate dose for a given patient.

Two major classes of sedatives are commonly used in airway management: analgesics and sedative-hypnotics **TABLE 16-14**. Analgesics decrease the perception of pain. Sedative-hypnotics induce sleep and decrease anxiety, but do not reduce pain.

Benzodiazepines

Benzodiazepines are sedative-hypnotic drugs. Diazepam (Valium) and midazolam (Versed) provide muscle relaxation and mild sedation and are used extensively as anxiolytic and antiseizure medications. They also produce **anterograde amnesia**, which is beneficial for patients undergoing invasive or uncomfortable procedures; the patient likely will not recall the event.

Midazolam is two to four times as potent as diazepam, is faster acting, and has a shorter duration of action. Some clinicians use midazolam to induce general anesthesia before beginning intubation; however, the likelihood of complications increases with this practice because of the large dose necessary to induce muscle relaxation. In general, neuromuscular blockers (paralytics) are the preferred means to achieve muscle relaxation because these medications require smaller doses to achieve the desired effect.

Respiratory depression and hypotension are potential side effects of benzodiazepine administration. Flumazenil (Romazicon) is a benzodiazepine antagonist that can reverse the effects of diazepam and midazolam; however, this drug is not commonly carried in the field. Thus, it is important to administer just enough benzodiazepine to produce the desired effect.

Dissociative Anesthetics

A **dissociative anesthetic** is a medication that produces anesthesia by distorting the patient's perception of sights and sounds and inducing a feeling of detachment (dissociation) from their environment and self. Unlike benzodiazepines, which primarily produce a sedative state, dissociative anesthetics induce anesthesia through hallucinogenic, amnestic, analgesic, and sedative effects.

Ketamine (Ketalar) is a dissociative anesthetic that is commonly used in emergency medicine; it is rapid-acting and has a relatively short duration of action. At lower (subdissociative) doses (0.2 to 0.3 mg/kg), ketamine is commonly used as an analgesic. Higher doses (2 mg/kg) induce sedation and are commonly given prior to a neuromuscular blocker to facilitate intubation. Ketamine produces a sympathomimetic effect, which makes it a hemodynamically stable choice among sedative induction agents when performing emergency airway management in patients with hypotension.

In some patients, a **reemergence phenomenon** may occur during the end of the half-life of ketamine, when the patient is awakening. Reemergence phenomena may range from pleasant dreams to vivid nightmares and delirium. Benzodiazepines have been shown to reduce the incidence of reemergence phenomena, as well as to calm the patient if a severe reemergence phenomenon occurs.

Opioids

Opioids are drugs that act as a CNS depressant and produce insensibility or stupor. An opioid can be a natural product derived from the opium or poppy plant (referred to more specifically as an opiate) or a synthetic product designed to produce similar effects. Opioids are used in emergency airway management as premedications, during induction, and in maintenance of sedation or amnesia. The two opioids most commonly used for airway management are fentanyl (Sublimaze) and alfentanil (Alfenta). Fentanyl is 70 to 150 times more potent than morphine. It has a rapid onset of action and a relatively short duration of action. Alfentanil is less potent than fentanyl but has a faster onset of action and a shorter duration of action. It is also eliminated from the body more quickly.

Opioids can cause profound respiratory and CNS depression and produce severe hypotension and bradycardia, especially in patients who are in hemodynamically unstable condition. These negative effects can be reversed with naloxone (Narcan), an opioid antagonist.

Non-opioids/Nonbarbiturates

Etomidate (Amidate) is a non-opioid, nonbarbiturate, hypnotic-sedative drug often used in the induction of general anesthesia. This fast-acting agent has a short duration. Etomidate has little effect on pulse rate, BP, and ICP, and does not cause the histamine release and bronchoconstriction that may occur with other agents. However, a high incidence of uncomfortable myoclonic muscle movement is associated with its use. Etomidate is a useful induction agent in patients with coronary artery disease, increased ICP, or borderline hypotension/hypovolemia.

> **Street Smarts**
>
> Consider combativeness, aggressiveness, and belligerence to be signs of cerebral hypoxia until proven otherwise. When faced with this presentation, be firm and direct, but still treat your patients with respect and empathy. Keep in mind that they are fighting for their lives, not with you.

Neuromuscular Blockade in Emergency Intubation

Cerebral hypoxia can make an ordinarily calm person combative, aggressive, belligerent, and uncooperative, resulting in a difficult and potentially dangerous situation, both for the patient and for the paramedic. A patient with cerebral hypoxia must be treated with aggressive oxygenation and ventilation, but combativeness or other resistive behavior often makes this task difficult, if not impossible. Clenching of the patient's teeth due to spasm of the jaw muscles (trismus) and laryngospasm can also hamper your efforts to obtain a definitive airway.

Historically, physical restraint of a combative patient was commonly used to enable providers to obtain a definitive airway. A safer, more effective approach is chemical paralysis with **paralytics**, collectively known as neuromuscular blocking agents. When the patient is chemically sedated and paralyzed, a loss of the protective airway reflexes occurs; you can then effectively perform oxygenation and ventilation, and the patient will not gag during insertion of an ET tube.

Neuromuscular Blocking Agents

Although sedatives alone can be used to facilitate intubation, especially in patients who already have a markedly depressed gag reflex, it is often necessary to administer a drug specifically designed to induce paralysis. Paralytic drugs affect every skeletal muscle in the body, including the diaphragm and the intercostal muscles. Within approximately 1 to 2 minutes of receiving an IV dose of a paralytic, a patient will become totally paralyzed. That is, the patient will stop breathing; the jaw muscles will go slack, and the base of the tongue will fall back against the posterior pharynx and obstruct the airway. Put bluntly, paralytics convert a breathing patient with a marginal airway into an apneic patient with no airway. Before you bring about such a change, you must be absolutely sure that you can protect the patient's airway and ensure adequate oxygenation and ventilation. Although it is optimal to insert an ET tube, you must have other airway devices (such as a King LT, LMA, or i-gel) readily available if ET intubation is unsuccessful. After a patient is paralyzed, you are completely responsible for the patient's breathing and well-being. Fortunately, paralytic agents do not affect cardiac or smooth muscle.

A paralyzed patient appears to be asleep or unresponsive, but is not! Paralytic agents, unlike sedatives, have no effect on LOC. The patient is fully

> **Words of Wisdom**
>
> While the use of sedative and paralytic agents has been shown to improve the conditions for performing intubation, these agents do *not* improve inherently poor intubation technique. Simply put, if your technique is poor before you paralyze a patient, it will be poor after you paralyze a patient. Ensure that the most experienced intubator performs the procedure.

aware and can hear, feel, and think. Do not administer a paralytic agent without aggressively treating pain and sedating the patient first!

Pharmacology of Neuromuscular Blocking Agents

To understand how medications induce paralysis, recall how skeletal muscles contract. All skeletal (striated) muscles are voluntary and require input from the somatic nervous system to initiate contraction. As an impulse to contract reaches the terminal end of a motor nerve, **acetylcholine (ACh)** is released into the synaptic cleft (the junction between the nerve cell and the muscle cell). This neurotransmitter diffuses across the short distance of the synaptic cleft and binds to receptor sites on the motor end plate. ACh occupying the receptor sites triggers changes in electrical properties of the muscle fiber, a process called depolarization. When enough motor end plates have been depolarized, a threshold is reached and the muscle fiber contracts. Depolarization lasts for only a few milliseconds because of the presence of acetylcholinesterase, an enzyme that quickly removes ACh from the synaptic cleft and from the receptors on the motor end plate.

Paralytic medications function at the neuromuscular junction and relax the muscle by impeding the action of ACh. They are classified into two categories: depolarizing and nondepolarizing agents. **TABLE 16-15** lists the standard doses for these agents used in the prehospital setting.

Words of Wisdom

Paralysis Versus Sedation

Imagine what it must be like to be completely paralyzed. You cannot blink, talk, move, or, most importantly, breathe! You are completely dependent on others to keep you alive. Paralytic agents do not induce sedation or amnesia. If you administer only a paralytic agent, then the patient will be fully responsive and remember the entire event. Therefore, unless contraindicated, you must manage pain and sedate the patient before administering a paralytic. Paralysis without sedation and pain control is a form of patient abuse!

Depolarizing Neuromuscular Blocking Agents

A **depolarizing neuromuscular blocker** competitively binds with the ACh receptor sites but is not affected as quickly by acetylcholinesterase. Therefore, it causes depolarization of the muscle and prevents future signals for depolarization from having an effect because all of the ACh receptor sites are already occupied.

Succinylcholine chloride (Anectine) is a depolarizing neuromuscular blocking agent. Because succinylcholine causes depolarization, **fasciculations**—characterized by brief, uncoordinated twitching of small muscle groups in the face, neck, trunk, and extremities—can be observed

TABLE 16-15 Neuromuscular Blocking Agent Doses

Drug	Standard Dose
Succinylcholine (depolarizing)	1–2 mg/kg via IV push (initial dose); a repeat dose can be given based on the patient's clinical response.
Vecuronium bromide[a] (nondepolarizing)	0.1–0.2 mg/kg via IV push (initial adult dose); maintenance dose within 45–60 minutes: 0.8–1.2 mg/kg. Initial pediatric dose: 0.1–0.3 mg/kg IV/IO; maintenance dose within 20–40 minutes: 0.01–0.015 mg/kg IV push.
Pancuronium bromide[a] (nondepolarizing)	0.06–0.1 mg/kg via slow IV (initial adult dose). Repeat every 30–60 minutes as needed. Pediatric: 0.04–0.1 mg/kg slow IV/IO.
Rocuronium bromide[a] (nondepolarizing)	0.6–1.2 mg/kg IV/IO. Pediatric (older than 3 months): 0.6–1.2 mg/kg IV/IO.

Abbreviations: IO, intraosseous; IV, intravenous

[a]Consider administering 10% of the initial dose (defasciculating dose) before administering succinylcholine.

during its administration. These fasciculations tend to cause generalized muscle pain at the termination of paralysis (when the succinylcholine wears off).

Depolarizing neuromuscular blockers are characterized by a very rapid onset (60 to 90 seconds) of total paralysis and a relatively short duration of action (5 to 10 minutes). For this reason, paramedics may choose succinylcholine as the initial paralytic. With this drug, if you are unable to secure the patient's airway, then you have to support ventilation for only a short period before the patient can breathe again independently.

Use succinylcholine with caution. This drug is contraindicated in patients with burns, crush injuries, and blunt trauma: conditions that can result in hyperkalemia. In addition, because its chemical structure is similar to that of ACh, succinylcholine can cause bradycardia, especially in pediatric patients. Administration of atropine sulfate, which may prevent succinylcholine-induced bradycardia, should be considered prior to administering succinylcholine to pediatric patients; follow your local protocols.

> **Words of Wisdom**
>
> Not all patients require additional doses of a paralytic medication after intubation. In many cases, additional doses of a sedative medication (ie, midazolam, ketamine) will facilitate patient compliance and allow you to continue to support oxygenation and ventilation. However, depending on the patient's clinical condition, you may need to administer additional doses of a paralytic. Remember to keep the patient adequately sedated.

Nondepolarizing Neuromuscular Blocking Agents

Nondepolarizing neuromuscular blockers also bind to ACh receptor sites; however, unlike depolarizing neuromuscular blockers, they do not cause depolarization of the muscle fiber. When a sufficient dose is given, the amount of nondepolarizing medication exceeds the amount of ACh in the synaptic cleft, and the critical threshold of depolarization cannot be achieved. Thus, when nondepolarizing paralytics are administered in small quantities before administering a depolarizing paralytic, they prevent fasciculations. The defasciculating dose is typically 10% of the normal dose; it does not induce paralysis, but causes weakness.

The most commonly used nondepolarizing neuromuscular blockers are vecuronium bromide (Norcuron), pancuronium bromide (Pavulon), and rocuronium bromide (Zemuron). All three agents have a duration of action longer than that of succinylcholine. **Vecuronium** has a rapid onset of action (2 minutes) and a duration of action of approximately 45 minutes. **Rocuronium** has a rapid onset of action (less than 2 minutes) and a duration of action of 30 to 60 minutes. **Pancuronium** also has a rapid onset of action (3 to 5 minutes) and a duration of action of approximately 60 minutes.

Nondepolarizing neuromuscular blockers, because of the longer duration of their action, are ideal choices when a patient requires extended periods of paralysis, such as during a prolonged transport or when the patient's airway has been secured and you need to manage other injuries or conditions. However, do not give these agents before you have secured the patient's airway.

Rapid Sequence Intubation

Rapid sequence intubation (RSI), also referred to as rapid sequence induction or drug-assisted intubation, represents the culmination and integration of all of your airway, problem-solving, and decision-making skills into one procedure. RSI consists of the safe, smooth, and rapid induction of sedation and paralysis, followed immediately by intubation. This procedure has been successfully performed in the operating room for years, and its use in the prehospital setting is common. It is generally used for responsive or combative patients who need to be intubated, but are otherwise unable to tolerate laryngoscopy.

Preparation of the Patient and Equipment

The experience of being intubated is frightening for patients, so you must explain what you are going to do and provide reassurance that the patient will be asleep during the procedure and will not feel or remember anything. Apply a cardiac monitor/defibrillator and pulse oximeter. Check, prepare, and assemble your equipment, and ensure that it is in good working order. In particular, have suction immediately available.

SAFETY

When the decision to perform RSI is made, it is critical for all team members to be aware of exactly what will occur. Side conversations should be avoided so that the entire team can focus on performing the procedure safely.

Preoxygenation

All patients undergoing RSI should be adequately preoxygenated before the procedure is begun. If the patient is breathing spontaneously and has adequate tidal volume, apply high-flow oxygen via nonrebreathing mask. However, if the patient is hypoventilating, assisted ventilations with a bag-mask device and high-flow oxygen may be necessary. Avoid bag-mask ventilation after administering a paralytic agent, when possible, to avoid gastric distention and the associated risks of regurgitation and aspiration.

Premedication

If your initial paralytic of choice is succinylcholine, then consider administering a defasciculating dose, typically 10% of the normal dose, of a nondepolarizing paralytic, if time permits. You may also consider administering atropine sulfate to decrease the risk of bradycardia associated with succinylcholine administration.

Sedation and Paralysis

Administer a sedative agent to induce sedation and amnesia. If the patient is hemodynamically unstable (systolic BP of less than 90 mm Hg), ketamine or etomidate should be considered rather than a benzodiazepine because of their minimal effect on BP. As soon as the patient is adequately sedated, administer the paralytic agent. The onset of paralysis will be quick and should be complete within 2 minutes. Observe for apnea and check for laxity (looseness) of the mandible; these are signs of adequate paralysis.

Intubation

The procedure of intubation is no different with RSI than it is in any other situation. "Rapid sequence" refers to the rapid administration of medications. If you cannot accomplish the intubation within a short period and/or if the patient's oxygen saturation level falls, then stop and ventilate the patient with a bag-mask device and 100% oxygen. When the patient's oxygen saturation level returns to an acceptable level, reattempt intubation. If you must ventilate the patient with a bag-mask device, then do so slowly (1 second per breath, just enough to produce visible chest rise).

After the tube is placed in the trachea, inflate the cuff, remove the stylet, and verify the correct position of the ET tube (by auscultation and continuous waveform capnography). Secure the tube in place as usual, and continue ventilations at the appropriate rate.

Words of Wisdom

You should attempt RSI only if you are confident that you will be able to intubate and ventilate the patient, or to keep the patient oxygenated and ventilated if intubation is unsuccessful. Otherwise, a patient who has been sedated and paralyzed will die. Above all, do no harm!

Maintenance of Paralysis and Sedation

When you are absolutely sure that you have successfully intubated the trachea, depending on your transport time and the patient's clinical status, additional paralytic administration may be necessary. If you administered succinylcholine (which has a short duration of action) initially, then administer a nondepolarizing agent (such as vecuronium or rocuronium) to maintain long-term paralysis. If you administered a long-acting paralytic initially, then additional dosing is usually not necessary for short transport times. Administer additional sedation as needed and continuously monitor the patient's BP.

Evidence-Based Medicine

Many patients who require ET intubation are hypoxemic, but you cannot preoxygenate them because of their mental status (ie, agitation, delirium, combativeness). In such cases, a procedure called **delayed sequence intubation (DSI)** should be performed. DSI is intended to facilitate the process of preoxygenation, allowing you to safely secure the patient's airway while avoiding oxygen desaturation. DSI is essentially a procedural sedation, with the procedure itself being preoxygenation.

To begin DSI, place the patient in a head-up position of at least 15°, ensuring the earlobes are aligned with the sternum. Continuous monitoring of the patient's ECG and oxygen saturation (Spo_2), $ETCO_2$, and BP values is essential.

After you have prepared the patient and all monitoring parameters are in place, administer a dissociative dose of ketamine (1 to 1.5 mg/kg). Ketamine is the ideal DSI induction agent because it preserves airway reflexes and does not suppress the patient's respiratory drive. You may give additional, smaller doses (0.5 mg/kg) of ketamine if needed, until the desired effect is achieved. After 10 to 15 seconds, administer oxygen at 15 L/min via nonrebreathing mask and nasal cannula to the patient, which initiates the process of denitrogenation. **Denitrogenation** attempts to replace alveolar nitrogen with oxygen; the goal is to achieve an intrapulmonary oxygen reserve that will allow apnea to be prolonged as long as possible with the least possible oxygen desaturation. If the patient's Spo_2 level is less than 95%, then use noninvasive positive-pressure ventilation with CPAP or a bag-mask device with a PEEP valve.

After ensuring that the patient's Spo_2 can be maintained at greater than 94% for 3 minutes, administer a paralytic (succinylcholine or rocuronium). Leave the nasal cannula in place at 15 L/min. The patient is intubated after approximately 90 seconds.

If the patient's Spo_2 cannot be maintained at greater than 94% during the intubation attempt, then repeat the process of denitrogenation for another 3 minutes. If several intubation attempts prior to desaturation prove unsuccessful, abort the DSI procedure and allow the patient to reassociate (ie, allow the ketamine to wear off).

TABLE 16-16 Rapid Sequence Intubation Checklist

Preoxygenation/Planning

• Cardiac, vital signs, and oxygen saturation monitoring in place
  • IV fluids or vasopressors given as needed for BP support
• Passive oxygenation
  • Nonrebreathing mask or nasal cannula at 15 L/min
  • If Spo_2 94% or less, use CPAP or bag-mask device with PEEP valve
• Head of bed elevated 15° to 30°, ensuring ear to sternal notch position

Equipment

• Suction on and immediately available
• Laryngoscope checked to ensure proper functioning
  • If using a video laryngoscope, turn it on early to allow the light to warm up; this helps reduce fogging of the video screen.
• ET tube checked and configured appropriately
  • Cuff is tested
  • Stylet is inserted
• Sedation and paralytic agents drawn up and doses confirmed
• Bougie and alternative airway devices immediately available

Induction/Intubation
• Induction agent administered • Paralytic administered • Suction the oropharynx as needed to facilitate the laryngoscopic view of the vocal cords • Perform intubation while continuously monitoring oxygen saturation • Immediate confirmation with quantitative waveform capnography and auscultation of breath sounds • Properly secure the ET tube in place
Postintubation
• Additional sedation as needed • Orogastric or nasogastric tube placed • Ventilator settings adjusted as needed

Abbreviations: BP, blood pressure; CPAP, continuous positive airway pressure; ET, endotracheal; IV, intravenous; PEEP, positive end-expiratory pressure; Spo_2, oxygen saturation

When performing RSI, providers should use a checklist to ensure that the procedure is carried out safely and efficiently. One person should be assigned to read the checklist aloud, ensuring that each step is completed before the team moves to the next. **TABLE 16-16** shows an example of an RSI checklist.

Evidence-Based Medicine

Oxygen uptake by the alveoli continues even when the diaphragm is not moving and the lungs are not expanding. In an apneic patient, approximately 250 mL/min of oxygen will move from the alveoli to the bloodstream. A much smaller amount of carbon dioxide (only 8 to 20 mL/min) moves into the alveoli; the remainder is buffered in the bloodstream. The difference in oxygen and carbon dioxide movement across the alveolar membrane reflects the difference in gas solubility in the blood, as well as the affinity of hemoglobin for oxygen. As a result of this movement, the net pressure in the alveoli becomes subatmospheric, which generates a flow of gas from the pharynx to the alveoli. This process, called **apneic oxygenation**, allows oxygenation to continue even though the patient is apneic. The administration of supplemental oxygen via nasal cannula at 15 L/min before and after the patient has been chemically sedated and paralyzed has been shown to extend the duration of normal oxygen saturation, thereby reducing the risk that hypoxic events will occur during the period of forced apnea induced by RSI.[12]

Alternative Advanced Airway Devices

Supraglottic Airway Devices

King LT Airway

The **King LT airway** is a latex-free, single-use, single-lumen airway that is blindly inserted into the esophagus **FIGURE 16-90**. You can use the King LT to provide positive-pressure ventilation to apneic patients and to maintain a patent airway in unresponsive patients who are breathing spontaneously but require advanced airway management. The King LT is available in both adult and pediatric sizes.

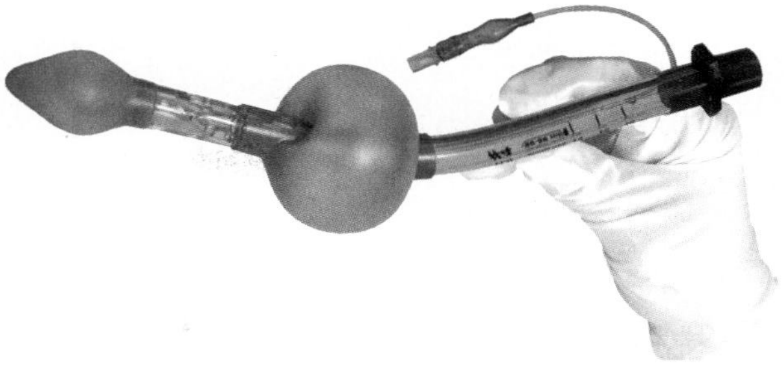

FIGURE 16-90 The King LT airway is a single-lumen airway that is blindly inserted into the esophagus. The King LT-D model is shown here.

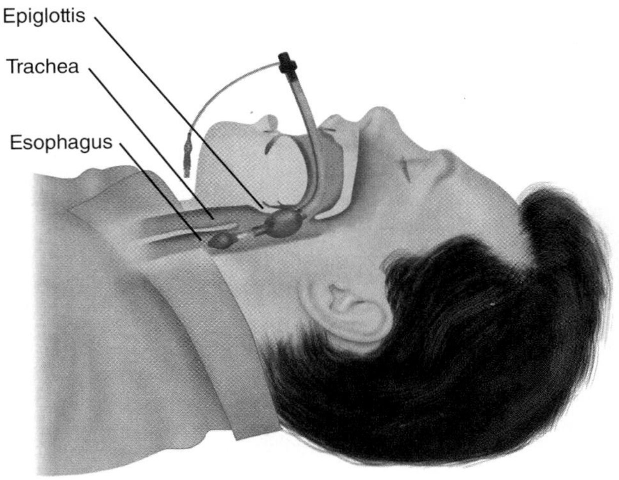

FIGURE 16-91 Placement of the King LT airway. When properly placed, the distal cuff seals the esophagus, and the proximal cuff seals the oropharynx.

The device consists of a curved tube with ventilation ports located between two inflatable cuffs. Both cuffs are inflated simultaneously using a single valve. When the airway is properly placed in the esophagus, the distal cuff seals the esophagus, and the proximal cuff seals the oropharynx **FIGURE 16-91**. Openings located between these two cuffs provide for ventilation of the lungs after positioning is confirmed.

Two types of King LT airways are available: the King LT-D and the King LTS-D. The King LTS-D is the more commonly used device; it is available in seven sizes, which are based on the patient's height and/or weight. Each size has a different color of proximal connector and requires different cuff inflation pressures. **TABLE 16-17** lists sizes and patient criteria for the King LTS-D. Each kit contains a single King LT, a syringe for cuff inflation, water-soluble gel, and instructions for use.

The King LT-D (see Figure 16-90) and the King LTS-D share most of the same features. Both have a proximal pharyngeal cuff and a distal cuff, as well as several ventilation outlets at the distal part of the tube. In both, an ET tube introducer (a gum bougie) can be inserted through the tube, where it exits at a "ramp" between the pharyngeal and distal cuffs. If you need to insert an ET tube, then simply insert the tube introducer through the King airway and into the patient's trachea. Next, remove the King

TABLE 16-17 Sizes and Patient Criteria for the King LTS-D

Size	Connector Color	Patient Criteria: Height and Weight[a]	Cuff Volume
0	Transparent	<11 lb (5 kg)	10 mL
1	White	11–26 lb (5–12 kg)	20 mL
2	Green	35–45 in. (90–115 cm) or 26–55 lb (12–25 kg)	35 mL
2.5	Orange	41–51 in. (105–130 cm) or 55–77 lb (25–35 kg)	40–45 mL
3	Yellow	4–5 ft (122–155 cm)	50–60 mL
4	Red	5–6 ft (155–180 cm)	70–80 mL
5	Purple	>6 ft (180 cm)	80–90 mL

[a]Sizes 0 and 1 are weight-based. Sizes 2 and 2.5 are weight- and/or height-based. Adult sizes (sizes 3–5) are height-based.

Data from: Ambu King LTS-D laryngeal tube. Ambu USA website. https://www.ambuusa.com/Files/Files/Downloads/Ambu%20USA/AirwayManagement/Laryngeal_Tubes/King%20LTS-D%20Disposable%20Laryngeal%20Tube/Datasheets/Ambu%20King%20LTS-D%20Datasheet.pdf. Updated August 2018. Accessed August 24, 2021.

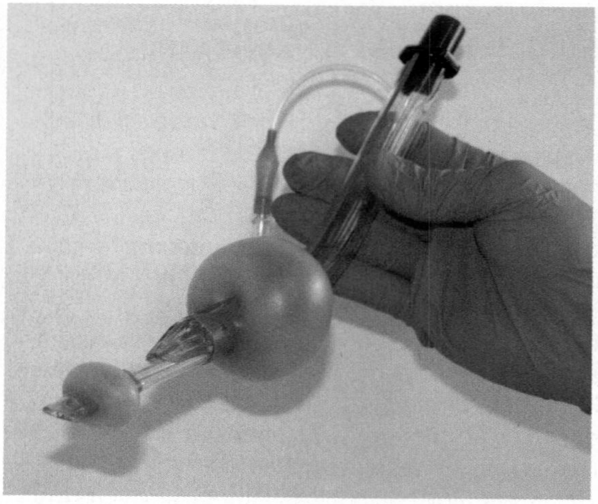

FIGURE 16-92 The King LTS-D.

Courtesy of Candice M. Thompson, NREMT-P.

airway, and direct an ET tube into the trachea by placing it over the tube introducer.

The distal end of the King LT-D is closed, whereas the distal end of the King LTS-D is open. This opening permits insertion of a suction catheter (up to size 18F) through a gastric access lumen on the proximal end of the King LTS-D to perform gastric decompression **FIGURE 16-92**.

Indications for the King LT Airway

The King LT airway is an alternative to bag-mask ventilation or ET intubation. This airway has the same advantages, disadvantages, complications, and special considerations as other ventilation devices inserted into the esophagus.

Contraindications for the King LT Airway

The King LT airway does not eliminate the risk of vomiting and aspiration. High airway pressures can cause air to leak into the stomach or out of the mouth. Do not use the King LT airway in patients with an intact gag reflex, patients with known esophageal disease (eg, tumors, varices, strictures), or patients who have ingested a caustic substance. As with other advanced airway devices, proper placement is confirmed by observing chest rise, auscultating the lungs and epigastrium, and using quantitative waveform capnography.

Complications of the King LT Airway

It is reasonable to assume that laryngospasm, vomiting, and possible hypoventilation may occur with introduction of the King LT airway. Improper insertion technique may also result in trauma. Ventilation may be difficult if the pharyngeal balloon pushes the epiglottis over the glottic opening. If this complication occurs, then gently withdraw the device without deflating the cuffs until ventilation becomes easier.

Words of Wisdom

It is important to follow the manufacturer's recommendation regarding the volume of air that is placed into the King LT. Too much air in the oropharyngeal cuff could compromise carotid artery blood flow and impair internal jugular venous return, resulting in inadequate cerebral perfusion and increased intracranial pressure.

Insertion Technique

As previously discussed, the King LT airway comes in seven sizes; the patient's height and weight will determine the size that you should use. The steps for inserting the King LT airway are shown in **SKILL DRILL 16-13**.

NR Skill

Skill Drill 16-13 Inserting a King LT Airway

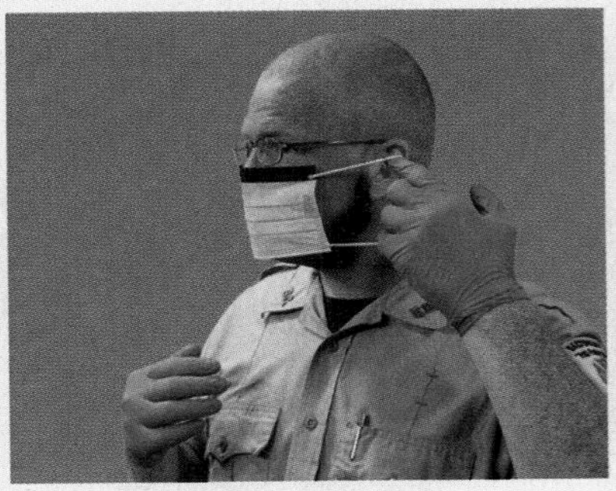

Step 1

Take standard precautions.

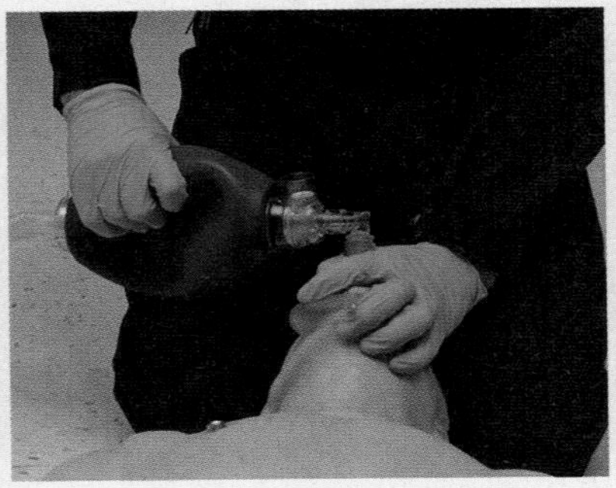

Step 2

Preoxygenate the patient with a bag-mask device and 100% oxygen.

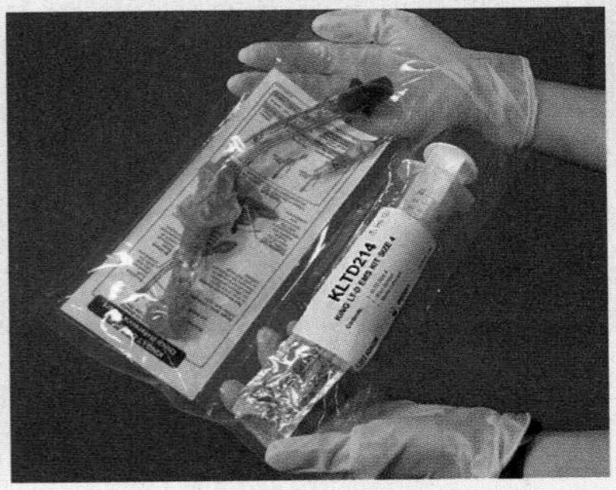

Step 3

Gather your equipment. Choose the proper size of King LT airway for the patient. Test the cuffs for proper inflation. Ensure all air is removed from the cuffs before insertion. Lubricate the tip of the device with a water-soluble gel for easy insertion and minimal airway damage.

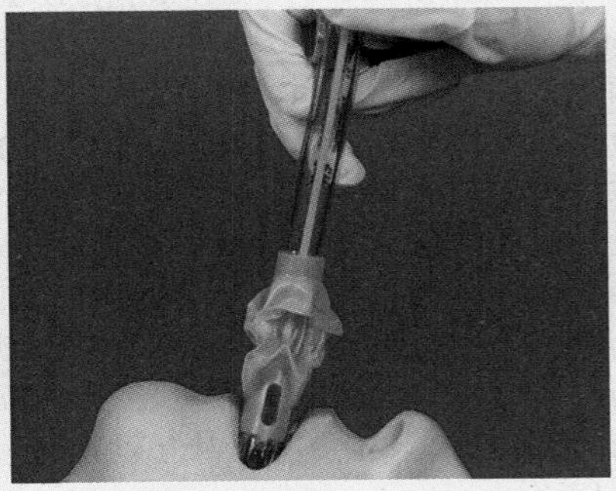

Step 4

Place the patient's head in a neutral position, unless contraindicated (use the jaw-thrust maneuver if you suspect trauma). In your dominant hand, hold the King LT airway at the connector. With your other hand, hold the patient's mouth open while positioning the head. Insert the tip of the King LT airway into the midline of the mouth.

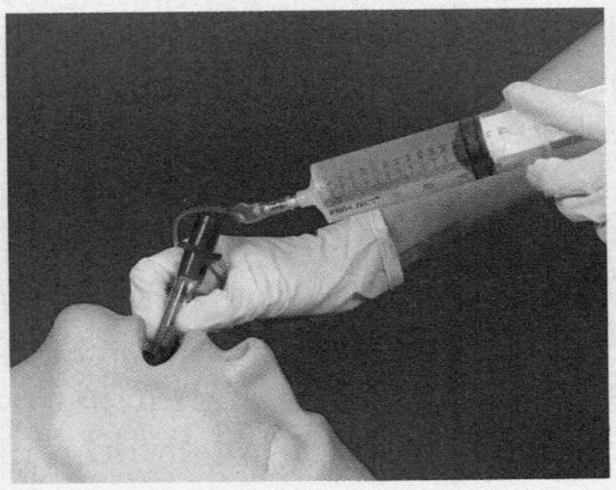

Step 5

Advance the tip beyond the base of the tongue. If you meet resistance, then rotate the airway slightly, change your angle, and advance it again. Continue to gently advance the airway until the base of the connector is aligned with the patient's teeth or gums. Do not use excessive force. Inflate the cuffs with the recommended amount of air or just enough to seal the airway.

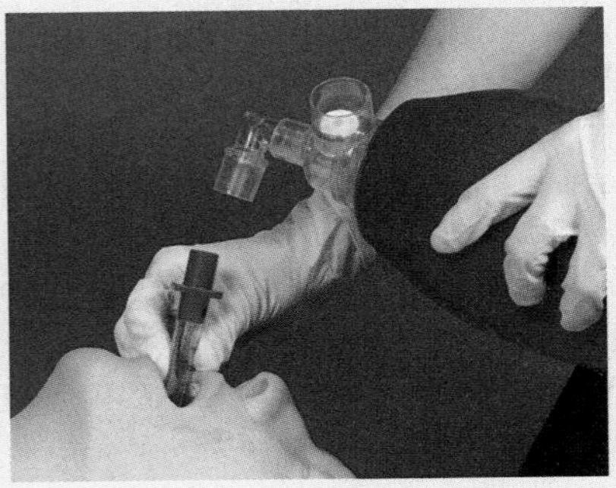

Step 6

Attach the tube to the ventilation device, and confirm tube placement by auscultating the lungs and epigastrium and monitoring waveform capnography. Add additional air to the cuffs to maximize the airway seal, if needed; however, avoid exceeding the manufacturer's recommended maximum amount of air. After placement is confirmed, continue to ventilate the patient.

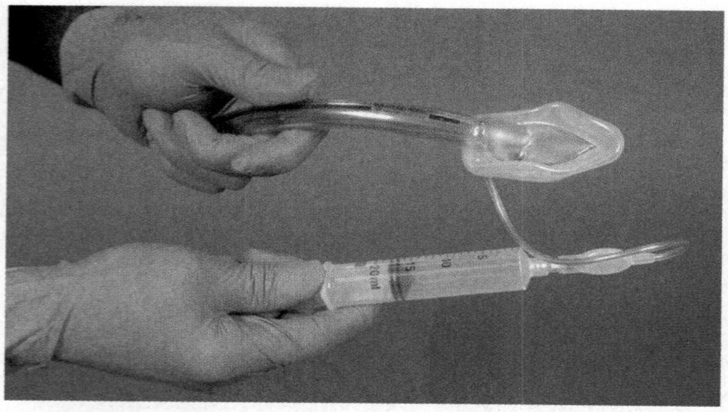

FIGURE 16-93 The laryngeal mask airway.

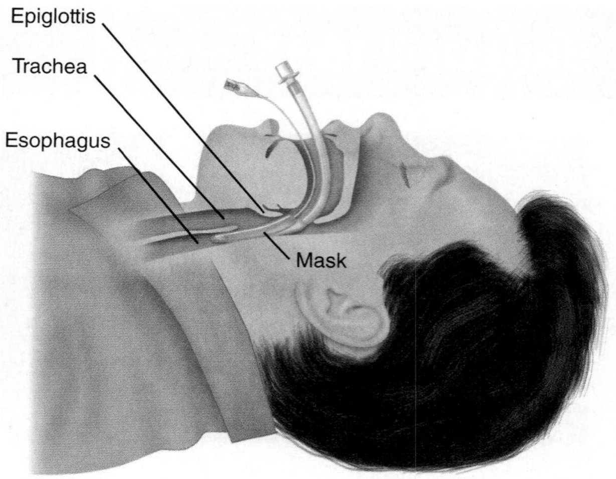

FIGURE 16-94 When properly positioned, the opening of the laryngeal mask airway is at the glottic opening, the tip is at the entrance of the esophagus, the lateral portions are in the piriform fossae, and the upper border is at the base of the tongue.

Laryngeal Mask Airway

The **laryngeal mask airway (LMA)** **FIGURE 16-93** was originally developed for use in the operating room. It represents a viable option for patients who require more airway and ventilatory support than bag-mask ventilation can provide. Like the King LT airway, the LMA does not require visualization of the airway.

The LMA is designed to provide a conduit from the glottic opening to the ventilation device. It surrounds the opening of the larynx with an inflatable silicone cuff positioned in the hypopharynx. When properly inserted, the opening of the LMA is positioned at the glottic opening, and the tip is inserted into the proximal esophagus, the lateral portions in the piriform fossae, and the upper border at the base of the tongue. The inflatable cuff conforms to the contours of the airway and forms a relatively airtight seal **FIGURE 16-94**.

Indications and Contraindications for the LMA

Consider the LMA as one possible alternative to bag-mask ventilation when the patient cannot undergo ET intubation. Do not consider the LMA as a primary airway in emergency situations.

The LMA is less effective in patients with obesity and should not be used at all in patients with morbid obesity. Pregnant patients and patients with a hiatal hernia are at an increased risk for regurgitation with this device; evaluate such patients carefully if you are considering use of the LMA. The LMA is ineffective for the ventilation of patients requiring high pulmonary pressures, such as patients with COPD or heart failure.

Advantages and Disadvantages of the LMA

The LMA has many advantages compared with ventilating an unprotected airway with a bag-mask device. This airway may provide better ventilation than a bag-mask device and an oral and/or nasal airway, and ventilation with an LMA does not require continual maintenance of a mask seal. Compared with ET intubation, LMA insertion is easier because it does not require laryngoscopy. Significantly less risk exists for soft-tissue, vocal cord, tracheal wall, and dental trauma than with ET intubation and other forms of intubation that rely on blocking the esophagus. In addition, the LMA provides protection from upper airway secretions, and the tip of the LMA wedged into the proximal esophagus most likely provides some obturation.

The main disadvantage of the LMA, especially in emergency situations, is that it does not protect against aspiration. In fact, this airway may increase the risk of aspiration if the patient regurgitates, because the stomach contents would most likely be directed into the trachea.

During prolonged LMA ventilation, some air may be insufflated into the stomach because the seal made in the airway is not airtight. Because of the risk of aspiration, it is unlikely that the LMA will ever replace ET intubation in prehospital emergency medical care.

Complications of the LMA

The most significant complications associated with use of the LMA involve regurgitation and subsequent aspiration. The product literature states that this airway should be used only in patients who are fasting. Unfortunately, this limitation would eliminate all patients in emergency situations, who should always be presumed to have full stomachs. You must weigh the risk of aspiration against the risk of hypoventilation with bag-mask ventilation in the context of the clinical scenario.

Observe the patient for clinical indications of adequate ventilation (ie, chest rise and breath sounds) during LMA ventilation. Hypoventilation of patients who require high ventilatory pressures can also occur, and patients should be monitored for evidence of upper airway swelling.

Equipment for the LMA

Several types of LMA are available, with the sizes being based on the patient's weight. Each device consists of a tube and an inflatable mask cuff. The cuff provides a collar that positions the opening of the tube at the glottic opening when inflated. Two vertical bars at the opening of the tube prevent occlusion. The proximal end of the tube is fitted with a standard 15/22-mm adapter that is compatible with any ventilation device. The cuff has a one-way valve assembly and should be inflated with a predetermined volume of air (based on the size of the airway) **FIGURE 16-95**.

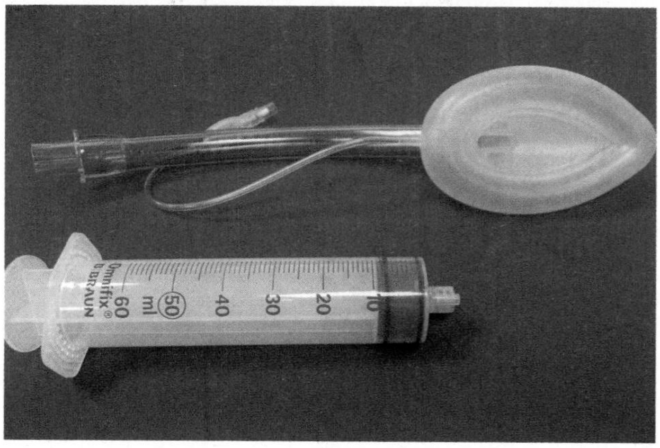

FIGURE 16-95 The laryngeal mask airway with the cuff inflated.

The LMA ProSeal has a built-in drain tube that allows expelled gastric contents to bypass the pharynx, thereby reducing the risk of aspiration **FIGURE 16-96**. The LMA Supreme is an anatomically shaped device that features a gastric access port, enabling a gastric tube to be inserted without interrupting ventilations **FIGURE 16-97**.

A 6.0-mm ET tube can be passed through a size 3 or 4 LMA, allowing for intubation. The vertical bars are designed to allow a well-lubricated tube to pass straight through; indeed, research in the operating room found a high success rate for ET intubation following this technique. The LMA Fastrach is designed to guide an ET tube into the trachea and may be a viable alternative to direct laryngoscopy **FIGURE 16-98**.

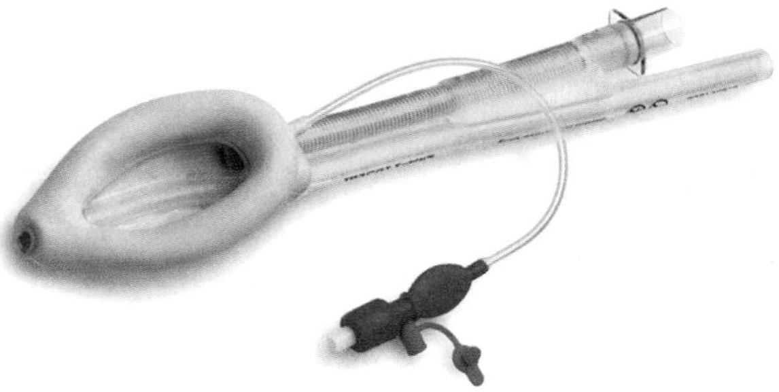

FIGURE 16-96 The ProSeal laryngeal mask airway.

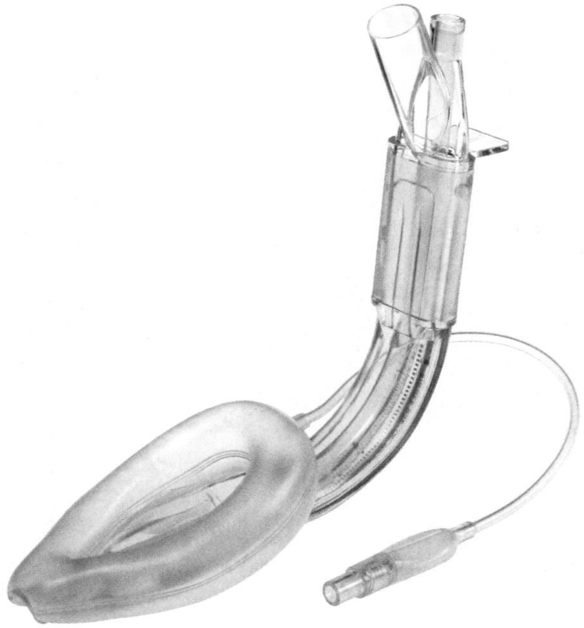

FIGURE 16-97 The Supreme laryngeal mask airway.

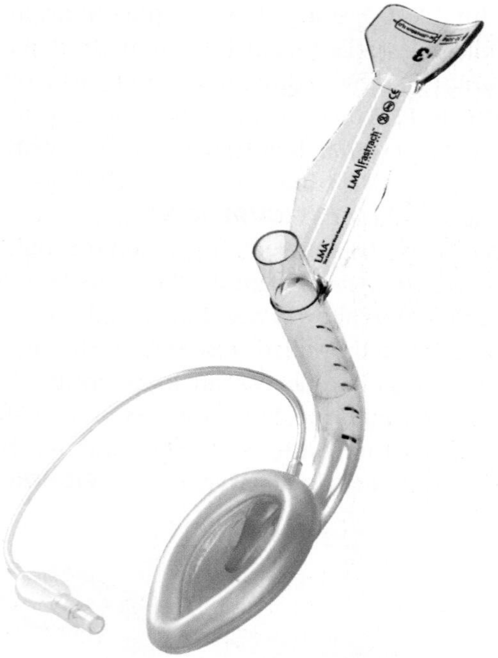

FIGURE 16-98 The Fastrach laryngeal mask airway can accommodate a 6.0-mm endotracheal tube.

Insertion Technique

Before beginning insertion of an LMA, check and prepare all equipment. The steps for inserting an LMA are shown in **SKILL DRILL 16-14**.

i-gel

The **i-gel** supraglottic airway is inserted in a manner similar to the LMA. This particular airway device was designed to create a noninflatable, anatomic seal of the pharyngeal, laryngeal, and perilaryngeal structures, while avoiding the compression trauma that may occur from devices with an inflatable cuff **FIGURE 16-99**. The i-gel is a commonly used supraglottic airway device and is a reasonable alternative to intubation.

The i-gel features an integral bite block, a gastric access channel that allows for passage of a 10-Fr gastric tube, a supplemental oxygen inlet port to facilitate passive oxygenation, and a support strap to secure the airway in position. A color-coded, proximal hook ring indicates the size of the i-gel and serves as an anchor for the support strap.

NR Skill

Skill Drill 16-14 Inserting an LMA

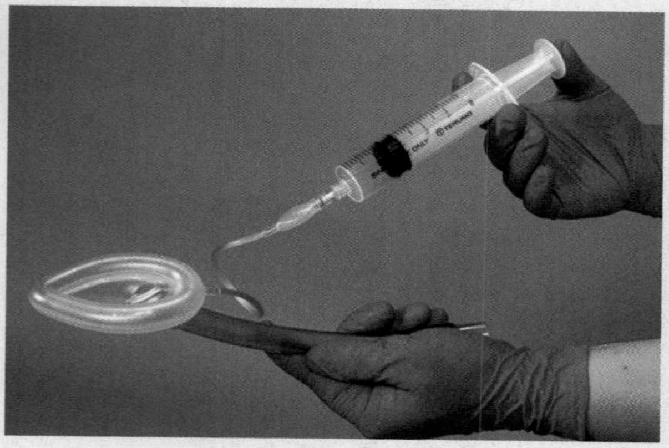

Step 1

Take standard precautions. Check the cuff of the LMA by inflating it with 50% more air than is required for the size of airway to be used.

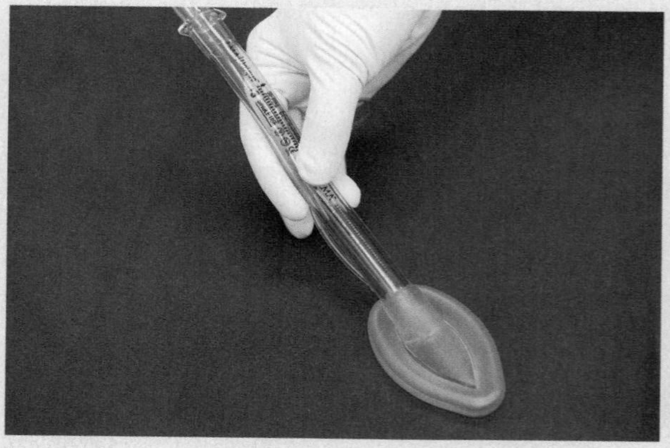

Step 2

Deflate the cuff completely, so that no folds appear near the tip. Deflation is best accomplished by pressing the device, cuff facing down, on a flat surface to remove all wrinkles from the cuff.

Skill Drill 16-14 Inserting an LMA (continued)

NR Skill

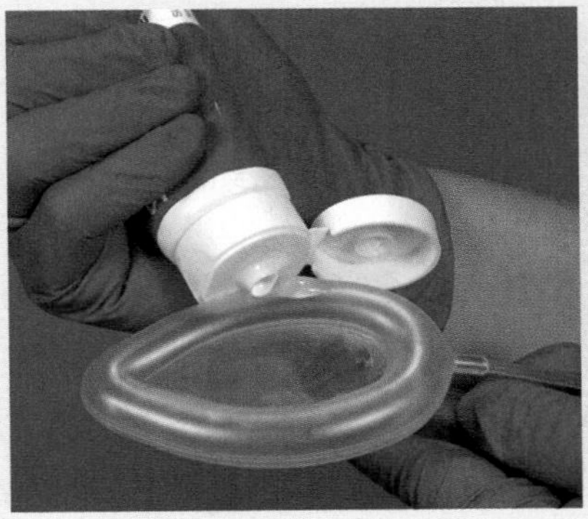

Step 3

Lubricate the outer rim of the device.

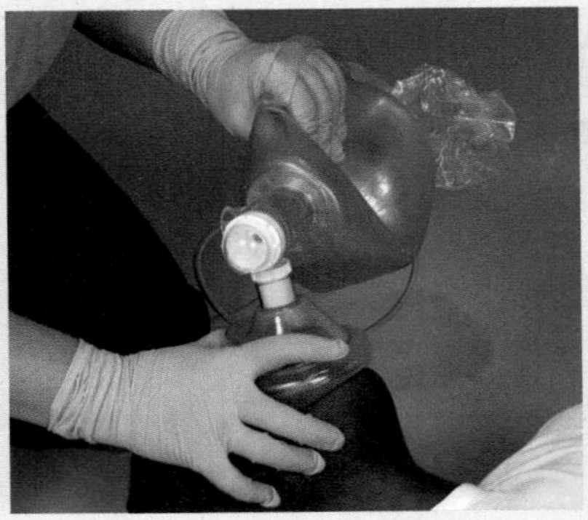

Step 4

Preoxygenate the patient before beginning the insertion attempt. Place the patient in the sniffing position. Insert the LMA as quickly, safely, and efficiently as possible.

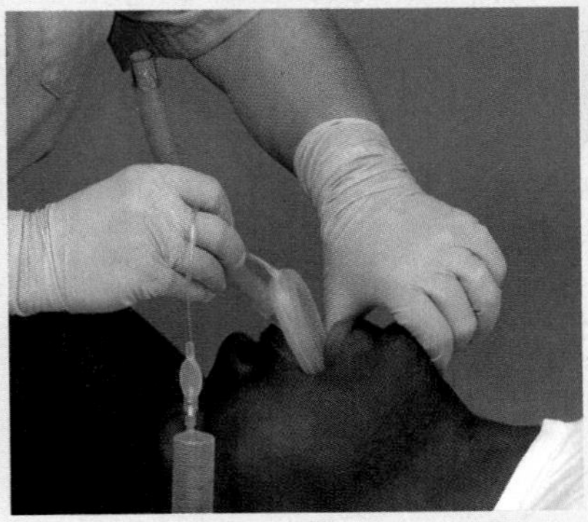

Step 5

Proper insertion of the LMA depends on holding the device properly. Insert your finger between the cuff and the tube. Place the index finger of your dominant hand in the notch between the tube and the cuff. Open the patient's mouth. Lift the jaw with one hand, and begin to insert the device with the other hand.

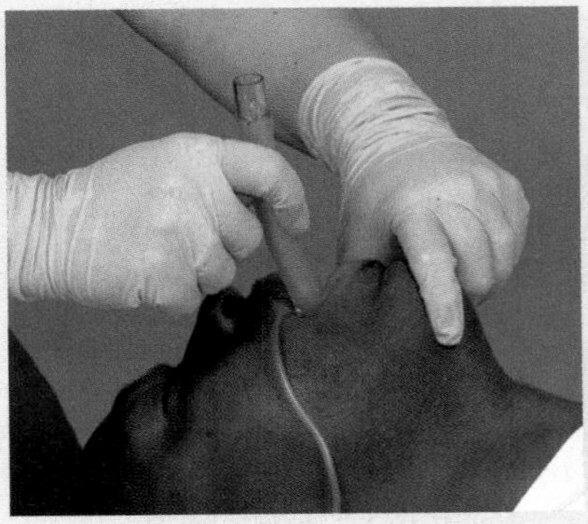

Step 6

Insert the LMA along the roof of the mouth. The key to proper insertion is to slide the convex surface of the airway along the roof of the mouth. Use your finger to push the airway against the hard palate. After it slides past the tongue, the LMA will move easily into position.

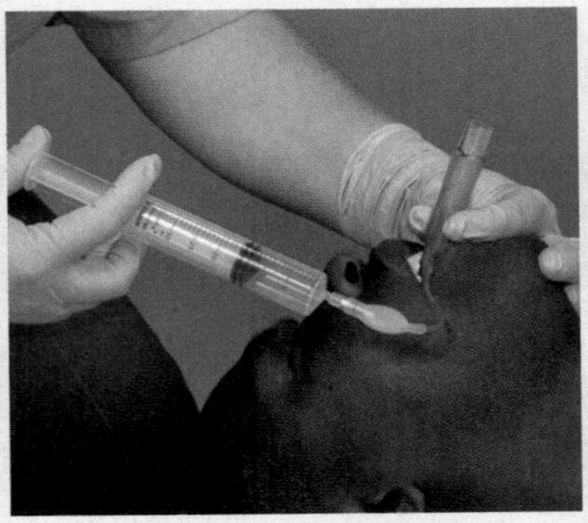

Step 7

Inflate the cuff with the amount of air indicated for the airway being used. If the LMA is properly positioned, it will move out of the airway slightly 0.5 to 0.75 inch (1 to 2 cm) as it moves into position (a good indication that the LMA is in the correct position).

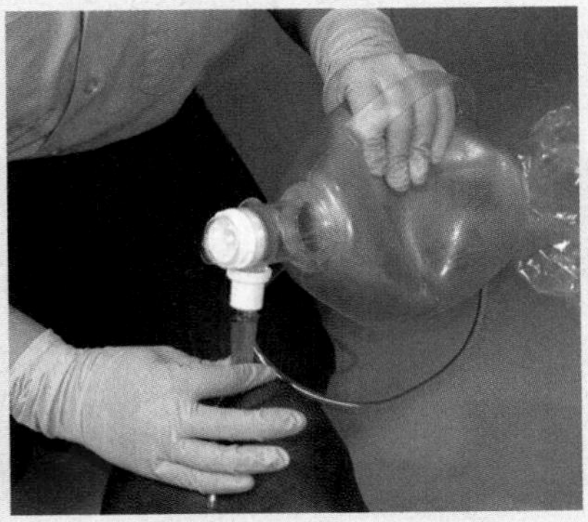

Step 8

Begin to ventilate the patient. Confirm chest rise and the presence of breath sounds. Ensure proper tube placement with waveform capnography. Continuously and carefully monitor the patient's condition.

Furthermore, the size and weight range for the i-gel is printed directly on the device.

As with the LMA, the tip of the i-gel is designed to fit into the proximal esophagus, while the sides and proximal parts of the device form a seal around the hypopharynx. This position facilitates air entry into the trachea **FIGURE 16-100**. **TABLE 16-18** lists three adult-size i-gel supraglottic airways and patient weight criteria.

The steps for inserting an i-gel supraglottic airway are shown in **SKILL DRILL 16-15**.

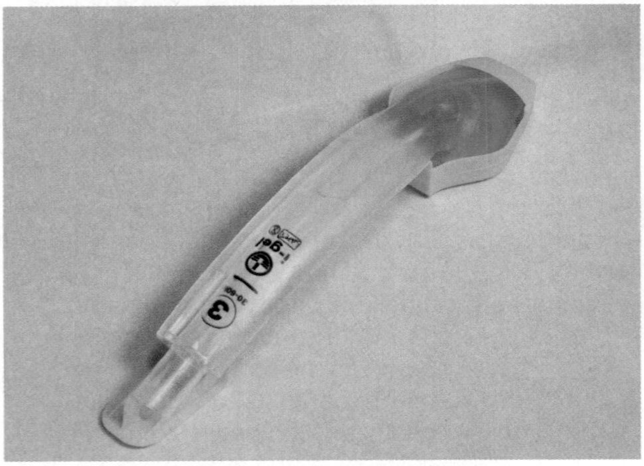

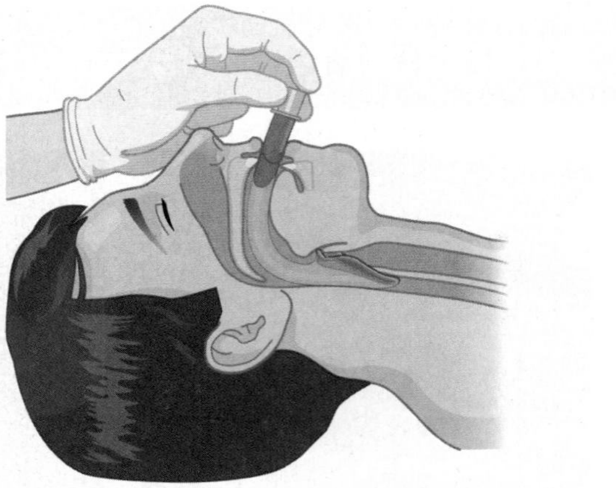

FIGURE 16-100 Correct position of the i-gel in the airway.

© Jones & Bartlett Learning.

FIGURE 16-99 The i-gel supraglottic airway.

© Photo Researchers, Inc./Science Source.

TABLE 16-18 Sizes and Patient Criteria for Adult i-gel Supraglottic Airway

Size	Connector Color	Weight Criteria
3	Yellow	66–132 lb (30–60 kg)
4	Green	110–198 lb (50–90 kg)
5	Orange	>198 lb (>90 kg)

Data from: i-gel information sheet (Issue 11). Intersurgical Ltd website. https://us.intersurgical.com/content/files /76110/183789915. Accessed August 16, 2021.

Skill Drill 16-15 Inserting an i-gel Supraglottic Airway

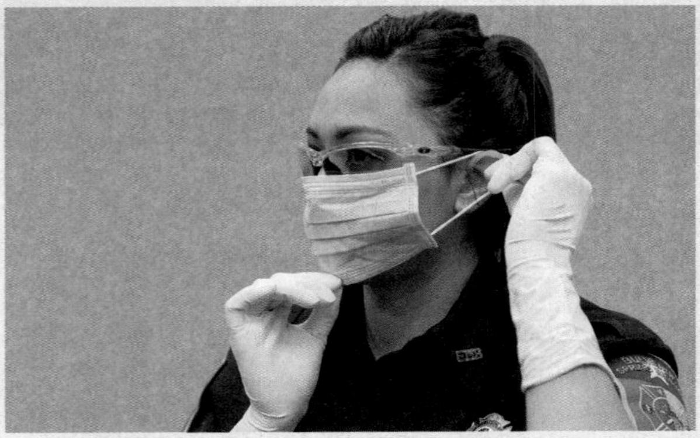

Step 1

Take standard precautions.

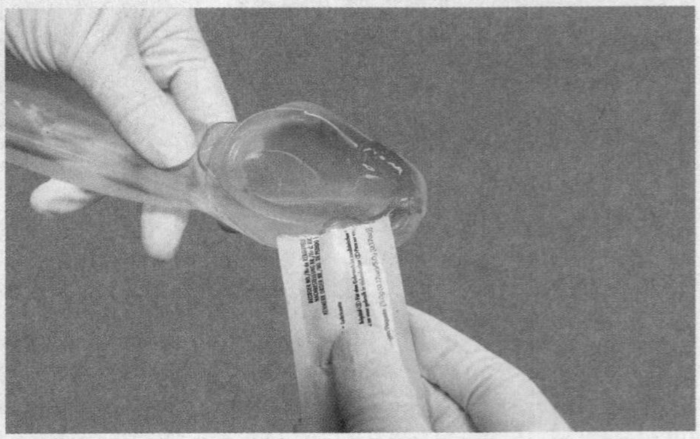

Step 2

Lubricate the back, sides, and front of the cuff with a thin layer of water-soluble gel.

Skill Drill 16-15 Inserting an i-gel Supraglottic Airway (continued)

NR Skill

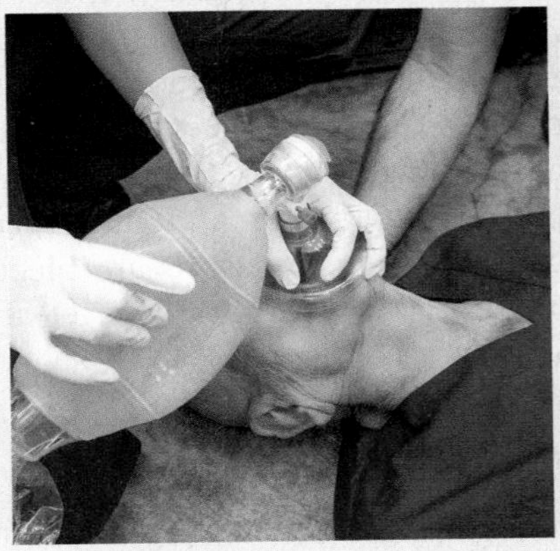

Step 3

Preoxygenate the patient before insertion. Place the patient in the sniffing position. Insert the i-gel as quickly, safely, and efficiently as possible.

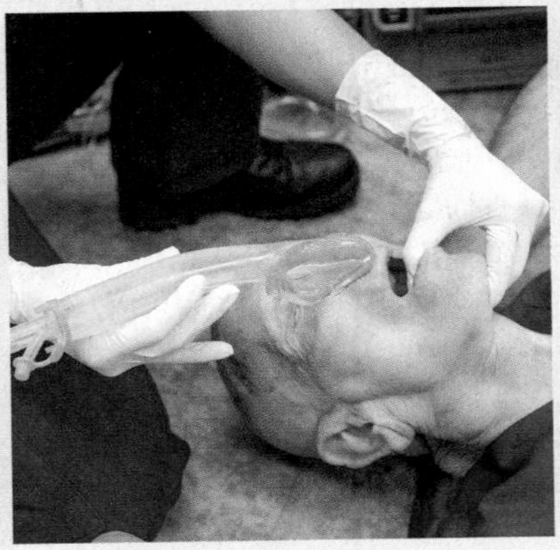

Step 4

Open the airway with the tongue-jaw lift maneuver and position the i-gel so that the cuff outlet faces toward the patient's chin.

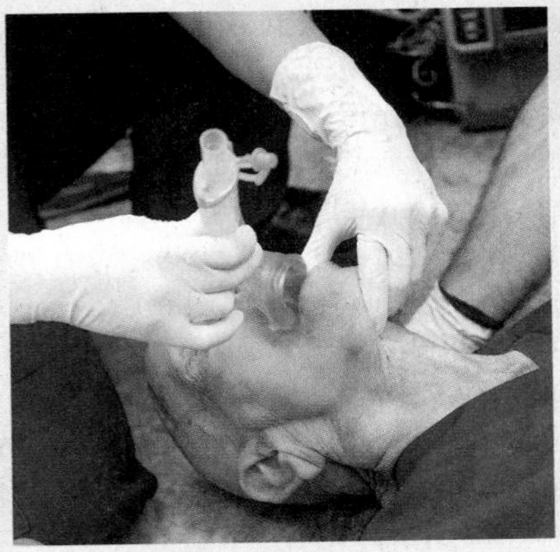

Step 5

Introduce the leading soft tip of the i-gel into the patient's mouth, directing it toward the hard palate.

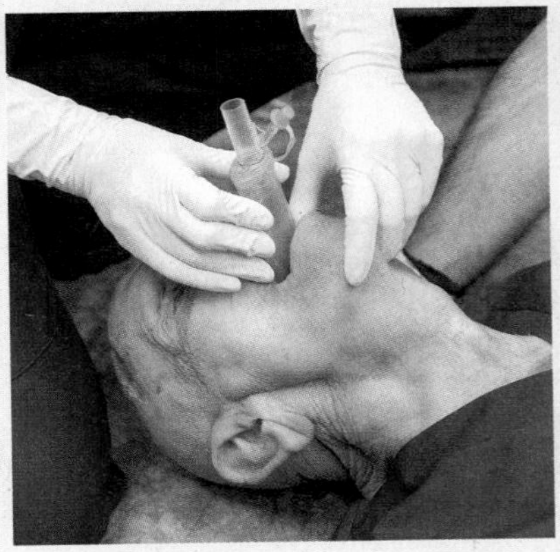

Step 6

Glide the i-gel downward and backward along the hard palate with a continuous but gentle push until a definitive resistance is felt.

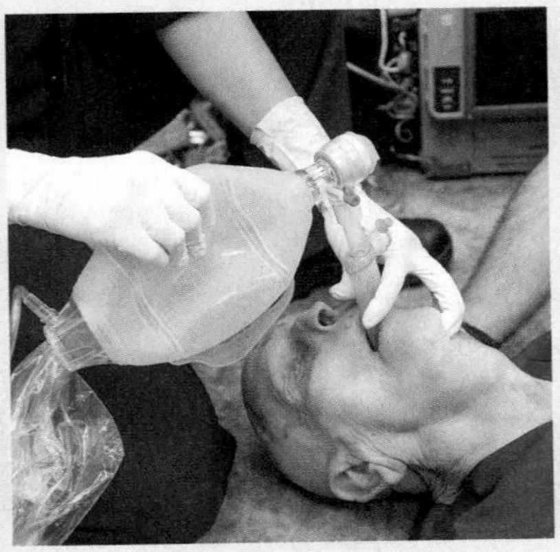

Step 7

Begin to ventilate the patient. Confirm chest rise and the presence of breath sounds. Ensure proper tube placement with waveform capnography. Continuously and carefully monitor the patient's condition.

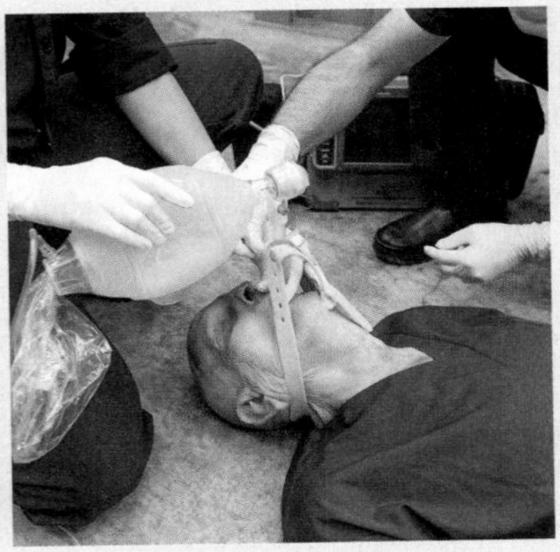

Step 8

Secure the i-gel in place with the provided strap.

Cricothyrotomy

In most cases, you can secure a patent airway using either basic methods (eg, bag-mask device with oral airway) or advanced methods (eg, ET intubation, supraglottic airway). Sometimes, however, the patient's condition or other factors preclude the use of conventional airway techniques, creating a situation in which you cannot intubate or ventilate the patient. In such cases, you must take a more aggressive and invasive approach to secure the patient's airway and maximize the patient's chances for survival.

Two methods of securing a patent airway are available when conventional techniques and methods fail: the surgical cricothyrotomy and the needle cricothyrotomy with translaryngeal catheter ventilation. To perform these procedures, you must be familiar with the key anatomic landmarks that lie in the anterior aspect of the neck **FIGURE 16-101**.

In addition, you must be familiar with the important blood vessels in this area. The superior cricothyroid vessels run at a transverse angle across the upper third of the cricothyroid membrane. The carotid arteries run vertically and are located lateral to the cricothyroid membrane. To avoid damaging these blood vessels, you must use great care when incising the cricothyroid membrane.

When performing a cricothyrotomy, it is important to know that the patient *will* bleed from the subcutaneous and small skin vessels as you incise down to the cricothyroid membrane. Although this bleeding is usually minor, it will impair your visual reference, making cricothyrotomy a tactile procedure. You should be able to easily control any bleeding with light pressure after you have inserted the tube into the trachea.

Surgical Cricothyrotomy

Surgical cricothyrotomy involves incising the cricothyroid membrane with a scalpel and inserting an ET or tracheostomy tube directly into the subglottic area (below the vocal cords) of the trachea. The cricothyroid membrane is the ideal site for making a surgical opening into the trachea because no important structures lie between the skin and the airway. The airway at this level lies relatively close to the skin (except in patients with obesity) and is easy to enter through the thin cricothyroid membrane.

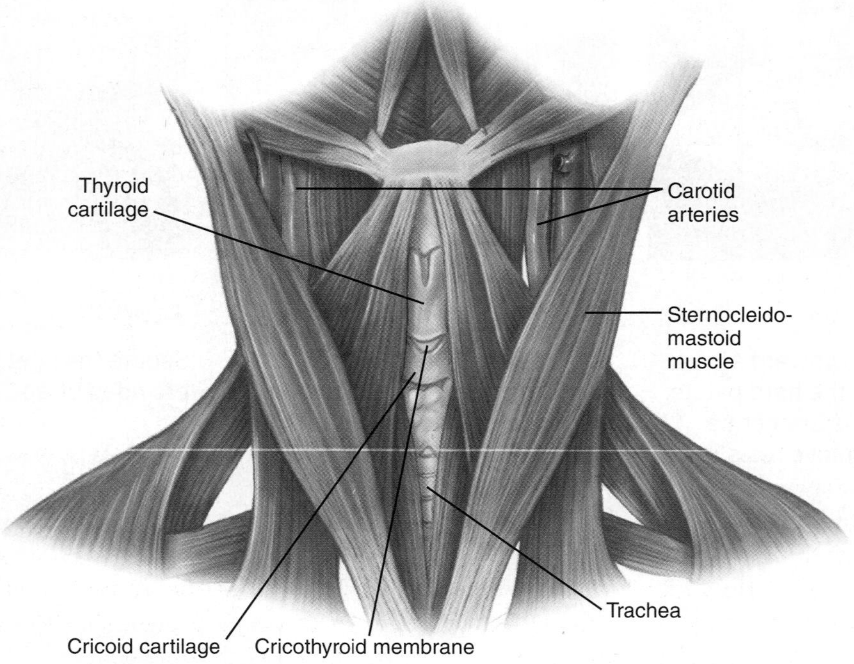

FIGURE 16-101 Anatomy of the anterior aspect of the neck.

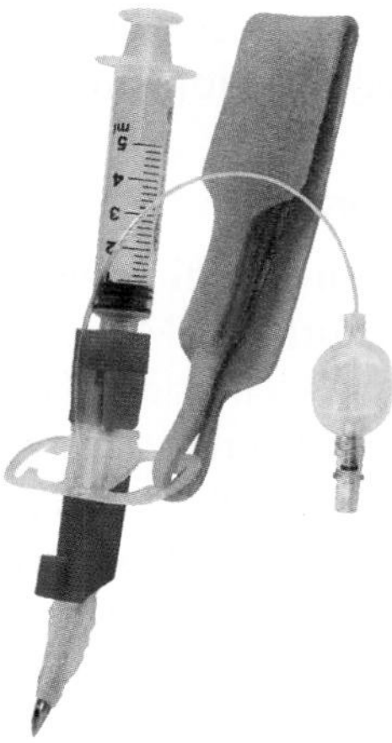

FIGURE 16-102 The Quicktrach II kit.

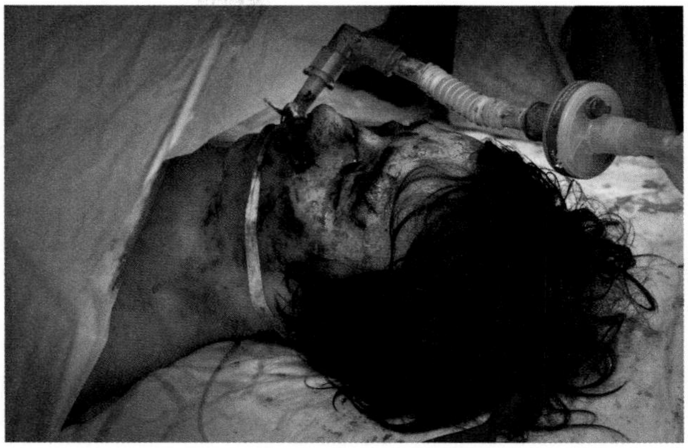

FIGURE 16-103 Patients with massive maxillofacial trauma often have mandibular fractures or profuse bleeding in the oropharynx, both of which can make bag-mask ventilation and intubation extremely difficult, if not impossible.

The posterior wall of the airway at this level is formed by the tough cricoid cartilage, which helps prevent accidental perforation through the back of the airway into the esophagus.

Several types of surgical cricothyrotomies exist. As previously discussed, surgical cricothyrotomy involves incising the patient's skin and cricothyroid membrane and inserting an ET tube or tracheostomy tube. A modified cricothyrotomy is another type of cricothyrotomy. Commercial modified cricothyrotomy kits are available, such as the Quicktrach, which may be used in the prehospital setting. The Quicktrach kit features a 4.0-mm cannula over a large-bore needle that punctures the cricothyroid membrane. A stopper prevents the needle from being inserted too deeply, reducing the risk of posterior tracheal wall perforation. The Quicktrach II kit includes all the features of the Quicktrach, but also has an inflatable cuff on the distal end of the cannula that minimizes the risk of aspiration **FIGURE 16-102**. No scalpel incision is necessary when using the Quicktrach kit.

Indications and Contraindications

Surgical cricothyrotomy is indicated when you cannot secure a patent airway by *any* other means: the "can't ventilate, can't oxygenate" scenario. It is not the preferred means of initially securing a patient's airway. For example, if you are unable to intubate a patient but can provide effective bag-mask ventilations, then cricothyrotomy is not indicated.

Situations that may preclude conventional airway management include severe foreign body obstruction of the upper airway that cannot be extracted with Magill forceps and direct laryngoscopy, airway obstruction from swelling (eg, epiglottitis, anaphylaxis, and upper airway burns), massive maxillofacial trauma, and inability to open the patient's mouth. Patients with massive maxillofacial trauma **FIGURE 16-103** often have associated mandibular fractures, which makes it extremely difficult to maintain an effective mask-to-face seal with a bag-mask device. Intubation in patients with these injuries may also be extremely difficult because of posterior tongue lacerations with profuse bleeding and oropharyngeal swelling. In such patients, frequent suctioning to prevent aspiration would delay intubation and increase hypoxia.

Patients with head injuries and trismus (clenched teeth) may require cricothyrotomy, especially if you do not have the resources or protocols to perform RSI. Furthermore, head injury, which is commonly accompanied by facial trauma, is a contraindication for nasotracheal intubation and placement of a nasal airway, especially if fluid is draining from the patient's nose **FIGURE 16-104**. If this fluid is CSF, then fracture of the cribriform plate is likely present. If you attempt nasotracheal intubation in this situation, the ET tube or nasal airway could inadvertently enter the cranial vault through the fractured plate; as previously discussed, this is a rare occurrence but is possible.

As noted earlier, the main contraindication to surgical cricothyrotomy is the ability to secure

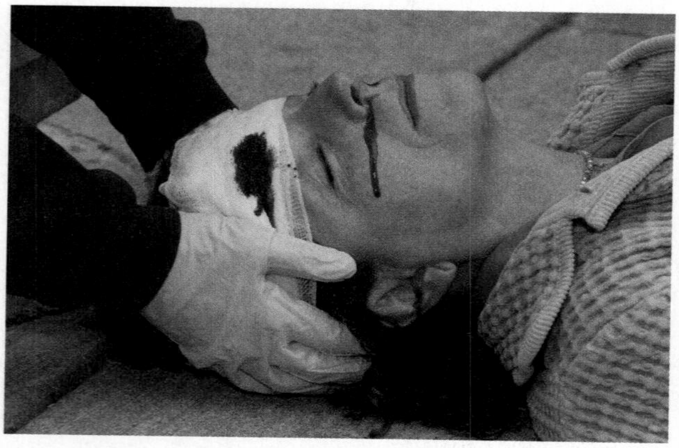

FIGURE 16-104 Endotracheal intubation may be impossible in patients with a head injury and trismus. Nasotracheal intubation is contraindicated in patients with head injury and fluid drainage from the nose.

a patent airway by any other means. Other contraindications include the inability to identify the correct anatomic landmarks (cricothyroid membrane), crushing injuries to the larynx and tracheal transection, underlying anatomic abnormalities (eg, trauma, tumors, or subglottic stenosis), and age younger than 8 years. The larynx of a small child is generally unable to support a tube large enough to produce effective ventilation without causing damage to the larynx; a needle cricothyrotomy (discussed later in this chapter) would be safer for young children.

In situations in which cricothyrotomy is contraindicated, promptly transport the patient to the closest appropriate facility, where an emergency tracheostomy can be performed.

Advantages and Disadvantages

Surgical cricothyrotomy can be performed quickly, and without manipulating the cervical spine. The latter characteristic is especially advantageous because many cricothyrotomies are performed in patients with massive facial trauma.

Disadvantages of cricothyrotomy include the difficulty encountered in performing the procedure in children, which is why it is contraindicated in children younger than 8 years. Compared to needle cricothyrotomy, surgical cricothyrotomy is more difficult to perform. However, inserting a large-bore tube (ie, an ET tube or a tracheostomy tube) can facilitate greater tidal volume, which facilitates more effective oxygenation and ventilation.

Complications

Expect some minor bleeding when an open cricothyrotomy is performed. More severe bleeding is usually the result of laceration of a larger vein. Incising the cricothyroid membrane vertically, instead of horizontally, will minimize the risk of this complication, as well as the risk of damaging the highly vascular thyroid gland. After the incision has been made, insert the tube gently to minimize the risks of perforating the esophagus and damaging the laryngeal nerves.

Words of Wisdom

Frequent practice on a cadaver, if available, or a special cricothyrotomy manikin will maximize your ability to perform cricothyrotomy quickly. In general, skills that are not frequently performed in the field should be routinely practiced to maintain proficiency and competence.

The decision to perform a surgical cricothyrotomy and execution of this procedure must be quick. Taking too long to decide that a cricothyrotomy is indicated will delay the procedure; as a result, the patient will become more hypoxic, which may result in cardiac dysrhythmias, permanent brain injury, and/or cardiac arrest.

It is possible to create a false passage if the tube undermines the subcutaneous tissue and never enters the trachea through the cricothyroid membrane. Although this complication can occur with any patient, the risk is greater when performing a surgical cricothyrotomy on a patient with obesity. Suspect tube misplacement when subcutaneous emphysema becomes apparent after performing a cricothyrotomy. Subcutaneous emphysema occurs when air infiltrates the subcutaneous (fatty) layers of the skin and is characterized by a "crackling" sensation when palpated.

Any invasive procedure performed in the prehospital setting is associated with the risk of infection for patients. Therefore, maintain aseptic technique to the extent possible when performing an open cricothyrotomy.

Equipment

If a commercially manufactured cricothyrotomy kit is unavailable, then you must prepare the following equipment and supplies:

- Scalpel (No. 10 blade)
- ET or tracheostomy tube (6.0 mm minimum)
- Commercial device (or tape) for securing the tube
- Suction apparatus
- Sterile gauze pads for bleeding control
- Bag-mask device attached to 100% oxygen
- $ETCO_2$ detector (quantitative waveform capnography)

Technique for Performing Surgical Cricothyrotomy

After you determine that a surgical cricothyrotomy is needed, you must proceed rapidly, yet cautiously. Identify the cricothyroid membrane by palpating for the V notch of the thyroid cartilage, which feels like a high, sharp bump. Stabilize the larynx between your thumb and middle fingers while you palpate with your index finger. When you have located the V notch, slide your index finger down over the thyroid prominence (Adam's apple) and into the depression between the thyroid and cricoid cartilage; that is the cricothyroid membrane.

Males have a prominent thyroid notch and thyroid prominence, whereas females do not. Because the cricoid ring is more prominent in females than it is in males, when palpating the anatomy in females, first locate the cricoid ring, then the cricothyroid membrane, and finally the thyroid cartilage.

While you are locating and preparing the site, your partner should prepare your equipment and ensure that the cardiac monitor/defibrillator and pulse oximeter are attached to the patient.

Maintain aseptic technique as you cleanse the area with iodine; avoid touching the area once cleansed. While stabilizing the larynx with one hand, make a vertical incision (approximately 0.5 to 0.75 inch [1 to 2 cm]) over the cricothyroid membrane; in patients with obesity, this vertical incision may need to be longer and deeper. A No. 10 scalpel is ideal because it has a pointed tip for puncturing and a beveled edge for incising.

After making the incision, remove the scalpel and immediately place your index finger on top of the cricothyroid membrane to reconfirm the anatomy. Remember, the patient will likely bleed after the first incision is made, so your visual reference may be reduced or lost. Therefore, it is critical to maintain stabilization of the larynx and to keep the cricothyroid membrane acquired. Puncture the cricothyroid membrane and make a horizontal incision (approximately 0.5 inch [1 cm]) in each direction from the midline; do not incise too far laterally. Remove the scalpel and immediately put your index finger through the cricothyroid membrane. At this point, you can use a tracheal hook or a Trousseau tracheal dilator (available in commercial cricothyrotomy kits) **FIGURE 16-105**. Your partner should be readily available to control any bleeding that might occur.

With the trachea exposed, gently insert a 6.0-mm cuffed ET tube or a 6.0 cuffed tracheostomy tube **FIGURE 16-106** and direct it into the trachea. After the

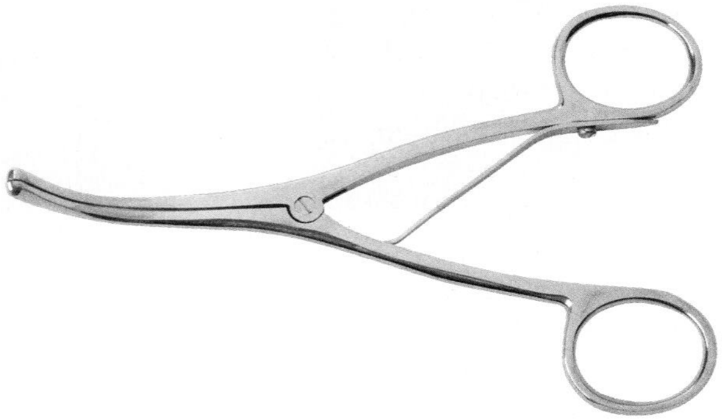

FIGURE 16-105 Trousseau tracheal dilator.

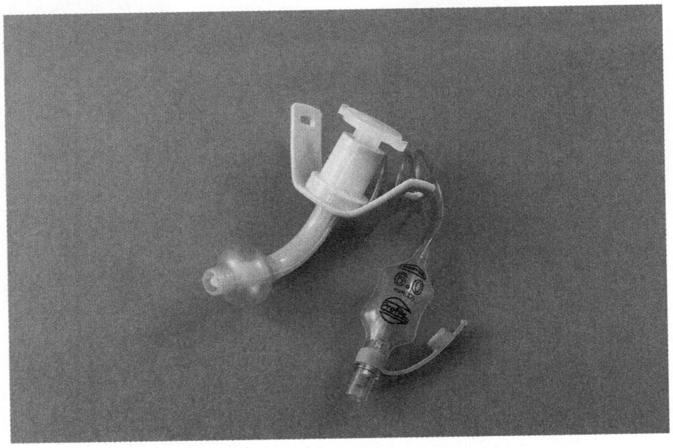

FIGURE 16-106 Cuffed tracheostomy tube.

tube is in place, stabilize it manually and inflate the distal cuff with the appropriate volume of air, typically 5 to 10 mL. Attach the bag-mask device to the standard 15/22-mm adapter on the tube, and ventilate the patient while your partner auscultates to ensure the presence of bilaterally clear breath sounds and the absence of epigastric sounds. If epigastric sounds are heard, then you have likely perforated the trachea and inserted the tube into the esophagus.

Additional confirmation of correct tube placement can be accomplished by attaching an $ETCO_2$ detector between the tube and ventilation device. After confirming proper tube placement, ensure that any minor bleeding has been controlled, properly secure the tube, and continue to ventilate the patient at the appropriate rate.

The steps for performing a surgical cricothyrotomy are shown in **SKILL DRILL 16-16**.

Skill Drill 16-16 Performing a Surgical Cricothyrotomy

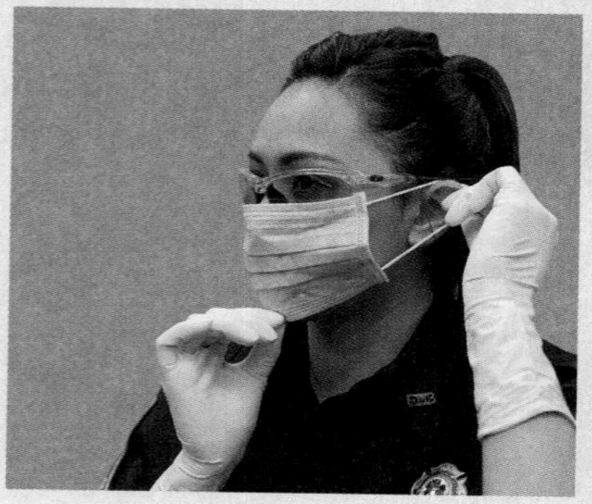

Step 1

Take standard precautions.

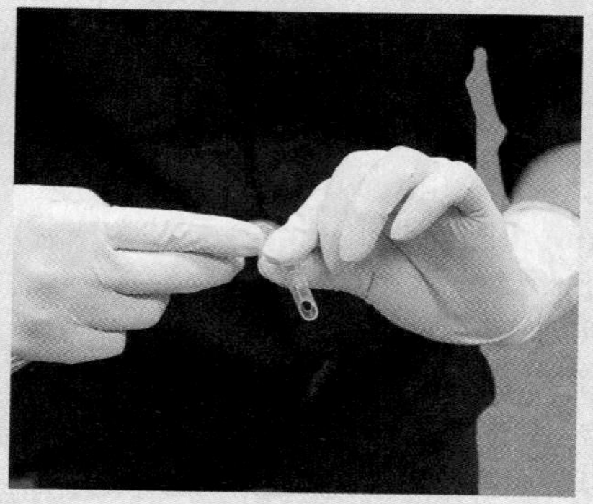

Step 2

Check, assemble, and prepare the equipment. Place a 90° bend in a 6.0-mm ET tube (with a stylet inserted), just proximal to the cuff.

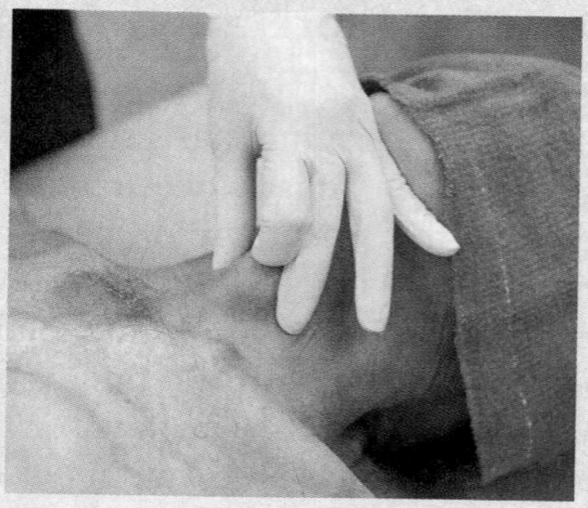

Step 3

With the patient's head in a neutral position, palpate for and locate the cricothyroid membrane.

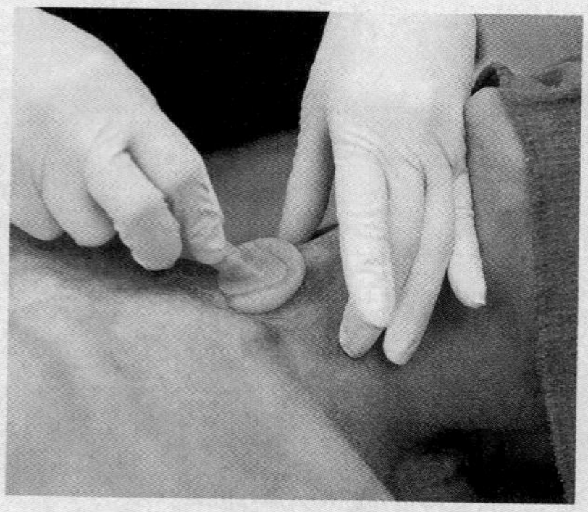

Step 4

Cleanse the area with an iodine- or chlorhexidine-containing solution.

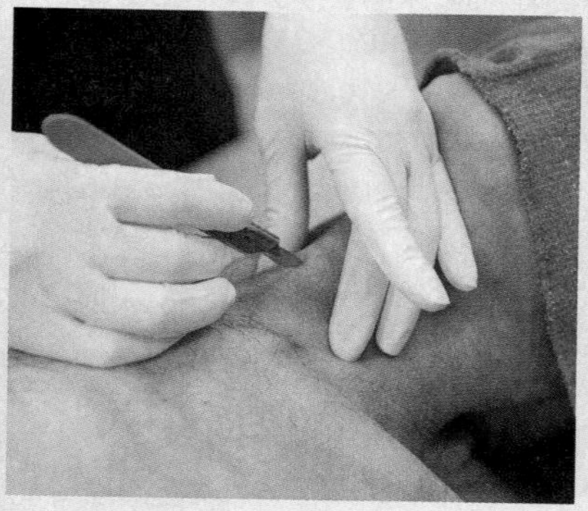

Step 5

Stabilize the larynx, and make a vertical incision (approximately 0.5 to 0.75 inch [1 to 2 cm]) over the cricothyroid membrane.

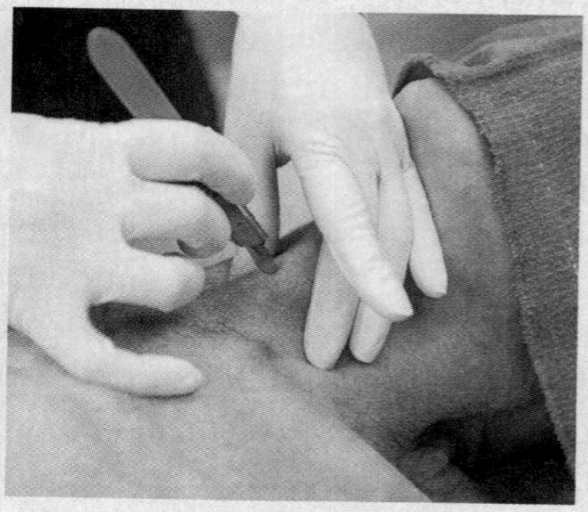

Step 6

Puncture the cricothyroid membrane.

Skill Drill 16-16 Performing a Surgical Cricothyrotomy (continued)

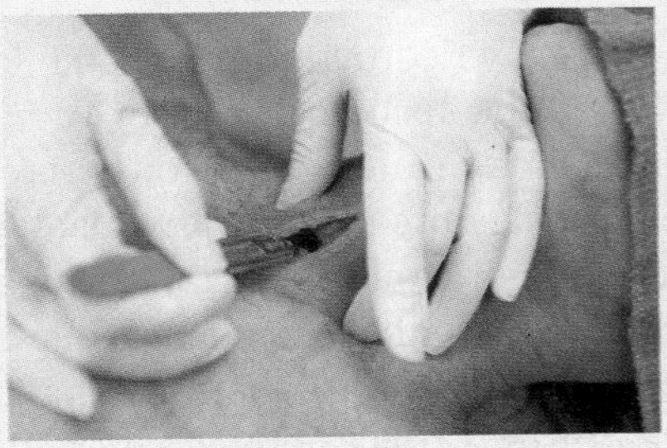

Step 7

Make a horizontal incision (approximately 0.5 inch [1 cm]) in each direction from the midline.

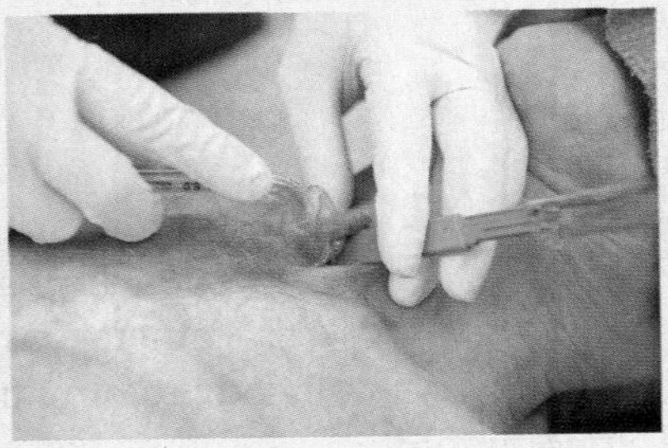

Step 8

Insert the tube until the cuff is completely inside the trachea and no more than approximately 1 to 2 cm to avoid going to deep past the carina and into the right main bronchus. To aid in inserting the tube, the knife handle can be introduced into the horizontal incision and rotated 90° to stent the opening for the tube.

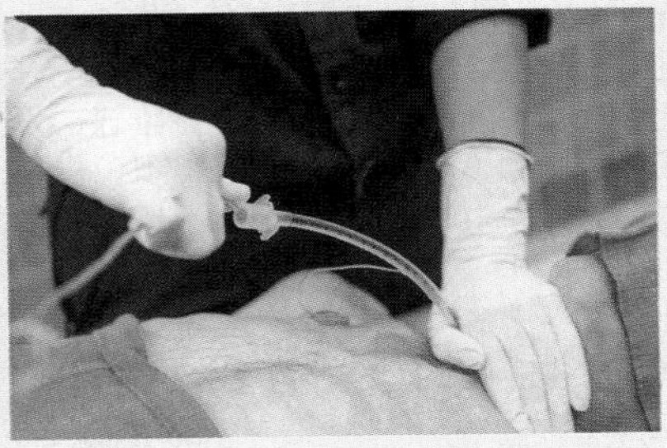

Step 9

Manually stabilize the ET tube between your thumb and index finger, carefully remove the stylet, and inflate the distal cuff.

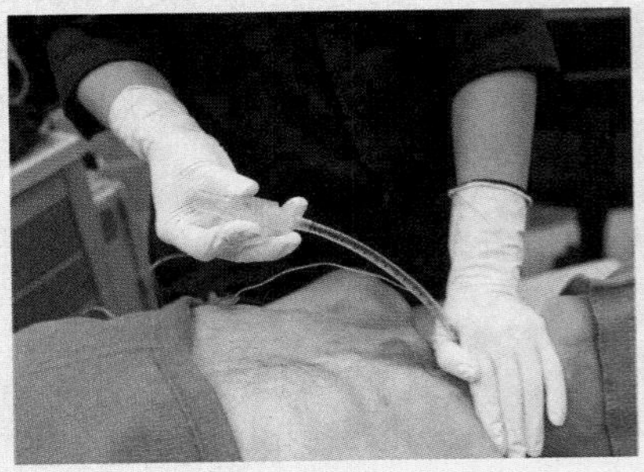

Step 10

Attach an $ETCO_2$ detector between the tube and the ventilation device.

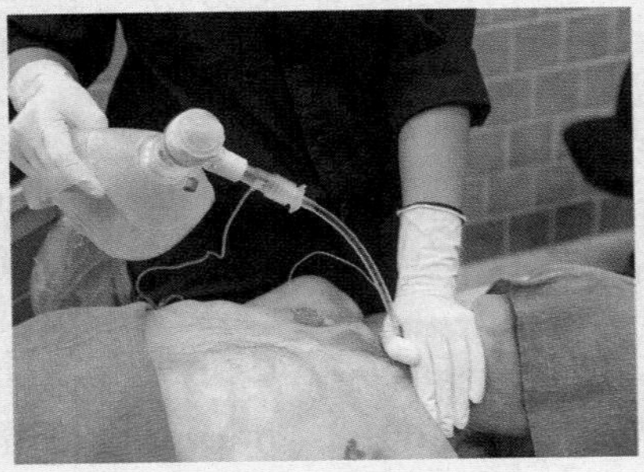

Step 11

Ensure proper tube placement with waveform capnography. Attach the $ETCO_2$ detector to the monitor. Ventilate the patient.

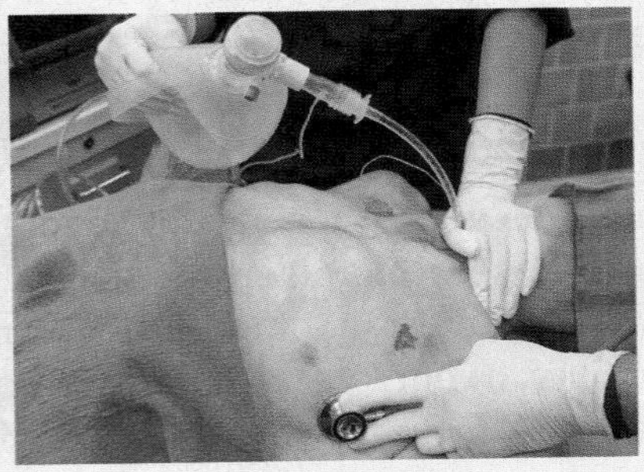

Step 12

Confirm correct tube placement by auscultating the apices and bases of both lungs and over the epigastrium.

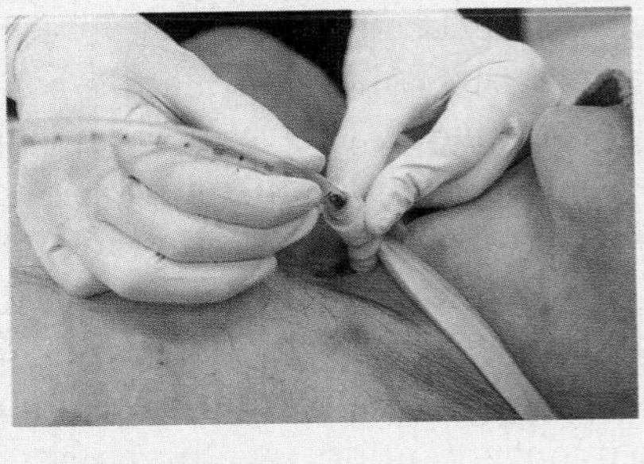

Step 13

Secure the tube with a commercial device or tape. Reconfirm correct tube placement, and resume ventilations at the appropriate rate.

> **Words of Wisdom**
>
> To avoid creating a false passage, insert a bougie into the cricothyroid membrane to confirm tactile appreciation of the tracheal rings, and then insert the ET or tracheostomy tube over the bougie. This can be accomplished with a regular bougie and 6.0-mm ET tube or with a commercial device that features a tracheostomy tube with a preinserted bougie.

Needle Cricothyrotomy

Needle cricothyrotomy also uses the cricothyroid membrane as an entry point into the airway. In this procedure, a 12- to 16-gauge over-the-needle IV catheter is inserted through the cricothyroid membrane and into the trachea. Adequate oxygenation and ventilation are then achieved by attaching a high-pressure jet ventilator to the hub of the catheter. Known as **translaryngeal catheter ventilation**, this procedure is commonly used as a temporary measure until a more definitive airway can be obtained (eg, surgical cricothyrotomy or tracheostomy). When using a high-pressure jet ventilator, watch the patient closely to avoid overinflation of the lungs.

Indications and Contraindications

The indications for needle cricothyrotomy and translaryngeal catheter ventilation are essentially the same as those for surgical cricothyrotomy: the inability to ventilate the patient by any other means, massive maxillofacial trauma, inability to open the patient's mouth, and uncontrolled oropharyngeal bleeding.

Needle cricothyrotomy is contraindicated in patients who have a severe airway obstruction above the site of catheter insertion. Exhalation cannot occur through the jet ventilation device, so it must occur via the glottic opening. If the airway is completely obstructed above the catheter insertion site, then exhalation will not be possible. As a result, the patient will become hypercapnic. The high-pressure jet ventilator used with needle cricothyrotomy causes an increase in intrathoracic pressure, potentially resulting in barotrauma and risk for a pneumothorax. Barotrauma can also be caused by overinflation of the lungs with the jet ventilator, so take care to open the release valve only until the patient's chest rise is adequate.

If the equipment necessary to perform translaryngeal catheter ventilation is not immediately available, then perform a surgical cricothyrotomy.

Advantages and Disadvantages

Compared with surgical cricothyrotomy, needle cricothyrotomy is faster and technically easier to perform. In particular, it is associated with a lower risk of causing damage to adjacent structures because you are puncturing the cricothyroid membrane with an IV catheter, not incising it with a scalpel. Needle cricothyrotomy also allows for subsequent intubation attempts because it uses a small-bore catheter, thus allowing an ET tube to easily pass beside it. This feature could be particularly beneficial if you do not have the equipment or protocols to perform a surgical cricothyrotomy. In addition, this procedure does not require manipulation of the patient's cervical spine.

However, disadvantages exist to performing a needle cricothyrotomy. Using a smaller-bore tube (such as an over-the-needle IV catheter) to ventilate the patient does not provide protection from aspiration like a cuffed ET tube or tracheostomy tube would during a surgical cricothyrotomy (a larger-bore tube, combined with the distal cuff, would fill the diameter of the trachea, protecting it from aspiration). Also, needle cricothyrotomy requires a specialized, high-pressure jet ventilator to provide adequate tidal volume. This jet ventilator will expend high volumes of oxygen rapidly.

Complications

Improper catheter placement during needle cricothyrotomy can result in severe bleeding if it damages adjacent structures. Even if the catheter is placed correctly, excessive air leakage around the insertion site can cause subcutaneous emphysema, especially if the patient has undetected laryngeal trauma. If too much air infiltrates into the subcutaneous space, compression of the trachea and subsequent obstruction may occur.

Exercise extreme care when ventilating a patient by using a jet ventilator. The ventilation valve should be depressed or occluded just long enough for adequate chest rise to occur. Overinflation of the lungs can result in barotrauma, which increases the risk of pneumothorax. Conversely, depressing or occluding the ventilation valve for too short a period could cause hypoventilation, resulting in inadequate oxygenation and ventilation.

Equipment

The following equipment is needed to perform needle cricothyrotomy and translaryngeal catheter ventilation:

- Large-bore IV catheter (12- to 16-gauge)
- 10-mL syringe
- 3 mL of sterile water or saline
- Oxygen source (50 psi)
- High-pressure jet ventilator device and oxygen tubing

Technique for Performing Needle Cricothyrotomy

When preparing your equipment, draw up approximately 3 mL of sterile water or saline into a 10-mL syringe and attach the syringe to the IV catheter. Next, place the patient's head in a neutral position, and locate the cricothyroid membrane. Cleanse the area with an iodine-containing solution.

While you are stabilizing the patient's thyroid cartilage, carefully insert the needle into the midline of the cricothyroid membrane at a 45° angle toward the feet (caudally). You should feel a pop as the needle penetrates the membrane. After the pop is felt, insert the needle approximately 0.5 inch (1 cm) farther, and then aspirate with the syringe. If the catheter has been correctly placed, then you should be able to easily aspirate air and see the saline or water bubbling within the syringe. If blood is aspirated or if you meet resistance, then reevaluate catheter placement because it is likely positioned outside the trachea.

After confirming correct placement, advance the catheter over the needle until the catheter hub is flush with the skin, then withdraw the needle and place it in a puncture-proof biohazard container. Next, attach one end of the oxygen tubing to the catheter and the other end to the jet ventilator.

Begin ventilations by opening the release valve on the jet ventilator and observing for adequate chest rise. Auscultation of breath and epigastric sounds will further confirm correct catheter placement. To prevent overexpansion of the lungs and subsequent barotrauma, release the ventilation valve as soon as you see the patient's chest rise. Exhalation will occur passively via the glottis. Ventilate the patient as dictated by the clinical condition.

Secure the catheter by placing a folded 4 × 4–inch (10 × 10–cm) gauze pad under the catheter and taping it in place. Continue ventilations while frequently reassessing the patient for adequacy of ventilations and for potential complications (eg, subcutaneous emphysema from incorrect placement).

The steps for performing needle cricothyrotomy with translaryngeal catheter ventilation are shown in **SKILL DRILL 16-17**.

Skill Drill 16-17 Performing Needle Cricothyrotomy and Translaryngeal Catheter Ventilation

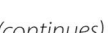

NR Skill

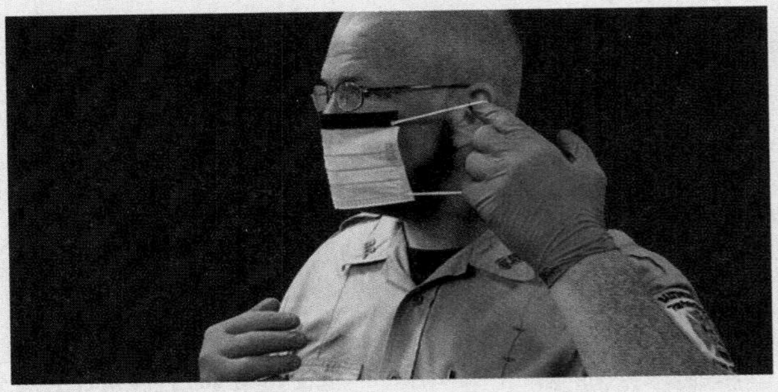

Step 1

Take standard precautions.

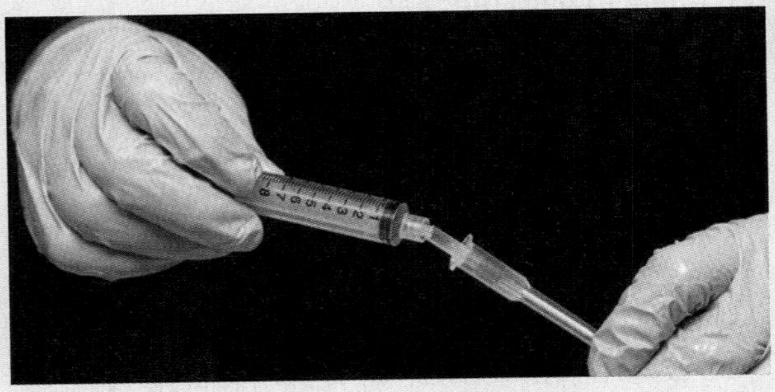

Step 2

Attach a 14- to 16-gauge IV catheter to a 10-mL syringe containing approximately 3 mL of sterile saline or water.

(continues)

NR Skill

Skill Drill 16-17 Performing Needle Cricothyrotomy and Translaryngeal Catheter Ventilation (continued)

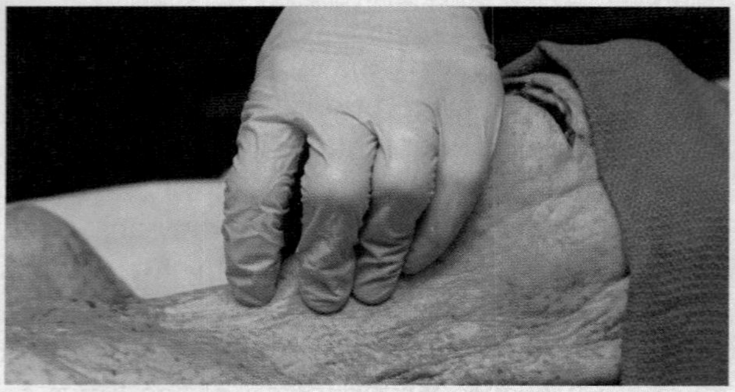

Step 3

With the patient's head in a neutral position, stabilize the thyroid cartilage, and palpate for and locate the cricothyroid membrane.

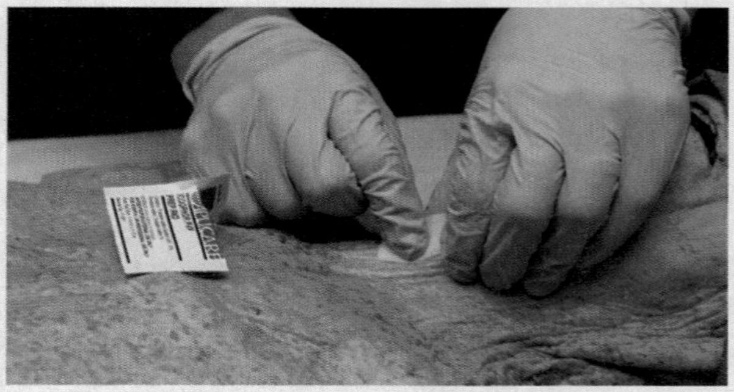

Step 4

Cleanse the area with an iodine-containing solution.

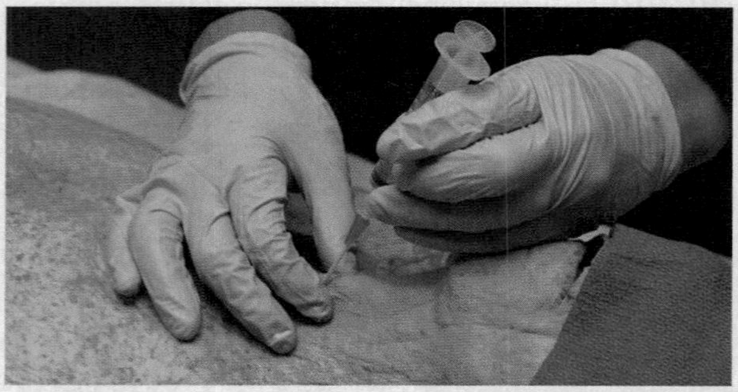

Step 5

While stabilizing the thyroid cartilage, insert the needle into the cricothyroid membrane at a 45° angle toward the feet.

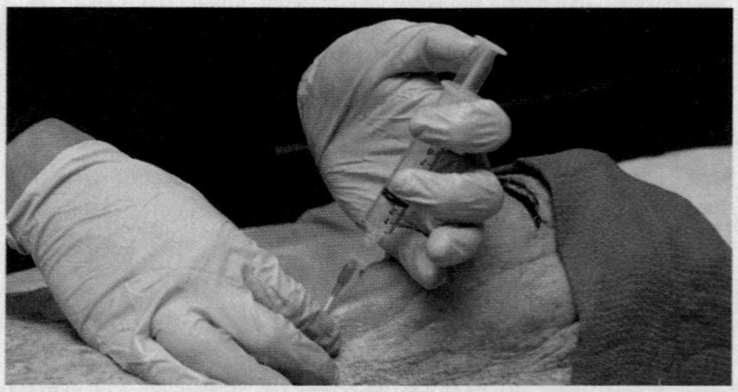

Step 6

Aspirate with the syringe to determine correct catheter placement.

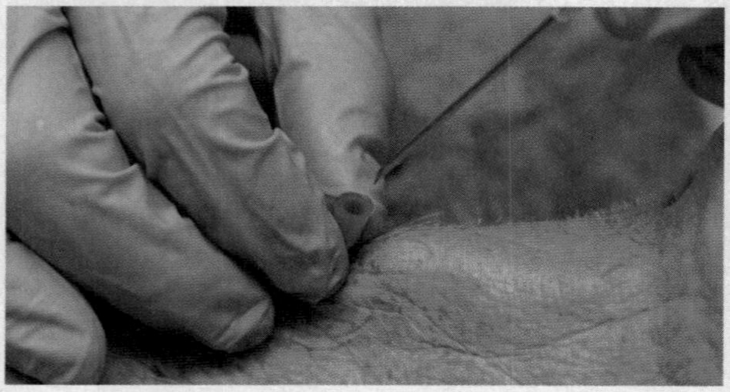

Step 7

Slide the catheter off of the needle until the hub of the catheter is flush with the patient's skin.

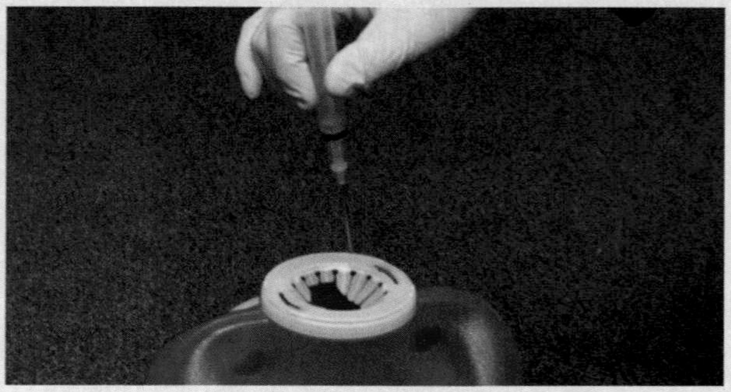

Step 8

Place the syringe and needle in a puncture-proof container.

Skill Drill 16-17 Performing Needle Cricothyrotomy and Translaryngeal Catheter Ventilation (continued)

NR Skill

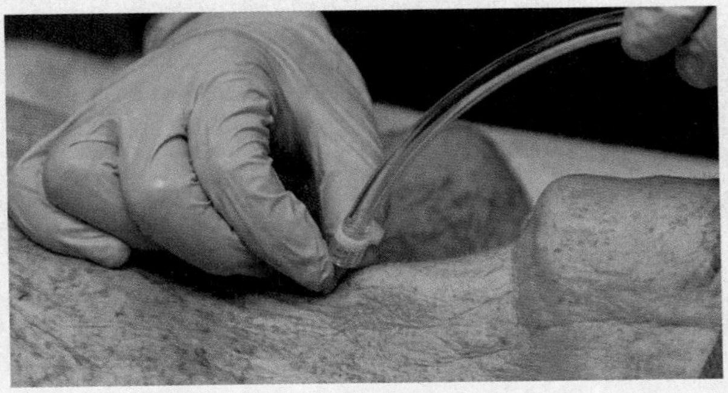

Step 9

Connect one end of the oxygen tubing to the catheter and the other end to the jet ventilator. Maintain manual stabilization of the catheter until it has been secured in place to avoid dislodgment with jet ventilation.

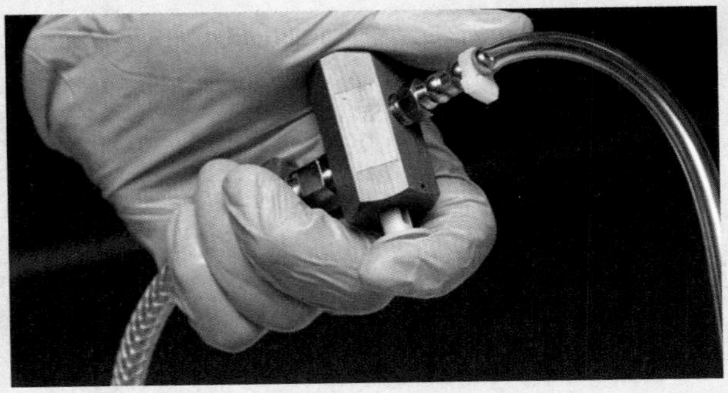

Step 10

Press or occlude the ventilation valve on the jet ventilator for 1 second while observing for chest rise. Release the ventilation valve for 2 to 3 seconds to allow for exhalation.

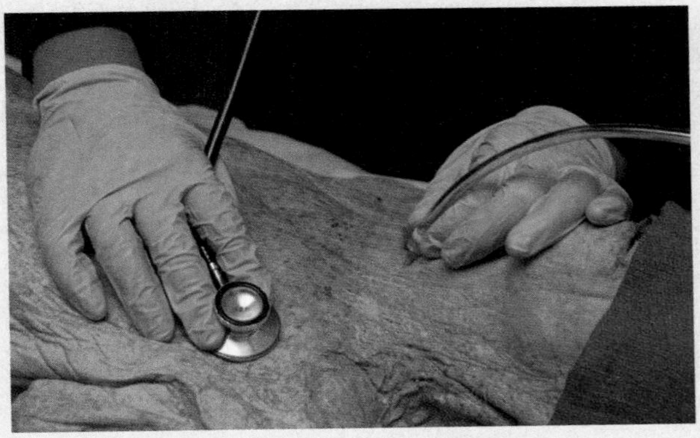

Step 11

Auscultate the apices and bases of both lungs and over the epigastrium to confirm correct catheter placement.

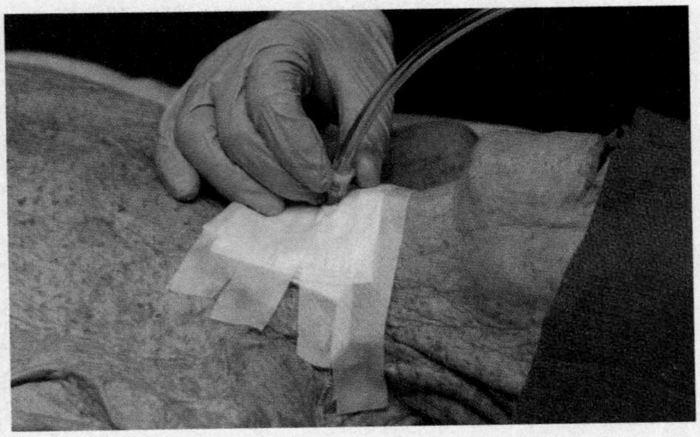

Step 12

Secure the catheter with a 4 × 4–inch (10 × 10–cm) gauze pad and tape. Continue ventilations while frequently reassessing for adequate ventilations and potential complications.

YOU are the Paramedic SUMMARY

1. What is the difference between respiratory distress and respiratory failure?

In respiratory distress, the patient is attempting to compensate for an underlying respiratory problem. Signs of physiologic compensation include retractions, which indicate increased work of breathing; increased respiratory rate and/or depth, which helps maintain adequate minute volume; accessory muscle use to increase the effectiveness of breathing; preferential positioning (ie, tripod positioning) to facilitate breathing; and tachycardia, which helps circulate oxygen faster. Patients with respiratory distress will exhibit increased work of breathing; if they are compensating effectively, their oxygen saturation and $ETCO_2$ levels may be near normal. It is important to quickly identify a patient in respiratory distress and initiate appropriate treatment. If the underlying cause is not corrected, the patient may develop respiratory failure.

Respiratory failure occurs when the body is no longer able to compensate for their respiratory problem. Signs of respiratory failure include physical exhaustion, decreased LOC, weakness with ineffective breathing and retractions, inadequate tidal volume, markedly low oxygen saturation, increased $ETCO_2$ levels, weak pulses, and bradycardia. Immediate intervention is required before the patient develops cardiopulmonary arrest. The survival rate for hypoxic cardiac arrest is very low.

2. Is it possible for a patient to ventilate, but not oxygenate? Why or why not?

Ventilation is the simple mechanical act of moving air into and out of the lungs. Therefore, when you observe a patient's chest rising and falling, all you can conclude is that ventilation is occurring; however, you cannot conclude that the patient is being oxygenated. If the patient is trapped in an area devoid of oxygen (ie, trench, grain silo, structural fire), ventilation may continue, despite the absence of oxygenation. Another example would be a pulmonary embolism: The patient may continue to ventilate, but the blood cannot be reoxygenated because of the blocked pulmonary artery. Therefore, it is possible to ventilate, but not oxygenate. For this reason, it is crucial to perform a thorough patient assessment to ensure that both ventilation and oxygenation occur.

3. How does oxygenation differ from respiration?

Oxygenation is the process of loading oxygen onto hemoglobin when blood circulates through the lungs. Respiration is the process by which gas exchange occurs. Pulmonary (external) respiration occurs when carbon dioxide is exchanged for oxygen in the lungs. Cellular (internal) respiration occurs when oxygen is exchanged for carbon dioxide at the cell and tissue level. Anything that impairs oxygenation will impair respiration. For example, if a patient has pulmonary edema or widespread alveolar collapse (atelectasis), oxygenation will be impaired; if the blood cannot be oxygenated, no oxygen will be delivered to the cells and tissues. Furthermore, oxygenation in the lungs does not guarantee oxygen delivery to the cells and tissues. For example, if a patient is bleeding severely, oxygenated blood will leak out of the vascular space before it gets to the cells and tissues.

4. What are some clinical signs of inadequate breathing?

If inadequate breathing is not quickly recognized and treated, the patient may soon experience respiratory failure, and potentially respiratory arrest. Clinical signs of inadequate breathing include a shallow depth of breathing (reduced tidal volume); a fast or slow respiratory rate; evidence of fatigue or physical exhaustion; a decreasing LOC; weak pulses (slow or fast); an increased (greater than 45 mm Hg) $ETCO_2$ level; and a decreased (less than 90%) oxygen saturation. Note that an otherwise healthy patient may maintain an oxygen saturation of greater than 90% for several minutes, even though breathing is not adequate. Furthermore, the pulse oximeter does not provide a real-time reading (it has a lag time of 90 to 120 seconds) and was designed to detect gross abnormalities, not subtle changes. Conversely, $ETCO_2$ monitoring provides real-time information on a patient's ventilation status. The patient's $ETCO_2$ level will increase within seconds when breathing becomes inadequate. Therefore, it is essential to correlate the patient's oxygen saturation and $ETCO_2$ with the findings from the physical assessment when determining the most appropriate treatment approach. Do not rely solely on numbers.

5. What underlying problem do you suspect is impairing this patient's ability to oxygenate?

Given the patient's history of "heart problems," as well as the clinical finding of coarse crackles in his lungs, you should suspect that the patient is experiencing pulmonary edema. Anything that creates a barrier to diffusion in the lungs will impair oxygenation and respiration. With pulmonary edema, the alveoli become filled with fluid; when gases attempt to move across the pulmonary capillary membrane, they are met with resistance. As a result, blood returns to the

YOU are the Paramedic SUMMARY continued

left side of the heart with essentially no more oxygen than when it entered the lungs. This condition, called intrapulmonary shunting, also occurs when there is widespread alveolar collapse (atelectasis).

6. Based on the patient's current clinical status, how should you proceed with your treatment?

It is evident that the patient's respiratory effort is inadequate (ie, labored breathing, cyanosis, low oxygen saturation, increased $ETCO_2$ level) and is not improving with supplemental oxygen alone. Given the coarse crackles in his lungs, the best course of treatment at this point would be CPAP, a noninvasive form of positive-pressure ventilation. CPAP is an effective therapy for patients with respiratory distress caused by conditions such as pulmonary edema and bronchospasm. With CPAP, the patient's exhalation is met with resistance, which is set by the clinician in a typical range of 2.5 to 15 cm H_2O to achieve the best clinical response. When the patient exhales against this resistance, an increase in PEEP occurs. PEEP is the residual pressure on the alveolar walls at the end of exhalation; it is what "splints" the alveoli open and keeps them from collapsing in between breaths. By increasing a patient's PEEP, more alveoli are recruited when fluid is forced from them; this results in improved pulmonary gas exchange. CPAP is also an effective therapy for patients with respiratory distress secondary to diffuse bronchospasm. In conjunction with administration of a nebulized bronchodilator, redirected positive pressure expands the bronchioles, thereby improving air flow through them.

7. Is RSI the best option for the patient at this point? Why or why not?

In a word, no! This patient is severely hypoxic and hypercarbic and has almost no respiratory reserve left. Sedating him and then administering a paralytic (which, of course, stops his breathing) would promptly take his respiratory reserve to zero, which could result in rapid decompensation to cardiopulmonary arrest. The process of RSI involves expediently, yet *safely*, taking control of a patient's airway and breathing in cases of respiratory failure, when the patient cannot maintain the airway, or when the patient is at high risk for aspiration. A critical component of the RSI procedure is ensuring that the patient is adequately oxygenated *before* administering a paralytic agent. By preoxygenating the patient, whether with high-flow supplemental oxygen, CPAP, or bag-mask ventilation, you provide the patient with an oxygen reserve, making it safer for them to be apneic during the intubation procedure. The higher and longer you can maintain the patient's oxygen saturation *before* administering a paralytic agent, the longer the "safe apneic" time will be.

8. Why is the patient's condition improving, even though you administered sedation?

When patients are significantly hypoxic and hypercarbic, they are often uncooperative; some patients can even be combative. Even though they desperately need oxygen, they will resist any and all attempts to administer it. Administering a sedative makes the patient less resistant, and therefore more tolerant of oxygenation. Ketamine is the ideal drug to use for sedation because it does not suppress the respiratory drive or cause the patient to lose their airway reflexes. The process being described is procedural sedation, where the procedure itself is oxygenation. If the patient is not fighting you, you can effectively oxygenate them. The increased oxygenation explains why the patient's condition is improving. Benzodiazepines, such as midazolam (Versed), lorazepam (Ativan), and diazepam (Valium), should not be used to sedate a hypoxic patient because they can suppress the respiratory drive.

9. What role does capnography play in assessing a patient's ventilation status?

Quantitative waveform capnography provides a numeric and graphic indicator of the amount of carbon dioxide detected at the end of exhalation ($ETCO_2$). Carbon dioxide is the by-product of aerobic metabolism, which takes place in the presence of oxygen and can be regarded as the body's exhaust. The only way to make carbon dioxide in the body is to deliver adequate oxygen to the cells. Capnography provides valuable information regarding a patient's ventilation status and information regarding their perfusion status. The less oxygen that reaches the cells, the less carbon dioxide that is produced and returned to the lungs; as a result, the $ETCO_2$ level would be low. $ETCO_2$ levels will also be low if the body eliminates carbon dioxide faster than it makes it, which is what happens in hyperventilating patients. A high $ETCO_2$ level would be expected if adequate carbon dioxide was produced in the cells and returned to the lungs, but a respiratory problem inhibited the body's ability to eliminate it. The patient in this scenario has a high $ETCO_2$ level because his pulmonary respiration is impaired, resulting in higher-than-normal amounts of carbon dioxide remaining in the lungs; this is exacerbated by his inability to eliminate carbon dioxide secondary to inadequate ventilation.

YOU are the Paramedic SUMMARY continued

10. How should you proceed with your treatment of this patient?

At this point, the most prudent decision would be to simply continue monitoring the patient. His condition has clearly improved with your treatment, as noted by his respiratory rate and quality, heart rate, oxygen saturation, and $ETCO_2$ level. Furthermore, the gray color of his lips and gums has resolved. Consider other treatments specific for his heart failure, as guided by your local protocols. However, at this point, no further airway or ventilatory support is indicated because you have accomplished your goal of improved oxygenation and ventilation.

11. How should you adjust your treatment of the patient?

The patient's acute deterioration underscores the importance of continuous monitoring. Your ultimate goal is to restore adequate oxygenation and ventilation; therefore, you should remove the CPAP device and begin assisting his ventilations with a bag-mask device attached to 100% oxygen. You should also consider inserting a nasopharyngeal airway to help maintain airway patency, as well as have suction immediately available. If possible, have your partner radio ahead to the hospital to inform them that you are bringing in a critical patient.

12. Why did you determine not to proceed with intubation?

As discussed in the answer to question 7, it is dangerous to give a hypoxemic patient a paralytic drug before you have ensured adequate oxygenation and ventilation. Furthermore, you are only a short distance from the hospital at this point. You will encounter situations like these as a paramedic, and you will have to make a decision. Even if you think the patient will be intubated in the ED, you must ask yourself, "Does the patient need to be intubated right now?" If you had a long transport time *and* you had achieved adequate oxygenation and ventilation, then it might be reasonable to proceed with RSI. Hypoxic patients improve because effective oxygenation and ventilation are restored; this process does not (and should not) always involve an ET tube.

EMS Patient Care Report (PCR)

Date: 03-11-22	**Incident No.:** 21030211	**Nature of Call:** Respiratory distress	**Location:** 212 E. Ave. B

Dispatched: 2125	**En Route:** 2126	**At Scene:** 2131	**Transport:** 2146	**At Hospital:** 2201	**In Service:** 2215

Patient Information

Age: 67 **Sex:** M **Weight (in kg [lb]):** estimated at 85 kg (187 lb)	**Allergies:** NKDA **Medications:** Unknown; information not available **Past Medical History:** "Heart problem" **Chief Complaint:** Respiratory distress

Vital Signs

Time: 2135	**BP:** 176/96	**Pulse:** 120	**Respirations:** 28	**SpO_2:** 76%	**$ETCO_2$:** 60	**ECG:** Sinus tachycardia
Time: 2138	**BP:** 182/94	**Pulse:** 140	**Respirations:** 28	**SpO_2:** 74%	**$ETCO_2$:** 63	**ECG:** Sinus tachycardia
Time: 2141	**BP:** 176/92	**Pulse:** 122	**Respirations:** 24 (with CPAP)	**SpO_2:** 87%	**$ETCO_2$:** 51	**ECG:** Sinus tachycardia
Time: 2145	**BP:** 169/88	**Pulse:** 114	**Respirations:** 22 (with CPAP)	**SpO_2:** 95%	**$ETCO_2$:** 46	**ECG:** Sinus tachycardia
Time: 2150	**BP:** 144/76	**Pulse:** 122	**Respirations:** 10 (with CPAP)	**SpO_2:** 79%	**$ETCO_2$:** 58	**ECG:** Sinus tachycardia
Time: 2155	**BP:** 148/80	**Pulse:** 100	**Respirations:** 14 (with PPV)	**SpO_2:** 97%	**$ETCO_2$:** 41	**ECG:** Sinus tachycardia

YOU are the Paramedic SUMMARY continued

EMS Treatment (circle all that apply)				
Oxygen @ 15 **L/min via (circle one):** NC (NRM) (Bag-mask device)		**Assisted Ventilation:** (CPAP BVM)	**Airway Adjunct:** Oral airway (Nasal airway)	**CPR**
Defibrillation	**Bleeding Control**	**Bandaging/Splinting**	**IV Therapy** **Time:** 2141 **Gauge:** 18 **Site:** Right arm **Fluid:** Normal saline **Rate:** TKO	**Other:** Cardiac monitoring, 12-lead ECG, $ETCO_2$ monitoring, pulse oximetry **Medication:** Ketamine **Time:** 2143 **Dose:** 170 mg **Route:** IM

Narrative

9-1-1 dispatch for a 67 y/o male with respiratory distress. Arrived on scene and found the pt in a tripod position on the edge of his couch. He was conscious and alert, but restless. Airway was patent but pt presented with marked respiratory distress and diaphoresis. Pt is dark-skinned; lips and gums were gray. Applied oxygen via NRM at 15 L/min, obtained baseline VS, and continued assessment. Despite NRM, pt remained hypoxemic and hypercarbic and became increasingly agitated. Pt stated, in broken sentences, that he has "heart problems" but has not seen his cardiologist in almost 2 years. Breath sounds revealed coarse crackles bilaterally. Pt resisted an attempt to apply CPAP and attempts to reapply the NRM. Administered 170 mg ketamine IM. Pt became compliant with CPAP. Oxygenation and ventilation improved, and pt responded to verbal stimuli. IV access was then established. After the pt was secured to the stretcher and loaded into the ambulance, a 12-lead ECG was acquired and showed no evidence of cardiac injury or ischemia. Transport was initiated and CPAP therapy continued en route. Acute pt deterioration was noted. Respiratory rate markedly diminished, pt was responsive only to pain, and his breathing became shallow. SpO_2 and $ETCO_2$ values indicated worsening hypoxemia and hypercarbia. Nasal airway inserted, and pt's breathing assisted with a BVM. Bag-mask ventilation continued because of short transport time, and a pt report called in to hospital. Reassessment revealed improvements in pt's work of breathing, SpO_2, $ETCO_2$, and mental status. VS indicated hemodynamic stability. Pt was delivered to the ED and handoff report was given to the attending physician. Medic 72 cleared the hospital and returned to service.

End of report

Prep Kit

Ready for Review

- The upper airway consists of all structures above the vocal cords: the larynx, oropharynx, nasopharynx, and tongue. Its functions include the warming, filtering, and humidification of inhaled air.
- The lower airway consists of all structures below the vocal cords: the trachea, main stem bronchi, bronchioles, pulmonary capillaries, and alveoli. Pulmonary gas exchange takes place at the alveolar level in the lungs.
- Ventilation, oxygenation, and respiration are crucial for the tissues to receive the needed nutrients.
- Ventilation is the act of moving air into and out of the lungs. For ventilation to occur, the diaphragm and intercostal muscles must function properly.

Prep Kit continued

- Negative-pressure ventilation is the drawing of air into the lungs due to changes in intrathoracic pressure. Positive-pressure ventilation is the forcing of air into the lungs and is provided via bag-mask device, pocket mask, or mechanical ventilation device to patients who are not breathing (apneic) or are breathing inadequately.
- In contrast to negative-pressure ventilation, which favors venous return to the heart, positive-pressure ventilation can impair venous return to the heart. Do not hyperventilate any patient; doing so can cause a significant increase in intrathoracic pressure, which can further impair venous return and reduce cardiac output.
- Oxygenation is the process of loading oxygen molecules onto hemoglobin in the bloodstream. Oxygenation may not occur if the environment is depleted of oxygen or if the environment contains carbon monoxide, which prevents oxygen from binding to hemoglobin.
- Respiration is the exchange of oxygen and carbon dioxide in the alveoli and tissues of the body.
- Many conditions can inhibit the body's ability to effectively deliver oxygen to the cells. With ventilation–perfusion ($\dot{V}/\dot{Q}$) mismatch, ventilation may be compromised but perfusion continues, leading to a lack of oxygen diffusing into the bloodstream, which can result in severe hypoxemia.
- Other factors that impede delivery of oxygen to cells include airway swelling, airway obstruction, medications that depress the CNS, neuromuscular disorders, respiratory and cardiac diseases, circulatory compromise, submersion, and trauma to the head, neck, spine, or chest.
- Hypoventilation and hyperventilation, along with hypoxia, can cause disruptions in the acid–base balance in the body that may lead to rapid deterioration in a patient's condition and death. When an excess of acid is present in the body, the fastest way to eliminate it is through the respiratory system. Excess acid can be expelled as carbon dioxide from the lungs. Conversely, slowing respirations will increase the level of carbon dioxide. Respiratory acidosis and respiratory alkalosis can result from a number of conditions and can be life threatening.
- Adequate breathing in the adult is characterized by a respiratory rate between 12 and 20 breaths/min, adequate depth (tidal volume), a regular pattern of inhalation and exhalation, symmetric chest rise, and bilaterally clear and equal breath sounds.
- Inadequate breathing in the adult is characterized by a respiratory rate that is too slow (less than 12 breaths/min) or too fast (greater than 20 breaths/min), a shallow depth of breathing (reduced tidal volume), an irregular pattern of inhalation and exhalation, asymmetric chest movement, adventitious (abnormal) breath sounds, cyanosis, and an altered mental status.
- It is important to be able to recognize abnormal breathing patterns when assessing a patient. These include Cheyne-Stokes respirations, Kussmaul respirations, Biot (ataxic) respirations, apneustic respirations, central neurogenic hyperventilation, and agonal gasps.
- While assessing breathing, auscultate breath sounds with a stethoscope. Breath sounds represent airflow into the alveoli. They should be clear and equal on both sides of the chest (bilaterally), anteriorly, and posteriorly. Abnormal breath sounds include wheezing, rhonchi, crackles, stridor, and pleural friction rub.
- The pulse oximeter measures the percentage of hemoglobin that is saturated with oxygen (Spo_2). This type of measurement depends on adequate perfusion to the capillary beds and can be inaccurate when the patient is cold, is in shock, or has been exposed to carbon monoxide.
- Peak expiratory flow is a fairly reliable assessment of the severity of bronchoconstriction. It is also used to gauge the effectiveness of treatments, such as administration of inhaled beta-2 agonists (eg, albuterol).

Prep Kit continued

- Carbon dioxide monitors detect the presence of carbon dioxide in exhaled air and are important adjuncts for determining ventilation adequacy and advanced airway placement. The colorimetric carbon dioxide detector is a qualitative device that attaches between an advanced airway and ventilation device; specially treated paper inside the detector turns yellow during exhalation, indicating the presence of exhaled carbon dioxide. The capnometer is a quantitative device that provides a numeric display of end-tidal carbon dioxide ($ETCO_2$). The capnographer, also a quantitative device, provides real-time objective data regarding $ETCO_2$ by displaying a waveform (waveform capnography) or a waveform and numeric display (digital/waveform capnography). The capnographer can be used to analyze air samples of a spontaneously breathing patient or when an advanced airway has been inserted and the patient is being manually or mechanically ventilated. Quantitative digital/waveform capnography is the most accurate (and preferred) method for monitoring a patient's $ETCO_2$ level.
- Patients who are apneic or are not breathing adequately require some form of positive-pressure ventilation, such as bag-mask ventilation. Patients who are breathing adequately, but have evidence of hypoxemia (SpO_2 level of 94% or less) or respiratory distress, should receive an appropriate concentration of oxygen via a nasal cannula or nonrebreathing mask. Never withhold oxygen from any patient suspected of being hypoxemic.
- Unrecognized inadequate breathing will lead to hypoxia, a dangerous condition in which the body's cells and tissues do not receive adequate oxygen.
- Regardless of the patient's condition, the airway must remain patent at all times. Therefore, the first step in airway management is to position the patient. The recovery position involves placing the patient in a left lateral recumbent position and is the preferred position to maintain the airway of unresponsive patients with adequate breathing and no evidence of injury to the spine, pelvis, or hips.
- The patient's head must be properly positioned. Manual airway maneuvers include the head tilt–chin lift, jaw-thrust, and the tongue-jaw lift maneuvers.
- Clearing the airway means removing obstructing material; maintaining the airway means keeping it open, either manually or with adjunctive devices.
- Oropharyngeal suctioning may be required after opening a patient's airway. Rigid (tonsil-tip, Yankauer, or DuCanto) catheters are preferred when suctioning the pharynx. Soft plastic (whistle-tip or French) catheters are used to suction secretions from the nose and can be passed down an ET tube to suction pulmonary secretions.
- Patients with secretions in the airway should be positioned on their side and the oropharynx should be suctioned until it is clear of secretions.
- Airway obstruction can be caused by choking on food (or, in children, on toys), epiglottitis, inhalation injuries, airway trauma with swelling, and anaphylaxis. It is critical to differentiate between a mild (partial) airway obstruction and a severe (complete) airway obstruction.
- The recommended sequence of events when attempting to remove a foreign body airway obstruction in an unresponsive adult is chest compressions, finger sweeps (only if the object can be seen and easily retrieved), manual removal of the object, and attempts to ventilate. Continuously perform abdominal thrusts in a responsive adult or child with an airway obstruction until the obstruction is relieved or the patient becomes unresponsive.
- If BLS maneuvers are not successful in relieving a foreign body airway obstruction in the unresponsive patient, visualize the airway with a laryngoscope. If you can see the foreign body, carefully grasp it with Magill forceps and slowly back it out of the airway.

Prep Kit continued

- Basic airway adjuncts include the oropharyngeal (oral) airway and the nasopharyngeal (nasal) airway. The oral airway keeps the tongue off the posterior pharynx; it is used only in unresponsive patients without a gag reflex. The nasal airway is better tolerated in patients with altered mental status who have an intact gag reflex.
- Administer supplemental oxygen to any patient with respiratory distress or evidence of hypoxemia (Spo_2 level of 94% or less). Be familiar with oxygen cylinder sizes and the duration of flow, and always take standard precautions when using oxygen.
- The nonrebreathing mask can deliver up to 90% oxygen when the flow rate is set at 15 L/min. A nasal cannula should be used if the patient cannot tolerate the nonrebreathing mask; it can deliver oxygen concentrations of 24% to 44% when the flowmeter is set at 1 to 6 L/min. Other types of oxygen-delivery devices include the partial rebreathing mask and Venturi mask.
- Methods of providing artificial ventilation include the one- and two-person bag-mask ventilation technique and mouth-to-mask ventilation with a one-way valve and supplemental oxygen attached. Artificial ventilation is indicated for patients who are apneic or are not breathing adequately.
- CPAP has been clinically proven to improve a patient's breathing by forcing fluid from the alveoli (in pulmonary edema) or dilating the bronchioles (in obstructive lung diseases and asthma). It involves the patient breathing against a certain amount of positive pressure during exhalation. CPAP has also been shown to reduce the need for intubation.
- Check for loose dental appliances in a patient before providing artificial ventilation. Loose dental appliances should be removed to prevent them from obstructing the airway; tight-fitting dental appliances should be left in place during artificial ventilation.
- If you are going to remove a patient's dental appliance, do so before intubation. Removing the appliance after the patient has been intubated may result in inadvertent extubation.
- Patients with massive maxillofacial trauma are at high risk for airway compromise due to oral bleeding. Assist ventilations and provide oral suctioning as needed.
- Ventilating too forcefully or too fast can cause gastric distention, which can cause regurgitation and aspiration. Administering ventilations over 1 second—just enough to produce visible chest rise—will reduce the incidence of gastric distention and the associated risks of regurgitation and aspiration.
- Invasive gastric decompression involves the insertion of a gastric tube into the stomach. A nasogastric tube is inserted into the stomach via the nose; an orogastric tube is inserted into the stomach via the mouth.
- Patients with a tracheal stoma or tracheostomy tube may require ventilation, suctioning, or tube replacement. Ventilation through a tracheostomy tube is performed by attaching the bag-valve device to the 15/22-mm adapter on the tube; ventilation of a patient with a stoma and no tracheostomy tube can be performed with a pocket mask or bag-mask device. Use pediatric-size masks when ventilating a patient through a stoma.
- Unresponsive patients or patients who cannot maintain their own airway should be considered candidates for ET intubation, the insertion of an ET tube into the trachea. In orotracheal intubation, the ET tube is inserted into the trachea via the mouth; in nasotracheal intubation (a blind technique), the ET tube is inserted into the trachea via the nose.
- Direct laryngoscopy involves directly visualizing the vocal cords with a laryngoscope. Video laryngoscopy involves visualizing the vocal cords on a video screen.
- A critical step in intubation is confirmation of correct tube placement. Continuous waveform capnography, in addition to a clinical assessment (such as auscultation of breath sounds and over the epigastrium and assessing for

Prep Kit continued

visible chest rise), is regarded as the most reliable method of confirming and monitoring correct placement of the ET tube.

- If an attempted intubation does not result in acceptable oxygen saturation levels, then perform BLS maneuvers with an oral airway and/or nasal airway and a bag-mask device, and consider using another airway device.
- Tracheobronchial suctioning is indicated if the condition of an intubated patient deteriorates because of pulmonary secretions in the ET tube.
- Do not perform extubation in the prehospital setting unless the patient is unreasonably intolerant of the tube. It is generally best to sedate an intubated patient who is becoming intolerant of the ET tube.
- RSI involves using pharmacologic agents to sedate and paralyze a patient to facilitate placement of an ET tube. It should be considered when a responsive or combative patient requires intubation but cannot tolerate laryngoscopy.
- Drugs used for RSI include sedatives, such as midazolam (Versed), diazepam (Valium), and ketamine (Ketalar), as well as neuromuscular blocking agents (paralytics) to induce complete paralysis. The latter agents are classified as either depolarizing (eg, succinylcholine) or nondepolarizing (eg, vecuronium, pancuronium, and rocuronium) paralytics.
- Alternative airway devices, which may be used if ET intubation is either impossible or unsuccessful, include the King LT, laryngeal mask airway, and i-gel supraglottic airway.
- Surgical cricothyrotomy involves incising the cricothyroid membrane, inserting a tracheostomy tube or ET tube into the trachea, and manually or mechanically ventilating the patient. Needle cricothyrotomy involves inserting a 14- to 16-gauge over-the-needle catheter through the cricothyroid membrane and ventilating the patient with a high-pressure jet ventilation device.
- Cricothyrotomy is indicated in situations where intubation is not possible and you cannot ventilate the patient by any other means.

Vital Vocabulary

3-3-2 rule A method used to predict difficult intubation. A mouth opening of less than three fingerbreadths, a mandible length of less than three fingerbreadths, and a distance from hyoid bone to thyroid notch of less than two fingerbreadths indicate a possibly difficult airway.

abdominal thrust maneuver Abdominal thrusts performed to relieve a foreign body airway obstruction.

accessory muscles The muscles not normally used during normal breathing; include the sternocleidomastoid muscles of the neck, the pectoralis major muscles of the chest, and the abdominal muscles.

acetylcholine (ACh) A chemical neurotransmitter of the parasympathetic nervous system.

adventitious Abnormal.

afterload The pressure gradient against which the heart must pump; an increase can decrease cardiac output.

agonal gasps Slow, shallow, irregular respirations or occasional gasping breaths that result from cerebral anoxia.

anoxia An absence of oxygen.

anterograde amnesia An inability to remember events after the onset of amnesia.

aphonia The inability to speak.

apneic oxygenation The continued alveolar uptake of oxygen, even when the patient is apneic; can be facilitated by administering oxygen via nasal cannula during intubation.

apneustic respirations Prolonged gasping inspirations followed by extremely short, ineffective expirations; associated with brainstem insult.

Prep Kit continued

asymmetric chest wall movement Unequal movement of the two sides of the chest; indicates decreased airflow into one lung.

automatic transport ventilator (ATV) A portable mechanical ventilator attached to a control box that allows the provider to set the variables of ventilation (eg, respiratory rate and tidal volume).

bag-mask device A manual ventilation device that consists of a bag, mask, reservoir, and oxygen inlet; capable of delivering up to 100% oxygen.

barotrauma Trauma resulting from excessive pressure.

benzodiazepines Sedative-hypnotic drugs that provide muscle relaxation and mild sedation; examples include diazepam (Valium) and midazolam (Versed).

bimanual laryngoscopy An effective technique to improve the laryngoscopic view of the vocal cords through external manipulation of the larynx.

bilevel positive airway pressure (BPAP) A noninvasive form of positive-pressure ventilation that delivers two pressures (a higher inspiratory positive airway pressure and a lower expiratory positive airway pressure).

Biot (ataxic) respirations Irregular pattern, rate, and depth of respirations with intermittent periods of apnea; result from increased intracranial pressure.

Bourdon-gauge flowmeter An oxygen flowmeter that is commonly used because it is not affected by gravity and can be placed in any position.

bronchovesicular sounds A combination of the tracheal and vesicular breath sounds; heard where the airways and alveoli are found, at the upper part of the sternum and between the scapulas.

BURP maneuver The backward, upward, and rightward pressure used during intubation to improve the laryngoscopic view of the glottic opening and vocal cords; also called external laryngeal manipulation.

capnographer A device that attaches between the endotracheal tube and the ventilation device; provides graphic information about the presence of exhaled carbon dioxide.

capnometer A device that performs the same function and attaches in the same way as a capnographer but provides a digital reading of the exhaled carbon dioxide.

carbon monoxide oximeter A device that measures absorption at several wavelengths to distinguish oxyhemoglobin from carboxyhemoglobin.

carboxyhemoglobin (COHb) Hemoglobin loaded with carbon monoxide.

Cheyne-Stokes respirations A gradually increasing rate and depth of respirations followed by a gradual decrease with intermittent periods of apnea; associated with brainstem insult.

colorimetric carbon dioxide detector A device that attaches between the endotracheal tube and the ventilation device; uses special paper that should turn from purple to yellow during exhalation, indicating the presence of exhaled carbon dioxide.

continuous positive airway pressure (CPAP) A method of ventilation that delivers a single pressure; used primarily in the treatment of critically ill patients with respiratory distress and can prevent the need for endotracheal intubation.

Cormack-Lehane classification A system used to predict intubation difficulty based on the airway structures observed during laryngoscopy.

crackles The breath sounds produced as fluid-filled alveoli pop open under increasing inspiratory pressure; can be fine or coarse; formerly called rales.

curved laryngoscope blade A blade designed to fit into the vallecula, indirectly lifting the epiglottis and exposing the vocal cords; also called the Macintosh blade.

cyanosis Blue or purple skin; indicates inadequate oxygen in the blood.

delayed sequence intubation (DSI) A procedure in which a patient is sedated for the purpose of

Prep Kit continued

preoxygenation prior to the administration of a paralytic agent and intubation.

denitrogenation The process of replacing nitrogen in the lungs with oxygen to maintain a normal oxygen saturation level during intubation.

depolarizing neuromuscular blocker A drug that competitively binds with acetylcholine receptor sites but is not affected as quickly by acetylcholinesterase; an example is succinylcholine chloride.

direct laryngoscopy Visualization of the airway with a laryngoscope.

dissociative anesthetic A medication that distorts perception of sights and sounds and induces a feeling of detachment from their environment and self.

dysphonia Difficulty speaking.

dyspnea Difficult or labored breathing.

endotracheal (ET) intubation Inserting an endotracheal tube through the glottic opening and sealing the tube with a cuff inflated against the tracheal wall.

endotracheal (ET) tube A tube that is inserted into the trachea for definitive airway maintenance; equipped with a distal cuff, a proximal inflation port, a 15/22-mm adapter, and centimeter markings on the side.

end-tidal carbon dioxide ($ETCO_2$) monitors Devices that detect the presence of carbon dioxide in exhaled air.

epiglottis A leaf-shaped cartilaginous structure that closes over the trachea during swallowing.

extubation The process of removing the endotracheal tube from an intubated patient.

face-to-face intubation Performing intubation at the same level as the patient's face; used when the standard position is not possible. In this position, the laryngoscope is held in the provider's right hand and the endotracheal tube in the left.

fasciculations Brief, uncoordinated twitching of small muscle groups in the face, neck, trunk, and extremities; may be seen after the administration of a depolarizing neuromuscular blocking agent (eg, succinylcholine chloride).

gag reflex An automatic reaction when something touches an area deep in the oral cavity, which helps protect the lower airway from aspiration.

gastric distention The enlargement or expansion of the stomach, often with air; can be a complication of ventilating the esophagus instead of the trachea.

gastric tube A tube that is inserted into the stomach to remove its contents.

gum bougie A flexible device that is inserted between the glottis under direct laryngoscopy; the endotracheal tube is threaded over the device, facilitating its entry into the trachea. Also called a tracheal tube introducer.

head tilt–chin lift maneuver Manual airway maneuver that involves tilting the head back while lifting up on the chin; used to open the airway of an unresponsive nontrauma patient.

hemoglobin An iron-containing protein found in red blood cells that has the ability to combine with oxygen.

hypercapnia Increased carbon dioxide content in arterial blood.

hyperventilation A condition in which an increased amount of air enters the alveoli; carbon dioxide elimination exceeds carbon dioxide production.

hypocapnia Decreased carbon dioxide content in arterial blood.

hypoventilation A condition in which a decreased amount of air enters the alveoli; carbon dioxide production exceeds the body's ability to eliminate it by ventilation.

hypoxemia A decrease in arterial oxygen level.

hypoxia A lack of oxygen to cells and tissues.

i-gel A supraglottic airway device that uses a noninflatable, gel-like mask to isolate the larynx and facilitate ventilation.

Prep Kit continued

inspiratory/expiratory (I/E) ratio An expression for comparing the length of inspiration with that of expiration, normally 1:2, meaning that expiration is twice as long as inspiration (not measured in seconds).

intrapulmonary shunting Bypassing of oxygen-poor blood past nonfunctional alveoli.

jaw-thrust maneuver A technique to open the airway by placing the fingers behind the angle of the jaw and bringing the jaw forward; used when a patient may have a cervical spine injury.

King LT airway A single-lumen airway that is blindly inserted into the esophagus; when properly placed in the esophagus, one cuff seals the esophagus and the other seals the oropharynx.

Kussmaul respirations A respiratory pattern characteristic of diabetic ketoacidosis, which features marked hyperpnea and tachypnea; represents the body's attempt to compensate for the acidosis.

laryngeal mask airway (LMA) A device that surrounds the opening of the larynx with an inflatable silicone cuff positioned in the hypopharynx; an alternative to bag-mask ventilation.

laryngectomy A surgical procedure in which the larynx is removed.

laryngoscope A device used in conjunction with a laryngoscope blade to perform direct laryngoscopy.

lung compliance The ability of the alveoli to expand when air is drawn into the lungs during negative-pressure ventilation or positive-pressure ventilation.

Magill forceps A special type of forceps that is curved, allowing paramedics to maneuver it in the airway.

Mallampati classification A system for predicting the relative difficulty of intubation based on the amount of oropharyngeal structures visible in an upright, seated patient who is able to fully open the mouth.

metabolism The chemical processes that provide the cells with energy from nutrients.

methemoglobin (metHb) A compound formed by oxidation of the iron on hemoglobin.

Murphy eye An opening on the side of an endotracheal tube at its distal tip that permits ventilation to occur even if the tip becomes occluded by blood, mucus, or the tracheal wall.

nasal cannula A device that delivers oxygen via two small prongs that fit into the patient's nostrils; with an oxygen flow rate of 1 to 6 L/min, an oxygen concentration of 24% to 44% can be delivered.

nasogastric (NG) tube A gastric tube that is inserted into the stomach through the nose.

nasopharyngeal (nasal) airway A soft rubber tube about 6 inches (15 cm) long that is inserted through the nose into the posterior pharynx behind the tongue, thereby allowing passage of air from the nose to the lower airway.

nasotracheal intubation Insertion of an endotracheal tube into the trachea through the nose.

needle cricothyrotomy Insertion of a 14- to 16-gauge over-the-needle intravenous catheter (such as an Angiocath) through the cricothyroid membrane and into the trachea.

negative-pressure ventilation Drawing of air into the lungs; airflow from a region of higher pressure (outside the body) to a region of lower pressure (the lungs); occurs during normal (unassisted) breathing.

nondepolarizing neuromuscular blockers Drugs that bind to acetylcholine receptor sites; they do not cause depolarization of the muscle fiber; examples include vecuronium (Norcuron) and pancuronium (Pavulon); also called paralytics.

nonrebreathing mask A combination mask and reservoir bag system in which oxygen fills a reservoir bag attached to the mask by a one-way valve, permitting a patient to inhale from the reservoir bag but not to exhale into it; at a flow rate of 15 L/min, it can deliver 90% to 100% inspired oxygen.

Prep Kit continued

opioids Drugs that act as a central nervous system depressant and produce insensibility or stupor. An opioid can be a natural product derived from the opium or poppy plant (referred to more specifically as an opiate) or a synthetic product designed to produce similar effects.

orogastric (OG) tube A gastric tube that is inserted into the stomach through the mouth.

oropharyngeal (oral) airway A hard plastic device that is curved so that it fits over the back of the tongue, with the tip in the posterior pharynx.

orotracheal intubation Insertion of an endotracheal tube into the trachea through the mouth.

orthopnea Positional dyspnea.

oxygen humidifier A small bottle of water through which the oxygen leaving the cylinder is moisturized before it reaches the patient.

oxyhemoglobin (Hbo_2) Hemoglobin that is occupied by oxygen.

pancuronium A nondepolarizing neuromuscular blocking agent; used to maintain paralysis following succinylcholine-facilitated intubation.

paradoxical motion The inward movement of the chest during inhalation and outward movement during exhalation; the opposite of normal chest wall movements during breathing.

paralytics Drugs that paralyze skeletal muscles; used in emergency situations to facilitate intubation; also called neuromuscular blocking agents.

partial laryngectomy Surgical removal of a portion of the larynx.

partial rebreathing mask A mask similar to the nonrebreathing mask but without a one-way valve between the mask and the reservoir; room air is not drawn in with inspiration; residual expired air is mixed in the mask and rebreathed.

patent Open.

peak expiratory flow An approximation of the extent of bronchoconstriction; used to determine whether therapy (such as with inhaled bronchodilators) is effective.

pleural friction rub The result of an inflammation that causes the pleura to thicken, decreasing the pleural space and allowing the pleurae to rub together.

positive end-expiratory pressure (PEEP) Mechanical maintenance of pressure in the airway at the end of expiration to increase the volume of gas remaining in the lungs.

positive-pressure ventilation Forcing of air into the lungs.

preload The pressure of blood in the heart at the end of diastole; affected by venous return.

pressure-compensated flowmeter An oxygen flowmeter that incorporates a float ball in a tapered calibrated tube; the float rises or falls according to the gas flow in the tube; is affected by gravity and must remain in an upright position for an accurate reading.

pulse oximeter A device that measures oxygen saturation level (Spo_2).

pulsus paradoxus A drop in the systolic blood pressure of 10 mm Hg or more; commonly seen in patients with pericardial tamponade or severe asthma.

rapid sequence intubation (RSI) A specific set of procedures, performed in rapid succession, to induce sedation and paralysis and intubate a patient quickly.

recovery position Left lateral recumbent position; used in all unresponsive nontrauma patients who are able to maintain their own airway spontaneously and are breathing adequately.

reduced hemoglobin Hemoglobin from which oxygen has been released to the cells.

reemergence phenomenon The occurrence of dreams, nightmares, or delirium that a person taking ketamine may experience as the drug approaches the end of its half-life.

respiratory acidosis A pathologic condition characterized by a blood pH of less than 7.35; caused by the accumulation of acids in the body from a respiratory cause.

Prep Kit continued

respiratory alkalosis A pathologic condition characterized by a blood pH of greater than 7.45; results from the accumulation of bases in the body from a respiratory cause.

retractions The drawing in of the intercostal muscles and the muscles above the clavicles that can occur in respiratory distress.

rhonchi A continuous, low-pitched sound; indicates mucus or fluid in the larger lower airways.

rocuronium A nondepolarizing neuromuscular blocking agent; used to maintain paralysis following succinylcholine-facilitated intubation.

safe residual pressure The pressure at which an oxygen cylinder should be replaced with a full one; often defined as 200 psi.

sedation Reduction of a patient's anxiety, induction of amnesia, and suppression of the gag reflex, usually by pharmacologic means.

stenosis A narrowing, such as of a blood vessel or stoma.

stoma In the context of the airway, the orifice of a tracheostomy that connects the trachea to the outside air; located in the midline of the anterior part of the neck.

straight laryngoscope blade A blade designed to lift the epiglottis and expose the vocal cords; also called a Miller blade.

stridor A high-pitched inspiratory sound created by air moving past an obstruction within or immediately above the glottic opening.

stylet In the context of intubation, a semirigid wire inserted into an endotracheal tube to mold and maintain the shape of the tube.

succinylcholine chloride A depolarizing neuromuscular blocker frequently used as the initial paralytic during rapid sequence intubation; causes muscle fasciculations.

surgical cricothyrotomy An emergency incision of the cricothyroid membrane with a scalpel and insertion of an endotracheal or a tracheostomy tube directly into the subglottic area of the trachea.

therapy regulator A device that attaches to the stem of the oxygen cylinder and reduces the high pressure of gas to a safe range (about 50 psi).

tongue-jaw lift maneuver A manual maneuver that involves grasping the tongue and jaw and lifting; commonly used to suction the airway and to place certain airway devices.

tonsil-tip catheter A hard or rigid suction catheter; also called a Yankauer catheter.

total laryngectomy Surgical removal of the entire larynx.

tracheal breath sounds Breath sounds heard by placing the stethoscope diaphragm over the trachea or sternum; also called bronchial breath sounds.

tracheobronchial suctioning Inserting a suction catheter into the endotracheal tube to remove pulmonary secretions.

tracheostomy A surgical opening into the trachea.

tracheostomy tube A plastic tube placed within the tracheostomy site (stoma).

translaryngeal catheter ventilation A method used in conjunction with needle cricothyrotomy to ventilate a patient; requires a high-pressure jet ventilator.

trismus Clenched teeth caused by spasms of the jaw muscles.

vecuronium A nondepolarizing neuromuscular blocking agent; used to maintain paralysis following succinylcholine-facilitated intubation.

Venturi mask A mask with a number of interchangeable adapters that draws room air into the mask along with the oxygen flow; allows for the administration of highly specific oxygen concentrations.

vesicular breath sounds Soft, muffled breath sounds in which the expiratory phase is barely audible.

video laryngoscopy Visualization of the epiglottis and vocal cords through a video monitor that is attached to a laryngoscope.

Prep Kit continued

V̇/Q̇ mismatch An imbalance between the anatomic portions of the lung being ventilated (V) and the anatomic portions being perfused (Q).

waveform capnography A waveform display of exhaled carbon dioxide.

wheezing A high-pitched whistling sound that may be heard on inspiration, expiration, or both; indicates air movement through a constricted lower airway, such as with asthma.

whistle-tip catheters Soft plastic, nonrigid catheters; also called French catheters.

References

1. Panchal AR, Bartos JA, Cabanas JG, et al. Part 3: adult basic and advanced life support: 2020 American Heart Association Guidelines update for cardiopulmonary resuscitation and emergency cardiovascular care. *Circulation*. 2020;142(suppl 2):S366-S468.
2. Hofmman R, James SK. Routine oxygen supplementation in acute cardiovascular disease. The end of a paradigm? *Circulation*. 2018;137(4):320-322.
3. O'Gara PT, Kushner FG, Ascheim DD, et al. 2013 ACCF/AHA guideline for the management of ST-elevation myocardial infarction: executive summary: a report of the American College of Cardiology Foundation/American Heart Association Task Force on Practice Guidelines. *J Am Coll Cardiol*. 2013;61:485-510.
4. O'Connor RE, Al Ali AS, Brady WJ, et al. Part 9: acute coronary syndromes: 2015 American Heart Association guidelines update for cardiopulmonary resuscitation and emergency cardiovascular care. *Circulation*. 2015;132 (suppl 2):S483-S500.
5. Link MS, Berkow LC, Kudenchuk PJ, et al. Part 7: adult advanced cardiovascular life support: 2015 American Heart Association guidelines update for cardiopulmonary resuscitation and emergency cardiovascular care. *Circulation*. 2015;132(suppl 2):S444-S464.
6. Atkins DL, Berger S, Duff JP, et al. Part 11: pediatric basic life support and cardiopulmonary resuscitation quality: 2015 American Heart Association guidelines update for cardiopulmonary resuscitation and emergency cardiovascular care. *Circulation*. 2015;132(suppl 2):S519-S525.
7. de Caen AR, Berg MD, Chameides L, et al. Part 12: pediatric advanced life support: 2015 American Heart Association guidelines update for cardiopulmonary resuscitation and emergency cardiovascular care. *Circulation*. 2015;132(suppl 2):S526-S542.
8. Nouruzi-Sedah P, Schumann M, Groeben H. Laryngoscopy via Macintosh blade versus GlideScope: success rate and time for endotracheal intubation in untrained medical personnel. *Anesthesiology*. 2009;110(1):32-37.
9. Jarvis JL, McClure SF, Johns D. EMS intubation improves with King vision video laryngoscopy. *Prehosp Emerg Care*. 2015;19(4):482-489.
10. Naito H, Guyette FX, Martin-Gill C, Callaway CW. Video laryngoscopic techniques associated with intubation success in a helicopter emergency medical service system. *Prehosp Emerg Care*. 2016;20(3):333-342.
11. Diggs LA, Yusuf JE, De Leo G. An update on out-of-hospital airway management practices in the United States. *Resuscitation*. 2014;85(7):885-892.
12. Weingart SD, Levitan RM. Preoxygenation and prevention of desaturation during emergency airway management. *J Ann Emerg Med*. 2012;59(3):165-175.

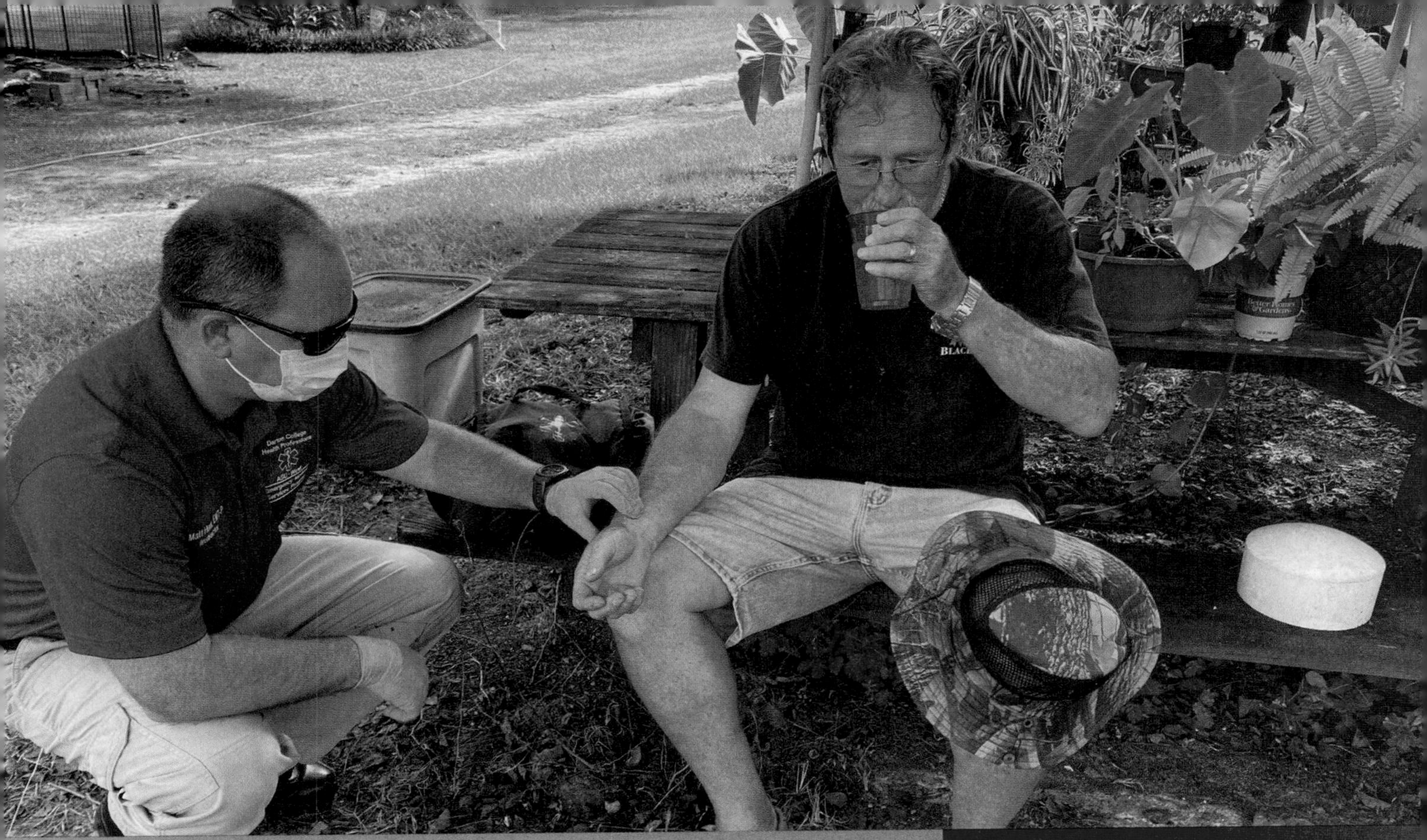

Medical

VOLUME 1

SECTION 6

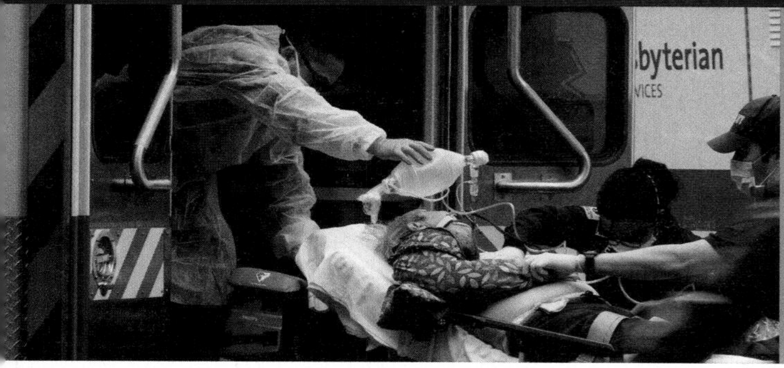

Chapter 17

Respiratory Emergencies

NATIONAL EMS EDUCATION STANDARD COMPETENCIES

Medicine

Integrates assessment findings with principles of epidemiology and pathophysiology to formulate a field impression and implement a comprehensive treatment/disposition plan for a patient with a medical complaint.

Respiratory

Anatomy, signs, symptoms, and management of respiratory emergencies, including those that affect the
- Upper airway (pp 1130–1133)
- Lower airway (pp 1133–1134)

Anatomy, physiology, pathophysiology, assessment, and management of
- Epiglottitis (see Chapter 44, *Pediatric Emergencies*)
- Spontaneous pneumothorax (p 1145)
- Pulmonary edema (pp 1143–1144)
- Asthma (pp 1134–1137)
- Chronic obstructive pulmonary disease (pp 1137–1140)
- Environmental/industrial exposure (p 1143)
- Toxic gas (p 1143)
- Pertussis (see Chapter 44, *Pediatric Emergencies*)
- Cystic fibrosis (see Chapter 46, *Patients With Special Challenges*)
- Pulmonary embolism (pp 1146–1147)
- Pneumonia (pp 1094,1137–1138, 1140–1141)
- Viral respiratory infections (pp 1102–1103, 1131)
- Obstructive/restrictive disease (pp 1130–1134, 1137)

Anatomy, physiology, epidemiology, pathophysiology, psychosocial effects, presentations, prognosis, and management of
- Acute upper airway infections (pp 1130–1133)
- Spontaneous pneumothorax (pp 1145)
- Obstructive/restrictive lung diseases (pp 1133–1134, 1137)
- Pulmonary infections (pp 1140–1141)
- Neoplasm (pp 1142–1143)
- Pertussis (see Chapter 46, *Pediatric Emergencies*)
- Cystic fibrosis (see Chapter 45, *Patients With Special Challenges*)

Shock and Resuscitation

Integrates comprehensive knowledge of causes and pathophysiology into the management of cardiac arrest and prearrest states.

Integrates a comprehensive knowledge of the causes and pathophysiology into the management of shock, respiratory failure, or arrest, with an emphasis on early intervention to prevent arrest.

KNOWLEDGE OBJECTIVES

1. Discuss the morbidity and mortality of respiratory illness in the United States. (p 1140)
2. Recall the primary structures of the respiratory system and the role of the respiratory system in breathing, cardiovascular regulation, and renal function. (pp 1095–1100)
3. Define hypoventilation and hyperventilation, including examples of conditions associated with each. (pp 1100–1102)
4. Describe the proper measures to ensure scene safety when called to care for a patient with dyspnea. (p 1102–1103)

5. Describe factors that contribute to a general impression of the patient's condition and an accurate estimation of the degree of respiratory distress. (pp 1117–1118)
6. Explain the typical presentation of a patient with dyspnea and the signs and symptoms that indicate a high level of respiratory distress. (pp 1104–1105)
7. Identify breathing alterations that may indicate respiratory distress and the signs of increased work of breathing. (pp 1105–1106)
8. Identify the signs of lung consolidation, including abnormal breath sounds associated with excessive fluid in the lungs. (pp 1107–1108)
9. Explain how to assess the adequacy of the circulation of a patient with dyspnea. (p 1113)
10. Describe the abnormal breathing patterns associated with neurologic insults that depress the respiratory center in the brain. (pp 1112–1113)
11. Discuss how transport decisions are made for patients with respiratory distress. (p 1114)
12. Describe how to investigate the chief complaint of a patient who is having trouble breathing. (pp 1114–1115)
13. Identify each component of the SAMPLE history as it applies to patients with dyspnea. (pp 1115–1117)
14. Describe the components of the physical examination of a patient with dyspnea. (pp 1117–1118)
15. Describe the devices used to monitor patients with respiratory complaints. (pp 1118–1121)
16. Describe interventions available for treating patients with dyspnea. (pp 1121–1128)
17. Explain the pathophysiology, assessment, and management of upper airway inflammation caused by infection. (pp 1131–1133)
18. Explain the pathophysiology, assessment, and management of an obstructive lower airway disease. (pp 1133–1134)
19. Explain the three features that characterize asthma and how each is treated. (pp 1135–1136)
20. Compare the signs and symptoms of asthma, emphysema, chronic bronchitis, and restrictive lung diseases. (pp 1134–1135, 1137)
21. Discuss complications that can cause a patient with chronic obstructive pulmonary disease (COPD) to decompensate. (pp 1137–1139)
22. Explain the concepts of hypoxic drive and auto-PEEP (positive end-expiratory pressure) as they relate to COPD. (pp 1139–1140)
23. Explain the pathophysiology, assessment, and management of pulmonary infections, atelectasis, cancer, toxic inhalations, pulmonary edema, and acute respiratory distress syndrome. (pp 1140–1145)
24. Explain the pathophysiology, assessment, and management of pneumothorax, pleural effusion, and pulmonary embolism. (pp 1145–1147)

SKILLS OBJECTIVES

1. Demonstrate the process of history taking for a patient with dyspnea. (pp 1114–1117)
2. Demonstrate the application of a CPAP/BPAP unit. (pp 1128–1130)

Introduction

Few reasons for dialing 9-1-1 are more compelling than the feeling of being unable to breathe (dyspnea). In most cases, respiratory distress originates within the respiratory system itself.

Respiratory disease is one of the most common pathologic conditions, making respiratory distress one of the most common emergency medical services (EMS) dispatches. Chronic lung conditions, such as asthma and chronic obstructive pulmonary disease (COPD), as among the leading causes of death and disability in the United States.[1] Approximately 16 million Americans have COPD, resulting in 156,979 deaths in 2019.[2] In addition, 25 million Americans have asthma,[3] resulting in 3,512 deaths in 2019 but contributing to several thousand more deaths.[4] **Pneumonia**, first described by Hippocrates in 400 BCE, remains one of the most common fatal illnesses in developing countries and accounts for 6% of inpatient deaths (50,000 per year) in the United States.[5] More than 30 causes of pneumonia have been identified.[6]

Some respiratory diseases, such as cystic fibrosis, have a genetic (or intrinsic) cause. Others, such as occupational lung diseases, are caused by external (or extrinsic) factors. Some respiratory diseases can be caused by either intrinsic or extrinsic factors. For example, approximately 80% of cases of COPD are related to cigarette smoking,[2] but 3% of cases can be attributed to the genetic absence of a critical enzyme (alpha-1 antitrypsin).[7]

Researchers have yet to fully decipher the multifactorial mechanism by which many respiratory diseases develop. Intrinsic factors, such as genetics, cardiac disease, and even stress, are thought to combine with extrinsic factors, such as smoking and environmental pollutants. For example, asthma may be affected by genetics, race, geographic location, diet, allergies, childhood illnesses, or some combination of these factors.

In this chapter, we examine these complex and sometimes puzzling respiratory conditions. We start by discussing how to assess a patient whose chief complaint is dyspnea, focusing on aspects to emphasize in obtaining the history and carrying out the physical examination. The chapter concludes with an in-depth look at some of the disorders that may affect each component of the respiratory system, from the respiratory control centers in the brain to the alveoli, the smallest functional units of respiration in the lung.

Anatomy and Physiology Review

The primary structures of the respiratory system are often compared with an inverted tree, with the trachea representing the trunk and the **alveoli**, the tiny saclike units in which gas exchange occurs resembling the leaves. That is a useful analogy, but in reality, a tree would have to branch 24 times and have nearly a billion leaves to rival the intricacy of the respiratory system **FIGURE 17-1**. Imagine attempting to pull fluid from the ground into the leaves by exerting negative pressure at the leaf ends, and the complexities of breathing become apparent.

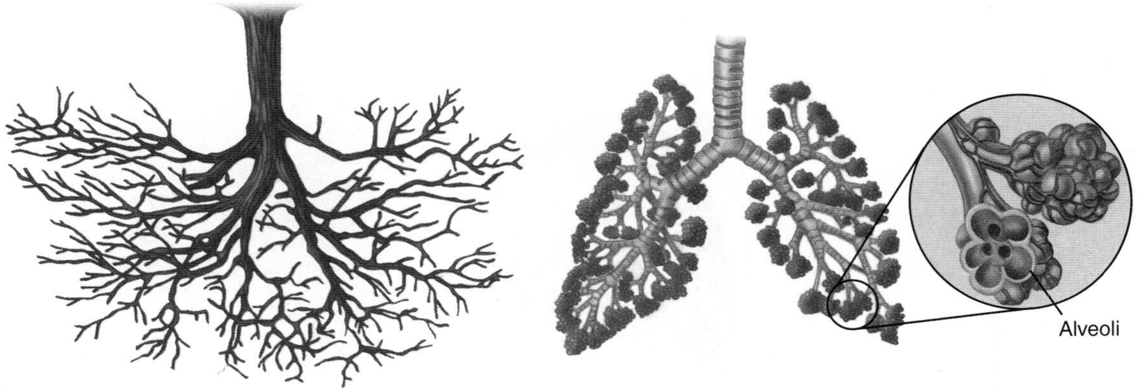

FIGURE 17-1 The tracheobronchial tree branches in much the same way as a real tree, except that even the most magnificent tree has only a small fraction of the number of branches in a single human lung.

YOU are the Paramedic

PART 1

You are dispatched to a medical alarm at a large apartment complex. When you arrive, you and your partner locate the correct building, grab your gear, and head to the closest entrance. You proceed to the fifth-floor apartment from which the call originated. There you find a 74-year-old man with ashen-gray skin who is diaphoretic and struggling to breathe. The patient lives alone and is speaking in one- to two-word sentences.

1. What initial, "from the door" findings make you concerned for this patient?
2. What are your priorities for this patient?

Tracheobronchial Tree

The trunk of the tracheobronchial tree is the trachea, or windpipe, which carries air to the lungs. The trachea serves only one function in the respiratory process: It acts as a pathway for air exchange. This is why many intubated patients who are hospitalized for an extended period receive a tracheostomy. The American College of Chest Physicians recommends transition to tracheostomy by 3 weeks to facilitate oral hygiene, decrease overall length of stay in the intensive care unit, and decrease the rate of complications.[8] The trachea extends about 4 to 5 inches (10 to 13 cm), from the larynx to the left and right main stem bronchi. The ridgelike point at which the tracheal cartilage bifurcates is called the **carina**. The carina is found at roughly the level of the fifth intercostal space **FIGURE 17-2**. In adults, the right main stem bronchus typically branches at a less-acute angle than the left. This anatomic peculiarity explains why an endotracheal (ET) tube advanced too far almost always goes into the right main stem bronchus in an adult. Similarly, aspirated foreign bodies often end up in the right main stem bronchus.

Bronchi

The right and left main stem bronchi continue to branch into the lobes of the lungs. The right lung has three lobes, and the left lung has two. These secondary or lobar bronchi divide into tertiary, or segmental, bronchi and then into subsegmental bronchi before ultimately becoming bronchioles. These conducting airways serve as pathways to the parts of the lung in which gas exchange occurs. Collectively, all airways that do not participate in gas exchange represent dead space. Patients with chronic respiratory disease may have increased dead space (physiologic dead space), indicating that an even larger proportion of each breath does not contribute to respiration.

Bronchioles

Gas transfer is most efficient in the alveoli, but a significant amount of gas is also exchanged across

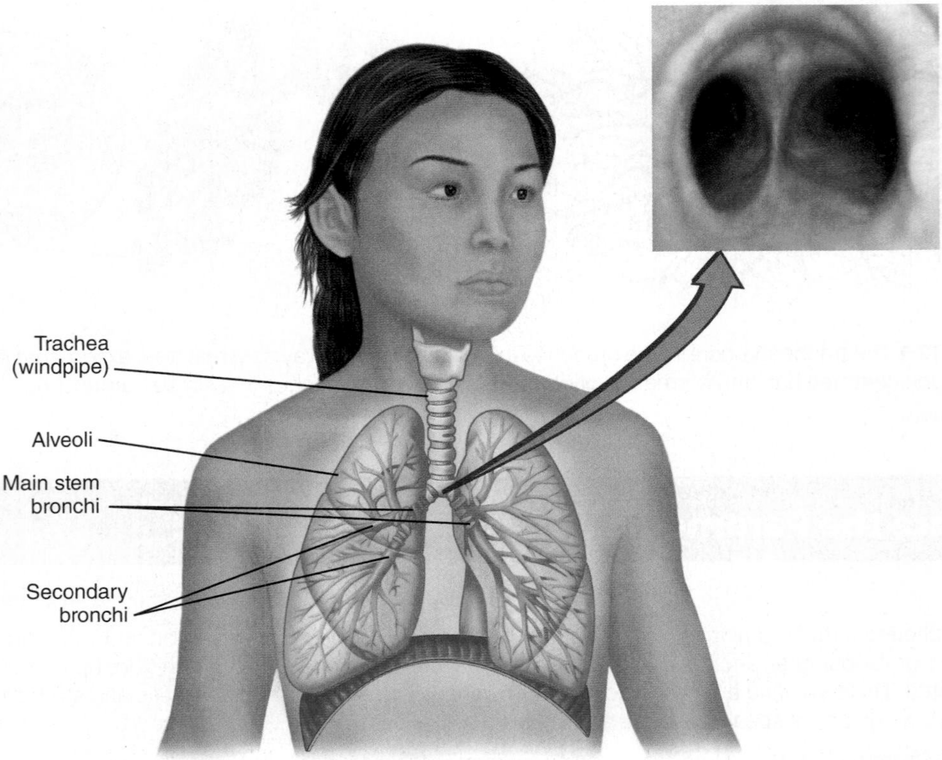

FIGURE 17-2 The right and left main stem bronchi bifurcate, or split, at the carina. In an adult, this point is at roughly the fifth intercostal space.

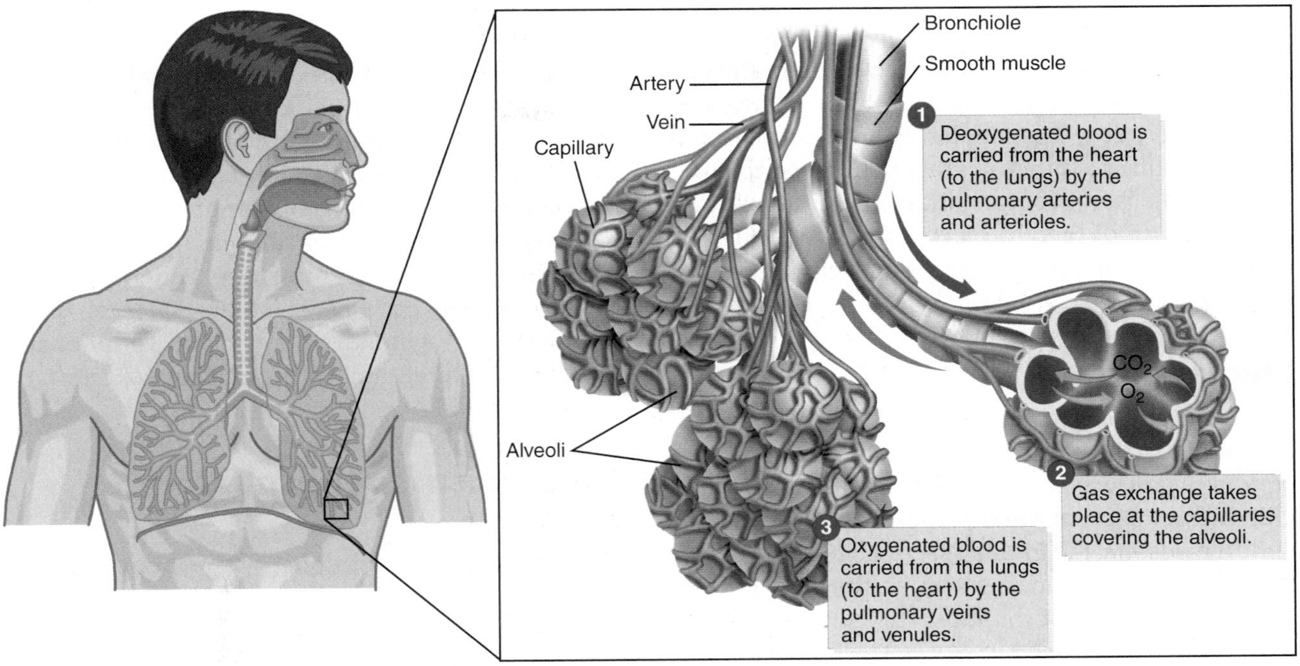

FIGURE 17-3 The respiratory bronchioles, sometimes called the terminal bronchioles, include the alveoli and the last several branches of the tracheobronchial tree. Gas exchange occurs over this entire area.

the respiratory bronchioles **FIGURE 17-3**. The terminal bronchioles are thin and have little cellular structure. This anatomic design is helpful for gas exchange, but it also means that the bronchioles lack cilia, have no protective blanket of mucus, and are not shielded by smooth muscle or more rigid structures.

With laminar airflow, particles approximately 5 micrometers in diameter are often carried this deep into the lungs (smaller particles are often exhaled without sticking). Once foreign material reaches the terminal bronchioles and alveoli, parts of the lung collectively known as the lung **parenchyma**, it may never come out. Common substances that break down to particles of this size include coal dust, asbestos fibers, and the contaminants in cigarette smoke. We all inhale small particulate matter during our lives. Most people have many small black spots on their lungs at autopsy from simply living in an industrialized society. Smokers and people who work around coal dust or other particulates may have significant areas of discoloration, or even completely blackened lungs **FIGURE 17-4**.

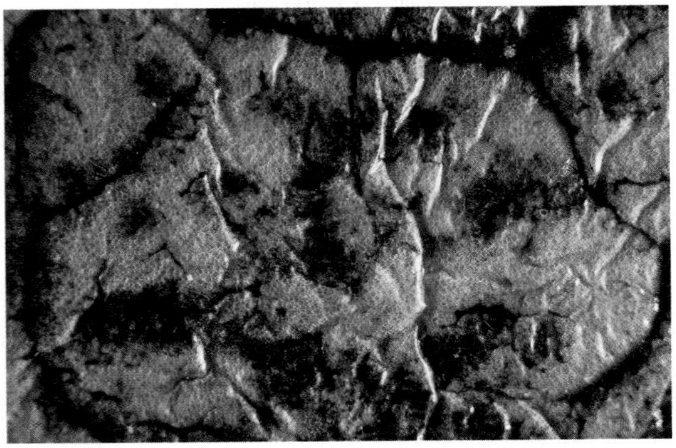

FIGURE 17-4 Smokers and people who work around coal dust or other particulates may have large areas of discoloration in their lungs.

Smooth muscle surrounds the conducting airways down to the subsegmental level. Bronchoconstriction occurs when the smooth muscle narrows these larger airways. Below the subsegmental level, bronchodilator medications have little effect. Wheezing that resolves with administration of bronchodilator medication was probably caused by constriction of the smooth muscle. Wheezing that is not resolved by these medications may have been caused by a pathologic condition deeper in the tracheobronchial tree.

Alveoli

The terminal airways and alveoli include branches 16 through 24 of the tracheobronchial tree, the so-called terminal bronchioles. The typical description of alveoli as a bunch of grapes clustered around a bronchiole is not completely accurate; rather, the entire surface of the alveoli and terminal bronchioles is covered in capillaries and participates in gas exchange.

Mediastinum

The heart and large blood vessels take up space in the middle of the chest between the lungs. The large conducting airways (trachea and main stem bronchi) and some other organs, such as the thymus in children, also reside in this space. Collectively, they appear on a chest radiograph as the large white area in the middle of the film. This middle ground is referred to as the *mediastinum*. The mediastinum can widen if the patient is bleeding from a ruptured aorta, or it might trap air from a traumatic injury, a condition called *pneumomediastinum*.

Pulmonary Blood Flow

Blood flows from the heart to the lungs via the pulmonary artery, which branches into smaller arteries, arterioles, and finally capillaries. The lung bases have a greater number of capillaries than the apices do, so more gas exchange occurs between the lung bases and the circulatory system than between the apices, tops of the lungs, and the circulatory system. Therefore, problems in the bases of the lungs (where most infectious processes occur and fluid may build up) impair **ventilation** more than do problems affecting the apices.

As with all capillaries in the body, the pulmonary capillaries are narrow and normally allow red blood cells to pass through only in single file. People with chronic lung disease and chronic **hypoxia** often generate a surplus of red blood cells over time, making their blood thick. Patients with **polycythemia**, for example, have viscous blood. The effort to push this blood through the tiny pulmonary capillaries can place a significant strain on the right side of the heart. When the alveoli become distended by COPD, they push against the capillary bed, further narrowing the capillaries and straining the right side of the heart. Right-side heart failure that occurs because of chronic lung disease is known as **cor pulmonale**.

Perfusion

Perfusion refers to the circulatory component of the respiratory system. If blood does not consistently flow through the pulmonary vessels, then good ventilation and diffusion are wasted, because an adequate supply of oxygen cannot come into contact with the blood. A large pulmonary embolus can block blood flow to an entire lung. Patients who are anemic (ie, who have a low **hemoglobin** level) or hypovolemic (ie, who have a low blood volume) also have an impaired ability to transport oxygen and carbon dioxide.

Mechanisms of Respiratory Control

The medulla and portions of the brainstem are involved in neurologic control of respiration, as described in Chapter 8, *Anatomy and Physiology*. Additional mechanisms of respiratory control are reviewed here.

Cardiovascular Regulation

The lungs are closely linked to cardiac function, so closely that some whimsically describe the lungs as an organ that lies between the right and left sides of the heart. While this description is not anatomically correct, it *is* true that changes in the right or left side of the heart can have dramatic pulmonary consequences. When you consider the prevalence of acute cardiac disorders and the total number of patients with respiratory disorders, it is easy to see why dispatches for shortness of breath are both common and diagnostically challenging.

Left-side heart failure typically progresses much faster than does right-side heart failure. Right-side heart failure may slowly worsen over many days, whereas left-side heart failure resulting from a massive acute myocardial infarction can kill a person in a matter of minutes. Thinking of the lungs as lying between the right and left sides of the heart (in terms of function) helps us understand why: The right side of the heart pumps blood to the lungs, whereas the left side of the heart receives blood from the lungs and then pumps it through the body to perfuse organs and tissues.

The body's immediate response to mild hypoxemia is to increase the heart rate, sometimes to higher than 130 beats/min, a rate that constitutes tachycardia. Severe hypoxia often causes bradycardia. Any uncorrected hypoxic insult may trigger a fatal cardiac dysrhythmia, such as ventricular fibrillation (VF) or ventricular tachycardia (VT). Changes in fluid balance, right-side heart pumping pressure, or left-side heart pumping pressure can cause various forms of heart failure. Given these many possibilities, a thorough evaluation of the cardiovascular system is essential to proper evaluation of a patient with a respiratory condition.

Muscular Control

The body is designed to take in air by means of negative pressure. Picture a vacuum cleaner at the base of the lungs that sucks in air during inhalation: This air is pulled in through the mouth and nose, over the turbinates, and around the complex terrain of the epiglottis and glottis. Air typically does not enter the esophagus and stomach because it is preferentially sucked into the trachea **FIGURE 17-5**.

This negative-pressure vacuum effect occurs because the thorax is essentially an airtight box, with the flexible diaphragm at the bottom and an open tube, the trachea, at the top. During quiet breathing, as the diaphragm flattens, the overall size of the container increases, and air is sucked in through the tube at the top, filling the increasing space within the thorax. The amount of air moved each minute is called *minute ventilation.* Minute ventilation can be increased by breathing deeply, which drops the diaphragm more aggressively, or by breathing more rapidly. Rapid breathing is called *tachypnea.*

Any traumatic opening of the thorax provides an alternative route for air to be drawn in. This air ends up in the pleural space, resulting in a sucking chest wound **FIGURE 17-6**. When multiple ribs are broken in more than one place (flail chest), free-floating sections of the thorax are pulled in as the patient breathes, limiting the amount of air that can be sucked in through the trachea.

Renal Status

Fluid balance, acid–base balance, and blood pressure (BP) are controlled, in part, by the kidneys, which receive approximately 25% of cardiac output. Each of these factors also affects the pulmonary mechanics and, therefore, oxygen delivery to

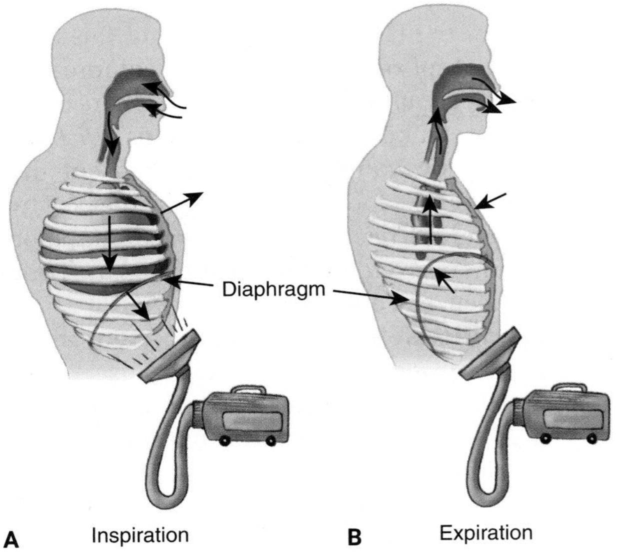

FIGURE 17-5 Normal ventilation is negative-pressure ventilation, meaning that air is sucked into the lungs, much as a vacuum cleaner sucks in air. When the diaphragm contracts, it pulls down into the abdomen, expanding the chest cavity and drawing in air **(A)**. When the pressure is released, the diaphragm relaxes and the lungs empty **(B)**. Compare with positive-pressure ventilation, shown in Figure 17-22.

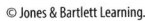

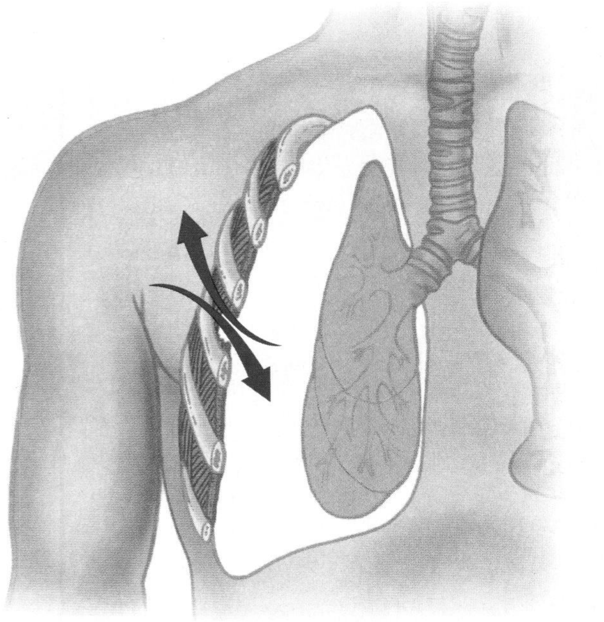

FIGURE 17-6 A sucking chest wound can compromise ventilation by allowing air to enter the thorax during the inspiratory or negative-pressure phase of ventilation.

the tissues. Patients with severe renal disease often present with respiratory signs and symptoms, so paramedics should always note signs of severe renal disease when evaluating a patient's condition. The condition of patients whose heart failure is associated with renal disease can be challenging to manage because **diuresis**, the production of large amounts of urine by the kidney, may be difficult or impossible. Patients with renal disease may also have acid–base disturbances that cause them to hyperventilate, giving the mistaken appearance of having respiratory disorders. Often, a patient's need for emergency dialysis may influence transport decisions and treatment options.

Hypoventilation

When the lungs fail to work properly, the body cannot efficiently dispose of carbon dioxide, so it accumulates in the blood. This excess carbon dioxide combines with water to form bicarbonate ions and hydrogen (H^+) ions, also known as *carbonic acid*, resulting in acidosis.

Acidosis can occur if hypoventilation is not recognized. Impaired ventilation can be attributed to a variety of factors, as shown in **TABLE 17-1**. We will examine each of these factors in detail later in the chapter.

TABLE 17-1 Selected Causes of Impaired Ventilation

Category	Conditions
Upper airway obstruction	Foreign body obstruction Infection Trauma
Lower airway obstruction	Trauma Obstructive disease Increased mucus production Airway swelling (edema)
Chest wall impairment	Pneumothorax Flail chest Pleural effusion Restrictive disease (scoliosis, kyphosis)
Neuromuscular impairment	Overdose Lou Gehrig disease (amyotrophic lateral sclerosis) Carbon dioxide narcosis

Recall that pH is an expression of how many free hydrogen ions (H^+) are present in a solution. Thus, the carbon dioxide level of the blood is directly related to pH (acid–base balance). Patients who are hypoventilating usually have respiratory acidosis. As their carbon dioxide level goes up, their pH level drops.

Many underlying conditions can cause patients to **hypoventilate**:

- **Conditions that impair lung function.** When a patient is breathing but gas exchange is impaired, the carbon dioxide level in the blood rises. This situation can occur in patients with severe atelectasis, pneumonia, pulmonary edema, asthma, or COPD.
- **Conditions that impair the mechanics of breathing.** Gas flow can be suppressed by a flail chest, diaphragmatic rupture, severe **retractions**, an abdomen full of air or blood, abdominal or chest binding (as may occur during spinal motion restriction), or anything else that restricts the pressure changes that facilitate respiration.

  Obesity hypoventilation syndrome (also known as Pickwickian syndrome) is respiratory compromise caused by morbid obesity. One of the earliest descriptions of this combination of obesity, respiratory compromise, and sleep apnea is found in the character of "Joe the fat boy" in Charles Dickens's *Pickwick Papers*. Joe would fall asleep in midsentence, snore loudly, and generally display signs of hypercapnia. This syndrome is becoming more common, given the nationwide increase in the prevalence of obesity.
- **Conditions that impair the neuromuscular apparatus.** A patient who has experienced head trauma, an intracranial infection, or a brain tumor may have sustained damage to the respiratory centers of the brain, which may in turn compromise ventilation. Other conditions also may impair the neuromuscular apparatus:
  - Serious injury to the spinal cord above the level of the fifth cervical vertebra (C5) may block the nerve impulses that stimulate breathing. The saying "C3, 4, and 5 keep the diaphragm alive" references the phrenic nerve, which originates from the spinal nerves in these areas and controls the diaphragm, which then controls breathing.

- **Guillain-Barré syndrome**, characterized by progressive muscle weakness and paralysis advancing up the body from the feet, can result in ineffective breathing if the paralysis reaches the diaphragm.
- Amyotrophic lateral sclerosis (ALS; also known as Lou Gehrig disease) also causes progressive muscle weakness. This disease is fatal, with death usually attributable to respiratory failure as the muscles of respiration become unable to maintain adequate ventilation.
- **Botulism** is caused by the bacterium *Clostridium botulinum.* This somewhat rare disease is usually caused by food poisoning or by giving infants raw (unpasteurized) honey, which may be contaminated with spores of the bacterium. Botulism can cause muscle paralysis and is usually fatal when it reaches the muscles of respiration.

- **Conditions that reduce respiratory drive.** The stimulus to breathe is often referred to as *respiratory drive.* In patients without respiratory-related disease, the drive to breathe is stimulated by chemoreceptors detecting increased carbon dioxide levels. In contrast, *hypoxic drive* refers to the stimulation to breathe from low oxygen levels in patients with chronic pulmonary disease due to their chronically increased carbon dioxide levels. Anything that interrupts or decreases the involuntary stimulus to breathe can result in hypoventilation or even apnea. Perhaps the hypoventilation crisis most commonly seen by paramedics is acute heroin overdose. Intoxication with alcohol, narcotics, or any of a host of other drugs and toxins can reduce the respiratory drive. Head injury, hypoxic drive, and asphyxia are all associated with grossly low respiratory rate and volume. The ultimate expression of hypoventilation is respiratory arrest followed by cardiac arrest.

In these circumstances, aggressive treatment must be initiated to assist the patient's respiratory efforts.

Hyperventilation

Hyperventilation occurs when people breathe in excess of their metabolic need by increasing the rate or depth of respiration, or both, expelling more carbon dioxide than normal. The result is alkalosis. As the patient's carbon dioxide level dips, the pH level rises. When this cycle is triggered by emotional distress or a panic attack, it may be called *hysterical hyperventilation* or *hyperventilation syndrome.* The falling carbon dioxide level may make the person feel short of breath, which results in even more anxiety and breathing even more rapidly and deeply. In acute hyperventilation syndrome, patients usually feel as if they cannot breathe at all. Hyperventilation that is not caused by some metabolic crisis is usually self-limiting.

Respiratory alkalosis causes numbness or tingling in the hands and feet and around the mouth. If it persists, then patients may complain of chest pain and will ultimately experience **carpopedal spasm**, in which the hands and feet become clenched into a clawlike position. These symptoms may frighten the patient even further and usually result in additional hyperventilation. A hysterical patient may eventually lose consciousness, but not before experiencing extreme distress. If the patient begins hyperventilating on awakening, then the process could repeat itself.

The traditional therapy for hyperventilation called for patients to rebreathe their own carbon dioxide from a paper bag or from a partial rebreathing mask set at 21% oxygen (not attached to supplemental oxygen). This practice can be dangerous for two important reasons:

1. Patients quickly exhaust the oxygen in the gas they are breathing (and rebreathing). Hyperventilation does not mean that the patient has too much oxygen, but rather that too much carbon dioxide is being exhaled. Rebreathing carbon dioxide can cause hypoxia, which is counterproductive when trying to terminate a relatively benign hyperventilation episode.
2. Hyperventilation in a patient with acidosis might represent the body's attempt to drive the pH level back up to normal. For example, in a patient with diabetic ketoacidosis, the body produces too much acid because of inadequate glucose metabolism. The body attempts to compensate for the acidosis through hyperventilation or **Kussmaul respirations**. A variety of overdoses, toxic exposures, and metabolic abnormalities, including shock and sepsis, can also produce acidosis and compensatory hyperventilation, and *none should be treated by rebreathing carbon dioxide.* Never conclude

that a patient is "just hyperventilating" until all possible causes of the presentation have been ruled out, which is difficult or perhaps impossible in the field. Hyperventilation is a diagnosis of exclusion; you cannot presume hyperventilation syndrome until all other medical causes have been ruled out.

Ultimately, treatment may include sedating a person who is truly hysterical and is hyperventilating, but such an extreme measure is rarely taken in the field. Hyperventilation is often triggered by an emotional stressor, such as having a family argument, being involved in a motor vehicle crash, or receiving bad news. Consider removing the patient from the environment and distancing them from the stressor. More often than not, psychological support is helpful. An important part of care is to help the patient understand that if the behavior that precipitated the hyperventilation is repeated, the hyperventilation will probably recur.

Other useful psychological support techniques include breathing with the patient, having the patient count to two between breaths (gradually increasing to higher numbers), and distracting the person in various ways, such as asking to hear the patient's life story. Singing a song with the patient may require the patient to use enough breath control to terminate the episode.

Patient Assessment

Evaluation of the respiratory organs is clearly an essential component of assessment during a respiratory emergency. However, the job performed by the respiratory system so dramatically affects other body systems that a thorough respiratory assessment includes much more than simply listening to the patient's lungs.

As always, recognizing and treating life threats, including life-threatening hemorrhage, is the priority during the primary survey and throughout the assessment. Because many respiratory ailments are life threatening, respiratory assessment is always an early step in patient assessment.

Scene Size-up

Paramedics should always think first about safety, including taking standard precautions. Using proper personal protective equipment (PPE) is vital whenever exposure to blood, body fluids, or respiratory secretions is possible. In addition, the patient may have a respiratory infection that could be communicable by sputum, respiratory droplets, or airborne particles (see Chapter 27, *Infectious Diseases*). When treating a patient with a respiratory complaint, the minimum PPE consists of disposable examination

YOU are the Paramedic

PART 2

It's evident to you that this patient is struggling to breathe. He tells you that he woke up suddenly with difficulty breathing and weakness. Your partner prepares to obtain vital signs and administer 100% oxygen via nonrebreathing mask. When you initially listen to the patient's lungs, you hear crackles in the apices and diminished lung sounds in the bases. No medication bottles are in obvious view.

Recording Time: 1 Minute	
Appearance	Ashen gray, poor
Level of consciousness	Alert (oriented to person, place, and time)
Airway	Patent
Breathing	Rapid and shallow with crackles
Circulation	Weak and rapid radial pulse

3. What is your working diagnosis at this time?

4. What assessment and treatment steps will you want to accomplish on scene?

gloves, a mask or face shield, and eye protection. A gown may also be used if the patient is suspected of having or is known to have a communicable respiratory infection, such as methicillin-resistant *Staphylococcus aureus* (MRSA), which could be transmitted in their sputum.

Pulmonary complaints are associated with a broad range of dangerous situations and toxins. The paramedic may be called to a scene where the atmosphere has a diminished oxygen concentration, such as a methamphetamine laboratory, a silo, or another enclosed, improperly ventilated space. The atmosphere on scene may contain carbon monoxide or irritant gases, or the patient may have a highly contagious respiratory illness. Therefore, it is essential to evaluate scene safety on every call, even on one that appears to be a routine dispatch for shortness of breath.

Respiratory disease can impair ventilation, diffusion, perfusion, or a combination of the three. The most common complaint of patients with a respiratory disease is dyspnea. The most common cause of dyspnea is hypercapnia, or too much carbon dioxide in the blood. This condition is caused by inadequate ventilation. Although dyspnea is often associated with hypoxia, some patients may be hypoxic without any associated dyspnea. Always evaluate the patient's oxygen saturation, even in the absence of a complaint of dyspnea.

Words of Wisdom

Respiratory illnesses are common community-acquired "minor" illnesses to which we are all subject. Paramedics are not immune to viruses and the common cold. Unfortunately, a minor illness in a young, healthy EMS provider might represent a deadly disease in very young, very old, or immunocompromised patients. For example, immunity conferred by the pertussis vaccination lasts for 5 to 10 years, so an adult who was vaccinated as a child can still contract this disease. An infected adult can transmit the infection to an unvaccinated child. As a paramedic, you must pay attention to your own health, including your vaccination history and immunity status. You will probably be exposed to tuberculosis, pertussis, hepatitis B, COVID-19 (coronavirus disease 2019), and various other pathogens and contagious diseases during your career (see Chapter 27, *Infectious Diseases*).

Rapid-onset dyspnea may be caused by acute **bronchospasm**, anaphylaxis, pulmonary embolism, or pneumothorax. **Paroxysmal nocturnal dyspnea** is dyspnea that comes on suddenly in the middle of the night and may be an ominous sign of left-side heart failure.

Factors that limit the ability of the diaphragm to move (such as advanced pregnancy, obesity, and air or blood in the abdomen), conditions that restrict chest wall movement (such as crush injuries, tightly applied immobilization devices, and an abnormal spinal curvature, like that associated with scoliosis or kyphosis), and injuries that disrupt the integrity of the thoracic cage (such as flail chest) hinder a patient's ability to move an adequate supply of air for ventilation.

Primary Survey

The priority in assessing and managing any respiratory condition is to establish and maintain an open airway. Food, gum, chewing tobacco, and the like should be removed from the patient's mouth. Suction should be applied if necessary and the airway kept in the optimal position, which is typically the position in which the patient feels most comfortable. See Chapter 16, *Airway Management*, for a more in-depth discussion of airway management techniques.

The following pages discuss signs associated with life-threatening respiratory distress. You may notice many other signs, both obvious and subtle, during the first few moments of every patient encounter.

One glance at a patient may suggest a body type associated with a particular pathologic condition. The classic presentation of a patient with **emphysema** includes a barrel chest (a chest that is larger in diameter from front to back than from side to side as a result of years of having air trapped in the thorax), muscle wasting (as a result of cannibalizing muscle mass for energy), and pursed-lip breathing (as a result of the obstructive disease). Patients with emphysema are often tachypneic and do not typically present with profound hypoxia and cyanosis.

Severely ill patients with immune system disorders and those with cancer or other end-stage diseases are often easily identified by their sickly appearance. They may have rigors and pneumonia with accompanying chills. Tall, thin young adults are predisposed to spontaneous pneumothorax, and women who smoke and take oral contraceptives are predisposed to pulmonary embolus.

Patients with **chronic bronchitis** tend to be more sedentary and may be obese as a result. You are likely to encounter such a patient in a chair or recliner, in which the patient sleeps in an upright position. A wastebasket nearby may overflow with tissues, and you may see an ashtray filled with cigarette butts or a cup into which the patient spits the copious secretions. A male patient might keep a urinal near the chair to avoid frequent trips to the bathroom. On a table next to the chair, you may see several medication bottles, inhalers, or an aerosol nebulizer. Such a scene can disclose volumes of information about the patient and the history long before you place a stethoscope on the patient's chest.

Clues to various pathologic conditions may be evident immediately, but keep in mind that they are only clues. Avoid constructing a hasty field impression based on minimal information. Patients with COPD often get pneumonia, an asthma attack can be triggered by an ongoing infection, and heart failure can develop in a patient who has cancer. In other words, the patient's presentation may suggest a particular condition, but a thorough assessment must confirm this suspicion.

Words of Wisdom

In the 1950s, John Hickam, MD, Duke University, coined the phrase that became known as Hickam's dictum. He found it necessary to remind medical students that patients often present with multiple pathologies, all of which must be considered during assessment. When evaluating respiratory distress, remember Hickam's advice: "Patients can have as many diseases as they damn well please."

Assess Oxygen Demand and Work of Breathing

Oxygen demand increases with exertion of any kind. If a patient's condition is stable at rest, then observe their condition during typical exertion. Ask if the patient becomes dyspneic when moving from the chair to the stretcher, when going to the bathroom, or while eating. Note the patient's oxygen saturation while at rest and during any simple exertion.

Increased work of breathing, anxiety, hypoxia, or fever can trigger a sympathetic nervous system response characterized by tachycardia, diaphoresis, and pallor. This effect can be so pronounced that the heart rate often decreases as patients respond to treatment even if they are treated with sympathetic stimulators that normally increase the heart rate.

Note Position and Determine Degree of Distress

Patients in respiratory distress tend to avoid the supine position and instead seek a sitting position. A person in the tripod position, for example, leans forward and rotates the scapulae outward by placing the arms on a table, elbows out, or by placing the hands on the knees **FIGURE 17-7**. This position opens up a little more space for airflow in the lung apices and draws the abdominal structures away

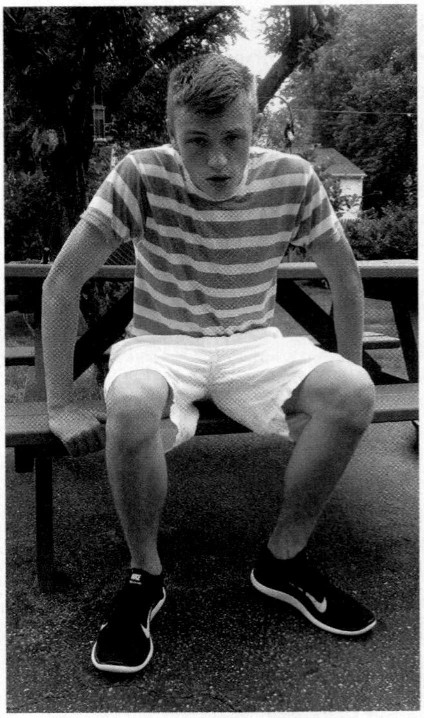

FIGURE 17-7 The tripod position (elbows out) improves diaphragmatic movement by getting the abdomen out of the way and rotating the scapulae laterally, allowing somewhat more air to flow to the apices. Unfortunately, this position takes work, which requires more oxygen, and may or may not ultimately benefit the patient.

from the diaphragm. Because considerably less perfusion occurs at the apex of the lung than at the base, the effort required for a person to assume the tripod position may offset the modest gain in oxygenation. Be wary if a patient in respiratory distress wants to lie flat; this could signify sudden deterioration in their condition.

A patient may try to maximize airflow through the upper airway by purposeful hyperextension, accomplished by holding the head in the head tilt–chin lift position, or so-called sniffing position. This position may also indicate upper airway swelling. Maintaining this position uses up valuable energy. A patient with severe respiratory disease who begins to feel fatigued may hold the head up in this position only during inhalation, letting the head and neck fall into flexion during exhalation. This "head bobbing" is an ominous sign of imminent decompensation and may be a clue to the severity of the situation.

Breathing Alterations

Breathing alterations can involve any of the following:

- The conducting airways (trachea, bronchi, and bronchioles), such as occurs in asthma or bronchitis
- The alveoli, as in pneumonia or emphysema
- The muscles and nerves that control breathing, as in Guillain-Barré syndrome or spinal cord injury
- The rigid structure of the thorax, thereby hampering the pressure changes that facilitate the breathing process, as occurs in flail chest

Increased Work of Breathing

Patients who rely on accessory muscles to breathe are in danger of tiring out, so noticing such muscle use is essential. For example, is the patient using the abdominal muscles to push air out (as in asthma or COPD), or using the muscles of the chest and neck to pull air in? Infants and small children have substantial chest wall elasticity; when they use accessory muscles to breathe, the flexible cartilage of the sternum or ribs often collapses, causing bony retractions **FIGURE 17-8**.

By the same mechanism, a patient of any age may pull the soft tissues in between the ribs, above or below the sternum or clavicles, causing

Words of Wisdom

Maintaining the airway and breathing for a patient are not the same thing. Many patients need assistance to establish a patent airway. However, having an open airway does not ensure an adequate volume of gas is moving into and out of the lungs. Proper ventilation is necessary to remove carbon dioxide and maintain acid–base balance. Increasing the amount of available oxygen ensures that even a patient who is not moving an adequate volume of gas (ie, a patient who is hypoventilating) can maintain adequate oxygen saturation. If ventilation remains inadequate in a hypoventilating patient, then the patient will become hypercapnic (the blood contains too much carbon dioxide) and acidotic (the arterial blood pH is too low). These conditions disrupt the balance of important body systems and will be fatal if uncorrected. While it is important to maintain an adequate oxygen saturation level, adequate oxygenation does not always equate to adequate ventilation. While closely related, maintaining an airway, maintaining adequate ventilation, and maintaining adequate oxygenation are three different things, and the paramedic must attend to each!

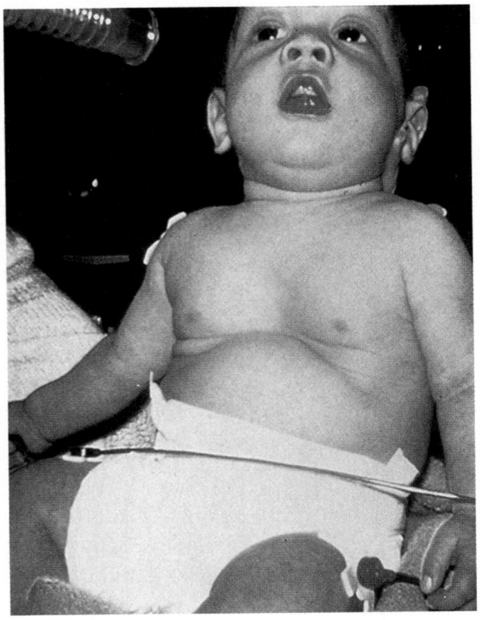

FIGURE 17-8 Bony retractions not only indicate severe distress and increased work of breathing, but also contribute to respiratory failure. With inhalation, the lower sternum is pulled into the lungs. Every cubic centimeter of space displaced by the retraction represents a cubic centimeter of air that cannot reach the airways.

soft-tissue retractions. In adults and children, profound intrathoracic pressure changes can make the peripheral pulse weak or imperceptible during inspiration but easier to palpate during exhalation, a state known as **pulsus paradoxus**, which is characteristic of conditions such as cardiac tamponade and severe asthma. Patients who are using accessory muscles to breathe may have dramatic pressure changes within the thorax and exhibit these and other signs of increased work of breathing, summarized in **TABLE 17-2**. Such signs may indicate life-threatening respiratory distress.

Altered Rate and Depth of Respiration

Assessing the rate and depth of breathing is an obvious component of respiratory assessment. Unfortunately, rate and depth both are sometimes inaccurately measured. The conscientious paramedic will observe the patient's respiratory rate and depth without being obvious (patients may breathe faster or deeper if they are aware that you are counting). Count the respiratory rate while you appear to be doing something else, such as checking the pulse or taking the BP. The rate may be a commonly "guessed" vital sign, but respiratory depth is even more commonly misjudged. The use of continuous end-tidal carbon dioxide ($ETCO_2$) monitoring provides documentation of the patient's respirations and makes it much easier to accurately determine rate and depth. A patient with an adequate rate but a low volume will still have an inadequate minute volume, which is calculated as follows:

$$\text{Respiratory rate} \times \text{Tidal volume} = \text{Minute volume}$$

The respiratory rate can vary significantly from minute to minute. Be sure to monitor trends in respiratory rate, whether it is increasing or decreasing, rather than concentrating on a specific rate from

TABLE 17-2 Signs of Increased Work of Breathing

Sign	Description
Bony retractions	During inhalation, the sternum or ribs pull back or recede (retract) into the chest, creating a visible deformity with each breath.
Soft-tissue retractions	Soft tissue is drawn in around the bones during inhalation. Dramatic retractions can be seen in the supraclavicular, intercostal, and subxiphoid areas.
Nasal flaring	The nostrils fan wide open during inhalation.
Tracheal tugging	During inhalation, the thyroid cartilage is drawn upward and the area just above the sternal notch is pulled in.
Paradoxical respiratory movement	During inhalation, the epigastrium is pulled in as the abdomen is pushed out, creating a seesaw effect as the two move in opposite directions.
Pulsus paradoxus	Peripheral pulses are weak or absent on inhalation, caused by extreme pressure changes in the thorax.
Pursed-lip breathing	Patients with obstructive diseases (such as COPD and acute asthma) have trouble pushing air out. It is more effective to exhale slowly over a longer period than to try to expel the air forcefully. Many patients learn to purse their lips (like a kiss) and exhale slowly through this restricted orifice. This technique allows more efficient exhalation and provides a diagnostic clue to the disease.
Grunting	In infants and young children with lower airway illness, the glottis closes at the end of exhalation and a grunt is emitted at the end of each breath. The grunting exerts a small amount of pressure that helps keep the alveoli open (as with positive end-expiratory pressure). The grunts may be audible, or a stethoscope may be required to hear them. Grunting is a classic sign of respiratory distress in infants.

Abbreviation: COPD, chronic obstructive pulmonary disease

the beginning of the assessment. While assessing the patient's respiration, note the pattern (see Table 17-5) and the inspiratory-to-expiratory (I:E) ratio. Is the patient working hard to inhale, exhale, or both? Does the breath have a peculiar odor (such as the acetone odor associated with diabetic ketoacidosis)? Are there any abnormal respiratory noises? As a general rule, *any* respiratory noises that are audible without a stethoscope are abnormal.

Abnormal Breath Sounds

Whenever possible, auscultate the lungs systematically. Although examiners tend to compare the left and right sides, recall that the lungs are not symmetric. For this reason, the paramedic must understand where to listen to hear each lobe **FIGURE 17-9**.

Many pathologic conditions are gravity dependent, meaning that most types of pneumonia and heart failure affect the lung bases. Wheezing is typically diffuse and spread throughout the lung fields. Wheezing confined to only one spot may indicate a foreign body or tumor. The bases are heard almost exclusively by listening with the stethoscope on the patient's back.

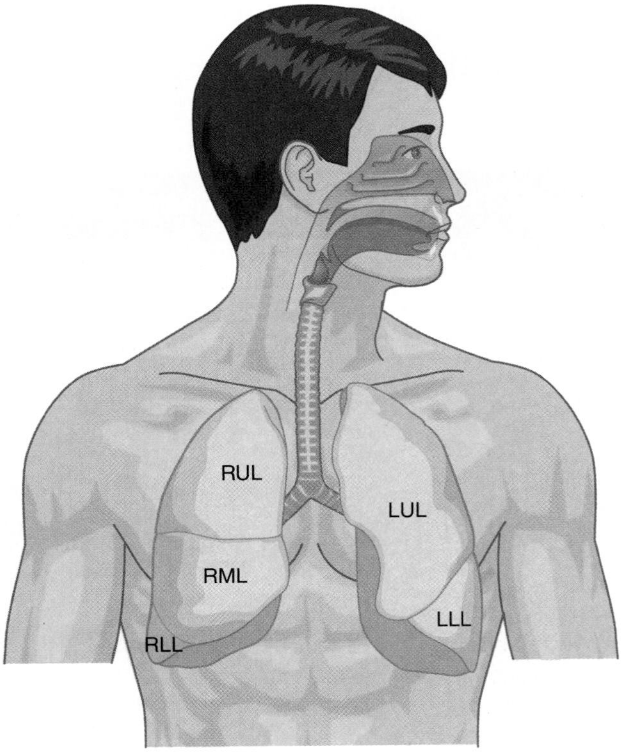

FIGURE 17-9 The lungs are not symmetric. Most acute pathologic conditions are best heard in the lung bases, requiring that the stethoscope be placed on the patient's back. The right middle lobe is best heard beneath the right breast or just lateral to it.

Abbreviations: LUL, left upper lobe; LLL, left lower lobe; RUL, right upper lobe; RML, right middle lobe; RLL, right lower lobe.

The upper lobes, which are less likely to have abnormalities, are heard by listening on the anterior part of the chest. The right middle lobe can best be heard by listening just beneath or lateral to the right breast. The best left-right differentiation can be noted at the midaxillary line; this is the best place to listen to confirm ET tube placement. Listening to the anterior part of the chest allows the paramedic to hear the noisemaker (the ET tube), whether it is in the trachea or the esophagus.

Breath sounds are made by turbulent airflow in the large airways. Using a stethoscope, you will hear these sounds as they are transmitted through the lung tissue. Tracheal breath sounds are not commonly auscultated, but note how harsh and tubular they sound. Bronchial breath sounds are also quite loud, but note that exhalation predominates. Farther toward the periphery, bronchovesicular sounds are softer and stay constant with inspiration and expiration. The most common breath sounds are the soft, breezy vesicular sounds heard in the periphery, which have a much more obvious inspiratory component. Listening to many healthy lungs can help you become familiar with these four different types of breath sounds **FIGURE 17-10**. However, some pathologic conditions cause normal breath sounds to be heard in abnormal places.

Sound moves better through fluid than it does through air. The more air in a patient's chest, then, the more distant or diminished the breath sounds are at the periphery, if they are audible at all. Patients with COPD and asthma, for example, may have diminished breath sounds. Conversely, the wetter the patient's lungs are, so to speak, the louder the sounds are at the periphery. Patients with wet lungs include those with pneumonia, heart failure, and **lung consolidation**, which occurs when fluid accumulation makes the lungs firm. Pneumonia in the right middle lobe produces bronchovesicular sounds (equal during inspiration and expiration). In the periphery, you may even hear bronchial sounds (louder during expiration than inspiration) instead of the expected vesicular sounds (louder during inspiration than expiration).

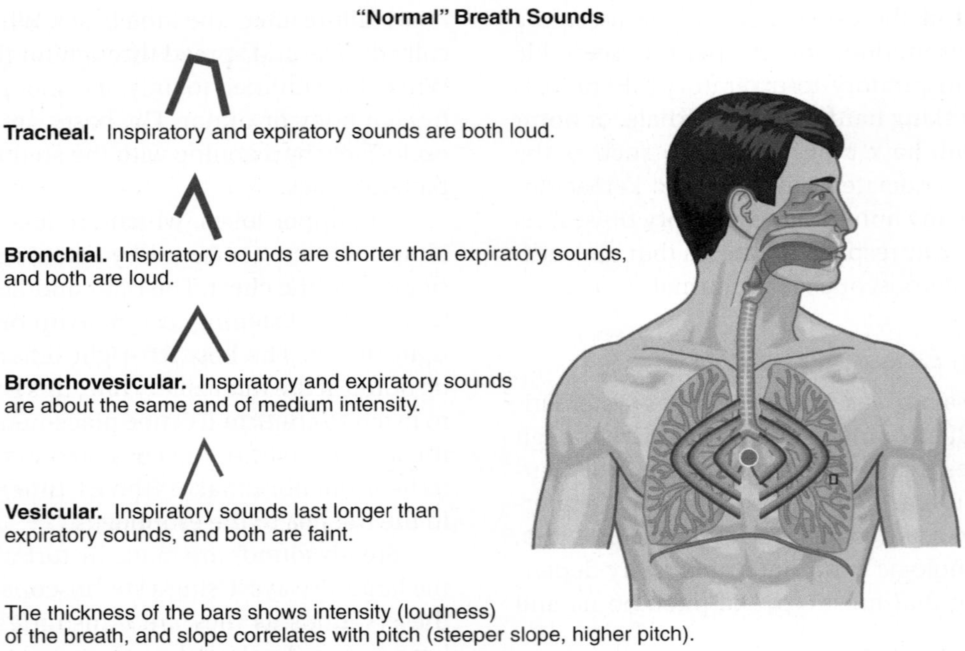

"Normal" Breath Sounds
Tracheal. Inspiratory and expiratory sounds are both loud.
Bronchial. Inspiratory sounds are shorter than expiratory sounds, and both are loud.
Bronchovesicular. Inspiratory and expiratory sounds are about the same and of medium intensity.
Vesicular. Inspiratory sounds last longer than expiratory sounds, and both are faint.
The thickness of the bars shows intensity (loudness) of the breath, and slope correlates with pitch (steeper slope, higher pitch).

FIGURE 17-10 Normal breath sounds are heard over different parts of the chest. As the stethoscope moves away from the largest airways, breath sounds become softer. The character of sounds during inspiration versus exhalation also changes.

The quality of the breath sounds also depends on how much extra tissue separates the stethoscope and the patient's respiratory structures. For this reason, it is often helpful to compare breath sounds on the right with those at approximately the same level on the left (keeping in mind that the lungs are not symmetric). In a patient with a one-sided pathologic condition such as pneumonia, the breath sounds may be *louder* over the side with the abnormality than over the healthy side.

Breath sounds and vocalizations travel more efficiently through a firm, fluid-filled lung than through a healthy lung, but they travel poorly through a hyperinflated lung. If a patient speaks during chest auscultation, then the examiner cannot usually understand what the patient is saying through the stethoscope. If the patient's words are audible, then it may mean the patient has consolidation from pneumonia or atelectasis. These sounds are most clearly audible directly over the consolidated lobe. **TABLE 17-3** lists signs of consolidation.

Adventitious (abnormal) breath sounds are the extra noises that can be heard on top of the breath sounds described previously. Continuous sounds (eg, a wheeze) can be heard across some portion of each breath. Discontinuous sounds consist of intermittent pops, snaps, and clicks known as **crackles** **FIGURE 17-11**.

TABLE 17-3 Signs of Lung Consolidation

Sign	Test
Bronchophony	When a patient says "99" repeatedly through a normal lung, it sounds like a hum. Through a consolidated lung, you can understand the word "99."
Egophony	The patient says "Eeeeee" while you are auscultating, and you hear "Aaaaaay" (as in "state"). The sound may be heard particularly well over a pleural effusion.
Whispered pectoriloquy	The patient whispers while you are auscultating, and you can understand what is said.

Wheezes are high-pitched whistling sounds that are produced when air is forced through narrowed airways, making them vibrate, much like the

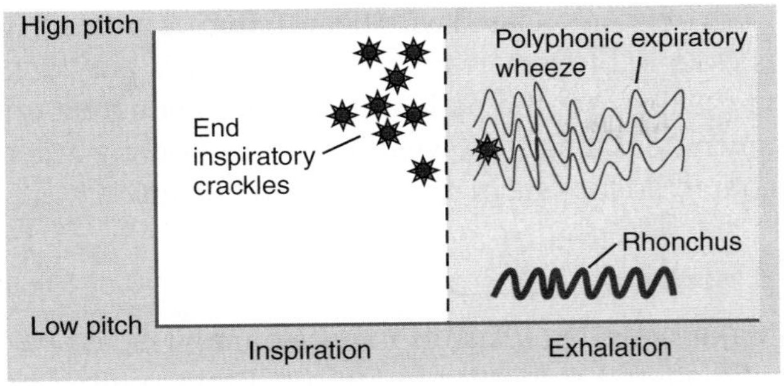

FIGURE 17-11 Adventitious sounds can be described as continuous (wheezes and rhonchi) or discontinuous (crackles). They can also be characterized by their pitch (such as high or low), by the point at which they occur in the respiratory cycle (end inspiration or forced exhalation), and by their complexity (monophonic versus polyphonic).

reed in a musical instrument. Wheezing may be diffuse, as in asthma and heart failure, or localized, as when a foreign body partially obstructs a bronchus. Pathologic conditions such as asthma rarely cause one-sided wheezing. Have the patient cough, and listen again. If the sound seems to originate on only one side, then it could be caused by the movement of secretions. If a single bronchus is vibrating, then the wheeze will produce a single note, known as a **monophonic** sound. If many bronchi are vibrating, then the wheeze may have many notes, like a bagpipe; this is called a **polyphonic** sound.

Also note when the sound is heard in the respiratory cycle. For example, does the wheeze occur during inspiration and exhalation? Just during exhalation? Or just at the end of exhalation?

During auscultation of the lungs, you may hear crackles (formerly known as rales), discontinuous sounds that are heard primarily on inspiration. Fine crackles are faint or low-intensity sounds made by the smaller airways snapping open, whereas coarse crackles are more pronounced deeper-pitched sounds made by the snapping open of larger airways. *Rhonchi* are loud, low-pitched sounds, often prominent on exhalation, caused by secretions trapped in the larger airways.

Certain sounds such as stridor from upper airway obstruction and grunting from lower airway obstruction are audible without a stethoscope. A low-pitched gurgling sound (sometimes called a "death rattle") is sometimes heard as the patient becomes unable to clear secretions. Wheezes and crackles that are audible when entering a room are more impressive than sounds requiring a stethoscope to hear. As a patient's condition worsens, the various emissions become louder and take on a musical character. As respiratory distress worsens, the noises may again diminish. The most ominous breath sounds are no breath sounds at all. An absence of breath sounds indicates that the patient is not moving enough air to ventilate the lungs. *Silence means danger.*

Noisy breathing is obstructed breathing. **Snoring** indicates partial obstruction of the upper airway by the tongue: a form of obstruction easily corrected by head-tilt maneuvers. Gurgling signals the presence of fluid in the upper airway. **Stridor**, a harsh, high-pitched sound heard during inhalation, indicates narrowing, usually as a result of swelling (laryngeal edema).

Quiet breathing can also be revealing. A patient with tachypnea and clear breath sounds may have hyperventilation syndrome but may also be breathing rapidly because of acidosis. Quiet tachypnea suggests possible shock. Paramedics occasionally assume that the patient's primary condition is tachypnea caused by pain, anxiety, or a metabolic disorder, when in fact the real cause is diabetic ketoacidosis or sepsis.

Sputum

Normally, a mucous blanket coats the upper tracheobronchial tree. As mucus moves up and out of the trachea, it is usually swallowed. Irritated airways secrete more mucus, which may be expelled as sputum. There is a difference between saliva from the mouth (oral secretions) and the thicker, sometimes color-tinged sputum from the lungs. This mucus may be mixed with blood, pulmonary edema fluid, aspirated food particles, or debris from dead infectious organisms. The sputum may be a variety of colors, which sometimes provides clues about the nature of the infection. The patient's level of hydration may affect the thickness of the sputum, with very thick secretions clogging the airways of dehydrated patients.

Note whether the patient is coughing up discolored sputum **TABLE 17-4**. Many smokers and people with chronic respiratory diseases cough up sputum every day (especially first thing in the morning). In such cases, try to determine if the color or amount of the sputum has changed.

TABLE 17-4 Classic Sputum Types

Type	Causes
Frothy, sometimes with a pink tinge	Heart failure
Thick	Dehydration or antihistamine use
Purulent	Infectious process (because the pus contains dead white blood cells)
Yellow, green, brown	Older secretions in various stages of decomposition
Clear or white	Bronchitis
Blood-streaked	Tumor, tuberculosis, pulmonary edema, or trauma from coughing

Increased sputum production coupled with fever and chills is a classic presentation of an infection such as pneumonia. Blood-tinged sputum may be a warning sign of **tuberculosis**, or it may mean the patient has been coughing forcefully enough to break small blood vessels in the airway. When air is forced through fluid-filled airways, the pink foam or froth often associated with heart failure is created. It is essential to note whether the mucus is **purulent**, or puslike. Ask the patient if they have coughed up any mucus and, if so, whether its color or any other characteristics seem different from normal.

Abnormal Breathing Patterns

Major neurologic insults may also manifest as specific altered respiratory patterns. Brain trauma or any event that disturbs brain function may depress the respiratory control centers in the medulla. For example, the increased intracranial pressure that occurs in patients with closed head trauma may literally put the squeeze on the medulla, producing a variety of respiratory abnormalities, including apnea. A stroke may have a similar effect by depriving portions of the brain of circulation, and therefore oxygenated blood (see Chapter 18, *Cardiovascular Emergencies*). Overdose with a central nervous system depressant, such as an opiate or barbiturate, may also severely depress respiratory center activity.

Severe traumatic brain injuries result in bizarre respiratory patterns when one or more of the brain's respiratory centers are damaged or deprived of adequate blood flow. **TABLE 17-5** summarizes various breathing patterns.

YOU are the Paramedic

PART 3

You have administered oxygen to the patient via a nonrebreathing mask, but this intervention does not seem to be improving his condition. His oxygen saturation level is still in the low 80s, so you decide to apply continuous positive airway pressure (CPAP). The patient is visibly anxious and is asking you to help him. Your partner helps assemble the CPAP equipment while you begin continuous electrocardiogram (ECG) monitoring. The 12-lead ECG shows ST elevation in leads 2 and 3. You inquire again if the patient has any chest pain or discomfort, which he denies.

Recording Time: 5 Minutes	
Respirations	34 breaths/min; shallow and rapid
Pulse	110 beats/min; weak
Skin	Gray and clammy
Blood pressure	140/100 mm Hg
Oxygen saturation (Spo_2)	80% with oxygen by nonrebreathing mask
Pupils	Pupils Equal, Round, and Reactive to Light and Accommodation (PERRLA)

5. Does this patient have an airway condition or a breathing disorder?

6. Does the absence of chest pain or discomfort indicate the patient is not having a heart attack?

TABLE 17-5 Breathing Patterns

Pattern	Description
Agonal	Slow, shallow, irregular, or occasional gasping breaths; results from cerebral anoxia. Agonal gasps may be observed when the heart has stopped but the brain continues to send signals to the muscles of respiration
Apneustic	Prolonged, gasping inhalation followed by extremely short, ineffective exhalation; associated with brainstem insult; an ominous sign of severe brain injury
Ataxic	Chaotically irregular respirations that indicate severe brain injury or brainstem herniation
Biot respirations	Irregular pattern, rate, and depth of breathing with intermittent periods of apnea; results from increased intracranial pressure and indicates severe brain injury or brainstem herniation
Bradypnea	Unusually slow respiration
Central neurogenic hyperventilation	Tachypneic hyperpnea; rapid, deep respirations caused by increased intracranial pressure or direct brain injury; drives the carbon dioxide level down and pH up, resulting in respiratory alkalosis
Cheyne-Stokes respirations	Gradual increase in rate and depth of respirations, followed by a gradual decrease of respirations with intermittent periods of apnea; associated with brainstem insult; not considered ominous unless it is grossly exaggerated or occurs in a patient with brain trauma
Cough	Forced exhalation against a closed glottis; an airway-clearing maneuver; also occurs when foreign substances irritate the airways; controlled by the cough center in the brain (antitussive medications work on the cough center to reduce this sometimes annoying physiologic response)
Eupnea	Normal breathing; regular rate and pattern; inspiration and expiration are equal
Hiccup	Spasmodic contraction of the diaphragm, causing short exhalations with a characteristic sound; sometimes seen in cases of diaphragmatic (or phrenic) nerve irritation from acute myocardial infarction, ulcerating disease, or endotracheal intubation
Hyperpnea	Abnormally increased rate and depth of breathing; seen in various neurologic and chemical disorders, including overdose with certain drugs
Hypopnea	Abnormally decreased rate and depth of breathing
Kussmaul respirations	Deep, gasping respirations; caused by the body's attempt, during metabolic acidosis, to rid itself of blood acetone via the lungs; observed in diabetic ketoacidosis; accompanied by a fruity (acetone) breath odor and, usually, cracked and dry mouth and lips
Sighing	Periodic deep breath of about twice the normal volume; forces open alveoli that routinely close from time to time
Tachypnea	Excessively rapid and shallow breathing; does not reflect the depth of respiration and does not mean a patient is hyperventilating (breathing too rapidly and deeply, resulting in a reduced carbon dioxide level); often involves moving only small volumes of air, or hypoventilation (much like a panting dog)
Yawning	Somewhat involuntary opening of the mouth and deep inhalation, followed by a slow exhalation; often stimulated by drowsiness or fatigue

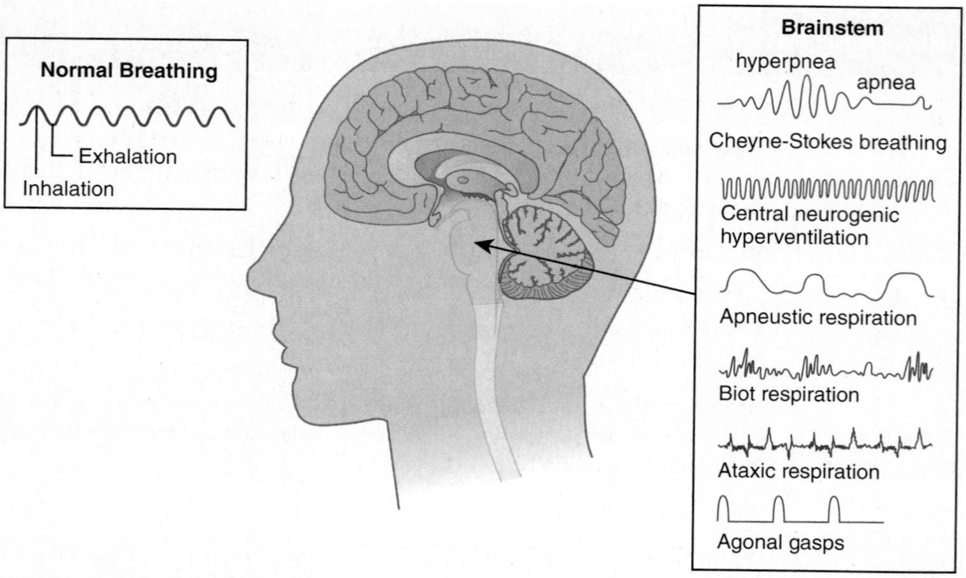

FIGURE 17-12 The neurologic control of respiration is complex, and many variations in the respiratory pattern may occur in a patient with brain injury. The respiratory patterns shown here, each recorded for 1 minute, were documented using an end-tidal carbon dioxide detector. Note that most irregular breathing patterns are controlled by the brainstem.

Most of the brain's respiratory centers are located in and around the brainstem **FIGURE 17-12**. Patients with serious trauma to the upper cerebral hemispheres, such as penetrating trauma from a gunshot wound, are often still breathing despite having mortal wounds. Apneustic breathing is caused by damage to the pneumotaxic center in the brain, which regulates the inspiratory pause. In a patient with apneustic respiration, each short, brisk inhalation is followed by a long pause before exhalation. This pattern indicates severe pressure within the cranium or direct trauma to the brain. Similarly, Biot respirations are seen when the center that controls breathing rhythm is damaged. This respiratory pattern is grossly irregular, sometimes including lengthy apneic periods.

Cheyne-Stokes respirations are more of a higher brain function. Many deep sleepers or intoxicated people have this respiratory pattern. The depth of breathing (or volume of snoring) gradually increases and then decreases (crescendo-decrescendo), followed by an apneic period. The apneic period is usually brief in a relatively healthy person. Exaggerated Cheyne-Stokes respirations, in which the crescendo-decrescendo cycle is much more pronounced, may be seen in patients with severe brain injury.

Words of Wisdom

Cheyne-Stokes respiration is clinically defined by specific time and cycle aspects. The American Academy of Sleep Medicine recommends scoring a respiratory event as Cheyne-Stokes breathing if the following two criteria are met[9]:

1. There are episodes of at least three consecutive central apneas and/or central hypopneas separated by a crescendo and decrescendo change in breathing amplitude with a cycle length of at least 40 seconds (typically 45 to 90 seconds).
2. There are five or more central apneas and/or central hypopneas per hour associated with the crescendo-decrescendo breathing pattern recorded over a minimum of 2 hours of monitoring.

Injury high in the spinal cord may paralyze the intercostal muscles and even the diaphragm. Whereas polio infection attacks the nerves that supply the respiratory muscles, certain chronic illnesses, such as myasthenia gravis, weaken the respiratory muscles themselves. The net effect of these conditions is inability of the respiratory muscles to function normally in response to the respiratory drive. As a consequence, tidal volume is shallow and is accompanied by a corresponding decrease in minute volume. Patients with such conditions often need assisted ventilation to boost their tidal volume, thereby increasing their minute volume.

Circulation Assessment in the Context of Respiratory Emergencies

Assessing skin color is a fast way to determine the adequacy of the patient's circulation **FIGURE 17-13**. Although it is important to note the generalized cyanosis of oxygen desaturation or the pallor of shock, more subtle information can be gained by assessing the mucous membranes. The tissue inside the mouth, under the eyelids, and even in the nail beds is usually the same pink color in all healthy patients. A few notable variations are as follows:

- **Cyanosis.** Healthy adults have a hemoglobin level of 12 to 14 g/dL. With a hemoglobin level in this range, the discoloration associated with cyanosis—typically blue in patients with light skin tone, gray-green in those with yellow skin tone, and ashen or gray in patients with darker skin tone—becomes apparent when approximately 5 g/dL of hemoglobin becomes desaturated (has no oxygen molecules attached). Such a person's oxygen saturation would be roughly 65%! If a person's hemoglobin level were only 10 g/dL, then 50% of the hemoglobin molecules (5 g/dL of the 10 g/dL) would have to become desaturated before the patient would look cyanotic. Similarly, in patients with high hemoglobin levels, such as those with chronic respiratory disease, cyanosis may develop earlier than in persons with normal hemoglobin levels. Of course, there are slight variations in what is considered normal. In addition, some patients with chronic respiratory conditions who have an artificially low oxygen saturation may also have a low level of chronic cyanosis. Patients with chronic bronchitis, for example, often have chronically low oxygen levels and relatively high hemoglobin levels, resulting in chronic peripheral cyanosis.
- **Dark brown skin.** High levels of methemoglobin derived from nitrates and specific toxic exposures may turn the mucous membranes brown. This transformation is typically more evident in the patient's venous blood than in the skin and mucous membranes.
- **Pallor.** Pallor of the skin and mucous membranes can be caused by several conditions, including hypoxia, shock, frostbite, lack of sun exposure, anemia, or the release of catecholamines, such as epinephrine or norepinephrine. Because skin pallor can be challenging to detect in patients with dark skin, check for pale mucous membranes inside the inner lower eyelid or oral mucosa. In patients with dark skin, pallor may appear as ashen or gray. Pallor may present as a shade of yellow in patients with brown skin and as a white color in patients with light skin. It is important to recognize that pallor is not always a sign of disease. For example, albinism is a genetic disorder that causes the skin to have little or no color.

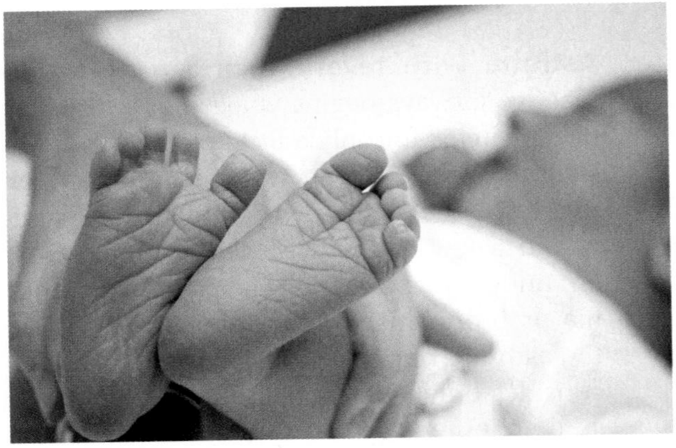

FIGURE 17-13 Skin color changes can be an early indicator of several disease processes. Skin color changes, such as the cyanosis seen here in an infant with light skin tone, can be an early indicator of several disease processes.

Note whether the patient's mucous membranes are moist or dry. Dehydration can be seen in the mucous membranes of the mouth and eyes. Dry, cracked lips; a dry, furrowed tongue; and dry, sunken eyes point to obvious dehydration. The skin of an older patient may always look dry because of reduced moisture.

Transport Decision

The treatment of acute cardiac and respiratory disorders is a fundamental component of care delivered in virtually all emergency departments (EDs). Patients with respiratory conditions are usually transported to the closest medical facility. Patients whose respiratory distress is related to renal failure would benefit from being taken to a facility that can provide emergency dialysis. (Not all centers that provide routine dialysis offer it on weekends or at night.)

Sometimes multiple EDs are available, separated by only a few minutes of additional travel time. In such cases, you must weigh the benefits of taking a patient to a preferred facility, where previous laboratory and radiograph results and the patient's own physician may be available, against the advantages of going to the closest facility. Patients with acute decompensation should usually be taken to the closest facility, but most patients with respiratory conditions can tolerate a few extra minutes during transport if the delay facilitates their care after arrival.

Special Populations

In some areas, specialty pediatric centers are an option for children, particularly children with tracheostomies, home ventilators, or other sophisticated ventilatory support.

History Taking

Ask patients to explain in their own words what they are feeling. Many patients can identify their conditions and explain the best way to treat it. A patient with a chronic respiratory condition is often knowledgeable about the disease or disorder and may have tried several treatment options before your arrival or might relate useful insights relating to past episodes, such as having been intubated and placed on a ventilator for a previous attack. Many patients with chronic respiratory disease have some symptoms all of the time. The pertinent question, then, is this: "What changed that made you call 9-1-1 today?" Increased cough, a change in the amount or color of sputum, fever, or wheezing may be some of the chief complaints, in addition to the usual dyspnea. Chest pain is also a common chief complaint. Its origin may range from myocardial ischemia leading to acute left-side heart failure, to pneumonia and pleural infection.

One challenge in assessing patients with respiratory conditions is that they may not be able to talk because of their difficulty breathing. Although it is usually best to ask open-ended questions and permit patients to tell their own stories, dyspneic patients may be able to speak only in short, choppy sentences. Some may be able to do no more than nod or shake their heads in response to a series of yes-or-no questions. In some cases, the bulk of the history taking may have to be hastily obtained from a family member or gleaned from the few clues immediately available, such as the medications present in the home. Interventions (such as oxygen or aerosol therapy) often must be instituted before getting the complete story from a patient. Sometimes, a patient must immediately be intubated, which precludes the possibility of obtaining a direct history from that point on.

When patients can discuss their chief complaints with you, they can often tell you exactly what condition they have. If they have one of the common respiratory illnesses (eg, asthma, COPD, or heart failure), then they may be having an acute flare-up (called an exacerbation). In other cases, they might have one of the following common disorders:

- **Asthma with fever.** When a patient with reactive airways begins wheezing, an inhaler usually helps for only a little while before the symptoms return. The typical asthma attack that responds to treatment but flares up again within a few hours is sometimes caused by an underlying infection (such as pneumonia or bronchitis), which repeatedly triggers the asthmalike symptoms. The asthma attack subsides only when the trigger is treated. Be sure to note signs of respiratory infection. Does the patient have a fever or chills? Is the patient coughing up sputum? What color is the sputum?
- **Nondelivery of medication.** Some inhalers indicate how many actuations (puffs) they are designed to deliver and how many doses

remain in the canister. If an automatic counter is not available, most patients do not keep close track of their use. Often the medication has been exhausted even though some propellant remains in the canister. A patient may have been inhaling nothing but propellant for days, which explains why the wheezing is not getting better. Similar difficulties can occur when patients use outdated medications or medications that have overheated or otherwise been stored improperly (eg, left in a hot automobile or similar environment). In such cases, the bronchodilator from your drug box may be effective, even though the patient's medication failed to produce results. Another possible scenario is that a patient does not fully understand how to use the device and does not inhale at an appropriate point, instead spraying the medicine on the inside of the mouth. This potential error is one reason that physicians often prescribe a spacer device to be used with an inhaler.

- **Travel-related conditions.** Advances in technology have given patients with chronic respiratory disease much more freedom to leave the house and to travel. Some patients present with significant pulmonary edema after a lengthy journey. The culprit: not wanting to take diuretics while traveling. Remember to ask the obvious ("What medications do you use?"), and follow up with "Did you take them during your trip?"

  In addition, paramedics may be called to assist someone whose oxygen tank has run dry, whose portable ventilator has suddenly malfunctioned, or whose medications were left behind or lost with the luggage.
- **Dyspnea triggers.** Just because a person knows the triggers for a reactive airway, such as pet dander, perfume, cigarette smoke or smog, pollen, or excessive heat, humidity, or cold, that does not mean these triggers can always be avoided. A social or family situation may be important enough to risk having an episode of dyspnea, and no one can prevent all contact with all triggers, many of which are present in public places.
- **Seasonal conditions.** Bacteria, mold, and fungi can grow in heating ducts or in air conditioning units during their respective off-seasons. When the weather suddenly changes and the use of heating or air conditioning systems begins, you can usually expect an increased number of calls from people with chronic respiratory diseases.
- **Noncompliance with therapy.** Some people with chronic respiratory disease rebel against therapy in an attempt to regain control over their lives. Other patients do not understand the long-term nature of the therapy and attempt to wean themselves off their medications, oxygen, or respiratory support devices. Unfortunately, these attempts may results in a crisis. Still other patients have been prescribed home oxygen, aerosol therapy, CPAP, bilevel positive airway pressure (BPAP), or a variety of medications that they do not use or that they take only sporadically. Dangerous complications can occur if certain medications, such as oral corticosteroids, are stopped abruptly.

The mnemonic SAMPLE (Signs and symptoms, Allergies, Medications, Pertinent past medical history, Last oral intake, Events preceding the onset of the complaint) helps paramedics systematically obtain information about the history of the present illness and the patient's medical history.

- **Signs and symptoms.** Respiratory difficulty must always be evaluated in light of the patient's cardiovascular and renal status. Many acute myocardial infarctions present as heart failure, for example, as do renal crises. Tachypnea can signal anxiety, diabetes, or shock. In addition, the vast majority of chronically ill patients have a respiratory component to their diseases. A whole host of pathologic conditions can masquerade as respiratory distress, especially in patients with underlying respiratory disease. Don't be too quick to conclude that the patient's *only* condition is a relatively straightforward respiratory disorder. Always dig deeper to determine what else may be triggering or worsening the patient's respiratory distress.
- **Allergies.** A person may know the triggers for the respiratory difficulties but be unable to avoid them. During your assessment, ask whether the patient has been exposed to a known trigger.

- **Medications.** Part of a thorough history includes reviewing the patient's prescribed and over-the-counter medications. Many patients take multiple medications. A common combination might include a rapid-acting **beta-2 agonist** (rescue inhaler), a corticosteroid, and a slow-acting bronchodilator.

  Dyspneic patients might resort to using (and sometimes misusing) over-the-counter medications in addition to their prescribed medications. The following is a list of over-the-counter medications that a patient may use in conjunction with any prescriptions:
  - Antihistamines dry out secretions and are a common ingredient in many over-the-counter cough and cold medications.
  - Antitussives are used to suppress cough. Because coughing helps clear secretions from the airways, suppressing a cough might not be helpful. Coughing can be annoying, particularly if it interrupts sleep. However, the need for comfort must be weighed against the need to rid the airway of excess secretions. Overuse of antitussives can cause sedation, reduce respiratory drive, and partially obstruct the airway with secretions. Many over-the-counter cough syrups also contain antihistamines that can cause respiratory symptoms if not used appropriately.
  - Some bronchodilators are available as over-the-counter preparations. They often produce a nonspecific response, meaning the medication may also have a significant effect on the heart and blood vessels, particularly when used in addition to a prescription bronchodilator. The most commonly encountered over-the-counter bronchodilators are simply attenuated (diluted) forms of epinephrine.
  - Expectorants thin out the pulmonary secretions so that they can be coughed up, and most of these medications can be purchased over the counter. Many products combine expectorants with antitussives or antihistamines. These combinations are often at odds with each other. People with increased mucus production should avoid antihistamine products, taking only products that contain the expectorant guaifenesin.

  By following a simple interviewing pattern, it becomes possible to determine which medications the patient is supposed to take (which often yields valuable clues about the patient's other conditions), whether the patient is taking the medications correctly, and whether the patient has any medication allergies.
- **Pertinent past medical history.** An asthma attack, heart failure, pneumonia in an immunocompromised patient, and even spontaneous pneumothorax are pathologic conditions that often occur repeatedly. A patient's experience with these types of events can serve as a baseline against which to assess the current condition. Ask these questions: Do you feel better or worse than last time? How often does this happen to you? What did the doctor tell you it was? What helped you or what happened last time?

  In addition, ask patients about tobacco use, secondhand smoke exposure, and other possible toxic exposures.
- **Last oral intake.** The typical reason for ascertaining the patient's last oral intake is concern about a full stomach should ET intubation be required. Patients with chronic respiratory disease also tend to eat and drink less when they become acutely ill, which can add dehydration, hypoglycemia, or malnutrition to the already complex picture of their illness.
- **Events preceding the onset of the complaint.** It is important to determine what was happening just before or when the patient began having symptoms. In addition, the speed with which the patient's distress has worsened is an important consideration in determining the underlying cause. Did the symptoms arise suddenly, or did they get worse over time? How long have the symptoms been this bad? The position of comfort and difficulty speaking may also indicate the degree of distress. A patient who is comfortable lying flat and who is speaking in full sentences can be assumed to be in little distress. A patient who is sitting in a **Fowler position** (sitting upright) and who is speaking only in two- or three-word statements is probably in considerable distress, possibly even life-threatening distress. Such a patient might be described as having "three-word dyspnea."

When respiratory disorders are chronic or recurring, patients may have already developed crisis management strategies. Determine what the patient may have already tried and whether it had any effect (positive or negative). Ask what the patient was doing when the dyspnea began. Patients often know exactly what set off the episode.

Secondary Assessment

By the time you have elicited a patient's history, you should have already gathered some important information about the patient's physical signs, such as level of consciousness, position, and degree of distress. This section presents the physical exam components in sequence, noting at each step the points of particular relevance to a patient with dyspnea.

Assessing the level of consciousness is imperative in patients with dyspnea. Although the patient's arterial blood gases cannot be measured in the field, the patient's brain is constantly doing precisely that. Any decline in the partial pressure of oxygen (Pao_2) constitutes hypoxemia and initially manifests as restlessness and confusion. In worst-case scenarios, it may progress to combative behavior. An increase in the partial pressure of carbon dioxide ($Paco_2$), by contrast, usually has sedative effects, making the patient sleepy and difficult to rouse.

If the lungs are not functioning properly, then oxygen delivery and carbon dioxide removal may be impaired. Failure to deliver oxygen efficiently results in cellular hypoxia. Hypoxia kills cells by making it impossible for them to produce enough energy to do their work; it also causes acidosis. Because the brain is highly sensitive to reduced levels of oxygen, any alteration in level of consciousness could represent some degree of respiratory compromise. Anxiety can be an early sign of hypoxia, whereas confusion, lethargy, and coma are typically later signs. A brief seizure often accompanies a hypoxic event or cardiac arrest. Dizziness and tingling extremities could signify hyperventilation.

In the neck, look for **jugular venous distention (JVD)** when a patient is in a semi-sitting position. JVD is a condition in which the jugular veins are engorged with blood. Healthy young adults often have JVD when they are supine, and it is common to see gross JVD when people are laughing or singing **FIGURE 17-14**.

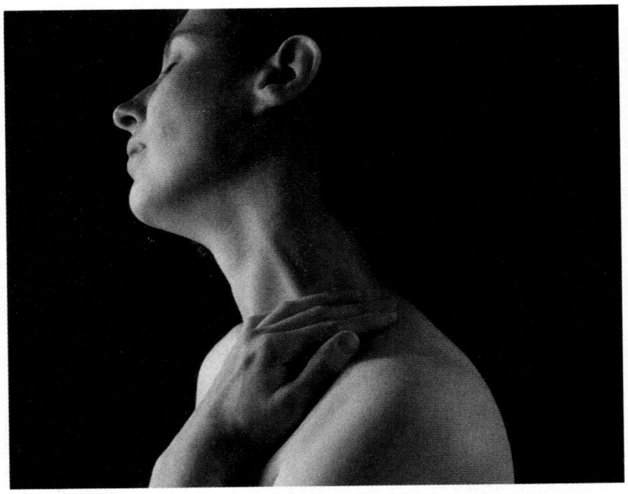

FIGURE 17-14 Jugular venous distention may be a normal finding in a healthy young adult who is supine or laughing. In an adult who is sitting upright, however, distention may indicate that blood is backing up as it tries to enter the thorax or the right atrium.

Cardiac tamponade, pneumothorax, heart failure, and COPD can all cause JVD. Distended neck veins may implicate cardiac failure as the source of dyspnea. JVD may also indicate that high pressure in the thorax is keeping the blood from draining out of the head and neck. In patients with normal blood flow, deoxygenated blood returns to the right side of the heart from the venae cavae and continues to the lungs to be oxygenated. Conditions that affect the functionality of the right side of the heart or lungs may prohibit the superior vena cava from draining due to the increased pressure. As blood backs up, the jugular vein becomes engorged, leading to distention.

JVD must be interpreted in the light of the patient's position and other vital signs. The presence of JVD in a patient who is sitting upright provides a rough measure of the pressure in the right atrium of the heart. Grossly distended jugular veins despite a BP of 80/40 mm Hg in a trauma patient should cause considerable concern; in contrast, JVD in a healthy 20-year-old person who is lying flat (but not while sitting) is of little concern.

While you are examining the neck, note the position of the trachea. Tracheal deviation is a classic, albeit late, sign of a tension pneumothorax **FIGURE 17-15**. The deviation occurs behind the sternum, so this sign is difficult to palpate except

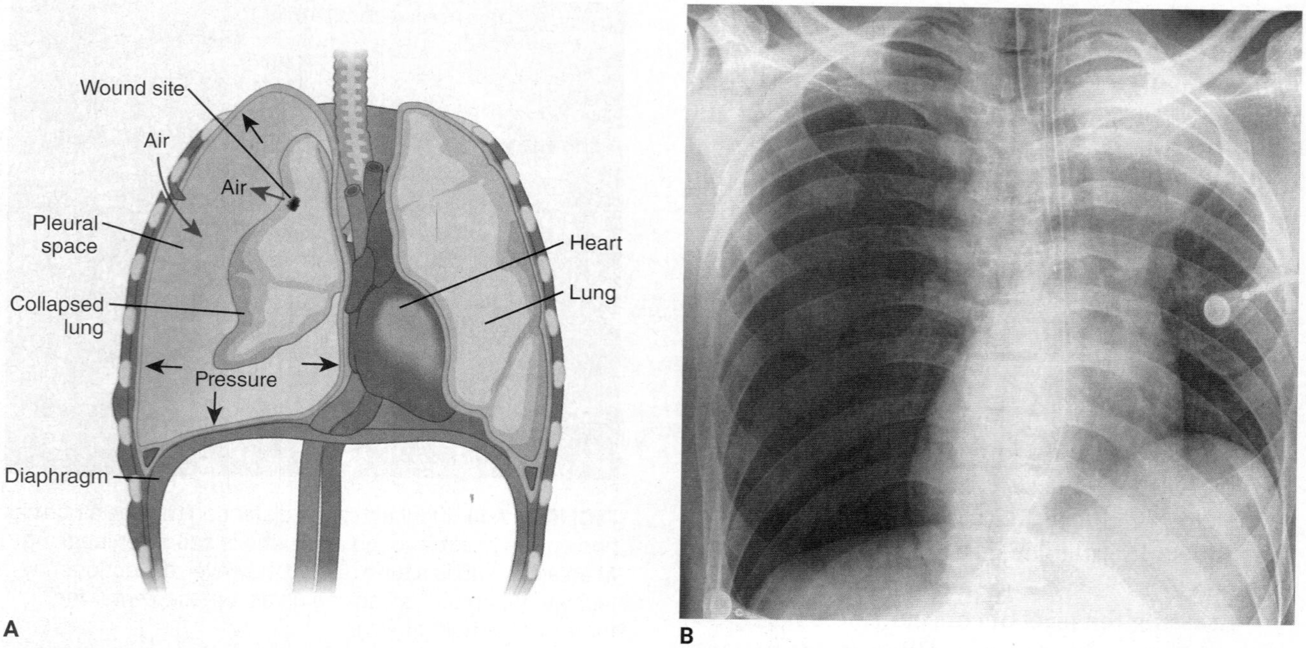

FIGURE 17-15 Pneumothorax occurs when air leaks into the pleural space between the lung and the chest wall **(A)**; radiograph **(B)** shows a collapsed right lung, which appears darker.

A: © Jones & Bartlett Learning; B: Courtesy of Stuart Mirvis, MD.

in extreme cases. Consider palpating the trachea at the suprasternal notch. On a radiograph, tracheal deviation caused by tension pneumothorax can be clearly identified.

Next, examine the chest and abdomen. When the right ventricle is not pumping effectively, blood backs up, making it difficult for the jugular veins and the large reservoir of blood in the liver to drain into the thorax. As a result, the combination of JVD and hepatomegaly (distended liver) may occur in patients with right-side heart failure. **Hepatojugular reflux** is distention of the jugular veins when the liver is gently pressed; it is specific to right-side heart failure. Assess for hepatojugular reflux by pressing gently on the liver while the patient is in a semi-Fowler (45° angle) position.

Feel the chest for vibrations as the patient breathes. Large-airway secretions produce obvious vibrations, called **tactile fremitus**, that are usually easy to feel and to hear. Some sources recommend performing chest percussion. With experience, the paramedic may be able to distinguish between the sound of a normal chest and the sound of a chest full of either blood (hemothorax) or air (pneumothorax), which will be hypertympanic to percussion. A chest tumor will be dull to percussion. Percussion remains a difficult procedure to use in the field, however, because of ambient noise.

Chest or abdominal trauma can cause respiratory distress by a variety of mechanisms (see Chapter 36, *Chest Trauma*, and Chapter 37, *Abdominal and Genitourinary Trauma*).

As you examine the patient's extremities, take note of anything unusual. Does the patient have edema of the ankles or lower back? If so, does it pit when you push a finger into the edematous tissue **FIGURE 17-16**? Is there peripheral cyanosis? Check the pulse. Does the patient have profound tachycardia as a result of exertion or hypoxia? Is there a weak or imperceptible peripheral pulse on inspiration (known as pulsus paradoxus)? Note the patient's skin temperature and check for any obvious fever. Is the patient's skin cool and clammy from shock? Is there distal clubbing as a result of chronic hypoxia **FIGURE 17-17**?

Vital Signs and Monitoring Devices

In addition to respiratory rate and quality of respirations, vital signs provide obvious clues to the respiratory workload. Patients under stress can be

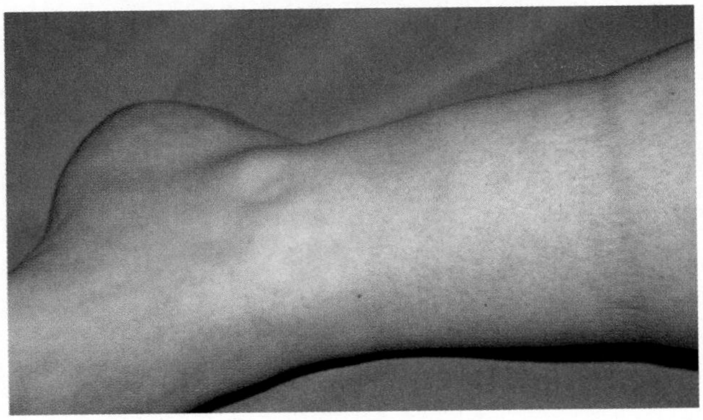

FIGURE 17-16 Pitting edema is present when the fingers leave a temporary depression in the tissue.

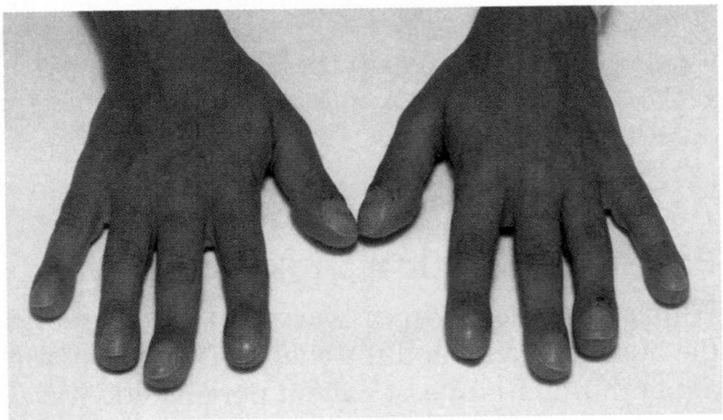

FIGURE 17-17 Digital clubbing is a sign of chronic hypoxia. It is seen in young people with congenital heart disease and in older people with severe chronic lung disease.

expected to have tachycardia because of hypoxemia, the use of sympathomimetic drugs, and the stress of dyspnea. They often also have hypertension for the same reasons. Bradycardia, hypotension, and a falling respiratory rate are ominous signs of impending arrest in patients with respiratory diseases.

As appropriate to the patient care plan, apply any monitors that are immediately available. Repeated vital signs, ECG, and pulse oximetry readings are the data most commonly collected. In some situations, depending on the available equipment, peak expiratory flow, $ETCO_2$, and transcutaneous carbon monoxide levels might also be recorded.

Stethoscope

Your stethoscope is one of the most important and frequently used tools at your command. Choose one that meets your needs and, of course, your budget. Make it a habit to clean your stethoscope between patient contacts. Check that the earpieces are clean and clear of earwax, and regularly wipe the length of the main tubing with an all-purpose cleaner to slow the breakdown of the tube from the oils picked up when the stethoscope is placed around the neck.

Pulse Oximeter

A pulse oximeter is a noninvasive device that measures the percentage of a patient's hemoglobin to which oxygen molecules are attached. Oxygen saturation greater than 94% is considered normal.

A pulse oximeter must "see" a pulsatile capillary bed to return an accurate reading. Inadequate peripheral perfusion, cold extremities, or the patient's movement (tremors or shivering) can make the reading inaccurate. A variety of pulse oximeter probes are available that may allow readings to be taken from the earlobe, forehead, or other areas of the body. Most pulse oximeters also display the patient's pulse rate; this reading should match the palpated heart rate.

If the patient's hemoglobin level is low, for example, as a consequence of trauma or hemorrhage, then the pulse oximetry result will be correspondingly high. If a patient's hemoglobin is only 6 g/dL (normal is 12 to 14 g/dL), then the oxygen saturation will probably be 100%. Such a patient needs more hemoglobin in the form of whole blood or packed red blood cells; providing additional oxygen would be of little value. Some people, such as those who live at high altitudes or have chronic hypoxia (eg, patients with COPD), have abnormally high hemoglobin levels, along with a correspondingly low oxygen saturation. For example, a patient with a combination of moderate hypoxia and polycythemia (excess red blood cell production) may have an oxygen saturation level that normally hovers around 90%.

While it is relatively easy to measure oxygenation, a favorable oxygen saturation result does not necessarily mean all is well. A pulse oximeter cannot differentiate between an oxygen molecule attached to hemoglobin and a carbon monoxide molecule attached to that same hemoglobin. Most people who live in an industrialized society have a 1% to 2% carbon monoxide level all the time. Smokers may have a level as high as 3% to 4%. Thus, a 97% pulse oximetry reading may actually represent 95% oxygen saturation and 2% carbon monoxide saturation. A patient whose hemoglobin has a toxic or even fatal level of carbon monoxide bound to it may nevertheless show a normal or high pulse oximetry value. Portable devices that specifically measure carbon monoxide levels enable paramedics to readily assess for carbon monoxide poisoning in the field **FIGURE 17-18**. These devices are available in some systems.

The oxyhemoglobin dissociation curve illustrates the relationship between oxygen saturation and the amount of oxygen dissolved in the plasma (Pao_2) **FIGURE 17-19**. It demonstrates that when oxygen molecules are scarce, they readily bind to hemoglobin, so that even small changes in Pao_2 bring about relatively large changes in oxygen saturation. As the hemoglobin receptors begin to fill up with oxygen molecules, larger changes in Pao_2 (shown on the horizontal axis of the curve) are required to produce changes in oxygen saturation.

Placing a nonrebreathing mask on a healthy patient may increase the saturation level from 96% to 99%, whereas giving oxygen by a nasal cannula at 2 L/min to a hypoxic patient may increase the oxygen saturation from 80% to 92%, a more significant change. Conversely, the more hypoxic a patient becomes, the faster desaturation will occur after the patient falls off the steep part of the oxyhemoglobin dissociation curve. Other factors, such as acid–base balance and body temperature, can also affect the entire system, shifting the curve to the left or right.

Words of Wisdom

In considering the differences between pulse oximetry and waveform capnography, keep in mind that oxygenation and ventilation are separate processes. Pulse oximetry accurately measures oxygen saturation but does not directly provide information about alveolar ventilation. The finding of decreased oxygenation may suggest a ventilation abnormality, but ventilation assessment is immediate and unambiguous when using capnography. Providers must remember that although pulse oximetry is currently the standard technique for measuring oxygen saturation, it does not provide early warning of hypoventilation, apnea, or airway obstruction in patients.[10]

End-Tidal Carbon Dioxide Monitor

With $ETCO_2$ detection, or waveform capnography, the absolute value and the shape of the waveform are both important assessment parameters. Waveform capnography can also be used to document unusual respiratory patterns and evaluate the

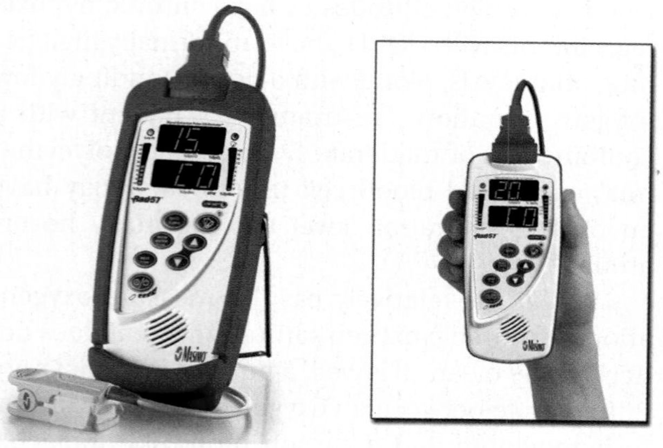

FIGURE 17-18 Devices are available that can measure oxygen saturation and carbon monoxide levels.

The Masimo® Rad-ST™ Pulse CO-Oximeter™courtesy of Masimo Corporation (www.masimo.com).

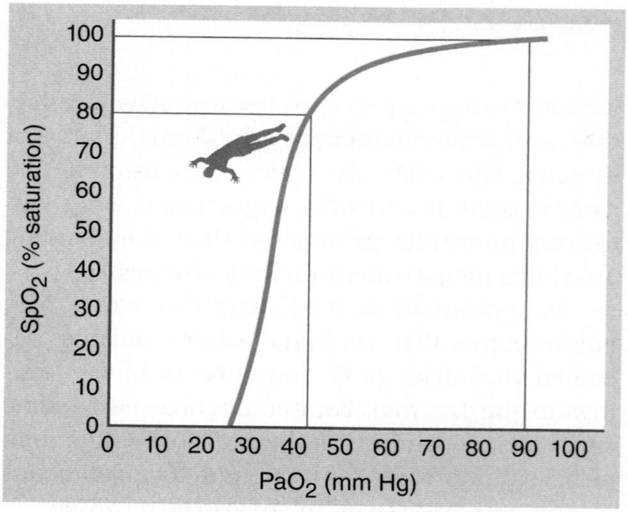

FIGURE 17-19 The oxyhemoglobin dissociation curve. As a patient becomes increasingly hypoxemic (lower Pao_2 [partial pressure of oxygen]), the patient may fall off the curve as saturation drops rapidly.

effectiveness of treatment. This technology is discussed in detail in Chapter 16, *Airway Management*.

Peak Expiratory Flowmeter

Peak flow is the maximum rate at which a patient can expel air from the lungs. (Chapter 16, *Airway Management*, describes the use of a peak expiratory flowmeter.) A lower value indicates that the patient's larger airways are narrowed by bronchial constriction or bronchial edema. Many patients with pulmonary disease check their peak flow twice per day and chart the results. They may present this chart when EMS personnel arrive. Normal peak flow values vary by age, sex, and height, but generally run from approximately 350 to 700 L/min. A peak flow less than 150 L/min is considered inadequate and signals significant distress, although some people with chronic asthma have a peak flow that never exceeds 100 L/min. Both bronchoconstriction and airway edema can reduce peak flow. If a bronchodilator is administered but peak flow does not improve, then airway edema may be the cause, in which case steroids may be indicated.

Reassessment

Contact medical control to report any change in the patient's level of consciousness or any increased difficulty breathing. Document any changes, noting the time at which they occurred, and document any orders given by medical control.

Emergency Medical Care

In this section, we discuss how to care for a patient with dyspnea. Later in the chapter, we consider how to manage specific diseases and conditions.

Paramedics have a relatively short list of tools to treat respiratory compromise. At the most basic level, your goal is to provide supportive care, administer supplemental oxygen therapy, and provide monitoring and transport. In actuality, you can do little in the field to alter the course of a pathologic condition (eg, COPD, pneumonia, or pulmonary contusion).

The primary exception is the treatment of bronchoconstriction. A host of bronchodilators are available to help relax bronchial smooth muscle. Such therapy can be beneficial if the patient's primary condition is bronchial muscle spasm caused by anaphylaxis or asthma. Bronchodilator therapy may be somewhat helpful to many other patients as well.

At the other end of the spectrum of care are patients with overt respiratory failure. The primary approach to their care is to take over the work of breathing completely by intubating and manually ventilating the patient. CPAP and BPAP have also proved to be effective strategies and may help avoid intubation in many patients.

Perform Standard Interventions

Before the paramedic administers the medications discussed in the following sections, several interventions should have already been implemented. Administering oxygen to keep the saturation greater than or equal to 94%[10] and establishing an intravenous (IV) line are common interventions for any patient who needs advanced life support. Psychological support is also an important consideration for a patient with dyspnea. Your efforts to reduce the patient's anxiety with a calm, professional, caring demeanor can help reduce the patient's heart rate and BP and promote maximum breathing effectiveness. Finally, allow the patient to assume a position of comfort. Most patients with dyspnea prefer to sit upright or lean forward, which can also help alleviate their distress.

Decrease the Work of Breathing

Even under normal circumstances, muscles must work to allow breathing, and they must work much harder during respiratory distress. This extra work comes at a cost. People with asthma, for example, can often compensate for respiratory distress by devoting substantial energy to breathing. They can maintain their oxygen and carbon dioxide levels in an acceptable range as long as they continue to recruit their muscles for this effort. Unfortunately, the tremendous workload involved consumes large amounts of energy, which must be fueled by even more oxygen and ventilation. A patient in such a condition typically is not able to eat and drink normally, so they become progressively more dehydrated, malnourished, and fatigued. At some point, the patient will tire and be unable to continue the necessary work of breathing; this patient will look sleepy, the rate and depth of respiration will decrease slowly, and decompensation (respiratory failure) will occur. Some patients with asthma may compensate for days, hoping that their steroids and bronchodilators will resolve an attack. By the time they realize that those approaches are not working, they may be in too much distress to seek care except by calling 9-1-1.

The Trendelenburg and supine positions, especially in a patient who is overweight, cause the abdominal organs to compress the diaphragm. With each breath, the patient must move the abdominal contents out of the way to expand the thorax and breathe. Abdominal distention with air or blood further complicates this situation. Shortness of breath induced by lying flat is called **orthopnea**. It explains why most people maintain a sitting position when they are short of breath. To decrease the work of breathing, help the patient sit up, if that is more comfortable. Remove constricting clothing, such as belts and tight collars. *Do not make the person walk.* Relieve gastric distention, perhaps with a nasogastric tube. Do not bind the chest or make the patient lie on the side of the unaffected lung.

Provide Supplemental Oxygen

It is essential to provide supplemental oxygen to any patient who needs it. As with any other medication, you must administer oxygen in the concentrations necessary to be effective. Patients who are not breathing adequately should receive bag-mask ventilation with supplemental oxygen, or more advanced airway management techniques. Closely reassess the patient's breathing status, and adjust the treatment accordingly. Pulse oximetry is a useful guide to oxygenation if it is accurate (ie, the pulse rate on the oximeter matches the palpated pulse) and if the patient's hemoglobin level is relatively normal.

It is safe to administer oxygen in concentrations less than 50% to almost anyone, and it is appropriate to do so when there is a reasonable chance the patient would benefit from it. Reserve oxygen concentrations higher than 50% for patients with hypoxia who do not respond to lower concentrations, and limit the use of 100% oxygen to the shortest period necessary.

Of the total amount of oxygen in the body, approximately 97% is bound to hemoglobin; the other 3% is dissolved in the plasma. Once all of the hemoglobin in the blood has become saturated with oxygen, further exposure to high oxygen concentrations begins to damage the lung tissue.

As a paramedic, you will treat many patients who require supplemental oxygen to maintain an acceptable oxygen saturation. Do not hesitate to administer oxygen to those patients who need it; however, most patients with good oxygen saturation (at least 94%) will not benefit from supplemental oxygen.[12–14] Even patients with trauma, stroke, and acute coronary syndrome derive no benefit from supplemental oxygen therapy if their oxygen saturation is already at or above 94%.[10] **Hyperoxia** (an excess of oxygen) should be avoided. Oxygen saturation of 100% should also be avoided, because it is impossible to predict how high the blood oxygen level may rise once the hemoglobin becomes completely saturated.

In a few situations, the pulse oximeter may not provide an accurate picture of oxygenation, such as in cases of carbon monoxide intoxication. In a pregnant patient, you might hyperoxygenate the pregnant woman in an attempt to deliver oxygen to a potentially compromised fetus. Be sure to follow your local protocol and consult medical control in such emergencies.

Words of Wisdom

The Renaissance physician Paracelsus observed that it is the dose of a substance, not its composition, that makes it poisonous. Even water, the most innocuous of all substances, can become toxic if a person ingests too much of it.

Just as any medication administered in high doses can kill a person, so, too, can the overzealous use of oxygen. Use moderation and common sense in deciding whether to administer or continue supplemental oxygen.

Administer a Bronchodilator

Many patients with respiratory distress will respond positively to bronchodilation, and some patients may benefit substantially. Today's aerosol bronchodilators rarely harm patients, so paramedics tend to use them aggressively in the field. Patients who do not have bronchospasm usually benefit only slightly from aerosol bronchodilators, however, and the oxygen concentration delivered is often reduced during a typical aerosol treatment. Under these circumstances, application of a nonrebreathing mask is a better choice than the aerosol treatment. Follow local protocol, but remember that bronchodilators are of little value in treating conditions such as pneumonia, pulmonary edema, and heart disease.

Bronchodilators relax the smooth muscle around the larger bronchi and are a significant therapy for bronchoconstriction. Fast-acting bronchodilators, which are administered using so-called rescue inhalers, provide almost instant relief: a property that sometimes leads to their misuse. Strictly speaking, bronchodilators do not reduce swelling, kill bacteria, push fluid out of the lungs, or open closed alveoli. However, patients with pneumonia, heart failure, or atelectasis may have a small amount of secondary bronchoconstriction that could be reversed with a bronchodilator.

Today, a medication specifically designed for aerosol use, ipratropium, is available. It is also available in an inhaler. In addition, the combination of albuterol (a beta-2 agonist) and ipratropium (an anticholinergic) is available as an aerosol spray or in a metered-dose inhaler (MDI). Popular long-acting bronchodilators have dramatically improved the quality of life for many patients with respiratory illness when they use these medications correctly.

Aerosol Therapy

An aerosol treatment is a simple method of delivering medications, such as bronchodilators. Aerosol nebulizers deliver liquid medications in the form of a fine mist **FIGURE 17-20**. Particles of approximately 5 micrometers ride the laminar airflow into the lower respiratory tract. Larger particles rain out in the mouth and pharynx and are swallowed, so they have little ultimate effect. Particles significantly smaller than 5 micrometers may be exhaled with the next breath. Most nebulizers need to have a gas flow of at least 6 L/min to generate the optimal particle size. Running the gas slower than that rate generates particles that are too large; running it significantly faster makes the particles smaller and makes the treatment go faster, with the potential for less medication delivery. While aerosol delivery is fast and convenient, only a small amount of the medication ultimately reaches the intended receptors. You should strive to maximize medication delivery by coaching the patient on proper technique.

In the home, most people run their aerosol treatments off of a small air compressor; in the ambulance, this therapy usually runs off of tanked oxygen or a wall unit attached to the main oxygen supply. As a result, the patient might receive only

YOU are the Paramedic

PART 4

While your partner prepares the patient for transport, you transmit the 12-lead ECG to the medical center and administer a dose of nitroglycerin paste. The patient's condition is still deteriorating. You have your partner begin positive-pressure ventilation with a bag-mask device, and you establish an IV line. The patient initially resists but eventually becomes more comfortable and tolerates the treatment. As soon as the patient is in the ambulance, you begin priority 1 transport to the medical facility. You contact medical control and request the use of additional nitroglycerin paste. The physician grants the request and also gives an order to administer 162 mg of chewable aspirin to the patient. During transport, the patient's oxygen saturation progressively increases with treatment.

Recording Time: 10 Minutes	
Respirations	28 breaths/min; assisted
Pulse	100 beats/min
Skin	Pallor and diaphoresis
Blood pressure	130/100 mm Hg
Oxygen saturation (Spo_2)	85% with oxygen by mask at 15 L/min and increasing
Pupils	PERRLA

7. What is the rationale for administering nitroglycerin if the patient has no chest pain or discomfort?

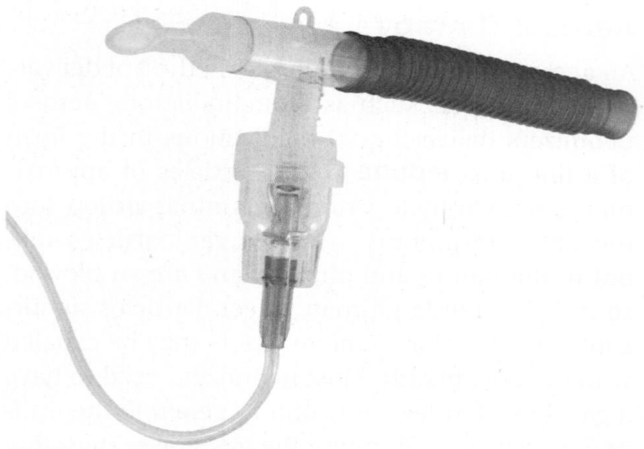

FIGURE 17-20 Aerosol nebulizers are often used to deliver medication directly to the respiratory tract. Unfortunately, they may supply only 30% to 40% oxygen during a treatment. Flow rate is an important factor in how much medication reaches the lungs. Do not confuse flow rate with oxygen concentration. Devices that work off the Venturi principle provide high flow rates but low to medium concentrations.

30% to 40% oxygen via an aerosol treatment; while this amount is still more than the 21% oxygen contained in room air, it may be less than the amount of supplemental oxygen required by a patient with significant hypoxia. The relative drop in the fraction of inspired oxygen that occurs when a patient's nonrebreathing mask is removed to administer an aerosol treatment may be a contraindication to this procedure, particularly if the aerosol therapy is relatively unlikely to improve the patient's condition.

A nebulizer can be attached to a mouthpiece (pipe), face mask, or **tracheostomy** collar, or it can simply be held in front of the patient's face: the so-called blow-by technique. The smaller the amount of mist the patient inhales, however, the less medication that is received. Blow-by and mouthpiece treatments are ineffective if patients continually turn their heads or remove the mouthpiece to answer questions. Once the decision has been made to deliver a breathing treatment, try to stop the conversation and let the patient focus on inhaling the medication.

The newer aerosol bronchodilators cause tachycardia far less often than is the case with the older, less beta-2–specific medications. As a result, it has become possible to give repeated treatments to patients with bronchospasm. Albuterol (Proventil, Ventolin), which is currently the most commonly used beta-2 agonist, is routinely given every 4 hours, but more frequent treatments and even continuous therapy for hours at a time are often administered without the occurrence of tachycardia. Continuous nebulizers that hold up to 10 times the usual medication dosages and run for an hour or more are available. However, they carry the potential for some beta-1 stimulation, causing tachycardia, so some physicians are concerned that the aerosol bronchodilators could worsen tachycardia in a patient with underlying cardiac disease. Tachycardia is almost always present in patients with dyspnea, so consult medical control or local protocols for guidance. The steps for administering medications via a small-volume nebulizer are shown in Chapter 14, *Medication Administration*.

Controversies

In some EMS systems, aerosol treatments are given to any patient who is dyspneic in the belief that they might help and are usually harmless; in other systems, use of aerosol bronchodilators is restricted to situations in which they are clearly indicated. Consult medical direction and your local protocols to keep abreast of how this class of medications is used in your region.

Metered-Dose Inhalers

When used correctly, an MDI delivers the same amount of medication as an aerosol treatment does. Because it does not require additional equipment (such as a nebulizer or air compressor), the MDI is usually the delivery method of choice for bronchodilators and corticosteroids in the home setting **FIGURE 17-21**. Because patients use (and may misuse) their own inhalers in the home, be sure to document how often the patient has been taking an extra puff. Do not forget to consult medical control before administering additional doses if this step is required in your system.

The MDIs in your drug box or on the emergency vehicle should ideally be equipped with **spacers**. A spacer is a device that collects the medication as it is released from the canister, allowing more to be delivered to the lungs and less to be lost to the environment. Remember, the mist coming out of

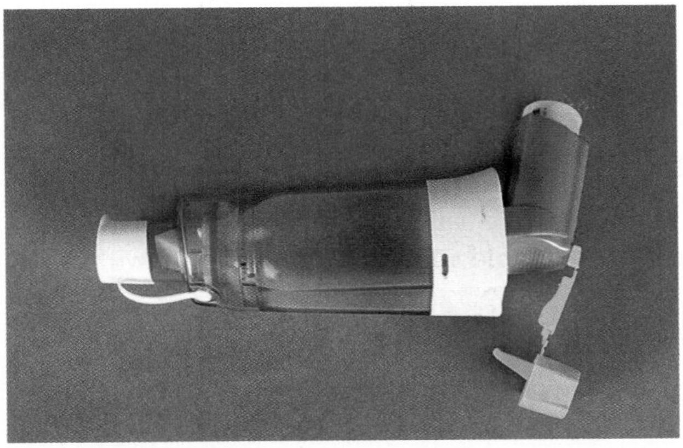

FIGURE 17-21 Metered-dose inhalers are a common delivery system for respiratory medications. Their effectiveness is greatly increased by using a spacer device (shown here), which regulates the release of medication into the inhaler.

the inhaler is not what reaches the patient's alveoli; rather, the 5-micrometer particles, which remain suspended in the spacer for several minutes, are pulled deep into the lungs by smooth laminar flow. When a spacer is used, the patient does not have to time the inhalation to coincide with the discharge of the inhaler. Spacers also reduce deposition of the medication into the mouth and oropharynx, which can occur with inexperienced users.

In addition to improving medication delivery, the spacer allows paramedics to use the same (expensive) inhaler for multiple patients. Each patient gets a new spacer, but the inhaler itself is used repeatedly. Be sure to establish a system to keep track of how many times an inhaler has been used so that patients receive the proper amount of medication, and not just propellant.

The correct technique when using a MDI is not difficult to master, but it requires constant reinforcement. The steps for administering medication with an MDI are shown in Chapter 14, *Medication Administration*. The following tips can help avoid common errors when using or administering a MDI:

- **The mist from an MDI must enter the lungs.** Therefore, patients must inhale deeply as they discharge the inhaler to draw the medication deep into their lungs. Placing the inhaler directly into the mouth (without a spacer) often causes much of the medication to fall on the posterior pharynx, where it is swallowed and subsequently digested, thereby negating its intended effect.
- **Some patients mistakenly blow into the spacer.** Tell them to think of the spacer as a big straw, from which they should try to suck the medication out of the bottom.
- **Many spacers make a harmonicalike sound if the patient sucks too hard.** The best particle deposition comes from smooth, low-pressure laminar flow. Inhaling too forcefully causes turbulent flow, making many of the particles stick to the trachea and large bronchi, where they are not as effective.
- **Patients should try to inhale the medication deeply and then hold their breath for a few seconds.** This is a lot to ask of someone who is dyspneic, and it is not always possible. Sometimes the inhalation causes the patient to cough immediately after inhaling the medication, which precludes delivery of a full dose but may be unavoidable.
- **Make sure the inhaler contains medication.** The labels of most inhalers list the number of puffs of medication in the canister. Patients should be encouraged to keep track of how many times they have used the inhaler and to discard it when they reach the recommended number of uses. The sound of fluid sloshing around when the canister is shaken is not a reliable indicator that it still contains medication.
- **Keep the spacer and canister holder clean.** Rinse off the spacer and canister holder occasionally to avoid inhaling dust and other particles. In addition, respiratory devices should be dried after they are cleaned to discourage the growth of microorganisms.
- **After using a corticosteroid inhaler, patients should rinse out the mouth with water or mouthwash.** Residual corticosteroid in the pharynx can predispose patients to thrush, an annoying fungal infection of the pharynx or mouth.

Failure of an MDI

MDIs have some drawbacks. Using such a device requires a cooperative patient who is willing and able to perform the maneuver correctly. Because the entire dose is delivered in one or two breaths, little or no medication will reach the lungs if incorrect technique is used to administer the dose. An inhaler may be contraindicated for a patient who is not moving enough air to effectively draw the medication into the lungs. In addition, the patient must be able to recognize when the inhaler is empty (when the canister contains some propellant, but no medication).

A patient who does not fully understand how to use the device may inhale at an inappropriate point and end up spraying medication on the inside of the mouth. This potential error is one reason that physicians often prescribe a spacer device to be used with an MDI.

Dry-Powder Inhalers

Some respiratory medications are most stable in the form of a fine powder. Notably, some corticosteroids and slow-acting bronchodilators are often dispensed by this means. For example, tiotropium (Spiriva), a once-per-day anticholinergic medication for the management of COPD, is delivered via dry-powder inhaler.

A dry-powder inhaler is a plastic disk that holds enough medication to last approximately 1 month. Each time the device is opened, the small plastic blister that holds the next dose is rotated into position. The patient then pushes a small lever to puncture the blister, presses the disk to the lips over the opening, and inhales deeply to suck the powder out of the device. Other dry-powder devices require the patient to insert a capsule of powdered medication, which is then pierced when the patient compresses a button or lever on the device. The patient sucks the powder out using a technique similar to that previously described.

Dry-powder inhalers are reasonably convenient and easy to use, but they are rarely used during emergency care. They deliver relatively expensive medications, so do not open and close the device repeatedly: Several days' worth of medication may be wasted as the blisters rotate into and then past the position in which they can be punctured.

Leukotriene Modifiers

In some patients, bronchoconstricting chemicals called leukotrienes are released during respiratory distress, particularly during an allergic response. In these cases, a leukotriene blocker, such as montelukast (Singulair), which is usually taken orally, may be effective.

Electrolytes

In severe asthma attacks, IV magnesium sulfate may be ordered or included in standard protocols. IV magnesium can cause hypotension if given too quickly, but it can encourage smooth muscle relaxation in severe asthma and is particularly useful in efforts to avoid intubation in patients with acute asthma.

Street Smarts

Teach patients to use their rescue inhalers before taking corticosteroids, slow-acting bronchodilators, or other medications. A rescue inhaler dilates the bronchi so that subsequent medications are delivered more effectively.

Corticosteroids

Corticosteroids are used to reduce bronchial swelling (edema). These corticosteroids are different from the anabolic corticosteroids that some athletes abuse. The corticosteroids used in respiratory medications have various adverse effects, and their long-term use can cause Cushing syndrome, which is characterized by the classic moon face and generalized edema. In addition, corticosteroids trigger rapid changes in blood glucose levels and can blunt the actions of the immune system, allowing infection to flourish. The use of corticosteroids such as prednisone must be discontinued gradually. Because of the long-term adverse effects, a course of corticosteroid therapy lasting only 1 or 2 weeks is usually prescribed.

Inhaled Corticosteroids

Inhaled corticosteroids do not seem to have the same adverse effects as their oral counterparts. For that reason, inhaled corticosteroids are becoming standard adjuncts to treat asthma and COPD. Two of the components in the asthma triad can be addressed by administering a slow-acting bronchodilator to reduce bronchospasm and an inhaled corticosteroid to reduce airway edema. (The third component of the triad is increased mucus production. Asthma is discussed in more detail later in the chapter.)

IV Corticosteroids

In a medical emergency, it is common practice to give IV corticosteroids. A single bolus of IV corticosteroids does not seem to cause negative long-term consequences and is reasonably safe. Methylprednisolone and hydrocortisone are IV corticosteroid preparations given as an IV bolus, usually for acute exacerbations of COPD or acute asthma attacks. Their onset of action is measured in hours, so no results will be seen in the field. As always, consult local protocols and medical control before administering these agents.

Administer a Vasodilator

Treatment options for pulmonary edema include strategies for promoting vasodilation, which sequesters more fluid in the venous circulation and decreases preload. Nitrates, in the form of sublingual nitroglycerin tablets or nitroglycerin drips, can be administered as long as the patient has an adequate BP and does not take a phosphodiesterase inhibitor such as sildenafil (Viagra) or tadalafil (Cialis). Morphine sulfate decreases anxiety but probably does not increase venous capacitance as much as was once thought. It is not used as often as it once was in treating pulmonary edema.

Restore Fluid Balance

Rehydration is supplemental therapy for patients with respiratory conditions who are dehydrated (eg, some patients with pneumonia or asthma). It is common to give a fluid bolus to younger patients who are dehydrated. In any older adult or other patient with cardiac dysfunction, administering too much fluid could cause pulmonary edema. Always assess breath sounds before and after giving a fluid bolus to be certain that the patient does not become overhydrated. Let the staff at the medical facility rehydrate the patient after they have more information, lab results, and radiographs. Because the condition of a patient with a respiratory complaint can deteriorate precipitously, placing an IV line is a wise precaution.

Administer a Diuretic

Not every patient with crackles has pulmonary edema. Giving diuretics to patients with pneumonia or asthma may worsen their overall condition by dehydrating them and causing secretions to further obstruct smaller airways.

Diuretics are used to help reduce BP and maintain fluid balance in patients with heart failure. Patients with pulmonary edema may benefit from a diuretic to remove excess fluid from the circulation, which ultimately keeps it out of the lungs. Loop diuretics (bumetanide [Bumex] and furosemide) are the most commonly used agents in emergencies. Thiazide diuretics are often taken orally to treat high BP and heart failure.

Many diuretics cause the loss of not only fluid, but also potassium. Patients who do not take potassium supplements may have low potassium levels and a resulting predisposition to cardiac dysrhythmias and chronic muscle cramping.

Do not give diuretics to patients with pneumonia or to those who are already dehydrated; reserve these agents for patients who clearly have pulmonary edema. Some EMS systems permit use of furosemide only in standing orders for patients with wet lungs and peripheral edema, and others have removed this medication from their prehospital formulary altogether.

Patients with some degree of renal failure may require sizable doses of diuretics or may not respond to them. If a patient requires dialysis for renal failure, then trying to induce diuresis is unlikely to be effective. Although the management of respiratory distress is routine care in virtually all EDs, a patient who is undergoing dialysis and has pulmonary edema may be best served in a medical facility with the ability to provide emergency dialysis. This is one of the few circumstances in which a paramedic may decide to transport a patient with respiratory difficulty to a specialty center instead of the local ED.

Support or Assist Ventilation

If the patient becomes fatigued, then their breathing might need to be supported more aggressively. Therapy with CPAP and BPAP is becoming increasingly common and can preclude the need for intubation in many patients. Some patients may simply require bag-mask ventilation for a short period to reoxygenate, improve hemoglobin saturation, and reduce the $Paco_2$ level.

Trying to assist breathing for a patient who is already breathing independently is one of the most difficult interventions. To avoid worsening a patient's condition, you must be confident in your bag-mask ventilation technique. Gastric distention and vomiting from overaggressive ventilation can complicate an already deteriorating situation. As always, *do no harm*. The same is true when providing sedation to anxious and possibly combative patients. The need to control a patient's behavior must be balanced against the possibility of further depressing respiration. It is almost always counterproductive to sedate a patient in the field to treat erratic behavior associated with dyspnea.

Continuous Positive Airway Pressure

CPAP is used in two distinctly different ways: to treat obstructive sleep apnea and to treat respiratory failure. Many people with obstructive sleep apnea wear a CPAP unit at night to maintain the airway during sleep. This type of CPAP may be applied via nasal pillows, a nasal mask, a face mask that resembles a typical mask used for bag-mask ventilation, or a mask that covers the entire face. This is *not* the same type of CPAP used to assist breathing in critically ill patients. In people who are not critically ill, the positive pressure delivered maintains the stability of the posterior pharynx, thereby preventing obstruction of the upper airway as the person sleeps. This pressure limits hypoxic episodes and snoring.

The CPAP used as therapy for respiratory failure is almost always delivered through a mask secured to the face by some type of strap. With positive-pressure ventilation (ie, with a pocket mask or bag-mask ventilation), air is forced into the upper airway and flows into the trachea and esophagus unless steps are taken to help direct it into the trachea **FIGURE 17-22**. Indeed, positive-pressure ventilation with bag-mask ventilation or a pocket mask is physiologically the opposite of normal (negative-pressure) ventilation.

Using a bag-mask device for ventilation produces positive pressure in the chest. The more forcefully the bag is squeezed, the higher the pressure will be. Pressure that is too high can be detrimental: Simple pneumothorax can evolve into tension pneumothorax, air leaks can produce huge amounts of subcutaneous air, and venous return can be impeded or even completely blocked. In recent years, prehospital providers have begun to understand the ramifications of using positive-pressure ventilation in patients with low-flow states such as shock and cardiac arrest. This understanding has led to

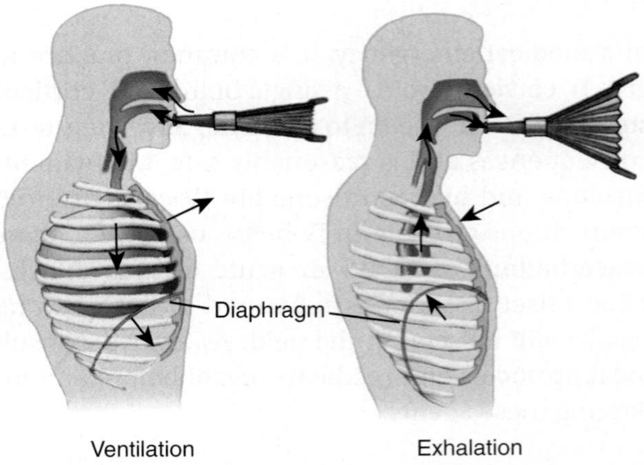

FIGURE 17-22 Positive-pressure ventilation is physiologically the opposite of normal ventilation. Air is pushed into the respiratory tract with bag-mask ventilation and can enter the esophagus, opening the normally flat tube and allowing air to enter the stomach, unless careful technique is used. Compare with negative-pressure ventilation, shown in Figure 17-5.

CPR guidelines that stress lower ventilation rates, smaller volumes, and lower pressures. CPR is based on hemodynamic principles, and the rate, volume, and pressure of delivered breaths can quickly do more harm than good during resuscitation if not calibrated correctly.

Similarly, administering CPAP increases pressure in the chest. If the patient's BP is already low, then too much CPAP can reduce venous return to the heart, causing a sudden drop in BP. This circumstance is uncommon with lower levels of CPAP, but the patient's BP must be carefully monitored whenever CPAP is used (especially at levels more than 10 cm H_2O). CPAP can turn a simple pneumothorax into a tension pneumothorax in only a few breaths.

When administering CPAP, remember to ensure a good seal with minimal leakage **FIGURE 17-23**. In the field, 100% supplemental oxygen is the most common gas driving the positive pressure. Be vigilant about monitoring the gas supply; depending on the flow rate and the patient's respiratory rate, some CPAP units may empty a D cylinder in as little as 5 or 10 minutes. The mask is fitted with a pressure-relief valve that determines the amount of pressure delivered (such as 5 cm H_2O). The effect is similar to being in a gale-force wind (high inspiratory flow) and having to push a pressure valve open by exhaling. This would seem to require a great deal

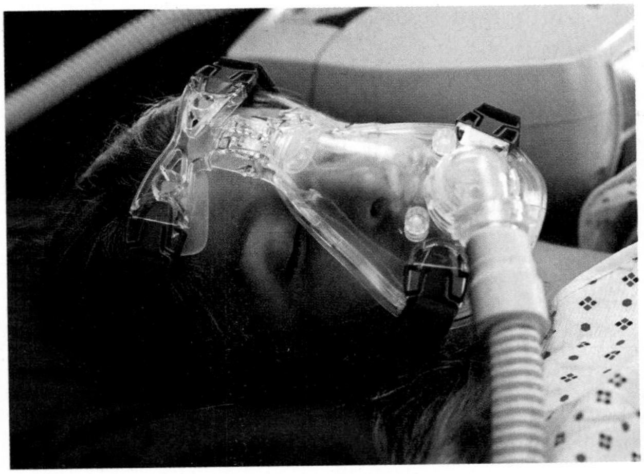

FIGURE 17-23 The continuous positive airway pressure used in the acute setting is usually administered via face mask, which must achieve a tight seal to function properly.

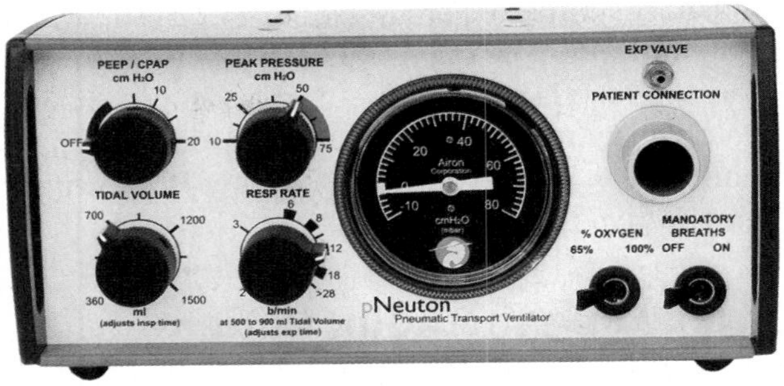

FIGURE 17-24 Portable versions of the automatic transport ventilator can be used in the field to dial in specific ventilation rates and volumes. This functionality can be useful in ensuring proper ventilation in a patient with cardiac arrest once an advanced airway has been inserted.

of effort and tire out a patient who has decompensating respiratory failure, but many patients in critical condition make a dramatic turnaround when CPAP is applied.

Sometimes patients find the CPAP mask claustrophobic and fight its application. Some patients can be talked through the mask application with good results, but others simply cannot tolerate this process. Don't struggle with a patient who is unwilling to use the mask; doing so will increase the patient's anxiety, cardiac workload, and cardiac oxygen consumption.

When CPAP works as intended, it can provide dramatic relief and avoid the need for intubation. When it fails, you must recognize the patient's deteriorating condition and be prepared to move to the next step (usually intubation). Within several minutes of application, the patient's oxygen saturation should increase, and the respiratory rate should decline. The outcome of CPAP is inversely related to the patient's respiratory rate soon after its application: If this rate *increases*, the therapy is likely to fail; if it *decreases*, the therapy is likely to succeed.

Indications, contraindications, application, and complications of CPAP administration are discussed in Chapter 16, *Airway Management*.

Bilevel Positive Airway Pressure

In BPAP, one level of pressure can be delivered during inspiration (inspiratory positive airway pressure) and a different level of pressure can be delivered during exhalation (expiratory positive airway pressure). Instead of delivering 20 cm H_2O as in CPAP, BPAP set at 20/8 delivers 20 cm H_2O pressure during inhalation and 8 cm H_2O pressure during exhalation. Because this type of positive airway pressure is more like normal breathing, it is often more comfortable for patients. It causes a pressure variation in the chest, which allows for more normal blood flow. The BPAP device is also more complex and expensive, and it is not commonly used in the field.

Automated Transport Ventilators

Automated transport ventilators are essentially flow-restricted, oxygen-powered ventilation devices with built-in timers. They can be set to deliver a particular volume of oxygen at a particular rate, which can be helpful when an extra pair of hands is needed **FIGURE 17-24**. These devices are a particularly good substitute for bag-mask ventilation for patients in cardiac or respiratory arrest. Basic automated transport ventilators may not offer advanced features, such as alarms, flow rate controls, and a selection of ventilatory modes. It is critical to recognize that they are *not* little ventilators and are *not* intended to ventilate patients without direct observation and attention by a skilled paramedic.

Conscious patients require up to 150 L/min of flow to breathe comfortably. Some automated transport ventilators are permanently set to deliver 40 L/min, which would be inadequate for a spontaneously breathing patient. Flow-restricted, oxygen-powered ventilation devices and automated transport ventilators are preset to 40 L/min, which is the optimal flow for ventilating a patient in cardiac arrest: via face mask and without causing gastric distention. A more detailed discussion of ventilators can be found in Chapter 46, *Patients With Special Challenges.*

Intubating the Adult Patient

Ultimately, patients who are in respiratory failure may need to be intubated and ventilated. Intubation can be lifesaving, and many patients can be extubated within a day or two and have an excellent outcome. However, some factors must be considered when intubating a patient. Paramedics must weigh these factors along with established protocol, medical direction, and any expression of the patient's wishes. Keep these guidelines in mind:

- **Patients with asthma are extremely difficult to ventilate and are susceptible to pneumothoraces.** Given these risks, intubation should be the last option for such patients.
- **Be proactive; ventilate patients *before* cardiac arrest occurs.** When in doubt, attempt to ventilate. A combative patient may not be ready for intubation. If a patient allows intubation, it was probably necessary. For patients who are conscious but in respiratory distress, sedation and neuromuscular blocking medications (through pharmacologically assisted intubation) are necessary to facilitate intubation.
- **Consider intubating a patient who has little or no gag reflex—for example, a patient who has had a stroke or is severely intoxicated.** The absence of a gag reflex poses a grave threat if the patient vomits. In this situation, consider intubating the patient to protect the airway even if ventilation is adequate.
- **Consider bag-mask ventilation.** Some patients who have diabetes or have overdosed are in obvious need of intubation. However, if an ampule of 50% dextrose or naloxone (Narcan) is likely to completely change that picture, it might be better to use bag-mask ventilation for a few minutes to monitor the effect of the initial medication therapy, assuming the patient can be ventilated without causing gastric distention and vomiting. Ventilate slowly (over 1 second), and use only enough ventilation to produce a visible chest rise.

Intubation is discussed in Chapter 16, *Airway Management.*

Inject a Beta Agonist Subcutaneously

Administration methods that require the patient to inhale medication may be unreliable or ineffective when the patient's breathing effort is inadequate, as evidenced by diminished tidal volume. In some circumstances, it may be beneficial to attempt beta agonist (beta-2) stimulation the old way, by administering subcutaneous or intramuscular terbutaline or epinephrine. These medications are not as specific to beta-2 as their aerosol cousins are, so they will also cause more tachycardia (beta-1 stimulation) and hypertension (alpha stimulation), but when a patient's airways are severely constricted, these agents are sometimes the more effective approach. Be particularly careful when using beta agonists in older adult patients, who may not easily tolerate the additional cardiac stimulation.

Pathophysiology, Assessment, and Management of Obstructive Upper Airway Diseases

Anatomic Obstruction

Pathophysiology

The most common source of upper airway obstruction in an unresponsive patient is the tongue. Every year, obstruction caused by the tongue results in the death of some trauma patients, patients in insulin shock, patients who have had a seizure, or patients who are intoxicated.

Assessment

Assessment of the airway is among the most foundational skills of paramedics. Anyone with a decreased level of consciousness, particularly a person in a supine position, is at risk of some upper airway obstruction. Sonorous (snoring) respiration is an obvious sign that breathing is at least partially obstructed. Other signs include gurgling, squeaking, or bubbling sounds during breathing. Stridor may be associated with accessory muscle use or retractions if the patient is attempting to breathe through an obstructed airway.

Management

Bystanders often place a pillow beneath the head of an unresponsive person, which exacerbates airway obstruction. If the patient is snoring, remove the pillow and reposition the patient's airway.

Excessive soft tissue in the airway is one cause of obstructive sleep apnea, and some people go so far as to have such tissue surgically removed from the pharynx to limit anatomic obstruction. Fortunately, the soft tissue of the upper airway can be manually displaced with a variety of basic maneuvers, as discussed in Chapter 16, *Airway Management*. If restriction of spinal motion is unnecessary, then place an unconscious patient in the recovery position to avoid blocking the airway. The recovery position is the safest position for many patients who have had a seizure or are hypoglycemic or intoxicated. It also reduces the risk of aspiration if the patient vomits.

Inflammation Caused by Infection

Pathophysiology

A variety of infections can cause swelling in the upper airway. Infection can lead to **laryngotracheobronchitis**, or inflammation of the larynx, trachea, and bronchi. An acute form of laryngotracheobronchitis is a common cause of **croup**, a condition characterized by stridor, hoarseness, and a barking cough that most commonly occurs in infants and small children. (Some authors consider laryngotracheobronchitis and croup to be the same.) The Poiseuille law holds that as the diameter of a tube decreases, resistance to flow increases exponentially. This law explains why children, who have narrow airways, often experience croup when an infection causes upper airway swelling, whereas adults with the same infection do not **FIGURE 17-25**. Viral infection is a more common underlying cause of croup than bacterial infection is. Croup may also be caused by allergies that result in airway swelling and obstruction, or by obstruction with a foreign body.

The **palatine tonsils** can also become impressively inflamed in children, though this condition is rarely life threatening. When a child is properly positioned for intubation, inflamed tonsils do not typically obstruct the view of the glottis. Take care to avoid injuring the tonsils with the laryngoscope, however, because they can swell and bleed if traumatized.

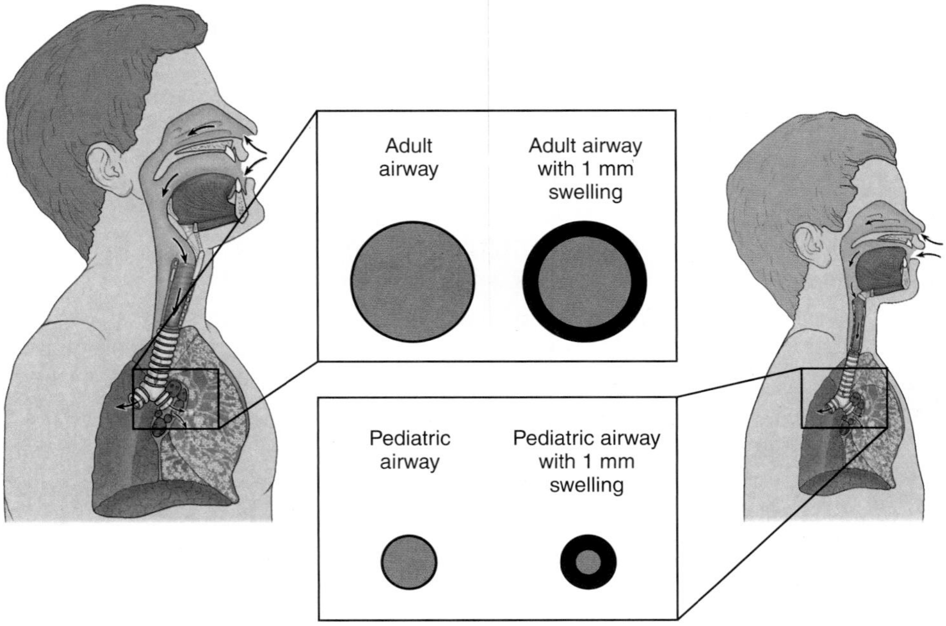

FIGURE 17-25 Any airway constriction (eg, in a condition such as asthma) can severely reduce the volume of airflow, especially in children. The Poiseuille law states that as the diameter of a tube decreases, resistance to flow increases exponentially.

Assessment

In recent decades, many deadly upper airway conditions, such as epiglottitis, have become rare as a result of widespread immunization efforts. Unfortunately, the rate of childhood immunization has begun to decline as the general public becomes complacent about such diseases. Paramedics must, therefore, remain vigilant for these pathologic conditions. **TABLE 17-6** lists the signs and symptoms of selected inflammatory conditions that can impair the upper airway.

Croup and tonsillitis are common, especially among children, but the other conditions mentioned in Table 17-6 are rare. When these pathologic conditions occur, they are critical emergencies, because swelling can rapidly obstruct the airway, making orotracheal intubation extremely difficult or impossible. *Avoid manipulating the airway* unless absolutely necessary. Ventilation can usually be accomplished with careful bag-mask technique.

Words of Wisdom

Immunization has significantly reduced the incidence of many infectious diseases, such as diphtheria; however, an increasing number of people in the United States are unable to obtain vaccinations (because of poverty, lack of access to health care, or geographic isolation, for example) or refuse to be vaccinated (because they fear that vaccines cause other diseases or believe that vaccinations are unnecessary). Lack of immunity among unvaccinated adults and children has led to the reemergence of certain diseases. In addition, because immunization does not last forever, conditions such as epiglottitis may be seen (albeit rarely) among adults in their 20s and 30s.

Management

If intubation is essential because the patient cannot be effectively ventilated with bag-mask technique, then the airway may already be entirely

TABLE 17-6 Inflammatory Conditions That Can Impair the Upper Airway

Condition	Comments
Croup	A condition most often found in children between 6 months and 6 years, but can occur at any age; in northern areas, most common between October and March; characterized by stridor, hoarseness, and a barking cough; distressing but not typically fatal; a viral infection is usually the underlying cause. Do not manipulate the airway.
Epiglottitis	Severe, rapidly progressive inflammation of the epiglottis and surrounding tissues, usually caused by infection (most commonly with *Haemophilus influenzae* type B); may be fatal because of sudden respiratory obstruction; a life-threatening emergency; signs and symptoms include sore throat, fever, drooling, hoarseness, and purposeful hyperextension of the neck; was once more common in children, but is now rare because of widespread immunization against *H influenzae*, leaving unvaccinated adults as the most common susceptible group. Fortunately, the pathology is less life threatening in adults.
Peritonsillar abscess	Uncommon in children, more common in young adults; abscess forms near one pharyngeal tonsil; symptoms include fever and sore throat; may be mistaken for epiglottitis until a lateral abscess (instead of enlarged epiglottis) is seen in the throat. Do not manipulate the airway.
Retropharyngeal abscess	Most common in children; caused by infection in the retropharyngeal lymph nodes and by direct pharyngeal trauma; signs and symptoms include fever and sudden stridor; may be mistaken for epiglottitis until laryngoscopic examination reveals retropharyngeal abscess (instead of cherry-red epiglottis). Do not manipulate the airway.
Diphtheria	Causative bacterium attacks and kills a layer of epithelial tissue, creating a **pseudomembrane**, often in the tonsillar area; this membrane (and swelling of upper airway associated with the disease) can obstruct the upper airway; no longer common because of diphtheria, tetanus, and pertussis (DTP) vaccination. Do not manipulate the airway.
Enlarged tonsils	The palatine tonsils can swell excessively, sometimes to the size of a golf ball; associated with fever, difficulty swallowing, and throat pain; enlarged tonsils rarely obstruct the airway but can cause snoring and stridor. Do not manipulate the airway.

obscured by the swelling. Attempts at laryngoscopy may worsen this swelling. Ask a partner to press on the patient's chest while you look for a stream of bubbles coming from the airway. Use an ET tube at least two full sizes smaller than would typically be appropriate for that patient. If this effort fails after a single attempt, then a needle or surgical cricothyrotomy is necessary. It is preferable to defer surgical attempts to create an airway to the staff at the closest medical facility, but time may force you to use an invasive airway approach if permitted in your system.

Aspiration

The inhalation of anything other than breathable gases is called **aspiration**. Patients can aspirate fresh or salt water, blood, vomitus, or food and beverages. Aspiration of foreign bodies, such as nuts or broken teeth, may also occur.

In older patients, chronic aspiration of food is a common cause of pneumonia from the bacteria in the aspirated material. The aspiration of stomach contents carries the additional risk of aspiration **pneumonitis**, in which gastric acid irritates lung tissue.

Pathophysiology

Most adults choke only when they are intoxicated or traumatized, or when the gag reflex has diminished after a stroke, as a result of other neurologic dysfunction, or as a consequence of aging. Many older adult patients have impaired swallowing. Patients who receive tube feedings are at risk of aspiration, particularly if they are placed supine immediately after receiving a large feeding.

Aspiration is associated with a high mortality rate. It is a common but profoundly dangerous complication in patients who have had a cardiac arrest and in patients who are unresponsive as a result of trauma or overdose. Such patients are at risk of aspirating vomitus.

Assessment

To assess a patient with a sudden onset of dyspnea, consider the circumstances. Did the breathing difficulty occur immediately after eating? Does the patient have a gastric feeding tube, and if so, when was the last feeding and how large was it? Is the material suctioned from the patient's airway the same color as the tube feeding? Is there particulate matter in the suctioned material? A fever and cough may present several hours after an event associated with increased risk of aspiration, such as a seizure or an episode of unresponsiveness. Some patients aspirate chronically and may have a history of aspiration pneumonia.

Management

Follow these guidelines when treating patients who are at risk of aspiration or who have aspirated:

1. Aggressively reduce the risk of aspiration by avoiding gastric distention when ventilating and by decompressing the stomach with a nasogastric tube whenever appropriate.
2. Aggressively monitor the patient's ability to protect the airway, and protect the patient's airway with an advanced airway when needed.
3. Aggressively treat aspiration with suctioning and airway control if steps 1 and 2 fail.

Patients at risk of aspiration should not eat when they are having difficulty breathing. If basic life support maneuvers fail to clear the obstructed airway, then use laryngoscopy and Magill forceps, and, if necessary, perform a needle or surgical cricothyrotomy if allowed by local protocol.

Pathophysiology, Assessment, and Management of Obstructive Lower Airway Diseases

Obstructive lower airway diseases are characterized by diffuse obstruction of airflow within the lungs. The most common obstructive lower airway diseases are emphysema, chronic bronchitis, and asthma, an acutely episodic syndrome; these three conditions collectively account for a large portion of the typical provider's calls for dyspnea. Emphysema and chronic bronchitis are collectively classified as COPD because the pulmonary structure and function changes that occur with these diseases are chronic, progressive, and irreversible. Asthma is considered a separate entity, at least in its early stages, because the airway narrowing is reversible.

Obstructive disease occurs when the positive pressure of exhalation causes the small airways to

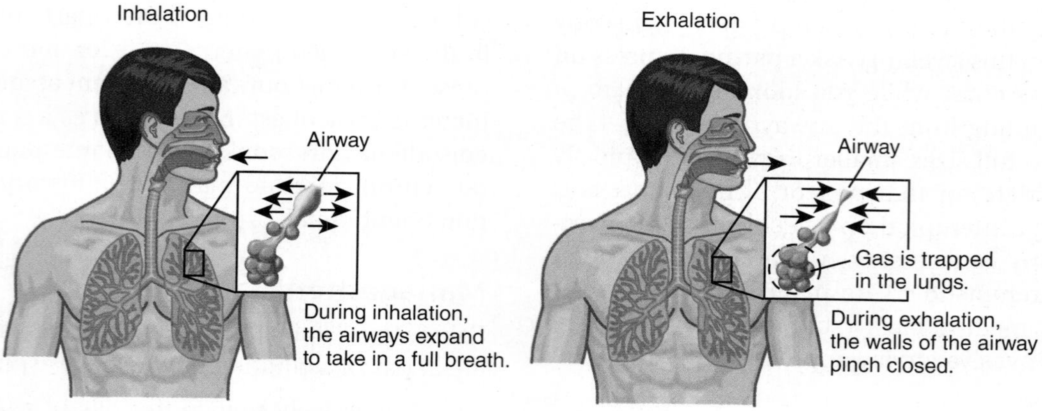

During inhalation, the airways expand to take in a full breath.

FIGURE 17-26 Obstructive disease is characterized by changes in the smaller airways that cause them to pinch closed during exhalation, trapping air inside the lungs. Healthy airways narrow during exhalation, but not enough to trap air or obstruct airflow.

pinch shut, trapping gas in the alveoli. The harder the patient tries to push air out, the more air becomes trapped in the alveoli **FIGURE 17-26**. Patients with obstructive disease learn that exhaling slowly at a low pressure is more effective than exhaling rapidly at high pressure.

Patients with obstructive airway disease may have a variety of physical findings that suggest the nature of their disease:

- **Pursed-lip breathing.** Breathing in this way allows patients to exhale slowly under controlled pressure.
- **Increased I:E ratio.** The I:E (inspiratory-to-expiratory) ratio is typically 1:2 in healthy people breathing quietly. In other words, it takes about twice as long to exhale as it does to inhale. Patients who are gravely ill with obstructive disease may have an I:E ratio as high as 1:6 or 1:8.
- **Abdominal muscle use.** Abdominal muscles help to push out air (during exhalation). Patients with obstructive disease must work to push out air with every breath. People with asthma, for example, may complain of abdominal pain after an attack because they do the equivalent of hundreds of sit-ups as they struggle to breathe.
- **JVD.** The trapped air in the lungs increases pressure in the thorax. Blood draining into the superior vena cava from the head and neck can back up in the jugular veins, causing JVD.

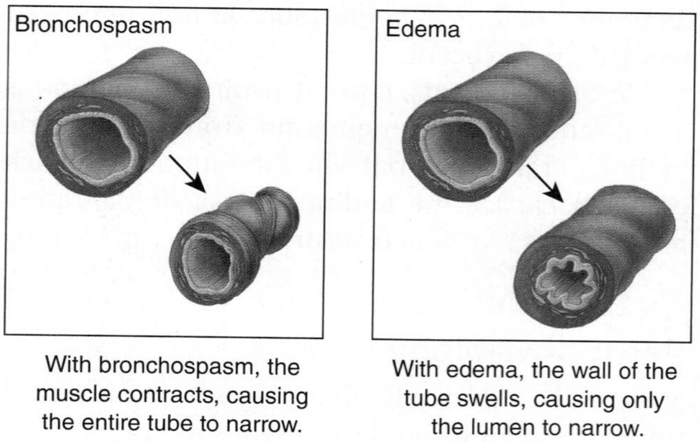

Bronchospasm
Edema
With bronchospasm, the muscle contracts, causing the entire tube to narrow.
With edema, the wall of the tube swells, causing only the lumen to narrow.

FIGURE 17-27 Bronchospasm is a constriction or narrowing of the diameters of both the inside and the outside portions of the airway. In contrast, in bronchial edema, only the diameter of the inside portion (the bronchial lumen) is constricted. Both conditions reduce the functional diameter of the airways.

Asthma

Pathophysiology

The name *asthma* (from a Greek word meaning "panting") was first given to this disease by the second-century Greek physician Areatus "because in the paroxysms [of an asthma attack], the patients also pant for breath." Bronchial asthma is characterized by increased reactivity of the trachea and bronchi to a variety of stimuli. This hyperreactivity results in widespread, reversible narrowing of the airways, or bronchospasm **FIGURE 17-27**. Asthma makes it difficult to exhale. Air becomes trapped in the distal portions of the lung, so that air from the next inhalation cannot enter the alveoli.

According to the Centers for Disease Control and Prevention, more than 24 million people in the United States reported having asthma in 2018, and the prevalence seems to be increasing.[15] Each year, 1.5 million people visit an ED because of asthma, and approximately 11% of them will be admitted to a medical facility.[15]

The fastest-growing asthma rates are observed in children younger than 5 years. Overall death rates from asthma are also higher in people younger than 35 years.[16] This disease is more common in men but tends to be more severe in women. African Americans, especially those who live in large urban areas, are three times more likely to be diagnosed with asthma and have death rates that are five times higher than those observed in other racial groups.[4]

Patients who have potentially fatal asthma often have severely compromised ventilation all the time. They are at serious risk if acute bronchospasm is triggered or if they have an infection. A patient with asthma is at high risk of respiratory arrest if their history includes any of the factors listed in **TABLE 17-7**. Not following the medication regimen and/or having a severe psychiatric disorder also increases the likelihood that a patient with asthma will have a fatal attack. Each day, approximately 10 people die of asthma in the United States.[4]

Sometimes asthma is referred to as **reactive airway disease**, a label indicating that the patient experiences bronchospasm when exposed to certain triggers, such as dust, cold, or smoke. In addition, edema and inflammation of the airways and increased mucus production can cause significant airway obstruction. Asthma characteristically produces acute attacks of variable duration. Between attacks, the person may be relatively asymptomatic.

TABLE 17-7 Factors Associated With an Increased Risk of Asthma-Related Death

- Previous intubation for respiratory failure or respiratory arrest
- Respiratory acidosis
- Two or more admissions to a medical facility despite oral corticosteroid use
- Two or more episodes of pneumothorax

Words of Wisdom

The term *asthma* describes a triad of airway alterations: bronchospasm, increased mucus production, and peripheral airway edema. It may present differently in different people, but it is a common pathologic condition.

Status asthmaticus is a severe, prolonged asthmatic attack that cannot be stopped with conventional treatment. *It is a true medical emergency.* Just as patients with COPD ordinarily do not call for EMS assistance unless their condition has changed markedly, patients with asthma do not usually dial 9-1-1 unless the attack is much worse than usual. It is reasonable to assume that *any person with asthma who feels sick enough to call 9-1-1 is in status asthmaticus until proven otherwise.*

Assessment

When patients begin wheezing, their inhalers usually help for only a short time before symptoms return. The typical asthma attack that responds to treatment but occurs again in a few hours is sometimes caused by an underlying infection, such as pneumonia or bronchitis, that continually triggers the asthmalike symptoms. The asthma attack will not subside until the trigger is removed or otherwise mitigated. Consider the potential triggers for each patient. Does the patient have a fever or chills? Is the patient coughing up colored sputum?

On examination, a patient in status asthmaticus will be desperately struggling to move air through the obstructed airways. You will see prominent use of the accessory muscles of breathing. The chest will be maximally hyperinflated. Breath sounds and wheezes may be entirely inaudible because air movement is negligible, and the patient will usually be exhausted, severely acidotic, and dehydrated.

Bronchospasm

Bronchospasm is caused by the constriction of the smooth muscle that surrounds the larger bronchi in the lungs **FIGURE 17-28**. Bronchospasm may be stimulated by an allergen or irritant such as dust, perfume, animal dander, or cold air, or by other

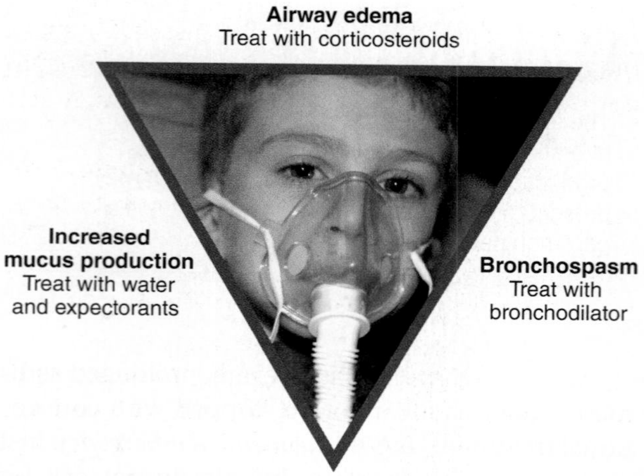
Airway edema
Treat with corticosteroids
Increased mucus production
Treat with water and expectorants
Bronchospasm
Treat with bronchodilator

FIGURE 17-28 The asthma triad consists of the three primary components of asthma and the respective treatments for each. Asthma presents differently in different people, so individual treatment must also vary.

stimuli, such as exercise or stress. When air is forced through the constricted airways, it causes them to vibrate, which provokes wheezing. Bronchospasm can also reduce the peak expiratory flow by causing turbulent airflow.

Bronchial Edema

Swelling of the bronchi and bronchioles also creates turbulent airflow and air trapping. Bronchodilator medications do little to reduce bronchial edema. If a patient takes such a medication and the peak flow does not dramatically improve, then some degree of bronchial edema is likely present.

Increased Mucus Production

Thick secretions may plug the distal airways and contribute to air trapping. People with asthma may be significantly dehydrated as a result of increased fluid loss from tachypnea and inadequate fluid intake. Dehydration makes secretions even thicker, further worsening the air trapping.

Management

Most people with asthma have a combination of these three pathologic conditions, although their predominance varies among individual patients:

- **Bronchospasm.** Bronchospasm is characterized primarily by bronchoconstriction, which tends to respond well to aerosol bronchodilators. Thus, the primary treatment for bronchospasm is nebulized bronchodilator medication. In patients who do not respond to nebulized bronchodilators, additional medications may be indicated. If severe bronchospasms are suspected, as indicated by a "shark-fin" appearance on waveform capnography, magnesium sulfate may be considered to relax smooth muscle. The use of epinephrine may be appropriate in extremis due to its strong beta-2 agonist properties.[17]
- **Bronchial edema.** Anticholinergic medications such as ipratropium bromide may be administered with nebulized bronchodilator medications to dry up fluid in the larger airways.[17] Bronchial edema is much less responsive to aerosol bronchodilators and usually shows significant improvement only after corticosteroids have been administered and taken effect. Corticosteroids may or may not be given in the field setting because, unlike bronchodilators, which can improve breathing immediately, corticosteroids take a few hours to reduce inflammation.
- **Excessive mucus secretion.** The primary approach to dealing with secretions in a person with asthma is to improve hydration. Mucolytics, which break down thick mucus, and expectorants, which loosen thick secretions so that they can be coughed out, are also sometimes used, most often in the inpatient setting.

Transport Considerations

Many patients routinely manage their asthma at home and may resist transport to a medical facility once their most acute symptoms have been relieved. Attempt to determine the trigger for an attack. If the patient has an underlying infection, indicated by fever, increased mucus production, or mucus that is green, yellow, or brown, or if the person will be continually exposed to a trigger (such as someone who wears a strong fragrance or smokes), then remove the patient from the environment for additional evaluation. A patient whose wheezing clears but whose peak flow does not improve may need corticosteroids. A patient who is undernourished or dehydrated may need additional IV fluids.

COPD: Emphysema and Chronic Bronchitis

Pathophysiology

COPD comprises at least two distinct clinical entities: emphysema and chronic bronchitis. Emphysema is thought to damage or destroy the fragile structure of the terminal bronchioles. In this disease, groups of alveoli merge into large blebs, or bullae, which are far less efficient at gas exchange than normal lung tissue because they have less surface area available. This part of the tracheobronchial tree becomes so weak that its branches collapse during exhalation, trapping air in the alveoli.

Restrictive Disease

Restrictive lung diseases comprise pathologies that limit the patient's ability to expand the lungs within the chest cavity. Examples include severe kyphosis and scoliosis **FIGURE 17-29**, sarcoidosis (an autoimmune disease), interstitial lung disease, obesity, and neuromuscular disease (eg, muscular dystrophy, amyotrophic lateral sclerosis). These disorders put patients at risk of infection and may severely limit their ability to compensate for any respiratory insult. Restrictive lung diseases by themselves do not generate many calls for EMS response. We mention them for the sake of comparison to obstructive diseases, which paramedics will encounter frequently.

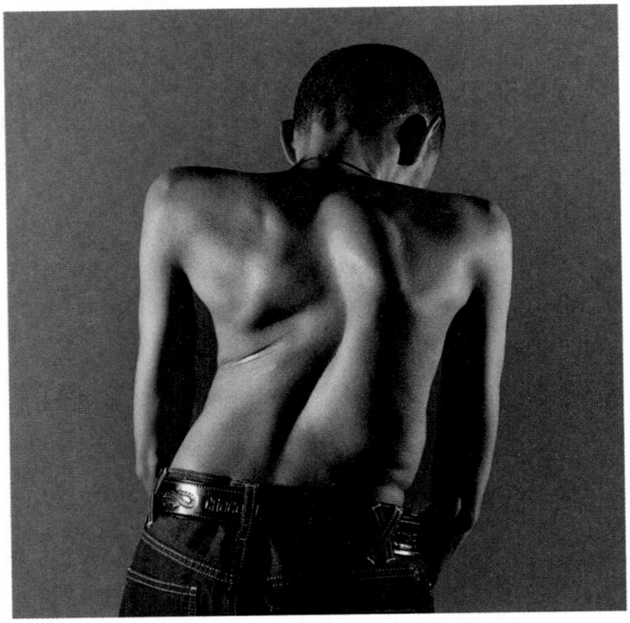

FIGURE 17-29 Diseases of the bones, such as scoliosis, can impair the patient's ability to move air because of chest compression.

Chronic bronchitis is defined as sputum production most days of the month for 3 or more months out of the year for more than 2 years. The hallmark of this disease is excessive mucus production in the bronchial tree, which is nearly always accompanied by a chronic or recurrent productive cough (a cough that produces phlegm). A typical patient with chronic bronchitis is almost invariably a heavy cigarette smoker, usually overweight and congested, and sometimes has a blue complexion. Blood gas levels tend to be abnormal, with elevated $Paco_2$ (hypercapnia) and decreased Pao_2 (hypoxemia) levels. Often, the patient has associated heart disease and right-side heart failure (cor pulmonale).

Assessment

Emphysema and chronic bronchitis represent two extremes of the COPD spectrum. In reality, as COPD progresses, most patients fall somewhere between these two clinical extremes, showing signs and symptoms of both disease processes.

Many patients with emphysema have a barrel chest caused by chronic lung hyperinflation. These patients are often tachypneic because they attempt to maintain a normal carbon dioxide level despite their dysfunctional lungs. They may consume extreme amounts of energy as they attempt to breathe, using their own muscle mass for energy in the process.

Among the causes of diffuse wheezing are acute left-side heart failure ("cardiac asthma"), smoke inhalation, chronic bronchitis, and acute pulmonary embolism. Localized wheezing suggests an obstruction, by foreign body or tumor, in a specific area. Only a careful history and physical examination will reveal the correct diagnosis.

The following are some common factors that cause decompensation in a patient with COPD.

COPD With Pneumonia

Because patients with COPD are chronically ill, have poor secretion clearance, and sometimes have excessive mucus production (which acts as a culture medium for pathogenic microorganisms), they often have lung infections. Assessment should ascertain whether fever is present, the color or amount of sputum production has changed, other signs of infection (eg, body aches, general malaise, or pain when breathing) are apparent, or auscultated breath sounds (eg, localized or one-sided crackles) are consistent with pneumonia. A patient who obviously has COPD might also have another condition, including another respiratory condition.

> **Words of Wisdom**
>
> Over the years, people with COPD learn how much exertion they can tolerate, in which position sleep is possible, and so forth. Thus, when a person with COPD calls for EMS assistance, it nearly always means something has changed for the worse.

COPD With Right-Side Heart Failure

It is a laborious task for the right side of the heart to push thick blood (thick because of polycythemia) through capillaries compressed by hyperinflated alveoli. This situation usually causes right-side heart failure as a result of lung disease (cor pulmonale). If patients take in too much salt or fluid or do not excrete sufficient amounts of fluid (because of renal failure or not using diuretics as prescribed), they may have an episode of heart failure. Assessment should look for peripheral edema, JVD with hepatojugular reflux, end-inspiratory crackles, a progressive increase in dyspnea over several days, a greater-than-usual fluid intake, and improper use of diuretics. Note that it can be difficult to differentiate the crackles of heart failure from the crackles always present because of COPD.

> **Words of Wisdom**
>
> In the 1930s, Chevalier Jackson, renowned laryngoscopist and airway management pioneer, coined the phrase "All that wheezes is not asthma."[18,19] It is particularly important to distinguish the wheezing of asthma from that caused by left-side heart failure because treatments for the two conditions are markedly different.

COPD With Left-Side Heart Failure

Patients with COPD are at high risk of sudden cardiac arrest. Any abrupt left ventricular dysfunction, such as an acute myocardial infarction or a cardiac rhythm disturbance (dysrhythmia), can cause rapid-onset, left-side heart failure. Do not allow an initial impression of COPD to preclude swift identification of an acute myocardial infarction.

Acute Exacerbation of COPD

In an acute exacerbation of COPD, no copathologic condition, such as heart failure or pneumonia, clearly accounts for the sudden decompensation. Instead, the patient's condition suddenly worsens, often because of some environmental change such as a sudden change in the weather, humidity, or recent seasonal activation of the heating or cooling system. An acute exacerbation can also be prompted by the inhalation of trigger substances, such as dust, mold, animal dander, or fresh paint.

Advances in technology have allowed people with chronic respiratory disease much more freedom to get out of the house and to travel. Paramedics may then be called to assist a person who has an acute exacerbation of COPD when an oxygen tank runs dry or a portable ventilator malfunctions, when medications are left at home or packed in checked baggage that is misdirected, or when therapy is deliberately discontinued because the person wants to regain some autonomy or does not understand the importance of the therapy.

End-Stage COPD

Patients with severe COPD eventually reach a point at which their lungs can no longer support oxygenation and ventilation. Their calls to 9-1-1 become more frequent as their condition deteriorates. Some will be in hospice care. In the end stages of the disease, it can be difficult to determine whether a patient has an exacerbation that can be resolved or has reached the end of the disease process. ET intubation may make it impossible for a patient to make their wishes known. In addition, the more frequently a patient requires intubation and mechanical ventilation, the more difficult ventilator weaning becomes. Apprehension about these bleak prospects heightens the patient's anxiety, thereby escalating cardiac workload and cardiac oxygen consumption, a potentially lethal series of events for a patient with end-stage COPD.

Each EMS system has its own ways of dealing with do-not-resuscitate orders. It is important to secure documentation of the patient's wishes as the terminal phase of the disease begins. Follow the local protocol or contact medical control as needed regarding such matters.

Documentation and Communication

Seek guidance from the medical director and observe local protocols when treating a patient with severe COPD or asthma who is in cardiac arrest or near-arrest.

COPD and Trauma

People with COPD are as susceptible to trauma as the rest of the population, but their disease lessens their ability to tolerate such trauma. Many patients with COPD must sit up to breathe, so strapping them to a long board can lead to decompensation. Anyone who has performed CPR compressions on a patient with chronic emphysema knows how poorly the chest wall tolerates trauma. Even when a patient with COPD survives the initial trauma, the patient is susceptible to pulmonary emboli and infection during recovery. Patients with COPD rarely have a "normal" oxygen saturation; their normal might be less than 90%. Providing supplemental oxygen in an effort to achieve a saturation of 98% is unrealistic and might be harmful.

Management

Although little can be done in the field to provide long-term relief for patients with COPD, the associated bronchospasm, edema, fluid, or hypoxia can often be relieved, helping to improve the patient's immediate situation.

Patients with COPD are often debilitated by the disease and have little or no respiratory reserve to help them deal with additional respiratory insults. Paramedics must actively try to determine the circumstances that tipped the precarious balance from relative stability to the state of respiratory insufficiency that prompted the 9-1-1 call. Effective management of COPD requires an understanding of the concepts of hypoxic drive and auto-PEEP (positive end-expiratory pressure).

Hypoxic Drive

Hypoxic drive is a state in which a person's stimulus to breathe comes from a decrease in PaO_2 rather than from the normal stimulus, an increase in $PaCO_2$. When a patient has chronic hypoventilation, bicarbonate ions (HCO_3^-) migrate into the cerebrospinal fluid, fooling the brain into thinking that acid and base are in balance. The patient's respiratory center might then switch to a hypoxic drive.

This phenomenon affects only a small percentage of patients: those with the most relentless forms of pulmonary disease. Hypoxic drive occurs during the end stage of the disease process. In such a case, you must decide whether the administration of oxygen is appropriate for any given patient. In making this decision, consider the following points:

1. Only a small subset of patients with COPD breathe because of hypoxic drive, but it is impossible to know who they are by just looking at them. Patients on home oxygen at very specific settings (such as 1.5 L/min) should arouse your suspicion.
2. Patients who breathe because of hypoxic drive do not suddenly become apneic after breathing oxygen. High levels of oxygen slowly depress the respiratory drive, and the respiratory rate slowly declines into the single digits before a patient becomes apneic. A paramedic is likely to recognize this phenomenon during a transport; the real concern is for a patient in a medical facility or an extended-care facility who is given 100% supplemental oxygen and left alone for a prolonged period.
3. Verbal and physical stimulation can encourage breathing. If the respiratory rate begins to drop, then gently shake the patient and yell "Breathe!" This technique works well in the early stages.
4. If a patient becomes apneic because of increased oxygenation, the skin may still appear perfused.
5. If the patient becomes apneic, provide artificial ventilation and consider intubation.
6. Although oxygen saturation (SpO_2) readings may be a valuable adjunct in deciding whether

to intubate, Spo_2 values are less useful in cases of COPD because they fail to shed light on the carbon dioxide level.

Supplemental oxygen is integral to therapy for many patients, so it does not make sense to withhold oxygen from someone who needs it for fear of decreasing the respiratory drive in those few patients who might have this complication. Keep in mind that an oxygen saturation of 93% is acceptable, and many patients with COPD routinely have even lower values. It is not necessary or desirable to oxygenate these patients to oxygen saturation levels of 99% or 100%.

Auto-PEEP

Not everyone should be ventilated the same way. When ventilating a patient with severe obstructive disease, such as decompensated asthma or COPD, remember that the person has difficulty exhaling. Complete exhalation must be allowed before the next breath is delivered, or else pressure in the thorax will continue to rise. This phenomenon, which is called auto-PEEP, can eventually cause a pneumothorax or cardiac arrest. If the pressure in the chest exceeds the pressure at which blood is returned to the heart, venous return will be limited and cardiac arrest may occur.

Patients in whom auto-PEEP is a concern should be ventilated at a rate of as little as 4 to 6 breaths/min. Such restraint is difficult, but is an absolute necessity to avoid the dire consequences of raising the thoracic pressure with each breath. Remember that the standard ventilation rate for adults in cardiac arrest is only 10 breaths/min in patients without COPD.

Pathophysiology, Assessment, and Management of Common Respiratory Conditions

Pulmonary Infections

Pathophysiology

Bacteria, viruses, fungi, protozoa, and a host of other organisms can cause infections. The respiratory tract is particularly vulnerable to a variety of airborne agents and to agents that reside in the nose or throat and may migrate into the lungs.

In general, infectious diseases cause swelling of the respiratory tissues, an increase in mucus production, and the production of pus. Swelling in well-perfused respiratory tissues can be dramatic, particularly in the upper airway. This swelling is problematic because of the Poiseuille law: The resistance to airflow increases exponentially when the airway diameter is narrowed. Alveoli can also become nonfunctional if they fill with fluid or pus, as occurs in pneumonia (consolidation).

Pneumonia may be caused by any of a variety of bacterial, viral, and fungal agents. Bacterial pneumonia is most often caused by *Streptococcus pneumoniae*, for which effective vaccines are now available. (At-risk patients older than 50 years are encouraged to get two different pneumonia vaccines annually.) Pneumonia is the second most common cause of admission to medical facilities in the United States, and 50,000 people die from pneumonia annually. In many other countries, pneumonia is the leading cause of death among children.[20]

Older adults, people with chronic illnesses, and people who smoke are at greater risk of pneumonia. Anyone who is not ventilating effectively, who has excessive secretions (such as a person with COPD or asthma, a postoperative patient, or a person who is bedridden or sedentary), or who is immunocompromised (from human immunodeficiency virus, other illnesses, posttransplantation immunosuppression, or chemotherapy) is at risk of the development of pneumonia. Patients with acquired immunodeficiency syndrome are particularly susceptible to *Pneumocystis jirovecii* pneumonia; it is a primary cause of morbidity and mortality. All high-risk patients are strongly encouraged to receive pneumonia vaccinations annually.

Another important consideration is that antibiotic-resistant organisms can colonize the respiratory tract. These organisms include, for example, MRSA and vancomycin-resistant enterococci, discussed in Chapter 27, *Infectious Diseases*. The aerosolization of these organisms when a patient coughs or during advanced airway procedures could be more dangerous to paramedics than when infections caused by these organisms exist in a pressure ulcer covered with a dressing. When presented with a patient in isolation because of an infection with MRSA (or a similar organism), always ask *where* the organism was found and wear proper respiratory protection if the organism is present in the patient's respiratory tract.

Assessment

A patient with pneumonia usually reports several hours to days of weakness, productive cough, fever, and sometimes chest pain worsened by coughing. The illness may have started abruptly, with shaking chills (rigors), or it might have come on more gradually, with progressive weakness. As you obtain the patient's history of recent illness, be particularly attuned to comments such as "I just got over the flu about a week ago." Pneumonia is often a secondary infection that follows a bout of influenza and is one of the leading causes of death under those circumstances.

Physical examination of a patient with pneumonia often reveals a grievously ill or toxic appearance. The patient may or may not be coughing. Crackles may be heard on auscultation of the chest, and the patient may have increased tactile fremitus and sputum production. Bronchial or bronchovesicular breath sounds may be noted over areas of consolidation; in advanced cases, breath sounds may become diminished or absent. Sputum may be either thick (because of dehydration) or purulent. If the infection also causes swelling of the pleural membranes, the patient may experience significant pain when breathing, especially when taking a deep breath or coughing. A pleural friction rub may be heard over the involved area.

Pneumonia often occurs in the lung bases, typically on only one side. Therefore, patients may have a "coughing fit" when turning from one side to the other. Sometimes patients' oxygen saturation will be significantly lower when they lie on one side versus the other. When the "good lung" is up, respiratory status may seem much better than when that lung is compressed by body weight.

> **Words of Wisdom**
>
> Adults sometimes have inflammation and plugging of the bronchioles, resulting in pneumonia distal to the blockages. This condition, known as bronchiolitis obliterans with organizing pneumonia, is referred to as "BOOP."

Patients with pneumonia are often dehydrated. Rehydration may temporarily worsen their condition as the thick secretions liquefy and expand in the chest. Supportive care includes oxygenation, secretion management (suctioning), and transport to the closest receiving facility. Bronchodilators will not help the pneumonia itself, but they may slightly improve the patient's ability to ventilate.

Management

Infections of the upper airway may require aggressive airway management approaches. Infections in the lower airway are usually treated with supportive care and by transport to a medical facility.

Atelectasis

Pathophysiology

The alveoli are vulnerable to several disorders. They may collapse from obstruction somewhere in the proximal airways or from external pressure produced, for example, by pneumothorax or hemothorax. They may fill with pus in pneumonia, with blood in pulmonary contusion, or with fluid in near drowning or heart failure. In addition, smoke or toxic gases may displace the fresh air that should be present in the alveoli.

Under normal conditions, most of the air that moves into and out of the lungs (approximately 79%) consists of the relatively inert gas nitrogen, which keeps the alveoli open. If a patient is given 100% oxygen, then any alveolus that becomes plugged will collapse once all of the oxygen diffuses out. Patients receiving high concentrations of oxygen are at increased risk of having this type of atelectasis.

The human body has billions of alveoli, and it is common for some of them to collapse from time to time. Humans (and most mammals) periodically sigh, cough, sneeze, and change positions, all actions that are thought to help open closed alveoli and avoid decreased ventilation to any one part of the lung. When people do not use these actions—for example, because they are sedated or in a coma, or because deep breathing or moving causes pain—increasing numbers of alveoli may collapse and not reopen. Like balloons, alveoli are more difficult to blow open once they have completely collapsed; eventually, entire lung segments may collapse. This condition, called **atelectasis**, increases the chance that pneumonia will develop in the affected areas.

Assessment

Although atelectasis can be a significant disease by itself, the larger concern is that the affected areas will become breeding grounds for pathogens, resulting in pneumonia. This risk is of concern in any patient who has a fever in the days following chest or abdominal surgery, particularly if breath sounds are decreased or abnormally colored sputum is produced.

Management

Postsurgical patients are encouraged to cough, deep breathe, and get out of bed with assistance, even if it is painful. Atelectasis may develop in people who cannot get out of bed, and the condition can lead to hypoxia or predispose a patient to lung infections and pneumonia.

At the medical facility, patients are constantly encouraged to take deep breaths. A device called an incentive spirometer helps patients quantify the depth of their breaths **FIGURE 17-30**. These devices are often sent home with patients for continued use after discharge from the medical facility (such as after rib fracture or chest surgery). Paramedics can reinforce deep breathing in patients who would benefit from it and can be watchful for atelectasis in patients who are sedentary or who take medications with sedative effects, including some analgesics.

Cancer

Pathophysiology

Lung cancer is one of the most common forms of cancer, especially among people who smoke cigarettes and those exposed to occupational lung hazards, such as asbestos, coal dust, or secondhand smoke. According to the American Lung Association, smoking contributes to 80% to 90% of new lung cancer cases.[21] Smokers are 13 to 23 times more likely to get lung cancer than are nonsmokers, and nonsmokers have a 20% to 30% greater risk of cancer if they are exposed to secondhand smoke at home or at work.[21] Although lung cancer was traditionally considered predominantly a disease of men, today 45% of new cases of lung cancer occur in women, most likely because of the increase in smoking among women.[21]

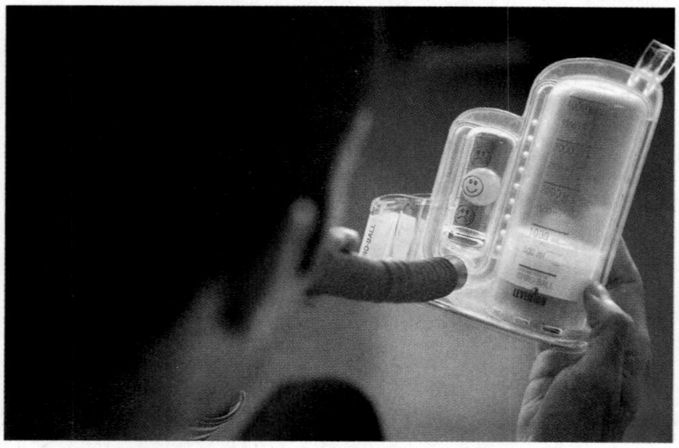

FIGURE 17-30 An incentive spirometer helps patients quantify how deep their breathing is. It helps them take deep breaths to avoid atelectasis.

Assessment

Lung cancer is often identified when tumors in the large airways bleed, causing **hemoptysis** (coughing up blood in the sputum) and uncontrollable coughing. It is frequently accompanied by COPD and impaired lung function. The lung is also a common site for the **metastasis** of cancer from other body sites.

Other types of cancer may invade the lymph nodes in the neck, producing tumors that threaten to occlude the upper airway. Patients with various types of cancer may have pulmonary complications from chemotherapy or radiation therapy. Lung irradiation, for example, may be associated with some degree of pulmonary edema. Tumors or treatment may also cause **pleural effusion**, which can present with rapidly progressing dyspnea.

Management

Paramedics can support oxygenation and ventilation and provide some amount of pain management, but there is little prehospital treatment specific to pleural effusion or hemoptysis other than transport to a medical facility. Paramedics are sometimes called to assist with end-of-life considerations for patients with cancer. Patients in hospice care, for example, may present with depressed respiration caused by the large amounts of narcotics used to relieve pain, anxiety, or other symptoms. In this type of narcotics overdose, titrate naloxone *only* enough to improve respiration; do not completely reverse the patient's primary pain control, or the patient may be plunged abruptly into complete misery. In the past, the respiratory depressant effects of narcotics and antianxiety agents may have been overemphasized, but now these agents are gaining increased popularity in the management of chronic pain, chronic cough, and anxiety in end-of-life scenarios. For example, fentanyl citrate (Sublimaze), a strong narcotic, is sometimes dispensed through an aerosol device to suppress chronic coughing in patients with end-stage lung cancer.

Toxic Inhalations

Pathophysiology

Many potentially toxic substances can be inhaled into the lungs. The type of damage from such an event depends largely on the water solubility of the toxic gas. **TABLE 17-8** shows how toxic gases are categorized.

Assessment

Highly water-soluble gases, such as ammonia, will react with the moist mucous membranes of the upper airway, causing swelling and irritation. If the substance gets into the patient's eyes, then the eyes will burn and feel inflamed and irritated.

Less water-soluble gases may get deep into the lower airway, where they may do damage over time. Such toxic gases have been used in war to disable the enemy, because they do not cause immediate distress, but rather cause pulmonary edema as long as 24 hours later. The gases phosgene and nitrogen dioxide behave in this manner.

Some common gases, such as chlorine, are moderately water soluble and produce signs and symptoms somewhere between the extremes of irritation and pulmonary edema. Severe exposure may present with upper airway swelling, whereas lower-level exposure may present with the classic delayed-onset lower airway damage. A common error is pouring household drain cleaner and chlorine bleach into a drain in an attempt to clear a clog, which may produce an irritant chlorine gas that can sicken the person and everyone else in the home or building. Industrial settings often use irritant gas–forming chemicals in large quantities and in higher concentrations than are available for home use, creating a possible scenario in which a larger number of people are exposed or a more toxic gas is produced. Paramedics should note industrial settings in their areas that present a high risk for this type of incident.

TABLE 17-8 Categorization of Toxic Gases

Category	Example	Effects
Highly water soluble	Ammonia	Acute upper airway irritation
Moderately water soluble	Chlorine	Effects depend on the concentration and amount of exposure, and range from coughing, wheezing, and crackles to pulmonary edema and chemical burns
Minimally water soluble	Phosgene	Delayed onset of pulmonary edema

Management

A patient who is exposed to a toxic gas must be immediately removed from contact with this substance and provided with 100% supplemental oxygen or assisted ventilation if breathing is impaired, as evidenced by reduced tidal volume. If the upper airway is compromised, then aggressive airway management (such as intubation or a cricothyrotomy) may be required.

Patients who have been exposed to slightly water-soluble gases may feel fine initially, only to have acute dyspnea many hours later. When such an exposure is suspected, patients should strongly consider transport to the closest ED for observation and further assessment.

Pulmonary Edema

Pathophysiology

Fluid buildup in lung tissue and air spaces occurs when fluid from the blood plasma migrates into the lung parenchyma. This pulmonary edema compromises gas exchange long before overt signs are present.

Pulmonary edema can be classified as high pressure (cardiogenic) or high permeability (noncardiogenic). Cardiogenic pulmonary edema (often called heart failure) can result from dysfunction of the right or left ventricle, chronic hypertension, dysrhythmias such as VT and supraventricular tachycardia, or cardiac diseases such as myocarditis. (These conditions are discussed in greater detail in Chapter 18, *Cardiovascular Emergencies*.)

Noncardiogenic pulmonary edema occurs in cases of acute hypoxemia, such as when inhaled toxins or near submersion damages alveolar tissue, causing fluid to seep into the lungs. Toxins or drugs in the bloodstream (such as toxins when a patient is in shock or using heroin) can damage the pulmonary capillaries and have the same effect. Sometimes trauma, severe shock, cardiac arrest, or even altitude changes can damage the alveoli and capillaries, causing acute respiratory distress syndrome or high-altitude pulmonary edema. See Chapter 39, *Environmental Emergencies*, for more information on high-altitude pulmonary edema.

Assessment

Some patients present with significant pulmonary edema after a lengthy journey, because they did not take diuretics while traveling. If a patient has been traveling, ask whether prescribed medications were taken regularly during that time.

Early in pulmonary edema, few signs are apparent. By the time fine crackles in the bases of the lungs become audible at the end of inspiration, fluid has leaked out of the capillaries, increased the diffusion space between the alveoli and capillaries, swollen the alveolar walls, and begun to seep into the alveoli. This sound is caused by fields of wet alveoli popping open as the lungs reach maximal inflation. Always listen to the lower lobes of the lungs through the patient's back, but never through clothing.

As pulmonary edema worsens, crackles may originate higher in the patient's lung fields, often described as "crackles up to the subscapular level" or "crackles up to the apices." As fluid migrates into the larger airways and mixes with mucus, coarse crackles will become audible during inspiration and exhalation, and tactile fremitus may be identified. Ultimately, the patient will begin to cough up watery sputum, which is often tinged pink by the presence of red blood cells. As air is forced into and out of the fluid-filled lungs, the fluid may bubble and foam. Coughing up pink, foamy, or blood-tinged sputum is a classic sign of severe pulmonary edema.

Management

The underlying cause of the pulmonary edema should be identified and treated. In all cases, it is essential to effectively manage the patient's airway and administer oxygen as appropriate to maintain recommended oxygen saturation levels. Noninvasive positive-pressure ventilation, such as CPAP or BPAP, may be indicated to stent the airway and allow the alveoli to inflate. Positive-pressure ventilation will also provide relief by reducing preload and afterload. Additionally, the use of nitrates may be considered to lower afterload and increase stroke volume, thereby improving cardiac output.

Acute Respiratory Distress Syndrome

Pathophysiology

Acute respiratory distress syndrome (ARDS; also known as shock lung, Da Nang lung, and, in neonates, hyaline membrane disease) is seldom seen in the field. Nevertheless, paramedics may have a vital role in preventing this devastating pathologic condition. This syndrome is caused by diffuse damage to the alveoli, perhaps as a result of shock, aspiration of gastric contents, pulmonary edema, barotrauma (from overly aggressive ventilation), or a hypoxic event. It seems to be worse when the patient has some direct damage to the lungs, as in trauma patients with severe pulmonary contusions.

Picture the alveoli as a beach surrounded by the sea of the bloodstream. During a near-death crisis, changes in permeability allow the tide to come in and wash over the beach. When the tide goes out, it washes away the surfactant from the alveoli and leaves behind debris, such as dead cells and bacteria, on the shore. The alveoli subsequently become stiff (noncompliant) and difficult to ventilate. Mechanical ventilation under extraordinarily high pressure is ultimately required, which causes even more damage. The delivery of high oxygen concentrations for prolonged periods causes additional destruction.

Assessment

Typically, ARDS is not seen in the field, but paramedics might be asked to transport a patient with ARDS between facilities. The assessment process is similar to that for any patient with a respiratory disorder. Document oxygen saturation, breath sounds, and any sudden change in the patient's condition. Patients with ARDS typically have stiff lungs (ie, low compliance). During manual ventilation, monitor the ventilation pressure to avoid overventilation and further lung damage. Various lung-protective strategies include low tidal volume, inverse I:E ratio, and permissive hypercapnia.

Pathophysiology, Assessment, and Management of Conditions Outside the Lung Parenchyma

Pneumothorax

Pathophysiology

When a patient has a simple pneumothorax, air typically collects between the visceral pleura and the parietal pleura lining the chest cavity. Air can enter the chest cavity via both traumatic (eg, open chest injury) and nontraumatic mechanisms. Some people have blebs in the lung parenchyma that are congenital or caused by COPD, which predisposes them to this condition. Blebs are weak spots that can rupture under stress, causing a spontaneous pneumothorax. The stress that ruptures the bleb may be as simple as coughing or as severe as aggressive bag-mask ventilation. People with severe asthma are susceptible to blebs, as are tall, thin people, especially those who smoke.

If the amount of air is small and no further complications occur, simple pneumothoraces can self-resolve. However, if air continues to build up, it could result in a tension pneumothorax, a more severe pneumothorax in which intrathoracic pressure is increased, causing decreased cardiac output due to reduced venous return caused by the increased pressure.

Assessment

Some patients who have had multiple simple pneumothoraces previously may actually say, "I'm having another pneumothorax." Patients may describe feeling a sharp pain after coughing, followed by increasing dyspnea during the subsequent minutes or hours.

Management

Most patients with pneumothorax will not require acute intervention, such as needle chest decompression, but they must at least receive oxygen and have their respiratory status closely monitored en route to the medical facility. If a tension pneumothorax is identified, immediate intervention with needle decompression to relieve intrathoracic pressure is typically indicated. See Chapter 36, *Chest Trauma*, for more on treating tension pneumothorax.

Pleural Effusion

Pathophysiology

When fluid collects between the visceral pleura and the parietal pleura, it produces a pleural effusion **FIGURE 17-31**. The sac of fluid formed is similar to a blister, and repeated trauma to the tissues causes even more fluid to collect there. Effusions can be caused by infections, tumors, or trauma.

To visualize how this condition arises, imagine a blister forming at the base of the lung. The tissues rub against each other breath after breath, causing inflammation and fluid accumulation in the space. Some pleural effusions can contain several liters of fluid. A large effusion decreases lung capacity and causes dyspnea.

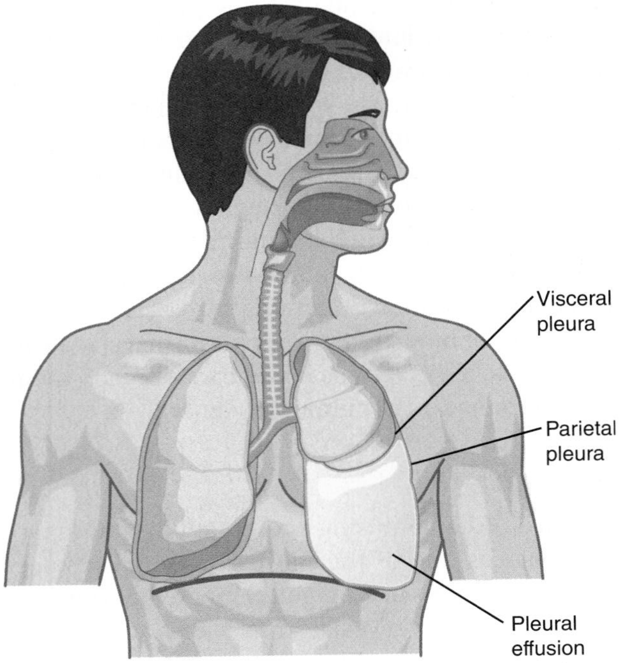

FIGURE 17-31 A pleural effusion is a buildup of fluid between the visceral pleura and the parietal pleura.

Assessment

It may be difficult to hear any breath sounds through the effusion. Because the effusion is filled with fluid, the patient's position may affect the ability to breathe.

Management

Shifting position may cause significantly more dyspnea, and patients usually resist being placed into anything other than the Fowler position. Supportive care, including proper positioning and aggressive supplemental oxygen administration, should be provided until the patient can be transported to a facility at which the effusion can be definitively treated. Large effusions may be drained at the medical facility in a procedure called *thoracentesis.* This procedure frequently provides immediate relief of symptoms.

Pulmonary Embolism

Pathophysiology

The pulmonary circulation may be compromised by a blood clot (embolism), a fat embolism from a broken bone, an amniotic fluid embolism from leakage of amniotic fluid during pregnancy, or an air embolism resulting from air entering the circulation via a laceration in the neck or an IV administration set that was improperly flushed or not flushed. A large embolism, of whatever type, usually lodges in a major branch of the pulmonary artery and prevents blood flow through that branch. Adequate gas exchange in the lungs requires functional alveoli to provide oxygen and take up carbon dioxide, along with intact pulmonary vessels to convey oxygen-poor blood to the alveoli. Normal alveoli are of little use if the venous blood cannot reach them, as is the situation in pulmonary embolism.

Assessment

Because of its confusing presentation, pulmonary embolism is one of the most frequently misdiagnosed conditions in emergency medicine. The early presentation may reveal normal breath sounds with good peripheral aeration, diverting attention away from a pulmonary pathology. The classic presentation is sudden dyspnea and cyanosis and, perhaps, a sharp pain in the chest. A hallmark of pulmonary embolism is that the cyanosis does not resolve with oxygen therapy.

Pulmonary emboli often originate in the large veins of the leg, particularly the greater saphenous vein. A clot can form there and then migrate through the venous circulation, passing through the right side of the heart and into the pulmonary circulation **FIGURE 17-32**. Patients with thrombophlebitis (inflammation of the veins in the legs) are at high risk for pulmonary embolism. They may have the Homan sign (calf pain during dorsiflexion of the foot caused by thrombophlebitis in the leg).

Clots also tend to form when a person is immobile for a prolonged period, such as during a long car trip or lengthy airplane flight, after removal of a lower extremity cast, or after major surgery.

Management

Bedridden patients are often prescribed anticoagulants, special stockings, or other devices to reduce the formation of blood clots in the legs. Especially

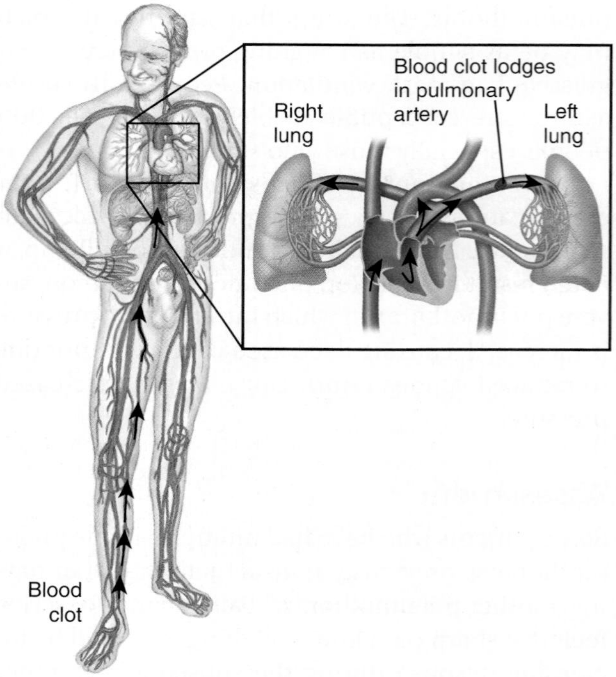

FIGURE 17-32 Pulmonary emboli are most common in sedentary people, in whom an embolus typically forms in the legs or pelvis. The embolus passes through the right side of the heart and lodges in the pulmonary artery, blocking blood flow to a portion of the lung.

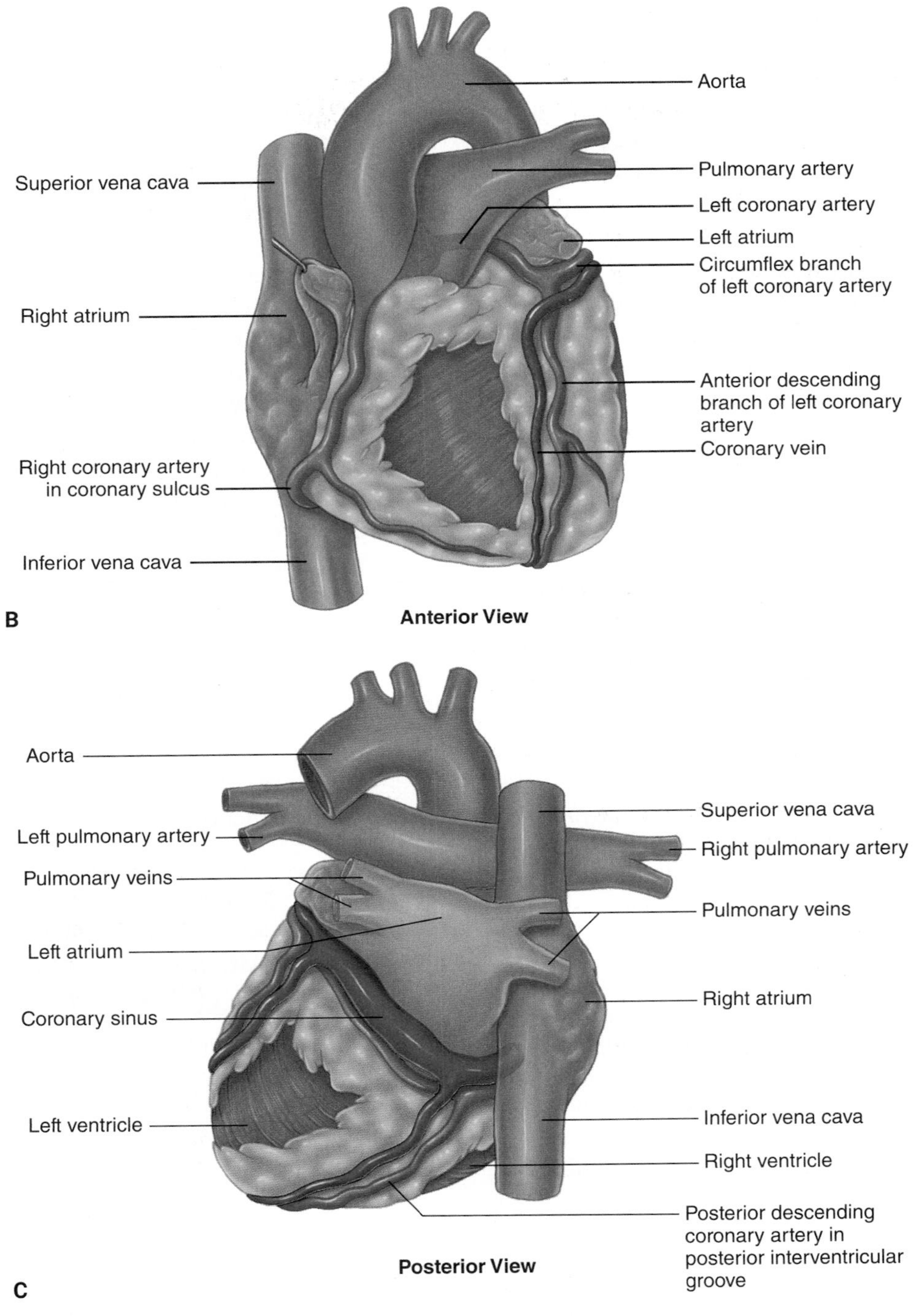

FIGURE 18-1 *Continued*

smaller coronary veins and then drains the blood into the right atrium. The left atrium receives freshly oxygenated blood from the lungs through the right and left pulmonary veins. Then the atria contract, pumping blood through the atrioventricular (AV) valve into the ventricles.

- The heart's two lower chambers are the right and left ventricles. The walls of the ventricles are much thicker than the atria walls. The right ventricle pumps deoxygenated blood to the lungs. The left ventricle pumps oxygenated blood throughout the body. When the left ventricle contracts, it normally produces an impulse that can be palpated at the heart's apex (apical impulse), which occurs because the left ventricle rotates forward as it contracts. In a normal heart, this rotation causes the apex of the left ventricle to strike the chest wall. The apical impulse is also called the **point of maximal impulse (PMI)** because it is the site at which the heartbeat is most strongly felt. The PMI usually is located on the left anterior part of the chest, at the fifth intercostal space (ICS) along the midclavicular line.

- An internal wall of connective tissue called the **septum** (plural *septa*) separates the heart's right and left sides. It is made up of two parts: The interatrial septum, which separates the right and left atria, and the interventricular septum, which separates the right and left ventricles.
- The septa separate the heart into two functional pumps. The right atrium and right ventricle comprise one pump. The left atrium and left ventricle comprise the other. The right side of the heart (sometimes called the "right heart") is a low-pressure system (pulmonary circulation). The left side of the heart (sometimes called the "left heart") is a high-pressure pump (systemic circulation).
- The myocardium is the middle layer of the heart wall. It is composed mostly of thick cardiac muscle tissue and is responsible for cardiac contraction and efficient ejection of blood from the heart.
- The **coronary arteries** supply blood to the tissues of the heart. There are two main coronary arteries: left and right. The left main coronary artery (LMCA) is the largest in diameter and the shortest of the myocardial blood vessels. It rapidly divides into the **left anterior descending artery (LAD)** and the **circumflex artery (Cx)**. Although the areas supplied by the coronary arteries can differ among patients, the LAD supplies blood to the left ventricle's anterior surface, part of the left ventricle's lateral surface, and a portion of the interventricular septum in most patients. The Cx artery supplies the left atrium, part of the lateral surface of the left ventricle, the inferior surface of the left ventricle in approximately 15% of people, the posterior surface of the left ventricle in 15% of people, the **sinoatrial (SA) node** in about 40% of people, and the AV bundle in 10% to 15% of people. Branches of the **right coronary artery (RCA)** supply blood to the walls of the right atrium and ventricle, a portion of the inferior part of the left ventricle, and portions of the conduction system (the SA node in approximately 60% of people and the AV bundle in 85% to 90% of people).
- Cardiac cells have four important properties that help the heart function efficiently: automaticity, excitability, conductivity, and contractility.
- The cardiac conduction system comprises six parts: the SA node, the AV node, the bundle of His, the right and left bundle branches, and the Purkinje fibers.
- Stimulation of sympathetic (accelerator) nerves strengthens the force of contraction and increases the heart rate. Stimulation of parasympathetic (inhibitory) nerve fibers slows the rate of discharge of the SA node, slows conduction through the AV node, weakens the strength of atrial contraction, and can cause a small reduction in the force of ventricular contraction.

Patient Assessment

Scene Size-up

A cardiac-related complaint is a common reason why a person seeks medical care. Patients with cardiovascular-related symptoms may be young, middle-aged, or older adults. They may be unresponsive, be awake and alert, or have an altered mental status. The patient may be stable or unstable and may or may not have a pulse. Regardless of the situation, a systematic approach to patient assessment is essential. This approach, including cardiac physical assessment, is discussed in Chapter 11, *Patient Assessment*. When used consistently, this type of approach will help ensure that you do not overlook physical findings or key questions pertinent to the patient's treatment plan. In this section, we focus on those areas of the assessment that require special attention for the patient who has a cardiovascular complaint or who is experiencing a cardiovascular emergency.

Primary Survey

The order of the steps for performing a primary survey differs depending on the type of cardiac patient. Whereas the order of steps in the primary survey is usually ABCDE (assess airway, breathing, and then circulation, disability, and exposure), if the patient is found unresponsive and is suspected of being in cardiac arrest, the order changes to CABDE (first assess circulation, then airway, breathing, disability, and exposure). In this section, we assume the patient is responsive, breathing, and has a pulse.

History Taking

Acute coronary syndromes (ACSs) are a series of cardiac conditions caused by an abrupt reduction in blood flow through a coronary artery. There are three major ACSs: **unstable angina**, non–ST-segment elevation myocardial infarction (NSTEMI), and ST-segment elevation myocardial infarction (STEMI). Common chief complaints in the patient experiencing an ACS include chest discomfort, dyspnea, fainting, palpitations, and fatigue.

Chest pain or discomfort is often the presenting symptom in a patient with an ACS. The patient's description of the discomfort is important for assessing its significance. You can use the OPQRST mnemonic (Onset, Provocation/palliation, Quality, Region/radiation, Severity, Timing) to elaborate on the patient's chief complaint.

Some patients may have more than one chief complaint. For example, a patient may report chest pain and difficulty breathing or palpitations and chest pain. If any of these symptoms occur, ask the patient which symptom started first and which bothers them the most. For example, further questioning of the patient who reports palpitations and chest pain may reveal that the patient felt the heart racing for a few minutes and then began having chest pain.

O What is the *Onset* or origin of the discomfort? Questions to ask include, how did it begin (suddenly or gradually)? Has anything like this ever happened before? Did a health care provider examine and treat the patient for the symptoms reported? If so, what was the diagnosis? How does the discomfort the patient is feeling right now compare with that?

P What *Provoked* the discomfort? Questions to ask include, what, if anything, brought it on? Is it exertional or nonexertional? What was the patient doing at the time? Sitting in a chair? Changing a tire? Shoveling snow? Arguing? **Angina pectoris** is chest discomfort that occurs when the heart muscle does not receive enough oxygen (myocardial **ischemia**). Examples of activities that increase the heart's demand for oxygen include experiencing emotional upset, smoking a cigarette, eating a heavy meal, walking up an incline or against a wind, working with the arms over the head, or being exposed to cold weather. An AMI may occur when a patient is at rest, after a serious illness or unusually vigorous exercise, in conjunction with severe emotional stress, or without warning. The circumstances that provoke the patient's symptoms can provide a clue to the cause of the pain or discomfort. For example, pain that worsens with exertion and resolves with rest may be related to myocardial ischemia. Pain that worsens after a meal may have a gastrointestinal (GI) cause. Pain that worsens when the patient takes a deep breath may be attributable to a respiratory or musculoskeletal cause. Does anything make the pain worse? What palliates the pain; that is, does anything make it better? Patients with **coronary artery disease (CAD)** may take nitroglycerin (NTG) for episodes of chest pain. Ask whether the patient took NTG. If so, how much did the patient take and did it help?

Q What is the *Quality* of the discomfort? Questions to ask include, what does it feel like? Get the patient's narrative description. Dull? Sharp? Crushing? Heavy? Squeezing? Note the exact words the patient uses to describe the discomfort, and observe the body language as the patient does so. Try not to lead patients' responses unless they are unable to describe the pain. In these cases, offer alternatives, such as "Is it sharp, dull, or crampy?" Use the word "discomfort" instead of "pain" in these questions. Although many patients having a cardiac-related event will tell you they have chest pain, some will not feel true pain. Some patients having a cardiac-related event present with signs and symptoms other than chest pain or discomfort, such as generalized weakness, sweating, light-headedness, shortness of breath, back pain, or nausea and vomiting.

R Does the discomfort *Radiate*? From where to where? To the jaw? Down the left arm? Into the back? Chest discomfort associated with myocardial ischemia usually begins in the central or left chest. It then radiates to the arm (especially the little finger [ulnar] side of the left arm), wrist, jaw, epigastrium, left shoulder, or between the shoulder blades. A similar pattern may also occur in **pericarditis** (inflammation of the pericardial sac). Severe ischemia may result in radiation to the right chest, right arm, and/or back. In a patient with a cardiac-related event, symptoms such as epigastric pain, nausea, and vomiting may be confused with the symptoms of a patient who has a GI disorder, such as a peptic ulcer. Aortic **dissection** or enlargement of an **aortic aneurysm** may produce pain that begins in the center of the chest and radiates to the back.

S What is the *Severity* of the discomfort? Questions to ask include, how bad is it? Assess the patient's discomfort using a 0-to-10 pain rating scale, with 10 being the worst. Although physical signs of pain may be obvious in many patients, some may feel severe pain and not show visible signs of discomfort. Remember, the patient is the authority regarding their pain. Using a pain rating scale allows you to evaluate the effectiveness of the emergency care you provide. Document the patient's initial rating of the pain or discomfort. Reassess (and document) the degree of discomfort after each treatment you perform and before transferring care at the receiving facility. If the patient has chronic angina, ask them to compare the pain with their "usual" angina pain.

T What was the *Timing* of the event? Questions to ask include, when did it start? How long did it last? What time did it get worse or better? Was it continuous or intermittent? Establishing when the patient's symptoms began is essential, particularly if the patient is a candidate for **reperfusion therapy** (ie, medications or procedures used to open a blocked coronary artery). Anginal symptoms usually last less than 20 minutes. Chest discomfort associated with AMI often lasts 20 minutes to several hours. Chest discomfort that lasts for hours may also be seen in patients with pericarditis and aortic dissection.

Another chief complaint among patients with an ACS is dyspnea (difficult or labored breathing). Dyspnea may vary in intensity from merely being aware of one's breathing to severe respiratory distress. Because dyspnea is not a sign but rather a symptom, assessing its severity is difficult. Ask the patient to rate the severity of the breathing difficulty on a scale of 0 to 10 or compare it to prior experiences.

Dyspnea that develops suddenly suggests **pulmonary embolism**, pneumothorax, acute **pulmonary edema**, pneumonia, or airway obstruction. Dyspnea that occurs on exertion or at rest suggests the presence of chronic obstructive pulmonary disease (COPD) or left ventricular failure. **Left ventricular failure (LVF)** causes fluid to build up in the lungs. In patients who have chronic LVF, dyspnea often develops slowly over weeks or months. Patients with chronic heart failure may have dyspnea when resting in a horizontal position because blood pools in the lungs when they lie down. Dyspnea that is relieved by a change in position (either sitting upright or standing) is called **orthopnea**. To avoid dyspnea, patients with orthopnea often sleep on two or more pillows to achieve an upright or semi-upright position.

Paroxysmal nocturnal dyspnea (PND) is a sudden onset of difficulty breathing in which the patient suddenly awakens from sleep. PND is often associated with LVF. PND usually begins 2 to 4 hours after the onset of sleep, and is often accompanied by coughing, wheezing, and sweating. The patient may awaken with a feeling of suffocation. The patient's condition usually improves after sitting up or standing for 15 to 30 minutes.

If the patient has a cough, then find out whether it is dry or productive. A dry cough is a nonproductive cough. A productive (or wet) cough clears the airway of mucus (sputum) and foreign material. The characteristics of the sputum produced may help you determine the cause of the cough. For example, pulmonary edema is often accompanied by frothy, pink-tinged sputum.

Fainting (**syncope**) is a brief loss of consciousness caused by a temporary decrease in the blood flow to the brain. In near syncope (also called presyncope), signs and symptoms of impending syncope occur, including dizziness with or without a blackout (called a gray-out), anxiety, pale mucous membranes, sweating, thready pulse, and low BP.

Fainting may occur while sitting, standing, walking, and occasionally during exercise. As part of history taking for a patient who has fainted, try to determine whether the patient fainted from cardiac or noncardiac causes. Cardiac causes of syncope include dysrhythmias, increased vagal tone, and heart lesions. Consider a cardiac cause if fainting occurs in a recumbent position, is provoked by exercise, or is associated with chest pain, or if a family history of fainting or sudden death is present. Noncardiac causes of syncope are discussed in Chapter 19, *Neurologic Emergencies.*

Patients with cardiac problems may present with a chief complaint of palpitations. **Palpitations** refer to the sensation of an abnormally fast or irregular heartbeat. Except after extreme exertion, a person usually remains blissfully unaware of their heartbeat. Palpitations can be caused by anxiety, lack of sleep, certain medicines, caffeine, stress, cocaine or amphetamine use, heavy cigarette smoking, or metabolic conditions, such as hyperthyroidism. Changes in the heart's rhythm or rate, including fast rhythms (tachycardias) and early beats, may also cause palpitations. A patient may not use the word palpitations but may report feeling the heart "skipping beats," "flip-flopping," "fluttering," or "racing," or use similar words. In such a case, ask about the onset, frequency, and duration of this symptom and previous episodes of palpitations. Ask about the presence of associated symptoms such as chest discomfort, dizziness, syncope, and dyspnea.

Fatigue is a common complaint in patients with impaired cardiovascular functions and is one of the vaguest of all symptoms. Many conditions can cause fatigue. Electrolyte disorders, such as unusually high or low potassium levels, are a common cause of generalized weakness and fatigue. Fatigue may precede or accompany other symptoms associated with ACS. Medications such as beta blockers, diuretics, or antihypertensives may also cause fatigue. Try to determine when the patient's fatigue began and how long it has been present. Ask about associated symptoms such as chest discomfort, nausea, dyspnea, syncope, or palpitations.

Patients may report a variety of other related symptoms as you explore the history of their present illness. They may have feelings of impending doom or sense that they will soon experience a life-changing event. Some patients report feeling nauseous or vomiting. Listen carefully to patients for indications that trauma may be involved or that their activity levels have been limited because of their conditions. Observe their faces as you listen to them tell their stories. Do you see a look of fear or anguish? Are they holding their chests? Most of the other associated complaints your patients may have will be related to hypoxia or poor perfusion resulting from inadequate cardiac output (CO), such as decreased level of responsiveness, diaphoresis, restlessness and anxiety, headache, behavioral changes, and syncope.

After exploring the patient's chief complaint, inquire briefly about pertinent aspects of the patient's other medical history. History taking provides an excellent opportunity to ask about medications prescribed and whether they are being taken as instructed. Ask when the patient last took their medications and whether they are taking medications prescribed for someone else (borrowed). Common cardiac medications include the following:

- Antidysrhythmics such as digoxin (Lanoxin), procainamide (Procan, Pronestyl), amiodarone (Cordarone), and verapamil (Calan, Isoptin, Verelan)
- Anticoagulants such as enoxaparin (Lovenox), clopidogrel (Plavix), and warfarin (Coumadin)
- Angiotensin-converting enzyme inhibitors such as captopril (Capoten), enalapril (Vasotec), and lisinopril (Prinivil, Zestril)
- Beta blockers such as atenolol (Tenormin), metoprolol (Lopressor), and propranolol (Inderal)
- Lipid-lowering agents such as gemfibrozil (Lopid), atorvastatin (Lipitor), fluvastatin (Lescol), lovastatin (Mevacor), pravastatin (Pravachol), rosuvastatin calcium (Crestor), and simvastatin (Zocor)
- Diuretics such as furosemide (Lasix) or hydrochlorothiazide (HCTZ)
- Vasodilators such as nitroglycerin (Nitrostat) or isosorbide (Isordil)

In addition to inquiring about prescription medications, ask about any over-the-counter medications or herbal supplements that the patient takes. Herbal supplements can cause serious, and even fatal, interactions when taken with certain cardiac medications. It may also be appropriate to ask about recreational drug use. Ask the patient whether they have taken a phosphodiesterase inhibitor such as sildenafil (Viagra) in the past 24 hours or tadalafil (Cialis), or vardenafil (Levitra) in the past 48 hours. When taken in combination with vasodilators such as NTG or isosorbide, these medications may cause a sudden and significant drop in BP. Common medications prescribed to patients with cardiovascular conditions are discussed in Chapter 13, *Principles of Pharmacology*.

Ask specifically whether the patient has ever been diagnosed with any of the following:

- Aneurysm
- Atherosclerotic heart disease: angina, previous MI, hypertension, heart failure
- Congenital anomalies
- CAD
- Diabetes
- Inflammatory cardiac disease
- Previous cardiac surgery (coronary artery bypass graft or valve replacement)
- Pulmonary disease
- Renal disease
- Valvular disease
- Vascular disease

Secondary Assessment

The physical exam during a secondary assessment is similar for many medical patients. Nevertheless, certain aspects warrant greater emphasis in the patient whose chief complaint suggests a cardiac problem.

Low CO results in inadequate tissue perfusion, which often results in pallor or skin that appears mottled or cyanotic. The skin of a patient having a heart attack may be cool and sweaty. The skin of a patient in cardiogenic shock may be cold and sweaty. This finding is a sympathetic response in which the blood within peripheral vessels is shunted to the vital organs to maintain adequate perfusion. Flushed, warm skin may be a sign of infection such as pericarditis. The body's response to pain may include restlessness, flushed skin, increased heart rate, increased respiratory rate, and/or elevated BP.

Inspect the neck and tracheal position. Is the trachea midline and mobile to gentle manipulation? Press down with your finger in the patient's suprasternal notch to verify that the trachea is midline. Inspect the neck veins for jugular venous distention (JVD). The external jugular veins reflect the pressure within the patient's systemic circulation. Normally, these veins are collapsed when a person is sitting or standing and are mildly distended when the patient is supine. Venous pressure increases with a significant increase in blood volume when the right ventricle fails or when increased pressure in the pericardial sac hinders the return of blood to the right atrium. Venous pressure decreases when blood volume is decreased significantly or ejection of blood occurs from the left ventricle. To estimate the patient's jugular venous pressure, place the patient in a semi-Fowler position (45° angle) with the head slightly rotated away from the jugular vein you are examining; observe the height of the distended fluid column within the vein, and note how far up the distention extends above the sternal angle.

Continue your assessment by inspecting and palpating the chest. Look for surgical scars that might indicate previous cardiac surgery. Look for other signs that suggest the patient has a history of cardiac disease. For example, the presence of a NTG patch on the patient's skin suggests a history of angina. A slight bulge under the skin of the patient's upper right or left chest or abdominal wall is probably a pacemaker or implantable defibrillator. Is the anterior-posterior diameter of the chest enlarged? This finding of an expanded chest that resembles a barrel's shape is called *barrel chest* and may be seen in patients with COPD. Palpating the chest may reveal areas of tenderness or crepitus. For example, costochondritis is a condition that may cause chest pain from inflammation of the cartilage and bones in the chest wall.

Listen carefully to the chest with your stethoscope. Crackles or wheezes may suggest LVF with pulmonary edema. A patient who has pulmonary edema may have foamy, blood-tinged sputum present in the mouth or nose.

Words of Wisdom

The word *pallor*, as used in this text, may apply to any patient whose skin presentation suggests reduced blood flow or oxygenation. It is distinguished from similar presentations, such as hypopigmentation (lack or loss of skin pigment) or simply a fair complexion. In general, the mucous membranes inside the inner lower eyelid and the oral mucosa will have a pink coloration in all healthy patients, regardless of skin color; thus, a white or pale appearance of these areas in any patient suggests reduced blood flow or oxygenation.

Inspect and lightly palpate the patient's abdomen for distention and pulsations. Strong pulsations in the epigastric area may be a sign of an abdominal aortic aneurysm. Look at the patient's arms, hands, legs, feet, and ankles for swelling. If the patient is confined to a bed, check for swelling in the lower back (sacral) area, as swelling occurs in the most dependent body areas. Bilateral pitting edema may be a sign of **right ventricular failure (RVF)**. Pitting edema limited to one side of the body suggests a blockage in a major vein.

When you obtain the vital signs, carefully assess the patient's pulse. A weak, thready pulse suggests a reduction in CO. A pulse that is very rapid (more than 150 beats per minute [beats/min]), very slow (less than 40 beats/min), or irregular may be one of the first indicators of a cardiac dysrhythmia and requires further evaluation. Place any patient who has a cardiac-related symptom on a cardiac monitor. Document the patient's initial rhythm and any changes in the rhythm.

One of the most important and widely used tools for paramedics is the cardiac monitor-defibrillator. This machine enables you to monitor and record 3-lead ECG tracings, and record 12-lead ECGs in the field. It also enables you to quickly identify suspected AMI, transmit the findings electronically to the receiving facility, and make sound transport decisions concerning patient destination based on the ECG findings. A monitor-defibrillator also enables you to treat cardiac dysrhythmias using electrical therapy, such as **defibrillation**, **synchronized cardioversion**, or **transcutaneous pacing (TCP)**, when such procedures are warranted.

While obtaining the vital signs, attach the cardiac monitor, waveform capnography, and pulse oximeter if you have not done so already. Use the ECG and oxygen saturation (Spo_2) measurement just as you do other vital signs—that is, as tools to help in the assessment and not as the only guide to treatment (treat the patient, not the monitor).

Pulse Findings in Cardiac Patients

Normally, the apical pulse rate is the same as the pulse rate in a peripheral location such as the radial pulse. Assess an apical pulse with a stethoscope. Place the stethoscope over the heart's apex, which is between the fifth and sixth ribs on the left side of the chest in adults. To assess for a pulse deficit, palpate a peripheral pulse while listening to the apical pulse. A difference between the apical pulse and the peripheral pulse rates indicates a pulse deficit. For example, if a patient's apical pulse rate is 100 beats/min and the radial pulse rate is 75 beats/min, a pulse deficit of 25 beats/min is present. Pulse deficit occurs with many abnormal heart rhythms or when the heart's contractions are too weak to propel blood through the peripheral arteries.

When the body is at rest, BP normally fluctuates during the respiratory cycle, falling with inspiration and rising with expiration. The accepted upper limit for a fall in systolic blood pressure (SBP) with inspiration is 10 mm Hg. Pulsus paradoxus occurs when the SBP falls more than 10 mm Hg with inspiration. Cardiac conditions in which this finding may be present include AMI, cardiogenic shock, **cardiac tamponade**, and constrictive pericarditis.

Finally, you might recognize a beat-to-beat difference in the strength of a pulse. This finding, called *pulsus alternans*, may be a sign of severe ventricular failure. It is believed the beat-to-beat changes in pulse strength are a result of a decrease in the number of myocardial cells contracting during alternate beats, resulting in decreased myocardial contractility.

BP Findings in Cardiac Patients

A normal SBP is less than 120 mm Hg and a normal diastolic blood pressure (DBP) is less than 80 mm Hg (these values were also identified in Chapter 11, *Patient Assessment*). Stage 2 hypertension exists when the SBP is 140 mm Hg or higher or the DBP is 90 mm Hg or higher.[3] In patients 30 years and older, higher SBP and DBP values are associated with increased risk of CVD incidence and angina, AMI, heart failure, stroke, peripheral artery disease, and abdominal aortic aneurysm.[3]

In emergency situations, an elevated BP may reflect the patient's anxiety or pain. A SBP of less than 90 mm Hg might suggest hypotension and shock, depending on the patient's overall condition and chief complaint. Markedly elevated BP values may contribute to aortic dissection, heart failure, or stroke. The pulse pressure reflects stroke volume and the elasticity of the arterial walls. Normal pulse pressure is 30 to 40 mm Hg. A widened (high) pulse pressure (more than 40 mm Hg) may be seen in conditions such as the later stages of shock.

A narrowed pulse pressure (less than 30 mm Hg) may be seen in conditions such as tachycardia and cardiac tamponade.

It may be beneficial to obtain BP readings in both arms and compare the readings. Some conditions such as stroke or aortic aneurysm may cause BP values to vary from the right to the left side.

Assessment of Heart Sounds

Assessing heart sounds requires a relatively quiet environment. As a result, detailed assessment of heart sounds is usually not always practical in the prehospital setting. However, the ability to recognize normal heart sounds can be useful. The purpose of listening to heart sounds is to identify the "lub-dub" that indicates the cardiac valves are operating properly. Chapter 8, *Anatomy and Physiology*, discusses heart sounds. Chapter 11, *Patient Assessment*, discusses how to auscultate heart sounds.

S_1 heart sounds occur near the beginning of ventricular contraction (systole), when the tricuspid and mitral valves close. The tricuspid valve's closing can be louder in patients experiencing pulmonary hypertension because of the increased pressure that exists past the valve. In patients with anemia, a fever, or hyperthyroidism, louder S_1 sounds may be heard because of the valves being open when the ventricles contract. A patient who has a stenosed mitral valve will also have a louder S_1. Patients with mitral valves that are subject to fibrosis or are calcified can have decreased S_1 heart sounds. Other conditions such as obesity, emphysema, and cardiac tamponade (fluid around the heart) can also diminish S_1 heart sounds. Any delay in the closing of these two valves, heard as a split sound, is considered abnormal.

S_2 heart sounds occur near the end of ventricular contraction (systole), when the pulmonary and aortic valves close. Patients with chronic high BP or pulmonary hypertension may experience a higher closing pressure for these valves, resulting in the aortic valve making a louder sound when it closes. Patients with hypotension will produce a decreased S_2 sound. The S_2 sound may be split if the patient has a right bundle branch, which results in a delay of the pulmonic valve closing. Left bundle branch blocks may cause the aortic valve to close more slowly than the pulmonic valve.

When an S_1, S_2, S_3 sequence is heard in adults, it is called a gallop rhythm because it sounds like a horse galloping. S_3 is heard in early ventricular diastole. This sound is caused by vibration of the ventricular walls during rapid ventricular filling and is often associated with heart failure.

S_4 is a rare heart sound heard just before S_1. It is caused by turbulent filling of a stiff ventricle, as seen in hypertrophy and possibly myocardial infarction (MI).

A murmur is an abnormal whooshing-like sound that is associated with turbulent blood flow through the heart valves. This turbulent blood flow can occur from increased blood flow across a normal valve, flow across an irregular or constricted valve, blood flow into an enlarged chamber of the heart, or blood flow going backward through a compromised valve.

Reassessment

Once the history and vital signs have been obtained and the physical exam has been completed, continue treating the patient and initiate transport to the most appropriate destination. The reassessment is accomplished en route to the hospital. It begins with a repeat of the primary survey (level of consciousness and ABCDEs). Obtain vital signs every 5 minutes for critical patients or every 15 minutes for patients determined to be in stable condition. Repeat the physical exam to see if any changes have occurred or if any conditions were missed in the initial physical exam.

Assess the effectiveness of all interventions implemented. For example, is the IV fluid still flowing? Has the pain diminish after NTG administration?

Prepare proper documentation of the call. Notify the receiving facility of any history findings, physical exam findings, and cardiac monitoring or ECG findings. Finally, part of the patient's care with STEMI should involve transmitting the 12-lead ECG to the catheterization lab to shorten the interval from the arrival time to treatment time.

Electrophysiology

The mechanical pumping action of the heart can occur only in response to an electrical stimulus. This impulse causes the heart to beat because of complex chemical changes within the myocardial cells.

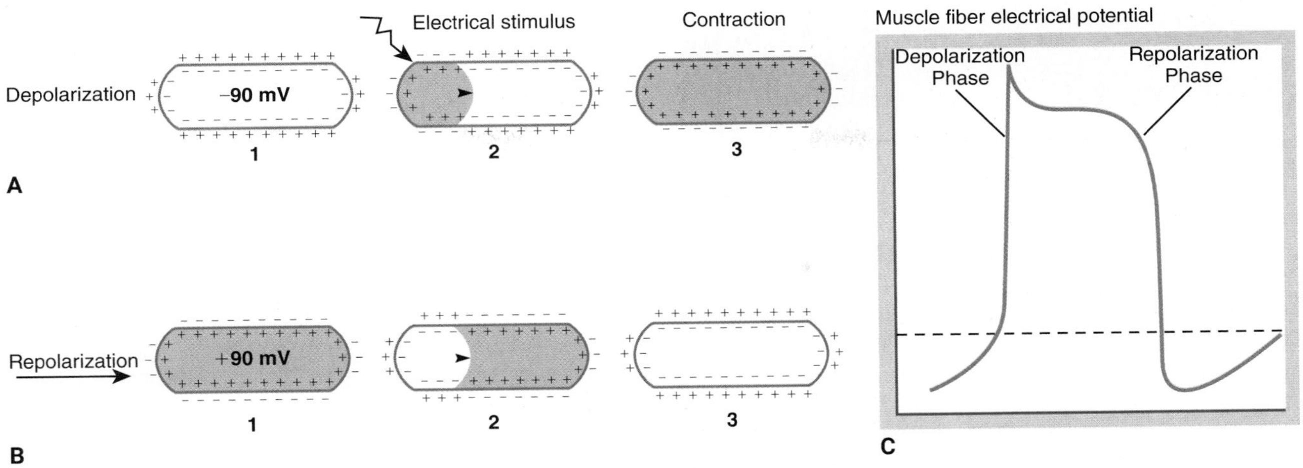

FIGURE 18-2 Movement of ions to produce a net current flow. **A.** Depolarization. (1) At rest, the cell's interior has a net charge of −90 mV. (2) The wave of depolarization begins as sodium ions pour into the cell. (3) Depolarized cell. **B.** Repolarization. (1) Depolarized cell. (2) The wave of repolarization begins as potassium ions leave the cell. (3) Repolarized cell. **C.** Changes in the electrical potential of muscle fiber associated with contraction.

Depolarization and Repolarization

An action potential is a sequence of changes in the membrane potential that occurs when an excitable cell is stimulated. In the heart, **depolarization** is the process of discharging resting cardiac muscle fibers by means of an electrical impulse that stimulates contraction **FIGURE 18-2A**.

Like all cells in the body, myocardial cells are bathed in an electrolyte solution. Chemical pumps inside the cell maintain the ion concentration within the cell, creating an electrical gradient across the cell membrane. Consequently, a resting (polarized) cell normally has a net internal charge of −90 millivolts (mV) relative to the outside of the cell (Figure 18-2, part A1). When a myocardial cell receives a stimulus from the conduction system (Figure 18-2, part A2), the cell wall becomes more permeable as specialized channels open, allowing sodium ions (Na^+) to rush into the cell. Thus, the inside of the cell becomes more positive. Calcium ions (Ca^{+2}) also enter the cell, albeit more slowly and through a different set of specialized channels. These ions help maintain the depolarized state of the cell membrane and allow cardiac muscle tissue to contract. This reversal of the cell's electrical charge begins at one point in the cell wall and spreads in a wave until the cell has been completely depolarized (Figure 18-2, part A3). As the cell depolarizes and calcium ions enter, mechanical contraction occurs.

If the cell remains depolarized, then it can never contract again! However, the cell can recover from depolarization through a process called *repolarization* **FIGURE 18-2B**. Repolarization begins as the sodium and calcium channels close, halting the rapid inflow of these ions. Next, special potassium channels open, allowing the rapid escape of potassium ions (K^+) from the cell, which helps restore a negative charge inside the cell; the proper electrolyte distribution is then reestablished as sodium ions are pumped out of the cell and potassium ions reenter. After the potassium channels close, this sodium-potassium pump helps move sodium and potassium ions back to their respective locations. For every three sodium ions this pump moves out of the cell, it moves two potassium ions into the cell, thereby maintaining the cell membrane's polarity.

TABLE 18-1 summarizes the roles of the various electrolytes in cardiac function.

Cardiac Action Potential

The action potential of a typical myocardial cell can be divided into five phases: phase 0 to phase 4 **FIGURE 18-3**:

- **Phase 0.** This phase begins when the cardiac muscle cell receives an impulse. Sodium moves into the cell through sodium channels, causing the cell's interior to become electrically positive relative to its exterior, resulting in a change in the transmembrane potential

TABLE 18-1 Role of Electrolytes in Cardiac Function

Electrolyte	Role in Cardiac Function
Sodium (Na^+)	Flows into the cell to initiate depolarization
Potassium (K^+)	Flows out of the cell to initiate repolarization Decreased or increased levels of potassium result in the following: • Hypokalemia → increased myocardial irritability • Hyperkalemia → decreased automaticity/conduction
Calcium (Ca^{+2})	Has a critical role in depolarization of pacemaker cells (maintains depolarization) and in myocardial contractility (involved in contraction of heart muscle tissue) Decreased or increased levels of calcium result in the following: • Hypocalcemia → decreased contractility and increased myocardial irritability • Hypercalcemia → increased contractility
Magnesium (Mg^{+2})	Stabilizes the cell membrane; acts in concert with potassium, and opposes the actions of calcium Decreased or increased levels of magnesium result in the following: • Hypomagnesemia → decreased conduction • Hypermagnesemia → increased myocardial irritability

(TMP) from −90 mV to about −70 mV. Still more sodium channels open at threshold, allowing a rapid influx of sodium and a rapid rise in membrane voltage to about +30 mV. At the same time, calcium enters more slowly through calcium channels. The influx of calcium causes the sarcoplasmic reticulum to release calcium for muscle contraction. The cell depolarizes and begins to contract. On an ECG, the QRS complex represents phase 0.

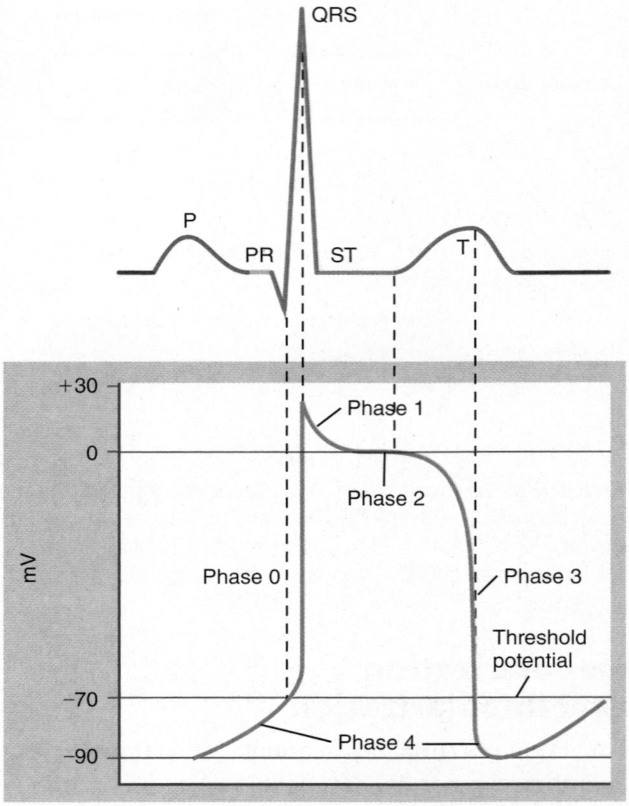

FIGURE 18-3 The components of an electrocardiogram rhythm correspond to the phases of myocyte stimulation.

- **Phase 1.** During this phase, inward sodium channels close and the cell begins to repolarize. Negatively charged chloride ions enter the cell. Outward potassium channels open briefly, allowing potassium to leave the cell and resulting in a decrease in the TMP.
- **Phase 2.** Called the plateau phase, this is the longest phase of the action potential. During this phase, sodium and calcium slowly enter the cell, while potassium flows out of the cell.[4] The presence of calcium prolongs depolarization of the membrane, creating a plateau. Contraction ends when the outward flow of potassium exceeds the inward flow of sodium and calcium. Phase 2 corresponds to the ST segment on the ECG.
- **Phase 3.** This is the final phase of repolarization. Slow calcium channels gradually close, and calcium is transported out of the cell. Potassium channels open, and potassium's rapid movement out of the cell causes the TMP to

become increasingly negative. By the end of this phase, the membrane potential has been restored to its resting value. With repolarization complete, the cell can now respond to a new stimulus. On an ECG, the T wave represents phase 3.

- **Phase 4.** This phase, called the resting phase, represents the normal working myocardial cell at its resting membrane potential of −90 mV.[4] Excess sodium is exchanged for potassium by means of the sodium-potassium pump, which restores the intracellular concentrations of sodium and potassium in readiness for the next depolarization.

Refractory Periods

A myocardial cell cannot respond to an electrical stimulus from the conduction system normally unless it is fully polarized. The period during which the cell is depolarized or in the process of repolarizing, the so-called **refractory period (RP)**, consists of two phases. In the **absolute refractory period (ARP)**, also called the effective refractory period, cardiac cells cannot respond to any stimulus. This period lasts from phase 0 to the middle of phase 3 of the cardiac action potential. A helpful analogy is a flushing toilet. If you flush a toilet and then immediately try to flush it again, does the toilet flush? No, because the tank has not yet filled back up with water.

The **relative refractory period (RRP)** extends from the middle of phase 3 to the beginning of phase 4 of the cardiac action potential. During this time, the heart muscle has been partially repolarized and may depolarize in response to an electrical stimulus. The RRP indicates that some cells have repolarized sufficiently to depolarize again. Returning to our flushing toilet analogy, if you waited 15 seconds before flushing again, what would happen? The result would be a partial flush because the tank had refilled with water perhaps halfway. So, during the ARP, nothing can stimulate the ventricles to contract again. However, during the RRP, a strong stimulus can initiate depolarization of those cells that have had enough time to repolarize.

The Conduction System

The network of cardiac tissue that initiates and conducts electrical impulses is called the **electrical conduction system**. The conduction system is composed of specialized pacemaker cells. These cells are found in the tissues of the SA node, internodal conduction pathways, AV node, bundle of His, and Purkinje fibers. The tissue in which the heart's electrical activity arises at any given time is called the pacemaker because it sets the pace (ie, rate) of cardiac contraction.

Theoretically, any cell within the heart's electrical conduction system can act as a pacemaker. In the normal heart, however, the dominant pacemaker is the SA node **FIGURE 18-4**. It normally fires at an intrinsic rate of 60 to 100 times per minute (times/min). The SA node lies at the junction of the superior vena cava and the right atrium, and, in most patients, the RCA supplies it with blood.

In approximately 0.08 second, electrical impulses generated in this node spread across the atria and advance through three **internodal pathways** in the atrial wall:

1. **Anterior internodal pathway.** The Bachmann bundle is the interatrial pathway connecting the right and left atria. A branch of the Bachmann bundle forms the anterior internodal pathway between the SA and AV nodes.
2. **Middle internodal tract.** The Wenckebach tract constitutes the middle internodal tract.
3. **Thorel tract.** The Thorel tract is the last of the internodal pathways and is represented by the posterior internodal pathway.

The **atrioventricular (AV) node** is a group of cells located in the floor of the right atrium behind the tricuspid valve, near the opening of the coronary sinus. In most people, its blood supply comes from a branch of the RCA; in others, it comes from a Cx artery branch. When the SA node's impulse enters the AV node, it is delayed for approximately 0.12 second before being relayed through the rest of the conduction system. This delay allows the atria to empty blood into the ventricles. Approximately 70% to 80% of the blood in the atria fills the ventricles by gravity; the remaining 20% to 30% comes from atrial contraction (atrial kick). The **atrioventricular (AV) junction**, which includes the AV node and the nonbranching portion of the **bundle of His**, also called the *AV bundle*, conducts impulses to the right and left bundle branches. In the normal heart, the AV junction can be thought of as a gatekeeper because it is the only electrical connection between the atria and ventricles.

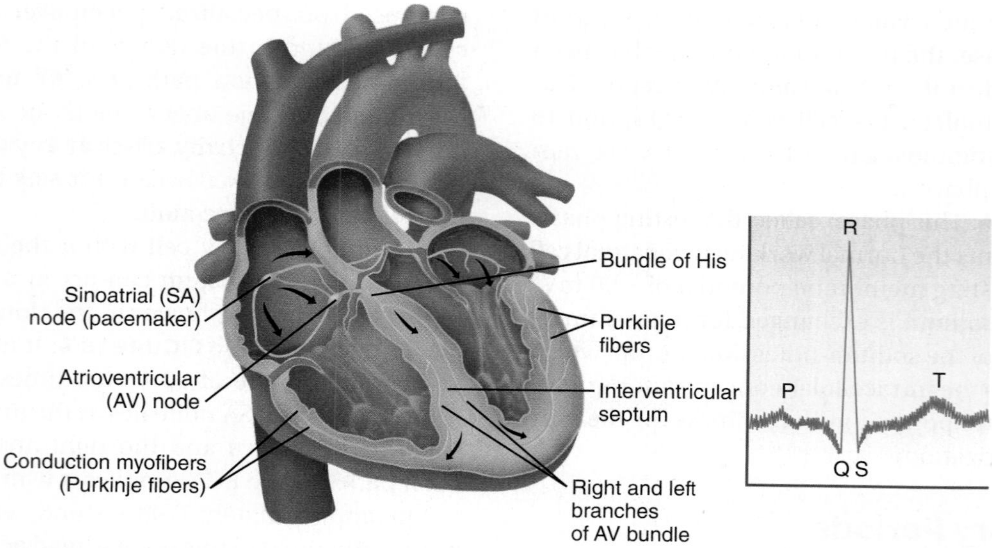

FIGURE 18-4 The electrical conduction system of the heart.

Normally, impulses pass through the AV junction into the bundle of His and then move rapidly into the right and left bundle branches on either side of the interventricular septum. If the atrial rate becomes very rapid, then the AV junction can regulate the number of impulses that reach the ventricles. The impulses that do proceed will spread from the bundle branches to the **Purkinje fibers**, cardiac muscle fibers distributed throughout the inner surfaces of the ventricular walls. It takes about 0.08 second for an electric impulse to spread across the ventricles, during which time the ventricles contract.

Secondary Pacemakers

If the SA node is damaged or suppressed, then any component of the conduction system can act as a secondary pacemaker. The farther removed the conduction tissue is from the SA node, however, the slower its intrinsic firing rate will be. Suppose the SA node were damaged by ischemia (tissue injury caused by hypoxemia) and consequently could not fire. If the AV node failed to receive an impulse from the SA node, then the AV junction should then begin firing at its own rate of 40 to 60 beats/min. If both the SA node and the AV junction failed to initiate an impulse, then the Purkinje fibers should initiate an impulse, generating a ventricular rhythm at a rate of 20 to 40 beats/min **TABLE 18-2**.

TABLE 18-2 Pacemaker Intrinsic Rates

Pacemaker	Rate (beats/min)
SA node	60–100
AV junction	40–60
Purkinje network	20–40

Abbreviations: AV, atrioventricular; SA, sinoatrial

Accessory Conduction Pathways

Some people are born with extra heart muscle tissue that connects the atria and ventricles, bypassing the AV node. This abnormal tissue is called an *accessory pathway* or a bypass tract:

- **James fibers.** James fibers in the atrial internodal pathways extend into the ventricles while bypassing the AV node.
- **Mahaim fibers.** The AV node, the bundle of His, and the bundle branches contain Mahaim fibers that extend into the ventricles and provide a common pathway for reentrant dysrhythmias.
- **Bundle of Kent.** The bundle of Kent is an accessory pathway typically located between the left atrium and the left ventricle, although it is sometimes found between the right atrium

and the right ventricle. The bundle of Kent enables the depolarization wave to bypass the AV node and trigger early depolarization of a section of ventricular tissue. Simultaneously, depolarization travels through the AV node and bundle of His to the bundle branches. These simultaneous depolarization events create a unique feature on the ECG tracing called a **delta wave**.

In certain instances, accessory pathways can trigger abnormally fast heart rates (tachydysrhythmias). Medical intervention is often required to terminate such rhythms.

The Autonomic Nervous System and the Heart

Both the sympathetic and parasympathetic divisions of the autonomic nervous system (ANS) affect the heart **FIGURE 18-5**. Sympathetic (accelerator) nerves supply specific areas of the heart's electrical system, atrial muscle, and ventricular myocardium. Sympathetic nerves transmit commands by releasing norepinephrine. Norepinephrine travels to the SA node, AV node, and ventricles, spreading the signal from the sympathetic nerves. The heart speeds up to prevent a buildup of lactic acid, thereby increasing CO and distributing more oxygen and nutrients throughout the body.

An accelerated heart rate shortens all phases of the **cardiac cycle**—the period from one cardiac contraction to the next. When the ventricles have less time to relax, less time is available for these chambers to fill adequately with blood. If the ventricles do not fill completely, then less blood is sent to the coronary arteries, less blood is pumped out of the ventricles, CO decreases, and signs of myocardial ischemia may appear. *Ischemia* is anoxia caused by diminished blood flow to tissue, usually because of an artery's narrowing or blockage.

Parasympathetic (inhibitory) nerve fibers supply the heart's SA node, atrial muscle, and AV junction by way of the vagus nerve. The vagus nerve, also called cranial nerve X (CN X), innervates

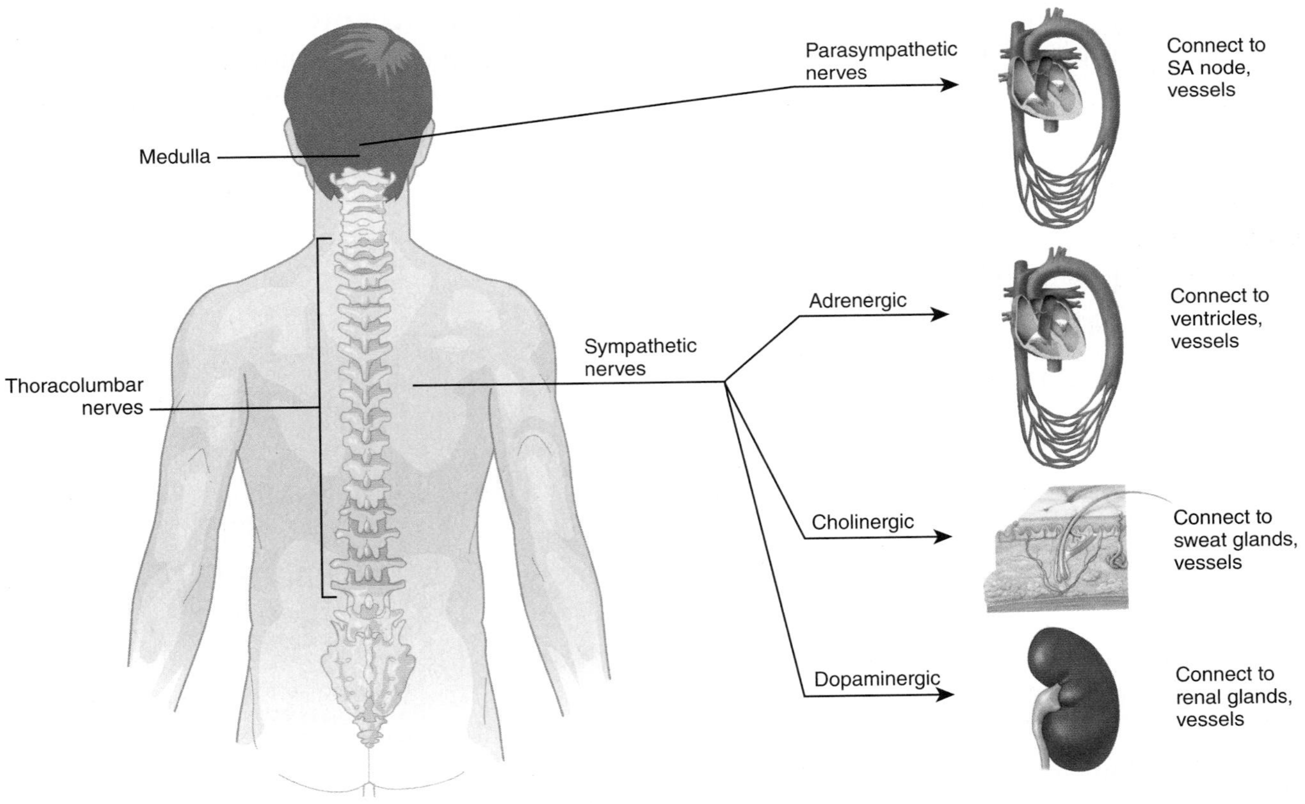

FIGURE 18-5 Sympathetic and parasympathetic nerve fibers, and their end organs (SA, sinoatrial).

functional areas ranging from the soft palate to the thoracic organs. It is also responsible for decreasing the heart rate. The vagus nerve can be stimulated in several ways, such as by increasing pressure on the carotid sinus, straining or forced exhalation against a closed glottis (Valsalva maneuver), or distention of a hollow organ, such as the bladder or stomach.

When pressure is applied over the carotid sinus or a person is straining during a bowel movement, the brain may sense that the heart should slow its pace. A message in the form of an electrical impulse will travel down the vagus nerve to the point where the nerve abuts the heart's SA node **FIGURE 18-6**. There, the electrical impulse stimulates the release of acetylcholine (ACh). This ACh crosses over to the SA node, signaling that the brain is calling for the heart rate to decelerate. Another ACh molecule travels to the AV node to ensure the message is received and acted on. In effect, this action reminds the SA node to slow down, ensuring no additional impulses get through to the ventricles. Afterward, ACh is escorted away from the SA and AV nodes by acetylcholinesterase (AChE), an enzyme that breaks down ACh so it can be recycled. Atropine is a commonly used parasympathetic blocker that opposes ACh's action, thereby accelerating the heart rate.

Baroreceptors and Chemoreceptors

Baroreceptors, or pressoreceptors, are sensors composed of specialized nerve tissue, found in the internal carotid arteries and aortic arch, that detect BP changes. When stimulated, they generate a reflex response in either the sympathetic or parasympathetic division of the ANS. For example, if BP falls, the body will attempt to compensate by constricting peripheral blood vessels, increasing the heart rate, and increasing the force of myocardial contraction. The sympathetic division orchestrates these compensatory responses, which are collectively called a *sympathetic* or *adrenergic response.* If BP rises, the body will decrease sympathetic stimulation and increase the parasympathetic division's response, resulting in a *parasympathetic* or *cholinergic response.*

Chemoreceptors in the internal carotid arteries, aortic arch, and medulla detect changes in the concentration of hydrogen ions (pH), oxygen, and carbon dioxide in the blood. The ANS may mount either a sympathetic or parasympathetic response to such changes.

Causes of Cardiac Dysrhythmia

A cardiac dysrhythmia is a disturbance in the normal cardiac rhythm, which may or may not be clinically

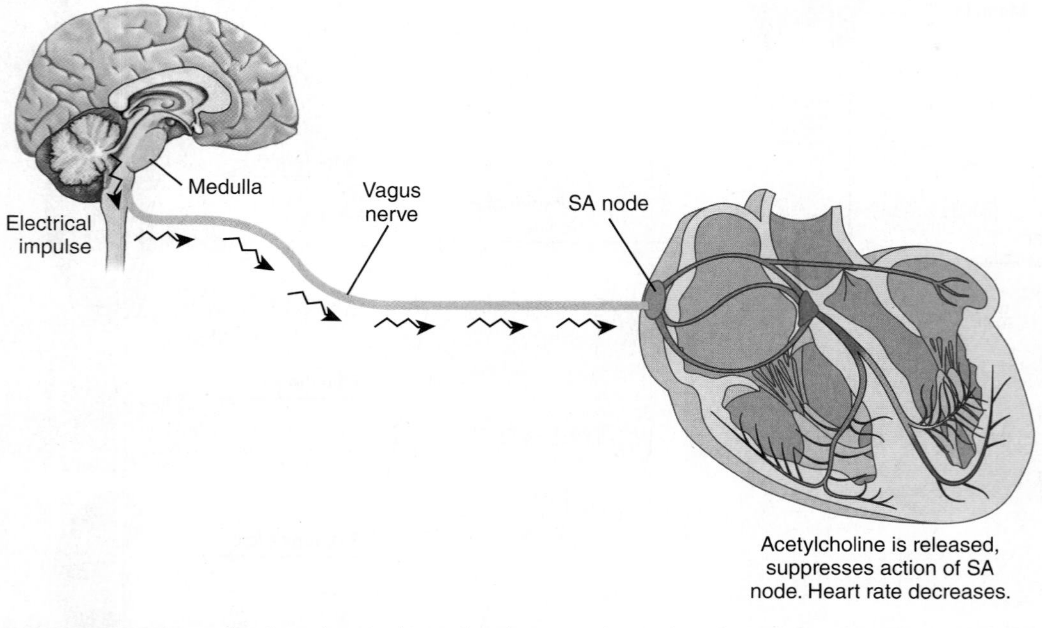
Medulla
Vagus nerve
SA node
Electrical impulse
Acetylcholine is released, suppresses action of SA node. Heart rate decreases.

FIGURE 18-6 Example of an electrical impulse that stimulates the release of a chemical. In this example, an electrical impulse travels from the brain down the vagus nerve, causing the release of acetylcholine (ACh) near the sinoatrial (SA) node. ACh suppresses the action of the SA node, slowing the heart rate.

Words of Wisdom

The following parable (a legacy of Dr. Nancy Caroline) demonstrates the effect of atropine on the parasympathetic nervous system.

"You're firing a little slowly today, aren't you?" says atropine.

"Just following instructions," replies the SA node. "The vagus told me to take it easy."

"Vagus, vagus—why are you always trying to slow everything down?"

"Hey, I'm just following orders from the brain," the vagus nerve explains. "You know a job can't be done well if you rush it."

"Yeah, well, chop chop, SA. We don't have time to slack off around here," says atropine.

"But what about the vagus?" protests the SA node.

"If you keep paying attention to the vagus, before you know it, you'll have slowed down so much that the brain will have to shut down for lack of blood and oxygen! Then where will you be? Take my advice, Bud, and open the gates wide. Let all impulses through, no questions asked."

"Are you sure that's a good idea? The vagus told me . . ."

"Forget about the vagus. He's just an old obstructionist."

"Okay, if you say so," says the SA node, always eager to please when atropine is around. So the SA node speeds up.

Atropine then blocks the vagus nerve so he can't interfere.

"Rats," says the vagus. "I guess I've been overruled."

significant. Cardiac rhythm disturbance or dysrhythmia may arise from a variety of causes **TABLE 18-3**. It is always necessary to evaluate the dysrhythmia in the context of the patient's overall clinical condition. It is the patient's clinical condition, not the lines or tracings on a screen or a piece of paper, that should ultimately determine whether treatment is necessary. Treat the patient, not the monitor!

The Electrocardiogram

An ECG is a graphic record of the voltage changes that occur in the heart muscle during depolarization and repolarization. The ECG monitor serves several functions in the prehospital setting **FIGURE 18-7**. You can use it to monitor the patient's cardiac rhythm continuously during transport, to print out a rhythm strip for interpretation, or to print out a 12-lead ECG for specific disease diagnosis.

Continuous ECG monitoring usually is performed using three **limb leads**: leads I, II, and III. You can use continuous ECG monitoring during transport to identify changes in the patient's heart rhythm. When analyzing cardiac monitoring ECGs, the tracing from lead II is often the most useful.

Because the heart is a three-dimensional organ, the use of only three leads limits the areas of the heart that can be viewed. A 12-lead ECG provides detailed information about the heart's conduction system and records its electrical activity from 12 separate angles. In virtually all cases when you record a 3-lead ECG, it will be because you suspect

YOU are the Paramedic

PART 2

You and your partner begin your assessment. The patient is alert and oriented, but he has diaphoretic skin, his inner lower eyelids are pale, and he is in visible respiratory distress. His initial vital signs are pulse, 150 beats/min; BP, 96/40 mm Hg; respirations, 20 breaths/min and deep; SpO_2 on room air, 88%. The patient denies any recent surgery or trauma.

Recording Time:	5 minutes
Appearance	Awake; moist skin; pale mucous membranes
Level of consciousness	Alert and oriented × 4
Airway	Open
Breathing	Inadequate; visible respiratory distress
Circulation	Inadequate; tachycardic

5. What interventions should you initiate at this time?

TABLE 18-3 Causes of Cardiac Dysrhythmias
Acid–base disturbance
ANS imbalance
Central nervous system damage
Certain poisons (eg, organophosphate insecticides)
Cor pulmonale (right ventricular failure caused by pulmonary disease)
Distention of cardiac chambers (as in heart failure)
Drug effects (phenothiazines, tricyclic antidepressants, and drugs used to treat dysrhythmias)
Electrolyte disturbances, especially those involving potassium, calcium, or magnesium
Endocrine disorders (hyperthyroidism, hypothyroidism)
Hypothermia
Hypoxemia from any cause
Increased sympathetic output
Increased vagal (parasympathetic) tone
Myocardial ischemia or infarction
Normal variation
Rheumatic heart disease
Trauma (eg, cardiac contusion)

Abbreviation: ANS, autonomic nervous system.

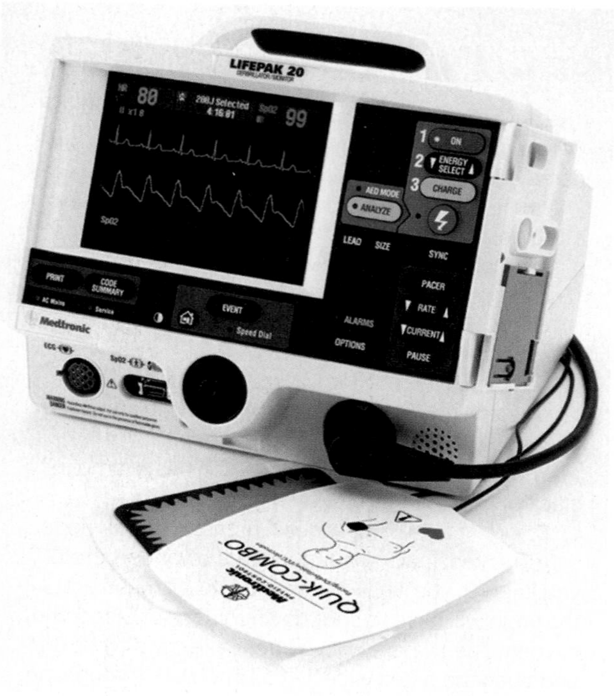

FIGURE 18-7 A commonly used monitor-defibrillator.

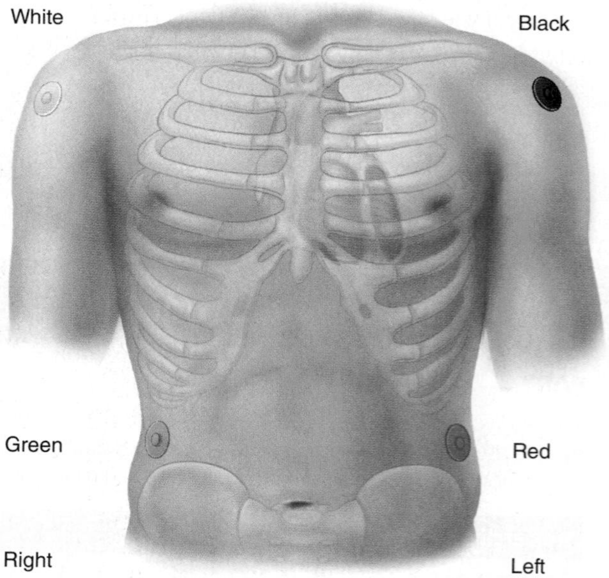

FIGURE 18-8 Electrode placement for cardiac monitoring.

the patient is experiencing a cardiac event; therefore, a 12-lead ECG should also be obtained.

Cardiac monitors are equipped with lead wires that are connected to electrodes, which are placed on the patient. Each **lead** offers an electrical snapshot of a specific part of the heart. The cardiac monitor records an ECG tracing for each lead used; health care professionals trained to interpret the findings can then review the tracings.

Electrode Placement

The electrodes must be placed in consistent, predetermined positions on each patient's body to obtain a reliable, useful ECG **FIGURE 18-8**.

Electrodes used in the prehospital setting are generally adhesive and have a gel center to aid in skin contact. Some manufacturers offer diaphoretic electrodes that adhere tightly to the skin of diaphoretic patients. Whichever type you use, following certain basic principles will help achieve the best skin contact and minimize signal distortion. Such distortion of an ECG tracing caused by interference, such as the patient's movement, is called an **artifact**.

- It may be necessary to shave the patient's body hair from the electrode site to maintain the correct lead placement. Do not be fooled by a hairy chest. It may initially appear that the electrode has good skin contact, but the electrode may later peel away from the skin and stick to the patient's hair.
- To remove oil and dead tissue from the skin's surface, rub the electrode site briskly with a dry gauze pad.
- Attach the electrodes to the ECG cables before placing them on the patient's body. Confirm that the electrode now attached to the cable is placed at the correct location on the patient's chest or limbs. Each cable is marked and color coded to indicate the correct location for its placement.
- Once all electrodes are in place, switch on the monitor and print a sample rhythm strip. If the strip shows any interference (artifact), verify that the electrodes are firmly attached to the skin and the monitor cable is plugged in correctly.

SKILL DRILL 18-1 shows the steps in performing cardiac monitoring.

Words of Wisdom

Artifact on the monitor can be tricky. A wavy baseline resembling ventricular fibrillation (VF) may be caused by patient movement or muscle tremor. Before you reach for the defibrillator paddles, look at the patient! If the patient is alert and in no apparent distress, then recheck the leads and equipment. Remember, treat the patient, not the monitor.

Skill Drill 18-1 Performing Cardiac Monitoring

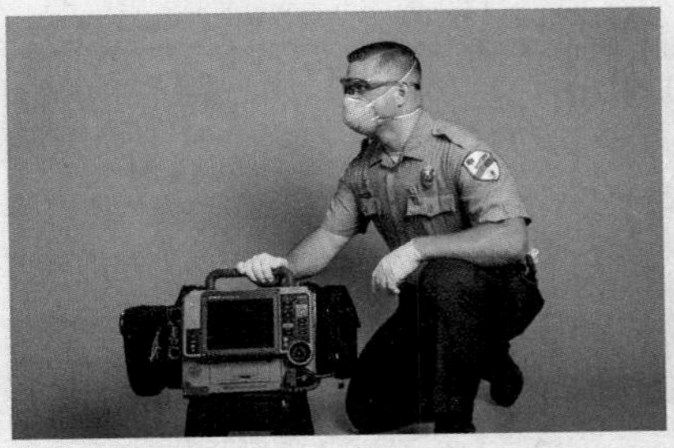

Step 1

Take standard precautions. Check your equipment. Ensure there are no loose pins at the end of the ECG cable and the cable or lead wires are intact. Ensure the monitor has an adequate paper supply. Connect the ECG cable to the machine. Connect the lead wires to the ECG cable (if not already connected). Turn on the power to the monitor. Adjust the screen contrast if necessary.

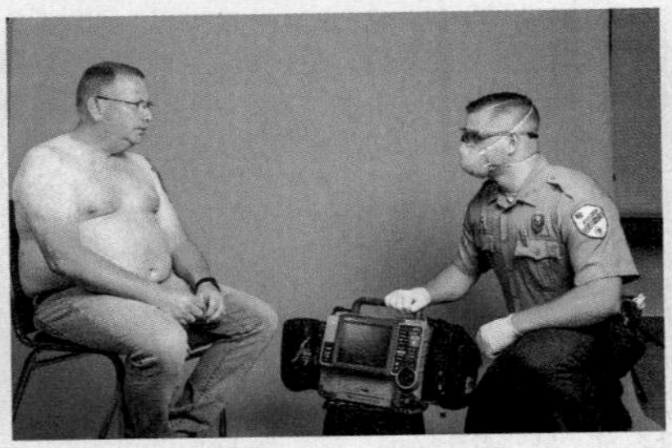

Step 2

Explain the procedure to the patient. To minimize ECG tracing distortion, prepare the skin for electrode placement by briskly rubbing it with a dry gauze pad to remove skin oils and improve impulse transmission. If you apply electrodes to the patient's chest, rather than to the limbs, ensure good contact by shaving small amounts of chest hair if needed.

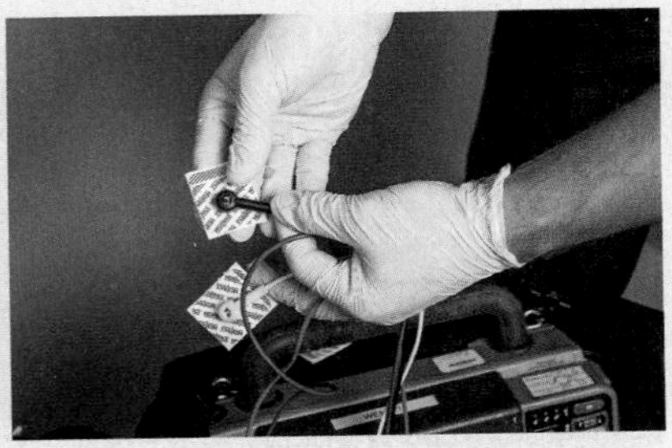

Step 3

Attach the electrodes to the lead wires before placing them on the patient.

(continues)

Skill Drill 18-1 Performing Cardiac Monitoring (continued)

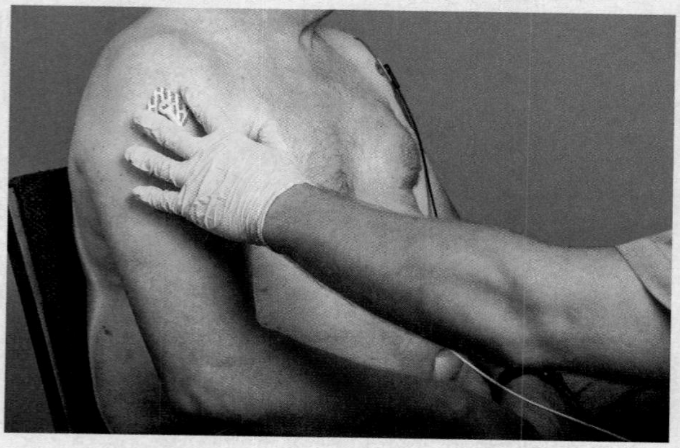

Step 4

One at a time, remove the backing from each electrode and apply it to the patient.

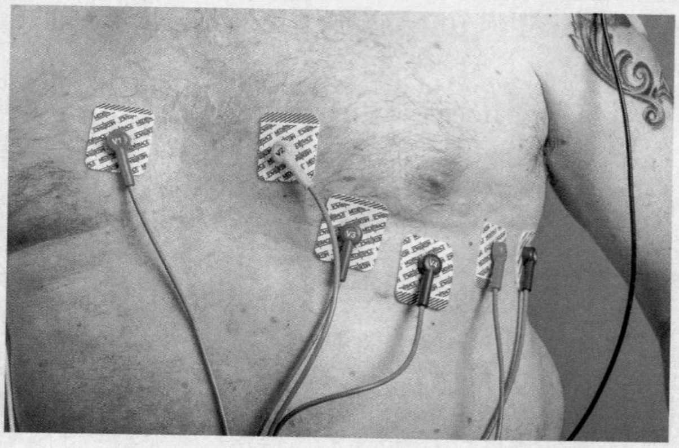

Step 5

If you plan to obtain a 12-lead tracing as well, then place the limb leads. Limb-lead electrodes are usually placed on the wrists and ankles but can be positioned anywhere on the appropriate limb. To reduce muscle tension and minimize artifact, ensure the patient's limbs are resting on a supportive surface. Do not apply electrodes over bony areas, broken skin, joints, skin creases, scar tissue, or rashes.

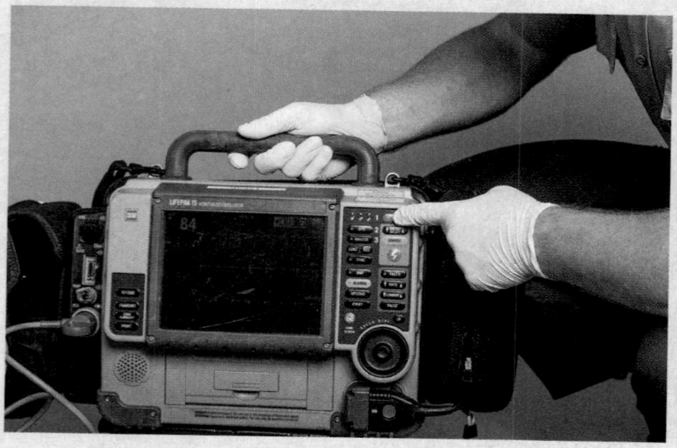

Step 6

Select the desired lead, which is typically lead II. Adjust the ECG size if necessary to ensure the machine detects the patient's QRS complexes. Feel the patient's pulse and compare it with the heart rate indicator on the monitor. If not already preset, set the heart rate alarms on the monitor according to your agency's policy.

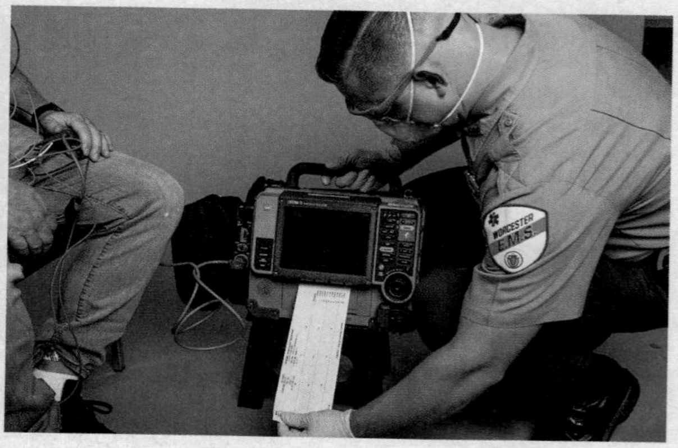

Step 7

Record the tracings, and label each strip.

The Leads

There are two main groups of leads: the limb leads and the **precordial leads**—that is, the chest leads. Leads I, II, and III are called limb leads, or standard limb leads, and leads aVR, aVL, and aVF are called **augmented limb leads**. The augmented limb leads contain only one true pole; the other end is a combination of information from other leads. A standard 12-lead ECG comprises the three standard limb leads, the three augmented limb leads, and the six precordial leads.

A lead wire is an electrical cable that attaches an electrode to the ECG monitor. A lead is an image of the heart, taken from a specified vantage point, that measures the electrical potential difference between two electrodes. An imaginary line joining the positive and negative poles of a lead is called the *lead axis*. The position of the positive electrode determines which area of the heart is viewed by each lead. Suppose you wanted to inspect the condition of a used vehicle you were considering buying. If you needed to know only whether the motor was running, you could stand anywhere near the car and listen. Likewise, you could use any single lead to monitor the cardiac rhythm. However, if you wanted to know the condition of the vehicle's body, you would have to walk around the vehicle and look at it from all sides. The driver's side might be in mint condition, but the entire doorframe on the passenger's side might be caved in from a wreck. Similarly, to localize the site of injury to the heart muscle and to identify other cardiac abnormalities, you need to look at the heart from several angles. One lead may detect significant damage that is invisible on another.

Leads I, II, and III view the heart from the front of the body; thus, they are called *frontal plane leads*. The precordial leads (V_1 to V_6) are called *unipolar chest leads* or *V leads*. These leads view the heart in the horizontal plane, so they provide images of the heart from the front (anterior wall of the heart) and from the left side (anterolateral view).

Limb Leads

Willem Einthoven is the physician and physiologist who discovered that every time the heart contracts, it emits a tiny amount of electrical energy that travels across the skin's surface. Einthoven found that these waves of energy could be recorded and plotted on a piece of grid paper; he assigned the letters P, Q, R, S, and T to the ECG deflections he observed. He initially recorded three leads: lead I, attached to the right and left arms; lead II, running between the right arm and left leg; and lead III, running between the left arm and left leg **FIGURE 18-9**.

Leads I, II, and III are **bipolar leads**. Bipolar leads contain a positive pole and a negative pole. With the standard limb leads, each lead measures the difference in electrical potential between electrodes placed on two extremities.

The left arm electrode is the positive terminal of lead I. This lead views the lateral surface of the left ventricle. The left leg electrode is the positive terminal of lead II. The left leg is the positive terminal of lead III **FIGURE 18-10**. Leads II and III look at the inferior surface of the left ventricle.

The augmented voltage (aV) leads (leads aVR, aVL, and aVF) are created by combining two of the limb leads, thereby forming a new lead, and using the remaining lead as the other pole. For example, lead aVR is created between the right arm and the combination of the left arm and leg electrodes **FIGURE 18-11**. The augmented leads are unipolar: they contain one true pole, while the other end

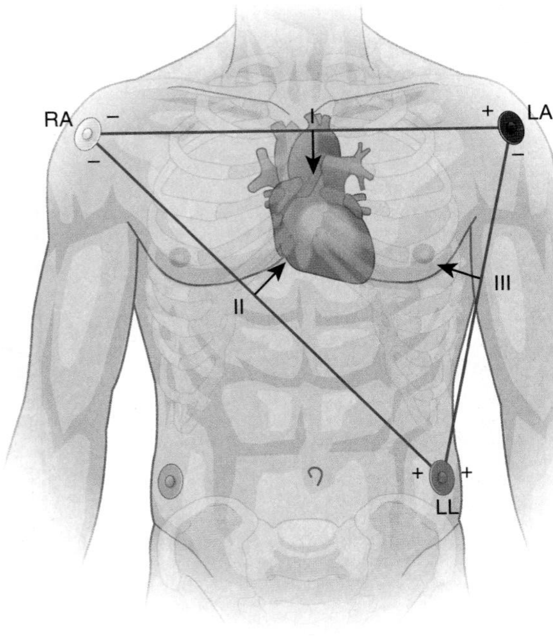

FIGURE 18-9 The Einthoven triangle. RA, right arm; LA, left arm; LL, left leg.

of the lead is referenced against a combination of other leads. For example, lead aVR is at the right arm, referenced against a combination of the left arm and the left leg. Lead aVL views the lateral surface of the left ventricle. Lead aVF views the inferior surface of the left ventricle.

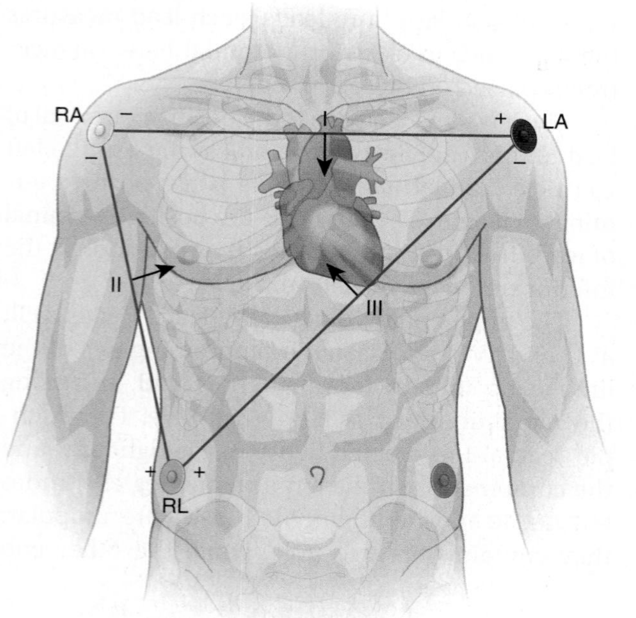

FIGURE 18-10 Each bipolar lead has a positive end and a negative end.

Reproduced from *12-Lead ECG: The Art of Interpretation*, courtesy of Tomas B. Garcia, MD.

If you are performing continuous cardiac monitoring, then place four electrodes on the patient's torso:

White—right upper chest near the shoulder
Black—left upper chest near the shoulder
Red—left lower abdomen
Green—right lower abdomen

If you are acquiring a 12-lead ECG, then place the four electrodes on the patient's limbs:

White—right wrist
Black—left wrist
Red—left ankle
Green—right ankle

Placing these four electrodes on the patient allows the ECG device to record all six limb leads using Einthoven's theory. The green lead serves as a ground in all cases and is electrically neutral.

Precordial Leads

The precordial leads V_1 to V_6 are unipolar. These leads are referenced against a calculated point known as *Wilson's central terminal* **FIGURE 18-12**. Wilson's central terminal is created by bisecting the limb leads in Einthoven's triangle.

The electrode for each unipolar lead is the positive terminal for that lead. Leads V_1 and V_2 view the septum, leads V_3 and V_4 look at the left ventricle's anterior wall, and leads V_5 and V_6 view the left ventricle's lateral wall.

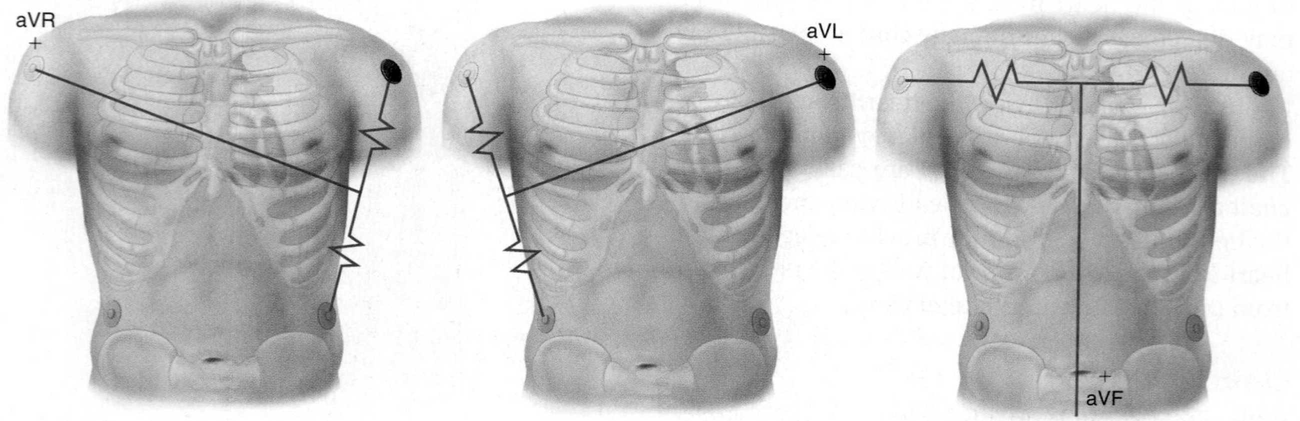

FIGURE 18-11 Augmented voltage leads analyze the limb leads, taking the data from one lead and synthesizing the information from the other two.

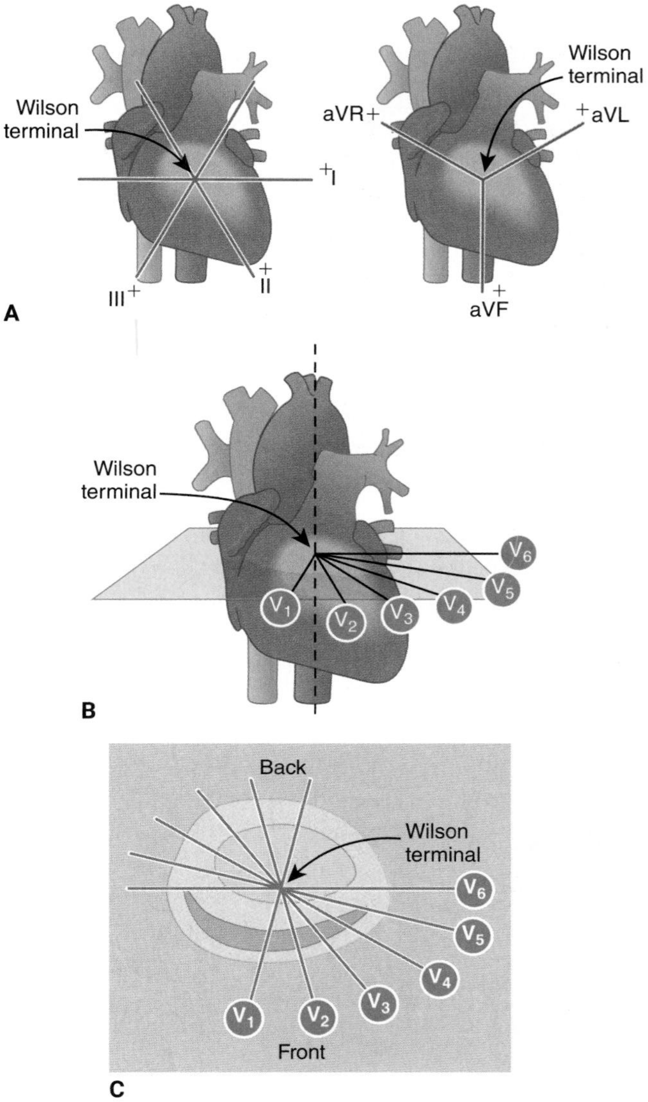

FIGURE 18-12 The Wilson central terminal, shown in relation to three types of leads: **A.** Bipolar leads. **B.** Augmented unipolar leads. **C.** Precordial leads.

Correct precordial electrode placement is essential to ensure the lead is viewing the heart from the intended angle each time an ECG is recorded. ECGs are often compared with previous ECGs. For this comparison to be reliable in identifying anything out of the ordinary, the precordial lead electrodes must be placed consistently **FIGURE 18-13** and **18-14**:

1. V_1—Right of the sternum, fourth ICS
2. V_2—Left of the sternum, fourth ICS
3. V_3—Precisely between leads V_2 and V_4
4. V_4—Left midclavicular line, fifth ICS
5. V_5—Left anterior axillary line at the level of lead V_4
6. V_6—Left midaxillary line at the level of lead V_4

Contiguous Leads

Contiguous leads view geographically similar areas of the myocardium, which can help localize areas of ischemia, injury, or **infarction**. Leads II, III, and aVF are contiguous. Leads V_1 and V_2, V_2 and V_3, V_3 and V_4, V_4 and V_5, and V_5 and V_6 are pairs of contiguous leads. Leads I and aVL, and aVL and V_5, are also contiguous pairs.

Right-Side Leads

Certain conditions require that you record a right-side ECG to evaluate the electrical activity of the right ventricle. In that case, place the precordial leads on the patient's right anterior thorax. Place the electrodes for the right-side ECG as follows **FIGURE 18-15**:

1. V_1R—Left of the sternum, fourth ICS
2. V_2R—Right of the sternum, fourth ICS
3. V_3R—Precisely between V_2R and V_4R
4. V_4R—Right midclavicular line, fifth ICS
5. V_5R—Right anterior axillary line at the level of lead V_4R
6. V_6R—Right midaxillary line at the level of lead V_4R

Note that lead V_4R is the most sensitive and specific for right ventricular AMI and is often the only lead recorded on a right-side ECG.

Posterior Leads

The posterior ECG is used to evaluate the electrical activity of the posterior wall of the left ventricle. In that case, place three of the precordial leads on the left posterior thorax **FIGURE 18-16**:

1. V_7—Between V_6 and V_8, fifth ICS
2. V_8—Midscapular, fifth ICS
3. V_9—Just to the left of the spine, fifth ICS

15- and 18-Lead ECGs

Because a standard 12-lead ECG does not view the right ventricle or the left ventricle's posterior surface, additional leads are needed to detect

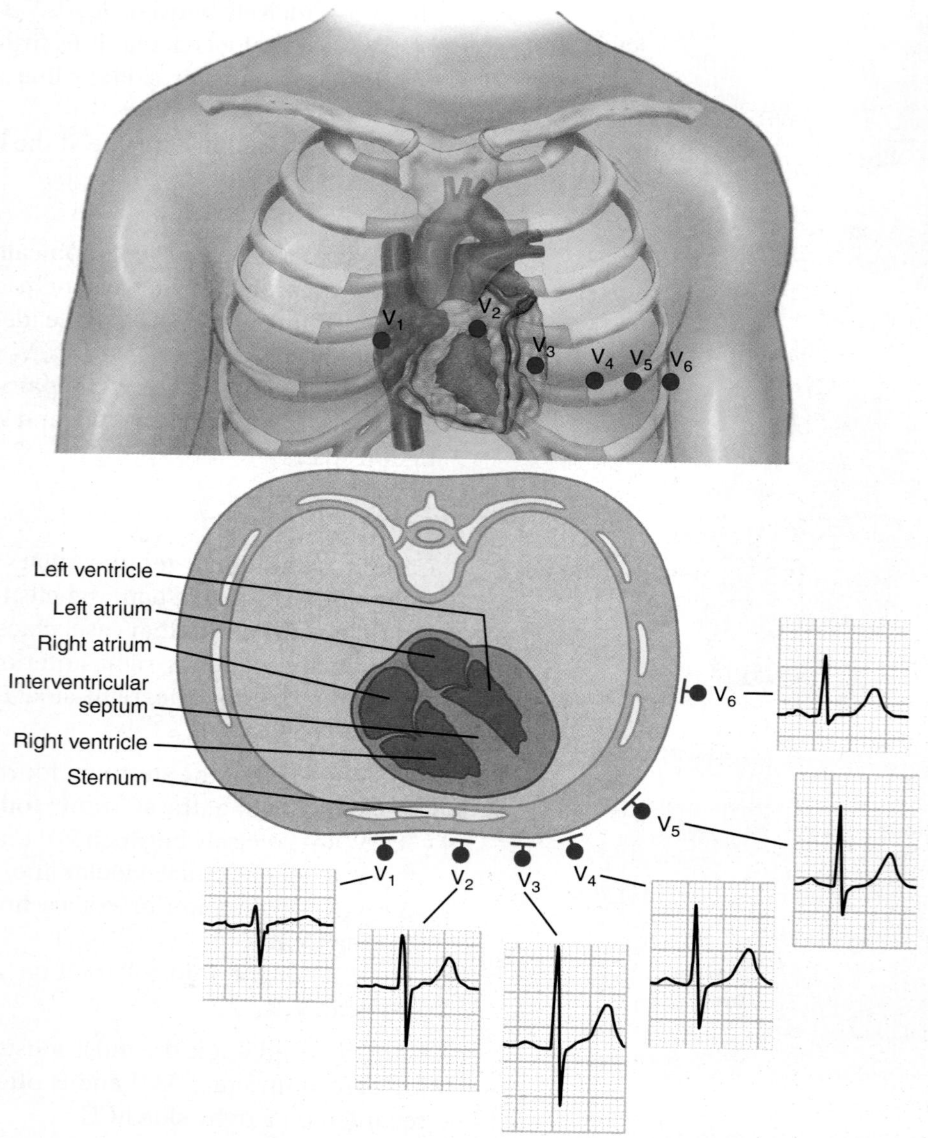

FIGURE 18-13 The precordial leads (chest leads) depict the heart in the horizontal plane. Inset: V_1 and V_2 view the interventricular septum. V_3 and V_4 view the anterior wall of the left ventricle. V_5 and V_6 represent the low lateral wall. The right ventricle cannot be seen on a standard tracing.

ischemia or infarction in those areas. A 15-lead ECG uses the standard 12-lead ECG, plus leads V_4R, V_7, and V_8. Obtaining a 15-lead ECG involves first recording a standard 12-lead ECG and then recording a second tracing containing the additional leads.

An 18-lead ECG uses the standard 12-lead ECG tracing plus leads V_4R through V_6R and V_7 through V_9. To obtain an 18-lead ECG, (1) record a standard 12-lead ECG, (2) record the right-side precordial leads, and (3) record the posterior leads.

ECG Concepts

As mentioned, the ECG uses electrodes placed on the body to detect minute electrical waves traveling across the skin's surface. The ECG baseline is generally a flat, straight, horizontal line that reflects a period of electrical silence in the myocardium **FIGURE 18-17**. Although the baseline is neither positive nor negative, there is still electrical activity (movement of ions) in the myocardium. Perhaps it would be more accurate to describe the baseline as

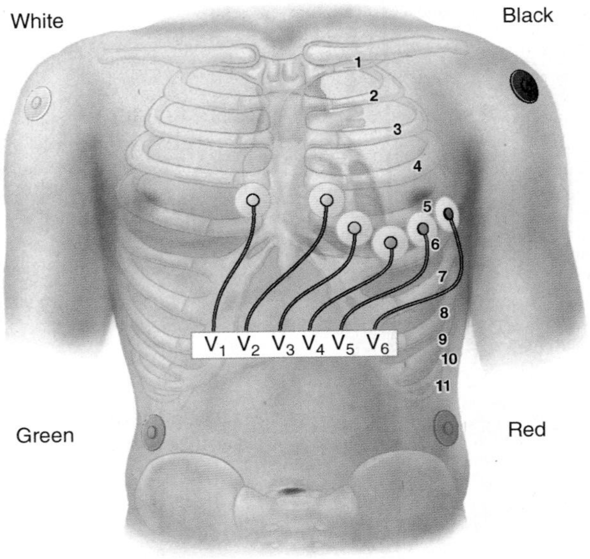

Lead	Location	View
V_1	4th intercostal space, right sternal border	Ventricular septum
V_2	4th intercostal space, left sternal border	Ventricular septum
V_3	Between V_2 and V_4	Anterior wall of left ventricle
V_4	5th intercostal space, midclavicular line	Anterior wall of left ventricle
V_5	Lateral to V_4 at the anterior axillary line	Lateral wall of left ventricle
V_6	Lateral to V_5 at the midaxillary line	Lateral wall of left ventricle

FIGURE 18-14 Placement of 12-lead electrodes.

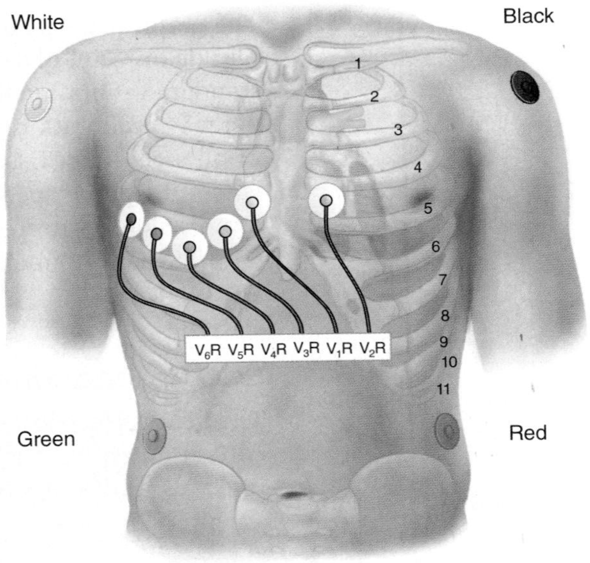

Lead	Location	View
V_1R	Left of sternum, 4th intercostal space (ICS)	Ventricular septum
V_2R	Right of sternum, 4th ICS	Ventricular septum
V_3R	Precisely between V_2 and V_4	Right ventricle
V_4R	Right midclavicular, 5th ICS	Right ventricle
V_5R	Precisely between V_4 and V_6	Right ventricle
V_6R	Right midaxillary, 5th ICS	Right ventricle

FIGURE 18-15 Placement of right-side leads.

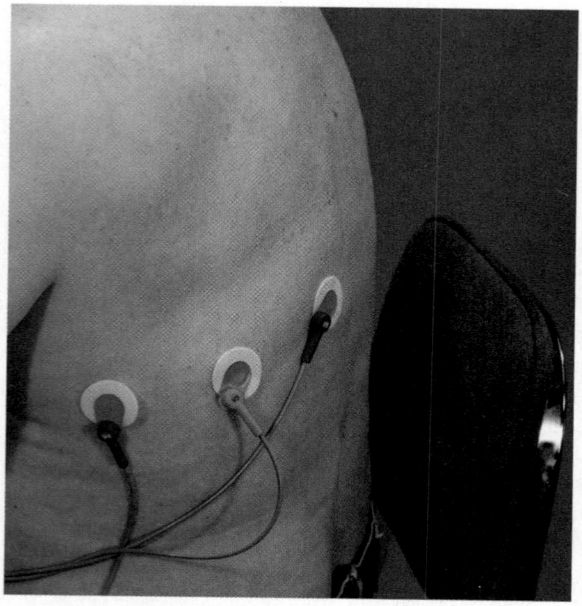

Lead	Location	View
V_7	Between V_6 and V_8, 5th intercostal space	Posterior wall of left ventricle
V_8	Midscapular, 5th intercostal space	Posterior wall of left ventricle
V_9	Just to the left of the spine, 5th intercostal space	Posterior wall of left ventricle

FIGURE 18-16 Placement of posterior leads.

© Jones & Bartlett Learning. Courtesy of MIEMSS.

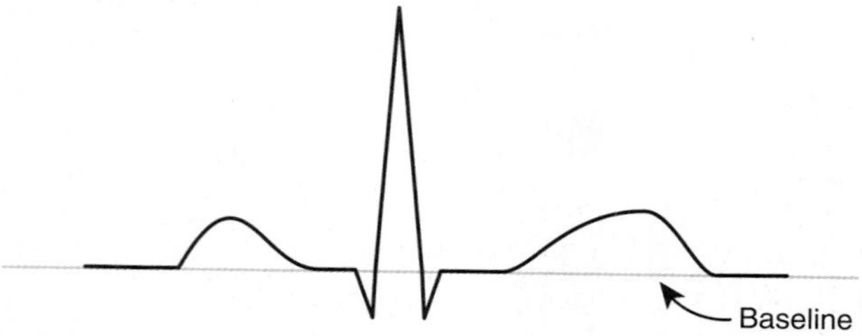

FIGURE 18-17 The electrocardiogram baseline.

Reproduced from *12-Lead ECG: The Art of Interpretation*, courtesy of Tomas B. Garcia, MD.

a period of electrical neutrality. The baseline is also referred to as the **isoelectric line**, *TP segment*, and *isomeric line*.

An electrical impulse moving in the direction of a negative electrode produces a deflection below the baseline. Conversely, an electrical impulse moving toward a positive electrode produces a deflection above the baseline **FIGURE 18-18**. Perpendicular movement of an impulse toward a positive electrode produces either a perfectly flat line or a waveform with both a positive and a negative component. Such waveforms are called *biphasic waves*.

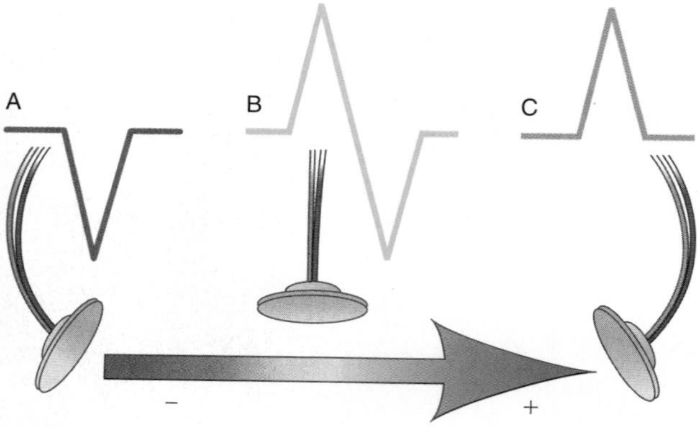

FIGURE 18-18 Negative, biphasic, and positive waveforms.

Reproduced from *12-Lead ECG: The Art of Interpretation*, courtesy of Tomas B. Garcia, MD.

ECG Paper

ECGs are recorded on graph paper that moves past a stylus at a constant speed (25 mm/s). Thus, the horizontal distance on the graph paper represents a given period. Specifically, one small (1 mm) box is the equivalent of 0.04 second (1/25th of a second), or 40 milliseconds, and one large box (which consists of five small boxes) is the equivalent of 0.20 second, or 200 milliseconds ($0.04 \times 5 = 0.20$) **FIGURE 18-19**. The graph paper's vertical axis represents the amplitude or "gain" of deflection, expressed in mV. The standard calibration for amplitude is 10 millimeters per mV. A calibration box is printed at the beginning of all 12-lead ECGs. The calibration box informs you of the paper speed and amplitude. It measures 5 mm wide by 10 mm tall, representing the standard 25-mm/s paper speed and 10-mm/mV gain **FIGURE 18-20**.

ECG Components

The heart's electrical conduction events can be recorded on an ECG as a series of waves, segments, intervals, and complexes **FIGURE 18-21**.

P Wave

The **P wave**, the first wave of an ECG complex, represents atrial depolarization and is characterized by a smooth, round, upright shape. A P wave's normal duration is less than 0.11 second (110 milliseconds), and its amplitude is less than 2.5 mm tall.

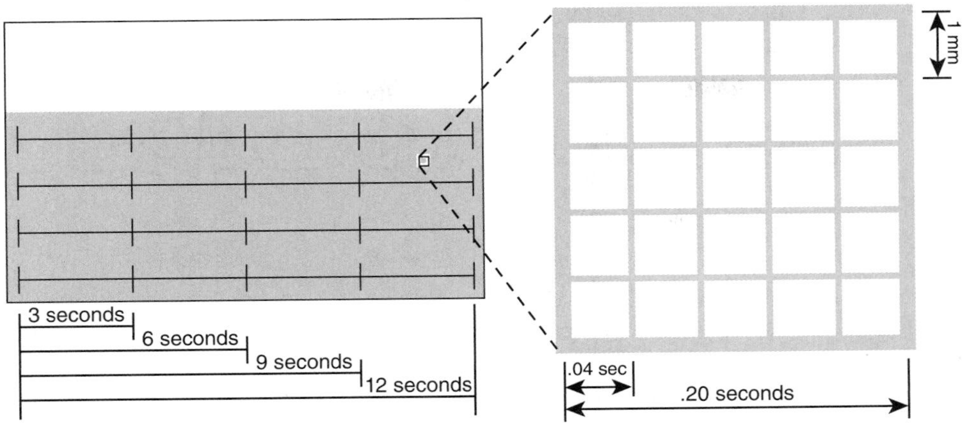

FIGURE 18-19 Electrocardiogram paper. Height, which indicates amplitude, is measured in millimeters (mm), and width is measured in milliseconds (ms) (0.04 second = 40 ms; 0.20 second = 200 ms).

Reproduced from *12-Lead ECG: The Art of Interpretation*, courtesy of Tomas B. Garcia, MD.

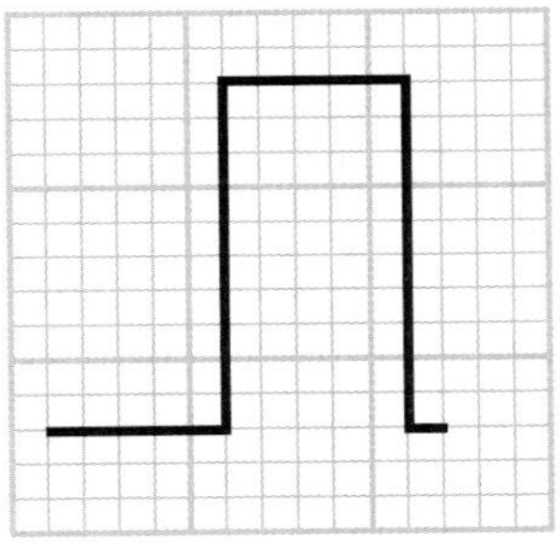

FIGURE 18-20 A calibration box is normally printed at the beginning of the electrocardiogram.

Reproduced from *12-Lead ECG: The Art of Interpretation*, courtesy of Tomas B. Garcia, MD.

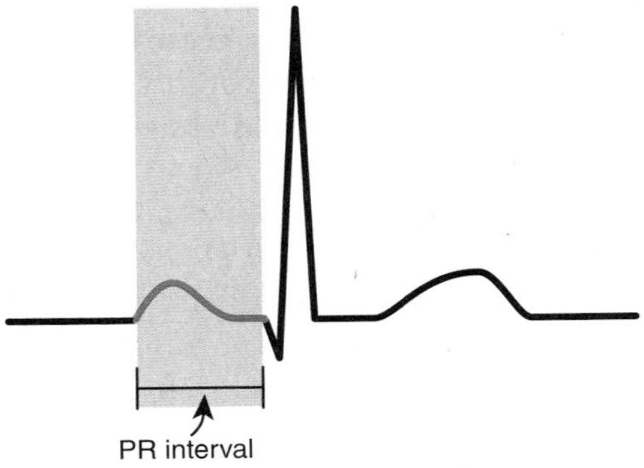

FIGURE 18-22 The normal PR interval is 0.12 to 0.20 second (120 to 200 milliseconds).

Reproduced from *12-Lead ECG: The Art of Interpretation*, courtesy of Tomas B. Garcia, MD.

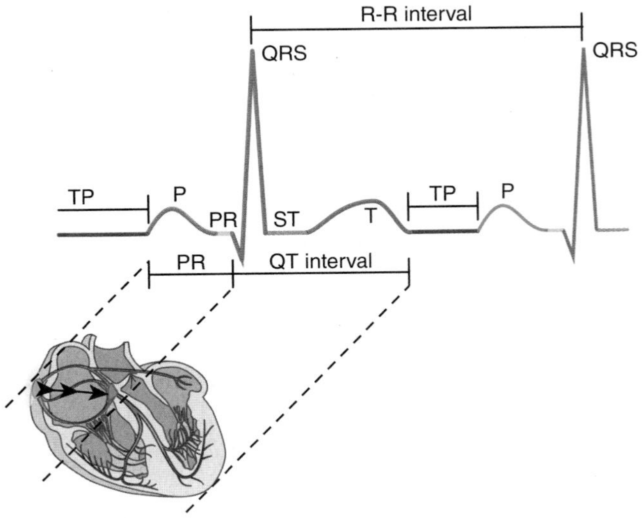

FIGURE 18-21 The electrocardiogram and cardiac events.

Reproduced from *12-Lead ECG: The Art of Interpretation*, courtesy of Tomas B. Garcia, MD.

PR Interval

The **PR interval (PRI)** is the distance from the beginning of the P wave to the beginning of the QRS complex. This distance represents the time required for an impulse to traverse the atria and AV junction, which normally ranges from 0.12 to 0.20 second (120 to 200 milliseconds). That period is equivalent to three to five small boxes on the ECG strip **FIGURE 18-22**. The PR segment represents the amount of time the AV node delays transmission of atrial activity to the ventricles. The wave produced by repolarization of the atria is too small to be seen on the ECG but occurs during the PR segment. When the AV node is diseased or hypoxic, the PR segment can become elongated **FIGURE 18-23**.

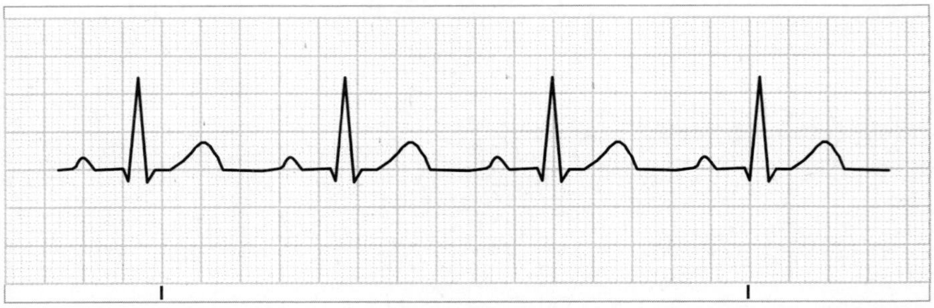

FIGURE 18-23 A PR interval greater than 0.20 second (200 ms) is considered prolonged.

Reproduced from *Arrhythmia Recognition: The Art of Interpretation*, courtesy of Tomas B. Garcia, MD.

Prolonged PRIs are discussed later in the chapter, when AV blocks are introduced.

QRS Complex

The **QRS complex**, which consists of three waveforms, represents ventricular depolarization. It is measured from the beginning of the Q wave to the end of the S wave and should consistently follow each P wave.

In healthy adults, the QRS complex is narrow, with a normal duration of 0.11 second or less.[5] Such a complex indicates that impulse conduction has proceeded from the AV junction, through the bundle of His, left and right bundles, and Purkinje system. If impulse conduction is abnormal, then the complex has a bizarre appearance and a duration of 0.12 second (120 milliseconds) or longer.

The first negative deflection in the QRS complex, the *Q wave*, represents conduction through the interventricular septum. The electrical impulse spreads from right to left through the septum. A normal Q wave should last no more than 0.04 second (40 milliseconds) and should be less than one-third of the QRS complex's overall height. Q waves are considered abnormal or pathologic if they are more than 0.03 second (30 milliseconds) wide or more than 30% of the following R-wave height in that lead, or both.[6] AMI is one possible cause of pathologic Q waves.

The first upward deflection of the QRS complex is referred to as the *R wave*. The S wave is any downward deflection after the R wave. A second upward deflection is called an R-prime (R′) wave. The R and S waves represent depolarization of the right and left ventricles.

As discussed earlier, as a current moves toward a lead, it creates a positive (upright) deflection on the lead's ECG tracing. Thus, in **FIGURE 18-24**, the current depolarizing the ventricles is moving toward lead II, so what you see in lead II is an upright QRS complex. If the depolarizing current is moving toward lead II, then it must be moving away from lead aVR, so you would expect to see a negative deflection in that lead. Indeed, in Figure 18-24, the QRS complex in aVR reveals a downward deflection. That makes intuitive sense. For example, if you and a friend are standing facing each other at opposite ends of a football field, then a ball thrown toward your friend will appear bigger and bigger as it approaches the friend; however, the same ball will appear smaller and smaller to you. Similarly, leads II and aVR, being nearly opposite each other, will present nearly opposite images of the same electrical depolarization wave. As in the football analogy, if a depolarizing wave is coming toward lead II, it will be going away from aVR.

J Point

The J point is the point in the ECG at which the QRS complex ends and the ST segment begins **FIGURE 18-25**. Thus, it represents the end of depolarization and the apparent beginning of repolarization. The J point is significant because it often becomes depressed or elevated when the myocardium is ischemic. J-point changes are discussed later in this chapter.

ST Segment

The **ST segment** begins at the J point and ends at the T wave. The ST segment represents early ventricular repolarization. It can fall below, rise above,

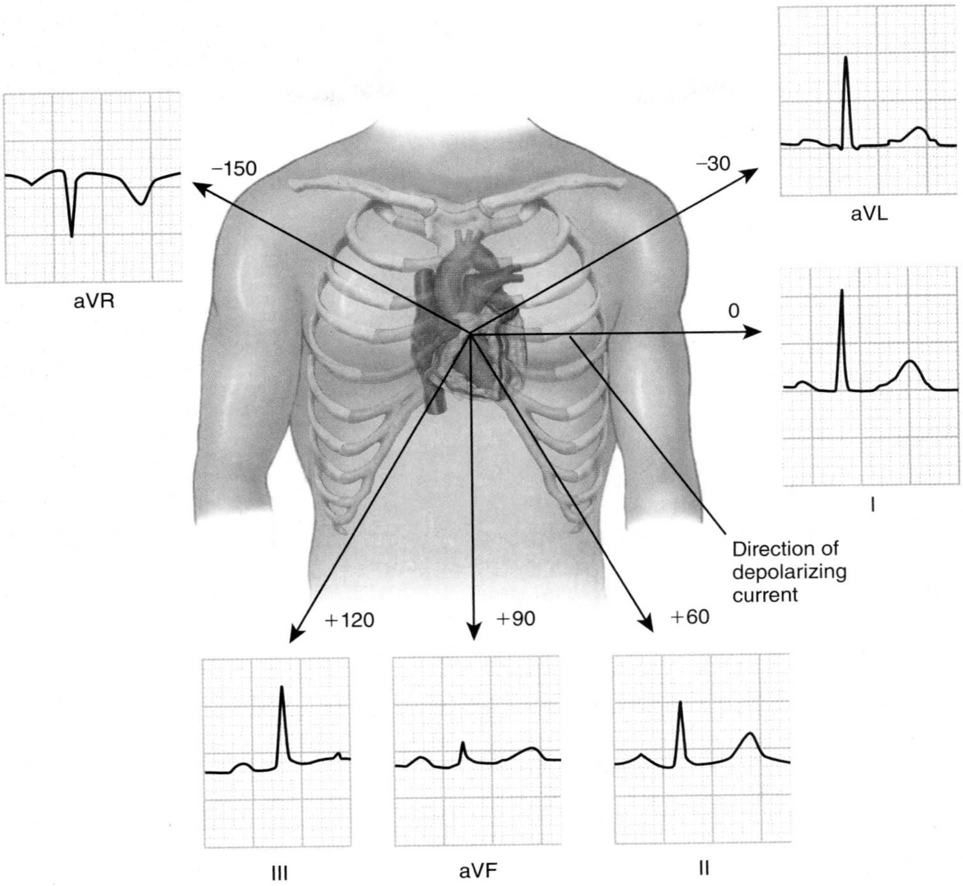

FIGURE 18-24 The morphology of the QRS complex depends on the lead position and in which direction the electrical impulse is moving within the heart. If the electrical impulse is moving primarily toward lead II, then it will be upright, as shown. However, lead aVR will be inverted because the impulse is moving away from it.

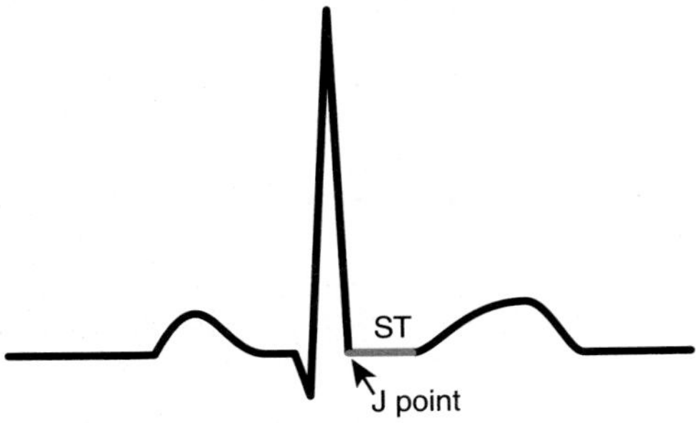

FIGURE 18-25 The J point.

or stay at the baseline during a myocardial event. An elevated ST segment may indicate myocardial injury. A depressed ST segment may indicate myocardial ischemia.

T Wave

A **T wave** is an upright, flat, or inverted wave following the QRS complex, which represents ventricular repolarization. The T wave should be asymmetric, less than one-half the overall height of the QRS complex, and oriented in the same overall direction **FIGURE 18-26**. For example, if the QRS complex is predominantly upright, the T wave should also be predominantly upright.

The T wave consists of two halves. The first half (closest to the QRS complex) represents the ARP. The second half represents the RRP.

During myocardial ischemia, injury, and infarction, the T wave becomes very large (hyperacute), peaked or tented in shape, symmetric, and broad. It is essential to look for these ECG

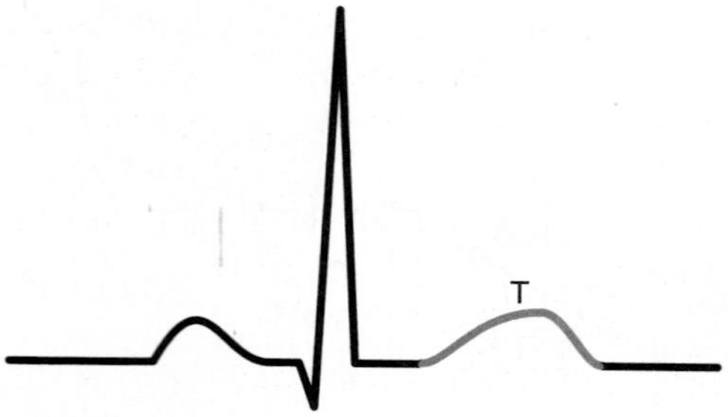

FIGURE 18-26 The T wave.

Reproduced from *Arrhythmia Recognition: The Art of Interpretation*, courtesy of Tomas B. Garcia, MD.

changes so you don't miss an ischemic event! Tall, pointed (peaked) T waves may be seen with **hyperkalemia** (excessive potassium concentration in the blood). Deeply inverted T waves may be seen with acute central nervous system (CNS) events, such as intracranial hemorrhage or massive stroke.[7]

Sometimes, a **U wave** may be seen after a T wave and before the next P wave. Experts think the U wave most likely represents the final stage of ventricular repolarization. When it is seen, the U-wave direction is usually the same as that of the preceding T wave in lead II. A U wave taller than 2 mm is considered abnormal and may be a sign of **hypokalemia** (low potassium concentration in the blood) or cardiomyopathy, among other conditions. When U waves occur, they are often mistaken for extra P waves or are misinterpreted as some other unknown abnormality.

QT Interval

The QT interval represents all the electrical activity of one complete ventricular cycle (ie, ventricular depolarization and repolarization). It begins at the onset of the Q wave and ends as the T wave returns to the baseline. If there is no Q wave, measurement begins with the R wave. The QT interval generally measures between 0.40 and 0.44 second, but varies with age, sex, and heart rate. Because of this variability, the QT interval can be measured more accurately if corrected (ie, adjusted) for the patient's heart rate. The corrected QT interval (QTc) is considered prolonged in adults if it measures 0.47 second or more in men and 0.48 second or more in women.[8,9] A prolonged QT interval can lead to ventricular dysrhythmias and SCA.

TABLE 18-4 Components of the ECG

ECG Representation	Cardiac Event
P wave	Depolarization of the atria
PR interval	Depolarization of the atria and delay at the AV junction
QRS complex	Depolarization of the ventricles
ST segment	Period between ventricular depolarization and beginning of repolarization
T wave	Ventricular repolarization
R-R interval	Time between two successive ventricular depolarizations

Abbreviations: AV, atrioventricular; ECG, electrocardiogram

TP Segment

The TP segment begins at the end of the T wave and ends at the start of the P wave. This portion of the ECG tracing is generally a flat, straight, horizontal line used as the baseline. The baseline is the reference point to which we compare the J point.

R-R Interval

The **R-R interval** is the period between two successive QRS complexes. It represents the interval between two ventricular depolarizations. The R-R interval can be used to calculate the heart rate and to determine the regularity of the patient's cardiac rhythm **TABLE 18-4**.

Approach to Dysrhythmia Interpretation

Part of your role as a paramedic will be to interpret ECG strips and be alert for dysrhythmias. Here we present a five-step method for performing this interpretation:

1. Identify the waves (P-QRS-T).
2. Measure the PRI.
3. Measure the QRS complex duration.
4. Determine rhythm regularity.
5. Measure the heart rate.

It is crucial to follow this method every time so you do not overlook any critical findings on the ECG tracing. Usually, you will exclusively use lead II for dysrhythmia interpretation.

We have already explained where P, QRS, and T waves appear; defined the PRI; and examined the QRS duration. If you can identify P waves, then note whether they are upright and fall within normal parameters. Is there only one P wave for every QRS complex? Next, we'll outline how to determine rhythm regularity and how to measure the heart rate.

Rhythm Regularity

Heart rhythm can be regular, regularly irregular, or irregularly irregular. Determining rhythm regularity can be as simple as measuring the distance between R waves. If the distance is the same, then the rhythm is regular **FIGURE 18-27**. If no two R waves are equidistant, then the rhythm is irregularly irregular **FIGURE 18-28**. If the R waves are irregular but appear to follow a pattern, then the rhythm is regularly irregular **FIGURE 18-29**. For example, suppose you obtain the following data when measuring the distance between R waves: 25, 27, 30, 25, 27, and 30 mm. This pattern represents a regularly irregular rhythm. You can also use ECG calipers to measure the distance between R waves, or use the edge of a piece of paper as a makeshift ruler.

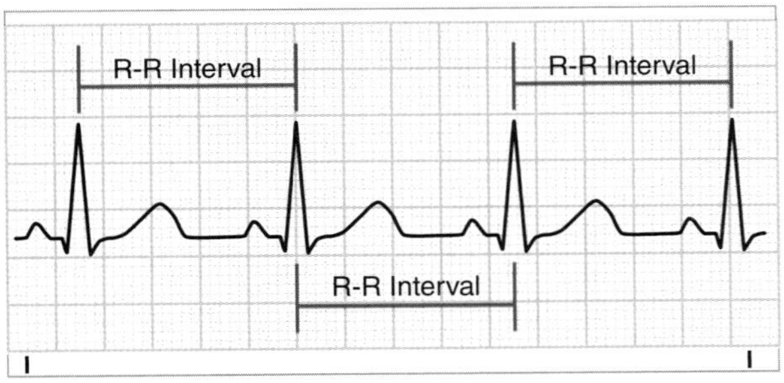

FIGURE 18-27 When the ventricular rhythm is regular, the R-R intervals are the same.

Reproduced from *Arrhythmia Recognition: The Art of Interpretation*, courtesy of Tomas B. Garcia, MD.

Determining Heart Rate

This section describes some of the more common ways of using a cardiac rhythm strip to determine heart rate.

The 6-Second Method

The 6-second method is the fastest way to measure heart rate from the ECG. Use this method for regular or irregular rhythms. In fact, it is the best method for calculating heart rate when the rhythm is irregular.

- Count the number of QRS complexes in a 6-second strip, and multiply that number by 10 to obtain the rate per minute **FIGURE 18-30**.

The Sequence Method

Use the sequence method **FIGURE 18-31** to determine the heart rate only when the rhythm is regular:

- First, memorize the following sequence: 300, 150, 100, 75, 60, 50.
- Find an R wave on a heavy line (large box), and count off "300, 150, 100, 75, 60, 50" for each large box you land on until you reach the next R wave. (Estimate the rate if the second R wave does not fall precisely on a heavy black line.)
- If the R-R interval spans fewer than three large boxes, the rate is greater than 100 (tachycardia).

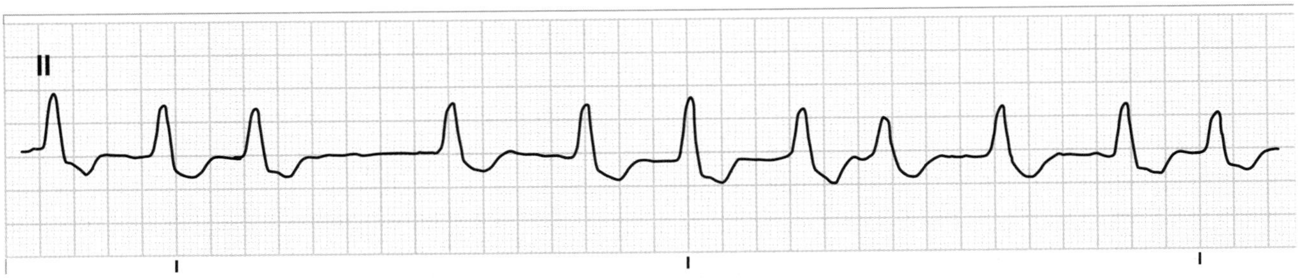

FIGURE 18-28 In an irregularly irregular rhythm, no two R-R intervals are the same. Note: The "II" in the upper left corner indicates this strip is from lead II.

Reproduced from *Arrhythmia Recognition: The Art of Interpretation*, courtesy of Tomas B. Garcia, MD.

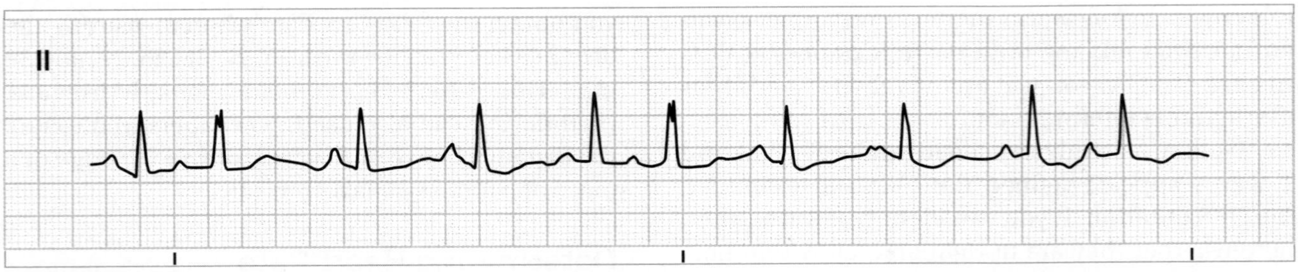

FIGURE 18-29 In a regularly irregular rhythm, the R-R intervals follow a discernible pattern.

Reproduced from *Arrhythmia Recognition: The Art of Interpretation*, courtesy of Tomas B. Garcia, MD.

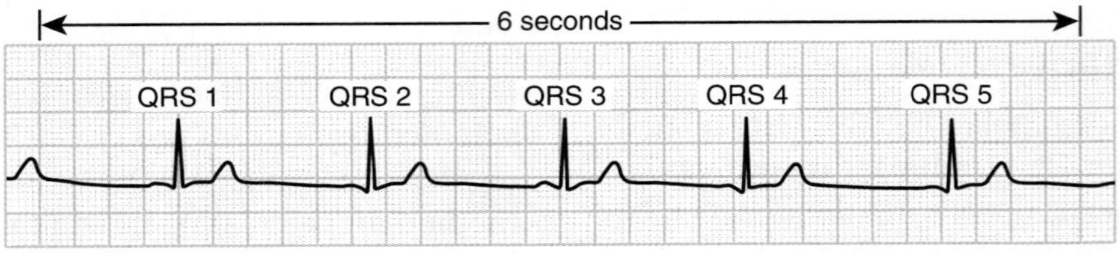

FIGURE 18-30 Calculation of heart rate. To calculate the rate, count the number of QRS complexes in a 6-second strip and multiply by 10.

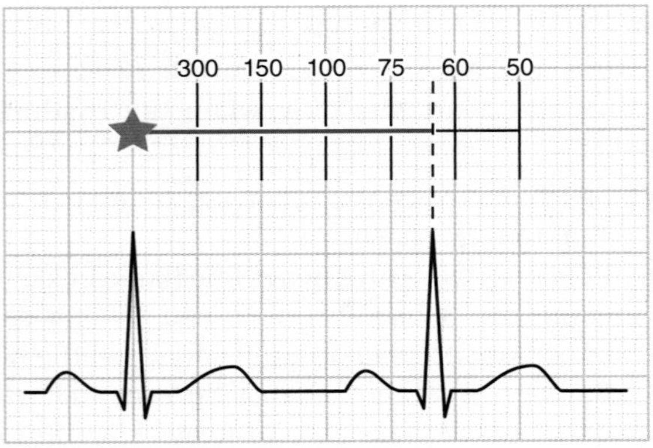

FIGURE 18-31 The sequence method.

Reproduced from *12-Lead ECG: The Art of Interpretation*, courtesy of Tomas B. Garcia, MD.

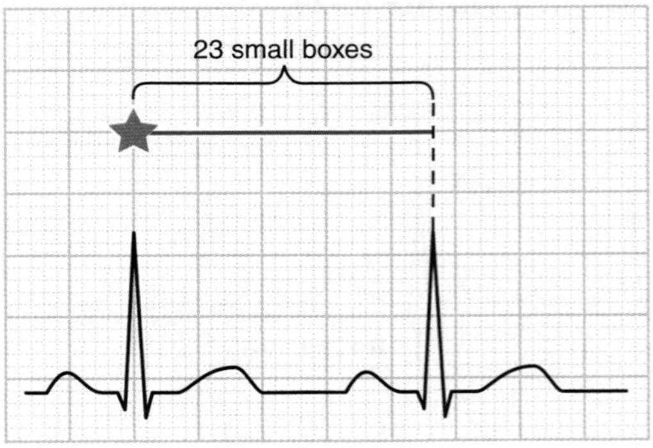

FIGURE 18-32 The 1,500 method.

Reproduced from *12-Lead ECG: The Art of Interpretation*, courtesy of Tomas B. Garcia, MD.

If it covers more than five large boxes, the rate is less than 60 (bradycardia).

The 1,500 Method

The 1,500 method is the most accurate way to calculate the heart rate from the ECG. It is typically used when the heart rate exceeds 150 beats/min, and only when the rhythm is regular:

- Calculate the rate by counting the number of small boxes between any two QRS complexes (the R-R interval); then divide 1,500 by that number.
- In **FIGURE 18-32**, for example, there are about 23 small boxes between two successive QRS complexes:

$$1{,}500 \div 23 = 65$$

- This calculation yields a rate of approximately 65 beats/min.

Specific Cardiac Dysrhythmias

Many different events can induce cardiac dysrhythmias. The flow of electricity through damaged or oxygen-deprived tissue is different from the flow through normal, well-oxygenated tissue, and this altered flow sometimes appears as an irregularity on the ECG. Many of these irregularities can be traced to ischemia, especially in areas of the heart responsible for conduction. Ischemia often causes spontaneous depolarization, generating a premature complex. These premature complexes then interfere with normal impulse conduction and induce dysrhythmia. In other situations, ischemia occurs within the conduction system and is the direct cause of its malfunction.

Many cardiac dysrhythmias are well tolerated and produce no serious symptoms, making it difficult to estimate the number of people affected by them. It is well documented, however, that cardiac dysrhythmias are the most common cause of cardiac arrest.

There are nearly as many ways of classifying cardiac dysrhythmias as there are books on the subject. Dysrhythmias can be characterized as disturbances of automaticity or disturbances of conduction. They can be separated into rhythms that are too fast (tachydysrhythmias) or too slow (bradydysrhythmias), or classified as life threatening or non–life threatening. In this section, cardiac dysrhythmias are categorized according to the site from which they arise (and as they appear in lead II). After looking at a sinus rhythm for comparison, we will cover the dysrhythmias that arise in the SA node, atrial tissue, AV junction, and ventricles. Finally, we will explore paced rhythms.

Rhythms Originating in the SA Node

Normal Sinus Rhythm

The SA node is the primary pacemaker for the heart. A **normal sinus rhythm** **FIGURE 18-33** arises in the SA node and has an intrinsic rate of 60 to 100 beats/min. The rhythm is regular, with minimal variation between R-R intervals. An upright P wave precedes each QRS complex. The PRI measures 0.12 to 0.20 second (120 to 200 milliseconds). The QRS complex measures 0.11 second (110 milliseconds) or less.

Sinus Bradycardia

The pacemaker is still the SA node with **sinus bradycardia**, but the rate is less than 60 beats/min **FIGURE 18-34**. The rhythm is regular, and an upright

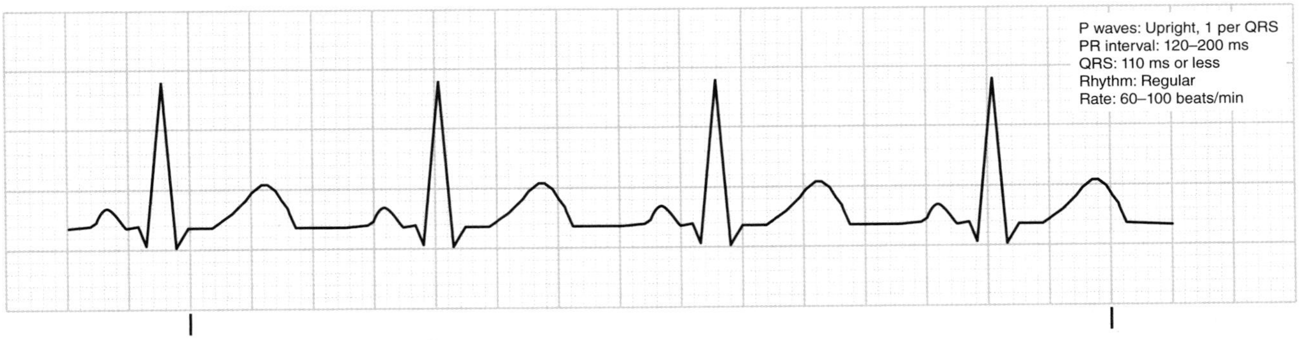

FIGURE 18-33 Normal sinus rhythm.

Reproduced from *Arrhythmia Recognition: The Art of Interpretation*, courtesy of Tomas B. Garcia, MD.

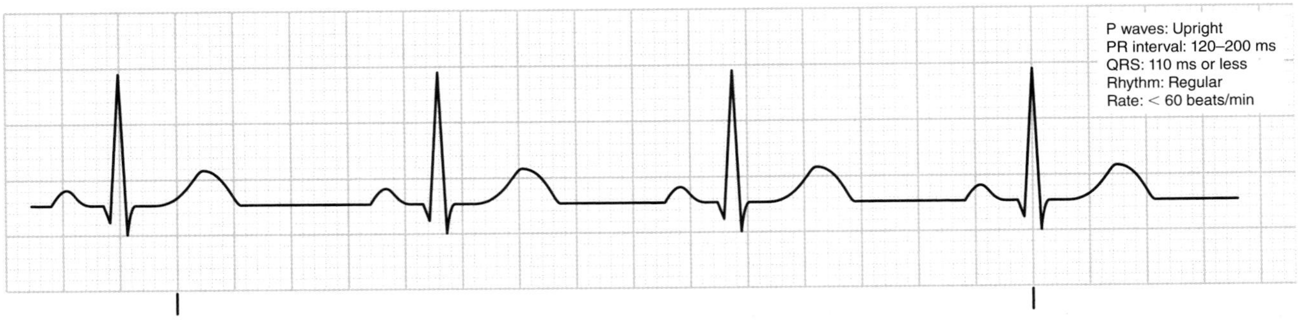

FIGURE 18-34 Sinus bradycardia.

Reproduced from *Arrhythmia Recognition: The Art of Interpretation*, courtesy of Tomas B. Garcia, MD.

P wave precedes each QRS complex. The PRI is 0.12 to 0.20 second (120 to 200 milliseconds). The QRS complex is 0.11 second (110 milliseconds) or less.

In many patients, a very slow heart rate (usually less than 50 beats/min) results in inadequate CO and often precipitates electrical instability of the heart. Furthermore, when the sinus rate becomes very slow, ectopic pacemakers in the AV junction or ventricles may fire, producing escape beats to assist in maintaining CO. The term **ectopic** refers to an impulse or rhythm originating from a site other than the SA node.

In healthy adults, especially well-conditioned athletes, sinus bradycardia can be an asymptomatic phenomenon and may occur during sleep. However, in other adults, bradycardia can cause altered mental status, ischemic chest discomfort, acute heart failure, seizures, syncope, or evidence of hemodynamic instability, such as diaphoresis or hypotension.[10] Treatment is indicated when these signs and symptoms persist despite adequate oxygenation and ventilation.

Management of Symptomatic Bradycardia

The emergency medical care of an adult patient with symptomatic bradycardia focuses on the following goals:

- Maintain adequate oxygenation, ventilation, and perfusion.
- Correct the rhythm disturbance and restore a stable perfusing rhythm.
- Search for the underlying cause, which may be hypoxia, hypothermia, hypoglycemia, shock, ACS, AV block, toxin exposure (beta blockers, calcium channel blockers, sodium channel blockers/antidepressants, organophosphates, digoxin, clonidine), an electrolyte disorder, increased intracranial pressure, or other factors.[10]

Follow these steps to administer emergency medical care for an adult with symptomatic bradycardia:

1. Maintain an open airway. Assist breathing as necessary. Administer supplemental oxygen as needed to target an Spo_2 of 95% to 98%. Target an oxygen saturation of 90% for patients with ACS and target an oxygen saturation of 92% to 98% during post–cardiac arrest care.[11]
2. Apply a cardiac monitor, BP monitor, and pulse oximeter. Obtain a 12-lead ECG, but do not delay emergency care to perform this step.
3. Establish an IV infusion of normal saline. Obtain a finger-stick blood glucose level. Treat hypoglycemia if present.
4. Administer an atropine IV bolus for symptomatic sinus bradycardia or a conduction block at the level of the AV node. Repeat atropine every 3 to 5 minutes until the desired heart rate is achieved (usually 60 beats/min or faster) or the dosage limit of 3 mg has been reached. Patients who have undergone cardiac transplant will not respond to atropine because they lack vagal nerve innervation. Cardiac-related medications are discussed in detail in Chapter 13, *Principles of Pharmacology*.
5. If atropine is ineffective and the patient's symptoms or hemodynamic instability persist, then consider TCP or the administration of a dopamine or epinephrine infusion. In cases of impending hemodynamic collapse, proceed directly to TCP.[10]
6. Transport the patient for definitive care.

The recommended treatment guidelines for adult bradycardia are shown in **FIGURE 18-35**.

Artificial pacemakers deliver repetitive bursts of electrical impulses to the heart. Like the tiny electrical signals generated by natural pacemakers, the current from an artificial pacemaker can depolarize the myocardial tissue. In this way, the artificial pacemaker can substitute for a blocked or nonfunctional natural pacemaker.

A **transcutaneous pacemaker** depolarizes the myocardium by delivering electrical energy through

Documentation and Communication

Key documentation elements for the patient with symptomatic bradycardia are as follows:[10]

- Initial cardiac rhythm and rate
- Time, dosage, and patient response to medications given
- Time at which pacing is started or stopped, rate (paced pulses per minute), energy setting, capture, and patient response
- History of an event supporting the treatment of underlying causes
- Monitor strips obtained before and during pacing and at the time of transfer

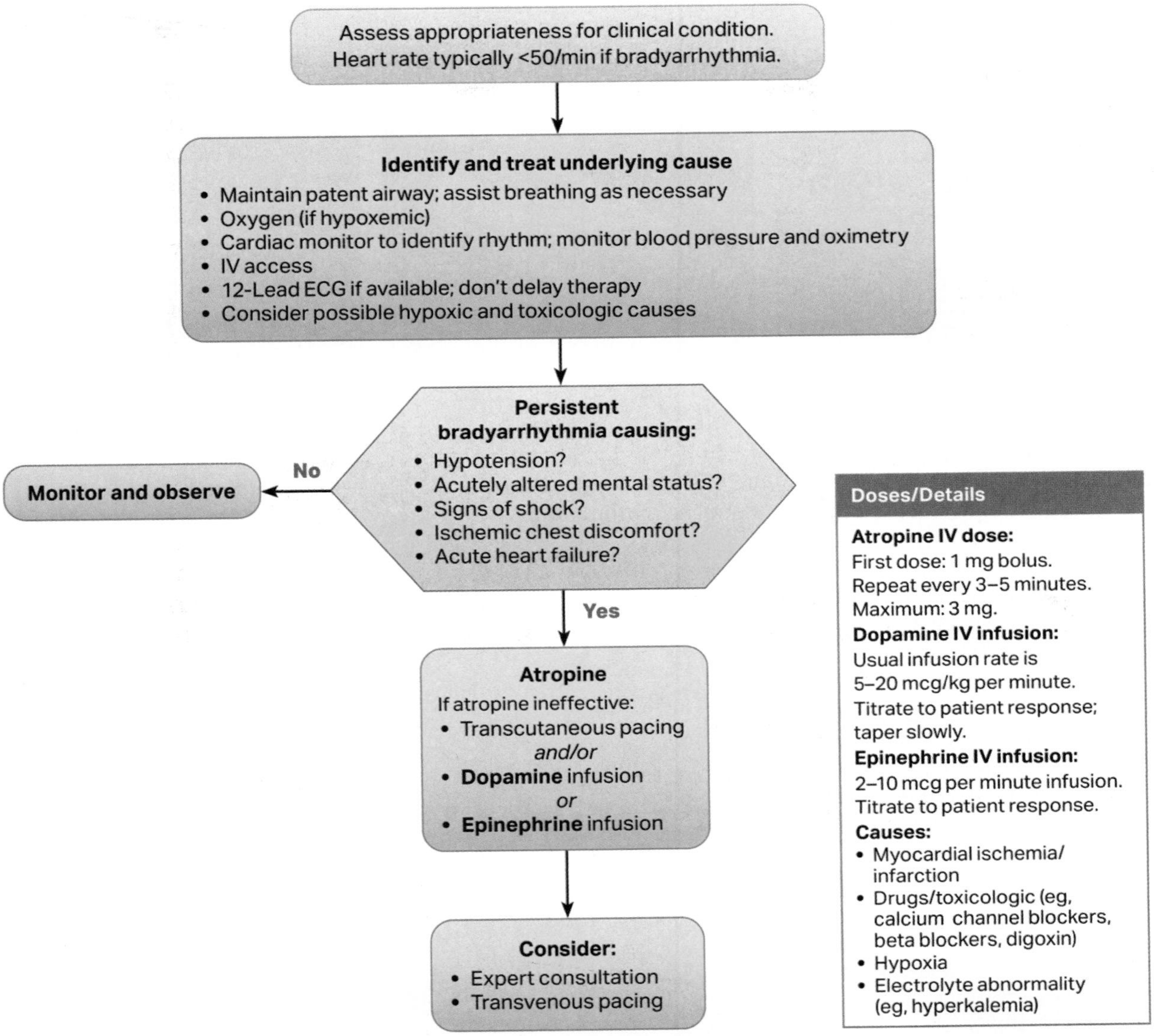

FIGURE 18-35 Adult bradycardia with a pulse algorithm.
Abbreviations: ECG, electrocardiogram; IV, intravenous.

the skin of the chest and is widely used. With a TCP, a small electrical charge passes through the patient's skin between one external pacing pad and another, spreading the signal across the heart. The pacer is set for a specific rate, and the energy is increased until the heart begins to react to the stimulus. This response, which is termed "capture," is usually associated with ventricular depolarization. It is characterized by a wide QRS complex on the ECG and should result in a corresponding palpable pulse.

In any of the following circumstances, TCP may allow enough time for the patient to reach a medical facility in a state of optimal perfusion, rather than in or near cardiac arrest:

- A patient with a bradydysrhythmia that severely reduces CO and does not respond to atropine
- A patient who requires interhospital transfer for permanent pacemaker implantation
- A symptomatic patient with artificial pacemaker failure

Many brands of TCPs are available, so you must become familiar with the specific device used in your local EMS system. The steps in initiating TCP are shown in **SKILL DRILL 18-2**.

Skill Drill 18-2 Performing TCP

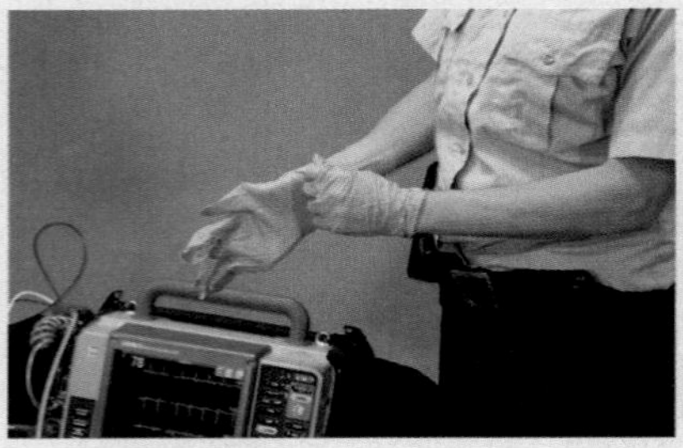

Step 1

Select, check, and assemble all necessary equipment, including a monitor-defibrillator with pacing capability, ECG electrodes, pacing pads, medication for pain or sedation (to be used if necessary), oxygen, and an appropriate oxygen administration device. Take standard precautions. Apply the ECG electrodes and assess the patient's vital signs. Ensure the patient is oxygenated adequately and establish a patent IV line.

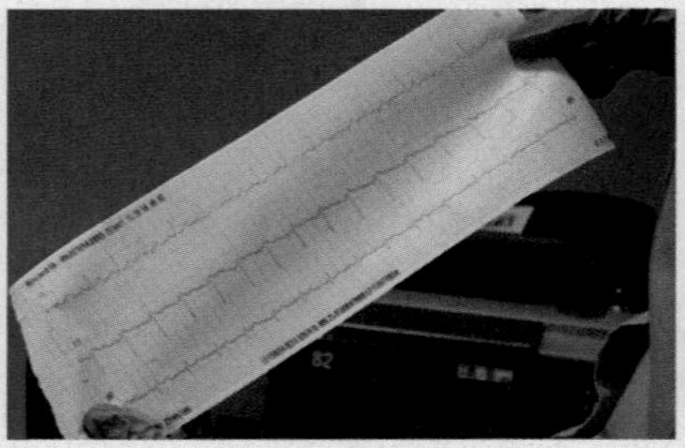

Step 2

Identify the rhythm and confirm TCP is warranted. Obtain a baseline rhythm strip.

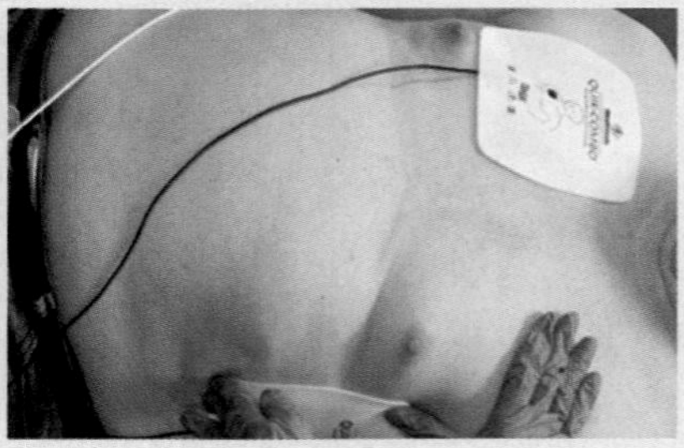

Step 3

Ensure the scene and environment are safe (evaluate risks such as sparks, combustibles, and an oxygen-rich atmosphere). Explain to the patient and the family the need for the procedure. Apply the pacing pads to the patient according to the manufacturer's recommendations. Sedation or analgesia may be needed to minimize the discomfort associated with this procedure. Ask the patient about any medication allergies before administering medications.

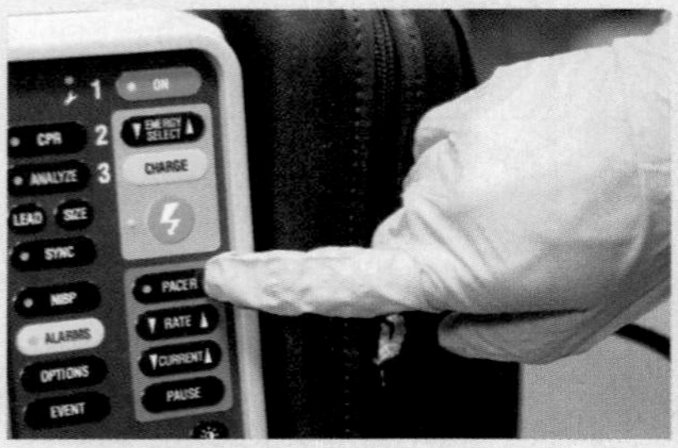

Step 4

Switch on the power to the pacer.

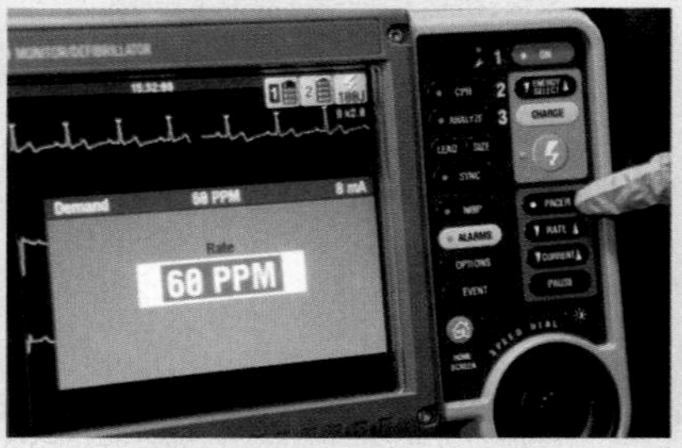

Step 5

Set the pacing rate to the desired number of paced pulses per minute (ppm). A rate between 60 and 80 beats/min is usually selected.

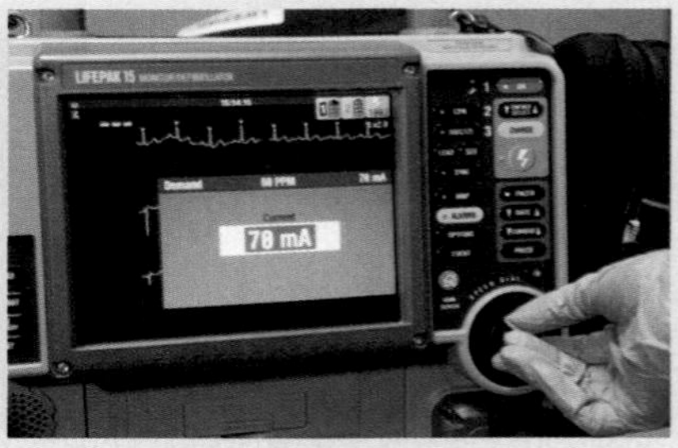

Step 6

Set the current (milliamps) to be delivered to the minimum setting. While watching the monitor screen, slowly but steadily increase the current until you achieve electrical capture (ie, a wide QRS complex follows each pacer spike).

Skill Drill 18-2 Performing TCP (continued)

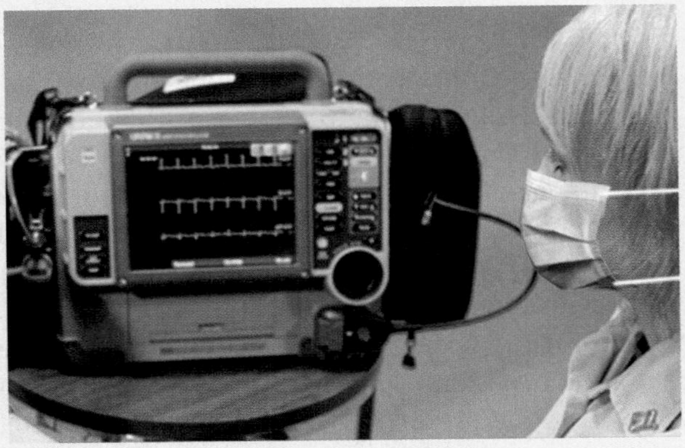

Step 7

Evaluate mechanical capture by assessing the patient's pulse and BP. Reassess the patient's mental status, Spo_2, color, and level of discomfort.

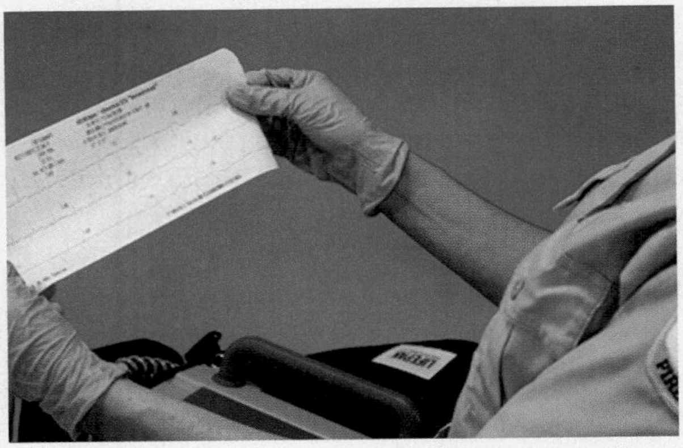

Step 8

Obtain rhythm strips for documentation and continuously monitor the patient's condition.

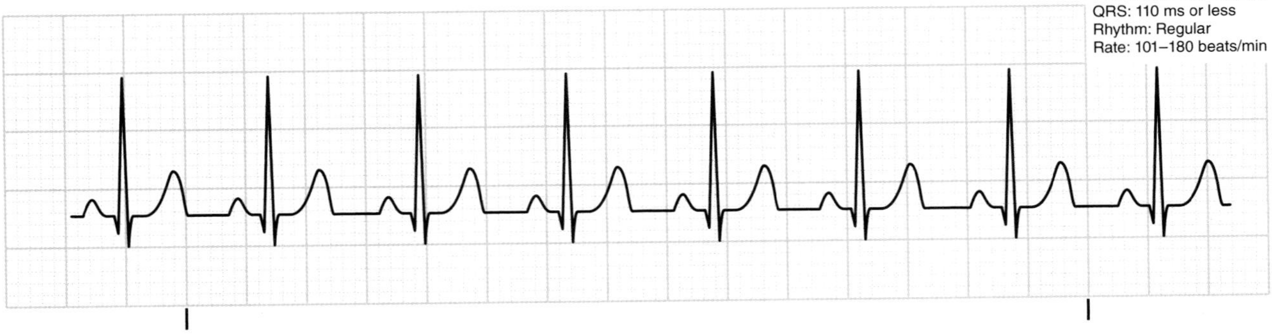

FIGURE 18-36 Sinus tachycardia.

Reproduced from *Arrhythmia Recognition: The Art of Interpretation*, courtesy of Tomas B. Garcia, MD.

Sinus Tachycardia

By definition, a tachycardia has a ventricular rate faster than 100 beats/min. The SA node is still the pacemaker with **sinus tachycardia**, but the heart rate is typically 101 to 180 beats/min in a resting adult **FIGURE 18-36**. The upper rate of sinus tachycardia is age related and can be calculated as approximately 220 beats/min minus the patient's age in years. The rhythm is regular, and an upright P wave precedes each QRS complex (although it is occasionally difficult to see if it is partially buried in the T wave of the preceding beat). The PRI is 0.12 to 0.20 second (120 to 200 milliseconds), and the QRS complex is 0.11 second (110 milliseconds) or less.

Sinus tachycardia has various causes, including pain, fever, hypoxia, hypovolemia, exercise, sympathetic nervous system stimulation (caused by stress, fright, or anxiety), AMI, pump failure, or anemia. In addition, caffeine, nicotine, alcohol, and certain other drugs, such as atropine, epinephrine, amphetamine, and cocaine, can cause tachycardia.

Hypoxia, metabolic alkalosis, hypokalemia, and **hypocalcemia** can lead to electrical instability, prompting the firing of cells that normally do not generate impulses.

Prolonged tachycardia increases the work of the heart, leading to further ischemia during an AMI. In addition, CO may be significantly reduced when the heart rate exceeds 150 beats/min because the ventricles have inadequate time to fill completely between contractions.

The treatment of sinus tachycardia depends on its underlying cause.

Sinus Dysrhythmia

Sinus dysrhythmia is a slight variation in the cycling of a sinus rhythm, usually exceeding 0.12 second (120 milliseconds) between the longest and shortest cycles, which is often associated with respiratory cycle fluctuations **FIGURE 18-37**. Specifically, the rate increases during inspiration and decreases during expiration. The SA node is still the pacemaker, and an upright P wave precedes each QRS complex. The PRI of 0.12 to 0.20 second (120 to 200 milliseconds) and the QRS complex of 0.11 second (110 milliseconds) or less are the same as in a normal sinus rhythm. Sinus dysrhythmia is often a normal finding in children and young adults and tends to diminish with age.

Sinus Arrest

Sinus arrest occurs when the SA node fails to initiate an impulse, eliminating the P wave, QRS complex, and T wave for one cardiac cycle **FIGURE 18-38**. After this missed set of waveforms, the SA node resumes normal functioning as if nothing ever happened. In sinus arrest, the atrial and ventricular rates are usually within normal limits and the rhythm is regular except for the absent complexes. P waves are present and upright, preceding every QRS complex, and the PRI, when present, is 0.12 to 0.20 second (120 to 200 milliseconds). The QRS complex, when present, is 0.11 second (110 milliseconds) or less.

Possible causes of sinus arrest include SA node ischemia, increased vagal tone, carotid sinus massage (discussed later in this chapter), and use of drugs such as digitalis and quinidine. Occasional episodes of sinus arrest are not significant; however, if the heart rate drops below 60 beats/min, CO may fall and an ectopic focus from either the AV junction or the ventricles may take over. In such

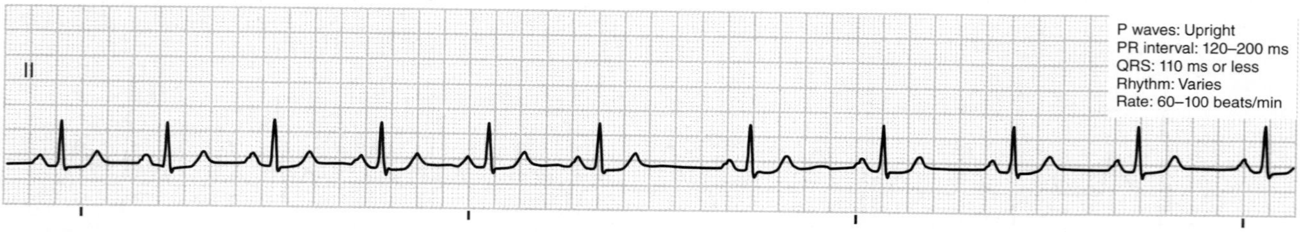

FIGURE 18-37 Sinus dysrhythmia.

Reproduced from *Arrhythmia Recognition: The Art of Interpretation*, courtesy of Tomas B. Garcia, MD.

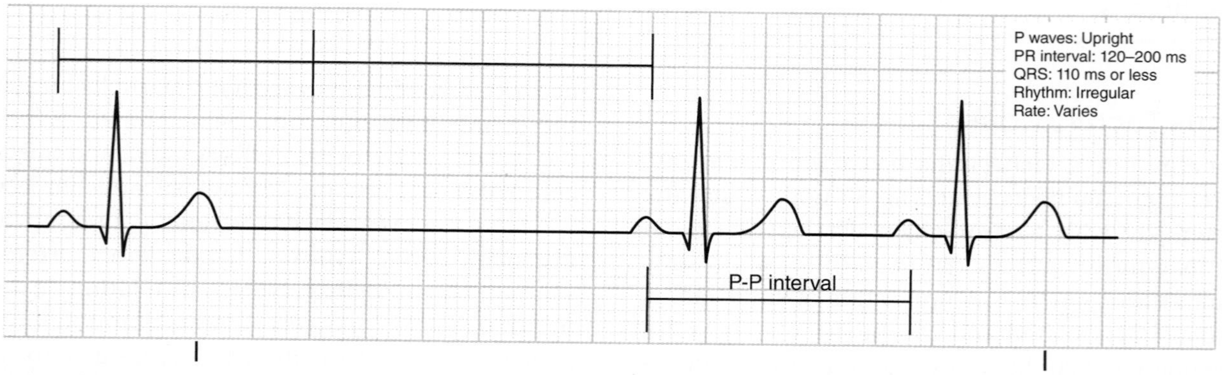

FIGURE 18-38 With a sinus arrest, at least one PQRST cycle is missing. The resulting P-P interval is not an exact multiple of the normal P-P interval.

Modified from *Arrhythmia Recognition: The Art of Interpretation*, courtesy of Tomas B. Garcia, MD.

circumstances, treatment is based on the patient's overall heart rate and tolerance. The patient may benefit from a temporary pacemaker (TCP in the field) or a permanent pacemaker after admission to the medical facility.

Sick Sinus Syndrome

Sick sinus syndrome (SSS) encompasses a variety of rhythms characterized by a poorly functioning SA node. This condition is common among older adults. Patients may remain asymptomatic, or they may have syncopal or near-syncopal episodes, dizziness, and palpitations. On an ECG, SSS may be evidenced by sinus bradycardia, sinus arrest, SA block, and alternating patterns of extreme bradycardia and tachycardia (bradycardia-tachycardia syndrome).

Rhythms Originating in the Atria

Although the SA node usually is the pacemaker for the heart, any area of the atria can originate an impulse, thereby superseding the SA node's pacemaking authority. Some rhythms originating from the atria produce upright P waves that precede each QRS complex, but are not as well rounded as those generated by the SA node.

Premature Atrial Complex

A premature atrial complex (PAC) is not, strictly speaking, a dysrhythmia, but rather an ectopic complex that appears within another rhythm **FIGURE 18-39**. A PAC occurs earlier than the next expected sinus complex, producing an abnormally short R-R interval between it and the previous complex. The presence of a PAC will make the rhythm irregular. An upright P wave precedes each QRS complex; however, its shape differs from the P waves originating from the SA node, indicating its different site of origin. The PRI measures 0.12 to 0.20 second (120 to 200 milliseconds), but may vary slightly based on the premature complex's origin. The QRS complex measures 0.11 second (110 milliseconds).

PACs are not always conducted to the ventricles. A P wave that occurs early on the ECG and is not followed by a QRS complex is called a *nonconducted PAC*. This phenomenon should not be confused with AV block. The two are easily differentiated because, unlike AV block, nonconducted PACs occur infrequently, in no particular pattern, producing a P wave that occurs early on the ECG. If you measure the P-P interval, then the P wave associated with a nonconducted PAC will be shorter than the other P-P intervals. However, in AV block, the P-P interval is constant.

PACs are very common and can be caused by stress, stimulants such as caffeine, or conditions such as heart failure or electrolyte imbalance. When PACs are frequent, treatment is focused on correcting the underlying cause.

Supraventricular Tachycardia

Supraventricular tachycardia (SVT) is a rhythm that originates from a site above the ventricles with a ventricular rate faster than 100 beats/min at rest.[12]

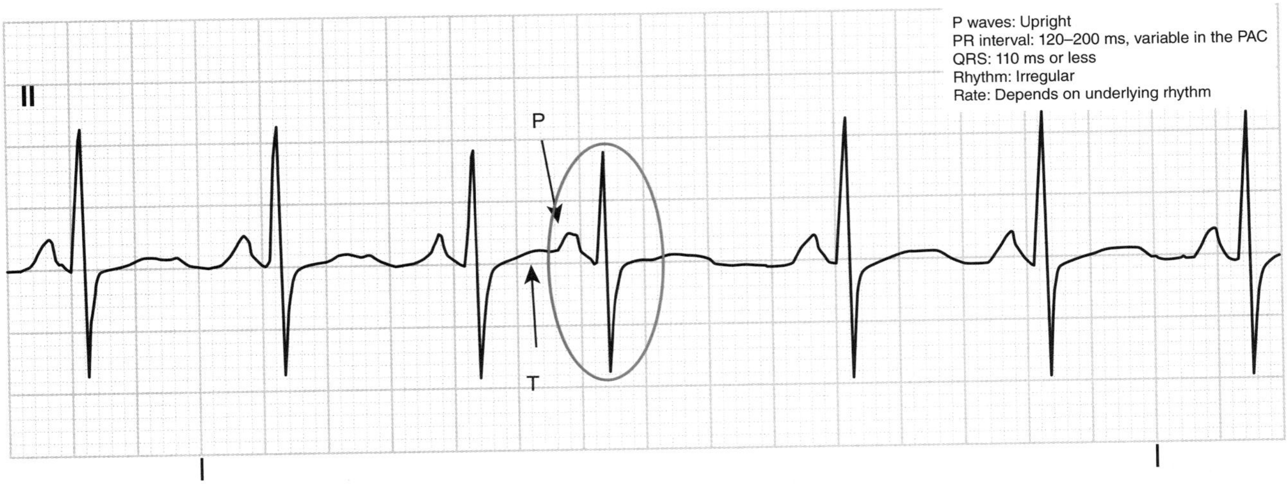

FIGURE 18-39 Premature atrial complex.

Reproduced from *Arrhythmia Recognition: The Art of Interpretation*, courtesy of Tomas B. Garcia, MD.

In patients with normal ventricular function, tachycardia with a rate of less than 150 beats/min rarely causes serious signs and symptoms. However, when the ventricular rate exceeds 150 beats/min, ventricular filling time is reduced, which can in turn reduce CO. When the ventricular rate reaches 150 to 180 beats/min, the P waves (if present) with SVT tend to be completely obscured by the T wave of the preceding beat **FIGURE 18-40**, making it impossible to measure the PRI. At a lower heart rate, P waves can be identified. The rhythm is regular, with essentially no variation between R-R intervals. The QRS complexes measure 0.11 second (110 milliseconds) or less, indicating that the rhythm originates above the ventricles.

The most common type of SVT is called *AV nodal reentrant tachycardia.* As its name implies, this type of SVT is associated with **reentry**, which is the spread of an impulse through tissue already stimulated by that same impulse **FIGURE 18-41**. Under the right conditions, such as when myocardial ischemia is present, a premature impulse can trigger a series of rapid beats. The AV node may be bombarded by more than one impulse, which can block one signal's pathway and allow another signal to stimulate cardiac cells that have already depolarized. The danger comes when these impulses get stuck in a repetitive pattern, generating multiple ectopic beats or a very rapid rhythm.

SVT is sometimes referred to as *paroxysmal SVT (PSVT)*, reflecting its tendency to begin and

Words of Wisdom

As you learn the criteria for cardiac dysrhythmias, you will notice the ventricular rate ranges for various dysrhythmias overlap. Carefully examine the ECG, identifying waveforms and calculating measurements, to aid in correctly identifying the dysrhythmia. If you are unsure about the origin of a rhythm, obtaining a 12-lead ECG can be helpful because you can observe the rhythm in multiple leads.

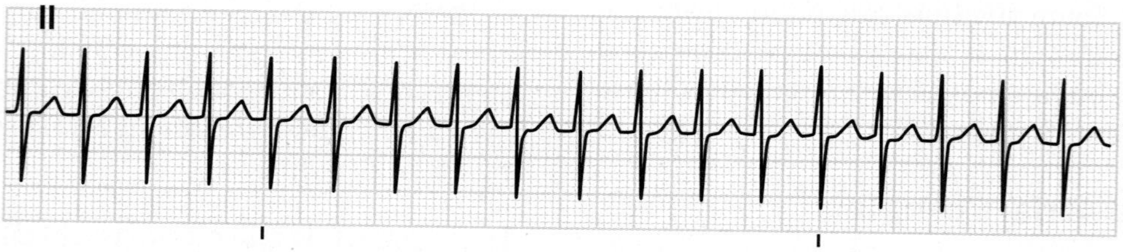

FIGURE 18-40 Supraventricular tachycardia.

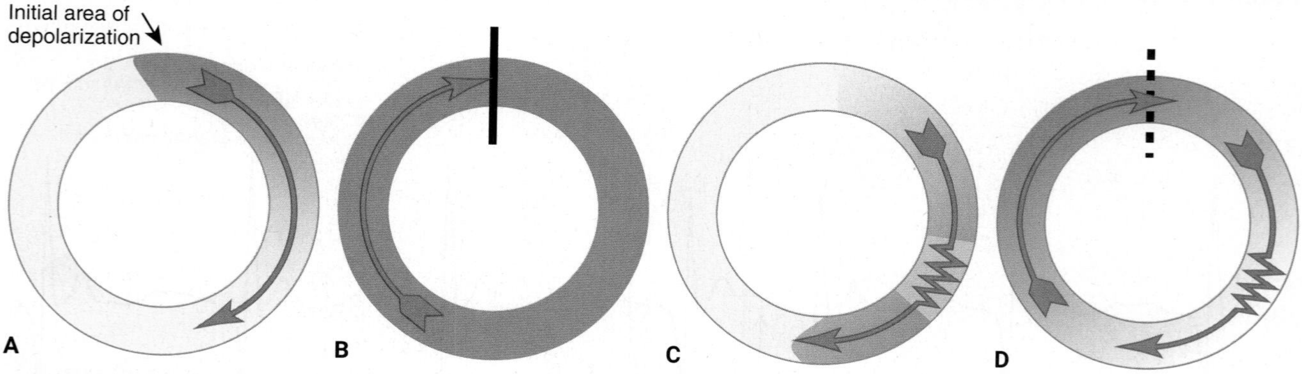

FIGURE 18-41 Reentry. **A.** The original impulse site fires, triggering a wave of depolarization that spreads over the remaining cells in the direction shown. **B.** When the depolarization wave returns to the original site (represented by the black line), the site is still refractory and cannot respond to the new impulse. The wave essentially subsides at this point. **C.** The yellow portion represents an area of slow conduction. The depolarization wave slows as it traverses this area. **D.** By the time the depolarization wave reaches the original site, represented by the dotted black line, the site is ready to receive a new impulse. The result is a self-perpetuating cyclical movement.

end abruptly (*paroxysmal* means "occurring in spasms"). Technically, to identify a dysrhythmia as a PSVT, you would need to witness the rhythm acceleration on the ECG.

Patients who present with SVT sometimes have a physical finding known as *cannon "A" waves*. Cannon "A" waves are created by a dissociation between the atria and ventricles. This sign can also occur with right atrial contraction against a closed tricuspid valve. Larger "A" waves can indicate deteriorating functionality of the right ventricle or increasing right ventricular end-diastolic pressure. A corresponding physical sign can be found where the jugular veins are located: During the cannon "A" wave, a depression of the jugular veins occurs, forming an "A."

The symptoms associated with SVT vary. The treatment for SVT depends on the severity of the patient's symptoms and may include medication or electrical therapy to slow the heart rate.

Management of Tachycardia With a Pulse

Treating a patient who presents with or develops tachycardia is more complicated than treating a patient with bradycardia. Tachycardia can originate from a supraventricular pacemaker site or may have a ventricular origin. Generally, wide QRS complexes are presumed to be of ventricular origin, whereas narrow QRS complexes (0.11 second [110 milliseconds] or less) are presumed to be of supraventricular origin. (Ventricular tachycardia [VT] is discussed later in this chapter.) Occasionally, a beat of supraventricular origin will follow an aberrant conduction pathway, making it difficult to determine whether the tachycardia is ventricular or supraventricular. In most cases, the rhythm is ventricular, rather than supraventricular, and should be treated as such.

Emergency medical care of a patient with tachycardia with a pulse focuses on the following goals:[10,11]

- Quickly identify and treat patients with signs or symptoms of hemodynamic instability (eg, ischemic chest pain, altered mental status, shock, hypotension, acute heart failure) or those who are symptomatic because of the dysrhythmia.
- Maintain adequate oxygenation, ventilation, and perfusion.
- Control the ventricular rate.
- Restore a sinus rhythm in an unstable patient.
- Search for the underlying causes, such as medications (caffeine, diet pills, thyroid agents, or decongestants), illicit drugs (cocaine, amphetamines), heart failure, or a history of dysrhythmia.

Because of the many possible variations in patients with tachycardia, you must make several judgments before starting treatment. First, determine the severity of the patient's signs or symptoms, and determine whether the tachycardia caused them or whether the tachycardia and its associated signs and symptoms occurred in response to another condition. For example, a patient who is experiencing an MI may be mildly tachycardic, but the MI obviously is responsible for the signs and symptoms, not the tachycardia. However, if a patient was previously asymptomatic but symptoms developed after the onset of the tachycardia, their symptoms can likely be attributed to this condition. Second, determine whether the QRS complex is narrow or wide. Third, determine whether the ventricular rhythm is regular or irregular. If time permits, obtain a 12-lead ECG.

Conservative therapies, such as vagal maneuvers and medications, are appropriate for an adult with stable vital signs and a regular narrow-complex tachycardia who is exhibiting symptoms related to the tachycardia, such as light-headedness or palpitations. However, suppose an adult with tachycardia presents with more serious signs and symptoms, such as acutely altered mental status, ischemic chest discomfort, acute heart failure, hypotension, or other signs of shock. In that case, you should consider the patient unstable, and the use of electrical therapy with synchronized cardioversion is recommended.

Follow this procedure to provide emergency care for an adult who has tachycardia with a pulse:

1. Maintain an open airway. Assist breathing as necessary, and administer supplemental oxygen as needed to maintain an Spo_2 between 95% and 98%. Target an oxygen saturation of 90% for patients with ACSs, and target an oxygen saturation of 92% to 98% during post–cardiac arrest care.[11]
2. Apply a cardiac monitor, BP monitor, and pulse oximeter. Obtain a 12-lead ECG, but do not delay emergency care.

3. Establish an IV infusion of normal saline and obtain a finger-stick blood glucose measurement. Treat hypoglycemia, if present.
4. If the QRS is narrow and regular, the patient is stable, and there are no contraindications, then perform vagal maneuvers. If the rhythm persists, then administer adenosine intravenously. Follow each dose with a 20-mL fluid bolus. Adenosine dosing and administration are discussed in Chapter 15, *Emergency Medications*.
5. If the QRS is narrow and regular and the patient is unstable, consider sedation before performing synchronized cardioversion.
6. Transport the patient for definitive care.

Recommended treatment guidelines for adult tachycardia with a pulse are shown in **FIGURE 18-42**.

Vagal maneuvers are attempted for stable patients with regular narrow-QRS tachycardia before starting medication therapy. Vagal maneuvers stimulate baroreceptors, which signal brainstem centers to stimulate the vagus nerve, thereby slowing the heart rate.

Many types of vagal maneuvers exist, including carotid sinus massage, also known as *carotid sinus pressure*. Recall that the carotid sinus is located in the neck **FIGURE 18-43**. Before performing this procedure, assess for carotid **bruits** by listening to each carotid artery with a stethoscope **FIGURE 18-44**. A bruit is an abnormal whooshing sound indicating

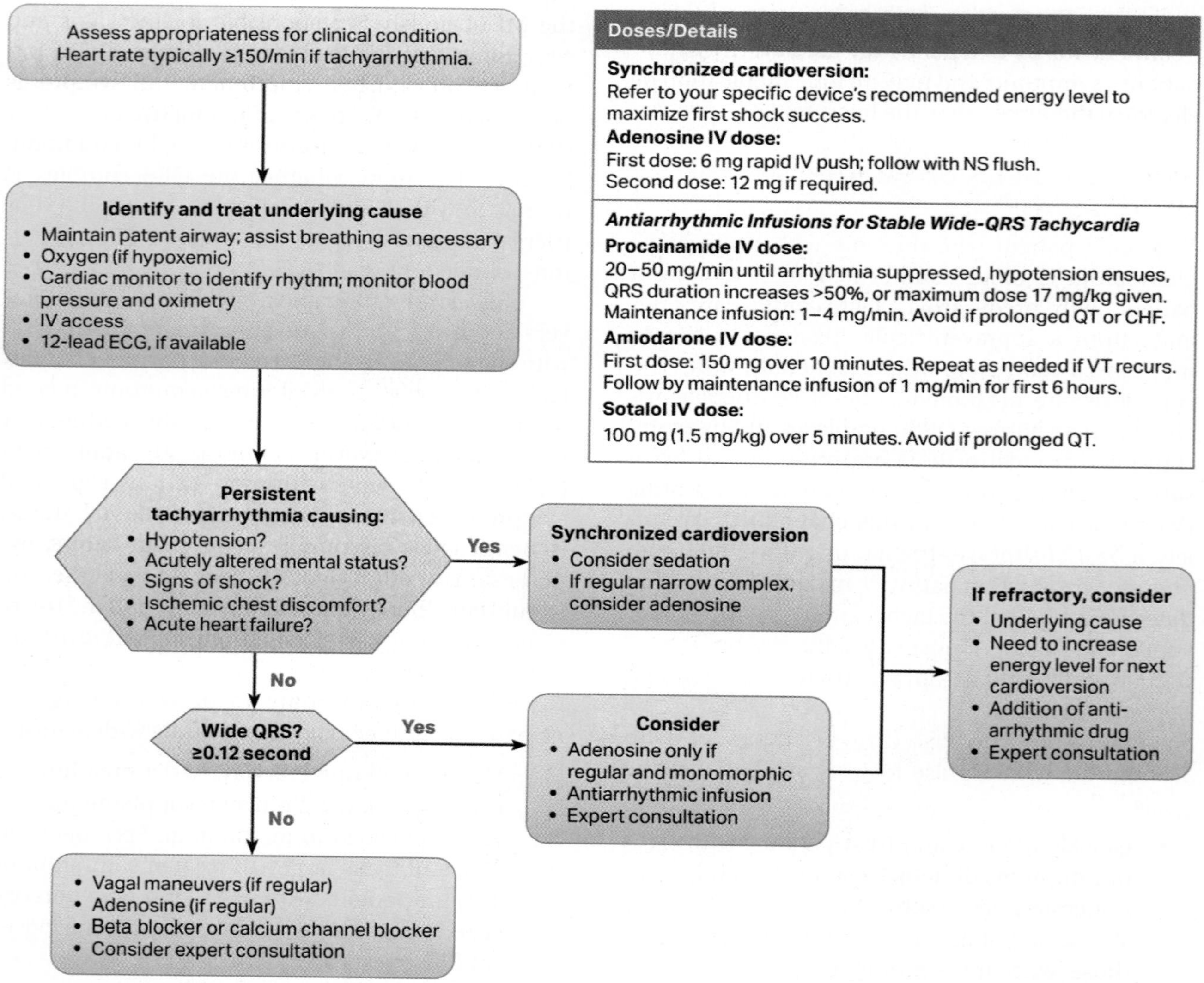

FIGURE 18-42 Algorithm for adult tachycardia with a pulse.
Abbreviations: CHF, congestive heart failure; ECG, electrocardiogram; IV, intravenous; NS, normal saline; VT, ventricular tachycardia.

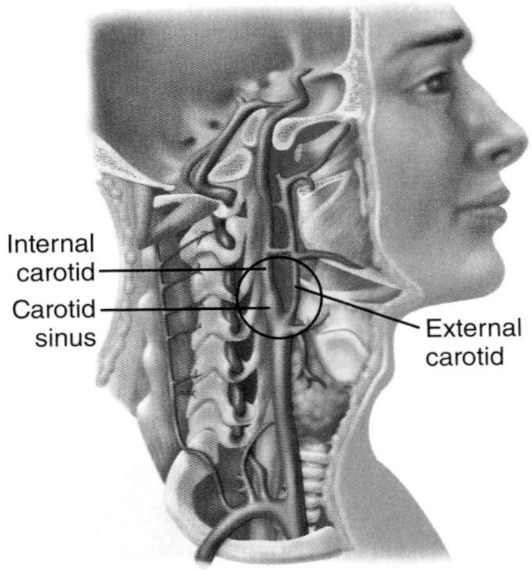

FIGURE 18-43 Location of the carotid sinus.

turbulent blood flow within a narrowed vessel. If you hear a bruit, then do not perform the procedure. If you do not hear a bruit and no contraindications are present, turn the patient's head to one side. Next, locate the carotid pulse and apply firm pressure to the carotid artery for 5 to 10 seconds. An older adult patient with a history of stroke, known carotid artery stenosis, or CAD and a high cholesterol level would not be a good candidate for carotid massage because of the high risk of **thromboembolism**. Because carotid sinus massage has been associated with many complications, including stroke, syncope (fainting), and dysrhythmias (including **asystole**), it is not permitted in all EMS systems. Check your local protocol about performing this procedure.

The Valsalva maneuver is a more commonly used vagal maneuver in which the patient bears down against a closed glottis for about 15 seconds. The patient is often instructed to bear down as if attempting to have a bowel movement. Valsalva maneuvers should not be attempted in patients with recent AMI, aortic stenosis, carotid artery stenosis, glaucoma, or retinopathy. Research has shown that performing a carotid sinus massage or a Valsalva maneuver with postural modifications, such as supine positioning and passive leg raising during the procedure, may increase the probability of successful rhythm conversion.[13,14]

If vagal maneuvers are ineffective and the patient with a regular narrow-QRS tachycardia remains stable, then administer adenosine. This medication is used to transiently induce AV nodal blockade, thereby interrupting the tachydysrhythmia. Before

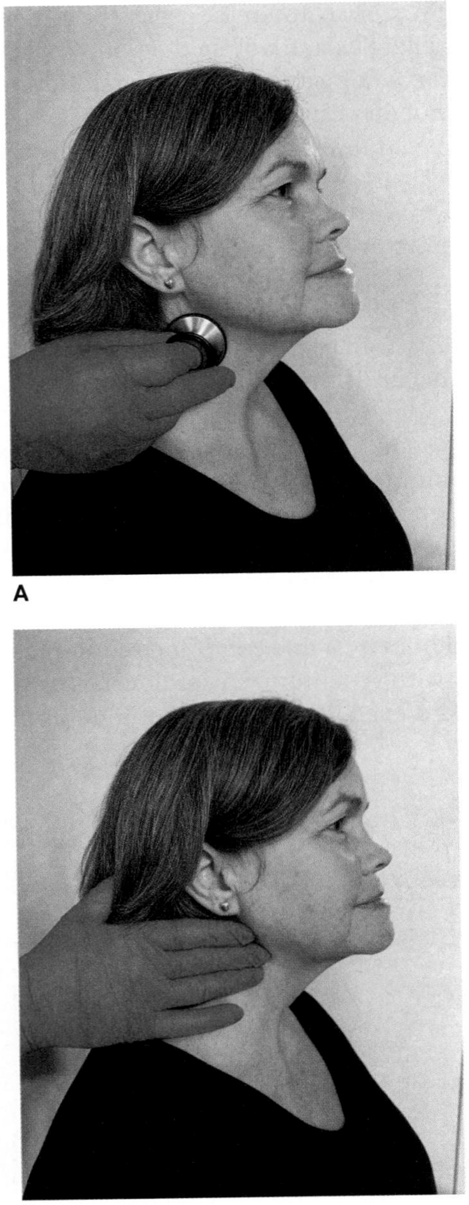

A

B

FIGURE 18-44 Carotid sinus pressure. **A.** Listen for bruits. **B.** Apply pressure to the carotid artery for 5 to 10 seconds.

Words of Wisdom

Ensure the patient is on a cardiac monitor and vascular access has been established before performing vagal maneuvers. Also, never massage the right and left carotid arteries at the same time, as doing so may cause significant bradycardia, stroke, or asystole.

you begin this treatment, recheck the patient's history for allergies and advise the patient of the possible adverse effects of adenosine administration. Because of the drug's very short half-life, adenosine should be administered at the IV site closest to the patient's heart. After clamping off the IV line above the site, push the adenosine as rapidly as possible, and then follow with a 20-mL flush of normal saline solution as soon as the plunger of the adenosine syringe hits bottom. Be prepared to see a short period of asystole, although this response does not always occur. If the tachycardia persists, a double dose of adenosine can be given after 1 to 2 minutes. If needed, the double dose can be repeated in 1 to 2 minutes. If adenosine does not convert the rhythm, transport the patient to the medical facility.

If the condition of a patient with SVT becomes unstable at any time, you should move to the unstable arm of the tachycardia algorithm. A tachycardic patient in unstable condition requires electrical therapy with synchronized cardioversion. Synchronized cardioversion is the use of a defibrillator to terminate a hemodynamically unstable tachydysrhythmia. Unlike defibrillation, a process in which energy may be delivered at any time during the cardiac cycle, synchronized cardioversion delivers timed bursts of electrical energy. The device identifies R waves on the ECG. When you press and hold the shock controls, the machine will discharge with the next detected R wave, avoiding the vulnerable period during the T wave of the cardiac cycle.

Cardioversion is indicated for VT and SVT associated with severely compromised CO. When cardioversion is performed on a responsive patient, the patient *must* be sedated first; cardioversion is a painful and terrifying experience for a patient who is awake. Benzodiazepines, such as diazepam (Valium) and midazolam (Versed), are commonly administered for sedation in these circumstances (follow your protocol).

The procedure for cardioversion is shown in **SKILL DRILL 18-3**. Ensure the patient is supine; be prepared for the possibility that the patient could go into cardiac arrest.

Skill Drill 18-3 Performing Synchronized Cardioversion

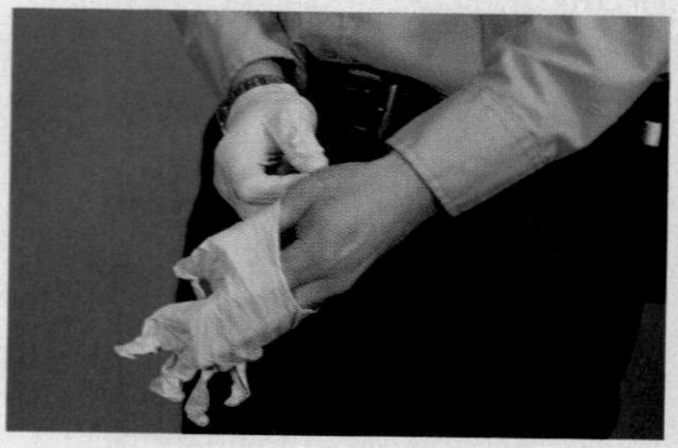

Step 1

Select, check, and assemble all necessary equipment, including a monitor-defibrillator with defibrillation pads, ECG electrodes, medication for pain or sedation (to be used if necessary), oxygen, and an appropriate oxygen administration device. Take standard precautions. Assess the patient's vital signs. Ensure the patient is oxygenated adequately and establish a patent IV line.

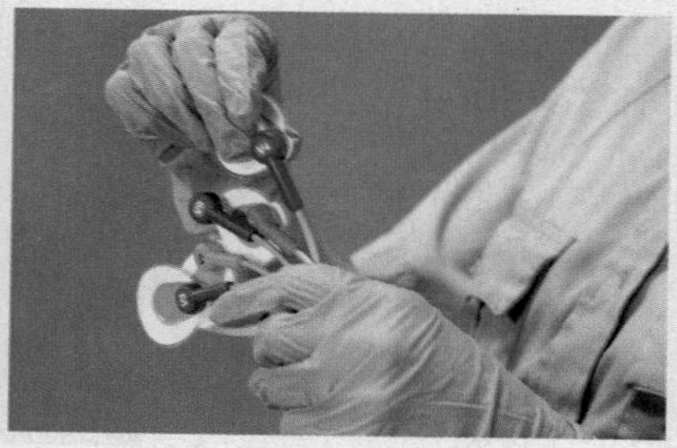

Step 2

Place the ECG electrodes in the same position as you would when performing cardiac monitoring. Obtain a baseline rhythm strip. Identify the rhythm and confirm that cardioversion is warranted. If the patient is responsive, consider the appropriate medication to sedate the patient. Ask about medication allergies before administering sedation.

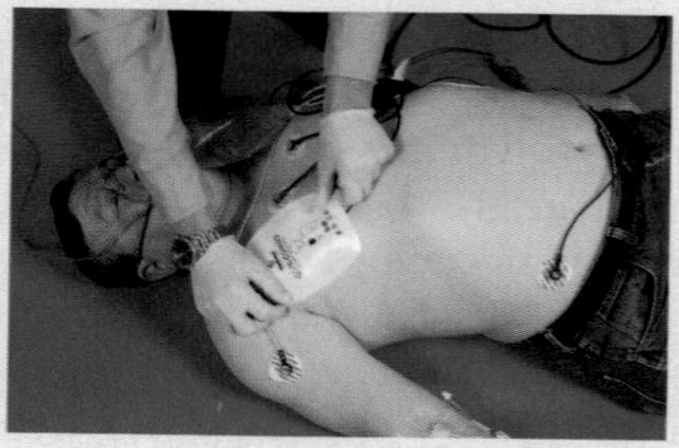

Step 3

Ensure the environment is safe (evaluate risks such as sparks, combustibles, and an oxygen-rich atmosphere). Explain to the patient and the family the need for the procedure. Apply the defibrillation pads to the patient according to the manufacturer's recommendations. Turn on the power to the defibrillator.

Skill Drill 18-3 Performing Synchronized Cardioversion (continued)

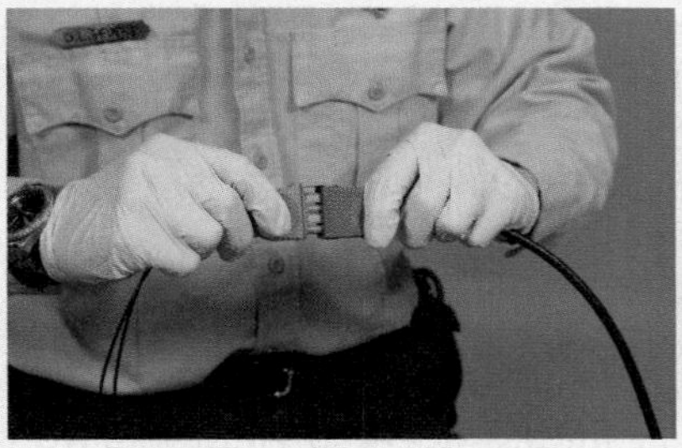

Step 4

Connect the pads to the monitor.

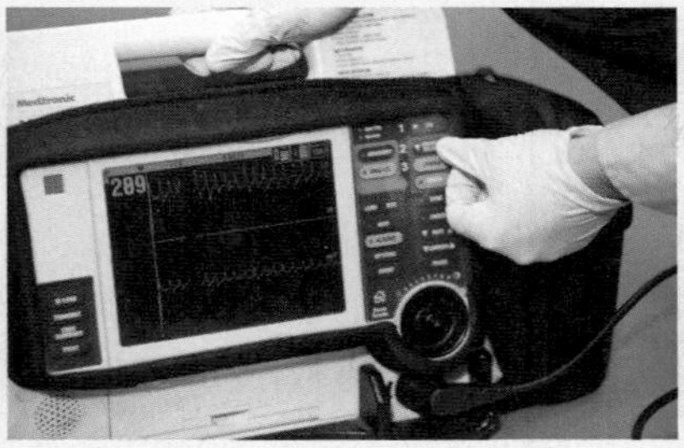

Step 5

Select the appropriate energy setting. Turn the synchronize control on the machine to the on position.

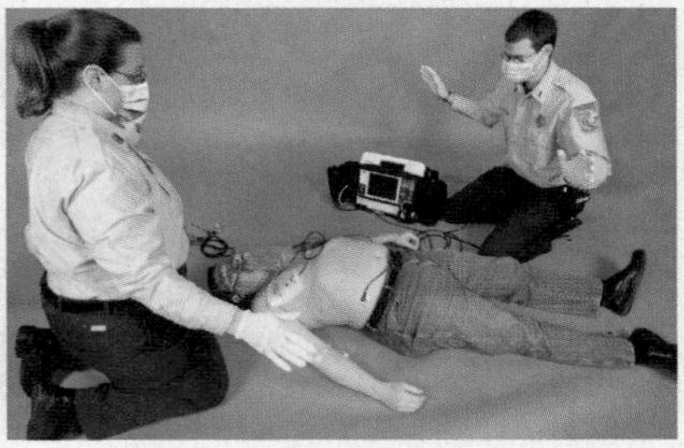

Step 6

Observe the ECG rhythm. Confirm that a sense marker appears near the middle of each QRS complex. If the sense markers are not visible or appear in the wrong location (eg, on the T wave), adjust the ECG size or select another lead until the machine reads the QRS complexes appropriately. Clear the area by announcing, "All clear!" and ensure everyone is clear of the patient.

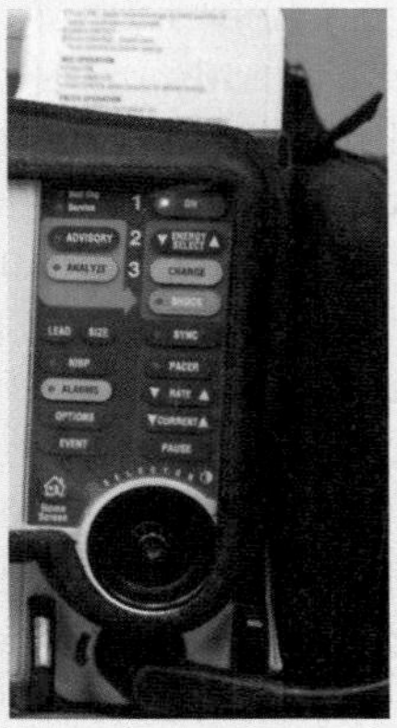

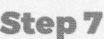

Step 7

Depress the *Shock* button. Keep it depressed until the defibrillator discharges.

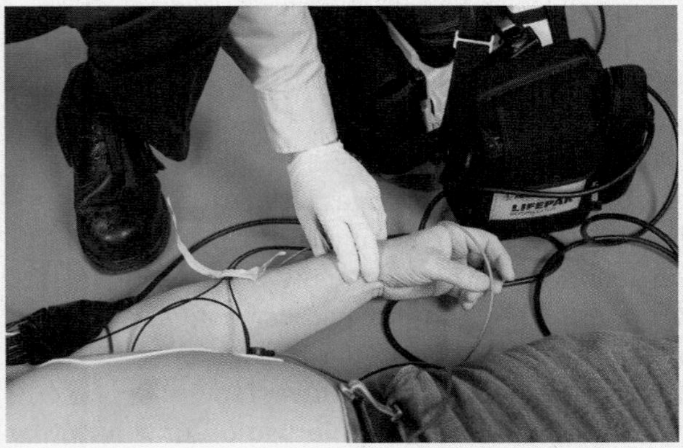

Step 8

Reassess the ECG rhythm and the patient (pulse and BP). If the tachycardia persists, ensure the machine is in sync mode before delivering another shock. If the rhythm changes to VF, ensure the patient has no pulse. If no pulse is present, ensure the sync control is off and proceed with defibrillation.

> **Documentation and Communication**
>
> Key documentation elements for the adult patient with a tachycardia and a pulse are as follows:[10]
>
> - Initial rhythm and all rhythm changes
> - Time, dose, and patient response to medications given
> - Cardioversion times, number of attempts, energy settings, and patient response
> - Monitor strips obtained before and after each intervention and at the time of transfer of patient care
> - History of an event supporting the treatment of underlying causes

Preexcitation

Preexcitation refers to the early depolarization of ventricular tissue through an accessory pathway between the atria and ventricles; an accessory pathway is an extra bundle of myocardial tissue that forms a connection between the atria and ventricles outside the normal conduction system. Patients with preexcitation syndromes are susceptible to tachydysrhythmias. A reentry SVT involving the AV node and an accessory pathway is called *AV reentrant tachycardia* (*AVRT*).

The most common preexcitation disorder is **Wolff-Parkinson-White (WPW) syndrome**. WPW syndrome is characterized by a short PRI (duration of less than 0.12 second [120 milliseconds]), nonspecific ST-T wave changes, a widened QRS complex, and the appearance of a *delta wave* on ECG. The delta wave, a slurring of the upstroke of the first part of the QRS complex, indicates an early departure from the PR segment as a result of conduction through the accessory pathway (bundle of Kent) and subsequent early depolarization of ventricular tissue **FIGURE 18-45**.

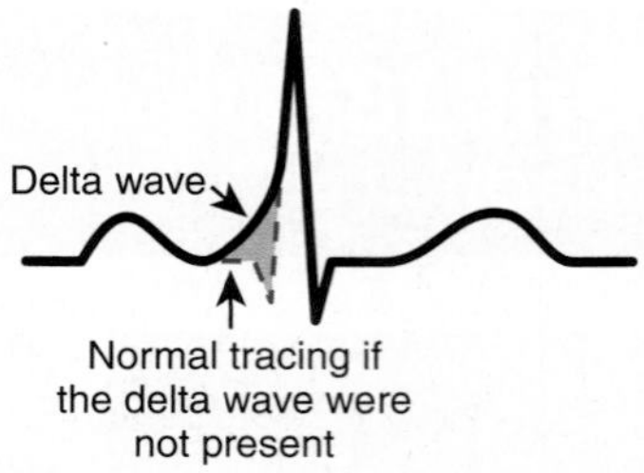

FIGURE 18-45 Delta wave: Wolff-Parkinson-White syndrome.

Reproduced from *12-Lead ECG: The Art of Interpretation*, courtesy of Tomas B. Garcia, MD.

Lown-Ganong-Levine syndrome is another disorder that causes preexcitation of ventricular tissue. The ECG signature of this syndrome is a short PRI and a normal QRS complex duration. Patients with WPW syndrome and those with Lown-Ganong-Levine syndrome are predisposed to tachydysrhythmias.

Seek the advice of a physician when caring for a symptomatic patient with a preexcitation syndrome. If the symptoms are attributable to the rapid ventricular rate, your treatment will depend on the gravity of the patient's instability, the width of the QRS complex, and the regularity of the ventricular rhythm. Do not administer medication that slows or blocks conduction through the AV node (eg, adenosine, calcium channel blockers, beta blockers) because it may accelerate conduction through the accessory pathway, further increasing the heart rate.

Atrial Fibrillation

Atrial fibrillation (AF) is a rhythm in which the atria no longer contract but instead fibrillate or quiver, with no organized contraction **FIGURE 18-46**. This condition occurs when multiple cells in the atria depolarize independently, rather than in response to an SA node impulse. The result of this random depolarization throughout the atria is a fibrillating or chaotic baseline. In AF, there are no clearly identifiable P waves on the ECG strip and, therefore, no PRI to measure. Instead, one of the hallmarks of this condition is its irregularly irregular appearance. Because the AV node is bombarded with impulses from the fibrillating atria, it allows impulses to pass on randomly to the ventricles, which produces a highly irregular ventricular rhythm. The QRS complex typically measures 0.11 second (110 milliseconds) or less.

AF is a common rhythm among older adult patients. One of the main hazards associated with this dysrhythmia is that the blood within the fibrillating atria tends to clot. These clots may become emboli that block circulation elsewhere in the body. Thus, AF increases the risk of stroke. Because of this risk, many older adult patients with AF are prescribed anticoagulant medications such

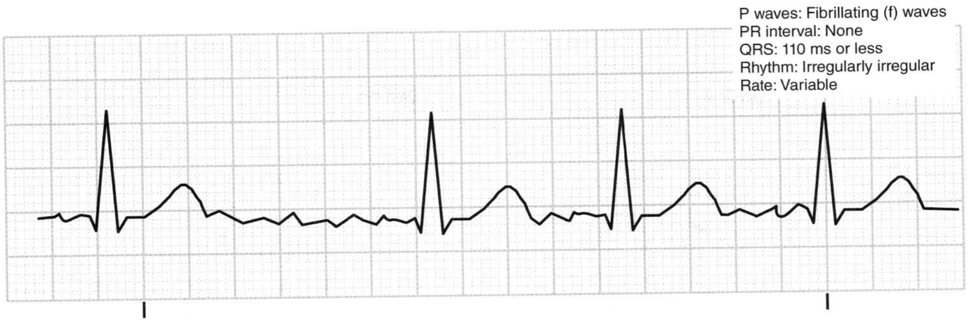

FIGURE 18-46 Atrial fibrillation.

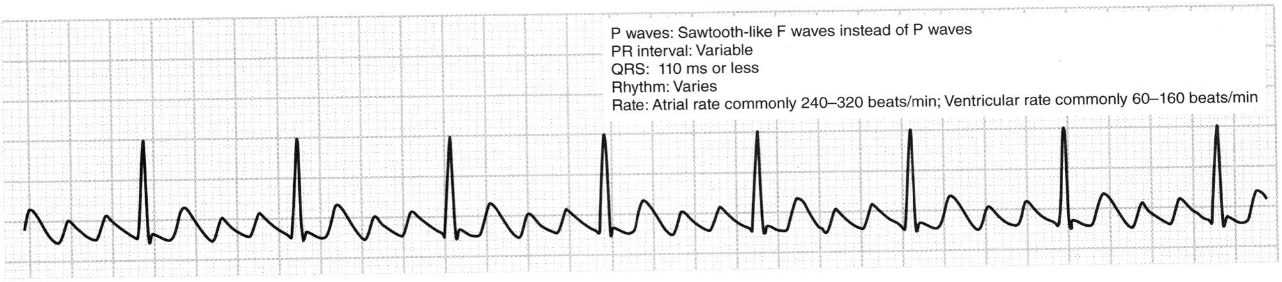

P waves: Sawtooth-like F waves instead of P waves
PR interval: Variable
QRS: 110 ms or less
Rhythm: Varies
Rate: Atrial rate commonly 240–320 beats/min; Ventricular rate commonly 60–160 beats/min

FIGURE 18-47 Atrial flutter (sawtooth flutter waves).

as warfarin (Coumadin). A beta blocker, calcium channel blocker, or digoxin may also be prescribed to regulate the ventricular response rate. AF accompanied by a rapid ventricular response is considered an irregular tachycardia. If the patient is stable but symptomatic, AF with a rapid ventricular response may be treated with a beta blocker or calcium channel blocker. If the patient is unstable, synchronized cardioversion may be necessary, although this is rarely done in the field because of the risk of a thromboembolic event.

Atrial Flutter

Atrial flutter is a rhythm in which an atrial impulse fires at a rate much too rapid for the ventricles to keep up **FIGURE 18-47**. The atrial complexes in atrial flutter are known as *flutter waves* or *F waves* rather than P waves. F waves have a distinctive sawtooth shape resembling a picket fence.

In atrial flutter, one or more of the F waves is blocked by the AV node, generating several flutter waves before each QRS complex. The rhythm is usually regular, with a constant (usually 2:1) conduction. The rhythm can be irregular if the conduction of atrial impulses to the ventricles varies. The QRS complex measures 0.11 second (110 milliseconds) or less.

Hypoxia, pneumonia, chronic lung disease, endocrine disorders, ischemic heart disease, valvular heart disease, and other conditions are associated with atrial flutter, which can degenerate into AF. It is common for atrial flutter and AF to coexist in the same patient.[12] Patients with atrial flutter are often prescribed anticoagulant medications because they are thought to have the same risk of thromboembolism as patients with AF.[12]

Like AF, atrial flutter accompanied by a rapid ventricular response is considered an irregular tachycardia. A beta blocker or calcium channel blocker may be administered if the patient is stable but symptomatic, although prehospital treatment of atrial flutter is uncommon in stable patients. Synchronized cardioversion may be necessary if the patient is unstable and generally requires less energy than that used for AF.[11]

Wandering Atrial Pacemaker

As the name suggests, in wandering atrial pacemaker, the heart's pacemaker site moves from the SA node to various areas within the atria or AV junction

FIGURE 18-48. This dysrhythmia usually has a rate of 60 to 100 beats/min. The rhythm is slightly irregular, with R-R intervals that vary depending on the site of the pacemaker for that particular complex. A P wave precedes each QRS complex; however, its shape varies, indicating multiple sites of origin. The definition of wandering atrial pacemaker requires at least three different P-wave shapes within one ECG strip. The PRI measures 0.12 to 0.20 second (120 to 200 milliseconds) and varies slightly based on the origin of a given complex. The QRS complex measures 0.11 second (110 milliseconds) or less.

Wandering atrial pacemaker is most often seen in children and athletes, presumably because of increased vagal tone. Treatment is usually not indicated in the prehospital setting unless the dysrhythmia is associated with a slow rate and the patient is symptomatic. Under those circumstances, treatment is the same as for symptomatic sinus bradycardia.

Multifocal Atrial Tachycardia

In multifocal atrial tachycardia (MAT), multiple ectopic sites within the atria depolarize at different but rapid rates FIGURE 18-49. MAT is characterized by a rate of more than 100 beats/min and is, in effect, a tachycardic wandering atrial pacemaker. The rhythm is irregular, with R-R intervals that vary depending on the site of the pacemaker for that particular complex. A P wave precedes each QRS complex; however, its shape varies, indicating multiple sites of origin. The PRI measures 0.12 to 0.20 second (120 to 200 milliseconds) and varies slightly based on the origin of a given complex. If the MAT increases to a rate exceeding 150 beats/min, then the P wave may no longer be visible; thus, the only indication of the rhythm may be the irregularity associated with the varying sites of origin within the atria. The QRS complex measures 0.11 second (110 milliseconds) or less.

MAT is most often seen in patients with significant lung disease, pulmonary hypertension, coronary disease, valvular heart disease, or hypomagnesemia, and in patients undergoing theophylline therapy.[12] Because therapies aimed at correcting SVT are usually ineffective with MAT, treatment is usually deferred until arrival at the emergency department (ED).

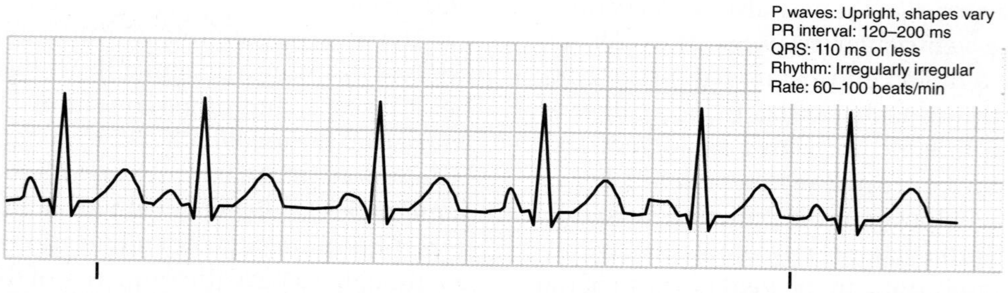

FIGURE 18-48 Wandering atrial pacemaker.

Reproduced from *Arrhythmia Recognition: The Art of Interpretation*, courtesy of Tomas B. Garcia, MD.

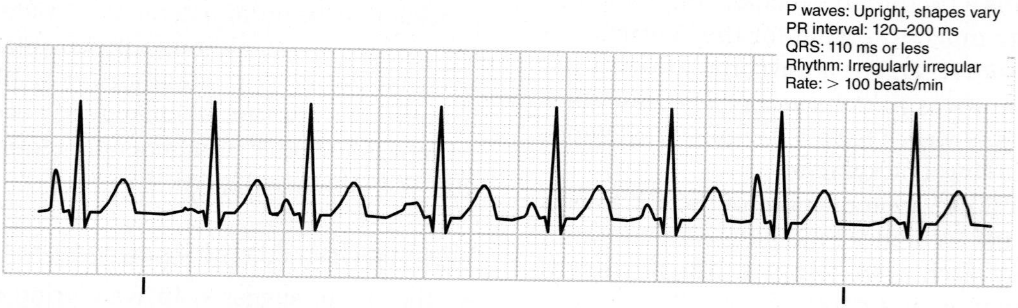

FIGURE 18-49 Multifocal atrial tachycardia.

Reproduced from *Arrhythmia Recognition: The Art of Interpretation*, courtesy of Tomas B. Garcia, MD.

Rhythms Originating at the AV Junction

If the SA node, the body's dominant pacemaker, fails to initiate an impulse, then the AV junction should take over as the heart's pacemaker. Because the AV junction is a secondary pacemaker, its intrinsic rate is slower than that of the SA node. As a result, junctional rhythms normally have a rate of 40 to 60 beats/min.

When an impulse is generated in the AV junction, it travels down through the conduction system into the ventricles as if it had come from the SA node, resulting in normal QRS complexes. The impulse also travels upward through the atria and the internodal pathways toward the SA node. Three possible circumstances, none associated with an upright P wave, exist in which the QRS complex appears normal:

- If the impulse begins moving upward through the atria before the other part of it enters the ventricles, an inverted P wave will be visible. (It is upside down because the impulse is traveling in the direction opposite of that which generates normal, upright P waves.) This P wave is usually followed immediately by a QRS complex.
- If the impulse moves through the atria at the same time as it travels through the ventricles, an inverted P wave will be buried within the QRS complex. As a result, the P wave will appear to be missing; that is, the baseline will remain flat until the next QRS complex begins.
- The impulse may begin late through the atria, resulting in an inverted P wave that appears after the QRS complex.

Premature Junctional Complex

A premature junctional complex (PJC) is not, strictly speaking, a dysrhythmia (just as PAC is not), but rather an early complex that appears within another rhythm **FIGURE 18-50**. PJCs are also known as *ectopic complexes*, meaning they arise from a site other than the SA node.

The rate depends on the underlying rhythm. Because a PJC is, by definition, an early beat, the underlying rhythm is irregular. If present, the P wave will be inverted and may either precede or follow the QRS complex. The PRI, if present, will measure less than 0.12 second (120 milliseconds). The QRS complex measures 0.11 second (110 milliseconds) or less.

PJCs can be caused by many of the same factors that cause PACs. PJCs do not normally require treatment since most people with the condition are asymptomatic. Some people with PJCs, however, may perceive skipped beats. Light-headedness, dizziness, and other signs of decreased CO can occur if PJCs occur frequently. Frequent PJCs may be a predictor of future cardiac dysrhythmias.

Junctional Escape Rhythm

A **junctional escape rhythm**, also called a *junctional rhythm*, can occur when the SA node ceases functioning and the AV junction takes over as the heart's pacemaker at a rate of 40 to 60 beats/min **FIGURE 18-51**. The ventricular rhythm is usually regular. The P wave may be absent or inverted before or after the QRS complex. If an inverted P wave is present before the QRS complex, the PRI will measure less than 0.12 second (120 milliseconds). The QRS complex measures 0.11 second (110 milliseconds) or less.

A junctional rhythm often accompanies SA node disease, increased vagal tone, valvular heart disease, inferior wall MI, and some other cardiac conditions, or it can occur after resuscitation from cardiac arrest. Because of the slow rate, treatment of symptomatic patients depends on the underlying cause and may require a surgically implanted

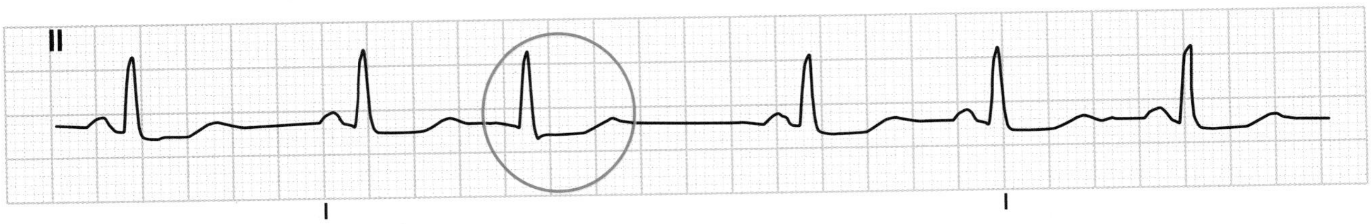

FIGURE 18-50 Sinus rhythm with a premature junctional complex.

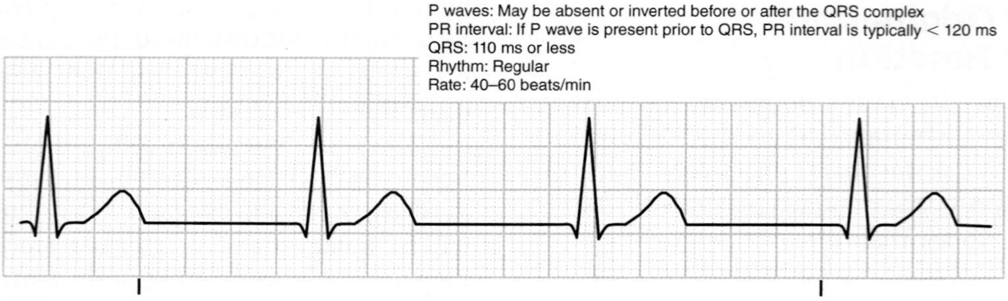

P waves: May be absent or inverted before or after the QRS complex
PR interval: If P wave is present prior to QRS, PR interval is typically < 120 ms
QRS: 110 ms or less
Rhythm: Regular
Rate: 40–60 beats/min

FIGURE 18-51 Junctional escape rhythm.

Reproduced from *Arrhythmia Recognition: The Art of Interpretation*, courtesy of Tomas B. Garcia, MD.

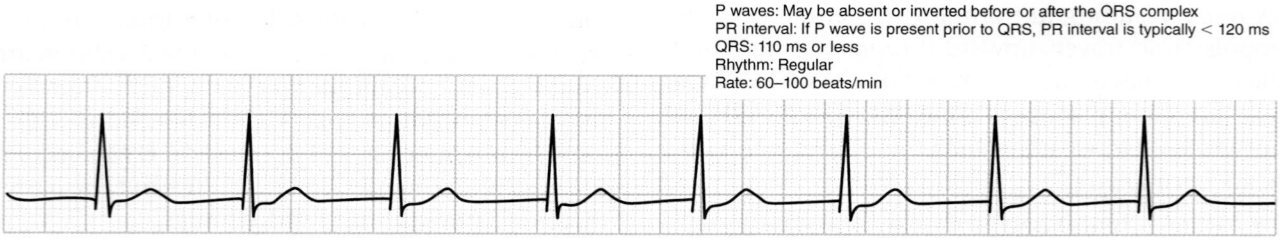

P waves: May be absent or inverted before or after the QRS complex
PR interval: If P wave is present prior to QRS, PR interval is typically < 120 ms
QRS: 110 ms or less
Rhythm: Regular
Rate: 60–100 beats/min

FIGURE 18-52 Accelerated junctional rhythm.

Reproduced from *Arrhythmia Recognition: The Art of Interpretation*, courtesy of Tomas B. Garcia, MD.

pacemaker. In the field, atropine should be considered, and TCP may be necessary if the patient's condition is severely compromised (see Figure 18-35).

Accelerated Junctional Rhythm

Occasionally, a junctional rhythm is accompanied by a heart rate that exceeds the normal upper rate of 60 beats/min but remains less than 100 beats/min. Such a rhythm is called an *accelerated junctional rhythm.* The ventricular rhythm is regular **FIGURE 18-52**. The P wave may be absent or, if present, may be inverted before or after the QRS complex. If an inverted P wave is present before the QRS complex, the PRI measures less than 0.12 second (120 milliseconds). The QRS complex measures 0.11 second (110 milliseconds) or less.

Accelerated junctional rhythms may be associated with digoxin toxicity (the most common cause), hypoxia, inferior wall MI, **rheumatic fever**, recent cardiac surgery, or an electrolyte imbalance, such as hypokalemia. Because the rate is fast enough to maintain a reasonable CO, the patient usually is asymptomatic. Nevertheless, patients with accelerated junctional rhythms should be monitored closely.

Junctional Tachycardia

Occasionally, a junctional rhythm is accompanied by a rate that exceeds 100 beats/min. Such a rhythm is termed *junctional tachycardia.* Its ECG characteristics are the same as those of an accelerated junctional rhythm, but the rate is faster than 100 beats/min **FIGURE 18-53**.

Junctional tachycardia is uncommon in adults but may be associated with ACS, heart failure, theophylline administration, or digoxin toxicity. Because the rate is fast enough to maintain a reasonable CO, it seldom requires treatment in the prehospital setting. However, if the rate exceeds 150 beats/min, CO could suffer. At a rapid ventricular rate, distinguishing junctional tachycardia from other regular narrow-QRS tachycardias is often difficult. Such a rhythm is referred to as *SVT.* If the patient is symptomatic, treatments should follow the tachycardia algorithm (see Figure 18-42).

Rhythms Originating in the Ventricles

If the SA node fails to initiate an impulse, the AV junction usually takes over as the heart's pacemaker. If the AV junction cannot perform this duty, then

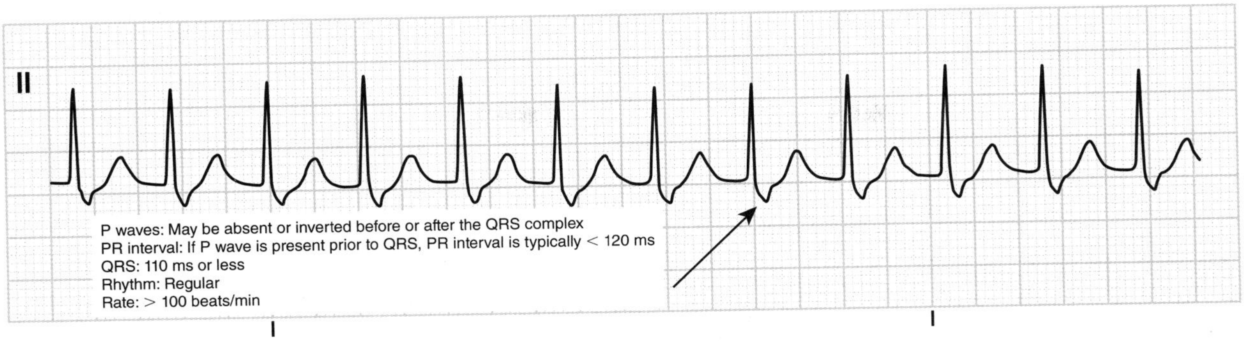

FIGURE 18-53 Junctional tachycardia. The blue arrow points to an inverted P wave after the QRS complex.

Reproduced from *Arrhythmia Recognition: The Art of Interpretation*, courtesy of Tomas B. Garcia, MD.

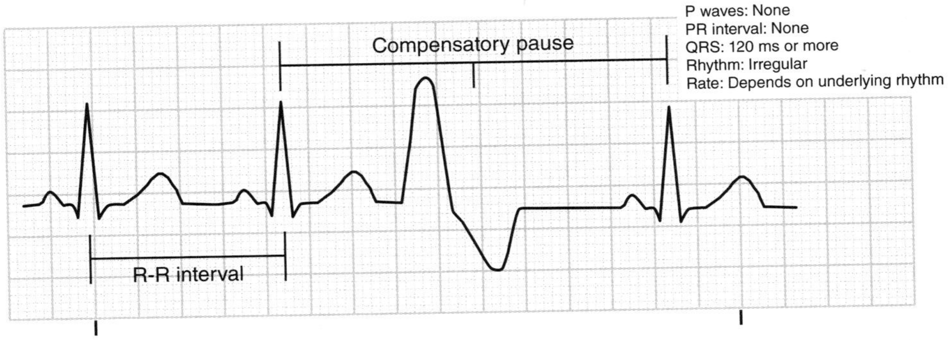

FIGURE 18-54 Sinus rhythm with a premature ventricular complex (PVC). A full compensatory pause usually follows a PVC. A pause is compensatory if the R-R interval that includes the PVC measures twice that of the underlying rhythm.

Modified from *Arrhythmia Recognition: The Art of Interpretation*, courtesy of Tomas B. Garcia, MD.

the ventricles may assume pacemaking responsibility. A missing P wave and wide QRS complex (0.12 second [120 milliseconds] or more in duration) are characteristic features of such ventricular beats or rhythms.

Premature Ventricular Complex

A premature ventricular complex (PVC) is not, strictly speaking, a dysrhythmia (just as premature atrial and junctional complexes are not), but rather an early complex that appears within another rhythm **FIGURE 18-54**. PVCs are considered ectopic complexes because they originate from a site other than the SA node. A PVC occurs earlier than the next expected sinus complex, producing an irregular ventricular rhythm. Because there is no P wave associated with the PVC, there is also no PRI. The QRS complex associated with the PVC measures 0.12 second (120 milliseconds) or more. The T wave is usually opposite in the direction of the QRS.

A full compensatory pause usually follows a PVC. A compensatory pause allows time to restore the underlying rhythm; that is, the pause compensates for the PVC. To determine if such a pause is present, measure an R-R interval of the underlying rhythm. Next, measure from the R wave of the QRS complex before the PVC to the R wave of the QRS complex after the PVC. A full compensatory pause has occurred if the R-R interval that includes the PVC measures twice that of the underlying rhythm.

PVCs may be further distinguished as unifocal or multifocal. **Unifocal** PVCs originate from the same area or "focus" within the ventricle and look alike on the ECG **FIGURE 18-55**. PVCs with a varied appearance are **multifocal**, meaning that more than one site is generating the ventricular impulses **FIGURE 18-56**.

Sometimes two consecutive PVCs occur, with no intervening pause. These paired PVCs constitute a ventricular **couplet** **FIGURE 18-57**. The occurrence of three or more PVCs in a row is called a "run" of VT;

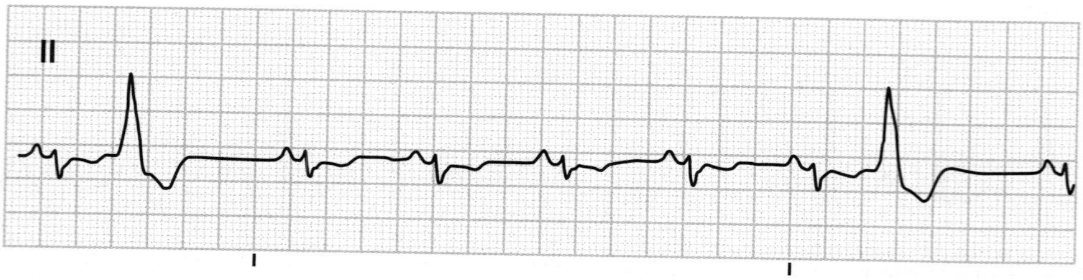

FIGURE 18-55 Unifocal premature ventricular complexes.

Reproduced from *Arrhythmia Recognition: The Art of Interpretation*, courtesy of Tomas B. Garcia, MD.

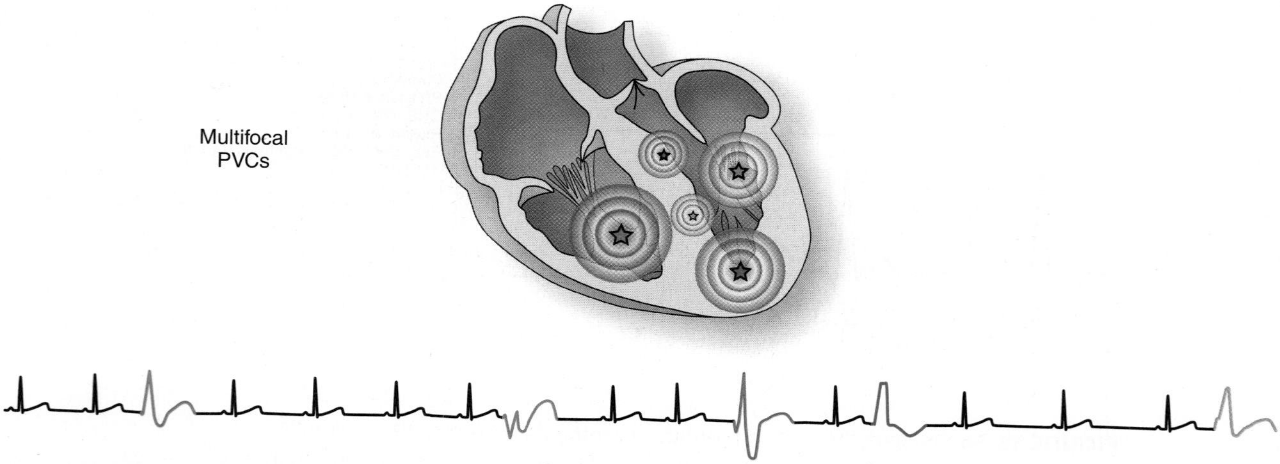

FIGURE 18-56 Multifocal premature ventricular complexes (PVCs).

Reproduced from *Arrhythmia Recognition: The Art of Interpretation*, courtesy of Tomas B. Garcia, MD.

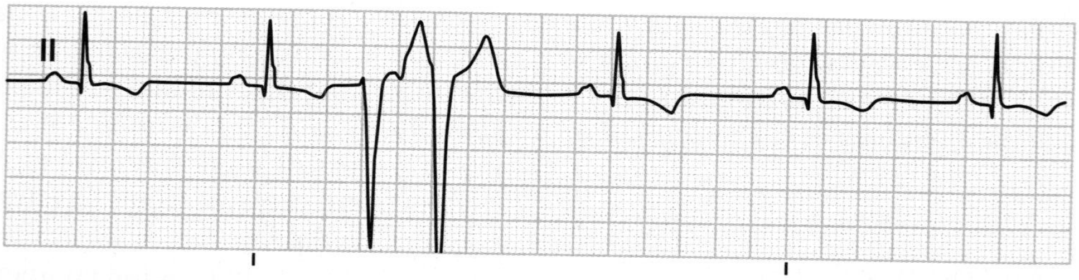

FIGURE 18-57 Ventricular couplet (paired premature ventricular complexes).

Reproduced from *Arrhythmia Recognition: The Art of Interpretation*, courtesy of Tomas B. Garcia, MD.

these surges are also referred to as *salvos* or *bursts*. Occasionally, the complexes become so frequent that they begin to alternate with normal complexes, generating a *normal–PVC–normal–PVC* pattern, called ventricular **bigeminy** **FIGURE 18-58**. If every third beat is a PVC (*normal–normal–PVC*), then the pattern is called ventricular **trigeminy**.

PVCs can arise in many of the same circumstances associated with premature atrial and junctional complexes, but they most often originate from ischemia in the ventricular tissue. These complexes are generally considered more serious than premature atrial or junctional complexes. Notably, multifocal PVCs, couplets, and ventricular bigeminy are considered more serious rhythm disturbances than unifocal PVCs.

When an R wave of a PVC occurs during the T wave of the preceding complex, the event is called an R-on-T PVC. Although this type of PVC is uncommon, it can lead to VT or VF because the ventricles

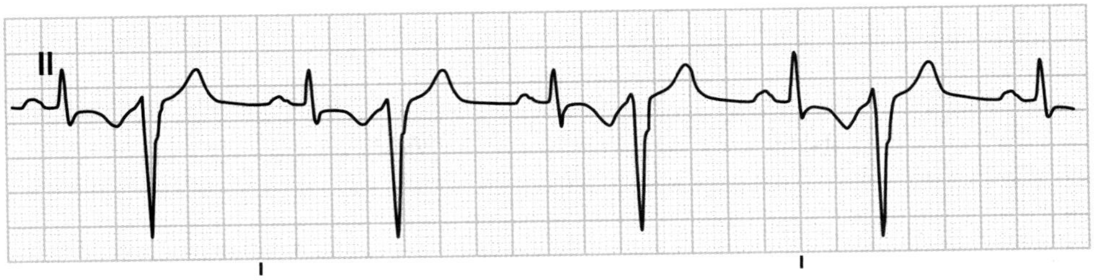

FIGURE 18-58 Ventricular bigeminy.

Reproduced from *Arrhythmia Recognition: The Art of Interpretation*, courtesy of Tomas B. Garcia, MD.

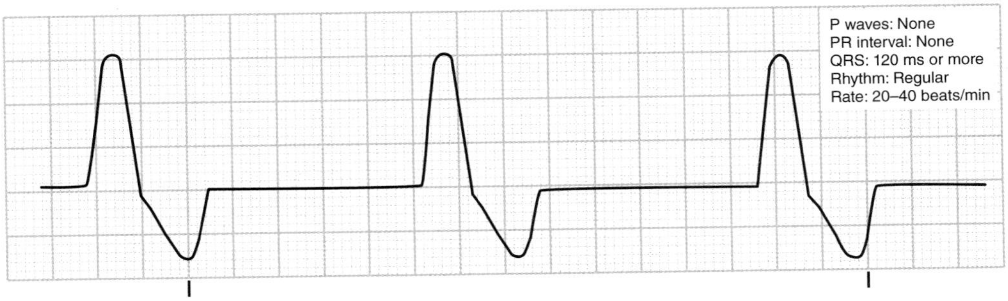

FIGURE 18-59 Idioventricular rhythm.

Reproduced from *Arrhythmia Recognition: The Art of Interpretation*, courtesy of Tomas B. Garcia, MD.

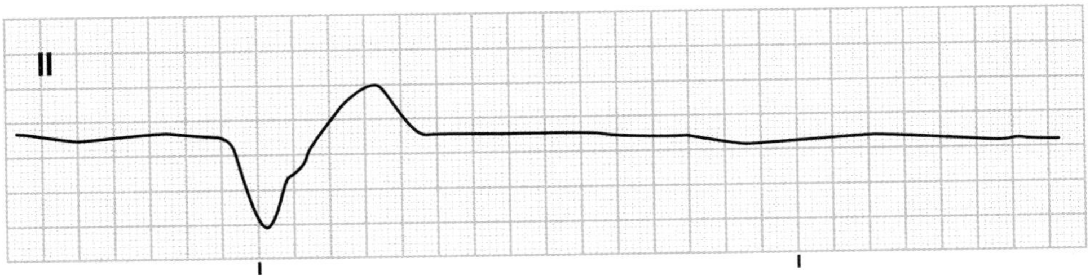

FIGURE 18-60 Agonal rhythm.

Reproduced from *Arrhythmia Recognition: The Art of Interpretation*, courtesy of Tomas B. Garcia, MD.

are stimulated before they have fully repolarized (ie, during the RRP).

Occasional PVCs are common and usually do not require treatment in otherwise healthy patients. PVCs that occur in patients with heart disease require close monitoring and a search for the underlying cause.

Idioventricular Rhythm

The term **idioventricular** means "only the ventricles" or "produced by the ventricles." An idioventricular rhythm (IVR), then, is one that occurs when the SA and AV nodes fail and the ventricles assume responsibility for pacing the heart **FIGURE 18-59**. An IVR is usually regular, with little variation between R-R intervals. P waves are absent owing to the failure of the SA and AV nodes. Because there is no P wave, there is also no PRI. The QRS complex will measure 0.12 second (120 milliseconds) or more because it originates in the ventricles. An IVR has a rate of 20 to 40 beats/min, which is the ventricles' intrinsic rate. When the ventricular rate slows to less than 20 beats/min, the pattern is called an **agonal rhythm** **FIGURE 18-60**. **Agonal** means "pertaining to the period of dying."

Because of the slow rate, the patient with an IVR is often symptomatic. IVRs may or may not be accompanied by a palpable pulse. Treatment is geared toward improving CO by increasing the rate and, if possible, treating the underlying cause, such as myocardial ischemia or electrolyte imbalances. If

IVR is associated with a pulse, then treat the rhythm using the bradycardia algorithm (see Figure 18-35). If there is no pulse associated with IVR, then the patient is in cardiac arrest. Treatment for cardiac arrest is discussed later in this chapter.

Accelerated IVR

Occasionally, an IVR exceeds the normal upper limit of 40 beats/min but remains less than 100 beats/min. Because the rate is faster than the ventricles' intrinsic rate but less than 100 beats/min, it is called *accelerated idioventricular rhythm* (*AIVR*).

AIVR usually begins and ends gradually and is regular, with little variation between R-R intervals. The P waves are absent, so there is no PRI **FIGURE 18-61**. The QRS complex measures 0.12 second (120 milliseconds) or more.

AIVR may be observed in patients with digitalis toxicity, electrolyte imbalances, cardiomyopathies, or heart disease, such as patients with AMI; after reperfusion therapy; or during resuscitation efforts. It is usually a transient rhythm, resolving when the sinus rate exceeds that of the ventricular rate. It rarely requires intervention because the rate is well tolerated.

Ventricular Tachycardia

VT is a series of three or more sequential ventricular beats at a rate exceeding 100 beats/min. VT is usually regular, but there may be a slight variation between R-R intervals. The P waves are absent, so the PRI is also absent. Because the QRS complex in VT measures 0.12 second (120 milliseconds) or more, VT is considered a wide-QRS tachycardia. When this dysrhythmia presents with QRS complexes that appear uniform, it is referred to as *monomorphic VT* because the QRS complex's shape remains constant **FIGURE 18-62**. Occasionally, VT presents with irregular QRS complexes of varied height and width in an alternating pattern, in which case it is called

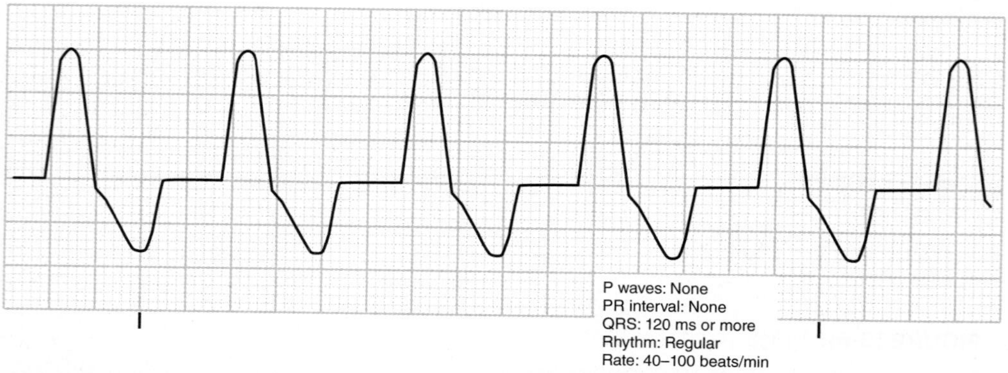

FIGURE 18-61 Accelerated idioventricular rhythm.

Reproduced from *Arrhythmia Recognition: The Art of Interpretation*, courtesy of Tomas B. Garcia, MD.

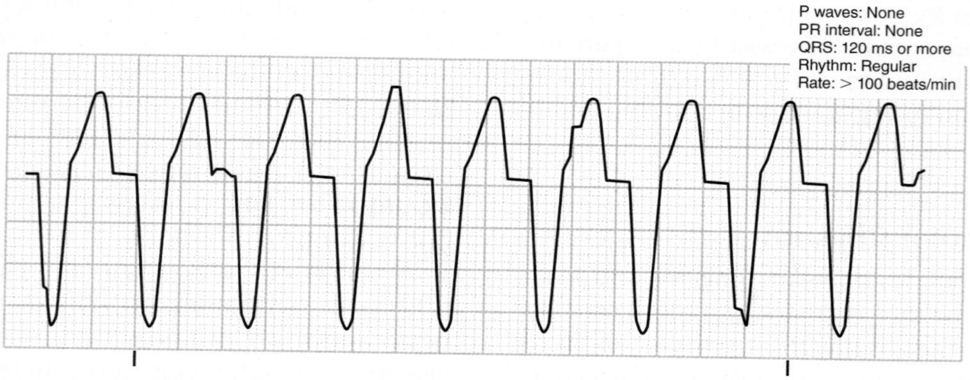

FIGURE 18-62 Monomorphic ventricular tachycardia.

Reproduced from *Arrhythmia Recognition: The Art of Interpretation*, courtesy of Tomas B. Garcia, MD.

polymorphic VT **FIGURE 18-63**. Polymorphic VT is a wide, irregular tachycardia.

Polymorphic VT with a prolonged QT interval is called *torsades de pointes.* A prolonged QT interval may be congenital or acquired (ie, medication induced). Examples of medications that prolong the QT interval include amiodarone (Cordarone), quinidine (Quinidex, Quinora), procainamide (Pronestyl), sotalol (Betapace), phenothiazines, and tricyclic antidepressants. Polymorphic VT may convert spontaneously to a normal rhythm, or it may degenerate into VF. Long-QT syndrome is discussed in more detail later in this chapter.

Because the rate is usually too fast to maintain adequate CO, VT is extremely serious and requires treatment. The reduced CO associated with this condition can lead to ventricular failure or fibrillation if not addressed promptly. If the patient is symptomatic but hemodynamically stable, emergency care should focus on treatment with antidysrhythmic medications (see Figure 18-42). If the patient is unstable and the cardiac monitor shows monomorphic VT, electrical therapy using synchronized cardioversion may be necessary. If the patient is unstable and the cardiac monitor shows polymorphic VT, defibrillation should be performed because the machine cannot synchronize QRS complexes of varying amplitude. If the cardiac monitor shows VT but the patient is pulseless, the patient is in cardiac arrest. Pulseless VT is treated the same as VF.

Ventricular Fibrillation

VF occurs when many different cells within the ventricles depolarize independently, rather than in response to an SA node impulse. As a result, the ventricles no longer contract, but rather fibrillate or quiver in no discernible pattern. Indeed, if you were to look at a fibrillating heart, you would see movement resembling that of a bag of energetic worms. The result of this random depolarization is a fibrillating or chaotic baseline with no evidence of organized electrical activity: no P waves, no PRI, no QRS complexes. When fibrillatory waves are greater than 3 mm in amplitude, the dysrhythmia is sometimes referred to as "coarse" VF **FIGURE 18-64**. When the fibrillatory waves are less than 3 mm in amplitude, the dysrhythmia is sometimes called "fine" VF **FIGURE 18-65**.

Defibrillation

VF and pulseless VT are shockable cardiac arrest rhythms, which means they are likely to respond to defibrillation. Defibrillation is the process by which a surge of unsynchronized direct current electrical energy is delivered to the heart to terminate VF. The goal of defibrillation is to administer a current powerful enough to depolarize all of the heart's

> **Words of Wisdom**
>
> Verapamil, a calcium channel blocker, may be used to control the rate of a tachydysrhythmia. This medication slows electrical impulse conduction through the AV node, protecting the ventricles from atrial tachydysrhythmias and slowing the overall heart rate. Wide QRS complexes on the ECG may indicate a bundle branch block, a ventricular dysrhythmia, or preexcitation. Administering verapamil to a patient with preexcitation can lead to VF or VT and sudden death. Therefore, this agent must be reserved for patients exhibiting narrow–QRS complex tachydysrhythmias and should never be given in wide-complex tachycardias.

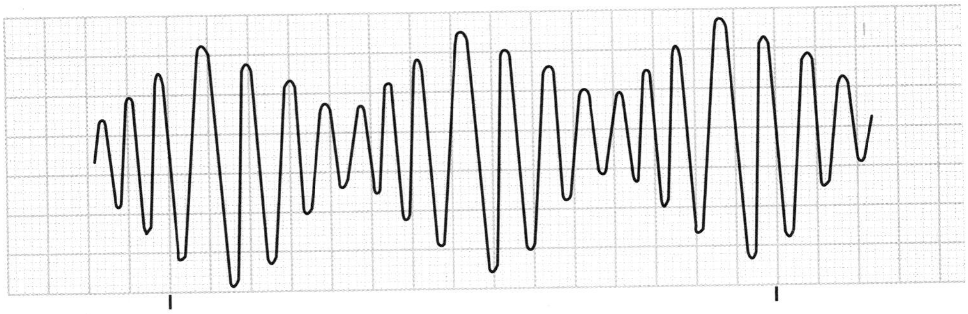

FIGURE 18-63 Polymorphic ventricular tachycardia.

Reproduced from *Arrhythmia Recognition: The Art of Interpretation*, courtesy of Tomas B. Garcia, MD.

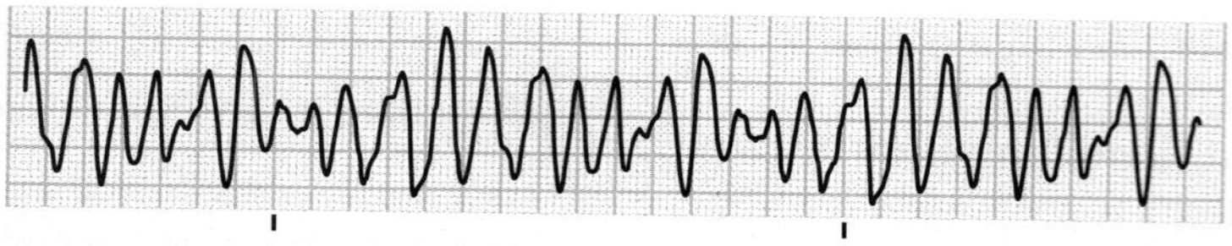

FIGURE 18-64 Coarse ventricular fibrillation.

Reproduced from *Arrhythmia Recognition: The Art of Interpretation*, courtesy of Tomas B. Garcia, MD.

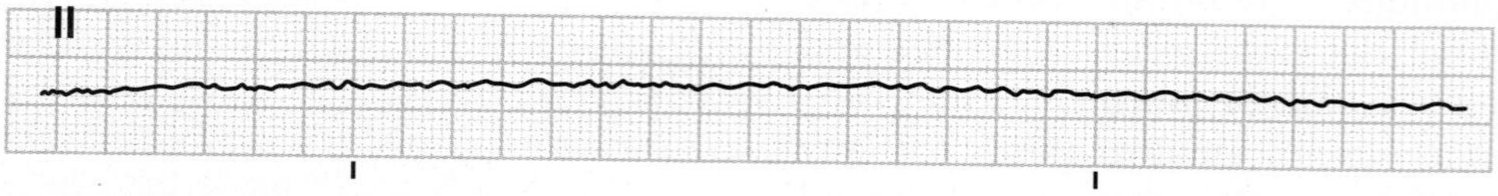

FIGURE 18-65 Fine ventricular fibrillation.

Reproduced from *Arrhythmia Recognition: The Art of Interpretation*, courtesy of Tomas B. Garcia, MD.

component muscle cells; ideally, when those cells repolarize after the shock, they will respond to an impulse from the SA node and resume organized depolarization, leading to cardiac contraction. Defibrillation is also called *unsynchronized countershock* or *asynchronous countershock* because, unlike in synchronized cardioversion, the timing of delivery of the current bears no relation to the cardiac cycle. When a shockable rhythm is identified, defibrillation must be carried out as soon as possible because the likelihood of its success declines rapidly.

An **automated external defibrillator (AED)** interprets the cardiac rhythm, determines whether defibrillation is needed, and guides the user through the resuscitation with audible prompts. A fully automated AED delivers a shock automatically if defibrillation is necessary. A **manual defibrillator** is a device that requires you, as a trained user, to interpret the cardiac rhythm and determine whether defibrillation is needed. Some defibrillators can perform defibrillation either manually or automatically, at the user's discretion. Regardless of which type of defibrillator you use, you must ensure high-quality CPR is ongoing while the defibrillator is readied for use. If you witness a patient's cardiac arrest, begin CPR starting with chest compressions, and attach the defibrillator as soon as it is available. For adults with an unmonitored cardiac arrest or in situations where a defibrillator is not readily available, start CPR while the machine is retrieved and then perform defibrillation, if indicated, as soon as the device is ready for use.

Adhesive pads are placed on the patient's chest wall to maximize the flow of current through the heart. They are placed on the patient's bare chest and connected to the defibrillator, enabling you to quickly assess the patient's cardiac rhythm and deliver an electrical shock, if indicated. It is crucial to follow the manufacturer's recommended placement on the chest. From here on, we will use the term *defibrillation pads* to refer to the adhesive pads used for defibrillation.

Special Populations

Remember to immediately note the patient's age. Use pediatric defibrillation pads when appropriate.

AEDs and manual defibrillators deliver energy in waveforms. Monophasic waveforms, used in older defibrillators, deliver energy through the heart from one defibrillation pad to the other in a single direction. With biphasic waveforms, energy travels through the heart from one defibrillation pad to the other and then reverses direction, flowing back through the heart from one pad to the other. Defibrillators equipped with biphasic waveforms are preferred over monophasic defibrillators because of their greater success in terminating dysrhythmias.[11] It is essential that you know the manufacturer's recommended energy levels for the type of defibrillator you are using **FIGURE 18-66**.

The same safety measures are used when performing manual defibrillation and when using an AED:

- Ensure no one is touching the patient.
- Do not defibrillate a patient who is lying in pooled water; doing so would be dangerous to

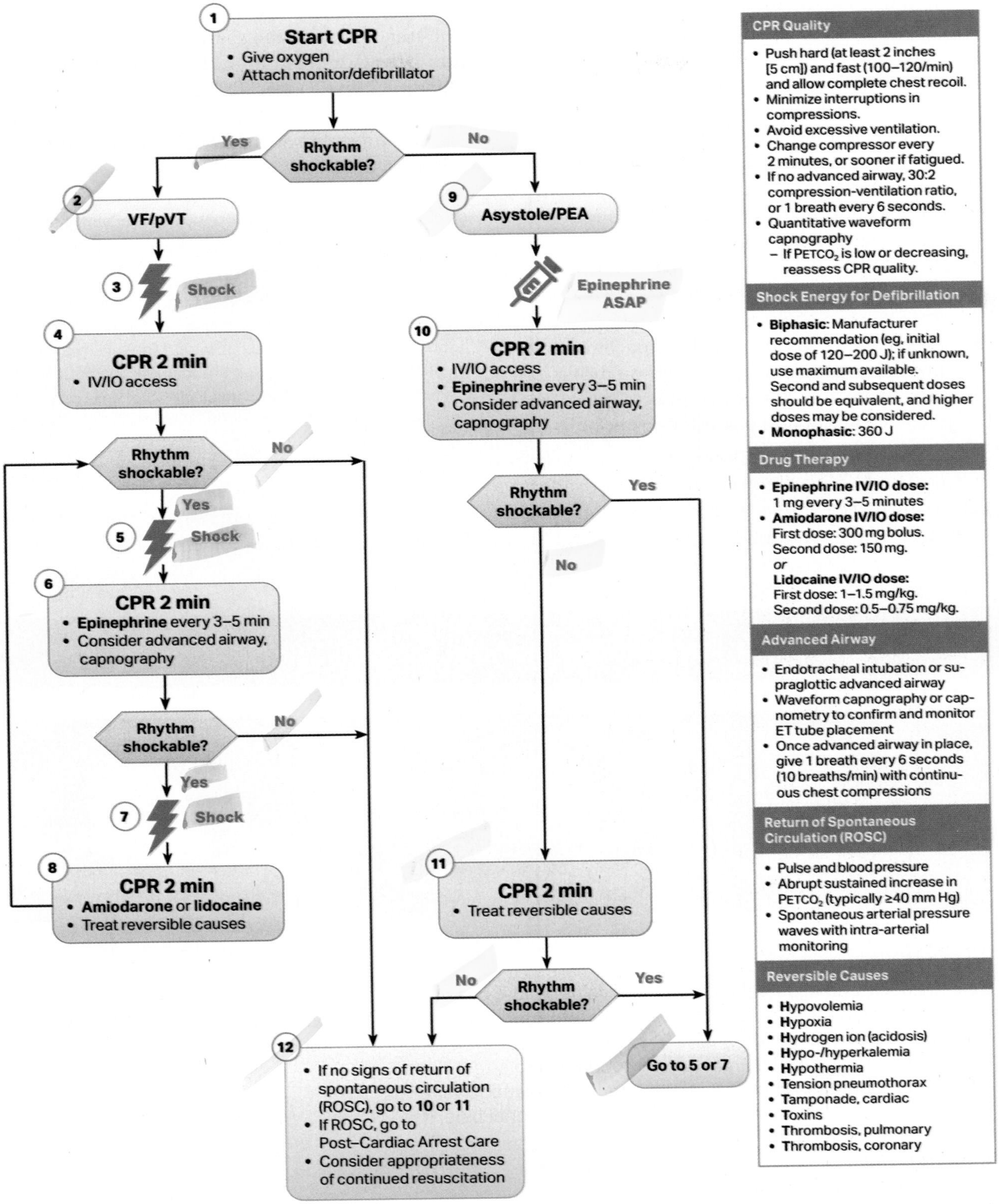

FIGURE 18-66 Adult cardiac arrest algorithm.

Abbreviations: ASAP, as soon as possible; CPR, cardiopulmonary resuscitation; ET, endotracheal; IO, intraosseous; IV, intravenous; PEA, pulseless electrical activity; P_{ETCO_2}, patient end-tidal carbon dioxide; pVT, pulseless ventricular tachycardia; VF, ventricular fibrillation.

both the patient and any providers who are in the water. The electricity will diffuse into the water instead of traveling between the defibrillation pads and through the patient's heart, so the heart will not receive enough electricity to cause defibrillation. You can defibrillate a soaking-wet patient, but first try to dry the patient's chest.

- Do not defibrillate someone who is touching metal that others are touching.
- Do not place a defibrillation pad over a medication patch or any metal objects such as jewelry. Doing so could result in burns.
- If the patient has an implanted pacemaker or internal defibrillator, place the defibrillation pad below the device/battery, or place the pads in anterior and posterior positions.

The defibrillator should be inspected at the beginning of each shift, using a checklist to cover all aspects of the device and its gear: defibrillation pads, cables and connectors, power supply, monitor, ECG recorder, and any ancillary supplies, such as extra defibrillation pads and spare batteries. The US Food and Drug Administration (FDA) has developed an Operator's Shift Checklist for inspecting defibrillators. The conscientious use of this checklist can significantly reduce the likelihood of defibrillator failure in the field.

Words of Wisdom

An implanted pacemaker, which may be detected by identifying the pacemaker-produced spikes on the ECG or by noticing the bulge where the pacemaker's battery pack has been implanted under the patient's skin, is not a contraindication to defibrillation. Just ensure not to place the defibrillation pads directly over the pacemaker battery.

SKILL DRILL 18-4 summarizes the procedures for manual defibrillation.

Skill Drill 18-4 Performing Manual Defibrillation

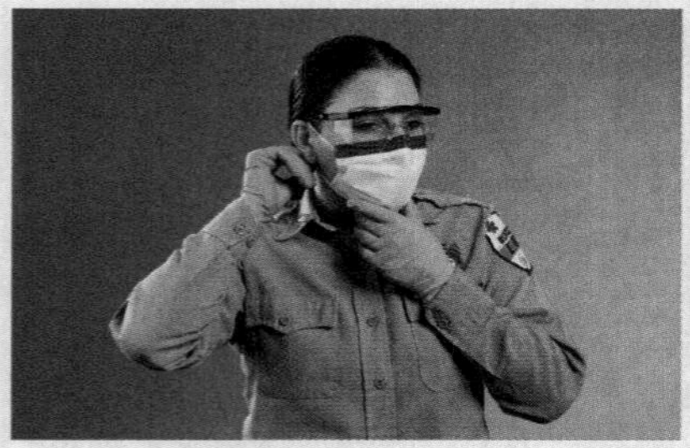

Step 1

Select, check, and assemble all necessary equipment, including a monitor-defibrillator with defibrillation pads, oxygen, and an appropriate oxygen administration device. Take standard precautions and ensure the scene and environment are safe (evaluate risks such as sparks, combustibles, and an oxygen-rich atmosphere).

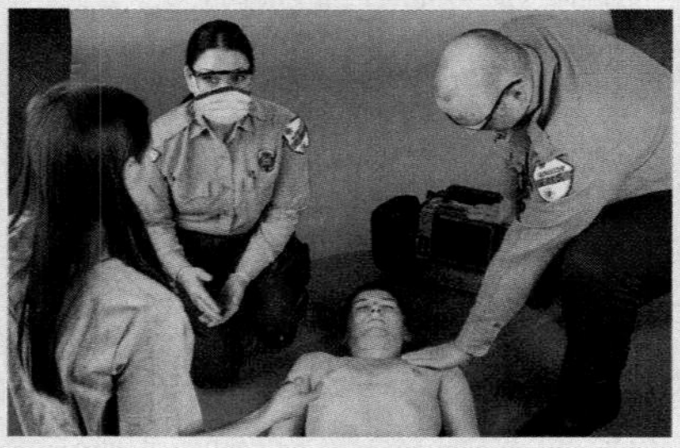

Step 2

If available (and if possible without interrupting care), ask bystanders about the events surrounding the arrest. Check the patient's responsiveness. Request additional help, if needed.

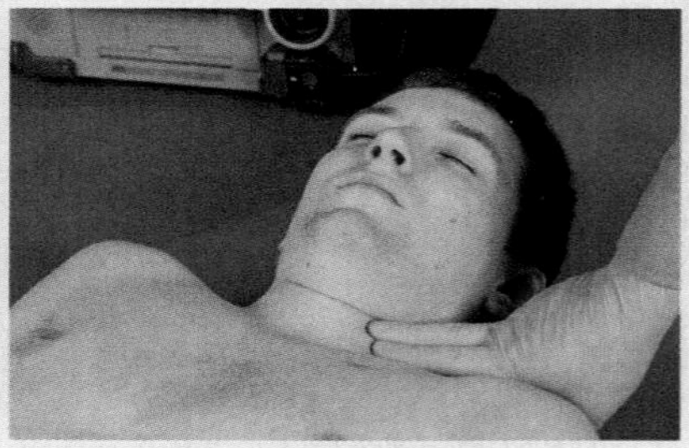

Step 3

Assess the patient for breathing while simultaneously checking for a carotid pulse.

Skill Drill 18-4 Performing Manual Defibrillation (continued)

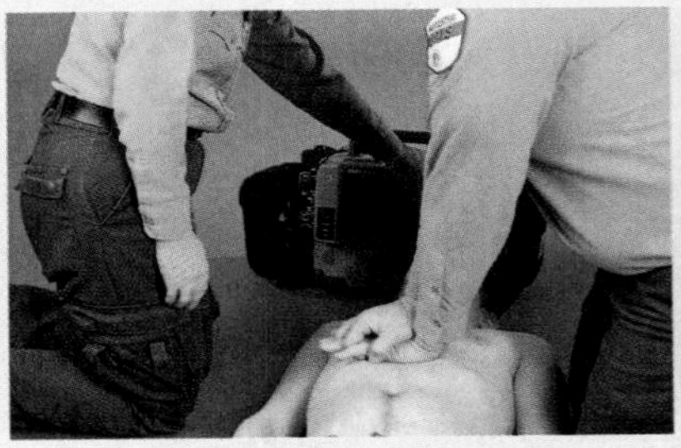

Step 4

Begin chest compressions if the patient is not breathing or is only gasping and has no pulse. Ensure an adequate depth and rate, use the correct compression-to-ventilation ratio, allow the chest to recoil completely, deliver an adequate volume for each breath, and keep interruption of chest compressions to 10 seconds or less throughout the resuscitation effort.

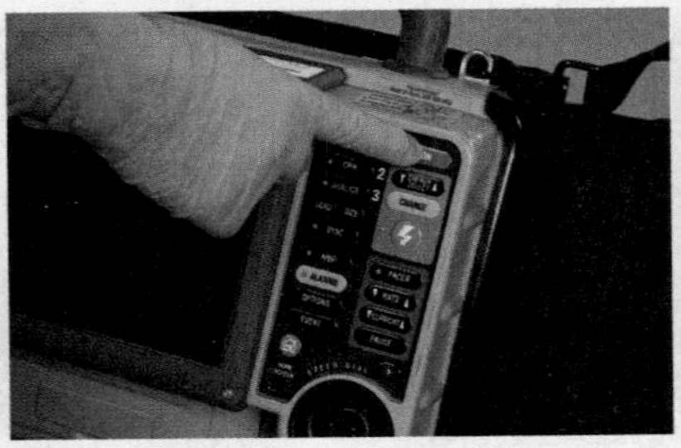

Step 5

Turn on the power to the defibrillator. If EMS providers have been using the machine in AED mode before your arrival, switch the machine to manual mode.

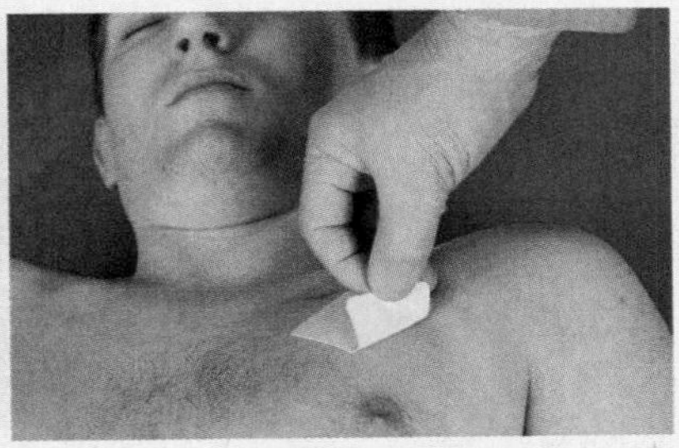

Step 6

Remove the clothing from the patient's upper body. With gloves, remove any medication paste or patches from the patient's chest and wipe away any residue.

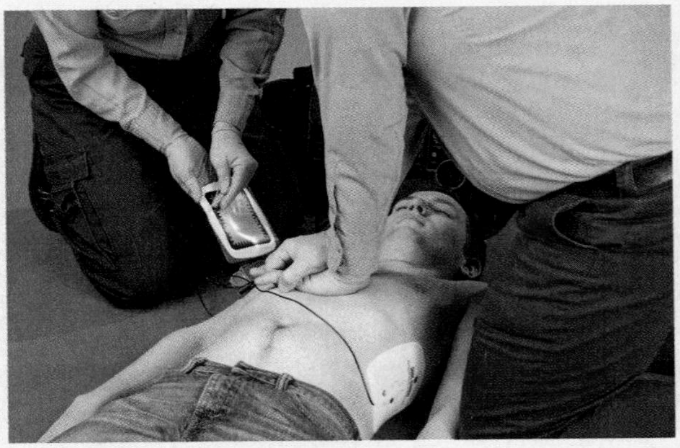

Step 7

Place the defibrillation pads on the patient's bare chest according to the manufacturer's recommendations. Do not place electrodes on top of breast tissue. If necessary, lift the breast out of the way and place the electrode underneath.

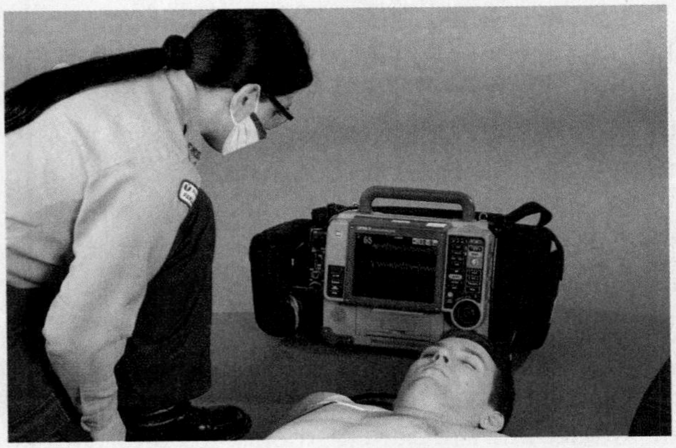

Step 8

Briefly interrupt CPR, identify the rhythm, and confirm that defibrillation is warranted. Note: Some newer defibrillators do not require interrupting CPR for rhythm identification. After verifying that a shockable rhythm is present, set the defibrillator to the proper energy setting.

(continues)

Skill Drill 18-4 Performing Manual Defibrillation (continued)

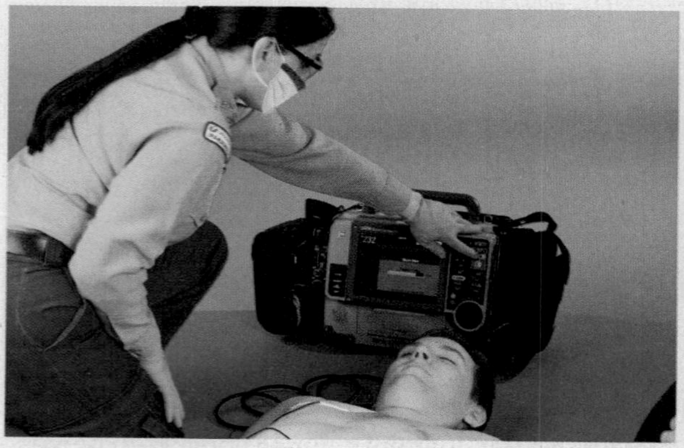

Step 9

Charge the defibrillator.

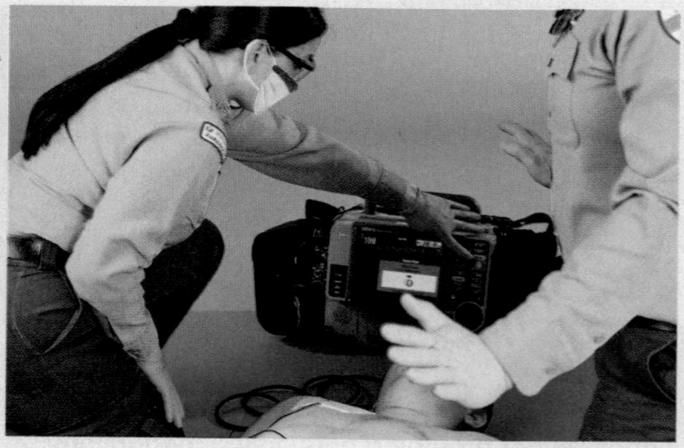

Step 10

Clear the area. Announce, "All clear!" and ensure no one is touching the patient. Press *Shock* on the machine and hold this button until the defibrillator discharges. Resume CPR immediately.

Although you will usually perform manual defibrillation, you may encounter a scene where law enforcement, first responders, or the public have already attached to the patient an AED set in AED mode. In such cases, use the AED, but switch it to manual mode. Manual mode allows for the use of all electrical therapy functions (such as TCP and synchronized cardioversion), as well as multiple-lead cardiac monitoring and 12-lead ECG acquisition.

You may also arrive at a scene where an AED is not in use, but the patient then goes into cardiac arrest. In that case, select manual mode on the defibrillator unit. You can then look at the monitor and determine whether the rhythm is shockable. If so, proceed with charging the unit and shocking the patient. Doing so saves time because CPR can continue until the moment the defibrillator is ready to provide a shock; you do not need to wait for the AED mode to analyze the rhythm and make a recommendation. Remember, it is essential to minimize the interruption of chest compressions with patients in cardiac arrest.

SAFETY

The US FDA Adverse Event Reporting System (FAERS) is used to report adverse medication or device malfunctions. For example, if a defibrillator failed to charge or deliver a shock during a call, the provider or agency could report the event directly to the FDA or the manufacturer. If a manufacturer receives an adverse report, it is required to report it to the FDA.

A fully automated AED (rarely used) can assess the patient's rhythm and, if VF or VT is present, charge the pads and defibrillate, with no intervention by the rescuer. However, a semiautomated AED (commonly used) detects VF and VT and uses visual and verbal prompts to indicate when a shock is advised. The rescuer must then depress the *Shock* button to defibrillate the patient. The steps for using an AED are shown in **SKILL DRILL 18-5**.

After the AED delivers a shock, care of the patient depends on your location and EMS system;

Skill Drill 18-5 Performing Defibrillation With an AED

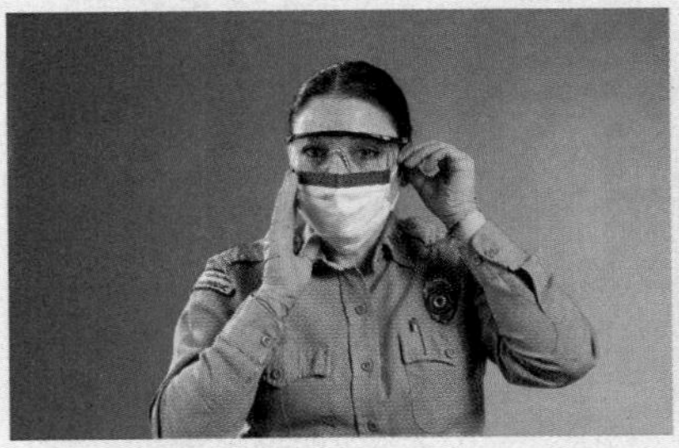

Step 1

Select, check, and assemble all necessary equipment, including the AED, AED pads, oxygen, and an appropriate oxygen administration device. Take standard precautions and ensure the scene and environment are safe (evaluate risks such as sparks, combustibles, and an oxygen-rich atmosphere).

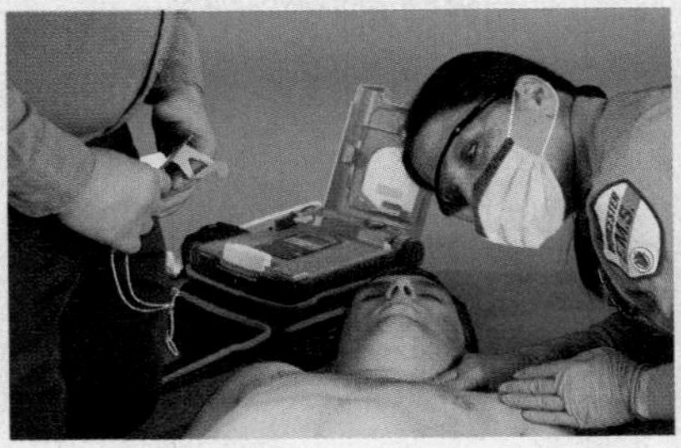

Step 2

If bystanders are present, ask them about the events surrounding the arrest (if doing so is possible without interrupting care). Check the patient's responsiveness. Request additional help, if needed. Assess for breathing while simultaneously checking for a carotid pulse.

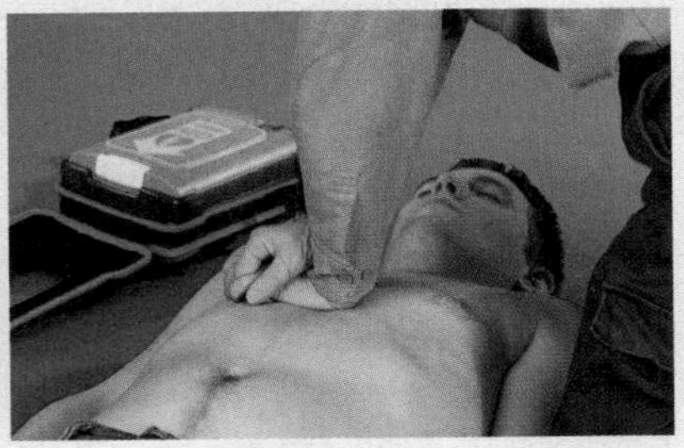

Step 3

If CPR is already in progress, then assess the effectiveness of chest compressions. If the patient is not breathing or is only gasping and has no pulse, and CPR has not been started, begin chest compressions and rescue breaths. Ensure an adequate depth and rate, use the correct compression-to-ventilation ratio, allow the chest to recoil completely, deliver an adequate volume for each breath, and keep interruption of chest compressions to 10 seconds or less throughout the resuscitation effort. Continue until the AED arrives and is ready for use.

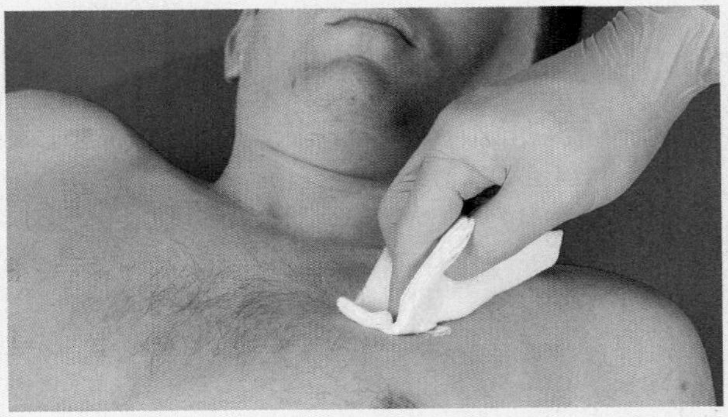

Step 4

Turn on the AED. Remove the clothing from the patient's upper body. With gloves, remove medication paste or patches from the patient's chest, if present, and wipe away any residue.

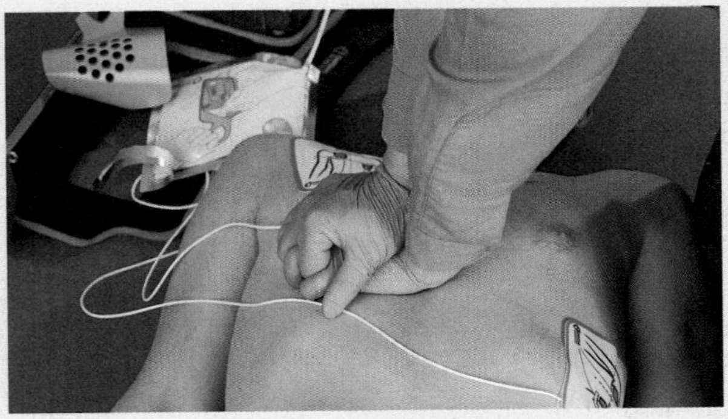

Step 5

Follow the machine's prompts; apply the AED pads to the patient's bare chest according to the manufacturer's recommendations. Attach the pads to the AED.

(continues)

Skill Drill 18-5 Performing Defibrillation With an AED (continued)

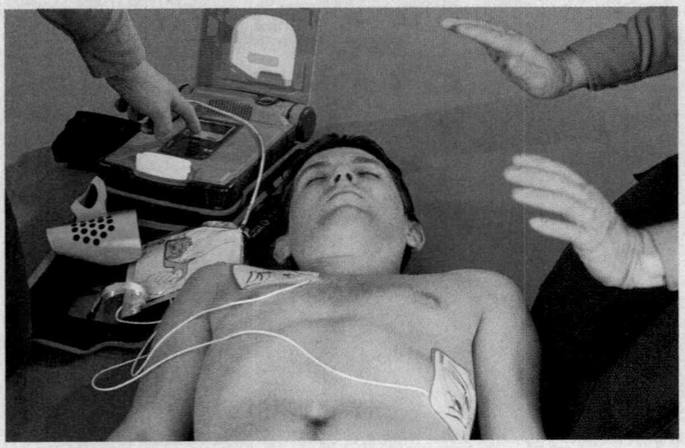

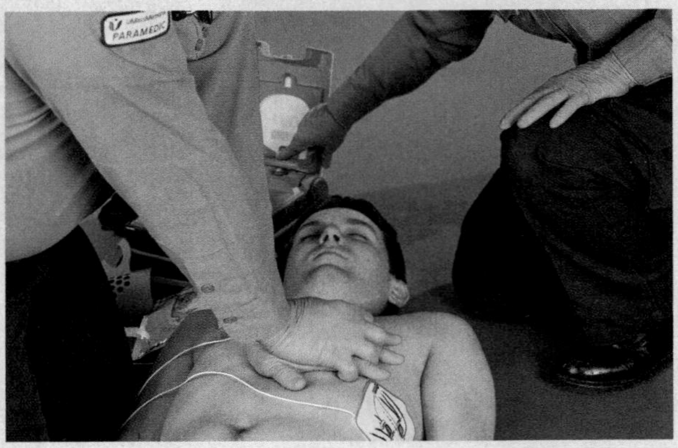

Step 6

Stop CPR and press the *Analyze* button (some AEDs will automatically begin analyzing the patient's rhythm). Ensure that everyone is clear of the patient. Wait for the AED to analyze the cardiac rhythm. If no shock is advised, then resume CPR, starting with chest compressions. Perform five cycles (about 2 minutes) of CPR and then reanalyze the cardiac rhythm. If a shock is advised, recheck that all rescuers are clear and press the *Shock* button.

Step 7

After the shock is delivered, immediately resume CPR, beginning with chest compressions. Do not interrupt chest compressions for more than 10 seconds. Do not turn off the AED during CPR. Continue to follow the AED prompts. To reduce the likelihood of rescuer fatigue, rotate the person delivering chest compressions every 2 minutes.

therefore, you should follow your local protocol. You will need to assess for a pulse, recognizing that one of the following outcomes is likely:

- The pulse is regained.
- The pulse is not regained, and the AED indicates that no shock is advised.
- The pulse is not regained, and the AED indicates that a shock is advised.

For each of these scenarios, the sequence of compressions and defibrillation is the same as described in the earlier section on manual defibrillation. The only difference is that the AED determines whether the rhythm is shockable.

Wearable Cardioverter-Defibrillators

You may encounter a patient with a wearable cardioverter-defibrillator (WCD). This device, which was first approved for use in 2002 by the FDA, is used for patients at high risk of SCD, but who are not immediate candidates for therapy with an implantable cardioverter-defibrillator; in early post-AMI patients with left ventricular dysfunction; and those with newly diagnosed nonischemic cardiomyopathy.[15] The LifeVest, manufactured by ZOLL, is currently the only commercially available WCD. It consists of a lightweight garment with a belt and shoulder straps and a battery-powered monitor-defibrillator; nonadhesive rhythm monitoring electrodes and defibrillation electrodes are embedded in the device. The WCD is worn under the patient's clothing to ensure adequate skin contact for the electrodes. The monitor continuously reads and records the patient's ECG. Patients are instructed to wear the device continuously, except when bathing or showering.

When VT or VF is detected, the patient is alerted using the WCD's alarm system, through vibration, sound alerts of increasing volume, and a verbal warning that states an electrical shock is possible. If the patient is responsive, they can respond by pressing two buttons to stop the treatment sequence. If the patient does not press these buttons, the device charges, the defibrillation electrodes exude gel, a bystander alert says, "Do not touch patient," and a shock is delivered.[16] A maximum of five biphasic energy shocks of up to 150 joules can be delivered for a single event. The LifeVest returns to monitoring mode if a normal rhythm is detected after the shock. If the dysrhythmia persists after the first defibrillation, then the cycle is repeated.

The WCD must be replaced after each series of defibrillations. Patient noncompliance with wearing the garment (primarily because of patient discomfort or dermatologic issues) and the lack of pacing capability for bradydysrhythmias are limitations of the WCD.[15,16]

Asystole

Asystole ("flat line"), the only true **arrhythmia**, is a rhythm in which the heart is no longer contracting and shows no evidence of organized activity **FIGURE 18-67**. Asystole is also known as *cardiac standstill.* This rhythm presents with a complete absence of ventricular electrical activity. Atrial activity, represented by P waves, may occasionally be seen, but they are not accompanied by QRS complexes or T waves when present. The terms *P-wave asystole, ventricular asystole,* or *ventricular standstill* are used when P waves are observed in the absence of ventricular electrical activity.

A flat line on an ECG monitor may or may not indicate asystole. Thus, one of the first things to do when you see a flat-line ECG is to rule out causes other than asystole. Possible causes of a flat-line ECG include leads that are not connected to the patient, loose leads, leads that are not connected to the monitor-defibrillator, an incorrect monitor setting, very-low-voltage VF, and true asystole.

Asystole is considered a nonshockable cardiac arrest rhythm (see Figure 18-66). Recall that the purpose of defibrillation is to deliver a shock of sufficient intensity to depolarize myocardial cells, enabling the SA node to resume pacemaking responsibility when the cells repolarize. In asystole, however, there is no electrical activity to reset.

Pulseless Electrical Activity

So far we have discussed three of four possible cardiac arrest rhythms: pulseless VT, VF, and asystole. The final cardiac arrest rhythm is **pulseless electrical activity (PEA)**, an organized cardiac rhythm (other than VT) on the monitor that is not accompanied by a detectable pulse. In the past, PEA was called *electromechanical dissociation.* With PEA, there is either no mechanical ventricular activity or the mechanical ventricular activity is simply too weak to produce a palpable pulse. This may occur, for example, in patients with cardiogenic or hypovolemic shock, cardiac tamponade, massive pulmonary embolism, electrolyte imbalance (including hyperkalemia in renal failure), or drug overdose. Providing the appropriate treatment for PEA, then, depends on identifying its cause. PEA is a nonshockable cardiac arrest rhythm (see Figure 18-66). Management of cardiac arrest is discussed in detail in the next section.

Management of Adult Cardiac Arrest

Nothing gets the adrenaline pumping more furiously (in paramedics, if not in patients) than a "code," or cardiac arrest. Although prior heart disease is a significant risk factor for cardiac arrest,

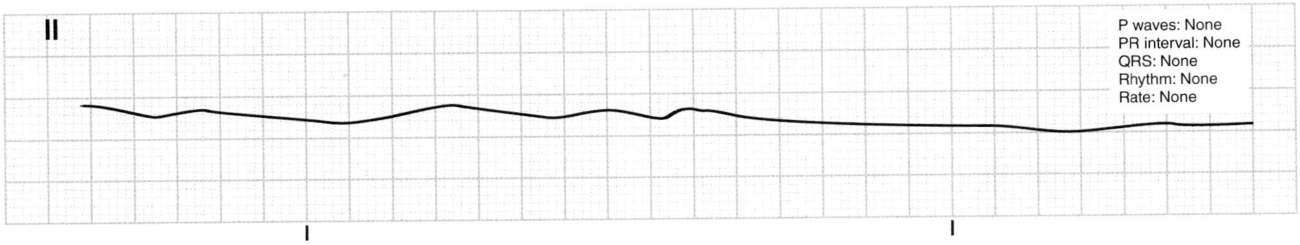

FIGURE 18-67 Asystole.

Reproduced from *Arrhythmia Recognition: The Art of Interpretation*, courtesy of Tomas B. Garcia, MD.

an SCA can also occur secondary to electrocution, a submersion incident, other traumatic events, or noncardiac conditions such as drug overdose, asthma, or anaphylaxis. Many people who experience cardiac arrest have no warning signs before the event occurs. No matter what the cause, cardiac arrest is stressful for all involved. The best way to reduce the stress among providers and increase the likelihood of returning spontaneous circulation in the patient is to practice, practice, and practice, so your team works as smoothly and efficiently as a race-car pit crew. This concept is discussed further in Chapter 40, *Responding to the Field Code*.

Managing a cardiac arrest requires you to deploy many of the advanced life support (ALS) skills you have learned and to do so under circumstances in which minutes may mean the difference between life and death. It is difficult to think clearly in such tense circumstances, especially when other distressed and panicky people are present at the scene (the patient's family, for example). For these reasons, you need to follow an orderly, systematic approach to cardiac arrest emergencies that must be rehearsed exhaustively, in a team setting, until it becomes nearly automatic.

Bring the following devices and equipment when you initially approach the scene:

- Defibrillator
- Portable oxygen cylinder
- Airway management equipment, including an intubation kit
- IV equipment
- Drug box

If you are shorthanded, don't spend time carrying every piece of equipment from the emergency vehicle to the patient. You can send someone to the vehicle later to retrieve other equipment, such as the backboard and stretcher.

The goals of emergency medical care for a patient in cardiac arrest include the return of spontaneous circulation (ROSC) and the preservation of neurologic function. The "no flow" phase of a cardiac arrest is when an arrest has occurred, but chest compressions have not begun. To minimize the duration of this phase, begin emergency medical care immediately on discovering pulselessness.

The National Association of State EMS Officials says that resuscitation should be started on all patients who are found apneic and pulseless unless one of the following conditions exists (does not apply to victims of lightning strikes, drowning, or hypothermia):[10]

- A medical cause or traumatic injury or body condition clearly indicates biologic death (irreversible brain death), limited to:
  - Decapitation
  - Decomposition or putrefaction
  - Transection of the torso
  - Incineration
  - Injuries incompatible with life (eg, massive crush injury, complete exsanguination, severe displacement of brain matter)
  - Futile and inhuman attempts as determined by agency policy/protocol related to "compelling reasons" for withholding resuscitation
  - Blunt or penetrating trauma in which the patient is apneic, pulseless, and without other signs of life on EMS arrival, including, but not limited to, spontaneous movement, ECG activity, or pupillary response
  - Nontraumatic arrest with obvious signs of death, including dependent lividity or rigor mortis

or

- The provider is presented with a valid do-not-resuscitate (DNR) order (eg, form, card, bracelet) or other actionable medical order (eg, physician order for life-sustaining treatment [POLST] form, medical order for life-sustaining treatment [MOLST] form) that conforms to the state specifications for color and construction, is intact (ie, has not been cut, broken, or obviously repaired), and displays the patient's name and the physician's name.

Words of Wisdom

Withholding Resuscitative Efforts

In situations where the patient's status is unclear and the appropriateness of withholding resuscitation efforts is uncertain, begin CPR and then contact medical control.[10] If you are presented with a valid do-not-intubate (DNI, MOLST, or POLST) advance directive, provide full treatment per protocols except for any intervention prohibited explicitly in the patient's advance directive. Contact medical control if an intervention that is prohibited by an advance directive is being considered.[10]

If bystanders have delivered adequate uninterrupted chest compressions before your arrival, or if the arrest was witnessed by EMS personnel, then proceed with rhythm analysis. If compressions have not been provided or the arrest was not witnessed by EMS personnel, begin chest compressions while a second rescuer sets up the AED or defibrillator. Proceed with rhythm analysis. Your initial efforts should focus on either creating a "low flow" state, in which the delivery of high-quality CPR begins and is continued throughout the resuscitation effort, or creating a "normal flow" state through the ROSC using defibrillation or other interventions. Components of high-quality adult CPR include the following:

- Perform chest compressions at a rate of at least 100/min and less than 120/min.
- Compress the chest to a depth of at least 2 inches (5 cm) and less than 2.4 inches (6 cm).
- Allow full chest recoil after each compression and avoid leaning on the chest between compressions.
- Minimize pauses in compressions and target a **chest compression fraction** of at least 60%.[11]
- Avoid excessive ventilation.
- Rotate the person delivering chest compressions every 2 minutes to minimize fatigue.

What you see on the monitor will determine which side of the cardiac arrest algorithm you should then follow (see Figure 18-66). Recall that there are four possible cardiac arrest rhythms: pulseless VT, VF, asystole, and PEA. Pulseless VT and VF are shockable rhythms; asystole and PEA are not. Key points to keep in mind include the following:

- If defibrillation is indicated, the provider giving chest compressions should continue while a second rescuer charges the defibrillator. Then pause CPR, clear the patient, and deliver the shock. Resume chest compressions immediately, without pausing for a rhythm or pulse check.
- After 2 minutes or five cycles of CPR, pause resuscitation efforts and check the rhythm on the monitor. If the rhythm is VF or VT, resume CPR while charging the defibrillator. Clear the patient and then defibrillate. If an organized rhythm appears on the monitor, identify this new rhythm and check for a pulse. If there is no pulse, move down the algorithm to the asystole-PEA pathway and immediately resume CPR. If there is a pulse, move to the appropriate algorithm for the new rhythm.
- Rescuer fatigue can reduce the effectiveness of chest compressions. Minimize rescuer fatigue by rotating rescuers at the end of each 2-minute session of CPR.
- To maximize the number of compressions delivered per minute, interruptions should not exceed 10 seconds.
- Using normal saline, attempt to establish vascular access only after beginning CPR and, when a shockable rhythm is present, after attempting defibrillation. If you cannot establish IV access, establish intraosseous (IO) access using an adult IO system. Vascular access should be achieved without interrupting chest compressions. In arrests associated with shockable rhythms, administer IV or IO epinephrine after the delivery of a second shock. In arrests associated with nonshockable rhythms, administer epinephrine as soon as possible. In all cardiac arrests, repeat epinephrine every 3 to 5 minutes until a pulse returns. When giving IV or IO medication during CPR, follow it immediately with a 20-mL flush of normal saline to facilitate the medication's delivery to the central circulation.
- Several options are available for airway management. In some EMS systems, passive ventilation using a nonrebreathing mask is initially used for three to four cycles of uninterrupted chest compressions, after which bag-mask ventilation or an advanced airway is considered. Another option is to use a bag-mask device throughout the resuscitation effort. For adults in cardiac arrest without an advanced airway, use a 30:2 compression to ventilation ratio. Ventilate with just enough volume to produce visible chest rise. Deliver each breath over about 1 second. If the decision is made to insert an advanced airway, verify its placement by multiple methods, including waveform capnography, and secure the tube. Deliver 1 breath every 6 seconds (10 breaths/min) without interrupting chest compressions.
- VF or pulseless VT that persists or recurs after one or more shocks is called refractory VF/VT.

An antidysrhythmic medication, such as amiodarone, may be considered for patients with VF/VT unresponsive to CPR, defibrillation, and epinephrine. Lidocaine may be considered as an alternative to amiodarone for patients with VF/VT. Antidysrhythmic medications are discussed in more detail in Chapter 13, *Principles of Pharmacology*.

- During the arrest, consider the Hs and Ts to identify possible reversible causes of the arrest and factors that may complicate the resuscitation effort **TABLE 18-5**.
- If ROSC occurs at any point, assess the patient's vital signs, support the airway and breathing as required, and give medications as indicated to manage cardiac dysrhythmias, and maintain the BP.

Patients who do not regain a pulse at the scene of a cardiac arrest usually do not survive. Whether and where you transport such patients depends on your EMS system and is dictated by your local protocol.

Administering CPR while a patient is being moved or transported is usually not effective. A patient has the best chance of survival when resuscitated at the scene, unless the location is unsafe. During transport, EMS providers will ideally provide care in the patient compartment while a third provider drives. It is not safe to defibrillate a patient in a moving ambulance; therefore, the vehicle should come to a complete stop if additional shocks are needed. Ensure you follow the local protocol established by your EMS system.

Special Circumstances in Cardiac Arrest

Some cardiac arrests occur in circumstances that require special considerations, treatments, or procedures beyond those typically applied or provided during a resuscitation effort. For example, you may

TABLE 18-5 Hs and Ts: Causes and Treatment of Cardiac Arrest Rhythms

Possible Reversible Cause	Clues	Treatment*
Hypovolemia	History, flat neck veins	Volume replacement
Hypoxemia	Cyanosis, airway compromise	Ventilation with 100% oxygen; consider advanced airway insertion
Hypothermia	History of exposure to cold	See the hypothermia algorithm in Chapter 39, *Environmental Emergencies*
Hyperkalemia, hypokalemia	History, ECG changes	Consider immediate transport
Hydrogen ions (acidosis)	History	Consider sodium bicarbonate if certain of acidosis
Tension pneumothorax	History (trauma, asthma, COPD), difficult to ventilate, unequal breath sounds with hyperresonance to percussion on affected side	Needle decompression of the affected side of the chest
Cardiac tamponade	History, jugular venous distention	Immediate transport for pericardiocentesis
Toxins (drug overdose)	History	Consider immediate transport, naloxone (Narcan) for opioid overdose
Thrombosis (massive MI, pulmonary embolism)	History	Immediate transport for possible emergent angiography or fibrinolysis

* Beyond managing the cardiac arrest

Abbreviations: ECG, electrocardiogram; COPD, chronic obstructive pulmonary disease; CPR, cardiopulmonary resuscitation; MI, myocardial infarction

Documentation and Communication

EMS systems regularly evaluate the emergency care provided to patients who have had a cardiac arrest. Key elements to document are the following:[10]

- Resuscitation attempts and all interventions performed
- Witnesses of the cardiac arrest
- Location of the cardiac arrest
- First monitored rhythm
- CPR efforts before EMS arrival
- Outcome or disposition (including any ROSC)
- Presumed etiology (presumed cardiac, trauma, submersion, respiratory, other noncardiac, unknown)

need to alter specific techniques to accommodate a patient with morbid obesity.

If the patient experiences anaphylaxis that results in cardiac arrest, standard resuscitative measures and immediate epinephrine administration are among the care priorities.[11] Close monitoring is essential, and advanced airway management, including planning for a possible surgical airway, may be required.

Patients with known or suspected opioid-associated cardiac arrest are managed per standard ACLS practices. However, you may need to administer naloxone during the post–cardiac arrest period to reverse the effects of long-acting opioids.

When cardiac arrest occurs in a patient with acute asthma and the patient becomes difficult to ventilate, you must watch for and be prepared to treat a tension pneumothorax.

Cardiac arrest associated with severe electrolyte disturbances or specific overdoses (eg, beta blockers, calcium channel blockers, tricyclic antidepressants) may require administering medications that paramedics do not routinely give during a resuscitation effort, such as sodium bicarbonate, calcium, or magnesium.

When cardiac arrest is associated with drowning, provide CPR, including rescue breathing, as soon as the unresponsive submersion victim is removed from the water. All drowning victims who require any form of resuscitation (including rescue breathing alone) should be transported to the hospital for evaluation and monitoring.[11]

Cardiac arrest in pregnant patients is discussed in Chapter 42, *Obstetrics*. Cardiac arrest in pediatric patients is discussed in Chapter 44, *Pediatric Emergencies*.

Words of Wisdom

Extracorporeal cardiopulmonary resuscitation (eCPR) is a technique in which a patient's large vein and artery are cannulated. A machine is used to pump the patient's blood through the machine and then return oxygenated blood to the patient. Currently, there is insufficient evidence to recommend the routine use of eCPR for patients in cardiac arrest. However, eCPR may be considered if the patient has a potentially reversible cause of cardiac arrest (eg, acute coronary artery occlusion, pulmonary embolism, refractory VF, profound hypothermia, drug toxicity) that would benefit from temporary mechanical cardiorespiratory support[10,11]

Words of Wisdom

Mechanical CPR devices deliver automated chest compressions, eliminating the need for rescuers to deliver manual chest compressions. Although the American Heart Association (AHA) does not recommend their routine use, mechanical CPR devices may be considered in specific settings where the delivery of high-quality manual compressions may be challenging or dangerous for the provider (eg, when an insufficient number of rescuers are available, during prolonged CPR, during hypothermic cardiac arrest, in a moving ambulance, in the angiography suite, during preparation for eCPR), provided that rescuers strictly limit the interruptions in CPR during deployment and removal of the device.[11] The use of a mechanical CPR device should also be considered in a patient in cardiac arrest who is known or suspected to have COVID-19.

Post–Cardiac Arrest Care

Post–cardiac arrest care is an essential component of the overall care of patients who experience cardiac arrest. The goals of post–cardiac arrest care are to optimize cardiopulmonary function and vital organ perfusion. If an effective cardiac rhythm is restored in the field, transport the patient immediately, ideally, to a facility with comprehensive post–cardiac arrest treatment, including acute coronary interventions, advanced neurologic monitoring and care, goal-directed critical care, and **targeted temperature management (TTM)**.

Begin by optimizing the patient's oxygenation and ventilation. Assess breath sounds (also known as lung sounds). After ROSC, most patients require ventilatory assistance. If not already done, consider early placement of an endotracheal tube. Be sure to use waveform capnography or capnometry to confirm and monitor tube placement. Titrate the oxygen therapy to achieve and maintain an Spo_2 of 92% to 98%. Provide 10 breaths/min if the patient requires assisted ventilation, and avoid hyperventilation.

Obtain a 12-lead ECG as soon as possible to determine whether acute ST-segment elevation is present. Assess the patient's BP, and aim to maintain an SBP of at least 90 mm Hg and a mean arterial pressure of at least 65 mm Hg.[11] Marked hypotension needs to be corrected rapidly because the patient's brain will not be adequately perfused if the BP is very low. Administer fluid boluses of normal saline or lactated Ringer solution per your local protocol. If the patient has marked hypotension and the transport time to the medical facility will be prolonged, consider administering a vasopressor infusion. If the rhythm is bradycardic or tachycardic, follow the bradycardia or tachycardia algorithm.

Perform a neurologic assessment and determine whether the patient can follow commands. If the patient does not follow commands, TTM, a therapy begun at the hospital, is recommended for at least 24 hours.

Regardless of the cause of a cardiac arrest, the hypoxemia, ischemia, and reperfusion that occurs during the arrest and resuscitation effort may damage multiple organ systems. During the post–cardiac arrest period, patients are often hemodynamically unstable, and many of them will re-arrest. Thus, the patient requires close monitoring following cardiac arrest. The adult post–cardiac arrest care algorithm is shown in **FIGURE 18-68**.

When to Stop CPR

On some calls, you may need to determine whether a patient is likely to benefit from ongoing resuscitative efforts or whether such efforts are futile. These decisions are often guided by the local protocol or direct communication with medical control.

When the patient does not respond to prehospital cardiac arrest treatment, it is acceptable and often preferable to cease futile resuscitation efforts in the field. This decision may be made for several reasons:[10]

- In most situations, ALS providers can perform an initial resuscitation equivalent to an in-hospital resuscitation attempt. In most cases, there is no additional benefit from ED resuscitation.
- CPR performed during patient packaging and transport is much less effective than CPR administered at the scene.
- EMS providers risk physical injury while attempting to perform CPR in a moving ambulance while unrestrained.
- Continuing resuscitation in futile cases places other motorists and pedestrians at risk, increases the amount of time during which the EMS crew is unavailable for other calls, impedes ED care of other patients, and incurs unnecessary medical facility charges.

The AHA has published criteria for BLS and ALS termination of resuscitation for adult OHCA **TABLE 18-6**.[11]

In some jurisdictions, state law does not permit paramedics to pronounce death at the scene. If legislation were enacted to permit such pronouncements in these jurisdictions, each EMS system would have to formulate its own criteria for terminating CPR in the prehospital setting.

Receiving permission to stop CPR in the field does not necessarily make your life easier. Complex issues that must be handled delicately are involved, such as the expectations of the patient's family and proper disposition of the body. In addition, you may face enormous pressure from bystanders to continue resuscitative efforts long after there is any medical justification for doing so. Stopping CPR may also be difficult for you; you may not be accustomed to explaining to a family that the person has died and nothing more can be done. It is much easier to transport the person to the medical facility and leave the ED staff with the unpleasant task of breaking the bad news.

Many jurisdictions have adopted protocols to help providers decide when resuscitation attempts are futile and should be terminated. If it is legal in

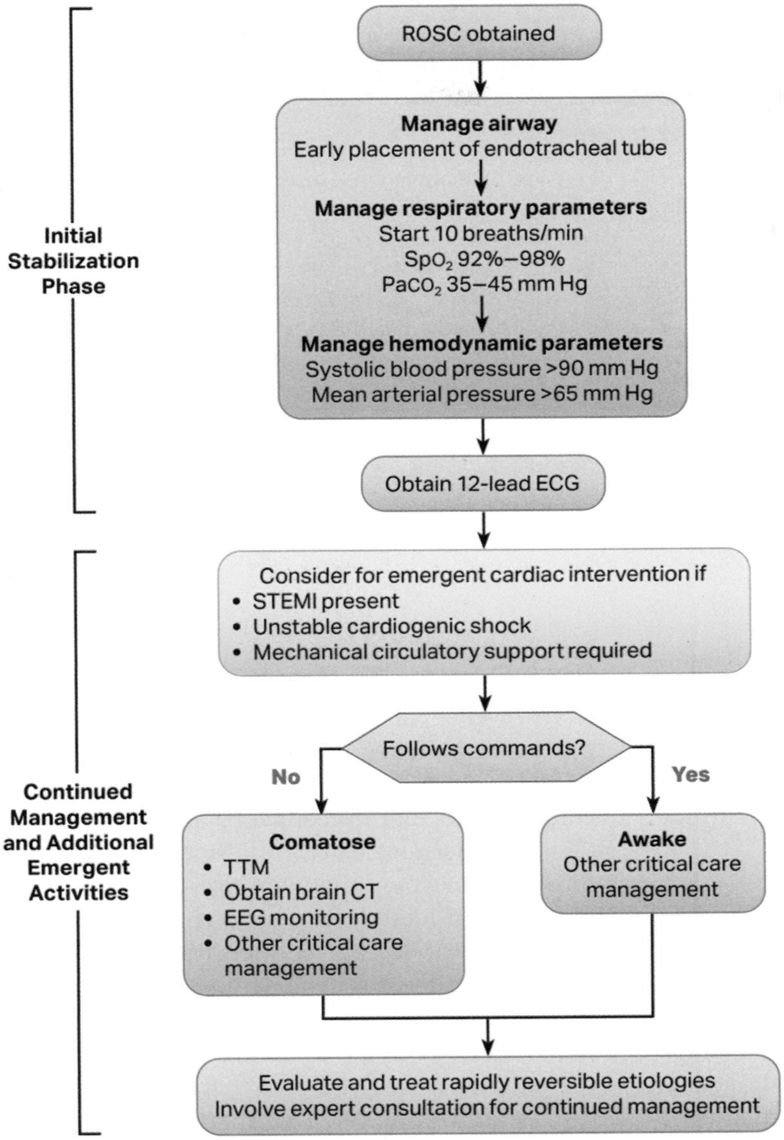

Initial Stabilization Phase

ROSC obtained

Manage airway
Early placement of endotracheal tube

Manage respiratory parameters
Start 10 breaths/min
SpO$_2$ 92%–98%
PaCO$_2$ 35–45 mm Hg

Manage hemodynamic parameters
Systolic blood pressure >90 mm Hg
Mean arterial pressure >65 mm Hg

Obtain 12-lead ECG

Continued Management and Additional Emergent Activities

Consider for emergent cardiac intervention if
• STEMI present
• Unstable cardiogenic shock
• Mechanical circulatory support required

Follows commands?

No — **Comatose**
• TTM
• Obtain brain CT
• EEG monitoring
• Other critical care management

Yes — **Awake**
Other critical care management

Evaluate and treat rapidly reversible etiologies
Involve expert consultation for continued management

Initial Stabilization Phase

Resuscitation is ongoing during the post-ROSC phase, and many of these activities can occur concurrently. However, if prioritization is necessary, follow these steps:
• Airway management: Waveform capnography or capnometry to confirm and monitor endotracheal tube placement
• Manage respiratory parameters: Titrate FIO$_2$ for SpO$_2$ 92%–98%; start at 10 breaths/min; titrate to PaCO$_2$ of 35–45 mm Hg
• Manage hemodynamic parameters: Administer crystalloid and/or vasopressor or inotrope for goal systolic blood pressure >90 mm Hg or mean arterial pressure >65 mm Hg

Continued Management and Additional Emergent Activities

These evaluations should be done concurrently so that decisions on targeted temperature management (TTM) receive high priority as cardiac interventions.
• Emergent cardiac intervention: Early evaluation of 12-lead electrocardiogram (ECG); consider hemodynamics for decision on cardiac intervention
• TTM: If patient is not following commands, start TTM as soon as possible; begin at 32–36°C for 24 hours by using a cooling device with feedback loop
• Other critical care management
 – Continuously monitor core temperature (esophageal, rectal, bladder)
 – Maintain normoxia, normocapnia, euglycemia
 – Provide continuous or intermittent electroencephalogram (EEG) monitoring
 – Provide lung-protective ventilation

H's and T's

Hypovolemia
Hypoxia
Hydrogen ion (acidosis)
Hypokalemia/**h**yperkalemia
Hypothermia
Tension pneumothorax
Tamponade, cardiac
Toxins
Thrombosis, pulmonary
Thrombosis, coronary

FIGURE 18-68 Adult post–cardiac arrest care algorithm.
Abbreviations: CT, computed tomography; Paco$_2$, partial pressure of carbon dioxide; ROSC, return of spontaneous circulation; Spo$_2$, pulse oximetry; STEMI, ST-segment elevation myocardial infarction.

TABLE 18-6 American Heart Association Rules for Terminating Resuscitation in Adults With OHCA

BLS Rule	ALS Rule
Consider terminating BLS resuscitation attempts for adults with OHCA before moving them to the ambulance for transport when all of the following criteria are met: 1. The arrest was not witnessed by EMS personnel. 2. No ROSC before transport. 3. No AED shocks were delivered before transport.	Consider terminating ALS resuscitation attempts for adults with OHCA before moving them to the ambulance for transport when all of the following criteria are met: 1. The arrest was not witnessed by EMS personnel. 2. No bystander CPR was provided. 3. No ROSC after full ALS care in the field before transport. 4. No AED shocks were delivered before transport.
If *all* criteria are present, consider termination of resuscitation. If *any* criteria are missing, continue resuscitation and transport.	

Abbreviations: AED, automated external defibrillator; ALS, advanced life support; BLS, basic life support; CPR, cardiopulmonary resuscitation; EMS, emergency medical services; OHCA, out-of-hospital cardiac arrest; ROSC, return of spontaneous circulation

Data from: Panchal AR, Bartos JA, Cabañas JG, et al. Part 3: adult basic and advanced life support: 2020 American Heart Association guidelines for cardiopulmonary resuscitation and emergency cardiovascular care. *Circulation.* 2020;142(16 suppl 2): S366-S468.

your EMS system to terminate CPR in the field, then meet with your medical director to walk through scenarios you may have to face. Role-play exercises can be beneficial to help you identify, in advance, situations in which you may feel uncomfortable and to help you develop strategies for coping with them.

AV Blocks

After the SA node initiates an impulse, it proceeds through the atria and ventricles, resulting in contraction of the heart. When the signal reaches the AV node, it is delayed to allow the atria to contract and fill the ventricles. This delay is a normal function of the AV node and usually causes no signs or symptoms. Occasionally, however, the impulse traveling through the AV node is delayed for a more extended period than usual or is completely blocked, resulting in an AV block, which is a type of heart block. This prolonged delay or block in impulse conduction can occur at the level of the AV node or below the bundle of His (infranodal), and it may involve one or more of the bundle branches and their fascicles.

AV blocks are classified into different degrees, depending on the block's seriousness and the amount of myocardial damage. The least serious is a first-degree AV block; the most serious is a third-degree block. In between, of course, is a second-degree block.

First-Degree AV Block

A **first-degree AV block**, also called *first-degree heart block*, occurs when each impulse reaching the AV node is delayed longer than normal, resulting in a constant PRI that exceeds 0.20 second (200 milliseconds). Because each impulse eventually passes through the AV node, generating a QRS complex, AV block is considered the least serious kind of heart block. Nevertheless, it is often the first indication that the AV node has been damaged.

Because first-degree AV block may occur with any rhythm in which a P wave precedes the QRS, the rate associated with it is that of the underlying rhythm **FIGURE 18-69**. This rhythm is usually regular, with minimal variation between R-R intervals, but its regularity depends on the underlying rhythm. An upright P wave precedes each QRS complex. Its size and shape may vary, depending on the underlying rhythm. The PRI measures greater than 0.20 second (200 milliseconds) and is constant in duration. The QRS complex measures 0.11 second (110 milliseconds) or less. The primary difference between first-degree AV block and normal sinus rhythm is the prolonged PRI.

First-degree AV block generally does not require treatment in the prehospital setting unless it is associated with symptomatic bradycardia. In such cases, the bradycardia is treated by following the bradycardia algorithm discussed earlier in this chapter.

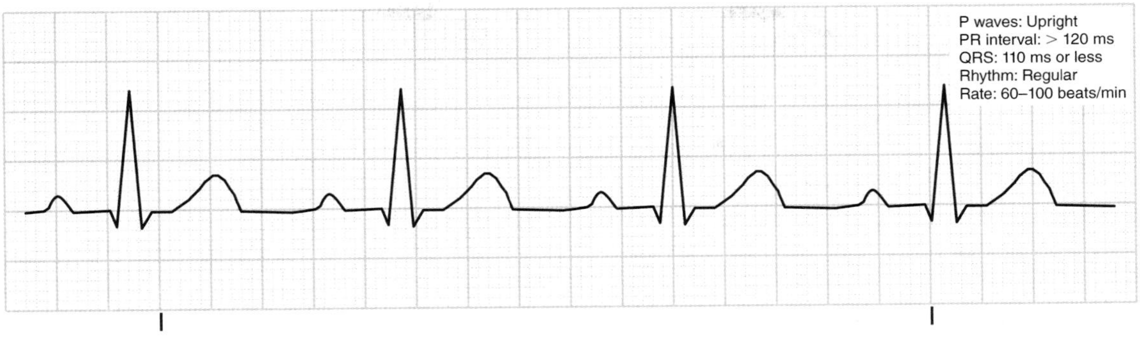

FIGURE 18-69 Sinus bradycardia with first-degree atrioventricular block.

Reproduced from *Arrhythmia Recognition: The Art of Interpretation*, courtesy of Tomas B. Garcia, MD.

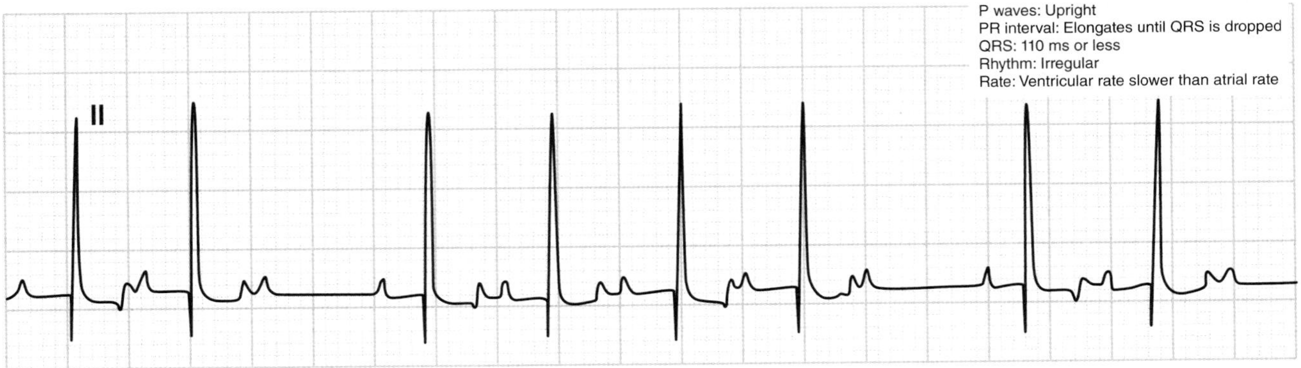

P waves: Upright
PR interval: Elongates until QRS is dropped
QRS: 110 ms or less
Rhythm: Irregular
Rate: Ventricular rate slower than atrial rate
II

FIGURE 18-70 Second-degree atrioventricular block type I.

Reproduced from *Arrhythmia Recognition: The Art of Interpretation*, courtesy of Tomas B. Garcia, MD.

Second-Degree AV Block Type I

A second-degree AV block occurs when an interruption in impulse conduction occurs within the AV node, bundle of His, or His-Purkinje system, preventing the impulse from proceeding to the ventricles and generating a QRS complex. Second-degree AV block type I, also called Mobitz type I second-degree block or Wenckebach, most often occurs because of impaired conduction through the AV node; however, it may occasionally occur below the AV node within the bundle of His or bundle branches.

With second-degree AV block type I, the interval between P waves is regular. An upright P wave precedes most QRS complexes. The ventricular rhythm is irregular, with a prolonged R-R interval between the last QRS complex before the blocked P wave and the QRS complex after the first unblocked P wave **FIGURE 18-70**. The PRI starts within the normal limits of 0.12 to 0.20 second (120 to 200 milliseconds) but grows longer with each successive P wave. Finally, a P wave appears that is followed not by a QRS complex, but rather by another P wave. This P wave is then followed by a QRS complex with a normal PRI. This pattern repeats over and over in the same rhythm. The QRS complex measures 0.11 second (110 milliseconds) or less.

The keys to recognizing second-degree AV block type I include (1) observing the presence of more P waves than QRS complexes, (2) noting P waves that occur at regular intervals, (3) identifying that the PRIs associated with the conducted P waves get longer and longer until a P wave appears that is not followed by a QRS complex, and (4) noting the ventricular rhythm is irregular.

Conditions in which second-degree AV block type I may be seen include ischemic heart disease, acute inferior wall or right ventricular MI, increased vagal tone, digoxin toxicity, and certain electrolyte imbalances. Administering amiodarone, beta blockers, and calcium channel blockers can cause second-degree AV block type I.

The patient with this type of AV block is usually asymptomatic because the ventricular rate often remains nearly normal and CO is not significantly compromised. However, if the ventricular rate slows and the patient becomes symptomatic because of the slow rate, the bradycardia should be treated per the bradycardia algorithm (see Figure 18-35). When this rhythm occurs in conjunction with AMI, continuously monitor the patient for increasing AV block.

Second-Degree AV Block Type II

Second-degree AV block type II, also called Mobitz type II second-degree block or type II AV block, is more serious than second-degree AV block type I. With AV block type II, impaired conduction usually occurs within the bundle of His or, more commonly, the bundle branches.

Second-degree AV block type II is an intermittent block characterized by regularly occurring P waves and the abrupt appearance of at least one P wave that is not followed by a QRS complex **FIGURE 18-71**. A P wave that occurs without a subsequent QRS complex indicates the SA node impulse was not conducted to the ventricles. The ventricular rhythm is irregular because of the dropped QRS complexes. The PRI is constant. The QRS complex will measure 0.11 second (110 milliseconds) or less if the block occurs above or within the bundle of His. If the block occurs below the bundle of His, then the QRS complex will be greater than 0.11 second (110 milliseconds).

Causes of second-degree AV block type II include ischemic heart disease, acute anterior wall MI, and infectious heart diseases. Second-degree type II AV block may also occur as a consequence of cardiac surgery. Second-degree type II AV block is often associated with a slow ventricular rate, and significantly reduced CO may be evident. Patients may experience dizziness, fatigue, dyspnea on exertion, or syncope. Because atropine is usually ineffective in reversing this type of block, emergency care may require the use of TCP (see Figure 18-35). Second-degree AV block type II can progress to third-degree AV block without warning, so patient monitoring is critical.

Second-degree AV blocks can occur in patterns. When two P waves appear for each QRS complex, a 2:1 AV block is present; when three P waves appear for one QRS complex, a 3:1 AV block is present. It can be challenging to determine whether the second-degree AV block is type I or type II in such situations. Although exceptions do occur, the duration of the QRS complex is usually within normal limits in type I blocks, but is usually longer than normal in type II blocks.

Third-Degree AV Block

A third-degree AV block occurs when all impulses reaching the AV junction are prevented from proceeding to the ventricles and generating a QRS complex. Consequently, this block is also known as a complete heart block or complete AV block. Because all impulses from the SA node are blocked, a secondary pacemaker (either junctional or ventricular) must assume responsibility for impulse conduction.

The traditional way to identify a third-degree AV block is to look for nonconducted P waves and the absence of any relationship between the P waves and the QRS complexes. There is no PRI because the atrial and ventricular rhythms occur independently of each other. The rhythm is usually regular, with consistent P-P and R-R intervals **FIGURE 18-72**. The P wave is present and upright. The atrial rate is faster than the ventricular rate. The ventricular rate, which depends on a secondary pacemaker's activity, is 40 to 60 beats/min if the pacemaker originates

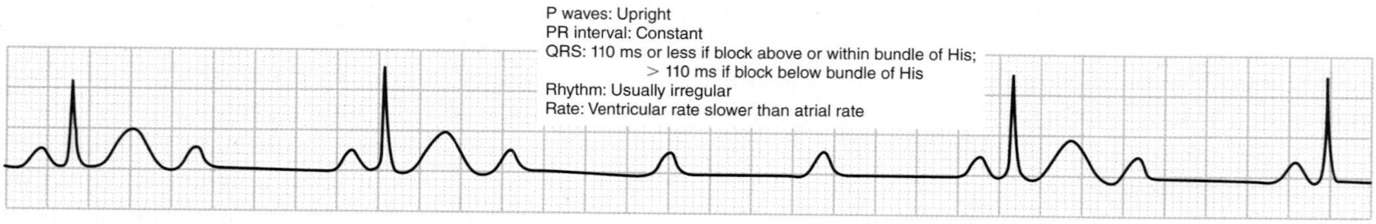

P waves: Upright
PR interval: Constant
QRS: 110 ms or less if block above or within bundle of His;
> 110 ms if block below bundle of His
Rhythm: Usually irregular
Rate: Ventricular rate slower than atrial rate

FIGURE 18-71 Second-degree atrioventricular block type II.

in the AV junction and 20 to 40 beats/min if it originates in the ventricles.

The QRS complexes seen in third-degree AV block may be of normal duration if they originate in the AV junction. They are generally 0.12 second (120 milliseconds) or more if the pacemaker site is in the ventricles.

Third-degree AV blocks can be produced by AMI, ischemic heart disease, hyperkalemia, or excessive doses of certain rate-control medications. Symptoms are related to the location of the block within the conduction system. The patient may be asymptomatic if the site of the block is in the AV node and a junctional rhythm is present, with a reasonable ventricular rate. However, fatigue, dyspnea, or syncope can occur if the site of the block is below the AV node, with a slow ventricular escape rhythm.[17] If the patient is symptomatic because of the slow rate, treat the bradycardia according to the bradycardia algorithm (see Figure 18-35).

Artificial Pacemaker Rhythms

Many patients encountered by paramedics will have experienced cardiac conduction system disorders for which an artificial pacemaker was implanted. An artificial pacemaker consists of a pulse generator, which is the battery-powered energy source, and wire electrodes attached to one or more chambers of the heart. The pulse generator of a permanent pacemaker contains programmable hardware. It is implanted in the subcutaneous tissue of the chest, below the right or left clavicle.

An artificial pacemaker firing generates a unique vertical spike on the ECG tracing **FIGURE 18-73**. A single-chamber pacemaker paces only one cardiac chamber, either the right atrium or the right ventricle. A dual-chamber pacemaker, also called an *AV sequential pacemaker*, paces both the right atrium and the right ventricle. This type of device produces a pacemaker spike followed by a P wave, and then another pacemaker spike followed by a wide QRS complex **FIGURE 18-74**. A biventricular pacemaker,

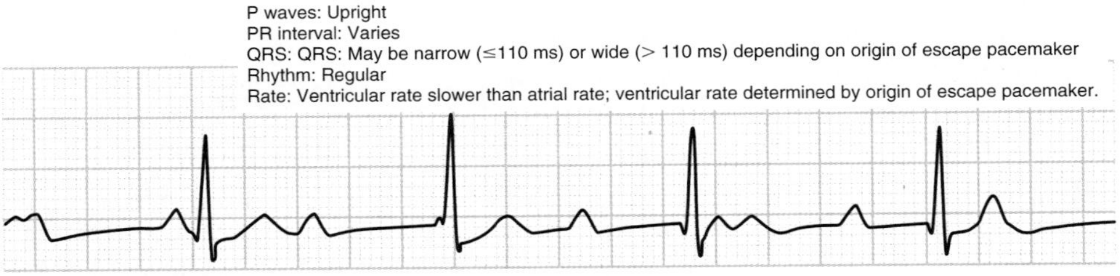

P waves: Upright
PR interval: Varies
QRS: QRS: May be narrow (≤110 ms) or wide (> 110 ms) depending on origin of escape pacemaker
Rhythm: Regular
Rate: Ventricular rate slower than atrial rate; ventricular rate determined by origin of escape pacemaker.

FIGURE 18-72 Third-degree atrioventricular block.

Reproduced from *Arrhythmia Recognition: The Art of Interpretation*, courtesy of Tomas B. Garcia, MD.

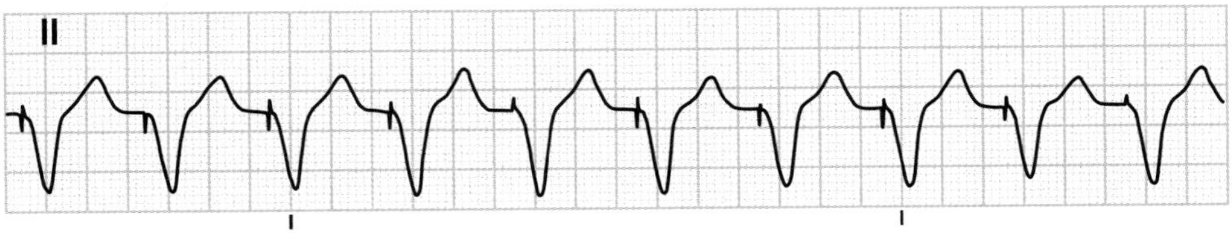

FIGURE 18-73 Ventricular paced rhythm.

Reproduced from *Arrhythmia Recognition: The Art of Interpretation*, courtesy of Tomas B. Garcia, MD.

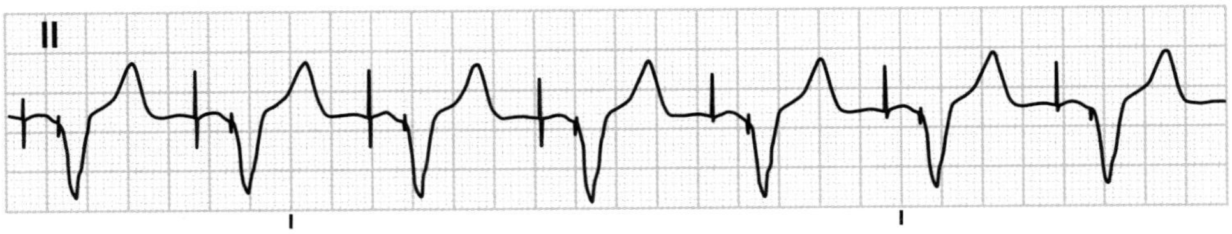

FIGURE 18-74 Dual-chamber (atrioventricular sequential) pacemaker rhythm.

Reproduced from *Arrhythmia Recognition: The Art of Interpretation*, courtesy of Tomas B. Garcia, MD.

which synchronizes the right and left ventricles' contraction, is used to treat patients with severe or moderately severe heart failure.

Pacemakers are available in two rate types. A fixed-rate pacemaker, which is seldom used today, generates a pacing impulse at a preprogrammed rate. In contrast, a demand pacemaker is equipped with a sensor that detects the rate of spontaneous cardiac depolarization. It generates a paced impulse only when it senses that the patient's heart rate has dropped below a predetermined rate (usually 60 beats/min) **FIGURE 18-75**.

Implanted Pacemaker Malfunction

Occasionally, a pacemaker fails. If the patient's pacemaker is failing, the pacemaker spikes may still be visible, but a QRS complex will not follow them. This failure to capture indicates the pacemaker is not operating properly. Failure to capture may occur if the wire connecting the pacemaker to the patient's heart dislodges. It may also occur because of battery depletion or ventricular perforation.

Failure to pace is a pacemaker malfunction indicated on the ECG by the absence of pacemaker spikes at expected times. Possible causes of failure to pace include pulse generator failure, a broken lead wire or dislodged lead, a disconnected wire or cable, or battery depletion.

Failure to sense is a malfunction in which the pacemaker competes with the patient's intrinsic rhythm. Pulse generator failure, a broken lead wire or dislodged lead, an excessively high sensitivity setting, or battery depletion can all cause undersensing. Undersensing is indicated on the ECG by the appearance of pacemaker spikes within the P wave, QRS complex, or T wave. Because pacemaker spikes occur inappropriately, this type of pacemaker malfunction poses a threat of VT or VF caused by pacemaker spikes occurring during the vulnerable period of the cardiac cycle.

When oversensing occurs, the pacemaker fails to generate an impulse because it has sensed extraneous signals (often muscular) and misinterpreted them as QRS complexes. It is indicated on the ECG by the occurrence of pacemaker spikes at a rate slower than the pacemaker's preset rate, or by the absence of paced beats even though the pacemaker's preset rate is faster than the patient's rate.

Another type of pacemaker failure is the so-called runaway pacemaker. A runaway pacemaker is indicated by a very tachycardic pacemaker rhythm that must be slowed to preserve the patient's cardiac function. Placing a strong magnet over the pacemaker will usually reset a runaway pacemaker. This recalibration would be done in the ED by a cardiologist.

If any of these malfunctions occur, the patient's heartbeat will depend on a natural pacemaker (usually the ventricles), causing significantly reduced CO. In such cases, TCP may be required to support the patient's CO until the pacemaker can be replaced.

12-Lead ECGs

For rhythm interpretation and identification of lethal rhythms, a single lead, typically lead II, is usually sufficient. However, a 12-lead ECG is useful when you want to see views of the heart from several angles to localize the site of cardiac injury or to identify dysrhythmias and other cardiac abnormalities. Examples of other indications for using a 12-lead ECG include the following:

- Before and after electrical therapy (defibrillation, cardioversion, pacing)
- Chest or upper abdominal discomfort
- Electrical injury

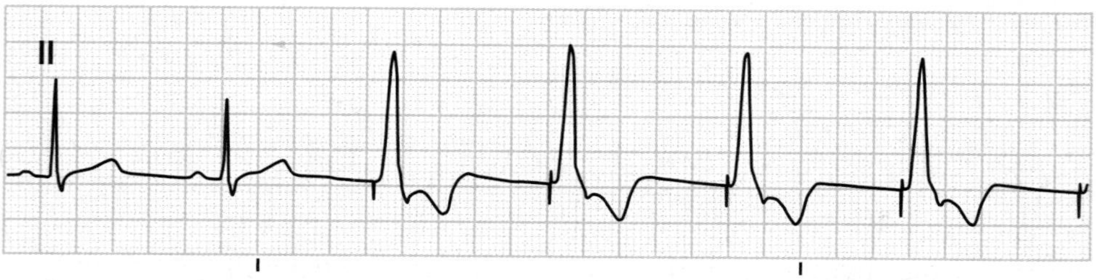

FIGURE 18-75 Ventricular demand pacemaker rhythm.

- Known or suspected electrolyte imbalance
- Known or suspected medication overdose
- RVF and/or LVF
- Post-syncope
- Stroke
- Syncope or near syncope
- Hemodynamic instability of unknown etiology

Devices capable of recording 12-lead ECGs contain interpretation software. Although this software is a useful tool and is generally very accurate in measuring intervals and durations, it has many limitations. When reading the ECG, it is best to rely on your interpretation instead of the automated findings. Think of automated interpretation software as a nudge or hint about what may be happening in the patient's heart, rather than as a definitive conclusion. Most devices can also transmit ECGs to the medical facility, allowing ED physicians to review the ECG before your arrival and prepare specialized resources in advance.

Acquisition Modes

The ECG device can record tracings using various electromagnetic frequency ranges in either of two acquisition modes: monitor mode or diagnostic mode. For rhythm interpretation, the ECG is recorded in monitor mode. This mode employs electronic filters to remove artifact and other unwanted information from the tracing. Unfortunately, monitor mode can also skew the shape and location of the ST segment and T wave. Monitor mode captures electrical information within the range of 1 to 30, 40, 100, or 150 hertz (Hz).

Diagnostic mode, the other acquisition mode, filters out very little electrical information, so more artifact may appear on the tracing. A bandwidth of 0.05 to 150 Hz is used for diagnostic ECGs, and the 12-lead ECG machine's interpretive analysis is performed using this bandwidth. Diagnostic mode is the default mode used to record a 12-lead ECG, and it cannot be changed. Many devices enable users to record 3-lead ECGs in diagnostic mode as well. However, the 3-lead ECG is usually acquired in the early minutes of patient contact, when there tends to be a lot of movement. The resulting crosstalk can create substantial artifact on the tracing, making it impossible to interpret the rhythm. Note that the frequency range is always printed near the bottom of the ECG tracing **FIGURE 18-76**.

FIGURE 18-76 The electromagnetic frequency range is printed near the bottom of the electrocardiogram (ECG). Diagnostic mode is always used in 12-lead ECG tracings.

Lead Placement

The best way to learn how to record a 12-lead ECG is to practice with the actual equipment. When positioning the electrodes, don't allow the patient to become chilled because shivering will produce artifact in the ECG tracing. **SKILL DRILL 18-6** outlines the steps in 12-lead ECG acquisition.

Approach to 12-Lead ECG Interpretation

Like dysrhythmia interpretation, 12-lead ECG interpretation requires a systematic approach to ensure nothing is missed. A seven-step method to 12-lead ECG interpretation is described here:

1. Review the snapshot.
2. Interpret the dysrhythmia.
3. Determine the axis.
4. Identify conduction system disturbances.
5. Evaluate chamber size.
6. Review for zones of ischemia, injury, and infarction.
7. Identify noncardiac causes.

Review the Snapshot

First, look at the tracing to see if anything stands out. For example, is the heart rate extremely slow or fast? This step is a quick overall look at the 12-lead ECG to see if all the leads printed, if artifact is present, and if the rate is at either extreme.

Interpret the Dysrhythmia

This interpretation relies on the same five-step process presented earlier in the chapter. Use these rules to identify the underlying rhythm:

1. Identify the waves (P-QRS-T).
2. Measure the PRI.
3. Measure the QRS duration.
4. Determine rhythm regularity.
5. Measure the heart rate.

Skill Drill 18-6 Acquiring a 12-lead ECG

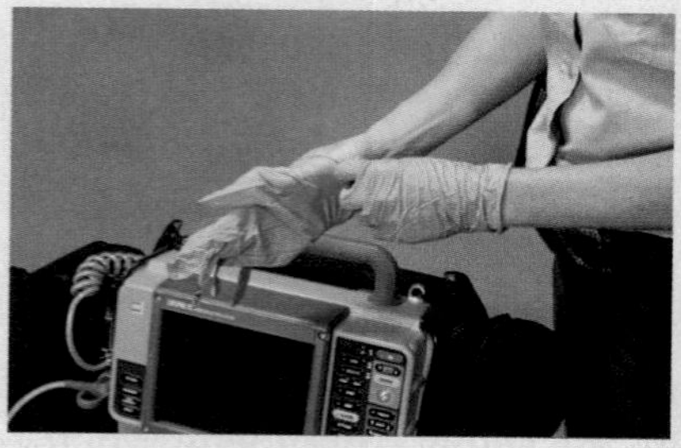

Step 1

Take standard precautions. Check your equipment. Ensure the ECG cable's end has no loose pins and the cable or lead wires are intact. Ensure the monitor has an adequate paper supply. Connect the ECG cable to the machine. Connect the lead wires to the ECG cable (if not already connected).

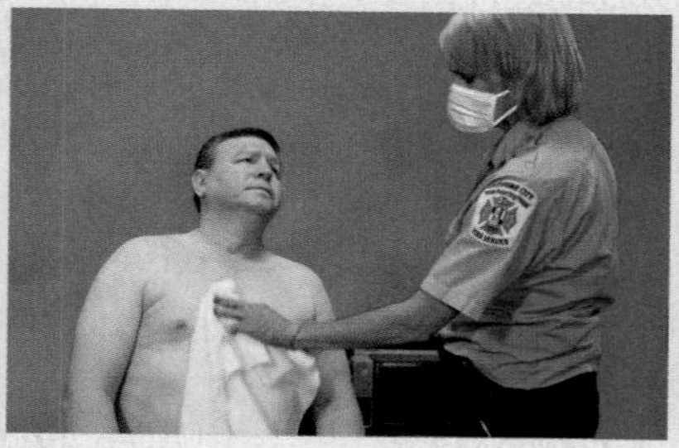

Step 2

Explain the procedure to the patient. Prepare the patient's skin for electrode placement; shave and cleanse the patient's skin as needed before placing the monitoring electrodes.

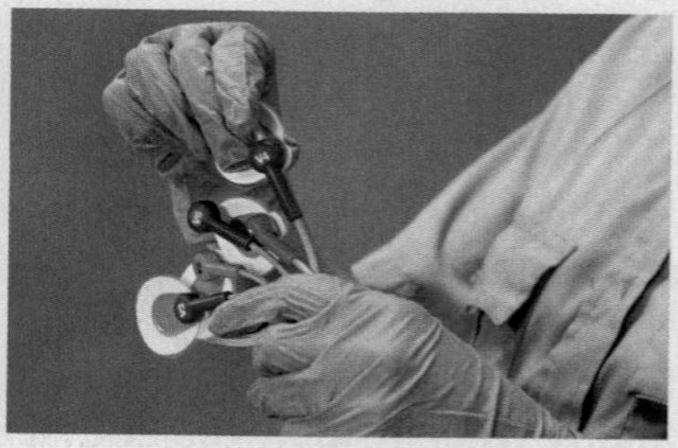

Step 3

Attach the electrodes to the leads before you place them on the patient.

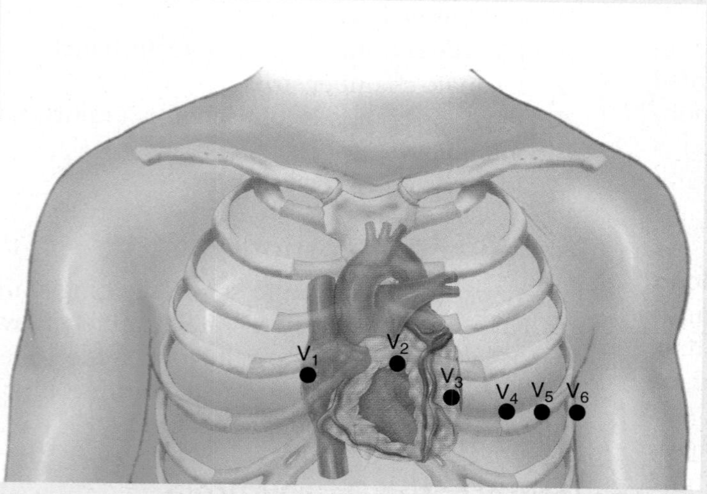

Step 4

Position the electrodes on the patient. Connect the four limb electrodes, and place them on the patient's arms and legs. Do not place the electrodes on the trunk of the body, as is sometimes done for ECG monitoring. Double-check to confirm the correct electrode has been positioned on each limb (the LA electrode on the left arm, the RA electrode on the right arm, and so on).

Once the limb electrodes have been secured, connect and apply the electrodes for the precordial leads:

V_1—Right of the sternum, fourth ICS
V_2—Left of the sternum, fourth ICS
V_3—Precisely between leads V_2 and V_4
V_4—Left midclavicular line, fifth ICS
V_5—Left anterior axillary line at the level of lead V_4
V_6—Left midaxillary line at the level of lead V_4

Skill Drill 18-6 Acquiring a 12-lead ECG (continued)

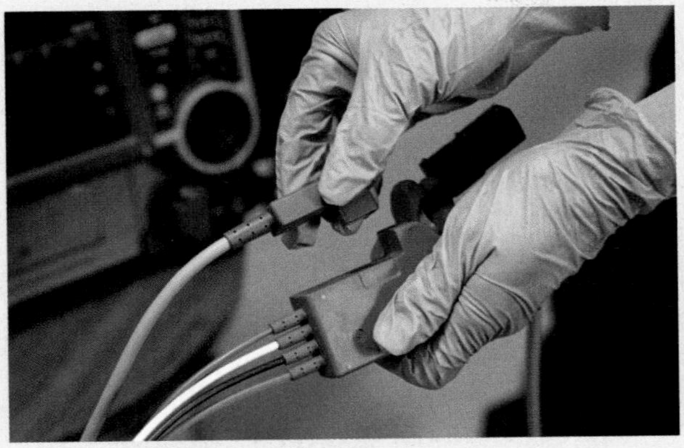

Step 5

Connect the cables to the monitor. Ensure the patient is sitting or lying still, the extremities are not crossed, and the patient is breathing normally and not talking. Turn on the power to the monitor and adjust the screen contrast if necessary. Ensure that all electrodes and cables are still connected and that no error message is displayed.

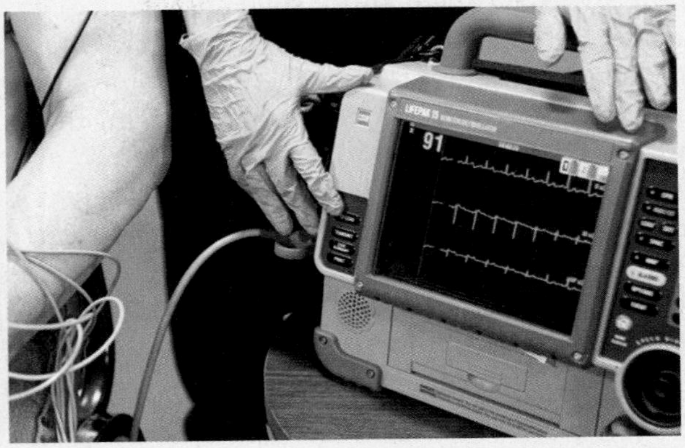

Step 6

Press the *12-Lead Analyze* button.

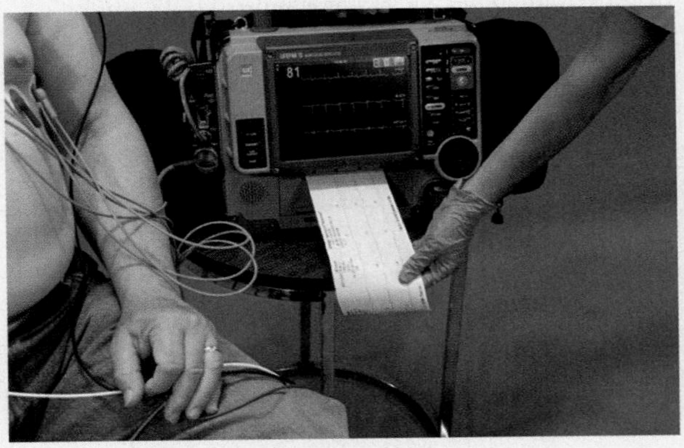

Step 7

Obtain the 12-lead ECG recording.

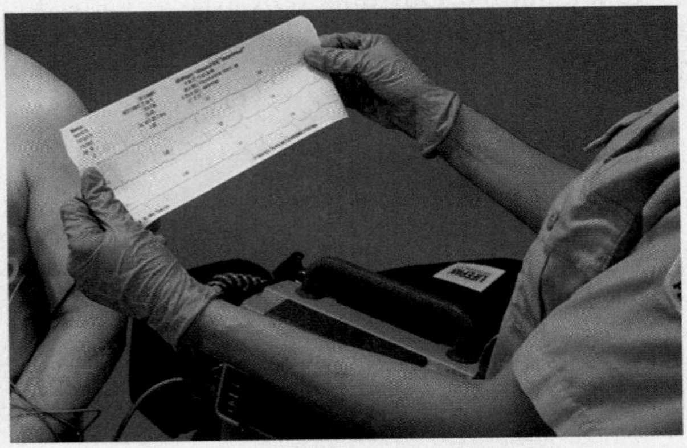

Step 8

Examine the tracing for acceptable quality. Interpret the 12-lead ECG, label it, and determine whether additional views of the right and posterior walls (15- or 18-lead tracings) are needed. Obtain a 12-lead ECG every 5 to 10 minutes in high-risk patients and post treatment.

Determine the Axis

Every myocyte emits a small electrical charge when it depolarizes. A vector, which is often illustrated using an arrow, is a quantity, such as force, that has both magnitude and direction. The **QRS axis** is a single vector that represents the mean (or average) of all vectors created by the ventricles during depolarization **FIGURE 18-77**.

A positive QRS deflection in lead I means the vector is heading toward the left arm, whereas a negative QRS deflection indicates the vector is heading toward the right arm **FIGURE 18-78**. A positive QRS deflection in lead aVF means the vector is moving toward the feet, whereas a negative QRS deflection indicates the vector is moving toward the head **FIGURE 18-79**.

Axis deviation refers to the movement of the QRS axis to the right or left of its normal position. Although axis deviation provides an important clue about electrical activity in the heart, it is not sensitive or specific to any particular diagnosis. Instead, clinicians use it in combination with other information to determine what is happening in the heart.

You can use several methods to determine the QRS axis. The easiest and fastest method entails creating a simple four-quadrant system using the QRS complexes in leads I and aVF **FIGURE 18-80**. These two leads are used because they are the only perfectly horizontal and vertical leads, respectively. The quadrants represent the space through which the impulse can travel. The center of the quadrants is the point at which the two lines intersect and represents the origin of the impulse. To determine the

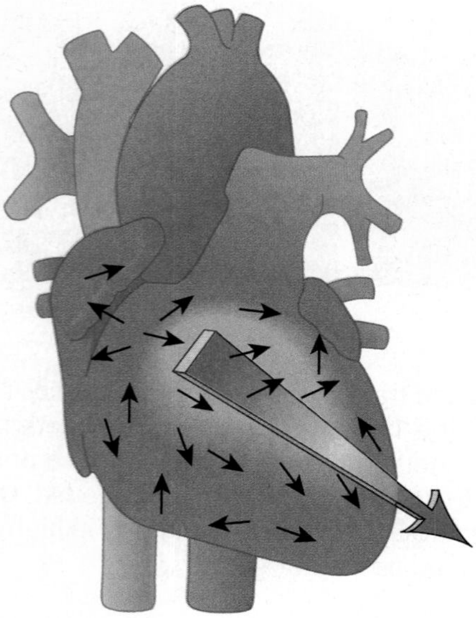

FIGURE 18-77 The QRS axis is the average of all ventricular vectors.

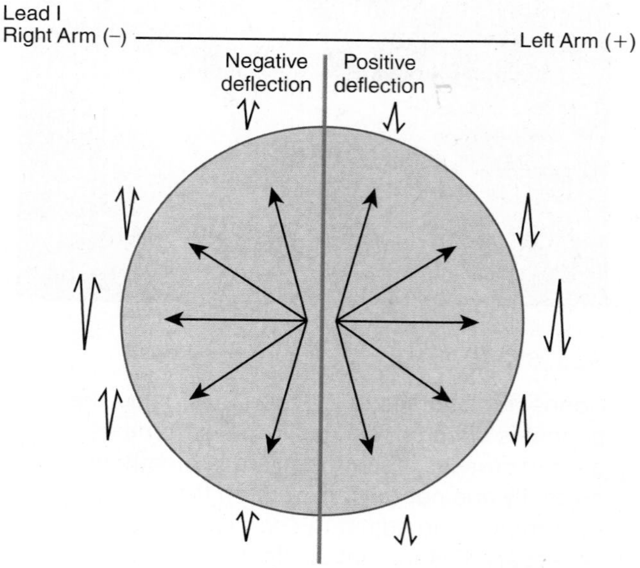

FIGURE 18-78 Viewed from lead I, the QRS will have a positive deflection if it is heading toward the left arm and a negative deflection if it is heading toward the right arm.

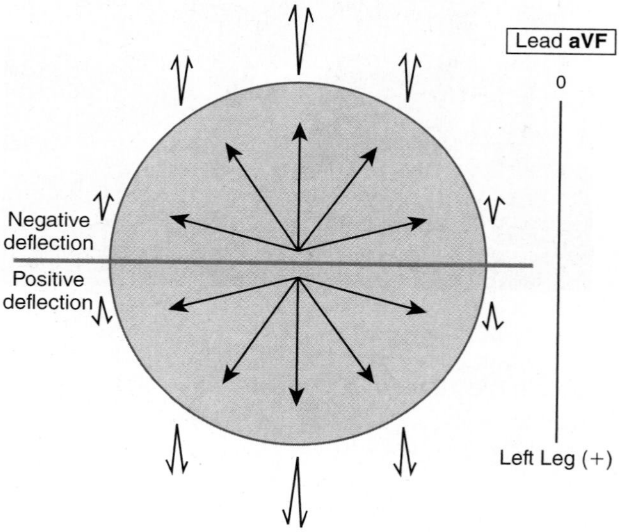

FIGURE 18-79 Viewed from lead aVF, the QRS will have a positive deflection if it is heading toward the patient's feet and a negative deflection if it is heading toward the patient's head.

QRS axis, use the direction of the QRS complexes in leads I and aVF.

First, look at the QRS complex in leads I and aVF and decide if it is positive or negative. If the QRS complex is positive in leads I and aVF, then the axis falls in quadrant 4 and lies between 0° and 90°. The normal QRS axis ranges from −30° to +90°, not 0° to 90°. This estimate of the QRS axis, however, is close enough. Left-axis deviation is present if the QRS complex is positive in lead I and negative in lead aVF. A negative QRS in lead I and a positive QRS complex in lead aVF suggest right-axis deviation. Finally, extreme right-axis deviation exists when the QRS complex is negative in leads I and aVF. **TABLE 18-7** summarizes how to determine the QRS axis using leads I and aVF.

Recall that the P wave represents electrical activity in the SA node, whereas the QRS complex indicates ventricular depolarization. Therefore, the direction of the QRS axis, or the axis deviation, corresponds to the ventricles' electrical activity. If one of the ventricles is enlarged (hypertrophic), it contributes more electrical energy than it normally would and the resulting electrical vector points in the direction of the hypertrophy. Conversely, an infarcted area is composed of dead tissue, which emits no electrical signal. Therefore, if a portion of the ventricle is infarcted, then the vector will point away from it.

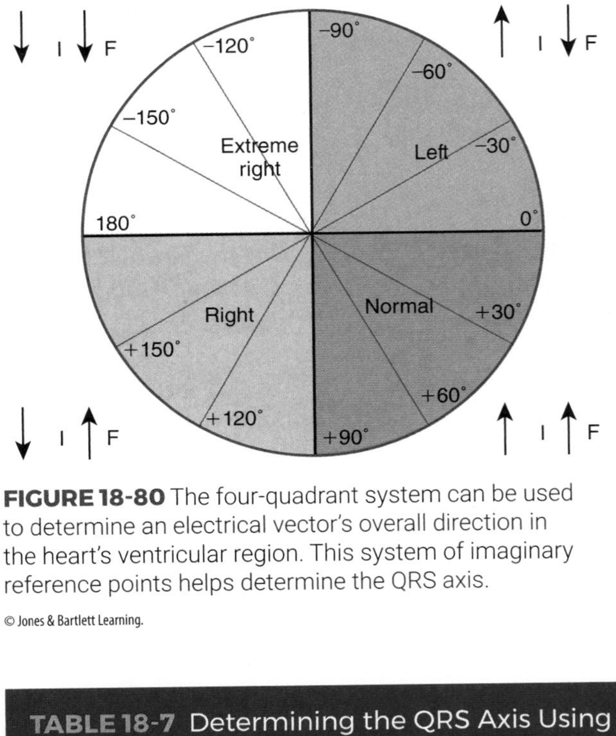

FIGURE 18-80 The four-quadrant system can be used to determine an electrical vector's overall direction in the heart's ventricular region. This system of imaginary reference points helps determine the QRS axis.

Identify Conduction System Disturbances

Next, look for conduction system disturbances on the 12-lead ECG. These include AV blocks and pre-excitation (discussed earlier in this chapter), the bundle branch blocks, and fascicular or hemiblocks.

Bundle Branch Block

Normally, the right and left ventricles depolarize at the same time. A QRS complex with a bizarre appearance and a duration of 0.12 second (120 milliseconds) or more signifies some abnormality in conduction through the ventricles. A **bundle branch block (BBB)** is a type of intraventricular conduction defect involving impaired conduction from the bundle of His to one or more of the bundle branches. A blockage at the level of the bundle branches affects the order in which they are activated, with the blocked bundle being the last to be depolarized.

Right bundle branch block (RBBB) and left bundle branch block (LBBB) are among the most common 12-lead ECG findings. The names of these electrical conduction abnormalities indicate where the electrical impulse is delayed. RBBB is characterized by a QRS complex duration of 0.12 second

TABLE 18-7 Determining the QRS Axis Using Leads I and aVF

	Lead I		Lead aVF		Position of QRS Axis
If	positive	*and*	positive	*then*	normal axis
If	positive	*and*	negative	*then*	left-axis deviation
If	negative	*and*	positive	*then*	right-axis deviation
If	negative	*and*	negative	*then*	extreme right-axis deviation

(120 milliseconds) or more and a terminal R wave in lead V_1 (the second half of the QRS complex terminates in an R wave) **FIGURE 18-81**. The QRS complex in lead V_1 typically appears as an rSR′ complex. (The ′ symbol represents an R-prime wave. An R-prime wave is never normal; it indicates trouble in the ventricular conduction system.) A terminal S wave also appears in leads I, aVL, and V_6.

LBBB is characterized by a QRS duration of 0.12 second (120 milliseconds) or more and a terminal S wave in lead V_1 (the second half of the QRS complex terminates in an S wave) **FIGURE 18-82**. Terminal R waves are also seen in leads I, aVL, and V_6.

The term RBBB or LBBB **aberration** describes the shape of the QRS complex in aberrantly (abnormally) conducted beats. For example, if a particular complex has an rSR′ shape, it is said to have RBBB morphology.

Fascicular Block (Hemiblock)

The left bundle branch divides into anterior and posterior fascicles. When these tissues become diseased or ischemic, one or both fascicles become unable to conduct electrical impulses, resulting in a **fascicular block (hemiblock)**. An anterior fascicular block is characterized by rS complexes in leads II, III, and aVF, and by qR complexes in leads I and aVL. A posterior fascicular block is rare and requires a diagnosis of exclusion. This kind of block is characterized by qR complexes in leads II, III, and aVF, and by rS complexes in lead I.

Descriptions of RBBB, LBBB, anterior hemiblock, and posterior hemiblock often mention the term *bifascicular block*. In a **bifascicular block**, two of the fascicles or conduction pathways are blocked. This combination can vary, producing different effects in different patients. The two blocked pathways might be RBBB with anterior hemiblock, RBBB with posterior hemiblock, or anterior hemiblock and posterior hemiblock (a combination known as *LBBB*). In a **trifascicular block**, all three components of the ventricular conduction system are blocked or impaired, but one still occasionally works to provide AV conduction.

QRS complexes in the precordial leads are said to have a **concordant precordial pattern** when they are all in the same direction. For example, if all the QRS complexes are upright in leads V_1 to V_6, then the QRS complexes exhibit concordance across the precordium. QRS concordance in the precordial leads can have several possible explanations, including improper lead placement, anterior wall MI, or VT.

Evaluate Chamber Size

The 12-lead ECG can also reveal the size of the heart's chambers. The right atrium is a small, thin structure

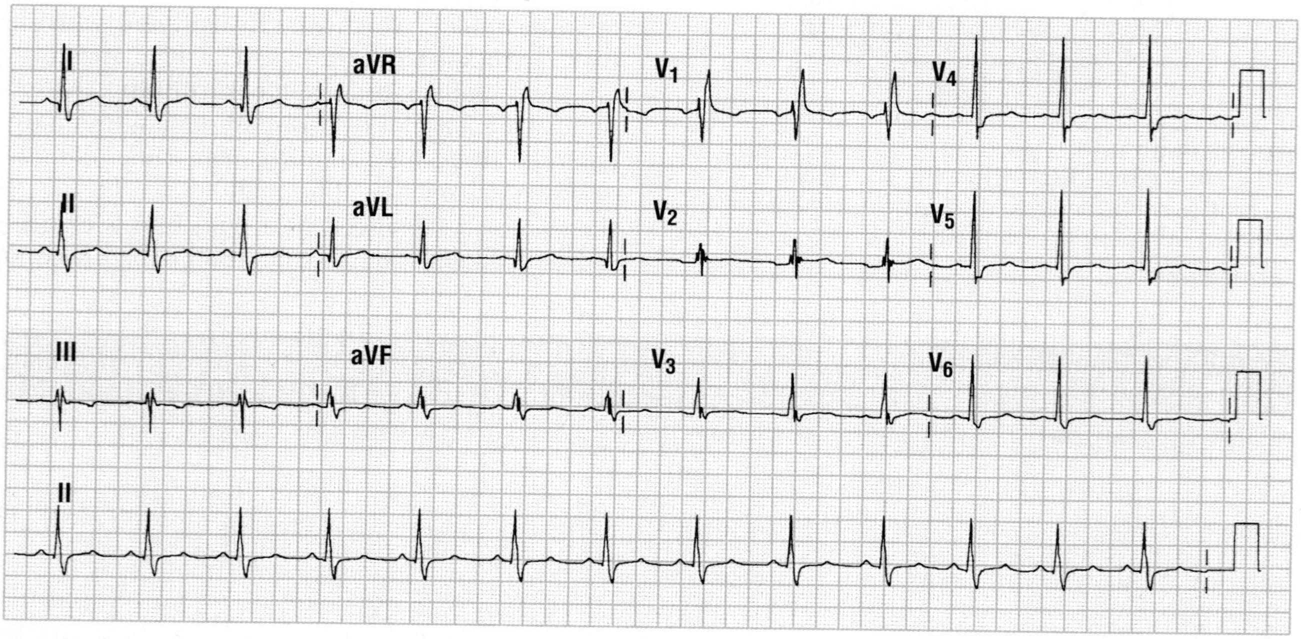

FIGURE 18-81 A 12-lead electrocardiogram showing right bundle branch block.

Reproduced from *12-Lead ECG: The Art of Interpretation*, courtesy of Tomas B. Garcia, MD.

designed to function efficiently in a low-pressure environment. If the returning venous pressure is elevated, or if pulmonary pressure is high, then the right atrium will dilate. **Right atrial abnormality**, formerly called *right atrial enlargement* or *right atrial hypertrophy*, is often associated with chronic pulmonary disorders. This abnormality is characterized by a P wave with an amplitude higher than 2.5 mm in lead II and/or higher than 1.5 mm in lead V_1 **FIGURE 18-83**. The duration of the P wave is usually normal.

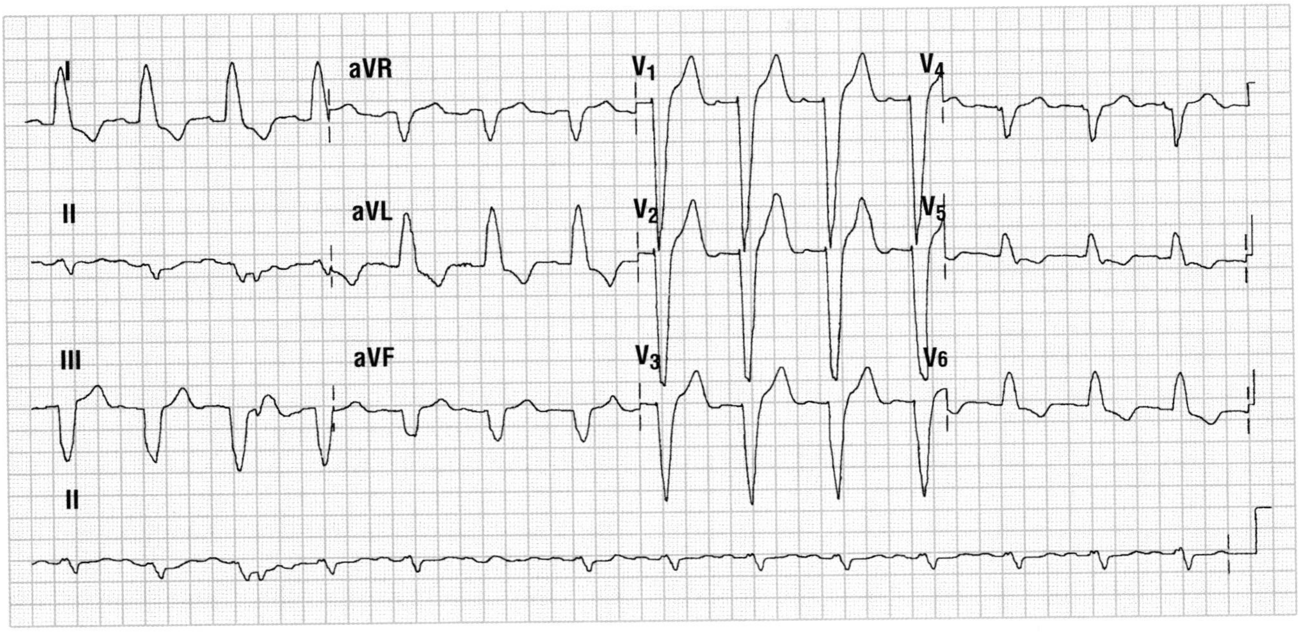

FIGURE 18-82 A 12-lead electrocardiogram showing left bundle branch block.

Reproduced from *12-Lead ECG: The Art of Interpretation*, courtesy of Tomas B. Garcia, MD.

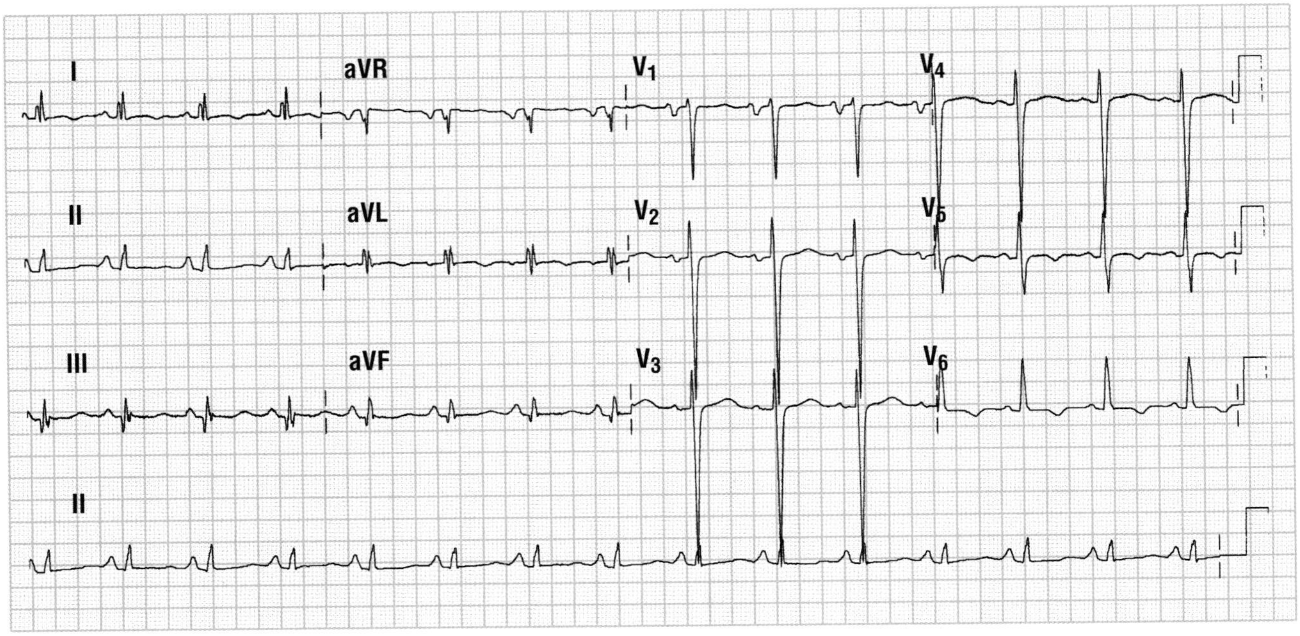

FIGURE 18-83 A 12-lead electrocardiogram showing right atrial abnormality.

Reproduced from *12-Lead ECG: The Art of Interpretation*, courtesy of Tomas B. Garcia, MD.

Left atrial abnormality is characterized by a P wave of normal height but prolonged duration, lasting 0.12 second (120 milliseconds) or more in lead II. A widely notched P wave may or may not be present **FIGURE 18-84**. Lead V_1 may show a biphasic P wave with a small initial positive deflection and a wide, negative terminal deflection. Left atrial abnormality may be seen in patients with valvular heart disease, particularly in those with mitral or aortic valve stenosis, hypertensive heart disease, cardiomyopathy, and CAD. It can also occur in an athletic heart.

In **right ventricular hypertrophy (RVH)**, the right ventricle becomes enlarged. This condition is usually caused by pulmonary hypertension. Normally, the R wave in lead V_1 is smaller than the S wave. An R wave that exceeds the S-wave height in this lead suggests RVH **FIGURE 18-85**.

In **left ventricular hypertrophy (LVH)**, the left ventricle becomes enlarged, most often due to systemic hypertension, although this condition can also arise with some cardiac abnormalities. The left ventricle becomes enlarged as the left ventricular wall thickens in response to the increased workload. The left ventricle will then lose elasticity and may fail to pump blood effectively, leading to heart failure. ECG criteria for identification of LVH are typically based on QRS voltages. A guideline commonly followed for adults older than 35 years is this: If the sum of the S-wave depth in lead V_1 and the R-wave height in either lead V_5 or V_6 exceeds 35 mm, then LVH should be considered **FIGURE 18-86**. LVH can produce tall R waves in lead aVL. An R wave with an amplitude greater than 11 mm in this lead suggests LVH.

Diagnosis of LVH is made by using an echocardiogram, not an ECG. It is inaccurate to say a patient has LVH if their ECG meets the criteria listed previously; it is more precise to say that the ECG meets the voltage criteria for LVH.

Review for Zones of Ischemia, Injury, and Infarction

Recall that ACSs are cardiac conditions precipitated by abruptly diminished blood flow through a coronary artery. Unstable angina, NSTEMI, and STEMI are the three major ACSs.

When a coronary artery becomes narrowed or blocked significantly, the tissue supplied by that vessel is deprived of oxygen and essential nutrients. Cells must resort to anaerobic metabolism, which results in acidosis. If this ischemic process is not interrupted, that is, if adequate blood flow is not

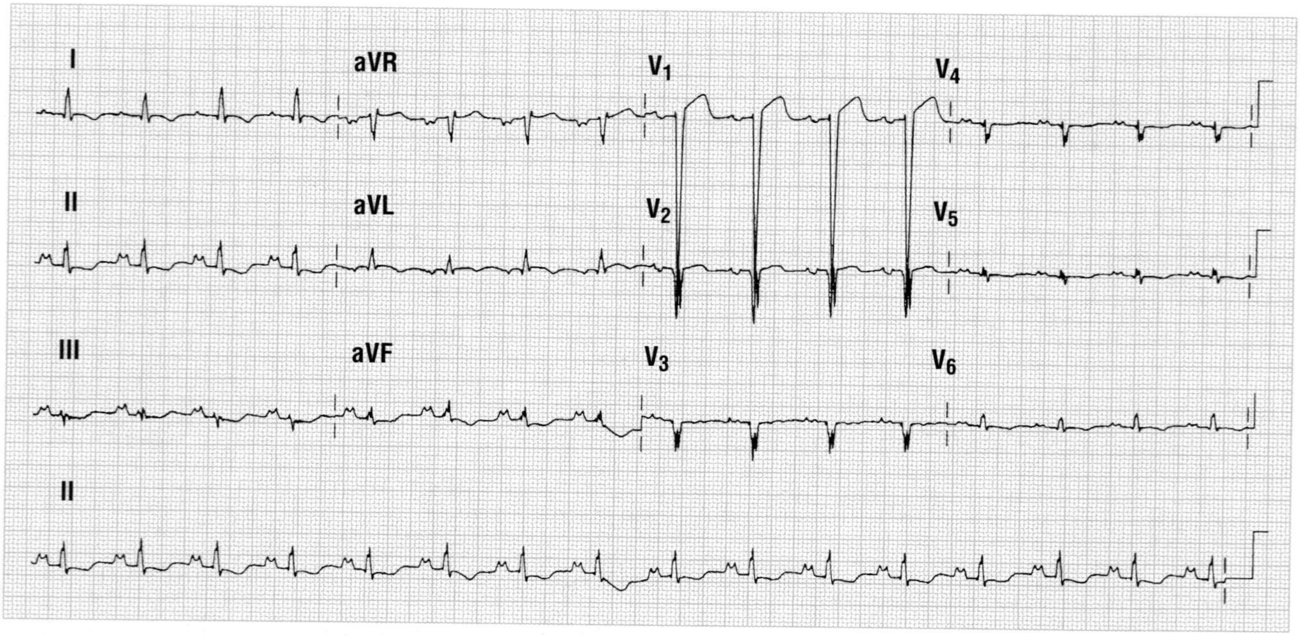

FIGURE 18-84 A 12-lead electrocardiogram showing left atrial abnormality.

Reproduced from *12-Lead ECG: The Art of Interpretation*, courtesy of Tomas B. Garcia, MD.

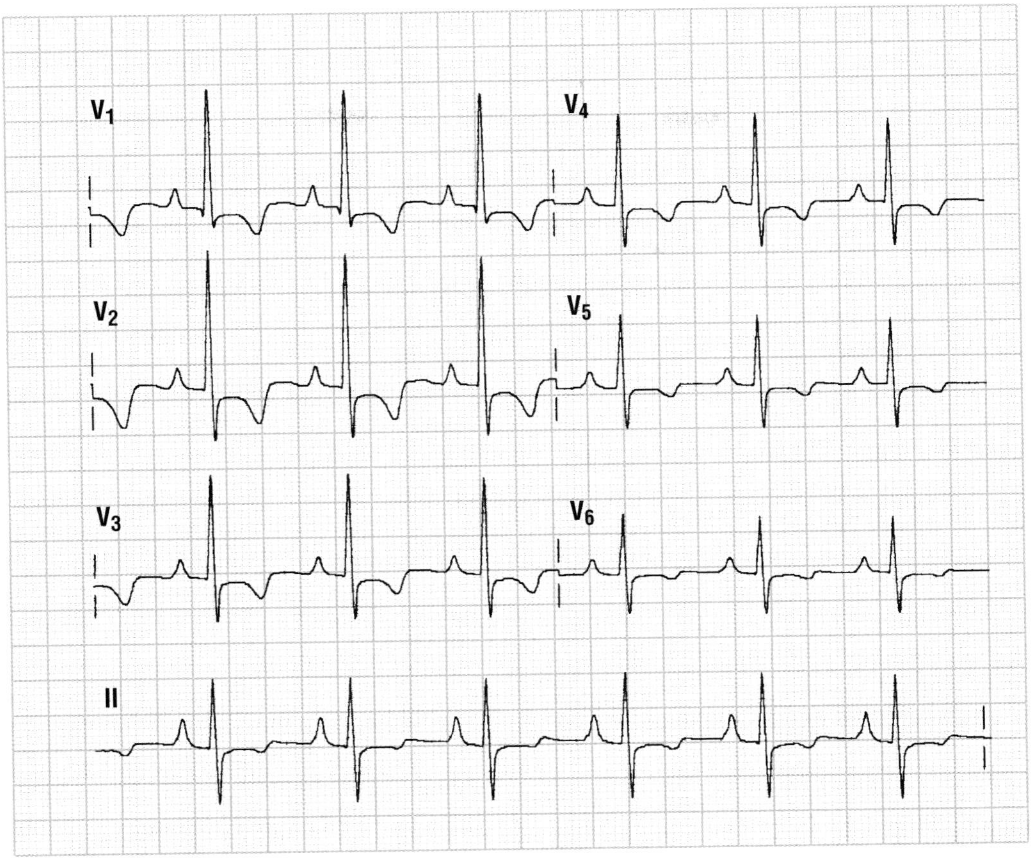

FIGURE 18-85 A 12-lead electrocardiogram showing right ventricular hypertrophy.

Reproduced from *12-Lead ECG: The Art of Interpretation*, courtesy of Tomas B. Garcia, MD.

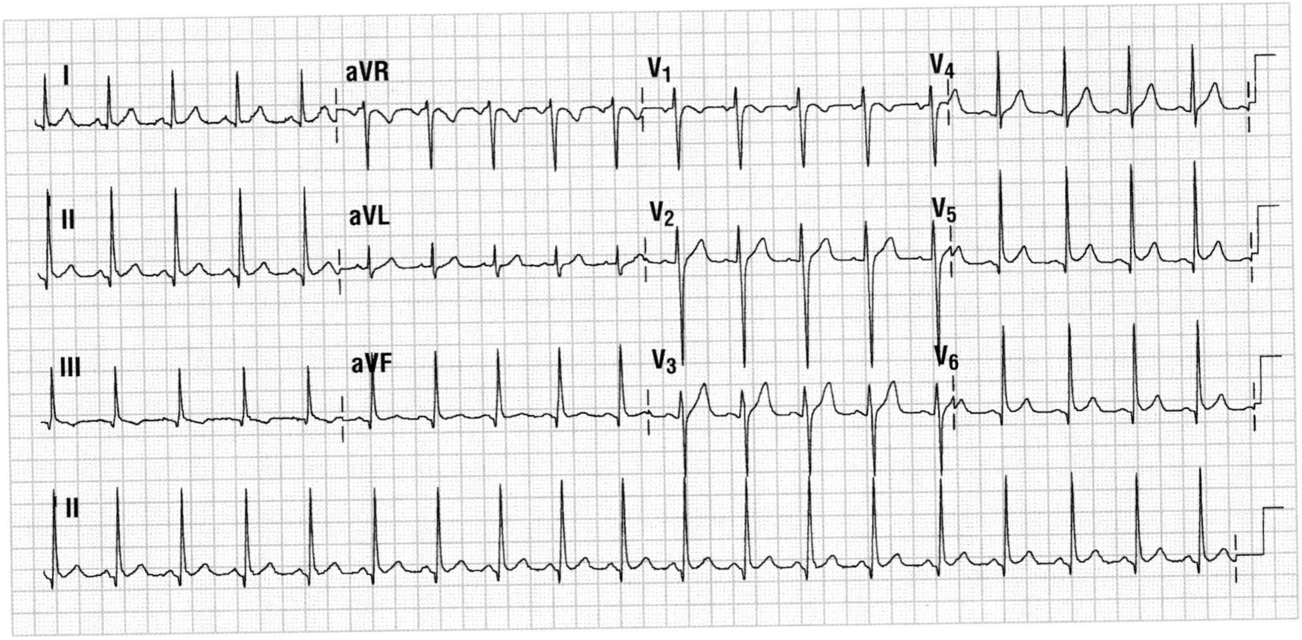

FIGURE 18-86 A 12-lead electrocardiogram showing left ventricular hypertrophy.

Reproduced from *12-Lead ECG: The Art of Interpretation*, courtesy of Tomas B. Garcia, MD.

restored, then signs of cellular injury will become evident. An *infarction* occurs when this ischemic process is not interrupted, resulting in tissue death. Because ischemia and injury are reversible processes, early recognition of ACS is critical in limiting heart tissue loss. Time is muscle.

When a coronary artery is blocked, the tissue it supplies undergoes characteristic changes that appear on the ECG in the leads facing the affected tissue. Ischemia is evidenced by ST-segment depression, and myocardial injury is evidenced by ST-segment elevation. Infarction may or may not be demonstrated by the appearance of pathologic Q waves. ST-segment depression of 0.5 mm or more in two or more contiguous leads in a patient with chest pain or discomfort indicates unstable angina or NSTEMI.[18] For leads V_2 and V_3, STEMI should be suspected if the ST-segment elevation is 2 mm or more in men 40 years and older, 2.5 mm or more in men younger than 40 years, 1.5 mm or more in women, or 1 mm or more at the J point in the other leads.[18] **FIGURE 18-87** shows the evolution of a heart from its normal state to ischemia to injury to infarction. An absence of ST-segment changes associated with an ACS presentation is referred to as a *nondiagnostic ECG.* Such a finding does not rule out acute myocardial ischemia, injury, or infarction, but merely means the tracing is nondiagnostic for those events. Serial blood work and additional testing are required to make a definitive diagnosis.

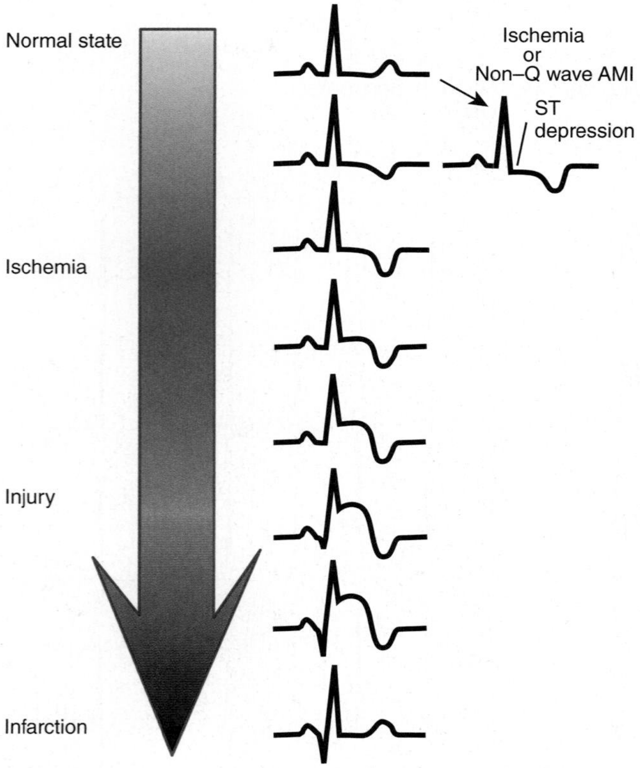

FIGURE 18-87 Evolutionary pattern of acute myocardial infarction.

Reproduced from *12-Lead ECG: The Art of Interpretation*, courtesy of Tomas B. Garcia, MD.

Because of its importance as a diagnostic tool, paramedics should acquire a 12-lead ECG within 10 minutes of patient contact for every patient who may be experiencing an ACS.[10] Treatment decisions are made based on the patient's presentation and history, the 12-lead ECG findings, and any laboratory test results (ie, cardiac biomarkers). For example, a patient with chest discomfort whose 12-lead ECG shows ST-segment elevation in two or more contiguous leads may be a candidate for immediate reperfusion therapy.

You must be able to correlate the patient's cardiovascular anatomy, including the areas supplied by each coronary artery, with the heart surface viewed by each ECG lead. Lead groups enable you to localize the ECG areas that show changes consistent with ischemia, injury, or infarction. **FIGURE 18-88** shows the colors associated with specific leads of the 12-lead ECG; each color corresponds to a specific heart surface. From this figure, you can see which leads provide views of the same area of the heart. For example, leads II, III, and aVF view the inferior wall. Lead aVR is not used for this purpose, so no color is assigned to it.

Reciprocal changes are mirror-image J-point, ST-segment, and T-wave changes seen on the ECG during an ACS. These ECG changes represent a location in the chest wall opposite the infarction. For example, if ST-segment elevation is present in a lead, then ST-segment depression and T-wave inversion are often seen in the reciprocal leads. The presence of reciprocal changes is evidence of AMI; however, the absence of such changes is not diagnostic. **TABLE 18-8** summarizes the heart surfaces, the facing leads, the leads likely to show reciprocal changes, and the coronary artery most likely to be affected.

FIGURE 18-89 shows an inferior infarction. An example of an anteroseptal infarction is shown in **FIGURE 18-90. FIGURE 18-91** depicts a lateral infarction, and **FIGURE 18-92** illustrates inferior and right

I High lateral wall LV Cx	aVR	V_1 Interventricular septum LAD	V_4 Anterior wall LV LAD
II Inferior wall LV RCA or Cx	aVL High lateral wall LV Cx	V_2 Interventricular septum LAD	V_5 Low lateral wall LV Cx
III Inferior wall LV RCA or Cx	aVF Inferior wall LV RCA or Cx	V_3 Anterior wall LV LAD	V_6 Low lateral wall LV Cx

FIGURE 18-88 The surfaces of the heart viewed by each lead of a standard 12-lead ECG. The coronary artery that typically supplies each surface is also listed.
Abbreviations: Cx, circumflex artery; LAD, left anterior descending artery; LV, left ventricle; RCA, right coronary artery.

TABLE 18-8 Facing Leads and Reciprocal Changes

Location	Facing Leads	Reciprocal Leads	Coronary Artery Involved
Inferior wall of the left ventricle	II, III, aVF	I, aVL	RCA or Cx
Septum	V_1 and V_2	None	LAD
Anterior wall of the left ventricle	V_3 and V_4	None	LAD
Lateral wall of the left ventricle	I, aVL, V_5, V_6	II, III, aVF	Cx
Right ventricle	V_4R	None	RCA or Cx
Posterior wall	V_7-V_9	V_1, V_2	RCA or Cx

Abbreviations: Cx, circumflex artery; LAD, left anterior descending artery; RCA, right coronary artery

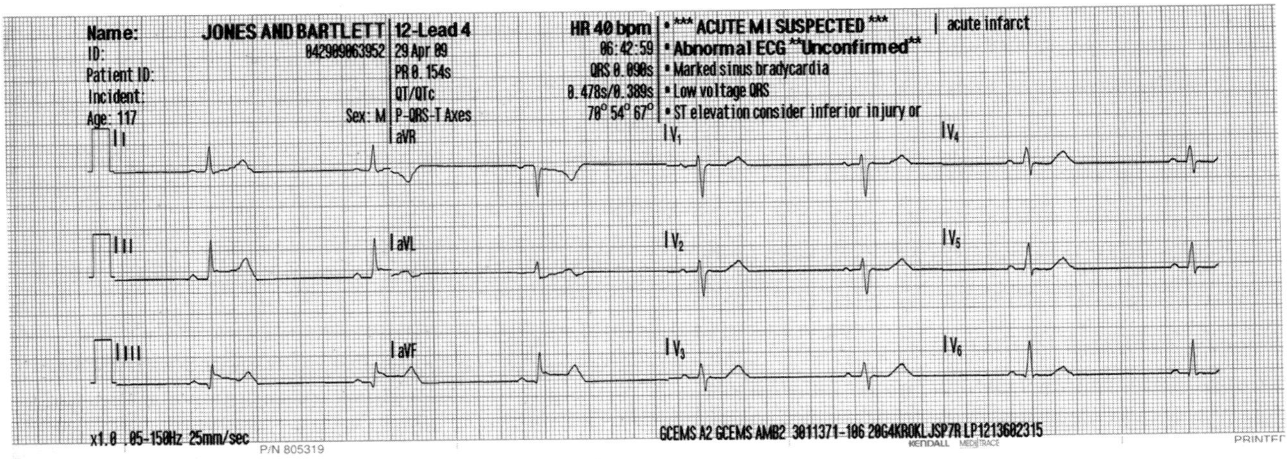

FIGURE 18-89 A 12-lead electrocardiogram showing inferior infarction.

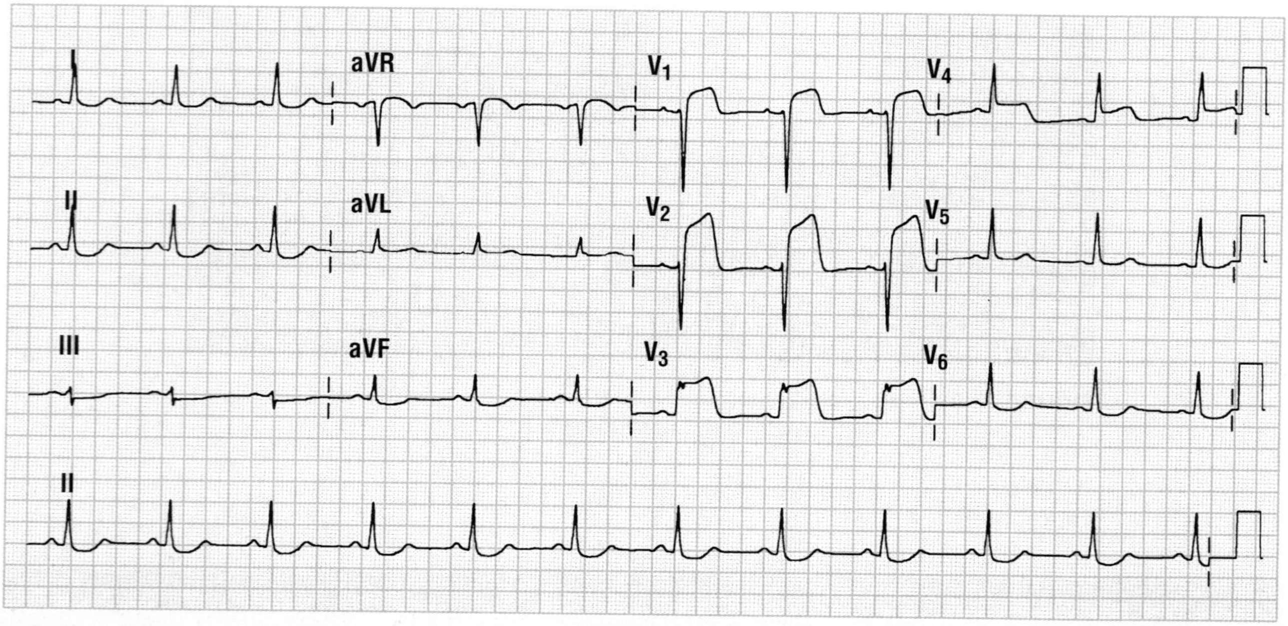

FIGURE 18-90 A 12-lead electrocardiogram showing anteroseptal infarction.

Reproduced from *12-Lead ECG: The Art of Interpretation*, courtesy of Tomas B. Garcia, MD.

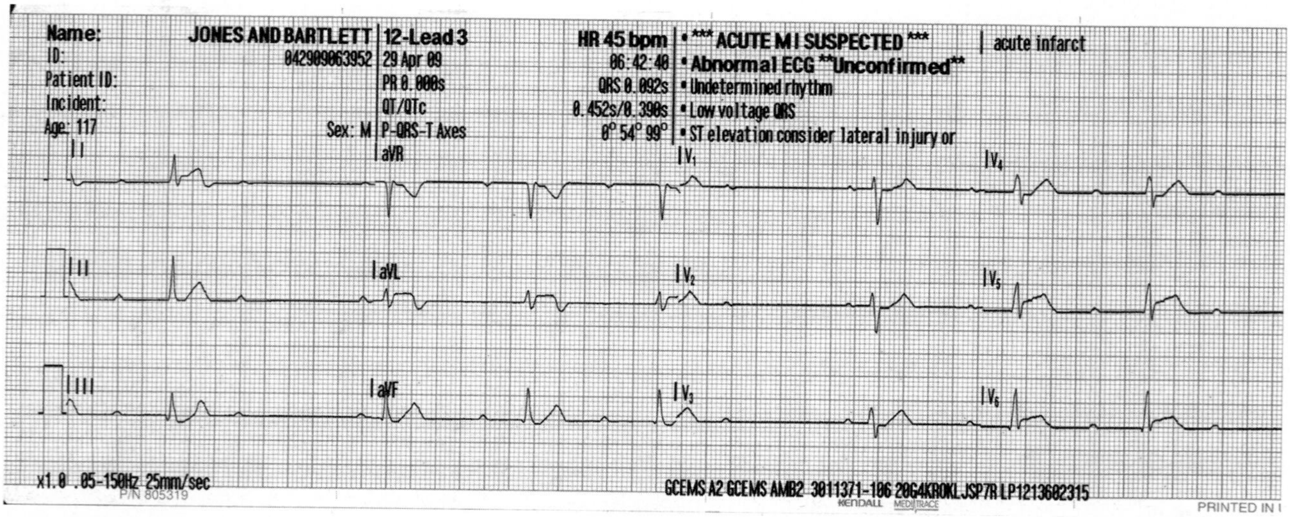

FIGURE 18-91 A 12-lead electrocardiogram showing lateral infarction.

Courtesy of Brian J. Williams.

ventricular infarction. Treating patients with an ACS is discussed in detail later in this chapter.

Other Cardiovascular Conditions

Benign early repolarization and pericarditis are two conditions that may produce ST-segment elevation, mimicking AMI. Benign early repolarization is characterized by ST-segment elevation, a J or fishhook appearance at the J point, and concave ST-segment morphology **FIGURE 18-93**. This pattern is thought to be a normal variant. Its diagnosis is almost always a coincidental finding made while recording an ECG during a routine physical exam or during testing for an unrelated condition. The changes are often seen exclusively in the left precordial leads (V_4 to V_6) and/or the inferior leads. Reciprocal changes are not seen in benign early repolarization.

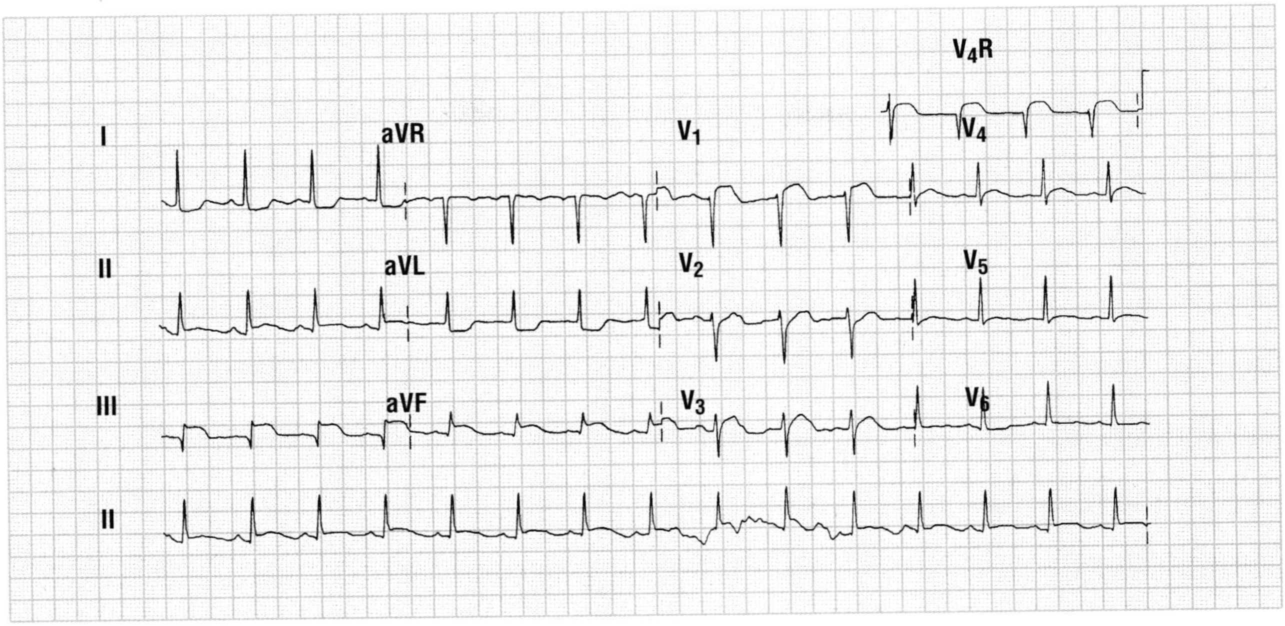

FIGURE 18-92 A 12-lead electrocardiogram showing inferior and right ventricular infarction.

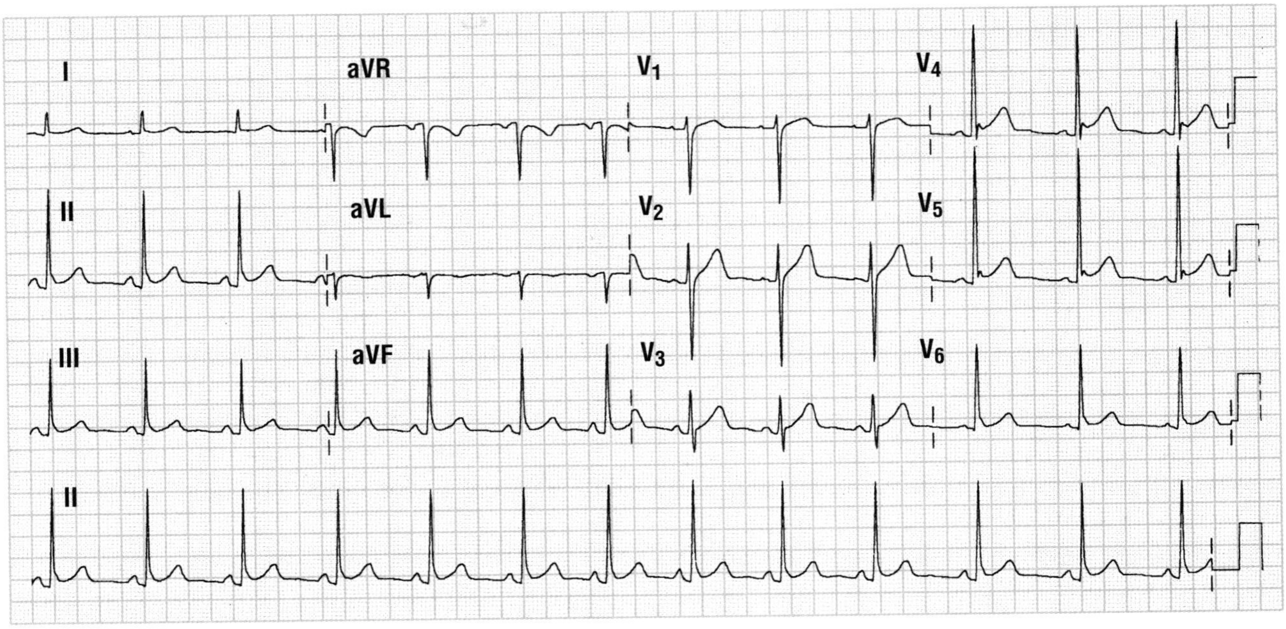

FIGURE 18-93 A 12-lead electrocardiogram showing benign early repolarization.

Pericarditis is the inflammation of the pericardial sac due to an infection (bacterial, viral, or fungal) or trauma. Patients can present with positional chest pain (which is often alleviated by sitting forward), shortness of breath, and history of recent infection or fever. The condition is characterized by ST-segment elevation (not exceeding 5 mm) present in multiple leads, a depressed or down-sloping PR segment **FIGURE 18-94**, a PR segment that is elevated or up-sloping in lead aVR, and a concave ST segment. Reciprocal ST-segment depression is not seen.

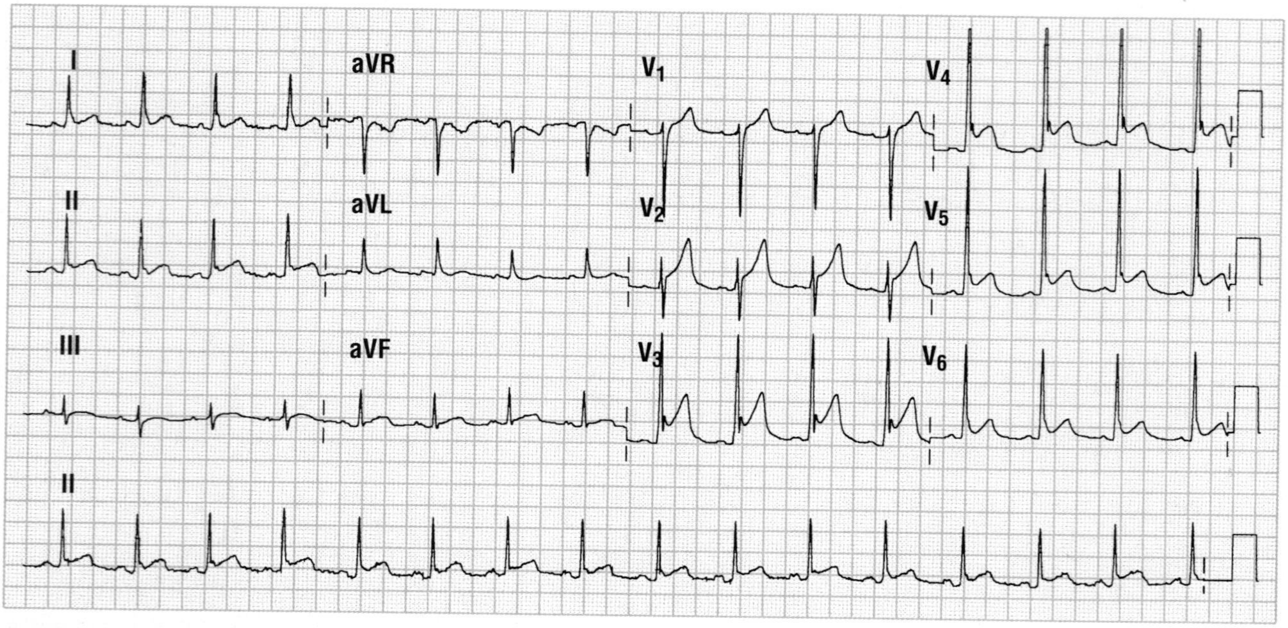

FIGURE 18-94 A 12-lead electrocardiogram showing pericarditis.

Reproduced from *12-Lead ECG: The Art of Interpretation*, courtesy of Tomas B. Garcia, MD.

Identify Noncardiac Causes of ECG Abnormalities

The 12-lead ECG can also provide information about noncardiovascular conditions, including pulmonary embolism, acute intracranial hemorrhage, electrolyte abnormalities, and genetic disorders that affect the heart's size or function.

Pulmonary Embolism

A pulmonary embolism, an obstruction in one or more of the pulmonary arteries, may also be identified on a 12-lead ECG. The criteria for suspecting a pulmonary embolism include the appearance of an S1Q3T3 pattern, new RBBB, and ST-segment depression in leads V_1 to V_3 **FIGURE 18-95**. The S1Q3T3 pattern refers to a deep S wave in lead I; a deep, narrow Q wave in lead III; and T-wave inversion in lead III. This pattern is sometimes seen in other conditions such as severe pneumonia, upper airway obstruction, COPD, asthma exacerbation, and pneumothorax. The absence of S1Q3T3 and RBBB on the surface ECG does not rule out pulmonary embolism, and it remains one of the most frequently missed conditions. It is crucial to perform a thorough physical exam and collect pertinent information about the patient's medical history, including any surgeries or medications, current health status, and family history.

Hypothermia

Patients with severe hypothermia may develop J waves (also called Osborne waves) on the ECG. The J wave is often a large, upright wave that appears on the terminal wave of the QRS complex. It may be accompanied by ST-segment depression and T-wave inversion. Generally, the more serious the hypothermia, the larger the J wave will be. The ECG of a patient with hypothermia also typically reveals a bradycardic rhythm and baseline containing artifact from shivering and poor electrode adhesion to cold skin **FIGURE 18-96**. Evidence of a J wave is only an indication of hypothermia; it is not enough to make a definitive diagnosis.

Electrolyte Imbalances

Electrolyte imbalances can also cause ECG changes. The two most common electrolyte imbalances involve potassium and calcium.

Hyperkalemia causes specific ECG changes. First, tall, peaked, asymmetric T waves develop. The P waves can become flattened and eventually disappear from the tracing. In severe cases, the QRS complex widens **FIGURE 18-97**. By contrast, hypokalemia usually presents with flat or absent T waves and a U wave **FIGURE 18-98**.

Hypercalcemia may produce a shortened QT interval, whereas hypocalcemia may slightly

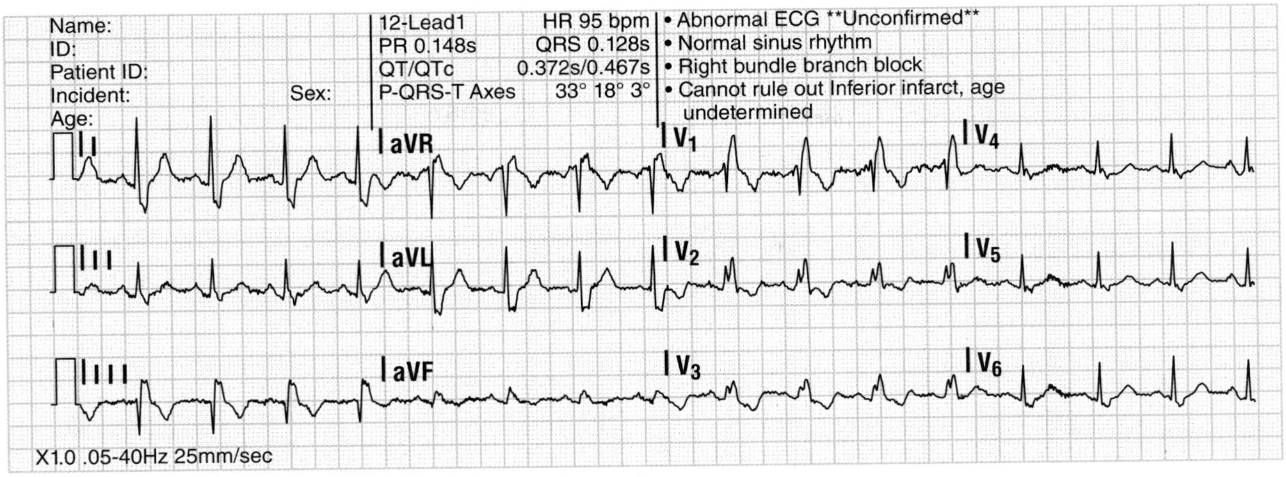

FIGURE 18-95 A 12-lead electrocardiogram showing pulmonary embolism.

© Jones & Bartlett Learning.

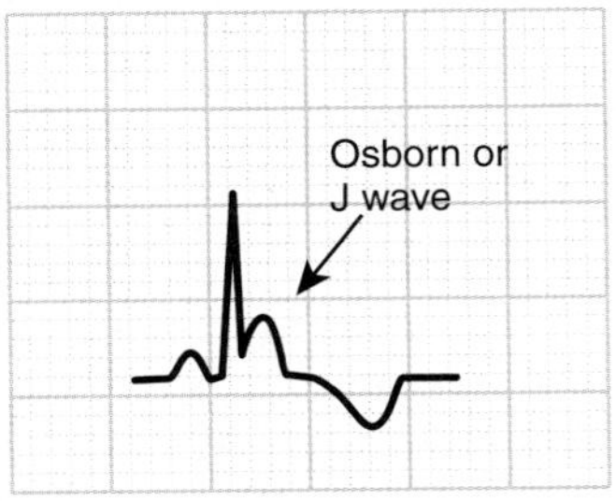

FIGURE 18-96 Osborne (J) wave.

Reproduced from *12-Lead ECG: The Art of Interpretation*, courtesy of Tomas B. Garcia, MD.

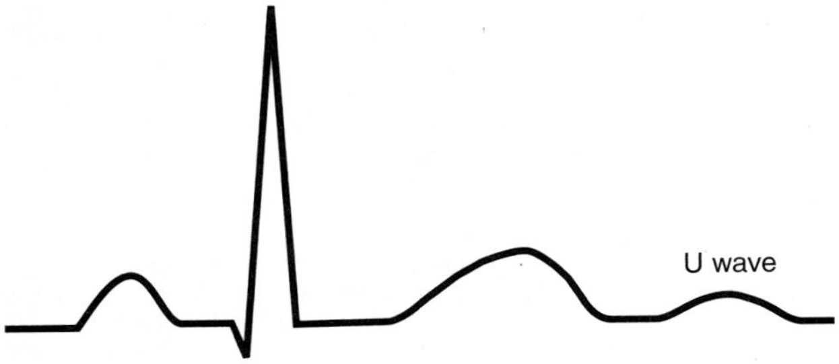

FIGURE 18-98 Hypokalemia.

Reproduced from *12-Lead ECG: The Art of Interpretation*, courtesy of Tomas B. Garcia, MD.

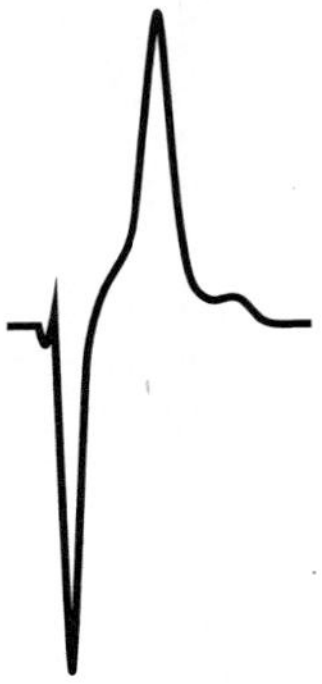

FIGURE 18-97 Hyperkalemia.

Reproduced from *12-Lead ECG: The Art of Interpretation*, courtesy of Tomas B. Garcia, MD.

lengthen the QT interval. The shortening or lengthening of the QT interval in hypercalcemia or hypocalcemia, respectively, is attributable entirely to the change in the length of the ST segment. The T wave itself is unaffected by changes in calcium concentration.

Cardiomyopathy

Cardiomyopathy is a disease of the heart muscle. The main types of cardiomyopathy are named for the types of muscle damage each causes: dilated, hypertrophic, and restrictive. With dilated cardiomyopathy, the heart muscle weakens, diminishing its ability to pump enough blood to the rest of the body. The pressure of the blood within the left ventricle causes the heart to enlarge and stretch. **Hypertrophic cardiomyopathy** is a genetic condition in which the myocardial wall becomes very thick. The greatest thickening tends to occur in the left ventricle. The thickened heart walls are stiff, which impairs ventricular filling. Inadequate filling can lead to left atrial enlargement and pulmonary congestion.

Patients with hypertrophic cardiomyopathy often experience shortness of breath, chest pain, or syncope. Such signs and symptoms are often associated with physical activity. Patients with this condition are often diagnosed in their 30s or 40s. In most cases, the disease is inherited; in the remaining cases, the cause is unclear or unknown. On ECG, hypertrophic cardiomyopathy is characterized by deep, narrow Q waves in the inferior leads and high lateral leads, and very tall R waves in the left precordial leads. These changes are similar to those seen in LVH **FIGURE 18-99**. The ventricular walls stiffen with restrictive cardiomyopathy because of abnormal substances deposited between heart muscle cells throughout the heart or because the heart's inner surface is lined with a layer of scar tissue. The rigidity of the ventricular walls hinders ventricular filling, and the heart eventually loses its ability to pump adequately.

Brugada Syndrome

Brugada syndrome is a rare inherited disorder involving the sodium channels in the heart. This condition is characterized by an RBBB pattern with ST-segment elevation in leads V_1 and V_2 (and possibly in V_3) **FIGURE 18-100**. Individuals of Asian

> **Words of Wisdom**
>
> Takotsubo cardiomyopathy, also called stress cardiomyopathy, is a temporary condition that can mimic AMI. Patients often present with chest pain or discomfort, ST-segment elevation, and elevated cardiac biomarkers, consistent with AMI. However, when they undergo cardiac angiography, the coronary arteries are found to be essentially normal. In some patients, weakening and ballooning of the left ventricular apex during systole has been found.
>
> This condition is often, but not always, associated with emotional or physical stress. Examples of triggers for stress cardiomyopathy that have been identified include the loss of a loved one, financial difficulties, relationship disagreements, earthquakes, lightning strikes, noncardiac surgery, seizures, trauma, anesthesia, and alcohol withdrawal. Although the exact etiology remains unknown, possible causes include spasms of multiple coronary arteries or stress-induced catecholamine release, among others. For most patients, normal heart function is restored within weeks of supportive therapy.

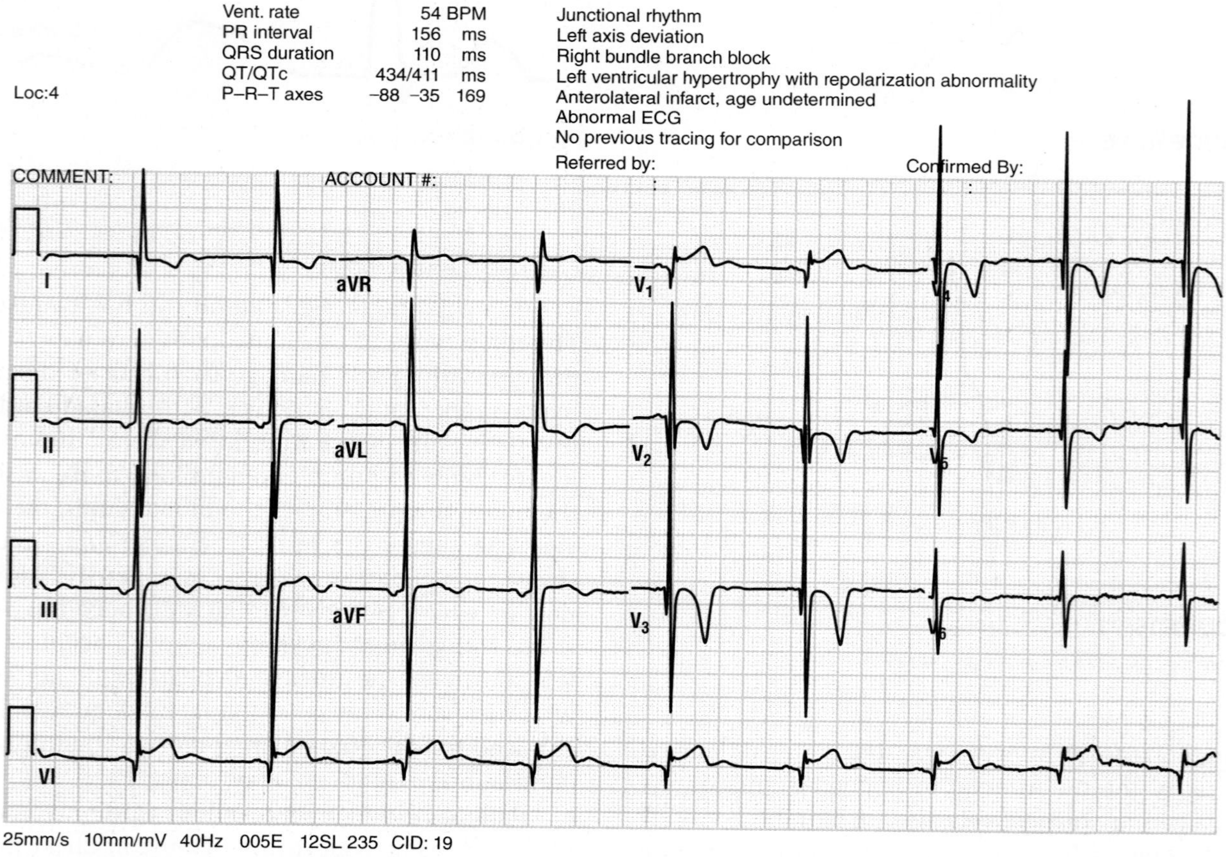

FIGURE 18-99 A 12-lead electrocardiogram showing evidence of hypertrophic cardiomyopathy.

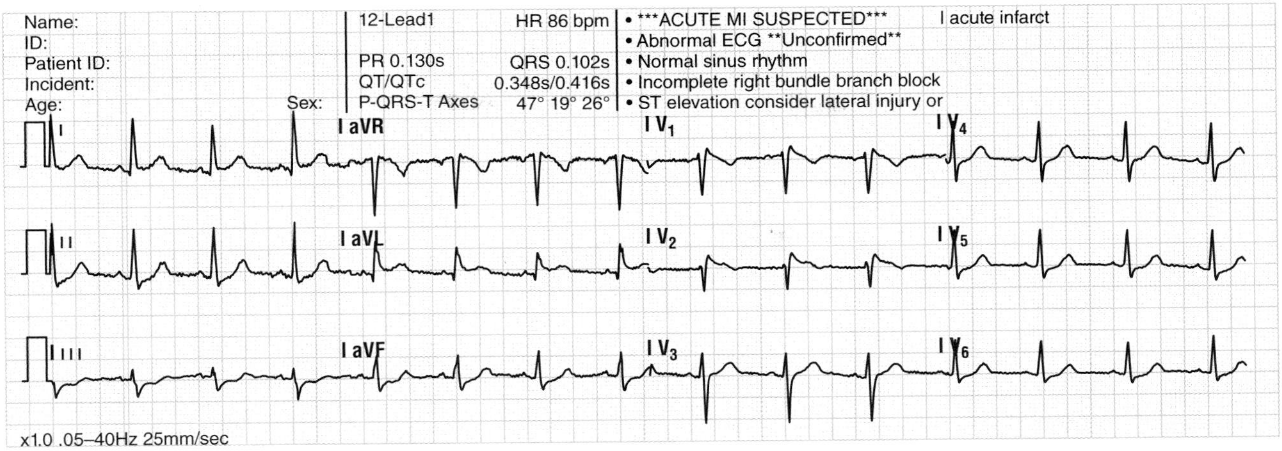

FIGURE 18-100 A 12-lead electrocardiogram showing evidence of Brugada syndrome.

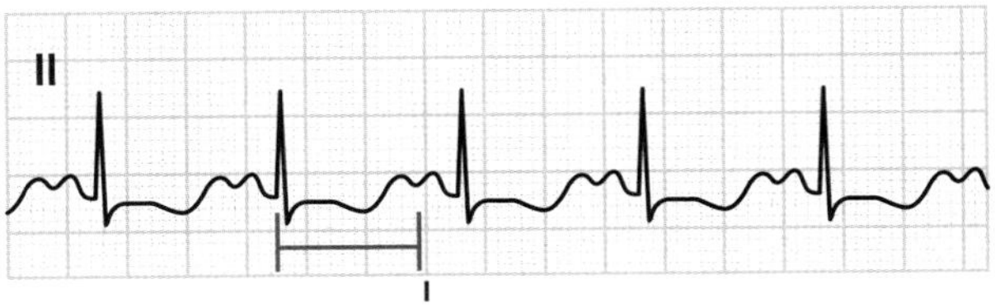

FIGURE 18-101 A 12-lead electrocardiogram showing long QT syndrome.

descent are at the most significant risk for this disorder, which occurs more often in young and middle-aged men than in women. Signs and symptoms can appear at any age, but usually develop during adulthood. Symptoms prompting medical care may include syncope, seizures, difficulty breathing, or SCA, which typically occurs during sleep. Although there is currently no cure for Brugada syndrome, treatment options may include the use of medications, catheter ablation, or an implanted cardioverter-defibrillator to help prevent sudden death.

Long QT Syndrome

Long QT syndrome (LQTS) is a repolarization abnormality characterized by a QT interval exceeding approximately 0.44 second (440 milliseconds) **FIGURE 18-101**. Patients with LQTS are at increased risk of developing ventricular dysrhythmias, such as torsades de pointes, a type of polymorphic VT. LQTS may be genetic, resulting from the mutation of several genes, or acquired. Acquired causes include AMI, electrolyte disorders, hypothyroidism, CNS injury (most often subarachnoid hemorrhage), hypothermia, and pericarditis. LQTS may also be caused by several medications, including antidysrhythmic medications (quinidine, procainamide), antipsychotics (lithium, phenothiazines), antihistamines (diphenhydramine), antibiotics (azithromycin), antidepressants (fluoxetine), and antiemetics (ondansetron, phenothiazines). Common symptoms include unexplained syncope, palpitations, or seizures. It is critical to record an ECG on all patients experiencing syncope, including younger patients.

Intracranial Hemorrhage

Intracranial hemorrhage can also cause ECG changes, although the mechanism by which these changes appear is not fully understood. Intracranial hemorrhage may cause deeply inverted, symmetric T waves in the precordial leads and a prolonged QT interval **FIGURE 18-102**. As a rule, patients with ECG changes resulting from intracranial hemorrhage almost always have neurologic symptoms or are unresponsive.

Pathophysiology, Assessment, and Management of Specific Cardiovascular Conditions

Epidemiology of CVD

CHD is the leading cause of CVD death in the United States.[2] Examples of cardiovascular diseases include angina pectoris, AMI, heart failure, hypertension, stroke, and diseases of the arteries.

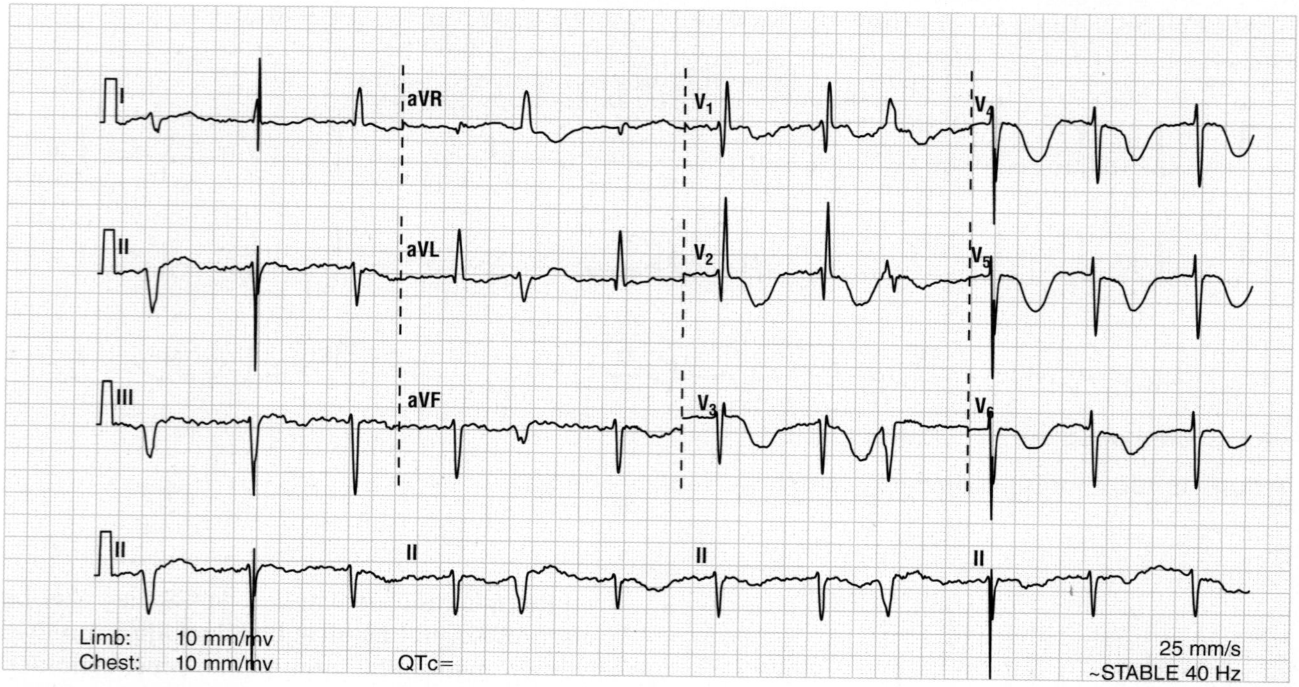

FIGURE 18-102 A 12-lead electrocardiogram showing deeply inverted T waves in a patient with an intracranial hemorrhage.

Acute Coronary Syndromes

The coronary arteries, of course, supply oxygen and nutrients to the myocardium. ACSs are characterized by an abrupt reduction in blood flow through one or more coronary arteries. If one of these blood vessels becomes blocked, then the muscle it supplies will be deprived of oxygen, a condition called ischemia. If the oxygen supply is not restored quickly, then the ischemic area of the heart muscle will eventually die. Such tissue death is known as *infarction.*

Etiology

The usual cause of ACS is the rupture of an atherosclerotic plaque. **Atherosclerosis** is of particular concern because it affects the inner lining of blood vessels, narrowing the vessels and reducing blood flow through them. The atherosclerotic process probably begins in childhood, when small amounts of fatty material are deposited along the inner wall (intima) of arteries. This usually occurs at turbulent blood flow points, such as where the arteries branch or where the arterial wall has been damaged. The streak of fatty material gradually enlarges, becoming a mass of fatty tissue called an **atheroma** or *atheromatous plaque.* This mass eventually calcifies, hardening into a lesion that infiltrates the arterial wall and diminishing its elasticity. At the same time, the expanding atheroma narrows the artery, decreasing the amount of blood flow through the **lumen**, the hollow interior space within the artery. The narrowed, roughened area of the arterial intima is an ideal site for forming a fixed blood clot, or **thrombus**, which may then obstruct the artery altogether. When such a clot forms in a coronary artery, it is known as a *coronary thrombosis.* In addition, calcium may precipitate from the bloodstream into the arterial walls, causing **arteriosclerosis**, a condition in which thickening and stiffening of the arterial walls greatly reduce the arteries' elasticity. Generally, obstructive CAD exists when an individual has stenosis of 50% or more of a coronary vessel; CAD is not considered to be present if there is stenosis of less than 20% in all vessels.[19]

Although obstructive coronary atherosclerosis and subsequent coronary thrombosis are the most common causes of myocardial ischemia, research shows that up to 50% of patients with stable angina who undergo diagnostic coronary angiography and 10% to 15% of those who present with ACS are found to have normal or near-normal coronary arteries.[19,20] In these patients, dysfunction of the coronary microvasculature (the smallest coronary arteries) may play an important role in causing myocardial ischemia.

Risk Factors for CHD

Risk factors are health conditions, lifestyle habits, and traits that may increase a person's chance of developing a disease. *Modifiable risk factors* can be controlled, modified, or treated, whereas *nonmodifiable risk factors* cannot be changed.

Examples of health conditions that increase CHD risk include diabetes, high levels of blood cholesterol and other lipids, high BP, and being obese or overweight.

- Diabetes increases the risk of CHD, cerebrovascular disease, peripheral vascular disease, and heart failure.
- A diet high in saturated fat, trans fat, and cholesterol increases the risk of atherosclerosis and heart disease. The level of serum cholesterol is at least in part a consequence of dietary intake of saturated fat. In populations with low fat intake, the incidence of CHD is also low. Furthermore, lowering the serum cholesterol level has been shown to reduce the risk of a heart attack. Cholesterol may also be controlled with medication, if necessary.
- High BP is a risk factor for heart disease, stroke, and end-stage renal disease. Hypertension cannot always be prevented or cured, but it can be controlled with diet and medication.
- Being obese or overweight is associated with an increased risk of CHD and developing other CHD risk factors, including high BP, diabetes, and high cholesterol. Weight reduction, using a sensible diet and increased physical activity, can bestow several lifelong and life-extending benefits. In particular, maintaining a healthy body weight can lower the risk of CHD.

Lifestyle habits that increase CHD risk include physical inactivity, excessive alcohol consumption, and tobacco smoking.

- People who are not physically active have a greater risk of CHD than those who participate in regular physical activity. Such activity improves overall fitness, cardiac reserve, and collateral coronary circulation. It can also help reduce stress.
- Excessive alcohol consumption can raise both BP and triglyceride levels. According to the US Centers for Disease Control and Prevention, women should limit their alcohol intake to no more than one drink per day and men to no more than two drinks per day.[21]
- Tobacco use increases the risk of damage to the heart and blood vessels, thereby increasing CHD and AMI risk. The chemicals in cigarettes increase levels of fibrinogen, promoting clotting. In addition, nicotine increases heart rate and BP. The good news is that smokers who quit return rapidly to the same risk level as nonsmokers.

Genetics and family history, increasing age, sex, and race are nonmodifiable risk factors that can affect a person's chance of developing CHD.

- A family history of heart disease increases a person's risk of developing CHD, particularly if a parent or sibling develops a heart or circulatory problem at an early age (younger than 55 years for men and younger than 65 years for women). Genetics also plays a role in other CHD risk factors, including high BP, diabetes, and obesity, and other CVDs, including heart failure, stroke, and AF.[2]
- Increasing age increases the risk of developing CHD. Generally, men are at greater risk of CHD than are premenopausal women, but a woman's CHD risk increases when she reaches menopause.
- In the United States, heart disease is the leading cause of death for African Americans, American Indians and Alaska Natives, and Caucasians.[21] African Americans are at greater risk of AMI, heart failure, stroke, and other cardiovascular events than are Caucasians, and CVD-related deaths occur earlier in African Americans than in Caucasians.[22]

Contributing risk factors are thought to increase heart disease and stroke risk, but their exact role has not been defined. Geography and socioeconomic status, stress, and some cancer therapies are examples of these risk factors.

- Geography and socioeconomic circumstances contribute to health disparities in the United States. Individual behaviors, including diet, exercise, and genetics, can contribute to these disparities. Additional factors include income, education, limited access to quality health care, a lack of insurance coverage, and communication barriers. Health system disparities include unintentional bias by health care providers and varying sensitivity to the needs and differences of patients from backgrounds that differ from their own.[22]

- Because every person manages stress differently, researchers are not sure how stress increases heart disease risk. It is clear, though, that hormones such as epinephrine are released during times of stress. The release of epinephrine accelerates the heart rate, raises BP, and increases the body's need for oxygen. Chronic stress exposes the body to persistent levels of epinephrine and increased BP. The body's response to stress can also worsen other risk factors. For example, a stressed person may be less active, overeat, start smoking, or smoke more than usual.
- Some cancer therapies, including chemotherapy medications and radiation treatments, may increase the risk of CVD.

Prevention

Education and early recognition are essential strategies to prevent CVD. Educating people about the risk factors of heart disease may decrease mortality and is an area of interest for EMS providers who are involved in community health promotion. **TABLE 18-9** lists methods to reduce CVD risk.

TABLE 18-9 Factors That Reduce the Risk of Cardiovascular Disease
• Awareness • Behavior modification • Blood pressure control • Cholesterol management • Diabetes management • Limit alcohol • Lipid management • Regular exercise • Smoking cessation • Stress management • Weight management

Angina Pectoris

The principal symptom of CAD is angina pectoris (literally, "choking in the chest"). Angina is the sudden pain that occurs when the supply of oxygen to the myocardium is insufficient to meet its demands. As a result, the cardiac muscle becomes ischemic, switching to anaerobic metabolism. This altered metabolism leads to the buildup of lactic acid and carbon dioxide.

Understanding the concept of "supply and demand" is crucial here: At rest, a person with heart disease who remains sedentary may have an adequate supply of oxygen to the myocardium despite some narrowing of the coronary arteries. However, when the same person exercises or experiences some other physiologic stress, blood flow to the myocardium may not satisfy the heart's increased oxygen demand; in that case, angina can result. Clearly, then, the patient with angina at rest, when oxygen needs are minimal, has more severe CAD than a person who reports angina only during vigorous exercise.

Stable Angina

Stable angina is episodic chest discomfort with a predictable location, intensity, and duration caused by myocardial ischemia. Symptom triggers may include emotional stress, exposure to extreme cold or heat, heavy meals, smoking, excessive alcohol consumption, and physical activity, such as climbing a flight of stairs or walking for a few blocks. The patient may report, for example, "Every time I walk up the hill to the bus stop, I get a squeezing pain under my breast bone, and I have to sit down for 2 or 3 minutes until it goes away."

Patients with chronic, stable angina often take NTG or some other nitrate agent to relieve anginal symptoms. NTG is supplied in several forms, including sublingual tablets, sustained-release capsules, a liquid that is sprayed under the tongue, an aerosol solution, a transdermal patch, and an ointment. Regardless of its form, NTG has a predictable effect in patients with stable angina, relieving symptoms within a few minutes.

ST-segment depression or inverted T waves may be observed on the ECG. These ECG changes usually resolve when the heart's oxygen demand is reduced to a level that can be supplied by the coronary artery (such as with rest) or when blood flow is increased by dilating the coronary arteries with NTG.

Unstable Angina

Unstable angina is more serious than stable angina. It is characterized by changes in the frequency, severity, and duration of pain and other symptoms. Other names for unstable angina include *preinfarction angina, crescendo angina, preocclusive syndrome, intermediate coronary syndrome,* and *ACS*. Unlike stable angina, unstable angina often occurs unpredictably. The patient may report that the anginal attacks have become more frequent and severe during the past several days or weeks, or the attacks may awaken the patient from sleep or otherwise occur when the patient is at rest. The anginal pain may or may not be relieved by rest or medications. Such attacks are often warning signs of an impending MI.

Variant Angina

Variant angina, also called Prinzmetal angina, is a type of angina caused by coronary artery vasospasm. It usually occurs at rest but may also be brought on by emotional stress, exertion, or cold weather. This type of angina can occur in patients with normal coronary arteries as well as in patients with CAD. Transient ST-segment elevation is often seen on the ECG. Symptoms may resolve on their own or with administration of NTG.

Microvascular Angina

Microvascular angina (MVA) is a type of angina caused by constriction or spasm within the walls of the heart's smallest coronary arteries. It often goes underrecognized and untreated because coronary angiography fails to show obstructive CAD or spasm of the epicardial coronary arteries. MVA is more common in women than in men and people with diabetes or hypertension. Chest discomfort may be more intense and prolonged with MVA, and it may take longer to resolve after the patient stops exercising or after the patient takes nitrates compared with other types of angina.[20] MVA may be accompanied by complaints of fatigue, shortness of breath, and sleep disturbances. ST-segment depression is usually seen on the ECG when episodes occur during exercise.[20]

Acute Myocardial Infarction

An AMI, or heart attack, occurs when a portion of the cardiac muscle is deprived of coronary blood flow long enough for portions of the muscle to die—in other words, to undergo **necrosis**, or infarct. The location and size of an MI depend on which coronary artery is blocked and where along its course the blockage occurs. Most infarcts involve the left ventricle. When the left ventricle's anterior, lateral, or septal wall is infarcted, the source is usually occlusion of the left coronary artery or one of its branches. Inferior wall infarcts are usually the result of RCA occlusion.

When the ischemic process affects only the inner layer of muscle, the infarct is called a **subendocardial myocardial infarction**. When the infarct extends through the ventricle's entire wall, it is described as a **transmural myocardial infarction**. The infarcted tissue is surrounded by a ring of ischemic tissue, an area that is relatively deprived of oxygen but still viable. This ischemic tissue tends to be electrically unstable and is often the source of cardiac dysrhythmias. The longer a segment of the myocardium remains ischemic, the less likelihood there is of salvaging the tissue and restoring its normal function. Thus, the sooner reperfusion therapy can begin after the onset of the blockage, the better the chances for saving the affected distal myocardium.

Patients with STEMI have ECG evidence of ST-segment elevation. As its name implies, NSTEMI produces no sign of myocardial injury (ST-segment elevation) on the patient's ECG. Distinguishing patients with unstable angina from those with AMI may be impossible during their initial presentation because the signs, symptoms, and ECG findings associated with these two conditions may be identical.

> **Words of Wisdom**
>
> For treatment purposes outside the medical facility, assume the patient with chest pain is having an AMI until proven otherwise.

Assessment

Time is muscle when caring for a patient experiencing an ACS, so you must rapidly and systematically assess the patient and provide necessary emergency care. Patient care goals include the following:[10]

- Identify quickly whether STEMI is present and, if so, notify the medical facility.

- Determine the time of symptom onset.
- Monitor the patient's cardiac rhythm and vital signs; be prepared to provide CPR and defibrillation, if needed.
- Administer appropriate medications.
- Transport the patient to an appropriate facility.

Symptoms

The most common symptom of an ACS is chest discomfort. Although some patients will have a history of angina, ACS will be the initial presentation of CAD in others.[7] A person with an ACS typically feels pain just beneath the sternum, variously described as heavy, squeezing, crushing, or tight. This pain may radiate to the arms (most often the left arm) and into the fingers; it may also radiate to the neck, jaw, upper back, or epigastrium. Ischemic chest discomfort is usually dull, rather than sharp, and is unaffected by deep inspiration, movement, or position. It may or may not be relieved by nitrates or rest. To convey the discomfort's squeezing nature, the patient may clench their fist and hold it against the sternum (Levine sign). Occasionally, a patient may mistake the pain of an ACS for indigestion and take antacids in an attempt to relieve the discomfort.

Not every patient with ACS will experience chest discomfort. Some have no chest pain, a phenomenon referred to as "silent MI." Others may present solely with dyspnea or with arm, shoulder, back, jaw, neck, epigastric, or ear discomfort.[7] Symptoms of myocardial ischemia other than chest pain or discomfort are called *anginal equivalents* **TABLE 18-10**.

TABLE 18-10 Anginal Equivalents

- Abdominal pain
- Acute change in mental status
- Diaphoresis
- Dizziness
- Dyspnea
- Dysrhythmia
- Epigastric pain
- Fatigue
- Generalized weakness
- Indigestion
- Isolated arm or jaw pain
- Light-headedness
- Palpitations
- Restlessness
- Syncope or near syncope
- Unexplained nausea or vomiting

Atypical or unusual symptoms are more common in women, older adults, and patients with diabetes. Women with an ACS often describe the discomfort as aching, tightness, pressure, sharpness, burning, fullness, or tingling. The location of the discomfort is often in the back, shoulder, or neck. Some women experience vague chest discomfort that tends to come and go, with no known aggravating factors. Frequently reported acute symptoms include shortness of breath, weakness, unusual fatigue, cold sweats, dizziness, and nausea or vomiting. Older adults may also have atypical symptoms, such as compromised mental status, generalized weakness, syncope, shortness of breath, fatigue, unexplained nausea, and abdominal or epigastric discomfort. Likewise, patients with diabetes may present atypically, with generalized weakness, syncope, light-headedness, or a diminished mental status.

When obtaining a history from a patient whose chief complaint is chest discomfort, ask the usual SAMPLE (Signs and symptoms, Allergies, Medications, Pertinent past medical history, Last oral intake, Events leading up to the illness or injury) and OPQRST questions to elaborate on the chief complaint. In addition, ask whether the patient has taken anything for the pain and, if so, whether it helped. If the patient reports having taken NTG without relief, then it is essential to establish *why* the pain was unrelieved. One of two reasons might explain this failure. First, the patient may be having an ACS, for which NTG did not provide complete pain relief. Second, the NTG may have gone stale. To distinguish between the two explanations, ask the patient whether the last few NTG doses have had the usual effects. Therapeutically active NTG tablets provoke a slight burning sensation under the tongue and may make the patient feel flushed or trigger a transient throbbing headache. If the patient confirms they felt some of those effects but their chest discomfort was not relieved, you know there was nothing wrong with the NTG. Nevertheless, there may be something very wrong with the patient.

When you assess the severity of the patient's discomfort, use a pain rating scale. Using a pain scale allows you to evaluate the effectiveness of your emergency care. Document the patient's initial rating of their discomfort. Reassess (and document) the degree of discomfort after each treatment you perform and before transferring care at the receiving facility.

Begin treatment as soon as you elicit a chief complaint of a cardiac nature; the more in-depth history taking and the secondary assessment can wait. For the purposes of this section, however, we will proceed through the history and secondary assessment. Besides pain (or sometimes instead of pain), several other symptoms are associated with ACSs:

- Diaphoresis (sweating), often profuse, is principally the result of massive discharge by the ANS. The sweat may soak through the patient's clothing, and they may report having a cold sweat.
- Dyspnea may be a warning sign of impending LVF.
- Anorexia (loss of appetite), nausea, vomiting, or belching frequently accompanies MI. Hiccups caused by diaphragmatic irritation in an inferior wall MI may occasionally occur as well.
- Weakness may be profound, and the patient may say they feel like "a limp rag" or something similar.
- If CO is diminished significantly, then the brain's reduced circulation may cause dizziness or acute mental status changes.
- Patients with cardiac dysrhythmias sometimes perceive palpitations as a sensation that the heart has skipped a beat.
- A feeling of impending doom is common among patients having an MI. The patient is frightened, appears frightened, and expresses their fear to others, all of which adds to a general atmosphere of panic and dread.

Words of Wisdom

Begin treatment immediately for any patient with chest discomfort or an anginal equivalent.

Signs

Although you may find some abnormalities in the physical exam for patients with ACS, many have relatively normal exam findings, and your field diagnosis will depend chiefly on the history and 12-lead ECG findings. Nevertheless, a few specific physical exam findings can help you detect AMI complications, such as heart failure or cardiogenic shock.

- Pay attention to the patient's general appearance. Does the patient appear anxious? Frightened? In obvious pain? Of course, not all chest pain is caused by ischemia, injury, or infarction. Many other conditions may cause chest pain that can mimic angina or an AMI.
- What is the patient's level of responsiveness? Is the patient fully alert? Confused? Remember, poor perfusion creates confusion. If the patient does not seem mentally sound, it may be because the heart is damaged and not enough oxygenated blood is reaching the brain.
- Does the skin present with pallor? Is it cold and clammy? A typical patient with an AMI is apprehensive, with ashen-gray pallor and cold, wet skin.
- Assess the patient's vital signs. Is the pulse strong or weak? Regular or irregular? Is the respiratory rate abnormally rapid? Is the BP abnormally high or low? In a patient with AMI, the heart rate may be normal, rapid, or slow. The BP may be decreased, reflecting decreased CO from the damaged heart or elevated from pain and anxiety.
- Are there signs of LVF (wheezes or crackles)? Signs of RVF (distended neck veins, pedal or presacral edema)?

You must perform a thorough physical exam, including history taking, to determine whether the

Words of Wisdom

As a general rule, it is safe to assume any patient who has called for medical assistance because of chest pain has, at the least, unstable angina and perhaps an evolving AMI. Patients with a history of angina rarely call for help unless something has changed, often dramatically, for the worse. Because it is difficult to differentiate between angina and an AMI in the field, the treatment of angina should be the same as that for an AMI. It is far better to overtreat angina as an AMI than to undertreat an AMI by assuming it is angina.

cause of the patient's signs and symptoms is likely cardiac in origin. **TABLE 18-11** shows differential diagnoses to consider throughout your assessment.

Management of ACSs

Among patients with an ACS, those with STEMI are most likely to benefit from reperfusion therapy, which is the restoration of blood flow either by mechanical means (such as **percutaneous coronary intervention [PCI]**) or by pharmacologic means (such as **fibrinolysis** [the process of dissolving blood clots]). PCI is a minimally invasive procedure performed under fluoroscopy to diagnose and treat blocked coronary arteries. With this therapy, a balloon, stent, or other device is passed through a peripheral artery catheter to reopen a blocked coronary artery by compressing the plaque against the vessel wall.

TABLE 18-11 Differential Diagnosis of Chest Pain and Discomfort

Classification	Possible Diagnoses
Cardiovascular causes	• Aneurysm • Aortic dissection • Myocardial ischemia • Myocarditis • Pericarditis
Gastrointestinal causes	• Cholecystitis • Esophageal spasm • Gastroesophageal reflux disease • Hiatal hernia • Indigestion • Pancreatitis • Peptic ulcer disease
Musculoskeletal causes	• Acromioclavicular disease • Chest wall trauma • Chest wall tumor • Costochondritis • Intercostal muscle cramps
Respiratory causes	• Pleurisy • Pneumonia • Pneumothorax • Pulmonary embolism • Respiratory infection
Other causes	• Anxiety disorder/panic attack • Herpes zoster (shingles)

Because reperfusion therapy benefits are time sensitive, start treatment at once on arrival at the scene for any patient with chest discomfort, even before you complete the history and secondary assessment. The ACS algorithm is shown in **FIGURE 18-103**.

Place the Patient at Physical and Emotional Rest

The stress response triggers a surge of catecholamines (epinephrine and norepinephrine) from the adrenal glands, sending the damaged heart racing. At the same time, the massive discharge throughout the fight-or-flight system puts the peripheral circulation in a state of severe vasoconstriction; thus, not only is the heart being pushed to go faster, but it must also work harder against the escalating afterload. Therefore, the heart's need for oxygen soars when it is already in a state of marked oxygen deprivation. This cycle can lead quickly to dysrhythmias and death.

Words of Wisdom

For the patient with an ACS, delays in prehospital care can occur during response time, on-scene time, and/or travel time to the receiving facility.[23] These delays prolong the time to treatment and can ultimately harm the patient's outcome. You can make a difference by working quickly and efficiently when providing emergency care to a patient with a suspected ACS.

One way to limit infarct size is to reduce the amount of work the heart must do, which decreases the patient's myocardial oxygen requirements. Begin your care by allowing the patient to assume a position of comfort. Most patients prefer a semi-Fowler position. From the time you arrive, the patient must not expend any effort, not even to walk to the stretcher.

Obtain Vital Signs and Perform Cardiac Monitoring

Obtain vital signs, including pulse, respiration, BP, and Spo_2. Measure the BP, and repeat that measurement at least every 5 minutes. Although the ECG monitor provides information about the heart's electrical activity, it reveals nothing about its

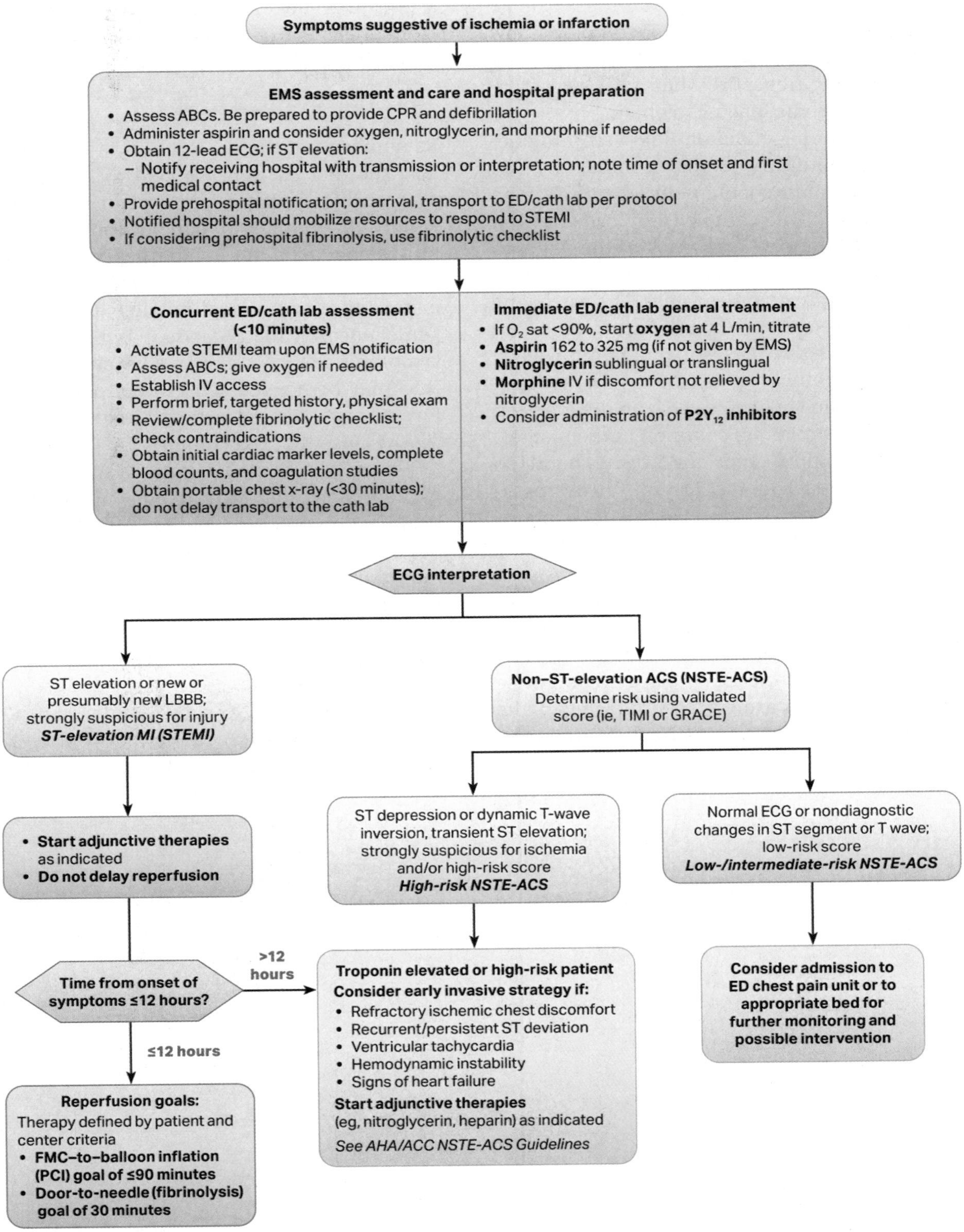

FIGURE 18-103 Acute coronary syndromes algorithm.

Abbreviations: ABC, airway, breathing, and circulation; ACS, acute coronary syndrome; CPR, cardiopulmonary resuscitation; ED, emergency department; FMC, first medical contact; LBBB, left bundle branch block; PCI, percutaneous coronary intervention; RBBB, right bundle branch block.

mechanical function. Therefore, you must palpate the patient's pulse to assess peripheral blood flow and the strength of the heartbeat. This is especially important during transport when vital sign measurements can be challenging to obtain.

Apply the cardiac monitor. Run a strip to document and identify the patient's initial rhythm. Ideally, your monitor should emit an audible tone or beep with each QRS complex (also called a "systole beep"), so you can keep track of the patient's cardiac rhythm even when you have to look away from the monitor to do other things. The ear, in any case, is far more sensitive than the eye in detecting slight rhythm irregularities, so you are more likely to hear the beginning of a cardiac dysrhythmia much sooner than you would see it on the monitor. Because dysrhythmias are common in the first few hours of an infarction, keep your drug box handy so you can quickly reach for medications if a dysrhythmia develops. Treat dysrhythmias using the appropriate algorithm and initiate CPR, defibrillation, or cardioversion, if indicated.

Administer Aspirin and Oxygen

In most EMS systems, as long as the patient has no aspirin allergy or GI bleeding, dispatchers advise patients to chew baby aspirin (160 to 325 mg). If the patient has not already taken aspirin before your arrival, give them 160 to 325 mg of non–enteric-coated aspirin to chew. Administer oxygen if the patient is dyspneic, is hypoxemic, or has obvious signs of heart failure. Target an Spo_2 level of 90%.

Obtain a 12-Lead ECG

Remember that the 12-lead ECG is the primary diagnostic tool used in the field to rapidly identify a cardiac event; therefore, obtain a 12-lead ECG within 10 minutes of patient contact while another team member establishes vascular access. Always acquire a 12-lead ECG *before* administering any medications (except possibly aspirin and oxygen). Repeating the 12-lead ECG when the patient's symptoms change is essential because the patient's ECG may be normal *between* episodes of discomfort but show signs of ischemia, injury, or infarction *during* episodes of discomfort.

In patients whose symptoms suggest ischemia or infarction, the 12-lead ECG allows for rapid stratification of the patient's condition into one of three categories: (1) STEMI (ST elevation in two or more contiguous leads, or new or suspected LBBB) **FIGURE 18-104**, (2) NSTEMI, or (3) normal (nondiagnostic). It is important to remember that a normal ECG does not rule out ischemia, injury, or infarction.

If the 12-lead ECG shows evidence of STEMI, your scene time goal is 10 minutes or less. Alert the receiving hospital and begin completing a

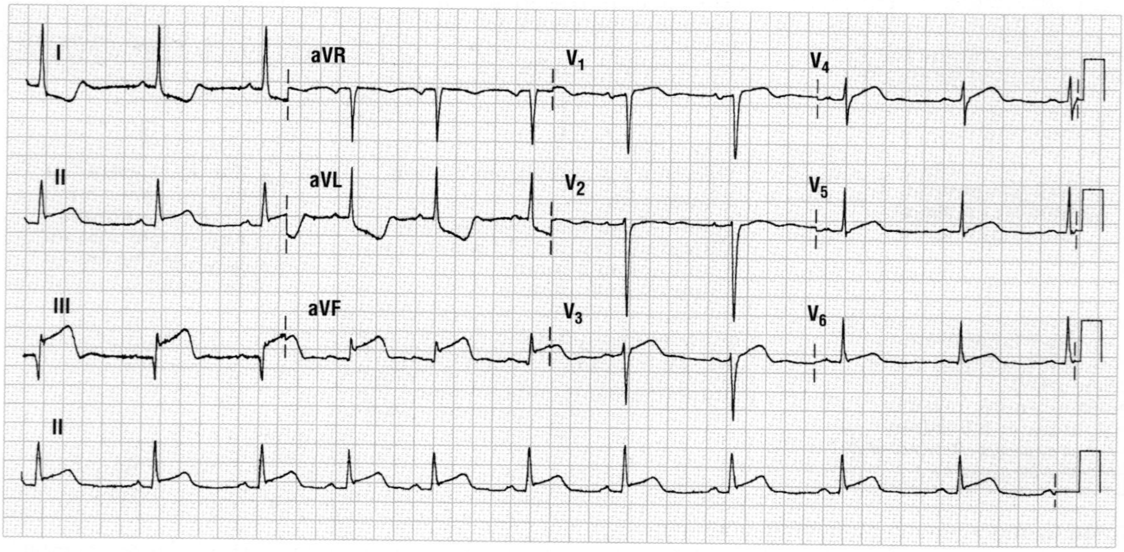

FIGURE 18-104 A 12-lead electrocardiogram showing ST-segment elevation in leads II, III, and aVF, with ST-segment depression and T-wave inversion in reciprocal leads I and aVL.

Reproduced from *Arrhythmia Recognition: The Art of Interpretation*, courtesy of Tomas B. Garcia, MD.

fibrinolytic checklist **FIGURE 18-105**. Prenotification allows medical facility personnel to assemble and begin preparations while the patient is in transit to the facility. Although several studies have proved that mechanical interventions produce better outcomes when performed promptly, fibrinolytic therapy plays a significant role in treating STEMI because only a minority of US hospitals

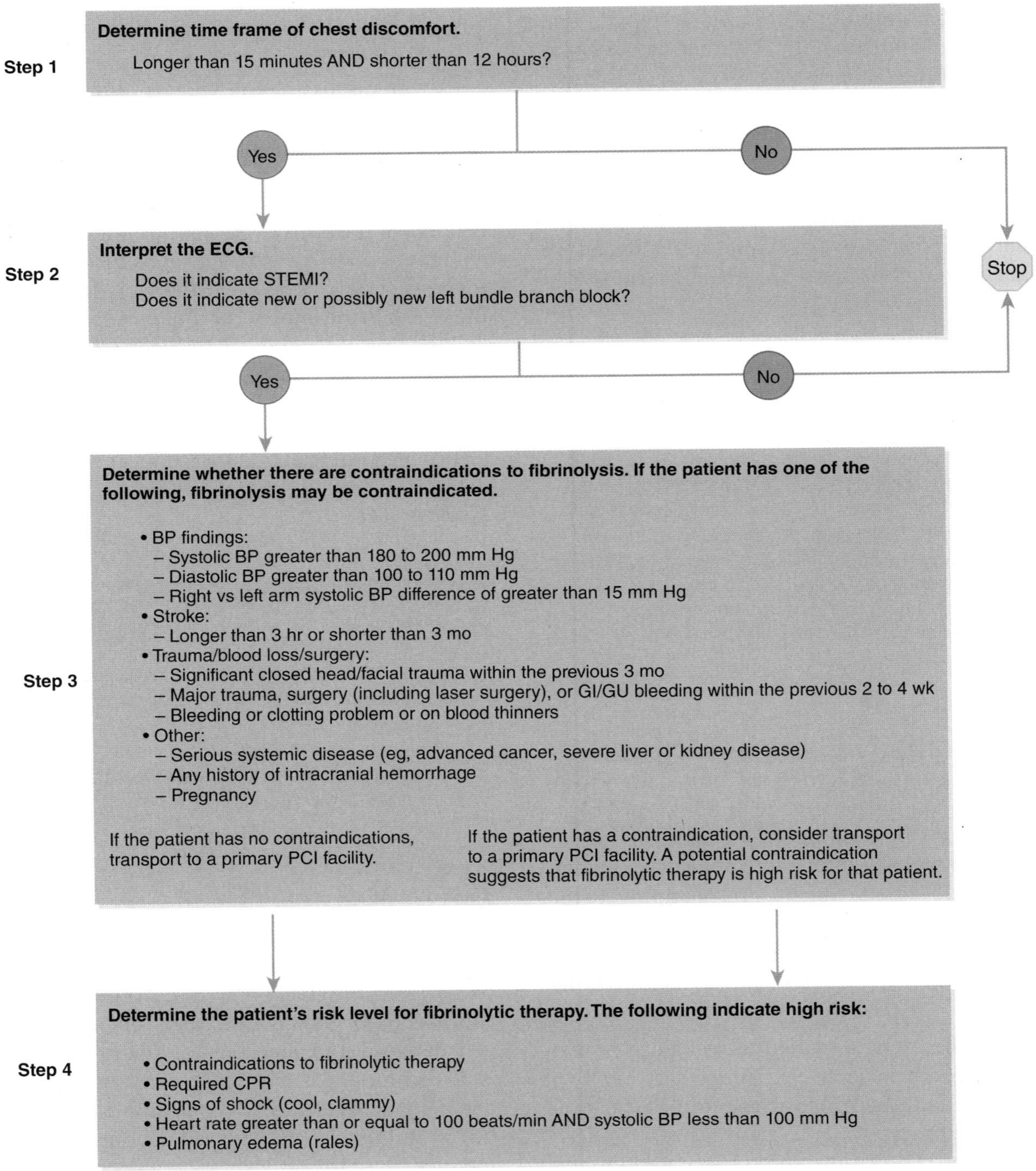

Step 1
Determine time frame of chest discomfort.
Longer than 15 minutes AND shorter than 12 hours?
Yes
No
Stop
Step 2
Interpret the ECG.
Does it indicate STEMI?
Does it indicate new or possibly new left bundle branch block?
Yes
No
Step 3
Determine whether there are contraindications to fibrinolysis. If the patient has one of the following, fibrinolysis may be contraindicated.
• BP findings:
– Systolic BP greater than 180 to 200 mm Hg
– Diastolic BP greater than 100 to 110 mm Hg
– Right vs left arm systolic BP difference of greater than 15 mm Hg
• Stroke:
– Longer than 3 hr or shorter than 3 mo
• Trauma/blood loss/surgery:
– Significant closed head/facial trauma within the previous 3 mo
– Major trauma, surgery (including laser surgery), or GI/GU bleeding within the previous 2 to 4 wk
– Bleeding or clotting problem or on blood thinners
• Other:
– Serious systemic disease (eg, advanced cancer, severe liver or kidney disease)
– Any history of intracranial hemorrhage
– Pregnancy
If the patient has no contraindications, transport to a primary PCI facility.
If the patient has a contraindication, consider transport to a primary PCI facility. A potential contraindication suggests that fibrinolytic therapy is high risk for that patient.
Step 4
Determine the patient's risk level for fibrinolytic therapy. The following indicate high risk:
• Contraindications to fibrinolytic therapy
• Required CPR
• Signs of shock (cool, clammy)
• Heart rate greater than or equal to 100 beats/min AND systolic BP less than 100 mm Hg
• Pulmonary edema (rales)

FIGURE 18-105 Prehospital fibrinolytic checklist.
Abbreviations: BP, blood pressure; CPR, cardiopulmonary resuscitation; ECG, electrocardiogram; GI, gastrointestinal; GU, genitourinary; PCI, percutaneous coronary intervention; STEMI, ST-segment elevation myocardial infarction.

have PCI capabilities. You must know which medical facilities in your area are equipped to administer **fibrinolytic therapy** and/or PCI. Fibrinolytic therapy involves administering a medication that converts the body's clot-dissolving enzyme from its inactive form, plasminogen, to its active form, **plasmin**, which then breaks down fibrinogen and fibrin clots. Unfortunately, if a medication capable of promoting clot dissolution is given intravenously, its effects cannot be limited to the clot in the coronary artery; the medication can act anywhere in the body where clots are being formed, which can lead to uncontrolled bleeding. Thus, the benefit of fibrinolytic therapy (ie, the possible salvage of myocardial tissue) must always be weighed against its risks—principally, the risk of bleeding.

Evidence-Based Medicine

Up to 20% of patients with STEMI do not present with chest pain or discomfort.[24] Research shows that more than 25% of patients with STEMI who present without chest pain do not receive prehospital ECGs and have significantly longer EMS-to-balloon times.[24] To avoid delays in reperfusion therapy when caring for a patient with a possible ACS, keep in mind the concepts of atypical presentation and anginal equivalents. When in doubt, obtain a 12-lead ECG.

As with the systems of care used for patients experiencing trauma, stroke, or cardiac arrest, the systems of care for patients with STEMI are coordinated efforts by health care providers and organizations to provide a full range of evidence-based care to these patients, with the aim of improving the timeliness of reperfusion, reducing mortality, and increasing the likelihood of a favorable outcome. The ideal STEMI system includes the following elements:

- EMS dispatchers trained to recognize probable signs of an acute cardiac event
- Well-established EMS triage and destination protocols
- 12-lead ECG acquisition, interpretation, and transmission capability with a STEMI alert
- ED protocols
- Staff experienced in ACLS
- Ability to communicate with the receiving institution
- Medical direction with training and experience in managing STEMI
- Interfacility transfer protocols
- Post–acute care capabilities
- Quality assurance/continuous quality improvement

When discussing STEMI, it is crucial to understand that EMS-to-balloon time, door-to-balloon time, and door-to-needle time must be minimized. These concepts refer to the time that elapses before the patient receives reperfusion therapy. EMS-to-balloon time starts at the first moment of patient contact by EMS providers. It ends when definitive therapy occurs (when a catheter passes through the lesion in the affected coronary vessel). Door-to-balloon time is the interval between patient presentation to the medical facility and definitive therapy. Door-to-needle time begins when the patient arrives at the ED and ends when a fibrinolytic medication is administered. Transport and destination decisions should be based on local resources and systems of care.[10]

Words of Wisdom

Your ability to identify candidates for reperfusion therapy plays a decisive role in helping medical facility personnel begin treatment early enough to make a difference. For this reason, you must ensure you have a thorough understanding of the principles of reperfusion therapy for ACS. Time is muscle!

Provide Pain Relief

Some form of pain relief is essential because the severe pain of AMI places enormous stress on the patient's ANS, which may contribute to complications. NTG, which decreases myocardial oxygen demand and increases coronary blood flow, is a common therapy used early in ACS management if there are no contraindications to its use. Administer NTG sublingually as a tablet or metered-dose spray.

NTG is contraindicated for patients with an initial SBP less than 90 mm Hg and in patients who have used a phosphodiesterase inhibitor within the past 48 hours. Examples of these medications include sildenafil (Viagra, Revatio), vardenafil (Levitra, Staxyn), and tadalafil (Cialis, Adcirca), which are used for erectile dysfunction and pulmonary hypertension. Also, avoid use of NTG in patients receiving IV epoprostenol (Flolan) or treporstenil (Remodulin), which are used to treat pulmonary hypertension.[10] Nitrates should be given with extreme caution, if at all, to patients with inferior STEMI or suspected right ventricular infarction (RVI). When an infarction involves these chambers, the effectiveness of the affected heart chamber is diminished, and the right heart becomes preload dependent. Hypotension can result if preload is reduced, which can occur with medications that decrease preload (eg, NTG, morphine, diuretics). If the 12-lead ECG indicates an inferior MI, then apply right-side chest leads to assess right ventricular involvement.

If the patient's discomfort is unrelieved by NTG and their vital signs remain stable, consider administering morphine sulfate. Morphine is the preferred analgesic for patients with STEMI and is considered a reasonable choice for patients with unstable angina/STEMI.[7] Fentanyl (Sublimaze) is favored over morphine for ischemic chest discomfort not relieved by NTG in some EMS systems because of its rapid onset, relatively short duration, and fewer side effects. Follow your local protocols.

Transport the Patient

Because time is muscle, obtain a more detailed history and perform the secondary assessment en route to the receiving facility. There is no reason to remain at the scene unless a cardiac arrest or dysrhythmia requires immediate treatment.

Transport the patient in a semi-Fowler position (unless the patient is in shock, in which case they should be supine). Do all you can to ensure the patient is as relaxed and as comfortable as possible. Depending on your local protocol, it may be necessary to perform some additional treatment measures in transit to reduce the patient's time in the ED. These measures may include establishing a second large-bore IV, applying defibrillation pads to the patient's chest, completing a fibrinolytic checklist (if not already done), and shaving the patient's wrist and groin areas.

On some calls, you may encounter patients who refuse treatment or transport despite having signs and symptoms consistent with an ACS. A person with chest discomfort who refuses care is an example of a "high-risk refusal"—in other words, there is a high risk of legal liability under these circumstances. Calmly and carefully, try to persuade the patient to accept the care you wish to provide, including transport. If you believe the patient may be having an MI, communicate in words they can easily understand. For example, use the phrase "heart attack" instead of MI. Let the patient know what emergency care you would like to provide and the benefits of accepting it. Explain the risks of turning away the care you have offered. Because an MI may be fatal, you must point out this possible outcome to the patient. The point is not to scare the patient, but rather to clearly outline the perils of refusing treatment, including transport. It may be helpful to contact medical direction in these situations. In some cases, the physician may ask to speak directly to the patient and be able to successfully persuade them to accept treatment and transport. If you are unable to convince the patient to accept care, carefully document the patient's refusal.

Words of Wisdom

AMI has many possible complications. Familiarize yourself with them. Electrical complications include bradycardia, AV block, bundle branch and fascicular blocks, tachycardia, and SCD. Ischemic complications include an extension of the infarction and reinfarction. Mechanical complications can also occur, including LVF, RVF, cardiogenic shock, and ventricular aneurysm. Pericarditis may be an inflammatory complication of AMI. Stroke, deep vein thrombosis (DVT), and pulmonary embolism are possible embolic complications.

Patient and Family Education

The time from symptom onset to emergency care can be shortened if patients, families, and bystanders recognize heart attack symptoms early and activate their EMS system promptly. Teach your patients and their families how to recognize the signs and symptoms of a heart attack. Instruct them to call 9-1-1 within 5 minutes of symptom onset. Explain that not all heart attacks are accompanied by sudden, crushing chest pain and a loss of responsiveness. Symptoms may begin gradually, or they may come and go. Advise patients who have had a previous heart attack that the signs and symptoms of a second or subsequent cardiac event may differ from those of the first.

Documentation and Communication

EMS systems regularly evaluate the care provided to patients with ACS. Key documentation elements are as follows:[10]

- Time of symptom onset
- Time of patient contact by EMS to the time of 12-lead ECG acquisition
- Time from first diagnostic 12-lead ECG to STEMI notification
- Time at which aspirin was administered (ie, taken before EMS arrival or given by EMS?); or reason why it was not given, substantiated by pertinent negatives
- Time of arrival at the receiving facility

Heart Failure

Heart failure occurs when the heart is unable, for any reason, to pump powerfully enough or fast enough to empty its chambers; as a result, blood backs up into the systemic circuit, the pulmonary circuit, or both. Heart failure is a syndrome, not a disease, and is characterized by volume overload and inadequate tissue perfusion. Common features include fatigue, dyspnea, edema, and exercise intolerance. Although lung congestion is common, it is not always heard, so the term *congestive heart failure* is no longer used.

Heart failure may be caused by any of several disorders that impair the ventricles' ability to fill with or eject blood, including CAD, long-standing high BP, and diabetes. Dysrhythmias, cardiomyopathy, valvular heart disease, and genetic conditions can also lead to heart failure. Cardiomyopathy is discussed in Chapter 44, *Pediatric Emergencies.* Factors that can contribute to heart failure include thyroid disorders, alcohol abuse, cocaine and other illegal substance abuse, cancer treatments that damage the myocardium (eg, chest radiation, chemotherapy),

YOU are the Paramedic

PART 3

You administer supplemental oxygen and then prepare the patient for transfer into the ambulance for further assessment and transport. As you lift the stretcher into the ambulance, the patient experiences a tonic-clonic seizure lasting 30 to 45 seconds, followed by agonal breathing at a rate of 4 to 6 breaths/min. He is unresponsive. A member of your crew begins bag-mask ventilation while you apply the cardiac monitor. The monitor shows a wide QRS third-degree AV block, with a ventricular rate of 36 beats/min. Before departing for the medical facility, you establish an IV line while another crew member gets a second set of vital signs.

Recording Time: 10 minutes	
Respirations	6 breaths/min; 10 breaths/min with bag-mask ventilation
Pulse	36 beats/min, regular
Skin	Cool, moist; pale mucous membranes
Blood pressure	62/40 mm Hg
Oxygen saturation (Spo_2)	99% with bag-mask ventilation
Pupils	Pupils Equal, Round, and Reactive to Light and Accommodation (PERRLA)

6. Is this patient high priority? Why or why not?
7. Given what you know at this time, what is the most likely cause of the seizure activity?
8. What is this patient's greatest life threat at this time? How will you treat it?
9. How will you manage the cardiac rhythm?

and infectious agents that cause inflammation, such as human immunodeficiency virus (HIV) or severe acute respiratory syndrome coronavirus 2 (SARS-CoV-2), which causes COVID-19.[25]

Heart failure can be identified based on symptom onset (acute versus chronic) and the ventricle initially involved (left versus right). In acute heart failure, symptoms occur suddenly. In chronic heart failure, symptoms develop more slowly. A person with chronic heart failure can develop acute heart failure. Although the failure of either ventricle can occur by itself, failure of both often occurs simultaneously: RVF is often a result of LVF.

Recall that CO is equal to stroke volume multiplied by the heart rate. Three main factors affect stroke volume: preload, afterload, and cardiac contractility. Thus, any condition that impairs preload, afterload, cardiac contractility, or heart rate can cause heart failure.

Left Ventricular Failure

Regardless of its cause, heart failure produces symptoms in most patients because the left ventricle does not pump blood effectively. When LVF occurs, blood backs up behind the left ventricle, causing a chain reaction **FIGURE 18-106**. Blood builds up in the lungs because the left ventricle is unable to eject all the blood within its walls. Consequently, the left atrium swells with blood because it cannot empty the blood within its walls into the left ventricle. The stretching of the atrial muscle fibers may cause atrial dysrhythmias. Likewise, the pulmonary veins cannot empty the blood from the pulmonary arteries into the left atrium because it is already full. Pressure within the pulmonary vessels increases, forcing fluid from the pulmonary capillaries across the alveolar walls into the alveoli, which can cause pulmonary edema. The buildup of fluid widens the gap between the alveolar-capillary membrane, impairing oxygen and carbon dioxide diffusion.

There are two types of LVF, and various diagnostic tests are used to view the cardiac anatomy and determine the type because their treatments differ. With systolic failure, the left ventricle is weak and has trouble pumping out all the blood in the chamber to the body. With diastolic heart failure, the left ventricle contracts normally but has become stiff, impeding its ability to relax and fill with blood between each contraction of the heart.

LVF may result from poorly controlled hypertension, which increases afterload and cardiac workload, and can lead to left ventricular hypertrophy. Tachydysrhythmias shorten the time for ventricular relaxation and impair ventricular filling, which can lead to decreased CO. CAD, including AMI, can cause permanent damage to the myocardium, resulting in impaired ventricular contractility and reduced CO. Increased demands on the heart associated with excessive volume or pressure can also cause heart failure. For example, giving a large volume of IV fluid over a short period (as in a runaway IV line) in a patient with a weakened left ventricle can cause volume overload. If a heart valve becomes thickened or narrowed, obstructing blood flow through it, pressure overload can occur.

Words of Wisdom

Pulmonary edema of cardiac origin is called cardiogenic pulmonary edema. Pulmonary edema attributable to climbing or living at a high altitude is called high-altitude pulmonary edema. Pulmonary edema can also be caused by other conditions such as toxic inhalation, excessive IV fluids, and some opioid medications. This type of pulmonary edema is called noncardiogenic pulmonary edema.

Right Ventricular Failure

The right ventricle must overcome high pressure and congestion within the pulmonary vessels to eject the blood within its walls. When it cannot keep up with the increased workload, the right ventricle's contractile function fails **FIGURE 18-107**. Blood backs up behind the right ventricle, raising the pressure in the right atrium. If the right atrium is unable to eject the blood within its walls, then blood backs up into the superior and inferior venae cavae. The veins become congested with blood because the superior and inferior venae cavae cannot drain into an already full right atrium. Because venous return is delayed, organs become congested with blood. For example, increased pressure in the hepatic veins enlarges the liver (hepatomegaly), making it tender. As venous congestion worsens, rising pressure within the veins forces serous fluid through

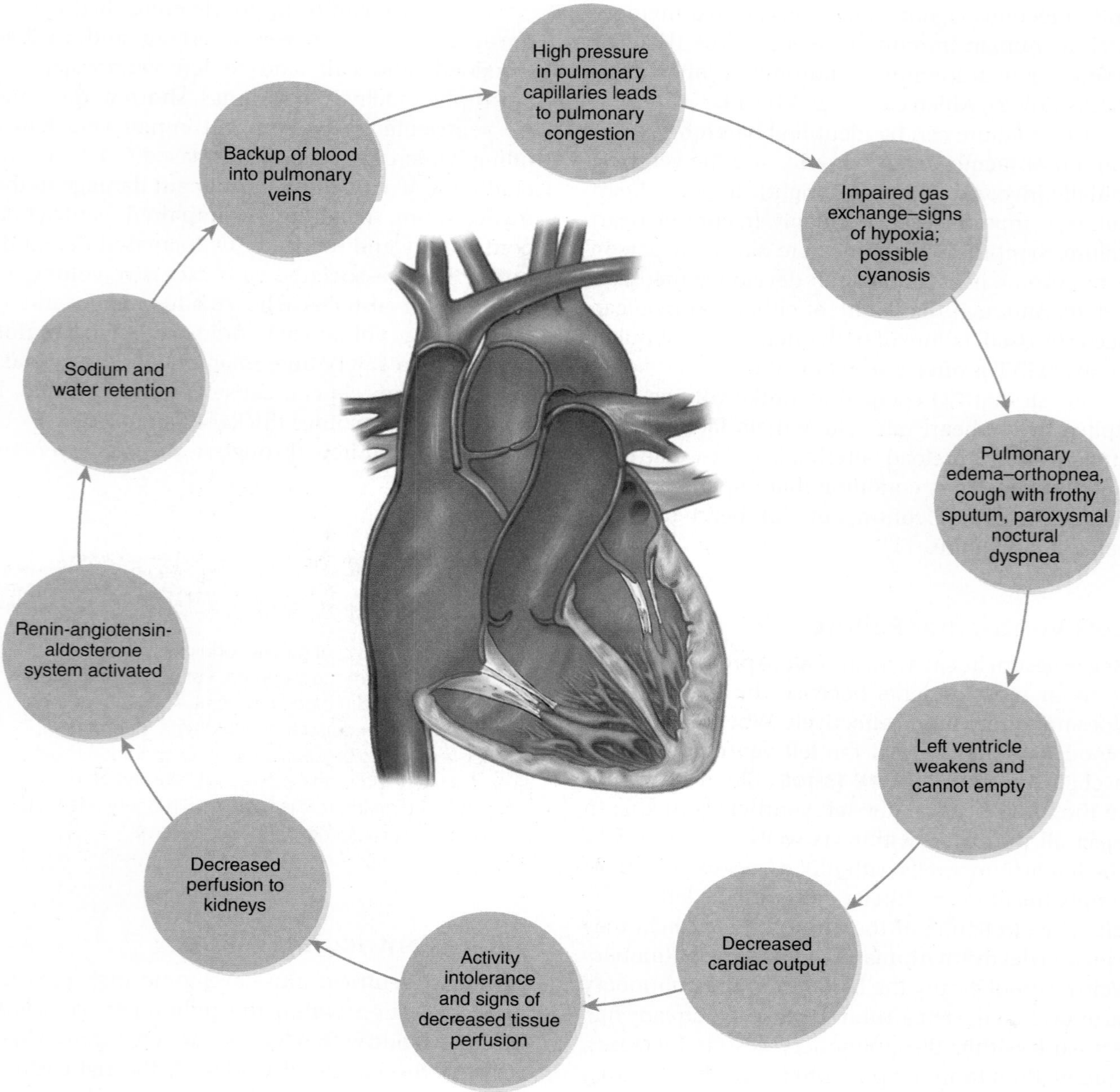

FIGURE 18-106 Left ventricular failure.

capillary walls and into the body's tissues, producing edema. Peripheral edema is most apparent in dependent areas of the body such as the feet and ankles. Serous fluid may also build up in the abdomen (ascites), pleural cavity (pleural effusion), and/or pericardial cavity (pericardial effusion). As RVF progresses, generalized edema of the entire body may occur; a condition called *anasarca*.

Cor Pulmonale

RVF may occur by itself (without LVF) in conditions such as RVI, pulmonary embolism, and pulmonary hypertension. Pulmonary hypertension is a disorder in which the pressure in the pulmonary arteries is higher than normal. The right ventricle must work hard to overcome this increased resistance to

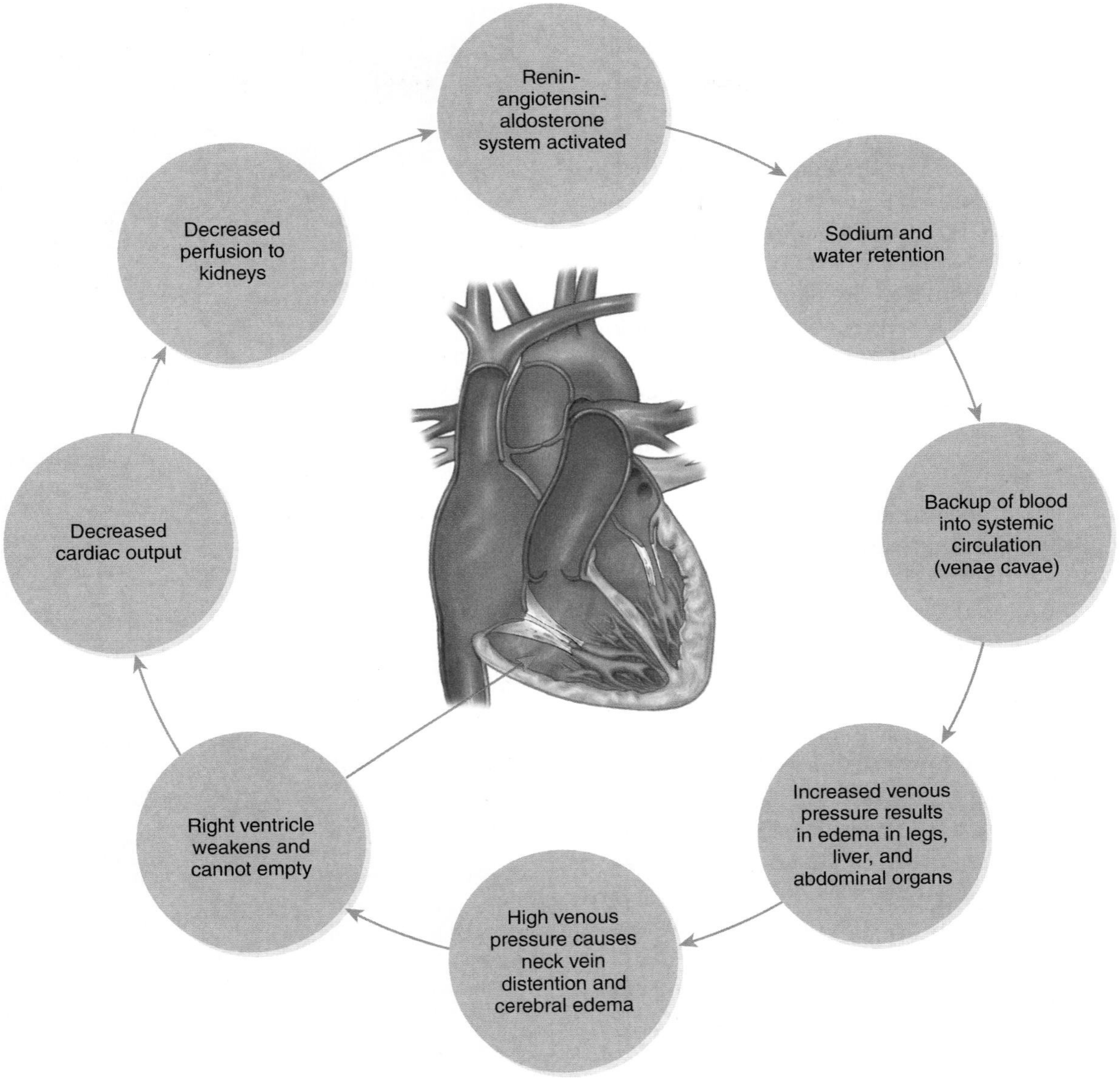

FIGURE 18-107 Right ventricular failure.

eject blood. Over time, the right ventricle enlarges and eventually fails. RVF caused by pulmonary disease is called *cor pulmonale,* which is usually the result of COPD.

Compensatory Mechanisms

As the heart begins to fail, the body's compensatory mechanisms attempt to improve CO by manipulating preload, afterload, cardiac contractility, and/or heart rate. Ultimately, these compensatory mechanisms may actually worsen heart failure. For example, the sympathetic nervous system boosts the heart rate, increases the force of contraction, and constricts blood vessels. The accelerated heart rate and stronger force of contraction increase the heart's oxygen demand, reduce the amount of time the ventricles have to fill, and decrease coronary artery perfusion time. Decreased blood flow to the kidneys stimulates the renin-angiotensin-aldosterone system. Angiotensin I forms angiotensin II, promoting more vasoconstriction. Constricted blood vessels (increased afterload) require the heart to work even harder to pump against high pressure. Angiotensin II encourages aldosterone release, which encourages sodium and water retention and increases blood volume (increasing preload).

These compensatory mechanisms are effective in increasing CO for a time, but eventually heart failure advances. Sodium and water retention enlarge the heart's chambers, thickening the ventricles' walls and ultimately weakening the force of ventricular contraction. As the force of contraction decreases, the weakened heart muscle cannot handle the increased volume of fluid, and CO decreases.

Assessment

The patient with heart failure may report a sudden onset of shortness of breath or shortness of breath that has worsened over hours or days. At first, the patient may have difficulty breathing only with activity or when lying down for a while (orthopnea). Respiratory or cardiac disorders can cause these symptoms. However, as LVF worsens, signs and symptoms also become evident at rest. The patient may instinctively assume a tripod position, because keeping the upper body elevated improves breathing by allowing for better chest expansion. The likelihood of a cardiac origin is greater if the patient reports having a previous heart attack or a history of high BP, valvular disease, or another cardiovascular condition.

The patient with heart failure may report having trouble sleeping and describe episodes of PND. During these nighttime episodes of shortness of breath, fluid pools in the lungs, literally drowning the patient in their own secretions. The patient awakens coughing and feeling as if they were suffocating.

In addition to shortness of breath or other breathing difficulties, patients with heart failure often report feeling tired or weak or having no energy. These symptoms, combined with a history of recent weight gain over a short period and/or progressive swelling of the lower extremities, are a red flag for heart failure **TABLE 18-12**.

The patient may report trouble concentrating recently, which may be the result of hypoxia. In addition, the patient may report nausea and a loss of appetite. Such symptoms usually arise from congestion of the liver and other abdominal organs. Some

patients may describe feeling faint, palpitations, or an irregular or rapid pulse. Ask the patient about the prescribed medications they are taking, specifically, beta blockers or calcium channel blockers, because these medications can affect the force with which the heart contracts.

Oxygenation is impaired when either side of the heart fails, decreasing the blood supply to the

TABLE 18-12 Signs and Symptoms of Heart Failure

Left Ventricular Failure	Right Ventricular Failure
Signs	
Restlessness, anxiety	Weight gain
Respiratory rate above normal for age	Dependent edema
Heart rate above normal for age	Ascites
Pulsus alternans	Anasarca
Crackles	Jugular venous distention
Cough with frothy sputum	Liver enlargement (hepatomegaly)
Third heart sound	Spleen enlargement (splenomegaly)
Retractions; accessory muscle use	
Labored breathing; tripod position	
Sweating	
Inability to speak in complete sentences; limited to phrases or words	
Symptoms	
Fatigue	Fatigue
Difficulty breathing	Nausea
Orthopnea	Loss of appetite
Paroxysmal nocturnal dyspnea	Right or left upper abdominal quadrant pain

© Jones & Bartlett Learning.

body's tissues. Restlessness, anxiety, or unexplained confusion (especially in older adults) may be signs of hypoxia. When talking with the patient, notice if they can speak in complete sentences. As heart failure worsens, the patient's shortness of breath will limit speech from sentences to phrases and then only to words. If the patient is too short of breath to answer your questions, you may be able to obtain the patient's history from a family member or neighbor at the scene.

The patient's respiratory rate and heart rate are often rapid. The skin may feel cool and have a pallor. Peripheral pulses may be diminished. These signs represent the sympathetic nervous system's response to hypoxia and the body's compensatory mechanism to maintain CO. You may see signs of increased work of breathing, including retractions and use of accessory muscles.

As hypoxia worsens, the patient may become cyanotic or may frequently cough as fluid irritates the airways. Coughing may produce pink, frothy sputum. As compensatory mechanisms fail, the progressive buildup of fluid in the lungs causes crackles (rales) that do not clear with coughing. This sound may be accompanied by wheezing if bronchospasm occurs. Crackles are heard first at the base of the lungs. As the fluid builds up, you will hear crackles farther up the chest. Pulsus paradoxus, pulsus alternans, and a third heart sound may be perceptible. The apical pulse may be displaced as enlargement of the left ventricle displaces the cardiac apex.

If RVF accompanies LVF, then JVD will be visible as the venous system becomes congested. Patients who can walk will have swelling of the ankles, feet, calves, or legs. Swelling of the sacral area may occur in patients confined to bed. If edema is present, note (and document) if it is pitting or nonpitting and localized in the ankles, to the mid-calf, or to the knees. Ascites, a buildup of fluid in the peritoneal cavity, may also occur. As the liver and spleen swell, the patient may report upper abdominal quadrant pain.

As the pump continues to fail, the heart rate begins to slow, BP falls, and CO decreases substantially. Cardiogenic shock occurs when heart failure is accompanied by hypotension.

Some of the signs and symptoms present with heart failure may also be present with other conditions. **TABLE 18-13** outlines the differential diagnosis of heart failure.

TABLE 18-13 Differential Diagnosis of Heart Failure

Classification	Possible Diagnoses
Cardiovascular causes	• Cardiac tamponade • Cardiogenic pulmonary edema • Cardiogenic shock • High-altitude pulmonary edema • Myocardial ischemia • Myocardial infarction
Respiratory causes	• Acute respiratory distress syndrome • Asthma • Chronic bronchitis • Chronic obstructive pulmonary disease • Pneumonia • Pneumothorax • Pulmonary embolism • Respiratory failure
Other causes	• Anaphylaxis • Aspiration • Noncardiogenic pulmonary edema • Toxin exposure

Words of Wisdom

JVD may be present in conditions other than RVF, but listening to breath sounds and heart sounds can help you identify the patient's underlying condition. For example, JVD in a patient with cardiac tamponade is usually characterized by clear breath sounds but muffled heart sounds. JVD in a patient with tension pneumothorax is usually characterized by diminished or absent breath sounds on the affected side. JVD in a patient with RVF associated with LVF will usually produce crackles in the lungs. In such patients, fluid administration is often limited and should be closely monitored. JVD in a patient with RVF associated with RVI usually produces clear breath sounds. A patient with RVI often requires IV fluid boluses to increase preload.

Management

A patient who is having difficulty breathing is usually quite anxious. Begin your care by offering the patient reassurance. Place the patient in a position of comfort as you work quickly to help relieve their symptoms. If pulmonary congestion is present and the patient's BP will tolerate it, place them in a sitting position with the feet dangling. This position encourages venous pooling in the legs, which will help decrease venous return, thereby decreasing the work of breathing.

Maintain adequate oxygenation and perfusion. Apply a pulse oximeter and provide supplemental oxygen as needed to maintain the patient's Spo_2 between 95% and 98%.[11] Noninvasive positive-pressure ventilation (NIPPV) has been proven useful in managing pulmonary edema associated with heart failure. NIPPV should not be used if the patient has a compromised airway, altered mental status, risk of aspiration, a pneumothorax, or SBP of less than 90 mm Hg. It may be necessary to insert an advanced airway if the patient is in severe distress. Assess breath sounds before and after each intervention. Monitor the patient's respiratory status using waveform capnography, or with pulse oximetry if waveform capnography is not available.

Limit the patient's physical activity. Do not allow the patient to walk up or down stairs or to the stretcher. Place the patient on a cardiac monitor and obtain a 12-lead ECG. A dysrhythmia may lead to heart failure. On the other hand, hypoxia and acidosis predispose patients with heart failure to dysrhythmias ranging from tachycardia to bradycardia.

Establish IV access. To help ensure the patient does not receive too much IV fluid, use a heparin lock or saline lock. If local protocol requires you to use an IV bag and tubing, infuse the fluid at a "to keep open" rate (30 mL/h). Check and recheck the volume of fluid in the bag while the patient is in your care. Document the amount of fluid in the bag when you start the IV line and the amount of fluid remaining when you transfer patient care at the receiving facility.

Pharmacologic therapy for heart failure may vary slightly by EMS system, so be sure to check your local protocol. Sublingual NTG may be given to reduce both preload and afterload, thereby supporting CO. Ask how much, if any, NTG the patient has already taken.

Furosemide (Lasix) is a diuretic that was used for many years in the prehospital management of heart failure. Currently, it is not recommended as a treatment for heart failure and acute pulmonary edema. It carries a risk of inducing hypokalemia, dysrhythmias, or increased systemic vascular resistance by enhancing the renin-angiotensin-aldosterone system. Any of these conditions may be harmful to the patient with acute heart failure. Misdiagnosis of heart failure and the subsequent inducement of inappropriate diuresis can increase the likelihood of morbidity and mortality.

If the patient's condition is stable, avoid using lights and siren during transport, as they may increase the patient's anxiety, heart rate, and BP. This response increases the heart's workload and oxygen demand and should be avoided if possible. Rapid transport is warranted if the patient's breathing worsens, if they have signs and symptoms of shock, or if a life-threatening dysrhythmia develops.

Surgically implanted ventricular assist devices (VADs) may be used in patients who have heart failure. A VAD acts as an artificial ventricle and does not depend on the contractility or electrical conduction of the patient's heart. A VAD can be placed in either the left ventricle (LVAD), the right ventricle (RVAD), or both (biventricular assist device) depending on which ventricle is failing. Because LVF is more common than RVF, the LVAD is the most common type of VAD.

A VAD may be used (1) to allow the heart to "rest" until the patient's heart can recover and resume its pumping function, (2) as a bridge to heart transplantation, and (3) as lifetime therapy, also called destination therapy, to maintain circulatory support in patients who are not candidates for a heart transplant. Several types of VADs are available, but they all typically consist of a blood pump, tubing (an inflow cannula and an outflow cannula), and an external power source connected to a controller. The controller regulates and monitors the VAD's functions. Alarms serve as reminders when the batteries require changing, when a connection is loose, or if the pump is malfunctioning.

VADs are categorized according to the type of blood flow (eg, continuous, pulsatile), the length of time the device can be used for circulatory support (eg, short-, intermediate-, or long-term), the source of driving power (eg, pneumatic or electric), and the device location (eg, internal or external). Pulsatile-flow VADs are rarely used today. Instead, current-generation VADs are continuous-flow devices that deliver flow throughout the entire cardiac cycle. Patients with a continuous-flow VAD typically do not have a palpable pulse, despite adequate perfusion.

In such patients, obtaining a BP measurement using a manual cuff and stethoscope and obtaining a pulse oximetry reading may be difficult or the results may be inaccurate because of reduced pulse pressure and the patient's weak or absent pulse.

With a transcutaneous VAD, both the pump and the power source are located externally. A tube from the pump goes through the patient's abdominal wall to the outside of the unit, connecting to the battery pack. With an implantable VAD, the pump is located inside the body and the power source is located externally. A cable connects the internal VAD to the power source via a small incision in the abdomen. With an LVAD, blood is withdrawn from the left atrium or the left ventricle's apex through a tube into the LVAD and then returned to the ascending aorta via a second tube. With an RVAD, blood is withdrawn from the right atrium into the RVAD and is returned to the pulmonary artery. The controller or batteries do not need to be disconnected to obtain a 12-lead ECG, defibrillate the patient, or perform synchronized cardioversion.

Many patients with VADs also have a permanent cardiac pacemaker or implantable cardioverter defibrillator in place. Complications associated with VADs include device malfunction or failure, thromboemboli (eg, stroke, AMI, or pulmonary embolism), bleeding (eg, nasal, GI, intracranial), heart failure, infection, dysrhythmias, cardiac tamponade, aortic insufficiency, and sepsis.[10] Because there are differences in VAD designs, methods for troubleshooting device failure are typically unique to each device. The patient with a VAD may be prescribed anticoagulant medications to prevent the development of clots within the VAD and bloodstream.

To assess for possible VAD pump malfunction, assess for alarms, auscultate for a "hum" from the pump, and assess for signs of hypoperfusion such as altered mental status, pallor, and diaphoresis. Use available resources to troubleshoot potential VAD malfunctions and determine the appropriate corrective actions to restore normal VAD function.[10] Contact the patient's VAD-trained companion (often a family member), if available. Using the phone number on the device, contact the patient's VAD coordinator to help you make treatment and transport destination decisions. Check all the system controller connections, change the VAD batteries, and/or change the system controller if indicated.[10] Have the patient stop all activity, and assess patient tolerance. Follow appropriate cardiovascular condition–specific protocols as indicated.

Contact the VAD coordinator if the patient with a VAD experiences a cardiac arrest while initiating initial emergency care. However, it is essential to recognize that not all patients with a VAD who are in VT or VF will be unresponsive. Evaluate perfusion by assessing mental status, breathing, skin color and temperature,[26] and capillary refill. If the VAD is not functioning, troubleshooting fails to identify the problem, and there are no signs of life, initiate chest compressions and begin defibrillation and administer medications according to current ACLS algorithms.[26] If defibrillation is required, be careful not to place the pads directly over the pump. Ideally, the patient should be transported to their VAD center. If you transport the patient to a non-VAD center, it is imperative that you bring all VAD-related equipment (eg, batteries, controllers, power module) because the equipment will be needed to mechanically support the patient and may aid the center in troubleshooting.[27]

Documentation and Communication

Key documentation elements for the patient with an implantable VAD include the following:[10]

- Vital signs and oxygen saturation
- Time of and patient response to interventions
- Information gained from the VAD control box indicating any specific device malfunctions
- Interventions performed to restore a malfunctioning VAD to normal function
- Time of notification to and instructions from the VAD-trained companion and/or VAD coordinator

Cardiac Tamponade

Pathophysiology

A pericardial effusion is an increase in the volume and/or a change in the character of the pericardial fluid, the fluid that surrounds the heart. The pressure within the pericardium increases as pericardial fluid builds up. The volume of blood or fluid in the pericardial space necessary to impair the heart's ability to fill depends on the rate at which the buildup of blood or fluid occurs and the pericardium's ability to stretch to accommodate the expanded fluid volume. If excess fluid builds up slowly, the pericardium will gradually expand and make room for a large volume before signs and symptoms appear. If the fluid builds up rapidly, the pressure within the pericardium significantly increases with a smaller volume of fluid.

Cardiac tamponade occurs when the buildup of pericardial fluid compresses the heart, impairing its contraction and restricting ventricular filling. Limited ventricular filling decreases stroke volume and CO, causing signs of shock.

Cardiac tamponade may develop gradually if caused by an infection or tumor. It can develop rapidly when caused by heart surgery, pacemaker or central venous catheter insertion, or cardiac trauma such as a stab wound or gunshot wound. **TABLE 18-14** shows some possible causes of cardiac tamponade.

Assessment

Patients with cardiac tamponade are usually too ill to answer questions about their medical history. They are likely to be anxious and restless, and to report shortness of breath, chest tightness, and/or dizziness. Family members may tell you of a recent invasive procedure, heart attack, chronic illness, or medications the patient is taking that may explain why the cardiac tamponade developed. Although tension pneumothorax is more common, suspect cardiac tamponade in any patient who has sustained a penetrating wound of the chest or upper abdomen. If the tamponade is not from trauma, the patient may relate a medical illness history such as pericarditis or end-stage renal disease. One way to differentiate between cardiac tamponade and tension pneumothorax is to remember that in cardiac tamponade, the breath sounds will be equal and the trachea will be midline because the lungs are not affected.

Signs of injury to the chest wall are usually present if cardiac tamponade occurs due to trauma. Cardiac tamponade produces a classic trio of signs known as **Beck triad**: JVD, hypotension, and muffled heart sounds. These signs, however, are present in fewer than one-half of all patients with the condition. JVD may be absent if the patient is hypovolemic. Heart sounds may be normal early on, becoming progressively more faint or muffled as the condition worsens. The patient may also have other signs of cardiac tamponade:

- Cold, mottled, or cyanotic skin; pallor
- Tachycardia
- Weak or absent peripheral pulses
- Narrowing pulse pressure (early sign)
- Pulsus paradoxus (late sign; may be absent if the patient has severe hypotension)
- Signs and symptoms mimicking heart failure (when cardiac tamponade develops slowly):
  - Dyspnea
  - Orthopnea
  - JVD

The ECG is of limited value in identifying cardiac tamponade. Low-amplitude QRS complexes and T waves, ST-segment elevation, or nonspecific T-wave changes may occur. Electrical alternans may be observed on the ECG in which the P wave, QRS complex, and T wave alternate in amplitude with every other beat because of the constant motion of the heart within the fluid-filled pericardium.

TABLE 18-14 Causes of Cardiac Tamponade

- Aortic dissection
- Autoimmune disease
- Blunt trauma to the chest (including CPR)
- Cardiac rupture after MI
- Cardiac tumors
- Chronic kidney failure
- End-stage lung cancer
- Heart surgery
- Hypothyroidism
- Penetrating trauma to the heart
- Pericarditis, pericardial effusion
- Radiation therapy to the chest (cancer treatment)
- Recent invasive heart procedures (angioplasty, central venous catheter insertion, pacemaker wire insertion)

Abbreviations: CPR, cardiopulmonary resuscitation; MI, myocardial infarction

Management

If trauma is the source of the patient's signs and symptoms, manage them as discussed in Chapter 36, *Chest Trauma.* Address any life-threatening hemorrhage. Ensure adequate oxygenation and ventilation. Apply a pulse oximeter and provide supplemental oxygen as needed to maintain the patient's Spo_2 between 95% and 98%. Apply the cardiac monitor. Avoid performing additional procedures on the scene that will delay transport to the medical facility.

Establish IV access en route to definitive care. Give IV fluids and medications per local protocol or medical direction. If the patient has no signs of heart failure, consider implementing an IV fluid challenge of normal saline to maintain circulating blood volume. Give IV fluids as a temporizing measure, but do not delay transport to initiate this intervention. Check the patient's response by assessing mental status, heart rate, respiratory effort, breath sounds, and BP. Explain all procedures to the patient and provide emotional support to the patient and family.

The definitive treatment for cardiac tamponade is in-hospital pericardiocentesis, a procedure in which a needle is inserted into the pericardial space to drain (aspirate) excess fluid through the needle. Often, the withdrawal of as little as 50 mL of fluid will significantly improve the patient's condition. If scarring is the cause of the tamponade, then surgery may be necessary to remove the affected area of the pericardium. When you are reporting to medical control, ensure you identify all signs and symptoms that led you to suspect the patient has cardiac tamponade, so the receiving medical facility will be prepared to perform the pericardiocentesis.

Words of Wisdom

To identify cardiac tamponade, you must perform a thorough assessment. Trends in BP measurements can be recognized only after obtaining at least three values, usually 5 to 10 minutes apart. Muffled heart sounds, pulsus alternans, electrical alternans, and pulsus paradoxus are uncommon signs, so they may be easily overlooked. However, if there was a penetrating injury in the area of the heart and the patient is symptomatic, this condition is highly likely.

Cardiogenic Shock

Cardiogenic shock is a condition in which heart muscle function is severely impaired, decreasing CO and resulting in inadequate tissue perfusion. The most common cause of cardiogenic shock is LVF secondary to AMI, which typically occurs with an infarction involving 40% or more of the left ventricle.

Pathophysiology

In most patients with cardiogenic shock, myocardial contractility is reduced, resulting in decreased CO, hypotension, and systemic vasoconstriction. Vasoconstriction initially increases coronary and peripheral perfusion, but this compensatory mechanism subsequently contributes to increased afterload, worsening cardiac performance and increasing myocardial oxygen demand. Ultimately, the damaged myocardium cannot overcome the increased resistance, resulting in end-organ hypoperfusion. Systemic inflammation triggered by acute cardiac injury may induce *vasodilation* and myocardial dysfunction in some patients with cardiogenic shock.[28]

Cardiogenic shock may occur as a complication of shock from any cause. In addition to myocardial damage from AMI, cardiogenic shock can result from heart failure, ventricular dysrhythmias, end-stage cardiomyopathy, acute myocarditis, blunt or penetrating cardiac trauma, or pulmonary embolism. It may also occur if myocardial contractility has diminished because of prolonged cardiac surgery, ventricular aneurysm, cardiac arrest, or ventricular wall rupture. When such a rupture occurs, blood leaks into the pericardial space, quickly leading to cardiac tamponade and cardiovascular collapse. Transient cardiogenic shock can occur after resuscitation.

Risk factors for developing cardiogenic shock include older age, anterior MI, diabetes, hypertension, multivessel CAD, previous MI, and peripheral vascular or cerebrovascular disease.

Assessment

A patient with cardiogenic shock can present in several different ways depending on its severity. For example, the patient may be "warm and dry," in which the skin is warm and signs of heart failure are present, but pulmonary congestion has not yet developed (ie, the lungs are dry). Tachycardia is also typically present. If a systemic inflammatory response syndrome develops after an MI, the patient may be "warm and wet," where the skin is warm because of vasodilation,[28] but pulmonary congestion has developed. Tachycardia and fever may also be present. The patient who is "cold and dry" has cool or cold skin because of peripheral vasoconstriction, but pulmonary congestion has not yet developed.

Additional signs and symptoms usually include tachycardia, narrowed pulse pressure, acute mental status changes, and dizziness.

Most patients with cardiogenic shock present as "cold and wet"; that is, the skin is cold and pulmonary crackles are heard on auscultation. The patient may appear ashen or cyanotic with mottled extremities. Altered mental status, dyspnea, orthopnea, JVD, and peripheral edema may be observed. Third and fourth heart sounds may be heard. As ventricular function worsens and CO falls, the SBP progressively decreases.

Because a patient in cardiogenic shock may be too ill to answer questions, be prepared to ask family members or others present about the patient's history. In addition to the usual questions asked when obtaining a SAMPLE history, use OPQRST to explore the patient's symptoms. Ask if the patient has been taking their medications as prescribed.

Management

Prehospital management of cardiogenic shock includes ensuring adequate oxygenation and ventilation, establishing vascular access, continuously monitoring the patient's ECG, and transporting for definitive care. In the hospital setting, cardiogenic shock treatment generally focuses on strengthening contractility without significantly increasing the heart rate, altering preload and afterload, and controlling any dysrhythmias contributing to shock.

Place a hypotensive patient in a supine position. Conversely, if pulmonary congestion is present and the patient's BP will tolerate it, place the patient in a sitting position with the feet dangling. Limit the patient's physical activity while they are in your care, including making sure the patient does not walk up or down stairs or to the stretcher.

Quickly obtain the patient's vital signs, apply a pulse oximeter, and administer supplemental oxygen as indicated. Closely monitor the patient's breathing effort and be prepared to provide bag-mask ventilation if needed. Advanced airway insertion may be necessary in some cases. Place the patient on a cardiac monitor and obtain a 12-lead ECG within 10 minutes of patient contact. Remember that AMI is a common cause of cardiogenic shock; therefore, it is critical to look for ECG evidence of MI and, if present, transport the patient to an appropriate facility for definitive care. Patients who are candidates for reperfusion therapy and receive prompt treatment may have an increased chance of survival.

Because other types of shock can present similarly to or can contribute to cardiogenic shock, it is best to consult medical direction before administering IV fluids or medications. Vasoactive IV medications may be ordered, such as dopamine, norepinephrine, or epinephrine. If you are instructed to give a vasoactive medication, be sure to check the IV site often during administration. Because these medications can cause significant vasoconstriction, tissue damage can occur if the medication leaks out of a vein. Check the patient's response to the medication by assessing their mental status, heart rate, respiratory effort, breath sounds, and BP.

Except for correcting a life-threatening dysrhythmia, there are no other measures you can take in the field to stabilize a patient in cardiogenic shock. Therefore, you must transport the patient expeditiously to the medical facility. En route, complete a fibrinolytic checklist.

If the patient refuses care, repeatedly urge the patient to accept your assistance, including transport. Explain to the patient that if their condition is not treated, symptoms are likely to worsen and could result in death. Consider contacting medical direction for advice. If you cannot persuade the patient to accept care, carefully document the patient's refusal and your attempts to persuade the patient to accept help.

Hypertensive Emergencies

Recall that stage 2 hypertension exists when the SBP is 140 mm Hg or higher or the DBP is 90 mm Hg or higher.[3] Hypertension is a modifiable risk factor for stroke, AMI, heart failure, dementia, peripheral vascular disease, aortic dissection, AF, and end-stage renal disease. Hypertension has been called the "silent killer" because this condition usually produces no signs or symptoms and therefore goes undetected and untreated, yet damages the heart, brain, eyes, blood vessels, and kidneys.

A **hypertensive emergency** is defined as an acute elevation of BP to 180/120 mm Hg or higher with evidence of end-organ damage (cardiovascular, neurologic, or renal). That last phrase is important, because it is the evidence of end-organ dysfunction, not the reading on the sphygmomanometer, which determines the urgency of the situation. A hypertensive emergency, formerly known as *hypertensive crisis* or *malignant hypertension*, usually occurs in patients with a history of hypertension. Failure to take BP medications or other treatments as prescribed is a common cause of such an emergency. Possible causes of hypertensive emergencies in patients with no known history of hypertension include the following:

- Acute aortic dissection
- Acute CNS events, such as subarachnoid hemorrhage, intracerebral hemorrhage, or stroke
- Acute kidney failure
- Drug-induced hypertension from recreational drug use, such as cocaine or amphetamines
- Pheochromocytoma (an adrenal tumor that raises BP)
- Toxemia of pregnancy

A **hypertensive urgency** exists when there is an acute elevation of BP to 180/120 mm Hg or higher *without* signs or symptoms of end-organ damage. Because the term *hypertensive urgency* can lead to overly aggressive management of patients with severe, uncomplicated hypertension, some experts prefer to use the phrase *asymptomatic markedly elevated BP* rather than hypertensive urgency.[29]

Words of Wisdom

The BP values used to define a hypertensive urgency or emergency are not universal. Experts note that the *rate of rise* of an individual's BP above their baseline is likely a more critical factor than the actual numbers. The rate of rise explains why patients without chronic hypertension may show signs of a hypertensive emergency at much lower levels and, in contrast, why those with longstanding hypertension may tolerate exceedingly high BP levels without developing acute end-organ damage.[30]

Pathophysiology

Most hypertension is the result of advanced atherosclerosis or arteriosclerosis, which narrows the lumen of the arteries and reduces their elasticity. The resulting high afterload on the heart expands filling volume and stimulates the Frank-Starling reflex, which raises the pressure at which blood is ejected from the heart.

YOU are the Paramedic

PART 4

You continue bag-mask ventilation with high-flow oxygen and then begin TCP, with mechanical capture verified by peripheral pulses. On arrival at the ED, the patient remains unresponsive, with a heart rate of 70 paced pulses/min; BP, 100/70 mm Hg; and spontaneous respirations, 0. The patient's wife informs the physician that her husband has been smoking crack cocaine regularly for the past year. His use has escalated during the past 2 months. The physician inserts a temporary pacemaker. The patient's mental status improves, and he is admitted to the ICU. Seven days after placement of a permanent pacemaker, the patient is discharged from the medical facility.

Recording Time:	15 minutes
Respirations	10 breaths/min with bag-mask ventilation
Pulse	70 paced pulses/min, regular
Skin	Warm, dry, and normal color
Blood pressure	100/70 mm Hg
Oxygen saturation (Spo_2)	99% with bag-mask ventilation
Pupils	PERRLA

10. Assume the patient remained unresponsive, with an unacceptably low BP despite pacing. What treatment would be appropriate under those circumstances?

11. Given the patient's final disposition, was your treatment appropriate? Why or why not?

Many conditions, such as anxiety or pain, can briefly elevate a person's BP (especially the SBP). "White coat hypertension" is a phrase used to describe a transient sympathetic nervous system response to BP measurement in a medical setting. In contrast, "masked hypertension" describes elevated self-measured BP readings but normal measurements obtained in a medical setting. Cigarette smoking, alcohol, physical activity, and job and mental stress are possible causes of masked hypertension. Clearly, a single BP measurement obtained during an emergency scarcely constitutes adequate grounds for telling a patient that they are hypertensive. Instead, you may say something like this: "Sir, your BP is a little high right now. That may be because of the stress you're under and may not have any real significance. To be safe, though, you should have your BP rechecked a couple of times in the next few weeks under less stressful circumstances."

If left untreated, hypertension significantly shortens a person's life span and predisposes them to various other medical conditions. The most common complications associated with hypertension are renal damage, stroke, and heart failure, resulting from the left ventricle having to pump for years against a markedly increased afterload.

A true hypertensive emergency requires a controlled lowering of BP with close monitoring to prevent or limit organ damage. If untreated, a hypertensive emergency may cause acute renal failure, AMI, stroke, or death within a few hours.

Assessment

Hypertensive emergencies often develop rapidly, and the patient typically appears sick. Signs and symptoms vary depending on the end organ(s) affected. Neurologic signs and symptoms can include headache, blurred vision, sudden blindness, aphasia (disturbances in speech production or comprehension), or unilateral numbness or weakness. Mental status changes may range from confusion to unresponsiveness. Widespread neuromuscular irritability may be signaled by muscle twitching or seizures. Cardiovascular signs and symptoms may include chest pain or tightness, shortness of breath, palpitations, dysrhythmias, or signs of heart failure. Complaints of sudden severe chest or upper back pain described as tearing or ripping may indicate aortic dissection. The patient may report a sudden decrease or absence of urine output, signaling renal involvement. Additional signs and symptoms may include nausea, vomiting, ringing in the ears (tinnitus), nosebleed, or muscle cramps.

Peripheral pulses may feel strong or bounding. Check (and document) the patient's BP in both arms in case aortic dissection has occurred. The patient may have seizures, signs of heart failure (such as JVD, crackles in the lungs, or peripheral edema), or signs consistent with AMI. Ischemic changes may be seen on the 12-lead ECG.

Ask the patient about prescribed and over-the-counter medications they are taking. Because noncompliance with BP medication is a common cause of hypertensive emergencies, determine if the patient has been prescribed BP medication and if so, has been taking it as prescribed. Ask the patient about recreational drug use, such as amphetamines, cocaine, and other sympathomimetic agents, which can cause severe hypertension. Differential diagnoses for hypertensive emergencies are shown in **TABLE 18-15**.

Management

Prehospital care of hypertensive emergencies includes supportive care. Give oxygen, if indicated; establish an IV line; and apply the cardiac monitor and pulse oximeter. Maintain the Spo_2 between 95% and 98%. Avoid performing additional procedures

TABLE 18-15 Differential Diagnosis of Hypertensive Emergencies

Classification	Possible Diagnoses
Cardiovascular	• Aortic dissection
Genitourinary	• Pheochromocytoma • Renal failure • Toxemia of pregnancy
Neurologic	• Epilepsy or postictal state • Head injury • Intracranial mass • Stroke • Subarachnoid hemorrhage
Other causes	• Acute anxiety • Cocaine or amphetamine use • Connective tissue disease • Drug overdose or withdrawal

on the scene that will delay transport to the medical facility. If the patient has heart failure or chest discomfort from myocardial ischemia, provide care according to your local protocol. Offer reassurance to the patient and family while providing care at the scene and during transport to the medical facility.

Paramedics working in rural areas or other circumstances in which long transport times to the medical facility are unavoidable may have to initiate drug therapy for a hypertensive emergency in the field. One widely accepted drug for this purpose is labetalol (Normodyne, Trandate), which has both alpha and beta blocking properties. As an alpha blocker, it prevents vasoconstriction, thereby decreasing overall peripheral vascular resistance. Meanwhile, its beta blocking actions prevent the reflex tachycardia that would otherwise occur in response to a drop in BP. As a beta blocker, however, labetalol is relatively contraindicated in patients with asthma and COPD. Keep the patient supine, and measure and document the BP at least every 2 to 3 minutes when giving a medication to lower the patient's BP. Cerebral hypoperfusion can occur if the BP is lowered too rapidly. Similarly, myocardial ischemia can result if the DBP is lowered too far, inhibiting coronary artery filling. Stop the infusion when the patient's BP has reached the target level specified by the physician.

A patient with a hypertensive emergency requires transport to the closest appropriate facility. If the patient refuses care, repeatedly urge the patient to accept your assistance, including transport. Explain that if their condition is not treated, symptoms are likely to worsen and could result in death. Consider contacting medical direction for advice. If you cannot persuade the patient to accept care, carefully document the patient's refusal and any patient education you provided.

Infectious Diseases of the Heart

Endocarditis

Endocarditis is an infection of the lining of the heart characterized by inflammation of the endocardium: the lining of the heart chambers, including the heart valves. If left untreated, endocarditis can damage the heart valves, causing them to malfunction.

Endocarditis is most often caused by a bacterial infection, and less commonly by a fungal infection. Most of these pathogenic organisms begin their journey to the heart from the skin, upper airway, or genitourinary or GI tract. The organism may initially gain access to the body in several ways, including minor skin infection, dental procedures (particularly tooth extractions), upper respiratory infection, endoscopic examinations, or a major operation. Body piercing and tattooing have also been linked to endocarditis. The severity of the patient's illness often reflects the virulence of the infecting organism. Less virulent organisms cause a low-grade fever and symptoms that usually develop over several weeks to months. Organisms that are more virulent cause high-grade fever and signs of serious illness that develop over days to weeks.

Endocarditis occurs most often in people with preexisting valvular disease such as mitral or aortic valve disease, or in those with mechanical (prosthetic) heart valves. It can also occur in people with congenital heart disease. Right-side endocarditis is a type of infective endocarditis that affects the tricuspid and pulmonary valves. This type of endocarditis is seen most often in people who use IV drugs and in patients with infected central venous catheters, dialysis shunts, or transvenous pacing wires.

Assessment

The most common symptoms of endocarditis are fever and chills. The patient may also report headache, loss of appetite, weight loss, muscle and joint aches and pains, night sweats, shortness of breath on exertion, or cough. Signs of heart failure may be present because of progressive heart valve destruction. If infective endocarditis invades the heart's conduction system, then ECG changes may be seen, including a prolonged PRI, third-degree AV block, or LBBB. Flat, painless, red-to-blue lesions (Janeway lesions) may appear on the palms and soles. Some patients develop small, tender nodules on the pads of the fingers or toes (Osler nodes).

Management

Prehospital care for the patient with endocarditis is mainly supportive. Allow the patient to assume a position of comfort, establish an IV line, and apply the cardiac monitor. Apply a pulse oximeter and administer oxygen, if indicated. If the patient has heart failure, proceed according to your local protocol or medical direction instructions. The patient will usually receive IV antibiotics at the medical facility. If a prosthetic valve is the infection site, then surgery will likely be necessary to remove the infected artificial valve. Most patients with endocarditis can be transported to the closest appropriate facility without lights and siren.

If the patient refuses care, repeatedly urge the patient to accept your assistance, including transport. Consider contacting medical direction for advice. If you are unable to persuade the patient to accept care, carefully document the patient's refusal.

Words of Wisdom

Blood flow through the heart can be compromised if a valve does not function properly. A malfunctioning heart valve is a type of valvular heart disease, which is classified as follows:

- **Valvular stenosis.** A valve is stenosed if it narrows, stiffens, or thickens. The heart must work harder to pump blood through a stenosed valve.
- **Valve prolapse.** If a valve flap becomes inverted, it is said to prolapse. Prolapse can occur if one valve flap is larger than the other. It can also occur if the chordae tendineae stretch markedly or rupture.
- **Valvular regurgitation.** Blood can flow backward, or regurgitate, if one or more of the heart's valves do not close properly.

Think about what might happen if a papillary muscle in the left ventricle were to tear or rupture. The mitral valve flaps may not completely close, and they may become inverted (prolapse), allowing blood from the left ventricle to leak into the left atrium (regurgitation) during ventricular contraction. Blood flow to the body (CO) may be diminished as a result.

Pericarditis

Pericarditis is an inflammation of the double-walled sac (pericardium) that envelops the heart. The pericardium helps anchor the heart, preventing excessive movement of this organ in the chest when body position changes, and protecting it from trauma and infection.

Pericarditis is caused by either a viral (most common), bacterial, or, occasionally, fungal infection. Pericarditis may develop days or weeks after a patient has a heart attack. It may also develop after blunt or penetrating chest trauma, open-heart surgery, or procedures such as coronary angioplasty or insertion of an implantable defibrillator or pacemaker. Radiation therapy may also cause pericarditis. It can develop in patients with kidney failure or inflammatory disorders, such as rheumatoid arthritis and lupus. It can also develop as a result of breast or lung cancer, lymphoma, or leukemia. In many cases, no cause for pericarditis can be identified (idiopathic pericarditis).

Assessment

Ask the patient about recent flulike signs and symptoms. Patients with pericarditis may relate a history of a recent upper respiratory infection. They may describe a recent fever with shaking chills, shortness of breath, coughing, skin rash, or weight loss. These patients may have a history of lupus, kidney disease, or recent MI, leukemia, Hodgkin disease, lymphoma, chest trauma, or heart surgery.

Chest discomfort is the most common symptom of pericarditis. The patient usually describes a sharp, stabbing pain, but sometimes reports a steady, constricting pain that radiates to the shoulder and to either or both arms, mimicking the discomfort of an ACS. However, unlike the pain of an ACS, the discomfort associated with pericarditis is usually made worse by deep inspiration, coughing, or lying flat. The discomfort often improves when the patient sits up and leans forward.

The patient's chest discomfort is most often located under the sternum but may be centered in the left anterior chest or epigastrium. It may persist for days. Listening to heart sounds may reveal a pericardial friction rub, although this sign is not always present. A pericardial friction rub is a scratchy or grating sound caused by contact between the visceral and parietal pericardium. It is best heard with the patient leaning forward as you listen at the third to fifth ICS to the left of the sternum. Ask the patient to hold their breath while you listen. If you hear a sound that resembles two pieces of dried leather rubbing together, or the sound made when walking on crunchy snow, then pericarditis is the probable cause.

The patient with pericarditis often has a fever, tachycardia, and tachypnea, and may have a pallor, and JVD may or may not be present. If JVD is present, it may indicate pericardial effusion (a buildup of fluid in the pericardial space) resulting from the infection. Breath sounds are usually normal unless

TABLE 18-16 Differential Diagnosis of Pericarditis

Classification	Possible Diagnoses
Cardiovascular	• ACS • Aortic dissection • Cardiomyopathy
Respiratory	• Pleurisy • Pneumothorax • Pulmonary embolism
Other causes	• Costochondritis • Gastroesophageal reflux disease • Lupus

Abbreviation: ACS, acute coronary syndrome

another condition, such as heart failure, exists. The ECG often reveals ST-segment elevation in multiple leads. Differential diagnoses to consider for pericarditis are shown in **TABLE 18-16**.

Management

Prehospital care of pericarditis is mainly supportive. Allow the patient to assume a position of comfort, establish an IV line, and apply the cardiac monitor. Apply a pulse oximeter and administer oxygen, if indicated. Obtain a 12-lead ECG. Pericarditis is usually treated with nonsteroidal anti-inflammatory drugs. Viral pericarditis usually resolves on its own. Bacterial pericarditis is treated with antibiotics, and fungal pericarditis is treated with antifungal medications. Most patients can be transported to the closest appropriate facility without lights and siren.

If the patient refuses care, repeatedly urge the patient to accept your assistance, including transport. Consider contacting medical direction for advice. If you are unable to persuade the patient to accept care, carefully document the patient's refusal.

Myocarditis

Myocarditis is an inflammation of the thickest layer of the heart, the myocardium. The myocardium, the heart's middle layer, contains the conduction system and the cardiac muscle fibers that allow the heart to contract. Myocarditis may or may not involve the endocardium or pericardium.

Myocarditis is usually benign and self-limiting. However, if inflammation in the heart muscle becomes widespread, the extensive destruction of heart muscle cells could impair the heart's ability to pump, resulting in RVF and LVF, dysrhythmias, or death. In some cases, myocarditis may lead to dilated cardiomyopathy.

Myocarditis can be caused by many different pathogens, including bacteria, viruses, and parasites. The most common cause of myocarditis is a viral infection. Other causes of myocarditis are heart transplant rejection; rheumatic fever; exposure to chemical poisons, such as heavy metals or in chronic alcoholism; and an adverse effect of radiation therapy for cancer, especially with large doses to the chest. In many cases, the cause of myocarditis is unknown.

Assessment

Most cases of myocarditis are associated with flulike symptoms for which the patient does not seek medical care. The patient may have fatigue, decreased appetite, mild shortness of breath, joint and muscle aches and pains, or fever.

Cardiac symptoms usually appear 10 to 14 days after the initial onset of symptoms. Complaints of palpitations are common. Some patients report chest discomfort, often described as a sharp, stabbing pain in the center of the chest. If a patient with myocarditis describes a complaint of squeezing chest discomfort, it may be challenging in the field to differentiate these symptoms from those associated with an ACS.

The patient's physical exam findings may range from mild or no signs to severe heart failure. Tachycardia and tachypnea are common. The ECG may show transient ECG changes such as low-voltage QRS complexes, pathologic Q waves, and nonspecific ST-segment and T-wave abnormalities. Although sinus tachycardia is probably the most common rhythm seen, patients sometimes have a second- or third-degree AV block. LBBB or RBBB also may be seen. JVD, crackles, ascites, and peripheral edema may be seen if heart failure is present. Differential diagnoses to consider for myocarditis include the following:

- ACS
- Aortic dissection
- Esophageal perforation, rupture, or tear

- Heart failure
- Kawasaki disease
- Pneumonia
- Pulmonary disease

Management

Prehospital care for patients with myocarditis is mainly supportive. Allow the patient to assume a position of comfort, establish an IV line, and apply the cardiac monitor. Apply a pulse oximeter and administer oxygen, if indicated. Obtain a 12-lead ECG. Be prepared to treat heart failure and dysrhythmia according to local protocol or instructions from medical direction.

Rheumatic Fever

Rheumatic fever is an inflammatory disease caused by streptococcal bacteria. This disease can cause stenosis of the mitral valve or aortic valve, leading to heart complications. Prehospital care is supportive.

Scarlet Fever

Scarlet fever is a disease caused by the bacterium *Streptococcus pyogenes*, which is the same bacterium responsible for causing strep throat. This disease is characterized by a sore throat, fever, rash, and "strawberry tongue" (a white tongue with red speckles). Patients younger than 1 year are at the greatest risk of developing the infection. Scarlet fever is treated with antibiotics, and prehospital care is supportive.

Vascular Disorders

Aortic Aneurysm

Like other arteries, the aorta is composed of three layers: The *adventitia* is the thin outer layer, the *media* is the thick, elastic middle layer, and the *intima* is the thin, innermost layer. The elastic tissue of the aorta's middle layer stretches as blood is forcefully ejected from the left ventricle. The tissue recoils as the heart relaxes. These efficient movements keep blood moving throughout the cardiac cycle.

Even in healthy adults, this ability of the arteries to stretch and recoil diminishes with age. In some people, the constant stress on the wall of the aorta weakens it. As a result, the aorta swells (dilates) gradually, called an aortic aneurysm. The word *aneurysm* refers to the dilation or outpouching of a blood vessel (or the wall of a chamber of the heart). The dilated area may leak or rupture if it stretches too far.

If the vessel wall tears, then its layers can separate in a process called dissection. Aortic dissection may begin with a tear in the aorta's inner lining (the intima) near the vessel's weakened area. As blood flows through this tear and between the vessel wall layers, it exposes the middle layer to blood under high pressure. Blood also fills the space between the layers of the vessel, causing them to separate (dissect). With each ventricular systole, a jet of blood is forced into the torn arterial wall, creating a false channel between the wall's intimal and medial layers. This channel is propagated distally and sometimes proximally along the length of the wall. If the dissection progresses back into the aortic valve, it may prevent the valve from closing. Blood will then be regurgitated back from the aorta into the left ventricle during systole. Recall that the coronary arteries branch off from the aorta just above the leaflets of the aortic valve; thus, if the valve is affected, coronary blood flow will likely be compromised as well. If the dissection involves the takeoff point of the innominate, left common carotid, or left subclavian artery, then blood flow through the affected artery or arteries will be diminished. Although an aortic dissection may occur anywhere along the aorta, most begin in the ascending aorta within 2 inches (5 cm) of the aortic valve or in the descending thoracic aorta just beyond the origin of the left subclavian artery at the site of the ligamentum arteriosum.

Several of the risk factors for atherosclerosis, such as tobacco smoking, high blood cholesterol, hypertension, and CHD, increase the risk of an aortic aneurysm. Of these, smoking is the most important modifiable risk factor for aortic aneurysm.[2]

Aneurysms of the ascending thoracic aorta are usually caused by cystic medial degeneration (formerly called cystic medial necrosis), a connective tissue disease characterized by degeneration of the elastic tissue and smooth muscle fiber of the middle (medial) layer of large arteries. The area of the vessel that was previously filled with normal elastic tissue is replaced with cystlike connective tissue.

A mild form of medial degeneration is often present in older adults' aortas and may occur as a natural consequence of aging. Aortic disease may have a genetic cause in younger people, such as Marfan syndrome, vascular Ehlers-Danlos syndrome, and

Loeys-Dietz syndrome, among others. These inherited connective tissue disorders affect the proteins responsible for the strength, elasticity, and integrity of the body's organs, skin, bones, and vasculature. If a connective tissue disease affects the aorta, the wall of the aorta becomes weak and dilates, increasing the risk of aneurysm development, aortic dissection, and rupture. Aortic aneurysms can also be congenital, the result of infective endocarditis or an untreated infection due to syphilis or salmonella, or may have a traumatic cause (usually a deceleration injury in a motor vehicle crash).

Assessment

An aneurysm does not always cause symptoms. If it does, the signs and symptoms will depend on the location of the aneurysm. As the aneurysm increases in size, stretching of the aortic wall produces pain. The pressure of a large amount of blood on surrounding organs may also produce symptoms. For example, difficulty swallowing (dysphagia) may occur as the esophagus is compressed. Laryngeal nerve compression may cause hoarseness. Heart failure or tracheal or bronchial compression may cause difficulty breathing. The sudden development of new or worsening pain may be a sign of impending aneurysm rupture.

The patient's description of the pain may provide clues to the location of the dissection. When the aorta dissects, almost all patients report the abrupt onset of constant, unbearable pain. This pain, which may last for hours to days, is described as tearing or ripping and sharp, stabbing, or knifelike. Common phrases used to describe the pain include "it feels like someone stabbed me in the chest with a knife" or "it feels like someone hit me in the back with an axe." Dissection of the ascending aorta is usually associated with pain that is either substernal or located in the neck, throat, jaw, or face. Descending aortic dissection usually produces flank pain, pain between the shoulder blades, or pain in the back, abdomen, or lower extremities. No matter where it begins, the pain may move as the dissection extends along the aorta.

Based on the patient's description, it may be difficult to distinguish the chest pain of a dissecting aneurysm from an AMI, but several distinctive features may help differentiate it. **TABLE 18-17** compares the clinical presentation of AMI with a dissecting aortic aneurysm.

The patient with aortic dissection is usually anxious and may describe a feeling of impending doom. Peripheral nerve ischemia may cause pain, weakness, or numbness and tingling in the extremities. Coronary artery compression may produce signs of myocardial ischemia. Although this presentation is less common, with or without accompanying chest pain, the patient may have signs and symptoms of heart failure, altered mental status, stroke, paraplegia, or cardiac arrest. Sudden death can occur. In some patients, increased vagal tone, hypovolemia, or dysrhythmia can lead to syncope.

In dissections of the ascending aorta, which tend to occur in younger patients previously in good health, one or more of the aortic arch vessels is compromised. Disruption of flow through the innominate artery, for example, is likely to produce a difference in BP between the two arms. Pressure

TABLE 18-17 Comparison of AMI With Dissecting Aortic Aneurysm

	AMI	Dissecting Aortic Aneurysm
Onset of pain	Gradual, with prodromal symptoms	Abrupt, without prodromal symptoms
Severity of pain	Increases with time	Maximal from the outset
Timing of pain	May wax and wane	Does not abate once it has started
Location of pain	Substernal; back is rarely involved	Back is often involved, between the shoulder blades
Clinical signs	Peripheral pulses equal	Blood pressure discrepancy between arms or a decrease in the femoral or carotid pulse

Abbreviation: AMI, acute myocardial infarction

differences greater than 20 mm Hg between the arms may indicate the presence of an aortic aneurysm. (If you do not routinely check the BP in both arms of a patient, you will never pick up that sign!) Suspect dissection if this finding is accompanied by other findings such as acute neurologic changes. Disruption of blood flow into the left common carotid artery may produce signs and symptoms of a stroke. When the dissection extends proximal to the coronary artery ostia, coronary blood flow is likely to be compromised, producing ECG changes characteristic of myocardial ischemia.

Dissection of the descending aorta is more common in older patients, especially in those with a history of hypertension. The pain is likely to be somewhat less severe when the descending aorta is involved. The patient may wait a few days before seeking help. Distal pulses may be hard to feel.

Rupture of a thoracic aneurysm usually occurs into the left intrapleural space or mediastinum or, less commonly, into the esophagus. Signs of a hemothorax may be present if the dissection ruptures into the pleural cavity. Signs of cardiac tamponade may be present if the dissection ruptures into the pericardial cavity.

Rupture of an abdominal aortic aneurysm is usually associated with sudden back pain accompanied by abdominal pain and tenderness. The patient may be hypotensive and have a pulsating abdominal mass between the xiphoid process and umbilicus. An aneurysm is often sensitive to palpation and may be quite tender if it is expanding rapidly or about to rupture. When an abdominal aortic aneurysm does rupture, distention of the abdominal cavity usually occurs. Massive GI hemorrhage may be present if the aneurysm ruptures into the duodenum.

Management

Aortic dissection is a medical emergency. The goal of prehospital management in a suspected dissecting aneurysm is to provide adequate pain relief and rapid transport. Contact medical direction as soon as you suspect the patient has a dissecting aneurysm. Relay this information to the receiving facility to allow the staff time to gather the necessary resources for the patient while you are in transit. Because nothing can be done to stabilize the patient's condition in the field, avoid performing any procedures on the scene that may delay transport to definitive care.

Establish an IV line, and apply the cardiac monitor. Apply a pulse oximeter and administer oxygen, if indicated. Give IV fluids and medications per local protocol or medical direction. Opioids may be ordered for pain control if the patient's BP can tolerate them; however, these medications may not be strong enough to relieve the patient's pain.

Reassess the patient at least every 5 minutes en route to the closest appropriate medical facility. The patient with aortic dissection will require aggressive therapy in the intensive care unit (ICU) and possibly surgery.

Acute Arterial Occlusion and Acute Limb Ischemia

An acute arterial occlusion is a sudden disruption of arterial blood flow because of a thrombus, embolus, tumor, direct trauma to an artery, or an unknown cause. Direct trauma to an artery may result from an extremity injury or diagnostic procedure such as cardiac catheterization. Less common causes of acute arterial occlusion include dissecting aneurysm, vasospasm (usually attributable to IV drug use), and a vascular graft blockage. Acute limb (extremity) ischemia results when an arterial occlusion suddenly stops or markedly reduces blood flow to an arm or leg.

In most cases, acute arterial occlusion is caused by an embolus that begins in the heart and travels to the extremities. Any of several conditions may favor the origination of an embolus in the heart, including AF, clot formation in the left ventricle after AMI, a rheumatic or prosthetic heart valve, and left ventricular aneurysm. Although arterial emboli can travel to various sites in the body, most lodge in the femoral artery, compromising lower-extremity circulation. Although less common, arterial emboli can also lodge in the brain, intestines, kidney, spleen, or upper extremities. Most emboli occur in patients with significant underlying heart disease.

When a thrombus blocks a previously open artery that has been narrowed by atherosclerosis, the area distal to the blockage becomes ischemic. When the blockage affects an extremity, blood flow to the muscle is limited. During exercise, blood flow to the area decreases further, and muscle contraction may stop blood flow. However, some patients have few symptoms because the process occurs gradually, allowing collateral circulation to develop as atherosclerosis causes the major vessel to narrow. If the patient develops extensive collateral circulation in the extremity, they may not notice any change or may perceive only a mild increase in symptoms when a major atherosclerotic vessel becomes blocked.

Individuals who have peripheral artery disease (PAD) are more likely to have atherosclerosis in other vessels such as the coronary, carotid, and renal arteries and the abdominal aorta.[2] Approximately 10% of patients with PAD have classic symptoms of intermittent **claudication**,[2] including pain, cramping, muscle tightness, fatigue, or weakness of the legs when walking or during exercise. These symptoms occur as a result of increased oxygen demand during activity. In such a case, the arteries that supply the muscles of the calves, hips, or buttocks are narrowed or blocked by atherosclerotic plaques that limit blood flow to the tissues. After a brief rest, symptoms disappear within a few minutes, and the patient can resume activity until the pain recurs. Approximately 40% of patients with PAD do not complain of leg pain and present with atypical symptoms such as leg tiredness or fatigue.[2] The remaining 50% are asymptomatic despite an abnormal pulse examination or have leg symptoms different from classic claudication (ie, exertional pain that either does not stop the individual from walking, does stop the individual from walking but does not involve the calves, or does not resolve within 10 minutes of rest).[2]

Assessment

You must gather an accurate history from a patient with acute limb ischemia. If the patient tells you the symptoms began suddenly, then suspect an embolus as the probable cause of the ischemia. If the patient tells you the symptoms have gradually worsened, then a thrombus is the more likely cause. Ask whether the patient has had similar symptoms in the past; if such a history is confirmed, determine if the episodes have become more frequent and how long each event lasts.

When obtaining the patient's history and performing the physical exam, keep in mind the five Ps of acute arterial occlusion: Pain, Pulselessness, Pallor, Paresthesia, and Paralysis. Pain associated with acute limb ischemia usually begins distal to the site of obstruction and gradually increases in severity. Ischemia of peripheral nerves in the affected limb causes motor impairment and sensory loss. The patient may report a decrease in pain as sensory loss progresses. Paralysis and paresthesia are signs and symptoms of limb-threatening ischemia.

Find out whether the patient has risk factors for developing a blood clot, such as a recent extremity injury, IV drug use, heart surgery or AMI, clotting disorder, pulmonary embolism, AF, contraceptive use, hormone replacement therapy, or rheumatic heart disease.

Assessing a patient with acute limb ischemia requires examining the limb for color and temperature abnormalities and feeling for arterial pulses. The skin of the affected limb usually appears pale or mottled distal to or over the affected area. If arterial blood flow to the limb is severely restricted, the foot will turn pale when raised and very red after 1 minute of placing it at a level lower than the heart. The skin of the affected limb may feel cool and may be either moist or dry. Feel the brachial, radial, femoral, posterior tibial, and dorsalis pedis arteries in pairs, and document your findings. Peripheral pulses may be absent or diminished in the affected limb.

Because advanced limb ischemia affects motor and sensory functions, assess movement and sensation in all extremities. Sensory deficits over the dorsum of the foot are often an early sign of vascular compromise.

Breath sounds are usually clear, but changes in heart rate and rhythm may occur. Check the patient's BP in both arms. Unequal BP readings may indicate a thoracic aneurysm. Listen for a bruit over the affected vessel or vessels. In general, information from the patient's ECG does not contribute significantly to emergency care for this condition.

If the patient has had PAD symptoms for some time, then signs of chronic limb ischemia may be present. These signs include muscle wasting, with shiny, scaly skin on the affected limb, cessation of hair growth over the dorsum of the toes and foot, and thickening of the toenails. The differential diagnosis of acute arterial occlusion and acute limb ischemia includes the following possible conditions:

- Abdominal aneurysm
- Arthritis
- DVT

- Scleroderma
- Soft-tissue injury
- Systemic lupus erythematosus

Management

Allow the patient to assume a position of comfort. If limb ischemia affects a lower extremity, place the patient in a sitting position if doing so is not contraindicated. Place the patient's feet lower than the chest to allow gravity to help perfuse the limb. Establish an IV line and apply the cardiac monitor. Apply a pulse oximeter and administer oxygen, if indicated. Give medications as instructed by medical direction. Medications to reduce pain may be ordered. Keep the patient compartment of the ambulance warm to avoid cold-induced vasoconstriction of the skin, but do not apply heat or cold to the affected limb. Ischemic tissue both burns at a lower temperature and is more susceptible to frostbite than nonischemic skin. The patient with acute limb ischemia requires rapid transport to the closest appropriate facility. Reassess the patient's condition frequently en route. Monitor the five Ps.

If the patient refuses care, repeatedly urge the patient to accept your assistance, including transport. Consider contacting medical direction for advice. If you are unable to persuade the patient to accept care, carefully document the patient's refusal.

Acute DVT

Thrombophlebitis is the development of a blood clot in an inflamed or damaged vein. Superficial thrombophlebitis occurs when a clot develops in a vein near the surface of the skin. If a clot develops in the deep veins of the extremities, then DVT is present. DVT is associated with an increased risk of pulmonary embolism.

Factors that predispose a person to thrombus formation include the following:

1. **Venous stasis, or sluggish blood flow.** Venous stasis is present in patients who are pregnant, who are immobile for long periods, and who have obesity or heart failure.
2. **Damage to the inner lining of the vessel.** Vascular damage can be caused by trauma, inflammation, venipuncture, or the action of agents given during IV therapy.
3. **Blood clotting disorders.** Conditions that promote blood clotting include dehydration, certain types of cancer, and the use of estrogen-based contraceptives, hormone replacement therapy, or infertility treatment.

Assessment

Patients with DVT may seek medical care because of swelling, pain, or tenderness in a limb. In some cases, they may seek help after the onset of symptoms from a pulmonary embolus. Ask the patient about the presence of risk factors for DVT.

Carefully assess the patient's upper and lower extremities. Compare the extremities in pairs. Classic signs of DVT include swelling of the affected limb, with pain or tenderness. However, these findings are present in only approximately one-half of patients with DVT. Look for signs of inflammation such as redness and warmth of the skin over the affected vein. Pain and tenderness of the calf muscle on dorsiflexion of the foot (Homan sign) may be present. As you assess the patient, be careful not to rub or massage the affected limb. Such action could dislodge a clot, at which point it would be termed a thromboembolism.

The differential diagnoses for DVT include arthritis, cellulitis, muscle or soft-tissue injury, and superficial thrombophlebitis.

Management

Prehospital care for DVT is supportive. Allow the patient to assume a position of comfort. Establish an IV line and apply the cardiac monitor. Apply a pulse oximeter and administer oxygen, if indicated. Monitor the patient closely for development of a pulmonary embolism.

Most patients with DVT can be transported to the closest appropriate facility without lights and siren. If the patient refuses care, repeatedly urge the patient to accept assistance, including transport. Consider contacting medical direction for advice. If you are unable to persuade the patient to accept care, carefully document the patient's refusal.

A few other cardiac conditions may lead to emergencies. These include congenital heart disease and cardiomyopathy. Congenital heart disease is discussed in Chapter 43, *Neonatal Care*. Cardiomyopathy is discussed in Chapter 44, *Pediatric Emergencies*.

YOU are the Paramedic SUMMARY

1. What is your initial impression of this patient's condition?

The patient is diaphoretic, with pale mucous membranes, tachycardia, and hypotension. Collectively, these signs suggest poor cellular perfusion, shock, and increased oxygen demand. The symptoms suggest a cardiac origin, and the onset at rest suggests an unstable condition. You should expedite your evaluation, stabilization, and transport to an appropriate facility.

2. What are some possible causes of the patient's symptoms?

Given the patient's description of the pain (crushing), you should consider a cardiac cause. Other possible causes of chest pain are trauma, pneumothorax, and pneumonia.

3. Although it is certainly possible, this patient is relatively young to be having an acute myocardial infarction (AMI). What factors might be associated with a cardiac event in a patient of this age?

Although an MI cannot be ruled out in a young adult, especially if the patient has a family history, use of stimulant drugs (cocaine or methamphetamine) is more commonly associated with acute MI in young people. However, your initial management is the same, so don't waste valuable time trying to identify a drug cause.

4. What additional assessment data will be necessary when evaluating this patient?

Evaluate and assess the skin and vital signs (to assess CO), the heart and lungs (to look for other causes and signs of heart failure), and the prior medical history. The ECG will also play an important role in evaluating this patient.

5. What interventions should you initiate at this time?

In this case, rapidly administer supplemental oxygen, establish IV access, and evaluate the ECG.

6. Is this patient high priority? Why or why not?

The patient was high priority before the seizure, and he is very high priority now. In addition to having had a tonic-clonic seizure, the patient has a compromised airway and ventilation, bradycardia, and decreased CO.

7. Given what you know at this time, what is the most likely cause of the seizure activity?

In the absence of other information, the two most likely causes of seizure are hypoxia (caused by a sudden drop in the pulse rate and cerebral perfusion) and stimulant drug use (given the risk for stimulant use related to cardiac symptoms in young people).

8. What is this patient's greatest life threat at this time? How will you treat it?

Shock poses the most significant threat at this point. The sudden drop in the patient's heart rate has resulted in a dramatic drop in BP. Overall, the strategy for treating this patient should begin with an attempt to restore normal cardiac rhythm and rate, followed by an effort to improve CO and BP.

9. How will you manage the cardiac rhythm?

Although atropine is the preferred drug for symptomatic bradycardia, it is unlikely to be effective in cases of third-degree AV block. Reasonable alternative treatment options include TCP or a dopamine or epinephrine IV infusion.

10. Assume the patient remained unresponsive, with an unacceptably low BP despite pacing. What treatment would be appropriate under those circumstances?

Once the pulse rate has been normalized, several strategies may be used to improve BP, depending on the local protocol. If the patient's breath sounds remain clear, then a fluid challenge (usually 250 mL) may be used to increase preload to improve cardiac contractility and output. Dopamine may also be considered to improve contractility and, depending on the dose, to increase afterload. A disadvantage of dopamine is it escalates myocardial oxygen demand, which may increase the size and severity of infarction.

11. Given the patient's final disposition, was your treatment appropriate? Why or why not?

A better choice may have been to attach the patient to the cardiac monitor before preparing him for transfer to the ambulance. Although this may have increased scene time, it could have allowed you to identify a lethal dysrhythmia (we do not know what the preseizure rhythm was). Early recognition and treatment may have prevented the onset of third-degree AV block.

YOU are the Paramedic SUMMARY continued

EMS Patient Care Report (PCR)

Date: 09-09-22	**Incident No.:** 889	**Nature of Call:** Cardiac		**Location:** 220 Halifax Ave	
Dispatched: 0828	**En Route:** 0828	**At Scene:** 0835	**Transport:** 0902	**At Hospital:** 0914	**In Service:** 0928

Patient Information

Age: 32 **Sex:** Male **Weight (in kg [lb]):** 89 kg (195 lb)	**Allergies:** NKDA **Medications:** None **Past Medical History:** None **Chief Complaint:** Chest pain

Vital Signs

Time: 0845	**BP:** 96/40	**Pulse:** 150 reg	**Respirations:** 20, deep	**Spo_2:** 88% on room air
Time: 0850	**BP:** 62/40	**Pulse:** 36 irreg	**Respirations:** 6 (10 with bag-mask ventilation)	**Spo_2:** 99% with bag-mask ventilation
Time: 0905	**BP:** 100/70	**Pulse:** 70 paced pulses/min; regular	**Respirations:** 10 with bag-mask ventilation	**Spo_2:** 99% with bag-mask ventilation

EMS Treatment (circle all that apply)

Oxygen @ 15 L/min via (circle one): **NC** **NRM** **(Bag-mask device)**		**(Assisted Ventilation)**	**Airway Adjunct**	**CPR**
Defibrillation	**Bleeding Control**	**Bandaging**	**Splinting**	**(Other: TCP)**

Narrative

Arrived to find a 32-year-old male who reports crushing chest pain (rated 9/10) with shortness of breath. Symptoms came on at rest and became more intense over 1 to 2 hours. Pt was initially awake, alert, and oriented, but he experienced a tonic-clonic seizure lasting 30 to 45 seconds while being loaded into the ambulance. Pt unresponsive, with no spontaneous breathing. Bag-mask ventilation begun. Cardiac monitor showed third-degree AV block with wide QRS at 36 beats/min. BP 62/40. Started IV of NS and began TCP. Electrical and mechanical capture achieved at 70 pulses/min with 60 mA. Patient remains unresponsive and apneic; bag-mask ventilation continued. BP 100/70, skin warm, dry, and normal color. Report to RMC on arrival to Susan RN.

End of report

Prep Kit

Ready for Review

- The cardiovascular system is composed of the heart and blood vessels. Its primary function is to deliver oxygenated blood and nutrients to every cell in the body. The cardiovascular system is also responsible for delivering chemical messengers (hormones) within the body and for transporting the waste products of metabolism from the cells to sites of recycling or disposal.
- CVD refers to a group of disorders of the heart and blood vessels. Examples include hypertension (high BP), peripheral vascular

Prep Kit continued

disease, heart failure, cardiomyopathies, and congenital heart disease. CHD is a type of CVD that includes disease of the coronary arteries and its associated signs, symptoms, and complications, such as angina pectoris and AMI. Recognizing and managing cardiovascular emergencies is an essential part of paramedic education.

- Acute coronary syndromes (ACSs) are a series of cardiac conditions caused by an abrupt reduction in blood flow through a coronary artery. There are three major ACSs: unstable angina, non–ST-segment elevation myocardial infarction (NSTEMI), and ST-segment elevation myocardial infarction (STEMI). Common chief complaints in patients experiencing an ACS often include chest discomfort, dyspnea, fainting, palpitations, and fatigue.
- Cardiac arrest is the cessation of cardiac mechanical activity, as confirmed by the absence of signs of circulation. Sudden cardiac arrest (SCA) is an unexpected cardiac arrest that results in attempts to restore circulation. If resuscitation attempts are unsuccessful, this situation is referred to as sudden cardiac death.
- The mechanical pumping action of the heart can occur only in response to an electrical stimulus. In the heart, depolarization is the process of discharging resting cardiac muscle fibers by means of an electrical impulse that stimulates contraction.
- A typical myocardial cell's cardiac action potential consists of five phases of electrical activity within the heart: phase 0 through phase 4. These phases reflect cardiac cell voltage changes, which correspond with the waveforms viewed on a rhythm strip.
- The heart's electrical conduction system comprises pacemaker cells found in the sinoatrial (SA) node tissues, internodal conduction pathways, atrioventricular (AV) node, bundle of His, and Purkinje fibers. An accessory conduction pathway allows electrical impulses to bypass the AV node and trigger ventricular depolarization in some patients.
- The body attempts to maintain a relatively constant BP to ensure perfusion of vital organs. When stimulated, baroreceptors in the internal carotid arteries and aortic arch generate compensatory responses that facilitate BP regulation by the autonomic nervous system's sympathetic division.
- A cardiac dysrhythmia is a disturbance in the normal cardiac rhythm, which may or may not be clinically significant. It is always necessary to evaluate the dysrhythmia in the context of the patient's overall clinical condition.
- An ECG is a graphic record of the voltage changes in the heart muscle during depolarization and repolarization. Cardiac monitors consist of lead wires connected to electrodes, which are then placed on the patient. The electrodes must be placed in consistent, predetermined positions on each patient's body to obtain a reliable, useful ECG. Each lead provides an electrical snapshot of a specific part of the heart. ECG analysis is indicated in any patient who might have a cardiac-related condition.
- A 12-lead ECG provides detailed information about the heart's conduction system and records its electrical activity from 12 separate angles. The 12 leads include three limb leads (I, II, and III), three augmented limb leads (aVR, aVL, and aVF), and six precordial leads (V_1 to V_6). Contiguous leads view geographically similar areas of the myocardium, which can help localize areas of ischemia, injury, or infarction.
- Because a standard 12-lead ECG does not view the right ventricle or the left ventricle's posterior surface, use additional leads to detect ischemia or infarction in those areas. Right-side precordial leads are positioned in specific locations on the right anterior thorax to analyze the right ventricle's electrical activity. If you need to view the left ventricle's posterior wall, place the three precordial leads in specific locations on the left posterior thorax.

Prep Kit continued

- Components of a rhythm strip produced by an ECG include the P wave, PRI, QRS complex, J point, ST segment, T wave, and QT interval.
- A systematic approach to analyzing and interpreting cardiac dysrhythmias includes identifying the P-QRS-T waves, measuring the PRI and QRS, determining rhythm regularity, and measuring the heart rate.
- A normal sinus rhythm arises in the SA node and has an intrinsic rate of 60 to 100 beats/min, a regular rhythm, and minimal variation between R-R intervals.
- Rhythms originating in the SA node include sinus bradycardia, sinus tachycardia, and sinus dysrhythmia. Sinus arrest occurs when the SA node fails to initiate an impulse.
- Treatment of symptomatic bradycardia may include an atropine IV bolus (for symptomatic sinus bradycardia or a conduction block at the level of the AV node), transcutaneous pacing (TCP), or a dopamine or epinephrine infusion, and supportive care.
- TCP is an intervention used to depolarize heart muscle using an external stimulus. Pads placed on the patient's chest deliver electrical energy to the heart, causing muscle contraction. The external pacemaker may serve as a bridge to permanent pacemaker implantation.
- Any area of the atria can originate an impulse, thereby superseding the SA node's pacemaking authority. The resulting rhythms include premature atrial complexes, supraventricular tachycardia (SVT), AV reentrant tachycardia (Wolff-Parkinson-White and Lown-Ganong-Levine syndromes), atrial fibrillation and atrial flutter, wandering atrial pacemaker, and multifocal atrial tachycardia.
- Conservative therapies, such as vagal maneuvers and medications, are appropriate for symptomatic adults with stable vital signs experiencing an SVT. However, if the patient becomes unstable, then electrical therapy using synchronized cardioversion is recommended.
- Synchronized cardioversion is an intervention used to interrupt rapid, organized, hemodynamically unstable rhythms, such as SVT and ventricular tachycardia (VT), and allow the SA node to resume its primary pacemaking function. Unlike defibrillation, in which energy may be delivered at any time during the cardiac cycle, synchronized cardioversion delivers timed bursts of electrical energy that are synchronized with the patient's cardiac rhythm. After identifying the R waves on the ECG, the machine will discharge with the next detected R wave, avoiding the vulnerable period during the T wave of the cardiac cycle.
- If the SA node fails to initiate an impulse, then the AV junction can take over as the heart's pacemaker. Rhythms that originate in the AV junction include premature junctional complexes, junctional escape rhythms, accelerated junctional rhythms, or junctional tachycardia. Treatment of symptomatic patients depends on the underlying cause.
- If the SA node and AV junction fail to pace the heart, the ventricles may assume pacing responsibility. Rhythms that originate in the ventricles include premature ventricular complexes, an idioventricular rhythm or accelerated idioventricular rhythm, VT, and ventricular fibrillation (VF).
- VF and pulseless VT are shockable cardiac arrest rhythms that may respond to defibrillation, an intervention used to interrupt rapid, chaotic rhythms. Defibrillation simultaneously depolarizes all cardiac tissue to allow the SA node to resume its primary pacing function.
- Nonshockable cardiac arrest rhythms include asystole, a complete absence of ventricular electrical activity, and pulseless electrical activity, an organized cardiac rhythm (other than VT) on the monitor that is not accompanied by a detectable pulse.
- Most adults who experience cardiac arrests have evidence of atherosclerosis or another

Prep Kit continued

underlying cardiac disease. However, SCA can also occur secondary to electrocution, a submersion incident, other traumatic events, or noncardiac conditions such as drug overdose, asthma, or anaphylaxis. Many people who experience SCA have no warning before the event.

- Taking a systematic, exhaustively rehearsed assessment approach in cardiac arrest emergencies is essential to achieve a return of spontaneous circulation and to preserve the patient's neurologic function. High-quality CPR, defibrillation, airway management, administration of fluid and medications, and rapid transport are essential emergency medical care elements for cardiac arrest patients.
- The goals of post–cardiac arrest care are to optimize cardiopulmonary function and vital organ perfusion.
- If an impulse traveling through the AV node is delayed more than usual or is completely blocked, it can result in an AV block. An AV block can occur at the level of the AV node or below the bundle of His (infranodal), involving one or more of the bundle branches and the fascicles. AV blocks are classified into degrees, from least to most serious: first-degree AV block, second-degree block, and third-degree block.
- A 12-lead ECG is useful for viewing the heart from several angles to localize the site of cardiac injury or to identify dysrhythmias and other cardiac abnormalities. Examples of other indications for performing a 12-lead ECG include electrical therapy (both before and after, including defibrillation, cardioversion, and pacing), chest or upper abdominal discomfort, electrical injury, electrolyte imbalance, overdose, right or left ventricular failure, stroke, syncope or near syncope, and hemodynamic instability of unknown etiology.
- The prompt transmission of 12-lead ECG findings to the receiving facility is a crucial step that can lead to a faster STEMI diagnosis, decrease the time from emergency onset to definitive therapy, and decrease mortality.
- A systematic approach to 12-lead ECG interpretation is essential. Steps include reviewing the snapshot; interpreting the dysrhythmia; determining the axis; recognizing conduction system disturbances; evaluating chamber size; reviewing for zones of ischemia, injury, and infarction; and investigating noncardiac causes. Twelve-lead interpretation is a vital paramedic skill and should be practiced regularly because equipment failure can occur.
- Injured, ischemic, or infarcted tissue undergoes characteristic changes that appear on the ECG in the facing leads. Ischemia is evidenced by ST-segment depression, and myocardial injury is evidenced by ST-segment elevation.
- ACSs are characterized by an abrupt reduction in blood flow through one or more coronary arteries. If one of these blood vessels becomes blocked, then the muscle it supplies will be deprived of oxygen, a condition called ischemia. Ischemia will lead to tissue death (infarction) if perfusion is not quickly restored. Time is muscle when caring for a patient experiencing an ACS, so you must rapidly and systematically assess the patient and provide necessary emergency care.
- Risk factors are health conditions, lifestyle habits, and traits that may increase a person's chance of developing a disease. Modifiable risk factors can be controlled, modified, or treated, whereas nonmodifiable risk factors cannot be changed. Contributing risk factors are thought to increase heart disease and stroke risk, but their exact role has not been defined.
- Patients may experience various symptoms when they have a cardiovascular condition, the most common of which are chest pain, dyspnea, fainting, palpitations, and fatigue. Symptoms of myocardial ischemia other than chest pain or discomfort are called anginal equivalents.

Prep Kit continued

- Older adults, women, and people with diabetes often have atypical symptoms of CVD. The location or quality of the discomfort or pain may be unusual. These patients may also have nausea, mental status changes, weakness, restlessness, or other symptoms that should be viewed as anginal equivalents.
- Rapid, systematic assessment of cardiovascular issues requires quick STEMI identification, determination of symptom onset, close monitoring of cardiac rhythm and the patient's vital signs, CPR and defibrillation if indicated, medication administration if appropriate, and rapid transport.
- Cardiac monitoring and ECG analysis are indicated in any patient who might have a cardiac-related condition. Any patient with chest pain or a history of a heart condition should undergo ECG analysis.
- STEMI treatment involves rapid reperfusion therapy to restore blood flow using mechanical means, such as percutaneous coronary intervention, or pharmacologic means (ie, using a fibrinolytic agent to dissolve blood clots).
- Heart failure occurs when the heart is unable to pump powerfully enough or fast enough to empty its chambers; as a result, blood backs up into the systemic circuit, the pulmonary circuit, or both. Heart failure may be caused by several disorders that impair the ventricles' ability to fill with or eject blood, including coronary artery disease, long-standing high BP, and diabetes. Dysrhythmias, cardiomyopathy, valvular heart disease, and genetic conditions can also lead to heart failure.
- Cardiac tamponade occurs when excess fluid accumulates within the pericardium and compresses the heart, thereby impairing the heart's contraction and restricting ventricular filling. Transport the patient to the closest emergency facility where an emergent pericardiocentesis can be performed to restore hemodynamic stability.
- Cardiogenic shock is a condition in which heart muscle function is severely impaired, decreasing cardiac output and resulting in inadequate tissue perfusion. Because the most common cause of cardiogenic shock is left ventricular failure secondary to acute myocardial infarction, it is critical to obtain a 12-lead ECG quickly, look for ECG evidence of myocardial infarction, and, if present, transport the patient to an appropriate facility for definitive care.
- A hypertensive emergency is an acute elevation of BP to 180/120 mm Hg or higher with evidence of end-organ dysfunction. A hypertensive urgency exists when the patient has an acute elevation of BP to 180/120 mm Hg or higher without signs or symptoms of end-organ damage. A patient with a hypertensive emergency requires transport to the closest appropriate facility.
- Infectious diseases of the heart include endocarditis, pericarditis, and myocarditis. Endocarditis is an inflammation of the lining of the heart, which is often caused by a bacterial infection. Pericarditis is an infection of the pericardial sac that envelops the heart; it may be caused by a viral, bacterial, or fungal infection. Myocarditis is an inflammation of the heart's thickest layer, the myocardium, which contains the conduction system and the cardiac muscle fibers that allow the heart to contract. Prehospital care for infectious diseases of the heart is mainly supportive.
- Aortic aneurysms, particularly acute dissecting aneurysms of the thoracic aorta and expanding or ruptured aneurysms of the abdominal aorta, are of critical concern to the EMS responder. Patients may describe sudden, severe ripping, tearing, or stabbing pain in the neck, throat, jaw, face, back, abdomen, chest, lower extremities, or between the shoulder blades. The pain may last hours or days. This condition is often characterized by a discrepancy between the BP in the arms, or a decrease in the femoral or carotid pulse.

Prep Kit continued

- An acute arterial occlusion is a sudden disruption of arterial blood flow because of a thrombus, embolus, tumor, direct trauma to an artery, or an unknown cause. Acute limb (extremity) ischemia occurs when an arterial occlusion suddenly stops or markedly reduces blood flow to an arm or leg. Patients with these conditions require frequent reassessment and rapid transport to the closest appropriate facility.

Vital Vocabulary

aberration A term describing the shape of the QRS complex in aberrantly (abnormally) conducted beats.

absolute refractory period (ARP) The early phase of cardiac repolarization, during which the heart muscle cannot be stimulated to depolarize; also known as the effective refractory period.

acute coronary syndromes (ACSs) A series of cardiac conditions caused by an abrupt reduction in coronary artery blood flow.

acute myocardial infarction (AMI) Cardiac ischemia that occurs when sudden narrowing or complete occlusion of a coronary artery leads to death (necrosis) of myocardial tissue.

agonal Pertaining to the period of dying.

agonal rhythm A ventricular rate of less than 20 beats/min; this rhythm is seen just before the heart stops beating altogether.

angina pectoris The sudden pain that occurs when the oxygen supply to the myocardium is insufficient to meet demand, causing ischemic changes in the tissue.

aortic aneurysm An outpouching or bulge in the wall of a portion of the aorta, caused by weakening and dilation of the vessel wall; a ruptured aortic aneurysm is life threatening.

arrhythmia The absence of any cardiac rhythm or organized activity; asystole or ventricular standstill.

arteriosclerosis A pathologic condition in which the thickening and stiffening of the arterial walls make the arteries less elastic.

artifact An artificial product; in cardiology, used to refer to noise or interference in an ECG tracing.

asystole The absence of ventricular contraction or electrical activity; a straight-line or flat-line ECG.

atheroma A mass of fatty tissue that gradually calcifies, hardening into an atheromatous plaque that infiltrates the arterial wall, diminishing its elasticity.

atherosclerosis An accumulation of fat inside a blood vessel that narrows the diameter of the lumen.

atrioventricular (AV) junction The portion of the conduction system of the heart that consists of the AV node and the nonbranching portion of the bundle of His.

atrioventricular (AV) node A group of cells that slows the electrical impulses from the sinoatrial node before relaying it to the ventricles; located in the floor of the right atrium immediately behind the tricuspid valve and near the opening of the coronary sinus.

augmented limb leads On an ECG, leads aVR, aVL, and aVF. They contain only one true pole; the other end is a combination of information from other leads. A standard 12-lead ECG consists of the three augmented leads, three standard limb leads, and the six precordial leads.

automated external defibrillator (AED) A smart defibrillator that can analyze the patient's ECG rhythm, determine whether a defibrillating shock is needed, and guide the user through the resuscitation effort via voice commands.

axis deviation Movement of the heart's QRS axis to the right or left of its normal position.

Beck triad The classic trio of signs associated with cardiac tamponade: narrowed pulse

Prep Kit continued

pressure, muffled heart tones, and jugular vein distention.

bifascicular block Blockage of any two fascicles or conduction pathways: a right bundle branch block (RBBB) with anterior hemiblock, RBBB with posterior hemiblock, or anterior hemiblock and posterior hemiblock (a combination known as left bundle branch block).

bigeminy A dysrhythmia in which every other complex is a premature complex, causing a *normal–early beat–normal–early beat* pattern; can be atrial, junctional, or ventricular.

bipolar leads On an ECG, leads that contain both a positive and a negative pole: leads I, II, and III.

bruits Abnormal whooshing sounds indicating turbulent blood flow within a narrowed vessel; usually heard in the carotid arteries.

bundle branch block (BBB) An intraventricular conduction disturbance involving impedance of electrical impulses from the bundle of His to the right or left bundle branch.

bundle of His The portion of the heart's conduction system located in the upper portion of the interventricular septum that conducts electrical impulses from the atrioventricular (AV) junction to the right and left bundle branches; also called the AV bundle.

cardiac arrest The cessation of cardiac mechanical activity, as confirmed by the absence of signs of circulation; also called cardiopulmonary arrest.

cardiac cycle The period from one cardiac contraction to the next. Each cardiac cycle consists of ventricular contraction (systole) and relaxation (diastole).

cardiac tamponade A pathologic condition characterized by restriction of cardiac contraction, falling cardiac output, and shock as a result of pericardial fluid accumulation.

cardiovascular disease (CVD) A group of disorders of the heart and blood vessels.

chest compression fraction The period during which compressions are delivered divided by the total time of the resuscitation attempt.

circumflex artery (Cx) One of the two branches of the left main coronary artery; branches of the Cx supply the left atrium, part of the lateral surface of the left ventricle, the inferior surface of the left ventricle in approximately 15% of people, the posterior surface of the left ventricle in 15%, the sinoatrial node in approximately 40%, and the atrioventricular bundle in 10% to 15%.

claudication Pain, cramping, muscle tightness, fatigue, or weakness of the legs during physical activity as a result of increased oxygen demand by the muscle tissue of the legs, hips, and buttocks.

concordant precordial pattern An ECG pattern in which the QRS complexes are all in the same direction in the precordial leads as a result of improper lead placement, anterior wall MI, VT, or other variables.

contiguous leads Leads that view geographically similar areas of the myocardium, such as leads II, III, and aVF; useful for localizing areas of ischemia.

coronary arteries The blood vessels that supply blood to the tissues of the heart.

coronary artery disease (CAD) A pathologic process characterized by progressive atherosclerotic narrowing and eventual obstruction of the coronary arteries.

coronary heart disease (CHD) Disease of the coronary arteries and its associated signs, symptoms, and complications, such as angina pectoris and acute myocardial infarction.

couplet Two consecutive (paired) premature ventricular complexes.

defibrillation The process by which an unsynchronized direct current (DC) electric shock is delivered to the heart to terminate ventricular fibrillation or pulseless ventricular tachycardia.

Prep Kit continued

delta wave The slurring of the upstroke of the first part of the QRS complex that occurs in Wolff-Parkinson-White syndrome.

depolarization The process of discharging resting cardiac muscle fibers by means of an electrical impulse that stimulates contraction.

dissection The process by which the intimal and medial layers of a vessel separate (dissect) after a tear occurs in an aneurysmal portion of the arterial wall. With each ventricular systole, a jet of blood is forced into the torn arterial wall, creating and propagating a false channel.

dysrhythmias Cardiac rhythm disturbances.

ectopic An impulse or rhythm that originates from a site other than the SA node.

electrical conduction system In the heart, the specialized cardiac tissue that initiates and conducts electric impulses; includes the SA node, internodal conduction pathways, atrioventricular node, bundle of His, and the Purkinje network.

endocarditis Inflammation of the endocardium as a result of infection.

fascicular block (hemiblock) Failure of the anterior or posterior fascicles of the heart to conduct electrical impulses because of disease or ischemia.

fibrinolysis The process of dissolving blood clots.

fibrinolytic therapy The use of medications that act to dissolve blood clots.

first-degree AV block A delay in the conduction of the depolarizing impulse from the SA node to the ventricles, prolonging the PR interval; also called first-degree heart block.

heart failure A syndrome that occurs when the heart is unable to pump powerfully enough or fast enough to empty its chambers; as a result, blood backs up into the systemic circuit, the pulmonary circuit, or both.

hyperkalemia A high concentration of potassium in the blood.

hypertension High blood pressure; stage 2 hypertension exists when the systolic blood pressure is 140 mm Hg or higher or the diastolic blood pressure is 90 mm Hg or higher.

hypertensive emergency An acute elevation of blood pressure to 180/120 mm Hg or higher with evidence of end-organ damage (cardiovascular, neurologic, or renal); formerly called hypertensive crisis or malignant hypertension.

hypertensive urgency An acute elevation of BP to 180/120 mm Hg or higher without signs or symptoms of end-organ damage.

hypertrophic cardiomyopathy A genetic condition in which the heart muscle wall is unusually thick, requiring the heart to pump harder to eject blood from the left ventricle.

hypocalcemia A low concentration of calcium in the blood.

hypokalemia A low concentration of potassium in the blood.

idioventricular Related to only the ventricles; produced by the ventricles.

infarction Death (necrosis) of a localized area of tissue caused by ischemia.

internodal pathways The three atrial pathways of electrical conduction that transmit impulses from the sinoatrial node to the atrioventricular node.

ischemia Tissue anoxia caused by diminished blood flow, usually as a result of narrowing or occlusion of an artery.

isoelectric line The baseline of the ECG; isoelectric means neither positive nor negative.

junctional escape rhythm A dysrhythmia arising from the atrioventricular junction with an intrinsic rate of 40 to 60 beats/min; also called junctional rhythm.

lead The electrical potential difference between two points. For example, lead I represents the difference in electrical potential between the right and left arm electrodes.

left anterior descending artery (LAD) One of the two branches of the left main coronary artery; branches of the LAD supply the left ventricle,

Prep Kit continued

interventricular septum, and part of the right ventricle.

left atrial abnormality Dilation of the left atrium that can occur in patients with valvular heart disease (particularly mitral or aortic valve stenosis), hypertensive disease, cardiomyopathy, or coronary artery disease; it can also occur in an athlete.

left ventricular failure (LVF) A condition in which the left ventricle must work harder to pump blood throughout the body. With systolic failure, the left ventricle does not contract normally and has trouble pumping all the blood in the chamber out to the body; with diastolic failure, the left ventricle contracts normally but has become stiff, impeding its ability to relax and fill with blood between each contraction of the heart.

left ventricular hypertrophy (LVH) A cardiac condition in which the left ventricle becomes enlarged, most often as a result of hypertension.

limb leads The ECG leads attached to the limbs; together, the standard limb leads (I, II, and III) and augmented limb leads (aVR, aVL, and aVF) form the hexaxial reference system along the frontal plane.

long QT syndrome (LQTS) A condition characterized by a QT interval exceeding approximately 0.44 second (440 milliseconds).

Lown-Ganong-Levine syndrome A disorder that causes preexcitation of ventricular tissue and is characterized on ECG by a short PR interval and a normal QRS duration.

lumen The hollow interior space within an artery or other hollow structure.

manual defibrillator A device that requires the paramedic or other trained rescuer to interpret the cardiac rhythm and determine whether defibrillation is needed (rather than relying on a device to make that determination automatically).

microvascular angina A type of angina caused by spasms within the walls of the heart's smallest coronary arteries.

multifocal Arising from or pertaining to many foci or locations.

myocarditis Inflammation of the myocardium.

necrosis The death of tissue, usually caused by a cessation of its blood supply.

normal sinus rhythm The normal rhythm of the heart that has an intrinsic rate of 60 to 100 beats/min; the rhythm is regular, with minimal variation between R-R intervals, and all measurements are within normal limits.

orthopnea Severe dyspnea experienced when lying down that is relieved by a change in position, such as sitting up or standing.

P wave The first wave of the ECG complex, representing depolarization of the atria.

palpitations The sensation of an abnormally fast or irregular heartbeat.

paroxysmal nocturnal dyspnea (PND) Severe shortness of breath occurring at night after several hours of recumbency, during which fluid pools in the lungs; the person is forced to sit up to breathe; caused by left heart failure or decompensation of chronic obstructive pulmonary disease.

percutaneous coronary intervention (PCI) A minimally invasive procedure performed under fluoroscopic guidance, in which a balloon, stent, or other device is advanced through a peripheral artery catheter and into an obstructed coronary vessel to diagnose and treat coronary artery obstruction.

pericarditis Inflammation of the pericardial sac.

plasmin A naturally occurring clot-dissolving enzyme.

point of maximal impulse (PMI) The palpable beat of the apex of the heart against the chest wall during ventricular contraction; normally palpated at the fifth left intercostal space along the midclavicular line.

PR interval (PRI) The distance between the beginning of the P wave (atrial depolarization) and the beginning of the QRS complex (ventricular

Prep Kit continued

depolarization), signifying the time required for the atria to depolarize and the excitation impulse to pass through the atrioventricular junction.

precordial leads A term used to describe the chest leads in an ECG.

preexcitation Early depolarization of ventricular tissue through an accessory pathway between the atria and ventricles.

pulmonary edema Congestion of the pulmonary air spaces with exudate and foam, often secondary to left ventricular failure.

pulmonary embolism Obstruction in one or more pulmonary arteries by a solid, liquid, or gas that has swept through the right side of the heart into the lungs.

pulseless electrical activity (PEA) An organized cardiac rhythm (other than ventricular tachycardia) on an ECG monitor that is not accompanied by a detectable pulse.

Purkinje fibers A network of cardiac muscle fibers distributed throughout the ventricular walls' inner surfaces that conduct the excitation impulse from the bundle branches to the ventricular myocardium.

QRS axis A single vector representing the mean (or average) of all vectors created by the ventricles during depolarization.

QRS complex Deflection of the ECG produced by ventricular depolarization.

reciprocal changes Mirror-image J-point, ST-segment, and T-wave changes seen on the ECG during an ACS.

reentry Spread of an impulse through tissue already stimulated by that same impulse.

refractory period (RP) A short period immediately after depolarization during which the myocytes have not yet repolarized and are unable to fire or conduct an impulse (the absolute refractory period) or have partially repolarized and may depolarize in response to an electrical stimulus (the relative refractory period).

relative refractory period (RRP) The portion of the cardiac action potential that extends from the middle of phase 3 to the beginning of phase 4; during this time, the heart muscle has been partially repolarized and may depolarize in response to an electrical stimulus.

reperfusion therapy Treatment intended to facilitate the resumption of blood flow through a blocked vessel; therapy may be either procedural, such as cardiac catheterization, or pharmacologic, such as administration of a fibrinolytic agent.

rheumatic fever An inflammatory disease caused by streptococcal bacteria; the disease can cause mitral or aortic valve stenosis.

right atrial abnormality Dilation of the right atrium that occurs when returning venous pressure is elevated or pulmonary pressure is high.

right coronary artery (RCA) Artery that provides oxygenated blood to the walls of the right atrium and ventricle, a portion of the inferior part of the left ventricle, and portions of the conduction system.

right ventricular failure (RVF) A condition in which the right side of the heart must work increasingly hard to pump blood into engorged pulmonary vessels; eventually, it cannot keep up with the increased workload.

right ventricular hypertrophy (RVH) A cardiac condition in which the right ventricle becomes enlarged, usually as a result of pulmonary hypertension.

R-R interval The period between the onset of one QRS complex and the onset of the next QRS complex.

scarlet fever A disease caused by the bacterium *Streptococcus pyogenes*, which is characterized by a sore throat, fever, rash, and "strawberry tongue."

septum A thick wall that separates the right and left sides of the heart.

Prep Kit continued

sinoatrial (SA) node The dominant pacemaker of the heart, located at the junction of the superior vena cava and the right atrium.

sinus bradycardia A sinus rhythm characterized by a heart rate of less than 60 beats/min.

sinus dysrhythmia A variation of the cycling of a sinus rhythm that is often associated with respiratory cycle fluctuations; the rate increases during inspiration and decreases during expiration.

sinus tachycardia A sinus rhythm characterized by a heart rate greater than 100 beats/min.

ST segment The interval between the end of the QRS complex (the J point) and the beginning of the T wave; when there is significant myocardial ischemia or injury, the ST segment is often depressed or elevated with respect to the isoelectric line.

stable angina Angina pectoris characterized by intermittent pain with a predictable pattern.

subendocardial myocardial infarction A type of acute myocardial infarction in which the ischemic process affects only the inner layer of muscle.

sudden cardiac arrest (SCA) An unexpected cardiac arrest that results in attempts to restore circulation.

sudden cardiac death (SCD) A sudden cardiac arrest in which the resuscitation attempt is unsuccessful.

synchronized cardioversion The use of a synchronized direct current (DC) electric shock to convert a tachydysrhythmia (such as supraventricular tachycardia) to a normal sinus rhythm.

syncope Fainting; brief loss of consciousness caused by transiently inadequate blood flow to the brain.

T wave The upright, flat, or inverted wave following the QRS complex of the ECG, representing ventricular repolarization.

targeted temperature management (TTM) The utilization of cool fluids to get the patient to a targeted hypothermic state during various critical conditions.

thromboembolism A blood clot that initially formed within a blood vessel but is now circulating through the bloodstream.

thrombus A fixed blood clot that can obstruct passage of blood flow through an artery.

transcutaneous pacemaker A device that depolarizes myocardial tissue by sending a small electrical charge through the skin of the chest between one externally placed pacing pad and another.

transcutaneous pacing (TCP) An intervention used to depolarize heart muscle using an external stimulus; pads placed on the patient's chest deliver electrical energy to the heart, causing muscle contraction.

transmural myocardial infarction A type of acute myocardial infarction in which the infarct extends through the entire wall of the ventricle.

trifascicular block Blockage or impairment of all three components of the ventricular conduction system, with one working occasionally to provide AV conduction.

trigeminy A dysrhythmia in which every third complex is a premature complex, causing a *normal– normal–early beat pattern*; can be atrial, junctional, or ventricular.

U wave A small, flat wave sometimes seen after the T wave and before the next P wave.

unifocal Arising from a single site.

unstable angina Angina pectoris characterized by a variable, unpredictable pain pattern, which may signal an impending acute myocardial infarction.

Valsalva maneuver Straining or forced exhalation against a closed glottis, the effect of which is to stimulate the vagus nerve, thereby slowing the heart rate.

variant angina A type of angina caused by coronary artery spasm that occurs when a person is at

Prep Kit continued

rest, when oxygen needs are minimal; also called Prinzmetal angina.

Wolff-Parkinson-White (WPW) syndrome A pre-excitation syndrome characterized by a short PR interval, a delta wave, a widened QRS complex, and nonspecific ST-T wave changes, indicating the presence of an accessory pathway.

References

1. Cardiovascular Disease. World Health Organization. www.who.int/cardiovascular_diseases/about_cvd/en/. Accessed December 17, 2020.
2. Virani SS, Alonso A, Benjamin EJ, et al. Heart disease and stroke statistics—2020 update: a report from the American Heart Association. *Circulation.* 2020;141(9):e139-e596.
3. Whelton PK, Carey RM, Aronow WS, et al. 2017 ACC/AHA/AAPA/ABC/ACPM/AGS/APhA/ASH/ASPC/NMA/PCNA guideline for the prevention, detection, evaluation, and management of high blood pressure in adults. *Hypertension.* 2018;71(6):1269-1324.
4. Grant AO. Cardiac ion channels. *Circ Arrhythm Electrophysiol.* 2009;2(2):185-194.
5. Surawicz B, Childers R, Deal BJ, et al. AHA/ACCF/HRS recommendations for the standardization and interpretation of the electrocardiogram: part III: intraventricular conduction disturbances: a scientific statement from the American Heart Association Electrocardiography and Arrhythmias Committee, Council on Clinical Cardiology; the American College of Cardiology Foundation; and the Heart Rhythm Society. Endorsed by the International Society for Computerized Electrocardiology. *J Am Coll Cardiol.* 2009;53(11):976-981.
6. Anderson JL, Fang JC. ST segment elevation acute myocardial infarction and complications of myocardial infarction. In: Goldman L, Schafer AI, eds. *Goldman-Cecil Medicine.* 26th ed. Philadelphia, PA: Elsevier; 2020:388-401.
7. Amsterdam EA, Wenger NK, Brindis RG, et al. 2014 AHA/ACC guideline for the management of patients with non–ST-elevation acute coronary syndromes: a report of the American College of Cardiology/American Heart Association Task Force on Practice Guidelines. *J Am Coll Cardiol.* 2014;64(24):e139-e228.
8. Drew BJ, Ackerman MJ, Funk M, et al. Prevention of torsade de pointes in hospital settings: a scientific statement from the American Heart Association and the American College of Cardiology Foundation. *J Am Coll Cardiol.* 2010;55(9):934-947.
9. Viskin S. The QT interval: too long, too short or just right. *Heart Rhythm.* 2009;6(5):711-715.
10. National Model EMS Clinical Guidelines, version 2.2. National Association of State EMS Officials. https://nasemso.org/projects/model-ems-clinical-guidelines/. Accessed December 19, 2020.
11. Panchal AR, Bartos JA, Cabañas JG, et al. Part 3: adult basic and advanced life support: 2020 American Heart Association guidelines for cardiopulmonary resuscitation and emergency cardiovascular care. *Circulation.* 2020;142(16 suppl 2):S366-S468.
12. Page RL, Joglar JA, Caldwell MA, et al. 2015 ACC/AHA/HRS guideline for the management of adult patients with supraventricular tachycardia: a report of the American College of Cardiology/American Heart Association Task Force on Clinical Practice Guidelines and the Heart Rhythm Society. *Circulation.* 2016;133(14):e506-e574.
13. Appelboam A, Reuben A, Mann C, et al. Postural modification to the standard Valsalva manoeuvre for emergency treatment of supraventricular tachycardias (REVERT): a randomised controlled trial. *Lancet.* 2015;386(10005):1747-1753.
14. Minczak BM, Laub GW. Techniques for supraventricular tachycardias. In: Robert JR, Custalow CB, Thomsen TW, eds. *Roberts and Hedges' Clinical Procedures in Emergency Medicine and Acute Care.* 7th ed. Philadelphia, PA: Elsevier; 2019:221-237.
15. Kahn PA, Gruen J, Thomas A, et al. Use and outcomes of wearable cardioverter-defibrillators in a large integrated academic health system. *Am Heart J.* 2020;226:232-234.
16. Chung MK. (2014). The role of the wearable cardioverter defibrillator in clinical practice. *Cardiol Clin.* 2014;32(2):253-270.
17. John RM. Atrioventricular block. In: Zipes DP, Jalife J, Stevenson WG, eds. *Cardiac Electrophysiology: From Cell to Bedside.* 7th ed. Philadelphia, PA: Elsevier; 2018:1003-1010.
18. Thygesen K, Alpert JS, Jaffe AS, et al. Fourth universal definition of myocardial infarction. *J Am Coll Cardiol.* 2018;72(18):2231-2264.
19. Patel MR, Peterson ED, Dai D, et al. (2010). Low diagnostic yield of elective coronary angiography. *N Engl J Med.* 2010;362(10):886-895.
20. Lanza GA, De Vita A, Kaski JC. "Primary" microvascular angina: clinical characteristics, pathogenesis and management. *Interv Cardiol.* 2018;13(3):108-111.
21. Heart disease. Centers for Disease Control and Prevention. www.cdc.gov/heartdisease/risk_factors.htm. Accessed December 29, 2020.
22. Graham G. Disparities in cardiovascular disease risk in the United States. *Curr Cardiol Rev.* 2015;11(3):238-245.

Prep Kit continued

23. Golden AP, Odoi A. Emergency medical services transport delays for suspected stroke and myocardial infarction patients. *BMC Emerg Med.* 2015;15(34):1-13.
24. Cannon AR, Lin L, Lytle B, et al. Use of prehospital 12-lead electrocardiography and treatment times among ST-elevation myocardial infarction patients with atypical symptoms. *Acad Emerg Med.* 2014;21(8):892-898.
25. Heart failure. National Heart, Lung, and Blood Institute. www.nhlbi.nih.gov/health-topics/heart-failure. Accessed January 2, 2021.
26. Peberdy MA, Gluck JA, Ornato JP, et al. Cardiopulmonary resuscitation in adults and children with mechanical circulatory support: a scientific statement from the American Heart Association. *Circulation*. 2017;135(24). www.ahajournals.org/doi/epub/10.1161/CIR.0000000000000504.
27. Singhvi A, Trachtenberg B. Left ventricular assist devices 101: shared care for general cardiologists and primary care. *J Clin Med*. 2019;8(10):1720.
28. van Diepen S, Katz JN, Albert NM, et al. Contemporary management of cardiogenic shock: a scientific statement from the American Heart Association. *Circulation*. 2017;136(16):e232-e268.
29. Wolf SJ, Lo B, Shih RD, et al. Clinical policy: critical issues in the evaluation and management of adult patients in the emergency department with asymptomatic elevated blood pressure. *Ann Emerg Med.* 2013;62(1):59-68.
30. Alley WD, Schick MA. Hypertensive emergency. *StatPearls*. www.ncbi.nlm.nih.gov/books/NBK470371/?report=classic. Accessed January 5, 2021.

Chapter 19

Neurologic Emergencies

NATIONAL EMS EDUCATION STANDARD COMPETENCIES

Medicine

Integrates assessment findings with principles of epidemiology and pathophysiology to formulate a field impression and implement a comprehensive treatment/disposition plan for a patient with a medical complaint.

Neurology

Anatomy, presentations, and management of
- Decreased level of responsiveness (p 1304)

Anatomy, physiology, pathophysiology, assessment, and management of
- Stroke/transient ischemic attack (pp 1318–1330)
- Seizure (pp 1304, 1334–1338)
- Status epilepticus (pp 1338–1339)
- Headache (pp 1340–1341)

Anatomy, physiology, epidemiology, pathophysiology, psychosocial impact, presentations, prognosis, and management of
- Stroke/intracranial hemorrhage/transient ischemic attack (pp 1318–1330)
- Seizure (pp 1304, 1334–1338)
- Status epilepticus (pp 1338–1339)
- Headache (pp 1340–1341)
- Dementia (pp 1341–1343)
- Neoplasms (p 1343)
- Demyelinating disorders (pp 1343–1345)
- Parkinson disease (pp 1345–1346)
- Cranial nerve disorders (pp 1347–1349)
- Movement disorders (pp 1314–1316, 1349–1350)
- Neurologic inflammation/infection (pp 1350–1352)
- Spinal cord compression (p 1343; see Chapter 35, *Head and Spine Trauma*)
- Hydrocephalus (see Chapter 44, *Pediatric Emergencies*)
- Wernicke encephalopathy (pp 1341–1342)

KNOWLEDGE OBJECTIVES

1. Describe the incidence, morbidity, and mortality of neurologic emergencies. (pp 1299–1300)
2. Review the anatomy and physiology of the organs and structures that make up the nervous system. (pp 1300–1302)
3. Explain the importance of taking standard precautions and ensuring scene safety when caring for a patient with a neurologic illness. (p 1304)
4. Describe how to determine level of consciousness (LOC) when assessing a patient with a neurologic illness. (p 1304)
5. Compare the characteristics of decorticate and decerebrate posturing, including the likely implications of each for the patient's outcome. (p 1305)
6. Identify the abnormal respiratory patterns associated with central nervous system illness. (pp 1306–1307)

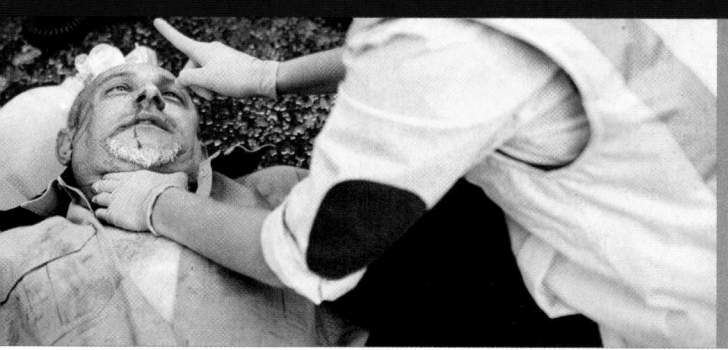

7. List the signs of increased intracranial pressure. (p 1307)
8. Compare how to investigate a chief complaint in an unresponsive patient with how you would do so in a responsive patient. (pp 1308–1309)
9. Review the components of the physical exam that are unique to a patient with a neurologic illness. (pp 1314–1315)
10. Identify speech and movement difficulties that can reveal a diminished LOC. (pp 1313–1315)
11. Review the standard guidelines and interventions for treating a patient with a neurologic illness. (pp 1316–1318)
12. Describe the factors that influence the development of multifactorial neurologic conditions. (p 1318)
13. Explain the pathophysiology, assessment, and management of stroke. (pp 1318–1329)
14. Compare the causes, signs, and symptoms of vascular neurologic conditions that occur suddenly with those that develop gradually. (p 1319)
15. Compare the pathophysiology of ischemic (occlusive) stroke with that of hemorrhagic stroke. (pp 1319–1321)
16. Specify how the cranial vault contents interact to increase intracranial pressure and the major conditions that result. (pp 1319–1321)
17. Describe several tools used to screen for stroke. (pp 1325–1327)
18. Explain transient ischemic attack as it relates to stroke. (pp 1329–1330)
19. Explain the pathophysiology, assessment, and management of seizure, including how to differentiate stroke from seizure. (pp 1334–1338)
20. Explain the three features by which seizures are classified. (pp 1334–1336)
21. Compare generalized seizures with focal seizures (pp 1335–1336)
22. Explain the pathophysiology, assessment, and management of status epilepticus. (pp 1338–1339)
23. Explain the pathophysiology, assessment, and management of syncope. (pp 1339–1340)
24. Explain the pathophysiology, assessment, and management of the most common types of headaches. (pp 1340–1341)
25. Explain the pathophysiology, assessment, and management of dementia, including the causes, signs and symptoms, and typical course of several common types. (pp 1341–1343)
26. Identify the types of neoplasms that affect the nervous system. (p 1343)
27. Analyze the common features of demyelinating conditions. (p 1343)
28. Explain the pathophysiology, assessment, and management of multiple sclerosis. (pp 1343–1345)
29. Explain the pathophysiology, assessment, and management of Guillain-Barré syndrome. (p 1345)
30. Explain the pathophysiology, assessment, and management of Parkinson disease. (p 1345–1346)
31. Explain the pathophysiology, assessment, and management of amyotrophic lateral sclerosis. (p 1346)
32. List several cranial nerve disorders, including the shared characteristics. (pp 1347–1348)
33. Explain the pathophysiology, assessment, and management of dystonia. (pp 1349–1350)
34. Describe the types of pathogenic organisms that can infect the nervous system, as well as the signs and symptoms of a nervous system infection. (pp 1350–1352)
35. Explain the pathophysiology, assessment, and management of an abscess. (p 1352)
36. Explain the pathophysiology, assessment, and management of poliomyelitis. (pp 1352–1353)
37. Explain the pathophysiology, assessment, and management of peripheral neuropathy. (p 1353)

SKILLS OBJECTIVES

1. Assess a patient's level of consciousness. (p 1304)
2. Apply several commonly used screening tools to screen a patient suspected of having had a stroke. (pp 1325–1327)

Introduction

According to the National Center for Health Statistics, two of the top 10 causes of death in 2019 were neurologic in nature.[1] **Stroke**, a serious medical condition in which blood supply to areas of the brain is interrupted, is the fifth leading cause of death in the United States.[1] The sixth leading cause of death is Alzheimer disease.[1] **TABLE 19-1** shows the occurrence of neurologic disorders throughout the United States. As you consider these statistics, it is important to place them in context. As of 2020, the US population was estimated to include 332.6 million people, and the world population, 7.8 billion.[2,3]

You may ask, "Why is it important to understand the prevalence of these conditions?" When you assess a patient, the signs and symptoms you record

TABLE 19-1 Neurologic Disorders in the United States

Disorder	Estimated Occurrence
Headache (chronic, recurring)	1 in 6 adults
Alzheimer disease	5.8 million cases (more than 90% of all cases occur in patients age 65 years or older)
Neoplasm, spinal	0.5–2.5 cases per 100,000 (primary spinal tumors) 5%–10% of all patients with cancer have metastasis to the spinal cord
Neoplasm, brain	7–19 cases per 100,000 population (primary brain tumors) 200,000 patients with metastatic brain tumors per year
Dystonia	Approximately 300,000 people affected within North America
Peripheral neuropathy	Approximately 14 million people with diabetes have neuropathy (almost one-half of all patients with diabetes)
Cerebral palsy	1 in 323 children

Data from: Burch R, Rizzoli, Loder E. The prevalence and impact of migraine and severe headache in the United States: figures and trends from government health studies. *Headache.* 2018;58(4):496-505; Alzheimer's disease information page. National Institute of Neurological Disorders and Stroke website. https://www.ninds.nih.gov/Disorders/All-Disorders/Alzheimers-Disease-Information-Page. Modified March 27, 2019. Accessed March 22, 2021; Borke J. Spinal cord neoplasms. Medscape website. http://emedicine.medscape.com/article/779872-overview. Updated July 17, 2019. Accessed March 22, 2021; Lo BM. Brain neoplasms. Medscape website. http://emedicine.medscape.com/article/779664-overview. Updated January 2, 2019. Accessed March 22, 2021; Types of dystonia. Dystonia Medical Research Foundation website. https://dystonia-foundation.org/what-is-dystonia/types-dystonia/. Accessed March 22, 2021; Quan D. Diabetic neuropathy. Medscape website. http://emedicine.medscape.com/article/1170337-overview. Updated July 28, 2020. Accessed March 22, 2021; and Cerebral palsy. Centers for Disease Control and Prevention website. https://www.cdc.gov/dotw/cerebral-palsy/index.html. Reviewed March 27, 2019. Accessed March 22, 2021.

YOU are the Paramedic

PART 1

You and your partner are dispatched for a patient experiencing a stroke. You arrive at a well-kept, three-story home in an urban setting. Police arrive with you. You are met by a concerned family member, who directs you to the basement, where you find a 49-year-old man sitting on a couch. His wife quickly tells you that she woke up about 15 minutes ago and found her husband sitting on the couch and unable to speak. The patient is more than 6 feet (2 m) tall and weighs approximately 240 pounds (109 kg). He is awake and tracking you with his eyes. He does not attempt to speak.

1. What are your next questions?
2. What assessment information do you need to gather?

may indicate many possible conditions. However, you must also take into account the likelihood of those conditions to help ground your conclusions. For example, a 10-year-old child with chest pain is unlikely to be experiencing a myocardial infarction (MI). Likewise, disease occurrence information helps you to expect that the patient with dementia is more likely to have Alzheimer disease than Creutzfeldt-Jakob disease.

Understanding a patient's neurologic condition will help you understand the person's potential vulnerability to secondary conditions. Many reflexes that protect an awake person can be temporarily inactive when the nervous system is depressed by any cause (eg, stroke, severe head injury). The eyelids do not blink away dust and irritants. The larynx does not cause gagging and coughing in reaction to secretions oozing down the airway. The body does not seek a more comfortable position in response to a limb's compression in an awkward position. The tongue goes slack. The airway is at risk.

A brief review of the nervous system's anatomy and physiology is presented next in this chapter to provide the proper foundation on which to begin a discussion of assessment and treatment of neurologic disorders.

Anatomy and Physiology Review

The basic structures of the nervous system are shown in **FIGURE 19-1**. The major structures of this system are divided into the central nervous system (CNS), which is responsible for thought, perception, feeling, and autonomic body functions, and the peripheral nervous system (PNS), which is responsible for transmitting commands from the brain to the body and receiving feedback from the body. The anatomy and physiology of the nervous system are discussed in detail in Chapter 8, *Anatomy and Physiology.*

To review the nervous system, it is helpful to consider the example of a child riding a bicycle. This common and seemingly simple activity actually requires many conscious and unconscious functions. The child has to do many things to avoid falling or riding into a tree.

On a summer morning, a young rider, Justin, goes to the garage to get his bike. His brain is already hard at work at this point. As Justin enters the garage, his brain must determine which object is a bike. As Justin scans the garage, the images produced by his eyes are transmitted via the optic nerve to the

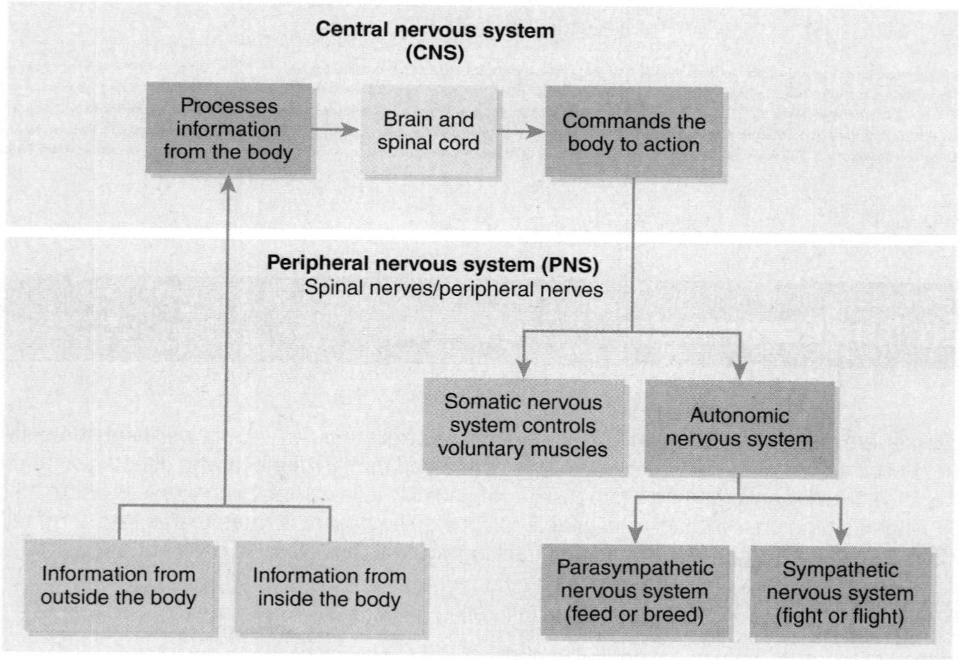

FIGURE 19-1 Basic organization of the nervous system.

occipital lobe of the brain. There, the image, which is transmitted upside down, needs to be reoriented. The occipital lobe then scans through tens of thousands of stored images to determine whether this image has been seen before.

After the image is recognized, an existing pathway is accessed to the temporal lobe, where language and speech are stored. As Justin walks through the garage, he can put names to what he sees: car, workbench, bike. When Justin was learning to speak, he often became confused about the correct names of objects. As he practiced, he received reinforcement for the correct names and redirection for the incorrect names. In his brain, more and more pathways were laid down that related to the image of an object with two wheels, a seat, and pedals. These pathways are stored in the occipital lobe as the word "bike."

As Justin reaches for his helmet, commands from the frontal lobe of his brain are sent to his arms so that he can pick up the helmet and place it on his head. The frontal lobe, which controls voluntary motion, sends signals out of the CNS to the arms, shoulders, chest, and hands to perform the task of picking up his helmet.

Which way should Justin apply the helmet? This motor memory is stored within the frontal lobe. The brain stores memories in the areas that were initially stimulated during their formation. While he applies the helmet, Justin needs to make fine adjustments to its position. During this process, his brain receives impulses from nerves within the skull and muscles of the head.

If the helmet is uncomfortable, then Justin will sense pressure and possibly pain from the improperly placed helmet. Signals of discomfort are sent to the parietal lobe, where the body's sense of touch and pain perception are found. More signals are then sent from the parietal lobe to the frontal lobe to tell the body to adjust the helmet until the pressure signals have stopped.

How does the brain manage a massive amount of information without suffering from confusion and misdirection? The information is divided into items that need to be managed consciously and those that can be handled unconsciously. This process is the responsibility of the diencephalon, which filters out unneeded information before it reaches the cerebral cortex. For example, the midbrain portion of the brainstem helps regulate level of consciousness (LOC). This function needs to occur constantly, but Justin could not ride his bike if he needed to devote time and energy to consciously controlling his LOC. The brainstem is one of the portions of the brain that frees the cerebral cortex to engage in higher-level activities.

YOU are the Paramedic

PART 2

The patient is mute; he neither makes nor attempts any sounds. He does follow commands. You note a slight weakness to his left hand and a slight facial droop to the left side of his face. You find no other cranial nerve deficits. The patient is not drooling and can swallow easily. You do not observe any evidence of respiratory distress or inability to protect his airway.

Recording Time: 0 Minutes	
Appearance	Awake
Level of consciousness	Alert and following commands, but mute
Airway	Patent
Breathing	Adequate
Circulation	Adequate

3. How can you determine whether the patient is oriented when he will not speak?
4. What vital signs or laboratory values are critical to gather for this patient?
5. What is this patient's Glasgow Coma Scale (GCS) score? Does it accurately depict this patient's acuity?

Justin now mounts his bike and begins to ride. The smile on his face indicates that he is having a good time. Emotions come from two main areas within the brain: the **limbic system**, where rage and anger are generated, and the hypothalamus, where pleasure, thirst, and hunger are found. The prefrontal cortex mediates all emotions so people can choose how they will respond to how they feel.

Justin begins to pick up speed. As he approaches a corner, he must turn or risk crashing into a tree. Justin can shift his weight and make the turn successfully due in large part to his cerebellum. This lobe of the brain, located in the posterior, inferior area of the skull, unconsciously manages complex motor activity. When Justin first learned to ride a bike, he had to think about what to do, where to shift his weight, and how to hold his upper body. Over time, and with practice, the brain's frontal lobe tired of sending the same commands repeatedly, so this task was transferred to the cerebellum.

TABLE 19-2 provides a basic reference to various portions of the nervous system.

TABLE 19-2 Structures and General Functions of the Nervous System

Major Structure	Subdivision	General Functions
CNS		
Brain	Occipital	• Vision and storage of visual memories
	Parietal	• Sense of touch and texture and storage of tactile memories
	Temporal	• Hearing and smell • Language • Storage of sound and odor memories
	Frontal	• Motor cortex: Voluntary muscle control and storage of spatial memories • Prefrontal cortex: Judgment and prediction of consequences of a person's actions, abstract intellectual functions
	Limbic system	• Basic emotions • Basic reflexes, such as chewing and swallowing
	Diencephalon (thalamus)	• Relay center that prioritizes signals to hone in on important messages
	Diencephalon (hypothalamus)	• Emotions • Temperature control • Interface with the endocrine system
Brainstem	Midbrain	• LOC • Location of the reticular activating system (RAS), which controls arousal and consciousness • Muscle tone and posture
	Pons	• Respiratory pattern and depth
	Medulla oblongata	• Pulse rate, blood pressure, and respiratory rate
Spinal cord		• Reflexes • Relay of information to and from the body
PNS		
Cranial nerves		• Special peripheral nerves that connect directly from the brain to body parts to relay information from the brain
Peripheral nerves		• Brain to spinal cord to body part • Receive stimulus from body; send commands to body

Major Structure	Subdivision	General Functions
CNS and PNS		
Neuron	Cell body	• Portion of the neuron where the nucleus resides; site of protein synthesis
	Axon	• Projection from the cell body that reaches out to connect with other neurons or target organs; signals are sent away from the cell body • Some axons are covered with insulation called myelin; myelin increases the speed of nerve conduction
	Dendrite	• A projection from the cell body that receives signals from axons of other neurons; most neurons have multiple dendrites
	Synapse	• The gap between an axon and a dendrite
	Neurotransmitter	• A chemical released into a synapse that helps make the connection between one neuron and another (eg, serotonin, dopamine, and epinephrine)

Abbreviations: CNS, central nervous system; LOC, level of consciousness; PNS, peripheral nervous system

Data from: Bailey R. Neuron anatomy, nerve impulses, and classifications. ThoughtCo website. https://www.thoughtco.com/neurons-373486. Updated July 10, 2019. Accessed March 22, 2021.

Patient Assessment

The brain is the most sensitive organ within the body to variable temperatures and fluctuating oxygen and glucose levels. Even small alterations can impair its function. Conversely, the brain is also surprisingly resilient to internal environmental changes. It does not simply shut down when the oxygen level falls.

Assessment of patients would most likely be easier if they were either fully awake or completely asleep. When you are trying to determine whether a patient has a neurologic condition, you need to look for both gross (obvious) changes and subtle, sometimes hidden changes that can indicate disease. You will still need to perform all of the general steps of patient assessment, such as considering scene safety, taking standard precautions, considering the mechanism of injury (MOI), and determining whether the patient has taken medications, alcohol, or other substances (and if so, then how much and when). The information in this section will allow you to focus on unique or important areas in the patient with a neurologic condition.

A good assessment is the backbone of excellent patient care. When assessing every patient, be curious, inquisitive, and adaptable. Rarely do patients demonstrate textbook disease presentations, showing every sign and symptom, every change in vital signs, and a perfect history of present illness. Use

SAFETY

Consider the following scenario in which you need to give a medication to a patient with a neurologic disorder. As a first step, you check for medical alert tags and find none. Patients with neurologic disorders may have speech difficulties, and they may sometimes choose the wrong word to answer your question. For example:

You ask, "Do you have any allergies?"

Although the patient may be aware that he has allergies and may intend to say yes, he responds, "No."

Unfortunately, you will often be unable to ascertain this issue in the context of a limited evaluation in the field. To attempt to do so, consider phrasing your question using at least two different formats. For example:

You ask, "Do you have any allergies?"

The patient states, "No."

You say, "Just to make sure, please tell me the names of medications to which you are allergic."

Now compare the patient's answers to the first and second questions. If they are not the same, then you need to ask more questions to ensure you do not give a medication that could harm the patient. Unfortunately, this approach is not feasible for all patients in the field, so it may not be possible to rely on all the information you receive from a patient with an apparent cognitive or communicative deficit.

the information you obtain during the assessment process to sharpen your focus, but avoid tunnel vision. If the patient reports chest pain and demonstrates a new-onset facial droop, for example, then you must assess both the cardiovascular and nervous systems.

Scene Size-up

Take standard precautions. A patient who has a **seizure** (the sudden, erratic firing of neurons) may be incontinent, and a patient with neurologic symptoms may have meningitis.

Your assessment of the physical environment begins at dispatch. The location of a neurologic patient can place you in scenes that may be unsafe. Some patients are unresponsive because of a drug overdose. When people use illegal drugs, weapons and crime may be close at hand. Ensure that no matter what type of event is taking place, you have a way to remove yourself from the scene. If an entire family in the same house reports a headache, then consider the possibility of carbon monoxide exposure and recognize that the house is an unsafe scene.

Finally, if the time needed to reach the nearest stroke center is greater than 1 hour, then request air medical transport early.

Primary Survey

Patients who state, "It hurts right here," provide evidence of a functioning nervous system. Patients found unresponsive should be evaluated as being in an unstable condition with obvious nervous system impairment. The answers to the following questions can give you clues to the overall functioning of the patient's nervous system:

- Where is the patient?
- Does the patient appear to be in distress or pain?
- Is the patient standing, sitting, or lying down?
- Is the patient outside or inside?
- Does the patient have obvious injuries?
- What does the environment look like?
- Do you see evidence of drug paraphernalia?
- What are the living conditions like: clean, cluttered, dirty?
- Is the patient able to ambulate within the home?
- Is the patient awake (aware of the surroundings) and alert (responding to the surroundings)?
- Is the patient in a stable or unstable condition?

Examining the living conditions can provide insight into the general functioning of the patient's brain. Cluttered or disorganized living conditions may be an indicator of a degenerative nervous system condition. Patients with progressive neurologic disease may initially care for themselves, but these tasks can become more difficult over time. With some conditions, such as amyotrophic lateral sclerosis (ALS; discussed later in this chapter), patients experience a loss of motor ability.

Assessing Level of Consciousness

Tools to assess the patient's LOC include the AVPU mnemonic, assessment of orientation, and the Glasgow Coma Scale (GCS). The GCS uses parameters that test a patient's eye opening, best verbal response, and best motor response. The three numeric scores are added together to form a total score that defines the patient's brain function. Refer to Chapter 11, *Patient Assessment*, to review how to perform and calculate the GCS.

The scores from tools to assess LOC can help you determine how to proceed with patient care, what care you should give, and where to transport the patient. Mildly ill patients need care that conforms to standard care guidelines; usually you can honor the patient's request to be transported to a particular hospital. Patients with moderate conditions require you to make more challenging decisions. They are not critically ill but are considered to be in an unstable condition; therefore, your most appropriate action should be to perform a careful assessment and provide prompt transport to the closest appropriate facility. Critically ill patients need airway management and prompt transport to the closest appropriate hospital.

As you determine a patient's level of orientation, note the speed and intensity at which the patient responds. As you are talking, does the patient appear to be sleepy or sluggish? Is the patient talking quickly and unable to sit still? How many words are in the sentences the patient uses? Do you have to speak loudly to the patient to get a response?

Words of Wisdom

Some patients may be confused. Such confusion may indicate a low blood glucose level, decreased oxygen level, overdose, or even decreased blood pressure (BP). Ask questions to which you know the answers if you are trying to determine the level of orientation, and use your training and the tools you have available to eliminate the causes of the altered level of consciousness.

Methods for Measuring Response to Pain

Imagine that you have walked up to a patient and announced yourself, and the patient has not responded. Now, the goal is to elicit a response to pain from the patient, if possible, but not cause any harm. A functioning brain, an intact spinal cord, and an intact peripheral nervous system are required for the patient to respond to pain. See Chapter 11, *Patient Assessment*, for a discussion of methods to evaluate a patient's response to pain.

While you generate a pain response from the patient, observe what happens. Does the patient wake up? Does the patient move away from the pain? Does the patient move in an abnormal fashion? Does the patient exhibit one of the two main abnormal postures that occur with any painful stimulation? It is essential to understand that abnormal **posturing** (abnormal body positioning that indicates damage to the brain) occurs involuntarily in patients who are otherwise unresponsive. You may notice these postures during the insertion of an intravenous (IV) line. The patient may move involuntarily after the painful stimulus occurs. The two abnormal postures indicate unresponsiveness; if you see either of them, then immediately consider the patient to be in critical condition.

The first abnormal posture is **decorticate posturing**, or abnormal flexion. In this posture, patients contract their arms and curl them toward their chests (remember bending the arms toward the "core" of the patient). At the same time, they point their toes. Finally, the wrists are flexed. Decorticate posturing is scored as a 3 on the motor section of the GCS. This posture may indicate damage to the area directly below the cerebral hemispheres **FIGURE 19-2**.

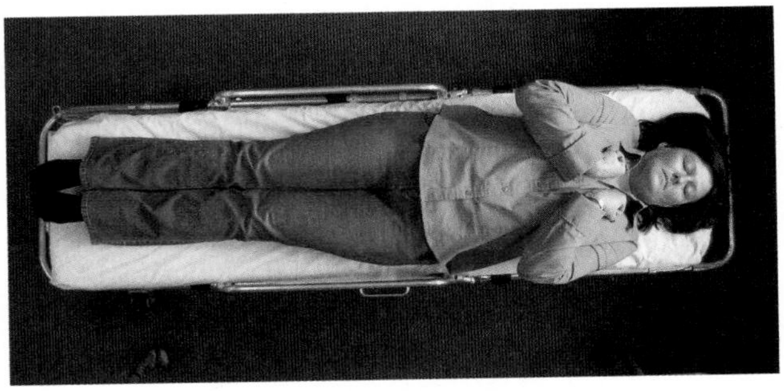

FIGURE 19-2 Decorticate posturing.

Courtesy of Chuck Sowerbrower, MEd, NREMT-P.

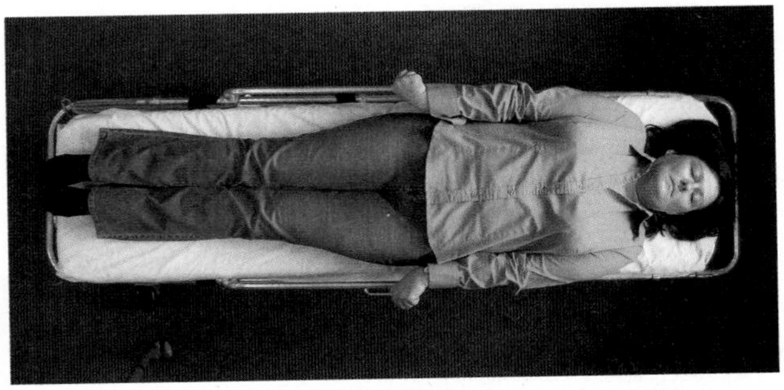

FIGURE 19-3 Decerebrate posturing.

Courtesy of Chuck Sowerbrower, MEd, NREMT-P.

The other abnormal posture is called **decerebrate posturing**, or abnormal extension. In this posture, patients again point their toes, but now extend their arms outward and rotate the lower arms in a palms-down manner (called **pronation**). The wrists are again flexed. Decerebrate posturing is scored as a 2 on the motor section of the GCS. This type of posturing is a more severe finding than decorticate posturing. In decerebrate posturing, the level of damage is within or near the brainstem (diencephalon/pons/midbrain) **FIGURE 19-3**.

Airway, Breathing, and Circulation Considerations

The trigeminal, glossopharyngeal, vagus, and hypoglossal nerves are responsible for airway control. These nerves allow for swallowing, controlling the tongue, and ensuring the hypopharynx muscles are slightly contracted. Alteration in the signals from these nerves can result in too much relaxation or too much constriction of the airway.

If the patient is not responding to stimuli, then carefully assess the airway. Tightly clenched teeth, called **trismus**, can make it challenging to manage the airway. Trismus can occur in either responsive or unresponsive patients. In the unresponsive patient, trismus can indicate a seizure in progress, severe head injury, and/or cerebral hypoxia. When trismus is present, the patient may need to be sedated/paralyzed to relax the facial muscles causing the clenched teeth, allowing you to better control the airway.

If you note trismus, then initially determine how effectively you can ventilate the patient with a bag-mask device. If ventilation is poor or unsuccessful, then attempt to insert a nasotracheal airway, as long as the patient is still breathing independently. If the introduction of a nasotracheal airway is unsuccessful, then consider a sedative/paralytic agent to relax the mouth and allow for airway management. If sedatives/paralytics are unavailable or contraindicated and you cannot ventilate the patient, then transtracheal airway management is the only remaining option to prevent hypoxia and death. For additional information on rapid sequence intubation or airway obstruction clearance, refer to Chapter 16, *Airway Management*.

Remember that routine hyperventilation of neurologic patients can be harmful. Thus, you should provide hyperventilation only to those patients with documented signs of increased intracranial pressure (ICP) and impending herniation. Follow your local protocols regarding hyperventilating a patient. The management of patients with elevated ICP is discussed later in this chapter.

Recall that the pons and the medulla oblongata control the functions of breathing. Check the rate and rhythm of the patient's breathing. Breathing patterns are summarized in **TABLE 19-3**. Notice how

TABLE 19-3 Respiratory Patterns

Pattern	Description	Causes
Eupnea	Regular rate and pattern; inspiration and expiration are equal	Normal breathing
Tachypnea	Excessively rapid and shallow breathing, regular pattern	Stimulants, exercise, excitement, lung disease or other medical cause (ie, anxiety, asthma, choking, chronic obstructive pulmonary disease, heart failure, or pulmonary embolus)
Bradypnea	Unusually slow respiratory rate, regular pattern	Opioids, sedatives, alcohol, pneumonia, sleep apnea, carbon monoxide exposure, traumatic brain injury
Apnea	Absence of breathing	Severe hypoxia, depressants, head injury, heart attack, irregular heartbeat, metabolic disorders (ie, a body's chemical, mineral, or acid–base imbalance), submersion, stroke
Hyperpnea	Abnormally increased rate and depth of breathing	Stimulants, overdose, exercise
Cheyne-Stokes respirations	Gradual increase in respiratory rate and depth, followed by a gradual decrease with intermittent periods of apnea	Pre-death pattern, brainstem injury, brain herniation syndrome
Biot/ataxic respirations	Irregular pattern, rate, and depth of respirations with periods of apnea	Brainstem injury, increased intracranial pressure
Kussmaul respirations	Deep, gasping respirations (extreme tachypnea and hyperpnea)	Acidosis Diabetic ketoacidosis
Apneustic respirations	Prolonged inspiratory phase with shortened expiratory phase and bradypnea	Brainstem injury

the rhythms can have subtle changes or can be dramatically different from normal. The greater the deviation from normal, the more severely affected the nervous system is likely to be.

Signs of Increased ICP

If a patient has increased pressure within the cranium, then the vital signs may change. Specifically, the BP rises and the pulse rate and respiratory rate fall in the setting of increased ICP **TABLE 19-4**. This response, which is called Cushing reflex, is indicated by the following signs:

- Decreased pulse rate (bradycardia)
- Decreased/irregular respiratory rate (bradypnea)
- Widened pulse pressure (systolic hypertension)

Cushing reflex is the opposite of what typically occurs in shock, when BP falls and the pulse rate and respiratory rate climb. The hallmarks of increased ICP are as follows:

- Cushing reflex
- Decorticate posturing
- Decerebrate posturing
- Biot respirations
- Apneustic respirations
- Cheyne-Stokes respirations
- Unresponsive and dilated pupils or **anisocoria** (unequal pupils with a greater than 1 mm difference)

As the ICP rises, blood flow to the brain diminishes. The medulla oblongata sends signals to the heart to increase the force of contraction to compensate for the reduced blood flow. This increase causes systolic blood pressure (SBP) to rise. If the ICP continues to increase, then downward forces on the brainstem begin to damage the medulla's ability to send signals to the body. As the blood vessels relax or dilate, diastolic BP decreases, resulting in a widened pulse pressure. This pressure also damages the ability to control the respiratory and pulse rates; consequently, they both decrease. Increased ICP is discussed in detail later in this chapter.

Special Populations

In the pediatric population, you must take the child's developmental stage into account during patient assessment. A 1-year-old child should cry when you conduct an assessment, because this is considered a normal reaction to strangers. A 5-year-old child who usually talks freely may be quiet with a stranger. Evaluate the child at the appropriate developmental level.

When you assess ICP in infants, consider the quality of the baby's cry. As ICP increases, the pitch of the cry rises as well until it resembles a shriek similar to that of a cat. At the same time, the shape of the pupils can change from round to more oval. These two findings are the basis of the mnemonic related to infants and ICP: "Cat's eyes and cat's cries."

The Rapid Full-Body Scan

When you have completed the primary survey, you need to decide how to proceed next. Is the patient in a stable or unstable condition? Do you suspect a major underlying problem? Consider how to transport this patient. At this point, you have the following two choices:

- Complete a rapid full-body scan, which would involve a head-to-toe approach, *or*
- Complete a secondary assessment and evaluate only the area(s) of the patient's chief complaint(s).

Perform a rapid full-body scan on any patient with an abnormal assessment, any patient with

TABLE 19-4 Vital Signs for Shock Versus Increased ICP

	Pulse Rate	Respiratory Rate	Blood Pressure	Pulse Pressure
Shock	↑	↑	↓	Narrowed
Increased ICP	↓	↓	↑	Widened

Abbreviation: ICP, intracranial pressure

a significant MOI/nature of illness (NOI), or any patient whom you suspect may have a significant problem. Examples would be a patient who is unresponsive, is experiencing a seizure, or has a sudden loss of body movement.

If the patient is in stable condition, then it is appropriate to conduct a secondary assessment based on the chief complaint(s). These patients, such as those with headaches or nontraumatic back pain, have a completely normal primary survey, have a minor MOI/NOI, and/or cause you to suspect a localized problem.

Be cautious, though: A headache is not always the result of a common cause, such as stress. Patients who have sustained a stroke can also have headaches. If you suspect a more complicated condition, then quickly perform the secondary assessment, covering the entire body. This expanded assessment will ensure you are giving the patient the best possible care.

History Taking

While taking the history, ask open-ended questions and listen carefully to the patient's response. Evaluate the patient's speech. Is it slurred? Does the patient make sense? At the same time, look for signs and symptoms that may indicate the cause of the altered mental status (eg, a stroke), as well as any evidence of the patient having had a seizure (eg, incontinence or a bitten tongue). The most important question to ask family members who may be present is "When was the patient last seen normal?" as this will help determine time frames for stroke alert activation.

Special Populations

Age will determine how much interaction a pediatric patient is able to have with you. If the child is able to speak and understands the concept of time, then talk to the child, in addition to the parents or caregivers, to gather information.

If you know that the patient has had a seizure and is now in a postictal state, then you will be unable to obtain a history from the patient. Look for any obvious explanation for why the patient had a seizure, such as trauma. If the patient has a headache, then try to determine the patient's level of stress, the likelihood of infection, and the patient's history of headaches. If you believe a more complicated condition may be present, then perform a more detailed evaluation.

Documentation and Communication

The patient's family or friends may report that the patient was last seen normal when going to bed the night before. If that is the case, report the time last seen normal was at bedtime, not when the patient awoke with symptoms.

Try to speak with family or friends who can explain the events leading to the patient's altered mental status. Remember, time can be critical in a neurologic emergency. As a paramedic in the field, you may be the only person with the opportunity to obtain crucial information about the time of onset.

Your SAMPLE history (Signs and symptoms, Allergies, Medications, Pertinent past history, Last oral intake, Events leading to injury or illness) should reveal whether the patient has a history of seizures. If so, then it is essential to find out what triggers them and whether this episode differs from previous ones. Also find out which medications the patient takes. A history of taking phenytoin (Dilantin) and phenobarbital (Solfoton), for example, points strongly toward a seizure disorder. Remember to ask about over-the-counter medications, including herbal products. Your history may reveal that the patient has run out of medication, recently adjusted the dosage, or stopped taking the medication. In addition, you may uncover coexisting conditions, such as diabetes. A patient who has diabetes and has a seizure may use up glucose in the body to fuel the seizure.

If a patient with no history of seizures is now experiencing a seizure for the first time, then suspect a grave condition, such as a brain tumor, intracranial bleeding, or a serious infection. Determine whether the patient takes medications that lower the blood glucose level, such as insulin or oral antihyperglycemic agents. Finally, inquire about drug use and exposure to toxins if appropriate.

Words of Wisdom

Although patients who have had a stroke might appear to be unresponsive and unable to speak, they may still be able to hear and understand what is taking place. As with any patient, avoid making any remarks that might cause the patient distress. Reassure the patient that you understand that verbal communication may be difficult at this time, but that you will keep the patient continually informed about what you and your team members are doing. Compassionate communication can help you calm the patient and ease these fears, which are undoubtedly intensified by the inability to communicate.

Special Populations

When you gather assessment findings and history of present illness information from members of the older adult population, also consider the patient's pertinent past medical history. Patients with a history of dementia (discussed later in this chapter) are complicated to manage. The primary question you need to answer is how much change has occurred in the patient's LOC. Do not evaluate the patient from the point of a normal LOC. Instead, speak to family, friends, or other caregivers to determine the patient's baseline LOC, and clearly document that level.

Medications can also create alterations in LOC. Explore all medications that the patient is taking: prescription, nonprescription, herbal, supplements, homeopathic, and illegal. Older adults are more likely to have many physicians, many conditions, and many medications (polypharmacy). Combinations of medications can result in unexpected neurologic effects.

Secondary Assessment

The head is the area in which you will spend the most time during a neurologic exam because you can gather critical information on the nervous system's functioning from this assessment. Notice the symmetry of the face: Do you observe any obvious facial droop? Look at the eyes: Are the eyelids even bilaterally? Drooping or sagging of the eyelids (**ptosis**) can indicate **Bell palsy** or a stroke. **FIGURE 19-4** demonstrates facial droop and ptosis.

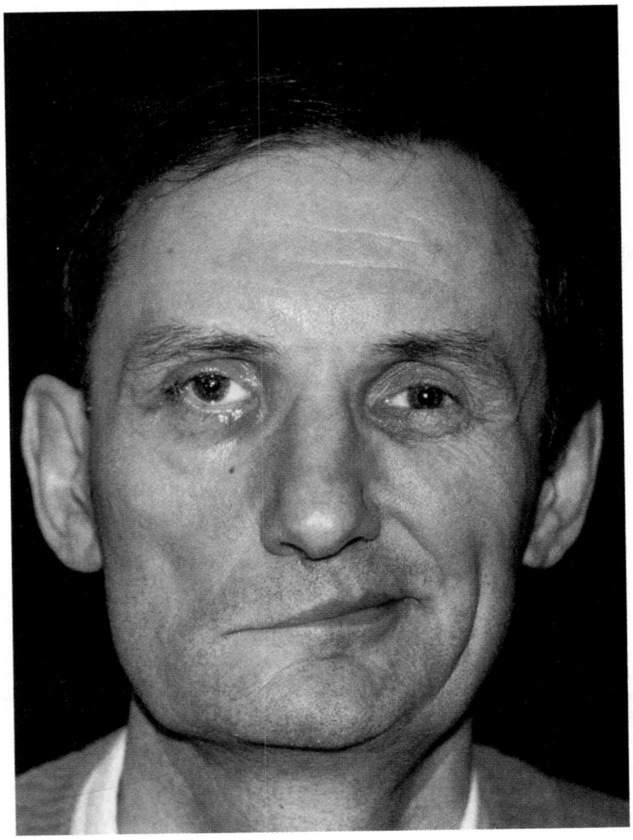

FIGURE 19-4 Facial droop and ptosis.

Chapter 11, *Patient Assessment,* covers the components of a neurologic exam.

The following findings during the neurologic exam are notable:

- Nausea and vomiting are common with some types of headaches.
- Urinary and/or fecal incontinence are common findings with seizures and fainting. Incontinence is also a relatively objective marker in determining the severity of illness in an unresponsive patient. Patients can control their bowel and bladder functions when they are asleep. If incontinence is present, then the LOC has decreased below that of sleep.
- Signs of recent venipuncture marks may indicate recent illegal drug use.

Many cardiac dysrhythmias can cause neurologic disorders by decreasing the amount of blood supplied to the brain. A 12-lead electrocardiogram (ECG) needs to be obtained for any patient experiencing a sudden loss of consciousness.

Level of Consciousness

A patient's LOC can vary widely. To help you better understand the many possible variations in LOC, **FIGURE 19-5** shows a continuum from a patient responding appropriately to the environment to a completely unresponsive patient. **Coma** is a state in which a person does not respond to either verbal or painful stimuli. The points in between are guide markings. Patients do not stop at every point, of course, as the LOC increases or decreases. Nevertheless, these points provide you with an idea of the relationships among various LOCs. Whereas the extremes of the scale are easy to understand, the middle points can be more challenging to interpret. The following section explains these questionable areas in more detail.

Common Reality

Some patients experience **hallucinations** or sensory stimulation that others cannot verify. People use their senses to determine what is real. If you see flames, smell smoke, and feel heat, then there must be a fire. But what if all of these sensations exist purely in your mind? One way to determine that the sensations you are experiencing are real is to ask others what they are experiencing. If others also see flames, smell smoke, and feel heat, then the fire is real. **Common reality** is sensory stimulation that others can confirm.

Hallucinations vary. Some patients can hear voices, see snakes, feel insects, smell burning paper, or taste metal. In such a case, the patient will respond as if the stimulus is real. Keep in mind that hallucinations are vivid and trigger strong reactions from the patient. For example, if a patient is afraid of snakes, then they will be frightened by the hallucination. Tell the patient that you do not see the snake but you understand that they see it. Do not reinforce the hallucination. Your task is to bring the patient back to a common reality, but do not argue if the patient insists on the validity of the hallucination. Provide reassurance that the patient is safe.

Delusions are similar to hallucinations. Delusions are thoughts, ideas, or perceived abilities that are not based in a common reality. Examples of delusions include patients who believe they can fly or that everyone is out to get them (paranoia). As with

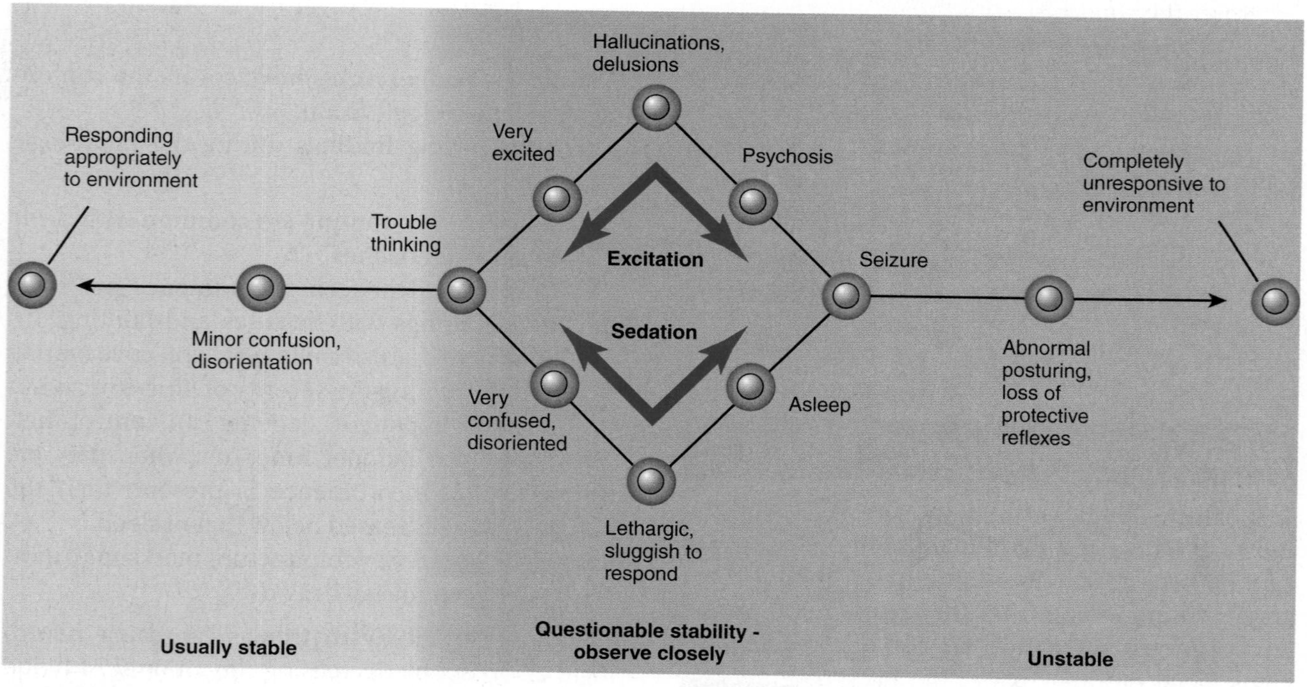

FIGURE 19-5 Level of consciousness continuum.

hallucinations, try to redirect patients, but do not argue with them.

As delusions and hallucinations increase, the patient may move further and further away from a common reality. Eventually, the amount of shared reality between you and the patient may become so minimal that the patient can no longer determine what is real and what is a product of the mind. This state is called **psychosis**. Patients with psychosis can be unpredictable, because they are responding to a barrage of stimulation that no one else is experiencing. They are also struggling to interact with a world in which the rules are constantly changing. Fear, anger, and helplessness are common emotions when a patient is in this state.

When you care for patients who are experiencing psychosis, first ensure your own safety. Because of the unpredictable nature of patients with psychosis, make sure you are not left alone with the patient and have a clear avenue of retreat. In this scenario, your job is to decrease the stimulation of the patient as much as possible. Limit the number of people talking to the patient to one person. Give clear, simple commands and be ready to patiently repeat those commands. Do not place the patient in a dimly lit room or ambulance, as the patient may interpret the shadows as harmful. The patient may need medication to help manage hallucinations, delusions, and psychosis. For more recommendations on managing patients with hallucinations, delusions, and/or psychosis, see Chapter 29, *Psychiatric Emergencies*.

Mood and Other Changes

Changes in the patient's mood or the tempo of the nervous system should alert you to changes in the patient's neurologic status. The oxygen level or BP could be falling. Body temperature could be climbing. A psychiatric condition might be escalating. The level of blood glucose could be either critically low or high. Regardless of the underlying cause, this observation of a change requires you to further evaluate the patient to ensure the appropriate level of care. Mood or affect is another attribute that provides insight into the patient. Ask how the patient feels. A low blood glucose or oxygen level can cause frustration, anger, or aggression.

A patient who has a decreased blood glucose level or is taking narcotics can have trouble concentrating. Low blood glucose levels and narcotics tend to sedate the nervous system. Patients who are taking cocaine can also have difficulty concentrating, because cocaine is a sympathomimetic that increases nervous system activity. These patients experience mania. Their thoughts can tumble in quickly, so they find it hard to concentrate. If the speed of nervous system activity continues to increase, then the patient may hallucinate, become delusional, or become psychotic.

Protective Reflexes

A patient's protective reflexes include the cough and gag reflexes, as well as the corneal reflex. The status of the patient's protective reflexes relates to the patient's LOC. A quick, simple way for you to determine indirectly whether the patient's cough and gag reflexes are intact is to assess the **corneal reflex**, which protects the eyes from trauma. This reflex causes blinking when an object touches the cornea of the eye.

If you tap lightly between the eyes and the patient does not blink or twitch, then assume that the patient does not have an intact cough or gag reflex and will not be able to protect the airway. If the patient does not cough or gag when you attempt to insert an oral airway, then you have confirmed that the airway is unprotected and you must take measures to protect it.

Words of Wisdom

Pupil size is measured in millimeters (mm). A quick way to determine this size is to imagine how many dimes can be stacked across the pupil. The width (thickness) of a dime is close to 1 mm. You can use the gauge on the side of the penlight (if present) to obtain a more accurate measurement.

Pupillary Response

When you assess the patient's eyes, ensure you are eliciting a reaction to light and not to movement. To avoid engaging the corneal reflex, take your penlight and approach the eyes from a 45° angle. This technique should ensure the pupils react to the light itself, rather than to the approach of the penlight.

Examine the pupils. They should be round, respond quickly to light by constricting, and be equal in size, shape, and response. Pupillary shape can be changed by trauma, glaucoma, or increased ICP.

Generally speaking, stimulants cause pupillary dilation. Recall the flight-or-fight sympathetic response caused by epinephrine. If someone is trying to attack you, then you need to see as much of your environment as possible to either defend yourself effectively or retreat. Your eyes, therefore, need as much light as possible. Cocaine, methamphetamines, and hallucinogens also tend to cause pupil dilation. Conversely, depressants tend to constrict the pupils.

Equality of pupils is an important observation. Unequal pupils (anisocoria) are a sign of increased ICP **FIGURE 19-6**. Many people have a slight inequality in pupillary size naturally; a difference greater than 1 mm is worth noting.

Blood Glucose Level

Recall that glucose is the fuel that runs the brain. The brain uses glucose faster than any other part of the body, but has no means to store it. All patients with a change in LOC should have their blood glucose level checked. Indeed, blood glucose monitoring is now the standard of care for the patient with an altered LOC. A normal blood glucose reading is 60 to 120 mg/dL. As the glucose level decreases, so does the LOC. A high blood glucose level also can affect the patient's LOC; however, the level must increase significantly before the LOC is diminished. A blood glucose level of less than 10 mg/dL is incompatible with brain functioning and is usually fatal. Generally, if the level of blood glucose falls below

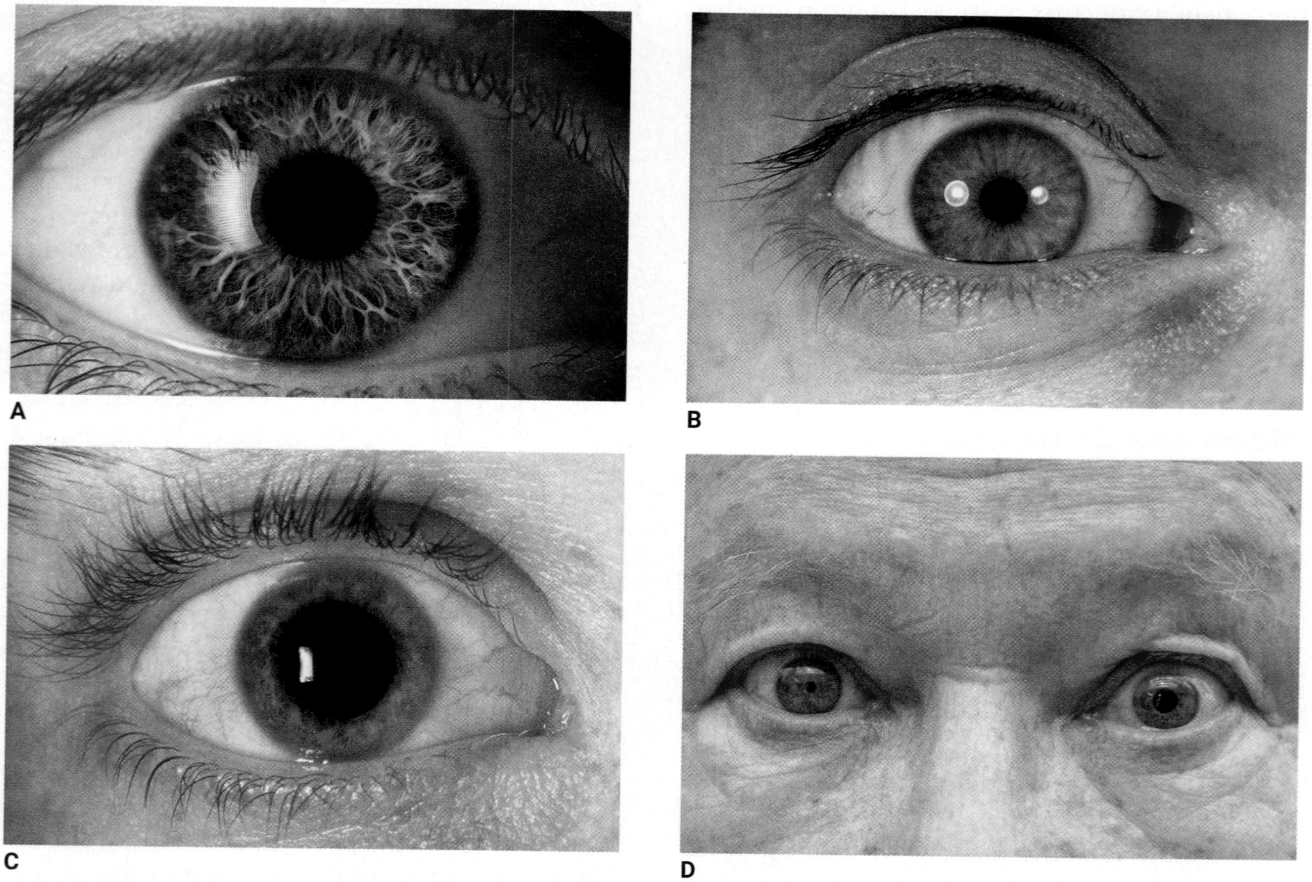

A B C D

FIGURE 19-6 Pupillary responses. **A.** Normal. **B.** Constricted. **C.** Dilated. **D.** Unequal (anisocoria).

30 mg/dL, then the patient will become confused or unresponsive.

Cranial Nerve Functioning

Assessment of the head includes gathering information on the functioning of the cranial nerves, which control various portions of the body **TABLE 19-5**. When you perform your assessment of the patient's cranial nerves, look for the patient's ability to respond, strength of response, and symmetry. Patients with stroke, trigeminal neuralgia, **myasthenia gravis**, or other conditions may demonstrate abnormal cranial nerve functioning. Refer to Chapter 11, *Patient Assessment*, for more information on how to assess the cranial nerves.

TABLE 19-5 The Cranial Nerves

Cranial Nerve	Function
I. Olfactory	Smell
II. Optic	Vision
III. Oculomotor	Movement of the eye, pupil, and eyelid
IV. Trochlear	Movement of the eye
V. Trigeminal	Chewing Pain Temperature Touch of the mouth and face
VI. Abducens	Movement of the eye
VII. Facial	Movement of the face Tears Salivation and taste
VIII. Auditory	Hearing and balance
IX. Glossopharyngeal	Glossopharyngeal: Swallowing, taste, and sensations in the mouth and pharynx
X. Vagus	Sensation and movement of the pharynx, larynx, thorax, and GI system
XI. Accessory	Movement of the head and shoulders
XII. Hypoglossal	Movement of the tongue

Abbreviation: GI, gastrointestinal

Speech

Listen to the quality of the patient's speech. Is it slurred? Slurring is a classic finding with stroke. Is the speech appropriate? To assess this quality, you need to focus not only on the spoken words but also on the words a patient chooses. Sometimes speech may be clear but word choice is incorrect. Also assess the patient's ability to recognize objects. Patients can have both slurred speech and object recognition difficulties.

Language can be affected by either injury or disease. In aphasia, a person's speech is affected. There are three primary forms of aphasia. Depending on the form, the patient may be unable to understand (receive) speech, but able to speak clearly; unable to speak (express oneself) clearly, but able to understand speech; or may have a combination of both.

Ask questions to which you and the patient know the answer, such as "Who is the president?" and "What month is it?" This strategy will enable you to verify that the patient understands the questions. Do not ask yes-or-no questions. Note whether the patient speaks clearly but gives incorrect answers.

Ask the patient to raise their arm. Complying with this request indicates that they can understand you. Then ask the patient's name. Note whether the patient does not respond or provides a slurred response.

Finally, if the patient can neither follow commands nor answer questions, then note these findings in your documentation.

Even when their speech is affected by a neurologic disorder, patients often can think clearly. They may have needs, anxieties, and discomforts, but no way to express them. This dysfunction can be frightening to patients who cannot understand what you are saying and cannot respond to your questions despite being able to formulate the answers in their minds. Be sensitive to this condition and reassure the patient by moving slowly and purposefully, using therapeutic touch, and maintaining good eye contact.

Patients may quickly tire of making the effort to communicate and become frustrated or emotionally exhausted. Be prepared for patients to shut down—and then gently encourage them to continue to try.

Words of Wisdom

The following approaches can be useful to facilitate communication with patients who have aphasia:

- **Use a communication board.** This tool can be purchased, handmade, or accessed via a smartphone or tablet in the form of an application. A communication board allows patients to select pictures or symbols to convey their meaning, thereby helping you to understand what they are thinking. It enables you to ask more complicated questions than the yes-or-no method. If the communication board is stored in the ambulance, then you may have to delay its use until the patient is loaded into the ambulance.
- **Writing.** Consider asking the patient to write down responses using a pencil and paper or type them using a mobile phone keypad. These tools must be on hand or else you may experience a delay in getting information.

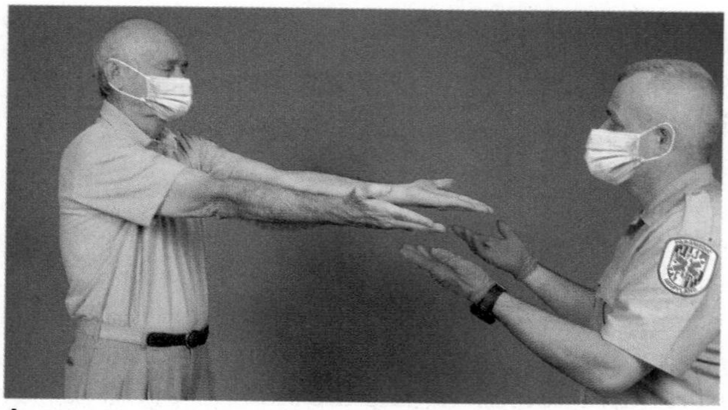

A

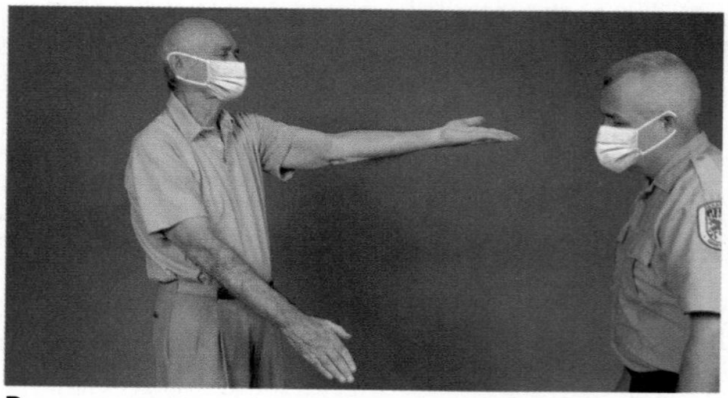

B

FIGURE 19-7 A. A person who has not had a stroke can hold both arms in front of the body even with their eyes closed. **B.** A person who has had a stroke might not be able to maintain this position. One arm will drift down and turn toward the body.

Body Movement

Hemiparesis and Hemiplegia

Patients with strokes can have weakness or paralysis of one side of the body. Weakness of one side of the body is called **hemiparesis**; paralysis of one side of the body is called **hemiplegia**. Sometimes, you will assess patients who have weakness on one side of the body but facial droop on the other side. A patient who has experienced a left cerebral stroke, for example, may have right-side arm and leg weakness, as well as loss of visual fields in the left eye, because the left side of the brain controls the right side of the body and the left eye.

Have the patient close their eyes and hold out the arms in front of the body at the same level. With the eyes closed, the patient's only way to tell where their arms are located is from the sensations being processed by the cerebellum. If the patient has had a stroke, then one of the arms may drift away from the other **FIGURE 19-7**.

Some patients have alterations in their **gait** (walking patterns). The term **ataxia** is used to describe alteration of a person's ability to perform coordinated motions such as walking. A person's gait can become slow, shuffling, or scissors-like, for example.

Unless you observe some medical reason to avoid it, have the patient walk for several steps. Assessing gait is another test of the cerebellum's activity. The cerebellum controls the mechanics of walking and allows you to focus on *where* you want to walk, rather than *how* to walk. Thus, a patient with damage to the cerebellum may walk erratically, stumble, or even experience a loss of the ability to walk.

In some cases, a patient's posture may become rigid. Have the patient stand up straight. Place one hand on the patient's chest and your other hand behind the patient's back, and then push on the chest. Normally, as you push backward, the patient compensates quickly by taking a step to keep from falling. In patients with certain disorders, such as **Parkinson disease** (discussed later in this chapter), the patient cannot compensate quickly enough, and you will push the patient over. It is essential to have a hand behind the patient to keep the patient from falling.

Bizarre Movement

Some patients may exhibit bizarre movement that indicates disruption within the nervous system. **Myoclonus** is a type of rapid, jerky muscle contraction that occurs involuntarily. Most people have experienced myoclonic jerks. A classic example of this phenomenon is the student who is about to fall asleep in class. As the student gets sleepier, the head begins to sag, until the head involuntarily jerks upward (myoclonic jerk) and the student wakes up.

Another form of bizarre movement is called **dystonia**. In this movement, a part of the body contracts and remains contracted. Dystonia is discussed later in this chapter.

Alterations in Smooth Motion

As you assess the patient, note whether their movement is smooth. When neurologic structures are functioning correctly, muscle groups alternately contract and relax, allowing the body to move. When this fine balance is upset, patients may develop **rigidity**, a condition in which muscles do not contract and relax smoothly, resulting in stiffness of motion.

Tremors are another example of an alteration in smooth motion. This oscillating (back and forth) movement usually occurs in the hands but can also affect the head, arms, torso, and legs. Tremors involve the motion of joints. They can occur at any age but are most common among middle-aged and older adults. Several types of tremor exist, named for the kind of activity that elicits them:

- **Rest tremor**. Occurs when the patient's arms, hands, or legs shake even while the muscles are relaxed (eg, hands resting on the lap). The tremor partly or completely disappears with voluntary movement.
- **Intention tremor**. Occurs when the patient is asked to demonstrate movement toward a target, such as touching the nose with a finger or reaching toward an object. The tremor typically increases as the patient gets closer to the target.
- **Postural tremor**. Occurs when a body part is placed in a particular position and required to maintain that position for an extended period. Most people have experienced this type of tremor when working hard for a long time. As fatigue sets in, the body parts being used the most begin to shake. A postural tremor can also occur when a person is standing. The body's muscles are constantly making tiny corrections to maintain posture. The head can oscillate back and forth as the person tries to keep it still.

Another type of movement that may appear similar to a tremor is a seizure. Seizures can be classified as either generalized (affecting large portions of the brain) or partial (affecting a limited area of the brain). Whereas a tremor is a fine movement, a generalized or tonic-clonic seizure (formerly called a grand mal seizure) is a larger, less focused type of movement. Generalized seizures affect a person's awareness and are associated with both tonic and clonic activity:

- **Tonic activity** is a rigid, contracted body posture. The arms, legs, neck, and back can contract so tightly that the body part shakes from the intensity of the contraction.
- **Clonic activity** is characterized by rhythmic contraction and relaxation of muscle groups. Clonic activity can be described as the bizarre, nonpurposeful movement of any body part. Arms and legs may flail, teeth may clench, the head may bob, and the torso may convulse wildly.

Seizures are discussed in more detail later in this chapter.

Sensation

The last area included in the assessment is sensation within the body. Many nervous system conditions can alter the ability to feel pain, temperature, pressure, or light touch. A sensation of numbness or tingling is called **paresthesia**. If the patient can feel nothing within a body part, then their condition is called **anesthesia**.

Vital Signs

In the patient who is having a stroke or seizure, check and document the pulse rate, rhythm, and quality; respiratory rate, rhythm, and quality; BP; skin temperature, color, and condition; and pupil size and reactivity. During most active seizures, however, it is impossible to evaluate vital signs, and doing so is not a priority. Unless the situation is unusual, vital signs obtained during the postictal state will be close to normal.

Words of Wisdom

Automatic, noninvasive BP cuffs can be inaccurate if used in moving ambulances. Check the patient's BP manually to have an accurate baseline before relying on automatic systems.

Given the critical importance of normal cerebral perfusion, you must closely monitor BP in any patient with the potential for increased ICP. Frequent reassessment becomes even more essential when the BP has dropped. Ensure the patient maintains an SBP of at least 110 to 120 mm Hg. Ensure adequate respiratory rate and pattern, and effective pulse rate and rhythm.

The patient's temperature can be difficult to determine in the prehospital setting. If you suspect hypothermia or hyperthermia, then the standard of care is to use a thermometer to establish the patient's temperature, as discussed in Chapter 11, *Patient Assessment.* Refer to Chapter 39, *Environmental Emergencies,* for guidance regarding active rewarming and cooling for environmentally induced temperature alterations.

Reassessment

Notify the receiving facility of the patient's chief complaint and your assessment findings. Most designated stroke centers will want you to call in a stroke alert for patients you have assessed and found to be having a stroke (check your local protocol). The American Stroke Association recommends that a stroke alert be activated if the onset time of the symptoms is less than 4.5 hours. Specialized stroke centers may extend those activation times up to 12 hours based on the procedures they have available for stroke care.[4] Forewarning the hospital about a patient with possible stroke will give the stroke team members at the hospital time to assemble their resources to treat the patient without delay. Be sure to communicate the time that the patient was last seen to be healthy, your neurologic exam findings, and the time you anticipate arriving at the hospital.

A key piece of information to document is the time of onset of the patient's signs and symptoms. If the diagnosis is an ischemic stroke, then this information is critical in determining whether the patient is a candidate for treatment with clot-dissolving (fibrinolytic) drugs. It is also essential to document your findings from administering the stroke scale and the patient's GCS score, along with any changes you found during your reassessment. As always, document interventions performed, the patient's response to those interventions, any change in patient condition during transport, and the reason for the choice of hospital.

For patients who have had a seizure, describe the seizure activity, if known, and include bystanders' comments if they witnessed it. Document the onset and duration of the seizure. Did the patient notice or express noticing an **aura** (visual changes such as flashing lights or blind spots in the field of vision)? Record any evidence of trauma and interventions performed. Document whether this is the patient's first seizure or whether the patient has a history of seizures. If the latter, determine how often the patient has them and whether the patient has any history of status epilepticus (discussed later in this chapter). Record the time of each intervention performed, how the patient responded to the intervention, and your reassessment findings.

You may be the only provider to witness some patient activity, so accurate documentation is critical to the continuity of care. Avoid using words that can have multiple meanings, such as "lethargic," "sleepy," "obtunded," and "out of it." Describe the patient using active language, as in the following examples:

"Arrived to find a male patient disoriented to place and time."

"Caring for a 43-year-old man who is slow to respond to verbal or painful stimulation."

Standard Care Guideline for the Neurologic Patient

The focus of care for a neurologic patient is to ensure the body has an adequate internal environment to allow for optimal brain function. Remember, the brain needs oxygen, glucose, and normal temperature to function properly. The following guidelines serve as the foundation on which additional care for specific neurologic conditions will be built. Through the remainder of this chapter, this guideline will be called the standard care guideline **TABLE 19-6**.

Administration of Dextrose

Follow your local protocol regarding what blood glucose reading is considered low. One possible guideline is that if the blood glucose level is less

TABLE 19-6 Standard Care Guideline for the Adult Neurologic Patient

Step	Description
Ensure scene safety and take standard precautions.	Ensure you and your partner are safe. Don appropriate personal protective equipment. Use masks and eye protection when managing the airway.
Assess airway and breathing.	Evaluate the airway and effectiveness of breathing. If needed, secure the airway and provide ventilatory support to ensure oxygen saturation is between 95% and 98%. • Hyperoxygenation (as evidenced by an oxygen saturation level of 100%) may be harmful. • Consider rapid sequence intubation, as appropriate. If respiratory failure or apnea is present, ventilate the patient at 10 breaths/min. • Routine hyperventilation may be harmful. Only provide hyperventilation to a patient with documented unresponsiveness and signs of increased ICP.
Assess circulation.	Establish IV access. Use your assessment findings about the patient's circulatory status as a guide to whether you should use a saline lock or hang a bag of fluids. If fluids are needed, then saline, normosol, or lactated Ringer solution are isotonic choices. • Do not use solutions containing dextrose. Consider drawing blood samples for later analysis at the hospital. Check blood pressure and heart rate. • Correct hypotension with IV fluids or vasopressors based on the cause of hypotension. Ensure continuous ECG monitoring. Perform a 12-lead ECG.

Check blood glucose level.	If <60 mg/dL and signs of decreased LOC, then determine:
	• Does the patient have a patent airway? Can the patient swallow?
	  • If yes, then consider oral glucose, candy, or orange juice. Closely monitor swallowing.
	  • If no, then administer dextrose or glucagon per your local protocol.
	  • Hyperglycemia can increase the morbidity of patients who have had a stroke.

Assess for increased ICP.	Look for the hallmarks of increased ICP. See Chapter 35, *Head and Spine Trauma*, for more information on increased ICP.
Check for drug use.	Survey the scene for pills and drug paraphernalia; assess the patient for track marks. Administer naloxone in case of a known or suspected opioid overdose.
Assess for seizures.	If the seizure is prolonged, then administer benzodiazepines.
Evaluate temperature.	If low, then cover the patient, turn on the heat in the patient compartment of the ambulance, and prevent heat loss. If high, then remove the patient's clothing and cover the naked patient in a sheet. Turn off the heat in the patient compartment.
Provide emotional support for the patient and family.	Neurologic emergencies can produce feelings of confusion, fear, anger, and helplessness. Provide a therapeutic, gentle touch on the shoulder. Touch can communicate compassion. Use a calm, reassuring voice. Assure the patient and family that you are there to help. If the patient is confused, then try to reorient the patient.

Abbreviations: ECG, electrocardiogram; ICP, intracranial pressure; IV, intravenous; LOC, level of consciousness

Modified from: National Model EMS Clinical Guidelines, Version 2.2. National Association of State EMS Officials. https://nasemso.org/wp-content/uploads/National-Model-EMS-Clinical-Guidelines-2017-PDF-Version-2.2.pdf. Updated January 2019. Accessed March 22, 2021.

than 60 mg/dL, then the patient needs glucose. Both IV dextrose and oral glucagon are available for the prehospital treatment of hypoglycemia. The effects of dextrose typically begin within 1 minute. If you cannot obtain IV access to administer dextrose, then administer glucagon. This naturally occurring body chemical is responsible for converting the body's stores of glycogen into glucose. You should see an increase in the LOC and blood glucose level within 20 minutes of administration. Chapter 24, *Endocrine Emergencies,* discusses how to administer dextrose.

If the patient's blood glucose level is high, then be aware that no safe way to decrease this level in the prehospital setting currently exists. Administration of insulin can be problematic because it is easy to overcorrect the imbalance, resulting in a hypoglycemic state. In such patients, ensure adequate support of BP. Patients with hyperglycemia are often dehydrated and may need volume support. In fact, rehydration alone in a severely dehydrated patient with hyperglycemia can dramatically lower the patient's blood glucose level. Note that hyperglycemia can increase the morbidity of patients who have had a stroke.

Finally, be cautious when caring for patients whose blood glucose level cannot be checked. If the patient is unresponsive or has decreased LOC and no blood glucose monitor is available, then contact medical direction or follow your local protocols.

Administration of Naloxone

Naloxone (Narcan) is used to reverse CNS and respiratory depression induced by opioids. This drug may be administered IV push, intramuscularly, endotracheally, or using a mucosal atomizer device. This intranasal (IN) device provides a safe, noninvasive, rapid-acting method of naloxone delivery. When on the scene of a known or suspected opioid overdose, ask bystanders if naloxone has been given (and if so, how much and when) because many states allow laypeople to administer it via nasal spray. For more information on the use of naloxone, see Chapter 28, *Toxicology.*

Interventions for Increased ICP

If the patient has signs of increased ICP, then establish vascular access and administer normal saline or lactated Ringer solution. Do not use solutions containing dextrose. Consider drawing blood samples for later analysis at the hospital. Also check the patient's BP and pulse rate. If the patient is hypotensive, support BP to ensure adequate cerebral perfusion pressure (CPP); normal CPP is 70 to 90 mm Hg. The target is an SBP of 110 mm Hg. Perform continuous heart monitoring with an ECG.

Pathophysiology, Assessment, and Management of Common Neurologic Emergencies

Most diseases or conditions, including neurologic disorders, are caused by more than one factor, so they are said to be *multifactorial.* If diseases had only one cause, then cause-effect relationships would be simple: Every person exposed to a particular pathogen would become infected, for example, and every person with a diet high in saturated fat would develop blocked arteries. In reality, disease susceptibility often depends on a multitude of factors, such as the following:

- How the body system was created during development of the embryo/fetus
- How effective the body's defense and repair functions are
- How severe or prolonged the body's exposure is to the pathogen, toxin, or other damaging factor

During the following discussions of some common neurologic conditions, keep in mind that disease development usually cannot be attributed to a single cause.

Stroke

A stroke, also called a brain attack or cerebrovascular accident (CVA), is a serious medical condition in which the blood supply to areas of the brain becomes interrupted, causing ischemia. People older than 65 years represent almost 75% of all patients who have strokes.[5]

The American Heart Association (AHA) reports that a significant number of patients who have strokes either deny their symptoms or do not understand what their symptoms mean.[6] Many patients fail to activate EMS when they experience stroke symptoms and consequently delay care for this condition. Public education on stroke awareness should be a function of your EMS agency. As recommended by the AHA, the goal of treatment is early recognition and rapid, appropriate intervention. The longer the stroke continues, the less likely the patient is to have a promising outcome, because "time is brain." Early recognition begins with an EMS system that can effectively identify potential strokes at dispatch and rapidly request the appropriate resources. As an EMS provider, do not delay your response to a patient with a potential stroke. According to the AHA, one-fifth of patients with an intracranial hemorrhage will have a significant decrease in their LOC between emergency medical care provided by EMS and care on transfer to the emergency department (ED). Again, time is brain!

Pathophysiology

Neurologic conditions can have a vascular origin, and vascular emergencies can occur either suddenly or gradually. Sudden occurrences are typically the result of emboli or aneurysms **FIGURE 19-8**. If a blood vessel is suddenly blocked, as in an embolism, then the cells beyond the blockage can become ischemic. As oxygen and glucose levels drop, brain cells turn to anaerobic metabolism in an effort to stay alive. This mechanism, however, is only a stopgap measure. Anaerobic metabolism creates only minuscule amounts of energy for the cell and produces acidic by-products. If circulation is not restored quickly, then the cell will not have enough fuel to survive.

Artery walls consist of three layers of tissue that lie on top of each other. An aneurysm is a weakness in one or more of those layers. The process of aneurysm development is as follows:

1. Small tears or defects occur within the arterial wall.
2. Blood enters between the layers of the artery.
3. Pressure builds up, and the initial small tear increases in size.

If this process continues, then the arterial wall will become so damaged that it can no longer withstand the normal pressure of blood flowing through the artery. The weakened wall will begin to bulge. If the damage is severe, then the bulging artery can leak or the wall can fail, causing an intracranial hemorrhage.

Pathophysiology of Stroke

The two basic types of strokes are **ischemic stroke**, which accounts for 87% of all strokes according to the AHA, and **hemorrhagic stroke**, which accounts for the remaining 13%.[7] Ischemic strokes are also called occlusive strokes because they are caused by an occlusion (blockage)—either a thrombus or an embolus.

The graph shown in **FIGURE 19-9** provides some insight into the evolution of a stroke. The two types of strokes have different presentation patterns. In an ischemic stroke, a blood vessel is blocked, so the tissue distal to the blockage becomes ischemic. Eventually that tissue will die if blood flow is not restored. But this pathology is self-limiting. Only the tissue beyond the blockage is affected, so the area or areas of the brain involved are limited.

In Figure 19-9, notice how the line representing signs and symptoms stops climbing and begins to stabilize. This stabilization does not imply that a patient cannot die from an ischemic stroke. The extent of the stroke and its severity are dictated by the artery involved and the portion of the brain being denied oxygen. For example, an ischemic stroke in which blood flow to the brainstem is blocked is life threatening. The plateau indicates that signs and symptoms have peaked and leveled off because the area of the brain affected is no longer working.

In contrast to ischemic strokes, hemorrhagic strokes tend to get worse over time because of ongoing bleeding within the cranium. This bleeding can cause increased ICP and brainstem herniation. One of the hallmarks of a hemorrhagic stroke is a chief complaint of "the worst headache of my life." If the patient reports a severe headache and later cannot speak, becomes difficult to arouse, and finally begins showing signs of increased ICP, then strongly consider a hemorrhagic stroke in the differential diagnosis.

To appreciate the effects of strokes, it is essential to understand the dynamics of ICP. The skull (cranial vault) is filled with three substances: brain, blood, and cerebrospinal fluid (CSF). These three substances exert pressure against the skull, and the skull exerts a reflected pressure **FIGURE 19-10**. This exchange is balanced, allowing the brain to fit snugly within the skull. If spaces or voids were present within the skull, then the brain would slam into the skull with only minimal head movement. The pressure of the various substances present within the skull constitutes ICP. Normally, ICP is less than

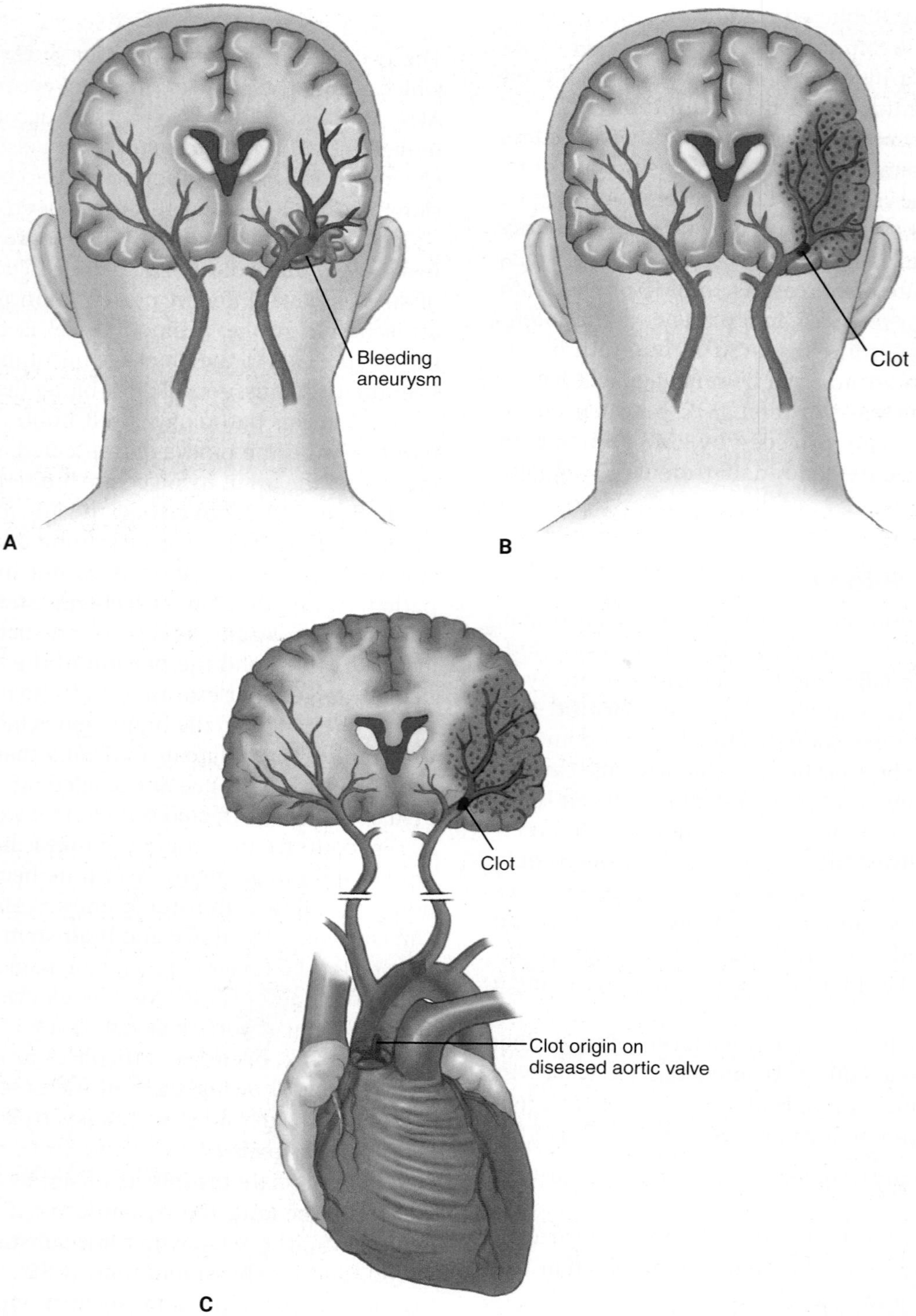

FIGURE 19-8 Vascular causes of neurologic conditions. **A.** An aneurysm is an area of weakness in an artery wall that can bulge out and eventually leak or rupture. **B.** Atherosclerosis can damage the wall of a cerebral artery, narrowing the artery or producing a clot. When the vessel is completely blocked, brain cells begin to die. **C.** An embolus is a blood clot formed elsewhere in the body, often on a diseased heart valve. It can travel through the vascular system and lodge in a cerebral artery, causing a stroke.

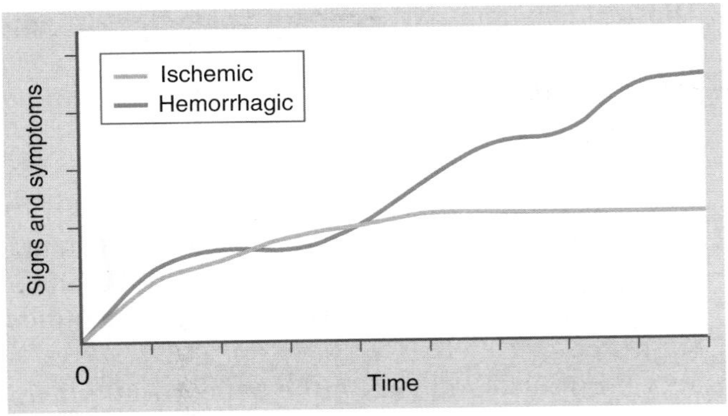

FIGURE 19-9 Symptom patterns for hemorrhagic compared with ischemic stroke.

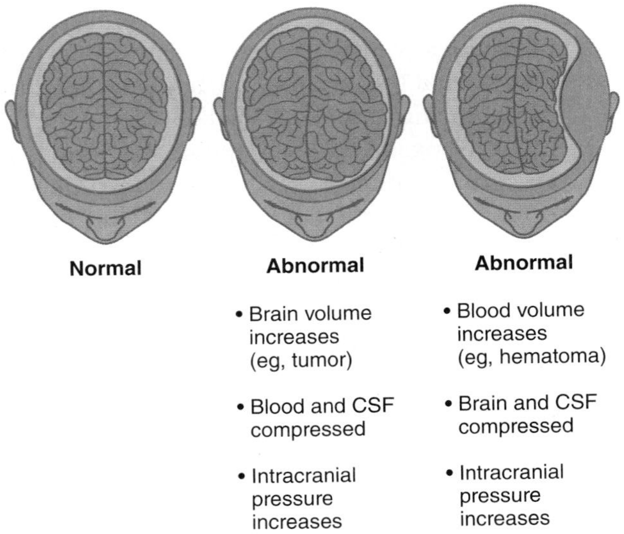

FIGURE 19-10 Normal and abnormal intracranial pressure.

Abbreviation: CSF, cerebrospinal fluid

10 to 15 mm Hg in adults and less than 3 to 7 mm Hg in young children.[8]

Two difficulties arise when the pressure within the cranial vault begins to climb and remains high: The brain may become ischemic because of a lack of blood supply and/or may herniate. **Herniation** is the movement of a structure from its normal location into another space. Portions of the brain can be pushed into different locations, causing tissue damage and potential death.

First, as ICP rises, the amount of blood available to the brain decreases. CPP, the pressure of blood within the cranial vault, begins to fall. (Recall that normal CPP is 70 to 90 mm Hg.) When the CPP decreases to less than 50 mm Hg, the brain begins to become ischemic. Chapter 35, *Head and Spine Trauma*, provides an in-depth discussion of this topic.

As is the case for most readings within the body, ICP is constantly changing. Coughing, vomiting, or bearing down, for instance, tends to increase ICP. These momentary spikes in ICP are not harmful. If blood, swelling, pus, or a tumor within the cranial vault are present, however, ICP will increase and remain high. The cranial vault volume is limited and inflexible, so the pressure increases as more and more substances are squeezed into this space. Patients can have life-threatening issues when ICP rises sharply and/or BP becomes critically low.

The second possible outcome of increased ICP is herniation; specifically, a shift of the intracranial contents within the cranial vault or displacement of the contents toward the foramen magnum, the large opening at the inferior portion of the skull through which the spinal cord exits. This shift will eventually compress the brainstem, at which point the patient will experience a loss of control of autonomic functions.

Large Vessel Occlusion

A large vessel occlusion is a type of ischemic stroke that results from a blockage in a major artery of the brain. Examples of these large vessels include the basilar artery, internal carotid artery terminus, and middle cerebral artery. When these major arteries are blocked, significant portions of the brain lose blood supply, resulting in higher-order brain function disruptions.[9,10] Patients with this condition will require advanced stroke care at a location that can perform endovascular therapy. In this surgical intervention, a neurospecialist removes the clot and attempts to restore blood flow. Prehospital evaluations, however, cannot differentiate between a large vessel occlusion and a small vessel occlusion.

Assessment

Stroke causes sudden-onset changes in neurologic status. As mentioned previously, patients can exhibit any combination of the following signs and symptoms:

- **Language effects.** Slurred speech, aphasia, agnosia (inability to identify people or objects), and apraxia (inability to perform purposeful actions; with speech apraxia, the person knows what they want to say but has difficulty pronouncing or sequencing the words)

- **Movement effects.** Hemiparesis, hemiplegia, arm drifting, facial droop, tongue deviation, swallowing difficulties, ptosis, and ataxia
- **Sensory effects.** Headache (hemorrhagic), sudden blindness, and sudden unilateral paresthesia
- **Cognitive effects.** Decreased LOC, difficulty thinking, seizures, and coma
- **Cardiac effects.** Hypertension

You can also use the BE-FAST mnemonic to assess for a stroke[11]:

B **Balance.** Sudden loss of balance, coordination, or dizziness
E **Eyesight.** Loss of vision (or change in vision) in one or both eyes
F **Face.** Facial droop
A **Arms.** Arm drift or weakness
S **Speech.** Speech impairment or inability to repeat a simple phrase
T **Time.** Time is critical—call 9-1-1; the T can also represent Thunderclap headache

Documentation and Communication

Patients with strokes can present with a wide range of communication difficulties.

- Patients who are multilingual may lose the ability to understand one language but not another.
- Patients may be able to understand the written word but not the spoken word.
- Patients may not be able to understand any form of communication.

Be open to trying various ways to communicate. Remember, communication challenges do not indicate that patients are not thinking. The problem is that they cannot get you to understand what they are thinking.

Vital signs may provide evidence of whether a patient has increased pressure within the cranium. The information in Table 19-4 can help you distinguish signs of increased ICP from those of shock. Recall that other signs of increased ICP include posturing, abnormal respiratory patterns, and unequal pupils.

Management

Management of the neurologic patient begins with the standard care guideline. Because "time is brain," prompt evaluation and transport to a stroke center are essential. Types of stroke centers are identified in **TABLE 19-7**.

It is crucial to monitor the patient with potential stroke. A significant number of patients who have had a stroke will also exhibit cardiac dysrhythmias. Continuous ECG monitoring will allow you to quickly intervene if the patient's rhythm destabilizes. Obtain a 12-lead ECG and draw blood for later laboratory evaluation; however, do not delay transport to accomplish these tasks. If the patient has a fever, then contact medical control. You may be ordered to give acetaminophen. Unless the patient is hypoxic, allow the patient to remain supine.[6]

In patients who are unresponsive *and* demonstrate other signs of increased ICP, administer fluids as needed to maintain near-normal SBP. Unless you suspect a possible cervical spine injury, elevate the patient's head 30°.[6] Keep the head and neck in neutral alignment without flexing the neck. This position will cause a slight decrease in ICP and allow the patient to better manage any airway secretions. Ensure the airway is clear, but do not vigorously suction because stimulating the cough and gag reflexes will increase ICP. Watch for seizures and be prepared to administer benzodiazepines. The patient may have bradycardia. However, atropine and transcutaneous pacing are not indicated because of the systolic hypertension that accompanies the bradycardia: The ICP is causing the bradycardia, not the other way around. Notify the hospital and provide prompt transport.

Closely monitor the BP of any patient with a potential problem with ICP. Frequent assessment becomes even more critical when a decrease in BP is also present. For any patient at risk for ICP, ensure the SBP remains at least 110 mm Hg.

Carbon dioxide (CO_2) levels are also important in patients with increased ICP. A high CO_2 level causes vasodilation of the cerebral arteries. This vasodilation allows more blood into the skull, increasing ICP. Conversely, a diminished level of CO_2 lowers ICP by causing vasoconstriction, decreasing blood

TABLE 19-7 Types of Stroke Centers

American Heart Association/ American Stroke Association Designation	Capabilities
Acute stroke–ready hospital (ASRH)	Stroke team available 24/7, CT scanner, acute stroke expertise available 24/7 or via telemedicine if needed, IV fibrinolytics, no designated stroke beds; anticipate transfer of patients who received fibrinolytics to PSC/TSC/CSC
Primary stroke center (PSC)	All ASRH functions plus dedicated stroke unit, stroke service, medical management of stroke, patient transfer for neurosurgical emergencies
Thrombectomy-capable stroke center (TSC)	All PSC functions plus MRI, dedicated neurointensive care beds, on-site critical care coverage 24/7, intra-arterial fibrinolytics, endovascular therapy, postprocedural care, patient transfer for neurosurgical emergencies
Comprehensive stroke center (CSC)	All TSC functions plus 24/7 availability of neurologist, neurosurgeon, neuroradiologist, neurointerventionist; neuroendovascular care, hemorrhagic stroke care

Abbreviations: CT, computed tomography; IV, intravenous; MRI, magnetic resonance imaging

Modified from: Stroke certification programs: program concept comparison. The Joint Commission website. https://www.jointcommission.org/-/media/tjc/idev-imports/topics-assets/comparison-grid-stroke-certification-programs/strokeprogramgrid_abbrev_010518pdf.pdf. Accessed March 31, 2021.

supply to the brain. Increasing ventilation, then, decreases ICP (good) by decreasing blood supply (bad). This incompatibility can make decision making difficult because prehospital treatment is simply not effective at decreasing ICP. Using end-tidal carbon dioxide ($ETCO_2$) readings, provide ventilatory support to maintain $ETCO_2$ at 30 to 35 mm Hg.[6]

The AHA has developed an algorithm showing goals for managing patients with suspected stroke **FIGURE 19-11**. Treatment at the hospital takes different paths of care for each type of stroke. One feature, however, is common to both paths: Time is essential. For ischemic strokes, fibrinolytics need to be administered within 3 to 4.5 hours of onset. This time limit may be extended as new and emerging approaches to stroke management continue to evolve. In hemorrhagic strokes, the more the patient bleeds into the cranium, the greater the potential for increased ICP and herniation becomes.

The AHA and the American Stroke Association (ASA) recommend a comprehensive approach to the emergency medical care of the patient experiencing a stroke. First, the general public needs to be educated about the signs and symptoms of stroke. The public then needs to call 9-1-1 so trained dispatchers can summon the appropriate prehospital resources. As an EMS provider, you need to have adequate training in delivering care to patients with strokes, including the ability to distinguish which patients would benefit from treatment at a stroke center. After the patient arrives in the ED, a coordinated and comprehensive approach to care is essential. Some patients will benefit from fibrinolytics, some may need intra-arterial clot removal, and others may need neurosurgery. After acute stroke care has been delivered, appropriate rehabilitation will likely be recommended to ensure the patient returns to the highest quality of life possible.

All EMS providers need to be involved in educating the community about stroke signs and symptoms, the effects of strokes, and how to activate EMS. Too many patients deny their symptoms or drive themselves to the ED. Patients need to understand that immediately on discovering stroke symptoms, they must call EMS for assistance.

Street Smarts

Neurologic emergencies can produce feelings of confusion, fear, anger, and helplessness. Therefore, you need to provide emotional support for the patient and family. A therapeutic, gentle touch on the shoulder can communicate your compassion to the patient. Use a calm, reassuring voice to reorient the patient and let them know that you are there to help.

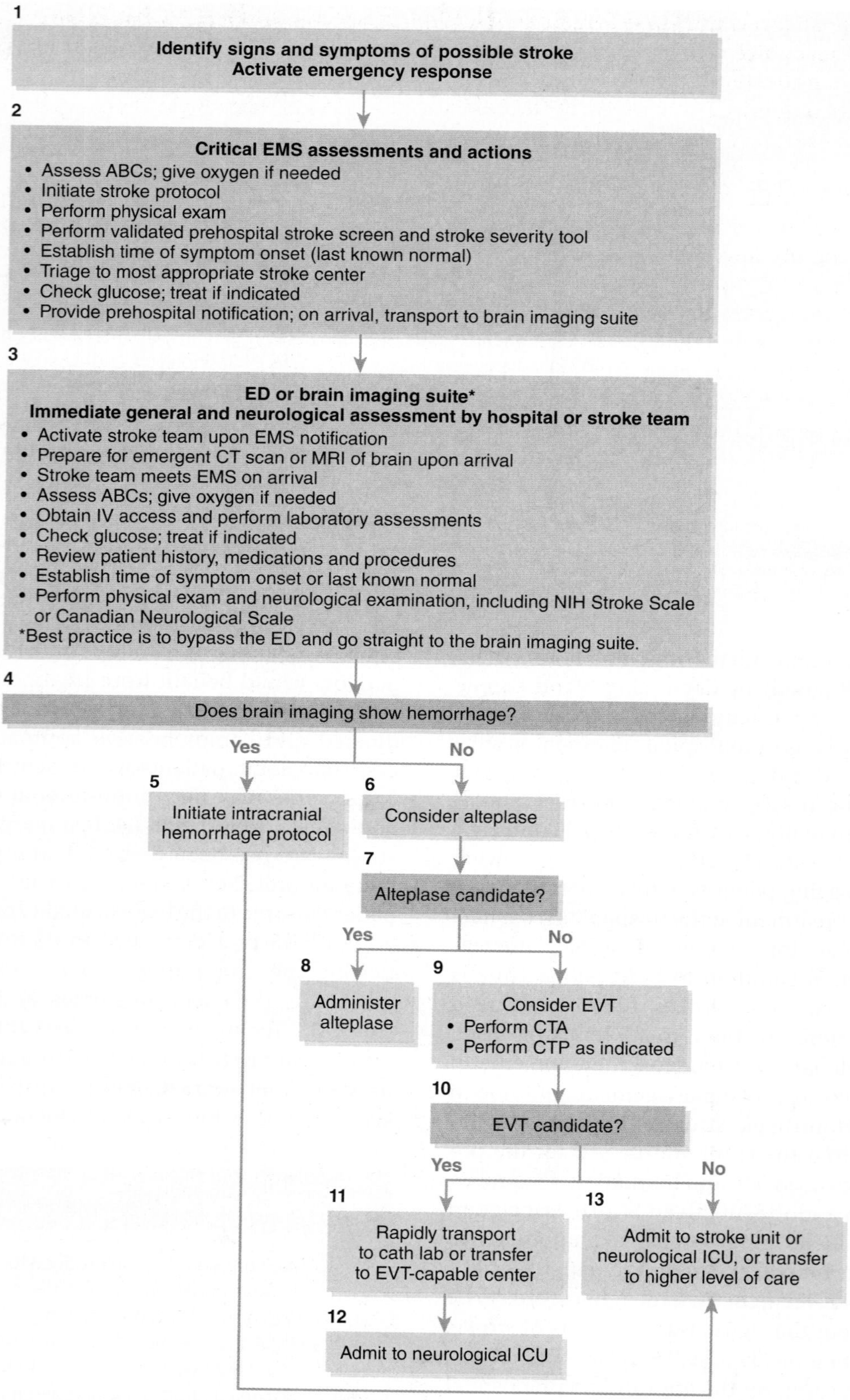

FIGURE 19-11 The Adult Suspected Stroke Algorithm from the American Heart Association. The steps in the initial boxes are intended for prehospital providers.

Abbreviations: ABC, airway, breathing, and circulation; CT, computed tomography; CTA, computed tomographic angiography; CTP, computed tomographic perfusion; ED, emergency department; EVT, endovascular thrombectomy; ICU, intensive care unit; IV, intravenous; MRI, magnetic resonance imaging

In addition, all levels of EMS providers should be trained to recognize stroke signs and symptoms. Rapid identification is imperative. Time is brain, and the administration of IV fibrinolytic agents is time-sensitive. The checklist presented in **TABLE 19-8** will help you focus on gathering the information that the ED physician will need before fibrinolytics can be considered. Patients who receive fibrinolytic therapy need to be evaluated to determine whether the medication will be helpful. Talk quickly with the family or caregivers to gather medical history, discharge instructions, all medications, allergy information, transfer orders, and other pertinent details. During the assessment phase, use a standard stroke assessment tool, such as the Cincinnati Prehospital Stroke Scale **TABLE 19-9** to increase the accuracy of your field impressions. You may also use the Los Angeles Prehospital Stroke Screen **TABLE 19-10** or the Miami Emergency Neurologic Deficit Prehospital Checklist **TABLE 19-11** to assess a patient with suspected stroke.

Assess the patient's oxygen saturation and titrate oxygen therapy to the patient's need. Supplemental oxygen is not recommended for nonhypoxic patients experiencing an acute ischemic stroke. If indicated, administer oxygen to maintain an oxygen saturation (Spo_2) level greater than 94%.[12]

Currently, no AHA/ASA guideline exists for the prehospital control of hypertension. Do not administer aspirin; it is helpful in patients with ischemic stroke but is harmful in patients with hemorrhagic

TABLE 19-8 Sample Prehospital Fibrinolytic Checklist for Stroke

Use this checklist for all patients suspected of having a stroke.

DATE: ______ TIME: ______		Time signs and symptoms began (record time). If unknown, answer the next question.
DATE: ______ TIME: ______		Time patient was last seen to be normal (record time)
______ mg/dL		Blood glucose level (record number)
____/____ Manual or Automatic Right arm or Left arm		Blood pressure (record readings; circle method and location)
Yes	No	(Check Yes or No for each item.)
❑	❑	Facial droop?
❑	❑	Slurred speech?
❑	❑	Arm drift (eyes closed and held for 10 seconds)?
❑	❑	In the past 7 days, has the patient had a procedure in which an artery was punctured?
❑	❑	In the past 14 days, has the patient had a major operation or serious trauma?
❑	❑	In the past 21 days, has the patient had any bleeding from the gastrointestinal or urinary tract?
❑	❑	In the past 3 months, has the patient experienced an MI, stroke, or head trauma?
❑	❑	When the signs and symptoms began, did the patient have a seizure?
❑	❑	Are current bleeding or clotting problems evident?
❑	❑	Is the patient taking anticoagulant medication?
❑	❑	Does the patient have intracranial bleeding—either now or in the past?
❑	❑	Are the patient's signs and symptoms of stroke rapidly improving?

TABLE 19-9 Cincinnati Prehospital Stroke Scale

Assessment	Normal	Abnormal
Facial Droop		
Ask the patient to smile and show the teeth.	Both sides of the face move equally.	One side of the face does not move as well as the other side.
Arm Drift		
Ask the patient to close the eyes and hold the arms out with palms up for 10 seconds.	Both arms move the same or neither arm moves. (If neither arm moves, then this may indicate the patient did not understand the instructions. Perform the test again.)	One arm does not move, or one arm drifts down compared with the other.
Speech		
Ask patient to say, "The sky is blue in Cincinnati."	The patient uses correct words with no slurring.	Patient slurs words, uses inappropriate words, or is unable to speak.

Interpretation: If any one item is abnormal, then the probability of a stroke is 72%.

TABLE 19-10 Los Angeles Prehospital Stroke Screen

Criteria	Yes	Unknown	No
1. Age >45 years	❑	❑	❑
2. History of seizures or epilepsy absent	❑	❑	❑
3. Symptoms <24 hours	❑	❑	❑
4. At baseline, patient does not use a wheelchair or is not bedridden.	❑	❑	❑
5. Blood glucose level between 60 and 400 mg/dL	❑	❑	❑
6. Obvious asymmetry (right versus left) in any of the following three exam categories (must be unilateral):	❑	❑	❑
	Equal	**Right Weak**	**Left Weak**
Facial smile/grimace	❑	❑ Droop	❑ Droop
Grip	❑	❑ Weak grip ❑ No grip	❑ Weak grip ❑ No grip
Arm strength	❑	❑ Drifts down ❑ Falls rapidly	❑ Drifts down ❑ Fall rapidly

Interpretation: If criteria 1–6 are marked yes, then the probability of a stroke is 97%.

TABLE 19-11 Miami Emergency Neurologic Deficit Prehospital Checklist

If Abnormal Time:		
Mental Status		
• Level of consciousness (AVPU)	❑	
• Speech (repeat "You can't teach an old dog new tricks") Abnormal = wrong words, slurred speech, no speech	❑	
• Questions (age, month)	❑	
• Commands (open and close eyes)	❑	
Cranial Nerves		
• Facial droop (show teeth and smile) Abnormal = one side does not move as well as other	❑ R	❑ L
• Visual fields (sees fingers in all four quadrants)	❑ R	❑ L
• Horizontal gaze (side to side)	❑ R	❑ L
Limbs		
Motor: arm drift (close eyes and hold out both arms) Abnormal = one side does not move as well as other	❑ R	❑ L
Motor: leg drift (open eyes and lift each leg separately)	❑ R	❑ L
Sensory: arm and leg (close eyes and touch, pinch)	❑ R	❑ L
Coordination: arm (finger to nose)	❑ R	❑ L
Coordination: leg (heel to shin)	❑ R	❑ L

Reprinted from *Advanced Stroke Life Support® Prehospital Provider Manual*, 11th edition, © 2015, with permission from the University of Miami Gordon Center for Simulation & Innovation in Medical Education, www.gordoncenter.miami.edu. The MEND checklist was created as part of the Advanced Stroke Life Support® curriculum to improve communication between healthcare providers throughout the continuum of care.

stroke. For this reason, it should be given only after obtaining a computed tomography (CT) or magnetic resonance imaging (MRI) study to confirm the type of stroke.

Because neurologic patients may be unable to feel or move their arms or legs, make sure to protect them from injury.

Complete a fibrinolytic checklist, focusing on when the signs and symptoms began or when the patient was last seen normal. Be aware that it can be difficult to pin down the exact time the stroke began. If possible, transport a family member or significant other who can speak to medical personnel in the ED.

Evidence-Based Medicine

According to age-old wisdom, "Oxygen is good and more oxygen is better." Oxygen is needed for cellular activity, but for patients in whom cells are being damaged and destroyed, more oxygen is not always better. After the cell membrane fails, cellular materials that were contained within that cell are able to move into the interstitial space. Some of these materials are chemicals (free radicals) that can cause damage to neighboring cells. In an oxygen-rich environment, these free radicals can increase their reactivity and "burn" hotter, causing damage or death to more neighboring cells.

As research continues into this concept, you can expect that conventional wisdom will continue to be challenged. The AHA and ASA report that patients who start with normal Spo_2 levels and receive high oxygen concentrations have similar outcomes compared with patients with normal Spo_2 levels who receive no supplemental oxygen when experiencing strokes.[6]

Words of Wisdom

Protocols are the beginning of patient care, not the totality of care.

The chronic medical patient is perhaps the most complicated type of patient you will encounter. Often, these patients have many diseases to manage and may take numerous medications. Your protocols are treatment guidelines that can provide you with a beginning framework to effectively care for patients. To be an effective paramedic, you must think critically and adapt to each patient's needs. For example, in the patient who has had a stroke, a history of chronic obstructive pulmonary disease (COPD) will complicate care. If a patient does not fit well into your protocol, then you need to reach out to your supervisor, your partner, or medical control. These resources can help you deliver safe and effective care to the patient.

Transport Decisions

When caring for a patient with suspected stroke, it is crucial to determine the appropriate facility for transport. You should transport patients with strokes to designated stroke centers (facilities with medical teams who are trained in the administration of fibrinolytics and in the diagnosis and

Controversies

Imagine the following scenario: You are unsure whether the patient is having an ischemic stroke or a hemorrhagic stroke. The patient wants to go to General Hospital, which does not have the appropriate resources to handle hemorrhagic strokes. Regional Hospital cares for patients with both types of strokes but is located 45 minutes away. To make the best decision, you need to determine which type of stroke is present.

In some parts of the country, EMS agencies are using an innovative system to answer this question.[13] Mobile stroke units—ambulances specifically equipped with a CT scanner—are typically operated by a paramedic, a critical care nurse, a CT technologist, and an EMS vehicle operator **FIGURE 19-12**. When a dispatch occurs for a patient with a possible stroke, the portable CT unit is dispatched as well. The team arrives, evaluates the patient, and then takes the patient, on the cot, into the mobile stroke unit. A quick scan is performed. This CT scan is transmitted to the hospital, where a neurosurgeon evaluates it to determine whether the patient is having a hemorrhagic or ischemic stroke. At the same time, a paramedic and critical care nurse perform a detailed assessment, including blood work. If appropriate, then fibrinolytics can be initiated while en route to the closest stroke center.

This novel approach to stroke care prompts many questions, such as the following:

- Does this system decrease the time from initial EMS contact to the administration of fibrinolytics?
- Are patients better triaged to the facilities that can best care for them?
- Does this system decrease the amount of neurologic deficit caused by strokes?
- What is the additional cost to the patient for this service?
- Which factors that affect stroke can best be mitigated using this system?

The only way for medicine to advance is to try something new and learn from the experience. This high-tech approach has many attractive aspects. Obviously, time is a significant contributor to the devastating effects related to stroke. How long until EMS arrives? How long until a physician evaluates the patient? How long until a CT scan is obtained? How long until fibrinolytics are administered? However, this intervention cannot help answer the critical question, "When was the patient last seen normal?"

The AHA and ASA report that fewer than one-half of all stroke patients who call 9-1-1 do so within 1 hour of the onset of signs and symptoms.[6] If the patient waits several hours before calling 9-1-1, then all the technology in the world may not prevent permanent neurologic damage. So, the real questions may be: How can services more quickly get medical care to patients who have had a stroke, and how can they better educate people about strokes so they call 9-1-1 sooner?

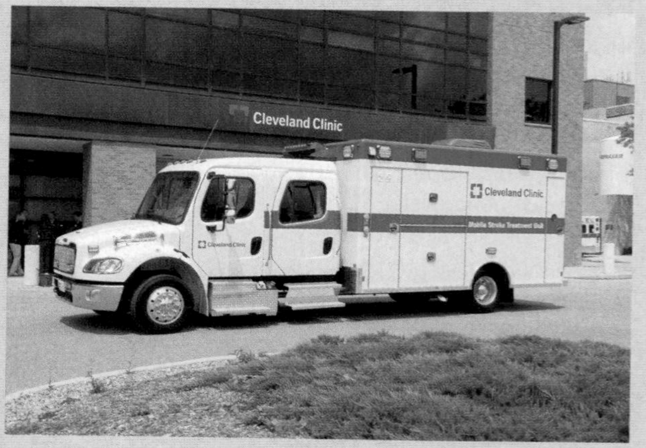

FIGURE 19-12 A mobile stroke unit.

management of various types of strokes). If you are more than 1 hour away from a stroke center, then consider air medical transportation. Contact the facility to ensure its CT/MRI capabilities are operational. Some facilities will need to contact imaging technicians who are on call during night hours or weekends. Early hospital notification to the ED can decrease the amount of time that elapses before the patient undergoes a CT/MRI. In fact, many facilities now allow ambulance patients to be transported directly to the CT scanner. This initial bypass of the ED can save valuable time, so call ahead to alert the ED. Typically, members of the ED team will meet you and guide you to the CT scanner. While you walk to the scanner, you will be asked to give your verbal report.

If a comprehensive stroke center is available in your region, based on the patient's presentation and needs, such as the need for endovascular therapy, you may be directed by protocol to transport your patient directly to one of these centers. Such stroke centers are staffed 24/7 with advanced stroke care specialists who can perform state-of-the-art procedures on stroke patients.

If the patient is rapidly decompensating or you suspect a hemorrhagic stroke, then consider transporting the patient to a facility that can perform neurosurgery. Again, call ahead to alert the hospital of the need for rapid evaluation.

Transient Ischemic Attacks

Pathophysiology

Transient ischemic attacks (TIAs) are episodes of cerebral ischemia that do not inflict any permanent damage. Any of the typical presentations associated with a stroke can occur with TIAs. What makes these events different from a stroke is the resolution of signs and symptoms. According to the AHA/ASA, many TIAs resolve completely within 1 hour—which can mean you are dispatched for stroke, but arrive to find a patient whose symptoms have resolved.[14]

No residual damage to brain tissue occurs with a TIA, and no signs and symptoms appear after the episode ends. However, these mini-strokes are often signs of a serious vascular condition that requires medical evaluation. It is estimated that one-third of patients with TIAs will experience an acute stroke sometime in the future.[15]

Words of Wisdom

Think of the relationship between TIA and stroke as the equivalent of the relationship between angina and MI.

Assessment

Because any of the signs and symptoms of strokes can occur with a TIA, your assessment will be the same.

Management

Patients may experience several TIAs. To manage patients with this condition, follow the stroke management guidelines discussed earlier. Close neurologic assessment is needed. Strongly encourage the patient to be transported, even if symptoms have resolved. If the patient refuses transportation, then appeal to the patient's family for assistance. If the patient still refuses, then encourage seeking medical care soon. It is important to reinforce with the patient that this TIA was a warning sign of a serious

YOU are the Paramedic

PART 3

The patient is calm, but you have to make multiple requests before he complies. When you ask him if he has a headache, he shakes his head "no." He also denies chest pain, shortness of breath, and abdominal pain. After many yes-or-no questions, you determine that he awoke about 2 hours ago. He has been unable to speak since that time. The patient's wife gave him 325 mg of aspirin before your arrival. His wife states that he had an episode of left-side weakness about a year ago. The cause was unclear, but his physician did not think he had experienced a stroke.

Recording Time: 5 Minutes	
Respirations	16 breaths/min, calm
Pulse	112 beats/min, regular
Skin	Warm, normal color, dry
Blood pressure	142/96 mm Hg
Oxygen saturation (Spo_2)	98% on room air
Pupils	Pupils Equal, Round, Reactive to Light and Accommodation (PERRLA)
Blood glucose level	164 mg/dL

6. Which portion of the neurologic assessment is inconsistent with the remainder of the exam?

7. If this patient is having a stroke, then how will the aspirin affect him?

and potentially deadly problem with the blood vessels within the brain. Hypertension is the number one preventable cause of strokes and TIAs. Encourage the patient to talk with a physician about BP control and to take antihypertensive medications as prescribed.

Coma

Pathophysiology

Paramedics are often called for an unresponsive person. One way to remember the most common causes of a decreased LOC is to use the mnemonic AEIOUTIPS **TABLE 19-12**. This memory aid will help you focus on general groups of causes. Note that each grouping has a different onset of signs and symptoms.

As with most medical complaints, the history of present illness is vital in determining the underlying cause of the patient's complaints. It would be unusual for a person to be healthy one minute and unresponsive the next because of an infection. A seizure, however, is an example of a condition that can cause unresponsiveness almost instantly.

TABLE 19-12 AEIOUTIPS: Altered Mental Status Causes

Letter	Name	Onset	Signs and Symptoms	Treatment Focus
A	Alcohol	Acute (hours) Chronic (days)	Intoxication; slurred speech; ataxia; odor of alcohol on breath; tremors; hallucinations	Ensure oxygen, glucose, and temperature for proper brain functioning. Consider thiamine with dextrose.
	Acidosis	Acute (hours)	Multiple causes; tachypnea and hyperpnea are common	Ventilation Sodium bicarbonate
E	Epilepsy (seizure)	Sudden (seconds)	Aura; hypertonic, tonic-clonic activity; postictal state	If prolonged, then diazepam (Valium) or lorazepam (Ativan)
	Endocrine	Chronic (days to weeks)	For thyroid conditions, increased metabolism (hyperthermia, hypertension, tachypnea, tachycardia) OR decreased metabolism (hypothermia, bradycardia, bradypnea, and hypotension)	Supportive care. See Chapter 24, *Endocrine Emergencies*, for more information.
	Electrolytes	Acute (hours) Chronic (days)	Dehydration; renal failure; liver failure; ECG changes, etc	Ensure adequate circulating volume; monitor ECG.
I	Insulin	Acute (hours)	Diaphoresis; tachycardia; tremors; ataxia	Dextrose or glucagon
O	Opiates	Acute (minutes to hours)	Constricted pupils; decreased LOC; bradypnea; cyanosis	Naloxone (Narcan); be prepared to administer additional doses as needed.
	Other drugs	Acute to gradual (hours to days, depending on agent)	Varies depending on agent involved; track marks; drug paraphernalia	Administration of selected drugs; consider naloxone (Narcan).
U	**Uremia** (kidney failure)	Gradual (days to weeks)	Nausea/vomiting; uremic frost; muscle cramping; dysrhythmias; pulmonary edema	Ensure oxygen, glucose, and temperature for proper brain functioning.

Letter	Name	Onset	Signs and Symptoms	Treatment Focus
T	Trauma	Sudden (seconds)	Generally, hypotension causes altered level of consciousness or direct head injury	Consider manual in-line stabilization; ensure adequate BP.
	Temperature	Acute to gradual (hours to days, depending on mechanism)	Hyperthermia (exertional, environmental, or endocrine); hypothermia (environmental, endocrine, situational [eg, immobile person lying on the floor for days])	Stop cooling or heating process—get patient inside, take off wet clothing, get off cold floor. Assess for trauma and other medical conditions. See Chapter 24, *Endocrine Emergencies*, and Chapter 39, *Environmental Emergencies*, for more information.
I	Infection	Gradual (hours to days)	Fever; rash; malaise; tachycardia; tachypnea; skin may be cold or warm depending on the degree of infection	Ensure adequate BP.
P	Poisoning	Acute to gradual (hours to days, depending on agent)	Varies depending on agent involved; empty pill bottles; chemical odors within a child's mouth; broken leaves of plants, open containers of pesticide	Supportive care based on the suspected agent involved. See Chapter 28, *Toxicology*, for more information.
	Psychogenic causes	Sudden (seconds) History of mental illness or substance abuse is typical	Delusions; hallucinations; disorganization; bizarre behavior or posture	Ensure oxygen, glucose, and temperature for proper brain functioning; restraints and sedation may be needed.
S	Shock	Acute to gradual (hours to days, depending on mechanism)	Decreased BP and other signs of poor perfusion	Ensure adequate circulating volume; administer vasopressors if needed.
	Stroke	Sudden (seconds to hours)	Facial droop; slurred speech; ataxia; abnormal/irregular respiratory pattern; potential bradycardia	Ensure oxygen, glucose, and temperature for proper brain functioning.
	Syncope	Acute onset	Prodrome of weakness or loss of peripheral vision, then loss of consciousness that resolves quickly	Ensure adequate circulating volume, oxygenation. Assess cardiac rhythm. Check for trauma that may have occurred during fall.
	Space-occupying lesion	Gradual, subtle changes	Headache; new-onset seizures; strokelike symptoms	Treat for stroke/seizure.
	Subarachnoid hemorrhage	Acute (minutes to hours)	Thunderclap headache; worst headache of life; signs and symptoms of stroke; seizures	Treat for stroke/seizure.

Abbreviations: BP, blood pressure; ECG, electrocardiogram; LOC, level of consciousness

Assessment

Determine when the patient was last seen functioning normally. Evaluate the speed of onset of the patient's altered LOC. Again, identifying the onset will help to distinguish one cause from another.

Common signs and symptoms of diminished LOC and imminent coma include the following:

- **Cognitive effects.** Decreasing LOC, confusion, hallucinations, delusions, psychosis, difficulty thinking, and sleepiness
- **Speech effects.** Slurred speech, agnosia, apraxia, and aphasia
- **Movement effects.** Ataxia, aphagia, seizures, and posturing
- **General CNS effects.** Total unresponsiveness (coma)

It can be difficult to determine the cause of an altered LOC. However, finding the cause will allow you to effectively treat the patient and focus your care. **FIGURE 19-13** provides an algorithm based on AEIOUTIPS, which may help you to progress to the correct area of your protocol.

Words of Wisdom

Technology such as the Pulsara platform can offer on-scene providers real-time contact with a stroke team using a smartphone. Pulsara includes video capabilities to enable enhanced assessment by the stroke team from a remote location.[16]

Management

The focus of care for patients who are comatose occurs in two stages. First, support vital functions. Following the standard care guideline should allow you to secure and maintain the ABCs effectively. Second, gather information about the possible cause of the altered LOC or coma and rule out what causes you can with the tools you have. Gather past medical history, evaluate medications, look for signs of trauma, and determine the history of the present illness. This information will help you direct your care to the most likely cause. As always, a good assessment is the foundation of excellent patient care.

It is not uncommon to have too little information to determine a cause—but this fact should not

YOU are the Paramedic

PART 4

The patient's condition does not change during transport to the hospital. Because you called ahead to the closest stroke center, a stroke team is awaiting your arrival. You are advised to take the patient directly to the CT scanner. You give your report to the emergency physician while you assist in transferring the patient from your cot onto the CT scanner. You then write your patient care report. As you leave, the emergency physician tells you the CT scan was unremarkable, with no sign of stroke or bleeding. She is beginning to consider nonstroke causes of this patient's muteness and other symptoms. The ED staff will continue to monitor the patient for several hours.

Recording Time:	15 Minutes
Respirations	20 breaths/min
Pulse	116 beats/min, regular
Skin	Warm, normal color, dry
Blood pressure	146/96 mm Hg
Oxygen saturation (Spo_2)	98% on room air
Pupils	PERRLA

8. What are other possible causes of strokelike presentations?

9. Were you correct to treat this patient as if he had experienced a stroke?

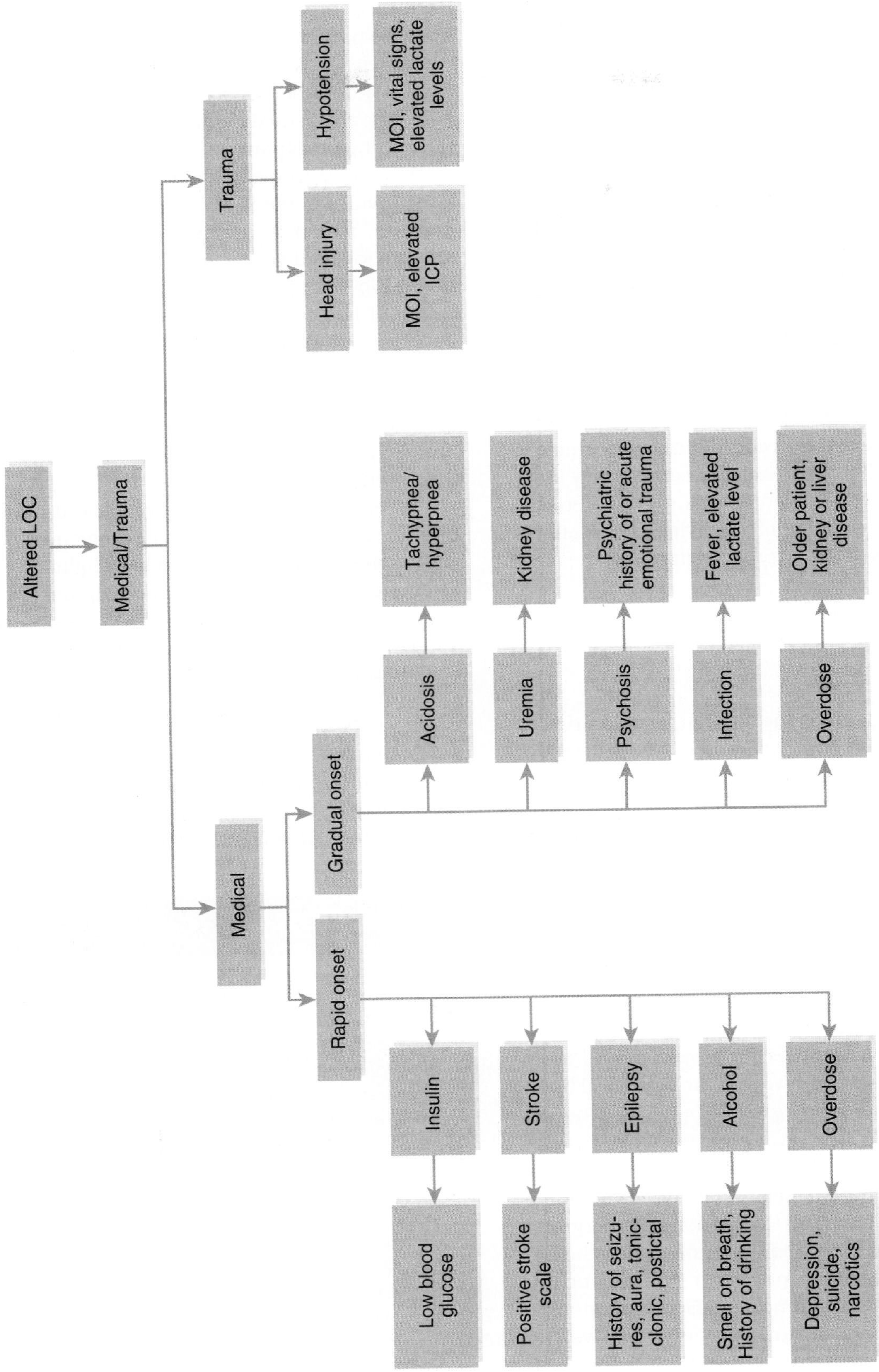

FIGURE 19-13 Altered level of consciousness algorithm.

Abbreviations: ICP, intracranial pressure; MOI, mechanism of injury deter you from looking for one. Is the patient wearing medical identification tags? How was the patient acting before you were called? Do you see drug paraphernalia near the patient? This information can be crucial to providing the continued, quality care this patient will need to return to health. Administer naloxone if you suspect an opioid overdose, as discussed in Chapter 28, *Toxicology*.

Finally, you may not be able to determine the cause of the patient's altered LOC. In such a case, report to the ED staff that you do not know what is wrong with the patient, and then report what is *not* wrong. For example, advise that you have checked the patient's blood glucose level, given naloxone, and gathered a large amount of information, and the patient does not appear to have had a stroke. The cause of the patient's condition may be unclear, but you can still provide excellent emergency medical care while you diligently attempt to determine the cause. The practice of medicine is sometimes more a process of ruling out conditions than ruling them in.

Seizures

Pathophysiology

Recall that a seizure is the sudden, erratic firing of neurons. Patients can experience a wide array of signs and symptoms when having seizures, such as muscle spasms, increased secretions, diaphoresis, and cyanosis. A seizure can be limited to the shaking of one hand or a metallic taste in the mouth, or it can involve the movement of every limb or the complete loss of consciousness. Patients may be aware of the seizure or they may wake up afterward not knowing what happened. Each of these experiences is defined as a seizure if it is brought on by the random firing of neurons.

If a seizure continues for a long period, then profound changes occur within the brain and body. Cerebral glucose and oxygen supplies can be depleted. Systemic (body-wide) hypoxia, hypercapnia, BP changes, and hyperthermia can occur. A single, short-duration seizure is typically not a life-threatening concern. However, if seizures group together and/or last for long periods, then the patient may experience long-term effects, including death. It is also common for EMS personnel to be dispatched on a seizure call, only to arrive and find the patient in cardiac arrest. What happened? The patient experienced a lethal dysrhythmia, BP decreased, blood flow to the brain decreased, and then the patient seized.

As with most medical patients, try to determine the cause of the problem—in this case, the seizure. Ask about medication compliance. Phenytoin (Dilantin), lorazepam (Ativan), carbamazepine (Tegretol), and valproic acid (Depakene) are common anticonvulsant medications. For various reasons, however, patients may have taken an insufficient amount of medication to prevent seizures. Some may stop taking their medication because they have not had a seizure in several months and believe they are cured. Patients who drink alcohol while on anticonvulsants are at an increased risk of having a drug interaction resulting in seizures. Children can outgrow their anticonvulsant medication dosage, and older adults may be unable to afford their medication.

Fever is a common cause of seizure in infants (febrile seizure). Seizure may also occur in people with diabetes who have a low blood glucose level. Knowing the cause of the seizure will help you direct management. Some common causes of seizure are listed in **TABLE 19-13**. Febrile seizures are covered in Chapter 44, *Pediatric Emergencies*.

Seizures are broadly classified based on three features: (1) where seizures begin in the brain, (2) the patient's level of awareness during a seizure, and (3) motor symptoms and other features associated with the seizure. The Epilepsy Foundation uses the term *awareness* instead of *consciousness*

TABLE 19-13 Common Causes of Seizures

- **Abscess**
- Alcohol
- Alcohol withdrawal (delirium tremens)
- Birth anomaly
- Brain infections (meningitis, encephalitis)
- Brain trauma
- Diabetes mellitus
- Fever (rapid rate of rise)
- Hypertension during pregnancy (eclampsia)
- **Idiopathic** (of no known cause)
- Inappropriate medication dosage
- Organic brain syndromes
- Recreational drug use (cocaine)
- Stroke or transient ischemic attack (TIA)
- Systemic infection
- Tumor
- Uremia (kidney failure)

when classifying seizures because it is simpler to evaluate.[17]

Generalized Seizures

Recall that generalized seizures affect awareness in some way and involve both sides of the brain at their onset. In contrast, focal seizures (formerly called partial seizures) begin on one side of the brain; awareness may remain intact or may be impaired. Two types of generalized seizures include tonic-clonic (generalized motor) and absence (generalized nonmotor) seizures.

Tonic-Clonic (Motor) Seizures. Tonic-clonic seizures, formerly called grand mal seizures, present you with the greatest assessment challenges. This type of seizure follows a specific pattern. Most tonic-clonic seizures proceed through each of the following steps in sequence (although some patients may not experience every step):

1. Loss of consciousness
2. Tonic phase: Systemic rigidity
3. Hypertonic phase: Arched back and rigidity
4. Clonic phase: Intermittent contractions of major muscle groups: arms, legs, and head movement; lip smacking, biting, clenching teeth. Contractions are chaotic, disorganized, and of small amplitude. Imagine ventricular fibrillation of the brain—that is what a seizure is electrically.
5. Postseizure: Major muscles relax, and **nystagmus** (an involuntary, rhythmic eye movement) may still be occurring. Eyes may be looking posterior (at the back of the head).
6. **Postictal** phase: Reset period of the brain. It can take several minutes to hours before the patient gradually returns to a preseizure LOC. During this time, the patient may display the following signs:
   - Initially aphasic (unable to speak)
   - Confused or unable to follow commands
   - Emotional
   - Tired
   - Headache
   - Gradual return of normal brain function

Tonic-clonic seizures are unsettling for both family and health care providers to watch. Breathing may be erratic and loud during a seizure. Alternatively, the patient may stop breathing and become cyanotic. These periods of apnea are usually short lived and do not require intervention. If the patient is apneic for more than 30 seconds, then immediately begin ventilatory assistance. Another distressing aspect of seizures, particularly for the patient, is incontinence.

Absence (Nonmotor) Seizures. In contrast to tonic-clonic seizures, nonmotor seizures (formerly called generalized absence or petit mal seizures) present with brief changes in awareness and little or no movement. The typical patient with a generalized nonmotor seizure is a child. Classically, the child will simply stop—stop walking, stop speaking mid-sentence, or stop playing and freeze with a toy in the hand. The child rarely falls. Generalized nonmotor seizures usually last no more than several seconds, with no postictal period and no confusion. Flashing lights or hyperventilation may bring on this type of seizure.

Focal Seizures

Focal seizures affect an area on one side of the brain. If a focal seizure progresses and subsequently involves both sides of the brain, it is considered a generalized seizure. With a focal aware seizure (formerly called simple partial seizure), the patient may be unable to talk or respond during the event, but their awareness remains intact. If the patient's awareness is affected or impaired at any time during a focal seizure, it is termed a *focal impaired-awareness seizure* (formerly called complex partial seizure). The terms *focal motor* and *focal nonmotor* are used to describe the behaviors associated with a focal seizure.

Because the patient experiencing a focal aware seizure is alert and can interact with you, you may be unable to tell they are having a seizure and need to rely on the patient to relay their symptoms to you. Some patients may experience a single seizure, whereas others may experience several seizures in a row. Seizures typically last less than 2 minutes. Signs and symptoms depend on where the nerve cell disruption occurs in the brain. Some patients experience motor symptoms such as involuntary jerking of the face, an arm, or a leg. Others experience sensory symptoms such as tingling, a funny taste, or the perception of seeing lights or hearing a high-pitched noise.

Focal impaired awareness seizures involve a change in awareness at some point during the seizure. The degree of loss varies, and most patients experience a postictal period afterward. Most seizures of this type last less than 2 minutes. Signs and symptoms depend on the brain area involved, and the patient may or may not experience automatisms, which are repetitive, involuntary muscle movements (eg, licking the lips, lip smacking, rubbing the hands). If the temporal lobe is affected, behaviors may include snapping the fingers, repeating phrases, or walking in circles. Gesturing, cycling, kicking movements, or a loud cry or scream may be noted if the frontal lobe is involved. Involvement of the parietal or occipital lobes is less common but can affect the patient's senses.

TABLE 19-14 summarizes the classification of seizures.

Pseudoseizures

Pseudoseizures are also called psychogenic nonepileptic seizures. Symptomatically, you may not notice any difference between these episodes and a tonic-clonic seizure. Tonic-clonic motion, loss of consciousness, and a postictal phase are all present during these events. The difference is that in pseudoseizures, the root cause is of psychiatric origin. It is important to understand that in most cases of pseudoseizure, the patient is not intentionally causing this behavior.

Patients with pseudoseizures present with loss of consciousness, which is usually triggered by some emotional event, stress, lights, or pain. Pseudoseizures conspicuously occur with witnesses, a fact that may lead health care providers to believe pseudoseizures are contrived. Motion that occurs during the seizure is relatively organized: side-to-side movement of the head, pedaling movements of the legs (like riding a bicycle), weeping, or stuttering. These patients often have a psychiatric history and/or other medical history, such as fibromyalgia, chronic pain, or chronic fatigue. Rarely does a pseudoseizure patient become incontinent.

Words of Wisdom

Tonic-clonic seizures are very difficult to mimic or fake. If you care for a patient who is demonstrating coordinated seizure activity, then suspect a pseudoseizure. The patient may also be faking the seizure. Report your findings to the ED before administering any benzodiazepines.

Assessment

Whether they are generalized or focal, most seizures are self-limiting. Thus, all you need to do is monitor and protect patients from injuring themselves. Other important characteristics of your assessment of a patient with a seizure are listed here:

- How long did the seizure last? What did it look like to bystanders or family?
- Describe the seizure as best as possible (unique body motions, regions of the body involved, body positions, etc).
- Does the patient have a history of seizures?
    - How many seizures does the patient usually have in a day or week? How long do they last? What do they look like?
    - Is the patient taking antiseizure medication as prescribed?

TABLE 19-14 Classification of Seizures

Onset	Awareness	Other Features
Generalized	All affect awareness in some way	Motor (tonic-clonic, other motor) Nonmotor
Focal	Aware (simple partial) Impaired awareness (complex partial) Awareness unknown	Motor Nonmotor
Unknown	May be unknown	Motor Nonmotor Unable to classify

 - Have any recent changes to medications occurred?
 - Did bystanders administer any medications?
 - Does the patient have a vagus nerve stimulator (VNS)? If yes, does the patient an activation magnet?
- Does the patient have a recent history of head trauma, overdose, pregnancy, diabetes, hypoglycemia, or heat exposure? Even if there is no history of diabetes, check the blood glucose level on all seizure patients.
- Does the patient have a fever?
- Was the patient apneic, cyanotic, and/or vomiting?
- Did the patient experience bowel or bladder incontinence?

Together with your thorough assessment, the answers to these questions will help the ED staff determine the cause of the seizure.

Management

To manage a seizure, begin with the standard care guideline for the neurologic patient. Quickly determine whether trauma is a concern. Where was the patient before the seizure? What was the patient doing before the seizure? How did the patient get to the current position? If trauma is unclear or confirmed, then perform manual in-line stabilization.

If you arrive while the seizure is still happening, then do not restrain the patient or try to stop the seizing movement. Remain calm and prevent the patient from striking objects and becoming injured. Do not place anything in the patient's mouth while the patient is seizing. If bystanders have placed an object in the patient's mouth (eg, a spoon or a butter knife inserted sideways), then remove it. If you believe the event is a pseudoseizure, then treat it like any other seizure; do not dismiss this behavior as a patient acting out. Correct hypoglycemia by giving IV glucose as needed. Otherwise, most seizures are self-limiting. You may need to provide ventilatory assistance if the patient's seizure or apnea is prolonged, but it is difficult to ventilate a patient who is actively having a seizure. It is next to impossible to perform oral or nasotracheal intubation during a seizure (see the discussion of status epilepticus).

After the seizure, provide emotional support. Ensure privacy for the patient and speak calmly and slowly. Be prepared to repeat yourself. Reorient the patient to place and time. If the seizure was febrile, then encourage the patient or parents or caregivers to administer fever reduction medications (eg, acetaminophen or ibuprofen). Consult your protocols for the appropriate administration of over-the-counter medications to patients.

Unless a clear and easily reversible cause for the seizure is found, transport all patients. Seizures can be a warning sign of more serious nervous system conditions such as stroke, brain tumor, or severe metabolic imbalance. If there is a known history of seizures, then the patient may not wish to go to the hospital. In such a case, advise the patient to follow up with a physician within 24 hours. The patient with diabetes who is awakened after administration of glucose may also not wish to be transported. Advise this patient to eat a good meal and follow up with a physician.

It may be challenging to differentiate a seizure from a stroke. When making this determination, consider your assessment findings and the past medical history. Patients with a history of seizures can have similar seizure patterns over time. Family can therefore anticipate what will happen. When a patient has a seizure caused by a stroke, however, it is unlikely that the pattern will be the same as that of the patient's baseline seizure. That difference can be a clue. Talk to the patient's family members and friends and determine whether the current seizure is the same as a typical seizure. **TABLE 19-15** provides additional guidelines for differentiating between a seizure and a stroke.

If you are concerned that a patient may have a seizure during transport, then establish vascular access so you are prepared to administer diazepam (Valium), lorazepam (Ativan), or midazolam (Versed)—the drugs of choice to stop seizures.

Words of Wisdom

When questioning patients after a seizure, discuss with them whether they experienced an aura before the seizure event. If the answer is yes, tell them that if they recognize the aura recurring during transport to advise you immediately so you can prepare for seizure activity.

TABLE 19-15 Differentiating Stroke From Seizure

Characteristic	Stroke	Seizure
Prodromal signs and symptoms	May have a headache	May have an odd taste in the mouth Seeing lights or hearing sounds Twitching
Activity during event	Muscle weakness that is often lateralized (one side)	Generalized body movement that typically stops within 12 minutes
Response after event	May completely resolve (eg, TIA) May have no change in muscle weakness May progress to worsening symptoms	Slow return of orientation

Abbreviation: TIA, transient ischemic attack

Place blankets over the rails of the ambulance cot and over any hard surfaces near the patient. Ensure the patient's cot straps are not too tight.

Status Epilepticus

Pathophysiology

Status epilepticus can be defined as a seizure that lasts longer than 4 to 5 minutes or consecutive seizures without a return to consciousness between seizures (no lucid interval). This time frame is arbitrary, however, and some authors suggest status epilepticus does not occur until after 30 minutes of uninterrupted seizure activity. Refer to your local protocols for guidelines related to how long a seizure can continue before you should intervene. Status epilepticus is a life-threatening neurologic disorder and should not be taken lightly.

During a seizure, neurons are in a hypermetabolic state (using large amounts of glucose and producing lactic acid). For a short period, this state does not produce long-term damage. If the seizure continues, then the body becomes unable to remove the waste products effectively or to ensure adequate glucose supplies. Status epilepticus can result in neurons being damaged or killed. The goal of prehospital care is to stop the seizure and to manage the ABCs.

Assessment

Assessment of the patient with status epilepticus is the same as that of the patient experiencing a seizure. The only difference is the length of time that the seizure lasts. In patients with status epilepticus, it is vital to ask bystanders or family if any antiseizure medication was administered before you arrived. Patients with epilepsy may have implanted IV access ports to allow for the administration of benzodiazepines. They may also have implanted devices such as a VNS to help control the nervous system's neurologic misfiring. You may need to adjust your dose of antiseizure medication based on the recent dose or doses given by the family.

Management

Follow the standard care guideline for the neurologic patient. Ensure the patient does not have hypoglycemia and administer a benzodiazepine. These medications may be administered via several routes depending on the drug. Generally speaking, if two doses of a benzodiazepine have not stopped the seizure, then contact medical control. This guideline applies to all doses, whether they were administered by family or EMS providers.

If you administer a benzodiazepine, be prepared to control the airway and ventilation completely because this medication can cause respiratory depression or arrest. Continue to use airway positioning and bag-mask ventilations until the medication has stopped the seizure. If the seizure cannot be quickly controlled by benzodiazepines and the patient cannot be ventilated, then administration of sedative/paralytics may be needed to allow for adequate airway management. Refer to your local protocols.

A subset of patients with tonic-clonic seizures will need a different medication. Specifically, pregnant patients experiencing eclampsia need to be managed with magnesium. More information about eclampsia and its treatment can be found in Chapter 42, *Obstetrics*.

Syncope

Pathophysiology

Syncope (fainting) is a sudden and temporary loss of consciousness with accompanying loss of postural tone. It can be a sign of life-threatening cardiac dysrhythmia, stroke, or other serious medical condition. Syncope accounts for 1% to 3% of all ED visits.[18] The brain uses glucose at an astounding rate and cannot store glucose, so even a 3- to 5-second interruption in blood flow can cause loss of consciousness. This interruption in blood flow is the typical underlying reason for syncope. The question is, what caused the sudden decrease in cerebral perfusion? **TABLE 19-16** lists the common causes of syncope.

TABLE 19-16 Common Causes of Syncope

General Cause	Specific Cause
Cardiac rhythm disturbances	Bradycardia of any type Sick sinus syndrome Supraventricular tachycardia Pacemaker malfunction Torsades de pointes Ventricular tachycardia (VT)
Other cardiac causes	Cardiomyopathy Myocardial infarction (MI) Cardiac medications (beta blockers, alpha blockers, nitrates, digitalis, diuretics) Cardiac valvular insufficiency
Noncardiac causes	Dehydration Hypoglycemia Vasovagal response Pulmonary embolism Situational (during urination, swallowing, or coughing) Other medications (alcohol, cocaine, opioid analgesics, tricyclic antidepressants)

Assessment

Classically, the patient with syncope is in a standing position when the event occurs. In younger adults, the pattern is usually one of vasovagal syncope. The adult experiences fear, emotional stress, or pain. The person then suddenly experiences a spinning sensation and passes out (which is why you should ensure a patient is seated before drawing blood or starting an IV line). In older adults, the more typical cause of syncope is a cardiac dysrhythmia. The patient experiences sudden VT, the BP drops, and the patient falls to the floor. The rhythm terminates, BP rises, and the patient feels fine.

Special Populations

Many older adults experience syncopal episodes while having a bowel movement due to straining and an already low heart rate. Vagus nerve stimulation leads to slowing of the heart rate and vasodilation.

Patients with syncope usually experience a **prodrome**. Prodromes are the signs or symptoms that precede a disease or condition. For syncope, the prodromal signs and symptoms include feelings of dizziness, weakness, shortness of breath, chest pain, a headache, or vision going black. Incontinence is possible with syncope. Gathering information about the situation can also help ED staff to diagnose the cause of syncope. Was the patient hot? Standing for an extended period? Performing a strenuous activity? Did the patient need to bear down while lifting something heavy? Was alcohol involved? The history of present illness is often invaluable when managing the patient with syncope.

Seizures and syncope can be difficult to differentiate if they are not witnessed. **TABLE 19-17** offers some guidance.

Management

The first step in managing syncope is to determine whether trauma might have occurred during the patient's fall and whether spinal stabilization is needed. Next, focus on BP and cardiac causes. Continuous ECG monitoring and 12-lead ECG evaluation are essential. Evaluate the blood glucose level

TABLE 19-17 Differentiating Syncope From Seizure

Characteristic	Syncope	Seizure
Position of patient before event	Standing	Any position
Prodromal signs and symptoms	Dizziness, visual changes, shortness of breath, weakness	Odd taste in the mouth Seeing lights or hearing sounds (hallucinations) Twitching
Activity during event	Relaxed	Generalized body movement
Response after event	Quick return of orientation	Slow return of orientation

and oxygen saturation level, and obtain orthostatic vital signs. If the patient's BP remains low, then provide fluids or vasopressors as appropriate, based on the cause of the hypotension. Provide emotional support—syncope can be embarrassing. Because you will not know the exact cause of the syncope, it is important to transport any patient with syncope to the hospital.

Headache

Everyone has had a headache at one time or another. But exactly what is hurting with this condition? The brain and skull do not have pain receptors. Headaches originate from the nerves within the scalp, face, blood vessels, and muscles of the neck and head. The most common types of headaches are discussed in this section. Other types of headaches, although rare, are caused by a tumor, inflammation of the temporal artery, stroke, CNS infection, or hypertension. Patients' presentation will vary depending on the underlying cause.

Pathophysiology and Assessment of Muscle Tension Headaches

Muscle tension headaches may be caused by stress, altered cortisol levels, and/or depression, which causes residual muscle contractions (tension) within the face and head. The majority of headaches are this type. The pain tends to be perceived on both sides of the head, traveling from back to front, and can be characterized as a dull ache or a squeezing pain. The jaw, neck, or shoulders may also be stiff or sore.

Pathophysiology and Assessment of Migraine Headaches

A migraine headache is a complex condition thought to be caused by minor instability within certain clusters of neurons as well as changes in the size of blood vessels at the base of the brain. The patient may report seeing an aura. The pain tends to be unilateral and focused, becoming more diffuse as the migraine headache progresses. The patient often describes throbbing, pounding, pulsating pain, and may have nausea and vomiting. The patient may prefer to remain in a dark (photophobia) and quiet environment. A migraine headache can last several days.

Pathophysiology and Assessment of Cluster Headaches

A cluster headache is a rare type of vascular headache that begins in the face as a minor pain around one eye. The pain—described as sharp and excruciating, or as if someone is pushing the eyeball out—quickly intensifies and spreads to one side of the face. These headaches occur in groups, or clusters, and last 30 to 45 minutes each. However, a person may have several cluster headaches per day. The headaches can recur for days and then stop entirely. They may return at the same time the following month or the same time the next day. It is unclear what triggers these headaches, but serotonin and histamine may play a role. The headaches are often accompanied by anxiety.

Pathophysiology and Assessment of Sinus Headaches

Sinus headaches are caused by inflammation or infection within the sinus cavities of the face. The pain is located in the superior portions of the face and increases when the patient bends over. Sinus headache pain is often worst on waking. This kind of headache may be accompanied by postnasal drip, a sore throat, and nasal discharge.

Management

When you care for a patient with a headache, be cautious because headaches can indicate a more serious condition. If other signs indicate that a stroke may be in progress, then treat the patient for stroke. Remember, a patient who reports the worst headache ever may be having a stroke.

Ask what medications the patient has taken, such as ibuprofen, acetaminophen, and aspirin. Determine how much the patient took and when the last dose or doses were taken.

Administer medications for pain management according to your local protocol. Most patients do not require narcotics. Also consider promethazine (Phenergan) or ondansetron (Zofran) for nausea and vomiting.

Dementia

Pathophysiology

Dementia is the chronic deterioration of memory, personality, language skills, perception, reasoning, or judgment, with no loss of consciousness. These changes can occur over weeks to years and can be subtle. The reasons for these neurologic changes can vary dramatically.

For example, Wernicke encephalopathy presents with dementia and is caused by a vitamin B_1 deficiency. This condition occurs in patients who are chronically malnourished. The classic presentation is a patient with chronic alcoholism who ingests a diet primarily consisting of simple sugars. Without vitamin B_1, brain neurochemistry will not work correctly.

In contrast to Wernicke encephalopathy, **Alzheimer disease**—the most common form of dementia—is a progressive, organic condition in which neurons die. When the affected brain tissue is examined under a microscope, it appears to be riddled with tangles and clumps of damaged tissue.

Do not confuse dementia with delirium. Delirium is a sudden state of confusion or disorientation. By definition, delirium is reversible, whereas many dementias are irreversible. If you have ever been to a bar and seen someone drunk, then you have witnessed delirium.

Assessment

In its initial stages, Alzheimer disease may be dismissed as forgetfulness or so-called old age. However, Alzheimer disease is not a natural part of aging. As the disease progresses, it becomes evident that this is not simple memory loss, as patients cannot remember names, addresses, directions, or how to perform tasks. Patients can become aggressive and violent because the disease damages their judgment centers. Confusion is the hallmark sign of Alzheimer disease. Eventually, the damage involves the ability to swallow. **TABLE 19-18** compares selected types of dementia.

Management

Prehospital management of patients with dementia follows the standard care guideline. Ensure no reversible cause is present. Check the blood glucose level and the oxygen level, as changes in these levels can cause confusion. In particular, you need to be compassionate and ready to repeat yourself. Dementia-related conditions can be frustrating for the patient. In the early stages, patients realize that they are not able to think as efficiently as in the past, and may experience depression and withdrawal.

Wernicke encephalopathy bears special mention. In this condition, the confusion and dementia are partially reversible. In patients with a vitamin B_1 deficit, giving glucose can cause confusion or worsen the patient's presentation if thiamine is not present. In some EMS systems, vitamin B_1 (thiamine) is given before the administration of dextrose 50% or glucagon to adults when alcoholism or malnourishment is suspected.

Patients with dementia may have other malnutrition concerns, including hypomagnesemia, hypokalemia, and hyponatremia. It would be prudent

Words of Wisdom

Do not assume that an older patient with a memory issue is suffering from dementia or Alzheimer disease. Your assessment should rule out possible causes that you can correct, such as hypoxia or hypoglycemia.

TABLE 19-18 Comparison of Selected Types of Dementia

Disease	Cause	Presentation	Typical Course of Disease
Alzheimer disease	Multifactorial: Gradual buildup of plaques within the brain, which cause neuronal death. Eventual decrease in brain mass. Process begins 10 to 20 years before signs and symptoms appear.	Chronic, insidious memory loss is the earliest finding. In moderate disease, a decrease in attention, judgment, and language functions occurs (people get lost, cannot balance a checkbook, repeat questions). In severe disease, patients cannot recognize people; eventually they cannot communicate and become bedridden.	3 to 10 years
Pick disease	Unknown. Disease has a genetic aspect. Its roots lie in damage to neurons in the frontal and temporal lobes.	Occurs in people between ages 55 and 65 years, with insidious presentation of socially inappropriate behavior, such as stealing and obsessive behaviors. Patients may be apathetic, depressed, or inappropriately elated. Additionally, rest tremors, difficulty naming common objects (anomia), and incontinence may be present.	6 years
Huntington disease (Huntington chorea)	An adult-onset genetic disorder marked by severe loss of neurons.	Initially fidgetiness, abnormal eye movements, tics, myoclonus, irritability, and loss of interest. As the disease progresses, bradykinesia, difficulty standing, ataxia, slowing of thinking, and memory loss occur.	19 years
Creutzfeldt-Jakob disease	Prions (proteins) clump together with resultant death of neurons.	Myoclonic jerking, major cognitive deterioration, visual impairment, unstable gait (ataxia). Disease is always fatal.	8 months
Wernicke encephalopathy	Thiamine (vitamin B_1) deficiency. Occurs in patients with longstanding malnutrition, such as those with chronic alcoholism.	Ataxia, confusion, agitation, memory loss, nystagmus, generalized weakness, foot drop, and peripheral neuropathy	Variable, depending on cause and extent of malnutrition
AIDS dementia	Infection with HIV and subsequent destruction of nervous system cells.	Blunted affect, impaired memory loss or slowed verbal response, and difficulty concentrating. Progresses to partial paralysis of the lower extremities, mutism, and eventually a vegetative state.	Untreated: 3–6 months Treated: approximately 3 years

Abbreviations: AIDS, acquired immunodeficiency syndrome; HIV, human immunodeficiency virus

Data from: Alzheimer's disease information page. National Institute of Neurological Disorders and Stroke (NINDS) website. https://www.ninds.nih.gov/Disorders/All-Disorders/Alzheimers-Disease-Information-Page. Accessed March 22, 2021; Lakhan SE. Alzheimer disease. Medscape website. http://emedicine.medscape.com/article/1134817-overview. Updated May 9, 2019. Accessed March 22, 2021; Barrett AM. Pick disease. Medscape website. http://emedicine.medscape.com/article/1135504-overview. Updated November 18, 2019. Accessed March 22, 2021; Revilla FJ. Huntington disease. Medscape website. http://emedicine.medscape.com/article/1150165-overview. Updated February 27, 2019. Accessed March 22, 2021; Creutzfeldt-Jakob disease fact sheet. National Institute of Neurological Disorders and Stroke website. http://www.ninds.nih.gov/disorders/cjd/detail_cjd.htm. Updated March 13, 2020. Accessed March 22, 2021; Salen PN. Wernicke encephalopathy. Medscape website. http://emedicine.medscape.com/article/794583-overview. Updated November 20, 2018. Accessed March 22, 2021; and Thomas FP. HIV encephalopathy and AIDS dementia complex. Medscape website. http://emedicine.medscape.com/article/1166894-overview. Updated February 23, 2016. Accessed March 22, 2021.

to perform ECG monitoring and obtain blood chemistries once in the ED.

In many dementias, no definitive treatment exists for the destroyed neurons.

Neoplasms

Pathophysiology

Neoplasm is the medical term for growths within the body that serve no useful purpose and are caused by errors that occur during cellular reproduction. Recall the discussion of neoplasm in Chapter 9, *Pathophysiology*. Within the context of the neurologic system, a neoplasm is a cancer of the brain or spinal cord.

Tumors can be classified according to whether they represent primary or metastatic disease. Primary neoplasms of the neurologic system are cancers that arise within the nervous system. Because mature neurons no longer divide, however, they rarely become cancerous. Primary CNS tumors, then, are usually caused by errors in mitosis within the support structures of the CNS, such as a meningioma.

The process by which cancerous cells move to sites distant from their site of origin is called **metastasis**. Metastatic neoplasms of the neurologic system are tumors that arise elsewhere in the body, travel through the bloodstream or lymphatic system, and take up residence within nervous system tissues. Lung and breast cancers are the types of cancer that most commonly metastasize to the CNS.

Assessment

Headache, nausea and vomiting, seizures, ataxia, change in mental status, and strokelike signs and symptoms are common in patients with brain tumors. The rate and intensity of these signs and symptoms depend on how quickly the cancer is growing and its location. Patients may have months of headaches or suddenly have a seizure without any prior signs or symptoms. Middle-aged to old adults with new-onset seizures should undergo CT or MRI imaging for possible brain tumors.

Patients with spinal tumors will have signs and symptoms related to compression of the spinal cord. Back pain is the most common symptom. Patients may also experience weakness, ataxia, loss of sensation in a limb, incontinence, and deformity along the spine. Other symptoms related to spinal cord compression are discussed in Chapter 35, *Head and Spine Trauma*.

Management

Prehospital management of patients with neoplasms is supportive. Watch for status epilepticus. If needed, administer a benzodiazepine according to your local protocol. These patients can have elevated ICP. All patients with new-onset seizures or chronic headaches that cannot be managed need medical evaluation. If the patient has a spinal tumor, then be prepared to protect the limbs from injury.

Pathophysiology, Assessment, and Management of Demyelinating, Degenerating, and Motor Neuron Disorders

The three neurologic conditions discussed in this section—demyelinating, degenerating, and motor neuron disorders—have similar presentations. Demyelinating conditions occur after damage is done to the myelin sheath surrounding the neuron, preventing smooth signal transmission from neuron to neuron. Degenerating conditions are incurable, and the major characteristics include progressive damage and/or death of neurons. Motor neuron diseases feature the destruction of the motor neuron. They tend to be progressive conditions in which patients experience difficulties with speech, ambulation, and general movement.

Multiple Sclerosis

Pathophysiology

Multiple sclerosis (MS) is an autoimmune condition in which the body attacks the myelin of the brain and spinal cord **FIGURE 19-14**. This process results in demyelination, or destruction of the myelin. The resulting areas of scarring led to the name *multiple sclerosis* (from the Greek word *skleros*, meaning "hard"). The body has the ability to determine

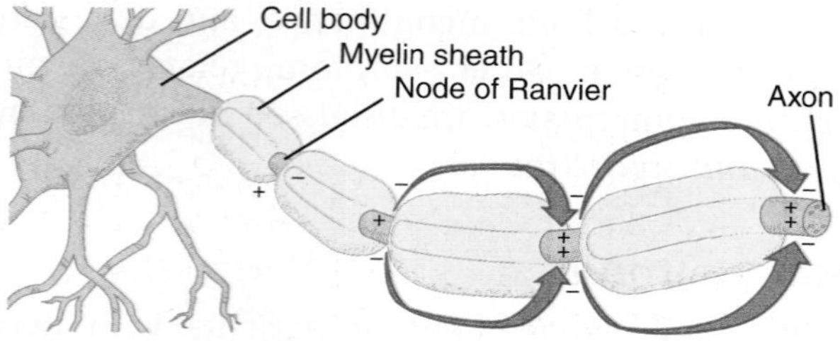

FIGURE 19-14 The myelin sheath insulates the axon, allowing impulses to jump from node to node, which accelerates the rate of signal transmission. In MS and other demyelinating conditions, this protective sheath is destroyed by inflammation, so that signals can no longer be transmitted smoothly.

which proteins are "self" and which are "non-self." In an autoimmune disorder, the body begins to attack its own cells, because the immune system is no longer able to distinguish friend from foe.

Consider the normal neuron. Myelin coats the axons of most nerve cells and allows for smooth transmission of signals to their target cell. In MS, the body believes that the proteins making up this insulation are foreign. The immune system subsequently attacks the myelin, creating gaps in the insulation that lead to characteristic signs and symptoms of MS. It is believed that some unknown environmental trigger, such as a virus, begins to focus the immune system's attention on the myelin. In some areas of the world and the United States, MS is more prevalent; for example, the Pacific Northwest has triple the case count compared to the prevalence in other areas of the United States.[19] While scientists do not know the exact cause of MS or understand its correlation with geographic factors, they believe that environmental factors such as temperature play a role.

Assessment

The presentation of MS follows a pattern of episodes and remissions. In the initial episode, double vision and blurred vision are common symptoms. The patient may have nystagmus.

The episodes can vary in intensity and remissions can vary in length. Patients may experience muscle weakness; impairment of pain, temperature, and touch senses; pain (moderate to severe); ataxia; intention tremors; speech and vision disturbances; vertigo; bladder and bowel dysfunction; sexual dysfunction; depression; euphoria; cognitive abnormalities; and fatigue during episodes **FIGURE 19-15**. They may also experience a strange electric sensation down the spine or extremities when the head is flexed forward (Lhermitte sign). Episodes may be brief, with little pattern to either their frequency or intensity. Subsequent episodes may involve other locations of the body.

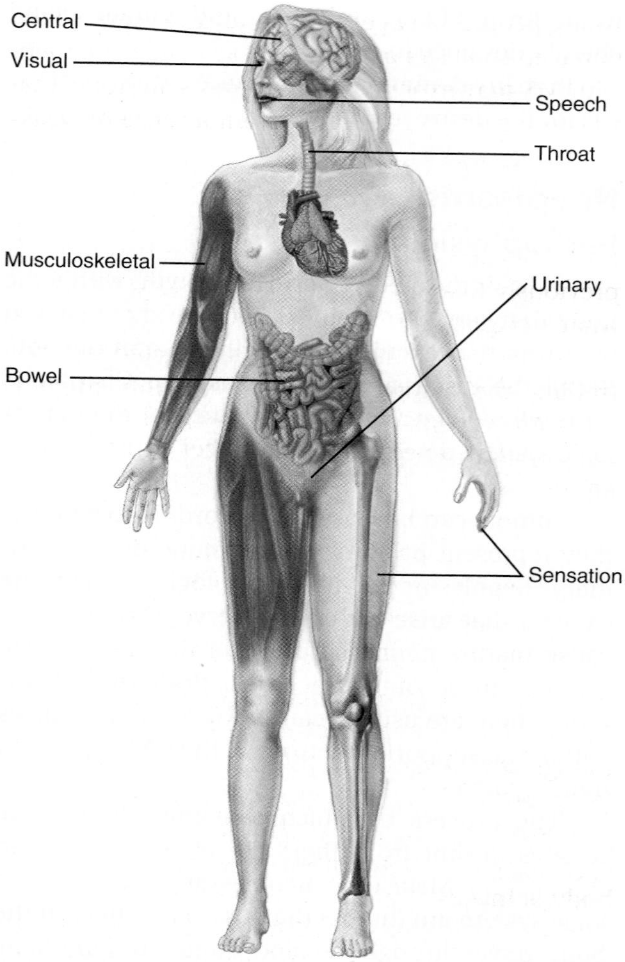

FIGURE 19-15 Areas of the body affected by the signs and symptoms of multiple sclerosis.

Management

Prehospital management of MS is supportive. This condition is typically diagnosed among relatively young people, between ages 20 and 50 years, so the initial episode can be especially alarming. A patient with MS may experience signs and symptoms that progress over several hours, from a sense of weakness to the inability to stand. Be prepared for possible trauma related to a fall. Additionally, the patient may have genuine confusion and anxiety—not because of some brain malfunction, but because this previously healthy person is trying to understand what is happening.

In-hospital management is directed at controlling the symptoms. Administration of anti-inflammatory medications may be used to decrease the length of the attack. Currently, no cure exists for MS.

Guillain-Barré Syndrome

Pathophysiology

Guillain-Barré syndrome is a rare disease in which the immune system attacks portions of the nervous system. The cause of this condition is unclear, although some degree of immune response appears to be present. Patients report having a minor respiratory or gastrointestinal infection before the beginning of the weakness. One theory is that the body is invaded by an infectious agent, which has a protein structure similar to that of myelin. When the body attacks the invading organism, it confuses normal myelin with the invader. Once triggered, the immune system attacks and damages the myelin, resulting in demyelination, which impairs signal transmission along the axon.

The reversal of Guillain-Barré syndrome can be almost as dramatic as its onset. Some patients recover completely without residual weakness in as little as several weeks.[20] Approximately one-third of all patients with this condition will need respiratory support at some point. Of patients who survive Guillain-Barré syndrome, 15% to 20% have permanent motor weakness.[20]

Assessment

Guillain-Barré syndrome is a rare condition that can be frightening for most patients. It begins as weakness and tingling sensations in the legs. This weakness moves up the legs and begins to affect the thorax and arms. The weakness can become severe and may lead to paralysis. The transition from walking and speaking to needing a ventilator to breathe can take as little as several hours. Most patients experience maximum muscle weakness or paralysis within 2 weeks of the disease's onset. In addition to the effects on the peripheral motor neurons, the autoregulatory system can become involved. Patients are susceptible to severe swings in pulse rate and BP.

Management

Prehospital management includes close assessment of the patient's ability to effectively protect the airway and ventilate. Monitor the patient closely with ECG and repeat vital signs. Continuous $ETCO_2$ readings can provide evidence of impending respiratory failure. Be prepared to administer IV fluids to maintain BP and treat hemodynamically significant bradycardia following AHA guidelines. Patients may experience terror as the condition progresses; therefore, use a comforting voice and a therapeutic touch as you care for the patient.

Some patients with Guillain-Barré have residual weakness that can be profound, requiring ventilatory support. Be prepared to manage a transport ventilator and assist with ambulation or other activities in these patients with chronic disease. Note that patients do not experience subsequent attacks, as occurs in MS. In-hospital management includes plasmapheresis (exchanging the plasma within the blood) and immunoglobulin injections. These therapies decrease the patient's recovery time.

Parkinson Disease

Pathophysiology

Parkinson disease is a neurologic condition in which environmental and genetic factors can place patients at risk for damage to certain neurons. A portion of the brain, the substantia nigra, is responsible for the production of dopamine. If this section is damaged or overused, then Parkinson disease can result. In some patients, the damage can be linked to past injuries; in other patients, the damage has no known cause. Dopamine is a neurotransmitter that, among other things, is needed for muscles to contract smoothly.

Assessment

A gradual onset of symptoms over months to years is typical with Parkinson disease. The initial signs are often unilateral tremors. Over time, as the dopamine level falls, more areas of the body are involved. Genetics plays an important role in this disease, but Parkinson-like activity can also be observed in patients with head injuries and some patients who have overdosed.

The classic presentation of Parkinson disease involves four characteristics:

- **Tremor.** Rest tremors and postural tremors are common among patients with Parkinson disease.
- **Postural instability.** Patients have a stiff posture in which they are stooped over, and the disease alters their gait. This stiffness, together with increased response times, makes these patients unsteady when walking and puts them at an increased risk of falling.
- **Rigidity.** Rigidity causes the patient to move in fits and starts.
- **Bradykinesia.** Patients with Parkinson disease have a classic gait presentation. They tend to shuffle in a straight line, with their feet close together. When asked to turn, they take small steps until the turn is complete. This is called **bradykinesia**, the slowing down of routine motions. Bradykinesia may also be demonstrated in slow blinking, a soft voice, or decreased facial expressions.

Other symptoms of Parkinson disease include depression, dementia, difficulty swallowing (aphagia), speech impairment, fatigue, and dystonia. Foot and leg contractions, in which the leg is arched, and adduction of the arm into a posture where the arm is flexed across the chest or abdomen are commonly seen. Prognosis is poor as the condition advances. Patients in later stages are at a much greater risk of death from aspiration, pneumonia, falls, or complications due to immobility.

Management

Prehospital management is supportive. Be aware that these patients may be depressed or even have some degree of dementia. Reorient the patient if needed. A compassionate gesture can be very helpful. If the patient has trauma, then those injuries will need to be managed as well.

Amyotrophic Lateral Sclerosis

Pathophysiology

Amyotrophic lateral sclerosis (ALS), also known as Lou Gehrig disease, is a disease that strikes the voluntary motor neurons. It is unclear what causes the death of the motor neurons, but one theory suggests that the body's immune system selectively attacks and kills them. Some evidence indicates that genetics may play a role. The condition is more common in middle-aged men of any race.

Assessment

Initially, ALS is subtle and progresses without being noticed. Fatigue, general weakness of muscle groups, fasciculations (muscle twitching), and difficulty doing routine activities such as eating, writing, and dressing eventually develop. Patients may also experience difficulty speaking. As the condition progresses, a loss of ability to walk, move the arms, eat, and speak occurs. The speed of progression differs for every patient. Because this condition affects only the motor neurons, the patient is completely aware of their surroundings and inability to move.

On average, a person diagnosed with this condition dies within 3 to 5 years. As the destruction of motor neurons continues, patients eventually require ventilatory assistance to breathe effectively. Patients die from respiratory infections or other complications related to immobility.

Management

Prehospital treatment for these patients follows the standard care guideline. Assess the patient's ability to swallow and monitor the airway closely. Patients may rely on various home medical technologies, including feeding pumps, IV pumps, long-term IV access ports, and ventilators. Thus, it can become complicated to transport such patients. Ask for guidance from the family or home health care provider to operate any unfamiliar devices. If necessary, disconnect the patient from the technology after consulting medical control and then transport.

In-hospital care for patients with ALS is geared toward supporting vital functions. Patients undergo physical therapy to help strengthen remaining neurons and muscles. Medications can be given to mitigate some of the symptoms; however, this condition has no cure.

Cranial Nerve Disorders

Pathophysiology

This portion of the chapter discusses relatively rare disorders, some of which can mimic other conditions. A patient with severe facial pain or sudden-onset facial paralysis is not necessarily having a stroke. Not everyone with chest pain is having an MI. Cranial nerve disorders are no different: They may not be as clear-cut as they first appear. The key to understanding these disorders is good assessment and detailed history-taking skills.

All of these conditions involve one or more of the cranial nerves, typically of the facial region. **TABLE 19-19** provides an overview of these disorders.

TABLE 19-19 Cranial Nerve Disorders

Disorder	Cause/Cranial Nerve Involved	Presentation	Treatment
Acoustic neuroma	Neoplasm (tumor) at the base of the brain. As the tumor grows, it can apply pressure to nerves, prevent movement of CSF, or compress blood vessels, causing ischemia. This process takes years because this tumor grows slowly. Affects the vestibulocochlear or facial nerves (cranial nerves VIII and VII, respectively).	Unilateral hearing loss, headache, tinnitus, facial numbness, and balance disorders. Hearing loss may be gradual or intermittent.	Provide supportive care. To prevent falls, ensure you walk with the patient due to balance disorders. Speak clearly and look directly at the patient.
Bell palsy	Minor infection of the facial nerve (cranial nerve VII).	The episode is sudden and can easily be confused with a stroke. Signs and symptoms are eyelid ptosis, facial droop or weakness, excessive salivation, and loss of the ability to taste. Episodes can last up to 2 weeks.	Consider CVA. If the patient is known to have Bell palsy, apply a dressing to the closed eyelid. This step will help to prevent drying of the eye.
Glossopharyngeal neuralgia	Irritation of the glossopharyngeal nerve (cranial nerve IX). Cause of the irritation is unknown.	Episodes of severe, sharp unilateral pain in the tongue, at the back of the throat, in the middle ear, and in the tonsil area. Pain can last from seconds to several minutes, with multiple episodes possible in one day. Swallowing, eating cold food or drinks, sneezing, or coughing can trigger attacks.	Provide supportive care.
Hemifacial spasm	Dilated blood vessels irritate the facial nerve (cranial nerve VII).	Involuntary unilateral facial movements. Tics, myoclonic contractions, jaw distortion, and facial tremors. No pain is associated with this condition.	Provide supportive care.

(continues)

TABLE 19-19 Cranial Nerve Disorders (continued)

Disorder	Cause/Cranial Nerve Involved	Presentation	Treatment
Ménière disease	Cause is unclear but the disease is believed to be related to an increase in fluid pressure within the inner ear. This pressure stimulates the vestibulocochlear nerve (cranial nerve VIII).	Recurrent and spontaneous unilateral tinnitus, dizziness, hearing loss, and a sensation of fullness in the ear. Episodes tend to last 2–4 hours. Repeated attacks can cause permanent deafness.	Provide supportive care. To prevent falls, ensure you walk with the patient due to balance disorders. Speak clearly and look directly at the patient.
Trigeminal neuralgia Also called tic douloureux (tik' doo-loo-roo')	The usual cause is irritation by an artery lying too close to the nerve. Over time, as the artery changes diameter to meet blood supply needs, this motion can grate the myelin sheath off of the nerve. With the insulation partially gone, the nerve can "short out," causing pain without trauma to the area. Involves the trigeminal nerve (cranial nerve V).	Severe, shocklike, or stabbing pain, usually on one side of the face. Episodes typically last several minutes and occur with a frequency of less than one per day to hundreds per day. Pain abates between attacks. Episodes are triggered by touching the face, speaking, brushing teeth, eating, putting on clothing, the wind—essentially any activity in which the face is stimulated.	Minimize touching while assessing the face. If small amounts of oxygen are needed for other reasons, then consider administering via blow-by technique directed at the unaffected side of the face. Masks or nasal cannula may trigger episodes. Episodes are severe but short lived. Opiate therapy is not typically needed.

Abbreviations: CSF, cerebrospinal fluid; CVA, cerebrovascular accident

Data from: Kutz JW Jr. Acoustic neuroma. Medscape website. http://emedicine.medscape.com/article/882876-overview. Updated April 29, 2020. Accessed March 22, 2021; Taylor DC. Bell palsy. Medscape website. http://emedicine.medscape.com/article/1146903-overview. Updated June 14, 2019. Accessed March 22, 2021; Glossopharyngeal neuralgia. MedlinePlus website. https://medlineplus.gov/ency/article/001636.htm. Accessed March 22, 2021; Singh PM, Manpreet K, Trikha A. An uncommonly common: glossopharyngeal neuralgia. *Ann Indian Acad Neurol.* 2013;16(1):1-8. https://www.ncbi.nlm.nih.gov/pmc/articles/PMC3644765/. Accessed March 22, 2021; Gulevich S. Hemifacial spasm. Medscape website. http://emedicine.medscape.com/article/1170722-overview. Updated September 16, 2019. Accessed March 22, 2021; Hemifacial spasm information page. National Institute of Neurological Disorders and Stroke website. https://www.ninds.nih.gov/Disorders/All-Disorders/Hemifacial-Spasm-Information-Page. Updated March 27, 2019. Accessed March 22, 2021; Li JC. Meniere disease (idiopathic endolymphatic hydrops). Medscape website. http://emedicine.medscape.com/article/1159069-overview. Updated May 7, 2020. Accessed March 22, 2021; and Singh MK. Trigeminal neuralgia. Medscape website. http://emedicine.medscape.com/article/1145144-overview. Updated July 11, 2019. Accessed March 22, 2021.

Assessment

Conduct the neurologic assessment described earlier in this chapter. Additionally, test for vertigo, albeit only in patients who are at no risk of cervical spine trauma or other neck disease. To perform this test, have the patient lie supine. Place your hands on either side of the head and move the head rapidly from side to side once. Then return the head to the neutral position. This maneuver causes the liquid within the inner ear to move. Next, look at the patient's eyes. If the patient has vertigo, then you should see nystagmus. Also, the motion of the head will typically increase the patient's sensation of vertigo.

Management

Prehospital management of cranial nerve disorders is mainly supportive. Patients may need promethazine (Phenergan) or ondansetron (Zofran) for

Documentation and Communication

When you consider cranial nerve disorders, it is important to clearly distinguish between vertigo and dizziness. Vertigo, which involves the cranial nerves, is the sensation that you are moving when you are not, like the feeling you had as a child rolling down a hill. It is typically caused by inner ear disease. Vertigo is not the same as dizziness. Dizziness is a sensation of light-headedness typically related to low BP in the brain. So how can you differentiate the two? Talk with the patient. Ask the patient to describe the sensation without using the word "dizzy." Listen carefully to the words the patient chooses. Words and phrases like "spinning," "whirling," and "off balance" point toward vertigo, whereas descriptors such as "fuzzy" and "blackout" suggest dizziness. Good communication with your patient can help you draw accurate conclusions.

the nausea and vomiting that may be present with some cranial nerve disorders. Benzodiazepines may provide some relief from vertigo. In most cases, nonsteroidal anti-inflammatory drugs (NSAIDs) and opiates have limited benefit in managing pain caused by cranial nerve disorders.

Dystonia

Pathophysiology

Dystonias are severe, abnormal muscle spasms that cause bizarre contortions, repetitive motions, or postures. Dystonia can be either a sign (occurring within another condition) or a condition in itself. Consider a patient with a headache: The headache could be a sign of a CVA, or the patient could simply have a headache. Patients with dystonia have normal intelligence, can think clearly, are not experiencing a seizure, and have normal LOC.

Primary dystonias occur for an unknown reason. A defect in the body's ability to process neurotransmitters is thought to be at the core of the problem. In these patients, dystonia would correctly be referred to as a condition. Some patients who take antipsychotic medications may have a sudden onset of bizarre contortions of the face or body. This finding would be a secondary dystonia and would more appropriately be considered a sign rather than a condition.

Spasmodic torticollis **FIGURE 19-16**, in which the neck muscles contract, twisting the head to one side and usually pulling it forward or backward, is a common example of a dystonia. The head then remains painfully frozen in that position. Facial dystonia can take several forms.

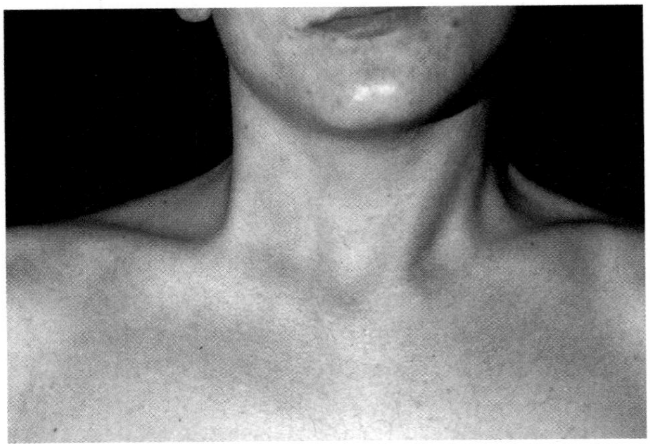

FIGURE 19-16 Example of torticollis or "wry neck" dystonia.

Assessment

Spasms due to dystonia are involuntary and are often painful. **TABLE 19-20** describes a wide variety of dystonias.

Management

Prehospital management of patients with dystonia focuses on ruling out other conditions, such

TABLE 19-20 Types of Dystonias

Type	Presentation
Cervical dystonia (torticollis)	Most common form of focal dystonia; intermittent, patterned, repetitive, spasmodic motion of the head in a twisting, flexing, extending, or tilting manner; can involve more than one motion type
Oculogyric crisis	Deviation of the eyes in any direction, usually with eyes strained toward the top of the head
Oromandibular	Forceful contractions of the face, which can involve the tongue darting in and out of the mouth
Blepharospasm	Eyelid spasms or uncontrollable blinking
Athetosis	Slow, writhing motions commonly involving the face and distal extremities
Upper limb dystonia	Cramping of the hands, elbows, and arms (eg, graphospasm [writer's cramp])
Choreiform movements	Quick, jerky, irregular, and unpredictable movements; often found in the face, arms, and hands
Spasmodic dysphonia	Involuntary contraction of the vocal cords, interrupting speech

as seizures, strokes, and reactions to medications prescribed for psychiatric conditions. If you suspect a dystonic reaction to an antipsychotic medication, then diphenhydramine (Benadryl) is the drug of choice to stop the contraction within 10 to 30 minutes. Dystonias tend to occur within 5 days of either starting a new psychotropic medication or changing the dosage of an existing psychotropic medication. Dystonic reactions secondary to psychiatric medications are not considered to be allergic in nature. Diphenhydramine is effective for this type of dystonia because of its anticholinergic properties.

Words of Wisdom

Regardless of the underlying cause, dystonias are socially upsetting because patients suddenly twist and writhe uncontrollably. It is critical that you provide compassionate care. The adverse effects of some medications can also be the underlying cause of dystonia.

Unfortunately, diphenhydramine is ineffective in primary dystonias. Regardless of the cause, dystonias can be very unnerving and even painful. Thus, pain management may be appropriate. Talk with the patient and state that you are trying to help. Be calm and reassuring. In-hospital management involves a variety of medication options to control the condition.

Central Nervous System Infections and Inflammation

Pathophysiology

To begin the discussion on CNS infections and inflammation, an understanding of some fundamental definitions is necessary. *Encephalitis* is inflammation of the brain. *Meningitis* is the inflammation of the meninges, the outer covering of the central nervous system. Clinically, these conditions are difficult, if not impossible, to distinguish in the prehospital setting. Both conditions can result from various causes, including infectious, chemical, and/or metabolic causes. Infectious pathology is the most common source of both conditions when it presents in the acute phase.

Infectious causes of encephalitis and meningitis may include bacteria, viruses, fungi, or prions gaining access to the body, which then reproduce and cause damage. These organisms have a basic goal—to continue to live. To do so, all organisms need food and must reproduce. As the organism begins to attack the body, it also looks for fuel that will enable it to create the next generation of bacteria, viruses, or other pathogens. The damage that these organisms create occurs due to several mechanisms, which can be characterized as involving either the body's reaction to the infection or the activities of the attacking organisms.

A common sign of infectious disease is the presence of a fever. Many pathogenic organisms prefer to grow within a narrow temperature range, so even a 2° to 3°F (1.2° to 1.8°C) climb in body temperature can slow the reproduction of some viruses or bacteria. This increase in temperature allows the immune system to gain control, providing valuable time for neutrophils (the body's defenses) to find and kill the invading organisms. It also signals the rest of the body that an attack is underway. More white blood cells are produced and chemical mediators are released to improve the body's effectiveness at finding and eliminating the foreign organisms. In this regard, fevers are good.

If the temperature of the body becomes too high, then the brain can be affected. Recall the last time you felt ill and had a fever: The increased temperature made your thinking dull, it was difficult to concentrate, and you may have developed a headache. These effects are common with fevers. Neurons are sensitive to temperature changes. Thus, as the body temperature rises, the effects on the neurons can become more profound. Eventually, a person may hallucinate, become delusional, or lose consciousness. Another possibility is random firing of neurons, leading to a febrile seizure.

Another mechanism by which infectious agents can cause damage to the body is through the destruction of cells. Organisms can produce either **endotoxins** or **exotoxins** that can damage nearby living cells, thereby providing the bacterium with a source of food. Endotoxins are proteins that are released by gram-negative bacteria when they die. *Neisseria meningitidis* is a bacterium that releases endotoxins; it is associated with meningitis.

Clostridium tetani is a bacterium that releases an exotoxin. *C tetani* causes tetanus (lockjaw), in which patients experience muscle contractions, stiff neck, difficulty moving the jaw, and dysphagia. Fortunately, this once-common condition is rare today because of the efforts of public health professionals and widespread immunization.

Assessment

As **TABLE 19-21** shows, encephalitis and meningitis have similar presentations. Both illnesses begin with flulike symptoms. As the pathogenic organism reproduces and causes more damage, a stiff neck, photophobia, lethargy, an altered LOC, and seizures are possible. Kernig sign or Brudzinski sign **FIGURE 19-17** may be elicited in meningitis.

Management

Prehospital management of these conditions is mainly supportive. For patients with suspected meningitis, place a mask over their mouths to limit the spread of organisms. Also wear a mask if the patient is coughing. Be prepared for seizures and treat accordingly. One risk associated with these conditions, particularly for bacterial meningitis, is increased ICP. Another risk is septicemia, which indicates the infection is present within the bloodstream. Septicemia can cause ruptures of capillaries and loss of vasomotor control of blood vessels. See Chapter 27, *Infectious Diseases,* for more information on septicemia.

TABLE 19-21 Comparison of Encephalitis and Meningitis

Condition	Organisms Usually Responsible	Presentation	Timeline
Encephalitis	Herpes simplex virus: Most common sporadic form. Arboviruses: Most common episodic form. These viruses are transmitted by vectors and cause outbreaks of illnesses. Examples include West Nile virus, rabies, and Japanese virus encephalitis.	First signs and symptoms are fever, headache, nausea/vomiting, and general malaise. As the condition progresses, changes in LOC occur, including behavioral and personality changes, nuchal rigidity (stiff neck), photophobia, lethargy, confusion, and seizure.	Several days, depending on the specific virus involved
Bacterial meningitis	Neonates: Group B streptococci and *Escherichia coli*. Infants/children: *Haemophilus influenzae* (more common in children), *Streptococcus pneumoniae*, and *Neisseria meningitidis*. Adults: *S pneumoniae*, *N meningitidis* (more common in young adults), and *Listeria monocytogenes*.	First signs and symptoms are upper respiratory infection (runny nose, cough, malaise). As the condition progresses, the patient may have headache, nuchal rigidity, and fever (the classic triad of symptoms). Chills, photophobia, vomiting, seizures, confusion, Kernig sign, and Brudzinski sign may also occur. Patients can experience life-threatening issues with increased ICP. Infants are irritable when held, and have a high-pitched cry (cat's cry) and bulging fontanelles.	Bacterial pathogen: presentation within 24 hours
Viral meningitis	Non-polio enterovirus is the most common viral type. Examples include echovirus and coxsackievirus.	Signs and symptoms are similar to bacterial meningitis. Viral meningitis does not cause increased ICP.	Viral pathogen: presentation in 1–7 days

Abbreviations: ICP, intracranial pressure; LOC, level of consciousness

Data from: Hasbun R. Meningitis. Medscape website. http://emedicine.medscape.com/article/232915-overview. Updated July 16, 2019. Accessed March 22, 2021; Howes DS. Encephalitis. Medscape website. http://emedicine.medscape.com/article/791896-overview. Updated August 7, 2018. Accessed March 22, 2021; and Bacterial meningitis. Centers for Disease Control and Prevention website. www.cdc.gov/meningitis/bacterial.html. Updated August 6, 2019. Accessed March 22, 2021.

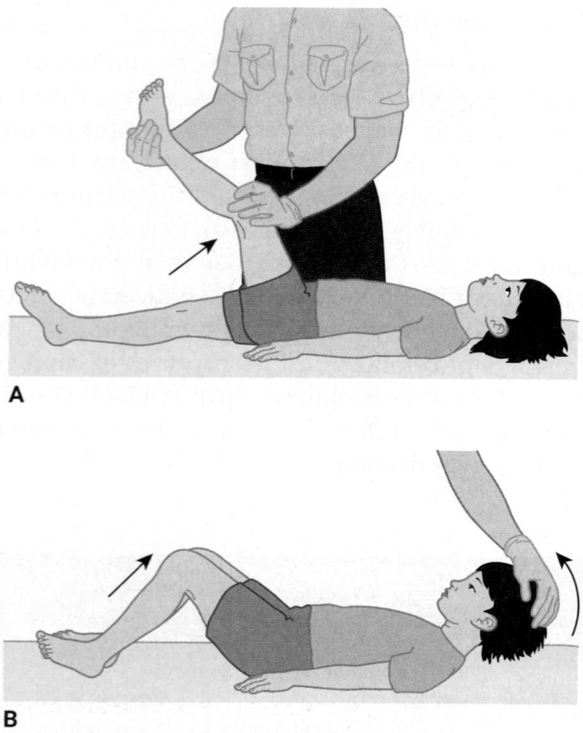

FIGURE 19-17 A. Kernig sign. Meningeal irritation results in pain when attempting to straighten the knee with the hips flexed. **B.** Brudzinski sign. Meningeal irritation results in an involuntary flexion of the knees when the head is flexed toward the chest. These classic signs do not occur frequently.

Encephalitis is not particularly contagious from person to person, but meningitis can be. As a paramedic, your follow-up care may involve preventive antibiotic treatment for possible bacterial meningitis. You (or your supervisor) need to stay in contact with the infection control officer from the hospital to which the patient was transported. In-hospital management is directed at decreasing swelling in the brain and spinal cord, fighting the infection, and supporting the patient's vital signs.

Abscesses

Pathophysiology

Abscesses are caused by an infectious agent within the brain or spinal cord. When an infectious agent attacks brain or spinal cord cells and destroys tissue, the immune system responds by attempting to kill the pathogen. If it cannot, then the body's second line of defense is to erect a "wall" to prevent the pathogen from spreading. This capsule envelops the infectious agent, as well as dead or dying brain or spinal cord cells, dead white blood cells, and white blood cells that are still fighting the infection. Over time, with continued tissue destruction and immune system response, swelling can occur. The result is an abscess.

The underlying reason for an infection within the brain or spinal cord may vary. Such an infection is often preceded by an infection of the sinuses, throat, gums, or ear. The pathogenic organism can also be introduced to the brain through head or spinal cord trauma.

Assessment

The two main consequences of the infection are damage to an area of the brain or spinal cord and the presence of an abscess within the cranial vault or spinal cord. These two factors dictate the presentation of a patient with a CNS abscess. Look for a low- or high-grade fever, persistent headache, drowsiness, confusion, generalized or focal seizures, nausea and vomiting, focal motor or sensory impairments, nuchal rigidity, and hemiparesis.

Management

Follow the standard care guideline. Pay close attention to evidence of increased ICP and take seizure precautions. Evaluate the patient's temperature; if it is high, then remove the patient's clothing, cover the patient with a sheet, and turn off the heat in the patient compartment of the ambulance. These patients may be critically ill and require prompt transport.

In-hospital management involves antibiotics, seizure precautions, and sometimes surgical removal of the abscess.

Poliomyelitis and Postpolio Syndrome

Pathophysiology

Poliomyelitis is a viral infection transmitted by the fecal–oral route. Its incidence peaked in the United States in the 1950s. Since then, an effective vaccine has been developed. No cases of wild polio within the United States have occurred since 1979, but the virus has been brought into the United States by outside travelers.[21] In the United States, people who contract the disease typically have not been immunized.

Assessment

Signs and symptoms for those people who become infected begin in as little as 1 week after exposure. In the most severe cases, they include sore throat, nausea, vomiting, diarrhea, stiff neck, and muscle weakness or paralysis.

Management

In-hospital care for patients with the acute illness is directed at hydration, ventilation, and calorie support until the infection has been managed by the immune system. The way the virus damages the nervous system places patients at risk for problems decades after the initial infection. The virus attacks motor neurons within the brain and brainstem, thereby causing the classic signs of weakness and paralysis. The remaining neurons then begin to send out new axons to try to compensate for this loss—a process that allows the patient to regain function.

Over time, these motor neurons must do more work than they are accustomed to handling, and can begin to break down and die. This process leads to **postpolio syndrome**. Patients who had polio in the early- to mid-20th century may now have difficulty swallowing, weakness, fatigue, or breathing conditions. Typically, the muscle groups affected by the postpolio syndrome are the same as those affected by the original polio infection, but they experience a milder level of weakness.

Prehospital management emphasizes managing possible airway obstruction due to swallowing difficulties. Remember that postpolio syndrome presents in older patients who contracted polio decades ago. Patients within extended care facilities may have this condition listed in their past medical history. Although postpolio syndrome does not specifically modify care for other conditions, it can affect the speed at which a patient decompensates. Consider a patient with congestive heart disease. As the patient struggles with fluid buildup in the alveoli, the patient has difficulty breathing. When coupled with decreased respiratory muscle strength due to postpolio syndrome, this patient may more quickly move into respiratory failure. Thus, you must consider the patient's past medical history and medications when delivering emergency medical care.

Peripheral Neuropathy

Pathophysiology

In **peripheral neuropathy**, the nerves leaving the spinal cord are damaged, so that the signals moving to or from the brain become distorted. The many causes for this group of conditions include trauma, toxins, tumors, autoimmune attacks, and metabolic disorders. Trigeminal neuralgia and Guillain-Barré syndrome are examples. The remainder of this discussion will be limited to the most common form of peripheral neuropathy—diabetic neuropathy.

Assessment

As the blood glucose level rises, damage can occur to the peripheral nerves. The result is misfiring and shorting of signals. Patients may have sensory or motor impairment. Loss of sensation, numbness, burning, pain, paresthesia, and muscle weakness are common. Patients may eventually lose the ability to feel their feet or other areas. This condition is progressive and is accelerated by high blood glucose levels.

Management

Management in the prehospital setting is supportive.

Special Populations

Neurologic conditions with special relevance to pediatric patients include hydrocephalus, spina bifida, and cerebral palsy.[22,23] These diseases are covered in Chapter 44, *Pediatric Emergencies*. You can also find information about patients with neurologic conditions requiring long-term care in Chapter 46, *Patients With Special Challenges*.

YOU are the Paramedic SUMMARY

1. What are your next questions?

It is paramount that you assess scene safety. This patient is physically imposing, but is he a potential safety risk? It is important to understand that his mere presence does not make him a threat. You need to make a more conscientious evaluation of the scene. A scene size-up involves more than simply listing the available risks. It also involves some degree of situational awareness—how likely is a certain risk to become a real threat?

In this scenario, the following questions can help you assess the level of risk:

- How would you describe the patient's mood?
- How would you describe his posture? Is he sitting or standing?
- What is his facial expression? Could you appropriately interpret it if he were having a stroke?
- Do you notice signs that he may be upset (eg, quick head movements, clenched fists, inability to sit still)?
- If you determine that the patient presents a real threat, then do you have enough help available? Are police officers present in the room with you?

As a paramedic, you cannot remove all risks from a situation. Your job is to use situational awareness to ensure you are constantly thinking about potential risks, weighing the probabilities, and then acting in the best interest of the patient while you keep yourself and your team safe.

2. What assessment information do you need to gather?

Initially, stroke should be high on the differential diagnosis list. Determine when the patient was last seen normal. Does the patient report a headache? A detailed neurologic assessment is appropriate.

3. How can you determine whether the patient is oriented when he will not speak?

To determine whether this patient is oriented, you can ask yes-or-no questions to which you know the answers; use a communication board; or ask the patient to either write down the responses using a pencil and paper, or type it using the keypad of a mobile phone.

4. What vital signs or laboratory values are critical to gather for this patient?

Obtain a full set of vital signs, including pulse oximetry. A blood glucose level is needed to rule out hypoglycemia. Focus on ensuring the BP reading is accurate. If you suspect a stroke, then transport the patient quickly.

5. What is this patient's Glasgow Coma Scale (GCS) score? Does it accurately depict this patient's acuity?

This patient's GCS score is 11. This score implies a diminished LOC. However, the only reason that this patient's score is 11 is that he cannot or will not speak.

6. Which portion of the neurologic assessment is inconsistent with the remainder of the exam?

The patient's inability to make any sound is inconsistent. The creation and processing of speech is complicated, and it involves multiples areas within the brain. The temporal lobe plays a major role in speech. Essentially, speech production can be broken down into a two-sided system: one that processes the auditory information coming in, and one that adjusts the vocal cords, breathing pattern, and mouth to create words. The latter side is impaired with this patient. His complete absence of sound generation is compelling. If this patient were having a stroke so severe as to completely impair his ability to make any sounds, you would expect him to have a decreased LOC. You would also expect an impaired ability to maintain the airway, such as swallowing difficulties. However, the patient appears to be functioning normally with the exception of his inability to make any sounds. His condition has removed his ability to make any sounds, yet it is not affecting his airway or LOC.

7. If this patient is having a stroke, then how will the aspirin affect him?

The three possible outcomes of aspirin administration are as follows:

1. If the patient is having an ischemic stroke, then aspirin may be beneficial.
2. If the patient is having a hemorrhagic stroke, then aspirin may be harmful. As the patient bleeds into his head, the body will attempt to

YOU are the Paramedic SUMMARY continued

form a clot. This clotting can curb the bleeding, thereby limiting the ICP. However, aspirin can also diminish the effectiveness of this clotting, thereby increasing the amount of bleeding. This process could result in a more significant hemorrhagic stroke.

3. If the patient is not having a stroke, then the effect of aspirin is unpredictable. If he is having is bleeding-related event, then the same problem just described could occur.

8. What are other possible causes of strokelike presentations?

Bell palsy can cause facial paralysis. Headaches can be caused by tension (stress), clusters, or migraine. Medications can cause mental status changes. A psychiatric condition called a conversion reaction can cause muteness.

9. Were you correct to treat this patient as if he had experienced a stroke?

Even though his presentation does not match the textbook description, this patient should still be treated as having a potential stroke. It is important to contact the closest stroke center and initiate a stroke alert. Because of the risk of brain damage if this patient is having a stroke, a CT/MRI scan is needed after he arrives at the ED.

EMS Patient Care Report (PCR)

Date: 11-06-22	**Incident No.:** 3986	**Nature of Call:** Stroke		**Location:** 1070 First St	
Dispatched: 0853	**En Route:** 0854	**At Scene:** 0858	**Transport:** 0916	**At Hospital:** 0923	**In Service:** 0938

Patient Information

Age: 49 **Sex:** M **Weight (in kg [lb]):** 109 kg (240 lb)	**Allergies:** NKDA **Medications:** Hydrochlorothiazide, exercise supplements **Past Medical History:** 1 year ago had an episode of left-side weakness that was not diagnosed as a stroke. Completely resolved. No diagnosis known. HTN. **Chief Complaint:** Unable to speak

Vital Signs

Time: 0903	**BP:** 142/96	**Pulse:** 112	**Respirations:** 16	**Spo_2:** 98% RA
Time: 0914	**BP:** 146/96	**Pulse:** 116	**Respirations:** 20	**Spo_2:** 98% RA
Time:	**BP:**	**Pulse:**	**Respirations:**	**Spo_2:**

EMS Treatment (circle all that apply)

Oxygen @ _____ L/min via (circle one): **NC NRM Bag-mask device**		**Assisted Ventilation**	**Airway Adjunct**	**CPR**
Defibrillation	**Bleeding Control**	**Bandaging**	**Splinting**	**Other:** IV started (circled)

YOU are the Paramedic SUMMARY *continued*

Narrative

Dispatched: Stroke.

CC: None stated by patient.

HPI: Pt was discovered by his wife this morning unable to speak. She administered 325 mg of aspirin. Pt admits to waking this morning about 2 hours ago and not being able to speak. He did alert his family.

PMH: HTN, 1 year ago had left-side weakness that completely resolved. Was not diagnosed as a stroke.

Meds: Hydrochlorothiazide.

Allergies: NKDA.

Physical Exam

General impression—Male patient sitting on couch in basement of home, with family in attendance. Pt has adequate hygiene and house is clean and organized.

Neuro—Awake, alert and appears to be oriented. Will answer yes/no questions by nodding. Slight facial droop noted to left face, neg ptosis, PERRLA, slight weakness noted to left arm. Able to stand and ambulate with minor assistance. Neg c/o headache. Cranial nerves II–XII are grossly intact unless otherwise noted, pt is able to swallow without difficulty, neg drooling noted, pt is mute without any sound generation or attempts at making words.

Cardiovascular—Skin is warm, dry, and normal color. Monitor shows sinus tach without obvious ST changes or ectopy noted, 12-lead shows no acute changes, neg c/o chest pain.

Respiratory—Lungs CTA bilaterally, neg use of accessory muscles, neg retractions noted, acyanotic, neg c/o difficulty breathing.

Gastrointestinal—Abd soft and non-tender without obvious masses or pulsation noted. Neg c/o nausea, neg vomiting noted.

Genitourinary—Stable pelvis to ambulation, neg overt incontinence noted.

Extr—Without obvious trauma, edema, or venipuncture marks noted.

Disposition—Transported pt to ABS hospital without incident, no change in patient condition or VS on arrival at hospital. Pt taken directly to CT scanner. Report to ED physician. Medic 123 available.

Impression—Potential stroke.
End of report

Prep Kit

Ready for Review

- Neurologic disorders can be dangerous because depressed reflexes leave the airway and other body systems vulnerable.
- A variety of disease processes can cause neurologic dysfunction, including cancer, degenerative conditions, developmental anomalies, infectious diseases, and vascular conditions. Most neurologic diseases are thought to be multifactorial—that is, a number of factors combine to induce vulnerability to a particular disease process.
- ICP is determined by the volume of the intracranial contents: the brain, blood, and CSF.
- The primary dangers of ICP are ischemia and brain herniation.

Prep Kit continued

- The neurologic assessment identifies small alterations that can impair nervous system function.
- Investigating the neurologic patient's chief complaint requires taking a history to determine the MOI or the NOI. This task is more difficult when the patient is unresponsive, but environmental clues and the reports of family, friends, and bystanders can be helpful.
- It is critical to determine when the patient was last seen normal because the amount of time elapsed since the onset of symptoms will dictate the treatments available.
- LOC can be evaluated using the GCS, the AVPU mnemonic, a test of corneal reflex or pupillary response, evaluation of cranial nerve functioning, assessment of the patient's orientation and alertness, assessment of the patient's speech and ability to recognize and name objects, evaluation of the patient's movement, testing of the patient's sensory perceptual abilities, testing of the blood glucose level, and measurement of vital signs.
- Following the standard care guideline can help you address common neurologic disorders in a systematic way.
- Stroke is a condition in which the blood supply to the brain is interrupted. In ischemic stroke, the blood supply may be blocked by a clot (thrombus or embolus). In hemorrhagic stroke, a damaged artery bleeds into the brain.
- Stroke causes sudden-onset changes in neurologic status, including effects on language, movement, sensation, LOC, and BP.
- Time is brain. To be effective, fibrinolytic agents must be administered in a time-sensitive manner after the onset of a stroke. Therefore, a stroke must be recognized and EMS dispatched quickly, and the patient must be transported promptly to a stroke center (if available in your region).
- TIAs are episodes of cerebral ischemia that resolve within 24 hours, leaving no permanent damage. Because they may signal an underlying vascular problem that can lead to a stroke, prompt medical evaluation is essential.
- A diminished LOC is marked by increasing deficits in cognition and speech and changes in movement and posture. The patient may become comatose without timely medical intervention.
- Seizures are caused by the sudden, erratic firing of neurons. They are broadly classified based on three features: (1) the location where seizures begin in the brain, (2) the patient's level of awareness during a seizure, and (3) motor symptoms and other features associated with the seizure.
- Generalized seizures affect awareness in some way and involve both sides of the brain at their onset. Focal seizures begin on one side of the brain; awareness may remain intact, or it may be impaired.
- Generalized seizures include tonic-clonic (generalized motor) and absence (generalized nonmotor) seizures. With a focal aware seizure (formerly called simple partial seizure), the patient may be unable to talk or respond during the event, but their awareness remains intact. If the patient's awareness is affected or impaired at any time during a focal seizure, it is termed a focal impaired awareness seizure (formerly called complex partial seizure). The terms "focal motor" and "focal nonmotor" are used to describe the behaviors associated with a focal seizure. Pseudoseizures have a psychiatric origin.
- Status epilepticus can be defined as a seizure that lasts longer than 4 to 5 minutes or consecutive seizures without a return to consciousness between seizures. Lengthy seizures can have devastating effects on the brain and body and may even be life threatening.
- Syncope (fainting) is caused by a brief interruption in cerebral blood flow that can be traced to cardiac rhythm disturbances, other cardiac causes, or noncardiac causes.

Prep Kit continued

- Headaches can be classified as muscle tension, migraine, cluster, or sinus headaches. Each has a different cause and a different presentation. Other types of headache may occur as well.
- Dementia is not a single illness, but a chronic process that can take many forms. It is characterized by deterioration of memory, personality, language skills, perception, reasoning, or judgment, with no loss of consciousness. Management is similar for the various dementias and is primarily supportive.
- Tumors of the neurologic system affect the brain and spinal cord and are classified as either primary or metastatic disease.
- Demyelinating conditions attack the insulating sheath that surrounds and protects the axon, so that nerve impulses can no longer travel smoothly.
- MS is an autoimmune condition in which episodes are followed by periods of remission. Patients with MS can have a range of neurologic deficits, from incontinence to significant sensory impairments.
- ALS (Lou Gehrig disease) is a disease that strikes the voluntary motor neurons, causing progressive paralysis and death.
- Parkinson disease damages the substantia nigra, the portion of the brain that produces dopamine, which is needed for muscle contraction.
- Cranial nerve disorders have a range of signs and symptoms and are often mistaken for other disorders.
- Dystonias are severe, abnormal muscle spasms that cause bizarre contortions, repetitive motions, or postures. They can affect the neck, face, jaw, or other muscles, and are often painful.
- Encephalitis and meningitis are CNS infections that cause inflammation of the brain and meninges, respectively.
- Abscesses indicate the presence of an infectious agent within the brain or spinal cord.
- Polio is a viral infection that can cause long-term damage to the brain and brainstem (postpolio syndrome), leading to muscle weakness and paralysis.
- In peripheral neuropathy, the nerves leaving the spinal cord are damaged by trauma, toxins, tumors, autoimmune attack, and metabolic disorders, or other processes. Diabetic neuropathy is the most common form.

Vital Vocabulary

abscess An area in the brain or spinal cord in which cells have been attacked, typically by an infectious agent. To prevent the spread of infection, the immune system "walls off" the area; pus may then collect in this pocket.

Alzheimer disease A progressive, organic condition in which neurons in the brain die, causing dementia.

amyotrophic lateral sclerosis (ALS) A condition that strikes the voluntary motor neurons, causing their death. The disease is characterized by fatigue and general weakness of muscle groups; eventually the patient becomes unable to walk, eat, or speak; also known as Lou Gehrig disease.

anesthesia Lack of feeling within a body part.

anisocoria Unequal pupils with a greater than 1 mm difference.

ataxia Alteration in the ability to perform coordinated motions such as walking.

aura Sensations commonly experienced before a seizure or migraine headache occurs; may include visual changes in addition to hallucinations.

Prep Kit continued

Bell palsy A temporary paralysis of the facial nerve (cranial nerve VII), which controls the muscles on each side of the face.

bradykinesia The slowing down of voluntary body movements; found in patients with Parkinson disease.

clonic activity Type of seizure movement involving the contraction and relaxation of muscle groups.

coma A state in which a person does not respond to either verbal or painful stimuli.

common reality Sensory stimulation that can be verified by others.

corneal reflex A protective movement that results in blinking, moving the head posteriorly, and pupillary constriction.

decerebrate posturing Abnormal extension of the arms with rotation of the wrists along with the toes pointed; this finding indicates brainstem damage.

decorticate posturing Abnormal flexion of the arms toward the chest with the toes pointed; this finding indicates lower cerebral damage.

delusions Thoughts, ideas, or perceived abilities that have no basis in common reality.

dementia The slow, progressive onset of disorientation, shortened attention span, and loss of cognitive function.

dystonia Contractions of body into bizarre positions.

endotoxins Toxins released by some bacteria when they die.

exotoxins Toxins secreted by living cells to aid in the death and digestion of other cells.

gait Patterns of walking or ambulating.

Guillain-Barré syndrome A rare condition that begins as a sensation of weakness and tingling in the legs, moving to the arms and thorax; the disorder can lead to paralysis within 2 weeks.

hallucinations Sensory stimulation that cannot be verified by others.

hemiparesis Weakness of one side of the body.

hemiplegia Paralysis of one side of the body.

hemorrhagic stroke One of the two main types of stroke; occurs as a result of bleeding inside the brain.

herniation The movement of a structure from its normal location into another space.

idiopathic Of no known cause.

intention tremor A tremor that occurs when trying to accomplish a task.

ischemic stroke One of the two main types of stroke, also called an occlusive stroke; occurs when blood flow to a particular part of the brain is cut off by a blockage, such as a blood clot, within an artery.

limbic system Structures within the cerebrum and diencephalon that influence emotions, motivation, mood, and sensations of pain and pleasure.

metastasis The process by which cells from a malignant neoplasm break away from the site of origin, such as the lung, and move through the bloodstream or lymphatic system to other body sites, such as the brain.

multiple sclerosis (MS) An autoimmune condition in which the body attacks the myelin that insulates the brain and spinal cord, causing scarring.

myasthenia gravis A condition in which the body generates antibodies against its own acetylcholine receptors, causing muscle weakness, often in the face.

myoclonus Involuntary jerking motions of the body.

neoplasm A tumor.

nystagmus Involuntary, rhythmic shaking of the eyes.

paresthesia Sensation of tingling or numbness in a body part.

Parkinson disease A neurologic condition in which the portion of the brain responsible for

Prep Kit continued

production of dopamine has been damaged or overused, resulting in tremors.

peripheral neuropathy A group of conditions in which the nerves that exit the spinal cord are damaged, distorting signals to or from the brain. One type is caused by diabetes; peripheral nerves are damaged as the blood glucose level rises, resulting in lack of sensation, numbness, burning, pain, paresthesia, and muscle weakness.

poliomyelitis A now-rare viral infection that attacks and destroys nerve axons, especially motor axons; the disease can cause weakness, paralysis, and respiratory arrest.

postictal The period after a seizure in which the brain is reorganizing activity.

postpolio syndrome The death of nerve fibers as a late consequence of poliomyelitis; characterized by swallowing difficulties, weakness, fatigue, and breathing problems.

postural tremor A tremor that occurs as the person holds a body part still.

posturing Abnormal body positioning that indicates damage to the brain.

prodrome An early sign or symptom that occurs before a disease or condition fully appears (eg, dizziness before fainting).

pronation Rotation of the lower arms in a palms-down manner.

psychosis A condition characterized by breaking with common reality and existing mainly within an internal world.

ptosis Prolapse of a body part; often refers to drooping of the eyelid.

rest tremor A tremor that occurs even when the patient's muscles are relaxed (eg, hands resting on the lap).

rigidity A condition in which muscles do not contract and relax smoothly, resulting in stiffness of motion; found in patients with Parkinson disease.

seizure The sudden, erratic firing of neurons; a neurologic episode caused by a surge of electric activity in the brain. It can be a convulsion characterized by generalized, uncoordinated muscular activity, and may be associated with loss of consciousness.

status epilepticus A condition in which seizures recur every few minutes, or consecutive seizures occur without a return to consciousness between seizures.

stroke An interruption of blood flow to the brain that results in the loss of brain function; also called a cerebrovascular accident.

syncope A fainting spell or transient loss of consciousness.

tonic activity A type of seizure movement involving the constant contraction and trembling of muscle groups.

transient ischemic attacks (TIAs) Disorder in which brain cells temporarily stop working because of insufficient oxygen, causing stroke-like symptoms that resolve completely within 24 hours of onset.

tremors Fine involuntary, rhythmic movements, usually involving the hands or head.

trismus The involuntary contraction of the mouth resulting in clenched teeth; occurs during seizures and head injuries.

uremia Severe renal failure resulting in the buildup of waste products within the blood; eventually impairs brain function.

References

1. Deaths and mortality. Centers for Disease Control and Prevention website. http://www.cdc.gov/nchs/fastats/deaths.htm. Reviewed March 1, 2021. Accessed April 8, 2021.
2. Jensen E. Demographic analysis uses birth and death records, international migration data and Medicare records to produce a range of population estimates as of April 1, 2020. US Census Bureau website.

Prep Kit continued

https://www.census.gov/library/stories/2020/12/census-bureau-provides-population-estimates-for-independent-evaluation-of-upcoming-census-results.html. Published December 15, 2020. Accessed April 8, 2021.

3. 2020 world population data sheet shows older populations growing, total fertility rates declining. Population Reference Bureau website. https://www.prb.org/2020-world-population-data-sheet/. Published July 10, 2020. Accessed April 8, 2021.
4. Top things to know: 2019 updated to the 2018 guidelines for the early management of acute ischemic stroke. American Heart Association website. https://professional.heart.org/en/science-news/2019-update-to-the-2018-acute-ischemic-stroke-guidelines/top-things-to-know. Published October 30, 2019. Accessed March 22, 2021.
5. Jauch EC. Ischemic stroke. Medscape website. http://emedicine.medscape.com/article/1916852-overview. Updated May 27, 2020. Accessed March 22, 2021.
6. Jauch EC, Saver JL, Adams HP Jr, et al; on behalf of American Heart Association Stroke Council, Council on Cardiovascular Nursing, Council on Peripheral Vascular Disease, and Council on Clinical Cardiology. Guidelines for the early management of patients with acute ischemic stroke: a guideline for healthcare professionals from the American Heart Association/American Stroke Association. *Stroke*. 2013;44:870-947.
7. Mozaffarian D, Benjamin EJ, Go AS, et al; on behalf of American Heart Association Statistics Committee and Stroke Statistics Subcommittee. Heart disease and stroke statistics—2016 update: a report from the American Heart Association. *Circulation*. 2016;133. https://www.ahajournals.org/doi/10.1161/cir.0000000000000350.
8. Rangel-Castillo L, Gopinath S, Robertson CS. Management of intracranial hypertension. *Neurol Clin*. 2008;26(2):521-541.
9. Beume L-A, Hieber M, Kaller CP, et al. Large vessel occlusion in acute stroke. *Stroke*. 2018;49:2323-2329.
10. Hulsman S. What every first responder should know about large vessel occlusion. EMS1 website. https://www.ems1.com/sponsored-article/articles/what-every-first-responder-should-know-about-large-vessel-occlusion-Q4RTOnGcL1AZ3gg4/. Published August 28, 2017. Accessed March 22, 2021.
11. Aroor S, Singh R, Goldstein LB. BE-FAST (balance, eyes, face, arm, speech, time): reducing the proportion of strokes missed using the FAST mnemonic. *Stroke*. 2017;48(2):479-481.
12. Powers WJ, Rabinstein AA, Ackerson T, et al. Guidelines for the early management of patients with acute ischemic stroke: 2019 update to the 2018 guidelines for the early management of acute ischemic stroke. *Stroke*. 50(12). https://doi.org/10.1161/STR.0000000000000211.
13. Mobile stroke unit. Cleveland Clinic website. http://my.clevelandclinic.org/services/neurological_institute/cerebrovascular-center/treatment-services/mobile-stroke-unit. Accessed March 22, 2021.
14. Sacco RL, Kasner SE, Broderick JP, et al; on behalf of American Heart Association Stroke Council, Council on Cardiovascular Surgery and Anesthesia, Council on Cardiovascular Radiology and Intervention, Council on Cardiovascular and Stroke Nursing, Council on Epidemiology and Prevention, Council on Peripheral Vascular Disease, and Council on Nutrition, Physical Activity and Metabolism. An updated definition of stroke for the 21st century: a statement for healthcare professionals from the American Heart Association/American Stroke Association. *Stroke*. 2013;44:2064-2089.
15. Transient ischemic attack information page. National Institute of Neurological Disorders and Stroke (NINDS) website. https://www.ninds.nih.gov/Disorders/All-Disorders/Transient-Ischemic-Attack-Information-Page. Accessed March 22, 2021.
16. Pulsara website [homepage]. https://www.pulsara.com. Accessed April 8, 2021.
17. Fisher RS, Shafer PO, D'Souza C. 2017 revised classification of seizures. Epilepsy Foundation website. https://www.epilepsy.com/article/2016/12/2017-revised-classification-seizures. Accessed April 8, 2021.
18. Morag R. Syncope. Medscape website. http://emedicine.medscape.com/article/811669-overview. Updated January 13, 2017. Accessed March 22, 2021.
19. Smith C. Search for cause of high rates of MS in Northwest would lead to new treatments. KUOW website. November 27, 2012. https://www.kuow.org/stories/search-cause-high-rates-ms-northwest-could-lead-new-treatments.
20. Andary MT. Guillain-Barré syndrome. Medscape website. http://emedicine.medscape.com/article/315632-overview. Updated June 24, 2020. Accessed March 22, 2021.
21. Polio elimination in the United States. Centers for Disease Control and Prevention website. https://www.cdc.gov/polio/what-is-polio/polio-us.html. Reviewed October 25, 2019. Accessed March 22, 2021.
22. Foster MR. Spina bifida. Medscape website. http://emedicine.medscape.com/article/311113-overview. Updated August 12, 2020. Accessed March 22, 2021.
23. Nelson SL Jr. Hydrocephalus. Medscape website. http://emedicine.medscape.com/article/1135286-overview. Updated June 4, 2018. Accessed March 22, 2021.

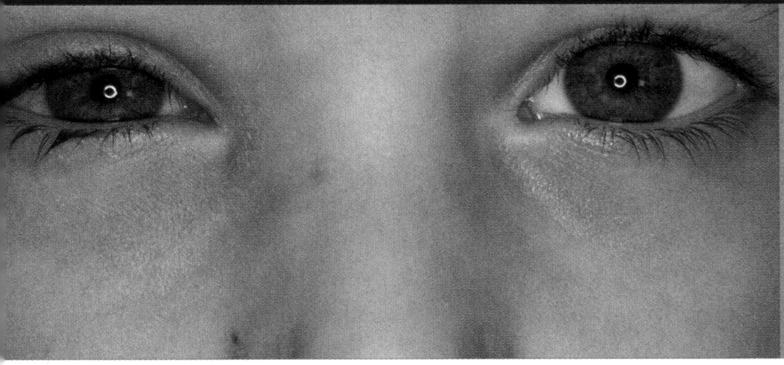

Chapter 20

Diseases of the Eyes, Ears, Nose, and Throat

NATIONAL EMS EDUCATION STANDARD COMPETENCIES

Medicine

Integrates assessment findings with principles of epidemiology and pathophysiology to formulate a field impression and implement a comprehensive treatment/disposition plan for a patient with a medical complaint.

Diseases of the Eyes, Ears, Nose, and Throat

Knowledge of the anatomy, physiology, epidemiology, pathophysiology, psychosocial effects, presentations, prognosis, and management of

- Common or major diseases of the eyes, ears, nose, and throat, including nose bleed (pp 1364–1389)

KNOWLEDGE OBJECTIVES

1. Explain facial anatomy and relate physiology to facial disorders. (pp 1364, 1374, 1378, 1379, 1382–1384)
2. Relate assessment findings associated with eye disorders to pathophysiology. (pp 1364–1369)
3. Describe assessment, treatment, and management of specific eye conditions. (pp 1369–1373)
4. Relate assessment findings associated with ear disorders to pathophysiology. (pp 1373–1375)
5. Describe assessment, treatment, and management of specific ear conditions. (pp 1375–1377)
6. Relate assessment findings associated with nose disorders to pathophysiology. (pp 1377–1379)
7. Describe assessment, treatment, and management of specific nose conditions. (pp 1379–1382)
8. Relate assessment findings associated with throat and mouth disorders to pathophysiology. (pp 1382–1384)
9. Describe assessment, treatment, and management of specific throat and mouth conditions. (pp 1385–1389)

SKILLS OBJECTIVES

There are no skills objectives for this chapter.

Introduction

Disorders of the eye, ear, nose, and throat (EENT) are a common focus of concern for paramedics who are treating medical patients. Therefore, understanding the basics of EENT diseases and injuries is an essential piece of your medical assessment and treatment knowledge base.

Many calls for emergency medical services (EMS) involving EENT structures result from trauma; such injuries are discussed in detail in Chapter 34, *Face and Neck Trauma*. This chapter covers medical conditions that could result in a call to 9-1-1 or that you could notice when you are assessing a patient who called 9-1-1 for an unrelated reason. During such calls, familiarity with EENT conditions will help you during assessment of the patient. Knowledge of these conditions also enables you to educate the patient about preventing or potentially caring for a condition that the patient may have.

Often, when you encounter a patient with an EENT disorder, it makes sense to transport the patient, possibly to an emergency department (ED) with access to an eye specialist or an ear, nose, and throat (ENT) specialist for further evaluation. For example, whenever an object is lodged in the eye, ear, nose, or throat, the patient must be transported to the hospital. In addition, patients with eye injuries should be transported to a Level 1 or 2 trauma center that offers ophthalmology services.

This chapter discusses general considerations when assessing a patient with a complaint related to an EENT condition. You will also learn about specific conditions and their field treatment, if any.

The Eye

The American College of Ophthalmology reports that more than 2.4 million Americans have eye emergencies each year.[1] Examples of eye disease emergencies include **glaucoma**, macular degeneration, and **diabetic retinopathy**. Patients with these diseases have a long-standing history of an underlying condition that predisposes them to the eye disorder (comorbidity). Mortality from eye disease is quite low, however.

Anatomy and Physiology Review

The eye is the body's window to the world. It is connected to the brain by two nerves. The **oculomotor nerve** (CN III), in addition to the trochlear (CN IV) and abducens (CN VI) nerves, innervate muscles that are involved in eye movement as well as the parasympathetic nerve fibers that cause constriction of the pupil and accommodation of the lens. The **optic nerve** (second cranial nerve) provides the sense of vision. **FIGURE 20-1** and **FIGURE 20-2** depict the anatomy of the eye and the lacrimal system, respectively.

Patient Assessment

Keeping your team safe from the often hidden dangers at medical scenes should be the first item on your priority list. In patients with eye disorders, fear and panic from vision loss can sometimes trigger dangerous and bizarre behavior. Keep the patient calm. The scene size-up is an opportunity to discover clues to the cause of the complaint while avoiding potential hazards.

YOU are the Paramedic

PART 1

On a blustery winter day, you are dispatched to a local acute care rehabilitation center for a 62-year-old woman experiencing a nosebleed. She is recovering from left-side weakness after a stroke. When you arrive on scene, you are directed to the dining area, where you find the patient seated at a table, with staff helping her hold a towel to her nose. Blood is visible on the table in front of the patient as well as on the towel. The patient is sitting upright and leaning slightly forward, breathing through her mouth. She is dark-skinned, and the mucous membranes of her eyelids and mouth appear pale. The staff advises you that the patient was eating lunch when suddenly her nose began to bleed.

1. What is your primary concern after scene safety is established?
2. Do you have concerns other than the nose bleed?

Special Populations

According to the US Centers for Disease Control and Prevention (CDC), vision disability is one of the top 10 disabilities among adults 18 years and older and one of the most prevalent disabling conditions among children.[2]

In the geriatric population, you are likely to encounter patients who have undergone laser-assisted eye surgery (Lasik surgery), a procedure that can reduce the need for corrective lenses. Traditional Lasik surgery uses a special laser to slice a flap in the cornea and adjust the shape of the middle section of the cornea (stroma); the latest techniques manipulate the stroma without creating the "flap" in the cornea. Immediately following the surgery and for the next few weeks, patients are instructed to avoid letting air blow directly into their eyes and to wear goggles while they sleep, so they do not scratch their cornea. Geriatric patients are also more likely to undergo **cataract** surgery and eye surgery for glaucoma.

Older people may also experience eye injuries from falls. Eye conditions and problems are among the many different comorbid conditions often found in the geriatric population.

Diabetic retinopathy is a disease that affects the small blood vessels in the retina. A common complication of diabetes, it is the leading cause of blindness in US adults.[3] More than 40% of Americans with diabetes have some degree of diabetic retinopathy.[4] The early stages of diabetic retinopathy usually are not associated with any symptoms, but in later stages of the disease, blood vessels in the retina start to bleed into the vitreous (the gel-like fluid in the center of the eye). This bleeding may be perceived by the patient as dark, floating spots; it may appear to others as streaks that look like cobwebs.[4] Currently, an estimated 4.1 million Americans are affected by retinopathy, with 899,000 experiencing vision-threatening retinopathy.[3]

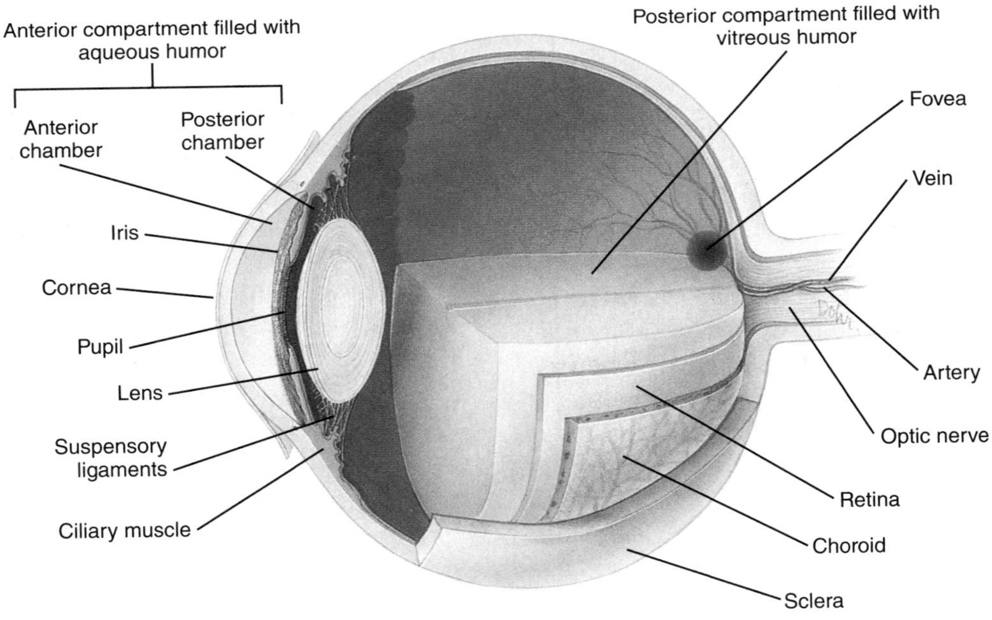

FIGURE 20-1 A review of the structures of the eye.

As you form a general impression of the patient, note environmental clues at the scene, the patient's evident sex and approximate age, and the degree of distress. Do not let the high degree of distress or concern over the potential visual impairment sidetrack your observations of the scene and cause you to miss the hazards that may have caused an injury or condition.

Do not become distracted by a swollen, irritated, or deformed eye to the extent that you bypass

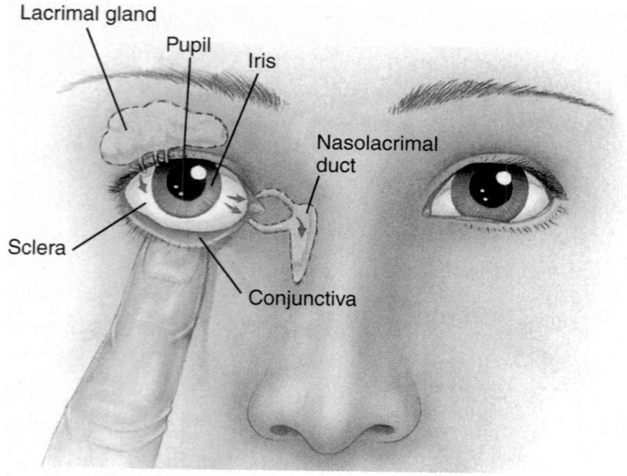

FIGURE 20-2 The lacrimal system of tear glands and ducts.

the highest-priority aspects of the patient's care. For example, you must first ensure the patient has an open and adequate airway, that the patient is breathing, that there are no threats to ventilation, that the patient has an adequate pulse, and that no life threats to the patient's circulation need immediate attention.

Depending on the severity of the eye condition, an early transport decision to an appropriate facility can improve outcomes. Level 1 trauma centers have the skilled services necessary to treat a serious eye problem.

Covering both eyes can limit damage to the affected eye by limiting conjugate eye movement (ie, synchronous movement of the injured eye when the uninjured eye moves). Consider pain treatments and, if necessary, mild sedation during transport for patients with eye emergencies. Cardiac monitoring is recommended in these patients as well. Ocular pressure can stimulate the vagus nerve, leading to a vagal response in the patient. Eye drops and eye medication can cause side effects such as low or high blood pressure (BP).

As a paramedic, your demeanor should be supportive and calm. Remember, a patient facing potential long-term vision loss will need emotional care as well; this can be a life-changing event for the patient.

Obtain the patient's chief complaint and elaborate on it using the OPQRST (Onset, Provocation/palliation, Quality, Region/radiation, Severity, Timing) mnemonic. When you obtain the history, determine how and when the symptoms began and which symptoms the patient is experiencing now. Are both eyes affected? Does the patient have any underlying diseases or conditions of the eye (such as glaucoma)? Does the patient take eye medications?

The following symptoms may indicate that the patient has a serious ocular condition:

- *Visual loss* that does not improve when the patient blinks is an important symptom. It may indicate damage to the globe or the optic nerve.
- *Double vision* usually points to trauma involving the extraocular muscles, such as a fracture of the orbit.
- *Severe eye pain* is a symptom of a significant eye injury.
- A *foreign body sensation* usually indicates superficial injury to the cornea or the presence of a foreign object trapped behind the eyelids.

Assessment of specific eye conditions begins with a thorough examination to determine the extent and nature of the situation. Always perform your examination while maintaining standard precautions, taking great care to avoid aggravating the affected area. Assess for pain or tenderness, swelling, abnormal or loss of movement, sensation changes, circulatory changes, deformity, visual changes, and airway compromise.

Physical examination of the eyes includes assessment of the visible ocular structures as well as ocular function. This evaluation is described in Chapter 11, *Patient Assessment*. Assess the ocular structures for the following findings:

- **Orbital rim.** Assess for ecchymosis, swelling, lacerations, and tenderness.
- **Eyelids.** Assess for ecchymosis, swelling, lacerations, and any abnormalities.
- **Corneas.** Assess for foreign bodies.
- **Conjunctivae.** Assess for redness, pus, inflammation, and foreign bodies.
- **Globes.** Assess for redness, abnormal pigmentation, and lacerations. Inspect the eye surface for growths, discoloration, and differences between the eyes.
- **Pupils.** Assess for PERRLA (pupils equal, round, reactive to light and accommodation). Note whether the pupils are symmetric.

When you are assessing ocular function, perform the following tests:

- **Visual acuity.** Assess the patient's ability to see large and small letters, such as by asking the patient to read the writing on a prescription bottle, or by using a hand-held visual acuity chart such as the Snellen chart (shown in Chapter 11, *Patient Assessment*). Test each eye separately and document the results.
- **Peripheral vision.** Evaluate the patient's peripheral vision by testing the ability to recognize an object entering the extremes of the visual field (confrontation).
- **Ocular motility.** Check the patient's ability to move the eyes in all directions. Check for paralysis of gaze or discoordination between the movements of the two eyes (**dysconjugate gaze**).

Obtain a full set of baseline vital signs during the secondary assessment. During reassessment, monitor vital signs every 5 to 15 minutes, depending on the severity of the patient's condition. Such an ongoing assessment allows you to track any trends in these indicators.

Use of multiple eye medications, or excessive use of any one medication, may produce both local and systemic adverse effects. Systemic effects are possible because the medication can enter the bloodstream via the nasolacrimal system, which drains tears from the eyes.

Ask the patient how they administered the eye medications. Sometimes part of the problem is that the patient did not follow the instructions for the specific medication. For example, it is usually recommended to wait approximately 5 minutes between administering the first and second drops of an eye medication. Of course, this 5-minute rule does not apply to emergency measures such as administering tetracaine before inserting a Morgan lens.

Many medications are available to address a variety of eye problems. Eye drops can be used for **conjunctivitis**, dry eyes, red eyes, eye pain, glaucoma, eye surgery, herpes simplex, itchy eyes, and corneal abrasions. Eye lubricants are available for protecting eyes that do not produce tears, resulting from conditions such as cranial nerve VII (facial nerve) damage. Eye drops and lubricants are most often applied by gently squeezing the lower eyelid to make a pouch and applying the medicine into the lower lid. The patient then should close their eyes and roll the eyes downward with eyes closed. Gentle pressure should be applied to the corner of the eyes to prevent drainage of the medicine from the eye.

Always ask patients which medications they have taken before your arrival on the scene. For the paramedic, administration of eye medications in the prehospital setting is usually limited to proparacaine (Alcaine, Ophthaine) or tetracaine (Pontocaine) for pain relief or emergency irrigation to remove a damaging or irritating substance from the eyes. However, as the population of geriatric patients increases, the scope of practice for the paramedic may change to include limited eye care, as these patients are more vulnerable to eye conditions such as glaucoma.

Irrigation of the eyes may be necessary in case of chemical burns or thermal burns. Such treatment consists of applying sterile water or isotonic saline solution to the eye, with the liquid being flushed from the inside corner to the outside of the eye, except when a Morgan lens is being used.

Words of Wisdom

Anisocoria, the condition in which the pupils are not of equal size, is a significant finding in patients with ocular injuries or closed head trauma. However, according to the American Association for Pediatric Ophthalmology and Strabismus, simple or physiologic anisocoria (difference in pupil size) occurs in up to 30% of the population.[5] Usually, the person's pupils differ in size by less than 1 mm, and the difference between the pupils does not change according to bright or dim lighting.[5]

Unilateral cataract surgery may also cause inequality of pupil size. The pupil of the eye affected by the cataract will be nonreactive to light.

Patients with eye injuries should be seen in the ED. Children with eye emergencies may need to be treated under anesthesia, and many patients with eye injuries will need a topical anesthetic and antibiotic. These medications are not generally administered by a paramedic but rather by hospital personnel.

Eye injuries may be irreversible, and patients may or may not be aware of the event's seriousness. Patients may exhibit denial, anger, fear, hysteria, and depression in response to the potential vision loss. Communication is key to keeping patients calm and informed. If they wear glasses, bring the glasses along to the ED. Remember that early decisions to transport to the appropriate facility can improve outcomes in some patients, and early communication with a medical control physician can help direct your care and inform transport decisions.

Patients Wearing Contact Lenses

You may encounter patients who wear contact lenses. In general, if the eye is injured, you should not attempt to remove contact lenses because you may further aggravate the injury. The only indication for removing contact lenses in the prehospital setting is a chemical burn of the eye (discussed in Chapter 34, *Face and Neck Trauma*). In this situation, the lens can trap the offending chemical and make irrigation difficult, thereby worsening the injury.

Use a small suction cup to remove a hard contact lens, moistening the end with saline **FIGURE 20-3A**. To remove soft lenses, place one to two drops of saline in the eye **FIGURE 20-3B**, gently pinch the lens between your gloved thumb and index finger, and lift it off the surface of the eye **FIGURE 20-3C**. Place the contact lens in a container with sterile saline solution. Always advise ED staff if a patient is wearing contact lenses.

Patients With an Eye Prosthesis

Occasionally, you may care for a patient who is wearing an eye prosthesis (artificial eye). You should suspect an eye is artificial if it does not respond to light, move in concert with the opposite eye, or appear quite the same as the opposite eye. If you are unsure whether the patient has an eye prosthesis, ask the patient. No harm will be done if you care for

Street Smarts

When patients ask you what you think is wrong, remember that you are serving them. Remind them that you do not have definitive answers and are not a physician, but tell them what you think is going on. Be honest and sincere about what you are telling them to keep patients both informed and calm.

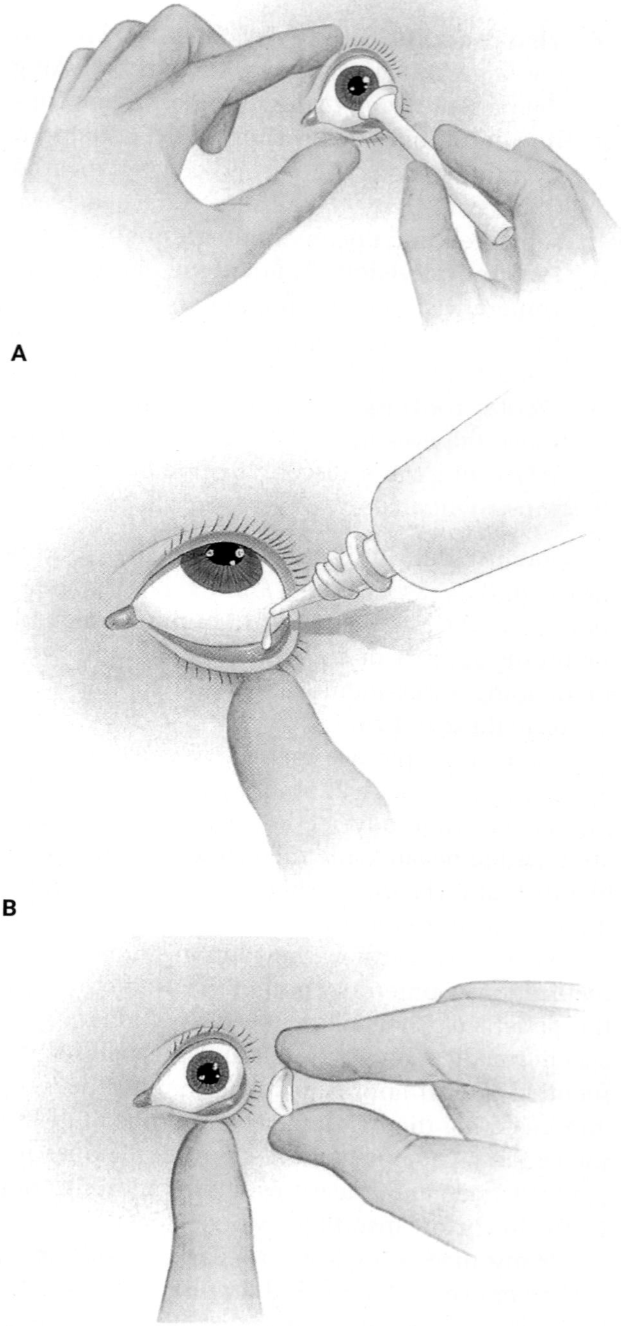

A

B

C

FIGURE 20-3 Removal of contact lenses should be limited to patients with chemical burns to the eye. **A.** To remove hard contact lenses, use a specialized suction cup moistened with sterile saline solution. **B.** Step 1: To remove soft contact lenses, instill 1 or 2 drops of saline or irrigating solution. **C.** Step 2: Pinch off the lens with your gloved thumb and index fingers.

an artificial eye as you would a normal one; however, you should make every attempt to accurately determine the patient's eye function.

Pathophysiology, Assessment, and Management of Specific Eye Conditions

This section covers specific eye conditions. Eye trauma (ie, adnexa, burns of the eye, corneal abrasion, foreign body in the eye, hyphema, retinal detachment and defect) is covered in Chapter 34, *Face and Neck Trauma.*

Conjunctivitis

Conjunctivitis, also known as "pink eye," is a condition in which the conjunctiva becomes inflamed and red **FIGURE 20-4**. The conjunctiva is a thin layer that lines the inside of the eyelids and the white part of the eye. Inflammation causes the white part of the eye to take on a red or pink tint.

Conjunctivitis most often starts in one eye and spreads to the other eye. This condition is often caused by bacteria, viruses, allergies, chemicals, or foreign bodies present in the eye. The viral and bacterial forms are highly contagious. Conjunctivitis has historically accounted for a significant number of absences in daycare and school settings; however, the CDC currently suggests that if the individual has conjunctivitis but no accompanying fever or symptoms, that person may be allowed to remain at work or school with a doctor's approval.[6]

Viral conjunctivitis is often associated with an upper respiratory virus or cold, whereas various bacterial infections cause bacterial conjunctivitis. Allergic conjunctivitis is caused by a trigger or irritating allergen, such as pollen. Chlorine in swimming pools and air pollution are potential causes of chemical conjunctivitis. If conjunctivitis is due to a foreign body, the eye will begin to produce tears in an attempt to flush out the object.

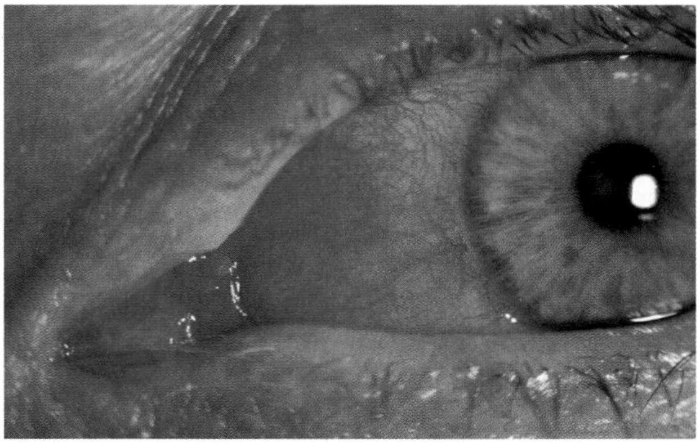

FIGURE 20-4 Conjunctivitis is inflammation of the eye. It may be associated with the presence of a foreign object in the eye.

Courtesy of John T. Halgren, MD, University of Nebraska Medical Center.

YOU are the Paramedic

PART 2

The patient seems tired and weak. While your partner is obtaining her vital signs, you ask the patient and care staff what happened. The patient states that she sat down to eat lunch, and blood started gushing from her nose. She is spitting up some blood as well.

Recording Time: 0 Minutes	
Appearance	Awake
Level of consciousness	Alert (oriented to person, place, time, and event)
Airway	Open
Breathing	Coughing; some gurgling in mouth as patient spits blood
Circulation	Adequate, epistaxis noted; pale mucous membranes of eyelids and mouth

3. What do you need to know about the patient's history?
4. What is the priority in managing this patient?

Assessment and Management

When conjunctivitis is suspected, a general assessment of the patient's vision should be performed, including visual acuity, the external eye, the pupils, peripheral vision, and eye movement.

Viral conjunctivitis typically resolves on its own. It can last up to 2 weeks but usually reaches its peak in 3 to 5 days. Bacterial conjunctivitis requires a topical antibiotic to eliminate the infection. Severe cases of allergic conjunctivitis may require nonsteroidal anti-inflammatory drugs (NSAIDs), antihistamines, and topical steroid eye drops prescribed by the physician in the ED.

Inflammation of the Eyelid (Chalazion and Hordeolum)

The eyelid contains oil glands and oil ducts that provide a protective film across the eye. A **chalazion** is a small, usually painless lump or pustule on the external eyelid that appears red and swollen, and that forms because of blockage and swelling of an oil gland in the eyelid **FIGURE 20-5**. A chalazion is often confused with a **hordeolum**. A hordeolum is an infection of an oil gland in the eyelid that produces a red, swollen, painful lump in the eyelid or at the lid margin **FIGURE 20-6**. It may be either internal (rare) or external. An external hordeolum is commonly called a stye.

Assessment and Management

A thorough assessment of vital signs, history, and transport for physician evaluation are warranted when a patient has an eyelid inflammation. The patient will usually be asked to apply warm compresses for 5 to 10 minutes several times per day to help soften the hardened oil blocking the ducts, thereby allowing the duct to drain. Topical or oral antibiotics may be prescribed.

Glaucoma

Glaucoma comprises a group of conditions that lead to increased intraocular pressure. It is one of the leading causes of blindness.

The aqueous humor is a clear, watery fluid that fills the eye's anterior chamber, as described in Chapter 8, *Anatomy and Physiology*. It maintains intraocular pressure, provides nutrients to the inner surface of the eye, and helps bend light.[7] The aqueous humor circulates through the pupil and drains into the venous system by the canal of Schlemm, a thin-walled vein extending around the eye.

Several types of glaucoma are distinguished. The most common form of glaucoma is *open-angle glaucoma*. With this form of glaucoma, the aqueous humor drains too slowly. Over time, pressure builds up within the eye (intraocular pressure), damaging the optic nerve. With *normal-tension glaucoma*, the optic nerve is damaged and vision changes occur, although there is no increase in intraocular pressure. In *narrow-angle glaucoma* (also called angle-closure glaucoma), access to the drainage channel is narrowed, preventing proper drainage of the aqueous humor. As a result, pressure builds up in the eye's posterior chamber, which pushes the lens forward. The lens then

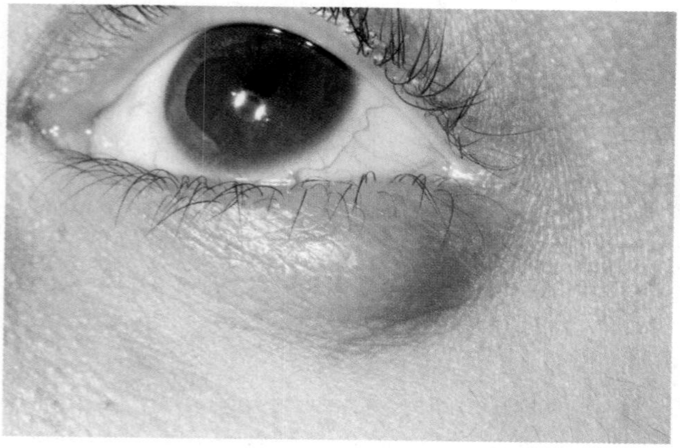

FIGURE 20-5 A chalazion is a small lump or pustule on the external eyelid.

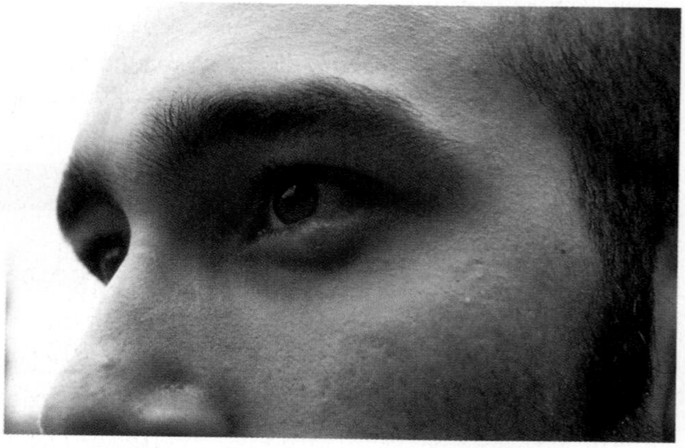

FIGURE 20-6 An external hordeolum, or stye, is a red, tender lump in the eyelid or at the lid margin.

pushes the iris into the drainage channel, completely blocking it.

Secondary glaucoma occurs as a result of conditions that damage the drainage channel in the eye. Examples of these conditions include diabetes, eye injuries, leukemia, sickle cell anemia, some types of arthritis, and cataracts.

The incidence of glaucoma increases with age, so that it is more common among older adults. Nevertheless, this condition can occur at any time from birth onward. Glaucoma is usually treated with eye drops that act to reduce ocular pressure.

Assessment and Management

Glaucoma usually affects a person's peripheral vision first. Eventually, the patient develops tunnel vision, in which they can see only what is directly ahead. With chronic glaucoma, the patient may have no symptoms until vision loss occurs.

A patient who experiences an acute attack of narrow-angle glaucoma may report severe eye pain, headache, photophobia, nausea, and vomiting. The cornea may look cloudy. The patient may report blurred vision and halos around lights because of corneal swelling. The pupils often have irregular margins and can be fixed in mid-position and dilated. An attack may be triggered by pupil dilation, such as eye drops given during an eye examination or dim lighting. Acute narrow-angle glaucoma is a medical emergency, and the patient needs evaluation by a physician. If intraocular pressure is not reduced, permanent vision loss can occur.

Assessment should rule out any trauma or physical injury to the eye. As described earlier, you should perform a general eye assessment, evaluating vision, movement, and any external eye or anterior surface abnormalities. Document any pertinent negatives and all abnormal findings. An ophthalmologist will later perform a much more comprehensive exam, assessing the intraocular pressure, the shape and color of the optic nerve viewed through a dilated pupil, the angle in the eye where the iris meets the cornea, and the thickness of the cornea. This physician will also perform a test to assess the entire field of vision. Because paramedics are generally not trained to conduct such a comprehensive eye exam, all patients with eye injuries or conditions should be transported to the ED for evaluation.

Words of Wisdom

In some areas, as part of an expanded-practice program, the medical director may train paramedics to use an ophthalmoscope and/or an otoscope **FIGURE 20-7**. Generally, however, these devices are reserved for use in a hospital or physician's office.

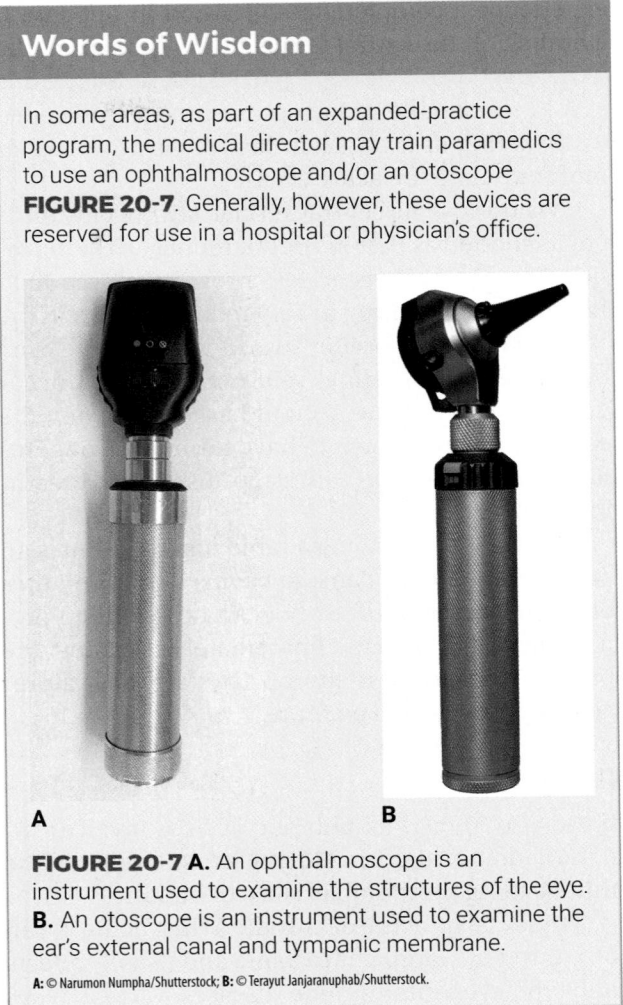

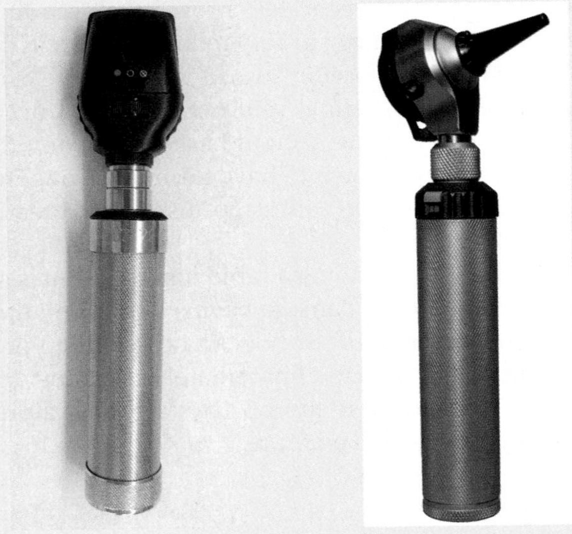

A B

FIGURE 20-7 A. An ophthalmoscope is an instrument used to examine the structures of the eye. **B.** An otoscope is an instrument used to examine the ear's external canal and tympanic membrane.

Central Retinal Artery Occlusion

Central retinal artery occlusion is a condition in which the blood supply to the retina becomes blocked because of a clot or embolus in the central retinal artery or one of its branches. Possible causes of central retinal artery occlusion include an embolus from the carotid artery, valvular heart disease, drug abuse, fat emboli, arterial spasm, and oral contraceptive use. Central retinal artery occlusion may cause partial blindness, which may be either temporary or permanent.

Assessment and Management

The patient with central retinal artery occlusion usually seeks medical assistance because of a sudden, painless loss of vision in one eye. If the central retinal artery is blocked, the patient will likely experience a complete loss of vision in one eye. If a branch of the central retinal artery is blocked, the patient will likely develop partial vision loss in one eye. In some patients, symptoms may be preceded by flickering or a transient loss of vision weeks or months before the acute event.

Vision loss in central retinal *vein* occlusion is not as sudden as that in central retinal artery occlusion. Instead, this vision loss progresses over 30 to 120 minutes, resulting in very reduced vision in the affected eye and possibly loss of vision in the eye.[8] Becauase central retinal vein occlusion can occur during sleep, providers should ascertain when the patient was last known to have normal vision. This disorder is associated with sleep-disordered breathing (apnea).[9]

A situation involving a rapid loss of vision is an emergency. Retinal damage begins within minutes of the cessation of blood flow and can lead to permanent visual deficits. Immediately transport the patient to the closest appropriate facility and provide supportive care en route.

Iritis

Iritis, also known as anterior uveitis, involves inflammation of the iris **FIGURE 20-8**. Uveitis is the third leading preventable cause of blindness.

Iritis can be acute or chronic. When acute, it can be caused by trauma or irritants and usually affects only one eye. Autoimmune diseases, various types of arthritis, irritable bowel disease, and Crohn disease can predispose patients to develop iritis. Infectious causes include Lyme disease, tuberculosis, and sexually transmitted diseases.

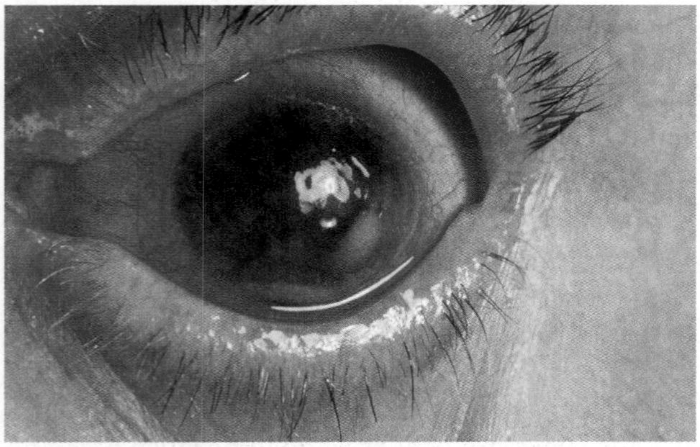

FIGURE 20-8 Iritis is inflammation of the iris.

Assessment and Management

Iritis presents as a red area surrounding the iris, cloudy vision, or an unusually shaped pupil. The assessment should focus on the history. Because many ophthalmologists are not trained to recognize iritis, patients suspected of having this condition should be directed to a uveitis specialist or an ocular immunologist.

Acute iritis usually responds well to topical corticosteroids as long as the cause is not fungal, viral, or bacterial. Failure to treat iritis can result in permanent disability.

Papilledema

Papilledema results from swelling or inflammation of the optic nerve at the rear part of the eye. The optic nerve communicates between the eyes and the brain. When it is affected by swelling or inflammation, patients may experience headaches, nausea and possibly vomiting, temporary vision loss, or narrowing vision fields. They may also experience a "graying" in their field of vision.

The increased pressure in the brain that causes optic nerve swelling and inflammation may have several different causes. Space-occupying lesions such as abscesses and tumors can create increased intracranial pressure (ICP). An inner ear infection, lung infection, or dental infection can lead to pus accumulation in the brain, causing an abscess that presses on the optic nerve. Meningitis, fever, brain tumors, hypertensive crisis, chronic high BP, and other diseases such as Guillain-Barré syndrome may increase cerebrospinal fluid (CSF) pressures, leading to papilledema.

Assessment and Management

The diagnosis of papilledema is made by a qualified clinician who has been trained to examine the patient's retina with an ophthalmoscope. If swelling is present, red spots will also indicate the presence of bleeding.

Prehospital management consists of treating the symptoms and transporting the patient. As always, assess the ABCDEs to ensure that there are no life threats. Depending on the severity of anxiousness or pain present, the patient may benefit from analgesics or a mild sedative. Vision loss can become permanent if treatment of papilledema does not begin within a few days of this condition's onset;

therefore, immediate treatment should be encouraged. Treatment is aimed at remedying the underlying cause of the ICP increase.

Cellulitis of the Orbit: Periorbital and Orbital Cellulitis

Periorbital and orbital cellulitis are most commonly caused by *Staphylococcus* and *Streptococcus* bacterial infections. The location of the infection determines which type is diagnosed.

Periorbital cellulitis is more prevalent in children than adults. Also known as preseptal cellulitis or eyelid cellulitis, it presents as a painful, red, swollen eyelid. Fever may also be a symptom, along with redness of the white part of the eyes (conjunctivitis). Insect bites, upper respiratory disorders, and trauma increase the patient's risk of developing periorbital cellulitis.

Orbital cellulitis is an infection within the eye socket that is considered a medical emergency because it can lead to permanent vision problems and blindness. The goal of treatment is to avoid the formation of an abscess. Risk factors that predispose individuals to develop orbital cellulitis include **sinusitis**, tooth infections, facial or middle ear infections, trauma, and sinus infections.

Assessment and Management

Prehospital management of cellulitis of the orbit is directed at ruling out life threats, taking a thorough history, and transporting the patient to an appropriate care site. Treatment of children usually consists of intravenous (IV) antibiotics for both forms of cellulitis. Adults are treated with oral antibiotics; however, if symptoms are severe, IV antibiotics may also be used.

Corneal Abrasion or Ulcer

The cornea, the transparent outer covering of the eye, is susceptible to injury and infection because of its location. A corneal abrasion is a common eye injury typically caused by direct trauma, foreign bodies, contact lenses, or exposure to ultraviolet radiation.[10] For example, traumatic corneal abrasions may result from fingernails, makeup applicators, tree branches, hand tools, sports injuries, or deployed air bags. Construction workers and mechanics are susceptible to corneal abrasions from foreign bodies such as pieces of metal, wood, glass, plastic, or fiberglass. Improperly fitted or maintained contact lenses can also cause a corneal abrasion. An ulcer can develop if an abrasion is not treated promptly. A corneal ulcer is always a medical emergency because it can cause blindness if left untreated.

Assessment and Management

Although some patients who have a corneal abrasion will be able to tell you precisely when the event occurred, others will be unable to do so because symptoms may not occur until hours after the injury. Signs and symptoms of corneal abrasion and ulcer include pain with extraocular movement, redness, and excessive tearing. The patient may describe a sensation of having something foreign in the eye, blurred vision or loss of vision, photophobia, and headache.

Prehospital management is directed at ruling out life threats, obtaining a thorough history, and transporting the patient promptly for definitive care.

The Ear

The ear is the primary structure for hearing and balance, but is also integral to self-protection. When you think of ear problems, you most likely think of hearing loss. In reality, hearing is not all the ear affects: The ear also plays an essential part in balance and orientation. Disorders and injury to the ear can leave a person unable to communicate, react, and maintain equilibrium. For example, scuba divers are susceptible to **vertigo** (dizziness) from cold water moving into the ear canal during pressure equalization. This transient vertigo is typically caused when cold water produces unequeal vestibular stimulation within the ear canals during immersion. Changes in air pressure when at levels higher than sea level (eg, in the mountains) and when flying can also cause ear discomfort. A tumor that grows on the eighth cranial nerve (acoustic neuroma) can affect the inner ear and balance. Such a tumor is usually slow growing, but other cranial nerves can be affected if it grows larger, including the fifth, sixth, and seventh cranial nerves. This kind of damage can affect facial sensation, eye movement, facial movement, taste, and hearing.

Loss of hearing is a significant health problem for adults, and is most likely to be associated with occupational noise injury. Hearing loss can affect a child's ability to develop communication, language, and social skills. The earlier children with hearing loss start receiving services, the more likely they are to reach their full potential.

Anatomy and Physiology Review

The ear is divided into three anatomic parts: external, middle, and inner **FIGURE 20-9**. Sound waves travel through the ear, and the internal ear structures form nerve impulses that travel to the brain via the auditory nerve. The brain then converts these impulses into sound.

Special Populations

Hearing loss is a common problem in the older population. With age, changes in the ear structures result in loss of high-frequency hearing or even deafness. If an older patient uses a hearing aid for everyday activity, it is best to keep this device in place to provide better communication during transport to the hospital. Even if the patient sustained an injury while not wearing their hearing aids, providing these devices to the patient will help you achieve a much more accurate assessment.

Consider learning American Sign Language so that you can better communicate with patients who are deaf.

Patient Assessment

Conditions affecting the ears may be due to either medical causes or trauma. Trauma is covered in Chapter 34, *Face and Neck Trauma.*

Foreign objects forced into the auditory canal can damage the eardrum. Ear infections may cause the eardrum to blister and bleed, and inner ear infections can cause excessive pressures to build up behind the eardrum. With rapidly changing altitudes, equalizing pressures can be difficult if the eustachian tubes are clogged from a cold, allergy, or inflammation. When a person moves to a higher altitude, expanding air needs to be released from the inner ear; swallowing and plugging the nose and blowing against a closed glottis can relieve this pressure. Blast pressure waves can burst the eardrum. If the ear damage is due to a blast injury, special considerations are warranted as to approach, staging, and scene safety; these issues are discussed in Chapter 30, *Trauma Systems and Mechanism of Injury.*

As you approach the patient with an ear condition, aside from determining the approximate age, evident sex, environmental conditions, and degree of distress, note whether the patient has a hearing aid. Sometimes patients do not sleep with their hearing aids in, and they may seem confused until you are told by someone else that the patient cannot hear you.

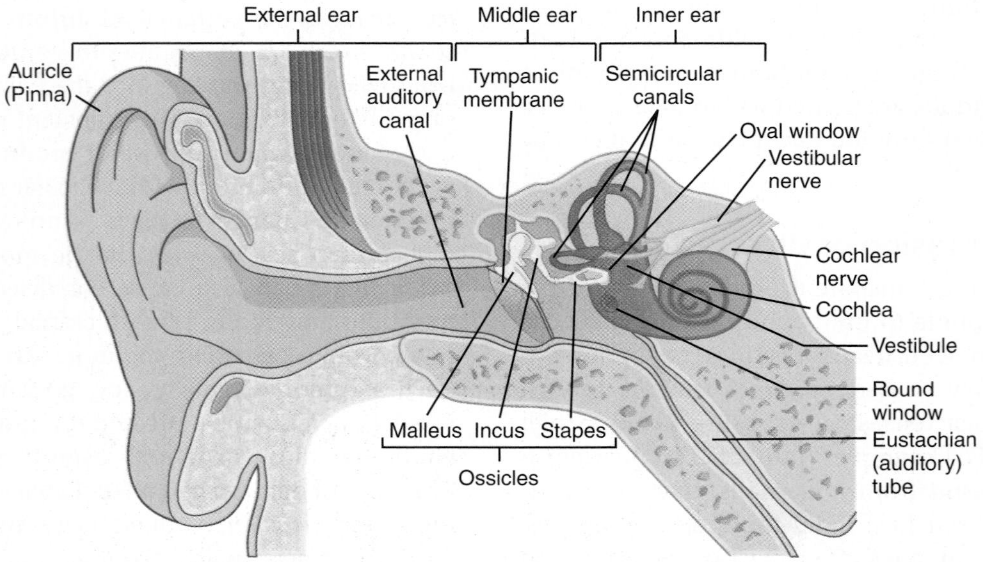

FIGURE 20-9 The structures of the ear.

Assessment and management of the patient with an ear condition begin with ensuring airway patency, assessing for adequate breathing and circulation, and managing any threats to life. Although patients with ear conditions may be in pain or have a hearing deficit, they generally are not considered the highest priority in a triage situation. Typically, medical conditions involving the ears are not life threatening unless the ear condition is a symptom of a much more serious problem (eg, ear damage from a blast injury or head trauma). These patients may be very uncomfortable, but their condition cannot be resolved in the field. Instead, you should transport these patients to the ED, where they can receive the appropriate physical examination, diagnosis, and treatment.

Take a complete history and find out if the patient has had this condition before. Observe the ears for drainage, excess **cerumen** (earwax), and inflammation or swelling. If the patient has pain, ask the patient to quantify it on a pain scale; identify the pain by region and cause. When asking OPQRST assessment questions, "P" (provocation) should include pertinent negatives, such as "Does it hurt when you swallow, sneeze, cough, or bend over?" The history of the events leading up to the complaint can help provide clues to the onset of symptoms. The patient may describe unusual pressure changes with "ear popping," itching in the ears, a recent respiratory infection or cold, or a scuba diving trip. Paramedics will generally treat only the discomfort caused by the symptoms and pass on the history to the treating facility.

Assess for new aberrations in hearing perception. If hearing is affected, changes should be noted and reassessed during transport. Ask the patient if they have experienced **tinnitus** (ringing in one or both ears) or dizziness. Inspect and palpate for wounds, swelling, or drainage (pus, blood, CSF). Often the mastoid process of the skull, which is palpated immediately posterior to the auricle, is assessed for discoloration and tenderness (**Battle sign**).

Words of Wisdom

Pulsatile tinnitus is a condition in which the patient hears a steady whooshing, thumping, or throbbing sound. Atherosclerosis, blood vessel disorders, hypertension, and head and neck tumors are among several possible causes. Transport may be needed to the hospital for imaging procedures and further examination by a physician.

Pathophysiology, Assessment, and Management of Specific Ear Conditions

This section covers specific ear conditions. Ear trauma (specifically, perforated tympanic membrane and foreign body in the ear) is covered in Chapter 34, *Face and Neck Trauma*.

Words of Wisdom

Ear pain is a common problem experienced by airplane travelers. It occurs when pressure builds on the eardrum as a result of changes in atmospheric pressure, which occur with increases or decreases in altitude. In such a case, the pressure is different in the middle ear than outside the ear.

Ear pain can also occur when diving deep under water. Patients often complain of pressure, feeling as if their ear is going to pop, or loss of hearing.

Patients can usually self-manage these feelings by sucking or swallowing (a reflex that is easily activated by chewing gum), which directs airflow from the nose to the ear's eustachian tube and helps balance the pressure. A patient can also be directed to perform a Valsalva maneuver (pinch the nose, blow out with the mouth closed), which helps force air into the eustachian tube. In rare cases, if the symptoms do not resolve and the patient is still experiencing severe pain, transport to the ED for physician evaluation may be needed.

Impacted Cerumen

Cerumen is the yellowish, oily substance found in the outer ear canal. It helps prevent dirt and water from entering the middle ear canal and protects the ear from bacteria or fungi. Cerumen may present as "wet," which is a sticky brown color, or "dry," which consists of a grayish flaky substance. Commonly known as "earwax," cerumen can become impacted and cause pressure against the eardrum. Impaction occurs when too much cerumen builds up and gets stuck in the outer ear canal.

Normally cerumen flows outward, toward the outer ear, and gets washed away. This process helps remove dead skin cells from the ear canal. Cerumen impaction is more common in older adults, in whom hearing aids may block the normal flow. Older adults also tend to produce cerumen that is dry and, therefore, more susceptible to buildup. Other risk factors for impaction include abnormal ear canal shape and diseases that cause more cerumen production, such as keratosis. In addition, improper use of cotton swabs and other hygiene tools or objects can block the flow and cause a cerumen plug.

Assessment and Management

Symptoms of impacted cerumen include the sensation of pressure or fullness in the ear, dizziness, ringing in the ears, loss of hearing, and pain or itching in the ear. Prehospital treatment should include a thorough history and visual inspection of the ear canal. Because an older adult may have many different medical conditions, it may be difficult to rule out other serious problems.

Treatment is aimed at removing the excess cerumen. Do not attempt to extract the material yourself. Rather, a physician will use an otoscope to identify the problem; the physician will then use specially designed tools to remove the wax. Suction and eardrops such as wax softeners may also be used. If left untreated, cerumen impaction can cause infection and irritation that can potentially damage the eardrum and hearing. The process of removing cerumen may also cause injury, so follow-up is necessary after the procedure.

Labyrinthitis

Labyrinthitis is most commonly recognized as the feeling of vertigo or loss of balance after an ear infection or upper respiratory infection. In this condition, irritation and swelling in the inner ear affect the inner ear's nerves and produce a loss of balance. Other symptoms include ringing in the ears (tinnitus), dizziness, temporary loss of hearing, nausea, and vomiting. Permanent hearing loss can occur as well.

Assessment and Management

Severe symptoms of labyrinthitis usually resolve within a week. Prehospital treatment is directed toward reducing the severity of nausea and vomiting and transporting the patient in a position of comfort. The differential diagnoses for vertigo with associated nausea include neurologic disorders such as Ménière disease and acoustic neuroma. These serious disorders will need to be ruled out at the hospital using computed tomography (CT) scan or magnetic resonance imaging (MRI). However, you should be able to recognize the serious implications of the symptoms and suggest the patient be seen at the ED.

Hospital treatment of labyrinthitis includes an antiemetic for nausea and vomiting, an antihistamine to reduce swelling, antivertigo medicine, and diazepam (Valium) as a sedative/muscle relaxant. Prompt treatment of respiratory and ear infections can reduce the risk of labyrinthitis.

Ménière Disease

Ménière disease is a chronic condition of the inner ear characterized by four symptoms that may or may not occur at the same time: (1) dizziness described as spinning vertigo, (2) low-frequency hearing loss, (3) tinnitus, and (4) a feeling of fullness in the affected ear.[11] It usually affects adults older than 50 years, although it can also occur in young children and older adults.

Ménière disease involves the overproduction and defective absorption of endolymphatic fluid, which increases the volume and pressure within the labyrinth of the inner ear until distention results in rupture and mixing of the endolymph and perilymph fluids **FIGURE 20-10**.[12] This mixture disrupts the balance of fluid and electrolytes within the labyrinth and damages the vestibular and cochlear hair cells. What causes the excessive fluid production is unclear; allergies, viral and bacterial infections, head trauma, metabolic disorders, and chronic stress have been suggested as potential causes.

In the early stages of this disease, attacks last less than 2 hours, although altered balance may last up to 2 days. Hearing loss fluctuates, returning to normal between episodes after the rupture heals. As the disease progresses, symptoms last for hours to days, the episodes occur with less warning and become more disabling, and recovery between attacks is incomplete. Permanent tinnitus, moderate to severe hearing loss, and chronic unsteadiness may result.[12]

Assessment and Management

The symptoms of hearing loss, ear pressure, vertigo, dizziness, nausea, and vomiting have many causes, including viral, bacterial, and neurologic causes, among others. In the prehospital setting, care is

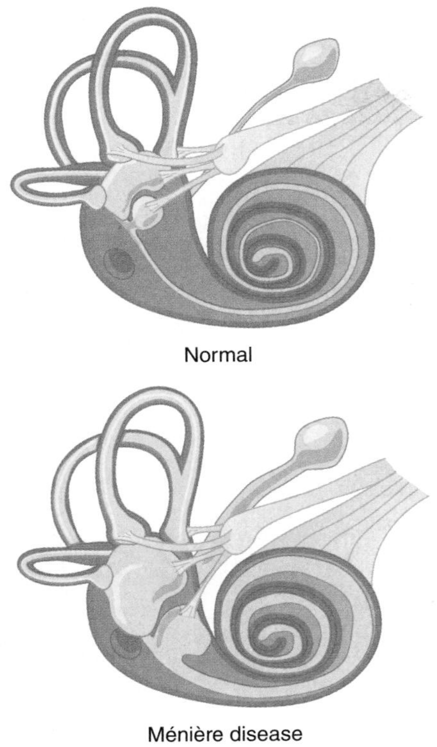

FIGURE 20-10 Ménière disease

focused on treating nausea and vomiting with an antiemetic. In the clinical setting, antiemetics and anticholinergics may be administered during an acute episode to manage symptoms. After diagnosing Ménière disease, the physician may prescribe diuretic medications to reduce the volume of endolymph and restore fluid balance in the inner ear. Some surgical procedures have shown limited success in treating this condition.

Otitis Externa and Media

Otitis is an infection that results from bacterial growth in the ear canal. It can be categorized as either otitis externa or otitis media: infection of the outer and middle ear cavity, respectively. Otitis is more common in children than in adults partially because as humans grow, the angle of the eustachian tube becomes more vertical, allowing it to drain more easily. By comparison, the angle of the eustachian tube in some children is almost horizontal, preventing the tube from adequately draining and allowing infective material to collect there. In children younger than 5 years, otitis media is the most common condition requiring medical intervention.

Otitis externa and otitis media are most commonly caused by bacteria. However, otitis externa can also be an allergic or fungal reaction, and otitis media can be virally induced, developing when sinusitis or **rhinitis** spreads along the eustachian tubes. In addition, auditory canal blockage from excessive cerumen or lack of enough cerumen can lead to bacterial growth that can cause infection.

Assessment and Management

Both otitis externa and otitis media are painful conditions. Allergic or fungal otitis externa may be accompanied by itching, and examination of the external ear canal will show edema and erythema. Patients with otitis media may experience diminished hearing acuity, and examination with an otoscope will reveal an inflamed, bulging tympanic membrane (eardrum). Both disorders are common in children. Before their language abilities develop, children will often indicate such ear pain by pulling at or rubbing the infected ear. In severe cases, the tympanic membrane may tear or rupture, revealing blood in the external ear canal. Untreated infections can cause permanent hearing loss.

Prehospital treatment should be directed at relieving unbearable symptoms. Monitor the patient's condition and administer pain medication when necessary.

The Nose

The nose is subject to increased rates of injury because of its prominent location on the human face. The nose is a filter, humidifier, and heater for the air that enters the body. Allergens, particles, and chemicals can all cause inflammation, infection, and injury to this structure. Because the sinus cavities are located in the forehead and face and drain to the back of the throat, complications from nasal disorders are common. Sinus headaches from pressure, scratchy throat from drainage, and respiratory infection from the aspiration of draining and infected material may all lead to other manifestations and systemic infections. You may encounter many symptoms that began as a nasal infection.

The inside of the nose is highly vascular. Although this characteristic can cause the nasal tissues to bleed, it makes intranasal administration an excellent route for giving some medicines. The intranasal route is also commonly used for delivering drugs of abuse such as cocaine; some abusers literally burn a hole in their nasal septum over time. In addition, the nasal mucosa offers a short route to the brain. The blood–brain barrier can be bypassed through the nasal mucosa, with substances passing through this mucosa and then entering the spinal fluid. Consequently, drug delivery via the intranasal route may proceed more rapidly than IV administration of some medicines.

Another major function of the nose is the ability to smell. Loss of smelling sensation may have many different causes, including aging, smoking, allergies, rhinitis, polyps, the flu, coronavirus disease 2019 (COVID-19), medications, and traumatic brain injury (damage to cranial nerve I [the olfactory nerve]). Types of smelling disorders include anosmia (total loss of sense of smell), dysosmia (distorted sense of smell, in which the person perceives unpleasant odors when the odors do not exist), hyperosmia (increased sensitivity to smell), hyposmia (decreased sense of smell), and presbyosmia (loss of smell from normal aging). Loss of smell also affects a person's sense of taste.

Anatomy and Physiology Review

The nose is one of the two primary entry points for oxygen-rich air to enter the body (the mouth is the other entry point). The nose warms and humidifies the air as it enters the body. It also contains bony structures **FIGURE 20-11** and is connected with the sinuses **FIGURE 20-12**.

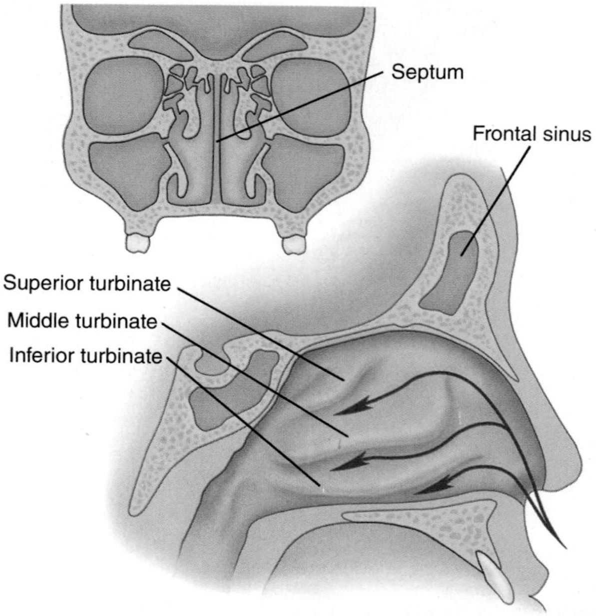

FIGURE 20-11 The nose has two chambers, which are divided by the septum.

YOU are the Paramedic

PART 3

You ask the patient, "Ma'am, what is your medical history? Are you taking any medications? Do you have any allergies?" Instead of answering your questions, she starts coughing up blood. This finding suggests that some blood has flowed from the back of her nose into her oropharynx, which could put her at risk for aspiration if the bleeding is not stopped. The staff explains that the patient has a history of ischemic stroke, high cholesterol, and high BP. She takes Pradaxa (dabigatran etexilate), Prinivil (lisinopril), Microzide (hydrochlorothiazide), and Lipitor (atorvastatin calcium). Her only known allergy is penicillin.

Recording Time: 3 Minutes	
Respirations	18 breaths/min
Pulse	115 beats/min
Skin	Warm, pale oral and eyelid mucous membranes
Blood pressure	98/70 mm Hg
Oxygen saturation (Spo_2)	95% room air
Pupils	Pupils Equal, Round, and Reactive to Light and Accommodation (PERRLA)

5. What do you suspect is wrong with the patient?

6. Do you have additional concerns other than stopping the bleeding?

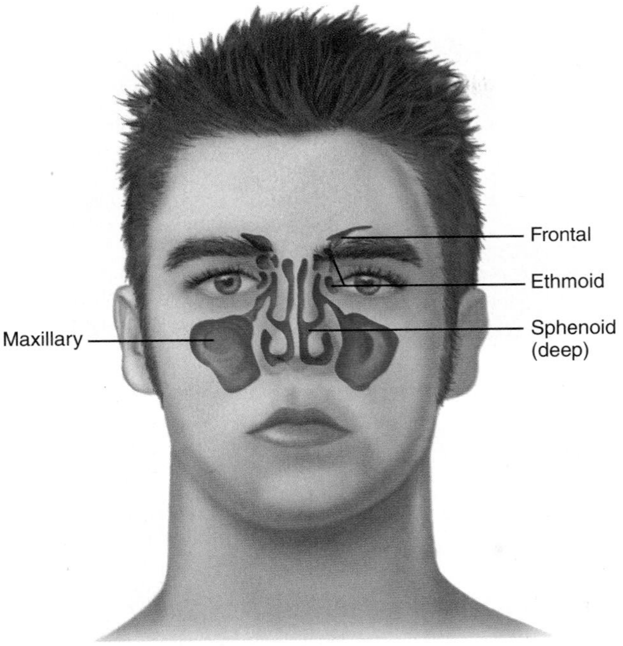

FIGURE 20-12 The paranasal sinuses.

Patient Assessment

A complaint related to the nose that is severe enough to warrant calling 9-1-1 could have several etiologies. The condition of the residence as you approach can give clues to exposure. A factory spewing toxins, the scent of cleaning agents in the hallway, or other unpleasant odors can alert you to possible dangers to you and your crew. Until the seriousness of the problem is known, standard precautions are vital to limit the spread of respiratory infections.

When the scene is determined to be safe for the crew to enter, your first impression of the patient can tell you if airway and breathing are sufficient, and you can note the amount of distress the patient is experiencing. Environmental clues, as well as your own nose, can identify possible irritants. Remember that a sneezing, sniffling, coughing patient easily spreads airborne germs in water droplets.

The vascular nature of the nasal cavities makes them susceptible to bleeding. A severe nosebleed or a condition that blocks the airway with swelling or blood is a life-threatening condition. In such a case, you must determine whether the patient has a general medical condition or if the condition is or could become life threatening.

Insert an airway adjunct as needed to maintain airway patency. However, *do not insert a nasopharyngeal airway or attempt nasotracheal intubation in any patient with suspected nasal fractures or in patients with CSF or blood leakage from the nose.* After establishing and maintaining a patent airway, assess the patient's breathing and intervene appropriately.

Inquire about a previous history of nose conditions or bleeding that needed to be packed and cauterized in the ED. Always consider hypertensive crisis when an older person has a nosebleed.

Pathophysiology, Assessment, and Management of Specific Nose Conditions

Epistaxis

Epistaxis, or nosebleed, is a common problem that can occur spontaneously or from trauma. Common causes of nosebleeds include digital trauma (picking the nose with a finger), which is more common in children; other causes include dry air (as in hot, low-humidity climates or heated indoor spaces) and hypertension. Nosebleeds are further classified into anterior and posterior epistaxis. Anterior nosebleeds are the most common, most typically occurring in the Kiesselbach plexus.[13] This plexus, which is formed by the convergence of branches of the external and internal carotid arteries, supplies an area on the anterior-inferior nasal septum known as Little's area, the most common site for epistaxis.[13] Anterior nosebleeds usually bleed relatively slowly, are usually self-limiting, and resolve quickly. Posterior nosebleeds are usually more severe and often cause blood to drain into the patient's throat, causing nausea and vomiting.

Words of Wisdom

Blood or CSF drainage from the nose (**cerebrospinal rhinorrhea**) suggests a skull fracture. This rare condition is typically found in patients who have sustained head trauma. Do not attempt to control this bleeding; doing so may increase ICP if the patient has a concomitant brain injury. Furthermore, the insertion of nasal airway adjuncts and nasotracheal intubation should be avoided in patients with suspected nasal fractures, especially if rhinorrhea is present. A nasally inserted airway device could enter the cranial vault through an occult fracture (such as a cribriform plate fracture) and penetrate the brain, further worsening the situation.

Assessment and Management

Try to estimate the amount of blood loss and relay this information to the staff at the receiving facility. For example, ask the patient if enough blood was lost to soak a handkerchief, facecloth, or towel and over what period the blood loss occurred.[14] With a non-trauma patient who is bleeding from the nose, you should place the patient in a sitting position, leaning forward with the mouth open over a container so that further blood loss can be estimated, and apply constant, firm pressure over the lower (nonbony) part of the nose for 20 minutes.[14] Alternatively, you may place pressure on the upper gums under the nose, or use a commercial nasal compression clip, if available **FIGURE 20-13**.[14] Direct the patient not to sniffle or blow their nose or to release the pressure too soon to check whether the bleeding has stopped. For a detailed discussion of the care for epistaxis in the context of trauma, see Chapter 31, *Bleeding*.

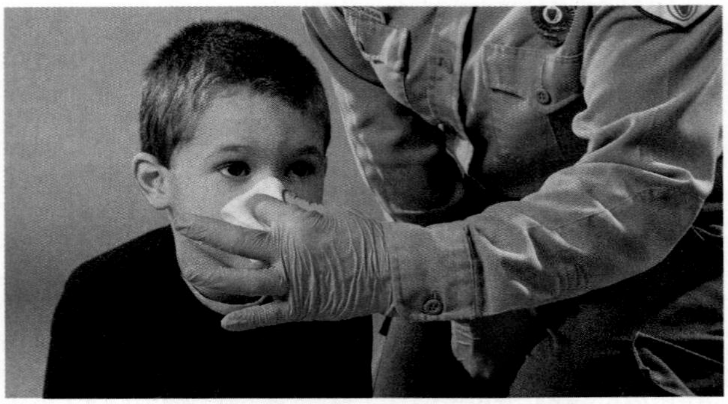

A

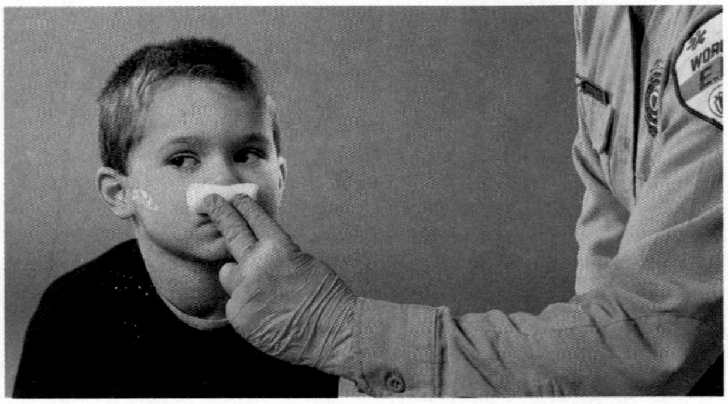

B

FIGURE 20-13 Control bleeding from the nose by one of the following methods: Either pinch the nostrils together **(A)** or apply pressure on the upper gums, beneath the nose, with gloved fingers and gauze **(B)**. If appropriate, take advantage of a teachable moment and have the child pinch their nostrils to control the bleeding. Alternatively, you may control bleeding with a commercial nasal compression clip.

Foreign Body

Foreign bodies in the nose are most likely to be seen in the pediatric population; these items are commonly solid objects, such as beads, stones, marbles, or small pieces of food. Young children have the greatest incidence of exploring their nasal cavities with foreign objects. At age 9 months, a child's grip is sufficient to grasp an object and direct it up one or both nares. Food, toys, rocks, and beads may become lodged or travel to the mouth through the nasopharyngeal cavity. Those objects that make it to the mouth become a risk for inhalation or may become lodged in the esophagus if swallowed. Sometimes these objects can be in place for several days before someone realizes something is wrong; by then, the drainage and smell may have become significant. Objects lodged in the nose can cause other complications as well. For example, pressure in the delicate nasal passage can cause tissue necrosis, inflammation, and swelling; the inflammatory process can cause tissue ulceration and epistaxis; and nasal blockage can lead to sinusitis.

Assessment and Management

In all patients, you must determine if the foreign body presents a life-threatening condition. Nasal foreign bodies are usually visible in the anterior nares, but some may be tucked far enough into the nares that they cannot be seen on visual examination. If you do see the object, only one end of it may be visible; the other end may be lodged in place. Any persistent, foul-smelling, purulent discharge from the nares should lead to suspicion of a foreign body. If you note a discharge from the nose, let it drain, treat it as potentially infective material, and transport the patient. Remember to always use standard precautions.

Transport the patient in the position of comfort, with an emphasis on limiting the risk of gravity moving the object farther into the cavity. Preventing aspiration is a priority. If the object is an extreme irritant, pain management may be necessary. Sedation may be necessary in rare cases. Consultation with medical control is advised.

Rhinitis

Rhinitis, or inflammation of the nasal cavity, is a common nasal disorder that may be caused by a bacterial or viral infection, allergens, medications, or changes in environmental temperature. Acute rhinitis most commonly occurs as a result of a viral infection. It is accompanied by symptoms of the "common cold:" nasal congestion and obstruction, increased nasal drainage, and a diminished sense of smell.[15] Allergic rhinitis may be triggered by allergens such as pollen, grasses, dust mites, or animal dander. Some patients, particularly older adults, experience rhinitis in association with eating or a change in the weather.[15] Rhinitis can also be caused by certain medications (eg, antihypertensive medications), foreign bodies, irritants in the air (eg, smoke, chemicals), and hormonal changes in pregnancy.

Assessment and Management

Signs and symptoms of rhinitis include nasal congestion, sneezing, itchy runny nose, itchy eyes, postnasal drip (which may feel like a tickle in the throat), and possibly cough. Prehospital care for rhinitis is primarily supportive. Keep the patient in Fowler position and provide transport. Physician-directed treatment is aimed at the cause of the rhinitis.

Sinusitis

Sinusitis (sinus inflammation) occurs when drainage from one or more of the sinuses (most often the paranasal sinuses) becomes disrupted, blocking drainage into the nasal cavity. The sinuses, which are normally sterile, then become colonized with nasal bacteria and infection results.[16] As mucus builds up inside the sinus cavity and thickens, pressure increases, causing facial pressure and pain. Sinusitis may be accompanied by a sore throat, nasal congestion, toothache (maxillary sinus), headache (ethmoid sinus), fever, chills, and muscle aches and pains.

Sinusitis affects 28.9 million adult Americans per year, or approximately 12% of the US population, according to the CDC.[17] Young children are especially susceptible to this disease due to their greater frequency of colds. Their smaller nasal air passages easily become clogged, providing the supportive environment necessary for bacterial growth. Older adults are also relatively more likely to experience sinusitis due to their dry nasal passages. Their weaker immune systems, coupled with a diminished cough and gag reflex, make them generally more susceptible to respiratory infections.

Assessment and Management

The duration of the symptoms determines whether sinusitis is characterized as chronic, acute, or recurrent. Prehospital management should include treatment of any respiratory compromise and transport for physician evaluation. Treatment is aimed at reducing inflammation and draining the sinuses.

YOU are the Paramedic

PART 4

Your partner places some gauze and an epistaxis nose clip on the patient, but she pulls on it and says it hurts. You explain that the clip will help control her bleeding, and attempt to calm her down. The patient insists that she cannot breathe with the nose clip on. You suction the patient's mouth and encourage her to breathe through her mouth.

Recording Time: 8 Minutes	
Respirations	24 breaths/min
Pulse	125 beats/min
Skin	Warm, pale oral and eyelid mucous membranes
Blood pressure	99/75 mm Hg
Oxygen saturation (Spo_2)	95% on room air
Pupils	PERRLA

7. Does this patient require any additional airway management?

8. Should you consider starting an IV line on this patient?

Mild to moderate symptoms lasting 7 to 10 days can be treated with a saline rinse and a decongestant. Note that decongestants can dry the nasal passages and delay healing if they are overused. Antibiotics are usually prescribed only after the sinusitis has persisted for 7 to 10 days without relief.

The Throat

Disorders of the pharynx and larynx may represent acute inflammation and infections, chronic inflammation, or abnormal growths. Specific disorders include vocal cord polyps and nodules, contact ulcers, vocal cord paralysis, laryngoceles, laryngeal papillomas, and cancer.

Throat infections (pharyngitis) are particularly common among children, although adults may be affected as well. Causes, symptoms, and treatment are similar in both groups, except that in adults and sexually abused children, gonorrhea (a sexually transmitted infection) may affect the throat.

Throat problems can be exacerbated by swallowing problems (**dysphagia**). Cranial nerves VI, VII, IX, and XII all play a role in swallowing. Neurologic problems associated with stroke or trauma can cause swallowing difficulty. Facial nerve paralysis (cranial nerve VII) can cause unilateral facial and gag reflex paralysis. People who have swallowing difficulty are at increased risk of aspiration pneumonia. This type of pneumonia may occur following the aspiration of vomitus in a patient with an altered mental status resulting from a seizure, drugs, alcohol, anesthesia, acute infection, or shock. It may also occur after the aspiration of a foreign body, or after aspiration of caustic substances such as gasoline. Prehospital care includes maintaining a patent airway, ensuring adequate breathing, close monitoring of vital signs, and prompt transport for definitive care.

Esophageal disorders can also affect the throat. The lower esophageal sphincter keeps the acidic stomach contents from coming back up the throat after swallowing. In the case of esophageal reflux, the lower sphincter only partially closes or opens too often. Symptoms of this condition include a burning sensation in the chest and indigestion. In addition, if the stomach acids come up the throat and reach the vocal cords, voice tone may change from inflammation and swelling. This phenomenon can cause a precancerous condition from tissue scarring in the esophagus.

Anatomy and Physiology Review

Your assessment of the patient's throat begins at the opening of the mouth with the teeth **FIGURE 20-14**. The hypoglossal, glossopharyngeal, trigeminal, and facial nerves supply the mouth and its structures **FIGURE 20-15**.

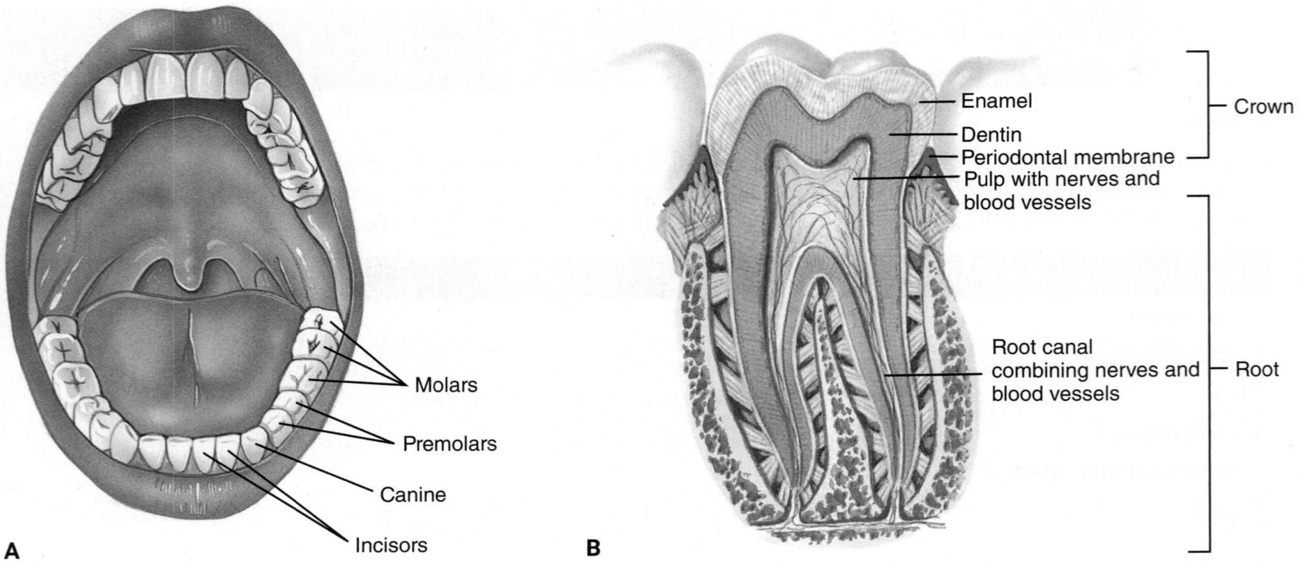

FIGURE 20-14 The teeth of the adult mouth. **A.** The incisors are used for biting. The canines are used for tearing food. The premolars and molars are used for grinding and crushing. **B.** Each tooth contains nerves and blood vessels.

The Neck

The principal structures of the anterior part of the neck include the thyroid and cricoid cartilage, trachea, and numerous muscles and nerves **FIGURE 20-16**. The major blood vessels in this area are the internal and external carotid arteries **FIGURE 20-17** and the internal and external jugular veins **FIGURE 20-18**. The vertebral arteries run laterally to the cervical vertebrae in the posterior part of the neck.

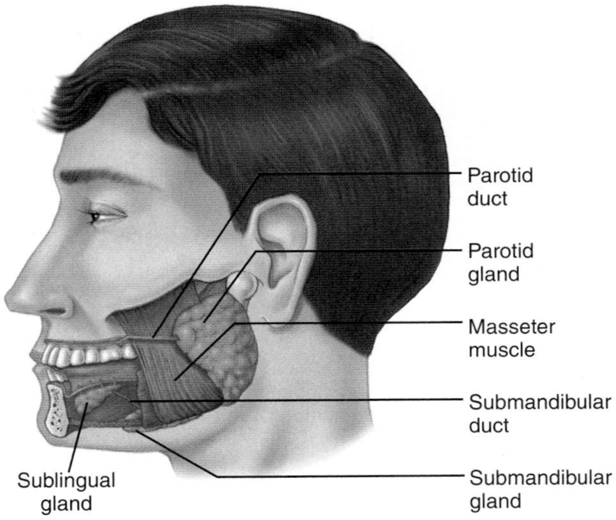

FIGURE 20-15 The glands and muscles of the mouth.

Patient Assessment

Patients with swallowing abnormalities or copious mucus production should be placed in a position to allow drainage. A lateral recumbent position or recovery position will allow mouth drainage and help protect the airway. Patients who have experienced a stroke may not be able to swallow as a result of neurologic deficit. Assessment of these patients must include early recognition of threats to their airway. When patients cannot protect their airways and are at risk for aspiration into the lungs, intubation should be considered.

Medical problems of the mouth, neck, and throat can seriously affect breathing. Consider epiglottitis as a possible cause if the patient's symptoms include sore throat, fever, drooling, and a head that is hung forward.

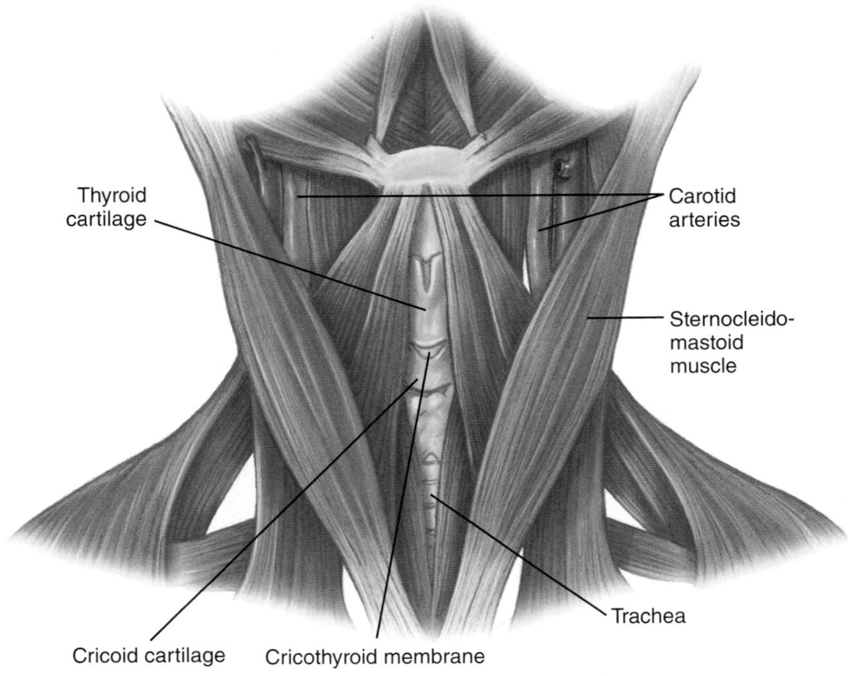

FIGURE 20-16 Anatomy of the anterior part of the neck.

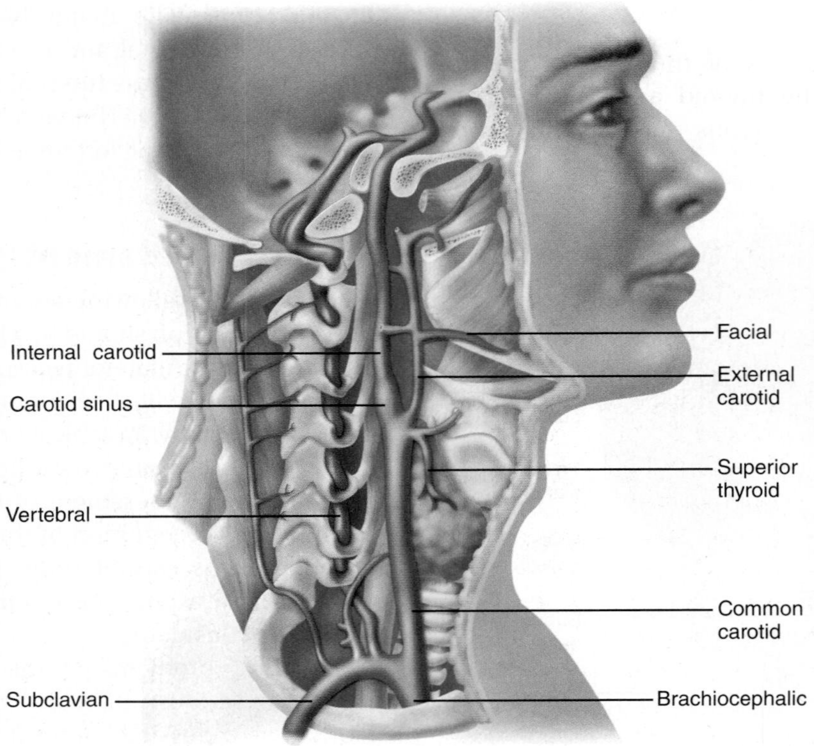

FIGURE 20-17 The arteries of the neck.

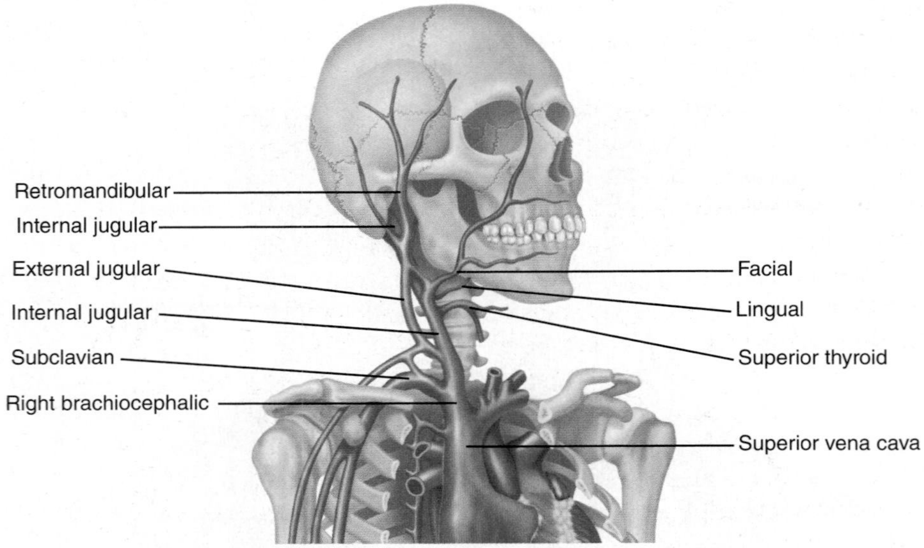

FIGURE 20-18 The veins of the neck.

Pathophysiology, Assessment, and Management of Specific Throat Conditions

This section covers specific throat conditions. Throat trauma (specifically, foreign body in the throat) is covered in Chapter 34, *Face and Neck Trauma*.

Dentalgia and Dental Abscess

Dentalgia or "toothache" can be the starting point for the development of a dental abscess. A cavity in a tooth harbors bacteria, resulting in rapid decay of the tooth. The tooth's integrity is eventually compromised, giving access to the tooth root and nerve, which can cause inflammation, swelling, and intense pain.

A **dental abscess** occurs when the bacteria growth spreads directly from the cavity into the gums, facial tissue, bones, and/or neck **FIGURE 20-19**. The pain is relieved somewhat when the abscess ruptures and drains pus, reducing the swelling. An abscess may have to be drained surgically.

Assessment and Management

If fever, chills, nausea, and vomiting are part of the dental abscess symptoms, the infection may have become systemic. In this case, a physician will prescribe antibiotics. An abscess in the throat, in the neck, or under the tongue can affect the ability to breathe, a true emergency condition. Depending on the abscess location, it may have to be surgically drained under anesthesia in the operating room.

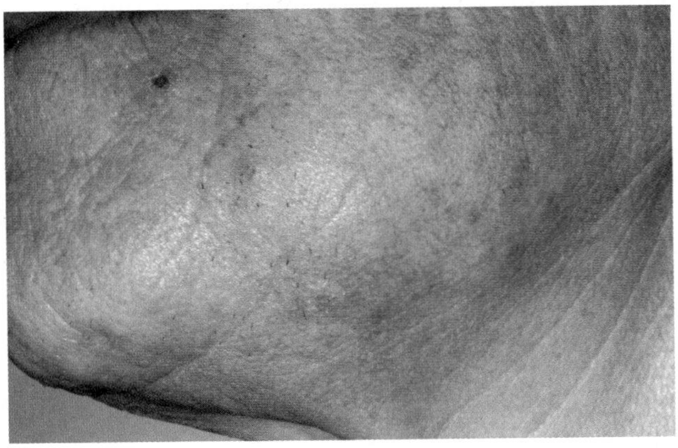

FIGURE 20-19 A dental abscess.

Prehospital treatment of a dental abscess or dentalgia is mostly aimed at relieving the symptoms. For example, the patient may take over-the-counter NSAIDs for relief of pain and inflammation. Any rupture and drainage of an abscess into the mouth should be rinsed with warm water.

Progression of the infection into the bone and surrounding tissue can have serious complications. For this reason, you should encourage patients to accept transport to an appropriate facility for further treatment.

Diseases of Oral Soft Tissue

Diseases of the soft tissues of the mouth can be the root causes of other health problems. For example, gum disease has been linked to heart disease, stroke, diabetes, osteoporosis, and low–birth-weight babies. Infective endocarditis, which affects the lining of the heart and heart valves, can be linked directly to a tooth infection and gum disease. The condition of the mouth reflects the condition of the human body. Indeed, many diseases affecting the human body may have oral manifestations, and a good dental examination may find these potential diseases in their early stages.[18] For example, diabetes, leukemia, cancer, heart disease, and kidney disease may manifest with mouth ulcers, swollen gums, and dry mouth. Poor oral health also affects the digestive system and may be a cause of irritable bowel syndrome.

Common mouth disorders include the following conditions:

- **Cold sores.** Painful sores on the lips and around the mouth caused by a type of herpesvirus.
- **Canker sores.** Shallow, painful ulcers in the mouth caused by stress or trauma (eg, braces, hot food, rough denture).
- **Oral candidiasis (thrush).** A yeast infection that causes white patches on the oral mucosa involving the mouth, tongue, palate, gums, and sometimes the throat (discussed further in Chapter 27, *Infectious Diseases*).
- **Leukoplakia.** Excess cell growth in the mouth, cheek, or gums that presents as white patches; it usually results from chronic irritation such

as that from tobacco smoke, chewing tobacco, cheek biting, or ill-fitting dentures.
- **Gingivitis.** Red swollen gums that bleed easily during brushing.
- **Bad breath.** Usually linked to impacted plaque and poor oral hygiene. Bacteria release sulfur compounds that account for the foul smell. A bowel obstruction can cause breath that smells like feces. Breath odor that smells of urine or that smells "fishy" may be caused by chronic renal failure.

Assessment and Management

Sores and diseases of the mouth can be embarrassing to the patient. Consequently, the patient may not want to tell you about them. Be sure to rule out urticaria and allergic reactions when assessing lumps and sores of the mouth.

Oral Candidiasis

More commonly called "thrush," **oral candidiasis** is a condition in which the fungus *Candida albicans* accumulates on the lining of the mouth. When a patient has oral thrush, creamy white lesions will appear on the tongue and inner cheeks that can spread to the roof of the mouth, gums, tonsils, or posterior pharynx **FIGURE 20-20**. These lesions may be painful and bleed if they are rubbed or scraped.

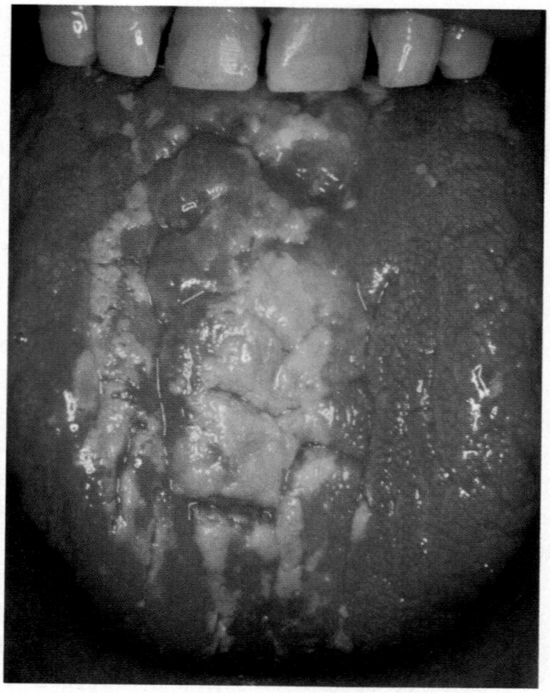

FIGURE 20-20 Oral candidiasis (thrush).

Assessment and Management

Thrush is most likely to be found in infants, patients with compromised immune systems, patients who wear dentures, and patients who use inhaled corticosteroids (eg, prednisone). In addition to the white lesions and slight bleeding, signs and symptoms of thrush include pain, cracking, and redness at the corners of the mouth, and a loss of taste. Patients often describe a "cottony" feeling in the mouth. In severe cases, the lesions can spread down the esophagus, causing the sensation that food is getting stuck in the throat when swallowing. Patients with a medical history of human immunodeficiency virus (HIV)/acquired immunodeficiency syndrome (AIDS), cancer, diabetes, and vaginal yeast infections are more likely to develop thrush.

Oral candidiasis is not a condition that requires paramedic care aside from treating higher priorities, making the patient comfortable, and encouraging the patient to follow up with a physician. You are likely to encounter patients with thrush when treating or transporting immune-deficient patients under physician care for the conditions mentioned earlier.

Ludwig Angina

Ludwig angina is a type of cellulitis caused by bacteria from an infected tooth root (tooth abscess) or mouth injury. It occurs on the floor of the mouth under the tongue. Because of the swelling associated with this infection, which may have a rapid onset, an airway obstruction may occur. A physical exam may show redness and swelling of the neck or under the chin. The tongue may also be swollen. In severe cases, the swelling caused by Ludwig angina is a potential life threat. You may have to insert an artificial airway through the nasal passages to avoid the affected and swollen tissue, and a tracheostomy may have to be surgically performed to adequately ventilate these patients. The abscess may also have to be surgically drained.

Assessment and Management

Symptoms of Ludwig angina may include difficulty breathing, difficulty swallowing, neck pain, neck swelling, fever, drooling, and altered speech sounds. Prehospital treatment requires aggressive management of the patient's airway in severe cases. Early treatment with steroids may slow the inflammatory process and reduce swelling. Early contact with a medical control physician is essential to determine your management options. Treatment may include dental surgery to repair the source of the infection at the tooth root.

Ludwig angina is painful and frightening for the patient because symptoms may develop rapidly. Remain calm and organized as you attend to the patient's ABCDEs while formulating a plan for aggressive airway management. Pay careful attention to the patient's condition and smells originating in the mouth to alert you to other disease processes that may be in progress.

Epiglottitis

Epiglottitis is an inflammation of the epiglottis (the flap at the base of the tongue that covers the trachea). As the epiglottis swells, it may begin to block the trachea and obstruct the airway. In the past, epiglottitis most commonly arose in pediatric patients (ages 1 to 5 years), but today it occurs more often in adults who did not receive inoculation for this disease. Because it often results from infection with the *Haemophilus influenzae* type b virus, this disease's incidence has decreased over time with widespread adoption of the Hib vaccine.

Assessment and Management

Patients with epiglottitis experience fever, sore throat, painful swallowing (dysphagia), stridor, and respiratory distress. A patient with epiglottitis looks sick and will be anxious, will sit upright in the classic "tripod" position or in the sniffing position with the chin thrust forward to allow for maximal air entry, and is often drooling because of an inability to swallow secretions. Work of breathing is increased, and skin color consistent with hypoxia may be present.

Transport a patient with suspected epiglottitis to an appropriate hospital while maintaining the patient's airway. Because this rapidly progressive disease carries a risk for acute airway obstruction and respiratory arrest, you should minimize your on-scene time and not attempt procedures that might agitate the patient. Remember not to attempt to look in the mouth, as doing so can precipitate complete airway obstruction. Alert personnel at the receiving facility to the suspected diagnosis and the patient's condition because they will need to mobilize a team to manage this difficult airway.

Laryngitis

Swelling and inflammation of the larynx are associated with hoarseness or loss of voice. These conditions can be the result of overuse, such that the vocal cords and larynx become inflamed, causing hoarseness. The most common form of **laryngitis** is caused by a virus, similar to the cold or flu, but it can also be caused by pneumonia, irritants and chemicals, gastroesophageal reflux disease (GERD), bronchitis, allergies, and bacterial infection. Typically laryngitis is not serious unless it leads to epiglottitis or croup; these conditions are covered in further depth in Chapter 44, *Pediatric Emergencies*.

Assessment and Management

A patient with laryngitis will present with fever, hoarseness, and swollen lymph nodes or glands in the neck. Obtain a good history to rule out evolving upper airway obstruction or an allergic reaction. A patient who speaks in a quiet tone and has a raspy voice may have sustained a hyoid bone fracture from a blow to the anterior neck. Otherwise, laryngitis is typically a symptom of an ongoing upper respiratory infection, and the patient should follow up with a physician.

Tracheitis

Tracheitis is an infection of the trachea, typically caused by *Staphylococcus aureus*. This condition frequently occurs in young children following a recent viral upper respiratory infection. In small children, the trachea is easily blocked by swelling, so this can be a life-threatening condition.

Assessment and Management

The symptoms of tracheitis include a deep "croup-like" (barking) cough, difficulty breathing, high fever, and high-pitched stridor with breathing. As the illness progresses, the child may exhibit tripod positioning and intercostal retractions. This condition can proceed from respiratory distress to respiratory failure if not managed quickly.

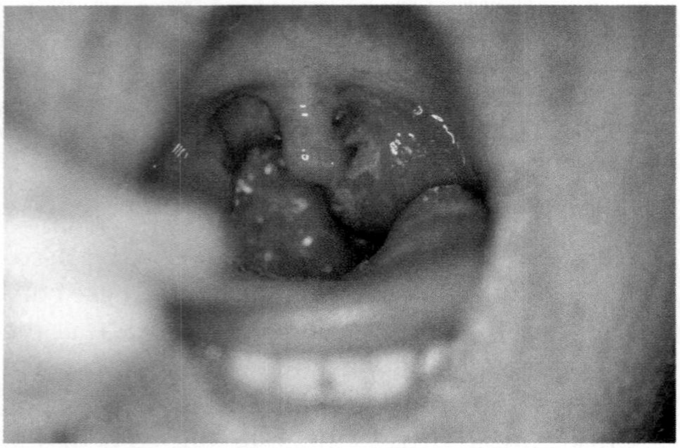

FIGURE 20-21 Tonsillitis.

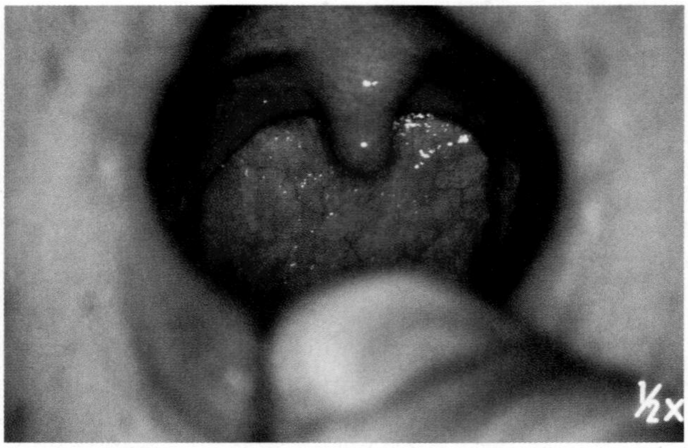

FIGURE 20-22 Pharyngitis.

Prehospital care is supportive, focusing on minimizing stress to the child and administering 100% oxygen. Use pulse oximetry and monitor vital signs en route. Be prepared for a difficult intubation and have the correct size of endotracheal (ET) tube and the next smaller size available. Transport the child as soon as possible to a facility capable of handling critically ill children.

Tonsillitis

Tonsillitis is swelling and inflammation of the tonsils, the two oval-shaped pads of tissue at the back of the throat **FIGURE 20-21**. Most cases of tonsillitis are caused by viral infections, although this condition may be caused by bacterial infections as well. As the tonsils become inflamed, they swell and cause difficulty swallowing.

Assessment and Management

The symptoms of tonsillitis include swollen tonsils, a sore throat, and difficulty swallowing. Patients will have red, swollen tonsils; white or yellow coating or patches on the tonsils; a fever; and a sore throat. Patients may also present with pain when swallowing, enlarged and tender lymph nodes in the neck, bad breath, headache, and a stiff neck. In severe cases, drooling indicates difficulty swallowing.

In the past, surgery to remove the tonsils was a common treatment for tonsillitis, but today this procedure is reserved for patients who have frequent bouts of tonsillitis that do not respond to drugs. Serious cases involving partial airway obstruction are also an indication for surgery. You should transport all patients with suspected tonsillitis to the ED for further evaluation.

Pharyngitis

Pharyngitis is an inflammation of the pharynx, the area at the back of the throat between the tonsils and the larynx **FIGURE 20-22**. Pharyngitis is often due to a rapid onset of sore throat with discomfort or pain on swallowing.

Assessment and Management

Symptoms of pharyngitis include a fever; pharyngeal erythema; headache; purulent, patchy yellow, gray, or white exudate; nasal congestion; hoarseness; cough; and ulcers on the soft palate.

When caring for a patient who is having difficulty swallowing, your priority in the prehospital setting is assessing for partial airway obstruction. Treatment involves follow-up in the ED, where the patient can be examined further and cultures can be obtained to assess for streptococcal infection; a decision will also be made regarding the use of antibiotics.

Peritonsillar Abscess

Peritonsillar abscess is a collection of infected material around one or both tonsils **FIGURE 20-23**. A complication of tonsillitis, it is most often caused by bacterial infection. Although this condition is usually found in older children and young adults, it has become relatively rare today due to the use of antibiotics to treat tonsillitis.

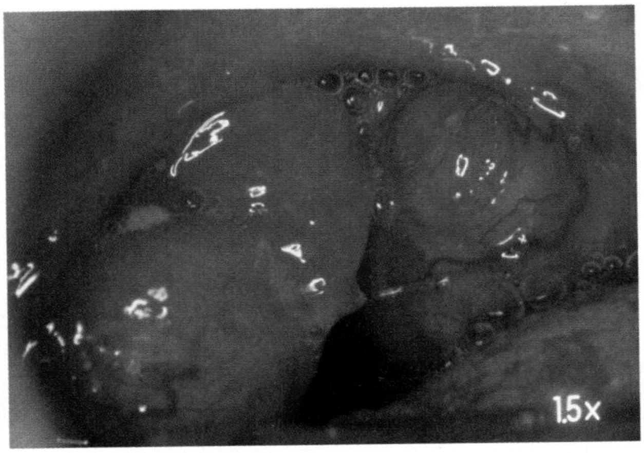

FIGURE 20-23 Peritonsillar abscess.

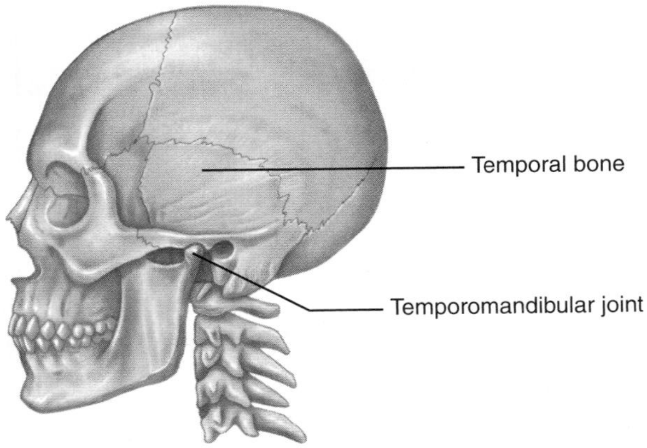

FIGURE 20-24 The temporomandibular joint articulates the mandible with the temporal bone.

Assessment and Management

With peritonsillar abscess, one or both tonsils are infected, and the roof of the mouth and the neck or chest may also be affected. The patient may have chills, difficulty opening the mouth, and pain when opening the mouth. Facial swelling, fever, drooling or inability to swallow saliva, headache, muffled voice, sore throat (usually on one side), and tender glands of the jaw and throat can develop.

Treatment involves administering antibiotics and draining the abscess. It may also include a tonsillectomy, so it is essential to take these patients to the hospital. In some cases, a peritonsillar abscess could be life threatening if the swollen tissues block the airway.

Temporomandibular Joint Disorders

The mandible is the large bone that forms the lower jaw and contains the lower teeth. Numerous muscles of chewing attach to the mandible and its rami. The posterior condyle of the mandible articulates with the temporal bone at the temporomandibular joint (TMJ), allowing movement of the mandible **FIGURE 20-24**. The actions of the TMJ allow a person to talk, chew, and yawn. When patients report jaw pain, clicking when they "jut" their jaw, or headaches, they often have been diagnosed, or may soon be, with a **temporomandibular joint (TMJ) disorder**.

Causes of TMJ disorders include arthritis-related damage to the joint's cartilage, jaw injury, and jaw muscle fatigue from grinding or clenching of the teeth, especially during sleep. The disk can erode or move out of its proper alignment, leading to TMJ disorder.

Assessment and Management

The symptoms of TMJ disorders include headache, jaw pain, aching around the ear, an uneven or painful bite, difficulty chewing, and locking of the joint that causes difficulty either opening or closing the mouth. Over-the-counter pain medications are used to manage symptoms. In severe cases, TMJ disorders may require dental or surgical intervention. As a paramedic, you should be aware of TMJ disorders, the symptoms they cause, and the fact that the patient's physician or dentist usually manages these conditions.

YOU are the Paramedic SUMMARY

1. What is your primary concern after scene safety is established?

The patient appears ill. She is bleeding profusely from the nose, and the bleeding needs to be controlled.

2. Do you have concerns other than the nose bleed?

Because the nose is part of the airway system, attention must be given to ensure the bleeding is not affecting the patient's ability to maintain a patent airway and breathe adequately. Remember the "A" (airway) and "B" (breathing) components of the ABCDEs, even though the bleeding is the most obvious sign.

3. What do you need to know about the patient's history?

Immediate thoughts about the patient's medical history should include questions about whether she has a history of nose bleeds, and if so, how the current incident compares to previous episodes. You should also seek to determine whether she has any associated medical conditions or takes any medications that could cause epistaxis or make it worse.

4. What is the priority in managing this patient?

In this patient, the priorities are managing the ABCDEs. Exerting immediate pressure by squeezing the nose and instructing the patient to lean forward to help reduce blood from going backward down into her mouth and near her airway are important. Other important priorities include continual assessment of the airway and suctioning to remove any blood from the mouth. In addition, assessing lung sounds and breathing to ensure the patient is not aspirating blood is important.

5. What do you suspect is wrong with the patient?

This patient has classic signs of epistaxis. While the cause appears to be nontraumatic and unknown, the fact that the patient is taking a blood thinner (Pradaxa) will make it more challenging to stop the bleeding in the field. In the ED, the patient may require medications or procedures to control the bleeding. Your efforts should focus on reducing the bleeding and protecting the patient's airway and breathing from aspiration.

6. Do you have additional concerns other than stopping the bleeding?

In tandem with stopping the bleeding, the primary concern with this patient will be suctioning and protecting the airway from aspiration of blood. Her history of hypertension and history of taking Pradaxa, which can cause bleeding, are additional concerns in this patient, as she is now borderline hypotensive. Given the amount of blood loss and ongoing bleeding, you should continue to assess the patient's vital signs, monitor for any signs or symptoms of hemorrhagic shock, and treat the patient accordingly if needed.

7. Does this patient require any additional airway management?

Given what you know here, this scenario does not clearly warrant any advanced airway procedures. As long as you can get the patient to lean forward and you can control the bleeding by pinching the patient's nose, keeping suction available and using it as needed, along with (perhaps) administering blow-by oxygen, should be sufficient. However, if the patient becomes unable to sit up or loses consciousness, rapid sequence intubation might be appropriate as a means to protect the airway from aspiration of blood.

8. Should you consider starting an IV on this patient?

If you can stop the bleeding and the patient's systolic BP remains greater than 90 mm Hg, an IV line is unnecessary unless other signs and symptoms of shock are present. Any risk of shock or a decline in BP would indicate the need for an IV line and fluid bolus. Establishing a saline lock as a precaution would be appropriate, as permitted by protocol. If you decide a fluid bolus is necessary to maintain a perfusing BP, keep in mind that letting the pressure rise too high may inhibit your ability to stop the bleeding or may cause any clots that have formed to dissolve or become dislodged, such that the bleeding will continue.

YOU are the Paramedic SUMMARY continued

EMS Patient Care Report (PCR)					
Date: 11-10-22	**Incident No.:** 99722	**Nature of Call:** Epistaxis		**Location:** Sunshine Acute Rehab Center	
Dispatched: 1218	**En Route:** 1220	**At Scene:** 1230	**Transport:** 1245	**At Hospital:** 1250	**In Service:** 1305

Patient Information	
Age: 62 **Sex:** F **Weight (in kg [lb]):** 69 kg (150 lb)	**Allergies:** Penicillin **Medications:** Lisinopril, hydrochlorothiazide, dabigatran etexilate, and atorvastatin calcium **Past Medical History:** HTN, high cholesterol, and history of ischemic stroke **Chief Complaint:** Severe nose bleed

Vital Signs				
Time: 1233	**BP:** 98/70	**Pulse:** 115	**Respirations:** 18	**Spo_2:** 95% RA
Time: 1238	**BP:** 99/75	**Pulse:** 125	**Respirations:** 24	**Spo_2:** 95% RA
Time: 1247	**BP:** 102/85	**Pulse:** 120	**Respirations:** 20	**Spo_2:** 95% RA

EMS Treatment (circle all that apply)				
Oxygen @ _____ L/min via (circle one): **NC NRM Bag-mask device**		**Assisted Ventilation**	**Airway Adjunct**	**CPR**
Defibrillation	**Bleeding Control**	**Bandaging**	**Splinting**	**Other:**

Narrative

Arrived to find 62 y/o F sitting at a lunch table in extended-care facility dining room with epistaxis. Blood was noted on a table and on a towel the care staff had been applying to patient's nose. We assumed care, applied gauze, pinched the patient's nose closed, and instructed her to lean forward. Patient's oral cavity was suctioned and breathing assessed. Patient vitals and medical history obtained. Patient assisted to cot, placed in upright position, and moved to truck. IV saline lock placed in patient's left forearm. Continued to assess airway, breathing, circulation, and vitals as noted en route. Report called to University Medical Center. Pt had no change during transport. Report and care transferred to Betty, RN, on arrival and patient left in ED bed 15.

End of report

Prep Kit

Ready for Review

- A patient may call EMS with an emergency related to a disorder of the eye, ear, nose, or throat, or paramedics may encounter patients with these disorders while assessing an unrelated emergency. Paramedics should be familiar with these important structures and the diseases that affect them.
- Be sure to assess for pain or tenderness, swelling, abnormal or loss of movement, sensation changes, circulatory changes, deformity, visual changes, and airway compromise. Obtain a thorough history of eye conditions, including how and when the symptoms began and which symptoms the

Prep Kit continued

patient is experiencing, whether both eyes are affected, if the patient has any underlying diseases or conditions of the eye (such as glaucoma), and if the patient takes eye medications.

- An early transport decision to the right facility can improve the outcome for a patient with eye disease. Consider transport to a Level 1 trauma center, which has the skilled services necessary to treat a serious eye problem. Consider pain management and, if necessary, mild sedation during transport.
- Remember to provide emotional care to patients with eye disorders. Fear and panic from loss of vision can cause dangerous and bizarre behavior. Keep the patient calm. The scene size-up is an opportunity to discover clues to the cause of the complaint while avoiding potential hazards.
- Specific medical conditions of the eye include conjunctivitis, inflammation of the eyelid, glaucoma, central retinal artery occlusion, iritis, papilledema, cellulitis of the orbit, and corneal abrasion or ulcer. Become familiar with these conditions so that you can recognize them in the field and transport the patient as needed.
- The ear is the primary structure for hearing and balance. Disorders and injury of the ear can leave a person unable to communicate, react, and maintain equilibrium. The patient will require transport to receive a complete assessment of the external ear canal and middle ear.
- Specific medical conditions of the ear include impacted cerumen, labyrinthitis, Ménière disease, and otitis.
- The nose is a highly vascular structure, which contains nasal mucosa that provides a short route to the brain.
- Never insert a nasopharyngeal airway or attempt nasotracheal intubation in any patient with suspected nasal fractures or in a patient with CSF or blood leakage from the nose.
- Specific medical problems related to the nose include epistaxis, foreign body obstruction, rhinitis, and sinusitis. Treatment of epistaxis focuses on controlling the bleeding. Treatment for foreign body obstruction is to transport the patient.
- Disorders of the throat (pharynx and larynx) may represent acute inflammation and infections, chronic inflammation, or abnormal growths. Specific disorders include vocal cord polyps and nodules, contact ulcers, vocal cord paralysis, laryngoceles, laryngeal papillomas, and cancer. Throat infections are particularly common among children, although adults may be affected as well.
- When you are assessing a patient with a throat complaint, note whether the patient is able to swallow. If not, position the patient to allow drainage. Be sure to assess for threats to the airway and breathing.
- The principal structures of the anterior part of the neck include the thyroid and cricoid cartilage, trachea, and numerous muscles and nerves. Specific medical disorders related to the throat include dentalgia, dental abscess, oral soft tissue diseases, oral candidiasis, Ludwig angina, epiglottitis, laryngitis, tracheitis, pharyngitis/tonsillitis, peritonsillar abscess, and temporomandibular joint disorders.

Vital Vocabulary

anisocoria A condition in which the pupils are not of equal size.

Battle sign Bruising over the mastoid bone behind the ear, commonly seen following a basilar skull fracture; also called retroauricular ecchymosis.

cataract A clouding of the lens of the eye that is normally a result of aging.

Prep Kit continued

cerebrospinal rhinorrhea Blood or cerebrospinal fluid drainage from the nose.

cerumen Earwax.

chalazion A small, usually painless lump or pustule on the external eyelid that appears red and swollen, and that forms because of blockage and swelling of an oil gland in the eyelid.

conjunctivitis An inflammation of the conjunctivae of the eye that usually is caused by bacteria, viruses, allergies, or foreign bodies; it should be considered highly contagious. Also called pink eye.

dental abscess A dental infection that occurs when bacterial growth spreads directly from the cavity into the gums, facial tissue, bones, and/or neck.

dentalgia Toothache.

diabetic retinopathy A condition associated with diabetes, in which the small blood vessels of the retina are affected; it can eventually lead to blindness.

dysconjugate gaze Paralysis of gaze or discoordination between the movements of the two eyes.

dysphagia Pain, discomfort, or difficulty in swallowing.

epiglottitis An inflammation of the epiglottis.

epistaxis Nosebleed.

glaucoma A group of conditions that lead to increased intraocular pressure, causing damage to the optic nerve; a leading cause of blindness.

hordeolum A red tender lump in the eyelid or at the lid margin; commonly known as a stye.

iritis Inflammation of the iris; also called anterior uveitis.

labyrinthitis Irritation and swelling in the inner ear that produce a loss of balance and possibly tinnitus, dizziness, temporary loss of hearing, nausea, and vomiting.

laryngitis Swelling and inflammation of the larynx that is associated with hoarseness or loss of voice.

Ludwig angina A type of cellulitis that occurs on the floor of the mouth under the tongue; it is caused by bacteria from an infected tooth root (tooth abscess) or mouth injury.

Ménière disease A chronic condition of the inner ear characterized by four symptoms that may or may not occur at the same time: (1) dizziness described as spinning vertigo, (2) low-frequency hearing loss, (3) tinnitus, and (4) a feeling of fullness in the affected ear.

oculomotor nerve Third cranial nerve; innervates the muscles that cause eye movement as well as the parasympathetic nerve fibers that cause constriction of the pupil and accommodation of the lens.

optic nerve Either of the second cranial nerves that enter the eyeball posteriorly, through the optic foramen.

oral candidiasis A condition that presents as creamy white lesions on the tongue and inner cheeks, caused by the fungus *Candida albicans*; also called thrush.

orbital cellulitis An infection within the eye socket.

otitis An infection of either the outer or middle ear cavity.

papilledema An eye condition that results from swelling or inflammation of the optic nerve at the rear part of the eye; symptoms include headaches, nausea with possible vomiting, temporary vision loss, or narrowing vision fields.

periorbital cellulitis An infection of the eyelid; also known as preseptal cellulitis or eyelid cellulitis.

peritonsillar abscess A collection of infected material around the tonsils.

pharyngitis Inflammation of the pharynx.

rhinitis A nasal disorder generally caused by bacterial or viral infection, allergens, medications, or changes in environmental temperature.

sinusitis An infection of the sinuses, characterized by thick nasal discharge, sinus and facial pressure, headache, and fever.

Prep Kit continued

temporomandibular joint (TMJ) disorder A collection of disorders that present with jaw pain, and that occur when the connection between the temporal bone and the TMJ erodes or moves out of proper alignment.

tinnitus The perception of sound in the inner ear with no external environmental cause; often reported as "ringing" in one or both ears, but may be roaring, buzzing, or clicking.

tonsillitis Swelling and inflammation of the tonsils.

tracheitis An infection of the trachea, typically caused by the bacterium *Staphylococcus aureus*.

vertigo A type of dizziness in which a person experiences the sensation of movement when standing still or of the environment moving; often due to an inner ear disorder.

References

1. Eye health statistics. American Academy of Ophthalmology website. https://www.aao.org/newsroom/eye-health-statistics. Accessed February 26, 2021.
2. Fast facts. Centers for Disease Control and Prevention, Vision Health Initiative website. https://www.cdc.gov/visionhealth/basics/ced/fastfacts.htm. Accessed February 26, 2021.
3. Common eye disorders and diseases. Centers for Disease Control and Prevention, Vision Health Initiative website. http://www.cdc.gov/visionhealth/basics/ced/index.html. Accessed February 27, 2021.
4. Diabetic retinopathy. National Eye Institute website. https://www.nei.nih.gov/learn-about-eye-health/eye-conditions-and-diseases/diabetic-retinopathy. Updated November 19, 2020. Accessed February 27, 2021.
5. What is anisocoria? American Association for Pediatric Ophthalmology and Strabismus website. https://aapos.org/glossary/anisocoria-and-horners-syndrome. Accessed February 27, 2021.
6. Conjunctivitis (pink eye) transmission. Centers for Disease Control and Prevention website. https://www.cdc.gov/conjunctivitis/about/transmission.html. Reviewed January 4, 2019. Accessed February 27, 2021.
7. Rizzo DC. The nervous system: the brain, cranial nerves, autonomic nervous system, and the special senses. In: *Fundamentals of Anatomy and Physiology*. 4th ed. Boston, MA: Cengage Learning; 2016:250-277.
8. Haine CL. The ophthalmic case historian. In: Benjamin WJ, ed. *Borish's Clinical Refraction*. 2nd ed. St. Louis, MO: Butterworth Heinemann; 2006:195-216.
9. Santos M, Hofmann RJ. Ocular manifestations of obstructive sleep apnea. *J Clin Sleep Med*. 2017;13(11):1345–1348.
10. Chang JS, Banta JT. Corneal surface defects and ocular surface foreign bodies. In: Buttaro TM, Trybulski J, Bailey PP, Sandberg-Cook J, eds. *Primary Care: A Collaborative Practice*. 4th ed. St. Louis, MO: Mosby; 2013:330-332.
11. Boodley CA, Buttaro TM. Inner ear disturbances. In: Buttaro TM, Trybulski J, Bailey PP, Sandberg-Cook J, eds. *Primary Care: A Collaborative Practice*. 4th ed. St. Louis, MO: Mosby; 2013:353-357.
12. Barnett TO. Problems of the ear. In: Monahan FD, Neighbors M, Sands JK, et al., eds. *Phipps' Medical–Surgical Nursing: Health and Illness Perspectives*. 8th ed. St. Louis, MO: Mosby; 2007:1845-1857.
13. Connelly A, Ramakrishnan VR. Epistaxis. In: Scholes MA, Ramakrishnan VR, eds. *ENT Secrets*. 4th ed. Philadelphia, PA: Elsevier; 2016:161-166.
14. Simmen DB, Jones NS. Epistaxis. In: Flint PW, Haughey BH, Lund V, et al., eds. *Cummings Otolaryngology*. 6th ed. Philadelphia, PA: Saunders; 2015:678-690.
15. Courey MS, Pletcher SD. Upper airway disorders. In: Broaddus VC, Mason RJ, Ernst JD, et al., eds. *Murray and Nadel's Textbook of Respiratory Medicine*. 6th ed. Philadelphia, PA: Saunders; 2016:877-896.
16. Wang EJ. Infections of the head and neck. In: Benjamin IJ, Griggs RC, Wing EJ, Fitz JG, eds. *Andreoli and Carpenter's Cecil Essentials of Medicine*. 9th ed. Philadelphia, PA: Saunders; 2016:867-871.
17. Chronic sinusitis. Centers for Disease Control and Prevention website. https://www.cdc.gov/nchs/fastats/sinuses.htm. Accessed February 27, 2021.
18. Babu NC, Gomes AJ. Systemic manifestations of oral diseases. *J Oral Maxillofac Pathol*. 2011;15(2):144-147.

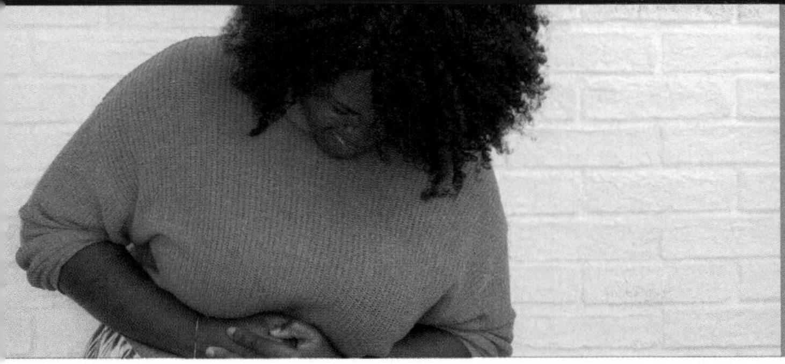

Chapter 21

Abdominal and Gastrointestinal Emergencies

NATIONAL EMS EDUCATION STANDARD COMPETENCIES

Medicine

Integrates assessment findings with principles of epidemiology and pathophysiology to formulate a working diagnosis and implement a comprehensive treatment/disposition plan for a patient with a medical complaint.

Abdominal and Gastrointestinal Disorders

Anatomy, presentations, and management of shock associated with abdominal emergencies

- Gastrointestinal bleeding (pp 1411–1417)

Anatomy, physiology, epidemiology, pathophysiology, psychosocial impact, presentations, prognosis, and management of

- Acute and chronic gastrointestinal hemorrhage (pp 1411–1417)
- Liver disorders (pp 1428–1431)
- Peritonitis (p 1420)
- Ulcerative diseases (p 1425)
- Irritable bowel syndrome (p 1426)
- Inflammatory disorders (pp 1419–1426)
- Pancreatitis (pp 1423–1425)
- Bowel obstruction (pp 1432–1433)
- Hernias (pp 1434–1435)
- Infectious disorders (pp 1427–1431)
- Gallbladder and biliary tract disorders (pp 1420–1421)
- Rectal abscess (p 1428)
- Rectal foreign body obstruction (p 1435)
- Mesenteric ischemia (pp 1435–1436)

KNOWLEDGE OBJECTIVES

1. Describe the incidence, morbidity, and mortality of gastrointestinal (GI) emergencies. (p 1397)
2. Identify the primary risk factors for GI disease. (p 1397)
3. Discuss the anatomy and physiology of the organs and structures of the GI system. (pp 1398–1401)
4. Explain how to size up scene safety when responding to a patient with a GI emergency. (p 1402)
5. List the personal protective equipment that is likely to be necessary during a call in response to a patient with a GI emergency. (p 1402)
6. Explain how to integrate pathophysiologic principles and assessment findings to formulate a field diagnosis and implement

a treatment plan for the patient with a GI emergency. (pp 1402–1403)

7. Evaluate the mechanisms by which airway patency might be compromised in the patient with a GI emergency. (pp 1402–1403)
8. Summarize assessment of breathing and circulation in a patient with a GI emergency. (p 1403)
9. Indicate the considerations that go into making a transport decision for the patient with a GI emergency. (p 1403)
10. Explore ways of investigating the chief complaint and taking the history of a patient with a GI disorder. (pp 1403–1405)
11. Describe the technique for performing a comprehensive physical examination on a patient with abdominal pain, including percussion and auscultation of bowel sounds and palpation to evaluate for pain and masses. (pp 1405–1407)
12. Discuss how orthostatic vital signs can help assess the extent of abdominal bleeding. (p 1407)
13. Consider the proper extent of pain management for the patient with an abdominal emergency. (pp 1408–1409)
14. Discuss the pathophysiologic mechanisms that can cause hypovolemia. (p 1410)
15. Compare the pathophysiology, assessment, and management of upper GI bleeding with that of lower GI bleeding. (pp 1411–1412)
16. Discuss the pathophysiology, assessment, and management of esophagogastric varices. (p 1412)
17. Discuss the pathophysiology, assessment, and management of Mallory-Weiss syndrome and Boerhaave syndrome. (pp 1412–1414)
18. Discuss the pathophysiology, assessment, and management of peptic ulcer disease and gastritis. (pp 1414–1415)
19. Discuss the pathophysiology, assessment, and management of gastroesophageal reflux disease and hiatal hernia. (pp 1415–1416)
20. Discuss the pathophysiology, assessment, and management of hemorrhoids. (p 1416)
21. Discuss the pathophysiology, assessment, and management of anal fissures. (pp 1416–1417)
22. Discuss the pathophysiology, assessment, and management of esophageal pathologies, including esophagitis, tracheoesophageal fistula, and esophageal stricture (or stenosis). (pp 1417–1419)
23. Explain how the immune system responds to acute and chronic inflammation within the GI tract. (pp 1419–1426)
24. Discuss the pathophysiology, assessment, and management of peritonitis. (p 1420)
25. Discuss the pathophysiology, assessment, and management of cholecystitis. (pp 1420–1421)
26. Discuss the pathophysiology, assessment, and management of appendicitis. (pp 1421–1422)
27. Discuss the pathophysiology, assessment, and management of diverticulitis. (pp 1422–1423)
28. Discuss the pathophysiology, assessment, and management of pancreatitis. (pp 1423–1425)
29. Discuss the pathophysiology, assessment, and management of ulcerative colitis. (p 1425)
30. Discuss the pathophysiology, assessment, and management of Crohn disease. (pp 1425–1426)
31. Discuss the pathophysiology, assessment, and management of irritable bowel syndrome. (p 1426)
32. Explain why the GI system is vulnerable to infection and how the immune system reacts to infection within the GI tract. (p 1427)
33. Discuss the pathophysiology, assessment, and management of acute gastroenteritis. (pp 1427–1428)
34. Discuss the pathophysiology, assessment, and management of rectal abscess. (p 1428)
35. Discuss the pathophysiology, assessment, and management of cirrhosis. (pp 1428–1430)
36. Discuss the pathophysiology, assessment, and management of hepatic encephalopathy. (pp 1430–1431)
37. Discuss the pathophysiology, assessment, and management of esophageal obstruction. (pp 1431–1432)
38. Discuss the pathophysiology, assessment, and management of small- and large-bowel obstruction. (pp 1432–1433)
39. Discuss the pathophysiology, assessment, and management of GI hernias. (pp 1434–1435)
40. Compare the four types of abdominal hernias: reducible, incarcerated, strangulated, and incisional. (p 1434)
41. Compare rectal foreign body obstructions caused by swallowed objects with obstructions caused by inserted objects. (p 1435)
42. Discuss the pathophysiology, assessment, and management of rectal foreign body obstructions. (p 1435)

43. Discuss the pathophysiology, assessment, and management of ischemic and neoplastic disorders, including mesenteric ischemia and tumors of the colon, pancreas, and liver. (pp 1435–1437)
44. Describe lifestyle changes that reduce the likelihood of developing GI disease. (p 1438)

SKILLS OBJECTIVES

1. Demonstrate how to auscultate the abdomen to assess for diminished, absent, or abnormal bowel sounds. (pp 1405–1406)
2. Demonstrate how to palpate the abdomen to assess for pain, rebound tenderness, and masses. (pp 1406–1407)
3. Demonstrate how to palpate the right upper quadrant to assess for Murphy sign, indicating cholecystitis. (p 1406)

Introduction

Gastrointestinal (GI) conditions can become life threatening because systemic consequences can result from untreated or undertreated disorders of the GI system. For example, when the appendix becomes infected, the consequences can be deadly if the condition goes unrecognized.

This chapter reviews the structures that perform **digestion**, including their functions and locations. After a brief review of the general assessment process for a patient with an **acute abdomen** (sudden onset of abdominal pain) or other abdominal emergency, the pathophysiology, assessment, and management of common GI conditions are discussed. To begin, you need to gain an appreciation for the scope of GI emergencies.

At one time or another, everyone has had abdominal pain or a case of GI distress. **Diarrhea**, nausea, and vomiting are the undesirable signs and symptoms of such an illness. They might cause intense discomfort and indicate an underlying condition. In other words, they cannot themselves be considered conditions or illnesses.

The number of disorders responsible for causing abdominal pain, diarrhea, and nausea is impressive. GI disorders account for 246,000 deaths and 21.7 million hospitalizations per year.[1] Fortunately, most GI disorders are not deadly. With the exception of **septicemia** (a generalized infection of the bloodstream that could be caused by a GI disorder), GI disorders are not among the top 10 diseases that cause death within the United States.

According to estimates by the US Census Bureau, the population of the United States included more than 330 million people in February 2021.[2] Of these individuals, 25% to 40% have **gastroesophageal reflux disease (GERD)**.[3] This certainly accounts for many advertisements for heartburn relief medications on television, in magazines, and on health-related websites. The National Institute of Diabetes and Digestive and Kidney Diseases, which is part of the National Institutes of Health, reports that 60 to 70 million people are affected by digestive diseases.[1] Given the widespread nature of these diseases, it is clear that paramedics will frequently be called to treat patients with GI disorders. As you explore these conditions, knowing which behaviors and characteristics may predispose patients to GI disorders can assist you with the care of these patients and the prevention of future GI disorders.

Two known behavioral risk factors for GI disorders are smoking and excessive alcohol consumption. Both nicotine and alcohol increase the release of gastric acid in the stomach. This is why a small amount of wine or a beer taken before a meal is known as an aperitif, from a French word meaning "to open": It primes the stomach for the forthcoming meal. However, smoking or chronic alcohol consumption increases the acidity of the stomach beyond the ability of the mucosal lining to protect it. The result is an increased risk for ulcers of the upper GI tract.

Other activities that place patients at increased risk for GI disorders are listed in **TABLE 21-1**. You can use this information to help educate patients about ways in which they can decrease or even eliminate their GI discomfort.

TABLE 21-1 Behaviors and Corresponding Association With GI Disease

Behavior	Association
Smoking	Functional dyspepsia and Crohn disease
Sleeping patterns	GERD, irritable bowel syndrome, and functional dyspepsia
Dietary behavior	Irritable bowel syndrome, cholecystitis, and GERD
Alcohol	Cirrhosis, pancreatitis, and peptic ulcer disease
Work behaviors (rotating shifts)	Irritable bowel syndrome, peptic ulcer disease
Exercise behavior	Constipation, nonalcoholic fatty liver disease
Stress	Disease throughout the GI tract

Abbreviations: GERD, gastroesophageal reflux disease; GI, gastrointestinal

Data from: Jia L, Jiang S-M, Lui J. Behavioral gastroenterology: an emerging system and new frontier of action. *World J Gastroenterol.* 2017;23(33):6059-6064. https://www.ncbi.nlm.nih.gov/pmc/articles/PMC5597497/. Accessed February 6, 2021.

Anatomy and Physiology Review

The anatomy and physiology of the GI system are covered in detail in Chapter 8, *Anatomy and Physiology*. **FIGURE 21-1** reviews the anatomy of the abdomen. The entire journey of food from mouth to anus, summarized in **TABLE 21-2**, takes 8 to 72 hours and involves the liver, pancreas, stomach, intestines, and other structures. At this pace, a normal number of bowel movements is between three per day and one every 3 days. Of course, this number varies according to the types of food you eat, the amount of water you consume, the amount of exercise you get, and how much stress your body is under.

Digestion begins with chewing, during which the molars crush and grind the food. Saliva is added to lubricate the food, allowing it to be more easily swallowed. Changing the consistency of food into a smooth bolus helps to prevent aspiration of food into the lungs. Saliva also contains enzymes that begin the chemical breakdown of starches, or complex carbohydrates, so the body can more easily absorb them.

Swallowed food is moved to the esophagus. The esophagus, which discourages a muscular hollow tube, lies in a collapsed position, discouraging air from entering it during breathing. Food is moved inferiorly toward the stomach with a wavelike muscular contraction called peristalsis.

In the stomach, hydrochloric acid is added to the food. As the stomach contracts, it mixes the food and acid. The acid begins the breakdown of food, transforming it into chyme. Substances of small molecular size are absorbed in the stomach, such as water, alcohol, caffeine, and some medications. The remaining chyme exits the pyloric sphincter and enters the duodenum, the first part of the small intestine. Here the pancreas, liver, and gallbladder connect to the digestive system.

YOU are the Paramedic

PART 1

Your unit is dispatched for an unresponsive person at a local residence. The dispatcher tells you the patient is a 64-year-old woman who became unresponsive in her bathroom. You arrive at the residence and are met at the door by the patient's husband. The husband leads you to the upstairs bathroom, where you find the patient lying next to the toilet. There is a foul odor in the room and you notice about 250 mL of melanotic stool covering the patient's clothing and around the floor near her buttocks. The patient is responsive when you approach. The husband explains that his wife had been sleeping, woke up, and asked him to help her to the bathroom because she had to have a bowel movement. When they reached the bathroom, he said she passed out, so he helped her to the floor next to the toilet. The patient said the last thing she remembers is walking to the bathroom with her husband. The patient has been feeling ill with stomach cramps for the past several days.

1. What is melena?
2. What part of the GI system do you believe might be affected?

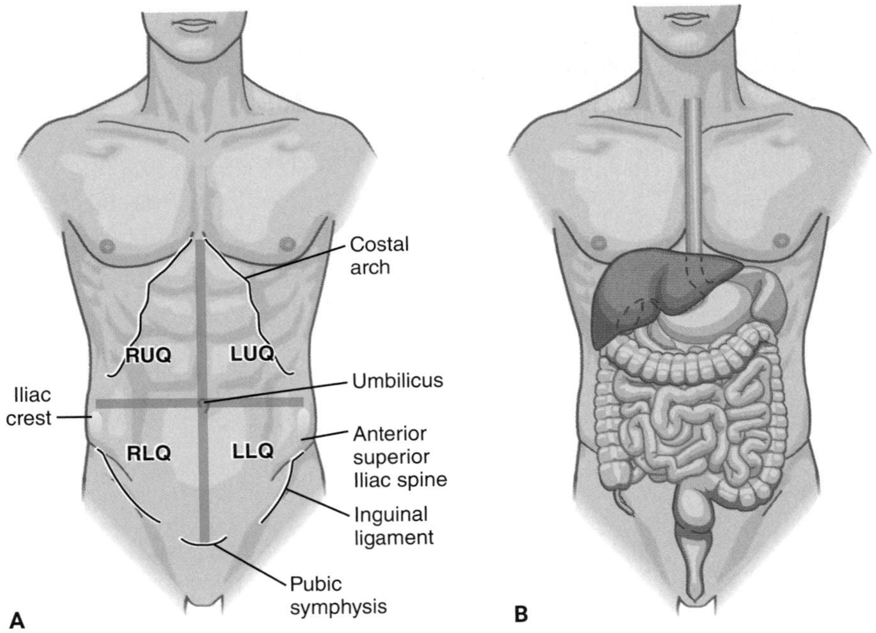

FIGURE 21-1 The anatomy of the abdomen. **A.** The four quadrants of the abdomen. **B.** Abdominal organs can lie in more than one quadrant. Although the kidneys are located in the abdomen (behind the structures shown here), they are considered part of the genitourinary system. (LLQ, left lower quadrant; LUQ; left upper quadrant; RLQ, right lower quadrant; RUQ, right upper quadrant)

TABLE 21-2 Location and Functions of the GI System-Related Organs

Organ/Structure	Location	Function
Mouth	Head	Mechanically breaks down food; begins chemical breakdown of food with saliva
Esophagus	Substernal, **epigastric**	Tube that moves food from the mouth to the stomach (muscular and vascular structure)
Stomach	Left upper quadrant, epigastric	Performs mechanical and chemical breakdown of food (food in, chyme out)
Liver	Upper abdomen; mainly right side of the central upper abdomen	Produces bile; assists with carbohydrate, protein, and fat metabolism; vitamin storage and manufacture; blood detoxification; waste elimination
Pancreas	Posterior to the stomach	
Exocrine		Produces enzymes for protein, carbohydrate, and fat breakdown within the duodenum
Endocrine		Produces insulin, somatostatin, and glucagon
Gallbladder	Inferior surface of the liver	Storage of bile
Spleen	Left upper abdomen	Filtering of blood; recycling of dead red blood cells
Aorta	Central upper abdomen	Main artery supplying blood to the lower body
Bladder	Suprapubic area	Storage of urine

(continues)

TABLE 21-2 Location and Functions of the GI System–Related Organs (continued)

Organ/Structure	Location	Function
Uterus	Suprapubic area	Reproduction
Iliac arteries	Central abdomen and lower right/left quadrants	Supply blood to the legs and pelvis
Small Intestine		
Duodenum	Central, upper **umbilical**	Major site for chemical breakdown of food; major site of water, fat, protein, carbohydrate, and vitamin absorption
Jejunum	Central, umbilical	Moves chyme forward, absorbs nutrients
Ileum	Central, hypogastric to lower right abdomen	Moves chyme forward, absorbs nutrients
Large Intestine		
Ascending colon	Right lower quadrant, hypogastric into epigastric	Water reabsorption, formation of feces, bacterial digestion of food
Transverse colon	Right to left upper quadrant, epigastric	Water reabsorption, formation of feces, bacterial digestion of food
Descending colon	Left upper and lower quadrant, epigastric to umbilical	Water reabsorption, formation of feces, bacterial digestion of food
Sigmoid colon	Left lower quadrant, hypogastric	Water reabsorption, formation of feces, bacterial digestion of food
Rectum	Suprapubic, hypogastric	Stores feces for later release
Anus	Most inferior portion of the large intestine	Sphincter to control release of feces
Peritoneum		
Parietal peritoneum	The lining or bag that contains abdominal organs	Protects and supports the organs within the abdomen
Visceral peritoneum	The lining that covers organs	
Peritoneal cavity	The space between the parietal and visceral peritoneum	
Mesentery	Double-layered fold of peritoneal tissue that attaches structures to the abdominal wall and anchors them in place	Attaches some organs (eg, stomach, small intestine, pancreas, spleen) to posterior abdominal wall; provides a passageway for blood and lymphatic vessels and nerves

Abbreviation: GI, gastrointestinal

The primary function of the GI system is to absorb the products of digestion to fuel the cells within the body. The real workhorse of the digestive system is the small intestine, where 90% of all absorption occurs. It would be difficult to stay adequately nourished if a section of your small intestine had to be removed because of **Crohn disease**, cancer, or some other disease process. The exocrine portion of the pancreas secretes several enzymes into the duodenum that assist with digestion of fats, proteins, and carbohydrates. Additionally, pancreatic juice helps to neutralize gastric acid.

The liver produces bile, which is stored in the gallbladder. Bile is an enzyme used by the body to help break down fats. Bile is released into the duodenum, where it helps to dissolve fats. The liver also promotes carbohydrate metabolism. If the blood glucose level falls, the liver can convert glycogen into glucose. Dramatic decreases in glucose stores will prompt the liver to convert fats and proteins into glucose. Remember, your brain cells can burn only one type of fuel: glucose. As blood flows through the liver, fat and protein metabolism continues. Without a functioning liver, you would be dead in a few days because your body would not be able to use any of the proteins absorbed through the GI system. The liver also detoxifies drugs, completes the breakdown of dead red and white blood cells, creates clotting factors, and stores vitamins and minerals.

Recall that the portal vein transports venous blood from the GI tract to the liver. For a variety of reasons, blood flow through the liver can be slow. The veins surrounding the stomach and esophagus can become dilated if blood backs up. Even a small amount of pressure can cause leaking or rupture of these vessels, resulting in minor or severe bleeding. This problem is discussed later in the pathology section for each condition.

The large intestine, or colon, contains the remaining waste products, called feces. The main role of the large intestine is to complete the reabsorption of water. Most water is reabsorbed in the small intestine. This osmotic function of the colon helps to solidify the stool. Failure of this bowel function results in soft stool, or diarrhea. Bacteria normally found in the colon help to complete the breakdown of chyme. Some bacteria produce gas as a byproduct called flatulence or flatus. Flatulence may be considered impolite, but it is normal.

Finally, the appendix is a small, saclike outcropping of the colon that contains T and B lymphocytes, secretes immunoglobulin A, and is thought to serve as a storage site for nonpathogenic (ie, "good") intestinal bacteria. It is theorized that the healthy bacteria stored in the appendix can migrate into the colon and restore balance if the bacterial balance within the colon becomes disrupted because of antibiotic use, infection, or diarrheal illness.

YOU are the Paramedic

PART 2

The patient states she has been ill for several days with dark, smelly stools twice every day for the past 3 days. She denies any vomiting but reports pain throughout her entire abdomen. According to the patient, this pain can be bad enough to wake her during sleep. She did not go to the hospital because she thought this was just a case of a stomach virus.

You obtain a set of orthostatic vital signs. As the patient sits up with your assistance, she reports being dizzy so you lay her back down right away. Assessment of the abdomen reveals normal bowel sounds. The abdomen is soft, but tender in all four quadrants.

Recording Time:	0 Minutes
Appearance	Awake, lying on bathroom floor
Level of consciousness	Alert and oriented to person, place, time, and event
Airway	Open
Breathing	Adequate
Circulation	Adequate

3. What do orthostatic vital signs indicate?
4. Do you expect the patient's blood pressure (BP) and pulse rate to increase or decrease when the patient is moved?

Patient Assessment

Because GI system emergencies often result from a medical condition rather than trauma, one of the most important areas of the assessment is the history of present illness. Ask the patient about dietary habits, fluid discharge from the body, and types of pain.

Scene Size-Up

Assessment of the GI system begins with the scene size-up. Standard precautions are essential when treating a patient with a GI emergency because of the high likelihood of contact with infectious agents. Whenever you might come in contact with vomitus, diarrhea, blood, and soiled patient clothing, additional personal protective equipment (PPE) may be necessary. Gowns can be helpful when dealing with patients who have become incontinent. Masks can help with noxious odors.

Street Smarts

Cleaning the patient with a GI disorder helps provide some degree of dignity to a person embarrassed by the circumstances of their disease.

Words of Wisdom

When responding to a patient with abdominal pain and diarrhea in a nursing home, suspect *Clostridioides difficile*. Wear proper PPE: gloves, gown, and mask. Limit the risk of transmission by cleaning the BP cuff, stethoscope, and ambulance cot well. Throw away any tape or tourniquet that was used. This disease can easily be transmitted to your next patient!

Primary Survey

As you begin to form your general impression of the patient, closely examine where the person is found. The patient's body posture or position can give you hints as to what happened. Was the patient walking to the bathroom when they passed out? Has the patient been in bed sick for several days? Was the patient at work when a sudden bout of pain caused them to double over? Look to the environment for clues as to the length and degree of illness the patient is experiencing.

One aspect of the general impression of the patient with a GI emergency is odor. As you enter the room, what do you smell? Is this odor coming from the patient, the room, animals, or something else? Few conditions create such a noxious odor as upper GI bleeding. The foul-smelling stool often present during these calls can make even experienced EMS providers nauseated.

Words of Wisdom

A tip when dealing with strong odors is to hold your ground. The sense of smell is the most acute for about 1 minute. After that time, more than 50% of the intensity of an odor is lost as the olfactory nerve becomes tired of sending the same signal. If you are faced with a strong odor on a call, stay in the environment. After about 2 to 5 minutes, your nose will tire of sending the same odor signal, and the smell may be hardly noticeable.

Closely inspect the patient's airway for foreign bodies. Remove or suction obstructions within the airway. While evaluating the airway, take note of any unusual odors from the mouth. Patients who have advanced bowel obstructions can have breath smelling of stool.

For the patient with a GI condition, airway concerns include possible aspiration or obstruction of the airway because of vomit or blood. Although rare, these situations do pose real concerns for the patient's health.

- Position the patient to ensure adequate drainage of material out of the mouth. If spinal motion restriction is needed, be prepared to tilt the long backboard. This requires ensuring that the patient is secured and padded well so spinal movement is minimized when the backboard is moved.
- Portable suction should be part of your "first in" equipment.
- Management of GI bleeding may require the use of a nasogastric tube. When placed in the stomach, this tube allows stomach contents to be removed with suction. Its use can

be beneficial in patients with severe upper GI bleeding or when decompressing the stomach of instilled air.

Monitoring the patient's capnography can assist with ensuring an effective respiratory pattern. Breathing management includes the following interventions:

- **Administer high-concentration oxygen.** Do not rely on oxygen saturation readings as evidence that oxygen is not needed. For example, patients with GI bleeding (especially those who do not have underlying respiratory disease) may have a decreased hemoglobin level and describe feeling tired and having shortness of breath that increases with exertion with no known cause. In these patients, the oxygen saturation may read 96%, but supplemental oxygen is still needed if their hemoglobin level is low.
- **Prevent aspiration.** Oxygen masks can cause some patients to experience a sense of confinement, which can be problematic for patients experiencing nausea. Monitor patients who are using a mask to ensure they can remove it quickly if they need to vomit.
- **Auscultate lung sounds.** Obtain baseline information and continue to monitor lung sounds to ensure the safe administration of fluids.

Words of Wisdom

When treating a patient who has had significant bleeding, remember that pulse oximetry measures the percentage of circulating hemoglobin saturated (typically with oxygen). If the patient's hemoglobin is 7 g/dL, the oxygen saturation may read 100%, indicating that 100% of the available hemoglobin is saturated; however, if the patient has lost one-half of their blood supply, they would have one-half the normal amount of hemoglobin. This reading, then, is dangerously misleading. When caring for a patient with a GI complaint, consider using capnography in addition to pulse oximetry. Reduced end-tidal carbon dioxide ($ETCO_2$) levels can help identify conditions such as hypovolemia and sepsis.

Assessment of the circulatory system is essential in understanding the effects of GI disease on the body. As with all patients, assess skin CTC: color, temperature, and condition. Note findings that would be consistent with shock. Determine the pulse rate. Evaluate the peripheral pulses and compare them with the central pulses.

When making your transport decision, integrate the information gathered from the primary survey. If the patient has positive orthostatic vital signs (vital signs that vary with a change in position), consider how the patient will be moved. Can the patient sit up in a stair chair, or will doing so cause them to pass out or suddenly vomit? Be cautious when transporting any patient in severe pain because syncope, simply from increased pain, is possible. Transportation of the patient with GI disease rarely requires lights and siren.

Documentation and Communication

When you are recording information about the patient's body substances, be as accurate as possible. Describe the substances in detail. Saying a patient had feces covering their legs is adequate if melena is not present. If you see diarrhea, use terms to describe how liquid it is. This information can help to determine the degree of dehydration the patient may be experiencing.

History Taking

Use the mnemonic SAMPLE (Signs and symptoms, Allergies, Medications, Pertinent past medical history, Last oral intake, Events leading up to the illness or injury) to gather information about the history of present illness and past medical history. Many people with GI emergencies have long-standing medical conditions, so the information obtained in the history can help you to formulate a working diagnosis. Many GI disorders can quickly increase in intensity after months of minimal signs and symptoms. Ask if this emergency has ever occurred before. When asking the patient about symptoms, you will need to discuss subjects that do not often come up in everyday conversation. You and your patient must have a common frame of reference. **TABLE 21-3** presents standardized language you can use so that the health care providers taking over care from you will have the same understanding of the patient's condition as you do.

TABLE 21-3 Body Substances Originating in the GI Tract

Substance	Description	Possible Cause
Vomitus	Food and partially digested food; strong acidic odor mixed with the odor of food	Influenza, food intolerance
Hematemesis or "coffee grounds" emesis	Black or very dark red granular material; this slurry may contain food, but the food and blood are indistinguishable	Blood from the mouth, esophagus, or stomach that has been digested by stomach acids and then vomited
Vomitus with gross blood	Vomitus in which red blood is obvious; food and blood are distinguishable	Bleeding from the mouth or esophagus that has not been exposed to stomach acids
Diarrhea	Frequent liquid stool with the consistency of water; can range in color from clear to dark brown	Intestinal infections, bowel obstructions; usually associated with small intestinal disorders; is always considered abnormal
Acholic stools	Tan-colored, formed stools; may be softer than typical	Liver disease: the liver releases bile into the small intestine; bile gives stool its normally dark color
Steatorrhea	Foamy, foul-smelling, mushy, yellow to gray stools; these oily stools usually float within water	Liver or pancreas disease causing excessive excretion of fat in the stool
Soft stool	Bowel movement that is the consistency of soft-serve ice cream; can range in color from tan to dark brown	Normal variant for some people; caused by new foods, a rapid change in diet, or use of stool softeners
Hematochezia	Stool and blood that are incorporated together into the same substance, yet are easily distinguished from each other	Bleeding from the lower GI tract
Melena	Black, tarry, sticky, and very odorous stool and blood blended together into one substance; blood cannot be distinguished from stool	Bleeding from the upper GI tract

Abbreviation: GI, gastrointestinal

Gather as much relevant information about the patient's history as possible:

- Ask about the foods ingested in the past 24 hours. Asking about foods eaten in the last 24 hours instead of focusing on the patient's most recent meal can help rule out potential food poisoning. Some types of meals are associated with particular conditions. For example, when a patient has a flare-up of cholecystitis, ingestion of a fatty meal is often followed by the onset of pain several hours later. Be sure to include the type and volume of fluids ingested.
- Ask about meal tolerance. Has the patient had any changes in appetite? Any recent weight gain or loss? Any nausea or vomiting? Ask the patient if these signs and symptoms have been occurring more often than usual. If vomiting has occurred, ask the patient to describe its amount, color, and odor. Does the patient have symptoms such as burping and flatulence that may indicate food intolerance?
- If the patient is of childbearing age, ask if pregnancy is a possibility.
- Ask if the patient is having difficulty swallowing or pain with swallowing.
- Ask the patient about their most recent bowel movement (including color and consistency) and stool frequency. Does the frequency reflect a change in their usual bowel habits? Does the patient use laxatives and stool softeners?

- Ask the patient about recent travel, which may have exposed them to an infectious agent unfamiliar to their body.
- Ask about additions or changes in prescribed and over-the-counter medications, including herbal supplements.

Secondary Assessment

The physical exam allows you to discover clues related to the patient's chief complaint. There should be no significant changes within the examination of the head, neck, or chest that directly relate to GI concerns. The major effects from GI disease on the nervous, cardiovascular, or respiratory systems result from pain, hypovolemia, and/or infection. If a patient has an esophageal pathology, throat pain is possible.

Examining the abdomen allows you to obtain more details about the patient's condition, but also requires more skill. This examination can sometimes be embarrassing for both you and the patient. Be professional and provide reassurance as you proceed with the examination. Place a pillow under the patient's knees if the patient is stable. Make sure your hands are warm before you touch the abdomen. Use the examination principles described in Chapter 11, *Patient Assessment*.

Look at the skin for irregularities. Are there scars indicating trauma or past surgery? Do you notice stretch marks, also called **striae** **FIGURE 21-2**? These indicate a change in the size of the abdomen over a short period, such as increases or decreases in weight, pregnancy, or severe abdominal edema.

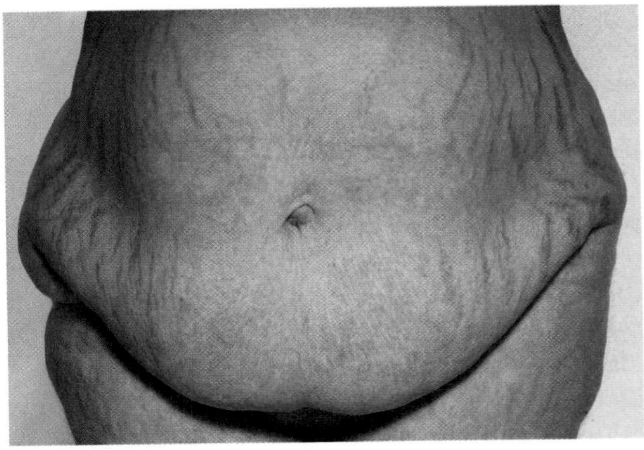

FIGURE 21-2 Striae. These vertical lines usually indicate a relatively rapid change in weight or a large amount of fluid accumulation in the abdomen.

Is the abdomen symmetric? Tumors, hernias, enlarged or distended organs, pregnancy, and other masses can cause asymmetry.

What is the appearance of the abdomen **FIGURE 21-3**? Is it flat, distended, or **scaphoid** (concave)? A scaphoid abdomen is the result of decreased abdominal volume, such as that associated with diaphragmatic hernia, dehydration, or malnutrition.

Auscultate the abdomen as appropriate given the time and noise level in your surroundings. Normal bowel sounds sound like gurgles and clicks. These sounds occur between 5 and 30 times per minute. In the secondary assessment, you are merely listening for the presence or absence of these sounds. Sometimes you will hear loud, prolonged sounds. This "stomach growling," called **borborygmi**, indicates strong contractions of the intestines, which can be normal or be present with diarrhea. Interestingly, increased activity in the bowel (**hyperperistalsis**) can also be present in patients with early bowel obstruction. In this case, the bowel is contracting forcefully in an effort to overcome the obstruction.

Decreased bowel sounds can indicate decreased peristalsis of the intestines (**hypoperistalsis**). This lack of movement can lead to bowel obstruction. Absent bowel sounds, defined as no sounds heard for 2 minutes, may be difficult to note in the

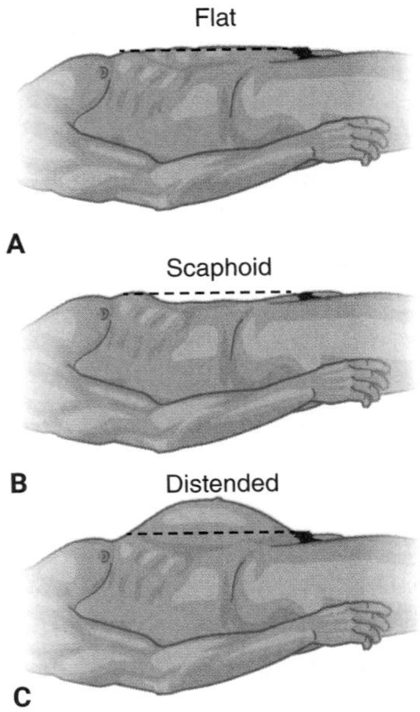

FIGURE 21-3 Appearance of abdomen. **A.** Flat. **B.** Scaphoid. **C.** Distended.

TABLE 21-4 Bowel Sounds

Name	Description	Possible Causes
Normal	Soft gurgles or clicks occurring at 5–30 per min	Normal movement of material through the intestines
Borborygmi	Loud gurgles, often heard without a stethoscope, and often occurring at greater than 30 per min	Hyperperistalsis Can be normal If prolonged, can indicate increased intestinal contractions, as with diarrhea of any cause
Decreased	Quiet sounds occurring at less than 1 sound per 15–20 seconds	Hypoperistalsis Can indicate impending intestinal obstruction
Absent	No sounds after 2 min of continuous listening	Bowel obstruction/intestinal paralysis

prehospital setting. An absence of bowel sounds indicates the intestines are not contracting; therefore, any material within them is not in motion. Bowel sounds are summarized in **TABLE 21-4**.

Percussion of the abdomen can reveal information about its contents. Typically, the abdomen should be **tympanic** (empty sounding) to percussion, due to the hollow organs in the abdominal cavity. A duller sound is generated around the upper left and upper right quadrants, due to the locations of the spleen and liver, respectively. Percussion of the epigastrium may reveal tympany (empty stomach) or dullness (full stomach).

Unfortunately, the intestines often mask or augment these findings based on their contents. Thus, you should consider the results of your percussion to be just one more piece of information, no more or less important than any other. Continue gathering information and comparing your assessment findings, looking for trends and associations to determine the correct working diagnosis.

Palpation of the abdomen can reveal important information. Recall the palpation principles discussed in Chapter 11, *Patient Assessment.* As you palpate the abdomen, it should be soft and nontender **FIGURE 21-4**. A rigid abdomen can indicate hemorrhage or infection. Pain is often an important finding in patients with abdominal emergencies. It can indicate trauma, hemorrhage, infection, obstruction, or other serious conditions. As blood volume begins to decrease, the body compensates by releasing catecholamines (ie, epinephrine and norepinephrine) to vasoconstrict the periphery, increase the pulse rate, and increase the force of left ventricular contraction. Pain stimulates similar body responses. Both pain and hemorrhage can cause tachycardia, diminished peripheral pulses, diaphoresis, and skin changes from baseline (ie, pallor, coolness, clamminess). Remember that compensatory responses, such as tachycardia, may be lessened or absent in patients taking medications meant to slow the heart rate, such as beta blockers. Types of abdominal pain include visceral, parietal, somatic, and referred pain **TABLE 21-5**.

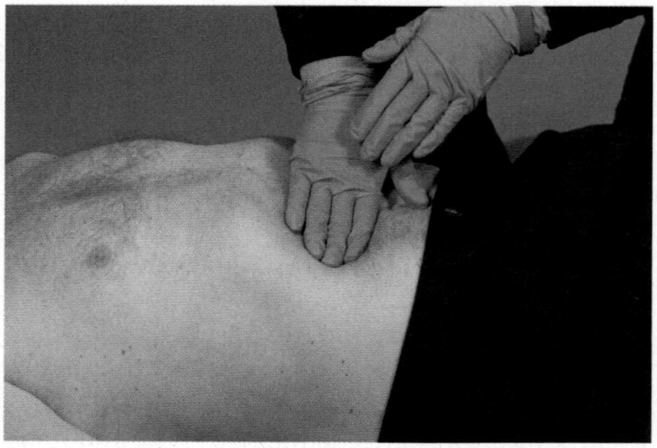

FIGURE 21-4 Palpating the four quadrants of the abdomen.

Rebound tenderness, also called **parietal pain**, can sometimes accompany abdominal pain. Rebound tenderness occurs when the peritoneum is

TABLE 21-5 Types of Abdominal Pain

Type	Origin	Description	Cause
Visceral pain	Hollow organs	May be steady or intermittent Poorly localized Described as dull, squeezing, burning, cramping, gnawing, or aching Usually felt superficially	Organ contracts too forcefully or is distended (stretched)
Parietal pain/ rebound pain	Peritoneum	Steady, achy pain Easier to localize than visceral pain Pain increases with movement	Inflammation of the peritoneum (caused by bleeding or infection)
Somatic pain	Peripheral nerve tracts	Localized pain, usually felt deeply Described as sharp, burning, aching, stabbing	Irritation of or injury to tissue, causing activation of peripheral nerve tracts
Referred pain	Peripheral nerve tracts	Pain originating in the abdomen and causing the perception of pain in distant locations Attributable to similar paths for the peripheral nerves of the abdomen and those in the distant location	Usually occurs after an initial visceral, parietal, or somatic pain

irritated because of either hemorrhage or infection, and it suggests serious and possibly life-threatening pathology. Because doing so is very painful, it is uncommon to check for rebound tenderness in the field.

As you palpate the abdomen, note the presence of any masses. These will feel like areas of increased density compared with the surrounding tissue. A mass may indicate an engorged liver, bowel distention, an aortic aneurysm, a cyst, or a tumor.

It is helpful to obtain the patient's orthostatic vital signs to gauge the extent of any bleeding. Normally, there should be little variation in the BP or pulse rate when the patient moves from a lying position to a sitting/standing position. When a patient has a significant loss of fluid within the vascular space, however, you will likely note a decrease in systolic BP of 20 mm Hg, an increase in diastolic BP (a narrowing pulse pressure) of 10 mm Hg, or a 20-beat increase in the pulse rate. Any of these findings indicate that the patient has experienced a significant volume loss.

Ultrasonography is an additional tool that may be available to the EMS provider; however, limited evidence has been found of improved patient outcomes in the small number of departments using this technology.[4] Ultrasonography is more typically seen in the critical care transport setting and on aeromedical craft. The information gathered from its use can be used to effectively triage patients to the correct medical facility, avoiding interfacility transfers. Patients who are assessed with this technology are also able to receive the definitive care they need more quickly.

Reassessment

Reassessment should include routine monitoring of the patient's pulse rate, BP, respiratory rate, pulse oximetry, and ECG. If the patient has GI bleeding, it is essential to continue to assess for signs of shock. Remember that capnography can provide some insight into the patient's degree of shock. It is equally important to determine the effects of your treatment on the patient. Before giving additional fluid boluses, for example, it is a good habit to auscultate lung sounds. This exam can provide valuable information about whether the patient is deteriorating into heart failure.

Many patients with abdominal pain are given pain medication. How effective was your treatment of the patient's pain? Does the patient need more medication? How is their BP and respiratory rate? These findings will help you evaluate the effectiveness of your treatment and form the foundation of future treatments.

When creating your documentation, try to be objective about your visual findings. Avoid terms like "covered in blood" when describing your visual findings of the patient and/or scene. Instead, you should use more descriptive sentences like, "Blood noted on the floor, toilet, and patient's clothing." A description like "Patient's clothing saturated with blood" also helps the reader understand the quantity of blood seen.

Street Smarts

Talk with the patient during your initial care and transport. Patients with GI disorders may be upset and embarrassed, so be kind and treat them with respect.

Emergency Medical Care

If there is a sudden dramatic change in the patient's condition, reassess the patient in the same manner that you would assess a new patient. Starting from the beginning will give you the best chance of modifying your care and managing any worrisome new developments.

As a paramedic, there is often little you can do about the GI disease itself, but you can address the effects of the disease. Patients may have severe pain; they may be experiencing severe dehydration, hypotension, or extreme nausea. Some may be thirsty, but you must inform them that they cannot eat or drink at this time. GI emergencies can result in the need for surgery, and ingestion of food or drink could delay needed medical treatment. Your primary goals are observation of standard precautions, maintenance of ABCs, and management of pain, nausea, and vomiting.

Management of Pain, Nausea, and Vomiting

When you provide pain management for GI conditions, the goal should be to make the patient more comfortable. Giving enough medication to eliminate the patient's pain may result in severe hemodynamic compromise. The following medications provide you with tools to manage abdominal pain. These and other medications, as well as dosages, are covered in Chapter 15, *Emergency Medications*.

- **Meperidine hydrochloride (Demerol).** This synthetic opioid is used for moderate to severe pain.
- **Morphine.** This opioid analgesic can cause hypotension and respiratory depression.
- **Ketorolac (Toradol).** This nonopioid analgesic is used for moderate to severe pain. It is contraindicated in patients who have renal

YOU are the Paramedic

PART 3

Your patient has a past medical history of diabetes, hypertension, and atrial fibrillation. She is currently taking propranolol, diltiazem, warfarin, and glyburide and has no allergies to medications. She has also been taking an over-the-counter bismuth solution (Pepto Bismol) hoping to relieve the pain.

Recording Time: 5 Minutes	
Respirations	20 breaths/min
Pulse	120 beats/min, lying down; 136 beats/min sitting
Skin	Cool, pale, moist
Blood pressure	106/82 mm Hg, lying down; 92/78 mm Hg, sitting
Oxygen saturation (Spo_2)	98% with oxygen at 15 L/min via nonrebreathing mask
Pupils	Pupils Equal, Round, and Reactive to Light and Accommodation (PERRLA)

5. On the basis of the patient's orthostatic vital signs, what is your suggested treatment?
6. Which of the patient's medications most concerns you?

disease, who have previous or recurrent GI bleeding, or who are pregnant.

- **Fentanyl (Sublimaze).** This potent, rapid-acting synthetic opioid has a short half-life. It can cause hypotension and respiratory depression.

Controversies

Should paramedics provide pain relief for patients with abdominal pain? This question may provoke some debate. In the past, surgeons relied on the location, quality, and intensity of abdominal pain to guide them during exploratory surgery. Today, technologies such as computed tomography (CT) and focused assessment with sonography in trauma (FAST) exams allow abdominal tissues to be viewed more clearly. The images provided by these technologies show incredibly detailed information about disease.

One reason often cited for withholding pain medication from a patient is the risk of addiction. The specter of drug addiction can be a powerful force that must be weighed when considering the appropriate means to alleviate pain. However, pain management can be provided without the risk of addiction because of the availability of non-narcotic medications.

With all of these advances, it is most humane to make a patient in pain more comfortable. Administer analgesia and antiemetics per your local medical control.

Fluid Resuscitation

Dehydration is also a concern in patients with GI emergencies. In patients who are dehydrated, the overall goal of treatment is to refill the cellular space. The degree of hemodynamic stability will dictate whether to use a hypotonic or isotonic solution. A patient in stable condition should receive a hypotonic solution. This treatment will effectively move fluids from the vascular space into the interstitial space and finally into the intracellular space, refilling the cells. In these patients, an infusion rate of 125 mL/h is usually sufficient to slowly rehydrate cells without causing dramatic swings in either fluid volume or electrolyte balance.

If the patient is more profoundly dehydrated, isotonic fluid will be needed to reexpand the vascular space first. Intravascular hypovolemia causes fluid to be pulled from the interstitial space. Consequently, fluid is pulled from the cellular space in an attempt to establish a new fluid balance point. Refilling the vascular space is essential to ensuring adequate perfusion to the vital organs of the body. The guidelines for emergent filling of the vascular space and refilling the vascular space due to hemorrhage are the same.

As with the severely dehydrated patient, care for the patient with hemorrhaging is directed at maintaining perfusion of vital organs. This can be a controversial subject. Internal hemorrhaging falls into the category of hemorrhaging that cannot be controlled. Volume replacement is critical to ensuring adequate circulation to the vital organs. However, very aggressive volume replacement can result in dramatic hemodilution (dilution of the blood). Without an adequate supply of blood, its oxygen supply, and clotting capabilities, the patient will die. As BP falls, the amount of bleeding decreases, so that the body actually retains more blood. Low pressure equals decreased perfusion, but retention of clotting factors and hemoglobin. Titrate fluids to a BP of 90 to 100 mm Hg; do not normalize the BP.

Fluids of choice in this setting are isotonic crystalloids. Normal saline, Normosol, Isolyte Plasmalyte, and lactated Ringer solution are all isotonic solutions, each of which has its own advantages and disadvantages. See Chapter 15, *Emergency Medications*, for a more in-depth discussion.

If the BP cannot be maintained at adequate levels to maintain peripheral perfusion, then you may need to consider the use of vasoactive medications. Dopamine, norepinephrine, and epinephrine are medications commonly used in the prehospital setting for BP support through vasoconstriction. Fluid resuscitation should be accomplished before these medications are considered.

Patients with GI bleeding often require blood replacement. If you are assisting with an interfacility transfer, be prepared to manage blood products.

Pathophysiology, Assessment, and Management of Specific Abdominal and GI Emergencies

You must have an understanding of many conditions to care effectively for a patient with an abdominal condition. Some of these conditions are difficult, if not impossible, to differentiate from one another in the prehospital setting. Even so, the patient care you will provide is important. Relieving pain, providing comfort, and easing nausea are all steps that the patient will value.

In some EMS systems, paramedics are asked to help online medical directors decide if the patient should be transported to a hospital, to a family physician, or to a clinic or pharmacy. The sophistication with which you assess patients must increase if you are to meet the demands of this role. It is less expensive to have a paramedic safely triage a patient to a family physician or a clinic than to transport every patient to the emergency department (ED).

Knowing more about each of these conditions puts the paramedic in a better place to provide patient education. How the body is maintained and how it functions are often key factors that affect whether a disease is well controlled or life threatening, and GI conditions are no different.

Consider patients with **cholecystitis** (inflammation of the gallbladder). Medical experts would agree that such patients should closely monitor the types of food they eat. If these patients eat very fatty meals, they are more likely to experience pain and discomfort. Patients may need to try small amounts of fatty food to see which ones they should avoid. This education is essential to improving the well-being of patients with cholecystitis. By learning about GI diseases, you may be able to help patients make better choices so they can stay healthy.

Remember to consider hypovolemia when managing a GI emergency. Hypovolemia is caused by either dehydration or hemorrhage. Dehydration occurs from vomiting and/or diarrhea. As the patient loses fluid, the body continues to shift water from inside the cells to interstitial space and finally into the vascular space to maintain adequate fluid volume in the blood vessels, until the patient has reached the limits of effectively moving fluid. During this process, electrolyte levels are also affected. Although persistent vomiting decreases the amount of food ingested, diarrhea causes more dramatic swings in the levels of electrolytes. The main electrolytes affected by diarrhea are sodium and potassium. Diarrhea can either increase or decrease electrolytes, depending on its water content. **TABLE 21-6** outlines the effects of electrolyte imbalances on the body.

The second cause of hypovolemia in patients with GI disorders is hemorrhage. Bleeding in the GI system typically occurs from either the rupture or the destruction of a structure. The GI system is well supplied with blood. This fact is essential to the underlying function of extracting nutrients from what is eaten and then transporting those nutrients to the cells that need replenishing. Without blood, the entire process of digestion would accomplish very little. This close proximity to the blood supply, however, makes damage to the GI system more likely to cause severe hemorrhage.

Trauma is an obvious mechanism for bleeding in the GI system. Other mechanisms include erosion of the protective mucosal layers, chemical destruction of tissue, and dilation of blood vessels. It is possible to experience a fatal hemorrhage from GI bleeding. The bleeding can occur slowly, over several days or weeks, or it can be sudden, with a large

TABLE 21-6 Electrolyte Imbalances Due to Diarrhea

Condition	Effects	Signs and Symptoms
Hyponatremia: Low sodium	Swelling of cells	Muscle weakness, cramps, coma, convulsions
Hypernatremia: High sodium	Shrinking of cells caused by excessive water loss	Coma, convulsions
Hypokalemia: Low potassium	More stimulation needed to fire nerve/muscle cells	Muscle cramps, weakness, paralysis, heart failure, dysrhythmias, flattened T waves, possible U waves
Hyperkalemia: High potassium	Less stimulation needed to fire nerve/muscle cells	Muscle weakness and cramps, dysrhythmias, tall T waves

volume of blood loss. In either case, assessment is the key to correctly identifying and treating these patients.

In patients with diarrhea or hemorrhage, an absolute loss of volume occurs. Consequently, classic signs and symptoms of shock are typically present. The brain is the first organ to show the effects of shock, with the patient becoming anxious and restless. Tachycardia and skin that is cool, clammy, or paler than the baseline color are common. The pulse pressure is usually narrowed because the epinephrine released into the bloodstream causes vasoconstriction. The respiratory rate increases. All of these changes occur with a near-normal BP. A drop in the patient's BP indicates that a significant volume of blood has been lost, and the body's efforts to compensate have failed. Such a patient is critically ill. See the management section of each condition for advice on how to manage these problems.

Pathophysiology, Assessment, and Management of GI Bleeding

Bleeding in the GI tract is a symptom of another disease, not a disease itself. **TABLE 21-7** lists possible causes of GI bleeding. The presentation differences between upper and lower GI bleeding are predominately related to the consistency and characteristics of the vomitus and stool that may be present. Upper GI bleeding is far more common than lower GI bleeding.

Generally speaking, upper GI bleeding causes **melena** (dark, tarry stool) and lower GI bleeding causes **hematochezia** (bright red blood in the stool). However, you must also consider the speed at which the blood is moving through the GI tract. If a patient is bleeding from a gastric ulcer and transit time of the blood to the rectum is short, instead of melena, the patient will have hematochezia. Copious bleeding can have a similar effect.

The presentation of GI bleeding varies. Each of the many conditions that can cause GI bleeding has its own pattern of disease progression. For example, diverticular disease has a rather gradual onset and tends to affect people in their 50s, 60s, or older. Mallory-Weiss syndrome has a sudden onset and affects people of any age. Gathering the information about how the patient moved from being healthy to needing an ambulance is critical in determining the correct working diagnosis.

The patient's past medical history and other possible events of abdominal pain or bleeding from the GI tract are also important information to obtain. Find out the medications the patient is taking. As previously mentioned, several medications can cause irritation of the GI tract, precipitating bleeding. Ask the patient how long they have been bleeding and whether they are taking any medications that affect coagulation. This information will help you to estimate how easily the bleeding can be controlled.

TABLE 21-7 GI Bleeding by Organ and Cause

Organ	Causes	Symptoms
Esophagus	Inflammation (esophagitis) Varices Tear (Mallory-Weiss syndrome) Cancer Dilated veins (cirrhosis, liver disease) GERD	Melena, hematemesis, vomitus with gross blood
Stomach	Ulcers Cancer Inflammation (gastritis)	Melena, hematemesis, vomitus with gross blood
Small intestine	Ulcer (duodenal) Cancer Inflammation (irritable bowel disease)	Melena, hematemesis, vomitus with gross blood
Large intestine	Infections Inflammation (ulcerative colitis) Colorectal polyps Colorectal cancer Diverticular disease	Hematochezia
Rectum	Hemorrhoids	Hematochezia, gross bleeding

Abbreviations: GERD, gastroesophageal reflux disease; GI, gastrointestinal

Treatment for patients with GI bleeding involves fluid resuscitation. In most patients, even those with stable vital signs, it is prudent to establish an intravenous (IV) line and provide 1,000 mL of an isotonic solution using a macrodrip tubing. This step will allow you to quickly resuscitate the patient with fluids should conditions change. Consider normal saline, Normosol, Isolyte, Plasma-Lyte, or lactated Ringer solution as options for fluid resuscitation. Refer to Chapter 14, *Medication Administration*, for a discussion of the various isotonic solutions. Specific conditions that cause GI bleeding are discussed next.

Upper GI Bleeding: Esophagogastric Varices

Pathophysiology

Esophagogastric varices are caused by pressure increases in the blood vessels that surround the esophagus and stomach. These esophageal blood vessels drain into the portal system. However, if the liver becomes damaged and blood cannot flow through it easily, the blood will begin to back up into the portal vessels, which can ultimately lead to their rupture. In the industrialized world, alcohol was once the main cause of **portal hypertension**. Today, hepatitis C is the primary cause. Men are more commonly diagnosed with esophageal varices, with 30% of patients bleeding within the first year after diagnosis; 30% of bleeding episodes involving esophageal varices are fatal.[5]

Assessment

Presentation of esophagogastric varices has a twofold appearance. Initially, the patient exhibits signs and symptoms of liver disease. Examples include fatigue, weight loss, jaundice, anorexia, an edematous abdomen, **pruritus** (itching), abdominal pain, nausea, and vomiting. The disease process, known as cirrhosis, is gradual, taking months to years to reach a state of extreme discomfort. (Cirrhosis is discussed in detail later in this chapter.)

Rupture of the varices is far more sudden. Patients will report an abrupt onset of discomfort in the throat. They may have severe dysphagia, vomiting of bright red blood, hypotension, and signs of shock. If the bleeding is less dramatic, **hematemesis** (vomit with blood) and melena are likely. Regardless of the speed of bleeding, damage to these vessels can be life threatening. The patient's hemoglobin level and hematocrit value will drop. These laboratory results can help determine the severity of the hemorrhaging. As with any patient who has liver disease, elevated levels of liver enzymes (alanine aminotransferase [ALT] and aspartate aminotransferase [AST]) should be expected.

Management

Expect large amounts of blood with rupture of esophagogastric varices. Owing to this aspect of the presentation, any health care provider can be unnerved by actively bleeding varices. Paramedics will need appropriate PPE, including mask and eye protection, because blood aerosolization is likely.

As with any GI bleeding disorder, accurate assessment of the degree of blood loss is critical. Be prepared for a hemodynamically unstable patient needing aggressive volume resuscitation and aggressive suctioning of the airway. Establish two large-bore IV lines with liter bags of isotonic solution. If the patient's level of consciousness (LOC) begins to decrease, consider securing the airway to prevent aspiration. This will be a difficult airway to manage due to the extreme amount of blood. Review Chapter 16, *Airway Management*, for guidance.

As with any emergent situation, communication with the team is essential. Fear can paralyze the novice. Openly discuss your concerns about the patient and management options. Talk yourself through the problem: airway, breathing, circulation. Coordinated, calm, calculated care will provide this patient with the best chance for survival.

Upper GI Bleeding: Mallory-Weiss Syndrome and Boerhaave Syndrome

Pathophysiology

Mallory-Weiss syndrome is a unique type of esophageal condition in which severe hemorrhage can occur. In this condition, the junction between the esophagus and the stomach tears, causing severe bleeding and potentially death. During the act of vomiting, pressure in the stomach can increase so greatly that it causes a failure of the structure of the esophagus. The tear that occurs is within the mucosal lining and does not travel entirely through the

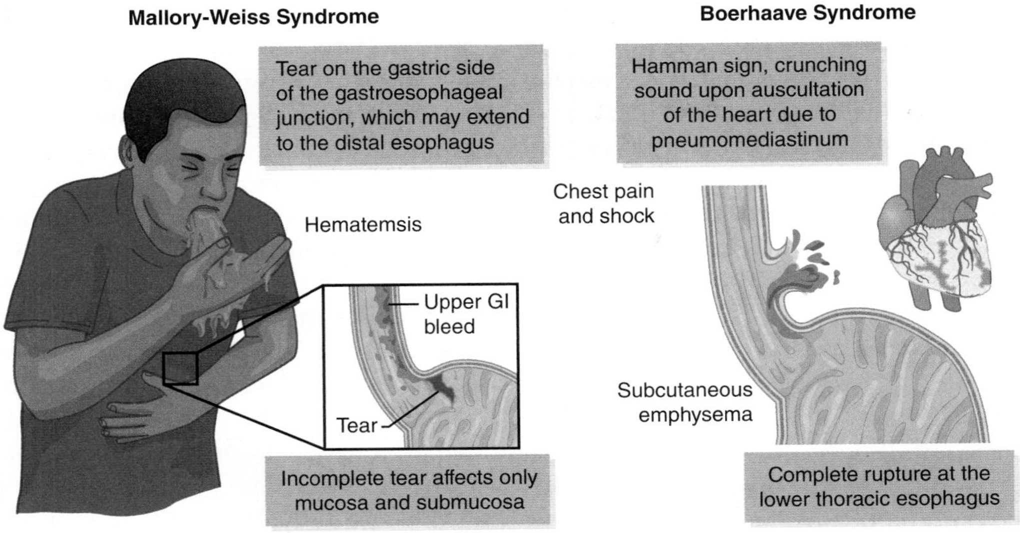

FIGURE 21-5 Mallory-Weiss syndrome versus Boerhaave syndrome.

wall of the esophagus. Mallory-Weiss syndrome occurs in men (most commonly between ages 40 and 50 years) more often than in women.[6] It has a mortality rate of as high as 8%.[6]

Similar to Mallory-Weiss syndrome, **Boerhaave syndrome** occurs during vomiting. In this case, the esophagus tears longitudinally and the tear travels entirely through the wall of the esophagus. This creates a passage for blood, air, and food out of the esophagus and into the mediastinum. Occurring more often in men, Boerhaave syndrome typically presents after a large meal that included alcohol consumption. If this condition is not treated within 2 days, mortality is approximately 90%.[7]

To summarize **FIGURE 21-5**, forceful vomiting that results in a tear in the esophagus near the stomach that *does not* go entirely through the esophageal wall is Mallory-Weiss syndrome. Forceful vomiting that results in a tear in the esophagus that extends entirely through the esophageal wall, creating a hole, is Boerhaave syndrome.

Assessment

Both conditions have a presentation linked to vomiting. In women, the vomiting may be associated with hyperemesis gravidarum, a condition of severe vomiting related to pregnancy. In men, the vomiting is typically associated with alcohol consumption. Mallory-Weiss syndrome classically presents with bleeding. The amount of the bleeding can range from small, resulting in little blood loss, to severe, leading to extreme hypovolemia. In extreme cases, patients will have signs and symptoms of shock, epigastric abdominal pain, hematemesis, and melena. It is nearly impossible to differentiate a severe Mallory-Weiss tear from bleeding esophageal varices in the field. Fortunately, the treatment is the same.

In contrast, Boerhaave syndrome presents with vomiting that is suddenly accompanied by upper chest pain. Swallowing often exacerbates the pain. There is little bleeding noted in this condition because any bleeding can travel into the newly created hole in the esophagus. This hole allows nonsterile materials, such as food and liquid, to enter into a sterile environment. The result is septicemia, pneumomediastinum (air in the mediastinum), mediastinitis (inflammation), empyema (a pocket of pus, in this case within the chest), or subcutaneous emphysema. Patients can have fever, sepsis (infection in the bloodstream), difficulty breathing, subcutaneous emphysema in the upper chest and neck region, and chest pain.

The time between when the tear occurs and when medical care is sought will determine the extent of the signs and symptoms. Mallory-Weiss syndrome's classical presentation is difficult to ignore: vomiting blood. Therefore, most people will seek medical care immediately after the tear occurs. Boerhaave syndrome, although a much more critical tear of the esophagus, has the unfortunate classical characteristic of causing chest pain after vomiting. This symptom is more easily ignored, especially by an individual who has consumed an excessive amount of alcohol. Often the patient will find a position of comfort and wait to feel better. The patient may drink some water or milk, which is now deposited into the chest, where it begins to cause infection. As the person breathes, small amounts of air can be trapped in the chest cavity. The longer the patient waits, the sicker they become and the more likely it is that sepsis will result in death.

Management

Management for Mallory-Weiss syndrome is the same as for esophagogastric varices and is directed at determining the extent of blood loss. In this case, the patient may be dehydrated from the repeated vomiting, so blood loss can have exaggerated effects.

Boerhaave syndrome requires management related to the potential for sepsis. Complicating this presentation is the symptom of chest pain. Because this condition tends to occur in men ages 50 to 70 years, the possibility of myocardial infarction (MI) is a reasonable conclusion.[7] The patient should be treated as if he had experienced an MI until proven otherwise. Be proactive in contacting medical control to help with these patients. Aspirin therapy is not desirable.

Upper GI Bleeding: Peptic Ulcer Disease and Gastritis

Pathophysiology

The stomach and duodenum are subjected to high levels of acidity. To help prevent damage, protective mucous layers line both organs. In **peptic ulcer disease (PUD)**, the protective layer has been eroded, allowing the acid to eat into the organ itself. This erosion typically occurs over weeks, months, or even years. Gastritis is caused by the same imbalance between stomach acid and the protective layers. **Gastritis** is a preulcerative state in which the stomach is inflamed, but erosion has not yet occurred.

PUD and gastritis, which affect men and women equally, are now known to have a variety of causes.[8] PUD was once thought to be related to eating a highly spiced diet; however, the most common cause is now recognized to be infection of the stomach with the bacterium *Helicobacter pylori*. Chronic use of NSAIDs is the most frequent cause of erosive gastritis, in which the mucosal lining of the stomach slowly erodes and ulcerates. Patients who have sustained severe burns or other types of trauma also are susceptible to gastritis, because these extreme stress states increase gastric acid production. Ulcers caused by the stress related to burns are called Curling ulcers. Those caused by head injuries or brain tumors are called Cushing ulcers. Remember the Cushing triad related to increased intracranial pressure? This is the same Cushing. Alcohol and smoking can also affect the severity of PUD by increasing gastric acidity. Zollinger-Ellison syndrome occurs when tumors within the pancreas and duodenum cause increased gastric acid production, leading to PUD. This syndrome has a genetic component and is most common in men 30 to 50 years of age.

All of the factors cited as risks for PUD can also cause gastritis. In addition, foodborne infections and food allergies also can cause inflammation of the stomach.

> **Special Populations**
>
> Older adults are more vulnerable to the primary and secondary causes of PUD. As a result, PUD tends to affect an older population. As people age, the immune system's ability to fight infection decreases, making infection with *Helicobacter pylori* more likely. In addition, older adults frequently use NSAIDs for arthritis and other musculoskeletal conditions. Thus, older adults are more likely to develop erosive gastritis; it occurs more often in people older than 60 years.[9]

Assessment

In both PUD and gastritis, patients will experience a classic sequence of pain in the epigastrium that subsides or diminishes immediately after eating and then reemerges 2 to 3 hours later. The pain is described as burning or gnawing. Nausea, vomiting, belching, and heartburn are common. In PUD, if the erosion is severe, gastric bleeding can occur with the result of hematemesis and melena. Both groups of patients may experience dyspepsia (belching, bloating, and fatty food intolerance), fatigue, and anemia. Many will complain of pain waking them from sleep.

In PUD, if the erosion has eaten through the wall of the stomach or duodenum, the ulcer is said to have *perforated*. The result is a sudden increase in the severity and quality of pain. What was epigastric now becomes more diffuse abdominal pain with any motion exacerbating the pain. At this point, the patient's stomach contents have access to the sterile peritoneum and infection can easily occur. **Peritonitis** (inflammation of the peritoneum) is the result, along with rebound tenderness and potential hypotension due to sepsis.

Management

The major focus for prehospital management of PUD and gastritis is accurate assessment of the degree of blood loss and preparation to manage any hypotension that is present. Orthostatic vital signs are critical in determining fluid needs and transportation/packaging issues. Because sudden vomiting of blood can occur with a change in position, these patients should be taken downstairs in a stair chair rather than walking.

IV fluids may be needed based on the amount of blood loss. Also, if you suspect a perforated gastric ulcer, then sepsis is a real concern. Management for gastritis is supportive. Consider administering antiemetics in patients with PUD and gastritis.

Upper GI Bleeding: Gastroesophageal Reflux Disease and Hiatal Hernia

Pathophysiology

Gastroesophageal reflux disease (GERD) is a condition in which the lower esophageal sphincter (LES)—the sphincter between the esophagus and the stomach, also called the cardiac sphincter—opens and allows stomach acid to move superiorly. This condition, also referred to as acid reflux disease, can cause a burning sensation within the chest (heartburn). Various factors can make some people more susceptible to this condition. Smoking, obesity, and pregnancy all increase the chances of GERD. Eating fatty fried foods, drinking alcohol, and eating citrus fruits are also associated with GERD. If the reflux continues over a long period, damage can occur to the esophageal wall. This damage could result in weakened portions that are more susceptible to bleeding.

A **hiatal hernia** is a protrusion of a portion of the stomach through the diaphragm. If there is a weakness in the diaphragm wall (through which the esophagus normally traverses), a portion of the stomach can become trapped superiorly to the diaphragm. This creates a small pocket in which the superior "door" is the LES and the inferior "door" is the diaphragm **FIGURE 21-6**. Food and acid can become temporarily stuck in this space, leading to GERD-like symptoms. However, most hiatal hernias are asymptomatic. Hiatal hernias are caused by increased intra-abdominal pressure. Hiatal hernias are more prevalent in older women.[10]

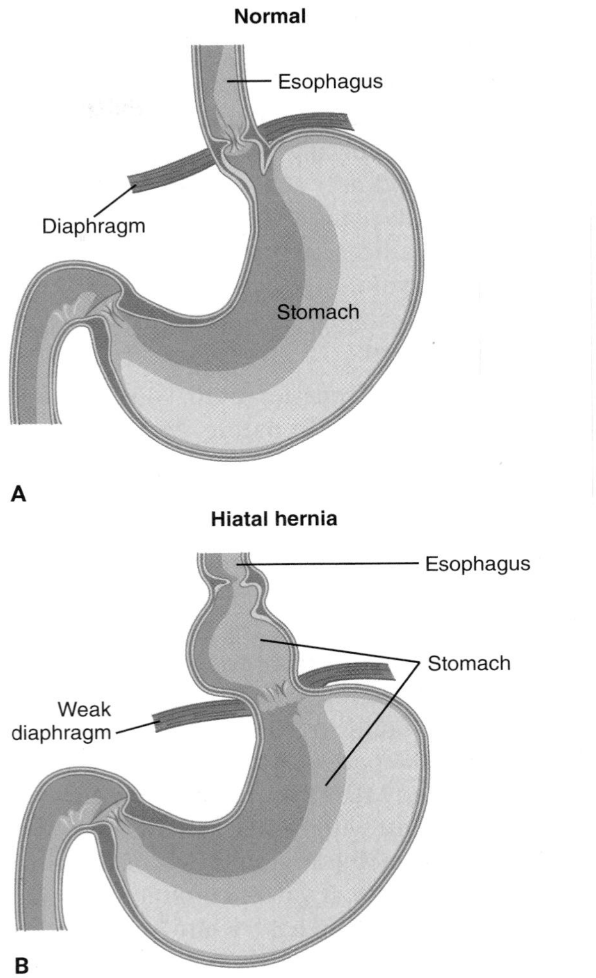

FIGURE 21-6 A. Normal configuration. **B.** Hiatal hernia.

One in four people in the United States has experienced GERD at some point in their lives, and nearly 1 in 10 experiences GERD symptoms daily.[3] EMS professionals will almost certainly encounter these patients.

Assessment

Heartburn is the predominant clinical finding for GERD. The pain may increase with positional changes; sitting upright is preferred, whereas lying flat makes the condition worse. Some patients may not have pain, but experience coughing or have difficulty swallowing. Bleeding can occur if the damage is long term, resulting in hematemesis and melena. Hiatal hernias typically do not become symptomatic unless food and acid cannot be flushed efficiently from the pocket. The retained acid can cause erosion of the herniated stomach wall, leading to bleeding and pain.

Management

Prehospital treatment for both GERD and hiatal hernia is supportive in nature. Medical treatment focuses on decreasing the acidity of the material within the esophagus by neutralizing it or preventing the acid from being produced. Antacids, proton pump inhibitors, and histamine H_2 receptor (H_2) blockers are the common classifications of medications used for this condition. If these medications fail to control the discomfort, then surgical repair may be needed.

One confounding circumstance that can occur is when the patient with a history of GERD begins to have an MI. Such a patient may confuse the pain in the chest with GERD. Patients may begin to self-medicate, taking large amounts of antacid to try to control the pain. If you encounter a patient who reports chest pain and has a white "milk mustache," the coating around the mouth may be an antacid. Ask how much antacid the patient has taken. Large amounts of antacid can cause metabolic alkalosis.

Lower GI Bleeding: Hemorrhoids

Pathophysiology

A number of conditions can cause lower GI bleeding. Hemorrhoids are a swelling and inflammation of the vascular cushions surrounding the rectum that can result in lower GI bleeding. These vascular cushions, or sinusoids, are made up of connections between arteries and veins along with their supportive muscle and connective tissue. Hemorrhoids are a common problem: An estimated 4% of the population has hemorrhoids, with 30% of those seeking medical care or using medication for their condition at some point.[11] Hemorrhoids can be caused by conditions that either increase pressure on the rectum or cause irritation of the rectum. Pregnancy, straining at stool, and chronic constipation cause increased pressure. Anal intercourse and diarrhea can cause irritation and lower GI bleeding.

Hemorrhoids are divided into two types: internal and external. Internal hemorrhoids are painless but can prolapse (protrude from the anal canal). External hemorrhoids are painful and tend to have an area of swelling and clot formation.

Assessment

Hemorrhoids present with bright red blood during defecation. This hematochezia, or frank bleeding, tends to be minimal and is easily controlled. Additionally, patients may experience itching and a small mass in the rectum. Typically this mass is a clot formed in response to the mild bleeding.

Management

Prehospital management is supportive. In isolation, hemorrhoids are more of an inconvenience than a life-threatening condition. Some patients may be at greater risk for serious consequences. Cautiously assess the patient who has any bleeding disorder or is taking anticoagulants. In this setting, even a minor bleeding disorder can become life threatening. To ensure the patient is hemodynamically stable, obtain orthostatic vital signs.

The best management for hemorrhoids is prevention, which includes eating a high-fiber diet and exercising.

Lower GI Bleeding: Anal Fissures

Pathophysiology

Anal fissures are linear tears to the mucosal lining in and near the anus that can cause lower GI bleeding. The exact reason why a fissure is created near the anus is unclear. It is thought to be precipitated by the passage of large, hard stools. Patients who have diets that are low in raw fruits and vegetables are at highest risk of anal fissures. Crohn disease, human immunodeficiency virus infection, trauma, and anorectal cancer are other causes of this painful condition. Anal fissures occur with equal frequency in men and women. The average age at onset is between 20 and 60 years.[12]

Assessment

Patients present with painful defecation. A small amount of bright red blood may be noted on the toilet paper, but rarely do these fissures cause significant blood loss. The pain persists for several minutes to several hours after the bowel movement.

Anytime this area is stretched, the fissure stretches, causing pain and more tearing. Pain is common with every bowel movement.

This pain creates a vicious cycle. Because it hurts to have a bowel movement, patients delay as long as possible. This delay causes the feces to become larger and harder, thus making them more difficult to pass. Eventually, when the movement is inevitable, the large stool causes more stretching, more tearing, and consequently more pain. This painful bowel movement precipitates an even greater reluctance to have a bowel movement, perpetuating the cycle.

Management

Treatment of anal fissures is the same as for hemorrhoids: supportive care. To facilitate patient comfort, a 5 × 9–inch dressing can be placed over the patient's anus to help pad the area. Do not under any circumstances pack dressings into the fissure or the anus. Remember, bleeding for this condition, as with hemorrhoids, is typically minimal and non–life threatening.

Most anal fissures heal without surgical intervention.

Pathophysiology, Assessment, and Management of Esophageal Pathologies

Esophagitis

Pathophysiology

As its name suggests, **esophagitis** is an inflammation of the esophagus. It can be caused by an infectious process or by reflux of gastric secretions into the esophagus. Additionally, some medications can be irritating, as can chemotherapy or radiation therapy. Esophagitis also is associated with eosinophils, a type of white blood cell.

Regardless of the underlying cause, the effects are irritation and swelling. Generally speaking, patients will present with dyspepsia (heartburn) or choking as their primary complaint. It can be difficult to distinguish GERD from esophagitis.

Assessment

Due to the irritation, patients experience dyspepsia and upper abdominal/lower chest pain. This pain tends to increase with bending over or lying supine. Water brash, the bitter taste of gastric acid in the mouth, may also occur. These symptoms are common with esophagitis caused by GERD. Other symptoms include dysphagia, odynophagia (painful dysphagia), and potential food impaction within the esophagus. These later symptoms are more common in eosinophilic, medication-related, and infectious esophagitis. There are few physical signs that are directly related to this condition. Most patients with esophagitis are adults.[13]

Management

Care for esophagitis is supportive in nature. One of the potentially confusing components of this condition is related to the symptom of chest pain. It can be difficult, if not impossible, to determine the exact cause of the chest pain. Be cautious: If your patient presents with chest pain, consider MI as the cause and treat accordingly. For patients who present with dyspepsia, see the section on GERD for management options. For patients with dysphagia, see the section on esophageal stricture for management options.

Tracheoesophageal Fistula

Pathophysiology

The trachea and the esophagus lie next to each other as they move inferiorly into the thorax. These two structures touch, which explains why patients frequently report coughing when they have something stuck in their esophagus. An opening between two portions of the body or between a body part and the outside of the body is called a **fistula**. The fistula allows communication of material between the two spaces. If a connection is made between the esophagus and the trachea, the opening is referred to as a **tracheoesophageal fistula (TEF)**.

Patients are either born with this atypical connection or acquire it during the life course. Common methods of acquiring TEF are through cancer, trauma, or iatrogenic (caused by a medical procedure such as endotracheal [ET] intubation) means. The cuff on the ET tube is used to isolate the trachea from secretions moving inferiorly and also to improve ventilation of the lungs. To perform its job, the cuff must have enough air pressure to seal around the circumference of the trachea. When you press your thumb against a hard surface, you squeeze the blood out, as evidenced by the blanching that occurs. Similarly, the pressure used to seal the ET tube can squeeze blood away from an area of the tracheal wall. Over many days, this area may become ischemic and can eventually die. An opening may be created through the weakened area of the trachea and the anterior portion of the esophagus. Similarly, a tumor within the esophagus or trachea can erode a hole between the two structures. A penetrating wound also can create an opening.

TEF allows food to move from the esophagus into the trachea and eventually into the lungs. Pneumonia and sepsis are two possible serious consequences of this aspiration. If TEF is left uncorrected, the patient can die. Fortunately, it takes many days to cause that degree of damage to the tracheal wall. This is the reason why patients are not typically intubated for longer than 7 to 14 days. To prevent TEF, patients receive a tracheotomy, which limits, but does not eliminate, the risk of TEF.

There are no racial or sexual predispositions for TEF. As people age, however, the likelihood they will need ventilator assistance increases. This use of artificial ventilation places older adults at greater risk for iatrogenic TEF. Patients with TEF have a high mortality, as they have an increased risk of developing sepsis, pneumonia, and acute respiratory distress syndrome (ARDS).[14]

Assessment

If TEF is due to cancer, patients will present with cough, fever, and aspiration. They may report excessive gas in the stomach and increased oral secretions. Patients who are intubated or have undergone a tracheostomy are more complicated. They may have a decreased LOC or may be fed via gastrostomy tubes. In these cases, the main presentation will be tachycardia, fever, and sepsis of unknown origin. Coughing may still be present.

Management

Acute care of patients with TEF focuses on ensuring adequate ventilation and managing potential sepsis. You may need to suction the patient due to increased oral secretions. If the patient needs ET intubation, it should be accomplished meticulously. Ensure proper tube placement and then reconfirm the correct positioning. Waveform capnography should provide early evidence of a misplaced tube. The fistula could allow the ET tube to be accidentally placed within the esophagus. If appropriate, elevating the head of the cot can help the patient manage secretions. IV fluids and appropriate vasopressors may be needed if the patient is septic. Ultimately, this condition will need surgical repair.

Esophageal Stricture or Stenosis

Pathophysiology

A **stricture** (or stenosis) is an abnormal narrowing of a structure. The esophagus can become narrowed as a result of inflammation, tumors, infection, scarring from acid reflux, and acid reflux. As the diameter of the esophagus diminishes, it becomes more difficult for the person to swallow **FIGURE 21-7**. This narrowing can occur along the entire length of the organ, but in 60% to 70% of cases it occurs at the distal portion of the esophagus.[15] Lower esophageal strictures are most often caused by GERD. Men have this condition more often than women.[15]

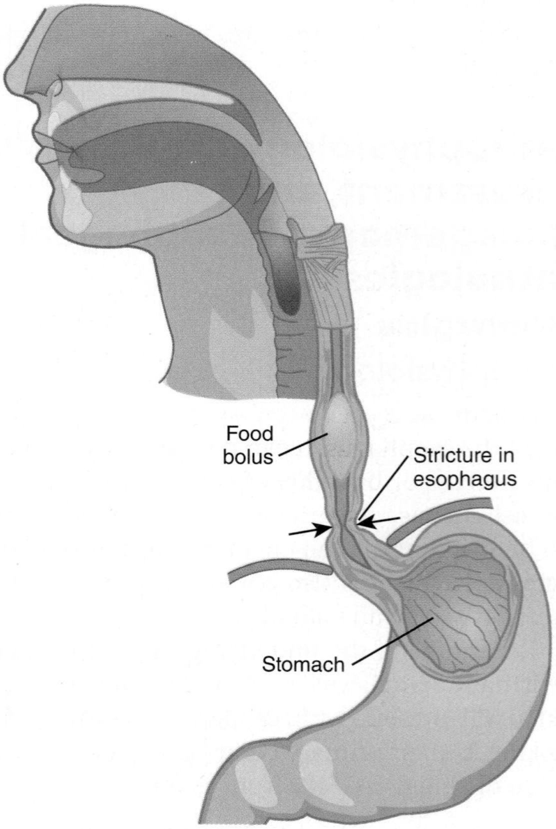

FIGURE 21-7 Esophageal stricture.

Assessment

Most patients with this condition have a history of multiple episodes of choking. They may have large volumes of secretions and the sensation of choking, with spitting up or gagging on a large quantity of saliva. They commonly report not being able to move a piece of food they just swallowed. This dysphagia can progress to odynophagia. There may be accompanying difficulty in breathing and hiccups that are painful, but cyanosis is rare, as the obstruction is in the esophagus. In the middle of an obstructive event, the patient may not be able to speak. Difficulty in managing oral secretions may also be present.

Management

As you might expect, the main concern with esophageal strictures is airway compromise. The patient may aspirate or have an obstruction that interferes significantly with airflow. Ensure the patient has a stable airway. If oxygen saturation is stable and the patient remains acyanotic, encourage the patient to remain calm; this sensation can lead to severe anxiety. If the airway is stable, then aggressive attempts at removal of the obstruction are not needed. If the patient is unable to move air effectively, then treat the situation as an airway obstruction and manage it appropriately.

Glucagon can be considered in patients with esophageal obstruction. This medication causes dilation of the esophagus and ideally will allow the obstruction to pass into the stomach. Glucagon has only a limited effect on strictures, so contact online medical direction before you administer it for this purpose. Have the patient sit upright and be prepared to assist with oral secretions. If you arrive and the patient has already cleared the obstruction, encourage the patient to go to the ED.

Pathophysiology, Assessment, and Management of Acute Inflammatory Conditions

Inflammation is a natural response to injury. If the body is attacked by an infectious agent, then vasodilation, mobilization of white blood cells, and changes in cellular metabolic processes will result. All of these effects allow the cell to move from a normal operating mode into one of being under siege. The purpose of inflammation is to assist the white blood cells in either destroying the invading agent or, at the least, sealing it off so it cannot spread.

The redness, swelling, and tenderness that occur during an infection are the result of inflammation. The change in vascular permeability and vasodilation will cause redness and swelling. Swelling can cause pressure, which causes pain. Vasodilation and increased capillary permeability enable white blood cells to more effectively reach the area of damage.

Inflammation in the GI system can occur at many levels. Localized inflammation will cause localized signs and symptoms. For example, patients with **hepatitis**, an inflammation of the liver, can experience pain in the right upper quadrant of the abdomen. This pain can be due to mild swelling of the liver. In peritonitis, inflammation and irritation affect the peritoneum throughout the abdomen, so the patient may experience generalized pain that is rebound in nature. If an infectious agent causes the inflammation, the peritonitis can be a sign of movement of bacteria into the abdomen and eventually into the bloodstream (sepsis).

The body will respond to sepsis with a more generalized inflammatory response. One of the severe consequences of sepsis is the depletion of resources to manage the infection. In sepsis, infection is almost literally everywhere in the body. The body is trying to fight many battles but does not have adequate white blood cells, histamine, blood, and energy to do so. Soon the defenses being mounted to infection diminish, resulting in possible detriment to the patient. If a balance between resource demand and supply cannot soon be restored, death will occur.

Conversely, the body may become hyperstimulated, as sepsis can trigger an exaggerated inflammatory response. This inflammation can damage portions of the body that are not infected. Consider the effects of COVID-19 (coronavirus disease 2019). This viral infection can trigger inflammation out of proportion to the level of infection. Thus, the virus starts a cascade of bodily defense reactions that can result in death.

Many diseases of the GI system are caused by inflammation, albeit with no defined reason for that inflammation to occur. In this case, the body begins attacking and killing its own cells, a process referred to as an autoimmune condition.

A variety of reasons have been postulated for this misdirected attack, but no definitive cause and effect relationship has been found. One theory is that the patient ingests food with a little-known antigen present. This protein substance is identified as foreign, with the body then creating antibodies against it. Another speculation is that the patient comes in contact with a virus that triggers an immune response. White blood cells then begin to destroy a portion of the GI system, causing damage. The body works to rebuild the damaged areas, but scarred portions of the GI tract may result.

Peritonitis

Pathophysiology

Recall that the peritoneum is the thin membrane that forms a sac containing all of the organs and structures within the abdominal cavity. If an infectious agent can gain access to it, this lining can become inflamed. The two main ways that peritoneal infections occur are through the rupture of an internal organ or the movement of bacteria out of the intestines. In **appendicitis**, if the appendix ruptures, purulent (pus-containing) material can leak into the peritoneal space, thus irritating the peritoneum. This can also happen with a ruptured bowel.

Spontaneous bacterial peritonitis refers to a condition in which bacteria migrate out of the intestine and enter the peritoneal space. **Ascites**, or abdominal edema, is associated with this condition in most adults. Cirrhosis is a common cause of ascites in these patients. The presence of excess fluid within the peritoneal space changes the permeability of the intestinal walls, allowing bacteria to exit.

In either case, the bacteria are able to flourish in the peritoneal space, and it does not take long until sepsis can occur. Uncomplicated peritonitis has a mortality rate of about 5%; however, if sepsis, ARDS, and multiorgan failure occur, the mortality rate jumps to nearly 70%.[16]

Assessment

Peritoneal irritation presents as abdominal pain. This pain tends to be diffuse, with a focal point over the area of greatest irritation. In patients with bowel rupture, the pain may be focused over the left upper quadrant if the transverse colon has failed. In appendicitis, the right lower quadrant of the abdomen will have greatest pain. A ruptured **diverticulum** will most commonly have the focal point in the left lower quadrant. Peritoneal pain will often increase with coughing (Dunphy sign) and pain will be rebound in nature. Patients tend to have board-hard abdomens and will not want to lie flat.

Pain associated with peritoneal irritation can range from dull to severe. Patients will often be febrile and want to lie in a fetal position, which relieves stress on the abdominal wall. Tachycardia, anorexia, nausea, vomiting, abdominal distention, and dehydration also occur. These patients are at risk for both hypovolemic shock and septic shock.

The presentation of peritonitis may be very subtle in patients who are immunocompromised or who otherwise have a decreased immune response. Elderly patients may present with unexplained new-onset changes in LOC and hypotension. Especially in these patients, a detailed history of present illness, past medical history, and current medications taken can assist you in exploring the possible causes of the recent changes.

Management

Patients with peritonitis are critically ill. Management of this condition is directed at supporting vital signs. Treat the patient for shock. Be prepared to administer several fluid boluses to maintain BP. Norepinephrine may be indicated if sepsis is present.

Managing these patients' pain is often tricky. Antiemetics are indicated. Many of the analgesics that you carry also cause vasodilation. In cases of sepsis, this adverse effect is undesirable.

Cholecystitis and Biliary Tract Disorders

Pathophysiology

Biliary tract disorders involve inflammation of the gallbladder. These disorders include the following conditions:

- **Cholangitis**. Inflammation of the bile duct
- **Cholelithiasis**. Presence of stones within the gallbladder
- Choledocholithiasis. Presence of at least one of the gallstones within the common bile duct
- Cholecystitis. Inflammation of the gallbladder
- Acalculous cholecystitis. Inflammation of the gallbladder without the presence of gallstones

Cholangitis can cause acalculous cholecystitis. These conditions have similar presentation patterns, so they will be discussed here as a group.

It is unclear why gallstones form; they are believed to be due to either increased bile production or decreased emptying of the gallbladder. Other causes of gallbladder inflammation arise from decreased flow of biliary materials, including major trauma, sepsis, sickle cell disease, and prolonged fasting.

Cholecystitis is more common in women than men. Caucasians have a higher prevalence than do African Americans.[17] Other persons at increased risk include older people and people who are overweight or obese or have had a recent extreme weight loss.[17] Remember the "five Fs" of cholecystitis related to people who have this condition most often:

- Fair (Caucasian)
- Fat
- Female
- Fertile
- Forty to fifty years old—the age at which diagnosis becomes more common

The gallbladder's function is to store bile, an enzyme used to break down fat, and then contract, releasing the bile. When fatty foods are present in the duodenum, the gallbladder contracts, but extreme pain will occur in the right upper quadrant and radiate to the right shoulder if a blockage is present.

Assessment

The classic pattern for cholecystitis is for the patient to have no pain until a fatty meal is eaten. Two to three hours later, the patient begins to develop severe upper right quadrant abdominal pain. However, this pattern is not absolute and may vary based on the consistency of the foods consumed. A fatty steak will remain in the stomach longer than a cheesy casserole. The faster the food is emptied from the stomach, the sooner the pain begins after the meal.

The abdominal pain associated with gallbladder disorders can be quite severe. In addition to the pain, the patient may demonstrate a positive Murphy sign. Ask the patient to breathe out. Then take the tips of your fingers and palpate deeply along the intercostal margin of the right upper quadrant. You are now applying pressure to the liver and subsequently to the gallbladder.

Next, ask the patient to inhale deeply. As inspiration continues, the diaphragm will drop and eventually come into contact with the gallbladder. A patient who has cholecystitis may suddenly stop inspiring because of a sharp increase in pain: a positive Murphy sign. Although not specific for cholecystitis, Murphy sign, along with additional assessment details, can provide valuable information.

Nausea, vomiting, fever, jaundice, epigastric pain, and tachycardia are also often present with this disease. Charcot triad—fever, right upper quadrant pain, and jaundice—may indicate an inflammation of the common bile duct in 15% to 20% of patients.[18]

Management

Prehospital treatment for cholecystitis is directed at making the patient comfortable. Rarely is this condition life threatening, though the pain from cholecystitis can cause the patient to experience vasovagal stimulation. Cholecystitis can cause pancreatitis due to the connection on the common bile duct into the pancreatic duct: If a stone is present, it can migrate and block the pancreatic duct.

Medications to control pain include opiates. Associated nausea typically subsides with relief of pain. If the patient experiences vomiting, IV fluid may be indicated.

Appendicitis

Pathophysiology

Appendicitis is a condition with which most people are familiar and a frequent cause of acute abdomen. The condition occurs when fecal matter or other material accumulates in the appendix. When the organ can no longer flush out this material normally, pressure builds. This pressure decreases the flow of blood and lymph fluid, hindering the body's ability to fight infection. The combination of bacteria in the feces and diminished ability to combat local infection creates an ideal environment for the uncontrolled reproduction of bacteria. If left unchecked, overpressurization of the appendix will eventually cause it to rupture, resulting in peritonitis, sepsis, and death.

Appendicitis occurs in every age group. Appendicitis most commonly occurs between the ages of 10 and 30 years.[19] Although older adults experience appendicitis less often, they have a higher mortality rate from it. Appendicitis is slightly more likely to develop in men than in women.[19]

> **Words of Wisdom**
>
> EMS can be a stressful, emotionally demanding career, and often our dietary choices are guided by these emotions. Paramedics may desire "comfort" foods and "rewards" with high levels of sugar and saturated fat, sugar- and caffeine-containing beverages for energy boosts, and maybe even a couple of alcoholic beverages after our shift to "unwind." Furthermore, paramedics are often pressed for time. Running from call to call does not make it easy to eat healthfully. What do you choose for lunch when you have only a few free minutes? Often, something unhealthy from a drive-through or convenience store seems like the only option.
>
> Don't overlook the importance of fiber in your diet. Fiber helps reduce the incidence of appendicitis by decreasing the transit time of stool through the bowel, thus flushing the appendix. Thus, one of the easiest ways to prevent appendicitis is to eat a high-fiber diet.
>
> You don't have to become a vegan, but eating a whole apple, having a salad instead of a burger, or adding baked beans to a dinner can go a long way toward increasing your fiber intake.
>
> Broccoli or barbeque? Why not both—better for your heart and better for your appendix!

> **Special Populations**
>
> As mentioned, appendicitis can be difficult to diagnosis. Consider that appendicitis occurs most often in young people, including young women who are pregnant. As the uterus expands to accommodate the growing fetus, it moves the appendix out of its normal position. A woman in her third trimester of pregnancy who has appendicitis is more likely to present with right upper quadrant or right flank pain instead of right lower quadrant pain. Even the most attentive paramedic will have difficulty determining if this pain is appendicitis, cholecystitis, or renal calculi.

Assessment

Appendicitis can be difficult to diagnose. The classic presentation of appendicitis can be divided into three stages: early, ripe, and rupture.

- **Early.** Periumbilical pain, nausea, vomiting, low-grade fever, loss of appetite
- **Ripe.** Pain in lower right quadrant (McBurney point)
- **Rupture.** Initial decrease in pain (decreased pressure), generalized severe abdominal pain, rebound tenderness

In early stages, patients classically present with poorly defined periumbilical pain. Nausea, vomiting, anorexia, and a low-grade fever are typically noted. The vomiting tends to occur after the pain starts, rather than before it emerges. Over several hours, the appendix will swell and eventually pressure will increase. This takes approximately 48 hours. The patient is now in the ripe stage. During this time, the pain will migrate to become localized right lower quadrant pain and will become more severe. If the appendix ruptures, the rupture stage is entered. In this stage, at first there may be a sudden decrease of pain with a sense of relief because of the sudden decreased pressure. Now the infectious material has access to the entire abdominal cavity. During this stage, the pain becomes generalized throughout the abdomen. Rebound tenderness is a sign of perforation of the appendix with resultant peritonitis.

Management

Prehospital management of appendicitis should include an assessment for septicemia. If this blood infection is present, septic shock can occur. Volume resuscitation may not be adequate to restore BP. Be prepared to use norepinephrine if crystalloids are not effective. Administration of pain and antinausea medications are indicated for these patients.

Diverticulitis

Pathophysiology

To understand **diverticulitis**, you must first know what a diverticulum is: a weak area in the colon that begins to have small outcroppings that turn into pouches. These pockets are called diverticula (the plural of *diverticulum*). The condition of having diverticula is referred to as diverticulosis. When these diverticula become inflamed, the patient is said to have diverticulitis. Diverticulitis is the most common diagnosis among patients with GI conditions treated in the ED.[20]

What causes diverticulitis is unclear, but research has shown that people in industrialized nations tend to have this condition more often than people from Africa and Asia.[20] The typical patient is older than 60 years. More important than sex or race is the amount of fiber in the patient's diet. Decreased amounts of fiber increase patients' risk for this disease.[21]

According to the proposed etiologic theory, as the amount of fiber in a person's diet decreases, the consistency of the normal stool becomes more solid. This hard stool takes more contractions to move and subsequently increases colon pressure. In this environment, small defects in the colonic wall that would otherwise never pose a problem now fail, resulting in bulges in the wall.

The next step in this process is similar to appendicitis. As feces travel through the colon, some may become trapped in the pouch. Bacteria can grow and cause localized inflammation and infection. As the body attempts to manage this infection, scarring, adhesions, and even fistulas can develop. A fistula, as noted earlier, is an abnormal connection between two cavities. The most common location for fistulas in diverticulitis is between the colon and the bladder. Significant infections can develop from having feces in the bladder.

Assessment

Presentation of diverticulitis is abdominal pain that tends to be localized to the left side of the lower abdomen. Classic signs of infection include fever, malaise, body aches, chills, nausea, and vomiting. Bleeding is rare with this condition. Patients can have diarrhea or constipation. Because of the local infections of the pouches on the colonic walls, adhesions can develop, thus narrowing the diameter of the colon. This can result in constipation, and potentially bowel obstruction. Although diverticulitis typically results in left-side pain, it can occur anywhere within the colon. Thus, diverticulitis can look like many other abdominal pain conditions.

Management

Management of diverticulitis is directed at making the patient comfortable. Examine the patient closely to ensure severe infection is not present. Sepsis can occur easily in patients with fistulas to the urinary bladder. These patients may need large amounts of fluids and/or norepinephrine to maintain BP. Work to improve the patient's comfort through positioning, pain medication, and antiemetics as needed.

Pancreatitis

Pathophysiology

The enzymes the pancreas creates are designed to break down the food ingested into substances that the intestines can absorb. If the pancreatic duct,

YOU are the Paramedic

PART 4

You establish an IV line and administer a 250-mL fluid challenge after listening to lung sounds in all fields. The patient continues to report abdominal pain, which she describes as an 8 on a scale of 0 to 10. The patient is still unable to sit up and appears restless.

Recording Time: 10 Minutes	
Respirations	18 breaths/min
Pulse	110 beats/min, lying down
Skin	Cool, pale, moist
Blood pressure	110/86 mm Hg, lying down
Oxygen saturation (Spo_2)	98% with oxygen at 15 L/min via nonrebreathing mask
Pupils	PERRLA

7. Knowing that this patient has postural vital signs, how will you move the patient downstairs?

8. Should you administer a pain medication to make the patient more comfortable?

the pathway through which these enzymes exit the pancreas, becomes blocked, the enzymes will perform their chemical processes on the protein and fat of the pancreas itself. This is referred to as autodigestion of the pancreas.

Autodigestion leads to inflammation of the pancreas, or **pancreatitis**. This process can occur suddenly or over many months. Patients can have single attacks or episodic attacks and remissions for a long time. Men tend to have this condition more commonly than women. It also occurs more often in African Americans ages 35 to 64 years.[22] The main causes of this condition are increased alcohol consumption (male patients) and gallstones (female patients). Other causes include medication reactions, trauma, cancer, and high triglyceride levels.[22]

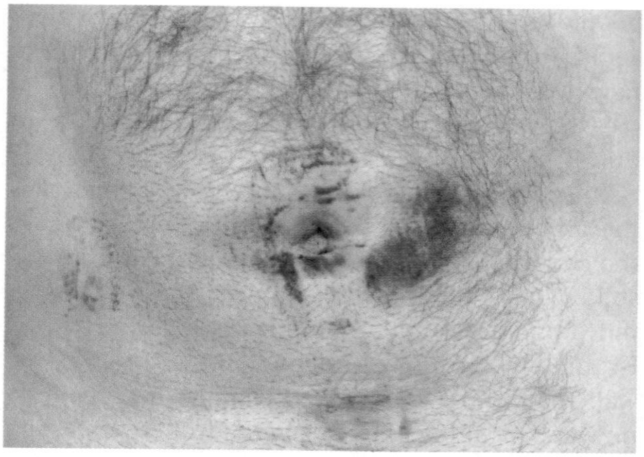

FIGURE 21-8 Periumbilical ecchymosis, or Cullen sign, indicating intraperitoneal hemorrhage.

Assessment

The pain of pancreatitis tends to be localized to the epigastric area, in the left upper quadrant. It can be a dull or steady, severe ache. Radiation of the pain to the back occurs in nearly one-half of patients. Patients typically obtain some relief by bending forward or assuming a fetal position. The pain tends to come on suddenly and is relatively constant. This unrelenting pain is what sends patients to a health care provider. In addition to the pain, patients may experience nausea, vomiting, fever, tachycardia, hypotension, and muscle spasms in the extremities. This condition tends to cause hypocalcemia, low blood calcium, which can lead to muscle spasms. Pancreatitis caused by gallstones can lead to jaundice.

The most alarming concern associated with pancreatitis is internal hemorrhage. If autodigestion is advanced, blood vessels in and near the pancreas can become compromised. Severe and uncontrolled hemorrhage can ensue. In these patients, hemodynamic instability can be present. In addition, Cullen sign (bruising around the umbilicus) **FIGURE 21-8** or Grey Turner sign (bruising in the flanks) **FIGURE 21-9** may be observed, indicating severe internal bleeding.

Patients with pancreatitis have a 10% to 15% mortality rate.[22] Sepsis and hemorrhage are the leading causes of death.

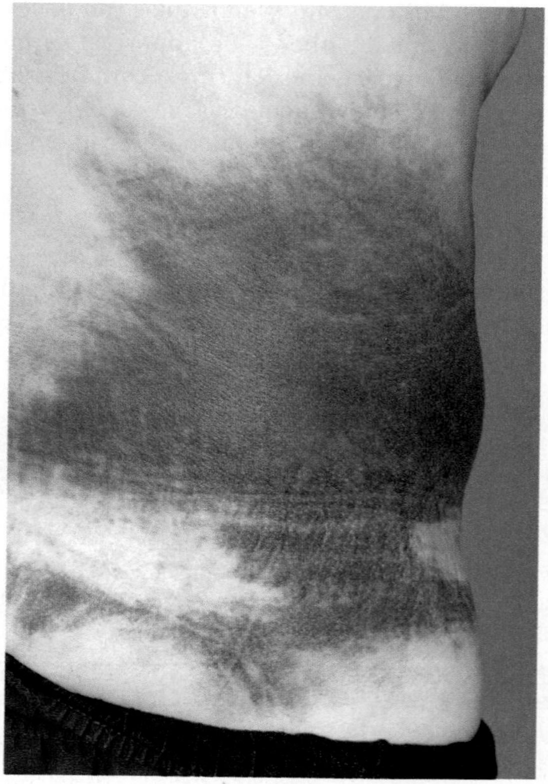

FIGURE 21-9 Flank ecchymosis, or Grey Turner sign, indicating retroperitoneal hemorrhage.

Management

Treatment for the prehospital patient with pancreatitis should be directed by general management guidelines. Pay special attention to assessing the patient for signs of severe hemorrhage. If present, begin fluid resuscitation. Opiate analgesics are often indicated in these patients. When narcotics are given, frequent reassessment of vital signs is essential to ensure hypotension and respiratory depression do not occur.

Pathophysiology, Assessment, and Management of Chronic Inflammatory Conditions

Patients who have chronic inflammation of all or part of the GI tract are said to have **inflammatory bowel disease (IBD)**. This broad definition covers both ulcerative colitis and Crohn disease. In both conditions, this inflammation damages the wall of the GI tract and places patients at greater risk for cancer. A similar-sounding condition, irritable bowel syndrome (IBS), produces similar symptoms but does not cause structural changes to the walls of the GI tract.

Ulcerative Colitis

Pathophysiology

Ulcerative colitis is caused by inflammation of the colon. The inflammation is generalized and does not occur in patches, as in Crohn disease. It is unclear what causes the chronic inflammation, though genetics, stress, and autoimmunity are speculated to be risk factors. In this condition, the chronic inflammation causes a thinning of the wall of the intestine, resulting in a weakened, dilated rectum. This damaged lining of the colon then becomes susceptible to infections by bacteria and bleeding. These two states establish the foundation on which the signs and symptoms develop.

In a typical patient with ulcerative colitis, the disease incidence peaks between ages 15 and 25 years and then again between 55 and 65 years.[23] It occurs slightly more often in women than men.[23] There is a strong family history component for this disease, with 1 in 6 patients reporting a family member with this disease.[23] Ulcerative colitis is also more prevalent among Caucasians than among other racial/ethnic groups.[23]

Assessment

The presentation of ulcerative colitis features a gradual onset of bloody diarrhea, discharge of mucus via the rectum, hematochezia, and mild to severe abdominal pain, usually in the left lower quadrant. Patients may also report a feeling of rectal fullness, known as *tenesmus*. Other signs and symptoms may include joint pain and skin lesions. These effects lend credence to the idea of an autoimmune component to the disease. Finally, the patient can experience fever, fatigue, and loss of appetite from the infection.

Management

Management consists of determining the degree of hemodynamic instability. Look for signs of shock. If the diarrhea and bleeding have caused sufficient volume loss to make the patient's condition unstable, administer fluids to return the patient to a near-normal volume balance. Otherwise, care is supportive.

Crohn Disease

Pathophysiology

Crohn disease is similar to ulcerative colitis; however, the entire GI tract can be involved. The main part of the GI tract that tends to be involved is the ileum. This is the last portion of the small intestine before it joins the large intestine. There are several theories as to the cause, though no definitive cause has been identified.

There are two peaks in the incidence of Crohn disease: between 15 and 30 years of age and then again between 60 and 70 years of age.[24] Men and women are diagnosed equally.[24] African Americans tend not to have this condition, whereas people of Jewish descent have an increased incidence.[24]

Of interest with Crohn disease and ulcerative colitis is the presence of signs and symptoms outside the GI system. This evidence helps to support the theory that there is an autoimmune component to these diseases, although it is unclear what causes this immune reaction. Another theory proposes that the immune system creates antibodies for an antigen that does not exist, thus creating a cascade of reactions to a nonexistent invader.

Family history and genetics play a role in the development of Crohn disease. Medical researchers are discovering that how the body is made (ie, genetics) and how it is able to function are important characteristics influencing whether a person gets a disease and how that disease progresses. The fact that many people with Crohn disease have family members who have some type of bowel disease suggests a familial or genetic component.

Regardless of the underlying causative factors, the result is a series of attacks by the immune system on the GI tract. This activity of white blood cells damages all layers of the portion of GI tract involved. The result is often a scarred, narrowed, stiff, and weakened portion of the small intestine. This patch of damage is found among normal areas of the intestine. This narrowing can cause bowel obstruction.

Assessment

Patients with Crohn disease present with chronic abdominal pain, often in the lower right area. This pain corresponds to the location of the ileum. Rectal bleeding, weight loss, diarrhea, arthritis, skin problems, and fever may also be present with this condition. Bleeding tends to occur in small amounts over a long period. Acute severe hemorrhage is rare, but chronic bleeding resulting in anemia and hypotension does occur. Patients can have episodes of mild to severe signs and symptoms. Among the key symptoms of Crohn disease that support the autoimmune theory are arthritis and arthralgia; patients tend to report hip, knee, and ankle pain.

Management

Management in the prehospital setting focuses on supporting the ABCs and providing comfort measures. Volume resuscitation may be needed if the patient has diarrhea and chronic hemorrhage. Patients with Crohn disease commonly require control of nausea and pain.

Irritable Bowel Syndrome

Pathophysiology

Irritable bowel syndrome (IBS) is a condition in which patients have abdominal pain and changes in their bowel habits. The current criteria for diagnosing this condition state that patients must have abdominal pain at least 1 day per week for the past 3 months. This pain needs to be associated with changes in the stool consistency or frequency, and it may be associated with defecation. The pathology of the disease is unclear. One theory is that the normal bacteria found within the small bowel begin to overgrow causing pain, distention, and changes in bowel habits.[25]

Three main factors are commonly observed in patients with IBS:

- **Hypersensitivity of bowel pain receptors.** Normal stretching of the bowel can be perceived as pain in these patients.
- **Hyperresponsiveness of the smooth muscles in the bowel.** This produces the cramping sensations and diarrhea.
- **Psychiatric disorder connection and IBS.** It is unclear if the bowel disorder causes the psychiatric disorder, or vice versa.

Hyperresponsiveness of the bowel in IBS can cause areas of spasm. These spasms can stop fecal movement, creating constipation and bloating. Conversely, if the spasms are more wavelike than localized, the patient can experience diarrhea as the feces are moved quickly through the bowel. The underlying causes of this syndrome are not clear.

Patients typically begin to have problems with bowel habits during childhood. In Western countries, young women are more susceptible to this disease.[25] IBS strikes members of most cultures at the same rate. It can be triggered by stress and is often associated with eating.

Assessment

IBS is a chronic condition that typically involves a flare-up. Signs and symptoms tend to be individualized. Patients may present with abdominal pain or discomfort that tends to be diffuse and nonradiating and is relieved by a bowel movement. When the pain starts, there is usually a change in the frequency and consistency of bowel movements. Patients may experience bloating, diarrhea, **steatorrhea**, or constipation.

Management

Management of these patients is supportive, and analgesia may be needed. You must understand that a coexisting psychiatric condition may be present and recognize that patients with IBS attacks commonly experience anxiety. Be kind and compassionate. Do not minimize the patient's pain or discomfort. Your assessment must include the patient's mood and thought content. Consider whether the patient is severely depressed and relay any concerns to the appropriate person when transferring patient care.

Pathophysiology, Assessment, and Management of Acute Infectious Conditions

Many foods are teeming with bacteria, viruses, and fungi. These microorganisms are present throughout the food chain. Infections in the GI system typically occur either when contaminated food is ingested or when the GI tract ruptures. When a person becomes ill from infection, either the number or complexity of the organisms overwhelms the immune system, or the immune system is weakened and cannot effectively defend the body.

Most people who become ill with foodborne illness have stomachaches, vomiting, or diarrhea. According to the Centers for Disease Control and Prevention (CDC), an estimated 48 million people will contract a foodborne illness in the United States every year.[26] Of this group, 3,000 will die; in other words, only 0.006% of those who become ill die.[26] So what makes that small group different from the vast majority? People who are immunocompromised, very old, and very young generally have a more difficult time combating an infection of any type. Types of patients who are immunocompromised would include those with acquired immunodeficiency syndrome or certain types of cancers, people undergoing chemotherapy, and transplant patients.

In the United States, the food chain is generally very clean. Thus, compared with other countries, the number of people who fall ill or die of foodborne disease is relatively small. Traveling to other countries can place patients at greater risk for food intolerances or foodborne infections. Traveler's diarrhea can occur in as many as 30% to 70% of all people who travel to countries where food cleanliness is less than adequate, as reported by the CDC.[27] Travel within North America and Europe is generally safer than travel throughout South America, Asia, and Africa in terms of the risk of foodborne illness.[27]

Damage to the GI system is another way infection can occur. A breach in the container allows GI contents filled with organisms to move into the surrounding tissues. In appendicitis, feces moving through the intestines become trapped in the appendix. The normal flushing of this structure is now prevented and fecal bacteria multiply. Pus and gas, by-products of bacterial activity, can cause pressure on the appendix. If the pressure is too high, the structure will fail, spilling material laden with pus and feces into the peritoneum and causing peritonitis. Sepsis can also occur. Sepsis and its hemodynamic complications are discussed in Chapter 27, *Infectious Diseases*.

Acute Gastroenteritis

Pathophysiology

Acute gastroenteritis is a family of conditions all revolving around a central theme of infection with fever, abdominal pain, diarrhea, nausea, and vomiting. These illnesses can be caused by a wide variety of organisms, as shown in **TABLE 21-8**. These agents typically enter the body via the fecal-oral route through contaminated food or water.

Cholera, though relatively unknown in the United States, is common in other parts of the world. Noroviruses are responsible for most cases of acute viral gastroenteritis in adults, whereas rotaviruses cause the same condition in children. Various parasites may be contracted by swimming in or drinking contaminated water. Most patients who die from gastroenteritis are infected with either norovirus or *Clostridium difficile*.[28] These patients tend to be older than 65 years.[28]

Assessment

Depending on the organism involved, patients may begin to experience GI upset and diarrhea in as little as hours or as long as days after contact with the

TABLE 21-8 Gastroenteritis: Causative Organisms

Type of Organism	Organism
Viruses	Norovirus: Norwalk virus Rotavirus
Parasites	*Giardia lamblia* (protozoan) *Cryptosporidium parvum* *Cyclospora cayetanensis*
Bacteria	*Escherichia coli* *Klebsiella pneumoniae* *Enterobacter* *Campylobacter jejuni* *Vibrio cholera* *Shigella* *Salmonella* *Clostridium difficile*

contaminated food or water. The disease can run its course in 2 to 3 days or continue for several weeks.

The presentation involves diarrhea of various types. Patients can experience large dumping-type diarrhea or frequent small liquid stools. The diarrhea can contain blood and/or pus, and it may have a foul odor or be odorless. Abdominal cramping is frequent as hyperperistalsis continues. Nausea and vomiting, fever, and anorexia are also present. The vomiting can occur quite suddenly. Sudden vomiting is typical in norovirus infections. Asking about recent travel history may reveal useful information; for example, norovirus has a reputation for spreading on cruise ships.

If the diarrhea continues, dehydration and hemodynamic instability will result. As the volume of fluid loss increases, the likelihood of potassium and sodium imbalance also increases. Watch these patients for changes in LOC and other profound signs of shock, which clearly indicate a critical volume loss. Severely dehydrated patients can demonstrate skin tenting, weight loss, tachycardia, orthostatic hypotension, and dry mucous membranes.

Management

Prehospital management is directed at managing dehydration. Fluid resuscitation may be needed; therefore, you should obtain the patient's orthostatic vital signs to determine the need for isotonic fluids. If the patient's condition is stable, half-normal saline solution may be indicated to begin rehydration. Additionally, patients often feel markedly better after rehydration. Performing cardiac monitoring is reasonable due to the risk of hypokalemia. Analgesic and antiemetic medications are also indicated for these patients. One of the most critical issues in managing this condition is patient education: You need to instruct patients about safe food and water use to prevent future infections.

As you are caring for these patients, consider your risk of being contaminated by vomit or stool. Gloves, gowns, and masks are appropriate when treating patients who are actively vomiting or have uncontrolled diarrhea.

Rectal Abscess

Pathophysiology

The rectum creates mucus to lubricate feces during defecation. If the ducts through which this mucus travels become blocked, a **rectal abscess** can result. This area has large amounts of bacteria present. The blockage can allow bacteria to grow and spread around the anus. Men are twice as likely to have this condition as women. The age groups most commonly affected by rectal abscesses are people in their 30s and 40s.[29]

Assessment

Patients present with rectal pain that increases with defecation and then diminishes. The pain will continue between defecations. Fever, pruritus, and rectal drainage are also common findings. Bleeding is typically not a problem. Patients may become constipated and unwilling to defecate because of increased pain.

Management

Management in the prehospital setting involves keeping the patient comfortable. Transport the patient in a position of comfort. The lateral position may be preferable to supine or the Fowler position. The pressure on the rectal area that occurs while in Fowler position may increase pain.

Liver Disease: Cirrhosis

Pathophysiology

The liver is a very resilient and important organ. Beyond its role in the metabolism of fats, proteins, and glucose, the liver is responsible for detoxifying the blood, creating coagulation factors, recycling dead red blood cells, storing vitamins, and creating hormones needed in growth. In consequence, damage to this organ can result in severe imbalances in the body. Few portions of the body are able to operate normally without a functioning liver.

When the liver is damaged by infection, the condition is referred to as hepatitis. This disease is discussed in detail in Chapter 27, *Infectious Diseases.* Other conditions that may damage the liver include direct trauma, toxic ingestion, and autoimmune disorders. Regardless of the cause, if the damage to the liver is severe, the patient will experience the beginning stages of liver failure. Early failure is referred to as **cirrhosis**.

As the liver is damaged, it works to rebuild itself. During the regeneration process, fibrotic tissue can result. This dense material will prevent proper filtering and flow of blood. Consequently, the hallmarks of cirrhosis are portal hypertension (discussed earlier in this chapter), deficiencies in coagulation, and diminished detoxification, which can result in hepatic encephalopathy. However, the liver is so resilient that adults can donate a portion of the liver to someone else. The donated portion will grow to normal size and the remaining portion will return to normal size and function. This regenerative property means most patients will take years to decades to demonstrate clinically significant liver failure.

Cirrhosis can be caused by alcohol, viral infections, toxins (acetaminophen and *Amanita phalloides*, the yellow death-cap mushroom, are examples), and nonalcoholic fatty liver disease (NAFLD). The specific cause of the cirrhosis will yield vastly different epidemiologic characteristics. Onset of signs and symptoms may occur over weeks to years, again depending on the etiology. The leading cause of cirrhosis in the United States is hepatitis C. Many patients who die from cirrhosis do so in their fifth and sixth decades of life.[30]

Assessment

Clinically, liver disease has two phases. In the first phase, patients experience joint aches, weakness, fatigue, nausea, vomiting, anorexia, **urticaria**, easy bruising, and pruritus. During this phase, the patient may be misdiagnosed as having influenza or gastroenteritis.

The second clinical phase involves more extensive damage to the liver. When the damage reaches a point where liver failure occurs, patients will be very sick. This phase is characterized by **acholic stools**, darkening of the urine, jaundice, **icteric** conjunctiva (yellow eyes) **FIGURE 21-10**, and ascites. Abdominal pain found in the right upper quadrant, along with an enlarged liver and spleen, are also present at this time. Patients may also have dilation of blood vessels on the surface of the abdomen. The term *caput medusa* refers to dilated blood vessels around the umbilicus. The literal translation of this term, "head of Medusa," reflects the snakelike appearance of the dilated blood vessels.

Portal hypertension prevents the esophageal blood vessels from dumping their blood into the liver effectively, which causes these blood vessels to become dilated. Such esophageal varices are at high risk of sudden rupture. Couple this with the decreased coagulation factors resulting from liver failure, and the result is a life-threatening bleeding risk.

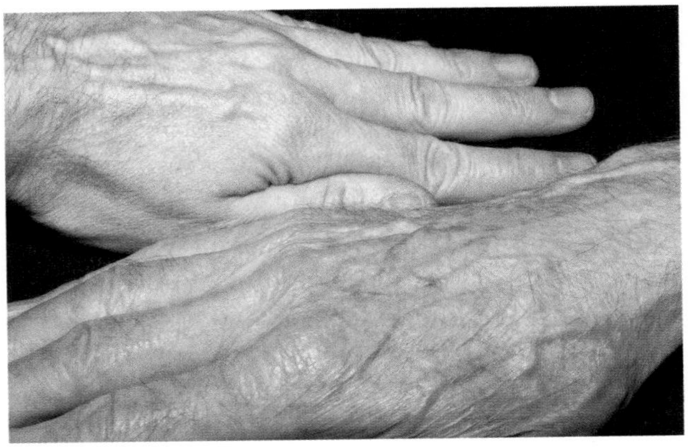

A

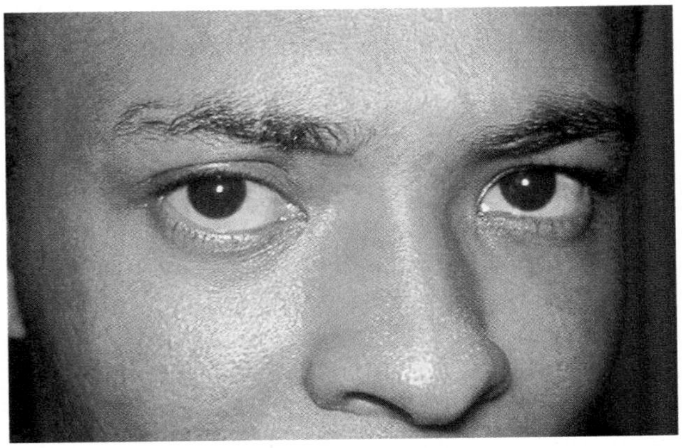

B

FIGURE 21-10 Jaundiced skin **(A)** and icteric sclera **(B)** caused by the buildup of bilirubin in the skin and conjunctiva.

A: © Dr P. Marazzi/Science Source; **B:** Courtesy of Dr. Thomas F. Sellers/Emory University/CDC.

Liver failure has cascading effects that affect multiple organs within the body. Albumin is a key intravascular protein that is responsible for fluid balance, particularly in the venous (as opposed to arterial) capillaries. The liver manufactures albumin. As albumin levels fall, fluid does not return into the vascular space after traveling through capillaries. Interstitial fluid levels rise throughout the body as intravascular fluid levels fall. At this point, patients may experience hypotension due to hypovolemia, ascites, body-wide peripheral edema, pulmonary edema, and cerebral edema. Simultaneously, renal failure occurs due to the same fluid shifts, so that patients can experience intravascular fluid overload. This contradictory state allows for unpredictable fluid levels within the vascular space. Examine the patient closely for signs of fluid overload or hypovolemia. As liver failure progresses, the patient's prospect for survival diminish.

Patients with severe liver disease are susceptible to hypoglycemia due to decreased carbohydrate metabolism. Liver failure will affect most blood values.

Management

The prehospital management for cirrhosis is supportive. These patients need a detailed head-to-toe assessment. Many possible complications of their underlying disease may need intervention. For example, patients can develop airway compromise due to bleeding. Respiratory distress can occur due to fluid shifts, so positive-pressure ventilation or continuous positive airway pressure may be needed. Ensure that patients have adequate circulating volume. Obtaining IV access with a large-bore catheter is desired. Any fluid administration must be preceded by meticulous evaluation of the patient's lung sounds. Ensure blood glucose levels are appropriate. Other important areas of focus involve bleeding control and medication administration. Because of damage to the liver, the blood's clotting ability may be impaired—so be cautious with all venipunctures. Because cirrhosis can be terminal, it is essential for you to abide by the patient's wishes related to their care. Determine if a living will or do-not-resuscitate (DNR) order has been discussed and/or established.

Because of the liver's detoxification functions, any drug that is given to a patient with a compromised liver will remain active in the body far longer than anticipated. Due to the inherent complexity of these patients, strongly consider contacting medical control for guidance. When administering medications to patients with signs of liver failure, use the lower ends of the normal dose range. Give medications at longer intervals and watch for signs of cumulative effects. These patients are often on antiemetics and analgesics. They have a significant risk for opiate overdose, so it is essential to consider the type and amount of analgesics that patients are taking at home before adding additional opiates to the body. Lactated Ringer solution should be avoided in these patients based on the same detoxification rationale.

Liver Disease: Hepatic Encephalopathy

Pathophysiology

As the functions of the liver continue to diminish, eventually brain function will be impaired. This state, which is called **hepatic encephalopathy**, is a continuation of cirrhosis instead of a separate disease. There are several theories as to the underlying cause of the brain dysfunction. Ammonia levels tend to rise as liver functions fail; ammonia can affect neurons by changing the flow of materials across the semipermeable membrane. Diminished functions of the nervous system may simply be due to diminished cellular energy supplies. The liver has a pivotal role in providing cellular substrates necessary for metabolism, so diminished liver function equals diminished metabolism. The decrease in function may also be caused by a change in the blood-brain barrier's permeability. If this barrier could be easily breached, neurotoxins could cause cellular damage resulting in an altered LOC. Regardless of the underlying cause, the brain is affected in hepatic encephalopathy.[30]

Assessment

The mental status of a patient with hepatic encephalopathy can range from mild loss of memory to coma. Patients may present with attention deficits, inability to concentrate, and impaired complex reasoning. These subtle changes can progress to disorientation, impaired behavior, and incomprehensible speech. Other signs and symptoms include bradykinesia, shuffling gait, and tremor. These last signs are reminiscent of Parkinson disease.

The patient's clinical findings are more important than the laboratory results. Most patients will have ammonia levels checked, but these results are not always a good indicator of the severity of brain impairment. The results of CT and magnetic resonance imaging are inconclusive for diagnosing this disease. Patients may have encephalopathy precipitated by an infection, renal failure, GI bleeding, or constipation. Opiates, benzodiazepines, and psychotropic medications can worsen the presentation.

Management

Treatment is primarily supportive. One of the most important issues for paramedics is to ensure that some other reversible cause for an altered LOC is not present. Check the patient's blood glucose level and vital signs. Assess for trauma and overdose. These patients will typically have a significant past medical history for cirrhosis. Gather detailed information about the history of present illness. What is normal for this patient? How long has the patient been sick? Focus on infections, renal function, bleeding, and constipation because these issues can precipitate hepatic encephalopathy.

Pathophysiology, Assessment, and Management of Obstructive Conditions

Obstructions within the GI system can occur anywhere from the oropharynx to the rectum. The reasons for these obstructions vary depending on the location. Rectal obstructions tend to occur in young men and are due to a foreign body. Esophageal obstructions also tend to be caused by foreign bodies, but the population affected tends to be children.

The cardinal sign of bowel obstruction is decreased intestinal motility, a condition in which the intestines cannot move material through the digestive tract. Two main reasons for this condition are paralysis of the intestines and a change in the diameter of their lumen. Paralysis can be caused by infection, kidney disease, impaired blood flow to the intestines, or medications. Narcotics and anesthetics are specific types of medications that can paralyze the intestinal muscles. This is why patients who have major surgery often will not be released from the hospital until they have had at least one bowel movement.

Intestinal lumen diameter compromise can be caused by neoplasms, tumors of the intestines, objects that the patient has swallowed, or strictures (narrowing of the lumen due to damage in the intestinal wall). Other causes include hernia (intestine trapped and compressed), **intussusception** (telescoping of the intestines into themselves), and **volvulus** (twisting of the intestines). The end result is that the diameter of the intestines is narrowed or blocked.

Esophageal Obstruction

Pathophysiology

Contractions of smooth muscles within the walls of the esophagus rhythmically move the food ingested. But, imagine a tube of toothpaste: As you squeeze the center, toothpaste moves in both directions: out toward the end of the tube and back deeper into the tube. Similarly, the esophagus has to manage both desired and undesired food motion resulting from its muscular contractions.

The upper esophageal sphincter (UES) is located at the superior end of the esophagus. As this ring of muscles tightens, it closes the superior portion of the esophagus to prevent food from moving superiorly back into the hypopharynx. As discussed earlier in the section on hiatal hernia, the LES closes to prevent food from exiting the stomach when the stomach contracts. It is undesirable to have food squeezed out of the stomach and back into the esophagus. To prevent this reflux, the LES closes.

Obstructions within the esophagus typically occur at either the upper or lower sphincter. When young children explore new objects, they like to place them in their mouth. This is one way for children to learn about their world. When unsupervised, a child can accidentally swallow an object, such as a coin, toy piece, button, or marble. The location of entrapment is at the UES. Adults, in contrast, tend to have entrapment at the LES, and the object can be almost anything that can fit in the mouth. Ingestion in adults may be either accidental, such as with a fruit pit or a denture plate, or intentional. Prisoners or psychiatric patients may swallow objects to hide or transport them. In 80% of cases, if the object reaches the stomach, it will pass through the remainder of the GI tract.[31]

Assessment

Dysphagia and drooling are the primary symptoms in these patients. How this is demonstrated will be markedly different if your patient is a 2-year-old child who swallowed a battery **FIGURE 21-11**, a 28-year-old man who is trying to conceal a key, or a 69-year-old woman who had some alcohol with dinner and swallowed her dentures. The UES is located close to the cricoid cartilage. The cricoid is the only cartilage within the trachea that forms a complete 360° ring, which prevents severe impingement from the esophagus in the event of obstruction.

Depending on the location of the object and its shape, it can generate a minor to severe sense of difficulty in breathing. If the object is inferior to the cricoid, it can impinge on the posterior wall of the trachea (which has no cartilage), and the patient will feel a strong sense of choking. Drooling, inability to swallow, pain, vomiting, and gagging can occur. In approximately one-third of children, there are no symptoms until they try to eat.

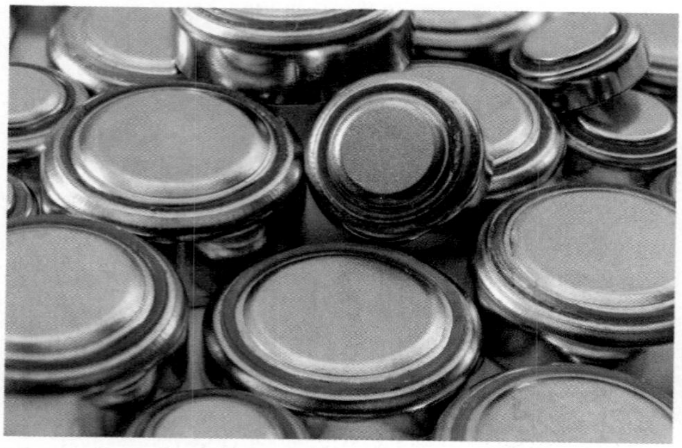

FIGURE 21-11 Button batteries may be swallowed by children. The leaking of the battery contents can cause necrosis of the esophagus.

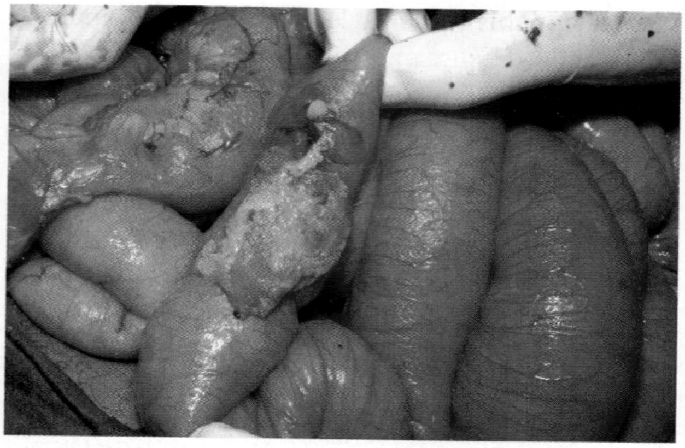

FIGURE 21-12 An adhesion between loops of small intestine.

Management

Airway patency is the primary concern for patients with esophageal obstruction. Allow the patient to sit in a high Fowler position. Be prepared to manage oral sections with suction and have an emesis basin ready. Eye protection, mask, and gowns will be needed if there is a reasonable risk of vomiting. Simply looking into the mouth to see if the object can easily be removed is reasonable. However, do not fight the patient to remove the object. It is better to keep the patient calm and allow health care providers in the ED to remove it.

If the patient has obvious airway compromise as evidenced by hypoxia, cyanosis, and altered LOC, then a more aggressive investigation of the hypopharynx is indicated. Refer to Chapter 16, *Airway Management,* to review use of Magill forceps and foreign body removal from the airway.

Glucagon can be considered in patients with esophageal obstruction. Due to its smooth muscle relaxation properties, this medication can potentially relax the LES. This may allow the object to pass into the stomach, relieving the patient of pain and dysphagia. Contact online medical direction or medical control if you are considering administration of glucagon for this purpose. Nitrates have a similar esophageal relaxation effect, but carry the risk of vasodilation.

Encourage patients to seek medical care even if the object is cleared when you arrive. Esophageal laceration and aspiration pneumonia are risks with esophageal obstruction, so medical follow-up is important.

Small-Bowel Obstruction

Pathophysiology

In the small intestine, postoperative adhesions are the most common cause of obstruction. When a patient undergoes a surgical procedure that requires opening the abdomen, the resulting inflammation results in scarring as the body heals. These weblike bands of tissue, called adhesions, can constrict the diameter of the intestine or decrease its ability to dilate **FIGURE 21-12**. Other causes of small-bowel obstruction include cancer, Crohn disease, hernias, and volvulus.[32]

Assessment

The presentation of a small-bowel obstruction begins with abdominal pain. The pain tends to be crampy and intermittent. Patients will initially experience diarrhea, nausea, and vomiting because of the increased pressure on the intestine. As the patient continues to eat, some food can advance beyond the blockage, causing increased intestinal pressure and increased peristalsis. Constipation will eventually occur because limited food will be able to get beyond the blockage. This leads to abdominal distention, and hyperactive bowel sounds in the early stages. Hypoactive bowel sounds are more common in late stages of the obstruction.

The material that is vomited may be feculent, having the smell of feces. Fever and tachycardia are also associated with small-bowel obstruction, and can indicate infection within the abdominal cavity. Untreated, this condition can lead to sepsis. Ask patients with suspected small-bowel obstruction if they have a history of abdominal surgery; if they are unresponsive or unreliable, look for a scar that could indicate such surgery. Patients can experience a small-bowel obstruction decades after undergoing abdominal surgery. Due to the vomiting and decreased ability to obtain nutrients, there may be changes in their electrolyte levels.

A blockage of the small intestine can cause several localized changes. The area involved becomes irritated, so that swelling occurs. This further complicates the blockage. If the bowel becomes twisted or for any other reason blood supply is compromised, ischemia can occur. This condition is referred to as a strangulated obstruction. Mortality in patients with untreated strangulated obstruction is near 100%.[32] If treated early, the mortality rate is markedly lower.

Management

Treatment is supportive. As with most conditions involving the GI tract, there is a concern related to sepsis. Monitor the patient's BP and be prepared to provide volume resuscitation and administer vasopressors as needed. A nasogastric tube may be used to decompress the stomach of any material. Antiemetics and analgesics are clearly indicated with small-bowel obstruction. Based on the length of time the patient has had the obstruction, IV fluids may be needed due to dehydration.

Large-Bowel Obstruction

Pathophysiology

As with small-bowel obstructions, large-bowel obstructions are caused by either mechanical obstruction or stricture of the colon resulting in decreased internal diameter. In the case of mechanical obstruction, the most common causes are colon cancer and diverticulitis. Both of these conditions are more closely associated with older patients; therefore, large-bowel obstructions are more common in that age group. Another cause is a volvulus, or twisting of the bowel until a kink occurs, blocking flow. In pediatric populations, intussusception is a more common diagnosis than in adults.[33]

Imaging studies are used to determine the location and extent of the obstruction. Finding the exact cause will direct eventual hospital treatment. Once located, many obstructions can be easily treated. Untreated, the mortality can be high if cancer is the cause of the obstruction. In addition, the blockage can lead to increased permeability of the intestinal wall, which allows intestinal bacteria to gain access to the bloodstream, and septicemia can occur.

If the obstruction is caused by cancer, an erosion of the bowel into adjacent cavities can occur. These fistulas can allow feces to enter the vagina or bladder. This results in patients with either feculent discharge from the vagina or fecaluria (feces in the bladder being discharged with the urine).

Assessment

In cases of large-bowel obstruction, the assessment will reveal a patient with abdominal pain. Nausea and vomiting are also common. The abdomen is distended and typically bowel sounds are absent. Percussion of the abdomen should reveal hyperresonance. If the obstruction has ruptured into the peritoneum, the classic signs of peritonitis (fever, tachycardia, and pain) will be present. Gather information about the patient's recent bowel habits and weight. If the obstruction is related to cancer, recent unexplained weight loss and gradually increasing difficulty in having bowel movements tend to occur.

These patients may demonstrate either constipation (a decrease in the frequency of bowel movements along with harder, drier stools) or obstipation. People with constipation are typically still able to pass gas. In contrast, obstipation is a complete blockage of the bowel, resulting in no bowel movements, little gas, and increased abdominal girth. The abdominal distention occurs due to the patient eating but not being able to empty the bowels. This creates backup of stool, causing anorexia and eventually feculent breath and/or vomiting feces. Dehydration is also associated with this condition.

Management

The treatment for large-bowel obstruction is the same as that for small-bowel obstruction. As a result of the elastic properties of the colon, it may be obstructed for a longer period with large-bowel obstructions versus small-bowel obstructions. This can lead to a greater degree of dehydration and need for fluid resuscitation. Pain management, antiemetics, and close observation for sepsis are indicated.

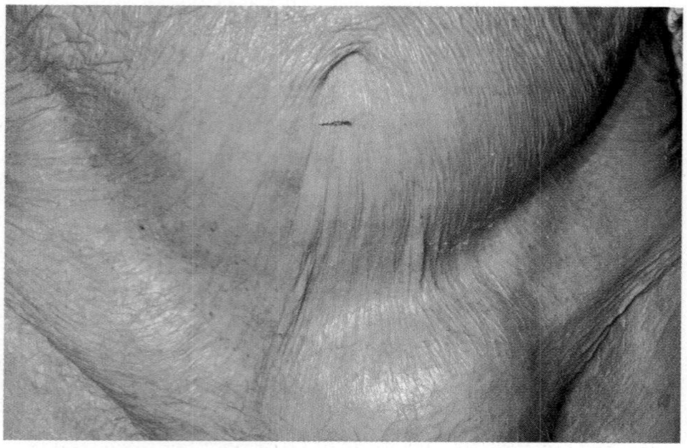

FIGURE 21-13 An inguinal hernia.

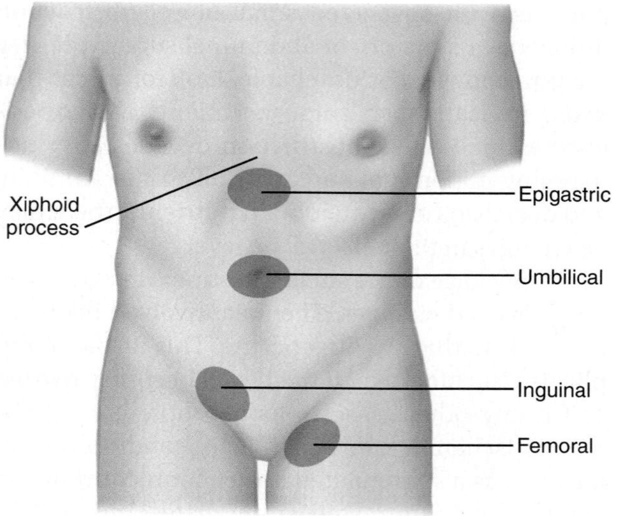

FIGURE 21-14 Common locations of abdominal hernias.

Abdominal Wall Hernia

Pathophysiology

A **hernia** is a protrusion of an organ or structure into an adjacent cavity. During a physical examination, a physician will often place their fingers on the wall of the lower abdomen as the patient is instructed to cough. Coughing increases intra-abdominal pressure. If there is a weakness in the wall of the abdomen, it can be felt as bulging during the cough. This procedure is done to check for an inguinal hernia. *Inguinal* simply refers to the location of the protrusion **FIGURE 21-13**. In this case, the intestines are typically the protruding organ. More than 1 million hernia repairs are done each year in the United States, with the inguinal hernia being the most common form.[34] Abdominal wall hernias are seven times more common in men than in women.[34]

Any condition or state that increases intra-abdominal pressure can facilitate the creation of a hernia. Obesity, standing for long periods, heavy lifting, straining during a bowel movement, or chronic obstructive pulmonary disease (COPD) can precipitate this condition. Chronic obstructive pulmonary disease is associated with hernias because of the increased work of breathing and subsequent use of the abdominal muscles.

Assessment

A typical assessment finding in a patient with abdominal wall hernia is a bulging of the area where the hernia is present. Four types of hernias may occur in the abdomen, and they tend to occur in several common locations **FIGURE 21-14**:

- **Reducible**. A hernia that will return to its normal location either spontaneously or by manual manipulation. The patient typically experiences little discomfort unless they have increasing intra-abdominal pressure. The patient may perceive a fullness or swelling, or report achiness at the hernia site.
- **Incarcerated**. Consider the nonmedical meaning of the word *incarcerate*: to place in jail. In this type of hernia, the organ is trapped in the new location. The most common consequence of this condition is bowel obstruction. Incarcerated hernias are more painful as a result of the obstruction.
- **Strangulated**. A strangulated hernia is one in which the intestine is trapped and squeezed to the point that blood supply to the area is diminished. Consequently, this kind of hernia is considered an emergency. Patients experience severe pain and sepsis and require urgent transport.
- **Incisional**. Patients recovering from abdominal surgery can have intestinal contents herniate through the incision. This is similar to the trauma condition known as evisceration.

Management

Prehospital treatment for hernias is supportive, with care directed at pain management. Place the patient in a comfortable position. Lying supine will probably not be comfortable because this stretches the abdominal wall. Closely assess the patient for sepsis. Though it is minimally to moderately painful, unless strangulated, a hernia is not a life-threatening emergency.

Rectal Foreign Body Obstruction

Pathophysiology

A foreign body in the rectum interferes with defecation. Objects can be introduced from the upper GI tract or by anal insertion. Indigestible swallowed objects may have difficulty passing. Chicken bones, toothpicks, and various other materials may pass through the entire GI tract without difficulty, only to become lodged in the rectum during defecation. Prisoners, for example, may swallow objects during an inspection or search. Fecaliths can also cause obstructions. A fecalith is a very hard piece of feces (*fecal* = feces, *lith* = stone). Finally, other objects that pass through the GI tract, such as gallstones, can cause obstructions.

Most rectal obstructions occur when an object is inserted into the rectum. Men are 28 times more likely to engage in this activity than are women, and the average age of these patients is in their 20s.[35] The primary reason for the activity is erotic stimulation. Older men may insert objects into their rectum to help relieve urinary difficulties caused by an enlarged prostate.

Assessment

The two types of causes create two very different patient presentations. If the rectal obstruction originated from the upper GI tract, the patient presents with a sudden onset of rectal pain with defecation. Rarely is bleeding or abdominal pain noted in the acute phase. If the object has perforated the rectum, peritonitis is possible. Peritonitis would in turn lead to fever, diffuse abdominal pain, and possible sepsis.

Most patients who have rectal obstructions seek medical care for removal of an intentionally placed object. Knowing what type of object was inserted and whether the patient has attempted to remove the object can be important. This information can help you determine whether the patient's rectum is perforated. During your history taking, ensure that the patient was not assaulted. Rectal insertion during an assault can cause severe and possibly life-threatening internal damage.

In either case, physical findings may be limited to the patient's report of rectal pain. If perforation has occurred, peritonitis and consequent sepsis may be present. Depending on the size and shape of the object, it may be apparent on physical examination.

Management

Even when the inserted object is visible on physical examination, you should not attempt to remove it. Treatment in the prehospital setting should be limited to ensuring that the patient is comfortable. Allow the patient to sit laterally, if possible, to reduce the pressure on the rectum. If the patient is in pain, analgesia is indicated. As with other abdominal emergencies in which peritonitis is a possibility, close monitoring of vital signs is important.

Street Smarts

Patients with rectal obstructions are often horribly embarrassed. Be compassionate and nonjudgmental, and recognize that it took courage for the patient to seek medical care.

Pathophysiology, Assessment, and Management of Ischemic and Neoplastic Disorders

Mesenteric Ischemia

Pathophysiology

Mesenteric ischemia is a condition in which the blood supply to the mesentery is interrupted. There are four main causes of this condition:

- **Acute arterial embolism.** These emboli tend to come from a cardiac thrombus (MI, atrial fibrillation, mitral stenosis, etc).
- **Acute arterial thrombosis.** These patients have underlying thrombotic disease in the mesenteric arteries. Plaque buildup narrows the lumen, which can suddenly close off. This process is very similar to how most MIs occur.
- **Profound vasospasm.** This condition can occur with the use of cocaine, with ergot poisoning, with administration of norepinephrine, or in severe shock.

- **Mesenteric venous thrombosis.** In this condition, a thrombus forms in one of the mesenteric veins, preventing blood from leaving the intestinal veins. Blood begins to pool. This creates back-pressure that prevents fresh blood from entering the area. Tissues are starved of oxygen.

Mesenteric ischemia occurs in both sexes and is more prevalent among older patients.[36] It is a rare but serious condition, with a mortality rate of 50% to 80%.[36] The primary cause of patient deterioration is sepsis.

Assessment

Depending on the exact cause of the abdominal pain, it may have a gradual or sudden onset. Early presentations offer few signs or symptoms. In later presentations, abdominal pain is the cardinal sign. The pain within the abdomen tends to be difficult to locate and severe. Nausea, vomiting, and diarrhea are also common. Blood may be present in the stool. The disease is difficult to diagnose. A thorough history is needed. If the patient has ingested something, this information will dramatically change the in-hospital therapy. Discovering the cause of the ischemia is essential to offering the correct life-saving therapy in the hospital.

Management

Patients with mesenteric ischemia require rapid transportation. Monitor these patients closely, checking vital signs for evidence of sepsis. If shock is present, initiate fluid resuscitation. If sepsis is the cause of hypotension, be prepared to use vasopressors to stabilize BP; these agents are warranted only after initial fluid therapy and, preferably, in consultation with medical direction or per local protocols. Analgesics may be indicated.

Neoplasms

Neoplasm is the medical term for growths or tumors within the body that serve no purpose and are caused by errors that occur during cellular reproduction. When an altered cell reproduces, it copies the error to its own daughter cells. The new cells may grow more rapidly and aggressively than the normal surrounding cells. Neoplasms can be categorized as either benign or malignant, and as primary or metastatic. Any portion of the GI system can develop a neoplasm or cancer. The most common forms are discussed next.

Tumors of the Colon

Pathophysiology

Colon, or colorectal, cancer is the third leading cause of cancer and the third leading cause of deaths related to cancer. It is the most common form of cancer within the GI system. As with many cancers, its cause is multifactorial. People with diets high in red meat and low in fiber and people who smoke are at greater risk of developing colon cancer. There is a strong correlation between heredity and colorectal cancer. One specific gene mutation that imparts a near-100% chance of developing colon cancer by age 40 has been identified.[37] Inflammatory bowel diseases, ulcerative colitis, and Crohn disease are also associated with increased risk for colorectal cancer.[37]

Assessment

Abdominal pain, rectal bleeding, anemia, abdominal mass, and changes in bowel habits are the most common signs of colon cancer. Fortunately, colorectal screening catches many cancers before symptoms begin. If the cancer is found on the right side of the colon, patients more commonly have bleeding and diarrhea. Left-side tumors tend to cause obstruction.

Management

Care is supportive. Many patients will require some degree of resection of the colon. This is currently the only curative measure for this cancer. Depending on the location and extent of the cancer, patients may require a colostomy. If caught early, patients with colon cancer have a survival rate of nearly 90%.[37]

Pancreatic Tumors

Pathophysiology

Pancreatic cancer is the fourth leading cause of death from cancer. Recall that the pancreas is located centrally in the upper abdomen and comprises both exocrine and endocrine cells. Most malignancies in this organ occur in the exocrine cells. Of all pancreatic cancers, 40% are sporadic in nature, with little evidence pointing to a direct cause.[38] Smoking causes 30% of cases, and 10% are related to heredity.[38] Patients with obesity and diabetes may have an increased risk of pancreatic cancer. This condition affects males more often than females and is also more prevalent in African Americans. The most common age for onset is the mid 60s.[38]

Assessment

Symptomatically, pancreatic cancer has a gradual, insidious presentation that is often mistaken for other benign conditions. Patients experience malaise, fatigue, nausea, vomiting, midepigastric pain, or back pain. As the cancer continues, anorexia and weight loss become apparent. It is rare that a patient with new-onset diabetes will have an occult pancreatic cancer.[38]

If the cancer is on the head of the pancreas, it can obstruct bile flow from the gallbladder. The common bile duct travels through the pancreas and then interconnects with the pancreatic duct. A growing tumor can block this structure, preventing bile from reaching the duodenum. This will result in darkening of the urine, pale-colored stool, and steatorrhea. Interestingly, depression is more common in patients with pancreatic cancer than in patients with any other abdominal cancer. Patients may have increased depression due to the poor prognosis of this disease or because they do not feel well.

If the cancer has metastasized, it can lead to hepatic cancer and resultant liver failure.

Management

Care for patients with pancreatic cancer is supportive in nature. This cancer is particularly fatal. The median survival time at diagnosis is 4 to 6 months.[38] Many of these patients will have a living will or a DNR order, or will be receiving hospice services, so it is important to understand the wishes of the patient and family.

Hepatic Tumors

Pathophysiology

Cancer of the liver is rare. Due to the liver's outstanding regenerative properties, it is able to repair most damage or cellular errors. Primary liver cancer accounts for only 2.4% of all new reported cancers. When it is present, liver cancer is more common among men (74% of cases), who are age 64 years, on average, when diagnosed.[39] Hispanics have the highest incidence. Frequently (approximately 75% of the time), primary liver cancers within the United States are associated with cirrhosis. Alcohol consumption and hepatitis B and C are known factors that increase risk of liver cancer.[39]

Assessment

Patients with liver cancer will be sick. This is not a condition that occurs overnight, so the patient will likely have already been diagnosed prior to EMS involvement. You can expect a patient with pruritus, jaundice, splenomegaly, hepatomegaly, cachexia (profound malnutrition and weight loss), ascites, caput medusae, and abdominal pain. Patients may also experience all of the signs and symptoms related to cirrhosis and hepatic encephalopathy. EMS may be dispatched for altered LOC or for bleeding. The liver is essential in the production of clotting factors, so with its deterioration, patients can develop GI bleeds.

Management

EMS care is directed at supporting vital signs and can be quite complicated. These patients will often have major fluid and electrolyte imbalances. This can create potentially lethal cardiac rhythm disturbances, so ECG monitoring is critical. Check potassium levels and hemoglobin/hematocrit levels, if possible. Patients will often have a severely altered LOC, so airway protection may be needed. Respiratory distress from pulmonary edema may require positive-pressure ventilation with positive end-expiratory pressure. Interpret these patients' pulse oximetry findings with caution, as they are chronically anemic. Patients with respiratory distress and anemia should receive oxygen despite normal oximetry readings. Remember that capnography can be helpful in these situations.

To complicate matters, because of damage to the liver, most medications that you administer will not be metabolized normally in patients with liver cancer. This may lead to potential medication toxicity issues. Generally speaking, if medications need to be administered, choose the lower end of the accepted range or increase the time between doses. Only about 5% of these patients are candidates for liver resectioning (removal of a portion of the liver).[39] Consequently, a large number of these patients are terminal. Talk with the patient and family to determine whether there is an advance directive. Ask to see the appropriate documentation (living will/DNR/medical power of attorney).

Prevention Strategies

As EMS evolves, it becomes more important for paramedics to consider disease prevention. EMS is moving from a service that is strictly related to delivering 9-1-1 services to a system that augments nonemergency aspects of health care. Many patient behaviors can either limit the intensity or entirely prevent the onset of many GI diseases. **TABLE 21-9** lists some of the behaviors and the diseases that can be affected.

Following a healthy diet is one of the best ways to prevent GI disorders. A diet that is high in fiber and low in fat will facilitate movement of materials through the GI tract. Good sources of dietary fiber are listed in **TABLE 21-10**. Not only does such a diet help improve bowel health, but it also has a strong connection to heart health. Another heart-healthy behavior that has a positive effect on the GI system is to eliminate smoking and to control the amount of alcohol consumed. Finally, the connection between stress and disease is clear. Meditating, exercising, and practicing relaxation techniques can have a profound effect on a person's quality and quantity of life.

TABLE 21-9 Prevention of Selected GI Conditions

Condition	Prevention Strategy
Constipation	Increase fiber and fluid content in diet Exercise Chew food fully
Diverticulitis	Increase fiber and fluid content in diet Exercise Chew food fully
Gallstones	Most gallstones cannot be prevented, but a lower-fat diet may provide some protection
Heartburn	Avoid smoking Avoid eating close to bedtime Avoid chocolate, peppermint, and caffeine
Hemorrhoids	Increase fiber and fluid content in the diet
Liver disease	Limit alcohol Avoid high doses of vitamins unless prescribed Follow directions on cleaning supplies (ventilation/gloves/masks)
Peptic ulcers	Manage stress well Limit caffeine Limit alcohol

Abbreviation: GI, gastrointestinal

TABLE 21-10 Selected Sources of Dietary Fiber

Fruits	Vegetables	Other Good Fiber Choices
Artichokes Apples, pears (with skin) Berries (blackberries, blueberries, raspberries) Dates Figs Prunes	Beans (navy, black, lima, pinto) Broccoli Chickpeas Lentils Parsnips Peas Pumpkin Rutabaga Squash (winter)	Barley Bread, muffins (whole wheat, bran) Cereals (bran flakes, bran, oatmeal, shredded wheat) Coconut Crackers (rye, whole wheat) Nuts (almonds, Brazil, peanuts, pecans, walnuts) Rice (brown) Seeds (pumpkin, sunflower)

YOU are the Paramedic SUMMARY

1. What is melena?

Melena is black, tarry, sticky, and very odorous stool and blood blended together into one substance. You are unable to distinguish blood from stool.

2. What part of the GI system do you believe might be affected?

Melena is common when there is bleeding from the esophagus, stomach, or proximal small intestine.

3. What do orthostatic vital signs indicate?

Orthostatic vital signs will help you determine the extent of bleeding that has occurred. Normally, there should be little change in the BP or pulse rate with this change.

4. Do you expect the BP and pulse rate to increase or decrease when the patient is moved?

A positive orthostatic change reflects a significant loss of fluid within the vascular space. There will be a 20-beat increase in the pulse rate, a decrease in systolic BP up to 20 mm Hg, and/or an increase in diastolic BP of more than 10 mm Hg.

5. On the basis of the patient's orthostatic vital signs, what is your suggested treatment?

The patient's vital signs indicate that she is hypovolemic. The patient should be given IV fluids as long as no findings are present that would contraindicate it. You should also attempt to keep the patient lying as flat as possible to minimize the postural effects.

6. Which of the patient's medications most concerns you?

You should be concerned with the warfarin because it is an anticoagulant. Volume replacement is still your treatment of choice, but warfarin should increase your suspicion of substantial bleeding somewhere in the GI tract. Bismuth solutions (Pepto Bismol) will also color stools black without any bleeding.

7. Knowing that this patient has postural vital signs, how will you move the patient downstairs?

The best method to help the patient's comfort level would be to allow her to maintain a lying position if at all possible. A stair chair would not be a good choice for this patient. A Reeves stretcher or a scoop stretcher may be your best choice.

8. Should you administer a pain medication to make the patient more comfortable?

Because this patient is already hemodynamically compromised, fentanyl or tramadol may be a better choice than morphine or meperidine (which cause vascular pooling), if your local protocols allow. Consult medical control regarding the best choice.

EMS Patient Care Report (PCR)

Date: 08-10-22	**Incident No.:** 73542	**Nature of Call:** Unresponsive		**Location:** 215 Brooks Street	
Dispatched: 0115	**En Route:** 0116	**At Scene:** 0121	**Transport:** 0146	**At Hospital:** 0153	**In Service:** 0201

Patient Information

Age: 64 **Sex:** F **Weight (in kg [lb]):** 91 kg (200 lb)	**Allergies:** NKDA **Medications:** Propranolol, diltiazem, warfarin, glyburide, bismuth OTC **Past Medical History:** Diabetes, HTN, AFib **Chief Complaint:** GI bleeding

Vital Signs

Time: 0126	**BP:** 106/82 lying, 92/78 sitting	**Pulse:** 120 lying, 136 sitting	**Respirations:** 20	**Spo_2:** 98% on 15 L/min
Time: 0134	**BP:** 110/86 lying	**Pulse:** 110 lying	**Respirations:** 18	**Spo_2:** 98% on 15 L/min
Time:	**BP:**	**Pulse:**	**Respirations:**	**Spo_2:**

YOU are the Paramedic SUMMARY continued

EMS Treatment (circle all that apply)				
Oxygen @ 15 L/min via (circle one): NC (NRM circled) Bag-mask device		Assisted Ventilation	Airway Adjunct	CPR
Defibrillation	Bleeding Control	Bandaging	Splinting	Other:

Narrative

Arrived to find 64 y/o woman in an upstairs bathroom at her residence. Husband states the pt has been feeling ill for a few days. Pt awoke and he assisted her to the bathroom when she became syncopal. Husband helped her to the floor and she did not fall. Pt has approx. 250 mL of melena on the floor near her position. Pt reports abd pain 8/10. Pt denies vomiting. Abd assessment equals soft, tender in all quads. Pt orthostatic vital signs show postural changes. IV established and 250-mL challenge administered. Pt lifted off floor with a scoop stretcher and carried down stairs to ambulance. Pt had no change during transport to Charity Hospital. Report given to charge nurse on arrival.

End of report

Prep Kit

Ready for Review

- GI conditions alone are rarely life threatening. This fact does not minimize the systemic disorders that can evolve from untreated or undertreated diseases of the GI system.
- The structures and functions of the GI system perform digestion, which begins in the mouth, and continues through a multitude of organs and structures: the esophagus, portal vein, stomach, duodenum, pancreas, liver, gallbladder, small intestine, large intestine, appendix, and anus.
- During calls for patients with suspected abdominal or GI emergencies, it is likely you will come into contact with blood, vomitus, urine, or feces. A complete size-up of scene safety requires a survey of the PPE required for protection against infectious agents.
- You form your general impression of the patient with a suspected abdominal or GI emergency by observing the patient's posture, the environment, any foul odors present, and the patient's LOC.
- Airway patency and adequate circulation must be maintained in patients with GI disorders, and you must assess the extent of any bleeding by obtaining their orthostatic vital signs.
- The transport decision is made by evaluating the patient's stability; use of rapid transport with lights and sirens is rarely necessary for abdominal emergencies.
- Your working diagnosis of the patient and the information you gather about the patient's medications, allergies, past medical history, and precipitating events can provide information about the cause of the patient's chief complaint.
- Secondary assessment is accomplished with a comprehensive physical examination in which you pay special attention to the appearance of the shape, size, color, and other characteristics of the abdomen; auscultate bowel sounds; and perform percussion and palpation to assess for dullness, rigidity, guarding, pain or discomfort, rebound tenderness, fluid accumulation, and masses.
- When taking a patient's orthostatic vital signs, a 20-beat increase in the pulse rate or a decrease in BP of 20 mm Hg indicates a significant volume loss caused by uncontrolled bleeding.

Prep Kit continued

- Reassessment includes monitoring for changes in pulse rate, ECG readings, BP, respiratory rate, oxygen saturation, or signs of shock.
- Advances in technology allow pain relief to be offered to most patients with abdominal or GI emergencies. It is also important to manage nausea and, by extension, vomiting.
- Talking with patients and their families to keep them calm and informed is the foundation of compassionate, high-quality care. Documenting your observations and the results of all assessments, examinations, and tests is also essential to delivering excellent patient care.
- Sudden, worrisome changes in a patient's condition warrant performing comprehensive and detailed new assessments and examinations.
- Airway management of patients with GI disorders includes delivery of high-concentration oxygen, prevention of aspiration, and auscultation of lung sounds, as dictated by the patient's condition.
- Circulation may be compromised in a patient with a GI emergency by dehydration or hemorrhage. Fluid resuscitation to replace volume and maintain perfusion may be a life-saving intervention.
- You must learn about individual GI diseases to keep pace with the rising stature of the EMS field and the increasing level of responsibility paramedics must be prepared to assume. Such knowledge is also necessary to educate patients about their own or a loved one's disease.
- Four major conditions are responsible for abdominal and GI emergencies:
  - Hypovolemia caused by dehydration or hemorrhage
  - Acute or chronic inflammation
  - Infection
  - Obstruction
- Bleeding within the GI tract is a symptom of another disease, and not a disease itself. Presentation of GI bleeding varies, as it can reflect the presence of a number of diseases. Each of these conditions has its own pattern of disease progression.
- Following a healthy diet, eliminating smoking, and reducing stress are all ways to prevent GI disorders. A diet that is high in fiber and low in fat will facilitate movement of materials through the GI tract.

Vital Vocabulary

acholic stools Light, clay-colored stools indicative of liver failure.

acute abdomen A sudden onset of pain within the abdomen, usually indicating peritonitis; demands immediate medical or surgical treatment.

acute gastroenteritis A family of conditions that revolve around a central theme of infection with fever, abdominal pain, diarrhea, nausea, and vomiting.

anal fissures Linear tears to the mucosal lining in and near the anus, possibly caused by the passage of large, hard stools; a cause of lower GI bleeding.

appendicitis Inflammation of the appendix.

ascites Abdominal edema typically signaling liver failure.

biliary tract disorders A group of disorders that involve inflammation of the gallbladder; these include cholangitis, cholelithiasis, cholecystitis, and acalculous cholecystitis.

Boerhaave syndrome Forceful vomiting that results in a tear in the esophagus that extends entirely through the esophageal wall, creating a hole.

borborygmi A bowel sound characterized by increased activity within the bowel; also called hyperperistalsis.

cholangitis Inflammation of the bile duct.

cholelithiasis The presence of stones within the gallbladder.

cholecystitis Inflammation of the gallbladder.

cirrhosis Early failure of the liver; characterized by portal hypertension, coagulation deficiencies, and diminished detoxification.

Prep Kit continued

Crohn disease Inflammation of the ileum and possibly other portions of the GI tract, in which the immune system attacks portions of the intestinal walls, causing them to become scarred, narrowed, stiff, and weakened.

diarrhea Liquid stool.

digestion The mechanical and chemical breakdown of the large molecules in food into small molecules that can be absorbed in the GI tract and converted to energy for cellular function.

diverticulitis Inflammation of pouches in the colon; these pouches form as a result of difficulty moving feces through the colon. Bacteria can become trapped in the pouches, leading to inflammation and infection.

diverticulum A weak area in the colon that begins to have small outcroppings that turn into pouches; plural is diverticula.

epigastric The region of the abdomen directly inferior to the xiphoid process and superior to the umbilicus.

esophagitis An inflammation of the esophagus.

esophagogastric varices Dilated blood vessels of the esophagus, commonly caused by difficulty in blood flow through the liver; the presence of these can lead to vessel rupture.

fistula An abnormal connection between two cavities.

gastritis A preulcerative state in which the stomach is inflamed, but erosion has not yet occurred.

gastroesophageal reflux disease (GERD) A condition in which the sphincter between the esophagus and the stomach opens, allowing stomach acid to move superiorly; can cause a burning sensation within the chest (heartburn); also called acid reflux disease.

hematemesis Vomit with blood; can either look like coffee grounds, indicating the presence of partially digested blood, or contain bright-red blood, indicating active bleeding.

hematochezia The passage of stool in which bright red blood can be distinguished; caused by lower gastrointestinal bleeding.

hepatic encephalopathy Impairment of brain function resulting from failure of the liver.

hepatitis Inflammation of the liver, usually caused by a virus, that causes fever, loss of appetite, jaundice, fatigue, and altered liver function.

hernia The protrusion of a loop of an organ or tissue through an abnormal body opening.

hiatal hernia The protrusion of a portion of the stomach through the diaphragm.

hyperperistalsis Increased activity within the bowel; also called borborygmi.

hypoperistalsis Decreased activity within the bowel.

icteric Yellowish coloration of the conjunctiva (the whites of the eyes) caused by the buildup of bilirubin in the blood during liver failure.

incarcerated A type of hernia in which an organ becomes trapped in the new location; most commonly obstructs the bowel.

incisional A type of hernia in which intestinal contents herniate through an incision; for example, after abdominal surgery.

inflammatory bowel disease (IBD) Chronic inflammation of all or part of the GI tract.

intussusception Telescoping of the intestines into themselves.

irritable bowel syndrome (IBS) A condition in which patients have abdominal pain and changes in their bowel habits; generally the pain and accompanying changes in bowel habits must be present for at least 3 days a month for at least 3 months to be considered this disease.

Mallory-Weiss syndrome A condition in which the junction between the esophagus and the stomach tears, causing severe bleeding and, potentially, death.

melena Dark, tarry, malodorous stools caused by upper GI bleeding.

mesenteric ischemia An interruption of the blood supply to the mesentery.

neoplasm A mass of tissue produced by abnormal cell growth and division that may be malignant (cancerous) or benign.

Prep Kit continued

pancreatitis Inflammation of the pancreas.

parietal pain Pain caused by inflammation of the parietal peritoneum that is generally described as steady, aching, and aggravated by movement.

peptic ulcer disease (PUD) A disease in which the mucous lining of the stomach and duodenum have been eroded, allowing the acid to eat into these organs.

peritonitis Inflammation of the peritoneum, the protective membrane that lines the abdominal and pelvic cavities.

portal hypertension Increased pressure in the portal veins; caused by the inability of blood to flow normally through the liver; can lead to rupture of these vessels.

pruritus Itching.

rebound tenderness Pain that the patient feels when pressure is released as opposed to when pressure is applied; characteristic of appendicitis.

rectal abscess An infection involving a collection of pus in the rectal walls that results from blockage of the rectal mucous ducts.

reducible A type of hernia that will return to its normal location either spontaneously or by manual manipulation.

scaphoid A concave shape of the abdomen; can be caused by evisceration.

septicemia A generalized infection of the bloodstream.

steatorrhea Foamy, fatty stools associated with liver failure or gallbladder conditions.

strangulated A type of hernia that causes complete obstruction of blood circulation in a given organ as a result of compression or entrapment; an emergency situation causing death of tissue.

striae Vertical stretch marks that occur when a person loses or gains weight rapidly.

stricture An abnormal narrowing of a structure; also called stenosis.

tracheoesophageal fistula (TEF) A connection between the esophagus and the trachea.

tympanic A loud, high-pitched sound, similar to the sound of a drum, heard on percussion of a hollow space (eg, the empty stomach or a puffed-out cheek).

ulcerative colitis Generalized inflammation of the colon that results in a weakened, dilated rectum, making it susceptible to infection and bleeding.

umbilical The region of the abdomen surrounding the umbilicus.

urticaria An itching rash.

volvulus Twisting of the bowel until a kink occurs; results in blocked flow.

References

1. Digestive diseases statistics for the United States. National Institute of Diabetes and Digestive and Kidney Diseases website. https://www.niddk.nih.gov/health-information/health-statistics/digestive-diseases. Published November 2014. Accessed February 6, 2021.
2. US Census Bureau. http://www.census.gov/. Published February 7, 2021. Accessed February 7, 2021.
3. Patti MG. Gastroesophageal reflux disease. *Medscape*. http://emedicine.medscape.com/article/176595-overview. Updated October 16, 2020. Accessed February 6, 2021.
4. Roantree RA, Furtado CS, Welch K, Lambert MJ. EMS ultrasound use. *StatPearls*. https://www.ncbi.nlm.nih.gov/books/NBK442034/. Updated September 19, 2020. Accessed February 6, 2021.
5. Carale J. Portal hypertension. *Medscape*. https://emedicine.medscape.com/article/182098. Updated November 30, 2017. Accessed February 7, 2021.
6. Wong Kee Song LM. Mallory-Weiss tear: overview of Mallory-Weiss syndrome. *Medscape*. https://emedicine.medscape.com/article/187134-overview. Updated October 2, 2019. Accessed February 7, 2021.
7. Roy PK. Boerhaave syndrome. *Medscape*. https://emedicine.medscape.com/article/171683-overview. Updated December 6, 2018. Accessed February 7, 2021.
8. Anand BS. Peptic ulcer disease. *Medscape*. https://emedicine.medscape.com/article/181753. Updated March 25, 2020. Accessed February 7, 2021.

Prep Kit continued

9. El-Nakeep S. Acute gastritis. *Medscape*. https://emedicine.medscape.com/article/175909-overview. Updated July 12, 2020. Accessed February 7, 2021.
10. Qureshi WA. Hiatal hernia. *Medscape*. https://emedicine.medscape.com/article/178393. Updated January 2, 2016. Accessed February 6, 2021.
11. Perry KR. Hemorrhoids. *Medscape*. https://emedicine.medscape.com/article/775407. Updated September 24, 2019. Accessed February 6 2021.
12. Lo BM. Anal fistulas and fissures. *Medscape*. https://emedicine.medscape.com/article/776150. Updated November 9, 2018. Accessed February 7, 2021.
13. Devuni D. Esophagitis. *Medscape*. https://emedicine.medscape.com/article/174223. Updated May 28, 2020. Accessed February 7, 2021.
14. Sharma S. Tracheoesophageal fistula. *Medscape*. https://emedicine.medscape.com/article/186735. Updated November 7, 2018. Accessed February 7, 2021.
15. Kumbum K. Esophageal stricture. *Medscape*. https://emedicine.medscape.com/article/175098. Updated August 20, 2019. Accessed February 7, 2021.
16. Daley B. Peritonitis and abdominal sepsis. *Medscape*. https://emedicine.medscape.com/article/180234-overview. Updated July 23, 2019. Accessed February 6, 2021.
17. Heuman DM. Gallstones (cholelithiasis). *Medscape*. https://emedicine.medscape.com/article/175667-overview. Updated April 1, 2019. Accessed February 6, 2021.
18. Scott TM. Acute cholangitis clinical presentation. *Medscape*. https://emedicine.medscape.com/article/774245-clinical#showall. Updated December 29, 2017. Accessed February 6, 2021.
19. Walker T. Emergency signs and symptoms of appendicitis. Healthline website. https://www.healthline.com/health/digestive-health/appendicitis-emergency-symptoms#1. Updated May 11, 2019. Accessed May 7, 2021.
20. Ghoulam EM. Diverticulitis. *Medscape*. https://emedicine.medscape.com/article/173388-overview. Updated August 6, 2019. Accessed February 6, 2021.
21. Commane DM, Arasaradnam RP, Mills S, et al. Diet, ageing and genetic factors in the pathogenesis of diverticular disease. *World J Gastroenterol*. 2009; 15(20):2479-2488. https://www.ncbi.nlm.nih.gov/pmc/articles/PMC2686906/. Accessed March 12, 2021.
22. Tang JCF. Acute pancreatitis: practice essentials, background, pathophysiology. *Medscape*. https://emedicine.medscape.com/article/181364-overview. Updated July 25, 2019. Accessed February 6, 2021.
23. Basson MD. Ulcerative colitis. *Medscape*. https://emedicine.medscape.com/article/183084-overview. Updated July 26, 2019. Accessed February 6, 2021.
24. Ghazi LJ. Crohn disease. *Medscape*. https://emedicine.medscape.com/article/172940-overview. Updated July 26, 2019. Accessed February 6, 2021.
25. Lehrer JK. Irritable bowel syndrome. *Medscape*. https://emedicine.medscape.com/article/180389-overview. Updated December 11, 2019. Accessed February 6, 2021.
26. Centers for Disease Control and Prevention. Estimates of foodborne illness in the United States. https://www.cdc.gov/foodborneburden/index.html. Updated November 5, 2018. Accessed January 30, 2021.
27. Connor BA. Travelers' diarrhea. https://wwwnc.cdc.gov/travel/yellowbook/2020/preparing-international-travelers/travelers-diarrhea. Updated November 22, 2019. Accessed February 6, 2021.
28. Diskin A. Emergent treatment of gastroenteritis. *Medscape*. https://emedicine.medscape.com/article/775277-overview. Updated February 10, 2017. Accessed January 30, 2021.
29. Hebra A. Anorectal abscess. *Medscape*. https://emedicine.medscape.com/article/191975-overview. Updated July 24, 2020. Accessed January 30, 2021
30. Wolf DC. Cirrhosis. *Medscape*. https://emedicine.medscape.com/article/185856-overview. Updated October 15, 2020. Accessed January 30, 2021.
31. Munter DW. Gastrointestinal foreign bodies. *Medscape*. https://emedicine.medscape.com/article/776566-overview. Updated January 4, 2018. Accessed January 30, 2021.
32. Ramnarine M. Small-bowel obstruction. *Medscape*. https://emedicine.medscape.com/article/774140-overview. Updated April 28, 2017. Accessed January 30, 2021.
33. Hopkins C. Large-bowel obstruction. *Medscape*. https://emedicine.medscape.com/article/774045-overview. Updated December 29, 2017. Accessed January 29, 2021.
34. Rather AA. Abdominal hernias. *Medscape*. https://emedicine.medscape.com/article/189563-overview. Updated July 23, 2019. Accessed January 29, 2021.
35. Munter DW. Rectal foreign bodies. *Medscape*. https://emedicine.medscape.com/article/776795-overview. Updated January 29, 2020. Accessed January 24, 2021.
36. Dang CV. Acute mesenteric ischemia. *Medscape*. https://emedicine.medscape.com/article/189146-overview. Updated March 26, 2020. Accessed January 24, 2021.
37. Dragovich T. Colon cancer. *Medscape*. https://emedicine.medscape.com/article/277496-overview. Updated February 11, 2021. Accessed January 24, 2021.
38. Dragovich T. Pancreatic cancer. *Medscape*. https://emedicine.medscape.com/article/280605-overview. Updated October 2, 2020. Accessed January 24, 2021.
39. Cicalese L. Hepatocellular carcinoma (HCC). *Medscape*. https://emedicine.medscape.com/article/197319-overview. Updated June 5, 2020. Accessed January 24, 2021.

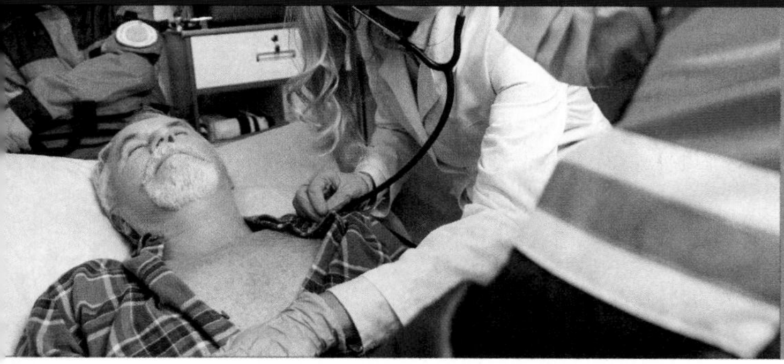

Chapter 22

Genitourinary and Renal Emergencies

NATIONAL EMS EDUCATION STANDARD COMPETENCIES

Medicine

Integrates assessment findings with principles of epidemiology and pathophysiology to formulate a field impression and implement a comprehensive treatment/disposition plan for a patient with a medical complaint.

Genitourinary/Renal

- Blood pressure assessment in hemodialysis patients (p 1450)

Anatomy, physiology, pathophysiology, assessment, and management of

- Complications related to
  - Renal dialysis (pp 1461–1464)
  - Urinary catheter management (not insertion) (p 1454)
- Kidney stones (pp 1455–1457)

Anatomy, physiology, epidemiology, pathophysiology, psychosocial impact, presentations, prognosis, and management of

- Complications of
  - Acute renal failure (pp 1457–1459)
  - Chronic renal failure (pp 1459–1460)
  - Dialysis (pp 1461–1464)
- Renal calculi (pp 1455–1457)
- Acid-base disturbances (p 1457)
- Fluid and electrolytes (pp 1461–1462)
- Infection (pp 1453–1454)
- Male genital tract conditions (pp 1464–1465)

KNOWLEDGE OBJECTIVES

1. Describe the anatomy and physiology of the male and female urinary systems: kidneys, ureters, urinary bladder, and urethra. (pp 1446–1447)
2. Describe the primary survey and secondary assessment processes for patients with renal and genitourinary emergencies. (pp 1447–1452)
3. Specify factors that influence transport decisions for patients with renal and genitourinary emergencies. (pp 1450–1453)
4. Discuss the questions that must be asked to obtain thorough historical information from a patient. (pp 1450–1451)
5. Specify best practices for documenting renal and genitourinary emergencies and communicating with the receiving facility. (p 1450)
6. Compare visceral pain with referred pain. (p 1451)
7. Explain how visceral pain and referred pain each contribute to the field diagnosis. (pp 1450–1451)
8. Indicate the components of the physical exam for a patient with a renal or genitourinary emergency. (p 1452)
9. Name the components of an effective treatment plan. (pp 1452–1453)

10. Outline the pathophysiology, assessment, and management of common diseases and conditions of the renal and genitourinary systems, including urinary tract infections, kidney stones, acute kidney injury, chronic kidney disease, and end-stage renal disease. (pp 1453–1461)
11. Discuss the purpose and types of renal dialysis. (pp 1461–1464)
12. Identify the possible complications of dialysis and the prehospital interventions associated with each. (pp 1461–1464)
13. Discuss the pathophysiology, assessment, and management of conditions related to the male genital tract, including epididymitis, orchitis, Fournier gangrene, priapism, phimosis, paraphimosis, benign prostate hypertrophy, testicular masses, and testicular torsion. (pp 1464–1465)

SKILLS OBJECTIVES

There are no skills objectives for this chapter.

Introduction

The urinary system performs the essential jobs of filtering the blood and removing metabolic wastes. In addition, the urinary system manages concentrations of electrolytes and maintains acid-base balance in the bloodstream. It also regulates fluid volume and blood pressure (BP).

Approximately 661,000 Americans have kidney failure, with more than 468,000 requiring dialysis, and an estimated 193,000 are living with a functioning kidney transplant.[1] More Americans die of kidney disease each year than die from breast or prostate cancer.[1] The most common acute renal disease is nephrolithiasis (kidney stones or renal calculi), which affects more than 11% of men and 6% of women in the United States.[2] Common urinary tract diseases include **urinary tract infections (UTIs)**, which occur in more than 50% of women,[3] and noncancerous enlargement of the prostate, which affects nearly 70% of men between 60 and 69 years and 80% of men age 70 years or older.[4]

Anatomy and Physiology Review

The urinary system **FIGURE 22-1** consists of the **kidneys**, which filter the blood and produce **urine**; the paired **ureters**, which transport urine from the kidneys to the bladder; the **urinary bladder**, which stores the urine until it is released from the body; and the **urethra**, the route by which urine leaves the bladder and exits the body. In females, the urethra is significantly shorter than in males, which increases their susceptibility to infections.

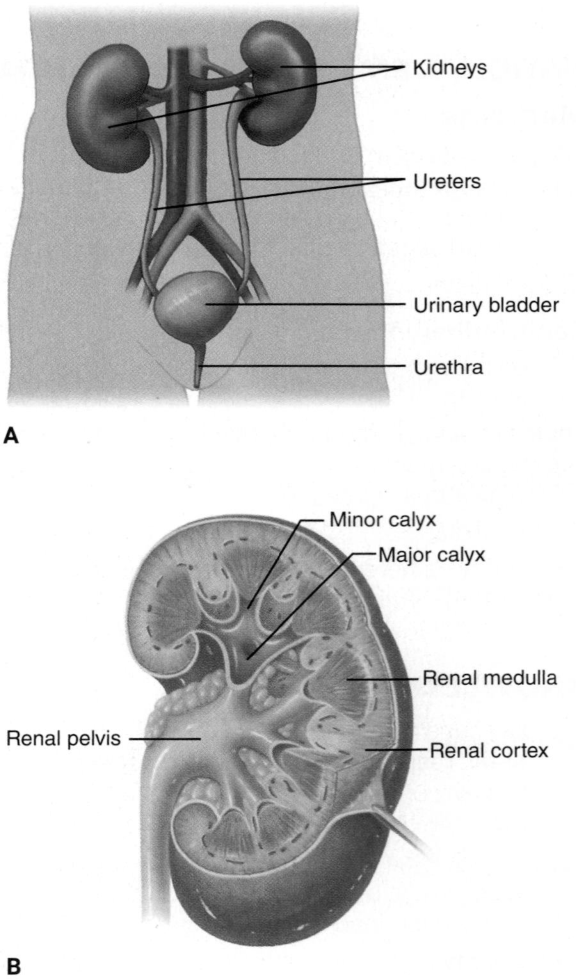

FIGURE 22-1 The urinary system. **A.** Anterior view showing the relationship of the kidneys, ureters, urinary bladder, and urethra. **B.** Cross section of the human kidney showing the renal cortex, renal medulla, and renal pelvis.

The kidney's internal anatomy can be divided into three distinct regions: the cortex, the medulla, and the pelvis, which drains urine into the ureter. **Nephrons** **FIGURE 22-2**, found in the cortex, are the structural and functional units of the kidney that form urine. Each nephron is composed of the glomerulus; the **glomerular (Bowman) capsule**, which surrounds the glomerulus; the **proximal convoluted tubule (PCT)**; the **loop of Henle**; and the **distal convoluted tubule (DCT)**, which connects with the kidney's collecting tubules.

The male genital system **FIGURE 22-3** is closely related to the urinary system, sharing the urethra as a conduit for urine as well as for semen and other secretions. The prostate gland surrounds the urethra and, along with the seminal vesicles, secretes fluids into the urethra during ejaculation. The testes are located in the scrotum and create spermatozoa, which are stored and mature in the epididymis. During ejaculation, the sperm travels from the epididymis into the vas deferens and through the ejaculatory ducts, where it mixes with fluid from the seminal vesicles, bulbourethral glands, and prostate to form semen. It then enters the urethra, through which it exits the body. The female genital system is discussed in detail in Chapter 23, *Gynecologic Emergencies.*

Patient Assessment

Assessment of a patient with a renal and genitourinary emergency is the same as for any other medical patient. Begin with the scene size-up, perform a primary survey, obtain a history, perform a secondary assessment including a physical exam, form a field impression, make a treatment decision, and reassess the patient continuously en route to the hospital.

Scene Size-up

During the scene size-up, you should ensure that the scene is safe for you and your fellow providers, consider the mechanism of injury, assess for hazards and the need for additional help, and determine the number of patients. Remember that urine is a body fluid, so you must take standard precautions to avoid contact with it.

Patients experiencing renal or genital conditions may exhibit many of the same symptoms as patients with other abdominal conditions—namely, nausea and vomiting, constipation or diarrhea, flank pain, and abdominal pain. Although pain is a common symptom in both abdominal and genitourinary ailments, it is often difficult to determine the pain's precise source. Genitourinary pain can have many origins, including bacterial infection, extension of the ureter by a kidney stone, or distention of the bladder because of prostate enlargement. Your assessment should focus on detecting and preventing life threats and providing supportive care for the patient. Be sure to keep a broad list of differential diagnoses in mind as you progress through your evaluation.

Primary Survey

In the primary survey, you form a general impression of the patient and check for life-threatening

YOU are the Paramedic

PART 1

At about 0600 hours, you are dispatched to 327 West Main Street for a woman reporting back pain. You arrive to find a slender, gray-haired man waiting for you at the front door of the turn-of-the-century residence. He motions for you and says, "It's my daughter. She's very sick. I would have taken her to the hospital myself, but I can't carry her. She's in the upstairs bedroom." The stairway is dark and narrow. As you walk up the steps, you hear a young woman say, "Dad, I'm going to be sick again."

1. What concerns may you have about the scene?
2. Although you have not seen your patient yet, what information do you already know that is part of the primary survey?

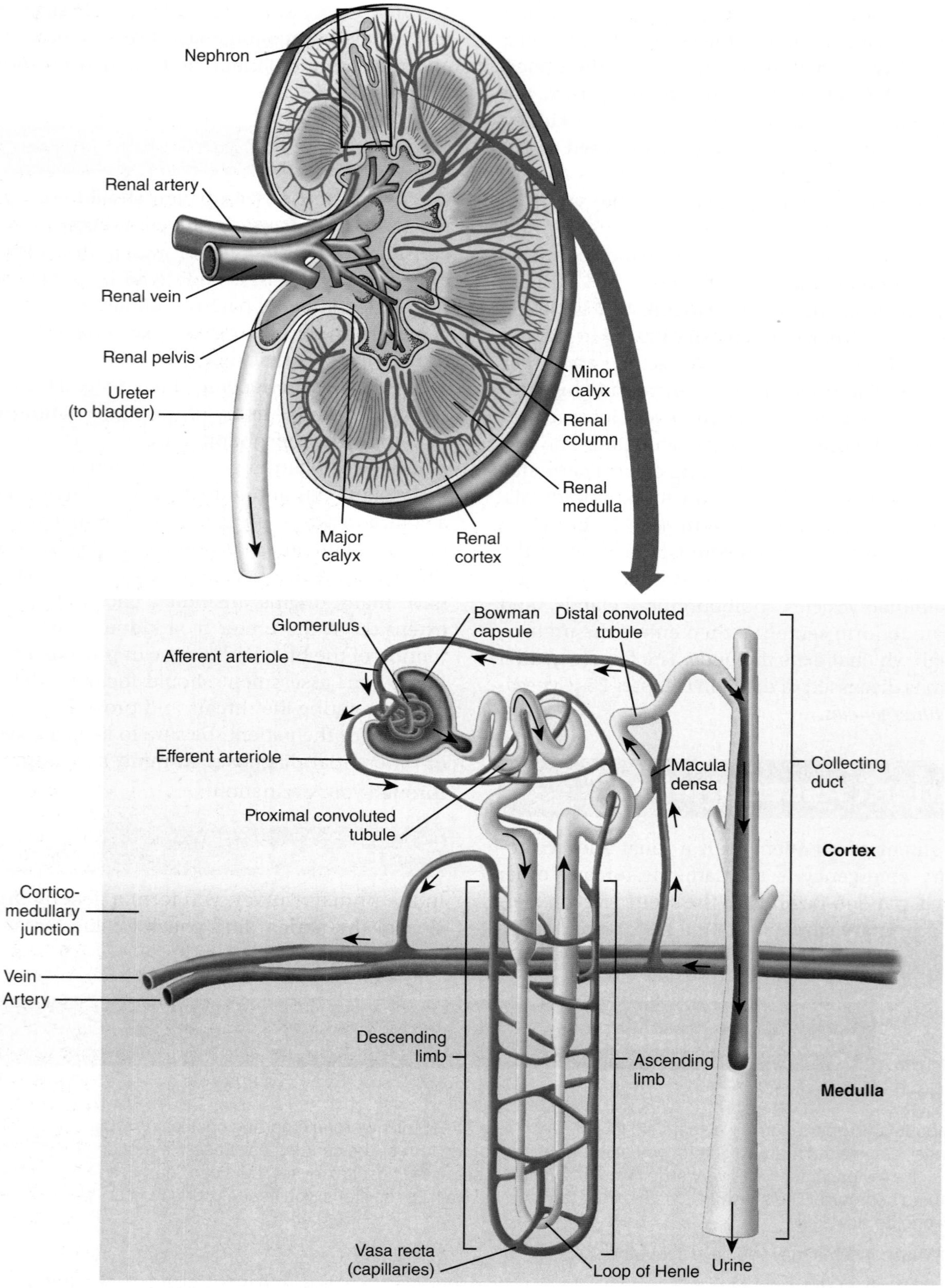

FIGURE 22-2 The nephrons of the kidney. Part of the nephron is located in the cortex, and part is located in the medulla.

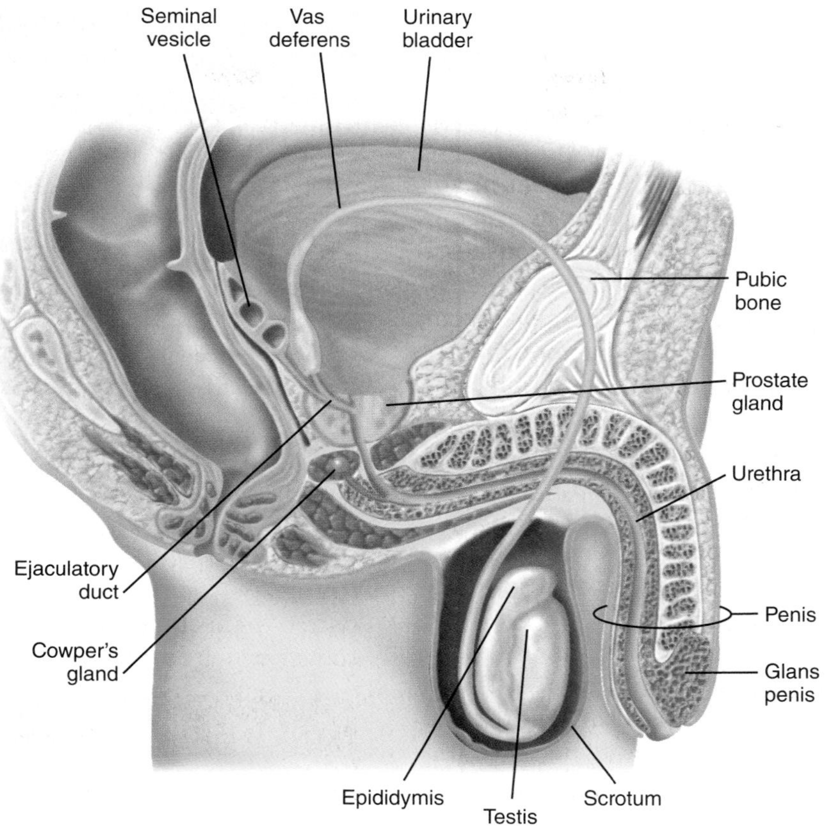

FIGURE 22-3 The male genital anatomy.

YOU are the Paramedic

PART 2

As you reach the bedroom door, you hear the sound of vomiting. You turn to your partner to request that he retrieve the stair chair. The father opens the door, and you see a woman in her early 20s in a bed covered with several blankets. The father tells you that she has been feeling ill for a few days, but she got worse last night around midnight. He said that she has been vomiting throughout the night and feels very dizzy when she tries to stand. You introduce yourself and ask if you can take her vital signs. She nods yes. You sit down and continue your assessment.

Recording Time: 0 Minutes	
Appearance	Lying on her right side, head hanging off the bed over a trash can
Level of consciousness	Alert
Airway	Patent with active vomiting
Breathing	Rapid
Circulation	Flushed, sweaty skin

3. What concerns do you have about her history, signs, and symptoms?
4. What should be done with the emesis?

conditions. A patient with a genitourinary or renal condition may exhibit extremes of activity. Is the patient changing position constantly in an attempt to find a comfortable position ("the kidney stone dance")? Or is the patient sitting very still with the knees drawn up to the chest? Is the patient in obvious pain? Does the patient appear pale or jaundiced? What is the patient's level of consciousness? Your observation of the patient's body movements, posture, skin color, breathing pattern, mental acuity, and other factors will give you a good overall sense of the severity of the patient's condition.

Check for life threats by assessing the patient's mental status and airway, breathing, and circulation (ABCs). Begin by observing the patient's breathing and ensure that the airway is patent. Look for signs of respiratory distress. Clear the airway and provide treatment as indicated by the patient's respiratory status.

Next, assess skin color, heart rate, and BP. Look for signs of shock, such as a rapid heart rate and low BP. Is the abdomen distended or rigid? If you discover any life-threatening conditions, take immediate steps to correct them and provide urgent transport to an appropriately equipped receiving facility. Advise the facility en route to begin mobilizing resources and staff so that they will be on standby at the time of transfer.

When making your transport decision, integrate the information you obtained in the primary survey. Determine as quickly as possible whether urgent transport is warranted for life threats such as **uremia** (excessive amounts of urea and other waste products in the blood), hyperkalemia, or testicular torsion. Consider how you will move the patient, especially if a change in position is likely to cause a decrease in the patient's BP. Take into account any special equipment needed to handle the patient, such as a bariatric stretcher. Also keep in mind which receiving facility has the diagnostic or treatment equipment that will be necessary after transfer, such as dialysis or a urologist on staff.

Street Smarts

Ensure that the ride during transport is as gentle as possible for the patient with a genitourinary or renal condition. Rapid driving can result in increased vehicle movement, potentially aggravating and possibly worsening the patient's pain.

Documentation and Communication

Establish and document your baseline impression early in the assessment process. Document any changes in mental status or level of consciousness as you reevaluate the patient, and note how the patient responds to the administration of supplemental oxygen, fluids, pain medication, and other interventions. Stay in close contact with medical control, and notify the receiving facility as soon as possible if life threats are apparent. Record the findings of your serial assessments in your report to the receiving facility, concluding with your overall impression of the patient's condition at the time of transfer.

History Taking

In patients with genitourinary issues, the history and physical exam will provide the information you need to successfully treat the patient. Because so many medical diagnoses are based on the patient's history, you must ask the right questions during this exam. Determining that the patient's pain started in the flank, for example, and not in its present location in the lower right quadrant, could mean the difference between a correct field diagnosis of a kidney stone and an incorrect field diagnosis of appendicitis. Similarly, determining that the patient has a history of diabetes and hypertension along with signs of uremia can help confirm your impression of chronic kidney failure.

The SAMPLE mnemonic (Signs and symptoms, Allergies, Medications, Pertinent past medical history, Last oral intake, Events leading up to the injury or illness) can guide you in obtaining pertinent historical information from the patient. For example, a patient who reports flank pain (S); who has had two previous kidney stone attacks (P); who ate bacon, eggs, and coffee for breakfast 7 hours ago (L); and who has been working in the sun all day (E) has presented a history that would lead you to suspect kidney stones. Before proceeding with treatment, you would also want to assess allergies (A) and any medications (M) the patient has taken.

Pain

Diseases and conditions of the renal and urologic systems range in severity from mild (UTIs) to emergent (acute kidney injury). Although the prehospital care for many urologic diseases is supportive, your ability to recognize the signs and symptoms of these conditions, especially when they are genuine emergencies, is critical to providing your patients with the best chance of a positive outcome.

Understanding the pathophysiology of pain, especially referred pain (ie, pain that feels as if it is originating from a body part other than the site being stimulated), is key to determining its origin. Visceral pain (ie, deep pain caused by activation of pain receptors in internal areas of the body enclosed within a cavity) is the type of pain most commonly associated with urologic conditions. It usually occurs when receptors in the hollow structures, such as the ureters, urinary bladder, and urethra, are stimulated. Pinpointing the source of such pain is challenging because only a few nerve fibers may be involved in the pain transmission. Because many different nerve fibers travel to the brain through the spinal cord, pain that originates in one area of the body (eg, the urinary bladder) may be perceived by the brain as coming from a different area of the body (eg, the neck or shoulder), resulting in the phenomenon of referred pain.

Pain Assessment Findings

The OPQRST (Onset, Provocation, Quality, Region/radiation/referral, Severity, Timing) mnemonic is used to elaborate on the chief complaint and evaluate the type and severity of pain. Determining the *onset* requires asking questions about when the pain started and what the patient was doing at the time. The patient may describe visceral pain, such as that caused by a kidney stone, as a crampy or aching sensation deep within the body. It often begins as a vague discomfort and then gradually increases. Next, determine what, if anything, *provokes* the pain (eg, the kidney stone dance or statue stillness). To help rule out other abdominal causes of pain, note any relationship between the patient's food consumption and the pain.

After determining the onset and provocation, assess the *quality* of the pain. As stated earlier, pain from a kidney stone usually begins as vague discomfort that becomes extremely sharp pain within an hour. The *R* in the mnemonic stands for *region* (location), *radiation*, or *referral*. For example, the pain from a kidney stone moves from the flank anteriorly, toward the groin. The fact that the pain has moved also suggests that a kidney stone is passing through the urinary system.

To evaluate the *severity* of the pain, ask the patient, "On a scale of 0 to 10, with 10 being the worst pain you have ever experienced, how would you rate the pain?" Although this number is helpful, by itself it tells you very little. The severity of the pain may not be consistent with the severity of the condition. It is essential to repeat the pain severity assessment to look for trends or verify treatment efficacy.

The final pain evaluation is to inquire about the *timing* of the pain. Did the pain come on suddenly, or did it emerge more gradually? Has it been constant, or does it come and go? In the case of a kidney stone, you would expect fairly constant pain that varies in severity and moves as the stone travels through the urinary system.

Special Populations

Older adults generally underreport pain for a variety of reasons.[5] Even mild atraumatic abdominal, back, or flank pain in an older patient should be taken seriously.

Secondary Assessment

The physical exam may focus on a specific area, or you may move from head to toe, depending on the presentation of signs and symptoms. For the purposes of assessment, the abdominal region is divided into either four quadrants overlying the internal organs **FIGURE 22-4A** or nine anatomic segments **FIGURE 22-4B**. A more detailed physical exam may be performed en route if one is not done at the scene. Be sure to assess for flank tenderness, which could imply kidney infection or distention. If a male patient reports lower abdominal pain without other clear cause, visually inspect the genitalia for signs of infection, swelling, or torsion.

Monitoring the patient's vital signs is part of the physical exam. You should obtain serial vital signs at least every 5 minutes if you suspect the patient

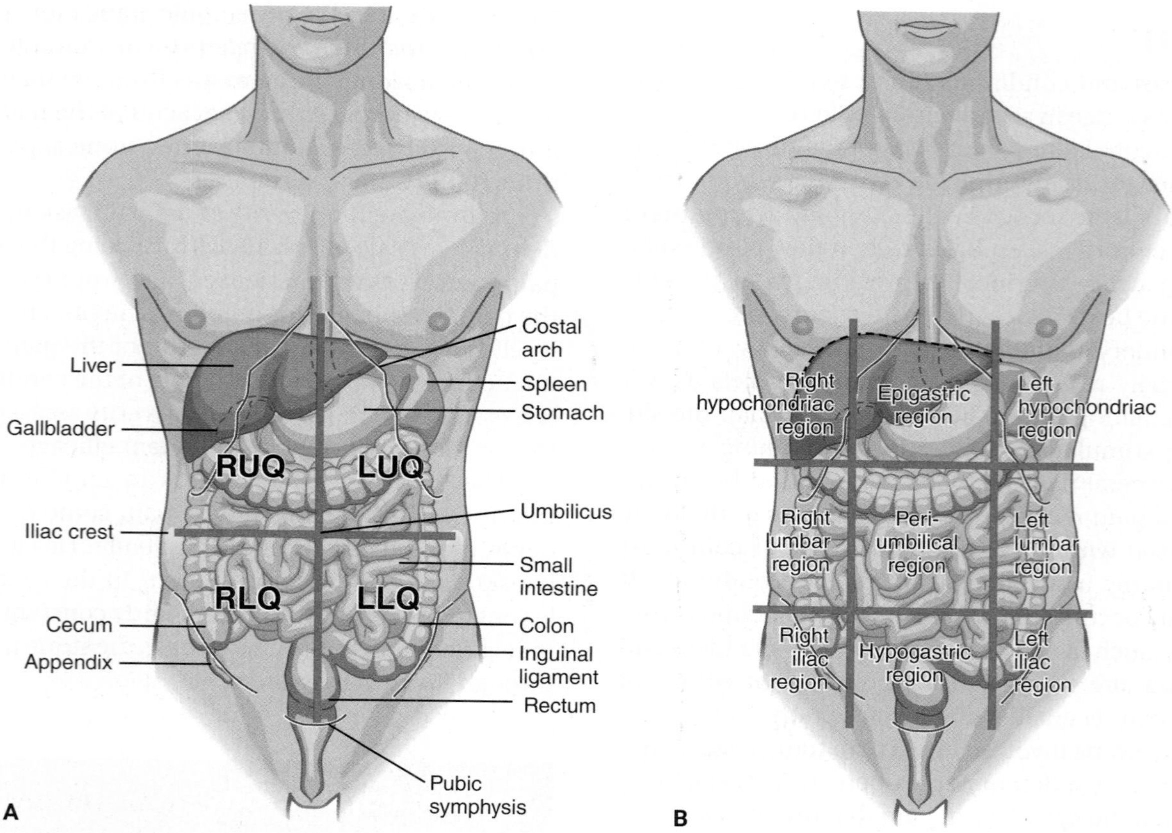

FIGURE 22-4 A. The four-quadrant system. **B.** Abdominal region mapping in nine sections.

has renal failure. Take prompt action if you note any deterioration in the patient's vital signs or level of consciousness.

Finally, consider the link between abnormal vital signs and the patient's history. For example, a diuretic or other medication might be responsible for a patient's low BP. Diabetes, chronic obstructive pulmonary disease, or another chronic condition noted in the patient's history might explain other abnormal findings and provide clues to the patient's current genitourinary diagnosis.

Electrocardiographic (ECG) monitoring is vital in any patient with a suspected urologic emergency because of the possibility of electrolyte imbalances that may affect the heart.

Special Populations

Abnormal vital signs in an older adult patient may be particularly worrisome. An older adult patient with a fever, for instance, should receive especially close scrutiny for other signs of infection. A UTI in an older adult can cause a recurrence of past stroke symptoms and significant mental status changes. Abdominal pain in the older patient is a serious complaint that is associated with a high mortality rate; such patients require thorough evaluation in the emergency department (ED).[6]

Reassessment

Patients with urologic emergencies, especially those with signs and symptoms of renal failure, require frequent reassessment. The electrolyte imbalances caused by the buildup of toxins can cause the functioning of the body's organs to deteriorate rapidly. The heart is particularly susceptible to electrolyte changes, so cardiac monitoring should be established for every renal patient.

The information obtained from the history and physical exam is used to update and refine the field impression and to select a treatment plan. The interventions chosen might be as simple as monitoring the ABCs and providing circulatory support to a patient with a UTI, or as complex as adjusting medications and providing support (with medical consultation and direction) for a patient with renal failure, based on ECG changes. The treatment plan also includes the transport decision, which may be made at any time during the assessment process. If the disease process requires immediate medical procedures (eg, removal of a urinary catheter, adjustment of a fistula or shunt) that go beyond the prehospital provider's scope of practice, perform the primary survey and transport the patient, reassessing the patient en route to the hospital.

Serial vital signs should be obtained and documented on the patient care report. Note any trends in the vital signs and level of consciousness, because they can indicate disease progression. Patients with a possible genitourinary disease should not be given anything by mouth because this may induce vomiting or complicate anesthesia administration for any necessary surgical procedures at the hospital. Document all vital signs and report any apparent trends to the receiving facility.

> **Words of Wisdom**
>
> Patients with renal failure who miss their dialysis treatments are susceptible to hyperkalemia (an elevated level of potassium in the blood), among other conditions. You should suspect hyperkalemia if the patient has muscle weakness and tall, peaked T waves appear on the ECG.

Emergency Medical Care

Pain Management

Once you have checked and established adequate ABCs, allow the patient to assume a position of comfort. Patients in severe pain may have nausea and vomiting, so be prepared to suction as needed. Establish an intravenous (IV) line if the patient has nausea or severe pain, and consider administering an antiemetic. If the patient has signs of dehydration or hemodynamic instability, administer an IV bolus of crystalloid fluid. Provide analgesia as necessary. Concerns about masking symptoms and reducing the accuracy of diagnosis made by the ED are not a reason to withhold pain control. Indeed, evidence has shown that the administration of pain medication does not reduce later diagnostic accuracy.[7]

Pathophysiology, Assessment, and Management of Specific Emergencies

Urinary Tract Infections

UTIs result in more than 2 million ED visits per year.[8] Such infections are most common in females after infancy. After the age of 50, there is an increase in UTIs in men because of obstruction of the urethra by the prostate, which commonly occurs with aging. Definitive treatment requires antibiotics. Mild cases respond well to oral antibiotics, whereas severe cases may require IV administration.

Pathophysiology

UTIs usually develop in the lower urinary tract (urethra and bladder), when normal flora (bacteria that naturally populate the skin) enter the urethra and grow there. These infections are more common in women because of their relatively short urethra and its proximity to the vagina and rectum. UTIs in the upper urinary tract occur most often when lower UTIs go untreated. Upper UTIs can lead to **pyelonephritis** (inflammation of the kidney linings) and even a perinephric abscess (a collection of pus around the kidney), which may result in the development of sepsis and become life threatening.

Assessment

Patients with UTIs display a classic triad of symptoms: painful urination, frequent urges to urinate, and difficulty in urination. The pain usually begins as a visceral discomfort, but soon evolves into an extreme, burning pain, especially during urination. The pain, which remains localized in the pelvis, is often perceived as bladder pain in women and as prostate pain in men. Sometimes the pain is referred to the shoulder or neck. In addition, the urine may have a foul odor or cloudy appearance, or may contain blood.

Patients with UTIs frequently appear to be restless and uncomfortable. Those with an uncomplicated UTI will appear well and have normal vital signs, but may have suprapubic tenderness. In contrast, a patient with pyelonephritis or a perinephric abscess will present as ill, have flank tenderness, generally have a fever, and may have unstable vital signs. UTIs are a common cause of sepsis in older adults and should be considered in any older patient with fever, shock, or unexplained mental status changes.

Management

Management of UTIs consists mainly of supportive care of the ABCs. Allow the patient to ride in a position of comfort, but be prepared for nausea and vomiting. Patients with pyelonephritis or sepsis will require more aggressive care, including IV fluids, antiemetics, and pain control. Transport the patient to the nearest appropriate facility for evaluation.

Urinary Catheters

Many patients who are hospitalized for a urinary condition or other medical disease receive catheterization with a Foley catheter. Bladder catheterization involves introducing a latex or plastic tube through the urethra and into the bladder. The tube is connected to a drainage bag, which is attached to the bed frame or wheelchair at a level below the bladder. The catheter allows a continuous outflow of urine and provides a means of measuring urine output.

When you are transporting a catheterized patient, urine backflow is a concern. If the drainage bag is raised above the level of the patient's bladder, urine can flow back into the bladder, increasing the chance of infection. Care should also be taken not to inadvertently pull out the catheter or kink it, obstructing flow. If a Foley catheter must be removed, ensure that the internal balloon is deflated.

Urinary Obstruction and Incontinence

Many conditions discussed in this section can cause **urinary retention**, defined as incomplete emptying of the bladder or a complete inability to empty the bladder. Conditions that may cause urinary retention are listed in **TABLE 22-1**. Patients with these conditions may present with extreme discomfort and should be transported to the nearest facility for urinary catheter placement.

YOU are the Paramedic

PART 3

Your partner returns with the stair chair. You ask him to obtain the patient's temperature while you finish taking the SAMPLE history and assemble your supplies to start an IV line. The patient tells you that she has had burning with urination for a few days and that she has had UTIs in the past. At one point, her physician put her on prophylactic ciprofloxacin (Cipro). She decided that was not a good idea, and now just takes herbal supplements containing cranberry when she feels an infection is starting.

Recording Time: 5 Minutes	
Respirations	24 breaths/min
Pulse	110 beats/min
Skin	Flushed, sweaty
Blood pressure	108/60 mm Hg; lying down
Oxygen saturation (Spo_2)	98%
Pupils	Pupils Equal, Round, and Reactive to Light and Accommodation (PERRLA)

5. What additional assessment techniques might you use?
6. Why is assessing the patient's body temperature important?

TABLE 22-1 Conditions That May Cause Urinary Retention
Kidney stones (renal calculi)
Acute kidney injury
Benign prostate hypertrophy
Urethral obstructions
Urinary tract infections
Nerve damage

Urinary incontinence is loss of bladder control: the inability to control the release of urine from the bladder. Whereas urinary incontinence can occur in anyone (eg, from sneezing or a forceful cough), it may also be a sign of a medical condition if it falls into one of the following two categories:

- **Urge incontinence.** This is a sudden, intense urge to urinate, followed within seconds to minutes by involuntary urine loss. Urination is frequent: for example, throughout the night. Urge incontinence has many potential medical causes, including UTI, medications, bladder irritants (eg, caffeine, carbonated drinks), bowel conditions, Parkinson disease, Alzheimer disease, stroke, cancers of the uterus and the urinary system, and nervous system damage associated with multiple sclerosis.
- **Overflow incontinence.** This is a constant, continual slow flow of urine. Overflow incontinence can have medical causes, such as a damaged bladder, blocked urethra, or nerve damage from diabetes, and prostate gland conditions in men.[9]

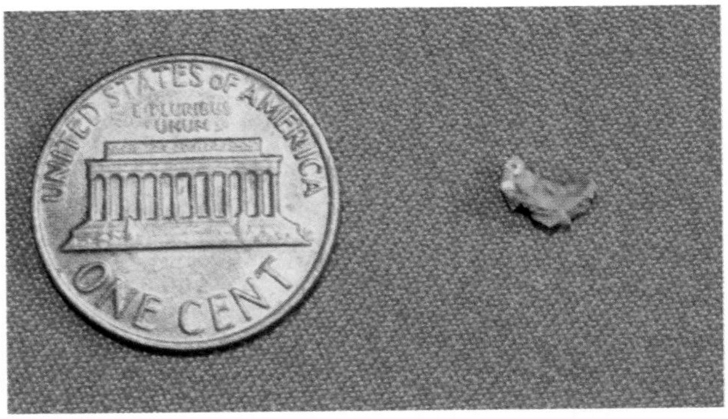

A

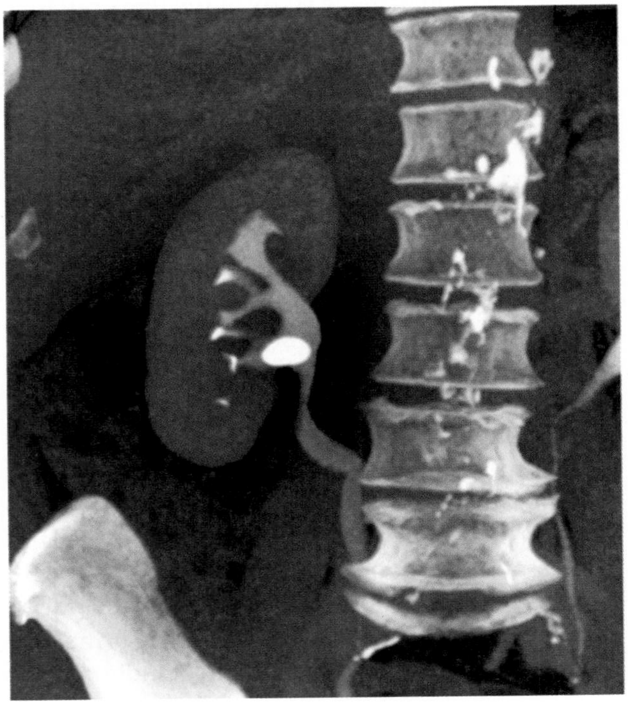

B

FIGURE 22-5 A. A kidney stone. **B.** A computed tomography scan of a kidney stone.

Kidney Stones (Renal Calculi)

Pathophysiology

Kidney stones are common and originate in the renal pelvis. They form when an excess of insoluble salts or uric acid crystallizes in the urine **FIGURE 22-5**. In the United States, roughly 10% of all people will experience a kidney stone, with men being affected more often than women.[10] The causes of kidney stones vary by type. Certain risk factors have been identified, including diet and hydration. General risk factors include a personal or family history of kidney stones, as well as hypertension.

The most common types of stones are calcium oxalate and calcium phosphate stones, which account for as many as 80% of kidney stones.[11] These stones are thought to form when the concentration of calcium oxalate or phosphate becomes too high in the urine, although other theories exist. Their formation may have a hereditary component, and risk is increased in people with a history of gout, gastric bypass surgery, and certain metabolic disorders.

Struvite stones are more common in women and are associated with chronic UTIs or frequent catheterization. Uric acid stones are most common in individuals with a history of gout and are more common in dry and arid regions of the United States. Cystine stones are associated with a condition that causes large amounts of amino acids and proteins to be excreted in the urine.

Assessment

Patients who have kidney stones are almost always in pain. The pain usually starts in the flank but may migrate forward, toward the groin, as the stone passes through the urinary system. The patient may feel vague discomfort that progresses to intense pain over time. Kidney stone pain can be severe, and it is frequently described as the worst pain of a person's life. The pain may cause increased BP and tachycardia. In older adults, these symptoms can lead to stroke or myocardial infarction.[12] Be sure to obtain a detailed patient and family history, which can supply clues about the stone's cause.

Some patients with kidney stones appear agitated and restless, pacing and moving about in an attempt to relieve the pain. Other patients try to remain motionless to guard the abdomen. Either behavior makes palpation of the abdomen difficult. Vital signs will vary according to the severity of pain. The greater the pain, the higher the patient's BP and pulse will be. These patients often present with **hematuria**, and if the stone is obstructing urine flow in the ureter **FIGURE 22-6**, with flank tenderness.

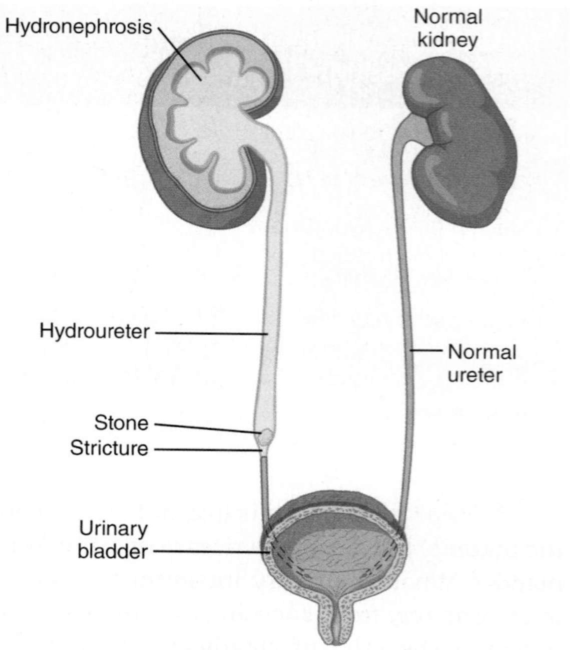

FIGURE 22-6 When a kidney stone obstructs the flow of urine, the patient may have blood in the urine (hematuria) and flank tenderness.

Words of Wisdom

Patients with kidney stones usually have severe, nearly unbearable pain, and should be given aggressive pain control, such as narcotic analgesics (ie, morphine, fentanyl). Because higher-than-usual doses are often required, naloxone (Narcan) must be readily available should central nervous system depression occur. Follow your local protocols or contact medical control as needed regarding pain relief for these patients.

Management

The prehospital management of kidney stones centers on pain relief. After ensuring the ABCs, allow the patient to assume a position of comfort. Administer analgesia; if your local protocols do not allow for this therapy, contact medical control regarding pain relief options. Nitrous oxide is an alternative treatment to narcotics. Establish an IV line and administer IV fluids for hydration, and give antiemetics as needed.

Some kidney stones will pass on their own, whereas others require surgery to remove them. An alpha (α)- blocker such as tamsulosin (Flomax) is often used to relax smooth muscle in the bladder neck and facilitate increased urine flow. When a UTI is present along with an obstructing kidney stone, the patient may have signs and symptoms of a UTI and can become quite ill and septic; this is an emergency requiring urologic intervention.

The treatment approach for persistent stones depends on the size, consistency, and location of the stones. Treatment options include the following:

- **Extracorporeal lithotripsy.** High-energy shock waves from outside the body are used to break up stones, resulting in much smaller stone fragments and dust that can pass easily.
- **Cystoscopy with stent placement.** Cystoscopy is the direct visualization of the ureter and

urinary collection system. It is accomplished by inserting a small camera through the urethra and into the ureter. A stent can be placed to enlarge the diameter of the ureter and allow for stone passage.

- **Percutaneous nephrostomy (PCN) tube placement.** A PCN tube is a small catheter that is placed from the outside of the body into the kidney to allow for drainage of material that is obstructed by a stone. This method is frequently used to decompress the kidney when the patient has an infection associated with a stone.

Acute Kidney Injury

Acute kidney injury (AKI) is a sudden decrease in the rate of filtration through the glomeruli, causing toxins to accumulate in the blood. This loss of function may occur over the course of several days. AKI most often occurs secondary to another disease process. As many as 50% of critically ill patients develop AKI,[13] and the mortality for these patients has been reported to be as high as 70%.[14]

Urine output of less than 500 mL/d in an adult or less than 0.5 mL/kg/h in an adult or child (less than 1 mL/kg/h in a neonate) is called **oliguria**, while complete cessation of urine production is called **anuria**. Whenever AKI occurs, the patient may experience generalized edema, acid buildup, and high levels of nitrogenous and metabolic wastes in the blood. If left untreated, AKI can lead to life-threatening volume overload, hyperkalemia, uremia, and metabolic acidosis.

AKI is classified into three types, based on the area in which the failure occurs: prerenal, intrarenal, and postrenal. The signs and symptoms of each type are summarized in **TABLE 22-2**.

TABLE 22-2 Signs and Symptoms of Acute Kidney Injury

Type of Acute Kidney Injury	Signs and Symptoms
Prerenal	Hypotension Tachycardia Dizziness Thirst
Intrarenal	Flank pain Joint pain Oliguria Hypertension Headache Confusion Seizure
Postrenal	Pain in lower flank, abdomen, groin, and genitalia Oliguria Distended bladder Hematuria Peripheral edema

Pathophysiology

The toxic buildup of nitrogenous wastes and salts in the blood associated with AKI causes impaired mentation, fluid retention, tachycardia, acid-base imbalances, and increased PR and QT intervals associated with hyperkalemia.

Prerenal acute kidney injury is caused by hypoperfusion of the kidneys. In other words, not enough blood passes into the glomeruli for them to produce filtrate. The most common causes of prerenal AKI are hypovolemia (low blood volume caused by hemorrhage or dehydration), trauma, shock, sepsis, and heart failure. Prerenal AKI is often reversible if the underlying condition can be treated and perfusion restored to the kidney. Hepatorenal syndrome is a specific type of AKI that occurs in patients with advanced liver disease, in which renal perfusion becomes severely decreased due to portal hypertension. The prognosis of patients with hepatorenal syndrome is linked to their recovery from the liver disease and is much worse than for patients with other forms of AKI.[15]

Intrarenal acute kidney injury (IAKI) involves damage to one of three areas in the kidney: the glomeruli capillaries and small blood vessels, the cells of the kidney tubules, or the renal parenchyma (the interstitial cells around the nephrons). Damage to the small vessels and glomeruli hinders blood flow through these vital parts of the nephrons. This damage is often caused by immune-mediated diseases, such as type 1 diabetes mellitus. Tubule damage can be caused by hypoperfusion leading to acute tubular necrosis or by toxins (eg, heavy metals). Rhabdomyolysis is another cause of IAKI, in which myoglobin released from muscle fibers damages the tubules. Chronic inflammation of the interstitial cells surrounding the nephrons (**interstitial nephritis**) can also produce IAKI. This type of renal failure may be caused by medications such as antibiotics, anticancer drugs, alcohol, and drugs of abuse (eg, cocaine).

Postrenal acute kidney injury is caused by obstruction of urine flow from the kidneys. The source of this obstruction is often a blockage of the urethra by an enlarged prostate, kidney stones, blood clots, or strictures. This blockage raises the pressure in the nephrons, which eventually causes them to shut down.

All forms of AKI lead to a common ending: the kidneys' inability to perform their cleansing functions. In turn, this can lead to the development of hyperkalemia (an increase in the blood's potassium level), metabolic acidosis (an increase in the blood's hydrogen ion content), and uremia (an increased level of urea in the blood). These conditions are life-threatening emergencies that can lead to fatal cardiac dysrhythmias secondary to hyperkalemia and acidosis, hypotension secondary to acidosis, and mental status changes secondary to uremia.

Assessment

The presentations of patients with AKI will vary based on the underlying cause. Patients with prerenal AKI will generally appear dehydrated or in shock with pale, cool, and moist skin. Frequently, decreased urine output or darkening of the urine will be reported. Flank pain may also be present, particularly in patients with intrarenal AKI. Patients with postrenal AKI usually report pain in the suprapubic area related to bladder distention or in the penis from obstruction. More severe cases of AKI may present with altered mental status or signs of heart failure.

During the physical exam, you should thoroughly evaluate the abdomen for other causes of discomfort or the presence of ascites. Assess flank tenderness. Perform an ECG to evaluate for dysrhythmias or signs of hyperkalemia. Evaluate for signs of infection, such as a fever or dysuria, and closely monitor vital signs for signs of shock.

Management

Because the metabolic changes caused by AKI can be life threatening, it is imperative that the treatment plan support and manage the ABCs as needed.

YOU are the Paramedic

PART 4

You explain to the patient that her condition requires that blood be drawn, and that it is necessary to establish an IV line to perform the blood draw and to administer fluids. Your partner has assembled the stair chair, listened to lung sounds, and placed the patient on the cardiac monitor. After you initiate the IV line and draw blood samples, you tell her, "We are going to put you in this chair with wheels to take you down the stairs." Her father tells you that is probably not a good idea because she "doesn't do well sitting up."

Recording Time: 10 Minutes	
Respirations	24 breaths/min
Pulse	112 beats/min
Skin	Flushed, sweaty
Blood pressure	108/60 mm Hg; lying down
Oxygen saturation (Spo_2)	98%
Pupils	PERRLA
Blood glucose level	96 mg/dL

7. What should you consider with regard to moving the patient to the ambulance based on the father's comment?

8. What other questions may you have for the patient?

Consider administering an IV bolus if the patient exhibits signs of shock, but use caution when giving fluids to prevent pulmonary edema. Patients in whom rhabdomyolysis is suspected may benefit from IV fluid boluses. If the ECG reveals signs of hyperkalemia, discuss these findings with medical control, who may instruct you to administer IV calcium and bicarbonate.

The increased levels of metabolites in patients with AKI may prove toxic to the kidneys. Many medications can be nephrotoxic (toxic to the kidneys), including many analgesics and antibiotics. Consult medical control if you suspect AKI and are transporting a patient with antibiotic or analgesic drips. Many patients with AKI have other comorbid diseases that also may need to be addressed in the treatment plan.

Chronic Kidney Disease

As mentioned earlier, in the United States, more than 468,000 people are on long-term dialysis.[1] In the US population, the number of patients with chronic kidney disease is increasing rapidly: According to Centers for Disease Control and Prevention (CDC) estimates, the prevalence of this disease in adults ages 30 years or older reached approximately 14% in 2020.[16] In the United States, more than 37 million people have some form of chronic kidney disease.[16]

Pathophysiology

Chronic kidney disease (CKD) is progressive and irreversible inadequate kidney function that is the result of permanent loss of nephrons. This disease develops over the course of months or years. More than one-half of all cases are a consequence of systemic disease, such as diabetes or hypertension. CKD can also be caused by congenital disorders or prolonged pyelonephritis.

As the damaged nephrons cease to function, scarring occurs in the kidneys. The tissue begins to shrink and waste away as the scarring progresses, leading to a loss of nephrons and renal mass. As kidney function diminishes, waste products and fluid build up in the blood. Uremia (an increased concentration of urea and other waste products in the blood) and **azotemia** (an increased level of nitrogenous wastes in the blood) develop, leading to systemic complications such as hypertension, heart failure, anemia, and electrolyte imbalances.

Assessment

Patients with CKD may have an altered mental status caused by electrolyte imbalances and their effects on nerve impulse transmission in the brain. Such patients may also present with lethargy, nausea, headaches, cramps, signs of anemia, weakness, vomiting, anorexia, increased thirst, pruritus, and hypertension. As part of the assessment, ask if the patient still produces urine, and ask the patient to describe the appearance of any urine. If CKD is present, urine volume may have decreased or the urine may appear rusty brown.

In a patient with CKD, the skin is pale, cool, and moist, and the patient may appear jaundiced because of the buildup of nitrogenous wastes. A powdery accumulation of uric acid called **uremic frost** may also be present, especially on the face. The skin may have bruises from coagulopathy, and muscle twitching may be observed.

Patients with CKD exhibit edema in the extremities and face because of fluid imbalances; they can also be hypotensive and tachycardic if they have dehydration or infection. If hyperkalemia develops, an ECG will show alterations in the waveforms and intervals. Pericarditis and pulmonary edema are also common in patients with CKD and should be evaluated during auscultation of the chest.

Documentation and Communication

In patients with CKD, you should frequently assess mental status, noting any apparent decline or improvement. Document your findings and include them in your report to the receiving facility.

Management

Because CKD is a chronic condition, managing a patient with CKD is generally not acutely performed in the field. However, some special considerations apply when treating a patient with CKD for other complaints. Specifically, patients with CKD may be at higher risk for pulmonary edema because they may not have the full ability to regulate their fluid balance; this possibility should be considered if a fluid bolus is planned. In addition, patients with CKD have an increased risk of cardiac disease, so any chest pain complaint should be taken seriously.

Transport should be undertaken calmly. Talk quietly and confidently with the patient to allay any fears. If the patient has an altered mental status, assess the patient's orientation frequently and record any changes.

Street Smarts

Do not give medications to patients with chronic kidney disease unless specifically instructed to do so by medical control.

End-Stage Renal Disease

Pathophysiology

If left untreated, acute or chronic kidney disease will progress to **end-stage renal disease (ESRD)**. In a patient with ESRD, the kidneys are unable to function and toxic waste materials build up in the patient's blood. ESRD is fatal unless treated by dialysis or renal transplantation. At the end of 2017, more than 746,000 people in the United States were undergoing treatment for ESRD.[17]

Words of Wisdom

Patients with ESRD who are on hemodialysis will sometimes require ambulance transportation between their home and the dialysis facility. These transports may become routine for prehospital providers; however, you must always complete a full assessment and be alert for changes in the patient's mental status or vital signs that could suggest an acute condition.

Assessment

The patient with ESRD is chronically ill, and assessment findings can change based on the amount of

YOU are the Paramedic

PART 5

Because family members serve as invaluable sources of information, you thank the patient's father. You explain that it is necessary to move his daughter to treat her properly, but that you will handle her gently and monitor her closely for changes in her condition. As you help the patient slowly sit up, she reports some dizziness, but seems to tolerate the position. You buckle her into the stair chair and explain how she will be moved down the stairs. You reach the front door, transfer her to the gurney, and cover her with blankets. You reassess the patient in the ambulance, and she tells you she feels better lying down. You note that her orthostatic vital signs are positive for change. After contacting medical control, you are advised to administer a 500-mL bolus of normal saline, give 4 mg of ondansetron (Zofran), and begin transport.

Recording Time: 15 Minutes	
Respirations	24 breaths/min
Pulse	120 beats/min
Skin	Flushed, sweaty
Blood pressure	100/50 mm Hg; lying down
Oxygen saturation (Spo_2)	98%
Pupils	PERRLA
IV fluids	500 mL normal saline

9. What may you consider requesting from medical control in addition to antiemetics?

10. How will her condition affect transport?

time from the last dialysis. After dialysis, patients can appear well, but occasionally they will be weak or dehydrated. If patients have missed dialysis appointments, they will frequently present with signs of volume overload: shortness of breath and peripheral edema. If toxins have accumulated, the patients may exhibit uremic frost, confusion, and muscle twitching. Most patients with ESRD will have some form of coagulopathy, and bruising may be apparent. Weakness and fatigue can be chronic and pronounced, and most patients with ESRD will be anemic.

Evaluate the ECG for signs of hyperkalemia, particularly if the patient missed the last scheduled dialysis session. As with patients with CKD, any chest pain should be taken seriously, and a full cardiac assessment should be performed. Patients with ESRD are susceptible to infections, pericarditis, and pericardial effusions; consider these in your differential diagnosis based on the complaint. If a patient with ESRD has been untreated for some time, significant confusion, seizures, and even coma can occur.

Management

Definitive treatment for patients with ESRD is limited to renal dialysis or kidney transplantation. When treating a patient with ESRD, ensure stability of the ABCs and provide supportive care as needed. In case of volume overload, consider administering a diuretic if the patient is still producing urine. If a patient appears dehydrated or in shock, medical control may instruct you to administer a fluid bolus while closely monitoring for signs of pulmonary edema. If the patient has chest pain or signs of cardiac ischemia, administer nitroglycerin and aspirin per your local protocol. If the patient has missed dialysis, be alert for hyperkalemia and treat it with calcium and bicarbonate as directed by your local protocol. Anytime a patient with ESRD is found in cardiac arrest, strongly consider hyperkalemia as the underlying cause.

Renal Dialysis

Although not truly a urologic disorder, **renal dialysis** and associated problems may require prehospital interventions. Renal dialysis is a technique for filtering toxic wastes from the blood, removing excess fluid, and restoring the normal balance of electrolytes **FIGURE 22-7**.

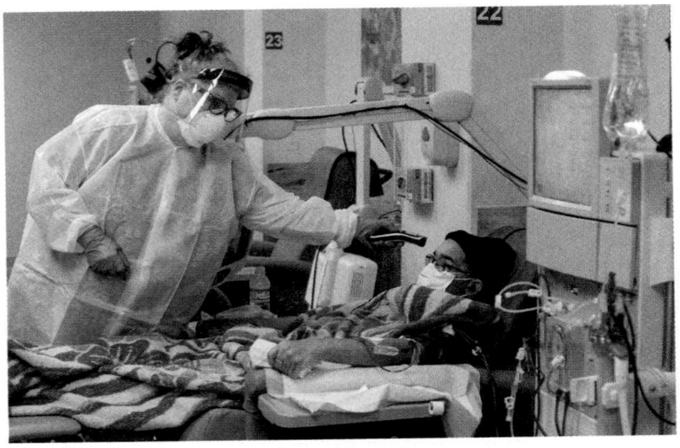

FIGURE 22-7 A patient undergoing dialysis.

Two types of dialysis are performed: peritoneal dialysis and hemodialysis. In peritoneal dialysis, large amounts of specially formulated dialysis fluid are infused into (and then drained from) the abdominal cavity. This fluid remains in the cavity for 1 to 2 hours, allowing equilibrium to occur as wastes diffuse across the peritoneal membrane and into the fluid. Peritoneal dialysis is very effective but is associated with a high risk of peritonitis; consequently, aseptic technique is essential. With proper training, however, peritoneal dialysis can be performed in the home.

In hemodialysis, the patient's blood circulates through a dialysis machine that functions in much the same way (albeit not as elegantly) as a normal kidney. Hemodialysis requires vascular access through either a fistula or an arteriovenous (AV) shunt, or in emergencies, a central venous catheter. A **fistula**, **shunt**, or **arteriovenous graft** is a surgically created arterial-to-venous vessel anastomosis tunneled through the subcutaneous tissue. It is usually located in the forearm or upper arm **FIGURE 22-8**. The patient is connected to the dialysis machine using this shunt, which allows blood to flow from the body into the dialysis machine and back into the body.

In patients with cardiac or respiratory arrest, when intraosseous access is difficult or impossible, the fistula or shunt may be used for IV access; this procedure should be performed only in accordance with local protocols. In all other instances, an IV site in the opposite arm should be selected. AV shunts should not be used for routine blood draws, and BP readings should be taken using the opposite arm.

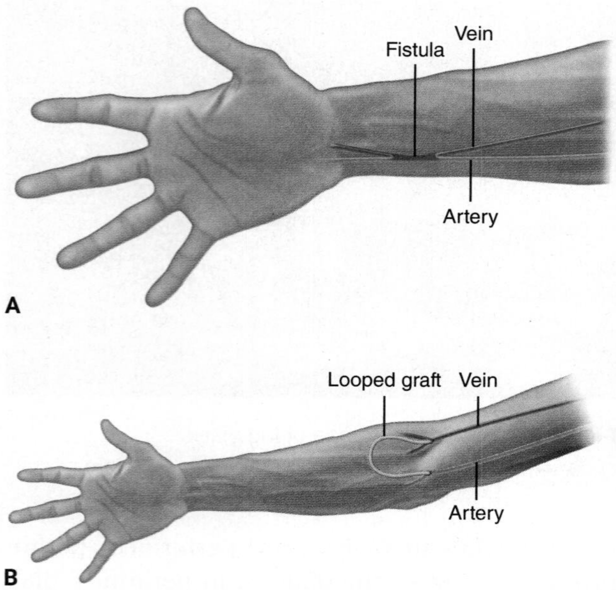

FIGURE 22-8 A. With an arteriovenous fistula, a bulge is created beneath the skin by arterial pressure at the site where the artery and vein have been directly connected. **B.** An arteriovenous graft creates a raised area beneath the skin that looks like a large vessel.

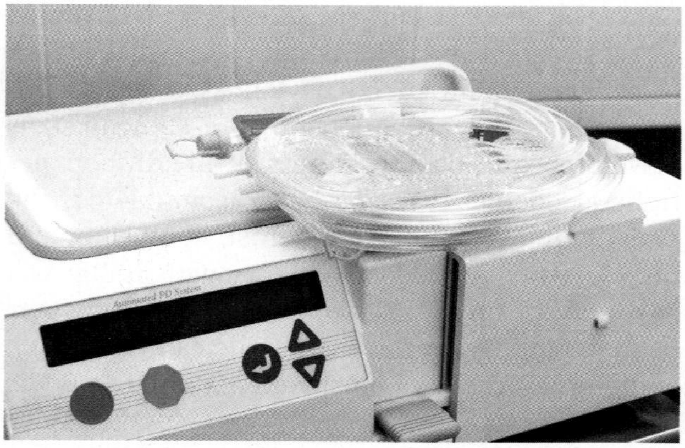

FIGURE 22-9 A home dialysis unit offers patients greater flexibility in their treatments.

The only time you are likely to see a dialysis machine is if your service transports patients to and from dialysis centers. If the patient has a dialysis machine in their private residence, treatments will most likely be performed by a trained dialysis technician or possibly by the patient or family members.

Patients requiring chronic dialysis in the hospital or in community dialysis facilities usually undergo this process every 2 or 3 days for 3 to 5 hours. In recent years, a significant number of patients have begun using home dialysis units (**FIGURE 22-9**). Patients undergoing dialysis at home usually have extensive training in these procedures, and often someone else in the home has also been trained. Home hemodialysis requires a patient to undergo sessions 5 to 6 times per week for 3 to 6 hours each time. Sessions can be performed either during the day or at night, allowing the patient greater autonomy in terms of lifestyle.[18] Most complications arising from home hemodialysis are associated with human error during cannulation of the shunt, connection to the machine, or disconnection from the machine.[19] If a problem with the machine occurs, the patient or family member may know more about it than you do, so always ask what the patient has done prior to your arrival.

Some patients can perform peritoneal dialysis at home. In such cases, patients have the option of continuous ambulatory peritoneal dialysis (CAPD) or automated peritoneal dialysis (APD). CAPD is performed by the patient, who instills dialysis solution into the abdomen and then removes it 4 to 6 hours later.[20] Fluid exchanges occur at least four times per day. The dialysis solution remains in the patient's abdomen during the night. An alternative method is automated peritoneal dialysis, which uses a machine to instill and remove the dialysis solution.[19] Patients who undergo peritoneal dialysis may experience peritonitis, weight gain, abdominal hernia, and inadequate dialysis. Both modalities of peritoneal dialysis can be performed in a clean, private place, allowing a patient to work and travel.[21]

Whereas patients undergoing chronic dialysis can experience the same spectrum of illnesses and injuries as other patients, they are particularly vulnerable to certain problems, either because of the dialysis itself or because of the underlying renal failure. Problems associated with dialysis may result from accidental disconnection from the machine, bleeding from a fistula or shunt, malfunction of the machine, or rapid shifts in fluids and electrolytes that produce hypotension, potassium imbalances, and disequilibrium syndrome. The management of medical emergencies resulting from dialysis is summarized in **TABLE 22-3**.

People who miss dialysis treatments will often present with signs of electrolyte imbalance,

TABLE 22-3 Medical Emergencies in Dialysis Patients

Problem	Prehospital Management
Problems related to dialysis itself:	
Hypotension	Administer 50 mL of normal saline intravenously.
Hemorrhage from the fistula or shunt	If the shunt cannot be reconnected, clamp it off; apply direct pressure to control bleeding; check for signs of shock.
Potassium imbalance	For hypokalemia: treat bradycardia with atropine. For hyperkalemia: calcium and bicarbonate may be considered if a lab value was obtained at the sending facility.
Disequilibrium syndrome	Provide only supportive treatment.
Air embolism	Position the patient in the left lateral recumbent position with about 10° of head-down tilt.
Machine dysfunction	Turn off the machine; clamp the ends of the shunt; disconnect the patient from the machine; transport.
Problems to which dialysis patients are more vulnerable:	
Heart failure	Administer oxygen; place in a sitting position; administer a diuretic if the patient is producing urine; provide rapid transport to a dialysis-capable facility.
Myocardial infarction and cardiac dysrhythmias	Treat as any other patient, but use caution when administering any medications.
Hypertension	Transport; provide supportive care.
Pericardial tamponade	Provide emergency transport as soon as detected.
Uremic pericarditis	Administer oxygen; allow the patient to assume a position of comfort; transport.

including muscle weakness, cramping, pulmonary edema, and uremic frost. Other general dialysis complications include muscle cramps, nausea and vomiting, and infections at the fistula or shunt site.

Hypotension and Shock

A sudden decrease in BP is not uncommon during or immediately after a patient undergoes dialysis, but it can lead to cardiac arrest if not promptly detected and treated.

The patient may feel light-headed or become confused, and often yawns more than usual. Because dialysis alters the blood's chemistry, the patient may experience an electrolyte imbalance. For this reason, you should always monitor dialysis patients for cardiac dysrhythmias. Shock secondary to bleeding is also possible from many causes, such as hypovolemia resulting from fluid shifts or bleeding due to less functional platelets. Bleeding may also occur at the site of the dialysis cannula and should be controlled with direct pressure.

Words of Wisdom

When you measure the BP in a dialysis patient, use the arm that does not have the shunt.

Potassium Imbalance

One consequence of renal impairment is the inability to excrete ingested potassium. Consequently, CKD patients are susceptible to the development of hyperkalemia. ECG changes to intervals and waveforms may be seen when such an imbalance occurs.

Hypokalemia may also occur as a consequence of overaggressive dialysis. The potassium level is most likely to fall during or immediately after a dialysis cycle. The patient may be hypotensive, and cardiac dysrhythmias may be present. Treat the dysrhythmia if it is hemodynamically significant or persistently symptomatic. For more detail, see Chapter 18, *Cardiovascular Emergencies.*

Disequilibrium Syndrome

Dialysis rapidly lowers the concentration of urea in the blood, whereas the concentration of solutes in the cerebrospinal fluid (CSF) remains high. Water, of course, moves by osmosis from a solution of lower concentration into a solution of higher concentration. Thus, dialysis can cause water to initially shift from the bloodstream into the CSF, thereby mildly increasing intracranial pressure. When this occurs, the patient may experience **disequilibrium syndrome**, a condition characterized by nausea, vomiting, headache, and confusion. Disequilibrium syndrome tends to occur in those starting dialysis or those who missed a few dialysis sessions and are restarting.[22] After a few hours, the fluid may re-equilibrate between the blood and CSF, and the patient's symptoms will improve. If it does not resolve by itself, a physician will need to provide treatment.

> **Words of Wisdom**
>
> In the field, it may be impossible to distinguish between disequilibrium syndrome and stroke or subdural hematoma—other conditions to which dialysis patients are particularly vulnerable. In such a case, transport the patient to the hospital immediately for a full neurologic evaluation.

Air Embolism

If any of the fittings and connections in the dialysis system are loose, air may enter the system, producing an **air embolism** in the patient. Symptoms of an air embolism include sudden dyspnea, hypotension, and cyanosis. If you suspect an air embolism, disconnect the patient from the dialysis machine, place the patient in the left lateral recumbent position with about 10° of head-down tilt, and transport immediately.

Male Genital Tract Conditions

Epididymitis and Orchitis

One possible complication of male UTI is **epididymitis**, an infection that causes inflammation of the epididymis along the posterior border of the testis. When one or both testes become infected, the condition is called **orchitis**. With orchitis, the infection causes one or both testes to become enlarged and tender, causing pain and swelling in the scrotum. Swelling may occur in the groin on the affected side. The pain may increase during bowel movements. The patient frequently will have a fever, and the urine will have a foul odor.

Prehospital management of these conditions is supportive. Because the patient likely is in pain, consider administering analgesics.

> **Words of Wisdom**
>
> A patient who has sustained blunt renal trauma often presents with flank pain and hematuria (blood in the urine) that usually goes undetected until evaluation in the ED. Obvious hematomas or ecchymoses over the upper abdomen, middle back, or lower rib cage may also suggest renal injuries. Keep this in mind when assessing a patient with a urologic emergency. For more detail, see Chapter 37, *Abdominal and Genitourinary Trauma*.

Fournier Gangrene

If bacteria enter the scrotum or perineum, **Fournier gangrene** may occur. This infection causes necrosis of the subcutaneous tissue and muscle in the scrotum. The patient will be febrile, and the scrotum and perineum will be tender, warm, and erythematous. Purulent drainage may be present, and if not addressed, skin in the area may become gray-black. This is a life-threatening emergency requiring prompt transport to the hospital. These patients can rapidly become septic and unstable, and will require aggressive treatment with IV fluids.

Priapism

Priapism, a painful, tender, persistent erection, can result from sickle cell disease, leukemia, spinal cord injury, and certain medications, such as antidepressants, anticonvulsants, and those used to treat erectile dysfunction. Be sure to maintain the patient's privacy and do not make assumptions about the cause of the condition. Whatever the cause, treat all patients with respect, and administer analgesics for pain. If a spinal cord injury is suspected, use proper immobilization techniques. Priapism is discussed in more detail in Chapter 37, *Abdominal and Genitourinary Trauma.*

Phimosis and Paraphimosis

Phimosis is the inability to retract the distal foreskin over the glans penis **FIGURE 22-10A**. This condition can be congenital or acquired, generally from poor hygiene or recurrent infections and scarring of the foreskin. Prehospital treatment includes cold compresses and transport.

Paraphimosis results when the foreskin is retracted over the glans penis and becomes entrapped **FIGURE 22-10B**. The tightness of the foreskin causes the glans to swell even further, making it even harder to slide the foreskin back into the normal position. Paraphimosis can occur after manual retraction of the foreskin, such as when a Foley catheter is placed. It can also occur after phimosis retraction or after piercings of the glans penis. Paraphimosis is a true emergency, and failure to relieve this condition can result in necrosis of the glans.

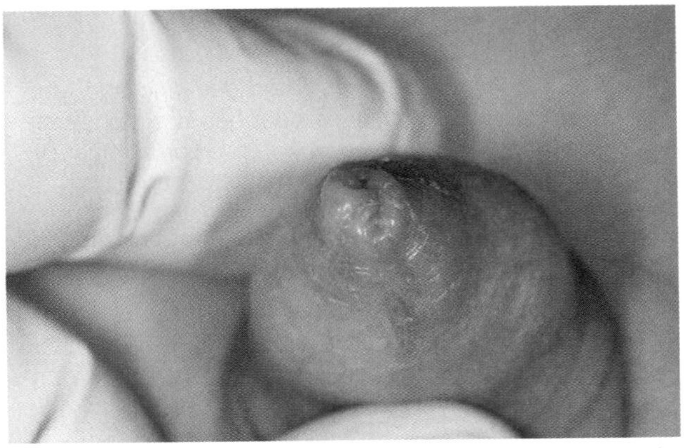

A

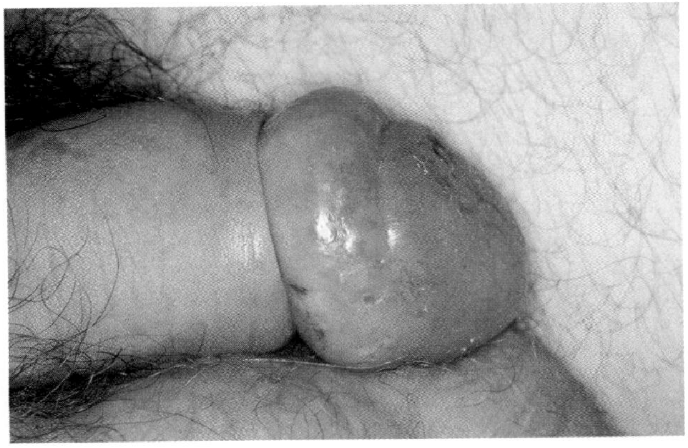

B

FIGURE 22-10 A. Phimosis. **B.** Paraphimosis.

Benign Prostate Hypertrophy

Benign prostate hypertrophy (BPH) is an age-related nonmalignant (noncancerous) enlargement of the prostate gland. It occurs in approximately 50% of men older than 50 years, and the prevalence continues to increase with age beyond that point.[23] It may be asymptomatic, or it may result in difficulty starting urine flow; a slow, weak urine flow once started; incomplete emptying of the bladder; increased urination at night; and urinary retention. If the prostate becomes infected, the patient is said to have **prostatitis**. This condition can present with symptoms similar to those of a UTI as well as with fever, tremors, or urinary obstruction.

Testicular Masses

Testicular masses, which may be either painful or painless, rarely require prehospital treatment. If they are painful, the pain may radiate up the spermatic cord or be localized to a specific scrotal point. Most are benign cystic masses or a varicocele: a painless mass of dilated veins posterior to the testicle. Testicular cancer usually presents as a painless solid lump on the testicle.

Testicular Torsion

Testicular torsion is a twisting of the testicle on the spermatic cord, from which it is suspended. This condition is associated with the sudden onset of scrotal pain and swelling. It is a medical emergency if the twisting of the vessels reduces blood flow to the testis. The torsion is usually unilateral, occurring in only one testis at a time. Torsions may occur with or without blunt trauma, a testicular lump, infection, or blood in the semen. Patients should be carefully and promptly transported and allowed to assume the position of greatest comfort. Analgesics may be given for pain control.

YOU are the Paramedic SUMMARY

1. What concerns may you have about the scene?

Performing a scene assessment is essential to ensure the safety of you and your crew. Knowing this is an older home with a narrow stairwell and the patient is on the second floor should prompt you to consider requesting additional personnel if needed for safe moving and lifting.

2. Although you have not seen your patient yet, what information do you already know that is part of the primary survey?

Because you heard your patient call out for her father, telling him she was about to "be sick again," you know that she is alert, has a patent airway, and is breathing. This information may change rapidly, but you have gathered a lot of information before you even see her.

3. What concerns do you have about her history, signs, and symptoms?

More information is needed to narrow your differential diagnosis. Causes for concern include the patient's skin signs, which point to fever/infection, as well as her dizziness while standing. She is likely to have positive orthostatic vital signs and be significantly dehydrated because of the vomiting.

4. What should be done with the emesis?

Do not forget to look at the emesis for any signs of blood. Follow your local protocols regarding the transport of specimens to the hospital.

5. What additional assessment techniques might you use?

One technique used to assess for kidney infection or pyelonephritis is to place your fist over the flank and gently tap with the other hand. If the kidney is infected, this will elicit a painful response; therefore, you should use this technique with caution.

6. Why is assessing the patient's body temperature important?

Assessing body temperature is essential and should not be forgotten in the prehospital setting. This patient's temperature and other assessment findings can assist you in treating and documenting infection.

7. What should you consider with regard to moving the patient to the ambulance based on the father's comment?

You should be prepared for the patient to exhibit neurologic symptoms, including syncope. In turn, you may have to adjust your method of moving the patient to the ambulance. Prehospital providers have a wide range of moving and lifting options to accommodate patient needs and to deal with access/egress challenges. In this scenario, moving the patient via a Reeves sleeve may be another option if she becomes too symptomatic while sitting up in a stair chair.

8. What other questions may you have for the patient?

Because she is a woman of childbearing age, you should ask her questions about her last menstrual cycle. Also ask about urination: color, frequency, odor, the presence of blood, or other symptoms.

9. What may you consider requesting from medical control in addition to antiemetics?

Pain management in a patient with a kidney emergency is an integral part of patient care. Many protocols will specifically address pain associated with kidney stones. Follow your local protocols.

10. How will her condition affect transport?

This patient is not demonstrating signs and symptoms of a life-threatening renal emergency. Therefore, she should be transported in a position of comfort with minimal jostling and slow, careful driving to avoid excessive bumps, sudden acceleration, deceleration, or turns.

YOU are the Paramedic SUMMARY continued

EMS Patient Care Report (PCR)

Date: 04-11-22	**Incident No.:** 20227	**Nature of Call:** Medical		**Location:** 327 West Main Street	
Dispatched: 0600	**En Route:** 0603	**At Scene:** 0608	**Transport:** 0632	**At Hospital:** 0645	**In Service:** 0655

Patient Information

Age: 23 **Sex:** F **Weight (in kg [lb]):** 70 kg (154 lb)	**Allergies:** NKDA **Medications:** Cipro, OTC cranberry supplement **Past Medical History:** UTIs **Chief Complaint:** Lower back pain

Vital Signs

Time: 0613	**BP:** 108/60	**Pulse:** 110	**Respirations:** 24	**Spo_2:** 98%
Time: 0618	**BP:** 108/60	**Pulse:** 112	**Respirations:** 24	**Spo_2:** 98%
Time: 0623	**BP:** 100/50	**Pulse:** 120	**Respirations:** 24	**Spo_2:** 98%

EMS Treatment (highlight all that apply)

Oxygen @ _____ L/min via (circle one): **NC NRM Bag-mask device**		**Assisted Ventilation**	**Airway Adjunct**	**CPR**
Defibrillation	**Bleeding Control**	**Bandaging**	**Splinting**	**Other:**

Narrative

Dispatched to female reporting lower back pain at 327 West Main Street. Pt 23 yo female lying on her right side in bed, vomiting into trash can. Alert, skin diaphoretic, very warm, flushed. Pt reporting lower back pain, stated she's been "feeling ill" for the past 2–3 days including burning with urination and n/v since last night around midnight. Urinating makes the pain worse. Pt describes lower back pain as "achy," radiating from flank to pubic bone. Pt rates severity as 4 on scale of 0 to 10, with 10 being the worst. Pt last ate yesterday 2100 hours.

Vital signs lying down as noted above. Temp 38.3°C, blood glucose level 96 mg/dL, PERRLA, HEENT atraumatic, breath sounds clear and equal bilaterally. Abd has overactive bowel sounds, soft, diffuse tenderness in all 4 quadrants with increased tenderness of both lower, right flank pain, p/m/s/ × 4. Suspect possible pyelonephritis.

Established IV 18 g NS 500 mL bolus. ECG ST w/o further ectopy. Moved pt with stair chair. Transported to WWMC. Continued to monitor en route w/o changes. Arrived at ED transfer of care to J. Smith, RN.

End of report

Prep Kit

Ready for Review

- Chronic kidney disease is the most common renal disorder. Kidney stones and UTIs also affect many people.
- The genitourinary system includes the kidneys, urinary bladder, ureters, urethra, male and female reproductive organs, and specific structures within the kidneys.
- Urine forms in the nephrons. The nephrons are composed of the glomerulus, the glomerular capsule, the proximal convoluted tubule, the loop of Henle, and the distal convoluted tubule.
- The anatomy of the urethra is different in males and females. The male urethra serves as a conduit for urine as well as semen and other secretions.
- Visceral pain is the type most often associated with genitourinary conditions. Referred pain originates in one organ or tissue but is perceived by the patient to be located in a different area of the body.
- The OPQRST (Onset, Provocation, Quality, Region/radiation/referral, Severity, Timing) mnemonic is used during assessments to elaborate on the chief complaint and to evaluate and reevaluate the type and severity of pain.
- In the physical exam, use the four-quadrant system and abdominal region mapping. Perform cardiac monitoring, and do not give patients with a possible genitourinary disease anything by mouth.
- Pain in patients with genitourinary conditions is managed with patient positioning, analgesics and fluids as indicated, and supportive care.
- Symptoms of UTI include painful urination, frequent urges to urinate, difficulty urinating, and possibly referred pain in the shoulder or neck. The urine may have a foul odor and be cloudy. Management of patients with UTIs consists mainly of supportive care of the ABCs, allowing the patient to remain in a position of comfort, and possibly administering analgesics.
- Catheterization of the bladder allows for a continuous outflow of urine and provides a means of measuring urine output in hemodynamically unstable patients. The drainage bag should not be lifted above the level of the patient's bladder to avoid the backflow of urine.
- Kidney stones form when an excess of insoluble salts or uric acid crystallizes in the urine. Symptoms include severe flank pain that may migrate to the groin. The pain may produce a spike in the patient's BP and pulse rate.
- Acute kidney injury is a sudden decrease in filtration through the glomeruli, resulting in a buildup of toxins in the blood. The three types of acute kidney injury are prerenal, intrarenal, and postrenal. Signs and symptoms range from hypotension, tachycardia, dizziness, and thirst, to pain, oliguria, distended bladder, hematuria, and peripheral edema.
- Chronic kidney disease is progressive and results in irreversible inadequate kidney function. Nephrons become damaged, losing their functionality and causing a buildup of wastes and fluid in the blood. Signs and symptoms can include an altered level of consciousness, lethargy, nausea, headaches, cramps, anemia, bruised skin, edema in the extremities and face, hypotension, and tachycardia.
- Patients with acute or chronic kidney disease require support of airway, breathing, and circulation; possibly administration of medications to regulate acidosis, electrolyte imbalances, and fluid volume; and calm transport with emotional support.
- If left untreated, acute or chronic kidney disease will progress to end-stage renal disease, meaning that the kidneys are unable to function. Toxic waste materials build

Prep Kit continued

up in the patient's blood, leading to many potential signs and symptoms and possibly dysrhythmias. Prehospital care is supportive, including treating for shock and, under medical direction, regulating fluid imbalances, electrolyte abnormalities, and cardiovascular function.

- Renal dialysis is a procedure for removing toxic wastes and excess fluid from the blood. Patients who are treated with dialysis usually have a fistula or shunt through which they are connected to the dialysis machine. Such patients are vulnerable to hypotension, potassium imbalances, disequilibrium syndrome, and air embolism.
- Many patients receive dialysis in the hospital or in community dialysis facilities, but a significant number have home dialysis units for performing either hemodialysis or peritoneal dialysis. Most complications arising from home hemodialysis are associated with human error during cannulation of the shunt, connection to the machine, and disconnection from the machine.
- Always monitor dialysis patients for cardiac dysrhythmias. Shock secondary to bleeding is also possible from any number of causes. Watch for peaked T waves on the ECG, a classic sign of hyperkalemia.
- Specific conditions that may occur in the male genital tract include epididymitis, Fournier gangrene, priapism, phimosis, paraphimosis, benign prostate hypertrophy, testicular masses, and testicular torsion. Prehospital management for most of these conditions is supportive. Because such a patient is likely to be in pain, consider administering analgesics and transport gently.

Vital Vocabulary

acute kidney injury (AKI) A sudden decrease in filtration through the glomeruli.

air embolism The presence of air in the venous circulation, which forms a gas bubble that can block the outflow of blood from the right ventricle to the lung; can lead to cardiac arrest, shock, or other life-threatening complications.

anuria A complete cessation of urine production.

arteriovenous graft A surgical connection between an artery and a vein.

azotemia Increased nitrogenous wastes in the blood.

benign prostate hypertrophy (BPH) Age-related nonmalignant (noncancerous) enlargement of the prostate gland.

chronic kidney disease (CKD) Progressive and irreversible inadequate kidney function caused by the permanent loss of nephrons.

disequilibrium syndrome A condition characterized by nausea, vomiting, headache, and confusion, which results when dialysis causes water to initially shift from the bloodstream into the cerebrospinal fluid, mildly increasing intracranial pressure.

distal convoluted tubule (DCT) Connects with the kidney's collecting tubules.

end-stage renal disease (ESRD) A condition in which the kidneys are unable to function, and toxic waste materials build up in the patient's blood; occurs after acute or chronic kidney injury.

epididymitis An infection that causes inflammation of the epididymis along the posterior border of the testis; a possible complication of male urinary tract infection.

fistula A surgically created connection between an artery and a vein, usually in the arm, for dialysis access.

Fournier gangrene A condition that results from bacteria entering the skin of the scrotum or perineum, causing infection and subsequent necrosis of the subcutaneous tissue and muscle in the scrotum.

Prep Kit continued

glomerular (Bowman) capsule A double-layered cup with the inner layer infiltrating and surrounding the capillaries of the glomerulus.

hematuria The presence of blood in the urine.

interstitial nephritis A chronic inflammation of the interstitial cells surrounding the nephrons.

intrarenal acute kidney injury (IAKI) A type of acute kidney injury characterized by damage in the kidney itself, often caused by immune-mediated diseases, prerenal acute kidney injury, toxins, heavy metals, some medications, or some organic compounds.

kidneys Solid, bean-shaped organs housed in the retroperitoneal space that filter blood and excrete body wastes in the form of urine.

kidney stones Solid crystalline masses formed in the kidney, resulting from an excess of insoluble salts or uric acid crystallizing in the urine; may become trapped anywhere along the urinary tract. Also called renal calculi.

loop of Henle The U-shaped portion of the renal tubule that extends from the proximal to the distal convoluted tubule; concentrates the filtrate and converts it to urine.

nephrons The kidney's structural and functional units that form urine; composed of the glomerulus, the glomerular (Bowman) capsule, the proximal convoluted tubule, the loop of Henle, and the distal convoluted tubule.

oliguria Urine output of less than 500 mL/d.

orchitis A complication of a male urinary tract infection in which one or both testes become infected, enlarged, and tender, causing pain and swelling in the scrotum.

paraphimosis A condition in which the foreskin is retracted over the glans penis and becomes entrapped; constriction of the glans causes it to swell even further.

phimosis Inability to retract the distal foreskin over the glans penis.

postrenal acute kidney injury A type of acute kidney injury caused by obstruction of urine flow from the kidneys, commonly caused by a blockage of the urethra by an enlarged prostate gland, blood clots, or strictures.

prerenal acute kidney injury A type of acute kidney injury caused by hypoperfusion of the kidneys, resulting from hypovolemia (hemorrhage, dehydration), trauma, shock, sepsis, or heart failure (secondary to myocardial infarction); often reversible if the underlying condition can be found and perfusion restored to the kidney.

priapism A painful, tender, persistent erection of the penis; can result from spinal cord injury, erectile dysfunction drugs, or sickle cell disease.

prostatitis Inflammation of the prostate gland.

proximal convoluted tubule (PCT) One of two complex sections of the nephron; the proximal convoluted tubule includes an enlargement at the end called the glomerular capsule.

pyelonephritis An upper urinary tract infection in which the kidneys are involved.

renal dialysis A technique for filtering the blood of its toxic wastes, removing excess fluids, and restoring the normal balance of electrolytes.

shunt A connection between the arterial and venous system in which no gas exchange occurs.

testicular torsion Twisting of the testicle on the spermatic cord, from which it is suspended; associated with scrotal pain and swelling, and is a medical emergency.

uremia The presence of excessive amounts of urea and other waste products in the blood.

uremic frost A powdery buildup of uric acid, especially on the skin of the face.

ureters A pair of thick-walled, hollow tubes that transport urine from the kidneys to the bladder.

urethra A hollow tubular structure that drains urine from the bladder, expelling it from the body.

Prep Kit continued

urinary bladder A hollow muscular sac in the midline of the lower abdominal area that stores urine until it is released from the body.

urinary incontinence The inability to control the release of urine from the bladder; loss of bladder control.

urinary retention Incomplete emptying of the bladder, or a complete lack of ability to empty the bladder.

urinary tract infections (UTIs) Infections, usually of the lower urinary tract (urethra and bladder), that occur when normal flora (bacteria that naturally populate the skin) enter the urethra and multiply.

urine Liquid waste products filtered out of the body by the urinary system.

References

1. National Institute of Diabetes and Digestive and Kidney Diseases. Kidney disease statistics for the United States. https://www.niddk.nih.gov/health-information/health-statistics/kidney-disease. Published December 2016. Accessed February 8, 2021.
2. National Institute of Diabetes and Digestive and Kidney Diseases. Definition and facts for kidney stones. https://www.niddk.nih.gov/health-information/urologic-diseases/kidney-stones/definition-facts#common. Published May 2017. Accessed February 8, 2021.
3. Medina M, Castillo-Pino E. An introduction to the epidemiology and burden of urinary tract infections. *Ther Adv Urol.* 2019;11:1756287219832172. doi:10.1177/1756287219832172.
4. McVary KT. Surgical treatment of benign prostatic hyperplasia (BPH). *UpToDate.* https://www.uptodate.com/contents/surgical-treatment-of-benign-prostatic-hyperplasia-bph#:~:text=Most%20procedures%20used%20in%20the,of%20the%20prostate%20%5BThuLEP%5D). Published July 9, 2020. Accessed February 8, 2021.
5. Leuthauser A, McVane B. Abdominal pain in the geriatric patient. *Emerg Med Clin North Am.* 2016;34:363-375. http://dx.doi.org/10.1016/j.emc.2015.12.009.
6. Long B. Stroke mimics: pearls and pitfalls. http://www.emdocs.net/stroke-mimics-pearls-and-pitfalls/. Published March 23, 2016. Accessed February 8, 2021.
7. Manterola C, Vial M, Moraga J, Astudillo P. Analgesia in patients with acute abdominal pain. *Cochrane Database Syst Rev.* 2011;1:CD005660.
8. Rui P, Kang K. National Hospital Ambulatory Medical Care Survey: 2017 emergency department summary tables. US Department of Health and Human Services, Centers for Disease Control and Prevention, National Center for Health Statistics. https://www.cdc.gov/nchs/data/nhamcs/web_tables/2017_ed_web_tables-508.pdf. Accessed February 8, 2021.
9. Michigan Medicine, University of Michigan. Overflow incontinence. https://www.uofmhealth.org/health-library/uh1227. Updated August 21, 2019. Accessed February 8, 2021.
10. Chewcharat A, Curhan G. Trends in the prevalence of kidney stones in the United States from 2007 to 2016. *Urolithiasis.* 2021;49:27-39. https://doi.org/10.1007/s00240-020-01210-w.
11. Kirkali Z, Rasooly R, Star RA, Rodgers GP. Urinary stone disease: progress, status, and needs. *Urology.* 2015;86(4):651-653.
12. Lin S-Y, Lin C-L, Chan Y-J, et al. Association between kidney stones and risk of stroke: a nationwide populations-based cohort study. *Medicine (Baltimore).* 2016;95(8):e2847. doi:10.1097/MD.0000000000002847.
13. Workeneh BT. Acute kidney injury. *Medscape.* https://emedicine.medscape.com/article/243492-overview#a5. Updated December 24, 2020. Accessed February 8, 2021.
14. Wiersema R, Eck RJ, Haapio M, et al. Burden of acute kidney injury and 90-day mortality in critically ill patients. *BMC Nephrol.* 2020;21:1. https://bmcnephrol.biomedcentral.com/articles/10.1186/s12882-019-1645-y. Accessed February 8, 2021.
15. Kanagasundaram S, Ashley C, Bohjani S, et al. Clinical practice guideline: acute kidney injury. Renal Association. https://renal.org/sites/renal.org/files/FINAL-AKI-Guideline.pdf. Published August 2019. Accessed February 8, 2021.
16. Centers for Disease Control and Prevention. *Chronic kidney disease in the United States, 2019.* Atlanta, GA: US Department of Health and Human Services, Centers for Disease Control and Prevention; 2019. https://www.cdc.gov/kidneydisease/publications-resources/2019-national-facts.html. Accessed February 8, 2021.
17. Michigan Medicine, University of Michigan. U.S. Renal Data System 2019 annual data report: epidemiology of

Prep Kit continued

kidney disease in the United States. https://www.uofmhealth.org/news/archive/201911/us-renal-data-system-2019-annual-data-report-epidemiology. Published November 5, 2019. Accessed February 8, 2021.

18. University of Florida, Division of Nephrology, Hypertension, and Renal Transplantation. Home dialysis and peritoneal dialysis. https://nephrology.medicine.ufl.edu/patient-care/renal-replacement-therpay/home-dialysis/. Accessed February 8, 2021.
19. Ibrahim I, Chan CT. Managing kidney failure with home hemodialysis. *Clin J Am Soc Nephrol.* 2019;14(8):1268-1273. https://cjasn.asnjournals.org/content/14/8/1268. Accessed February 8, 2021.
20. National Institute of Diabetes and Digestive and Kidney Diseases. Peritoneal dialysis. https://www.niddk.nih.gov/health-information/kidney-disease/kidney-failure/peritoneal-dialysis. Published January 2018. Accessed February 8, 2021.
21. Mayo Clinic. Peritoneal dialysis. https://www.mayoclinic.org/tests-procedures/peritoneal-dialysis/about/pac-20384725. Accessed February 8, 2021.
22. Zepeda-Orozco D, Quigley R. Dialysis disequilibrium syndrome. *Pediatric Nephrol.* 2012;27(12):2205-2211.
23. Vuichoud C, Loughlin KR. Benign prostatic hyperplasia: epidemiology, economics and evaluation. *Urol Clin North Am.* 2009;36(4):403-415.

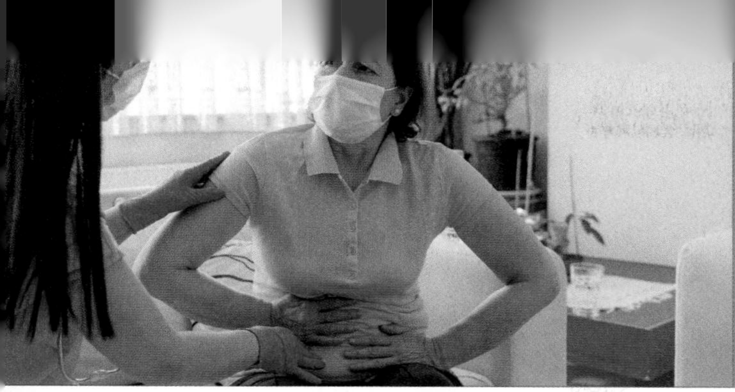

Chapter 23

Gynecologic Emergencies

NATIONAL EMS EDUCATION STANDARD COMPETENCIES

Medicine

Integrates assessment findings with principles of epidemiology and pathophysiology to formulate a field impression and implement a comprehensive treatment/disposition plan for a patient with a medical complaint.

Gynecology

Recognition and management of shock associated with

- Vaginal bleeding (pp 1484–1485)

Anatomy, physiology, assessment findings, and management of

- Vaginal bleeding (pp 1483–1485)
- Sexual assault (to include appropriate emotional support) (pp 1485–1487)
- Infections (pp 1479–1481)

Anatomy, physiology, epidemiology, pathophysiology, psychosocial impact, presentations, prognosis, and management of common or major gynecologic diseases and/or emergencies

- Vaginal bleeding (pp 1477, 1479, 1483–1485)
- Sexual assault (pp 1485–1487)
- Infections (pp 1479–1481)
- Pelvic inflammatory disease (pp 1479–1481)
- Ovarian cysts (pp 1481–1482)
- Dysfunctional uterine bleeding (p 1483)
- Vaginal foreign body (p 1488)

KNOWLEDGE OBJECTIVES

1. Recall the anatomy and physiology of the female reproductive system. (pp 1474–1475)
2. Identify the normal events of the menstrual cycle. (pp 1475–1476)
3. Describe the assessment process for patients with gynecologic emergencies. (pp 1476–1477)
4. Discuss the importance of history taking when assessing a patient with a gynecologic emergency. (pp 1477–1478)
5. Describe how to treat a patient with significant vaginal bleeding. (pp 1477–1482)
6. Discuss the general management of a patient with a gynecologic emergency. (pp 1478–1479)
7. Discuss the management of a patient with gynecologic trauma. (p 1479)
8. Discuss the pathophysiology, assessment, and management of infections related to the gynecologic system. (pp 1479–1481)
9. Discuss the pathophysiology, assessment, and management of ovarian disorders. (pp 1481–1482)
10. Discuss the pathophysiology, assessment, and management of uterine disorders. (pp 1482–1483)
11. Discuss the pathophysiology, assessment, and management of ectopic pregnancy. (pp 1484–1485)
12. Discuss special concerns, assessment, and management, when caring for a suspected sexual assault patient. (pp 1485–1488)

SKILLS OBJECTIVES

There are no skills objectives for this chapter.

Introduction

Gynecology is the branch of medicine that deals with the diseases and routine physical care of the female reproductive system. This chapter first reviews the female anatomy and physiology, and then outlines issues unique to female patients, including conditions that may be encountered in the emergency setting. In addition, it covers the gynecologic causes of abdominal pain and looks in detail at life-threatening conditions. Also discussed are the topics of vaginal bleeding and sexual assault, and how these two emergencies should be managed in the field.

Anatomy and Physiology Review

The female reproductive structures include the external female genitalia, uterus, vagina, cervix, fallopian tubes, ovaries, and the mammary glands **FIGURE 23-1**. The **ovaries** are a pair of organs that release eggs, or ova (singular, *ovum*), as well as

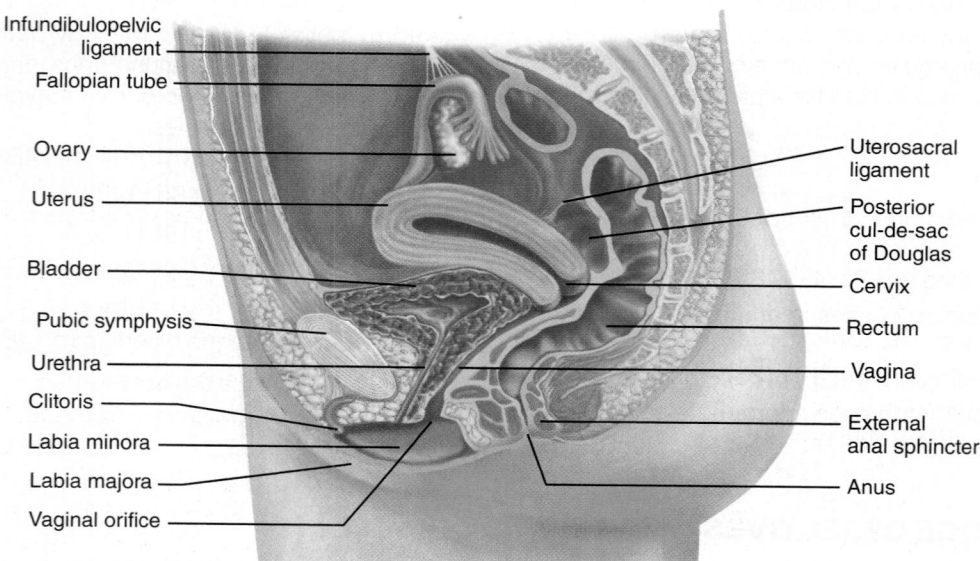

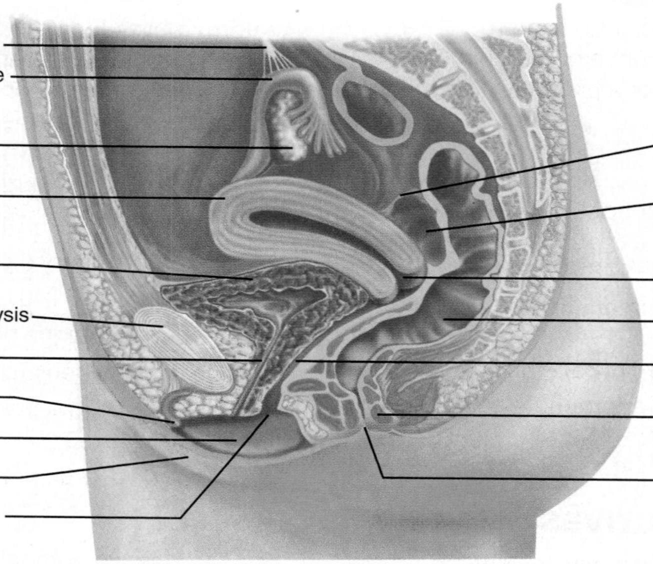

FIGURE 23-1 Anatomy of the female genital tract and pelvis.

YOU are the Paramedic

PART 1

Your unit is dispatched for a patient with abdominal pain. While you are en route, the dispatcher tells you the patient is a 24-year-old woman who is reporting lower abdominal pain and vaginal bleeding. When you arrive at the residence, the patient's husband meets you. He tells you that his wife has had "problems with her period for months." He called 9-1-1 because she is in a lot of pain today.

1. What are you looking for in your scene size-up?
2. What are you looking for in your primary survey?

reproductive hormones. After its release, an egg travels down the adjacent **fallopian tube** into the uterus.

> ## Words of Wisdom
>
> Although this chapter discusses gynecologic conditions as pertaining to female patients, providers should be mindful that a patient who does not identify as female can have gynecologic issues. Thus, the paramedic must consider conditions relating to the female reproductive system regardless of the patient's presenting gender.
>
> Because there are unique medical risks associated with being a genotypic male or female, it is important to know this information for the medical record, but it should be ascertained in a sensitive manner. For instance, you may use questions such as, "What gender do you currently identify yourself as?", "What gender were you identified as at birth?", or "Have you had any gender-specific surgeries?"

The **uterus** is a pear-shaped organ where the **embryo**, or fertilized egg, implants and grows. The upper, convex portion of the uterus, called the fundus, contains an internal uterine cavity. The uterine wall consists of two layers: the myometrium (the muscular layer) and the **endometrium** (the nutrient-rich inner layer that is shed during **menstruation**, the monthly flow of blood). If an egg is fertilized (which usually occurs within the fallopian tube) after its release, it travels to the uterine cavity and implants into the endometrium, where it will grow and mature. The neck of the uterus, called the **cervix**, inserts into the **vagina**, which leads to the outside of the body. Together, the lower part of the uterus, the cervix, and the vagina are referred to as the birth canal. The **perineum** comprises the tissue between the vaginal opening and the anus.

The external female genitalia **FIGURE 23-2** (also known as the vulva) include the **mons pubis**, a hair-covered fat pad overlying the symphysis pubis; the **labia majora**, rounded folds of external adipose tissue; and the **labia minora**, thinner, pink-red folds that extend anteriorly to surround the **clitoris**, the region of sexual stimulation. Coarse, dark hair normally appears on the mons pubis in early puberty, becoming sparser later in life with the advent of menopause. The urethral meatus opens into the area between the clitoris and the vagina. Below the urethral meatus lies the opening to the vagina. This vaginal orifice is protected by the **hymen**. This membrane forms a border around the vaginal orifice, partially enclosing it. The hymen ruptures during the first intercourse, but may also be ruptured before first intercourse by trauma or by events such as horseback riding, gymnastics, or other sports. Pain and vaginal bleeding may be present in such an event.

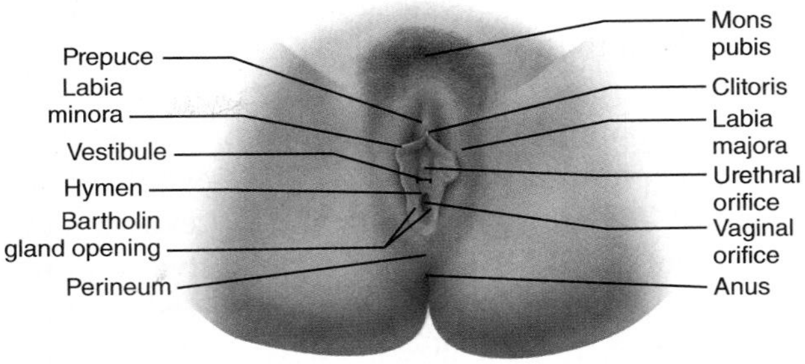

FIGURE 23-2 Anatomy of the external female genitalia.

In some cases, the hymen may completely cover the vaginal orifice, a condition called *imperforate hymen*. If it remains undetected until puberty, this condition will block the flow of first menses, resulting in relatively acute pain, with severe constipation and low back pain. Imperforate hymen may lead to endometriosis or cause other secondary painful effects. In some cases, this condition is caused by childhood sexual abuse, with the imperforation resulting from scarring from digital or penile penetration.

Menstruation

Menstruation, also called the menses, period, or menstrual cycle, is the normal discharge of blood, epithelial cells, mucus, and tissue from the uterine cavity. **Menarche** is the onset of the first menses, when a girl reaches childbearing age. **Menopause**, also called the female climacteric, is the cessation of ovarian function and of the menstrual cycle.

The menstrual cycle is divided into two phases: the ovarian cycle (ovarian changes) and the uterine cycle (changes in the uterus). The ovarian cycle is divided into the follicular phase (days 1 to 13) and the luteal phase (days 14 to 28). The uterine cycle is divided into the proliferative phase (days 5 to 14) and the secretory phase (days 15 to 28).

Ovulation occurs when an ovum, or egg, is released from an ovarian follicle. This event usually occurs 14 days after the start of the previous menstrual period. If fertilization occurs, the endometrium is prepared to receive the fertilized ovum. If the ovum is not fertilized, menstruation ensues, including discharge of the endometrial lining. Menstruation lasts 4 to 6 days, with blood loss of approximately 25 to 65 mL. The menstrual cycle, along with the hormones released during each of its phases, is discussed in more detail in Chapter 8, *Anatomy and Physiology*.

Some women may experience abdominal pain and cramping in the middle of the menstrual cycle. This pain and its accompanying symptoms result from the physiologic rupture of an ovarian follicle and are collectively called *mittelschmerz* (pronounced "MITT-ul-shmurz"; German for "middle pain"). In most cases, the pain is not severe; it may last only a few minutes or as long as 48 hours (average, 6 to 8 hours). Signs and symptoms include sharp, cramping pain in the lower abdomen, localized to one side, beginning mid-cycle, with a history of similar pain episodes during previous periods. The pain may also be reported as "switching sides" from month to month. The condition itself is not serious, and the pain can often be relieved by over-the-counter analgesics.

Amenorrhea is the absence or cessation of menses. Although a number of factors may lead to this condition, the most common cause is pregnancy. Exercise-induced amenorrhea is common in female athletes, particularly those who participate in physically intense sports. Amenorrhea may occur when a woman's body fat drops below a certain percentage. It can also be caused by emotional problems or extreme stress. In an adolescent or young adult, the condition may originate in anorexia nervosa; in this case, it is a symptom of the patient's malnutrition and emotional state.

Patient Assessment

Many of the same conditions that cause abdominal pain in men may occur in women—for example, renal colic, ulcers, gastroenteritis, cholecystitis, diverticulitis, pancreatitis, appendicitis, and dissecting aneurysm. In addition, there are numerous gynecologic causes of abdominal pain. Gynecologic emergencies are usually associated with one or more of the following signs or symptoms: vaginal bleeding, abdominal pain or tenderness, vomiting, fever, tachycardia, hypotension, diaphoresis, syncope, changes in stool pattern, dyspareunia (pain during intercourse), or urinary symptoms **FIGURE 23-3**.

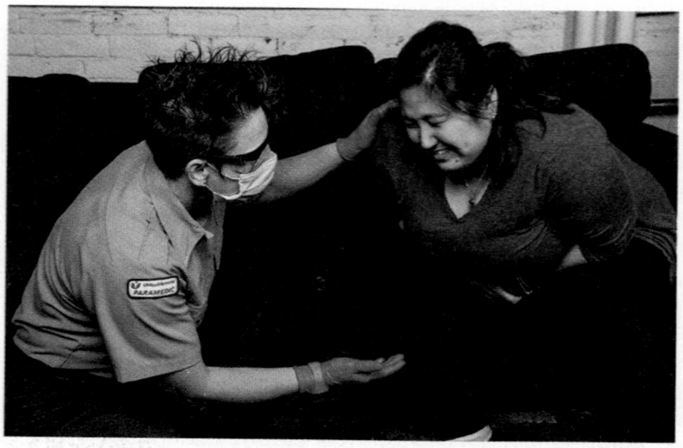

FIGURE 23-3 A patient experiencing a gynecologic emergency may be uncomfortable discussing her symptoms. Be professional and respectful so you can obtain the information needed to provide appropriate care.

Street Smarts

Any patient of childbearing years with abdominal pain should be considered to have a gynecologic emergency until proven otherwise.

Scene Size-up

As always, begin with a thorough scene size-up. Is the scene safe? Will you need assistance? Gynecologic emergencies can involve large amounts of blood and body fluids that can be contaminated with pathogens.

All information you obtain will contribute to your assessment of the patient's overall health and the safety of the scene. In case of a crime scene, you may also be required to testify in court regarding the conditions at the scene.

Primary Survey

When evaluating a patient with a potential gynecologic emergency, assess the ABCDEs (airway, breathing, circulation, disability, and exposure), and manage life threats. Provide pain management and fluid resuscitation as indicated by the patient's condition. Even if bleeding from the vagina is significant, do not pack any dressings inside the vagina. Make note of the amount, color, and type of discharge or bleeding, including the presence of clots or tissue. Transport the patient to a hospital for further evaluation. If the patient passed any clots or tissue before or during transport, bring these with the patient to the hospital in a sealed container if possible.

Words of Wisdom

In a woman with abdominal pain, the most important things to look for are signs of shock.

Words of Wisdom

Vaginal bleeding is a sign of internal bleeding and should not be taken lightly. Apply a pad over the vaginal area, and transport all used pads with the patient to the hospital.

History Taking

A complete gynecologic history should include the chief complaint as well as associated symptoms. If vaginal bleeding has occurred, try to quantify it in terms of pads per hour or in comparison with the patient's normal menstrual period. Ask about the date of the last normal menstrual period, regularity of menstrual cycles, whether a current pregnancy exists, number of previous pregnancies, number of pregnancies carried to term, number of miscarriages or abortions, history of prior gynecologic problems or surgeries, current sexual activity, type of birth control, and history of sexually transmitted infections (STIs) **TABLE 23-1**. (STIs are covered in Chapter 27, *Infectious Diseases.*)

TABLE 23-1 Elements of the Gynecologic History

Current symptoms: Vaginal bleeding? Amount? Any tissue passed?
Current symptoms: Abdominal pain? Onset, duration, character, location, radiation, severity?
Current symptoms: Vaginal discharge? Color, amount, odor, itching?
Currently pregnant?
Current sexual activity? Birth control?
Last menstrual period (LMP)?
Prior pregnancies (gravidity)?
Prior births (parity)?
Prior pregnancy complications or losses?
Prior cesarean sections or other abdominal surgery?
Other past medical history, medications, allergies
Prior or current sexually transmitted infections

Gynecologic emergencies can be embarrassing for the patient, and many women may be uncomfortable discussing their sexual history in front of strangers or even close family members. A teenage or adolescent girl may want to keep her sexual history from her parents. Few women are comfortable with having their genitals exposed to a crowd of family, neighbors, paramedics, law enforcement officers, or firefighters. Protect the patient's modesty at all times while obtaining the gynecologic history and conducting your assessment.

Documentation and Communication

Your attempts to acquire, truthful information from the patient may be hindered by the presence of family members, loved ones, or bystanders. Removing nonessential personnel from the area will increase the likelihood that you obtain accurate information from the patient.

Obtaining an accurate and detailed patient assessment is of utmost importance when dealing with gynecologic issues. You may not be able to make a specific diagnosis in the field, but a thorough assessment and patient history will help you determine whether the patient is experiencing a life-threatening emergency.

Secondary Assessment

When possible, the paramedic performing the physical examination should be the same gender as the patient. Limit the crowd in the room to only those personnel required to perform the necessary tasks, and show the patient you respect her by advocating for her modesty. You will also serve as a role model for other EMS providers when you act in this way.

During the secondary assessment, you should examine and assess the patient's abdomen. Inspect the abdomen for signs of abuse, such as bruising. Also note bruising in other areas, which could indicate possible abuse. The abdomen is a favorite target of abusers, especially if a woman is pregnant. Because clothing hides the evidence, the abdomen is also a favorite injection spot for chronic drug abusers. Look for a positive Cullen sign (ecchymosis at the umbilicus) or Grey Turner sign (ecchymosis at the flanks); both signal the presence of internal bleeding.

Palpate the abdomen, starting at the quadrant farthest from the pain and working toward the quadrant where the pain is located. Examine this quadrant last. Is the abdomen rigid (possibly indicative of internal bleeding)? Is there point tenderness? Does the palpation elicit more pain? Is rebound tenderness present (indicative of infection, such as may be associated with appendicitis)? Are there masses present? If yes, are they pulsating (abdominal aortic aneurysm)?

What are the patient's vital signs? Is the blood pressure normal, low, or elevated? Check the pressure in both the sitting and standing positions, provided the patient is not dizzy. Do you observe significant orthostatic changes? If yes, assume that the patient is in shock.

Street Smarts

Communication and documentation are important, but in gynecologic cases, do not focus on your documentation during the call. Your main focus must be on the patient, including providing emotional care. Documentation can wait until the patient has been delivered to the receiving facility.

YOU are the Paramedic

PART 2

The patient is lying on the sofa and is conscious, alert, and cooperative. She tells you that she has been having lower back and pelvic pain for at least 3 months. She has had a very heavy menstrual flow with spotting between periods. She adamantly denies any possibility she could be pregnant.

Recording Time: 0 Minutes	
Appearance	Awake
Level of consciousness	Alert and oriented to person, place, time, and event
Airway	Open
Breathing	Adequate
Circulation	Adequate

3. Which gynecologic emergencies present with pain?

4. What steps will you take in your further assessment of this patient?

Reassessment

En route to the hospital, recheck your interventions and remember to obtain serial vital signs. Pay specific attention to the needs of the patient and accommodate her desire for conversation or silence.

Emergency Medical Care

Primary management of a gynecologic patient is directed at mitigating life threats, being supportive and compassionate, and protecting the patient's modesty. In most gynecologic emergencies, your role will be largely investigatory. The more accurate and detailed the history and examination are, the better you will be at differentiating gynecologic and nongynecologic pathology. For all patients, assess oxygenation status and administer oxygen as needed. Obtain an initial set of vital signs, and continue to monitor these signs throughout your patient care.

Street Smarts

You likely will not carry the necessary supplies and equipment to make a definitive diagnosis of a gynecologic problem in the field. Instead, focus on life threats, treat for shock, provide emotional support, and transport the patient in a position of comfort.

Consider gaining intravenous (IV) access in any woman of childbearing age with abdominal pain. Initiate fluid therapy, providing for pharmacologic interventions (pain management) or volume replacement as necessary. General management of abdominal or pelvic pain is primarily supportive. Local protocols may allow for administration of pain management medications, including narcotics. Eliminating or reducing the patient's pain during transport will significantly reduce the patient's anxiety.

Provide transport. Protect the patient's modesty and provide emotional care with a supportive attitude.

Management of Gynecologic Trauma

The female genital area is highly vascular and susceptible to trauma. Motor vehicle crashes, sporting events, assault, and even consensual sex are common mechanisms of injury. Bleeding from genital trauma may be profuse (and very painful). If the patient is currently having her period, trying to differentiate between menstrual blood and trauma-related blood can be difficult.

Applying simple external pressure over the area of the laceration is usually sufficient to control bleeding. Bleeding from the internal genitalia, by contrast, can be massive and very difficult to control. Blindly packing the vagina is dangerous and is not recommended or even beneficial. A woman with exsanguinating vaginal hemorrhage must be treated as any other injured patient with exsanguinating hemorrhage—that is, she must be treated for shock and rapidly transported to the hospital, preferably one with obstetric and gynecologic services.

Do *not* perform an internal vaginal examination. Examination of the external genitalia is only warranted in the presence of genital trauma.

Pathophysiology, Assessment, and Management of Specific Emergencies

Infections

Pelvic Inflammatory Disease

Pelvic inflammatory disease (PID) is an infection of a woman's reproductive organs. Although PID is a complication often caused by an STI, such as chlamydia or gonorrhea, other infections that are not sexually transmitted can also cause this disease.[1] Many women who have PID either have no signs or symptoms or have symptoms but do not seek treatment. The disease is most prevalent in sexually active women who are age 25 years or younger.[1]

With PID, disease-causing organisms enter the vagina, generally via the process of sexual activity, and migrate through the opening of the cervix and into the uterine cavity, where they invade the mucosa. The infection may then expand to the fallopian tubes, where the tubal walls swell and the lumen of the tube fills with purulent fluid that obstructs the tube. The purulent fluid drips out of the tube and onto the ovary and surrounding tissue. Peritonitis may develop and pelvic abscesses may form as the inflammatory response attempts to contain the infection. If the infection spreads, it may eventually lead to sepsis. Because PID can affect the fallopian tubes and ovaries, long-term complications of PID can include infertility and an increased risk of ectopic pregnancy.

If a patient with PID has symptoms, she may report pain that generally starts during or after normal menstruation, so eliciting the last menstrual period (LMP) is an essential component of the history. The pain is typically diffuse and is spread over both quadrants of the lower abdomen. It may be described as "achy," and the patient may volunteer that the pain is made worse by walking or by sexual intercourse. The latter revelation usually indicates cervical involvement in the infective process. Pain localized to the right upper quadrant (RUQ) indicates infection that has spread to the abdominal cavity. Associated symptoms may include vaginal discharge, fever and chills, and pain or burning on urination (dysuria).

Risk factors for PID include an untreated STI, sexual activity with multiple partners, douching, and a history of previous PID. This disease may also be associated with abortion, childbirth, or the insertion of an intrauterine device (IUD), which is used to prevent pregnancy, or another instrument contaminated by organisms from the lower reproductive tract or other source. With regard to IUD use, the increased risk of PID is mostly limited to the first 3 weeks after placement of this device **FIGURE 23-4**.

Any woman with PID who feels sick enough to seek medical assistance probably has a severe infection and is likely to present as febrile and look sick. Physical examination findings may be sparse or may include the entire textbook profile. Be alert for signs of peritoneal irritation—for example, a patient who winces on palpation of the abdomen or every time the ambulance hits a bump. Be very gentle should you decide to palpate this patient's abdomen as part of the examination.

PID generally requires administration of an appropriate antibiotic for 10 to 14 days. Prehospital care is primarily supportive, but may include supplemental oxygen, IV fluids, or both, depending on the patient's presentation. Make the patient as comfortable as possible and transport with as gentle a ride as can be managed.

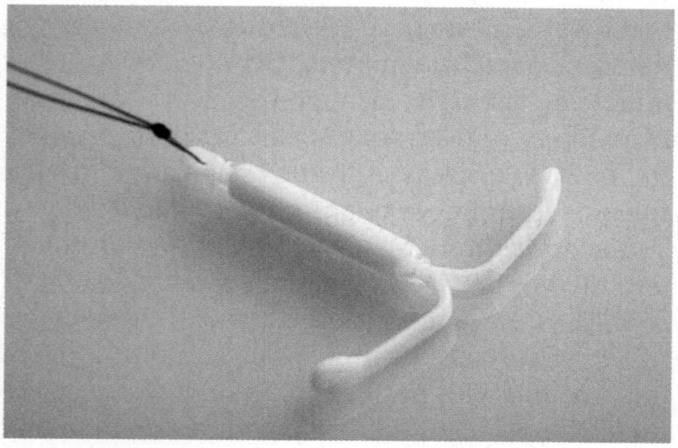

FIGURE 23-4 Insertion of an intrauterine device can increase a woman's risk of developing pelvic inflammatory disease for a brief time after insertion.

Bartholin Abscess

Just inside the lower vagina are two small ducts, one on each side, that lead to the **Bartholin glands**. These glands secrete mucus that acts as a lubricant during intercourse. A cyst may form if one of these ducts becomes blocked, causing the duct and gland to swell. A Bartholin abscess can develop if the cyst or the gland itself becomes infected.

A Bartholin cyst is typically small. A large cyst or a cyst that becomes infected can cause vulvar pain, pain with intercourse, and a painful lump in the vulvar area. A Bartholin abscess may be unilateral or bilateral.[2] If a cyst is infected or if an abscess is present, a surgical incision to drain the infected gland is usually required. Prehospital care is primarily supportive.

Vaginitis

Vaginitis, by definition, is an inflammation of the vagina that is caused by an infection. Vaginitis can spread upward to the cervix, uterus, fallopian tubes, and ovaries to cause PID. Although some patients may be asymptomatic, common symptoms include itching, irritation, discharge, odor, painful intercourse, and lower abdominal pain. Vaginal foreign bodies such as retained tampons, condoms, or other devices may predispose women to vaginitis. A physician can usually remove them easily. Several different types of vaginitis are possible, including vaginal yeast infections.

Vaginal yeast infection is typically caused by the *Candida albicans* fungus. Yeasts are tiny organisms that normally live in small numbers inside the vagina and on the skin. The normal acidic environment of the vagina helps keep yeast from growing. However, if the vaginal environment becomes less acidic, the yeast population may increase dramatically and result in infection. Conditions that may alter the acidic balance of the vagina include the use of oral contraceptives, menstruation, pregnancy, diabetes, some antibiotics, deodorant tampons, and the excessive use of vaginal sprays or douches.[3] Moisture and irritation of the vagina also seem to encourage yeast growth. Stress from lack of sleep, illness, or poor diet are other contributing factors. Women with immunosuppressive diseases such as human immunodeficiency virus (HIV) infection or diabetes are also at increased risk. Symptoms may include itching, burning, soreness in the vagina and around the vulva, and vulvar swelling. Some women may report a thick, white vaginal discharge ("cottage cheese" appearance), pain during sexual intercourse, and burning on urination.

Vulvovaginitis is an inflammation of the external vulva. Its symptoms include redness, pain, swelling, discharge, burning, and itching. A physician should evaluate patients with this condition.

If not treated, vaginitis can lead to infertility, preterm birth, endometritis, PID, and an increased risk for STIs. Prehospital management is generally limited to supportive care, as antibiotics are required for definitive treatment. Treatment of vulvovaginitis may also include topical creams.

Cystitis

Cystitis (bladder infection) is usually caused by bacteria that ascend from the perineum through the genital tract into the urethral opening. With this condition, infection is isolated in the bladder. Patients often present with suprapubic pain, cloudy urine, urinary frequency, hematuria, and dysuria. If untreated, cystitis may lead to **pyelonephritis**, or infection of the kidneys. Pyelonephritis is more serious than cystitis, and patients with this infection may be severely ill, with fevers, chills, and vomiting. Treatment of cystitis and pyelonephritis includes antibiotics and pain relief.

Ovarian Disorders

An **ovarian cyst** is a fluid-filled sac located on or within an ovary. Ovarian cysts are common, developing in both ruptured and unruptured ovarian follicles.[4] Cysts may be solitary or multiple, and they can occur unilaterally or bilaterally.[5] Most are asymptomatic, generally lasting about 8 to 12 weeks before disappearing on their own without complications.[4]

Sometimes, a cyst will become large enough to cause pelvic discomfort, urinary retention or urinary frequency, or menstrual irregularities.[4] Symptom onset is usually gradual, and the patient may report a feeling of heaviness in the pelvis. An ovarian cyst may rupture spontaneously or after mild abdominal injury, intercourse, or exercise. If rupture occurs, the patient may have either no symptoms, mild symptoms, or severe symptoms. The patient may report a sudden onset of moderate to severe lower abdominal discomfort, which may radiate to the back. If internal bleeding is severe, the patient may experience light-headedness and signs of shock, including hypotension and tachycardia. Patients also may have a small amount of vaginal bleeding. Possible assessment findings associated with a **ruptured ovarian cyst** are shown in **TABLE 23-2**.

Ovarian torsion, or twisting of the ovary such that its blood supply is interrupted, must be considered if lower abdominal pain is severe or symptoms worsen. Ovarian torsion is more common in patients with a history of ovarian cysts, as a cyst may make the ovary more susceptible to twisting on its axis. A surgical emergency, torsion can lead to permanent damage to the ovary. This condition is associated with an acute onset of moderate to severe unilateral pain in the lower abdomen that increases over hours. The pain may be intermittent and may radiate to the back, pelvis, or thigh. Although nausea and vomiting are common with ovarian torsion, these are nonspecific findings. The affected side will be tender to palpation, and often a mass may be felt. However, the absence of these findings does not rule out the possibility of ovarian torsion. Prehospital treatment for a ruptured ovarian cyst and

TABLE 23-2 Ruptured Ovarian Cyst: Assessment Findings
Possible sudden onset of moderate to severe lower abdominal discomfort
Typically affects one side, pain may radiate to back
Possible vaginal bleeding

for suspected ovarian torsion involves recognition, quick transport to the ED, and treatment of any symptoms.

Uterine Disorders

Endometritis is an inflammation of the endometrium (uterine lining) and is the most common cause of infection following childbirth.[6] In most cases, the signs and symptoms of endometritis occur within 36 hours after childbirth.[7] They include fever, chills, vomiting, tachycardia, lower abdominal or pelvic pain and cramping, and a foul-smelling vaginal discharge. When this condition is suspected, reassure the patient and transport in a position of comfort. If necessary, start an IV line and titrate to the patient's vital signs. Most patients fully recover after antibiotic treatment, but severe infection and sepsis may occur if endometritis goes untreated.

Endometriosis is the presence of tissue outside the uterus that resembles the endometrium in both structure and function. This tissue is usually found on pelvic structures around the uterus such as the ovaries, fallopian tubes, bowel, or rectum. This condition can be extremely painful, but sometimes does not produce any symptoms. In fact, many women do not even realize they have endometriosis until they encounter difficulties trying to get pregnant. In women who experience symptoms, the most common complaint is pain (sometimes chronic pain), generally localized in the lower back, pelvic, and abdominal regions. The pain is often described as constant and deep; it may be unilateral or bilateral, and either sharp or dull.[8] Other symptoms may include heavy or prolonged menstrual flow, excruciating and escalating menstrual cramping, pain with intercourse, sensations of rectal pressure or urgency, and fatigue (perhaps leading to misdiagnosis as chronic fatigue syndrome). Patients may also experience bleeding between periods or report premenstrual spotting. Prehospital care for endometriosis is based on the patient's signs and symptoms. If the patient reports severe pain, provide pain relief with analgesics if allowed in your protocol. Let the patient position herself so she is as comfortable as possible. Use dressings or towels as needed to absorb any significant vaginal bleeding.

Within the pelvic cavity, fascia, muscles, tendons, and ligaments support the pelvic organs. If these structures weaken, they may no longer be able to hold an organ in place. **Uterine prolapse** is the protrusion of part, or all, of the uterus outside the vagina. In addition to genetics, factors predisposing patients to this condition include obesity, weakening of pelvic support because of decreased estrogen, increased intra-abdominal pressure related to pregnancy, and difficult childbirth including prolonged labor, multiple births, birth of a large baby, or repeated pregnancies separated by short intervals.[9] Although the early stages of uterine prolapse may

YOU are the Paramedic

PART 3

Your partner begins assessing the patient's vital signs. The patient states that she is not under a physician's care for this problem because it seemed normal at first. She tells you that she has been taking ibuprofen to alleviate the pain, but it has not been working. She describes the pain as a constant dull ache in her pelvis and lower back.

Recording Time: 5 Minutes	
Respirations	18 breaths/min
Pulse	80 beats/min
Skin	Warm, dry, and normal color
Blood pressure	128/60 mm Hg
Oxygen saturation (Spo_2)	98% on room air
Pupils	Pupils Equal, Round, and Reactive to Light and Accommodation (PERRLA)

5. What is the next question you should ask this patient?

be asymptomatic, more advanced stages can cause a feeling of pelvic heaviness or fullness, fatigue, and low back pain. Symptoms typically become worse after prolonged standing, but are relieved when lying down. If vaginal tissue is visibly prolapsed outside the vaginal orifice, cover it with sterile, moist gauze and transport the patient to the closest appropriate facility for further care.

TABLE 23-3 summarizes assessment findings associated with uterine disorders.

Vaginal Bleeding

Although vaginal bleeding is a normal part of the monthly menstrual cycle, sometimes it may be quite heavy or irregular. It also may be accompanied by severe, cramping pain. Vaginal bleeding in a nonpregnant patient is not usually life threatening. However, a woman may not yet realize she is pregnant if the bleeding occurs early in the pregnancy.

Dysfunctional Uterine Bleeding

Dysfunctional uterine bleeding is uterine bleeding that is abnormal in amount or frequency (more than every 21 days). A diagnosis of dysfunctional uterine bleeding is made after ruling out anatomic or systemic conditions such as medication therapy or disease.[10] This type of bleeding occurs when the hormonal events responsible for the menstrual cycle balance are interrupted. Such a disruption occurs most often at the beginning or end of a woman's reproductive years, when ovulation is becoming established or when it is becoming irregular at or after menopause.[10] Risk factors associated with dysfunctional uterine bleeding include extreme weight loss or gain, age greater than 40 years, high stress levels, polycystic ovary disease, long-term medication use (eg, oral contraceptives), excessive exercise, and anatomic abnormalities such as uterine fibroids.[10] A woman with dysfunctional uterine bleeding may require hormone therapy or, if she does not respond to medical management, surgery.

Prehospital care for the patient with dysfunctional uterine bleeding is supportive. Allow the patient to assume a position of comfort. If necessary, use dressings or towels to absorb any significant vaginal bleeding.

Words of Wisdom

Assume that any woman of childbearing age with vaginal bleeding has a potentially life-threatening condition until proven otherwise.

Traumatic Vaginal Bleeding

Traumatic vaginal bleeding is common after vigorous voluntary intercourse, although violent involuntary sexual activity should be considered as a cause. **TABLE 23-4** lists other causes of traumatic vaginal bleeding. The posterior vaginal wall behind the cervix is most commonly injured, although all pelvic organs can be involved. Complications can include bleeding, organ rupture, and hypovolemic shock.

Treat these patients as you would any other patient with the potential for hemorrhagic shock. Keep the patient warm, give oxygen, obtain IV acess, and administer IV fluids as indicated. Carefully monitor vital signs and give this patient high priority for transport and treatment.

TABLE 23-3 Uterine Disorders: Assessment Findings

Endometritis	Endometriosis	Uterine Prolapse
Fever Chills Vomiting Tachycardia Lower abdominal or pelvic pain and cramping Foul-smelling vaginal discharge	Constant and deep pain generally localized in the lower back, pelvic, and abdominal regions Heavy or prolonged menstrual flow Extremely painful and escalating menstrual cramping Pain with intercourse Sensations of rectal pressure or urgency Fatigue	Protrusion of tissue Feeling of pelvic heaviness or fullness Fatigue Low back pain

TABLE 23-4 Possible Causes of Traumatic Vaginal Bleeding
Vigorous intercourse
Straddle-type injury
Pelvic fracture
Direct blow to perineum
Blunt force to lower abdomen from assault or seat belt
Foreign body inserted into vagina
Abortion attempts

Ectopic Pregnancy

An **ectopic pregnancy** occurs outside the uterus. Ectopic pregnancies are often called *tubal pregnancies* because most are located in the fallopian tube **FIGURE 23-5**.[11] Other possible sites for implantation of a fertilized oocyte, although much less common, include the abdominal cavity, on an ovary, or on the cervix.

An ectopic pregnancy is a life-threatening cause of vaginal bleeding in early pregnancy. Risk factors include anything that may promote scarring or inflammation in the pelvis, such as previous surgical adhesions or ectopic pregnancies, PID, and tubal ligation, and use of an IUD to prevent pregnancy.

If a fertilized oocyte becomes implanted in the fallopian tube instead of the uterus, it will stretch the tube as it grows. The fallopian tube lacks the expansive muscle capacity of the uterus, however, so the developing embryo soon runs out of growing room. When this occurs, the tube is likely to rupture, causing pain and possibly life-threatening bleeding.

When the site of oocyte implantation is a fallopian tube, most cases are diagnosed before rupture based on three classic findings: (1) abdominal pain, (2) delayed menses, and (3) abnormal vaginal bleeding (spotting) that occurs about 6 to 8 weeks after the last normal menstrual period.[12] Most patients with an ectopic pregnancy will report abdominal pain. If the tube is unruptured, the pain begins as a dull, lower quadrant pain on one side. As the tube stretches, the pain changes to a colicky pain, then a sharp, stabbing pain, and, with tube rupture, to a sudden, excruciating pain that is felt throughout the lower abdomen. Referred shoulder pain is possible as the abdomen fills with blood. Most women report having a period that is delayed by 1 to 2 weeks, a lighter period than usual, or an irregular period. As many as 80% of women experience mild to moderate dark red or brown intermittent vaginal bleeding.[13]

Words of Wisdom

In ectopic pregnancy, bleeding usually occurs after the onset of pain.

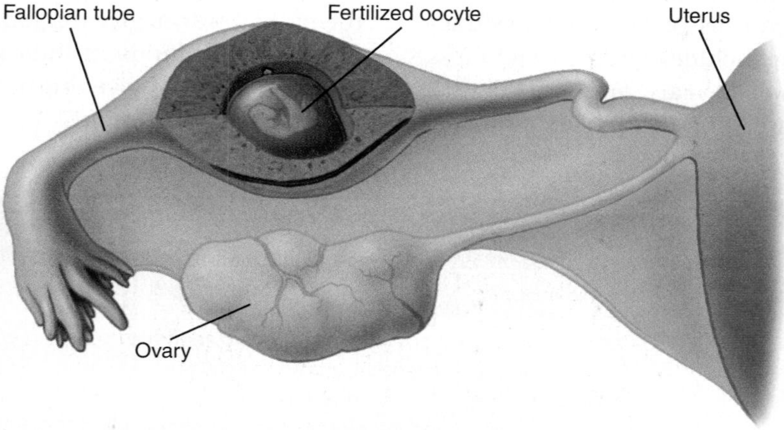

FIGURE 23-5 In an ectopic pregnancy, a fertilized oocyte implants somewhere other than the uterus. Here it is implanted in one of the fallopian tubes.

Follow these steps when caring for a patient with a suspected ectopic pregnancy **FIGURE 23-6**:

- Ensure an adequate airway and administer supplemental oxygen if indicated. Give nothing by mouth, including water.
- Keep the patient left laterally recumbent, even if unconscious and intubated.
- Initiate IV fluid therapy with an 18-gauge IV line according to your local protocol.
- Anticipate vomiting. Have an emesis bag and suction within arm's reach.
- Keep the patient warm.
- Place the patient on a cardiac monitor.
- Transport the patient to the nearest facility with surgical capabilities. Notify the receiving hospital of the patient's suspected diagnosis, her condition, and your estimated time of arrival.
- Recheck vital signs frequently during transport.

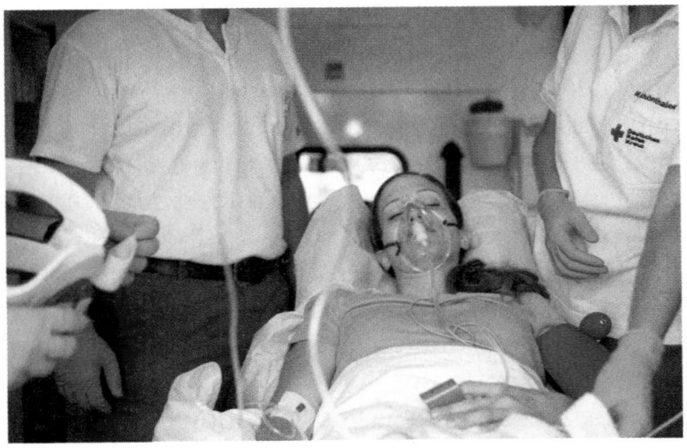

FIGURE 23-6 Treat any woman with abdominal pain and vaginal bleeding as if she has shock.

Sexual Assault

The US Department of Justice defines **sexual assault** as "any nonconsensual sexual act proscribed by federal, tribal, or state law, including when the victim lacks capacity to consent."[14] The Centers for Disease Control and Prevention defines *sexual violence* as a sexual act that is committed or attempted by another person without freely given consent of the victim or against someone who is unable to consent or refuse.[15,16] Although definitions vary by state, the National Institute of Justice notes that most statutes define **rape** as nonconsensual oral, anal, or vaginal penetration of the victim by body parts or objects using force or threats of bodily harm, or by taking advantage of a victim who is incapacitated or otherwise incapable of giving consent.[17]

Unfortunately, sexual assault and rape are all too common. EMS providers called to treat a victim

YOU are the Paramedic

PART 4

The patient tells you her LMP was 7 days ago. The flow was very heavy and she was in a great deal of pain. She is still having the pain, but now she is also spotting. You determine the hospital of choice for the patient and she agrees to transport. Before placing the patient on your stretcher, you have your partner assess her vital signs, which show no change. En route, the patient rests comfortably with no change in signs or symptoms.

Recording Time:	10 Minutes
Respirations	18 breaths/min
Pulse	80 beats/min, lying; 82 beats/min, sitting
Skin	Normal color, warm, dry
Blood pressure	128/60 mm Hg, lying; 124/56 mm Hg, sitting
Oxygen saturation (Spo_2)	98% on room air
Pupils	PERRLA

6. What is the general patient care for this patient?

7. Can you accurately diagnose a difference between a gynecologic and abdominal problem in the field?

of sexual assault, sexual abuse, or actual or alleged rape face many complex issues, ranging from obvious medical conditions to serious psychological and legal issues. You may be the first person with whom the victim has contact after the encounter. How you manage the situation from first contact throughout treatment and transport may have a lasting effect for both the patient and you. Being professional, respectful, and sensitive is very important.

Both men and women can be victims of sexual assault. A rape victim has just experienced a "major vehicle crash" of their mind and body. The act was most likely perpetrated by someone they knew and trusted. The last thing the victim wants to do is give a concise, detailed report of what they have just experienced, and attempting to elicit information in this manner most likely will cause the victim to shut down. Whenever possible, a female rape victim should be given the option of being treated by a female paramedic because the patient may be experiencing ambivalent feelings toward men in general; these feelings will hinder assessment and the patient's well-being.

Documentation and Communication

Just as you might be uncomfortable talking about your last sexual encounter with a total stranger, so your patient might feel a mix of emotions, including shame and frustration, after being assaulted. A calm, nonjudgmental approach from a same-gender paramedic will be helpful.

Street Smarts

Work with law enforcement to preserve the scene whenever possible. However, your primary responsibility is to attend to the physical and emotional needs of your patient.

Because sexual assault and rape are crimes, you can expect law enforcement to be involved early in the situation. In many cases, EMS may be called by law enforcement. While law enforcement personnel usually have basic medical training, their primary focus is on the criminal investigation, not patient care. As a paramedic, you are responsible for managing the medical aspects of the case and acting as the patient's advocate.

Assessment

Begin your assessment by asking the patient whether they would be more comfortable with a female or male paramedic, and make every effort to fulfill this request.

Limit any physical examination to a brief survey for life-threatening injuries. Expose and examine the vaginal area only if there is evidence of bleeding that needs to be treated. Do everything possible to protect the patient's privacy and give some sense of control back to the patient. Examine and interview the patient with a minimum of people present, moving the patient to the ambulance if necessary to ensure privacy.

The first issue is the medical treatment of the patient. Is the patient physically injured? Are any life-threatening injuries present? Does the patient complain of any pain?

The second issue is your emotional care of the patient. Do not cross-examine or attempt to elicit information for the benefit of law enforcement. These issues will be handled later in the ED. Do not pass judgment on the patient, and protect the patient from the judgment of others on the scene. Many victims report feeling "re-raped" when subjected to interrogation, criticism, or disbelief.

When performing your assessment, take note of any information suggesting the potential use of date rape or *club* drugs. The patient may or may not be aware of the use of drugs in the assault, but an inability to remember the event should heighten your suspicion regarding their administration. Along with alcohol, flunitrazepam (Rohypnol; roofies), gamma-hydroxybutyrate (GHB; liquid E or liquid ecstasy), ketamine (Special K), clonazepam (Klonopin), and alprazolam (Xanax) are drugs that are frequently used during sexual assault and rape for the intended purpose of incapacitating a person. These drugs can be put into a person's drink and may go undetected because they often do not have a color, smell, or taste. Their effects may be immediate and are made more active with alcohol. The patient may become weak and confused and may even have a loss of consciousness. These drugs cause muscle relaxation and loss of muscle compliance, making the victim more compliant during a sexual assault. If the drugs are still in the patient's system during your assessment, you may see hypotension, bradycardia, difficulty breathing, seizures, coma, and even death.

Street Smarts

Treat any patient who has experienced a sexual assault with respect, dignity, and empathy. The patient has undergone a traumatic event and requires emotional support.

Management

Remember that you are at a crime scene. Although your job is to treat the medical aspects of the incident and not to collect evidence, you still have a responsibility to preserve evidence. Do not cut through any clothing or throw away anything from the scene. Place bloodstained articles in separate paper (not plastic) bags. Paper bags allow wet items to dry naturally, whereas plastic allows mold to grow and may destroy biologic evidence. Obtain evidentiary bags from law enforcement if necessary.

It may also be necessary to gently persuade the patient not to clean up. This will be a natural desire on the part of the patient, stemming from the desire to "wash away" the humiliation and embarrassment of the assault. Valuable evidence can be destroyed in this process. The patient also needs to be discouraged from using hand sanitizer, urinating, changing clothes, having a bowel movement, or rinsing out their mouth. Respect the patient's feelings.

Some patients may refuse transport. For mentally competent adults, this is the patient's right. In such cases, follow your system's refusal-of-treatment policy or procedure for sexual assault victims without judging or being condescending to the patient. In no instance should you simply accept the patient's refusal and leave. Offer to call the local rape crisis center for the patient. Many communities have rape crisis centers, with victim advocates available on an on-call basis. Getting a professional advocate to the scene may help the patient deal with the trauma, and the advocate can better explain the necessities of evidence preservation in more compassionate detail. Many victim advocates are rape-trauma survivors themselves. Most rape victims are photographed and examined by nurses or physicians trained in sexual assault examination and management (sometimes called Sexual Assault Nurse Examiners, or SANE nurses).

Follow your protocol concerning this type of call. Some EMS systems may consider administering a sedative to a patient in this situation.

The patient care report is a legal document and, should the case result in an arrest and subsequent trial, may be subpoenaed. Keep your report concise, and record only what the patient stated in their own words. Use quotation marks to indicate that you are reporting the patient's version of events. Do not insert your own opinion as to whether the patient was raped or offer any conclusions that would either validate or invalidate the patient's account of the event. Document the facts. Record your observations during the physical examination—the patient's emotional state, the condition of their clothing, and any apparent injuries.

Words of Wisdom

Rape is a legal diagnosis, not a medical diagnosis. The medical team can only establish whether sexual intercourse occurred; a court must decide whether intercourse was inflicted forcibly or without consent of the victim.

Intimate Partner Violence

Intimate partner violence refers to physical, sexual, or psychological harm inflicted by a current or former partner or spouse. This type of violence can occur among heterosexual or same-sex couples and does not require sexual intimacy.[18] As the first member of the health care team to contact the patient outside the hospital or at the patient's home, you may be able to gather valuable information not available to hospital personnel. If you arrive at an uncontrolled scene where you suspect intimate partner violence has occurred, avoid confronting the parties involved. Your top priority should always be safety—yours, your partner's, and your patient's.

Sexual Practices and Vaginal Foreign Bodies

Men and women engage in sexual acts in a variety of ways. Your exposure to these practices will most likely occur when these private sexual practices go bad, resulting in an embarrassing call to 9-1-1.

The most common sexual gynecologic emergency you may encounter is simply a foreign object (a soda pop or beer bottle or a sex toy) that has become stuck in the vagina or anus. For example, a bottle may develop a vacuum inside the body and stick to an interior structure. Attempts at removal by the patient may result in intense pain or even vaginal bleeding as internal structures tear. Bleeding and pain typically cause the patient to panic. With this type of call, keep the patient calm, protect their dignity as much as possible, and transport. Do not attempt to remove any foreign objects from the vagina or anus. If at all possible, do not let the patient walk. Overpenetration of any item may lead to internal injury.

Some cases of bottle insertion may be associated with rape, so bear in mind that the patient may be an assault victim. Some gangs have been known to insert beer bottles in a woman's vagina after rape, then take turns punching the woman in the lower abdomen until the bottle breaks. If this is the case, use extreme care and do not move the patient more than necessary to prevent even more internal damage.

Another alternative sexual practice you may encounter is the technique known as "fisting," which involves placing the closed fist and wrist into a body orifice (vagina or rectum) for sexual stimulation. Whether the patient is male or female, organ rupture (rectum, vagina) is likely, and life-threatening peritonitis may result. Another sexual practice is the insertion of live animals into the vagina or anus, including fish, eels, snakes, and worms. The patient is likely to become alarmed if the animal goes in but does not come out.

Assessment

Assessment in this situation is sensitive. Maintain your patient's privacy. Depending on the circumstances, you may need to inspect the genital area for bleeding, wounds, or objects that may need to be stabilized. Avoid focusing on only one part of your patient; you still need to conduct a thorough patient assessment, including vital signs and history.

Management

Treat such a case as you would with any other foreign object, remain nonjudgmental, and transport. Do not attempt to retrieve the object, even if it is an animal, from inside the vagina or anus. Transport the patient in a knees-flexed, legs-together position.

YOU are the Paramedic SUMMARY

1. What are you looking for in your scene size-up?

Look for the same elements of scene size-up as you would with any call: scene safety, need for additional resources, initial impression (medical, trauma, or both), and number of patients. Take standard precautions. Note the conditions at the scene; this information may be helpful should you be asked to testify in court.

2. What are you looking for in your primary survey?

Answer the following questions during your primary survey: What is the overall presentation of the patient? Does your rapid scan reveal any obvious life threats? Is she conscious? Does she have obvious breathing difficulty or evidence of injury? Does she appear pale, cyanotic, red, or gray? Is she alert and oriented or confused? Is she calm or distraught? What is her emotional state? What is her physical appearance—well kempt or dirty? Do you find the patient sitting up, lying down, prone, supine, in the fetal position, in the tripod position, in the bathtub, or on all fours?

Once you have answered these basic questions and treated any immediate threats to airway, breathing, or circulation, you can proceed with a secondary assessment and obtain a more detailed history of the present illness.

YOU are the Paramedic SUMMARY continued

3. Which gynecologic emergencies present with pain?

Most gynecologic emergencies can present with pain (eg, abdominal pain, pelvic pain, low back pain, pain during intercourse, cramping). Ectopic pregnancy and ruptured ovarian cyst are two conditions that are potentially life threatening. Although other gynecologic causes of pain may not be life threatening, any manifestation of pain will naturally be worrisome to the patient.

4. What steps will you take in your further assessment of this patient?

What is the patient's chief complaint? If it is excessive bleeding, you can move on to obtaining the gynecologic history. If the chief complaint is abdominal pain, you need to find out more about the pain itself, using the OPQRST method (Onset; Provoking factors; Quality of pain; Region of pain and whether it radiates or refers; Severity; and Time [duration]).

5. What is the next question you should ask this patient?

Proceed to obtain a gynecologic history. Probably the most critical question to ask is, "When did you have your last menstrual period?" If the patient is certain, record the beginning and ending dates of the LMP. If she is unsure, record the approximate dates. Ask the patient whether she noticed anything unusual about the LMP.

6. What is the general patient care for this patient?

The management of a gynecologic patient is generally supportive because definitive care cannot be provided in the field. Primary management will be directed at managing life threats, being supportive and compassionate, and protecting the patient's modesty. Assess and supply the appropriate oxygen needs. Obtain the patient's vital signs, and continue to monitor her vital signs throughout her care.

7. Can you accurately diagnose a difference between a gynecologic and abdominal problem in the field?

No. Gynecologic emergencies often have the same signs and symptoms as emergencies involving other abdominal organs. Assess the patient carefully to determine the nature and extent of the problem. Be sure to follow the SAMPLE (Signs and symptoms, Allergies, Medications, Pertinent past medical history, Last oral intake, Events leading up to the illness or injury) mnemonic. What, if any, associated signs and symptoms are noted: fever, diaphoresis, syncope, diarrhea, constipation, and dysuria? Other medical problems may present as an abdominal problem. For example, cardiac pain may be misinterpreted as epigastric pain.

EMS Patient Care Report (PCR)

Date: 05-31-22	**Incident No.:** 78865	**Nature of Call:** Abdominal pain		**Location:** 1065 Meadow Lane	
Dispatched: 1005	**En Route:** 1005	**At Scene:** 1010	**Transport:** 1040	**At Hospital:** 1047	**In Service:** 1058

Patient Information

Age: 24 **Sex:** F **Weight (in kg [lb]):** 91 kg (200 lb)	**Allergies:** NKDA **Medications:** OTC ibuprofen **Past Medical History:** Denies **Chief Complaint:** Abd/pelvic pain

Vital Signs

Time: 1015	**BP:** 128/60	**Pulse:** 80	**Respirations:** 18	**Spo_2:** 98%
Time: 1025	**BP:** 128/60 lying, 124/56 sitting	**Pulse:** 80 lying, 82 sitting	**Respirations:** 18	**Spo_2:** 98%

YOU are the Paramedic SUMMARY *continued*

EMS Treatment (circle all that apply)				
Oxygen @ _____ L/min via (circle one): NC NRM Bag-mask device		Assisted Ventilation	Airway Adjunct	CPR
Defibrillation	Bleeding Control	Bandaging	Splinting	Other:

Narrative
Arrived to find 24 y/o woman complaining of abd and pelvic pain. Pt states the pain is a dull ache located in her pelvis and lower back that has been present for 3 months. Pt also c/o increased menstrual flow with spotting between periods. Pt states LMP was 7 days ago. Pt states pain is constant and does not change with movement or OTC medication. Pt is not under a doctor's care for same. Pt states she is not pregnant. Orthostatic vital signs assessed, which show no change. Pt agreed to transport to Community Hospital. Pt rested comfortably during transport with no change in condition noted. Report to Dr. Sullivan on arrival in ED bed 4. **End of report**

Prep Kit

Ready for Review

- Gynecology is the study and care of diseases of the female reproductive system.
- The internal female genitalia include the ovaries, fallopian tubes, uterus, cervix, and vagina. The external female genitalia include the mons pubis, labia majora, labia minora, perineum, and clitoris.
- Menstruation is the cyclical shedding of the endometrial lining from the uterine cavity. Menarche refers to the onset of the first menses, when a girl reaches childbearing age. Menopause is the period when a woman's reproductive cycle ceases.
- Ovulation occurs when an ovum, or egg, is released from an ovarian follicle. This usually occurs 14 days after the start of the previous menstrual period. Some women experience abdominal pain and cramping (mittelschmerz) in the middle of the menstrual cycle.
- Amenorrhea is the absence or cessation of menses. The most common cause is pregnancy. Amenorrhea can also occur in athletes, and in people with anorexia nervosa, emotional problems, extreme stress, or low body fat.
- Signs and symptoms of gynecologic emergencies generally include one or more of the following: vaginal bleeding, abdominal pain, vomiting, fever, tachycardia, hypotension, diaphoresis, syncope, changes in stool pattern, dyspareunia (pain during intercourse), or urinary symptoms.
- When assessing a patient with a gynecologic emergency, begin by focusing on the ABCDEs and assessing for shock. Additional care includes obtaining IV access, monitoring vital signs, providing pain management and fluid resuscitation as indicated by the patient's condition, and transport.
- While taking the patient's history, determine when the patient had her LMP, if it is unusual in any way, whether she could be pregnant, and whether she uses contraception. Also note any previous pregnancies, miscarriages, or abortions. If the patient has a vaginal discharge, ask about the color, amount, and whether there is any odor.
- General management for gynecologic emergencies is supportive, including addressing life threats, providing emotional

Prep Kit continued

support, and protecting the patient's modesty. When possible, the paramedic performing the physical examination should be the same gender as the patient.

- The female genital area is highly vascular and very susceptible to trauma. If the patient has sustained trauma to the external genitalia, apply pressure to control bleeding. Do not perform an interior vaginal examination.
- Pelvic inflammatory disease (PID) is an infection of a woman's female reproductive organs. Because PID can affect the fallopian tubes and ovaries, long-term complications of PID include infertility and a high risk of ectopic pregnancy.
- A patient with a large Bartholin cyst or abscess may report vulvar pain, pain with intercourse, or a painful lump in the vulvar area. If the cyst is infected or if an abscess is present, a surgical incision to drain the infected gland is usually required. Prehospital care is primarily supportive.
- Vaginitis and vulvovaginitis are inflammations of the vaginal tissues and external vulva caused by an infection. Symptoms include itching, irritation, discharge, odor, painful intercourse, and lower abdominal pain. Both of these common conditions are treated with antibiotics.
- Ovarian disorders include ovarian cysts and ovarian torsion. If an ovarian cyst ruptures, the patient may have no symptoms, mild symptoms, or severe symptoms. If internal bleeding is severe, the patient may experience light-headedness, accompanied by hypotension and tachycardia. Ovarian torsion must be considered if lower abdominal pain is severe or symptoms worsen; it is a surgical emergency that can lead to permanent damage to the ovary. Prehospital treatment for a ruptured ovarian cyst and for suspected ovarian torsion involves recognition, quick transport to the ED, and treatment of any symptoms.
- Uterine disorders include endometritis, endometriosis, and uterine prolapse. Endometritis is inflammation of the endometrium. Its signs and symptoms may include fever, chills, vomiting, tachycardia, lower abdominal or pelvic pain and cramping, and a foul-smelling vaginal discharge. Endometriosis is the presence of tissue outside the uterus that resembles the endometrium in both structure and function; it can cause infertility. In women who experience symptoms, the most common complaint is pain (sometimes chronic pain), generally localized in the lower back, pelvic, and abdominal regions. Uterine prolapse is the protrusion of part or all of the uterus outside the vagina. If vaginal tissue is visibly prolapsed outside the vaginal orifice, cover it with sterile, moist gauze and transport the patient.
- Vaginal bleeding that does not occur during the course of regular menstruation is cause for concern. Consider whether there is a mechanism of injury. Dysfunctional uterine bleeding is uterine bleeding that is abnormal in amount or frequency (more than every 21 days). Treat these patients as if they have the potential for hemorrhagic shock.
- In ectopic pregnancy, a fertilized oocyte implants somewhere other than the uterus, usually in a fallopian tube, which can lead to rupture of the fallopian tube. This condition can be life threatening. Treat the patient for shock, and transport.
- In sexual assault, sexual violence, and rape cases, your professionalism, respect, and sensitivity are of the utmost importance.
- It may be difficult to obtain a history from a victim of rape. Have a same-gender paramedic treat the patient when possible.
- Remember that your job is to medically treat the patient who has experienced sexual assault. Ask only medical questions, and do not judge the patient. Limit the physical examination to addressing life-threatening injuries.

Prep Kit continued

- Preserve evidence when possible. Try to persuade the rape victim not to clean up.
- Document cases of sexual assault properly and professionally. On your PCR, report the patient's exact words in quotation marks. Record facts obtained from the physical examination, and document any information suggesting the potential use of date rape or club drugs.
- In scenes involving intimate partner violence, do not confront the parties involved. Remember that safety is your top priority.
- Sexual emergencies may involve foreign objects stuck in the vagina or anus, which may potentially lead to internal injury. In such a case, do not remove the object. Remain professional, and transport the patient.

Vital Vocabulary

amenorrhea Absence of menstruation.

Bartholin glands The glands that secrete mucus for sexual lubrication.

cervix The narrowest portion (lower third of the neck) of the uterus that opens into the vagina.

clitoris A small, cylindrical mass of erectile tissue and nerves located at the anterior junction of the labia minora, similar to the glans penis of the male.

cystitis Infection caused by bacteria that travel from the perineum, through the genital tract, into the urethral opening; also called bladder infection.

dysfunctional uterine bleeding Uterine bleeding that is abnormal in amount or frequency (more than every 21 days).

ectopic pregnancy A pregnancy in which the fertilized oocyte implants somewhere other than the uterus.

embryo A fertilized egg.

endometriosis The presence of tissue outside the uterus that resembles the endometrium in both structure and function.

endometritis An inflammation of the endometrium that often is associated with a bacterial infection.

endometrium The inner layer of the uterine wall.

fallopian tube The anatomic structure that connects each ovary with the uterus and provides a passageway for the ova.

hymen A membrane that protects the vaginal orifice before first intercourse.

labia majora A pair of prominent, rounded folds of skin covered with pubic hair that protect the vagina.

labia minora A pair of skin folds devoid of pubic hair that protect the vagina.

menarche The first menstrual cycle; the onset of menses.

menopause The period when a woman's reproductive cycle ceases; also called the female climacteric.

menstruation Cyclical shedding of the endometrial lining from the uterine cavity.

mons pubis A rounded pad of fatty tissue that overlies the symphysis pubis and is anterior to the urethral and vaginal openings.

ovarian cyst A fluid-filled sac that forms on or within an ovary.

ovarian torsion A painful condition in which the ovary becomes twisted.

ovaries A pair of female reproductive organs that release eggs (ova) that, if fertilized, will develop into a fetus.

ovulation Midcycle release of an egg (ovum) during the menstrual cycle.

pelvic inflammatory disease (PID) An infection of the female reproductive organs.

perineum The area between the vaginal opening and the anus.

Prep Kit continued

pyelonephritis Kidney infection.

rape Nonconsensual oral, anal, or vaginal penetration of the victim by body parts or objects using force, threats of bodily harm, or by taking advantage of a victim who is incapacitated or otherwise incapable of giving consent.

ruptured ovarian cyst A fluid-filled sac within the ovary that bursts from internal pressure.

sexual assault Any nonconsensual sexual act proscribed by federal, tribal, or state law, including when the victim lacks capacity to consent.

uterine prolapse A condition in which the uterus moves or drops into the vagina.

uterus The muscular inverted pear-shaped organ where the fetus grows.

vagina The genital canal in the female that serves as a passageway for the elimination of menstrual fluids, receives the penis during sexual intercourse, holds the spermatozoa before their passage into the uterus, and serves as the passageway for childbirth.

vaginal yeast infection An infection caused by the fungus, *Candida albicans*, in which fungi overpopulate the vagina.

vaginitis An inflammation of the vagina that is caused by an infection.

vulvovaginitis An inflammation of the external vulva.

References

1. Pelvic inflammatory disease (PID): CDC fact sheet. Centers for Disease Control and Prevention website. https://www.cdc.gov/std/PID/STDFact-PID.htm. Reviewed November 19, 2020. Accessed March 4, 2021.
2. Lobo RA, Gershenson DM, Lentz GM, Valea FM. *Comprehensive Gynecology.* 7th ed. Philadelphia, PA: Elsevier; 2017:371-372, 525. http://gynecology.sbmu.ac.ir/uploads/4_5825615235666412577.pdf. Accessed March 4, 2021.
3. Yeast infection (vaginal). Mayo Clinic website. https://www.mayoclinic.org/diseases-conditions/yeast-infection/symptoms-causes/syc-20378999. Updated January 8, 2021. Accessed March 4, 2021.
4. VanMeter KC, Hubert RJ. Reproductive system disorders. In: VanMeter KC, Hubert RJ. *Gould's Pathophysiology for the Health Professions*. 6th ed. St. Louis, MO: Saunders; 2018: Chapter 19.
5. Mobeen S, Apostol R. Ovarian cyst. *StatPearls*. https://www.ncbi.nlm.nih.gov/books/NBK560541/#_NBK560541_pubdet_. Updated July 8, 2020. Accessed March 4, 2021.
6. Taylor M, Pillarisetty LS. Endometritis. *StatPearls*. https://www.ncbi.nlm.nih.gov/books/NBK553124/. Updated December 21, 2020. Accessed March 4, 2021.
7. Rivlin ME. Endometritis clinical presentation. *Medscape*. https://emedicine.medscape.com/article/254169-clinical. Updated April 25, 2019. Accessed March 4, 2021.
8. Davila GW. Endometriosis clinical presentation. *Medscape*. https://emedicine.medscape.com/article/271899-clinical. Updated July 25, 2018. Accessed March 4, 2021.
9. Uterine prolapse. Mayo Clinic website. https://www.mayoclinic.org/diseases-conditions/uterine-prolapse/symptoms-causes/syc-20353458. Updated September 19, 2020. Accessed March 4, 2021.
10. Davis E, Sparzak PB. Abnormal uterine bleeding. *StatPearls*. https://www.ncbi.nlm.nih.gov/books/NBK532913/. Updated February 10, 2021. Accessed March 4, 2021.
11. FAQs: Ectopic pregnancy. American College of Obstetricians and Gynecologists website. https://www.acog.org/womens-health/faqs/ectopic-pregnancy. Published February 2018. Accessed March 4, 2021.
12. Ectopic pregnancy. Cedars Sinai website. https://www.cedars-sinai.org/health-library/diseases-and-conditions/e/ectopic-pregnancy.html. Accessed March 4, 2021.
13. Cashion K. Hemorrhagic disorders. In: Lowdermilk DL, Perry SE, Cashion K, Alden KR, eds. *Maternity and Women's Health Care*. 11th ed. St. Louis, MO: Elsevier; 2016:669-686.
14. Sexual assault. US Department of Justice website. https://www.justice.gov/ovw/sexual-assault. Accessed March 4, 2021.

Prep Kit continued

15. Sexual violence. Centers for Disease Control and Prevention website. https://cdc.gov/violenceprevention/sexualviolence/. Reviewed February 5, 2021. Accessed March 4, 2021.
16. Basile KC, Smith SG, Breiding MJ, Black MC, Mahendra R. *Sexual Violence Surveillance: Uniform Definitions and Recommended Data Elements, Version 2.0*. Atlanta, GA: National Center for Injury Prevention and Control, Centers for Disease Control and Prevention; 2014. https://www.cdc.gov/violenceprevention/pdf/sv_surveillance_definitionsl-2009-a.pdf. Accessed March 4, 2021.
17. Overview of rape and sexual violence. National Institute of Justice website. https://nij.ojp.gov/topics/articles/overview-rape-and-sexual-violence. October 25, 2010. Accessed March 8, 2017.
18. Intimate partner violence. Centers for Disease Control and Prevention website. https://www.cdc.gov/violenceprevention/intimatepartnerviolence/index.html. Reviewed October 9, 2020. Accessed March 4, 2021.

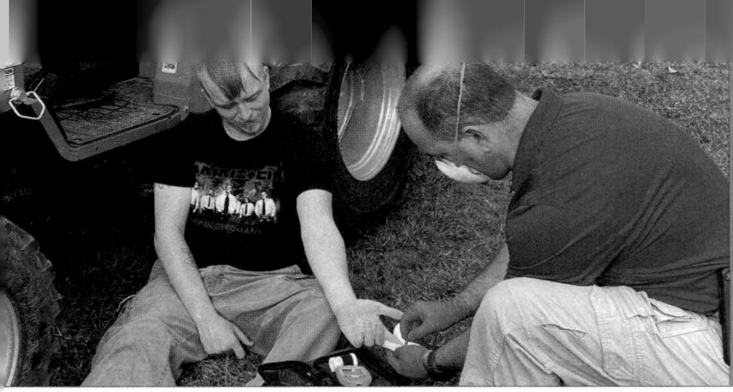

Chapter 24

Endocrine Emergencies

NATIONAL EMS EDUCATION STANDARD COMPETENCIES

Medicine

Integrates assessment findings with principles of epidemiology and pathophysiology to formulate a field impression and implement a comprehensive treatment/disposition plan for a patient with a medical complaint.

Endocrine Disorders

Awareness that

- Diabetic emergencies cause altered mental status (pp 1501, 1503–1504, 1508, 1511, 1516)

Anatomy, physiology, pathophysiology, assessment, and management of

- Acute diabetic emergencies (pp 1504–1520)

Anatomy, physiology, epidemiology, pathophysiology, psychosocial impact, presentations, prognosis, and management of

- Acute diabetic emergencies (pp 1504–1520)
- Diabetes (pp 1500–1504)
- Adrenal disease (pp 1521–1523)
- Pituitary and thyroid disorders (pp 1523–1527)

KNOWLEDGE OBJECTIVES

1. Review the anatomy and physiology of the organs and structures of the endocrine system. (pp 1497–1499)
2. Discuss the role of glucose as a major energy source for the body, including the relationship of glucose to insulin. (pp 1498–1499)
3. Describe the patient assessment process for a broad range of endocrine disorders. (pp 1499–1504)
4. Specify how to manage airway, breathing, and circulation in patients with endocrine system emergencies. (pp 1500–1501)
5. Define the term *diabetes*. (pp 1500, 1504)
6. Describe the factors that lead to glucose metabolic derangements. (p 1504)
7. Describe the incidence, morbidity, and mortality of diabetic emergencies. (pp 1505, 1514)
8. Identify the common characteristics of the various types of diabetes. (p 1504)
9. Describe the chronic and acute complications associated with diabetes mellitus. (pp 1505–1507)
10. Explain some age-related considerations to keep in mind when treating an older adult patient who is thought to have undiagnosed diabetes. (p 1507)
11. Compare the pathophysiology, assessment, and management of type 1 diabetes mellitus with that of type 2 diabetes. (pp 1507–1510)
12. Identify risk factors associated with prediabetes, including the role of hemoglobin A1c blood tests, in distinguishing prediabetes from diabetes. (p 1510)
13. Explain how to diagnose and manage gestational diabetes. (pp 1510–1511)

14. Compare hyperglycemic and hypoglycemic diabetic emergencies, including their pathophysiology, assessment, and management. (pp 1511–1518)
15. Describe the interventions for providing emergency medical care during a hypoglycemic crisis to conscious and unconscious patients who have a history of diabetes. (pp 1513–1514)
16. Provide the generic and trade names, form, dose, indications, contraindications, and procedure for administering 50% dextrose to a patient with hypoglycemia. (pp 1503, 1514)
17. Define hyperglycemia and discuss its pathophysiology, assessment, and management. (pp 1514–1518)
18. Describe the relationship between diabetic ketoacidosis (DKA) and hyperglycemia. (pp 1515–1518)
19. List the signs and symptoms of DKA. (p 1517)
20. Describe the interventions for providing emergency medical care during a hyperglycemic crisis to conscious and unconscious patients who have a history of diabetes. (pp 1518–1520)
21. Define hyperosmolar hyperglycemic nonketotic syndrome (HHNS) and the findings characteristic of this condition. (pp 1518–1520)
22. Describe the pathophysiology, assessment, and management of pancreatitis. (p 1520)
23. Compare primary and secondary adrenal insufficiency, including their incidence, morbidity and mortality, pathophysiology, assessment, and management. (pp 1521–1522)
24. Identify addisonian crisis, triggers of this emergency, its chief clinical manifestation and other signs and symptoms, and its management. (p 1522)
25. Identify Cushing syndrome, the physical manifestations characteristic of the disorder, and its pathophysiology, assessment, and management. (pp 1522–1523)
26. Discuss the clinical presentation of a patient with an adrenal gland tumor. (p 1523)
27. Compare the effects of hypothyroidism and hyperthyroidism on the body. (pp 1523–1524)
28. Explain the pathophysiology of Graves disease, including the characteristic signs and symptoms of the disease. (pp 1500, 1524)
29. Explain the pathophysiology of Hashimoto disease, including how it compares with Graves disease. (p 1524)
30. Outline the characteristic signs and symptoms of myxedema coma, as well as its management. (pp 1524–1525)
31. Describe thyrotoxicosis and thyroid storm, and their relationship to hyperthyroidism. (pp 1525–1526)
32. Describe hyperparathyroidism, including its pathophysiology, presentation, and management. (p 1526)
33. Differentiate between diabetes insipidus and syndrome of inappropriate antidiuretic hormone secretion (SIADH). (pp 1526–1527)

SKILLS OBJECTIVES

1. Demonstrate the assessment and care of a patient with hypoglycemia and a decreased level of consciousness. (pp 1512–1514)
2. Demonstrate how to administer glucose to a patient with an altered mental status. (pp 1503, 1513)
3. Demonstrate how to administer dextrose to a patient with hypoglycemia. (p 1514)
4. Demonstrate how to administer glucagon to a patient with hypoglycemia. (pp 1503, 1514)

Introduction

Few other systems in the body share the level of responsibility assigned to the endocrine system. This system directly or indirectly influences almost every cell, organ, and function of the body. Consequently, patients with an endocrine disorder often have a broad range of signs and symptoms, necessitating a thorough assessment and immediate treatment to avert life-threatening emergencies.

Anatomy and Physiology Review

The endocrine system controls and regulates all body systems. It works with the nervous system to maintain internal homeostasis and coordinate responses to environmental changes and stress.

Components of the Endocrine System

The endocrine system's major components include the hypothalamus, pineal gland, pituitary gland, thyroid gland, thymus gland, parathyroid gland, adrenal glands, pancreas, and gonads, including the ovaries and testes. The pancreas has a role in hormone production as well as in digestion.

Hormones are chemical messengers that are secreted into the bloodstream by endocrine glands. Hormones circulate throughout the body and target organs to maintain homeostasis. The action triggered by a hormone depends on the specific organ affected. Chapter 8, *Anatomy and Physiology*, discusses the hormones produced by the endocrine system.

Hypothalamus

The hypothalamus is not a gland, but rather a small region of the brain that contains several control centers for body functions and emotions. It is the primary link between the endocrine system and the nervous system.

The hypothalamus also produces regulatory (releasing and inhibitory) hormones, which control the release of hormones by the pituitary gland. The hypothalamus and pituitary gland are intimately related through the vascular system. The hypothalamic–pituitary system controls the function of multiple peripheral endocrine organs (eg, thyroid, adrenal cortex, gonads, and breasts).

Some of the hormones produced by the hypothalamus have physiologic effects that depend on their concentration. For example, a decrease in the body's water content triggers the release of **antidiuretic hormone (ADH)**. The hypothalamus senses salt concentration in body fluids; when this concentration increases, it signals the posterior pituitary gland to increase ADH secretion. Increased levels of ADH stimulate the renal tubules to reabsorb sodium and water. At the same time, ADH acts as a vasopressor.

Pituitary Gland

Located at the base of the brain, the pituitary gland is divided into anterior and posterior regions.

Six of the hormones secreted by the pituitary gland stimulate other endocrine glands; thus, they are referred to as "tropic" (from the Greek *tropos*, meaning "to turn" or "change") hormones. These include **adrenocorticotropic hormone (ACTH)**, follicle-stimulating hormone, growth hormone, **luteinizing hormone**, prolactin,

YOU are the Paramedic

PART 1

You are dispatched to a local grocery store for a woman "sitting in the butter." When you arrive, you are greeted by an older man, who tells you there is a large woman sitting in one of the store's refrigerated sections. The man points down the dairy aisle and says, "There she is. We found her like that. She was shaking all over and is very hot to the touch. I tried to help her, but now I have to go."

From a distance, you see an obese woman with a ruddy complexion casually sitting on top of a refrigerated dairy case. As you approach, you notice her bulging eyes and observe that she is diaphoretic. There are numerous large white tablets scattered on the aisle floor and what appears to be a food wrapper next to her feet. There is emesis on the floor nearby. When you call out to her, she does not respond.

1. Which key information is provided from the dispatch and scene size-up?
2. Which types of medical conditions can cause an altered mental status?

and thyroid-stimulating hormone. The other two hormones, ADH and oxytocin, control other body functions.

During times of stress, the hypothalamus secretes a hormone that stimulates the anterior pituitary to release ACTH. ACTH targets the adrenal cortex, causing it to secrete cortisol (a glucocorticoid and adrenocorticoid). Cortisol stimulates most body cells to increase their energy production.

Thyroid Gland

Thyroid hormones, which affect metabolism, are secreted in response to the stimulation of the thyroid gland by the anterior pituitary gland. The anterior pituitary gland secretes thyroid-stimulating hormone (TSH) in response to the hypothalamus's secretion of thyrotropin-releasing hormone (TRH).

The thyroid gland secretes thyroxine (T_4) when the body's metabolic rate decreases. Thyroxine, the body's major metabolic hormone, stimulates energy production in cells, thereby increasing the rate at which cells consume oxygen and use carbohydrates, fats, and proteins. Production of thyroxine depends on the proper intake level of dietary iodine, however, and lack of thyroxine will diminish the patient's physical and mental growth.

The thyroid gland also secretes calcitonin, which helps maintain normal calcium levels in the blood. This hormone is secreted when the thyroid detects high levels of calcium. Calcitonin travels to the bones, where it stimulates the bone-building cells to absorb the excess calcium. It also stimulates the kidneys to absorb and excrete excess calcium.

Parathyroid Glands

The parathyroid glands assist in the regulation of calcium. Specifically, parathyroid hormone, when secreted by the parathyroid, acts as an antagonist to calcitonin. Parathyroid hormone is secreted when calcium blood levels are low. It stimulates the bone-dissolving cells to break down bone and release calcium into the bloodstream. In the kidneys, parathyroid hormone decreases the amount of calcium released in the urine.

Thymus Gland

The function of the thymus gland, or *thymus*, is to help the immune system identify and destroy foreign intruders. In studies involving organ transplantation in baby mice that had their thymus removed, the transplanted organ was not rejected; however, the mice became highly susceptible to disease-causing pathogens and various pathogenic processes such as cancer.

Pancreas

The pancreas is considered both an endocrine gland and an exocrine gland. As an exocrine gland, it secretes digestive enzymes into the duodenum via the pancreatic duct. As an endocrine gland, it secretes three hormones from groups of cells called the islets of Langerhans. In essence, the islets of Langerhans within the pancreas act like "an organ within an organ," secreting glucagon from alpha cells, insulin from beta cells, and somatostatin from delta cells **FIGURE 24-1**. Somatostatin inhibits insulin and glucagon secretion.

In a healthy patient, the body regulates blood glucose levels using both insulin and glucagon. When the body's blood glucose level falls, glucagon is secreted to raise the glucose level. When it enters the bloodstream, glucagon stimulates the liver to convert glycogen into sugar (glucose) and secrete it into the bloodstream, which transports it to cells that can use the glucose for energy.

When blood glucose levels are elevated, the islets of Langerhans also secrete insulin, which is carried by the bloodstream to the cells. Insulin increases the cell membrane's permeability, allowing for easier movement of glucose into the cells. The cells then take in more glucose and use it to produce energy. Insulin also stimulates the liver to take

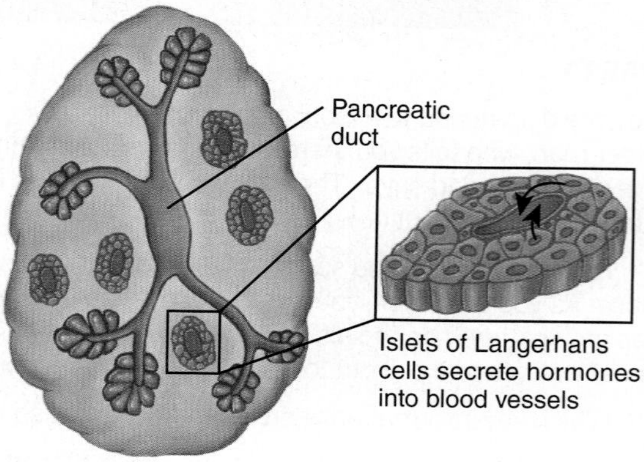

FIGURE 24-1 The islets of Langerhans secrete hormones into blood vessels.

in more glucose and store it as glycogen for later use by the body.

Insulin is the *only* hormone that decreases the blood glucose levels. It is essential for glucose to enter and nourish the cells. Once the blood glucose levels have returned to normal, the islets of Langerhans discontinue insulin secretion.

Adrenal Glands

The adrenal glands, located on each side of the body on the superior aspect of each kidney, are divided into two distinct sections: the adrenal cortex and the adrenal medulla. The adrenal cortex surrounds the inner adrenal medulla.

If the body experiences a drop in blood pressure (BP) or volume, a decrease in the sodium level, or an increase in the potassium level, the adrenal cortex is stimulated to secrete **aldosterone** (a mineralocorticoid). Aldosterone stimulates the kidneys to reabsorb sodium from the urine and excrete potassium by altering the blood's osmotic gradient. When sodium is reabsorbed into the blood, water follows, increasing both blood volume and BP. Aldosterone also reduces the amount of salt and water lost through the sweat and salivary glands.

When the hypothalamus is stimulated as part of the "fight-or-flight" response, the adrenal medulla secretes small amounts of **norepinephrine** and large amounts of **epinephrine**. Norepinephrine raises BP by causing contraction of the smooth muscle that lines the arterioles and relaxation of the smooth muscle that lines the bronchioles. Epinephrine stimulates sympathetic nervous system receptors throughout the body. In addition, it stimulates the liver to convert glycogen to glucose, which the cells can use as energy. The actions of both hormones result in increased levels of oxygen and glucose in the blood and faster circulation of blood to the brain, heart, and muscles, which in turn enables the body to respond to the short-term emergency situation.

Gonads

In both men and women, the primary functions of the gonads are to promote sexual maturation during puberty and to fulfill any subsequent reproductive needs. The gonads are the body's primary source of sex hormones.

In men, the interstitial cells of the testes produce male hormones known as **androgens**. Androgens regulate body changes associated with sexual development (puberty), including growth spurts, deepening of the voice, growth of facial and pubic hair, and muscle growth and strength. The most prominent of these hormones is **testosterone**. Testosterone promotes healthy sperm production, determines secondary male sex characteristics such as hair production, and stimulates growth. This hormone is responsible for male secondary characteristics such as increased muscle and bone mass as well as aggressive behavior.

In women, the gonads are the ovaries. The anterior pituitary gland directs the actions of the ovaries through the follicle-stimulating hormone (FSH) and luteinizing hormone (LH). The ovaries release eggs and secrete the hormones **estrogen** and **progesterone**, along with a small amount of testosterone. Estrogen signals the anterior pituitary gland to secrete LH when an egg is developing in an ovarian follicle. Estrogen and progesterone also assist in the regulation of the menstrual cycle. At puberty, estrogen supports development of the female secondary sex characteristics: enlargement of the breasts, uterine enlargement, fat deposits in the hips and thighs, and development of hair under the arms and in the pubic area. Progesterone prepares the uterus for implantation of the fertilized egg. During pregnancy, this hormone ensures that the uterine wall maintains functionality and prepares the mammary glands for activity.

Words of Wisdom

Although the specific pathophysiology varies for each disease, endocrine emergencies are usually caused by one of the following conditions:

- Failure of normal hormone production
- Excessive hormone production
- Failure of feedback inhibition systems involving the hypothalamus, pituitary gland, endocrine gland, and the target organ

Patient Assessment

The difficult part of assessing patients with endocrine emergencies is that their problems tend to affect many organ systems and the seriousness of their presentations varies greatly. Many patients will have had their conditions for some time and may already be receiving treatment. When you are talking to them, these patients or their family members will likely share the patient's history of an endocrine problem; this information, in addition to the common signs and symptoms associated with each endocrine emergency, should help you determine the cause of the current problem. In any event, do not take these calls lightly, because poor outcomes can happen quickly.

Scene Size-up

Scene safety should always be a primary concern as you arrive at the patient's location. Make sure that all hazards are addressed and that you take standard precautions.

Your observations of the scene can also give valuable information regarding what might have happened. Check bureau tops, bedside tables, and medicine cabinets for medications that might explain the patient's underlying illness. Also, check the refrigerator for insulin.

Primary Survey

The primary survey begins with the basics: airway, breathing, circulation, disability, and exposure (ABCDE). Patients experiencing an endocrine emergency may be in serious distress, so you must immediately identify and manage any life threats. In patients with an altered mental status, check for a medical identification bracelet or necklace that may list allergies or known conditions.

Your general impression, combined with a thorough physical assessment and patient history, plays an essential role in helping to identify the causes of the patient's distress. Endocrine diseases present with signs and symptoms that will depend on which type of hormone production or secretion is affected. Is the patient alert, or is there a change in their mental status? An unresponsive patient is obviously in a critical state and may be experiencing an endocrine crisis, such as **hypoglycemia** (abnormally low blood glucose level), **hyperglycemia** (abnormally high blood glucose level), or **myxedema coma** (a rare condition that can occur in patients who have severe, untreated hypothyroidism) with severe thyroid deficiency. Diaphoresis is usually a sign of severe distress; along with pulmonary edema, it occurs in patients experiencing **thyrotoxicosis** (a toxic condition caused by excessive levels of circulating thyroid hormone).

Your general impression can assist you in initiating the process of forming a field impression. A "buffalo hump," "moon face," and acne are telltale signs of **Cushing syndrome**, discussed later in this chapter. Mottled skin may be associated with pancreatitis. Enlarged or abnormal-appearing body parts may occur in combination with conditions such as edema in patients with **syndrome of inappropriate antidiuretic hormone secretion (SIADH)** (an endocrine disorder in which an excess of ADH results in decreased urinary output and, therefore, systemic fluid overload) or anasarca (extreme, generalized edema) with myxedema coma. Weight changes (underweight or overweight) may indicate an endocrine dysfunction such as hypothyroidism, hyperthyroidism, or **diabetes**—a group of complex metabolic disorders with many causes. **Exophthalmos** (protruding eyeballs) is present in **Graves disease**, an autoimmune disorder that causes thyroid gland hypertrophy and severe hyperthyroidism. Children with **panhypopituitarism** (inadequate production or absence of the pituitary hormones) may have abnormal development.

Check the patient's airway to ensure that it is patent and there are no obstructions. When patients present with an altered level of consciousness, they may be unable to protect their airway. Also, many will be very ill and have chronic episodes of vomiting. Maintain the airway as needed through patient positioning, suctioning, or use of basic airways.

Patients with endocrine emergencies may present with differences in their levels of breathing rate, rhythm, quality, and effort. You should immediately assess the patient's effort of breathing—breathing should be effortless—and administer supplemental oxygen as necessary.

Assess the color, moisture, and temperature of the patient's skin, and obtain the patient's BP. Skin condition can assist you in determining the patient's medical status. A patient with pale, cool, moist skin may be in shock or have hypoglycemia, whereas a patient with hot, dry skin may have a fever or hyperglycemia. A patient in hypoglycemic crisis will have a rapid, weak pulse. Because endocrine emergencies may affect the body's compensating systems, intravenous (IV) fluid administration may be necessary. Follow your local protocols.

Many patients with endocrine disorders are already being treated by specialists, and they should be transported to a facility specializing in these conditions. If the patient's condition is unstable or shows signs of becoming unstable, such as a diminished level of consciousness, transport the patient rapidly to the closest facility for stabilization first.

History Taking

Particularly in diabetic emergencies, the family history can provide important information. Because diabetes is a genetic disease (passed down through family members), learning that a parent or grandparent has a history of diabetes is a major clue and can prove invaluable in your treatment decision. This is especially true if the patient is a child and has a new onset of altered mental status.

Investigate the chief complaint or the history of the present illness. While you are assessing the chief complaint, you should consider the patient's signs and symptoms and any pertinent negatives.

If a patient is unresponsive, obtain a blood glucose level and manage any abnormalities appropriately. Just because a patient does not have a history of diabetes, you should not assume the person does not have a new onset of the disease.

Follow the SAMPLE mnemonic (Signs and symptoms, Allergies, Medications, Pertinent past medical history, Last oral intake, Events leading up to the illness or injury). Gather as much information as possible from the scene and any family members or bystanders present.

Observe the patient for any signs that may assist you in confirming the patient's reported symptoms. Signs and symptoms of endocrine disorders include those mentioned earlier as well as symptoms such as polyphagia, polyuria, and polydipsia in patients with undiagnosed or poorly managed diabetes. Tachycardia, premature ventricular complexes, and atrial dysrhythmias, including premature atrial complexes, can occur in patients with hyperthyroidism and thyrotoxicosis.

It is essential to ascertain any allergies the patient may have before administering medication. Document all medications the patient is currently taking regularly and whether the patient has been compliant with the regimen. Is the patient taking medications associated with diabetes (eg, insulin, oral antidiabetic agents)? Is the patient undergoing thyroid hormone replacement therapy for hypothyroidism or using glucocorticoids to manage Cushing syndrome?

Pertinent past medical history is important when diagnosing and managing a patient with an endocrine condition. Many of these conditions will have been diagnosed before your arrival, and the patient may have a substantial amount of

YOU are the Paramedic

PART 2

As you introduce yourself and ask the patient what is wrong, you see she has chocolate all over her mouth and an ice cream sandwich melting in her hand. She does not respond to you until you pinch the back of her hand. She then pushes your hand away.

Recording Time: 0 Minutes	
Appearance	Sitting upright with a blank stare
Level of consciousness	P (responsive to painful stimulus)
Airway	Open
Breathing	Adequate chest rise and volume
Circulation	Weak, rapid radial pulse; skin cool, pale, diaphoretic

3. Although the patient is cooperative, what do you need to consider when treating any patient with an altered mental status?
4. What could be the cause of the patient's reported shaking?

information regarding their condition. Likewise, family members are often well informed about these conditions.

In addition to inquiring about last oral intake, ask women of childbearing age about their last menstrual period. Patients with hypothyroidism, for example, may have a history of light or absent periods.

The patient, family members, or bystanders may be able to provide additional information about the events that preceded the current situation. For example, a patient with diabetes may not have eaten that day or may have been under a high level of emotional stress or physical activity.

Secondary Assessment

Begin the physical exam by observing the patient's general appearance. Note whether the patient exhibits decorticate or decerebrate posturing; both are signs of serious illness.

Your physical exam should be geared toward identifying as many atypical findings as possible. Unless the patient had an endocrine emergency that caused some form of trauma, a focused exam is rarely necessary. Instead, a full-body exam is usually more appropriate, although life threats always should be managed first.

The physical exam will reveal the finer abnormalities that will help determine your treatment. For example, the condition of the patient's skin provides essential information. Cold, clammy skin is a classic sign of shock but may also signal severe hypoglycemia, as from an insulin reaction and the body's response to catecholamine release. Cold, dry skin can indicate an overdose of sedative drugs or alcohol intoxication. Hot, dry skin suggests hyperglycemia, fever, or possibly heatstroke.

The goals of the physical exam in the comatose patient are twofold. First, you want to determine the patient's level of consciousness with precision, so that later assessments can readily determine whether the patient's condition is improving or deteriorating. Second, you should look for signs that might provide clues about the cause of the coma.

When you check the patient's vital signs, look for the combination of hypertension and bradycardia, which suggests increased intracranial pressure. Be alert for abnormal respiratory patterns. Cheyne-Stokes breathing usually points to a non-neurologic cause of the coma. Kussmaul respirations are often present in patients experiencing

YOU are the Paramedic

PART 3

Your protocol requires obtaining a blood glucose reading for any patient with a decreased level of consciousness. You record this patient's blood glucose level as 30 mg/dL. You obtain IV access and prepare to administer dextrose 50% per your protocols. A bystander comes up to you and says, "Is she going to be okay? When another shopper and I found her there, I called 9-1-1. An older gentleman said she probably has diabetes, so he tried to shove ice cream in her mouth, but it didn't seem to help."

Recording Time: 5 Minutes	
Respirations	24 breaths/min
Pulse	100 beats/min, weak, and regular
Skin	Cool, pale, and diaphoretic
Blood pressure	160/94 mm Hg
Oxygen saturation (Spo_2)	97% on room air
Pupils	Pupils Equal, Round, and Reactive to Light and Accommodation (PERRLA)

5. What concerns you about the bystander's statement?
6. If your partner was unable to obtain IV access, which additional treatment options exist for correcting the patient's blood glucose level?

diabetic ketoacidosis (DKA), a form of acidosis in uncontrolled diabetes in which certain acids accumulate when insulin is not available; such respirations are one of the body's compensatory mechanisms to "blow off" the excess acid that is produced in this condition.

More worrisome are other abnormal breathing patterns, such as central neurogenic ventilation or huffing and puffing that do not seem to move much air. Look for respiratory-related motions such as sneezing and yawning. An intact brainstem is required to produce a sneeze or a yawn, so both actions have positive prognostic importance. Hiccupping and coughing, by contrast, can indicate brainstem damage.

Reassessment

After initiating your treatment plan, continually reassess the patient to check for obvious and subtle changes. For every action you take, there should be a response. No response *is* a response. Document your findings along the way.

The ABCs should be managed during the primary survey. Remember that a patient whose gag reflex is absent cannot protect their airway from aspiration, so be prepared to suction the airway in an unresponsive patient. If the patient does not regain consciousness with treatment (eg, a patient with hypoglycemia receives glucose and remains unresponsive), consider whether to intubate the patient. Be sure to obtain blood specimens early in patients with diabetes, because any administration of prehospital dextrose or other medications will substantially change the chemical makeup of subsequent blood samples.

An essential aspect of patient care is to address the patient's emotional needs. Diabetes can be a stressful condition to manage, and patients with this disease have an increased risk of depression. Be empathetic and responsive to the patient's needs and provide emotional support as needed.

Monitor the cardiac rhythm of every comatose patient. During the neurologic assessment, the most crucial consideration is not one measurement obtained at a single time but rather the *trend* shown by several measurements you obtained. Recheck the patient's vital signs, pupils, and level of consciousness (every 5 minutes in unstable patients and every 15 minutes in stable patients) and *record your findings* immediately. Every patient you transport should have at least two sets of vital signs documented, regardless of the length of the transport.

Documentation and Communication

Communication with hospital staff is vital to ensure continuity of care. Hospital personnel need to be informed about the patient's history, present situation, assessment findings, your interventions, and the results. Your PCR is the only legal document that will reflect the appropriate care you provided. Document your assessment findings clearly, as they serve as the basis for your treatment. Patients who refuse transport because you "cured" them with oral glucose may require even more thorough documentation. Follow your local protocols for patients who refuse treatment or transport.

Emergency Medical Care

If the patient has an altered mental status, establish an IV line with 0.9% normal saline (NS) or a saline lock. Measure the blood glucose level immediately and initiate treatment if the reading is less than 60 mg/dL. Giving D_{50} (50 g of dextrose per every 100 mL, or 50% concentration) at a dose per your local protocols will reverse most cases of hypoglycemia. Some EMS systems no longer carry D_{50}; instead, they may use glucagon or D_{10} (10% dextrose concentration). When used to treat hypoglycemia, glucagon is administered intramuscularly (IM) or intranasally (IN). Patients who receive this treatment have a significantly increased recovery time relative to those given IV D_{50} or D_{10}. D_{50} causes greater fluctuations in blood glucose levels after administration. D_{10} is a lesser concentration and is not

Words of Wisdom

Glucagon can also be administered intranasally and is supplied as a powder in a prefilled autoinjector for home use. As part of your assessment, determine whether the patient or a lower-level EMS provider has administered this medicine prior to your arrival on scene.

hypertonic; its decreased osmolarity is less caustic to the veins and tissues. Document reassessment of vital signs and mental status after administration of dextrose or glucagon.

If the patient's condition does not improve after a dose of dextrose, and if you have reason to suspect a narcotic overdose (based on signs of pinpoint pupils, needle tracks on the arms, or depressed respirations), consider administering naloxone (Narcan).

Transport the comatose patient *supine* with a cervical collar in place if the patient is intubated to decrease the risk of unintentional extubation during transport. Otherwise, you can transport the patient in the lateral recumbent or recovery position, unless any injuries preclude that position. If the patient shows signs of increasing intracranial pressure such as the Cushing reflex (slowing pulse, rising BP, and an erratic respiratory pattern), posturing, or unequal pupils, transport with the head elevated to a 30° to 45° angle and the head midline to assist in venous return and to minimize intracranial pressure. Suction as necessary to keep the mouth and pharynx free of secretions, vomitus, and blood.

Pathophysiology, Assessment, and Management of Glucose Metabolic Derangements

Endocrine disorders are caused by either hypersecretion or insufficient secretion of hormones by a gland. Hypersecretion presents as overactivity of the target organ regulated by the gland. Insufficient secretion results in underactivity of the organ controlled by the gland. The effects of a disturbance of endocrine gland function are determined by the degree of dysfunction of the gland and by the patient's age and sex.

Glucose metabolic derangements, or disorders, are caused by dysfunction of the pancreas, which impairs the body's ability to metabolize glucose. Pancreatic dysfunction can range from barely detectable to extreme. Most glucose derangements and other clinically important endocrine emergencies result in compromise of the ABCs, improper fluid balance, deteriorating mental status, and abnormal vital signs and blood glucose levels.

Diabetes Mellitus

Diabetes is a metabolic disorder that is now considered to encompass a group of complex diseases with many causes:

- **Diabetes mellitus**—a disease characterized by the body's inability to sufficiently metabolize glucose
- **Gestational diabetes**—diabetes that develops during pregnancy in women who did not have diabetes before pregnancy
- Hypoglycemia/hyperglycemia
- Diabetic ketoacidosis
- Hyperosmolar hyperglycemic nonketotic syndrome

These pathologic conditions reflect a flaw in the production or function of insulin, or both. Insulin, a hormone produced in the pancreas, assists in the metabolism of carbohydrates and glucose transport into the cells. The end result of diabetes is hyperglycemia, also known as high blood sugar.

Medically, the term *diabetes* refers to a metabolic disorder in which the body's ability to metabolize simple carbohydrates (glucose) is impaired. It is characterized by the following symptoms:

- **Polyphagia**, an increased appetite caused by the inability of glucose to be transported across the cell membrane.
- **Polydipsia**, a significant thirst caused by dehydration brought about by an increase in **diuresis** (the production of large amounts of urine by the kidney).
- **Polyuria**, the passage of large quantities of urine. In diabetes, excess glucose is excreted in the urine (**glycosuria**) and attracts water, resulting in excessive diuresis.

Glucose (also known as *dextrose*) is one of the basic sugars in the body; along with oxygen, it is the primary fuel for cellular metabolism. *Diabetes mellitus* is characterized by the body's inability to sufficiently metabolize glucose. *Mellitus*, from the Greek word for honeybee, means "sweet"—a reference to the presence of glucose in the urine. In people with this disease, either the pancreas does not produce enough insulin or the body's cells do not respond to the effects of the insulin that is produced. The result is the same in both cases: elevated glucose levels in the blood and the urine. Glucose builds up in the blood, overflows into the urine, and flows out of the body. Thus, cells can "starve," or be deprived of glucose, even when the blood contains large amounts of glucose **FIGURE 24-2**.

According to the 2020 National Diabetes Statistics Report, 34.2 million people in the United States (approximately 10.5% of the population) have diabetes; of these, 7.3 million remain undiagnosed. Thus, one in five people with diabetes is unaware of their disease status.[1,2]

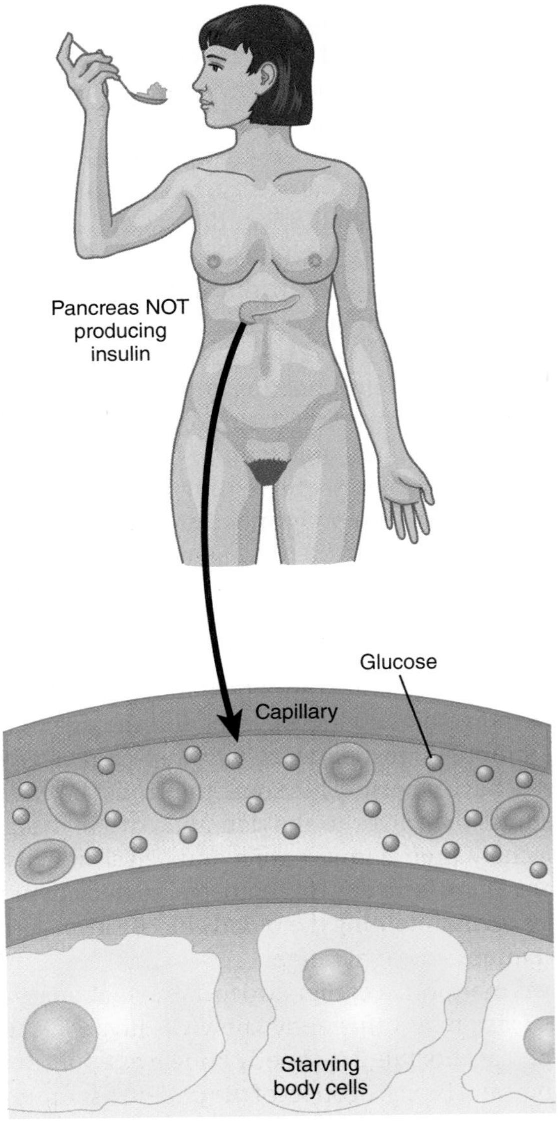

FIGURE 24-2 Diabetes is defined as a lack of or ineffective action of insulin. Without insulin, cells begin to "starve" because insulin is needed to allow glucose to enter and nourish them.

In 2017, diabetes was the seventh leading cause of death in United States, although the Centers for Disease Control and Prevention (CDC) suggests diabetes may be underreported as a source of mortality.[1] Diabetes produces a major financial burden for millions of Americans every year and, more generally, for the US economy through direct medical costs and indirect costs such as disability, work loss, and premature death.[2–4]

Diabetes mellitus is responsible for myriad life-altering complications, some of which are listed here:

- **Kidneys.** Diabetes is the principal cause of kidney failure, accounting for 38.6% of new cases in 2017.[4] In this disease, the glomeruli of the kidney become sclerotic, causing necrosis of the papillary tissue and leading to nephropathy (end-stage renal disease) and renal failure. High glucose levels in the blood cause the kidneys to work harder than normal and decrease kidney function over time.
- . Adults with diabetes are approximately two times more likely to die of heart disease or to have a stroke than those who do not have diabetes.[5] When diabetes is poorly controlled, the process of **lipolysis** (from *lipo-*, meaning "fat," and *-lysis*, meaning "breakdown") raises the level of fat in the blood. As a result of the increased fat level (known as **dyslipidemia**), the risk of atherosclerosis and coronary artery disease increases. The fat circulating through the bloodstream adheres to the vessel walls, eventually causing them to become stiff and brittle. In addition, glucose crystals have sharp edges, so they can damage the blood vessels when present in higher-than-normal levels. Over time, the microscopic deterioration of the vessel walls, called **microangiopathy**, leads to swelling of basement membrane cells, restricting blood flow to organs and tissues. Inadequate blood flow (ischemia) causes necrosis, or tissue death. Chronic heart failure develops over several years.[5] Central nervous system damage can cause cardiac dysrhythmias, which can then lead to cardiac arrest and sudden death. Microangiopathy and neuropathy both contribute to an increased risk of *silent* myocardial infarction in patients with diabetes: The combination of these pathologies may

result in the patient with diabetes not perceiving the common signs of chest pain, pressure, or tightness often associated with an acute myocardial infarction (AMI). Therefore, an AMI should always be assumed until proven otherwise. A 12-lead electrocardiogram should always be obtained and interpreted for any patient with diabetes who complains of a syncopal episode, fainting, weakness, fatigue, malaise, or dyspnea on exertion.

- **Cerebrovascular disease, stroke, and hypertension.** Vessels damaged by microangiopathy are common in patients with cerebrovascular disease and are associated with an increased incidence of stroke. Peripheral artery disease is also common in people with diabetes and impairs circulation to the lower extremities. Two out of three people with diabetes report having high BP or take prescription medications to lower their BP.[6] Hypertension is associated with an increased risk of heart disease, stroke, kidney disease, and blindness.
- **Eyes.** In adults age 18 to 64 years, diabetes is the chief cause of new cases of blindness as a result of retinopathy.[4] High glucose levels in the blood damage the vessels of the eye, causing swelling, wall weakness, and obstruction. Scar tissue can form that causes a pulling of the retina from the eye, or retinal detachment. Cataracts are a cloudy film that forms when fructose and sorbitol are deposited in the lens of the eye.
- **Neuropathy.** Neuropathy is nerve damage that results in a loss of sensation and function in the area innervated by the affected nerves. Such damage can cause sexual impotence, neurogenic bladder, constipation, or diarrhea. Neuropathy associated with diabetes often affects peripheral nerves, causing diminished sensation and function in the extremities. Patients with peripheral neuropathy often have paresthesia, a tingling or prickling sensation in the hands, feet, arms, or legs. Paresthesia and dysesthesia (painful burning, prickling, or aching sensation) can blunt pain perception, making it possible for foot ulcers to go unnoticed until they become seriously infected. Because many of these patients also have poor circulation in the extremities, gangrene can develop in adjacent tissues, and infection may spread to the bone. It is estimated that every 30 seconds a leg is amputated throughout the world, and 85% of these amputations are attributed to diabetes.[7]

Because of diabetes' widespread effects on all body systems, any preexisting condition will be more complex to manage after diabetes develops in the patient. The more closely patients adhere to the recommended management of their diabetes, the better the outcomes of their other conditions will be. Conditions that develop after the onset of diabetes will respond more effectively when diabetes is managed appropriately. Many conditions associated with diabetes can be delayed or prevented with appropriate lifestyle changes and continued management of diabetes. Conversely, any kind of distress can negatively affect the patient and result in a 9-1-1 call because blood glucose levels are more challenging to control in the setting of increased physical activity or emotional stress.

Both chronic and acute complications are associated with diabetes mellitus. Although these complications are present in both forms of the disease (type 1 and type 2), they tend to be more severe in people with diabetes who require insulin. Diabetes leads to organ system dysfunction, wasting of body tissues, and death if left untreated. Even with excellent medical care, some patients with particularly aggressive forms of diabetes will die at a relatively young age from complications of the disease. The severity of diabetic complications correlates with the average blood glucose level and the age of onset. Although most patients with well-controlled diabetes have a normal life span, they must be willing to adjust their lives to the demands of the disease, especially their eating habits and physical activity levels. There is no cure for diabetes, so treatment focuses on maintaining the blood glucose level within the patient's normal range.

As mentioned earlier, two forms of diabetes mellitus exist: type 1 (formerly known as juvenile-onset diabetes) and type 2 (formerly known as adult-onset diabetes). The age of onset of the patient's symptoms is less important than whether the patient requires insulin to survive. Both types of diabetes mellitus are serious conditions that affect many tissues and functions other than the glucose-regulating mechanism, and both require lifelong medical management. In addition, the condition known as **prediabetes** is now recognized as a warning sign that may precede the development of **type 2 diabetes**, and is discussed later in this chapter.

The Diabetes Control and Complications Trial (DCCT) and its follow-up study, Epidemiology of Diabetes Interventions and Complications (EDIC), both of which were funded by the National Institute of Diabetes and Digestive and Kidney Diseases, have emphasized the need for intensive control of diabetes to prevent and minimize long-term complications from this disease.[8] The initial study noted that patients who maintained intensive diabetes control significantly reduced nephropathy, neuropathy, and retinopathy.[8] The follow-up study demonstrated a significant reduction in the incidence of cardiovascular disease in patients who implemented intensive glucose control.[8]

Special Populations

You might encounter an older adult patient who has undiagnosed diabetes. These patients report that they have not been feeling well for a while but have not seen a physician. A patient with undiagnosed diabetes or one who is in denial or ignores their physician's advice may call 9-1-1 when the signs and symptoms get worse. Nonhealing wounds, blindness, renal failure, and other complications are associated with poorly controlled or uncontrolled diabetes. You must recognize the signs and symptoms of diabetes because you might be the first health care provider to suggest medical treatment to an older adult patient who might otherwise ignore this condition.

Older adult patients and individuals with diabetes who experience an AMI commonly present atypically. They often do not report the classic crushing substernal chest pain or pressure because of the neuropathy associated with increasing age and diabetes. Older adults also generally have a higher pain tolerance compared with younger patients. Other causes of an altered perception of pain can include impaired cognition or slowed nerve conduction. You should maintain a high index of suspicion when members of these populations experience a syncopal episode, fatigue, shortness of breath, or nausea and diaphoresis.

Older adult patients are also more susceptible to dehydration and infections. As we age, we naturally have a lower volume of water in our bodies.[9] Older adult patients may not become thirsty or react to thirst until they are extremely dehydrated. Medications can also cause an increase in diuresis, compounding the problem.

Type 1 Diabetes Mellitus

Pathophysiology

Type 1 diabetes has historically been referred to as insulin-dependent diabetes mellitus (IDDM) or juvenile-onset diabetes because it generally becomes apparent during childhood. Although type 1 diabetes has a hereditary predisposition, it is believed that environmental factors may play a role in its development; for example, an infection may trigger an autoimmune disorder. In patients with type 1 diabetes, the body develops autoantibodies that incorrectly identify the body's own tissues or substances as foreign invaders to be destroyed. Contributing to pancreatic destruction are autoantibodies to the insulin-secreting beta cells in the islets of Langerhans, to insulin, and to other pancreatic substances. The rate of beta cell destruction varies, occurring rapidly in some patients (primarily children) and slowly in others (primarily adults).[10] Eventually, the pancreatic beta cells become incapable of secreting insulin and regulating intracellular glucose. Because beta cells are the body's only insulin source, this hormone must be administered by injection or with a pump when these cells are destroyed.

Latent autoimmune diabetes in adults is a variant of type 1 diabetes that occurs in adults older than 30 years. The pathophysiology is the same as that of young-onset diabetes, with the body's immune system destroying the beta cells. Thus, patients with latent autoimmune diabetes in adults will ultimately require insulin therapy.

When the endocrine system (or pancreas) fails to produce insulin (as is the case in most patients with type 1 diabetes), patients require daily injections of supplementary, synthetic insulin throughout their lives to control their blood glucose levels. In addition to daily insulin injections, strict dietary control must be observed, which can be challenging to achieve with young children. Both increased activity and alcohol consumption can lead to low blood glucose levels—alcohol depletes glycogen stores in the liver. Therefore, in adults with type 1 diabetes, alcohol consumption also must be controlled.

Assessment

Assessment of a patient with a history of diabetes will be similar to your assessment of any other medical patient; however, there are some special considerations you will want to keep in mind. Begin by determining whether the patient is compliant with the management of their disease.

If the patient has an altered mental status, you should suspect a low blood glucose level. Hypoglycemia is a potentially life-threatening event. Patients with diabetes may also have other chronic conditions such as renal failure, heart failure, coronary artery disease, hypertension, and vision and hearing impairment. Because they may have an altered perception of pain, particularly in their extremities, it is essential to assess for any signs of sores or infections. It is also important to ask about tingling, numbness, or swelling of the extremities. Patients with long-standing diabetes may have undergone amputation, and their residual limb may become infected or septic.

Ask the patient about any vision changes, headaches, dizziness, bleeding, or sores in the mouth. Also ask whether there has been a recent change in the patient's bowel movements or eating habits.

Evidence-Based Medicine

Research suggests that lethal cardiac dysrhythmias may be triggered by hypoglycemia and may lead to the sudden death of patients with type 1 diabetes who experience hypoglycemia.[11]

Management

Type 1 diabetes always requires insulin administered by injection or an insulin pump, also called continuous subcutaneous insulin infusion therapy. Insulin cannot be ingested orally because the digestive process will render it inactive.

You will likely encounter patients with diabetes who use insulin pumps to treat their disease. An alternative to multiple daily injections of insulin, insulin pumps provide improved control of blood glucose levels and better quality of life for many patients. These small devices consist of an infusion set, a reservoir for insulin, and the pump itself. The pump is approximately the size of a deck of cards, weighs approximately 3 ounces, and can be worn on a belt or carried in a pocket **FIGURE 24-3**. Insulin is administered through a catheter under the skin. The pump is often set to deliver a basal amount of insulin continuously throughout the day. Alternatively, the pump can be set to deliver a bolus of insulin at specific times such as mealtimes, when blood glucose levels are high.

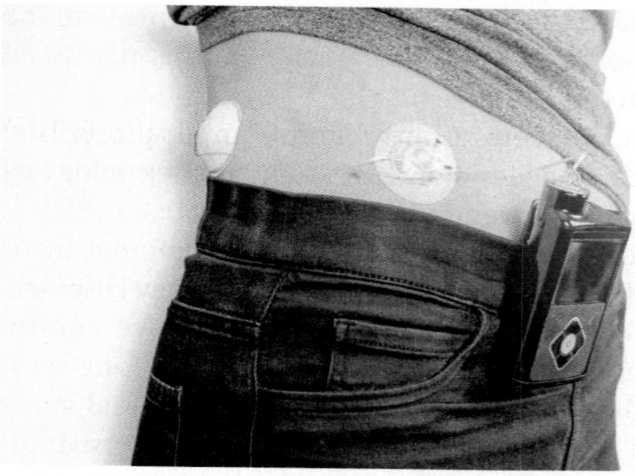

FIGURE 24-3 An insulin pump is a small electronic device that automatically delivers insulin to maintain the desired blood glucose level.

Several different types of insulin are available in the United States: rapid-acting insulin, regular or short-acting insulin, intermediate-acting insulin, and long-acting insulin. The various types differ in their onset of action, duration, and peak time. All of the US versions of insulin are synthetic; however, animal insulin can be imported.

Type 2 Diabetes Mellitus

Pathophysiology

The most common form of diabetes is *type 2 diabetes*, a condition in which blood glucose levels are elevated because the body cannot produce enough insulin to compensate for the inability to utilize insulin effectively. In many people with type 2 diabetes, the pancreas actually produces enough insulin; however, for reasons not fully understood, the body cannot effectively use it—a condition known as **insulin resistance**. One possible explanation is that the insulin receptors located on the target cells have changed in some way and are no longer able to receive the insulin when it arrives at the target cell.

In some cases, an abnormal increase in the liver's glucose production causes an increase in blood glucose levels. Typically, when blood glucose and insulin levels are low, the pancreas releases glucagon and stimulates the liver to produce and release glucose into the blood. In some people, however, the levels of glucagon stay high. When glucagon levels remain high, excess amounts of glucose are produced, leading to high blood glucose levels. Metformin, the medication most commonly prescribed for the management of type 2 diabetes, causes a decrease in glucose production.

According to the World Health Organization, 8.5% of the world's population is affected by diabetes, mostly type 2, making it a global health concern.[12] Approximately 90% to 95% of all people with diabetes in the United States have type 2 diabetes, which typically develops in middle-aged adults.[1] The development of type 2 diabetes has been associated with obesity and physical inactivity, two characteristics becoming more common in today's younger population. Type 2 diabetes may also be related to *metabolic syndrome*, a cluster of characteristics including excessive fat in the abdominal area, elevated BP, and high blood lipid levels. Risk factors for developing metabolic syndrome include excess weight, lack of physical activity, and genetic factors.

Assessment

Symptoms of type 2 diabetes may include the following:

- Fatigue
- Nausea
- Frequent urination
- Thirst
- Unexplained weight loss
- Blurred vision
- Frequent infections and slow healing of wounds
- Being cranky, confused, or shaky
- Unresponsiveness
- Seizure

These symptoms tend to develop gradually and usually become noticeable in middle age. In fact, the onset of type 2 diabetes may be so subtle that patients may not realize they have the disease. In some instances, the symptoms can develop over several years in overweight adults older than 40 years. A small percentage of patients do not display any symptoms.

Management

Weight loss is an essential factor in helping to control type 2 diabetes. Exercise and a well-balanced, nutritious diet are vital components in combating the complications of diabetes. Food intake must be spread throughout the day in coordination with daily medications/insulin injections to maintain glucose levels within the normal range. You can help patients by reinforcing this message to the patient and by helping the family understand how to reduce the patient's risk of diabetic complications.

Oral medications indicated to manage type 2 diabetes can be used alone or in combination because they exhibit different mechanisms of action. As with all medications, there is always the risk of interaction with other medications. A physician or pharmacist should be consulted before adding any medication, whether an over-the-counter or prescription agent, to the patient's treatment regimen. Oral antidiabetic agents are discussed in Chapter 15, *Emergency Medications.*

Evidence-Based Medicine

According to the National Institutes of Health, most of the genetic risk for type 2 diabetes can be attributed to common, shared genetic variants—each contributing a small amount to a patient's overall risk of the disease—rather than to rare variants unique to a single patient.[12] This multifactorial nature resolves a question about the genetics of type 2 diabetes that has puzzled researchers for decades. It suggests the need to account for both environmental factors and the patient's genetic profile when developing a plan of treatment or prevention.[13]

Street Smarts

New-onset weakness in a patient known to have diabetes must be considered a myocardial infarction until proved otherwise. Many patients with either type 1 or type 2 diabetes have an acquired dysfunction in the peripheral nervous system (neuropathy). Also, increased insulin levels result in increased blood lipid levels. This combination often leads to an earlier onset of coronary artery disease. Note that people with diabetes do not always have typical clinical symptoms of acute coronary syndrome because of an alteration in sensation; instead, they are more likely to present with general body weakness.

Prediabetes

Prediabetes is a condition identified in people who have certain risk factors associated with type 2 diabetes. It exists when blood glucose levels or hemoglobin A1c levels are higher than normal, yet not high enough to be diagnosed as diabetes. The A1c blood test reveals information regarding the patient's blood glucose levels over the previous 3 months. A normal A1c level is less than 5.7%, prediabetes is diagnosed with an A1c level between 5.7% and 6.4%, and type 2 diabetes is diagnosed with an A1c level greater than 6.4%.

According to the CDC, prediabetes affects 1 out of 3 adults in the United States, or approximately 88 million people, and 84% are unaware of their status.[14,15] Within 5 years of developing prediabetes and with no intervention, many people will be diagnosed with type 2 diabetes. Risk factors for experiencing this disease course include the following characteristics:[16]

- Being overweight
- Being older than 45 years of age
- Having a parent or sibling with type 2 diabetes
- Being physically active fewer than three times per week
- Giving birth to a baby who weighed more than 9 pounds (4 kg)
- Having a history of diabetes while pregnant (gestational diabetes)
- Having polycystic ovary syndrome

Although some of the risk factors affecting the pathway from prediabetes to type 2 diabetes cannot be altered, others can. According to the CDC, interventions affecting two specific factors can help prevent or delay the onset of type 2 diabetes by 58%: (1) losing 5% to 7% of the patient's body weight and (2) getting at least 150 minutes of physical activity per week.[16]

Words of Wisdom

The hemoglobin A1c test does not require fasting and can be performed at any time of the day. Unfortunately, it can be inaccurate in people of African, Mediterranean, or Southeast Asian descent and in individuals with a family history of sickle cell anemia. People with kidney or liver failure may also have inaccurate A1c results.

Gestational Diabetes

Pathophysiology

Gestational diabetes does not have a pancreatic component, but rather is a form of glucose intolerance that can occur during pregnancy. This condition has been identified more often in African American, Hispanic/Latino, and Native American populations and in women with obesity or who have a family history of diabetes. Women who experience gestational diabetes during pregnancy have a 40% to 60% increased risk of developing type 2 diabetes within 1 decade.[17,18] For most women, gestational diabetes will resolve before delivery. In a few women, however, diabetes will not resolve or type 2 diabetes will develop.

Blood glucose crosses the placental barrier. When a pregnant woman is hyperglycemic, high levels of glucose enter the fetus, causing increased insulin production by the fetus in an attempt to normalize blood glucose levels. The extra glucose is converted into fat in the fetus, such that women experiencing gestational diabetes often deliver large babies (macrosomia) and may encounter difficult deliveries. Often, cesarean sections are required.

Gestational diabetes is usually diagnosed at 28 weeks' gestation and peaks in the third trimester of pregnancy. It is thought that two hormones produced by the placenta, progesterone and estrogen, result in increased sensitivity to insulin. Because this condition does not occur until later in pregnancy, it does not produce congenital disabilities. Infants of mothers in whom gestational diabetes developed are at higher risk for obesity and diabetes in their lifetime.

Assessment

The oral glucose tolerance test is used to diagnose gestational diabetes. This test should be used until the pregnant woman is within 12 weeks of delivery. The hemoglobin A1c test can be used during the first pregnancy visit to identify the presence of preexisting diabetes or prediabetes.

Management

Management of gestational diabetes should be initiated as soon as possible to stabilize blood glucose levels and minimize potential complications to both mother and baby. Management includes diet modification, exercise, and blood glucose testing. Oral medications are not prescribed for this form of diabetes, but insulin injections may be required.

Hypoglycemia

Normal blood glucose levels range from approximately 60 to 120 mg/dL; *hypoglycemia* (a low blood glucose level) occurs when blood glucose levels drop to 45 mg/dL or less. Hypoglycemia is a common problem associated with both type 1 and type 2 diabetes. These patients must closely monitor and intensively control their diabetes to prevent long-term complications. According to the CDC, approximately 235,000 US emergency department (ED) visits made by adults 18 years or older in 2016 involved hypoglycemia as the diagnosis.[4]

Although hypoglycemia is relatively common and not completely preventable, it can be treated easily. This condition can be detected with regular blood glucose monitoring and rarely results in complications for the patient.

In contrast, severe hypoglycemia, resulting in loss of consciousness or altered mental status, is a more common reason for a call to 9-1-1, and requires intervention and treatment. As an EMS professional, you will need to promptly provide treatment to these patients. If untreated or not detected, serious hypoglycemia can lead to coma or death.

Pathophysiology

Hypoglycemia in people with type 1 diabetes often results from having taken too much insulin, too little food, or both. Many body tissues can usually metabolize fat or protein in addition to sugar. However, central nervous system tissues (including the brain) depend entirely on glucose as their energy source. If the glucose level in the blood drops dramatically, the brain is literally starved.

Counter-regulation is the body's natural defensive ability geared toward maintaining blood glucose at an appropriate level. Understanding this concept is critical, as it will help you treat (and ideally prevent) severe hypoglycemia.

The body's first line of defense against low blood glucose is to reduce insulin production by the pancreas and to increase glucagon production by the alpha cells. The body's second line of defense is the adrenal gland's secretion of catecholamines, including epinephrine and norepinephrine. The effects of this catecholamine release can be seen in the hypoglycemic patient as tachycardia and diaphoresis. The second line of defense also includes production of cortisol, an adrenocorticoid (ie, a steroid produced in the adrenal gland). Cortisol release leads to an increased level of glucose in the blood, which in turn counteracts insulin's actions. Other hormones produced by the intestine and growth hormone produced by the pituitary gland also increase blood glucose levels.

Lastly, stimulation of the autonomic nervous system generates signals that allow production of counter-regulatory hormones to increase. The same stimulation also triggers symptoms telling the body that the blood glucose level is low; ideally, the affected patient will recognize these symptoms and consume a source of sugar to remedy the imbalance. In response to the actions of these hormones, the body mobilizes fatty acids and amino acids from adipose and muscle, respectively. The liver uses these products to make new glucose for the body in a process called *gluconeogenesis.*

In patients with type 1 diabetes, the islets of Langerhans do not make insulin. As a result, the body's first line of defense against hypoglycemia is lost because it cannot decrease insulin levels via this mechanism. A low blood glucose level in a patient with diabetes is often caused by an elevated level of exogenous insulin from inaccurate dosing, intentional overdose, or perhaps a mismatch between carbohydrate intake and exogenous insulin intake. In addition, increased use of glucose, such as occurs during exercise, may cause the blood glucose level to drop sharply, resulting in hypoglycemia.

In patients with type 2 diabetes, the pancreas can generate insulin, so these patients can suppress insulin production from within their own bodies. However, their bodies may be resistant to the effects of insulin, or they may not make enough insulin over time to lower the blood glucose level adequately. Medications given to treat type 2 diabetes act by either stimulating the body's ability to secrete insulin or by improving insulin's actions. These medications also tend to contribute to hypoglycemia, especially in patients such as older adults and those who are not metabolizing these medications properly because of liver or kidney disease. Often, if the hypoglycemia is caused by excessive insulin dosing by the patient or by the prolonged or exaggerated effects of oral diabetes medications, the low blood glucose level will have a prolonged effect and more long-term treatment may be needed.

In some patients who have had type 1 diabetes for many years, and to a lesser degree in patients who have had type 2 diabetes for many years, the pancreas may not release glucagon in response to hypoglycemia.[19] Lack of glucagon response makes the body more dependent on epinephrine to overcome the effects of hypoglycemia, yet the diabetic patient's body may not respond to epinephrine normally.[20,21] Prolonged disease can also decrease a patient's ability to recognize the presence of a low blood glucose level (a state called *hypoglycemic unawareness*), preventing them from taking the necessary self-treatment measures.

Assessment

A patient with hypoglycemia will tremble, have a rapid pulse rate, sweat, and feel hungry. The brain is highly sensitive to glucose levels, so the signs and symptoms associated with this condition reflect the disordered function of the brain cells and the alarm reaction (sympathetic nervous system discharge) set off by the brain's distress signals. If hypoglycemia persists, cerebral dysfunction progresses quickly to permanent brain damage.

The most common signs and symptoms of hypoglycemia include the following:

- Blood glucose level less than 60 mg/dL
- Hunger
- Agitation, irritability, or combative behavior that cannot be explained
- Altered mentation or confusion
- Nausea
- Weakness
- Tachycardia
- Cool, clammy skin

Additional signs and symptoms associated with hypoglycemia include headache, memory loss, incoordination, slurred speech, dilated pupils, and seizures and coma in severe cases.

Hypoglycemia develops *rapidly,* over a period ranging from minutes to a few hours, and should be suspected in any patient with diabetes who presents with bizarre behavior, neurologic signs, or coma. Often the hypoglycemic patient appears intoxicated because of slurred speech and lack of coordination and may be paranoid, hostile, and aggressive.

Of course, people with diabetes are not the only ones likely to have hypoglycemic episodes. Patients with alcoholism, patients who have ingested certain poisons or overdosed with certain drugs (notably aspirin), and patients with certain cancers, liver disease, kidney disease, and some other conditions may also experience hypoglycemic episodes. Do not discount the possibility of hypoglycemia in a comatose patient just because the patient is not known to have diabetes. Conversely, do not let a known diagnosis of diabetes prevent you from considering other causes of coma. People with diabetes can also experience head injury, stroke, seizures, meningitis, and other traumatic injuries or conditions. Keep an open mind and assess the patient thoroughly.

Words of Wisdom

The longer a patient remains unconscious from hypoglycemia, the more likely it becomes that permanent brain damage will occur! If more than 20 to 30 minutes pass, toxic compounds (free radicals) in the brain are produced that can cause permanent neuronal damage. Therefore, once you have determined that a patient has a low blood glucose level, you must fix it right away. Do not wait until after you have moved the patient to the ambulance, or until you are en route to the ED.

SAFETY

A patient experiencing a hypoglycemic event may be confused with a patient having a stroke. D_{50} is contraindicated in stroke in the presence of normal blood glucose levels. Thus, the blood glucose level should be assessed and verified carefully in patients with signs associated with stroke before administering D_{50}. The hypertonic properties of D_{50} may result in increased cerebral edema in the event of a cerebrovascular event.

Management

Management of hypoglycemia includes immediately increasing blood glucose levels, with the precise treatment depending on several factors. It is always preferable to implement the least invasive treatment method possible that will successfully address the condition.

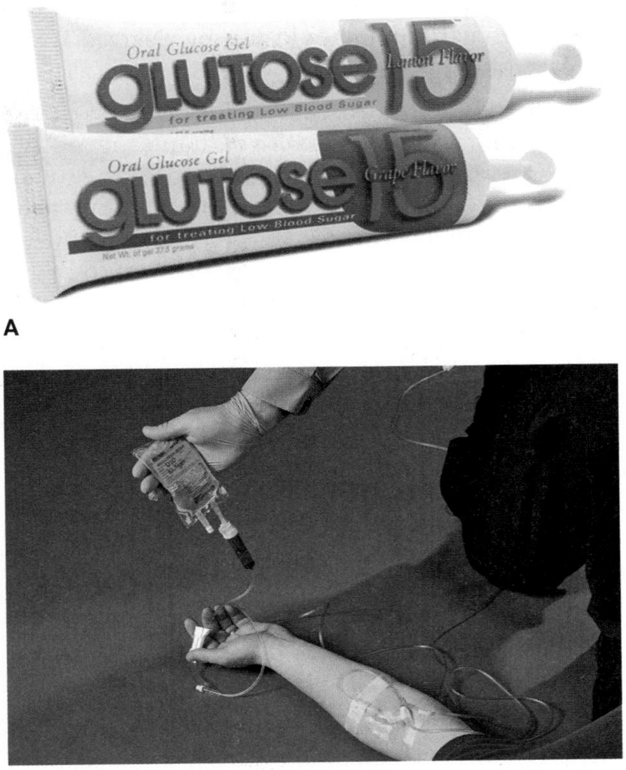

A

B

FIGURE 24-4 Administering glucose is appropriate in diabetic emergencies unless you have a reliable blood glucose measurement indicating normal or high blood glucose levels. Available forms include oral glucose paste **(A)** and glucose solution for intravenous infusion **(B)**.

Measure the patient's blood glucose level, especially if you are treating an older adult or a patient whose clinical history suggests that the problem may be stroke; administration of concentrated glucose solutions in a suspected stroke situation may exacerbate cerebral damage **FIGURE 24-4**. When the comatose patient is older than 55 years or the family reports a history of recent transient ischemic attacks, perform a field glucose test to rule out hypoglycemia.

A field glucose test involves obtaining a small amount of blood and using a blood glucose monitor to determine the patient's blood glucose level. This test is summarized here. It is discussed in detail in Chapter 11, *Patient Assessment.*

1. Take appropriate infection control precautions.
2. Verify the device is calibrated appropriately.
3. Clean the site to be punctured with alcohol.
4. Allow the patient's arm to hang briefly to allow blood to flow to the fingertips.
5. Grasp the finger near the area to be pricked (the side of the finger is less painful to prick than the top) and squeeze for 3 seconds.
6. Use a sterile lancet device and quickly prick the side of the fingertip. Apply adequate pressure to puncture the skin.
7. Properly dispose of the lancet.
8. Keep the hand down, and squeeze gently until you obtain a drop of blood. Be careful not to squeeze too hard.
9. Place a sterile dressing on the wound as needed.
10. Apply the blood to the test strips according to the manufacturer's instructions.
11. Accurately read and document the results.

If the patient is alert, can swallow, and has an intact gag reflex, encourage the patient to take glucose tablets. If glucose tablets are not available, household sources of glucose may be used. For example, you may administer sugar by mouth. Provide a candy bar, a glass of warm water to which a few teaspoons of sugar have been added, or a non-diet cola drink—any of those should improve the patient's condition. An unresponsive patient should *never* be given oral glucose or anything by mouth because of the risk of choking and aspiration.

If the patient has an altered level of consciousness or you are potentially unable to manage the airway, aspiration may result with administration of oral substances. In that case, you will need to manage the airway and breathing as you would with any patient with an altered level of consciousness. Placement of an advanced airway should be avoided until the patient has received dextrose. If the patient remains unresponsive, an advanced airway can be considered.

SAFETY

Before you give a conscious patient glucose tablets, anything to eat or drink, or instant glucose, you must ensure that there is no danger of aspiration. One rule of thumb: If patients can lift the cup or squirt the glucose into their own mouths, they are most likely not in danger of aspiration. Watch them carefully!

The steps for performing an IV infusion are covered in Chapter 14, *Medication Administration.* To administer dextrose to a patient with altered level of consciousness, follow these steps:

1. Insert an IV line and ensure it is patent. An 18-gauge catheter is preferable in a large vein due to the viscosity of dextrose. If you are using D_{50}, note that this solution is hypertonic and acidic, so any extravasation may lead to tissue necrosis.
2. Administer a 0.9% NS flush of 10 to 20 mL to confirm patency of the IV line.
3. Administer 50% dextrose [D_{50}], 25% dextrose, or 10% dextrose [D_{10}]) at a dose per your local protocols over a minimum of 3 minutes while continuously assessing the patient's response.
4. If the coma is caused by hypoglycemia, the patient will often awaken rapidly. In cases of severe hypoglycemia, another dose of D_{50} may be required to restore a normal level of consciousness.

If the patient has a decreased level of consciousness and you are unable to obtain a patent IV line, administer glucagon IM or IN in adults. Hypoglycemia is a life-threatening event, and glucose administration should not be delayed if you cannot establish an IV line.

Glucagon increases blood glucose levels and relaxes the smooth muscle located in the gastrointestinal tract if administered parenterally. Patients with type 1 diabetes may not experience as great an increase in blood glucose levels as those with stable type 2 diabetes. Therefore, patients with type 1 diabetes require immediate access to oral carbohydrates or additional glucose administration. See Chapter 15, *Emergency Medications*, for more information on glucagon.

Hyperglycemia and Diabetic Ketoacidosis

According to the CDC, approximately 224,000 ED visits made by adults in the United States in 2016 involved a hyperglycemic crisis.[1]

Pathophysiology

Hyperglycemia (a high blood glucose level) is one of the classic symptoms of diabetes mellitus. Typical

YOU are the Paramedic

PART 4

As you administer dextrose, you notice the patient begins to look around. After a few minutes, she says, "Oh! That one snuck up on me!" She tells you that she has type 1 diabetes, and she felt her blood glucose level dropping. She tried to open her package of glucose tablets, and that was the last thing she remembers. You assist her from the refrigerator case and reassess her vital signs, including her blood glucose level, which is now 120 mg/dL.

The patient's 21-year-old son arrives. The patient tells you, "Thanks very much. I'll be fine now." After discussing the case with medical control and receiving their agreement to leave the patient with her son, you inform dispatch that the patient refused further treatment and transport and that your medic unit is now available for calls. You assist the patient to the food court, where she orders a hamburger and fries.

Recording Time: 10 Minutes	
Respirations	20 breaths/min; regular
Pulse	90 beats/min, regular
Skin	Slightly cool, pale, diaphoretic
Blood pressure	156/92 mm Hg
Oxygen saturation (Spo_2)	98% on room air
Pupils	PERRLA

7. Which challenges often occur on calls such as this one?

8. How would you document this patient contact?

early signs include frequent and excessive thirst accompanied by frequent and excessive urination. Hyperglycemia occurs when blood glucose levels exceed the normal range (60 to 120 mg/dL). In patients with diabetes, physicians try to maintain glucose levels at less than 160 mg/dL. Hyperglycemia can be caused by excessive food intake, insufficient insulin dosages, infection or illness, injury, surgery, and emotional stress. Reassess the patient frequently for the presence of these underlying causes so that definitive treatment can be given. Onset may be rapid (within minutes) or gradual (hours to days), depending on the cause. For example, excessive food intake may cause blood glucose to rise quickly, whereas an infection or illness will result in hyperglycemia over several days.

Other causes of hyperglycemia include the *dawn phenomenon* and the *Somogyi effect*. The dawn phenomenon occurs in the hours before waking. As the body prepares for a new day, it releases hormones such as cortisol and catecholamines. These hormones trigger a release of glucose from the liver, resulting in hyperglycemia. In contrast, the Somogyi effect occurs when a low blood glucose level generates a release of hormones that then trigger a release of glucose from the liver, causing hyperglycemia.

Some patients with type 2 diabetes may go undiagnosed for several years. Over time, however, repeated hyperglycemia episodes will cause several physiologic changes that have detrimental long-term effects. Largely because of the increased hyperosmolarity it causes, hyperglycemia puts undue strain on the cardiovascular system, kidneys, and other end organs that are sensitive to increased serum viscosity and the subsequent pressures exerted by the thicker serum. The eventual result is an increased incidence of renal failure, heart failure, retinopathy, coronary artery disease, and neuropathy.

When serum glucose levels rise above tolerable levels, other physiologic changes occur. These changes signal the presence of actual pathologic conditions called diabetic ketoacidosis (blood glucose level greater than approximately 350 mg/dL) and **hyperosmolar hyperglycemic nonketotic syndrome (HHNS)** (blood glucose level greater than approximately 600 mg/dL) **FIGURE 24-5**.

DKA is associated predominately with type 1 diabetes. A life-threatening condition, it occurs when certain acids accumulate in the body because insulin is not available. Common causes of DKA include

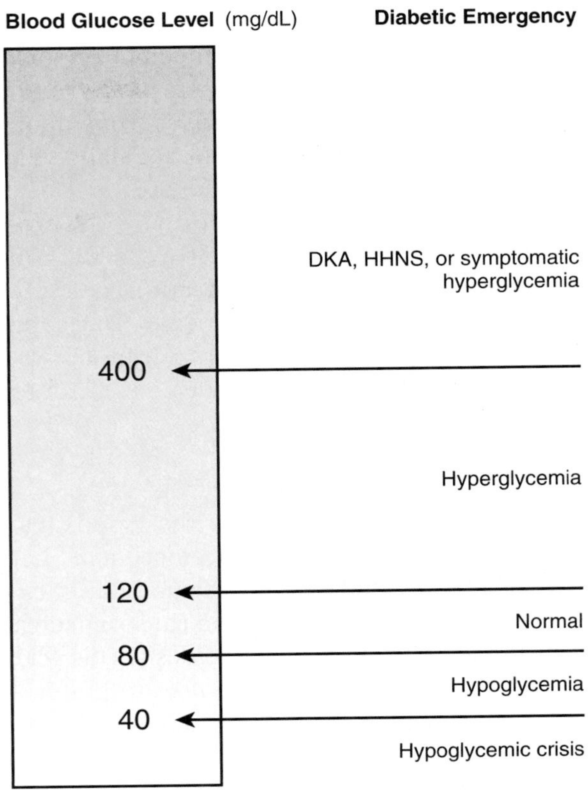

FIGURE 24-5 The two most common diabetic emergencies, diabetic ketoacidosis and hypoglycemic crisis, occur when the patient has too much or too little glucose in the blood, respectively. The left column illustrates blood glucose levels; the right column illustrates the conditions associated with that particular level of blood glucose. Notice that the normal range is rather small in comparison with the other ranges.

(*Abbreviations*: DKA, diabetic ketoacidosis; HHNS, hyperosmolar hyperglycemic syndrome).

infection, injury, alcohol use, emotional distress, and illness such as stroke or myocardial infarction. Patients who have this condition tend to be young—teenagers and young adults.

In patients with DKA, hyperglycemia continues—that is, glucose continues to accumulate in the blood. Eventually, the patient undergoes massive osmotic diuresis (passing large amounts of urine because of the high solute concentration of the blood); this, together with vomiting, causes dehydration and even shock.

In DKA, a deficiency of insulin prevents cells from taking up the extra glucose. The cells are starving, and a distress signal goes out over the sympathetic nervous system, causing the release of various stress hormones. Because the body cannot use glucose, it turns instead to other energy sources—principally, fat. The metabolism of fat generates *acids* and *ketones* as waste products. (The ketone bodies give the characteristic fruity odor to the breath of a patent in DKA, but not all providers can detect this odor.) Because glucose must be excreted in the urine in solution, the body loses excessive amounts of water and electrolytes (sodium and potassium), which may lead to disturbances in water balance and acid–base balance. (Disturbances in acid-base balance and the compensatory role of the kidneys are covered in more detail in Chapter 9, *Pathophysiology*.)

Fatty acids are broken down primarily by the mitochondria in liver cells. As part of this process, ketone bodies are released into the bloodstream. Ketone bodies consist of acetoacetate, beta-hydroxybutyrate, and acetone. Large quantities of ketone bodies in the bloodstream cause a decrease in the blood's pH and result in acidosis. This acidosis then triggers the body's attempts to buffer the acidity with bicarbonate (HCO_3^-), and the blood pH decreases because of the inability to keep up with the ongoing acidity. In addition to fat tissue breaking down its stores of energy, muscle tissue mobilizes its stores to create more glucose for the body. This process creates amino acids that the liver may use to make glucose (gluconeogenesis). Lactate levels in the bloodstream also increase, which contributes to lowering the body's pH level.

In patients with type 2 diabetes, DKA is rare because insulin is still present, at least early in the disease. Despite the elevated blood glucose levels, the insulin level is sufficient to prevent the uncontrolled breakdown of glycogen, adipose tissue, and muscle. In all patients with type 2 diabetes, regardless of the duration of the disease, ketone bodies can be found in the urine when the patient experiences hyperglycemia. With increased duration of type 2 diabetes, a loss of pancreatic insulin production may occur. In fact, patients can develop elevated serum ketone levels, reduced blood pH, and DKA—much like patients with type 1 diabetes.

Assessment

A hyperglycemic condition without other classic symptoms is not conclusive evidence of the presence of diabetes mellitus. That is, hyperglycemia can be an independent medical condition with other causes.

The signs and symptoms of hypoglycemia and hyperglycemia can be similar **TABLE 24-1**. The signs and symptoms of simple hyperglycemia are usually mild, if present at all. They may include blurred vision, polyuria, polydipsia, polyphagia, orthostatic syncope, frequent infections, and skin ulcerations. If you encounter a patient with simple hyperglycemia who has not progressed to a more serious syndrome, treatment should include supportive care and transport.

Hyperglycemia usually progresses slowly, over 12 to 48 hours, with the patient's level of consciousness deteriorating only gradually. The higher-than-normal load of glucose present within the kidneys during hyperglycemia results in glucose spilling into the urine, causing the body to become hyperosmotic. As the kidneys remove the excess glucose, water is removed via increased urination, leading to dehydration. The kidneys also help clear ketone bodies from the blood. Along with the substantial amount of water lost through diuresis, patients lose excessive amounts of sodium, potassium, and phosphates in the urine. This combination of effects leads to both dehydration and metabolic acidosis with associated electrolyte imbalances.

The resulting signs and symptoms reflect these etiologic factors:

- Polyuria (excessive urine output), because of osmotic diuresis
- Polydipsia (excessive thirst), because of dehydration
- Polyphagia (excessive eating), probably related to inefficient utilization of nutrients
- Nausea and vomiting, with the latter worsening the patient's dehydration
- Tachycardia, as a consequence of dehydration
- Deep, rapid respirations (Kussmaul respirations)—the body's attempt to compensate for acidosis by blowing off carbon dioxide (CO_2)
- Warm, dry skin and dry mucous membranes, also reflecting dehydration
- Fruity odor of ketones (acetone smell) on the breath
- Abdominal pain
- Sometimes fever

Patients usually appear thin or dehydrated and have warm, dry skin. Some may exhibit orthostatic hypotension, supine hypotension, fatigue, altered mental status, and, with time, weight loss from the

TABLE 24-1 Comparison of Hypoglycemia and Hyperglycemia

	Hypoglycemia	Hyperglycemia: Diabetic Ketoacidosis[a]	Hyperglycemia: HHNS[b]
Food intake	Insufficient	Excessive	Excessive
Insulin dosage	Excessive	Insufficient	Insufficient
Onset	Rapid, within minutes	Gradual—hours to days	Gradual—days to weeks
Skin	Pale and moist	Warm and dry	Warm and dry
Infection	Uncommon	Common	Usual
Thirst	Absent	Intense	Very intense
Hunger	Intense	Excessive	Excessive
Vomiting	Uncommon	Common	Uncommon
Breathing	Normal or rapid	Rapid, deep (Kussmaul respirations)	Tachypnea
Odor of breath	Normal	Sweet, fruity (nail polish remover/acetone smell)	No ketone bodies are produced; therefore, there is no fruity odor
Blood pressure	Low	Normal to low	Hypotension
Pulse	Rapid, weak	Normal or rapid and full	Rapid, weak
Level of consciousness	Irritability, confusion, seizure, or coma	Restless merging to coma	Restless merging to coma
Urine: Sugar	Absent	Present	Present
Urine: Acetone	Absent	Present	Absent
Blood glucose level (mg/dL)	<60	>250	>600
Response to treatment	Immediately after administration of glucose	Gradual, within 6 to 12 hours following medical treatment	

Abbreviation: HHNS, hyperosmolar hyperglycemic nonketotic syndrome.

[a] Usually associated with type 1 diabetes.
[b] Usually associated with type 2 diabetes.

hypermetabolic state. However, patients in DKA are seldom deeply comatose; thus, if the patient is unresponsive, look for another source of the coma, such as head injury, stroke, or drug overdose.

In patients with DKA, the respiratory rate is usually elevated and the tidal volume is increased (Kussmaul respirations) because of **ketonemia** (excess amounts of ketone bodies in the blood), acidosis, and the body's attempt to relieve itself of the excessive burden of CO_2. These respiratory changes result in hypocapnia, which can be recognized by lower than normal end-tidal CO_2 levels. Because end-tidal CO_2 levels are affected, capnography is another tool you can use to confirm your diagnosis. DKA results in both Kussmaul respirations and metabolic acidosis; a capnography value less than 25 mm Hg corroborates your suspicions.[22]

There is no predictable correlation between the increase in a patient's blood glucose level and the degree of ketoacidosis in the blood. Rely on the patient's clinical presentation rather than on test results to assess this condition.

Management

The treatment of DKA in the field depends on making the correct diagnosis. If the patient's history and physical exam are consistent with DKA and your field measurement of the patient's glucose level reveals that it is markedly elevated (more than 250 mg/dL), the physician will probably order treatment for DKA. Prehospital treatment goals are to begin rehydration and correct the patient's electrolyte and acid-base abnormalities. In most instances, specific treatment with insulin should await the patient's arrival at the hospital, where therapy can be closely monitored with laboratory determinations of blood glucose and ketone levels.

Follow the procedure for any comatose patient with regard to airway maintenance and oxygen. Be particularly alert for vomiting, and have suction ready.

- Start an IV line and infuse up to 1 L of NS during the first half-hour or at the rate suggested by your local protocol or online medical control. Remember, a patient in DKA is severely dehydrated, often to the point of shock, and needs volume, usually at a rate of about 1 L/h for at least the first few hours. (See Chapter 44, *Pediatric Emergencies*, for information specific to treatment of pediatric patients.)
- If the patient is hypotensive, rapidly administer isotonic fluids until the systolic pressure is 80 mm Hg, then slow the infusion. As with any patient in whom fluid boluses are being administered, closely monitor the patient for the development of pulmonary edema.
- Monitor cardiac rhythm. Changes in serum potassium caused by DKA can lead to marked myocardial instability. Note the contour of the T waves on the rhythm strip; if they are sharply peaked, the patient's potassium level may be dangerously high. Sodium bicarbonate ($NaHCO_3$) may be administered, typically in the ED, after laboratory tests confirm the presence of hyperkalemia. As potassium levels rise, the QRS complex will widen and may blend with the T wave, and the heart rate may become bradycardic. At this point, management with calcium chloride or gluconate may be indicated to antagonize potassium at the receptor site. If you are ordered to administer calcium, proceed with caution—even a slight excess can cause serious problems or death.

Controversies

The administration of $NaHCO_3$ as part of the management of metabolic acidosis in DKA remains controversial. $NaHCO_3$ is generally not considered unless the patient's pH is less than 7.0. $NaHCO_3$ should not be used in a prehospital setting and must be deemed necessary by the medical team. Arbitrary administration of $NaHCO_3$ can cause a paradoxical acidosis in the cerebrospinal fluid as well as several other complications that can worsen the patient's condition and outcome. The patient's vital signs should be closely monitored, including BP, heart rate, respiratory rate, and neurologic status.[23,24]

Hypomagnesemia (a low level of magnesium in the blood) is commonly associated with DKA due to the loss of magnesium through the urine. This electrolyte imbalance can worsen vomiting, cause alterations in mental status, induce other electrolyte abnormalities, and lead to potentially fatal cardiac dysrhythmias. Magnesium deficiency from DKA is generally not treated in the prehospital setting.

Complications of DKA are frequently associated with its management. The infusion of insulin can lead to hypoglycemia, so blood glucose levels should be monitored continuously. Hypokalemia may result when insulin shifts potassium into cells, lowering blood serum levels; therefore, management of hyperkalemia should be considered cautiously. Cerebral edema may occur if blood glucose levels shift too rapidly; however, this complication is more prevalent in pediatric patients, particularly newborns and premature infants. Children are less likely to have cardiovascular complications secondary to hyperkalemia.

Hyperosmolar Hyperglycemic Nonketotic Syndrome

Pathophysiology

Hyperosmolar hyperglycemic nonketotic syndrome (HHNS), formerly called hyperosmolar nonketotic coma (HONK) and sometimes called hyperosmolar hyperglycemic syndrome (HHS), is a metabolic derangement that occurs principally in patients with type 2 diabetes.[25–28] This condition is characterized by hyperglycemia, hyperosmolarity, and an absence of significant ketosis. The term *hyperosmolarity* describes highly concentrated blood as a result of relative dehydration. Key signs and symptoms of HHNS include the following:

- Hyperglycemia
- Altered mental status, drowsiness, and lethargy
- Severe dehydration, thirst, and dark urine
- Visual or sensory deficits
- Partial paralysis or muscle weakness
- Seizures

Oddly enough, fewer than 20% of patients with HHNS present in a comatose state.[29] Instead, most patients have severe dehydration and focal or global neurologic deficits. In addition, AMI is frequently associated with HHNS. The clinical features of HHNS and DKA tend to overlap and are often observed simultaneously.

TABLE 24-2 Comparison of Hyperglycemic Conditions

	HHNS	Diabetic Ketoacidosis
Glucose	>600 mg/dL	>250 mg/dL
Arterial pH	>7.3	<7.3
Ketone bodies	Absent	Present
Type of diabetes mellitus	Type 2	Type 1

Abbreviations: HHNS, hyperosmolar nonketotic hyperglycemic syndrome.

Street Smarts

Certain medications—including diuretics, beta blockers, and histamine-2 (H_2) blockers—as well as dialysis, total parenteral nutrition, and dextrose-containing fluids, may contribute to the development of HHNS by raising serum glucose levels, inhibiting insulin release, or causing dehydration. Hyperglycemia and hyperosmolarity lead to osmotic diuresis and an osmotic shift of fluid to the intravascular space, resulting in further intracellular dehydration.

HHNS often develops in patients with diabetes who have a secondary illness that leads to reduced fluid intake. Although infection (particularly pneumonia and urinary tract infection) is the most common cause, many other conditions can cause altered mentation or dehydration. In most cases, the secondary illness is not identified.

Assessment

Unlike patients with DKA, patients with HHNS do not experience ketoacidosis. The onset of DKA can occur in as little as a few hours, whereas HHNS may take several weeks to develop. Blood glucose levels tend to be substantially higher in HHNS as compared to DKA **TABLE 24-2**. Although most patients diagnosed with HHNS have a known history of diabetes (usually type 2), approximately 30% do not have a prior diagnosis of diabetes. The stress response to any acute illness tends to increase hormones that favor elevated glucose levels; cortisol, catecholamines (epinephrine and norepinephrine), glucagon, and many other hormones have effects that tend to counter those of insulin. Various neurologic changes may be found in patients with HHNS, including drowsiness and lethargy, delirium and coma, focal or generalized seizures, visual disturbances, hemiparesis, and sensory deficits.

Not all patients with increased blood glucose levels have DKA or HHNS. Many people have glucose intolerance and hyperglycemia with no symptoms. To determine the precise condition, look at the patient, not at the number.

Management

The treatment of HHNS in the prehospital setting follows the pathway for dehydration and altered mental status. Airway management is the priority because the comatose patient is often unable to maintain and protect their airway. For this reason, advanced airway management may be indicated and should be completed as early as possible. Spinal motion restriction should be used for all unresponsive patients found lying down, unless witnesses can validate that no fall occurred. Large-bore IV access should be gained as soon as possible, but do not delay transfer while initiating the IV line. If necessary, obtain IV access en route to the ED. Also, obtain a blood glucose level as soon as possible.

After you have initiated the IV line, a bolus of 500 mL 0.9% NS is appropriate for almost all clinically dehydrated adults. In patients with a history of congestive heart failure and/or renal insufficiency, a 250-mL bolus may be a more appropriate starting point. Fluid deficits in patients with HHNS may amount to 10 L or more. These patients may receive 1 to 2 L of fluids within the first hour of treatment.

Pathophysiology, Assessment, and Management of Other Disorders of the Pancreas

Pancreatitis

Pathophysiology

Pancreatitis—an inflammation of the pancreas—can occur as either an acute or a chronic condition, and is more common in men than in women. Acute pancreatitis is a medical emergency and can lead to dehydration and hypotension. The most common causes of pancreatitis are gallstones, which cause bile duct obstruction, and chronic alcohol abuse. Similarly, years of alcohol abuse is the most common cause of chronic pancreatitis. These two etiologies account for 60% to 80% of acute pancreatitis cases, with alcohol abuse being more common in younger patients and obstruction more common in older adults.[30,31] Other potential causes of pancreatitis include the use of certain medications, trauma, pancreatic cancer, and genetic predisposition.

Chronic pancreatitis refers to a progressive disease that destroys the pancreas, eventually leading to the loss of all endocrine and exocrine functions. It often causes chronic pain. Computed tomography is used to diagnosis the presence of this condition.

Assessment

Patients with acute pancreatitis present with what is described as a constant dull, boring flank and/or epigastric pain that worsens if the patient is placed in a supine position. Tachycardia, fever, and jaundice also can be present. Typically, a pancreatic attack is a result of a large, heavy meal or excessive drinking. Symptoms include nausea and vomiting, abdominal distention or muscle spasms, and less frequently, necrosis and organ failure. Laboratory tests used to diagnose acute pancreatitis include determinations of serum amylase, lipase, and trypsin, if available.

Management

After pancreatitis has been diagnosed, most patients are treated with supportive care. Patients should not eat until nausea and vomiting have subsided. They should be transported and pain management can be considered, although it is not always effective with pancreatitis. Endoscopic retrograde cholangiopancreatography is used for patients who have cholelithiasis. No other treatments have been shown to decrease pain or hospital stay length.

For patients with chronic pancreatitis, lifestyle changes, including dietary changes and termination of alcohol and tobacco use, are critical to treatment. Analgesics are used to control pain, pancreatic enzymes can help mitigate steatorrhea (excessive fat in the stool) and malabsorption, and ultimately surgical intervention may be considered. Patients should be monitored for pancreatic cancer because a higher incidence of this disease is noted in patients with chronic pancreatitis.

Words of Wisdom

Adenocarcinoma is a type of cancer that affects the epithelial cells lining glandular tissue. This type of cancer can affect the pancreas. Pancreatic cancer is a common cause of cancer death in the United States. Signs and symptoms, which are vague and nondifferential, include pain, weight loss, and jaundice. These manifestations usually are not present in the early stages of pancreatic cancer, making early diagnosis uncommon.

Cystadenoma refers to benign cysts that are present in glandular tissue and can affect the pancreas. Secretion function is maintained when a cyst is present; however, it may result in more cysts.

Neuroendocrine tumors affect the endocrine and nervous systems and begin in the endocrine-secreting cells. These tumors can be found anywhere in the body; however, gastroenteropancreatic endocrine tumors affect the gastrointestinal tract and the pancreas. These tumors are rare and slow growing.

Pathophysiology, Assessment, and Management of Adrenal Insufficiency

Adrenal insufficiency is characterized by decreased function of the adrenal cortex and consequent underproduction of cortisol and aldosterone. A decrease in either of these adrenal hormones will result in weakness, dehydration, and the body's inability to maintain adequate BP or to properly respond to stress.

Cortisol affects almost every organ and tissue in the body. Although its primary role is to assist with the body's response to stress, this adrenal hormone also helps maintain BP and cardiovascular function; regulates the metabolism of carbohydrates, proteins, and fats; modulates glucose levels in the blood by balancing the effects of insulin; and functions as an anti-inflammatory agent by slowing the inflammatory response.

The secretion of aldosterone is regulated chiefly by the renin–angiotensin system, but is also stimulated by increased serum potassium concentrations. Abnormal adrenal cortical function produces abnormalities in the metabolism of carbohydrates and protein as well as disturbances in salt and water metabolism.

Adrenal insufficiency is usually well tolerated unless the clinical picture is complicated by coexisting factors such as infection or stress. This condition affects approximately 4 people per 100,000 in the United States, occurs equally in men and women, and is found in patients of all races and ages. Adrenal insufficiency is classified as either primary or secondary.

Primary Adrenal Insufficiency

Pathophysiology

Primary adrenal insufficiency (also known as Addison disease) is caused by atrophy or destruction of both adrenal glands, leading to deficiencies of all steroid hormones produced by these glands. A rare disease (occurring in approximately 1 per 100,000 people in the United States), primary adrenal insufficiency is usually the result of idiopathic atrophy, an autoimmune process in which the immune system creates antibodies that attack the adrenal cortex, leading to its gradual destruction.[32] This phenomenon accounts for approximately 70% of all cases of Addison disease in the United States.[32] Adrenal insufficiency occurs when at least 90% of the adrenal cortex has been destroyed. Less commonly (approximately 30% of cases), the adrenal destruction is caused by tuberculosis; a bacterial, viral, or fungal infection; adrenal hemorrhage; or cancer of the adrenal glands.[32] Treatment can enable patients with Addison disease to have a normal life expectancy.

Assessment

Signs of chronic adrenal insufficiency include unexplained weight loss, fatigue, vomiting, diarrhea, anorexia, salt craving, muscle and joint pain, abdominal pain, postural dizziness, and increased pigmentation in the extensor surfaces, palmar creases, and oral mucosa **FIGURE 24-6**. In patients with Addison disease, the body improperly regulates the concentrations of sodium, potassium, and water in body fluids. Blood volume and BP fall, as does the blood's sodium concentration; blood potassium level rises. The blood volume may become reduced to such a low level that the circulation can no longer be maintained efficiently.

Management

Treatment of patients experiencing an adrenal crisis includes assessment and management of the ABCs. If needed, use the coma protocol of glucose, thiamine, and naloxone, as indicated. Aggressive

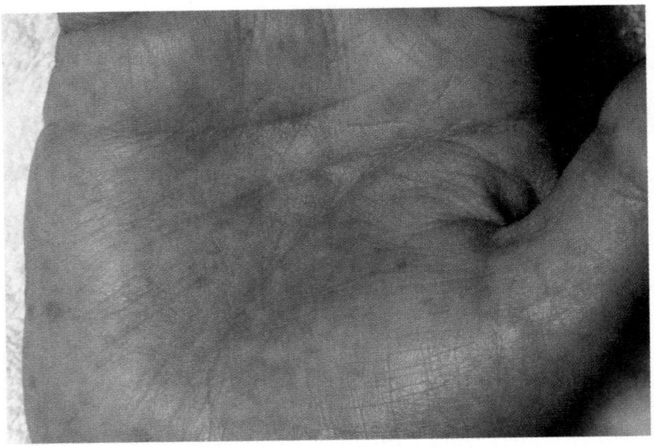

FIGURE 24-6 The hand of a patient with Addison disease.

fluid replacement using 5% dextrose in normal saline should be initiated. Hydrocortisone, 100 mg IV, is indicated in the acute management of a crisis. Electrolyte imbalances are common in patients with adrenal emergencies, but may not be evident in the prehospital environment.

Secondary Adrenal Insufficiency

Pathophysiology

Secondary adrenal insufficiency is a relatively common condition characterized by a lack of adrenocorticotropic hormone (ACTH) secretion from the pituitary gland. ACTH, a pituitary messenger, stimulates the adrenal cortex to manufacture and secrete cortisol. If ACTH secretion is insufficient, cortisol production is not stimulated. Patients who abruptly stop taking **corticosteroids** (eg, prednisone) may also experience secondary adrenal insufficiency. Corticosteroid treatments suppress natural cortical production; however, aldosterone production is usually not affected in this form of adrenal insufficiency.

Words of Wisdom

Although oral corticosteroid therapy is the most common cause of exogenous adrenal suppression, inhaled corticosteroids (used for asthma or chronic obstructive pulmonary disease) may have a similar effect.

Assessment

Signs and symptoms of acute adrenal insufficiency can appear suddenly, creating an **addisonian crisis**. An acute exacerbation of chronic insufficiency may trigger an addisonian crisis, usually brought on by stress, trauma, surgery, or severe infection. Corticosteroid withdrawal is the most common cause.

Although most patients with acute adrenal insufficiency have symptoms severe enough to prompt them to seek medical treatment before a crisis occurs, approximately 25% first experience symptoms during an addisonian crisis.[32] Shock is the chief clinical manifestation of adrenal crisis. Patients also may manifest nonspecific symptoms, including weakness; lethargy; confusion or loss of consciousness; low BP (vascular collapse); elevated temperature; severe pain in the lower back, legs, or abdomen; and severe vomiting and diarrhea that leads to dehydration.

Management

An unrecognized, untreated episode of acute adrenal insufficiency can be fatal. Death usually is attributable to hypotension or cardiac dysrhythmias caused by hyperkalemia. Treatment depends on the patient's clinical presentation and findings and is geared toward maintaining the ABCs until the patient's arrival at the ED. Regarding airway maintenance and supplemental oxygen, follow the procedure for a patient who has altered mental status or is comatose. Be alert for vomiting and have suction ready.

Other goals of prehospital treatment are to begin rehydrating the patient and to correct the electrolyte and acid-base abnormalities. Start an IV line and infuse up to 1 L of 0.9% NS. If the patient is hypotensive, administer an NS bolus at 20 mL/kg. Remember, a patient in adrenal insufficiency may be severely dehydrated, often to the point of shock, and needs fluid volume replenishment.

Check the patient's blood glucose level. Administer dextrose or glucose per your protocols to correct the hypoglycemia. Although D_5NS is the preferred IV fluid, it is rarely carried in the field. Administering D_5W through a second IV can help maintain the patient's blood glucose level. Monitor cardiac rhythm, because changes in serum electrolytes can lead to marked myocardial instability.

Pathophysiology, Assessment, and Management of Other Adrenal Emergencies

Cushing Syndrome

Pathophysiology

Cushing syndrome is caused by overproduction of cortisol by the adrenal glands or by excessive use of cortisol or other similar corticosteroid (glucocorticoid) hormones. Tumors of the pituitary gland or adrenal cortex can stimulate the production of excess hormone, for example, and lead to Cushing syndrome. Administration of large amounts of cortisol or other glucocorticoid hormones (eg, hydrocortisone, prednisone, methylprednisolone, or dexamethasone) to treat life-threatening illnesses, such as asthma, rheumatoid arthritis, systemic lupus, inflammatory bowel disease, and some allergies, can also cause this syndrome.

Regardless of the cause, excess cortisol causes characteristic changes in many body systems. Metabolism of carbohydrates, proteins, and fats is disturbed such that the blood glucose level rises. Protein synthesis is impaired so that body proteins are broken down, which leads to loss of muscle fibers and muscle weakness. Bones become weaker and more susceptible to fracture.

Assessment

Other common signs and symptoms related to excess cortisol include the following:

- Weakness and fatigue
- Depression and mood swings
- Increased thirst and urination
- High blood glucose level
- Weight gain, especially on the abdomen, face ("moon face"), neck, and upper back ("buffalo hump")
- Thinning of the skin, with easy bruising and pink or purple stretch marks (striae) on the abdomen, thighs, breasts, and shoulders
- Increased acne, facial hair growth, and scalp hair loss in women, and cessation of menstrual periods
- Darkening of skin (acanthosis) on the neck
- Obesity and poor growth in height in children

Management

Management is designed to decrease the level of cortisol in the body, which is difficult in the prehospital environment. Assess and manage the patient's ABCs and treat any life-threatening conditions immediately. Prehospital treatment is generally supportive. Obtain a blood glucose level.

Adrenal Gland Tumor

Pheochromocytoma is a rare condition of the adrenal gland in which a tumor, usually in the medulla, causes excessive release of the hormones epinephrine and norepinephrine. Approximately 10% of such tumors are malignant (cancerous).[33]

These tumors can occur at any age, but are most common in young adult to mid-adult life. A common clinical presentation involves a combination of symptoms (ie, hypertension, anxiety, chest pain, abdominal pain, fatigue, weight loss, vision problems, and sometimes seizures) that may be frequent but sporadic, and may increase in frequency, duration, and severity.

Pathophysiology, Assessment, and Management of Thyroid, Parathyroid, and Pituitary Gland Disorders

Growth Hormone Pathologies

The anterior pituitary gland secretes growth hormone. Problems associated with growth hormone secretion include both oversecretion or undersecretion, are rare, and usually result from a tumor. Oversecretion results in *acromegaly*, a condition usually diagnosed in young adulthood. This disease leads to gigantism and abnormally large hands and face, as well as specific facial characteristics: an enlarged jaw, and a brow and teeth that are abnormally widely spaced.[34] Undersecretion of growth hormone is a rare event and is characterized by delayed development and growth. A lack of treatment may lead to *dwarfism*.[35] Proportionate dwarfism presents with normal body proportions and mental functions.

Hypothyroidism and Hyperthyroidism

Approximately 20 million people in the United States have some kind of thyroid disorder, and many are unaware of their condition. Graves disease, the most common type of hyperthyroidism, increases metabolism. In contrast, hypothyroidism, often a result of autoimmune disease, decreases metabolism. **TABLE 24-3** summarizes the major effects of hypothyroidism and hyperthyroidism.

Patients with hyperthyroidism and hypothyroidism are likely to require supplemental oxygen. Hyperthyroid metabolic activity increases oxygen demand. Hypothyroid conditions may lead to diminished respiratory effort, such that patients may require positive-pressure ventilation.

TABLE 24-3 Comparison of the Major Effects of Hypothyroidism and Hyperthyroidism

	Hypothyroidism	Hyperthyroidism
Cardiovascular effects	Slow pulse, reduced cardiac output	Rapid pulse, increased cardiac output
Metabolic effects	Decreased metabolism, cold skin, weight gain	Increased metabolism, skin hot and flushed, weight loss
Neuromuscular effects	Weakness, sluggish reflexes	Tremor, hyperactive reflexes
Mental, emotional effects	Mental processes sluggish, personality placid	Restlessness, irritability, emotional lability
Gastrointestinal effects	Constipated	Diarrhea
General somatic effects	Cold, dry skin	Warm, moist skin

Graves Disease

The most severe and common cause of hyperthyroidism is Graves disease. This disorder is 10 times more common in women than in men; the overall incidence in women is 0.4 case per 1,000.[36] Graves disease tends to follow a chronic course of remission and relapse. If left untreated, it can be fatal.

Graves disease is an autoimmune disorder in which the thyroid gland hypertrophies, or enlarges, as its activity increases. The hypertrophied thyroid gland produces a visible mass called a **goiter** in the anterior part of the neck. The overactive gland secretes an excessive amount of thyroxine, causing the hyperthyroidism that characterizes Graves disease. In addition to the presence of a goiter, signs and symptoms of this condition include a substantially increased appetite with marked weight loss that may progress to cachexia (wasting of muscle and tissue). Patients also have polydipsia as a result of dehydration caused by diarrhea and excessive sweating. Some may present with exophthalmos, a condition caused by edema of the tissue behind the eyes. Another sign of Graves disease is **pretibial myxedema**, an "orange peel" appearance and nonpitting edema of the skin on the anterior part of the leg below the knee. Finally, the hypermetabolism that accompanies Graves disease increases stress on the heart and may lead to heart failure.

Hashimoto Disease

Hashimoto disease is another cause of hyperthyroidism that is also more common in women. In this case, the thyroid gland is enlarged as a result of the infiltration of T lymphocytes and plasma cells. Like Graves disease, Hashimoto disease is an autoimmune disorder that affects the TSH receptors; however, it is milder than Graves disease. The hyperthyroidism is transient, with subsequent hypothyroidism developing after antibodies destroy the follicles.

Myxedema Coma

Thyroid hormones are critical for cell metabolism and organ function. If their supply becomes inadequate, organ tissues do not grow or mature (due to the decreased metabolic rate), energy production declines (a cause of the decreased metabolic rate), and the actions of other hormones are affected.

Adult hypothyroidism is sometimes called *myxedema*. Frequently, patients have localized accumulations of mucinous material in the skin, which gives this disease its name (the prefix *myx-* refers to "mucin," and *edema* means "swelling") **FIGURE 24-7**. Hypothyroidism is manifested as a general slowing of the body's metabolic processes due to the reduction or absence of thyroid hormone. All organ systems may exhibit symptoms of the disorder, and the severity of the symptoms will reflect the degree of the hormone deficiency.

Symptoms of hypothyroidism include fatigue, feeling cold, weight gain, dry skin, and sleepiness. Because these symptoms are often subtle and can be mistaken for other conditions, the disease may go undiagnosed. Continued decreases in hormone levels may lead to myxedema coma, an extreme

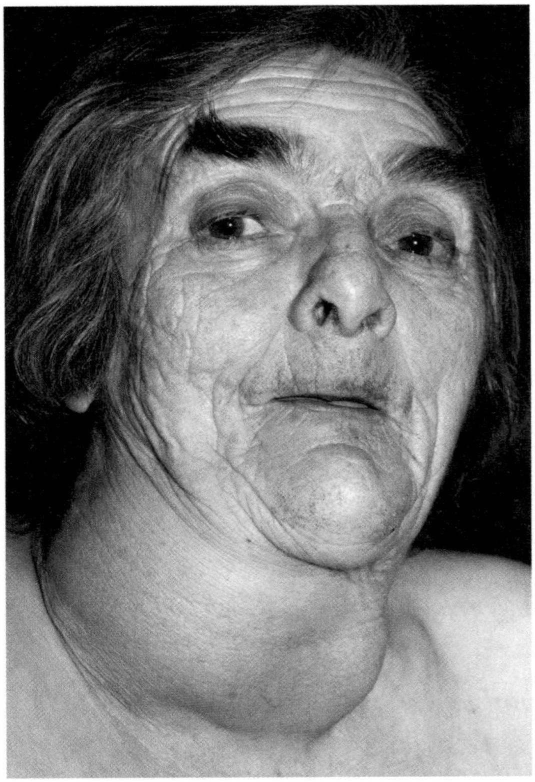

FIGURE 24-7 Localized accumulations of mucinous material in the neck of a patient with hypothyroidism.

manifestation of untreated hypothyroidism that is accompanied by physiologic decompensation. When hypothyroidism is long-standing, physiologic adaptations occur, such as reduced metabolic rate and decreased oxygen consumption, which in turn lead to peripheral vasoconstriction. Triggers such as infection (especially pulmonary and urinary tract infections), exposure to cold, trauma, surgery, and certain medications are often precipitating factors in the progression to myxedema coma.

The hallmark of myxedema coma is deterioration of the patient's mental status. Although family members may not be overly concerned about more subtle changes, such as apathy or decreased intellectual function, more obvious changes, such as confusion, psychosis, and coma, will most certainly elicit a call for emergency assistance.

Most cases of myxedema coma occur during the winter in women older than 60 years. This disorder is more common in women than in men. Just as the incidence of hypothyroidism increases with age, myxedema coma occurs primarily in older adult patients. One consistent finding is hypothermia, and you may need to use a thermometer that records body temperatures less than 90°F in cases of myxedema coma. Thus, the absence of fever in the presence of infection is a common finding.

Hypothyroidism decreases intestinal motility, and the decreased metabolic rate associated with this condition can lead to drug toxicity, especially in older adults. A slower metabolic rate causes the levels of medications, especially those that affect the central nervous system, to rise to toxic levels in the blood. This kind of accidental overdose in the patient with hypothyroidism can precipitate myxedema coma.

Myxedema coma is a metabolic and cardiovascular emergency. If not diagnosed and treated immediately, mortality rates are estimated to be as high as 40%.[37] Thus, the patient's condition must be stabilized as soon as possible.

Administer supplemental oxygen therapy to correct hypoxia. Intubation and ventilation are indicated for patients with diminished respiratory drive or those who cannot protect their airway; these measures will help prevent respiratory failure.

Monitor the patient's cardiac status. Hypotension may respond to crystalloid therapy, and vasopressor agents (eg, dopamine) may be necessary. Administer dextrose or glucagon per local protocols if blood glucose levels are less than 60 mg/dL.

Treat hypothermia with passive rewarming methods, because aggressive rewarming may lead to vasodilation and hypotension. Hemodynamically unstable patients with profound hypothermia, however, will require active rewarming. Avoid sedatives, narcotics, and anesthetics because of the delayed metabolism.

Thyrotoxicosis

Thyrotoxicosis is a toxic condition caused by excessive levels of circulating thyroid hormone. Although hyperthyroidism can cause thyrotoxicosis in some patients, the two conditions are not identical. Thyrotoxicosis also may be caused by goiters, autoimmune disorders such as Graves disease, or thyroid cancer.

Thyroid storm is a rare, life-threatening condition that may occur in patients with thyrotoxicosis. This condition is usually triggered by a stressful event or increased volume of thyroid hormones in the circulation. In addition to the usual signs and symptoms of hyperthyroidism, patients may present with fever, severe tachycardia, nausea, vomiting, altered mental status, and possibly heart failure.

> **Words of Wisdom**
>
> Both hyperthyroidism and hypothyroidism can adversely affect the electrical status of the myocardium. Application of the cardiac monitor may reveal tachydysrhythmias in hyperthyroidism or bradydysrhythmias in hypothyroidism. Treat all dysrhythmias according to your local protocol, while keeping in mind that these dysrhythmias may be difficult to correct without first fixing the underlying disorder.

Hyperparathyroidism

The increased parathyroid hormone level that characterizes hyperparathyroidism will result in hypercalcemia and decreased phosphate blood levels. Causes of hyperparathyroidism can be divided between primary and secondary causes. Primary causes result from the gland itself, whereas secondary causes occur elsewhere in the body and affect gland secretion. The most common cause of hyperparathyroidism is a benign tumor on the gland, called an adenoma.

Signs and symptoms of hyperparathyroidism can be vague, as is the case for many endocrine conditions. Fatigue, weakness, nausea, vomiting, and confusion may be present. Occasionally, pathologic fractures can occur secondary to thinning bones, or kidney stones can occur due to an increase in calcium and phosphorus levels in the urine. Surgery to remove the enlarged gland is definitive management and has a 95% success rate.[38] Patients with mild forms of the disease require monitoring of calcium blood levels. Prehospital management involves management of ABCs and supportive care as indicated.

Panhypopituitarism

Panhypopituitarism is the inadequate production or absence of the pituitary hormones, including adrenocorticotropic hormone, cortisol, thyroxine, LH, FSH, growth hormone, and ADH. The anterior pituitary gland is responsible for producing several different hormones; therefore, the clinical presentation of panhypopituitarism varies depending on the hormone or hormones that are lacking. **FIGURE 24-8** summarizes these hormones and the symptoms associated with each deficiency.

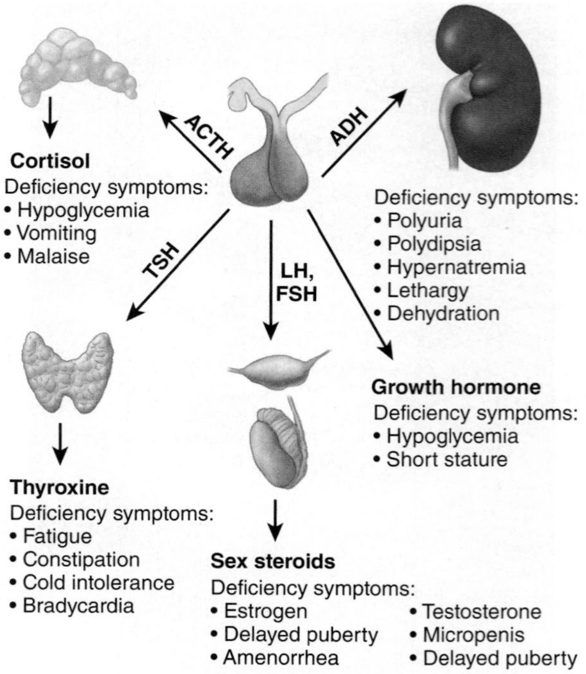

FIGURE 24-8 Panhypopituitarism.

Courtesy of Leonard Crowley.

Diabetes Insipidus and SIADH

Diabetes insipidus (DI) has some of the same characteristics as diabetes mellitus, such as polyuria and polydipsia. DI is a relatively uncommon disorder; however, unlike diabetes mellitus, it is not a pancreatic pathology. In diabetes insipidus, either the body cannot regulate fluid due to a lack of ADH (central DI) or the kidneys are unable to respond appropriately (nephrogenic diabetes insipidus). ADH causes the kidneys to retain water; therefore, a lack of ADH will cause increased urination (polyuria), like that seen in diabetes mellitus. One difference between DI and diabetes mellitus is the amount of glucose present in the urine. In DI, the urine is very dilute; in contrast, excessive glucose is present in the urine of patients with diabetes mellitus. It seems obvious that dehydration and electrolyte imbalances may occur in DI, but there is also the risk of water intoxication and hyponatremia. In extreme cases, hypotension can occur. Management may include synthetic ADH.

In SIADH, an excess of ADH results in decreased urinary output and, therefore, systemic fluid overload. This condition may cause hypertension, tachycardia, hyponatremia, seizures, and confusion. Management may include loop diuretics and hypertonic fluids. **TABLE 24-4** compares DI and SIADH.

TABLE 24-4 Comparison of Diabetes Insipidus and SIADH Secretion

Diabetes Insipidus	Syndrome of Inappropriate ADH Secretion
Decreased levels of ADH	Increased levels of ADH
Polyuria	Oliguria
Dehydration, hypotension	Systemic fluid overload

Abbreviations: ADH, antidiuretic hormone; SIADH, syndrome of inappropriate antidiuretic hormone.

YOU are the Paramedic SUMMARY

1. Which key information is provided from the dispatch and scene size-up?

The dispatch information indicated unusual circumstances or bizarre behavior. Your scene size-up has confirmed a patient with an altered mental status. The presence of medication and an ice cream wrapper lead you to suspect the patient could have hypoglycemia.

2. Which types of medical conditions can cause an altered mental status?

Numerous medical emergencies can cause an altered mental status, including seizure, stroke, or drug overdose.

3. Although the patient is cooperative, what do you need to consider when treating any patient with an altered mental status?

Patients with an altered mental status can become combative, particularly those experiencing hypoglycemia. Some patients may stare off into space, whereas others may curse and exhibit bizarre or sometimes violent behavior. When you are in doubt about scene safety, wait until law enforcement personnel declare the scene safe before you begin treatment.

4. What could be the cause of the patient's reported shaking?

In addition to epilepsy, the patient could be having a seizure from an extremely low blood glucose level or merely be shivering from sitting on a refrigeration unit. Look for a medical identification bracelet for additional information and perform a thorough assessment, noting the presence or absence of incontinence. Seizures due to hypoglycemia are an ominous sign.

5. What concerns you about the bystander's statement?

Often, laypeople are well intentioned but do not know what to do. Patients with an altered mental status frequently have airway problems and sometimes require airway management. It is possible that in addition to hypoglycemia, the patient has aspirated food into their lungs.

6. If your partner were unable to obtain IV access, which additional treatment options exist for correcting the patient's blood glucose level?

Patients with diabetes often have fragile veins. Also, this patient is obese, and obtaining IV access could be difficult. Another treatment option is to administer glucagon IM. Administering glucagon requires the patient to have adequate glycogen stores in the liver to be effective

7. Which challenges often occur on calls such as this one?

Often, patients with diabetes do not wish to be transported. It is vitally important that the patient eat a meal as soon as possible. Administration of IV dextrose is only a temporary measure. If the patient does not eat a meal containing complex carbohydrates,

YOU are the Paramedic SUMMARY continued

their blood glucose level will likely drop again, and another 9-1-1 call will be necessary.

8. How would you document this patient contact?

It is imperative to thoroughly document the patient assessment findings and interventions provided, the consequences of refusal of treatment and/or transport, and that the patient's refusal was an informed decision. Document the contact and discussion with medical control in which you obtained authorization to refuse transport (or treatment). Also document that you left the patient in her son's care, with instructions to call back if needed.

EMS Patient Care Report (PCR)

Date: 05-30-22	**Incident No.:** 53011	**Nature of Call:** Altered mental status		**Location:** Walt's Grocery	
Dispatched: 0900	**En Route:** 0901	**At Scene:** 0903	**Transport:** N/A	**At Hospital:** N/A	**In Service:** 0930

Patient Information

Age: 40 **Sex:** F **Weight (in kg [lb]):** 160 kg (353 lb)	**Allergies:** Penicillin **Medications:** Insulin **Past Medical History:** IDDM **Chief Complaint:** Hunger

Vital Signs

Time: 0908	**BP:** 160/94	**Pulse:** 100	**Respirations:** 24	**Spo_2:** 97% on room air
Time: 0913	**BP:** 156/92	**Pulse:** 90	**Respirations:** 20	**Spo_2:** 98% on room air
Time:	**BP:**	**Pulse:**	**Respirations:**	**Spo_2:**

EMS Treatment (highlight all that apply)

Oxygen @ ____ L/min via (circle one): **NC NRM Bag-mask device**		**Assisted Ventilation**	**Airway Adjunct**	**CPR**
Defibrillation	**Bleeding Control**	**Bandaging**	**Splinting**	**Other:**

Narrative

Dispatched to "woman sitting in the butter" at a grocery store. Pt, a 40-year-old woman, was found sitting in the refrigerated section by a man bystander. Man reported the pt was "shaking all over." On arrival, pt was found sitting upright in the dairy section with chocolate all over her face and an ice cream sandwich melting in her hand. Medication tablets were on the floor. Airway was open and breathing adequate. Weak, rapid radial pulse present. Pt responsive to pain (a pinch to the back of her hand); skin cool, pale, and diaphoretic; no trauma noted to HEENT; PERRLA; chest rise and volume adequate, no apparent trauma and bilateral breath sounds present/no adventitious lung sounds; no trauma noted to abd. Pt had an altered mental status secondary to hypoglycemia. Initial blood glucose 30 mg/dL, IV line started with 18-gauge R AC, NS KVO. Gave 25 g of D_{50}. Glucose level increased to 120 mg/dL. Pt's 21-year-old son arrived. Pt refused transport; IV and oxygen discontinued. Pt advised IV dextrose will not prevent glucose level from dropping again and she could have aspirated food into her lungs. Pt assisted to food court, where she ordered a hamburger and fries. Contacted medical control and obtained approval for refusal. Refusal of care signature obtained; pt advised to call back if she changed her mind. Pt released to self and left in care of 21-year-old son; notified dispatch.

End of report

Prep Kit

Ready for Review

- The endocrine system directly or indirectly influences almost every cell, organ, and body function.
- The endocrine system comprises a network of glands that produce and secrete hormones. The main function of the endocrine system and its hormonal messengers is to maintain homeostasis.
- The endocrine system's major components include the hypothalamus, pituitary gland, pineal gland, thyroid, parathyroid, thymus, pancreas, adrenal glands, pancreas, and gonads, including the ovaries and testes.
- Endocrine emergencies can be challenging to assess because they affect many organ systems, and the seriousness of their presentations varies greatly. Do not take these calls lightly because poor outcomes can happen quickly.
- Management of an endocrine emergency may require intubation, administration of supplemental oxygen, infusion of dextrose, or other measures. All findings must be thoroughly documented.
- Endocrine disorders are caused by either hypersecretion or insufficient secretion of a gland. Hypersecretion presents as overactivity of the target organ regulated by the gland; insufficient secretion results in underactivity of the organ controlled by the gland.
- Diabetes is a metabolic disorder that encompasses a group of complex diseases with many causes (ie, diabetes mellitus, gestational diabetes, hypoglycemia/hyperglycemia, diabetic ketoacidosis, hyperosmolar hyperglycemic nonketotic syndrome); in all cases, the body's ability to metabolize glucose is impaired. Diabetes is characterized by the passage of large quantities of urine containing glucose, significant thirst, an increased appetite, and deterioration of body function.
- In type 1 diabetes mellitus, the beta cells in the islets of Langerhans have been destroyed and no longer produce insulin. Patients with this type of diabetes require close monitoring of blood glucose and at least daily insulin administration by injection or pump.
- In type 2 diabetes mellitus (the most common form of diabetes), the blood glucose level is elevated because the body cannot produce enough insulin to compensate for the inability to utilize insulin effectively.
- Prediabetes is a condition in which blood glucose levels or hemoglobin A1c levels are higher than normal, yet not high enough to be diagnosed as diabetes. Prediabetes is often a precursor condition to type 2 diabetes.
- Gestational diabetes is a form of glucose intolerance that usually manifests itself late in pregnancy.
- Hypoglycemia (abnormally low blood glucose level) in a patient with insulin-dependent diabetes is often the result of having taken too much insulin, too little food, or both. As a result of the actions of epinephrine, the patient will tremble, have a rapid pulse rate, sweat, and feel hungry.
- Hyperglycemia (abnormally high blood glucose level) is a classic symptom of diabetes mellitus. Typical early signs include frequent and excessive thirst accompanied by frequent and excessive urination.
- If left untreated, hyperglycemia may progress to the life-threatening condition known as diabetic ketoacidosis (DKA). DKA occurs when certain acids accumulate in the body because insulin is not available.
- Hyperosmolar hyperglycemic nonketotic syndrome (HHNS) is a metabolic derangement that occurs principally in patients with type 2 diabetes. This condition is characterized by hyperglycemia, hyperosmolarity, and an absence of significant ketosis.
- Acute pancreatitis is a medical emergency and can lead to dehydration and hypotension. By comparison, chronic pancreatitis is a progressive disease that destroys the pancreas, eventually leading to the loss of all endocrine and

Prep Kit continued

exocrine functions, and often causing chronic pain.
- Adrenal insufficiency is characterized by the underproduction of cortisol and aldosterone, leading to weakness, dehydration, and the body's inability to maintain adequate BP or respond properly to stress.
- Primary adrenal insufficiency (Addison disease) is caused by atrophy or destruction of both adrenal glands, leading to deficiencies of all the steroid hormones produced by these glands.
- Secondary adrenal insufficiency is defined as a lack of ACTH secretion from the pituitary gland.
- Acute adrenal insufficiency, referred to as addisonian crisis, may be triggered by an acute exacerbation of chronic adrenal insufficiency, usually brought on by stress, trauma, surgery, or severe infection.
- Cushing syndrome is caused by overproduction of cortisol by the adrenal glands or by excessive use of cortisol or other similar corticosteroid (glucocorticoid) hormones.
- Pheochromocytoma is generally a nonmalignant tumor of the adrenal gland, usually in the medulla, that causes excessive release of the hormones epinephrine and norepinephrine.
- Graves disease is the most severe and common cause of hyperthyroidism. This disease can produce goiter, exophthalmos, and pretibial myxedema.
- Hashimoto disease, another cause of hyperthyroidism, is an autoimmune disorder in which the thyroid gland becomes enlarged due to the infiltration of T lymphocytes and plasma cells. The hyperthyroidism is transient, with subsequent hypothyroidism developing after antibodies destroy the follicles.
- Symptoms of hypothyroidism include feeling fatigued, feeling cold, weight gain, dry skin, and sleepiness. Continued decrease of thyroid hormone levels may lead to myxedema coma, an extreme manifestation of untreated hypothyroidism that is accompanied by physiologic decompensation.
- Thyrotoxicosis is a toxic condition caused by excessive levels of circulating thyroid hormone.
- Thyroid storm is a rare, life-threatening condition that may occur in patients with thyrotoxicosis.
- In hyperparathyroidism, blood calcium levels increase, resulting in hypercalcemia and decreased phosphate blood levels.
- Panhypopituitarism is the inadequate production or absence of the pituitary hormones.
- Diabetes insipidus is a result of decreased levels of ADH, which leads to polyuria. Dehydration and electrolyte imbalances may occur in diabetes insipidus, as well as an increased risk of water intoxication and hyponatremia. In extreme cases, hypotension can occur.
- SIADH is caused by an excess of ADH, which results in a decrease in urinary output and, in turn, systemic fluid overload.

Vital Vocabulary

addisonian crisis Acute adrenal insufficiency.

adrenocorticotropic hormone (ACTH) Hormone that stimulates the adrenal cortex to manufacture and secrete cortisol (a glucocorticoid).

aldosterone Hormone that stimulates the kidneys to reabsorb sodium from the urine and excrete potassium by altering the osmotic gradient in the blood.

androgens Male sex hormones that regulate body changes associated with sexual development (puberty), including growth spurts, deepening of the voice, growth of facial and pubic hair, and muscle growth and strength.

antidiuretic hormone (ADH) Hormone secreted by the posterior pituitary lobe of the pituitary

Prep Kit continued

gland that constricts blood vessels and raises the blood pressure; also called *vasopressin.*

calcitonin Hormone secreted by the thyroid gland that helps maintain normal calcium levels in the blood.

corticosteroids Hormones that regulate the body's metabolism, the balance of salt and water in the body, the immune system, and sexual function.

cortisol Hormone that stimulates most body cells to increase their energy production.

Cushing syndrome A condition caused by overproduction of cortisol by the adrenal glands or by excessive use of cortisol or other similar corticosteroid (glucocorticoid) hormones.

diabetes A group of complex metabolic disorders with many causes; includes diabetes mellitus, gestational diabetes, hypoglycemia/hyperglycemia, diabetic ketoacidosis, and hyperosmolar hyperglycemic syndrome.

diabetes insipidus (DI) A relatively uncommon disorder that has some of the same characteristics as diabetes, such as polyuria and polydipsia, in which the body is unable to regulate fluid owing to a lack of antidiuretic hormone (central diabetes insipidus) or the kidneys are unable to respond appropriately (nephrogenic diabetes insipidus).

diabetes mellitus Disease characterized by the body's inability to sufficiently metabolize glucose; occurs either because the pancreas does not produce enough insulin or because the cells do not respond to the effects of the insulin that is produced.

diabetic ketoacidosis (DKA) A form of acidosis in uncontrolled diabetes in which certain acids accumulate when insulin is not available.

diuresis The production of large amounts of urine by the kidney.

dyslipidemia An excessive level of lipids (fats) circulating in the blood, which increases the risk of atherosclerosis and coronary artery disease.

epinephrine Hormone produced by the adrenal medulla that plays a vital role in the function of the sympathetic nervous system.

estrogen A primary female hormone that brings about secondary sex characteristics at puberty.

exophthalmos Protrusion of the eyes from the normal position within the socket.

gestational diabetes Diabetes that develops during pregnancy in women who did not have diabetes before pregnancy.

glucagon Hormone produced by the pancreas that is vital to the control of the body's metabolism and blood glucose level. Glucagon stimulates the breakdown of glycogen to glucose.

glycosuria The passage of large quantities of urine containing glucose.

goiter A visible mass in the anterior part of the neck caused by enlargement of the thyroid gland.

Graves disease An autoimmune disorder that causes thyroid gland hypertrophy and severe hyperthyroidism.

Hashimoto disease A type of hyperthyroidism in which the thyroid gland becomes enlarged as it is infiltrated by T lymphocytes and plasma cells.

hyperglycemia Abnormally high blood glucose level.

hyperosmolar hyperglycemic nonketotic syndrome (HHNS) A metabolic derangement that occurs principally in patients with type 2 diabetes; it is characterized by hyperglycemia, hyperosmolarity, and an absence of significant ketosis. Formerly known as hyperosmolar nonketotic coma (HONK).

hypoglycemia Abnormally low blood glucose level.

insulin Hormone produced by the pancreas that is vital to the control of the body's metabolism and blood glucose level; it causes sugar, fatty acids, and amino acids to be absorbed and metabolized by cells.

insulin resistance Condition in which the pancreas produces enough insulin but the body cannot effectively use it.

Prep Kit continued

islets of Langerhans A specialized group of cells within the pancreas that act like an organ within an organ, secreting glucagon from alpha cells, insulin from beta cells, and somatostatin from delta cells.

ketonemia Excess amounts of ketone bodies in the blood.

lipolysis The metabolism (breakdown or destruction) of stored fat that has been released into the circulation.

luteinizing hormone (LH) Hormone that regulates the production of both eggs and sperm, as well as production of reproductive hormones.

microangiopathy Microscopic deterioration of vessel walls caused primarily by adherence of blood lipids to vessel walls.

myxedema coma A rare condition that can occur in patients who have severe, untreated hypothyroidism.

norepinephrine Hormone produced by the adrenal glands that is vital in the function of the sympathetic nervous system.

panhypopituitarism Inadequate production or absence of the pituitary hormones, including adrenocorticotropic hormone, cortisol, thyroxine, luteinizing hormone, follicle-stimulating hormone, estrogen, testosterone, growth hormone, and antidiuretic hormone.

parathyroid hormone A hormone secreted by the parathyroids that acts as an antagonist to calcitonin; secreted when calcium blood levels are low.

pheochromocytoma A tumor of the adrenal gland, usually in the medulla, that causes excessive release of the hormones epinephrine and norepinephrine.

polydipsia Significant thirst.

polyphagia Increased appetite.

polyuria Frequent and plentiful urination.

prediabetes A condition identified in people who have certain risk factors associated with type 2 diabetes; exists when blood glucose levels or hemoglobin A1c levels are higher than normal, yet not high enough to be diagnosed as diabetes.

pretibial myxedema An "orange peel" appearance and nonpitting edema of the skin on the anterior part of the leg below the knee.

primary adrenal insufficiency A rare disease in which the adrenal glands atrophy or are destroyed, leading to deficiencies of all steroid hormones produced by these glands; also known as Addison disease.

progesterone A primary female hormone that assists in the regulation of the menstrual cycle.

secondary adrenal insufficiency A relatively common condition characterized by a lack of adrenocorticotropic hormone (also called corticotrophin) secretion from the pituitary gland.

somatostatin Hormone that inhibits insulin and glucagon secretion by the pancreas.

syndrome of inappropriate antidiuretic hormone secretion (SIADH) An endocrine disorder in which an excess of antidiuretic hormone results in decreased urinary output and, in turn, systemic fluid overload.

testosterone An androgen in men that promotes healthy sperm production, determines secondary male sex characteristics such as hair production, and stimulates growth.

thyroid-stimulating hormone (TSH) Hormone that controls the release of thyroid hormone from the thyroid gland.

thyroid storm A rare, life-threatening condition that may occur in patients with thyrotoxicosis; usually triggered by a stressful event or increased volume of thyroid hormones in the circulation.

thyrotoxicosis A toxic condition caused by excessive levels of circulating thyroid hormone.

thyroxine (T_4) The body's major metabolic hormone. Thyroxine stimulates energy production in cells, which increases the rate at which the cells consume oxygen and use carbohydrates, fats, and proteins.

Prep Kit continued

type 1 diabetes The type of diabetic disease that usually starts in childhood and requires daily injections of supplemental synthetic insulin to control blood glucose levels; formerly called insulin-dependent diabetes mellitus (IDDM) or juvenile-onset diabetes.

type 2 diabetes The type of diabetic disease that typically develops in middle-age adult patients and often can be controlled through diet and oral medications; formerly called adult-onset diabetes.

References

1. National diabetes statistics report. Centers for Disease Control and Prevention website. https://www.cdc.gov/diabetes/data/statistics-report/index.html. Last reviewed August 28, 2020. Accessed February 9, 2021.
2. Statistics about diabetes. American Diabetes Association website. https://www.diabetes.org/resources/statistics/statistics-about-diabetes. Updated March 22, 2018. Accessed February 9, 2021.
3. Economic costs of diabetes in the U.S. in 2017. American Diabetes Association website. https://care.diabetesjournals.org/content/early/2018/03/20/dci18-0007. Accessed February 9, 2021.
4. Coexisting conditions and complications. Centers for Disease Control and Prevention website. https://www.cdc.gov/diabetes/data/statistics-report/coexisting-conditions-complications.html. Last reviewed July 21, 2020. Accessed February 9, 2021.
5. Diabetes and your heart. Centers for Disease Control and Prevention website. https://www.cdc.gov/diabetes/library/features/diabetes-and-heart.html. Last reviewed January 31, 2020. Accessed February 9, 2021.
6. Conquer high blood pressure. American Diabetes Association website. https://www.diabetes.org/diabetes-risk/prevention/high-blood-pressure. Accessed February 9, 2021.
7. Caffrey M. Diabetic amputations may be rising in the United States. AJMC website. https://www.ajmc.com/view/diabetic-amputations-may-be-rising-in-the-united-states. Published December 13, 2018. Accessed February 9, 2021.
8. Nathan DM, Cleary PA, Backlund JY, et al. Diabetes Control and Complications Trial/Epidemiology of Diabetes Interventions and Complications (DCCT/EDIC) Study Research Group. Intensive diabetes treatment and cardiovascular disease in patients with type 1 diabetes. *N Engl J Med*. 2005;353:2643-2653.
9. Dehydration. Mayo Clinic website. https://www.mayoclinic.org/diseases-conditions/dehydration/symptoms-causes/syc-20354086. Accessed February 25, 2021.
10. Lough ME. Endocrine disorders and therapeutic management. In: Urden LD, Stacy KM, Lough ME, eds. *Critical Care Nursing: Diagnosis and Management*. 9th ed. St. Louis, MO: Mosby; 2022:750-790.
11. Reno CM, Daphna-Iken D, Chen S, et al. Severe hypoglycemia-induced lethal cardiac arrhythmias are mediated by sympathoadrenal activation. *Diabetes*. 2013;62(10):3570-3581.
12. Diabetes Fact Sheet. World Health Organization website. http://www.who.int/mediacentre/factsheets/fs312/en/. Reviewed June 8, 2020. Accessed February 9, 2021.
13. Fuchsberger C, Flannick J, Teslovich TM, et al. The genetic architecture of type 2 diabetes. *Nature*. 2016;536;41-47.
14. Diabetes 2019 report card. Centers for Disease Control and Prevention website. https://www.cdc.gov/diabetes/pdfs/library/Diabetes-Report-Card-2019-508.pdf. Accessed February 9, 2021.
15. Prediabetes: your chance to prevent type 2 diabetes. Centers for Disease Control and Prevention website. https://www.cdc.gov/diabetes/basics/prediabetes.html. Last reviewed June 11, 2020. Accessed February 9, 2021.
16. About prediabetes & type 2 diabetes. Centers for Disease Control and Prevention website. http://www.cdc.gov/diabetes/prevention/prediabetes-type2/index.html. Updated April 4, 2019. Accessed February 9, 2021.
17. Gestational diabetes and pregnancy. Centers for Disease Control and Prevention website. https://www.cdc.gov/pregnancy/diabetes-gestational.html. Updated July 14, 2020. Accessed February 9, 2021.
18. Diabetes and pregnancy: gestational diabetes. Centers for Disease Control and Prevention website. https://www.cdc.gov/pregnancy/documents/diabetes_and_pregnancy508.pdf. Accessed February 9, 2021.
19. Gerich JE, Langlois M, Noacco C, et al. Lack of glucagon response to hypoglycemia in diabetes: evidence for an intrinsic pancreatic alpha cell defect. *Science*. 1973;182(4108):171-173.
20. Sandoval DA, Guy DL, Richardson MA, et al. Effects of low and moderate antecedent exercise on counterregulatory responses to subsequent hypoglycemia in type 1 diabetes. *Diabetes*. 2004;53(7):1798-1806.
21. Cryer P. Hypoglycemia during therapy of diabetes. In: DeGroot LJ, Chrousos G, Dungan K, et al., eds. *Endotext [Internet]*. South Dartmouth, MA: MDText.com; 2000.

Prep Kit continued

https://www.ncbi.nlm.nih.gov/books/NBK279100/. Updated June 18, 2018. Accessed February 9, 2021.

22. Soleimanpour H, Taghizadieh A, Niafar M, et al. Predictive value of capnography for suspected diabetic ketoacidosis in the emergency department. *West J Emerg Med.* 2013;14(6):590-594.
23. Sabatini S, Kurtzman NA. Bicarbonate therapy in severe metabolic acidosis. *J Am Soc Nephrol.* 2008;20(4):692-695.
24. Umpierrez GE, Kitabchi AE. Diabetic ketoacidosis. *Treat Endocrinol.* 2003;2(2):95-108.
25. Diabetic hyperglycemic hyperosmolar syndrome. US National Library of Medicine Medline website. https://medlineplus.gov/ency/article/000304.htm. Updated January 5, 2021. Accessed February 9, 2021.
26. Crandall JP, Shamoon H. Diabetes mellitus. In: Goldman L, Schafer AI, eds. *Goldman-Cecil Medicine.* 26th ed. Philadelphia, PA: Elsevier; 2020:1490-1510.
27. Maloney GE, Glauser JM. Diabetes mellitus and disorders of glucose homeostasis. In: Wall RN, Hockberger RS, Gausche-Hill M, eds. *Rosen's Emergency Medicine: Concepts and Clinical Practice.* 9th ed. Philadelphia, PA: Elsevier; 2018:1533-1547.
28. Whitlatch HB. Hyperosmolar hyperglycemic syndrome. In: Ferri FF, ed. *Ferri's Clinical Advisor 2017.* Philadelphia, PA: Elsevier; 2017:632-633.
29. Collopy K, Kivlehan S, Snyder S. Prehospital treatment of hyperglycemia. http://www.emsworld.com/article/11112993/prehospital-treatment-of-hyperglycemia. Published September 1, 2013. Accessed February 9, 2021.
30. Forsmark CE, Vaillie J, AGA Institute Clinical Practice and Economics Committee, AGA Institute Governing Board. AGA Institute technical review on acute pancreatitis. *Gastroenterology. 2007;*132(5):2022-2044.
31. Yang AL, Vadhavkar S, Singh G, Omary MB. Epidemiology of alcohol-related liver and pancreatic disease in the United States. *Arch Intern Med.* 2008;168(6):649-656.
32. Corrigan EK. Adrenal insufficiency (Addison's disease). Pituitary Network Association website. https://pituitary.org/knowledge-base/disorders/adrenal-insuffieciency-addison-s-disease. Accessed February 9, 2021.
33. Scholz T, Eisenhofer G, Pacak K, et al. Clinical review: current treatment of malignant pheochromocytoma. *J Clin Endocrinol Metab.* 2007;92(4):1217-1225.
34. Acromegaly. National Institutes of Diabetes and Digestive and Kidney Diseases website. https://www.niddk.nih.gov/health-information/endocrine-diseases/acromegaly. Published April 2012. Accessed February 9, 2021.
35. Growth hormone deficiency. National Organization of Rare Diseases website. https://rarediseases.org/rare-diseases/growth-hormone-deficiency/. Accessed February 9, 2021.
36. Vanderpump MPJ. The epidemiology of thyroid disease. *Br Med Bull.* 2011;99(1):39-51.
37. Beynon J, Akhtar S, Kearney T. Predictors of outcome in myxoedema coma. *Crit Care.* 2008;12(1):111.
38. Silverberg SJ, Bilezikian JP. Primary hyperparathyroidism. In: Jameson JL, DeGroot LJ, de Kretser DM, et al., eds. *Endocrinology: Adult and Pediatric.* 7th ed. (online version). Philadelphia, PA: Saunders; 2016:1105-1124.

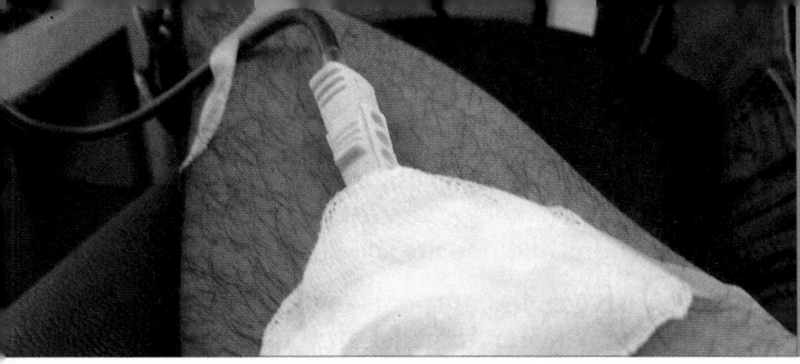

Chapter 25

Hematologic Emergencies

NATIONAL EMS EDUCATION STANDARD COMPETENCIES

Medicine

Integrates assessment findings with principles of epidemiology and pathophysiology to formulate a field impression and implement a comprehensive treatment/disposition plan for a patient with a medical complaint.

Hematology

Anatomy, physiology, pathophysiology, assessment, and management of
- Sickle cell crisis (pp 1544–1546)
- Clotting disorders (pp 1536–1541)

Anatomy, physiology, epidemiology, pathophysiology, psychosocial impact, presentations, prognosis, and management of common or major hematological diseases and/or emergencies
- Sickle cell crisis (pp 1544–1546)
- Blood transfusion complications (pp 1552–1554)
- Hemostatic disorders (pp 1536–1541)
- Lymphomas (pp 1549–1550)
- Red blood cell disorders (pp 1546–1547, 1550–1552)
- White blood cell disorders (pp 1547–1550, 1552)
- Coagulopathies (pp 1540, 1551)

KNOWLEDGE OBJECTIVES

1. Discuss the composition and functions of blood's essential components. (p 1536)
2. Summarize the role of white blood cells in the normal inflammatory process. (pp 1538–1539)
3. Define hemostasis and mechanisms essential to its maintenance in the body. (pp 1539–1540)
4. Outline the steps in the primary survey and management of a patient with a hematologic disorder. (p 1542)
5. Summarize general emergency care for a patient with a hematologic disorder. (p 1544)
6. Describe pathophysiology, assessment, and management of sickle cell disease. (pp 1544–1546)
7. Describe three types of sickle cell crisis. (pp 1544–1545)
8. Outline pathophysiology, assessment, and management of other common diseases and conditions of the blood, including anemia, leukopenia, thrombocytopenia, leukemia, lymphomas, polycythemia, disseminated intravascular coagulation, hemophilia, and multiple myeloma. (pp 1546–1552)
9. Discuss the causes, symptoms, assessment, and management of blood transfusion complications. (pp 1552–1554)

SKILLS OBJECTIVES

There are no skills objectives for this chapter.

Introduction

Hematology is, by definition, simply the study of blood; however, it addresses not only the blood, but also how its constituent parts are involved in health and disease. These components include red blood cells (RBCs), white blood cells (WBCs), platelets, and other proteins involved in the bleeding and clotting cascades, as well as the **hematopoietic system**—that is, the organs and tissues involved in the production of blood components (primarily bone marrow, spleen, and lymph nodes). Emergency medical services (EMS) personnel rarely respond to a new onset of hematologic emergencies. Instead, most calls involve an exacerbation of existing issues.

The blanket term **hematologic disorder** refers to any blood disorder. Within this general category, **hemolytic disorders** refer to disease processes that cause the breakdown of RBCs, and **hemostatic disorders** refer to bleeding and clotting abnormalities. These disorders can be complex, difficult to assess, and challenging to treat in the prehospital setting.

As a paramedic, you should understand the hematopoietic system and hematologic disorders and know how to respond to these kinds of emergencies appropriately. Although you may be able to provide only limited interventions in the field for patients with hematologic disorders, your actions may not just offer support, but save the patient's life.

Anatomy and Physiology Review

Blood and Plasma

Blood is a connective tissue. It is made up of cells and cell fragments suspended in **plasma**, the liquid portion of blood. In the adult body, blood accounts for approximately 8% of the total body weight, and the total blood volume is in the range of approximately 5 to 6 L for an average weight adult. The primary functions of blood are as follows:

- Supply oxygen and nutrients to the cells.
- Transport carbon dioxide and nitrogenous wastes from the tissues to the lungs and kidneys, where the wastes can be removed from the body.
- Carry hormones from the endocrine glands to the target tissues.
- Regulate body temperature.
- Regulate pH through the buffering components in the blood.
- Keep fluid and electrolytes balanced through sodium and plasma proteins.
- Regulate the immune system through the actions of WBCs and antibodies.
- Form clots through the action of platelets.

Blood comprises two main components: plasma and formed elements (cells). Plasma is 92% water, with the remaining 8% being made up of various solutes, including proteins, electrolytes, clotting factors, and glucose. Plasma accounts for 55% of the total blood volume, and the formed elements make up the remaining 45%. The formed elements include RBCs, also called **erythrocytes**; WBCs, also called **leukocytes**; and platelets, also called **thrombocytes**. Most of these elements (99%) are RBCs **FIGURE 25-1**.

FIGURE 25-2 shows the development of the cells of the hematologic system. The production of RBCs occurs within **stem cells**, or cells that develop into other types of cells in the body; this production is stimulated by erythropoietin, a protein that is secreted by the kidneys in response to circulatory need. The RBCs may take as long as 5 days to

YOU are the Paramedic

PART 1

Your unit is dispatched to a private residence for a "general medical" complaint. The dispatcher informs you that the patient is a 73-year-old man with a history of leukemia who is feeling "poorly." When you arrive on scene, you find a man who appears frail. Family members confirm the patient was diagnosed with leukemia years ago. A family member states that the patient has a fever (temperature of 102°F [39°C]) and is feeling pain all over. You notice bruising on the patient's arms.

1. Why is a fever significant in this patient?
2. What do you need to know about this patient's status?

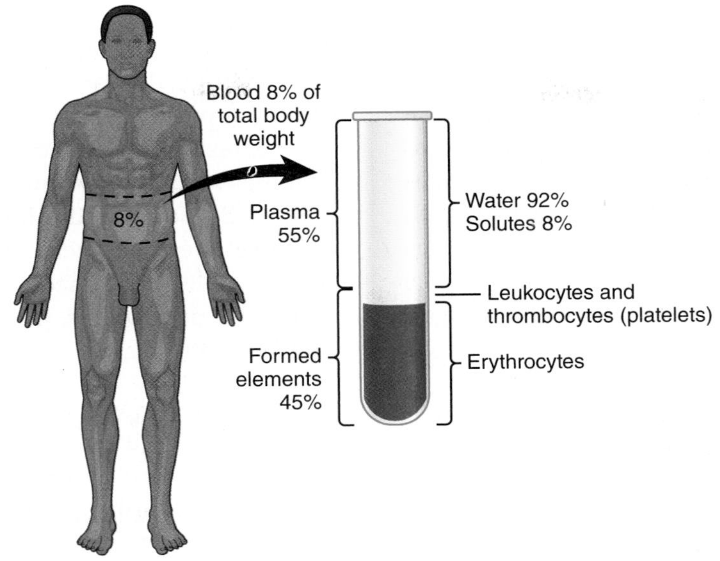

FIGURE 25-1 Components of a spun-down blood sample.

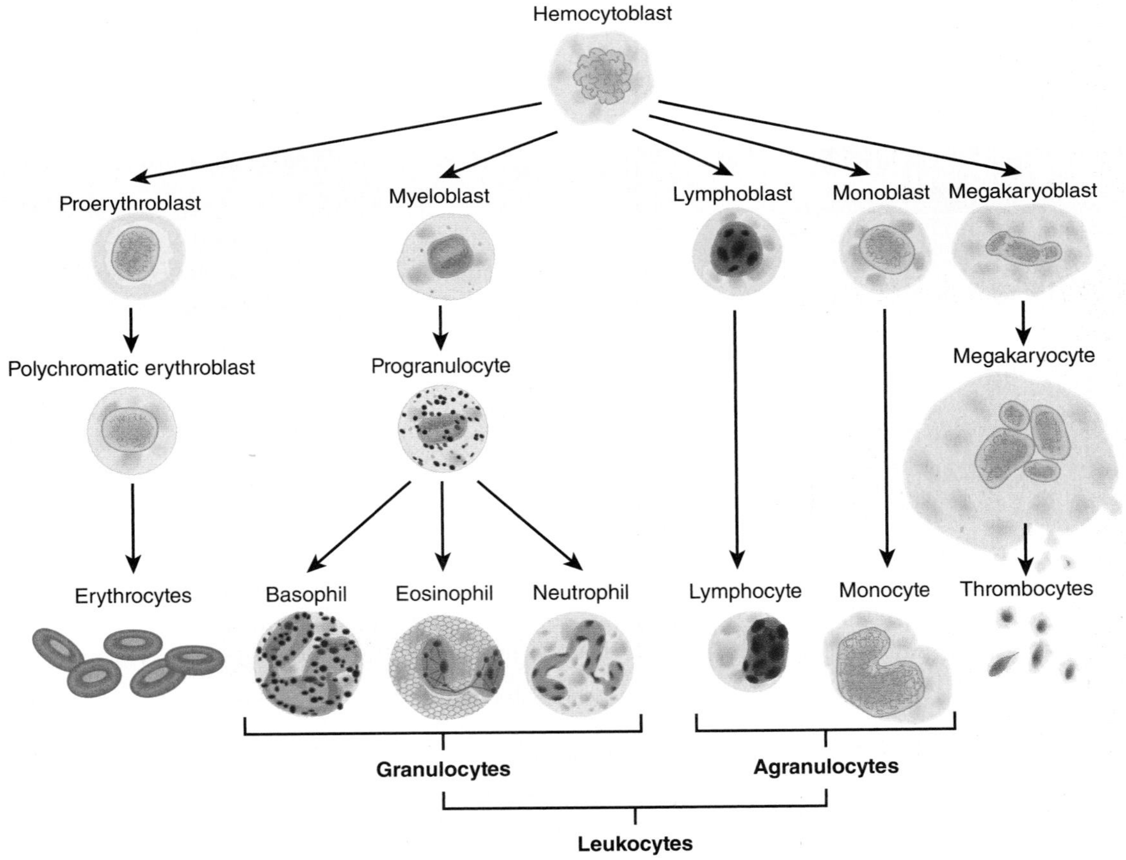

FIGURE 25-2 Development of the cells of the hematologic system.

mature and have an average life of 120 days. Within the RBCs, iron-rich **hemoglobin** is responsible for carrying oxygen to the tissues. Oxygen attached to hemoglobin gives blood its characteristic red color, although many other factors can change the color of blood (eg, carbon monoxide poisoning changes blood's color to bright red). When the oxygen-rich RBCs encounter an environment that contains a higher concentration of carbon dioxide (and is therefore more acidotic), they release the oxygen there. This physiologic phenomenon is called the Bohr effect.

Three laboratory tests are commonly performed on blood: RBC counts, hemoglobin levels, and hematocrit measurements. The RBC count measures the number of RBCs in a blood sample, whereas the hemoglobin level identifies the amount of hemoglobin found within the RBCs. The measurement of **hematocrit** identifies the overall proportion of RBCs in the blood. The patient's blood is considered balanced (even if the numbers are too high or low) if the hemoglobin level is one-third of the hematocrit value and the RBC count is one-third of the hemoglobin level. **TABLE 25-1** describes these tests in more detail.

The WBCs, which are larger than RBCs, provide the body with immunity against "foreign invaders." Just like RBCs, they are derived from stem cells. Several types of WBCs exist, each of which performs a specific task in relation to maintaining the immune system; **TABLE 25-2** summarizes the components of the WBC count and differential. Certain disease processes are also specific to the differential WBCs. For example, **neutropenia** is an abnormally low number of neutrophils, which make up most of the circulating WBCs.

Words of Wisdom

In a normal adult, the WBC count initially increases in response to infection. As the infection continues, the WBC count may drop as the WBCs are exhausted more rapidly than they can regenerate. Thus a low WBC count does not necessarily indicate absence of infection.

Immune system responses can be categorized into humoral immunity and cell-mediated immunity. *Humoral immunity* refers to the secretion of

TABLE 25-1 RBC and Platelet Counts

Name	Normal Values[a]	Examples of Conditions Associated With Low Readings	Examples of Conditions Associated With High Readings
RBC count ($\times 10^6$/mcL)	4.5–6 in adults; 3.3–5.5 in children	Anemia, hemorrhage, certain leukemias, overhydration, chronic infections	Polycythemia, cardiovascular disease, hemoconcentration, dehydration
Hemoglobin (g/dL)	12–16 in females; 14–18 in males; 10.7–17.1 in children	Anemia, hyperthyroidism, liver disease, hemorrhage, hemolytic reactions	COPD, HF, polycythemia, high-altitude sickness
Hematocrit (%)	35–45 in females; 40–50 in males; 32–55 in children	Same as for RBCs and hemoglobin, including leukemia, lupus, endocarditis, rheumatic fever, nutritional disorders	Polycythemia and usually anything that produces severe dehydration
Thrombocytes (platelets)	150,000–400,000 cells/mcL	Thrombocytopenia, certain cancers, certain leukemias, sickle cell disease, systemic lupus erythematosus	Pulmonary embolism, polycythemia, acute hemorrhage, metastatic cancer, surgical stress

Abbreviations: COPD, chronic obstructive pulmonary disease; HF, heart failure; RBC, red blood cell.

[a] The normal ranges provided are not intended to be definitive. Each laboratory determines its own values, and normal ranges are method dependent.

TABLE 25-2 WBC Count and Differential

Name	Normal Values[a]	Examples of Conditions Associated With Low Readings	Examples of Conditions Associated With High Readings
WBC count	4,500–10,000 cells/mm^3 in adults; 4,500–15,500 cells/mm^3 in children; 9,400–34,000 cells/mm^3 in infants	Viral infections, bone marrow diseases or disorders, leukemia, radiation, late-stage AIDS	Viral and bacterial infections, hemorrhage, traumatic tissue injuries, leukemia, cigarette smoking
Neutrophils (segmented and unsegmented)	50%–60%;[b] 2,500–8,000 cells/mm^3	Leukemia, infections, rheumatoid arthritis, vitamin B_{12} deficiency, enlarged spleen	Bacterial infections, tissue breakdown, hemolytic reactions, tumors, MI, surgical stress, cancer
Basophils (also known as mast cells)	0.5%–1%[a]; 25–100 cells/mm^3	Allergic reactions, hyperthyroidism, MI, bleeding ulcers, stress	Certain leukemias, inflammations, allergy, polycythemia, hemolytic anemia
Eosinophils	1%–4%[a]; 50–500 cells/mm^3	Mononucleosis, HF, Cushing disease	Addison disease, tumors, skin infections, allergies
Lymphocytes	20%–40%[a]; 1,000–4,000 cells/mm^3	Hodgkin disease, burns, trauma, lupus, Cushing disease, immunodeficiency states	Numerous bacterial and viral infections, hepatitis, leukemia, toxoplasmosis, Graves disease
Monocytes	2%–6%[a]; 100–700 cells/mm^3	Corticosteroid use, infections, rheumatoid arthritis, HIV	Numerous bacterial and parasitic infections, recovery from acute infections, TB, hematologic disorders

Abbreviations: AIDS, acquired immunodeficiency syndrome; HF, heart failure; HIV, human immunodeficiency virus; MI, myocardial infarction, TB, tuberculosis; WBC, white blood cell.

[a] The normal ranges provided are not intended to be definitive. Each laboratory determines its own values, and normal ranges are method dependent.

[b] Percentage of the total WBC count. Example: If the WBC is 5,000, then neutrophils should account for 2,500–3,000 of this count.

Words of Wisdom

The life cycle of a WBC begins when the bone marrow releases cells called granulocytes. Granulocytes remain in the circulation for 6 to 12 hours. If these cells travel to tissues, then they live for a few more days. At the end of their lives, WBCs are recycled by the **reticuloendothelial system**, as are RBCs.

antibodies called immunoglobulins, which recognize a specific antigen. In *cell-mediated immunity*, macrophages and T cells attack and destroy pathogens or foreign substances.

Platelets are the smallest of the formed elements. They are derived from stem cells and have an average life span of approximately 7 to 10 days. Approximately two-thirds of the platelets circulate throughout the blood; the rest are stored in the spleen.

Platelets are responsible for the clotting of the blood. These cells form the initial plug following vascular injury; the clotting proteins then toughen and complete the blood clot. Without platelets, our bodies would not be able to stop bleeding. There can be too much of a good thing with platelets, however: Conditions such as **thrombocytosis**, in which the body produces too many platelets, can lead to other dangerous medical conditions, such as coagulation or clotting of blood inside of a blood vessel, called **thrombosis**.

Hemostasis is a highly complex process that allows the body to stop bleeding through vascular spasm, coagulation, and platelet plugging. The opposite of hemostasis is hemorrhage.

The clots themselves are made up of fibrin. When injury is detected, thrombin converts fibrinogen to fibrin, and the clotting process begins. Calcium acts as a binding agent, holding fibrin fibers close together to form the clot's meshwork.

The **clotting cascade**—that is, the process by which clotting factors work together to form fibrin, also called the coagulation cascade—can be initiated through either an intrinsic or an extrinsic pathway **FIGURE 25-3**. Any process that interferes with the activation or continuation of the clotting cascade or hemostasis is known as a **coagulopathy**. Coagulopathies can lead to heavy or prolonged bleeding. One such bleeding disorder is **von Willebrand disease**, in which the blood's ability to clot is decreased due to the absence of a key protein, von Willebrand factor, that is necessary for platelet adhesion.

Words of Wisdom

"Clot busters"—fibrinolytic therapy given in cases of acute myocardial infarction and acute ischemic stroke—activate the body's fibrinolytic system, resulting in clot decomposition (also known as lysis). Such therapy must be monitored closely in patients with hematologic disorders, because clot busters may cause excess bleeding in these individuals.

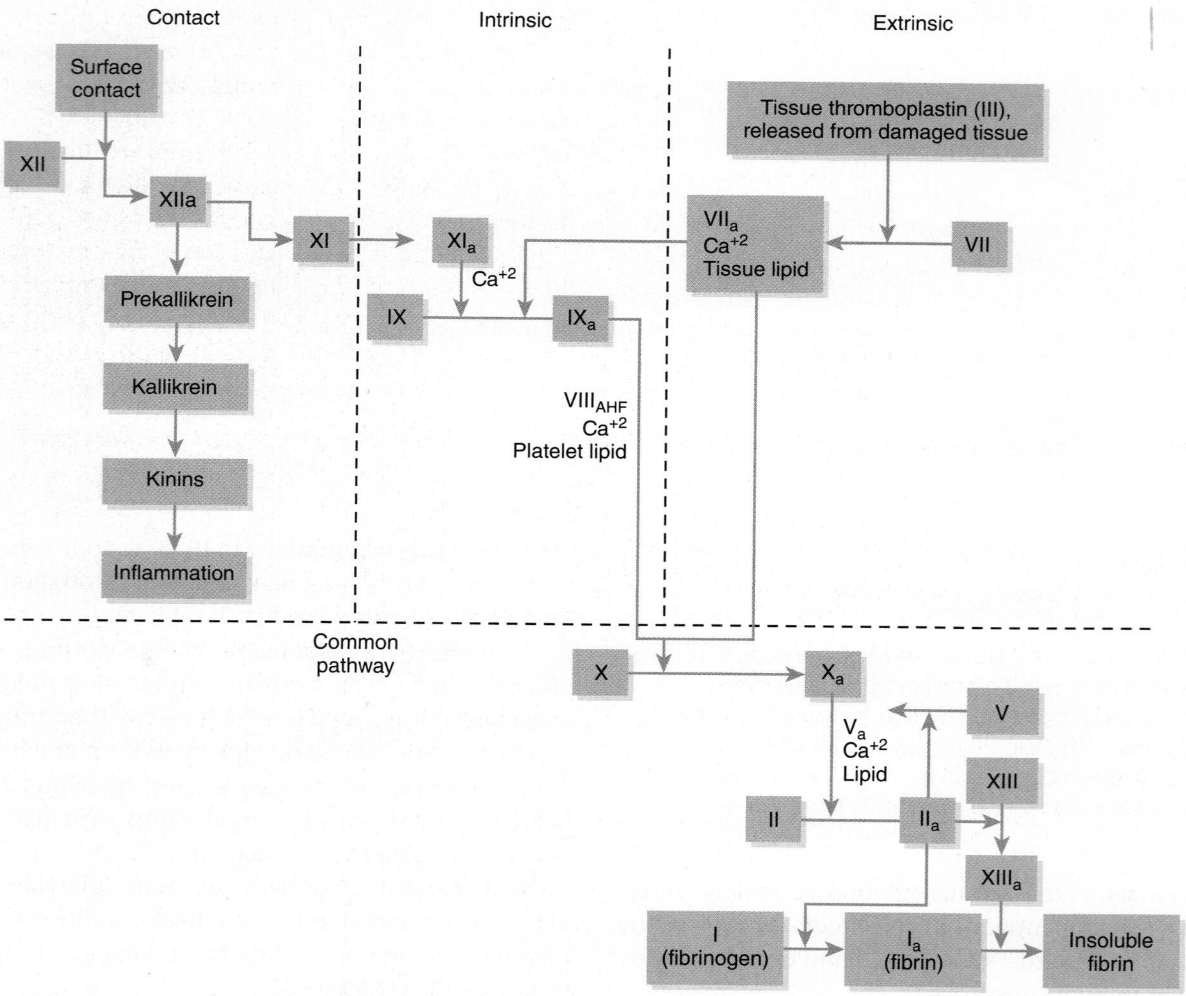

FIGURE 25-3 The clotting cascade.

Blood-Forming Organs and RBC Production

Although many parts and organs of the human body can alter or affect the hematologic system, the major players are the bone marrow, liver, and spleen **FIGURE 25-4**.

The bone marrow is the primary site for cell production within the human body. It is found in most of the long bones plus the pelvis, skull, and vertebrae.

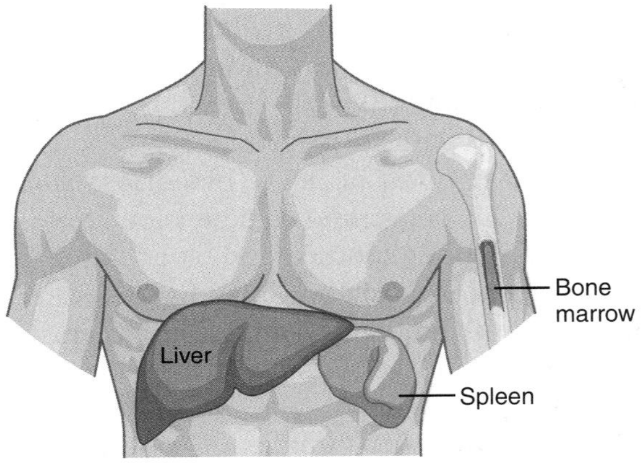

FIGURE 25-4 The bone marrow, liver, and spleen are instrumental in producing and regulating the blood and its components.

The liver produces the **clotting factors** found in the blood. This organ filters the blood, removing toxins, and is essential to normal metabolism and homeostasis. As old RBCs enter the liver, they are broken down into bile. The liver is a highly vascular organ that also stores blood.

Like the liver, the spleen is quite vascular. It is involved with the filtering and breakdown of RBCs, assists with the production of lymphocytes, and plays a vital role in providing homeostasis and infection control. The spleen stores about one-third of the platelets. If the spleen is removed, then the platelets formed after that time remain in the blood throughout their life span.

Patient Assessment

A patient suspected of having a hematologic disorder should be assessed in the same way as every other patient, with a few additional items to consider and questions to ask. During the primary survey, note any signs and symptoms that may be immediately life threatening. Unusual bleeding or uncontrolled hemorrhage can indicate underlying pathology. A major purpose of taking a history and performing the secondary assessment is to clearly and thoroughly understand the chief complaint, which requires asking in-depth and relevant

YOU are the Paramedic

PART 2

You begin your assessment of the patient while your partner obtains more information from the family. The patient is alert and cooperative with your questioning. You ask the patient what he is experiencing right now. The patient states, "My bones hurt, and I do not feel well." The patient also tells you that he takes chemotherapy and his most recent treatment was 4 days ago. You notice numerous used facial tissues that appear to have blood on them.

Recording Time: 0 Minutes	
Appearance	Awake, frail
Level of consciousness	Alert and oriented
Airway	Open
Breathing	Adequate
Circulation	Adequate

3. Which signs or symptoms is the patient showing that could indicate thrombocytopenia?
4. How will a patient with leukemia typically present?

questions about the patient's history and SAMPLE (Signs and symptoms, Allergies, Medications, Pertinent past history, Last oral intake, Events leading to injury or illness) history and following up on the responses to these questions. Because some patients with a blood disorder may be unwilling to disclose their conditions for fear of being treated differently from people without the disorder, a nonjudgmental approach is essential.

Street Smarts

Question patients with multiple bruises about the potential for bleeding disorders and/or the use of blood-thinning medications.

Scene Size-up

As always, ensure the scene is safe for entry, consider the mechanism of injury, determine the number of patients, and assess for hazards and the need for additional help. Standard precautions should consist of gloves, mask, and eye protection, at a minimum. Remember to evaluate each situation quickly and make sure you have the necessary personal protective equipment readily available.

Primary Survey

Perform cervical spine stabilization, if necessary. Do not dismiss a pain complaint of the spine as insignificant, because it could be a manifestation of the patient's current disease state. For example, even though a person has a history of **sickle cell disease**, that disease may not be causing the current problem; trauma or another type of medical emergency may be the actual cause of the patient's pain. For this reason, you must always perform a thorough, careful primary survey, paying attention to assess the ABCDEs (Airway, Breathing, Circulation, Disability, and Exposure), and immediately correct any life-threatening issues.

Perform a rapid full-body scan of the patient to form an initial general impression. How does the patient look? Does the patient appear anxious, restless, or listless? Is the patient apathetic or irritable? Determine the patient's level of consciousness.

As you are forming your general impression, assess the patient's airway and breathing. Patients showing signs of inadequate breathing or altered mental status should receive appropriate oxygen therapy. Depending on the severity of the patient's condition, this may be accomplished with a nasal cannula, nonrebreathing mask, or even assisted ventilation with a bag-mask device as needed. If you need to provide additional airway support with suctioning and/or use of basic or advanced airways, be aware that even minor trauma inflicted during these procedures can lead to bleeding into the airway and increase the risk of airway compromise.

Once you have assessed the airway and breathing and have performed the necessary interventions, check the patient's circulatory status. Assess for signs of shock, such as a rapid pulse rate and low blood pressure (BP).

In patients with suspected **hemophilia**, be alert for signs of hypoxia or acute blood loss such as pallor, a weak pulse, and hypotension. Note any nosebleeds, bloody sputum, and blood in the urine or stool. Fluid resuscitation may be necessary for these patients; however, it must be administered with care so as not to "wash out" the clots that are forming.

If you find any life-threatening conditions, take immediate steps to manage them and provide urgent transport to an appropriately equipped receiving facility. Whether you decide to rapidly transport the patient will depend on the severity of the patient's condition and the patient's wishes. Transport to the closest, most appropriate facility should always be recommended for any patient experiencing a **sickle cell crisis** or uncontrolled bleeding.

History Taking

You may need to ask a lot of questions about the patient's history to fully understand their chief complaint today. When you are obtaining the patient's history, keep in mind that hematologic disorders may present with multiple symptoms that at first glance seem unrelated, such as pneumonia in a patient with sickle cell disease or abdominal pain in a patient with **polycythemia**. You must put these pieces together to get a complete picture of the patient.

During history taking, look for changes in level of consciousness and symptoms such as vertigo, feelings of fatigue, and syncopal episodes. Has the patient had dyspnea, chest pain, changes in pulse rate and rhythm, or coughing up blood? Has the patient experienced visual disturbances, muscle pain, or stiffness? Are these complaints related to a more extensive disease process, or are they simply multiple unrelated complaints? If the patient has a complaint of pain, then ascertain whether the pain is isolated to a single location or whether it is felt throughout the entire body.

Has the patient had episodes of unexpected, significant, or recurrent bleeding? If so, what was the source? How often has it occurred? Has the patient experienced skin changes such as color changes, burning, or itching? Ask about bleeding from the nose, gums, or mouth. Problems with the genitourinary system (eg, excessive menstrual bleeding, unusual urine color)? Is the patient experiencing any gastrointestinal problems (eg, liver problems, gastritis, ulcers, tarry stools, hemorrhoidal bleeding, abdominal cramping)?

Documentation and Communication

Many anti-inflammatory medications (eg, aspirin and ibuprofen) and some herbal products (eg, ginkgo, garlic, ginger, ginseng, and feverfew) decrease platelet aggregation. Although this effect may be beneficial (as in the prevention of myocardial infarction and stroke), these medications may also increase the tendency to bleed. Always ask patients about the medications they are taking, including over-the-counter and herbal medications.

Secondary Assessment

The secondary assessment may be performed on scene, en route to the emergency department, or not at all. Your decision to perform this assessment will depend on the transport time and the patient's condition.

When treating a patient with a known or suspected blood disorder, you will need to perform a physical exam and recognize some of the common findings associated with blood disorders **TABLE 25-3**. Obtain the patient's baseline vital signs, including lung sounds and oxygen saturation level. Keep in mind that the oxygen saturation reading you obtain may be inaccurate in a patient with a hematologic disorder.

TABLE 25-3 Common Findings With Blood Disorders

System	Examples of Common Findings
Level of consciousness	Alterations may range from excitability, agitation, and combativeness to unresponsiveness
Skin	Uncontrolled bleeding, easy bruising, petechiae, itching, pallor, jaundice (yellow appearance usually indicates liver problems), leg ulcers (may be seen with sickle cell disease)
Head and neck	Epistaxis (bloody nose), bleeding gums, blurred vision, diplopia (double vision), complete or partial vision loss, seeing black or gray spots, retinal hemorrhage, vertigo, tinnitus
Chest	Dyspnea, tachycardia, palpitations, chest pain, hemoptysis (coughing up blood), sternal tenderness (may be seen with leukemia, myeloma, or lymphoma)
Back and extremities	Chronic joint or bone pain or rigidity, edema
Gastrointestinal	Ulcers, melena (blood in the stool), liver failure (causes jaundice), abdominal pain
Genitourinary	Hematuria, menorrhagia, chronic or recurring infections

Reassessment

Reassess the patient frequently to identify any changes in condition. For example, has the patient's mental status changed? Are the ABCs still intact? How is the patient responding to the interventions performed? Should you adjust or change those interventions? In many patients, you will note marked improvement with appropriate treatment.

Communication with hospital staff is essential to ensure continuity of care. Hospital personnel need to be informed about the patient's history, the present situation, your assessment findings, and your interventions and their results.

Document your assessment findings thoroughly, any treatments administered and the patient's response, the time of the interventions, and any changes in the patient's condition. Follow your local protocols for patients who refuse treatment or transport.

Emergency Medical Care

Emergency medical care for any patient with problems related to a blood disorder should include the following measures:

- **Oxygen.** The amount needed and how it is given (ie, via nasal cannula, nonrebreathing mask, or bag-mask device) depend on the severity of the patient's condition and respiratory status.
- **Fluids.** Initiate intravenous (IV) fluid replacement as indicated for the specific disorder or chief complaint.
- **Electrocardiogram (ECG).** Monitor and treat symptomatic cardiac rhythm disturbances as needed.
- **Transport.** Transport the patient to the closest, most appropriate facility.
- **Comfort.** Place the patient in a position of comfort, and cover the patient with a blanket to maintain body temperature.
- **Pharmacology.** Pain management is often necessary, especially in a sickle cell crisis.
- **Psychological support.** Be supportive of and communicate therapeutically with the patient.

Street Smarts

Remember to treat the patient, not the diagnostic tool! Pulse oximeter readings may be inaccurate in the presence of hematologic disorders.

Pathophysiology, Assessment, and Management of Specific Emergencies

The general emergency medical care steps apply to all patients with an emergency related to a blood disorder. Depending on the specific blood disorder, you will then need to refine your assessment and management of the patient, as discussed in the next sections. While hematologic disorders are not the most common complaints encountered by prehospital care providers, they can be serious and are often life threatening.

Sickle Cell Crisis

Pathophysiology

Sickle cell disease is the most common inherited blood disorder. Although it primarily affects African American, Puerto Rican, and European populations, it can occur in anyone. As of 2016, approximately 100,000 people in the United States had sickle cell disease.[1] Mortality at younger ages is common with this condition, with the average life expectancy being 42 years for males with sickle cell anemia and 48 years for females with this disorder.[2]

Sickle cell disease starts with a gene defect of the adult-type hemoglobin (HbA). This mutation can be inherited from both parents (HbSS) or from just one parent (HbS). When the gene is inherited from both parents, there is a high probability that their offspring will be susceptible to sickle cells (ie, the person actually has the disease) or the sickle cell trait (ie, the person is a carrier of the mutation).

The defective RBCs have an oblong shape instead of a smooth, round shape **FIGURE 25-5**. This shape makes the RBCs poor carriers of oxygen, which means a patient with this disease is highly susceptible to hypoxia. Because sickle cells also have a much shorter life span than normal RBCs, the patient is more susceptible to developing **anemia**.

Sickle cell disease may lead to either an **aplastic crisis** or a **hemolytic crisis**. In an aplastic crisis, the body temporarily stops RBC production, causing the patient to become easily tired, anemic, pale, and short of breath. In contrast, a hemolytic crisis arises when acute RBC destruction leads to jaundice. In both cases, the patient may have rapidly evolving anemia, **leukocytosis**, and fever. The odd shape of the RBCs may also cause these cells to become lodged in small blood vessels, leading to thrombosis. A sickle cell crisis may manifest in several ways:

- **Vasoocclusive crisis** occurs when blood flow to an organ becomes restricted, causing pain, ischemia, and often organ damage. Most vasoocclusive crises last between 5 and 7 days. Frequently, circulation to the spleen becomes

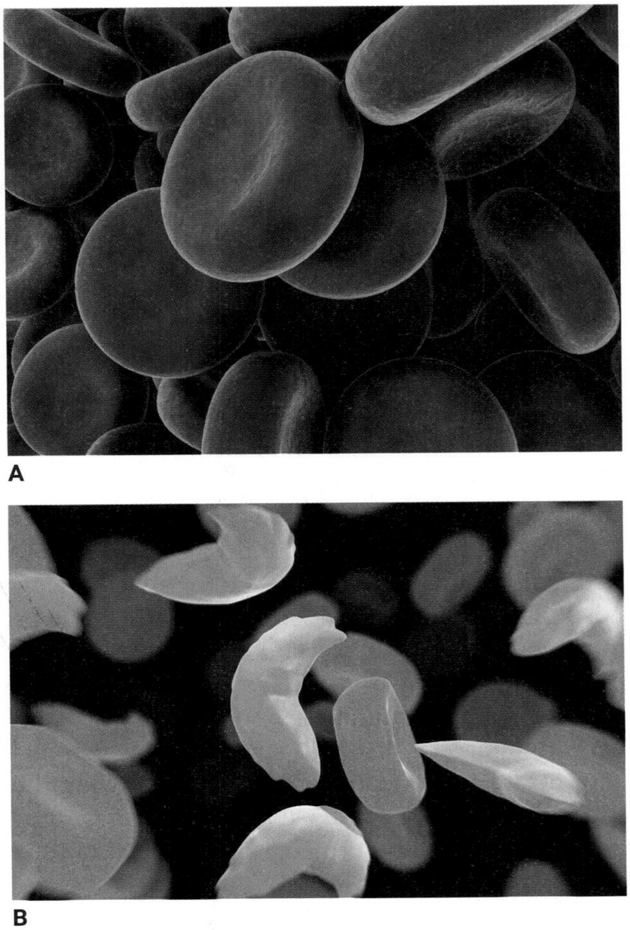

FIGURE 25-5 A. Normal red blood cells. **B.** Sickle cells.

obstructed as a result of this organ's narrow vessels and function of removing damaged RBCs. The spleen may swell to the point of rupture—an event that can lead to death. Vasoocclusion in the brain may result in a cerebrovascular accident (stroke).

- **Acute chest syndrome** is a vasoocclusive crisis that can be associated with pneumonia and pulmonary embolism. Consider the possibility of acute chest syndrome in patients with sickle cell disease accompanied by signs and symptoms including chest pain, fever, and respiratory signs and symptoms, such as a cough.
- **Splenic sequestration crisis** refers to sickle cells trapping blood within the spleen, resulting in acute enlargement of this organ and a hard, bloated, painful abdomen. This condition usually occurs in infants and toddlers and may be accompanied by nausea, vomiting, lethargy, or irritability. **Acute splenic sequestration syndrome** is a life-threatening complication in which RBCs become trapped in the spleen, causing a dramatic decline in the amount of hemoglobin available in the circulation. Patients present with not only a painful abdomen, but also sudden weakness, pallor, tachypnea, and tachycardia. Acute splenic sequestration syndrome can rapidly progress to shock.

Assessment

Do not take a call for a person having a sickle cell crisis lightly. These patients are often in life-threatening crises, characterized by shortness of breath and signs of pneumonia. Their skin may be jaundiced and show signs of inadequate perfusion, accompanied by hypotension. Yellowing in the eye (icteric sclera) may be evident. Signs of mild dehydration and many other complaints are often present as well.

Words of Wisdom

Treatment for a patient with a sickle cell crisis focuses on adequate oxygenation, fluid administration, and pain relief.

In acute crises, patients may have significant pain resulting from congested blood vessels that do not allow the passage of oxygen and nutrients into their tissues and joints. Some may report multiple system involvement, including chest, abdominal, and arthritic-type pain, while others report only fatigue or achiness along with fever. Pediatric patients will typically present with initial pain in the hands and feet, whereas adult patients will report back and proximal extremity pain.

Management

Distinguishing a sickle cell crisis from other nonspecific causes of pain can be difficult. In these situations, perform a thorough assessment and seek medical direction to help sort out the patient's signs and symptoms, problem-solve the situation, and obtain guidance on caring for the patient.

Place the patient in a position of comfort and cover the patient with a blanket to maintain body temperature. It is essential to maintain the patient's body temperature; cold can contribute to sickling of the cells, whereas warm compresses may reduce the likelihood of further sickling.

Supplemental oxygen should be administered via nonrebreathing mask in an attempt to saturate the remaining hemoglobin and increase the level of perfusion that has been decreased by the sickled cells. Ventilation should be provided if the patient's respirations are insufficient. You may also need to give IV fluid therapy to counter the patient's dehydration and flush damaged RBCs from the organs and peripheral tissues. Administer nitrous oxide or other analgesics for pain as allowed by your local protocol. Many patients will have lived with their disease for a long time and, therefore, may have a very high pain threshold. As a consequence, they often require a higher level of analgesia due to developed tolerance. Recommend that the patient rest as much as possible during transport.

Once the patient has arrived at the hospital, care for sickle cell disease may include additional analgesics, antibiotics to prevent infection, and a blood transfusion depending on the severity of the crisis.

Anemia

Pathophysiology

Anemia is defined as a hemoglobin or RBC level that is lower than normal. Usually, this condition is associated with some type of underlying disease process. Anemia may also result from acute or chronic blood loss, or from a decrease in production or an increase in destruction of erythrocytes. In some cases, it may be an outcome of a preexisting hemolytic disorder (ie, a disorder related to the breakdown of RBCs).

Iron-deficiency anemia is the most common type of anemia. Typical causes include gastrointestinal blood loss, menstrual bleeding (the most common cause in US women, affecting primarily African American women), and blood loss due to frequent donations or diagnostic tests for patients hospitalized for long periods. In children, this type of anemia is most often related to premature birth or low birth weight.

Anemia may sometimes be caused by an inherited hemolytic disorder, such as sickle cell disease or **thalassemia**. In these disorders, when the RBCs are first developing their membranes, they become rigid and deformed. As a result, the RBCs

YOU are the Paramedic

PART 3

Your partner returns and tells you the family was unsure of what to do. A home health care agency that has been assisting with the patient's supportive care was contacted, and their staff suggested general comforting methods for the patient. The patient has a do-not-resuscitate order and documents show supportive measures should be undertaken as required. The family is concerned that the patient is not responding well to "supportive measures" and wants the patient transported to the Downtown Hospital oncology unit.

Recording Time: 5 Minutes	
Respirations	20 breaths/min
Pulse	100 beats/min
Skin	Cool, pale, and moist
Blood pressure	100/60 mm Hg
Oxygen saturation (Spo_2)	90% while breathing room air
Pupils	Pupils Equal, Round, and Reactive to Light and Accommodation (PERRLA)

5. Are you concerned with the patient's vital signs at this point?

6. What are "supportive measures" for this patient?

may become lodged in small blood vessels, leading to a thrombosis (blood clot).

Anemia may also be caused by hematologic disorders resulting from a deficiency of an enzyme known as glucose-6-phosphate dehydrogenase. This enzyme helps protect RBCs during infections. When levels of this enzyme are low, cells can become damaged. Although glucose-6-phosphate dehydrogenase deficiency is most commonly seen in African Americans, it can occur in people of any race.

The most common type of acquired anemia develops when the flow of RBCs is disrupted because of problems with the blood vessel linings (such as aneurysms and weaknesses) or blood clots. In autoimmune disorders, RBCs are destroyed by the body's own antibodies, which erroneously perceive the normal blood cells as foreign invaders. Microorganisms can also destroy RBCs in the blood.

Anemia can have serious consequences for people who travel to high-altitude areas. For example, the combination of a smaller number of RBCs and the reduced partial pressure of oxygen in the atmosphere can lead to hypoxia, difficulty breathing, and chest pain.

Assessment

Patients with anemia will often complain of feeling worn down, having no energy, or feeling as if they have overexerted themselves. They may also report that they "can't catch their breath." Because of their abnormally low hemoglobin level, some may have anginal-type chest discomfort related to decreased oxygen supply to the heart muscle. The reduction in functional RBCs can result in skin color changes, such that subtle variations are noted when assessing the conjunctiva of the eyes, the inside of the lips, and the creases of the palms of the hand. These areas can be instrumental in identifying pallor, especially in patients with darker skin. Other conditions that are common in patients with anemia include **leukopenia** (reduction in WBCs) and **thrombocytopenia** (reduction in platelets); both conditions can induce more frequent infections, fevers, cutaneous bleeding, and nosebleeds.

Words of Wisdom

When abnormalities of the blood cells are suspected, note the following points:

- Anemia commonly results in complaints of fatigue, lethargy, and dyspnea.
- Low WBC counts (leukopenia) often lead to infection and fever.
- Low platelet counts (thrombocytopenia) often cause cutaneous bleeding (including petechiae) and bleeding from mucous membranes (such as nosebleeds and rectal bleeding).

Management

Allow the patient to assume a position of comfort while closely monitoring the patient's airway and breathing. Because the patient with anemia has a limited oxygen-carrying capacity, administer oxygen when indicated to ensure that the RBCs that are present are saturated. Check vital signs frequently. Apply a cardiac monitor and closely observe the rhythm if the patient has chest discomfort; a 12-lead ECG may also be warranted. BP management may be needed, along with fluid replacement therapy. Monitor patients closely during fluid replacement. IV fluids do not contain RBCs or blood components, so they may induce unwanted or unexpected bleeding. Do not be surprised if you have to control significant nosebleeds in any patient with anemia.

Transport the patient with anemia to the closest, most appropriate facility. In most cases, gentle transport is appropriate. However, if the patient experiences an abrupt change in mental status, hypotension develops, or other significant changes arise, consider rapid transport.

Words of Wisdom

Remember that IV fluid does not carry oxygen. Consider using vasopressors to increase BP if the patient does not require rehydration and if such treatment is consistent with your local protocols.

Leukemia

Pathophysiology

Leukemia is cancer that develops in the **lymphoid system**, resulting in increased production of immature and/or abnormal blood cells, particularly

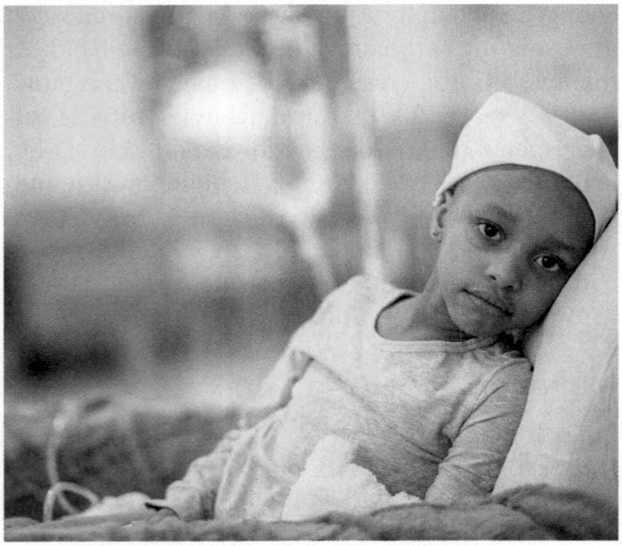

FIGURE 25-6 People with leukemia may have frequent bleeding, bruising, infections, and fever.

WBCs. Leukemia can cause anemia, thrombocytopenia (decrease in platelets), and leukocytosis (increased WBCs). The chemotherapy used to treat this condition typically leads to leukopenia (decreased WBCs). Patients with leukemia experience frequent bleeding, bruising, infections, and fever **FIGURE 25-6**.

Leukemia is classified as either acute or chronic. In most situations, but especially in chronic cases, the disease tends to develop more frequently in older adults (65 years or older). In acute leukemia, bone marrow is replaced with abnormal **lymphoblasts**. In chronic leukemia, abnormal mature lymphoid cells accumulate in the bone marrow, lymph nodes, spleen, and peripheral blood. This form of leukemia is typically found by chance during routine blood tests; suspicions are raised when the tests reveal a high lymphocyte count.

Survival of a person with leukemia depends on factors such as the stage at which the disease is detected, the patient's underlying medical condition, and the response to treatment. Both acute and chronic leukemia are treated with chemotherapy and radiation therapy. In most cases, treatment results in remission, especially when the condition was identified early. According to the National Cancer Institute, children younger than 15 years with acute lymphoblastic leukemia have a 5-year survival rate of more than 90%.[3]

Assessment

Assessment starts with appropriate standard precautions, including gloves and a mask. The presentation of patients with leukemia depends on the stage of the leukemia and the patient's current treatment. Most will complain of fatigue, headaches, or dyspnea, and they may have signs of neurologic defects. During the physical exam, fever, bone pain, and diaphoresis may be found. Patients may report feeling full, soreness in the midpart of the chest, and unexplained bleeding. Assess all vital signs and the cardiac rhythm. Hypotension and tachycardia are often present; therefore, vital signs may be consistent with signs of shock.

Management

Management of leukemia includes providing airway support and oxygen therapy as appropriate. IV fluid therapy and analgesics for comfort may also be necessary. Patients typically need constant positive support because many have a negative outlook on their condition. The patient's loved ones may be quite concerned, especially during advanced stages of the disease; be supportive of them as well. In some cases, you may be called because the patient's condition has deteriorated and the family is uncertain about what to do. In such a scenario, your assessment may indicate normal findings for the patient. The patient or family may change their minds about transport, or they may not have wanted transport at all, but rather professional insight and support. Discuss this situation with medical control, document all findings before leaving, and get a refusal and/or release form signed if the patient or family member decides against transport.

Few calls for patients with leukemia require extreme measures or rapid transport; however, you should be alert to rapid changes in the patient's condition. If you do transport the patient, be aware that the patient could go into arrest en route to the hospital. Make sure you find out the patient's and family's wishes about what to do in this situation.

Lymphomas

Pathophysiology

Lymphomas are malignant diseases that arise within the lymphoid system. They are classified into two categories: non-Hodgkin lymphoma (which accounts for the majority of cases) and Hodgkin lymphoma.

Non-Hodgkin lymphoma can occur at any age in any person and can be hereditary. Furthermore, these types of cancer may be characterized based on the progression of the disease: indolent, aggressive, or highly aggressive. With very slow (indolent) progression, the disease may never leave the lymphoid system. In the highly aggressive form, the disease may affect multiple organs in a relatively short period, usually within several months. How well the disease responds to treatment depends on the specific type of non-Hodgkin lymphoma and how early it is recognized and classified.

Hodgkin lymphoma is a painless, progressive enlargement of the lymphoid glands, most commonly affecting the spleen and the lymph nodes. A rare form of lymphoma, it is suspected to have some hereditary components. Hodgkin lymphoma incidence has two peaks: a first peak between 10 and 35 years of age and a second peak in late life.[4] Patients may not show any symptoms for many years, with the disease being found only after patients complain of night sweats, chills, persistent cough, and swelling of various lymph nodes (usually in the neck first). They may also note a loss of appetite for an unknown reason, significant weight loss, generalized itching, fatigue, and bone pain. According to the American Cancer Society, with treatment, symptoms may disappear for long periods; 65% to 90% of patients may be cured, increasing the 5-year survival rate.[5]

Assessment

Generally speaking, lymphomas require specialized levels of treatment involving some form of chemotherapy or radiation therapy. How well the disease responds to these treatments depends on the stage of the disease and its classification. As a rule, lymphomas respond well to chemotherapy; in fact, aggressive lymphomas respond better than indolent ones. Even if an indolent lymphoma is not cured with chemotherapy, many patients may survive as long as 10 years.

When you are assessing patients with lymphoma, ask specific questions such as "Which type of lymphoma (cancer) do you have?" and "Which type of treatment are you receiving?" As you perform

YOU are the Paramedic

PART 4

Your partner administers oxygen to the patient at 2 L/min via nasal cannula and establishes IV access. The patient agrees to be transported to the hospital for evaluation; he is still feeling considerable pain throughout his body. You lift the patient onto the stretcher and move the patient to the ambulance for transport.

Recording Time: 10 Minutes	
Respirations	20 breaths/min
Pulse	100 beats/min
Skin	Cool, pale, and moist
Blood pressure	98/60 mm Hg
Oxygen saturation (Spo_2)	96% on 2 L/min nasal cannula
Pupils	PERRLA

7. Do you think the patient's family has called you unnecessarily?
8. Would you classify this patient as having acute or chronic leukemia?
9. If this patient were 7 years old instead of 73, what would be different about the course of the disease process?

your assessment of the patient's skin, you will usually note pallor. The patient's airway will usually be patent and the breathing adequate, although sometimes you may note some congestion in the lower lung fields. The patient may describe being first hot and then cold, or even both hot and cold in different areas of the body. Signs of inadequate perfusion are common, including low BP accompanied by an elevated pulse rate. Abnormal ECG rhythms may also be evident.

Management

Patients with lymphoma may be in constant, extreme pain; therefore, if pain management is needed and available, it may have to be aggressive because the patient will likely already be receiving a high-dose analgesic regimen. Treat inadequate perfusion with fluid therapy, and provide supplemental oxygen **FIGURE 25-7**. If necessary, then treat abnormal heart rhythms. If the patient's condition does not improve or even deteriorates following these measures, then initiate rapid transport to the closest facility. As in cases involving patients with leukemia, you may be called to offer support but no transport. Be supportive, discuss your findings with medical control, explain the options to the patient and family, and allow them to make a decision.

Polycythemia

Pathophysiology

Polycythemia is characterized by an overabundance or overproduction of RBCs, resulting in increased blood viscosity and volume. This hyperviscosity and hypervolemia can result in congestion of tissues and organs. Hyperviscosity of the blood increases the risk of thrombus formation. The increased RBC production can be caused by a rare disorder originating in a single stem cell or by an existing disease, such as heart failure or hypertension. Polycythemia can also arise in people who live in high-altitude areas for long periods.

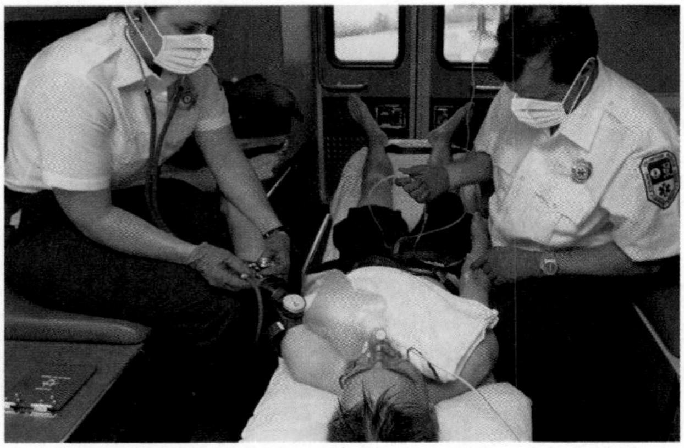

FIGURE 25-7 Patients with lymphoma who are in extreme pain should receive fluid therapy, oxygen, and analgesia.

The overabundance of the blood components associated with polycythemia may lead to many other conditions, such as stroke, transient ischemic attacks, deep vein thrombosis, pulmonary embolism, myocardial infarction, headaches, and abdominal pain (usually associated with an enlarged spleen). This disease is often found incidentally when blood cell counts are performed after a patient reports frequently experiencing signs and symptoms associated with hematologic diseases.

Clinical treatment usually includes phlebotomy to try to maintain hematocrit levels at less than 45% in men and less than 42% in women. Other treatments may include cancer-type therapy intended to slow the production of new RBCs within the bone marrow.

Assessment

Assessment findings may vary widely in patients with polycythemia. An altered level of consciousness may be evident due to stroke or transient ischemic attack–like events; hypoxia may occur due to poor circulation. Respiratory distress can occur, as can changes in peripheral pulses, pulse rate, and skin color. Tachycardia is the most common change in heart rhythm.

As you assess the patient, note the extent and duration of dyspnea, if present. Has the patient experienced uncontrolled itching (pruritus) or noted changes in skin temperature? Make sure to obtain a thorough medical history in patients with known or suspected polycythemia.

Management

Prehospital treatment should initially focus on the chief complaint. Although the underlying pathology may be polycythemia, the patient may now be experiencing a different medical emergency, such as a stroke or cardiac event. Otherwise, treatment primarily consists of supportive care and transporting the patient to an appropriate facility. Administer oxygen as needed. Establish IV access for possible pharmacologic interventions for pain as appropriate. Be supportive of the patient and family.

Disseminated Intravascular Coagulation

Pathophysiology

Disseminated intravascular coagulation (DIC) may result from any number of life-threatening conditions, including massive injury and hypotension due to trauma. Sepsis and obstetric complications also may cause DIC.

This condition progresses in two stages. In the first stage, free thrombin and fibrin deposits in the blood increase, and platelets begin to aggregate. In this stage, defibrination—that is, a breakdown of the fibrin clots—occurs owing to excessive bleeding, massive blood loss, or tissue injury. In the second stage, the patient develops uncontrolled hemorrhage owing to the severe reduction in clotting factors.

Determining the mortality rate for patients with DIC is difficult because they often have additional conditions that can cause signs and symptoms similar to those of DIC.[6] The primary causes of death relate to uncontrolled bleeding, hypotension, and shock.

Words of Wisdom

Patients with DIC experience the simultaneous failure of multiple organs (eg, kidneys, lungs, and heart), accompanied by bleeding from IV sites, bleeding into joints, and, possibly, intracranial hemorrhage.

Assessment

As you assess and care for critically injured or ill patients, keep in mind the issues that may lead to DIC. Your goal is to identify the signs and symptoms commonly associated with DIC or progression toward this coagulopathy. In cases involving severe trauma, patients may have episodes of respiratory difficulty, signs of shock, and skin changes ranging from cold and clammy to pallor to small black-and-blue marks (purpura) on the chest and abdomen.

Management

Maintain the patient's airway, administer supplemental oxygen, and treat the patient for shock (keep the patient warm, control bleeding, and administer IV fluids or vasopressors for hypotension) per your local protocol. Pharmacologic interventions may entail pain management and treatment for abnormal heart rhythms, although interventions for altered heart rhythms should come last. Patients with DIC resulting from severe trauma have a poor survival rate; both they and their family members need support. Be optimistic but honest with patients and family, and do not give false hope regarding survival.

Hemophilia

Pathophysiology

Hemophilia is a bleeding disorder in which clotting either does not occur or is insufficient (as in von Willebrand disease). It is usually associated with an X-linked recessive inheritance pattern, albeit one that is poorly understood. This disease is classified into two primary types: type A, which is due to low levels of factor VIII (antihemophilic globulin and antihemophilic factor), and type B, which is associated with a deficiency of factor IX (plasma thromboplastin component, also known as the Christmas factor). Hemophilia primarily affects males. The levels of factors VIII and IX determine the severity of the disease.

Both type A and type B hemophilia have the same signs and symptoms. Acute and chronic bleeding can occur at any time and may or may not be life threatening. Any injury or illness that can cause bleeding should not be taken lightly in a person with hemophilia. Spontaneous intracranial bleeding is common in patients with hemophilia and is a major cause of death. Patients with significant acute bleeding episodes require hospitalization for transfusion and often require infusion of factors VIII and IX.

Assessment

When you are obtaining the patient's history, you may learn that the patient has a history of conditions associated with hemophilia. In addition to managing the ABCs, be alert for signs of acute blood loss, including pallor, weak pulse, and hypotension.

Note any nosebleeds, bloody sputum, or patient reports of hematuria or melena. Owing to blood loss, patients may exhibit signs of hypoxia due to the reduction in their RBCs' oxygen-carrying capacity.

Management

Administer oxygen if indicated. Note the ECG findings, and treat symptomatic dysrhythmias as appropriate. Prehospital care for a patient with hemophilia may include IV therapy to treat hypotension; definitive care typically involves the transfusion of blood or plasma, which will occur at the hospital. Some patients will have significant pain, so analgesics may be appropriate. Cover patients to maintain their body temperatures. Although you may be called to treat someone with bleeding of unknown cause, only to find that the bleeding stopped before you arrived on scene, you should suggest that the patient get prompt hospital or physician follow-up.

Multiple Myeloma

Pathophysiology

In **multiple myeloma**, the number of plasma cells (B cells that form antibodies) in the bone marrow increases abnormally, leading to the formation of tumors in the bone. These tumors impair the bone marrow's ability to function normally, decreasing RBC, WBC, and platelet formation. Anemia and susceptibility to infection result. Neoplastic (cancerous) cells may also accelerate protein development in the bloodstream, leading to organ failure (primarily the kidneys) and eventually death. Multiple myeloma rarely occurs early in life; most patients are older than 40 years. This disease occurs more frequently in men than in women.

As the disease progresses further and tumors grow or become more numerous, patients may develop weakness in the bones, resulting in spontaneous fractures and pain in the bones and back. Other potential complications include renal failure and recurrent infections. In advanced myeloma cases, treatment options to prolong survival may include stem cell transplant, chemotherapy, and radiotherapy, though these measures may not cure the disease. Morbidity and mortality primarily depend on the extent of the disease and any underlying medical conditions.

Assessment

Because of their susceptibility to infection, be vigilant about using appropriate standard precautions, including wearing a mask and gloves, to help keep patients with multiple myeloma safe. Findings during your assessment and management of these patients will depend on the stage of disease. Early-stage complaints may include fatigue or mild pain, whereas later-stage disease may produce unexplained hemorrhage and significant weight loss, frequent bone fractures, and pain in any number of locations.

Management

Management of multiple myeloma is similar to that for other blood disorders: oxygen (if indicated), IV fluid therapy, pain management, and supportive care. Definitive care at an appropriate facility may improve the patient's condition.

Transfusion Reactions

Pathophysiology

Emergency care may be required if a patient reacts badly to a blood transfusion. **Transfusion reactions** occur in approximately 0.2% to 10% of blood transfusions.[7] Such reactions are similar to an anaphylactic reaction—they occur rapidly and can cause severe circulatory collapse and even death. When a patient undergoes a blood transfusion, it is important to closely monitor the individual for the first 30 to 60 minutes because transfusion reactions typically begin within this time frame.

It is essential to determine the patient's blood type and the type of blood received. When a patient receives blood or plasma that matches the patient's blood type (eg, A+ given to an A+ patient) or the universal donor blood type (O), problems rarely arise. However, administration of an incompatible blood type to a patient—for example, if a patient with type A blood receives type B blood—may cause a potentially fatal transfusion reaction. Also, if a patient with A− blood receives an A+ transfusion, a transfusion reaction could occur. Such reactions are rare, however, because the response to the Rh factor (indicated by the "+" or "−" after the blood type) is not as prevalent and the reaction is not as significant. **TABLE 25-4** summarizes the ABO and Rh compatibility rules.

TABLE 25-4 ABO Rh Type and Preferred and Alternative Donor Types

Recipient Blood Type	Preferred Donor Type	Additional Permissible Types
A+	A+	A−, O+, O−
A−	A−	O−
AB+	AB+	AB−, A+, A−, B+, B−, O+, O−
AB−	AB−	A−, B−, O−
B+	B+	B−, O+, O−
B−	B−	O−
O+	O+	O−
O−	O−	None

Data from: Applegate EJ. *The Anatomy and Physiology Learning System.* 4th ed. Philadelphia, PA: Saunders; 2011.

Assessment

Signs and symptoms of transfusion reactions are generally easy to spot in a responsive patient, but they may be more subtle in an unresponsive or intubated patient. In an acute reaction, the patient experiences a rapid onset of chills, fever, back pain, vomiting, tachycardia, and hypotension. Transfusion reactions may also be delayed up to 7 days after the transfusion, although these events tend to be less severe than the typical acute reaction.

Complications generally fall into the following categories:

- **Hemolytic reaction.** An acute hemolytic reaction is the greatest threat to the patient during a blood transfusion. The primary cause is incompatibility between the recipient and the donor blood. The recipient's immune system is activated by the donor blood, with the new RBCs being destroyed as a result of this reaction. Not only does this outcome return the patient to the state that required the transfusion, but the patient's body has the added burden of managing and clearing all of the destroyed RBCs. Careful screening of the patient and the blood product can typically prevent a hemolytic reaction from occurring.
- **Febrile reaction.** A simple febrile reaction is the most common transfusion complication. It is usually benign and is treated with an antipyretic and observation.
- **Allergic reaction.** In addition to the transfusion reaction, a patient may experience an anaphylactic reaction to preservatives or other agents in the product being transfused. This kind of allergic reaction typically begins within the first few minutes of transfusion and is accompanied by classic signs and symptoms of an anaphylactic state, adding to the patient's already compromised state.
- **Transfusion-related lung injury.** Transfusion-related lung injury is a noncardiogenic pulmonary edema caused by increased capillary permeability post transfusion. Treatment of this condition focuses on supporting the ABCs. Because this type of lung injury does not involve a cardiac failure or fluid overload issue, diuretics are generally ineffective in remedying it.
- **Circulatory overload.** The rapid infusion of blood products can lead to circulatory overload, mimicking heart failure. This type of reaction typically occurs in patients with preexisting cardiomyopathy or ventricular dysfunction. Treatment consists of relieving the system of its excess fluids through diuresis and oxygen, nitrates, and morphine.
- **Bacterial infection.** Bacterial infection is typically a result of poor blood product handling or contamination during the infusion process. It occurs most commonly with platelet transfusions because platelets are kept at room temperature. This kind of infection can lead to systemic sepsis, requiring antibiotic administration and supportive care.

Street Smarts

Immediately discontinue administration of any blood or blood products when the patient shows signs of a transfusion reaction. Take the remainder of the bag and all tubing to the receiving hospital for analysis.

Management

In general, the severity of the transfusion reaction is directly correlated to the amount of blood volume transfused. If the patient develops signs of a transfusion reaction, immediately stop the transfusion, check identifying information on the donor blood to determine whether the wrong blood was given, contact medical control, and provide supportive care to counteract shock. Replace the existing IV tubing and bag with normal saline. Follow your local protocols for allergic reactions or medical control instructions. Retain the blood products and tubing, and transfer them to the blood bank at the hospital.

YOU are the Paramedic SUMMARY

1. Why is a fever in this patient significant?

When a patient has abnormally functioning WBCs, the body is more susceptible to infections. This patient's fever indicates that he now has an infection of some sort in addition to leukemia. The excessive production of the abnormal WBCs can also interfere with production of the other blood cells, resulting in additional hematologic complications.

2. What do you need to know about this patient's status?

The family and patient should be prepared to provide you with written documentation concerning the patient's status. This documentation should include the patient's "code" status and what care should be provided to the patient. Many states have standard forms that are designed for use by medical care providers. Make sure you know the legal requirements for documentation of patients receiving home care in your area.

3. Which signs or symptoms is the patient showing that could indicate thrombocytopenia?

The clearest sign is the presence of the bloody tissues. Under normal conditions, blowing the nose does not cause bleeding. If bleeding starts, then the formation of a platelet plug early in the cascade triggers several other biochemical reactions. However, in this patient, the decreased number of circulating platelets results in less clotting and reduced signaling in the rest of the cascade that follows.

4. How will a patient with leukemia typically present?

Patients with leukemia experience frequent bleeding, bruising, infections, and fever.

5. Are you concerned with the patient's vital signs at this point?

Although the vital signs obtained in this case would commonly indicate shock or impending shock, they may be "normal" for this patient. Anemia can lead to an increased pulse rate and respirations as the body tries to compensate for the inadequate number of RBCs, which carry hemoglobin (the oxygen-carrying component of blood). It is essential to carefully observe the patient's vital signs throughout your care and to contact medical control for analgesic dose advice. Nevertheless, unless a substantial or sudden change in the patient's condition occurs, symptomatic treatment—such as oxygen, IV fluids, and analgesics—is sufficient.

6. What are "supportive measures" for this patient?

Management of this patient includes providing airway support and oxygen therapy as appropriate. In this case, oxygen therapy at 2 L/min via nasal cannula to maintain the patient's oxygen saturation at greater than 94% is warranted. IV fluid therapy and analgesics for comfort may be needed as well. Also, provide positive support; the patient may feel discouraged about his condition. Be honest and do not give false hope.

7. Do you think the patient's family has called you unnecessarily?

You should not think this call for service was unwarranted. The patient's loved ones are concerned, especially because the patient is in the advanced stages of leukemia; be supportive of the family members and the patient. In some cases, you may be called because the patient's condition has deteriorated and the family is uncertain about what to do.

8. Would you classify this patient as having acute or chronic leukemia?

Based on the patient's age and the family's comment that he was "diagnosed years ago," this case appears to involve chronic leukemia.

9. If this patient were 7 years old instead of 73, what would be different about the course of the disease process?

A 7-year-old would typically be experiencing acute leukemia, whereas this patient likely has chronic leukemia. Although the symptoms are the same, the outcome in patients with acute leukemia can be remission and even a cure if treatment is initiated early; by comparison, the cure rate for patients with chronic leukemia is lower.

YOU are the Paramedic SUMMARY continued

EMS Patient Care Report (PCR)					
Date: 11-06-21	**Incident No.:** 9875	**Nature of Call:** General medical		**Location:** 11384 Castle Rock Road	
Dispatched: 1840	**En Route:** 1841	**At Scene:** 1845	**Transport:** 1908	**At Hospital:** 1918	**In Service:** 1930

Patient Information	
Age: 73 **Sex:** M **Weight (in kg [lb]):** 59 kg (130 lb)	**Allergies:** NKDA **Medications:** Numerous, see list **Past Medical History:** Leukemia **Chief Complaint:** Fever/body pain

Vital Signs				
Time: 1850	**BP:** 100/60	**Pulse:** 100	**Respirations:** 20	**Spo_2:** 90%, room air
Time: 1855	**BP:** 98/60	**Pulse:** 100	**Respirations:** 20	**Spo_2:** 96%, 2 L/min NC
Time:	**BP:**	**Pulse:**	**Respirations:**	**Spo_2:**

EMS Treatment (circle all that apply)				
Oxygen @ 2 L/min via (circle one): **(NC)** **NRM** **Bag-mask device**		**Assisted Ventilation**	**Airway Adjunct**	**CPR**
Defibrillation	**Bleeding Control**	**Bandaging**	**Splinting**	**Other:**

Narrative

Dispatched for a 73-year-old man with a history of leukemia. Pt is experiencing general body pain and temp of 102°F. Pt is receiving chemotherapy; last treatment was on 11-02-21. Pt is under home health agency care and has advance directive for supportive care only. Family presented appropriate written documentation verifying same. Family contacted home health agency and received instructions to reduce fever and manage pt's pain. Family stated they became concerned when these measures were ineffective and called 9-1-1. Pt is responsive, alert, oriented, and cooperative. Spo_2 initially 90% room air; now 96% with 2 L/min by NC. IV established TKO. Pt agreed to transport to Downtown Hospital. Because BP was low, medical control contacted concerning administration of analgesic. Medical control advised to administer 2 mg of morphine sulfate IV titrated to effect. Pain decreased, and pt rested comfortably during transport. Report to charge nurse on arrival.

End of report

Prep Kit

Ready for Review

- Most EMS systems rarely respond to hematologic emergencies.
- Blood performs respiratory, nutritional, excretory, regulatory, and defensive functions.
- Blood is made up of plasma and formed elements, or cells, including RBCs, WBCs, and platelets.
- Laboratory tests commonly performed on blood include red blood cell counts, hemoglobin levels, and hematocrit measurements.
- During the primary survey of a patient with a hematologic disorder, it is important to note any signs and symptoms that may be immediately life threatening.

Prep Kit continued

- While taking a history and during the secondary assessment of a patient with a hematologic disorder, look for changes in the level of consciousness, vertigo, feelings of fatigue, or syncopal episodes.
- General management for any patient with problems related to a blood disorder should include the following elements: oxygen (if indicated), fluids, ECG, transport, medications, and psychological support.
- Hematologic disorders include sickle cell crisis, anemia, leukopenia, thrombocytopenia, leukemia, lymphomas, polycythemia, disseminated intravascular coagulation, hemophilia, multiple myeloma, and complications of blood transfusions.
- A patient experiencing a sickle cell crisis will experience significant pain due to congested vessels and may have a serious infection that can lead to sepsis and death.
- A patient with anemia has a hemoglobin or red blood cell level that is lower than normal. Anemia may be caused by an underlying hematologic or hemolytic disorder.
- Leukopenia is a reduction in the number of white blood cells; thrombocytopenia is a reduction in the number of platelets. Both of these conditions are often seen in patients with anemia or leukemia.
- Leukemia is a type of cancer that affects the production of WBCs. Patients often experience bleeding, bruising, infections, and fever.
- Lymphomas are a group of malignant disorders that arise within the lymphoid system. The two types distinguished are non-Hodgkin lymphoma (which accounts for the majority of cases) and Hodgkin lymphoma.
- Polycythemia is characterized by an overabundance or overproduction of RBCs, which leads to hyperviscosity of the circulatory system.
- Disseminated intravascular coagulation may result from a massive injury, sepsis, or obstetric complications. In the first stage, too much blood clotting results from an overactivated coagulation system. In the second stage, the body's natural reaction to break up these clots causes uncontrolled hemorrhage.
- Hemophilia is a bleeding disorder found primarily in males, in which clotting does not occur or occurs insufficiently. Type A hemophilia is due to a low level of factor VIII; type B hemophilia is due to a deficiency in factor IX.
- Multiple myeloma is a cancer of the bone marrow caused by malignant plasma cells.
- Complications of blood transfusions are similar to anaphylactic reactions; they are caused by a mismatch of the patient's blood type to that received or an allergic reaction to preservatives or agents in the transfused product.

Vital Vocabulary

acute chest syndrome A vasoocclusive crisis that can be associated with pneumonia; common signs and symptoms include chest pain, fever, and cough; associated with sickle cell disease.

acute splenic sequestration syndrome A condition in which red blood cells become trapped in the spleen, causing a dramatic decline in the amount of hemoglobin available in the circulation; it usually occurs in infants or toddlers.

anemia A lower than normal hemoglobin or erythrocyte level.

aplastic crisis A temporary halt in the production of red blood cells; it may occur as a result of sickle cell disease.

clotting cascade The process by which clotting factors work together to ultimately form fibrin.

clotting factors Substances in the blood that are necessary for clotting; also called coagulation factors.

coagulopathy Any type of bleeding disorder that interferes with the activation or continuation of the clotting cascade or hemostasis.

Prep Kit continued

disseminated intravascular coagulation (DIC) A condition that begins with widespread activation of the clotting cascade, which depletes the clotting factors and platelets, and eventually results in uncontrolled hemorrhage.

erythrocytes Red blood cells.

hematocrit The proportion of red blood cells in the total blood volume.

hematologic disorder Any disorder of the blood.

hematology The study of the physiology of blood.

hematopoietic system The system that includes all blood components and the organs involved in their development and production.

hemoglobin The iron-rich protein in the blood that carries oxygen.

hemolytic crisis A condition in which red blood cells break down quickly; it may occur as a result of sickle cell disease.

hemolytic disorders Disorders relating to the breakdown of red blood cells.

hemophilia A bleeding disorder that is primarily hereditary, in which clotting does not occur or occurs insufficiently.

hemostasis The body's natural blood-clotting mechanism.

hemostatic disorders Bleeding and clotting abnormalities.

iron-deficiency anemia The most common type of anemia, in which iron stores are low or lacking and the serum iron concentration is low.

leukemia A cancer (malignancy) of the blood-forming organs that particularly affects the white blood cells, which develop abnormally and/or excessively at the expense of normal blood cells.

leukocytes White blood cells.

leukocytosis An increase in the total number of white blood cells.

leukopenia A reduction in the number of white blood cells.

lymphoblasts Lymphocytes that have been transformed because of stimulation by an antigen.

lymphoid system The system primarily made up of the bone marrow, lymph nodes, and spleen, which participates in formation of lymphocytes and immune responses; also called the lymphatic system.

lymphomas Malignant diseases that arise within the lymphoid system; they include non-Hodgkin and Hodgkin lymphomas.

multiple myeloma A disease in which the number of plasma cells in the bone marrow increases abnormally, causing tumors to form in the bones.

neutropenia An abnormally low number of neutrophils.

plasma A component of blood, made of 92% water, 6% to 7% proteins, and electrolytes, clotting factors, and glucose; plasma accounts for 55% of the total blood volume.

polycythemia An overabundance or overproduction of red blood cells, white blood cells, and platelets.

reticuloendothelial system The body system that is primarily used to defend against infection.

sickle cell crisis A condition in which a patient with sickle cell disease experiences significant pain due to insufficient passage of oxygen and nutrients into tissues and joints because of vessel congestion.

sickle cell disease A disease that causes the red blood cells to be misshapen, resulting in poor oxygen-carrying capability and potentially resulting in red blood cells becoming lodged in the blood vessels or the spleen.

splenic sequestration crisis An acute, painful enlargement of the spleen caused by sickle cell disease.

stem cells Cells that can develop into other types of cells in the body.

Prep Kit continued

thalassemia A type of anemia in which either not enough hemoglobin is produced or the hemoglobin is defective.

thrombocytes Platelets.

thrombocytopenia A reduction in the number of platelets.

thrombocytosis A condition in which the body produces too many platelets.

thrombosis Coagulation or clotting of blood in a blood vessel.

transfusion reactions Physiologic responses that are similar to anaphylactic reactions, in which the body reacts to the infusion of blood; they occur rapidly and can cause severe circulatory collapse and death.

transfusion-related lung injury A transfusion reaction characterized by increased pulmonary capillary permeability, resulting in noncardiogenic pulmonary edema.

vasoocclusive crisis Ischemia and pain caused by sickle-shaped red blood cells that obstruct blood flow to a portion of the body.

von Willebrand disease A bleeding disorder in which the patient is missing the von Willebrand factor (a protein essential for platelet adhesion); its absence means that the blood does not clot well.

References

1. Sickle cell disease (SCD). Centers for Disease Control and Prevention website. https://www.cdc.gov/ncbddd/sicklecell/data.html. Last reviewed December 16, 2020. Accessed February 9, 2021.
2. Platt OS, Brambilla DJ, Rosse WF, et al. Mortality in sickle cell disease: life expectancy and risk factors for early death. *N Engl J Med.* 1994;330:1639-1644. http://www.nejm.org/doi/full/10.1056/NEJM199406093302303#t=article. Accessed February 9, 2021.
3. Childhood acute lymphoblastic leukemia treatment (PDQ®)—health professional version. National Cancer Institute website. https://www.cancer.gov/types/leukemia/hp/child-all-treatment-pdq. Updated February 4, 2021. Accessed February 9, 2021.
4. Harris NL. Hodgkin's lymphomas: classification, diagnosis, and grading. *Semin Hematol.* 1996;36(3):220-232.
5. Survival rates for Hodgkin disease by stage. American Cancer Society website. https://www.cancer.org/cancer/hodgkin-lymphoma/detection-diagnosis-staging/survival-rates.html. Revised May 23, 2016. Accessed February 9, 2021.
6. Costello RA, Nehring SM. Disseminated intravascular coagulation. *StatPearls.* https://www.ncbi.nlm.nih.gov/books/NBK441834/. Updated July 17, 2020. Accessed March 10, 2021.
7. Kumar R, Gupta M, Gupta V, et al. Acute transfusion reactions (ATRs) in intensive care unit (ICU): a retrospective study. *J Clin Diagn Res.* 2014;8(2):127-129. https://www.ncbi.nlm.nih.gov/pmc/articles/PMC3972528/. Accessed February 9, 2021.

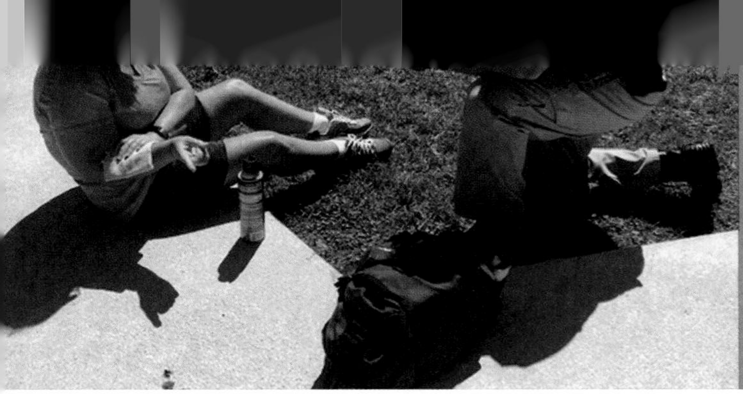

Chapter 26

Immunologic Emergencies

NATIONAL EMS EDUCATION STANDARD COMPETENCIES

Medicine

Integrate assessment findings with principles of epidemiology and pathophysiology to formulate a field impression and implement a comprehensive treatment/disposition plan for a patient with a medical complaint.

Immunology

Recognition and management of shock and difficulty breathing related to

- Anaphylactic reactions (pp 1560, 1568, 1572–1574)

Anatomy, physiology, pathophysiology, assessment, and management of hypersensitivity disorders and/or emergencies

- Allergic and anaphylactic reactions (pp 1561–1576)

Anatomy, physiology, epidemiology, pathophysiology, psychosocial effects, presentations, prognosis, and management of common or major immunologic system disorders and/or emergencies

- Hypersensitivity (pp 1561–1562)
- Allergic and anaphylactic reactions (pp 1561–1576)
- Anaphylactoid reactions (pp 1562, 1569)
- Collagen vascular diseases (pp 1576–1579)
- Transplantation-related problems (pp 1579–1581)

KNOWLEDGE OBJECTIVES

1. Describe the purpose of the immune system. (pp 1561–1562)
2. Define the terms allergic reaction, anaphylaxis, biphasic reaction, prolonged (persistent) reaction, and anaphylactoid reaction. (pp 1561–1562)
3. Explain the difference between a local and a systemic response to allergens. (pp 1561, 1568, 1571)
4. Discuss the process that begins when a foreign substance is detected in the body (primary response). (p 1565)
5. Describe the process that occurs when the body undergoes a secondary response. (p 1565)
6. Explain the role of basophils and mast cells in the immune response process. (pp 1565–1567)
7. Explain the roles of chemical mediators, including histamines and leukotrienes, in the immune response process. (pp 1565–1567)
8. Describe the assessment process for a patient with an allergic reaction. (pp 1567–1572)
9. Explain the importance of managing the care of a patient who is having an allergic reaction. (pp 1571–1572)
10. Compare the signs and symptoms of an allergic reaction with those of anaphylaxis. (pp 1573–1574)

11. Review the process for providing emergency medical care to a patient who is experiencing an allergic reaction. (p 1572)
12. Describe the administration of epinephrine to a patient who is having an allergic reaction, including different forms of epinephrine. (pp 1575–1576)
13. Explain the various treatment options and pharmacologic interventions used to manage anaphylaxis. (pp 1569–1572, 1574–1576)
14. Explain the factors involved when making a transport decision for a patient having an allergic reaction. (pp 1569, 1576)
15. Discuss autoimmune disorders and collagen vascular diseases, including systemic lupus erythematosus and scleroderma. (pp 1576–1579)
16. Describe the principles of organ transplantation and disorders related to organ transplantations. (pp 1579–1581)
17. Explain the importance of patient education in the management of anaphylaxis and allergic reactions. (p 1568)

SKILLS OBJECTIVES

1. Demonstrate how to remove a stinger from a bee sting and proper patient care following its removal. (pp 1574–1575)
2. Demonstrate how to administer epinephrine using an auto-injector. (p 1575)

Introduction

"Please respond to an allergic reaction." Hearing this request from dispatch tends to make emergency medical services (EMS) providers uncomfortable. It is not the care of the patient's **allergic reaction** that causes concern, but rather the potential for a life-threatening anaphylactic reaction. The good news about **anaphylaxis** is that the incidence is relatively low. According to survey results reported by Wood et al., less than 6% of the US population has experienced an anaphylactic reaction.[1] Most of these anaphylaxis incidents were due to medications, followed by foods, and then insect stings **FIGURE 26-1**.[1] The bad news is that the incidence of anaphylactic reactions has been increasing.[2,3] One study found that the greatest incidence of increase was in children and young adults, and that food allergies were the most frequently cited causes.[2] Of the deaths from anaphylaxis studied, the risk of drug-related anaphylactic deaths was higher in the older adult and African American populations.[4]

In dealing with allergy-related emergencies, you must prepare for the possibility of acute airway obstruction and cardiovascular collapse. Because allergic reactions and anaphylaxis often begin similarly, you must be able to distinguish between the body's natural response to a sting or bite, an allergic reaction, and a severe anaphylactic reaction. It is crucial to identify an anaphylactic reaction and be prepared to administer epinephrine. Your ability to recognize and manage anaphylactic reactions may be the difference between life and imminent death for a patient.

This chapter begins by reviewing the physiology of the body's immune response and the pathophysiology of an allergic reaction: how an immune response can become a potentially life-threatening event. You will explore hypersensitivity, allergic reactions, anaphylaxis, biphasic allergic reactions, anaphylactoid reactions, collagen vascular diseases, and transplantation-related disorders.

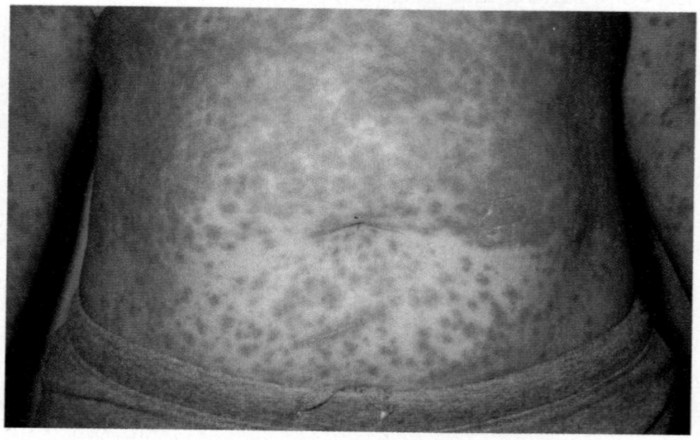

FIGURE 26-1 A patient with a severe allergic reaction to medication. This patient was allergic to penicillin and several other antibiotics.

Courtesy of Carol B. Guerrero.

Anatomy and Physiology Review

The immune system protects the human body from substances and organisms that are considered foreign. Without the immune system for protection, life as we know it would not exist. The body would be under constant attack from any bacterium, virus, or other type of exposure it encountered. Luckily, for most of the population, the body is equipped with an amazing immune system that is on patrol 24 hours a day, 7 days a week, to detect unauthorized visits or invading attacks by foreign substances.

The body protects itself via two types of systems: cell-mediated immunity and humoral immunity (as discussed in Chapter 9, *Pathophysiology*). In cell-mediated immunity, also called *cellular immunity*, the body produces special white blood cells called T cells that attack and destroy invaders. In humoral immunity, B cell lymphocytes produce antibodies that dissolve in the plasma and lymph and wage war on invading organisms. The cells producing immunity are located throughout the body, in the lymph nodes, spleen, and gastrointestinal (GI) tract. Their goal is to intercept foreign forces as they enter the body, thereby limiting the spread and damage of invaders.

Immune Response

There are many terms associated with the various immune system reactions. An **allergen** is a foreign substance that produces allergic symptoms in a patient. Most allergens are usually harmless substances that do not pose a threat to other people; for example, eggs, peanuts, antibiotics, and insect venom. An **antibody** is a protein the body produces in response to an **antigen**. This protein (globulin) is found in the plasma, and is referred to as *immunoglobulin* (Ig). The immunoglobulin E (IgE) antibody is the primary antibody responsible for allergic reactions. (An in-depth discussion of globulins can be found in Chapter 9, *Pathophysiology*.)

When the body is exposed to a foreign substance, the immune system responds, resulting in a localized or systemic reaction. In a **local reaction**, the body limits its response to a specific area after exposure to a foreign substance such as the swelling around an insect bite. A **systemic reaction** occurs throughout the body, possibly affecting multiple body systems. An example of this type of reaction is seen when a person who is allergic to strawberries develops swelling and hives all over the body after eating strawberry shortcake.

Hypersensitivity occurs when a person's immune system reacts with exaggerated or inappropriate symptoms after coming in contact with a substance perceived by the body to be harmful. Hypersensitivity is typically divided into four types.

1. **Allergic reaction.** An abnormal immune response that the body develops when the person has been previously exposed or sensitized to a substance or allergen. In most people, exposure to this substance would produce no reaction or a minor reaction; in a person who is sensitive to the allergen, a significant local or systemic reaction may occur.
2. **Anaphylaxis.** An extreme systemic form of an allergic reaction involving one, two, or

YOU are the Paramedic

PART 1

Your unit is dispatched to a local clinic for a 50-year-old man with an altered mental status and difficulty speaking. The dispatcher tells you the patient was initially seen for an upper respiratory infection, but there is no further information because the call was made from the front desk. When you enter the clinic, you are directed to an examination room, where you find an older African American man lying on the exam table. The head of the bed is elevated. The patient's wife, a nurse, and a physician's assistant (PA) are present. When you look at the man, his mouth looks swollen. He is responsive but does not focus on you as you address him.

1. What is your first impression of this patient?
2. Do you need to take any immediate actions?
3. What differential diagnoses are you considering?

more body systems. In anaphylactic reactions, life-threatening effects are the greatest concern.

3. **Biphasic reaction.** A two-phase allergic reaction in which the patient's symptoms improve and then reappear without exposure to the trigger (allergen) for a second time. The symptoms can resurface up to 8 or more hours after the initial incident. The literature reports a wide variance in incidence of biphasic reactions, from less than 1% to up to 23%.[5–8]
4. **Prolonged (persistent) reactions.** Anaphylaxis symptoms that continue over time, with time frames from 5 to 32 hours.[5] Again, there is an inconsistent report of incidence, from uncommon to up to 23% to 28%.[5]

Anaphylaxis is classified as a response mediated by IgE antibodies, while an **anaphylactoid reaction** is a response that does not involve IgE antibody mediation. The exact mechanism is unknown, but an anaphylactoid event may occur without the patient being previously exposed to the offending agent. Examples of causes of anaphylactic reactions are nuts, fish, and latex. Causes of anaphylactoid reactions include some contrast agents given before radiography, morphine-derivative medications, and aspirin. Even though the process that causes the reaction is different, the patient presentation is the same.

Words of Wisdom

Anaphylactic and anaphylactoid responses are clinically indistinguishable and should be treated in the same manner because both can be life threatening.

Words of Wisdom

The term *anaphylaxis* is not really accurate; the fundamental problem in an anaphylactic reaction is not a lack of protection, but rather overprotection. That is, anaphylaxis is an extreme and devastating form of allergy in which the body's protective immune system goes overboard. This term was first used in 1902, when Portier and Richet were experimenting with vaccinating dogs with sea anemone toxin. After the second dose of the toxin, one of the dogs died due to a severe allergic response. Because this response was mounted against a substance given as protection, it was referred to as anaphylaxis (meaning "without protection").

Routes of Entry for Allergens

Substances can enter and invade the body through the skin, the respiratory tract, or the GI tract. Invasion through the skin may come in the form of injection or absorption. In **injection**, the invading substance pierces the skin and deposits foreign material into the skin. Bees and hornets are often the cause of this type of invasion. Intravenous (IV) or parenteral administration of medications are other examples. **Absorption** occurs when foreign material is deposited on and absorbed through the skin. Absorption can also occur through the vaginal wall. Instances of anaphylactic response to seminal fluid have been documented, so asking patients about recent sexual activity may be necessary.[9] Invasion by allergens does not stop at the skin; substances may also enter the respiratory tract as the patient quietly breathes. This is referred to as an **inhalation** exposure: The foreign substance advances through the respiratory system and launches its attack from the lungs. Cat hair and dander, peanuts, and many plants are involved in this type of exposure. The final way allergens enter the body is through the GI tract via **ingestion**. Foods such as strawberry shortcake, a mushroom and cheese omelet, or peanut butter pie can cause an allergic reaction.

Although it is estimated that millions of Americans are at risk for anaphylaxis, no exact cause or route of exposure or entry for this life-threatening event can be determined in up to two-thirds of patients.[1] Furthermore, no one route of exposure is identified as leading to a greater risk of anaphylaxis. In addition, people with high sensitivity can be at risk from routes of exposure not commonly associated with an antigen. For example, you would expect someone with a peanut allergy to react to ingesting peanuts or peanut-containing foods. However, a patient with a food allergy may have a reaction simply through airborne exposure, such as if the antigen is released in vapor while cooking.

To anticipate anaphylaxis, of course, it would be useful to identify people at greatest risk. Neither race nor sex seems to affect the incidence of anaphylaxis; however, certain ages and sexes tend to have a greater incidence of anaphylaxis associated with specific types of exposure.[10] The incidence of anaphylaxis from insect stings tends to be higher in men.[11] Women have a greater incidence of anaphylactic reactions to latex, aspirin, and IV muscle relaxants.[11,12] Anaphylactic reactions have been documented in children as young as 4 months and in the geriatric population.[4,13] Children are more likely to have severe food allergies, whereas adults tend to have anaphylactic reactions to insect stings, anesthetics, radiocontrast media, and medications. **TABLE 26-1** lists common substances associated with anaphylaxis.

TABLE 26-1 Causes of Anaphylactic Reactions

Antigen, General Category	Comments
Foods	• Most common prehospital cause of anaphylactic reactions; associated with high incidence of fatalities • Peanuts: As little as 100 mcg can cause a reaction. • Peanuts, tree nuts, and shellfish allergies: Common to all ages • Cow's milk, wheat, soy, eggs: Common in children • Eggs: Formerly a contraindication for receiving the flu vaccine (affected individuals now encouraged to receive a single dose of influenza vaccine)

Medications	• Penicillin, beta lactam antibiotics, and cephalosporins are the most common causes of anaphylactic reactions.
	  • Those with penicillin allergy are more likely to have a reaction when administered cephalosporins (especially with cephalothin, cephalexin, cefadroxil, or cefazolin).
	    • May have a higher incidence of allergies to other medications
	• Other medications that can cause reactions:
	  • Antibiotics: ampicillin and sulfa drugs (sulfonamide, sulfisoxazole)
	  • Muscle relaxants: Neuromuscular blocking agents are most common cause (50% to 70%) of anaphylaxis during anesthesia.
	  • Induction agents: Barbiturates may cause IgE response; allergies to soy and eggs are contraindications to propofol use.
	  • Opioids: IV administration of opioids is often associated with flushing and **urticaria**; slowing IV administration usually decreases the effect.
	  • Plasma expanders: dextran, hydroxyethyl starch. If the expander is gelatin based, reaction is possible with gelatin sensitivity.
	  • Insulin isophane suspension (NPH) (Humulin N, Novolin N) may increase anaphylaxis potential.
	  • Salicylates and NSAIDs: Aspirin and NSAIDs are common causes of anaphylactic reactions; cross-allergies may occur.
	  • Local anesthetics
	  • Enzymes (eg, chymotrypsin, penicillinase)
	  • Biologic extracts (eg, insulin and heparin)
	  • Vaccines: Monitor the patient for reactions.

Latex (gloves, supplies, or materials containing latex)	• Use latex-free supplies. Some moulage/simulation supplies contain latex. • The rate of incidence is decreasing. • Cross-reactions may occur with banana, kiwi, and strawberry allergies. • Risk factors: Patients with frequent exposure to latex, sensitized health care workers
Blood transfusions (mismatched)	• Administering A-positive blood to a B-negative recipient • IV immunoglobulin or animal antiserum

(continues)

TABLE 26-1 Causes of Anaphylactic Reactions (continued)

Antigen, General Category	Comments
Hymenoptera stings (bees, yellow jackets, hornets, wasps, and fire ants)	• Systemic reactions occur in 0.5% to 3% of people after being stung. • Adults who develop generalized urticaria are at greater risk for anaphylactic reactions. • Localized reactions are not considered risk factors for anaphylaxis.
Animals	• Dander (long-haired animals) • Animal serum products (eg, horse serum and gamma globulins)
Seminal fluid	• Anaphylactic reactions to seminal fluid have been reported.
Allergen-specific SCIT (allergy injections and skin testing)	• Common cause of anaphylaxis, but rarely cause fatal reactions • Risk factors: Poorly controlled asthma, concurrent use of beta blockers, high allergen dose, errors in administration, and lack of a sufficient observation period following the injection, atopic disease history
Chlorhexidine (antiseptic)	• Used in dental rinses and for a surgical scrub

Anticancer drugs	• Chemotherapy
	  • Encountered more often
	  • Platinum-containing medications are more commonly associated with reactions.
	• Monoclonal antibodies
	  • Omalizumab often results in a delayed and prolonged reaction. Monitor for 3 hours after the first three injections and for 30 minutes after subsequent injections.

Radio contrast media (iodinated radiocontrast dyes used in obtaining radiographs)	• Both anaphylactic and anaphylactoid reactions have been reported. • Risk factors for more severe reactions: Patients with asthma, beta blocker use, cardiovascular disease • No evidence that seafood or iodine-containing solutions applied topically are related to anaphylactoid radio contrast media reactions.

Other	• Rare incidents of anaphylaxis coinciding with menstruation have been reported.
	• Exercise-induced physical activity has been reported to cause anaphylaxis.
	  • Risk factors or co-triggers: Ingestion of foods (may be specific foods or general ingestion); NSAID use, especially aspirin; high pollen count (rare)
	  • Reactions/incidents do not consistently recur with similar incidents.

Idiopathic (unknown cause)	• Patients may experience anaphylaxis without an identifiable cause. • Treatment should be initiated; a cause can be determined later. • Patients may have multiple episodes of idiopathic anaphylaxis per year.

Abbreviations: IgE, immunoglobulin E; IV, intravenous; NPH, neutral protamine Hagedorn; NSAID, nonsteroidal anti-inflammatory drug; SCIT, subcutaneous immunotherapy

Data from: Mustafa S. Anaphylaxis. Medscape website. http://emedicine.medscape.com/article/135065-overview#a4. Updated May 16, 2018. Accessed February 11, 2021; and Peroni DG, Sansotta N, Bernardini R, et al. Muscle relaxants allergy. *Int J Immunopathol Pharmacol.* 2011;24(suppl 3):S35-S46. Pub Med Abstract. https://www.ncbi.nlm.nih.gov/pubmed/22014924. Accessed February 11, 2021.

SAFETY

EMS providers must be prepared for latex allergies in the field and consider the need to provide a latex-free or latex-safe environment. The National Institute for Occupational Safety and Health offers publications on preventing allergic reactions to latex in the workplace.

Diseases related to allergies, also referred to as atopic diseases, include allergic rhinitis, asthma, and atopic dermatitis. The presence of atopic diseases increases the potential for anaphylactic reactions. Anaphylaxis recurrence has a higher incidence in patients with atopic diseases.[14]

It is important to note the route of exposure, although a severe reaction can occur by any route.

The time between exposures to a substance should be noted as well, because the more time that passes between exposures, the less likely it is that a severe anaphylactic reaction will occur. This relationship is thought to be due to the decreased production of the specific Ig or antibody cells in the body over time. It is *not* the case for anaphylactoid reactions, so being prepared for intervention is key, as it may not be possible to differentiate between the two reactions in the field.

Words of Wisdom

The severity of a future allergic reaction cannot be predicted based on the severity of a past reaction. A mild allergic reaction can be followed by a life-threatening reaction.[15]

Physiology of Immune Response

Once a foreign substance enters the body, the body initiates a series of responses. The first encounter with the foreign substance begins the **primary response**. Cells (macrophages) immediately confront and engulf the foreign substances to determine if they are allowed in the body. If the body cannot identify the substance, it uses immune cells to record the salient features of the outside substance. These cells record one or two of the proteins on the surface of the invading substance and then design specific proteins to match each substance. These proteins (called antibodies) are intended to match up with the antigen and inactivate it.

Through the primary response, the body develops **sensitivity**, that is, the ability to recognize the antigen the next time it is encountered. To determine whether the substance is "one of us," the body records enough details to assist in future identification of the substance and production of antibodies to perfectly fit the invading antigen. The **secondary response** occurs with reexposure to a foreign substance.

The **basophils** and **mast cells** produce the body's **chemical mediators** **TABLE 26-2**. These cells contain granules filled with a host of powerful substances ready to be released to fight invading antigens. As

TABLE 26-2 Chemical Mediators

Mediator	Physiologic Effects
Histamine	• Systemic vasodilation • Increased permeability of blood vessels • Decreased cardiac contractility • Decreased coronary blood flow • Dysrhythmias • Bronchoconstriction • Pulmonary vasoconstriction
Eosinophil chemotactic factor	• Attracts eosinophils and neutrophils

Arachidonic acid (precursor of the following):
Prostaglandin
Leukotrienes (SRS-A)
	These factors act to produce other inflammatory mediators:
	• Smooth muscle contraction
	• Vascular permeability
	• Bronchoconstriction
	• Increased mucus secretion
	• Decreased force of cardiac contraction
	• Decreased coronary blood flow
	• Dysrhythmias
	  • More potent than histamine (thousands of times)
	  • React more slowly than histamine

Platelet-activating factor	• Platelet aggregation • Causes histamine release
Serotonin	• Pulmonary vasoconstriction

(continues)

TABLE 26-2 Chemical Mediators (continued)

Mediator	Physiologic Effects
Proteoglycans Heparin Chondroitin sulfate	• Control the release of histamine. These mediators as a whole work to activate the kinin system and are thought to contribute to prolonged and biphasic reactions.
Chemokines Cytokines	• These mediators trigger inflammatory pathways and increase the recruitment of inflammatory cells.
Kinins	• Kinins are proteins produced at sites of tissue injury or inflammation, causing vasodilation and smooth muscle contraction. Bradykinin is one of the stronger kinins and is responsible for increased vascular permeability.

Abbreviation: SRS-A, slow-reacting substance of anaphylaxis

long as the body is not invaded by one of the previously identified foreign substances, the granules are kept encapsulated in their protective walls and remain inactive. If an antigen invades the body and combines with one of the antibodies, however, the granules are ejected from the mast cells, and the chemical mediators are then released into the surrounding tissue and the bloodstream **FIGURE 26-2**. (An in-depth review of the immune system is included in Chapter 9, *Pathophysiology*.)

YOU are the Paramedic

PART 2

While your partner sets up the oxygen equipment to start treating the patient, you ask what happened. The PA shares that the patient came to the clinic for an upper respiratory infection. The patient was diagnosed with an ear and sinus infection, he was administered penicillin and given an albuterol inhaler for bronchitis. You ask if the patient has ever had this type of reaction before. The nurse replies, "No," and adds, "He has an allergy to aspirin, but not to penicillin." The wife agrees with these statements. She says they were in the waiting room after her husband got his shot when he started having trouble talking and started acting funny. She called the nurse, and the nurse called you. The nurse also states the patient has a history of hypertension and takes an angiotensin-converting enzyme (ACE) inhibitor. The staff administered diphenhydramine (Benadryl) and 0.3 mg of epinephrine via the intramuscular (IM) route before your arrival. You ask your partner to attach the patient to the cardiac monitor.

Recording Time: 0 Minutes	
Appearance	Awake
Level of consciousness	Not alert
Airway	Open with swelling of the lips
Breathing	Audible stridor and wheezing without stethoscope, which develops as you are applying oxygen and collecting an initial report
Circulation	Weak, rapid radial pulse

4. Can this be an allergic reaction if the patient has not had a previous reaction?
5. What are the implications of a history of hypertension and taking an ACE inhibitor for this case?
6. Was the administration route and dose of epinephrine appropriate, and should you allow them to administer a second dose? Defend your decision.

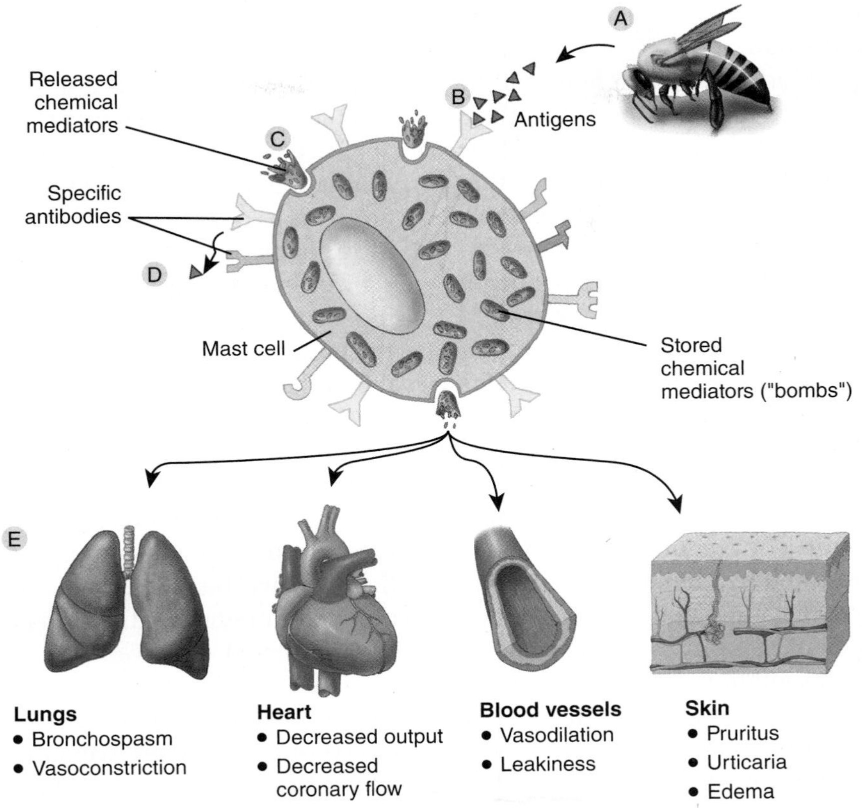

FIGURE 26-2 The sequence of events in anaphylaxis. **A.** The antigen is introduced into the body. **B.** The antigen–antibody reaction at the surface of a mast cell. **C.** Release of mast cell chemical mediators. **D.** A specific antibody reacts with its corresponding antigen. **E.** Chemical mediators exert their effects on end organs.

Patient Assessment

Scene Size-up

Assess the scene for safety issues, such as a swarm of bees, which may put you, your crew, and the patient at risk. Once you have ensured that the scene is safe, determine the nature of the illness by observing for any potential exposure problems. For example, if the patient was gardening, a bee sting might be a cause of the problem. Dinner at a seafood restaurant should make you suspicious of the shellfish menu items or food fried in peanut oil. Because anaphylaxis is a life-threatening event, taking the time to survey the scene for potential hazards for anaphylaxis is important.

Primary Survey

Assessment of a patient with an allergic or anaphylactic reaction can be challenging. To save the patient's life, you may have to simultaneously assess the patient, identify the problem, and intervene within seconds of arriving on the scene. Index of suspicion for anaphylaxis must be high on your list if any of the symptoms discussed previously are present. You may not have a second opportunity because the patient's condition may deteriorate quickly.

Allergic symptoms are almost as varied as the allergens themselves. A patient may have bite or sting marks that may accompany other signs and symptoms of an allergic reaction. Your assessment of a patient experiencing an allergic reaction should include evaluations of the level of consciousness, the respiratory system, the circulatory system, mental status, and the skin.

As mentioned earlier, allergic reactions can be either local or systemic. They can be categorized as mild, moderate, or severe. Mild reactions affect a local area of the body and do not spread to other areas. Itchy, watery eyes or a rash are examples of a mild reaction. Slight congestion would also be considered a mild reaction. Moderate reactions begin as mild reactions, but the symptoms do spread to other parts of the body. For example, the patient initially reports itchy, watery eyes and then develops tightness in the chest with trouble breathing. Severe reactions are considered anaphylactic reactions, and they result in potentially life-threatening emergencies. Severe reactions are systemic; for example, the patient may report congestion that progresses to respiratory distress and hypotension. Onset may be sudden and affect the entire body.

Observe the patient to form a general impression. The patient's presentation will give you an indication of the severity of the problem. If the patient is unable to speak, edema may be affecting the vocal cords. Level of consciousness is an indicator of the patient's severity and a reflection of the patient's oxygenation and circulatory status. Restlessness, confusion, anxiety, and combativeness are common signs of hypoxia. Any change in mental status in an anaphylactic patient should direct you to begin immediate epinephrine administration and airway evaluation and management.

Part of forming a general impression involves evaluating the airway and breathing. A noisy upper airway is a concern in any patient, but even more so in an anaphylactic patient because it may be an early sign of impending airway occlusion due to swelling. Listen for stridor and hoarseness. In addition, the patient may report a tight feeling or a "lump in the throat." Observe the patient for difficulty speaking, noisy airway, tachypnea, labored breathing, accessory muscle use, abnormal retractions, and prolonged expiration. The severity of these findings predicts the stability of the patient's condition. Breath sounds are also a predictor of severity. Initially, you will hear wheezing. As the patient's condition deteriorates and the lungs become tighter and less ventilated (hypoventilation), lung sounds will diminish and the chest may become silent. A silent chest is an ominous finding and requires immediate intervention. Early intervention is key in these patients. Not all patients will have respiratory issues, so maintain a high index of suspicion.

Monitor the patient closely for changes in circulation. Evaluate the skin for erythema, rashes,

YOU are the Paramedic

PART 3

You elect to administer a second dose of epinephrine IM. Your partner administers oxygen to the patient, who is starting to focus and is complaining of trouble breathing. Stridor can be heard clearly. Wheezing is still present on auscultation. The PA recommends sitting the patient upright to assist with his breathing. Your partner recommends initiation of albuterol via nebulizer while you start an IV line.

Recording Time: 5 Minutes	
Respirations	26 breaths/min, very shallow
Pulse	120 beats/min
Skin	Urticaria forming across the chest and arms, warm, dry
Blood pressure	90/58 mm Hg
Oxygen saturation (Spo_2)	92% on room air, 94% on oxygen via nonrebreathing mask
Pupils	Pupils Equal, Round, and Reactive to Light and Accommodation (PERRLA)

7. Are there concerns with allowing this patient to sit upright, and would you position the patient in an upright position?
8. What effect can you expect the albuterol to have on this patient?
9. What type of fluid should you administer, and how much fluid is indicated? Are there any concerns with fluid administration for this patient?

edema, moisture, **pruritus** (itching), and urticaria (hives). Urticaria may appear as reddened, elevated patches on the skin (eg, welts) in individuals with pale skin. Urticaria can be difficult to recognize in individuals with dark skin because although patches of elevated skin may be present and the skin may appear inflamed, it is unlikely to be red. Instead the skin may appear slightly lighter or darker than usual. These symptoms are more commonly associated with an anaphylactic reaction due to histamine release; however, anaphylaxis can occur without these common skin signs. Pallor and cyanosis may be present as well. (Because pallor and cyanosis may be challenging to detect in patients with dark skin, check the mucous membranes [lips, tongue, conjunctivae], nail beds, or palms of the hands for an ashen, gray, or blue color.) A weak, thready, or absent radial pulse is indicative of potential cardiovascular collapse. Recall that anaphylaxis can present with hypotension alone or that hypotension may not be present even in life-threatening cases. Do not wait for the signs of shock to develop. Early recognition and initiation of immediate treatment are a priority.

As you are completing the primary survey, you should be making transport decisions. You must decide whether to remain on the scene, load the patient and initiate treatment during transport, or call for air transport. In addition, you should determine which facility the patient should be transported to based on the patient's need for services.

Words of Wisdom

In patients with high sensitivity to an allergen, always ask about less traditional routes of exposure as you collect the history. For example, ask about inhalation exposure in a patient with a peanut allergy.

History Taking

The patient history should include investigation of the chief complaint, SAMPLE (Signs and symptoms, Allergies, Medications, Pertinent past history, Last oral intake, Events leading to injury or illness), and OPQRST (Onset, Provocation/palliation, Quality, Region/radiation, Severity, Timing). The history should be specifically directed at this incident. Some steps may be skipped or data may be collected later if a life threat exists. Does the patient have any allergies? Has the patient ever had an allergic or anaphylactic reaction? If so, how severe was the incident and how rapidly did it progress? Comparing it to this incident by asking how severe this incident is and how rapidly it is progressing is a useful tool as well.

Ask whether any interventions have been performed. Determine whether the patient had a previous exposure to the antigen; for example, if the patient just ate peanuts, asking about previous ingestions may be useful. A severe reaction may occur at the first or second exposure to an antigen, so the patient might not know about the allergy. Asking about medications, particularly new medications, may help identify the antigen. In addition, ask questions regarding risk factors for severe anaphylaxis, such as the following:[16]

- Peanut and tree nut allergy history (especially in adolescents)
- Preexisting respiratory or cardiovascular disease
- Asthma
- Delayed administration of epinephrine
- Previous biphasic anaphylactic reactions
- Advanced age
- Mast cell disease

In some anaphylactoid (non-IgE) reactions, a previous exposure may not be present. Additionally, there will be cases in which you cannot identify the offending antigen. In the presence of a severe reaction, intervention takes priority over identifying the antigen. To help determine where the patient is in the reaction process, ask when the symptoms began. Direct your assessment to potential signs of life threats, such as feelings of tightness in the throat, feelings of dyspnea, syncopal events, or hypotension.

Also determine whether the patient or first responders have administered any treatment before your arrival. This may include using an EpiPen, taking diphenhydramine, or using an inhaler with a beta agonist (such as albuterol or metaproterenol) or aerosolized epinephrine (such as Primatene Mist) **FIGURE 26-3**. If the patient has an EpiPen or has used one, be aware that some EpiPens come with two doses. Do not discard the second dose.

Ask about less-common causes of anaphylaxis, such as exercise-induced reactions. In the rare case of seminal fluid reaction, ask about recent sexual activity. Do not delay treatment to find the cause.

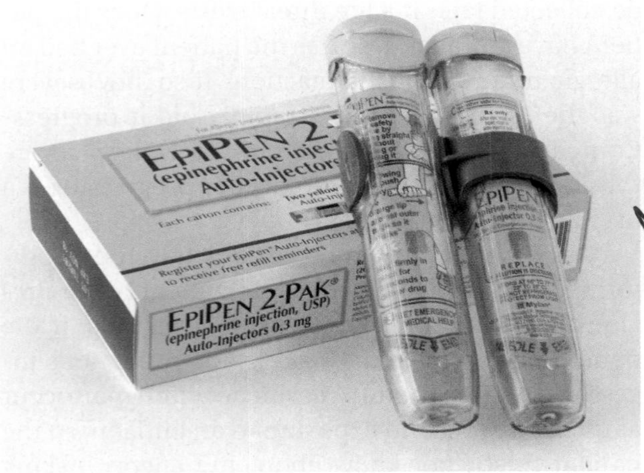

FIGURE 26-3 Patients who experience severe allergic reactions often carry prescription epinephrine, which comes predosed in an auto-injector or a prefilled syringe.

Patients may have idiopathic anaphylaxis, so you may not be able to identify the cause. **TABLE 26-3** shows a guideline for identifying anaphylaxis.

Secondary Assessment

As time and conditions allow, perform a physical examination. The classic presentation of anaphylaxis includes respiratory symptoms and hypotension. In addition, GI symptoms such as abnormal cramping, nausea, vomiting, and diarrhea may be present. If the patient is identified as having a life-threatening condition, perform a physical examination; however, it should be done after life threats are addressed and you are en route to the hospital.

The secondary assessment may help direct treatment. As in all emergencies, your assessment

TABLE 26-3 Diagnosis of Anaphylaxis

Anaphylaxis is likely when any one of the three criteria is fulfilled.

Criterion 1 Acute onset of an illness (minutes to several hours) with involvement of:	**Criterion 2** Two or more of the following that occur rapidly after exposure to a likely allergen for that patient:	**Criterion 3** After exposure to a known allergen for that patient (minutes to several hours):
Skin and/or mucosa: • Pruritus • Flushing • Hives • Angioedema And either: Respiratory compromise: • Dyspnea • Wheeze-bronchospasm • Decreased peak expiratory flow • Stridor • Hypoxemia Or: Decreased blood pressure or end-organ dysfunction: • Collapse • Syncope • Incontinence	Skin and/or mucosa: • Pruritus • Flushing • Hives • Angioedema Respiratory compromise: • Dyspnea • Wheeze-bronchospasm • Decreased peak expiratory flow • Stridor • Hypoxemia Decreased blood pressure or end-organ dysfunction: • Collapse • Syncope • Incontinence Persistent gastrointestinal symptoms: • Vomiting • Crampy abdominal pain • Diarrhea	Decreased blood pressure

Modified from: Manivannan V, Decker WW, Stead LG, et al. Visual representation of National Institute of Allergy and Infectious Disease and Food Allergy and Anaphylaxis Network criteria for anaphylaxis. *Int J Emerg Med.* 2009;2:3-5. doi:10.1007/s12245-009-0093-z. https://link.springer.com/article/10.1007%2Fs12245-009-0093-z. Accessed February 11, 2021.

of a patient experiencing an allergic reaction should include a systematic head-to-toe or focused assessment to determine hidden trauma or other unrelated medical conditions.

Perform evaluations of the respiratory system. Thoroughly assess the airway and breathing, including stridor, increased work of breathing, use of accessory muscles, head bobbing, tripod positioning, nostril flaring, and grunting. Carefully auscultate the trachea and the chest.

Stridor and wheezing may be present during an allergic reaction. Stridor occurs when swelling in the upper airway closes off the airway and can lead to total obstruction. Wheezing occurs because excessive fluid and mucus are secreted into the bronchial passages, and muscles around these passages tighten in response to the release of histamines and leukotrienes induced by the allergen. As a result, exhalation becomes increasingly difficult as the patient tries to cough up the secretions or move air past the constricted airways. Breathing becomes more difficult, and the patient may even stop breathing. Prolonged respiratory difficulty can cause tachycardia, shock, respiratory failure, and death.

Assess the circulatory system. Monitor for signs of hemodynamic compromise, including blood pressure (BP), pulse rate, cardiac monitoring, and pulse oximetry. Remember, the presence of hypoperfusion (shock) or respiratory distress indicates that the patient's reaction is severe and may result in death.

Carefully assess the skin for swelling, rash, hives, and signs of the source of the reaction: bite, sting, or contact marks. A rapidly spreading rash can be concerning because it may indicate a systemic reaction and quickly proceed to anaphylaxis. In individuals with light skin, red, hot skin may also indicate a systemic reaction as the blood vessels lose their ability to constrict and blood moves to the extremities.

Words of Wisdom

Even though cutaneous signs such as urticaria and flushing are common in anaphylaxis, it is important to remember that rapid and severe cardiovascular collapse may occur without cutaneous signs being present.

In people with dark skin, it may be necessary to rely on skin temperature changes rather than changes in skin color. If this reaction continues, the body will have difficulty supplying blood and oxygen to the vital organs. One of the first signs will be altered mental status as the organs are deprived of oxygen and glucose.

Assess baseline vital signs, including pulse, respirations, BP, skin, pupils, and oxygen saturation. Rapid, labored breathing indicates airway compromise. Rapid respiratory and pulse rates may indicate respiratory distress or systemic shock. Fast pulse rates and hypotension are ominous signs, indicating systemic vascular collapse and shock. Skin signs may not be consistent with signs of hypoperfusion because of rashes and swelling.

Use tools such as a cardiac monitor in your assessment because dysrhythmias may be associated with anaphylaxis. Consider a 12-lead electrocardiogram (ECG) to monitor for cardiac ischemia. This step is especially important in patients with a history of cardiovascular or pulmonary disease. End-tidal carbon dioxide ($ETCO_2$) levels may be elevated in anaphylaxis. Watch for a "shark fin" waveform on the $ETCO_2$ monitor, which indicates bronchoconstriction. $ETCO_2$ may be decreased with hypoperfusion and should improve as the patient's BP and hemodynamic status improve. Monitoring pulse oximetry may alert you to low oxygen saturation levels, which will assist in identifying the degree of respiratory distress. Oxygen administration should be considered for patients with signs of anaphylaxis, or cardiovascular or respiratory compromise, based on analysis of respiratory distress, pulse oximetry, and your protocols.

Reassessment

Reassessment typically is conducted en route to the emergency department (ED). Be vigilant in monitoring a patient experiencing a suspected allergic reaction because deterioration of the patient's condition can be rapid and fatal. Give special attention to any signs of airway compromise, including increasing work of breathing, stridor, and wheezing. Monitor the patient's anxiety level because increased anxiety suggests that the reaction may be progressing. Observe the skin for signs of shock, including pallor and diaphoresis, as well as for flushing. Obtain serial vital signs and note any increase in the respiratory or pulse rate or any decrease in BP. Continue to reassess the chief complaint.

Once you have performed interventions, recheck them. If you administered epinephrine, what was the effect? Is the patient's condition improving? Do you need to consider a second dose? You may need to give more than one epinephrine injection or consider an infusion if you note that the patient has decreasing mental status, increasing breathing difficulty, or a decreasing BP. Be sure to consult medical control or your protocols first. Identify and treat changes in the patient's condition.

Remember, when the patient has a severe condition, the more time you can give the staff at the facility to prepare for the patient, the better. Communicate and document the patient's status, interventions completed, and the patient's response.

Emergency Medical Care

To treat allergic reactions, you must first identify how much distress the patient is experiencing. Some allergic reactions will produce severe signs and symptoms in a matter of minutes and threaten the patient's life. Early epinephrine administration is a priority in care of the patient experiencing an anaphylactic reaction. Ventilatory support and/or fluid resuscitation are required for severe reactions. Other allergic reactions have a slower onset, cause less severe distress, and may resolve without intervention. Milder reactions, without respiratory or cardiovascular distress, may require only supportive care, such as oxygen. In either situation, the patient should be transported to a medical facility for further evaluation.

Pathophysiology, Assessment, and Management of Specific Emergencies

Anaphylactic Reactions

Pathophysiology

As discussed earlier, an overzealous immune system can result in problems that range in severity from a simple annoyance to a life-threatening crisis. This variation occurs because the immune cells of the person with allergy are more sensitive than the immune cells of a person without allergies. Although these cells can recognize and react to dangerous invaders, such as bacteria and viruses, they also identify harmless substances as posing a threat.

When the invading substance enters the body, the mast cells recognize it as potentially harmful and release chemical mediators. Histamine, one of the primary chemical weapons, causes the blood vessels in the local area to dilate and the capillaries to leak. Leukotrienes, which are even more powerful, are released and cause additional dilation and leaking. White blood cells are called to the area to help engulf and destroy the enemy, and platelets begin to collect and clump together. In most cases, this overreaction to harmless invaders is restricted to the local area being invaded. The runny, itchy nose and swollen eyes associated with hay fever are examples of a local allergic reaction.

With anaphylaxis, the person is not so lucky. Chemical mediators are released, and the effect involves more than one system throughout the body. An initial effect may be seen from the histamine release, with secondary effects following a few hours later when additional chemicals are released.

Histamine release causes immediate vasodilation, which often presents as erythematous skin and hypotension. It also increases vascular permeability, which results in edema, fluid secretion, and fluid loss. The edema can present as urticaria **FIGURE 26-4**, airway constriction, and increased

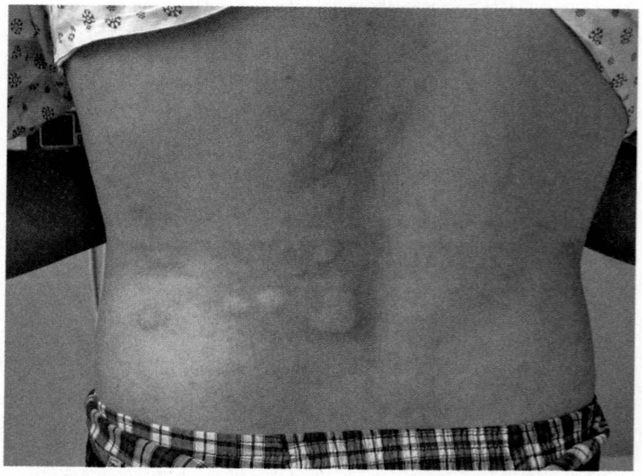

FIGURE 26-4 Urticaria, or hives, may appear following a sting and are characterized by multiple, small, raised areas on the skin.

fluids in the airway. Histamine causes smooth muscle contraction as well, especially in the respiratory and GI systems, resulting in laryngospasm or bronchospasm and abdominal cramping. Finally, histamine decreases the inotropic effects of the heart. When this effect is coupled with vasodilation, the person may experience profound hypotension. Dysrhythmias due to hypoperfusion and hypoxia are also common.

Later responses from the much more powerful leukotrienes compound the effects of histamine. Thus, the person's respiratory status will become even more dire as these highly potent bronchoconstrictors are released. In addition, leukotriene release causes coronary vasoconstriction, contributing to a worsening cardiac condition and myocardial irritability. Leukotrienes are also associated with increased vascular permeability, contributing to a further state of hypoperfusion.

The remaining chemical mediators continue to worsen the situation as they take steps to protect the body from this foreign invader. As a result of these activities, when the body has an anaphylactic reaction, the person may not survive without immediate intervention. (For a more in-depth discussion, see Chapter 9, *Pathophysiology*.)

Clinical Symptoms of Anaphylaxis

The skin is the body's first line of defense against would-be invaders, so skin symptoms are often the first indications of anaphylaxis. Initially, the person may be aware of feeling warm and flushed. Pruritus is another early sign that is due to vasodilation and capillary leaking. The area around the eyes is often susceptible to this effect, which causes swollen, red eyes. Swelling of the face and tongue (angioedema) may contribute to airway compromise. Edema of the hands and feet may also be noted. Histamine is responsible for the urticaria (hives) experienced by the patient with anaphylaxis.

Common complaints include respiratory symptoms, which often present as shortness of breath or dyspnea and tightness in the throat and chest. Stridor and/or hoarseness may also be noted. These signs and symptoms are often due to upper airway swelling in the laryngeal and epiglottic areas. Affected patients may report a lump in the throat or have difficulty speaking. The lower airway is often involved as well. Bronchoconstriction and increased secretions may result in wheezing and crackles (rales). It is not uncommon for the patient to cough or sneeze as the body tries to clear the airway. These symptoms may progress slowly or alarmingly fast. You may have only 1 to 3 minutes to halt this rapid, life-threatening process.

Cardiovascular symptoms are serious complications of anaphylaxis. As noted earlier, histamine and leukotrienes work directly on the heart to decrease its contractility. The resulting decrease in cardiac output is complicated by vasodilation and increased capillary permeability, decreasing the amount of fluid returned to the heart. As cardiac output declines, perfusion decreases, leading to ischemia and bringing the potential for cardiac dysrhythmias. As the fluid leaks out of the capillaries, the intravascular system is left short on fluid. (As much as 50% of the vascular volume can be shifted to the extravascular space within 10 minutes of exposure to an antigen.[17] This situation is analogous to having 3 L of blood in a 6-L container.) Instead of responding normally to the fluid loss and constricting, the blood vessels do just the opposite: They dilate. The already low vascular volume becomes inadequate, and hypotension sets in. The heart rate increases in response to the low BP, putting stress on the already compromised heart. In this situation, tachycardia, flushed skin, and hypotension are synonymous with anaphylactic shock.

GI symptoms may also be part of an anaphylactic response, particularly if the offending antigen has been ingested. Abdominal cramping is a common presentation, but nausea, bloating, vomiting, abdominal distention, and profuse, watery diarrhea may be present as well.

Patients may present with central nervous system symptoms in response to decreased cerebral perfusion and hypoxia. These symptoms include headache, dizziness, confusion, syncopal events, and anxiety. A sense of "impending doom" aptly represents the patient's sense of being near death. A patient who expresses a sense of impending doom requires rapid assessment and treatment.

Anaphylaxis may affect any two or more of these body systems, so the picture can be confusing at times. Think of a patient with anaphylaxis as experiencing three types of shock: (1) cardiogenic shock due to decreased cardiac output, (2) hypovolemic shock due to fluids leaking into the tissues, and (3) neurogenic shock due to inability of the blood vessels to constrict. You will need to use your assessment skills to identify the potential for anaphylaxis and take aggressive action to manage the situation and stop the anaphylactic process as rapidly as possible.

Assessment

You will need to rapidly differentiate between anaphylaxis and other conditions with similar symptoms. Questioning the patient about allergy history and exposure to triggers is the key to identifying the diagnosis of anaphylaxis. Time is of the essence, so be familiar with other possibilities, such as the following:

- **Syncope.** Consider vasovagal incidents or other causes of syncope or shock.
- **Flushing.** Ask about a history of cancer or mast cell disease.
- **Red man syndrome.** Ask about vancomycin infusions, as they can cause this condition, which is characterized by a flushing pruritus and a rash to the upper body.
- **Severe anxiety and respiratory distress.** This can be associated with panic attacks.
- **Wheezing and respiratory distress.** Ask about chronic obstructive pulmonary disease, foreign body aspiration, and asthma history, and whether current symptoms are different than usual.
- **Monosodium glutamate poisoning.** This condition should also be considered. Signs and symptoms include headache, hives, numbness around the mouth, sweating, and upset stomach. With high doses, palpitations, chest pain, and shortness of breath may be present.
- **Scombroid fish poisoning.** This condition can mimic food-induced anaphylactic reactions. The bacteria found in the spoiled fish release enzymes that are capable of mast cell degranulation.
- **Transfusion-related acute lung injury.** This injury may occur up to 6 hours after administration of blood products and presents with hypoxia, shortness of breath, and hypotension.
- **ACE inhibitor angioedema.** Angioedema is a common side effect of ACE inhibitor use and is more common in African Americans.[18] Swelling of the tongue, lips, and face is common. Bronchoconstriction is not commonly seen in ACE inhibitor angioedema. Most patients respond to antihistamine administration and discontinuation of the medication.[18] Close monitoring and preparation for airway management is essential in these patients.

If you are unable to determine another cause of the symptoms and the patient continues to present with anaphylactic symptoms, do not delay treatment for a more complete diagnosis.

Management

People having allergic reactions are separated into two groups for treatment purposes. The first group includes patients with signs of an allergic reaction (for example, urticaria) but no respiratory distress or dyspnea. The drug of choice for these patients is diphenhydramine. Continue to monitor for changes in the patient's condition, but most patients in this group will recover with no further problems.

The second group includes patients who are not stable initially, are deteriorating, or have a history of deterioration. These are the patients with anaphylaxis or the potential to develop anaphylaxis.

Eliminate the offending agent. When possible, remove the patient from the situation involving the antigen or remove the antigen from the patient. For example, if the patient is allergic to peanuts and is being exposed to peanuts through inspiration, you may need to remove the patient from the room, because you may not be able to eliminate the peanut allergen from the air. If the patient has a stinger from a bee sting still in place, you need to remove the stinger. Remember to scrape the stinger off, because you can inject more venom into the patient if you pinch or squeeze the stinger **FIGURE 26-5**.

Maintain the airway. The airway is always a priority in every situation. Be prepared to assist breathing as needed. Assessing for the presence of stridor and hoarseness should indicate the severity of the airway compromise. Be cautious in changing the position of an anaphylactic patient from supine to an upright or standing position. Upright positions have been associated with an increased mortality rate.[16] Use an appropriate oxygen device for supplemental oxygen administration, and consider early transport. *Early administration of epinephrine should be a priority.*

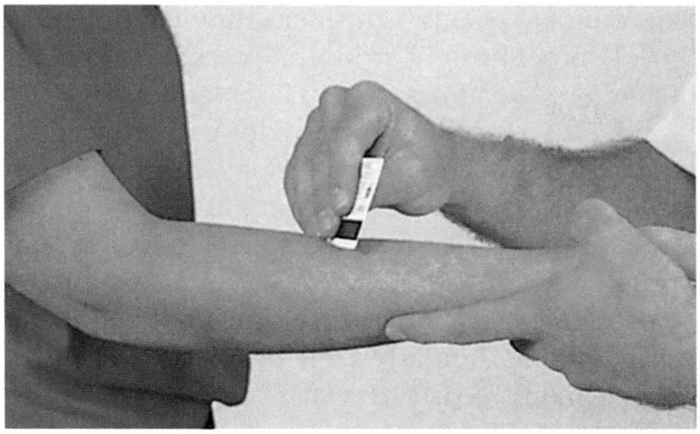

FIGURE 26-5 To remove the stinger of a honeybee, gently scrape the skin with the edge of a sharp, stiff object such as a credit card.

Words of Wisdom

IM administration of epinephrine is preferred over subcutaneous administration of epinephrine because it provides for more rapid absorption. If the patient does not respond to IM administration, IV or intraosseous (IO) infusion of epinephrine is recommended.[19]

IM administration of epinephrine in the anterolateral thigh is the drug and route of choice for anaphylaxis and must be considered early **FIGURE 26-6**. Do not delay administration of epinephrine; delay is considered the major contributing factor to fatalities.[15] Some patients will require more than one dose of epinephrine to reverse the reaction. Additional IM doses may be repeated every 5 to 15 minutes as needed. If there is no response to the IM doses, an IV infusion of epinephrine should be administered in conjunction with an IV fluid bolus to support the hemodynamic status as needed. IV or IO boluses are recommended only if you are unable to quickly deliver infusions of epinephrine, for impending cardiovascular collapse, or if initial infusions are not effective. Endotracheal administration may be considered if other routes are not available.

Epinephrine is the drug of choice for anaphylactic reactions because it stops the process of mast cell degranulation. The action of epinephrine is immediate; it can rapidly reverse the effects of anaphylaxis. In addition, epinephrine reverses the effects of the chemical mediators released via degranulation. Its alpha adrenergic properties cause the blood vessels to constrict, which reverses vasodilation and hypotension. This, in turn, elevates the diastolic BP and improves coronary blood flow. The beta-1 adrenergic effects increase cardiac contractility, reversing the depressing effects on the heart and improving the strength of cardiac contractions. The beta-2 adrenergic effects cause bronchodilation, relieving bronchospasm in the lungs.

Many patients and emergency medical technicians carry epinephrine in the form of an EpiPen, and they may have administered a dose before your arrival. The patient may have taken other medications as well, so it is important to obtain a medication history. See Chapter 15, *Emergency Medications*, for recommended epinephrine doses.

Maintain circulation. Insert at least one 18-gauge IV catheter to administer an isotonic solution (lactated Ringer or normal saline). Ideally, you should place two IV lines en route to the ED. If IV access is not available, obtain IO access. This step is crucial, especially if the patient is hypotensive and does not respond to the epinephrine. Initially, administer 20 mL/kg of isotonic fluid (normal saline

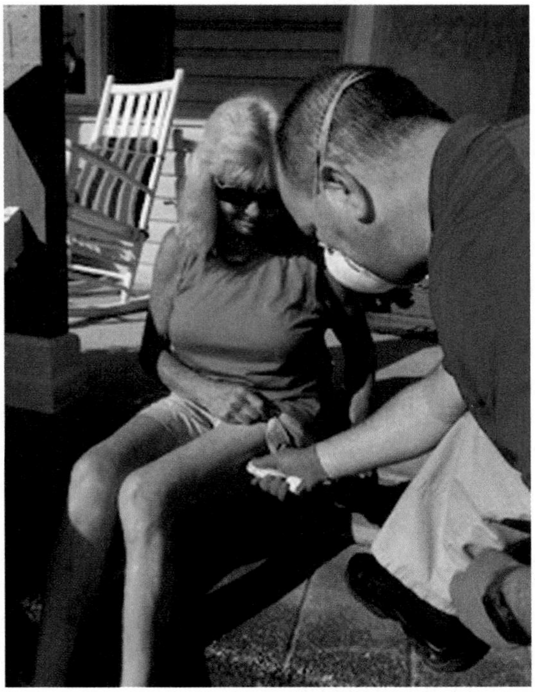

FIGURE 26-6 Administration of epinephrine with an auto-injector.

Evidence-Based Medicine

Take steps to ensure the patient's leg does not move during the administration of epinephrine with an auto-injector. The injection time (the time the device is held against the leg) is 3 seconds. Both of these actions (the act of ensuring the patient's leg does not move and the short injection time) are recommended to decrease the chance of patient harm during the administration process.[19]

Evidence-Based Medicine

You must weigh the risks versus benefits when choosing to administer epinephrine to patients with cardiovascular disease. In a 2017 study, researchers observed that cardiovascular complications (eg, ventricular dysrhythmias, ischemic ECG findings, elevated cardiac biomarkers, stroke) were rare in both young patients (ages 17 to 49 years in this study) and older adults (defined as 50 years or older in this study) who received IM epinephrine for anaphylaxis. The authors concluded that IM epinephrine administration appears safe in all patients with anaphylaxis; however, the use of IV epinephrine should be avoided, especially in older patients, because of the potential of developing serious cardiac complications.[20]

or lactated Ringer) rapidly over 15 minutes IV or IO, repeating as needed.[21] If there is no response, consult medical control or consider administering a vasopressor in conjunction with fluid administration according to your local protocols. Take caution to avoid fluid overload, especially in the cardiac patient.

Following the administration of epinephrine, administer diphenhydramine if urticaria or pruritus is present. Diphenhydramine is an antihistamine that blocks histamine-1 (H_1) and histamine-2 (H_2) receptor sites. This medication does not prevent histamine release, but rather blocks histamine effects at the H_1 receptor sites. H_2 blockers such as cimetidine (Tagamet) and famotidine (Pepcid) can be given orally or IV in conjunction with diphenhydramine for urticaria.[21]

Inhaled beta adrenergic agents such as albuterol (Ventolin) and/or nebulized epinephrine may be considered if respiratory distress with wheezing is present. Consider administering nebulized epinephrine if stridor is present.[21] Reassess the patient's response to your interventions.

Maintain a supine position for patients in anaphylaxis with hypotension. For patients with respiratory distress, reassess the patient's lung sounds and consider slight head elevation, but avoid an upright position.

Research shows no proven benefit from using steroids in the management of allergic reactions and/or anaphylaxis.[21] However, corticosteroid use may be indicated in certain situations, such as for prevention of idiopathic reactions or recurrent anaphylactic reactions to radiocontrast media.

Emotional support is a crucial component of patient care. Anaphylaxis can progress rapidly and has the potential to be a life-threatening event. Patients and their families will need reassurance as you perform the necessary interventions. Many of these patients have experienced similar events in the past and may recognize how serious their condition has become. For others, this may be a first-time event. You need to be professional and reassuring and focus on early intervention and transport.

Initiate early transport if the patient needs resources beyond your capabilities. Even if you are able to stop the reaction and the patient begins to recover, it is recommended that patients be observed in a medical facility. As many as 20% of patients will have a recurrence of the symptoms within the next 8 hours, even if they have been free of symptoms for a time.[16]

Autoimmune Disorders and Collagen Vascular Diseases

In anaphylactic and allergic reactions, the body responds to a foreign invader as the enemy, but the same is not true with autoimmune disorders. In an autoimmune disorder, the immune system inappropriately attacks its own host tissue. Many disorders and conditions are considered to be autoimmune, including those listed in **TABLE 26-4**; those that are not discussed in this section are discussed in other chapters.

Collagen vascular diseases are considered autoimmune diseases; that is, the body perceives its own tissues or cells (in this case, collagen tissue) as a dangerous invader and attacks that tissue.

The attack can be chronic, causing long-term inflammation, or severe enough to result in death. The next sections address two collagen vascular diseases: systemic lupus erythematosus and scleroderma.

TABLE 26-4 Autoimmune Disorders and Conditions

Addison disease	Myasthenia gravis
Cardiomyopathy	Myositis
Celiac disease (also called gluten-sensitive enteropathy or nontropical sprue)	Narcolepsy
Chronic active hepatitis	Neutropenia
Chronic persistent hepatitis	Peripheral neuropathy
Crohn disease	Psoriasis
Demyelinating neuropathies	Raynaud phenomenon
Endometriosis	Restless legs syndrome
Glomerulonephritis	Rheumatic fever
Graves disease	Rheumatoid arthritis
Guillain-Barré syndrome	Thrombocytopenic purpura (TTP)
Hemolytic anemia	Ulcerative colitis
Lyme disease	Scleroderma
Ménière disease	Systemic lupus erythematosus
Multiple sclerosis	Type 1 diabetes mellitus
	Vasculitis

Data from: Autoimmune disease list. American Autoimmune Related Diseases Association website. https://www.aarda.org/diseaselist//. Accessed February 11, 2021.

Pathophysiology

Systemic Lupus Erythematosus

Systemic lupus erythematosus (often referred to simply as lupus or by the abbreviation SLE) is a chronic, progressive, multisystem autoimmune disease. Immune complexes lodged in various body areas can cause inflammation, loss of tissue integrity, and permanent damage. Disease onset is slow and initial symptoms are typically mild and vague, making diagnosis difficult. Patients generally experience periods of active symptoms, called flares, and intervals where symptoms appear to resolve for long periods (remission). The effects of lupus on body symptoms and their prehospital implications are outlined in **TABLE 26-5**.

Lupus occurs more commonly in women than in men. In the United States, it affects an estimated 1.5 million Americans.[22] African American women are four times more likely to have lupus than Caucasian women, and Asian women also have a higher incidence of lupus than Caucasian women.[22] Lupus is most often diagnosed in young women, particularly young African American women of childbearing age.[23]

Patients with lupus tend to die of kidney failure, infection, or cardiovascular disease.[23]

Your priority when caring for these patients should be directed at monitoring for life threats. In addition, because these patients may be on

YOU are the Paramedic

PART 4

The patient indicates improved breathing. The PA recommends another dose of epinephrine. You agree that additional epinephrine may be indicated if there has been no improvement in the BP after administering a fluid bolus of 20 mL/kg. You agree to initiate an epinephrine infusion en route if needed. The patient stabilizes.

Recording Time: 10 Minutes	
Respirations	20 breaths/min; wheezes continue
Pulse	126 beats/min
Skin	Urticaria on upper body and arms resolving, warm, dry
Blood pressure	122/76 mm Hg
Oxygen saturation (Spo_2)	98% on oxygen via nonrebreathing mask
Pupils	PERRLA

10. If the patient deteriorates, how would you mix and administer the epinephrine drip?

TABLE 26-5 Signs, Symptoms, and Prehospital Implications of Lupus

System	Signs and Symptoms	Prehospital Implications
Cutaneous	• Rash that is aggravated by sunlight • Butterflylike rash across the cheeks and nose • Sores or lesions in the mouth • Hair loss • Bruising	• Patients are sensitive to the sun; protect them from prolonged exposure to the sun.
Musculoskeletal	• Joint pain and swelling • Muscle aches and pain • Inflammation of the hands causing symmetric hand pain • Lesions on the extremities that result in gangrene	• Do not let the complaints of joint and muscle pain distract you from assessing for a life threat. • Assess potential for infection.
Pleural	• Pleurisy, pleural effusions, or pleural rub • Pulmonary hemorrhage with hemoptysis • Pneumonia • Pulmonary emboli • Pulmonary hypertension	• Assess for any of these conditions if a patient reports fever, tachypnea, cough, or worsening of chest pain.
Pericardial	• Pericarditis (most common) • Myocardial infarction • Pericardial effusion • Hypertension • Endocarditis • Myocarditis • Vasculitis • Valvular heart disease	• Obtain a 12-lead ECG and assess for signs of pericarditis or ischemia. • Patients with lupus have an increased risk of AMI and post-AMI mortality.
Neurologic	• Stroke • Seizures • Behavioral changes • Psychosis • Migraines • Peripheral neuropathies • Meningitis	• Monitor for stroke and initiate seizure precautions when neurologic symptoms are present.
Renal	• Nephritis • Proteinuria • Renal failure that may require dialysis • Urinary tract infection • Fluid and electrolyte imbalance • Edema	• Assess for history of renal failure and electrolyte imbalance. • Assess for urinary tract infections.
Hematologic	• Anemia • Decreased white blood cell count • Thrombocytopenia	• Recognize potential for hypoxia due to anemia, and risk for infection and bleeding (usually not severe).
Gastrointestinal	• Oral ulcers • Abdominal cramping • Pseudo-obstruction • Pancreatitis • Vasculitis that may result in perforation • Gangrene and peritonitis	• Collect a history to include bloody stools. • Maintain a high index of suspicion.

Abbreviations: AMI, acute myocardial infarction; ECG, electrocardiogram

Data from: Lin C-Y, Shih C-C, Yeh C-C, et al. Increased risk of acute myocardial infarction and mortality in patients with systemic lupus erythematosus: two nationwide retrospective cohort studies. *Int J Cardiol.* 2014;176(3):847-851.

medications to suppress their immune system, slight changes such as fever, cough, or increased pain should alert you to be prepared to treat these patients aggressively as their condition warrants.

Scleroderma

Scleroderma (from *sclero*, meaning "hard," and *derma*, meaning "skin") is an autoimmune connective tissue disease. There are two main classifications of scleroderma: localized scleroderma and systemic scleroderma (also called systemic sclerosis). Changes associated with localized scleroderma are usually found in only a few places on the skin or muscles and rarely spread elsewhere. With this form of scleroderma, the internal organs are usually unaffected, and individuals rarely develop the systemic form of the disease.[24] Systemic scleroderma causes fibrotic (similar to scar tissue) changes to the many parts of the body, including the blood vessels, muscles, joints, skin, GI tract, lungs, kidneys, heart, and other internal organs. Women have a higher incidence of scleroderma than do men.[25]

Patients with systemic scleroderma will often have symptoms of Raynaud phenomenon (pain, blanching, cyanosis, or redness of the fingers and toes when stress occurs or when exposed to the cold or stress). Patients with dark skin will often notice changes in the pigmentation (either lighter or darker) of the hands, arms, or face. Common complaints of systemic scleroderma include musculoskeletal aches and pains, decreased joint motion, and decreased hand function. Stiffness of the lungs and blood vessels can result in shortness of breath, pulmonary fibrosis, and pulmonary hypertension. Cardiac involvement may result in dysrhythmias and damage to the heart muscle, leading to heart failure. Decreased blood flow to the kidneys can result in the release of hormones that cause an increase in BP, which triggers a further reduction in renal blood flow (ie, renal crisis), worsening kidney function.

Assessment

Assessment of patients with lupus or scleroderma should focus on ruling out life threats. These patients may have extensive multisystem problems; do not overlook urgent conditions by attributing their complaints to their chronic conditions.

Management

Treatment of lupus and scleroderma may include administering medications to suppress the patient's overactive immune system. Priority is given to treating any life threats. Be aware that pulse oximetry readings may be inaccurate in patients with Raynaud phenomenon if the sensor is applied to a finger (because of vasospasm and reduced blood flow). If the patient has pulmonary fibrosis or pulmonary hypertension, you may not observe a significant improvement in the patient's oxygen saturation despite supplemental oxygen administration because of impaired oxygen transport between the lungs and blood. Establishing IV access in a patient with scleroderma can be challenging because of the effects of the disease on the blood vessels and the skin over the intended puncture site. Provide supportive care during transport.

Organ Transplantation Disorders

Pathophysiology

When a patient's organs are severely damaged, a transplantation may be performed. The problem with a transplanted organ is that the body sees the replacement organ as foreign; thus, even though the body could not survive without the new organ, the immune system will work to eliminate or "reject" the organ. Patients who receive transplants are placed on medications that prevent the immune system from attacking the new organs to prevent their rejection. These medications, however, place the person at greater risk for infection. In addition, the medications cause the body's self-defense mechanism to either not recognize other threats or to shut down portions of its function, putting them at risk for infection and sepsis.

As a paramedic, you will encounter patients who have undergone organ transplantations. The organs most likely to be transplanted include the heart, liver, kidney, pancreas, and lungs. As you care for these patients, it is important to address the priorities in caring for the specific organ that has been transplanted.

Heart Transplantation

Approximately 3,500 heart transplantations are performed in the United States each year.[26] In the most common procedure used, the recipient's heart is removed and replaced by the donor heart. On the ECG, you may notice an increase in heart rate or tachycardia at the rate of 100 to 110 beats/min due to denervation of the vagus nerve. Chest pain is uncommon because the denervated heart cannot generate anginalike pain. Therefore, a patient with ischemia tends to present with signs of heart failure or dysrhythmias rather than angina. Atropine is not indicated for bradycardia or heart blocks (a delay or disruption of the normal electrical signals that cause the heart to beat). Because the implanted heart does not have vagus nerve innervation, the heart would not respond to the vagolytic action of atropine. Sympathomimetic drugs tend to work well for patients who undergo heart transplantation. If hypertension occurs, antihypertensive medications tend to work even in crisis situations. Norepinephrine and isoproterenol (Isuprel) may have a slightly increased response in these patients.

The majority of rejections occur in the first 3 months post transplantation.[27] Approximately 10% to 15% of patients will experience one episode of rejection, but additional episodes are possible.[28] The signs and symptoms may be subtle and require a biopsy for confirmation. Dysrhythmias have also been associated with rejection. Common problems include sepsis and pneumonia. Assess for fever, shortness of breath, hypoxia, hypotension, poorly controlled hypertension, or the development of a new dysrhythmia, as these are indicators of infection.

Liver Transplantation

Liver transplantations are the second most common solid-organ transplantation procedure. If rejection occurs, the loss of function results in rapid deterioration of the patient and possibly death. Infection, especially opportunistic infection, is a problem for patients who undergo liver transplantation. Observe for jaundice and palpate for tenderness over the site. Patients may present with symptoms that range from vague to complete fulminant hepatic failure. Monitor for hyperkalemia caused by immunosuppressive drugs.

Kidney Transplantation

Kidney transplantations are the most common type of transplantation in the United States and have proved extremely successful. Infection is one of the major concerns for these patients, as it is with all patients who receive transplants. These patients also have a tendency to develop hepatitis C and later liver disease. Rejection of the graft presents as fever, with tenderness and swelling over the implanted kidney, which is located in the anterior area of the retroperitoneal pelvis. Monitor for hypovolemia because hypotension is a common complication. Up to 90% of these patients have hypertension, so ask about their normal BP as part of your assessment.[29] When dealing with patients who have undergone renal transplantation, it is important to understand that many of them are extremely knowledgeable about their condition and can provide you with valuable information. Your assessment should include observation of the site for infection, auscultation for the development of a bruit, and evaluation for other signs of infection. Ask whether the patient has had the spleen removed, because this increases the risk for infection progressing more rapidly.

Lung Transplantation

Lung transplantations may be performed either alone or in conjunction with a heart transplantation. Three types of lung transplantations are performed: bilateral, unilateral, and lobar. In the case of single-lung transplantations, unequal breath sounds are a common finding. Adhesions may be present that complicate the placement of the chest tube on the side of the lung transplantation. Hemothorax is an early complication of lung transplantation. Signs of rejection include cough, dyspnea, vomiting, fever, crackles, rhonchi, and a decrease in oxygenation. Infection presents similarly to the signs of rejection and requires immediate intervention.

Pancreas Transplantation

Pancreas transplantations have a high rate of complications and a lower survival rate than the other single-organ transplantations at 1 year. Most pancreas transplantations are performed in patients with diabetes, and these procedures are often performed in tandem with kidney transplantations. The pancreas has an exocrine function, so a route to drain the exocrine component must be placed. The secretions may be drained into the intestine or the bladder. When drained into the bladder, monitor for urinary tract signs and symptoms such as infections and hematuria. In addition, these patients have a chronic non–anion gap acidosis because the bicarbonate produced by the pancreas drains directly into the bladder for excretion. Remember this point when evaluating the patient and the patient's arterial blood gases, to avoid confusing this condition with lactic acidosis. These patients take oral bicarbonate supplements. Assess for compliance with these medications, as well as other medications. Patients with pancreas transplants are also at risk for dehydration and may present with orthostatic hypotension. Infection and rejection are common problems for these patients.

Assessment

Assessment of the patient who has undergone organ transplantation requires an awareness of subtle signs and symptoms. Keep a high index of suspicion for infection and rejection. Signs and symptoms of organ rejection vary depending on the organ; for example, rejection of a transplanted kidney may cause the patient to excrete less urine. Patients who are experiencing organ transplant rejection will usually have general discomfort and feel ill. Remember that if a transplantation patient calls for EMS, the condition is usually serious. Consider contacting the patient's transplantation center if you have any questions regarding the assessment or findings in these patients. Monitor the cardiac rhythm for indications of hyperkalemia caused by the antirejection drugs and for dysrhythmias in general, particularly in the heart transplantation patients.

Management

The priorities of care for patients who have undergone organ transplantation are focused on the organ transplanted, the medications, recognition of infection or rejection, and transport to the most appropriate facility. Care for these patients varies depending on the organ that was transplanted. Therefore, it is essential that you familiarize yourself with the priorities of patient care with each type of transplantation. Before administering medication, make sure you know how the medication will interact with the medications the patient is taking and how the medication will be metabolized to ensure that toxicity will not develop. Because patients who have undergone transplantations may be immunosuppressed, monitor them for signs and symptoms of infection or organ rejection. Remember, missing even one dose of their immunosuppressive medications is an emergency. Finally, consider transporting the patient to a transplantation facility when possible, or consulting the facility about care when transport to the facility is not possible.

Patients who have undergone organ transplantations must take immunosuppressant medications; suppression of the immune system is key to their survival. Solid-organ transplantations include the heart, liver, kidney, pancreas, and lungs. No matter what type of transplant the patient has received, you must understand the anatomic considerations, and you must be prepared to identify signs of rejection, infection, and medication toxicity.

When the body receives a new organ, that organ comes without its previous connections and message-relaying ability. In consequence, the organ may not behave "normally" when it is having problems. For example, pain is a symptom; however, the organ cannot relay this information to its new host, so pain, such as angina, is not as reliable an indicator of problems as it may be in patients without organ transplants. In addition, the new organs will be tethered to the structures in the body such as blood vessels, other organs, and tissues. Knowing where and how an organ is placed and attached may be useful in identifying problems.

With any organ transplantation, infection is the greatest threat to the patient's survival, so you must be constantly alert to the potential for infection. Rejection of the organ immediately after the surgery is less common today than it was in the past because of improved donor–recipient matching. It is essential that patients take their immunosuppressant medications; however, failure to take even one dose may result in rejection of the organ. Drug toxicity is also a problem for patients who undergo transplantation.

YOU are the Paramedic SUMMARY

1. What is your first impression of this patient?

Looking at the patient can give you an indication of the severity of the problem. In this case, the patient has been having trouble speaking, and although he is responsive, he is not following you with his eyes. This suggests that his level of consciousness is beginning to decrease.

2. Do you need to take any immediate actions?

Due to the swelling of the patient's lips, the recent receipt of an antibiotic, and the change in level of consciousness, you need to act quickly to address possible airway compromise and determine the cause of this patient's condition. Because he just received an antibiotic, is older, and is African American, anaphylaxis is a concern, as drug-related anaphylactic reactions occur at a higher incidence in this population.

3. What differential diagnoses are you considering?

Besides anaphylaxis, you should also consider angioedema because the patient is on an ACE inhibitor. The difficulty speaking should make you evaluate this patient for a possible stroke, and cardiac issues altering his level of consciousness cannot be ruled out because he is older and has a history of hypertension.

4. Can this be an allergic reaction if the patient has not had a previous reaction?

Yes, although patients may need to be sensitized to the allergen before an anaphylactic reaction will occur, in some cases of anaphylaxis or anaphylactoid reactions, previous sensitization may not be present.

5. What are the implications of a history of hypertension and taking an ACE inhibitor for this case?

The swelling of the patient's lips and possible angioedema due to ACE inhibitor ingestion are a concern; however, this appears to be an anaphylactic issue and care should focus on anaphylaxis treatment. This patient will need close cardiac monitoring due to concerns about his cardiovascular history.

6. Was the administration route and dose of epinephrine appropriate, and should you allow them to administer a second dose? Defend your decision.

IM injection into the lateral thigh is the recommended route for initial epinephrine administration. The benefits are rapid access and rapid and more reliable absorption. The IM adult dose is 0.01 mg/kg (maximum dose of 0.5 mg) per single dose.

7. Are there concerns with allowing this patient to sit upright, and would you position the patient in an upright position?

Yes, an increase in mortality has occurred in patients who have been moved to an upright position. Helping patients in anaphylaxis to sit upright or stand is not recommended. The supine position is the position of choice, but slight elevation of the head for ventilation may be considered.

8. What effect can you expect the albuterol to have on this patient?

The beta-2 effect of the albuterol decreases bronchospasm in most patients and typically relieves respiratory distress. It will not affect angioedema or hypotension, so epinephrine administration is still indicated.

9. What type of fluid should you administer, and how much fluid is indicated? Are there any concerns with fluid administration for this patient?

This patient should receive an isotonic crystalloid. A bolus of 20 mL/kg should be administered to address the hypotension. Due to this patient's possible cardiovascular history, close monitoring for possible fluid overload is necessary, especially if additional fluids are needed. If necessary, administering epinephrine via IV infusion is preferred. Intravenous bolus administration is associated with dysrhythmias, which may be a concern for this patient. The patient was beginning to improve and you had time to mix the infusion, so the infusion was preferred over the bolus, but close cardiac monitoring is still necessary due to his history.

10. If the patient deteriorates, how would you mix and administer the epinephrine drip?

The infusion or drip would be prepared by adding 1 mg/1 mL (1:1,000) epinephrine concentration to 1,000 mL of 5% dextrose in water (D_5W) or normal saline. This produces a 1 mcg/mL concentration.

YOU are the Paramedic SUMMARY continued

EMS Patient Care Report (PCR)					
Date: 06-30-22	**Incident No.:** 4563	**Nature of Call:** Altered mental status		**Location:** Main Street Clinic, 100 N. Main Street	
Dispatched: 1810	**En Route:** 1810	**At Scene:** 1818	**Transport:** 1832	**At Hospital:** 1841	**In Service:** 1853
Patient Information					
Age: 50 **Sex:** M **Weight (in kg [lb]):** 78 kg (172 lb)			**Allergies:** Aspirin **Medications:** ACE inhibitor **Past Medical History:** Hypertension, upper airway infection **Chief Complaint:** Altered mental status with difficulty speaking		

Vital Signs				
Time: 1823	**BP:** 90/58	**Pulse:** 120	**Respirations:** 26	**Spo_2:** 92% on room air
Time: 1828	**BP:** 122/76	**Pulse:** 126	**Respirations:** 20	**Spo_2:** 98% O_2
Time:	**BP:**	**Pulse:**	**Respirations:**	**Spo_2:**
EMS Treatment (circle all that apply)				
Oxygen @ 15 L/min via (circle one): **NC** **(NRM)** **Bag-mask device**		**Assisted Ventilation**	**Airway Adjunct**	**CPR**
Defibrillation	**Bleeding Control**	**Bandaging**	**Splinting**	**Other:**

Narrative

Arrived at the Main Street Clinic for a reported altered mental status. On arrival, we found a 50-year-old man lying on an exam table with his head slightly elevated. PA, nurse, and pt's wife are present. The medical personnel report the pt was being seen for an upper respiratory infection and bronchitis, and was administered penicillin and albuterol. During his observation period, he started to have difficulty speaking and his LOC changed. The patient is allergic to aspirin, but no other known allergies. He takes an ACE inhibitor for hypertension. The staff administered 0.3 mg of epinephrine IM. Attached pt to cardiac monitor, which shows sinus tachycardia. The pt has edema around the lips and does not respond to verbal stimuli. His skin was warm and dry initially and then developed urticaria. Wheezing presented but began to reverse after a second dose of epinephrine 0.3 mg IM. Patient's mental status improved and he reported improved breathing. Albuterol nebulizer was administered with an improvement in respiratory status. Wheezing continued. IV with an 18-gauge catheter in the left forearm was obtained and a 20 mL/kg fluid bolus of normal saline was administered en route. Continued improvement noted until arrival at ED. Report to Dr. Morrison on arrival.

End of report

Prep Kit

Ready for Review

- An antigen is a substance the body recognizes as foreign. This recognition causes the body to produce antibodies to destroy the foreign substance.
- The immune system protects the human body from substances and organisms that are considered foreign.
- An allergic response occurs when the body produces an antigen–antibody reaction when exposed to a substance that is usually harmless. An allergic response is usually limited to one body system or a local area.
- Hypersensitivity occurs when a person's immune system reacts with exaggerated or

Prep Kit continued

inappropriate symptoms after coming in contact with a substance perceived by the body to be harmful. Hypersensitivity is typically divided into four types: allergic reaction, anaphylaxis, biphasic reaction, and prolonged (persistent) reactions.

- Most often a person has been sensitized to an antigen before an allergic or anaphylactic reaction occurs; however, patients may present with anaphylaxis without prior exposure.
- Anaphylaxis is an extreme form of systemic allergic response typically involving two or more body systems. However, it may present in a single system, such as the respiratory system.
- An anaphylactoid reaction may occur without the patient being previously exposed to the offending agent.
- The routes of exposure to an antigen include injection, absorption, inhalation, and ingestion.
- Assess for nontraditional causes of anaphylaxis, such as seminal fluid exposure, exercise-induced reaction, or idiopathic.
- Mast cells release chemical mediators that stimulate the allergic reaction.
- Chemical mediators produce signs and symptoms through their effects on the skin, cardiovascular, respiratory, neurologic, and gastrointestinal systems.
- Skin effects of anaphylaxis include erythema, urticaria, and pruritus. Cyanosis and pallor may also be present.
- Cardiovascular effects include vasodilation, hypotension, decreased cardiac output, cardiac ischemia, and dysrhythmias.
- Respiratory effects include upper airway edema and stridor, hoarseness, bronchoconstriction, increased bronchial secretions, wheezes, and hypoxia.
- Neurologic symptoms include syncope, altered level of consciousness, anxiety, restlessness, combativeness, and unresponsiveness.
- Gastrointestinal symptoms include nausea, vomiting, diarrhea, and cramping.
- As part of your assessment, you should evaluate the scene; the patient history; and the patient's level of consciousness, upper airway, lower airway, skin, and vital signs.
- Treatment of anaphylaxis includes removing the offending agent; maintaining the airway; administering medications such as epinephrine, antihistamines (diphenhydramine, cimetidine, ranitidine), corticosteroids, inhaled beta adrenergic agents, and vasopressors; resuscitating with intravenous fluids; and initiating rapid transport.
- IM epinephrine is first-line drug therapy for anaphylaxis.
- Collagen vascular diseases and other autoimmune diseases may require treatment that involves administering medications to suppress the immune system and decrease the attack.
- Organ transplantation disorders can present a multitude of problems in patients. It is important to know the treatment priorities when you care for patients who have undergone organ transplantations.

Vital Vocabulary

absorption In allergic reactions, when foreign material is deposited on and moves into the skin.

allergen A substance that produces allergic symptoms in a patient.

allergic reaction An abnormal immune response the body develops when reexposed to a substance or allergen.

anaphylactoid reaction An extreme allergic response that does not involve immunoglobulin E antibody mediation. The exact mechanism is unknown, but an event of this type may occur without the patient being previously exposed to the offending agent.

Prep Kit continued

anaphylaxis An extreme systemic form of an allergic reaction involving one, two, or more body systems.

antibody A protein that the body produces in response to an antigen; an immunoglobulin.

antigen An agent that, when taken into the body, stimulates the formation of specific protective proteins called antibodies.

basophils White blood cells that work to produce chemical mediators during an immune response.

biphasic reaction A two-phase allergic reaction in which the patient's symptoms improve and then reappear without being exposed to the trigger (allergen) for a second time; the symptoms can resurface up to 8 or more hours after the initial incident.

chemical mediators Chemicals that work to cause the immune or allergic response; for example, histamine.

collagen vascular diseases A group of autoimmune disorders that affect the collagen in tendons, bones, and connective tissues.

histamine A chemical found in mast cells that, when released, causes vasodilation, capillary leaking, and bronchiole constriction.

hypersensitivity Occurs when a patient reacts with exaggerated or inappropriate allergic symptoms after coming in contact with a substance the body perceives as harmful.

ingestion Eating or drinking materials for absorption through the gastrointestinal tract.

inhalation In allergic reactions, when foreign substances are breathed in through the respiratory system.

injection In allergic reactions, when the skin is pierced and foreign material is deposited into the skin.

local reaction When the body limits a response to a specific area after being exposed to a foreign substance.

mast cells Basophils that are located in the tissues.

primary response The first encounter with the foreign substance that begins the immune response.

prolonged (persistent) reactions Anaphylaxis symptoms that continue over time, with the time frame ranging from 5 to 32 hours.

pruritus Itching.

scleroderma An autoimmune connective tissue disease that causes fibrotic (scar tissue–like) changes to the skin, blood vessels, muscles, and internal organs.

secondary response The body's reaction when it is exposed to an antigen for which it already has antibodies, in which it responds by killing the invading substance.

sensitivity The ability to recognize a foreign substance the next time it is encountered.

systemic lupus erythematosus A multisystem autoimmune disease.

systemic reaction A reaction that occurs throughout the body, possibly affecting multiple body systems.

urticaria Hives. In individuals with pale skin, it typically appears as reddened, elevated patches on the skin (eg, welts); in individuals with dark skin, it may appear as patches of elevated, inflamed skin and skin coloration that is slightly lighter or darker than usual.

References

1. Wood RA, Camargo CA, Lieberman P, et al. Anaphylaxis in America: the prevalence and characteristics of anaphylaxis in the United States. *J Allergy Clin Immunol.* 2014;133(2):461-467.
2. Lin RY, Anderson AS, Shah SN, et al. Increasing anaphylaxis hospitalizations in the first 2 decades of life: New York State, 1990–2006. *Ann Allergy Asthma Immunol.* 2008;101(4):387-393.

Prep Kit continued

3. Mulla ZD, Lin RY, Simon MR. Perspectives on anaphylaxis epidemiology in the United States with new data and analyses. *Curr Allergy Asthma Rep*. 2001;11(1):37-44.
4. Jerschow E, Lin RY, Scaperotti MM, et al. Fatal anaphylaxis in the United States, 1999–2010: temporal patterns and demographic associations. *J Allergy Clin Immunol*. 2014;134(6):1318-1328.
5. Mustafa S. Anaphylaxis. Medscape website. https://emedicine.medscape.com/article/135065-overview#a4. Updated May 16, 2018. Accessed February 11, 2021.
6. Grunau BE, Li J, Stenstrom R, et al. Incidence of clinically important biphasic reactions in emergency department patients with allergic reactions or anaphylaxis. *Ann Emerg Med*. 2014;63(6):736-744.
7. Tole JW, Lieberman P. Biphasic anaphylaxis: review of incidence, clinical predictors, and observation recommendations. *Immunol Allergy Clin North Am*. 2007;27(2):309-326.
8. Scranton SE, Gonzalez EG, Waibel KH. Incidence and characteristics of biphasic reactions after allergen immunotherapy. *J Allergy Clin Immunol*. 2009;123(2):493-498.
9. Bernstein DI. Allergic reactions to seminal plasma. UpToDate website. http://www.uptodate.com/contents/allergic-reactions-to-seminal-plasma. Updated June 21, 2019. Accessed February 11, 2021.
10. Allergy facts and figures. Asthma and Allergy Foundation website. http://www.aafa.org/page/allergy-facts.aspx. Accessed February 11, 2021.
11. Hsieh F. Anaphylaxis. Cleveland Clinic Center for Continuing Education website. https://www.clevelandclinicmeded.com/medicalpubs/diseasemanagement/allergy/anaphylaxis/. Reviewed December 2017. Accessed February 11, 2021.
12. Peroni DG, Sansotta N, Bernardini R, et al. Muscle relaxants allergy. *Int J Immunopathol Pharmacol*. 2011;24(suppl 3):S35-S46.
13. Dosanjh A. Infant anaphylaxis: the importance of early recognition. *J Asthma Allergy*. 2013;6:103-107.
14. Alonso T, Moro Moro M, García M. Epidemiology of anaphylaxis. *Clin Exp Allergy*. 2015;45(6):1027-1039.
15. Lieberman P, Nicklas RA, Randolph C, et al. Anaphylaxis—a practice parameter update 2015. *Ann Allergy Asthma Immunol*. 2015;115:348. https://www.aaaai.org/Aaaai/media/MediaLibrary/PDF%20Documents/Practice%20and%20Parameters/2015-Anaphylaxis-PP-Update.pdf. Accessed February 11, 2021.
16. Campbell RL, Li JT, Nicklas RA, et al. Emergency department diagnosis and treatment of anaphylaxis: a practice parameter. *Ann Allergy Asthma Immunol*. 2014;113:603.
17. Kaplan MS. Anaphylaxis. *Perm J*. 2007;11(3):53-56.
18. Sica DA, Black HR. ACE inhibitor–related angioedema: can angiotensin-receptor blockers be safely used? MedScape website. http://www.medscape.com/viewarticle/443226. Accessed February 11, 2021.
19. EPIPEN—epinephrine injection; EPIPEN JR—epinephrine injection. DailyMed, US National Library of Medicine website. https://dailymed.nlm.nih.gov/dailymed/fda/fdaDrugXsl.cfm?setid=7560c201-9246-487c-a13b-6295db04274a&type=display. Revised December 2020. Accessed February 11, 2021.
20. Kawano T, Scheuermeyer FX, Stenstrom R, et al. Epinephrine use in older patients with anaphylaxis: clinical outcomes and cardiovascular complications. *Resuscitation*. 2017;112:53-58.
21. National Model EMS Clinical Guidelines. Version 2.2. National Association of State EMS Officials website. https://nasemso.org/wp-content/uploads/National-Model-EMS-Clinical-Guidelines-2017-PDF-Version-2.2.pdf. Published November 2019. Updated November 3, 2020. Accessed July 31, 2021.
22. Lupus facts and statistics. Lupus Foundation of America website. https://www.lupus.org/resources/lupus-facts-and-statistics. Accessed February 11, 2021.
23. Lupus detailed fact sheet. Centers for Disease Control and Prevention website. https://www.cdc.gov/lupus/facts/detailed.html. Reviewed October 17, 2018. Accessed February 11, 2021.
24. What is scleroderma. Scleroderma Foundation website. https://www.scleroderma.org/site/SPageServer/?pagename=patients_whatis#.YRaHCi1h0W9. Accessed August 13, 2021.
25. Jimenez SA. Scleroderma. Medscape website. http://emedicine.medscape.com/article/331864-overview#a5. Updated June 24, 2020. Accessed February 11, 2021.
26. Everly MJ. Cardiac transplantation in the United States: an analysis of the UNOS registry. *Clin Transpl*. 2008:35-43.
27. Transplant trends. United Network for Organ Sharing website. https://unos.org/data/transplant-trends/. Updated January 17, 2021. Accessed February 11, 2021.
28. Preventing organ and tissue rejection. Donor Alliance website. https://www.donoralliance.org/newsroom/donation-essentials/preventing-organ-and-tissue-rejection. October 5, 2020. Accessed February 11, 2021.
29. Tantisattamo E, Molnar MZ, Ho BT, et al. Approach and management of hypertension after kidney transplantation. *Front Med*. 2020;7:229.

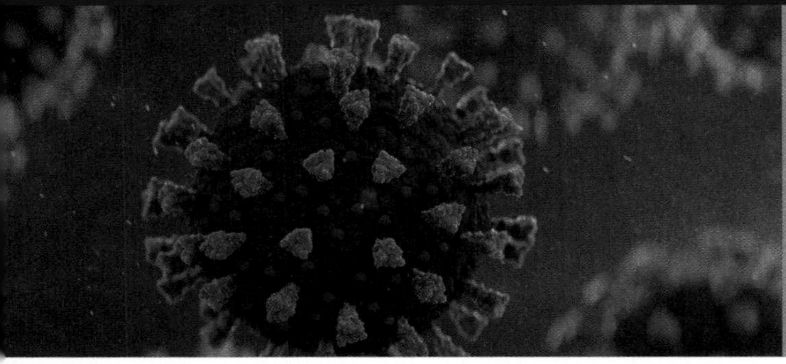

Chapter 27

Infectious Diseases

NATIONAL EMS EDUCATION STANDARD COMPETENCIES

Medicine

Integrates assessment findings with principles of epidemiology and pathophysiology to formulate a field impression and implement a comprehensive treatment/disposition plan for a patient with a medical complaint.

Infectious Diseases

Awareness, assessment, and management of
- A patient who may have an infectious disease (p 1589)
- How to decontaminate equipment after treating a patient (p 1591)

Assessment and management of
- How to decontaminate the ambulance and equipment after treating a patient (p 1591)
- A patient who may be infected with a bloodborne pathogen (pp 1598, 1619–1624)
- Bloodborne diseases (pp 1619–1624)
- Human immunodeficiency virus (HIV) (pp 1622–1624)
- Hepatitis B virus (pp 1619–1621)
- Hepatitis C virus (pp 1621–1622)
- Syphilis (pp 1615–1616)
- Antibiotic-resistant infections (pp 1635–1639)
- Current infectious diseases prevalent in the community (pp 1592–1601)

Anatomy, physiology, epidemiology, pathophysiology, psychosocial impact, presentations, prognosis, and management of
- HIV-related disease (pp 1622–1624)
- Hepatitis (pp 1619–1622)
- Pneumonia (see Chapter 17, *Respiratory Emergencies*)
- Droplet-transmitted diseases (pp 1605–1610)
- Meningococcal meningitis (pp 1605–1606)
- Pertussis (pp 1607–1608)
- Influenza (pp 1606–1607)
- COVID-19 (pp 1609–1610)
- Airborne-transmitted diseases (pp 1610–1614)
- Tuberculosis (pp 1610–1611)
- Chickenpox (Varicella) (pp 1611–1612)
- Measles (pp 1612–1614)
- Tetanus (p 1635)
- Viral diseases (pp 1608–1609, 1611–1614, 1630–1631, see also Chapter 17, *Respiratory Emergencies*, and Chapter 44, *Pediatric Emergencies*)
- Sexually transmitted infections (pp 1615–1619)
- Gastroenteritis (p 1628)
- Fungal infections (p 1624)
- Rabies (pp 1633–1634)
- Scabies and lice (pp 1617–1618)
- Lyme disease (pp 1631–1632)
- Rocky Mountain spotted fever (pp 1632–1633)
- Antibiotic-resistant infections (pp 1635–1639)

KNOWLEDGE OBJECTIVES

1. Define communicable disease. (p 1589)
2. Outline the functions of the agencies responsible for protecting the public health in the United States at the national, state, and local levels. (pp 1589–1590)
3. Describe the paramedic's obligation to protect the public from infection and what steps the paramedic can take to meet it. (pp 1590–1591)
4. Describe how communicable diseases are transmitted by direct and indirect contact, droplet transmission, and airborne transmission. (pp 1592–1593)
5. Discuss the importance of work restriction guidelines. (p 1592)
6. Discuss transmission-based precautions. (pp 1593–1594)
7. Recall the standard precautions the paramedic must take to prevent exposure during patient care activities. (p 1593)
8. List the personal protective equipment (PPE) a paramedic may need in specific circumstances to prevent exposure to communicable and other infectious diseases. (p 1594)
9. Describe the steps to take for personal protection from airborne/droplet and bloodborne pathogens. (pp 1594, 1598)
10. Describe how to remove PPE properly. (p 1596)
11. Explain proper follow-up after exposure to a patient's blood or other potentially infectious materials (OPIM), including documentation of the event and communication with a designated infection control officer and public health authorities. (pp 1596–1601)
12. List the general assessment and management principles for a patient with a communicable disease. (pp 1601–1602)
13. Discuss the importance of obtaining travel histories for all patients. (p 1601)
14. List the general management principles when caring for a patient with a suspected communicable disease. (pp 1601–1602)
15. Describe the cycle of infection, including factors that affect susceptibility to communicable diseases. (pp 1602–1604)
16. Discuss the pathophysiology, assessment, and management of a patient with sepsis. (pp 1604–1605)
17. Discuss the pathophysiology, assessment, and management of a patient with meningitis. (pp 1605–1606)
18. Discuss the pathophysiology, assessment, and management of a patient with influenza. (pp 1606–1607)
19. Discuss the pathophysiology, assessment, and management of patients with seasonal influenza, pertussis, mumps, and rubella (pp 1606–1609)
20. Discuss the pathophysiology, assessment, and management of a patient with tuberculosis. (pp 1610–1611)
21. Discuss precautions paramedics should take to protect themselves from exposure to tuberculosis. (p 1611)
22. Discuss the pathophysiology, assessment, and management of a patient with chickenpox. (pp 1611–1612)
23. Discuss the pathophysiology, assessment, and management of a patient with measles. (pp 1612–1614)
24. Discuss the pathophysiology, assessment, and management of a patient with mononucleosis. (p 1614)
25. Discuss general principles of assessment and management for a patient with a possible sexually transmitted infection. (p 1615)
26. Discuss the pathophysiology, assessment, and management of patients with gonorrhea, syphilis, genital herpes, and chlamydia. (pp 1615–1617)
27. Describe the risk factors, incidence, pathophysiology, assessment, and management of patients with scabies and lice infestation. (pp 1617–1618)
28. Discuss other sexually transmitted infections and conditions. (pp 1618–1619)
29. Discuss the pathophysiology, assessment, and management of a patient with a fungal skin infection. (p 1624)
30. Compare the types of viral hepatitis, including general assessment findings and management principles for the patient with hepatitis. (pp 1619–1622, 1628–1629)
31. Discuss precautions paramedics should take to protect themselves from exposure to hepatitis, and postexposure follow-up. (pp 1619–1622)
32. Discuss the pathophysiology, assessment, and management of a patient with human immunodeficiency virus/acquired immunodeficiency syndrome (HIV/AIDS). (pp 1622–1624)

33. Discuss precautions paramedics should take to protect themselves from exposure to HIV, and postexposure follow-up. (pp 1623–1624)
34. Discuss the pathophysiology, assessment, and management of a patient with suspected Ebola. (pp 1626–1627)
35. Discuss precautions paramedics should take to protect themselves from exposure to Ebola, and postexposure follow-up. (p 1627)
36. Discuss the pathophysiology, assessment, and management of a patient with gastroenteritis. (pp 1627–1628)
37. Discuss the pathophysiology, assessment, and management of patients with non-bloodborne hepatitis viruses. (pp 1628–1629)
38. Discuss the pathophysiology, assessment, and management of patients with West Nile virus, dengue fever, chikungunya fever, and Zika virus. (pp 1629–1631)
39. Discuss the pathophysiology, assessment, and management of patients with Lyme disease, Rocky Mountain spotted fever, hantavirus, rabies, Middle East respiratory syndrome (MERS), and tetanus. (pp 1631–1633, 1634–1635)
40. Compare the most common antibiotic-resistant organisms and multidrug-resistant organisms, including what steps paramedics and patients can take to curb their spread. (pp 1635–1639)
41. Discuss general principles of assessment and management for patients with severe acute respiratory syndrome (SARS), avian flu, and COVID-19. (pp 1639–1640, 1609–1610)

SKILLS OBJECTIVES

1. Demonstrate how to clean and disinfect the ambulance interior and equipment. (p 1591)

Introduction

In 1913, Randolph Bourne said, "We can become as much slaves to precaution as we can to fear." This statement is particularly relevant to EMS care today, because many health care providers are fearful when caring for patients who have or are suspected of having a **communicable disease**—that is, an **infectious disease** that can be passed from one person to another. A paramedic who does not understand how communicable diseases are transmitted and how to take sensible precautions will be hesitant in caring for some patients, no matter what the cause of their illness. This chapter explores how such diseases are transmitted and outlines some measures paramedics can take to protect against them. The communicable diseases that paramedics are most likely to encounter in their work are examined, as are the illnesses that create the greatest anxiety among EMS personnel and the public.

Protecting Public Health

Responsibilities of Public Health Agencies

Several government agencies are responsible for protecting the health of the general public.

YOU are the Paramedic

PART 1

Your unit is dispatched to an assisted care facility for a patient who is vomiting and has had diarrhea for a few days. While you are en route, the dispatcher states that the nurse on scene says the patient has watery diarrhea, low-grade fever, and nausea. When you arrive on scene, staff members meet you at the door. As they guide you to the room, one of the nurses tells you that the staff physician thinks the patient may have *Clostridioides difficile* (previously known as *Clostridium difficile* and commonly referred to as *C diff*) infection due to antibiotic treatment.

1. What is your first concern at this scene?
2. What is *C diff* and what precautions should you put in place for transport?

Agencies at the national level include the Occupational Health and Safety Administration (OSHA), which promulgates rules and regulations designed to protect the employees of public and private organizations. This chapter refers to several OSHA regulations—for example, CFR 1910.1030, commonly known as the Bloodborne Pathogen Standard. (Recall that **bloodborne pathogens** are pathogenic microorganisms that are present in human blood and can cause disease in humans.) OSHA also enforces several of the Centers for Disease Control and Prevention (CDC) guidelines based on its General Duty Clause; these guidelines are identified later in this chapter. Data on the number of patients infected with particular diseases and research and guidance for health care providers and the general public are available from the CDC.

The Ryan White Comprehensive AIDS Resources Emergency (CARE) Act, Part G, is a federal law that requires medical facilities to notify emergency response personnel of airborne and droplet-transmitted diseases diagnosed or suspected in patients they transported. This notification must happen as soon as possible and no longer than 48 hours from the time the facilities have a "suspect" case. The diseases listed in the original act included human immunodeficiency virus (HIV), hepatitis B virus (HBV), tuberculosis, meningococcal disease, diphtheria, pneumonic plague, viral hemorrhagic fevers, and rabies. Subsequently, in August 2011, the CDC published an expanded list of diseases covered under this mandate. The diseases added include hepatitis C virus (HCV), measles, rubella, severe acute respiratory syndrome coronavirus 2 (CoV-2, the virus that causes coronavirus disease 2019), pertussis, cutaneous anthrax, chickenpox, mumps, vaccinia, novel influenza A viruses, and potentially life-threatening diseases caused by biologic agents. Coronavirus disease 2019 (COVID-19) was formally added in 2020.[1] Through these expansions of the mandated list, there is now much broader coverage for emergency responders to be notified of and followed for exposures to infectious diseases.

State and county public health departments bear the responsibility for protecting the public from disease, preventing epidemics, and managing outbreaks at the state and local levels. Although paramedics may not believe that supervision of water quality and cleanliness of restaurants relate directly to emergency care, it is beneficial for EMS agencies to know their local public health officials and to work closely with them. When potential threats to a community's health exist—such as in the aftermath in Hurricane Katrina, during the anthrax and smallpox scares, and following the emergence of avian flu, influenza A virus subtype H1N1 (H1N1), and COVID-19 virus outbreaks—a close working relationship between EMS providers and public health agencies is essential. If you do not know the public health professionals and officials in your county or parish, the designated infection control officer (DICO) will act as your liaison. In the case of an outbreak, public health officials will notify the DICO in an affected area.

In addition, with the reemergence of common childhood diseases, routine vaccination and immunization programs are essential for protecting EMS personnel and their patients. Today, many EMS training programs require candidates to show proof of vaccinations before entering the programs. Similarly, medical facilities may not permit students to do clinical rotations until they have signed declination forms.

State and local public health departments are responsible for many activities related to infectious and/or communicable diseases, including collecting data on disease incidence, performing contact follow-up, and conducting immunization clinics. The public health department monitors reportable diseases on a weekly, monthly, and annual basis. This surveillance helps public health officials identify any upswing in the incidence of a particular disease. If the incidence of cases of a specific disease in a particular geographic area remains steady over time, that figure is said to be the **endemic** number of cases for that area. A rising caseload may signal the beginning of an outbreak or **epidemic**. When a disease infects large numbers of people and spreads worldwide, it is considered a **pandemic**. Public health departments have a significant role in investigating epidemics and pandemics.

The public health department collects all disease statistics for each locality and shares the information with the state health department, which then sends the state totals to the CDC.

Responsibilities of Paramedics

Paramedics have an obligation to protect patients from **health care–associated infection** (ie, infection acquired from a health care setting). Health care–associated infections occur in all types of care settings. These infections can be associated with procedures and the devices used in medical procedures (eg, catheters), community paramedicine, and mobile integrated health care. One way to protect patients is by participating in protective vaccine and immunization programs; another is by complying with work restriction guidelines.

Reporting for work when you have a sore throat or the flu is *not* in the best interest of your patients, your coworkers, or yourself. Today, OSHA's General Duty Clause is being used to enforce the CDC work restriction guidelines. In Section 5(a)(1), the General Duty Clause states that each employer is required to furnish to each of its employees a workplace that is free from recognized hazards that are causing or likely to cause death or serious physical harm. Most of us are familiar with this employer responsibility. However, Section 5(b) of the General Duty Clause addresses employee responsibilities: "Each employee shall comply with occupational safety and health standards and all rules, regulations, and orders issued pursuant to this Act which are applicable to his own actions and conduct." Thus, infection control focuses on both patient protection and care provider protection.

Another way to protect patients from health care–associated infections is to keep the ambulance interior and its equipment clean and disinfected. When cleaning and disinfecting equipment, select the cleaning solutions appropriate to the equipment category:

- **Critical equipment.** Items that come in contact with mucous membranes, such as laryngoscope blades and bag-valve masks. High-level disinfection (ie, use of Environmental Protection Agency [EPA]–registered chemical "sterilants") is the minimum level of cleaning for this equipment.
- **Semicritical equipment.** Items that come in direct contact with intact skin, such as stethoscopes, blood pressure (BP) cuffs, splints, uniforms, and personal protection equipment (PPE). Clean with solutions that have a label claiming to kill HBV. Bleach and water at a 1:100 dilution fits this requirement.
- **Noncritical equipment.** Cleaning surfaces, floors, ambulance seats, and work surfaces. For this equipment, a mixture of EPA-registered hospital-grade cleaner or bleach and water is effective at a 1:100 dilution (¼ cup (62 mL) bleach to 1 gallon (4 L) of water.

General cleaning routines and brand names of cleaning agents need to be listed in the department's exposure control plan. A rule of thumb is to follow these steps after *every* call:

1. Remove used linens from the stretcher immediately after use, and place them in a plastic bag or the designated receptacle in the emergency department (ED).
2. In an appropriate receptacle, discard all disposable equipment used to care for a patient that meets your state's definition of medical waste. Most items will be considered general trash. Refer to your state law's definitions related to medical waste disposal.
3. Wash contaminated areas with soap and water. For disinfection to be effective, cleaning must be done first.
4. Disinfect all reusable equipment used in patient care (eg, glucometer, BP cuff) according to agency policies and manufacturer recommendations.
5. Clean the stretcher with an EPA-registered germicidal-virucidal solution or bleach and water at a 1:100 dilution. Wear heavy-duty utility gloves for all cleaning activities. This is an OSHA requirement.
6. If any spillage or other contamination occurred in the ambulance, clean it up with the same germicidal-virucidal or bleach-water solution. No special cleaning solution or system is needed for any diseases, including Ebola and COVID-19.
7. Create a schedule for routine full cleaning for the vehicle, as required by the exposure control plan. Identify the brands of solution to be used for this purpose.
8. Have a written policy and procedure for cleaning each piece of equipment. Refer to the manufacturer's recommendations as a guide.
9. Cleaning should focus on high-touch items—items used for patient care and items with which the patient was in contact.

Protecting Health Care Providers

Risks for contracting a communicable disease have been determined by the National Institute for Occupational Safety and Health (NIOSH), the CDC, and the World Health Organization (WHO).[2] These data reveal that providers have a low risk of contracting these diseases. OSHA's Compliance Directive (CPL 02-02.069) lists specific requirements for training newly hired personnel about protecting themselves and others from communicable diseases. OSHA also has a requirement for annually updating training to keep personnel informed of new disease research developments that will deepen their understanding of these diseases.

Following the work restriction guidelines developed by the CDC—which OSHA enforces using the General Duty Clause, Section A, under duties—is essential for the protection of care providers, their coworkers, and the patients served in their community.[3] These guidelines should be formally incorporated into department policies, presented in new-hire training, and included in the department's exposure control plan. In the face of the COVID-19 pandemic, the need for strictly adhering to these guidelines has come to the forefront, and all providers should willingly comply with them.

Communicable Disease Transmission

By the very nature of their work, health care providers come in contact with sick people; a certain proportion of those sick people have communicable diseases. Communicable diseases are diseases that can be transmitted from one person to another under certain conditions. These conditions factor into the formula for infection and reflect the infectious agent's dose, virulence, and mode of entry, as well as the host's health status. Although infectious diseases may cause illness in the patient, they do not always pose an immediate risk to the health care provider.

To understand the principles of prevention, you must first understand how diseases are spread. Infectious diseases are caused by pathogenic microorganisms—usually **bacteria** or **viruses**, but sometimes **fungi** and **parasites**. They spread from person to person by several specific mechanisms:

- **Contact transmission**. Direct contact with an infected person may be brief, such as touching a patient. Most cases of the common cold are thought to be transmitted through casual direct contact. Venereal diseases, such as syphilis and gonorrhea, are transmitted principally by direct sexual contact and, therefore, are referred to as sexually transmitted infections (STIs).

  Direct contact also includes puncture by a contaminated needle or other sharp instrument. Punctures may occur if a health care provider is not using a needle-safe or needleless device.

  Another form of direct contact is transfusion of contaminated blood products from one patient to another. Screening tests for bloodborne disease have vastly reduced the risks of contracting illnesses from contaminated blood. Even so, donated blood is not 100% safe from bloodborne pathogens.

  Indirect contact occurs by touching or handling an infected object or by coming in contact with a person who is contaminated with pathogens from an infected person or their secretions. For example, you can become infected if you touch a bloody stretcher railing and have an open cut or sore on your hand, or if you do not wash your hands after touching a contaminated surface. Objects that harbor microorganisms and can transmit them to others, such as the stretcher railing in the preceding example, are called **fomites**.
- **Droplet transmission**. Droplet transmission occurs with inhalation of infected droplets, such as those released into the surroundings when a person with influenza or COVID-19 coughs or sneezes. With these diseases, transmission is most likely to occur when someone is within about 6 feet (2 m) of the infected person.[4]
- **Airborne transmission**. Pathogens transmitted by the airborne route are carried in microscopic particles that become aerosolized when an infected person coughs or sneezes. These infectious particles can remain suspended in the air for some time (usually hours).

Disease transmission can also occur by means other than person-to-person transmission. A **vector** is an organism that harbors pathogens that are harmless to the organism but cause disease when transmitted to a human host. For example, a mosquito infected with West Nile virus or Zika virus that bites a person may transmit the disease.

Once it is established how a disease is transmitted, it is easy to know what PPE is needed

SAFETY

A study by Greek scientists, published in the journal *Physics of Fluids*, argues that with a breeze of as little as 2.5 mph, it takes only 5 seconds for tiny aerosolized droplets to travel 18 feet.[5] Indeed, the common assumption that pathogens larger that 5 microns fall to ground quickly may be flawed, with studies showing that pathogens as large as 100 microns may be airborne.[6] Based on these results, standard social distancing of 6 feet may not offer needed protection from exposure.

SAFETY

A single cough can launch virus-laden secretions at a speed of 50 mph, expelling nearly 3,000 respiratory droplets. Coughing has long been recognized as a key vector of respiratory infections. A sneeze is even more powerful, forcing 100,000 droplets into the immediate environment at a speed of 100 mph.[7]

Place a surgical mask on the patient and an N95 mask or high-efficiency particulate air (HEPA) respirator on yourself!

when rendering care. This concept is termed **transmission-based precautions**.

Transmission-Based Precautions

Standard Precautions

The term **standard precautions** describes infection control practices that reduce the opportunities for an exposure to occur in the daily care of patients. It replaces the older terms *universal precautions* and *body substance isolation (BSI)*. BSI precautions have been taught to EMS providers for several years; this approach assumes that all blood and body fluids are infectious. Standard precautions add another element: protection from moist body substances that may transmit other bacterial or viral infections. For example, a paramedic with a cut on a finger who suctions a patient with oral herpes lesions and does not wear a glove could become infected with herpes whitlow. Standard precautions apply to all body substances *except* sweat.

In addition to standard precautions, three other categories of precautions have been identified: airborne, droplet, and contact. Some diseases may require a combination of precautions. For example, when caring for a patient with Ebola disease, the recommendations for providers include taking standard, contact, and droplet precautions.

Words of Wisdom

Standard precautions are used with all transmission-based categories.

Airborne Precautions

In the context of EMS, **airborne precautions** apply to infections that spread through exposure to virus-containing respiratory droplets, which encompass both small droplets and particles. For example, airborne precautions apply when working with patients suspected of having or diagnosed with tuberculosis, chickenpox, or measles. Airborne precautions involve placing a surgical mask on the patient and ensuring good airflow in the vehicle (exhaust system). Avoid using the vehicle's recirculated air option during patient transport; instead bring in fresh air by using the vehicle's vents or lowering the windows. If the patient cannot wear a mask, the health care provider should wear a surgical mask or N95 respirator. Although it is best if both the patient and the health care provider are masked, masking only one person suffices.[8] Health care workers should wear N95 respirators if they are performing **aerosol-generating procedures**.

Droplet Precautions

Droplet precautions are appropriate with diseases that spread through exposure to large and small droplets and particles generated when an infected person coughs or sneezes. Such diseases include influenza, meningitis, pertussis (whooping cough), mumps, rubella (German measles), Ebola, and COVID-19. To apply droplet precautions, EMS providers should place a surgical mask on the patient.[9] Basic infection control is to contain at the source. As with airborne precautions, use the airflow system in the vehicle as a means to prevent transmission: Ventilation is the key to risk reduction.

Contact Precautions

Contact precautions are appropriate with all patients presenting with draining wounds, multidrug-resistant infection, lice, norovirus, and Ebola. Contact precautions include the use of gloves, a gown if clothing could be contaminated, and cleaning of **high-touch items**. High-touch items include areas with which the patient was in contact and all equipment used during patient care.

Personal Protective Equipment and Practices: Task Based

PPE serves as a secondary protective barrier beyond what your body provides. The selection and use of PPE depend on the task and procedure at hand or, as mentioned, on how the disease is transmitted (transmission-based precautions). Your department's exposure control plan should list the various risk-associated procedures and the PPE recommended for use during these procedures. The CDC has also developed guidelines for PPE use.

Performing hand hygiene, including handwashing, both before and after patient care activities is your primary protective measure. The current standard for handwashing is to use antimicrobial, alcohol-based foams or gels, and to scrub vigorously for at least 20 seconds before rinsing with clean water.[10–12] The friction used to get alcohol-based foams and gels to evaporate removes surface organisms and kills viruses but leaves the normal protective flora intact.

Evidence-Based Medicine

Several studies on handwashing compliance in EMS reveal that this critical practice has a low compliance rate for EMS providers.[11,12]

Words of Wisdom

Wash your hands before and after every call—and after glove removal!

According to the CDC, OSHA, and National Fire Protection Association (NFPA) 1581, *Standard on Fire Department Infection Control Program*, health care providers who have open cuts or sores on their hands should cover those areas with a dressing.[13–15] If the area is too large to cover, the provider should not perform high-risk tasks and procedures. Tattoos are considered an open area anywhere from 1 week to approximately 1 month after the tattooing procedure is done. The health care provider should be placed on work restriction until the areas have healed. Health care providers are not permitted to wear artificial nail extensions and gel nails, as studies reported in the CDC Hand Hygiene Guidelines have documented the transmission of bacterial and fungal infections from health care workers wearing these nails to their patients.[16]

PPE should include, but is not be limited to, disposable gloves, protective eyewear, cover gowns, surgical masks, N95 respirators (or N100 respirators, which are required in California under certain circumstances), waterless handwashing alcohol-based foam or gel, needle-safe or needleless devices, biohazard bags, and resuscitative equipment.

A particulate respirator filters particles that come in through the mask. Never place a respirator on a patient. A full respiratory protection program that complies with the OSHA respiratory protection program 1910.134 must be in place if N95 or P100 respirators are carried on EMS vehicles.[14]

Evidence-Based Medicine

Surgical masks protect against spatter into the mouth or nose. Patients thought to have airborne- or droplet-transmitted diseases may be asked to wear them because they filter what goes out through the mask. This precaution is termed *source control*.

According to the CDC, N95 or P100 respirators are indicated for providers performing emergency intubation and open suctioning.[17] Some health officials suggest that these procedures generate aerosols that could transmit airborne/droplet particles. No evidence-based studies support the assertion that using an N95 or P100 respirator offers more protection than wearing a surgical mask in most cases. In fact, well-controlled studies indicate that surgical masks are as effective as respirators in protecting against infection.[18–21]

The CDC also downgraded its recommendation for Ebola protection from N95 respirators to surgical masks in December 2014.[9] Ebola is not an airborne disease, but rather is transmitted via droplets.

Words of Wisdom

Respirators are rated according to their ability to filter airborne particles and resist oil aerosols. The CDC describes the rating system as follows[17]:

> Respirator filters that collect at least 95% of the challenge aerosol are given a "95" rating. Those that collect at least 99% receive a "99" rating. And those that collect at least 99.97% (essentially 100%) receive a "100" rating. Respirator filters are rated as N, R, or P for their level of protection against oil aerosols. This rating is important in industry because some industrial oils can remove electrostatic charges from the filter media, thereby degrading (reducing) the filter efficiency performance. Respirators are rated "N" if they are not resistant to oil, "R" if somewhat resistant to oil, and "P" if strongly resistant (oil proof). Thus, there are nine types of particulate respirator filters:
>
> - N95, N99, and N100
> - R95, R99, and R100
> - P95, P99, and P100
>
> These characteristics are tested and approved by NIOSH.

Gloves are not needed for intramuscular or subcutaneous injections or contact with sweat. However, according to the CDC and OSHA, they are recommended for starting intravenous (IV) lines, suctioning, intubation or use of an advanced airway, contact with blood or **other potentially infectious materials (OPIM)**, and contact with a patient's mucous membranes or nonintact skin.[22] OPIM includes cerebrospinal fluid (CSF), pericardial fluid, amniotic fluid, synovial fluid, peritoneal fluid, and any fluid containing visible blood. For cleaning activities, OSHA requires the use of utility-style gloves (dishwashing gloves); these gloves are washable and reusable as long as they are free of tears and holes **FIGURE 27-1**. Hands should be washed *after* glove removal because gloves are not a primary protection. Many gloves contain holes and absorb viruses and bacteria, a process termed *viral penetration*.

Protective eyewear blocks spatter into the eye. If the health care provider uses prescription eyeglasses, they may be worn with disposable or reusable side shields. Goggles should not be worn over prescription eyeglasses because they can distort the wearer's vision **FIGURE 27-2**.

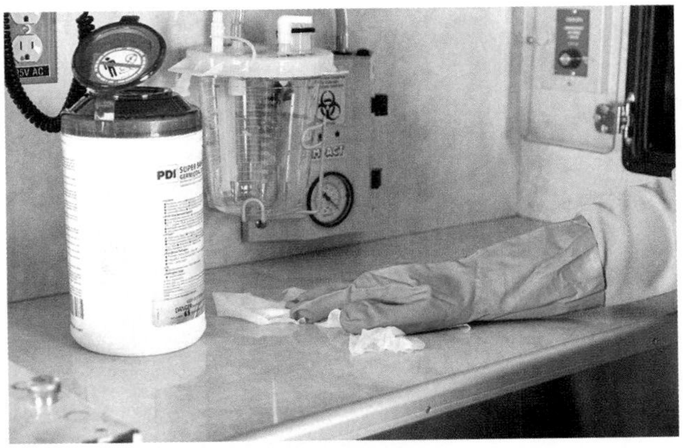

FIGURE 27-1 Utility-style gloves are washable and reusable as long as they are free of tears and holes.

Words of Wisdom

Blood is not the only fluid that poses a threat of infection. OPIM include semen, vaginal secretions through sexual contact, CSF, synovial fluid, pleural fluid, pericardial fluid, peritoneal fluid, amniotic fluid, saliva in dental procedures, any body fluid that is visibly contaminated with blood, and all body fluids in situations where it is difficult or impossible to differentiate between body fluids.[23]

According to the CDC and OSHA, tears, sweat, saliva, stool, urine, vomitus, nasal secretions, and sputum do not pose a risk for transmission of HIV, HBV, or HCV unless they contain visible blood.[24]

Cover garments are recommended for large-splatter situations. These garments could be washable or disposable jackets or gowns. Uniforms may also serve as PPE if the employer purchases, maintains, and launders them. Booties and hair covers are not routinely needed in the prehospital setting, but pocket masks and/or respiratory assistive devices (ie, bag-mask devices) must be readily available.

As defined by the CDC, a sharps injury is a penetrating stab wound from a needle, scalpel, or other sharp object that may result in exposure to blood or other body fluids.[25] In 2000, Congress passed the Needlestick Safety and Prevention Act, which required that all sharps be needle-safe or **needleless systems**.[26] The EMS systems that have adopted

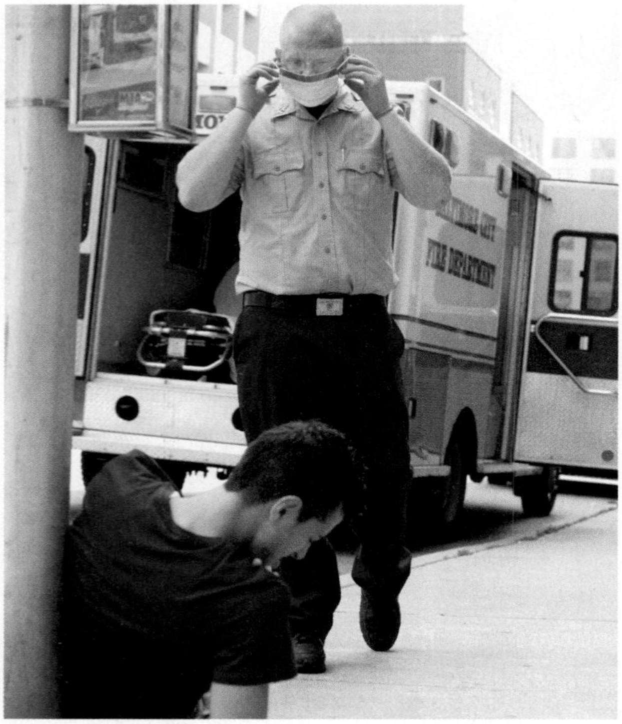

FIGURE 27-2 Wear eye protection and a mask to prevent blood and oral secretions from spattering into your eyes, nose, and mouth.

needle-safe and needleless devices have reported no sharps injuries from their use. All sharps must be placed into sharps containers that are puncture-resistant, closable, and leakproof, and that are labeled with the biohazard symbol **FIGURE 27-3**. Sharps containers must be located at the site of use.

Removal of PPE

No matter how high tech PPE might be, it will be effective only if proper removal techniques are employed. **FIGURE 27-4** shows the proper removal procedures for PPE as identified by the CDC. Note that the procedure for removing PPE donned as protection against pathogens differs from the procedure for removing hazardous materials (hazmat) PPE. Remember, handwashing after glove removal is always important!

Postexposure Medical Follow-up

Postexposure medical follow-up is your third line of defense against the effects of communicable diseases.

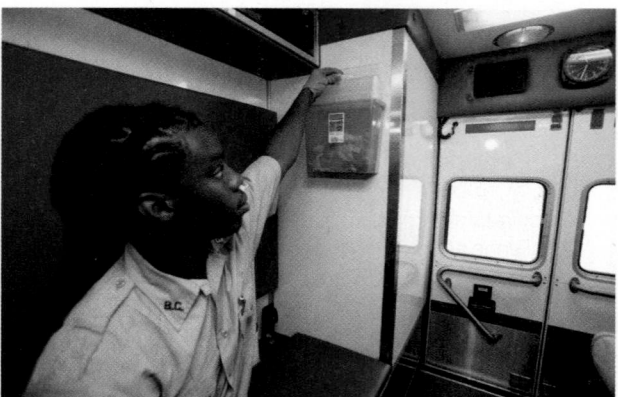

FIGURE 27-3 For proper disposal, all sharps must be placed in containers that are puncture-resistant, closable, and leakproof, and that bear the biohazard symbol. This disposal should be performed at the site of use.

Designated Infection Control Officer

The federal Ryan White CARE Act, Part G, requires that every emergency response agency have a **designated infection control officer (DICO)**. This person is charged with ensuring that proper postexposure medical treatment and counseling are provided to any exposed employee or volunteer.

Postexposure medical treatment is offered to reduce the chances of an exposed health care provider contracting the disease. Treatment should be offered within 24 to 48 hours following exposure, with the actual time frame being based on the diagnosis. Exposure to bacterial meningitis, for example, would require treatment within 24 hours.

The DICO tracks and monitors compliance with the correct time frames, serves as a liaison between the exposed employee and the medical facility, ensures that confidentiality is maintained, and ensures that documentation adheres to guidelines. The DICO role is vital for handling workers' compensation issues, and ensures that an exposed employee/volunteer receives proper care and counseling. In addition, this service offers liability protection for both the care provider and the department.

The communication network for exposure reporting involves three people: the exposed paramedic, the DICO, and the treating physician. A paramedic who believes an exposure has occurred should call the DICO directly. It is the DICO's job to determine whether an actual exposure occurred. Each department must have a reporting

HOW TO SAFELY REMOVE PERSONAL PROTECTIVE EQUIPMENT (PPE)

EXAMPLE 1

There are a variety of ways to safely remove PPE without contaminating your clothing, skin, or mucous membranes with potentially infectious materials. Here is one example. Remove all PPE before exiting the patient room except a respirator, if worn. Remove the respirator after leaving the patient room and closing the door. Remove PPE in the following sequence:

1. GLOVES

- Outside of gloves are contaminated!
- If your hands get contaminated during glove removal, immediately wash your hands or use an alcohol-based hand sanitizer
- Using a gloved hand, grasp the palm area of the other gloved hand and peel off first glove
- Hold removed glove in gloved hand
  - Slide fingers of ungloved hand under remaining glove at wrist and peel off second glove over first glove
- Discard gloves in a waste container

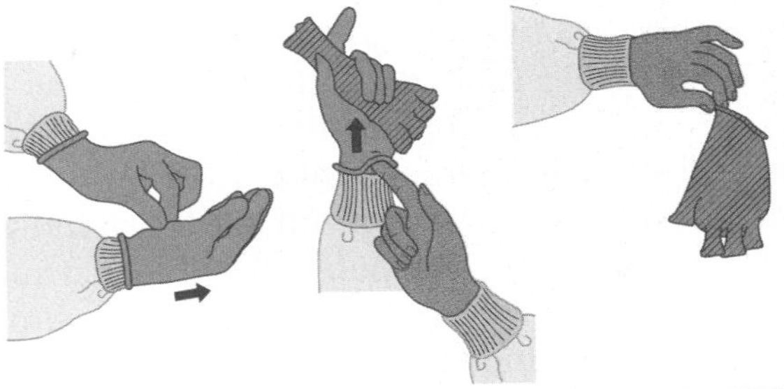

2. GOGGLES OR FACE SHIELD

- Outside of goggles or face shield are contaminated!
- If your hands get contaminated during goggle or face shield removal, immediately wash your hands or use an alcohol-based hand sanitizer
- Remove goggles or faceshield from the back by lifting head band or ear pieces
- If the item is reusable, place in designated receptacle for reprocessing. Otherwise, discard in a waste container

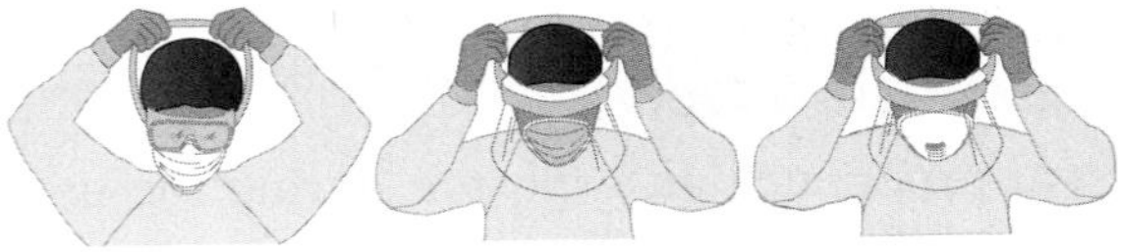

3. GOWN

- Gown front and sleeves are contaminated!
- If your hands get contaminated during gown removal, immediately wash your hands or use an alcohol-based hand sanitizer
- Unfasten gown ties, taking care that sleeves don't contact your body when reaching for ties
- Pull gown away from neck and shoulders, touching inside of gown only
- Turn gown inside out
- Fold or roll into a bundle and discard in a waste container

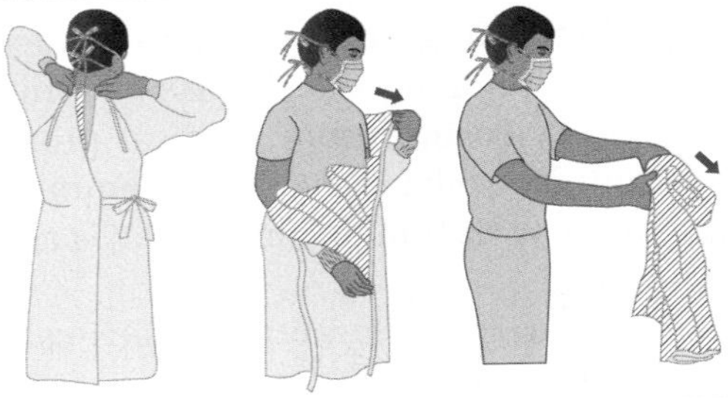

4. MASK OR RESPIRATOR

- Front of mask/respirator is contaminated — DO NOT TOUCH!
- If your hands get contaminated during mask/respirator removal, immediately wash your hands or use an alcohol-based hand sanitizer
- Grasp bottom ties or elastics of the mask/respirator, then the ones at the top, and remove without touching the front
- Discard in a waste container

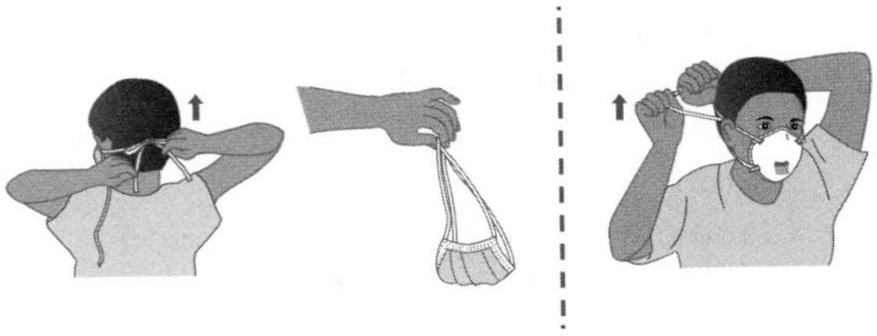

5. HAND HYGIENE

- Wash hands or use an alcohol-based hand sanitizer immediately after removing all PPE.

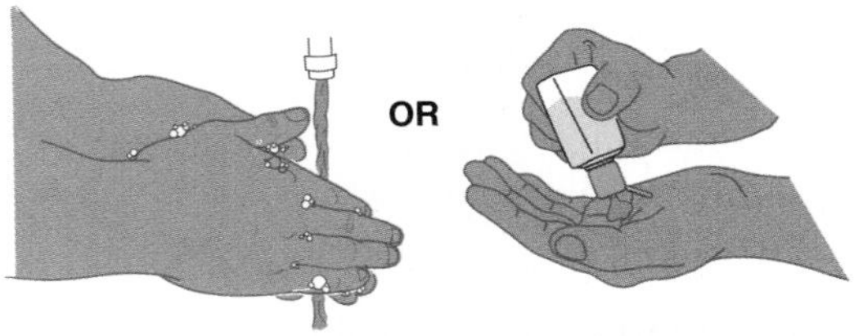

Perform hand hygiene between steps if hands become contaminated and immediately after removing all PPE.

FIGURE 27-4 Centers for Disease Control and Prevention chart on proper removal of personal protective equipment (PPE). Note that for incidents involving hazardous materials, the sequence is different than that shown here.

Modified from Centers for Disease Control and Prevention.

system that complies with the Ryan White notification law and the OSHA-required exposure control plan. The DICO must be available 24 hours per day, 7 days per week, and must work outside of the usual chain of command for confidentiality reasons.

The public health department acts as a backup for exposure notification and determination of the need for medical follow-up treatment. Under the Ryan White notification law, the local public health department must know the DICO's identity for each EMS department and be able to reach that individual on a 24/7 basis. The public health department director serves as a liaison for problems regarding exposure notification by the medical facility and the sharing of source-patient testing results.

The Process When an Exposure Occurs

If you experience an exposure during the course of your duties, the DICO will ensure the source patient is tested. If the test is positive, you will receive baseline testing and proper postexposure medical treatment, including counseling, to reduce your chances of developing the disease to which you were exposed. Postexposure medical prophylaxis (prevention) is available for many communicable diseases, except HCV infection. If HCV is acquired, it can be cured.

Exposure to bloodborne pathogens can occur in several different ways[27]:

- A contaminated needlestick injury. (The sharp has been in the patient's body.)
- Blood or OPIM spattered into the eye, nose, or mouth.
- Blood or OPIM in contact with an open area of the skin (eg, a fresh cut, an abrasion, an area of dermatitis).
- Cuts with a sharp object covered with blood or OPIM.
- Human bites involving blood exposure. (The source is the person who is bleeding, not the biter.)

If any of these events occur, you should immediately contact your DICO. This contact is essential because the DICO determines whether an exposure has occurred. If an event is deemed an exposure, the DICO will have the medical facility begin source-patient testing. The exposed employee does not need to sign in and have baseline tests performed. A baseline is not needed immediately and is performed only if the source tests positive. A baseline establishes the care provider's history; it does not offer any information about the exposure event.

For airborne- and/or droplet-transmissible diseases, the DICO receives notice from the medical facility and reviews the following criteria: the organism involved, the amount of time spent with the patient, the provider's distance from the patient, the procedure or task being performed, and the ventilation present.

Words of Wisdom

An ambulance has an air exchange rate of every 2 minutes. In the 1970s, the US General Services Administration built a requirement for air exchangers into the KKK-A-1822F ambulance specifications. In some vehicles, this risk reduction mechanism is manually engaged, and in others, it is automatic.

Postexposure medical management includes identification of the **source individual**,[28] as the source is the key to identifying whether risk is actually present. Employee baseline testing is only needed if the source tests positive. According to the OSHA Compliance Directive for Bloodborne Pathogens, employers must pay for all costs related to exposure events, including testing the source individual.[29]

The source patient's bloodwork should include rapid HIV testing, testing for HBV surface antigen, rapid HCV antibody, and rapid syphilis testing. The HIV, HCV, and syphilis results should be available in less than 1 hour, and HBV surface antigen results usually are available by the following day. Because most health care providers have been vaccinated against some diseases already, this time frame is not a major concern. Testing for HIV requires patient consent in roughly one-half of all states in the United States, but state law often makes exceptions for occupational exposure of health care providers. The other states rely on "deemed consent"; that is, the state assumes consent to be tested. Each EMS department should be aware of its state testing law.

Under the Ryan White CARE Act (otherwise known as the Ryan White notification law), the medical facility must release the source patient's test results to the DICO; this release is not considered a violation of privacy under the Health Insurance Portability and Accountability Act. The Ryan White CARE Act, Part G, also requires medical facilities to notify the DICO if a patient who is suspected of having or is known to have an airborne- or droplet-transmitted disease is transported.[1]

This information is shared with the exposed employee, and if the source patient tests positive, proper care and counseling begin. Baseline blood work done on an exposed paramedic does not yield information on the exposure that just occurred; rather, it documents whether the paramedic already has one of these diseases. As mentioned, postexposure medical counseling and treatment should begin within 24 to 48 hours, unless the source patient's testing yields information that necessitates more rapid follow-up.

CDC-Recommended Immunizations and Vaccinations

Vaccines are suspensions of whole (live or inactivated) or fractionated bacteria or viruses that have been rendered nonpathogenic; they bring about immunity by causing the immune system to produce antibodies. Some vaccines are made using DNA technology, which removes the risks of a person experiencing an allergic reaction or developing Guillain-Barré syndrome. Guillain-Barré syndrome is a temporary paralysis that usually resolves over time. Messenger RNA (mRNA) vaccines train the body's cells to recognize the proteins produced by disease-causing organisms (such as the COVID-19 virus), trigger an immune response, and then produce antibodies to protect the individual from the disease. Keeping current with recommended **vaccinations** boosts host resistance and the immune response.

In 1999, OSHA began enforcing the CDC guidelines on immunization of health care personnel. In 2011, the CDC published an updated **immunization** schedule for health care providers. A tetanus, diphtheria, and pertussis (Tdap) booster is required because of the increasing incidence of pertussis (whooping cough) in the United States. **TABLE 27-1** lists the CDC's current recommendations for health care providers.

Each employer must offer the CDC-recommended vaccinations to staff and pay for them. This includes volunteer departments, because the CDC defines health care personnel as "all paid and unpaid persons." Individual paramedics have the right to decline being vaccinated but will be required to sign a declination form.[15] However, medical facilities will not permit students to participate in clinical rotations if declination forms have

YOU are the Paramedic

PART 2

You and your partner arrive at the patient's room, which is shared with another resident. The patient is an 86-year-old woman who appears very ill. She is pale and appears weak, but is alert and able to answer questions. The staff member tells you the patient has been vomiting and having watery, nonbloody diarrhea for 2 days. The patient leans forward to vomit into a basin, and nothing comes up. The staff member, who is not wearing gloves, takes a tissue from a container, wipes the patient's mouth, and discards the tissue in the trash can.

Recording Time: 1 Minute	
Appearance	Awake
Level of consciousness	Alert (oriented to person, place, time, and event)
Airway	Open
Breathing	Adequate
Circulation	Adequate

3. What can you determine about the patient's condition now?
4. Because a diagnosis of *C diff* infection has not been confirmed for this patient, are you concerned about exposure?

TABLE 27-1 Recommended Vaccinations for Health Care Providers

Hepatitis B
Measles, mumps, rubella (MMR)
Varicella (chickenpox)
Tuberculosis (TB) testing on hire and following exposure
Tetanus, diphtheria, and pertussis (Tdap): one-time dose[a]
Influenza (annually)
Coronavirus disease 2019 (COVID-19)
Meningococcal

[a] Tetanus and diptheria boosters are needed every 10 years. It has not yet been determined when pertussis boosters are needed.

Data from: Recommended Vaccines for Healthcare Workers. Centers for Disease Control and Prevention. https://www.cdc.gov/vaccines/adults/rec-vac/hcw.html. Accessed March 23, 2021.

TABLE 27-2 Exposure Control Plan Components

Exposure determination
Education and training
Hepatitis B vaccine program
Tuberculosis testing program
Expanded vaccine program: MMR, chickenpox vaccine, Tdap booster
Personal protective equipment
Engineering controls and work practices
Postexposure medical treatment and documentation
Medical waste management
Compliance monitoring
Record keeping

Abbreviations: MMR, measles, mumps, rubella; Tdap, tetanus, diphtheria, and pertussis

been signed. Most training programs now require that vaccinations be up-to-date before candidates enter the program, and many departments mandate vaccines for current employees.

All new employees and volunteers need to obtain their vaccination records and childhood disease history, whether from a personal physician, high school, college, training program, previous employer, or Veterans Affairs clinic. Current staff members also need to obtain these records. To comply with privacy regulations, records must be requested by the employee or volunteer from one of the aforementioned sources. This information is reviewed to determine who is and is not protected from a vaccine-preventable disease. If the employee is not protected, the department must offer to pay for preventive vaccines. If the employee declines, they must sign a declination form. This action does not remove any employee rights, but rather documents that the employer met the responsibility to offer the vaccine.

Department Responsibilities

Under the OSHA mandate and the Ryan White CARE Act, Part G, to protect staff from exposure to bloodborne pathogens and airborne and droplet diseases, each EMS department must establish a comprehensive exposure control plan. This document lays out the specifics of how the department plans to reduce the risk of exposure to infectious agents and provide postexposure medical follow-up, if needed. Key elements of the exposure control plan include proper education and training related to bloodborne pathogens and airborne and droplet diseases, and establishment of postexposure medical follow-up procedures **TABLE 27-2**.

Another key component of the plan is compliance monitoring. Management must make spot checks to ensure that staff members are following the exposure control plan and that the plan is working effectively. Although management is responsible for developing and implementing the plan, OSHA has made it clear that the employees must follow the plan. This requirement is addressed in the General Duty Clause (b), which states, "Each employee shall comply with occupational safety and health standards and all rules, regulations, and orders issued pursuant to this Act which are applicable to his own actions and conduct."

One notable part of the exposure control plan that benefits both department personnel and patients is the work restriction guidelines. These guidelines, which the CDC published and OSHA enforces, indicate when employees with various illnesses may or may not be at work and when they may not care for high-risk patients. The work restriction guidelines require employees to use sick time for these absences unless the illness results from an occupational exposure, in which case it is covered under workers' compensation. Following the work restriction guidelines is of particular importance during the flu (respiratory influenza) season.

Infection is defined as the invasion of a host or host tissue by pathogenic organisms such as bacteria, viruses, or parasites that produces illness that may or may not have clinical manifestations. It is essential to distinguish between contamination and infection. An object that has microorganisms on or in it is **contaminated**. This term applies to water, food, dressing materials, linens, sharps, equipment, and even the ambulance. A person is not infected, however, unless the microorganisms produce an illness. With some diseases, such as HBV or HCV infection, a person may have the disease and not be aware of it; there are no signs or symptoms, and the person is not ill. However, such **carriers** can pass the disease to others through their blood and through sexual contact.

Words of Wisdom

Safe EMS practice depends largely on the dispatcher's ability to relay accurate and sufficient information to responders. Information provided during the 9-1-1 call may raise concerns that the patient has been exposed to an infectious disease. This information must be shared with responders so they may take appropriate precautions before patient contact, such as donning appropriate PPE, limiting the number of providers who come in contact with the patient, or placing a surgical mask on the patient immediately on arrival. When a patient's condition is suggestive of exposure to a highly infectious pathogen, the dispatcher should try to determine whether the patient has recently visited an endemic area or is experiencing other tell-tale signs and symptoms of that disease. During a community outbreak of an infectious disease, screening questions can be incorporated into the dispatch algorithm that are targeted at identifying infectious patients.[30]

Patient Assessment

The assessment of a patient suspected of having an infectious or communicable disease should be approached much like that of any other medical patient. First, perform a scene size-up and take standard precautions. Once you have ensured that the scene is safe (there is no threatening person or animal), proceed with the primary survey by following the ABCDE process—assess the patient's airway, breathing, circulation, disability, and exposure—to identify all injuries. Include mental status assessment, and prioritize treatment of the patient. With most patients who have a potentially communicable disease and are being seen in the prehospital setting, the next step is to obtain the patient's history, using OPQRST (Onset, Provocation/palliation, Quality, Radiation, Severity, Time of onset) to elaborate on the chief complaint. Typical chief complaints include fever, nausea, rash, pleuritic chest pain, and difficulty breathing. Be sure to obtain a SAMPLE (Signs and symptoms, Allergies, Medications, Pertinent past history, Last oral intake, Events leading to injury or illness) history and a set of baseline vital signs, paying particular attention to medications the patient is currently taking, the events leading up to the patient's problem today, and whether the patient has recently traveled. The importance of travel history has been demonstrated with SARS, Ebola, H1N1, carbapenem-resistant *Enterobacteriaceae* (CRE), and Zika infections, so it should be a routine assessment question. Always show respect for the feelings of patients, family, and others at the scene. After completing these steps, proceed to the secondary assessment, including the physical exam.

General Management Principles

The general care for a patient with a suspected communicable disease first focuses on any life-threatening conditions identified in the primary survey (airway maintenance, oxygen and ventilatory assistance, and circulatory support). Remember to be empathetic. Because most patients with a communicable disease will have a fever of an unexplained origin or mild breathing problems, place the patient in a position of comfort on the stretcher and keep them warm. If the patient has early signs of dehydration, establishing a preliminary IV line and a fluid infusion of normal saline or lactated Ringer solution may be appropriate. Remember to take standard precautions and to properly dispose of sharps, even needle-safe devices.[6] Always follow your agency's exposure control plan for cleaning the suction unit and any reusable equipment, and properly discard any disposable supplies and linens.

Chain of Infection

Infection involves a chain of events through which the communicable disease spreads. In some cases, solving the puzzle of why a specific disease developed in a particular person or group of people may be as simple as retracing their steps to find the source of exposure. In other cases, the puzzle is more challenging to solve, with infectious disease experts taking years to find a pattern in the spread of a disease and then plan a strategy to break the chain of the infection. The study of communicable diseases considers population demographics that can affect the spread of a disease, such as age distributions; genetic factors; income levels; ethnic groups; workplaces and schools; geographic boundaries; and the expansion, decline, or movement of the disease.

SAFETY

Here is a scenario that illustrates how easily disease may spread. In a local hospital pediatric unit, a visitor brought a box of candy for a child. Because of the "no food" rule, an attentive nurse placed the candy at the nurses' station. Another nurse had emptied a bedpan of stool from a child admitted for a hepatitis A virus (HAV) infection but was in such a rush that she forgot to wash her hands. She then noticed the box of candy, poked at a few selections with her fingernails, and finally found one she wanted to eat. The candy was consumed throughout the morning. Subsequently, another nurse came down with HAV, a disease typically spread by the oral-fecal route. The chain of infection in this scenario could have been broken by handwashing.

Exposure and the Risk of Infection

Several factors determine a person's risk of contracting an infection following an exposure. An organism's mere presence creates a risk, but other factors then influence the precise level of risk, including the dose of the organism, the virulence of the organism, its mode of entry, and the host resistance of the exposed person.

Type of Organism

Pathogenic organisms include bacteria, viruses, fungi, and parasites. They differ in how they infect the host, grow and reproduce within host tissues, and cause illness. **TABLE 27-3** compares these organisms.

Dose of the Organism

A certain number of organisms must be present for infection to occur. For example, the laboratory report on a urine specimen sent for culture may note "greater than 100,000 colonies of bacteria per milliliter" of urine indicating infection. A value of equal to or less than 100,000 is considered as not indicating infection.

Virulence of the Organism

Virulence is an organism's ability to invade and create disease in a host. It also encompasses the organism's ability to survive outside the living host. For example, HIV does not pose a risk outside the human body because it dies when it is exposed to light and air. By contrast, a bacterium like *Salmonella* can multiply every 15 to 20 minutes in the presence of the right temperature and nutrients.

Mode of Entry

If the organism does not enter the body by the "correct" route, infection cannot occur. For example, a respiratory virus that enters the body through a cut will not cause a respiratory infection and likely will not cause any infection. Conversely, an inhaled respiratory droplet could cause respiratory illness. Thus, if you apply a mask to a patient who might have a communicable respiratory disease, you are less likely to inhale the droplets.

Host Resistance

The healthier you are, the less susceptible you are to infection. Your ability to fight off infection is called **host resistance**. A strong immune system will help protect you from acquiring disease even though all

TABLE 27-3 Comparison of Selected Pathogenic Organisms

Organism	Life Cycle	Effect on Host	Example
Bacteria	Grow and reproduce outside the human cell in an environment characterized by the appropriate temperature and nutrients	Cause disease when they invade and multiply within the host's tissues	*Salmonella* bacteria can multiply in potato salad that has been unrefrigerated, leading to human illness when the food is eaten.
Viruses	Much smaller than bacteria and can multiply only inside a host; die when exposed to the environment	Cause disease when they invade and multiply within the host's tissues	HIV does not multiply or maintain its infectiousness outside a living host.
Fungi	Similar to bacteria in that they can grow rapidly in the presence of nutrients and organic material	Most infections acquired from contact with decaying organic matter or airborne spores in the environment; often cause opportunistic infections in people with compromised immune systems	Range from relatively harmless infections of the skin, such as athlete's foot (*Tinea pedis*), to life-threatening systemic infections, such as pneumonia (*Pneumocystis jirovecii*, formerly known as *Pneumocystis carinii*) in people with AIDS.
Parasites	Live in or on another living creature	Take advantage of their host by feeding off the host cells and tissues	Scabies and lice. **Protozoa**: single-celled, usually microscopic, eukaryotic organisms such as amoebas, ciliates, flagellates, and sporozoans. *Entamoeba histolytica*, for example, causes dysentery. Helminths (commonly called worms): invertebrates with long, flexible, rounded, or flattened bodies. *Ascaris lumbricoides*, for example, causes hookworm.

Abbreviations: AIDS, acquired immunodeficiency syndrome; HIV, human immunodeficiency virus

of the other risk factors may be present. Wellness programs and immunization programs serve to boost host resistance.

Once a susceptible person has been exposed to an organism, it takes time for the organism to multiply within the body and produce symptoms. That period between exposure to the organism and the first symptoms of illness is called the **incubation period**. For example, it usually takes 12 to 26 days from a susceptible person's exposure to the mumps virus until the person begins to feel feverish and ill. The incubation period for the influenza virus is much shorter—usually 24 to 72 hours.

Most communicable diseases are contagious only during a portion of the illness. A person may be sick with chickenpox for 2 to 3 weeks but can transmit the virus to another person for only about 1 week—from 1 day before the **vesicles** appear on the skin to about 6 days after their emergence. The period during which a person can transmit the illness to someone else is called the **communicable period**.

In the context of communicable disease, a **reservoir** is a place where organisms may live and multiply. For example, in institutional settings, air-conditioning systems and showerheads have been identified as reservoirs for the bacterium that causes Legionnaires' disease. In ambulances, the oxygen humidifier is commonly implicated as a reservoir for infection. Health care personnel are responsible not only for protecting themselves from contracting communicable diseases, but also ensuring, to the extent possible, that they and their equipment do not transmit illness to others. This responsibility is significant: If a patient with Medicare or Medicaid insurance acquires an infection after being cared for by EMS and is hospitalized, the government may term it a health care–associated infection and refuse to reimburse its cost. Medical facilities are monitoring EMS as a possible source for some patient infections.

Host Defense Mechanisms

The human body provides built-in protection from pathogenic organisms through several defenses that protect against infection. Skin, which covers the entire exterior of the body, represents a primary protective barrier, blocking pathogens' ability to enter through the intact surface. The normal secretions of the skin also have an antibacterial property that protects against pathogen entry. Antibacterial handwashing solutions should not be used because they kill all bacteria on the skin, including normal flora, and contribute to the development of resistant bacteria.

Mucous membranes represent another protective barrier. For example, the eyes produce tears that dilute and remove foreign substances. The mucous membranes that line the urinary, respiratory, and gastrointestinal (GI) tracts also trap and remove organisms. The cells that line the respiratory tract secrete lysozymes that destroy bacteria, while macrophages trap and destroy bacteria; thus, these mucous membranes serve as a first line of defense against airborne- and droplet-transmitted diseases. Goblet cells lining the GI tract produce highly acidic and alkaline secretions, forming barriers that guard against penetration by bacteria and some viruses.

The immune system also contains proteins that kill viruses. Triggering of the immune response ignites the production of antibodies that are directed against specific invading organisms. As part of this process, B cells and T cells work together to fight infection.

Infection and Sepsis

The CDC is working to raise awareness of **sepsis**. A CDC report published in August 2016 stated that 80% of patients with sepsis developed the infection that led to sepsis in a setting outside the hospital, and that 7 of 10 patients diagnosed with sepsis had received recent health care services or had a chronic disease that required frequent medical care visits.[31]

The CDC report also suggested the importance of EMS providers, in recognizing sepsis and alerting the receiving facility when a patient with possible sepsis is being transported, as key to improving patient outcomes. In recent years, the definitions of sepsis and **septic shock** have been revised by an international task force and presented at the Society of Critical Care Medicine's 45th Critical Care Congress. A Surviving Sepsis Campaign (SSC) has also been launched to improve the diagnosis and management of sepsis.[32] Finally, evidence-based interventions called bundles have been developed in an attempt to increase patient survival rates; one of these bundles addresses resuscitation, while a second addresses management of care.

Pathophysiology

Sepsis is the body's overreaction to an infection or virus, which can progress to shock. A medical emergency, it requires rapid treatment to prevent tissue damage, organ failure, and death. People identified as being at increased risk for sepsis include those age 65 and older, infants younger than 1 year, people with compromised immune systems, and those with chronic medical conditions such as diabetes.

Assessment

In a patient with suspected sepsis, perform a primary survey and obtain a focused history and appropriate physical exam. Signs and symptoms of sepsis include one or more of the following:

- Shivering, fever, or feeling very cold
- Extreme pain or discomfort
- Clammy or discolored skin
- Confusion or disorientation
- Shortness of breath
- Elevated heart rate

You have learned that the feasibility of definitive care and optimal patient outcomes depend on timely recognition of trauma, myocardial infarction, and stroke in patients experiencing these conditions. Similarly, the early identification of patients with sepsis and prompt emergency care in the initial hours after sepsis develops can improve these patients' outcomes.[32] The quick Sepsis-related Organ Failure Assessment (qSOFA) is a rapid scoring system that can be used to identify patients who have an infection and may be at risk of dying from sepsis. The objective of early identification of sepsis is to begin treatment before the syndrome worsens. The qSOFA score is easy to calculate because it has only three components, each of which is easily identified: (1) respiratory rate (≥22 breaths/min), (2) altered mentation (Glasgow Coma Scale score <15), and (3) systolic blood pressure (≤100 mm Hg).[33] One point is assigned for each component, so the total score ranges from 0 to 3 points. A score of 2 or more is associated with poor outcomes due to sepsis.

Management

If you suspect sepsis or septic shock, initiate pulse oximetry and cardiac and BP monitoring. Give supplemental oxygen if indicated. Bag-mask ventilation may be necessary if the patient's breathing is inadequate.

Obtain vascular access and begin fluid resuscitation. If sepsis-induced hypoperfusion is present, the Surviving Sepsis Campaign recommends administering at least 30 mL/kg of IV crystalloid within the first 3 hours.[32] In addition to monitoring oxygen saturation, heart rate, and BP, carefully monitor the patient for increased work of breathing or the development of crackles. If hypotension persists despite fluid administration, consult medical direction for advice about giving additional fluids versus the use of vasopressors. Transport the patient to the closest appropriate facility.

Pathophysiology, Assessment, and Management of Droplet-Transmitted Diseases

Meningitis

Meningitis is an inflammation of the *meninges*—that is, the membranes that cover the brain and spinal cord. Two types of meningitis are distinguished: bacterial and viral. The bacterial form is communicable, whereas the viral form is not. More than 90% of meningitis cases in the United States are viral and do not pose a risk to health care providers.[34] Meningitis is spread through droplets, so transmission occurs by direct contact with a patient's oral or nasal secretions. The most common bacterial organisms implicated in meningitis are *Neisseria meningitidis, Streptococcus pneumoniae, Haemophilus influenzae,* group B *Streptococcus,* and *Listeria monocytogenes.*

The most severe type of meningitis is **meningococcal meningitis**, which is caused by *N meningitidis.* In the past, sporadic cases of meningococcal meningitis occurred most frequently during winter and spring, especially when people lived together in crowded conditions, such as in college dorms, homeless shelters, or military barracks. Currently, all preteens, high school students, and college students entering dormitory living are vaccinated against the primary types of meningitis, which has resulted in a decrease in cases on a national level. New meningitis B vaccines have been approved for young adults ages 16 to 23 years to prevent disease caused by *N meningitidis.* The meningitis vaccine is not recommended for any health care provider group, only for college students entering dormitory living for the first time, military recruits, and middle school and high school students.

Pathophysiology

Transmission occurs following direct contact with an infected person's nasopharyngeal secretions (mouth-to-mouth, suctioning, or intubation with spraying of secretions) or prolonged contact time of 8 or more hours. The incubation period for meningococcal meningitis is between 2 and 10 days. The communicable period varies; it lasts as long as meningococcal bacteria are present in the patient's nasal and oral secretions. The microorganisms generally disappear from the patient's upper respiratory tract within 24 hours after antibiotic treatment begins.

Words of Wisdom

Meningitis is not transmitted by airborne means. Viral meningitis is infectious but not communicable.

Assessment

The classic signs and symptoms of meningitis are the same for the viral and bacterial forms: sudden-onset fever, severe headache, stiff neck, Kernig sign (the patient cannot extend their leg at the knee when the thigh is flexed because of pain or resistance), Brudzinski sign (involuntary flexion of the knees when the head is flexed toward the chest), photosensitivity, and a pink rash that becomes purple. The patient almost always experiences changes in mental status, ranging from apathy to delirium. Projectile vomiting is common. Diagnosis is made by Gram stain, a simple test in which CSF (obtained through a procedure known as a lumbar puncture) is placed on a slide, crystal violet stain is added to the CSF, and there is an initial identification of whether a bacterium is present. A Gram stain gives a quick result and can help distinguish viral from bacterial infection, often in just a few minutes after a CSF sample is obtained.

Management

When you are treating a patient with meningitis, ask the patient to wear a surgical mask or a nonrebreathing mask. If this is not possible, you should wear a surgical mask. Routine standard precautions, including gloves and good handwashing technique, are also necessary. Diagnosis is not made until a lumbar puncture is performed, so precautions must be maintained throughout your patient interactions.

The health care provider must assess the patient for signs and symptoms suggestive of meningitis, including fever, vomiting, irritability, and lethargy. In infants, a bulging fontanelle may also be noted. Assess the patient for respiratory distress, which may indicate the need for intubation en route, oxygen administration, and rapid transport.

Other treatments will be added based on the patient's symptoms—for example, oxygen, airway management, and ventilation support. Medical control may order IV fluids based on the patient's signs and symptoms, and medications may be ordered en route if seizures occur or the patient shows signs of shock. Only patients with severe signs and symptoms require rapid transport to a medical facility.

Transmission of meningitis from patient to health care provider is rare. Postexposure treatment typically includes ciprofloxacin (one dose given orally). Counseling is essential, however, because there are many contraindications for prescribing ciprofloxacin. Ciprofloxacin-resistant bacterial meningitis has been documented within the United States, so postexposure treatment should be offered only when an actual exposure has occurred.

As an alternative to ciprofloxacin, rifampin is given orally for 2 days. This treatment is not appropriate if the person is taking birth control pills, and it should not be offered to pregnant patients. Ceftriaxone (Rocephin) is the drug of choice if an exposed health care provider is pregnant.

Special Populations

Meningitis in infants and children has decreased in incidence and mortality with the development and widespread administration of vaccines. Vaccines protect against *H influenzae* type b, *S pneumoniae*, and *N meningitidis*. Vaccine administration is started at age 2 months. However, in a child who has not been vaccinated, meningitis remains a major emergency that requires antibiotic treatment.

Respiratory Conditions

Several respiratory conditions may (or may not) be associated with a fever and may (or may not) be infectious. These conditions run the gamut from mildly annoying symptoms to potentially life-threatening conditions. Notably, respiratory syncytial virus (RSV) is the leading cause of lower respiratory tract infections in infants, older adults, and immunocompromised people. It and other communicable diseases relevant to the pediatric population (such as bronchiolitis and croup) are discussed in Chapter 44, *Pediatric Emergencies*.

Seasonal Influenza

Influenza (flu) viruses cause acute respiratory illnesses generally presenting as winter epidemics. In the United States, the flu causes approximately 36,000 deaths each year.[20]

nH1N1 (novel H1N1) influenza began in California and was first believed to be poised to cause a major pandemic. Fortunately, it proved to be a new seasonal flu virus that, compared with the normal seasonal flu, did not result in a significant number of deaths either in the United States or worldwide.[35,36] This disease is now called H1N1.

Special Populations

Influenza infection rates are high in children, but the largest number of deaths from this cause occur among adults older than 65 years, especially people with medical conditions such as chronic pulmonary or heart disease. Death is preventable with vaccination.

Pathophysiology

For this droplet-transmitted disease, transmission was thought to be airborne. However, further research has shown transmission to be hand-to-nose-to-mouth-to-eye. The incubation period is about 1 to 4 days following exposure. The communicable period in adults lasts from the day before symptoms begin until about 5 days after the onset of the illness.

Assessment

Signs and symptoms of influenza include systemic fever, shaking chills, headache, muscle pain, malaise, and loss of appetite. Respiratory symptoms include dry, often protracted coughing; hoarseness; and nasal discharge. The duration of illness is about 3 to 4 days, and complications may include viral or bacterial pneumonia.

Management

Prevention of influenza, which has been a mild disease during the past 4 years, involves placing a surgical mask or nonrebreathing mask on the patient. Very few patients with this disease require IV fluids for dehydration or ventilation assistance during transport. The key preventive measure, however, is an annual flu shot. Each year, a new vaccine is developed based on the anticipated strains for that year. The vaccine's injectable form does not contain live virus, so you cannot get the disease from the flu shot. As an alternative to the injectable form, the nasal spray vaccine contains live attenuated virus. A vaccine is also available for people who have egg, mercury, and antibiotic allergies.

Words of Wisdom

A paramedic with a cold or flu can be extremely hazardous to a patient who is immunocompromised.

An effort is underway to make seasonal flu vaccination mandatory for all health care providers as a patient safety issue. Many medical facilities have already made flu shots a condition of employment for their employees. If you do not take a flu shot, you must sign a declination form—a provision established by OSHA, NFPA 1581, and the CDC. In addition, unvaccinated health care providers must wear a mask whenever they are working around patients. If EMS providers decline the flu shot, they will be required to wear a mask when entering the medical facility.

If you have not been vaccinated against influenza and have an exposure, antiviral drugs may be offered within 48 hours to reduce the flu's severity should you contract it.

Pertussis (Whooping Cough)

Pertussis is a disease caused by the *Bordetella pertussis* bacterium. Cases have been increasing in the United States over the past several years because of unvaccinated children and waning protection for adults. Currently, pertussis is a disease with one of the largest case numbers in this country. The CDC recommends that all health care providers receive a booster for pertussis.[37] To guard against infection, all pregnant women in the United States are given Tdap boosters with each pregnancy.

Pathophysiology

Pertussis is a large-droplet–transmitted disease and is considered to be highly contagious. The incubation period is 7 to 10 days following an exposure.

Assessment

The patient with pertussis presents with fever, thick nasal discharge, and a cough that progresses to coughing spasms. The patient is not able to take a breath. Children often develop black eyes from the coughing. When the patient can finally take a breath, a "whoop" sound is heard. Vomiting generally follows.

Management

Pertussis in children must be treated quickly. This illness also must be reported to the public health department to prevent additional cases. Patients are considered to be infectious at the time of presentation of the runny nose, sneezing, and low-grade fever. This period is referred to as the catarrhal stage. The second stage, known as paroxysms, is when the coughing attacks occur.

The recommended treatment for pertussis is a 5-day course of azithromycin, but other antibiotics may be prescribed, such as erythromycin. In 2013, the Food and Drug Administration (FDA) warned that azithromycin could cause abnormal changes in cardiac electrical activity. Another drug should be considered for people with known cardiac disease.

For health care providers, protection via the recommended Tdap booster is important.

Mumps

Mumps (infectious parotitis) is a droplet-transmitted disease. Before a vaccine became available in 1967, many children sustained permanent deafness, encephalitis, and death from mumps. Prior to the vaccine's launch, approximately 186,000 cases were reported each year in the United States.[38]

As a side effect of the success of the US vaccination program, many health care providers are now unaware of the complications of childhood diseases like mumps. In recent years, outbreaks of mumps have occurred in colleges, corporations, and even the National Hockey League (2015). These outbreaks are related to people not being vaccinated or not receiving two doses of the mumps vaccine. Case numbers began to decrease in 2015 as more people, including health care providers, became vaccinated. However, data from the CDC for 2016 through 2019 show an increase in mumps cases. This increase is significant because 20% to 40% of infected people may not show signs or symptoms of this disease.[38]

Pathophysiology

Mumps virus multiplies in the upper respiratory tract and is transmitted through direct contact with saliva or respiratory secretions. Fomites can also transmit mumps virus. The incubation period for this illness is 16 to 18 days following exposure.

Complications from acquiring mumps occur more often in adults than in children. According to the CDC,[39] the most common complication is orchitis (inflammation of one testis), which can occur in 3% to 10% of males. Other complications in adults may include deafness, meningitis, encephalitis, and pancreatitis. These complications have occurred in fewer than 1% of cases in recent US outbreaks. Complications may also occur in women who acquire mumps when pregnant.

Assessment

Mumps presents with fever, headache, muscle aches, loss of appetite, and swelling of the salivary glands under the ears. This swelling can occur either on one side or bilaterally.

Management

Treatment is supportive. Age-appropriate pain management and cold packs may offer some relief. All mumps cases must be reported to the public health department.

Vaccination is the key to protection. If no history of mumps or confirmation of receipt of two doses of the measles, mumps, rubella (MMR) vaccine can be produced, the person should be considered nonimmune and offered the vaccine. Titers (tests that detect the presence and measure the amount of antibodies within a person's blood) do not need to be performed unless they are deemed cost-effective. Generally, titers cost more than the vaccine.[13]

Vaccination before an exposure occurs is essential. The vaccine is *not* effective postexposure. If an exposure occurs in a nonimmune person, that person will be placed on work restrictions from days 12 to 25 following the exposure event.

Rubella (German Measles)

Rubella is caused by a virus. Although it is also called the German measles, this disease is actually caused by a different virus than the one that causes measles. The rubella vaccination program started in 1969. Once the vaccine became widely used, the number of people infected with rubella in the United States dropped significantly. It is thought that rubella was eliminated from the United States in 2004. Although it is no longer endemic (constantly present) in the United States, this disease continues to be brought into the United States from other countries.

During the last major rubella epidemic in the United States from 1964 to 1965, an estimated 12.5 million people acquired rubella, 11,000 pregnant women miscarried, 2,100 newborns died, and 20,000 babies were born with congenital rubella syndrome.[40] The congenital disabilities seen in congenital rubella syndrome are very much like those seen with Zika virus infection. Because of recent decreases in vaccination rates, congenital rubella again poses a threat. EMS personnel, in turn, are now required to ask pregnant women if they have had prenatal care.

Pathophysiology

Rubella is transmitted through droplets and spreads when an infected person coughs or sneezes. An individual with rubella may spread the disease to others up to 1 week before the rash appears. The incubation period is from 12 to 23 days following an exposure event. An infected person can remain contagious up to 7 days after the rash appears. Approximately 25% to 50% of people infected with rubella do not develop a rash or have any symptoms.[41] This makes vaccination a critical factor for exposure protection.

Assessment

Rubella is generally a mild disease. Infected individuals present with a rash that usually begins on the face and then spreads to the rest of the body. Other signs and symptoms include headache, mild pink eye, swollen and enlarged lymph nodes, cough, and a runny nose.

Management

There is no specific treatment for rubella.

> **Street Smarts**
>
> Prevention is important. Know your childhood disease history and if you are not protected, get vaccinated. If you are not protected, put a surgical mask on the patient. If you are not able to mask the patient, then you should wear a mask.

COVID-19

COVID-19 is a new **coronavirus** that is believed to have originated in China in 2019. According to the CDC and WHO, it is transmitted by droplets and by direct contact. In 2020, COVID-19 was formally declared a pandemic. Transmission likely first occurred from animal to human, with the strongest evidence suggesting that a bat may have been the original source. Bats are a common source of virus transmission. The first outbreak of this new illness occurred in a market in Wuhan, China; however, new data suggest that cases in the Wuhan area may have actually predated the outbreak in the market and the virus may have been developed in a virology lab. COVID-19 was present in the United States before the discovery of the person who was called the first case; that is, testing of donated blood has shown that this virus was present in seven states before December 2019. More information about the origins, spread, and nature of this disease is becoming available as research into COVID-19 continues.[42]

Pathophysiology

Early in the pandemic, both the CDC and WHO stated that the method of transmission was droplet and direct contact. Close contact with both infected respiratory secretions and saliva has been documented as a means of transmission. Droplets can be expelled through coughing, sneezing, talking, and singing. COVID-19 is also thought to be transmitted by indirect contact, such as contact with a contaminated surface or object; however, it has been determined that this is not a primary method for disease transmission.[43]

Airborne transmission of COVID-19 can occur during aerosol-generating procedures. The potential for buildup of suspended small respiratory droplets and particles is particularly concerning in indoor settings with inadequate ventilation or poor air handling. This risk factor illustrates the importance of using the ambulance's rear exhaust fan.[44]

Assessment

Persons suspected of having COVID-19 should be assessed for fever, cough, shortness of breath, headache, loss of sense of smell or taste, muscle aches, sore throat, and chills. Source control is the focus of blocking disease transmission. According to the CDC guidelines for EMS personnel, dispatch should advise patients with symptoms suggestive of COVID-19 to don a mask before EMS providers arrive to the scene.

Management

If the patient cannot wear a surgical mask to prevent the spread of airborne droplets, then an oxygen mask may be used. N95 or higher-level respirators and eye protection are indicated when performing aerosol-generating procedures. These procedures are to be performed with guidance from medical control. If transport is needed for the patient, the ambulance's rear exhaust fan should be placed on the high setting and the heating system set to a non-recirculating cycle.

COVID-19 is an enveloped virus. When an enveloped virus lands on a surface, the envelope opens, leaving the viral components susceptible to any low-level disinfectant. Thus, after transport of a patient with COVID-19, no special cleaning solution is needed for the ambulance; any EPA-registered cleaning/disinfectant agent is appropriate.

Medical facilities are required to notify the DICO if a crew transported a patient with COVID-19. The DICO will then interview the crew to determine if an exposure occurred.

Pathophysiology, Assessment, and Management of Airborne-Transmitted Diseases

Tuberculosis

Tuberculosis (TB) has been an important cause of disability and death in much of the developing world. This disease was once widespread in the United States, but no longer poses such a great risk. In 2019, the lowest TB incidence in US history was documented, with 8,916 cases reported nationwide.[45] WHO and the CDC are working together to eliminate this disease worldwide. Their original target date of 2019 was not achieved due to medication shortages and wars in areas where disease cases are the highest. Their new target date for disease elimination is 2030.

Pathophysiology

TB is not a highly communicable disease. Three types of TB exist: *typical*, which is communicable, and *atypical* and *extrapulmonary* (TB of the bone, kidney, lymph glands, and so on), which are not communicable. For statistical purposes, TB incidence includes all three types of TB. The TB case rate is high in the incarcerated population due to overcrowded conditions and inadequate health care. Immunocompromised people, homeless people, and residents in long-term care facilities are also at increased risk for TB. In the United States, the highest rate of this disease is found in the Asian population.[46]

TB *infection* (latent TB) means a person has tested positive for TB exposure but does not have, and may never develop, active disease. People with TB infection do not pose a risk to others. TB *disease* means the person has active TB disease verified by laboratory testing, a positive chest radiograph, and a confirmatory laboratory test. Rapid testing, with results being produced in 2 hours, is now available.

Drug-resistant TB can occur with misuse or mismanagement of the medications used to treat this disease. Multidrug-resistant TB (MDR TB) means that the bacterium is resistant to two or more of the first-line medications (of several available) used to treat TB. Extensively drug-resistant TB (XDR TB) is an uncommon type of TB that is resistant to two of the first-line oral medications and at least one of three injectable second-line medications.[47] Both MDR TB and XDR TB are still treatable diseases.

Transmission of TB occurs by large, airborne particles from a person with active untreated disease. In general, that type of spread occurs among people who have prolonged contact with or

Words of Wisdom

Noncompliance with TB treatment has been addressed by implementing directly observed therapy, which involves health nurses watching patients take their medications. With advances in technology, medication compliance can also be monitored using telehealth apps. Because TB patients are now cared for while living in their own homes, family members often shoulder the responsibility of ensuring medication compliance.

intimate exposure to the infected person (primarily people living in the same household). For paramedics, such intense exposure is likely to occur only when mouth-to-mouth ventilation is given to a patient with active untreated TB or when intubation and suctioning are performed while the provider is not wearing PPE.

The incubation period for TB is 4 to 12 weeks. This disease is communicable only when an active lesion develops in the lungs and bacteria are expelled into the air by coughing. Of patients who are treated, 10% are no longer communicable after 2 days of treatment. After 14 days of treatment, virtually all patients are no longer communicable.

Street Smarts

Notify your DICO if you believe you may have been exposed to TB. The medical facility is required to notify the DICO if a patient you have transported may have or is suspected of having TB.

Early infection with TB can be detected by a **tuberculin skin test** or by the **tuberculosis blood test**. Two TB blood tests are available in the marketplace: QuantiFERON-TB Gold blood test and T-spot TB.

The TB blood test is a one-time blood draw for which accurate results become available in 24 hours. Health departments and fire/EMS agencies across the United States are now using the TB blood test because it is reliable and convenient. All health care providers, including paramedics, should have a tuberculin test at the beginning of employment and not again unless there is a documented exposure.[48] If a known positive history is present when a person is hired, the employee must complete a questionnaire, which the designated physician then reviews. As mentioned, TB develops in only 10% of persons with a positive TB test. Disease activation depends on the overall health status of the person later in life. Chest radiography is indicated only for a first positive test. Additional or routine chest radiography is not needed.

Assessment

The classic presentation of TB includes a persistent cough for more than 3 weeks, plus one or more of the following: night sweats, headache, fever, fatigue, weight loss, hemoptysis, hoarseness, or chest pain. This clinical presentation should raise a red flag.

Management

As a preventive measure, place a surgical mask on a patient suspected of having TB. If the patient cannot be masked, place a mask on yourself to reduce the risk of TB transmission. According to the CDC's 2005 TB Guidelines and OSHA's enforcement of those guidelines, N95 or HEPA respirators are not needed or required for EMS transport of a patient with suspected TB.[49] The patient may require oxygen administration and/or airway or ventilation support based on assessment. If the patient requires supplemental oxygen, consider using an oxygen mask instead of a nasal cannula. You can administer the same fraction of inspired oxygen while limiting the spread of droplets when the patient coughs.

If preventive measures were not taken, report the incident to your DICO. Given that the incubation period for TB ranges from 4 to 12 weeks, if you suspect you have been exposed to TB, work with the department DICO to assess the need for baseline testing and then be retested in 8 to 10 weeks. If a subsequent test is positive during that time, you will need to have a chest radiograph to rule out infection and usually will be offered a 12-week course of antibiotic therapy, per the WHO/CDC recommendations.[50] Because the antibiotics are toxic to the liver, you should not consume alcohol while taking these drugs, and liver function tests should be conducted monthly.

No special measures are required after transporting a patient suspected of having active TB. The vehicle should be cleaned as usual. No airing is required.

Varicella Zoster (Chickenpox)

Varicella zoster (chickenpox) is a highly contagious disease. Varicella zoster virus (VZV) is a member of the herpes virus family. Reactivation of latent infection with VZV causes herpes zoster (shingles).

A chickenpox vaccine became available in 1995. Fewer outbreaks have been reported since the inception of the two-dose chickenpox vaccination program, which effectively prevents severe cases.[51] People who take the vaccine are also protected from developing shingles later in life. Unfortunately, chickenpox cases have been on the rise in the United States over the past several years, owing to some parents' reluctance to vaccinate their children against this disease.

Pathophysiology

Primary infection with VZV causes varicella. After the primary infection, VZV stays in the body (in the sensory nerve ganglia) as a latent infection.

Transmission of the virus can occur in two ways: via direct contact or by inhalation of aerosols from the lesions. Respiratory secretions can also transmit this disease. The incubation period ranges from 14 to 16 days after exposure, but the average time frame is between 10 and 21 days.

Assessment

People who had chickenpox develop lifelong immunity to the virus. Obtain a thorough history if the patient presents with rash beginning on the abdomen that spreads to other parts of the body, or has a fever and photosensitivity (wants to be in the dark) **FIGURE 27-5**.

Management

Use airborne precautions and contact precautions when caring for a patient diagnosed with or suspected of having chickenpox. There is no specific treatment for chickenpox, but antipruritic agents may help relieve the itching. The patient should be observed for signs of secondary infection of the lesions. Group A *Streptococcus* infection (flesh-eating strep) is often the cause of secondary infection with chickenpox.

Exposure to chickenpox is defined as greater than 5 minutes to 1 hour in the same room (indoors) or face-to-face contact. If an unprotected exposure occurs, contact the DICO. The vaccine may be administered within 72 hours to prevent infection from occurring in a nonimmune health care provider. However, if the exposed health care provider is pregnant or immunocompromised, the vaccine cannot be given. A special immunoglobulin (varicella zoster immune globulin), VariZig, must be ordered to achieve protection. Work restrictions will also need to be implemented for 18 days following the exposure event.

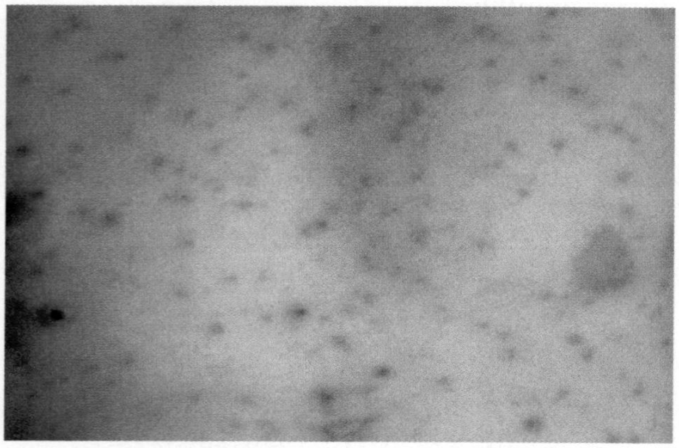

FIGURE 27-5 The distinctive rash produced by chickenpox is composed of small, blisterlike vesicles that arise in clusters.

Courtesy of Centers for Disease Control and Prevention.

Measles

Measles (rubeola, not to be confused with German measles [rubella]) is considered highly communicable. Outbreaks have occurred in many states over the years. A vaccine for measles became available in 1963, but approximately 500,000 cases were documented each year before it was available. Among those 500,000 cases, about 500 deaths occurred, 48,000 were hospitalized, and about 1,000 people sustained brain damage due to encephalitis. Outbreaks of measles still occur; several were documented between 2015 and 2019.[52]

Pathophysiology

Measles is caused by a virus that is transmitted when an infected person coughs or sneezes. The measles virus can remain in the air for 2 hours. The incubation period for measles is 7 to 18 days following an exposure event.

Assessment

In the early (prodromal) phase, measles is characterized by fever, conjunctivitis, and coryza (acute rhinitis). The onset of coughing, a blotchy red rash (which often starts on the head), and white-gray spots on the buccal (mouth) mucosa (known as Koplik spots) then follow **FIGURE 27-6**. The rash spreads from the head to the trunk to the lower extremities. Patients are considered to be contagious from 4 days before to 4 days after the rash appears.

FIGURE 27-6 A blotchy red rash is characteristic of measles.

Courtesy of Dr. Heinz F. Eichenwald/CDC.

Common complications from measles include otitis media, bronchopneumonia, laryngotracheobronchitis, and diarrhea.

Management

Care of a patient with measles is supportive. There is no treatment for measles other than reducing fever and maintaining comfort. Although placing a mask on the patient may prevent transmission, the only certain protection against measles is immunity. Exposure is defined as transport of a patient or being in the same room as the patient. In an ambulance, use of the rear exhaust fan is essential for risk reduction.

Words of Wisdom

People who were vaccinated between 1963 and 1967 need to be revaccinated with the live measles vaccine. During those years, a killed virus vaccine was used and has proved not to be protective.

People who were born during or after 1957 who do not have evidence of immunity against measles should receive at least one dose of the MMR vaccine.[53]

Prevention relies on vaccination. All health care workers should receive measles vaccinations. Anyone who has had measles or who received two doses of live virus measles vaccine after 1968 should be able to document immunity to measles. If you received a vaccine between 1963 and 1967, you need to be revaccinated with a live measles vaccine. The immunity status of all fire department and EMS employees must be assessed. Postexposure treatment includes vaccination if you are not immune. If an unprotected exposure occurs, the MMR vaccine can be given within 72 hours of the exposure event.

YOU are the Paramedic

PART 3

You begin your assessment of the patient. When asked, she says that she has been nauseated and having diarrhea for a few days. She also says she is too weak to stand and has not been able to keep water down. When your partner feels for the patient's pulse, there is obvious tenting when the skin on her forearm is pinched.

Recording Time: 5 Minutes	
Respirations	18 breaths/min
Pulse	106 beats/min
Skin	Pale, cool, dry; tenting noted
Blood pressure	98/58 mm Hg
Oxygen saturation (Spo_2)	97% on room air
Pupils	Pupils Equal, Round, and Reactive to Light and Accommodation (PERRLA)

5. What is your first choice of treatment for this patient?

6. Are there any notifications you should make concerning the scene?

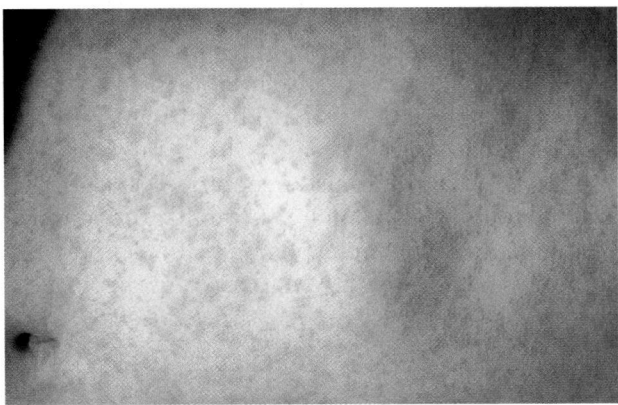

Special Populations

Because of their relatively immature immune systems, infants and young children are especially susceptible to infectious diseases. Pediatric immunizations prevent disease in children who receive them and protect those who contact unvaccinated people. Although this incidence of vaccine-preventable diseases has decreased in the United States, the viruses and bacteria that cause them still exist. According to the CDC, the following immunizations are recommended for all children[54]:

- Diphtheria, pertussis, and tetanus
- *H influenzae* type b
- Hepatitis A
- Hepatitis B
- Human papillomavirus
- Inactivated poliovirus
- Measles, mumps, and rubella
- Meningococcal ACWY
- Meningococcal B
- Pneumococcal conjugate
- Pneumococcal polysaccharide
- Rotavirus
- Influenza
- Varicella

No special disinfection measures are required for the ambulance after transporting a patient known to have measles. Simply washing patient contact areas and laundering any soiled linens are sufficient. The vehicle does not need to be taken out of service or aired out.

Other Infections of the Respiratory Tract

Mononucleosis

Pathophysiology

Mononucleosis (mono) is caused by the Epstein-Barr virus. This virus is also suspected of causing a related disease, chronic fatigue syndrome. Epstein-Barr virus grows in the epithelium of the oropharynx and is shed into saliva—hence the nickname "kissing disease" for mononucleosis. Most cases of mononucleosis do not result in symptoms, which means the infection is subclinical. At least one in every four teens and young adults who acquires Epstein-Barr virus becomes infected with mono.[55] This illness is not reportable in all states.

Transmission of Epstein-Barr virus occurs via direct contact with the saliva of an infected person. Some cases have also been linked to contaminated blood transfusions. The incubation period is 4 to 6 weeks following exposure, with a prolonged communicable period. Most cases resolve in 2 to 4 weeks.

Assessment

Signs and symptoms of mononucleosis include sore throat, fever, secretions from the pharynx, swollen lymph glands (especially the posterior cervical glands), malaise, anorexia, headache, rash, muscle pain, and an enlarged liver and/or spleen. Pharyngeal secretions may persist for 1 year or more after infection. In severe cases, complications may include anemia, dehydration, spleen rupture, seizures, or pneumonia.

Management

Prevention of mononucleosis involves using gloves and good handwashing techniques when in direct contact with a patient's oral secretions (standard precautions). No special cleaning solutions are required to clean the ambulance following patient transport. Moreover, no medical follow-up is indicated or recommended for an exposure.

Words of Wisdom

Cases of pneumococcal pneumonia are decreasing due to widespread use of the pneumonia vaccine. The key to preventing cases of pneumonia is vaccination for people in the recommended age groups. Pneumococcal conjugate vaccine (PCV) is recommended for all children younger than 5 years, all adults older than 65 years, and people 6 years or older with certain risk factors. Pneumococcal polysaccharide vaccine (PPSV) is recommended for all adults 65 years or older. Vaccine programs are geared toward reducing or eliminating vaccine-preventable diseases.

Pneumonia is discussed in Chapter 17, *Respiratory Emergencies*.

Pathophysiology, Assessment, and Management of STIs

As the name implies, **sexually transmitted infections (STIs)** are usually acquired by sexual contact. Although the term *STI* ordinarily conjures up diagnoses such as gonorrhea or syphilis, the range of diseases transmitted sexually is vast and includes such conditions as herpes, hepatitis, and HIV infection. Hepatitis, HIV infection, and syphilis are bloodborne diseases. This section reviews the features of gonorrhea, syphilis, scabies, and genital herpes infections, as well as other STIs. In most cases, you will not know that a patient has an STI; therefore, standard precautions and good handwashing are appropriate with all patients.

In general, there is no specific prehospital treatment for STIs. Protect the patient's privacy and modesty. Your assessment will reveal the signs and symptoms that require treatment—most commonly, pain, nausea and vomiting, bleeding, and fever. If indicated, start an IV line (titrate to the patient's vital signs), and administer analgesics and antiemetics.

Gonorrhea

Pathophysiology

Gonorrhea is an infection caused by a gonococcal bacterium, *Neisseria gonorrhoeae*. Gonorrhea is especially prevalent in people ages 15 to 24 years. Transmission occurs sexually, by contact with the pus-containing fluid from the mucous membranes of infected people. In consequence, anyone who engages in unprotected sexual contact is at risk. The incubation period is usually 2 to 7 days but may be longer. This infection is communicable for months if not treated; if treated, the disease is noncommunicable within hours. In 2019, 580,000 cases of gonorrhea were reported in the United States, representing a 5% increase in the number of cases since 2018.[56] A new antibiotic-resistant strain has also been found in the US population.

Assessment

Signs and symptoms of gonorrhea differ between males and females. Males usually experience a pus-containing discharge from the urethra and often report pain on urination (dysuria) starting a few days after exposure. In women, the initial inflammation of the urethra or cervix may be so mild that it passes unnoticed, and the illness may progress to pelvic inflammatory disease (PID), with signs and symptoms of an acute abdomen. Depending on the patient's sexual practices, gonorrheal infection may also involve the anus and throat.

Management

The risk of acquiring any STI through a route other than sexual contact is remote. Prevention (standard precautions) includes glove use if touching drainage from the genital area and thorough handwashing. Providing care for a person with gonorrhea would not be considered an occupational health risk or an exposure event.

Syphilis

Pathophysiology

Syphilis is caused by the spiral-shaped bacterium *Treponema pallidum*. Because this disease progresses in three stages, it is considered both an acute disease and a chronic disease. Its incidence has been increasing in the United States for the past 10 years. In 2019, approximately 37,000 cases were reported in the United States.[57] The group with the highest incidence rate consists of people ages 20 to 69 years. A high incidence rate in this age group has been identified across the country, and senior communities have been added to the high-risk-group listing. The CDC initially published a plan to eliminate this disease in the United States by 2010. However, due to new STI guidelines, this goal was reset, and the new target is 2025. Syphilis testing is now a routine part of health care, and testing for syphilis is part of postexposure testing of a source patient.

Transmission of *T pallidum* occurs by direct contact with infectious fluids from the primary lesion or chancre. The bacteria can be transmitted across the placenta from an infected mother to her fetus, by sexual contact, or through blood transfusion. The incubation period is 10 days to 3 months; the communicable period varies. If treated with penicillin, an infected person is considered noncontagious within 48 hours.

Assessment

The primary infection with syphilis produces an ulcerative lesion, called a **chancre**, of the skin or mucous membrane at the infection site. Chancres are most commonly located in the genital region. *Secondary infection* is the term used to describe the presence of skin rash, patchy hair loss, and swollen lymph glands. Complications of syphilis in the tertiary (third) stage can include cardiac, ophthalmic, auditory, and central nervous system complications and lesions of the tissues and bone. The most tragic health consequence is newborn deaths related to congenital syphilis, which increased 22% from 2017 to 2018 (from 77 to 94 deaths).[56]

Management

Preventive measures against transmission of syphilis include taking standard precautions—gloves and good handwashing techniques. No special cleaning precautions are required. The occupational risk for transmission to a health care provider is from a contaminated needlestick injury. If a contaminated needlestick injury occurs, notify your DICO. Treatment is available with procaine penicillin G. If you are allergic to penicillin, tetracycline and doxycycline are alternatives. Rapid fingerstick tests for syphilis give results in 10 to 15 minutes and can be performed in the ED.

Syphilis is a common coinfection in persons infected with HIV. Likewise, coinfection is often seen in people with HCV infection.

Genital Herpes

Pathophysiology

Genital herpes is a chronic, recurrent illness produced by infection with the herpes simplex virus. The herpes simplex virus is further classified into two types: Type 1 is generally transmitted via contact with oral secretions, and type 2 is spread through sexual contact. All sexually active persons are at risk for this infection. Cases of genital herpes do not have to be reported to the CDC, so official data on this disease's incidence are not available.

Herpes simplex type 1 infection is usually activated from a dormant status by stress and febrile illness. It causes a blisterlike sore, usually on the lips or inside the mouth. Infants may become infected if delivered through the birth canal of a woman with active disease.

The incubation period is 2 to 12 days. Secretion of the virus in saliva has been noted to persist for as long as 7 weeks following a lesion's appearance. Genital lesions remain infectious for 4 to 7 days. This disease is elusive; it can suddenly become reactivated, often repeatedly, over many years. Outbreaks are often stress-related.

Assessment

Genital herpes is characterized by vesicular lesions **FIGURE 27-7**. In women, the vesicles occur initially on the cervix; during recurrent infections, vesicles may also appear around the vulva, legs, and buttocks. In men, lesions commonly occur on the penis and around the anus, depending on sexual practices. Herpes type 1 oral lesions may be present on the patient's mouth.

Management

There is no cure for genital herpes. However, treatment with acyclovir, valacyclovir, or famciclovir for 7 to 10 days can reduce outbreaks. Preventive measures include standard precautions—the use

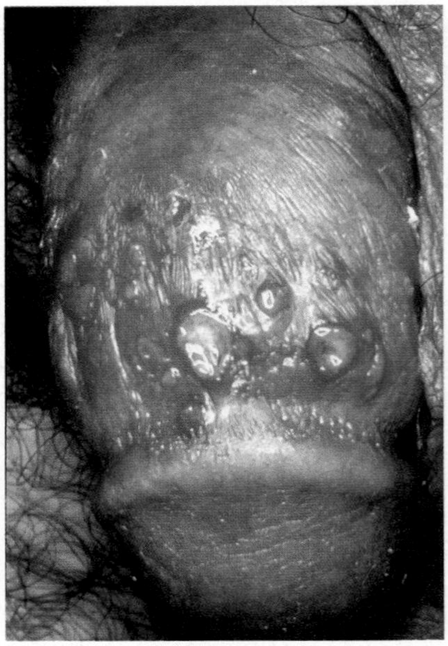

FIGURE 27-7 Genital herpes.

Courtesy of Dr. N. J. Fumara and Dr. Gavin Hart/CDC.

of gloves when touching drainage from lesions and good handwashing techniques. No special cleaning precautions are necessary.

If you have an open cut on your hand or finger and contact the drainage from a herpes type 1 oral lesion, you may develop herpetic whitlow (herpes infection of the finger), which is considered an occupational risk. To avoid such risks, use of gloves is essential when suctioning or intubating a patient with oral lesions. There is no postexposure treatment for this infection.

Chlamydia

Pathophysiology

Chlamydia infections are the most frequently reported bacterial STI in the United States.[58] In 2019, more than 1.7 million cases were reported to the CDC, a 3% increase from 2018. This increase is attributed to the availability of more sensitive screening tests and the trend toward routine screening.

Transmission of chlamydia occurs through sexual contact. Perinatal infections may result in premature rupture of membranes, premature birth, or stillbirth. The incubation period is believed to be 7 to 14 days or longer. The communicable period is unknown.

Assessment

In most women with chlamydia, the infection initially remains asymptomatic. However, PID eventually develops in many women infected with *Chlamydia trachomatis*. In men, infection may lead to epididymitis, prostatitis, proctitis, and proctocolitis.

Signs and symptoms include inflammation of the urethra, epididymis, cervix, and fallopian tubes when the infection is acquired through sexual transmission. Urethral discharge may be gray or white. The amount of discharge varies.

Management

Chlamydia infection is treated with antibiotics. Preventive measures include wearing gloves when in contact with discharge from the genital area and using good handwashing techniques. There are no special cleaning requirements for the EMS vehicle or linens.

Scabies

Pathophysiology

Scabies is caused by infection with *Sarcoptes scabiei*, a parasite. The incidence of this disease has been increasing during the past few years in the United States and Europe. This infection commonly affects families, children, sexual partners, chronically ill patients, and people in group homes. People of every race and social class are vulnerable to scabies infection.

Transmission occurs via direct skin-to-skin contact, such as through wrestling, during sexual contact, and by sharing undergarments, towels, and linens. The incubation period is 4 to 6 weeks for people with no prior exposure to the pathogen. A second or subsequent infestation may appear in only a few days. The communicable period lasts until the mites and eggs are destroyed by treatment. The female mite can live on a human host for several weeks. Without a host, however, the parasite dies in 2 to 4 days. Transmission generally requires direct prolonged contact.

Assessment

Signs and symptoms of scabies include a rash of small, raised red bumps where the mite has burrowed into the skin, causing intense itching, especially at night. The rash appears on the hands, flexor aspects of the wrists, axillary folds, ankles, toes, genital area, buttocks, and abdomen. A rash between the fingers is a common sign of scabies. **FIGURE 27-8**. The patient may develop sores from scratching the rash.

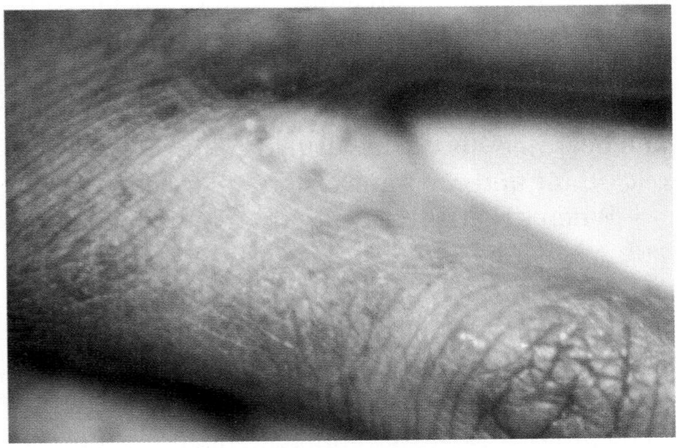

FIGURE 27-8 Rash produced by scabies.

Courtesy of Centers for Disease Control and Prevention.

Management

Prevention of scabies using standard precautions consists of wearing gloves and practicing good handwashing techniques. Vehicle linens require only routine washing in hot water, with routine cleaning of the vehicle after patient transport. The products used to treat scabies are called *scabicides* because they kill scabies mites; some also kill mite eggs. These medications require a prescription. No treatment cream or lotion should be applied on a routine basis because of reports of toxicity. In case of documented exposure, treatment will be undertaken and work restrictions from patient care may be ordered.

Scabies is considered an occupational health risk. In turn, exposure should be reported to the DICO.

Lice

Pathophysiology

Lice are small insects that crawl through the hair and feed on blood through the skin. They cannot hop or fly. There are three types of lice: the head louse (*Pediculus humanus capitis*), body louse (*Pediculus humanus corporis*), and pubic louse (*Phthirus pubis*).

All types of lice are acquired through direct contact with an infested person. Head and body lice can also be acquired from objects such as hats, combs, or clothes infested with lice. Lice eggs look like small white or tan dots on the skin. The eggs hatch after about 1 week, and the new lice mature in 1 to 2 weeks. Thereafter, an adult louse will begin to reproduce and will lay eggs over the next 28 days. Head lice can be found in the hair and in other hairy areas of the head, such as eyebrows, eyelashes, mustaches, and beards. Body lice are usually found in the seams of clothing and can transfer certain diseases.

When discussing lice as an STI, the focus is on pubic lice. The *P pubis* parasite usually has a gray color. Lice are common in people with poor hygiene, people living in group homes, and people with multiple sexual partners.

Transmission of pubic lice occurs through intimate physical or sexual contact. The incubation period lasts approximately 8 to 10 days after the eggs hatch. The communicable period ends when all lice and eggs are destroyed by treatment.

Assessment

Signs and symptoms of pubic lice include slight to severe itching and irritation and, possibly, sores. Nits (eggs) can be seen clinging to the pubic, perianal, or perineal hair. Pubic lice can also infest eyelashes, eyebrows, axillae, scalp, and other body hairs.

Management

Preventive measures include standard precautions—namely, wearing gloves and practicing good handwashing techniques. Routine cleaning of the vehicle after transport is sufficient. In case of documented exposure, treatment with permethrin cream may be prescribed, and restrictions from patient care may be indicated until the paramedic is free of lice.

Lice are considered an occupational health risk. Any exposure to them should be reported to the DICO.

Other STIs and Related Conditions

Genital Warts and Human Papillomavirus

Genital warts (also called condylomata acuminata and venereal warts) are caused by the **human papillomavirus (HPV)**. Of the more than 100 types of HPV that have been identified (most are harmless), approximately 30 types are spread through sexual contact. HPV is the most common STI, with millions of new cases being reported every year. Sources estimate that 75% to 80% of all people in the United States will be infected with HPV at some time in their lives.[59] Some people infected with HPV have no symptoms. In others, multiple growths develop in the genital areas—that is, the vagina, vulva, cervix, or rectum, or the penis and scrotum in men. HPV has been identified as a causative agent in cervical, vulvar, and anal cancers. In pregnant women, warts may develop that become large enough to impede urination or obstruct the birth canal. If the virus is passed to the fetus, the child may develop *laryngeal papillomatosis* (throat warts that block the airway), a potentially life-threatening condition.

Chancroid

Chancroid is caused by infection with the bacterium *Haemophilus ducreyi*. This is a highly contagious yet curable disease. Chancroid is known to facilitate the transmission of HIV. It causes painful sores (ulcers), usually of the genitals. Swollen, painful lymph glands or inguinal buboes in the groin area may be present as well. Women may be asymptomatic and, therefore, unaware they have the disease. Prehospital treatment is supportive only.

Trichomoniasis

Trichomoniasis is a parasitic infection caused by *Trichomonas vaginalis*, a single-cell parasite that is transmitted through sexual contact. According to the CDC,[60] in men, the urethra is the most commonly infected body part; in women, the lower genital tract (eg, vulva, vagina, cervix, urethra) are most frequently infected. Approximately 70% of infected people are asymptomatic. When present, symptoms usually appear within 5 to 28 days of exposure, but can occur much later after exposure. In men, signs and symptoms may include a feeling of itching or irritation inside the penis, frequent urination, burning after urination or ejaculation, and, possibly, a purulent discharge from the penis. In women, signs and symptoms may include a foul-smelling vaginal discharge that is clear, white, yellow, gray, or green in color. Women may also complain of vaginal itching and tenderness, frequent urination, and spotting.

Trichomoniasis can be treated with oral medication. Left untreated, the infection can lead to low birth weight or premature birth in pregnant women and to increased susceptibility to HIV infection.

Bacterial Vaginosis

Bacterial vaginosis is one of the most common conditions that affects women. In this infection, normal bacteria in the vagina are replaced by an overgrowth of other bacterial forms. Symptoms may include itching, burning, or pain, which may be accompanied by a fishy, foul-smelling discharge. Left untreated, bacterial vaginosis can lead to premature birth or low birth weight in cases of pregnancy, make the patient more susceptible to more serious infections, and result in PID.

Bacterial vaginosis is treated with metronidazole, an antibiotic. If the patient consumes alcohol while taking this therapy, severe nausea and vomiting may develop.

Candidiasis

Candidiasis or *thrush* can develop after having sex with someone who is also infected with this disease. It is not technically defined as an STI, but is more commonly known as a yeast infection. Candidiasis occurs in both pregnant and nonpregnant females, although it seems to be more common during pregnancy due to the chemical changes in the vagina (increased glycogen facilitates growth). Risk factors include poorly controlled diabetes and gestational diabetes, taking antibiotics, wearing tight-fitting clothing (which increases warmth and decreases airflow), menstruation, excessive use of vaginal sprays or douches, and other activities as insignificant as a bubble bath (which can cause an irritation that leads to an infection).[61]

Treatment involves the use of prescription creams and over-the-counter medications. In the context of pregnancy, the fetus will not be affected by this infection while in utero. An infant may potentially develop thrush in the mouth after delivery if the infection is active during a vaginal delivery or if the woman breastfeeds.

Pathophysiology, Assessment, and Management of Common Bloodborne Diseases

Types of Viral Hepatitis

Viral hepatitis is an inflammation of the liver produced by a virus. Five distinct forms of viral hepatitis (A, B, C, D, and E) exist. They are produced by different viruses and vary somewhat in their means of transmission. However, all types present with the same signs and symptoms, so the type causing illness is ultimately determined by blood testing. HAV and hepatitis E virus (HEV) are discussed as enteric (intestinal) diseases in this chapter because they are not bloodborne infections. HEV is not widely found in the United States.

Hepatitis B Virus Infection

Hepatitis type B virus (HBV), also known as **serum hepatitis**, is transmitted through infectious blood, semen, and other body fluids primarily through sexual contact, blood transfusion, or puncture of the skin with contaminated needles or other contaminated sharp instruments.[62] In the United States, the rate of new HBV infections has declined by about 82% since 1991, when a national immunization program to eliminate HBV infection was implemented.[63] Occupationally acquired hepatitis B infections are now a rare event. There is no recommendation for routine titer testing or boosters.

Pathophysiology

Needles, including those used for tattooing and acupuncture, and occasionally other objects, such as shared razors, have been implicated in transmission of HBV. Type B hepatitis is prevalent among IV drug users who share needles.

One study suggested that the HBV can survive outside the body in the medium of dried blood for as long as 7 days—for example, in the presence of dried blood on stainless steel in a hemodialysis center. The incubation period for HBV varies widely, from 60 to 90 days, with symptom onset beginning an average of 90 days after exposure to HBV. In 2016, according to the WHO,[64] fewer than 5% of all people infected with HBV became chronic carriers; 20% to 30% of people chronically infected with HBV were expected to experience cirrhosis of the liver and/or liver cancer.

Assessment

Signs and symptoms of HBV infection include loss of appetite, nausea, vomiting, general fatigue and malaise, low-grade fever, vague abdominal discomfort, and, sometimes, aching in the joints. The very smell of food may provoke nausea, and smokers often notice a sudden distaste for cigarettes. At this point, signs and symptoms subside for 50% to 60% of infected persons, which explains why many infected people never know that they have acquired the disease. For people whose disease progresses into the second phase, their urine begins to turn dark. A day or two later, **jaundice**, a yellowing of the skin, and scleral **icterus**, a yellowing of the sclera (the whites of the eyes), develop in the patient **FIGURE 27-9**.

HBV symptoms usually lasts several weeks, although complete recovery may take 3 to 4 months. Some individuals become chronically infected. Medications that limit replication of the virus can protect the liver and improve the person's overall health, but there is no cure at this time.

Management

Prevention of HBV transmission focuses on practicing standard precautions—that is, using gloves when handling blood, OPIM, or materials containing visible blood. Good handwashing technique is also essential. Paramedics should be immunized against HBV when hired, if not previously vaccinated. Vaccination, which is safe and effective, protects against HBV for life; it also indirectly protects against hepatitis D virus (HDV) infection (because a person must be infected with type B to acquire type D).

OSHA requires that employers of health care workers offer the HBV immunization at no cost to

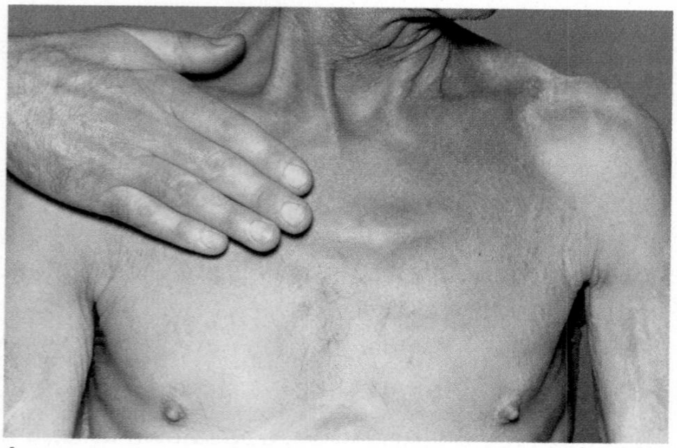

A

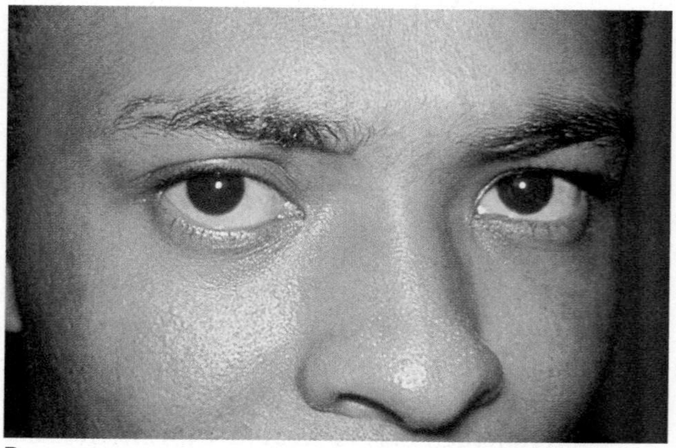

B

FIGURE 27-9 Signs of infection caused by hepatitis type B virus. **A.** Jaundice. **B.** Scleral icterus.

A: Courtesy of Centers for Disease Control and Prevention; **B:** © SPL/Science Source.

at-risk staff members. If you are allergic to yeast, notify the vaccine administrator, and arrangements will be made to obtain the proper vaccine to meet your needs. Traditionally, the vaccine has been administered in a three-dose series over a 6-month time frame. However, a two-dose vaccine (Heplisav-B) is now available that is more protective; this series is completed in 2 months. For both vaccine types, a second dose is given 4 weeks after the first dose. However, the original vaccine requires a third dose 6 months after the first, whereas Heplisav-B does not require a third dose.[65] With either type of vaccine, when the series has been completed, you should have a blood test (titer) performed 1 to 2 months later to ensure that your immune system responded. Periodic titer testing is neither required nor recommended. It is essential to complete all doses to achieve protection.

To guard against HBV transmission, practice routine standard precautions. If you are exposed, notify your DICO. The DICO will verify the source patient's test results. If you have a positive titer on file, no follow-up treatment is needed. If you do not have a titer report on file and the patient is positive for HBV infection, a titer test will be ordered for you. Treatment will depend on the results of the titer testing. If you have not been vaccinated and the patient is positive for HBV, you will be offered one dose of hepatitis B immunoglobulin (HBIG) and the vaccine series.

Hepatitis C Virus Infection

HCV is spread primarily through contact with the blood of an infected person. The resulting infection can be either acute or chronic. An acute HCV infection occurs within the first 6 months after exposure to the HCV. An acute infection often leads to a chronic infection; in fact, it is estimated that 75% to 85% of people who become infected with HCV will experience chronic infection.[66] Chronic HCV occurs when the virus remains present in a person's body. It can lead to serious liver problems, including cirrhosis (scarring of the liver) or liver cancer. HCV is the leading cause of liver transplantation in the United States, Europe, and Japan.[67]

Approximately 15% to 25% of HCV infections resolve on their own.[68] In recent years, new testing methods and new treatment medications have changed the diagnosis and treatment options for HCV infection, and this disease can now be cured. Rapid fingerstick testing for HCV is the standard of care for source-patient testing, with results becoming available in 20 to 30 minutes.

Pathophysiology

Transmission of HCV most often occurs by sharing needles, syringes, or other equipment to inject drugs; needlestick injuries in health care settings; and being born to a mother who has HCV. HCV was once commonly spread through the transfusion of blood and blood products and organ transplants. This method of HCV transmission is now rare in the United States because of blood screening for the virus that became available in 1992. HCV is less commonly spread by sharing personal care items that may have come in contact with another person's blood, such as razors or toothbrushes, or having sexual contact with a person infected with HCV.

Two cases of HCV transmission via blood splash to the eye have been reported.[69] The last, reported in 2003, occurred in a laboratory. Studies have not shown HCV to be spread through licensed, commercial tattooing facilities; however, transmission of HCV (and other infectious diseases) is possible when poor infection-control practices are used during tattooing or piercing.[70]

This virus can survive on environmental surfaces for up to 16 hours at room temperature if not properly cleaned.

Assessment

It is estimated that 70% to 80% of people with acute HCV do not have any symptoms.[71] When signs and symptoms do occur, they generally appear within 6 to 9 weeks after exposure, though this period can range from 4 to 12 weeks. Signs and symptoms are the same as those for HBV infection: lack of appetite, nausea and vomiting, low-grade fever, abdominal distress, joint discomfort, dark urine, clay-colored bowel movements, jaundice, and a general feeling of illness and listlessness. The diagnosis is established by testing for HCV antibody and genotype testing. There are six genotypes that cause HCV infection.

Management

To prevent HCV transmission, take standard precautions—wear gloves when in direct contact with blood or OPIM, and use needle-safe or needleless devices. Any blood spills, including dried blood, should be cleaned using a dilution of 1 part household bleach to 100 parts water.[72]

If you have sustained an exposure, testing will begin with the source patient; permission to test for HCV is not required. Rapid HCV testing should be performed on the source, with results in 1 hour. If the source is HCV positive, a second test for viral load will be performed; its results will be available in about 3 hours. Testing for viral load is important because infection resolves in 15% of people, meaning antibody testing alone will not reveal infection. If the patient has a viral load, you will have a baseline HCV antibody test and liver function test. You should also have an HCV-RNA test (test for the virus) 3 weeks following the exposure event.[73,74] If it is negative, you did not acquire HCV from the exposure. If it is positive, you will be offered 8 to 12 weeks of treatment.

The treatment now available is highly successful in resolving this infection and can cure all six genotypes of HCV. However, there is currently no medication that can be offered after exposure to prevent infection. A vaccine for prevention of HCV infection is now in human clinical trials; it is considered a therapeutic vaccine because it is given only to newly diagnosed persons. Workers' compensation covers all of the FDA-approved treatments.

Hepatitis D Virus Infection

A host must be infected with HBV before HDV (also called delta hepatitis) infection can occur. For this reason, HDV is considered a parasite for HBV. There are three known genotypes of HDV. Genotype 1 has a worldwide distribution; genotype 2 exists in Taiwan, Japan, and northern Asia; and genotype 3 is found in South America. This viral infection is rare in the United States.

Pathophysiology

Transmission generally occurs by percutaneous exposure, because HDV is not effectively transmitted through sexual contact. Perinatal transmission is rare. The incubation period for HDV infection ranges from 30 to 180 days. Blood is considered to be infectious during all phases of the illness.

Assessment

Signs and symptoms are the same as those associated with HBV infection.

Management

The first step in protecting against HDV transmission is receiving the HBV vaccine. If you are protected from HBV, you cannot acquire HDV. In addition, use standard precautions: Wear gloves when in contact with blood or OPIM, use needle-safe or needleless devices, and perform routine cleaning of the vehicle following patient transport. Do not go through the pockets of known IV drug users who are found unconscious because they may contain contaminated sharps. If a documented exposure occurs, notify your DICO. Testing begins with the source patient in accordance with state testing laws. Consent is not needed to test for hepatitis viruses. If the source is positive for HDV and you are protected against HBV, no further treatment is indicated.

Human Immunodeficiency Virus Infection and Acquired Immunodeficiency Syndrome

Human immunodeficiency virus (HIV), type 1, has existed in the United States since at least the mid to late 1970s. In 2015, the CDC reported that there were approximately 40,000 newly diagnosed cases of HIV infection in the United States.[75] Worldwide, an estimated 2.1 million new cases of HIV occurred in 2015.[76] Reporting HIV infection to public health authorities is not legally mandated in all states in the United States. Because of advances in testing and treatment, persons with HIV and AIDS can now live 50 years or longer after diagnosis as productive members of society.[77]

Special Populations

HIV is a bloodborne disease that can be transmitted from mother to infant in the birthing process. In the United States, all pregnant women who receive prenatal care are tested for HIV infection. The rate of infection from mother to child is only 1% to 2% because infected mothers are treated with antiretroviral drugs beginning in the second trimester of pregnancy.[78]

Pathophysiology

In addition to being spread through contact with blood or OPIM, including sexual transmission, HIV can be transmitted through blood transfusions. Although all blood donated is tested for HIV, it is not 100% safe. However, such transmissions have occurred at a very low rate since testing was implemented for the presence of P24 (a protein present from the beginning of the HIV life cycle) in donated blood. With P24 testing of donated blood, the virus can now be detected 1 to 6 days after infection.

HIV is not transmitted through casual or even household contact. Even among people who routinely share eating utensils, toothbrushes, and razors with HIV-infected patients, there is no evidence of an increased rate of HIV infection. This disease is not transmitted by airborne or droplet means.

The HIV pathogen envelops into infected cells and attacks the immune system and other body organs. As a result, the immune system cannot assist in protecting an infected person from other diseases. It takes approximately 7 days for the virus to envelop into a cell, and this process may occur 4 to 6 weeks after the exposure event. The communicable period is unknown but is believed to span from the onset of infection until about 48 weeks after treatment with medications begins. After 48 weeks of treatment, replicated studies show there is no circulating virus and, therefore, no risk for disease transmission.[79] One of the newest medications has been shown to produce an undetectable viral load after 8 weeks of treatment. Further, a reduced or absent viral load means the patient's infection is less likely to progress to **acquired immunodeficiency syndrome (AIDS)**, the end-stage disease process.

A patient with AIDS is vulnerable to numerous **opportunistic infections** that would not affect a person with an intact immune system. Patients who respond to the cocktail drug treatment (96% of all patients who receive this therapy) render the virus unable to multiply, meaning they cannot transmit the disease. Thus, prevention through treatment is possible.

The incubation period of AIDS spans the time between documented infection (ie, becoming HIV-positive) and development of the end-stage disease; it is determined by the CD4 cell count and the presence of opportunistic infections. The Ryan White CARE Act (1990) makes HIV therapy available to all people in the United States with or without the ability to pay.

Assessment

Signs and symptoms may include acute febrile illness, malaise, swollen lymph glands, headache, and, possibly, rash. Following initial infection with HIV, most people present with enlargement of the lymph nodes but appear otherwise healthy. However, if the infection is left untreated, the number of T-helper lymphocytes (CD4 cells) gradually declines. T-helper cells are essential components of the immune system that mediate cellular and humoral immunity. Seroconversion—meaning that antibodies can be detected in the blood—usually occurs within the first 3 months following exposure. However, rapid testing can detect two proteins present at the beginning of this virus's life cycle. People who are **seropositive** for HIV are prescribed antiretroviral drug treatment (combined double-drug treatment). The rapid fingerstick tests give results in 1 minute. To diagnose people who may not be aware of their infection, the US Preventive Services Task Force recommends that clinicians screen all patients ages 15 to 65 years.[80]

The development of specific opportunistic bacterial, viral, and fungal infections defines the transition from HIV infection to AIDS. These conditions are known accordingly as *AIDS-defining* or *AIDS-related conditions*. They include *Pneumocystis jirovecii* (formerly known as *Pneumocystis carinii*) pneumonia in infants or people with compromised immune systems; cytomegalovirus, which can cause blindness; red or purple skin cancers known as Kaposi sarcoma; atypical TB; and cryptococcal meningitis. Development of these opportunistic infections is now rare due to the availability of medications and medical care for HIV-infected individuals.

Management

Prevention focuses on standard precautions—use of gloves when in direct contact with patient blood or OPIM, use of needle-safe or needleless devices, good handwashing technique, and routine cleaning of the vehicle after transport. There is no need to restrict pregnant health care providers from contact with patients with known HIV infection or AIDS.

The risk for acquiring HIV infection for health care providers is related to handling and disposal of sharps. As of September 5, 2020, occupationally acquired HIV infection had been documented in 58 health care providers; none were fire or EMS personnel.[81] Of these occupational infections, 50 were the result of a needlestick injury exposure. A needlestick exposure to HIV includes *all* of the following elements: a deep stick with a large-gauge hollow-bore needle, visible blood on the device, an HIV-positive patient with a high viral load, and a device that had been in the patient's vein or artery. Following this type of exposure, the risk of transmission is 0.23% for exposure to the mucous membrane of the eye and 0.09% for nonintact skin (only one case has been reported and documented).

If an exposure occurs, notify your DICO. The source patient will be tested in accordance with state law, ideally using the rapid HIV testing method. Its results are accurate and available in less than 1 hour. If the test is negative, no further testing is indicated. If the source is positive, a blood sample is sent for assessment of viral load, with results becoming available in 2 to 3 hours. If the source patient is positive for HIV and has circulating virus, and the type of exposure meets the CDC criteria, the provider may be offered postexposure antiretroviral medications. However, based on the new data related to viral load, the need for these drugs after an exposure has diminished. The CDC sets the criteria for use of these drugs; they are not given automatically. OSHA enforces the CDC guidelines for postexposure prophylaxis under the bloodborne pathogens regulation (CFR 1910.1030). The CDC recommends that a physician knowledgeable in the use of these drugs be consulted. If one is not available, then the physician should contact the 24-hour Post-Exposure Prophylaxis (PEP) Hotline at 1-888-448-4911 before prescribing these drugs. The PEP hotline is staffed by infectious disease physicians who will determine if PEP is appropriate.[82,83]

Words of Wisdom

Unless they contain visible blood, the following body fluids do not transmit bloodborne disease: saliva, tears, sweat, urine, stool, vomitus, nasal secretions, and sputum.

As noted earlier, the newest antiretroviral medications offer protection from transmission through treatment. Antiretroviral drugs are toxic, so careful and complete counseling should be provided to exposed health care providers. Before initiating antiretroviral therapy, baseline laboratory testing should be done—specifically, a complete blood count and liver and kidney function tests. For a female of childbearing age, pregnancy testing is appropriate. These tests should be repeated every 2 weeks during drug therapy.

Street Smarts

Diseases acquired through contact with bloodborne pathogens are considered protected conditions under the Americans with Disabilities Act.

Fungal Skin Infections

Dermatophyte Infections

Pathophysiology

Fungal infections of the skin are common and usually superficial. In most cases, they result from a group of fungi called *dermatophytes*. Most are identified by the word *tinea*, followed with a term that denotes the location of the lesion. **TABLE 27-4** lists the most common tinea infections and their locations.

Assessment

The history and physical findings will vary depending on the type of tinea. In most cases, the patient has a scaly rash and associated itching. The differential diagnosis varies with the type of tinea (see Table 27-4), as other types of dermatitis may mimic tinea.

Management

Because most dermatophyte infections involve limited areas, they respond well to topical antifungal agents. Complications are rare.[84]

Helminths

A helminth is a worm classified as a parasite that lives in humans. Helminth eggs can contaminate

TABLE 27-4 Tinea Infection Sites

Name	Location	Appearance
Tinea capitis	Head, scalp	Round, scaly area where no hair is growing; diffuse scaling
Tinea corporis	Body	Round lesion appears in a small area; ringworm
Tinea cruris	Groin, genitalia	Sharply demarcated area with elevated scaling, geographic borders
Tinea pedis	Feet	Thinning of tissue between the toes, scaling on soles or sides of the foot, sometimes vesicles and/or pustules **FIGURE 27-10**
Tinea manuum	Hands	Dry, diffuse scaling, usually on palm
Tinea unguium	On or under fingernails or toenails	Dark debris under nails
Tinea versicolor	Trunk	Pink, tan, or white patches with scaly skin areas

FIGURE 27-10 Tinea pedis.

pets, livestock, and water. Humans can come in contact with helminths by touching contaminated water or an animal and not washing their hands afterward. They may then ingest the eggs, which hatch in the intestine. Common symptoms of helminthic infections include fatigue, weight loss, abdominal cramps, nausea, and vomiting. Treatment includes medications such as albendazole, ivermectin, mebendazole, and pyrantel pamoate. Although the toxicity of these medications varies, they may cause side effects including GI distress, headache, weakness, tachycardia, and hypotension.

Hookworm

Ancylostoma duodenale and *Necator americanus* are two hookworms known to infect humans. In the infection process, the larva (immature worms) of these parasites penetrate intact skin, enter the circulation, travel to the lungs, are coughed up and swallowed, and develop to adulthood in the small intestine.[85] The adult worms then lay eggs, which are released into the feces. Egg laying begins 4 to 8 weeks after exposure and can last as long as 5 years. The primary method of transmission occurs by walking barefoot on contaminated soil. *A duodenale* can also be transmitted through the ingestion of larvae.[86]

Although some people may have no symptoms, possible early signs of infection include itching and a localized rash. As the infection worsens, the patient may have abdominal pain, diarrhea, loss of appetite, weight loss, and fatigue. The diagnosis is made by stool examination for ova and parasites.

Pinworm

Pinworm infection, which is caused by a small roundworm called *Enterobius vermicularis*, is common in crowded conditions such as daycare centers, schools, and mental institutions.[85] This infection is spread by the fecal-oral route. Larvae hatch in the small intestine and travel to the large intestine, where they mature in 2 to 6 weeks. Female pinworms

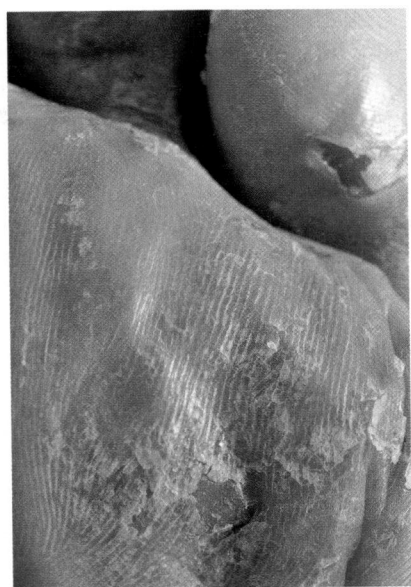

leave the intestine through the anus during sleep and deposit their eggs on the surrounding skin.[87] These egg deposits can cause itching and may be transmitted from hand to mouth when the infected person scratches the inflamed area. Pinworms can survive for long periods in the dust that builds up over doors, on windowsills, and under beds in the rooms of infected people. Indirect transmission can occur when handling contaminated clothing, bedding, food, or play objects.

Diagnosis is usually made by the tape test, in which transparent tape is applied to the skin around the anus. This tape is then examined for eggs using a microscope. Pinworm infection can be treated with over-the-counter or prescription medication.

Words of Wisdom

Bedbugs are small, red-brown insects about the size of a tick that feed on the blood of humans as well as other warm-blooded animals such as dogs, cats, birds, and rodents. They hide in the cracks and crevices of beds, particularly along mattress seams, and in luggage, overnight bags, folded clothing, and furniture. Bedbug infestations generally occur around the areas where people sleep, including suburban homes, apartments, hotels, and dormitories. They sometimes appear in movie theaters, health care facilities, and office buildings.

Bedbugs typically bite humans at night during sleep and crawl to a secluded area to digest their meal after feeding. Bites are usually found on the face, neck, shoulder, back, arms, and legs. Because a bedbug injects an anesthetic and an anticoagulant when biting, a person may not realize they have been bitten. Although some people develop a red, itchy welt within a day or so of the bite, others have little or no reaction. Topical corticosteroids are used to treat bites. Bedbugs can harbor various pathogens, but disease transmission to humans has not been proven; therefore, bed bugs do not pose a risk for disease transmission.[88]

Eradicating bedbugs can be accomplished using a spray bottle and 90% alcohol, which can be purchased at a hardware store or local pharmacy. The bugs are killed on contact when sprayed. Heavy extermination, which is sometimes necessary, involves washing and drying of all bedding on a hot setting, and placing the mattress and box spring in a zippered plastic case.

Words of Wisdom

Some diseases require a combination of precautions based on how the disease is transmitted. For example, Ebola requires taking standard precautions, droplet precautions, and contact precautions..

Ebola

Ebola is a disease that falls in two categories for precautions: contact and droplet. Ebola is not a new disease; health care workers have been dealing with Ebola for more than 40 years. However, its presence has been limited to West Africa for most of the outbreaks. Where this virus hides between outbreaks has not been determined, but it is now known that the African fruit bat plays a significant role in its transmission. In the past, outbreaks were limited to one local area, but the recent outbreak in 2013–2014 occurred on the border between three countries, which was problematic. The most recent outbreak of Ebola in the Democratic Republic of Congo ended in June 2020. An Ebola vaccine has been approved by the FDA and is 100% effective.

The Ebola virus is an enveloped virus, which means it can readily be killed by application of many common EPA-registered agents. This virus dies after a few hours on surfaces.

Pathophysiology

Ebola virus can be spread to others through direct contact via nonintact skin or mucous membranes. The incubation period is 2 to 21 days following exposure. Sources of transmission include the following[89]:

- Direct contact through nonintact skin or mucous membranes
- Infected fruit bats or primates (apes and monkeys) when butchered and used as food
- Blood or body fluids (including, but not limited to, urine, saliva, sweat, feces, vomit, breast milk, and semen) of a person who is sick with or has died from Ebola
- Needles and syringes that have been contaminated with body fluids of a person who is sick with Ebola
- The body of a person who has died from Ebola
- Contact with contaminated surfaces

People coming from West Africa into the United States enter the country through airports that are designated treatment centers; if found to be infected with Ebola, they would be transported by medical units trained by those facilities. This system lessens the number of people who might come in contact with the virus.

Assessment

Travel history is important for Ebola and many other diseases. Determine whether the patient has come from West Africa or been in contact with a person with Ebola. Assess for fever. Initial symptoms include a sudden onset of fever (101.5°F [38.6°C]), intense weakness, muscle pain, headaches, and sore throat. As the disease progresses, the patient often experiences profuse diarrhea and vomiting, rash, and impaired kidney and liver function. Some infected people experience internal and external bleeding.

Management

Follow EMS guidelines, not hospital guidelines, for patient care during the transport of a patient suspected to have Ebola. Limit the use of sharps, and limit invasive procedures. Keep a list of names of people involved in patient care for contact follow-up, if needed.

There is no specific treatment for Ebola. Instead, treatment is supportive: rehydration, balance of fluids and electrolytes, and maintenance of oxygen and BP status. The CDC recommends taking standard, droplet, and contact precautions when within 3 feet (1 m) of the patient.[89] A surgical mask should be placed on the patient when possible; otherwise, the health care provider should wear a surgical mask. A cover gown and protective eyewear should be worn as well. Shoe covers and double gloves are needed only in case of profuse vomiting and diarrhea. If the patient is vomiting, give them a biohazard bag to contain any emesis. If the patient has profuse diarrhea, consider wrapping the patient in an impermeable sheet to reduce contamination of other surfaces. When transporting a patient with suspected Ebola, notify the receiving facility in advance, so that proper infection control precautions can be initiated at the facility before your arrival.

Care should be taken when removing contaminated PPE. No special cleaning solution is needed for Ebola, as this virus can be killed with many common chemical agents, including household bleach. There are no special laundry requirements. Follow state medical waste regulations for disposal of medical waste.

> **Words of Wisdom**
>
> PPE is only as effective as its proper removal. The procedure for removing PPE in case of pathogens differs from the procedure for removing hazmat PPE. Handwashing after glove removal is always important!

Should an exposure event such as contaminated needlestick injury or mucous membrane contact with body fluids occur, perform first aid and notify your DICO. Work restrictions may need to be addressed as long as 21 days.

Pathophysiology, Assessment, and Management of Enteric (Intestinal) Diseases

Norovirus Infection

Pathophysiology

Previously termed Norwalk agent, norovirus causes an estimated 90% of epidemic nonbacterial outbreaks of **gastroenteritis** in the world. Norovirus may be responsible for as many as 50% of all foodborne outbreaks in the United States. This virus affects people of all ages. Noroviruses are classified into six genogroups, three of which cause human disease (GI, GII, and GIV).[90]

When norovirus (a spore-forming organism) enters the body, it begins to multiply in the small intestines. Transmission can occur from person to person, by ingestion of food or water that has been contaminated by infected feces (the fecal-oral route), or by contaminated surfaces. Symptoms may appear within 1 to 2 days. Acute symptoms usually begin in 24 to 28 hours and may last 24 to 60 hours. The virus can be shed for weeks after infection.

Assessment

Patients will present with nausea, forceful vomiting, watery diarrhea, abdominal pain, weakness, and low-grade fever. They are rarely admitted to the hospital.

Management

Standard precautions include wearing gloves and practicing good handwashing technique using soap and warm water. Alcohol sanitizers are not considered effective against norovirus. This virus is enclosed by a structure called a capsid; therefore, cleaning after transport requires the use of a chlorine-based product such as bleach diluted with water to kill the spores.

Pathophysiology, Assessment, and Ma-nagement of Non-Bloodborne Hepatitis Viruses

Hepatitis A Virus Infection

Pathophysiology

HAV, or **infectious hepatitis**, was formerly one of the most common types of hepatitis in the United States. In the past, outbreaks of this disease have been reported in multiple states. Transmission is by the fecal-oral route. Epidemic outbreaks are most often traced to contaminated drinking water, milk, sliced meats, and undercooked shellfish. In recent years, however, outbreaks have been largely related to infected food handlers and the homeless population. No cases related to flood water have been reported since the early 1980s. As a result of programs focused on vaccination of children against all vaccine-preventable diseases, HAV case numbers have been falling each year. In addition, vaccination of homeless populations has undertaken to control the source, given the current trends in outbreaks.

HAV is often described as a benign disease because acquiring it provides lifelong immunity to it. Since 2000, children in the United States have been immunized to protect them from contracting this disease. The vaccine is usually administered at age 12 months (with a range between 12 and 23 months of age). Children who have not been vaccinated by 2 years of age should be vaccinated as soon as possible.

The incubation period is usually about 2 to 4 weeks, although it can range from 15 to 50 days after ingestion of the virus. The communicable period probably starts toward the end of the incubation period and continues for a few days after the patient becomes jaundiced.

Assessment

Signs and symptoms in phase 1 of HAV infection include fatigue, loss of appetite, fever, nausea, and abdominal pain; smokers lose their interest in smoking. In phase 2, patients have jaundice, dark-colored urine, and pale, clay-colored stools.

As noted earlier, chronic liver disease or liver cancer may develop in patients with HBV and HCV. In contrast, HAV is not associated with long-term disease and is considered a "mild" disease because it resolves after several weeks.

Management

Prevention includes taking standard precautions: using good handwashing technique, and, if in contact with patient stool, wearing gloves. No special cleaning of the vehicle is needed. HAV vaccine is recommended for Federal Emergency Management Agency response team members who may respond *outside* the United States, but not for any other health care provider groups or emergency response teams who respond inside the United States.

Hepatitis E Virus Infection

Pathophysiology

HEV is also referred to as enterically transmitted non-A, non-B hepatitis. HEV is most common in developing countries with inadequate water supplies and poor environmental sanitation. When symptomatic HEV occurs in the United States, it is usually the result of travel to a developing country where this disease is endemic. A few sporadic HEV cases not associated with travel have been identified in developed countries.[91] For these non–travel-related domestically acquired cases, no clear exposure has been found.

Transmission typically occurs via the fecal-oral route by ingestion of fecally contaminated drinking water. Animals may also spread HEV; some cases of HEV have occurred after eating uncooked or undercooked pork or deer meat.

This disease has an incubation period of about 15 to 60 days, with the average being 40 days after exposure. The communicable period has not been determined.

Assessment

Signs and symptoms of HEV infection are the same as for other forms of hepatitis.

Management

HEV usually requires only symptomatic treatment and resolves on its own. Patients are typically asked to maintain adequate nutrition and fluids, avoid alcohol, and obtain their physicians' advice before taking any medications that can damage the liver, especially acetaminophen. Prevention includes the use of gloves when in contact with stool, good handwashing technique, and cleaning contaminated equipment.

Pathophysiology, Assessment, and Management of Vector-Borne and Zoonotic (Animal-Borne) Diseases

Diseases that are transmitted through a vector (vector-borne diseases) are usually spread by ticks or mosquitoes. They include diseases such as Rocky Mountain spotted fever, Lyme disease, West Nile virus, dengue fever, and Zika. Such diseases may also be referred to as **zoonotic** diseases.

Mosquito-Borne Diseases

West Nile Virus

West Nile virus (WNV) has been present in the United States for several years. This virus was discovered in Uganda in the 1930s and was first detected in North America in 1999. In the United States, the only states that have not reported cases of WNV are Alaska and Hawaii.

Pathophysiology

Transmission of WNV most often occurs via a bite from a mosquito carrying the virus, which it obtained by feeding on infected birds. However, a small number of human infections have been documented following blood transfusions, organ transplants, exposure in a laboratory setting, and from mother to baby during pregnancy, delivery, or breastfeeding.[92] This infection is not transmitted from person to person, so there is no period of communicability. The incubation period is usually 2 to 6 days but ranges from 2 to 14 days after transmission.

YOU are the Paramedic

PART 4

After starting an IV line and administering fluid, you move the patient to your unit for transport. The transport is uneventful, and you report to the receiving facility staff on arrival. The patient's BP improves slightly in response to the fluid administration. After you transfer your patient to the hospital bed, you notice the sheets on your stretcher are wet.

Recording Time: 10 Minutes	
Respirations	18 breaths/min
Pulse	96 beats/min
Skin	Cool, pale, and dry
Blood pressure	102/60 mm Hg
Oxygen saturation (Spo_2)	97% on room air
Pupils	PERRLA

7. What decontamination measures should you use for your stretcher?
8. What measures should you use for handwashing?

Assessment

In most cases, WNV disease is mild and uneventful; 80% of people who acquire this infection remain unaware that they have it.[93] Many cases are identified when an individual goes to donate blood. Those who are symptomatic tend to exhibit a fever, along with headache, fatigue, weakness, joint pain, vomiting, diarrhea, or rash. Mild symptoms appear in older people and immunocompromised people. In healthy people, the immune system fights off the disease. Serious neurologic illness, such as encephalitis or meningitis, develops in fewer than 1% of people who are infected.[93]

Management

Use needle-safe devices to avoid a contaminated sharps injury when WNV infection is suspected. If you sustain a contaminated sharps injury while caring for a patient with WNV, notify your DICO. There is no recommended medical follow-up treatment. No special cleaning of the vehicle is needed or recommended.

Dengue Fever

Dengue is transmitted between people by the mosquitoes *Aedes aegypti* and *Aedes albopictus*, which are found throughout the world. This mosquito is also a vector for chikungunya and the Zika virus. There are four dengue viruses (DENV-1, -2, -3, and -4). If one is contracted, you have acquired immunity to the one you contracted, but not to the other three. According to the CDC, nearly all dengue cases reported in the 48 contiguous US states have involved travelers who were infected elsewhere.[94]

Pathophysiology

As just noted, transmission is usually by the bite of a mosquito. From 8 to 12 days after a mosquito becomes infected, it can transmit the virus by biting a healthy person; this is its incubation period. Although a mosquito bite is the most common method of dengue transmission, reports have also cited transmission via organ transplantation, blood transfusions from infected donors, and from an infected pregnant woman to her fetus.

Assessment

Signs and symptoms begin about 4 to 7 days after the mosquito bite and usually last 3 to 10 days. The primary signs and symptoms of dengue are a high fever that is accompanied by two or more of the following: severe headache, severe pain behind the eyes, joint pain, muscle and/or bone pain, rash, or mild bleeding (eg, bleeding from nose or gums, petechiae, easy bruising).

In some patients, dengue fever may progress to dengue hemorrhagic fever. Warning signs may emerge as the patient's fever declines, heralding the start of a 24- to 48-hour period when capillaries become leaky, allowing fluid to escape from the blood vessels into the peritoneum (causing ascites) and into the pleural cavity (leading to pleural effusions). This may lead to hemorrhage, hypovolemic shock, and possibly death without prompt, appropriate treatment.

Management

There is no specific treatment for dengue fever. There is no occupational health risk for health care providers caring for a patient with dengue fever. In 2019, the FDA approved a vaccine for use in children ages 9 to 16 years living in areas where dengue is common, including the US territories of American Samoa, Puerto Rico, and the US Virgin Islands.[95]

Chikungunya Fever

Chikungunya virus appears to have originated in Africa. Its discovery occurred nearly 200 years ago, and the virus made its most recent appearance in 2013. In Cuba, it was called dengue, but the two viruses have since been differentiated. The mosquito that transmits dengue fever, *Aedes aegypti*, also transmits chikungunya virus. These mosquitoes breed in the rain-filled containers that are commonly found around homes and workplaces, such as water storage containers, saucers under potted plants, and drinking bowls for domestic animals, as well as in discarded tires, birdbaths, and food containers. In 2019, 192 cases of chikungunya were reported in the United States in people who had traveled from areas where this disease is common.[96]

Pathophysiology

Transmission of chikungunya occurs by the bite of the *A aegypti* mosquito. It is rarely life threatening.

Assessment

Complaints include fever that typically lasts from 5 to 7 days, and severe, possibly incapacitating joint pain. The patient may not be aware of a mosquito bite.

Management

There is no specific treatment for chikungunya, but analgesics and nonsteroidal anti-inflammatory drugs (NSAIDs) may be used to reduce the pain and swelling. Aspirin should be avoided.

Chikungunya virus is not an occupational health risk related to patient care. Clinical trials evaluating an experimental chikungunya vaccine are ongoing.[97]

Zika Virus

Zika virus is relatively new to the United States, having first appeared in mid-2015. Thus far, cases have been related to travel to areas where this infection is prevalent. Zika is transmitted by the bite of the *Aedes aegypti* mosquito—a mosquito known for biting more often in the daylight hours than in the evening hours. Most cases in the United States have been acquired elsewhere; however, some de novo cases have occurred in the Miami, Florida, area.

Transmission from an infected mother to her fetus, resulting in microcephaly, difficulty swallowing, and learning disabilities, has been documented. Also, sexual transmission from an infected male to his sexual partners has been documented. There is also a well-documented correlation between Zika virus and the onset of Guillain-Barré syndrome, as described earlier in this chapter.

No cases of Zika virus transmission through blood transfusions have been reported. To protect against this possibility, people who have traveled to areas where Zika is found are not allowed to donate blood for 28 days after returning to the United States. Currently, all donated blood in the United States is tested for Zika virus. In 2019, there were no documented cases confirmed.[98]

Pathophysiology

The incubation period is 3 to 14 days following the mosquito bite. The virus is then present in urine, saliva, and semen. There is an approved test for Zika, and it is believed that urine testing is the most accurate means of identifying the presence of infection.

Assessment

Many people infected with Zika virus are asymptomatic.[99] For those who have symptoms, the most common are fever, rash, joint pain, conjunctivitis (no drainage), muscle pain, and headache. When assessing a patient for this infection, note any travel history to areas where Zika virus is prevalent.

Management

Care for patients with Zika infection is supportive—rest, fluids, analgesics, and antipyretics. Take standard precautions for patient care. There are currently no recommendations for special protective equipment for medical personnel, except to prevent person-to-person transmission through blood or body fluids. Routine standard precautions are all that is needed or recommended. If wounds and skin sites have been exposed to blood or body fluids, they should be washed promptly with soap and water. Mucous membranes should be flushed with copious amounts of clean water.

> **Words of Wisdom**
>
> Mosquito control is an essential part of risk reduction for mosquito-borne diseases. Remove standing pools of water. Wear clothing to cover exposed areas of the body, and use insect repellent.

Standard precautions should be used when caring for a patient with suspected Zika. Occupational risk may be related to a contaminated sharps injury. Report all sharps injuries directly to the DICO.

Tick-Borne Diseases

Lyme Disease

Lyme disease is named for Lyme, Connecticut, the town where the disease was first identified. It is the most common tick-borne disease in the United States. The deer tick can be a vector for the bacterium *Borrelia burgdorferi*; the tick's bite injects the pathogen into the bloodstream of a human host. In 1982, a national reporting system was established for this infection. The highest prevalence of Lyme disease is found in states in the US Northeast. The peak season for this disease is between June and August, with incidence rates decreasing in the early fall. Each year, approximately 30,000 cases are reported in the United States—making Lyme disease the most commonly reported vector-borne illness in this country. In 2014, it was the fifth most common nationally notifiable disease (each state has a list of diseases that the public health department requires to be reported); however, this disease does *not* occur nationwide, but rather is concentrated heavily in the Northeast and upper Midwest.[77]

Pathophysiology

Lyme disease occurs more often in children younger than 10 years and in middle-aged adults. It is not transmitted from person to person. The incubation period ranges from 3 to 32 days.

Assessment

Lyme disease primarily affects the skin, heart, joints, and nervous system. Some patients remain asymptomatic. For patients in whom signs and symptoms develop, the disease is usually divided into three stages: early localized, early disseminated, and late manifestations:

1. **Early localized stage.** The early stage is characterized by a round, red skin lesion. This bull's-eye rash (so called because it extends outward with a ring in the center) is most common in the area of the groin, thigh, or axilla **FIGURE 27-11**. If present, it is warm to the touch and may blister or scab.
2. **Early disseminated stage.** In the early disseminated stage, secondary lesions may develop within days, and the patient may report flulike symptoms—fever, chills, headache, malaise, and muscle pain. Nonproductive cough, testicular swelling, sore throat, enlarged spleen, and enlarged lymph nodes may be present. Neurologic involvement, including meningoencephalitis and cranial and peripheral neuropathy, occurs in untreated patients within 2 to 8 weeks. Cardiac involvement, including pericarditis, myocarditis, and atrioventricular conduction difficulties, occurs in untreated patients.
3. **Late manifestations.** In the third stage of the illness, arthritis may occur in untreated patients, beginning days to years after the initial infection. Intermittent joint pain may affect patients and lasts from days to months. Chronic neurologic symptoms are uncommon. In the United States, memory impairment, depressed mood, and severe fatigue are the most common symptoms of Lyme disease.

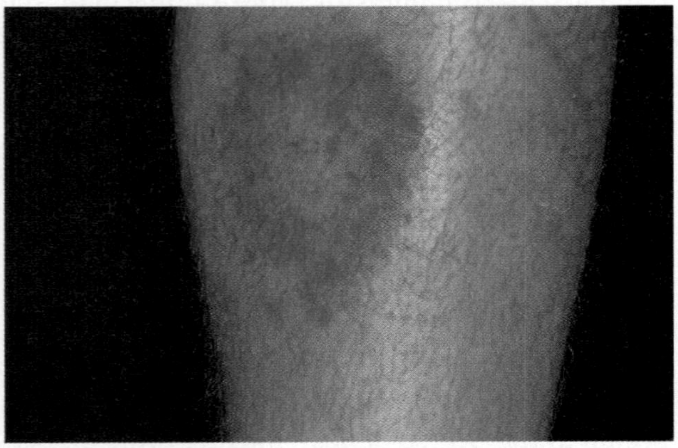

FIGURE 27-11 The bull's-eye rash of Lyme disease is most commonly seen in the area of the groin, thigh, or axilla.

Management

Prevention includes wearing long sleeves and pants when in tick-infested areas, and using insecticides that contain carabaril, diazinon, chlorpyrifos, or cyfluthrin. If you sustain a tick bite, use proper technique for removing ticks. Postexposure treatment with antibiotics is not warranted or recommended.

Rocky Mountain Spotted Fever

Rocky Mountain spotted fever (RMSF) is a tick-borne disease caused by the bacterium *Rickettsia rickettsii.* This organism is a cause of potentially fatal human illness in North and South America. Transmission to humans occurs by the bite of infected tick species. In the United States, these include the American dog tick (*Dermacentor variabilis*), Rocky Mountain wood tick (*Dermacentor andersoni*), and brown dog tick (*Rhipicephalus sanguineous*).

As of January 1, 2010, cases of RMSF are reportable. There were approximately 1,985 cases in 2010, but only 156 were confirmed, with the highest incidence in Missouri and Tennessee.[77] In the last 20 years, incidence went from 495 cases in 2000 to a peak of 6,248 in 2017. However, fewer cases were reported in 2018.[100]

Pathophysiology

RMSF can be a severe or even fatal illness if not treated in the first few days of symptoms. Patients who have a particularly severe infection requiring prolonged hospitalization may experience long-term health problems caused by this disease.

Assessment

Typical symptoms include fever, headache, abdominal pain, vomiting, and muscle pain. A rash may also develop, but is often absent in the first few days. In some patients, a rash never develops.

The initial diagnosis is made based on clinical signs and symptoms and medical history and can later be confirmed by using specialized laboratory tests. However, the inability to differentiate between spotted fever group *Rickettsia* species using commonly available serologic tests makes it unclear how many cases are RMSF and how many result from other spotted fevers. RMSF and other tick-borne diseases can be prevented by protecting oneself against tick bites.

Management

Doxycycline is the first-line treatment for adults and children of all ages. This therapy is most effective if started before the fifth day of symptoms.

RMSF is not a communicable disease. It is not transmitted from patient to health care provider. To be exposed, a person needs to be bitten by the tick.

Hantavirus Infection

Hantavirus infection, also known as *hemorrhagic fever with pulmonary syndrome,* is associated with the deer mouse, white-footed mouse, and cotton rat, but has also been found in rats in urban areas. Hantavirus pulmonary syndrome may occur as well; it is characterized by flulike symptoms that can progress rapidly to potentially life-threatening breathing problems.

Hantavirus infection was first identified in Korea in the early 1950s and in the southwestern United States in 1993. According to the CDC,[101] by 2017 about 728 cases had been reported in the United States. In 2017, most of these cases were reported in Colorado, Arizona, New Mexico, and California. In Canada and the United States, the deer mouse, which carries the Sin Nombre hantavirus, is responsible for the majority of cases of hantavirus.

Pathophysiology

Hantavirus is found in the urine, feces, and saliva of chronically infected rodents. Transmission occurs via direct contact with rodent waste matter, often through aerosol inhalation, which can occur when cleaning up infested areas such as households, barns, and sheds. The incubation period usually lasts 12 to 16 days following exposure, but has been noted to range from 5 to 42 days. This disease is not transmitted from person to person, so there is no period of communicability.

Assessment

Signs and symptoms of hantavirus infection begin with the sudden onset of fever, which lasts 3 to 8 days. It is accompanied by headache, abdominal pain, loss of appetite, and vomiting. In the pulmonary syndrome, signs and symptoms present in two stages. In stage 1, complaints may include fever, chills, headaches, muscle aches, vomiting, diarrhea, and abdominal pain. In stage 2, the patient may develop a cough that produces secretions, shortness of breath, and fluid accumulation within the lungs. Low BP and cardiac insufficiency may also be noted.

Management

Prevention focuses on standard precautions. Routine cleaning of the vehicle is all that is indicated. Depending on the patient's stage of illness and presenting symptoms, other supportive measures may be needed as part of EMS care. Assisted respiration, through advanced airway management or mechanical ventilation, may be indicated. Oxygen therapy may also be needed. Rapid transport is paramount, as a diagnosis will be made at the medical facility following antibody testing for hantavirus.

Hantavirus is not an occupationally acquired disease because it is not transmitted person to person.

Rabies

Rabies (hydrophobia) is found worldwide. In the United States, human cases have been declining since rabies control programs began in the 1940s. Over the years, deaths from rabies reported in the United States have declined from more than 100 per year to 1 or 2 per year.[102] The vaccination of domestic animals and the development of a vaccine and rabies immunoglobulin have greatly reduced the number of deaths in humans who contract rabies.

Pathophysiology

Transmission of rabies is primarily related to the direct bite of an infected animal. The virus is shed in the saliva of the infected animal from the time it becomes infected. Animals most commonly identified as having rabies include raccoons, skunks, foxes, coyotes, and insectivorous bats. Other (rare) routes of transmission include contamination of mucous membranes (ie, eyes, nose, mouth), aerosol transmission, and corneal and organ transplantations. In general, however, nonbite exposures to rabies—scratches, abrasions, open wounds, or mucous membranes contaminated with saliva or OPIM from a rabid animal—are rare. There are no documented cases of human-to-human transmission of rabies. The incubation period is usually 2 to 8 weeks but varies depending on the severity of the bite and the location of the wound.

Assessment

Signs and symptoms of rabies in humans are generally nonspecific, generally resembling signs associated with the flu: fever, chills, sore throat, malaise, headache, and weakness. Paresthesia (tingling skin sensation with no apparent cause) may develop at or near the site of exposure. Following these initial signs, the neurologic phase of the disease begins—hyperactivity, seizures, bizarre behavior, and hydrophobia. Patients may also have fear of the sight of water or while drinking it as a result of severe spasms of the throat and masseter (chewing) muscles. As the disease progresses, paralysis may develop and mental status may deteriorate, leading to coma. Although rabies is generally viewed as a fatal disease, several cases of survival have been reported recently even after symptoms had appeared.

Management

As a preventive measure, take standard precautions for patient care and cleaning of the vehicle. If you are bitten or scratched by a suspect animal, you will be offered an injection of human immunoglobulin and started on human rabies vaccine if deemed appropriate. The CDC does not recommend rabies vaccination for EMS personnel on a routine basis. Follow-up would include wound care. Remember, first aid always comes before reporting to your DICO.

Middle East Respiratory Syndrome

Middle East respiratory syndrome (MERS) is a viral disease that presents a very low risk to health care providers and the general public in the United States. In May 2014, two cases of MERS were identified and treated in the United States—one case in Florida and a second in Indiana. Both cases involved health care providers who worked and lived in Saudi Arabia. They acquired this disease in Saudi Arabia, were diagnosed and treated, and then discharged in the United States.

Pathophysiology

MERS-CoV (MERS-related coronavirus) is a coronavirus, a type of pathogen that has been associated with patients developing severe acute respiratory illness. Studies have linked this disease to the nasal secretions and urine of camels. Transmission occurs through close contact with an infected person and may occur even in the health care setting. Research has not documented any ongoing transmission in communities. Infected people have, for the most part, shown symptoms much like those associated with the common cold. People with underlying medical conditions have experienced pneumonia or kidney failure. The incubation period appears to be 5 to 6 days, but can last as long as 14 days.

A reduced level of lymphocytes in the blood (lymphopenia) has been noted in most patients infected with MERS-CoV, as was also noted in SARS infections.

Laboratory testing for MERS-CoV is not routinely available. However, polymerase chain reaction tests for MERS-CoV are available at state health departments, the CDC, and some international laboratories.

Assessment

If this infection is suspected, obtain the patient's travel history to identify travel to or from the Arabian Peninsula and possible contact with camels (urine or nasal secretions), camel milk, or meat. Assess for fever, cough, and shortness of breath. GI disturbances, including nausea and vomiting, may be reported as well. People who develop severe disease may require ventilation assistance for acute respiratory distress syndrome.

Management

No specific antiviral treatment exists for MERS-CoV; instead, medical care focuses on relief of symptoms. Health care providers who are caring for patients with this infection should take standard precautions, contact precautions, and airborne precautions. Airborne precautions for EMS involve the use of the air exchange system and a surgical mask.

If an unprotected exposure occurs, notify your DICO directly. No vaccine currently exists for MERS, and no specific treatment has been recommended. Current treatment is supportive.

Tetanus

According to the CDC,[103] reported **tetanus** cases have declined more than 95%, and deaths from tetanus have declined more than 99% in the United States since 1947, when the disease became reportable nationally. Tetanus is more common in agricultural areas and in underdeveloped areas, where contact with animal waste is more likely and immunization is inadequate. Tetanus is a vaccine-preventable disease. Vaccinations are given at ages 2 months, 4 months, 6 months, and 18 months, followed by doses at 4 and 6 years of age. A booster is recommended for children between ages 11 and 12; thereafter a booster should be given every 10 years. Occasional cases of tetanus continue to occur in adults, especially in those who were not vaccinated in childhood or did not remain current on their 10-year booster shots.

Pathophysiology

The tetanus bacillus is found in the intestines of horses and other animals, but some cases have been linked to use of IV drugs. Transmission occurs when tetanus spores enter the body by either of two means: (1) a puncture wound contaminated with animal feces, street dust, or soil; or (2) contaminated street drugs. Tetanus is not transmitted from person to person. Occasionally, cases have occurred postoperatively or following seemingly minor injuries.

The incubation period is usually about 14 days from the exposure but has been documented to be as short as 3 days. The cases that have short incubation periods tend to have a higher level of contamination.

Assessment

Signs and symptoms begin at the site of the wound, followed by painful muscle contractions or rigidity (tetany) in the neck, face, jaw, and trunk muscles. The key sign that suggests tetanus, particularly in children, is abdominal rigidity, although this rigidity may be confined to the location of the injury. Dysphagia, hydrophobia, drooling, and respiratory distress may also occur.

Management

Prevention involves taking standard precautions: wearing gloves when treating any patient wounds and management of drainage. A patient with tetanus may require airway and ventilation support en route. Oxygen may be ordered, along with IV fluids. Tetanus immune globulin is recommended for treatment of tetanus. A single intramuscular dose of 3,000 to 5,000 units is generally recommended for children and adults, with part of the dose infiltrated around the wound if it can be identified.

Paramedics should be offered tetanus booster doses every 10 years to protect them against this infection. No special cleaning routines are necessary after transport of a patient with tetanus.

Pathophysiology, Assessment, and Management of Infection With Antibiotic-Resistant Organisms and Multidrug-Resistant Organisms

The overuse and misuse of antibiotics have led some pathogens to develop resistance to the antibiotic drugs commonly prescribed to eradicate them. In the past, the medical community has been concerned that some infections might become untreatable due to resistance. This situation has now occurred. Currently, no new antibiotics are under development. Consequently, medical facility pharmacies and the CDC now restrict the use of many antibiotics, an approach termed antibiotic stewardship.

Patients infected with some types of antibiotic-resistant organisms, particularly vancomycin-resistant enterococci (VRE) and methicillin-resistant

Staphylococcus aureus (MRSA), may be protected by the Americans with Disabilities Act (infection with these organisms is discussed in the sections that follow), depending on the definition of "disability" used in their state's law.

Methicillin-Resistant *Staphylococcus aureus*

Staphylococcus aureus became resistant to penicillin in the late 1950s. In the early 1960s, the drug methicillin became available to treat *S aureus* infections. By the mid-1970s, MRSA was present in US hospitals; it has since moved into the community. Today, most cases involve community-acquired MRSA. The number of health care–associated cases of MRSA is starting to decline with the increased focus on infection control in all health care settings. In 2010, encouraging results from a CDC study showed that life-threatening MRSA infections in health care settings are declining.[104] MRSA infections that began in hospitals declined 54% between 2005 and 2011, with 30,800 fewer severe MRSA cases being reported.[105] Decreases in infection rates were even greater for patients with bloodstream infections. However, a recent study conducted by the CDC and the Centers for Medicare and Medicaid Services (CMS) showed that 30% to 50% of antibiotic prescriptions from EDs and urgent care centers are unnecessary.[106]

Strains of MRSA are also resistant to some other antibiotics, including cephalosporins, erythromycins, clindamycin (Cleocin), tetracyclines, and aminoglycosides. Although vancomycin (Vancocin) has been shown to treat MRSA effectively, some strains have shown resistance to this drug as well. Other drugs used to treat MRSA include a quinupristin-dalfopristin combination (Synercid), linezolid (Zyvox), and daptomycin (Cubicin).

Special Populations

Community-acquired MRSA infection with clone USA300 is a major cause of infectious disease in children. This disease presents primarily as a superficial soft-tissue infection and can be easily treated by incision and drainage without the use of antibiotics.

Pathophysiology

In health care settings, it is believed that MRSA is transmitted from patient to patient via the unwashed hands of health care providers. Studies have shown that 33% of people carry staphylococci in their nose and 2 in 100 people carry MRSA.[107] The pathogen can subsequently be transferred to skin and other areas of the body through a break in the skin, leading to infection **FIGURE 27-12**. Surfaces contaminated with MRSA do not seem to be important in transmission. The presence of MRSA in ambulances and fire stations has been documented, which suggests that cleaning routines and good handwashing techniques are not being followed. Factors that increase the risk for developing MRSA include antibiotic therapy, prolonged hospital stays, a stay in an intensive care unit or a burn unit, and exposure to an infected patient. Many patients who contract MRSA live in long-term care facilities.

Assessment

Patients with MRSA may be **colonized** with this organism or infected. The incubation period seems to be between 5 and 45 days. The communicable period varies; patients who have active infection may carry MRSA for months. In community-acquired cases, MRSA results in soft-tissue infections. Manifestations may include localized skin abscesses and cellulitis, empyema, and endocarditis. Sepsis

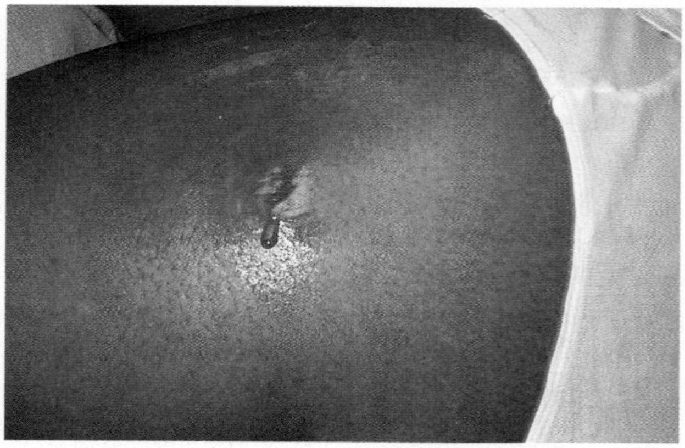

FIGURE 27-12 A draining, purulent skin abscess on the thigh caused by methicillin-resistant *Staphylococcus aureus*. Consider any drainage from a wound to be potentially infectious and use appropriate contact precautions.

Courtesy of Bruno Coignard, MD/Jeff Hageman, MHS/CDC.

is found in older patients with *S aureus* infections. After bloodstream infection with MRSA, secondary infections such as osteomyelitis and septic arthritis may develop at sites other than the initial site of MRSA infection.

Management

Patients with soft-tissue infections are treated by carrying out incision and drainage of those sites. No antibiotics need to be prescribed. This treatment is in accordance with the guidelines published by the Infectious Disease Society of America. Most MRSA soft-tissue infections will clear following incision and drainage alone.

To prevent MRSA transmission, take standard precautions (gloves and good handwashing technique) and contact precautions when in contact with wounds and nonintact skin. If you are in direct contact with wound drainage but your skin is intact, no exposure will occur. No special cleaning is required and normal laundry of linens is appropriate. If you have a true exposure, notify your DICO. No postexposure treatment is recommended.

Vancomycin-Resistant *S aureus*

Vancomycin is one of the leading drugs for treating *Staphylococcus* infections. However, once the organism has become resistant to this drug, it is no longer effective in treating the infections. Like MRSA, vancomycin-resistant *S aureus* (VRSA) infections present as pimples, boils, and other skin conditions. VRSA infections can become severe, resulting in sepsis, a dangerous systemic bloodstream infection. Presently, the incidence of this infection is rare in the United States.

Pathophysiology

People at risk for development of VRSA infections include those with multiple underlying health conditions (eg, diabetes and kidney disease), previous infections with MRSA, indwelling catheters (eg, indwelling urinary catheters), recent hospitalizations, and recent exposure to vancomycin or other antimicrobial agents.

Assessment

Signs and symptoms may include localized skin abscesses and cellulitis, pneumonia, bloodstream infections, meningitis, or osteomyelitis. Fever, chills, body weakness and pain, cough, chest pain, and trouble breathing are often present, but other signs and symptoms will depend on the location of the infection.

Management

VRSA infection is currently treatable with antibiotics. Standard and contact precautions and routine cleaning of the vehicle and patient care equipment after each call are important, as is routine handwashing. Make sure all open cuts on your skin are covered. No postexposure treatment is recommended, but if you are exposed, notify your DICO.

Vancomycin-Resistant Enterococci

Enterococcus is a common organism that is normally found in the GI tract, urinary tract, and genitourinary tract. More than 450 species of enterococci exist, many of which are resistant to antimicrobial agents. These organisms grow under reduced oxygen and oxygenated conditions. When they become resistant to vancomycin—the main drug used for treating enterococcal infection—the patient is said to have vancomycin-resistant enterococci (VRE).

According to recent National Nosocomial Infections Surveillance surveys,[108] enterococci remain one of the top three pathogens that cause health care–associated infections in the United States. These infections have occurred in the general hospitalized population. An estimated 20,000 to 85,000 cases of VRE occur each year in US hospitals.

Pathophysiology

Infection with VRE is primarily a health care–associated infection. Patients identified with VRE infections outside the hospital setting typically reside in nursing homes or visit hemodialysis centers. In fact, individuals are not susceptible to VRE infection unless they are already ill or immunocompromised. Patients in the ICU and transplant recipients are especially vulnerable to this disease.

VRE may be found in urinary tract infections (UTIs) and bloodstream infections; these pathogens have also been identified in livestock stool, uncooked chicken, and people who work at farms or processing plants. The infectious organisms can live on surfaces for long periods, so transmission may occur by direct contact with contaminated surfaces or equipment.

A person can be colonized or infected with VRE, but only infected patients can transmit the organism. Thus, transmission may occur when you have direct contact with wound drainage and an open cut or sore allows entry of the organism into your body. VRE infection can be treated with a new synthetic antibiotic, linezolid.

Assessment

VRE can cause UTIs, particularly in patients who have urinary catheters. Other kinds of catheters, such as central lines, can serve as a port of entry for VRE, causing bacteremia that sometimes evolves into sepsis. Surgical wounds, especially in patients who have had abdominal or chest surgery, may also become infected with VRE.

Management

Prevention relies on taking standard/contact precautions, wearing gloves, and practicing good handwashing technique when in contact with wound drainage. A cover gown is necessary only if your uniform may come in contact with wound drainage. Post-transport cleaning of all areas that came in contact with the patient is important, but no special cleaning solution is required. If you sustain direct contact with an open wound and body fluids from a patient with a VRE infection, notify your DICO and complete an exposure report. No postexposure medical treatment is indicated.

Clostridioides difficile

C diff is not a multidrug-resistant organism but is treated like one. Infection with this pathogen can occur after antibiotic treatment—some antibiotics can destroy the normal bacteria in the intestine, allowing the *C diff* organisms to take over. In the past, infections with *C diff* were generally related to a stay in a health care facility, but now they are mainly found in the community setting, largely because of issues with antibiotic prescribing.

Pathophysiology

The spore-forming bacterium *C diff* produces two endotoxins that cause watery diarrhea, the chief symptom of infection. Transmission occurs by contact with surfaces contaminated with feces. In particular, the bacterium can be transmitted to patients by contact with the unwashed hands of health care providers. Diagnosis is usually made by stool culture. The illness resolves 2 to 3 days after discontinuing antibiotics. Recurrence is common, however, especially in people ages 65 years and older.

Assessment

Infection with *C diff* causes frequent watery, green, foul-smelling diarrhea; nausea and vomiting; fever; loss of appetite; and abdominal discomfort. Diseases associated with *C diff* infection include pseudomembranous colitis, sepsis, and colonic perforation. For patients presenting with these signs and symptoms, a paramedic should ask about the patient's medications, especially any current use of antibiotics.

Management

Standard/contact precautions for *C diff* include wearing gloves and using good handwashing technique. In addition, cleaning of contaminated surfaces with an appropriate cleaning agent is important in managing *C diff*. Because this bacterium is a spore-forming agent, a chlorine-based cleaning solution is required to eradicate it. Also, alcohol-based foams and gels for handwashing will not kill spores, so soap and warm water should be used. Report contamination of open skin areas to your DICO. No medical follow-up is recommended after exposure to *C diff*.

Carbapenem-Resistant Enterobacteriaceae

Carbapenem-resistant Enterobacteriaceae (CRE) are bacteria that are highly resistant to most antibiotics. This group of antibiotics includes the carbapenem agents, which are used as a last resort for treating infections. CRE came to the United States via medical tourism (people leaving the United States to obtain health care at a lower cost); it is believed to have originated in India. Obviously, this factor makes the patient's travel history very important information to obtain. The question to ask is: "Have you been hospitalized overnight outside the United States in the past 6 months?" The death rate from CRE infection is estimated to be approximately 40%, but could be higher.[109]

Pathophysiology

Enterobacteriaceae are bacteria normally found in the GI and vaginal tracts, but many have acquired the ability to counteract antibiotics. These bacteria—either *Klebsiella* or *Escherichia coli*—develop resistance due to antibiotic treatment. Transmission occurs through unwashed hands and contaminated surfaces. It has not been determined how long CRE can live on a surface. CRE is a spore-forming organism, a characteristic that affects the selection of cleaning and handwashing products.

Assessment

Symptoms of CRE infection may vary from patient to patient depending on the location of the bacteria. Observe the patient for signs of sepsis and an indwelling device (ie, IV catheter, indwelling urinary catheter, ventilators). Patients may present with fever, UTI, fatigue, chills, and sepsis. Also ask about the use of over-the-counter antibiotic treatments for open sores. Assess whether the patient has been on long-term antibiotic treatment.

Management

Take standard precautions and contact precautions if the patient has draining wounds. Use soap and warm water for handwashing; alcohol-based cleaners do not kill spores. Use a chlorine-based cleaning solution for vehicles and equipment used for patient care.

Pathophysiology, Assessment, and Management of Newly Recognized Diseases

In the past, a disease would "jump" from animals to humans every 20 to 30 years. Today, this kind of leap occurs much more frequently. Recent examples include HIV infection, monkeypox, severe acute respiratory syndrome (SARS), and avian flu. The latter two are discussed here.

Severe Acute Respiratory Syndrome

Severe acute respiratory syndrome (SARS) is a new disease that arose from the merger of two viruses, one from mammals and one from birds. The source of this virus has been identified as bats found in Hong Kong. SARS was first reported in Asia in February 2003. Within a few months, the disease had spread from Asia to Canada, South America, and Europe. By spring 2003, WHO reported a total of 8,098 cases worldwide and 774 deaths.[110] In the United States, there were 8 confirmed cases (all mild) and no deaths; all of the US cases involved people who had traveled to areas where SARS cases had been reported.[110] The last cases of SARS were reported in April 2004 in China and resulted from a laboratory accident. In the United States, no health care providers have contracted SARS.

Pathophysiology

Transmission of SARS occurs by close personal contact—that is, living with and caring for a person with the disease or having direct contact with the respiratory secretions or body fluids of an infected person (eg, by kissing or hugging, sharing eating utensils, or standing within 3 feet [1 m] of an infected person who is talking). The incubation period is about 10 days from the date of exposure; the communicable period has not been well defined.

Assessment

Signs and symptoms include a fever of greater than 100.4°F (38°C), headache, overall feeling of discomfort, and body aches. Initially, SARS resembles any general flulike illness. However, after 2 to 7 days, a dry cough appears, and severe cases may progress to pneumonia. In this phase, patients may need respiratory support.

Management

If you care for a person suspected of having SARS, you should use adequate PPE, notify the DICO, complete an exposure form, and perhaps be placed on a 10-day quarantine. The public health department is responsible for contact follow-up.

> **Words of Wisdom**
>
> The most important action for you to take if you believe you have been exposed to a multidrug-resistant organism is to wash your hands immediately and to clean any contaminated equipment or clothing. Report the incident to your DICO. There is no medical follow-up needed or recommended for any infections from multidrug-resistant organisms.

Avian Flu

The first cases of **avian (bird) flu** in humans were reported in Hong Kong in 1997; 18 people became infected and 6 died in this outbreak.[111] There have been two cases of avian flu in Canada. Patients acquired the disease from their flocks but recovered, and no additional transmission was reported. New strains have been identified, but recent outbreaks have been limited to poultry. Even so, these developments remain of concern to WHO and the United Nations. Sustained person-to-person transmission has not been noted to occur with avian flu.

Pathophysiology

Avian flu is caused by a virus that occurs naturally in the bird population. This virus is carried in the intestinal tract of wild birds and does not usually cause illness in humans. However, it is very contagious in domestic bird populations (eg, chickens, ducks, turkeys). Birds acquire the virus from contact with contaminated excretions or surfaces that are contaminated with excretions. If an infected bird is used for food and is cooked, it does not pose a risk to the people who eat it.

No rapidly spread human-to-human cases of this disease have been reported. Instead, the cases occurring in humans have involved close contact with infected birds. The transmission risk for humans is quite low.

Some concern exists that someone infected with a regular type A flu virus may become coinfected with avian flu, allowing the two viruses to merge and form a new virus. In August 2011, the United Nations reported that avian flu was once again on the rise in Asia. In 2013, an outbreak in China involved a new strain of the virus. Other outbreaks occurred in China in 2016–2017 and 2019.

Assessment

For patients with suspected avian flu, it is important to obtain a travel history. Signs and symptoms of avian flu include fever, sore throat, cough, and muscle aches; some eye infections have also been noted. Illness may eventually progress to pneumonia and severe respiratory distress.

Management

Preventive measures include placing a surgical mask on the patient to contain secretions. If the patient's condition does not permit this action, you can wear a surgical mask for your own protection. Follow current CDC guidelines regarding protection for health care providers. Under the current information-sharing system, a medical facility is required to notify the DICO if a patient who is transported by an EMS agency is later diagnosed with avian flu. If an exposure is documented, an antiviral drug may be offered within 48 hours of exposure. Antiviral drugs do not prevent the flu, but can reduce the severity of the illness. It is also important to get an annual flu shot to ensure protection from type A viruses. A vaccine for avian flu is currently available.

YOU are the Paramedic SUMMARY

1. What is your first concern at this scene?

Because *C diff* infection is a possibility, you should immediately don gloves during this call.

2. What is *C diff* and what precautions should you put in place for transport?

Clostridioides difficile is a bacterium that is shed in feces. To prevent contamination with *C diff*, use

YOU are the Paramedic SUMMARY continued

good handwashing technique with soap and warm water, and clean contaminated surfaces with a chlorine-based cleaning solution. Use contact precautions in addition to standard precautions.

3. What can you determine about the patient's condition now?

Staff members have advised that the patient has been ill for a few days and has been vomiting and having diarrhea. You witnessed the patient attempt to vomit, and nothing was produced. This information, along with the tenting of the skin on the forearm, should lead you to believe that substantial dehydration exists.

4. Because a diagnosis of *C diff* infection has not been confirmed for this patient, are you concerned about exposure?

Yes, you should be concerned about exposure. However, it is important to note that no postexposure treatment is recommended. Gastroenteritis, also known as the stomach flu, encompasses many types of infections and irritations of the GI tract, including those caused by norovirus. Patients experience symptoms such as nausea and vomiting, fever, abdominal cramps, and diarrhea. In healthy people, gastroenteritis is usually not serious. In children, older adults, and patients with chronic illness, however, severe complications such as dehydration may develop. Some of the viral strains are extremely contagious.

5. What is your first choice of treatment for this patient?

You should focus on fluid replacement because of the evidence of dehydration. You should consider a fluid challenge after assessing lung sounds. Consider starting at 250 mL and repeating the fluid administration until the desired effect is reached or whatever is appropriate in your protocol.

6. Are there any notifications you should make concerning the scene?

The federal Ryan White Law, Part G (2009), requires that every emergency response agency have a designated infection control officer (DICO). This person is charged with ensuring that proper postexposure medical treatment and counseling are provided to exposed employees and volunteers. Postexposure medical treatment is offered to prevent exposed health care providers from contracting the disease to which they were exposed. Treatment should be offered within 24 to 48 hours following an exposure, with the actual time frame based on the diagnosis. Exposure to bacterial meningitis, for example, would require treatment within 24 hours.

7. What decontamination measures should you use for your stretcher?

Remove the used linens from the stretcher immediately after use, and place them in a plastic bag or in the designated receptacle in the emergency department. Clean the stretcher with an EPA-registered germicidal-virucidal solution or a 1:100 bleach/water solution.

8. What measures should you use for handwashing?

You should have already been using standard/contact precautions. These precautions apply to all body substances except sweat. You should also wash your hands well, using warm water and soap, because alcohol-based handwashing solutions do not kill a spore-forming organism. If your uniform was contaminated, you should change into a clean uniform and wash exposed skin. If you have a significant exposure, notify your DICO or follow your agency's policy.

EMS Patient Care Report (PCR)

Date: 07-30-22	**Incident No.:** 9678	**Nature of Call:** Vomiting		**Location:** 550 Health Care Blvd	
Dispatched: 0950	**En Route:** 0950	**At Scene:** 0955	**Transport:** 1015	**At Hospital:** 1020	**In Service:** 1035

Patient Information

Age: 86 **Sex:** F **Weight (in kg [lb.]):** 54 kg (120 lb)	**Allergies:** Denies **Medications:** Diltiazem (Cardizem) **Past Medical History:** Heart disease, diabetes **Chief Complaint:** N/V for 48 h

YOU are the Paramedic SUMMARY continued

Vital Signs				
Time: 1000	**BP:** 98/58	**Pulse:** 106	**Respirations:** 18	**Spo_2:** 97% on room air
Time: 1005	**BP:** 102/60	**Pulse:** 96	**Respirations:** 18	**Spo_2:** 97% on room air

EMS Treatment (circle all that apply)				
Oxygen @ _____ L/min via (circle one): **NC NRM Bag-mask device**	**Assisted Ventilation**	**Airway Adjunct**	**CPR**	
Defibrillation	**Bleeding Control**	**Bandaging**	**Splinting**	**Other:** IV established, 250 mL

Narrative

Arrived at The Springs assisted living facility for an 86 y/o woman reporting n/v for 48 h. Staff member reports a staff physician believes the patient may have *C diff*. Pt appears weak and reports she is unable to stand because of weakness. Pt attempted to vomit, but nothing was produced. Assessment revealed tenting of skin on the pt's forearm. IV established with a 250-mL challenge per protocol. Lung sounds were clear in all fields before and after challenge. Pt had slight improvement in VS during transport to receiving hospital. Report given to A. Baxter, RN.

End of report

Prep Kit

Ready for Review

- Government agencies such as the Occupational Safety and Health Administration (OSHA), the Centers for Disease Control and Prevention (CDC), and state and county public health departments bear the responsibility for protecting the public from disease, preventing epidemics, and managing outbreaks.
- Clean and disinfect the ambulance and your equipment to protect patients from infection. Focus on high-touch items.
- Communicable diseases can be transmitted from one person to another under certain conditions.
- Infectious diseases are caused by pathogenic microorganisms, usually bacteria or viruses, but sometimes fungi and parasites.
- Infectious diseases may be spread from person to person by several specific mechanisms: contact transmission (either direct or indirect), droplet transmission, and airborne transmission.
- Transmission-based precautions refer to infection control practices that reduce the opportunity for an exposure to occur in the daily care of patients. Standard precautions add the element of protection from moist body substances that may transmit bacterial or viral infections.
- It is critical to remove personal protective equipment (PPE) properly. Handwashing after glove removal is always important.
- Protection against and reduction of the occurrence of communicable diseases involve the DICO, the public health department, standard precautions, immunizations and vaccinations, PPE, postexposure medical follow-up, and an exposure control plan.

Prep Kit continued

- A patient suspected of having an infectious or communicable disease is assessed like any other medical patient.
- The general management of a patient with a suspected communicable disease first focuses on treating any life-threatening conditions, placing the patient in a position of comfort, administering IV fluid if needed, treating the patient with empathy, taking standard precautions and properly disposing of sharps, and following your agency's exposure control plan.
- Infection involves a typical chain of events through which a communicable disease spreads.
- The risk of infection depends on the type and dose of the organism, its virulence, its mode of entry, and the host's resistance.
- The human body uses several defenses to protect against infection, such as skin, the mucous membranes, and the immune system.
- Droplet-transmitted diseases include meningitis, various respiratory conditions, seasonal influenza, pertussis, mumps, rubella, and COVID-19. Droplet precautions include placing a surgical mask on the patient, implementing basic infection control measures, and using the ambulance's airflow system.
- Airborne-transmitted diseases include tuberculosis, chickenpox, and measles.
- Airborne precautions include placing a surgical mask on the patient and using the ambulance's airflow system. Ventilation is key to risk reduction. Airborne diseases involve small droplets and particles that can travel over long distances, generally 6 feet (2 m) or more, before dropping to the ground. In droplet diseases, large and small droplets and particles are generated when an infected person coughs or sneezes that generally travel 6 feet (2 m) or less before falling to the ground.
- Other infections of the respiratory tract include mononucleosis and chronic fatigue syndrome.
- Sexually transmitted infections (STIs) are usually acquired by sexual contact and are caused by a wide range of organisms.
- Common bloodborne diseases include viral hepatitis and human immunodeficiency virus (HIV), acquired immunodeficiency syndrome (AIDS), hepatitis C virus (HCV), and syphilis.
- Caring for patients infected with Ebola virus requires both contact and droplet precautions. Contact precautions include the use of gloves, a cover gown if clothing could be contaminated, and cleaning of high-touch items.
- Enteric diseases are infectious diseases that affect the GI tract. The organisms that cause enteric infections include parasites and bacteria.
- Non-bloodborne hepatitis viruses include the hepatitis A and E viruses.
- A vector is an organism that harbors pathogens that are harmless to the organism but cause disease when transmitted to a human host. The pathogen can be transmitted to humans by means of a bite, inhalation of contaminated animal feces, or other means.
- Mosquito-borne diseases include West Nile virus, dengue fever, chikungunya fever, and Zika virus.
- Tick-borne diseases include Lyme disease and Rocky Mountain spotted fever.
- Zoonotic diseases include hantavirus infection, rabies, Middle East respiratory syndrome, and tetanus.
- The overuse and misuse of antibiotics has led some pathogens to develop resistance to the drugs commonly prescribed to eradicate them. Some examples include methicillin-resistant *S aureus*, vancomycin-resistant *S aureus*, vancomycin-resistant enterococci, and carbapenem-resistant Enterobacteriaceae.
- *Clostridioides difficile* is not a multidrug-resistant organism but is treated like one. Infection with this pathogen can occur after antibiotic treatment because some antibiotics can destroy the normal bacteria in the

Prep Kit continued

intestine, allowing the *C diff* organisms take over.
- In the past, a disease would "jump" from animals to humans every 20 to 30 years. Today, this transmission occurs much more frequently, with recent examples including HIV infection, monkeypox, severe acute respiratory syndrome (SARS), and avian flu.

Vital Vocabulary

acquired immunodeficiency syndrome (AIDS) The end-stage disease process caused by the human immunodeficiency virus; it results in extreme vulnerability to numerous opportunistic bacterial, viral, and fungal infections that would not affect a person with an intact immune system.

aerosol-generating procedures Procedures that can increase the number and load of droplets from the patient. Examples include intubation and suctioning or performing mouth-to-mouth resuscitation.

airborne precautions Placement of a surgical mask on the patient and the use of airflow measures to prevent airborne transmission; apply to infections that spread through exposure to respiratory droplets composed of small droplets and particles that can travel over long distances, generally 6 feet (2 m) or more, before dropping to the floor.

airborne transmission The transmission of an infectious agent by inhalation of small particles that become aerosolized when the infected person coughs, sneezes, talks, or exhales; particles can remain suspended in the air for some period and can travel 6 feet (2 m) or more.

avian (bird) flu A disease caused by a virus that occurs naturally in the bird population; signs and symptoms include fever, sore throat, cough, and muscle aches.

bacteria Small organisms that can grow and reproduce outside the human cell in the presence of the appropriate temperature and nutrients; they cause disease by invading and multiplying in the tissues of the host.

bacterial vaginosis An overgrowth of bacteria in the vagina, characterized by itching, burning, or pain, which may be accompanied by a fishy, foul-smelling discharge.

bloodborne pathogens Pathogenic microorganisms that are present in human blood and can cause disease in humans. These pathogens include, but are not limited to, hepatitis B virus, human immunodeficiency virus, hepatitis C virus, and syphilis.

candidiasis A vaginal infection that is not technically a sexually transmitted infection; it can occur in pregnant and nonpregnant females, but is more common in pregnancy; also called thrush or a yeast infection.

carriers People who harbor an infectious agent and, although not personally ill, can pass the disease to others through their blood and through sexual contact.

chancre The primary hard lesion or ulcer of syphilis that occurs at the entry site of the infection.

chancroid A highly contagious sexually transmitted infection caused by the bacteria *Haemophilus ducreyi,* which causes painful sores (ulcers), usually of the genitals.

chikungunya A virus that originated in Africa and is transmitted by the *Aedes aegypti* mosquito; signs and symptoms include fever that typically lasts from 5 to 7 days, and possibly incapacitating joint pain.

chlamydia A sexually transmitted infection caused by the bacterium *Chlamydia trachomatis,* which is the most frequently reported sexually transmitted infection; signs and symptoms include inflammation of the urethra, epididymis, cervix, and fallopian tubes, and discharge from the urethra.

Prep Kit continued

colonized A pathogen is present but has produced no illness in the host; often progresses to active infection. A colonized host is often called a *carrier* because the host can transmit the pathogen to others.

communicable disease An infectious disease that can be transmitted from one person to another by direct contact or by indirect contact through a vector or fomite; also called contagious disease.

communicable period The period during which an infected person can transmit a communicable disease to someone else.

contact precautions The use of precautions (gloves, gown, and cleaning of high-touch items) to prevent contact transmission; used for patients presenting with draining wounds, multidrug-resistant infection, lice, norovirus, or Ebola.

contact transmission The transmission of an infectious agent through direct or indirect contact with the infected persons, such as skin-to-skin contact or contact with the patient's environment and/or equipment.

contaminated The presence of blood or other potentially infectious materials on an item or surface.

coronavirus Any of a group of RNA viruses that cause a variety of respiratory, gastrointestinal, and neurologic diseases in humans and other animals.

dengue A virus transmitted by the mosquitos *Aedes aegypti* and *Aedes albopictus*, found throughout the world. The majority of people with dengue are asymptomatic; if the severe form develops, it is characterized by hemorrhage, hypovolemic shock, and potentially death.

designated infection control officer (DICO) A person charged with ensuring that proper post-exposure medical treatment and counseling are provided to an exposed employee or volunteer.

droplet precautions Use of a surgical mask on the patient and airborne precautions to prevent droplet transmission; used for patients with possible influenza, meningitis, pertussis (whooping cough), mumps, rubella (German measles), Ebola, and COVID-19; also called "source control."

droplet transmission The transmission of an infectious agent through exposure to large and small droplets and particles generated when an infected person coughs or sneezes, which generally travel 6 feet (2 m) or less before falling to the ground.

Ebola A virus formerly limited to West Africa, which is spread through direct contact through nonintact skin or mucous membranes, and whose initial symptoms include fever, intense weakness, muscle pain, headaches, and sore throat; some infected people experience internal and external bleeding. Both contact and droplet precautions are needed with this disease.

endemic Consistently present or prevalent in a population or geographic area.

Enterococcus A common, normal organism of the gastrointestinal tract, urinary tract, and genitourinary tract that can be pathogenic and become resistant to vancomycin.

epidemic An outbreak of disease that substantially exceeds what is expected based on recent experience.

fomites Inanimate objects contaminated with microorganisms that serve as a means of transmitting an illness.

fungi Small organisms that can grow rapidly in the presence of the needed nutrients and organic material and can cause infection related to contact with decaying organic matter or from airborne spores in the environment such as molds; singular, *fungus*.

gastroenteritis A term that comprises many types of infections and irritations of the gastrointestinal tract; symptoms include nausea and forceful vomiting, low-grade fever, abdominal pain, and diarrhea; also called stomach flu.

Prep Kit continued

genital warts Warts caused by the human papillomavirus, a sexually transmitted infection; also called condylomata acuminata or venereal warts.

gonorrhea A sexually transmitted infection that results in infection caused by the gonococcal bacterium *Neisseria gonorrhea*; signs and symptoms include pus-containing discharge from the urethra and painful urination in males, and signs and symptoms of an acute abdomen in females.

hantavirus A type of virus found in wild rodents, which can also cause disease in humans; characterized by fever, headache, abdominal pain, loss of appetite, and vomiting. Diseases caused include hemorrhagic fever with renal syndrome and hantavirus pulmonary syndrome.

health care–associated infection An infection acquired 2 days after admission to a health care setting or 30 days after discharge from such a facility.

high-touch items Items that are used to care for the patient or surfaces that are in contact with the patient.

host resistance One's ability to fight off infection.

human immunodeficiency virus (HIV) The virus that may lead to acquired immunodeficiency syndrome; cells in the immune system are killed or damaged so that the body is unable to fight infections and certain cancers.

human papillomavirus (HPV) The most common sexually transmitted infection, which can cause genital warts and some types of cancer.

icterus Jaundice; the yellow appearance of the skin and other tissues caused by an accumulation of bile pigments.

immunization The process of producing widespread immunity to a specific infectious disease among a targeted group by inoculating individual members of the population; can also refer to a set of vaccinations given together or on a recommended schedule.

incubation period The period between exposure to an organism and the first symptoms of illness, during which the organism multiplies within the body and starts to produce symptoms.

infection The invasion of a host or host tissue by pathogenic organisms such as bacteria, viruses, or parasites that produces illness that may or may not have clinical manifestations.

infectious disease A disease caused by pathogenic organisms.

infectious hepatitis Another name for hepatitis A; an inflammation from a virus that causes mild fatigue, loss of appetite, fever, nausea, abdominal pain, and, eventually, jaundice, dark-colored urine, and pale, clay-colored stools.

influenza The flu; a respiratory infection caused by a variety of viruses. It differs from the common cold in that the flu involves a fever, shaking chills, headache, muscle pain, malaise, and loss of appetite. Respiratory symptoms include dry, often protracted coughing; hoarseness; and nasal discharge.

jaundice The presence of excessive bile pigments in the bloodstream that give the skin, mucous membranes, and eyes a distinct yellow color; often associated with liver disease.

lice Tiny, wingless, parasitic insects that feed on blood; an infestation is easily spread through close personal contact. Types include head, body, and pubic lice.

Lyme disease A tick-borne disease that primarily affects the skin, heart, joints, and nervous system and is characterized by a round, red lesion or bull's-eye rash.

measles An infectious viral disease that occurs most often in late winter and spring. It begins with a fever, conjunctivitis, and coryza (acute rhinitis); an onset of coughing; and a blotchy red rash that spreads from the head to the trunk to the lower extremities.

meningitis An inflammation of the membranes that cover the brain and spinal cord; usually caused by a virus or bacterium. The viral type is

Prep Kit continued

not communicable and is less severe than the bacterial type, which can result in brain damage, hearing loss, learning disability, or death.

meningococcal meningitis A type of meningitis caused by the meningococcal bacterium, *Neisseria meningitidis.*

Middle East respiratory syndrome (MERS) A disease originating from the Arabian peninsula, which is transmitted by close contact with camel urine or nasal secretions, milk, or meat. Symptoms include fever, cough, and shortness of breath, and gastrointestinal disturbances; health care providers should take standard precautions, contact precautions, and airborne precautions.

mononucleosis Infectious mononucleosis or mono (glandular fever); caused by the Epstein-Barr virus and often called the kissing disease; also spread by coughing or sneezing.

mumps A viral infection that primarily affects the parotid glands, which are one of the three pairs of salivary glands; causes swelling in front of the ears.

needleless systems Devices that do not use needles for the collection of body fluids or withdrawal of body fluids after initial venous or arterial access is established, the administration of medication or fluids, or any other procedure involving the potential for occupational exposure to bloodborne pathogens by percutaneous injuries from contaminated sharps.

opportunistic infections Infections in which the invading organism thrives because the immune system has been compromised by illness, chemotherapeutic medications, or antirejection drugs in an organ transplant recipient. These fungi, bacteria, viruses, and parasites are normally held in check by a healthy immune system.

other potentially infectious materials (OPIM) Cerebrospinal fluid, pericardial fluid, amniotic fluid, synovial fluid, peritoneal fluid, and any fluid containing visible blood.

pandemic An outbreak of disease that occurs on a global scale.

parasites Organisms living in or on any other living creature; they take advantage of the host by feeding off cells and tissues.

pertussis An acute communicable disease caused by the *Bordetella pertussis* bacterium and characterized by a catarrhal stage, followed by a paroxysmal cough that ends in a whooping inspiration; also called whooping cough.

protozoa Single-celled, usually microscopic, eukaryotic organisms such as amoebas, ciliates, flagellates, and sporozoans; a type of parasite.

rabies A fatal infection of the central nervous system caused by a bite from an animal that has been infected with the rabies virus.

reservoir In the context of communicable disease, a place where organisms may live and multiply.

rubella A viral disease similar to measles, best known by the distinctive red rash on the skin; not nearly as infectious or severe as measles.

scabies An infestation of the skin with the mite *Sarcoptes scabiei*; spreads rapidly with skin-to-skin contact.

sepsis Life-threatening organ dysfunction caused by a dysregulated host response to infection.

septic shock Sepsis accompanied by circulatory and cellular/metabolic abnormalities profound enough to substantially increase mortality.

seropositive Having a positive blood test for an infectious agent, such as human immunodeficiency virus or hepatitis B or C virus.

serum hepatitis Infection with the hepatitis B virus, which is transmitted through sexual contact, blood transfusion, or puncture of the skin with contaminated needles or other contaminated sharp instruments. Signs and symptoms include loss of appetite, nausea, vomiting, general fatigue and malaise, low-grade fever, vague abdominal discomfort, and sometimes aching in the joints; eventually, jaundice occurs.

Prep Kit continued

severe acute respiratory syndrome (SARS) A potentially life-threatening viral infection that usually starts with flulike symptoms.

sexually transmitted infections (STIs) A group of diseases usually acquired by sexual contact; include gonorrhea, syphilis, chlamydia, scabies, pubic lice, herpes, hepatitis, and human immunodeficiency virus infection.

source individual Any person, living or dead, whose blood or other potentially infectious materials may be a source of occupational exposure to another person. Examples include, but are not limited to, hospital and clinic patients, clients in institutions for the developmentally disabled, trauma victims, clients of drug and alcohol treatment facilities, residents of hospices and nursing homes, human remains, and people who donate or sell blood or blood components.

standard precautions The term currently used to describe infection control practices that reduce the opportunity for exposure to occur in the daily care of patients; considers all body substances, except sweat, to present a possible risk. Replaced the older terms "universal precautions" and "body substance isolation" in 2005.

Staphylococcus aureus A strain of bacteria that became resistant to the drug methicillin, creating a new strain; symptoms include soft-tissue infections and possibly localized skin abscesses and cellulitis, empyema, and endocarditis.

syphilis A sexually transmitted infection caused by the spiral-shaped bacterium *Treponema pallidum*; signs and symptoms include an ulcerative lesion or chancre of the skin or mucous membrane at the site of infection, commonly in the genital region.

tetanus A disease caused by spores that enter the body through a puncture wound contaminated with animal feces, street dust, or soil, or through contaminated street drugs; signs and symptoms begin at the wound site, followed by painful muscle contractions in the neck, face, jaw, and trunk muscles.

transmission-based precautions Precautions beyond standard precautions that are designed to interrupt specific disease transmission routes; the three types are airborne, droplet, and contact. Can be used alone or in combination; always used in conjunction with standard precautions.

trichomoniasis A parasitic infection caused by *Trichomonas vaginalis*, a single-cell parasite that is transmitted through sexual contact.

tuberculin skin test A test to determine if a person has ever been infected with tuberculosis.

tuberculosis (TB) An infection that can progress to a disease characterized by a persistent cough lasting longer than 3 weeks plus one or more of the following: night sweats, headache, fever, fatigue, weight loss, hemoptysis, hoarseness, or chest pain.

tuberculosis blood test Measurement via interferon-gamma release assays of how the immune system reacts to the bacteria that cause tuberculosis; offers accurate results in 24 hours; also called blood analysis *Mycobacterium tuberculosis.*

vaccinations Inoculations with a vaccine, usually by injection or inhalation, to bring about immunity to a specific disease in a person.

vaccines The products formulated to bring about immunity by introducing into the body a killed or weakened virus to which the immune system produces antibodies.

varicella zoster A highly contagious disease caused by the varicella zoster virus, which is part of the herpes virus family, and which occurs most often in the winter and early spring; also called chickenpox.

vector An organism that harbors pathogens that are harmless to the organism but cause disease when transmitted to a human host.

vesicles Tiny fluid-filled sacs; small blisters.

viral hepatitis An inflammation of the liver produced by one of five distinct forms of hepatitis virus—A, B, C, D, and E. The types differ in their

Prep Kit continued

mode of transmission but present with the same signs and symptoms.

virulence The ability of an organism to invade and create disease in a host; also refers to the ability of an organism to survive outside the living host.

viruses Small organisms that can multiply only inside a host, such as a human, and cause disease.

West Nile virus (WNV) A type of virus that is transmitted by mosquitos. It usually causes only mild disease in humans but can cause encephalitis, meningitis, and death; symptoms, if any, include fever, headache, fatigue, weakness, joint pain, vomiting, diarrhea, or rash.

Zika A type of virus that is transmitted by the *Aedes aegypti* mosquito; the majority of infected persons are asymptomatic. Transmission can occur from an infected mother to her fetus, and from an infected male to his sexual partners; related to onset of Guillain-Barré syndrome.

zoonotic Refers to infectious diseases of animals that can be transmitted to humans and cause disease.

References

1. Infectious Diseases and Circumstances Relevant to Notification of Emergency Response Employees: Implementation of Sec. 2695 of the Ryan White HIV/AIDS Treatment Extension Act of 2009, March, 2020. Infectious diseases and circumstances relevant to notification requirements. Centers for Disease Control and Prevention website. https://www.cdc.gov/niosh/docs/2020-119/default.html. Accessed March 22, 2021.
2. Centers for Disease Control and Prevention. Notes from the field: occupationally acquired HIV infection among health care workers—United States, 1985–2013. *MMWR.* 2015;63(53):1245-1246.
3. Recommended work restrictions for communicable diseases in health care workers. Association of Occupational Health Professionals in Healthcare website. https://aohp.org/aohp/Portals/0/Documents/MemberServices/templateandform/WR4CD-HCW.pdf. Published October 24, 2014. Accessed March 22, 2021.
4. Science brief: SARS-CoV-2 and potential airborne transmission. Centers for Disease Control and Prevention website. https://www.cdc.gov/coronavirus/2019-ncov/science/science-briefs/scientific-brief-sars-cov-2.html. Updated October 5, 2020. Accessed April 10, 2021.
5. Dbouk T, Drikakis D. On coughing and airborne droplet transmission to humans. *Phys Fluids.* https://aip.scitation.org/doi/10.1063/5.0011960. Published May 19, 2020. Accessed December 6, 2020.
6. I. Review of scientific data regarding transmission of infectious agents in healthcare settings. Centers for Disease Control and Prevention website. https://www.cdc.gov/infectioncontrol/guidelines/isolation/scientific-review.html. Reviewed July 22, 2019. Accessed July 7, 2021.
7. How fast is a sneeze versus a cough? Cover your mouth either way. American Lung Association website. https://www.lung.org/blog/sneeze-versus-cough. Updated April 9, 2020. Accessed April 10, 2021.
8. Transmission-based precautions. Centers for Disease Control and Prevention website. https://www.cdc.gov/infectioncontrol/basics/transmission-based-precautions.html. Reviewed January 6, 2016. Accessed April 10, 2021.
9. Interim guidance for emergency medical services (EMS) systems and 9-1-1 public safety answering points (PSAPs) for management of patients under investigation (PUIs) for Ebola virus disease (EVD) in the United States. Centers for Disease Control and Prevention website. http://www.cdc.gov.vhf/ebola/hep/interim-guidance-emergency-medical-services-systems. Updated September 10, 2015. Accessed March 22, 2021.
10. Handwashing: clean hands save lives. Centers for Disease Control and Prevention website. https://www.cdc.gov/handwashing/when-how-handwashing.html. Last reviewed November 24, 2020. Accessed March 22, 2021.
11. Bucher J, Donovan C, Ohman-Strickland P, McCoy J. Hand washing practices among emergency medical services providers. *Western J Emerg Med.* 2015;16(5):727-735. doi:10.5811/westjem.2015.7.25917.
12. Teter J, Millin MG, Bissell R. Hand hygiene in emergency medical services. *Prehosp Emerg Care.* 2015;19(2):313-319. doi:10.3109/10903127.2014.967427.
13. Centers for Disease Control and Prevention. Immunization of health-care personnel: recommendations of the Advisory Committee on Immunization Practices (ACIP), 2011. *MMWR.* 2011;60(7):1-72.
14. OSHA Act 1970 General Duty Clause. US Department of Labor, Occupational Safety and Health Administration website. https://www.osha.gov/laws-regs/oshact/section5-duties. Accessed March 22, 2021.
15. National Fire Protection Association. *NFPA 1581: Standard on Fire Department Infection Control Program.* Quincy, MA: National Fire Protection Association; 2015.

Prep Kit continued

16. Hand hygiene in healthcare settings. Centers for Disease Control and Prevention website. https://www.cdc.gov/handhygiene/index.html. Reviewed January 30, 2020. Accessed March 22, 2021.
17. N95 respirators and surgical masks. Centers for Disease Control and Prevention website. https://blogs.cdc.gov/niosh-science-blog/2009/10/14/n95. Accessed March 22, 2021.
18. Ang B, Fong Poh B, Win Kyaw M, Chow A. Surgical masks for protection of health care personnel against pandemic novel swine-origin influenza A (H1N1)–2009: results from an observational study. *Clin Infect Dis.* 2010;50(7):1011-1014.
19. Influenza (flu): prevention strategies for seasonal influenza in healthcare settings. Centers for Disease Control and Prevention website. https://www.cdc.gov/flu/professionals/infectioncontrol/healthcaresettings.htm. Last reviewed October 30, 2018. Accessed March 22, 2021.
20. Diaz K, Smaldone GC. Quantifying exposure risk: surgical mask and respirators, *Am J Infect Control.* 2010;38(7):501-508. doi:10.1016/j.ajic.2010.06.002.
21. Loeb M, Dafoe N, Mahoney J, et al. Surgical mask vs N95 respirator for preventing influenza among health care workers. *JAMA.* 2009;302(17):1865-1871. doi:10.1001/jama.2009.1466.
22. Standard interpretations. US Department of Labor, Occupational Safety and Health Administration website. https://www.osha.gov/laws-regs/standardinterpretations/publicationdate/currentyear. Accessed March 22, 2021.
23. Waseem M. Body fluid exposures. https://emedicine.medscape.com/article/782611-overview. Updated June 19, 2019. Accessed March 30, 2021.
24. Occupational and safety health standards. US Department of Labor, Occupational Safety and Health Administration website. https://www.osha.gov/pls/oshaweb/owastand.display_standard_group?p_part_number=1910&p_toc_level=1. Accessed March 23, 2021.
25. Stop sticks campaign. Centers for Disease Control and Prevention website. https://www.cdc.gov/nora/councils/hcsa/stopsticks/default.html. Accessed March 23, 2021.
26. PL 106-430: Needlestick Safety and Prevention Act. US Government Publishing Office website. https://www.govinfo.gov/content/pkg/PLAW-106publ430/html/PLAW-106publ430.htm. Accessed March 23, 2021.
27. Bloodborne pathogen exposure. Centers for Disease Control and Prevention website. https://www.cdc.gov/niosh/docs/2007-157/default.html. Accessed August 17, 2021.
28. Bloodborne pathogen exposure incidents. US Department of Labor, Occupational Safety and Health Administration website. https://www.osha.gov/OshDoc/data_BloodborneFacts/bbfact04.html. Accessed March 23, 2021.
29. Enforcement procedures for the occupational exposure to bloodborne pathogens. CPL 02-02.069: November 27, 2001; paragraph (d)(3)(ii). US Department of Labor, Occupational Safety and Health Administration website. https://www.osha.gov/pls/oshaweb/owadisp.show_document?p_table=directives&p_id=2570. Accessed March 23, 2021.
30. Assistant Secretary for Preparedness and Response, US Department of Health and Human Services. *EMS Infectious Disease Playbook*. EMS.gov website. https://www.ems.gov/pdf/ASPR-EMS-Infectious-Disease-Playbook-June-2017.pdf. Accessed April 10, 2021.
31. Centers for Disease Control and Prevention. Vital signs: epidemiology of sepsis. Prevalence of health care factors and opportunities for prevention. *MMWR*. 2016;65(33):864-869.
32. Rhodes A, Evans L, Alhazzani W, et al. Surviving Sepsis Campaign: international guidelines for management of sepsis and septic shock: 2016. *Crit Care Med.* 2017;45(3):486-552.
33. Lamontagne F, Harrison DA, Rowan KM. qSOFA for identifying sepsis among patients with infection. *JAMA.* 2017;317(3):267-268. doi:10.1001/jama.2016.19684.
34. Centers for Disease Control and Prevention. Prevention and control of meningococcal disease: recommendations of the Advisory Committee on Immunization Practices (ACIP). *MMWR*. 2013;62(2):1-22.
35. The 2009 H1N1 pandemic: summary highlights, April 2009–April 2010. Centers for Disease Control and Prevention website. https://cdc.gov/h1n1flu/cdcresponse.htm. Accessed March 23, 2021.
36. Estimated influenza illnesses, medical visits, hospitalizations, and deaths in the United States—2018–2019 influenza season. Centers for Disease Control and Prevention website. https://www.cdc.gov/flu/about/burden/2018-2019.html. Accessed March 23, 2021.
37. Pertussis: summary of vaccine recommendations. Centers for Disease Control and Prevention website. https://www.cdc.gov/vaccines/vpd/pertussis/recs-summary.html. Accessed March 23, 2021.
38. Mumps cases and outbreaks. Centers for Disease Control and Prevention website. https://www.cdc.gov/mumps/outbreaks.html. Accessed March 29, 2021.
39. Mumps. Centers for Disease Control and Prevention website. https://www.cdc.gov/mumps/hcp.html. Accessed March 23, 2021.
40. Rubella (German measles, three-day measles). Centers for Disease Control and Prevention website. https://www.cdc.gov/rubella/about/in-the-us.html. Accessed March 23, 2021.
41. Rubella (German measles, three-day measles): for healthcare professionals. Centers for Disease Control and Prevention website. https://www.cdc.gov/rubella/hcp.html. Reviewed December 31, 2020. Accessed March 23, 2021.

Prep Kit continued

42. Modes of transmission of virus causing COVID-19: implications for ICP precaution recommendations: scientific brief. World Health Organization website. https://www.who.int/publications/i/item/modes-of-transmission-of-virus-causing-covid-19-implications-for-ipc-precaution-recommendations. March 29, 2020. Accessed March 25, 2021.
43. Science brief: SARS-CoV-2 and surface (fomite) transmission for indoor community environments. Centers for Disease Control and Prevention website. https://www.cdc.gov/coronavirus/2019-ncov/more/science-and-research/surface-transmission.html. Updated October 5, 2020. Accessed April 11, 2021.
44. Coronavirus disease (COVID-19): ventilation and air conditioning in public spaces and buildings. World Health Organization; July 29, 2020. https://www.who.int/news-room/q-a-detail/coronavirus-disease-covid-19-ventilation-and-air-conditioning-in-public-spaces-and-buildings. Updated March 2, 2021. Accessed March 25, 2021.
45. Centers for Disease Control and Prevention. Tuberculosis trends—United States, 2014. *MMWR*. 2015;64(10): 265-269.
46. Health disparities in HIV/AIDS, viral hepatitis, STDs, and TB. Centers for Disease Control and Prevention website. https://www.cdc.gov/nchhstp/healthdisparities/asians.html. Accessed March 23, 2021.
47. Tuberculosis: drug-resistant TB. Centers for Disease Control and Prevention website. https://www.cdc.gov/tb/topic/drtb/default.htm. Accessed March 23, 2021.
48. Tuberculosis screening, testing, and treatment of U.S. health care personnel: recommendations from the National Tuberculosis Controllers Association and CDC, 2019. *MMWR*. 2019;68(19):439-443.
49. Enforcement procedures and scheduling for occupational exposure to tuberculosis. US Department of Labor, Occupational Safety and Health Administration website. https://www.osha.gov/OshDoc/Directive_pdf/CPL_02-02-078.pdf. Accessed March 23, 2021.
50. TB elimination: treatment options for latent tuberculosis infection. Centers for Disease Control and Prevention website. https://www.cdc.gov/tb/publications/factsheets/treatment/ltbitreatmentoptions.pdf. Accessed March 23, 2021.
51. Chickenpox (varicella): outbreak identification, investigation, and control. Centers for Disease Control and Prevention website. http://www.cdc.gov/chickenpox/outbreaks.html. Accessed March 23, 2021.
52. Centers for Disease Control and Prevention. Measles—United States, January 4–April 2, 2015. *MMWR*. 2015;64(14):373-376.
53. Vaccines and preventable diseases: measles, mumps, rubella (MMR) vaccination—what everyone should know. Centers for Disease Control and Prevention website. https://www.cdc.gov/vaccines/vpd/mmr/public/index.html. Accessed March 24, 2021.
54. Immunization schedules: child and adolescent schedule. Centers for Disease Control and Prevention. https://www.cdc.gov/vaccines/schedules/hcp/imz/child-adolescent.html. Accessed March 23, 2021.
55. Epstein-Barr virus and infectious mononucleosis: about infectious mononucleosis. Centers for Disease Control and Prevention website. https://www.cdc.gov/Epstein-barr/about-mono.html. Accessed March 24, 2021.
56. NCHHSTP newsroom: new CDC report: STDs continue to increase in the U.S. Centers for Disease Control and Prevention website. https://www.cdc.gov/nchhstp/newsroom/2019/2018-STD-surveillance-report-press-release.html. Released October 8, 2019. Accessed March 24, 2021.
57. 2015 STD surveillance report press release. Centers for Disease Control and Prevention website. https://www.cdc.gov/nchhstp/newsroom/2016/std-surveillance-report-2015-press-release.html. Updated October 19, 2016. Accessed March 24, 2021.
58. Chlamydia: chlamydia—CDC fact sheet. Centers for Disease Control and Prevention website. https://www.cdc.gov/std/chlamydia/stdfact-chlamydia-detailed.htm. Accessed March 24, 2021.
59. Centers for Disease Control and Prevention. Sexually transmitted diseases treatment guidelines, 2015: recommendations and reports. *MMWR*. 2015;64(3):1-137.
60. Trichomoniasis: CDC fact sheet. Centers for Disease Control and Prevention website. https://www.cdc.gov/std/trichomonas/stdfact-trichomoniasis.htm. Accessed March 24, 2021.
61. Leifer G. Reproductive anatomy and physiology. In: *Maternity Nursing: An Introductory Text*. 11th ed. St. Louis, MO: Saunders; 2012:16-28.
62. Viral hepatitis—hepatitis B information: the ABCs of hepatitis fact sheet. Centers for Disease Control and Prevention website. https://www.cdc.gov/hepatitis/hbv/profresourcesb.htm. Accessed March 24, 2021.
63. Viral hepatitis—hepatitis B information: hepatitis B questions and answers for health professionals. Centers for Disease Control and Prevention website. https://www.cdc.gov/hepatitis/hbv/hbvfaq.htm#overview. Accessed March 24, 2021.
64. Hepatitis B: fact sheet. World Health Organization website. https://www.who.int/news-room/fact-sheets/detail/hepatitis-b. Updated July 2020. Accessed March 24, 2021.
65. Heplisav-B (HepB-CpG) vaccine. Centers for Disease Control and Prevention website. https://www.cdc.gov/vaccines/schedules/vacc-updates/heplisav-b.html. Reviewed April 24, 2018. Accessed April 10, 2021.
66. Viral hepatitis—hepatitis C information: hepatitis C questions and answers. Centers for Disease Control and Prevention website. https://www.cdc.gov/hepatitis/hcv/cfaq.htm. Accessed March 24, 2021.

Prep Kit continued

67. Tsoulfas G, Goulis I, Giakoustidis D, et al. Hepatitis C and liver transplantation. *Hippokratia.* 2009;13(4):211-215.
68. Centers for Disease Control and Prevention. Recommendations for prevention and control of hepatitis C virus (HCV) infection and HCV-related chronic disease. *MMWR.* 1998;47(19):1-39.
69. Hosoqlu S, Celen MK, Akalin S, et al. Transmission of hepatitis C by blood splash into conjunctiva in a nurse. *Am J Infect Control.* 2003;31(8):502-504.
70. Hepatitis C and tattoos. Hepatitis Central website. www.hepatitiscentral.com/hcv/hepatitis/tattoos/. Accessed March 24, 2021.
71. Viral hepatitis—hepatitis C information: hepatitis C questions and answers for the public. Centers for Disease Control and Prevention website. https://www.cdc.gov/hepatitis/hcv/cfaq.htm. Accessed March 24, 2021.
72. Healthcare Infection Control Practices Advisory Committee (HICPAC). Guideline for disinfection and sterilization in healthcare facilities, 2008. Centers for Disease Control and Prevention website. https://www.cdc.gov/hicpac/disinfection_sterilization/6_0disinfection.html. Accessed March 24, 2021.
73. Interpretation of results of tests for hepatitis C virus (HCV) infection and further actions. Centers for Disease Control and Prevention website. https://www.cdc.gov/hepatitis/hcv/HCVTestResults-InterpretationAndActions.htm. Reviewed May 2, 2019. Accessed March 30, 2021.
74. Viral hepatitis and liver disease. U.S. Department of Veterans Affairs website. https://www.hepatitis.va.gov/patient/hcv/testing/time-required-to-test-positive.asp. Accessed March 24, 2021.
75. HIV: basic statistics. Centers for Disease Control and Prevention website. https://www.cdc.gov/hiv/basics/statistics.html. Accessed March 24, 2021.
76. Fact sheet November 2020 global HIV & AIDS statistics. UNAIDS website. www.unaids.org/en/resources/fact-sheet. Accessed March 24, 2021.
77. Centers for Disease Control and Prevention. Final 2015 reports of nationally notifiable infectious diseases and conditions. *MMWR.* 2016;65(46):1306-1321.
78. Centers for Disease Control and Prevention. Revised recommendations for HIV screening of pregnant women. *MMWR.* 2001;50(19)59-86.
79. Guidelines for the use of antiretroviral agents in adults and adolescents with HIV. Clinical Info HIV.gov. https://clinicalinfo.hiv.gov/sites/default/files/guidelines/documents/AdultandAdolescentGL.pdf. Updated December 18, 2019. Accessed March 24, 2021.
80. Final recommendation statement. Human immunodeficiency virus (HIV) infection: screening. US Preventive Services Task Force. https://www.uspreventiveservicestaskforce.org/uspstf/recommendation/human-immunodeficiency-virus-hiv-infection-screening. Published June 11, 2019. Accessed March 24, 2021.
81. Centers for Disease Control and Prevention. Notes from the field: occupationally acquired HIV infection among health care workers—United States, 1985-2013. *MMWR.* 2015;63(53):1245-1246.
82. Centers for Disease Control and Prevention. Updated US Public Health Service guidelines for the management of occupational exposures to HBV, HCV, and HIV and recommendations for postexposure prophylaxis. *MMWR.* 2001;50(11):1-42.
83. Centers for Disease Control and Prevention. *Updated U.S. Public Health Service Guidelines for the Management of Occupational Exposures to Human Immunodeficiency Virus and Recommendations for Postexposure Prophylaxis.* Chicago, IL: University of Chicago Press; July 6, 2015. https://npin.cdc.gov/publication/updated-us-public-health-service-guidelines-management-occupational-exposures-human. Accessed March 24, 2021.
84. Lookingbill DP, Marks JG. *Principles of Dermatology.* 3rd ed. Philadelphia, PA: Saunders; 2000.
85. Nematodes. In: Murray PR, Rosenthal KS, Pfaller MA, eds. *Medical Microbiology.* 6th ed. St. Louis, MO: Mosby; 2009:853-870.
86. Parasites—hookworm: hookworm FAQs. Centers for Disease Control and Prevention website. https://www.cdc.gov/parasites/hookworm/gen_info/faqs.html. Accessed March 24, 2021.
87. Parasites—enterobiasis (also known as pinworm infection): pinworm infection FAQs. Centers for Disease Control and Prevention website. https://www.cdc.gov/parasites/pinworm/gen_info/faqs.html. Accessed March 24, 2021.
88. Parasites—bed bugs: bed bugs FAQs. Centers for Disease Control and Prevention website. https://www.cdc.gov/parasites/bedbugs/faqs.html. Accessed March 24, 2021.
89. Ebola—Ebola virus disease: interim guidance for emergency medical services (EMS) systems and 9-1-1 public safety answering points (PSAPs) for management of patients under investigation (PUIs) for Ebola virus disease (EVD) in the United States. Centers for Disease Control and Prevention website. https://www.cdc.gov/vhf/ebola/healthcare-us/emergency-services/ems-systems.html. Updated September 10, 2015. Accessed March 24, 2021.
90. Rooney BL, Pettipas J, Grudeski E, et al. Detection of circulating norovirus genotypes: hitting a moving target. *Virol J.* 2014;11:129. doi:10.1186/1743-422X-11-129.
91. Viral hepatitis—hepatitis E information: hepatitis E questions and answers for health professionals. CDC website. Centers for Disease Control and Prevention website. https://www.cdc.gov/hepatitis/hev/hevfaq.htm. Accessed March 24, 2021.
92. West Nile virus: transmission. Centers for Disease Control and Prevention website. https://www.cdc.gov/westnile/transmission/index.html. Accessed March 24, 2021.

Prep Kit continued

93. West Nile virus. Centers for Disease Control and Prevention website. https://www.cdc.gov/westnile/index.html. Accessed March 24, 2021.
94. Dengue: dengue in the US states and territories. Centers for Disease Control and Prevention website. https://www.cdc.gov/dengue/areaswithrisk/in-the-us.html. Accessed March 24, 2021.
95. Dengue vaccine. Centers for Disease Control and Prevention website. https://www.cdc.gov/dengue/prevention/dengue-vaccine.html. Reviewed September 23, 2019. Accessed April 10, 2021.
96. Chikungunya virus. Centers for Disease Control and Prevention website. https://www.cdc.gov/chikungunya/geo/united-states-2019.html. Reviewed December 2, 2020. Accessed April 10, 2021.
97. National Institute of Allergy and Infectious Diseases. Experimental chikungunya vaccine is safe and well-tolerated in early trials. National Institutes of Health website. https://www.niaid.nih.gov/news-events/experimental-chikungunya-vaccine-safe-and-well-tolerated-early-trial. Published April 17, 2020. Accessed April 10, 2021.
98. Statistics and maps. Centers for Disease Control and Prevention website. https://www.cdc.gov/zika/reporting/index.html. Reviewed March 3, 2021. Accessed April 10, 2021.
99. Zika virus: symptoms. Centers for Disease Control and Prevention website. https://www.cdc.gov/zika/symptoms/symptoms.html. Accessed March 24, 2021.
100. Epidemiology and statistics: Rocky Mountain spotted fever (RMSF). Centers for Disease Control and Prevention. https://www.cdc.gov/rmsf/stats/index.html. Last reviewed April 7, 2020. Accessed March 24, 2021.
101. Hantavirus: hantavirus disease, by state of reporting. Centers for Disease Control and Prevention website. https://www.cdc.gov/hantavirus/surveillance. Accessed March 24, 2021.
102. Rabies: rabies in the U.S. Centers for Disease Control and Prevention website. https://www.cdc.gov/rabies/location/usa/index.html. Accessed March 24, 2021.
103. Tetanus: surveillance. Centers for Disease Control and Prevention website. https://www.cdc.gov/tetanus/surveillance.html. Accessed March 24, 2017.
104. Malani PN. National burden of invasive methicillin-resistant *Staphylococcus aureus* infection. *JAMA.* 2014;311(14):1438-1439. doi:10.1001/jama.2014.1666.
105. Methicillin-resistant *Staphylococcus aureus* (MRSA). Centers for Disease Control and Prevention website. https://www.cdc.gov/mrsa/tracking/index.html. Accessed March 24, 2021.
106. Antibiotic use in the United States: progress and opportunities. Centers for Disease Control and Prevention; 2017. https://www.cdc.gov/antibiotic-use/stewardship-report/pdf/stewardship-report.pdf. Accessed March 24, 2021.
107. Methicillin-resistant *Staphylococcus aureus* (MRSA): healthcare settings. Centers for Disease Control and Prevention website. https://www.cdc.gov/mrsa/healthcare/index.html. Accessed March 24, 2021.
108. VRE has a domino effect among regional hospitals. Infection Control Today website. https://www.infectioncontroltoday.com/view/vre-has-domino-effect-among-regional-hospitals. Accessed March 24, 2021.
109. New carbapenem-resistant Enterobacteriaceae warrant additional action by healthcare providers. Infectious Diseases Society of America website. http://www.idsociety.org/CDCHAN341.htm. February 14, 2013. Accessed March 24, 2024.
110. Severe acute respiratory syndrome (SARS). Centers for Disease Control and Prevention website. https://www.cdc.gov/sars/about/fs-sars.html. Reviewed December 6, 2017. Accessed April 10, 2021.
111. Highly pathogenic Asian avian influenza A (H5N1) virus. Centers for Disease Control and Prevention website. https://www.cdc.gov/flu/avianflu/h5n1-virus.htm. Reviewed December 8, 2018. Accessed March 30, 2021.

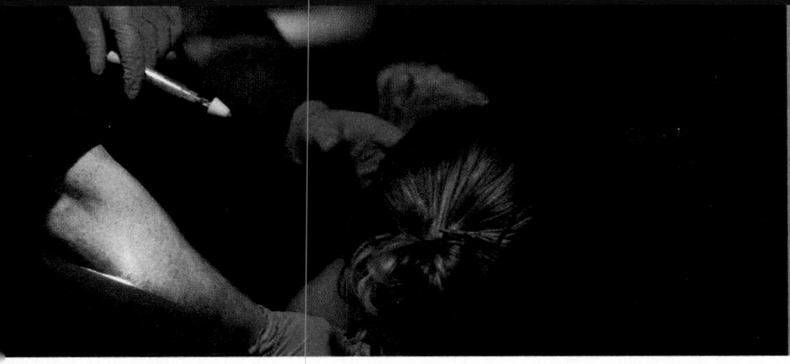

Chapter 28

Toxicology

NATIONAL EMS EDUCATION STANDARD COMPETENCIES

Medicine

Integrates assessment findings with principles of epidemiology and pathophysiology to formulate a field impression and implement a comprehensive treatment/disposition plan for a patient with a medical complaint.

Toxicology

Recognition and management of
- Carbon monoxide poisoning (pp 1690–1691)
- Nerve agent poisoning (pp 1689–1690)

How and when to contact a poison control center (pp 1658–1659)

Anatomy, physiology, pathophysiology, assessment, and management of
- Inhaled poisons (pp 1660–1662)
- Ingested poisons (pp 1659–1660)
- Injected poisons (p 1662)
- Absorbed poisons (pp 1662–1663)
- Alcohol intoxication and withdrawal (pp 1673–1674)
- Opioid toxidrome (pp 1663–1664)

Anatomy, physiology, epidemiology, pathophysiology, psychosocial impact, presentations, prognosis, and management of the following toxidromes and poisonings:
- Cholinergics (p 1664)
- Anticholinergics (p 1664)
- Sympathomimetics (p 1664)
- Sedative-hypnotics (pp 1682–1685)
- Opioids (pp 1685–1686)
- Serotonin syndrome (pp 1664, 1704)
- Alcohol intoxication and withdrawal (pp 1673–1674)
- Over-the-counter and prescription medications (pp 1659–1660, 1676–1677, 1704–1706)
- Carbon monoxide (pp 1690–1691)
- Illegal drugs (pp 1674–1682)
- Herbal preparations (p 1710)

KNOWLEDGE OBJECTIVES

1. Define toxicology, poison, and overdose. (pp 1656–1657)
2. Describe routes of entry of toxic substances into the body, including ingestion, inhalation, injection, and absorption. (pp 1659–1663)
3. Explain the appropriate use of activated charcoal, including situations when it may be most beneficial to the patient. (pp 1660, 1683–1684)
4. Explain the importance of situational awareness and an accurate scene size-up when responding to a toxicologic emergency. (pp 1661, 1667–1668, 1675)
5. Discuss the major toxidromes and their use in the assessment and management of toxicologic emergencies. (pp 1663–1664)
6. Identify the common signs and symptoms of poisoning. (p 1665)

7. Discuss substance misuse and concepts associated with it. (pp 1663, 1666–1667)
8. Describe the assessment and treatment of the patient with suspected poisoning or overdose. (pp 1667–1670)
9. Recognize the role of airway management in the patient with suspected poisoning or overdose. (p 1668)
10. Identify the main types of specific poisons and their effects. (pp 1689–1690, 1707–1710)
11. Discuss emergencies related to severe intoxication, including alcohol use disorder. (pp 1670–1674)
12. Describe the assessment and treatment of the patient with suspected plant or mushroom poisoning. (pp 1707–1711)
13. Describe the assessment and treatment of the patient with suspected food poisoning. (pp 1711–1712)

SKILLS OBJECTIVES

1. Demonstrate the steps in the assessment and treatment of the patient with suspected poisoning. (pp 1689–1701)
2. Demonstrate the steps in the assessment and treatment of the patient with suspected overdose. (pp 1667–1668)

Introduction

Toxicologic emergencies are some of the most challenging situations you will face as a paramedic. Toxicologic emergencies require you to think critically to identify the substances involved, determine the differential diagnosis, and formulate a treatment plan based on the anticipated clinical course of the patient. **Licit** (legal) or **illicit** (illegal) drugs will frequently play a role in situations you encounter in the field **FIGURE 28-1**, even when drug use is not the primary reason for the 9-1-1 call. One of the cornerstones of prehospital emergency medicine is a solid understanding of various substances and medications, as well as pharmacokinetics (the activity of drugs in the body over time, including the processes of absorption, distribution, and elimination). In this chapter, you will form a working knowledge of common substances to which patients may have been exposed and their effects on patients. This foundation will allow you to initiate appropriate treatment of patients with poisoning or drug overdose. Although illicit drugs such as heroin and methamphetamine are still common on the streets, waves of new, chemically engineered drugs may be finding their way into your local community as well.

First, some key terms must be defined. **Toxicology** is the study of toxic or poisonous substances. A **poison** is a substance whose chemical action could damage structures or impair function when introduced into the body. Even a small amount of poison may cause serious symptoms and possible death. By contrast, a **drug** is a substance that has some therapeutic effect (such as reducing inflammation,

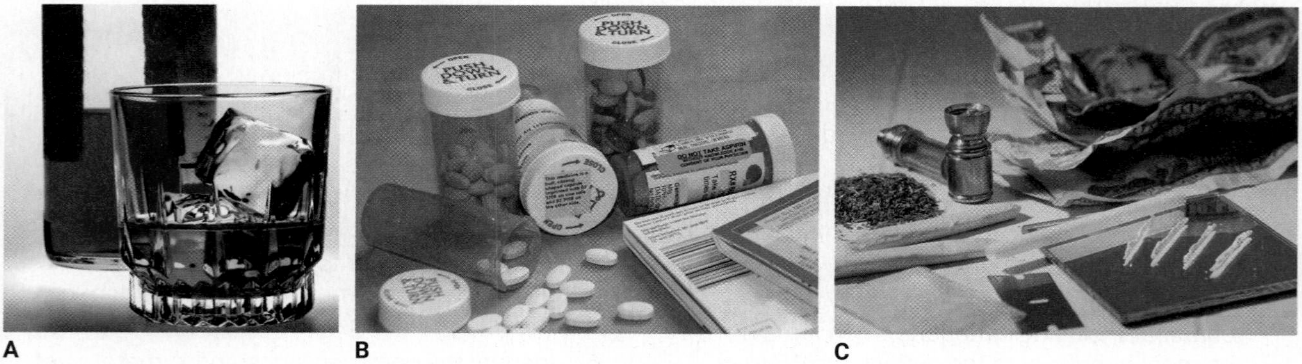

FIGURE 28-1 A. Alcohol is a legal substance that is a drug. **B.** Medications are legal substances that can be misused. **C.** Illegal drugs can also be misused.

A: © Ed Isaacs/Shutterstock; B: © Anne Kitzman/Shutterstock; C: © Comstock Images/Getty Images.

fighting bacteria, or producing euphoria) when given in the appropriate circumstances and in the appropriate dose. A **toxin** is a poison or harmful substance produced by bacteria, animals, or plants. An **overdose** occurs when a drug (either licit or illicit) is taken in excess. An overdose can be a true medical emergency because of the profound effects of the overwhelming presence of the drug in the body.

Words of Wisdom

A poison is always a poison, whereas a licit or illicit substance may poison a person if taken to excess.

Bioavailability describes the percentage of unchanged substance that is present in the systemic circulation. *Half-life* describes the amount of time needed for the average person to metabolize or eliminate 50% of a substance in the plasma. The half-life of a drug is commonly expressed in minutes, but the half-life can last for hours or even days. Lastly, *excretion* is used to describe how a drug is removed from the body.

Types of Toxicologic Emergencies

Toxicologic emergencies usually fall under one of two general headings: intentional and unintentional. According to the National Capital Poison Center, 76.6% of all poison exposures reported in 2019 were unintentional. However, intentional exposures were over 30 times more likely to have serious outcomes (ie, major or fatal effects) than unintentional exposures.[1] Analgesic substances are the most common source of both adult poison exposures and pediatric deaths from poisoning. Intentional toxicologic emergencies frequently involve a person who is depressed and may be attempting to die by suicide. The patient may have ingested several different substances, so you need to be thorough in your interview and assessment. Emergency medical services (EMS) providers have also encountered increased rates of chemical suicides in recent years (discussed later in this chapter). Such situations may pose a significant threat to you and other responders who are unaware of toxic gases in enclosed spaces.

Intentional overdoses may also play a role in criminal activities. Historically, drugs such as flunitrazepam (Rohypnol) and gamma-hydroxybutyric acid (GHB) have been used to facilitate sexual assault. These medications may cause both antegrade and retrograde amnesia, so the patient's ability to recall the events surrounding the assault may be significantly impaired. Flunitrazepam is discussed later in this chapter. Finally, another type of intentional poisoning is that caused by chemical warfare, which is covered in Chapter 51, *Terrorism Response*.

An unintentional toxicologic emergency can occur in many ways, such as neglect, oversight, an idiosyncratic reaction, or confusion about one's drug regimen. (Idiosyncratic reactions are discussed in Chapter 13, *Principles of Pharmacology*.) For example, consider an older man who forgets that he has already taken his daily dose of a prescription beta blocker to control his hypertension. He then takes a

YOU are the Paramedic

PART 1

At 1430 hours, your unit is dispatched to a single-family residence. The dispatcher tells you that a woman was found unresponsive by family members. Fire department personnel are responding with you, but no law enforcement officers have been dispatched. When you arrive, you find a middle-aged woman lying supine in bed. The room is neat and well-kept. Nothing looks obviously out of place or suspicious. Your primary survey reveals that the patient is barely breathing but has a strong pulse. The family reports that the patient underwent back surgery 4 days earlier. The family says she was last seen acting normal for her about 6 hours earlier when she laid down for a nap. The patient had trouble sleeping during the previous night because of pain in her back.

1. What is your first impression of this patient?
2. What is your priority for patient care?

second dose, which leaves him feeling weak and dizzy as his heart rate and blood pressure drop in response to the increased level of the medication in his system.

You must be able to decipher the patient's list of medications while paying particular attention to any new medications or changes to the dosage. If the patient has multiple physicians, then check whether the patient is taking multiple medications prescribed by different physicians for the same indication. The patient may not understand that two similar medications with different trade names, such as the beta blockers carvedilol (Coreg) and metoprolol (Toprol XL), could result in a dangerous drug interaction if mixed. Recent changes in pharmacy policies and procedures have attempted to prevent such situations. You will also want to consider over-the-counter (OTC) medications, home remedies, and herbal therapies to obtain a complete picture of what the patient has been taking. The potential for a polypharmacy overdose (one involving multiple medications) should be considered with any toxicologic emergency.

SAFETY

To avoid creating an unintentional overdose in patients, you must be diligent in administering all medications. A simple miscalculation in volume or dose can cause you to give 10 mg of morphine to a pediatric patient instead of the 1 mg you had planned to administer. This error can be the difference between therapeutic relief of pain and quickly scrambling for a bag-mask device to support the patient with acute respiratory depression. Whenever possible, confirm pediatric and high-risk medication doses with another trained health care provider or a reliable reference source.

Unintentional toxic exposures commonly occur with children. Anyone who has spent any length of time around young children knows they explore the world using their mouths, which may result in unintentional ingestions **FIGURE 28-2**. From holly berries around the winter holidays to brightly colored prenatal gummy vitamins, innocent toddlers may become seriously ill after deciding to taste their newfound treasure.

Finally, unintentional toxicologic emergencies can occur in the workplace. For example, during their daily duties, employees at an airplane

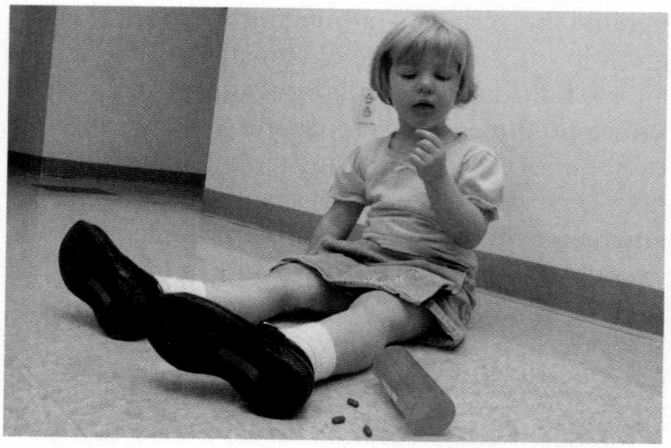

FIGURE 28-2 A toddler may mistake brightly colored pills for candy. This unintentional exposure can lead to a life-threatening illness, even with ingestion of very small amounts of the substance.

assembly plant may work in several areas that contain chemicals, including hydrocarbons and hydrofluoric acid. A patient experiencing shortness of breath could have been exposed to either chemical, so a thorough scene size-up and history taking would be prudent to help identify the specific toxins to which the patient may have been exposed.

Poison Control Centers

Given the variety of illicit drugs and the continued growth of prescription drug misuse, even veteran paramedics may find it challenging to keep current with the various drugs sold in the streets today. For this reason, the American Association of Poison Control Centers (AAPCC) may be an indispensable aid. The AAPCC supports the nation's poison control centers in their efforts to prevent and treat poison exposures. The phone number for the Poison Control Center hotline is 1-800-222-1222 (available 24 hours a day, 7 days a week). Some mobile device apps, such as Epocrates, can assist with pill identification. If you input basic information about the pills (size, shape, color, or markings), the software may help to narrow down the list of potential medications. The National Capital Poison Center has an online tool and mobile device app called webPOISONCONTROL that both laypeople and health care providers can use.

Suppose you are called to a home where a frantic mother is hovering over a toddler who sits beside an empty packet that contained the dog's flea medication. Is the medication poisonous? How poisonous? Is an **antidote** (something to counteract the effect of the poison) available? In such a scenario, you can call the poison control center and get a fast rundown on the ingestion, its toxic potential, and steps to negate its effects. With this information in hand, you can initiate proper patient care while contacting online medical control, if needed, for specific orders or instructions if they go beyond the range of your standing orders.

Poison control centers are a veritable goldmine of information that you should add to your paramedic toolbox. Never hesitate to tap these resources when you are confronted with any toxin with which you have limited or no familiarity. When in doubt, call!

At the same time, your call helps the center's staff to collect data on poisonings in your region. These data may be analyzed to help detect trends, spot developing public health problems, and evaluate current treatment protocols for different poisonings.

Words of Wisdom

The National Capital Poison Center was founded in 1980 to help prevent poisonings, limit injuries from poisonings, and save lives. The organization is accredited by the AAPCC and offers around-the-clock guidance for poisoning by certified specialists in poison information. Board-certified physician toxicologists back up the team of specialists and help manage each case.

In addition to knowing how to reach the National Capital Poison Center, familiarize yourself with the information on poisoning available at the Centers for Disease Control and Prevention (CDC) website. This website documents recent trends and current statistics to help health care providers stay informed.

Words of Wisdom

In toxicology, it is important to observe and record all of the patient's symptoms and clinical signs. Do not dismiss subtle changes or seemingly benign symptoms that the patient may report. Thorough documentation may be the key in determining the substances to which the patient has been exposed.

Pathophysiology

Routes of Entry

A substance must first enter the body to have an effect. The four primary methods of entry are ingestion, inhalation, injection, and absorption. The rate at which the toxin is absorbed into the body varies based on the route of entry. After a toxin has entered the body, the combination of the amount of toxin and the relative speed at which it is metabolized affect both the bioavailability of the toxin and the excretion rate.

Poisoning by Ingestion

Ingested poisons may produce immediate damage to tissues, or the toxic effects may be delayed for several hours. Damage can occur rapidly when a caustic substance is ingested. A household cleaner that contains a strong acid or alkali substance will immediately cause significant damage to local tissues. Personal care products and cleaning products remain the most common ingestions for pediatric patients. Analgesics account for most ingestions by patients older than 20 years.[1]

For a patient who has ingested a toxic substance, you must consider all possibilities regarding the substance and whether the ingestion was intentional or unintentional. For example, consider a child who eats a liquid laundry detergent capsule after mistakenly thinking it is candy **FIGURE 28-3**. Now consider a person who is taking prescription medication for pain relief following a surgical procedure. To control the pain, the patient may take several doses of more than one opioid-containing medication. Both of these scenarios are considered unintentional ingestions.

Assessment clues pointing toward ingestion can be as obvious as a plant with partially chewed leaves or a section of plant with berries missing. Look for stained fingers, lips, or tongues. Any patient reporting the sudden onset of stomach cramps with or without nausea, vomiting, or diarrhea may have an ingestion-related condition. Prescription and OTC pill bottles can provide you with valuable information in your assessment of the patient and the scene. Pay particular attention to the date when the prescriptions were filled. Does it make sense that the pill bottle is empty 4 weeks after being filled? Possibly. What if the prescription was filled only

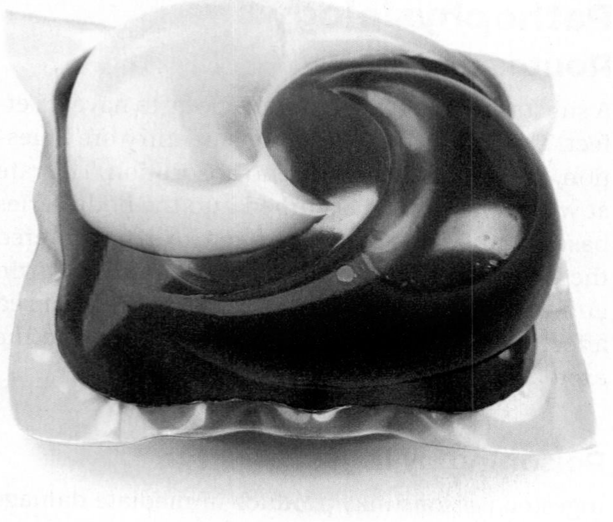

FIGURE 28-3 Although companies have created new safety features on detergent containers and have repackaged laundry detergent capsules (pictured) to make them less visually appealing to children, unintentional ingestions can still occur.

2 days earlier? These clues can paint vastly different pictures.

After a substance is ingested, the amount of time that it spends in the stomach may vary from person to person. Because little absorption occurs in the stomach, you have time to work on identifying the ingested substance. The goal of treatment is to develop a plan to either remove or neutralize the toxin before it has a chance to enter the small intestine, where most absorption takes place. The practice of forced vomiting via administration of ipecac is not indicated in any patient. Activated charcoal with sorbitol may be appropriate, depending on the substance, because it helps prevent the body from absorbing the poison. Activated charcoal is most effective when given close to the time of ingestion, and it may be more beneficial when treating an ingestion of extended-release capsules. Activated charcoal will not bind to certain substances, such as alcohols, so it should not be administered for ingestions of those substances. Gastric decontamination may occur at the hospital after an accurate clinical assessment and anticipated course of treatment has been determined.

Poisoning by ingestion may also occur in individuals attempting to hide or transport illicit drugs. "Body packers" hide drugs in their body cavities to secretly transport them, typically over international borders. The drugs are usually carefully packaged in selected materials, such as latex or condoms. "Body stuffers" (sometimes called "mules") rapidly swallow drugs in whatever packaging is immediately available to avoid imminent discovery by law enforcement. This packaging is susceptible to failure. Body packers and stuffers are susceptible to massive, life-threatening overdoses if drug packages unexpectedly open inside the body. Suspect body packing or body stuffing in situations where a massive overdose occurs in individuals traveling from abroad or attempting to flee law enforcement.

Poisoning by Inhalation

A person can be poisoned by inhalation when the toxic agent is present in the surrounding atmosphere. This situation also poses a high risk to you as a responder. Similar to ingestion, poisoning by inhalation can be either unintentional or intentional. Your scene size-up should include extra precautions when dealing with the possibility of an inhaled toxin. If the patient remains in the potentially hazardous environment, then any responder who attempts to move the patient should be fitted with an appropriate self-contained breathing apparatus. Do not make the mistake of rushing to the patient's aid only to become a patient yourself.

Even if an inhaled toxin was not included in your initial dispatch information, you must remain alert to this possibility as the cause of the patient's symptoms. For example, you are called to assess a man who has passed out at a swimming pool. En route, you may be thinking that the patient could have heat exhaustion or a cardiac condition. When you arrive, the fire department personnel inform you that they found two other people who had passed out behind a building next to the pool. At this point, warning sirens should be going off inside your head, and you should immediately reevaluate the safety of the scene. If you do not include the possibility of an inhaled poison, then you run the risk of missing this critical decision point. If you do not think about it, then you cannot catch it.

Also be aware of a method of suicide in the United States that places EMS, fire, and law enforcement officers at risk.[2] **Chemical suicide**, also called detergent suicide, is a method that involves mixing certain household chemicals in an enclosed space to create toxic gases (such as hydrogen sulfide and hydrogen cyanide), which are then inhaled. The resulting chemical vapors are often colorless and may or may not have a recognizable odor.

In scenarios involving chemical suicide, emergency responders are at risk of serious injury when attempting to access the vehicle, area, or patient after observing an unresponsive person inside. In some instances, the suicidal person has left a note, warning bystanders and emergency responders of the presence of toxic chemicals. Therefore, maintain your situational awareness and, before opening any door, be sure to read any note you come across. In other instances, bystanders attempting to render aid and emergency responders have been exposed to extremely hazardous chemicals while trying to access and assess a person who is already dead.

From a physiologic perspective, inhaled toxins are quick to produce signs and symptoms. The toxin enters the body through the respiratory tract and rapidly reaches the alveoli, where simple diffusion allows the toxin to cross the alveolar-capillary membrane and be readily transported through the cardiovascular system.

Carbon monoxide is an example of an inhaled toxin. It has a high affinity for hemoglobin and severe carbon monoxide poisoning is often fatal. In addition, rapid systemic distribution of carbon monoxide can occur with an equally rapid onset of signs and symptoms. For this reason, the window of opportunity for problem identification and subsequent treatment is limited. Carbon monoxide poisoning is discussed later in this chapter.

Words of Wisdom

Your diagnostic equipment is only one piece of the puzzle. Be aware that carbon monoxide and cyanide poisoning may result in falsely high pulse oximeter readings. Carbon monoxide binds to hemoglobin and does not let go, and cyanide impairs the offloading of oxygen at the cellular level. Therefore, do not get a false sense of security from an oxygen saturation reading of 100% in an acutely ill patient. If a patient is acutely short of breath following an exposure or suspected exposure, then administer a high concentration of oxygen. Consider using a handheld carbon monoxide oximeter (if available) to immediately assess for carbon monoxide in the patient's bloodstream.

When you are managing an inhalation incident, the first general consideration is that of scene safety. Only personnel fitted with the appropriate breathing apparatus should consider removing the patient or patients to a safe environment before beginning any assessment or treatment.

SAFETY

Scene safety is your primary concern when you are called to an inhalation incident. Be suspicious of some form of poisoning whenever you have multiple patients with similar complaints. It is your critical thinking that will save you; do not rely on your sense of sight or smell alone. Toxic fumes may be odorless and colorless, and they do not discriminate between responders and patients.

After you have identified the possibility of an inhalation incident, do not allow your emotions to cloud your ability to make sound decisions regarding your safety and that of your fellow responders. You cannot help your patient if you become a patient yourself.

Inhaled toxins produce a wide range of signs and symptoms, many of which are unique to the toxin involved. It is critical to use all of the information available to you to determine the toxins involved. For residential calls, rely on your suspicions and gut instincts. Ask appropriate questions regarding recent events and the potential substances involved. If you are in an industrial environment or a large workplace, search for clues such as a safety data sheet (SDS), a shipping manifest, a bill of lading, or transportation placards.

The National Library of Medicine has developed the Wireless Information System for Emergency Responders (WISER). WISER is available for download via personal computers, as well as smartphone applications. WISER provides information about hazardous chemicals and other substances, including human health and treatment information.[3]

Talk to the patient's coworkers about substances that may be located in the patient's work area or stored at the facility. That information, coupled with the assistance of the poison control center and direction from the medical control physician, will drive your treatment plan. Correction of hypoxia is a must; deliver a high concentration of oxygen and support adequate ventilation, if needed. Establish vascular access, apply an electrocardiogram (ECG) monitor, and perform pulse oximetry and capnography.

> **Words of Wisdom**
>
> E-cigarettes are popular due to their relatively low cost, myriad flavor options, and ability to be used indoors, but they are becoming a rare but emerging type of poisoning. The liquid nicotine contained in the e-cigarette is often the offending agent. The most common route of exposure is inhalation, but cases of ingestion and absorption through the skin or eyes have also been reported. Nausea, vomiting, and eye irritation are common symptoms following an exposure.[4]

Poisoning by Injection

Injected poisons usually gain access to the body due to stings or bites from various insects and animals. Depending on your geographic location, possibilities for poisoning by injection frequently exist in the environment. For example, snakebites and scorpion stings are more prevalent in the southwestern United States, whereas people in coastal areas are more likely to be stung by jellyfish, Portuguese man-of-wars, sea urchins, or sea anemones. Wasps, yellow jackets, and hornets have a wider geographic distribution.

Some of these injected poisons produce localized or systemic reactions, whereas others may be neurotoxic. When a bite or sting hits a blood vessel, the injected toxin immediately enters the bloodstream. The outcome is much more dangerous than when the same toxin enters a muscle mass, from which the toxin has a much slower rate of absorption and distribution.

When you assess bites and stings, physical findings will usually provide the most obvious clues, especially local reactions such as pain at the wound site. The patient's signs and symptoms can vary depending on the specific toxin. Occasionally, the patient may be able to identify the culprit, greatly simplifying the assessment process. Chapter 39, *Environmental Emergencies*, discusses bites and stings in detail.

Misuse of intravenous (IV) drugs such as heroin, cocaine, and amphetamines may prompt a call for EMS. *Speedballing* refers to the simultaneous use of heroin and cocaine. Although the patient or bystanders may not be forthcoming with information about the substances involved, you can focus your attention on the physical assessment, signs, and symptoms to help with possible identification. In addition, the patient's presentation will likely help guide you in identifying the type of drug involved. For example, drugs that are injected directly into the bloodstream will have a more rapid onset than those injected into the muscle or subcutaneous tissue.

> **SAFETY**
>
> All tools used to inject substances or puncture the skin should be considered biohazards. These needles, blades, or injection devices may have been shared with drug users and may carry the human immunodeficiency virus, hepatitis, or other pathogens. Make sure you do your part in disposing of hazardous materials by placing all sharps into a sharps container.

Poisoning by Absorption

Some poisons gain access to the body by being absorbed through the skin. When you consider the time from exposure to the emergence of symptoms, remember that substances that are absorbed through the skin have a longer time until onset of their effects compared to substances that are inhaled or injected. Poisonings caused by pesticides such as organophosphates and similar substances are often the most serious of the poisonings that occur by absorption. Because of the highly toxic nature of organophosphates, scene safety remains paramount when exposure to these substances is suspected. These patients may need to be decontaminated. Follow your agency's decontamination protocols, which may include using a hazardous materials (hazmat) team. Organophosphates are discussed in detail later in this chapter.

In 2017, the American College of Medical Toxicology (ACMT) and the American Academy of Clinical Toxicology (AACT) released a joint position statement addressing concerns related to possible occupational exposure to fentanyl and fentanyl analogs for emergency responders, including law enforcement, fire, and EMS personnel. This paper concluded that the risk of serious opioid toxicity is unlikely with proper education, training, and the use of standard EMS personal protective equipment (PPE), including nitrile examination gloves. If aerosolized particles are potentially present, the authors recommended that responders wear either an N-95 or a P-100 respirator mask to prevent inhalation.[5]

> **Words of Wisdom**
>
> Absorption of toxic substances through the skin is a common problem in the agriculture and manufacturing industries. Most solvents, insecticides, herbicides, and pesticides are toxic and can be readily absorbed through the skin.

Understanding and Using Toxidromes

When you consider the growing list of thousands of potentially harmful substances, OTC drugs, and prescription medications, you may feel overwhelmed. Fortunately, many different drugs react similarly after they enter the body. While performing a thorough patient assessment, you may be able to note a pattern in the signs and symptoms. For example, consider the category of stimulants. Regardless of whether the stimulant is a natural product derived from the coca plant (cocaine) or a synthetic compound created in a makeshift laboratory (methamphetamine), all drugs in this group work in a similar manner by stimulating the central nervous system (CNS), so they produce similar signs and symptoms. The syndromelike symptoms associated with a class or group of similar poisonous agents are termed a toxic syndrome, or **toxidrome**. Knowledge of common toxidromes can help guide your assessment and management of conditions involving different substances that fall under the same clinical umbrella. Six major toxidromes exist: opioid, sympathomimetic, sedative-hypnotic, cholinergic, anticholinergic, and serotonin syndrome **TABLE 28-1**. Toxidrome signs and symptoms can be masked or obscured in polypharmacy events.[6]

Common signs and symptoms of poisoning are listed in **TABLE 28-2**. If you consider the patient's history and physical exam findings in conjunction with their vital signs, you can develop a working diagnosis that will enable you to provide appropriate emergency medical care until you deliver the patient to the receiving facility. For example, suppose a patient has respiratory depression, bradycardia, hypotension, and constricted pupils. Using **TABLE 28-1**, you could see that opioids produce all of those signs and symptoms. Now imagine that a similar patient presents with the same symptoms, but has dilated pupils. Would that finding change your working diagnosis for the patient? If yes, which causative agent would be a better fit? Consider a barbiturate as the offending agent.

Overview of Substance Misuse

During your career as a paramedic, you will undoubtedly come in contact with patients who have substance use disorders. Apart from the physical effects of substance misuse, addiction carries a social stigma that can lead to feelings of isolation, paranoia, and depression. Innovative methods of synthesizing new drugs or altering existing drugs are constantly being developed to improve their effects. Because of these ongoing changes in the array of drugs that patients may be taking and the sheer number of drugs available today, scientists and researchers are faced with the never-ending task of documenting the effects of each substance and the potential for misuse.

In recent years, one of the most interesting discussions regarding the definition of substance misuse involves marijuana. For centuries, this drug was used recreationally for its euphoric and psychoactive properties. However, recent research has demonstrated medicinal uses for marijuana. For example, a marijuana extract called cannabidiol can be effective at controlling seizure activity. A specific type of marijuana has been designed to have a high cannabidiol content and a low tetrahydrocannabinol (THC; the psychoactive component of marijuana) content. The US Food and Drug Administration (FDA) has approved its use for treatment of severe forms of childhood epilepsy. The FDA has also approved the medications dronabinol and nabilone for the treatment of nausea and vomiting caused by chemotherapy and for the treatment of anorexia associated with weight loss in people with AIDS. Ongoing debate continues about whether its use for medical conditions outweighs the potential negatives associated with recreational use.

Another component of the discussion around substance misuse points out that the societal

TABLE 28-1 Major Toxidromes

Toxidrome	Drug Examples	Signs and Symptoms
Opioid	Morphine, codeine, heroin, methadone, opium, morphine, hydromorphone, fentanyl, oxycodone, and aspirin combination	Altered mental status, hypoventilation, respiratory arrest, constricted (pinpoint) pupils, bradycardia, hypotension, track marks (intravenous substance use disorder), drowsiness, coma
Sympathomimetic	Pseudoephedrine, phenylephrine, phenylpropanolamine, amphetamine, methamphetamine, cocaine, caffeine, nasal decongestants, synthetic cathinones (bath salts)	Hypertension, diaphoresis, tachycardia, tachypnea, dilated pupils (mydriasis), agitation, seizures, hyperthermia, delusions/paranoia
Sedative-hypnotic	Phenobarbital, secobarbital, diazepam, thiopental, midazolam, lorazepam, propofol, ethanol, flunitrazepam, zolpidem tartrate	Hypoventilation, respiratory arrest, drowsiness, disinhibition, ataxia, slurred speech, mental confusion, respiratory depression, progressive CNS depression, hypotension
Cholinergic	Organophosphates, acephate, diazinon, malathion, parathion, sarin, tabun, V agent	**DUMBELS** (Diarrhea, Urination, Miosis [constriction of the pupils]/Muscle weakness, Bradycardia/Bronchospasm/Bronchorrhea [discharge of mucus from the lungs], Emesis [vomiting], Lacrimation [excessive tearing of the eyes], Seizures/Salivation/Sweating), respiratory depression, apnea, coma, and tachycardia can occur early, with bradycardia developing as toxicity progresses
Anticholinergic	Atropine, scopolamine, antihistamines, diphenhydramine, chlorpheniramine, tricyclic antidepressants, antipsychotics, jimson weed	Red as a beet (flushed skin) Dry as a bone (dry skin) Mad as a hatter (altered mental status) Blind as a bat (mydriasis) Hot as a pistol (hyperthermia) Full as a flask (urinary retention) "Tachy" like a pink flamingo (tachycardia and hypertension)
Serotonin syndrome	Usually caused by the use of two or more serotonergic substances including SSRIs, SNRIs, MAOIs, tricyclic antidepressants, bupropion, illicit drugs (LSD, amphetamines, ecstasy, cocaine), opioids, herbal supplements (St. John's wort, ginseng, nutmeg), OTC medications containing dextromethorphan, antimigraine medications	Presentation with at least three of the following: agitation, ataxia, diaphoresis, diarrhea, hyperreflexia, mental status changes, myoclonus, shivering, tremor, hyperthermia, tachycardia

Abbreviations: CNS, central nervous system; LSD, lysergic acid diethylamide; MAOIs, monoamine oxidase inhibitors; OTC, over-the-counter; SNRIs, serotonin and norepinephrine reuptake inhibitors; SSRIs, selective serotonin reuptake inhibitors

Data from *National Model EMS Clinical Guidelines: Version 2.2.* National Association of State EMS Officials website. https://nasemso.org/wp-content/uploads/National-Model-EMS-Clinical-Guidelines-2017-PDF-Version-2.2.pdf. Published January 2019. Accessed September 30, 2021.

TABLE 28-2 Common Signs and Symptoms of Poisoning

Sign or Symptom	Type	Possible Causative Agents
Odor	Bitter almonds	Cyanide
	Garlic	Arsenic, organophosphates, phosphorus
	Acetone	Methyl alcohol, isopropyl alcohol, aspirin, acetone, diabetes
	Wintergreen	Methyl salicylate
	Pears	Chloral hydrate
	Violets	Turpentine
	Camphor	Camphor
	Alcohol	Alcohol
Pupils	Constricted	Opioids, organophosphates, jimson weed, nutmeg, propoxyphene (Darvon)
	Dilated	Barbiturates, atropine, amphetamine, glutethimide (Doriden), LSD, cyanide, carbon monoxide
Mouth	Salivation	Organophosphates, arsenic, strychnine, mercury, salicylates
	Dry mouth	Atropine (belladonna), amphetamines, diphenhydramine (Benadryl), opioids
	Burns in mouth	Formaldehyde, iodine, lye, toxic plants, phenols, phosphorus, pine oil, silver nitrate, acids
Skin	Pruritus	Jimson weed, belladonna, boric acid
	Dry, hot skin	Atropine (in belladonna), botulism, nutmeg
	Sweating	Organophosphates, arsenic, aspirin, amphetamines, barbiturates, mushrooms, naphthalene
Respiratory	Depressed respirations	Opioids, alcohol, propoxyphene, carbon monoxide, barbiturates
	Increased respirations	Aspirin, amphetamines, boric acid, cyanide, kerosene, methyl alcohol, nicotine
	Pulmonary edema	Organophosphates, petroleum products, opioids, carbon monoxide
Cardiovascular	Tachycardia	Alcohol, amphetamines, arsenic, atropine, aspirin, cocaine, some antiasthma drugs
	Bradycardia	Beta blockers, calcium channel blockers, digitalis, gasoline, nicotine, mushrooms, opioids, cyanide, mistletoe, rhododendron
	Hypertension	Amphetamines, lead, nicotine, antiasthma drugs
	Hypotension	Beta blockers, calcium channel blockers, barbiturates, opioids, tranquilizers, house plants, mistletoe, nitroglycerin, antifreeze
Central nervous system	Seizures	Amphetamines, camphor, cocaine, strychnine, arsenic, carbon monoxide, petroleum products, scorpion sting
	Coma	All depressant drugs (such as opioids, barbiturates, tranquilizers, alcohol), carbon monoxide, cyanide
	Hallucinations	Atropine, LSD, mushrooms, organic solvents, PCP, nutmeg
	Headache	Carbon monoxide, alcohol, disulfiram (Antabuse)
	Tremors	Organophosphates, carbon monoxide, amphetamines, tranquilizers, poisonous marine animals
	Weakness or paralysis	Organophosphates, botulism, eel, hemlock, pufferfish, pine oil, rhododendron
Gastrointestinal	Cramps, nausea, vomiting, and/or diarrhea	Many, if not most, ingested poisons

Abbreviations: LSD, lysergic acid diethylamide; PCP, phencyclidine

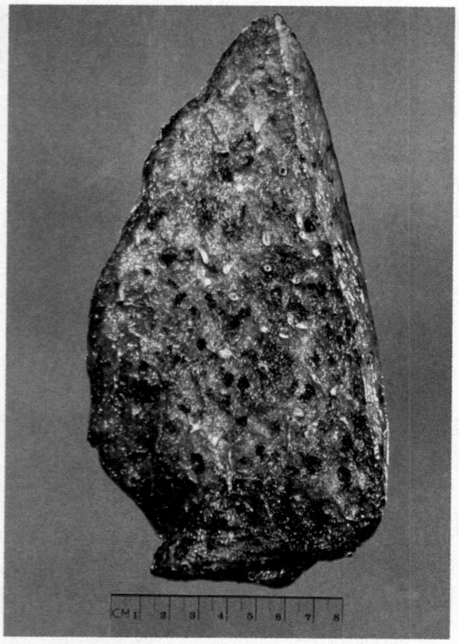

FIGURE 28-4 A diseased lung due to frequent tobacco use.

Street Smarts

As a key health advocate in your community, be mindful of the words you use to describe substance use disorders. Words that negatively characterize a person, such as "addict," "alcoholic," or "substance abuser," can reinforce a person's feelings of shame and guilt. Individuals who do not feel worthy of treatment or who fear the social judgment that might result from seeking treatment are obviously less likely to receive the treatment they need. Moreover, when these biased words are used in legal proceedings, the person is more likely to be deemed a criminal and punished more severely.[7] Using nonjudgmental wording, such as "substance use disorder," "substance misuse," and "addiction to alcohol," has been shown to decrease stigma around these disorders and improve a person's likelihood of seeking treatment.[7] Choose your words carefully, and encourage your coworkers and other members of your community to do likewise.

definition of misuse may have little relation to the potential harm from the misused substance. For example, other than states' decision to set a legal age for purchasing tobacco, our culture places no restrictions on the long-term and compulsive use of this substance, even though it is a significant contributor to cardiovascular and respiratory disease **FIGURE 28-4**. By comparison, use of marijuana is less likely to cause long-term lung and heart problems (when used in an occasional, recreational context), yet it is often punishable by fines or imprisonment. There is a growing movement to decriminalize or legalize recreational marijuana use in many jurisdictions.

Words of Wisdom

Substance use disorder is not limited to members of the younger generation or to any particular section of society. It occurs in all age groups and at all social levels.

The following list defines some basic terms and concepts related to substance misuse:

- **Drug misuse**. Any use of a drug that causes physical, psychological, economic, legal, or social harm to the user or others affected by the user's behavior.
- **Habituation**. A physical and psychological dependence on a drug.
- **Physical dependence**. A physiologic state of adaptation to a drug caused by chronic use, usually characterized by tolerance to the effects of the drug and withdrawal if use of the drug is stopped (especially abruptly).
- **Psychological dependence**. The emotional state of craving a drug to maintain a feeling of well-being.
- **Tolerance**. Physiologic adaptation to the effects of a drug such that increasingly larger doses of the drug are required to achieve the same effect.
- **Withdrawal syndrome**. A predictable set of signs and symptoms, usually involving altered CNS activity, that occurs after the abrupt cessation of a drug or after a rapid decrease in the usual dosage of a drug.
- **Drug addiction**. A chronic disorder characterized by the compulsive use of a substance that results in physical, psychological, economic, legal, or social harm to the user; the user continues to use the substance despite the harm.
- **Antagonist**. A molecule that blocks the ability of a given chemical to bind to its receptor, preventing a biologic response.

- **Potentiation**. The enhancement of the effect of one drug by another drug.
- **Synergism**. The action of two substances such as drugs, in which the total effects are greater than the sum of the independent effects of the two substances.

Patient Assessment

The general assessment approach is the same for all patients: scene size-up, primary survey, history taking, secondary assessment, and reassessment. If the patient's mental status is altered, diligently monitor the patient's airway and breathing to prevent aspiration and ensure adequate minute ventilation. Prepare your suction equipment. Ensure you get a good overall clinical picture of the patient. For example, is the patient able to maintain the airway, or is the patient struggling to swallow and clear secretions? If the patient is unresponsive, obtain vital signs and complete a rapid full-body scan; obtain the patient history from bystanders and family members, if possible. If the patient is responsive, then use the OPQRST mnemonic (Onset, Provocation/palliation, Quality, Region/radiation, Severity, Timing) to elaborate on the chief complaint. Next, obtain the patient's vital signs and a SAMPLE history (Signs and symptoms, Allergies, Medications, Pertinent past history, Last oral intake, Events leading up to the illness or injury). Then perform a rapid full-body scan before moving on to a thorough physical exam.

Do not forget that patients with toxicologic emergencies may also have sustained traumatic injuries before your arrival.

Scene Size-up

Scene safety is paramount with toxicologic emergencies. Continually reevaluate your surroundings from the moment you arrive at the scene. As you approach the patient, look for clues such as pill bottles, household cleaners, or handwritten notes that may be useful to you **FIGURE 28-5**. Be aware that patients who have taken an overdose may be

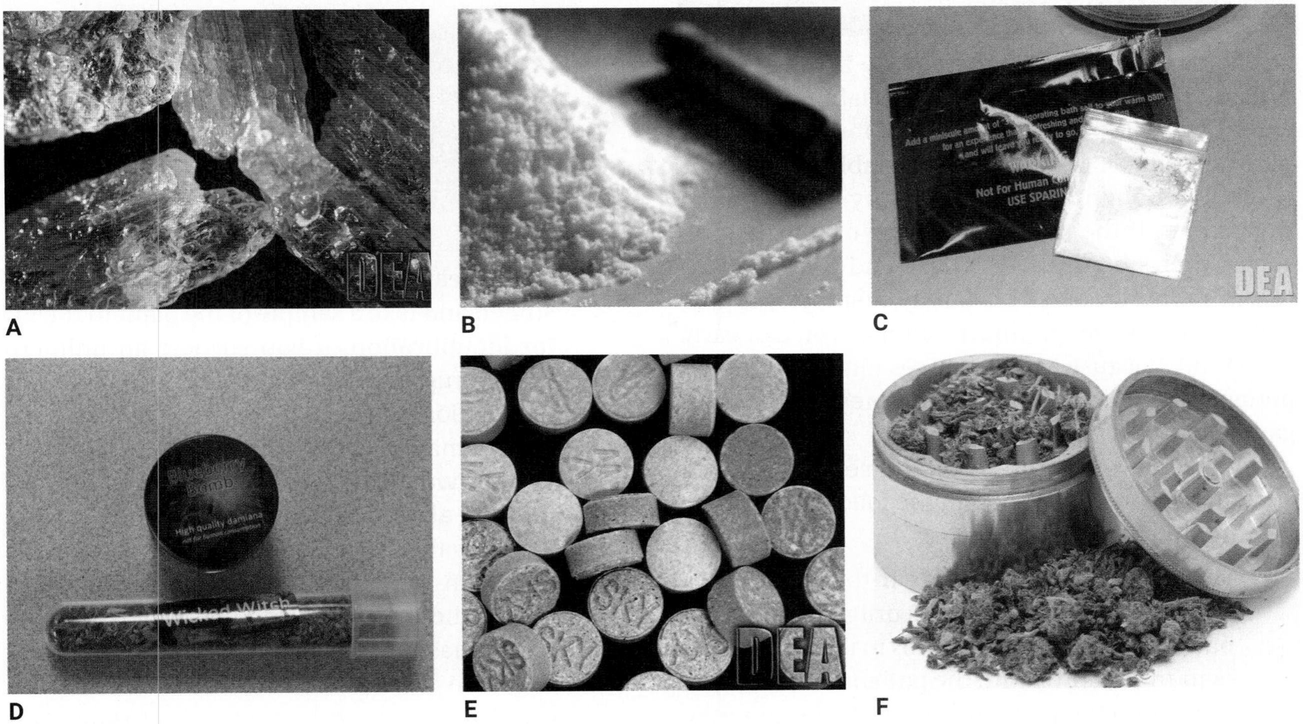

FIGURE 28-5 Misused substances include a wide and ever-evolving range of street drugs such as methamphetamine **(A)**, cocaine **(B)**, bath salts (Flakka) **(C)**, synthetic cannabinoids (Spice) **(D)**, Ecstasy **(E)**, and marijuana **(F)**.

A, C, D, and **E:** Courtesy of US Department of Justice, Drug Enforcement Administration; **B:** © Andrew Burns/Shutterstock; **F:** © iStock/Thinkstock/Getty Images.

extremely dangerous. If necessary, call for law enforcement backup or a crisis unit to minimize the potential for injury to you and your team.

Primary Survey

The primary survey of a patient who has overdosed on drugs or has been poisoned begins with forming your general impression. It can be as simple as "an adult woman lying prone on the bed." The primary survey seeks to rapidly identify life threats: any concerns with mental status, airway, breathing, and circulation that require rapid intervention. By the end of your primary survey, you should be able to identify the nature of illness (NOI) or possible mechanism of injury (MOI). Based on your findings, you can determine the severity of the patient's condition and begin to establish your priorities for the rest of the call.

Basic airway management is a crucial skill that will allow you time to obtain the information needed to make the appropriate patient treatment decisions. If you can ventilate the patient effectively, then you have time to decide what needs to be done.

History Taking

Toxicologic emergencies frequently involve symptomatic patients, so you need to elaborate on the chief complaint using the OPQRST mnemonic as part of history taking. Work to establish a rapport while you obtain a SAMPLE history directly from the patient. If the patient is unable or unwilling to speak, then obtain the OPQRST and SAMPLE history from bystanders and family members, if possible. Obtain as much information as you can early in the call, because acute changes may occur in the patient's mental status that could prevent you from gathering additional information.

To choose the appropriate course of action in a toxicologic emergency, obtain the following specific information at a minimum:

- **What is the substance?** If the patient has overdosed on a prescription drug, bring the pill bottle and the remaining pills to the emergency department (ED) with the patient **FIGURE 28-6**. Consider taking the SDS if available. You may also copy or photograph the drug label information for review by the hospital staff if you cannot safely transport the container. If the patient ingested a plant, then find out what part (roots, leaves, stem, flower, or fruit) was consumed and take a sample of the plant to the ED for identification. If you suspect an unintentional drug overdose, ask questions about any medications, OTC drugs, or home remedies the patient may have been taking.
- **When was the substance ingested, injected, absorbed, or inhaled?** Time often works against you when treating a patient who has been exposed to a toxic substance. The longer the toxin is inside the body, the more time it has to cause its effects. It is important to obtain an accurate timeline for the poisoning. As a general rule, acute-onset symptoms often indicate a more serious patient scenario than delayed-onset symptoms; for example, if the patient immediately began to have crushing chest pain after smoking crack cocaine.

FIGURE 28-6 If the patient has overdosed on a prescription drug, bring the medication container and its remaining contents to the emergency department.

Special Populations

In an unintentional overdose or poisoning, an older adult patient may have become confused about their drug regimen. The person may have forgotten if a dose of medication had been taken and may repeat the dose one or more times. The patient may also have forgotten the physician's instructions to discard leftover medication and might have taken both the current medication and the older drug, resulting in increased effects or unwanted drug interactions.

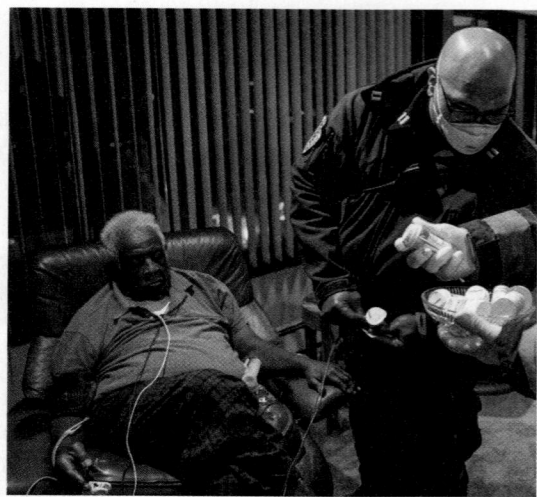

- **How much was taken, injected, absorbed, or inhaled?** In almost all cases, the toxin dosage is directly proportional to its toxic effects on the body. An unintentional overdose commonly involves taking too much of a medication. It may be more difficult for you to determine the quantity that was taken in an intentional overdose. The patient may be unwilling or unable to tell you how much was taken, so you must rely on your observational skills. Observe the drug label to determine how much of the medication would have been in the container when it was full, and compare that quantity with the amount that remains.
- **What else was taken?** The majority of intentional self-poisonings (suicide attempts) or illicit drug overdoses involve polydrug ingestions, often with alcohol as one of the drugs. The patient may also have tried to take an antidote. This information can be invaluable to ED staff when deciding which laboratory tests to order.

Documentation and Communication

When you document the contents of any medication bottle, be specific about the number and type of pills that you counted, even if several different types of pills are present in one bottle. Consider having another individual, such as a nurse at the ED, count the pills on your arrival at the hospital. This practice will help to account for all of the medications that were present when you delivered the patient to the hospital. Include the details of this count (including who was present) in your documentation. This step is considered a best practice and will help mitigate any claims if medications go missing.

Documentation and Communication

As a paramedic, you are the only reliable link between the emergency scene and the hospital. The hospital staff will look to you to provide them with relevant information from the scene. Ensure you have obtained all of the pertinent details about the substance involved in a poisoning while you are on scene. Write down the type and amount of substances involved. Finally, ensure your verbal and written reports are complete and thorough.

- **Has the patient vomited or aspirated?** If so, then how soon after the ingestion or exposure? How much? Inspect the vomitus for pill fragments. If the patient vomited into a clear emesis bag, then consider transporting the contents to the ED.
- **Why was the substance taken?** Ask this question of every patient. Do not make assumptions. The patient may have taken the substance mistakenly, or it could be a suicide attempt caused by severe depression. Whenever possible, use quotation marks to record the patient's own words in the patient care report.

Secondary Assessment

After completing the primary survey, begin the secondary assessment. Toxicologic emergencies are often medical emergencies only. Complete the appropriate secondary assessment for every patient. Recall that the secondary assessment is a systematic scan that allows you to observe any abnormalities that may be present. Toxins can either target a single body system or result in a critical systemic event. You must be able to appreciate the differences that may be present based on the interactions of the toxin with the body. These interactions may range from subtle tachypnea to obvious organophosphate poisoning with abnormal findings in almost every body system. Do not hesitate to use the major toxidromes (see Table 28-1) or mnemonics to help you remember the wide variety of abnormal presentations associated with toxicologic emergencies.

Patients with a toxicologic emergency may have alterations in mental status and may be suscpetible to nausea and vomiting. Nausea and vomiting may result in a critical airway problem, so be sure to perform a thorough assessment and develop a plan of action based on your findings.

Controversies

If a pediatric patient is in stable condition and has a history of a single, small ingestion of a low-risk agent, then some EMS systems allow the transport to be canceled after agreement from medical control. Although this approach may be medically sound, it eliminates an opportunity for assessment of psychosocial and risk factors in the ED.

If trauma is also present, perform the appropriate trauma assessment (rapid full-body scan or focused exam) based on whether the patient has a significant MOI. Because some patients with a toxicologic emergency may have gruesome self-inflicted injuries (eg, self-evisceration), focus on completing your entire exam. You must be able to properly prioritize your treatment and interventions.

Reassessment

Reassessment focuses on monitoring the patient's condition, reprioritizing the patient's status if necessary, and checking the effectiveness of the interventions provided. Reassessment is typically done in the ambulance while en route to the ED. Continually monitor all patients who have ingested, injected, absorbed, or inhaled a poisonous substance.

Emergency Medical Care

From a management perspective, advanced life support care for toxicologic emergencies builds on the following basics:

- Ensure the scene is safe for access and egress.
- Maintain the airway.
- Ensure breathing is adequate.
- Ensure circulation is not compromised (ie, either by hypoperfusion or a dysrhythmia).
- Administer supplemental oxygen to maintain saturation levels greater than 94%.
- Establish vascular access.
- Consider administration of an antidote or mitigating medication, if available.
- Prepare to manage shock, coma, seizures, and dysrhythmias.
- Transport the patient as soon as possible. If any risk of vomiting exists, then place the patient in the left lateral recumbent position to reduce the risk of aspiration.

Pathophysiology, Assessment, and Management of Misuse of and Overdose With Specific Substances

Alcohol

The form of alcohol consumed by humans in alcoholic beverages is ethyl alcohol (or ethanol). It is not conventionally recognized as a poison, even though it has many properties of a poison when ingested in sufficient quantities. Nevertheless, alcohol is undeniably part of human society. People commonly drink alcohol to relax, socialize, and celebrate. According to a 2019 study by the National Institute

YOU are the Paramedic

PART 2

You check the patient's carotid pulse and note it is strong and regular at a rate of 100 beats/min. The patient is breathing at a rate of about 4 breaths/min, so you ask your partner to place a nasopharyngeal airway and assist the patient's respirations with a bag-mask device connected to supplemental oxygen. While you consider a list of differential diagnoses, you turn to the family members to ask about the events leading up to the 9-1-1 call.

Recording Time: 2 Minutes	
Appearance	Unconscious
Level of consciousness	Unresponsive
Airway	Open
Breathing	4 breaths/min
Circulation	Carotid pulse strong and regular at 100 beats/min

3. If this patient has overdosed, then which drug classification would be your focus?
4. Give some examples of drugs that would meet this classification.

on Alcohol Abuse and Alcoholism (NIAAA), approximately 86% of people age 18 years or older have consumed alcohol at some point in their lives. Furthermore, almost 26% of people age 18 years or older reported that they had engaged in binge drinking (occasional heavy use) within the past month.[8]

The NIAAA describes alcohol misuse as "drinking in a manner, situation, amount, or frequency that could cause harm to the person who is engaging in drinking or to those around them."[9] Thus, alcohol use by individuals younger than the minimum legal drinking age or by pregnant individuals constitutes alcohol misuse.[9] With increased alcohol use comes an increased risk of developing **alcohol use disorder**, a medical condition characterized by a physical and psychological addiction to ethanol that can range from mild to severe. This condition is considered a brain disorder. Changes in the brain resulting from alcohol misuse perpetuate the condition, making the individual susceptible to relapse.[10] Alcohol use disorder encompasses the conditions formerly referred to as alcohol abuse, alcohol dependence, alcohol addiction, and alcoholism.

From million-dollar gated communities to low-income housing developments, alcohol use disorder occurs in all social strata and in almost every culture. The American Psychiatric Association's *Diagnostic and Statistical Manual of Mental Disorders, Fifth Edition,* outlines criteria used to diagnose someone with an alcohol use disorder. Common warning signs include the following:[11]

- Consuming alcohol in large quantities or over a long period
- Spending considerable time in activities necessary to obtain alcohol, use alcohol, or recover from its effects
- Causing or exacerbating social or interpersonal problems due to alcohol use
- Reducing social, occupational, or recreational activities due to alcohol use
- Continuing to use alcohol even after acknowledging the physical or psychological problems that are caused or exacerbated by alcohol use

Pathophysiology

As mentioned previously, psychological dependence on alcohol involves drinking to function "normally" and feel good. Alcohol acts as a depressant in the frontal lobe and can alter the decision-making process and/or decrease a person's inhibitions. Because of the disinhibition and euphoria that can accompany alcohol consumption, people often use alcohol as a "social lubricant" to feel more comfortable in social situations. In some people, the perception of social acceptance or increased social ease may influence them to drink more. People may feel as though they can escape their worries or become more likeable while they are under the influence of alcohol. The psychological dependence may escalate to a point where people feel they require alcohol to survive socially or emotionally.

Physical dependence results from the regular consumption of large quantities of alcohol. At this level of dependence, should a person abruptly stop consuming alcohol, withdrawal symptoms will result. The severity of the withdrawal can vary according to the severity of the dependence. Minor withdrawal is characterized by restlessness, anxiousness, difficulty sleeping, agitation, and tremors. For those with a more serious physical dependence, sudden abstinence can cause significant symptoms, such as hypertension, tachycardia, vomiting, hallucinations, and delirium tremens (discussed later in this chapter).

Words of Wisdom

You will commonly encounter patients who have consumed alcohol. When you assess a patient with an altered mental status and a history of recent alcohol consumption, never assume that the patient is "just intoxicated." Perform the appropriate assessments and remember to consider other possible causes for the altered mental status.

People with severe dependence may go to extreme lengths to obtain alcohol. People with chronic alcohol use disorder (or those without the financial means to afford alcoholic beverages) may resort to drinking hazardous products with alcohol content (eg, mouthwash, hand sanitizer). When you treat a patient who has ingested a toxic substance just for the alcohol content, always consider the other ingredients of those substances. For example, the toxic chemical methanol is sometimes used in hand sanitizers and can cause critical illness or death when consumed.

A person with alcohol use disorder is susceptible to many serious illnesses and injuries **TABLE 28-3**. Alcohol has profound effects on the neurologic, cardiovascular, and gastrointestinal (GI) systems.

The CNS is particularly vulnerable to alcohol misuse. From neurotransmitter imbalances to structural breakdown of the cells, the body will experience slower cognitive and motor function capabilities when a person consumes alcohol. You may note slurred speech, memory loss, and an unsteady gait in a severely intoxicated patient because of alcohol's effects on neurotransmitters (such as glutamate).

As alcohol travels through the digestive system, it irritates the tissues there and can damage the stomach lining by causing acid imbalances, inflammation, and acute gastric distress. Often, the result is gastritis (an inflamed stomach), gastroesophageal reflux disease, or heartburn. The more frequently someone drinks, the more likely it is that the GI system will be irritated. Alcohol misuse is also a risk factor for some cancers, specifically cancer of the mouth and esophagus. The National Cancer Institute reports that approximately 3.5% of all cancer deaths are related to alcohol use. People who consume alcohol are up to five times more likely to develop certain types of cancer than those who do not consume alcohol.[12]

The toxic effects of alcohol on the liver produce a variety of complications, such as coagulopathies (easy bleeding and poor clotting ability), hypoglycemia, and GI bleeding. Through manifestations ranging from fatty liver disease to cirrhosis, alcohol can significantly affect the body's ability to metabolize and filter harmful substances. This impairment also causes a fluid backup and may lead to elevated pressures in the hepatic system. As pressures rise, smaller vessels leading into the liver can become

TABLE 28-3 Medical Conditions to Which People With Alcohol Use Disorder Are Particularly Susceptible

Condition	Contributing Factors
Subdural hematoma	Frequent falls; impaired clotting mechanisms; brain atrophy allows for significant movement during impact
Gastrointestinal bleeding	Irritation of stomach lining (leading to gastritis); impaired clotting mechanisms; cirrhosis (excess scar tissue) of the liver, leading to engorgement of esophageal veins (esophageal varices)
Pancreatitis	Secretion of enzymes, causing inflammation
Hypoglycemia	Damage to the liver; impairs gluconeogenesis
Pneumonia	Aspiration of vomitus occurring during intoxication and coma; suppression of immune system by alcohol
Burns	Risky behaviors during intoxication; decreased pain sensitivity during intoxication
Hypothermia	Insensitivity to extremes of temperatures while intoxicated; falling asleep outside in the cold; impaired thermoregulation
Seizures	Effect of withdrawal from alcohol; neurotransmitter or electrolyte imbalance
Dysrhythmias (atrial fibrillation or ventricular tachycardia)	Toxic effects of alcohol on the heart; hypertension; electrolyte imbalance
Cancer	Products of alcohol metabolized by the liver are toxic to cells; may cause alterations in normal cellular pathways
Esophageal varices	Develop when normal blood flow to the liver is blocked and blood backs up into smaller, more fragile blood vessels in the esophagus

engorged with blood and swell. This swelling is the pathology behind esophageal varices, which can rupture and cause bleeding into the esophagus and oropharynx. This condition requires rapid suctioning and effective airway management.

Acute Alcohol Intoxication

Alcohol suppresses excitatory neurotransmitters, so it acts as a CNS depressant. When you consider the amount of alcohol that someone has consumed, you must also account for the person's size. For example, a 240-pound (109-kg) man may consume three drinks and have a blood alcohol content (BAC) of 0.07% (note that most states define legal intoxication as a BAC of 0.08% or more). However, a woman weighing 140 pounds (64 kg) may consume the same three drinks and have a BAC of 0.14%. Always look at the entire clinical picture. Keep in mind the concept of proportion.[13] Symptoms usually progress proportionately to BAC. Death from alcohol intoxication can occur with blood alcohol levels of 0.40% (400 mg/dL).[14]

SAFETY

You should remain alert for unexpected violent or bizarre behavior from individuals with alcohol intoxication. Take steps to keep you and your team safe during encounters with intoxicated individuals, especially at scenes where multiple intoxicated individuals are present.

One of the most significant risks to an acutely intoxicated person is from respiratory depression and/or aspiration of vomitus, secondary to the inability to protect the airway. If an intoxicated patient is unconscious, then treat them as you would any unconscious patient. Assess the patency of the airway. Is the patient able to maintain their airway? Is the patient swallowing spontaneously? Are secretions pooled in the oropharynx (a clear indicator of a markedly depressed or absent gag reflex)? Because of the high risk for aspiration, consider advanced airway management if the patient is unable to maintain their airway. Always have suction equipment prepared and within arm's reach.

In addition, provide supplemental oxygen to maintain adequate oxygen saturation levels. Assist ventilations as needed. Do not use excessive force when ventilating the patient. Gastric insufflation may cause vomiting and further complicate airway management if you ventilate with excessive force or too quickly. Establish vascular access. Monitor the ECG rhythm. Assess the patient's blood glucose level, and treat hypoglycemia if it is found. Local protocols or online medical control may direct the administration of IV thiamine to prevent Wernicke-Korsakoff syndrome (acute onset of confusion and delirium secondary to thiamine deficiency). Finally, transport the patient to an appropriate facility.

Words of Wisdom

Alcohol may be one small piece of the clinical puzzle. Although the odor of ethyl alcohol on the breath of an intoxicated patient may be one of the most obvious signs during your assessment, remember that alcohol is often used in conjunction with other substances in both unintentional and intentional overdoses.

Withdrawal Seizures

A person who has been drinking heavily for an extended period and suddenly stops drinking may experience a variety of withdrawal phenomena. Seizures usually occur within about 12 to 48 hours, but may occur as quickly as 6 hours after the last drink or as late as 72 hours after. The approach to a patient with withdrawal seizures should be similar to your treatment of an intoxicated patient. Short, isolated seizures do not require treatment, but medical control may direct the administration of a benzodiazepine as prophylaxis against another seizure. Prolonged seizures usually respond to lorazepam. Keep in mind that patients with chronic alcohol use disorder may have cross-tolerance to medications used to treat withdrawal or seizure activity.[14]

Words of Wisdom

Alcohol can impair an individual's ability to make health care decisions such as refusal of treatment or transport. Carefully assess the patient's decision-making capacity when alcohol use is suspected and consult medical direction as needed.

Delirium Tremens

One of the most serious and potentially lethal complications of alcohol withdrawal is **delirium tremens (DTs)**. Symptoms usually start 48 to 72 hours after the last alcohol intake, although the onset could be delayed by several days. Signs and symptoms include confusion, tremors, restlessness, fever, diaphoresis, tachycardia, and hypotension, often secondary to dehydration. The patient experiencing DTs is susceptible to vivid hallucinations and is extremely responsive to external stimuli. Cognitive function often decreases as the heart rate and temperature increase. The condition may result in increased mortality if the patient is not treated aggressively.

The treatment of a patient with DTs aims to protect the patient from injury and support the cardiovascular system. Try to keep the patient calm. Minimize external stimuli if possible. Do not position yourself in a dark area because the patient may confuse you for something else (such as a threat) during the hallucinations. Follow local protocols for benzodiazepine administration if the patient is agitated or combative. Physical restraints may cause additional agitation and could worsen the patient's condition, but always consider your safety first. Consider contacting online medical control to discuss aggressive benzodiazepine use. In addition, administer supplemental oxygen and establish vascular access. Manage hypotension with an infusion of normal saline; this administration may also help to manage increasing body temperature. Maintain an ongoing dialogue with the patient throughout transport to help orient and reassure the patient.

Stimulants

Stimulants, in both licit and illicit forms, can have devastating effects on those people who misuse them. Stimulants may range from smokable cocaine (crack) and methamphetamine (meth) to prescription diet aids and medications for attention-deficit disorder. At some point in your career as a paramedic, you will undoubtedly care for a patient who is under the influence of stimulants.

Stimulants come in various forms that allow for absorption by ingestion, inhalation, or injection. Most stimulants work to enhance the release of catecholamines, which stimulate the CNS (specifically, alpha and beta receptors). This CNS stimulation can increase alertness and create a sense of euphoria.

YOU are the Paramedic

PART 3

Your partner has placed a nasopharyngeal airway and is assisting the patient's breathing with a bag-mask device and supplemental oxygen while you finish the rapid full-body scan. You note that the patient is unresponsive with respiratory depression and pinpoint pupils. The pulse oximeter reading was initially 90%, but has been steadily rising. The family members report that the patient was prescribed 10 mg of hydrocodone for pain control after her surgical procedure. The prescription was filled 4 days earlier, and only two tablets are missing from the bottle. You wonder if two tablets could have produced such a dramatic patient presentation.

Recording Time: 5 Minutes	
Respirations	Assisted via bag-mask device
Pulse	100 beats/min
Skin	Cyanosis around lips; dry and cool
Blood pressure	92/58 mm Hg
Oxygen saturation (Spo_2)	90% room air; rising with bag-mask ventilation
Pupils	Pinpoint, nonreactive

5. Should you intubate this patient?

6. What is your next step in treating this patient after the airway is controlled?

However, increased catecholamine release can also lead to agitation, hyperthermia, tachycardia, hypertension, and seizures.

CNS excitation can create agitation, anxiousness, delirium, and dilated pupils. You may observe the patient struggling to sit still and fidgeting frequently. Hyperthermia and tachycardia will cause the patient to be hypermetabolic. You may note profuse sweating while assessing the skin. Because the body is constantly running at a faster rate and depleting energy stores, the person who chronically uses stimulants may appear thin. You may observe signs of drug misuse, such as track marks from IV injection or burns to the fingers from a crack cocaine pipe. Remember that patients who use or misuse stimulants may be sleep deprived, anxious, and even paranoid. Always maintain your situational awareness to ensure a safe environment for you and your partner.

SAFETY

While treating a patient experiencing the effects of a potent sympathomimetic, sedatives may be used to help safely treat and transport the patient. Do not allow the patient's agitation or combativeness to distract you while calculating an appropriate dose for the patient. Take the time to double check the dose and the volume that you are preparing to administer. Before administering the sedative, communicate the dose to your partner. This step could help prevent a serious medication error.

Cocaine

Cocaine is a naturally occurring alkaloid that is extracted from the leaves of the *Erythroxylon coca* plant, which grows in South America. After the leaves are processed into cocaine hydrochloride, the active ingredient in the leaves increases in potency. In the 19th and early 20th centuries, elixirs often contained cocaine as an active ingredient to treat various illnesses. Ear, nose, and throat physicians once used cocaine as a local anesthetic. The euphoric and addictive qualities of cocaine have contributed to its demand on the streets.

According to the 2019 National Survey on Drug Use and Health, cocaine use has declined slightly among people ages 12 to 25 years, but the overall use among people age 26 years and older has remained largely the same.[15] The amount of biologically active cocaine present may vary from one form to another. Some variance may exist based on the amount of filler (which potentially may consist of toxic adulterants) used to dilute or "cut" the drug. The higher the purity of the cocaine, the more serious the potential for dependence becomes. In other words, people who occasionally use a less pure solution of the drug will not be as psychologically or physiologically dependent as someone who is using a purer solution. Cocaine users with serious dependence problems may have significant health conditions as well as social and psychological challenges.

Pathophysiology

Cocaine is a local anesthetic and a nervous system stimulant. It enhances the release and activity of neurotransmitters in the body, including norepinephrine, dopamine, and serotonin. The enhanced dopamine activity is responsible for the euphoria experienced with cocaine use, which features enhanced alertness and a tremendous sense of well-being. Collectively, this constellation of effects makes cocaine one of if not the most psychologically addictive drugs available. The enhanced norepinephrine activity results in stimulation of the sympathetic nervous system. The physical manifestation of this stimulation accounts for many of the common adverse effects associated with cocaine use, such as tachycardia, hypertension, and hyperthermia. In addition, this sympathetic nervous system stimulation can place every organ system at risk due to significant vasoconstriction, along with increased cellular metabolic and oxygen demands.

One chemical form of cocaine, water-soluble hydrochloride salt, is quickly absorbed across all mucosal membranes, allowing it to be applied topically, insufflated (snorted), swallowed, or injected intravenously. Another form of cocaine, crack cocaine, is simply cocaine mixed with two inexpensive ingredients, baking soda and water. After the ingredients are mixed together into a pastelike slurry and cooked or baked, the end result is smokable cocaine.

When cocaine is snorted nasally, the patient may begin to feel high within 1 to 5 minutes. When crack cocaine is smoked and the alveoli are bathed in cocaine-laden smoke, the onset of effects is much more rapid (in the 8- to 10-second range). Injection of cocaine has a similarly rapid onset as it enters the cerebral circulation. Smoking and injecting cocaine are known to produce a rush followed by a high.[16] The duration of the effects will depend on the patient's tolerance level and the purity of the drug. People who have a high tolerance level or commonly use higher-purity cocaine may seek to repeat their doses more frequently due to the body's dependence on higher levels of the drug.

When the effects of cocaine wear off, the user experiences a so-called crash, which is characterized by depression, irritability, and exhaustion. Depending on the amount and length of cocaine use, the person may experience a cascade of adverse effects collectively referred to as *cocaine washout syndrome*. This syndrome presents as a hypoactive state related to a lack of synaptic neurotransmitters. Large quantities of neurotransmitters interact with the central and peripheral nervous systems while the user is experiencing the high. After the effects of cocaine wear off, all of those neurotransmitters become less active or unavailable for use by the body.

The patient who is experiencing cocaine washout syndrome may be difficult to assess. Signs of hyperactivity may have already dissipated. However, the patient may be on the downward slope of the high, so the patient may be hypoactive. Remember to assess for other pathology during your assessment. Consider other potential and far more ominous causes of the patient's hypoactive state, such as stroke or myocardial infarction (MI) with profound shock.

Adding to the problem, a person with cocaine addiction who is trying to avoid the unpleasant effects of a crash may take more cocaine or a sedative (such as diazepam [Valium], alcohol, or heroin). This could result in the patient having several types of drugs in their system when they require assistance from EMS. People with heroin addiction may use cocaine to withdraw or detoxify themselves from heroin by gradually decreasing the amounts of heroin taken while increasing the amounts of cocaine used.

Assessment

A person who has overdosed on cocaine may exhibit any of the signs and symptoms of stimulant misuse, including chest pain, shortness of breath, diaphoresis, and psychosis. Cardiac effects may be observed in the form of ventricular dysrhythmias, MI, or sudden cardiac arrest. Because of the sodium channel–blocking properties of cocaine, you may observe a widened QRS complex or a prolonged QT interval on an ECG tracing. Chronic users may exhibit significant left ventricular hypertrophy.

As mentioned earlier, the significant vasoconstriction triggered by cocaine use means that the drug may affect any organ system. During your assessment, be alert for signs of neurologic insult and renal failure. Always assess your patient based on the clinical presentation and symptoms.

Amphetamine, Methamphetamine, and Amphetaminelike Drugs

Amphetamines are structurally similar to the derivatives of phenylethylamine; they include methamphetamine (crank or ice), methylenedioxyamphetamine (MDA, Adam), and methylenedioxymethamphetamine (MDMA, Eve, Ecstasy). Amphetamine and amphetaminelike drugs have several legitimate clinical applications, including as nasal decongestants and in the treatment of narcolepsy, attention-deficit disorder, and attention-deficit/hyperactivity disorder **FIGURE 28-7**. Increased amphetamine misuse has been noted in schools. Adolescents with attentional disorders may be prescribed amphetamines for increased alertness and focus, but may misuse the prescription

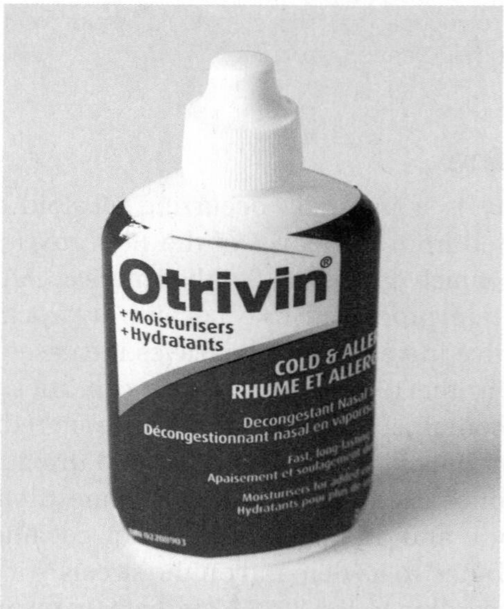

FIGURE 28-7 Drugs such as nasal decongestants and diet pills generally fall into the category of amphetamines.

medication and/or participate in drug diversion (ie, transferring a prescription medication from the person for whom it was prescribed to another person) for financial gain.

Molly, the "chemically pure" crystal powder form of MDMA, is highly desired on the streets because of its incredible high. Most drug users fail to realize that this substance may be tainted with other additives that could produce adverse effects and significant medical conditions. Research has shown that the actual prevalence of MDMA use is underreported because of confusion or lack of awareness that Molly is a type of MDMA.[17]

Methamphetamine is a low-cost, long-acting stimulant that is highly addictive. The ingredients required to manufacture methamphetamine can be purchased in stores. However, federal regulations are intended to make obtaining large quantities of pseudoephedrine and other required ingredients more difficult. The process of manufacturing methamphetamine involves using hazardous chemicals that could present a health and safety hazard to you and your fellow responders. Keep scene safety uppermost in your mind when you are assessing a patient who may have been involved in the manufacturing process.

The clinical presentation of the patient who is abusing amphetamine or methamphetamine is almost identical to that of a person who is abusing cocaine, with the primary exception that the effects of amphetamines last longer than those of cocaine. Be alert to the potential for emotional and psychological instability in individuals with a drug use disorder, particularly in patients who have been on a binge. With each passing day of no sleep and little or no food, they become increasingly paranoid. Their behavior can quickly become violent, so always be mindful of your exit strategy when on scene. Do not hesitate to ask for law enforcement support if the scene seems likely to destabilize.

Synthetic Cathinones (Bath Salts)

Synthetic cathinones, also known as bath salts, comprise an emerging group of drugs similar to MDMA. Synthetic cathinones are psychoactive substances related to a chemical compound derived from the khat plant, which is native to East Africa. Khat leaves are traditionally chewed for a stimulant and euphoric effect. Synthetic cathinones are chemically engineered to have a higher potency than the natural compound. However, bath salts should not be confused with bathing products such as Epsom salt (magnesium sulfate).

Some of the chemical components used in synthetic cathinones enter the United States from countries such as China. In early 2015, three to four people were hospitalized every day in areas of south Florida following the use of a synthetic cathinone called Flakka. International pressure for governments to ban the substances used to make synthetic cathinones have curbed some of the production and, therefore, the frequency with which these drugs appear on the street.[18] However, people have found replacement substances and ingredients that are chemically similar to synthetic cathinones.

Synthetic cathinones are popular because they offer effects similar to stimulants such as cocaine and amphetamines, but usually cost less. Bath salts are sometimes sold as plant food or cleaners, and are labeled as "not for human consumption." Synthetic cathinones often have a white or brown crystallike appearance and come in foil packages with names like Flakka, Cloud Nine, or White Lightning. They may be sold in convenience stores or gas stations, making them more accessible than other illicit drugs. It is difficult to identify new psychoactive substances and their unique characteristics, which in turn creates huge challenges in recognizing and treating patients who have used these substances.

As with other stimulants, synthetic cathinones can be ingested, insufflated (snorted), smoked, or injected. The speed of onset depends on the route of absorption. According to the National Institute on Drug Abuse (NIDA), the two routes associated with the highest mortality rates are insufflation and needle injection.[19] Synthetic cathinone use has been associated with significant paranoia, hallucinations, incredible strength, excited delirium, and other bizarre behaviors. Tachycardia, diaphoresis, nausea, and hyperthermia may also be present.

Management of Stimulant Misuse

The most life-threatening presentations of stimulant misuse include dysrhythmias, vascular events, hypertension, hyperthermia, seizures, and agitation. Treatment of stimulant misuse and toxicity includes supportive care, maintaining oxygenation, proper monitoring, and assessing the need for appropriate intervention with IV fluids and/or medications, as follows:

- Establish and maintain the airway. Consider an advanced airway as needed.
- Provide supplemental oxygen to maintain saturation levels of greater than 94%.
- Establish vascular access.
- Apply the ECG monitor, pulse oximeter, and capnometer.
- To control anxiety and seizures, administer benzodiazepines per local protocols.
- Manage hypotension with serial fluid infusions of normal saline.
- For patients who demonstrated violent behavior, follow local protocols or contact medical control for sedation.
- Transport to the appropriate facility.

Fluid resuscitation may be required for patients with signs of hypoperfusion. Assess the patient for cardiac dysrhythmias that may require treatment. Treat chest pain as an acute coronary syndrome and consider other symptoms (such as respiratory distress) as an atypical presentation of acute coronary syndrome. If an acute coronary syndrome is suspected, consider the administration of sublingual nitroglycerin, if not contraindicated. Follow your local protocols and consult medical control as needed for the patient experiencing a stimulant overdose.

Severe agitation and excited delirium are thought to be linked to stimulant overdose. If the patient exhibits bizarre behavior, is inappropriately clothed for the environment, or has a history of noncompliance with psychiatric medications, then this finding may elevate the suspicion of stimulant overdose and excited delirium. Chemical restraints and sedation may be indicated to keep both the patient and yourself safe. Local protocols may dictate which agent you use for this purpose. Antipsychotics, benzodiazepines, and dissociative agents are commonly used in the field.

Aggressive cooling may be indicated if the patient is hyperthermic and signs of delirium or severe agitation are present. Consider placing external cooling packs on the groin, axilla, and forearms. Follow your local protocols. Throughout the resuscitation process, it is essential to maintain urine output with aggressive fluid therapy.

If the patient has a seizure, then benzodiazepines remain the treatment of choice. In addition, neuromuscular blockade may be needed to control motor activity to avoid hyperthermia, acidosis, and, potentially, **rhabdomyolysis** (the destruction of muscle tissue leading to a release of potassium and myoglobin). Online medical control will usually be required before reaching this step in the treatment algorithm.

Marijuana and Cannabis Compounds

When the leaves and flower buds of the *Cannabis sativa* plant are harvested and dried, the end product is referred to as **marijuana** (also known as weed, pot, dope, and bud) **FIGURE 28-8**. The resin produced by the maturing flower tops can also be harvested and used to produce hashish (also known as hash). Over the past decade, some states have legalized marijuana and some of its compounds for medical use; other states have made it legal for any use. This action has created many controversial discussions about marijuana use. According to results from the National Survey on Drug Use and Health from the NIDA, marijuana remains the most commonly used illicit drug in the United States, with approximately 32% of people ages 18 to 25 years using marijuana within the past year.[15] For these reasons, it is important to have a thorough understanding of marijuana and cannabis compounds.

Marijuana contains several cannabis compounds, which may have different therapeutic effects. Cannabidiol (CBD) is one of the main active

FIGURE 28-8 A marijuana plant.

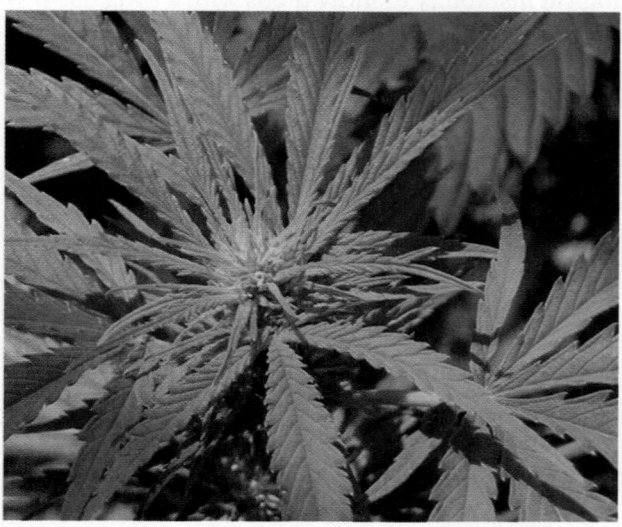

chemical compounds. While its reported therapeutic benefits are far ranging, from analgesia to treatment of mental illnesses, clinical research into its effects is limited. One condition for which it has been thoroughly studied, and for which the FDA has approved its use, is intractable epilepsy syndromes.[20] CBD does not have the euphoric or intoxicating effects of THC, and it has served as the driving force for some states to enact laws to allow access to cannabidiol oil or high-CBD strains of marijuana.

Pathophysiology

As mentioned earlier, the primary psychoactive ingredient in marijuana and hashish is delta 9-tetrahydrocannabinol, or THC. THC binds to cannabinoid receptors throughout the brain. Marijuana use may cause the user to have enhanced sensory perception and euphoria. These unusual effects may cause anxiety or panic. Common short-term effects of marijuana use include tachycardia, balance and coordination problems, increased appetite, conjunctival injection, dry mouth, and possible memory loss. Drowsiness and relaxation may also occur following use of this drug. Chronic use of marijuana may result in pulmonary symptoms without the obstructive airway disease that is commonly seen with tobacco use.[21]

Smoking marijuana usually causes euphoria and relaxation that can last as long as 4 to 6 hours. Fine motor skills, concentration, and depth perception can be altered for up to 24 hours, affecting the person's ability to safely perform activities such as driving or operating heavy machinery.[21] Marijuana products may also be ingested, insufflated, vaporized, and applied topically to the skin.

> **SAFETY**
>
> Because of the relative length of time that marijuana use could impair an EMS provider's ability to perform job duties and THC remaining in the blood, EMS agencies should consider adopting zero-tolerance policies for marijuana use.

Assessment and Management

When you assess the patient who has used marijuana or cannabis compounds, know that although intoxication and withdrawal from marijuana are not life threatening, it can cause tachycardia that can impair myocardial perfusion in older individuals.[22] Novice users may become panicked or anxious due to the euphoria, spatial disorientation, and altered sense of reality that can occur. Emotional support and supportive care are often all that is required. Benzodiazepines may be considered for sedation if the patient has significant anxiety. If the patient has severe or life-threatening signs and symptoms, then consider whether another substance or drug may be at work as you continue your assessment and search for other causes.

Sometimes patients may be unaware of their exposure, such as when someone has unknowingly ingested marijuana in a brownie. Pediatric patients may experience more serious signs and symptoms after ingesting an edible food source that has been adulterated with marijuana (eg, lollipops, brownies, or gummy bears). In such a case, contact the poison control center and provide prompt transport to the hospital, as the child will likely require hospitalization based on their symptoms.[23]

Occasionally, you may encounter a patient with cannabinoid hyperemesis syndrome. This syndrome involves cyclic episodes of nausea and vomiting in chronic cannabis users. IV fluids and antiemetics are indicated during transport to the appropriate facility.[21]

Spice

Similar to synthetic cathinones, **spice** is a synthetic cannabinoid that falls into the category of new psychoactive substances. Because the cannabinoids act on the same cellular receptors as THC, spice is often marketed as synthetic marijuana. However, the active substance is a blend of chemicals that is either sprayed onto plantlike material for smoking, or sold as a liquid for vaporizing in electronic cigarettes. Some users report euphoria similar to that associated with marijuana use; however, these chemicals can be more dangerous than marijuana. Adverse effects of spice use may include psychosis, hallucinations, tachycardia, vomiting, renal conditions, and seizures.

As with synthetic cathinones, it can be challenging to obtain a good assessment and form a treatment plan for someone who has used spice. Remember that various chemicals may have been used in the spice, so patient presentations may vary. Supportive care with fluids and antiemetics is often appropriate. If the patient is experiencing a seizure, then benzodiazepines are the medication of choice.

Hallucinogens

A **hallucinogen** is a substance that can impair judgment, alter the user's perception of reality, and create a realistic sensation of images or sounds that are not actually present. Experiences with hallucinogens are unpredictable and can vary markedly from person to person. The overall drug experience is affected by the user's previous drug experience, the dose taken, and the social setting. Keep this information in mind when you move the patient into an environment with bright lights, loud sirens, and significant bumps and vibrations, such as the ambulance.

Hallucinogenic substances can be classified into two categories: synthetic and naturally occurring. The synthetic class of hallucinogens includes lysergic acid diethylamide (LSD), phencyclidine (PCP), and ketamine. Naturally occurring hallucinogens include mescaline, psilocybin mushrooms, and the seeds of the jimson weed plant.

LSD

LSD is derived from a fungus that contaminates rye flour and wheat. It is usually ingested orally and is sold on the street in tablets, capsules, or liquid form. Small, colorful squares of paper may also be dipped in LSD and then placed on the tongue. A single dose is represented by one square of paper. The time until onset of the effects is usually 30 to 60 minutes, and duration of the effects can last up to 24 hours. LSD is considered a non–habit-forming drug, although tolerance can occur if it is taken for several days in a row.

Pathophysiology

LSD is a serotonin receptor agonist. It has the ability to distort reality, change a person's mood, and alter perceptions. LSD may also result in the user experiencing synesthesias. Synesthesias, a crossing of the senses, often prompt a user to respond to the question "What were you doing?" with a bizarre reply, such as "I was tasting the colors shining from that traffic light." Users may experiment with LSD for self-exploration or for religious reasons.

Because of the potency of LSD, even small doses may create a significant experience for the first-time user. Higher doses may lead to a longer-duration or more intense experience. Tolerance can develop to LSD, requiring chronic users to take higher doses, but almost no evidence exists of a physical dependence or withdrawal syndrome if the user stops using the drug.

From a physiologic perspective, the effects of LSD are mostly sympathomimetic, often consisting of mild tachycardia, palpitations, mydriasis, and sweating. In a "bad trip," the user has a vivid, frightening experience similar to a nightmare, resulting in an acute anxiety attack and physical effects secondary to increased anxiety. The bad trip does not end until the drug wears off.

Assessment and Management

The treatment of a patient using LSD is primarily supportive, focusing on the psychological aspects of the drug experience. Follow local protocols when considering administration of anxiolytics for patients with severe anxiety.

During transport of a patient who has taken LSD, try to limit sensory stimulation as much as possible; for example, by avoiding the use of the emergency lights and siren. Routine transport to the appropriate facility and providing emotional support are usually all that is required for these patients.

Phencyclidine

PCP, also called angel dust or rocket fuel, is a dissociative anesthetic that has hallucinogenic properties. It was developed for use in the 1950s as an IV anesthetic, but patients experienced significant delirium following its administration. It is no longer used for any medical purpose in the United States. Although it is commonly sold in powder, crystal, or tablet form, some users dip marijuana cigarettes in PCP (known as wets or super grass). PCP is commonly added to other illicit drugs to create a more intense high. This practice can occur without the user's knowledge. Users may believe they are going to relax after smoking a marijuana joint (rolled cigarette), only to find that it has been laced with PCP.

Pathophysiology

Phencyclidine works at the *N*-methyl-D-aspartate (NMDA) receptors. As a dissociative drug, PCP can distort sight and sound and make users feel separated from their own body. It is typically smoked or snorted, although it can be injected. Doses of 5 to

10 mg can produce signs and symptoms of intoxication in an adult. Slurred speech, staggering gait, tachycardia, hypertension, staring blankly for extended periods, and horizontal nystagmus (involuntary, rhythmic movement of the eyes) are common with PCP use. Users may also display extraordinary strength, have a sense of invincibility, or seem to lack awareness of pain, continuing to function despite significant orthopaedic injuries. A small, thin man on PCP may be able to successfully attack several larger people despite sustaining injuries, which can become a significant issue when considering scene safety and management of a combative patient.

Assessment and Management

PCP can cause some of the most violent and difficult behavior you will encounter in the field. The patient's moods may change rapidly, and the patient may attack other people without warning. For that reason, the safety of the EMS team is a continuous concern when responding to calls involving PCP users. Emergency care focuses on trying to calm the patient and addressing any wounds. Intramuscular (IM) sedatives may be considered for an aggressive or combative patient. Coordinate your efforts with your fellow responders to ensure that everyone knows the plan before moving to administer the medication. It may be feasible to obtain IV access after the patient has initially been sedated. Administer oxygen, monitor vital signs, and provide safe transport to an appropriate facility.

Ketamine

Ketamine (special K, vitamin K) is another dissociative anesthetic (discussed further in Chapter 29, *Psychiatric Emergencies*). This medication is relatively short acting and has clinical uses in the veterinary and medical fields for procedural sedation, management of agitated or violent behavior, and pain control. Ketamine is at risk for drug diversion from veterinary clinics or hospitals, and a significant amount of illicit ketamine has been smuggled into the United States from Mexico. Ketamine is sometimes added to other illicit drugs to produce a more intense user experience.

Pathophysiology

Like PCP, ketamine works at the NMDA receptors. It also binds to mu-opioid receptors, giving it analgesic properties. At low doses, a user presents with mild inebriation, euphoria, and increased sociability. At higher doses, a patient may have pronounced nausea, difficulty moving, and significant hallucinations, as well as other systemic effects.[24]

Assessment and Management

Although outbreaks of violence in patients are much less likely with ketamine than with PCP, management principles are the same for patients who have used either drug. Secure the patient well, assess the ABCDEs and manage any life threats, provide oxygen therapy, establish vascular access if the patient is receptive, and provide safe transport to the appropriate facility. Watch the patient closely because violent behavior can occur suddenly. Benzodiazepines may help calm an agitated patient who is experiencing significant delirium.

Peyote and Mescaline

Native tribes in the southwestern United States and Mexico have been using hallucinogens for thousands of years, primarily for religious purposes, with mescaline as the substance of choice. Mescaline is the hallucinogenic agent found in the small peyote cactus. Peyote and mescaline are Schedule I substances with a high potential for misuse and no currently accepted medical use in the United States.

Pathophysiology

The exact mechanism of action for mescaline has not been determined. The dried flower "buttons" may be ingested or soaked in water to produce a liquid infused with mescaline **FIGURE 28-9**. The buttons have a bitter taste and are a potent gastric irritant, with profound vomiting occurring shortly after ingestion. The psychedelic experience then typically begins with feelings of increased sensitivity to sensory stimulation. Flashes of color, commonly in geometric patterns, are noted. As with use of other hallucinogens, the experience may be guided by the user's social environment; reports of hallucinations involving talking animals and vivid nature-based experiences are common. Users experience a distortion of time and space, and out-of-body experiences are commonly reported.

Structurally, mescaline looks more like amphetamine, which accounts for its physical

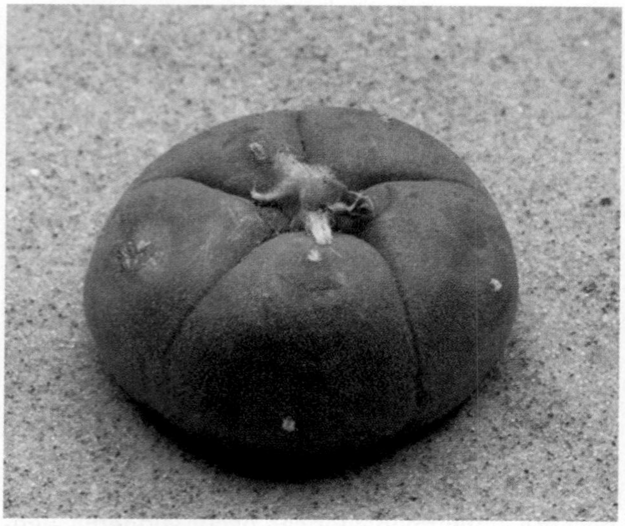

FIGURE 28-9 Dried flower buttons of the peyote cactus contain mescaline and produce a hallucinogenic effect if ingested.

FIGURE 28-10 Mushrooms containing psilocybin are hallucinogenic if ingested.

effects: dilated pupils, increased pulse rate, mild hypertension, and increased body temperature.

Assessment and Management

Emergency medical care in the field setting is primarily supportive. Administer supplemental oxygen, monitor vital signs, provide positive emotional support, and arrange safe transport to the receiving facility. Consider fluids and antiemetics if the patient has nausea and intense vomiting.

Psilocybin Mushrooms

Certain mushrooms contain the hallucinogenic substances psilocybin and psilocyn **FIGURE 28-10**. In the United States, the most commonly misused mushrooms are *Psilocybe mexicana* and *Psilocybe cyaescens,* but several varieties containing psilocybin and psilocyn are also indigenous to tropical and subtropical climates in North, Central, and South America. These mushrooms typically have a bitter taste, and they may be combined with other liquids or foods to disguise the foul flavor.

Pathophysiology

The onset of symptoms and hallucinogenic effects (similar to LSD but less intense) occurs within 30 minutes of ingestion, and effects usually last 4 to 6 hours. Signs and symptoms include muscle weakness, drowsiness, nausea and vomiting, mydriasis, mild tachycardia, and mild hypertension. The likelihood of serious adverse effects is low, although seizures and hyperthermia have occurred in some patients.

Assessment and Management

Provide supportive care. Hallucinations are likely to subside quickly if the patient is in a secure, safe environment. Managing the ABCs and monitoring vital signs are usually all that is required, along with safe transport to the appropriate facility. If time and circumstances allow, then establish vascular access to facilitate seizure control with benzodiazepines, if necessary.

Sedatives and Hypnotics

The drugs in the **sedative-hypnotic** category have a wide range of applications and well-established therapeutic benefits. These drugs work as CNS depressants and can produce a range of effects, from light sedation to total anesthesia. Drugs with sedative qualities are used to reduce anxiety and to calm agitated patients. Drugs with hypnotic qualities are used as sleep aids, helping to produce drowsiness and sleep. Because of the effectiveness of sedative and hypnotic medications, they have a high potential for misuse and are at high risk for drug diversion in the medical field.

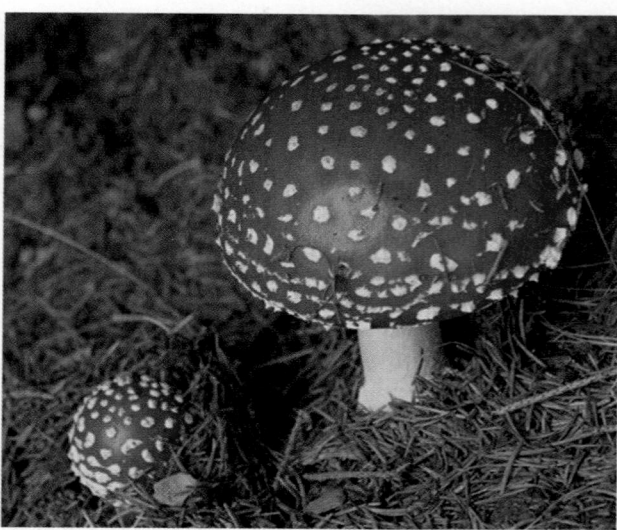

Barbiturates

Barbiturates are a class of medications that act as CNS depressants. As such, they have established therapeutic uses as anxiolytics, anticonvulsants, and hypnotics. Analgesic effects are associated with barbiturate use, but these effects are often minimal. Clinically speaking, barbiturates are similar to alcohol in terms of dependence and withdrawal symptoms.

The frequent combination of alcohol and barbiturates as a suicide mechanism, coupled with the high incidence of unintentional overdoses, pushed researchers to develop sedative-hypnotic drugs that had fewer depressive effects on the respiratory system and were less lethal. Today, the likelihood of death after the ingestion of a single-entity sedative-hypnotic such as diazepam (Valium) is small.

Pathophysiology

Barbiturates potentiate gamma-aminobutyric acid (GABA) at specific receptors to inhibit cellular excitation. As the dose increases, barbiturates bind to other receptor sites and cause more widespread CNS depression. Barbiturates come in four basic configurations: long-acting, intermediate-acting, short-acting, and ultra–short-acting. Ultra–short acting barbiturates are highly lipid-soluble and have a rapid onset because they quickly cross the blood–brain barrier. These substances are preferred when time is of the essence, such as with airway management or for stopping an active seizure. Long-acting barbiturates are less lipid-soluble; therefore, they have a delayed onset of action and are preferred when a sustained therapeutic level of a medication is required over a long period. The liver metabolizes most barbiturates into inactive waste products, although barbiturates that bind less tightly to proteins tend to be excreted unchanged in the urine.

Assessment

The patient assessment findings will reflect the dosing and the configuration of the barbiturate. Mild to moderate barbiturate intoxication is similar to alcohol intoxication; symptoms include decreased alertness, nystagmus, ataxia, mental confusion, and slurred speech. As the dose increases, the patient moves further down the scale of CNS depression, becoming increasingly lethargic and eventually unresponsive. Be aware of the potential for respiratory depression.

> **Evidence-Based Medicine**
>
> Administration of activated charcoal for barbiturate overdose has not been shown to decrease overall morbidity and mortality.[25] Historically, the process of gastric lavage (or gastric emptying) was regularly practiced in emergency medicine. This practice may have been considered for substances that were ingested several hours earlier or could not be bound by activated charcoal. Research has failed to demonstrate the benefits of gastric lavage for gastric decontamination.[26]

Management

Because some degree of CNS depression is likely with barbiturate overdose, these patients are often at risk for vomiting and aspiration. Therefore, pay particular attention to the patency of the patient's airway. If the patient is unable to protect the airway, then move to secure the airway. Proper oxygenation and proper ventilation should be monitored with pulse oximetry and capnometry.

> **Words of Wisdom**
>
> Activated charcoal can be a messy drug to administer. Consider covering the cup and providing a straw through which the patient may drink the solution. Often, patients will not continue to drink the solution after they see or smell it. Keep an emesis bag or large receptacle handy should the patient vomit during or following administration.

If signs of shock are evident, administer fluid support in 250-mL increments (up to 2 L) of crystalloids. Perform a frequent reevaluation of breath sounds to ensure pulmonary edema is not developing. If hypotension persists despite adequate fluid replacement, consider administering a vasopressor according to local protocols.

If you are treating a conscious patient within 1 hour of ingestion of a barbiturate overdose, consider administering activated charcoal. Ensure the patient can maintain the airway before this administration. Activated charcoal may prove more beneficial for overdoses involving long-acting barbiturates.

> **Words of Wisdom**
>
> Consider the possibility of a drug-related condition in any patient presenting with unexplained behavioral changes, stupor, coma, or seizures.

Individuals who use barbiturates quickly develop tolerance and require ever-larger doses to produce the desired effects. Long-term use results in physical addiction. Abrupt cessation in a person who has been a long-term barbiturate user will produce typical signs and symptoms of withdrawal syndrome in approximately 24 hours. In case of minor withdrawal, the patient may present with symptoms similar to those observed in a patient with alcohol withdrawal: restlessness, tremulousness, insomnia, diaphoresis, abdominal cramping, and nausea and vomiting. With patients in severe withdrawal, you may also see delirium, hallucinations, psychosis, hyperthermia, and cardiovascular collapse. Life-threatening withdrawal, similar to DTs, is possible with abrupt cessation of large doses of barbiturates.

If you encounter barbiturate withdrawal syndrome in the prehospital setting, focus your treatment efforts on preventing seizures (IV benzodiazepines are a common choice) and cardiovascular collapse (serial fluid boluses). Rapid transport to the ED, with subsequent intensive care, will be required to best manage the patient over the long term.

Benzodiazepines

Benzodiazepines are also members of the sedative-hypnotic family. They are most commonly used to treat anxiety, seizures, and withdrawal symptoms. In recent years, the use of fast-acting benzodiazepines, such as zolpidem tartrate (Ambien) for treatment of insomnia, has grown rapidly. These drugs are often readily available online or from people selling their prescription medications for financial gain.

Pathophysiology

Similar to barbiturates, benzodiazepines exert their effects by stimulating the GABA pathways, resulting in sedation and reduced anxiety. When taken orally, these medications are readily absorbed from the GI tract. IV administration allows for more rapid onset of action and more controlled dosing. IM injections may have a variable rate of absorption. These drugs are metabolized primarily by the liver.

Assessment

In a single-entity overdose, benzodiazepines have a relatively low rate of morbidity and mortality. The most common clinical effects of benzodiazepine overdose include altered mentation, drowsiness, confusion, slurred speech, ataxia, and general loss of coordination. Benzodiazepine overdose rarely causes hypotension and has not been known to cause dysrhythmias. If either of these conditions is present, then search for another cause.[25] In the case of intentional overdose, it is likely that the patient has taken multiple substances. Use your investigative skills and assessment to guide the clinical care of the patient. On occasion, extrapyramidal reactions may occur in tandem with hepatotoxic or hematologic reactions.

Withdrawal from benzodiazepines may lead to tachycardia, tremulousness, confusion, and possibly seizures. While benzodiazepine withdrawal is rarely a life-threatening event, it can be complicated by withdrawal from other substances, such as alcohol. Flumazenil (Romazicon), a benzodiazepine receptor antagonist, is not indicated in a suspected benzodiazepine overdose because it can precipitate refractory/intractable seizures if the patient is benzodiazepine dependent.[6]

Management

Treatment of benzodiazepine overdose includes the following steps:

- Assess and manage the airway, providing ventilatory support as needed.
- Administer supplemental oxygen.
- Establish vascular access.
- Apply the ECG monitor, pulse oximeter, and capnometer.
- Consider a fluid challenge for hypotension.
- Consider vasopressor administration if hypotension persists despite adequate fluid resuscitation.
- Consider activated charcoal administration (in consultation with poison control or medical control), especially with extended-release medications.
- Transport to the appropriate facility.

Opioids

An **opioid** is a drug that acts as a CNS depressant and produces insensibility or stupor. An opioid can be a natural product derived from the opium or poppy plant (referred to more specifically as an **opiate**) or a synthetic product designed to produce similar effects. In recent years, street use of incredibly potent drugs such as carfentanil and desomorphine has increased. Carfentanil is an animal tranquilizer used for large mammals, such as elephants. It is far more potent than morphine or fentanyl, and its use by persons with substance use disorder seeking a quick opioid high can be fatal.

> **Words of Wisdom**
>
> The term *narcotic* originally referred to a substance that dulled the senses and relieved pain. In everyday speech, it is often used to mean all illegal drugs, but technically, it refers only to opioids. To avoid confusion, *opioid* is the preferred term in the medical community.

Prehospital providers have seen a significant increase in the number of opioid overdoses since 2000. According to the CDC, more than 70,000 drug overdose deaths occurred in the United States in 2019, two-thirds of which (49,860) involved opioids.[27] Prescription opioids and heroin were the primary drugs associated with these overdose deaths.[28] The medical community has responded to these alarming statistics with changes in practices regarding the use of opioid medications. In 2016, the FDA published a special report that outlined a multifaceted approach to help combat this epidemic. The FDA's approach works to address the issues of individual needs and societal risks. It creates clear guidelines for opioid use, addresses the lack of nonopioid alternatives for pain management, identifies guidelines for writing opioid prescriptions, and creates a better evidence base to guide the use of opioid medications.[29]

An FDA-approved auto-injector device can deliver an IM or subcutaneous injection of naloxone (Narcan) to reverse opioid overdose. The FDA has also approved intranasal devices, allowing for rapid administration of naloxone to treat overdose. Local pharmacies may sell this reversal agent to people with or without a prescription. Law enforcement officers may administer naloxone before EMS arrival. Always ask whether naloxone has been administered by family members, bystanders, or other responders. Expanded access to naloxone is one approach to deal with the deadly opioid epidemic. It is important to remember that a dose of naloxone may not permanently reverse the effects of an opioid, and the patient may lapse into unconsciousness due to the shorter half-life of naloxone compared to the opioid.

As a paramedic, what role do you play in this epidemic? The rapid recognition of opioid overdose followed by appropriate treatment is critical. Patient education and the identification of persons who are at high risk for abusing opioids is important. This risk of addiction or misuse should not, however, influence your decision to treat acute pain in the prehospital environment. A significant portion of the opioid misuse epidemic is caused by misuse of prescription pain medication. For the treatment of severe pain in an emergency, opioid administration is currently the most commonly available option in the field. However, many EMS agencies have developed protocols using ketamine (a nonopioid) to treat severe pain.

Never forget the basics in terms of splinting, positioning, and supportive care, but do not withhold opioid pain medication because of concerns about making the patient susceptible to addiction. Consider your options when choosing how to treat a patient's pain. For example, does the patient have a stubbed toe that may be best treated with an ice pack? Or does the patient have an open femur fracture with severe pain? Conduct a thorough exam and attempt to relieve the pain with basic maneuvers before considering opioid administration.

Pathophysiology

Opioids affect the CNS by binding with three main opioid receptor sites: delta, kappa, and mu. These receptor sites can produce analgesia and a euphoric sensation. The highest concentrations of opioid receptor sites are found in the limbic system, frontal and temporal cortices, thalamus, hypothalamus, midbrain, and spinal cord.

Opioids can be ingested, insufflated (ie, blown into a body cavity), inhaled, and injected. As with other substances, the route of absorption will help determine the speed of onset and duration of effects. When taken orally, the effects of these drugs are lessened because of their significant first-pass metabolism through the liver compared with their effects when given parenterally. Opioids can also be absorbed through the skin via transdermal patches.

SAFETY

Remember the importance of performing a rapid full-body scan on patients who have overdosed on opioids. Recall that people may use multiple routes of administration when abusing opioids. In particular, look for transdermal patches. Missing a fentanyl patch that was covered by clothing could lead to the patient lapsing back into respiratory arrest. If you have not found and removed the patch, then you may not be successful in treating the life-threatening overdose.

Morphine and fentanyl are two commonly used analgesics in the prehospital setting. Fentanyl is a far more potent drug than morphine. This potency does not mean that fentanyl is a stronger or better medication; it simply takes less of the medication to create a therapeutic effect. Morphine has some vasodilatory properties due to histamine release, and fentanyl has a shorter half-life. Based on the clinical situation, one of these medications may be more appropriate for the patient than the other.

Assessment

The classic presentation of opioid use features euphoria, hypotension, respiratory depression, and pinpoint pupils. Depending on the particular agent, nausea, vomiting, and constipation may occur as well. With increased doses, coma, seizures (usually secondary to hypoxia), and cardiac arrest (usually secondary to respiratory arrest) are common.

Morphine and heroin produce a dreamlike state. Shortly after injecting heroin, a user will appear to pass out. However, the user is typically lucid and remains acutely aware of what is being done or said even though it appears as though the user has dozed off.

Management

Because of the CNS depressant effects of opioids, patient management initially focuses on establishing and maintaining a patent airway and providing adequate ventilation. A patient experiencing an opioid overdose is usually hypoventilating with slow and shallow respirations. Hypoventilation will create increased carbon dioxide retention (hypercapnia) and respiratory acidosis. Rather than moving immediately to intubation, place a nasopharyngeal or oropharyngeal airway and provide bag-mask ventilation with 15 L/min of supplemental oxygen.

Next, establish vascular access and administer naloxone. Remember that naloxone is given to improve the patient's spontaneous respiratory effort. You can titrate IV naloxone to improve the respiratory status without bringing the patient back to a fully conscious and alert state. Adverse effects of rapid naloxone administration include hypotension, vomiting, and potential agitation associated with the patient regaining consciousness. The IM and intranasal routes are also valid options for administration of naloxone if IV access is unavailable.

Sometimes the patient may not respond to the initial dose of naloxone and may remain unconscious. The patient may be under the influence of a very potent and/or large dose of the opioid. Follow local protocols or consider contacting medical control if you believe the patient may require higher doses of naloxone. Alternatively, the coma may be from another source altogether, such as a stroke or a polypharmacy overdose. In either scenario, you should insert an advanced airway, provide supportive care as needed, and transport the patient to an appropriate facility.

When a cardiac arrest occurs with an opioid overdose, it is usually the result of a loss of airway patency and inadequate ventilation.[30] Therefore, initial care should focus on opening the airway and providing bag-mask ventilation. Because no studies have demonstrated improved patient outcomes from administering naloxone during cardiac arrest, high-quality chest compressions should be performed next.[30] If you have a high index of suspicion that opioid poisoning may have precipitated the cardiac arrest, naloxone administration is indicated, in addition to standard resuscitative measures, if its administration will not delay the delivery of CPR **FIGURE 28-11**.

Cardiac Medications

Pathophysiology

Cardiac medications can benefit patients with chronic cardiovascular disorders involving blood

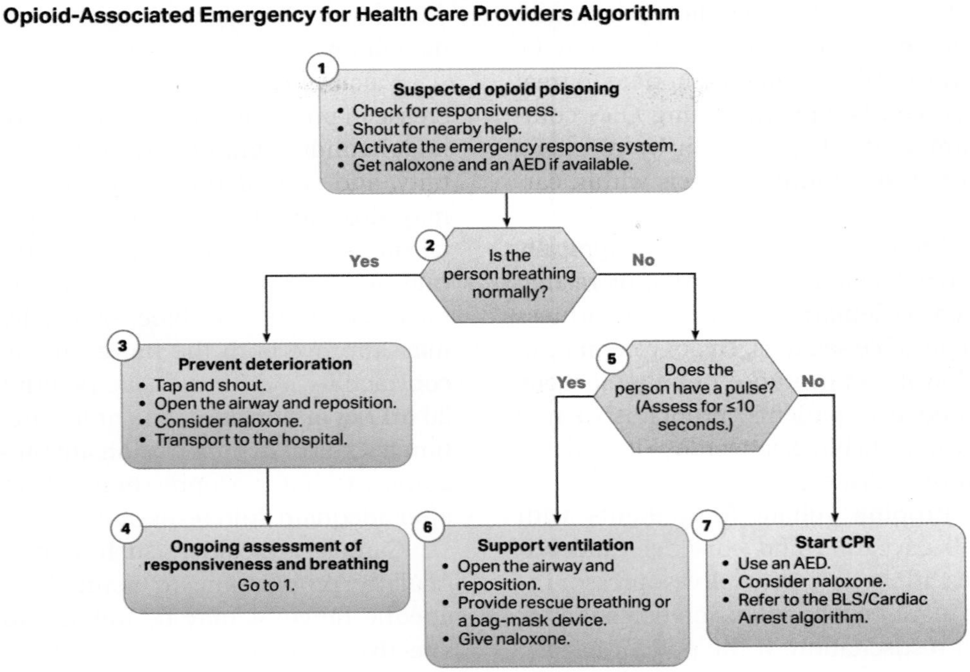

FIGURE 28-11 The American Heart Association's algorithm for life-threatening opioid overdose (Abbreviations: AED, automated external defibrillator; BLS, basic life support; CPR, cardiopulmonary resuscitation).

pressure, heart rate, or dysrhythmias. As a paramedic, you also have the ability to treat life-threatening events with appropriate doses of these medications. However, these medications can produce severe effects on the body when they reach toxic levels. The major classes of cardiac drugs include antidysrhythmics, beta blockers, calcium channel blockers, cardiac glycosides, and angiotensin-converting enzyme inhibitors. These medications are classified using the Vaughan-Williams system. Medications that have similar mechanisms of action are grouped as Class I, Class II, Class III, or Class IV, as discussed in Chapter 13, *Principles of Pharmacology*.

Overdoses of cardiac medications are usually unintentional. A single pill or tablet of many of these cardiac medications can cause serious effects or death in small children and infants who unintentionally ingest them.

Assessment and Management

Because of the wide variety of presentations associated with the different classes of antidysrhythmics, use the patient's history and list of medications as a guide in identifying what substances are involved in the overdose. Identification is key because many standard treatments may be ineffective due to the toxic levels of the medication. Work to minimize the negative effects of the overdose while determining whether an antidote is available. As with all emergencies, ensure a patent airway and adequate ventilation, and administer supplemental oxygen as needed.

With overdoses of most cardiac medications, you should contact a poison control center or medical control early in your treatment of the patient. You may receive an order from medical control to administer activated charcoal without sorbitol if the patient is within the first hour of ingestion. If you are able to confirm that an extended-release medication has been ingested, then this information may create additional consideration for activated charcoal. Do not administer activated charcoal if the patient is at risk for a rapidly declining mental status.

With sodium channel blockers, overdoses can cause QRS prolongation, QT prolongation, hypotension secondary to depressed myocardial contractility, and ventricular dysrhythmias. Consider atropine sulfate for the bradycardic patient who is symptomatic. In certain instances, you may be asked to administer IV sodium bicarbonate to treat slowed impulse conduction (widening QRS complex), bradycardia, and hypotension by reversing the inhibition of fast sodium channels within cardiac cells.

Patients with beta blocker toxicity typically present with hypotension, bradycardia, or related symptoms such as lethargy, weakness, shortness of breath, and possible seizures. Hypoglycemia can also occur following an overdose of beta blockers, especially in pediatric patients. Bronchospasm is possible following beta blocker overdose in patients with reactive airway disease.

Consider atropine sulfate for patients with symptomatic bradycardia and consider fluid boluses for those with hypotension. A vasopressor infusion may be required if hypotension persists after adequate fluid resuscitation. If the patient experiences seizure activity, then midazolam is the medication of choice.

Acute toxicity from potassium channel blockers may present as hypotension, bradycardia, or certain ventricular dysrhythmias. One of the predominant effects observed on the ECG is a prolonged QT interval. The treatment of acute potassium channel blocker toxicity is primarily supportive, although you may use IV magnesium sulfate to treat torsades de pointes.

Calcium channel blocker toxicity causes a decrease in pulse rate, decreased atrioventricular (AV) nodal conduction, decreased myocardial contractility, and vasodilation. Calcium channel blockers may also cause nausea and vomiting, altered mental status, and metabolic acidosis. IV calcium chloride or calcium gluconate is the initial treatment for calcium channel blocker toxicity. IV glucagon may improve both the pulse rate and myocardial contractility. Administer an IV fluid challenge of 20 mL/kg of normal saline or lactated Ringer solution if signs of hypoperfusion are present. Consider administering a vasopressor if hypotension persists after adequate fluid resuscitation.

Cardiac glycosides (such as digoxin) are particularly problematic to maintain within a therapeutic range. It may be difficult to maintain an effective therapeutic level of these medications without increasing the dose to a toxic level. Acute digoxin toxicity presents with nausea, vomiting, GI distress, and lethal hyperkalemia. Digoxin immune fab (Digibind) is the definitive treatment for acute digoxin toxicity and is usually administered in a hospital setting. Supportive care and the consideration of calcium gluconate may be reasonable in a patient with suspected digoxin toxicity. Because of

YOU are the Paramedic

PART 4

You place the patient on the cardiac monitor and observe sinus tachycardia. You wonder whether any other drugs could be present in the patient's system, so you ask the family to search the bathroom again. As you prepare to initiate IV access, you feel something underneath the patient's shirt. You log roll the patient to discover that her entire back is covered with fentanyl patches.

Recording Time: 10 Minutes	
Respirations	Assisted
Pulse	100 beats/min
Skin	Cyanosis is resolving
Blood pressure	98/56 mm Hg
Oxygen saturation (Spo_2)	96% (assisted with bag-mask device and 100% oxygen)
Pupils	Pinpoint and nonreactive

7. What is your medication choice and dosage to treat this patient?

8. What should you do if this medication does not correct the overdose?

the sophistication of cardiac drugs and the likelihood that the patient may be taking multiple cardiac and other medications, it is prudent to make contact with medical control.

Organophosphates

Organophosphates are a major component in many insecticides used in commercial agriculture and in the home. Organophosphates were developed in the early 1900s when German scientists were trying to reduce dependence on food imports by creating new insecticides that would increase domestic crop yields. The people exposed to these insecticides experienced serious adverse effects, and the potential for using organophosphates as chemical weapons was quickly recognized. Organophosphates are classified as acetylcholinesterase inhibitors. This classification also includes acephate (Orthene), diazinon (Spectracide), malathion (Cythion), carbamates, and nerve agents (sarin, soman, V agent).

Suicide attempts account for a considerable share of organophosphate poisonings, with ingestions accounting for most of these exposures.[31] Unintentional agricultural exposure is another common cause of organophosphate poisoning, and people involved in the manufacture of organophosphates and similar compounds are also at risk.

Pathophysiology

Organophosphates exert toxic effects at junctions (synapses) of the nerve cells of the autonomic nervous system. The conduction of an impulse from one nerve to another occurs through the release of acetylcholine (ACh) at the synapse. ACh works as a chemical messenger, crossing the synapse to depolarize the nerve on the other side of the junction. Organophosphates and carbamates are potent inhibitors of acetylcholinesterase, which serves to terminate synaptic transmissions. This termination creates an abundance of ACh in the CNS and peripheral nervous system. When the muscarinic and nicotinic receptors are overstimulated, a predictable response occurs in the body.

Regardless of whether the poison was ingested, inhaled, or absorbed, the symptoms of organophosphate poisoning are fundamentally the same. Patients who have ingested an organophosphate may have a delayed onset of symptoms, whereas vapor exposure will cause nearly immediate symptoms. The predictable response is the basis for the toxidrome represented by the mnemonic DUMBELS (see Table 28-1). In patients with moderate to severe organophosphate poisoning, the following symptoms may also be present: muscle fasciculations, severe respiratory distress, seizures, and flaccid paralysis.

Assessment and Management

The first component of patient assessment and treatment is decontamination, which is likely to be performed by a hazmat crew according to local protocol. If possible, position the nonambulatory patient in a lateral recumbent position to allow for passive drainage of oral secretions, and help prevent unintentional aspiration. Recognize that contaminated clothing can provide a source of continued toxin exposure.

After proper decontamination, the patient may be assessed. Consider the following measures for a patient with organophosphate poisoning:

- Establish and maintain the airway. Consider an advanced airway as needed.
- Suction as needed.
- Administer oxygen to maintain saturation levels of greater than 94%.
- Establish vascular access (IV or intraosseous [IO]), if possible without delaying further care.
- Administer atropine IV/IO push or by autoinjector, and repeat until easing of ventilation and reduction of secretions (atropinization) occur.
- Administer pralidoxime (2-PAM) concurrently with atropine in the first hour after exposure. Multiple doses may be required for patients with severe exposure.
- Apply the ECG monitor, pulse oximeter, and capnometer.
- Notify the receiving hospital early, and transport to the appropriate facility.

Atropine is the primary antidote for acetylcholinesterase inhibitor poisoning. Liberally administer repeat doses to symptomatic patients. Relief of bronchospasm and lessening of bronchorrhea indicate clinical improvement. Do not rely on the patient's pupillary response or heart rate to determine the clinical end point of atropine administration. The patient's heart rate may be within normal

> **Words of Wisdom**
>
> Most paramedic EMS vehicles do not routinely carry enough atropine to treat a patient with significant organophosphate poisoning, or multiple patients with moderate symptoms. EMS and other responders in high-risk settings for accidental exposures or terrorist activities should follow local protocols, which may include keeping larger quantities of atropine readily available.

limits, bradycardic, or tachycardic during the exposure. Treat seizures with benzodiazepines.

Carbon Monoxide

As mentioned previously, carbon monoxide is one of the most common causes of fatal poisonings. Carbon monoxide is produced during the incomplete combustion of organic fuels, such as in a motor vehicle engine, generator, or home-heating device. Carbon monoxide poisoning may occur more frequently in colder climates as a result of the use of gas-powered heaters in poorly ventilated areas.[32] A motor vehicle running in a closed garage can quickly generate a lethal concentration of carbon monoxide, making carbon monoxide inhalation a common method of suicide. When caring for these patients, remember that individuals who attempt suicide often take other substances (eg, alcohol, pills) before attempted carbon monoxide poisoning. Carbon monoxide is also a major contributor to death in house fires.

> **Words of Wisdom**
>
> Carbon monoxide can be hazardous to responders. If multiple patients from the same residence are sick, warning bells should be going off in your head. Consider evacuating everyone to a safe location. Allow fire department personnel equipped with self-contained breathing apparatus to check the air quality of that location.

Pathophysiology

According to the CDC, more than 400 deaths occur each year from accidental (non–fire-related) carbon monoxide poisoning.[32] Carbon monoxide is a colorless, odorless, tasteless gas, so people exposed to this toxin have no idea that they are inhaling a toxic substance until it is too late. Carbon monoxide displaces oxygen from the hemoglobin molecule in red blood cells because of its greater affinity for binding to hemoglobin. Even relatively small concentrations of this gas in the atmosphere can convert a significant proportion of hemoglobin into carboxyhemoglobin (COHb, hemoglobin combined with carbon monoxide) making it ineffective as an oxygen carrier.

Any increase in the body's metabolic or oxygen demands, such as fever, tachycardia, or exertion, will increase the severity of the poisoning. Children, whose metabolic rates are intrinsically higher than those of adults, tend to have more severe symptoms at any given level of exposure.

Assessment

Carbon monoxide poisoning can be difficult to diagnose in the field. Consider the patient's environment. Was adequate ventilation available? Was a source of combustion present (eg, gasoline engine)? Are other individuals present with similar signs and symptoms? Given the difficulty in detecting this gas, many EMS organizations have placed carbon monoxide detectors on portable equipment carried into emergency scenes to alert the crew of the hazard.

The signs and symptoms of carbon monoxide poisoning vary. Headache, nausea, vertigo, lightheadedness, and fatigue may be experienced with mild carbon monoxide intoxication. With moderate to severe carbon monoxide intoxication, the patient may experience altered mental status, confusion, tachypnea, tachycardia, and cardiac arrest. The cherry red color that can be seen in light-skinned people is a late sign of carbon monoxide poisoning; that is, it may be seen in the morgue.

Adequately assessing patients with suspected exposure requires removing them from the toxic environment as quickly as possible. Assess the patient's ABCDEs and vital signs, including pulse oximetry, temperature, and capnometry, if available. Note that pulse oximetry will not provide a true assessment of arterial oxygenation under these circumstances because the device cannot determine whether carbon monoxide or oxygen is bound to the hemoglobin. Therefore, do not trust an Spo_2 level of 99% in a patient who is symptomatic because of suspected carbon monoxide poisoning.

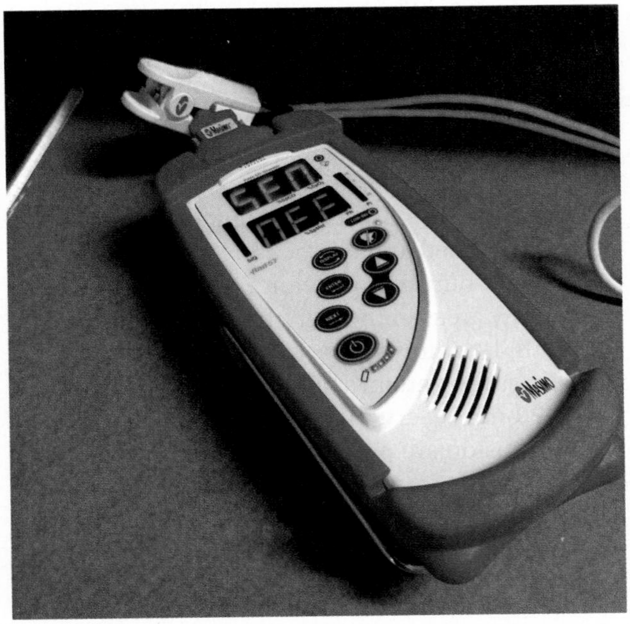

FIGURE 28-12 When using a handheld carbon monoxide oximeter, like the one shown here, be sure to document the level detected.

Apply a cardiac monitor, obtain a 12-lead ECG reading if that equipment is available, and assess the patient's blood glucose level. Noninvasive measuring of blood carbon monoxide (Spco) levels that indicate poisoning can be performed in the field (similar to pulse oximetry), which helps address the problem of delayed diagnosis. A high reading on a carbon monoxide oximeter **FIGURE 28-12** may help confirm suspicions of carbon monoxide poisoning; however, do not allow a low reading to exclude carbon monoxide poisoning from your differential diagnosis. Research is ongoing to determine the correlation between carbon monoxide oximeter readings and COHb values in a blood sample.

Management

Field treatment of carbon monoxide poisoning is aimed at providing the highest concentration of oxygen possible to attempt to displace carbon monoxide molecules from the hemoglobin. For patients with mild symptoms, the elimination half-life of COHb is roughly 4 hours. By comparison, if the patient is breathing 100% oxygen, then the half-time can be reduced to approximately 1.5 hours. Hyperbaric oxygen therapy at 2.5 atmospheres of pressure can further reduce the elimination time to 15 to 20 minutes. Early and serial reassessment of a patient's mental status and motor function can be extremely useful in determining the response to interventions and the need for hyperbaric therapy.[6] Because maternal COHb levels do not accurately reflect fetal levels of COHb, pregnant patients with suspected carbon monoxide poisoning may be more likely to receive hyperbaric oxygen therapy.

If you suspect carbon monoxide poisoning, take the following actions:

- Remove the patient from the exposure environment.
- Establish and maintain the airway, inserting an advanced airway as needed.
- Administer high-flow oxygen with a tight-fitting nonrebreathing mask.
- Establish vascular access.
- Keep the patient calm and at rest to minimize oxygen demand.
- Monitor the patient's ECG rhythm, mental status, and motor function.
- Transport to the appropriate facility. If the patient is unresponsive or has signs of serious carbon monoxide poisoning, then direct transport to a facility capable of providing hyperbaric medicine is preferred.
- For patients with injuries or illness from a structural or vehicular fire, consider the possibility of combined carbon monoxide and cyanide poisoning, especially if the patient has signs of shock or altered mental status. Contact medical control for an order to administer hydroxocobalamin or sodium thiosulfate, if available.

Carbon monoxide poisoning can be reversed if it is diagnosed and treated in time. You can have a significant effect on the patient's recovery with early recognition and early intervention. However, even if the patient recovers, acute carbon monoxide poisoning may permanently damage vital organs and lead to mild to severe neurologic deficits.

Chlorine Gas

Incidents involving chlorine gas are relatively common because of the widespread use of chlorine compounds in the home and occupational settings. Household exposures can occur when someone mixes a cleaning agent containing sodium hypochlorite (such as bleach) with a strong acid or with ammonia in an overzealous attempt at cleaning or disinfecting. The resulting chemical reaction releases chlorine gas, often in concentrations high enough to be toxic. Household ingestions can occur if chlorine-containing solutions are kept in unlabeled containers. Most cases of chlorine gas exposure occur outside the home, however. Acute exposures are often caused by faulty industrial valves or pumps that dump large amounts of gas into the environment, possibly exposing many people. Leakage of chlorine gas from an industrial storage tank, truck, or rail car can also result in a mass-casualty incident.

Pathophysiology

The signs and symptoms of chlorine gas exposure depend on the concentration of the inhaled gas and the duration of exposure. Chlorine gas is extremely irritating to all mucous membranes. When it comes in contact with the moisture on those surfaces, it can form hydrochloric acid and other substances that are damaging to human tissue. With a minor exposure, the patient will experience burning sensations in the eyes, nose, and throat along with a slight cough. More intense exposure to chlorine gas causes chest tightness, choking, paroxysmal cough, headache, nausea and vomiting, and diffuse wheezing. Patients with more severe exposures may also develop cyanosis, pulmonary edema, shock, seizures, and loss of consciousness.

Assessment and Management

When you treat patients who have been exposed to chlorine gas, your priority is to remove them from the area of exposure. Use the same precautions that would apply in a hazmat situation when choosing where to position your vehicle and selecting your PPE.

After moving the patients to a safe environment and performing decontamination, quickly triage the patients (triage is discussed in Chapter 48, *Incident Management and Mass-Casualty Incidents*). Rapidly assess the patient's respiratory status, mental status, and oxygenation. Monitor pulse oximetry and capnometry for signs of decompensation. People with dyspnea, wheezing, severe cough, or other signs of respiratory distress are priority patients; administer oxygen (humidified, if available) by mask. Nebulized bronchodilators (eg, albuterol, ipratropium) should be administered to patients in respiratory distress with signs of bronchospasm. Noncardiogenic pulmonary edema may develop in patients within 6 to 24 hours of significant exposure. The use of continuous positive airway pressure/bilevel positive airway pressure may benefit these patients. Consider early intubation for patients with airway burns, stridor, or airway edema or those who become fatigued and can no longer compensate.

Irrigate burning or itching eyes with water, as well as any areas of the skin that have come in contact with the chlorine gas. Establish vascular access and assess the patient's blood glucose level. Administer a 20-mL/kg crystalloid IV fluid bolus if signs of hypoperfusion are present. Transport to the appropriate facility.

Cyanide

Cyanide is a chemical substance that is a by-product of the combustion of synthetic materials that contain carbon and nitrogen. The combustion of household goods such as insulation, carpeting, upholstery, plastic, and synthetic rubber can release a significant amount of cyanide. Hydrogen cyanide is a colorless or pale blue liquid at temperatures less than 78°F (25.6°C) and a colorless gas at higher temperatures.[33] Sodium cyanide and potassium cyanide are white powders.

Historically, cyanide has been used in warfare as a chemical weapon. Cyanide and cyanide-containing compounds are also used in pesticides and fumigants, in mining to extract gold, and in manufacturing of plastics, paper, and textiles. Cyanide poisoning has been used as a method of execution, genocide, and suicide.

The pits and seeds of some common fruits (eg, apricots, apples, peaches) may have substantial amounts of chemicals that are metabolized to cyanide.[34] In addition, some foods and plants, such as lima beans, almonds, and apple seeds, contain small amounts of cyanide. Although cyanide has been reported to have a "bitter almond" scent, many individuals cannot detect it, and the odor's presence does not provide adequate warning of hazardous concentrations.

Pathophysiology

Cyanide is one of the most rapid-acting and deadly poisons and can affect the body by ingestion, inhalation, skin contact, or eye contact. A mitochondrial toxin, it does its damage by combining with a crucial cellular enzyme, cytochrome oxidase, which blocks the use of oxygen at the cellular level. As a result, cellular hypoxia can rapidly develop throughout the body, causing cardiovascular collapse and death. The brain is the most sensitive target organ of cyanide poisoning, followed by the heart, because these organs require the most significant amounts of oxygen.[34]

Depending on its form, cyanide can enter the body through inhalation, ingestion, or absorption through the skin **TABLE 28-4**. The rapidity of symptom onset is related to the concentration, duration, and route of exposure. For example, symptoms begin within seconds to minutes after inhalation exposure, and death may occur within minutes. Ingestion of hydrogen cyanide solutions or cyanide salts can be rapidly fatal. Symptom onset may be either immediate or delayed for 30 to 60 minutes after absorption through the skin.[34]

Assessment and Management

After moving the patient to a safe environment and performing decontamination if indicated, quickly assess the patient's respiratory status, mental status, and oxygenation. Initiate treatment as quickly as possible, including the administration of 100% oxygen via nonrebreathing mask or bag-mask ventilation. The aim of treatment is to displace the cyanide from the cytochrome oxidase by introducing another chemical that will "attract" the cyanide and bind to it. Assess the patient's vital signs, including temperature, pulse oximetry, and capnometry. Because cyanide impairs the body's ability to properly offload the oxygen molecules at a cellular level, recognize that the pulse oximeter reading may be high despite true hypoxia being present at a cellular level. Monitor the patient closely for signs of decompensation regardless of the pulse oximetry readings obtained.

Attach a cardiac monitor and obtain a 12-lead ECG. Establish vascular access, and assess the patient's blood glucose level. Contact medical control for an order to administer hydroxocobalamin or sodium thiosulfate, if available. Hydroxocobalamin is a member of the vitamin B_{12} family and is the only agent considered safe for treating cyanide poisoning in the pregnant patient. Some EMS agency kits with hydroxocobalamin are available, which include tubes to obtain a blood sample (if feasible). Hydroxocobalamin is considered a relatively safe antidote, with allergy and anaphylaxis being the primary concern with its use. Patients will also experience some temporary effects such as redness of the skin, eyes, and urine, as well as itching, after its administration.

TABLE 28-4 Effects of Cyanide Exposure

Exposure Route	Cyanide Effects
Ingestion exposure	Abdominal pain, nausea/vomiting, burning sensation in the mouth and throat
Skin exposure	Irritation Rapid absorption that occurs even more readily when ambient temperature and relative humidity are high
Inhalation exposure, mild to moderate exposure	Central nervous system: altered mental status (confusion), headache, restlessness, anxiety, dizziness, weakness, and loss of consciousness Cardiovascular system: palpitations, chest tightness Respiratory system: dyspnea, tachypnea/hyperpnea (early), bradypnea/apnea (late) Gastrointestinal system: nausea/vomiting
Inhalation exposure, severe exposure	Central nervous system: seizures, coma, fixed and dilated pupils Cardiovascular system: dysrhythmias, hypotension, shock, cardiac arrest Respiratory system: tachypnea/hyperpnea (early), bradypnea/apnea (late), pulmonary edema, respiratory arrest Eyes: fixed and dilated pupils, eye surface inflammation, temporary blindness Other: muscle spasms in which the head, neck, and spine are arched backward

Modified from: About cyanide poisoning. Cyanokit website. https://www.cyanokit.com/about-cyanide-poisoning. Accessed October 4, 2021; Facts about cyanide. Centers for Disease Control and Prevention website. https://emergency.cdc.gov/agent/cyanide/basics/facts.asp. Reviewed April 4, 2018. Accessed October 4, 2021; and Hydrogen cyanide (AC): systemic agent. Centers for Disease Control and Prevention website. https://www.cdc.gov/niosh/ershdb/emergencyresponsecard_29750038.html. Reviewed May 12, 2011. Accessed October 4, 2021.

Amyl nitrite and sodium nitrite are no longer used as cyanide antidotes and are no longer available in commercial kits.[6]

Transport the patient without delay to an appropriate facility. Ingested cyanide reacts with stomach acids, generating hydrogen cyanide gas that may be released when the patient vomits or belches. During transport, maximize air circulation in the patient compartment to reduce exposure risk.

Words of Wisdom

The most important aspect of treatment for patients with toxic inhalations is to remove the patient from the toxic environment. You cannot help the patient if you become ill yourself, so always ensure the rescue is performed by someone using an appropriate self-contained breathing apparatus.

Caustics

Caustics include strong acids (pH <2.0) and strong alkalis (pH >12.0). Both types of chemicals are commonly used in industry, in agriculture (anhydrous ammonia), and in the home as cleaning agents **TABLE 28-5** and **FIGURE 28-13**. According to the 2019 Annual Report of the AAPCC's National Poison Data System, almost 185,000 exposures to caustic agents occurred in adults and children.[35] Again, pediatric ingestions are generally unintentional. If the patient is an adult, then oral ingestion of caustics is usually a suicide attempt.

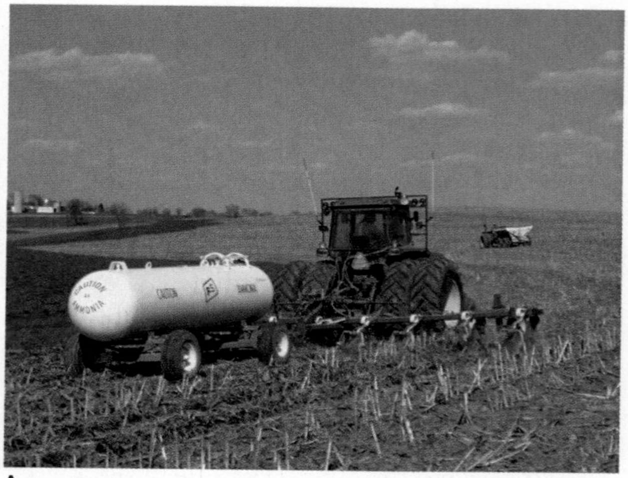

A

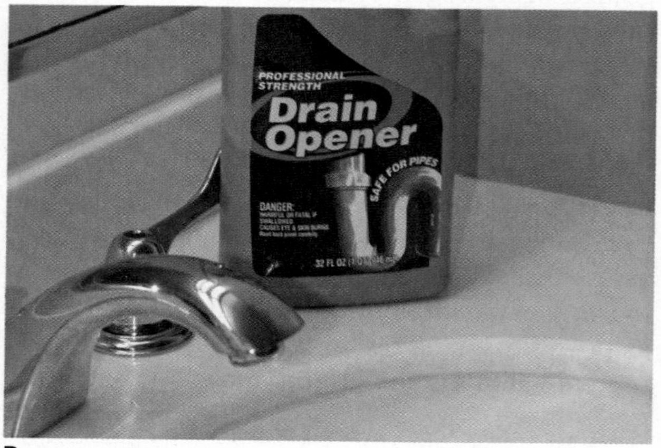

B

FIGURE 28-13 Caustic chemicals are commonly used in industry. **A.** Anhydrous ammonia tank used in agriculture. **B.** Plumbing agents used in the home.

A: Courtesy of Lynn Betts/NRCS; B: © Jones & Bartlett Learning. Photographed by Kimberly Potvin.

TABLE 28-5 Common Caustic Substances

Substance	Example	Source
Acids	Hydrochloric acid	Toilet bowl cleaners, swimming pool cleaners
	Sulfuric acid	Battery acid, toilet bowl cleaners (such as bisulfate)
	Others	Bleach disinfectants, slate cleaners
Alkalis	Lye (sodium or potassium hydroxide)	Paint removers, washing powders, drain cleaners (such as Drano, Liquid-Plumr, Plunge), button-shaped batteries, Clinitest tablets
	Sodium hypochlorite	Bleach (Clorox)
	Sodium carbonate	Bleach (Purex), nonphosphate detergents
	Ammonia	Hair dyes, jewelry cleaners, metal cleaners or polishes, antirust agents
	Potassium permanganate	Electric dishwasher detergents

> **Words of Wisdom**
>
> If a patient who swallowed a caustic agent is in respiratory distress, provide prompt transport to the hospital. Coughing, tachypnea, and stridor are ominous signs. Significant hypopharyngeal edema may develop and require consideration of a surgical airway.

Pathophysiology

Caustic substances cause direct chemical injury to the tissues they contact. Acids cause coagulation necrosis. Normally, a layer of eschar (leathery scar tissue) forms and contains the damaged tissue. Alkalis cause liquefaction necrosis, a breakdown of tissue to pus and the liquid contents of the involved cells. Dilution or neutralization is usually required to slow or stop the damage process. Signs and symptoms of a caustic exposure include drooling, burns, difficulty talking or swallowing (with oral ingestions), and hypoperfusion or shock (rarely, usually secondary to internal bleeding).

> **Words of Wisdom**
>
> Some chemicals react vigorously with water, so be sure to check the relevant warnings or placard for information. When you decontaminate a patient with water, do your best to avoid secondary exposures to surrounding tissues while the substances are washed from the primary point of contact.

In the home, caustic liquids may start to leak from the original containers and the homeowner may choose to store the product in a plastic soda bottle, or to keep a small amount in an open plastic cup while using it. These practices increase the likelihood that someone may unintentionally drink from the container and ingest a caustic substance. As the liquid enters the mouth and begins to burn, the patient may simultaneously remove the bottle and turn the head, resulting in burns to the mouth, tongue, face, and neck.

As noted earlier, the intentional mixing of different household chemicals may also result in the release of toxic vapors (ie, chlorine, chloramine).

Assessment and Management

Most patients who have swallowed caustic substances present with severe pain in the mouth, throat, or chest. Respiratory distress, if present, is most probably due to soft-tissue swelling in the larynx, epiglottis, or vocal cords, which means that the patient is in immediate danger of complete airway obstruction. Identify the specific substance and call the poison control center or contact online medical control. For a caustic ingestion, dilution with milk or water is only useful in the minutes immediately following the exposure. Do not attempt dilution in patients with respiratory distress, altered mental status, severe abdominal pain, or nausea or vomiting, or in patients who cannot swallow or protect their airway.[6] Gastric tube placement is contraindicated because it can cause further tissue damage. Establish vascular access, usually en route, because prompt transport to the ED is indicated.

With dermal exposure to a strong acid, the result is immediate and excruciating pain. For a strong alkali, the onset of pain is somewhat delayed, allowing more time before the patient reacts and increasing the severity of the burn. In such an injury, diluting and flushing away the caustic substance is the main goal of field treatment. Acids tend to be more water-soluble than alkalis, so they can often be diluted relatively quickly. It is more important to keep water continually flowing with alkalis because it usually takes much longer to rinse away the substance.

For an eye exposure, cut off the prong section of a nasal cannula, place it on the bridge of the patient's nose, plug in a macrodrip IV administration set, and run it wide open to provide continuous irrigation. This practice also frees you up to perform other tasks. You may also use a Morgan lens after the initial gross flushing has been accomplished. Use of a Morgan lens is covered in Chapter 34, *Face and Neck Trauma*.

One of the most common caustic exposures in the agricultural setting involves anhydrous ammonia. Such an exposure usually occurs during the hookup or disconnection of a tank. Eye exposure to anhydrous ammonia can cause devastating damage in less than 1 minute, resulting in cataracts or blindness. In addition, inhalation exposure can create respiratory distress secondary to pulmonary edema. After the patient has been appropriately decontaminated, start appropriate airway management and supportive care.

Keep the following points in mind for patients with caustic ingestions:

- *Do not* give any "neutralizing substances" orally. Now-outdated recommendations incorrectly advised the administration of an acid after an alkali ingestion, or vice versa. Mixing an acid and an alkali may produce an *exothermic reaction,* adding a thermal injury to the chemical injury.
- *Do not* induce vomiting. Reexposure to a caustic substance will worsen the damage.
- *Do not* perform gastric lavage.
- *Do not* give activated charcoal. It is ineffective in acid or alkali ingestion, and it may interfere with the patient's subsequent medical care by blackening the field of vision when an endoscope is used to inspect the esophagus and stomach for damage.

Common Household Items

From a toxicologic perspective, the average home is full of dangerous substances: from colorful plants to sweet-smelling cleaning products. Identification of the substance involved is the most important part of the history of the ingestion. It is not possible within the scope of this chapter to discuss all of the possibilities when it comes to household poisonings. As always, keep in mind that the poison control center is an invaluable resource.

Drugs Misused for Sexual Purposes

Drugs that are misused for sexual purposes include those that increase sexual gratification and those that are used to facilitate sexual assault.

Drugs That Increase Sexual Gratification

Phosphodiesterase type 5 (PDE5) inhibitors (ie, sildenafil, tadalafil, and vardenafil) are among the most commonly prescribed drugs to treat erectile dysfunction. Unintentional toxic levels are usually the result of aggressive dosing to achieve maximum sexual performance. Occasionally, the patient may have unknowingly received a dose of a PDE5 inhibitor as a prank. Elevated levels may produce hypotension, tachycardia, ischemic chest pain, tachydysrhythmias, and prolonged priapism requiring urologic evaluation. Supportive care is usually all that is required for overdose of PDE5 inhibitors. If you are treating a patient with acute coronary syndrome, then avoid nitrates because they may cause significant hypotension.

Cocaine and other stimulant drugs (such as amphetamines and methamphetamine) are popular choices for people seeking a more intense sexual experience. Treatment is identical to the treatment detailed earlier in this chapter regarding stimulant misuse. Be aware that the stimulant may have been laced with another drug to intensify the patient's response.

Another drug that increases sexual gratification is amyl nitrite (also known as poppers, rush, and happy snaps). This organic nitrate drug can be crushed and inhaled to produce an intense sexual experience. As mentioned earlier, its use may cause methemoglobinemia, affecting the oxygen-carrying ability of blood, and result in the associated ischemic effects. As with any nitrate, hypotension may result from blood pooling in the periphery owing to the drug's vasodilatory effects.

One of the unique drugs in this group is MDMA (Ecstasy, Adam), which was mentioned earlier in the section on stimulants. MDMA is an analog of methamphetamine, and it may have similar toxic effects on a smaller scale. The release of serotonin, a sensation of euphoria, and disinhibition are the effects associated with its use when taken to enhance a person's sexual experience. More significant adverse effects (such as hyperthermia) and electrolyte abnormalities (such as hyponatremia) may also occur. Supportive care is appropriate during transport.

Dextromethorphan (DXM), which is found in several OTC cough suppressants, can produce a euphoric floating sensation or out-of-body experience. Structurally related to codeine, DXM produces a mild stimulant effect that may enhance a sexual experience. Consuming large quantities of DXM can lead to hallucinations, psychedelic visions, loss of motor control, confusion, blurred vision, dreamlike euphoria, and out-of-body sensations.

Drugs Used to Facilitate Sexual Assault

Drugs used to facilitate sexual assault are often administered to an unsuspecting person, frequently dissolved in an alcoholic drink. Sexual predators use these substances to incapacitate others, which explains why they are called "date rape" drugs. They are discussed further in Chapter 23, *Gynecologic Emergencies.*

GHB

Gamma-hydroxybutyrate (GHB) is an endogenous metabolite of gamma-aminobutyric acid that causes intoxication similar to alcohol use. In the late 1980s, GHB gained popularity with young people as a club drug, earning the name "Liquid Ecstasy" from its euphoric effects at raves (all-night dance parties). By the mid-1990s, GHB had become increasingly associated with sexual assaults. In 1990, the FDA banned this drug from OTC sales.

GHB is a colorless and odorless liquid that may go undetected when placed in a drink. Once ingested, it quickly crosses the blood–brain barrier, exerting its effects within 30 to 60 minutes. Ingestion may produce disinhibition, severe passivity (ie, a lack of the will to resist), and antegrade amnesia. Associated use with alcohol increases the risk of respiratory depression, coma, and death. GHB also has a withdrawal presentation similar to that of alcohol or benzodiazepine use.[36]

Treatment of GHB intoxication focuses on supportive care. The patient may be unable to protect the airway. First, establish and maintain the airway, inserting an advanced airway as needed. Monitor oxygenation and ventilation. Administer supplemental oxygen as needed. Establish vascular access. Apply the ECG monitor, pulse oximeter, and capnometer. Finally, provide rapid transport to the ED.

Flunitrazepam (Rohypnol)

Also known as roofies, this drug is a potent benzodiazepine that is also used to facilitate sexual assault. When combined with another drug that works to depress the CNS, flunitrazepam may cause the patient to experience profound effects including unconsciousness, respiratory depression, and death. This drug is illegal to make or distribute, so most of the supply found in the United States enters the country from Mexico.

Poisonous Alcohols

As mentioned previously, the form of alcohol consumed by humans in alcoholic beverages (ethanol) is not conventionally recognized as a poison. Instead, poisonous alcohols are generally considered to encompass alcohols manufactured for industrial or nongastronomic purposes, such as methyl alcohol and ethylene glycol.

Methyl Alcohol

Methyl alcohol (also known as wood alcohol or methanol) is present in paints, paint remover, windshield washer fluids, varnishes, antifreeze, and canned fuels such as Sterno **FIGURE 28-14**.

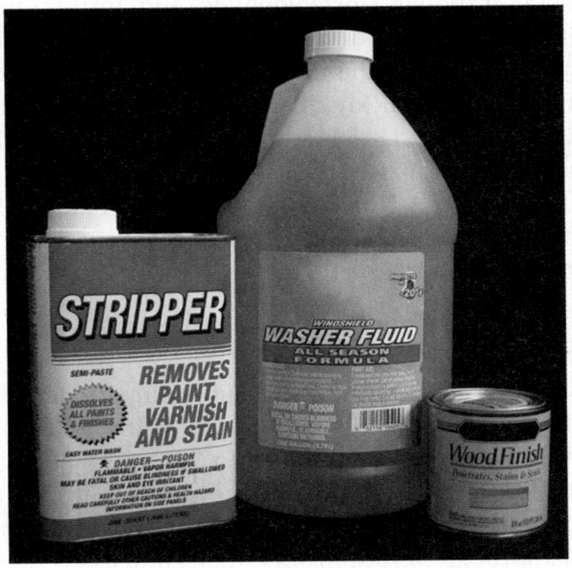

A

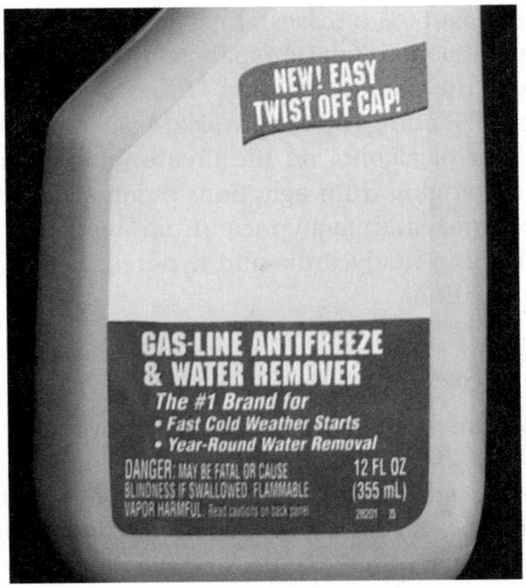

B

FIGURE 28-14 Methyl alcohol is present in paints, paint remover, windshield washer fluids, and varnishes **(A)** and in antifreeze and canned fuels **(B)**.

Methanol may be a popular substitute for ethanol among people with alcohol use disorder when they do not have the means to obtain ethanol. This colorless liquid has a unique odor. Ingestion of as little as 60 to 250 mL in adults or 8 to 10 mL in children is associated with severe toxicity.

Pathophysiology

When methanol is ingested, its metabolic breakdown products (formaldehyde and formic acid) are responsible for the characteristic signs and symptoms of methanol poisoning. Once ingested, methanol is quickly absorbed from the GI tract, with peak blood levels attained within 30 to 90 minutes. In mild toxicity, the half-life of methanol is 14 to 20 hours. As toxicity increases, the half-life increases to 24 to 30 hours. The liver eliminates 90% to 95% of the methanol.

Assessment

The symptoms of methanol poisoning do not usually appear immediately but begin from 12 to 18 hours, and occasionally up to 72 hours, after ingestion. Because of this latency period, it may be difficult to determine the source of the symptoms. Be thorough in your history taking and assessment. Patient complaints include nausea and vomiting (in almost 50% of cases), headache or vertigo, abdominal pain (often from pancreatitis), and blurred vision (the patient may say, "It looks like a snowstorm"). Findings on the physical exam may include an odor of alcohol on the breath, altered mental status ranging from agitation to coma, mydriasis, hyperpnea and tachypnea (from metabolic acidosis), and bradycardia and hypotension as a late presentation.

Management

Field care for methanol poisoning is primarily supportive. Establish and manage the airway, considering advanced airway placement as needed. Establish vascular access. Assess the blood glucose level, and administer glucose if the patient has hypoglycemia. Activated charcoal does not bind well to alcohol, and methanol is rapidly absorbed in the stomach. For these reasons, activated charcoal is often contraindicated unless you have identified other substances that were ingested for which activated charcoal may be beneficial.[37]

Sodium bicarbonate may be ordered by medical control to assist with ion trapping and counteracting metabolic acidosis. Morbidity and mortality are often driven by the amount of methanol ingested and the speed with which the patient receives definitive treatment. Provide prompt transport to an appropriate facility.[38]

Ethylene Glycol

Ethylene glycol is a colorless, odorless liquid found in a variety of commercial products, including antifreeze, coolant, deicers, polishes, and paints. Similar to methanol, it may be used by people with alcohol use disorder who cannot obtain ethanol. The lethal dose of ethylene glycol is estimated to be 2 mL/kg, or as little as 150 mL in the average-size adult.

Pathophysiology

Ethylene glycol is water-soluble. With oral intake, it is absorbed rapidly, with peak blood levels attained within 1 to 4 hours after ingestion. The liver and kidneys metabolize ethylene glycol into a number of toxic metabolites, including aldehydes, lactate, oxalate, and glycolate. In turn, these metabolites inhibit cellular respiration and glucose metabolism; they also impair cellular function through an anion gap metabolic acidosis.

Assessment

Toxicity from ethylene glycol occurs in three stages, so the signs and symptoms will vary depending on when you encounter the patient relative to the time of ingestion:

- **Stage 1.** CNS depression is the hallmark of the initial stage. The patient may appear intoxicated, as evidenced by slurred speech and ataxia, without an obvious odor of alcohol present. These symptoms progress to include nausea, vomiting, seizures, or coma as metabolites begin to accumulate in the body. Stage 1 begins soon after ingestion and can last up to 12 hours.
- **Stage 2.** Cardiopulmonary symptoms begin to appear as the patient enters the second stage. The patient may exhibit hypertension, hypotension, or tachycardia. Pulmonary injury may

- Be alert for agitation or violence. Provide reassurance and administer benzodiazepines, if needed.
- Treat seizures with benzodiazepines.
- Provide rapid transport to the appropriate facility.

Monoamine Oxidase Inhibitors

Pathophysiology

Monoamine oxidase inhibitors (MAOIs) are used primarily to treat atypical depression. Norepinephrine, serotonin, and dopamine are the primary neurotransmitters that assist with improving mood and affect when they are present in certain cells and circuits in the brain. Monoamine oxidase (MAO) is an enzyme that removes these neurotransmitters from the brain. MAOIs prevent the regular removal of the neurotransmitters, resulting in increased levels in circulation. When they reach toxic levels, MAOIs can block these enzymes for a short or long duration based on the medication. With some ingestions, a new series of enzymes can be synthesized by the body only after several days. Examples of MAOIs include phenelzine and tranylcypromine.

Assessment

Symptoms of MAOI toxicity are often delayed, occurring 6 to 12 hours after ingestion of the medication. Cardiovascular effects of MAOI toxicity include hypertension, tachycardia, palpitations, chest pain, diaphoresis, and atrial dysrhythmias. Marked hyperthermia, muscle rigidity, respiratory failure, delirium, and seizures may occur in patients with severe toxicity. After signs and symptoms begin to appear, prepare to manage a life-threatening event. When death occurs from an MAOI overdose, it is usually secondary to multiple-system organ failure.

Management

In a patient with suspected MAOI overdose, establish and maintain the airway, inserting an advanced airway as needed. In addition, administer oxygen. If rapid sequence intubation is required, use of a nondepolarizing paralytic such as rocuronium is recommended during this procedure because MAOIs may enhance the actions of succinylcholine. Establish large-bore vascular access. Monitor the ECG rhythm, staying alert for changes indicative of hyperkalemia. Consult with medical control for additional guidance or follow local protocols.

If the patient's condition is deteriorating, treat hypotension with sequential fluid boluses of normal saline. If seizures occur, treat them with benzodiazepines per local protocol; otherwise, persistent seizures may contribute to the combined problems of metabolic acidosis, hyperkalemia, and rhabdomyolysis. Consider midazolam administration if the patient is hyperthermic.

Selective Serotonin Reuptake Inhibitors

Pathophysiology

Their larger therapeutic window has helped make **selective serotonin reuptake inhibitors (SSRIs)** a common pharmacologic choice for managing depression. SSRIs work by enhancing serotonergic neurotransmission and inhibiting the breakdown of serotonin. SSRIs have few cardiac effects or anticholinergic effects, so they are a safer option for the management of depression compared to TCAs. Popular SSRIs include fluoxetine (Prozac), paroxetine (Paxil), citalopram (Celexa), and sertraline (Zoloft).

Assessment

When SSRIs are taken in conjunction with alcohol, look for tachycardia, mild hypotension, and lethargy as the most common signs and symptoms. Other symptoms include nausea, vomiting, and tremors. Dilated pupils, agitation, hypotension or hypertension, seizures, and hallucinations may be less commonly noted. Dysrhythmias are also rare but may include QT prolongation and torsades de pointes.

Management

A pure SSRI overdose with no other drugs or alcohol involved usually produces limited toxic effects, with the exception of seizures or serotonin syndrome (discussed later in this section). As such, management of an SSRI overdose follows the general approach for poisoned patients:

- Establish and maintain the airway.
- Administer oxygen to maintain blood saturation levels at greater than 94%.
- Establish vascular access.
- Provide continuous ECG monitoring and treat dysrhythmias according to current resuscitation guidelines.

- Control hyperthermia with cooling measures.
- Administer a crystalloid IV fluid challenge (20 mL/kg) for hypotension; consider vasopressor administration if hypotension persists despite adequate fluid resuscitation.
- Treat seizure activity and agitation with benzodiazepines per local protocol.
- Transport to the appropriate facility.

Serotonin Syndrome

Serotonin syndrome is an idiosyncratic complication that occasionally occurs with antidepressant therapy. This condition is not limited to patients taking SSRIs, but can also occur when patients take St. John's wort or any combination of drugs that increase central serotonin neurotransmission (see Table 28-1). The onset of serotonin syndrome is commonly within 6 hours of ingestion (and possibly the result of something as simple as an increased dosage of a medication). Prehospital treatment is supportive. Consider cooling measures if hyperthermia is present. Symptoms may persist beyond 24 hours in severe cases or if extended-release medications are involved.

Lithium

Despite the major advances made in many areas of psychiatric medicine, **lithium** remains a common mood stabilizer used in the treatment of bipolar disorder. In 1949, lithium salts made their debut for the treatment of mania. Eventually, they were found to be much more efficacious for the treatment of bipolar disorder, and they retain their position as the main treatment of this condition. Lithium assists with dampening mood swings rather than affecting the normal mood.

Pathophysiology

Lithium is almost completely absorbed in the GI tract roughly 8 hours after ingestion. Bioelimination occurs relatively slowly, with approximately one-third of the dose remaining in the body for roughly 2 weeks after administration. Given its small therapeutic window and slow excretion process, the threats of toxic levels and overdosing are ever present.

Assessment

Early signs and symptoms of lithium overdose include nausea, vomiting, headache, hand tremors, excessive thirst, and slurred speech. With increased toxicity come increased neurologic symptoms: ataxia, muscle weakness and incoordination, abnormal thermoregulation, blurred vision, and hyperreflexia (twitching). Eventually, the patient may have seizures and become comatose.

Management

Management of a patient suspected of a lithium overdose is mostly supportive. Establish and maintain the airway, inserting an advanced airway as needed. Provide high-concentration supplemental oxygen, and establish vascular access. If the patient experiences hypotension, administer serial boluses of normal saline. Maintain continuous ECG monitoring, being alert for AV blocks and ventricular dysrhythmias. Finally, transport the patient to an appropriate facility. Hemodialysis and continuous renal replacement therapy may be indicated at the hospital, so consider these possibilities when determining your transport destination.

Nonprescription Pain Medications

Medications used for pain management make up a large part of the OTC drug market. In the OTC and prescription drug markets, nonsteroidal anti-inflammatory drugs (NSAIDs) are some of the most popular options for pain relief, fever control, and anti-inflammatory action. Their convenient dosing schemes and large therapeutic windows, coupled with their safe track records relative to acute ingestion and overdose, enhance their popularity.

Pathophysiology

NSAIDs are rapidly absorbed from the GI tract before being eliminated from the body in urine and feces. The half-lives of these agents vary widely, ranging from 2 to 4 hours for ibuprofen, to approximately 15 hours for selective cyclooxygenase-2 inhibitors, to 50 hours for some long-acting agents. Patients who take both lithium and NSAIDs have slowed renal clearance of the lithium, increasing the likelihood that they will inadvertently reach a toxic lithium level.

Most of the conditions associated with NSAID use involve long-term use; patients may experience GI bleeding and kidney dysfunction. Acute ingestion and overdoses are rare, with ibuprofen being the NSAID most commonly encountered in the acute setting.

Assessment

Many NSAID overdoses remain asymptomatic. Very large doses are usually required before any signs or symptoms of toxicity occur. At toxic levels, the signs and symptoms of NSAID overdose may include nausea with vomiting and abdominal pain. Metabolic acidosis can occur with severe NSAID toxicity.

Management

For symptomatic patients, emergency medical care is usually supportive. Establish and maintain the airway, inserting an advanced airway as needed. Administer high-concentration supplemental oxygen, and establish vascular access. Administer crystalloid fluid boluses for hypotensive patients. Treat seizures with benzodiazepines per local protocol. Finally, transport the patient to an appropriate facility.

A unique adverse effect of NSAID use is aseptic meningitis, in which a patient presents with reports of a stiff neck, headache, and fever within several hours after taking an NSAID. Discontinuing the NSAID therapy generally resolves this condition, but patients must be evaluated at the hospital to rule out other causes.

Salicylates

Although aspirin (acetylsalicylic acid [ASA]) can be involved in a toxic event, it is more typical for OTC products containing **salicylates** to cause unintentional toxicity. For example, a single 30-mL dose of bismuth subsalicylate (Pepto-Bismol) contains 261 mg of salicylate (two-thirds the total dose of one aspirin). Aggressive dosing of salicylates for analgesia or fever control may lead to toxic levels of the substance.

Pathophysiology

Ingestion of 150 mg/kg or less will usually result in mild toxicity. At this level, chief complaints are usually nausea, vomiting, and abdominal pain. With a dosing range of 150 to 300 mg/kg, signs and symptoms may include ringing in the ears (tinnitus), pulmonary edema, and acid–base disturbances. At levels of 300 mg/kg, severe toxicity may produce metabolic acidosis. Although you may be unable to analyze an actual blood gas level in the field, you may note that the patient has tachypnea and hyperpnea: the body's compensatory mechanism for correcting metabolic acidosis.

An acute salicylate event with an adult usually involves an intentional overdose, with a common patient profile being young women with a history of drug misuse or psychiatric conditions. A fatal event is possible if an adult with suspected salicylate overdose is unresponsive during the primary survey and presents with a high fever, seizures, or cardiac dysrhythmias.

Assessment and Management

No salicylate antidote or antagonist is available, so field management is primarily supportive. Establish and maintain the airway, inserting an advanced airway as needed. Provide supplemental oxygen and monitor carbon dioxide levels with capnometry. If you are ventilating the patient, then you may consider not immediately correcting hypocapnia. The patient was compensating by breathing fast. Failure to provide a ventilation rate similar to the compensatory rate may result in rising carbon dioxide levels that worsen the acidosis. Obtain vascular access. If hypotension develops, then administer serial boluses of normal saline. Medical control may ask you to administer activated charcoal because of aspirin's erratic absorption. Finally, transport the patient to an appropriate facility.

Acetaminophen

Acetaminophen is a well-tolerated OTC drug with few adverse effects. These characteristics have made this drug one of the best-selling analgesics in the United States and a common culprit in toxic exposures. Similar to the case for other NSAIDs, many OTC medications have acetaminophen as an active ingredient. Unintentional overdoses may occur when several medications containing acetaminophen are taken together. These unintentional overdoses may occur several times throughout the course of a day or several days, and the patient may unknowingly build up a toxic level.

Pathophysiology

After it is ingested, acetaminophen is rapidly absorbed from the GI tract, producing peak serum levels in 30 to 120 minutes. Absorption slows when the drug is combined with diphenhydramine (Tylenol PM) or with propoxyphene (Darvocet). One unique

TABLE 28-7 Signs and Symptoms of Acetaminophen Toxicity

Stage	Time Frame	Signs and Symptoms
I	<24 h	Nausea, vomiting, loss of appetite, pallor, malaise
II	24–72 h	Right upper quadrant abdominal pain; abdomen tender to palpation
III	72–96 h	Metabolic acidosis, renal failure, coagulopathies, recurring GI symptoms
IV	4–14 d (or longer)	Recovery slowly begins, or liver failure progresses and the patient dies

Abbreviation: GI, gastrointestinal

aspect of acetaminophen toxicity is that the signs and symptoms appear in four distinct stages **TABLE 28-7**.

Assessment and Management

It is important to accurately estimate the time of ingestion because this information drives the decision-making process for patient care both in the field and in the hospital. An antidote for acetaminophen toxicity exists: acetylcysteine (Acetadote). Ideally, this drug should be given less than 8 hours after the ingestion. Typically, however, it is administered based on the patient's laboratory results; as such, it is not a field intervention.

Management of the patient in the field first focuses on establishing and maintaining the airway, with an advanced airway being inserted as needed. Establish vascular access. Consider activated charcoal administration after consulting with medical control for recent (within the first hour) ingestions and prolonged transport times to definitive care. Transport the patient to an appropriate facility.

Metals and Metalloids

Although acute metal and metalloid toxic exposures are relatively rare, when they occur, they can produce devastating results, usually because of delayed diagnosis or misdiagnosis. Asymptomatic patients or patients who have vague, nonspecific symptoms can be difficult to diagnose. This difficulty in reaching the correct diagnosis may contribute to increased mortality or morbidity because of delayed or inadequate treatment. Toxic exposures involving metals or metalloids usually manifest by affecting four body systems: neurologic, hematologic, renal, and GI.

Iron

Although only a small amount of iron is required as part of a healthy diet, many adult and pediatric multivitamins contain iron. Children younger than 6 years have frequent iron exposures, usually secondary to ingesting chewable vitamins. Many chewable vitamins are marketed to look and taste like candy. Prenatal vitamins are a common source for lethal pediatric iron ingestions. By comparison, most toxic exposures in adults are intentional.

Pathophysiology

In the average 155-pound (70-kg) adult, the body's entire iron supply consists of only about 4 g. Of that total, roughly 65% is found in hemoglobin. Excessive amounts of iron in the body can speed up the formation of oxygen free radicals, creating a metabolic acidosis. They may also affect the coagulation cascade and the liver, causing significant coagulopathy.

From a practical perspective, the toxic effects of an iron exposure reflect the amount of elemental iron ingested. With ingestion of 20 to 60 mg/kg, mild to moderate toxicity should be expected. With dosing of more than 60 mg/kg, severe and potentially lethal toxicity is a possibility.

Assessment and Management

From the time of ingestion, iron poisoning will usually cause symptoms within the first 6 hours. If patients do not have symptoms during this time, then it is unlikely they will experience serious toxicity. Early stages of iron poisoning may include vomiting, diarrhea, abdominal pain, hematemesis, tachycardia, hypotension, and altered mental status. Patients commonly experience metabolic acidosis and become tachypneic as the body attempts to correct the pH by increasing the elimination of carbon dioxide. A patient in the later stages of iron poisoning will present with profound shock, seizures, hyperthermia, liver failure, and coagulopathy.

Unfortunately, you can do little in the field for iron poisoning, other than provide attention to the ABCs and transport the patient to the hospital for further evaluation and laboratory studies. Provide supportive care directed at maintaining adequate perfusion and oxygenation. Activated charcoal does not adsorb iron and should not be used unless other toxins were ingested.

Arsenic

In 2019, the AAPCC reported that arsenic (not contained in pesticides) was involved in approximately 8% of all heavy metal poisonings.[33] This metal is used in various industries and appears in many compounds, so it is often the source of unintentional exposures. Intentional exposures include the use of arsenic in homicide and suicide.

Pathophysiology

Arsenic can enter the body by ingestion, inhalation, and absorption and dermally through a wound. It is eliminated from the body through the kidneys.

Assessment

The clinical presentation of arsenic poisoning depends on the type, amount, and concentration of arsenic that enters the body and the rate of absorption and elimination. In general, symptoms appear within 30 minutes to several hours of arsenic ingestion. Arsenic poisoning should be suspected with patients who present with hypotension of unknown cause following a bout of severe gastroenteritis.

Signs and symptoms of arsenic poisoning include severe abdominal pain, nausea, explosive diarrhea, "metallic taste" in the mouth, dysphagia, general malaise, weakness, hypotension, pulmonary edema, rhabdomyolysis, metabolic acidosis, and renal failure. ECG changes and dysrhythmias (usually supraventricular tachycardia) may be apparent, but nonspecific ST-segment and T-wave changes are also possible, as is QT prolongation. Ventricular tachycardia and torsades de pointes can occur as well.

Management

A patient with acute arsenic toxicity is in critical condition and requires aggressive interventions. Establish and maintain the airway, inserting an advanced airway as needed. Administer supplemental oxygen, and establish vascular access. For patients with hypotension, administer sequential boluses of normal saline. If the hypotension proves refractory to fluid therapy, then administer a vasopressor. Continuously monitor the ECG, and follow the advanced cardiac life support algorithms for dysrhythmias. Finally, provide rapid transport to an appropriate facility.

Poisonous Plants

Of the thousands of plant varieties, only a few are poisonous **FIGURE 28-16**. Oddly enough, poisonous plants represent some of the most common ornamental garden shrubs and houseplants. Perhaps for that reason, approximately 58% of plant-related exposures involve children age 5 years or younger. In the AAPCC's 2019 Annual Report, plant ingestions were listed in the top 25 substance categories most frequently involved in human exposures and in the top 10 substances for pediatric exposures.[33] Thankfully, deaths from plant ingestions are rare; in 2019, only three fatal ingestions were reported in more than 45,000 reported cases. Most plant ingestions result in minimal symptoms unless a large amount is ingested or the substance has been concentrated in a tea or paste. **TABLE 28-8** lists plants that can cause toxic results and, in some cases, death.

Pathophysiology

The ubiquitous **dieffenbachia** is a lovely green plant with broad, variegated leaves. It is nicknamed "dumb cane," because eating dieffenbachia can result in a person being unable to speak. All parts of the dieffenbachia plant (leaves, stems, and roots) contain sharp calcium oxalate crystals. When ingested, these crystals cause burns of the mouth and tongue and, sometimes, paralysis of the vocal cords. In severe cases, edema of the tongue and larynx may lead to airway compromise. **Caladium**, with its stunning multicolored leaves, is another hazardous plant; poisoning with caladium has a similar presentation to poisoning with dieffenbachia.

Azaleas and rhododendrons have a similar mechanism of toxicity based on grayanotoxins that are present in the plants. Ingestion of the leaves or flowers of the plants, as well as the nectar of honey

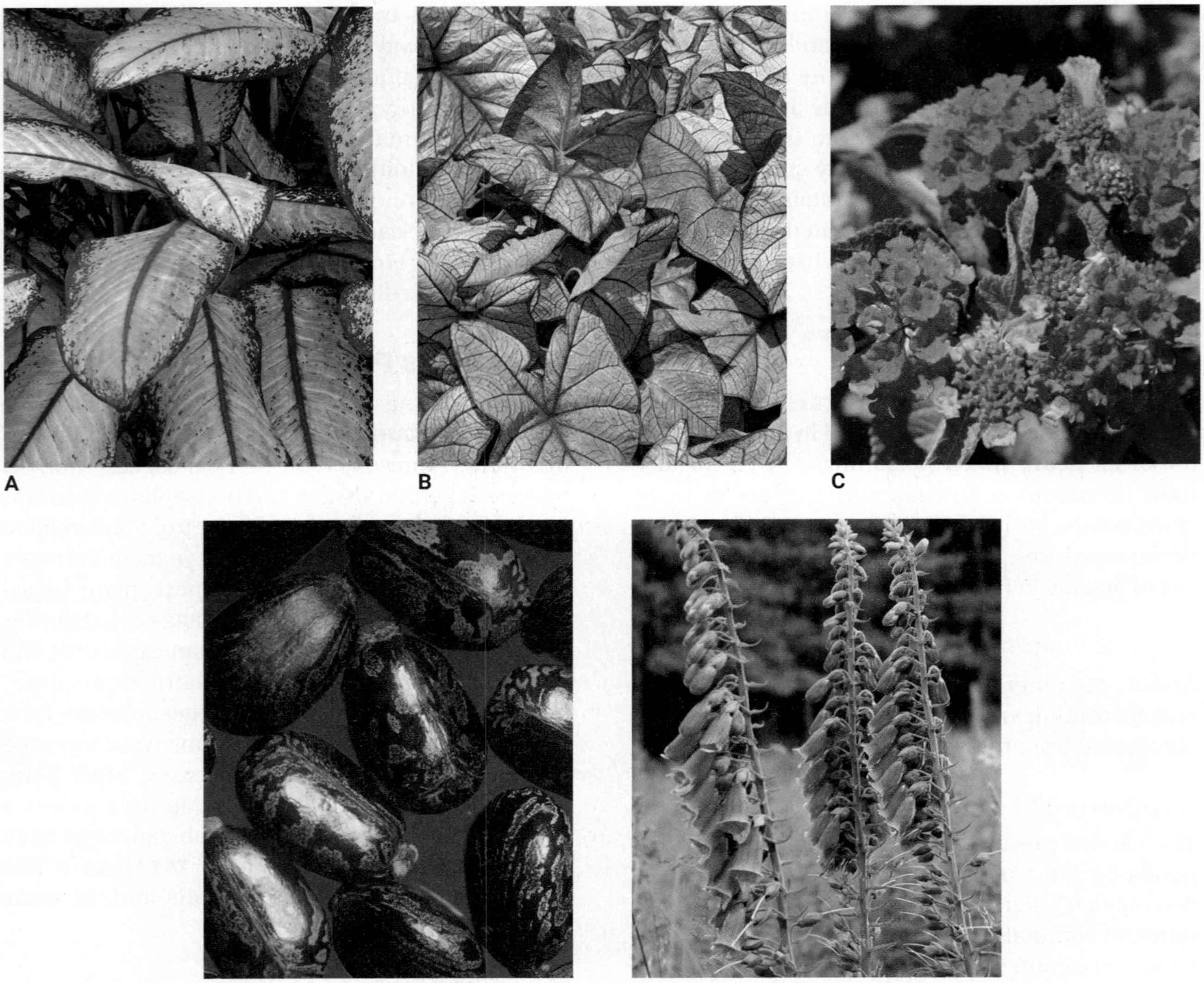

A B C D E

FIGURE 28-16 Poisonous plants. **A.** Dieffenbachia. **B.** Caladium. **C.** Lantana. **D.** Castor beans. **E.** Foxglove.

A: © Andriy Doriy/Shutterstock; B: © Hatem Eldoronki/Shutterstock; C: © MaxFX/Shutterstock; D: Courtesy of Brian Prechtel/USDA; E: © Jean Ann Fitzhugh/Shutterstock.

TABLE 28-8 Poisons in Some Common Plants

Plant	Poisonous Part	Poison	Signs and Symptoms of Poisoning
Apricot	Seeds	Cyanide	Headache, dizziness, weakness, nausea, vomiting, coma, seizures, metabolic acidosis
Autumn crocus	Entire plant	Colchicine	Delayed cramps, nausea, diarrhea, dehydration, coagulopathy, multiple organ failure
Azalea	Entire plant	Grayanotoxin	Nausea, salivation, vomiting, dizziness, dyspnea, cholinergic symptoms
Bloodroot	Roots	Sanguinarine	Cramps, diarrhea, dizziness, paralysis, coma

Plant	Poisonous Part	Poison	Signs and Symptoms of Poisoning
Buttercup	Entire plant	Protoanemonin	Gastroenteritis, seizures
Caladium	Leaves and roots	Calcium oxalate	Burning of mucous membranes, swelling of the tongue and throat, salivation, gastroenteritis
Cherry tree	Bark, leaves, seeds	Amygdalin	Stupor, vocal cord paralysis, seizures, coma
Chinaberry	Berries; leaves and bark to a lesser extent	Tetranortriterpenoid neurotoxins	Vomiting, diarrhea, sometimes excitement or depression
Daffodil	Bulb	Multiple	Gastroenteritis
Deadly nightshade	Berries, leaves, roots	Atropine	Hyperthermia, seizures, hallucinations, anticholinergic symptoms
Dieffenbachia	Leaves and roots	Calcium oxalate	Mucosal damage similar to caladium
Elderberry	Leaves, shoots, bark	Sambunigrin	Gastroenteritis
Holly	Berries	Ilicin	Gastroenteritis, coma
Hyacinth	Bulb	Multiple	Severe gastroenteritis
Jack-in-the-pulpit	All parts	Calcium oxalate	Severe gastroenteritis
Jimson weed	All parts	Atropine	Dry mouth; hot, red skin; headache; hallucinations; tachycardia; hypertension; delirium; seizures
Laurel	All parts	Andromedotoxin	Salivation, lacrimation, rhinorrhea, vomiting, seizures, bradycardia, hypotension, paralysis
Lily of the valley	Leaves, flowers	Glycosides	Hyperkalemia, cardiac dysrhythmias, gastroenteritis, altered mental status
Mistletoe	All parts	Tyramine	Bradycardia, gastroenteritis, hypertension, dyspnea, delirium, sweating, shock
Morning glory	Seeds	LSD	Hallucinations
Narcissus	Bulb	Multiple	Gastroenteritis
Oleander	Entire plant	Oleanin	Cramps, bradycardia, dilated pupils, bloody diarrhea, coma, apnea (one leaf is lethal)
Philodendron	Entire plant	Calcium oxalate	Edema of tongue, throat
Poinsettia	Leaves, stems, sap	Multiple	Contact dermatitis, gastroenteritis
Potato	Green tubers, new sprouts	Solanine	Severe gastroenteritis, headache, apnea, shock
Rhododendron	Entire plant	Grayanotoxin	Nausea, salivation, vomiting, dizziness, dyspnea, cholinergic symptoms
Rhubarb	Leaves only	Oxalic acid	Cramps, nausea, vomiting, anuria
Wisteria	Pods	Glycoside	Severe gastroenteritis, shock

Abbreviation: LSD, lysergic acid diethylamide

made by the bees that feed on them, can cause cholinergic symptoms.[39]

Lantana (also known as red sage or wild sage) is a perennial flowering shrub with clusters of little red berries. These berries can lead to serious poisoning, particularly when ripe. Even when still green, the berries contain lantadene A, a poison that causes GI upset, muscle weakness, shock, and sometimes death.

Another dangerous plant is the **castor bean**. The seeds of this attractive shrub are highly poisonous: chewing on just a few seeds (and, in some cases, just one) can kill a child. Ricin, the poison in castor beans, causes a variety of toxic effects: burning of the mouth and throat; nausea, vomiting, diarrhea, and severe stomach pains; prostration; failing vision; and kidney failure (the usual cause of death).

Foxglove, which has beautiful trumpetlike flowers, contains cardiac glycosides and is used in making the drug digitalis. Along with nausea, vomiting, diarrhea, and abdominal cramps, ingestion of foxglove can produce hyperkalemia and cardiac dysrhythmias, usually bradydysrhythmias.

Assessment

When you encounter a pediatric patient with plant poisoning, get all the information you can from the parent and/or caregiver, and then consult your regional poison control center for advice:

- **When was the plant ingested?** If it was more than 12 hours ago and the patient is still asymptomatic, it is likely that the patient will not experience any medical emergencies. Most plant poisonings produce signs and symptoms of toxicity, if they are going to do so, within 4 hours of ingestion. One notable exception is the castor bean, for which symptoms may not appear until 1 to 3 days after ingestion.
- **What, exactly, did the child eat?** Try to find out not just which type of plant, but also which parts of the plant (leaf, root, stem, flower, or fruit) were eaten. If possible, estimate how much was ingested (such as a bite or two from a leaf, or three or four leaves). If you transport the child to the hospital, also take the offending plant (or whatever is left of it) with you.
- **What signs or symptoms, if any, does the child have?**

Management

If the patient is symptomatic, then treat this ingestion like any other and initiate transport to the most appropriate facility. However, most plant-related exposures require no treatment, a decision that can be made after consulting with the poison control center and medical control per local protocol. If a responsible adult is present who can keep a close eye on the child for at least 4 to 6 hours after the ingestion, then there is no need to transport the child to the hospital.

Poisonous Mushrooms

Four groups of people are most likely to experience poisoning related to mushroom ingestion: wild mushroom pickers, people looking for hallucinogenic mushrooms to get high, people attempting suicide or homicide, and young children who eat them by accident. Even among educated people who like to gather their own mushrooms in the wild, mistakes can happen. In 2019, poison control centers received more than 5,700 calls related to mushroom ingestions, with 55% of these ingestions occurring in children younger than 5 years. Thankfully, most of these events result in limited or no toxic effects; only two fatal ingestions were reported.[33]

Pathophysiology

A variety of factors determine whether a mushroom ingestion will produce toxic results: the age of the mushroom, the season in which it was gathered, the amount ingested, and the preparation method. Toxic effects vary from mild GI signs and symptoms to severe cytotoxic, even lethal, effects. In the United States, deaths from mushroom ingestion usually involve the *Amanita* species (*Amanita phalloides*, *Amanita virosa*, and *Amanita verna*) **FIGURE 28-17**.

Words of Wisdom

Herbal preparations can cause potentially serious interactions with traditional medications. Cases of overdose that involved herbal preparations have been reported. Be sure to determine all medications the patient may have taken, including herbal medications or supplements.

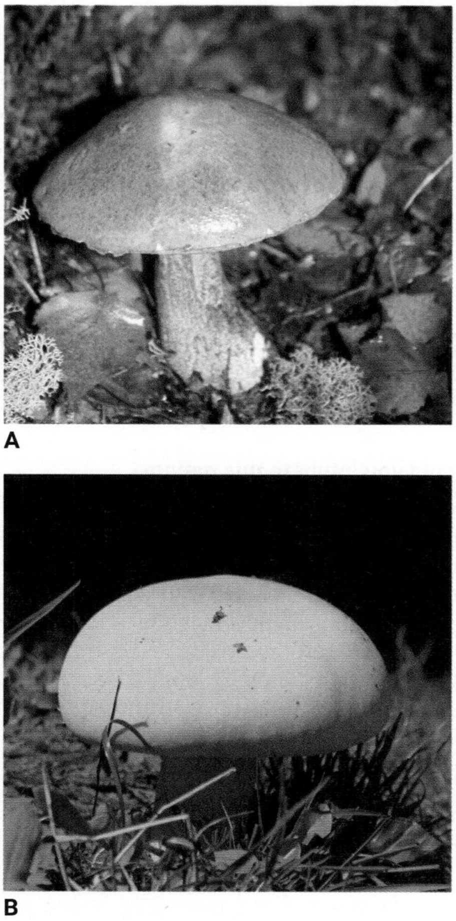

FIGURE 28-17 A. The deadly *Amanita* mushroom. **B.** A nonpoisonous, edible mushroom.

A: © Ivor Toms/Alamy Stock Photo; B: © paul prescott/Shutterstock.

Mushrooms are classified according to the toxins they produce. These classifications include cyclopeptides (amatoxins), gyromitrin, orellanine, muscarine, muscimol, coprine, psilocybin, and GI irritants.

Assessment

Time of symptom onset can serve as a predictor of potential severity. If the patient presents with symptoms within approximately 2 hours of ingestion, then the event will most likely be non–life-threatening. By comparison, if symptom onset occurs 6 hours or later, a much greater likelihood exists that the event will be serious and potentially fatal. The most common patient complaints involve abdominal pain, diarrhea, vomiting, GI bleeding, anuria, and headache. Depending on the toxins involved, multiple organ failure may occur approximately 24 hours after ingestion. Hemodialysis may be required following kidney failure.

Management

Management for a symptomatic patient with a toxic mushroom ingestion includes supportive measures. Establish and maintain the airway, and establish vascular access. For hypotension secondary to vomiting and diarrhea, administer fluid boluses of normal saline. Contact the poison control center and medical control per local protocol and transport the patient to an appropriate facility.

Food Poisoning

Whenever you encounter two or more people sick at the same time and at the same scene with similar symptoms, think food poisoning or carbon monoxide poisoning: your hunch will likely be correct. You also may be asked to evaluate patients who have grown concerned after being notified of food recalls by local grocery stores or restaurant chains.

Pathophysiology

Three toxins, *Salmonella*, *Listeria*, and *Toxoplasma*, are frequently associated with food-related deaths. Poisoning with *Clostridium botulinum*, an extremely deadly toxin, is usually the result of improper food storage or canning. In addition, the toxins produced by dinoflagellates in "red tides" may contaminate bivalve shellfish such as oysters, clams, and mussels and produce life-threatening or fatal paralytic shellfish poisoning. Cooking does not kill these toxins.

Assessment

Depending on the toxin, onset of signs and symptoms can range from several hours after ingestion to days or weeks. This delayed onset may make it difficult to isolate the offending agent while interviewing the patient. GI complaints are the most common and include abdominal pain, cramping, nausea, vomiting, and diarrhea. With prolonged episodes of vomiting or diarrhea, hypotension secondary to fluid loss and electrolyte imbalance becomes likely. Respiratory distress or arrest can occur with toxins such as *C botulinum* or those found in paralytic shellfish poisoning.

Management

Care of patients with food poisoning is usually supportive because most cases will not be life threatening, and the signs and symptoms of acute gastroenteritis are typically self-limiting. Manage the patient's airway or support respirations with supplemental oxygen as needed. Establish vascular access and treat hypotension secondary to fluid loss with fluid boluses of normal saline. Consider administration of antiemetics, per local protocol. For patients with facial flushing (most likely secondary to histamine release), consider administration of diphenhydramine per local protocol. Finally, transport the patient to an appropriate facility.

YOU are the Paramedic SUMMARY

1. What is your first impression of this patient?

The patient is in critical condition. As you begin your assessment and interview, you will likely have several thoughts regarding the possible cause of her condition. Stroke, hypoglycemia, sepsis, and overdose could be among the possible causes. After you have determined that the patient is acutely ill, begin setting priorities for patient care and searching for any reversible causes.

2. What is your priority for patient care?

The patient has a strong carotid pulse with respiratory depression. Take appropriate measures to maintain a patent airway while ensuring a proper ventilatory rate and tidal volume. Have suction prepared and ready at the patient's side. Placement of a nasopharyngeal or an oropharyngeal airway would be appropriate based on the patient's clinical presentation.

3. If this patient has overdosed, then which drug classification would be your focus?

The patient's most critical issues are hypoventilation and respiratory depression. These issues are components of two major toxidromes: opioid and sedative-hypnotic. You can refine your differential diagnosis based on additional physical findings or by performing a thorough patient interview and scene survey to determine what drugs or medications may be present in the home.

4. Give some examples of drugs that would meet this classification.

Opioid agents include morphine, codeine, heroin, fentanyl (Sublimaze), oxycodone (OxyContin), meperidine (Demerol), propoxyphene (Darvon), and dextromethorphan. Opioids are used primarily in clinical medicine for analgesia, whereas the illicit drug heroin is used for the unique euphoria it produces. Sedative-hypnotics include barbiturates and benzodiazepines.

5. Should you intubate this patient?

Advanced airway management may be in this patient's future, but start with the basics first. Your initial action should be to provide supplemental oxygen and assisted ventilations with a bag-mask device. The patient has hypoventilation and hypercapnia. The elevated carbon dioxide levels may cause the patient to have an altered mental status. First correct the issues that you can have an immediate effect on, and then determine your next step after evaluating the patient's response to the treatment.

6. What is your next step in treating this patient after the airway is controlled?

As a paramedic, you should always be moving with purpose and trying to anticipate the future needs of the patient. Ensure the patient is connected to all of the appropriate monitoring equipment, including the cardiac monitor, noninvasive blood pressure monitor, pulse oximeter, and carbon dioxide detector (sidestream or connected to the bag-mask device). Obtain IV access and continue to search for the underlying cause of the patient's condition. While you will have a list of priorities for treatment, always be thinking, "If it is not this, then next I will search for that." Seizure, stroke, hypoglycemia, sepsis, and toxins should all be in your mind while treating this patient.

7. What is your medication choice and dosage to treat this patient?

Administer 0.4 to 2 mg of naloxone (Narcan). The best approach is to draw up 2 mg of naloxone in a 10-mL syringe and fill the rest of the syringe with normal saline. Administer the naloxone just to the point that the patient's respirations improve. You do not have to "wake the patient up" all the way; you simply need to improve the patient's respiratory status. Pushing too large of a dose or even an appropriate dose too rapidly may cause the patient to vomit or experience withdrawal. Both situations could harm the patient.

YOU are the Paramedic SUMMARY continued

8. What should you do if this medication does not correct the overdose?

Sometimes the patient may not respond to naloxone, and some opioids may require higher doses of naloxone to combat the respiratory depression. This situation may also be a mixed overdose in which more than one drug was taken. If allowed by protocol, then repeat the naloxone dose or call for orders to increase the dose. Remember that basic airway maneuvers and successful bag-mask ventilation allow you more time to determine your next course of action. This patient may require advanced airway management. If the patient remains at high risk for aspiration, then protect the patient's airway and perform endotracheal intubation.

EMS Patient Care Report (PCR)

Date: 08-10-22	**Incident No.:** 4563	**Nature of Call:** OD		**Location:** Edenvale Rd	
Dispatched: 1430	**En Route:** 1431	**At Scene:** 1438	**Transport:** 1450	**At Hospital:** 1510	**In Service:** 1525

Patient Information

Age: 45 **Sex:** F **Weight (in kg [lb]):** 70 kg (154 lb)	**Allergies:** Unknown **Medications:** Hydrocodone **Past Medical History:** Back surgery **Chief Complaint:** Possible overdose

Vital Signs

Time: 1443	**BP:** 92/58	**Pulse:** 100	**Respirations:** 4	**Spo_2:** 90% on room air
Time: 1448	**BP:** 98/56	**Pulse:** 100	**Respirations:** Assisted	**Spo_2:** 96% O_2
Time: 1454	**BP:** 100/60	**Pulse:** 98	**Respirations:** 12	**Spo_2:** 97% O_2
Time: 1505	**BP:** 112/64	**Pulse:** 94	**Respirations:** 12	**Spo_2:** 98% O_2
Time: 1510	**BP:** 108/84	**Pulse:** 92	**Respirations:** 14	**Spo_2:** 98% O_2

EMS Treatment (circle all that apply)

Oxygen @ __15__ L/min via (circle one): **NC NRM Bag-mask device** (circled)		**Assisted Ventilation:** (circled)	**Airway Adjunct:** NPA (circled)	**CPR**
Defibrillation	**Bleeding Control**	**Bandaging**	**Splinting**	**Other:**

Narrative

Arrived on scene to find female pt lying supine in bed. Pt has PMH of recent back surgery and prescription opioids use (hydrocodone 10 mg). Last seen normal time @ 0800 this morning. Pt is unconscious with a resp of 4 per min. The pt has a strong carotid pulse. Airway maintained with NPA and bag-mask device at 15 L/min assisted to a rate of 12 breaths/min. Sinus tachycardia on the monitor. IV established, BGL is 120 mg/dL. Found fentanyl patches on pt's back and removed. Naloxone (Narcan) administered at 0.4 mg IVP without change. Dose repeated × 2 per protocol with an increase in respiratory effort noted. Pt responds to painful stimuli post Narcan and is able to maintain airway. Pt transported emergency to regional hospital. Report to Dr. Phillips on arrival.

End of report

Prep Kit

Ready for Review

- Toxicologic emergencies can be categorized as either unintentional or intentional.
- Both licit and illicit drugs are constantly evolving. You may also encounter patients with complex presentations involving multiple substances that have different pharmacokinetics. For these reasons, poison control centers may be an indispensable aid.
- The four primary methods whereby a toxin commonly enters the body are ingestion, inhalation, injection, and absorption.
- Toxidromes can help you work toward identifying the toxic substance in situations where that information is not readily available. After you conduct your assessment and have identified the presentation, you can proceed with a focused treatment plan.
- As a paramedic, you will encounter patients involved with substance use disorder. The physiologic and societal effects of alcohol use disorder are well known and thoroughly documented. Effects of new drugs and new variations are more difficult to know and document due to their continual evolution.
- Generally, patients with toxicologic emergencies are considered medical patients, although toxicologic emergencies may also lead to trauma as well.
- Maintain a high level of situational awareness when responding to toxicologic emergencies. Patients who have taken an overdose may be extremely dangerous.
- Basic airway management is important in these patients and is a mainstay of the primary survey.
- Obtain as much information about the substance as possible, early in the call.
- Management for toxicologic emergencies includes advanced life support care built on the basics:
  - Ensure the scene is safe for access and egress.
  - Maintain the airway; secure it as needed.
  - Ensure that breathing is adequate.
  - Ensure that circulation is not compromised (by hypoperfusion or dysrhythmia).
  - Maintain adequate blood/oxygen saturation levels (95%).
  - Establish vascular access.
  - Consider administration of an antidote, if available.
  - Be prepared to manage shock, coma, seizures, and dysrhythmias.
  - Transport the patient as soon as possible. Place the patient in the left lateral recumbent position if any risk of vomiting exists to reduce the risk of aspiration.
- Additional management for stimulant misuse includes obtaining an electrocardiogram (ECG), pulse oximetry level, and capnography reading; administering benzodiazepines per local protocol for anxiety and seizures; and managing hypotension with fluid resuscitation.
- Marijuana use is legal in some states for medical purposes and in other states for any purpose. Management of these patients is primarily supportive and may include benzodiazepines for sedation.
- Hallucinogens include lysergic acid diethylamide (LSD), phencyclidine (PCP), and ketamine. Emergency medical care is primarily supportive, with scene safety remaining a concern; intramuscular sedatives may be necessary. Benzodiazepines may be helpful in calming a patient who is delirious because of ketamine use.
- Sedative-hypnotics include barbiturates and benzodiazepines. In patients who have used barbiturates, central nervous system depression is likely, making airway management critical. Benzodiazepines, while also used as a prehospital agent for sedation, are also potential substances of misuse. A reversal agent is available for benzodiazepine overdose.
- Opioids have become the driving cause of most overdose deaths. Management of a patient with opioid overdose focuses on airway management. Naloxone (Narcan) may be

Prep Kit continued

administered to improve the patient's spontaneous respiratory effort. Follow the American Heart Association algorithm for management of a life-threatening opioid overdose.
- An additional step when a patient has organophosphate poisoning is to perform decontamination prior to assessment and management. Specific medications such as atropine and pralidoxime may be required. Also perform pulse oximetry, capnometry, and ECG monitoring.
- If a patient has carbon monoxide poisoning, then remove the patient from the exposure environment, provide the highest concentration of oxygen possible, establish intravenous access, and perform ECG monitoring.
- For a caustic ingestion, identify the specific substance and contact the poison control center or online medical control for further instructions.
- Contact medical control regarding use of activated charcoal; it is often contraindicated when the exact ingested substance(s) is unknown. This therapy typically may be used with 1 hour of ingestion in the following overdoses: known long-acting barbiturate, tricyclic antidepressant, selective serotonin reuptake inhibitor, salicylate, or acetaminophen. It also may be used with most cardiac medication overdoses. The patient must be able to maintain the airway prior to and during administration.
- Hydrocarbons may be inhaled or ingested. The primary treatment goals for a patient who has inhaled hydrocarbons are removal from the exposure environment, administration of high-concentration oxygen, and prompt transport. The primary treatment goals for a patient who has ingested hydrocarbons are decontamination, high-flow oxygen administration, ECG monitoring, and fluid resuscitation if hypotension is present.
- Most ingested plant poisonings are treated like any other ingestion. Most plant-related exposures require no treatment, but this decision should be determined by poison control.

Vital Vocabulary

alcohol use disorder A condition characterized by a physical and psychological addiction to ethanol that can range from mild to severe.

amphetamines A class of drugs that increase alertness and excitation (stimulants); include methamphetamine (crank or ice), methylenedioxyamphetamine (MDA, Adam), and methylenedioxymethamphetamine (MDMA, Eve, Ecstasy).

antagonist A molecule that blocks the ability of a given chemical to bind to its receptor, preventing a biologic response.

antidote Something to counteract the effect of a poison.

barbiturates Potent sedative-hypnotics historically used as sleep aids, as antianxiety drugs, and as part of the regimen for seizure control; include drugs such as thiopental (Pentothal, Trapanal) and methohexital (Brevital).

benzodiazepines The family of sedative-hypnotics that provide muscle relaxation and mild sedation; most commonly used to treat anxiety, seizures, and alcohol withdrawal; include drugs such as diazepam (Valium) and midazolam (Versed).

caladium A common houseplant that contains calcium oxalate crystals; ingestion leads to nausea, vomiting, and diarrhea.

castor bean A seed that contains the poison ricin. Its ingestion causes a variety of toxic effects: burning of the mouth and throat; nausea, vomiting, diarrhea, and severe stomach pains; prostration; failing vision; and kidney failure, which is the usual cause of death.

caustics Chemicals that are acids or alkalis; cause direct chemical injury to the tissues they contact.

Prep Kit continued

chemical suicide A method of suicide that involves mixing certain household chemicals in an enclosed space to create toxic gases, such as hydrogen sulfide and hydrogen cyanide, as the chemicals combine; also called detergent suicide.

cocaine A stimulant; a naturally occurring alkaloid that is extracted from the leaves of the *Erythroxylon coca* plant, which is found in South America.

delirium tremens (DTs) A severe withdrawal syndrome seen in people with alcohol use disorder who are deprived of ethyl alcohol; characterized by restlessness, fever, sweating, disorientation, agitation, and seizures; can be fatal if untreated.

dieffenbachia A common houseplant that is also called dumb cane; ingestion leads to burns of the mouth and tongue and, possibly, paralysis of the vocal cords and nausea and vomiting; in severe cases, edema of the tongue and larynx may occur, leading to airway compromise.

drug A substance that has some therapeutic effect (such as reducing inflammation, fighting bacteria, or producing euphoria) when given in the appropriate circumstances and in the appropriate dose.

drug addiction A chronic disorder characterized by the compulsive use of a substance that results in physical, psychological, or social harm to the user who continues to use the substance despite the harm.

drug misuse Any use of drugs that causes physical, psychological, economic, legal, or social harm to the user or others affected by the user's behavior.

DUMBELS An acronym that represents the symptoms of organophosphate poisoning: Diarrhea, Urination, Miosis, Bradycardia/Bronchospasm/Bronchorrhea, Emesis, Lacrimation, and Seizures/Salivation/Sweating.

foxglove A plant that contains cardiac glycosides and is used in making digitalis; ingestion of leaves causes nausea, vomiting, diarrhea, abdominal cramps, hyperkalemia, and a variety of dysrhythmias.

habituation A physical tolerance and psychological dependence on a drug or drugs.

hallucinogen An agent that produces false perceptions in any one of the five senses.

hydrocarbons Compounds made up principally of hydrogen and carbon atoms; mostly obtained from the distillation of petroleum.

illicit In relation to drugs, illegal drugs such as marijuana, cocaine, and lysergic acid diethylamide.

lantana A perennial flowering shrub with clusters of red berries that can lead to serious and even fatal poisoning. Also known as red sage or wild sage; ingestion causes stomach upsets, muscle weakness, shock, and, sometimes, death.

licit In relation to drugs, legalized drugs such as coffee, alcohol, and tobacco.

lithium A common mood stabilizer used in the treatment of bipolar disorder.

marijuana The dried leaves and flower buds of the *Cannabis sativa* plant, which are smoked to achieve a high.

methamphetamine A highly addictive drug in the amphetamine family.

monoamine oxidase inhibitors (MAOIs) Psychiatric medications used primarily to treat atypical depression by increasing norepinephrine and serotonin levels in the central nervous system.

opiate Various alkaloids derived from the opium or poppy plant.

opioid A drug that acts as a central nervous system depressant and produces insensibility or stupor. An opioid can be a natural product derived from the opium or poppy plant or a synthetic product designed to produce similar effects.

organophosphates A class of chemicals found in many insecticides used in agriculture and in the home.

overdose A condition that occurs when a drug (either licit or illicit) is taken in excess; can have toxic or lethal consequences.

Prep Kit continued

physical dependence A physiologic state of adaptation to a drug, usually characterized by tolerance to the effects of the drug and a withdrawal syndrome if use of the drug is stopped, especially abruptly.

poison A substance whose chemical action could damage structures or impair function when introduced into the body.

potentiation Enhancement of the effect of one drug by another drug.

psychological dependence The emotional state of craving a drug to maintain a feeling of well-being.

rhabdomyolysis The destruction of muscle tissue leading to a release of potassium and myoglobin.

salicylates Chemicals found in plants; a primary ingredient in aspirin.

sedative-hypnotic A drug used to reduce anxiety, calm agitated patients, and help produce drowsiness and sleep; a central nervous system depressant.

selective serotonin reuptake inhibitors (SSRIs) A class of antidepressants that inhibit the reuptake of serotonin.

serotonin syndrome An idiosyncratic complication that occurs with antidepressant therapy in which patients have lower extremity muscle rigidity, confusion or disorientation, and/or agitation.

spice An illicit drug consisting of a blend of synthetic cannabinoids; it can produce delirium and short- and long-term psychotic effects.

synergism The action of two substances such as drugs, in which the total effects are greater than the sum of the independent effects of the two substances.

tolerance Physiologic adaptation to the effects of a drug such that increasingly larger doses of the drug are required to achieve the same effect.

toxicologic emergencies Medical emergencies caused by toxic agents such as poison; may be intentional or unintentional.

toxicology The study of toxic or poisonous substances.

toxidrome The syndromelike symptoms of any given class or group of poisonous agents.

toxin A poison or harmful substance produced by bacteria, animals, or plants.

tricyclic antidepressants (TCAs) A group of drugs used to treat severe depression and manage pain; minimal dosing errors can cause toxic results.

withdrawal syndrome A predictable set of signs and symptoms, usually involving altered central nervous system activity that occurs after the abrupt cessation of a drug or after rapidly decreasing the usual dosage of a drug.

References

1. Poison statistics: national data 2019. National Capital Poison Center website. http://www.poison.org/poison-statistics-national. Accessed September 1, 2021.
2. Chemical suicides: the risk to emergency responders. Chemical Hazards Emergency Medical Management website. https://chemm.hhs.gov/chemicalsuicide.htm. Accessed September 1, 2021.
3. WebWISER home. US National Library of Medicine, National Institutes of Health, Department of Health and Human Services. https://webwiser.nlm.nih.gov. Accessed September 1, 2021.
4. New CDC study finds dramatic increase in e-cigarette–related calls to poison centers. Centers for Disease Control and Prevention website. https://www.cdc.gov/media/releases/2014/p0403-e-cigarette-poison.html. Published April 3, 2014. Accessed September 1, 2021.
5. Moss MJ, Warrick BJ, Nelson LS, et al. ACMT and AACT position statement: preventing occupational fentanyl and fentanyl analog exposure to emergency responders. *J Med Toxicol*. 2017;13(4):347-351. doi:10.1007/s13181-017-0628-2.
6. *National Model EMS Clinical Guidelines: Version 2.2*. National Association of State EMS Officials website. https://nasemso.org/wp-content/uploads/National-Model-EMS-Clinical-Guidelines-2017-PDF-Version-2.2.pdf. Published January 2019. Accessed September 30, 2021.

Prep Kit continued

7. Volkow ND, Gordon JA, Koob GF. Choosing appropriate language to reduce the stigma around mental illness and substance use disorders. *Neuropsychopharmacology*. 2021. https://doi.org/10.1038/s41386-021-01069-4.
8. Alcohol facts and statistics. National Institute on Alcohol Abuse and Alcoholism website. https://www.niaaa.nih.gov/publications/brochures-and-fact-sheets/alcohol-facts-and-statistics. Updated June 2021. Accessed September 2, 2021.
9. When it comes to reducing alcohol-related stigma, words matter. National Institute on Alcohol Abuse and Alcoholism website. https://www.niaaa.nih.gov/alcohols-effects-health/reducing-alcohol-related-stigma. Accessed October 4, 2021.
10. Understanding alcohol use disorder. National Institute on Alcohol Abuse and Alcoholism website. https://www.niaaa.nih.gov/publications/brochures-and-fact-sheets/understanding-alcohol-use-disorder. Accessed October 4, 2021.
11. American Psychiatric Association. *Diagnostic and Statistical Manual of Mental Disorders,* 5th ed. Washington, DC: American Psychiatric Association; 2013.
12. Alcohol and cancer risk. National Cancer Institute website. http://www.cancer.gov/about-cancer/causes-prevention/risk/alcohol/alcohol-fact-sheet. Updated July 14, 2021. Accessed September 2, 2021.
13. State of California Department of Motor Vehicles. *California Driver Handbook: Alcohol and Drugs.* https://www.dmv.ca.gov/portal/handbook/california-driver-handbook/alcohol-and-drugs/. Accessed September 2, 2021.
14. O'Malley GF, O'Malley R. Alcohol toxicity and withdrawal. *Merck Manuals Professional Edition.* https://www.merckmanuals.com/professional/special-subjects/recreational-drugs-and-intoxicants/alcohol-toxicity-and-withdrawal. Published January 2016. Accessed September 2, 2021.
15. Key substance use and mental health indicators in the United States: results from the 2019 National Survey on Drug Use and Health. Substance Abuse and Mental Health Services Administration website. https://www.samhsa.gov/data/report/2019-nsduh-annual-national-report. Published September 2020. Accessed September 2, 2021.
16. Cocaine overview: pharmacology. MethOIDE: Methamphetamine and Other Illicit Drug Education website. http://methoide.fcm.arizona.edu/infocenter/index.cfm?stid=170. Accessed September 1, 2021.
17. Communications NYU. Rolling on Molly: US high school seniors underreport Ecstasy use when not asked about Molly. https://www.nyu.edu/about/news-publications/news/2016/june/rolling-on-molly-us-high-school-seniors-underreport-ecstasy-use-when-not-asked-about-molly.html. Published June 9, 2016. Accessed September 1, 2021.
18. Stores C. Is Flakka gone for good? http://www.cnn.com/2016/04/18/health/flakka-drug-disappearance/. Published April 18, 2016. Accessed September 1, 2021.
19. Synthetic cathinones ("bath salts"). *DrugFacts.* National Institute on Drug Abuse website. https://www.drugabuse.gov/publications/drugfacts/synthetic-cathinones-bath-salts. Published July 2020. Accessed September 2, 2021.
20. VanDolah HJ, Bauer BA, Mauck KF. Clinicians' guide to cannabidiol and hemp oils. *Mayo Clin Proc.* August 21, 2019. https://www.mayoclinicproceedings.org/article/S0025-6196(19)30007-2/fulltext. Accessed October 4, 2021.
21. O'Malley GF, O'Malley R. Marijuana (cannabis). *Merck Manuals Professional Edition.* https://www.merckmanuals.com/professional/special-subjects/recreational-drugs-and-intoxicants/marijuana-cannabis. Revised May 2020. Accessed September 6, 2021.
22. Zukkoor Zorn S. Cardiovascular risk of marijuana. American College of Cardiology website. https://www.acc.org/latest-in-cardiology/articles/2021/06/10/03/08/cardiovascular-risk-of-marijuana#:~:text=Data%20analyzed%20from%20the%20US,lenient%20approaches%20to%20cannabis%20dispensing. Published June 10, 2021. Accessed November 5, 2021.
23. Acute marijuana intoxication. Children's Hospital Colorado website. https://www.childrenscolorado.org/conditions-and-advice/conditions-and-symptoms/conditions/acute-marijuana-intoxication/. Accessed September 6, 2021.
24. Orhurhu VJ, Vashisht R, Claus LE, Cohen SP. Ketamine toxicity. *StatPearls [Internet]*. https://www.ncbi.nlm.nih.gov/books/NBK541087/. Updated July 25, 2021. Accessed November 5, 2021.
25. O'Malley GF, O'Malley R. Anxiolytics and sedatives. *Merck Manuals Professional Edition.* http://www.merckmanuals.com/professional/special-subjects/recreational-drugs-and-intoxicants/anxiolytics-and-sedatives. Revised May 2020. Accessed September 6, 2021.
26. Benson BE, Hoppu K, Troutman WG, et al. Position paper update: gastric lavage for gastrointestinal decontamination. *Clin Toxicol*. 2013;51(3):140-146.
27. Drug overdose deaths. Centers for Disease Control and Prevention website. https://www.cdc.gov/drugoverdose/data/statedeaths.html. Last reviewed March 3, 2021. Accessed September 6, 2021.
28. Rudd RA, Aleshire N, Zibbell JE, Gladden RM. Increases in drug and opioid overdose deaths—United States, 2000–2014. *Morb Mortal Wkly Rep*. 2016;64(50-51):1378-1382.
29. Cliff RM, Woodcock J, Ostroff S. A proactive response to prescription opioid abuse. *NEJM*. 2016;374(15):1480-1485.

Prep Kit continued

30. Panchal AR, Bartos JA, Cabañas JG, et al. Part 3: adult basic and advanced life support: 2020 American Heart Association guidelines for cardiopulmonary resuscitation and emergency cardiovascular care. *Circulation*. 2020;142(16 suppl 2):S366-S468.
31. Bertolote JM, Fleischmann A, Eddleston M, Gunnell D. Deaths from pesticide poisoning: are we lacking a global response? *Br J Psychiatry*. 2006;189:201-203.
32. Preventing carbon monoxide poisoning after an emergency. Centers for Disease Control and Prevention website. https://www.cdc.gov/disasters/cofacts.html. Reviewed September 27, 2017. Accessed September 6, 2021.
33. Hydrogen cyanide (AC): systemic agent. Centers for Disease Control and Prevention website. https://www.cdc.gov/niosh/ershdb/emergencyresponsecard_29750038.html. Reviewed May 12, 2011. Accessed October 4, 2021.
34. Facts about cyanide. Centers for Disease Control and Prevention website. https://emergency.cdc.gov/agent/cyanide/basics/facts.asp. Reviewed April 4, 2018. Accessed October 4, 2021.
35. Gummin DD, Mowry JB, Beuhler MC, et al. 2019 Annual report of the American Association of Poison Control Centers' National Poison Data System (NPDS): 36th annual report. *Clin Toxicol.* 2020;58(12):1360-1541.
36. O'Malley GF, O'Malley R. Gamma hydroxybutyrate. *Merck Manuals Professional Edition.* https://www.merckmanuals.com/professional/special-subjects/recreational-drugs-and-intoxicants/gamma-hydroxybutyrate. Revised May 2020. Accessed September 6, 2021.
37. McMartin K, Jacobsen D, Hovda KE. Antidotes for poisoning by alcohols that form toxic metabolites. *Br J Clin Pharmacol*. 2016;81(3):505-515.
38. O'Malley GF, O'Malley R. Specific poisons. *Merck Manuals Professional Edition.* http://www.merckmanuals.com/professional/injuries-poisoning/poisoning/specific-poisons. Updated April 2020. Accessed September 6, 2021.
39. Mekonnen S. Azaleas and rhododendrons. http://www.poison.org/articles/2015-mar/azaleas-and-rhododendrons. Accessed September 6, 2021.

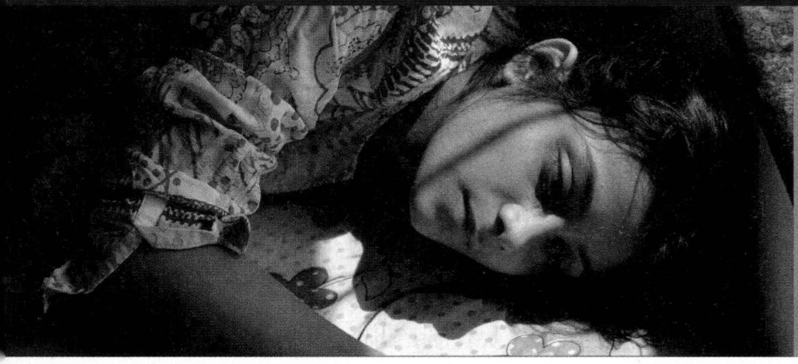

Chapter 29

Psychiatric Emergencies

NATIONAL EMS EDUCATION STANDARD COMPETENCIES

Medicine

Integrates assessment findings with principles of epidemiology and pathophysiology to formulate a field impression and implement a comprehensive treatment/disposition plan for a patient with a medical complaint.

Psychiatric

Recognition of

- Behaviors that pose a risk to the EMS provider, patient, or others (pp 1728–1729)

Assessment and management of

- Basic principles of the mental health system (pp 1727–1732)
- Suicidal/risk (pp 1745–1746)

Anatomy, physiology, epidemiology, pathophysiology, psychosocial impact, presentations, assessment, prognosis, and management of

- Acute psychosis (pp 1740–1742)
- Excited delirium (pp 1743–1745)
- Cognitive disorders (pp 1743–1745)
- Thought disorders (pp 1740–1742, 1750)
- Mood disorders (pp 1748–1750)
- Neurotic disorders (pp 1750–1752)
- Substance-related disorders/addictive behavior (pp 1752–1753)
- Somatoform disorders (pp 1753–1754)
- Factitious disorders (pp 1754–1755)
- Personality disorders (p 1755)
- Patterns of violence/abuse/neglect (pp 1746–1748)
- Organic psychoses (p 1750)

KNOWLEDGE OBJECTIVES

1. Discuss the possible causes of behavioral emergencies, including drug overdoses, violent behavior, and mental illness. (pp 1725–1726)
2. Define normal, abnormal, overt, and covert behavior. (p 1722)
3. Identify the prevalence of mental illness in the United States. (p 1724)
4. Discuss medicolegal considerations and their role in psychiatric emergencies. (pp 1724–1725)
5. Discuss the organic and environmental causes of abnormal behavior. (pp 1725–1726)
6. Explain how psychiatric signs and symptoms are categorized. (pp 1726–1727)
7. Describe the assessment process for patients with psychiatric emergencies, including safety guidelines and specific questions to ask. (pp 1727–1732)
8. Discuss the importance of history taking in assessing a patient with a psychiatric emergency. (pp 1730–1731)

9. Identify strategies for communicating with patients during behavioral crises. (pp 1732–1733)
10. Discuss general care of a patient with a psychiatric emergency. (pp 1733–1734)
11. Compare physical restraint with chemical restraint, including examples of when each might be used and situations in which restraint might be justified. (pp 1734–1739)
12. Describe the emergency medical care of a patient with psychosis. (p 1742)
13. Describe the emergency medical care of a patient with excited delirium. (p 1745)
14. Explain how to recognize the behavior of a patient at risk of suicide, including the emergency medical care of such a patient. (pp 1745–1746)
15. Discuss factors indicating that a patient is at risk of becoming violent. (p 1747)
16. Explain the approach to safely caring for a potentially violent patient. (pp 1747–1748)
17. List specific psychiatric disorders that can be characterized by a state of acute psychosis or excited delirium. (p 1740)
18. Discuss assessment and management of specific psychiatric emergencies, including those related to mood disorders, schizophrenia, neurotic disorders, substance use, somatoform disorders, factitious disorders, impulse control disorders, and personality disorders. (pp 1748–1755)
19. Discuss medications used to treat psychiatric disorders and manage behavioral emergencies. (pp 1755–1757)
20. Recognize issues specific to posttraumatic stress disorder and the returning combat veteran. (pp 1726, 1757–1759)

SKILLS OBJECTIVES

1. Demonstrate the technique used to perform four-point physical restraint of a patient. (p 1737, Skill Drill 29-1)

Introduction

The mind and the body are not separate entities; they are inseparable parts of a whole human being. When a person becomes ill with any disease, that illness will inevitably affect the person's behavior, often making the person anxious or depressed. Similarly, changes in mental state affect the body's physical health. Persons with depression, for example, may lose their appetite or become more susceptible to bodily disease. Thus, whenever you examine a patient, you must view the patient as a whole person. Try to learn about both the physical and the mental factors that are contributing to the patient's distress.

As a paramedic, you can expect to care for patients undergoing a psychological or behavioral crisis. This chapter covers various kinds of behavioral emergencies. These emergencies can involve overdoses, violent behavior, and mental illness. This chapter also addresses legal concerns in the emergency medical care of patients who are disturbed.

Definition of Behavioral Emergency

The concept of **behavior** has been debated over the years, with most experts defining it as the way people act or perform, such as how they respond to a situation. Behavior includes all the things people do and the reasons they do those things. Who defines abnormal and normal behavior is a source of debate. These concepts can be defined by society in general, a particular community or social group, a parent, a boss, a friend, or even a stranger. Both normal and abnormal behavior may be overt. **Overt behaviors** are open and generally understood by those around the person. **Covert behaviors** are those that have hidden meanings or intentions that only the person displaying the behavior understands.

Abnormal behavior in itself may not be a medical condition and is hardly cause for alarm. The real questions are, "When does abnormal behavior require medical intervention?" and "When does it require an emergency medical services (EMS) response?" Almost all disordered behavior represents the person's effort to adapt to some internal or external stress. The disruptive behavior usually is temporary, fading when the person has managed to mobilize their psychological defense mechanisms.

Behavioral emergencies are situations in which the patient's presenting problem is some disorder of mood, thought, or behavior that interferes with **activities of daily living (ADLs)**. ADLs are everyday activities such as getting dressed and taking out the garbage. When a person becomes so depressed that getting up in the morning, showering, and making breakfast are impossible, or when someone has **delusions** (false beliefs) or **hallucinations** (sensory perceptions not founded on objective reality) that prohibit them from holding a job, the condition becomes a behavioral emergency.

A **psychiatric emergency** occurs when the abnormal behavior threatens a person's health and safety or the health and safety of another person. In the most extreme cases, a person has a suicidal, homicidal, or psychotic episode. In a psychotic episode, a person often experiences delusions or hallucinations and illusions (errors in perception) that result in loss of contact with reality. For example, a patient who has taken illicit drugs may experience an alteration of reality: a "bad trip." Psychotic episodes can be dangerous for the patient, bystanders, and you as a responder because the patient may display violent behavior, usually from exaggerated fear or paranoia.

Street Smarts

When called for a psychiatric emergency, keep in mind that you will rarely be encountering a new-onset condition. The patient or others on scene may offer helpful insights, such as what treatments the patient is currently undergoing or how a similar situation was resolved in the past. Consider asking questions such as the following to guide your approach:

- What is different today?
- Have you taken your prescribed medication?
- Has something happened to upset you?

While compassion is imperative when dealing with a behavioral problem, remain alert for potential episodes of violence, especially when responding to calls involving illicit drug use. If the patient is becoming increasingly agitated, leave the scene and call for additional assistance.

Regardless of how textbooks define a psychiatric emergency, the operative definition of a behavioral or psychiatric emergency is given by the person who dials 9-1-1. A behavioral or psychiatric emergency often becomes an "emergency" because of panic experienced by the patient, the family, bystanders, or all of these parties. That panic, in turn, may translate into a demand for action on your part, and you may therefore face intense pressure to do something. For example, you may be pressured to transport the patient to the emergency department (ED).

YOU are the Paramedic

PART 1

You are dispatched to the third floor of an apartment building for a 44-year-old man who says he fears for his life. You learn that law enforcement personnel have been on scene with this patient for 20 minutes, and the patient will not leave his apartment. The apartment building is known to house residents with psychiatric disorders. As you arrive at the building, an officer directs you to the elevator and tells you that the patient is not armed, but officers are remaining on scene in case he becomes violent.

You go to the third floor, where another officer meets you. He informs you that law enforcement personnel were called to the scene by the patient, who had stated that someone was trying to kill him. He told officers that he had overheard information that was not meant for him, and now someone is planning to kill him. The door to the apartment is open, and the patient is visible. He doesn't appear to have a weapon but refuses to leave the apartment or let anyone in.

1. What are the initial components of the assessment for this patient?
2. What are your safety concerns in dealing with this patient?

Paradoxically, it is precisely in a situation, during which the patient is behaving strangely and bystanders are clamoring for action, that you may feel least able to do something.

You may have difficulty performing to the best of your ability when you are trying to understand the confused and frayed feelings that the patient often presents during a psychiatric emergency. Some paramedics may feel more comfortable dealing with straightforward problems such as fractures of the legs, cardiac dysrhythmias, or narcotic overdoses. Paramedics tend to be action-oriented people who like to see tangible results, such as a patient with hypoglycemia improving after a bolus of glucose, or a clinically dead patient restored to life by cardiopulmonary resuscitation (CPR) and defibrillation. What tangible rewards can you gain in escorting a confused, hallucinating patient to a medical facility, or caring for a belligerent and violent patient who is screaming obscenities?

Prehospital behavioral intervention *is* possible and often critical in these emergencies. You can make a difference in the life of a patient who is disturbed, and you can learn the skills just like any other skill. Indeed, these skills you learn for dealing with abnormal behavior ultimately may be much more critical to your work than skills such as endotracheal intubation. For example, how many of your calls require you to place an advanced airway? Many more calls will require you to care for people who are angry, depressed, agitated, panicky, or out of control. Clearly, you will benefit greatly by learning how to take an organized and systematic approach to emergencies that involve abnormal behavior.

Prevalence

According to the Centers for Disease Control and Prevention (CDC), the average number of mentally unhealthy days (those including stress, **depression**, and problems with emotions) for Americans has increased. In 2013, Americans reported an average of 3.7 mentally unhealthy days per month, but by 2019, this number had increased to 4.3 days.[1]

In any given year, an estimated 43.5 million adults age 18 years or older have had a mental illness in the past year.[2] This figure represents 18.1% of all adults in the United States.[2] Almost 10 million adults age 18 years or older, representing 4.2% of the US population, are estimated to have had a serious mental illness within the past year. Serious mental illness is generally defined as a diagnosis of a psychiatric disorder, for example, with serious functional impairment.[2] The prevalence of serious mental illness among specific age groups and ethnicities is shown in **TABLE 29-1**. According to the National Institute of Drug Abuse, 7.7 million US adults have both mental illness and a substance use disorder, which can complicate their assessment and treatment.[3]

TABLE 29-1 Prevalence of Serious Mental Illness in Selected US Population Subgroups, 2018

Population	Prevalence of Serious Mental Illness (% of population)
Sex	
Women, 18 years or older	5.7
Men, 18 years or older	3.4
Employment	
Unemployed adults	7.9
Employed adults, part-time	5.8
Employed adults, full-time	3.9
Race	
White	5.1
American Indian or Alaska Native	6.4
Hispanic or Latino	3.6
Black or African American	3.6
Asian	2.1

Data from: Results from the 2018 National Survey on Drug Use and Health: Mental Health Detailed Tables. Substance Abuse and Mental Health Services Administration website. https://www.samhsa.gov/data/sites/default/files/cbhsq-reports/NSDUHDetailedTabs2018R2/NSDUHDetTabsSect8pe2018.htm. Accessed November 3, 2021.

Medicolegal Considerations

Every call has potential legal complications, especially calls for behavioral emergencies. When a patient's behavior, speech, and thoughts are erratic and disorganized, you may encounter difficulty in communicating clearly and understanding the situation. Be prepared to spend time with the patient. Don't be in a hurry; instead, convey the message that you have the time and concern to learn what is bothering the patient. Obtain consent, just as with any other patient, when possible. If the patient refuses to engage with you, then continue to talk about the situation. Explain your responsibilities now that you have been called to the scene and have responded.

If the patient refuses transportation, then follow local protocols and standing orders for providing transport against the patient's will. You will often need help from law enforcement personnel. In most jurisdictions, paramedics (and others) are not allowed to restrain or transport people against their will except possibly at the express order of a county mental health physician.

Be clear in explaining the treatments and medications you will administer. Don't assume that the patient cannot understand what you're doing, regardless of the patient's state of mind. As always, include the patient as much as possible. As you assess and manage a patient with mental health concerns, you must take extra time to thoroughly record the call. Be objective and factual, and include comments the patient makes. Communicating well, following standards and protocols, and having patience will be your best protection against legal action.

Pathophysiology

Causes of Abnormal Behavior

Abnormal behavior typically results from a complex interaction of biologic or organic causes, developmental factors, psychological stressors, emotional stimuli, and sociocultural influences. These causes can be classified into four broad categories: (1) causes that are biologic or organic, (2) causes resulting from the person's environment, (3) causes resulting from acute injury or illness, and (4) causes that are substance-related.

Biologic or Organic Causes

Many patients who present with psychiatric symptoms are actually affected by biologic or organic factors that interfere with normal cerebral function. Such patients were previously described as having **organic brain syndrome**. This term encompassed disorders that were due to organic or physiologic causes as opposed to purely psychiatric causes. However, the distinction was somewhat arbitrary; it is now understood that many people with what were previously thought to be nonorganic abnormalities have physiologic dysfunction in the brain that is causing their psychiatric illness. Examples of biologic or organic causes of abnormal behavior include conditions such as chronic hypoxia, seizure, traumatic brain injury (TBI), chronic alcohol and substance use disorder, and brain tumors **TABLE 29-2**. These conditions alter the normal

TABLE 29-2 Selected Disease States That May Produce Psychotic Symptoms

Disease State	Psychotic Symptoms
Toxic and deficiency states	Drug-induced psychoses, especially from: • Digitalis • Steroids • Disulfiram • Amphetamines • LSD, PCP, and other psychedelics Nutrition disorders: • Alcohol use disorder • Vitamin deficiencies Poisoning with bromide or other heavy metals: • Kidney failure • Liver failure
Infections	• Syphilis • Parasites • Viral encephalitis (eg, after measles) • Brain abscess
Neurologic disease	• Seizure disorders (especially temporal lobe seizures) • Primary and metastatic tumors of the brain • Dementia • Stroke • Closed head injury
Cardiovascular disorders	• Low cardiac output (eg, in heart failure)
Endocrine disorders	• Thyroid hyperfunction (thyrotoxicosis) • Adrenal hyperfunction (Cushing syndrome)
Metabolic disorders	• Electrolyte imbalances (eg, after severe diarrhea) • Hypoglycemia • Diabetic ketoacidosis

Abbreviations: LSD, lysergic acid diethylamide; PCP, phencyclidine functioning of the brain and may cause derangements in behavior. The most common offenders are probably alcohol and drugs, but you also should consider dementia and delirium.

Environmental Causes

A person's environment exerts a tremendous influence on behavior. Typically, that environment includes both psychosocial and sociocultural influences on behavior.

When people are consistently exposed to stressful psychosocial events (eg, childhood trauma) or developmental influences (eg, parents who deprived them of love, caring, support, and encouragement), they may develop abnormal reactions. When a person's basic needs are threatened, that person faces a crisis. People in crisis have two alternatives for dealing with this threat: (1) cope with it by finding ways to alter the situation or their perception of it so that it is no longer as stressful, or (2) attempt to alleviate the discomfort by escaping from the stress. Escape may take many forms, including alcohol, drugs, psychiatric symptoms, and even suicide (discussed later in this chapter).

Humans are social animals, preferring to live in groups. Thus, it's not surprising that sociocultural factors directly affect biology, behavior, and responses to the stress of emergencies. For example, assault, rape, racial violence, or the death of a loved one may produce significant changes in a person's behavior.

Injury and Illness as Causes

Acute illness can overwhelm a person, causing changes in behavior. Medical conditions such as severe infections, electrolyte abnormalities, and many types of metabolic disorders stress coping mechanisms and can cause abnormal behaviors.

Traumatic events occurring in the general population have increased in both frequency and intensity in recent years. An acutely traumatic situation creates a great deal of stress for the person experiencing the trauma as well as those around that person. As a paramedic, you are not immune to this stress. **Posttraumatic stress disorder (PTSD)** is a severe form of anxiety that stems from a traumatic experience. In this condition, the individual relives the stress of the original situation. Causes of PTSD can include military combat, terrorist attacks, car crashes, domestic violence, and sexual assault **FIGURE 29-1**. PTSD is discussed in more detail later in this chapter.

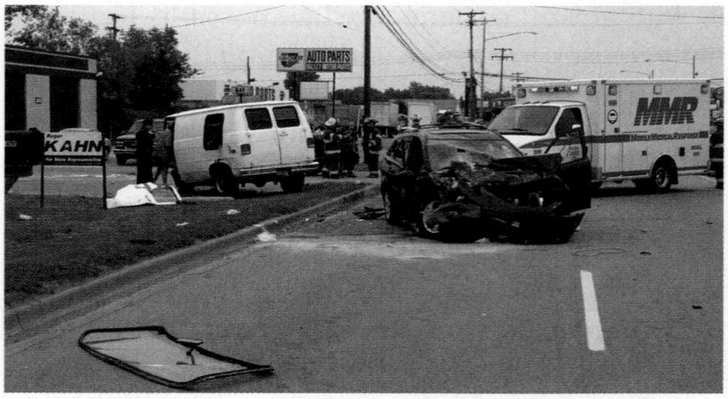

FIGURE 29-1 Posttraumatic stress disorder can be caused by a traumatic event such as a fatal car crash.

Courtesy of Captain David Jackson, Saginaw Township Fire Department.

Substance-Related Causes

Substance-related disorders include the use of alcohol, cigarettes, illicit drugs, and other substances to change the way a person feels, behaves, or thinks. These disorders cost thousands of lives and billions of dollars annually. Substance-related disorders are now recognized to be a complex biologic and psychological problem rather than a sign of moral weakness.

Psychiatric Signs and Symptoms

When a person's physical health is challenged, the body mobilizes various defenses to correct the abnormality. The patient experiences the effects of those abnormalities and corrective measures as symptoms, and you observe these effects as signs. Physical symptoms and signs reveal the body's attempt to maintain its balance in the face of physical stress. When a person's mental health is challenged, similar psychological mechanisms or behaviors are mobilized to help return the person's mental state to homeostasis. These defense mechanisms present various psychiatric signs, symptoms, or behaviors that you may observe.

Like the symptoms and signs of physical illness, psychiatric symptoms and signs can be grouped according to the "systems" they affect. Here, however, the focus is on systems of psychological (rather than physiologic) functioning. The psychological functions that can be affected are consciousness, motor activity, speech, thought, **affect** (the outward expression of a person's inner feelings, such as happy, sad, angry, fearful, or withdrawn), memory, orientation, and perception. Psychiatric signs and symptoms include these areas, as well as changes in thought progression, thought content, mood, and intelligence **TABLE 29-3**.

TABLE 29-3 Classification of Psychiatric Signs and Symptoms

Function Affected	Psychiatric Signs and Symptoms
Consciousness	• Distractibility and inattention • Confusion • Delirium • Stupor and coma
Motor activity	• Restlessness • **Stereotyped movements** (repetition of movements that do not seem to serve any useful purpose) • **Compulsions** (repetitive actions that are carried out to relieve the anxiety of obsessive thoughts) • Slow movements
Speech	• Slow speech • Acceleration or **pressure of speech** (the pouring out of words like water escaping under pressure) • **Neologisms** (words the patient invents) • **Echolalia** (the patient echoes words that they hear) • **Mutism** (the patient does not speak at all)
Thought progression	• **Flight of ideas** (accelerated thinking in which the mind skips very rapidly from one thought to the next) • Slowness of thought • **Perseveration** (repetition of the same idea over and over again) • **Circumstantial thinking** (the inclusion of many irrelevant details)
Thought content	• Delusions • Obsessions • **Phobias** (obsessive, irrational fears of specific things or situations, such as fear of heights, fear of open places, fear of confined spaces, or fear of certain animals)
Mood and affect	• Anxiety • Euphoria • Depression • **Inappropriate affect** (emotion that is out of sync with the situation; eg, wearing a smile while discussing a parent's death) • **Flat affect** (the absence of emotion; appearing to feel no emotion at all)
Memory	• Amnesia • **Confabulation** (inventing experiences to fill gaps in memory)
Orientation	• Disorientation to person, place, and time
Perception	• Illusions • Hallucinations
Intelligence	• Difficulty learning

Patient Assessment

Your assessment of the patient with a psychiatric emergency differs in at least two ways from the typical methods of patient assessment you have studied so far. First, when assessing the patient with trauma or acute illness, you use diagnostic instruments to measure vital functions and detect abnormalities, such as a stethoscope to evaluate breath sounds and a sphygmomanometer to measure blood pressure. When you assess a patient who is disturbed, however, *you* are the diagnostic instrument. You must use your thinking processes to evaluate someone else's thinking processes, your perceptions to test the validity of someone else's perceptions, and your feelings to measure someone else's feelings. This skill takes practice because most EMS providers are not accustomed to using their feelings in this way. For example, if you feel angry at something someone says, your instinct may be to respond angrily. In working an emergency call, however, a more useful paradigm is "I feel infuriated with that patient, so it's likely he is paranoid, because paranoid patients often elicit anger in others."

A second way the assessment in a behavioral emergency differs from the assessment in acute illness or trauma is that the assessment is part of the treatment. As soon as you speak, your voice and manner will affect the patient's condition, for better or worse. Your process of listening to the patient describe the issue at hand can also mitigate it.

Assess the patient at the site of the emergency. Do not immediately rush the patient to the medical facility, because the medical facility is likely to be a strange, intimidating place for the patient. Your haste to get to a medical facility may reinforce the patient's belief that something is terribly wrong. Let the patient attempt to recover in familiar surroundings when medically possible.

Scene Size-up

The safety concerns at a behavioral emergency may not appear as threatening as a hazardous chemical spill or a motor vehicle crash on a busy highway. However, a situation involving a distraught person with severe depression or a person with a drug addiction experiencing an acute psychotic break poses its own unique threats. Although every situation you encounter has the potential for surprises, situations with a strong behavioral component are those most likely to present unexpected findings. At first, these calls may appear to be simple "injury with bleeding" or "breathing difficulty" calls, but the superficial problem may actually result from the patient's erratic behavior. Follow the general guidelines listed in **TABLE 29-4** to ensure your safety at the scene of a behavioral emergency.

Assessing the environment can give you clues to the patient's condition or the cause of the emergency. In a behavioral crisis, it is especially important to look for clues from the patient's social history; general living conditions; availability of social and family support; activity level; medications; overall appearance with respect to nutrition, general health, cleanliness, and personal hygiene; and attitude and mental well-being.

Finally, consider the mechanism of injury and/or nature of illness. For example, a patient with diabetes may have an altered mental status because of a low blood glucose level.

Primary Survey

Clearly identify yourself. Tell the patient who you are and what you are trying to do. If the patient is confused or delusional, then you may have to explain who you are at frequent intervals. Do so in a nonargumentative, emotionally neutral tone of voice. ("No, Mr. Jones, I'm not from the Central Intelligence Agency. I'm a paramedic with the city ambulance service, and I'm here to help you.")

The patient's overall condition and the nature of the psychiatric emergency will determine how much of the assessment you can perform. A patient who is disturbed may prefer not to be touched. You must respect that wish unless a compelling medical reason exists for doing otherwise (eg, profuse bleeding from slashed wrists or a decreased level of consciousness from an overdose). At the very least, you should be able to assess the patient's general appearance, such as the patient's dress, cleanliness, and grooming. All of these factors are clues to the patient's self-perception. Note the patient's posture. Does the patient appear frustrated, angry, grief-stricken, or **catatonic** (lacking expression or movement, or appearing rigid)?

You must also carefully assess the pupils because they may indicate other causes of altered mental status. For example, constricted pupils may indicate opiate ingestion, and unequal pupils may indicate cerebral trauma.

When performing your assessment, limit the number of people around the patient. Remember to stay alert to potential danger. A patient in unstable

TABLE 29-4 Safety Guidelines for Behavioral Emergencies
Assess the scene. If the patient is armed or in possession of potentially harmful objects, then have law enforcement personnel remove these objects before you provide emergency medical care.
Be prepared to spend extra time. You may need more time than usual to assess, listen to, and prepare the patient for transport.
Have a definitive plan of action. Decide who will do what. If restraint is needed, then how will it be implemented?
Know where the exits are. Identify your exit strategy in case the situation becomes volatile. Never let a patient get between you and the door! Park your emergency vehicle in a location that gives you a safe and easy way out should it become necessary for you to leave the scene.
Don personal protective equipment (PPE). An agitated patient may try to spit on you or worse. Anticipate such a threat by wearing the necessary PPE.
Urgently de-escalate the patient's level of agitation. It is critical to keep a high-pressure situation from erupting into violence.
Identify yourself calmly. Try to gain the patient's confidence. If you begin shouting, then the patient is likely to shout louder or become more excited. Maintain a calm voice and demeanor to ensure a quieting influence.
Be direct. State your intentions and what you expect of the patient.
Stay with the patient. *Do not let the patient leave the area, and do not leave the area yourself unless law enforcement personnel can and will stay with the patient.* Otherwise, the patient may go to another room and obtain weapons, lock doors to keep health care providers out, or take pills.
Encourage purposeful movement. Help the patient get dressed and gather appropriate belongings to take to the medical facility.
Express interest in the patient's story. Let the patient tell you in their own words what happened or what is going on now. However, don't play along with auditory or visual disturbances, as doing so may reinforce the patient's delusion or hallucination.
Keep a safe distance from the patient. Everyone needs personal space. Be sure you can move quickly if the patient becomes violent or tries to run away. Don't physically talk down to or directly confront the patient. A squatting, 45° angle approach is usually not confrontational, but may hinder your movements. Do not allow the patient to get between you and the exit.
Avoid arguing or fighting with the patient. Do not get into a power struggle. Remember, the patient is not responding to you in a normal manner; this person may be wrestling with internal forces over which neither of you has control. You and others may be unknowingly stimulating these inner forces. If you can respond with understanding to the feeling that the patient is expressing, whether it is anger, fear, or desperation, then you may be able to gain their cooperation. If you must use force, then ensure that you have adequate help and move toward the patient quietly and with assured firmness.
Be honest and reassuring. If the patient asks whether transport to the medical facility is necessary, then your answer should be "Yes, that is where you can receive medical help."
Don't judge. You may see behavior that you dislike. Set those feelings aside and concentrate on providing emergency medical care.

condition may become violent at any time. Watch for signs of agitation or aggression. Separate the patient from bystanders or family members who seem to be worsening the patient's condition. You may ask those people to step into another room and speak to your partner, or you may take the patient to the ambulance before beginning your primary survey, if appropriate.

Attend first to the patient's airway, breathing, and circulation (ABCs). Assess the airway to make sure it is patent and adequate. Next, evaluate the patient's breathing. Provide appropriate interventions based on your assessment findings. In most patients with behavioral emergencies, however, the problem will be more psychiatric than physiologic. During your assessment, look for signs and symptoms of abnormal functioning or behavior and remain alert for threatening gestures.

Assess the patient's pulse rate, quality, and rhythm. Obtain the systolic and diastolic blood pressures when possible. Evaluate for the presence of shock and bleeding. Assess the patient's perfusion level by evaluating skin color, temperature, condition, and capillary refill time.

Patients who are seriously disturbed should be seen by a physician and evaluated for possible hospitalization. Many such patients will consent to be transported to the medical facility. Others will not want your help and will try to prevent you from taking them to a medical facility. Because transporting patients against their will deprives them of their civil liberties, you must never make this decision lightly. Even an experienced psychiatrist may have difficulty defining behavior that justifies removal from society or that constitutes so-called dangerous behavior. Furthermore, laws vary from region to region, so know the legal requirements in your community.

As a general rule, an alert adult must consent to be taken to a medical facility. If the patient withholds this consent, then the patient may be taken only at the express request of law enforcement personnel or the county mental health physician (in many jurisdictions). The same policy applies to the use of forcible restraints. If such measures are deemed necessary, then summon law enforcement officers.

In addition, every EMS system should have clearly defined protocols, drawn up with legal advice, for dealing with patients who require involuntary commitment. Follow those protocols without deviation and consult medical control as necessary.

History Taking

The **mental status exam (MSE)** is a key part of your assessment of a patient who is experiencing an acute psychiatric emergency. To conduct the MSE,

YOU are the Paramedic

PART 2

As you approach the apartment, you note the patient is pacing back and forth just inside the doorway. He is clenching and unclenching his fists. You hear him repeating, "They're coming for me," in a low voice. Speaking calmly, you ask the patient his name and tell him that you're with emergency medical services and are here to help him. He stops pacing, turns to you, and tells you his name. He tells you that you cannot help him because "they" are going to kill him.

You repeat that you want to help him and ask the patient to tell you why he feels this way. He looks around nervously and says he must whisper because "they" can hear him. He continues to refuse to come into the hall because he says he would be an easier target there. You ask if you can come in and sit with him. He allows you in, and you sit in a chair near the door so that your access to the exit is not blocked. The apartment appears neat. No visible evidence of alcohol in the kitchen or living area is present. The patient is fully dressed in wrinkled clothes that appear clean. You don't notice any unusual odors. You are limited to a visual assessment of the patient at this time.

Recording Time: 0 Minutes	
Appearance	Agitated, anxious
Level of consciousness	Alert and oriented to person and place; distracted by delusions
Airway	Patent
Breathing	Appears adequate; occasionally rapid
Circulation	Skin color appears appropriate for baseline skin color

3. What is your initial impression of this patient? What factors, signs, or symptoms lead you to this conclusion?

4. Does this patient need to be evaluated at a medical facility?

you must check each of the "systems" of mental function in order. A helpful mnemonic for the elements of the MSE is COASTMAP:

- **Consciousness.** Determine the patient's level of consciousness (alert, confused, responds to pain, unresponsive). Note the patient's ability to pay attention to a discussion and concentrate. Is the patient easily distracted, or is the patient able to focus on the events at hand?
- **Orientation.** Ask the patient the current year or month and location (country, state, town, or specific location). If the patient is not sure, then have the patient make a best guess.
- **Activity.** Examine the patient's behavior. Is the patient restless and agitated, pacing up and down? Experiencing tremors? Sitting still, scarcely moving at all? Making any strange or repetitive movements (scanning of the environment, odd or repetitive gestures)?
- **Speech.** Identify the form, rather than the content, of the patient's speech. Note the rate, volume, flow, articulation, and intonation of speech. Is it too fast or too slow? Too loud or too soft? Is the speech garbled or slurred (dysarthria)? Is the patient stuttering or mumbling? Using any strange words?
- **Thought.** Listen to the patient's story. Is the person thinking clearly? Making sense? Expressing apparently false ideas (delusions), such as a belief that they are being followed? Experiencing any false sensory impressions (hallucinations), such as hearing voices? Experiencing a flight of ideas (rapid shifting of ideas)?
- **Memory.** Develop a general impression of the patient's memory, including for recent, remote, and immediate events. If the patient has memory loss, then determine whether it is constant or variable. Some patients may create memories to take the place of things they cannot recall (confabulation).
- **Affect and mood.** The patient's mood may be objectively noted via body language. Is the mood euphoric or sad? Is it **labile** (rapidly shifting among different emotional states)? Does the affect seem appropriate to the situation or is it animated, angry, flat, or withdrawn?
- **Perception.** Detecting perception disorders may be difficult because patients often hesitate to answer direct questions about hallucinations or illusions. Sometimes it is helpful to ask the patient, "Do you ever hear things that other people cannot hear?"

You can conduct nearly all of the MSE just by watching and listening (and knowing what to watch and listen for). Only the assessment of memory, orientation, and perhaps perception requires you to ask some direct questions.

Words of Wisdom

Practice being an observer. As you sit in a restaurant, eavesdrop on the waitress talking to other customers and systematically go through the COASTMAP sequence to evaluate her mental status. Get into the habit of noticing how other people talk, move, and express their feelings, and practice describing those elements to your partner.

Secondary Assessment

While much of your assessment focuses on interviewing the patient about their psychiatric history and performing the MSE, you must also look for signs of an organic cause of the patient's behavior:

- Obtain the patient's vital signs to identify fever or indications of increased intracranial pressure.
- Examine the skin temperature and moisture. Scars may indicate self-mutilation in patients with **borderline personality disorder**.
- Inspect the head for evidence of trauma.
- Check the pupils for size, equality, and reaction to light. Pupillary abnormalities may indicate a toxic ingestion or an intracranial process as the source of the patient's behavior.
- Note any unusual odors on the patient's breath, such as poisons, alcohol, or ketones from diabetic ketoacidosis.
- As you examine the extremities, check for needle tracks, tremors, and unilateral weakness or loss of sensation.

Reassessment

Reassess the patient during transport. This is a good time to further explore the patient's mental status or confirm findings you have already obtained.

Patients with abnormal behavior often settle down physically by the time you start your assessment. However, their minds may still be in a state of flux, which could lead to impulsive behavior. Monitor patients vigilantly for sudden changes in thought or behavior, particularly in transit as you near the medical facility. If patients don't want help, then they may try to jump from the ambulance or hurt themselves in an attempt to complete a suicide attempt before arriving at the medical facility. They may even turn that aggressive and impulsive behavior toward you.

Your radio report to the medical facility should include your usual report of medical and mental health history, medications prescribed, and assessment findings based on local protocols and guidelines. In addition, include pertinent information from the MSE to create a clear picture of the patient.

Discuss the need for restraints or medications to control behavior with the medical facility before instituting these interventions when possible. If such measures have already been used or other standing orders have been instituted to protect the patient and providers, inform the medical facility staff.

If the patient is aggressive or potentially violent, then give the ED staff advance notice so they can mobilize security or additional help before your arrival.

Emergency Medical Care

Care of the patient with a psychiatric emergency follows the approach used throughout this text. First, ensure scene safety and focus on life-threatening conditions. Second, if the erratic behavior might be caused by a medical disorder (eg, hypoglycemia, overdose, or hypoxia), then treat the patient for the medical disorder before assuming that the patient's behavior has an emotional or psychiatric cause. These measures may include oxygen therapy, testing of the blood glucose level, and administration of dextrose, as well as general interventions for hypothermia or shock.

Communication Techniques

As always, good communication is part of treating a patient with a psychiatric emergency.

When evaluating a trauma patient, you can generally obtain enough information to select the appropriate initial treatment based only on the physical exam findings, even if the patient is unresponsive and cannot provide a history. However, when you evaluate a patient with a behavioral emergency, virtually all of the diagnostic information, and much of the therapeutic benefit, comes from your communication with the patient. Therefore, your skill in interviewing a patient with a behavioral crisis is central to treating psychiatric emergencies.

Set some ground rules for your interview. Let the patient know what you expect and what the patient may expect of you. ("It's okay to cry or even scream, but we aren't going to let you hurt yourself or anyone else.") Allow the patient to tell the story in their own way. Don't attempt to direct the conversation, but allow the patient to vent. Following are some communication guidelines:

- **Begin with an open-ended question.** An open-ended question does not give the patient possible answers, but rather allows the patient to form an answer. For example, you might say, "It's clear you've been feeling bad. Tell me something about the kind of troubles you've been having." (Begin with more direct questioning when you must obtain specific information quickly, such as "What kind of pills did you take? How many?")
- **Let the patient talk and tell the story in their own way, even if it takes a little more time.** Letting patients talk allows them to gain some control over themselves and their situations. At the same time, it enables you to assess the patient's speech, affect, and thought processes.
- **Listen, and show that you are listening.** Your facial expression, posture, eye contact, an occasional nod; all of these things can show the patient that you are paying close attention to what is being said **FIGURE 29-2**.
- **Don't be afraid of silent pauses, even if they seem intolerably long.** Maintain an attentive and relaxed attitude until the patient takes up the story again. It's essential to be silent when the patient stops speaking because of overwhelming emotion. Avoid the temptation to jump into the silence to comfort the patient or forestall expressions of emotion, such as crying. The expression of feelings is often therapeutic in itself, and the patient will probably be better able to describe what is happening after this emotional release.

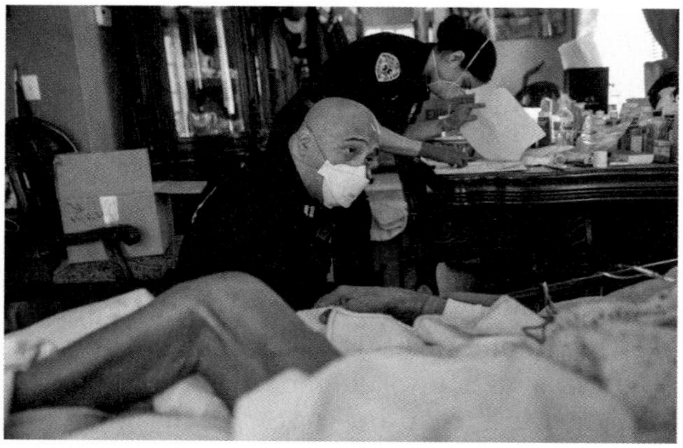

FIGURE 29-2 Making eye contact with a patient can yield useful clues about the patient's emotional state. Be careful, though, not to stare at the patient.

- **Acknowledge and label the patient's feelings.** The patient who is disturbed may feel overwhelmed by intense and chaotic feelings. Identifying those feelings and giving them a name (eg, "You seem angry") can help the patient gain control over them.
- **Don't argue.** If the patient misperceives reality, then note the misperceptions, but don't try to talk the patient out of them. When a misperception frightens or distresses the patient, you may try once to make a factual statement, in a neutral tone of voice ("Yes, that does look a lot like a snake, but it's just a shadow"). But don't get into a dispute about the nature of reality.
- **Facilitate communication.** Facilitation is a technique used to encourage the patient to communicate by using gestures or noncommittal words, such as a nod of the head or a phrase such as "Go on," "I see," or "What happened after that?" You can also use facilitation to return the patient to a topic on which you would like some elaboration. For example, a patient may have made a passing reference to suicidal thoughts and then moved on to another subject. When the patient finishes, you might comment, "You say you've had thoughts of suicide?" This remark tells the patient that you have been paying attention to the story and would like to learn more.
- **Direct the patient's attention.** Confrontation means pointing out something of interest in the patient's conversation or behavior, thereby directing the patient's attention to something they may not have noticed. Confrontations describe the way the patient appears to the interviewer and are based on observations, *not* judgments. For example, you might remark, "You seem worried" or "You look sad." Such comments often elicit a freer expression of feelings from the patient. Confrontations must be carefully phrased so that they don't sound nagging or condescending.
- **Ask questions.** When the patient finishes giving the initial account of the problem, you will want to ask questions. Keep them as open-ended as possible. Avoid asking questions that can be answered with a yes or no ("Are you angry?") or asking leading questions ("Do you think that your husband is a part of the problem?"). Instead, pose open-ended *how* and *what* questions ("How did you feel when that happened?" "What factors have contributed to how you're feeling right now?").
- **Adjust your approach as needed.** Some patients have difficulty with the lack of structure in open-ended questioning and may become anxious during silences. This reaction is especially common among adolescents, individuals with severe depression, and confused or disorganized patients. When your open-ended questions meet with uncomprehending silence, try another approach and perform a more structured interview.

Crisis Intervention Skills

The following guidelines apply to the care of any patient with a psychiatric emergency:

- **Be as calm and direct as possible.** Patients who are disturbed are often afraid of losing self-control. Your behavior should show that you have confidence in the patient's ability to maintain control. One of the primary purposes of the interview is to help the patient reestablish some self-mastery. If you show anxiety or panic, then you merely affirm the patient's conviction that the situation is overwhelming.
- **Exclude disruptive people.** In most cases, you should interview the patient alone. Relatives and bystanders should wait in another room, where your partner can interview them. Some patients, however, become anxious if

separated from an important person, such as a parent or a friend. If another person has a calming effect on the patient, then ask that person to remain present.

- **Sit down.** Sit down to interview the patient, preferably at a 45° angle from the patient, so you don't encroach on their personal space **FIGURE 29-3**.
- **Maintain a nonjudgmental attitude.** Accept the patient's right to have feelings about things, and don't blame, judge, or criticize the patient for those feelings.
- **Give honest reassurance.** Give supportive, truthful information. For example, you might say, "Many people go through periods of hopelessness like you're having, but today we have effective treatments for those feelings." At the same time, avoid excessive reassurances, such as "Everything's going to be all right." Such statements merely convince patients that you don't understand how bad things are for them.
- **Develop a plan of action.** After the patient has finished talking and you have concluded your assessment, you can develop a specific plan of action. This step gives the patient the feeling that something is being done to help, which can relieve anxiety. In addition, people in crisis need direction. Don't give the patient an array of choices (eg, "Do you want to go to the medical facility, or would you rather stay at home and call your physician tomorrow?"). Rather, state what you think is the best course of action ("I think it's important for you to go to the medical facility. There are physicians there who can help you."). When the plan has been determined and you have begun to carry it out, allow the patient to make choices and thereby exercise some control over the situation. You might ask, for example, whether the patient prefers to be carried on a stretcher or to walk to the ambulance. These small decisions may seem minor, but they allow the patient to attain a measure of autonomy and self-respect.
- **Encourage some motor activity.** Moving about can help ease anxiety. If you are taking the patient to the medical facility, then help the patient gather things to bring along. Let patients do as much for themselves as possible.
- **Stay with the patient at all times.** When you have responded to the emergency, the patient's safety becomes your responsibility. Therefore, do not allow the patient to leave you. For example, allowing the patient to go to the bathroom alone might allow the patient to swallow the contents of a bottle of pills.
- **Bring all of the patient's medications to the medical facility.** If the patient is currently receiving treatment for a psychiatric disorder, knowing the medications that have already been prescribed can help physicians identify the condition for which the patient has been treated. Medications for other medical conditions may cause adverse effects or unusual interactions that alter behavior.
- **Don't assume that it is impossible to talk with any patient until you have tried to do so.** Even if the patient sits silently and appears unaware of your presence, assume that the patient can hear and understand everything you say.

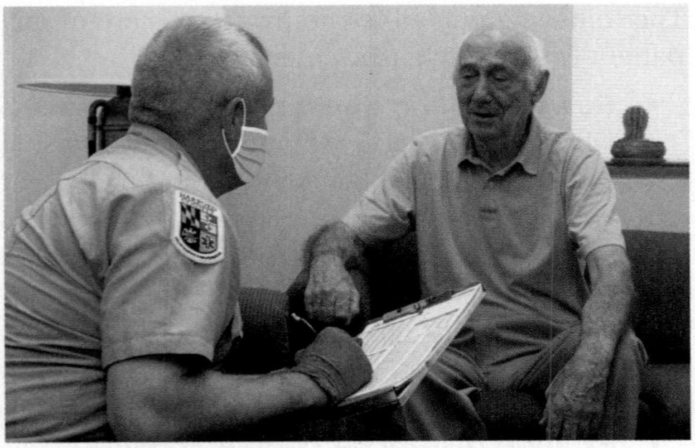

FIGURE 29-3 When interviewing the patient, sitting at a 45° angle is one way to avoid encroaching on the patient's personal space.

Use of Force and Types of Restraint

When verbal interventions fail to reduce severe agitation in a patient, consider the use of physical or chemical restraint.

Physical Restraint

Some devices used for physical restraint may be improvised from materials on the emergency vehicle; others are commercially made from leather or nylon that is padded for comfort and safety. Most commercial restraints are applied to the wrists and ankles to prevent movement of the arms and legs. Some are placed around the waist to restrict movement of the torso.

Vest-type restraints are applied from the front of the patient and may include sleeves to prevent the arms from moving. Make sure you are familiar with the restraints used by your agency before you need to use them.

Before attempting to restrain the patient, ensure you have enough personnel to effectively overpower and restrain the patient. You must have overwhelming force to apply a physical restraint, which means a minimum of five trained people: one for each limb and one for the head. Assign a specific limb in advance to each emergency responder. Appoint one leader to direct the team and maintain verbal contact with the patient.

Before you begin, discuss the plan of action. Law enforcement personnel are often trained in both verbal and physical techniques used to subdue violent people. They should be included in any plan to physically restrain a violent patient. They can also offer an objective view of the situation. However, law enforcement personnel will sometimes refuse to help restrain a patient without a warrant for the subject's arrest or evidence that the individual poses an immediate threat to others. Therefore, paramedics must be prepared to physically restrain patients on their own when necessary and should practice these techniques regularly.

When subduing a patient who is disturbed, use the minimum force necessary. Avoid acts of physical force that may injure the patient. Do not move toward the patient immediately; give the patient a chance to choose a nonviolent alternative behavior.

If the show of force does not calm the patient, then emergency responders must prepare to restrain the patient. Remove any equipment or jewelry from your own body that could be used as a weapon (eg, name badge, scissors worn on the belt, key chain, earrings). Make sure you have adequate restraining devices immediately available, preferably padded leather or nylon restraints.

YOU are the Paramedic

PART 3

The patient agrees to sit in a chair opposite you. You ask the patient if he knows what day it is. He replies with the correct day of the week. You use the COASTMAP method to continue your mental status assessment of this patient. The patient is restless in his seat. He is gripping the edge of the chair and rocking back and forth. You ask the patient if he has any medical conditions. He tells you that he sees his physician regularly because he has schizophrenia. He is supposed to take medication every day, but he has not taken any for the past week. He says he overheard "them" at the drug store when he was refilling his prescriptions. When he realized that they knew he overheard them, he stopped taking his medications because they were poisoned. He explains to you that he wanted to take the medications, but he is afraid. He says he cannot go out to get more.

You ask the patient if your partner can check his vital signs while you look at the medications he takes. He consents and directs you to a basket on the table with medicine bottles. You locate two new bottles indicated for the treatment of schizophrenia: (1) thioridazine (Mellaril), 200 mg twice daily, and (2) mesoridazine (Serentil), 50 mg twice daily.

Recording Time: 8 Minutes	
Respirations	20 breaths/min
Pulse	110 beats/min
Skin	Warm, dry, and color typical for baseline
Blood pressure	130/84 mm Hg
Oxygen saturation (Spo_2)	99% on room air
Pupils	Pupils Equal, Round, Reactive to Light and Accommodation (PERRLA)

5. What conclusions might you make about medication compliance and the patient's medical history?

6. If the patient refuses to be transported, then what options should you, as a paramedic, consider?

The best position in which to secure the patient to the stretcher is the supine position, with both legs and both arms secured to one side of the stretcher and with the patient's head turned to the side. This position prevents aspiration in case of vomiting. *Never* place a patient facedown, because you cannot adequately monitor the patient in this position. This position also may inhibit the breathing of an impaired or exhausted patient. Be careful not to place restraints in a way that compromises the patient's respirations. Never tie the patient's ankles and wrists together as one; this type of restraint has been known to result in death. Never "hobble tie" a patient (tying just the feet together). Placing a patient facedown in a Reeves stretcher can also be dangerous and lead to positional asphyxia or aspiration.

Throughout the process, someone (preferably you or your partner) should talk with the patient. Remember to treat the patient with dignity and sensitivity at all times. Keeping the patient informed in a calm, respectful manner reduces the amount of stimuli the patient experiences. After the restraints are in place, do not remove them. Don't negotiate or make deals.

Words of Wisdom

During the process of restraining an agitated patient, the patient may try to bite you or spit at you. Take appropriate precautions to avoid either action. A surgical mask may be used to protect against spitting. Consider the use of a nonrebreathing mask for the patient who may be hypoxic.

Continuously monitor the patient for a clear airway and breathing, vomiting, airway obstruction, and cardiovascular stability. Drug or alcohol intoxication initially may cause violent behavior but then can lead to physical problems such as vomiting and aspiration or respiratory depression.

Check the patient's peripheral circulation every few minutes to ensure that the restraints are not too tight **FIGURE 29-4**. Check the radial pulses in the arms and the dorsalis pedis pulses in the feet.

Be careful if a combative patient suddenly becomes calm and cooperative. Such an abrupt change in behavior does not signal a time to relax; instead, remain vigilant. The patient may suddenly become combative again and injure someone.

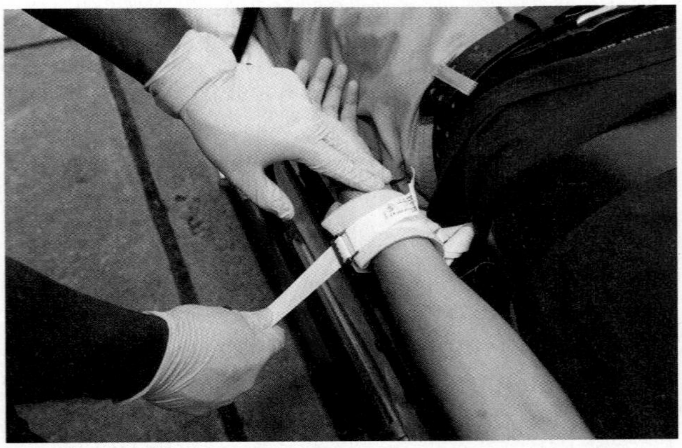

FIGURE 29-4 Assess circulation frequently while a patient is restrained.

Your documentation should include the reasons for using restraints. Be specific, giving examples of the patient's behavior and indicators of the patient's potential for violence; the number of people used to subdue the patient; the restraining devices used; and the status of the patient's airway, breathing, and peripheral circulation after restraints were applied. Remember that you may use reasonable force to defend yourself against an attack by a patient who is emotionally disturbed. Having witnesses in attendance, even during transport, and documenting their presence, may be extremely helpful in protecting you from false accusations.

Proper use of the four-point physical restraint technique is shown in **SKILL DRILL 29-1**. Caution is required when considering this technique. Because providers cannot roll the patient and suction vomit with this technique, it is typically used only if there is no medical concern and the patient is alert. Many services secure the patient to a backboard or scoop stretcher, which can be tipped to the side to assist with clearing the airway as needed while still keeping the patient restrained.

A two-point restraint technique is an option if allowed per local protocols. This technique is performed in the same way as four-point restraint, but instead of restraining all four extremities to the stationary frame of the stretcher, one arm is placed upward toward the head, and the other is placed downward toward the waist.

Chemical Restraint

Physical restraint of a patient for aggressive and psychotic behavior can be complicated and dangerous

Skill Drill 29-1 Restraining a Patient

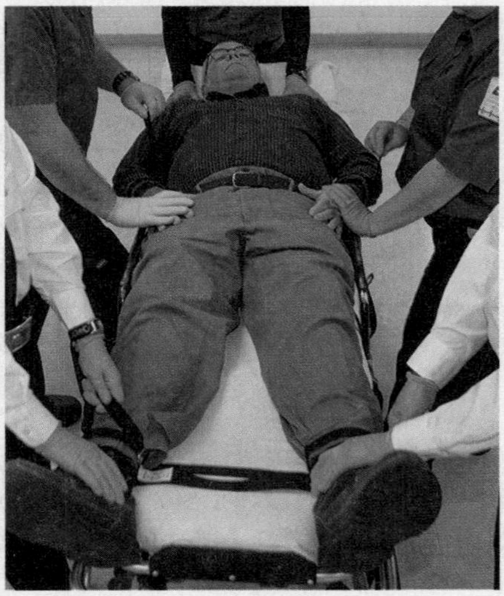

Step 1

Make sure you have enough personnel to perform this skill (five trained responders). Bring down the patient into the prone position. Then, acting at the same time, secure the patient in the supine or left lateral position with wrist and ankle restraints. Some services require using a backboard for restraint so a patient who becomes unresponsive or who vomits can be turned onto the side quickly to manage the airway.

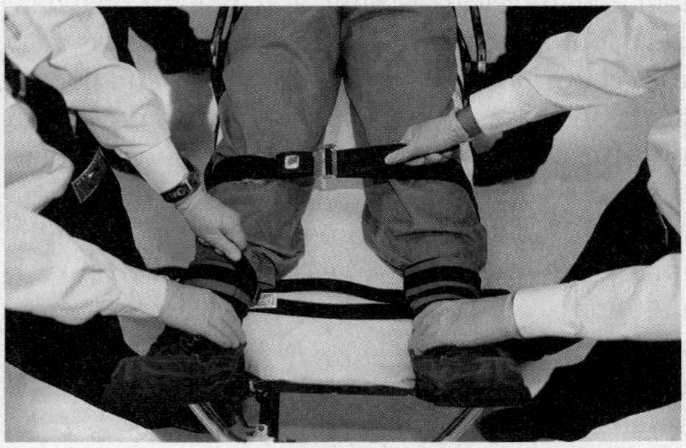

Step 2

Use stretcher straps or sheets to secure the patient's legs.

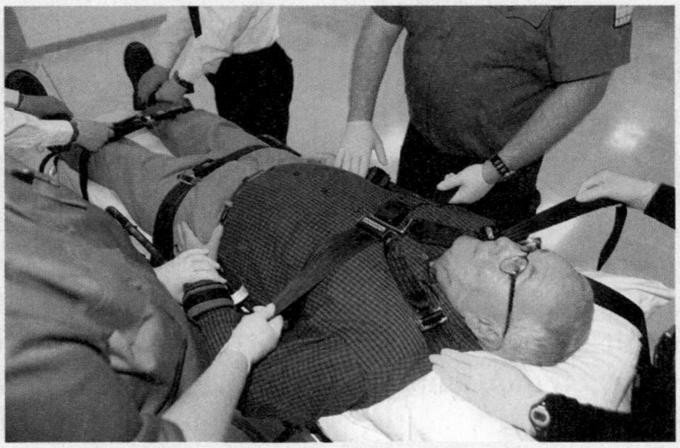

Step 3

Fasten the remaining stretcher straps. Continue to verbally reassure and calm the patient following physical restraint. Regularly check circulation to the extremities.

for both you and the patient. One alternative to physical restraint is **chemical restraint**, the use of medication to subdue a patient. This option should be used only with approval from medical control and by following clearly established local protocols and guidelines.

Chemical restraint is not always easier to implement than physical restraint, and it has its own hazards. Combinations of sedative medications may produce unexpected drug interactions and should be avoided. Use physical and/or chemical restraint only after verbal attempts to de-escalate a patient with excited delirium have failed. Giving the patient a blanket or pillow, or otherwise trying to make the patient comfortable, may help to reduce the anxiety that often accompanies **psychosis** (a state of delusion in which a person is out of touch with reality). Both excited delirium and psychosis are discussed later in this chapter.

Special Populations

When you administer psychiatric medications to older patients, begin with lower doses (as with any medication). Repeat the dose based on the advice of medical control.

Benzodiazepines

Benzodiazepines such as diazepam (Valium), lorazepam (Ativan), and midazolam (Versed) can be given as either intramuscular (IM) or intravenous (IV) injections. However, only midazolam and lorazepam have reliable IM absorption. Drowsiness, decreased mental alertness, sedation, and ataxia are the most common adverse effects. However, respiratory depression is possible. Although infrequent, paradoxical responses to benzodiazepines, such as insomnia and agitation, are more common among older adults.

Because aggressive and dangerous behaviors are often caused by the use of illicit drugs (eg, cocaine, methamphetamines, phencyclidine [PCP]), benzodiazepines are usually a safer and more effective form of chemical restraint when compared with other medications.

Short-acting benzodiazepines, such as midazolam, may be given intranasally using a mucosal atomizer device. This method provides easy preparation and quick administration with less risk to health care providers compared with IM or IV injections. When you deliver midazolam by an atomizer device, administer one-half the total dose in each nostril. Consider a more concentrated solution because of the limited volume of medication the nares can reliably absorb.

The onset of action for the various benzodiazepines varies depending on the route of administration and the dose. Diazepam, lorazepam, and midazolam can be administered to pediatric or adult patients. Doses for these and the other medications discussed in this section are listed in Chapter 15, *Emergency Medications.*

Antipsychotic Medications

You may also use antipsychotic medications, such as droperidol (Inapsine), haloperidol (Haldol), and ziprasidone (Geodon), in the treatment of agitated patients. However, the FDA has issued a black box warning for droperidol because of its association with prolonged QT syndromes.[4] Higher doses and IV administration of haloperidol, a typical antipsychotic agent, also appear to be associated with a higher risk of QT prolongation and torsades de pointes.

SAFETY

Exercise caution when administering droperidol and haloperidol in patients with suspected electrolyte imbalances or known cardiac abnormalities, or in patients who are taking drugs that affect the QT interval. When either medication is administered intravenously, electrocardiographic (ECG) monitoring is recommended.

Typical antipsychotics, including droperidol and haloperidol, may cause seizures or a wide array of extrapyramidal symptoms, including involuntary movements, tremors, rigidity, muscle contractions, restlessness, and changes in breathing and pulse rate. Newer atypical antipsychotics such as olanzapine (Zyprexa) and ziprasidone have fewer extrapyramidal symptoms. The incidence of anticholinergic effects also may be lower with the atypical agents. Combined use of these medications with alcohol and other central nervous system (CNS) depressants may worsen CNS depression. Monitor for hypotension, bradycardia, and glucose levels in patients receiving atypical antipsychotics.

Special Populations

Exercise caution when administering antipsychotics to pediatric patients. Droperidol is not routinely recommended, but haloperidol may be used in pediatric patients. Limited data are available regarding the use of olanzapine and ziprasidone in pediatric patients.

Older patients with dementia-related psychosis treated with antipsychotic medications have an increased risk of death.[5] Administration of parenteral olanzapine and a benzodiazepine to the same patient can lead to severe orthostatic hypotension, as well as cardiac or respiratory depression. Avoid this combination of medications in geriatric patients.

Evidence-Based Medicine

The medications used most often for chemical restraint include short-acting benzodiazepines, antipsychotics, dissociative agents, and antihistamines. Many of these medications have not been approved by the US Food and Drug Administration (FDA) for chemical restraint. In addition, the FDA has issued black box warnings for some of these medications. A black box warning indicates that the drug may be associated with serious adverse effects.[6]

Because of its rapid onset of action and multiple routes of administration, ketamine has emerged as a potentially preferred drug for the control of patient agitation in the prehospital environment.[7] However, ketamine has been associated with emesis, tachycardia, hypertension, palpitations, respiratory depression, laryngospasm, hypersalivation, and emergence reaction; therefore, consider the risk versus benefits before administering this medication. For example, a reduced dose may be warranted to minimize the risk of respiratory problems.[8]

Antihistamines

Antihistamines, specifically diphenhydramine (Benadryl), have been used for many years in the treatment of psychiatric patients. Although diphenhydramine is best known for its sedative properties, it also produces an anticholinergic effect that affects neurotransmitters in the brain that affect behavior. It can be used for both adult and pediatric patients.

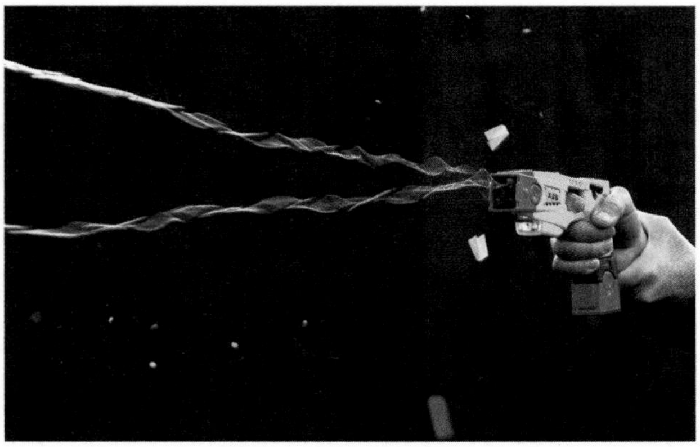

FIGURE 29-5 TASER X26P. When deployed, compressed nitrogen projects two small probes up to 25 feet (7.6 m), delivering a 5-second electric shock as the probes make contact with the body or clothing. This shock is intended to result in an immediate but temporary incapacitation.

SAFETY

Many law enforcement agencies use a conducted-energy weapon (CEW), such as a TASER, as a less-lethal force measure to immobilize people who are behaving in a violent or aggressive manner **FIGURE 29-5**.

Patients subjected to the deployment of a CEW may sustain a variety of injuries, including abrasions, bruises, lacerations, strained muscles, marks from the application of the CEW, trauma to the head and torso, dislocations, or fractures.[9] In addition, the patient may be at risk for medical complications resulting from an underlying condition. You must identify these underlying conditions and ensure appropriate emergency medical care. Such conditions include drug overdose syndromes, excited delirium, acute psychiatric decompensation, hypoglycemia, heatstroke, hepatic encephalopathy, seizure disorders, dementia, and encephalitis. Law enforcement officers are not routinely trained to recognize these conditions. They rely on you to make appropriate medical decisions at the scene.

Pathophysiology, Assessment, and Management of Specific Emergencies

Many factors contribute to behavior disturbances. Some of these influences are easily identified and treated, but others may never be clearly understood. The causes, signs, symptoms, and management of abnormal behavior can be grouped into several common areas, shown in **TABLE 29-5**. The areas most relevant to paramedicine are acute psychosis, excited delirium, suicide, and patterns of violence, abuse, and neglect. Finally, we will discuss specific psychiatric disorders.

Acute Psychosis

Pathophysiology

Recall that psychosis is a state of delusion in which a person is out of touch with reality. Affected people are tuned into their own internal reality of ideas and feelings, which they mistake for the reality of the external world. To the person experiencing an acute psychotic episode, the line differentiating reality from fantasy is blurred rather than distinct, as it is in people without psychoses. That internal reality may make patients belligerent and angry toward others. Alternatively, these patients may become mute and withdrawn as they give all their attention to the voices and feelings within.

Psychoses or psychotic episodes result from many causes. These causes may be biologic or

TABLE 29-5 Categorization of Psychiatric Disorders

Type of Disorder	Specific Disorder
Cognitive	• Excited delirium
Thought	• Schizophrenia • Acute psychosis
Mood	• Bipolar mood disorder • Manic behavior • Depression
Neurotic	• Generalized anxiety disorder • Phobias • Panic disorder
Substance-related disorders and addictive behavior	• Substance use • Substance intoxication • Substance misuse • Substance dependence • Eating disorders (bulimia nervosa, anorexia nervosa)
Somatoform	• Hypochondriasis • Conversion disorder (physical problem that has no identifiable pathophysiology; results from a psychological conflict)
Factitious	Condition in which a person deliberately produces or feigns symptoms of an illness • Münchausen syndrome (most severe type of factitious disorder; most symptoms are physical) • Münchausen syndrome by proxy (mental illness in which caregiver makes up or produces illness or injury in a person to whom care is given; eg, a parent intentionally makes a child sick; also called factitious disorder by proxy)
Impulse control	• Intermittent explosive disorder (acting on aggressive impulses involving the destruction of property) • Kleptomania (acting on the urge to steal things) • Pyromania (acting on the urge to set fires) • Pathologic gambling
Personality	• Odd or eccentric disorders • Dramatic, erratic, or emotional disorders • Anxious or fearful disorders

Street Smarts

Terms that negatively characterize a person, such as "crazy," "psycho," or "EDP" (an abbreviation often used in EMS and law enforcement for *emotionally disturbed person*), can be stigmatizing, affecting how people with mental health disorders view themselves, but also how others perceive and treat them. When diagnostic wording seems to describe the person's character (eg, "he's a schizophrenic"), rather than the person's disorder (eg, "he has schizophrenia"), the person is less likely to receive the help they need. After all, we are conditioned to regard disorders as treatable, but personalities as fixed. As a key health advocate in your community, be careful to use wording that does not label patients by their condition.

organic, or may result from mental illness or substance misuse. The use of mind-altering substances is one of the most common causes, and that psychotic episode may be limited to the time during which the substance is being metabolized within the body. Other causes may be more related to the patient's environment or mental illness. These causes can include intense stress, delusional disorders, and, more often, schizophrenia (discussed later in this chapter). Some psychotic episodes last for brief periods; others last a lifetime.

Disorganization and **disorientation** are not diagnoses, but rather ways in which various conditions such as schizophrenia or organic brain syndromes may present themselves. These presentations account for many EMS calls, particularly for older people. Although you need not make a specific diagnosis in such cases, you do need to know how to care for these patients in the field.

Assessment

The most characteristic feature of psychosis is a profound thought disorder, often accompanied by disturbances in mood and perception. Patients are usually incoherent or rambling in their speech, although they may be oriented to person and place. They often wander down a street, dressed oddly, and utter meaningless words and sentences. A thorough exam of the patient is rarely possible, and your principal objective is to transport the patient to the medical facility without trauma.

Using the COASTMAP mnemonic, the following list describes the common signs and symptoms of the patient with psychosis:

- **Consciousness.** The patient with psychosis is awake and alert, but may be easily distracted, especially if paying attention to hallucinations. If the level of consciousness fluctuates, suspect an organic brain syndrome.
- **Orientation.** Disturbances in orientation are more common in organic disorders than in psychoses, but the patient with severe psychosis may be disoriented as to time and place.
- **Activity.** Activity is most often accelerated, characterized by agitation and hyperactivity, but also may be reduced. Bizarre, stereotyped movements are common.
- **Speech.** Speech may be pressured or sound strange because of unusual words that the patient has invented (neologisms).
- **Thought.** Thought is disturbed in progression and content and may show any of the following disorders:
  - Flight of ideas, with the patient's mind plunging from one thought to another.
  - **Loosening of associations**, in which the logical connection between one idea and the next becomes obscure, at least to the listener. In extreme cases, the patient's speech may be entirely incomprehensible.
  - Delusions, especially of persecution.
  - **Thought broadcasting** (the belief that thoughts are broadcast aloud and can be heard by others).
  - **Thought insertion** (the belief that thoughts are being thrust into the patient's mind by another person) and **thought withdrawal** (the belief that thoughts are being removed).
- **Memory.** Memory can be relatively or entirely intact in psychosis. You may encounter difficulty in obtaining the patient's cooperation for formal memory testing.
- **Affect and mood.** Mood is likely to be disturbed in psychosis. The disturbance may take the form of euphoria, sadness, or wide swings in mood; affect may reflect those inner states or be flat.
- **Perception.** Auditory hallucinations are common in psychosis. Patients hear voices commenting on their behavior or telling them

what to do. Suspect that patients are hearing such voices when they seem to be attending a conversation other than yours or talking to themselves.

Management

Dealing with a patient with acute psychosis is difficult. The usual methods of reasoning with a patient are unlikely to be effective because the person has their own rules of logic that may be very different from those that govern nonpsychotic thinking.

In addition, you are likely to feel uncomfortable in the presence of a person with psychosis. Those uncomfortable feelings are one of your built-in diagnostic instruments. They are elicited by the fear, suspicion, and hostility that the patient is broadcasting through body language. Use your uncomfortable feelings to help make a tentative diagnosis of a psychotic problem.

The patient experiencing disorganization needs structure. Explain in plain language what you are doing and what the patient's role is. Directions should be simple, consistent, and firm. It may be impossible to obtain a detailed history; a name and address may be the only information you can gather. Explain to such patients that they need to be seen by a physician and that you will take them to the medical facility to get help.

In caring for the patient experiencing disorientation, the key is to orient the patient to time, place, and the people in the environment as often as necessary. Tell the patient who you are and explain what you are doing. You may have to repeat that information several times en route. Reassure the patient and point out landmarks to help orient them.

Words of Wisdom

Be forewarned! The patient who hears voices that command them to cause harm to self or others must be considered dangerous.

When a patient's behavior becomes so excited that it threatens the patient's well-being or the safety of others, you must take more aggressive steps to prevent injury. These steps can include either physical or chemical restraint and, at times, both. When evaluating the need for restraint, also consider calling for law enforcement if you have not already contacted them.

Special Populations

Some communities have crisis intervention teams (CIT) staffed by law enforcement officers with specialized training in recognizing and responding to people experiencing a mental health crisis. The primary role of the CIT is to keep patients from revolving through the criminal justice system and the medical facility. As an alternative to this pattern, the program seeks to establish long-term care and other solutions for people with chronic and persistent mental health conditions. These patients might otherwise lack the resources or support to get that help.

People experiencing a psychotic episode often do not comply with treatments, especially medication administration. Such patients often leave before an IV line can be started and a sedative agent administered. They might have the delusion that you are injecting them with something harmful. You should employ nonpharmacologic interventions first, as discussed earlier. Developing trust is an important therapy, but doing so may be difficult to achieve with a patient in an acutely agitated state.

When these methods fail, safely restraining the patient and administering a medication to treat the behavior may be appropriate. If safe administration is possible, then an antianxiety medication such as a benzodiazepine (eg, midazolam) given intranasally, or an antipsychotic medication such as haloperidol given intramuscularly, should help calm the patient. Follow your medical control direction and standing orders when using medications to control behavior.

Delirium

Pathophysiology

Delirium is a condition of impairment in cognitive function that can present with disorientation, hallucinations, or delusions. Symptoms typically begin over hours or a few days and usually, but not always, affect older adults. **Dementia** is a more chronic process that produces severe deficits in memory,

Street Smarts

Patient-Centered Communication

Your personal style of interacting with people (manner of speech, values, beliefs, and ability to listen) is integral to treating patients with psychiatric disorders. It is vital to suspend any judgment of the patient and to provide the patient with a sense of emotional safety. Patients with psychiatric disorders may not know why they feel agitated, tense, depressed, or chaotic and out of control. You must provide a sense of safety in this situation so the patient will trust you and allow you and the other providers to help. Unfortunately, many patients have life experiences that have eroded their sense of the world as a safe place, which means the burden falls on the paramedic to go the extra mile.

To help establish trust with the patient, use several techniques, including maintaining cultural sensitivity. Psychiatric disorders are viewed differently across cultures, and norms of interpersonal space and eye contact vary widely. Be sensitive to these differences. In addition, extend respect to earn the patient's trust. Most patients recognize when you approach them with genuine compassion. In contrast, if your first thought is "This patient is an irresponsible jerk," chances are the patient has just as quickly decided that you are insincere and cannot be of help. Regardless of their appearance or demeanor, approach each patient as a fellow human in the grip of something they cannot escape without assistance.

When an individual has a psychiatric disorder, acknowledge their distress. Identify with the patient's internal struggle. Convey the message that while you do not feel what the patient is feeling, you do understand that they feel that way (eg, "That must be very frustrating," "Let's talk more about that"). Listen actively, and respond rather than react. Focus on what the patient is saying and respond by paraphrasing their words and emotions. The goal is to make sure the patient feels understood. Keep at it, clarifying where necessary.

Above all, do not offer solutions and give advice. You might be tempted to jump ahead with answers or options before the patient is ready to hear them, but resist this urge. Active listening does not mean probing or bombarding the patient with questions that are answered with a simple "yes" or "no." It does not mean offering false reassurance ("This will all work out fine"). It does not mean identifying with the patient with inappropriate self-disclosure ("I can relate to your situation. I just argued with my spouse yesterday"). Instead, active listening means understanding the patient, engaging them in the treatment process, exploring the problem, acknowledging their feelings (particularly as a way of defusing negative feelings), and even responding to delusions and hallucinations.

Take these steps to promote active listening:[10]

- Sit upright and face the patient.
- Lean slightly forward toward the patient.
- Maintain an open posture (arms and legs uncrossed).
- Make comfortable, nonstaring eye contact.
- Relax.
- Be attentive.
- Nod and encourage the patient (eg, "Go on").
- Avoid interruptions.

abstract thinking, and judgment. There are three main types of delirium:

- Hyperactive delirium involves periods of agitation and restlessness.
- Hypoactive delirium, associated with inactivity, may occur in individuals taking CNS depressants or who have fever or liver or kidney failure.
- Mixed delirium is characterized by hyperactive and hypoactive delirium.

Hyperactive delirium is often treated with haloperidol. Delirium symptoms that begin suddenly should prompt a search for reversible causes such as hypoglycemia, hypoxia, sepsis, thiamine deficiency, and medication overdose.

Although patients experiencing delirium are generally not dangerous, they may strike out irrationally if they exhibit agitation, a behavior characterized by restless and irregular physical activity. Therefore, one of the most important factors to consider in these situations is your safety. People experiencing delirium may become agitated and violent when stressors overwhelm them. The result is similar to that in a patient who is experiencing an acute psychotic state.

Excited delirium is a term used to describe a potentially fatal state of extreme agitation and delirium.[11] Clinical features of excited delirium include an acute onset of agitation, aggressiveness, tolerance to significant pain, inappropriate clothing for the environment (which may reflect the patient's hyperthermia), acute psychotic behavior, bizarre behaviors, noncompliance with instructions from law enforcement or medical personnel, profuse sweating, incoherent speech, superhuman strength, hyperactivity, respiratory arrest, and death. Autopsy studies have not revealed findings that uniquely indicate a diagnosis of excited delirium; further, intoxicant levels tend to be at a recreational level rather than a fatally toxic level. As such, the diagnosis is one of exclusion.[11] Conditions that may be associated with, or mimic, excited delirium include hypoglycemia, thyroid storm, some types of seizures, head injury, or cocaine, hallucinogen, or methamphetamine intoxication.

Controversies

The primary characteristics that define excited delirium (ie, agitation and delirium) increase the likelihood that law enforcement, medical, and institutional personnel will use physical force, possibly including pharmacologic interventions, when responding to the person.[11] Use of forceful restraint can cause death from positional or compressive asphyxia, and administration of sedative-hypnotic and dissociative drugs in a person whose medication history may be completely unknown is a dangerous, potentially fatal, practice. The American Medical Association (AMA) released a statement to address the concern that law enforcement and other responders are unnecessarily employing dangerous methods when responding to individuals presenting with a behavioral emergency. Following a special meeting of its House of Delegates in 2021, the AMA adopted a policy opposing the use of *excited delirium* as a medical diagnosis until a clear set of diagnostic criteria has been established.[12] Further, it reasserts the need for physician-led medical oversight in out-of-hospital situations deemed medical emergencies. The AMA emphasizes the risk posed by sedative-hypnotic and dissociative drugs when given without an adequate understanding of the patient. The AMA's policy is guided by a concern for the violent policing practices born of institutional racism. By calling for an end to the use of the term excited delirium, the AMA hopes to delegitimize a concept that they believe is often used as a "cover-up" for dangerous policing practices that tend to target members of marginalized and minority communities who would be better served by behavioral interventions, such as de-escalation.[11,12]

The term *agitated delirium* is often used synonymously with excited delirium. Although the medical literature uses the same terms and risk factors for both conditions, the term excited delirium is primarily used when cases involve fatalities. Both excited delirium and agitated delirium describe the same premortem patient characteristics, including both nonlethal and lethal cases.[1] Neither of these terms currently appears in the International Classification of Diseases or in the *Diagnostic and Statistical Manual of Mental Disorders, Fifth Edition*, and nearly all of the published research regarding these conditions is limited to retrospective case studies and series.[11]

Assessment

If you can safely approach the patient with delirium, be calm, supportive, and empathetic. Be an active listener by nodding, indicating understanding, and limiting your interruptions of the patient's comments. It is vital to approach the patient slowly and purposefully and to respect the patient's territory. Limit physical contact with the patient as much as possible. Do not leave the patient unattended unless the situation becomes unsafe for you or your partner.

Depending on the level of impairment, you should first try to reorient patients to their surroundings and circumstances. Then, carefully use interviewing techniques to assess the patient's cognitive functioning. Try to indirectly determine the patient's orientation, memory, concentration, and judgment by asking simple questions such as "When did you first begin to notice these feelings?" Through interviewing, try to determine what the patient is thinking. Are the patient's thoughts disorganized? For example, does the patient begin to answer your question and then drift off, only to begin discussing a childhood friend? Is the patient experiencing delusions or hallucinations? Does the patient have any unusual worries or fears?

Perform a thorough assessment, including past medical history and medications, to help differentiate delirium from dementia or identify other causes. Pay particular attention to the patient's ability to communicate clearly, and make notes on the patient's apparent mood. Is the patient anxious, depressed, or joyful under inappropriate circumstances? Is the patient agitated? Pay attention to the patient's appearance, dress, and personal hygiene. If you determine that the patient requires restraint because the person poses a threat to self or others, ensure you have adequate, well-trained personnel available to help you before approaching the patient. If the patient appears to be experiencing an overdose, take all medication bottles or illegal substances with you to the medical facility. Transport the patient to a hospital with psychiatric facilities capable of handling their condition. Whenever possible, refrain from using lights and siren because these sights and sounds may aggravate the patient's condition.

Management

Patients with excited delirium often do not respond to attempts to verbally de-escalate the situation. As a result, law enforcement personnel are often necessary to provide restraint. EMS should be allowed access to the patient as soon as it is safe. An ongoing struggle can increase the patient's temperature, prompt the fight-or-flight response, cause acid–base imbalances, and increase the risk of sudden death.

Identifying the stressor or metabolic condition may help identify possible treatments (eg, reducing fever, administering glucose for hypoglycemia, treating dysrhythmias to improve hypoperfusion). Follow local protocols for treating each condition. Sedation is considered the primary treatment for excited delirium.[13] Options include ketamine, benzodiazepines (eg, midazolam, lorazepam), and antipsychotics (eg, haloperidol, droperidol). Provide cardiac monitoring and advanced airway management when giving any of these medications. Follow local protocols and consult medical control for further direction.

Suicidal Ideation

Pathophysiology

Suicide is any willful act designed to end one's own life. It is the 10th leading overall cause of death in the United States.[14] Suicide is more common among men than women, especially those who are Caucasian and single, widowed, or divorced. In addition, patients with depression are at higher risk of suicide. Alcohol use disorder is another important risk factor. Though many suicide attempts are not reported, it is estimated that more than 1 million people in the United States intentionally harm themselves each year.[15] **TABLE 29-6** summarizes the risk factors for suicide.

TABLE 29-6 Risk Factors for Suicide

• Depression, or sudden improvement in depression	• Expresses suicidal thoughts and concrete plans for carrying them out
• Male sex, age <55 years	• Caucasian
• Single, widowed, or divorced	• Social isolation
• Alcohol or other substance misuse	• Previous suicide attempt(s)
• Recent loss of spouse or significant relationship	• Financial setback or job loss
• Chronic, debilitating illness	• Family history of suicide
• Schizophrenia	

Suicide attempts typically occur when the person feels that close emotional attachments are endangered or when the person has lost someone or something important. The person who is suicidal also may have feelings characteristic of depression: feelings of worthlessness, lack of self-esteem, and a sense of being unable to manage life.

SAFETY

When caring for a patient who is exhibiting or acknowledging suicidal ideation, do not neglect your own safety, or that of others on scene. A patient experiencing this level of distress may also be considering harm to others. Similarly, a suicide attempt may unintentionally place others at risk.

Assessment

Your assessment of *every* patient with depression must include an evaluation of suicide risk. Unfortunately, many paramedics are reluctant to ask a patient directly about suicidal thoughts because they fear putting ideas into the patient's head. Remember, however, that suicide is not an original idea and that a patient with depression will have thought of it. Furthermore, most patients with depression are relieved when you bring up the topic because it gives them "permission" to talk about their suicidal ideas.

You and the patient may find the subject easier to broach using a stepwise approach. For example, you might start by asking, "Have you ever thought that life wasn't worth living?" From there, you may proceed by degrees by asking the following questions:

- Did you ever feel that you would be better off dead?
- Have you ever thought of harming yourself? Do you feel that way now?
- Do you have a plan for going about it? Do you have the things you need to carry out the plan?
- Has anyone in your family ever died by suicide?
- Have you ever tried to kill yourself before?

Patients who have made previous attempts; those who have fashioned detailed, concrete plans for suicide; and those with a history of suicide among close relatives are at higher risk and must be evaluated at a medical facility.

Many patients make last-minute efforts to communicate their suicidal intentions. When a person telephones to threaten suicide, someone should stay on the line until the rescue squad has reached the scene. On arrival, ensure your safety and quickly survey the area for any implements that the patient might use for self-injury and discreetly remove them. Encourage the patient to discuss their feelings. Ask about the patient's suicidal ideas and plans.

Management

Whenever you find a patient with severe depression or you have another reason to suspect that a patient is at risk of suicide, follow these guidelines:

- **Do not leave the patient alone.** The patient's well-being is your responsibility until they are transferred to the care of another medical professional.
- **Collect implements.** Bring any implements of potential self-destruction you may have found at the scene (pill bottles, weapons) to the medical facility.
- **Acknowledge the patient's feelings.** Don't argue with the wish to die, but provide honest reassurance. For example, you might say, "It's not unusual for a person to feel like you do after losing someone close to them. Sometimes it helps to talk about it."
- **Encourage transport.** If the patient refuses transport, then try to get the people who are close to the patient to help the patient cooperate. If the patient continues to resist, then you may need to call for assistance from law enforcement.

When a person has attempted suicide, medical treatment takes priority. The patient who has taken an overdose of sedative or depressant drugs must be managed for possible respiratory depression or circulatory collapse. The patient who has slashed their wrists must be treated to control bleeding and restore circulating volume. Nonetheless, if the patient is still alert, try to establish communication and ask the patient to talk about the situation.

A person who attempts suicide is in enormous distress. One of the most important skills you can acquire is seeing beyond a person's behavior to the underlying distress. For example, when called to treat a person who has attempted suicide, say something to communicate empathy to the patient, such as "Life must have seemed unbearable for you to do something like this. It's time to get some help." Such a statement is also a good reminder to yourself to be compassionate in such situations.

Patterns of Violence, Abuse, and Neglect

Few situations are as complex as dealing with a hostile, angry patient, or a person who has been abused or neglected. You will need a great deal of maturity and experience to understand your own feelings, remain professional and positive, and provide the best possible emergency medical care to all parties.

Abuse and Neglect

Perpetrators of violence and abuse or their targets may themselves have a mental illness that contributes to the situation. As an astute paramedic, you must assess the patient and the environment as well as other involved people. Look for indications of abuse, neglect, or violence. Document your findings so that they can be used to support a legal charge of neglect or abuse. Report your concerns about possible abuse or neglect according to local protocols. In these situations, your priorities are safety and management of acute medical and trauma conditions.

Violence

Anger may be a response to illness. The patient may use aggressive behavior to deal with feelings of helplessness, as if to say, "There's something wrong with me, and you're not doing everything possible to help." You may be tempted to respond with anger, but doing so rarely serves any useful purpose.

You can calm most angry patients by conveying an attitude of confidence that the patient will behave well. You may find it helpful to ask the patient directly about their anger: "Can you explain why you're angry with me?" Giving the patient a chance to talk about these feelings often provides an opportunity to overcome them.

One of the most difficult challenges you will face is a patient who is violent or threatening violence. You must prepare yourself beforehand, both psychologically and tactically, to deal with hostile or violent behavior. An encounter with a violent patient always carries the risk that someone will get hurt, including the patient, a bystander, the paramedics, or all of the above.

Assessing the potential for violence is not just an academic exercise. Most paramedics are exposed to some form of violence during their careers. Such violence can take the form of verbal intimidation, verbal abuse, physical abuse, sexual harassment, or sexual assault. Stay alert for possible violent encounters and take measures to prevent them.

Identifying Situations With the Potential for Violence

Begin your preventive action by psychologically preparing for a possible violent encounter. Be aware of that possibility during your response to every call. Do not rely entirely on the information your dispatcher gives you.

Being psychologically prepared for violence does *not* mean becoming paranoid or treating every patient with distrust. However, it does mean developing a "nose for danger," also known as situational awareness.

Risk Factors for Violence

While providers should ensure their personal safety on all calls, certain warning signs, such as the following, should raise their level of concern for scene violence:

- Situations where alcohol or illicit drugs are being consumed (eg, tavern, party)
- Incidents involving large crowds (eg, political rallies, protest marches, sporting events)
- Incidents in which violence has already occurred (eg, shooting, stabbing, domestic disturbances)

People who are more likely to be violent include those who are intoxicated with alcohol or drugs (especially PCP, lysergic acid diethylamide [LSD], amphetamines, and cocaine), experiencing withdrawal from alcohol or drugs, experiencing psychosis (especially manic and paranoid types), or experiencing delirium from any cause (eg, hypoglycemia, sepsis).

The most important clues to the patient's potential for violence are found in the person's behavior and body language. Look for the following warning signals:

- **Posture:** The patient sits tensely at the edge of the chair or grips at the armrest.
- **Speech:** The patient's speech is loud, critical, threatening, and/or full of profanity.
- **Motor activity:** The patient cannot sit still, paces back and forth or in circles, or is easily startled.
- **Other body language:** The patient displays clenched fists, avoids eye contact, and turns away when spoken to.
- **Your own feelings:** Be mindful of your own "gut" response to the patient. If your instinct tells you that you're in danger, then pay attention!

Treatment of the Violent Patient

After you have concluded, for any reason, that a situation carries a potential for violence, you must act quickly.

Assess the entire situation. Are factors in the surroundings contributing to the escalation of violence (eg, friends who are encouraging the patient's behavior)? Can those factors be removed? Does evidence suggest drug use, alcohol use, or head injury? Can any bystanders give you some background information? For example, did the patient's behavior come on gradually or suddenly? Does the patient have a history of violent behavior? Are there any known medical conditions, such as diabetes?

Observe your surroundings. Make sure you have an escape route. Place yourself between the patient and the door, but do not move behind an agitated patient. Do not turn your back on the patient, even for a moment. Note any furniture or other potential barriers. Scan the area for anything that could be used as a weapon (eg, heavy or sharp objects) if the level of violence escalates.

If a violent patient is armed with a weapon, then don't try to deal with the situation yourself. Back off and notify law enforcement. Make sure that others at the scene are not endangered while you await the arrival of law enforcement.

Even if the patient is unarmed, you should maintain a safe distance. Moving too close to a potentially violent patient is likely to increase the patient's anxiety level. Maintain a safety zone of two arm lengths. If the patient is backing away from you, then you are too close. Let the patient find a comfortable distance. Don't position yourself directly face-to-face with the patient, but rather slightly to the side at a 45° angle, with your escape route unobstructed.

Try verbal interventions first. Anger and aggressive behavior are often responses to illness or feelings of helplessness. Simply talking to the angry person in a calm, sympathetic way may defuse some of the anger. Consider the following guidelines:

- Take a moment to concentrate your own thoughts so that you can convey an impression of calmness and self-control to the patient.
- Identify yourself as a medical professional who is there to help. Keep your voice low, a technique that forces the patient to stop and focus on what you are saying.
- Acknowledge the patient's behavior, and restate your willingness to help. ("You look upset. How can we help you?")
- Encourage the patient to talk about what is bothering them. Listen to what is said, and show that you are listening by paraphrasing the words back to the patient. ("I think I understand. Are you saying that . . .?")
- Ask the patient specifically about any sort of weapon or the possibility of losing control.
- Define your expectations of the patient's behavior. Acknowledge the person's potential to do harm ("You could really hurt someone with that crowbar . . ."), but emphasize to the patient that losing control is not permitted.
- If verbal de-escalation is not working, then back off and get help. ("Sir, I think we need to take a break to see if you can get hold of yourself, but I'm not leaving. We'll try talking again in a few minutes. If that doesn't work, then I'm going to have some people with me to keep you from hurting anyone.")

Specific Psychiatric Disorders

As a paramedic, you will not diagnose the following disorders, but you should be familiar with them as possible causes of acute psychosis or excited delirium. Assessment and treatment of patients with these conditions follow the general principles discussed earlier in this chapter.

Mood Disorders

Mood disorders, formally known as affective disorders, are among the most common psychiatric disorders. Approximately 20% of the US population will experience a mood disorder, such as a **manic-depressive illness** or major depression, at some point in their lives.[16] As many as 45% of these disorders are classified as severe.[16]

Although feelings such as depression and joy are universal, mood disorders differ from normal bouts of sadness or happiness. In these disorders, the changes in affect are accompanied by other symptoms, and the net effect is to cause a major disturbance in the person's ability to function. Patients who experience either depression or mania have a unipolar mood disorder. That is, their mood remains at only one pole of the depression–mania continuum. In contrast, patients who alternate between mania and depression (both poles of the continuum) have **bipolar mood disorder**. Most patients with a unipolar mood disorder have depression. Unipolar mania is relatively rare.

Manic Behavior

Mania is one of the most striking psychiatric conditions. A patient with mania is unlikely to believe that anything is wrong, so it is typically a bystander or family member who calls for EMS assistance. In fact, the patient with mania is apt to report being "on top of the world—I've never felt better in my life." People experiencing mania typically have an exaggerated perception of happiness, joy, or euphoria, with hyperactivity and insomnia.

Patients with mania are typically awake and alert but are easily distracted. They are also often markedly hyperactive and may report being unable to concentrate. Almost all patients with mania report a significantly decreased need for sleep, and they may go for days without sleeping.

In conversation, people experiencing mania are talkative, and demonstrate pressured and rapid speech. Flight of ideas (rapid shifting of thoughts) and delusions of grandeur (inflated belief about one's own fame, wealth, power, or intelligence) make it difficult for them to focus on one thing. Patients may report that their thoughts are racing. Their monologues may demonstrate **tangential thinking**, which is characterized by skipping rapidly from one topic to another. (Tangential thinking differs from circumstantial thinking, which refers to including many irrelevant details.) Their ideas are often grandiose. For example, they may have unrealistic plans to embark on a large business venture or to run for high public office. Patients may also believe that they have special powers or are famous and wealthy.

The memory of a patient with mania is usually intact but may be distorted by underlying delusions. The affect is elated (the hallmark of mania). The patient seems to be on a "high," and is unusually and infectiously cheerful. The good cheer may be fragile, however, and the person may quickly become irritable, sarcastic, and hostile with little provocation. A person having an acute manic episode may also show psychotic symptoms such as hallucinations.

People experiencing acute manic episodes often get themselves into trouble of one sort or another. For example, they may go on wild spending sprees, make foolish business investments, drive recklessly, commit sexual indiscretions, or pick fights. Generally, EMS responders are summoned when the person has gotten into some sort of trouble, or when the behavior has become intolerably disruptive.

Because patients with mania are unlikely to consider themselves ill, they may not agree that they need treatment. When dealing with such a patient, be calm, firm, and patient. Don't argue or get into a power struggle. Minimize external stimulation. Talk to the patient in a quiet place, away from other people. Meanwhile, have your partner obtain the medical history separately from relatives or bystanders. When you transport the patient, do not use sirens.

If the patient refuses transport, then consult medical control. Obtain assistance from law enforcement for transport if your medical director indicates that medical facility evaluation is necessary.

Depression

In 2019, an estimated 19.4 million adults age 18 years or older in the United States reported that they had experienced at least one major depressive episode in the past year.[17] That number represents 7.8% of all adults in the United States.[17] Patients with depression are often readily identified by a sad expression, bouts of crying, and listless or apathetic behavior. They express feelings of worthlessness, guilt, and pessimism. These patients may want to be left alone, asserting that no one understands or cares about them and that their problems are hopeless.

Depression may occur in episodes that have a sudden onset and limited duration. This finding is common in major depressive disorder, in which the patient feels substantial suffering and pain that interfere with social or occupational functioning. In other patients, depression may be subtle in onset and chronic in nature. When a person experiences signs and symptoms of depression for most days over at least 2 years, they may have a chronic form of depression known as dysthymic disorder. The signs and symptoms of dysthymic disorder cause social and occupational distress but rarely require hospitalization unless the person becomes suicidal.

The diagnostic features of depression are most easily remembered by the mnemonic GAS PIPES:

- **Guilt and self-reproach are characteristic features of depression.** One way to explore the patient's guilt feelings is to ask a question such as "Are you down on yourself?" or "Do you ever feel as if you're worthless?"
- **Appetite is abnormal in depression.** Usually it is decreased, but a minority of patients with depression may report increased appetite.
- **Sleep disturbance usually takes the form of insomnia.** The typical patient with depression reports waking up at 0300 or 0400 hours and being unable to get back to sleep.

- **Paying attention.** The patient with depression has an impaired ability to concentrate. The impairment is sometimes severe. Ask the patient, "When you're reading a book or a newspaper, can you get all the way through what you're reading, or does your mind start to wander after a couple of minutes?"
- **Interest.** The patient with depression loses interest in things that were once important. The patient can no longer summon enthusiasm for work or hobbies. You might ask, "Are you a [local team name] fan?" If the answer is yes, then ask, "How are they doing this season?" The patient will tell you, "Well, I haven't really been following them lately."
- **Psychomotor abnormalities.** In the patient with depression, psychomotor abilities can be either increased (from agitation) or slowed. Although many patients seem to do everything in slow motion, a significant percentage of patients with depression show agitated behavior, such as pacing, wringing their hands, or picking at themselves.
- **Energy.** People with depression have no energy. They are tired all the time and don't feel like doing anything.
- **Suicidal thoughts.** Most worrisome, people with depression tend to have pervasive and recurrent thoughts of suicide.

Schizophrenia

Schizophrenia is a complex disorder that is neither easily defined nor readily treated, yet dramatically affects society. Precise schizophrenia prevalence numbers are difficult to obtain because of medical and data collection factors, but schizophrenia and related disorders are estimated to affect between 0.25% and 0.64% of the US population.[18] Globally, prevalence estimates range from 0.3% to 0.75%.[18] The typical onset occurs during early adulthood, with dysfunctional symptoms becoming more prominent over time.

Some people diagnosed with schizophrenia display signs during early childhood. Their disease may be associated with brain damage sustained early in life. Other influences thought to contribute to this disorder include genetics, neurobiologic influences, and psychological and social influences.

People with schizophrenia may experience delusions, hallucinations, apathy, mutism, a flat affect, a lack of interest in pleasure, erratic speech, overly emotional responses, and extreme motor behavior (either a lack of motor behavior or excessive motor behavior).

Neurotic Disorders

Neurotic disorders are a collection of psychiatric disorders without psychotic symptoms and lacking

YOU are the Paramedic

PART 4

The patient appears to have tolerated having his vital signs taken, but he continues to glance nervously at the law enforcement personnel outside his apartment. You explain to the patient that you can help him by transporting him to the medical facility, where he can obtain safe medication and treatment. You explain that he needs to continue taking his medication to treat his illness. You offer to drive him in the ambulance where he'll be safe. He appears to consider this option but remains apprehensive.

The patient becomes more agitated and refuses transport to the medical facility. He tells you that it's dangerous for him to leave his apartment. The officers express concern about allowing him to refuse transport because of the potential for harm to himself or others should his condition worsen.

You consider your options and contact medical control for recommendations. The physician orders administration of haloperidol (Haldol) 5 mg IM. You are concerned about how the patient may react to this decision, but you explain to the patient that the physician at the medical facility feels he should be evaluated and treated for his condition and has ordered some medications to help him relax.

7. What are your considerations and concerns about administering this medication to an uncooperative patient?

8. What are some legal implications of taking this patient to the medical facility without his consent?

the intense psychopathology of other mood disorders. These disorders cause many problems for people, their families, and society in general. Treating neurotic disorders carries a large price; however, the cost to society of not treating these disorders (in terms of lost production and lost efficiency) is probably higher.

The neurotic category of conditions includes **anxiety disorders**, mental disorders in which the dominant moods are fear and apprehension. Everyone experiences anxiety occasionally, and a certain amount of anxiety helps people adapt constructively to stress. Patients with anxiety disorders, however, experience persistent, incapacitating anxiety in the absence of external threat. In the United States, the prevalence of adults with any anxiety disorder in the last 12 months is 19.1%.[19] Several types of anxiety disorders, including generalized anxiety disorder, phobias, and panic disorder, are likely to elicit a call for EMS assistance or affect your delivery of prehospital care.

Generalized Anxiety Disorder

Although some anxiety in everyday life is normal, when a person worries about everything for no particular reason, or if that worrying is unproductive and the person cannot decide what to do about an upcoming situation, the person may be experiencing **generalized anxiety disorder (GAD)**. For a person to be diagnosed with GAD, symptoms (anxiety and worry) must be present more days than not for at least 6 months, and the worry must be difficult to turn off or control. GAD is one of the most common anxiety disorders. Patients experiencing GAD may not require treatment until their symptoms prevent them from carrying out ADLs. Treatment often involves both pharmacologic agents and counseling. The acute symptoms of anxiety and worry can become overwhelming in GAD, prompting a family member or coworker to call for EMS assistance.

When caring for a patient with GAD, identify yourself in a calm, confident manner. Listen attentively to the patient and talk with the person generally about their feelings.

Phobias

Phobic disorders are an unreasonable fear, apprehension, or dread of a specific situation or thing. The patient with a **simple phobia** focuses all anxieties onto one class of objects (eg, mice, spiders, dogs) or situations (eg, high places, darkness, flying). Research suggests that approximately 7% of Americans are affected by social anxiety disorder or social phobia.[20] People with social phobias fear everyday social situations, such as going to parties, meeting new people, speaking, or eating in public.

When confronted with the feared object or situation, the person with a phobia experiences intolerable anxiety and all of the autonomic symptoms that anxiety brings. The patient usually recognizes that the fear is unreasonable but cannot do anything about it.

When you are caring for a patient with a phobia, explain each step of treatment in detail before you carry it out **FIGURE 29-6**: "First we'll give you oxygen to help you breathe. Then we're going to move you onto the stretcher, so that we can carry you downstairs."

Panic Disorder

Panic disorder is characterized by sudden, usually unexpected, and overwhelming feelings of fear and

Street Smarts

GAD can present with serious symptoms (eg, dyspnea, chest pain) promping a call for EMS. Such symptoms should not be dismissed as passing "flare-ups" of the person's GAD. Nor should a patient's history of GAD cause providers to overlook other causes for such symptoms.

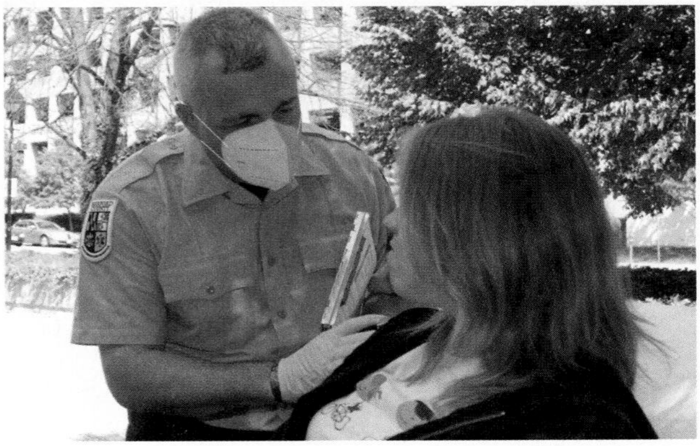

FIGURE 29-6 When caring for a patient with a phobia, explain each step of treatment in detail before carrying it out.

dread, accompanied by various other symptoms produced by a massive activation of the autonomic nervous system. Women are more likely to be affected by this condition than are men.[21]

The attacks usually begin between 20 and 29 years of age. Most affected people can identify a stressful event that preceded their first attack, such as an illness or loss of a loved one. Thereafter, the attacks may come "out of the blue," without any apparent precipitating stressor. If allowed to continue, panic attacks may severely limit the patient's lifestyle. The person becomes afraid to go to work, to go shopping, or to leave the house at all, out of fear that an attack will occur away from home. The fear of going into public places is called **agoraphobia** (literally, "fear of the marketplace").

The classic signs and symptoms of panic disorder are summarized in **TABLE 29-7**. A large percentage of these signs and symptoms, such as palpitations and sweating, result from autonomic nervous system discharge, while some others (eg, chest discomfort, paresthesias) reflect hyperventilation. The symptoms usually peak in intensity within about 10 minutes and last about an hour.

By the time you arrive at the scene, the patient having a panic attack may be surrounded by many anxious and excited people, who may themselves contribute to the problem. Accordingly, you must take the following steps to control the situation quickly:

- **Separate the patient from panicky bystanders.** However, if you can find a calm friend or member of the patient's family, having this person present may be helpful.
- **Create a calm environment.** The environment should be as calm as possible as you transport the patient to the medical facility.
- **Tolerate the patient's disability.** The patient having an anxiety attack may not cooperate or answer questions at first because of intense fear and distress. Your manner must convey that everything is under control.
- **Provide reassurance of the patient's safety.** The word *safe* can often reduce symptoms to a more manageable level: "We're going to take you down these stairs on the stretcher. It's going to be okay. We'll go slowly and be careful to keep you safe while we move you."
- **Give the patient's symptoms a name.** After you have checked the patient's vital signs and the ECG, reassure the patient that there is no immediate danger of dying: "I know that the sense of panic you're feeling is distressing, but it's not life-threatening."
- **Help the patient regain control.** Encourage the patient to do things to the extent possible, so as to help regain a sense of control.

A panic attack may mimic a range of physical disorders in its presentation. Conversely, anxiety symptoms may be the presenting complaint in medical conditions such as cardiac dysrhythmias, withdrawal states, anaphylaxis, hyperthyroidism, and certain tumors. Therefore, any patient experiencing a panic attack, especially a first-time panic attack, should be fully evaluated in a medical facility.

TABLE 29-7 Signs and Symptoms of a Panic Attack

• Shortness of breath or a sensation of being smothered • Palpitations or tachycardia • Sweating • Nausea or abdominal distress • Chills or hot flashes • Fear of dying • Feelings of unreality or of being detached from oneself	• Feeling dizzy, unsteady, light-headed, or faint • Trembling or shaking • Feeling of choking • Paresthesias • Chest pain or discomfort • Fear of losing control or going crazy

Data from: American Psychiatric Association. *Diagnostic and Statistical Manual of Mental Disorders.* 5th ed. Washington, DC: American Psychiatric Association; 2013.

Words of Wisdom

A patient who is hyperventilating should not be treated with "paper bag therapy." Use of a paper bag when breathing can cause serious complications or even death from hypoxemia in patients whose anxiety results from an unsuspected pulmonary embolism or cardiac problem. You can best manage hyperventilation by coaching patients to slow their breathing until they regain control.

Substance-Related Disorders and Addictive Behavior

Disorders of substance use, addiction, and personal control generally evolve over a relatively long time. Because of the chronic nature of these problems, EMS typically will be called when an underlying problem becomes acutely exacerbated. For example, a patient with bulimia may experience electrolyte imbalances that produce a sudden onset of weakness, dizziness, cardiac or respiratory problems, or seizures, or a patient with alcoholism may experience respiratory depression from binge drinking. Emergency medical care for these patients typically focuses on treating symptomatic complaints and the presenting signs and symptoms.

Substance-Related Disorders

Substance-related disorders include psychological disorders associated with the use of alcohol, tobacco, illicit drugs, and other substances that change the way a person feels, behaves, or thinks. These disorders cost thousands of lives and billions of dollars annually.[22–24] An estimated 20.8% of the US population used illicit drugs in 2019.[17]

Substance-related disorders are grouped into four levels:

- In **substance use**, a person may use moderate amounts of a substance without seriously affecting their ADLs (eg, a social drinker).
- **Substance intoxication** describes use of a substance that results in impaired thinking and motor function (eg, a drunk driver).
- **Substance use disorder** describes use of a substance that disrupts ADLs (eg, a person has difficulty with work, school, or relationships).
- **Substance dependence** describes an addiction to a substance. The person is physiologically dependent and requires increasingly larger amounts to produce the same effect. A person with a substance dependence may display drug-seeking behaviors, such as repeated use of the substance, taking desperate measures to ingest more of the substance, stealing money, or standing out in the cold to smoke a cigarette.

Determining the most effective treatment for substance-related disorders requires an integrative approach that accounts for the social, biologic, cultural, cognitive, and psychological dimensions of the problem. As a paramedic, you may be unable to explore all these areas during a short transport to the medical facility, particularly because much of your time will be devoted to ensuring the safety of your crew and managing the patient's ABCs. Understanding the complex nature of substance-related disorders is your first step in providing professional, competent, and compassionate care to all affected people.

Eating Disorders

The reported incidence of eating disorders began to increase rapidly in the 1950s and 1960s. Today, eating disorders are common in the developed world and are emerging as a problem in developing countries. Some countries are experiencing a fourfold increase in eating disorders.[25] The people most likely to be affected by these disorders are women between the ages of 12 and 25 years.[26]

The two major types of eating disorders are **bulimia nervosa** and **anorexia nervosa**. In both forms, severe electrolyte imbalances may occur, leading to cardiac conditions, seizures, and renal failure, as well as erosion of dental enamel and salivary gland enlargement. Anxiety, depression, and substance use disorders are also often present in patients diagnosed with eating disorders.[27]

Bulimia nervosa is characterized by consumption of large amounts of food, typically more junk food than fruits and vegetables. Many people with this disorder describe their eating as "out of control." Most patients compensate for the binge eating by purging through vomiting, laxatives, diuretics, or excessive exercise. Individuals with bulimia may feel humiliated by both the problem and the lack of control.

People with anorexia differ from those with bulimia in one important way: They lose so much weight that they jeopardize their health and even their lives. They may even binge, albeit on smaller quantities of food. People with anorexia lose weight by exerting extraordinary control over their food consumption. The typical person with anorexia has a low body weight for age and height, and demonstrates an intense fear of obesity despite being underweight. If the person with an eating disorder is a woman of child-bearing age, then she may experience amenorrhea (the absence of menstruation).

Somatoform Disorders

People who are overly concerned with their physical health and appearance may have a **somatoform disorder** if that preoccupation dominates their lives. Hypochondriasis is the classic example of a somatoform disorder. In hypochondriasis, patients have extreme anxiety or fear that they may have a serious disease. They are so convinced that they are ill that even a physician will be unable to convince them otherwise. Although the main problem in hypochondriasis is anxiety, the person is preoccupied with other imagined symptoms. With somatization disorder, patients also have multiple complaints, but they are more concerned with the symptoms than with their meaning.

In conversion disorders, a physical condition (eg, paralysis, blindness, or seizures) has no identifiable pathophysiology but results from malingering or faking a physical disorder.

Factitious Disorders

A **factitious disorder**, also called Münchausen syndrome, is a condition in which a person intentionally produces or feigns physical or psychological signs or symptoms. In such cases, the patient wishes to be sick. Patients can have various motives for such behavior, such as avoiding legal responsibility or gaining attention. The symptoms the patient is experiencing are under voluntary control, and no obvious physiologic cause of the symptoms is present.

The symptoms the patient experiences may be physical, psychological, or both; are usually dramatic; and indicate an immediate need for medical care. Patients will typically present at night or on weekends in hopes of finding less skilled health care providers or of preventing their insurance or medical records from being found.

One type of factitious disorder is factitious disorder by proxy, also called Münchausen syndrome by proxy. In this condition, a parent or caregiver intentionally makes a child sick to garner attention

YOU are the Paramedic

PART 5

The patient attempts to rise and move past you as you prepare the medication. Your partner has already explained the medication that has been ordered to the law enforcement personnel. The officers quickly move to restrain the patient to the chair. They continue to secure him while you administer the medication to a site on the rectus femoris muscle through his slacks.

You expect to see changes in the patient within 10 minutes, so the officers continue to restrain the patient to the chair while your partner prepares the stretcher and you obtain another set of vital signs, including a blood glucose level. You continue to tell the patient what is happening, and you collect his medications and identification. The patient has become much more relaxed and is secured to the stretcher.

You and your partner move the patient to the ambulance with the assistance of two officers. During transport, you reassess the patient's vital signs every 5 minutes, watching for adverse effects from the medication. On arrival, you give your report to the receiving nurse and place the patient in the psychiatric treatment area of the ED. You complete your patient care report, understanding the importance of good documentation for the patient with a behavioral emergency.

Recording Time:	20 Minutes
Respirations	14 breaths/min
Pulse	88 beats/min
Skin	Warm, dry, and color typical for baseline
Blood pressure	118/78 mm Hg
Oxygen saturation (Spo_2)	98% on room air
Pupils	PERRLA
Blood glucose level	96 mg/dL

9. Why must you check blood glucose levels in a patient with a behavioral emergency?

10. What is the most common adverse effect of haloperidol, and how do you treat it?

11. What are some important elements of documentation for a patient having a behavioral emergency that you should include in your report?

and pity. This condition is considered an atypical form of child abuse.

Impulse Control Disorders

People who have **impulse control disorders** lack the ability to resist a temptation or cannot avoid acting on a drive. Examples of impulse control disorders include intermittent explosive disorder, kleptomania, pyromania, and pathologic gambling.

Of course, not every arsonist has pyromania, and not everyone who steals has kleptomania. Impulse control disorders are typically associated with other disorders, such as depression, antisocial or borderline personality disorders, and Alzheimer disease. This group of disorders is rare.

Treatment of impulse control disorders at a medical facility relies on cognitive and behavioral interventions to identify underlying triggers and influences.

Personality Disorders

According to the American Psychiatric Association, **personality disorders** are described as "a way of thinking, feeling, and behaving that deviates from the expectations of the culture, causes distress or problems functioning, and lasts over time."[28] Common definitions of personality include an individual's distinctive character. How people think or behave in the world and with others may be suspicious, outgoing, fearful, or overly dramatic. When these ways of relating to others become dysfunctional or cause distress to other people, the person is considered to have a personality disorder.

True personality disorders are rare in the general population. When a person does have a personality disorder, another psychiatric illness is also likely to be present at the same time. Such patients tend to do poorly during treatment. For example, patients who are depressed in addition to having a personality disorder usually have more difficulty managing the depression compared with patients who do not have a personality disorder.

You may have difficulty treating patients with personality disorders because of your limited interactions with these patients. Nevertheless, you must understand these abnormal behaviors so that you can respond appropriately when you encounter them. For example, a patient with an antisocial personality will not hesitate to hurt you if agitated, and a patient with a histrionic personality may be demanding and dictate the level of emergency medical care. Be calm and professional in your interactions with patients exhibiting these traits.

> **Words of Wisdom**
>
> Psychotropic medications target the autonomic nervous system by either inhibiting or stimulating the sympathetic or parasympathetic nervous systems. You must thoroughly understand these two systems and know how the medications in your paramedic's kit might interact with psychotropic medications.

Medications for Psychiatric Disorders and Behavioral Emergencies

Patients with psychiatric emergencies may take several types of **psychotropic medications**, which affect mood, thought, or behavior. During your assessment, identify the medications that have been prescribed to the patient and determine whether the patient is actually taking them.

Refer to Chapter 28, *Toxicology*, for coverage of psychiatric medications as well as other psychiatric-related topics such as substance use disorders, street drugs, and withdrawal symptoms.

Psychiatric Medication Types

Antidepressants

Antidepressants are prescribed to combat the symptoms of depressive illness. The main types of antidepressants are selective serotonin reuptake inhibitors (SSRIs), serotonin-norepinephrine reuptake inhibitors (SNRIs), tricyclic antidepressants (TCAs), and monoamine oxidase inhibitors (MAOIs), which are discussed in Chapter 15, *Emergency Medications*. Most antidepressants work by altering levels of neurotransmitters (eg, serotonin, norepinephrine, or dopamine) in the autonomic nervous system.

The most commonly prescribed antidepressant in the United States is citalopram (Celexa), an SSRI.[29] Other SSRIs include fluoxetine, sertraline, and paroxetine. SSRIs are primarily used to treat major depressive episodes but are also useful in anxiety disorders, including GAD, panic disorder, and obsessive-compulsive disorder.

Heterocyclic (tricyclic and tetracyclic) antidepressants are a group of medications, some in use since the 1950s, that have been primarily used for major depression but also may be effective for panic disorder, agoraphobia, obsessive-compulsive disorder, enuresis, and school phobia. Examples include amitriptyline, desipramine, imipramine, and nortriptyline. Heterocyclic antidepressants are not often prescribed today because of their potentially serious adverse effects.

A third class of antidepressant, MAOIs, are recommended for atypical major depressive episodes. MAOIs also are sometimes useful in selected cases of heterocyclic-refractory major depression and panic disorder.

Benzodiazepines

Benzodiazepines are not a substitute for more formal therapy, but a physician may prescribe benzodiazepines for a person experiencing severe emotional distress, even if the patient does not have psychosis or is not an imminent threat to self or others. Short-term medication therapy may help the anxious patient experiencing crisis or acute panic reactions.

Other uses of benzodiazepines include muscle relaxation; control of seizures; and treatment of alcohol, sedative, or hypnotic withdrawal.

Antipsychotics

Antipsychotic medications were introduced in the 1950s to treat mental health illnesses such as schizophrenia and other psychoses. They revolutionized the management of these types of disorders through their effect on the patient's neurologic function, which led to the name *neuroleptics.* These older medications, which are called typical antipsychotic drugs, are still in use today, but are known to have varying degrees of adverse effects. Newer antipsychotic medications, known as atypical antipsychotic (AAP) drugs, are associated with less risk of adverse effects and are more effective at treating the cognitive dysfunction associated with psychoses. The pharmacokinetics of all antipsychotic medications are similar. **TABLE 29-8** lists antipsychotic medications.

TABLE 29-8 Antipsychotic Medications

Type	Generic Name	Trade Name
Atypical antipsychotic agents	Aripiprazole	Abilify
	Clozapine	Clozaril
	Olanzapine	Zyprexa
	Quetiapine	Seroquel
	Risperidone	Risperdal
	Ziprasidone	Geodon
Traditional (typical) antipsychotic agents	Chlorpromazine	Thorazine
	Chlorprothixene	Taractan
	Fluphenazine	Prolixin, Permitil
	Haloperidol	Haldol
	Loxapine	Loxitane, Daxolin
	Mesoridazine	Serentil
	Molindone	Moban
	Perphenazine	Trilafon
	Thioridazine	Mellaril
	Thiothixene	Navane
	Trifluoperazine	Stelazine

The AAP agents often are used as first-line therapy because they not only relieve symptoms such as delusions and hallucinations, but also improve the patient's quality of life by reducing the affective symptoms of anxiety and depression and reducing suicidal tendencies. However, the AAP medications may cause adverse metabolic effects such as glucose deregulation, hypercholesterolemia, and hypertension.

The cardiovascular effects of both typical and atypical antipsychotics depend on the specific medication. These agents directly affect the heart and blood vessels, but also act indirectly through CNS and autonomic reflexes to produce other cardiovascular changes. The results can range from simple orthostatic hypotension to conditions as complex as ECG changes.

A subcategory of traditional antipsychotics, known as phenothiazines, may reduce contractility of the heart. Haloperidol, which is commonly used in paramedicine for treatment of acute psychosis, is a member of this class. ECG changes seen with phenothiazines may include prolongation of the QT and PR intervals, blunting of T waves, and depression of the ST segment.

Patients taking antipsychotic agents may occasionally experience an **acute dystonic reaction** in which the patient develops muscle spasms of the neck, face, and back within a few days of starting treatment with the medication. You can rapidly correct an acute dystonic reaction by giving IV diphenhydramine (Benadryl), 25 to 50 mg. However, the muscle spasms are likely to recur after the diphenhydramine wears off.

Typical antipsychotic medications also have **atropine-like effects** (anticholinergic effects). Thus, patients taking antipsychotic medications may experience the adverse effects associated with atropine use, such as dry mouth, blurred vision, urinary retention, and cardiac dysrhythmias.

Amphetamines

Amphetamines are powerful CNS and parasympathetic nervous system (PNS) stimulants similar to other sympathomimetic medications (eg, epinephrine). Amphetamines (eg, Adderall) are prescribed as treatments for attention-deficit disorder with hyperactivity in both adults and children. In addition, they are used to treat narcolepsy in adults. These medications raise both systolic and diastolic blood pressure while often slowing the pulse rate. Cardiac dysrhythmias may occur with large doses. The psychological effects depend on the dose, the patient's mental state, and the patient's personality, but may include alertness, reduced sense of fatigue, elevated mood, increased concentration, euphoria, and increased motor and speech activities.

Problems Associated With Medication Noncompliance

Most psychotropic medications are designed to alter a patient's mental state, most often to sedate or calm the patient. Dulling of the senses and slowing of thinking are common reasons why patients choose not to comply with these medications (ie, not stay on their medications).

Another factor in **medication noncompliance** may be the cost of the medications. For example, patients who have been prescribed amphetamines but who cannot afford them or do not have health insurance may consume energy drinks with high doses of caffeine or herbal supplements containing ephedra (ma huang) to compensate. This medication noncompliance often results in conflict with others when the patient exhibits abnormal behaviors.

Changes in behavior are not always a result of a substance use disorder. Behavior changes may also result from noncompliance with medications prescribed and dispensed to treat mental health symptoms.

Noncompliance with medications combined with substance misuse increases the risk that a person with a severe mental illness will commit a violent act. When obtaining the patient's medication history, always try to identify previously prescribed medications and missed doses.

Emergency Use of Medications

To some degree, every call you handle has a behavioral component in addition to the patient's trauma or medical problem. For example, the businessman having a heart attack may appear calm and collected, but he is still anxious.

If a behavioral crisis, such as an acute psychotic episode, is likely to escalate, the threat to the patient, bystanders, and health care professionals may be too great not to intervene, and emergency use of medications may be indicated. The intensity of the situation, the patient's response to you, and your protocols will determine whether verbal, physical, or chemical intervention is necessary.

Before you decide to administer medications to control the patient's behavior, carry out a complete assessment. Make sure you thoroughly understand the patient's chief complaint, allergies, and medical and medication history. Administration of antipsychotics or benzodiazepines may be beneficial in situations involving aggression, but you must weigh their benefits against the possible risks.

The specific concerns and approaches to managing behavioral or psychiatric emergencies in pediatric and geriatric patients are discussed in Chapter 44, *Pediatric Emergencies*, and Chapter 45, *Geriatric Emergencies*.

The Psychological Effects of War: Returning Combat Veterans

One final topic warrants attention in this chapter. Stressful events such as divorce, failure, rejection, and financial setback are often part of the human experience. These experiences help to shape who we are and what our behavior will be like. In 1980, the third edition of the *Diagnostic and Statistical Manual of Mental Disorders* introduced the concept that traumatic stressful events outside of an individual's control, such as war, torture, sexual assault, natural disasters, airplane crashes, and factory explosions, can lead to trauma of a psychological nature, not just a physical nature.[31]

Military personnel who experienced combat have a high incidence of PTSD. PTSD occurred in as many as 20% of veterans of the Iraq and Afghanistan Wars, 10% of Gulf War veterans, and 30% of Vietnam War veterans.[32,33] Reminders of their experiences in the military, such as news coverage or gatherings of veterans, can also be emotional triggers.

A 2008 study explored the effects of war on service members deployed for Operation Enduring Freedom in Afghanistan and Operation Iraqi Freedom in Iraq.[34] The study results focused on PTSD, major depression, and TBI. These three conditions are important not only because of the high-level policy interest in them, but also because unlike the physical wounds of war, they are often unrecognized and unacknowledged by other service members, family members, and society in general.[34] All three of these conditions affect mood, thoughts, and behavior.[34]

According to the US Department of Veterans Affairs (VA), PTSD can occur after someone goes through a traumatic event such as combat, assault, or disaster.[35] According to data about VA health care utilization from 2002 through 2015, the three most frequent diagnoses among veterans were (1) musculoskeletal ailments (principally joint and back disorders), (2) mental disorders, and (3) symptoms, signs, and ill-defined conditions.[36] On average, 57% of these patient encounters were for mental health disorders, of which PTSD and depressive disorders were number one and two on the list, respectively.[36]

Symptoms of PTSD vary in severity but are usually classified into four categories:[37]

- **Intrusive thoughts**, such as distressing dreams, flashbacks, or nightmares. These thoughts may include a feeling of reliving the experience.
- **Avoiding reminders** of the event, including people, places, objects, situations, etc. The patient may refuse to talk about the event or feelings related to it.
- **Negative thoughts and feelings**, such as fear, anger, guilt, and shame, or a feeling of detachment from others.
- **Arousal and reactive symptoms** related to the event that cause problems sleeping or focusing on activities, or even self-destructive behaviors.

People experiencing intense distress will often develop symptoms within days of the event, a condition known as *acute stress disorder*. The diagnosis of acute stress disorder is made within the first month of the appearance of symptoms.[38] The symptoms differ from those of PTSD in that they are dissociative symptoms, such as amnesia, depersonalization, or a feeling of emotional numbness.[38] Acute stress disorder is considered a precursor to PTSD; if symptoms continue beyond 1 month, further evaluation may lead to a diagnosis of PTSD.[38]

Street Smarts

PTSD affects those working in EMS, fire services, and law enforcement agencies. In a 2016 report published by the National Association of EMTs, *National Survey on EMS Mental Health Services*, most EMS providers surveyed felt personally affected by mental health issues.[30] Take care of yourself and watch for signs of depression and other mental illnesses in your coworkers. As EMS providers, we need to take care of each other. Helpful resources on this subject include EMS Strong (www.emsstrong.org) and the Code Green Campaign (codegreencampaign.org).

Words of Wisdom

A hope box is a small container physically kept with a person. It may be a shoe box, envelope, or plastic bag that holds meaningful pictures, quotes, or mementos of happy times and pleasant memories. Hope boxes are used to provide encouragement and hope when a veteran is feeling anxious or stressed. They may provide distraction from more negative behaviors.

A hope box application is also available for smartphones. Like a physical hope box, a virtual hope box can assist the patient in shifting distressing thoughts or behaviors. Examples of items that can be included in a virtual hope box include videos, sound recordings, photos, or games.

When working with a combat veteran, ask if the patient has a hope box or virtual hope box to bring with them to the hospital. The hope box can be a useful tool when working with this population.[39]

Symptoms of PTSD include feelings of helplessness, anxiety, anger, and fear. People with PTSD may avoid things that remind them of the original trauma, including loud noises or smells, and sometimes they may avoid interactions with other people. This emotional and physical distancing from others can negatively affect the individual's quality of life. Memories of the trauma linger and continue to be disruptive. Symptoms of PTSD may be made worse in the context of other mental health challenges.

The sympathetic nervous system provides the fight-or-flight response to help protect us in situations perceived to be dangerous. This mechanism is not intended to be activated for any longer than it takes to mitigate the threat. People with PTSD, however, experience nervous system arousal that is ongoing and not easily suppressed. Heart rate increases to channel more blood into the heart, lungs, and brain; pupils dilate; and systolic blood pressure increases. Senses are sharpened, and mental acuity is heightened. The patient may be hypervigilant or display an exaggerated startle response to perceived danger.

Symptoms of PTSD can develop within several months of the original event, but their onset may sometimes be delayed even longer. PTSD causes significant problems functioning or the inability to respond normally to everyday situations, which is why you may be called to a situation as a paramedic.

People with PTSD can relive the traumatic event through intrusive thoughts, nightmares, or even flashbacks. Flashbacks are uncontrollable events triggered by a sound, sight, or smell. The patient may experience the same visceral response that occurred during the initial encounter with the stress. These episodes can last for seconds or hours and can occur at any time, even years after the exposure. The person fears the inability to control a flashback and worries that it will present as irrational behavior. Recent traumatic events may also trigger old memories and create a reflex reaction of preparing for the worst. A person who has experienced flashbacks may become preoccupied with the perception of danger. Hypervigilance and trouble sleeping are not unusual.

With dissociative PTSD, the person attempts to find an escape from constant internal distress or a particularly disturbing event. The individual's altered consciousness allows for continued functioning under adverse conditions. Some people may undergo an out-of-body experience; others experience delusions. Other psychological conditions such as personality disorders and increased functional impairment can develop in those individuals with a dissociative subtype of PTSD.

Guilt, shame, paranoia, hostility, and depression are not uncommon in combat veterans. Alcohol and/or drug use often represents an attempt to suppress the sympathetic nervous system's activity and slow down the body. This attempt at anesthesia can quickly become addictive.

Another consideration when caring for combat veterans is their higher incidence of TBI sustained from trauma secondary to the explosion of an improvised explosive device (IED). In some cases, the TBI may go undiagnosed because its manifestations are similar to the symptoms of PTSD or because the patient downplays the symptoms. People with TBI can experience sensory dysfunction, confusion headaches, memory loss, and general disorientation. Memory loss can include retrograde and anterograde amnesia (affecting memories formed before and after the event, respectively).

When treating a combat veteran with PTSD, try to eliminate excess noise. Do not touch or do anything to the veteran without an explanation. Interestingly, diesel fumes can be a trigger for combat veterans, so keep your diesel equipment far enough away that its odors are not noticeable by the patient.

The returning combat veteran is a patient who requires a unique level of understanding, compassion, and specialized attention. These patients experience pain that is emotional as well as physical. Developing military cultural competency is a specific skill that can help you identify the sometimes subtle indicators that a patient is a discharged military member. Military culture, beliefs, and ideals of defending a nation or national identity are influenced by courage, loyalty, sacrifice above self (also known as *selfless service*), and a commitment to society. These beliefs can be a source of strength during stressful situations, but they can also cause distress when a sense of failure or injustice challenges the patient's military values. When you encounter military service members who are experiencing acute medical or behavioral problems, use the same compassion, understanding, and protocols as you would use with civilians, but be cognizant of their cultural background.[40]

YOU are the Paramedic SUMMARY

1. What are the initial components of the assessment for this patient?

Provider safety is essential. Carefully assess the scene for hazards or weapons. Forming your general impression of the scene is important for identifying clues to the patient's condition/behavior. Also form a general impression of the patient, including behavior, personal hygiene, and posture. Visually assess the patient for life threats, such as signs of alteration in breathing, inadequate circulation, or obvious hemorrhage.

2. What are your safety concerns in dealing with this patient?

This patient is exhibiting behaviors suggestive of an acute psychotic episode. He is experiencing delusions and has an altered perception of reality. He is exhibiting signs of risk for violence, such as refusal to allow law enforcement personnel in his apartment, refusal to come out of his apartment, delusions of violence against himself, and low socioeconomic status/potential for history of psychiatric illness based on his residence.

3. What is your initial impression of this patient? What factors, signs, or symptoms would lead you to this conclusion?

The patient appears to be having an acute psychotic episode, possibly related to schizophrenia. He appears agitated, as demonstrated by his pacing. He is exhibiting repetitive behavior by clenching and unclenching his fists. He is having paranoid delusions of people wanting to kill him. His mood appears anxious, and he is wary of strangers.

4. Does this patient need to be evaluated at a medical facility?

This patient needs to be evaluated at a medical facility because he is having an acute episode. Because of his delusions, he may be a threat to himself or others. He may not be competent to refuse treatment and transport in his current condition.

5. What conclusions might you make about medication compliance and the patient's medical history?

Based on the fact that the patient is aware of his illness, states that he sees a physician regularly, and filled his prescription recently, it is likely the patient is normally compliant with his medications. Based on the results seen with medication noncompliance, the patient's current episode of psychotic behavior is probably a result of not taking medications for about a week. Therapeutic levels may have fallen to a degree that this patient's condition has worsened or his behavior has become abnormal.

6. If the patient refuses to be transported, then what options should you, as a paramedic, consider?

Local protocols may address the use of restraint or law enforcement intervention in this situation. Local statutes may require that law enforcement personnel intervene out of concern for the patient and the safety of others based on his condition. Consider the legal implications, including the competence of the patient to make decisions. Medical control is an excellent resource. Medical control may grant orders to apply physical restraints or administer medications for the purposes of chemical restraint.

7. What are your considerations and concerns for administration of this medication to an uncooperative patient?

Benzodiazepines are typically considered to be the safest class of medications for this purpose because of their ability to be administered intranasally. Administering a medication such as IM haloperidol means that you will expose a large needle. If the patient is unrestrained or restrained ineffectively, then you could be harmed during the administration attempt. The patient may view any medication administered as dangerous or a threat to his person. All medications have risks of adverse effects. A potential advantage of this course of action is that you may administer haloperidol through clothing in this type of situation.

8. What are some legal implications of taking this patient to the medical facility without his consent?

The patient may be determined to be competent later, and your actions may constitute a violation of his rights. Adverse outcomes may generate other potential grounds for litigation as well as harm to the patient.

9. Why must you check blood glucose levels in a patient with a behavioral emergency?

You can obtain blood glucose levels easily and thereby rule out a medical disorder such as hypoglycemia as a cause for the abnormal behavior. Patients experiencing psychiatric disturbances may not be maintaining adequate nutrition; hypoglycemia may be present and may contribute to the patient's condition.

YOU are the Paramedic SUMMARY continued

10. What is the most common adverse effect of haloperidol, and how do you treat it?

The most common adverse effect is extrapyramidal symptoms. If such symptoms occur, then you may administer diphenhydramine hydrochloride in a dose of 25 to 50 mg, depending on local protocols. Because of the risk of this adverse effect, and assuming protocols allow diphenhydramine hydrochloride, you should have this medication readily available after you administer haloperidol (Haldol).

11. What are some important elements of documentation for a patient having a behavioral emergency that you should include in your report?

Take extra care and time to complete a thorough patient care report. Document all assessment findings. Be objective in your findings and factual in your statements. Use direct quotes to incorporate any comments the patient makes. Identify all personnel who cared for the patient, including the name of the physician giving any orders. Document all efforts to convince the patient to consent to treatment and/or transport.

EMS Patient Care Report (PCR)

Date: 08-14-22	**Incident No.:** 201035684	**Nature of Call:** Psychiatric emergency	**Location:** 906 Abbott Street, Apt 312

Dispatched: 1528	**En Route:** 1529	**At Scene:** 1535	**Transport:** 1604	**At Hospital:** 1610	**In Service:** 1625

Patient Information

Age: 44 **Sex:** M **Weight (in kg [lb]):** 76.4 kg (168 lb)	**Allergies:** NKDA **Medications:** Mellaril 200 mg twice daily, Serentil 50 mg twice daily **Past Medical History:** Schizophrenia **Chief Complaint:** Paranoid delusions

Vital Signs

Time: 1543	**BP:** 130/84	**Pulse:** 110	**Respirations:** 20	**Spo_2:** 99%
Time: 1555	**BP:** 118/78	**Pulse:** 88	**Respirations:** 14	**Spo_2:** 98%
Time:	**BP:**	**Pulse:**	**Respirations:**	**Spo_2:**

EMS Treatment (circle all that apply)

Oxygen @ ____ L/min via (circle one): **NC NRM Bag-mask device**		**Assisted Ventilation**	**Airway Adjunct**	**CPR**
Defibrillation	**Bleeding Control**	**Bandaging**	**Splinting**	**Other:** 5 mg haloperidol (circled)

Narrative

EMS requested to above location for a man fearing for his life. On arrival, pt found inside apartment, anxious and agitated, pacing in the living area. Multiple officers on scene in the hallway. Pt refused to leave apartment. Pt stating repeatedly, "They're coming for me." EMS allowed into apartment by pt. Pt sat in chair, continuing to clench hands, and appeared restless. Pt reported he has a history of schizophrenia but has not taken his medications for approximately 1 week because he "knows it's poisoned." EMS advised pt of need for transport to medical facility for evaluation and treatment. Pt refused transport. Medical direction contacted. Dr. Jones ordered administration of 5 mg haloperidol IM for agitation and transport to City Memorial Medical Center for further evaluation and treatment. 5 mg haloperidol IM was given as ordered. Pt placed on stretcher and loaded into ambulance for nonemergent transport. Blood glucose level was 96 mg/dL. Pt became more relaxed and was calm during transport. Pt reassessed en route without changes. Report called to ED before arrival, which included pt's current condition and ETA. On arrival, pt was placed on the ED stretcher, rails up both sides, and report given to RN. Physician signature obtained for medication order.

End of report

Prep Kit

Ready for Review

- Behavioral emergencies such as drug overdoses, violent behavior, and mental illness can present unique challenges in patient care. Panic by the patient, the family, bystanders, or all of these parties may create a demand for action on your part. Focus on reducing the patient's stress without exposing yourself to unnecessary risks.
- A behavioral or psychiatric emergency is any reaction to events that interferes with activities of daily living. A person who is no longer able to respond appropriately to the environment and whose abnormal behavior threatens the health and safety of self or others may be having a true psychiatric emergency.
- Not all behavioral emergencies involve a mental health problem. Some emergencies are a temporary response to a traumatic event.
- Calls for behavioral emergencies have special medical and legal considerations. These considerations can include the need to obtain consent, to follow local guidelines and standing orders for transporting patients against their will, and to obtain law enforcement assistance when appropriate to do so.
- You have limited legal authority to require a patient to undergo emergency medical care in the absence of a life-threatening emergency. Most states have provisions allowing law enforcement personnel to place mentally impaired people in custody so that such care can be provided. Always involve law enforcement personnel any time you are called to assist a patient with a severe behavioral or psychiatric crisis.
- If a patient poses an immediate threat, then leave the area until law enforcement personnel secure the scene. Always consult medical control and contact law enforcement for help.
- Underlying causes of behavioral emergencies fall into four broad categories: biologic (organic) causes, causes resulting from the person's environment, causes resulting from acute injury or illness, and causes that are substance related.
- Psychiatric signs and symptoms occur when a person's mental health is challenged and psychological mechanisms or behaviors are mobilized to help return the person's mental state to homeostasis. Psychiatric signs and symptoms can be grouped according to the systems of psychological (rather than physiologic) functioning they affect: consciousness, motor activity, speech, thought, affect, memory, orientation, and perception.
- Assessing a patient with a behavioral emergency differs from other methods of patient assessment in that with the patient who is disturbed, you are the diagnostic instrument, using your thinking processes, perceptions, and feelings to evaluate and measure the patient. With a behavioral emergency, assessment is also part of the treatment because your voice and manner affect the patient's response.
- When providing emergency medical care to a patient having a behavioral emergency, be direct, honest, and calm; have a definitive plan of action; stay with the patient at all times, but do not get too close; and express interest in the patient's story, but don't judge the behavior. Always treat patients with respect.
- When you are assessing the scene, pay special attention to potential dangers and threats (objects that may be used as weapons, hazardous chemicals, and the like). Remove potentially harmful objects. Situations with a strong behavioral component have great potential for sudden and unexpected turns of events, so follow established safety guidelines when responding.
- The primary survey in case of a behavioral emergency includes identifying yourself clearly, forming a general impression of the patient's overall condition and the nature of the psychiatric emergency, performing the primary survey, making a decision about

Prep Kit continued

transport, and taking a history via the mental status exam. A useful mnemonic for the exam is COASTMAP: consciousness, orientation, activity, speech, thought, memory, affect/mood, and perception.

- Secondary assessment includes looking for signs of an organic cause of the patient's behavioral emergency. This includes inspecting the patient for head trauma, checking pupil size, noting any unusual odors on the patient's breath, and examining the extremities for needle tracks, tremors, or unilateral weakness/loss of sensation.
- Care of the patient with a behavioral emergency focuses on ensuring scene safety and maintaining awareness of life-threatening conditions, while treating the patient for any medical disorders before assuming an emotional or psychiatric cause for the problem.
- Effective communication techniques for a behavioral emergency include beginning with an open-ended question, allowing the patient to talk, showing that you are listening, allowing silence when appropriate, acknowledging and labeling the patient's feelings, avoiding argument, facilitating communication, directing the patient's attention, asking questions, and adjusting your approach as needed.
- Crisis intervention skills include staying calm and being as direct as possible, excluding any disruptive people from the scene, sitting down to interview the patient, maintaining a nonjudgmental attitude, providing honest reassurance, developing a plan of action, encouraging some motor activity, staying with the patient at all times, bringing all of the patient's medications to the medical facility, and assuming that the patient can hear and understand everything you say.
- Use of physical or chemical restraints is reserved for times when verbal intervention fails to reduce severe agitation. Be familiar with the type of restraints and medications used by your agency before you encounter a situation in which they are needed. If restraints are required, then use the minimum force necessary. Assess the ABCs (airway, breathing, circulation) often while the patient is restrained, and maintain a constant dialogue with the patient throughout the restraining process. Maintain constant vigilance to protect safety and document everything that is done.
- Pathophysiologic factors that contribute to behavioral disturbances include cognitive impairment (excited delirium), thought disorders (including schizophrenia and psychosis), mood disorders (bipolar mood disorder, manic behavior, and depression), neurotic disorders (generalized anxiety disorder, phobias, and panic disorder), substance-related disorders and addictive behavior, somatoform disorders (hypochondriasis and conversion disorder), factitious disorders, impulse control disorders, and personality disorders. Each condition has its own unique pathophysiology as well as standards for assessment and management, so be familiar with each.
- You may encounter patients with psychosis, a thought disorder characterized by a state of delusion in which the person is out of touch with reality. Patients may be belligerent and angry, or silent and withdrawn. The usual methods of reasoning with a patient are unlikely to be effective with patients with psychoses, so be sure to learn the guidelines for caring for these patients. These guidelines include being calm, direct, straightforward, and nonconfrontational.
- You may also encounter patients with excited delirium, which is impairment of cognitive function that can present with disorientation, hallucinations, or delusions, and is characterized by restless and irregular physical activity. One of the most important factors to consider when caring for these patients is your personal safety. Use careful interviewing

Prep Kit continued

techniques and refrain from upsetting the patient further.

- The threat of suicide requires immediate intervention. Depression is the most significant risk factor for suicide, but other risk factors include personal or family history of suicide attempts, chronic debilitating illness, financial setback, and severe mental illness. Guidelines for managing the suicidal patient include never leaving the patient alone, collecting any implements of self-destruction, acknowledging the patient's feelings, and providing transport.
- Situations involving violence, abuse, and neglect can present a particular challenge because of their potential for escalation and for evoking emotional responses in you. Violent patients make up only a small percentage of those persons experiencing a behavioral or psychiatric crisis, but you must assess for risk factors for such a patient. Risk factors for violence include history, posture, the scene, speech patterns and other vocal activity, agitation, depression, and physical activity. Managing the violent patient requires you to assess the entire situation, observe your surroundings, maintain a safe distance, try verbal interventions first, and of course request law enforcement personnel if they are not already present.
- Patients with psychiatric emergencies may be taking any of several types of psychotropic medications. During assessment, you must identify which medications the patient has been prescribed and whether the patient is actually taking them. Types of psychiatric medications include antidepressants, benzodiazepines, antipsychotics, and amphetamines. Patients' medication noncompliance often results in abnormal behaviors and confrontational behavior toward others.
- Returning combat veterans have a high incidence of PTSD. Develop military cultural competency, and treat these patients with compassion and understanding.

Vital Vocabulary

activities of daily living (ADLs) The basic activities a person usually accomplishes during a normal day, such as eating, dressing, and washing.

acute dystonic reaction A syndrome that may occur in patients taking typical antipsychotic agents; characterized by the development of muscle spasms of the neck, face, and back within a few days of starting treatment with the medication.

affect The outward expression of a person's inner feelings (eg, happy, sad, angry, fearful, withdrawn).

agoraphobia Literally, "fear of the marketplace"; fear of entering a public place from which escape may be impeded.

anorexia nervosa An eating disorder in which a person diets by exerting extraordinary control over eating, and loses weight to the point of jeopardizing health and life.

anxiety disorders Mental disorders in which the dominant mood is fear and apprehension.

atropine-like effects Adverse effects similar to those seen with atropine, including dry mouth, blurred vision, urinary retention, and cardiac dysrhythmias; may occur with the use of some antipsychotic medications.

behavior How a person functions or acts in response to the environment.

behavioral emergencies Points at which a person's reactions to events interfere with activities of daily living; they become psychiatric emergencies when they cause a major life interruption, such as attempted suicide.

bipolar mood disorder A disorder in which a person alternates between mania and depression.

Prep Kit continued

borderline personality disorder A disorder characterized by disordered images of self, impulsive and unpredictable behavior, marked shifts in mood, and instability in relationships with others.

bulimia nervosa An eating disorder characterized by consumption of large amounts of food, for which the patient often compensates by using purging techniques.

catatonic Lacking expression or movement, or appearing rigid.

chemical restraint The use of medication to subdue a patient.

circumstantial thinking Situation in which the patient includes many irrelevant details in an account of things.

compulsions Repetitive actions carried out to relieve the anxiety of obsessive thoughts.

confabulation The invention of experiences to cover gaps in memory, seen in patients with certain organic brain syndromes.

confrontation Act of pointing out something of interest in the patient's conversation or behavior, thereby directing the patient's attention to something.

covert behaviors Behaviors that have a hidden meaning or intention that only the person understands.

delusions Fixed beliefs that are not shared by other people with the same culture or background and that cannot be changed by reasonable argument; false beliefs.

dementia A chronic process that produces severe deficits in memory, abstract thinking, and judgment.

depression A mental health disorder characterized by a persistent mood of sadness, despair, and discouragement; it may be a symptom of many different mental and physical disorders, or it may be a disorder on its own.

disorganization A condition in which a person demonstrates uncontrolled and disconnected thoughts, is usually incoherent or rambling in speech, and may or may not be oriented to person and place.

disorientation A condition in which a person may be confused about person, place, or time; one of the ways in which conditions such as schizophrenia or organic brain syndrome may present.

echolalia Meaningless echoing of the interviewer's words by the patient.

excited delirium An acute confrontational state characterized by global impairment of thinking, perception, judgment, and memory.

factitious disorder A disorder in which a person wishes to be sick and intentionally produces or feigns physical or psychological signs or symptoms. Symptoms are under voluntary control, with no obvious physiologic reason.

flat affect The absence of emotion; appearing to feel no emotion at all.

flight of ideas Accelerated thinking in which the mind skips very rapidly from one thought to the next.

generalized anxiety disorder (GAD) A disorder in which a person worries about everything for no particular reason, or in which the worrying is unproductive and the person cannot decide what to do about an upcoming situation.

hallucinations Sensory perceptions not founded on objective reality; false perceptions.

impulse control disorders Conditions in which a person lacks the ability to resist a temptation or cannot stop acting on a drive.

inappropriate affect Emotion that is out of sync with the situation (eg, wearing a smile while discussing a parent's death).

labile Rapidly shifting among different emotional states.

loosening of associations A situation in which the logical connection between one idea and the next becomes obscure, at least to the listener.

Prep Kit continued

mania A mental disorder characterized by abnormally exaggerated happiness, joy, or euphoria with hyperactivity, insomnia, and grandiose ideas.

manic-depressive illness A bipolar disorder in which mood fluctuates between depression and mania; the alterations in mood are usually episodic and recurrent.

medication noncompliance A situation in which a patient chooses not to take medications as prescribed, for reasons that may include undesirable adverse effects or prohibitive cost.

mental status exam (MSE) A tool for measuring the "mental vital signs" in a patient who is disturbed. The mnemonic COASTMAP can be used to conduct this exam, assessing consciousness, orientation, activity, speech, thought, memory, affect and mood, and perception.

mood disorders Disorders in which the disturbance of mood is accompanied by full or partial manic or depressive syndrome.

mutism The absence of speech.

neologisms Invented words that have meaning only to their inventor.

neurotic disorders A collection of psychiatric disorders without psychotic symptoms and lacking the intense psychopathology of other mood disorders; includes anxiety disorders, phobias, and panic disorder.

organic brain syndrome Temporary or permanent dysfunction of the brain, caused by a disturbance in the physical or physiologic functioning of brain tissue.

overt behaviors Behaviors that are open and generally understood by those around the person.

panic disorder A disorder characterized by sudden, usually unexpected, and overwhelming feelings of fear and dread, accompanied by a variety of other symptoms produced by a massive activation of the autonomic nervous system.

perseveration Repeating the same idea over and over again.

personality disorders Conditions in which a person behaves or thinks in a way that is dysfunctional or causes distress to other people.

phobias Abnormal and persistent dread of specific objects or situations.

phobic disorders Disorders involving an unreasonable fear, apprehension, or dread of a specific situation or thing.

posttraumatic stress disorder (PTSD) A severe form of anxiety that stems from a traumatic experience; characterized by the reliving of the stress and nightmares of the original situation.

pressure of speech Speech in which words seem to tumble out under immense emotional pressure.

psychiatric emergency An emergency in which abnormal behavior threatens a person's health and safety or the health and safety of another person, such as with a person who becomes suicidal or homicidal, or who has a psychotic episode.

psychosis A mental disorder characterized by a loss of contact with reality.

psychotropic medications Medications that affect mood, thought, or behavior.

schizophrenia A complex mental disorder that is difficult to identify and whose typical onset is during early adulthood. Dysfunctional symptoms typically become more prominent over time and include delusions, hallucinations, apathy, mutism, flat affect, lack of interest in pleasure, erratic speech, dysfunctional emotional responses, and dysfunctional motor behavior.

simple phobia A fear that is focused on one class of objects (eg, mice, spiders, dogs) or situations (eg, high places, darkness, flying).

somatoform disorder A condition in which a person is overly concerned with physical health and appearance to the point that it dominates everything (eg, hypochondria).

Prep Kit continued

stereotyped movements Repetitive movements that do not appear to serve any purpose.

substance dependence Use of a substance that results in addiction and physiologic dependence on the substance.

substance intoxication Use of a substance that results in impaired thinking and motor function.

substance use Use of moderate amounts of a substance without seriously affecting activities of daily living.

substance use disorder Use of a substance that disrupts activities of daily living.

tangential thinking A tendency to leave the current topic in conversation to talk about something else, thereby inhibiting interpersonal communication.

thought broadcasting The belief that thoughts are broadcast aloud and can be heard by others.

thought insertion The belief that thoughts are being thrust into one's mind by another person.

thought withdrawal The belief that thoughts are being removed from one's mind.

References

1. Average number of poor mental health days reported in the last 30 days among all adults by sex. Kaiser Family Foundation website. https://www.kff.org/other/state-indicator/poor-mental-health-by-sex/?currentTimeframe=0&sortModel=%7B%22colId%22:%22Location%22,%22sort%22:%22asc%22%7D. Accessed July 14, 2021.
2. Mental health and mental disorders. Healthy People 2020. Office of Disease Prevention and Health Promotion website. https://www.healthypeople.gov/2020/topics-objectives/topic/mental-health-and-mental-disorders. Accessed July 14, 2021.
3. Comorbidity: substance use and other mental disorders. National Institute on Drug Abuse website. https://www.drugabuse.gov/drug-topics/trends-statistics/infographics/comorbidity-substance-use-other-mental-disorders. Published August 15, 2018. Accessed July 14, 2021.
4. Ristich K. FDA strengthens warnings and precautions for droperidol. Medscape website. https://www.medscape.com/viewarticle/786350. Published December 6, 2001. Accessed July 14, 2021.
5. Marcinkowska M, Sniecikowska J, Fajkis N, et al. Management of dementia-related psychosis, agitation and aggression: a review of the pharmacology and clinical effects of potential drug candidates. *CNS Drugs.* 2020;34(3):243-268.
6. Mattingly BB, Schraga ED. Chemical restraint. Medscape website. https://emedicine.medscape.com/article/109717-overview Updated March 2, 2021. Accessed September 30, 2021.
7. Report 2 of the Council on Science and Public Health (June 2021): use of drugs to chemically restrain agitated individuals outside of hospital settings (Reference Committee E). American Medical Association website. https://www.ama-assn.org/system/files/2021-05/j21-csaph02.pdf. Published 2021. Accessed September 30, 2021.
8. O'Brien ME, Fuh L, Raja AS, White BA, Yun BJ, Hayes BD. Reduced-dose intramuscular ketamine for severe agitation in an academic emergency department. *Clin Toxicol (Phila).* 2020;58(4):294-298.
9. Winslow JE, Bozeman WP, Fortner MC, Alson RL. Conducted energy weapon: a case report. *Ann Emerg Med.* 2007;50(5):584-586.
10. Sheldon LK. *Communication for Nurses Talking With Patients*. 2nd ed. Sudbury, MA: Jones and Bartlett; 2009.
11. Strommer EMF, Leith W, Zeegers MP, Freeman MD. The role of restraint in fatal excited delirium: a research synthesis and pooled analysis. *Forens Sci Med Pathol.* 2020;16:680-692.
12. Takeuchi A, Ahern TL, Henderson SO. Excited delirium. *West J Emerg Med.* 2011;12(1):77-83.
13. Roach B, Echols K, Burnett A. Excited delirium and the dual response. Federal Bureau of Investigation website. https://leb.fbi.gov/articles/featured-articles/excited-delirium-and-the-dual-response-preventing-in-custody-deaths. Published July 8, 2014. Accessed July 14, 2021.
14. National Center for Health Statistics. Leading causes of death. Centers for Disease Control and Prevention website. https://www.cdc.gov/nchs/fastats/leading-causes-of-death.htm. Reviewed March 1, 2021. Accessed September 30, 2021.
15. Suicide statistics. American Foundation for Suicide Prevention website. https://afsp.org/suicide-statistics/. Accessed September 30, 2021.
16. Any mood disorder among adults. National Institute of Mental Health website. https://www.nimh.nih.gov/health/statistics/any-mood-disorder. Updated November 2017. Accessed July 14, 2021.
17. Substance Abuse and Mental Health Services Administration. *Key Substance Use and Mental Health Indicators in the United States: Results From the 2019 National*

Prep Kit continued

Survey on Drug Use and Health (HHS Publication No. PEP20-07-01-001, NSDUH Series H-55). Washington, DC: Center for Behavioral Health Statistics and Quality, Substance Abuse and Mental Health Services Administration; 2020.

18. Schizophrenia. National Institute of Mental Health website. https://www.nimh.nih.gov/health/statistics/prevalence/schizophrenia.shtml. Updated May 2018. Accessed July 14, 2021.
19. Any anxiety disorder. National Institute of Mental Health website. https://www.nimh.nih.gov/health/statistics/prevalence/any-anxiety-disorder-among-adults.shtml. Updated November 2017. Accessed July 14, 2021.
20. Social anxiety disorder: more than just shyness. National Institute of Mental Health website. https://www.nimh.nih.gov/health/publications/social-anxiety-disorder-more-than-just-shyness/index.shtml. Accessed September 30, 2021.
21. Panic disorder. National Institute of Mental Health website. https://www.nimh.nih.gov/health/statistics/panic-disorder. Updated November 2017. Accessed July 14, 2021.
22. National Drug Intelligence Center. *The Economic Impact of Illicit Drug Use on American Society*. Washington, DC: US Department of Justice; April 2011.
23. Excessive drinking is draining the U.S. economy. Centers for Disease Control and Prevention website. https://www.cdc.gov/features/alcoholconsumption/. Reviewed December 30, 2019. Accessed July 14, 2021.
24. US Department of Health and Human Services. *The Health Consequences of Smoking—50 Years of Progress. A Report of the Surgeon General*. Atlanta, GA: US Department of Health and Human Services, Centers for Disease Control and Prevention, National Center for Chronic Disease Prevention and Health Promotion, Office on Smoking and Health; 2014. Printed with corrections, January 2014.
25. Pike KM, Dunne PE. The rise of eating disorders in Asia: a review. *J Eat Disord*. 2015;3:33.
26. Child and Adolescent Eating Disorders Program. Anorexia nervosa. University of Rochester Medicine Golisano Children's Hospital website. https://www.urmc.rochester.edu/childrens-hospital/adolescent/eating-disorders/teens/anorexia-nervosa.aspx. Accessed July 14, 2021.
27. Eating disorders. Anxiety and Depression Association of America website. https://www.adaa.org/understanding-anxiety/related-illnesses/eating-disorders. Accessed September 30, 2021.
28. American Psychiatric Association. *Diagnostic and Statistical Manual of Mental Disorders*. 5th ed. Washington, DC: American Psychiatric Association; 2013.
29. Coupland C. Antidepressant use and risk of suicide and attempted suicide or self harm in people aged 20 to 64: cohort study using a primary care database. *Brit Med J*. 2015;350:h517.
30. NAEMT national survey finds EMS mental health services lacking. National Association of Emergency Medical Technicians website. http://www.naemt.org/docs/default-source/member-resources-documents/naemt-news/2016/fall-2016-issue-low-res.pdf. Published Fall 2016. Accessed September 27, 2021.
31. Friedman MJ. PTSD history and overview. US Department of Veterans Affairs website. https://www.ptsd.va.gov/professional/treat/essentials/history_ptsd.asp. Accessed July 14, 2021.
32. How common is PTSD in veterans? US Department of Veterans Affairs website. https://www.ptsd.va.gov/understand/common/common_veterans.asp. Accessed July 15, 2021.
33. Gradus JL. Epidemiology of PTSD. US Department of Veterans Affairs website. https://www.ptsd.va.gov/professional/treat/essentials/epidemiology.asp. Accessed July 14, 2021.
34. Tanielian T, Jaycox LH, Adamson DM, et al. Invisible wounds of war: psychological and cognitive injuries, their consequences, and services to assist recovery. RAND Corporation website. http://www.rand.org/pubs/monographs/MG720.html. Accessed July 14, 2021.
35. PTSD basics. US Department of Veterans Affairs website. https://www.ptsd.va.gov/understand/what/ptsd_basics.asp. Accessed July 14, 2021.
36. Epidemiology Program, Post-Deployment Health Group, Office of Patient Care Services, Veterans Health Administration, Department of Veterans Affairs. *Analysis of VA Health Care Utilization Among Operation Enduring Freedom (OEF), Operation Iraqi Freedom (OIF), and Operation New Dawn (OND) Veterans: Cumulative From 1st Qtr FY 2002 Through 3rd Qtr FY 2015*. Washington, DC: US Department of Veterans Affairs; 2017. http://www.publichealth.va.gov/docs/epidemiology/healthcare-utilization-report-fy2015-qtr3.pdf. Accessed July 114, 2021.
37. What is posttraumatic stress disorder? American Psychiatric Association website. https://www.psychiatry.org/patients-families/ptsd/what-is-ptsd?_ga=1.133267214.1055821636.1488863540. Accessed July 14, 2021.
38. Gibson LE. Acute stress disorder. US Department of Veterans Affairs website. https://www.ptsd.va.gov/professional/treat/essentials/acute_stress_disorder.asp. Accessed July 14, 2021.
39. Smartphone virtual "hope box" could help reduce suicidal thoughts. US Department of Veterans Affairs website. https://www.research.va.gov/news/research_highlights/hope_box-012913.cfm. Accessed July 14, 2021.
40. Convoy S, Westphal RJ. The importance of developing military cultural competence. *J Emerg Nurs*. 2013;39(6):591-594.

Glossary: Volume 1

3-3-2 rule: A method used to predict difficult intubation. A mouth opening of less than three fingerbreadths, a mandible length of less than three fingerbreadths, and a distance from hyoid bone to thyroid notch of less than two fingerbreadths indicate a possibly difficult airway.
abandonment: Termination of medical care for the patient without giving the patient sufficient opportunity to find another qualified health care professional to take over medical treatment. In the context of child welfare, a type of child maltreatment in which a parent or guardian physically leaves a child without regard to the child's health, safety, or welfare.
abdominal thrust maneuver: Abdominal thrusts performed to relieve a foreign body airway obstruction.
abduction: Movement of a limb away from the midline.
aberration: A term describing the shape of the QRS complex in aberrantly (abnormally) conducted beats.
ABO system: The commonly used blood classification system, based on the antigens present or absent in the blood.
abscess: An area in the brain or spinal cord in which cells have been attacked, typically by an infectious agent. To prevent the spread of infection, the immune system "walls off" the area; pus may then collect in this pocket.
absolute refractory period (ARP): The early phase of cardiac repolarization, during which the heart muscle cannot be stimulated to depolarize; also known as the effective refractory period.
absorption: The process by which the molecules of a substance are moved from the site of entry or administration into systemic circulation; in allergic reactions, movement of a foreign material into the skin. In the context of decontamination, use of large pads to soak up liquid and remove it from the patient.
accessory muscles: The muscles not normally used during quiet breathing; examples include the sternocleidomastoid muscles of the neck, the chest pectoralis major muscles, and the abdominal muscles.
access port: A sealed hub on an administration set designed to provide sterile access to the intravenous fluid.
accommodation: The ability of the lens of the eye to change its shape to focus on a close object.
acetabulum: The socket formed by the coxal (hip) bone into which the ball-shaped femoral head fits snugly.
acetylcholine (ACh): A neurotransmitter released at synapses within the autonomic nervous system and by motor neurons to stimulate skeletal muscle contraction.
acetylcholinesterase: An enzyme found in the central nervous system, in red blood cells, and in motor endplates of skeletal muscle that causes the decomposition of acetylcholine.
acholic stools: Light, clay-colored stools indicative of liver failure.
acidosis: A pathologic condition resulting from the accumulation of acids in the body (blood pH less than 7.35).
acids: Molecules that can give up a hydrogen ion, and therefore increase the concentration of hydrogen ions in a water solution.
acquired immunity: The immunity that occurs when the body is exposed to a foreign substance or disease and produces antibodies to the invader; also called acquired immunity.
acquired immunodeficiency syndrome (AIDS): The end-stage disease process caused by the human immunodeficiency virus; it results in extreme vulnerability to numerous opportunistic bacterial, viral, and fungal infections that would not affect a person with an intact immune system.
acromion process: The tip of the shoulder and the site of attachment for the clavicle and various shoulder muscles.
actin: A contractile protein found in the thin filaments of skeletal muscle cells.
action potentials: Sequences of changes in the membrane potential that occur when an excitable cell (neuron or muscle) is stimulated.
activation: In the inflammatory response, the stage in which mediators of inflammation trigger the appearance of selectins and integrins on the surfaces of endothelial cells and polymorphonuclear neutrophils, respectively.
active metabolites: Medications that have undergone biotransformation and are able to alter a cellular process or body function.
active transport: A method used to move compounds across a cell membrane to create or maintain an imbalance of charges, usually against a concentration gradient and requiring the expenditure of energy.
activities of daily living (ADLs): The basic activities a person usually accomplishes during a normal day, such as eating, dressing, and washing.
acute abdomen: A sudden onset of pain within the abdomen, usually indicating peritonitis; demands immediate medical or surgical treatment.
acute chest syndrome: A vasoocclusive crisis that can be associated with pneumonia; common signs and symptoms include chest pain, fever, and cough; associated with sickle cell disease.
acute coronary syndromes (ACSs): A series of cardiac conditions caused by an abrupt reduction in coronary artery blood flow.
acute dystonic reaction: A syndrome that may occur in patients taking typical antipsychotic agents; characterized by the development of muscle spasms of the neck, face, and back within a few days of starting treatment with the medication.
acute gastroenteritis: A family of conditions that revolve around a central theme of infection with fever, abdominal pain, diarrhea, nausea, and vomiting.
acute kidney injury (AKI): A sudden decrease in filtration through the glomeruli.
acute myocardial infarction (AMI): Cardiac ischemia that occurs when sudden narrowing or complete occlusion of a coronary artery leads to death (necrosis) of myocardial tissue.
acute splenic sequestration syndrome: A condition in which red blood cells become trapped in the spleen, causing a dramatic decline in the amount of hemoglobin available in the circulation; it usually occurs in infants or toddlers.

acute stress reaction: Reaction to stress that occurs during a stressful situation.
adaptation: The temporary or permanent reduction of sensitivity to a particular stimulus.
addisonian crisis: Acute adrenal insufficiency.
adduction: Movement of a limb toward the midline.
adenosine triphosphate (ATP): The nucleotide formed from the metabolism of nutrients in the cell; involved in energy metabolism; used to store energy.
adhesion: In the inflammatory response, the stage characterized by attachment of polymorphonuclear neutrophils to endothelial cells, mediated by selectins and integrins.
administration set: Tubing that connects to the intravenous bag access port and the catheter to deliver intravenous fluid.
adolescents: People who are 13 through 18 years of age.
adrenal cortex: The outer layer of the adrenal gland; it produces hormones that are important in regulating the water and salt balance of the body.
adrenal glands: Paired endocrine glands located on top of the kidneys, which release epinephrine and norepinephrine when stimulated by the sympathetic nervous system; each adrenal gland consists of an inner adrenal medulla and an adrenal cortex.
adrenergic: Having the characteristics of the sympathetic division of the autonomic nervous system.
adrenocorticotropic hormone (ACTH): Hormone that stimulates the adrenal cortex to manufacture and secrete cortisol (a glucocorticoid).
advance directive: A written document or oral statement that expresses the wants, needs, and desires of a patient in reference to future medical care; examples include living wills, do not resuscitate orders, and organ donation orders.
adventitious: Abnormal.
adventitious breath sounds: Abnormal breath sounds, such as wheezing, rhonchi, crackles, stridor, and pleural friction rubs.
adverse effects: Abnormal or harmful effects to an organism caused by exposure to a chemical; indicated by some result such as death, a change in food or water consumption, altered body and organ weights, altered enzyme levels, or visible illness.
aerobic metabolism: Metabolism that can proceed only in the presence of oxygen.
aerosol-generating procedures: Procedures that can increase the number and load of droplets from the patient. Examples include intubation and suctioning or performing mouth-to-mouth resuscitation.
affect: The outward expression of a person's inner feelings (eg, happy, sad, angry, fearful, withdrawn).
affinity: The ability of a medication to bind with a particular receptor site.
afterimage: The perception that a stimulus is still present after the stimulus has been removed.
afterload: The pressure in the aorta against which the left ventricle must pump blood; increasing this pressure can decrease cardiac output.
agonal: Pertaining to the period of dying.
agonal gasps: Slow, shallow, irregular respirations or occasional gasping breaths that result from cerebral anoxia.
agonal rhythm: A ventricular rate of less than 20 beats/min; this rhythm is seen just before the heart stops beating altogether.
agonist medications: A group of medications that initiates or alters a cellular activity by attaching to receptor sites, prompting a cellular response.
agoraphobia: Literally, "fear of the marketplace"; fear of entering a public place from which escape may be impeded.
airborne precautions: Placement of a surgical mask on the patient and the use of airflow measures to prevent airborne transmission; apply to infections that spread through exposure to respiratory droplets composed of small droplets and particles that can travel over long distances, generally 6 feet (2 m) or more, before dropping to the floor.
airborne transmission: The transmission of an infectious agent by inhalation of small particles that become aerosolized when the infected person coughs, sneezes, talks, or exhales; particles can remain suspended in the air for some period and can travel 6 feet (2 m) or more.
air embolism: The presence of air in the venous circulation, which forms a gas bubble that can block the outflow of blood from the right ventricle to the lung; can lead to cardiac arrest, shock, or other life-threatening complications.
albumins: The smallest of plasma proteins; they make up approximately 60% of the plasma proteins and are responsible for the oncotic pressure in the vasculature, thereby controlling the movement of water into and out of the circulation.
alcoholic ketoacidosis: A metabolic acidotic state that manifests because of inadequate nutritional habits associated with chronic alcohol abuse. The liver and body experience inadequate fuel reserves of glycogen and, therefore, have to switch to fatty acid metabolism.
alcohol use disorder: A condition characterized by a physical and psychological addiction to ethanol that can range from mild to severe.
aldosterone: Hormone that stimulates the kidneys to reabsorb sodium from the urine and excrete potassium by altering the osmotic gradient in the blood.
alert and oriented (A&O): A determination made when assessing mental status by looking at whether the patient is oriented in four areas: person, place, time, and the event itself. Each element provides information about different aspects of the patient's memory.
alkalosis: A pathologic condition resulting from the accumulation of bases in the body (blood pH greater than 7.45).
alleles: Variant forms of a gene, which can be identical or slightly different in a sequence of deoxyribonucleic acid.
allergen: Any substance that causes a hypersensitivity reaction.
allergic reaction: An abnormal immune response the body develops when reexposed to a substance or allergen.
allergy: A hypersensitivity reaction to the presence of an agent (allergen).
alternative time sampling: Time parameters that are set during a research project.
alveoli: The air sacs of the lungs in which the exchange of oxygen and carbon dioxide takes place; also, the bony sockets for the teeth that reside in the mandible and maxilla (singular, *alveolus*).
Alzheimer disease: A progressive, organic condition in which neurons in the brain die, causing dementia.
amenorrhea: Absence of menstruation.
amphetamines: A class of drugs that increase alertness and excitation (stimulants); include methamphetamine (crank or ice), methylenedioxyamphetamine (MDA, Adam), and methylenedioxymethamphetamine (MDMA, Eve, Ecstasy).
ampules: Small glass containers that are sealed and whose contents are sterilized.
amyotrophic lateral sclerosis (ALS): A condition that strikes the voluntary motor neurons, causing their death. The disease is characterized by fatigue and general weakness of muscle groups; eventually the patient becomes unable to walk, eat, or speak; also known as Lou Gehrig disease.
anabolism: The building of larger substances from smaller substances, such as the building of proteins from amino acids.

anaerobic metabolism: Metabolism that occurs in the absence of oxygen.

anal fissures: Linear tears to the mucosal lining in and near the anus, possibly caused by the passage of large, hard stools; a cause of lower gastrointestinal bleeding.

analgesia: The state of being insensible to pain while still conscious.

anaphylactic shock: A severe hypersensitivity reaction that involves bronchoconstriction and cardiovascular collapse; also called anaphylaxis.

anaphylactoid reaction: An extreme allergic response that does not involve immunoglobulin E antibody mediation. The exact mechanism is unknown, but an event of this type may occur without the patient being previously exposed to the offending agent.

anaphylaxis: An extreme systemic form of an allergic reaction involving one, two, or more body systems.

anatomic position: The position of reference, in which the patient stands facing you, arms at the side, with the palms of the hands facing forward.

anatomy: The study of the structure of an organism and its parts.

androgens: Male sex hormones that regulate body changes associated with sexual development (puberty), including growth spurts, deepening of the voice, growth of facial and pubic hair, and muscle growth and strength.

anemia: A lower-than-normal hemoglobin or erythrocyte level.

anesthesia: Lack of feeling within a body part.

anesthetic: A medication that causes the inability to feel sensation.

aneurysm: A swelling or enlargement of part of a blood vessel, resulting from weakening of the vessel wall.

angina pectoris: The sudden pain that occurs when the oxygen supply to the myocardium is insufficient to meet demand, causing ischemic changes in the tissue.

angiogenesis: The growth of new blood vessels.

angle of Louis: A prominence of the sternum that indicates the point where the second rib joins the sternum; also called the sternal angle or manubriosternal junction.

anisocoria: Unequal pupils with a greater than 1-mm difference.

anorexia nervosa: An eating disorder in which a person diets by exerting extraordinary control over eating, and loses weight to the point of jeopardizing health and life.

anoxia: An absence of oxygen.

antagonist: A molecule that blocks the ability of a given chemical to bind to its receptor, preventing a biologic response.

antagonist medications: A group of medications that prevent endogenous or exogenous agonist chemicals from reaching cell receptor sites and initiating or altering a particular cellular activity.

antecubital: The anterior aspect of the elbow.

anterior: The front surface of the body; the side facing you in the anatomic position.

anterograde amnesia: An inability to remember events after the onset of amnesia.

anteroposterior axis: The axis that runs perpendicular to the coronal plane.

antibiotics: Medications used to fight infection by killing the microorganisms or preventing their multiplication to allow the body's immune system to overcome them.

antibody: A protein secreted by certain immune cells that bind antigens to make them more visible to the immune system; an immunoglobulin.

anticoagulants: Substances that prevent blood from clotting.

antidiuretic hormone (ADH): Hormone secreted by the posterior pituitary lobe of the pituitary gland that constricts blood vessels and raises the blood pressure; also called *vasopressin.*

antidote: Something to counteract the effect of a poison.

antifungals: Medications used to treat fungal infections.

antigen: A protein, polysaccharide, glycoprotein, or glycolipid commonly found on the surface of a red blood cell that stimulates an immune system response and causes formation of antibodies; cells learn to recognize antigens as either "self" or "nonself" (foreign).

antimicrobials: Medications used to kill or suppress the growth of microorganisms.

antiseptics: Chemicals used to cleanse an area before performing an invasive procedure, such as starting an intravenous line; they are not toxic to living tissues. Examples include chlorhexidine, isopropyl alcohol, and iodine.

antonyms: Pairs of word roots, prefixes, or suffixes that have opposite meanings.

anuria: A complete cessation of urine production.

anxiety disorders: Mental disorders in which the dominant mood is fear and apprehension.

anxious avoidant attachment: A bond formed between an infant and the parent or caregiver in which the infant is repeatedly rejected and develops an isolated lifestyle that does not depend on the support and care of others.

aorta: The principal artery leaving the left side of the heart and carrying freshly oxygenated blood to the body; the largest artery in the body.

aortic aneurysm: An outpouching or bulge in the wall of a portion of the aorta, caused by weakening and dilation of the vessel wall; a ruptured aortic aneurysm is life threatening.

aortic valve: The semilunar valve that regulates blood flow from the left ventricle to the aorta.

apex: The pointed extremity of a conical structure.

aphasia: The language impairment that affects the production or understanding of speech and the ability to read or write.

aphonia: The inability to speak.

aplastic crisis: A temporary halt in the production of red blood cells; it may occur as a result of sickle cell disease.

apneic oxygenation: The continued alveolar uptake of oxygen, even when the patient is apneic; can be facilitated by administering oxygen via nasal cannula during intubation.

apneustic center: A portion of the pons that is thought to work with the pontine respiratory group to regulate the length and depth of inspiration.

apneustic respirations: Prolonged gasping inspirations followed by extremely short, ineffective expirations; associated with brainstem insult.

apoptosis: Normal cell death.

apparent life-threatening event (ALTE): An episode characterized by some combination of apnea (central or obstructive), skin color change (cyanotic, pallid, erythematous, or plethoric), change in muscle tone (usually diminished), and choking or gagging.

appendicitis: Inflammation of the appendix.

appendicular skeleton: The portion of the skeletal system made up of the upper extremities, shoulder girdle, pelvic girdle, and lower extremities.

aqueous humor: Watery fluid filling the anterior eye cavity; its quantity determines the intraocular pressure, which is critical to sight.

areolar tissue: A type of loose connective tissue that binds skin to underlying organs and fills in spaces between muscles.

arrhythmia: The absence of any cardiac rhythm or organized activity; asystole or ventricular standstill.

arteriosclerosis: A pathologic condition in which the thickening and stiffening of the arterial walls make the arteries less elastic.

arteriovenous graft: A surgical connection between an artery and a vein.

artifact: An artificial product; in cardiology, used to refer to noise or interference in an electrocardiographic tracing.

arytenoid cartilages: Six paired cartilages stacked on top of each other in the larynx.

ascites: Abnormal accumulation of fluid in the peritoneal cavity, causing abdominal edema; typically signals liver failure.

aseptic technique: A method of cleansing used to prevent contamination of a site from pathogens when you are performing an invasive procedure, such as starting an intravenous line.

aspiration: The drawing in or out by suction. In the lungs, aspiration of food, liquids, blood, or foreign objects can occur when a patient is unable to protect the airway.

assault: To create in another person a fear of immediate bodily harm or invasion of bodily security (including loss of freedom).

asthma: A chronic inflammatory lower airway condition resulting in intermittent wheezing and excess mucus production.

astigmatism: Condition where parts of the image are out of focus and others are in focus; caused by irregularities in the shape of the eye lens.

asymmetric chest wall movement: Unequal movement of the two sides of the chest; indicates decreased airflow into one lung.

asystole: The absence of ventricular contraction or electrical activity; a straight-line or flat-line electrocardiogram.

ataxia: Inability to properly coordinate the muscles; often used to describe a staggering gait.

atelectasis: Alveolar collapse that prevents use of that portion of the lungs for ventilation and oxygenation.

atheroma: A mass of fatty tissue that gradually calcifies, hardening into an atheromatous plaque that infiltrates the arterial wall, diminishing its elasticity.

atherosclerosis: A disorder in which cholesterol and calcium build up inside the walls of the blood vessels, forming plaque, which eventually leads to partial or complete blockage of blood flow.

atlas: The first cervical vertebra (C1), which provides support for the head.

atopic: An allergic tendency.

atria: The two upper chambers of the heart (singular, *atrium*).

atrial natriuretic peptide: Hormone produced by the atria when they are distended by increased blood volume; it inhibits the absorption of water and sodium in the renal tubules, thereby increasing the elimination of water.

atrioventricular (AV) junction: The portion of the conduction system of the heart that consists of the AV node and the nonbranching portion of the bundle of His.

atrioventricular (AV) node: A group of cells that slows the electrical impulses from the sinoatrial node before relaying it to the ventricles; located in the floor of the right atrium immediately behind the tricuspid valve and near the opening of the coronary sinus.

atrioventricular (AV) valves: The mitral and tricuspid valves, through which blood flows on its way from the atria to the ventricles.

atrophy: A decrease in cell size due to a loss of subcellular components.

atropine-like effects: Adverse effects similar to those seen with atropine, including dry mouth, blurred vision, urinary retention, and cardiac dysrhythmias; may occur with the use of some antipsychotic medications.

augmented limb leads: On an electrocardiogram, leads aVR, aVL, and aVF. They contain only one true pole; the other end is a combination of information from other leads. A standard 12-lead electrocardiogram consists of the three augmented leads, three standard limb leads, and the six precordial leads.

aura: Sensations commonly experienced before a seizure or migraine headache occurs; may include visual changes in addition to hallucinations.

aural: Pertaining to the ear.

auscultation: The act of using a stethoscope to listen to sounds within the body.

authoritarian: A parenting style that demands absolute obedience.

authoritative: A parenting style that balances parental authority with the child's freedom by setting and enforcing rules, but also allowing the child to have some freedom.

autoantibodies: Antibodies directed against the self.

autoimmunity: The production of antibodies or T cells that work against the tissues of one's own body, producing hypersensitivity reactions or autoimmune disease.

automated external defibrillator (AED): A defibrillator that can analyze the patient's heart rhythm and determine whether a defibrillating shock is needed to terminate ventricular fibrillation or ventricular tachycardia.

automatic crash notification (ACN): Specialized onboard computer systems in motor vehicles that automatically send telemetry data to a monitoring station in the event of a crash, which then relays the data to emergency responders; also called advanced automatic crash notification.

automaticity: Ability of cardiac pacemaker cells to initiate an electrical impulse spontaneously without being stimulated from another source (such as a nerve).

automatic transport ventilator (ATV): A portable mechanical ventilator attached to a control box that allows the provider to set the variables of ventilation (eg, respiratory rate and tidal volume).

autonomic nervous system (ANS): A subdivision of the nervous system that controls primarily involuntary body functions; composed of the sympathetic and parasympathetic nervous systems.

autosomal dominant: A pattern of inheritance that involves genes located on autosomes (any chromosome other than sex chromosomes). Inheritance of only one copy of a particular form of a gene is needed to show the trait.

autosomal recessive: A pattern of inheritance that involves genes located on autosomes (any chromosome other than sex chromosomes). Inheritance of two copies of a particular form of a gene is needed to show the trait.

autosomes: The chromosomes that do not carry genes that determine sex.

avian (bird) flu: A disease caused by a virus that occurs naturally in the bird population; signs and symptoms include fever, sore throat, cough, and muscle aches.

AVPU: A method of assessing mental status by determining whether a patient is Awake and alert, responsive to Verbal stimuli or Pain, or Unresponsive; used principally in the primary survey.

axial skeleton: The portion of the skeleton made up of the skull, thoracic cage, and vertebral column.

axis: An imaginary line joining the positive and negative electrodes of a lead; also the second cervical vertebra.

axis deviation: Movement of the heart's QRS axis to the right or left of its normal position.

axon: A long, slender extension of a neuron (nerve cell) that conducts electrical impulses away from the nerve cell body to adjacent cells.

azotemia: Increased nitrogenous wastes in the blood.

bacterial vaginosis: An overgrowth of bacteria in the vagina, characterized by itching, burning, or pain, which may be accompanied by a fishy, foul-smelling discharge.

bacteria: Small organisms that can grow and reproduce outside the human cell in the presence of the appropriate temperature and nutrients; they cause disease by invading and multiplying in the tissues of the host.

bag-mask device: A manual ventilation device that consists of a bag, mask, reservoir, and oxygen inlet; capable of delivering up to 100% oxygen.

barbiturates: Potent sedative-hypnotics historically used as sleep aids, as antianxiety drugs, and as part of the regimen for seizure control; include drugs such as thiopental (Pentothal, Trapanal) and methohexital (Brevital).

baroreceptors: Receptors in the blood vessels, kidneys, brain, and heart that respond to changes in pressure in the heart or main arteries to help maintain homeostasis.

barotrauma: Trauma resulting from pressure disequilibrium across body surfaces; for example, from too much pressure in the lungs.

Bartholin glands: The glands that secrete mucus for sexual lubrication.

basal ganglia: Structures located deep within the cerebrum, diencephalon, and midbrain that have an important role in coordination of motor movements and posture.

basal metabolic rate (BMR): The heat energy produced at rest from normal body metabolic reactions, determined mostly by the liver and skeletal muscles.

base station: A radio at a fixed location (ie, hospital or dispatch center) consisting of a transmitter, receiver, and antenna.

basophils: White blood cells that contain histamine granules and other substances that are released during inflammatory and allergic responses.

battery: The act of carrying out a physical threat; the use of force against another person, resulting in harmful, offensive, or sexual contact.

Battle sign: Bruising over the mastoid bone behind the ear, often seen after a basilar skull fracture; also called retroauricular ecchymosis.

Beck triad: The classic trio of signs associated with cardiac tamponade: narrowed pulse pressure, muffled heart tones, and jugular vein distention associated with cardiac tamponade; usually caused by penetrating chest trauma.

behavior: How a person functions or acts in response to the environment.

behavioral emergencies: Points at which a person's reactions to events interfere with activities of daily living; they become psychiatric emergencies when they cause a major life interruption, such as attempted suicide.

Bell palsy: A temporary paralysis of the facial nerve (cranial nerve VII), which controls the muscles on each side of the face.

benign prostate hypertrophy (BPH): Age-related nonmalignant (noncancerous) enlargement of the prostate gland.

benzodiazepines: The family of sedative-hypnotics that provide muscle relaxation and mild sedation; most commonly used to treat anxiety, seizures, and alcohol withdrawal; include drugs such as diazepam (Valium) and midazolam (Versed).

beta-2 agonist: A pharmacologic agent that stimulates the beta-2 receptor sites found in smooth muscle; includes common bronchodilators such as albuterol and levalbuterol.

bifascicular block: Blockage of any two fascicles or conduction pathways: a right bundle branch block (RBBB) with anterior hemiblock, RBBB with posterior hemiblock, or anterior hemiblock and posterior hemiblock (a combination known as left bundle branch block).

bigeminy: A dysrhythmia in which every other complex is a premature complex, causing a *normal–early beat–normal–early beat* pattern; can be atrial, junctional, or ventricular.

bilateral: In anatomy, a body part or condition that appears on both sides of the midline.

bilevel positive airway pressure (BPAP): A noninvasive form of positive-pressure ventilation that delivers two pressures (a higher inspiratory positive airway pressure and a lower expiratory positive airway pressure).

biliary tract disorders: A group of disorders that involve inflammation of the gallbladder; these include cholangitis, cholelithiasis, cholecystitis, and acalculous cholecystitis.

bilirubin: A waste product of red blood cell destruction that undergoes further metabolism in the liver.

bimanual laryngoscopy: An effective technique to improve the laryngoscopic view of the vocal cords through external manipulation of the larynx.

binocular vision: The merging of two images into one.

bioavailability: The percentage of the unchanged medication that reaches systemic circulation.

Biot (ataxic) respirations: Irregular pattern, rate, and depth of respirations with intermittent periods of apnea; result from increased intracranial pressure.

biotelemetry: Transmission of physiologic data, such as an electrocardiogram, from the patient to a distant point of reception (commonly known as telemetry in EMS).

biotransformation: A process with four possible effects on a medication absorbed into the body: (1) An inactive substance can become active, capable of producing desired or unwanted clinical effects. (2) An active medication can be changed into another active medication. (3) An active medication may be completely or partially inactivated. (4) A medication is transformed into a substance (active or inactive) that is easier for the body to eliminate.

biphasic reaction: A two-phase allergic reaction in which the patient's symptoms improve and then reappear without being exposed to the trigger (allergen) for a second time; the symptoms can resurface up to 8 or more hours after the initial incident.

bipolar leads: On an electrocardiogram, leads that contain both a positive and a negative pole: leads I, II, and III.

bipolar mood disorder: A disorder in which a person alternates between mania and depression.

blinding: A research design in which the patient and providers do not know if the subject (patient) is receiving the intervention being evaluated or a placebo. All other aspects of the study (ie, consent) must follow the requirements of the approving institutional review board.

blind panic: A fear reaction in which a person's judgment seems to disappear entirely; it is particularly dangerous because it may cause mass panic among others.

bloodborne pathogens: Pathogenic microorganisms that are present in human blood and can cause disease in humans. These pathogens include, but are not limited to, hepatitis B virus, human immunodeficiency virus, hepatitis C virus, and syphilis.

bloodborne pathogens: Pathogenic microorganisms that are present in human blood and can cause disease in humans; they include, but are not limited to, hepatitis B virus and human immunodeficiency virus.

blood–brain barrier: A layer of tightly adhered cells that protects the brain and spinal cord from exposure to medications, toxins, and infectious particles.

blood pressure (BP): The measurement of the force exerted against the walls of the blood vessels as the heart contracts and relaxes; it is calculated as the product of cardiac output and peripheral vascular resistance.

blood tubing: A special type of macrodrip administration set designed to facilitate rapid fluid replacement by manual infusion of multiple intravenous bags or intravenous–blood replacement combinations.

B lymphocytes: Lymphocytes that exist in the blood, and are abundant in the lymph nodes, bone marrow, intestinal lining, and spleen; also called B cells.

Boerhaave syndrome: Forceful vomiting that results in a tear in the esophagus that extends entirely through the esophageal wall, creating a hole.
bolus: "In one mass"; in medication administration, a single dose given by the intravenous or intraosseous route; may be a small or large quantity of the drug.
bonding: The formation of a close, personal relationship.
Bone Injection Gun (BIG): A spring-loaded device that is used for inserting an intraosseous needle into the proximal tibia in adult and pediatric patients.
bone marrow: Soft tissue that fills the inside of bones and is the site of production of red blood cells, platelets, and most white blood cells.
bony labyrinth: The collection of hollows in the bone of the inner ear that provide protection to the structures of the inner ear from damage and from extraneous stimulation.
borborygmi: A bowel sound characterized by increased activity within the bowel; also called hyperperistalsis.
borderline personality disorder: A disorder characterized by disordered images of self, impulsive and unpredictable behavior, marked shifts in mood, and instability in relationships with others.
borrowed servant doctrine: A principle that absolves an institution of liability when one of its members acts beyond the scope of certification or training by following someone else's orders.
botulism: Poisoning characterized by severe muscle paralysis and usually caused by eating food containing the botulinum toxin.
Bourdon-gauge flowmeter: An oxygen flowmeter that is commonly used because it is not affected by gravity and can be placed in any position.
Boyle's law: Gas law that demonstrates that as pressure increases, volume decreases; at a constant temperature, the volume of a gas is inversely proportional to its pressure (if the pressure on a gas is doubled, then its volume is halved); written as $PV = k$, where P = pressure, V = volume, and k = a constant.
bradykinesia: The slowing down of voluntary body movements; found in patients with Parkinson disease.
bradypnea: A slow respiratory rate.
brain: The part of the central nervous system located within the cranium; contains billions of neurons that serve a variety of functions, including consciousness, perception, control of reactions to the environment, emotional responses, and judgment.
brainstem: The area of the brain between the spinal cord and the cerebrum that contains the midbrain, pons, and medulla; controls functions that are necessary for life, such as breathing.
bronchial sounds: Hollow, tubular, lower-pitched sounds heard over the trachea.
bronchoconstriction: Narrowing of the bronchial tubes.
bronchodilation: Widening of the bronchial tubes.
bronchophony: A test of decreased breath sounds performed by placing the diaphragm of the stethoscope over the area in question while the patient says "ninety-nine"; a loud, clear sound indicates lung consolidation.
bronchospasm: Severe constriction of smooth muscle surrounding the bronchial tree.
bronchovesicular sounds: A combination of the tracheal and vesicular breath sounds; heard where the airways and alveoli are found, in the upper part of the sternum and between the scapulae.
bruit: Abnormal *whooshing* sounds indicating turbulent blood flow within a narrowed blood vessel, usually heard in the carotid arteries.
buccal: Between the cheek and gums.
buffer systems: Fast-acting defenses against acid–base changes, which provide almost immediate protection against changes in the hydrogen ion concentration of extracellular fluid.
bulimia nervosa: An eating disorder characterized by consumption of large amounts of food, for which the patient often compensates by using purging techniques.
bundle branch block (BBB): An intraventricular conduction disturbance involving impedance of electrical impulses from the bundle of His to the right or left bundle branch.
bundle of His: The portion of the heart's conduction system located in the upper portion of the interventricular septum that conducts electrical impulses from the atrioventricular junction to the right and left bundle branches; also called the AV bundle.
burnout: The exhaustion of physical or emotional strength.
BURP maneuver: The backward, upward, and rightward pressure used during intubation to improve the laryngoscopic view of the glottic opening and vocal cords; also called external laryngeal manipulation.
bursa: A small, padlike sac or cavity filled with a small amount of synovial fluid that helps reduce the amount of friction between a tendon and a bone or between a tendon and a ligament, usually located near a joint.
butterfly catheter: A rigid, hollow, venous cannulation device identified by its plastic "wings" that act as anchoring points for securing the catheter.
caladium: A common houseplant that contains calcium oxalate crystals; ingestion leads to nausea, vomiting, and diarrhea.
calcaneus: The heel bone; the largest of the tarsal bones.
calcitonin: Hormone secreted by the thyroid gland that helps maintain normal calcium levels in the blood.
calorie: The amount of heat needed to raise the temperature of 1 gram of water by 1°C; the amount of energy that can be obtained from the nutrients taken in through the diet; also called a kilocalorie.
candidiasis: A vaginal infection that is not technically a sexually transmitted infection; it can occur in pregnant and nonpregnant females, but is more common in pregnancy; also called thrush or a yeast infection.
cannulation: The insertion of a catheter into a body cavity, duct, or vessel to allow for fluid flow.
cape cyanosis: Deep cyanosis of the face and neck that extends across the chest and back; associated with little or no blood flow; a particularly ominous sign.
capillary refill time: A test performed on the fingernails or toenails that involves briefly squeezing the toenail or fingernail and evaluating the time it takes for the color to return.
capnographer: A device that attaches between the endotracheal tube and the ventilation device; provides graphic information about the presence of exhaled carbon dioxide.
capnography: The use of a noninvasive diagnostic tool that can quickly and efficiently provide information on a patient's ventilatory and circulatory status with a graphic and digital depiction similar to an electrocardiogram.
capnometer: A device that performs the same function and attaches in the same way as a capnographer but provides a digital reading of the exhaled carbon dioxide.
capnometry: The use of a capnometer, which is a monitoring device used to measure amount of expired carbon dioxide. The reading is usually given as a digital reading.
carbohydrates: Substances (including sugars and starches) that provide much of the energy required by the body's cells and help build cell structures.

carbon monoxide oximeter: A device that measures absorption at several wavelengths to distinguish oxyhemoglobin from carboxyhemoglobin.

carboxyhemoglobin (COHb): Hemoglobin loaded with carbon monoxide.

cardiac arrest: The cessation of cardiac mechanical activity, as confirmed by the absence of signs of circulation; also called cardiopulmonary arrest.

cardiac cycle: The period from one cardiac contraction to the next. Each cardiac cycle consists of ventricular contraction (systole) and relaxation (diastole).

cardiac tamponade: A condition in which the atria and right ventricle are collapsed by a collection of blood or other fluid within the pericardial sac, resulting in diminished cardiac output.

cardiogenic shock: A condition caused by loss of 40% or more of the functioning myocardium; the heart cannot circulate enough blood to maintain adequate peripheral oxygen delivery.

cardiovascular disease (CVD): A group of disorders of the heart and blood vessels.

carina: A ridgelike projection of tracheal cartilage located where the trachea bifurcates into the right and left main stem bronchi.

carpal bones: The eight small bones of the wrist.

carpopedal spasm: A contorted position in which the fingers or toes flex in a clawlike manner; may result from hyperventilation or hypocalcemia.

carriers: People who harbor an infectious agent and, although not personally ill, can pass the disease to others through their blood and through sexual contact.

cartilaginous joints: Joints connected by hyaline cartilage, or fibrocartilage, such as the joints that separate the vertebrae.

case study: A type of research in which a single case is investigated and documented over a specified period.

castor bean: A seed that contains the poison ricin. Its ingestion causes a variety of toxic effects: burning of the mouth and throat; nausea, vomiting, diarrhea, and severe stomach pains; prostration; failing vision; and kidney failure, which is the usual cause of death.

catabolism: The breakdown of larger molecules into smaller ones.

cataract: A clouding of the lens of the eye that is normally a result of aging.

catatonic: Lacking expression or movement, or appearing rigid.

catecholamines: Amine substances such as dopamine, epinephrine, and norepinephrine that function as neurotransmitters, hormones, or both.

catheter shear: An event in which a needle is reinserted into the catheter and slices through the catheter, creating a free-floating segment.

caustics: Chemicals that are acids or alkalis; cause direct chemical injury to the tissues they contact.

cell-mediated immunity: The immune process by which T cell lymphocytes (1) recognize antigens and then secrete cytokines (specifically lymphokines) that attract other cells or (2) become cytotoxic cells themselves and kill infected or abnormal cells.

cell membrane: The cell wall; a selectively permeable layer that surrounds the intracellular contents and controls movement of substances into and out of the cell; also called the cytoplasmic membrane or plasma membrane.

cell phones: Wireless telephones that communicate via radio waves with the telephone system through an interconnected network of repeater stations called cells.

cellular respiration: A biochemical process resulting in the production of energy in the form of adenosine triphosphate.

Celsius scale: A scale for measuring temperature, where water freezes at 0° and boils at 100°.

central nervous system (CNS): The brain and spinal cord.

central shock: A type of shock caused by central pump failure, including cardiogenic shock and obstructive shock.

cerebellum: Area of the brain involved in fine and gross muscle coordination; responsible for interpretation of actual movement and correction of any movements that interfere with coordination and the body's position.

cerebral cortex: The outer covering of gray matter that covers the cerebral hemispheres; regulates voluntary skeletal movement and plays an important role in the individual's level of awareness.

cerebral perfusion pressure (CPP): Pressure inside the cerebral arteries and an indicator of brain perfusion; calculated by subtracting intracranial pressure from mean arterial pressure.

cerebrospinal fluid (CSF): Fluid produced in the ventricles of the brain that flows in the subarachnoid space and bathes the meninges.

cerebrospinal rhinorrhea: Blood or cerebrospinal fluid drainage from the nose.

cerebrum: The largest part of the brain; made up of several lobes that control movement, hearing, balance, speech, visual perception, emotions, and personality; divided into right and left hemispheres; also called gray matter.

certification: A process in which a person, an institution, or a program is evaluated and recognized as meeting certain predetermined standards to provide safe and ethical care.

cerumen: Earwax.

cervical canal: The interior of the cervix.

cervix: The narrowest portion (lower third of the neck) of the uterus that opens into the vagina.

chalazion: A small, usually painless lump or pustule on the external eyelid that appears red and swollen, and that forms because of blockage and swelling of an oil gland in the eyelid.

chancre: The primary hard lesion or ulcer of syphilis that occurs at the entry site of the infection.

chancroid: A highly contagious sexually transmitted infection caused by the bacteria *Haemophilus ducreyi*, which causes painful sores (ulcers), usually of the genitals.

CHARTE method: A narrative writing method that allows the narrative to be broken down into logical sections similar to the steps of the patient assessment; components include chief complaint, history (ie, history of the event as well as patient medical history), assessment, treatment, transport, and exceptions.

chelating agents: Medications that bind with heavy metals in the body and create a compound that can be eliminated; used in cases of ingestion or poisoning.

chemical mediators: Chemicals that work to cause the immune or allergic response; for example, histamine.

chemical restraint: The use of medication to subdue a patient.

chemical suicide: A method of suicide that involves mixing certain household chemicals in an enclosed space to create toxic gases, such as hydrogen sulfide and hydrogen cyanide, as the chemicals combine; also called detergent suicide.

chemoreceptors: Sense organs that monitor the levels of oxygen and carbon dioxide and the pH of cerebrospinal fluid and blood; they provide feedback to the respiratory centers to modify the rate and depth of breathing based on the body's needs at any given time.

chemotaxins: Components of the activated complement system that attract leukocytes from the circulation to help fight infections.
chemotaxis: The movement of polymorphonuclear neutrophils toward the site of inflammation in response to chemotactic factors released by bacteria or formed from activated complement, chemokines, or arachidonic acid derivatives (such as leukotrienes) in response to cell injury.
chest compression fraction: The period during which compressions are delivered divided by the total time of the resuscitation attempt.
Cheyne-Stokes respirations: A gradually increasing rate and depth of respirations followed by a gradual decrease with intermittent periods of apnea; associated with brainstem insult.
chief complaint: The reason the patient is seeking help.
chikungunya: A virus that originated in Africa and is transmitted by the *Aedes aegypti* mosquito; signs and symptoms include fever that typically lasts from 5 to 7 days, and possibly incapacitating joint pain.
chlamydia: A sexually transmitted infection caused by the bacterium *Chlamydia trachomatis*, which is the most frequently reported sexually transmitted infection; signs and symptoms include inflammation of the urethra, epididymis, cervix, and fallopian tubes, and discharge from the urethra.
cholangitis: Inflammation of the bile duct.
cholecystitis: Inflammation of the gallbladder.
cholelithiasis: The presence of stones within the gallbladder.
cholinergic: Having the characteristics of the parasympathetic division of the autonomic nervous system; also refers to other structures or functions that are related to acetylcholine.
chordae tendineae: Thin bands of fibrous tissue that attach to the atrioventricular valves in the heart and prevent them from inverting.
choroid: The vascular, pigmented middle layer of the eye wall.
choroid plexus: Group of specialized cells in the ventricles of the brain; filters blood through cerebral capillaries to create cerebrospinal fluid.
chromosomes: Structures formed from condensed fibers and protein of deoxyribonucleic acid; these threadlike structures are found in the nucleus of the cells.
chronic bronchitis: A chronic inflammatory condition affecting the bronchi that is characterized by excessive mucus production as a result of overgrowth of the mucous glands in the airways.
chronic kidney disease (CKD): Progressive and irreversible inadequate kidney function caused by the permanent loss of nephrons.
chronotropic effect: Related to the effect of the rate of contraction of the heart.
ciliary body: The structure associated with the choroid layer of the eye that secretes aqueous humor and contains the ciliary muscle.
circulatory system: The complex arrangement of connected tubes, including the arteries, arterioles, capillaries, venules, and veins, that moves blood, oxygen, nutrients, carbon dioxide, and cellular waste throughout the body.
circumflex artery (Cx): One of the two branches of the left main coronary artery; branches of the Cx supply the left atrium, part of the lateral surface of the left ventricle, the inferior surface of the left ventricle in approximately 15% of people, the posterior surface of the left ventricle in 15%, the sinoatrial node in approximately 40%, and the atrioventricular bundle in 10% to 15%.
circumflex coronary artery: One of two branches of the left main coronary artery.
circumstantial thinking: Situation in which the patient includes many irrelevant details in an account of things.
cirrhosis: Early failure of the liver; characterized by portal hypertension, coagulation deficiencies, and diminished detoxification.
citric acid cycle: A sequence of enzymatic reactions involving the metabolism of carbon chains of glucose, fatty acids, and amino acids to yield carbon dioxide, water, and high-energy phosphate bonds; also known as the Krebs cycle or tricarboxylic acid cycle.
civil lawsuit: An action instituted by a person or entity against another person or entity.
claudication: Pain, cramping, muscle tightness, fatigue, or weakness of the legs during physical activity as a result of increased oxygen demand by the muscle tissue of the legs, hips, and buttocks.
clear text: Using regular language (plain English) and accepted terms to enhance clarity of communication, rather than using ten-codes or other code systems.
clitoris: A small, cylindrical mass of erectile tissue and nerves located at the anterior junction of the labia minora, similar to the glans penis of the male.
clonic activity: Type of seizure movement involving the contraction and relaxation of muscle groups.
closed-ended question: A question that is specific and focused, requiring either a yes or no answer, or an answer chosen from specific options; this type of question is helpful for patients who report shortness of breath.
clotting cascade: A set of interactions that lead to the formation of a fibrin clot; also called the coagulation cascade.
clotting factors: Substances in the blood that are necessary for clotting; also called coagulation factors.
coagulation system: A system that serves a vital role in the formation of blood clots in blood vessels. Inflammation triggers the coagulation cascade, initiating a complex series of reactions that encourage fibrin formation.
coagulopathy: Any type of bleeding disorder that interferes with the activation or continuation of the clotting cascade or hemostasis.
cocaine: A stimulant; a naturally occurring alkaloid that is extracted from the leaves of the *Erythroxylon coca* plant, which is found in South America.
cochlea: The portion of the inner ear that has hearing receptors.
cohort research: A type of research that examines patterns of change, a sequence of events, or trends over time within a certain population of study subjects.
collagen vascular diseases: A group of autoimmune disorders that affect the collagen in tendons, bones, and connective tissues.
colloid solutions: Solutions that contain molecules (usually proteins) that are too large to pass out of the capillary membranes and, therefore, remain in the vascular compartment.
colonized: A pathogen is present but has produced no illness in the host; often progresses to active infection. A colonized host is often called a *carrier* because the host can transmit the pathogen to others.
colorimetric carbon dioxide detector: A device that attaches between the endotracheal tube and the ventilation device; uses special paper that should turn from purple to yellow during exhalation, indicating the presence of exhaled carbon dioxide.
coma: A state in which a person does not respond to either verbal or painful stimuli.
combining form: A word root, prefix, or suffix followed by a vowel.
combining vowel: The vowel used to combine two word roots or a word root and a prefix or suffix.

common law: A decision that a judge has made through a court case based on interpretation of statutes and constitutions; it can be overturned either by another court with a higher authority or the issuing court at a later time. Also called case law.

common reality: Sensory stimulation that can be verified by others.

communicable disease: An infectious disease that can be transmitted from one person to another by direct contact or by indirect contact through a vector or fomite; also called contagious disease.

communicable period: The period during which an infected person can transmit a communicable disease to someone else.

comorbidity: The existence of two or more chronic diseases or conditions in a patient.

compassion fatigue: Also known as secondary stress disorder; a disorder characterized by gradual lessening of compassion over time.

competitive antagonists: Medications that temporarily bind with cellular receptor sites, displacing agonist chemicals.

competitive depolarizing: A term used to describe paralytic agents that act at the neuromuscular junction by binding with nicotinic receptors on muscles, causing fasciculations and preventing additional activation by acetylcholine.

complement system: A group of plasma proteins that attract white blood cells to sites of inflammation, activate white blood cells, and directly destroy cells.

compound: A substance that can be broken down into the two or more elements contained within it.

compound words: Words containing more than one word root.

compulsions: Repetitive actions carried out to relieve the anxiety of obsessive thoughts.

computer-assisted dispatch (CAD): Linked dispatch center computer consoles and vehicle-mounted mobile data terminals.

concentration: The total weight of a drug contained in a specific volume of liquid.

concept formation: Pattern of understanding based on initially obtained information; the first stage of the critical thinking process in prehospital care.

concordant precordial pattern: An electrocardiographic pattern in which the QRS complexes are all in the same direction in the precordial leads as a result of improper lead placement, anterior wall myocardial infarction, ventricular tachycardia, or other variables.

conductivity: The property that allows a cardiac cell to receive an electrical impulse and pass it on to an adjoining cardiac cell.

cones: One of the two kinds of photoreceptors within the retina that can distinguish colors; it requires a greater amount of light to activate and create an image.

confabulation: The invention of experiences to cover gaps in memory, seen in patients with certain organic brain syndromes.

confrontation: Act of pointing out something of interest in the patient's conversation or behavior, thereby directing the patient's attention to something.

conjunctivae: The membranous coverings on the anterior surface of the eye, and which also line the eyelids.

conjunctivitis: An inflammation of the conjunctivae that usually is caused by bacteria, viruses, allergies, or foreign bodies; should be considered highly contagious if infectious in origin; also called pinkeye.

connective tissues: Tissues that bind, support, protect, frame, and fill body structures; they also store fat, produce blood cells, repair tissues, and protect against infection.

consent: Agreement by the patient to accept a medical intervention.

contact precautions: The use of precautions (gloves, gown, and cleaning of high-touch items) to prevent contact transmission; used for patients presenting with draining wounds, multidrug-resistant infection, lice, norovirus, or Ebola.

contact transmission: The transmission of an infectious agent through direct or indirect contact with the infected persons, such as skin-to-skin contact or contact with the patient's environment and/or equipment.

contaminated: The presence of blood or other potentially infectious materials on an item or surface.

contaminated stick: The puncturing of an emergency care provider's skin with a needle or catheter that was used on a patient.

contiguous leads: Leads that view geographically similar areas of the myocardium, such as leads II, III, and aVF; useful for localizing areas of ischemia.

continuous positive airway pressure (CPAP): A method of ventilation that delivers a single pressure; used primarily in the treatment of critically ill patients with respiratory distress and can prevent the need for endotracheal intubation.

continuous quality improvement (CQI): A system of internal and external reviews and audits of all aspects of an EMS system.

contractility: The ability of myocardial cells to shorten in response to an impulse, which results in contraction.

contraindications: Any conditions, especially any diseases, that render some particular line of treatment improper or undesirable.

contralateral: On the opposite side of the body.

contributory negligence: Act(s) committed by a plaintiff that contribute to adverse outcomes.

convenience sampling: A type of research in which subjects are manually assigned to a specific person or crew, rather than being randomly assigned; the least-preferred component of research.

conventional reasoning: A type of reasoning in which a child looks for approval from peers and society.

conversion hysteria: A reaction in which a person subconsciously transforms their anxiety into a bodily dysfunction; the person may be unable to see or hear or may become partially paralyzed.

cookbook medicine: Blindly following a protocol or algorithm without thinking about what is being done and whether it is working.

Cormack-Lehane classification: A system used to predict intubation difficulty based on the airway structures observed during laryngoscopy.

cornea: The transparent anterior portion of the eye that overlies the iris and pupil.

corneal reflex: A protective movement that results in blinking, moving the head posteriorly, and pupillary constriction.

coronal (frontal) plane: An imaginary plane in which the body is cut into front and back portions.

coronary arteries: The blood vessels that supply blood to the tissues of the heart.

coronary artery disease (CAD): A pathologic process characterized by progressive atherosclerotic narrowing and eventual obstruction of the coronary arteries.

coronary heart disease (CHD): Disease of the coronary arteries and its associated signs, symptoms, and complications, such as angina pectoris and acute myocardial infarction.

coronary sinus: Venous drain for the coronary circulation into the right atrium.

coronavirus: Any of a group of RNA viruses that cause a variety of respiratory, gastrointestinal, and neurologic diseases in humans and other animals.

cor pulmonale: Heart disease that develops because of chronic lung disease and affects primarily the right side of the heart.

corpus callosum: A deep bridge of nerve fibers connecting the brain hemispheres.
corticosteroids: Hormones that regulate the body's metabolism, the balance of salt and water in the body, the immune system, and sexual function; any of several steroids secreted by the adrenal gland.
cortisol: A glucocorticoid released by the middle adrenal cortex that influences protein and fat metabolism and stimulates synthesis of glucose from noncarbohydrates. This hormone stimulates most body cells to increase their energy production.
couplet: Two consecutive (paired) premature ventricular complexes.
covert behaviors: Behaviors that have a hidden meaning or intention that only the person understands.
crackles: Abnormal breath sounds produced as fluid-filled alveoli pop open under increasing inspiratory pressure; can be fine or coarse; formerly called rales.
cranial nerves: The 12 pairs of nerves that arise from the base of the brain.
cranial vault: The bones that encase and protect the brain, including the parietal, temporal, frontal, occipital, sphenoid, and ethmoid bones; the roof of the skull (cranium).
cranium: The area of the head above the ears and eyes; the part of the skull that houses the brain.
credentialing: The process of obtaining, verifying, and assessing a practitioner's qualifications to provide care for a specific health care agency.
crepitus: A grating sensation caused when two pieces of broken bone rub together or subcutaneous emphysema is palpated.
crew resource management (CRM): An operational practice designed to enhance communication and teamwork, and to thereby reduce preventable errors.
cribriform plate: A horizontal bone perforated with numerous openings for the passage of the olfactory nerve filaments from the nasal cavity.
cricoid cartilage: A firm ridge of cartilage that forms the lower part of the larynx; the first ring of the trachea and the only upper airway structure that forms a complete ring; also called the cricoid ring.
cricothyroid membrane: A thin sheet of fascia located between the thyroid and cricoid cartilage that is relatively avascular and contains few nerves; the site for emergency access to the airway.
criminal prosecution: An action instituted by the government against a person for violation of criminal law.
critical incident: An event that overwhelms the ability to cope with the experience, either at the scene or later.
critical incident stress management (CISM): A process that utilizes trained counselors who confront responses to critical incidents and help to defuse them, directing emergency services personnel toward physical and emotional equilibrium.
Crohn disease: Inflammation of the ileum and possibly other portions of the gastrointestinal tract, in which the immune system attacks portions of the intestinal walls, causing them to become scarred, narrowed, stiff, and weakened.
cross section: The product of slicing an object crosswise, perpendicular to its long axis.
cross-sectional design: A data collection method in which all data at one point in time are collected, essentially serving as a "snapshot" of events and information.
cross-tolerance: A process in which repeated exposure to a medication within a particular class causes a tolerance that may be "transferred" to other medications in the same class.
croup: A common disease of infancy and childhood caused by upper airway obstruction and characterized by stridor, hoarseness, and a barking cough.
crystalloid solutions: Solutions of dissolved crystals (eg, salts or sugars) in water; contain compounds that quickly dissociate in solution.
cultural competence: An understanding of the predominant cultures that exist in the geographic area in which the paramedic provides patient care.
cultural intelligence: Ability to function effectively across various cultural contexts, interacting with people of all nationalities and getting along with those of all ethnic, political, and generational differences.
culture: The system of beliefs, attitudes, and behaviors that are learned and shared by members of a group.
cumulative action: Several smaller doses of a particular medication capable of producing the same clinical effects as a single larger dose of that same medication.
cumulative stress reaction: Prolonged or excessive stress.
current health status: A composite picture of a number of factors in a patient's life, such as dietary habits, current medications, allergies, exercise, alcohol or tobacco use, recreational drug use, sleep patterns and disorders, and immunizations.
curved laryngoscope blade: A blade designed to fit into the vallecula, indirectly lifting the epiglottis and exposing the vocal cords; also called the Macintosh blade.
Cushing reflex: The combination of a slowing pulse, rising blood pressure, and an erratic respiratory pattern; a grave sign for patients with head trauma or cerebrovascular accident.
Cushing syndrome: A condition caused by overproduction of cortisol by the adrenal glands or by excessive use of cortisol or other similar corticosteroid (glucocorticoid) hormones.
cyanosis: A blue-gray skin color that is caused by inadequate levels of oxygen in the blood.
cystitis: Infection caused by bacteria that travel from the perineum, through the genital tract, into the urethral opening; also called bladder infection.
cytochrome P-450 system: A hemoprotein involved in the detoxification of many drugs.
cytokines: The products of cells that affect the function of other cells.
cytoplasm: The gellike material that fills out a cell and in which the organelles are suspended; it makes up most of the volume of the cell.
D_5W: An intravenous solution made up of 5% dextrose in water.
damages: Compensation for injury awarded by a court.
data interpretation: The process of reaching conclusions based on comparing the patient's presentation with information from your training, education, and past experiences; the second stage of the critical thinking process in prehospital care.
decerebrate posturing: Abnormal extension of the arms with rotation of the wrists along with the toes pointed; this finding indicates brainstem damage.
decision-making capacity: The patient's ability to understand and process the information given and the proposed treatment plan.
decorticate posturing: Abnormal flexion of the arms toward the chest with the toes pointed; this finding indicates lower cerebral damage.
deep: Farther inside the body and away from the skin.
deep fascia: A dense layer of fibrous tissue below the subcutaneous tissue; composed of tough bands of tissue that surround muscles and other internal structures.

defamation: Intentionally making a false statement, through written or verbal communication, that injures a person's good name or reputation.

defendant: In a civil lawsuit, the person against whom a legal action is brought.

defense mechanisms: Psychological ways to relieve stress, which are usually automatic or subconscious; they include denial, regression, projection, and displacement.

defibrillation: The use of an unsynchronized direct current electric shock to terminate ventricular fibrillation or pulseless ventricular tachycardia.

dehydration: Depletion of the body's systemic fluid volume.

delayed sequence intubation (DSI): A procedure in which a patient is sedated for the purpose of preoxygenation prior to the administration of a paralytic agent and intubation.

delayed stress reaction: Reaction to stress that occurs after a stressful situation.

delirium: An acute confusional state characterized by global impairment of thinking, perception, judgment, and memory.

delirium tremens (DTs): A severe withdrawal syndrome seen in people with alcohol use disorder who are deprived of ethyl alcohol; characterized by restlessness, fever, sweating, disorientation, agitation, and seizures; can be fatal if untreated.

delta wave: The slurring of the upstroke of the first part of the QRS complex that occurs in Wolff-Parkinson-White syndrome.

delusions: Thoughts, ideas, or perceived abilities that have no basis in common reality.

dementia: A chronic process that produces severe deficits in memory, abstract thinking, and judgment.

dendrites: Branchlike projections of nerve cells that receive impulses or sensory information from nearby cells and conduct impulses toward the nerve cell body.

dengue: A virus transmitted by the mosquitos *Aedes aegypti* and *Aedes albopictus*, found throughout the world. The majority of people with dengue are asymptomatic; if the severe form develops, it is characterized by hemorrhage, hypovolemic shock, and potentially death.

denial: An early response to a serious medical emergency, in which the severity of the emergency is diminished or minimized. Denial is the first coping mechanism for people who believe they are going to die.

denitrogenation: The process of replacing nitrogen in the lungs with oxygen to maintain a normal oxygen saturation level during intubation.

dental abscess: A dental infection that occurs when bacterial growth spreads directly from the cavity into the gums, facial tissue, bones, and/or neck.

dentalgia: Toothache.

deoxyribonucleic acid (DNA): Specialized structure within the cell that carries genetic material for reproduction.

dependence: The physical, behavioral, or emotional need for a medication or chemical to maintain "normal" physiologic function.

depolarization: In response to an action potential, the rapid movement of electrolytes across a cell membrane that changes the overall charge of the cell. This rapid shifting of electrolytes and cellular charges is the main catalyst for muscle contractions and neural transmissions.

depolarizing neuromuscular blocker: A drug that competitively binds with acetylcholine receptor sites but is not affected as quickly by acetylcholinesterase; an example is succinylcholine chloride.

depressant: A chemical or medication that decreases the performance of the central nervous system or sympathetic nervous system.

depression: A mental health disorder characterized by a persistent mood of sadness, despair, and discouragement; it may be a symptom of many different mental and physical disorders, or it may be a disorder on its own.

dermatome: An area of the body innervated by sensor components of spinal nerves.

descending aorta: The portion of the aorta that extends through the thorax and abdomen into the pelvis.

descriptive: A research format in which an observation of an event is made, but without attempts to alter or change it.

designated infection control officer (DICO): A person charged with ensuring that proper postexposure medical treatment and counseling are provided to an exposed employee or volunteer.

desired dose: The amount of a drug that the physician orders for a patient; the drug order.

despair phase: The second phase of an infant's response to a situational crisis; characterized by monotonous wailing.

diabetes: A group of complex metabolic disorders with many causes; includes diabetes mellitus, gestational diabetes, hypoglycemia/hyperglycemia, diabetic ketoacidosis, and hyperosmolar hyperglycemic syndrome.

diabetes insipidus (DI): A relatively uncommon disorder that has some of the same characteristics as diabetes, such as polyuria and polydipsia, in which the body is unable to regulate fluid because of a lack of antidiuretic hormone (central diabetes insipidus) or the kidneys are unable to respond appropriately (nephrogenic diabetes insipidus).

diabetes mellitus: Disease characterized by the body's inability to sufficiently metabolize glucose; occurs either because the pancreas does not produce enough insulin or because the cells do not respond to the effects of the insulin that is produced.

diabetic ketoacidosis (DKA): A form of acidosis in uncontrolled diabetes in which certain acids accumulate when insulin is not available.

diabetic retinopathy: A condition associated with diabetes, in which the small blood vessels of the retina are affected; it can eventually lead to blindness.

diagnosis: The identification of a disease based on its signs and symptoms.

diapedesis: A process whereby leukocytes move through the wall of a capillary and out to the tissues where they are needed most.

diaphoresis: Excessive sweating; it is often associated with shock.

diaphragm: Large skeletal muscle that plays a major role in breathing and separates the chest cavity from the abdominal cavity.

diaphysis: The shaft of a long bone.

diarrhea: Liquid stool.

diastole: Phase of the cardiac cycle in which the atria and ventricles relax between contractions and blood enters these chambers.

diastolic pressure: The result of residual pressure in the circulatory system while the left ventricle is relaxing (ie, in diastole).

dieffenbachia: A common houseplant that is also called dumb cane; ingestion leads to burns of the mouth and tongue and, possibly, paralysis of the vocal cords and nausea and vomiting; in severe cases, edema of the tongue and larynx may occur, leading to airway compromise.

diencephalon: Portion of the brain between the brainstem and cerebrum; contains the epithalamus, the thalamus, the hypothalamus, and the subthalamus.

differential diagnosis: The process of weighing the probability of one disease versus other diseases by comparing clinical findings that could account for a patient's illness; also refers to the list of possible conditions considered based on the patient's signs and symptoms.

differentiation: The process of specialization of a cell.

diffusion: The process of particles moving from an area of higher concentration to an area of lower concentration along a concentration gradient until equilibrium is achieved.

digestion: The mechanical and chemical breakdown of the large molecules in food into small molecules that can be absorbed in the gastrointestinal tract and converted to energy for cellular function.

digitalis preparations: Drugs used in the treatment of heart failure and certain atrial dysrhythmias.

digital radio: The transmission of information via radio waves using native digital (computer) data or analog (voice) signals that have been converted to a digital signal and compressed.

diluent: A solution (usually water or normal saline) used for diluting a medication.

diploid cells: Cells that carry two of each of the 23 chromosomes—one from the father and one from the mother.

diplopia: Double vision.

direct contact: Exposure to or transmission of a communicable disease from one person to another by physical contact.

direct laryngoscopy: Visualization of the airway with a laryngoscope.

disequilibrium syndrome: A condition characterized by nausea, vomiting, headache, and confusion, which results when dialysis causes water to initially shift from the bloodstream into the cerebrospinal fluid, mildly increasing intracranial pressure.

disinfectants: Chemicals used on nonliving objects to kill organisms; they are toxic to living tissues.

disorganization: A condition in which a person demonstrates uncontrolled and disconnected thoughts, is usually incoherent or rambling in speech, and may or may not be oriented to person and place.

disorientation: A condition in which a person may be confused about person, place, or time; one of the ways in which conditions such as schizophrenia or organic brain syndrome may present.

dispatch: To send to a specific destination or to send on a task.

displacement: A defense mechanism characterized by redirection of an emotion from one person to another.

dissection: The process by which the intimal and medial layers of a vessel separate (dissect) after a tear occurs in an aneurysmal portion of the arterial wall. With each ventricular systole, a jet of blood is forced into the torn arterial wall, creating and propagating a false channel.

disseminated intravascular coagulation (DIC): A condition that begins with widespread activation of the clotting cascade, which depletes the clotting factors and platelets, and eventually results in uncontrolled hemorrhage.

dissociative anesthetic: A medication that distorts perception of sights and sounds and induces a feeling of detachment from their environment and self.

distal: Farther from the trunk and nearer to the free end of the extremity.

distal convoluted tubule (DCT): Connects with the kidney's collecting tubules.

distal traction: Gentle downward or lateral traction on the skin.

distribution: The movement and transportation of a medication throughout the bloodstream to tissues and cells and, ultimately, to its target receptor.

distributive shock: A type of shock caused by widespread dilation of the resistance vessels (small arterioles), the capacitance vessels (small venules), or both.

diuresis: The production of large amounts of urine by the kidney.

diuretic: A chemical that increases urinary output.

diverticulitis: Inflammation of pouches in the colon; these pouches form as a result of difficulty moving feces through the colon. Bacteria can become trapped in the pouches, leading to inflammation and infection.

diverticulum: A weak area in the colon that begins to have small outcroppings that turn into pouches; plural is diverticula.

do not resuscitate (DNR) order: A type of advance directive that describes which life-sustaining procedures should be performed in the event of a sudden deterioration in the patient's medical condition.

dorsal respiratory group (DRG): The portion of the medulla oblongata that functions as a respiratory integration center; it receives input from several sources including the pontine respiratory group, the glossopharyngeal and vagus nerves, central chemoreceptors in the medulla, and peripheral chemoreceptors.

dorsal: The posterior surface of the body, including the back of the hand.

dose-response curve: A graphic illustration of the response of a drug according to the dose administered.

dosing: The specified amount of a medication to be given at specific intervals.

double documentation: The act of documenting the care and treatment provided at an incident more than once, which increases the risk of errors and inconsistencies.

down-regulation: The process in which a mechanism reducing available cell receptors for a particular medication results in tolerance.

drip chamber: The area of the administration set where fluid accumulates so that the tubing remains filled with fluid.

droplet precautions: Use of a surgical mask on the patient and airborne precautions to prevent droplet transmission; used for patients with possible influenza, meningitis, pertussis (whooping cough), mumps, rubella (German measles), Ebola, and COVID-19; also called "source control."

droplet transmission: The transmission of an infectious agent through exposure to large and small droplets and particles generated when an infected person coughs or sneezes, which generally travel 6 feet (2 m) or less before falling to the ground.

drug: A substance that has some therapeutic effect (such as reducing inflammation, fighting bacteria, or producing euphoria) when given in the appropriate circumstances and in the appropriate dose.

drug addiction: A chronic disorder characterized by the compulsive use of a substance that results in physical, psychological, or social harm to the user who continues to use the substance despite the harm.

drug class: The grouping to which a medication belongs. Medications are grouped according to their characteristics, traits, or primary components.

drug misuse: Any use of drugs that causes physical, psychological, economic, legal, or social harm to the user or others affected by the user's behavior.

drug reconstitution: Injecting sterile water or saline from one vial into another vial containing a powdered form of the drug.

due process: The right to a fair procedure for a legal action against a person or agency. It has two components: notice and opportunity to be heard.

DUMBELS: An acronym that represents the symptoms of organophosphate poisoning: Diarrhea, Urination, Miosis,

Bradycardia/Bronchospasm/Bronchorrhea, Emesis, Lacrimation, and Seizures/Salivation/Sweating.

duplex: Radio system using paired frequencies to permit the use of remote repeaters or simultaneous transmission and reception.

dura mater: The outermost layer of the three meninges that enclose the brain and spinal cord; the toughest meningeal layer.

duration (of action): In a pharmacologic context, the time a medication concentration can be expected to remain above the minimum level needed to provide the intended action.

duty: Legal obligation of public and certain other ambulance services to respond to a call for help in their jurisdiction.

dysconjugate gaze: Paralysis of gaze or lack of coordination between the movements of the two eyes.

dysfunctional uterine bleeding: Uterine bleeding that is abnormal in amount or frequency (more than every 21 days).

dyslipidemia: An excessive level of lipids (fats) circulating in the blood, which increases the risk of atherosclerosis and coronary artery disease.

dysphagia: Pain, discomfort, or difficulty in swallowing.

dysphonia: Difficulty speaking.

dysplasia: An alteration in the size, shape, and organization of cells.

dyspnea: Difficult or labored breathing.

dysrhythmias: Cardiac rhythm disturbances.

dystonia: Contractions of body into bizarre positions.

dystonic: Pertaining to voluntary muscle movements that are distorted or impaired because of abnormal muscle tone.

early adults: People who are 19 to 40 years of age.

Ebola: A virus formerly limited to West Africa, which is spread through direct contact through nonintact skin or mucous membranes, and whose initial symptoms include fever, intense weakness, muscle pain, headaches, and sore throat; some infected people experience internal and external bleeding. Both contact and droplet precautions are needed with this disease.

ecchymosis: Localized bruising or collection of blood within or under the skin.

echolalia: Meaningless echoing of the interviewer's words by the patient.

ectopic: An impulse or rhythm that originates from a site other than the SA node.

ectopic foci: Sites of generation of electrical impulses other than normal pacemaker cells.

ectopic pregnancy: A pregnancy in which the fertilized oocyte implants somewhere other than the uterus.

edema: Swelling caused by excessive fluid trapped in the body tissues.

efficacy: In a pharmacologic context, the ability of a medication to produce the desired effect.

egophony: A test of decreased breath sounds performed by placing the diaphragm of the stethoscope over the area in question while the patient says a drawn-out "ee"; an "A" sound indicates lung consolidation.

electrical conduction system: In the heart, the specialized cardiac tissue that initiates and conducts electric impulses; includes the SA node, internodal conduction pathways, atrioventricular node, bundle of His, and the Purkinje network.

electrolytes: Salt or acid substances that become ionic conductors when dissolved in a solvent (such as water); chemicals dissolved in the blood.

elimination: In a pharmacologic context, the removal of a medication or its by-products from the body.

emancipated minor: A person who is younger than the legal age (generally 18 years) in a given state, but is legally considered an adult because of other circumstances.

embryo: A fertilized egg.

emergency medical dispatch (EMD): A system that assists dispatchers in selecting appropriate units to respond to a particular call for assistance and provides callers with vital instructions until the arrival of EMS crews.

emergency medical services (EMS): A health care system designed to bring immediate on-scene care to those in need, along with transport to a definitive medical care facility.

Emergency Medical Treatment and Active Labor Act (EMTALA): A federal law enacted in 1986 to combat the practice of patient dumping—that is, hospitals refusing to admit seriously ill patients or women in labor who could not pay, forcing EMS providers to dump the patients at another hospital. Issues are regulated by the Centers for Medicare and Medicaid Services, and the law carries severe monetary penalties—up to and including loss of Medicare funding—for hospitals and physicians that fail to comply.

emphysema: The infiltration of any tissue by air or gas; a chronic obstructive pulmonary disease characterized by distention of the alveoli and destructive changes in the lung parenchyma.

employee assistance program (EAP): A counseling program to help with situations that may affect the health and well-being of EMS professionals.

encoded radio signals: Embedded signals that allow multiple users to share frequencies and repeaters.

endemic: Consistently present or prevalent in a population or geographic area.

endocarditis: Inflammation of the endocardium as a result of infection.

endocardium: The thin membrane lining the inside of the heart.

endocrine glands: Glands that have no ducts and secrete directly into tissue fluid or blood.

endocrine system: The complex message and control system that integrates many body functions, including the release of hormones.

endogenous: Originating from within the organism (body).

endolymph: A fluid containing nerve receptors that resides inside the membranous labyrinth. Sound waves converted into pressure waves are transmitted through this fluid to the auditory nerves.

endometriosis: The presence of tissue outside the uterus that resembles the endometrium in both structure and function.

endometritis: An inflammation of the endometrium that often is associated with a bacterial infection.

endometrium: The inner layer of the uterine wall.

endotoxins: Toxins released by some bacteria when they die.

endotracheal (ET) intubation: Inserting an endotracheal tube through the glottic opening and sealing the tube with a cuff inflated against the tracheal wall.

endotracheal (ET) tube: A tube that is inserted into the trachea for definitive airway maintenance; equipped with a distal cuff, a proximal inflation port, a 15/22-mm adapter, and centimeter markings on the side.

end-stage renal disease (ESRD): A condition in which the kidneys are unable to function, and toxic waste materials build up in the patient's blood; occurs after acute or chronic kidney injury.

end-tidal carbon dioxide ($ETCO_2$) monitors: Devices that detect the presence of carbon dioxide in exhaled air.

enema: A fluid solution, possibly containing supplemental medications, that can be administered rectally to aid in a variety of gastrointestinal complications.

enhanced 9-1-1 systems: Emergency communications systems that collect information about 9-1-1 calls from the telephone network, such as the caller's phone number and location, and display this information on the computer dispatch terminal.

enteral medications: Medication administration that involves the medication passing through a portion of the gastrointestinal tract.

enteric nervous system (ENS): The subdivision of the autonomic nervous system that controls the digestive system.

***Enterococcus*:** A common, normal organism of the gastrointestinal tract, urinary tract, and genitourinary tract that can be pathogenic and become resistant to vancomycin.

enzymes: Substances designed to speed up the rate of specific biochemical reactions.

eosinophils: Leukocytes that may play a role following infection in various areas in the body.

epicardium: The layer of the serous pericardium that lies closely against the heart; also called the visceral pericardium.

epidemic: An illness or disease that affects or tends to affect a disproportionately large number of people within a specific population, community, or region at the same time.

epidemiologists: Public health professionals who investigate patterns and causes of disease and injury in a given population, and seek to reduce the risk, occurrence, and negative effects of these threats through research, public education, and legislative change.

epidemiology: A scientific field devoted to studying the distribution and determinants of health-related events and conditions in a population in an attempt to address health problems.

epididymitis: An infection that causes inflammation of the epididymis along the posterior border of the testis; a possible complication of male urinary tract infection.

epigastric: The region of the abdomen directly inferior to the xiphoid process and superior to the umbilicus.

epiglottis: A thin, flaplike cartilaginous structure that allows air to pass into the trachea but prevents food and liquid from entering it.

epiglottitis: An inflammation of the epiglottis.

epinephrine: A hormone produced by the adrenal medulla that has a vital role in the function of the sympathetic division of the autonomic nervous system; mediates the fight-or-flight response; also called adrenaline.

epiphyseal plate: The growth plate of a long bone; a major site of bone development during childhood; also called the physis.

epiphyses: The ends of a long bone.

epistaxis: Nosebleed.

epithelial tissues: Body tissues that cover organs, form the inner lining of cavities, and line hollow organs.

eponym: The name of a disease, device, procedure, or drug that is based on the person who invented, discovered, or first described it.

erythrocytes: Red blood cells.

esophagitis: An inflammation of the esophagus.

esophagogastric varices: Dilated blood vessels of the esophagus, commonly caused by difficulty in blood flow through the liver; the presence of these can lead to vessel rupture.

estrogen: A primary female hormone released from the ovaries that brings about secondary sex characteristics at puberty and stimulates the uterine lining during the menstrual cycle.

ethical: A behavior expected by a person or group following a set of rules.

ethics: A set of values in society that differentiates right from wrong.

ethnocentrism: Viewing other cultures based solely on the standards and values of one's own culture; a belief in the inherent superiority of one's own culture or ethnic group.

eustachian tube: A branch of the internal auditory canal that connects the middle ear to the oropharynx.

evaluation: Application of the appropriate methods, skills, and activities to determine whether a service or program is needed, likely to be used, conducted as planned, and actually helps people.

evidence-based practice: The use of practices that have been proven to be effective in improving patient outcomes; strongly relies on the reviewed literature but incorporates the provider's experience and training, and characteristics of the population.

excitability: The ability of cardiac muscle cells to respond to an electrical, chemical, or mechanical stimulus.

excited delirium: An acute confrontational state characterized by global impairment of thinking, perception, judgment, and memory.

exhalation: The passive part of the breathing process in which the diaphragm and the intercostal muscles relax, forcing air out of the lungs.

exocrine glands: Glands that secrete chemicals into ducts that open onto a surface for elimination.

exogenous: Originating outside the organism (body).

exophthalmos: Protrusion of the eyes from the normal position within the socket.

exotoxins: Toxins secreted by living cells to aid in the death and digestion of other cells.

expiratory reserve volume: The amount of air that can be exhaled following a normal exhalation; average volume is about 1,200 mL.

expressed consent: A type of informed consent that occurs when the patient does something, either through words (verbal or written) or by taking some sort of action, that demonstrates permission to provide emergency medical care.

extension: The straightening of a joint.

external jugular (EJ) vein: Large neck vein that is lateral to the carotid artery.

external rotation: Rotating an extremity at its joint away from the midline.

extracellular fluid (ECF): Fluid outside of the cell, which contains most of the body's supply of sodium; accounts for 15% to 20% of body weight.

extravasation: Seepage of blood and medication into the tissue surrounding the blood vessel.

extrinsic muscles: In the eye, these are the six muscles that attach to the exterior of the globe and are controlled by the cranial nerves.

extubation: The process of removing the endotracheal tube from an intubated patient.

EZ-IO: A handheld, battery-powered driver to which a special intraosseous needle is attached; used for insertion of the intraosseous needle into the proximal tibia of children and adults.

face-to-face intubation: Performing intubation at the same level as the patient's face; used when the standard position is not possible. In this position, the laryngoscope is held in the provider's right hand and the endotracheal tube in the left.

facilitated diffusion: The process of medication molecules binding with carrier proteins when no energy is expended.

factitious disorder: A disorder in which a person wishes to be sick and intentionally produces or feigns physical or psychological signs or symptoms. Symptoms are under voluntary control, with no obvious physiologic reason.

Fahrenheit scale: A scale for measuring temperature, where water freezes at 32° and boils at 212°.

fallopian tube: The anatomic structure that connects each ovary with the uterus and provides a passageway for the ova.

false imprisonment: Intentionally or unjustifiably detaining a person. Examples include transporting a patient without consent, or wrongfully using restraints.
fascia: A sheet or band of tough fibrous connective tissue that covers, supports, and separates muscles, and that also covers arteries, veins, tendons, and ligaments.
fascicular block (hemiblock): Failure of the anterior or posterior fascicles of the heart to conduct electrical impulses because of disease or ischemia.
fasciculations: Brief, uncoordinated twitching of small muscle groups in the face, neck, trunk, and extremities; may be seen after the administration of a depolarizing neuromuscular blocking agent (eg, succinylcholine chloride).
FAST devices: First Access for Shock and Trauma devices; manual sternal intraosseous devices used in patients age 12 years and older; include an infusion tube, subcutaneous portal, an introducer, a target/strain relief patch, and a protective dome.
Federal Communications Commission (FCC): The independent government agency that regulates interstate and international communications by radio, television, wire, satellite and cable in all 50 states, the District of Columbia, and US territories.
fibrin: A white, insoluble protein formed by the action of thrombin on fibrinogen during the blood clotting process; forms the matrix of a blood clot.
fibrinogen: A plasma protein that is important for blood clotting.
fibrinolysis: The process of dissolving blood clots.
fibrinolysis cascade: The breakdown of fibrin in blood clots and the prevention of the polymerization of fibrin into new clots.
fibrinolytic therapy: The use of medications that act to dissolve blood clots.
fibrous joints: Joints that lie between bones that closely contact each other, and are joined by thin, dense connective tissue.
field impression: A field conclusion about the patient's problem based on the clinical presentation and the exclusion of other possible causes through considering the differential diagnoses.
fight-or-flight response: A physiologic response to a profound stressor that helps a person deal with the situation at hand; features increased sympathetic tone and results in dilation of the pupils, increased heart rate, dilation of the bronchi, mobilization of glucose, shunting of blood away from the gastrointestinal tract and cerebrum, and increased blood flow to the skeletal muscles.
filtration: The movement of fluid from intravascular fluid under high pressure to interstitial fluid, which is generally under lower pressure.
first-degree AV block: A delay in the conduction of the depolarizing impulse from the sinoatrial node to the ventricles, prolonging the PR interval; also called first-degree heart block.
first-order elimination: The process in which the rate of elimination is directly influenced by plasma levels of a substance.
first-pass effect: The alteration of a medication via metabolism within the gastrointestinal tract before it reaches systemic circulation.
fistula: A surgically created connection between an artery and a vein, usually in the arm, for dialysis access; also, an abnormal connection between two cavities.
flash chamber: The area of an intravenous catheter that fills with blood to help indicate when a vein is cannulated.
flat affect: The absence of emotion; appearing to feel no emotion at all.
flexion: The bending of a joint.
flight of ideas: Accelerated thinking in which the mind skips very rapidly from one thought to the next.
fluid balance: The process of maintaining homeostasis through equal intake (water taken into the body) and output (water excreted from the body) of fluids.
focused exam: A type of physical exam that is typically performed on responsive patients who have sustained an isolated injury; it is based on the chief complaint and focuses on one body system or part.
fomites: Inanimate objects contaminated with microorganisms that serve as a means of transmitting an illness.
fontanelles: Sheets of tough connective tissue between the flat bones of the skull that soften and expand when the newborn passes through the birth canal; they are gradually replaced as the bones of the skull fuse together and form suture joints by age 2 years; also called soft spots.
Fournier gangrene: A condition that results from bacteria entering the skin of the scrotum or perineum, causing infection and subsequent necrosis of the subcutaneal tissue and muscle in the scrotum.
Fowler position: A sitting position, with the head elevated at a 90° angle (sitting straight upright).
foxglove: A plant that contains cardiac glycosides and is used in making digitalis; ingestion of leaves causes nausea, vomiting, diarrhea, abdominal cramps, hyperkalemia, and a variety of dysrhythmias.
fraction of inspired oxygen (FIO_2): The percentage of oxygen in inhaled air.
free radicals: Molecules that are missing one electron in their outer shell.
frequency: The number of oscillations (or cycles) per second of a radio signal.
full-body exam: A systematic head-to-toe exam performed during the secondary assessment of a patient who has sustained a significant mechanism of injury, is unresponsive, or is in critical condition.
fungi: Small organisms that can grow rapidly in the presence of the needed nutrients and organic material and can cause infection related to contact with decaying organic matter or from airborne spores in the environment such as molds; singular, *fungus.*
gag reflex: A normal neural reflex elicited by touching the soft palate or posterior pharynx; it leads to symmetric elevation of the palate, retraction of the tongue, and contraction of the pharyngeal muscles.
gait: Patterns of walking or ambulating.
gallstones: Stonelike masses in the gallbladder or its ducts caused by precipitation of substances contained in bile, such as cholesterol and bilirubin; also known as choleliths.
gastric distention: The enlargement or expansion of the stomach, often with air; can be a complication of ventilating the esophagus instead of the trachea.
gastric tube: A tube that is inserted into the stomach to decompress the stomach; can also be used to administer certain enteral medications.
gastritis: A preulcerative state in which the stomach is inflamed, but erosion has not yet occurred.
gastroenteritis: A term that comprises many types of infections and irritations of the gastrointestinal tract; symptoms include nausea and forceful vomiting, low-grade fever, abdominal pain, and diarrhea; also called stomach flu.
gastroesophageal reflux disease (GERD): A condition in which the sphincter between the esophagus and the stomach opens, allowing stomach acid to move superiorly; can cause a burning sensation within the chest (heartburn); also called acid reflux disease.

gauge: The internal diameter of an intravenous catheter or needle.

general adaptation syndrome: A three-stage reaction to stressors, either physical (such as injury) or emotional (such as loss of a loved one). The stages include alarm, resistance or adaptation, and exhaustion.

general impression: The overall initial impression that determines the priority of patient care; based on the patient's surroundings, the mechanism of injury, signs and symptoms, and the chief complaint.

generalized anxiety disorder (GAD): A disorder in which a person worries about everything for no particular reason, or in which the worrying is unproductive and the person cannot decide what to do about an upcoming situation.

general senses: Sensations monitored throughout the body by receptors scattered throughout many different tissues.

genital warts: Warts caused by the human papillomavirus, a sexually transmitted infection; also called condylomata acuminata or venereal warts.

genotype: The arrangement of a person's genes and their characteristics is based on the combination of alleles, for one gene or many.

geographic information system (GIS): Technology that uses global positioning system and other data to (1) track and predict ambulance response times, (2) determine the distance to the closest trauma center or other hospitals from specific locations, (3) track the frequency of motor vehicle crashes and the severity of injuries from different geographic locations, (4) determine the location of emergency helipads, and (5) provide other information useful in EMS system operations and planning.

gestational diabetes: Diabetes that develops during pregnancy in women who did not have diabetes before pregnancy.

Glasgow Coma Scale (GCS): An evaluation tool used to determine level of consciousness by evaluating and assigning point values (scores) for eye opening, verbal response, and motor response, which are then totaled; effective in helping predict patient outcomes.

glaucoma: A disease of the eye caused by an increase in intraocular pressure; when severe enough, it may damage the optic nerve and potentially cause permanent loss of vision.

globulins: Antibodies made by the liver or lymphatic tissues that represent approximately 36% of the plasma proteins.

glomerular (Bowman) capsule: A double-layered cup with the inner layer infiltrating and surrounding the capillaries of the glomerulus.

glottis: The true vocal cords and the opening between them.

glucagon: Hormone produced by the pancreas that is vital to the control of the body's metabolism and blood glucose level. Glucagon stimulates the breakdown of glycogen to glucose.

gluconeogenesis: A process that stimulates both the liver and the kidneys to produce glucose from noncarbohydrate molecules.

glycogen: A long polymer from which glucose is converted in the liver (animal starch).

glycogenolysis: The breakdown of glycogen to glucose.

glycolysis: Process by which glucose and other sugars are broken down to yield lactic acid (anaerobic glycolysis) or pyruvic acid (aerobic glycolysis). The breakdown releases energy in the form of adenosine triphosphate.

glycosuria: The passage of large quantities of urine containing glucose.

goiter: A visible mass in the anterior part of the neck caused by enlargement of the thyroid gland.

gonorrhea: A sexually transmitted infection that results in infection caused by the gonococcal bacterium *Neisseria gonorrhoeae*; signs and symptoms include pus-containing discharge from the urethra and painful urination in males, and signs and symptoms of an acute abdomen in females.

Good Samaritan law: A statute providing limited immunity from liability to people responding voluntarily and in good faith to the aid of an injured person outside the hospital.

gram-negative: A reaction of bacteria to a Gram stain in which the bacteria do not retain the dark purple stain; such bacteria have cell walls that consist largely of lipids, and have pathogenic qualities that make them especially problematic for humans.

gram-positive: A reaction of bacteria to a Gram stain in which the bacteria retain the dark purple stain; such bacteria have thick cell walls composed of many layers peptidoglycan (amino acids and glucose).

Graves disease: An autoimmune disorder that causes thyroid gland hypertrophy and severe hyperthyroidism.

gross negligence: Negligence that is willful, wanton, intentional, or reckless; a serious departure from the accepted standards.

growth plates: Structures located on either end of long bones, which are the centers of longitudinal bone growth during childhood.

gtt: A unit of measure that indicates drops.

guarding: Contraction of the abdominal muscles indicating peritoneal irritation.

Guillain-Barré syndrome: A disease of unknown cause characterized by progressive paralysis moving from the feet to the head (ascending paralysis); if paralysis reaches the diaphragm, the patient may require respiratory support.

gum bougie: A flexible device that is inserted between the glottis under direct laryngoscopy; the endotracheal tube is threaded over the device, facilitating its entry into the trachea. Also called a tracheal tube introducer.

habituation: A physical tolerance to the therapeutic and adverse clinical effects of a medication or chemical.

Haddon matrix: A framework developed by William Haddon, Jr, MD, as a method to generate ideas about injury prevention that address the host, agent, and environment and their impact in the pre-event, event, and post-event phases of the injury process.

half-life: The time needed in an average person for metabolism or elimination of 50% of a substance in the plasma.

hallucinations: Sensory perceptions not founded on objective reality; false perceptions.

hallucinogen: An agent that produces false perceptions in any one of the five senses.

hantavirus: A type of virus found in wild rodents, which can also cause disease in humans; characterized by fever, headache, abdominal pain, loss of appetite, and vomiting. Diseases caused include hemorrhagic fever with renal syndrome and hantavirus pulmonary syndrome.

haploid cells: Cells that carry genetic instructions via 23 individual chromosomes.

hapten: A substance that normally does not stimulate an immune response but can be combined with an antigen and, at a later time, initiate a specific antibody response on its own.

hard palate: The anterior portion of the palate that is supported by bone (primarily the maxillary bone).

Hashimoto disease: A type of hyperthyroidism in which the thyroid gland becomes enlarged as it is infiltrated by T lymphocytes and plasma cells.

head tilt–chin lift maneuver: Manual airway maneuver that involves tilting the head back while lifting up on the chin; used to open the airway of an unresponsive nontrauma patient.

health care–associated infection: An infection acquired 2 days after admission to a health care setting or 30 days after discharge from such a facility.

health care power of attorney: A legal document that allows another person to make health care decisions for the patient, including withdrawal or withholding of care, when the patient is incapacitated.

health care professional: A person who follows specific professional attributes that are outlined in this profession.

Health Insurance Portability and Accountability Act (HIPAA): A federal law enacted in 1996 that provides for criminal sanctions and civil penalties for releasing a patient's protected health information in a way not authorized by the patient.

heart failure: A syndrome that occurs when the heart is unable to pump powerfully enough or fast enough to empty its chambers; as a result, blood backs up into the systemic circuit, the pulmonary circuit, or both.

heave: The perception that the heart is beating very strongly; felt on palpation of the chest wall, this finding suggests hypertrophy; also called lift.

helper T cells: A type of T lymphocyte that is involved in cell-mediated and antibody-mediated immune responses; it secretes cytokines that stimulate the B cells and other T cells.

hematemesis: Vomit with blood; can either look like coffee grounds, indicating the presence of partially digested blood, or contain bright-red blood, indicating active bleeding.

hematochezia: The passage of stool in which bright red blood can be distinguished; caused by lower gastrointestinal bleeding.

hematocrit: A measure of the relative percentage of blood cells (mainly erythrocytes) in a given volume of whole blood.

hematologic disorder: Any disorder of the blood.

hematology: The study of the physiology of blood.

hematoma: A mass of blood in the soft tissues beneath the skin; it indicates bleeding into soft tissues and may be the result of a minor or a severe injury.

hematopoietic system: The system that includes all blood components and the organs involved in their development and production.

hematuria: The presence of blood in the urine.

hemiparesis: Weakness of one side of the body.

hemiplegia: Paralysis of one side of the body.

hemochromatosis: An inherited (autosomal recessive) disease in which the body absorbs more iron than it needs, which it then stores in the liver, kidneys, and pancreas.

hemoglobin: An iron-containing pigment found in red blood cells that carries oxygen to the cells from the lungs and carbon dioxide away from the cells to the lungs.

hemolysis: The destruction of red blood cells by disruption of the cell membrane.

hemolytic anemia: A disease characterized by increased destruction of the red blood cells. This disorder has several causes, such as an Rh factor blood transfusion reaction (most likely to occur in the neonate population), a disorder of the immune system, and exposure to bacterial toxins or chemicals such as benzene.

hemolytic crisis: A condition in which red blood cells break down quickly; it may occur as a result of sickle cell disease.

hemolytic disorders: Disorders relating to the breakdown of red blood cells.

hemophilia: A bleeding disorder that is primarily hereditary, in which clotting does not occur or occurs insufficiently.

hemoptysis: Coughed-up blood.

hemorrhagic stroke: One of the two main types of stroke; occurs as a result of bleeding inside the brain.

hemostasis: The body's natural blood-clotting mechanism. It involves the steps of blood vessel spasm, platelet plug formation, and blood clotting.

hemostatic disorders: Bleeding and clotting abnormalities.

Henry's law: A gas law that states that the amount of a gas in a solution varies directly with the partial pressure of a gas over a solution.

hepatic encephalopathy: Impairment of brain function resulting from failure of the liver.

hepatic portal system: A specialized part of the venous system that carries blood from the digestive tract to the liver and then to the inferior vena cava.

hepatitis: Inflammation of the liver, usually caused by a virus, that causes fever, loss of appetite, jaundice, fatigue, and altered liver function.

hepatojugular reflux: Engorgement of the jugular veins when the liver is gently pressed; this finding is specific to right-side heart failure.

Hering-Breuer reflex: A protective mechanism that terminates inhalation, thereby preventing overexpansion of the lungs.

hernia: The protrusion of a loop of an organ or tissue through an abnormal body opening.

herniation: A process in which tissue is forced out of its normal position, such as when the brain is forced from the cranial vault, either through the foramen magnum or over the tentorium.

hertz (Hz): Unit of measure of a frequency equal to 1 cycle per second; 1 million Hz equals one megahertz and 1,000 megahertz equals one gigahertz.

hiatal hernia: The protrusion of a portion of the stomach through the diaphragm.

high-touch items: Items that are used to care for the patient or surfaces that are in contact with the patient.

histamine: A vasoactive amine found in basophils that increases vascular permeability, causes vasodilation, and can cause bronchoconstriction, nausea, and vomiting.

history of the present illness: A narrative detail of the symptoms that a patient is experiencing, usually obtained using the OPQRST mnemonic.

homeostasis: A tendency toward constancy or stability in the body's internal environment; processes that balance the supply and demand of the body's needs.

homologous chromosome: A chromosome of the same numbered pair from the opposite parent.

homonyms: Words that sound alike but are spelled differently and have different meanings.

hordeolum: A red tender lump in the eyelid or at the lid margin; commonly known as a stye.

horizontal axis: The axis that runs perpendicular to the sagittal plane; also called the mediolateral axis.

hormones: Substances that are produced in one tissue or organ and are released into the blood and carried to other (target) organs, where they act to produce a specific response.

hostile environment: Situation in which an employer or an employer's agent either creates an offensive practice or allows it to continue, making it uncomfortable or impossible for an employee to continue working.

host resistance: One's ability to fight off infection.

human immunodeficiency virus (HIV): The virus that may lead to acquired immunodeficiency syndrome; cells in the immune system are killed or damaged so that the body is unable to fight infections and certain cancers.

human papillomavirus (HPV): The most common sexually transmitted infection, which can cause genital warts and some types of cancer.

humoral immunity: A type of immunity in which B cell lymphocytes produce antibodies called immunoglobulins, which recognize a specific antigen and then react with it.

hydrocarbons: Compounds made up principally of hydrogen and carbon atoms; mostly obtained from the distillation of petroleum.

hydrophilic: Attracted to water molecules.

hydrostatic pressure: The pressure of water against the walls of its container.

hymen: A membrane that protects the vaginal orifice before first intercourse.

hyoid bone: A small, horseshoe-shaped bone to which the jaw, tongue, epiglottis, and thyroid cartilage attach.
hypercalcemia: An increased serum calcium level.
hypercapnia: Increased carbon dioxide levels in the bloodstream.
hypercholesterolemia: An elevated blood cholesterol level.
hyperextension: Extension of a limb or other body part beyond its usual range of motion.
hyperflexion: Maximum flexion or flexion beyond the normal range of motion.
hyperglycemia: Abnormally high blood glucose level.
hyperkalemia: An abnormally elevated level of potassium in the blood.
hypermagnesemia: An increased serum magnesium level.
hypernatremia: A serum sodium level greater than or equal to 143 mEq/L.
hyperopia: Farsighted; the ability to see distant objects, combined with difficulty focusing on up-close objects.
hyperosmolar hyperglycemic nonketotic syndrome (HHNS): A metabolic derangement that occurs principally in patients with type 2 diabetes; it is characterized by hyperglycemia, hyperosmolarity, and an absence of significant ketosis. Formerly known as hyperosmolar nonketotic coma (HONK).
hyperoxia: An excess of oxygen.
hyperperistalsis: Increased activity within the bowel; also called borborygmi.
hyperphosphatemia: An abnormally elevated serum phosphate; often associated with decreased calcium. Normal phosphate levels are between 0.81 and 1.45 mmol/L.
hyperplasia: An increase in the actual number of cells in an organ or tissue, usually resulting in an increase in the size of the organ or tissue.
hypersensitivity: Exaggerated or inappropriate responses of the body to a substance to which a patient has increased sensitivity (ie, a substance the body perceives as harmful).
hypertension: High blood pressure; stage 2 hypertension exists when the systolic blood pressure is 140 mm Hg or higher or the diastolic blood pressure is 90 mm Hg or higher.
hypertensive emergency: An acute elevation of blood pressure to 180/120 mm Hg or higher with evidence of end-organ damage (cardiovascular, neurologic, or renal); formerly called hypertensive crisis or malignant hypertension.
hypertensive urgency: An acute elevation of blood pressure to 180/120 mm Hg or higher without signs or symptoms of end-organ damage.
hypertonic: Concentration of solute is higher compared with another solution.
hypertonic solution: A solution that has a greater concentration of sodium than does the cell; the increased osmotic pressure can draw out water from the cell and cause it to collapse.
hypertrophic cardiomyopathy: A genetic condition in which the heart muscle wall is unusually thick, requiring the heart to pump harder to eject blood from the left ventricle.
hypertrophy: An increase in the size of the cells due to synthesis of more subcellular components, which in turn leads to an increase in tissue and organ size.
hyperventilation: A condition in which an increased amount of air enters the alveoli; carbon dioxide elimination exceeds carbon dioxide production.
hypocalcemia: A low concentration of calcium in the blood.
hypocapnia: Decreased carbon dioxide content in arterial blood.
hypoglycemia: Abnormally low blood glucose level.
hypokalemia: A low concentration of potassium in the blood.
hypomagnesemia: A decreased serum magnesium level.
hyponatremia: A serum sodium level that is less than or equal to 135 mEq/L.
hypoperfusion: A condition in which the level of tissue perfusion decreases below that needed to maintain normal cellular functions; also called shock.
hypoperistalsis: Decreased activity within the bowel.
hypophosphatemia: A decreased serum phosphate level.
hypothalamic-pituitary-adrenal axis: A major part of the neuroendocrine system that controls reactions to stress; the mechanism for a set of interactions among glands, hormones, and parts of the midbrain that mediate the general adaptation syndrome.
hypothalamus: An area of the diencephalon that is the primary link between the endocrine system and the nervous system; responsible for control of many body functions, including heart rate, digestion, sexual development, temperature regulation, emotion, hunger, thirst, and regulation of the sleep cycle.
hypotonic: Concentration of solute is lower compared with another solution.
hypotonic solution: A solution that has a lower concentration of sodium than does the cell; the increased osmotic pressure lets water flow into the cell, causing it to swell and possibly burst.
hypoventilate: To move inadequate volumes of air into the lungs.
hypoventilation: A condition in which a decreased amount of air enters the alveoli; carbon dioxide production exceeds the body's ability to eliminate it by ventilation.
hypovolemic shock: A type of shock that occurs when the circulating blood volume is insufficient to deliver adequate oxygen and nutrients to the body.
hypoxemia: A decrease in arterial oxygen level.
hypoxia: A dangerous condition in which the supply of oxygen to the tissues is reduced.
hypoxic drive: A state in which the stimulus to breathe comes from a decrease in Pao_2, rather than from the normal stimulus, an increase in $Paco_2$.
iatrogenic: Related to a side effect or complication of medications or other medical treatment.
icteric: Yellowish coloration of the conjunctiva (the whites of the eyes) caused by the buildup of bilirubin in the blood during liver failure.
icterus: Jaundice; the yellow appearance of the skin and other tissues caused by an accumulation of bile pigments.
idiopathic: Of no known cause.
idiosyncratic: In a pharmacologic context, abnormal susceptibility to a medication, possibly due to genetic traits or dysfunction of a metabolic enzyme, that is peculiar to an individual patient (and usually unexplained).
idioventricular: Related to only the ventricles; produced by the ventricles.
i-gel: A supraglottic airway device that uses a noninflatable, gel-like mask to isolate the larynx and facilitate ventilation.
illicit: In relation to drugs, illegal drugs such as marijuana, cocaine, and lysergic acid diethylamide.
immune response: The body's defense reaction to any substance it recognizes as foreign.
immune system: The body system that includes all of the structures and processes associated with the body's defense against foreign substances and disease-causing agents.
immunity: The body's ability to protect itself from acquiring a disease; in the legal context, protection from penalties that could normally be incurred under the law.
immunization: The process of producing widespread immunity to a specific infectious disease among a targeted group by inoculating individual members of the population; can also refer to a set of vaccinations given together or on a recommended schedule.

immunodeficiency: An abnormal condition in which some part of the body's immune system is inadequate, and, consequently, resistance to infectious disease is decreased.

immunogen: An antigen capable of generating an immune response.

immunoglobulins: Antibodies secreted by B cells.

implanted vascular access devices: Devices that are implanted in surgery, sutured under the skin, for the purpose of long-term medication administration, total parenteral nutrition, chemotherapy, blood product administration, and venous blood sampling; an arteriovenous fistula is an example.

implied consent: Assumption on behalf of a person unable to give consent that the person would have done so.

impulse control disorders: Conditions in which a person lacks the ability to resist a temptation or cannot stop acting on a drive.

inactive metabolites: Medications that have undergone biotransformation and are no longer able to alter a cell process or body function; not pharmacologically active.

inappropriate affect: Emotion that is out of sync with the situation (eg, wearing a smile while discussing a parent's death).

incarcerated: A type of hernia in which an organ becomes trapped in the new location; most commonly obstructs the bowel.

incidence: The number of new cases of a disease in a population.

incisional: A type of hernia in which intestinal contents herniate through an incision; for example, after abdominal surgery.

incubation period: The period between exposure to an organism and the first symptoms of illness, during which the organism multiplies within the body and starts to produce symptoms.

indication: A circumstance that points to or shows the cause, pathology, treatment, or issue of an attack of disease; that which points out; that which serves as a guide or warning.

indirect contact: Exposure or transmission of disease from one person to another by contact with a contaminated, inanimate object.

infants: Babies from age 1 month to 1 year.

infarction: Death (necrosis) of a localized area of tissue caused by ischemia.

infection: The invasion of a host or host tissue by pathogenic organisms such as bacteria, viruses, or parasites that produces illness that may or may not have clinical manifestations.

infection control: Procedures to reduce transmission of infection among patients and health care personnel.

infectious disease: A disease that is caused by growth and spread of small, harmful organisms within the body, or that is capable of being transmitted with or without direct contact.

infectious hepatitis: Another name for hepatitis A; an inflammation from a virus that causes mild fatigue, loss of appetite, fever, nausea, abdominal pain, and, eventually, jaundice, dark-colored urine, and pale, clay-colored stools.

inferential: A research format that uses a hypothesis to prove one finding from another.

inferior: Below or closer to the feet.

inferior vena cava filter: A mesh filter placed in the inferior vena cava to catch blood clots in patients who are at high risk of pulmonary embolus.

infiltration: The escape of fluid into the surrounding tissue; the result of vein perforation during intravenous cannulation.

inflammatory bowel disease (IBD): Chronic inflammation of all or part of the gastrointestinal tract.

inflammatory response: A reaction by tissues of the body to irritation or injury, characterized by pain, swelling, redness, and heat.

influenza: The flu; a respiratory infection caused by a variety of viruses. It differs from the common cold in that the flu involves a fever, shaking chills, headache, muscle pain, malaise, and loss of appetite. Respiratory symptoms include dry, often protracted coughing; hoarseness; and nasal discharge.

informed consent: A patient's voluntary agreement to be treated after being told about the nature of the disease, the risks and benefits of the proposed treatment, alternative treatments, or the choice of no treatment at all.

infusion pump: A mechanical device that infuses a precise intravenous volume programmed by the clinician.

ingestion: Eating or drinking materials for absorption through the gastrointestinal tract.

inhalation: The active process of moving air into the lungs; also called inspiration; also a route of medication delivery.

injection: In allergic reactions, when the skin is pierced and foreign material is deposited into the skin.

in loco parentis: Phrase meaning "in the place of the parent"; used to describe situations in which a designated authority figure makes medical treatment and transport decisions for a minor child when a parent or guardian is unavailable.

inotropic effect: The effect on the contractility of muscle tissue, especially cardiac muscle.

insertion: A movable part of the body to which a skeletal muscle is fastened at a movable joint; its action opposes that at the origin.

inspection: Looking at the patient, either in general or at a specific area (ie, a patient's overall appearance from the doorway versus looking specifically at the chest wall for abnormalities/deformities).

inspiratory/expiratory (I/E) ratio: An expression for comparing the length of inspiration with that of expiration, normally 1:2, meaning that expiration is twice as long as inspiration (not measured in seconds).

inspiratory reserve volume: The additional amount of air that can be inhaled after the normal tidal volume has been reached.

institutional review board (IRB): A group or institution that follows a set of requirements for reviewing proposed research that the US Public Health Service devised.

insulin: Hormone produced by the pancreas that is vital to the control of the body's metabolism and blood glucose level; it causes sugar, fatty acids, and amino acids to be absorbed and metabolized by cells.

insulin resistance: Condition in which the pancreas produces enough insulin but the body cannot effectively use it.

integumentary system: The largest organ system in the body, consisting of the skin and accessory structures (eg, hair, nails, glands).

intentional injuries: Injuries that are purposefully inflicted by a person on themselves or on another person; examples include suicide or attempted suicide, homicide, rape, assault, domestic abuse, elder abuse, and child abuse.

intention tremor: A tremor that occurs when trying to accomplish a task.

interference: A situation in which one medication or chemical taken by a patient undermines the effectiveness of another medication taken by or administered to a patient.

interferon: A protein produced by cells in response to viral invasion that is released into the bloodstream or intercellular fluid to induce healthy cells to manufacture an enzyme that counters the infection.

interleukins: Chemical substances that attract white blood cells to the sites of injury and bacterial invasions.

internal rotation: Rotating the anterior surface of an extremity toward the midline.

internodal pathways: The three atrial pathways of electrical conduction that transmit impulses from the sinoatrial node to the atrioventricular node.
interoperability: Public safety communications systems that are compatible across all local, tribal, state, and federal agencies.
interstitial fluid: The fluid located outside of the blood vessels in the spaces between the body's cells.
interstitial nephritis: A chronic inflammation of the interstitial cells surrounding the nephrons.
interstitial space: The space in between the cells.
interventions: In the context of prevention, specific measures or activities designed to meet a program objective; categories include education/behavior change, enforcement/legislation, engineering/technology, and economic incentives.
intracellular fluid (ICF): Fluid within cells in which most of the body's supply of potassium is contained; accounts for 40% to 45% of body weight.
intradermal: The layer of the dermis, just beneath the epidermis; a medication delivery route.
intramuscular (IM): Into a muscle; a medication delivery route.
intranasal: Within the nose.
intraosseous (IO): Within the bone.
intraosseous infusion: A technique of administering fluids, blood and blood products, and medications into the intraosseous space of a long bone, usually the proximal tibia.
intraosseous space: The spongy cancellous bone of the epiphyses and the medullary cavity of the diaphysis, collectively.
intrapulmonary shunting: Bypassing of oxygen-poor blood past nonfunctional alveoli.
intrarenal acute kidney injury (IAKI): A type of acute kidney injury characterized by damage in the kidney itself, often caused by immune-mediated diseases, prerenal acute kidney injury, toxins, heavy metals, some medications, or some organic compounds.
intravascular fluid: Fluid outside cells but inside the circulatory system; the majority of it consists of plasma, the fluid component of blood.
intravenous (IV): Within a vein.
intravenous therapy: Cannulation of a vein with an intravenous catheter to access the patient's vascular system.
intussusception: An event in which one part of the intestine folds into another part of the intestines, leading to a blockage.
involuntary consent: An oxymoron, because consent is never involuntary; often used to describe a scenario in which a figure of authority dictates that medical care be given to someone who is in custody or incapacitated, or a minor.
ionic bond: A chemical bond in which oppositely charged ions attract each other.
ionic concentration: The amount of charged particles found in a particular area.
ions: Atoms that have become positively or negatively charged, by either giving up or acquiring an electron.
ipsilateral: On the same side of the body.
iritis: Inflammation of the iris; also called anterior uveitis.
iron-deficiency anemia: The most common type of anemia, in which iron stores are low or lacking and the serum iron concentration is low.
irritable bowel syndrome (IBS): A condition in which patients have abdominal pain and changes in their bowel habits; generally the pain and accompanying changes in bowel habits must be present for at least 3 days a month for at least 3 months to be considered this disease.
ischemia: Tissue anoxia caused by diminished blood flow, usually as a result of narrowing or occlusion of an artery.
ischemic stroke: One of the two main types of stroke, also called an occlusive stroke; occurs when blood flow to a particular part of the brain is cut off by a blockage, such as a blood clot, within an artery.
islets of Langerhans: A specialized group of cells within the pancreas that act like an organ within an organ, secreting glucagon from alpha cells, insulin from beta cells, and somatostatin from delta cells.
isoelectric line: The baseline of the electrocardiogram; isoelectric means neither positive nor negative.
isoimmunity: The formation of antibodies or T cells that are directed against the antigens on another person's cells (typically after the transplantation of an organ or tissues).
isotonic crystalloid solution: An intravenous solution that does not cause a fluid shift into or out of the cell; examples include normal saline and lactated Ringer solution.
isotonic solution: A solution containing an equal concentration of solutes and water on either side of a semipermeable membrane. In this case, water does not shift across the membrane, and no change in cell shape occurs.
jaundice: The presence of excessive bile pigments in the bloodstream that give the skin, mucous membranes, and eyes a distinct yellow color; often associated with liver disease.
jaw-thrust maneuver: A technique to open the airway by placing the fingers behind the angle of the jaw and bringing the jaw forward; used when a patient may have a cervical spine injury.
joint capsule: A saclike envelope that encloses the cavity of a synovial joint.
jugular venous distention (JVD): The visible bulging of the jugular veins when a patient is in semi-Fowler or full Fowler position; indicates inadequate blood movement through the heart and/or lungs.
junctional escape rhythm: A dysrhythmia arising from the atrioventricular junction with an intrinsic rate of 40 to 60 beats/min; also called junctional rhythm.
ketoacidosis: An acidotic state created by the production of ketones via fat metabolism.
ketonemia: Excess amounts of ketone bodies in the blood.
ketones: Acidic by-products of fat metabolism.
kidneys: Solid, bean-shaped organs housed in the retroperitoneal space that filter blood and excrete body wastes in the form of urine.
kidney stones: Solid crystalline masses formed in the kidney, resulting from an excess of insoluble salts or uric acid crystallizing in the urine; may become trapped anywhere along the urinary tract. Also called renal calculi.
killer T cells: The cells released during a type IV allergic reaction that kill antigen-bearing target cells.
kilocalorie: The amount of energy that can be obtained from the nutrients taken in through the diet; typically referred to simply as a calorie in the nutritional setting.
King LT airway: A single-lumen airway that is blindly inserted into the esophagus; when properly placed in the esophagus, one cuff seals the esophagus and the other seals the oropharynx.
kinin system: A group of polypeptides that mediate inflammatory responses by stimulating visceral smooth muscle and relaxing vascular smooth muscle to produce vasodilation.
Korotkoff sounds: Sounds related to blood pressure measurement that are heard by stethoscope.
Kussmaul respirations: A respiratory pattern characteristic of diabetic ketoacidosis, which features marked hyperpnea and tachypnea; represents the body's attempt to compensate for the acidosis.
kyphosis: Outward curve of the thoracic spine.

labia majora: A pair of prominent, rounded folds of skin lateral to the labia minora of the female external genitalia that protect the vagina.
labia minora: A pair of skin folds that border the vestibule in the female external genitalia and that protect the vagina.
labile: Rapidly shifting among different emotional states.
labyrinthitis: Irritation and swelling in the inner ear that produce a loss of balance and possibly tinnitus, dizziness, temporary loss of hearing, nausea, and vomiting.
lacrimal glands: The glands that produce fluids to keep the eye moist; also called tear glands.
lactated Ringer (LR) solution: A sterile, isotonic, crystalloid solution containing specified amounts of calcium chloride, potassium chloride, sodium chloride, and sodium lactate in water.
lactic acid: A metabolic end product of the breakdown of glucose that accumulates when metabolism proceeds in the absence of oxygen.
lactic acidosis: The product of anaerobic cellular respiration, which occurs when tissues and organs are inadequately perfused, as in shock and cardiac arrest.
landline: Communications system linked by wires, usually in reference to a conventional telephone system.
lantana: A perennial flowering shrub with clusters of red berries that can lead to serious and even fatal poisoning. Also known as red sage or wild sage; ingestion causes stomach upsets, muscle weakness, shock, and, sometimes, death.
laryngeal mask airway (LMA): A device that surrounds the opening of the larynx with an inflatable silicone cuff positioned in the hypopharynx; an alternative to bag-mask ventilation.
laryngectomy: A surgical procedure in which the larynx is removed.
laryngitis: Swelling and inflammation of the larynx that is associated with hoarseness or loss of voice.
laryngoscope: A device used in conjunction with a laryngoscope blade to perform direct laryngoscopy.
laryngotracheobronchitis: Inflammation of the larynx, trachea, and bronchi.
larynx: A complete structure formed by the epiglottis, thyroid cartilage, cricoid cartilage, arytenoid cartilage, corniculate cartilage, and cuneiform cartilage; also called the voice box.
late adults: People who are 61 years of age or older.
lateral: In anatomy, parts of the body that lie farther from the midline.
lead: The electrical potential difference between two points. For example, lead I represents the difference in electrical potential between the right and left arm electrodes.
left anterior descending (LAD) artery: One of the two branches of the left main coronary artery; branches of the LAD artery supply the left ventricle, interventricular septum, and part of the right ventricle.
left atrial abnormality: Dilation of the left atrium that can occur in patients with valvular heart disease (particularly mitral or aortic valve stenosis), hypertensive disease, cardiomyopathy, or coronary artery disease; it can also occur in an athlete.
left ventricular failure (LVF): A condition in which the left ventricle must work harder to pump blood throughout the body. With systolic failure, the left ventricle does not contract normally and has trouble pumping all the blood in the chamber out to the body; with diastolic failure, the left ventricle contracts normally but has become stiff, impeding its ability to relax and fill with blood between each contraction of the heart.
left ventricular hypertrophy (LVH): A cardiac condition in which the left ventricle becomes enlarged, most often as a result of hypertension.
legal obligation: A duty that is enforceable in a court of law.
lens: The transparent disc within the eye that refracts light to focus images on the retina.
lesions: Localized areas of the skin that do not resemble the area surrounding them.
leukemia: A cancer (malignancy) of the blood-forming organs that particularly affects the white blood cells, which develop abnormally and/or excessively at the expense of normal blood cells.
leukocytes: White blood cells.
leukocytosis: An increased number of leukocytes in the blood, often due to inflammation.
leukopenia: A reduction in the number of white blood cells.
leukotrienes: Arachidonic acid metabolites that function as chemical mediators of inflammation; also known as slow-reacting substances of anaphylaxis.
liability: A finding in civil cases that most of the evidence shows the defendant was responsible for the plaintiff's injuries.
libel: A false statement in written form that could be harmful to a person's current or future reputation.
licensure: The process whereby a state allows qualified people to perform a regulated act.
lice: Tiny, wingless, parasitic insects that feed on blood; an infestation is easily spread through close personal contact. Types include head, body, and pubic lice.
licit: In relation to drugs, legalized drugs such as coffee, alcohol, and tobacco.
life expectancy: The average number of years a person can be expected to live.
lift: A sensation felt on palpation of the chest wall, in which the heart beats extremely strongly; suggests hypertrophy; also called heave.
limbic system: Structures within the cerebrum and diencephalon that influence emotions, motivation, mood, and sensations of pain and pleasure.
limb leads: The electrocardiographic leads attached to the limbs; together, the standard limb leads (I, II, and III) and augmented limb leads (aVR, aVL, and aVF) form the hexaxial reference system along the frontal plane.
lipids: Fats, fatlike substances (cholesterol and phospholipids), and oils that supply energy for body processes and building of certain structures.
lipolysis: The metabolism (breakdown or destruction) of stored fat that has been released into the circulation.
lipophilic: Attracted to fats and lipids.
literature review: A form of research in which the existing literature is reviewed, and the researcher analyzes the collection of research to draw a conclusion.
lithium: A common mood stabilizer used in the treatment of bipolar disorder.
living will: A type of advance directive, generally requiring a precondition for withholding resuscitation when the patient is incapacitated.
local reaction: When the body limits a response to a specific area after being exposed to a foreign substance.
longitudinal axis: The axis that runs perpendicular to the transverse plane.
longitudinal design: A data collection method in which information is collected at various set time intervals, and not just at one time.
longitudinal section: The view of an object cut along its long axis.
long QT syndrome (LQTS): A condition characterized by a QT interval exceeding approximately 0.44 second (440 milliseconds).
loop of Henle: The U-shaped portion of the renal tubule that extends from the proximal to the distal convoluted tubule; concentrates the filtrate and converts it to urine.

loosening of associations: A situation in which the logical connection between one idea and the next becomes obscure, at least to the listener.

lordosis: Inward curve of the lumbar spine just above the buttocks. An exaggerated form results in the condition known as swayback.

Lown-Ganong-Levine syndrome: A disorder that causes preexcitation of ventricular tissue and is characterized on electrocardiogram by a short PR interval and a normal QRS duration.

Ludwig angina: A type of cellulitis that occurs on the floor of the mouth under the tongue; it is caused by bacteria from an infected tooth root (tooth abscess) or mouth injury.

lumen: The hollow interior space within an artery or other hollow structure.

lung compliance: The ability of the alveoli to expand when air is drawn into the lungs during negative-pressure ventilation or positive-pressure ventilation.

lung consolidation: Firming of the lungs as a result of fluid accumulation.

luteinizing hormone (LH): Hormone that regulates the production of both eggs and sperm, as well as production of reproductive hormones.

Lyme disease: A tick-borne disease that primarily affects the skin, heart, joints, and nervous system and is characterized by a round, red lesion or bull's-eye rash.

lymph: A thin liquid formed from interstitial fluid that flows through the lymphatic vessels and lymph nodes; it aids in immune response and debris removal.

lymphatic system: A network of capillaries, vessels, ducts, nodes, and organs that helps to maintain the body's fluid environment by producing lymph and transporting it through the body.

lymph nodes: Round or bean-shaped structures interspersed along the course of the lymph vessels, which filter the lymph and serve as a source of lymphocytes.

lymphoblasts: Lymphocytes that have been transformed because of stimulation by an antigen.

lymphocytes: White blood cells that have an important role in immunity.

lymphoid system: The system primarily made up of the bone marrow, lymph nodes, and spleen, which participates in formation of lymphocytes and immune responses; also called the lymphatic system.

lymphokines: Cytokines released by lymphocytes, including many of the interleukins, gamma interferon, tumor necrosis factor beta, and chemokines.

lymphomas: Malignant diseases that arise within the lymphoid system; they include non-Hodgkin and Hodgkin lymphomas.

lymph vessels: Unidirectional, thin-walled vessels through which lymph circulates in the body; they travel close to the major veins.

macrodrip sets: Intravenous administration sets named for the large orifice between the piercing spike and the drip chamber; they allow for rapid fluid flow into the vascular system; the maximum flow rate is 10 or 15 gtt/mL, depending on the manufacturer.

macrophages: Large cells, usually derived from monocytes, that are specialized for phagocytosis; they kill pathogens, absorb foreign materials, and slow infections and infectious agents.

macula: A yellow depression in the retina where acute vision arises; also known as the macula lutea.

Magill forceps: A special type of forceps that is curved, allowing paramedics to maneuver it in the airway.

malfeasance: Unauthorized act committed outside the scope of medical practice defined by law.

Mallampati classification: A system for predicting the relative difficulty of intubation based on the amount of oropharyngeal structures visible in an upright, seated patient who is able to fully open the mouth.

Mallory-Weiss syndrome: A condition in which the junction between the esophagus and the stomach tears, causing severe bleeding and, potentially, death.

mania: A mental disorder characterized by abnormally exaggerated happiness, joy, or euphoria with hyperactivity, insomnia, and grandiose ideas.

manic-depressive illness: A bipolar disorder in which mood fluctuates between depression and mania; the alterations in mood are usually episodic and recurrent.

manual defibrillator: A device that requires the paramedic or other trained rescuer to interpret the cardiac rhythm and determine whether defibrillation is needed (rather than relying on a device to make that determination automatically).

margination: In the inflammatory response, the stage in which the loss of fluid from blood vessels into the inflamed or infected tissue increases the viscosity of the blood remaining in the vessels, which slows the flow of blood and produces stasis.

marijuana: The dried leaves and flower buds of the *Cannabis sativa* plant, which are smoked to achieve a high.

mast cells: Basophils that are located in connective tissues to which antibodies, formed in response to allergens, attach; the cells burst and release chemical mediators in response to an antigen-antibody reaction.

measles: An infectious viral disease that occurs most often in late winter and spring. It begins with a fever, conjunctivitis, and coryza (acute rhinitis); an onset of coughing; and a blotchy red rash that spreads from the head to the trunk to the lower extremities.

mechanism of action: The way in which a medication produces the intended response.

mechanism of injury (MOI): The way in which traumatic injuries occur; the forces that act on the body to cause damage.

medial: Closer to the midline.

median effective dose (ED_{50}): The weight-based dose of a medication that was effective in 50% of the humans and animals tested.

median lethal dose (LD_{50}): The weight-based dose of a medication that caused death in 50% of the animals tested.

median toxic dose (TD_{50}): The weight-based dose of a medication that demonstrated toxicity in 50% of the animals tested.

mediastinum: The space between the lungs, in the center of the chest, that contains the heart, great vessels, part of the esophagus, lymphatic channels, trachea, primary bronchi, and paired vagus and phrenic nerves.

medical ambiguity: Vague or unclear aspects of medicine.

medical asepsis: The practice of preventing contamination of the patient by using aseptic technique.

medical direction: Direction given to an EMS system or provider by a physician.

medical necessity: A standard used by Medicare to determine whether a patient's condition requires ambulance transport in a particular situation.

Medical Practice Act: An act that usually defines the minimum qualifications of those who may perform various health services, defines the skills that each type of practitioner is legally permitted to use, and establishes a means of licensure or certification for different categories of health care professionals.

medical priority dispatch system (MPDS): A dispatch system using a specific format to indicate the nature of the emergency (emergency medical dispatch protocol) and its priority (determinant level/number).

medication: A substance used to treat an illness or condition.

medication monograph: A document that gives detailed information about drugs, such as their indications and uses, dosing information, precautions, contraindications, and adverse effects.

medication noncompliance: A situation in which a patient chooses not to take medications as prescribed, for reasons that may include undesirable adverse effects or prohibitive cost.

medication sensitivity: A mild to severe reaction after the first exposure to a medication or other substance, which often features many of the same signs and symptoms as an immune-mediated reaction.

medulla oblongata: Inferior part of the brainstem that is continuous inferiorly with the spinal cord; serves as a conduction pathway for the ascending and descending nerve tracts; responsible for maintenance of basic life functions, such as heart rate and breathing.

meiosis: A type of cell division that occurs in the production of eggs and sperm.

melanin: The pigment that gives skin its color.

melena: Dark, tarry, malodorous stools caused by upper gastrointestinal bleeding.

membrane attack complex: Molecules that insert themselves into the bacterial membrane, weakening those areas in the membrane.

menarche: A female's first menstrual cycle; the onset of menses.

Ménière disease: A chronic condition of the inner ear characterized by four symptoms that may or may not occur at the same time: (1) dizziness described as spinning vertigo, (2) low-frequency hearing loss, (3) tinnitus, and (4) a feeling of fullness in the affected ear.

meninges: A set of three tough membranes—the dura mater, arachnoid, and pia mater—that enclose the entire brain and spinal cord.

meningitis: Inflammation of the meningeal coverings of the brain and spinal cord; usually caused by a virus or bacterium. The viral type is less severe than the bacterial type; the bacterial type can result in brain damage, hearing loss, learning disability, or death.

meningococcal meningitis: A type of meningitis caused by the meningococcal bacterium, *Neisseria meningitidis.*

menopause: The cessation of menstruation, which begins in a woman's late 40s or early 50s, and which marks the end of the reproductive years; also called the female climacteric.

menstruation: Cyclical shedding of the endometrial lining from the uterine cavity.

mental status exam (MSE): A tool for measuring the "mental vital signs" in a patient who is disturbed. The mnemonic COASTMAP can be used to conduct this exam, assessing consciousness, orientation, activity, speech, thought, memory, affect and mood, and perception.

mesenteric ischemia: An interruption of the blood supply to the mesentery.

metabolic acidosis: A pathologic condition characterized by a blood pH of less than 7.35 and caused by an accumulation of acids in the body from a metabolic cause.

metabolic alkalosis: A pathologic condition characterized by a blood pH of greater than 7.45 and caused by an accumulation of bases in the body from a metabolic cause.

metabolism: The chemical processes that provide the cells with energy from nutrients.

metacarpals: The five bones that form the palm and back of the hand.

metaplasia: A reversible, cellular adaptation in which one adult cell type is replaced by another adult cell type.

metastasis: The process by which cells from a malignant neoplasm break away from the site of origin, such as the lung, and move through the bloodstream or lymphatic system to other body sites, such as the brain.

metered-dose inhaler (MDI): A pressurized canister that delivers a specific dose of a medication; commonly used for beta agonist bronchodilators.

methamphetamine: A highly addictive drug in the amphetamine family.

methemoglobin (metHb): A compound formed by oxidation of the iron on hemoglobin.

metric system: A measurement system based on multiples of 10 (ie, a decimal system) that is used for the measurement of length, weight, and volume.

microangiopathy: Microscopic deterioration of vessel walls caused primarily by adherence of blood lipids to vessel walls.

microdrip sets: Intravenous administration sets named for the small needlelike orifice between the piercing spike and the drip chamber; they allow for carefully controlled fluid flow and are ideally suited for medication administration; the maximum flow rate is 60 gtt/mL.

microvascular angina: A type of angina caused by spasms within the walls of the heart's smallest coronary arteries.

midbrain: The most superior portion of the brainstem; it works with the pons to route information from higher within the brain to the spinal cord, and vice versa.

middle adults: People who are 41 to 60 years of age.

Middle East respiratory syndrome (MERS): A disease originating from the Arabian peninsula, which is transmitted by close contact with camel urine or nasal secretions, milk, or meat. Symptoms include fever, cough, and shortness of breath, and gastrointestinal disturbances; health care providers should take standard precautions, contact precautions, and airborne precautions.

midsagittal plane (midline): An imaginary vertical line drawn from the middle of the forehead through the nose and the umbilicus (navel) to the floor.

mineral: An inorganic element essential for human metabolism.

minimum data set: The mandatory clinical assessment standard information that must be documented on every emergency call, as determined by Medicare and Medicaid, and per the National Highway Traffic Safety Administration for the purpose of informing the national data system.

minor: A person younger than 18 years of age who does not have the legal authority to refuse or consent to emergency care.

minute volume: The amount of air that moves in and out of the lungs per minute minus the dead space; also called minute ventilation.

misfeasance: An appropriate act performed in an improper manner, such as a medication administered at the wrong dose.

mitosis: The division of chromosomes in a cell nucleus.

mitral valve: The atrioventricular valve in the heart, which separates the left atrium from the left ventricle.

Mix-o-Vial: A single vial divided into two compartments by a rubber stopper; methylprednisolone sodium succinate (Solu-Medrol) is stored this way.

mobile intensive care units (MICUs): An early title given to an ambulance-style unit.

monoamine oxidase inhibitors (MAOIs): Psychiatric medications used primarily to treat atypical depression by increasing norepinephrine and serotonin levels in the central nervous system.

monocytes: White blood cells that mature in the blood and then travel to the tissues, where they differentiate into macrophages; function primarily as scavengers for the tissues.

mononucleosis: Infectious mononucleosis or mono (glandular fever); caused by the Epstein-Barr virus and often called the kissing disease; also spread by coughing or sneezing. Signs and symptoms include sore throat, fever, secretions from the pharynx, swollen lymph glands, malaise, anorexia, headache, rash, muscle pain, and an enlarged liver and/or spleen.

monophonic: The sound of one note during wheezing, caused by the vibration of a single bronchus.

monosaccharides: The simplest carbohydrate molecules.

mons pubis: A rounded pad of fatty tissue that overlies the symphysis pubis and is anterior to the urethral and vaginal openings.

mood disorders: Disorders in which the disturbance of mood is accompanied by full or partial manic or depressive syndrome.

morality: Pertaining to conscience, conduct, and character.

morbidity: Number of nonfatally injured or disabled people; usually expressed as a rate, calculated as the number of nonfatal injuries in a certain population in a given time period divided by the size of the population.

morbid obesity: An excessively unhealthy accumulation of body fat, defined as a body mass index greater than or equal to 40 kg/m^2.

Moro reflex: A reflex in which an infant opens the arms wide, spreads the fingers, and seems to grab at things when caught off guard.

mortality: The number of deaths in each population caused by injury and disease; usually expressed as a rate, calculated as the number of deaths in a certain population in a given time period divided by the size of the population.

motor nerve: Nerve that carries information from the central nervous system to the muscles of the body.

motor neurons: Nerve cells that transmit instructions from the central nervous system to end organs; also known as efferent neurons.

mottling: A blotchy pattern on the skin; a typical finding in states of severe protracted hypoperfusion and shock.

mucosal atomizer device (MAD): A device that attaches to the end of a syringe that is used to spray (atomize) certain medications via the intranasal route.

mucous membrane: The lining of body cavities and passages that communicates directly or indirectly with the environment outside the body.

mucus: The opaque, sticky secretion of mucous membranes that lubricates the body openings.

multifocal: Arising from or pertaining to many foci or locations.

multiple myeloma: A disease in which the number of plasma cells in the bone marrow increases abnormally, causing tumors to form in the bones.

multiple organ dysfunction syndrome (MODS): A progressive condition usually characterized by combined failure of several organs, such as the lungs, liver, and kidneys, along with some clotting mechanisms, which occurs after severe illness or injury.

multiple sclerosis (MS): An autoimmune condition in which the body attacks the myelin that insulates the brain and spinal cord, causing scarring.

multiplex: Simultaneous transmission of multiple data streams, most often voice and electrocardiogram signals.

mumps: A viral infection that primarily affects the parotid glands, which are one of the three pairs of salivary glands; causes swelling in front of the ears.

murmur: An abnormal *whooshing* sound heard over the heart that indicates turbulent blood flow around a cardiac valve.

Murphy eye: An opening on the side of an endotracheal tube at its distal tip that permits ventilation to occur even if the tip becomes occluded by blood, mucus, or the tracheal wall.

muscle tissue: Contractile tissue consisting of filaments of actin and myosin, which slide past each other, shortening cells.

musculoskeletal: The bones and voluntary muscles of the body.

mutism: The absence of speech.

mutual aid: Agreements with neighboring or regional jurisdictions to back up each other in the event of a large-scale incident.

myasthenia gravis: A condition in which the body generates antibodies against its own acetylcholine receptors, causing muscle weakness, often in the face.

myocarditis: Inflammation of the myocardium.

myocardium: The middle, thickest layer of the heart; it contains the cardiac muscle fibers that cause contraction of the heart, as well as the conduction system and blood supply.

myoclonus: Involuntary jerking motions of the body.

myoglobin: A pigment synthesized in the muscles that gives skeletal muscles their red-brown color.

myopia: Nearsighted; the ability to see objects nearby combined with difficulty seeing objects far away.

myosin: A contractile protein found in the thick filaments of skeletal muscle cells.

myxedema coma: A rare condition that can occur in patients who have severe, untreated hypothyroidism, resulting in toxic levels of medication in the blood.

narrow band: Reassignment of frequencies by the Federal Communications Commission to a 12.5 megahertz spacing, now required for all EMS and public safety radio systems.

nasal cannula: A device that delivers oxygen via two small prongs that fit into the patient's nostrils; with an oxygen flow rate of 1 to 6 L/min, an oxygen concentration of 24% to 44% can be delivered.

nasogastric (NG) tube: A gastric tube that is inserted into the stomach through the nose.

nasopharyngeal (nasal) airway: A soft rubber tube about 6 inches (15 cm) long that is inserted through the nose into the posterior pharynx behind the tongue, thereby allowing passage of air from the nose to the lower airway.

nasopharynx: The part of the pharynx that lies above the level of the palate.

nasotracheal intubation: Insertion of an endotracheal tube into the trachea through the nose.

natural immunity: A nonspecific cellular and humoral (antibody) response that operates as the body's first line of defense against pathogens; also called native immunity.

nature of illness (NOI): The general type of illness a patient is apparently experiencing.

near miss: An unplanned event that did not cause an injury, illness, or damage, but had the potential to do so.

nebulizer: A device for producing a fine spray or mist that is used to deliver inhaled medications.

necrosis: The death of tissue, usually caused by a cessation of its blood supply.

needle cricothyrotomy: Insertion of a 14- to 16-gauge over-the-needle intravenous catheter (such as an Angiocath) through the cricothyroid membrane and into the trachea.

needleless systems: Devices that do not use needles for the collection of body fluids or withdrawal of body fluids after initial venous or arterial access is established, the administration of medication or fluids, or any other procedure involving the potential for occupational exposure to bloodborne pathogens by percutaneous injuries from contaminated sharps.

negative feedback: The concept that once the desired effect of a process has been achieved, further action is inhibited until it is needed again; also called feedback inhibition.

negative-pressure ventilation: Drawing of air into the lungs; airflow from a region of higher pressure (outside the body) to a region of lower pressure (the lungs); occurs during normal (unassisted) breathing.

negligence: Professional action or inaction on the part of the health care practitioner that does not meet the standard of ordinary care expected of similarly trained and prudent health care practitioners, resulting in injury to the patient.

negligence per se: Inexcusable violation of a statute, such as practicing paramedicine without a valid license or certification.

neologisms: Invented words that have meaning only to their inventor.

neoplasm: A mass of tissue produced by abnormal cell growth and division that may be malignant (cancerous) or benign.

neoplasm: A mass of tissue produced by abnormal cell growth and division that may be malignant (cancerous) or benign.

nephrons: The kidney's structural and functional units that form urine; composed of the glomerulus, the glomerular (Bowman) capsule, the proximal convoluted tubule, the loop of Henle, and the distal convoluted tubule.

nervous system: The system that controls virtually all activities of the body, both voluntary and involuntary.

nervous tissues: Tissues composed of neurons and neuroglia.

neurogenic shock: A type of shock that usually results from spinal cord injury; loss of normal sympathetic nervous system tone and vasodilation occur.

neuroglia: Supporting cells that provide a supporting skeleton for neural tissues, isolate and protect the cell membranes of neurons, regulate the composition of interstitial fluid, defend neural tissues from pathogens, and aid in the repair of injury.

neuromuscular junction: The connection between a motor neuron and a muscle fiber.

neurons: The basic nerve cells of the nervous system, which contain a nucleus within a cell body and one or more processes extending from the cell body; masses of these cells form nervous tissue.

neurotic disorders: A collection of psychiatric disorders without psychotic symptoms and lacking the intense psychopathology of other mood disorders; includes anxiety disorders, phobias, and panic disorder.

neurotransmitters: Chemicals released from one nerve that crosses the synaptic cleft to reach a receptor.

neutropenia: An abnormally low number of neutrophils.

neutrophils: One of the three types of granulocytes; these cells have multilobed nuclei that resemble a string of baseballs held together by a thin strand of thread; they destroy bacteria, antigen-antibody complexes, and foreign matter.

New Intraosseous (NIO) device: A spring-loaded device that contains neither a drill nor a battery; used for inserting an intraosseous needle into the proximal tibia of an adult patient.

noise: Interference in a radio signal.

noncompetitive antagonists: Medications that permanently bind with receptor sites and prevent activation by agonist chemicals.

nondepolarizing: A term used to describe drugs that produce muscle relaxation by interfering with impulses between the nerve ending and the muscle receptor.

nondepolarizing neuromuscular blockers: Drugs that bind to acetylcholine receptor sites; they do not cause depolarization of the muscle fiber; examples include vecuronium (Norcuron) and pancuronium (Pavulon); also called paralytics.

nonfeasance: Failing to perform a required or expected act.

nonionic: Uncharged.

nonrebreathing mask: A combination mask and reservoir bag system in which oxygen fills a reservoir bag attached to the mask by a one-way valve, permitting a patient to inhale from the reservoir bag but not to exhale into it; at a flow rate of 15 L/min, it can deliver 90% to 100% inspired oxygen.

nontunneling vascular access devices: Devices that have been inserted by direct venipuncture through the skin directly into a selected vein, for the purpose of long-term medication administration, total parenteral nutrition, chemotherapy, and venous blood sampling; peripheral inserted central catheters and central venous catheters are examples.

norepinephrine: A naturally occurring catecholamine that functions as a neurotransmitter and adrenal hormone; it is synthesized by the adrenal medulla, the peripheral sympathetic nerves, and the central nervous system, and produces vasoconstriction through its alpha-stimulator properties. It is also available as a drug that is sometimes used in the treatment of severe hypotension.

normal saline: A solution of 0.9% sodium chloride; an isotonic crystalloid.

normal sinus rhythm: The normal rhythm of the heart that has an intrinsic rate of 60 to 100 beats/min; the rhythm is regular, with minimal variation between R-R intervals, and all measurements are within normal limits.

nucleic acids: Large organic molecules, or macromolecules, that carry genetic information or form structures within cells; they include deoxyribonucleic acid and ribonucleic acid.

nucleus: In the context of the cell, a cellular organelle that contains the genetic information; it controls the function and structure of a cell. In the context of an atom, the central portion of an atom that contains protons and neutrons.

nutrients: Substances that provide nourishment for growth such as carbohydrates, lipids, proteins, vitamins, minerals, and water.

nystagmus: Involuntary, rhythmic shaking of the eyes.

obesity: An unhealthy accumulation of body fat; a body mass index of greater than or equal to 30 kg/m^2.

objective information: Information that is observable and measurable, such as a patient's blood pressure.

obstructive shock: A type of shock that occurs when blood flow becomes blocked in the heart or great vessels.

ocular: Pertaining to the eye.

oculomotor nerve: The third cranial nerve; it innervates the muscles that cause eye movement as well as the parasympathetic nerve fibers that cause constriction of the pupil and accommodation of the lens.

off-line (indirect) medical control: Patient care orders in the form of protocols or standing orders that do not require direct contact with the medical control physician.

oligosaccharides: Simple sugars composed of 2 to 10 monosaccharides.

oliguria: Urine output of less than 500 mL/d.

oncotic pressure: The pressure of water to move, typically into the capillary, as the result of the presence of plasma proteins.

online (direct) medical control: Patient care orders provided directly (in real time) to the paramedic by the medical control physician by radio or telephone.

onset: The time needed for the concentration of the medication at the target tissue to reach the minimum effective level.

oocytes: Immature female sex cells produced in the ovary that may develop by meiosis into ova (eggs).

oogenesis: The process of egg cell formation, which begins at puberty.

open-ended question: A question that does not have a yes or no answer, and that does not give the patient specific options from which to choose.

ophthalmoscope: An instrument used to examine a patient's eyes and view the retina and aqueous fluid; consists of a concave mirror and a battery-powered light that is usually contained in the handle.

opiate: Various alkaloids derived from the opium or poppy plant.

opioid: A drug that acts as a central nervous system depressant and produces insensibility or stupor. An opioid can be a natural product derived from the opium or poppy plant (referred to more specifically as an opiate) or a synthetic product designed to produce similar effects.

opportunistic infections: Infections in which the invading organism thrives because the immune system has been compromised by illness, chemotherapeutic medications, or antirejection drugs in an organ transplant recipient. These fungi, bacteria, viruses, and parasites are normally held in check by a healthy immune system.

opsonization: The process by which an antibody coats an antigen to facilitate its recognition by immune cells.

optic chiasm: Location where approximately one-half of the nerve fibers from each eye cross over to the opposite side of the brain.

optic nerve: Either of the second cranial nerves that enter the eyeball posteriorly, through the optic foramen.

oral candidiasis: A condition that presents as creamy white lesions on the tongue and inner cheeks, caused by the fungus *Candida albicans*; also called thrush.

orbital cellulitis: An infection within the eye socket.

orbits: Bony cavities in the frontal part of the skull that enclose and protect the eyes.

orchitis: A complication of a male urinary tract infection in which one or both testes become infected, enlarged, and tender, causing pain and swelling in the scrotum.

ordinary negligence: Negligence that involves a failure to act, or a simple mistake that causes harm to a patient.

organelles: Structures within cells that have specialized functions.

organic brain syndrome: Temporary or permanent dysfunction of the brain, caused by a disturbance in the physical or physiologic functioning of brain tissue.

organ of Corti: The organ that is the primary receptor for sound; made up of thousands of individual cilia, each with its own associated nerve.

organophosphates: A class of chemicals found in many insecticides used in agriculture and in the home. Nerve agents fall into this class.

origin: A relatively immovable part of the body where a skeletal muscle is fastened at a movable joint; its action opposes that of an insertion.

orogastric (OG) tube: A gastric tube that is inserted into the stomach through the mouth.

oropharyngeal (oral) airway: A hard plastic device that is curved so that it fits over the back of the tongue, with the tip in the posterior pharynx.

oropharynx: A tubular structure that extends vertically from the back of the mouth to the esophagus and trachea.

orotracheal intubation: Insertion of an endotracheal tube into the trachea through the mouth.

orthopnea: Severe dyspnea experienced when lying down that is relieved by a change in position, such as sitting up or standing.

orthostatic hypotension: A fall in blood pressure when changing to a standing position.

orthostatic vital signs: Multiple sets of vital signs taken with the patient in different positions. (eg, in supine and sitting or standing positions) to determine the degree of hypovolemia; also called a tilt test.

osmolarity: The ability to influence the movement of water across a semipermeable membrane.

osmosis: The movement of a solvent, such as water, from an area of low solute concentration to one of high concentration through a selectively permeable membrane to equalize concentrations of a solute on both sides of the membrane.

osmotic: Characterized by the movement of a solvent, such as water, across a semipermeable membrane (eg, the cell wall) from an area of lower solute concentration to an area of higher concentration.

osmotic pressure: The pressure exerted by the concentration of the solutes in a given space to stop the flow of solvent across a semipermeable membrane.

ossification: The formation of bone by osteoblasts.

osteoclasts: Macrophages of the bone surface that dissolve the matrix and return minerals to the extracellular fluid.

osteocytes: Mature bone cells.

osteogenesis imperfecta: A congenital bone disease that results in fragile bones.

osteomyelitis: Inflammation of the bone and muscle caused by infection.

other potentially infectious materials (OPIM): Cerebrospinal fluid, pericardial fluid, amniotic fluid, synovial fluid, peritoneal fluid, and any fluid containing visible blood.

otitis: An infection of either the outer or middle ear cavity.

otoliths: A pair of fluid-filled sacs within the inner ear that are used by the central nervous system to collect information about movement and orientation in space.

otoscope: An instrument used to examine the ears of a patient; consists of a head and a handle. The head contains an electric light source and a low-power magnifying lens.

outcome (impact) objective: A statement of the intended effect of the program on participants or on the community in such terms as the participants' increased knowledge, changed behaviors or attitudes, or decreased injury rates.

oval window: The opening between the stapes and inner ear.

ovarian cyst: A fluid-filled sac that forms on or within an ovary.

ovarian torsion: A painful condition in which the ovary becomes twisted.

ovaries: A pair of female reproductive organs that release eggs (ova) that, if fertilized, will develop into a fetus.

overdose: A condition that occurs when a drug (either licit or illicit) is taken in excess; can have toxic or lethal consequences.

overhydration: An increase in the body's systemic fluid volume.

overt behaviors: Behaviors that are open and generally understood by those around the person.

over-the-needle catheter: A Teflon (plastic) catheter inserted over a hollow needle.

overweight: An unhealthy accumulation of body fat; a body mass index of 25 to 29.9 kg/m^2.

ovulation: Midcycle release of an egg (ovum) during the menstrual cycle.

oxygenation: The process of loading oxygen molecules onto hemoglobin molecules in the bloodstream.

oxygen humidifier: A small bottle of water through which the oxygen leaving the cylinder is moisturized before it reaches the patient.

oxyhemoglobin (Hbo_2): Hemoglobin to which oxygen molecules are bound.

palate: The roof of the nasal cavity; separates the nasal cavity from the oral cavity.

palatine tonsils: One of three sets of lymphatic organs that constitute the tonsils; located in the back of the throat, on each side of the posterior opening of the oral cavity; help protect the body from bacteria and other pathogens introduced into the mouth and nose.

palliative care: Medical care aimed at relief of pain and suffering in terminally ill patients; may or may not involve curative efforts.

pallor: Skin coloration that diverges from the patient's baseline skin tone and suggests reduced blood flow or oxygenation.

palmar: The forward-facing part of the hand in the anatomic position.

palmar grasp: An infant reflex that occurs when something is placed in the infant's palm, and the infant grasps the object.

palpation: Physical touching for the purpose of obtaining information (eg, to detect tenderness).

palpitations: The sensation of an abnormally fast or irregular heartbeat.

pancreas: An organ with both endocrine and exocrine functions; it is a major source of digestive enzymes and produces the hormone insulin.

pancreatitis: Inflammation of the pancreas.

pancuronium: A nondepolarizing neuromuscular blocking agent; used to maintain paralysis following succinylcholine-facilitated intubation.

pandemic: An illness or disease that affects a high proportion of the population over a broad or potentially worldwide geographic area.

panhypopituitarism: The inadequate production or absence of the pituitary hormones, including adrenocorticotropic hormone, cortisol, thyroxine, luteinizing hormone, follicle-stimulating hormone, estrogen, testosterone, growth hormone, and antidiuretic hormone.

panic disorder: A disorder characterized by sudden, usually unexpected, and overwhelming feelings of fear and dread, accompanied by a variety of other symptoms produced by a massive activation of the autonomic nervous system.

papillary muscles: Muscles attached to the chordae tendineae of the atrioventricular heart valves and the ventricular muscle of the heart.

papilledema: An eye condition that results from swelling or inflammation of the optic nerve at the rear part of the eye; symptoms include headaches, nausea with possible vomiting, temporary vision loss, or narrowing vision fields.

paradoxical: Opposite from expected.

paradoxical motion: The inward movement of the chest during inhalation and outward movement during exhalation; the opposite of normal chest wall movements during breathing.

paralytics: Drugs that paralyze skeletal muscles; used in emergency situations to facilitate intubation; also called neuromuscular blocking agents.

parameters: Outlined measures that may be difficult to obtain in a research project.

paranasal sinuses: The sinuses, or hollowed sections of bone in the front of the head, which are lined with mucous membrane and drain into the nasal cavity; the frontal, ethmoid, sphenoid, and maxillary sinuses.

paraphimosis: A condition in which the foreskin is retracted over the glans penis and becomes entrapped; constriction of the glans causes it to swell even further.

parasites: Organisms living in or on any other living creature; they take advantage of the host by feeding off cells and tissues.

parathyroid glands: Four glands that are embedded in the posterior portion of each lobe of the thyroid; they produce and secrete parathyroid hormone.

parathyroid hormone (PTH): A hormone produced and secreted by the parathyroid glands that acts as an antagonist to calcitonin; secreted when calcium blood levels are low; it maintains normal levels of calcium in the blood and supports normal neuromuscular function.

parenchyma: The functional portions of a gland or solid organ.

parenteral route: A route of medication administration that involves any route other than the gastrointestinal tract.

paresthesias: Abnormal sensations such as burning, numbness, or tingling.

parietal pain: Pain caused by inflammation of the parietal peritoneum that is generally described as steady, aching, and aggravated by movement.

parietal pleura: The lining of the pleural cavity, which is attached tightly to the interior of the chest cage.

Parkinson disease: A neurologic condition in which the portion of the brain responsible for production of dopamine has been damaged or overused, resulting in tremors.

paroxysmal nocturnal dyspnea (PND): Severe shortness of breath occurring at night after several hours of recumbency, during which fluid pools in the lungs; the person is forced to sit up to breathe; caused by left heart failure or decompensation of chronic obstructive pulmonary disease.

partial agonist: A chemical that binds to the receptor site but does not initiate as much cellular activity or change as other agonists do; lowers the efficacy of other agonist chemicals present at the cells.

partial laryngectomy: Surgical removal of a portion of the larynx.

partial pressure: The pressure exerted by an individual gas in a mixture.

partial rebreathing mask: A mask similar to the nonrebreathing mask but without a one-way valve between the mask and the reservoir; room air is not drawn in with inspiration; residual expired air is mixed in the mask and rebreathed.

passive interventions: Something that offers automatic protection from injury or illness, often without requiring any conscious change of behavior by the person; child-resistant bottles and airbags are examples.

past medical history: Information obtained during the history-taking process, such as the patient's general state of health, childhood and adult diseases, surgeries and hospitalizations, psychiatric and mental illnesses, or traumatic injuries, which may relate to the patient's current condition.

patent: Open.

pathologic fracture: A fracture that occurs in an area of abnormally weakened bone.

pathophysiology: The study of the physiology of altered functioning in the presence of disease.

patient autonomy: The right to direct one's own medical care, and to decide how end-of-life medical care should be provided.

patient care report (PCR): A legal document used to record all patient care activities during an incident; a handwritten or electronic report that describes the nature of the patient's injuries or illness at the scene and the treatment provided; also known as the prehospital care report.

patient history: Information about the patient's chief complaint, present symptoms, and previous illnesses.

patient safety: Reduction of the risk of unnecessary harm associated with emergency medical services care to an acceptable minimum, which is defined by the limits of the best available medical evidence, equipment, technology, and human skill.

peak: In a pharmacologic context, the point of maximum effect of a drug.

peak expiratory flow: An approximation of the extent of bronchoconstriction; used to determine whether therapy (such as with inhaled bronchodilators) is effective.

peer review: The process used by medical magazines, journals, and other publications to ensure the quality and validity of an article before it is published, and which involves sending the article to subject-matter experts for review of the content and research methods.

pelvic inflammatory disease (PID): An infection of the female reproductive organs.

pelvis: The attachment of the lower extremities to the body, consisting of the sacrum and two pelvic bones.

penis: The cylindrical male sex organ; it conveys urine and semen through the urethra.

Penrose drain: A type of surgical drain often used as a constricting band.

peptic ulcer disease (PUD): A disease in which the mucous lining of the stomach and duodenum have been eroded, allowing the acid to eat into these organs.

peptides: Protein molecules consisting of amino acids held together by peptide bonds.

perception: Becoming aware of or understanding something using the senses.

percussion: Gently striking the surface of the body, typically overlying various body cavities, to detect changes in the densities of the underlying structures.

percutaneous: Through the skin or mucous membrane.

percutaneous coronary intervention (PCI): A minimally invasive procedure performed under fluoroscopic guidance, in which a balloon, stent, or other device is advanced through a peripheral artery catheter and into an obstructed coronary vessel to diagnose and treat coronary artery obstruction.

perfusion: The delivery of oxygen and nutrients and removal of wastes from the cells, organs, and tissues by the circulatory system.

pericardial tamponade: The impairment of diastolic filling of the right and left ventricles due to significant amounts of fluid in the pericardial sac surrounding the heart, leading to a decrease in the cardiac output.

pericarditis: Inflammation of the pericardial sac.

pericardium: In the heart, a thin, double-layered membrane made up of the fibrous pericardium and serous pericardium.

perilymph: Fluid within the bony labyrinth that surrounds and protects the membranous labyrinth while allowing transmission of pressure waves caused by sound.

perineum: The area between the vaginal opening and the anus.

periorbital cellulitis: An infection of the eyelid; also known as preseptal cellulitis or eyelid cellulitis.

peripheral nervous system (PNS): The part of the nervous system that consists of 31 pairs of spinal nerves and 12 pairs of cranial nerves, which are responsible for communication between the central nervous system and the rest of the body. It includes sensory nerves, motor nerves, and connecting nerves.

peripheral neuropathy: A group of conditions in which the nerves that exit the spinal cord are damaged, distorting signals to or from the brain. One type is caused by diabetes; peripheral nerves are damaged as the blood glucose level rises, resulting in lack of sensation, numbness, burning, pain, paresthesia, and muscle weakness.

peripheral shock: Shock caused by peripheral circulatory abnormalities; includes hypovolemic shock and distributive shock.

peripheral vein cannulation: A technique in which a cannula (tube) is inserted into veins of the peripheral areas—that is, veins that can be seen and/or palpated. Examples of peripheral veins include those of the hand, arm, and lower extremity and the external jugular vein.

peristalsis: The wavelike contraction of smooth muscle by which the ureters or other tubular organs propel their contents along their length.

peritoneum: The double-layered serous membrane that lines the abdominal cavity and covers the organs located in the abdominopelvic cavity.

peritonitis: Inflammation of the peritoneum, the protective membrane that lines the abdominal and pelvic cavities.

peritonsillar abscess: A collection of infected material around the tonsils.

permissive: A parenting style in which the parent does not impose many rules, if any, on the child; two subcategories include indifferent and indulgent.

perseveration: Repeating the same idea over and over again.

personality disorders: Conditions in which a person behaves or thinks in a way that is dysfunctional or causes distress to other people.

pertinent negatives: The absence of certain signs and symptoms normally expected of specific illnesses or conditions; these findings warrant no medical care or intervention, but demonstrate the thoroughness of the patient exam and history.

pertussis: An acute communicable disease caused by the *Bordetella pertussis* bacterium and characterized by a catarrhal stage, followed by a paroxysmal cough that ends in a whooping inspiration; also called whooping cough.

pervasive developmental disorders (PDDs): A group of disorders that cause delays in many areas of childhood development, such as the development of skills to communicate and interact socially, and may include repetitive body movements and difficulty with changes in routine; include autism and Asperger syndrome, among others.

phagocytes: White blood cells that engulf and consume foreign material such as microorganisms and cellular debris.

phagocytosis: A form of endocytosis in which a cell surrounds a foreign particle and engulfs it.

pH: A measure of the acidity or alkalinity of a solution.

phantom pain: A sensation of pain in a part of the body that is no longer present.

pharmacodynamics: The biochemical and physiologic effects and mechanism of action of a medication in the body.

pharmacokinetics: The activity of medications in the body over time, such as absorption, distribution, and elimination.

pharmacology: The scientific study of how various substances interact with or alter the function of living organisms.

pharyngitis: Inflammation of the pharynx.

pharynx: The area between the nasal cavity and the larynx, located posterior to the oral cavity; the throat.

phenotype: The appearance, health condition, or other characteristics associated with a particular genotype.

pheochromocytoma: A tumor of the adrenal gland, usually in the medulla, that causes excessive release of the hormones epinephrine and norepinephrine.

phimosis: Inability to retract the distal foreskin over the glans penis.

phobias: Abnormal and persistent dread of specific objects or situations.

phobic disorders: Disorders involving an unreasonable fear, apprehension, or dread of a specific situation or thing.

phospholipids: Lipid molecules that make up the cell membrane.

physical dependence: A physiologic state of adaptation to a drug, usually characterized by tolerance to the effects of the drug and a withdrawal syndrome if use of the drug is stopped, especially abruptly.

physiology: The study of the processes and functions of the living organism.

pia mater: The innermost and thinnest of the three meninges that enclose the brain and spinal cord; rests directly on the brain and spinal cord.

piercing spike: The hard, sharpened plastic spike on the end of the administration set designed to pierce the sterile membrane of the intravenous bag.

pineal gland: A gland in the brain that synthesizes and secretes melatonin, a hormone that affects patterns of sleep and wakefulness.

pinna: The external ear; the cartilage formation that protects the ear and collects sounds into the ear canal, while allowing some perception of the direction from which the sound comes; also called the auricle.

pinocytosis: A form of endocytosis in which the cell membrane sinks inward and ingests droplets of extracellular fluid.

pituitary gland: An endocrine gland responsible for directly or indirectly affecting all body functions; also called the hypophysis.

placebo effect: In a pharmacologic context, the positive and negative effects of an inactive medication on a person that are related to the person's expectations and other factors.

plaintiff: In a civil lawsuit, the person who brings a legal action against another person.

plantar: The sole or bottom surface of the foot.

plasma: A watery, yellow fluid that carries the blood cells and nutrients and transports cellular waste material to the organs of excretion; made of 92% water, 6% to 7% proteins, and electrolytes, clotting factors, and glucose. Plasma accounts for 55% of the total blood volume.

plasma cells: Cells that produce antibodies (immunoglobulins) to destroy antigens or antigen-containing particles; formed from divided and differentiated B cells.

plasma protein binding: A process in which medication molecules temporarily attach to proteins in the blood plasma, significantly altering medication distribution in the body.

plasmin: A naturally occurring enzyme that dissolves the fibrin fibers in blood clots; usually present in the body in its inactive form, plasminogen.

platelets: Formed elements of the blood that function in blood clotting; also called thrombocytes.

pleura: The serous membranes covering the lungs and lining the thoracic cavity.

pleural effusion: Excessive accumulation of fluid in the pleural space.

pleural friction rubs: Squeaking or grating sounds that occur when the pleural linings thicken and rub together, which may be heard on inspiration, expiration, or both; commonly caused by inflammation of the pleura.

pleural space: The potential space between the parietal pleura and the visceral pleura.

plexus: A cluster of nerve roots that permits peripheral nerve roots to rejoin and function as a group.

pneumonia: An inflammation of the lungs caused by bacterial, viral, or fungal infections or infections with other microorganisms..

pneumonitis: Lung inflammation from an irritant, such as a chemical, dust, or radiation, or from aspiration, such as aspiration of gastric contents.

point of maximal impulse (PMI): The palpable beat of the apex of the heart against the chest wall during ventricular contraction; normally palpated at the fifth left intercostal space along the midclavicular line.

poison: A substance whose chemical action could damage structures or impair function when introduced into the body.

polarized: A condition in which active transport of ions into and out of the resting cell creates an electrochemical gradient across the cell membrane.

poliomyelitis: A viral infection that attacks and destroys motor axons; it can cause weakness, paralysis, and respiratory arrest. Because an effective vaccine has been developed, the incidence of this disease is now rare.

polycythemia: The production of too many red blood cells over time, which makes the blood thick; a characteristic of people with chronic lung disease and chronic hypoxia.

polydipsia: Significant thirst.

polymorphonuclear neutrophils (PMNs): A type of white blood cell formed by bone marrow tissue that has a nucleus consisting of several parts or lobes connected by fine strands.

polypeptide: A peptide formed from many amino acids bound into a chain. When it has more than 100 molecules, it is considered to be a protein.

polyphagia: Increased appetite.

polyphonic: The sound of multiple notes during wheezing; caused by the vibrations of multiple bronchi.

polysaccharides: Complex carbohydrates that contain many simple joined sugar units, such as plant starch. Some, such as cellulose, cannot be broken down for nutrition in humans but play important roles in digestion.

polyuria: Frequent and plentiful urination.

pons: Area of the brainstem that contains the sleep and respiratory centers for the body and that, along with the medulla, controls breathing.

pontine respiratory group (PRG): A portion of the pons that communicates information to both the ventral and dorsal respiratory groups; it is thought to smooth the transition between each phase of the ventilatory cycle and alter breathing by making each breath shorter and shallower or longer and deeper, depending on the body's needs.

portal hypertension: Increased pressure in the portal veins; caused by the inability of blood to flow normally through the liver; can lead to rupture of these vessels.

positive end-expiratory pressure (PEEP): Mechanical maintenance of pressure in the airway at the end of expiration to increase the volume of gas remaining in the lungs.

positive-pressure ventilation: Forcing of air into the lungs.

postconventional reasoning: A type of reasoning in which a child makes decisions guided by the child's conscience.

posterior: In anatomy, the body's back surface; the side away from you in the standard anatomic position.

postictal: The period after a seizure in which the brain is reorganizing activity.

postpolio syndrome: The death of nerve fibers as a late consequence of poliomyelitis; characterized by swallowing difficulties, weakness, fatigue, and breathing problems.

postrenal acute kidney injury: A type of acute kidney injury caused by obstruction of urine flow from the kidneys, commonly caused by a blockage of the urethra by an enlarged prostate gland, blood clots, or strictures.

posttraumatic stress disorder (PTSD): A severe form of anxiety that stems from a traumatic experience; characterized by the reliving of the stress and nightmares of the original situation.

postural tremor: A tremor that occurs as the person holds a body part still.

posturing: Abnormal body positioning that indicates damage to the brain.

potency: The relationship between the desired response of a medication and the dose required to achieve the response.

potentiation: Enhancement of the effect of one drug by another drug.

precapillary sphincter: Smooth muscle located at the entrance to a capillary; responsive to local tissue needs.

preconventional reasoning: A type of reasoning in which a child acts almost purely to avoid punishment and to get what the child wants.

precordial leads: A term used to describe the chest leads in an electrocardiogram.

prediabetes: A condition identified in people who have certain risk factors associated with type 2 diabetes; exists when blood glucose levels or hemoglobin A1c levels are higher than normal, yet not high enough to be diagnosed as diabetes.

preexcitation: Early depolarization of ventricular tissue through an accessory pathway between the atria and ventricles.

prefilled syringes: Medication syringes that are prepackaged and prepared with a specific concentration.

prefix: Part of a term that appears before a word root, changing the meaning of the term.

preload: The volume of blood in the ventricle at the end of diastole; it is primarily a reflection of venous return (the blood returned to the heart).

prerenal acute kidney injury: A type of acute kidney injury caused by hypoperfusion of the kidneys, resulting from hypovolemia (hemorrhage, dehydration), trauma, shock, sepsis, or heart failure (secondary to myocardial infarction); often reversible if the underlying condition can be found and perfusion restored to the kidney.

presbyopia: The increased difficulty in focusing on objects that occurs with aging.

preschoolers: Children ages 3 to 5 years.

pressure-compensated flowmeter: An oxygen flowmeter that incorporates a float ball in a tapered calibrated tube; the float rises or falls according to the gas flow in the tube; is affected by gravity and must remain in an upright position for an accurate reading.

pressure infuser device: A sleeve that is placed around the intravenous bag and inflated to force fluid to flow from the intravenous bag and into the tubing.

pressure of speech: Speech in which words seem to tumble out under immense emotional pressure.

pretibial myxedema: An "orange peel" appearance and nonpitting edema of the skin on the anterior part of the leg below the knee.

prevalence: The number of cases of a disease or condition in a particular population within a particular period.

priapism: A painful, tender, persistent erection of the penis; can result from spinal cord injury, erectile dysfunction drugs, or sickle cell disease.

primary adrenal insufficiency: A rare disease in which the adrenal glands atrophy or are destroyed, leading to deficiencies of all steroid hormones produced by these glands; also known as Addison disease.

primary prevention: Keeping an injury or illness from occurring.

primary response: The first encounter with the foreign substance that begins the immune response.

primary survey: The part of the assessment process that focuses on identifying immediate or potential life-threatening conditions so you can initiate lifesaving care.

primitive reflexes: Reflex reactions such as Babinski, grasping, and sucking signs normally found in infants.

PR interval (PRI): The distance between the beginning of the P wave (atrial depolarization) and the beginning of the QRS complex (ventricular depolarization), signifying the time required for the atria to depolarize and the excitation impulse to pass through the atrioventricular junction.

process objective: A statement of how a program will be implemented, describing the service to be provided, the nature of the service, and to whom it will be directed.

prodrome: An early sign or symptom that occurs before a disease or condition fully appears (eg, dizziness before fainting).

profession: A specialized set of knowledge, skills, and/or expertise.

progesterone: A female hormone released from the ovaries that promotes changes in the uterus during the reproductive cycle, affects the mammary glands, and helps regulate gonadotropin secretion.

projection: A defense mechanism characterized by blaming unacceptable feelings, motives, or desires on others.

prolonged (persistent) reactions: Anaphylaxis symptoms that continue over time, with the time frame ranging from 5 to 32 hours.

pronation: Rotation of the lower arms in a palms-down manner.

pronator drift: The drifting of one arm downward toward a patient's feet while they hold out their arms, palm side up, with their eyes shut; can be a sign of a stroke.

prone: Lying flat, facedown.

proprioception: The ability to perceive the position and movement of one's body or limbs.

prospective research: A type of research that gathers information as events occur in real time.

prostaglandins: A group of lipids that usually act more locally than hormones and that are very potent chemical messengers in reproduction, the inflammatory response to infection, pain perception.

prostatitis: Inflammation of the prostate gland.

protected health information (PHI): Any identifiable health information created, disclosed, used, maintained, stored, or transmitted related to providing a health care service.

proteins: Large peptides created from amino acids; they include enzymes, plasma proteins, muscle components (actin and myosin), hormones, and antibodies.

protest phase: An infant's initial response to a situational crisis; characterized by loud crying.

prothrombin: A protein made in the liver and released into the blood, where it is converted into thrombin during the process of blood clotting.

protocol: A treatment plan developed for a specific illness or injury.

protozoa: Single-celled, usually microscopic, eukaryotic organisms such as amoebas, ciliates, flagellates, and sporozoans; a type of parasite.

proximal: Closer to the trunk.

proximal convoluted tubule (PCT): One of two complex sections of the nephron; the proximal convoluted tubule includes an enlargement at the end called the glomerular capsule.

proximate cause: The specific reason that an injury occurred; one of the items that must be proven for a paramedic to be held liable for negligence.

pruritus: Itching.

pseudomembrane: A false membrane formed by a dead tissue layer; seen in the posterior pharynx of patients with diphtheria.

psychiatric emergency: An emergency in which abnormal behavior threatens a person's health and safety or the health and safety of another person, such as with a person who becomes suicidal or homicidal, or who has a psychotic episode.

psychological dependence: The emotional state of craving a drug to maintain a feeling of well-being.

psychosis: A condition characterized by breaking with common reality and existing mainly within an internal world.

psychotropic medications: Medications that affect mood, thought, or behavior.

ptosis: Prolapse of a body part; often refers to drooping of the eyelid.

public health: An industry whose mission is to prevent disease and promote good health within groups of people.

public safety answering point (PSAP): The location to which 9-1-1 calls are routed, which may or may not serve as the dispatch center.

pulmonary artery: One of two arteries that carry deoxygenated blood from the right ventricle to the lungs.

pulmonary circulation: The flow of blood from the right ventricle through the pulmonary arteries and all of their branches and capillaries in the lungs, and back to the left atrium through the venules and pulmonary veins; also called the lesser circulation.

pulmonary edema: Congestion of the pulmonary air spaces with exudate and foam, often secondary to left ventricular failure.

pulmonary embolism: Obstruction in one or more pulmonary arteries by a solid, liquid, or gas that has swept through the right side of the heart into the lungs.

pulmonary veins: The four veins that return oxygenated blood from the lungs to the left atrium of the heart.

pulmonic valve: The semilunar valve that regulates blood flow between the right ventricle and the pulmonary artery; also called the pulmonary semilunar valve.

pulse: The wave of pressure created as the heart contracts and forces blood out the left ventricle and into the major arteries; palpated at a point where an artery passes close to a bone.

pulseless electrical activity (PEA): An organized cardiac rhythm (other than ventricular tachycardia) on an electrocardiographic monitor that is not accompanied by a detectable pulse.

pulse oximeter: A device that measures oxygen saturation level (Spo_2).

pulse oximetry: An assessment tool used to measure oxygen saturation of hemoglobin in the capillary beds.

pulse pressure: The difference between the systolic blood pressure and the diastolic blood pressure.

pulsus paradoxus: A drop in the systolic blood pressure of 10 mm Hg more than during inspiration; commonly; also defined as weakening or loss of a palpable pulse during inspiration; characteristic of conditions that cause profound pressure changes in the thorax, such as cardiac tamponade and severe asthma.

punitive damages: Compensation, usually monetary, awarded to a plaintiff for intentional or reckless acts committed by the defendant.

Purkinje fibers: A network of cardiac muscle fibers distributed throughout the ventricular walls' inner surfaces that conduct the excitation impulse from the bundle branches to the ventricular myocardium.

purulent: Full of pus; having the character of pus.

P wave: The first wave of the electrocardiographic complex, representing depolarization of the atria.

pyelonephritis: An upper urinary tract infection in which the kidneys are involved.

pyrogenic reaction: A reaction characterized by an abrupt temperature elevation (as high as 106°F [41°C]) with severe chills, backache, headache, weakness, nausea, and vomiting; a potential complication of intravenous or intraosseous therapy.

pyrogens: Chemicals or proteins that travel to the brain, where they affect the hypothalamus and stimulate a rise in the body's core temperature.

QRS axis: A single vector representing the mean (or average) of all vectors created by the ventricles during depolarization.

QRS complex: Deflection of the ECG produced by ventricular depolarization.

quadrants: The four sections of the abdominal cavity shown by two imaginary lines intersecting at the umbilicus, dividing the abdomen into four equal areas.

qualified immunity: Protection in which the paramedic is only held liable when the plaintiff can show that a clearly established law, of which the paramedic should have known, has been violated.

qualitative: A type of descriptive statistic in research that does not use numeric information.

quality control: The medical director's responsibility to ensure the appropriate medical care standards are met by EMS personnel on each call.

quantitative: A type of measurement in research that uses numerical data and statistics, including the mean, median, mode, and standard deviation.

quid pro quo: Circumstance in which a person in authority attempts to exchange some work-related benefit, such as a raise or promotion, for an inappropriate employee action (eg, sexual favors); literal translation from Latin is "this for that."

rabies: A fatal infection of the central nervous system caused by a bite from an animal that has been infected with the rabies virus.

radio dead spots: Areas where mobile or portable radios are unable to communicate with a repeater or each other.

range of motion (ROM): The arc of movement of an extremity at a joint in a particular direction.

rape: Nonconsensual oral, anal, or vaginal penetration of the victim by body parts or objects using force, threats of bodily harm, or by taking advantage of a victim who is incapacitated or otherwise incapable of giving consent.

rapid full-body scan: A 60- to 90-second nonsystematic review and palpation of the patient's body to identify injuries that must be managed or protected immediately; also called a rapid full-body sweep.

rapid sequence intubation (RSI): A specific set of procedures, performed in rapid succession, to induce sedation and paralysis and intubate a patient quickly.

reactive airway disease: Any condition that causes hyperreactive bronchioles and bronchospasm in response to certain triggers.

reassessment: The portion of the assessment process in which a patient's condition is reevaluated and responses to treatment are assessed.

rebound tenderness: Pain that the patient feels when pressure is released as opposed to when pressure is applied; characteristic of appendicitis.

receptor: A specialized area in tissues that initiates certain actions after specific stimulation.

reciprocal changes: Mirror-image J-point, ST-segment, and T-wave changes seen on the electrocardiogram during an acute coronary syndrome.

reciprocity: The process of granting licensure or certification to a provider from another state or agency.

recovery position: Left lateral recumbent position; used in all unresponsive nontrauma patients who are able to maintain their own airway spontaneously and are breathing adequately.

rectal abscess: An infection involving a collection of pus in the rectal walls that results from blockage of the rectal mucous ducts.

reduced hemoglobin: Hemoglobin from which oxygen has been released to the cells.

reducible: A type of hernia that will return to its normal location either spontaneously or by manual manipulation.

reemergence phenomenon: The occurrence of dreams, nightmares, or delirium that a person taking ketamine may experience as the drug approaches the end of its half-life.

reentry: Spread of an impulse through tissue already stimulated by that same impulse.

referred pain: Pain that feels as if it is originating from a body part other than the site being stimulated.

reflex arc: A sensory message that reaches the spinal cord and meets with a motor nerve to cause an action; the reflex action occurs without the message first having to reach the brain to voluntarily cause the action.

reflexes: Involuntary motor responses to specific sensory stimuli, such as a tap on the knee or stroking the eyelash.
refracting system: A series of transparent structures within the eye that redirect light as it passes through media of different densities.
refractory period (RP): A short period immediately after depolarization during which the myocytes have not yet repolarized and are unable to fire or conduct an impulse (the absolute refractory period) or have partially repolarized and may depolarize in response to an electrical stimulus (the relative refractory period).
registration: Providing information to an entity that stores it in some form of record book. In the context of EMS, records of your education, state or local licensure, and recertification are held by a recognized board.
regression: A defense mechanism characterized by a return to more childlike behavior while under stress.
relative refractory period (RRP): The portion of the cardiac action potential that extends from the middle of phase 3 to the beginning of phase 4; during this time, the heart muscle has been partially repolarized and may depolarize in response to an electrical stimulus.
remote terminal: A terminal that receives transmissions of telemetry and voice from the field and transmits messages back, usually through the base station.
renal corpuscle: The initial blood-filtering component of the nephron.
renal cortex: The outer portion of each kidney; it forms renal columns and has tiny tubules associated with the nephrons.
renal dialysis: A technique for filtering the blood of its toxic wastes, removing excess fluids, and restoring the normal balance of electrolytes.
renal medulla: The inner portion of each kidney; it is made of conical renal pyramids, and has striations.
renal pelvis: A cone-shaped collecting area that connects the ureter and the kidney.
renal tubules: Portions of the nephron containing the tubular fluid that has been filtered through the glomerulus.
renin: A hormone produced by cells in the juxtaglomerular apparatus when the blood pressure is low.
repeater: Remote radio transceiver that receives radio signals and rebroadcasts them at a higher power, extending the range of a radio communications system.
reperfusion therapy: Treatment intended to facilitate the resumption of blood flow through a blocked vessel; therapy may be either procedural, such as cardiac catheterization, or pharmacologic, such as administration of a fibrinolytic agent.
repolarization: The process by which ions move across the cell membrane to return the cell to a polarized state.
reproductive system: The system in males and females that controls the reproductive processes via organs and glands that create sex cells and transport them to areas where fertilization can occur.
research agenda: The specific questions that a study aims to answer, and the precise methods through which the data will be gathered.
research consortium: A group of agencies working together to study a particular topic.
research domain: The area (clinical, basic science, systems, or education) that a study will impact.
reservoir: In the context of communicable disease, a place where organisms may live and multiply.
residual volume: The amount of air remaining in the lungs and airway passages that is unable to be expelled after a maximal forced exhalation.
res ipsa loquitur: Theory of negligence that assumes an injury can only occur when a negligent act occurs.
respiration: The exchange of gases between a living organism and its environment.
respiratory acidosis: A pathologic condition characterized by a blood pH of less than 7.35 and caused by an accumulation of acids in the body from a respiratory cause.
respiratory alkalosis: A pathologic condition characterized by a blood pH of greater than 7.45 and caused by an accumulation of bases in the body from a respiratory cause.
respiratory membrane: The site where gas exchange takes place; at this point of contact, oxygen is picked up in the bloodstream and carbon dioxide is eliminated through the lungs.
respiratory system: All the structures of the body that contribute to the process of breathing, consisting of the upper and lower airways and their component parts.
restrictive lung diseases: Diseases that limit the lungs' ability to expand appropriately. Skeletal abnormalities such as kyphosis and scoliosis are common examples of conditions that can cause these diseases.
rest tremor: A tremor that occurs even when the patient's muscles are relaxed (eg, hands resting on the lap).
reticular activating system (RAS): Group of specialized neurons in the brainstem; involved in sleep-wake cycles; maintains consciousness.
reticuloendothelial system: The body system that is primarily used to defend against infection.
retina: A delicate 10-layered structure of nervous tissue located in the rear of the interior of the globe; it receives light and generates nerve signals that are transmitted to the brain through the optic nerve.
retractions: The drawing in of the intercostal muscles and the muscles above the clavicles, which can occur in respiratory distress.
retrospective research: Research performed from currently available information.
rhabdomyolysis: The destruction of muscle tissue leading to a release of potassium and myoglobin.
rheumatic fever: An inflammatory disease caused by streptococcal bacteria; the disease can cause mitral or aortic valve stenosis.
Rh factor: A protein found on the red blood cells of most people; when a woman without this protein is impregnated by a man with this protein, the woman's body can create antibodies against the protein that attack future fetal red blood cells.
rhinitis: A nasal disorder generally caused by bacterial or viral infection, allergens, medications, or changes in environmental temperature.
rhonchi: A continuous, low-pitched sound; indicates mucus or fluid in the larger lower airways.
right atrial abnormality: Dilation of the right atrium that occurs when returning venous pressure is elevated or pulmonary pressure is high.
right coronary artery (RCA): The artery that provides oxygenated blood to the walls of the right atrium and ventricle, a portion of the inferior part of the left ventricle, and portions of the conduction system.
right ventricular failure (RVF): A condition in which the right side of the heart must work increasingly hard to pump blood into engorged pulmonary vessels; eventually, it cannot keep up with the increased workload.
right ventricular hypertrophy (RVH): A cardiac condition in which the right ventricle becomes enlarged, usually as a result of pulmonary hypertension.
rigidity: A clinically important sign characterized by marked peritoneal irritation and guarding, indicating an injury or illness for which urgent surgical intervention may be required; in

patients with Parkinson disease, a condition in which muscles do not contract and relax smoothly, resulting in stiffness of motion.

risk: A potentially hazardous situation that puts people in a position in which they could be harmed.

risk factors: Characteristics of people, behaviors, or environments that increase the chances of disease or injury; examples include alcohol use, poverty, smoking, and sex.

rocuronium: A nondepolarizing neuromuscular blocking agent; used to maintain paralysis following succinylcholine-facilitated intubation.

rods: One of two types of photoreceptors of the retina that are sensitive to light, but do not discriminate colors; they produce a picture that is somewhat less focused and essentially black and white.

rooting reflex: A reflex that occurs when something touches an infant's cheek, and the infant instinctively turns the head toward the touch.

R-R interval: The period between the onset of one QRS complex and the onset of the next QRS complex.

rubella: A viral disease similar to measles, best known by the distinctive red rash on the skin; not nearly as infectious or severe as measles.

rubor: Redness; one of the classic signs of inflammation.

ruptured ovarian cyst: A fluid-filled sac within the ovary that bursts from internal pressure.

sacroiliac joints: The points of attachment of the ilium to the sacrum.

saddle joint: Two saddle-shaped articulating surfaces oriented at right angles to each other so that complementary surfaces articulate with each other; an example is found in the thumb.

safe residual pressure: The pressure at which an oxygen cylinder should be replaced with a full one; often defined as 200 psi.

safety culture: In an EMS organization, a system of beliefs and practices that (1) acknowledges that organizations engage in high-risk activities, (2) determines the importance of consistent, safe operations to counteract these activities, (3) supports a blame-free environment where errors can be reported without fear of punishment, and (4) maintains organizational commitment to address reported errors and safety concerns.

sagittal (lateral) plane: A plane of the body that passes vertically from front to back, dividing the body into left and right portions.

salicylates: Chemicals found in plants; a primary ingredient in aspirin.

saline locks: Special types of intravenous devices that eliminate the need to hang a bag of intravenous fluid; also called a buff cap or INT (intermittent); commonly used for patients who do not require fluid boluses but may require medication therapy.

sampling errors: Expected errors that occur in the sampling phase of research.

scabies: An infestation of the skin with the mite *Sarcoptes scabiei*; spreads rapidly with skin-to-skin contact.

scaffolding: An instructional technique that builds on what has already been learned.

scaphoid: The wrist bone that is found just beyond the most distal portion of the radius; also, a concave shape of the abdomen; can be caused by evisceration.

scarlet fever: A disease caused by the bacterium *Streptococcus pyogenes*, which is characterized by a sore throat, fever, rash, and "strawberry tongue."

scene size-up: A step in the patient assessment process involving a quick assessment of the scene and its surroundings to gather information about the overall safety and stability of the scene and the mechanism of injury or nature of illness. This process is carried out before you enter the scene and begin patient care.

schizophrenia: A complex mental disorder that is difficult to identify and whose typical onset is during early adulthood. Dysfunctional symptoms typically become more prominent over time and include delusions, hallucinations, apathy, mutism, flat affect, lack of interest in pleasure, erratic speech, dysfunctional emotional responses, and dysfunctional motor behavior.

school-age children: Children ages 6 to 12 years.

Schwann cells: Neuroglial cells in the peripheral nervous system that form a myelin sheath around axons.

sclera: The white, fibrous outer layer of the eyeball.

scleroderma: An autoimmune connective tissue disease that causes fibrotic (scar tissue–like) changes to the skin, blood vessels, muscles, and internal organs.

scoliosis: Sideways curvature of the spine.

scope of practice: Describes what a state permits a paramedic practicing under a license or certification to do.

scrotum: A pouch of skin and subcutaneous tissue hanging from the lower abdominal region, posterior to the penis.

sebaceous glands: Glands that produce an oily substance called sebum, which is discharged along the shafts of the hairs.

secondary adrenal insufficiency: A relatively common condition characterized by a lack of adrenocorticotropic hormone (also called corticotrophin) secretion from the pituitary gland.

secondary assessment: The process by which more detailed, quantifiable, objective information is obtained from the patient about their overall state of health.

secondary prevention: Reducing the effects of an injury or illness that has already happened.

secondary response: The body's reaction when it is exposed to an antigen for which it already has antibodies, in which it responds by killing the invading substance.

secure attachment: A bond formed between an infant and the parent or caregiver, in which the infant understands that parents and/or caregivers will be responsive to the infant's needs and provide care when help is needed.

sedation: Reduction of a patient's anxiety, induction of amnesia, and suppression of the gag reflex, usually by pharmacologic means.

sedative-hypnotic: A drug used to reduce anxiety, calm agitated patients, and help produce drowsiness and sleep; a central nervous system depressant.

seizure: The sudden, erratic firing of neurons; a neurologic episode caused by a surge of electric activity in the brain. It can be a convulsion characterized by generalized, uncoordinated muscular activity, and may be associated with loss of consciousness.

selective serotonin reuptake inhibitors (SSRIs): A class of antidepressants that inhibit the reuptake of serotonin.

self-concept: A person's perception of oneself.

self-esteem: How people feel about themselves and how they fit in with peers.

semilunar (SL) valves: The aortic and pulmonic valves, which are shaped like half-moons and separate the heart from the aorta and pulmonary arteries.

semipermeable: Property of the cell membrane that describes the ability to allow certain elements to pass through while blocking the passage of others.

sensitivity: The ability to recognize a foreign substance the next time it is encountered.

sensory nerves: The nerves that carry sensations of touch, taste, heat, cold, pain, and other modalities from the body to the central nervous system.

sensory receptors: Structures located in the dermis that initiate nerve impulses that can reach the individual's conscious awareness.

sepsis: A pathologic state, usually in a febrile patient, resulting from the presence of invading microorganisms or their poisonous products in the bloodstream.

septicemia: A generalized infection of the bloodstream.

septic shock: A type of shock that occurs as a result of widespread infection, usually bacterial; if left untreated, the result is multiple organ dysfunction syndrome and often death.

septum: A thick wall that separates the right and left sides of the heart.

seropositive: Having a positive blood test for an infectious agent, such as human immunodeficiency virus or hepatitis B or C virus.

serotonin: A vasoactive amine that increases vascular permeability, causes vasodilation, and can cause bronchoconstriction, nausea, and vomiting.

serotonin syndrome: An idiosyncratic complication that occurs with antidepressant therapy in which patients have lower extremity muscle rigidity, confusion or disorientation, and/or agitation.

serum hepatitis: Infection with the hepatitis B virus, which is transmitted through sexual contact, blood transfusion, or puncture of the skin with contaminated needles or other contaminated sharp instruments. Signs and symptoms include loss of appetite, nausea, vomiting, general fatigue and malaise, low-grade fever, vague abdominal discomfort, and sometimes aching in the joints; eventually, jaundice occurs.

serum sickness: A condition in which antigen–antibody complexes formed in the bloodstream become deposited in sites around the body, most notably the kidneys, resulting in inflammatory reactions there.

severe acute respiratory syndrome (SARS): A potentially life-threatening viral infection that usually starts with flulike symptoms.

sex chromosomes: The X and Y chromosomes, which determine sex.

sexual assault: Any nonconsensual sexual act proscribed by federal, tribal, or state law, including when the victim lacks capacity to consent.

sexually transmitted infections (STIs): A group of diseases usually acquired by sexual contact; include gonorrhea, syphilis, chlamydia, scabies, pubic lice, herpes, hepatitis, and human immunodeficiency virus infection.

sharps: Any contaminated item that can cause injury; includes intravenous needles and catheters, broken ampules or vials, or anything else that can penetrate or lacerate the skin.

shunt: A connection between the arterial and venous system in which no gas exchange occurs.

sickle cell crisis: A condition in which a patient with sickle cell disease experiences significant pain due to insufficient passage of oxygen and nutrients into tissues and joints because of vessel congestion.

sickle cell disease: A disease that causes the red blood cells to be misshapen, resulting in poor oxygen-carrying capability and potentially resulting in red blood cells becoming lodged in the blood vessels or the spleen.

signs: Objective observations that can be seen, heard, felt, smelled, or measured.

simple phobia: A fear that is focused on one class of objects (eg, mice, spiders, dogs) or situations (eg, high places, darkness, flying).

simplex: Radio communication using a single frequency.

sinoatrial (SA) node: The normal site of the origin of electrical impulses; located high in the right atrium, it is the natural pacemaker of the heart.

sinus bradycardia: A sinus rhythm characterized by a heart rate of less than 60 beats/min.

sinus dysrhythmia: A variation of the cycling of a sinus rhythm that is often associated with respiratory cycle fluctuations; the rate increases during inspiration and decreases during expiration.

sinuses: Cavities formed by the cranial bones that trap contaminants from entering the respiratory tract and act as tributaries for fluid to and from the eustachian tubes and tear ducts.

sinusitis: An infection of the sinuses, characterized by thick nasal discharge, sinus and facial pressure, headache, and fever.

sinus tachycardia: A sinus rhythm characterized by a heart rate greater than 100 beats/min.

situational crisis: A crisis caused by a specific set of circumstances.

situation, background, assessment, and recommendation (SBAR): A structured patient report format designed to convey important information in a concise manner.

skeletal muscle tissue: Voluntary muscle tissue attached to bones and composed of long, threadlike cells that have light and dark striations.

slander: A false verbal statement that injures a person's good name.

sliding filament theory: An explanation of the action of muscle contraction focusing on how sarcomeres shorten, with thick and thin filaments sliding past each other toward the center of the sarcomere from both ends.

smooth muscle: The nonstriated involuntary muscle found in vessel walls, glands, and the gastrointestinal tract.

snoring: A noise made during inhalation when the upper airway is partially obstructed by the tongue.

SOAP method: A narrative writing method in which information is organized into four categories: Subjective information, Objective information, Assessment, and Plan (for treatment).

social history: A subsection of the patient history that provides valuable information regarding the patient's overall health status and helps to identify risk factors for various disease processes; includes items such as tobacco use, alcohol and drug use, sexual behavior, diet, travel history, living environment, and occupation.

sodium-potassium pump: The mechanism by which the cell brings in two potassium ions and releases three sodium ions.

soft palate: The posterior portion of the palate, which is made up of mucous membrane, muscular fibers, and mucous glands; it is so named because it has no bony support.

solute: The dissolved particles contained in a solvent.

solution: A mixture of a solvent and a solute.

solvent: The fluid that dissolves a solute, or the substance in which a solute is dissolved or mixed.

somatic nervous system: The part of the nervous system that regulates activities over which there is voluntary control.

somatic pain: Pain caused by the activation of pain receptors in the body's superficial tissues, such as the skin, bones, muscles, and joints; compared to visceral pain, it is generally more intense and more precisely localized.

somatoform disorder: A condition in which a person is overly concerned with physical health and appearance to the point that it dominates everything (eg, hypochondria).

somatostatin: Hormone that inhibits insulin and glucagon secretion by the pancreas.

source individual: Any person, living or dead, whose blood or other potentially infectious materials may be a source of occupational exposure to another person. Examples include, but are not limited to, hospital and clinic patients, clients in institutions for the developmentally disabled, trauma victims, clients of drug and alcohol treatment facilities, residents of hospices and nursing homes, human remains, and people who donate or sell blood or blood components.

spacers: Devices that collect medication as it is released from the canister of a metered-dose inhaler, allowing more medication to be delivered to the lungs and less to be lost to the environment.

spermatogenesis: The process by which sperm cells are formed.

sphincters: Circular muscular walls of capillaries that constrict and dilate, acting as gates to either increase or decrease blood flow.

sphygmomanometer: A device to measure blood pressure; a blood pressure cuff.

spice: An illicit drug consisting of a blend of synthetic cannabinoids; it can produce delirium and short- and long-term psychotic effects.

spinal nerves: The 31 pairs of nerves that originate from the spinal cord and exit the spine on either side between vertebrae; each has a sensory root and a motor root, and is responsible for sending and receiving sensory and motor messages to and from the central nervous system from a portion of the body.

splenic sequestration crisis: An acute, painful enlargement of the spleen caused by sickle cell disease.

splitting: In the context of heart sounds, a situation in which events on the right side of the heart occur slightly later than those on the left side, creating two discernible sounds rather than one heart sound.

squelch: Filtering system to block out background noise, but still allow radio signals to be heard.

stable angina: Angina pectoris characterized by intermittent pain with a predictable pattern.

standard deviation: A measure of the range of scores in a set of data relative to the mean score.

standard of care: Describes what a reasonable paramedic with training would do in the same or a similar situation.

standard precautions: Protective measures that have traditionally been developed by the Centers for Disease Control and Prevention for use in dealing with objects, blood, body fluids, or other potential exposure risks of communicable disease; replaced the older terms "universal precautions" and "body substance isolation" in 2005.

standing order: A type of written protocol signed by the EMS system's medical director that outlines specific directions, permissions, and sometimes prohibitions regarding patient care that is rendered before contacting medical control.

***Staphylococcus aureus*:** A strain of bacteria that became resistant to the drug methicillin, creating a new strain; symptoms include soft-tissue infections and possibly localized skin abscesses and cellulitis, empyema, and endocarditis.

status asthmaticus: A severe, prolonged asthma attack that cannot be stopped with conventional treatment, such as the administration of epinephrine.

status epilepticus: A seizure that lasts longer than 4 to 5 minutes or consecutive seizures without a return to consciousness between seizures.

statutes of limitations: Laws that limit the period within which a lawsuit may be filed.

steatorrhea: Foamy, fatty stools associated with liver failure or gallbladder conditions.

stem cells: Cells that retain the ability to divide repeatedly without specializing, and that allow for continual growth and renewal.

stenosis: A narrowing, such as of a blood vessel or stoma.

stereotyped movements: Repetitive movements that do not appear to serve any purpose.

sterile: Devoid of all living organisms; achieved by using heat, gas, or chemicals.

Stevens-Johnson syndrome: A severe, possibly fatal reaction that mimics a burn; may be due to a medication.

stimulant: A medication or chemical that temporarily enhances central nervous system and sympathetic nervous system functioning.

stoma: In the context of the airway, the resultant orifice of a tracheostomy that connects the trachea to the outside air; located in the midline of the anterior part of the neck.

strabismus: Loss of perception of depth and overlapping or doubled images.

straight laryngoscope blade: A blade designed to lift the epiglottis and expose the vocal cords; also called a Miller blade.

strangulated: A type of hernia that causes complete obstruction of blood circulation in a given organ as a result of compression or entrapment; an emergency situation causing death of tissue.

stratum corneum: The outermost or dead layer of the skin.

stress: A reaction of the body to any agent or situation that requires the person to adapt.

stressor: Any agent or situation that causes stress, whether good or bad.

striae: Vertical stretch marks that occur when a person loses or gains weight rapidly.

stricture: An abnormal narrowing of a structure; also called stenosis.

stridor: A harsh, high-pitched inspiratory sound representing air moving past an obstruction within or immediately above the glottic opening; associated with severe upper airway obstruction, such as that caused by laryngeal edema.

stroke: An interruption of blood flow to the brain that results in the loss of brain function; also called a cerebrovascular accident.

stroke volume (SV): The amount of blood that the left ventricle ejects into the aorta per contraction.

ST segment: The interval between the end of the QRS complex (the J point) and the beginning of the T wave; when there is significant myocardial ischemia or injury, the ST segment is often depressed or elevated with respect to the isoelectric line.

stylet: In the context of intubation, a semirigid wire inserted into an endotracheal tube to mold and maintain the shape of the tube.

subarachnoid space: The space located between the pia mater and the arachnoid membrane.

subcutaneous: Into the tissue between the skin and muscle; a medication delivery route.

subendocardial myocardial infarction: A type of acute myocardial infarction in which the ischemic process affects only the inner layer of muscle.

subjective information: Information that is obtained from the patient but cannot be seen, such as the symptoms a patient describes.

sublingual: Under the tongue; a medication delivery route.

substance dependence: Use of a substance that results in addiction and physiologic dependence on the substance.

substance intoxication: Use of a substance that results in impaired thinking and motor function.

substance use: Use of moderate amounts of a substance without seriously affecting activities of daily living.

substance use disorder: Use of a substance that disrupts activities of daily living.

succinylcholine chloride: A depolarizing neuromuscular blocker frequently used as the initial paralytic during rapid sequence intubation; causes muscle fasciculations.

sucking reflex: A reflex in which an infant starts sucking when the lips are stroked.

sudden cardiac arrest (SCA): An unexpected cardiac arrest that results in attempts to restore circulation.

sudden cardiac death (SCD): A sudden cardiac arrest in which the resuscitation attempt is unsuccessful.

suffix: The part of a term that comes after the word root, at the end of the term.

superficial: Closer to or on the surface of the skin.

superior: Above or closer to the head.

supination: Turning the palms upward (toward the sky).

supine: Lying faceup.

suppository: A drug mixed in a firm base that melts at body temperature and is shaped to fit the rectum.

suprasternal notch: The indentation formed by the superior border of the manubrium and the clavicles, which is often used as a landmark for procedures such as subclavian vein access; also known as the jugular notch.

surfactant: A liquid protein substance that coats the alveoli in the lungs, decreases alveolar surface tension, and keeps the alveoli expanded; a low level in a premature infant contributes to respiratory distress syndrome.

surgical cricothyrotomy: An emergency incision of the cricothyroid membrane with a scalpel and insertion of an endotracheal or a tracheostomy tube directly into the subglottic area of the trachea.

surrogate decision maker: A person legally authorized to make health care decisions on behalf of a patient who is incapable of making or communicating the decision on their own.

surveillance: The ongoing systematic collection, analysis, and interpretation of injury data essential to the planning, implementation, and evaluation of public health practice.

sutures: Seams that occur only between the bones of the skull; they are a type of fibrous joint.

sweat glands: The glands that secrete sweat, which are located in the dermal layer of the skin.

sympathomimetics: Medications administered to stimulate the sympathetic nervous system.

symptoms: Subjective information the patient feels, such as pain, discomfort, or other abnormality.

synapse: A functional connection where neurons communicate with other cells.

synaptic cleft: The space between neurons; also called the synaptic gap.

synaptic vesicles: Small sacs that contain neurotransmitters.

synchronized cardioversion: The use of synchronized direct-current electric shock to convert tachydysrhythmias (such as atrial fibrillation) to normal sinus rhythm.

syncope: Fainting; brief loss of consciousness caused by transiently inadequate blood flow to the brain.

syndrome of inappropriate antidiuretic hormone secretion (SIADH): An endocrine disorder in which an excess of antidiuretic hormone results in decreased urinary output and, in turn, systemic fluid overload.

syndromic surveillance: The monitoring, usually by local or state health departments, of patients presenting to emergency departments and alternative care facilities, the recording of emergency medical services call volume, and the use of over-the-counter medications.

synergism: The action of two substances such as drugs, in which the total effects are greater than the sum of the independent effects of the two substances.

synonyms: Pairs of word roots, prefixes, or suffixes that have the same or almost the same meaning.

synovial fluid: The fluid secreted by synovial membranes that lubricates synovial joints.

synovial joints: Complex joints that allow free movement of the component bones and are lubricated with synovial fluid.

synovial membrane: The lining of a joint that secretes synovial fluid into the joint space.

synthesize: To combine several things, such as history elements, into a coherent whole.

syphilis: A sexually transmitted infection caused by the spiral-shaped bacterium *Treponema pallidum*; signs and symptoms include an ulcerative lesion or chancre of the skin or mucous membrane at the site of infection, commonly in the genital region.

systematic sampling: A computer-generated list of subjects or groups for research.

systemic complications: Reactions that affect systems of the body.

systemic lupus erythematosus: A multisystem autoimmune disease.

systemic reaction: A reaction that occurs throughout the body, possibly affecting multiple body systems.

systemic vascular resistance (SVR): The resistance that blood must overcome to be able to move within the blood vessels; related to the amount of dilation or constriction in the blood vessel.

systolic pressure: Blood pressure created by the left ventricle as it contracts (ie, in systole).

tachyphylaxis: A condition in which repeated doses of medication within a short period rapidly cause tolerance, making the medication virtually ineffective.

tactile fremitus: Vibrations in the chest that can be felt with a hand on the chest as the patient breathes.

tangential thinking: A tendency to leave the current topic in conversation to talk about something else, thereby inhibiting interpersonal communication.

targeted temperature management (TTM): The use of cool fluids to get the patient to a targeted hypothermic state during various critical conditions, such as to lower body temperature in patients who are in a coma after return of spontaneous circulation; ideally performed in the hospital setting; formerly called therapeutic hypothermia.

telemedicine: Computer-based system permitting real-time two-way transmission of sound, video, vital signs, electrocardiographic tracings, and other diagnostic data between the paramedic and medical control physician.

temporomandibular joint (TMJ) disorder: A collection of disorders that present with jaw pain, and that occur when the connection between the temporal bone and the TMJ erodes or moves out of proper alignment.

ten-code: A radio code system using the number 10 plus another number. No longer used in many EMS systems.

tenting: A sign of dehydration in which the skin slowly retracts after being pinched and pulled away slightly from the body.

tentorium: A horizontal projection of the dura that separates the cerebellum from the cerebrum.

terminal drop hypothesis: The theory that a person's mental function declines in the last 5 years of life.

testicular torsion: Twisting of the testicle on the spermatic cord, from which it is suspended; associated with scrotal pain and swelling, and is a medical emergency.

testosterone: An androgen in men that promotes healthy sperm production, determines secondary male sex characteristics such as hair production, and stimulates growth.

tetanus: A disease caused by infection with an anaerobic bacterium, *Clostridium tetani*; it has become a rare occurrence because of the availability of a vaccine.

thalamus: Structure of the diencephalon that acts as the sensory switchboard of the brain, through which almost all signals travel on their way in or out of the brain.
thalassemia: A type of anemia in which either not enough hemoglobin is produced or the hemoglobin is defective.
therapeutic communication: Communicating with the patient using specific strategies to encourage the patient to express ideas and feelings, and to convey respect and acceptance.
therapeutic index: The relationship between the median effective dose and the median lethal dose or median toxic dose; also known as the therapeutic ratio.
therapy regulator: A device that attaches to the stem of the oxygen cylinder and reduces the high pressure of gas to a safe range (about 50 psi).
thermoregulation: The process by which the body maintains temperature through a combination of heat gain by metabolic processes and muscular movement and heat loss through breathing, evaporation, conduction, convection, and perspiration.
third spacing: The shifting of fluid into the tissues, creating edema.
thoracic duct: One of two great lymph vessels; it empties into the superior vena cava.
thought broadcasting: The belief that thoughts are broadcast aloud and can be heard by others.
thought insertion: The belief that thoughts are being thrust into one's mind by another person.
thought withdrawal: The belief that thoughts are being removed from one's mind.
threshold level: In a pharmacologic context, the concentration of medication at which initiation or alteration of cellular activity begins.
thrill: A humming vibration that can be palpated through the chest wall, suggesting an underlying bruit or murmur.
thrombin: An enzyme that causes the conversion of fibrinogen to fibrin, which binds to a platelet plug, forming a final mature clot.
thrombocytes: Platelets.
thrombocytopenia: A reduction in the number of platelets in the blood.
thrombocytosis: A condition in which the body produces too many platelets.
thromboembolism: A blood clot that initially formed within a blood vessel but is now circulating through the bloodstream.
thrombophlebitis: Inflammation of a vein related to a thrombus (blood clot).
thromboplastin: A chemical that stimulates blood clotting.
thrombosis: Coagulation or clotting of blood in a blood vessel.
thrombus: A fixed blood clot that can obstruct passage of blood flow through an artery.
thymus: A lymphatic organ located in the thorax that is important in early immunity; it shrinks with age and is eventually replaced by other types of tissue.
thyroid cartilage: A firm prominence of cartilage that forms the upper part of the larynx; the Adam's apple.
thyroid gland: A large endocrine gland located at the base of the neck; it produces and excretes hormones that influence growth, development, and metabolism.
thyroid-stimulating hormone (TSH): Hormone that controls the release of thyroid hormone from the thyroid gland.
thyroid storm: A rare, life-threatening condition that may occur in patients with thyrotoxicosis; usually triggered by a stressful event or increased volume of thyroid hormones in the circulation.
thyrotoxicosis: A toxic condition caused by excessive levels of circulating thyroid hormone.
thyroxine (T_4): The body's major metabolic hormone. Thyroxine stimulates energy production in cells, which increases the rate at which the cells consume oxygen and use carbohydrates, fats, and proteins.
tidal volume: The amount of air moved in and out of the lungs in one relaxed breath; approximately 500 mL for an adult.
tinnitus: The perception of sound in the inner ear with no external environmental cause; often reported as "ringing" in one or both ears, but may be roaring, buzzing, or clicking.
tissues: Groups of cells that share a similar structure and function.
titin: A noncontractile protein found in sarcomeres of cardiac and skeletal muscle.
T lymphocytes: Lymphocytes that interact directly with antigens, producing the cellular immune response; they also stimulate the B lymphocytes to produce antibodies; also called T cells.
toddlers: Children ages 1 to 3 years.
tolerance: Physiologic adaptation to the effects of a drug such that increasingly larger doses of the drug are required to achieve the same effect.
tongue-jaw lift maneuver: A manual maneuver that involves grasping the tongue and jaw and lifting; commonly used to suction the airway and to place certain airway devices.
tonic activity: A type of seizure movement involving the constant contraction and trembling of muscle groups.
tonsillitis: Swelling and inflammation of the tonsils.
tonsil-tip catheter: A hard or rigid suction catheter; also called a Yankauer catheter.
topographic anatomy: Superficial landmarks of the body that serve as guides to the structures that lie beneath them.
tort: A wrongful act that gives rise to a civil lawsuit.
total body water (TBW): Total amount of fluid in the human body; accounts for approximately 60% of the weight of a healthy adult male; divided into various compartments within the body.
total laryngectomy: Surgical removal of the entire larynx.
toxicologic emergencies: Medical emergencies caused by toxic agents such as poison; may be intentional or unintentional.
toxicology: The study of toxic or poisonous substances.
toxidrome: The syndromelike symptoms of any given class or group of poisonous agents.
toxin: A poison or harmful substance produced by bacteria, animals, or plants.
tracheal breath sounds: Breath sounds heard by placing the stethoscope diaphragm over the trachea or sternum; also called bronchial breath sounds.
tracheitis: An infection of the trachea, typically caused by the bacterium *Staphylococcus aureus*.
tracheobronchial suctioning: Inserting a suction catheter into the endotracheal tube to remove pulmonary secretions.
tracheoesophageal fistula (TEF): A connection between the esophagus and the trachea.
tracheostomy: The surgical opening into the trachea created during a tracheotomy procedure.
tracheostomy tube: A plastic tube placed within the tracheostomy site (stoma).
track marks: The visible scars from repeated cannulation of a vein; commonly associated with illicit drug use.
transceivers: Radios containing both a transmitter and a receiver; two-way radios.
transcellular fluid: Fluid classified as extracellular, but which is formed from the transport activities of cells. Examples include cerebrospinal fluid, bladder urine, aqueous humor, and synovial fluid of the joints.

transcutaneous pacemaker: A device that depolarizes myocardial tissue by sending a small electrical charge through the skin of the chest between one externally placed pacing pad and another.

transcutaneous pacing (TCP): An intervention used to depolarize heart muscle using an external stimulus; pads placed on the patient's chest deliver electrical energy to the heart, causing muscle contraction.

transdermal: Across the skin; a medication delivery route.

transfusion reactions: Physiologic responses that are similar to anaphylactic reactions, in which the body reacts to the infusion of blood; they occur rapidly and can cause severe circulatory collapse and death.

transfusion-related lung injury: A transfusion reaction characterized by increased pulmonary capillary permeability, resulting in noncardiogenic pulmonary edema.

transient ischemic attacks (TIAs): Disorder in which brain cells temporarily stop working because of insufficient oxygen, causing strokelike symptoms that resolve completely within 24 hours of onset.

translaryngeal catheter ventilation: A method used in conjunction with needle cricothyrotomy to ventilate a patient; requires a high-pressure jet ventilator.

transmigration (diapedesis): In the inflammatory response, the stage in which polymorphonuclear neutrophils permeate the vessel wall, passing into the interstitial space.

transmission: The spread of an infectious agent from one organism to another; mechanisms of transmission may be classified as contact (direct or indirect), airborne, foodborne, or vector-borne.

transmission-based precautions: Precautions beyond standard precautions that are designed to interrupt specific disease transmission routes; the three types are airborne, droplet, and contact. Can be used alone or in combination; always used in conjunction with standard precautions.

transmural myocardial infarction: A type of acute myocardial infarction in which the infarct extends through the entire wall of the ventricle.

transverse (axial) plane: An imaginary plane passing horizontally through the body at the waist, dividing it into top and bottom halves.

trauma systems: The collaboration of prehospital and in-hospital medicine that focuses on optimizing the use of resources and assets of each, with a primary goal of reducing the mortality and morbidity of trauma patients.

traumatic fracture: A fracture that occurs when abnormal forces are applied to normal bone structures.

tremors: Fine involuntary, rhythmic movements, usually involving the hands or head.

trichomoniasis: A parasitic infection caused by *Trichomonas vaginalis*, a single-cell parasite that is transmitted through sexual contact.

tricuspid valve: The atrioventricular valve that separates the right atrium from the right ventricle.

tricyclic antidepressants (TCAs): A group of drugs used to treat severe depression and manage pain; minimal dosing errors can cause toxic results.

trifascicular block: Blockage or impairment of all three components of the ventricular conduction system, with one working occasionally to provide AV conduction.

trigeminy: A dysrhythmia in which every third complex is a premature complex, causing a *normal–normal–early beat pattern*; can be atrial, junctional, or ventricular.

trismus: The involuntary contraction of the mouth resulting in clenched teeth; occurs during seizures and head injuries.

trocar: A solid boring needle.

tropomyosin: An actin-binding protein that regulates muscle contraction and other actin-related mechanical functions of the body.

troponin: A regulatory protein in the actin filaments of skeletal and cardiac muscle that attaches to tropomyosin.

trunked radio systems: Computerized sharing of radio frequencies by multiple units, agencies, or systems.

trust and mistrust: A phrase that refers to a stage of development from birth to about 18 months of age, during which infants learn to trust their parents and/or caregivers if their world is planned, organized, and routine.

tuberculin skin test: A test to determine if a person has ever been infected with tuberculosis.

tuberculosis (TB): A chronic bacterial disease caused by *Mycobacterium tuberculosis* that usually affects the lungs but can also affect other organs, such as the brain and kidneys; characterized by a persistent cough lasting longer than 3 weeks plus one or more of the following: night sweats, headache, fever, fatigue, weight loss, hemoptysis, hoarseness, or chest pain.

tuberculosis blood test: Measurement via interferon-gamma release assays of how the immune system reacts to the bacteria that cause tuberculosis; offers accurate results in 24 hours; also called blood analysis *Mycobacterium tuberculosis.*

tubular reabsorption: The process that moves substances from the tubular fluid into the blood, within the peritubular capillary.

tubular secretion: The process that moves substances from the blood in the peritubular capillary into the renal tubule.

tunica adventitia: The outer layer of tissue of a blood vessel wall, composed of elastic and fibrous connective tissue.

tunica intima: The smooth, thin, inner lining of a blood vessel.

tunica media: The middle, thickest layer of tissue of a blood vessel wall, composed of elastic tissue and smooth muscle cells that allow the vessel to expand or contract in response to changes in blood pressure and tissue demand.

tunnel vision: A situation in which a paramedic becomes so completely involved with patient care that they fail to see the possibility of physical harm to the patient or other care providers.

turgor: Loss of skin elasticity.

T wave: The upright, flat, or inverted wave following the QRS complex of the electrocardiogram, representing ventricular repolarization.

tympanic: A loud, high-pitched sound, similar to the sound of a drum, heard on percussion of a hollow space (eg, the empty stomach or a puffed-out cheek).

type 1 diabetes: The type of diabetic disease that usually starts in childhood and requires daily injections of supplemental synthetic insulin to control blood glucose levels; formerly called insulin-dependent diabetes mellitus (IDDM) or juvenile-onset diabetes.

type 2 diabetes: The type of diabetic disease that typically develops in middle-age adult patients and often can be controlled through diet and oral medications; formerly called adult-onset diabetes.

ulcerative colitis: Generalized inflammation of the colon that results in a weakened, dilated rectum, making it susceptible to infection and bleeding.

ultra high frequency (UHF) band: The portion of the radio frequency spectrum between 300 and 3,000 megahertz.

umbilical: The region of the abdomen surrounding the umbilicus.

unblinded study: A type of study in which the subjects are advised of all aspects of the study.

unifocal: Arising from a single site.

unilateral: Occurring or appearing on only one side of the body.

unintentional injuries: Injuries that occur without intent to harm (commonly called accidents); examples include motor vehicle collisions, poisonings, drownings, falls, and most burns.

universal timeout: A planned pause before the beginning of a procedure that improves safety and communication among all personnel, and helps prevent human errors.

unstable angina: Angina pectoris characterized by a variable, unpredictable pain pattern, which may signal an impending acute myocardial infarction.

untoward effects: Clinical changes caused by a medication that cause harm or discomfort to a patient; also known as adverse effects.

uremia: Severe renal failure resulting in the buildup of waste products within the blood; eventually impairs brain function.

uremic frost: A powdery buildup of uric acid, especially on the skin of the face.

ureters: A pair of thick-walled, hollow tubes that transport urine from the kidneys to the bladder.

urethra: A hollow tubular structure that drains urine from the bladder, expelling it from the body.

urinary bladder: A hollow muscular sac in the midline of the lower abdominal area that stores urine until it is released from the body.

urinary incontinence: The inability to control the release of urine from the bladder; loss of bladder control.

urinary retention: Incomplete emptying of the bladder, or a complete lack of ability to empty the bladder.

urinary system: The organs that control the discharge of certain waste materials filtered from the blood and excreted as urine.

urinary tract infections (UTIs): Infections, usually of the lower urinary tract (urethra and bladder), that occur when normal flora (bacteria that naturally populate the skin) enter the urethra and multiply.

urine: Liquid waste products filtered out of the body by the urinary system.

urticaria: An itching rash that may be one of the warning signs of impending anaphylaxis; also known as hives. In individuals with pale skin, it typically appears as reddened, elevated patches on the skin (eg, welts); in individuals with dark skin, it may appear as patches of elevated, inflamed skin and skin coloration that is slightly lighter or darker than usual.

uterine prolapse: A condition in which the uterus moves or drops into the vagina.

uterus: A muscular, inverted pear-shaped organ that lies situated between the urinary bladder and the rectum.

U wave: A small, flat wave sometimes seen after the T wave and before the next P wave.

$\dot{V}/\dot{Q}$ mismatch: An imbalance between the anatomic portions of the lung being ventilated (V) and the anatomic portions being perfused (Q).

vaccinations: Inoculations with a vaccine, usually by injection or inhalation, to bring about immunity to a specific disease in a person.

vaccines: The products formulated to bring about immunity by introducing into the body a killed or weakened virus to which the immune system produces antibodies.

Vacutainer: A cylindrical device that attaches to an 18- or 20-gauge sampling needle; accommodates self-sealing blood tubes when blood samples are being obtained.

vagina: The genital canal in the female that serves as a passageway for the elimination of menstrual fluids, receives the penis during sexual intercourse, holds the spermatozoa before their passage into the uterus, and serves as the passageway for childbirth.

vaginal yeast infection: An infection caused by the fungus, *Candida albicans*, in which fungi overpopulate the vagina.

vaginitis: An inflammation of the vagina that is caused by an infection.

Valsalva maneuver: Straining or forced exhalation against a closed glottis, the effect of which is to stimulate the vagus nerve, thereby slowing the heart rate.

variant angina: A type of angina caused by coronary artery spasm that occurs when a person is at rest, when oxygen needs are minimal; also called Prinzmetal angina.

varicella zoster: A highly contagious disease caused by the varicella zoster virus, which is part of the herpes virus family, and which occurs most often in the winter and early spring; also called chickenpox.

varicose veins: Veins on the leg that are large, twisted, and rope-like and can cause pain, swelling, or itching.

vasculitis: An inflammation of the blood vessels.

vasoactive amines: Substances such as histamine and serotonin that increase vascular permeability, cause vasodilation, and can cause bronchoconstriction, nausea, and vomiting.

vasoconstriction: Narrowing of the diameter of a blood vessel.

vasodilation: Widening of the diameter of a blood vessel.

vasoocclusive crisis: Ischemia and pain caused by sickle-shaped red blood cells that obstruct blood flow to a portion of the body.

Vaughan-Williams classification: A classification scheme for medications based on the mechanism of action rather than on specific medication groups.

vector: An organism that harbors pathogens that are harmless to the organism but cause disease when transmitted to a human host.

vecuronium: A nondepolarizing neuromuscular blocking agent; used to maintain paralysis following succinylcholine-facilitated intubation.

venous thrombosis: The development of a stationary blood clot in the venous circulation.

ventilation: The mechanical process of moving air into and out of the lungs in two separate phases: inhalation (inspiration) and exhalation (expiration).

ventral: The anterior surface of the body.

ventral respiratory group (VRG): An area of the medulla oblongata that can cause inspiration or expiration depending on which motor neurons are stimulated.

Venturi mask: A mask with a number of interchangeable adapters that draws room air into the mask along with the oxygen flow; allows for the administration of highly specific oxygen concentrations.

vertigo: A type of dizziness in which a person experiences the sensation of movement when standing still or of the environment moving; often due to an inner ear disorder.

very high frequency (VHF) band: The portion of the radio frequency spectrum between 30 and 300 megahertz.

vesicles: Tiny fluid-filled sacs; small blisters.

vesicular breath sounds: Soft, muffled breath sounds in which the expiratory phase is barely audible.

vesicular sounds: Normal breath sounds made by air moving in and out of the alveoli.

vestibule: The structure into which the vagina opens posteriorly, and into which the female urethra opens in the midline; also, the central part of the labyrinth of the ear, behind the cochlea and in front of the semicircular canals.

vials: Small glass or plastic bottles that contain medication; may contain single or multiple doses.

video laryngoscopy: Visualization of the epiglottis and vocal cords through a video monitor that is attached to a laryngoscope.

viral hepatitis: An inflammation of the liver produced by one of five distinct forms of hepatitis virus—A, B, C, D, and E.

The types differ in their mode of transmission but present with the same signs and symptoms.

virulence: The ability of an organism to invade and create disease in a host; also refers to the ability of an organism to survive outside the living host.

virus: A small organism that can multiply only inside a host, such as a human, and cause disease.

visceral pain: Deep pain caused by activation of pain receptors in internal areas of the body that are enclosed within a cavity, such as the chest, abdomen, or pelvis; common with genitourinary problems.

visceral pleura: The lining of the pleural cavity, which adheres tightly to the surface of the lung.

visual acuity: Determined by the ability or inability to see, and by how far.

vital capacity: The amount of air moved in and out of the lungs with maximum inspiration and exhalation.

vitamins: Organic compounds required for normal metabolism.

vitreous humor: A jellylike fluid filling the posterior eye cavity that helps the globe maintain its shape without distorting light.

volume of distribution: The extent to which a medication will spread within the body.

volume on hand: The amount of fluid you have on hand, such as the amount of fluid in an intravenous bag or the amount of fluid in a vial of medication.

Volutrol: A special type of microdrip set that features a 100- or 200-mL calibrated drip chamber; used for fluid regulation in patients susceptible to circulatory overload, such as pediatric and older patients; also called a Buretrol.

volvulus: Twisting of the bowel until a kink occurs; results in blocked flow.

von Willebrand disease: A bleeding disorder in which the patient is missing the von Willebrand factor (a protein essential for platelet adhesion), preventing the blood from clotting well.

vulvovaginitis: An inflammation of the external vulva.

water soluble: A property that indicates a material can be dissolved in water.

waveform capnography: A waveform display of exhaled carbon dioxide.

West Nile virus (WNV): A type of virus that is transmitted by mosquitos. It usually causes only mild disease in humans but can cause encephalitis, meningitis, and death; symptoms, if any, include fever, headache, fatigue, weakness, joint pain, vomiting, diarrhea, or rash.

wheezing: A high-pitched whistling sound that may be heard on inspiration, expiration, or both; indicates air movement through a constricted lower airway, such as with asthma.

whispered pectoriloquy: A test of decreased breath sounds performed by placing the diaphragm of the stethoscope over the area in question as the patient whispers "ninety-nine"; a loud, clear sound indicates lung consolidation.

whistle-tip catheters: Soft plastic, nonrigid catheters; also called French catheters.

white matter: Bundles of myelinated nerves.

withdrawal: In the context of infant behavior, the final phase of an infant's response to a situational crisis; characterized by apathy and boredom.

withdrawal syndrome: A predictable set of signs and symptoms, usually involving altered central nervous system activity that occurs after the abrupt cessation of a drug or after rapidly decreasing the usual dosage of a drug.

Wolff-Parkinson-White (WPW) syndrome: A preexcitation syndrome characterized by a short PR interval, a delta wave, a widened QRS complex, and nonspecific ST-T wave changes, indicating the presence of an accessory pathway.

word root: The foundation of a word; establishes the basic meaning of a word.

working diagnosis: The one diagnosis from a differential diagnosis list used as the basis for the patient's treatment plan.

years of potential life lost (YPLL): A way of measuring and comparing the overall impact of deaths resulting from different causes.

zero-order elimination: A process in which a fixed amount of a substance is removed during a certain period, regardless of the total amount in the body.

Zika: A type of virus that is transmitted by the *Aedes aegypti* mosquito; the majority of infected persons are asymptomatic. Transmission can occur from an infected mother to her fetus, and from an infected male to his sexual partners; related to onset of Guillain-Barré syndrome.

zoonotic: Refers to infectious diseases of animals that can be transmitted to humans and cause disease.

Index: Volume 1

Note: Figures and tables are indicated with *f* and *t* following the page numbers.

B

D

E

G

H

I

J

K

O

S

T

W

X

Y

Z